Davidson's
Principles and Practice of
Medicine

Sir Stanley Davidson (1894–1981)

This famous textbook was the brainchild of one of the great Professors of Medicine of the 20th century. Stanley Davidson was born in Sri Lanka and began his medical undergraduate training at Trinity College, Cambridge; this was interrupted by World War I and later resumed in Edinburgh. He was seriously wounded in battle, and the carnage and shocking waste of young life that he encountered at that time had a profound effect on his subsequent attitudes and values.

In 1930 Stanley Davidson was appointed Professor of Medicine at the University of Aberdeen, one of the first full-time Chairs of Medicine anywhere and the first in Scotland. In 1938 he took up the Chair of Medicine at Edinburgh and was to remain in this post until retirement in 1959. He was a renowned educator and a particularly gifted teacher at the bedside, where he taught that everything had to be questioned and explained. He himself gave most of the systematic lectures in Medicine, which were made available as typewritten notes that emphasised the essentials and far surpassed any textbook available at the time.

Principles and Practice of Medicine was conceived in the late 1940s with its origins in those lecture notes. The first edition, published in 1952, was a masterpiece of clarity and uniformity of style. It was of modest size and price, but sufficiently comprehensive and up to date to provide students with the main elements of sound medical practice. Although the format and presentation have seen many changes in 22 subsequent editions, Sir Stanley's original vision and objectives remain. More than half a century after its first publication, his book continues to inform and educate students, doctors and health professionals all over the world.

Davidson's
Principles and Practice of

Medicine

23rd Edition

Edited by

Stuart H Ralston
MD, FRCP, FMedSci, FRSE, FFPM(Hon)

Arthritis Research UK Professor of Rheumatology,
University of Edinburgh; Honorary Consultant Rheumatologist,
Western General Hospital, Edinburgh, UK

Ian D Penman
BSc(Hons), MD, FRCPE

Consultant Gastroenterologist,
Royal Infirmary of Edinburgh;
Honorary Senior Lecturer, University of Edinburgh, UK

Mark WJ Strachan
BSc(Hons), MD, FRCPE

Consultant Endocrinologist,
Metabolic Unit, Western General Hospital, Edinburgh;
Honorary Professor, University of Edinburgh, UK

Richard P Hobson
LLM, PhD, MRCP(UK), FRCPath

Consultant Microbiologist,
Harrogate and District NHS Foundation Trust;
Honorary Senior Lecturer, University of Leeds, UK

Illustrations by Robert Britton

ELSEVIER   Edinburgh   London   New York   Oxford   Philadelphia   St Louis   Sydney   2018

ELSEVIER

First edition 1952
Second edition 1954
Third edition 1956
Fourth edition 1958
Fifth edition 1960
Sixth edition 1962
Seventh edition 1964
Eighth edition 1966

Ninth edition 1968
Tenth edition 1971
Eleventh edition 1974
Twelfth edition 1977
Thirteenth edition 1981
Fourteenth edition 1984
Fifteenth edition 1987
Sixteenth edition 1991

Seventeenth edition 1995
Eighteenth edition 1999
Nineteenth edition 2002
Twentieth edition 2006
Twenty-first edition 2010
Twenty-second edition 2014
Twenty-third edition 2018

ISBN   978-0-7020-7028-0
International ISBN   978-0-7020-7027-3

Notices

your source for books,
journals and multimedia
in the health sciences

www.elsevierhealth.com

Working together
to grow libraries in
developing countries

www.elsevier.com • www.bookaid.org

The
publisher's
policy is to use
**paper manufactured
from sustainable forests**

Printed in China

Last digit is the print number: 9 8 7 6 5 4 3

Content Strategist: Laurence Hunter
Content Development Specialist: Wendy Lee
Content Coordinator: Susan Jansons
Project Manager: Louisa Talbott
Designer: Miles Hitchen

Contents

Preface	ix
Contributors	xi
International Advisory Board	xv
Acknowledgements	xvii
Introduction	xix

PART 1   FUNDAMENTALS OF MEDICINE   1

1. Clinical decision-making — 1
N Cooper, AL Cracknell

2. Clinical therapeutics and good prescribing — 13
SRJ Maxwell

3. Clinical genetics — 37
K Tatton-Brown, DR FitzPatrick

4. Clinical immunology — 61
SE Marshall, SL Johnston

5. Population health and epidemiology — 91
H Campbell, DA McAllister

6. Principles of infectious disease — 99
JAT Sandoe, DH Dockrell

PART 2   EMERGENCY AND CRITICAL CARE MEDICINE   131

7. Poisoning — 131
SHL Thomas

8. Envenomation — 151
J White

9. Environmental medicine — 163
M Byers

10. Acute medicine and critical illness — 173
VR Tallentire, MJ MacMahon

| PART 3 | CLINICAL MEDICINE | 215 |

11.	**Infectious disease**	215
	DH Dockrell, S Sundar, BJ Angus	
12.	**HIV infection and AIDS**	305
	G Maartens	
13.	**Sexually transmitted infections**	329
	GR Scott	
14.	**Clinical biochemistry and metabolic medicine**	345
	A Mather, L Burnett, DR Sullivan, P Stewart	
15.	**Nephrology and urology**	381
	B Conway, PJ Phelan, GD Stewart	
16.	**Cardiology**	441
	DE Newby, NR Grubb	
17.	**Respiratory medicine**	545
	PT Reid, JA Innes	
18.	**Endocrinology**	629
	MWJ Strachan, JDC Newell-Price	
19.	**Nutritional factors in disease**	691
	AG Shand, JPH Wilding	
20.	**Diabetes mellitus**	719
	ER Pearson, RJ McCrimmon	
21.	**Gastroenterology**	763
	E El-Omar, MH McLean	
22.	**Hepatology**	845
	QM Anstee, DEJ Jones	
23.	**Haematology and transfusion medicine**	911
	HG Watson, DJ Culligan, LM Manson	
24.	**Rheumatology and bone disease**	981
	GPR Clunie, SH Ralston	
25.	**Neurology**	1061
	JP Leach, RJ Davenport	
26.	**Stroke medicine**	1147
	P Langhorne	
27.	**Medical ophthalmology**	1163
	J Olson	
28.	**Medical psychiatry**	1179
	RM Steel, SM Lawrie	
29.	**Dermatology**	1209
	SH Ibbotson	
30.	**Maternal medicine**	1269
	L Mackillop, FEM Neuberger	

31.	**Adolescent and transition medicine** R Mann	**1287**
32.	**Ageing and disease** MD Witham	**1301**
33.	**Oncology** GG Dark	**1313**
34.	**Pain and palliative care** LA Colvin, M Fallon	**1337**
35.	**Laboratory reference ranges** SJ Jenks	**1357**
	Index	**1365**

Preface

Well over two million copies of *Davidson's Principles and Practice of Medicine* have been sold since it was first published in 1952. Now in its 23rd Edition, *Davidson's* is regarded as a 'must-have' textbook for thousands of medical students, doctors and health professionals across the world, describing the pathophysiology and clinical features of the most important conditions encountered in the major specialties of adult medicine and explaining how to investigate, diagnose and manage them. The book is the winner of numerous prizes and awards and has been translated into many languages. Taking its origins from Sir Stanley Davidson's much-admired lecture notes, the book has endured because it continues to keep pace with how modern medicine is taught and to provide a wealth of information in an easy-to-read, concise and beautifully illustrated format.

Davidson's strives to ensure that readers can not only recognise the clinical features of a disease but also understand the underlying causes. To achieve this, each chapter begins with a summary of the relevant pre-clinical science, linking pathophysiology with clinical presentation and treatment so that students can use the book from the outset of their medical studies right through to their final examinations and beyond.

The regular introduction of new authors and editors is important for maintaining freshness. On this occasion, Professor Mark Strachan and Dr Richard Hobson have come on board as editors, and 26 new authors have joined our existing contributors to make up an outstanding team of authorities in their respective fields. As well as recruiting authors from around the globe, particularly for topics such as infectious diseases, HIV and envenomation, we welcome members from 17 countries on to our International Advisory Board. These leading experts provide detailed comments that are crucial to our revision of each new edition. A particularly important aspect in planning the revision is for the editors to meet students and faculty in medical schools in those countries where the book is most widely read, so that we can respond to the feedback of our global readership and their tutors. We use this feedback, along with the information we gather via detailed student reviews and surveys, to craft each edition. The authors, editors and publishing team aim to ensure that readers all over the world are best served by a book that integrates medical science with clinical medicine to convey key knowledge and practical advice in an accessible and readable format. The amount of detail is tailored to the needs of medical students working towards their final examinations, as well as candidates preparing for Membership of the Royal Colleges of Physicians (MRCP) or its equivalent.

With this new edition we have introduced several changes in both structure and content. The opening six chapters provide an account of the principles of genetics, immunology, infectious diseases and population health, along with a discussion of the core principles behind clinical decision-making and good prescribing. Subsequent chapters discuss medical emergencies in poisoning, envenomation and environmental medicine, while a new chapter explores common presentations in acute medicine, as well as the recognition and management of the critically ill. The disease-specific chapters that follow cover the major medical specialties, each one thoroughly revised and updated to ensure that readers have access to the 'cutting edge' of medical knowledge and practice. Two new chapters on maternal and adolescent/transition medicine now complement the one on ageing and disease, addressing particular problems encountered at key stages of patients' lives. Medical ophthalmology is also now included as a direct response to readers' requests.

The innovations introduced in recent editions have been maintained and, in many cases, developed. The highly popular 'Clinical Examination' overviews have been extended to the biochemistry, nutrition and dermatology chapters. The 'Presenting Problems' sections continue to provide an invaluable overview of the most common presentations in each disease area. The 'Emergency' and 'Practice Point' boxes have been retained along with the 'In Old Age', 'In Pregnancy' and 'In Adolescence' boxes, which emphasise key practical points in the presentation and management of the elderly, women with medical disorders who are pregnant or planning pregnancy, and teenagers transitioning between paediatric and adult services.

Education is achieved by assimilating information from many sources and readers of this book can enhance their learning experience by using several complementary resources. We are delighted to have a new self-testing companion book entitled *Davidson's Assessment in Medicine*, containing over 1250 multiple choice questions specifically tailored to the contents of *Davidson's*. The long-standing association of *Davidson's* with its sister books, *Macleod's Clinical Examination* (now in its 14th Edition) and *Principles and Practice of Surgery* (7th Edition), still holds good. Our 'family' has also expanded with the publication of *Davidson's Essentials of Medicine*, a long-requested pocket-sized version of the main text; *Davidson's 100 Clinical Cases*, which contains scenarios directly based on our 'Presenting Problems'; and *Macleod's Clinical Diagnosis*, which describes a systematic approach to the differential diagnosis of symptoms and signs. We congratulate the editors and authors of these books for continuing the tradition of easily digested and expertly illustrated texts.

We all take immense pride in continuing the great tradition first established by Sir Stanley Davidson and in producing an outstanding book for the next generation of doctors.

SHR, IDP, MWJS, RPH
Edinburgh 2018

Contributors

Brian J Angus BSc(Hons), DTM&H, FRCP, MD, FFTM(Glas)
Associate Professor, Nuffield Department of Medicine, University of Oxford, UK

Quentin M Anstee BSc(Hons), PhD, FRCP
Professor of Experimental Hepatology, Institute of Cellular Medicine, Newcastle University, Newcastle upon Tyne; Honorary Consultant Hepatologist, Freeman Hospital, Newcastle upon Tyne, UK

Leslie Burnett MBBS, PhD, FRCPA, FHGSA
Chief Medical Officer, Genome.One, Garvan Institute of Medical Research, Sydney; Conjoint Professor, St Vincent's Clinical School, UNSW; Honorary Professor in Pathology and Genetic Medicine, Sydney Medical School, University of Sydney, Australia

Mark Byers OBE, FRCGP, FFSEM, FIMC, MRCEM
Consultant in Pre-Hospital Emergency Medicine, Institute of Pre-Hospital Care, London, UK

Harry Campbell MD, FRCPE, FFPH, FRSE
Professor of Genetic Epidemiology and Public Health, Centre for Global Health Research, Usher Institute of Population Health Sciences and Informatics, University of Edinburgh, UK

Gavin PR Clunie BSc, MD, FRCP
Consultant Rheumatologist and Metabolic Bone Physician, Cambridge University Hospitals NHS Foundation Trust, Addenbrooke's Hospital, Cambridge, UK

Lesley A Colvin BSc, FRCA, PhD, FRCPE, FFPMRCA
Consultant, Department of Anaesthesia, Critical Care and Pain Medicine, Western General Hospital, Edinburgh; Honorary Professor in Anaesthesia and Pain Medicine, University of Edinburgh, UK

Bryan Conway MB, MRCP, PhD
Senior Lecturer, Centre for Cardiovascular Science, University of Edinburgh; Honorary Consultant Nephrologist, Royal Infirmary of Edinburgh, UK

Nicola Cooper FAcadMEd, FRCPE, FRACP
Consultant Physician, Derby Teaching Hospitals NHS Foundation Trust, Derby; Honorary Clinical Associate Professor, Division of Medical Sciences and Graduate Entry Medicine, University of Nottingham, UK

Alison L Cracknell FRCP
Consultant, Medicine for Older People, Leeds Teaching Hospitals NHS Trust, Leeds; Honorary Clinical Associate Professor, University of Leeds, UK

Dominic J Culligan BSc, MD, FRCP, FRCPath
Consultant Haematologist, Aberdeen Royal Infirmary; Honorary Senior Lecturer, University of Aberdeen, UK

Graham G Dark FRCP, FHEA
Senior Lecturer in Medical Oncology and Cancer Education, Newcastle University, Newcastle upon Tyne, UK

Richard J Davenport DM, FRCPE, BMedSci
Consultant Neurologist, Royal Infirmary of Edinburgh and Western General Hospital, Edinburgh; Honorary Senior Lecturer, University of Edinburgh, UK

David H Dockrell MD, FRCPI, FRCPG, FACP
Professor of Infection Medicine, Medical Research Council/ University of Edinburgh Centre for Inflammation Research, University of Edinburgh, UK

Emad El-Omar BSc(Hons), MD(Hons), FRCPE, FRSE, FRACP
Professor of Medicine, St George and Sutherland Clinical School, University of New South Wales, Sydney, Australia

Marie Fallon MD, FRCP
St Columba's Hospice Chair of Palliative Medicine, University of Edinburgh, UK

David R FitzPatrick MD, FMedSci
Professor, Medical Research Council Human Genetics Unit, Institute of Genetics and Molecular Medicine, University of Edinburgh, UK

Neil R Grubb MD, FRCP
Consultant in Cardiology, Royal Infirmary of Edinburgh; Honorary Senior Lecturer in Cardiovascular Sciences, University of Edinburgh, UK

Sally H Ibbotson BSc(Hons), MD, FRCPE
Professor of Photodermatology, University of Dundee; Honorary Consultant Dermatologist and Head of Photobiology Unit, Ninewells Hospital and Medical School, Dundee, UK

J Alastair Innes BSc, PhD, FRCPE
Consultant, Respiratory Unit, Western General Hospital, Edinburgh; Honorary Reader in Respiratory Medicine, University of Edinburgh, UK

Sara J Jenks BSc(Hons), MRCP, FRCPath
Consultant in Metabolic Medicine, Department of Clinical Biochemistry, Royal Infirmary of Edinburgh, UK

Sarah L Johnston FCRP, FRCPath
Consultant Immunologist, Department of Immunology and Immunogenetics, North Bristol NHS Trust, Bristol, UK

David EJ Jones MA, BM, PhD, FRCP
Professor of Liver Immunology, Institute of Cellular Medicine, Newcastle University, Newcastle upon Tyne; Consultant Hepatologist, Freeman Hospital, Newcastle upon Tyne, UK

Peter Langhorne PhD, FRCPG, FRCPI
Professor of Stroke Care, Institute of Cardiovascular and Medical Sciences, University of Glasgow, UK

Stephen M Lawrie MD(Hons), FRCPsych, FRCPE(Hon)
Professor of Psychiatry, University of Edinburgh, UK

John Paul Leach MD, FRCPG, FRCPE
Consultant Neurologist, Institute of Neuroscience, Queen Elizabeth University Hospital, Glasgow; Head of Undergraduate Medicine and Honorary Associate Clinical Professor, University of Glasgow, UK

Gary Maartens MBChB, FCP(SA), MMed
Professor of Clinical Pharmacology, University of Cape Town, South Africa

Lucy Mackillop MA(Oxon), FRCP
Consultant Obstetric Physician, Oxford University Hospitals NHS Foundation Trust, Oxford; Honorary Senior Clinical Lecturer, Nuffield Department of Obstetrics and Gynaecology, University of Oxford, UK

Michael J MacMahon FRCA, FICM, EDIC
Consultant in Anaesthesia and Intensive Care, Victoria Hospital, Kirkcaldy, UK

Rebecca Mann BMedSci, MRCP, FRCPCh
Consultant Paediatrician, Taunton and Somerset NHS Foundation Trust, Taunton, UK

Lynn M Manson MD, FRCPE, FRCPath
Consultant Haematologist, Scottish National Blood Transfusion Service, Department of Transfusion Medicine, Royal Infirmary of Edinburgh, UK

Sara E Marshall FRCP, FRCPath, PhD
Professor of Clinical Immunology, Medical Research Institute, University of Dundee, UK

Amanda Mather MBBS, FRACP, PhD
Consultant Nephrologist, Department of Renal Medicine, Royal North Shore Hospital, Sydney; Conjoint Senior Lecturer, Faculty of Medicine, University of Sydney, Australia

Simon RJ Maxwell BSc, MD, PhD, FRCP, FRCPE, FBPhS, FHEA
Professor of Student Learning – Clinical Pharmacology and Prescribing, and Medical Director, UK Prescribing Safety Assessment, Clinical Pharmacology Unit, University of Edinburgh, UK

David A McAllister MSc, MD, MRCP, MFPH
Wellcome Trust Intermediate Clinical Fellow and Beit Fellow, Senior Clinical Lecturer in Epidemiology, and Honorary Consultant in Public Health Medicine, University of Glasgow, UK

Rory J McCrimmon MD, FRCPE
Professor of Experimental Diabetes and Metabolism, University of Dundee, UK

Mairi H McLean BSc(Hons), MRCP, PhD
Senior Clinical Lecturer in Gastroenterology, School of Medicine, Medical Sciences and Nutrition, University of Aberdeen; Honorary Consultant Gastroenterologist, Aberdeen Royal Infirmary, UK

Francesca EM Neuberger MRCP(UK)
Consultant Physician in Acute Medicine and Obstetric Medicine, Southmead Hospital, Bristol, UK

David E Newby BA, BSc(Hons), PhD, BM DM DSc, FMedSci, FRSE, FESC, FACC
British Heart Foundation John Wheatley Professor of Cardiology, British Heart Foundation Centre for Cardiovascular Science, University of Edinburgh, UK

John DC Newell-Price MA, PhD, FRCP
Professor of Endocrinology and Consultant Endocrinologist, Department of Oncology and Metabolism, University of Sheffield, UK

John Olson MD, FRPCE, FRCOphth
Consultant Ophthalmic Physician, Aberdeen Royal Infirmary; Honorary Reader, University of Aberdeen, UK

Ewan R Pearson MA, PhD, FRCPE
Professor of Diabetic Medicine, University of Dundee, UK

Paul J Phelan MD, FRCPE
Consultant Nephrologist and Renal Transplant Physician, Royal Infirmary of Edinburgh; Honorary Senior Lecturer, University of Edinburgh, UK

Stuart H Ralston MD, FRCP, FMedSci, FRSE, FFPM(Hon)
Arthritis Research UK Professor of Rheumatology, University of Edinburgh; Honorary Consultant Rheumatologist, Western General Hospital, Edinburgh, UK

Peter T Reid MD, FRCPE
Consultant Physician, Respiratory Medicine, Lothian University Hospitals, Edinburgh, UK

Jonathan AT Sandoe PhD, FRCPath
Associate Clinical Professor, University of Leeds; Consultant Microbiologist, Leeds Teaching Hospitals NHS Trust, UK

Gordon R Scott BSc, FRCP
Consultant in Genitourinary Medicine, Chalmers Sexual Health Centre, Edinburgh, UK

Alan G Shand MD, FRCPE
Consultant Gastroenterologist, Western General Hospital, Edinburgh, UK

Robby M Steel MA, MD, FRCPsych
Consultant Liaison Psychiatrist, Department of Psychological Medicine, Royal Infirmary of Edinburgh; Honorary (Clinical) Senior Lecturer, Department of Psychiatry, University of Edinburgh, UK

Grant D Stewart BSc(Hons), FRCSEd(Urol), PhD
University Lecturer in Urological Surgery, Academic Urology Group, University of Cambridge; Honorary Consultant Urological Surgeon, Department of Urology, Addenbrooke's Hospital, Cambridge; Honorary Senior Clinical Lecturer, University of Edinburgh, UK

Peter Stewart MBBS, FRACP, FRCPA, MBA
Associate Professor in Chemical Pathology, University of Sydney; Area Director of Clinical Biochemistry and Head of the Biochemistry Department, Royal Prince Alfred and Liverpool Hospitals, Sydney, Australia

Mark WJ Strachan BSc(Hons), MD, FRCPE
Consultant Endocrinologist, Metabolic Unit, Western General Hospital, Edinburgh; Honorary Professor, University of Edinburgh, UK

David R Sullivan MBBS, FRACP, FRCPA, FCSANZ
Clinical Associate Professor, Faculty of Medicine, University of Sydney; Physician and Chemical Pathologist, Department of Chemical Pathology, Royal Prince Alfred Hospital, Sydney, Australia

Shyam Sundar MD, FRCP(London), FAMS, FNASc, FASc, FNA
Professor of Medicine, Institute of Medical Sciences, Banaras Hindu University, Varanasi, India

Victoria R Tallentire BSc(Hons), MD, FRCPE
Consultant Physician, Western General Hospital, Edinburgh; Honorary Clinical Senior Lecturer, University of Edinburgh, UK

Katrina Tatton-Brown BA, MD, FRCP
Consultant in Clinical Genetics, South West Thames Regional Genetics Service, St George's Universities NHS Foundation Trust, London; Reader in Clinical Genetics and Genomic Education, St George's University, London, UK

Simon HL Thomas MD, FRCP, FRCPE
Professor of Clinical Pharmacology and Therapeutics, Medical Toxicology Centre, Newcastle University, Newcastle upon Tyne, UK

Henry G Watson MD, FRCPE, FRCPath
Consultant Haematologist, Aberdeen Royal Infirmary; Honorary Professor of Medicine, University of Aberdeen, UK

Julian White MB, BS, MD, FACTM
Head of Toxinology, Women's and Children's Hospital, North Adelaide; Professor, University of Adelaide, Australia

John PH Wilding DM, FRCP
Professor of Medicine, Obesity and Endocrinology, University of Liverpool, UK

Miles D Witham PhD, FRCPE
Clinical Reader in Ageing and Health, University of Dundee, UK

International Advisory Board

Acknowledgements

Following the publication of the 22nd edition of *Davidson's*, Professor Brian Walker and Dr Nicki Colledge retired as editors. We would like to express our gratitude for the immense contribution they both made to the continuing success of this textbook.

The current editors would like to acknowledge and offer grateful thanks for the input of all previous editions' contributors, without whom this new edition would not have been possible. In particular we are indebted to those former authors who step down with the arrival of this new edition. They include Assistant Professor Albiruni Ryan Abdul-Razak, Professor Andrew Bradbury, Dr Jenny Craig, Professor Allan Cumming, Dr Robert Dawe, Emeritus Professor Michael Field, Dr Jane Goddard, Professor Philip Hanlon, Dr Charlie Lees, Dr Helen Macdonald, Professor Iain McInnes, Dr Graham Nimmo, Dr Simon Noble, Dr David Oxenham, Professor Jonathan Seckl, Professor Michael Sharpe, Professor Neil Turner, Dr Simon Walker and Professor Timothy Walsh.

We are grateful to members of the International Advisory Board, all of whom provided detailed suggestions that have improved the book. Several members have now retired from the Board and we are grateful for their support during the preparation of previous editions. They include Professor OC Abraham, Professor Tofayel Ahmed, Professor Samar Banerjee, Professor Tapas Das, Professor Tsuguya Fukui, Professor Saman Gunatilake, Professor Wasim Jafri, Professor Saraladevi Naicker, Professor Nardeep Naithani, Professor Prem Pais, Professor A Ramachandran, the late Professor (Mrs) Harsha R Salkar and Professor Subhash Varma.

Detailed chapter reviews were commissioned to help plan this new edition and we are grateful to all those who assisted, including Professor Rustam Al-Shahi, Dr David Enoch, Dr Colin Forfar, Dr Richard Herriot and Dr Robert Lindsay.

The Editors and Publisher would like to thank all those who have provided valuable feedback on this textbook and whose comments have helped shape this new edition. We would particularly like to extend our thanks to the many readers who contact us with suggestions for improvements. This input has been invaluable and is much appreciated; we regret the names are too numerous to mention individually.

As part of the Publisher's review, 360 readers from over 200 universities and colleges around the world supplied many innovative ideas on how to enhance the book. We are deeply indebted to the following for their enthusiastic support and we trust we have listed all those who contributed; we apologise if any names have been accidentally omitted. Rabab Hasan Abbasi, Ayesha Abdul Aziz, Ahmed Al Abdullah, Osama Abuzagaia, Humaira Achakzai, Sajan Acharya, Anurag Adhikari, Esha Agarwal, Avin Aggarwal, Dorothy Agrapidis, Sakir Ahmed, Iman Akhtar, Muhammad Faizan Ali, Syeda A Rfa Ali, M Amogh, Ramprasath Anbazhagan, Anju George C, Vamseedhar Annam, Muhammad Ehtisham Ansar, David C Antoney, Hina Arif, Sriharsha Athota, Muhammed Ali Azher, Bilal Al Azzawi, Janak Bahirwani, Devyani Bahl, Mohammed Naseem Baig, Deepak Kumar Bandari, Sagnik Banerjee, Tapastanu Banerjee, Kieran Bannerman, Emily Bart, Suranjana Basak, Saravana Bavan, Mark Beeston, Andrew Beverstock, Jeetendra Bhandari, Navin Bhatt, Soumyadeep Bhaumik, Rajrsh Bhawani, Kriti Bhayana, Praveen Bhugra, Amit Bisht, Rahul Bisht, Rudradeep Biswas, Tamoghna Biswas, Moira Bradfield, S Charles Bronson, Rosie Jane Campbell, Anup Chalise, Subhankar Chatterjee, Chiranjivi Chaudhari, Lok Bandhu Chaudhary, Muhammad Hamid Chaudhary, Umar Iftikhar Chaudhry, Himshree Gaurang Chhaya, Smitha Chirayil, Alexandra Choa, Rahul Choudhary, Guy Conlon, Gabriel Metcalf-Cuenca, Jack Cuningham, Gopal Dabade, Saraswata Das, Rahul Dev, Muinul Islam Dewan, Sree Divya, Muhammad Dizayee, Lucy Drummond, Simon Dryden, Fiona Drysdale, Kaitlin Duell, Gemma Dwyer, Md Khader Faheem N, Mahedi Hasan Faisal, Ali Mokhtari Farivar, Mohammed Omar Farooq, Ten Fu Fatt, Muhammad Zubair Fazal, Rebecca Ferris, Rebecca Fisher, Kartik Nimish Gandhi, Vibhav Gandhi, James Gao, Ella Gardner, Ankit Kumar Garg, Vibhuti Garg, Vishal Garg, Rakesh Garlapati, Partha Sarathi Ghosh, Prattay Ghosh, Muhammad Umer Gill, Madelaine Gimzewska, Nikolaos D Giotis, Evan Goh, Iain Gow, Bharatiram Guduri, Aantriksha Gupta, Shiwam Kumar Gupta, Michael Hagarty, Md Rashid Haider, Iqra Haq, Abdalla A Hassan, Fatima Hemani, Bianca Honnekeri, Prerana Huddar, Sandip Hulke, Mohammed Laique Hussain, Syahir Ibrahim, Victor Ilubaera, Sushrut Ingawale, Aroobah Iqbal, Tooba Irshad, Nagib Ul-Islam, Sehra Jabeen, Jeevan Jacob, Samreen Jaffar, Ankita Jain, Anukriti Jain, Ghazfa Jamil, Karan Jatwani, Surani Dilhani Jayawickrema, Pcr-Kristian Jensen, Love Kapil, Ishwor Karki, Ewan D Kennedy, Amit Keshri, Haider Ali Khalid, Ali Khaliq, Hina Khan, Md Taha Ali Khan, Raazia Khan, Priya Khetarpal, Robert Kimmitt, Navneet Kishore, Narendranath Reddy Konda, Kirsten Kramers, Ajay Kumar, Gaurav Kumar, Karun Kumar, Mudit Kumar, Sathish Kumar A, Sonu Kumar, Ramasamy Shakthi Kumaran, Joachim Langhans, Keith Leung, Ang Li, Lai Nai Lim (Jeremiah), Marlene Da Vitoria Lobo, Bo Løfgren, Sham Kumar Lulla, Apurva Lunia, Arslan Luqman, Faizan Luqman, Mithilesh Chandra Malviya, Sudhir Mane, Sachin Mangal, G. Manju, Adupa Manupranay, Ussama Maqbool, Zahid Marwat, Ronny John Mathew, Ross Mclaren, Lucy Mcnally, Varshil Mehta, Kamran Younis Memon, Nisha Menon, Varun Menon P, Jessica Mills, Asim Abid Minhas,

Mohd Nasir Mohiuddin, Matshidiso Mokgwathi, Kristin Monk, Joseph Raja Mony, Sudeb Mukherjee, Sadaf Nadeem, Huda Naim, B Abhilash Nair, Ramya Narasimhan, Rahul Navani, Ayesha Nazir, Prakhar Nigam, Sripriya Nopany, Prakash Raj Oli, Chieh Yin Ooi, Muhammad Osama, Kate O'Sullivan, Hajer Oun, Ashwin Pachat, Akshay Pachyala, Kannan Padma, Gregory Page, Vishal Krishna Pai, Dhiman Pal, Vidit Panchal, Madhav Pandey, Ambikapathi Panneerselvam, Rakesh Singh Panwar, Prakash Parida, Ashwin Singh Parihar, Kunal Parwani, Riya Patel, Himanshu Pathak, Prathamesh Pathrikar, Samanvith Patlori, Gary Paul, Harris Penman, Lydia B Peters, Kausthubha Puttalingaiah, Muneeb Qureshi, Sidra Qureshi, Varun Venkat Raghavan MS, Raghavendra MS, Abdur Rahaman, Ajmal Rahman Km, SM Tajdit Rahman, Ankit Raj, Solai Raj, Namita Raja, Revathi Rajagopal, Aswathy Raju B, Nagarajan Raju, Al-Amin Hossain Rakib, Abhiraj Ramchandani, Varun Ramchandani, Viviktha Ramesh, Jai Ranjan, Ganga Raghava Rao, Gomathi Ravula, Aneeqa Abdul Rehman, Neeha Abdul Rehman, Varun Bhaktarahalli Renukappa, Rosalind Revans, Madina Riaz, Lachlan Rodd, Jan Ross, Pritam Roy, Jazeel Sa, Iqra Saeed, Israel Safiriyu, Partha Saha, Mohammed Sulaiman Sait J, Ribha Salman, Souvik Samaddar, Juliane Rf Sanner, Abhinav Sathe, Smarter Sawant, Jeff Schwartz, Somanshi Sehgal, Arbind Shah, Basit Shah, Rakesh Kumar Shah, Mohith Shamdas, Abhishek Sharma, Anmol Sharma, Deepak Sharma, Pawan Kumar Sharma, Nisha Sharoff, Alsba Sheikh, Haris Sheikh, Nujood Al Shirawi, William Shomali, Pratima Shrestha, Suhana Shrestha, Ajay Shukla, Prithiv Siddharth, Arpit Sikri, Ankita Singh, Avinash Singh, Deepali Singh, Jeevika Singh, Prince Singh, Rajshree Singh, Shruti Singh, Vikas Singh, Yogita Singh, Ayush Keshav Singhal, Dattatreya Sitaram, Brooke Smith, Yeshwanth Sonnathi, Soundarya Soundararajan, Nicola Stuber, Maleeha Subhan, Udayasree Sagar Surampally, Monika Surana, Jason Suresh, Salman Ali Syed, Mohammad Hasnain Tahir, Syeda Sara Tamkanath, Areeba Tariq, Saipriya Tatineni, Ghias Un Nabi Tayyab, Arul Qubert Thaya, Jolley Thomas, Stephanie Tristram, Neelanchal Trivedi, Vaibhav Trivedi, Kriti Upadhyay, Sanjaya Kumar Upadhyaya, Rukhsar Vankani, Rajkumar Krishnan Vasanthi, D Vijayaraju, R Vinayak, Neelakantan Viswanathan, Joarder Wakil, Syed Hamza Bin Waqar, Waiz A Wasey, William Wasif, Kiran Wasti, Donald Waters, Katherine Weir, Clinton White, Aalok Yadav, Loong Yee Yew, Shahwar Yousuf, Amal Yusof and Hassam Zulfiqar.

The authors of Chapter 20 would like to thank Dr Drew Henderson, who reviewed the 'Diabetic nephropathy' section.

Two short sections in Chapter 3 on array comparative genomic hybridisation and single-molecule sequencing are adapted from Dr K Tatton-Brown's Massive Open Online Course for FutureLearn. We would like to thank the Open University and St George's, University of London, for permission to use this material.

We are especially grateful to all those working for Elsevier, in particular Laurence Hunter, Wendy Lee and Robert Britton, for their endless support and expertise in the shaping, collation and illustration of this edition.

SHR, IDP, MWJS, RPH
Edinburgh 2018

Introduction

The opening six chapters of the book, making up Part 1 on 'Fundamentals of Medicine', provide an account of the principles of genetics, immunology, infectious diseases and population health, along with a discussion of the core principles behind clinical decision-making and good prescribing. Subsequent chapters in Part 2, 'Emergency and Critical Care Medicine', discuss medical emergencies in poisoning, envenomation and environmental medicine, while a new chapter explores common presentations in acute medicine, as well as the recognition and management of the critically ill. The third part, 'Clinical Medicine', is devoted to the major medical specialties. Each chapter has been written by experts in the field to provide the level of detail expected of trainees in their discipline. To maintain the book's virtue of being concise, care has been taken to avoid unnecessary duplication between chapters.

The system-based chapters in Part 3 follow a standard format, beginning with an overview of the relevant aspects of clinical examination, followed by an account of functional anatomy, physiology and investigations, then the common presentations of disease, and details of the individual diseases and treatments relevant to that system. In chapters that describe the immunological, cellular and molecular basis of disease, this problem-based approach brings the close links between modern medical science and clinical practice into sharp focus.

The methods used to present information are described below.

Clinical examination overviews

The value of good clinical skills is highlighted by a two-page overview of the important elements of the clinical examination at the beginning of most chapters. The left-hand page includes a mannikin to illustrate key steps in examination of the relevant system, beginning with simple observations and progressing in a logical sequence around the body. The right-hand page expands on selected themes and includes tips on examination technique and interpretation of physical signs. These overviews are intended to act as an aide-mémoire and not as a replacement for a detailed text on clinical examination, as provided in our sister title, *Macleod's Clinical Examination.*

Presenting problems

Medical students and junior doctors must not only assimilate a great many facts about various disorders but also develop an analytical approach to formulating a differential diagnosis

and a plan of investigation for patients who present with particular symptoms or signs. In *Davidson*'s this is addressed by incorporating a 'Presenting Problems' section into all relevant chapters. Nearly 250 presentations are included, which represent the most common reasons for referral to each medical specialty.

Boxes

Boxes are a popular way of presenting information and are particularly useful for revision. They are classified by the type of information they contain, using specific symbols.

 ### General Information

These include causes, clinical features, investigations, treatments and other useful information.

 ### Practice Point

There are many practical skills that students and doctors must master. These vary from inserting a nasogastric tube to reading an ECG or X-ray, or interpreting investigations such as arterial blood gases or thyroid function tests. 'Practice Point' boxes provide straightforward guidance on how these and many other skills can be acquired and applied.

 ### Emergency

These boxes describe the management of many of the most common emergencies in medicine.

 ### In Old Age

In many countries, older people comprise 20% of the population and are the chief users of health care. While they contract the same diseases as those who are younger, there are often important differences in the way they present and how they are best managed. Chapter 32, 'Ageing and disease', concentrates on the principles of managing the frailest group who suffer from multiple comorbidity and disability, and who tend to present with non-specific problems such as falls or delirium. Many older people, though, also suffer from specific single-organ pathology. 'In Old Age' boxes are thus included in each chapter and describe common presentations, implications of physiological changes of ageing, effects of age on investigations, problems of treatment in old age, and the benefits and risks of intervention in older people.

 ### *In Pregnancy*

Many conditions are different in the context of pregnancy, while some arise only during or shortly after pregnancy. Particular care must be taken with investigations (for example, to avoid radiation exposure to the fetus) and treatment (to avoid the use of drugs that harm the fetus). These issues are highlighted by 'In Pregnancy' boxes distributed throughout the book, which complement the new chapter on maternal medicine.

 ### *In Adolescence*

Although paediatric medicine is not covered in *Davidson's*, many chronic disorders begin in childhood and adult physicians often contribute to multidisciplinary teams that manage young patients 'in transition' between paediatric and adult health-care services. This group of patients often presents a particular challenge, due to the physiological and psychological changes that occur in adolescence and which can have a major impact on the disease and its management. Adolescents can be encouraged to take over responsibility from their parents/carers in managing their disease, but are naturally rebellious and often struggle to adhere to the impositions of chronic treatment. To highlight these issues, we have introduced a new chapter on adolescent and transition medicine to accompany the 'In Adolescence' boxes that appear in relevant chapters.

Terminology

The recommended International Non-proprietary Names (INNs) are used for all drugs, with the exception of adrenaline and noradrenaline. British spellings have been retained for drug classes and groups (e.g. amphetamines not amfetamines).

Units of measurement

The International System of Units (SI units) is the recommended means of presentation for laboratory data and has been used throughout *Davidson's*. We recognise, though, that many laboratories around the world continue to provide data in non-SI units, so these have been included in the text for the commonly measured analytes. Both SI and non-SI units are also given in Chapter 35, which describes the reference ranges used in Edinburgh's laboratories. It is important to appreciate that these reference ranges may vary from those used in other laboratories.

Finding what you are looking for

A contents list is given on the opening page of each chapter. In addition, the book contains numerous cross-references to help readers find their way around, along with an extensive index. A list of up-to-date reviews and useful websites with links to management guidelines appears at the end of each chapter.

Giving us your feedback

The Editors and Publisher hope that you will find this edition of *Davidson's* informative and easy to use. We would be delighted to hear from you if you have any comments or suggestions to make for future editions of the book. Please contact us by e-mail at: davidson. feedback@elsevier.com. All comments received will be much appreciated and will be considered by the editorial team.

N Cooper
AL Cracknell

1

Clinical decision-making

Introduction 2

The problem of diagnostic error 2

Clinical reasoning: definitions 2

Clinical skills and decision-making 3

Use and interpretation of diagnostic tests 3
Normal values 3
Factors other than disease that influence test results 4
Operating characteristics 4
Sensitivity and specificity 4
Prevalence of disease 5

Dealing with uncertainty 5

Cognitive biases 6
Type 1 and type 2 thinking 7
Common cognitive biases in medicine 7
Human factors 9

Reducing errors in clinical decision-making 9
Cognitive debiasing strategies 9
Using clinical prediction rules and other decision aids 10
Effective team communication 10

Patient-centred evidence-based medicine and shared decision-making 10

Clinical decision-making: putting it all together 10

Answers to problems 12

Introduction

A great deal of knowledge and skill is required to practise as a doctor. Physicians in the 21st century need to have a comprehensive knowledge of basic and clinical sciences, have good communication skills, be able to perform procedures, work effectively in a team and demonstrate professional and ethical behaviour. But how doctors think, reason and make decisions is arguably their most critical skill. Knowledge is necessary, but not sufficient on its own for good performance and safe care. This chapter describes the principles of clinical decision-making, or clinical reasoning.

The problem of diagnostic error

It is estimated that diagnosis is wrong 10–15% of the time in specialties such as emergency medicine, internal medicine and general practice. Diagnostic error is associated with greater morbidity than other types of medical error, and the majority is considered to be preventable. For every diagnostic error there are a number of root causes. Studies of misdiagnosis assign three main categories, shown in Box 1.1; however, errors in clinical reasoning play a significant role in the majority of diagnostic adverse events.

i	**1.1 Root causes of diagnostic error in studies**	
Error category	**Examples**	
No fault	Unusual presentation of a disease Missing information	
System error	Inadequate diagnostic support Results not available Error-prone processes Poor supervision of inexperienced staff Poor team communication	
Human cognitive error	Inadequate data-gathering Errors in reasoning	

Adapted from Graber M, Gordon R, Franklin N. Reducing diagnostic errors in medicine: what's the goal? Acad Med 2002; 77:981–992.

i	**1.2 Reasons for errors in clinical reasoning**	
Source of error	**Examples**	
Knowledge gaps	Telling a patient she cannot have biliary colic because she has had her gallbladder removed – gallstones can form in the bile ducts in patients who have had a cholecystectomy	
Misinterpretation of diagnostic tests	Deciding a patient has not had a stroke because his brain scan is normal – computed tomography and even magnetic resonance imaging, especially when performed early, may not identify an infarct	
Cognitive biases	Accepting a diagnosis handed over to you without question (the 'framing effect') instead of asking yourself 'What is the evidence that supports this diagnosis?'	

Diagnostic error has been defined as 'a situation in which the clinician has all the information necessary to make the diagnosis but then makes the wrong diagnosis'. Why does this happen? Studies reveal three main reasons:

- knowledge gaps
- misinterpretation of diagnostic tests
- cognitive biases.

Examples of errors in these three categories are shown in Box 1.2.

Clearly, clinical knowledge is required for sound clinical reasoning, and an incomplete knowledge base or inadequate experience can lead to diagnostic error. However, this chapter focuses on other elements of clinical reasoning: namely, the interpretation of diagnostic tests, cognitive biases and human factors.

Clinical reasoning: definitions

'Clinical reasoning' describes the thinking and decision-making processes associated with clinical practice. It is a clinician's ability to make decisions (often with others) based on all the available clinical information, starting with the history and physical examination. Our understanding of clinical reasoning derives from the fields of education, cognitive psychology and studies of expertise.

Figure 1.1 shows the different elements involved in clinical reasoning. Good clinical skills are fundamental, followed by understanding how to use and interpret diagnostic tests. Other essential elements include an understanding of cognitive biases and human factors, and the ability to think about one's own thinking (which is explained in more detail later). Other key elements of clinical reasoning include patient-centred evidence-based medicine (EBM) and shared decision-making with patients and/or carers.

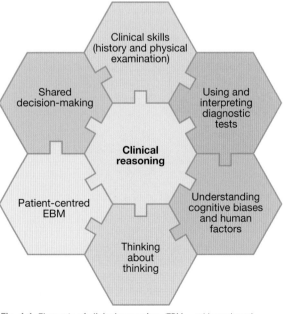

Fig. 1.1 Elements of clinical reasoning. (EBM = evidence-based medicine)

Clinical skills and decision-making

Even with major advances in medical technology, the history remains the most important part of the clinical decision-making process. Studies show that physicians make a diagnosis in 70–90% of cases from the history alone. It is important to remember that a good history is gathered not only from the patient but also, if necessary (and with consent if required), from all available sources: for example, paramedic and emergency department notes, eye-witnesses, relatives and/or carers.

Clinicians need to be aware of the diagnostic usefulness of clinical features in the history and examination. For example, students are taught that meningitis presents with the following features:

- headache
- fever
- meningism (photophobia, nuchal rigidity).

However, the frequency with which patients present with certain features and the diagnostic weight of each feature are important in clinical reasoning. For example, many patients with meningitis do not have classical signs of meningeal irritation (Kernig's sign, Brudzinski's sign and nuchal rigidity). In one prospective study, they had likelihood ratios of around 1, meaning they carried little diagnostic weight (Fig. 1.2).

Likelihood ratios (LR) are clinical diagnostic weights. An LR of greater than 1 increases the probability of disease (the higher the value, the greater the probability). Similarly, an LR of less than 1 decreases the probability of disease. LRs are developed against a diagnostic standard (e.g. in the case of meningitis, lumbar puncture results), so do not exist for all clinical findings. LRs illustrate how an individual clinical finding changes the probability of a disease. For example, in a person presenting with headache and fever, the clinical finding of nuchal rigidity (neck stiffness) may carry little weight in deciding whether to perform a lumbar puncture because LRs do not determine the prior probability of disease; they reflect only how a single clinical finding changes it. Clinicians have to take all the available information from the history and physical examination into account. If the overall clinical probability is high to begin with, a clinical finding with an LR of around 1 does not change this.

'Evidence-based history and examination' is a term used to describe how clinicians incorporate knowledge about the prevalence and diagnostic weight of clinical findings into their history and physical examination. This is important because an estimate of clinical probability is vital in decision-making and the interpretation of diagnostic tests.

Use and interpretation of diagnostic tests

There is no such thing as a perfect diagnostic test. Test results give us test probabilities, not real probabilities. Test results have to be interpreted because they are affected by the following:

- how 'normal' is defined
- factors other than disease
- operating characteristics
- sensitivity and specificity
- prevalence of disease in the population.

Normal values

Most tests provide quantitative results (i.e. a value on a continuous numerical scale). In order to classify quantitative results as normal or abnormal, it is necessary to define a cut-off point. Many quantitative measurements in populations have a Gaussian or 'normal' distribution. By convention, the normal range is defined as those values that encompass 95% of the population, or 2 standard deviations above and below the mean. This means that 2.5% of the normal population will have values above, and 2.5% will have values below the normal range. For this reason, it is more appropriate to talk about the 'reference range' rather than the 'normal range' (Fig. 1.3).

Test results in abnormal populations also have a Gaussian distribution, with a different mean and standard deviation. In some diseases there is no overlap between results from the abnormal and normal population. However, in many diseases there is overlap; in these circumstances, the greater the difference between the test result and the limits of the reference range, the higher the chance that the person has a disease.

However, there are also situations in medicine when 'normal' is abnormal and 'abnormal' is normal. For example, a normal $PaCO_2$ in the context of a severe asthma attack is abnormal and means the patient has life-threatening asthma. A low ferritin in a young menstruating woman is not considered to be a disease at all. Normal, to some extent, is therefore arbitrary.

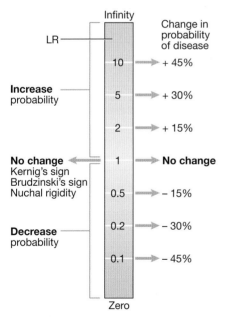

Fig. 1.2 Likelihood ratio (LR) of Kernig's sign, Brudzinski's sign and nuchal rigidity in the clinical diagnosis of meningitis.

$$LR = \frac{\text{probability of finding in patients } \textbf{with} \text{ disease}}{\text{probability of finding in patients } \textbf{without} \text{ disease}}$$

LRs are also used for diagnostic tests; here a physical examination finding can be considered a diagnostic test. *Data from Thomas KE, Hasbun R, Jekel J, Quagliarello VJ. The diagnostic accuracy of Kernig's sign, Brudzinski's sign, and nuchal rigidity in adults with suspected meningitis. Clin Infect Dis 2002; 35:46–52.*

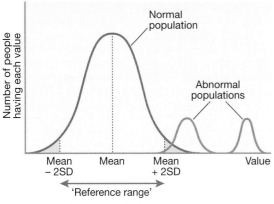

Fig. 1.3 Normal distribution and reference range. For many tests, the frequency distribution of results in the normal healthy population (red line) is a symmetrical bell-shaped curve. The mean ±2 standard deviations (SD) encompasses 95% of the normal population and usually defines the 'reference range'; 2.5% of the normal population have values above, and 2.5% below, this range (shaded areas). For some diseases (blue line), test results overlap with the normal population or even with the reference range. For other diseases (green line), tests may be more reliable because there is no overlap between the normal and abnormal population.

1.3 Examples of factors other than disease that influence test results	
Factor	**Examples**
Age	Creatinine is lower in old age (due to relatively lower muscle mass) – an older person can have a significantly reduced eGFR rate with a 'normal' creatinine
Ethnicity	Healthy people of African ancestry have lower white cell counts
Pregnancy	Several tests are affected by late pregnancy, due to the effects of a growing fetus, including: Reduced urea and creatinine (haemodilution) Iron deficiency anaemia (increased demand) Increased alkaline phosphatase (produced by the placenta) Raised D-dimer (physiological changes in the coagulation system) Mild respiratory alkalosis (physiological maternal hyperventilation) ECG changes (tachycardia, left axis deviation)
Sex	Males and females have different reference ranges for many tests, e.g. haemoglobin
Spurious (in vitro) results	A spurious high potassium is seen in haemolysis and in thrombocytosis ('pseudohyperkalaemia')

(ECG = electrocardiogram; eGFR = estimated glomerular filtration rate, a better estimate of renal function than creatinine)

Factors other than disease that influence test results

A number of factors other than disease influence test results:

- age
- ethnicity
- pregnancy
- sex
- spurious (in vitro) results.

Box 1.3 gives some examples.

Operating characteristics

Tests are also subject to operating characteristics. This refers to the way the test is performed. Patients need to be able to comply fully with some tests, such as spirometry (p. 569), and if they cannot, then the test result will be affected. Some tests are very dependent on the skill of the operator and are also affected by the patient's body habitus and clinical state; ultrasound of the heart and abdomen are examples. A common mistake is when doctors refer to a test result as 'no abnormality detected' when, in fact, the report describes a technically difficult and incomplete scan that should more accurately be described as 'non-diagnostic'.

Some conditions are paroxysmal. For example, around half of patients with epilepsy have a normal standard electroencephalogram (EEG). A normal EEG therefore does not exclude epilepsy. On the other hand, around 10% of patients who do *not* have epilepsy have epileptiform discharges on their EEG. This is referred to as an 'incidental finding'. Incidental findings are common in medicine, and are increasing in incidence with the greater availability of more sensitive tests. Test results should always be interpreted in the light of the patient's history and physical examination.

Sensitivity and specificity

Diagnostic tests have characteristics termed 'sensitivity' and 'specificity'. Sensitivity is the ability to detect true positives; specificity is the ability to detect true negatives. Even a very good test, with 95% sensitivity, will miss 1 in 20 people with the disease. Every test therefore has 'false positives' and 'false negatives' (Box 1.4).

A very sensitive test will detect most disease but generate abnormal findings in healthy people. A negative result will therefore reliably exclude disease but a positive result does not mean the disease is present – it means further evaluation is required. On the other hand, a very specific test may miss significant pathology but is likely to establish the diagnosis beyond doubt when the result is positive. All tests differ in their sensitivity and specificity, and clinicians require a working knowledge of the tests they use in this respect.

In choosing how a test is used to guide decision-making there is a trade-off between sensitivity versus specificity. For example, defining an exercise electrocardiogram (p. 449) as abnormal if there is at least 0.5 mm of ST depression would ensure that very few cases of coronary artery disease are missed but would generate many false-positive results (high sensitivity, low specificity). On the other hand, a cut-off point of 2.0 mm of ST depression would detect most cases of important coronary artery disease with far fewer false positives. This trade-off is illustrated by the receiver operating characteristic curve of the test (Fig. 1.4).

An extremely important concept is this: the probability that a person has a disease depends on the pre-test probability, and the sensitivity and specificity of the test. For example, imagine that an elderly lady has fallen and hurt her left hip. On examination,

i	**1.4 Sensitivity and specificity**	
	Disease	**No disease**
Positive test	A (True positive)	B (False positive)
Negative test	C (False negative)	D (True negative)
	Sensitivity = A/(A+C) × 100 Specificity = D/(D+B) × 100	

Fig. 1.4 Receiver operating characteristic graph illustrating the trade-off between sensitivity and specificity for a given test. The curve is generated by 'adjusting' the cut-off values defining normal and abnormal results, calculating the effect on sensitivity and specificity and then plotting these against each other. The closer the curve lies to the top left-hand corner, the more useful the test. The red line illustrates a test with useful discriminant value and the green line illustrates a less useful, poorly discriminant test.

the hip is extremely painful to move and she cannot stand. However, her hip X-rays are normal. Does she have a fracture?

The sensitivity of plain X-rays of the hip performed in the emergency department for suspected hip fracture is around 95%. A small percentage of fractures are therefore missed. If our patient has (or is at risk of) osteoporosis, has severe pain on hip movement and cannot bear weight on the affected side, then the clinical probability of hip fracture is high. If, on the other hand, she is unlikely to have osteoporosis, has no pain on hip movement and is able to bear weight, then the clinical probability of hip fracture is low.

Doctors are continually making judgements about whether something is true, given that something else is true. This is known as 'conditional probability'. Bayes' Theorem (named after English clergyman Thomas Bayes, 1702–1761) is a mathematical way to describe the post-test probability of a disease by combining pre-test probability, sensitivity and specificity. In clinical practice, doctors are not able to make complex mathematical calculations for every decision they make. In practical terms, the answer to the question of whether there is a fracture is that in a high-probability patient a normal test result does not exclude the condition, but in a low-probability patient it makes it very unlikely. This principle is illustrated in Figure 1.5.

Sox and colleagues (see 'Further information') state a fundamental assertion, which they describe as a profound and subtle principle of clinical medicine: the interpretation of

new information depends on what you believed beforehand. In other words, the interpretation of a test result depends on the probability of disease before the test.

Prevalence of disease

Consider this problem that was posed to a group of Harvard doctors: if a test to detect a disease whose prevalence is 1 : 1000 has a false-positive rate of 5%, what is the chance that a person found to have a positive result actually has the disease, assuming you know nothing about the person's symptoms and signs? Take a moment to work this out. In this problem, we have removed clinical probability and are only considering prevalence. The answer is at the end of the chapter.

Predictive values combine sensitivity, specificity and prevalence. Sensitivity and specificity are characteristics of the test; the population does not change this. However, as doctors, we are interested in the question, 'What is the probability that a person with a positive test actually has the disease?' This is illustrated in Box 1.5.

Post-test probability and predictive values are different. Post-test probability is the probability of a disease after taking into account new information from a test result. Bayes' Theorem can be used to calculate post-test probability for a patient in any population. The pre-test probability of disease is decided by the doctor; it is a judgement based on information gathered prior to ordering the test. Predictive value is the proportion of patients with a test result who have the disease (or no disease) and is calculated from a table of results in a specific population (see Box 1.5). It is not possible to transfer this value to a different population. This is important to realise because published information about the performance of diagnostic tests may not apply to different populations.

In deciding the pre-test probability of disease, clinicians often neglect to take prevalence into account and this distorts their estimate of probability. To estimate the probability of disease in a patient more accurately, clinicians should anchor on the prevalence of disease in the subgroup to which the patient belongs and then adjust to take the individual factors into account.

i	**1.5 Predictive values: 'What is the probability that a person with a positive test actually has the disease?'**	
	Disease	**No disease**
Positive test	A (True positive)	B (False positive)
Negative test	C (False negative)	D (True negative)
	Positive predictive value = A/(A+B) × 100 Negative predictive value = D/(D+C) × 100	

Dealing with uncertainty

Clinical findings are imperfect and diagnostic tests are imperfect. It is important to recognise that clinicians frequently deal with uncertainty. By expressing uncertainty as probability, new information from diagnostic tests can be incorporated more accurately. However, subjective estimates of probability can sometimes be unreliable. As the section on cognitive biases will demonstrate (see below), intuition can be a source of error.

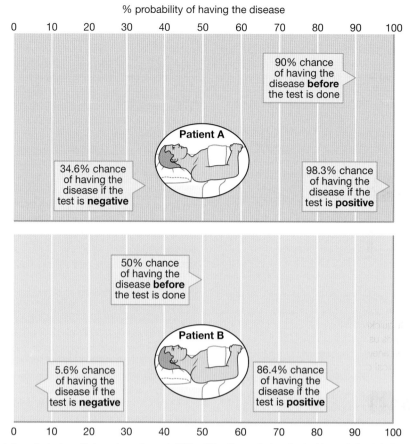

Fig. 1.5 **The interpretation of a test result depends on the probability of the disease before the test is carried out.** In the example shown, the test being carried out has a sensitivity of 95% and a specificity of 85%. Patient A has very characteristic clinical findings, which make the pre-test probability of the condition for which the test is being used very high – estimated as 90%. Patient B has more equivocal findings, such that the pre-test probability is estimated as only 50%. If the result in Patient A is negative, there is still a significant chance that he has the condition for which he is being tested; in Patient B, however, a negative result makes the diagnosis very unlikely.

Knowing the patient's true state is often unnecessary in clinical decision-making. Sox and colleagues (see 'Further information') argue that there is a difference between knowing that a disease is present and acting as if it were present. The requirement for diagnostic certainty depends on the penalty for being wrong. Different situations require different levels of certainty before starting treatment. How we communicate uncertainty to patients will be discussed later in this chapter (p. 10).

The treatment threshold combines factors such as the risks of the test, and the risks versus benefits of treatment. The point at which the factors are all evenly weighed is the threshold. If a test or treatment for a disease is effective and low-risk (e.g. giving antibiotics for a suspected urinary tract infection), then there is a lower threshold for going ahead. On the other hand, if a test or treatment is less effective or high-risk (e.g. starting chemotherapy for a malignant brain tumour), then greater confidence is required in the clinical diagnosis and potential benefits of treatment first. In principle, if a diagnostic test will not change the management of the patient, then careful consideration should be given to whether it is necessary to do the test at all.

In summary, test results shift our thinking, but rarely give a 'yes' or a 'no' answer in terms of a diagnosis. Sometimes tests shift the probability of disease by less than we realise. Pre-test probability is key, and this is derived from the history and physical examination, combined with a sound knowledge of medicine and an understanding of the prevalence of disease in the particular care setting or the population to which the patient belongs.

Cognitive biases

Advances in cognitive psychology in recent decades have demonstrated that human thinking and decision-making are prone to error. Cognitive biases are subconscious errors that lead to inaccurate judgement and illogical interpretation of information. They are prevalent in everyday life; as the famous saying goes, 'to err is human.'

Take a few moments to look at this simple puzzle. Do not try to solve it mathematically but listen to your intuition:

A bat and ball cost £1.10.

The bat costs £1 more than the ball.

How much does the ball cost?

The answer is at the end of the chapter. Most people get the answer to this puzzle wrong. Two things are going on: one is that humans have two distinct types of processes when it comes to thinking and decision-making – termed 'type 1' and 'type 2' thinking. The other is that the human brain is wired to jump to conclusions sometimes or to miss things that are obvious. British psychologist and patient safety pioneer James

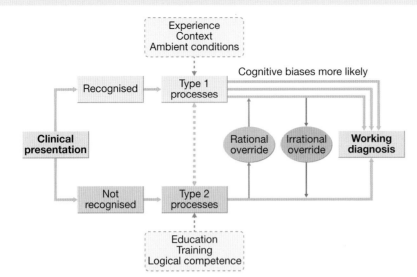

Fig. 1.6 **The interplay between type 1 and type 2 thinking in the diagnostic process.** *Adapted from Croskerry P. A universal model of diagnostic reasoning. Acad Med 2009; 84:1022–1028.*

Reason said that, 'Our propensity for certain types of error is the price we pay for the brain's remarkable ability to think and act intuitively – to sift quickly through the sensory information that constantly bombards us without wasting time trying to work through every situation anew.' This property of human thinking is highly relevant to clinical decision-making.

Type 1 and type 2 thinking

Studies of cognitive psychology and functional magnetic resonance imaging demonstrate two distinct types of processes when it comes to decision-making: intuitive (type 1) and analytical (type 2). This has been termed 'dual process theory'. Box 1.6 explains this in more detail.

Psychologists estimate that we spend 95% of our daily lives engaged in type 1 thinking – the intuitive, fast, subconscious mode of decision-making. Imagine driving a car, for example; it would be impossible to function efficiently if every decision and movement were as deliberate, conscious, slow and effortful as in our first driving lesson. With experience, complex procedures become automatic, fast and effortless. The same applies to medical practice. There is evidence that expert decision-making is well served by intuitive thinking. The problem is that although intuitive processing is highly efficient in many circumstances, in others it is prone to error.

Clinicians use both type 1 and type 2 thinking, and both types are important in clinical decision-making. When encountering a problem that is familiar, clinicians employ pattern recognition and reach a working diagnosis or differential diagnosis quickly (type 1 thinking). When encountering a problem that is more complicated, they use a slower, systematic approach (type 2 thinking). Both types of thinking interplay – they are not mutually exclusive in the diagnostic process. Figure 1.6 illustrates the interplay between type 1 and type 2 thinking in clinical practice.

Errors can occur in both type 1 and type 2 thinking; for example, people can apply the wrong rules or make errors in their application while using type 2 thinking. However, it has been argued that the common cognitive biases encountered in medicine tend to occur when clinicians are engaged in type 1 thinking.

For example, imagine being asked to see a young woman who is drowsy. She is handed over to you as a 'probable overdose' because she has a history of depression and a packet of painkillers

i 1.6 **Type 1 and type 2 thinking**	
Type 1	**Type 2**
Intuitive, heuristic (pattern recognition)	Analytical, systematic
Automatic, subconscious	Deliberate, conscious
Fast, effortless	Slow, effortful
Low/variable reliability	High/consistent reliability
Vulnerable to error	Less prone to error
Highly affected by context	Less affected by context
High emotional involvement	Low emotional involvement
Low scientific rigour	High scientific rigour

was found beside her at home. Her observations show she has a Glasgow Coma Scale score of 10/15, heart rate 100 beats/min, blood pressure 100/60 mmHg, respiratory rate 14 breaths/min, oxygen saturations 98% on air and temperature 37.5°C. Already your mind has reached a working diagnosis. It fits a pattern (type 1 thinking). You think she has taken an overdose. At this point you can stop to think about your thinking (rational override in Fig. 1.6): 'What is the evidence for this diagnosis? What else could it be?'

On the other hand, imagine being asked to assess a patient who has been admitted with syncope. There are several different causes of syncope and a systematic approach is required to reach a diagnosis (type 2 thinking). However, you recently heard about a case of syncope due to a leaking abdominal aortic aneurysm. At the end of your assessment, following evidence-based guidelines, it is clear the patient can be discharged. Despite this, you decide to observe the patient overnight 'just in case' (irrational override in Fig. 1.6). In this example, your intuition is actually availability bias (when things are at the forefront of your mind), which has significantly distorted your estimate of probability.

Common cognitive biases in medicine

Figure 1.7 illustrates the common cognitive biases prevalent in medical practice. Biases often work together; for example, in

Anchoring
The common human tendency to rely too heavily on the first piece of information offered (the 'anchor') when making decisions

Diagnostic momentum
Once a diagnostic label has been attached to a patient (by the patient or other health-care professionals), it can gather momentum with each review, leading others to exclude other possibilities in their thinking

Premature closure
The tendency to close the decision-making process prematurely and accept a diagnosis before it, and other possibilities, have been fully explored

Ascertainment bias
We sometimes see what we expect to see ('self-fulfilling prophecy'). For example, a frequent self-harmer attends the emergency department with drowsiness; everyone assumes he has taken another overdose and misses a brain injury

Framing effect
How a case is presented – for example, in handover – can generate bias in the listener. This can be mitigated by always having 'healthy scepticism' about other people's diagnoses

Psych-out error
Psychiatric patients who present with medical problems are under-assessed, under-examined and under-investigated because problems are presumed to be due to, or exacerbated by, their psychiatric condition

Availability bias
Things may be at the forefront of your mind because you have seen several cases recently or have been studying that condition in particular. For example, when one of the authors worked in an epilepsy clinic, all blackouts were possible seizures

Hindsight bias
Knowing the outcome may profoundly influence the perception of past events and decision-making, preventing a realistic appraisal of what actually occurred – a major problem in learning from diagnostic error

Search satisficing
We may stop searching because we have found something that fits or is convenient, instead of systematically looking for the best alternative, which involves more effort

Base rate neglect
The tendency to ignore the prevalence of a disease, which then distorts Bayesian reasoning. In some cases, clinicians do this deliberately in order to rule out an unlikely but worst-case scenario

Omission bias
The tendency towards inaction, rooted in the principle of 'first do no harm.' Events that occur through natural progression of disease are more acceptable than those that may be attributed directly to the action of the health-care team

Triage-cueing
Triage ensures patients are sent to the right department. However, this leads to 'geography is destiny'. For example, a diabetic ketoacidosis patient with abdominal pain and vomiting is sent to surgery. The wrong location (surgical ward) stops people thinking about medical causes of abdominal pain and vomiting

Commission bias
The tendency towards action rather than inaction, on the assumption that good can come only from doing something (rather than 'watching and waiting')

Overconfidence bias
The tendency to believe we know more than we actually do, placing too much faith in opinion instead of gathered evidence

Unpacking principle
Failure to 'unpack' all the available information may mean things are missed. For example, if a thorough history is not obtained from either the patient or carers (a common problem in geriatric medicine), diagnostic possibilities may be discounted

Confirmation bias
The tendency to look for confirming evidence to support a theory rather than looking for disconfirming evidence to refute it, even if the latter is clearly present. Confirmation bias is common when a patient has been seen first by another doctor

Posterior probability
Our estimate of the likelihood of disease may be unduly influenced by what has gone on before for a particular patient. For example, a patient who has been extensively investigated for headaches presents with a severe headache, and serious causes are discounted

Visceral bias
The influence of either negative or positive feelings towards patients, which can affect our decision-making

Fig. 1.7 Common cognitive biases in medicine. *Adapted from Croskerry P. Achieving quality in clinical decision-making: cognitive strategies and detection of bias. Acad Emerg Med 2002; 9:1184–1204.*

overconfidence bias (the tendency to believe we know more than we actually do), too much faith is placed in opinion instead of gathered evidence. This bias can be augmented by the availability bias and finally by commission bias (the tendency towards action rather than inaction) – sometimes with disastrous results.

The mark of a well-calibrated thinker is the ability to recognise what mode of thinking is being employed and to anticipate and recognise situations in which cognitive biases and errors are more likely to occur.

Human factors

'Human factors' is the science of the limitations of human performance, and how technology, the work environment and team communication can adapt for this to reduce diagnostic and other types of error. Analysis of serious adverse events in clinical practice shows that human factors and poor team communication play a significant role when things go wrong.

Research shows that many errors are beyond an individual's conscious control and are precipitated by many factors. The discipline of human factors seeks to understand interactions between:

- people and tasks or technology
- people and their work environment
- people in a team.

An understanding of these interactions makes it easier for health-care professionals, who are committed to 'first do no harm,' to work in the safest way possible. For example, performance is adversely affected by factors such as poorly designed processes and equipment, frequent interruptions and fatigue. The areas of the brain required for type 2 processing are most affected by things like fatigue and cognitive overload, and the brain reverts to type 1 processing to conserve cognitive energy. Figure 1.8 illustrates some of the internal and external factors that affect human judgement and decision-making.

Various experiments demonstrate that we focus our attention to filter out distractions. This is advantageous in many situations, but in focusing on what we are trying to see we may not notice the unexpected. In a team context, what is obvious to one person may be completely missed by someone else. Safe and effective team communication therefore requires us never to assume, and to verbalise things, even though they may seem obvious.

Reducing errors in clinical decision-making

Knowledge and experience do not eliminate errors. Instead, there are a number of ways in which we can act to reduce errors in clinical decision-making. Examples are:

- adopting 'cognitive debiasing strategies'
- using clinical prediction rules and other decision aids
- engaging in effective team communication.

Cognitive debiasing strategies

There are some simple and established techniques that can be used to avoid cognitive biases and errors in clinical decision-making.

History and physical examination

Taking a history and performing a physical examination may seem obvious, but these are sometimes carried out inadequately. This is the 'unpacking principle': failure to unpack all the available information means things can be missed and lead to error.

Problem lists and differential diagnosis

Once all the available data from history, physical examination and (sometimes) initial test results are available, these need to be synthesised into a problem list. The ability to identify key clinical data and create a problem list is a key step in clinical reasoning. Some problems (e.g. low serum potassium) require action but not necessarily a differential diagnosis. Other problems (e.g. vomiting) require a differential diagnosis. The process of generating a problem list ensures nothing is missed. The process of generating a differential diagnosis works against anchoring on a particular diagnosis too early, thereby avoiding search satisficing and premature closure (see Fig. 1.7).

Mnemonics and checklists

These are used frequently in medicine in order to reduce reliance on fallible human memory. ABCDE (airway, breathing, circulation, disability, exposure/examination) is probably the most successful checklist in medicine, used during the assessment and treatment of critically ill patients (ABCDE is sometimes prefixed with 'C' for 'control of any obvious problem'; see p. 188). Checklists ensure that important issues have been considered and completed, especially under conditions of complexity, stress or fatigue.

Red flags and ROWS ('rule out worst case scenario')

These are strategies that force doctors to consider serious diseases that can present with common symptoms. Red flags in back pain are listed in Box 24.19 (p. 996). Considering and investigating for possible pulmonary embolism in patients who

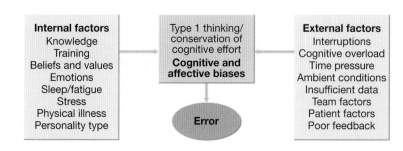

Fig. 1.8 **Factors that affect our judgement and decision-making.** Type 1 thinking = fast, intuitive, subconscious, low-effort.

present with pleuritic chest pain and breathlessness is a common example of ruling out a worst-case scenario, as pulmonary embolism can be fatal if missed. Red flags and ROWS help to avoid cognitive biases such as the 'framing effect' and 'premature closure'.

Newer strategies to avoid cognitive biases and errors in decision-making are emerging. These involve explicit training in clinical reasoning and human factors. In theory, if doctors are aware of the science of human thinking and decision-making, then they are more able to think about their thinking, understand situations in which their decision-making may be affected, and take steps to mitigate this.

Using clinical prediction rules and other decision aids

A clinical prediction rule is a statistical model of the diagnostic process. When clinical prediction rules are matched against the opinion of experts, the model usually outperforms the experts, because it is applied consistently in each case. However, it is important that clinical prediction rules are used correctly – that is, applied to the patient population that was used to create the rule. Clinical prediction rules force a scientific assessment of the patient's symptoms, signs and other data to develop a numerical probability of a disease or an outcome. They help clinicians to estimate probability more accurately.

A good example of a clinical prediction rule to estimate pre-test probability is the Wells score in suspected deep vein thrombosis (see Box 10.15, p. 187). Other commonly used clinical prediction rules predict outcomes and therefore guide the management plan. These include the GRACE score in acute coronary syndromes (see Fig. 16.62, p. 494) and the CURB-65 score in community-acquired pneumonia (see Fig. 17.32, p. 583).

Effective team communication

Effective team communication and proper handovers are vital for safe clinical care. The SBAR system of communication has been recommended by the UK's Patient Safety First campaign. It is a structured way to communicate about a patient with another health-care professional (e.g. during handover or when making a referral) and increases the amount of relevant information being communicated in a shorter time. It is illustrated in Box 1.7.

In increasingly complex health-care systems, patients are looked after by a wide variety of professionals, each of whom has access to important information required to make clinical decisions. Strict hierarchies are hazardous to patient safety if certain members of the team are not able to speak up.

Patient-centred evidence-based medicine and shared decision-making

'Patient-centred evidence-based medicine' refers to the application of best-available research evidence while taking individual patient factors into account; these include both clinical and non-clinical factors (e.g. the patient's social circumstances, values and wishes). For example, a 95-year-old man with dementia and a recent gastrointestinal bleed is admitted with an inferior myocardial infarction. He is clinically well. Should he be treated

i	**1.7 The SBAR system of communicating**	
SBAR	**Example (a telephone call to the Intensive Care team)**	
Situation	I am [name] calling from [place] about a patient with a NEWS of 10.	
Background	[Patient's name], 30-year-old woman, no past medical history, was admitted last night with community-acquired pneumonia. Since then her oxygen requirements have been steadily increasing.	
Assessment	Her vital signs are: blood pressure 115/60 mmHg, heart rate 120 beats/min, temperature 38°C, respiratory rate 32 breaths/min, oxygen saturations 89% on 15 L via reservoir bag mask. An arterial blood gas shows pH 7.3 (H^+ 50 nmol/L), $PaCO_2$ 4.0 kPa (30 mmHg), PaO_2 7 kPa (52.5 mmHg), standard bicarbonate 14 mmol/L. Chest X-ray shows extensive right lower zone consolidation.	
Recommendation	Please can you come and see her as soon as possible? I think she needs admission to Intensive Care.	

(NEWS = National Early Warning Score; a patient with normal vital signs scores 0)
From Royal College of Physicians of London. National Early Warning Score: standardising the assessment of illness severity in the NHS. Report of a working party. RCP, July 2012; www.rcplondon.ac.uk/projects/outputs/national-early-warning-score-news (accessed March 2016).

with dual antiplatelet therapy and low-molecular-weight heparin as recommended in clinical guidelines?

As this chapter has described, clinicians frequently deal with uncertainty/probability. Clinicians need to be able to explain risks and benefits of treatment in an accurate and understandable way. Providing the relevant statistics is seldom sufficient to guide decision-making because a patient's perception of risk may be influenced by irrational factors as well as individual values.

Research evidence provides statistics but these can be confusing. Terms such as 'common' and 'rare' are nebulous. Whenever possible, clinicians should quote numerical information using consistent denominators (e.g. '90 out of 100 patients who have this operation feel much better, 1 will die during the operation and 2 will suffer a stroke'). Visual aids can be used to present complex statistical information (Fig. 1.9).

How uncertainty is conveyed to patients is important. Many studies demonstrate a correlation between effective clinician–patient communication and improved health outcomes. If patients feel they have been listened to and understand the problem and proposed treatment plan, they are more likely to follow the plan and less likely to re-attend.

Clinical decision-making: putting it all together

The following is a practical example that brings together many of the concepts outlined in this chapter:

A 25-year-old woman presents with right-sided pleuritic chest pain and breathlessness. She reports that she had an upper

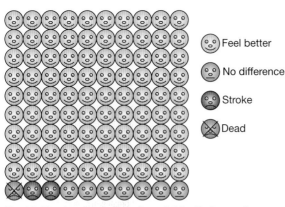

Feel better
No difference
Stroke
Dead

Fig. 1.9 Visual portrayal of benefits and risks. The image refers to an operation that is expected to relieve symptoms in 90% of patients, but cause stroke in 2% and death in 1%. *From Edwards A, Elwyn G, Mulley A. Explaining risks: turning numerical data into meaningful pictures. BMJ 2002; 324:827–830, reproduced with permission from the BMJ Publishing Group.*

respiratory tract infection a week ago and was almost back to normal when the symptoms started. The patient has no past medical history and no family history, and her only medication is the combined oral contraceptive pill. On examination, her vital signs are normal (respiratory rate 19 breaths/min, oxygen saturations 98% on air, blood pressure 115/60 mmHg, heart rate 90 beats/min, temperature 37.5°C) and the physical examination is also normal. You have been asked to assess her for the possibility of a pulmonary embolism.

(More information on pulmonary embolism can be found on page 619.)

Evidence-based history and examination

Information from the history and physical examination is vital in deciding whether this could be a pulmonary embolism. Pleurisy and breathlessness are common presenting features of this disease but are also common presenting features in other diseases. There is nothing in the history to suggest an alternative diagnosis (e.g. high fever, productive cough, recent chest trauma). The patient's vital signs are normal, as is the physical examination. However, the only feature in the history and examination that has a negative likelihood ratio in the diagnosis of pulmonary embolism is a heart rate of less than 90 beats/min. In other words, the normal physical examination findings (including normal oxygen saturations) carry very little diagnostic weight.

Deciding pre-test probability

The prevalence of pulmonary embolism in 25-year-old women is low. We anchor on this prevalence and then adjust for individual patient factors. This patient has no major risk factors for pulmonary embolism. To assist our estimate of pre-test probability, we could use a clinical prediction rule: in this case, the modified Wells score for pulmonary embolism, which would give a score of 3 (low probability – answering yes only to the criterion 'PE is the number one diagnosis, an alternative is less likely').

Interpreting test results

Imagine the patient went on to have a normal chest X-ray and blood results, apart from a raised D-dimer of 900 (normal <500 ng/mL). A normal chest X-ray is a common finding in pulmonary embolism. Several studies have shown that the D-dimer assay has at least 95% sensitivity in acute pulmonary embolism but it has a low specificity. A very sensitive test will detect most disease but generate abnormal findings in healthy people. On the other hand, a negative result virtually, but not completely, excludes the disease. It is important at this point to realise that a raised D-dimer result does not mean this patient has a pulmonary embolism; it just means that we have not been able to exclude it. Since pulmonary embolism is a potentially fatal condition we need to rule out the worst-case scenario (ROWS), and the next step is therefore to arrange further imaging. What kind of imaging depends on individual patient characteristics and what is available.

Treatment threshold

The treatment threshold combines factors such as the risks of the test, and the risks versus benefits of treatment. A CT pulmonary angiogram (CTPA) could be requested for this patient, although in some circumstances ventilation–perfusion single-photon emission computed tomography (V̇/Q̇ SPECT, p. 620) may be a more suitable alternative. However, what if the scan cannot be performed until the next day? Because pulmonary embolism is potentially fatal and the risks of treatment in this case are low, the patient should be started on treatment while awaiting the scan.

Post-test probability

The patient's scan result is subsequently reported as 'no pulmonary embolism'. Combined with the low pre-test probability, this scan result reliably excludes pulmonary embolism.

Cognitive biases

Imagine during this case that the patient had been handed over to you as 'nothing wrong – probably a pulled muscle'. Cognitive biases (subconscious tendencies to respond in a certain way) would come into play, such as the 'framing effect', 'confirmation bias' and 'search satisficing'. The normal clinical examination might confirm the diagnosis of musculoskeletal pain in your mind, despite the examination being entirely consistent with pulmonary embolism and despite the lack of history and examination findings (e.g. chest wall tenderness) to support the diagnosis of musculoskeletal chest pain.

Human factors

Imagine that, after you have seen the patient, a nurse hands you some blood forms and asks you what tests you would like to request on 'this lady'. You request blood tests including a D-dimer on the wrong patient. Luckily, this error is intercepted.

Reducing cognitive error

The diagnosis of pulmonary embolism can be difficult. Clinical prediction rules (e.g. modified Wells score), guidelines (e.g. from the UK's National Institute for Health and Care Excellence, or NICE) and decision aids (e.g. simplified pulmonary embolism severity index, or PESI) are frequently used in combination with the doctor's opinion, derived from information gathered in the history and physical examination.

Person-centred EBM and information given to patient

The patient is treated according to evidence-based guidelines that apply to her particular situation. Tests alone do not make a diagnosis and at the end of this process the patient is told that the combination of history, examination and test results mean she is extremely unlikely to have a pulmonary embolism. Viral pleurisy is offered as an alternative diagnosis and she is reassured that her symptoms are expected to settle over the coming days with analgesia. She is advised to re-present to hospital if her symptoms suddenly get worse.

Answers to problems

Harvard problem (p. 5)

The problem originates from a 1978 article in the New England Journal of Medicine (Casscells et al, see 'Further information'). Almost half of doctors surveyed said 95%, but they neglected to take prevalence into account. If 1000 people are tested, there will be 51 positive results: 50 false positives and 1 true positive (assuming 100% sensitivity). The chance that a person found to have a positive result actually has the disease is therefore only 1/51 or ~2%.

Bat and ball problem (p. 6)

This puzzle is from the book, *Thinking, Fast and Slow*, by Nobel laureate Daniel Kahneman (see 'Further information'). He writes,

'A number came to your mind. The number, of course, is 10p. The distinctive mark of this easy puzzle is that it evokes an answer that is intuitive, appealing – and wrong. Do the math, and you will see.' The correct answer is 5p.

Further information

Books and journal articles

Cooper N, Frain J (eds). ABC of clinical reasoning. Oxford: Wiley–Blackwell; 2016.

Kahneman D. Thinking, fast and slow. Harmondsworth: Penguin; 2012.

Casscells W, Schoenberger A, Graboys TB. Interpretation by physicians of clinical laboratory results. N Engl J Med 1978; 299:999–1001.

McGee S. Evidence-based physical diagnosis, 3rd edn. Philadelphia: Saunders; 2012.

Scott IA. Errors in clinical reasoning: causes and remedial strategies. BMJ 2009; 338:b186.

Sox H, Higgins MC, Owens DK. Medical decision making, 2nd edn. Chichester: Wiley–Blackwell; 2013.

Trowbridge RL, Rencic JJ, Durning SJ. Teaching clinical reasoning. Philadelphia: American College of Physicians; 2015.

Vincent C. Patient safety. Edinburgh: Churchill Livingstone; 2006.

Websites

chfg.org *UK Clinical Human Factors Group.*

clinical-reasoning.org *Clinical reasoning resources.*

creme.org.uk *UK Clinical Reasoning in Medical Education group.*

improvediagnosis.org *Society to Improve Diagnosis in Medicine.*

vassarstats.net/index.html *Suite of calculators for statistical computation (Calculator 2 is a calculator for predictive values and likelihood ratios).*

SRJ Maxwell

2

Clinical therapeutics and good prescribing

Principles of clinical pharmacology 14

Pharmacodynamics 14

Pharmacokinetics 17

Inter-individual variation in drug responses 19

Adverse outcomes of drug therapy 21

Adverse drug reactions 21

Drug interactions 23

Medication errors 24

Drug regulation and management 26

Drug development and marketing 26

Managing the use of medicines 27

Prescribing in practice 28

Decision-making in prescribing 28

Prescribing in special circumstances 31

Writing prescriptions 33

Monitoring drug therapy 34

Prescribing medicines is the major tool used by doctors to restore or preserve the health of patients. Medicines contain drugs (the specific chemical substances with pharmacological effects), either alone or in combination with additional drugs, in a formulation mixed with other ingredients. The beneficial effects of medicines must be weighed against their cost and potential adverse drug reactions and interactions. The latter two factors are sometimes caused by injudicious prescribing decisions and by prescribing errors. The modern prescriber must meet the challenges posed by the increasing number of drugs and formulations available and of indications for prescribing them, and the greater complexity of treatment regimens followed by individual patients ('polypharmacy', a particular challenge in the ageing population). The purpose of this chapter is to elaborate on the principles and practice that underpin good prescribing (Box 2.1).

---

i | **2.1 Steps in good prescribing**

- Make a diagnosis
- Consider factors that might influence the patient's response to therapy (age, concomitant drug therapy, renal and liver function etc.)
- Establish the therapeutic goal*
- Choose the therapeutic approach*
- Choose the drug and its formulation (the 'medicine')
- Choose the dose, route and frequency
- Choose the duration of therapy
- Write an unambiguous prescription (or 'medication order')
- Inform the patient about the treatment and its likely effects
- Monitor treatment effects, both beneficial and harmful
- Review/alter the prescription

*These steps in particular take the patient's views into consideration to establish a therapeutic partnership (shared decision-making to achieve 'concordance').

Principles of clinical pharmacology

Prescribers need to understand what the drug does to the body (pharmacodynamics) and what the body does to the drug (pharmacokinetics) (Fig. 2.1). Although this chapter is focused on the most common drugs, which are synthetic small molecules, the same principles apply to the increasingly numerous 'biological' therapies (sometimes abbreviated to 'biologics') now in use, which include peptides, proteins, enzymes and monoclonal antibodies (see Box 4.2, p. 65).

Pharmacodynamics

Drug targets and mechanisms of action

Modern drugs are usually discovered by screening compounds for activity either to stimulate or to block the function of a specific molecular target, which is predicted to have a beneficial effect in a particular disease (Box 2.2). Other drugs have useful but less selective chemical properties, such as chelators (e.g. for treatment of iron or copper overload), osmotic agents (used as diuretics in cerebral oedema) or general anaesthetics (that alter the biophysical properties of lipid membranes). The following characteristics of the interaction of drugs with receptors illustrate some of the important determinants of the effects of drugs:

- *Affinity* describes the propensity for a drug to bind to a receptor and is related to the 'molecular fit' and the

Fig. 2.1 Pharmacokinetics and pharmacodynamics.

strength of the chemical bond. Some drug–receptor interactions are *irreversible*, either because the affinity is so strong or because the drug modifies the structure of its molecular target.
- *Selectivity* describes the propensity for a drug to bind to one target rather than another. Selectivity is a relative term, not to be confused with absolute specificity. It is common for drugs targeted at a particular subtype of receptor to exhibit some effect at other subtypes. For example, β-adrenoceptors can be subtyped on the basis of their responsiveness to the endogenous agonist noradrenaline (norepinephrine): the concentration of noradrenaline required to cause bronchodilatation (via β_2-adrenoceptors) is ten times higher than that required to cause tachycardia (via β_1-adrenoceptors). 'Cardioselective' β-blockers have anti-anginal effects on the heart (β_1) but may still cause bronchospasm in the lung (β_2) and are contraindicated for asthmatic patients.
- *Agonists* bind to a receptor to produce a conformational change that is coupled to a biological response. As agonist concentration increases, so does the proportion of receptors occupied, and hence the biological effect. *Partial agonists* activate the receptor but cannot produce a maximal signalling effect equivalent to that of a full agonist, even when all available receptors are occupied.
- *Antagonists* bind to a receptor but do not produce the conformational change that initiates an intracellular signal. A *competitive antagonist* competes with endogenous ligands to occupy receptor-binding sites, with the resulting antagonism depending on the relative affinities and concentrations of drug and ligand. *Non-competitive antagonists* inhibit the effect of an agonist by mechanisms other than direct competition for receptor binding with the agonist (e.g. by affecting post-receptor signalling).

Dose–response relationships

Plotting the logarithm of drug dose against drug response typically produces a sigmoidal dose–response curve (Fig. 2.2). Progressive increases in drug dose (which, for most drugs, is proportional to the plasma drug concentration) produce increasing

i 2.2 Examples of target molecules for drugs

Drug target	Description	Examples
Receptors		
Channel-linked receptors	Ligand binding controls a linked ion channel, known as 'ligand-gated' (in contrast to 'voltage-gated' channels that respond to changes in membrane potential)	Nicotinic acetylcholine receptor GABA receptor Sulphonylurea receptor
G-protein-coupled receptors (GPCRs)	Ligand binding affects one of a family of 'G-proteins' that mediate signal transduction either by activating intracellular enzymes (such as adenylate or guanylate cyclase, producing cyclic AMP or GMP, respectively) or by controlling ion channels	Muscarinic acetylcholine receptor β-adrenoceptors Dopamine receptors 5-Hydroxytryptamine (5-HT, serotonin) receptors Opioid receptors
Kinase-linked receptors	Ligand binding activates an intracellular protein kinase that triggers a cascade of phosphorylation reactions	Insulin receptor Cytokine receptors
Transcription factor receptors	Intracellular and also known as 'nuclear receptors'; ligand binding promotes or inhibits gene transcription and hence synthesis of new proteins	Steroid receptors Thyroid hormone receptors Vitamin D receptors Retinoid receptors PPARγ and α receptors
Other targets		
Voltage-gated ion channels	Mediate electrical signalling in excitable tissues (muscle and nervous system)	Na$^+$ channels Ca^{2+} channels
Enzymes	Catalyse biochemical reactions. Drugs interfere with binding of substrate to the active site or of co-factors	Cyclo-oxygenase ACE Xanthine oxidase
Transporter proteins	Carry ions or molecules across cell membranes	5-HT re-uptake transporter Na$^+$/K$^+$ ATPase
Cytokines and other signalling molecules	Small proteins that are important in cell signalling (autocrine, paracrine and endocrine), especially affecting the immune response	Tumour necrosis factors Interleukins
Cell surface antigens	Block the recognition of cell surface molecules that modulate cellular responses	Cluster of differentiation molecules (e.g. CD20, CD80)

(ACE = angiotensin-converting enzyme; AMP = adenosine monophosphate; ATPase = adenosine triphosphatase; GABA = γ-aminobutyric acid; GMP = guanosine monophosphate; PPAR = peroxisome proliferator-activated receptor)

Fig. 2.2 Dose–response curve. The green curve represents the beneficial effect of the drug. The maximum response on the curve is the E_{max} and the dose (or concentration) producing half this value ($E_{max}/2$) is the ED_{50} (or EC_{50}). The red curve illustrates the dose–response relationship for the most important adverse effect of this drug. This occurs at much higher doses; the ratio between the ED_{50} for the adverse effect and that for the beneficial effect is the 'therapeutic index', which indicates how much margin there is for prescribers when choosing a dose that will provide beneficial effects without also causing this adverse effect. Adverse effects that occur at doses above the therapeutic range are normally called 'toxic effects', while those occurring within the therapeutic range are 'side-effects' and those below it are 'hyper-susceptibility effects'.

response but only within a relatively narrow range of dose; further increases in dose beyond this range produce little extra effect. The following characteristics of the drug response are useful in comparing different drugs:

- *Efficacy* describes the extent to which a drug can produce a target-specific response when all available receptors or binding sites are occupied (i.e. E_{max} on the dose–response curve). A full agonist can produce the maximum response of which the receptor is capable, while a partial agonist at the same receptor will have lower efficacy. *Therapeutic efficacy* describes the effect of the drug on a desired biological endpoint and can be used to compare drugs that act via different pharmacological mechanisms (e.g. loop diuretics induce a greater diuresis than thiazide diuretics and therefore have greater therapeutic efficacy).
- *Potency* describes the amount of drug required for a given response. More potent drugs produce biological effects at lower doses, so they have a lower ED_{50}. A less potent drug can still have an equivalent efficacy if it is given in higher doses.

The dose–response relationship varies between patients because of variations in the many determinants of pharmacokinetics and pharmacodynamics. In clinical practice, the prescriber is unable to construct a dose–response curve for each individual patient. Therefore, most drugs are licensed for use within a recommended range of doses that is expected to reach close to the top of the dose–response curve for most patients. However, it is sometimes possible to achieve the desired therapeutic efficacy at doses towards the lower end of, or even below, the recommended range.

Therapeutic index

The adverse effects of drugs are often dose-related in a similar way to the beneficial effects, although the dose–response curve for these adverse effects is normally shifted to the right (Fig. 2.2). The ratio of the ED_{50} for therapeutic efficacy and for a major adverse effect is known as the 'therapeutic index'. In reality, drugs have multiple potential adverse effects, but the concept of therapeutic index is usually based on adverse effects that might require dose reduction or discontinuation. For most drugs, the therapeutic index is greater than 100 but there are some notable exceptions with therapeutic indices of less than 10 (e.g. digoxin, warfarin, insulin, phenytoin, opioids). The doses of such drugs have to be titrated carefully for individual patients to maximise benefits but avoid adverse effects.

Desensitisation and withdrawal effects

Desensitisation refers to the common situation in which the biological response to a drug diminishes when it is given continuously or repeatedly. It may be possible to restore the response by increasing the dose of the drug but, in some cases, the tissues may become completely refractory to its effect.

- *Tachyphylaxis* describes desensitisation that occurs very rapidly, sometimes with the initial dose. This rapid loss of response implies depletion of chemicals that may be necessary for the pharmacological actions of the drug (e.g. a stored neurotransmitter released from a nerve terminal) or receptor phosphorylation.
- *Tolerance* describes a more gradual loss of response to a drug that occurs over days or weeks. This slower change implies changes in receptor numbers or the development of counter-regulatory physiological changes that offset the actions of the drug (e.g. accumulation of salt and water in response to vasodilator therapy).
- *Drug resistance* is a term normally reserved for describing the loss of effectiveness of an antimicrobial (p. 116) or cancer chemotherapy drug.
- In addition to these pharmacodynamic causes of desensitisation, reduced response may be the consequence of lower plasma and tissue drug concentrations as a result of altered *pharmacokinetics* (see below).

When drugs induce chemical, hormonal and physiological changes that offset their actions, discontinuation may allow these changes to cause 'rebound' withdrawal effects (Box 2.3).

i 2.3 **Examples of drugs associated with withdrawal effects**			
Drug	**Symptoms**	**Signs**	**Treatment**
Alcohol	Anxiety, panic, paranoid delusions, visual and auditory hallucinations	Agitation, restlessness, delirium, tremor, tachycardia, ataxia, disorientation, seizures	Treat immediate withdrawal syndrome with benzodiazepines
Barbiturates, benzodiazepines	Similar to alcohol	Similar to alcohol	Transfer to long-acting benzodiazepine then gradually reduce dosage
Glucocorticoids	Weakness, fatigue, decreased appetite, weight loss, nausea, vomiting, diarrhoea, abdominal pain	Hypotension, hypoglycaemia	Prolonged therapy suppresses the hypothalamic–pituitary–adrenal axis and causes adrenal insufficiency requiring glucocorticoid replacement. Withdrawal should be gradual after prolonged therapy (p. 670)
Opioids	Rhinorrhoea, sneezing, yawning, lacrimation, abdominal and leg cramping, nausea, vomiting, diarrhoea	Dilated pupils	Transfer addicts to long-acting agonist methadone
Selective serotonin re-uptake inhibitors (SSRIs)	Dizziness, sweating, nausea, insomnia, tremor, delirium, nightmares	Tremor	Reduce SSRIs slowly to avoid withdrawal effects

Pharmacokinetics

Understanding 'what the body does to the drug' (Fig. 2.3) is extremely important for prescribers because this forms the basis on which the optimal route of administration and dose regimen are chosen and explains the majority of inter-individual variation in the response to drug therapy.

Drug absorption and routes of administration

Absorption is the process by which drug molecules gain access to the blood stream. The rate and extent of drug absorption depend on the route of administration (Fig. 2.3).

Enteral administration

These routes involve administration via the gastrointestinal tract:

- *Oral*. This is the most common route of administration because it is simple, convenient and readily used by patients to self-administer their medicines. Absorption after an oral dose is a complex process that depends on the drug being swallowed, surviving exposure to gastric acid, avoiding unacceptable food binding, being absorbed across the small bowel mucosa into the portal venous system, and surviving metabolism by gut wall or liver enzymes ('first-pass metabolism'). As a consequence, absorption is frequently incomplete following oral administration. The term 'bioavailability' describes the proportion of the dose that reaches the systemic circulation intact.
- *Buccal, intranasal and sublingual (SL)*. These routes have the advantage of enabling rapid absorption into the systemic circulation without the uncertainties associated with oral administration (e.g. organic nitrates for angina pectoris, triptans for migraine, opioid analgesics).
- *Rectal (PR)*. The rectal mucosa is occasionally used as a site of drug administration when the oral route is compromised because of nausea and vomiting or unconsciousness (e.g. diazepam in status epilepticus).

Parenteral administration

These routes avoid absorption via the gastrointestinal tract and first-pass metabolism in the liver:

- *Intravenous (IV)*. The IV route enables all of a dose to enter the systemic circulation reliably, without any concerns about absorption or first-pass metabolism (i.e. the dose is 100% bioavailable), and rapidly achieve a high plasma concentration. It is ideal for very ill patients when a rapid, certain effect is critical to outcome (e.g. benzathine benzylpenicillin for meningococcal meningitis).
- *Intramuscular (IM)*. IM administration is easier to achieve than the IV route (e.g. adrenaline (epinephrine) for acute anaphylaxis) but absorption is less predictable and depends on muscle blood flow.
- *Subcutaneous (SC)*. The SC route is ideal for drugs that have to be administered parenterally because of low oral bioavailability, are absorbed well from subcutaneous fat, and might ideally be injected by patients themselves (e.g. insulin, heparin).
- *Transdermal*. A transdermal patch can enable a drug to be absorbed through the skin and into the circulation (e.g. oestrogens, nicotine, nitrates).

Other routes of administration

- *Topical* application of a drug involves direct administration to the site of action (e.g. skin, eye, ear). This has the advantage of achieving sufficient concentration at this site while minimising systemic exposure and the risk of adverse effects elsewhere.
- *Inhaled (INH)* administration allows drugs to be delivered directly to a target in the respiratory tree, usually the small airways (e.g. salbutamol, beclometasone). However, a significant proportion of the inhaled dose may be absorbed from the lung or is swallowed and can reach the systemic circulation. The most common mode of delivery is the metered-dose inhaler but its success depends on some degree of manual dexterity and timing (see Fig. 17.23, p. 571). Patients who find these difficult may use a 'spacer' device to improve drug delivery. A special mode

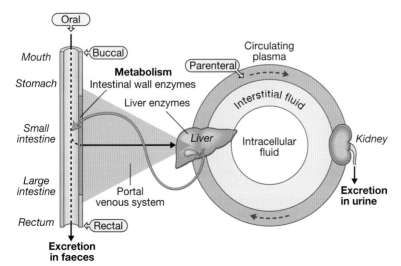

Fig. 2.3 **Pharmacokinetics summary.** Most drugs are taken orally, are absorbed from the intestinal lumen and enter the portal venous system to be conveyed to the liver, where they may be subject to first-pass metabolism and/or excretion in bile. Active drugs then enter the systemic circulation, from which they may diffuse (or sometimes be actively transported) in and out of the interstitial and intracellular fluid compartments. Drug that remains in circulating plasma is subject to liver metabolism and renal excretion. Drugs excreted in bile may be reabsorbed, creating an enterohepatic circulation. First-pass metabolism in the liver is avoided if drugs are administered via the buccal or rectal mucosa, or parenterally (e.g. by intravenous injection).

of inhaled delivery is via a nebulised solution created by using pressurised oxygen or air to break up solutions and suspensions into small aerosol droplets that can be directly inhaled from the mouthpiece of the device.

Drug distribution

Distribution is the process by which drug molecules transfer into and out of the blood stream. This is influenced by the drug's molecular size and lipid solubility, the extent to which it binds to proteins in plasma, its susceptibility to drug transporters expressed on cell surfaces, and its binding to its molecular target and to other cellular proteins (which can be irreversible). Most drugs diffuse passively across capillary walls down a concentration gradient into the interstitial fluid until the concentration of free drug molecules in the interstitial fluid is equal to that in the plasma. As drug molecules in the blood are removed by metabolism or excretion, the plasma concentration falls, drug molecules diffuse back from the tissue compartment into the blood and eventually all will be eliminated. Note that this reverse movement of drug away from the tissues will be prevented if further drug doses are administered and absorbed into the plasma.

Volume of distribution

The apparent volume of distribution (V_d) is the volume into which a drug appears to have distributed following intravenous injection. It is calculated from the equation

$$V_d = D/C_0$$

where D is the amount of drug given and C_0 is the initial plasma concentration (Fig. 2.4A). Drugs that are highly bound to plasma proteins may have a V_d below 10 L (e.g. warfarin, aspirin), while those that diffuse into the interstitial fluid but do not enter cells because they have low lipid solubility may have a V_d between 10 and 30 L (e.g. gentamicin, amoxicillin). It is an 'apparent' volume because those drugs that are lipid-soluble and highly tissue-bound may have a V_d of greater than 100 L (e.g. digoxin, amitriptyline). Drugs with a larger V_d have longer half-lives (see below), take longer to reach steady state on repeated administration and are eliminated more slowly from the body following discontinuation.

Drug elimination

Drug metabolism

Metabolism is the process by which drugs are chemically altered from a lipid-soluble form suitable for absorption and distribution to a more water-soluble form that is necessary for excretion. Some drugs, known as 'prodrugs', are inactive in the form in which they are administered but are converted to an active metabolite in vivo.

Phase I metabolism involves oxidation, reduction or hydrolysis to make drug molecules suitable for phase II reactions or for excretion. Oxidation is by far the most common form of phase I reaction and chiefly involves members of the cytochrome P450 family of membrane-bound enzymes in the endoplasmic reticulum of hepatocytes.

Phase II metabolism involves combining phase I metabolites with an endogenous substrate to form an inactive conjugate that is much more water-soluble. Reactions include glucuronidation, sulphation, acetylation, methylation and conjugation with glutathione. This is necessary to enable renal excretion, because lipid-soluble metabolites will simply diffuse back into the body after glomerular filtration (p. 349).

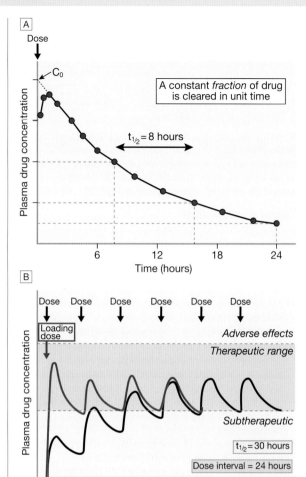

Fig. 2.4 Drug concentrations in plasma following single and multiple drug dosing. **A** In this example of first-order kinetics following a single intravenous dose, the time period required for the plasma drug concentration to halve (half-life, $t_{1/2}$) remains constant throughout the elimination process. **B** After multiple dosing, the plasma drug concentration rises if each dose is administered before the previous dose has been entirely cleared. In this example, the drug's half-life is 30 hours, so that with daily dosing the peak, average and trough concentrations steadily increase as drug accumulates in the body (black line). Steady state is reached after approximately 5 half-lives, when the rate of elimination (the product of concentration and clearance) is equal to the rate of drug absorption (the product of rate of administration and bioavailability). The long half-life in this example means that it takes 6 days for steady state to be achieved and, for most of the first 3 days of treatment, plasma drug concentrations are below the therapeutic range. This problem can be overcome if a larger loading dose (red line) is used to achieve steady-state drug concentrations more rapidly.

Drug excretion

Excretion is the process by which drugs and their metabolites are removed from the body.

Renal excretion is the usual route of elimination for drugs or their metabolites that are of low molecular weight and sufficiently water-soluble to avoid reabsorption from the renal tubule. Drugs bound to plasma proteins are not filtered by the glomeruli. The pH of the urine is more acidic than that of plasma, so that some drugs (e.g. salicylates) become un-ionised and tend to be reabsorbed. Alkalination of the urine can hasten excretion (e.g. after a salicylate overdose; p. 138). For some drugs, active secretion into the proximal tubule lumen, rather than glomerular filtration, is the predominant mechanism of excretion (e.g. methotrexate, penicillin).

Faecal excretion is the predominant route of elimination for drugs with high molecular weight, including those that are excreted in the bile after conjugation with glucuronide in the liver, and any drugs that are not absorbed after enteral administration. Molecules of drug or metabolite that are excreted in the bile enter the small intestine, where they may, if they are sufficiently lipid-soluble, be reabsorbed through the gut wall and return to the liver via the portal vein (see Fig. 2.3). This recycling between the liver, bile, gut and portal vein is known as 'enterohepatic circulation' and can significantly prolong the residence of drugs in the body.

Elimination kinetics

The net removal of drug from the circulation results from a combination of drug metabolism and excretion, and is usually described as 'clearance', i.e. the volume of plasma that is completely cleared of drug per unit time.

For most drugs, elimination is a high-capacity process that does not become saturated, even at high dosage. The rate of elimination is therefore directly proportional to the drug concentration because of the 'law of mass action', whereby higher drug concentrations will drive faster metabolic reactions and support higher renal filtration rates. This results in 'first-order' kinetics, when a constant fraction of the drug remaining in the circulation is eliminated in a given time and the decline in concentration over time is exponential (Fig. 2.4A). This elimination can be described by the drug's half-life ($t_{1/2}$), i.e. the time taken for the plasma drug concentration to halve, which remains constant throughout the period of drug elimination. The significance of this phenomenon for prescribers is that the effect of increasing doses on plasma concentration is predictable – a doubled dose leads to a doubled concentration at all time points.

For a few drugs in common use (e.g. phenytoin, alcohol), elimination capacity is exceeded (saturated) within the usual dose range. This is called 'zero-order' kinetics. Its significance for prescribers is that, if the rate of administration exceeds the maximum rate of elimination, the drug will accumulate progressively, leading to serious toxicity.

Repeated dose regimens

The goal of therapy is usually to maintain drug concentrations within the therapeutic range (see Fig. 2.2) over several days (e.g. antibiotics) or even for months or years (e.g. antihypertensives, lipid-lowering drugs, thyroid hormone replacement therapy). This goal is rarely achieved with single doses, so prescribers have to plan a regimen of repeated doses. This involves choosing the size of each individual dose and the frequency of dose administration.

As illustrated in Figure 2.4B, the time taken to reach drug concentrations within the therapeutic range depends on the half-life of the drug. Typically, with doses administered regularly, it takes approximately 5 half-lives to reach a 'steady state' in which the rate of drug elimination is equal to the rate of drug administration. This applies when starting new drugs and when adjusting doses of current drugs. With appropriate dose selection, steady-state drug concentrations will be maintained within the therapeutic range. This is important for prescribers because it

means that the effects of a new prescription, or dose titration, for a drug with a long half-life (e.g. digoxin – 36 hours) may not be known for a few days. In contrast, drugs with a very short half-life (e.g. dobutamine – 2 minutes) have to be given continuously by infusion but reach a new steady state within minutes.

For drugs with a long half-life, if it is unacceptable to wait for 5 half-lives until concentrations within the therapeutic range are achieved, then an initial 'loading dose' can be given that is much larger than the maintenance dose and equivalent to the amount of drug required in the body at steady state. This achieves a peak plasma concentration close to the plateau concentration, which can then be maintained by successive maintenance doses.

'Steady state' actually involves fluctuations in drug concentrations, with peaks just after administration followed by troughs just prior to the next administration. The manufacturers of medicines recommend dosing regimens that predict that, for most patients, these oscillations result in troughs within the therapeutic range and peaks that are not high enough to cause adverse effects. The optimal dose interval is a compromise between convenience for the patient and a constant level of drug exposure. More frequent administration (e.g. 25 mg 4 times daily) achieves a smoother plasma concentration profile than 100 mg once daily but is much more difficult for patients to sustain. A solution to this need for compromise in dosing frequency for drugs with half-lives of less than 24 hours is the use of 'modified-release' formulations. These allow drugs to be absorbed more slowly from the gastrointestinal tract and reduce the oscillation in plasma drug concentration profile, which is especially important for drugs with a low therapeutic index (e.g. levodopa).

Inter-individual variation in drug responses

Prescribers have numerous sources of guidance about how to use drugs appropriately (e.g. dose, route, frequency, duration) for many conditions. However, this advice is based on average dose–response data derived from observations in many individuals. When applying this information to an individual patient, prescribers must take account of inter-individual variability in response. Some of this variability is predictable and good prescribers are able to anticipate it and adjust their prescriptions accordingly to maximise the chances of benefit and minimise harm. Inter-individual variation in responses also mandates that effects of treatment should be monitored (p. 34).

Some inter-individual variation in drug response is accounted for by differences in pharmacodynamics. For example, the beneficial natriuresis produced by the loop diuretic furosemide is often significantly reduced at a given dose in patients with renal impairment, while delirium caused by opioid analgesics is more likely in the elderly. Differences in pharmacokinetics more commonly account for different drug responses, however. Examples of factors influencing the absorption, metabolism and excretion of drugs are shown in Box 2.4.

It is hoped that a significant proportion of the inter-individual variation in drug responses can be explained by studying genetic differences in single genes ('pharmacogenetics'; Box 2.5) or the effects of multiple gene variants ('pharmacogenomics'). The aim is to identify those patients most likely to benefit from specific treatments and those most susceptible to adverse effects. In this way, it may be possible to select drugs and dose regimens for individual patients to maximise the benefit-to-hazard ratio ('personalised medicine').

2.4 Patient-specific factors that influence pharmacokinetics

Age

- Drug metabolism is low in the fetus and newborn, may be enhanced in young children, and becomes less effective with age
- Drug excretion falls with the age-related decline in renal function

Sex

- Women have a greater proportion of body fat than men, increasing the volume of distribution and half-life of lipid-soluble drugs

Body weight

- Obesity increases volume of distribution and half-life of lipid-soluble drugs
- Patients with higher lean body mass have larger body compartments into which drugs are distributed and may require higher doses

Liver function

- Metabolism of most drugs depends on several cytochrome P450 enzymes that are impaired in patients with advanced liver disease
- Hypoalbuminaemia influences the distribution of drugs that are highly protein-bound

Kidney function

- Renal disease and the decline in renal function with ageing may lead to drug accumulation

Gastrointestinal function

- Small intestinal absorption of oral drugs may be delayed by reduced gastric motility
- Absorptive capacity of the intestinal mucosa may be reduced in disease (e.g. Crohn's or coeliac disease) or after surgical resection

Food

- Food in the stomach delays gastric emptying and reduces the rate (but not usually the extent) of drug absorption
- Some food constituents bind to certain drugs and prevent their absorption

Smoking

- Tar in tobacco smoke stimulates the oxidation of certain drugs

Alcohol

- Regular alcohol consumption stimulates liver enzyme synthesis, while binge drinking may temporarily inhibit drug metabolism

Drugs

- Drug–drug interactions cause marked variation in pharmacokinetics (see Box 2.11)

2.5 Examples of pharmacogenetic variations that influence drug response

Genetic variant	Drug affected	Clinical outcome
Pharmacokinetic		
Aldehyde dehydrogenase-2 deficiency	Ethanol	Elevated blood acetaldehyde causes facial flushing and increased heart rate in ~50% of Japanese, Chinese and other Asian populations
Acetylation	Isoniazid, hydralazine, procainamide	Increased responses in slow acetylators, up to 50% of some populations
Oxidation (CYP2D6)	Nortriptyline	Increased risk of toxicity in poor metabolisers
	Codeine	Reduced responses with slower conversion of codeine to more active morphine in poor metabolisers, 10% of European populations
		Increased risk of toxicity in ultra-fast metabolisers, 3% of Europeans but 40% of North Africans
Oxidation (CYP2C18)	Proguanil	Reduced efficacy with slower conversion to active cycloguanil in poor metabolisers
Oxidation (CYP2C9)	Warfarin	Polymorphisms known to influence dosages
Oxidation (CYP2C19)	Clopidogrel	Reduced enzymatic activation results in reduced antiplatelet effect
Sulphoxidation	Penicillamine	Increased risk of toxicity in poor metabolisers
Human leucocyte antigen (HLA)-B*1502	Carbamazepine	Increased risk of serious dermatological reactions (e.g. Stevens–Johnson syndrome) for 1 in 2000 in Caucasian populations (much higher in some Asian countries)
Pseudocholinesterase deficiency	Suxamethonium (succinylcholine)	Decreased drug inactivation leads to prolonged paralysis and sometimes persistent apnoea requiring mechanical ventilation until the drug can be eliminated by alternate pathways; occurs in 1 in 1500 people
Pharmacodynamic		
Glucose-6-phosphate dehydrogenase (G6PD) deficiency	Oxidant drugs, including antimalarials (e.g. chloroquine, primaquine)	Risk of haemolysis in G6PD deficiency
Acute intermittent porphyria	Enzyme-inducing drugs	Increased risk of an acute attack
SLC01B1 polymorphism	Statins	Increased risk of rhabdomyolysis
HLA-B*5701 polymorphism	Abacavir	Increased risk of skin hypersensitivity reactions
HLA-B*5801 polymorphism	Allopurinol	Increased risk of rashes in Han Chinese
HLA-B*1502 polymorphism	Carbamazepine	Increased risk of skin hypersensitivity reactions in Han Chinese
Hepatic nuclear factor 1 alpha (HNF1A) polymorphism	Sulphonylureas	Increased sensitivity to the blood glucose-lowering effects
Human epidermal growth factor receptor 2 (HER2)-positive breast cancer cells	Trastuzumab	Increased sensitivity to the inhibitory effects on growth and division of the target cancer cells

Adverse outcomes of drug therapy

The decision to prescribe a drug always involves a judgement of the balance between therapeutic benefits and risk of an adverse outcome. Both prescribers and patients tend to be more focused on the former but a truly informed decision requires consideration of both.

Adverse drug reactions

Some important definitions for the adverse effects of drugs are:
- *Adverse event.* A harmful event that occurs while a patient is taking a drug, irrespective of whether the drug is suspected of being the cause.
- *Adverse drug reaction (ADR).* An unwanted or harmful reaction that is experienced following the administration of a drug or combination of drugs under normal conditions of use and is suspected to be related to the drug. An ADR will usually require the drug to be discontinued or the dose reduced.
- *Side-effect.* Any effect caused by a drug other than the intended therapeutic effect, whether beneficial, neutral or harmful. The term 'side-effect' is often used interchangeably with 'ADR', although the former usually implies an ADR that occurs during exposure to normal therapeutic drug concentrations (e.g. vasodilator-induced ankle oedema).
- *Hypersensitivity reaction.* An ADR that occurs as a result of an immunological reaction and often at exposure to subtherapeutic drug concentrations. Some of these reactions are immediate and result from the interaction of drug antigens with immunoglobulin E (IgE) on mast cells and basophils, which causes a release of vasoactive biomolecules (e.g. penicillin-related anaphylaxis). 'Anaphylactoid' reactions present similarly but occur through a direct non-immune-mediated release of the same mediators or result from direct complement activation (p. 75). Hypersensitivity reactions may occur via other mechanisms such as antibody-dependent (IgM or IgG), immune complex-mediated or cell-mediated pathways.
- *Drug toxicity.* Adverse effects of a drug that occur because the dose or plasma concentration has risen above the therapeutic range, either unintentionally or intentionally (drug overdose; see Fig. 2.2 and p. 137).
- *Drug abuse.* The misuse of recreational or therapeutic drugs that may lead to addiction or dependence, serious physiological injury (such as liver damage), psychological harm (abnormal behaviour patterns, hallucinations, memory loss) or death (p. 1184).

Prevalence of ADRs

ADRs are a common cause of illness, accounting in the UK for approximately 3% of consultations in primary care and 7% of emergency admissions to hospital, and affecting around 15% of hospital inpatients. Many 'disease' presentations are eventually attributed to ADRs, emphasising the importance of always taking a careful drug history (Box 2.6). Factors accounting for the rising prevalence of ADRs are the increasing age of patients, polypharmacy (higher risk of drug interactions), increasing

2.6 How to take a drug history

Information from the patient (or carer)

Use language that patients will understand (e.g. 'medicines' rather than 'drugs', which may be mistaken for drugs of abuse) while gathering the following information:
- Current prescribed drugs, including formulations (e.g. modified-release tablets), doses, routes of administration, frequency and timing, duration of treatment
- Other medications that are often forgotten (e.g. contraceptives, over-the-counter drugs, herbal remedies, vitamins)
- Drugs that have been taken in the recent past and reasons for stopping them
- Previous drug hypersensitivity reactions, their nature and time course (e.g. rash, anaphylaxis)
- Previous ADRs, their nature and time course (e.g. ankle oedema with amlodipine)
- Adherence to therapy (e.g. 'Are you taking your medication regularly?')

Information from GP medical records and/or pharmacist
- Up-to-date list of medications
- Previous ADRs
- Last order dates for each medication

Inspection of medicines
- Drugs and their containers (e.g. blister packs, bottles, vials) should be inspected for name, dosage, and the number of dosage forms taken since dispensed

(ADR = adverse drug reaction)

2.7 Risk factors for adverse drug reactions

Patient factors
- Elderly age (e.g. low physiological reserve)
- Gender (e.g. ACE inhibitor-induced cough in women)
- Polypharmacy (e.g. drug interactions)
- Genetic predisposition (see Box 2.5)
- Hypersensitivity/allergy (e.g. β-lactam antibiotics)
- Diseases altering pharmacokinetics (e.g. hepatic or renal impairment) or pharmacodynamic responses (e.g. bladder instability)
- Adherence problems (e.g. cognitive impairment)

Drug factors
- Steep dose–response curve (e.g. insulin)
- Low therapeutic index (e.g. digoxin, cytotoxic drugs)

Prescriber factors
- Inadequate understanding of principles of clinical pharmacology
- Inadequate knowledge of the patient
- Inadequate knowledge of the prescribed drug
- Inadequate instructions and warnings provided to patients
- Inadequate monitoring arrangements planned

(ACE = angiotensin-converting enzyme)

availability of over-the-counter medicines, increasing use of herbal or traditional medicines, and the increase in medicines available via the Internet that can be purchased without a prescription from a health-care professional. Risk factors for ADRs are shown in Box 2.7.

ADRs are important because they reduce quality of life for patients, reduce adherence to and therefore efficacy of beneficial treatments, cause diagnostic confusion, undermine the confidence of patients in their health-care professional(s) and consume health-care resources.

Retrospective analysis of ADRs has shown that more than half could have been avoided if the prescriber had taken more care in anticipating the potential hazards of drug therapy. For example, non-steroidal anti-inflammatory drug (NSAID) use accounts for many thousands of emergency admissions, gastrointestinal bleeding episodes and a significant number of deaths. In many cases, the patients are at increased risk due to their age, interacting drugs (e.g. aspirin, warfarin) or a past history of peptic ulcer disease. Drugs that commonly cause ADRs are listed in Box 2.8.

Prescribers and their patients ideally want to know the frequency with which ADRs occur for a specific drug. Although this may be well characterised for more common ADRs observed in clinical trials, it is less clear for rarely reported ADRs when the total numbers of reactions and patients exposed are not known. The words used to describe frequency can be misinterpreted by patients but widely accepted meanings include: very common (10% or more), common (1–10%), uncommon (0.1–1%), rare (0.01–0.1%) and very rare (0.01% or less).

Classification of ADRs

ADRs have traditionally been classified into two major groups:

- *Type A ('augmented') ADRs*. These are predictable from the known pharmacodynamic effects of the drug and are dose-dependent, common (detected early in drug development) and usually mild. Examples include constipation caused by opioids, hypotension caused by antihypertensives and dehydration caused by diuretics.
- *Type B ('bizarre') ADRs*. These are not predictable, are not obviously dose-dependent in the therapeutic range, are rare (remaining undiscovered until the drug is marketed) and often severe. Patients who experience type B reactions are generally 'hyper-susceptible' because of unpredictable immunological or genetic factors (e.g. anaphylaxis caused by penicillin, peripheral neuropathy caused by isoniazid in poor acetylators).

This simple classification has shortcomings, and a more detailed classification based on dose (see Fig. 2.2), timing and susceptibility (DoTS) is now used by those analysing ADRs in greater depth (Box 2.9). The AB classification can be extended as a reminder of some other types of ADR:

- *Type C ('chronic/continuous') ADRs*. These occur only after prolonged continuous exposure to a drug. Examples include osteoporosis caused by glucocorticoids, retinopathy caused by chloroquine, and tardive dyskinesia caused by phenothiazines.
- *Type D ('delayed') ADRs*. These are delayed until long after drug exposure, making diagnosis difficult. Examples include malignancies that may emerge after immunosuppressive treatment post-transplantation (e.g. azathioprine, tacrolimus) and vaginal cancer occurring many years after exposure to diethylstilboestrol.
- *Type E ('end-of-treatment') ADRs*. These occur after abrupt drug withdrawal (see Box 2.3).

A teratogen is a drug with the potential to affect the development of the fetus in the first 10 weeks of intrauterine life (e.g. phenytoin, warfarin). The thalidomide disaster in the early 1960s highlighted the risk of teratogenicity and led to mandatory testing of all new drugs. Congenital defects in a live infant or aborted fetus should

---

i | **2.8 Drugs that are common causes of adverse drug reactions**

Drug or drug class	Common adverse drug reactions
ACE inhibitors (e.g. lisinopril)	Renal impairment Hyperkalaemia
Antibiotics (e.g. amoxicillin)	Nausea Diarrhoea
Anticoagulants (e.g. warfarin, heparin)	Bleeding
Antipsychotics (e.g. haloperidol)	Falls Sedation Delirium
Aspirin	Gastrotoxicity (dyspepsia, gastrointestinal bleeding)
Benzodiazepines (e.g. diazepam)	Drowsiness Falls
β-blockers (e.g. atenolol)	Cold peripheries Bradycardia
Calcium channel blockers (e.g. amlodipine)	Ankle oedema
Digoxin	Nausea and anorexia Bradycardia
Diuretics (e.g. furosemide, bendroflumethiazide)	Dehydration Electrolyte disturbance (hypokalaemia, hyponatraemia) Hypotension Renal impairment
Insulin	Hypoglycaemia
NSAIDs (e.g. ibuprofen)	Gastrotoxicity (dyspepsia, gastrointestinal bleeding) Renal impairment
Opioid analgesics (e.g. morphine)	Nausea and vomiting Delirium Constipation

(ACE = angiotensin-converting enzyme; NSAID = non-steroidal anti-inflammatory drug)

---

i | **2.9 DoTS classification of adverse drug reactions**

Category	Example
Dose	
Below therapeutic dose	Anaphylaxis with penicillin
In the therapeutic dose range	Nausea with morphine
At high doses	Hepatotoxicity with paracetamol
Timing	
With the first dose	Anaphylaxis with penicillin
Early stages of treatment	Hyponatraemia with diuretics
On stopping treatment	Benzodiazepine withdrawal syndrome
Significantly delayed	Clear-cell cancer with diethylstilboestrol
Susceptibility	See patient factors in Box 2.7

(INR = international normalised ratio)

provoke suspicion of an ADR and a careful exploration of drug exposures (including self-medication and herbal remedies).

Detecting ADRs – pharmacovigilance

Type A ADRs become apparent early in the development of a new drug. By the time a new drug is licensed and launched on to a possible worldwide market, however, a relatively small number of patients (just several hundred) may have been exposed to it, meaning that rarer but potentially serious type B ADRs may remain undiscovered. Pharmacovigilance is the process of detecting ('signal generation') and evaluating ADRs in order to help prescribers and patients to be better informed about the risks of drug therapy. Drug regulatory agencies may respond to this information by placing restrictions on the licensed indications, reducing the recommended dose range, adding special warnings and precautions for prescribers in the product literature, writing to all health-care professionals or withdrawing the product from the market.

Voluntary reporting systems allow health-care professionals and patients to report suspected ADRs to the regulatory authorities. A good example is the 'Yellow Card' scheme that was set up in the UK in response to the thalidomide tragedy. Reports are analysed to assess the likelihood that they represent a true ADR (Box 2.10). Although voluntary reporting is a continuously operating and effective early-warning system for previously unrecognised rare ADRs, its weaknesses include low reporting rates (only 3% of all ADRs and 10% of serious ADRs are ever reported), an inability to quantify risk (because the ratio of ADRs to prescriptions is unknown), and the influence of prescriber awareness on likelihood of reporting (reporting rates rise rapidly following publicity about potential ADRs).

More systematic approaches to collecting information on ADRs include 'prescription event monitoring', in which a sample of prescribers of a particular drug are issued with questionnaires concerning the clinical outcome for their patients, and the collection of population statistics. Many health-care systems routinely collect patient-identifiable data on prescriptions (a surrogate marker of exposure to a drug), health-care events (e.g. hospitalisation, operations, new clinical diagnoses) and other clinical data (e.g. haematology, biochemistry). As these records are linked, with appropriate safeguards for confidentiality and data protection, they are providing a much more powerful mechanism for assessing both the harms and benefits of drugs.

All prescribers will inevitably see patients experiencing ADRs caused by prescriptions written by themselves or their colleagues. It is important that these are recognised early. In addition to the features in Box 2.10, features that should raise suspicion of an ADR and the need to respond (by drug withdrawal, dosage reduction or reporting to the regulatory authorities) include:

* concern expressed by a patient that a drug has harmed them
* abnormal clinical measurements (e.g. blood pressure, temperature, pulse, blood glucose and weight) or laboratory results (e.g. abnormal liver or renal function, low haemoglobin or white cell count) while on drug therapy
* new therapy started that could be in response to an ADR (e.g. omeprazole, allopurinol, naloxone)
* the presence of risk factors for ADRs (see Box 2.7).

Drug interactions

A drug interaction has occurred when the administration of one drug increases or decreases the beneficial or adverse responses to another drug. Although the number of potential interacting drug combinations is very large, only a small number are common in clinical practice. Important drug interactions are most likely to occur when the affected drug has a low therapeutic index, steep dose–response curve, high first-pass or saturable metabolism, or a single mechanism of elimination.

Mechanisms of drug interactions

Pharmacodynamic interactions occur when two drugs produce additive, synergistic or antagonistic effects at the same drug target (e.g. receptor, enzyme) or physiological system (e.g. electrolyte excretion, heart rate). These are the most common interactions in clinical practice and some important examples are given in Box 2.11.

Pharmacokinetic interactions occur when the administration of a second drug alters the concentration of the first at its site of action. There are numerous potential mechanisms:

* *Absorption interactions.* Drugs that either delay (e.g. anticholinergic drugs) or enhance (e.g. prokinetic drugs) gastric emptying influence the rate of rise in plasma concentration of other drugs but not the total amount of drug absorbed. Drugs that bind to form insoluble complexes or chelates (e.g. aluminium-containing antacids binding with ciprofloxacin) can reduce drug absorption.
* *Distribution interactions.* Co-administration of drugs that compete for protein binding in plasma (e.g. phenytoin and diazepam) can increase the unbound drug concentration, but the effect is usually short-lived due to increased elimination and hence restoration of the pre-interaction equilibrium.

i	**2.10 TREND analysis of suspected adverse drug reactions**	
Factor	**Key question**	**Comment**
Temporal relationship	What is the time interval between the start of drug therapy and the reaction?	Most ADRs occur soon after starting treatment and within hours in the case of anaphylactic reactions
Re-challenge	What happens when the patient is re-challenged with the drug?	Re-challenge is rarely possible because of the need to avoid exposing patients to unnecessary risk
Exclusion	Have concomitant drugs and other non-drug causes been excluded?	ADR is a diagnosis of exclusion following clinical assessment and relevant investigations for non-drug causes
Novelty	Has the reaction been reported before?	The suspected ADR may already be recognised and mentioned in the SPC approved by the regulatory authorities
De-challenge	Does the reaction improve when the drug is withdrawn or the dose is reduced?	Most, but not all, ADRs improve on drug withdrawal, although recovery may be slow

(SPC = summary of product characteristics)

i   **2.11 Common drug interactions**

Mechanism	Object drug	Precipitant drug	Result
Pharmaceutical*			
Chemical reaction	Sodium bicarbonate	Calcium gluconate	Precipitation of insoluble calcium carbonate
Pharmacokinetic			
Reduced absorption	Tetracyclines	Calcium, aluminium, and magnesium salts	Reduced tetracycline absorption
Reduced protein binding	Phenytoin	Aspirin	Increased unbound and reduced total phenytoin plasma concentration
Reduced metabolism:			
CYP3A4	Amiodarone	Grapefruit juice	Cardiac arrhythmias because of prolonged QT interval (p. 476)
	Warfarin	Clarithromycin	Enhanced anticoagulation
CYP2C19	Phenytoin	Omeprazole	Phenytoin toxicity
CYP2D6	Clozapine	Paroxetine	Clozapine toxicity
Xanthine oxidase	Azathioprine	Allopurinol	Azathioprine toxicity
Monoamine oxidase	Catecholamines	Monoamine oxidase inhibitors	Hypertensive crisis due to monoamine toxicity
Increased metabolism (enzyme induction)	Ciclosporin	St John's wort	Loss of immunosuppression
Reduced renal elimination	Lithium	Diuretics	Lithium toxicity
	Methotrexate	NSAIDs	Methotrexate toxicity
Pharmacodynamic			
Direct antagonism at same receptor	Opioids	Naloxone	Reversal of opioid effects used therapeutically
	Salbutamol	Atenolol	Inhibits bronchodilator effect
Direct potentiation in same organ system	Benzodiazepines	Alcohol	Increased sedation
	ACE inhibitors	NSAIDs	Increased risk of renal impairment
Indirect potentiation by actions in different organ systems	Digoxin	Diuretics	Digoxin toxicity enhanced because of hypokalaemia
	Warfarin	Aspirin, NSAIDs	Increased risk of bleeding because of gastrotoxicity and antiplatelet effects
	Diuretics	ACE inhibitors	Blood pressure reduction (may be therapeutically advantageous) because of the increased activity of the renin–angiotensin system in response to diuresis

*Pharmaceutical interactions are related to the formulation of the drugs and occur before drug absorption.
(ACE = angiotensin-converting enzyme; NSAID = non-steroidal anti-inflammatory drug)

- *Metabolism interactions.* Many drugs rely on metabolism by different isoenzymes of cytochrome P450 (CYP) in the liver. CYP enzyme inducers (e.g. phenytoin, rifampicin) generally reduce plasma concentrations of other drugs, although they may enhance activation of prodrugs. CYP enzyme inhibitors (e.g. clarithromycin, cimetidine, grapefruit juice) have the opposite effect. Enzyme induction effects usually take a few days to manifest because of the need to synthesise new CYP enzyme, in contrast to the rapid effects of enzyme inhibition.
- *Excretion interactions.* These primarily affect renal excretion. For example, drug-induced reduction in glomerular filtration rate (e.g. diuretic-induced dehydration, angiotensin-converting enzyme (ACE) inhibitors, NSAIDs) can reduce the clearance and increase the plasma concentration of many drugs, including some with a low therapeutic index (e.g. digoxin, lithium, aminoglycoside antibiotics). Less commonly, interactions may be due to competition for a common tubular organic anion transporter (e.g. methotrexate excretion may be inhibited by competition with NSAIDs).

Avoiding drug interactions

Drug interactions are increasing as patients are prescribed more medicines (polypharmacy). Prescribers can avoid the adverse consequences of drug–drug interactions by taking a careful drug history (see Box 2.6) before prescribing additional drugs, only prescribing for clear indications, and taking special care when prescribing drugs with a narrow therapeutic index (e.g. warfarin). When prescribing an interacting drug is unavoidable, good prescribers will seek further information and anticipate the potential risk. This will allow them to provide special warnings for the patient and arrange for monitoring, either of the clinical effects (e.g. coagulation tests for warfarin) or of plasma concentration (e.g. digoxin).

Medication errors

A medication error is any *preventable* event that may lead to inappropriate medication use or patient harm while the medication is in the control of the health-care professional or patient. Errors may occur in prescribing, dispensing, preparing solutions, administration or monitoring. Many ADRs are considered in retrospect to have been 'avoidable' with more care or forethought; in other words, an adverse event considered by one prescriber to be an unfortunate ADR might be considered by another to be a prescribing error.

Medication errors are very common. Several thousand medication orders are dispensed and administered each day in a medium-sized hospital. Recent UK studies suggest that

ℹ 2.12 Hospital prescribing errors	
Error type	Approximate % of total
Omission on admission	30
Underdose	11
Overdose	8
Strength/dose missing	7
Omission on discharge	6
Administration times incorrect/missing	6
Duplication	6
Product or formulation not specified	4
Incorrect formulation	4
No maximum dose	4
Unintentional prescribing	3
No signature	2
Clinical contraindication	1
Incorrect route	1
No indication	1
Intravenous instructions incorrect/missing	1
Drug not prescribed but indicated	1
Drug continued for longer than needed	1
Route of administration missing	1
Start date incorrect/missing	1
Risk of drug interaction	<0.5
Controlled drug requirements incorrect/missing	<0.5
Daily dose divided incorrectly	<0.5
Significant allergy	<0.5
Drug continued in spite of adverse effects	<0.5
Premature discontinuation	<0.5
Failure to respond to out-of-range drug level	<0.5

ℹ **2.13 Causes of prescribing errors**

Systems factors
- Working hours of prescribers (and others)
- Patient throughput
- Professional support and supervision by colleagues
- Availability of information (medical records)
- Design of prescription forms
- Distractions
- Availability of decision support
- Checking routines (e.g. clinical pharmacy)
- Reporting and reviewing of incidents

Prescriber factors

Knowledge
- Clinical pharmacology principles
- Drugs in common use
- Therapeutic problems commonly encountered
- Knowledge of workplace systems

Skills
- Taking a good drug history
- Obtaining information to support prescribing
- Communicating with patients
- Numeracy and calculations
- Prescription writing

Attitudes
- Coping with risk and uncertainty
- Monitoring of prescribing
- Checking routines

7–9% of hospital prescriptions contain an error, and most are written by junior doctors. Common prescribing errors in hospitals include omission of medicines (especially failure to prescribe regular medicines at the point of admission or discharge, i.e. 'medicines reconciliation'), dosing errors, unintentional prescribing and poor use of documentation (Box 2.12).

Most prescription errors result from a combination of failures by the individual prescriber and the health-service systems in which they work (Box 2.13). Health-care organisations increasingly encourage reporting of errors within a 'no-blame culture' so that they can be subject to 'root cause analysis' using human error theory (Fig. 2.5). Prevention is targeted at the factors in Box 2.13, and can be supported by prescribers communicating and cross-checking with colleagues (e.g. when calculating doses adjusted for body weight, or planning appropriate monitoring after drug administration), and by health-care systems providing clinical pharmacist support (e.g. for checking the patient's previous medications and current prescriptions) and electronic prescribing (which avoids errors due to illegibility or serious dosing mistakes, and may be combined with a clinical decision support system to take account of patient characteristics and drug history, and provide warnings of potential contraindications and drug interactions).

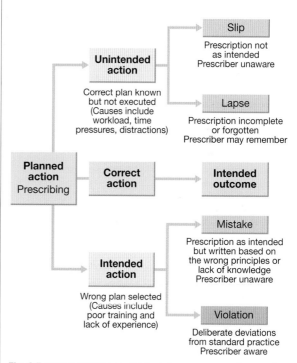

Fig. 2.5 Human error theory. Unintended errors may occur because the prescriber fails to complete the prescription correctly (a slip; e.g. writes the dose in 'mg' not 'micrograms') or forgets part of the action that is important for success (a lapse; e.g. forgets to co-prescribe folic acid with methotrexate); prevention requires the system to provide appropriate checking routines. Intended errors occur when the prescriber acts incorrectly due to lack of knowledge (a mistake; e.g. prescribes atenolol for a patient with known severe asthma because of ignorance about the contraindication); prevention must focus on training the prescriber.

Responding when an error is discovered

All prescribers will make errors. When they do, their first duty is to protect the patient's safety. This will involve a clinical review and the taking of any steps that will reduce harm (e.g. remedial treatment, monitoring, recording the event in the notes, informing colleagues). Patients should be informed if they have been exposed to potential harm. For errors that do not reach the patient, it is the prescriber's duty to report them, so that others can learn from the experience and take the opportunity to reflect on how a similar incident might be avoided in the future.

Drug regulation and management

Given the powerful beneficial and potentially adverse effects of drugs, the production and use of medicines are strictly regulated (e.g. by the Food and Drug Administration in the USA, Medicines and Healthcare Products Regulatory Agency in the UK, and Central Drugs Standard Control Organisation in India). Regulators are responsible for licensing medicines, monitoring their safety (pharmacovigilance; p. 23), approving clinical trials, and inspecting and maintaining standards of drug development and manufacture.

In addition, because of the high costs of drugs and their adverse effects, health-care services must prioritise their use in light of the evidence of their benefit and harm, a process referred to as 'medicines management'.

Drug development and marketing

Naturally occurring products have been used to treat illnesses for thousands of years and some remain in common use today. Examples include morphine from the opium poppy (*Papaver somniferum*), digitalis from the foxglove (*Digitalis purpurea*), curare from the bark of a variety of species of South American trees, and quinine from the bark of the *Cinchona* species. Although plants and animals remain a source of discovery, the majority of new drugs come from drug discovery programmes that aim to identify small-molecule compounds with specific interactions with a molecular target that will induce a predicted biological effect.

The usual pathway for development of these small molecules includes: identifying a plausible molecular target by investigating pathways in disease; screening a large library of compounds for those that interact with the molecular target in vitro; conducting extensive medicinal chemistry to optimise the properties of lead compounds; testing efficacy and toxicity of these compounds in vitro and in animals; and undertaking a clinical development programme (Box 2.14). This process typically takes longer than 10 years and may cost up to US$1 billion. Manufacturers have a defined period of exclusive marketing of the drug while it remains protected by an original patent, typically 10–15 years, during which time they must recoup the costs of developing the drug. Meanwhile, competitor companies will often produce similar 'me too' drugs of the same class. Once the drug's patent has expired, 'generic' manufacturers may step in to produce cheaper formulations of the drug. Paradoxically, if a generic drug is produced by only one manufacturer, the price may actually rise, sometimes substantially. Newer 'biological' products are based on large molecules (e.g. human recombinant antibodies) derived from complex manufacturing processes involving specific

Phase I

- Healthy volunteers (20–80)
- These involve initial single-dose, 'first-into-man' studies, followed by repeated-dose studies. They aim to establish the basic pharmacokinetic and pharmacodynamic properties, and short-term safety
- Duration: 6–12 months

Phase II

- Patients (100–200)
- These investigate clinical effectiveness ('proof of concept'), safety and dose–response relationship, often with a surrogate clinical endpoint, in the target patient group to determine the optimal dosing regimen for larger confirmatory studies
- Duration: 1–2 years

Phase III

- Patients (100s–1000s)
- These are large, expensive clinical trials that confirm safety and efficacy in the target patient population, using relevant clinical endpoints. They may be placebo-controlled studies or comparisons with other active compounds
- Duration: 1–2 years

Phase IV

- Patients (100s–1000s)
- These are undertaken after the medicine has been marketed for its first indication to evaluate new indications, new doses or formulations, long-term safety or cost-effectiveness

cell lines, molecular cloning and purification processes. After the patent for the originator product expires, other manufacturers may develop similar products ('biosimilars') that share similar pharmacological actions but are not completely identical. 'Biosimilars' are considered distinct from 'generic' medications, as complex biological molecules are more susceptible to differences in manufacturing processes than conventional small-molecule-type pharmaceuticals.

The number of new drugs produced by the pharmaceutical industry has declined in recent years. The traditional approach of targeting membrane-bound receptors and enzymes with small molecules (see Box 2.2) is now giving way to new targets, such as complex second-messenger systems, cytokines, nucleic acids and cellular networks. These require novel therapeutic agents, which present new challenges for 'translational medicine', the discipline of converting scientific discoveries into a useful medicine with a well-defined benefit–risk profile (Box 2.15).

Licensing new medicines

New drugs are given a 'market authorisation', based on the evidence of quality, safety and efficacy presented by the manufacturer. The regulator not only will approve the drug but also will take great care to ensure that the accompanying information reflects the evidence that has been presented. The summary of product characteristics (SPC), or 'label', provides detailed information about indications, dosage, adverse effects, warnings, monitoring and so on. If approved, drugs can be made available with different levels of restriction:

- *Controlled drug (CD)*. These drugs are subject to strict legal controls on supply and possession, usually due to their abuse potential (e.g. opioid analgesics).

i	2.15 Novel therapeutic alternatives to conventional small-molecule drugs		
Approaches	**Therapeutic indications**		**Challenges**
Monoclonal antibodies Targeting of receptors or other molecules with relatively specific antibodies	Cancer Chronic inflammatory diseases (e.g. rheumatoid arthritis, inflammatory bowel disease)		Selectivity of action Complex manufacturing process
Small interfering RNA (siRNA) Inhibition of gene expression	Macular degeneration		Delivery to target
Gene therapy Delivery of modified genes that supplement or alter host DNA	Cystic fibrosis Cancer Cardiovascular disease		Delivery to target Adverse effects of delivery vector (e.g. virus)
Stem cell therapy Stem cells differentiate and replace damaged host cells	Parkinson's disease Spinal cord injury Ischaemic heart disease		Delivery to target Immunological compatibility Long-term effects unknown

- *Prescription-only medicine (PoM).* These are available only from a pharmacist and can be supplied only if prescribed by an appropriate practitioner.
- *Pharmacy (P).* These are available only from a pharmacist but can be supplied without a prescription.
- *General sales list (GSL).* These medicines may be bought 'over the counter' (OTC) from any shop and without a prescription.

Although the regulators take great care to agree the exact indications for prescribing a medicine, based on the evidence provided by the manufacturer, there are some circumstances in which prescribers may direct its use outside the terms stated in the SPC ('off-label' prescribing). Common situations where this might occur include prescribing outside the approved age group (e.g. prescribing for children) or using an alternative formulation (e.g. administering a medicine provided in a solid form as an oral solution). Other important examples might include prescribing for an indication for which there are no approved medicines or where all of the approved medicines have caused unacceptable adverse effects. Occasionally, medicines may be prescribed when there is no marketing authorisation in the country of use. Examples include when a medicine licensed in another country is imported for use for an individual patient ('unlicensed import') or when a patient requires a specific preparation of a medicine to be manufactured ('unlicensed special'). When prescribing is 'off-label' or 'unlicensed', there is an increased requirement for prescribers to be able to justify their actions and to inform and agree the decision with the patient.

Drug marketing

The marketing activities of the pharmaceutical industry are well resourced and are important in the process of recouping the massive costs of drug development. In some countries, such as the USA, it is possible to promote a new drug by direct-to-consumer advertising, although this is illegal in the countries of the European Union. A major focus is on promotion to prescribers via educational events, sponsorship of meetings, advertisements in journals, involvement with opinion leaders, and direct contact by company representatives. Such largesse has the potential to cause significant conflicts of interest and might tempt prescribers to favour one drug over another, even in the face of evidence on effectiveness or cost-effectiveness.

Managing the use of medicines

Many medicines meet the three key regulatory requirements of quality, safety and efficacy. Although prescribers are legally entitled to prescribe any of them, it is desirable to limit the choice so that treatments for specific diseases can be focused on the most effective and cost-effective options, prescribers (and patients) gain familiarity with a smaller number of medicines, and pharmacies can concentrate stocks on them.

The process of ensuring optimal use of available medicines is known as 'medicines management' or 'quality use of medicines'. It involves careful evaluation of the evidence of benefit and harm from using the medicine, an assessment of cost-effectiveness, and support for processes to implement the resulting recommendations. These activities usually involve both national (e.g. National Institute for Health and Care Excellence (NICE) in the UK) and local organisations (e.g. drug and therapeutics committees).

Evaluating evidence

The principles of evidence-based medicine are described on page 10. Drugs are often evaluated in high-quality randomised controlled trials, the results of which can be considered by systematic review (Fig. 2.6). Ideally, data are available not only for comparison with placebo but also for 'head-to-head' comparison with alternative therapies. Trials are conducted in selected patient populations, however, and are not representative of every clinical scenario, so extrapolation to individual patients is not always straightforward. Other subtle bias may be introduced because of the sources of funding (e.g. pharmaceutical industry) and the interests of the investigators in being involved in research that has a 'positive' impact. These biases may be manifest in the way the trials are conducted or in how they are interpreted or reported. A common example of the latter is the difference between relative and absolute risk of clinical events reported in prevention trials. If a clinical event is encountered in the placebo arm at a rate of 1 in 50 patients (2%) but only 1 in 100 patients (1%) in the active treatment arm, then the impact of treatment can be described as either a 50% relative risk reduction or 1% absolute risk reduction. Although the former sounds more impressive, it is the latter that is of more importance to the

Odds ratio

Fig. 2.6 Systematic review of the evidence from randomised controlled clinical trials. This forest plot shows the effect of warfarin compared with placebo on the likelihood of stroke in patients with atrial fibrillation in five randomised controlled trials that passed the quality criteria required for inclusion in a meta-analysis. For each trial, the purple box is proportionate to the number of participants. The tick marks show the mean odds ratio and the black lines indicate its 95% confidence intervals. Note that not all the trials showed statistically significant effects (i.e. the confidence intervals cross 1.0). However, the meta-analysis, represented by the black diamond, confirms a highly significant statistical benefit. The overall odds ratio is approximately 0.4, indicating a mean 60% risk reduction with warfarin treatment in patients with the characteristics of the participants in these trials.

individual patient. It means that the number of patients that needed to be treated (NNT) for 1 to benefit (compared to placebo) was 100. This illustrates how large clinical trials of new medicines can produce highly statistically significant and impressive relative risk reductions and still predict a very modest clinical impact.

Evaluating cost-effectiveness

New drugs often represent an incremental improvement over the current standard of care but are usually more expensive. Health-care budgets are limited in every country and so it is impossible to fund all new medicines. This means that very difficult financial decisions have to be taken with due regard to the principles of ethical justice. The main approach taken is cost-effectiveness analysis (CEA), where a comparison is made between the relative costs and outcomes of different courses of action. CEA is usually expressed as a ratio where the denominator is a gain in health and the numerator is the cost associated with the health gain. A major challenge is to compare the value of interventions for different clinical outcomes. One method is to calculate the quality-adjusted life years (QALYs) gained if the new drug is used rather than standard treatment. This analysis involves estimating the 'utility' of various health states between 1 (perfect health) and 0 (dead). If the additional costs and any savings are known, then it is possible to derive the incremental cost-effectiveness ratio (ICER) in terms of cost/QALY. These principles are exemplified in Box 2.16. There are, however, inherent weaknesses in this kind of analysis: it usually depends on modelling future outcomes well beyond the duration of the clinical trial data that are available; it assumes that QALYs gained at all ages are of equivalent value; and the appropriate standard care against which the new drug should be compared is often uncertain.

These pharmacoeconomic assessments are challenging and resource-intensive, and are undertaken at national level in most countries, e.g. in the UK by NICE.

---

i ### 2.16 Cost-effectiveness analysis

A clinical trial lasting 2 years compares two interventions for the treatment of colon cancer:
- Treatment A: standard treatment, cost £1000/year, oral therapy
- Treatment B: new treatment, cost £6000/year, monthly intravenous infusions, often followed by a week of nausea.

The new treatment (B) significantly increases the average time to progression (18 months versus 12 months) and reduces overall mortality (40% versus 60%). The health economist models the survival curves from the trial in order to undertake a cost–utility analysis and concludes that:
- Intervention A: allows an average patient to live for 2 extra years at a utility 0.7 = 1.4 QALYs (cost £2000)
- Intervention B: allows an average patient to live for 3 extra years at a utility 0.6 = 1.8 QALYs (cost £18 000).

The health economists conclude that treatment B provides an extra 0.4 QALYs at an extra cost of £16 000, meaning that the ICER = £40 000/QALY. They recommend that the new treatment should not be funded on the basis that their threshold for cost acceptability is £30 000/QALY.

(ICER = incremental cost-effectiveness ratio; QALY = quality-adjusted life year)

Implementing recommendations

Many recommendations about drug therapy are included in clinical guidelines written by an expert group after systematic review of the evidence. Guidelines provide recommendations rather than obligations for prescribers and are helpful in promoting more consistent and higher-quality prescribing. They are often written without concern for cost-effectiveness, however, and may be limited by the quality of available evidence. Guidelines cannot anticipate the extent of the variation between individual patients who may, for example, have unexpected contraindications to recommended drugs or choose different priorities for treatment. When deviating from respected national guidance, prescribers should be able to justify their practice.

Additional recommendations for prescribing are often implemented locally or imposed by bodies responsible for paying for health care. Most health-care units have a drug and therapeutics committee (or equivalent) comprised of senior and junior medical staff, pharmacists and nurses, as well as managers (because of the implications of the committee's work for governance and resources). This group typically develops local prescribing policy and guidelines, maintains a local drug formulary and evaluates requests to use new drugs. The local formulary contains a more limited list than any national formulary (e.g. *British National Formulary*) because the latter lists all licensed medicines that can be prescribed legally, while the former contains only those that the health-care organisation has approved for local use. The local committee may also be involved, with local specialists, in providing explicit protocols for management of clinical scenarios.

Prescribing in practice

Decision-making in prescribing

Prescribing should be based on a rational approach to a series of challenges (see Box 2.1).

Making a diagnosis

Ideally, prescribing should be based on a confirmed diagnosis but, in reality, many prescriptions are based on the balance of probability, taking into account the differential diagnosis (e.g. proton pump inhibitors for post-prandial retrosternal discomfort).

Establishing the therapeutic goal

The goals of treatment are usually clear, particularly when relieving symptoms (e.g. pain, nausea, constipation). Sometimes the goal is less obvious to the patient, especially when aiming to prevent future events (e.g. ACE inhibitors to prevent hospitalisation and extend life in chronic heart failure). Prescribers should be clear about the therapeutic goal against which they will judge success or failure of treatment. It is also important to establish that the value placed on this goal by the prescriber is shared by the patient (concordance).

Choosing the therapeutic approach

For many clinical problems, drug therapy is not absolutely mandated. Having taken the potential benefits and harms into account, prescribers must consider whether drug therapy is in the patient's interest and is preferred to no treatment or one of a range of alternatives (e.g. physiotherapy, psychotherapy, surgery). Assessing the balance of benefit and harm is often complicated and depends on various features associated with the patient, disease and drug (Box 2.17).

Choosing a drug

For most common clinical indications (e.g. type 2 diabetes, depression), more than one drug is available, often from more than one drug class. Although prescribers often have guidance about which represents the rational choice for the average patient, they still need to consider whether this is the optimal choice for the individual patient. Certain factors may influence the choice of drug:

Absorption

Patients may find some formulations easier to swallow than others or may be vomiting and require a drug available for parenteral administration.

Distribution

Distribution of a drug to a particular tissue sometimes dictates choice (e.g. tetracyclines and rifampicin are concentrated in the bile, and lincomycin and clindamycin in bones).

Metabolism

Drugs that are extensively metabolised should be avoided in severe liver disease (e.g. opioid analgesics).

> **i** | **2.17 Factors to consider when balancing benefits and harms of drug therapy**
>
> - Seriousness of the disease or symptom
> - Efficacy of the drug
> - Seriousness of potential adverse effects
> - Likelihood of adverse effects
> - Efficacy of alternative drugs or non-drug therapies
> - Safety of alternative drugs or non-drug therapies

Excretion

Drugs that depend on renal excretion for elimination (e.g. digoxin, aminoglycoside antibiotics) should be avoided in patients with impaired renal function if suitable alternatives exist.

Efficacy

Prescribers normally choose drugs with the greatest efficacy in achieving the goals of therapy (e.g. proton pump inhibitors rather than H_2-receptor antagonists). It may be appropriate, however, to compromise on efficacy if other drugs are more convenient, safer to use or less expensive.

Avoiding adverse effects

Prescribers should be wary of choosing drugs that are more likely to cause adverse effects (e.g. cephalosporins rather than alternatives for patients allergic to penicillin) or worsen coexisting conditions (e.g. β-blockers as treatment for angina in patients with asthma).

Features of the disease

This is most obvious when choosing antibiotic therapy, which should be based on the known or suspected sensitivity of the infective organism (p. 116).

Severity of disease

The choice of drug should be appropriate to disease severity (e.g. paracetamol for mild pain, morphine for severe pain).

Coexisting disease

This may be either an indication or a contraindication to therapy. Hypertensive patients might be prescribed a β-blocker if they also have left ventricular impairment but not if they have asthma.

Avoiding adverse drug interactions

Prescribers should avoid giving combinations of drugs that might interact, either directly or indirectly (see Box 2.11).

Patient adherence to therapy

Prescribers should choose drugs with a simple dosing schedule or easier administration (e.g. the ACE inhibitor lisinopril once daily rather than captopril 3 times daily for hypertension).

Cost

Prescribers should choose the cheaper drug (e.g. a generic or biosimilar) if two drugs are of equal efficacy and safety. Even if cost is not a concern for the individual patient, it is important to remember that unnecessary expenditure will ultimately limit choices for other prescribers and patients. Sometimes a more costly drug may be appropriate (e.g. if it yields improved adherence).

Genetic factors

There are already a small number of examples where genotype influences the choice of drug therapy (see Box 2.5).

Choosing a dosage regimen

Prescribers have to choose a dose, route and frequency of administration (dosage regimen) to achieve a steady-state drug concentration that provides sufficient exposure of the target tissue without producing toxic effects. Manufacturers draw up dosage recommendations based on average observations in many patients but the optimal regimen that will maximise the benefit to harm ratio for an individual patient is never certain.

Rational prescribing involves treating each prescription as an experiment and gathering sufficient information to amend it if necessary. There are some general principles that should be followed, as described below.

Dose titration

Prescribers should generally start with a low dose and titrate this slowly upwards as necessary. This cautious approach is particularly important if the patient is likely to be more sensitive to adverse pharmacodynamic effects (e.g. delirium or postural hypotension in the elderly) or have altered pharmacokinetic handling (e.g. renal or hepatic impairment), and when using drugs with a low therapeutic index (e.g. benzodiazepines, lithium, digoxin). There are some exceptions, however. Some drugs must achieve therapeutic concentration quickly because of the clinical circumstance (e.g. antibiotics, glucocorticoids, carbimazole). When early effect is important but there may be a delay in achieving steady state because of a drug's long half-life (e.g. digoxin, warfarin, amiodarone), an initial loading dose is given prior to establishing the appropriate maintenance dose (see Fig. 2.4).

If adverse effects occur, the dose should be reduced or an alternative drug prescribed; in some cases, a lower dose may suffice if it can be combined with another synergistic drug (e.g. the immunosuppressant azathioprine reduces glucocorticoid requirements in patients with inflammatory disease). It is important to remember that the shape of the dose–response curve (see Fig. 2.2) means that higher doses may produce little added therapeutic effect and might increase the chances of toxicity.

Route

There are many reasons for choosing a particular route of administration (Box 2.18).

Frequency

Frequency of doses is usually dictated by a manufacturer's recommendation. Less frequent doses are more convenient for patients but result in greater fluctuation between peaks and troughs in drug concentration (see Fig. 2.4). This is relevant if the peaks are associated with adverse effects (e.g. dizziness with antihypertensives) or the troughs are associated with troublesome loss of effect (e.g. anti-Parkinsonian drugs). These problems can be tackled either by splitting the dose or by employing a modified-release formulation, if available.

Timing

For many drugs the time of administration is unimportant. There are occasionally pharmacokinetic or therapeutic reasons, however, for giving drugs at particular times (Box 2.19).

Formulation

For some drugs there is a choice of formulation, some for use by different routes. Some are easier to ingest, particularly by children (e.g. elixirs). The formulation is important when writing repeat prescriptions for drugs with a low therapeutic index that come in different formulations (e.g. lithium, phenytoin, theophylline). Even if the prescribed dose remains constant, an alternative formulation may differ in its absorption and bioavailability, and hence plasma drug concentration. These are examples of the small number of drugs that should be prescribed by specific brand name rather than 'generic' international non-proprietary name (INN).

i	2.18 Factors influencing the route of drug administration	
Reason	**Example**	
Only one route possible	Dobutamine (IV) Gliclazide (oral)	
Patient adherence	Phenothiazines and thioxanthenes (2 weekly IM depot injections rather than daily tablets, in schizophrenia)	
Poor absorption	Furosemide (IV rather than oral, in severe heart failure)	
Rapid action	Haloperidol (IM rather than oral, in acute behavioural disturbance)	
Vomiting	Phenothiazines (PR or buccal rather than oral, in nausea)	
Avoidance of first-pass metabolism	Glyceryl trinitrate (SL, in angina pectoris)	
Certainty of effect	Amoxicillin (IV rather than oral, in acute chest infection)	
Direct access to the site of action (avoiding unnecessary systemic exposure)	Bronchodilators (INH rather than oral, in asthma) Local application of drugs to skin, eyes etc.	
Ease of access	Diazepam (PR, if IV access is difficult in status epilepticus) Adrenaline (epinephrine) (IM, if IV access is difficult in acute anaphylaxis)	
Comfort	Morphine (SC rather than IV in terminal care)	

(IM = intramuscular; INH = by inhalation; IV = intravenous; PR = per rectum; SC = subcutaneous; SL = sublingual)

Duration

Some drugs require a single dose (e.g. thrombolysis post myocardial infarction), while for others the duration of the course of treatment is certain at the outset (e.g. antibiotics). For most, the duration will be largely at the prescriber's discretion and will depend on response and disease progression (e.g. analgesics, antidepressants). For many, the treatment will be long-term (e.g. insulin, antihypertensives, levothyroxine).

Involving the patient

Patients should, whenever possible, be engaged in making choices about drug therapy. Their beliefs and expectations affect the goals of therapy and help in judging the acceptable benefit/harm balance when selecting treatments. Very often, patients may wish to defer to the professional expertise of the prescriber. Nevertheless, they play key roles in adherence to therapy and in monitoring treatment, not least by providing early warning of adverse events. It is important for them to be provided with the necessary information to understand the choice that has been made, what to expect from the treatment, and any measurements that must be undertaken (Box 2.20).

A major drive to include patients has been the recognition that up to half of the drug doses for chronic preventative therapy are not taken. This is often termed 'non-compliance' but is more appropriately called 'non-adherence', to reflect a less paternalistic view of the doctor–patient relationship; it may or may not be intentional. Non-adherence to the dose regimen reduces the likelihood of benefits to the patient and can be costly in terms

2.19 Factors influencing the timing of drug therapy

Drug	Recommended timing	Reasons
Diuretics (e.g. furosemide)	Once in the morning	Night-time diuresis undesirable
Statins (e.g. simvastatin)	Once at night	HMG CoA reductase activity is greater at night
Antidepressants (e.g. amitriptyline)	Once at night	Allows adverse effects to occur during sleep
Salbutamol	Before exercise	Reduces symptoms in exercise-induced asthma
Glyceryl trinitrate Paracetamol	When required	Relief of acute symptoms only
Regular nitrate therapy (e.g. isosorbide mononitrate)	Eccentric dosing regimen (e.g. twice daily at 8 a.m. and 2 p.m.)	Reduces development of nitrate tolerance by allowing drug-free period each night
Aspirin	With food	Minimises gastrotoxic effects
Alendronate	Once in the morning before breakfast, sitting upright	Minimises risk of oesophageal irritation
Tetracyclines	2 hours before or after food or antacids	Divalent and trivalent cations chelate tetracyclines, preventing absorption
Hypnotics (e.g. temazepam)	Once at night	Maximises therapeutic effect and minimises daytime sedation
Antihypertensive drugs (e.g. amlodipine)	Once in the morning	Blood pressure is higher during the daytime

(HMG CoA = 3-hydroxy-3-methylglutaryl-coenzyme A)

2.20 What patients need to know about their medicines*

Knowledge	Comment
The reason for taking the medicine How the medicine works	Reinforces the goals of therapy
How to take the medicine	May be important for the effectiveness (e.g. inhaled salbutamol in asthma) and safety (e.g. alendronate for osteoporosis) of treatment
What benefits to expect	May help to support adherence or prompt review because of treatment failure
What adverse effects might occur	Discuss common and mild effects that may be transient and might not require discontinuation Mention rare but serious effects that might influence the patient's consent
Precautions that improve safety	Explain symptoms to report that might allow serious adverse effects to be averted, monitoring that will be required and potentially important drug–drug interactions
When to return for review	This will be important to enable monitoring

*Many medicines are provided with patient information leaflets, which the patient should be encouraged to read.

of wasted medicines and unnecessary health-care episodes. An important reason may be lack of concordance with the prescriber about the goals of treatment. A more open and shared decision-making process might resolve any misunderstandings at the outset and foster improved adherence, as well as improved satisfaction with health-care services and confidence in prescribers. Fully engaging patients in shared decision-making is sometimes constrained by various factors, such as limited consultation time and challenges in communicating complex numerical data.

Writing the prescription

The culmination of the planning described above is writing an accurate and legible prescription so that the drug will be dispensed and administered as planned (see 'Writing prescriptions' below).

Monitoring treatment effects

Rational prescribing involves monitoring for the beneficial and adverse effects of treatment so that the balance remains in favour of a positive outcome (see 'Monitoring drug therapy' below).

Stopping drug therapy

It is also important to review long-term treatment at regular intervals to assess whether continued treatment is required. Elderly patients are keen to reduce their medication burden and are often prepared to compromise on the original goals of long-term preventative therapy to achieve this.

Prescribing in special circumstances

Prescribing for patients with renal disease

Patients with renal impairment are readily identified by having a low estimated glomerular filtration rate (eGFR <60 mL/min) based on their serum creatinine, age, sex and ethnic group (p. 386). This group includes a large proportion of elderly patients. If a drug (or its active metabolites) is eliminated predominantly by the kidneys, it will tend to accumulate and so the maintenance dose must be reduced. For some drugs, renal impairment makes patients more sensitive to their adverse pharmacodynamic effects.

2.21 Some drugs that require extra caution in patients with renal or hepatic disease

Kidney disease	Liver disease
Pharmacodynamic effects enhanced	
ACE inhibitors and ARBs (renal impairment, hyperkalaemia)	Warfarin (increased anticoagulation because of reduced clotting factor synthesis)
Metformin (lactic acidosis)	
Spironolactone (hyperkalaemia)	Metformin (lactic acidosis)
NSAIDs (impaired renal function)	Chloramphenicol (bone marrow suppression)
Sulphonylureas (hypoglycaemia)	
Insulin (hypoglycaemia)	NSAIDs (gastrointestinal bleeding, fluid retention)
	Sulphonylureas (hypoglycaemia)
	Benzodiazepines (coma)
Pharmacokinetic handling altered (reduced clearance)	
Aminoglycosides (e.g. gentamicin)	Phenytoin
Vancomycin	Rifampicin
Digoxin	Propranolol
Lithium	Warfarin
Other antibiotics (e.g. ciprofloxacin)	Diazepam
	Lidocaine
Atenolol	Opioids (e.g. morphine)
Allopurinol	
Cephalosporins	
Methotrexate	
Opioids (e.g. morphine)	

(ACE = angiotensin-converting enzyme; ARB = angiotensin receptor blocker; NSAID = non-steroidal anti-inflammatory drug)

Examples of drugs that require extra caution in patients with renal disease are listed in Box 2.21.

Prescribing for patients with hepatic disease

The liver has a large capacity for drug metabolism and hepatic insufficiency has to be advanced before drug dosages need to be modified. Patients who may have impaired metabolism include those with jaundice, ascites, hypoalbuminaemia, malnutrition or encephalopathy. Hepatic drug clearance may also be reduced in acute hepatitis, in hepatic congestion due to cardiac failure, and in the presence of intrahepatic arteriovenous shunting (e.g. in hepatic cirrhosis). There are no good tests of hepatic drug-metabolising capacity or of biliary excretion, so dosage should be guided by the therapeutic response and careful monitoring for adverse effects. The presence of liver disease also increases the susceptibility to adverse pharmacological effects of drugs. Some drugs that require extra caution in patients with hepatic disease are listed in Box 2.21.

Prescribing for elderly patients

The issues around prescribing in the elderly are discussed in Box 2.22.

Prescribing for women who are pregnant or breastfeeding

Prescribing in pregnancy should be avoided if possible to minimise the risk of adverse effects in the fetus. Drug therapy in pregnancy may, however, be required either for a pre-existing problem (e.g. epilepsy, asthma, hypothyroidism) or for problems that arise during pregnancy (e.g. morning sickness, anaemia, prevention of neural tube defects, gestational diabetes, hypertension). About 35% of women take drug therapy at least once during

2.22 Prescribing in old age

- **Reduced drug elimination**: partly due to impaired renal function.
- **Increased sensitivity to drug effects**: notably in the brain (leading to sedation or delirium) and as a result of comorbidities.
- **More drug interactions**: largely as a result of polypharmacy.
- **Lower starting doses and slower dose titration**: often required, with careful monitoring of drug effects.
- **Drug adherence**: may be poor because of cognitive impairment, difficulty swallowing (dry mouth) and complex polypharmacy regimens. Supplying medicines in pill organisers (e.g. dosette boxes or calendar blister packs), providing automatic reminders, and regularly reviewing and simplifying the drug regimen can help.
- **Some drugs that require extra caution, and their mechanisms**:
  Digoxin: increased sensitivity of Na^+/K^+ pump; hypokalaemia due to diuretics; renal impairment favours accumulation → increased risk of toxicity.
  Antihypertensive drugs: reduced baroreceptor function → increased risk of postural hypotension.
  Antidepressants, hypnotics, sedatives, tranquillisers: increased sensitivity of the brain; reduced metabolism → increased risk of toxicity.
  Warfarin: increased tendency to falls and injury and to bleeding from intra- and extracranial sites; increased sensitivity to inhibition of clotting factor synthesis → increased risk of bleeding.
  Clomethiazole, lidocaine, nifedipine, phenobarbital, propranolol, theophylline: metabolism reduced → increased risk of toxicity.
  Non-steroidal anti-inflammatory drugs: poor renal function → increased risk of renal impairment; susceptibility to gastrotoxicity → increased risk of upper gastrointestinal bleeding.

2.23 Prescribing in pregnancy

- **Teratogenesis**: a potential risk, especially when drugs are taken between 2 and 8 weeks of gestation (4–10 weeks from last menstrual period). Common teratogens include retinoids (e.g. isotretinoin), cytotoxic drugs, angiotensin-converting enzyme inhibitors, antiepileptics and warfarin. If there is inadvertent exposure, then the timing of conception should be established, counselling given and investigations undertaken for fetal abnormalities.
- **Adverse fetal effects in late gestation**: e.g. tetracyclines may stain growing teeth and bones; sulphonamides displace fetal bilirubin from plasma proteins, potentially causing kernicterus; opioids given during delivery may be associated with respiratory depression in the neonate.
- **Altered maternal pharmacokinetics**: extracellular fluid volume and V_d increase. Plasma albumin falls but other binding globulins (e.g. for thyroid and steroid hormones) increase. Glomerular filtration increases by approximately 70%, enhancing renal clearance. Placental metabolism contributes to increased clearance, e.g. of levothyroxine and glucocorticoids. The overall effect is a fall in plasma levels of many drugs.
- **In practice**:
  Avoid any drugs unless the risk:benefit analysis is in favour of treating (usually the mother).
  Use drugs for which there is some record of safety in humans.
  Use the lowest dose for the shortest time possible.
  Choose the least harmful drug if alternatives are available.

pregnancy and 6% take drug therapy during the first trimester (excluding iron, folic acid and vitamins). The most commonly used drugs are simple analgesics, antibacterial drugs and antacids. Some considerations when prescribing in pregnancy are listed in Box 2.23.

Drugs that are excreted in breast milk may cause adverse effects in the baby. Prescribers should always consult the summary of product characteristics for each drug or a reliable formulary when treating a pregnant woman or breastfeeding mother.

Writing prescriptions

A prescription is a means by which a prescriber communicates the intended plan of treatment to the pharmacist who dispenses a medicine and to a nurse or patient who administers it. It should be precise, accurate, clear and legible. The two main kinds of prescription are those written, dispensed and administered in hospital and those written in primary care (in the UK by a GP), dispensed at a community pharmacy and self-administered by the patient. The information supplied must include:

- the date
- the identification details of the patient
- the name of the drug
- the formulation
- the dose
- the frequency of administration
- the route and method of administration
- the amount to be supplied (primary care only)
- instructions for labelling (primary care only)
- the prescriber's signature.

Prescribing in hospital

Although GP prescribing is increasingly electronic, most hospital prescribing continues to be based around the prescription and administration record (the 'drug chart') (Fig. 2.7). A variety of charts are in use and prescribers must familiarise themselves with the local version. Most contain the following sections:

- *Basic patient information*: will usually include name, age, date of birth, hospital number and address. These details are often 'filled in' using a sticky addressograph label but this increases the risk of serious error.
- *Previous adverse reactions/allergies*: communicates important patient safety information based on a careful drug history and/or the medical record.
- *Other medicines charts*: notes any other hospital prescription documents that contain current prescriptions being received by the patient (e.g. anticoagulants, insulin, oxygen, fluids).
- *Once-only medications*: for prescribing medicines to be used infrequently, such as single-dose prophylactic antibiotics and other pre-operative medications.
- *Regular medications*: for prescribing medicines to be taken for a number of days or continuously, such as a course of antibiotics, antihypertensive drugs and so on.
- *'As required' medications*: for prescribing for symptomatic relief, usually to be administered at the discretion of the nursing staff (e.g. antiemetics, analgesics).

Prescribers should be aware of the risks of prescription error (Box 2.24 and see Box 2.13), ensure they have considered the rational basis for their prescribing decision described above, and then follow the guidance illustrated in Figure 2.7 in order to write the prescription. It is a basic principle that a prescription will be followed by a judgement as to its success or failure and any appropriate changes made (e.g. altered dosage, discontinuation or substitution).

---

i **2.24 High-risk prescribing moments**

- Trying to amend an active prescription (e.g. altering the dose/timing) – *always avoid and start again*
- Writing up drugs in the immediate presence of more than one prescription chart or set of notes – *avoid*
- Allowing one's attention to be diverted in the middle of completing a prescription – *avoid*
- Prescribing 'high-risk' drugs (e.g. anticoagulants, opioids, insulin, sedatives) – *ask for help if necessary*
- Prescribing parenteral drugs – *take care*
- Rushing prescribing (e.g. in the midst of a busy ward round) – *avoid*
- Prescribing unfamiliar drugs – *consult the formulary and ask for help if necessary*
- Transcribing multiple prescriptions from an expired chart to a new one – *take care to review the rationale for each medicine*
- Writing prescriptions based on information from another source such as a referral letter (the list may contain errors and some of the medicines may be the cause of the patient's illness) – *review the justification for each as if it is a new prescription*
- Writing up 'to take out' drugs (because these will become the patient's regular medication for the immediate future) – *take care and seek advice if necessary*
- Calculating drug doses – *ask a colleague to perform an independent calculation or use approved electronic dose calculators*
- Prescribing sound-alike or look-alike drugs (e.g. chlorphenamine and chlorpromazine) – *take care*

Hospital discharge ('to take out') medicines

Most patients will be prescribed a short course of their medicines at discharge. This prescription is particularly important because it usually informs future therapy at the point of transfer of prescribing responsibility to primary care. Great care is required to ensure that this list is accurate. It is particularly important to ensure that any hospital medicines that should be stopped are not included and that those intended to be administered for a short duration only are clearly identified. It is also important for any significant ADRs experienced in hospital to be recorded and any specific monitoring or review identified.

Prescribing in primary care

Most of the considerations above are equally applicable to primary care (GP) prescriptions. In many health-care systems, community prescribing is electronic, making issues of legibility irrelevant and often providing basic decision support to limit the range of doses that can be written and highlight potential drug interactions. Important additional issues more relevant to GP prescribing are:

- *Formulation*. The prescription needs to carry information about the formulation for the dispensing pharmacist (e.g. tablets or oral suspension).
- *Amount to be supplied*. In the hospital the pharmacist will organise this. Elsewhere it must be specified either as the precise number of tablets or as the duration of treatment. Creams and ointments should be specified in grams and lotions in mL.
- *Controlled drugs*. Prescriptions for 'controlled' drugs (e.g. opioid analgesics, with potential for drug abuse) are subject to additional legal requirements. In the UK, they

A

PRESCRIPTION AND ADMINISTRATION RECORD

Standard Chart

Hospital/Ward: *W26*	Consultant: *Maxwell*	Name of patient: *John Smith*
Weight: *78 Kg*	Height: *1.84 m*	Hospital number: *WGH5522589*
If rewritten, date: *14.2.18*		D.O.B.: *16/10/64*
DISCHARGE PRESCRIPTION Date completed:–	Completed by:–	(Attach printed label here)

OTHER MEDICINES CHARTS	PREVIOUS ADVERSE REACTIONS				
	(This must be completed before prescribing on this chart)				
Date	Type of chart	Medicine	Description of reaction	Completed by	Date
14.2.18	*Oxygen*	*Penicillin*	*Serious reaction (hospitalised) age 15*	*S. Jones*	*14.2.18*
14.2.18	*Warfarin*	*Cefalexin*	*Rash (discontinued) 2006*	*S. Jones*	*14.2.18*

CODES FOR NON-ADMINISTRATION OF PRESCRIBED MEDICINE

If a dose is not administered as prescribed, intial and enter a code in the column with a circle drawn round the code according to the reason as shown below. **Inform the responsible doctor of the appropriate timescale.**

1. Patient refuses
2. Patient not present
3. Medicines not available – CHECK ORDERED
4. Asleep/drowsy
5. Administration route not available – CHECK FOR ALTERNATIVE

6. Vomiting/nausea
7. Time varied on doctor's instructions
8. Once-only/as-required medicine given
9. Dose withheld on doctor's instructions
10. Possible adverse reaction/side-effect

B

ONCE-ONLY MEDICINES

Date	Time	Medicine (approved name)	Dose	Route	Prescriber – sign and print	Time given	Given by
14.2.18	*16.00*	MORPHINE SULFATE	*5 mg*	*IV*	*S. JONES*	*16.20*	*ST*
14.2.18	*16.00*	GLYCERYL TRINITRATE	*2 mg*	*Buccal*	*S. JONES*	*16.10*	*DK*
14.2.18	*16.00*	METOCLOPRAMIDE	*10 mg*	*IV*	*S. JONES*	*16.20*	*ST*

Fig. 2.7 Example of a hospital prescription and administration record ('drug chart'). A *Front page.* The correct identification of the patient is critical to reducing the risk of an administration error. This page also clearly identifies other prescriptions charts in use and previous adverse reactions to drugs to minimise the risk of repeated exposure. Note also the codes employed by the nursing staff to indicate reasons why drugs may not have been administered. The patient's name and date of birth should be written on each page of the chart. The patient's weight and height may be required to calculate safe doses for many drugs with narrow therapeutic indices. B *'Once-only medicines'.* This area is used for prescribing medicines that are unlikely to be repeated on a regular basis. Note that the prescriber has written the **names of all drugs** legibly in block capitals. The generic international non-proprietary name (INN) should be used in preference to the brand name (e.g. write 'SIMVASTATIN', not 'ZOCOR'). The only exceptions are when variation occurs in the properties of alternative branded formulations (e.g. modified-release preparations of drugs such as lithium, theophylline, phenytoin and nifedipine) or when the drug is a combination product with no generic name (e.g. Kliovance). The only acceptable abbreviations for **drug dose** units are 'g' and 'mg'. 'Units' (e.g. of insulin or heparin) and 'micrograms' must always be written in full, never as 'U' or 'μg' (nor 'mcg', nor 'ug'). For liquid preparations write the dose in mg; 'mL' can be written only for a combination product (e.g. Gaviscon liquid) or if the strength is not expressed in weight (e.g. adrenaline (epinephrine) 1 in 1000). Use numbers/figures (e.g. 1 or 'one') to denote use of a sachet/enema but avoid prescribing numbers of tablets without specifying their strength. Always include the dose of inhaled drugs in addition to stating numbers of 'puffs', as strengths can vary. Widely accepted abbreviations for **route of administration** are: intravenous – 'IV'; intramuscular – 'IM'; subcutaneous – 'SC'; sublingual – 'SL'; per rectum – 'PR'; per vaginam – 'PV'; nasogastric – 'NG'; inhaled – 'INH'; and topical – 'TOP'. 'ORAL' is preferred to per oram – 'PO'. Care should be taken in specifying 'RIGHT' or 'LEFT' for eye and ear drops. The prescriber should sign and print their name clearly so that they can be identified by colleagues. The prescription should be dated and have an administration time. The nurse who administered the prescription has signed to confirm that the dose has been administered.

must contain the address of the patient and prescriber (not necessary on most hospital forms), the form and the strength of the preparation, and the total quantity of the preparation/number of dose units in both words and figures.

- *'Repeat prescriptions'.* A large proportion of GP prescribing involves 'repeat prescriptions' for chronic medication. These are often generated automatically, although the prescriber remains responsible for regular review and for ensuring that the benefit-to-harm ratio remains favourable.

Monitoring drug therapy

Prescribers should measure the effects of the drug, both beneficial and harmful, to inform decisions about dose titration (up or down), discontinuation or substitution of treatment. Monitoring can be achieved subjectively by asking the patient about symptoms or, more objectively, by measuring a clinical effect. Alternatively, if the pharmacodynamic effects of the drug are difficult to assess, the plasma drug concentration may be measured, on the basis that it will be closely related to the effect of the drug (see Fig. 2.2).

C

REGULAR MEDICINES	Date → Time ↓	February 2018 14	15	16	17	18	19	20	21			
Drug (approved name) **AMOXICILLIN**	6											
Dose *500 mg* / Route ORAL	⑧	X	DK	RB	RB	DK		X	X	X	X	X
	12											
Prescriber–sign and print *S. JONES* / Start date 14. 02.18	⑭	X	DK	2	RB			X	X	X	X	X
	18											
Notes *For chest infection* / Pharmacy	㉒	X	DK	RB	RB			X	X	X	X	X
Drug (approved name) **AMLODIPINE**	6											
Dose *5 mg* / Route ORAL	⑧	X	DK	RB								
	12				*Discontinued due to*							
Prescriber–sign and print *S. JONES* / Start date 14. 02.18	14				*persistent ankle*							
	18				*oedema*							
Notes *For hypertension* / Pharmacy	22				*S. Maxwell 16.02.18*							
Drug (approved name) **LISINOPRIL**	6											
Dose *20 mg* / Route ORAL	⑧	X	DK	RB	RB	DK						
	12											
Prescriber–sign and print *S. JONES* / Start date 14. 02.18	14											
	18											
Notes *Review renal function on 16. 2.18* / Pharmacy	22											

D

AS-REQUIRED THERAPY			
Drug (approved name) **PARACETAMOL**	Date	16.2	
	Time	11.15	
Dose and frequency *1g 4-hrly* / Route ORAL	Dose	*1 g*	
	Initials	DK	
Prescriber–sign and print *S. JONES* / Start date 16. 02.18	Date		
	Time		
Indication/notes *For pain Maximum 4g/24 hr* / Pharmacy	Dose		
	Initials		
Drug (approved name) **GLYCERYL TRINITRATE**	Date		
	Time		
Dose and frequency *500 micrograms* / Route Sublingual	Dose		
	Initials		
Prescriber–sign and print *S. JONES* / Start date 16. 02.18	Date		
	Time		
Indication/notes *For cardiac ischaemia* / Pharmacy	Dose		
	Initials		

Fig. 2.7, cont'd C *'Regular medicines'.* This area is used for prescribing medicines that are going to be given regularly. In addition to the name, dose and route, a **frequency of administration** is required for each medicine. Widely accepted Latin abbreviations for dose frequency are: once daily – 'OD'; twice daily – 'BD'; 3 times daily – 'TDS'; 4 times daily – 'QDS'; as required – 'PRN'; in the morning – 'OM' (omni mane); at night – 'ON' (omni nocte); and immediately – 'stat'. The hospital chart usually requires specific times to be identified for regular medicines that coincide with nursing drug rounds and these can be circled. If treatment is for a known time period, cross off subsequent days when the medicine is not required. The **'notes' box** can be used to communicate additional important information (e.g. whether a medicine should be taken with food, type of inhaler device used, and anything else that the drug dispenser should know). State here the times for peak/trough plasma levels for drugs requiring therapeutic monitoring. Prescriptions should be **discontinued** by drawing a vertical line at the point of discontinuation, horizontal lines through the remaining days on the chart, and diagonal lines through the drug details and administration boxes. This action should be signed and dated and a supplementary note written to explain it (e.g. describing any adverse effect). In this example, amlodipine has been discontinued because of ankle oedema. There is room for the ward pharmacist to sign to indicate that the prescription has been reviewed and that a supply of the medicine is available. The administration boxes allow the nurse to sign to confirm that the dose has been given. Note that these boxes also allow for recording of reasons for non-administration (in this example '2' indicates that the patient was not present on the ward at the time) and the prevention of future administration by placing an 'X' in the box. D *'As-required medicines'.* These prescriptions leave the administration of the drug to the discretion of the nursing staff. The prescription must describe clearly the indication, frequency, minimal time interval between doses, and maximum dose in any 24-hour period (in this case, the maximum daily dose of paracetamol is 4 g).

Clinical and surrogate endpoints

Ideally, clinical endpoints are measured directly and the drug dosage titrated to achieve the therapeutic goal and avoid toxicity (e.g. control of ventricular rate in a patient with atrial fibrillation). Sometimes this is impractical because the clinical endpoint is a future event (e.g. prevention of myocardial infarction by statins or resolution of a chest infection with antibiotics); in these circumstances, it may be possible to select a 'surrogate' endpoint that will predict success or failure. This may be an intermediate step in the pathophysiological process (e.g. serum cholesterol as a surrogate for risk of myocardial infarction) or a

i	**2.25 Drugs commonly monitored by plasma drug concentration**	
Drug	**Half-life (hrs)***	**Comment**
Digoxin	36	Steady state takes several days to achieve. Samples should be taken 6 hrs post dose. Measurement is useful to confirm the clinical impression of toxicity or non-adherence but clinical effectiveness is better assessed by ventricular heart rate. Risk of toxicity increases progressively at concentrations >1.5 µg/L, and is likely at concentrations >3.0 µg/L (toxicity is more likely in the presence of hypokalaemia)
Gentamicin	2	Measure pre-dose trough concentration (should be <1 µg/mL) to ensure that accumulation (and the risk of nephrotoxicity and ototoxicity) is avoided; see Fig. 6.18 (p. 122)
Levothyroxine	>120	Steady state may take up to 6 weeks to achieve (p. 640)
Lithium	24	Steady state takes several days to achieve. Samples should be taken 12 hrs post dose. Target range 0.4–1 mmol/L
Phenytoin	24	Measure pre-dose trough concentration (should be 10–20 mg/L) to ensure that accumulation is avoided. Good correlation between concentration and toxicity. Concentration may be misleading in the presence of hypoalbuminaemia
Theophylline (oral)	6	Steady state takes 2–3 days to achieve. Samples should be taken 6 hrs post dose. Target concentration is 10–20 mg/L but its relationship with bronchodilator effect and adverse effects is variable
Vancomycin	6	Measure pre-dose trough concentration (should be 10–15 mg/L) to ensure clinical efficacy and that accumulation and the risk of nephrotoxicity are avoided (p. 123)

*Half-lives vary considerably with different formulations and between patients.

measurement that follows the pathophysiology, even if it is not a key factor in its progression (e.g. serum C-reactive protein as a surrogate for resolution of inflammation in chest infection). Such surrogates are sometimes termed 'biomarkers'.

Plasma drug concentration

The following criteria must be met to justify routine monitoring by plasma drug concentration:

- Clinical endpoints and other pharmacodynamic (surrogate) effects are difficult to monitor.
- The relationship between plasma concentration and clinical effects is predictable.
- The therapeutic index is low. For drugs with a high therapeutic index, any variability in plasma concentrations is likely to be irrelevant clinically.

Some examples of drugs that fulfil these criteria are listed in Box 2.25.

Measurement of plasma concentration may be useful in planning adjustments of drug dose and frequency of administration; to explain an inadequate therapeutic response (by identifying subtherapeutic concentration or incomplete adherence); to establish whether a suspected ADR is likely to be caused by the drug; and to assess and avoid potential drug interactions.

Timing of samples in relation to doses

The concentration of drug rises and falls during the dosage interval (see Fig. 2.4B). Measurements made during the initial absorption and distribution phases are unpredictable because of the rapidly changing concentration, so samples are usually taken at the end of the dosage interval (a 'trough' or 'pre-dose' concentration). This measurement is normally made in steady state, which usually takes five half-lives to achieve after the drug is introduced or the dose changed (unless a loading dose has been given).

Interpreting the result

A target range is provided for many drugs, based on average thresholds for therapeutic benefit and toxicity. Inter-individual variability means that these can be used only as a guide. For instance, in a patient who describes symptoms that could be consistent with toxicity but has a drug concentration in the top half of the target range, toxic effects should still be suspected. Another important consideration is that some drugs are heavily protein-bound (e.g. phenytoin) but only the unbound drug is pharmacologically active. Patients with hypoalbuminaemia may therefore have a therapeutic or even toxic concentration of unbound drug, despite a low 'total' concentration.

Further information

Websites

bnf.org *The British National Formulary (BNF) is a key reference resource for UK NHS prescribers, with a list of licensed drugs, chapters on prescribing in renal failure, liver disease, pregnancy and during breastfeeding, and appendices on drug interactions.*

cochrane.org *The Cochrane Collaboration is a leading international body that provides evidence-based reviews (around 7000 so far).*

evidence.nhs.uk *NHS Evidence provides a wide range of health information relevant to delivering quality patient care.*

icp.org.nz *The Interactive Clinical Pharmacology site is designed to increase understanding of principles in clinical pharmacology.*

medicines.org.uk/emc/ *The electronic Medicines Compendium (eMC) contains up-to-date, easily accessible information about medicines licensed by the UK Medicines and Healthcare Products Regulatory Agency (MHRA) and the European Medicines Agency (EMA).*

nice.org.uk *The UK National Institute for Health and Care Excellence makes recommendations to the UK NHS on new and existing medicines, treatments and procedures.*

who.int/medicines/en/ *The World Health Organisation Essential Medicines and Pharmaceutical Policies.*

K Tatton-Brown
DR FitzPatrick

3

Clinical genetics

The fundamental principles of genomics 38

The packaging of genes: DNA, chromatin and chromosomes 38
From DNA to protein 38
Non-coding RNA 40
Cell division, differentiation and migration 40
Cell death, apoptosis and senescence 41

Genomics, health and disease 42

Classes of genetic variant 42
Consequences of genomic variation 44
Normal genomic variation 45
Constitutional genetic disease 46
Somatic genetic disease 50

Interrogating the genome: the changing landscape of genomic technologies 51

Looking at chromosomes 51
Looking at genes 52

Genomics and clinical practice 56

Genomics and health care 56
Treatment of genetic disease 58
Ethics in a genomic age 59

We have entered a genomic era. Powerful new technologies are driving forward transformational change in health care. Genetic sequencing has evolved from the targeted sequencing of a single gene to the parallel sequencing of multiple genes. In addition to improving the chances of identifying a genetic cause of rare diseases, these technologies are increasingly directing therapies and, in the future, are likely to be used in the diagnosis and prevention of common diseases such as diabetes. In this chapter we explore the fundamentals of genomics, the basic principles underlying these new genomic technologies and how the data generated can be applied safely for patient benefit. We will review the use of genomic technology across a breadth of medical specialties, including obstetrics, paediatrics, oncology and infectious disease, and consider how health care is likely to be transformed by technology over the coming decade. Finally, we will consider the ethical impact that these technologies are likely to have, both for the individual and for their wider family.

The fundamental principles of genomics

The packaging of genes: DNA, chromatin and chromosomes

Genes are functional units encoded in double-stranded deoxyribonucleic acid (DNA), packaged as chromosomes and located in the nucleus of the cell: a membrane-bound compartment found in all cells except erythrocytes and platelets (Fig. 3.1). DNA consists of a linear sequence of just four bases: adenine (A,) cytosine (C), thymine (T) and guanine (G.) It forms a 'double helix', a twisted ladder-like structure formed from two complementary strands of DNA joined by hydrogen bonds between bases on the opposite strand that can form only between a C and a G base and an A and a T base. It is this feature of DNA that enables faithful DNA replication and is the basis for many of the technologies designed to interrogate the genome: when the DNA double helix 'unzips', one strand can act as a template for the creation of an identical strand.

A single copy of the human genome comprises approximately 3.1 billion base pairs of DNA, wound around proteins called histones. The unit consisting of 147 base pairs wrapped around four different histone proteins is called the nucleosome. Sequences of nucleosomes (resembling a string of beads) are wound and packaged to form chromatin: tightly wound, densely packed chromatin is called heterochromatin and open, less tightly wound chromatin is called euchromatin.

The chromatin is finally packaged into the chromosomes. Humans are diploid organisms: the nucleus contains two copies of the genome, visible microscopically as 23 chromosome pairs (known as the karyotype). Chromosomes 1 through to 22 are known as the autosomes and consist of identical chromosomal pairs. The 23rd 'pair' of chromosomes are the two sex chromosomes: females have two X chromosomes and males an X and Y chromosome. A normal female karyotype is therefore written as 46,XX and a normal male is 46,XY.

From DNA to protein

Genes are functional elements on the chromosome that are capable of transmitting information from the DNA template

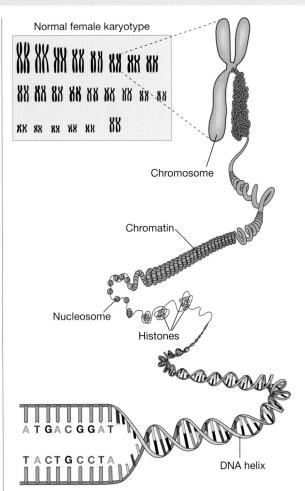

Normal female karyotype

Chromosome

Chromatin

Nucleosome

Histones

A T G A C G G A T

T A C T G C C T A

DNA helix

Fig. 3.1 The packaging of DNA, genes and chromosomes. From bottom to top: the double helix and the complementary DNA bases; chromatin; and a normal female chromosome pattern – the karyotype.

via the production of messenger ribonucleic acid (mRNA) to the production of proteins. The human genome contains over 20 000 genes, although many of these are inactive or silenced in different cell types, reflecting the variable gene expression responsible for cell-specific characteristics. The central dogma is the pathway describing the basic steps of protein production: transcription, splicing, translation and protein modification (Fig. 3.2). Although this is now recognised as an over-simplification (contrary to this linear relationship, a single gene will often encode many different proteins), it remains a useful starting point to explore protein production.

Transcription: DNA to messenger RNA

Transcription describes the production of ribonucleic acid (RNA) from the DNA template. For transcription to commence, an enzyme called RNA polymerase binds to a segment of DNA at the start of the gene: the promoter. Once bound, RNA polymerase moves along one strand of DNA, producing an RNA molecule complementary to the DNA template. In protein-coding genes this is known as messenger RNA (mRNA). A DNA sequence close to the end of the gene, called the polyadenylation signal, acts as a signal for termination of the RNA transcript (Fig. 3.3).

3

| DNA | 5' CGATTC3'
3' GCTAAG5' |

Transcription

| RNA | 5' CGAUUC3' |

Translation

| Protein | N_ArgPhe_C |

Fig. 3.2 The central dogma of protein production. Double-stranded DNA as a template for single-stranded RNA, which codes for the production of a peptide chain of amino acids. Each of these chains has an orientation. For DNA and RNA, this is 5′ to 3′. For peptides, this is N-terminus to C-terminus.

RNA differs from DNA in three main ways:
- RNA is single-stranded.
- The sugar residue within the nucleotide is ribose, rather than deoxyribose.
- It contains uracil (U) in place of thymine (T).

The activity of RNA polymerase is regulated by transcription factors. These proteins bind to specific DNA sequences at the promoter or to enhancer elements that may be many thousands of base pairs away from the promoter; a loop in the chromosomal DNA brings the enhancer close to the promoter, enabling the bound proteins to interact. The human genome encodes more than 1200 different transcription factors. Mutations within transcription factors, promoters and enhancers can cause disease. For example, the blood disorder alpha-thalassaemia is usually caused by gene deletions (see p. 954 and Box 3.4). However, it can also result from a mutation in an enhancer located more than 100 000 base pairs (bp) from the α-globin gene promoter, leading to greatly reduced transcription.

Gene activity, or expression, is influenced by a number of complex interacting factors, including the accessibility of the gene promoter to transcription factors. DNA can be modified by the addition of a methyl group to cytosine molecules (methylation). If DNA methylation occurs in promoter regions, transcription is silenced, as methyl cytosines are usually not available for transcription factor binding. A second mechanism determining promoter accessibility is the structural configuration of chromatin. In open chromatin, called euchromatin, gene promoters are accessible to RNA polymerase and transcription factors; therefore it is transcriptionally active. This contrasts with heterochromatin, which is densely packed and transcriptionally silent. The chromatin configuration is determined by modifications (such as methylation or acetylation) of specific amino acid residues of histone protein tails.

Modifications of DNA and histones are termed epigenetic ('epi-' meaning 'above' the genome), as they do not alter the primary sequence of the DNA code but have biological significance in chromosomal function. Abnormal epigenetic changes are increasingly recognised as important events in the progression of cancer, allowing expression of normally silenced genes that result in cancer cell de-differentiation and proliferation. They also afford therapeutic targets. For instance, the histone deacetylase inhibitor vorinostat has been successfully used to treat cutaneous T-cell lymphoma, due to the re-expression of genes that had

Fig. 3.3 RNA synthesis and its translation into protein. Gene transcription involves binding of RNA polymerase II to the promoter of genes being transcribed with other proteins (transcription factors) that regulate the transcription rate. The primary RNA transcript is a copy of the whole gene and includes both introns and exons, but the introns are removed within the nucleus by splicing and the exons are joined to form the messenger RNA (mRNA). Prior to export from the nucleus, a methylated guanosine nucleotide is added to the 5′ end of the RNA ('cap') and a string of adenine nucleotides is added to the 3′ ('polyA tail'). This protects the RNA from degradation and facilitates transport into the cytoplasm. In the cytoplasm, the mRNA binds to ribosomes and forms a template for protein production. (tRNA = transfer RNA; UTR = untranslated region)

previously been silenced in the tumour. These genes encode transcription factors that promote T-cell differentiation as opposed to proliferation, thereby causing tumour regression.

RNA splicing, editing and degradation

Transcription produces an RNA molecule that is a copy of the whole gene, termed the primary or nascent transcript. This nascent transcript then undergoes splicing, whereby regions not required to make protein (the intronic regions) are removed while those segments that are necessary for protein production (the exonic regions) are retained and rejoined.

Splicing is a highly regulated process that is carried out by a multimeric protein complex called the spliceosome. Following splicing, the mRNA molecule is exported from the nucleus and used as a template for protein synthesis. Many genes produce more than one form of mRNA (and thus protein) by a process termed alternative splicing, in which different combinations of exons are joined together. Different proteins from the same gene can have entirely distinct functions. For example, in thyroid C cells the calcitonin gene produces mRNA encoding the osteoclast inhibitor calcitonin (p. 634), but in neurons the same gene produces an mRNA with a different complement of exons via alternative splicing that encodes a neurotransmitter, calcitonin-gene-related peptide (p. 772).

Translation and protein production

Following splicing, the segment of mRNA containing the code that directs synthesis of a protein product is called the open reading frame (ORF). The inclusion of a particular amino acid in the protein is specified by a codon composed of three contiguous bases. There are 64 different codons with some redundancy in the system: 61 codons encode one of the 20 amino acids, and the remaining three codons – UAA, UAG and UGA (known as stop codons) – cause termination of the growing polypeptide chain. ORFs in humans most commonly start with the amino acid methionine. All mRNA molecules have domains before and after the ORF called the 5′ untranslated region (UTR) and 3′UTR, respectively. The start of the 5′UTR contains a cap structure that protects mRNA from enzymatic degradation, and other elements within the 5′UTR are required for efficient translation. The 3′UTR also contains elements that regulate efficiency of translation and mRNA stability, including a stretch of adenine bases known as a polyA tail (see Fig. 3.3).

The mRNAs then leave the nucleus via nuclear pores and associate with ribosomes, the sites of protein production (see Fig. 3.3). Each ribosome consists of two subunits (40S and 60S), which comprise non-coding rRNA molecules (see Fig. 3.9, p. 50) complexed with proteins. During translation, a different RNA molecule known as transfer RNA (tRNA) binds to the ribosome. The tRNAs deliver amino acids to the ribosome so that the newly synthesised protein can be assembled in a stepwise fashion. Individual tRNA molecules bind a specific amino acid and 'read' the mRNA ORF via an 'anticodon' of three nucleotides that is complementary to the codon in mRNA (see Fig. 3.3). A proportion of ribosomes is bound to the membrane of the endoplasmic reticulum (ER), a complex tubular structure that surrounds the nucleus.

Proteins synthesised on these ribosomes are translocated into the lumen of the ER, where they undergo folding and processing. From here, the protein may be transferred to the Golgi apparatus, where it undergoes post-translational modifications, such as glycosylation (covalent attachment of sugar moieties), to form the mature protein that can be exported into the cytoplasm or packaged into vesicles for secretion. The clinical importance of post-translational modification of proteins is shown by the severe developmental, neurological, haemostatic and soft tissue abnormalities that are associated with the many different congenital disorders of glycosylation. Post-translational modifications can also be disrupted by the synthesis of proteins with abnormal amino acid sequences. For example, the most common mutation in cystic fibrosis (ΔF508) results in an abnormal protein that cannot be exported from the ER and Golgi (see Box 3.4).

Non-coding RNA

Approximately 4500 genes in humans encode non-coding RNAs (ncRNA) rather than proteins. There are various categories of ncRNA, including transfer RNA (tRNA), ribosomal RNA (rRNA), ribozymes and microRNA (miRNA). The miRNAs, which number over 1000, have a role in post-translational gene expression: they bind to mRNAs, typically in the 3′UTR, promoting target mRNA degradation and gene silencing. Together, miRNAs affect over half of all human genes and have important roles in normal development, cancer and common degenerative disorders. This is the subject of considerable research interest at present.

Cell division, differentiation and migration

In normal tissues, molecules such as hormones, growth factors and cytokines provide the signal to activate the cell cycle: a controlled programme of biochemical events that culminates in cell division. In all cells of the body, except the gametes (the sperm and egg cells, also known as the germ line), mitosis completes cell division, resulting in two diploid daughter cells. In contrast, the sperm and eggs cells complete cell division with meiosis, resulting in four haploid daughter cells (Fig. 3.4).

The stages of cell division in the non-germ-line, somatic cells are shown below:

- *Cells not committed to mitosis* are said to be in G_0.
- *Cells committed to mitosis* must go through the preparatory phase of interphase consisting of G_1, S and G_2:
  - G_1 (first gap): synthesis of the cellular components necessary to complete cell division
  - S (synthesis): DNA replication producing identical copies of each chromosome called the sister chromatids
  - G_2 (second gap): repair of any errors in the replicated DNA before proceeding to mitosis.
- *Mitosis* (M) consists of four phases:
  - Prophase: the chromosomes condense and become visible, the centrioles move to opposite ends of the cell and the nuclear membrane disappears.
  - Metaphase: the centrioles complete their migration to opposite ends of the cell and the chromosomes – consisting of two identical sister chromatids – line up at the equator of the cell.
  - Anaphase: spindle fibres attach to the chromosome and pull the sister chromatids apart.
  - Telophase: the chromosomes decondense, the nuclear membrane reforms and two daughter cells – each with 46 chromosomes – are formed.

The progression from one phase to the next is tightly controlled by cell-cycle checkpoints. For example, the checkpoint between

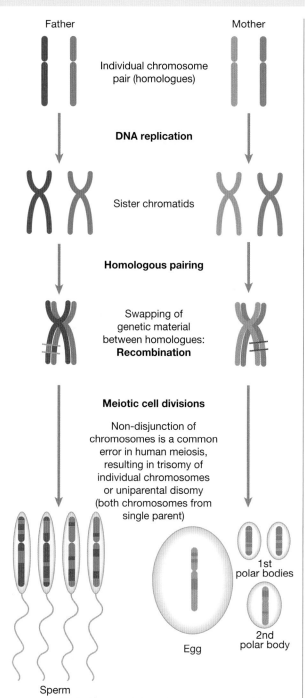

Father   Mother

Individual chromosome
pair (homologues)

DNA replication

Sister chromatids

Homologous pairing

Swapping of
genetic material
between homologues:
Recombination

Meiotic cell divisions

Non-disjunction of
chromosomes is a common
error in human meiosis,
resulting in trisomy of
individual chromosomes
or uniparental disomy
(both chromosomes from
single parent)

1st
polar bodies

2nd
polar body

Egg

Sperm

Fig. 3.4 Meiosis and gametogenesis: the main chromosomal stages of meiosis in both males and females. A single homologous pair of chromosomes is represented in different colours. The final step is the production of haploid germ cells. Each round of meiosis in the male results in four sperm cells; in the female, however, only one egg cell is produced, as the other divisions are sequestered on the periphery of the mature egg as peripheral polar bodies.

G_2 and mitosis ensures that all damaged DNA is repaired prior to segregation of the chromosomes. Failure of these control processes is a crucial driver in the pathogenesis of cancer, as discussed on page 1316.

• *Meiosis* is a special, gamete-specific, form of cell division (Fig. 3.4). Like mitosis, meiosis consists of four phases (prophase, metaphase, anaphase and telophase) but differs from mitosis in the following ways:

• It consists of two separate cell divisions known as meiosis I and meiosis II.
• It reduces the chromosome number from the diploid to the haploid number via a tetraploid stage, i.e. from 46 to 92 (MI S) to 46 (MI M) to 23 (MII M) chromosomes, so that when a sperm cell fertilises the egg, the resulting zygote will return to a diploid, 46, chromosome complement. This reduction to the haploid number occurs at the end of meiosis II.
• The 92 chromosome stage consists of 23 homologous pairs of sister chromatids, which then swap genetic material, a process known as recombination. This occurs at the end of MI prophase and ensures that the chromosome that a parent passes to his or her offspring is a mix of the chromosomes that the parent inherited from his or her own mother and father.

The individual steps in meiotic cell division are similar in males and females. However, the timing of the cell divisions is very different. In females, meiosis begins in fetal life but does not complete until after ovulation. A single meiotic cell division can thus take more than 40 years to complete. As women become older, the separation of chromosomes at meiosis II becomes less efficient. That is why the risk of trisomies (p. 44) due to non-disjunction grows greater with increasing maternal age. In males, meiotic division does not begin until puberty and continues throughout life. In the testes, both meiotic divisions are completed in a matter of days.

Cell death, apoptosis and senescence

With the exception of stem cells, human cells have only a limited capacity for cell division. The Hayflick limit is the number of divisions a cell population can go through in culture before division stops and enters a state known as senescence. This 'biological clock' is of great interest in the study of the normal ageing process. Rare human diseases associated with premature ageing, called progeric syndromes, have been very helpful in identifying the importance of DNA repair mechanisms in senescence (p. 1034). For example, in Werner's syndrome, a DNA helicase (an enzyme that separates the two DNA strands) is mutated, leading to failure of DNA repair and premature ageing. A distinct mechanism of cell death is seen in apoptosis, or programmed cell death.

Apoptosis is an active process that occurs in normal tissues and plays an important role in development, tissue remodelling and the immune response. The signal that triggers apoptosis is specific to each tissue or cell type. This signal activates enzymes, called caspases, which actively destroy cellular components, including chromosomal DNA. This degradation results in cell death, but the cellular corpse contains characteristic vesicles called apoptotic bodies. The corpse is then recognised and removed by phagocytic cells of the immune system, such as macrophages, in a manner that does not provoke an inflammatory response.

A third mechanism of cell death is necrosis. This is a pathological process in which the cellular environment loses one or more of the components necessary for cell viability. Hypoxia is probably the most common cause of necrosis.

Genomics, health and disease

Classes of genetic variant

There are many different classes of variation in the human genome, categorised by the size of the DNA segment involved and/or by the mechanism giving rise to the variation.

Nucleotide substitutions

The substitution of one nucleotide for another is the most common type of genomic variation. Depending on their frequency and functional consequences, these changes are known as point mutations or single nucleotide polymorphisms (SNPs). They occur by misincorporation of a nucleotide during DNA synthesis or by chemical modification of the base. When these substitutions occur within ORFs of a protein-coding gene, they are further classified into:

- *synonymous* – resulting in a change in the codon without altering the amino acid
- *non-synonymous* (also known as a missense mutation) – resulting in a change in the codon and the encoded amino acid
- *stop gain* (or *nonsense mutation*) – introducing a premature stop codon and resulting in truncation of the protein
- *splicing* – taking place at splice sites that most frequently occur at the junction between an intron and an exon.

These different types of mutation are illustrated in Box 3.1 and examples are shown in Figures 3.5 and 3.6.

Insertions and deletions

One or more nucleotides may be inserted or lost in a DNA sequence, resulting in an insertion/deletion (indel) polymorphism or mutation (Box 3.1 and Fig. 3.5). If a multiple of three nucleotides is involved, this is in-frame. If an indel change affects one or two nucleotides within the ORF of a protein-coding gene, this can have serious consequences because the triple nucleotide sequence of the codons is disrupted, resulting in a frameshift mutation. The effect on the gene is typically severe because the amino acid sequence is totally disrupted.

i	3.1 Classes of genetics variant	
The classes of genetic variant can be illustrated using the sentence 'THE FAT FOX WAS ILL COS SHE ATE THE OLD CAT'		
Synonymous Silent polymorphism with no amino acid change		THE FAT FOX WAS ILL COS SHE ATE THE OLD KAT where the C is replaced with a K but the meaning remains the same
Non-synonymous Causing an amino acid change		THE FAT BOX WAS ILL COS SHE ATE THE OLD CAT where the F of FOX is replaced by a B and the original meaning of the sentence is lost
Stop gain (also called a nonsense mutation) Causing the generation of a premature stop codon		THE CAT where the F of FAT is replaced by a C generating a premature stop codon
Indel Where bases are either inserted or deleted; disruption of the reading frame is dependent on the number of bases inserted or deleted		THE FAT FOX WAS ILL ILL COS SHE ATE THE OLD CAT where the insertion of three bases results in maintenance of the reading frame THE FAT FOX WAW ASI LLC OSS HEA TET HEO LDC AT where the insertion of two bases results in disruption of the reading frame

Fig. 3.5 **Different types of mutation affecting coding exons.** A Normal sequence. B A synonymous nucleotide substitution changing the third base of a codon; the resulting amino acid sequence is unchanged. C A missense mutation in which the nucleotide substitution results in a change in a single amino acid from the normal sequence (AAG) encoding lysine to glutamine (CAG). D Insertion of a G residue (boxed) causes a frameshift mutation, completely altering the amino acid sequence downstream. This usually results in a loss-of-function mutation. E A nonsense mutation resulting in a single nucleotide change from a lysine codon (AAG) to a premature stop codon (TAG).

Fig. 3.6 Splice site mutations. [A] The normal sequence is shown, illustrating two exons, and intervening intron (blue) with splice donor (AG) and splice acceptor sites (GT) underlined. Normally, the intron is removed by splicing to give the mature messenger RNA that encodes the protein. [B] In a splice site mutation the donor site is mutated. As a result, splicing no longer occurs, leading to read-through of the mRNA into the intron, which contains a premature termination codon downstream of the mutation.

ⓘ 3.2 Diseases associated with triplet and other repeat expansions*

		No. of repeats				
	Repeat	**Normal**	**Mutant**	**Gene**	**Gene location**	**Inheritance**
Coding repeat expansion						
Huntington's disease	[CAG]	6–34	>35	*Huntingtin*	4p16	AD
Spinocerebellar ataxia (type 1)	[CAG]	6–39	>40	*Ataxin*	6p22–23	AD
Spinocerebellar ataxia (types 2, 3, 6, 7)	[CAG]	Various	Various	Various	Various	AD
Dentatorubral-pallidoluysian atrophy	[CAG]	7–25	>49	*Atrophin*	12p12–13	AD
Machado–Joseph disease	[CAG]	12–40	>67	*MJD*	14q32	AD
Spinobulbar muscular atrophy	[CAG]	11–34	>40	Androgen receptor	Xq11–12	XL recessive
Non-coding repeat expansion						
Myotonic dystrophy	[CTG]	5–37	>50	*DMPK-3′UTR*	19q13	AD
Friedreich's ataxia	[GAA]	7–22	>200	*Frataxin-intronic*	9q13	AR
Progressive myoclonic epilepsy	[CCCCGCCCCGCG]₄₋₈	2–3	>25	*Cystatin B-5′UTR*	21q	AR
Fragile X mental retardation	[CGG]	5–52	>200	*FMR1–5′UTR*	Xq27	XL dominant
Fragile site mental retardation 2 (FRAXE)	[GCC]	6–35	>200	*FMR2*	Xq28	XL, probably recessive

*The triplet repeat diseases fall into two major groups: those with disease stemming from expansion of [CAG]ₙ repeats in coding DNA, resulting in multiple adjacent glutamine residues (polyglutamine tracts), and those with non-coding repeats. The latter tend to be longer. Unaffected parents usually display 'pre-mutation' allele lengths that are just above the normal range. (AD/AR = autosomal dominant/recessive; UTR = untranslated region; XL = X-linked)

Simple tandem repeat mutations

Variations in the length of simple tandem repeats of DNA are thought to arise as the result of slippage of DNA during meiosis and are termed microsatellite (small) or minisatellite (larger) repeats. These repeats are unstable and can expand or contract in different generations. This instability is proportional to the size of the original repeat, in that longer repeats tend to be more unstable. Many microsatellites and minisatellites occur in introns or in chromosomal regions between genes and have no obvious adverse effects. However, some genetic diseases are caused by microsatellite repeats that result in duplication of amino acids within the affected gene product or affect gene expression (Box 3.2).

Copy number variations

Variation in the number of copies of an individual segment of the genome from the usual diploid (two copies) content can be categorised by the size of the segment involved. Rarely, individuals may gain (trisomy) or lose (monosomy) a whole chromosome. Such numerical chromosome anomalies most commonly occur by a process known as non-disjunction, where pairs of homologous chromosomes do not separate at meiosis II (p. 40). Common trisomies include Down's syndrome (trisomy 21), Edward's syndrome (trisomy 18) and Patau's syndrome (trisomy 13). Monosomy of the autosomes (present in all the cells, as opposed to in a mosaic distribution) does not occur but Turner's syndrome, in which there is monosomy for the X chromosome, affects approximately 1 in 2500 live births (Box 3.3).

Large insertions or deletions of chromosomal DNA also occur and are usually associated with a learning disability and/or congenital malformations. Such structural chromosomal anomalies usually arise as the result of one of two different processes:

- non-homologous end-joining
- non-allelic homologous recombination.

Random double-stranded breaks in DNA are a necessary process in meiotic recombination and also occur during mitosis at a predictable rate. The rate of these breaks is dramatically increased by exposure to ionising radiation. When such breaks take place, they are usually repaired accurately by DNA repair mechanisms within the cell. However, in a proportion of breaks, segments of DNA that are not normally contiguous will be joined ('non-homologous end-joining'). If the joined fragments are from different chromosomes, this results in a translocation. If they are from the same chromosome, this will result in either inversion, duplication or deletion of a chromosomal fragment (Fig. 3.7). Large insertions and deletions may be cytogenetically visible as chromosomal deletions or duplications. If the anomalies are too small to be detected by microscopy, they are termed microdeletions and microduplications. Many microdeletion syndromes have been described and most result from non-allelic homologous recombination between repeats of highly similar DNA sequences, which leads to recurrent chromosome anomalies – and clinical syndromes – occurring in unrelated individuals (Fig. 3.7 and Box 3.3).

Consequences of genomic variation

The consequence of an individual mutation depends on many factors, including the mutation type, the nature of the gene product and the position of the variant in the protein. Mutations can have profound or subtle effects on gene and cell function. Variations that have profound effects are responsible for 'classical' genetic diseases, whereas those with subtle effects may contribute to the pathogenesis of common disease where there is a genetic component, such as diabetes.

- *Neutral variants* have no effect on quality or type of protein produced.
- *Loss-of-function mutations* result in loss or reduction in the normal protein function. Whole-gene deletions are the archetypal loss-of-function variants but stop-gain or indel mutations (early in the ORF), missense mutations affecting a critical domain and splice-site mutations can also result in loss of protein function.

i 3.3 Chromosome and contiguous gene disorders

Disease	Locus	Incidence	Clinical features
Numerical chromosomal abnormalities			
Down's syndrome (trisomy 21)	47,XY,+21 or 47,XX+21	1 in 800	Characteristic facies, IQ usually <50, congenital heart disease, reduced life expectancy
Edwards' syndrome (trisomy 18)	47,XY,+18 or 47,XX,+18	1 in 6000	Early lethality, characteristic skull and facies, frequent malformations of heart, kidney and other organs
Patau's syndrome (trisomy 13)	47,XY,+13 or 47, XX,+13	1 in 15 000	Early lethality, cleft lip and palate, polydactyly, small head, frequent congenital heart disease
Klinefelter's syndrome	47,XXY	1 in 1000	Phenotypic male, infertility, gynaecomastia, small testes (p. 660)
XYY	47,XYY	1 in 1000	Usually asymptomatic, some impulse control problems
Triple X syndrome	47,XXX	1 in 1000	Usually asymptomatic, may have reduced IQ
Turner's syndrome	45,X	1 in 5000	Phenotypic female, short stature, webbed neck, coarctation of the aorta, primary amenorrhoea (p. 659)
Recurrent deletions, microdeletions and contiguous gene defects			
Di George/velocardiofacial syndrome	22q11.2	1 in 4000	Cardiac outflow tract defects, distinctive facial appearance, thymic hypoplasia, cleft palate and hypocalcaemia. Major gene seems to be *TBX1* (cardiac defects and cleft palate)
Prader–Willi syndrome	15q11–q13	1 in 15 000	Distinctive facial appearance, hyperphagia, small hands and feet, distinct behavioural phenotype. Imprinted region, deletions on paternal allele in 70% of cases
Angelman's syndrome	15q11–q13	1 in 15 000	Distinctive facial appearance, absent speech, electroencephalogram (EEG) abnormality, characteristic gait. Imprinted region, deletions on maternal allele encompassing *UBE3A*
Williams' syndrome	7q11.23	1 in 10 000	Distinctive facial appearance, supravalvular aortic stenosis, learning disability and infantile hypercalcaemia. Major gene for supravalvular aortic stenosis is *elastin*
Smith–Magenis syndrome	17p11.2	1 in 25 000	Distinctive facial appearance and behavioural phenotype, self-injury and rapid eye movement (REM) sleep abnormalities. Major gene seems to be *RAI1*

A How structural chromosomal anomalies are described

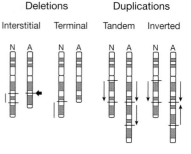

B Mechanism underlying recurrent deletions and duplication: non-allelic homologous recombination

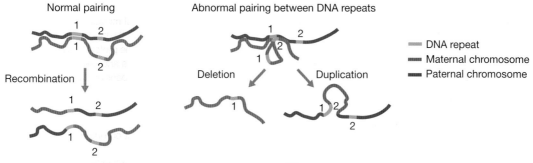

Fig. 3.7 Chromosomal analysis and structural chromosomal disorders. A Human chromosomes can be classed as metacentric if the centromere is near the middle, or acrocentric if the centromere is at the end. The bands of each chromosome are given a number, starting at the centromere and working out along the short (p) arm and long (q) arm. Translocations and inversions are balanced structural chromosome anomalies where no genetic material is missing but it is in the wrong order. Translocations can be divided into reciprocal (direct swap of chromosomal material between non-homologous chromosomes) and Robertsonian (fusion of acrocentric chromosomes). Deletions and duplications can also occur due to non-allelic homologous recombination (illustrated in part B). Deletions are classified as interstitial if they lie within a chromosome, and terminal if the terminal region of the chromosome is affected. Duplications can be either in tandem (where the duplicated fragment is inserted next to the region that is duplicated and orientated in the correct direction) or inverted (where the duplicated fragment is in the wrong direction). (N = normal; A = abnormal) B A common error of meiotic recombination, known as non-allelic homologous recombination, can occur (right panel), resulting in a deletion on one chromosome and a duplication in the homologous chromosome. The error is induced by tandem repeats in the DNA sequences (green), which can misalign and bind to each other, thereby 'fooling' the DNA into thinking the pairing prior to recombination is correct.

- *Gain-of-function mutations* result in a gain of protein function. They are typically non-synonymous mutations that alter the protein structure, leading to activation/alteration of its normal function through causing either an interaction with a novel substrate or a change in its normal function.
- *Dominant negative mutations* are the result of non-synonymous mutations or in-frame deletions/duplications but may also, less frequently, be caused by triplet repeat expansion mutations. Dominant negative mutations are heterozygous changes that result in the production of an abnormal protein that interferes with the normal functioning of the wild-type protein.

Normal genomic variation

We each have 5–50 million variants in our genome, occurring approximately every 300 bases. These variants are mostly polymorphisms, arising in more than 1% of the population; they have no or subtle effects on gene and cell function, and are not associated with a high risk of disease. Polymorphisms can occur within exons, introns or the intergenic regions that comprise 98–99% of the human genome. Each of the classes of genetic variant discussed on page 42 is present in the genome

as a common polymorphism. However, the most frequent is the single nucleotide polymorphism, or SNP (pronounced 'snip'), describing the substitution of a single base.

Polymorphisms and common disease

The protective and detrimental polymorphisms associated with common disease have been identified primarily through genome-wide association studies (GWAS, p. 56) and are the basis for many direct-to-consumer tests that purport to determine individual risk profiles for common diseases or traits such as cardiovascular disease, diabetes and even male-pattern baldness! An example is the polymorphism in the gene *SLC2A9* that not only explains a significant proportion of the normal population variation in serum urate concentration but also predisposes 'high-risk' allele carriers to the development of gout. However, the current reality is that, until we have a more comprehensive understanding of the full genomic landscape and knowledge of the complete set of detrimental and protective polymorphisms, we cannot accurately assess risk.

Evolutionary selection

Genetic variants play an important role in evolutionary selection, with advantageous variants resulting in positive selection via improved reproductive fitness, and variations that decrease reproductive fitness becoming excluded through evolution. Given this simple paradigm, it would be tempting to assume that common mutations are all advantageous and all rare mutations are pathogenic. Unfortunately, it is often difficult to classify any common mutation as either advantageous or deleterious – or, indeed, neutral. Mutations that are advantageous in early life and thus enhance reproductive fitness may be deleterious in later life. There may be mutations that are advantageous for survival in particular conditions (e.g. famine or pandemic) that may be disadvantageous in more benign circumstances by causing a predisposition to obesity or autoimmune disorders.

Constitutional genetic disease

Familial genetic disease is caused by constitutional mutations, which are inherited through the germ line. However, different mutations in the same gene can have different consequences, depending on the genetic mechanism underlying that disease. About 1% of the human population carries constitutional mutations that cause disease.

Constructing a family tree

The family tree – or pedigree – is a fundamental tool of the clinical geneticist, who will routinely take a three-generation family history, on both sides of the family, enquiring about details of all medical conditions in family members, consanguinity, dates of birth and death, and any history of pregnancy loss or infant death. The basic symbols and nomenclature used in drawing a pedigree are shown in Figure 3.8.

Patterns of disease inheritance

Autosomal dominant inheritance

Take some time to draw out the following pedigree:

Anne is referred to Clinical Genetics to discuss her personal history of colon cancer (she was diagnosed at the age of 46 years) and family history of colon/endometrial cancer: her mother was diagnosed with endometrial cancer at the age of 60 years and her cousin through her healthy maternal aunt was diagnosed with colon cancer in her fifties. Both her maternal grandmother and grandfather died of 'old age'. There is no family history of note on her father's side of the family. He has one brother and both his parents died of old age, in their eighties. Anne has two healthy daughters, aged 12 and 14 years, and a healthy full sister.

This family history is typical of an autosomal dominant condition (Fig. 3.8): in this case, a colon/endometrial cancer susceptibility syndrome known as Lynch's syndrome, associated with disruption of one of the mismatch repair genes: *MSH2*, *MSH6*, *MLH1* and *PMS2* (see p. 830 and Box 3.11, p. 57).

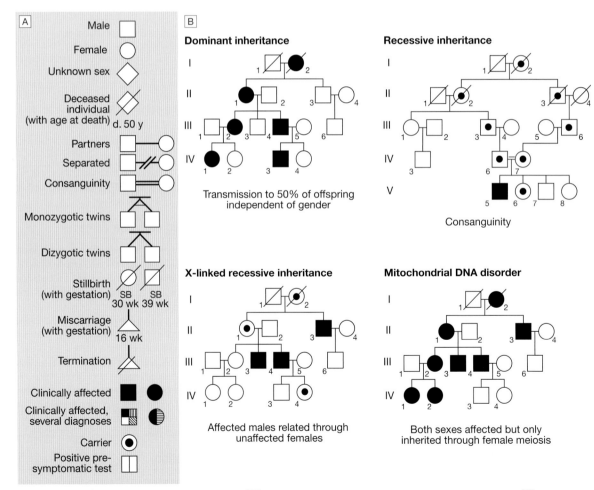

Fig. 3.8 **Drawing a pedigree and patterns of inheritance.** [A] The main symbols used to represent pedigrees in diagrammatic form. [B] The main modes of disease inheritance (see text for details).

Features of an autosomal dominant pedigree include:

- There are affected individuals in each generation (unless the mutation has arisen de novo, i.e. for the first time in an affected individual). However, variable penetrance and expressivity can influence the number of affected individuals and the severity of disease in each generation. Penetrance is defined as the proportion of individuals bearing a mutated allele who develop the disease phenotype. The mutation is said to be fully penetrant if all individuals who inherit a mutation develop the disease. Expressivity describes the level of severity of each aspect of the disease phenotype.

- Males and females are usually affected in roughly equal numbers (unless the clinical presentation of the condition is gender-specific, such as an inherited susceptibility to breast and/or ovarian cancer).

The offspring risk for an individual affected with an autosomal dominant condition is 1 in 2 (or 50%). This offspring risk is true for each pregnancy, since half the affected individual gametes (sperm or egg cells) will contain the affected chromosome/gene and half will contain the normal chromosome/gene.

There is a long list of autosomal dominant conditions, some of which are shown in Box 3.4.

i 3.4 Genetic conditions dealt with by clinicians in other specialties

Name of condition	Gene	Reference
Autosomal dominant conditions		
Autosomal dominant polycystic kidney disease (ADPKD)	PKD1 (85%), PKD2 (15%)	p. 405
		Box 15.28, p. 415
Tuberous sclerosis	TSC1	p. 1264
	TSC2	p. 1264
Marfan's syndrome	FBN1	p. 508
Long QT syndrome	KCNQ1	p. 476
Brugada's syndrome	SCN5A	p. 477
Neurofibromatosis type 1	NF1	p. 1131
		Box 25.77, p. 1132
Neurofibromatosis type 2	NF2	p. 1131
		Box 25.77, p. 1132
Hereditary spherocytosis	ANK1	p. 947
Vascular Ehlers–Danlos syndrome (EDS type 4)	COL3A1	p. 970
Hereditary haemorrhagic telangiectasia	ENG, ALK1, GDF2	p. 970
Osteogenesis imperfecta	COL1A1, COL1A2	p. 1055
Charcot–Marie–Tooth disease	PMP22, MPZ, GJB1	p. 1140
Hereditary neuropathy with liability to pressure palsies	PMP22	
Autosomal recessive conditions		
Familial Mediterranean fever	MEFV	p. 81
Mevalonic aciduria (mevalonate kinase deficiency)	MVK	p. 81
Autosomal recessive polycystic kidney disease (ARPKD)	PKHD1	Box 15.28, p. 415
Kartagener's syndrome (primary ciliary dyskinesia)	DNAI1	Box 17.30, p. 578
Cystic fibrosis	CFTR1	p. 580
		Box 17.30, p. 578
		p. 842
Pendred's syndrome	SLC26A4	p. 650
Congenital adrenal hyperplasia-21 hydroxylase deficiency	CYP21A	p. 676
		Box 18.27, p. 658
Haemochromatosis	HFE	p. 895
Wilson's disease	ATP7B	p. 896
Alpha₁-antitrypsin deficiency	SERPINA1	p. 897
Gilbert's syndrome	UGT1A1	p. 897
Benign recurrent intrahepatic cholestasis	ATP8B1	p. 902
Alpha-thalassaemia	HBA1, HBA2	p. 951
		p. 954
Beta-thalassaemia	HBB	p. 951
		p. 953
Sickle cell disease	HBB	p. 951
Spinal muscular atrophy	SMN1	p. 1117
X-linked conditions		
Alport's syndrome	COL4A5	Box 15.28, p. 415
		p. 403
Primary agammaglobulinaemia	BTK	p. 78
Haemophilia A (factor VIII deficiency)	F8	p. 971
Haemophilia B (factor IX deficiency)	F9	p. 973
Duchenne muscular dystrophy	DMD	p. 1143 and Box 25.91

Autosomal recessive inheritance

As above, take some time to draw a pedigree representing the following:

Mr and Mrs Kent, a non-consanguineous couple, are referred because their son, Jamie, had severe neonatal liver disease. Included among the many investigations that the paediatric hepatologist undertook was testing for α_1-antitrypsin deficiency (Box 3.5). Jamie was shown to have the PiZZ phenotype. Testing confirmed both parents as carriers with PiMZ phenotypes. In the family, Jamie has an older sister who has no medical problems. Mr Kent is one of four children with two brothers and a sister and Mrs Kent has a younger brother. Both sets of grandparents are alive and well. There is no family history of α_1-antitrypsin deficiency.

This family history is characteristic of an autosomal recessive disorder (Fig. 3.8), where both alleles of a gene must be mutated before the disease is manifest in an individual; an affected individual inherits one mutant allele from each of their parents, who are therefore healthy carriers for the condition. An autosomal recessive condition might be suspected in a family where:

- Males and females are affected in roughly equal proportions.
- Parents are blood related; this is known as consanguinity. Where there is consanguinity, the mutations are usually homozygous, i.e. the same mutant allele is inherited from both parents.

3.5 Alpha₁-antitrypsin deficiency

Inheritance pattern

- Autosomal recessive

Genetic cause

- Two common mutations in the *SERPINA1* gene: p.Glu342Lys and p.Glu264Val

Prevalence

- 1 in 1500–3000 of European ancestry

Clinical presentation

- Variable presentation from neonatal period through to adulthood
- Neonatal period: prolonged jaundice with conjugated hyperbilirubinaemia or (rarely) liver disease
- Adulthood: pulmonary emphysema and/or cirrhosis. Rarely, the skin disease, panniculitis, develops

Disease mechanism

- *SERPINA1* encodes α_1-antitrypsin, which protects the body from the effects of neutrophil elastase. The symptoms of α_1-antitrypsin deficiency result from the effects of this enzyme attacking normal tissue

Disease variants

- M variant: if an individual has normal *SERPINA1* genes and produces normal levels of α_1-antitrypsin, they are said to have an M variant
- S variant: p.Glu264Val mutation results in α_1-antitrypsin levels reduced to about 40% of normal
- Z variant: p.Glu342Lys mutation results in very little α_1-antitrypsin
- PiZZ: individuals who are homozygous for the p.Glu342Lys mutation are likely to have α_1-antitrypsin deficiency and the associated symptoms
- PiZS: individuals who are compound heterozygous for p.Glu342Lys and p.Glu264Val are likely to be affected, especially if they smoke, but usually to a milder degree

- Individuals within one sibship in one generation are affected and so the condition can appear to have arisen 'out of the blue'.

Approximately 1 in 4 children born to carriers of an autosomal recessive condition will be affected. The offspring risk for carrier parents is therefore 25% and the chances of an unaffected child, with an affected sibling, being a carrier is 2/3.

Examples of some autosomal recessive conditions, discussed elsewhere in this book, are shown in Box 3.4.

X-linked inheritance

The following is an exemplar of an X-linked recessive pedigree (Fig. 3.8):

Edward has a diagnosis of Duchenne muscular dystrophy (DMD, Box 3.6). His parents had suspected the diagnosis when he was 3 years old because he was not yet walking and there was a family history of DMD: Edward's maternal uncle had been affected and died at the age of 24 years. Edward's mother has no additional siblings. After Edward demonstrated a very high creatinine kinase level, the paediatrician also requested genetic testing, which identified a deletion of exons 2–8 of the dystrophin gene. Edward has a younger, healthy sister and grandparents on both sides of the family are well, although the maternal grandmother has recently developed a cardiomyopathy. Edward's father has an older sister and an older brother who are both well.

Genetic diseases caused by mutations on the X chromosome have specific characteristics:

- X-linked diseases are mostly recessive and restricted to males who carry the mutant allele. This is because males

3.6 Duchenne muscular dystrophy*

Inheritance pattern

- X-linked recessive

Genetic cause

- Mutations or deletions encompassing/within the *DMD* (dystrophin) gene located at Xp21

Prevalence

- 1 in 3000–4000 live male births

Clinical presentation

- Delayed motor milestones
- Speech delay
- Grossly elevated creatine kinase (CK) levels (in the thousands)
- Ambulation is usually lost between the ages of 7 and 13 years
- Lifespan is reduced with a mean age of death, usually from respiratory failure, in the mid-twenties
- Cardiomyopathy affects almost all boys with Duchenne muscular dystrophy and some female carriers

Disease mechanism

- *DMD* encodes dystrophin, a major structural component of muscle
- Dystrophin links the internal cytoskeleton to the extracellular matrix

Disease variants

- Becker muscular dystrophy, although a separate disease, is also caused by mutations in the dystrophin gene
- In Duchenne muscular dystrophy, there is no dystrophin protein, whereas in Becker muscular dystrophy there is a reduction in the amount or alteration in the size of the dystrophin protein

*See also page 1143.

have only one X chromosome, whereas females have two (see Fig. 3.1). However, occasionally, female carriers may exhibit signs of an X-linked disease due to a phenomenon called skewed X-inactivation. All female embryos, at about 100 cells in size, stably inactivate one of their two X chromosomes in each cell. Where this inactivation is random, approximately 50% of the cells will express the genes from one X chromosome and 50% of cells will express genes from the other. Where there is a mutant gene, there is often skewing away from the associated X chromosome, resulting in an unaffected female carrier. However, if, by chance, there is a disproportionate inactivation of the normal X chromosome with skewing towards the mutant allele, then an affected female carrier may be affected (albeit more mildly than males).

- The gene can be transmitted from female carriers to their sons: in families with an X-linked recessive condition, there are often a number of affected males related through unaffected females.
- Affected males cannot transmit the condition to their sons (but all their daughters would be carriers).

The risk of a female carrier having an affected child is 25% or half of her male offspring.

Mitochondrial inheritance

The mitochondrion is the main site of energy production within the cell. Mitochondria arose during evolution via the symbiotic association with an intracellular bacterium. They have a distinctive structure with functionally distinct inner and outer membranes. Mitochondria produce energy in the form of adenosine triphosphate (ATP). ATP is mostly derived from the metabolism of glucose and fat (Fig. 3.9). Glucose cannot enter mitochondria directly but is first metabolised to pyruvate via glycolysis. Pyruvate is then imported into the mitochondrion and metabolised to acetyl-co-enzyme A (acetyl-CoA). Fatty acids are transported into the mitochondria following conjugation with carnitine and are sequentially catabolised by a process called β-oxidation to produce acetyl-CoA. The acetyl-CoA from both pyruvate and fatty acid oxidation is used in the citric acid (Krebs) cycle – a series of enzymatic reactions that produces CO_2, the reduced form of nicotinamide adenine dinucleotide (NADH) and the reduced form of flavine adenine dinucleotide ($FADH_2$). Both NADH and $FADH_2$ then donate electrons to the respiratory chain. Here these electrons are transferred via a complex series of reactions, resulting in the formation of a proton gradient across the inner mitochondrial membrane. The gradient is used by an inner mitochondrial membrane protein, ATP synthase, to produce ATP, which is then transported to other parts of the cell. Dephosphorylation of ATP is used to produce the energy required for many cellular processes.

Each mitochondrion contains 2–10 copies of a 16-kilobase (kB) double-stranded circular DNA molecule (mtRNA). This mtDNA contains 13 protein-coding genes, all involved in the respiratory chain, and the ncRNA genes required for protein synthesis within the mitochondria (Fig. 3.9). The mutational rate of mtDNA is relatively high due to the lack of protection by chromatin. Several mtDNA diseases characterised by defects in ATP production have been described. Mitochondria are most numerous in cells with high metabolic demands, such as muscle, retina and the basal ganglia, and these tissues tend to be the ones most severely affected in mitochondrial diseases (Box 3.7). There are many other mitochondrial diseases that are caused by mutations in nuclear genes, which encode proteins that are then imported into the mitochondrion and are critical for energy production, e.g. most forms of Leigh's syndrome (although Leigh's syndrome may also be caused by a mitochondrial gene mutation).

The inheritance of mtDNA disorders is characterised by transmission from females, but males and females generally are equally affected (see Fig. 3.8). Unlike the other inheritance patterns mentioned above, mitochondrial inheritance has nothing to do with meiosis but reflects the fact that mitochondrial DNA is transmitted by oöcytes: sperm do not contribute mitochondria to the zygote. Mitochondrial disorders tend to be variable in penetrance and expressivity within families, and this is mostly accounted for by the fact that only a proportion of multiple mtDNA molecules within mitochondria contain the causal mutation (the degree of mtDNA heteroplasmy).

Imprinting

Several chromosomal regions (loci) have been identified where gene expression is inherited in a parent-of-origin-specific manner;

---

i 3.7 The structure of the respiratory chain complexes and the diseases associated with their dysfunction

Complex	Enzyme	nDNA subunits[1]	mtDNA subunits[2]	Diseases
I	NADH dehydrogenase	38	7	MELAS, MERRF bilateral striatal necrosis, LHON, myopathy and exercise intolerance, Parkinsonism, Leigh's syndrome, exercise myoglobinuria, leucodystrophy/myoclonic epilepsy
II	Succinate dehydrogenase	4	0	Phaeochromocytoma, Leigh's syndrome
III	Cytochrome bc₁ complex	10	1	Parkinsonism/MELAS, cardiomyopathy, myopathy, exercise myoglobinuria, Leigh's syndrome
IV	Cytochrome c oxidase	10	3	Sideroblastic anaemia, myoclonic ataxia, deafness, myopathy, MELAS, MERRF mitochondrial encephalomyopathy, motor neuron disease-like, exercise myoglobinuria, Leigh's syndrome
V	ATP synthase	14	2	Leigh's syndrome, NARP, bilateral striatal necrosis

[1]nDNA subunits. [2]mtDNA subunits = number of different protein subunits in each complex that are encoded in the nDNA and mtDNA, respectively.
(ATP = adenosine triphosphate; LHON = Leber hereditary optic neuropathy; MELAS = myopathy, encephalopathy, lactic acidosis and stroke-like episodes; MERRF = myoclonic epilepsy and ragged red fibres; mtDNA = mitochondrial DNA; NADH = the reduced form of nicotinamide adenine dinucleotide; NARP = neuropathy, ataxia and retinitis pigmentosa; nDNA = nuclear DNA)

Fig. 3.9 Mitochondria. **A** Mitochondrial structure. There is a smooth outer membrane surrounding a convoluted inner membrane, which has inward projections called cristae. The membranes create two compartments: the inter-membrane compartment, which plays a crucial role in the electron transport chain, and the inner compartment (or matrix), which contains mitochondrial DNA and the enzymes responsible for the citric acid (Krebs) cycle and the fatty acid β-oxidation cycle. **B** Mitochondrial DNA. The mitochondrion contains several copies of a circular double-stranded DNA molecule, which has a non-coding region, and a coding region that encodes the genes responsible for energy production, mitochondrial transfer RNA (tRNA) molecules and mitochondrial ribosomal RNA (rRNA) molecules. (ATP = adenosine triphosphate; NADH = the reduced form of nicotinamide adenine dinucleotide) **C** Mitochondrial energy production. Fatty acids enter the mitochondrion conjugated to carnitine by carnitine-palmityl transferase type 1 (CPT I) and, once inside the matrix, are unconjugated by CPT II to release free fatty acids (FFA). These are broken down by the β-oxidation cycle to produce acetyl-co-enzyme A (acetyl-CoA). Pyruvate can enter the mitochondrion directly and is metabolised by pyruvate dehydrogenase (PDH) to produce acetyl-CoA. The acetyl-CoA enters the Krebs cycle, leading to the production of NADH and flavine adenine dinucleotide (reduced form) ($FADH_2$), which are used by proteins in the electron transport chain to generate a hydrogen ion gradient across the inter-membrane compartment. Reduction of NADH and $FADH_2$ by proteins I and II, respectively, releases electrons (e), and the energy released is used to pump protons into the inter-membrane compartment. Coenzyme Q_{10}/ubiquinone (Q) is an intensely hydrophobic electron carrier that is mobile within the inner membrane. As electrons are exchanged between proteins in the chain, more protons are pumped across the membrane, until the electrons reach complex IV (cytochrome oxidase), which uses the energy to reduce oxygen to water. The hydrogen ion gradient is used to produce ATP by the enzyme ATP synthase, which consists of a proton channel and catalytic sites for the synthesis of ATP from ADP. When the channel opens, hydrogen ions enter the matrix down the concentration gradient, and energy is released that is used to make ATP.

these are called imprinted loci. Within these loci the paternally inherited gene may be active while the maternally inherited may be silenced, or vice versa. Mutations within imprinted loci lead to an unusual pattern of inheritance where the phenotype is manifest only if inherited from the parent who contributes the transcriptionally active allele. Examples of imprinting disorders are given in Box 3.8.

Somatic genetic disease

Somatic mutations are not inherited but instead occur during post-zygotic mitotic cell divisions at any point from embryonic development to late adult life. An example of this phenomenon is polyostotic fibrous dysplasia (McCune–Albright syndrome), in

i	**3.8 Imprinting disorders**			
Disorder	**Locus**	**Genes**	**Notes**	
Beckwith–Wiedemann syndrome	11p15	*CDKN1C, IGF2, H19*	Increased growth, macroglossia, hemihypertrophy, abdominal wall defects, ear lobe pits/creases and increased susceptibility to developing childhood tumours	
Prader–Willi syndrome	15q11–q13	*SNRPN, Necdin* and others	Obesity, hypogonadism and learning disability. Lack of paternal contribution (due to deletion of paternal 15q11–q13, or inheritance of both chromosome 15q11–q13 regions from the mother)	
Angelman's syndrome (AS)	15q11–q13	*UBE3A*	Severe mental retardation, ataxia, epilepsy and inappropriate laughing bouts. Due to loss-of-function mutations in the maternal *UBE3A* gene. The neurological phenotype results because most tissues express both maternal and paternal alleles of *UBE3A*, whereas the brain expresses predominantly the maternal allele	
Pseudohypoparathyroidism (p. 664)	20q13	*GNAS1*	Inheritance of the mutation from the mother results in hypocalcaemia, hyperphosphataemia, raised parathyroid hormone (PTH) levels, ectopic calcification, obesity, delayed puberty and shortened 4th and 5th metacarpals (the syndrome known as Albright's hereditary osteodystrophy, AHO). When the mutation is inherited from the father, PTH, calcium and phosphate levels are normal but the other features are present (pseudopseudohypoparathyroidism, p. 664). These differences are due to the fact that, in the kidney (the main target organ through which PTH regulates serum calcium and phosphate), the paternal allele is silenced and the maternal allele is expressed, whereas both alleles are expressed in other tissues.	

which a somatic mutation in the G_S alpha gene causes constitutive activation of downstream signalling, resulting in focal lesions in the skeleton and endocrine dysfunction (p. 1055).

The most important example of human disease caused by somatic mutations is cancer (see Ch. 33). Here, 'driver' mutations occur within genes that are involved in regulating cell division or apoptosis, resulting in abnormal cell growth and tumour formation. The two general categories of cancer-causing mutation are gain-of-function mutations in growth-promoting genes (oncogenes) and loss-of-function mutations in growth-suppressing genes (tumour suppressor genes). Whichever mechanism is acting, most tumours require an initiating mutation in a single cell that can then escape from normal growth controls. This cell replicates more frequently or fails to undergo programmed death, resulting in clonal expansion. As the size of the clone increases, one or more cells may acquire additional mutations that confer a further growth advantage, leading to proliferation of these subclones, which may ultimately result in aggressive metastatic cancer. The cell's complex self-regulating machinery means that more than one mutation is usually required to produce a malignant tumour (see Fig. 33.3, p. 1318). For example, if a mutation results in activation of a growth factor gene or receptor, then that cell will replicate more frequently as a result of autocrine stimulation. However, this mutant cell will still be subject to normal cell cycle checkpoints to promote DNA integrity in its progeny. If additional mutations in the same cell result in defective cell-cycle checkpoints, however, it will rapidly accumulate further mutations, which may allow completely unregulated growth and/ or separation from its matrix and cellular attachments and/or resistance to apoptosis. As cell growth becomes increasingly dysregulated, cells de-differentiate, lose their response to normal tissue environment and cease to ensure appropriate mitotic chromosomal segregation. These processes combine to generate the classical malignant characteristics of disorganised growth, variable levels of differentiation, and numerical and structural chromosome abnormalities. An increase in somatic mutation rate can occur on exposure to external mutagens, such as ultraviolet

light or cigarette smoke, or if the cell has defects in DNA repair systems. Cancer is thus a disease that affects the fundamental processes of molecular and cell biology.

Interrogating the genome: the changing landscape of genomic technologies

Looking at chromosomes

The analysis of metaphase chromosomes by light microscopy was the mainstay of clinical cytogenetic analysis for decades, the aim being to detect gain or loss of whole chromosomes (aneuploidy) or large chromosomal segments (>4 million bp). More recently, genome-wide microarrays (array comparative genomic hybridisation or array CGH) have replaced chromosome analysis, allowing rapid and precise detection of segmental gain or loss of DNA throughout the genome (see Box 3.3). Microarrays consist of grids of multiple wells containing short DNA sequences (reference DNA) that are complementary to known sequences in the genome. Patient and reference DNA are each labelled with a coloured fluorescent dye (generally, patient DNA is labelled with a green fluorescent dye and reference DNA with a red fluorescent dye) and added to the microarray grid. Where there is an equal quantity of patient and reference DNA bound to the spot, this results in yellow fluorescence. Where there is too much patient DNA (representing a duplication of a chromosome region), the spot will be greener; it will be more red (appears orange) where there is 2:1 ratio of the control:patient DNA (representing heterozygous deletion of a chromosome region; Fig. 3.10).

Array CGH and other array-based approaches can detect small chromosomal deletions and duplications. They are also generally more sensitive than conventional karyotyping at detecting mosaicism (where there are two or more populations of cells, derived from a single fertilised egg, with different genotypes).

Fig. 3.10 Detection of chromosome abnormalities by comparative genomic hybridisation (CGH). Deletions and duplications are detected by looking for deviation from the 1:1 ratio of patient and control DNA in a microarray. Ratios in excess of 1 indicate duplications, whereas ratios below 1 indicate deletions.

However, array-based approaches will not detect balanced chromosome rearrangements where there is no loss or gain of genes/chromosome material, such as balanced reciprocal translocations, or a global increase in copy number, such as triploidy.

The widespread use of array-based approaches has brought a number of challenges for clinical interpretation, including the identification of copy number variants (CNVs) of uncertain clinical significance, CNVs of variable penetrance and incidental findings. A CNV of uncertain clinical significance describes a loss or gain of chromosome material where there are insufficient data to conclude whether or not it is associated with a learning disability and/or medical problems. While this uncertainty can be difficult to prepare families for and can be associated with considerable anxiety, it is likely that there will be greater clarity in the future as we generate larger CNV datasets.

A CNV of variable penetrance, also known as a neurosusceptibility locus, describes a chromosome deletion or duplication associated with a lower threshold for manifesting a learning disability or autistic spectrum disorder. CNVs of variable penetrance are therefore identified at greater frequencies among individuals with a learning disability and/or autistic spectrum disorder than in the general population. The current understanding is that additional modifying factors (genetic, environmental or stochastic) must influence the phenotypic expression of these neurosusceptibility loci.

Finally, an incidental CNV finding describes a deletion or duplication encompassing a gene or genes that are causative of a phenotype or risk unrelated to the presenting complaint. For instance, if, through the array CGH investigation for an intellectual disability, a deletion encompassing the *BRCA1* gene were identified, this would be considered an incidental finding.

Looking at genes

Gene amplification: polymerase chain reaction

The polymerase chain reaction (PCR) is a fundamental laboratory technique that amplifies targeted sections of the human genome for further analyses – most commonly, DNA sequencing. The method utilises thermal cycling: repeated cycles of heating and cooling allow the initial separation of double-stranded DNA into two single strands (known as denaturation), each of which serves as a template during the subsequent replication step, guided by primers designed to anneal to a specific genomic region. This cycle of heating/cooling and denaturation/replication is repeated many times, resulting in the exponential amplification of DNA between primer sites (Fig. 3.11).

Gene sequencing

In the mid-1970s, a scientist called Fred Sanger pioneered a DNA sequencing technique ('Sanger sequencing') that determined the precise order and nucleotide type (thymine, cytosine, adenine and guanine) in a molecule of DNA. Modern Sanger sequencing uses fluorescently labelled, chain-terminating nucleotides that are sequentially incorporated into the newly synthesised DNA, generating multiple DNA chains of differing lengths. These DNA chains are subject to capillary electrophoresis, which separates them by size, allowing the fragments to be 'read' by a laser and producing a sequence chromatogram that corresponds to the target sequence (Fig. 3.12). Although transformative, Sanger sequencing was difficult and costly to scale, as exemplified by the Human Genome Project, which took 12 years to sequence the entire human genome at a cost approaching 3 billion dollars. Recently, DNA sequencing has been transformed again by a group of technologies collectively known as 'next-generation sequencing' (NGS; Fig. 3.13). This refers to a family of post-Sanger sequencing technologies that utilise the same five basic principles:

- *Library preparation*: DNA samples are fragmented (by enzyme cleavage or ultrasound) and then modified with a custom adapter sequence.
- *Amplification*: the library fragment is amplified to produce DNA clusters, each originating from a single DNA fragment. Each cluster will act as a single sequencing reaction.
- *Capture*: if an entire genome is being sequenced, this step will not be included. The capture step is required if targeted resequencing is necessary, such as for a panel gene test or an exome (Box 3.9).
- *Sequencing*: each DNA cluster is simultaneously sequenced and the data from each captured; this is known as a 'read' and is usually between 50 and 300 bases long sequenced (see Box 3.10 for a detailed description of the three most commonly used sequencing methods: synthesis, ligation and ion semiconductor sequencing).
- *Alignment and variant identification*: specialised software analyses read sequences and compares the data to a reference template. This is known as 'alignment' or 'mapping' and, although there are 3 billion bases in the

3

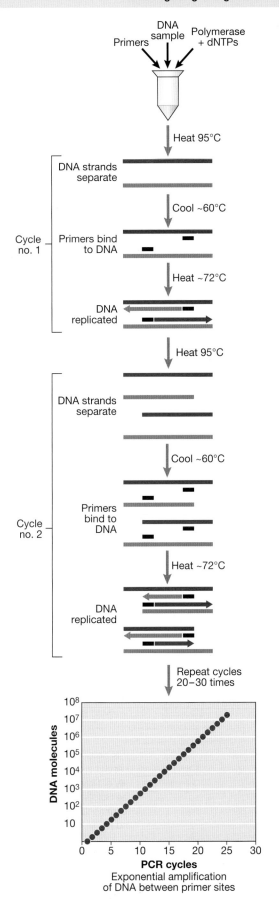

Fig. 3.11 The polymerase chain reaction (PCR). PCR involves adding a tiny amount of the patient's DNA to a reaction containing primers (short oligonucleotides 18–21 bp in length, which bind to the DNA flanking the region of interest) and deoxynucleotide phosphates (dATP, dCTP, dGTP, dTTP), which are used to synthesise new DNA and a heat-stable polymerase. The reaction mix is first heated to 95°C, which causes the double-stranded DNA molecules to separate. The reaction is then cooled to 50–60°C, which allows the primers to bind to the target DNA. The reaction is then heated to 72°C, at which point the polymerase starts making new DNA strands. These cycles are repeated 20–30 times, resulting in exponential amplification of the DNA fragment between the primer sites. The resulting PCR products can then be used for further analysis – most commonly, DNA sequencing (see Fig. 3.12).

human genome, allows the remarkably accurate determination of the genomic origin where a read consists of 25 nucleotides or more. Variants are identified as differences between the read and the reference genome. For instance, if there is a different nucleotide in half the reads at a given position compared to the reference genome, this is likely to represent a heterozygous base substitution. The number of reads that align at a given point is called the 'depth' or 'coverage'. The higher the read depth, the more accurate the variant call. However, in general, a depth of 30 or more reads is generally accepted as producing diagnostic-grade results.

Rather than sequencing only one small section of DNA at a time, NGS allows the analysis of many hundreds of thousands of DNA strands in a single experiment and so is also commonly referred to as multiple parallel sequencing technology. Today's NGS machines can sequence the entire human genome in a single day at a cost approaching 1000 US dollars.

NGS capture

Although we now have the capability to sequence the entire genome in a single experiment, whole-genome sequencing is not always the optimal use of NGS. NGS capture refers to the 'pull-down' of a targeted region of the genome and may constitute several to several hundred genes associated with a given phenotype (a gene panel), the exons of all known coding genes (an exome), or the exons of all coding genes known to be associated with disease (a clinical exome). Each of these targeted resequencing approaches is associated with a number of advantages and disadvantages (see Box 3.9). In order for NGS to be used for optimal patient benefit, it is essential for the clinician to have a good understanding of which test is the best one to request in any given clinical presentation.

Challenges of NGS technologies

Genomic technologies have the potential to transform the way that we practise medicine, and ever faster and cheaper DNA sequencing offers increasing opportunities to prevent, diagnose and treat disease. However, genomic technologies are not without their challenges: for instance, storing the enormous quantities of data generated by NGS. While the A, C, T and G of our genomic code could be stored on the memory of a smartphone, huge computers, able to store several petabytes of data (where 1 petabyte is 1 million gigabytes of data), are required to store the information needed to generate each individual's genome.

Even if we can store and handle these huge datasets successfully, we then need to be able to sift through the millions of

Fig. 3.12 Sanger sequencing of DNA, which is very widely used in DNA diagnostics. This is performed using PCR-amplified fragments of DNA corresponding to the gene of interest. The sequencing reaction is carried out with a combination dNTP and fluorescently labelled di-deoxy-dNTP (ddATP, ddTTP, ddCTP and ddGTP), which become incorporated into the newly synthesised DNA, causing termination of the chain at that point. The reaction products are then subject to capillary electrophoresis and the different-sized fragments are detected by a laser, producing a sequence chromatogram that corresponds to the target DNA sequence.

i 3.9 The advantages and disadvantages of whole-genome sequencing, whole-exome sequencing and gene panels

Test	Advantages	Disadvantages
Whole-genome sequencing (WGS)	The most comprehensive analysis of the genome available. More even coverage of genes, allowing better identification of dosage abnormalities. Will potentially detect all gene mutations, including intronic mutations	More expensive to generate and store. Will detect millions of variants in non-coding DNA, which can be very difficult to interpret. Associated with a greater risk of identifying incidental findings. Shallow sequencing (few reads per gene) and so less sensitive and less able to detect mosaicism
Whole-exome sequencing (WES)	Cheaper than whole-genome sequencing. Analysis is not restricted to only those genes known to cause a given condition. Fewer variants detected than in WGS and so easier interpretation. Deeper sequencing than WGS increases sensitivity and detection of mosaicism	Less even coverage of the genome and so dosage abnormalities are more difficult to detect. Less comprehensive analysis (1–2% of the genome) than WGS. Increased risk of identifying incidental findings over targeted gene sequencing
Gene panels	Cost-effective. Very deep sequencing, increasing the chances of mosaicism being detected. Fewer variants detected and so data easier to interpret. As analysis is restricted to known genes, the likelihood of a variant being pathogenic is greatly increased	Will only detect variation in genes known to cause a given condition. Difficult to add new genes to the panel as they are discovered

normal variants to identify the single (or, rarely, several) pathogenic, disease-causing mutation. While this can, to an extent, be achieved through the application of complex algorithms, these take time and considerable expertise to develop and are not infallible.

Furthermore, even after these data have been sifted by bioinformaticians, it is highly likely that clinicians will be left with some variants for which there are insufficient data to enable their definitive categorisation as either pathogenic or non-pathogenic. This may be because we simply do not know enough about the gene, because the particular variant has not previously been reported and/or it is identified in an unaffected parent. These variants must be interpreted with caution and, more usually,

their interpretation will require input from a genetics expert in the context of the clinical presentation, where an 'innocent until proven guilty' approach is often adopted.

Finally, if we are to interrogate the entire genome or even the exome, it is foreseeable that we will routinely identify 'incidental' or secondary findings – in other words, findings not related to the initial diagnostic question. The UK has so far advocated a conservative approach to incidental findings.

Uses of NGS

NGS is now frequently used, within diagnostic laboratories, to identify base substitutions and indels (although the latter were

1 Library preparation

Genomic DNA

Fragmentation

Adapter ligation

2 Cluster amplification

Flow cell

Amplification

3 Sequencing

G   A
   T   C

4 Alignment and variant interpretation

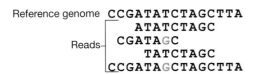

Reference genome CCGATATCTAGCTTA

Reads—
   ATATCTAGC
   CGATAGC
   TATCTAGC
   CCGATAGCTAGCTTA

Fig. 3.13 Sequencing by synthesis as used in the Illumina system.
(1) Library preparation: DNA is fragmented and specialist adapters are ligated to the fragmented ends. (2) Cluster amplification: the library is loaded to a flow cell and the adapters hybridise to the flow-cell surface. Each bound fragment is hybridised. (3) Sequencing. (4) Alignment and variant interpretation: reads are aligned to a reference sequence using complex software and differences between reference and case genomes are identified.

---

i 3.10 Next-generation sequencing methods

Sequencing by synthesis (Fig. 3.13)

- The most frequently used NGS method
- Used in Illumina systems (commonly used in diagnostic laboratories)
- Uses fluorescently labelled, terminator nucleotides that are sequentially incorporated into a growing DNA chain
- Library DNA samples (fragmented DNA flanked by DNA adapter sequences) are anchored to a flow cell by hybridisation of the DNA adapter sequence to probes on the flow-cell surface
- Amplification occurs by washing the flow cell in a mixture containing all four fluorescently labelled terminator nucleotides: A, C, T and G
- Once the nucleotide, complementary to the first base of the DNA template, is incorporated, no further nucleotides can be added until the mixture is washed away
- The nucleotide terminator is shed and the newly incorporated nucleotide reverts to a regular, non-fluorescent nucleotide that can be extended
- The process is then repeated with the incorporation of a second base etc.
- Sequencing by synthesis is therefore space- and time-dependent: a sensor will detect the order of fluorescent emissions for each spot on the plate (representing the cluster) and determine the sequence for that read

Sequencing by ligation

- Used in SOLiD systems
- Uses DNA ligase rather than DNA polymerase (as is used in sequencing by synthesis) and short oligonucleotides (as opposed to single nucleotides)
- Library DNA samples are washed in a mixture containing oligonucleotide probes representing 4–16 dinucleotide sequences. Only one nucleotide in the probe is fluorescently labelled
- The complementary oligo probes will hybridise, using DNA ligase, to the target sequence, initially at a primer annealed to the anchor site and then progressively along the DNA strand
- After incorporation of each probe, fluorescence is measured and the dye is cleaved off
- Eventually, a new strand is synthesised (composed of a series of the oligo probes)
- A new strand is then synthesised but is offset by one nucleotide
- The process is repeated a number of times (5 rounds in the SOLiD system), providing overlapping templates that are analysed and a composite of the target sequence determined

Ion semiconductor sequencing

- When a nucleotide is incorporated into a growing DNA strand, a hydrogen ion is released that can be detected by an alteration in the pH of the solution. This hydrogen ion release forms the basis of ion semiconductor sequencing
- Each amplified DNA cluster is located above a semiconductor transistor, capable of detecting differences in the pH of the solution
- The DNA cluster is washed in a mixture containing only one type of nucleotide
- If the correct nucleotide, complementary to the next base on the DNA template, is in the mixture and incorporated, a hydrogen ion is released and detected
- If a homopolymer (sequence of two or more identical nucleotides) is present, this will be detected as a decrease in pH proportionate to the number of identical nucleotides in the sequence

---

initially problematic). The current NGS challenge is to detect large deletions or duplications spanning several hundreds or thousands of bases and therefore exceeding any single read. Increasingly, however, this dosage analysis is being achieved using sophisticated computational methods, negating the need for more traditional technologies such as array CGH. Additional potential uses of NGS include detection of balanced and unbalanced translocations and mosaicism: NGS has proved remarkably sensitive at detecting the latter when there is high read coverage for a given region. Of note, however,

NGS is still not able to interrogate the epigenome (and so will not identify conditions caused by a disruption of imprinting, such as Beckwith–Wiedemann, Silver–Russell, Angelman's and Prader–Willi syndromes) and will not detect triplet repeat expansions such as those that cause Huntington's disease, myotonic dystrophy and fragile X syndrome (see Boxes 3.8 and 3.2).

Third-generation sequencing

Increasingly, third-generation or single-molecule sequencing is entering the diagnostic arena. As with next- or second-generation sequencing, a number of different platforms are commercially available. One of the most successful is SMRT technology (single-molecule sequencing in real time), developed by Pacific Biosciences. This system utilises a single-stranded DNA molecule (as compared to the amplified clusters used in NGS), which acts as a template for the sequential incorporation, using a polymerase, of fluorescently labelled nucleotides. As each complementary nucleotide is added, the fluorescence (and therefore the identity of the nucleotide) is recorded before it is removed and another nucleotide is added.

A key advantage of third-generation sequencing is the long length of the read it generates: in the region of 10–15 kilobases. It is also cheaper than NGS, as fewer reagents are required. Given these inherent advantages, third-generation sequencing is likely to supersede NGS in the near future. Given the confusion surrounding the terminology of NGS and third-generation sequencing, these technologies are increasingly referred to as 'massively parallel sequencing'.

Genomics and clinical practice

Genomics and health care

Genomics in rare neurodevelopmental disorders

Although, by definition, the diagnosis of a rare disorder is made infrequently, rare diseases, when considered together, affect about 3 million people in the UK, the majority of whom are children. NGS has transformed the ability to diagnose individuals affected by a rare disease. Whereas previously, when we were restricted to the sequential analysis of single genes, a clinician would need to make a clinical diagnosis in order to target testing, NGS allows the interrogation of multiple genes in a single experiment. This might be done through a gene panel, a clinical exome or an exome (see Box 3.9 and p. 53), and has increased the diagnostic yield in neurodevelopmental disorders to approximately 30%. Not only does the identification of the genetic cause of a rare disorder potentially provide families with answers, prognostic information and the opportunity to meet and derive support from other affected families but also it can provide valuable information for those couples planning further children and wishing to consider prenatal testing in the future.

Genomics and common disease

Most common disorders are determined by interactions between a number of genes and the environment. In this situation, the genetic contribution to disease is termed polygenic. Until recently, very little progress had been made in identifying the genetic variants that predispose to common disorders, but this has been changed by the advent of genome-wide association studies. A GWAS typically involves genotyping many (> 500 000) genetic markers (SNPs) spread across the genome in a large group of individuals with the disease and in controls. By comparing the SNP genotypes in cases and controls, it is possible to identify regions of the genome, and therefore genes, more strongly associated with a given SNP profile and therefore more likely to contribute to the disease under study.

Genomics and obstetrics

Prenatal genetic testing may be performed where a pregnancy is considered at increased risk of being affected with a genetic condition, either because of the ultrasound/biochemical screening results or because of the family history. While invasive tests, such as amniocentesis and chorionic villus sampling, have been the mainstay of prenatal diagnosis for many years, they are increasingly being superseded by non-invasive testing of cell-free fetal DNA (cffDNA), originating from placental trophoblasts and detectable in the maternal circulation from 4–5 weeks' gestation; it is present in sufficient quantities for testing by 9 weeks.

- *Non-invasive prenatal testing (NIPT)*: the sequencing and quantification, using NGS, of cffDNA chromosome-specific DNA sequences to identify trisomy 13, 18 or 21. The accuracy of NIPT in detecting pregnancy-specific aneuploidy approaches 98%. A false-negative result can occur when there is too little cffDNA (possibly due to early gestation or high maternal body mass index) or when aneuploidy has arisen later in development and is confined to the embryo and not represented in the placenta. False positives can occur with confined placental mosaicism (describing aneuploidy in the placenta, not the fetus) or with an alternative cause of aneuploidy in the maternal circulation, such a cell-free tumour DNA.
- *Non-invasive prenatal diagnosis (NIPD)*: the identification of a fetal single-gene defect that either has been paternally inherited or has arisen de novo and so is not identifiable in the maternal genome. Examples of conditions that are currently amenable to NIPD include achondroplasia and the craniosynostoses. Increasingly, however, NIPD is being used for autosomal recessive conditions such as cystic fibrosis, where parents are carriers for different mutations. The free fetal DNA is tested to see whether the paternal mutation is identified and, if absent, the fetus is not affected. If the paternal mutation is identified, however, a definitive invasive test is required to determine whether the maternal mutation has also been inherited and the fetus is affected.

Where a genetic diagnosis is known in a family, a couple may opt to undertake pre-implantation genetic diagnosis (PGD). PGD is used as an adjunct to in vitro fertilisation and involves the genetic testing of a single cell from a developing embryo, prior to implantation.

Genomics and oncology

Until recently, individuals were stratified to genetic testing if they presented with a personal and/or family history suggestive of an inherited cancer predisposition syndrome (Box 3.11). Relevant clinical information included the age of cancer diagnosis and number/type of tumours. For example, the diagnosis of bilateral breast cancer in a woman in her thirties with a mother who had ovarian cancer in her forties is suggestive of *BRCA1/2*-associated familial breast/ovarian cancer. In many familial cancer syndromes, somatic mutations act together with an inherited mutation to cause specific cancers (p. 50). Familial cancer syndromes may be due to germ-line loss-of-function mutations in tumour suppressor genes encoding DNA repair enzymes or proto-oncogenes. At the cellular level, loss of one copy of a tumour suppressor

3

i 3.11 Inherited cancer predisposition syndromes

Syndrome name	Gene	Associated cancers	Additional clinical features
Birt–Hogg–Dubé syndrome	*FLCN*	Renal tumour (oncocytoma, chromophobe (and mixed), renal cell carcinoma)	Fibrofolliculoma Trichodiscoma Pulmonary cysts
Breast/ovarian hereditary susceptibility	*BRCA1* *BRCA2*	Breast carcinoma Ovarian carcinoma Pancreatic carcinoma Prostate carcinoma	
Cowden's syndrome	*PTEN*	Breast carcinoma Thyroid carcinoma Endometrial carcinoma	Macrocephaly Intellectual disability/autistic spectrum disorder Trichilemmoma Acral keratosis Papillomatous papule Thyroid cyst Lipoma Haemangioma Intestinal hamartoma
Gorlin's syndrome/basal cell naevus syndrome	*PTCH1*	Basal cell carcinoma Medulloblastoma	Odontogenic keratocyst Palmar or plantar pits Falx calcification Rib abnormalities (e.g. bifid, fused or missing ribs) Macrocephaly Cleft lip/palate
Li–Fraumeni syndrome	*TP53*	Sarcoma (e.g. osteosarcoma, chondrosarcoma, rhabdomyosarcoma) Breast carcinoma Brain cancer (esp. glioblastoma) Adrenocortical carcinoma Brain	
Lynch's syndrome/ hereditary non-polyposis colon cancer	*MLH1* *MSH2* *MSH6* *PMS2*	Colorectal carcinoma (majority right-sided) Endometrial carcinoma Gastric carcinoma Cholangiocarcinoma Ovarian carcinoma (esp. mucinous)	
Multiple endocrine neoplasia 1	*MEN1*	Parathyroid tumour Endocrine pancreatic tumour Anterior pituitary tumour	Lipoma Facial angiofibroma
Multiple endocrine neoplasia 2 and 3 (also known as 2a and 2b, respectively)	*RET*	Medullary thyroid tumour Phaeochromocytoma Parathyroid tumour	
Polyposis, familial adenomatous (FAP)	*APC*	Colorectal adenocarcinoma (FAP is characterised by thousands of polyps from the second decade; without colectomy, malignant transformation of at least one of these polyps is inevitable) Duodenal carcinoma Hepatoblastoma	Desmoid tumour Congenital hypertrophy of the retinal pigment epithelium (CHRPE)
Polyposis, MYH-associated	*MYH (MUTYH)*	Colorectal adenocarcinoma Duodenal adenocarcinoma	
Retinoblastoma, familial	*RB1*	Retinoblastoma Osteosarcoma	

gene does not have any functional consequences, as the cell is protected by the remaining normal copy. However, a somatic mutation affecting the normal allele is likely to occur in one cell at some point during life, resulting in complete loss of tumour suppressor activity and a tumour developing by clonal expansion of that cell. This two-hit mechanism (one inherited, one somatic) for cancer development is known as the Knudson hypothesis. It explains why tumours may not develop for many years (or ever) in some members of these cancer-prone families. In DNA repair diseases, the inherited mutations increase the somatic mutation rate. Autosomal dominant mutations in genes encoding components of specific DNA repair systems are relatively common causes of familial colon cancer and breast cancer (e.g. *BRCA1*).

Increasingly, genetics is moving into the mainstream, becoming integrated into routine oncological care as new gene-specific treatments are introduced. Testing for a genetic predisposition to cancer is therefore moving from the domain of clinical genetics, where it has informed diagnosis, cascade treatment and screening/prophylactic management, to oncology, where it is informing the immediate management of the patient following cancer diagnosis. This is exemplified by *BRCA1* and *BRCA2* (*BRCA1/2*)-related breast cancer. Previously, women with a mutation in either the *BRCA1* or *BRCA2* gene would have received similar first-line chemotherapy to women with a sporadic breast cancer without a known genetic association. More recently, it has been shown that *BRCA1/2* mutation-positive tumours are sensitive to poly ADP ribose polymerase (PARP) inhibitors. PARP inhibitors block the single-strand break-repair pathway. In a *BRCA1/2* mutation-positive tumour – with compromised double-strand break repair – the additional loss of the single-strand break-repair pathway will drive the cell towards apoptosis. Indeed, PARP inhibitors have been shown to be so effective at destroying *BRCA1/2* mutation-positive tumour cells, and with such minimal side-effects, that *BRCA1/2* gene testing is increasingly determining patient management. It is likely, with a growing understanding of the genomic architecture of tumours, increasing accessibility of NGS and an expanding portfolio of gene-directed therapies, that testing for many of the other inherited cancer susceptibility genes will, in time, move into the mainstream.

Genomics in infectious disease

NGS technologies are also transforming infectious disease. Given that a microbial genome can be sequenced within a single day at a current cost of less than 100 US dollars, microbiologists are able to identify a causative microorganism and target effective treatment rapidly and accurately. Moreover, microbial genome sequencing enables the effective surveillance of infections to reduce and prevent transmission. Finally, an understanding of the microbial genome will drive the development of vaccines and antibiotics, essential in an era characterised by increasing microbial resistance to established antibiotic agents.

Treatment of genetic disease

Pharmacogenomics

Pharmacogenomics is the science of dissecting the genetic determinants of drug kinetics and effects using information from the human genome. For more than 50 years, it has been appreciated that polymorphic mutations within genes can affect individual responses to some drugs, such as loss-of-function mutations in *CYP2D6* that cause hypersensitivity to debrisoquine, an adrenergic-blocking medication formerly used for the treatment of hypertension, in 3% of the population. This gene is part of a large family of highly polymorphic genes encoding cytochrome P450 proteins, mostly expressed in the liver, which determine the metabolism of a host of specific drugs. Polymorphisms in the *CYP2D6* gene also determine codeine activation, while those in the *CYP2C9* gene affect warfarin inactivation. Polymorphisms in these and other drug metabolic genes determine the persistence of drugs and, therefore, should provide information about dosages and toxicity. With the increasing use of NGS, genetic testing for assessment of drug response is seldom employed routinely, but in the future it may be possible to predict the best specific drugs and dosages for individual patients based on genetic profiling: so-called 'personalised medicine'. An example is the enzyme thiopurine methyltransferase (TPMT), which catabolises azathioprine, a drug that is used in the treatment of autoimmune diseases and in cancer chemotherapy. Genetic screening for polymorphic variants of TPMT can be useful in identifying patients who have increased sensitivity to the effects of azathioprine and who can be treated with lower doses than normal.

Gene therapy and genome editing

Replacing or repairing mutated genes (gene therapy) is challenging in humans. Retroviral-mediated ex vivo replacement of the defective gene in bone marrow cells for the treatment of severe combined immune deficiency syndrome (p. 79) has been successful. The major problems with clinical use of virally delivered gene therapy have been oncogenic integration of the exogenous DNA into the genome and severe immune response to the virus.

Other therapies for genetic disease include PTC124, a compound that can 'force' cells to read through a mutation that results in a premature termination codon in an ORF with the aim of producing a near-normal protein product. This therapeutic approach could be applied to any genetic disease caused by nonsense mutations.

The most exciting development in genetics for a generation has been the discovery of accurate, efficient and specific techniques to enable editing of the genome in cells and organisms. This technology is known as CRISPR/Cas9 (clustered regularly interspaced short palindromic repeats and CRISPR-associated) genome editing. It is likely that ex vivo correction of genetic disease will become commonplace over the next few years. In vivo correction is not yet possible and will take much longer to become part of clinical practice.

Induced pluripotent stem cells and regenerative medicine

Adult stem-cell therapy has been in wide use for decades in the form of bone marrow transplantation. The identification of adult stem cells for other tissues, coupled with the ability to purify and maintain such cells in vitro, now offers exciting therapeutic potential for other diseases. It was recently discovered that many different adult cell types can be trans-differentiated to form cells (induced pluripotent stem cells or iPS cells) with almost all the characteristics of embryonal stem cells derived from the early blastocyst. In mammalian model species, such cells can be taken and used to regenerate differentiated tissue cells, such as in heart and brain. They have great potential both for the development of tissue models of human disease and for regenerative medicine.

Pathway medicine

The ability to manipulate pathways that have been altered in genetic disease has tremendous therapeutic potential for Mendelian disease, but a firm understanding of both disease pathogenesis and drug action at a biochemical level is required. An exciting example has been the discovery that the vascular pathology associated with Marfan's syndrome is due to the defective fibrillin molecules causing up-regulation of transforming growth factor (TGF)-β signalling in the vessel wall. Losartan is an antihypertensive drug that is marketed as an angiotensin II receptor antagonist. However, it also acts as a partial antagonist of TGF-β signalling and is effective in preventing aortic dilatation in a mouse model of Marfan's syndrome, showing promising effects in early human clinical trials.

Ethics in a genomic age

As genomic technology is increasingly moving into mainstream clinical practice, it is essential for clinicians from all specialties to appreciate the complexities of genetic testing and consider whether genetic testing is the right thing to do in a given clinical scenario. To exemplify the ethical considerations associated with genetic testing, it may be helpful to think about them in the context of a clinical scenario. As you read the scenario, try to think what counselling/ethical issues might arise.

A 32-year-old woman is referred to discuss *BRCA2* testing; she is currently pregnant with her second child (she already has a 2-year-old daughter) and has an identical twin sister. Her mother, a healthy 65-year-old with Ashkenazi Jewish ancestry, participated in direct-to-consumer testing (DCT) for 'a bit of fun' and a *BRCA2* mutation – common in the Ashkenazi Jewish population – was identified. There is no significant cancer family history of note.

Consider the following issues:

- *Pre-symptomatic/predictive testing*: this describes testing for a known familial gene mutation in an unaffected individual (compared with diagnostic testing, where genetic testing is undertaken in an affected individual). Although this could be considered for the unaffected patient, in the current scenario any testing would also have implications for her identical twin sister. This needs to be fully explored with the patient and her sister prior to testing. There is also the potential issue of predictive testing in the patient's first child. A fundamental tenet in clinical genetics is that predictive genetic testing should be avoided in childhood for adult-onset conditions. This is because, if no benefit to the patient is accrued through childhood testing, it is better to retain the child's right to decide for herself, when she is old enough, whether she wishes to participate in genetic testing or not.
- *Prenatal testing*: the principles behind predictive genetic testing in childhood can be extended to prenatal testing, i.e. if a pregnancy is being continued, a baby should not be tested for an adult-onset condition that cannot be prevented or treated in childhood. However, prenatal testing itself is hugely controversial and there is much debate as to how severe a condition should be to justify prenatal diagnosis, which would determine ongoing pregnancy decisions.
- *DCT*: while DCT can be interesting and empowering for individuals wishing to find out more about their genetic backgrounds, it also has several drawbacks. Perhaps the main one is that, unlike face-to-face genetic counselling (which usually precedes any genetic testing, certainly where there are serious health implications for the individual and their family, such as is associated with

BRCA1/2 mutations), DCT is undertaken in isolation with no direct access to professional support. Furthermore, in addition to some (common) single-gene mutations, such as the founder *BRCA1/2* mutations frequently identified in the Ashkenazi Jewish population and discussed in this example, current DCT packages utilise a series of SNPs to determine an overall risk profile; they evaluate the number of detrimental and protective SNPs for a given disease. However, given that only a minority of the risk SNPs have so far been characterised, this is often inaccurate. Individuals may be falsely reassured that they are not at increased risk of a genetic condition despite a family history suggesting otherwise, resulting in inadequate surveillance and/or management.

The ethical considerations listed in this clinical scenario give just a flavour of some of the issues frequently encountered in clinical genetics. They are not meant to be an exhaustive summary and whole textbooks and meetings are devoted to the discussion of hugely complex ethical issues in genetics. However, a guiding principle is that, although each counselling situation will be unique with specific communication and ethical challenges, a genetic result is permanent and has implications for the whole family, not just the individual. Where possible, therefore, an informed decision regarding genetic testing should be taken by a competent adult following counselling by an experienced and appropriately trained clinician.

Further information

Books and journal articles

Alberts B, Bray D, Hopkin K et al. Essential cell biology, 4th edn. New York: Garland Science; 2013.

Firth H, Hurst JA. Oxford desk reference: clinical genetics. Oxford: Oxford University Press; 2005.

Read A, Donnai D. New clinical genetics, 2nd edn. Banbury: Scion; 2010.

Strachan T, Read A. Human molecular genetics, 4th edn. New York: Garland Science; 2010.

Websites

bsgm.org.uk *British Society for Genetic Medicine; has a report on genetic testing of children*.

decipher.sanger.ac.uk *Excellent, comprehensive genomic database*.

ensembl.org *Annotated genome databases from multiple organisms*.

futurelearn.com/courses/the-genomics-era *Has a Massive Open Online Course on genomics, for which one of the authors of the current chapter is the lead educator*.

genome.ucsc.edu *Excellent source of genomic information*.

ncbi.nlm.nih.gov *Online Mendelian Inheritance in Man (OMIM)*.

ncbi.nlm.nih.gov/books/NBK1116/ Gene Reviews: *excellent US-based source of information about many rare genetic diseases*.

orpha.net/consor/cgi-bin/index.php *Orphanet: European-based database on rare disease*.

Clinical immunology

Functional anatomy and physiology 62
The innate immune system 62
The adaptive immune system 67

The inflammatory response 70
Acute inflammation 70
Chronic inflammation 71
Laboratory features of inflammation 71

Presenting problems in immune disorders 73
Recurrent infections 73
Intermittent fever 74
Anaphylaxis 75

Immune deficiency 77
Primary phagocyte deficiencies 77
Complement pathway deficiencies 78
Primary antibody deficiencies 78
Primary T-lymphocyte deficiencies 79
Secondary immune deficiencies 80

Periodic fever syndromes 81

Amyloidosis 81

Autoimmune disease 81

Allergy 84

Angioedema 87

Transplantation and graft rejection 88
Transplant rejection 88
Complications of transplant immunosuppression 89
Organ donation 90

Tumour immunology 90

The immune system has evolved to identify and destroy pathogens while minimising damage to host tissue. Despite the ancient observation that recovery from an infectious disease frequently results in protection against that condition, the existence of the immune system as a functional entity was not recognised until the end of the 19th century. More recently, it has become clear that the immune system not only protects against infection but also regulates tissue repair following injury, and when dysregulated, governs the responses that can lead to autoimmune and auto-inflammatory diseases. Dysfunction or deficiency of the immune response can lead to a wide variety of diseases that may potentially involve every organ system in the body.

The aim of this chapter is to provide a general understanding of the immune system, how it contributes to human disease and how manipulation of the immune system can be put to therapeutic use. A review of the key components of the immune response is followed by sections that illustrate the clinical presentation of the most common forms of immune dysfunction: immune deficiency, inflammation, autoimmunity and allergy. More detailed discussion of individual conditions can be found in the relevant organ-specific chapters of this book.

Functional anatomy and physiology

The immune system consists of an intricately linked network of lymphoid organs, cells and proteins that are strategically placed

to protect against infection (Fig. 4.1). Immune defences are normally categorised into the innate immune response, which provides immediate protection against an invading pathogen, and the adaptive or acquired immune response, which takes more time to develop but confers exquisite specificity and long-lasting protection.

The innate immune system

Innate defences against infection include anatomical barriers, phagocytic cells, soluble molecules such as complement and acute phase proteins, and natural killer cells. The innate immune system recognises generic microbial structures present on non-mammalian tissue and can be mobilised within minutes. A specific stimulus will elicit essentially identical responses in different individuals, in contrast with adaptive antibody and T-cell responses, which vary greatly between individuals.

Physical barriers

The tightly packed keratinised cells of the skin physically limit colonisation by microorganisms. The hydrophobic oils that are secreted by sebaceous glands further repel water and microorganisms, and microbial growth is inhibited by the skin's low pH and low oxygen tension. Sweat also contains lysozyme, an enzyme that destroys the structural integrity of bacterial cell walls; ammonia, which has antibacterial properties; and several

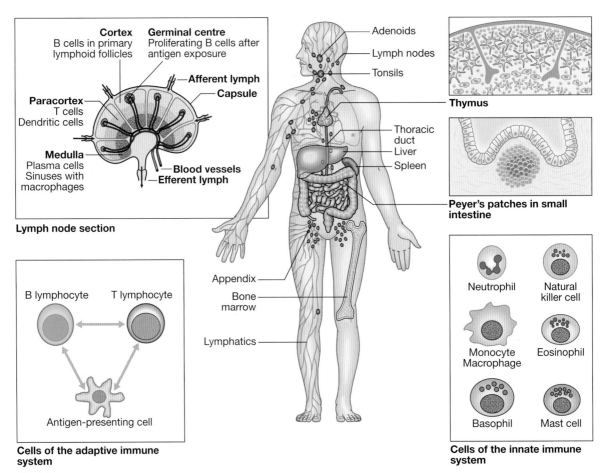

Lymph node section

Cells of the adaptive immune system

Cells of the innate immune system

Fig. 4.1 Anatomy of the immune system.

antimicrobial peptides such as defensins. Similarly, the mucous membranes of the respiratory, gastrointestinal and genitourinary tracts provide a physical barrier to infection. Secreted mucus traps invading pathogens, and immunoglobulin A (IgA), generated by the adaptive immune system, prevents bacteria and viruses attaching to and penetrating epithelial cells. As in the skin, lysozyme and antimicrobial peptides within mucosal membranes directly kill invading pathogens, and lactoferrin acts to starve invading bacteria of iron. Within the respiratory tract, cilia directly trap pathogens and contribute to removal of mucus, assisted by physical manœuvres such as sneezing and coughing. In the gastrointestinal tract, hydrochloric acid and salivary amylase chemically destroy bacteria, while normal peristalsis and induced vomiting or diarrhoea assist clearance of invading organisms.

The microbiome, which is made up of endogenous commensal bacteria, provides an additional constitutive defence against infection. Approximately 10^{14} bacteria normally reside at epithelial surfaces in symbiosis with the human host (p. 102). They compete with pathogenic microorganisms for scarce resources, including space and nutrients, and produce fatty acids and bactericidins that inhibit the growth of many pathogens. In addition, recent research has demonstrated that commensal bacteria help to shape the immune response by inducing specific regulatory T cells within the intestine. Eradication of the normal flora with broad-spectrum antibiotics commonly results in opportunistic infection by organisms such as *Clostridium difficile*, which rapidly colonise an undefended ecological niche.

These constitutive barriers are highly effective, but if external defences are breached by a wound or pathogenic organism, the specific soluble proteins and cells of the innate immune system are activated.

Phagocytes

Phagocytes ('eating cells') are specialised cells that ingest and kill microorganisms, scavenge cellular and infectious debris, and produce inflammatory molecules that regulate other components of the immune system. They include neutrophils, monocytes and macrophages, and are particularly important for defence against bacterial and fungal infections. Phagocytes express a wide range of surface receptors, including pattern recognition receptors (PRRs), which recognise pathogen-associated molecular patterns (PAMPs) on invading microorganisms, allowing their identification. The PRRs include Toll-like receptors, nucleotide oligomerisation domain (NOD) protein-like receptors and mannose receptors, whereas the PAMPs they recognise are molecular motifs not present on mammalian cells, including bacterial cell wall components, bacterial DNA and viral double-stranded RNA. While phagocytes can recognise microorganisms through PRRs alone, engulfment of microorganisms is greatly enhanced by opsonisation. Opsonins include acute phase proteins produced by the liver, such as C-reactive protein and complement. Antibodies generated by the adaptive immune system also act as opsonins. They bind both to the pathogen and to phagocyte receptors, acting as a bridge between the two to facilitate phagocytosis (Fig. 4.2). This is followed by intracellular pathogen destruction and downstream activation of pro-inflammatory genes, resulting in the generation of pro-inflammatory cytokines as discussed below.

Fig. 4.2 Phagocytosis and opsonisation. Phagocytosis of microbes can be augmented by several opsonins, such as C-reactive protein, antibodies and complement fragments like C3b, which enhance the ability of phagocytic cells to engulf microorganisms and destroy them. Phagocytes also recognise components of microbes, such as lipopolysaccharide, peptidoglycans, DNA and RNA, collectively as pathogen-associated molecular patterns (PAMPs). These activate pattern recognition receptors (PRRs), such as Toll-like receptors and nucleotide oligomerisation domain (NOD)-like receptors, which promote inflammatory gene expression through the nuclear factor kappa beta (NFκB) pathway. Uric acid and other crystals can also promote inflammation through the NOD pathway.

Neutrophils

Neutrophils, also known as polymorphonuclear leucocytes, are derived from the bone marrow and circulate freely in the blood. They are short-lived cells with a half-life of 6 hours, and are produced at the rate of 10^{11} cells daily. Their functions are to kill microorganisms, to facilitate rapid transit of cells through tissues, and to amplify the immune response non-specifically. These functions are mediated by enzymes contained in granules, which also provide an intracellular milieu for the killing and degradation of microorganisms.

Two main types of granule are recognised: primary or azurophil granules, and the more numerous secondary or specific granules. Primary granules contain myeloperoxidase and other enzymes important for intracellular killing and digestion of ingested microbes. Secondary granules are smaller and contain lysozyme, collagenase and lactoferrin, which can be released into the extracellular space. Enzyme production is increased in response to infection, which is reflected by more intense granule staining on microscopy, known as 'toxic granulation'.

Changes in damaged or infected cells trigger local production of inflammatory molecules and cytokines. These cytokines stimulate the production and maturation of neutrophils in the bone marrow, and their release into the circulation. Neutrophils are recruited to specific sites of infection by chemotactic agents, such as interleukin 8 (IL-8), and by activation of local endothelium. Up-regulation of cellular adhesion molecules on neutrophils and the endothelium also facilitates neutrophil migration. The transit of neutrophils through the blood stream is responsible for the rise in neutrophil count that occurs in early infection. Once present within infected tissue, activated neutrophils seek out and engulf invading microorganisms. These are initially enclosed within membrane-bound vesicles, which fuse with cytoplasmic granules to form the phagolysosome. Within this protected compartment, killing of the organism occurs through a combination of oxidative and non-oxidative killing. Oxidative killing, also known as the respiratory burst, is mediated by the nicotinamide adenine dinucleotide phosphate (NADPH)–oxidase enzyme complex, which converts oxygen into reactive oxygen species such as hydrogen peroxide and superoxide that are lethal to microorganisms. The myeloperoxidase enzyme within neutrophils produces hypochlorous acid, which is a powerful oxidant and antimicrobial agent. Non-oxidative (oxygen-independent) killing occurs through the release of bactericidal enzymes into the phagolysosome. Each enzyme has a distinct antimicrobial spectrum, providing broad coverage against bacteria and fungi.

An additional, recently identified form of neutrophil-mediated killing is neutrophil extracellular trap (NET) formation. Activated neutrophils can release chromatin with granule proteins such as elastase to form an extracellular matrix that binds to microbial proteins. This can immobilise or kill microorganisms without requiring phagocytosis. The process of phagocytosis and NET formation (NETosis) depletes neutrophil glycogen reserves and is followed by neutrophil death. As the cells die, their contents are released and lysosomal enzymes degrade collagen and other components of the interstitium, causing liquefaction of closely adjacent tissue. The accumulation of dead and dying neutrophils results in the formation of pus, which, if extensive, may lead to abscess formation.

Monocytes and macrophages

Monocytes are the precursors of tissue macrophages. They are produced in the bone marrow and enter the circulation, where they

i	**4.1 Functions of macrophages**

Amplification of the inflammatory response

- Stimulate the acute phase response (through production of IL-1 and IL-6)
- Activate vascular endothelium (IL-1, TNF-α)
- Stimulate neutrophil maturation and chemotaxis (IL-1, IL-8)
- Stimulate monocyte chemotaxis

Killing of microorganisms

- Phagocytosis
- Microbial killing through oxidative and non-oxidative mechanisms

Clearance, resolution and repair

- Scavenging of necrotic and apoptotic cells
- Clearance of toxins and other inorganic debris
- Tissue remodelling (elastase, collagenase, matrix proteins)
- Down-regulation of inflammatory cytokines
- Wound healing and scar formation (IL-1, platelet-derived growth factor, fibroblast growth factor)

Link between innate and adaptive immune systems

- Activate T cells by presenting antigen in a recognisable form
- T cell-derived cytokines increase phagocytosis and microbicidal activity of macrophages in a positive feedback loop

(IL = interleukin; TNF = tumour necrosis factor)

constitute about 5% of leucocytes. From the blood stream they migrate to peripheral tissues, where they differentiate into tissue macrophages and reside for long periods. Specialised populations of tissue macrophages include Kupffer cells in the liver, alveolar macrophages in the lung, mesangial cells in the kidney, and microglial cells in the brain. Macrophages, like neutrophils, are capable of phagocytosis and killing of microorganisms but also play an important role in the amplification and regulation of the inflammatory response (Box 4.1). They are particularly important in tissue surveillance and constantly survey their immediate surroundings for signs of tissue damage or invading organisms.

Dendritic cells

Dendritic cells are specialised antigen-presenting cells that are present in tissues in contact with the external environment, such as the skin and mucosal membranes. They can also be found in an immature state in the blood. They sample the environment for foreign particles and, once activated, carry microbial antigens to regional lymph nodes, where they interact with T cells and B cells to initiate and shape the adaptive immune response.

Cytokines

Cytokines are signalling proteins produced by cells of the immune system and a variety of other cell types. More than 100 have been identified. Cytokines have complex and overlapping roles in cellular communication and regulation of the immune response. Subtle differences in cytokine production, particularly at the initiation of an immune response, can have a major impact on outcome. Cytokines bind to specific receptors on target cells and activate downstream intracellular signalling pathways, ultimately leading to changes in gene transcription and cellular function. Two important signalling pathways are illustrated in Figure 4.3. The nuclear factor kappa B (NFκB) pathway is activated by tumour necrosis factor (TNF), by other members of the TNF superfamily such as receptor activator of nuclear kappa B ligand

Fig. 4.3 Cytokines signalling pathways and the immune response. Cytokines regulate the immune response through binding to specific receptors that activate a variety of intracellular signalling pathways, two of which are shown. Members of the tumour necrosis factor (TNF) superfamily and the Toll-like receptors and NOD-like receptors (Fig. 4.2) signal through the nuclear factor kappa B (NFκB) pathway. Several other cytokines, including interleukin-2 (IL-2), IL-6 and interferons, employ the Janus kinase/signal transducer and activator of transcription (JAK-STAT) pathway to regulate cellular function (see text for more details). (IκB = inhibitor of kappa B; IKK = I kappa B kinase; P = phosphorylation of the signalling protein; TRAF = tumour necrosis factor receptor-associated factor)

4

i 4.2 Important cytokines in the regulation of the immune response

Cytokine	Source	Actions	Biologic therapies
Interferon-alpha (IFN-α)	T cells and macrophages	Antiviral activity Activates NK cells, CD8+ T cells and macrophages	Recombinant IFN-α used in hepatitis C and some malignancies
Interferon-gamma (IFN-γ)	T cells and NK cells	Increases antimicrobial activity of macrophages Regulates cytokine production by T cells and macrophages	Used in chronic granulomatous disease
Tumour necrosis factor alpha (TNF-α)	Macrophages, NK cells and others, including T cells	Pro-inflammatory Increases expression of other cytokines and adhesion molecules Causes apoptosis of some target cells Directly cytotoxic	TNF-α inhibitors used in rheumatoid arthritis, inflammatory bowel disease, psoriasis and many other inflammatory conditions
Interleukin-1 (IL-1)	Macrophages and neutrophils	Stimulates neutrophil recruitment, fever, and T-cell and macrophage activation as part of the inflammatory response	IL-1 inhibitors used in systemic juvenile rheumatoid arthritis, periodic fever syndromes and acute gout
Interleukin-2 (IL-2)	CD4+ T cells	Stimulates proliferation and differentiation of antigen-specific T lymphocytes	
Interleukin-4 (IL-4)	CD4+ T cells	Stimulates maturation of B and T cells, and production of IgE antibody	Antibodies to IL-4 receptor used in severe atopic dermatitis
Interleukin-6 (IL-6)	Monocytes and macrophages	Stimulates neutrophil recruitment, fever, and T-cell and macrophage activation as part of the inflammatory response, stimulates maturation of B cells into plasma cells	Antibodies to IL-6 receptor used in rheumatoid arthritis
Interleukin-12 (IL-12)	Monocytes and macrophages	Stimulates IFN-γ and TNF-α release by T cells Activates NK cells	Antibody to p40 subunit of IL-12 used in psoriasis and psoriatic arthritis
Interleukin-17 (IL-17)	Th17 cells (T helper), NK cells, NK-T cells	Pro-inflammatory cytokine Involved in mucosal immunity and control of extracellular pathogens, synergy with IL-1 and TNF	Antibody to IL-17 used in psoriasis, psoriatic arthritis and ankylosing spondylitis
Interleukin-22 (IL-22)	Th17 cells	Induction of epithelial cell proliferation and antimicrobial proteins in keratinocytes	

(IgE = immunoglobulin E; NK = natural killer)

(RANKL; p. 985), and by the Toll-like receptors and NOD-like receptors (see Fig. 4.2). In the case of TNF superfamily members, receptor binding causes the inhibitor of kappa B kinase (IKK) complex of three proteins to be recruited to the receptor by binding TNF receptor-associated proteins (TRAF). This activates IKK, which in turn leads to phosphorylation of the inhibitor of nuclear factor kappa B protein (IκB), causing it to be degraded, and allowing NFκB to translocate to the nucleus and activate gene transcription. The Janus kinase/signal transducers and activators of transcription (JAK-STAT) pathway is involved in transducing signals downstream of many cytokine receptors, including those for IL-2, IL-6 and interferon-gamma (IFN-γ). On receptor binding, JAK proteins are recruited to the intracellular portion of the receptor and are phosphorylated. These in turn phosphorylate STAT proteins, which translocate to the nucleus and activate gene transcription, altering cellular function. The function and disease associations of several important cytokines are shown in Box 4.2. Cytokine inhibitors are now routinely used in the treatment of autoimmune diseases, most of which are monoclonal antibodies to cytokines or their receptors. In addition, small-molecule inhibitors have been developed that inhibit the intracellular signalling pathways used by cytokines. These include the Janus kinase inhibitors tofacitinib and baracitinib, which are used in rheumatoid arthritis (p. 1026), and the tyrosine kinase inhibitor imatinib, which is used in chronic myeloid leukaemia (p. 959).

Integrins

Integrins are transmembrane proteins that play important roles in cell–cell and cell–matrix interactions. They mediate attachment of the cell to the extracellular matrix, signal transduction and cell migration. Their role in autoimmune disease has been extensively studied. Targeted therapy with a recombinant humanised anti-α4 integrin antibody, natalizumab, is an effective treatment for multiple sclerosis, which works by preventing immune cells from traversing the vascular endothelium and entering the central nervous system (p. 1109).

Complement

The complement system comprises a group of more than 20 tightly regulated, functionally linked proteins that act to promote inflammation and eliminate invading pathogens. Complement proteins are produced in the liver and are present in inactive form in the circulation. When the complement system is activated, it sets in motion a rapidly amplified biological cascade analogous to the coagulation cascade (p. 918).

There are three mechanisms by which the complement cascade can be activated (Fig. 4.4):

- *The alternate pathway* is triggered directly by binding of C3 to bacterial cell-wall components, such as lipopolysaccharide of Gram-negative bacteria and teichoic acid of Gram-positive bacteria.
- *The classical pathway* is initiated when two or more IgM or IgG antibody molecules bind to antigen. The associated conformational change exposes binding sites on the antibodies for the first protein in the classical pathway, C1, which is a multiheaded molecule that can bind up to six antibody molecules. Once two or more 'heads' of a C1 molecule are bound to antibody, the classical cascade is triggered. An important inhibitor of the classical pathway is C1 inhibitor (C1inh), as illustrated in Figure 4.4.
- *The lectin pathway* is activated by the direct binding of mannose-binding lectin to microbial cell surface carbohydrates. This mimics the binding of C1 to immune complexes and directly stimulates the classical pathway, bypassing the need for immune complex formation.

Activation of complement by any of these pathways results in activation of C3. This in turn activates the final common pathway, in which the complement proteins C5–C9 assemble to form the membrane attack complex (MAC). This can puncture the cell wall, leading to osmotic lysis of target cells. This step is particularly

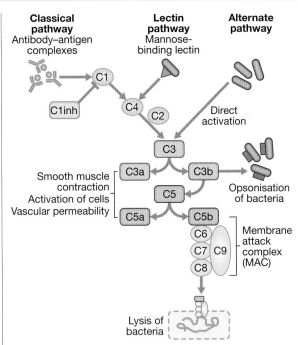

Fig. 4.4 The complement pathway. The classical pathway is activated by binding of antigen–antibody complexes to C1 but is blocked by C1 inhibitor (C1inh), whereas mannose-binding lectins, which are macromolecules that bind to various microorganisms, activate the pathway by binding C4. Bacteria can directly activate the pathway through C3, which plays a pivotal role in complement activation through all three pathways.

important in the defence against encapsulated bacteria such as *Neisseria* spp. and *Haemophilus influenzae*.

Complement fragments generated by activation of the cascade can also act as opsonins, rendering microorganisms more susceptible to phagocytosis by macrophages and neutrophils (see Fig. 4.2). In addition, they are chemotactic agents, promoting leucocyte trafficking to sites of inflammation. Some fragments act as anaphylotoxins, binding to complement receptors on mast cells and triggering release of histamine, which increases vascular permeability. The products of complement activation also help to target immune complexes to antigen-presenting cells, providing a link between the innate and the acquired immune systems. Finally, activated complement products dissolve the immune complexes that triggered the cascade, minimising bystander damage to surrounding tissues.

A monoclonal antibody directed against the central complement molecule C5, eculizumab, has been developed for therapeutic use in paroxysmal nocturnal haemoglobinuria and atypical haemolytic uraemic syndromes (p. 408). Invasive infection, including meningococcal sepsis, has been reported with eculizumab therapy, highlighting the importance of the complement system in preventing such infections.

Mast cells and basophils

Mast cells and basophils are bone marrow-derived cells that play a central role in allergic disorders. Mast cells reside predominantly in tissues exposed to the external environment, such as the skin and gut, while basophils circulate in peripheral blood and are recruited into tissues in response to inflammation. Both contain large cytoplasmic granules that enclose vasoactive substances such as histamine (see Fig. 4.14). Mast cells and basophils express IgE receptors on their cell surface, which bind IgE antibody. On encounter with specific antigen, the cell is triggered to release histamine and other mediators present within the granules and to synthesise additional mediators, including leukotrienes, prostaglandins and cytokines. An inflammatory cascade is initiated that increases local blood flow and vascular permeability, stimulates smooth muscle contraction, and increases secretion at mucosal surfaces.

Natural killer cells

Natural killer (NK) cells are large granular lymphocytes that play a major role in defence against tumours and viruses. They exhibit features of both the adaptive and the innate immune systems in that they are morphologically similar to lymphocytes and recognise similar ligands, but they are not antigen-specific and cannot generate immunological memory. NK cells express a variety of cell surface receptors, some of which are stimulatory and others inhibitory. The effects of inhibitory receptors normally predominate. These recognise human leucocyte antigen (HLA) molecules that are expressed on normal nucleated cells, preventing NK cell-mediated attack, whereas the stimulatory receptors recognise molecules that are expressed primarily when cells are damaged. This allows NK cells to remain tolerant to healthy cells but not to damaged ones. When cells become infected by viruses or undergo malignant change, expression of HLA class I molecules on the cell surface can be down-regulated. This is an important mechanism by which these cells then evade adaptive T-lymphocyte responses. In this circumstance, however, NK cell defences becomes important, as down-regulation of HLA class I abrogates the inhibitory signals that normally prevent NK activation. The net result is NK attack on the abnormal target cell. NK cells can also be activated by binding of antigen–antibody complexes to surface receptors. This physically links the NK cell to its target in a manner analogous to opsonisation and is known as antibody-dependent cellular cytotoxicity (ADCC).

Activated NK cells can kill their targets in various ways. They secrete pore-forming proteins such as perforin into the membrane of the target cell, and proteolytic enzymes called granzymes into the target cell, which cause apoptosis. In addition, NK cells produce a variety of cytokines such as TNF-α and IFN-γ, which have direct antiviral and anti-tumour effects.

The adaptive immune system

If the innate immune system fails to provide effective protection against an invading pathogen, the adaptive immune system is mobilised (see Fig. 4.1). This has three key characteristics:

- It has exquisite specificity and can discriminate between very small differences in molecular structure.
- It is highly adaptive and can respond to an almost unlimited number of molecules.
- It possesses immunological memory, and changes consequent to initial activation by an antigen allow a more effective immune response on subsequent encounters.

There are two major arms of the adaptive immune response. Humoral immunity involves the production of antibodies by B lymphocytes, and cellular immunity involves the activation of T lymphocytes, which synthesise and release cytokines that affect other cells, as well as directly killing target cells. These interact closely with each other and with the components of the innate immune system to maximise effectiveness of the immune response.

Lymphoid organs

The primary lymphoid organs are involved in lymphocyte development. They include the bone marrow, where T and B lymphocytes differentiate from haematopoietic stem cells (p. 914) and where B lymphocytes also mature, and the thymus, the site of T-cell maturation (see Fig. 4.1). After maturation, lymphocytes migrate to the secondary lymphoid organs. These include the spleen, lymph nodes and mucosa-associated lymphoid tissue. These trap and concentrate foreign substances and are the major sites of interaction between naïve lymphocytes and microorganisms.

The thymus

The thymus is a bi-lobed structure in the anterior mediastinum, and is organised into cortical and medullary areas. The cortex is densely populated with immature T cells, which migrate to the medulla to undergo selection and maturation. The thymus is most active in the fetal and neonatal period, and involutes after puberty. Failure of thymic development is associated with profound T-cell immune deficiency (p. 79) but surgical removal of the thymus in childhood (usually during major cardiac surgery) is not associated with significant immune dysfunction.

The spleen

The spleen is the largest of the secondary lymphoid organs. It is highly effective at filtering blood and is an important site of phagocytosis of senescent erythrocytes, bacteria, immune complexes and other debris, and of antibody synthesis. It is important for defence against encapsulated bacteria, and asplenic individuals are at risk of overwhelming *Streptococcus pneumoniae* and *H. influenzae* infection (see Box 4.5).

Lymph nodes

These are positioned to maximise exposure to lymph draining from sites of external contact, and are highly organised (Fig. 4.1)

- The *cortex* contains primary lymphoid follicles, which are the site of B-lymphocyte interactions. When B cells encounter antigen, they undergo intense proliferation, forming germinal centres.
- The *paracortex* is rich in T lymphocytes and dendritic cells.
- The *medulla* is the major site of antibody-secreting plasma cells.
- Within the medulla there are many *sinuses,* which contain large numbers of macrophages.

Mucosa-associated lymphoid tissue

Mucosa-associated lymphoid tissue (MALT) consists of diffusely distributed lymphoid cells and follicles present along mucosal surfaces. It has a similar function to the more organised, encapsulated lymph nodes. They include the tonsils, adenoids and Peyer's patches in the small intestine.

Lymphatics

Lymphoid tissue is connected by a network of lymphatics, with three major functions: it provides access to lymph nodes, returns interstitial fluid to the venous system, and transports fat from the small intestine to the blood stream (see Fig. 14.13, p. 372). The lymphatics begin as blind-ending capillaries, which come together to form lymphatic ducts, entering and leaving regional lymph nodes as afferent and efferent ducts, respectively. They eventually coalesce and drain into the thoracic duct and left subclavian vein. Lymphatics may be either deep or superficial, and follow the distribution of major blood vessels.

Humoral immunity

Humoral immunity is mediated by B lymphocytes, which differentiate from haematopoietic stem cells in the bone marrow. Their major functions are to produce antibody and interact with T cells, but they are also involved in antigen presentation. Mature B lymphocytes can be found in the bone marrow, lymphoid tissue, spleen and, to a lesser extent, the blood stream. They express a unique immunoglobulin receptor on their cell surface, the B-cell receptor, which binds to soluble antigen targets (Fig. 4.5). Encounters with antigen usually occur within lymph nodes. If provided with appropriate cytokines and other signals from nearby T lymphocytes, antigen-specific B cells respond by rapidly proliferating in a process known as clonal expansion (Fig. 4.5). This is accompanied by a highly complex series of genetic rearrangements known as somatic hypermutation, which generates B-cell populations that express receptors with greater affinity for antigen than the original. These cells differentiate into either long-lived memory cells, which reside in the lymph nodes, or plasma cells, which produce antibody. Memory cells allow production of a more rapid and more effective response on subsequent exposure to that pathogen.

Fig. 4.5 B-cell activation. Activation of B cells is initiated through binding of an antigen with the immunoglobulin receptor on the cell surface. For activation to proceed, an interaction with T-helper cells is also required, providing additional signals through binding of CD40 ligand (CD40L) to CD40; an interaction between the T-cell receptor (TCR) and processed antigenic peptides presented by human leucocyte antigen (HLA) molecules on the B-cell surface; and cytokines released by the T-helper cells. Fully activated B cells undergo clonal expansion with differentiation towards plasma cells that produce antibody. Following activation, memory cells are generated that allow rapid antibody responses when the same antigen is encountered on a second occasion. (CD = cluster of differentiation; IL = interleukin)

Immunoglobulins

Immunoglobulins (Ig) play a central role in humoral immunity. They are soluble proteins produced by plasma cells and are made up of two heavy and two light chains (Fig. 4.6). The heavy chain determines the antibody class or isotype, such as IgG, IgA, IgM, IgE or IgD. Subclasses of IgG and IgA also occur. The antigen is recognised by the antigen-binding regions (F_{ab}) of both heavy and light chains, while the consequences of antibody binding are determined by the constant region of the heavy chain (F_c) (Box 4.3). Antibodies have several functions.

Fig. 4.6 The structure of an immunoglobulin (antibody) molecule. The variable region is responsible for antigen binding, whereas the constant region can interact with immunoglobulin receptors expressed on immune cells.

4.3 Classes and properties of antibody

Antibody	Concentration in adult serum	Complement activation*	Opsonisation	Presence in external secretions	Other properties
IgG	6.0–16.0 g/L	IgG1 +++ IgG2 + IgG3 +++	IgG1 ++ IgG3 ++	++	Four subclasses: IgG1, IgG2, IgG3, IgG4 Distributed equally between blood and extracellular fluid, and transported across placenta IgG2 is particularly important in defence against polysaccharides antigens
IgA	1.5–4.0 g/L	–	–	++++	Two subclasses: IgA1, IgA2 Highly effective at neutralising toxins Particularly important at mucosal surfaces
IgM	0.5–2.0 g/L	++++	–	+	Highly effective at agglutinating pathogens
IgE	0.003–0.04 g/L	–	–	–	Majority of IgE is bound to mast cells, basophils and eosinophils Important in allergic disease and defence against parasite infection
IgD	Not detected	–	–	–	Function in B-cell development

*Activation of the classical pathway, also called 'complement fixation'.

They facilitate phagocytosis by acting as opsonins (see Fig. 4.2) and facilitate cell killing by cytotoxic cells, particularly NK cells by antibody-dependent cellular cytotoxicity. Binding of antibodies to antigen can trigger activation of the classical complement pathway (see Fig. 4.4). In addition, antibodies can directly neutralise the biological activity of their antigen target. This is a particularly important feature of IgA antibodies, which act predominantly at mucosal surfaces.

The humoral immune response is characterised by immunological memory, in which the antibody response to successive exposures to an antigen is qualitatively and quantitatively improved from the first exposure. When a previously unstimulated or 'naïve' B lymphocyte is activated by antigen, the first antibody to be produced is IgM, which appears in the serum after 5–10 days. Depending on additional stimuli provided by T lymphocytes, other antibody classes (IgG, IgA and IgE) are produced 1–2 weeks later. If the memory B cell is subsequently re-exposed to the same antigen, the lag time between exposure

and production of antibody is decreased to 2–3 days, the amount of antibody produced is increased, and the response is dominated by IgG antibodies of high affinity. Furthermore, in contrast to the initial antibody response, secondary antibody responses do not require additional input from T lymphocytes. This allows the rapid generation of highly specific responses on re-exposure to a pathogen and is an important mechanism in vaccine efficacy.

Cellular immunity

Cellular immunity is mediated by T lymphocytes, which play important roles in defence against viruses, fungi and intracellular bacteria. They also play an important immunoregulatory role, by orchestrating and regulating the responses of other components of the immune system. T-lymphocyte precursors differentiate from haematopoietic stem cells in the bone marrow and are exported to the thymus when they are still immature (see Fig. 4.1). Individual T cells express a unique receptor that is highly

Fig. 4.7 T-cell activation. Activation of T cells is initiated when an antigenic peptide bound to a human leucocyte antigen (HLA) molecule on antigen-presenting cells interacts with the T-cell receptor expressed by T lymphocytes. Additional signals are required for T-cell activation, however. These include binding of the co-stimulatory molecules CD80 and CD86 with CD28 on the T cell, and interleukin 2 (IL-2), which is produced in an autocrine manner by T cells that are undergoing activation. Other molecules are present that can inhibit T-cell activation, however, including cytotoxic T-lymphocyte-associated protein 4 (CTLA4), which competes with CD28 for binding to CD80 and CD86; and PD1, which, by binding PDL1, is also inhibitory. Following activation, T cells proliferate and, depending on their subtype, have various functions with distinct patterns of cytokine production, as indicated. Memory cells are also generated that can mount a rapid immune response on encountering the same antigen. (CD = cluster of differentiation; CD40L = CD40 ligand; IFN-γ = interferon-gamma; IL = interleukin; PD1 = programmed cell death 1; PDL1 = programmed death ligand 1; TGF-β = transforming growth factor beta; TNF-α = tumour necrosis factor alpha)

specific for a single antigen. Within the thymus T cells undergo a process of stringent selection to ensure that autoreactive cells are destroyed. Mature T lymphocytes leave the thymus and expand to populate other organs of the immune system. It has been estimated that an individual possesses 10^7–10^9 T-cell clones, each with a unique T-cell receptor, ensuring at least partial coverage for any antigen encountered.

Unlike B cells, T cells cannot recognise intact protein antigens in their native form. Instead, the protein must be broken down into component peptides by antigen-presenting cells for presentation to T lymphocytes in association with HLA molecules on the antigen-presenting cell surface. This process is known as antigen processing and presentation, and it is the complex of peptide and HLA together that is recognised by individual T cells (Fig. 4.7). The structure of HLA molecules varies widely between individuals. Since each HLA molecule has the capacity to present a subtly different peptide repertoire to T lymphocytes, this ensures enormous diversity in recognition of antigens by the T-cell population. All nucleated cells have the capacity to process and present antigens, but cells with specialised antigen-presenting functions include dendritic cells, macrophages and B lymphocytes. These carry additional co-stimulatory molecules, such as CD80 and CD86, providing the necessary 'second signal' for full T-cell activation.

T lymphocytes can be divided into two subgroups on the basis of function and recognition of HLA molecules. These are designated CD4+ and CD8+ T cells, according to the 'cluster of differentiation' (CD) antigen number of key proteins expressed on their cell surface.

CD8+ T lymphocytes

These cells recognise antigenic peptides in association with HLA class I molecules (HLA-A, HLA-B, HLA-C). They kill infected cells directly through the production of pore-forming molecules such as perforin and release of digesting enzymes triggering apoptosis of the target cell, and are particularly important in defence against viral infection.

CD4+ T lymphocytes

These cells recognise peptides presented on HLA class II molecules (HLA-DR, HLA-DP and HLA-DQ) and have mainly immunoregulatory functions. They produce cytokines and provide co-stimulatory signals that support the activation of CD8+ T lymphocytes and assist the production of mature antibody by B cells. In addition, their close interaction with phagocytes determines cytokine production by both cell types. CD4+ lymphocytes can be further subdivided into subsets on the basis of the cytokines they produce:

- Th1 (T helper) cells typically produce IL-2, IFN-γ and TNF-α, and support the development of delayed-type hypersensitivity responses (p. 83).
- Th2 cells typically produce IL-4, IL-5, IL-10 and IL-13, and promote allergic responses (p. 84).
- T-regulatory cells (T regs) are a further subset of specialised CD4+ lymphocytes that are important in actively suppressing activation of other cells and preventing autoimmune disease.
- Th17 cells are pro-inflammatory cells defined by their production of IL-17. They are related to regulatory T cells, and play a role in immune defence at mucosal surfaces

T-cell activation is regulated by a balance between co-stimulatory molecules, the second signal required for activation, and inhibitory molecules that down-regulate T-cell activity. One such inhibitory molecule, CTLA4, has been harnessed therapeutically in the form of abatacept, which is a fusion protein comprised of the Fc fragment of immunoglobulin linked to CTLA4. This is used to inhibit T-cell activation in rheumatoid arthritis and solid organ transplantation.

The inflammatory response

Inflammation is the response of tissues to injury or infection, and is necessary for normal repair and healing. This section focuses on the general principles of the inflammatory response and its multisystem manifestations. The role of inflammation in specific diseases is discussed in many other chapters of this book.

Acute inflammation

Acute inflammation is the result of rapid and complex interplay between the cells and soluble molecules of the innate immune system. The classical external signs include heat, redness, pain and swelling (Fig. 4.8). The inflammatory process is initiated by local tissue injury or infection. Damaged epithelial cells produce cytokines and antimicrobial peptides, causing early infiltration of phagocytic cells. Production of leukotrienes, prostaglandins, histamine, kinins, anaphylotoxins and inducible nitric oxide synthase also occurs within inflamed tissue. These mediators cause vasodilatation and increased vascular permeability, causing trafficking of fluid and cells into the affected tissue. In addition, pro-inflammatory cytokines, such as IL-1, TNF-α and IL-6 produced at the site of injury, are released systemically and act on the hypothalamus to cause fever, and on the liver to stimulate production of acute phase proteins.

The acute phase response

The acute phase response refers to the production of a variety of proteins by the liver in response to inflammatory stimuli. These proteins have a wide range of activities. Circulating levels of C-reactive protein (CRP) and serum amyloid A may be increased 1000-fold, contributing to host defence and stimulating repair and regeneration. Fibrinogen plays an essential role in wound healing, and α_1-antitrypsin and α_1-antichymotrypsin control the pro-inflammatory cascade by neutralising the enzymes produced by activated neutrophils, preventing widespread tissue destruction. In addition, antioxidants such as haptoglobin and manganese superoxide dismutase scavenge for oxygen free radicals, while increased levels of iron-binding proteins such as ferritin and lactoferrin decrease the iron available for uptake by bacteria (p. 941). Immunoglobulins are not acute phase proteins but are often increased in chronic inflammation.

Septic shock

Septic shock is the clinical manifestation of overwhelming inflammation (p. 196). It is characterised by excessive production of pro-inflammatory cytokines by macrophages, causing hypotension, hypovolaemia and tissue oedema. In addition, uncontrolled neutrophil activation causes release of proteases and oxygen free radicals within blood vessels, damaging the vascular endothelium and further increasing capillary permeability. Direct activation of the coagulation pathway combines with endothelial cell disruption to form clots within the damaged vessels. The

4

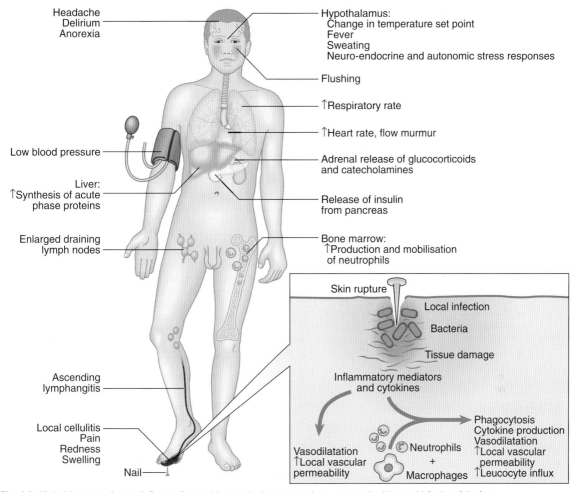

Fig. 4.8 **Clinical features of acute inflammation.** In this example, the response is to a penetrating injury and infection of the foot.

clinical consequences include cardiovascular collapse, acute respiratory distress syndrome, disseminated intravascular coagulation, multi-organ failure and often death. Septic shock most frequently results from infection with Gram-negative bacteria, because lipopolysaccharide produced by these organisms is particularly effective at activating the inflammatory cascade. Early recognition and appropriate early intervention can improve patient outcome (p. 196).

Resolution of inflammation

Resolution of an inflammatory response is crucial for normal healing. This involves active down-modulation of inflammatory stimuli and repair of bystander damage to local tissues. Extravasated neutrophils undergo apoptosis and are phagocytosed by macrophages, along with the remains of microorganisms. Macrophages also synthesise collagenase and elastase, which break down local connective tissue and aid in the removal of debris. Normal tissue homeostasis is also associated with reversion of parenchymal cells to a non-inflammatory phenotype. Macrophage-derived cytokines, including transforming growth factor-beta (TGF-β) and platelet-derived growth factor, stimulate fibroblasts and promote the synthesis of new collagen, while angiogenic factors stimulate new vessel formation.

Chronic inflammation

In most instances, the development of an active immune response results in clearance and control of the inflammatory stimulus and resolution of tissue damage. Failure of this process may result in chronic inflammation, with significant associated bystander damage, known as hypersensitivity responses. Persistence of microorganisms can result in ongoing accumulation of neutrophils, macrophages and activated T lymphocytes within the lesion. If this is associated with local deposition of fibrous tissue, a granuloma may form. Granulomas are characteristic of tuberculosis and leprosy (Hansen's disease), in which the microorganism is protected by a robust cell wall that shields it from killing, despite phagocytosis.

Laboratory features of inflammation

Inflammation is associated with changes in many laboratory investigations. Leucocytosis is common, and reflects the transit of activated neutrophils and monocytes to the site of infection. The platelet count may also be increased. The most widely used laboratory measure of acute inflammation is CRP. Circulating levels of many other acute phase reactants, including fibrinogen, ferritin and complement components, are also increased in response to acute inflammation, while albumin levels are reduced. Chronic inflammation is frequently associated with a normocytic normochromic anaemia (p. 943).

C-reactive protein

C-reactive protein (CRP) is an acute phase reactant synthesised by the liver, which opsonises invading pathogens. Circulating concentrations of CRP increase within 6 hours of the start of an inflammatory stimulus. Serum concentrations of CRP provide a direct biomarker of acute inflammation and, because the serum half-life of CRP is 18 hours, levels fall promptly once the inflammatory stimulus is removed. Sequential measurements are useful in monitoring disease activity (Box 4.4). For reasons that remain unclear, some diseases are associated with only minor elevations of CRP despite unequivocal evidence of active inflammation. These include systemic lupus erythematosus (SLE), systemic sclerosis, ulcerative colitis and leukaemia. An important practical point is that if the CRP is raised in these conditions, it suggests intercurrent infection rather than disease activity. Since the CRP is a more sensitive early indicator of the acute phase response, it is generally used in preference to the erythrocyte sedimentation rate (ESR). If both ESR and CRP are used, any discrepancy should be resolved by assessing the individual determinants of the ESR, which are discussed below.

Erythrocyte sedimentation rate

The ESR is an indirect measure of inflammation. It measures how fast erythrocytes fall through plasma, which is determined by the composition of plasma proteins and the morphology of circulating erythrocytes. These factors govern the propensity of red cells to aggregate, the major determinant of the ESR. Erythrocytes are inherently negatively charged, which prevents them from clumping together in the blood stream. Since plasma proteins are positively charged, an increase in plasma protein concentrations neutralises the negative charge of erythrocytes, overcoming their inherent repulsive forces and causing them aggregate, resulting in rouleaux formation. Rouleaux have a higher mass-to-surface area ratio than single red cells, and therefore sediment faster. The most common reason for an increased ESR is an acute phase response, which causes an increase in the concentration of acute phase proteins, including CRP. However, other conditions that do not affect acute phase proteins may alter the composition and concentration of other plasma protein (Box 4.4). For example, immunoglobulins comprise a significant proportion of plasma proteins but do not participate in the acute phase response. Thus any condition that causes an increase in serum immunoglobulins will increase the ESR without a corresponding increase in CRP. In addition, abnormal red cell morphology can make rouleaux formation impossible. For these reasons, an inappropriately low ESR occurs in spherocytosis and sickle-cell anaemia.

Plasma viscosity

Plasma viscosity is another surrogate measure of plasma protein concentration. Like the ESR, it is affected by the concentration of large plasma proteins, including fibrinogen and immunoglobulins. It is not affected by properties of erythrocytes and is generally considered to be more reliable than the ESR as a marker of inflammation.

4.4 Conditions commonly associated with abnormal C-reactive protein (CRP) and/or erythrocyte sedimentation rate (ESR)			
Condition	Consequence	Effect on CRP[1]	Effect on ESR[2]
Acute bacterial, fungal or viral infection	Stimulates acute phase response	Increased (range 50–150 mg/L; in severe infections may be >300 mg/L)	Increased
Necrotising bacterial infection	Stimulates profound acute inflammatory response	Greatly increased (may be >300 mg/L)	Increased
Chronic bacterial or fungal infection Localised abscess, bacterial endocarditis or tuberculosis	Stimulates acute and chronic inflammatory response with polyclonal increase in immunoglobulins, as well as increased acute phase proteins	Increased (range 50–150 mg/L)	Increased disproportionately to CRP
Acute inflammatory diseases Crohn's disease, polymyalgia rheumatica, inflammatory arthritis	Stimulates acute phase response	Increased (range 50–150 mg/L)	Increased
Systemic lupus erythematosus, Sjögren's syndrome, ulcerative colitis	Chronic inflammatory response	Normal	Increased
Multiple myeloma	Monoclonal increase in serum immunoglobulin without acute inflammation	Normal	Increased
Pregnancy, old age, end-stage renal disease	Increased fibrinogen	Normal	Moderately increased
[1]Reference range <10 mg/L. [2]Reference range: adult males <10 mm/hr, adult females <20 mm/hr.			

Presenting problems in immune disorders

Recurrent infections

Infections can occur in otherwise healthy individuals but recurrent infection raises suspicion of an immune deficiency. Depending on the component of the immune system affected, the infections may involve bacteria, viruses, fungi or protozoa, as summarised in Box 4.5. T-cell deficiencies can involve pathogens from all groups.

Aetiology

Infections secondary to immune deficiency occur because of defects in the number or function of phagocytes, B cells, T cells or complement, as described later in this chapter.

Clinical assessment

Clinical features that may indicate immune deficiency are listed in Box 4.6. Frequent or severe infections, or ones caused by unusual organisms or at unusual sites are typical of immune deficiency.

Investigations

Initial investigations should include full blood count and white cell differential, CRP, renal and liver function tests, urine dipstick, serum immunoglobulins with protein electrophoresis, and HIV testing. Additional microbiological tests, virology and imaging are required to identify the causal organism and localise the site of infection, as outlined in Box 4.7. If primary immune deficiency is suspected on the basis of initial investigations, more specialised tests should be considered, as summarised in Box 4.8.

Management

If an immune deficiency is suspected but has not yet been formally characterised, patients should not receive live vaccines because of the risk of vaccine-induced disease. Further management depends on the underlying cause and details are provided later.

i 4.6 Warning signs of primary immune deficiency*

In children	In adults
≥4 new ear infections within 1 year	≥2 new ear infections within 1 year
≥2 serious sinus infections within 1 year	≥2 new sinus infections within 1 year, in the absence of allergy
≥2 months on antibiotics with little effect	Recurrent viral infections
≥2 pneumonias within 1 year	≥1 pneumonia per year for more than 1 year
Failure of an infant to gain weight or grow normally	Chronic diarrhoea with weight loss
Recurrent deep skin or organ abscesses	Recurrent deep skin or organ abscesses
Persistent thrush in mouth or elsewhere on skin after infancy	Persistent thrush or fungal infection on skin or elsewhere
Need for intravenous antibiotics to clear infections	Recurrent need for intravenous antibiotics to clear infections
≥2 deep-seated infections such as sepsis, meningitis or cellulitis	Infection with atypical mycobacteria
A family history of primary immune deficiency	A family history of primary immune deficiency

*The presence of two or more of the above features may indicate the presence of an underlying primary immunodeficiency.
© Jeffrey Modell Foundation.

i 4.5 Immune deficiencies and common patterns of infection

Phagocyte deficiency	Complement deficiency	Antibody deficiency	T-lymphocyte deficiency
Bacteria			
Staphylococcus aureus	Neisseria meningitidis	Haemophilus influenzae	Mycobacterium tuberculosis
Pseudomonas aeruginosa	Neisseria gonorrhoeae	Streptococcus pneumoniae	Atypical mycobacteria
Serratia marcescens	Haemophilus influenzae	Staphylococcus aureus	
Burkholderia cenocepacia	Streptococcus pneumoniae		
Nocardia			
Mycobacterium tuberculosis			
Atypical mycobacteria			
Fungi			
Candida spp.	–	–	Candida spp.
Aspergillus spp.			Aspergillus spp.
			Pneumocystis jirovecii
Viruses	–	–	Cytomegalovirus (CMV)
			Enteroviruses
			Epstein–Barr virus (EBV)
			Herpes zoster virus
			Human papillomavirus
			Human herpesvirus 8
Protozoa	–	Giardia lamblia	Toxoplasma gondii
			Cryptosporidia

i 4.7 Initial investigations in suspected immune deficiency

Test	Value	Comment
Full blood count	Full white cell differential	May define pathway for further investigation
Acute phase reactants	Help determine presence of active infection	
Serum immunoglobulins	Detection of antibody deficiency	
Serum protein electrophoresis	Detection of paraprotein	May be the cause of immune paresis; paraprotein should be excluded prior to diagnosis of primary antibody deficiency
Serum free light chains/Bence Jones proteins	Detection of paraprotein	
Human immunodeficiency virus (HIV) test	To exclude HIV as cause of secondary immune deficiency	
Imaging according to history and examination findings	Detection of active infection/end-organ damage	May support treatment decisions, e.g. if there is evidence of bronchiectasis

i 4.8 Specialist investigations in suspected immune deficiency

Test	Value	Comment
Complement (C3/C4/CH50/AP50)	Investigation of recurrent pyogenic bacterial infection	Inherited complement deficiency likely to give low/absent results on functional assays
Test vaccination	Determination of functional humoral immune response	Helpful in patients with borderline low or normal immunoglobulins but confirmed recurrent infection
Neutrophil function	Investigation of recurrent invasive bacterial and fungal infection, especially with catalase-positive organisms Investigation of leucocyte adhesion deficiency	Respiratory burst low/absent in chronic granulomatous disease Leucocytosis with absent CD11a, b, c expression
Lymphocyte immunophenotyping (by flow cytometry)	Determination of specific lymphocyte subsets, T cell, B cell, NK cell	May define specific primary immune deficiency, e.g. absent B cells in X-linked agammaglobulinaemia
Lymphocyte proliferation	Determination of lymphocyte proliferation in response to mitogenic stimulation	Poor responses seen in certain T-cell immune deficiencies
Cytokine production	To determine T-cell immune function in response to antigen stimulation; limited availability, not routine	Can be helpful, for example, in investigation of atypical mycobacterial infection
Genetic testing	Under specialist supervision when specific primary immune deficiency suspected	May confirm genetic cause, with implications for family members and future antenatal testing

(NK = natural killer)

Intermittent fever

Intermittent fever has a wide differential diagnosis, including recurrent infection, malignancy and certain rheumatic disorders, such as Still's disease, vasculitis and SLE (pp. 1040 and 1034), but a familial fever syndrome is a potential cause.

Aetiology

Familial fever syndromes are genetic disorders caused by mutations in genes responsible for regulating the inflammatory response. The symptoms are caused by activation of intracellular signalling pathways involved in the regulation of inflammation, with over-production of pro-inflammatory cytokines such as IL-1.

Clinical assessment

A full clinical history and physical examination should be performed, paying attention to the patient's ethnic background and any family history of a similar disorder. If this assessment shows no evidence of underlying infection, malignancy or a rheumatic disorder and there is a positive family history and early age at onset, then the likelihood of a familial fever syndrome is increased.

Investigations

Blood should be taken for a full blood count, measurement of ESR and CRP, and assessment of renal and liver function. Serum ferritin should be checked, as very high levels support the diagnosis of Still's disease. Blood and urine cultures should also be performed, along with an autoimmune screen that includes measurement of antinuclear antibodies and consideration of antineutrophil cytoplasmic antibodies to check for evidence of SLE or vasculitis, respectively. Imaging may be required to exclude occult infection. If these investigations provide no evidence of infection or another cause, then genetic analysis should be considered to confirm the diagnosis of a familial fever syndrome (p. 81). Negative genetic testing does not, however, entirely exclude a periodic fever syndrome.

Management

Symptomatic management with non-steroidal anti-inflammatory drugs (NSAIDs) should be initiated, pending the results of investigations. If the response to NSAIDs is inadequate, glucocorticoids can be tried, provided that infection has been excluded. If a familial fever syndrome is confirmed, then definitive therapy should be initiated, depending on the underlying diagnosis (p. 81).

Anaphylaxis

Anaphylaxis is a potentially life-threatening, systemic allergic reaction characterised by circulatory collapse, bronchospasm, laryngeal stridor, often associated with angioedema, and urticaria. The risk of death is increased in patients with pre-existing asthma, particularly if this is poorly controlled, and in situations where treatment with adrenaline (epinephrine) is delayed.

Aetiology

Anaphylaxis occurs when an allergen binds to and cross-links membrane-bound IgE on mast cells in a susceptible individual, causing release of histamine, tryptase and other vasoactive mediators from mast cells. These mediators have a variety of effects, including vasodilatation, increased capillary permeability leading to hypotension, and bronchoconstriction, as summarised in Box 4.9. It can be difficult to distinguish IgE-mediated anaphylaxis clinically from non-specific degranulation of mast cells on exposure to drugs, chemicals or other triggers where IgE is not involved, previously known as anaphylactoid reactions. Common triggers are shown in Box 4.10.

Clinical assessment

The clinical features of anaphylaxis and 'anaphylactoid' reactions are indistinguishable and are summarised in Figure 4.9. Several other conditions can mimic anaphylaxis and these are listed in Box 4.11.

It is important to assess the severity of the reaction, and the time between allergen exposure and onset of symptoms provides

---

i | **4.9 Clinical features of mast cell degranulation**

Mediator	Biological effects
Pre-formed and stored within granules	
Histamine	Vasodilatation, chemotaxis, bronchoconstriction, increased capillary permeability and increased mucus secretion
Tryptase	Bronchoconstriction, activates complement C3
Eosinophil chemotactic factor	Eosinophil chemotaxis
Neutrophil chemotactic factor	Neutrophil chemotaxis
Synthesised on activation of mast cells	
Leukotrienes	Increase vascular permeability, chemotaxis, mucus secretion and smooth muscle contraction
Prostaglandins	Bronchoconstriction, platelet aggregation and vasodilatation
Thromboxanes	Bronchoconstriction
Platelet-activating factor	Bronchoconstriction, chemotaxis of eosinophils and neutrophils

---

i | **4.10 Common causes of systemic allergic reactions**

Anaphylaxis: IgE-mediated mast cell degranulation

Foods
- Peanuts
- Tree nuts
- Fish and shellfish
- Milk
- Eggs
- Soy products

Insect stings
- Bee venom
- Wasp venom

Chemicals, drugs and other foreign proteins
- Intravenous anaesthetic agents (suxamethonium)
- Penicillin and other antibiotics
- Latex

Anaphylactoid: non-IgE-mediated mast cell degranulation

Drugs
- Aspirin and non-steroidal anti-inflammatory drugs (NSAIDs)
- Opiates
- Radiocontrast media

Physical
- Exercise
- Cold

Idiopathic
- No cause is identified in 20% of patients with anaphylaxis

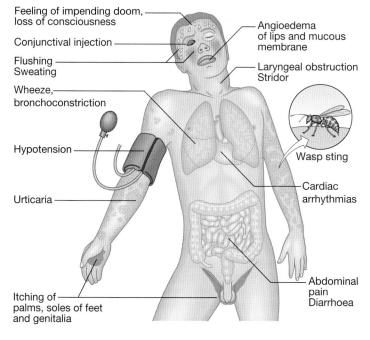

Feeling of impending doom, loss of consciousness

Conjunctival injection

Flushing
Sweating

Wheeze, bronchoconstriction

Hypotension

Urticaria

Itching of palms, soles of feet and genitalia

Angioedema of lips and mucous membrane

Laryngeal obstruction
Stridor

Wasp sting

Cardiac arrhythmias

Abdominal pain
Diarrhoea

Fig. 4.9 Clinical manifestations of anaphylaxis. In this example, the response is to an insect sting containing venom to which the patient is allergic. This causes release of histamine and other vasoactive mediators, which cause the characteristic features of anaphylaxis that are illustrated.

4.11 Differential diagnosis of anaphylaxis

Causes of hypotension

- Vasovagal syncope
- Cardiac arrhythmia
- Cardiogenic shock

Causes of respiratory distress

- Status asthmaticus
- Pulmonary embolus

Causes of laryngeal obstruction

- C1 inhibitor deficiency
- Idiopathic angioedema

Causes of generalised flushing

- Systemic mastocytosis
- Carcinoid syndrome
- Phaeochromocytoma

✚ **4.12 Emergency management of anaphylaxis**

Treatment	Comment
Prevent further contact with allergen	Prevents ongoing mast cell activation
Ensure airway patency	Prevents hypoxia
Administer adrenaline (epinephrine) promptly: 0.3–1.0 mL 1 : 1000 solution IM in adults Repeat at 5–10-min intervals if initial response is inadequate	Intramuscular route important because of peripheral vasoconstriction Acts within minutes Increases blood pressure Reverses bronchospasm
Administer antihistamines: Chlorphenamine 10 mg IM or slow IV injection	Blocks effect of histamine on target cells
Administer glucocorticoids: Hydrocortisone 200 mg IV	Reduces cytokine release Prevents rebound symptoms in severe cases
Provide supportive treatment: Nebulised β₂-agonists IV fluids Oxygen	Reverses bronchospasm Restores plasma volume Reverses hypoxia

(IM = intramuscular; IV = intravenous)

---

a guide. Enquiry should be made about potential triggers. If none is immediately obvious, a detailed history of the previous 24 hours may be helpful. The most common triggers of anaphylaxis are foods, latex, insect venom and drugs (see Box 4.10). A history of previous local allergic responses to the offending agent is common. The route of allergen exposure may influence the principal clinical features of a reaction; for example, if an allergen is inhaled, the major symptom is frequently wheezing. Features of anaphylaxis may overlap with the direct toxic effects of drugs and venoms (Chs 7 and 8). Potentiating factors, such as exercise or alcohol, can lower the threshold for an anaphylactic event. It is important to identify precipitating factors so that appropriate avoidance measures may be taken in the longer term.

Investigations

Measurement of serum mast cell tryptase concentrations is useful to confirm the diagnosis but cannot distinguish between anaphylaxis and non-IgE-mediated anaphylactoid reactions. Specific IgE tests may be useful in confirming hypersensitivity and may be preferable to skin-prick tests when investigating patients with a history of anaphylaxis.

 4.13 How to prescribe self-injectable adrenaline (epinephrine)

Prescription (normally initiated by an immunologist or allergist)

- Specify the brand of autoinjector, as they have different triggering mechanisms
- Prescribe two devices

Indications

- Anaphylaxis to allergens that are difficult to avoid:
  Insect venom
  Foods
- Idiopathic anaphylactic reactions
- History of severe localised reactions with high risk of future anaphylaxis:
  Reaction to trace allergen
  Likely repeated exposure to allergen
- History of severe localised reactions with high risk of adverse outcome:
  Poorly controlled asthma
  Lack of access to emergency care

Patient and family education

- Know when and how to use the device
- Carry the device at all times
- Seek medical assistance immediately after use
- Wear an alert bracelet or necklace
- Include the school in education for young patients (see 'Further information')

Other considerations

- Caution with β-blockers in anaphylactic patients as they may increase the severity of an anaphylactic reaction and reduce the response to adrenaline (epinephrine)

 4.14 Allergy in adolescence

- **Resolution of childhood allergy**: most children affected by allergy to milk, egg, soybean or wheat will grow out of their food allergies by adolescence but allergies to peanuts, tree nuts, fish and shellfish are frequently life-long.
- **Risk-taking behaviour and fatal anaphylaxis**: serious allergy is increasingly common in adolescents and this is the highest risk group for fatal, food-induced anaphylaxis. This is associated with increased risk-taking behaviour, and food-allergic teenagers are more likely than adults to eat unsafe foods, deny reaction symptoms and delay emergency treatment.
- **Emotional impact of food allergies**: some adolescents may neglect to carry a prescribed adrenalin autoinjector because of the associated nuisance and/or stigma. Surveys of food-allergic teens reveal that many take risks because they feel socially isolated by their allergy.

Management

The principles of management of the acute event are summarised in Box 4.12. Individuals who have recovered from an anaphylactic event should be referred for specialist assessment. The aim is to identify the trigger factor, to educate the patient regarding avoidance and management of subsequent episodes, and to establish whether specific treatment, such as immunotherapy, is indicated. If the trigger factor cannot be identified or avoided, recurrence is common. Patients who have previously experienced an anaphylactic event should be prescribed self-injectable adrenaline (epinephrine) and they and their families or carers should be instructed in its use (Box 4.13). The use of a MedicAlert (or similar) bracelet will increase the likelihood of the injector being administered in an emergency. Allergy in adolescence requires additional consideration and management, as set out in Box 4.14.

Immune deficiency

The consequences of immune deficiency include recurrent infection, autoimmunity as a result of immune dysregulation, and increased susceptibility to malignancy, especially malignancy driven by viral infections such as Epstein–Barr virus. Immune deficiency may arise through intrinsic defects in immune function but is much more commonly due to secondary causes, including infection, drug therapy, malignancy and ageing. This section gives an overview of primary immune deficiencies. More than a hundred such deficiencies have been described, most of which are genetically determined and present in childhood or adolescence. The presentation of immune deficiency depends on the component of the immune system that is defective (see Box 4.5). There is considerable overlap and redundancy in the immune network, however, and some diseases do not fall easily into this classification.

Primary phagocyte deficiencies

Primary phagocyte deficiencies typically present with recurrent bacterial and fungal infections, which may involve unusual sites. Affected patients require aggressive management of infections, including intravenous antibiotics and surgical drainage of abscesses, and long-term prophylaxis with antibacterial and antifungal agents. The most important examples are illustrated in Figure 4.10 and discussed below.

Chronic granulomatous disease

This is caused by mutations in genes that encode NADPH oxidase enzymes, which results in failure of oxidative killing. The defect leads to susceptibility to catalase-positive organisms such as *Staphylococcus aureus*, *Burkholderia cenocepacia* and *Aspergillus*. Intracellular killing of mycobacteria in macrophages is also impaired. Infections most commonly involve the lungs, lymph nodes, soft tissues, bone, skin and urinary tract, and are characterised histologically by granuloma formation. Most cases are X-linked (p. 48).

Leucocyte adhesion deficiencies

These very rare disorders of phagocyte migration occur because of failure to express adhesion molecules on the surface of leucocytes, resulting in their inability to exit the blood stream. The most common cause is loss-of-function mutations affecting the *ITGB2* gene, which encodes the integrin β-2 chain, a component of the adhesion molecule LFA1. They are characterised by recurrent bacterial infections but sites of infection lack evidence of neutrophil infiltration, such as pus formation. Peripheral blood neutrophil counts may be very high during acute infection because of the failure of mobilised neutrophils to exit blood vessels. Specialised tests show reduced or absent expression of adhesion molecules on neutrophils.

Normal

Neutrophils traverse endothelium through binding of LFA1 to ICAM1

Cytokines activate macrophages

Destruction of microorganisms through NADPH oxidase-mediated killing

Primary phagocyte deficiency

Leucocyte adhesion deficiency

Neutrophils cannot traverse endothelium due to defects in ITGB2, a component of LFA1

Cytokine defects

Phagocytes cannot be activated due to defects in cytokines or their receptors

Chronic granulomatous disease

Microorganisms cannot be destroyed in lysosomes due to NADPH oxidase deficiency

Fig. 4.10 Normal phagocyte function and mechanisms of primary phagocyte deficiency. Under normal circumstances, neutrophils traverse the endothelium to enter tissues by the cell surface molecule lymphocyte function-associated antigen 1 (LFA1), which binds to intercellular adhesion molecule 1 (ICAM1) on endothelium. In order for macrophages to engulf and kill microorganisms, they need to be activated by cytokines and also require nicotinamide adenine dinucleotide phosphate (NADPH) oxidase to generate free radicals. Primary phagocyte deficiencies can occur as the result of leucocytes being unable to traverse endothelium due to defects in LFA1, because of mutations in cytokines or their receptors, or because of defects in NADPH oxidase. (IFN-γ = interferon-gamma; IL = interleukin)

Defects in cytokines and cytokine receptors

Mutations of the genes encoding cytokines such as IFN-γ, IL-12, IL-23 or their receptors result in failure of intracellular killing by macrophages, and affected individuals are particularly susceptible to mycobacterial infections.

Complement pathway deficiencies

Loss-of-function mutations have been identified in almost all the complement pathway proteins (see Fig. 4.4). While most complement deficiencies are rare, mannose-binding lectin deficiency is common and affects about 5% of the northern European population, many of whom are asymptomatic (see below).

Clinical features

Patients with deficiency in complement proteins can present in different ways. In some cases, the presenting feature is recurrent infection with encapsulated bacteria, particularly *Neisseria* spp., reflecting the importance of the membrane attack complex in defence against these organisms. However, genetic deficiencies of the classical complement pathway (C1, C2 and C4) also present with an increased risk of autoimmune disease, particularly SLE (p. 1034). Individuals with mannose-binding lectin deficiency have an increased incidence of bacterial infections if subjected to an additional cause of immune compromise, such as premature birth or chemotherapy. The significance of this condition has been debated, however, since population studies have shown no overall increase in infectious disease or mortality in patients with this disorder. Deficiency of the regulatory protein CI inhibitor is not associated with recurrent infection but causes recurrent angioedema (p. 87).

Investigations

Screening for complement deficiencies usually involves specialised functional tests of complement-mediated haemolysis. These are known as the CH50 (classical haemolytic pathway 50) and AP50 (alternative pathway 50) tests. If abnormal, haemolytic tests are followed by measurement of individual complement components.

Management

Patients with complement deficiencies should be vaccinated with meningococcal, pneumococcal and *H. influenzae* B vaccines to boost their adaptive immune responses. Lifelong prophylactic penicillin to prevent meningococcal infection is recommended, as is early access to acute medical assessment in the event of infection. Patients should also carry a MedicAlert or similar. At risk family members should be screened for complement deficiencies with functional complement assays. The management of C1 esterase deficiency is discussed elsewhere.

Primary antibody deficiencies

Primary antibody deficiencies occur as the result of abnormalities in B-cell function, as summarised in Figure 4.11. They are characterised by recurrent bacterial infections, particularly of the respiratory and gastrointestinal tract. The most common causative organisms are encapsulated bacteria such as *Streptococcus pneumoniae* and *H. influenzae*. These disorders usually present in infancy, when the protective benefit of placental transfer of maternal immunoglobulin has waned. The most important causes are discussed in more detail below.

X-linked agammaglobulinaemia

This rare X-linked disorder (p. 48) is caused by mutations in the *BTK* gene, which encodes Bruton tyrosine kinase, a signalling protein that is required for B-cell development. Affected males present with severe bacterial infections during infancy. There is a marked reduction in B-cell numbers and immunoglobulin levels are low or undetectable. Management is with immunoglobulin replacement therapy and antibiotics to treat infections.

Selective IgA deficiency

This is the most common primary antibody deficiency, affecting 1:600 northern Europeans. Although IgA deficiency is usually asymptomatic with no clinical sequelae, about 30% of individuals experience recurrent mild respiratory and gastrointestinal infections. The diagnosis can be confirmed by measurement of IgA levels, which are low or undetectable (<0.05 g/L). In some

Fig. 4.11 B lymphocytes and primary antibody deficiencies (green boxes). (Ig = immunoglobulin)

4

4.15 Investigation of primary antibody deficiencies

	Serum immunoglobulin (Ig) concentrations				Circulating lymphocyte numbers		
	IgM	IgG	IgA	IgE	B cells	T cells	Test immunisation
Selective IgA deficiency	Normal	Often elevated	Absent	Normal	Normal	Normal	Not applicable*
Common variable immune deficiency	Normal or low	Low	Low or absent	Low or absent	Variable	Variable	No antibody response
Specific antibody deficiency	Normal	Normal	Normal	Normal	Normal	Normal	No antibody response to polysaccharide antigens

*Test immunisation is not usually performed in IgA deficiency but some patients may have impaired responses.

patients, there is a compensatory increase in serum IgG levels. Specific treatment is generally not required.

Common variable immune deficiency

Common variable immune deficiency (CVID) is characterised by low serum IgG levels and failure to make antibody responses to exogenous pathogens. It is a heterogeneous adult-onset primary immune deficiency of unknown cause. The presentation is with recurrent infections, and bronchiectasis is a recognised complication. Paradoxically, antibody-mediated autoimmune diseases, such as idiopathic thrombocytopenic purpura and autoimmune haemolytic anaemia, are common in CVID. It is also associated with an increased risk of malignancy, particularly lymphoproliferative disease.

Functional IgG antibody deficiency

This is a poorly characterised condition resulting in defective antibody responses to polysaccharide antigens. Some patients are also deficient in the antibody subclasses IgG2 and IgG4, and this condition was previously called IgG subclass deficiency. There is overlap between specific antibody deficiency, IgA deficiency and CVID, and some patients may progress to a more global antibody deficiency over time.

Investigations

Serum immunoglobulins (Box 4.15) should be measured in conjunction with protein and urine electrophoresis to exclude secondary causes of hypogammaglobulinaemia, and B- and T-lymphocyte subsets should be measured. Specific antibody responses to known pathogens should be assessed by measuring IgG antibodies against tetanus, *H. influenzae* and *S. pneumoniae* (most patients will have been exposed to these antigens through infection or immunisation). If specific antibody levels are low, immunisation with the appropriate killed vaccine should be followed by repeat antibody measurement 6–8 weeks later; failure to mount a response indicates a significant defect in antibody production. These functional tests have generally superseded IgG subclass quantitation.

Management

Patients with antibody deficiencies generally require aggressive treatment of infections and prophylactic antibiotics may be indicated. An exception is deficiency of IgA, which usually does not require treatment. The mainstay of treatment in most patients with antibody deficiency is immunoglobulin replacement therapy. This is derived from plasma from hundreds of donors and contains IgG antibodies to a wide variety of common organisms. Replacement immunoglobulin may be administered either intravenously or subcutaneously, with the aim of maintaining trough IgG levels (the

IgG level just prior to an infusion) within the normal range. This has been shown to minimise progression of end-organ damage and improve clinical outcome. Treatment may be self-administered and is life-long. Benefits of immunisation are limited because of the defect in IgG antibody production, and as with all primary immune deficiencies, live vaccines should be avoided.

Primary T-lymphocyte deficiencies

These are a group of diseases characterised by recurrent viral, protozoal and fungal infections (see Box 4.5). Many T-cell deficiencies are also associated with defective antibody production because of the importance of T cells in providing help for B cells. These disorders generally present in childhood. Several causes of T-cell deficiency are recognised. These are summarised in Figure 4.12 and discussed in more detail below.

DiGeorge syndrome

This results from failure of development of the third and fourth pharyngeal pouches, and is usually caused by a deletion of chromosome 22q11. The immune deficiency is accounted for by failure of thymic development; however, the immune deficiency can be very heterogeneous. Affected patients tend to have very low numbers of circulating T cells despite normal development in the bone marrow. It is associated with multiple developmental anomalies, including congenital heart disease, hypoparathyroidism, tracheo-oesophageal fistulae, cleft lip and palate.

Bare lymphocyte syndromes

These rare disorders are caused by mutations in a variety of genes that regulate expression of HLA molecules or their transport to the cell surface. If HLA class I molecules are affected, CD8+ lymphocytes fail to develop normally, while absent expression of HLA class II molecules affects CD4+ lymphocyte maturation. In addition to recurrent infections, failure to express HLA class I is associated with systemic vasculitis caused by uncontrolled activation of NK cells.

Severe combined immune deficiency

Severe combined immune deficiency (SCID) results from mutations in a number of genes that regulate lymphocyte development, with failure of T-cell maturation, with or without accompanying B- and NK-cell maturation. The most common cause is X-linked SCID, resulting from loss-of-function mutations in the interleukin-2 receptor gamma (*IL2RG*) gene. The gene product is a component of several interleukin receptors, including those for IL-2, IL-7 and IL-15, which are absolutely required for T-cell and NK development. This results in T-cell-negative, NK-cell-negative,

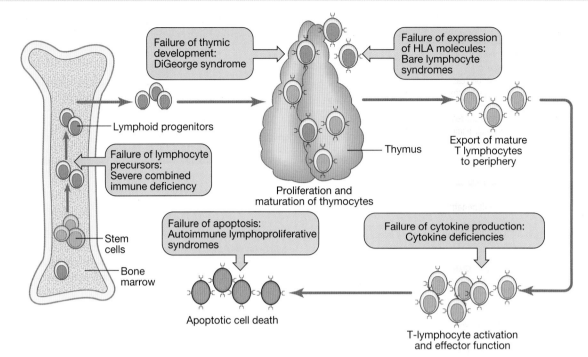

Fig. 4.12 T-lymphocyte function and dysfunction (green boxes). (HLA = human leucocyte antigen)

B-cell-positive SCID. Another cause is deficiency of the enzyme adenosine deaminase (ADA), which causes lymphocyte death due to accumulation of toxic purine metabolites intracellularly, resulting in T-cell-negative, B-cell-negative and NK-cell-negative SCID.

The absence of an effective adaptive immune response causes recurrent bacterial, fungal and viral infections soon after birth. Bone marrow transplantation (BMT; p. 936) is the treatment option of first choice. Gene therapy has been approved for treatment of ADA deficiency when there is no suitable donor for BMT and is under investigation for a number of other causes of SCID.

Investigations

The principal tests for T-lymphocyte deficiencies are a total lymphocyte count and quantitation of individual lymphocyte subpopulations. Serum immunoglobulins should also be measured. Second-line, functional tests of T-cell activation and proliferation may be indicated. Patients in whom T-lymphocyte deficiencies are suspected should be tested for HIV infection (p. 310).

Management

Patients with T-cell deficiencies should be considered for anti-*Pneumocystis* and antifungal prophylaxis, and require aggressive management of infections when they occur. Immunoglobulin replacement is indicated for associated defective antibody production. Stem cell transplantation (p. 936) or gene therapy may be appropriate in some disorders. Where a family history is known and antenatal testing confirms a specific defect, stem cell therapy prior to recurrent invasive infection can improve outcome.

Autoimmune lymphoproliferative syndrome

This rare disorder is caused by failure of normal lymphocyte apoptosis, most commonly due to mutations in the *FAS* gene, which encodes Fas, a signalling protein that regulates programmed cell death in lymphocytes. This results in massive accumulation of autoreactive T cells, which cause autoimmune-mediated anaemia, thrombocytopenia and neutropenia. Other features

include lymphadenopathy, splenomegaly and a variety of other autoimmune diseases. Susceptibility to infection is increased because of the neutropenia.

Secondary immune deficiencies

Secondary immune deficiencies are much more common than primary immune deficiencies and occur when the immune system is compromised by external factors (Box 4.16). Common causes include infections, such as HIV and measles, and cytotoxic

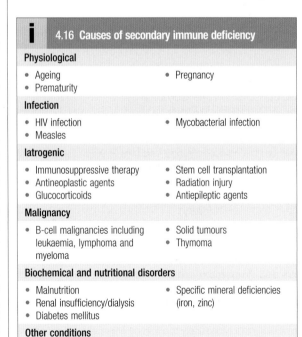

i 4.16 Causes of secondary immune deficiency	
Physiological	
• Ageing	• Pregnancy
• Prematurity	
Infection	
• HIV infection	• Mycobacterial infection
• Measles	
Iatrogenic	
• Immunosuppressive therapy	• Stem cell transplantation
• Antineoplastic agents	• Radiation injury
• Glucocorticoids	• Antiepileptic agents
Malignancy	
• B-cell malignancies including leukaemia, lymphoma and myeloma	• Solid tumours • Thymoma
Biochemical and nutritional disorders	
• Malnutrition	• Specific mineral deficiencies (iron, zinc)
• Renal insufficiency/dialysis	
• Diabetes mellitus	
Other conditions	
• Burns	• Asplenia/hyposplenism

4.17 Immune senescence

- **T-cell responses**: decline, with reduced delayed-type hypersensitivity responses.
- **Antibody production**: decreased for many exogenous antigens. Although autoantibodies are frequently detected, autoimmune disease is less common.
- **Response to vaccination**: reduced; 30% of healthy older people may not develop protective immunity after influenza vaccination.
- **Allergic disorders and transplant rejection**: less common.
- **Susceptibility to infection**: increased; community-acquired pneumonia by threefold and urinary tract infection by 20-fold. Latent infections, including tuberculosis and herpes zoster, may be reactivated.
- **Manifestations of inflammation**: may be absent, with lack of pyrexia or leucocytosis.
- **Secondary immune deficiency**: common.

and immunosuppressive drugs, particularly those used in the management of transplantation, autoimmunity and cancer. Physiological immune deficiency occurs at the extremes of life; the decline of the immune response in the elderly is known as immune senescence (Box 4.17). Management of secondary immune deficiency is described in the relevant chapters on infectious diseases (Ch. 11), HIV (Ch. 12), haematological disorders (Ch. 23) and oncology (Ch. 33).

Periodic fever syndromes

These rare disorders are characterised by recurrent episodes of fever and organ inflammation, associated with an elevated acute phase response (p. 74).

Familial Mediterranean fever

Familial Mediterranean fever (FMF) is the most common of the familial periodic fevers, predominantly affecting Mediterranean people, including Arabs, Turks, Sephardic Jews and Armenians. It results from mutations of the *MEFV* gene, which encodes a protein called pyrin that regulates neutrophil-mediated inflammation by indirectly suppressing the production of IL-1. FMF is characterised by recurrent painful attacks of fever associated with peritonitis, pleuritis and arthritis, which last for a few hours to 4 days and are associated with markedly increased CRP levels. Symptoms resolve completely between episodes. Most individuals have their first attack before the age of 20. The major complication of FMF is AA amyloidosis (see below). Colchicine significantly reduces the number of febrile episodes in 90% of patients but is ineffective during acute attacks.

Mevalonic aciduria (mevalonate kinase deficiency)

Mevalonate kinase deficiency, previously known as hyper-IgD syndrome, is an autosomal recessive disorder that causes recurrent attacks of fever, abdominal pain, diarrhoea, lymphadenopathy, arthralgia, skin lesions and aphthous ulceration. Most patients are from Western Europe, particularly the Netherlands and northern France. It is caused by loss-of-function mutations in the gene encoding mevalonate kinase, which is involved in the metabolism of cholesterol. It remains unclear why this causes an inflammatory periodic fever. Serum IgD and IgA levels may be persistently elevated, and CRP levels are increased during acute

attacks. Standard anti-inflammatory drugs, including colchicine and glucocorticoids, are ineffective in suppressing the attacks but IL-1 inhibitors, such as anakinra, and TNF inhibitors, such as etanercept, may improve symptoms and can induce complete remission in some patients.

TNF receptor-associated periodic syndrome

TNF receptor-associated periodic syndrome (TRAPS) also known as Hibernian fever, is an autosomal dominant syndrome caused by mutations in the *TNFRSF1A* gene. The presentation is with recurrent attacks of fever, arthralgia, myalgia, serositis and rashes. Attacks may be prolonged for 1 week or more. During a typical attack, laboratory findings include neutrophilia, increased CRP and elevated IgA levels. The diagnosis can be confirmed by low serum levels of the soluble type 1 TNF receptor and by mutation screening of the *TNFRSF1A* gene. As in FMF, the major complication is amyloidosis, and regular screening for proteinuria is advised. Acute episodes respond to systemic glucocorticoids. Therapy with IL-1 inhibitors, such as anakinra, can be effective in preventing attacks.

Amyloidosis

Amyloidosis is the name given to a group of acquired and hereditary disorders characterised by the extracellular deposition of insoluble proteins.

Pathophysiology

Amyloidosis is caused by deposits consisting of fibrils of the specific protein involved, linked to glycosaminoglycans, proteoglycans and serum amyloid P. Protein accumulation may be localised or systemic, and the clinical manifestations depend on the organ(s) affected. Amyloid diseases are classified by the aetiology and type of protein deposited (Box 4.18).

Clinical features

The clinical presentation may be with nephrotic syndrome (p. 395), cardiomyopathy (p. 538) or peripheral neuropathy (p. 1138). Amyloidosis should always be considered as a potential diagnosis in patients with these disorders when the cause is unclear.

Investigations

The diagnosis is established by biopsy, which may be of an affected organ, rectum or subcutaneous fat. The pathognomonic histological feature is apple-green birefringence of amyloid deposits when stained with Congo red dye and viewed under polarised light. Immunohistochemical staining can identify the type of amyloid fibril present. Quantitative scintigraphy with radiolabelled serum amyloid P is a valuable tool in determining the overall load and distribution of amyloid deposits.

Management

The aims of treatment are to support the function of affected organs and, in acquired amyloidosis, to prevent further amyloid deposition through treatment of the primary cause. When the latter is possible, regression of existing amyloid deposits may occur.

Autoimmune disease

Autoimmunity can be defined as the presence of immune responses against self-tissue. This may be a harmless phenomenon, identified

i 4.18 Causes of amyloidosis

Disorder	Pathological basis	Predisposing conditions	Other features
Acquired systemic amyloidosis			
Reactive (AA) amyloidosis (p. 81)	Increased production of serum amyloid A as part of prolonged or recurrent acute inflammatory response	Chronic infection (tuberculosis, bronchiectasis, chronic abscess, osteomyelitis) Chronic inflammatory diseases (untreated rheumatoid arthritis, familial Mediterranean fever)	90% of patients present with non-selective proteinuria or nephrotic syndrome
Light chain amyloidosis (AL)	Increased production of monoclonal light chain	Monoclonal gammopathies, including myeloma, benign gammopathies and plasmacytoma	Restrictive cardiomyopathy, peripheral and autonomic neuropathy, carpal tunnel syndrome, proteinuria, spontaneous purpura, amyloid nodules and plaques Macroglossia occurs rarely but is pathognomonic Prognosis is poor
Dialysis-associated ($A\beta_2M$) amyloidosis	Accumulation of circulating β_2-microglobulin due to failure of renal catabolism in kidney failure	Renal dialysis	Carpal tunnel syndrome, chronic arthropathy and pathological fractures secondary to amyloid bone cyst formation Manifestations occur 5–10 years after the start of dialysis
Senile systemic amyloidosis	Normal transthyretin protein deposited in tissues	Age >70 years	Feature of normal ageing (affects >90% of 90-year-olds) Usually asymptomatic
Hereditary systemic amyloidosis			
>20 forms of hereditary systemic amyloidosis	Production of protein with an abnormal structure that predisposes to amyloid fibril formation. Most commonly due to mutations in *transthyretin* gene	Autosomal dominant inheritance	Peripheral and autonomic neuropathy, cardiomyopathy Renal involvement unusual 10% of gene carriers are asymptomatic throughout life

only by the presence of low-titre autoantibodies or autoreactive T cells. However, if these responses cause significant organ damage, autoimmune diseases occur. These are a major cause of chronic morbidity and disability, affecting up to 1 in 30 adults at some point during life.

Pathophysiology

Autoimmune diseases result from the failure of immune tolerance, the process by which the immune system recognises and accepts self-tissue. Central immune tolerance occurs during lymphocyte development, when T and B lymphocytes that recognise self-antigens are eliminated before they develop into fully immunocompetent cells. This process is most active in fetal life but continues throughout life as immature lymphocytes are generated. Some autoreactive cells inevitably evade deletion and escape into the circulation, however, and are controlled through peripheral tolerance mechanisms. Peripheral immune tolerance mechanisms include the suppression of autoreactive cells by regulatory T cells; the generation of functional hyporesponsiveness (anergy) in lymphocytes that encounter antigen in the absence of the co-stimulatory signals that accompany inflammation; and cell death by apoptosis. Autoimmune diseases develop when self-reactive lymphocytes escape from these tolerance mechanisms.

Multiple genetic and environmental factors contribute to the development of autoimmune disease. Autoimmune diseases are much more common in women than in men, for reasons that remain unclear. Many are associated with genetic variations in the HLA loci, reflecting the importance of HLA genes in shaping lymphocyte responses. Other important susceptibility genes include

i 4.19 Association of specific gene polymorphisms with autoimmune diseases

Gene	Function	Diseases
HLA complex	Key determinants of antigen presentation to T cells	Most autoimmune diseases
PTPN22	Regulation of T- and B-cell receptor signalling	Rheumatoid arthritis, type 1 diabetes, systemic lupus erythematosus
CTLA4	Important co-stimulatory molecule that transmits inhibitory signals to T cells	Rheumatoid arthritis, type 1 diabetes
IL23R	Cytokine-mediated control of T cells	Inflammatory bowel disease, psoriasis, ankylosing spondylitis
TNFRSF1A	Control of tumour necrosis factor network	Multiple sclerosis
ATG5	Autophagy	Systemic lupus erythematosus

those determining cytokine activity, co-stimulation (the expression of second signals required for full T-cell activation; see Fig. 4.7) and cell death. Many of the same gene variants underlie multiple autoimmune disorders, reflecting their common pathogenesis (Box 4.19). Even though some of these associations are the strongest that have been identified in complex genetic diseases, they have very limited predictive value and are generally not useful in determining management of individual patients. Several environmental factors may be associated with autoimmunity in genetically predisposed individuals, including infection, cigarette smoking and hormone levels. The most widely studied of these is infection, as occurs in acute rheumatic fever following streptococcal infection or reactive arthritis following bacterial infection. Several mechanisms have been invoked to explain the autoimmunity that occurs after an infectious trigger. These include cross-reactivity between proteins expressed by the pathogen and the host (molecular mimicry), such as Guillain–Barré syndrome and *Campylobacter* infection (p. 1140); release of sequestered antigens from tissues that are damaged during infections that are not usually visible to the immune system; and production of inflammatory cytokines that overwhelm the normal control mechanisms that prevent bystander damage. Occasionally, autoimmune disease may be an adverse effect of drug treatment. For example, metabolic products of the anaesthetic agent halothane can bind to liver enzymes, resulting in a structurally novel protein that is recognised as a foreign antigen by the immune system. This can provoke the development of autoantibodies and activated T cells, which can cause hepatic necrosis.

Clinical features

The clinical presentation of autoimmune disease is highly variable. Autoimmune diseases can be classified by organ involvement or by the predominant mechanism responsible for tissue damage. The Gell and Coombs classification of hypersensitivity is the most widely used, and distinguishes four types of immune response that result in tissue damage (Box 4.20).

- *Type I hypersensitivity* is relevant in allergy but is not associated with autoimmune disease.
- *Type II hypersensitivity* causes injury to a single tissue or organ and is mediated by specific autoantibodies.
- *Type III hypersensitivity* results from deposition of immune complexes, which initiates activation of the classical complement cascade, as well as recruitment and activation of phagocytes and CD4+ lymphocytes. The site of immune complex deposition is determined by the relative amount of antibody, size of the immune complexes, nature of the antigen and local haemodynamics. Generalised deposition of immune complexes gives rise to systemic diseases such as SLE.
- *Type IV hypersensitivity* is mediated by activated T cells and macrophages, which together cause tissue damage.

Investigations

Autoantibodies

Many autoantibodies have been identified and are used in the diagnosis and monitoring of autoimmune diseases, as discussed elsewhere in this book. Antibodies can be quantified either by titre (the maximum dilution of the serum at which the antibody can be detected) or by concentration in standardised units using an enzyme-linked immunosorbent assay (ELISA) in which the antigen is used to coat microtitre plates to which the patient's serum is added (Fig. 4.13A). Qualitative tests are also employed for antinuclear antibodies in which the pattern of nuclear staining is recorded (Fig. 4.13B).

Fig. 4.13 Autoantibody testing. **A** Measurement of antibody levels by enzyme-linked immunosorbent assay (ELISA). The antigen of interest is used to coat microtitre plates to which patient serum is added. If autoantibodies are present, these bind to the target antigen on the microtitre plate. The amount of bound antibody is quantitated by adding a secondary antibody linked to an enzyme that converts a colourless substrate to a coloured one, which can be detected by a plate reader. **B** Qualitative analysis of autoantibodies by patterns of nuclear staining. In this assay, patient serum is added to cultured cells and a secondary antibody is added with a fluorescent label to detect any bound antibody. If antinuclear antibodies are present, they are detected as bright green staining. Different antinuclear antibody patterns may be seen in different types of connective tissue disease (Ch. 24). *B (Nucleolar and Homogenous), Courtesy of Juliet Dunphy, Biomedical Scientist, Royal United Hospital Bath, previously of Bath Institute of Rheumatic Diseases, UK; (Speckled), Courtesy of Mr Richard Brown, Clinical Scientist in Immunology, Southwest Pathology Services, UK.*

i 4.20 Gell and Coombs classification of hypersensitivity diseases

Type	Mechanism	Example of disease in response to exogenous agent	Example of autoimmune disease
Type I Immediate hypersensitivity	IgE-mediated mast cell degranulation	Allergic disease	None described
Type II Antibody-mediated	Binding of cytotoxic IgG or IgM antibodies to antigens on cell surface causes cell killing	ABO blood transfusion reaction Hyperacute transplant rejection	Autoimmune haemolytic anaemia Idiopathic thrombocytopenic purpura Goodpasture's disease
Type III Immune complex-mediated	IgG or IgM antibodies bind soluble antigen to form immune complexes that trigger classical complement pathway activation	Serum sickness Farmer's lung	Systemic lupus erythematosus Cryoglobulinaemia
Type IV Delayed type	Activated T cells, and phagocytes	Acute cellular transplant rejection Nickel hypersensitivity	Type 1 diabetes Hashimoto's thyroiditis

	4.21 Classification of cryoglobulins		
	Type I	**Type II**	**Type III**
Immunoglobulin (Ig) isotype and specificity	Isolated monoclonal IgM paraprotein with no particular specificity	Immune complexes formed by monoclonal IgM paraprotein directed towards constant region of IgG	Immune complexes formed by polyclonal IgM or IgG directed towards constant region of IgG
Prevalence	25%	25%	50%
Disease association	Lymphoproliferative disease, especially Waldenström macroglobulinaemia (p. 966)	Infection, particularly hepatitis C; lymphoproliferative disease	Infection, particularly hepatitis C; autoimmune disease, including rheumatoid arthritis and systemic lupus erythematosus
Symptoms	*Hyperviscosity:* Raynaud's phenomenon Acrocyanosis Retinal vessel occlusion Arterial and venous thrombosis	*Small-vessel vasculitis:* Purpuric rash Arthralgia Neuropathy Cutaneous ulceration, hepatosplenomegaly, glomerulonephritis, Raynaud's phenomenon	*Small-vessel vasculitis:* Purpuric rash, arthralgia Cutaneous ulceration Hepatosplenomegaly, glomerulonephritis Raynaud's phenomenon
Protein electrophoresis	Monoclonal IgM paraprotein	Monoclonal IgM paraprotein	No monoclonal paraprotein
Rheumatoid factor	Negative	Strongly positive	Strongly positive
Complement	Usually normal	Decreased C4	Decreased C4
Serum viscosity	Raised	Normal	Normal

Complement

Measurement of complement components can be useful in the evaluation of immune complex-mediated diseases. Classical complement pathway activation leads to a decrease in circulating C4 levels and is often also associated with decreased C3 levels. Serial measurement of C3 and C4 is a useful surrogate measure of disease activity in conditions such as SLE.

Cryoglobulins

Cryoglobulins are antibodies directed against other immunoglobulins, forming immune complexes that precipitate in the cold. They can lead to type III hypersensitivity reactions, with typical clinical manifestations including purpuric rash, often of the lower extremities, arthralgia and peripheral neuropathy. Cryoglobulins are classified into three types, depending on the properties of the immunoglobulin involved (Box 4.21). Testing for cryoglobulins requires the transport of a serum specimen to the laboratory at 37°C. Cryoglobulins should not be confused with cold agglutinins; the latter are autoantibodies specifically directed against the I/i antigen on the surface of red cells, which can cause intravascular haemolysis in the cold (p. 950).

Management

The management of autoimmune disease depends on the organ system involved and further details are provided elsewhere in this book. In general, treatment of autoimmune diseases involves the use of glucocorticoids and immunosuppressive agents, which are increasingly used in combination with biologic agents targeting disease-specific cytokines and their receptors. Not all conditions require immune suppression, however. For example, the management of coeliac disease involves dietary gluten withdrawal, while autoimmune hypothyroidism requires appropriate thyroxine supplementation.

Allergy

Allergic diseases are a common and increasing cause of illness, affecting between 15% and 20% of the population at some time.

They comprise a range of disorders from mild to life-threatening and affect many organs. Atopy is the tendency to produce an exaggerated IgE immune response to otherwise harmless environmental substances, while an allergic disease can be defined as the clinical manifestation of this inappropriate IgE immune response.

Pathophysiology

The immune system does not normally respond to the many environmental substances to which it is exposed on a daily basis. In allergic individuals, however, an initial exposure to a normally harmless exogenous substance (known as an allergen) triggers the production of specific IgE antibodies by activated B cells. These bind to high-affinity IgE receptors on the surface of mast cells, a step that is not itself associated with clinical sequelae. However, re-exposure to the allergen binds to and cross-links membrane-bound IgE, which activates the mast cells, releasing a variety of vasoactive mediators (the early phase response; Fig. 4.14 and see Box 4.9). This type I hypersensitivity reaction forms the basis of an allergic reaction, which can range from sneezing and rhinorrhoea to anaphylaxis (Box 4.22). In some individuals, the early phase response is followed by persistent activation of mast cells, manifest by ongoing swelling and local inflammation. This is known as the late phase reaction and is mediated by mast cell metabolites, basophils, eosinophils and macrophages. Long-standing or recurrent allergic inflammation may give rise to a chronic inflammatory response characterised by a complex infiltrate of macrophages, eosinophils and T lymphocytes, in addition to mast cells and basophils. Once this has been established, inhibition of mast cell mediators with antihistamines is clinically ineffective in isolation. Mast cell activation may also be non-specifically triggered through other signals, such as neuropeptides, anaphylotoxins and bacterial peptides.

The increasing incidence of allergic diseases is largely unexplained but one widely held theory is the 'hygiene hypothesis'. This proposes that infections in early life are critically important in maturation of the immune response and bias the immune system against the development of allergies; the high prevalence

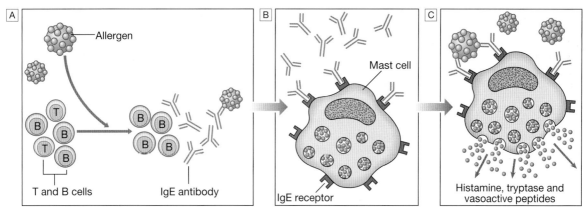

Fig. 4.14 Type I (immediate) hypersensitivity response. [A] After an encounter with allergen, B cells produce immunoglobulin E (IgE) antibody against the allergen. [B] Specific IgE antibodies bind to circulating mast cells via high-affinity IgE cell surface receptors. [C] On re-encounter with allergen, the allergen binds to the IgE antibody-coated mast cells. This cross-linking of the IgE triggers mast cell activation with release of vasoactive mediators (see Box 4.9).

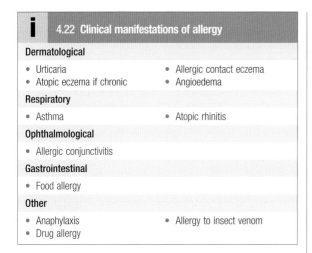

i 4.22 Clinical manifestations of allergy	
Dermatological	
• Urticaria	• Allergic contact eczema
• Atopic eczema if chronic	• Angioedema
Respiratory	
• Asthma	• Atopic rhinitis
Ophthalmological	
• Allergic conjunctivitis	
Gastrointestinal	
• Food allergy	
Other	
• Anaphylaxis	• Allergy to insect venom
• Drug allergy	

of allergic disease is the penalty for the decreased exposure to infection that has resulted from improvements in sanitation and health care. Genetic factors also contribute strongly to the development of allergic diseases. A positive family history is common in patients with allergy, and genetic association studies have identified a wide variety of predisposing variants in genes controlling innate immune responses, cytokine production, IgE levels and the ability of the epithelial barrier to protect against environmental agents. The expression of a genetic predisposition is complex; it is governed by environmental factors, such as pollutants and cigarette smoke, and the incidence of bacterial and viral infection.

Clinical features

Common presentations of allergic disease are shown in Box 4.22. Those that affect the respiratory system and skin are discussed in more detail in Chapters 17 and 29, respectively. Here we focus on general principles of the approach to the allergic patient, some specific allergies and anaphylaxis.

Insect venom allergy

Local non-IgE-mediated reactions to insect stings are common and may cause extensive swelling around the site lasting up to 7 days. These usually do not require specific treatment. Toxic reactions to venom after multiple (50–100) simultaneous stings may mimic anaphylaxis. In addition, exposure to large amounts

of insect venom frequently stimulates the production of IgE antibodies, and thus may be followed by allergic reactions to single stings. Allergic IgE-mediated reactions vary from mild to life-threatening. Antigen-specific immunotherapy (desensitisation; see below) with bee or wasp venom can reduce the incidence of recurrent anaphylaxis from 50–60% to approximately 10% but requires up to 5 years of treatment.

Peanut allergy

Peanut allergy is the most common food-related allergy. More than 50% of patients present before the age of 3 years and some individuals react to their first known exposure to peanuts, thought to result from sensitisation to arachis oil in topical creams. Peanuts are ubiquitous in the Western diet, and every year up to 25% of peanut-allergic individuals experience a reaction as a result of inadvertent exposure.

Birch oral allergy syndrome

This syndrome is characterised by the combination of birch pollen hay fever and local oral symptoms, including itch and angioedema, after contact with certain raw fruits, raw vegetables and nuts. Cooked fruits and vegetables are tolerated without difficulty. It is due to shared or cross-reactive allergens that are destroyed by cooking or digestion, and can be confirmed by skin prick testing using fresh fruit. Severe allergic reactions are unusual.

Diagnosis

When assessing a patient with a complaint of allergy, it is important to identify what the patient means by the term, as up to 20% of the UK population describe themselves as having a food allergy; in fact, less than 1% have true allergy, as defined by an IgE-mediated hypersensitivity reaction confirmed on double-blind challenge. The nature of the symptoms should be established and specific triggers identified, along with the predictability of a reaction, and the time lag between exposure to a potential allergen and onset of symptoms. An allergic reaction usually occurs within minutes of exposure and provokes predictable, reproducible symptoms such as angioedema, urticaria and wheezing. Specific enquiry should be made about other allergic symptoms, past and present, and about a family history of allergic disease. Potential allergens in the home and workplace should be identified. A detailed drug history should always be taken, including details of adherence to medication, possible adverse effects and the use of over-the-counter or complementary therapies.

Investigations

Skin-prick tests

Skin-prick testing is a key investigation in the assessment of patients suspected of having allergy. A droplet of diluted standardised allergen is placed on the forearm and the skin is superficially punctured through the droplet with a sterile lancet. Positive and negative control material must be included in the assessment. After 15 minutes, a positive response is indicated by a local weal and flare response 2 mm or more larger than the negative control. A major advantage of skin-prick testing is that patient can clearly see the results, which may be useful in gaining adherence to avoidance measures. Disadvantages include the remote risk of a severe allergic reaction, so resuscitation facilities should be available. Results are unreliable in patients with extensive skin disease. Antihistamines inhibit the magnitude of the response and should be discontinued for at least 3 days before testing; low-dose glucocorticoids do not influence test results. A number of other prescribed medicines can also lead to false-negative results, including amitriptyline and risperidone.

Specific IgE tests

An alternative to skin-prick testing is the quantitation of IgE directed against the suspected allergen. The sensitivity and specificity of specific IgE tests (previously known as radioallergosorbent tests, RAST) are lower than those of skin-prick tests. However, IgE tests may be very useful if skin testing is inappropriate, such as in patients taking antihistamines or those with severe skin disease or dermatographism. They can also be used to test for cross-reactivity – for example, with multiple insect venoms, where component-resolved diagnostics, using recombinant allergens, is increasingly used rather than crude allergen extract. Specific IgE tests can also be used post-mortem to identify allergens responsible for lethal anaphylaxis.

Supervised exposure to allergen

Tests involving supervised exposure to an allergen (allergen challenge) are usually performed in specialist centres on carefully selected patients, and include bronchial provocation testing, nasal challenge, and food or drug challenge. These may be particularly useful in the investigation of occupational asthma or food allergy. Patients can be considered for challenge testing when skin tests and/or IgE tests are negative, as they can be helpful in ruling out allergic disease.

Mast cell tryptase

Measurement of serum mast cell tryptase is extremely useful in investigating a possible anaphylactic event. Ideally, measurements should be made at the time of the reaction following appropriate resuscitation, and 3 hours and 24 hours later. The basis of the test is the fact that circulating levels of mast cell degranulation products rise dramatically to peak 1–2 hours after a systemic allergic reaction. Tryptase is the most stable of these and is easily measured in serum.

Serum total IgE

Serum total IgE measurements are not routinely indicated in the investigation of allergic disease, other than to aid in the interpretation of specific IgE results, as false-positive specific IgEs are common in patients with atopy, who often have a high total IgE level. Although atopy is the most common cause of an elevated total IgE in developed countries, there are many other causes, including parasitic and helminth infections (pp. 299 and 288), lymphoma (p. 961), drug reactions and eosinophilic granulomatosis with polyangiitis (previously known as Churg–Strauss vasculitis; p. 1043). Normal total IgE levels do not exclude allergic disease.

Eosinophilia

Peripheral blood eosinophilia is common in atopic individuals but lacks specificity. Eosinophilia of more than 20% or an absolute eosinophil count over 1.5×10^9/L should initiate a search for a non-atopic cause, such as eosinophilic granulomatosis with polyangiitis or parasitic infection (p. 928).

Management

Several approaches can be deployed in the management of allergic individuals, as discussed below.

Avoidance of the allergen

This is indicated in all cases and should be rigorously attempted, with the advice of specialist dietitians and occupational physicians if necessary.

Antihistamines

Antihistamines are useful in the management of allergy as they inhibit the effects of histamine on tissue H_1 receptors. Long-acting, non-sedating preparations are particularly useful for prophylaxis.

Glucocorticoids

These are highly effective in allergic disease, and if used topically, adverse effects can be minimised.

Sodium cromoglicate

Sodium cromoglicate stabilises the mast cell membrane, inhibiting release of vasoactive mediators. It is effective as a prophylactic agent in asthma and allergic rhinitis but has no role in management of acute attacks. It is poorly absorbed and therefore ineffective in the management of food allergies.

Antigen-specific immunotherapy

This involves the sequential administration of increasing doses of allergen extract over a prolonged period of time. The mechanism of action is not fully understood but it is highly effective in the prevention of insect venom anaphylaxis and of allergic rhinitis secondary to grass pollen. The traditional route of administration is by subcutaneous injection, which carries a risk of anaphylaxis and should be performed only in specialised centres. Sublingual immunotherapy is also increasingly used. Clinical studies to date do not support the use of allergen immunotherapy for food hypersensitivity, although this is an area of active investigation.

Omalizumab

Omalizumab is a monoclonal antibody directed against IgE; it inhibits the binding of IgE to mast cells and basophils. It is licensed for treatment of refractory chronic spontaneous urticaria and also for severe persistent allergic asthma that has failed to respond to standard therapy (p. 572). The dose and frequency are determined by baseline IgE (measured before the start of treatment) and body weight. It is under investigation for allergic rhinitis but not yet approved for this indication.

Adrenaline (epinephrine)

Adrenaline given by injection in the form of a pre-loaded self-injectable device can be life-saving in the acute management of anaphylaxis (see Box 4.12).

Angioedema

Angioedema is an episodic, localised, non-pitting swelling of submucous or subcutaneous tissues.

Pathophysiology

The causes of angioedema are summarised in Box 4.23. It may be a manifestation of allergy or non-allergic degranulation of mast cells in response to drugs and toxins. In these conditions the main cause is mast cell degranulation with release of histamine and other vasoactive mediators. In hereditary angioedema, the cause is C1 inhibitor deficiency, which causes increased local release of bradykinin. Angiotensin-converting enzyme (ACE) inhibitor-induced angioedema also occurs as the result of increased bradykinin levels due to inhibition of its breakdown.

Clinical features

Angioedema is characterised by soft-tissue swelling that most frequently affects the face (Fig. 4.15) but can also affect the extremities and genitalia. Involvement of the larynx or tongue may cause life-threatening respiratory tract obstruction, and oedema of the intestinal mucosa may cause abdominal pain and distension.

Investigations

Differentiating the mechanism of angioedema is important in determining the most appropriate treatment. A clinical history of allergy or drug exposure can give clues to the underlying diagnosis. If no obvious trigger can be identified, measurement of complement C4 is useful in differentiating hereditary and acquired angioedema from other causes. If C4 levels are low, further investigations should be initiated to look for evidence of C1 inhibitor deficiency.

Management

Management depends on the underlying cause. Angioedema associated with allergen exposure generally responds to antihistamines and glucocorticoids. Following acute management of angioedema secondary to drug therapy, drug withdrawal

Fig. 4.15 Angioedema. This young man has hereditary angioedema. **A** Normal appearance. **B** During an acute attack. *From Helbert M. Flesh and bones of immunology. Edinburgh: Churchill Livingstone, Elsevier Ltd; 2006.*

i	**4.23 Types of angioedema**			
	Allergic reaction to specific trigger	**Idiopathic angioedema**	**Hereditary angioedema**	**ACE-inhibitor associated angioedema**
Pathogenesis	IgE-mediated degradation of mast cells	Non-IgE-mediated degranulation of mast cells	C1 inhibitor deficiency, with resulting increased local bradykinin concentration	Inhibition of breakdown of bradykinin
Key mediator	Histamine	Histamine	Bradykinin	Bradykinin
Prevalence	Common	Common	Rare autosomal dominant disorder	0.1–0.2% of patients treated with ACE inhibitors
Clinical features	Usually associated with urticaria History of other allergies common Follows exposure to specific allergen, in food, animal dander or insect venom	Usually associated with urticaria May be triggered by physical stimuli such as heat, pressure or exercise Dermatographism common Occasionally associated with underlying infection or thyroid disease	Not associated with urticaria or other features of allergy Does not cause anaphylaxis May cause life-threatening respiratory tract obstruction Can cause severe abdominal pain	Not associated with urticaria Does not cause anaphylaxis Usually affects the head and neck, and may cause life-threatening respiratory tract obstruction Can occur years after the start of treatment
Investigations	Specific IgE tests or skin-prick tests	Specific IgE tests and skin-prick tests often negative Hypothyroidism should be excluded	Complement C4 (invariably low in acute attacks) C1 inhibitor levels	No specific investigations
Treatment	Allergen avoidance Antihistamines	Antihistamines are mainstay of treatment and prophylaxis	Unresponsive to antihistamines Anabolic steroids C1 inhibitor concentrate or icatibant for acute attacks	ACE inhibitor should be discontinued ARBs should be avoided if possible unless there is a strong indication
Associated drug reactions	Specific drug allergies	NSAIDs Opioids, radiocontrast media		ACE inhibitors, ARBs

(ACE = angiotensin-converting enzyme; ARBs = angiotensin II receptor blockers; NSAIDs = non-steroidal anti-inflammatory drugs)

should prevent further attacks, although ACE inhibitor-induced angioedema can continue for a limited period post drug withdrawal. Management of angioedema associated with C1 inhibitor deficiency is discussed below.

Hereditary angioedema

Hereditary angioedema (HAE), also known as inherited C1 inhibitor deficiency, is an autosomal dominant disorder caused by decreased production or activity of C1 inhibitor protein. This complement regulatory protein inhibits spontaneous activation of the classical complement pathway (see Fig. 4.4). It also acts as an inhibitor of the kinin cascade, activation of which increases local bradykinin levels, giving rise to local pain and swelling.

Clinical features

The angioedema in HAE may be spontaneous or triggered by local trauma or infection. Multiple parts of the body may be involved, especially the face, extremities, upper airway and gastrointestinal tract. Oedema of the intestinal wall causes severe abdominal pain and many patients with undiagnosed HAE undergo exploratory laparotomy. The most important complication is laryngeal obstruction, often associated with minor dental procedures, which can be fatal. Episodes of angioedema are self-limiting and usually resolve within 48 hours. Patients with HAE generally present in adolescence but may go undiagnosed for many years. A family history can be identified in 80% of cases. HAE is not associated with allergic diseases and is specifically not associated with urticaria.

Investigations

Acute episodes are accompanied by low C4 levels; a low C4 during an episode of angioedema should therefore trigger further investigation. The diagnosis can be confirmed by measurement of C1 inhibitor levels and function.

Management

Severe acute attacks should be treated with purified C1 inhibitor concentrate or the bradykinin receptor antagonist icatibant. Anabolic steroids, such as danazol, can be used to prevent attacks and act by increasing endogenous production of complement proteins. Tranexamic acid can be helpful as prophylaxis in some patients. Patients can be taught to self-administer therapy and should be advised to carry a MedicAlert or similar.

Acquired C1 inhibitor deficiency

This rare disorder is clinically indistinguishable from HAE but presents in late adulthood. It is associated with autoimmune and lymphoproliferative diseases. Most cases are due to the

4.24 Immunological diseases in pregnancy

Allergic disease

- **Maternal dietary restrictions during pregnancy or lactation**: current evidence does not support these for prevention of allergic disease.
- **Breastfeeding for at least 4 months**: prevents or delays the occurrence of atopic dermatitis, cow's milk allergy and wheezing in early childhood, as compared with feeding formula milk containing intact cow's milk protein.

Autoimmune disease

- **Suppressed T-cell-mediated immune responses in pregnancy**: may suddenly reactivate post-partum. Some autoimmune diseases may improve during pregnancy but flare immediately after delivery. Systemic lupus erythematosus (SLE) is an exception, however, as it is prone to exacerbation in pregnancy or the puerperium.
- **Passive transfer of maternal antibodies**: can mediate autoimmune disease in the fetus and newborn, including SLE, Graves' disease and myasthenia gravis.
- **Antiphospholipid syndrome** (p. 977): an important cause of fetal loss, intrauterine growth restriction and pre-eclampsia.
- **HIV in pregnancy**: see p. 326.

development of autoantibodies to C1 inhibitor, but the condition can also be caused by autoantibodies that activate C1. Treatment of the underlying disorder may induce remission of angioedema. As with HAE, a low C4 is seen during acute episodes.

Transplantation and graft rejection

Transplantation provides the opportunity for definitive treatment of end-stage organ disease. The major complications are graft rejection, drug toxicity and infection consequent to immunosuppression. Transplant survival continues to improve, as a result of the introduction of less toxic immunosuppressive agents and increased understanding of the processes of transplant rejection. Stem cell transplantation and its complications are discussed on page 936.

Transplant rejection

Solid organ transplantation inevitably stimulates an aggressive immune response by the recipient, unless the transplant is between monozygotic twins. The type and severity of the rejection response is determined by the genetic disparity between the donor and recipient, the immune status of the host and the nature of the tissue transplanted (Box 4.25). The most important genetic determinant

i 4.25 Classification of transplant rejection

Type	Time	Pathological findings	Mechanism	Treatment
Hyperacute rejection	Minutes to hours	Thrombosis, necrosis	Pre-formed antibody to donor antigens results in complement activation (type II hypersensitivity)	None – irreversible graft loss
Acute cellular rejection	5–30 days	Cellular infiltration	CD4+ and CD8+ T cells (type IV hypersensitivity)	Increase immunosuppression
Acute vascular rejection	5–30 days	Vasculitis	Antibody and complement activation	Increase immunosuppression
Chronic allograft failure	>30 days	Fibrosis, scarring	Immune and non-immune mechanisms	Minimise drug toxicity, control hypertension and hyperlipidaemia

is the difference between donor and recipient HLA proteins (p. 67). The extensive polymorphism of these proteins means that donor HLA antigens are almost invariably recognised as foreign by the recipient immune system, unless an active attempt has been made to minimise incompatibility.

- *Hyperacute rejection* results in rapid and irreversible destruction of the graft (Box 4.25). It is mediated by pre-existing recipient antibodies against donor HLA antigens, which arise as a result of previous exposure through transplantation, blood transfusion or pregnancy. It is very rarely seen in clinical practice, as the use of screening for anti-HLA antibodies and pre-transplant cross-matching ensures the prior identification of recipient–donor incompatibility.
- *Acute cellular rejection* is the most common form of graft rejection. It is mediated by activated T lymphocytes and results in deterioration in graft function. If allowed to progress, it may cause fever, pain and tenderness over the graft. It is usually amenable to increased immunosuppressive therapy.
- *Acute vascular rejection* is mediated by antibody formed de novo after transplantation. It is more curtailed than the hyperacute response because of the use of intercurrent immunosuppression but it is also associated with reduced graft survival. Aggressive immunosuppressive therapy is indicated and physical removal of antibody through plasmapheresis may be indicated in severe causes. Not all post-transplant anti-donor antibodies cause graft damage; their consequences are determined by specificity and ability to trigger other immune components, such as the complement cascade.
- *Chronic allograft failure*, also known as chronic rejection, is a major cause of graft loss. It is associated with proliferation of transplant vascular smooth muscle, interstitial fibrosis and scarring. The pathogenesis is poorly understood but contributing factors include immunological damage caused by subacute rejection, hypertension, hyperlipidaemia and chronic drug toxicity.

Investigations

Pre-transplantation testing

HLA typing determines an individual's HLA polymorphisms and facilitates donor–recipient matching. Potential transplant recipients are also screened for the presence of anti-HLA antibodies. The recipient is excluded from receiving a transplant that carries these alleles.

Donor–recipient cross-matching is a functional assay that directly tests whether serum from a recipient (which potentially contains anti-donor antibodies) is able to bind and/or kill donor lymphocytes. It is specific to a prospective donor–recipient pair and is done immediately prior to transplantation. A positive cross-match is a contraindication to transplantation because of the risk of hyperacute rejection.

Post-transplant biopsy: C4d staining

C4d is a fragment of the complement protein C4 (see Fig. 4.4). Deposition of C4d in graft capillaries indicates local activation of the classical complement pathway and provides evidence of antibody-mediated damage. This is useful in the early diagnosis of vascular rejection.

Complications of transplant immunosuppression

Transplant recipients require indefinite treatment with immunosuppressive agents. In general, two or more immunosuppressive drugs are used in synergistic combination in order to minimise adverse effects (Box 4.26). The major complications of long-term immunosuppression are infection and malignancy. The risk of some opportunistic infections may be minimised through the use of prophylactic medication, such as ganciclovir for cytomegalovirus prophylaxis and trimethoprim–sulfamethoxazole for *Pneumocystis* prophylaxis. Immunisation with killed vaccines is appropriate, although the immune response may be curtailed. Live vaccines should not be given.

i 4.26 Immunosuppressive drugs used in transplantation

Drug	Mechanism of action	Major adverse effects
Anti-proliferative agents Azathioprine, mycophenolate mofetil	Inhibit lymphocyte proliferation by blocking DNA synthesis May be directly cytotoxic at high doses	Increased susceptibility to infection Leucopenia Hepatotoxicity
Calcineurin inhibitors Ciclosporin, tacrolimus	Inhibit T-cell signalling; prevent lymphocyte activation; block cytokine transcription	Increased susceptibility to infection Hypertension Nephrotoxicity Diabetogenic (especially tacrolimus) Gingival hypertrophy, hirsutism (ciclosporin)
Glucocorticoids	Decrease phagocytosis and release of proteolytic enzymes; decrease lymphocyte activation and proliferation; decrease cytokine production; decrease antibody production	Increased susceptibility to infection Multiple other complications (p. 670)
Anti-thymocyte globulin (ATG)	Antibodies to cell surface proteins deplete or block T cells	Profound non-specific immunosuppression Increased susceptibility to infection
Basiliximab	Monoclonal antibody directed against CD25 (IL-2Rα chain), expressed on activated T cells	Increased susceptibility to infection Gastrointestinal side-effects
Belatacept	Selectively inhibits T-cell activation through blockade of CTLA4	Increased susceptibility to infection and malignancy Gastrointestinal side-effects Hypertension Anaemia/leucopenia

The increased risk of malignancy arises because T-cell suppression results in failure to control viral infections associated with malignant transformation. Virus-associated tumours include lymphoma (associated with Epstein–Barr virus), Kaposi's sarcoma (associated with human herpesvirus 8) and skin tumours (associated with human papillomavirus). Immunosuppression is also linked with a small increase in the incidence of common cancers not associated with viral infection (such as lung, breast and colon cancer), reflecting the importance of T cells in anti-cancer surveillance.

Organ donation

The major problem in transplantation is the shortage of organ donors. Cadaveric organ donors are usually previously healthy individuals who experience brainstem death (p. 211), frequently as a result of road traffic accidents or cerebrovascular events. Even if organs were obtained from all potential cadaveric donors, though, their numbers would be insufficient to meet current needs. An alternative is the use of living donors. Altruistic living donation, usually from close relatives, is widely used in renal transplantation. Living organ donation is inevitably associated with some risk to the donor and it is highly regulated to ensure appropriate appreciation of the risks involved. Because of concerns about coercion and exploitation, non-altruistic organ donation (the sale of organs) is illegal in most countries.

Tumour immunology

Surveillance by the immune system is critically important in monitoring and removing damaged and mutated cells as they arise. The ability of the immune system to kill cancer cells effectively is influenced by tumour immunogenicity and specificity. Many cancer antigens are poorly expressed and specific antigens can mutate, either spontaneously or in response to treatment, which can result in evasion of immune responses. In addition, the inhibitory pathways that are used to maintain self-tolerance and limit collateral tissue damage during antimicrobial immune responses can be co-opted by cancerous cells to evade immune destruction. Recognition and understanding of these immune checkpoint pathways has led to the development of a number of new treatments for cancers that are otherwise refractory to treatment. For example, antibodies to CTLA4, a co-stimulatory molecule normally involved in down-regulation of immune responses, have been licensed for refractory melanoma, and antibodies to PD1 (programmed cell death protein 1) are used in melanoma, non-small-cell lung cancer and renal cell carcinoma. Potential risks include the development of autoimmunity, reflecting the importance of these pathways in the control of self-tolerance.

Further information

allergy.org.au *An Australasian site providing information on allergy, asthma and immune diseases.*

allergyuk.org *UK site for patients and health-care professionals.*

anaphylaxis.org.uk *Provides information and support for patients with severe allergies.*

info4pi.org *A US site managed by the non-profit Jeffrey Modell Foundation, which provides extensive information about primary immune deficiencies.*

niaid.nih.gov *National Institute of Allergy and Infectious Diseases: provides useful information on a variety of allergic diseases, immune deficiency syndromes and autoimmune diseases.*

H Campbell
DA McAllister

5

Population health and epidemiology

Global burden of disease and underlying risk factors 92
Life expectancy 92
Global causes of death and disability 92
Risk factors underlying disease 93

Social determinants of health 93
The hierarchy of systems – from molecules to ecologies 93
The life course 93
Preventive medicine 93

Principles of screening 94

Epidemiology 95
Understanding causes and effect 95

Health data/informatics 97

The UK Faculty of Public Health defines public health as 'the science and art of promoting and protecting health and well-being, preventing ill-health and prolonging life through the organised efforts of society'. This definition recognises that there is a collective responsibility for the health of the population that requires partnerships between government, health services and others to promote and protect health and prevent disease. Population health has been defined as 'the health outcomes of a group of individuals, including the distribution of such outcomes within the group'. Medical doctors can play a role in all these efforts to improve health both through their clinical work and through their support of broader actions to improve public health.

Global burden of disease and underlying risk factors

The Global Burden of Disease (GBD) exercise was initiated by the World Bank in 1992, with first estimates appearing in 1993. Regular updated figures have been published since, together with projections of future disease burden. The aim was to produce reliable and internally consistent estimates of disease burden for all diseases and injuries, and to assess their physiological, behavioural and social risk factors, so that this information could be made available to health workers, researchers and policy-makers.

The GBD exercise adopted the metric 'disability adjusted life year' (DALY) to describe population health. This combines information about premature mortality in a population (measured as Years of Life Lost from an 'expected' life expectancy) and years of life lived with disability (Years of Life lived with Disability, which is weighted by a severity factor). The International Classification of Disease (ICD) rules, which assign one cause to each death, are followed. All estimates are presented by age and sex groups and by regions of the world. Many countries now also report their own national burden of disease data.

Life expectancy

Global life expectancy at birth increased from 61.7 years in 1980 to 71.8 years in 2015, an increase of 0.29 years per calendar year. This change is due to a substantial fall in child mortality (mainly caused by common infections), partly offset by rises in mortality from adult conditions such as diabetes and chronic kidney disease. Some areas have not shown these increases in life expectancy in men, often due to war and interpersonal violence.

Global causes of death and disability

Box 5.1 shows a ranked list of the major causes of global premature deaths in 2015. Communicable, maternal, neonatal and nutritional causes accounted for about one-quarter of deaths worldwide, down from about one-third in 1990. In contrast, deaths from non-communicable diseases are increasing in importance and now account for about two-thirds of all deaths globally, including about 13 million from ischaemic heart disease and stroke, and about 8 million from cancer. The age-standardised death rates for most diseases globally are falling. However, despite this, the numbers of deaths from many diseases are rising due to global population growth and the change in age structure of

---

i | **5.1 Global premature mortality: top 15 ranked causes, 2015[1,2]**

1. Ischaemic heart disease (4)
2. Cerebrovascular disease (5)
3. Lower respiratory infections (1)
4. Neonatal preterm birth complications (2)
5. Diarrhoeal diseases (3)
6. Neonatal encephalopathy (6)
7. HIV/AIDS (29)
8. Road injuries (10)
9. Malaria (7)
10. Chronic obstructive pulmonary disease (12)
11. Congenital anomalies (9)
12. Tuberculosis (11)
13. Lung cancer[3] (20)
14. Self-harm (16)
15. Diabetes (>30)

[1]By Years of Life Lost (YLL). [2]Rank in 1990 is shown in brackets. [3]'All cancers combined' would rank in the top three causes.

---

i | **5.2 Global disability: top 15 ranked causes, 2015[1,2]**

1. Lower back and neck pain (1)
2. Sense organ diseases (3)
3. Depressive disorders (4)
4. Iron deficiency anaemia (2)
5. Skin diseases (5)
6. Diabetes (9)
7. Migraine (6)
8. Other musculoskeletal conditions[3] (7)
9. Anxiety disorders (8)
10. Oral disorders (11)
11. Asthma (10)
12. Schizophrenia (13)
13. Osteoarthritis (19)
14. Chronic obstructive pulmonary disease (14)
15. Falls (12)

[1]By Years of Life lived with Disability (YLD). [2]Rank in 1990 is shown in brackets. [3]Not otherwise classified as specific conditions such as osteoarthritis.

---

the population to older ages, and this is placing an increasing burden on health systems. For a few conditions (e.g. HIV/AIDS, diabetes mellitus and chronic kidney disease), age-standardised death rates continue to rise. Within this overall pattern, significant regional variations exist: for example, communicable, maternal, neonatal and nutritional causes still account for about two-thirds of premature mortality in sub-Saharan Africa.

GBD also provides estimates of disability from disease (Box 5.2). This has raised awareness of the importance of conditions like depression, low back and neck pain, and asthma, which account for a relatively large disease burden but relatively few deaths. This, in turn, has resulted in greater health policy priority being given to these conditions. Since the policy focus in national health systems is increasingly on keeping people healthy rather than only on reducing premature deaths, it is important to have measures of these health outcomes.

It is also essential to recognise that, although these estimates represent the best overall picture of burden of disease, they are based on imperfect data. Nevertheless, the quality of data underlying the estimates and the modelling processes are

i 5.3 Global risk factors: top 15 ranked causes, 2015[1-3]

1. High blood pressure (3)
2. Smoking/second-hand smoke exposure (5)
3. High fasting blood glucose (10)
4. High body mass index (13)
5. Childhood underweight (1)
6. Ambient particulate matter pollution (6)
7. High total cholesterol (12)
8. Household air pollution (4)
9. Alcohol use (11)
10. High sodium intake (14)
11. Low wholegrain intake (15)
12. Unsafe sex (20)
13. Low fruit intake (16)
14. Unsafe water (2)
15. Low glomerular filtration rate (21)

[1]By percentage of burden of disease they cause. [2]Rank in 1990 is shown in brackets. [3]All dietary risk factors and physical inactivity combined accounted for 10% of global burden of disease. Low physical activity was ranked 21, iron deficiency 16 and suboptimal breastfeeding 22 in 2015.

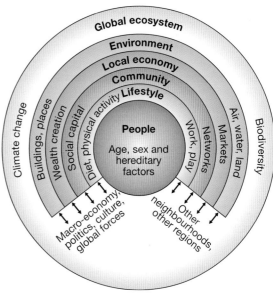

Fig. 5.1 Hierarchy of systems that influence population health.
Adapted from an original model by Whitehead M, Dahlgren G. What can be done about inequalities in health? Lancet 1991; 338:1059–1063.

improving over time and provide an increasingly robust basis for evidence-based health planning and priority setting.

Risk factors underlying disease

Box 5.3 shows a ranked list of the main risk factors that underlay GBD in 2015 and how this ranking has changed in recent years.

Social determinants of health

Health emerges from a highly complex interaction between a person's genetic background and environmental factors (aspects of the physical, biological (microbes), built and social environments, and also distant influences such as the global ecosystem; Fig. 5.1).

The hierarchy of systems – from molecules to ecologies

Influences on health exist at many levels and extend beyond the individual to include the family, community, population and ecology. Box 5.4 shows an example of this for determinants of coronary heart disease and demonstrates the importance of considering not only the disease process in a patient but also its context. Health care is not the only determinant – and is usually not the major determinant – of health status in the population. The concept of 'global health' recognises the global dimension of health problems, whether these be emerging or pandemic infections or global economic influences on health.

The life course

The determinants of health operate over the whole lifespan. Values and behaviours acquired during childhood and adolescence have a profound influence on educational outcomes, job prospects and risk of disease. These can have a strong influence, for example, on whether a young person takes up damaging behaviour like smoking, risky sexual activity and drug misuse. Influences on health can operate even before birth. Low birth weight can lead

i 5.4 'Hierarchy of systems' applied to ischaemic heart disease

Level in the hierarchy	Example of effect
Molecular	ApoB mutation causing hypercholesterolaemia
Cellular	Macrophage foam cells accumulate in vessel wall
Tissue	Atheroma and thrombosis of coronary artery
Organ	Ischaemia and infarction of myocardium
System	Cardiac failure
Person	Limited exercise capacity, impact on employment
Family	Passive smoking, diet
Community	Shops and leisure opportunities
Population	Prevalence of obesity
Society	Policies on smoking, screening for risk factors
Ecology	Agriculture influencing fat content in diet

to higher risk of hypertension and type 2 diabetes in young adults, and of cardiovascular disease in middle age. It has been suggested that under-nutrition during middle to late gestation permanently 'programs' cardiovascular and metabolic responses. This 'life course' perspective highlights the cumulative effect on health of exposures to illness, adverse environmental conditions and behaviours that damage health.

Preventive medicine

The complexity of interactions between physical, social and economic determinants of health means successful prevention is often difficult. Moreover, the life-course perspective illustrates that it may be necessary to intervene early in life or even before birth, to prevent important disease later. Successful prevention is likely to require many interventions across the life course and at several levels in the hierarchy of systems. The examples below illustrate this.

Alcohol

Alcohol use is an increasingly important risk factor underlying GBD (see Box 5.3). Reasons for increasing rates of alcohol-related harm vary by place and time but include the falling price of alcohol (in real terms), increased availability and cultural change fostering higher levels of consumption. Public, professional and governmental concern has now led to a minimum price being charged for a unit of alcohol, tightening of licensing regulations and curtailment of some promotional activity in many countries. However, even more aggressive public health measures will be needed to reverse the levels of harm in the population. The approach for individual patients suffering adverse effects of alcohol is described elsewhere (e.g. pp. 1184 and 880).

Smoking

Smoking is one of the top three risk factors underlying GBD (see Box 5.3). It is responsible for a substantial majority of cases of chronic obstructive pulmonary disease (COPD) and lung cancer (pp. 573 and 598), and most smokers die either from these or from ischaemic heart disease. Smoking also causes cancers of the upper respiratory and gastrointestinal tracts, pancreas, bladder and kidney, and increases risks of peripheral vascular disease, stroke and peptic ulceration. Maternal smoking is an important cause of fetal growth retardation. Moreover, there is evidence that passive ('second-hand') smoking has adverse effects on cardiovascular and respiratory health.

The decline in smoking in many high-income countries has been achieved not only by warning people of the health risks but also by increasing taxation of tobacco, banning advertising, legislating against smoking in public places and giving support for smoking cessation to maintain this decline. However, smoking rates remain high in many poorer areas and are increasing among young women. In many developing countries, tobacco companies have found new markets and rates are rising.

A complex hierarchy of systems interacts to cause smokers to initiate and maintain their habit. At the molecular and cellular levels, nicotine acts on the nervous system to create dependence and maintain the smoking habit. There are also strong influences at the personal and social level, such as young female smokers being motivated to 'stay thin' or 'look cool' and peer pressure. Other important influences include cigarette advertising, with the advertising budget of the tobacco industry being much greater than that of health services. Strategies to help individuals stop smoking (such as nicotine replacement therapy, anti-smoking advice and behavioural support) are cost-effective and form an important part of the overall strategy.

Obesity

Obesity is an increasingly important risk factor underlying GBD (see Box 5.3). The weight distribution of almost the whole population is shifting upwards: the slim are becoming less slim while the fat are getting fatter (p. 698). In the UK, this translates into a 1 kg increase in weight per adult per year (on average over the adult population). The current obesity epidemic cannot be explained simply by individual behaviour and poor choice but also requires an understanding of the obesogenic environment that encourages people to eat more and exercise less. This includes the availability of cheap and heavily marketed energy-rich foods, the increase in labour-saving devices (e.g. lifts and remote controls) and the rise in passive transport (cars as opposed to walking, cycling, or walking to public transport hubs). To combat the health impact of obesity, therefore, we not only need to help those who are already obese but also develop strategies that impact on the whole population and reverse the obesogenic environment.

Poverty and affluence

The adverse health and social consequences of poverty are well documented: high birth rates, high death rates and short life expectancy. Typically, with industrialisation, the pattern changes: low birth rates, low death rates and longer life expectancy. Instead of infections, chronic conditions such as heart disease dominate in an older population. Adverse health consequences of excessive affluence are also becoming apparent. Despite experiencing sustained economic growth for the last 50 years, people in many industrialised countries are not growing any happier and the litany of socioeconomic problems – crime, congestion, inequality – persists.

Many countries are now experiencing a 'double burden'. They have large populations still living in poverty who are suffering from problems such as diarrhoea and malnutrition, alongside affluent populations (often in cities) who suffer from chronic illness such as diabetes and heart disease.

Atmospheric pollution

Emissions from industry, power plants and motor vehicles of sulphur oxides, nitrogen oxides, respirable particles and metals are severely polluting cities and towns in Asia, Africa, Latin America and Eastern Europe. Burning of fossil and biomass fuels, with production of short-lived carbon pollutants (SLCPs – methane, ozone, black carbon and hydrofluorocarbons), contributes to increased death rates from respiratory and cardiovascular disease in vulnerable adults, such as those with established respiratory disease and the elderly, while children experience an increase in bronchitic symptoms. Developing countries also suffer high rates of respiratory disease as a result of indoor pollution caused mainly by heating and cooking using solid biomass fuels.

Climate change and global warming

Climate change is arguably the world's most important environmental health issue. A combination of habitat destruction and increased production of carbon dioxide and SLCPs, caused primarily by human activity, seems to be the main cause. The temperature of the globe is rising, and if current trends continue, warming by 4°C is predicted by 2050. The climate is being affected, putting millions of people at risk of rising sea levels, flooding, droughts and failed crops These have already claimed millions of lives during the past 20 years and have adversely affected the lives of many more. The economic costs of property damage and the impact on agriculture, food supplies and prosperity have also been substantial. Global warming will also include changes in the geographical range of some vector-borne infectious diseases. Currently, politicians cannot agree an effective framework of actions to tackle the problem, but reducing emissions of CO_2 and SLCPs is essential.

Principles of screening

Screening is the application of a test to a large number of asymptomatic people with the aim of reducing morbidity or mortality from a disease. The World Health Organisation (WHO) has identified a set of ('Wilson and Jungner') criteria to guide health systems in deciding when it is appropriate to implement screening programmes. The essential criteria are:

- Is the disease an important public health problem?
- Is there a suitable screening test available?
- Is there a recognisable latent or early stage?
- Is there effective treatment for the disease at this stage that improves prognosis?

A suitable screening test is one that is cheap, acceptable, easy to perform and safe, and gives a valid result in terms of sensitivity and specificity (p. 4). Screening programmes should always be evaluated in trials so that robust evidence is provided in favour of their adoption. These evaluations are prone to several biases – self-selection bias, lead-time bias and length bias – and these need to be accounted for in the analysis. Examples of large-scale programmes in the UK include breast, colorectal and cervical cancer national screening programmes and a number of screening tests carried out in pregnancy and in the newborn, such as the:

- diabetic eye screening programme
- fetal anomaly screening programme
- infectious diseases in pregnancy screening programme
- newborn and infant physical examination screening programme
- newborn blood spot screening programme
- newborn hearing screening programme
- sickle-cell and thalassaemia screening programme.

These are illustrated in Figure 5.2.

Problems with screening include:

- over-diagnosis (of a disease that would not have come to attention on its own or would not have led to death)
- false reassurance
- diversion of resources from investments that could control the disease more cost-effectively.

An example of these problems is the use of prostate-specific antigen (PSA) testing as a screening test for the diagnosis of prostate cancer (p. 438).

Epidemiology

Epidemiologists study disease in free-living humans, seeking to describe patterns of health and disease and to understand how different exposures cause or prevent disease (Box 5.5).

Chronic diseases and risk factors (e.g. smoking, obesity etc.) are often described in terms of their prevalence. A prevalence is simply a proportion: e.g. the prevalence of diabetes in people aged 80 and older in developed countries is around 10%.

Events such as deaths, hospitalisations and first occurrences of a disease are described using incidence rates: e.g. if there are 100 new cases of a disease in a single year in a population of 1000, the incidence rate is 105 per 1000 person-years, not 100, because of the effect of 'person-time'. Person-time is the sum of the total 'exposed' time for the population and in this example is 950 person-years. The reason person-time is less than 1000 is that 100 people experienced the event. These 100 people are assumed to have had an event, on average, halfway through the time period, removing 100×0.5 person-years from the exposure time (as it is not possible to have a first occurrence of a disease twice). Hence, the incidence per 1000 person-years is 105, not 100.

5.5 Calculation of risk using descriptive epidemiology

Prevalence

- The ratio of the number of people with a longer-term disease or condition, at a specified time, to the number of people in the population

Incidence

- The number of events (new cases or episodes) occurring in the population at risk during a defined period of time

Attributable risk

- The difference between the risk (or incidence) of disease in exposed and non-exposed populations

Attributable fraction

- The ratio of the attributable risk to the incidence

Relative risk

- The ratio of the risk (or incidence) in the exposed population to the risk (or incidence) in the non-exposed population

A similar measure is the cumulative incidence or risk, which is the number of new cases as a proportion of the total people at risk at the beginning of the exposure time. If, in the example above, the same 1000 people were observed for a year (i.e. with no one joining or leaving the group), then the 1-year risk is 10% (100/1000). The time period should always be specified.

These rates and proportions are used to describe how diseases (and risk factors) vary according to time, person and place. Temporal variation may occur seasonally (e.g. malaria occurs in the wet season but not the dry) or as longer-term 'secular' trends (e.g. malaria may re-emerge due to drug resistance). Person comparisons include age, sex, socioeconomic status, employment, and lifestyle characteristics. Place comparisons include the local environment (e.g. urban versus rural) and international comparisons.

Understanding causes and effect

Epidemiological research complements that based on animal, cell and tissue models, the findings of which do not always translate to humans. For example, only a minority of drug discoveries from laboratory research are effective when tested in people.

However, differentiating causes from mere non-causal associations is a considerable challenge for epidemiology. This is because while laboratory researchers can directly manipulate conditions to isolate and understand causes, such approaches are impossible in free-living populations. Epidemiologists have developed a different approach, based around a number of study designs (Box 5.6). Of these, the clinical trial is closest to the laboratory experiment. An early example of a clinical trial is shown in Figure 5.3, along with 'effect measures', which are used to quantify the difference in rates and risks.

In clinical trials, patients are usually allocated randomly to treatments so that, on average, groups are similar, apart from the intervention of interest. Nevertheless, for any particular trial, especially a small trial, the laws of probability mean that differences can and do occur by chance. Poorly designed or executed trials can also limit comparability between groups. Allocation may not be truly random (e.g. because of inadequate concealment of the randomisation sequence), and there may

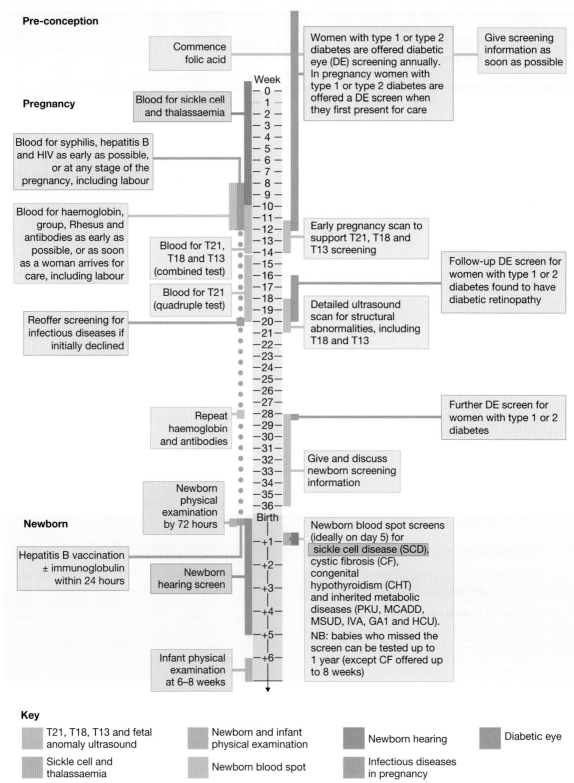

Pre-conception

Commence folic acid

Women with type 1 or type 2 diabetes are offered diabetic eye (DE) screening annually. In pregnancy women with type 1 or type 2 diabetes are offered a DE screen when they first present for care

Give screening information as soon as possible

Pregnancy

Blood for sickle cell and thalassaemia

Blood for syphilis, hepatitis B and HIV as early as possible, or at any stage of the pregnancy, including labour

Blood for haemoglobin, group, Rhesus and antibodies as early as possible, or as soon as a woman arrives for care, including labour

Blood for T21, T18 and T13 (combined test)

Blood for T21 (quadruple test)

Reoffer screening for infectious diseases if initially declined

Early pregnancy scan to support T21, T18 and T13 screening

Follow-up DE screen for women with type 1 or 2 diabetes found to have diabetic retinopathy

Detailed ultrasound scan for structural abnormalities, including T18 and T13

Repeat haemoglobin and antibodies

Further DE screen for women with type 1 or 2 diabetes

Give and discuss newborn screening information

Newborn physical examination by 72 hours

Newborn

Hepatitis B vaccination ± immunoglobulin within 24 hours

Newborn hearing screen

Infant physical examination at 6–8 weeks

Newborn blood spot screens (ideally on day 5) for sickle cell disease (SCD), cystic fibrosis (CF), congenital hypothyroidism (CHT) and inherited metabolic diseases (PKU, MCADD, MSUD, IVA, GA1 and HCU).
NB: babies who missed the screen can be tested up to 1 year (except CF offered up to 8 weeks)

Week 0–36, Birth, +1 to +6

Key

T21, T18, T13 and fetal anomaly ultrasound

Newborn and infant physical examination

Newborn hearing

Diabetic eye

Sickle cell and thalassaemia

Newborn blood spot

Infectious diseases in pregnancy

Fig. 5.2 UK NHS Pregnancy and Newborn Screening Programmes: optimum times for testing. (GA1 = glutaric aciduria type 1; HCU = homocystinuria; IVA = isovaleric acidaemia; MCADD = medium-chain acyl-CoA dehydrogenase deficiency; MSUD = maple syrup urine disease; PKU = phenylketonuria; T13, 18, 21 = trisomy 13, 18 and 21) *Based on Version 8.1, March 2016, Gateway ref: 2014696, Public Health England.*

i	**5.6 Epidemiological study designs**	
Design	**Description**	**Example**
Clinical trial	Enrols a sample from a population and compares outcomes after randomly allocating patients to an intervention	Medical Research Council (MRC) Streptomycin Trial – demonstrated effectiveness of streptomycin in tuberculosis
Cohort	Enrols a sample from a population and compares outcomes according to exposures	Framingham Study – identified risk factors for cardiovascular disease
Case–control	Enrols cases with an outcome of interest and controls without that outcome and compares exposures between the groups	Doll R, Hill AB. Smoking and carcinoma of the lung. British Medical Journal 1950 – demonstrated that smoking caused lung cancer
Cross-sectional	Enrols a cross-section (sample) of people from the population of interest; obtains data on exposures and outcomes	World Health Organisation Demographic and Health Survey – captures risk factor data in a uniform way across many countries

Effect measures

Risk ratio (relative risk, RR)	0.25
Odds ratio (OR)	0.30
Absolute risk reduction (ARR)	21.6%
Relative risk reduction (RRR)	74.8%
Number needed to treat to prevent one death (NNT= 1/ARR)	4.6

Fig. 5.3 An example of a clinical trial: streptomycin versus bed rest in tuberculosis. Both prevalences and risks are, in fact, proportions, and are therefore frequently expressed as odds. The reasons for doing so are beyond the scope of this text.

be systematic differences (biases) in the way people allocated to different groups are treated or studied.

Such biases also occur in observational epidemiological study designs, such as cohort, case–control and cross-sectional studies (Box 5.6). These designs are also much more subject to the problem of confounding than are randomised trials.

Confounding is where the relationship between an exposure and outcome of interest is confused by the presence of some other causal factor. For example, coffee consumption may be associated with lung cancer because smoking is more common among coffee-drinkers. Here, smoking is said to confound the association between coffee and lung cancer.

Despite these limitations, for most causes of diseases, randomised controlled trials are not feasible because of ethical,

or more often practical, considerations. Epidemiologists therefore seek to minimise bias and confounding by good study analysis and design. They subsequently make causal inferences by balancing the probability that an observed association has been caused by chance, bias and/or confounding against the alternative probability that the relationship is causal. This weighing-up requires an understanding of the frequency and importance of different sources of bias and confounding, as well as the scientific rationale of the putative causal relationship. It was this approach, collectively and over a number of years, that settled the fact that smoking causes lung cancer and, subsequently, heart disease.

Health data/informatics

As patients pass through health and social care systems, data are recorded concerning their family background, lifestyle and disease states, which is of potential interest to health-care organisations seeking to deliver services, policy-makers concerned with improving health, scientific researchers trying to understand health, and also pharmaceutical and other commercial organisations aiming to identify markets.

There is a long tradition of maintaining health information systems. In most countries, registration of births and deaths is required by law, and in the majority, the cause of death is also recorded (Fig. 5.4). There are many challenges in ensuring such data are useful, especially for comparisons across time and place:

- A system of standard terminologies is needed, such as the WHO International Classification of Diseases (ICD-10), which provides a list of diagnostic codes attempting to cover every diagnostic entity.
- These terms must be understood to refer to the same, or at least similar, diseases in different places.
- Access to diagnostic skill and facilities is required.
- Standard protocols for assigning clinical diagnoses to ICD-10 codes are needed
- Robust quality control processes are needed to maintain some level of data completeness and accuracy.

Many countries employ similar systems for hospitalisations, to allow recovery of health-care utilisation costs or to manage and plan services. Similar data are rarely collected for community-based health care, nor are detailed data on health-care processes generally included in national data systems. Consequently, there has been considerable interest in using data from information technology systems used to deliver care, such as electronic

INTERNATIONAL FORM OF MEDICAL CERTIFICATE OF CAUSE OF DEATH

	Cause of death		Approximate interval between onset and death
I Disease or condition directly leading to death*	(a) *Acute myocardial infarction*	I21.9	*2 days*
	due to (or as a consequence of)		
Antecedent causes Morbid conditions, if any, giving rise to the above cause, stating the underlying condition last	(b) *Familial hypercholesterolaemia*	E78.0	*30 years*
	due to (or as a consequence of)		
	(c)		
	due to (or as a consequence of)		
	(d)		
II Other significant conditions contributing to the death, but not related to the disease or condition causing it	*Brochiectasis*	J47	*10 years*

This does not mean the mode of dying, e.g. heart failure, respiratory failure. It means the disease, injury, or complication that caused death.

Fig. 5.4 Completed death certificate. International Classification of Diseases 10 (ICD-10) codes are appended in red. *WHO ICD-10, vol. 2; 1990.* Available at *https://commons.m.wikimedia.org/wiki/File:International_form_of_medical_certificate_of_cause_of_death.png.*

patient records, drug-dispensing databases, radiological software and clinical laboratory information systems.

Data from such systems are, of course, much less structured than those obtained from vital registrations. Moreover, the completeness of such data depends greatly on local patterns of health-care utilisation, as well as how clinicians and others use information technology systems within different settings. As such, deriving useful, unbiased information from such data is a considerable challenge.

Much of the discipline of health informatics is concerned with addressing this challenge. One approach has been to develop comprehensive standard classification systems such as SNOMED-CT, 'a standardised, multilingual vocabulary of terms relating to the care of the individual', which has been designed for electronic health-care records.

An alternative has been to use statistical methods such as natural language processing to derive information automatically from free text (such as culling diagnoses from radiological reports), or to employ 'machine learning', in which software algorithms are applied to data in order to derive useful insights. Such approaches are suited to large, messy data where the costs of systematisation would be prohibitive. It is likely that such innovations will, over the coming years, provide useful information to complement that obtained from more traditional health information systems.

Further information

Books and journal articles

GBD 2015 Disease and Injury Incidence and Prevalence Collaborators. Global, regional, and national incidence, prevalence, and years lived with disability for 310 diseases and injuries, 1990–2015: a systematic analysis for the Global Burden of Disease Study 2015. Lancet 2016; 388:1545–1602.

GBD 2015 Mortality and Causes of Death Collaborators. Global, regional, and national life expectancy, and cause-specific mortality for 249 causes of death, 1980–2015: a systematic analysis for the Global Burden of Disease Study 2015. Lancet 2016; 388:1459–1544.

GBD 2015 Risk Factors Collaborators. Global, regional, and national comparative risk assessment of 79 behavioural, environmental and occupational, and metabolic risks or clusters of risks, 1990–2015: a systematic analysis for the Global Burden of Disease Study 2015. Lancet 2016; 388:1659–1724.

Kindig D, Stoddart G. What is population health? Am J Public Health 2003; 93:380–383.

Websites

fph.org.uk *UK Faculty of Public Health: What is public health?*

gov.uk *UK Government: population screening programmes.*

JAT Sandoe
DH Dockrell

Principles of infectious disease

Infectious agents 100

Normal microbial flora 102

Host–pathogen interactions 104

Investigation of infection 105
Direct detection of pathogens 105
Culture 106
Indirect detection of pathogens 106
Antimicrobial susceptibility testing 109

Epidemiology of infection 110

Infection prevention and control 111
Health care-associated infection 111
Outbreaks of infection 114
Immunisation 114

Antimicrobial stewardship 115

Treatment of infectious diseases 116
Principles of antimicrobial therapy 116
Antibacterial agents 120
Antimycobacterial agents 125
Antifungal agents 125
Antiviral agents 126
Antiparasitic agents 128

'Infection' in its strict sense describes the situation where microorganisms or other infectious agents become established in the host organism's cells or tissues, replicate, cause harm and induce a host response. If a microorganism survives and replicates on a mucosal surface without causing harm or illness, the host is said to be 'colonised' by that organism. If a microorganism survives and lies dormant after invading host cells or tissues, infection is said to be 'latent'. When the infectious agent, or the host response to it, is sufficient to cause illness or harm, then the process is termed an 'infectious disease'. Most pathogens (infectious agents that can cause disease) are microorganisms but some are multicellular organisms. The manifestations of disease may aid pathogen dissemination (e.g. diarrhoea).

The term 'infection' is often used interchangeably with 'infectious disease' but not all infections are 'infectious', i.e. transmissible from person to person. Infectious diseases transmitted between hosts are called communicable diseases, whereas those caused by organisms that are already colonising the host are described as endogenous. The distinction is blurred in some situations, including health care-associated infections such as meticillin-resistant *Staphylococcus aureus* (MRSA) or *Clostridium difficile* infection (CDI), in which colonisation precedes infection but the colonising bacteria may have been recently transmitted between patients. The chain of infection (Fig. 6.1) describes six essential elements for communicable disease transmission.

Despite dramatic advances in hygiene, immunisation and antimicrobial therapy, infectious agents still cause a massive burden of disease worldwide. Key challenges remain in tackling infection in resource-poor countries. Microorganisms are continually mutating and evolving; the emergence of new infectious agents and antimicrobial-resistant microorganisms is therefore inevitable. This chapter describes the biological and epidemiological principles of infectious diseases and the general approach to their prevention, diagnosis and treatment. Specific infectious diseases are described in Chapters 11–13 and many of the organ-based chapters.

Infectious agents

The concept of an infectious agent was established by Robert Koch in the 19th century (Box 6.1). Although fulfilment of 'Koch's postulates' became the standard for the definition of an infectious agent, they do not apply to uncultivable organisms (e.g. *Mycobacterium leprae*, *Tropheryma whipplei*) or members of the normal human flora (e.g. *Escherichia coli*, *Candida* spp.). The following groups of infectious agents are now recognised.

Viruses

Viruses are incapable of independent replication. Instead, they subvert host cellular processes to ensure synthesis of their nucleic acids and proteins. Viruses' genetic material (the genome) consists of single- or double-stranded DNA or RNA. Retroviruses transcribe their RNA into DNA in the host cell by reverse transcription. An antigenically unique protein coat (capsid) encloses the genome, and together these form the nucleocapsid. In many viruses, the nucleocapsid is packaged within a lipid envelope. Enveloped viruses are less able to survive in the environment and are spread by respiratory, sexual or blood-borne routes, including arthropod-based transmission. Non-enveloped viruses survive better in the environment and are predominantly transmitted by faecal–oral or, less often, respiratory routes. A generic virus life cycle is shown in Figure 6.2. A virus that infects a bacterium is a bacteriophage (phage).

Prokaryotes: bacteria (including mycobacteria and actinomycetes)

Prokaryotic cells are capable of synthesising their own proteins and nucleic acids, and are able to reproduce autonomously, although they lack a nucleus. The bacterial cell membrane is bounded by a peptidoglycan cell wall, which is thick (20–80 nm) in Gram-positive organisms and thin (5–10 nm) in Gram-negative ones. The Gram-negative cell wall is surrounded by an outer membrane containing lipopolysaccharide. Genetic information is contained within a chromosome but bacteria may also contain rings of extra-chromosomal DNA, known as plasmids, which can be transferred between organisms, without cells having to divide. Bacteria may be embedded in a polysaccharide capsule,

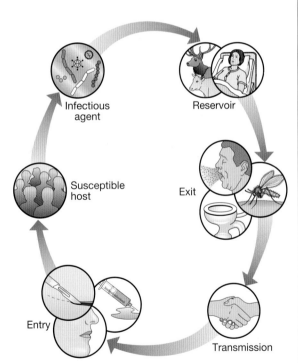

Fig. 6.1 Chain of infection. The infectious agent is the organism that causes the disease. The reservoir is the place where the population of an infectious agent is maintained. The portal of exit is the point from which the infectious agent leaves the reservoir. Transmission is the process by which the infectious agent is transferred from the reservoir to the human host, either directly or via a vector or fomite. The portal of entry is the body site that is first accessed by the infectious agent. Finally, in order for disease to ensue, the person to whom the infectious agent is transmitted must be a susceptible host.

i	6.1 Definition of an infectious agent – Koch's postulates

1. The same organism must be present in every case of the disease
2. The organism must be isolated from the diseased host and grown in pure culture
3. The isolate must cause the disease, when inoculated into a healthy, susceptible animal
4. The organism must be re-isolated from the inoculated, diseased animal

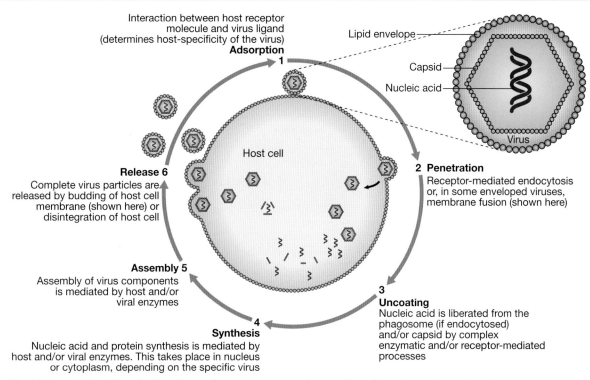

Fig. 6.2 A generic virus life cycle. Life cycle components common to most viruses are host cell attachment and penetration, virus uncoating, nucleic acid and protein synthesis, virus assembly and release. Virus release is achieved either by budding, as illustrated, or by lysis of the cell membrane. Life cycles vary between viruses.

---

i	**6.2 How bacteria are identified**

Gram stain reaction (see Fig. 6.3)	**Motility**
• Gram-positive (thick peptidoglycan layer), Gram-negative (thin peptidoglycan) or unstainable	• Motile or non-motile
	Antibiotic susceptibility
Microscopic morphology	• Identifies organisms with invariable susceptibility (e.g. to optochin in *Streptococcus pneumoniae* or metronidazole in obligate anaerobes)
• Cocci (round cells) or bacilli (elongated cells)	
• Presence or absence of capsule	**Matrix-assisted laser desorption/ionisation time-of-flight mass spectrometry (MALDI-TOF-MS)**
Cell association	
• Association in clusters, chains or pairs	• A rapid technique that identifies bacteria and some fungi from their specific molecular composition
Colonial characteristics	**Sequencing bacterial 16s ribosomal RNA gene**
• Colony size, shape or colour	
• Effect on culture media (e.g. β-haemolysis of blood agar in haemolytic streptococci; see Fig. 6.4)	• A highly specific test for identification of organisms in pure culture and in samples from normally sterile sites
Atmospheric requirements	**Whole-genome sequencing**
• Strictly aerobic (requires O_2), strictly anaerobic (requires absence of O_2), facultatively aerobic (grows with or without O_2) or micro-aerophilic (requires reduced O_2)	• Although not yet in routine use, whole-genome sequencing (WGS) offers the potential to provide rapid and simultaneous identification, sensitivity testing and typing of organisms from pure culture and/or directly from clinical samples. As such, WGS is likely to replace many of the technologies described above over the next few years (p. 58)
Biochemical reactions	
• Expression of enzymes (oxidase, catalase, coagulase)	
• Ability to ferment or hydrolyse various biochemical substrates	

---

and motile bacteria are equipped with flagella. Although many prokaryotes are capable of independent existence, some (e.g. *Chlamydia trachomatis*, *Coxiella burnetii*) are obligate intracellular organisms. Bacteria that can grow in artificial culture media are classified and identified using a range of characteristics (Box 6.2); examples are shown in Figures 6.3 and 6.4.

Eukaryotes: fungi, protozoa and helminths

Eukaryotic cells contain membrane-bound organelles, including nuclei, mitochondria and Golgi apparatus. Pathogenic eukaryotes are unicellular (e.g. fungi, protozoa) or complex multicellular organisms (e.g. nematodes, trematodes and cestodes, p. 288).

Gram stain

Gram-positive cocci	Gram-positive bacilli	Gram-negative cocci	Gram-negative bacilli

Colony morphology (e.g. haemolysis), Gram stain appearance, agglutination reactions, coagulase test, catalase

Colony morphology, growth characteristics (e.g. growth in anaerobic atmosphere), Gram stain appearance, MALDI-TOF-MS identification

Colony morphology, growth characteristics, oxidase reaction, sugar fermentation/MALDI-TOF-MS identification

Colony morphology, growth characteristics, lactose fermentation, oxidase reaction, MALDI-TOF-MS identification

Gram-positive cocci–clusters

Examples
Staphylococcus aureus
Coagulase-negative staphylococci

or

Gram-positive cocci–chains

Examples
Oral streptococci
Streptococcus pneumoniae (often pairs)
Beta-haemolytic strepto-cocci
Enterococci (short chains)

Examples
Actinomycetes
Arcanobacterium haemo-lyticum
Bacillus spp.
Corynebacterium diphtheriae
Lactobacillus spp.
Listeria monocytogenes
Nocardia spp.
Clostridium spp.

Examples
Neisseria meningitidis
Neisseria gonorrhoeae
Moraxella catarrhalis

Examples
Escherichia coli
Klebsiella pneumoniae
Proteus spp.
Enterobacter spp.
Serratia spp.
Salmonella spp.
Shigella spp.
Yersinia spp.
Vibrio spp.
Pseudomonas aeruginosa

Fig. 6.3 Flow chart for bacterial identification, including Gram film appearances on light microscopy (×100). (MALDI-TOF-MS = matrix-assisted laser desorption/ionisation time-of-flight mass spectroscopy)

Fig. 6.4 Beta-haemolytic streptococci (A) and alpha-haemolytic streptococci (B) spread on each half of a blood agar plate (backlit). This image is half life size. ×0.5. Beta-haemolysis renders the agar transparent around the colonies (A) and alpha-haemolysis imparts a green tinge to the agar (B).

Fungi exist as either moulds (filamentous fungi) or yeasts. Dimorphic fungi exist in either form, depending on environmental conditions (see Fig. 11.59, p. 300). The fungal plasma membrane differs from the human cell membrane in that it contains the sterol, ergosterol. Fungi have a cell wall made up of polysaccharides, chitin and mannoproteins. In most fungi, the main structural component of the cell wall is β-1,3-D-glucan, a glucose polymer. These differences from mammalian cells are important because they offer useful therapeutic targets.

Protozoa and helminths are often referred to as parasites. Many parasites have complex multi-stage life cycles, which involve animal and/or plant hosts in addition to humans.

Prions

Although prions are transmissible and have some of the characteristics of infectious agents, they are not microorganisms and are not diagnosed in microbiology laboratories. Prions are covered on page 250.

Normal microbial flora

The human body is colonised by large numbers of microorganisms (collectively termed the human microbiota). These colonising

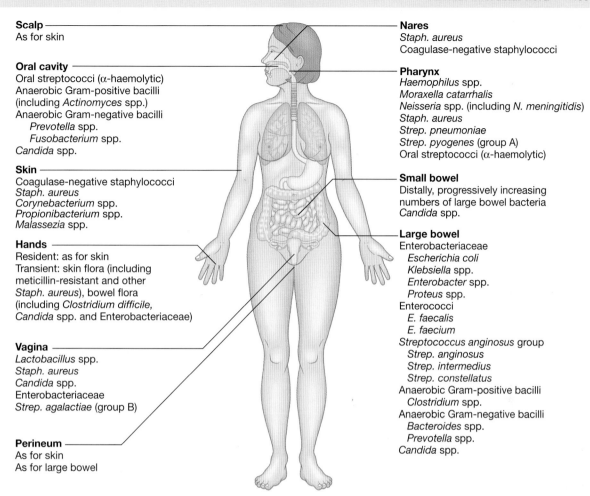

Scalp
As for skin

Oral cavity
Oral streptococci (α-haemolytic)
Anaerobic Gram-positive bacilli
(including *Actinomyces* spp.)
Anaerobic Gram-negative bacilli
    Prevotella spp.
    Fusobacterium spp.
Candida spp.

Skin
Coagulase-negative staphylococci
Staph. aureus
Corynebacterium spp.
Propionibacterium spp.
Malassezia spp.

Hands
Resident: as for skin
Transient: skin flora (including
meticillin-resistant and other
Staph. aureus), bowel flora
(including *Clostridium difficile*,
Candida spp. and Enterobacteriaceae)

Vagina
Lactobacillus spp.
Staph. aureus
Candida spp.
Enterobacteriaceae
Strep. agalactiae (group B)

Perineum
As for skin
As for large bowel

Nares
Staph. aureus
Coagulase-negative staphylococci

Pharynx
Haemophilus spp.
Moraxella catarrhalis
Neisseria spp. (including *N. meningitidis*)
Staph. aureus
Strep. pneumoniae
Strep. pyogenes (group A)
Oral streptococci (α-haemolytic)

Small bowel
Distally, progressively increasing
numbers of large bowel bacteria
Candida spp.

Large bowel
Enterobacteriaceae
    Escherichia coli
    Klebsiella spp.
    Enterobacter spp.
    Proteus spp.
Enterococci
    E. faecalis
    E. faecium
Streptococcus anginosus group
    Strep. anginosus
    Strep. intermedius
    Strep. constellatus
Anaerobic Gram-positive bacilli
    Clostridium spp.
Anaerobic Gram-negative bacilli
    Bacteroides spp.
    Prevotella spp.
Candida spp.

Fig. 6.5 Human non-sterile sites and normal flora in health.

bacteria, also referred to as the 'normal flora', are able to survive and replicate on skin and mucosal surfaces. The gastrointestinal tract and the mouth are the two most heavily colonised sites in the body and their microbiota are distinct, in both composition and function. Knowledge of non-sterile body sites and their normal flora is required to inform microbiological sampling strategies and interpret culture results (Fig. 6.5).

The microbiome is the total burden of microorganisms, their genes and their environmental interactions, and is now recognised to have a profound influence over human health and disease. Maintenance of the normal flora is beneficial to health. For example, lower gastrointestinal tract bacteria synthesise and excrete vitamins (e.g. vitamins K and B_{12}); colonisation with normal flora confers 'colonisation resistance' to infection with pathogenic organisms by altering the local environment (e.g. lowering pH), producing antibacterial agents (e.g. bacteriocins (small antimicrobial peptides/proteins), fatty acids and metabolic waste products), and inducing host antibodies that cross-react with pathogenic organisms.

Conversely, normally sterile body sites must be kept sterile. The mucociliary escalator transports environmental material deposited in the respiratory tract to the nasopharynx. The urethral sphincter prevents flow from the non-sterile urethra to the sterile bladder.

Physical barriers, including the skin, lining of the gastrointestinal tract and other mucous membranes, maintain sterility of the submucosal tissues, blood stream and peritoneal and pleural cavities, for example.

The normal flora contribute to endogenous disease mainly by translocation to a sterile site but excessive growth at the 'normal' site (overgrowth) can also cause disease. Overgrowth is exemplified by dental caries, vaginal thrush and 'blind loop' syndrome (p. 808). Translocation results from spread along a surface or penetration though a colonised surface, e.g. urinary tract infection caused by perineal/enteric flora, and surgical site infections, particularly of prosthetic materials, caused by skin flora such as staphylococci. Normal flora also contribute to disease by cross-infection, in which organisms that are colonising one individual cause disease when transferred to another, more susceptible, individual.

The importance of limiting perturbations of the microbiota by antimicrobial therapy is increasingly recognised. Probiotics are microbes or mixtures of microbes that are given to a patient to prevent or treat infection and are intended to restore a beneficial profile of microbiota. Although probiotics have been used in a number of settings, whether they have demonstrable clinical benefits remains a subject of debate.

Host–pathogen interactions

'Pathogenicity' is the capability of an organism to cause disease and 'virulence' is the extent to which a pathogen is able to cause disease. Pathogens produce proteins and other factors, termed virulence factors, which contribute to disease.

- *Primary pathogens* cause disease in a proportion of individuals to whom they are exposed, regardless of the host's immunological status.
- *Opportunistic pathogens* cause disease only in individuals whose host defences are compromised, e.g. by an intravascular catheter, or when the immune system is compromised, by genetic susceptibility or immunosuppressive therapy.

Characteristics of successful pathogens

Successful pathogens have a number of attributes. They compete with host cells and colonising flora by various methods, including sequestration of nutrients and production of bacteriocins. Motility enables pathogens to reach their site of infection, often sterile sites that colonising bacteria do not reach, such as the distal airway. Many microorganisms, including viruses, use 'adhesins' to attach to host cells initially. Some pathogens can invade through tissues. Many bacterial and fungal infections form 'biofilms'. After initial adhesion to a host surface, bacteria multiply in biofilms to form complex three-dimensional structures surrounded by a matrix of host and bacterial products that afford protection to the colony and limit the effectiveness of antimicrobials. Biofilms forming on man-made medical devices such as vascular catheters or grafts can be particularly difficult to treat.

Pathogens may produce toxins, microbial molecules that cause adverse effects on host cells, either at the site of infection, or remotely following carriage through the blood stream. Endotoxin is the lipid component of Gram-negative bacterial outer membrane lipopolysaccharide. It is released when bacterial cells are damaged and has generalised inflammatory effects. Exotoxins are proteins released by living bacteria, which often have specific effects on target organs (Box 6.3).

Intracellular pathogens, including viruses, bacteria (e.g. *Salmonella* spp., *Listeria monocytogenes* and *Mycobacterium tuberculosis*), parasites (e.g. *Leishmania* spp.) and fungi (e.g. *Histoplasma capsulatum*), are able to survive in intracellular environments, including after phagocytosis by macrophages. Pathogenic bacteria express different genes, depending on environmental stress (pH, iron starvation, O_2 starvation etc.) and anatomical location.

Genetic diversity enhances the pathogenic capacity of bacteria. Some virulence factor genes are found on plasmids or in phages and are exchanged between different strains or species. The ability to acquire genes from the gene pool of all strains of the species (the 'bacterial supragenome') increases diversity and the potential for pathogenicity. Viruses exploit their rapid reproduction and potential to exchange nucleic acid with host cells to enhance diversity. Once a strain acquires a particularly effective combination of virulence genes, it may become an epidemic strain, accounting for a large subset of infections in a particular region. This phenomenon accounts for influenza pandemics (see Box 6.10).

The host response

Innate and adaptive immune and inflammatory responses, which humans use to control the normal flora and respond to pathogens, are reviewed in Chapter 4.

Pathogenesis of infectious disease

The harmful manifestations of infection are determined by a combination of the virulence of the organism and the host response to infection. Despite the obvious benefits of an intact host response, an excessive response is undesirable. Cytokines and antimicrobial factors contribute to tissue injury at the site of infection, and an excessive inflammatory response may lead to hypotension and organ dysfunction (p. 196). The contribution of the immune response to disease manifestations is exemplified by the immune reconstitution inflammatory syndrome (IRIS). This is seen, for example, in human immunodeficiency virus (HIV) infection, post-transplantation neutropenia or tuberculosis (which causes suppression of T-cell function): there is a paradoxical worsening of the clinical condition as the immune dysfunction is corrected, caused by an exuberant but dysregulated inflammatory response.

The febrile response

Thermoregulation is altered in infectious disease, which may cause both hyperthermia (fever) and hypothermia. Fever is mediated mainly by 'pyrogenic cytokines' (e.g. interleukins IL-1 and IL-6, and tumour necrosis factor alpha (TNF-α)), which are released in response to various immunological stimuli including activation of pattern recognition receptors (PRRs) by microbial pyrogens (e.g. lipopolysaccharide) and factors released by injured cells. Their ultimate effect is to induce the synthesis of prostaglandin E_2, which binds to specific receptors in the preoptic nucleus of the hypothalamus (thermoregulatory centre), causing the core temperature to rise.

Rigors are a clinical symptom (or sign if they are witnessed) characterised by feeling very cold ('chills') and uncontrollable shivering, usually followed by fever and sweating. Rigors occur when the thermoregulatory centre attempts to correct a core temperature to a higher level by stimulating skeletal muscle activity and shaking.

There are data to support the hypothesis that raised body temperature interferes with the replication and/or virulence of pathogens. The mechanisms and possible protective role of infection-driven hypothermia, however, are poorly understood, and require further study.

i 6.3 Exotoxin-mediated bacterial diseases

Disease	Organism
Antibiotic-associated diarrhoea/pseudomembranous colitis	*Clostridium difficile* (p. 230)
Botulism	*Clostridium botulinum* (p. 1126)
Cholera	*Vibrio cholerae* (p. 264)
Diphtheria	*Corynebacterium diphtheriae* (p. 265)
Haemolytic uraemic syndrome	Enterohaemorrhagic *Escherichia coli* (*E. coli* 0157 and other strains) (p. 263)
Necrotising pneumonia	*Staphylococcus aureus* (p. 250)
Tetanus	*Clostridium tetani* (p. 1125)
Toxic shock syndrome	*Staphylococcus aureus* (p. 252) *Streptococcus pyogenes* (p. 253)

Investigation of infection

The aims of investigating a patient with suspected infection are to confirm the presence of infection, identify the specific pathogen(s) and identify its susceptibility to specific antimicrobial agents in order to optimise therapy. The presence of infection may be suggested by identifying proteins that are produced in response to pathogens as part of the innate immune and acute phase responses (p. 70). Pathogens may be detected directly (e.g. by culturing a normally sterile body site) or their presence may be inferred by identifying the host response to the organism, ('indirect detection', Box 6.4). Careful sampling increases the likelihood of diagnosis (Box 6.5). Culture results must be interpreted in the context of the normal flora at the sampled site (see Fig. 6.5). The extent to which a microbiological test result supports or excludes a particular diagnosis depends on its statistical performance (e.g. sensitivity, specificity, positive and negative predictive value, p. 4). Sensitivity and specificity vary according to the time between infection and testing, and positive and negative predictive values depend on the prevalence of the condition in the test population. The complexity of test interpretation is illustrated in Figure 6.8 below, which shows the 'windows of opportunity' afforded by various testing methods. Given this complexity, effective communication between the clinician and the microbiologist is vital to ensure accurate test interpretation.

Direct detection of pathogens

Some direct detection methods provide rapid results and enable detection of organisms that cannot be grown easily on artificial culture media, such as *Chlamydia* spp.; they can also provide information on antimicrobial sensitivity, e.g. *Mycobacterium tuberculosis*.

Detection of whole organisms

Whole organisms are detected by examination of biological fluids or tissue using a microscope.

- *Bright field microscopy* (in which the test sample is interposed between the light source and the objective lens) uses stains to enhance visual contrast between the

organism and its background. Examples include Gram staining of bacteria and Ziehl–Neelsen or auramine staining of acid- and alcohol-fast bacilli (AAFB) in tuberculosis (the latter requires an ultraviolet light source). In histopathological examination of tissue samples, multiple stains are used to demonstrate not only the presence of microorganisms but also features of disease pathology.
- *Dark field microscopy* (in which light is scattered to make organisms appear bright on a dark background) is used, for example, to examine genital chancre fluid in suspected syphilis.
- *Electron microscopy* may be used to examine stool and vesicle fluid to detect enteric and herpesviruses, respectively, but its use has largely been supplanted by nucleic acid detection (see below).
- *Flow cytometry* can be used to analyse liquid samples (e.g. urine) for the presence of particles based on properties such as size, impedance and light scatter. This technique can detect bacteria but may misidentify other particles as bacteria too.

6.5 How to provide samples for microbiological sampling

Communicate with the laboratory

- Discuss samples that require processing urgently or that may contain hazardous or unusual pathogens with laboratory staff *before* collection
- Communication is key to optimising microbiological diagnosis. If there is doubt about any aspect of sampling, it is far better to discuss it with laboratory staff beforehand than to risk diagnostic delay by inappropriate sampling or sample handling

Take samples based on a clinical diagnosis

- Sampling in the absence of clinical evidence of infection is rarely appropriate (e.g. collecting urine, or sputum for culture)

Use the correct container

- Certain tests (e.g. nucleic acid and antigen detection tests) require proprietary sample collection equipment

Follow sample collection procedures

- Failure to follow sample collection instructions precisely can result in false-positive (e.g. contamination of blood culture samples) or false-negative (e.g. collection of insufficient blood for culture) results

Label sample and request form correctly

- Label sample containers and request forms according to local policies, with demographic identifiers, specimen type and time/date collected
- Include clinical details on request forms
- Identify samples carrying a high risk of infection (e.g. blood liable to contain a blood-borne virus) with a hazard label

Use appropriate packaging

- Close sample containers tightly and package securely (usually in sealed plastic bags)
- Attach request forms to samples but not in the same compartment (to avoid contamination, should leakage occur)

Manage storage and transport

- Transport samples to the microbiology laboratory quickly
- If pre-transport storage is required, conditions (e.g. refrigeration, incubation, storage at room temperature) vary with sample type
- Notify the receiving laboratory prior to arrival of unusual or urgent samples, to ensure timely processing

---

i | **6.4 Tests used to diagnose infection**

Non-specific markers of inflammation/infection

- e.g. White cell count in blood sample (WCC), plasma C-reactive protein (CRP), procalcitonin, serum lactate, cell counts in urine or cerebrospinal fluid (CSF), CSF protein and glucose

Direct detection of organisms or organism components

- Microscopy
- Detection of organism components (e.g. antigen, toxin)
- Nucleic acid amplification (e.g. polymerase chain reaction)

Culture of organisms

- ± Antimicrobial susceptibility testing

Tests of the host's specific immune response

- Antibody detection
- Interferon-gamma release assays (IGRA)

Detection of components of organisms

Components of microorganisms detected for diagnostic purposes include nucleic acids, cell wall molecules, toxins and other antigens. Commonly used examples include *Legionella pneumophila* serogroup 1 antigen in urine and cryptococcal polysaccharide antigen in cerebrospinal fluid (CSF). Most antigen detection methods are based on in vitro binding of specific antigen/antibody and are described below. Other methods may be used, such as tissue culture cytotoxicity assay for *C. difficile* toxin. In toxin-mediated disease, detection of toxin may be of greater relevance than identification of the organism itself (e.g. stool *C. difficile* toxin).

Nucleic acid amplification tests

In a nucleic acid amplification test (NAAT), specific sequences of microbial DNA and RNA are identified using a nucleic acid primer that is amplified exponentially by enzymes to generate multiple copies of a target nucleotide sequence. The most commonly used amplification method is the polymerase chain reaction (PCR; see Fig. 3.11, p. 53). Reverse transcription (RT) PCR is used to detect RNA from RNA viruses (e.g. hepatitis C virus and HIV-1). The use of fluorescent labels in the reaction enables 'real-time' detection of amplified DNA; quantification is based on the principle that the time taken to reach the detection threshold is proportional to the initial number of copies of the target nucleic acid sequence. In multiplex PCR, multiple primer pairs are used to enable detection of several different organisms at once.

Determination of nucleotide sequences in a target gene(s) can be used to assign microorganisms to specific strains, which may be relevant to treatment and/or prognosis (e.g. in hepatitis C infection, p. 877). Genes that are relevant to pathogenicity (such as toxin genes) or antimicrobial resistance can also be detected; for example, the *mecA* gene is used to screen for MRSA.

NAATs are the most sensitive direct detection methods and are also relatively rapid. They are used widely in virology, where the possibility of false-positive results from colonising or contaminating organisms is remote, and are applied to blood, respiratory samples, stool and urine. In bacteriology, PCR is used to examine CSF, blood, tissue and genital samples, and multiplex PCR is being developed for use in faeces. PCR is particularly helpful for microorganisms that cannot be readily cultured, e.g. *Tropheryma whipplei*, and is being used increasingly in mycology and parasitology.

Culture

Microorganisms may be both detected and further characterised by culture from clinical samples (e.g. tissue, swabs and body fluids).

- *Ex vivo culture* (tissue or cell culture) was widely used in the isolation of viruses but has been largely supplanted by NAAT.
- *In vitro culture* (in artificial culture media) of bacteria and fungi is used to confirm the presence of pathogens, allow identification, test antimicrobial susceptibility and subtype the organism for epidemiological purposes.

Culture has its limitations: results are not immediate, even for organisms that are easy to grow, and negative cultures rarely exclude infection. Organisms such as *Mycobacterium tuberculosis* are slow-growing, typically taking at least 2 weeks, even in rapid-culture systems. Certain organisms, such as *Mycobacterium leprae* and *Tropheryma whipplei*, cannot be cultivated on artificial media, and others (e.g. *Chlamydia* spp. and viruses) grow only in culture systems, which are slow and labour-intensive.

Blood culture

The terms 'bacteraemia' and 'fungaemia' describe the presence of bacteria and fungi in the blood. 'Blood-stream infection' (p. 225) is the association of bacteraemia/fungaemia with clinical evidence of infection. The presence of bacteraemia/fungaemia can be determined by inoculating a liquid culture medium with freshly drawn blood, which is then incubated in a system that monitors it constantly for growth of microorganisms (e.g. by detecting products of microbial respiration using fluorescence; Fig. 6.6). If growth is detected, organisms are identified and sensitivity testing is performed. Traditionally, identification has been achieved by Gram stain appearance and biochemical reactions. However, matrix-assisted laser desorption/ionisation time-of-flight mass spectroscopy (MALDI-TOF-MS; see Box 6.2) is being used increasingly to identify organisms. MALDI-TOF-MS produces a profile of proteins of different sizes from the target microorganism and uses databases of such profiles to identify the organism (Fig. 6.7). It is rapid and accurate. Taking multiple blood samples for culture at different times allows differentiation of transient (one or two positive samples) and persistent (majority are positive) bacteraemia. This can be clinically important in the identification of the source of infection (p. 530).

Indirect detection of pathogens

Tests may be used to detect the host's immune (antibody) response to a specific microorganism, and can enable the diagnosis of infection with organisms that are difficult to detect by other methods or are no longer present in the host. The term 'serology' describes tests carried out on serum and includes both antigen (direct) and antibody (indirect) detection.

Antibody detection

Organism-specific antibody detection is applied mainly to blood (Fig. 6.8). Results are typically expressed as titres: that is, the reciprocal of the highest dilution of the serum at which antibody is detectable (for example, detection at serum dilution of 1:64 gives a titre of 64). 'Seroconversion' is defined as either a change from negative to positive detection or a fourfold rise in titre between acute and convalescent serum samples. An acute sample is usually taken during the first week of disease and the convalescent sample 2–4 weeks later. Earlier diagnosis can be achieved by detection of immunoglobulin M (IgM) antibodies, which are produced early in infection (p. 68). A limitation of these tests is that antibody production requires a fully functional host immune system, so there may be false-negative results in immunocompromised patients. Also, other than in chronic infections and with IgM detection, antibody tests usually provide a retrospective diagnosis.

Antibody detection methods are described below (antigen detection methods are also described here as they share similar methodology).

Enzyme-linked immunosorbent assay

The principles of the enzyme-linked immunosorbent assay (ELISA, EIA) are illustrated in Figure 6.9. These assays rely on linking

1 Patient sampling

Contamination minimised by aseptic technique. Maximise sensitivity by sampling correct volume

2 Sample handling

Follow local instructions for safety, labelling, and numbers of samples and bottles required

3 Specimen transport

Transport samples to laboratory as quickly as possible. Follow manufacturer's instructions for the blood culture system used if temporary storage is required

6

4 Incubation

Incubate at 35–37°C for 5–7 days. Microbial growth is usually detected by constant automatic monitoring of CO_2. **If no growth, specimen is negative and discarded**

5 Growth detection

Time to positivity (TTP) is usually 12–24 hrs in significant bacteraemia, but may be shorter in overwhelming sepsis or longer with fastidious organisms (e.g. *Brucella* spp.)

6 Preliminary results*

A Gram film of the blood culture medium is examined and **results are communicated immediately to the clinician** to guide antibiotic therapy

7 Incubation

A small amount of the medium is incubated on a range of culture media. Preliminary susceptibility testing may be carried out

8 Culture results*

Preliminary susceptibility results are communicated to the clinician

9 Definitive results

Further overnight incubation is often required for definitive identification of organisms (by biochemical testing) and additional susceptibility testing; identification by MALDI-TOF MS (Fig. 6.7) is more rapid

10 Reporting

A final summary is released when all testing is complete. For clinical care, communication of interim results (Gram film, preliminary identification and susceptibility) is usually more important than the final report. **Effective clinical–laboratory communication is vital**

 Overnight incubation required

 Urgent communication required

Fig. 6.6 An overview of the processing of blood cultures. *In laboratories equipped with MALDI-TOF-MS (p. 106), rapid definitive organism identification may be achieved at stage 6 and/or stage 8.

an antibody with an enzyme that generates a colour change on exposure to a chromogenic substrate. Various configurations allow detection of antigens or specific subclasses of immunoglobulin (e.g. IgG, IgM, IgA). ELISA may also be adapted to detect PCR products, using immobilised oligonucleotide hybridisation probes and various detection systems.

Immunoblot (Western blot)

Microbial proteins are separated according to molecular weight by polyacrylamide gel electrophoresis (PAGE) and transferred (blotted) on to a nitrocellulose membrane, which is incubated with patient serum. Binding of specific antibody is detected with an enzyme–anti-immunoglobulin conjugate similar to that used in ELISA, and specificity is confirmed by its location on the membrane. Immunoblotting is a highly specific test, which may be used to confirm the results of less specific tests such as ELISA (e.g. in Lyme disease, p. 255).

Immunofluorescence assays

Indirect immunofluorescence assays (IFAs) detect antibodies by incubating a serum sample with immobilised antigen (e.g. cells known to be infected with virus on a glass slide); any virus-specific antibody present in the serum binds to antigen and is then detected using a fluorescent-labelled anti-human immunoglobulin ('secondary' antibody). Fluorescence is visualised using a microscope. This method can also detect organisms in clinical samples (usually tissue or centrifuged cells) using a specific antibody in place of immobilised antigen to achieve capture.

Complement fixation test

In a complement fixation test (CFT), patient serum is heat-treated to inactivate complement and mixed with the test antigen. Any specific antibody in the serum will complex with the antigen. Complement is then added to the reaction. If antigen–antibody complexes are present, the complement will be 'fixed' (consumed). Sheep erythrocytes, coated with an anti-erythrocyte antibody, are added. The degree of erythrocyte lysis reflects the remaining complement and is inversely proportional to the quantity of the specific antigen–antibody complex present.

Agglutination tests

When antigens are present on the surface of particles (e.g. cells, latex particles or microorganisms) and cross-linked with antibodies, visible clumping (or 'agglutination') occurs.

- In *direct agglutination*, patient serum is added to a suspension of organisms that express the test antigen.

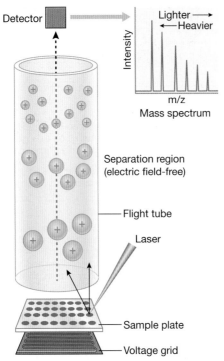

Fig. 6.7 The workings of matrix-assisted laser desorption/ionisation time-of-flight mass spectrometry (MALDI-TOF MS). *Adapted from Sobin K, Hameer D, Ruparel T. Digital genotyping using molecular affinity and mass spectrometry. Nature Rev Genet 2003; 4:1001–1008.*

For example, in the Weil–Felix test, if a patient's serum contains antibodies to rickettsial species they cause agglutination when *Proteus* spp. surface (O) antigens are added because the antibodies cross-react with the *Proteus* antigens. The test lacks sensitivity and specificity but is still used to diagnose rickettsial infection in resource-limited settings. The Widal test reaction uses a suspension of *Salmonella typhi* and *S. paratyphi* 'A' and 'B', treated to retain only 'O' and 'H' antigens. These antigens are kept to detect corresponding antibodies in serum from a patient suspected of having typhoid fever. The test is not specific but is still used in some parts of the world.

- In *indirect (passive) agglutination*, specific antigen is attached to the surface of carrier particles, which agglutinate when incubated with patient samples that contain specific antibodies.
- In *reverse passive agglutination* (an antigen detection test), the carrier particle is coated with antibody rather than antigen.

Other tests

Immunodiffusion involves antibodies and antigen migrating through gels, with or without the assistance of electrophoresis, and forming insoluble complexes where they meet. The complexes are seen on staining as 'precipitin bands'. Immunodiffusion is used in the diagnosis of dimorphic fungi (p. 300) and some forms of aspergillosis (p. 596).

Immunochromatography is used to detect antigen. The system consists of a porous test strip (e.g. a nitrocellulose membrane), at one end of which there is target-specific antibody, complexed with coloured microparticles. Further specific antibody is immobilised in a transverse narrow line some distance along the strip. Test material (e.g. blood or urine) is added to the antibody–particle complexes, which then migrate along the strip by capillary action. If these are complexed with antigen, they will be immobilised by the specific antibody and visualised as a transverse line across the strip. If the test is negative, the antibody–particle complexes will bind to a line of immobilised anti-immunoglobulin antibody placed further along the strip, which acts as a negative control. Immunochromatographic tests are rapid and relatively cheap to perform, and are appropriate for point-of-care testing, e.g. in HIV 1 and malaria (p. 276).

Fig. 6.8 Detection of antigen, nucleic acid and antibody in infectious disease. The acute sample is usually taken during the first week of illness, and the convalescent sample 2–4 weeks later. Detection limits and duration of detectability vary between tests and diseases, although in most diseases immunoglobulin M (IgM) is detectable within the first 1–2 weeks.

Fig. 6.9 Antibody (Ab) and antigen (Ag) detection by enzyme-linked immunosorbent assay (ELISA). This can be configured in various ways. **A** Patient Ab binds to immobilised specific Ag and is detected by addition of anti-immunoglobulin–enzyme conjugate and chromogenic substrate. **B** Patient Ab binds to immobilised Ig subclass-specific Ab and is detected by addition of specific Ag, followed by antibody–enzyme conjugate and chromogenic substrate. **C** Patient Ab and antibody–enzyme conjugate bind to immobilised specific Ag. Magnitude of colour change reaction is inversely proportional to concentration of patient Ab. **D** Patient Ag binds to immobilised Ab and is detected by addition of antibody–enzyme conjugate and chromogenic substrate. In A, the conjugate Ab is specific for human immunoglobulin. In B–D, it is specific for Ag from the disease-causing organism.

Antibody-independent specific immunological tests

The interferon-gamma release assay (IGRA) is being used increasingly to diagnose latent tuberculosis infection (LTBI). The principle behind IGRA is discussed on page 594. IGRA cannot distinguish between latent and active tuberculosis infection and is therefore appropriate for use only in countries where the background incidence of tuberculosis is low.

Antimicrobial susceptibility testing

If growth of microorganisms in culture is inhibited by the addition of an antimicrobial agent, the organism is considered to be susceptible to that antimicrobial. Bacteriostatic agents cause reversible inhibition of growth and bactericidal agents cause cell death; the terms fungistatic/fungicidal are equivalent for antifungal agents, and virustatic/virucidal for antiviral agents. The lowest concentration of antimicrobial agent at which growth is inhibited is the minimum inhibitory concentration (MIC), and the lowest concentration that causes cell death is the minimum bactericidal concentration (MBC). If the MIC is less than or equal to a predetermined breakpoint threshold, the organism is considered susceptible, and if the MIC is greater than the breakpoint, it is resistant.

Breakpoints are determined for each antimicrobial agent from a combination of pharmacokinetic (p. 17) and clinical data. The relationship between in vitro antimicrobial susceptibility and clinical response is complex, as response also depends on immune status, pharmacokinetic variability (p. 17), comorbidities that may influence pharmacokinetics or pharmacodynamics, and antibiotic dosing, as well as MIC/MBC. Thus, although treating a patient according to the results of susceptibility testing increases the likelihood of recovery, it does not guarantee therapeutic success.

Susceptibility testing is often carried out by disc diffusion (Fig. 6.10). Antibiotic-impregnated filter paper discs are placed on agar plates containing bacteria; antibiotic diffuses into the agar, resulting in a concentration gradient centred on the disc. Bacteria are unable to grow where the antibiotic concentration exceeds the MIC, which may therefore be inferred from the size of the zone of inhibition. The MIC is commonly measured in diagnostic laboratories using 'diffusion strips'.

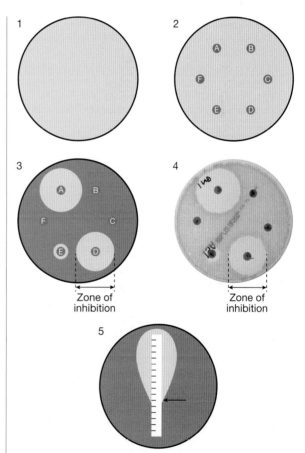

Fig. 6.10 Antimicrobial susceptibility testing by disc diffusion (panels 1-4) and minimum inhibitory concentration (MIC, panel 5).
1. The test organism is spread over the surface of an agar plate.
2. Antimicrobial-impregnated discs (A–F) are placed on the surface and the plate is incubated (e.g. overnight). 3–4. After incubation, zones of growth inhibition may be seen. The organism is considered susceptible if the diameter of the zone of inhibition exceeds a pre-determined threshold.
5. In a 'diffusion strip' test, the strip is impregnated with antimicrobial at a concentration gradient that decreases steadily from top to bottom. The system is designed so that the MIC value is the point at which the ellipse cuts a scale on the strip (arrow). *4, Kindly supplied by Charlotte Symes.*

Epidemiology of infection

The communicability of infectious disease means that, once a clinician has diagnosed an infectious disease, potential exposure of other patients must also be considered. The patient may require separation from other patients ('isolation'), or an outbreak of disease may need to be investigated in the community (Ch. 5). The approach will be specific to the microorganism involved (Chs 11–13) but the principles are outlined below.

Geographical and temporal patterns of infection

Endemic disease

Endemic disease has a constant presence within a given geographical area or population. The infectious agent may have a reservoir, vector or intermediate host that is geographically restricted, or may itself have restrictive environmental requirements (e.g. temperature range, humidity). The population affected may be geographically isolated or the disease may be limited to unvaccinated populations. Factors that alter geographical restriction include:

- expansion of an animal reservoir (e.g. Lyme disease from reforestation)
- vector escape (e.g. airport malaria)
- extension of host range (e.g. schistosomiasis from dam construction)
- human migration (e.g. carbapenemase-producing *Klebsiella pneumoniae*)
- public health service breakdown (e.g. diphtheria in unvaccinated areas)
- climate change (e.g. dengue virus and Rift Valley fever).

Emerging and re-emerging disease

An emerging infectious disease is one that has newly appeared in a population, or has been known for some time but is increasing in incidence or geographical range. If the disease was previously known and thought to have been controlled or eradicated, it is considered to be re-emerging. Many emerging diseases are caused by organisms that infect animals and have undergone adaptations that enable them to infect humans. This is exemplified by HIV-1, which is believed to have originated in higher primates in Africa. The geographical pattern of some recent emerging and re-emerging infections is shown in Figure 6.11.

Reservoirs of infection

The US Centers for Disease Control (CDC) define a reservoir of infection as any person, other living organism, environment or combination of these in which the infectious agent lives and replicates and on which the infectious agent is dependent for its survival. The infectious agent is transmitted from this reservoir to a susceptible host.

Human reservoirs

Both colonised individuals and those with infection can act as reservoirs, e.g. with *Staph. aureus* (including MRSA), *Strep. pyogenes* and *C. difficile*. For infected humans to act as reservoirs, the infections caused must be long-lasting in at least a proportion of those affected, to enable onward transmission (e.g. tuberculosis, sexually transmitted infections). Humans are the only reservoir for some infections (e.g. measles).

Animal reservoirs

The World Health Organization (WHO) defines a zoonosis as 'a disease or infection that is naturally transmissible from vertebrate animals to humans'. Infected animals may be asymptomatic. Zoonotic agents may be transmitted via any of the routes described below. Primary infection with zoonoses may be transmitted onward between humans, causing secondary disease (e.g. Q fever, brucellosis, Ebola).

Environmental reservoirs

Many infective pathogens are acquired from an environmental source. However, some of these are maintained in human or animal reservoirs, with the environment acting only as a conduit for infection.

Fig. 6.11 Geographical locations of some infectious disease outbreaks, with examples of emerging and re-emerging diseases. (CPE = carbapenemase-producing Enterobacteriaceae; MDR-TB = multidrug-resistant tuberculosis; MERS-Co-V = Middle East respiratory syndrome coronavirus; XDR-TB = extensively drug-resistant tuberculosis)

i 6.6 Incubation periods of important infections[1]	
Infection	Incubation period
Short incubation periods	
Anthrax, cutaneous[3]	9 hrs to 2 weeks
Anthrax, inhalational[3]	2 days[2]
Bacillary dysentery[5]	1–6 days
Cholera[3]	2 hrs to 5 days
Dengue haemorrhagic fever[6]	3–14 days
Diphtheria[6]	1–10 days
Gonorrhoea[4]	2–10 days
Influenza[5]	1–3 days
Meningococcaemia[3]	2–10 days
Norovirus[1]	1–3 days
SARS coronavirus[3]	2–7 days[2]
Scarlet fever[5]	2–4 days
Intermediate incubation periods	
Amoebiasis[6]	1–4 weeks
Brucellosis[4]	5–30 days
Chickenpox[5]	11–20 days
Lassa fever[3]	3–21 days
Malaria[3]	10–15 days
Measles[5]	6–19 days
Mumps[5]	15–24 days
Poliomyelitis[6]	3–35 days
Psittacosis[4]	1–4 weeks
Rubella[5]	15–20 days
Typhoid[6]	5–31 days
Whooping cough[5]	5–21 days
Long incubation periods	
Hepatitis A[5]	3–7 weeks
Hepatitis B[4]	6 weeks to 6 months
Leishmaniasis, cutaneous[6]	Weeks to months
Leishmaniasis, visceral[6]	Months to years
Leprosy (Hansen's disease)[3]	5–20 years
Rabies[4]	2–8 weeks[2]
Trypanosoma brucei gambiense infection[6]	Months to years
Tuberculosis[5]	1–12 months

[1]Incubation periods are approximate and may differ from local or national guidance. [2]Longer incubation periods have been reported. [3]WHO. [4]Health Protection Agency (now Health Protection England). [5]Richardson M, Elliman D, Maguire H, et al. Pediatr Infect Dis J 2001; 20:380–388. [6]Centers for Disease Control, USA.
(SARS = severe acute respiratory syndrome)

Transmission of infection

Communicable diseases may be transmitted by one or more of the following routes:

- *Respiratory route*: inhalation.
- *Faecal–oral route*: ingestion of material originating from faeces.
- *Sexually transmitted infections*: direct contact between mucous membranes.
- *Blood-borne infections*: direct inoculation of blood or body fluids.
- *Direct contact*: very few organisms are capable of causing infection by direct contact with intact skin. Most infection by this route requires contact with damaged skin (e.g. surgical wound).
- *Via a vector or fomite*: the vector/fomite bridges the gap between the infected host or reservoir and the uninfected host. Vectors are animate, and include mosquitoes in malaria, dengue and Zika virus infection, fleas in plague

i 6.7 Periods of infectivity in common childhood infectious diseases	
Disease	Infectious period
Chickenpox[1]	From 4 days before until 5 days after appearance of the rash (transmission before 48 hrs prior to the onset of rash is rare)[4]
Measles[2]	From 4 days before onset to 4 days after onset of the rash
Mumps[3]	From 2–3 days before to 5 days after disease onset[5]
Rubella[3]	From 10 days before until 15 days after the onset of the rash, but most infectious during prodromal illness[4]
Scarlet fever[1]	Unknown[6]
Whooping cough[1]	Unknown[6,7]

[1]From Richardson M, Elliman D, Maguire H, et al. Pediatr Infect Dis J 2001; 20:380–388. [2]Centers for Disease Control, USA; cdc.gov/measles/hcp/. [3]Bennett JE, Dolin R, Blaser MJ. Mandell, Douglas and Bennett's Principles and practice of infectious diseases, 8th edn. Philadelphia: Elsevier; 2015. [4–6]Exclude from contact with non-immune and immunocompromised people for 5 days from [4]onset of rash, [5]onset of parotitis, or [6]start of antibiotic treatment. [7]Exclude for 3 weeks if untreated.
Durations are approximate and vary between information sources, and these recommendations may differ from local or national guidance.

and humans in MRSA. Fomites are inanimate objects such as door handles, water taps and ultrasound probes, which are particularly associated with health care-associated infection (HCAI).

The likelihood of infection following transmission of a pathogen depends on organism factors (virulence, p. 104) and host susceptibility. The incubation period is the time between exposure and development of symptoms, and the period of infectivity is the period after exposure during which the patient is infectious to others. Knowledge of incubation periods and of periods of infectivity is important in controlling the spread of disease, although for many diseases these estimates are imprecise (Boxes 6.6 and 6.7).

Deliberate release

Deliberate release of pathogens with the intention of causing disease is known as biological warfare or bioterrorism, depending on the scale and context. Deliberate release incidents have included a 750-person outbreak of *Salmonella typhimurium* caused by contamination of salads in 1984 (Oregon, USA) and 22 cases of anthrax (five fatal) from the mailing of finely powdered (weaponised) anthrax spores in 2001 (New Jersey, USA). Diseases with high potential for deliberate release include anthrax, plague, tularaemia, smallpox and botulism (through toxin release).

Infection prevention and control

Infection prevention and control (IPC) describes the measures applied to populations with the aim of breaking the chain of infection (see Fig. 6.1, p. 100).

Health care-associated infection

The risk of developing infection following admission to a health-care facility (health care-associated infection, HCAI) in

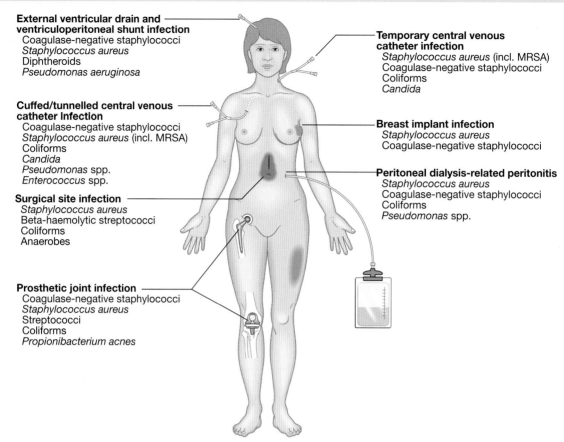

External ventricular drain and ventriculoperitoneal shunt infection
Coagulase-negative staphylococci
Staphylococcus aureus
Diphtheroids
Pseudomonas aeruginosa

Cuffed/tunnelled central venous catheter Infection
Coagulase-negative staphylococci
Staphylococcus aureus (incl. MRSA)
Coliforms
Candida
Pseudomonas spp.
Enterococcus spp.

Surgical site infection
Staphylococcus aureus
Beta-haemolytic streptococci
Coliforms
Anaerobes

Prosthetic joint infection
Coagulase-negative staphylococci
Staphylococcus aureus
Streptococci
Coliforms
Propionibacterium acnes

Temporary central venous catheter infection
Staphylococcus aureus (incl. MRSA)
Coagulase-negative staphylococci
Coliforms
Candida

Breast implant infection
Staphylococcus aureus
Coagulase-negative staphylococci

Peritoneal dialysis-related peritonitis
Staphylococcus aureus
Coagulase-negative staphylococci
Coliforms
Pseudomonas spp.

Fig. 6.12 Commonly encountered health care-associated infections (HCAIs) and the factors that predispose to them.

---

i | **6.8 Measures used in infection prevention and control (IPC)**

Institutions	Clinical practice
• Handling, storage and disposal of clinical waste	• Antibiotic stewardship (p. 115)
• Containment and safe removal of spilled blood and body fluids	• Aseptic technique
• Cleanliness of environment and medical equipment	• Perioperative antimicrobial prophylaxis
• Specialised ventilation (e.g. laminar flow, air filtration, controlled pressure gradients)	• Screening patients for colonisation or infection (e.g. MRSA, GRE, CPE)
• Sterilisation and disinfection of instruments and equipment	**Response to infections**
• Food hygiene	• Surveillance to detect alert organism (see text) outbreaks and antimicrobial resistance
• Laundry management	• Antibiotic chemoprophylaxis in infectious disease contacts, if indicated (see Box 6.18)
Health-care staff	• Isolation (see Box 6.9)
• Education	• Reservoir control
• Hand hygiene, including hand-washing (see Fig. 6.13)	• Vector control
• Sharps management and disposal	
• Use of personal protective equipment (masks, sterile and non-sterile gloves, gowns and aprons)	
• Screening health workers for disease (e.g. tuberculosis, hepatitis B virus, MRSA)	
• Immunisation and post-exposure prophylaxis	

(CPE = carbapenemase-producing Enterobacteriaceae; GRE = glycopeptide-resistant enterococci; MRSA = meticillin-resistant *Staphylococcus aureus*)

---

the developed world is about 10%. Many nosocomial bacterial infections are caused by organisms that are resistant to numerous antibiotics (multi-resistant bacteria), including MRSA, extended-spectrum β-lactamases (ESBLs) and carbapenemase-producing Enterobacteriaceae (CPE), and glycopeptide-resistant enterococci

(GRE). Other infections of particular concern in hospitals include *C. difficile* (p. 264) and norovirus (p. 249). Some examples are shown in Figure 6.12.

IPC measures are described in Box 6.8. The most important is maintenance of good hand hygiene (Fig. 6.13). Hand

Wash hands only when visibly soiled! Otherwise use handrub! Duration of the entire procedure: 40–60 sec.

| 1 Wet hands with water using elbow-operated or non-touch taps (if available) | 2 Apply enough soap to cover all hand surfaces | 3 Rub hands palm to palm | 4 Right palm over left dorsum with interlaced fingers and vice versa | 5 Palm to palm with fingers interlaced | 6 Backs of fingers to opposing palms with fingers interlaced |

| 7 Rotational rubbing of left thumb clasped in right palm and vice versa | 8 Rotational rubbing, backwards and forwards with clasped fingers of right hand in left palm and vice versa | 9 Rinse hands with water | 10 Dry thoroughly with a single-use towel | 11 If hand-operated taps have been used, use towel to turn off tap | 12 ...and your hands are clean |

Fig. 6.13 Hand-washing. Good hand hygiene, whether with soap/water or alcohol handrub, includes areas that are often missed, such as fingertips, web spaces, palmar creases and the backs of hands. *Adapted from the 'How to Handwash' URL: who.int/gpsc/5may/How_To_Handwash_Poster.pdf © World Health Organization 2009. All rights reserved.*

i 6.9 Types of isolation precaution[1]

Airborne transmission	Contact transmission	Droplet transmission
Precautions		
Negative pressure room with air exhausted externally or filtered. N95 masks or personal respiratiors for staff; avoid using non-immune staff	Private room preferred (otherwise, inter-patient spacing ≥ 1 m). Gloves and gown for staff in contact with patient or contaminated areas	Private room preferred (otherwise, inter-patient spacing ≥ 1 m). Surgical masks for staff in close contact with patient
Infections managed with these precautions		
Measles. Tuberculosis, pulmonary or laryngeal, confirmed or suspected	Enteroviral infections in young children (diapered or incontinent). Norovirus[2]. *C. difficile* infection. Multidrug-resistant organisms (e.g. MRSA, ESBL, GRE, VRSA, penicillin-resistant *Strep. pneumoniae*)[3]. Parainfluenza in infants and young children. Rotavirus. RSV in infants, children and immunocompromised. Viral conjunctivitis, acute	Diphtheria, pharyngeal. *Haemophilus influenzae* type B infection. Herpes simplex virus, disseminated or severe. Influenza. Meningococcal infection. Mumps. *Mycoplasma pneumoniae*. Parvovirus (erythrovirus) B19 (erythema infectiosum, fifth disease). Pertussis. Plague, pneumonic/bubonic. Rubella. *Strep. pyogenes* (group A), pharyngeal

Infections managed with multiple precautions

← Smallpox, monkeypox, VZV (chickenpox or disseminated disease)[4] →
← Adenovirus pneumonia →
← SARS, viral haemorrhagic fever[2] →

[1]Recommendations based on 2007 CDC guideline for isolation precautions. May differ from local or national recommendations. [2]Not a CDC recommendation. [3]Subject to local risk assessment. [4]Or in any immunocompromised patient until possibility of disseminated infection excluded. (ESBL = extended-spectrum β-lactamase; GRE = glycopeptide-resistant enterococci; MRSA = meticillin-resistant *Staph. aureus*; RSV = respiratory syncytial virus; SARS = severe acute respiratory syndrome; VRSA = vancomycin-resistant *Staph. aureus*; VZV = varicella zoster virus)

decontamination (e.g. using alcohol gel or washing) is mandatory before and after every patient contact. Decontamination with alcohol gel is usually adequate but hand-washing (with hot water, liquid soap and complete drying) is required after any procedure that involves more than casual physical contact, or if hands are visibly soiled. In situations where the prevalence of *C. difficile* is high (e.g. a local outbreak), alcohol gel decontamination between patient contacts is inadequate as it does not kill *C. difficile* spores, and hands must be washed.

Some infections necessitate additional measures to prevent cross-infection (Box 6.9). To minimise risk of infection, invasive procedures must be performed using strict aseptic technique.

Outbreaks of infection

Descriptive terms are defined in Box 6.10. Confirmation of an infectious disease outbreak usually requires evidence from 'typing' that the causal organisms have identical phenotypic and/or genotypic characteristics. If this is found not to be the case, the term pseudo-outbreak is used. When an outbreak of infection is suspected, a case definition is agreed. The number of cases that meet the case definition is then assessed by case-finding, using methods ranging from administration of questionnaires to national reporting systems. Case-finding usually includes microbiological testing, at least in the early stages of an outbreak. Temporal changes in cases are noted in order to plot an outbreak curve, and demographic details are collected to identify possible sources of infection. A case–control study, in which recent activities (potential exposures) of affected 'cases' are compared to those of unaffected 'controls', may be undertaken to establish the outbreak source, and measures are taken to manage the outbreak and control its spread. Good communication between relevant personnel during and after the outbreak is important to inform practice in future outbreaks.

Surveillance ensures that disease outbreaks are either prevented or identified early. In hospitals, staff are made aware of the isolation of alert organisms, which have the propensity to cause outbreaks, and alert conditions, which are likely to be caused by such organisms. Analogous systems are used nationally; many countries publish lists of organisms and diseases, which, if detected (or suspected), must be reported to public health authorities (reportable or notifiable diseases). Reasons for a disease to be classified as reportable are shown in Box 6.11.

i	6.10 Terminology in outbreaks of infection	
Term	**Definition**	
Classification of related cases of infectious disease*		
Cluster	An aggregation of cases of a disease that are closely grouped in time and place, and may or may not exceed the expected number	
Epidemic	The occurrence of more cases of disease than expected in a given area or among a specific group of people over a particular period of time	
Outbreak	Synonymous with epidemic. Alternatively, a localised, as opposed to generalised, epidemic	
Pandemic	An epidemic occurring over a very wide area (several countries or continents) and usually affecting a large proportion of the population	
Classification of affected patients (cases)		
Index case	The first case identified in an outbreak	
Primary cases	Cases acquired from a specific source of infection	
Secondary cases	Cases acquired from primary cases	
Types of outbreak		
Common source outbreak	Exposure to a common source of infection (e.g. water-cooling tower, medical staff member shedding MRSA). New primary cases will arise until the source is no longer present	
Point source outbreak	Exposure to a single source of infection at a specific point in time (e.g. contaminated food at a party). Primary cases will develop disease synchronously	
Person-to-person spread	Outbreak with both primary and secondary cases. May complicate point source or common source outbreak	

*Adapted from cdc.gov. (MRSA = meticillin-resistant *Staphylococcus aureus*)

i	6.11 Reasons for including an infectious disease on a regional/national list of reportable diseases*	
Reason for inclusion	**Examples**	
Endemic/local disease with the potential to spread and/or cause outbreaks	Influenza, *Salmonella*, tuberculosis	
Imported disease with the propensity to spread and/or cause outbreaks	Typhoid, cholera (depending on local epidemiology)	
Evidence of a possible breakdown in health protection/public health functions	*Legionella*, *Cryptosporidium*	
Evidence of a possible breakdown in food safety practices	Botulism, verotoxigenic *E. coli*	
Evidence of a possible failure of a vaccination programme	Measles, poliomyelitis, pertussis	
Disease with the potential to be a novel or increasing threat to human health	SARS, MERS-CoV, multi-resistant bacteria	
Evidence of expansion of the range of a reservoir/vector	Lyme disease, rabies, West Nile encephalitis	
Evidence of possible deliberate release	Anthrax, tularaemia, plague, smallpox, botulism	

*Given the different geographical ranges of individual diseases and wide national variations in public health services, vaccination programmes and availability of resources, reporting regulations vary between regions, states and countries. Many diseases are reportable for more than one reason. (MERS-CoV = Middle East respiratory syndrome coronavirus; SARS = severe acute respiratory syndrome)

Immunisation

Immunisation may be passive or active. Passive immunisation is achieved by administering antibodies targeting a specific pathogen. Antibodies are obtained from blood, so confer some of the risks associated with blood products (p. 933). The protection afforded by passive immunisation is immediate but of short duration (a few weeks or months); it is used to prevent or attenuate infection before or after exposure (Box 6.12).

Vaccination

Active immunisation is achieved by vaccination with whole organisms or organism components (Box 6.13).

Types of vaccine

Whole-cell vaccines consist of live or inactivated (killed) microorganisms. Component vaccines contain only extracted or synthesised components of microorganisms (e.g. polysaccharides or proteins). Live vaccines contain organisms with attenuated (reduced) virulence, which cause only mild symptoms but induce T-lymphocyte and humoral responses (p. 68) and are therefore more immunogenic than inactivated whole-cell vaccines. The use of live vaccines in immunocompromised individuals is not generally recommended, but they may be used by specialists following a risk/benefit assessment.

Component vaccines consisting only of polysaccharides, such as the pneumococcal polysaccharide vaccine (PPV), are poor activators of T lymphocytes and produce a short-lived antibody response without long-lasting memory. Conjugation of polysaccharide to a protein, as in the *Haemophilus influenzae* type B (Hib) vaccine and the protein conjugate pneumococcal

6.12 Indications for post-exposure prophylaxis with immunoglobulins

Human normal immunoglobulin (pooled immunoglobulin)

- Hepatitis A (unvaccinated contacts*)
- Measles (exposed child with heart or lung disease)

Human specific immunoglobulin

- Hepatitis B (sexual partners, inoculation injuries, infants born to infected mothers)
- Tetanus (high-risk wounds or incomplete or unknown immunisation status)
- Rabies
- Chickenpox (immunosuppressed children and adults, pregnant women)

*Active immunisation is preferred if contact is with a patient who is within 1 week of onset of jaundice.

6.13 Vaccines in current clinical use

Live attenuated vaccines

- Measles, mumps, rubella (MMR)
- Oral poliomyelitis (OPV, not used in UK)
- Rotavirus
- Tuberculosis (bacille Calmette–Guérin, BCG)
- Typhoid (oral typhoid vaccine)
- Varicella zoster virus

Inactivated (killed) whole-cell vaccines

- Cholera
- Hepatitis A
- Influenza
- Poliomyelitis (inactivated polio virus, IPV)
- Rabies

Component vaccines

- Anthrax (adsorbed extracted antigens)
- Diphtheria (adsorbed toxoid)
- Hepatitis B (adsorbed recombinant hepatitis B surface antigen, HBsAg)
- *Haemophilus influenzae* type B (conjugated capsular polysaccharide)
- Human papillomavirus (recombinant capsid proteins)
- Meningococcal, quadrivalent A, C, Y, W135 (conjugated capsular polysaccharide)
- Meningococcal, serogroup C (conjugated capsular polysaccharide)
- Pertussis (adsorbed extracted antigens)
- Pneumococcal conjugate (PCV; conjugated capsular polysaccharide, 13 serotypes)
- Pneumococcal polysaccharide (PPV; purified capsular polysaccharide, 23 serotypes)
- Tetanus (adsorbed toxoid)
- Typhoid (purified Vi capsular polysaccharide)

6.14 Guidelines for vaccination against infectious disease

- The principal contraindication to inactivated vaccines is an anaphylactic reaction to a previous dose or a vaccine component
- Live vaccines should not be given during an acute infection, to pregnant women or to the immunosuppressed, unless the immunosuppression is mild and the benefits outweigh the risks
- If two live vaccines are required, they should be given either simultaneously in opposite arms or 4 weeks apart
- Live vaccines should not be given for 3 months after an injection of human normal immunoglobulin (HNI)
- HNI should not be given for 2 weeks after a live vaccine
- Hay fever, asthma, eczema, sickle-cell disease, topical glucocorticoid therapy, antibiotic therapy, prematurity and chronic heart and lung diseases, including tuberculosis, are not contraindications to vaccination

---

vaccinated to curtail further spread. Vaccination is aimed mainly at preventing infectious disease. However, vaccination against human papillomavirus (HPV) was introduced to prevent cervical and other cancers that complicate HPV infection. Vaccination guidelines for individuals are shown in Box 6.14.

Vaccination becomes successful once the number of susceptible hosts in a population falls below the level required to sustain continued transmission of the target organism (herd immunity). Naturally acquired smallpox was declared to have been eradicated worldwide in 1980 through mass vaccination. In 1988, the WHO resolved to eradicate poliomyelitis by vaccination; the number of cases worldwide has since fallen from approximately 350 000 per annum to 74 in 2015. Recommended vaccination schedules vary between countries. In addition to standard vaccination schedules, catch-up schedules are specified for individuals who join vaccination programmes later than the recommended age.

Antimicrobial stewardship

Antimicrobial stewardship (AMS) refers to the systems and processes applied to a population to optimise the use of antimicrobial agents. The populations referred to here may be a nation, region, hospital, or a unit within a health-care organisation (e.g. ward or clinic). AMS aims to improve patient outcomes and reduce antimicrobial resistance (AMR). IPC and AMS complement each other (Fig. 6.14). Elements of AMS include treatment guidelines, antimicrobial formularies and ward rounds by infection specialists.

---

vaccine (PCV), activates T lymphocytes, which results in a sustained response and immunological memory. Toxoids are bacterial toxins that have been modified to reduce toxicity but maintain antigenicity. Vaccine response can be improved by co-administration with mildly pro-inflammatory adjuvants, such as aluminium hydroxide.

Use of vaccines

Vaccination may be applied to entire populations or to subpopulations at specific risk through travel, occupation or other activities. In ring vaccination, the population immediately surrounding a case or outbreak of infectious disease is

Fig. 6.14 The relationship between infection prevention and control (IPC) and antimicrobial stewardship (AMS).

Treatment of infectious diseases

Key components of treating infection are:

- optimising antimicrobial therapy while minimising selection for antimicrobial resistance and the impact on commensal flora
- addressing predisposing factors, e.g. glycaemic control in diabetes mellitus; viral load control in HIV-1-associated opportunistic infection
- considering source control, e.g. removal of an infected medical device or necrotic tissue
- managing complications, e.g. severe sepsis (systemic inflammatory response syndrome, or SIRS, p. 196) and acute kidney injury (p. 411).

For communicable disease, treatment must also take into account contacts of the infected patient, and may include IPC interventions such as isolation, antimicrobial prophylaxis, vaccination and contact tracing.

Principles of antimicrobial therapy

In some situations (e.g. pneumonia) it is important to start appropriate antimicrobial therapy promptly, whereas in others prior confirmation of the diagnosis and pathogen is preferred. The principles underlying the choice of antimicrobial agent(s) are discussed below. The WHO 'World Antibiotic Awareness Week' campaign is a yearly event aimed at highlighting the importance of prudent antimicrobial prescribing (see 'Further information').

Antimicrobial action and spectrum

Antimicrobial agents may kill or inhibit microorganisms by targeting essential and non-essential cellular processes, respectively. The range, or spectrum, of microorganisms that is killed or inhibited by a particular antimicrobial agent needs consideration when selecting therapy. Mechanisms of action of the major classes of antibacterial agent are listed in Box 6.15 and appropriate agents for some common infecting organisms are shown in Box 6.16. In severe infections and/or immunocompromised patients, it is customary to use bactericidal agents in preference to bacteriostatic agents.

Empiric versus targeted therapy

Empiric antimicrobial therapy is selected to treat a suspected infection (e.g. meningitis) before the microbiological cause is known. Targeted or 'directed' therapy can be prescribed when the pathogen(s) is known. Empirical antimicrobial regimens need to have activity against the range of pathogens that could be causing the infection in question; because broad-spectrum agents affect many more bacteria than needed, they select for antimicrobial resistance. 'Start Smart – Then Focus' (Fig. 6.15) describes the principle of converting from empiric therapy to narrow-spectrum targeted therapy. Optimum empiric therapy depends on the site of infection, patient characteristics and local antimicrobial resistance patterns. National or local guidelines are often used to inform antimicrobial prescribing decisions.

Combination therapy

It is sometimes appropriate to combine antimicrobial agents:

- when there is a need to increase clinical effectiveness (e.g. biofilm infections)

6.15 Target and mechanism of action of common antibacterial agents

Aminoglycosides, chloramphenicol, macrolides, lincosamides, oxazolidinones
- Inhibition of bacterial protein synthesis by binding to subunits of bacterial ribosomes

Tetracyclines
- Inhibition of protein synthesis by preventing transfer RNA binding to ribosomes

Beta-lactams
- Inhibition of cell wall peptidoglycan synthesis by competitive inhibition of transpeptidases ('penicillin-binding proteins')

Cyclic lipopeptide (daptomycin)
- Insertion of lipophilic tail into plasma membrane causing depolarisation and cell death

Glycopeptides
- Inhibition of cell wall peptidoglycan synthesis by forming complexes with D-alanine residues on peptidoglycan precursors

Nitroimidazoles
- The reduced form of the drug causes strand breaks in DNA

Quinolones
- Inhibition of DNA replication by binding to DNA topoisomerases (DNA gyrase and topoisomerase IV), preventing supercoiling and uncoiling of DNA

Rifamycins
- Inhibition of DNA synthesis by inhibiting DNA-dependent RNA polymerase

Sulphonamides and trimethoprim
- Inhibition of folate synthesis by dihydropteroate synthase (sulphonamides) and dihydrofolate reductase (trimethoprim) inhibition

- when no single agent's spectrum covers all potential pathogens (e.g. polymicrobial infection)
- when there is a need to reduce development of antimicrobial resistance in the target pathogen, as the organism would need to develop resistance to multiple agents simultaneously (e.g. antituberculous chemotherapy, p. 592; antiretroviral therapy (ART), p. 324).

Antimicrobial resistance

Microorganisms have evolved in the presence of naturally occurring antibiotics and have therefore developed resistance mechanisms (categorised in Fig. 6.16) to all classes of antimicrobial agent (antibiotics and their derivatives). Intrinsic resistance is an innate property of a microorganism, whereas acquired resistance arises by spontaneous mutation or horizontal transfer of genetic material from another organism (e.g. via a plasmid, p. 100). Plasmids often encode resistance to multiple antibiotics.

The *mecA* gene encodes a penicillin-binding protein, which has a low affinity for penicillins and therefore confers resistance to β-lactam antibiotics in staphylococci. Extended-spectrum β-lactamases (ESBLs) are frequently encoded on plasmids, which are transferred relatively easily between bacteria, including Enterobacteriaceae. Plasmid-encoded carbapenemases have been detected in strains of *Klebsiella pneumoniae* (e.g. New Delhi metallo-β-lactamase 1, NDM-1). Strains of MRSA have been described that also have reduced susceptibility to glycopeptides through the development of a relatively impermeable cell wall.

i 6.16 Antimicrobial options for common infecting bacteria

Organism	Antimicrobial options*
Gram-positive organisms	
Enterococcus faecalis	Ampicillin, vancomycin/teicoplanin
Enterococcus faecium	Vancomycin/teicoplanin, linezolid
Glycopeptide-resistant enterococci	Linezolid, tigecycline, daptomycin
MRSA	Clindamycin, vancomycin, rifampicin (never used as monotherapy), linezolid, daptomycin, tetracyclines, tigecycline, co-trimoxazole
Staphylococcus aureus	Flucloxacillin, clindamycin
Streptococcus pyogenes	Penicillin, clindamycin, vancomycin
Streptococcus pneumoniae	Penicillin, cephalosporins, levofloxacin, vancomycin
Gram-negative organisms	
Escherichia coli, 'coliforms' (enteric Gram-negative bacilli)	Amoxicillin, trimethoprim, cefuroxime, ciprofloxacin, co-amoxiclav
Enterobacter spp., *Citrobacter* spp.	Ciprofloxacin, meropenem, ertapenem, aminoglycosides
ESBL-producing Enterobacteriaceae	Ciprofloxacin, meropenem, ertapenem (if sensitive), temocillin, aminoglycosides
Carbapenemase-producing Enterobacteriaceae	Ciprofloxacin, aminoglycosides, tigecycline, colistin
Haemophilus influenzae	Amoxicillin, co-amoxiclav, macrolides, cefuroxime, cefotaxime, ciprofloxacin
Legionella pneumophila	Azithromycin, levofloxacin, doxycycline
Neisseria gonorrhoeae	Ceftriaxone/cefixime, spectinomycin
Neisseria meningitidis	Penicillin, cefotaxime/ceftriaxone, chloramphenicol
Pseudomonas aeruginosa	Ciprofloxacin, piperacillin–tazobactam, aztreonam, meropenem, aminoglycosides, ceftazidime/cefepime
Salmonella typhi	Ceftriaxone, azithromycin (uncomplicated typhoid), chloramphenicol (resistance common)
Strict anaerobes	
Bacteroides spp.	Metronidazole, clindamycin, co-amoxiclav, piperacillin–tazobactam, meropenem
Clostridium difficile	Metronidazole, vancomycin (oral), fidaxomicin
Clostridium spp.	Penicillin, metronidazole, clindamycin
Fusobacterium spp.	Penicillin, metronidazole, clindamycin
Other organisms	
Chlamydia trachomatis	Azithromycin, doxycycline
Treponema pallidum	Penicillin, doxycycline

*Antibiotic selection depends on multiple factors, including local susceptibility patterns, which vary enormously between geographical areas. There are many appropriate alternatives to those listed. (ESBL = extended-spectrum β-lactamase; MRSA = meticillin-resistant *Staphylococcus aureus*)

Fig. 6.15 Stages in the selection and refinement of antimicrobial therapy: 'Start Smart – Then Focus'.

Active efflux of antimicrobial agent
Tetracycline resistance in Gram-positive and Gram-negative bacteria
Fluconazole resistance in *Candida* spp.

Target modification
β-lactam resistance in MRSA – altered penicillin-binding protein
Glycopeptide resistance in enterococci – altered peptidoglycan amino acid sequence
Rifampicin resistance in *M. tuberculosis* – RNA polymerase mutation
Ciprofloxacin resistance in Enterobacteriaceae – DNA gyrase mutation
Linezolid resistance in staphylococci and enterococci – 23S rRNA methylation

Impermeability/reduced permeability
Carbapenem resistance in *Pseudomonas* spp.
Aminoglycoside resistance in anaerobes (uptake requires O_2-dependent transport mechanism)

Enzymatic degradation of agent
β-lactam resistance in many organisms (penicillinase in *Staph. aureus*; ESBLs, *ampC* and NDM-1 in Enterobacteriaceae)
Chloramphenicol resistance in staphylococci (CAT)

Antimicrobial target   Antimicrobial agent

Fig. 6.16 Examples of mechanisms of antimicrobial resistance. (CAT = chloramphenicol acetyltransferase; ESBLs = extended-spectrum β-lactamases; MRSA = meticillin-resistant *Staph. aureus*; NDM-1 = New Delhi metallo-β-lactamase 1).

Factors promoting antimicrobial resistance include the inappropriate use of antibiotics (e.g. to treat viral infections), inadequate dosage or unnecessarily prolonged treatment, and use of antimicrobials as growth promoters in agriculture. However, *any* antimicrobial use exerts a selection pressure that favours the development of resistance. Combination antimicrobial therapy may reduce the emergence of resistance in the target pathogen but not in the normal flora that it also affects. Despite use of combination therapy for *M. tuberculosis*, multidrug-resistant tuberculosis (MDR-TB, resistant to isoniazid and rifampicin) and extremely drug-resistant tuberculosis (XDR-TB, resistant to isoniazid and rifampicin, any fluoroquinolone and at least one injectable antimicrobial antituberculous agent) have been reported worldwide and are increasing in incidence.

The term 'post-antibiotic era' has been coined to describe a future in which the acquisition of resistance by bacteria will have been so extensive that antibiotic therapy is rendered useless. A more realistic scenario, which is currently being experienced, is a gradual but inexorable progression of resistance, necessitating the use of ever more toxic and expensive antimicrobials.

Duration of therapy

Treatment duration reflects the severity of infection and accessibility of the infected site to antimicrobial agents. For most infections, there is limited evidence available to support a specific duration of treatment (Box 6.17). Depending on the indication, initial intravenous therapy can often be switched to oral as soon as the patient is apyrexial and improving. In the absence of specific guidance, antimicrobial therapy should be stopped when there is no longer any clinical evidence of infection.

Pharmacokinetics and pharmacodynamics

Pharmacokinetics of antimicrobial agents determine whether adequate concentrations are obtained at the sites of infection. Septic patients often have poor gastrointestinal absorption, so the preferred initial route of therapy is intravenous. Knowledge of anticipated antimicrobial drug concentrations at sites of infection is critical. For example, achieving a 'therapeutic' blood level of gentamicin is of little practical use in treating meningitis, as CSF penetration of the drug is poor. Knowledge of routes of antimicrobial elimination is also critical; for instance, urinary tract infection is ideally treated with a drug that is excreted unchanged in the urine.

Pharmacodynamics describes the relationship between antimicrobial concentration and microbial killing. For many agents, antimicrobial effect can be categorised as 'concentration-dependent' or 'time-dependent'. The concentration of antimicrobial achieved after a single dose is illustrated in Figure 6.17. The maximum concentration achieved is C_{max} and the measure of overall exposure is the area under the curve (AUC). The efficacy of antimicrobial agents whose killing is concentration-dependent (e.g. aminoglycosides) increases with the amount by which C_{max} exceeds the minimum inhibitory concentration (C_{max} : MIC ratio). For this reason, it has become customary to administer aminoglycosides (e.g. gentamicin) infrequently at high doses (e.g. 7 mg/kg) rather than frequently at low doses. This has the added advantage of minimising toxicity by reducing the likelihood

6.17 Duration of antimicrobial therapy for some common infections*	
Infection	**Duration of therapy**
Viral infections	
Herpes simplex encephalitis	2–3 weeks
Bacterial infections	
Gonorrhoea	Single dose
Infective endocarditis (streptococcal, native valve)	4 weeks ± gentamicin for first 2 weeks
Infective endocarditis (prosthetic valve)	6 weeks
Osteomyelitis	6 weeks
Pneumonia (community-acquired, severe)	7–10 days (no organism identified), 14–21 days (*Staph. aureus* or *Legionella* spp.)
Septic arthritis	2–4 weeks
Urinary tract infection (male)	2 weeks
Urinary tract infection, upper tract, uncomplicated (female)	7 days
Urinary tract infection, lower (female)	3 days
Mycobacterial infections	
Tuberculosis (meningeal)	12 months
Tuberculosis (pulmonary)	6 months
Fungal infections	
Invasive pulmonary aspergillosis	Until clinical/radiological resolution and reversal of predisposition
Candidaemia (acute disseminated)	2 weeks after last positive blood culture and resolution of signs and symptoms

*All recommendations are indicative. Actual duration takes into account predisposing factors, specific organisms and antimicrobial susceptibility, adjuvant therapies, current guidelines and clinical response.

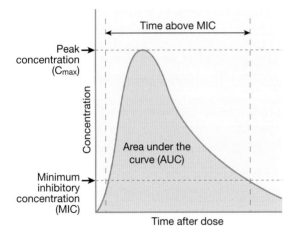

Fig. 6.17 Antimicrobial pharmacodynamics. The curve represents drug concentrations after a single dose of an antimicrobial agent. Factors that determine microbial killing are C_{max} : MIC ratio (concentration-dependent killing), time above MIC (time-dependent killing) and AUC : MIC ratio.

of drug accumulation. Conversely, the β-lactam antibiotics and vancomycin exhibit time-dependent killing, and their efficacy depends on C_{max} exceeding the MIC for a certain time (which is different for each class of agent). This is reflected in the dosing interval of benzylpenicillin, which is usually given every 4 hours in severe infection (e.g. meningococcal meningitis), and may be administered by continuous infusion. For other antimicrobial agents, the pharmacodynamic relationships are more complex and often less well understood. With some agents, bacterial inhibition persists after antimicrobial exposure (post-antibiotic and post-antibiotic sub-MIC effects).

Therapeutic drug monitoring

Therapeutic drug monitoring is used to confirm that levels of antimicrobial agents with a low therapeutic index (e.g. aminoglycosides) are not excessive, and that levels of agents with marked pharmacokinetic variability (e.g. vancomycin) are adequate. Specific recommendations for monitoring depend on individual clinical circumstances; for instance, different pre- and post-dose levels of gentamicin are recommended, depending on whether it is being used in traditional divided doses, once daily or for synergy in endocarditis (p. 530).

Antimicrobial prophylaxis

Antimicrobial prophylaxis is the use of antimicrobial agents to prevent infection. Primary prophylaxis is used to reduce the risk of infection following certain medical procedures (e.g. colonic resection or prosthetic hip insertion), following exposure to a specific pathogen (e.g. *Bordetella pertussis*) or in specific situations such as post-splenectomy (Box 6.18). It should be

6.18 Recommendations for antimicrobial prophylaxis in adults*	
Infection risk	**Recommended antimicrobial**
Bacterial	
Diphtheria (prevention of secondary cases)	Erythromycin
Gas gangrene (after high amputation or major trauma)	Penicillin or metronidazole
Lower gastrointestinal tract surgery	Cefuroxime + metronidazole, gentamicin + metronidazole, or co-amoxiclav (single dose only)
Meningococcal disease (prevention of secondary cases)	Rifampicin or ciprofloxacin
Rheumatic fever (prevention of recurrence)	Phenoxymethylpenicillin or sulfadiazine
Tuberculosis (prevention of secondary cases)	Isoniazid ± rifampicin
Whooping cough (prevention of secondary cases)	Erythromycin
Viral	
HIV, occupational exposure (sharps injury)	Combination tenofovir/emtricitabine and raltegravir. Modified if index case's virus known to be resistant
Influenza A (prevention of secondary cases in adults with chronic respiratory, cardiovascular or renal disease, immunosuppression or diabetes mellitus)	Oseltamivir
Fungal	
Aspergillosis (in high-risk haematology patients)	Posaconazole (voriconazole or itraconazole alternatives if intolerant)
Pneumocystis pneumonia (prevention in HIV and other immunosuppressed states)	Co-trimoxazole, pentamidine or dapsone
Protozoal	
Malaria (prevention of travel-associated disease)	Specific antimalarials depend on travel itinerary (p. 278)

*These are based on current UK practice. Recommendations may vary locally or nationally. Antimicrobial prophylaxis for infective endocarditis during dental procedures is not currently recommended in the UK.

associated with minimal adverse effects. In the case of exposure, it may be combined with passive immunisation (see Box 6.12). Secondary prophylaxis is used in patients who have been treated successfully for an infection but remain predisposed to it. It is used in haemato-oncology patients in the context of fungal infection and in HIV-positive individuals with an opportunistic infection until a defined level of immune reconstitution is achieved.

Antibacterial agents

For details of antibacterial usage in pregnancy and old age, see Boxes 6.19 and 6.20.

 6.19 Antimicrobial agents in pregnancy[1]

Contraindicated

- Chloramphenicol: neonatal 'grey baby' syndrome – collapse, hypotension and cyanosis
- Fluconazole: teratogenic in high doses
- Quinolones: arthropathy in animal studies
- Sulphonamides: neonatal haemolysis and methaemoglobinaemia
- Tetracyclines, glycylcyclines: skeletal abnormalities in animals in first trimester; fetal dental discoloration and maternal hepatotoxicity with large parenteral doses in second or third trimesters
- Trimethoprim: teratogenic in first trimester

Relatively contraindicated

- Aminoglycosides: potential damage to fetal auditory and vestibular nerves in second and third trimesters
- Metronidazole: avoidance of high dosages is recommended[2]

Not known to be harmful; use only when necessary

- Aciclovir
- Cephalosporins
- Clarithromycin
- Clindamycin
- Erythromycin
- Glycopeptides
- Linezolid
- Meropenem
- Penicillins

[1]Data extracted from Joint Formulary Committee. British National Formulary (online). London: BMJ Group and Pharmaceutical Press; (medicinescomplete. com) [accessed on 16 March 2013]. [2]Theoretical risk of teratogenicity, not supported by available clinical evidence.

 6.20 Problems with antimicrobial therapy in old age

- **_Clostridium difficile_ infection**: all antibiotics predispose to some extent, but second- and third-generation cephalosporins, co-amoxiclav and fluoroquinolones (e.g. ciprofloxacin) especially so.
- **Hypersensitivity reactions**: rise in incidence due to increased previous exposure.
- **Renal impairment**: may be significant in old age, despite 'normal' creatinine levels (p. 386).
- **Nephrotoxicity**: more likely, e.g. first-generation cephalosporins, aminoglycosides.
- **Accumulation of β-lactam antibiotics**: may result in myoclonus, seizures or coma.
- **Reduced gastric acid production**: gastric pH is higher, which causes increased penicillin absorption.
- **Reduced hepatic metabolism**: results in a higher risk of isoniazid-related hepatotoxicity.
- **Quinolones**: associated with delirium and may increase the risk of seizures.

Beta-lactam antibiotics

These antibiotics have a β-lactam ring structure and exert a bactericidal action by inhibiting enzymes involved in cell wall synthesis (penicillin-binding proteins, PBPs). They are classified in Box 6.21.

Pharmacokinetics

- Good drug levels are achieved in lung, kidney, bone, muscle and liver, and in pleural, synovial, pericardial and peritoneal fluids.
- CSF levels are low, except when meninges are inflamed.
- Activity is not inhibited in abscess (e.g. by low pH and PO_2, high protein or neutrophils).
- Beta-lactams are subject to an 'inoculum effect' – activity is reduced in the presence of a high organism burden (PBP expression is down-regulated by high organism density).
- Generally safe in pregnancy (except imipenem/cilastatin).

Adverse effects

Immediate (IgE-mediated) allergic reactions are rare but life-threatening. Approximately 90% of patients who report a penicillin allergy do not have a true IgE-mediated allergy. Other reactions, such as rashes, fever and haematological effects (e.g. low white cell count), usually follow more prolonged therapy (more than 2 weeks). A large proportion of patients with infectious mononucleosis develop a rash if given aminopenicillins; this does not imply lasting allergy. The relationship between allergy to penicillin and allergy to cephalosporins depends on the specific cephalosporin used; there is significant cross-reactivity with first-generation cephalosporins but cross-reactivity to second-/third-generation cephalosporins is less common. Avoidance of cephalosporins, however, is recommended in patients who have IgE-mediated penicillin allergy (p. 84). Cross-reactivity between penicillin and carbapenems is rare (approximately 1% by skin testing) and carbapenems may be administered if there are no suitable alternatives and appropriate resuscitation facilities are available. The monobactam aztreonam (p. 121) is the β-lactam least likely to cross-react in patients with penicillin allergy.

Gastrointestinal upset and diarrhoea are common, and a mild reversible hepatitis is recognised with many β-lactams. More severe forms of hepatitis can be observed with flucloxacillin and co-amoxiclav. Leucopenia, thrombocytopenia, coagulation

---

 6.21 Beta-lactam antibiotics

Penicillins

- Natural penicillins: benzylpenicillin, phenoxymethylpenicillin
- Penicillinase-resistant penicillins: meticillin, flucloxacillin, nafcillin, oxacillin
- Aminopenicillins: ampicillin, amoxicillin
- Carboxy- and ureido-penicillins: ticarcillin, piperacillin, temocillin

Cephalosporins

- See Box 6.22

Monobactams

- Aztreonam

Carbapenems

- Imipenem, meropenem, ertapenem, doripenem

deficiencies, interstitial nephritis and potentiation of aminoglycoside-mediated kidney damage are also recognised (p. 122). Seizures and encephalopathy have been reported, particularly with high doses in the presence of renal insufficiency. Thrombophlebitis occurs in up to 5% of patients receiving parenteral β-lactams.

Drug interactions

Synergism occurs in combination with aminoglycosides in vitro. Ampicillin decreases the biological effect of oral contraceptives and the whole class is significantly affected by concurrent administration of probenecid, producing a 2–4-fold increase in the peak serum concentration.

Penicillins

Natural penicillins are primarily effective against Gram-positive organisms (except staphylococci, most of which produce a penicillinase) and anaerobic organisms. *Strep. pyogenes* has remained sensitive to natural penicillins worldwide. According to the European Antimicrobial Resistance Surveillance Network (EARS-Net), the prevalence of non-susceptibility to penicillin in *Strep. pneumoniae* in Europe in 2014 varied widely from 0% (Cyprus) to 46.7% (Romania).

Penicillinase-resistant penicillins are the mainstay of treatment for infections with *Staph. aureus*, other than MRSA. However, EARS-Net data from 2014 indicate that MRSA rates in Europe vary widely from 0.9% (Netherlands) to 56% (Romania).

Aminopenicillins have the same spectrum of activity as the natural penicillins, with additional Gram-negative cover against Enterobacteriaceae. Amoxicillin has better oral absorption than ampicillin. Unfortunately, resistance to these agents is widespread (57.1% of *E. coli* Europe-wide in 2014, range 34.7–73%), so they are no longer appropriate for empirical use in Gram-negative infections. In many organisms, resistance is due to β-lactamase production, which can be overcome by the addition of β-lactamase inhibitors (clavulanic acid or sulbactam).

Carboxypenicillins (e.g. ticarcillin) and ureidopenicillins (e.g. piperacillin) are particularly active against Gram-negative organisms, especially *Pseudomonas* spp., which are resistant to the aminopenicillins. Beta-lactamase inhibitors may be added to extend their spectrum of activity (e.g. piperacillin–tazobactam). Temocillin is derived from ticarcillin; it has good activity against Enterobacteriaceae, including those that produce ESBL enzymes, but poor activity against *Pseudomonas aeruginosa* and Gram-positive bacteria.

Cephalosporins and cephamycins

Cephalosporins are broad-spectrum agents. Unfortunately, their use is associated with CDI (p. 264). With the exception of ceftobiprole, the group has no activity against enterococci. Only the cephamycins have anti-anaerobic activity. All cephalosporins are inactivated by ESBL. Cephalosporins are arranged in 'generations' (Box 6.22).

- *First-generation compounds* have excellent activity against Gram-positive organisms and some activity against Gram-negatives.
- *Second-generation drugs* retain Gram-positive activity but have extended Gram-negative activity. Cephamycins (e.g. cefoxitin), included in this group, are active against anaerobic Gram-negative bacilli.
- *Third-generation agents* further improve anti-Gram-negative cover. For some (e.g. ceftazidime), this is extended to include *Pseudomonas* spp. Cefotaxime and ceftriaxone have excellent Gram-negative activity and

i	**6.22 Cephalosporins**	
First generation		
• Cefalexin, cefradine (oral)	• Cefazolin (IV)	
Second generation		
• Cefuroxime (oral/IV) • Cefaclor (oral)	• Cefoxitin (IV)	
Third generation		
• Cefixime (oral) • Cefotaxime (IV)	• Ceftriaxone (IV) • Ceftazidime (IV)	
Fourth generation		
• Cefepime (IV)		
Fifth generation (also referred to as 'next generation')		
• Ceftobiprole (IV)	• Ceftaroline (IV)	

retain good activity against *Strep. pneumoniae* and β-haemolytic streptococci. Ceftriaxone is administered once daily and is therefore a suitable agent for outpatient intravenous (parenteral) antimicrobial therapy (OPAT).
- *Fourth-generation agents*, e.g. cefipime, have a broad spectrum of activity, including streptococci and some Gram-negatives, including *P. aeruginosa.*
- *Fifth-generation agents*, such as ceftobiprole and ceftaroline, have an enhanced spectrum of Gram-positive activity that includes MRSA, and also have activity against Gram-negative bacteria; some, such as ceftobiprole, are active against *P. aeruginosa*.

The spectrum of cephalosporins has also been enhanced by adding β-lactamase inhibitors.

Monobactams

Aztreonam is the only available monobactam. It is active against Gram-negative bacteria, except ESBL-producing organisms, but inactive against Gram-positive organisms or anaerobes. It is a parenteral-only agent and may be used safely in most penicillin-allergic patients other than those with an allergy to ceftazidime, which shares a common side chain with aztreonam.

Carbapenems

These intravenous agents have the broadest antibiotic activity of the β-lactam antibiotics, covering most clinically significant bacteria, including anaerobes (e.g. imipenem, meropenem, ertapenem).

Macrolide and lincosamide antibiotics

Macrolides (e.g. erythromycin, clarithromycin and azithromycin) and lincosamides (e.g. clindamycin) are bacteriostatic agents. Both classes bind to the same component of the ribosome, so they are not administered together. Macrolides are used for *Legionella*, *Mycoplasma*, *Chlamydia* and *Bordetella* infections. Azithromycin is employed for single-dose/short-course therapy for genitourinary *Chlamydia/Mycoplasma* spp. infections. Clindamycin is used primarily for skin, soft tissue, bone and joint infections.

Pharmacokinetics

Macrolides

- Variable bioavailability (intravenous and oral preparations available).

- Frequency of administration: erythromycin is administered 4 times daily, clarithromycin twice daily, azithromycin once daily.
- High protein binding.
- Excellent intracellular accumulation.

Lincosamides (e.g. clindamycin)

- Good oral bioavailability.
- Food has no effect on absorption.
- Good bone/joint penetration; limited CSF penetration.

Adverse effects

- Gastrointestinal upset, especially in young adults (erythromycin 30%).
- Cholestatic jaundice with erythromycin estolate.
- Prolongation of QT interval can cause torsades de pointes (p. 476).
- Clindamycin predisposes to CDI.

Aminoglycosides and spectinomycin

Aminoglycosides are effective mainly in Gram-negative infections and are therefore commonly used in regimens for intra-abdominal infection. Some aminoglycosides, e.g. amikacin, are important components of therapy for MDR-TB. Because they act synergistically with β-lactam antibiotics they are used in combinations to treat biofilm infections, including infective endocarditis and orthopaedic implant infections. They cause very little local irritation at injection sites and negligible allergic responses. Oto- and nephrotoxicity must be avoided by monitoring of renal function and drug levels and by use of short treatment regimens. Aminoglycosides are not subject to an inoculum effect (p. 120) and they all exhibit a post-antibiotic effect (p. 119).

Pharmacokinetics

- Negligible oral absorption.
- Hydrophilic, so excellent penetration to extracellular fluid in body cavities and serosal fluids.
- Very poor intracellular penetration (except hair cells in cochlea and renal cortical cells).
- Negligible CSF and corneal penetration and may require intrathecal administration during neurosurgical infections.
- Peak plasma levels 30 minutes after infusion.
- Monitoring of therapeutic levels required.

Gentamicin dosing

- Except in certain forms of endocarditis, pregnancy, severe burns, end-stage renal disease and paediatric patients, gentamicin is administered at 7 mg/kg body weight. The appropriate dose interval depends on drug clearance and is determined by reference to the Hartford nomogram (Fig. 6.18).
- In streptococcal and enterococcal endocarditis, gentamicin is used with a cell wall active agent (usually a β-lactam), to provide synergy. Commonly used doses are 1 mg/kg 2–3 times daily for enterococcal endocarditis and 3 mg/kg once daily for most strains of oral streptococci. Target pre- and post-dose levels are <1 mg/L and 3–5 mg/L, respectively, when gentamicin is dosed 3 times daily.
- When not used according to the Hartford regimen or for endocarditis, gentamicin is administered twice or 3 times daily at 3–5 mg/kg/day. Target pre- and post-dose levels

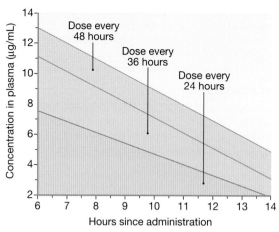

Fig. 6.18 Dosing of aminoglycosides using the Hartford nomogram. The nomogram is used to determine the dose interval for 7 mg doses of gentamicin or tobramycin, using measurements of drug levels in plasma 6–14 hours after a single dose.

are <1 mg/L and 5–10 mg/L (7–10 mg/L with less sensitive organisms, e.g. *P. aeruginosa*), respectively.
- For other aminoglycosides, consult local guidance.

Adverse effects

- Renal toxicity (usually reversible) accentuated by other nephrotoxic agents.
- Cochlear toxicity (permanent) more likely in older people and those with a predisposing mitochondrial gene mutation.
- Neuromuscular blockade after rapid intravenous infusion (potentiated by calcium channel blockers, myasthenia gravis and hypomagnesaemia).

Spectinomycin

Chemically similar to the aminoglycosides and given intramuscularly, spectinomycin was developed to treat strains of *Neisseria gonorrhoeae* resistant to β-lactam antibiotics. Unfortunately, resistance to spectinomycin is very common. Its only indication is the treatment of gonococcal urethritis in pregnancy or in patients allergic to β-lactam antibiotics.

Quinolones and fluoroquinolones

These are effective and generally well-tolerated bactericidal agents. The quinolones have purely anti-Gram-negative activity, whereas the fluoroquinolones are broad-spectrum agents (Box 6.23). Ciprofloxacin has anti-pseudomonal activity but resistance emerges rapidly. In 2014, European surveillance showed that resistance to fluoroquinolones in *E. coli* ranged between 7.8% (Iceland) and 46.4% (Cyprus). Quinolones and fluoroquinolones are used for a variety of common infections, including urinary tract infection and pneumonia, and less common problems like MDR-TB.

Pharmacokinetics

- Well absorbed after oral administration but delayed by food, antacids, ferrous sulphate and multivitamins.
- Wide volume of distribution; tissue concentrations twice those in serum.
- Good intracellular penetration, concentrating in phagocytes.

i	6.23 Quinolones and fluoroquinolones		
Agent	Route of administration	Typical antimicrobial spectrum	
Quinolones			
Nalidixic acid	Oral	Enteric Gram-negative bacilli (not *Pseudomonas aeruginosa*)	
Fluoroquinolones			
Ciprofloxacin	IV/oral	Enteric Gram-negative bacilli, *P. aeruginosa*, *Haemophilus* spp., 'atypical' respiratory pathogens*	
Norfloxacin	Oral		
Ofloxacin	IV/oral/topical		
Levofloxacin (L-isomer of ofloxacin)	IV/oral	*Haemophilus* spp., *Strep. pneumoniae*, 'atypical' respiratory pathogens*	
Moxifloxacin	Oral	*Strep. pneumoniae*, *Staph. aureus*, 'atypical' respiratory pathogens*, Mycobacteria and anaerobes	

*'Atypical' pathogens include *Mycoplasma pneumoniae* and *Legionella* spp. Fluoroquinolones have variable activity against *M. tuberculosis* and other mycobacteria.

Adverse effects

- Gastrointestinal side-effects in 1–5%.
- Rare skin reactions (phototoxicity).
- Tendinitis and Achilles tendon rupture, especially in older people.
- Central nervous system effects (delirium, tremor, dizziness and occasional seizures in 5–12%), especially in older people.
- Reduces clearance of xanthines and theophyllines, potentially inducing insomnia and increased seizure potential.
- Prolongation of QT interval on ECG, cardiac arrhythmias.
- Ciprofloxacin use is associated with the acquisition of MRSA and emergence of *C. difficile* ribotype 027 (p. 264).

Glycopeptides

Glycopeptides (vancomycin and teicoplanin) are effective against Gram-positive organisms only, and are used against MRSA and ampicillin-resistant enterococci. Some staphylococci and enterococci demonstrate intermediate sensitivity or resistance. Vancomycin use should be restricted to limit emergence of resistant strains. Teicoplanin is not available in all countries. Neither drug is absorbed after oral administration but vancomycin is used orally to treat CDI.

Pharmacokinetics

Vancomycin

- Administered by slow intravenous infusion, good tissue distribution and short half-life.
- Enters the CSF only in the presence of inflammation and may require intrathecal administration during neurosurgical infections.
- Therapeutic monitoring of intravenous vancomycin is recommended, to maintain pre-dose levels of >10 mg/L (15–20 mg/L in serious staphylococcal infections).

Teicoplanin

- Long half-life allows once-daily dosing.

Adverse effects

- Histamine release due to rapid vancomycin infusion produces a 'red man' reaction (rare with modern preparations).
- Nephrotoxicity is rare but may occur with concomitant aminoglycoside use, as may ototoxicity.
- Teicoplanin can cause rash, bronchospasm, eosinophilia and anaphylaxis.

Lipopeptides

Daptomycin is a cyclic lipopeptide with bactericidal activity against Gram-positive organisms (including MRSA and GRE) but not Gram-negatives. It is not absorbed orally, and is used intravenously to treat Gram-positive infections, such as soft tissue infections and *Staph. aureus* infective endocarditis. Daptomycin is not effective for community-acquired pneumonia. Treatment can be associated with increased levels of creatine kinase and eosinophilic pneumonitis.

Polymyxins

Colistin is a polymyxin antibiotic that binds and disrupts the outer cell membrane of Gram-negative bacteria, including *P. aeruginosa* and *Acinetobacter baumannii*. Its use has increased with the emergence and spread of multi-resistant Gram-negative bacteria, including CPEs. It can be administered by oral, intravenous and nebulised routes. Significant adverse effects include neurotoxicity, including encephalopathy, and nephrotoxicity.

Folate antagonists

These are bacteriostatic antibacterials (p. 109). A combination of a sulphonamide and either trimethoprim or pyrimethamine is most commonly used, which interferes with two consecutive steps in the metabolic pathway. Available combinations include trimethoprim/sulfamethoxazole (co-trimoxazole) and pyrimethamine with either sulfadoxine (used to treat malaria) or sulfadiazine (used in toxoplasmosis). Co-trimoxazole is the first-line drug for *Pneumocystis jirovecii* infection, the second-line drug for treatment and prevention of *B. pertussis* (whooping cough) infection, and is also used for a variety of other infections, including *Staph. aureus*. Dapsone is used to treat leprosy (Hansen's disease) and to prevent toxoplasmosis and pneumocystis when patients are intolerant of other medications. Folinic acid should be given to prevent myelosuppression if these drugs are used long-term or unavoidably in early pregnancy.

Pharmacokinetics

- Well absorbed orally.
- Sulphonamides are hydrophilic, distributing well to the extracellular fluid.
- Trimethoprim is lipophilic with high tissue concentrations.

Adverse effects

- Trimethoprim is generally well tolerated, with few adverse effects.
- Sulphonamides and dapsone may cause haemolysis in glucose-6-phosphate dehydrogenase deficiency (p. 948).
- Sulphonamides and dapsone cause skin and mucocutaneous reactions, including Stevens–Johnson syndrome and 'dapsone syndrome' (rash, fever and lymphadenopathy).
- Dapsone causes methaemoglobinaemia (p. 135) and peripheral neuropathy.

Tetracyclines and glycylcyclines

Tetracyclines

Of this mainly bacteriostatic class, the newer drugs doxycycline and minocycline show better absorption and distribution than older ones. Many streptococci and Gram-negative bacteria are now resistant, in part due to their use in animals (which is banned in Europe). Tetracyclines are indicated for *Mycoplasma* spp., *Chlamydia* spp., *Rickettsia* spp., *Coxiella* spp., *Bartonella* spp., *Borrelia* spp., *Helicobacter pylori*, *Treponema pallidum* and atypical mycobacterial infections. Tetracyclines can also be used for malaria prevention.

Pharmacokinetics

- Best oral absorption is in the fasting state (doxycycline is 100% absorbed unless gastric pH rises) and absorption is inhibited by cations, e.g. calcium or iron, which should not be administered at the same time.

Adverse effects

- All tetracyclines except doxycycline are contraindicated in renal failure.
- Dizziness with minocycline.
- Binding to metallic ions in bones and teeth causes discoloration (avoid in children and pregnancy) and enamel hypoplasia.
- Oesophagitis/oesophageal ulcers with doxycycline.
- Phototoxic skin reactions.

Glycylcyclines (tigecycline)

Chemical modification of tetracycline has produced tigecycline, a broad-spectrum, parenteral-only antibiotic with activity against resistant Gram-positive and Gram-negative pathogens, such as MRSA and ESBL (but excluding *Pseudomonas* spp.). Re-analysis of trial data has shown that there was excess mortality following tigecycline treatment as opposed to comparator antibiotics, so tigecycline should be used only when there has been adequate assessment of risk versus benefit.

Nitroimidazoles

Nitroimidazoles are highly active against strictly anaerobic bacteria, especially *Bacteroides fragilis*, *C. difficile* and other *Clostridium* spp. They also have significant antiprotozoal activity against amoebae and *Giardia lamblia*.

Pharmacokinetics

- Almost completely absorbed after oral administration (60% after rectal administration).
- Well distributed, especially to brain and CSF.
- Safe in pregnancy.

Adverse effects

- Metallic taste (dose-dependent).
- Severe vomiting if taken with alcohol – 'Antabuse effect'.
- Peripheral neuropathy with prolonged use.

Phenicols

Chloramphenicol is the only example in clinical use. In developed countries its use tends to be reserved for severe and life-threatening infections when other antibiotics are either unavailable or impractical, largely because of concerns about toxicity. It is bacteriostatic to most organisms but apparently bactericidal to *H. influenzae*, *Strep. pneumoniae* and *N. meningitidis*. It has a very broad spectrum of activity against aerobic and anaerobic organisms, spirochaetes, *Rickettsia*, *Chlamydia* and *Mycoplasma* spp. It competes with macrolides and lincosamides for ribosomal binding sites, so should not be used in combination with these agents. Significant adverse effects are 'grey baby' syndrome in infants (cyanosis and circulatory collapse due to inability to conjugate drug and excrete the active form in urine); reversible dose-dependent bone marrow depression in adults receiving high cumulative doses; and severe aplastic anaemia in 1 in 25 000–40 000 exposures (unrelated to dose, duration of therapy or route of administration).

Oxazolidinones

Linezolid and tedizolid are examples and their good activity against Gram-positive organisms means they are often used to treat skin and soft tissue infections. They may also be used in infection caused by resistant Gram-positive bacteria, including MRSA and GRE. Administration can be intravenous or oral. Common linezolid adverse effects include mild gastrointestinal upset and tongue discoloration. Myelodysplasia and peripheral and optic neuropathy can occur with prolonged use. Linezolid has monoamine oxidase inhibitor (MAOI) activity, and co-administration with other MAOIs or serotonin re-uptake inhibitors should be avoided, as this may precipitate a 'serotonin syndrome' (p. 1199).

Other antibacterial agents

Fusidic acid

This antibiotic, active against Gram-positive bacteria, is available in intravenous, oral or topical formulations. It is lipid-soluble and distributes well to tissues. Its antibacterial activity is, however, unpredictable. Fusidic acid is used in combination, typically with antistaphylococcal penicillins, or for MRSA with clindamycin or rifampicin. It interacts with coumarin derivatives and oral contraceptives.

Nitrofurantoin

This drug has very rapid renal elimination and is active against aerobic Gram-negative and Gram-positive bacteria, including enterococci. It is used only for treatment of urinary tract infection, being generally safe in pregnancy and childhood. With prolonged treatment, however, it can cause eosinophilic lung infiltrates, fever, pulmonary fibrosis, peripheral neuropathy, hepatitis and haemolytic anaemia so its use must be carefully balanced against risks.

Fidaxomicin

Fidaxomicin is an inhibitor of RNA synthesis, and was introduced for the treatment of CDI in 2012. In non-severe CDI it is non-inferior to oral vancomycin and is associated with a lower recurrence rate. Its effectiveness has not been assessed in severe CDI.

Fosfomycin

Fosfomycin acts by inhibiting cell wall synthesis. It has activity against Gram-negative but also Gram-positive bacteria and can demonstrate in vitro synergy against MRSA when combined with other antimicrobials. It is used for treatment of urinary tract infections but can be employed in other situations against multi-resistant bacteria.

Antimycobacterial agents

Isoniazid

Isoniazid is bactericidal for replicating bacteria and bacteriostatic for non-replicating bacteria. It is activated by mycobacterial catalase-peroxidase (KatG) and inhibits the *InhA* gene product, a reductase involved in mycolic acid synthesis. Mutations in *KatG* or *InhA* result in isoniazid resistance, which was reported in 15% of cases of *M. tuberculosis* infection globally in 2013. Isoniazid is well absorbed orally and metabolised by acetylation in the liver. The major side-effects are hepatitis, neuropathy (ameliorated by co-administration of pyridoxine) and hypersensitivity reactions.

Rifampicin

Rifampicin inhibits DNA-dependent RNA polymerase and is bactericidal against replicating bacteria. It is also active in necrotic foci, where mycobacteria have low levels of replication, and is therefore important in sterilisation and sputum conversion. Resistance most often involves the β-subunit of RNA polymerase and most often occurs with isoniazid-resistant MDR-TB. Rifampicin is well absorbed orally. It is metabolised by the liver via the microsomal cytochrome P450 system and is one the most potent inducers of multiple P450 isoenzymes, so is subject to extensive drug–drug interactions. Common side-effects include hepatitis, influenza-like symptoms and hypersensitivity reactions. Orange discoloration of urine and body secretions is expected.

Pyrazinamide

The mechanism of action of pyrazinamide is incompletely defined but includes inhibition of fatty acid synthase and ribosomal trans-translation. Pyrazinamide is often bacteriostatic but can be bactericidal and is active against semidormant bacteria in a low-pH environment. Primary resistance is rare but MDR-TB strains are frequently pyrazinamide-resistant and intrinsic resistance is a feature of *Mycobacterium bovis* strains. Pyrazinamide is well absorbed orally and metabolised by the liver. Side-effects include nausea, hepatitis, asymptomatic elevation of uric acid and myalgia.

Ethambutol

Ethambutol is a bacteriostatic agent. It inhibits arabinosyl transferase, which is involved in the synthesis of arabinogalactan, a component of the mycobacterial cell wall. Resistance is usually seen when resistance to other antimycobacterial agents is also present, e.g. in MDR-TB strains. It is orally absorbed but, in contrast to the first-line agents described above, it achieves poor CSF penetration and is renally excreted. The major side-effect is optic neuritis with loss of red–green colour discrimination and impaired visual acuity. It can also cause hepatitis.

Streptomycin

Streptomycin is an aminoglycoside whose mechanism of action and side-effects are similar to those of other aminoglycosides. It is administered intramuscularly.

Other antituberculous agents

Second-line agents used in MDR or XDR strains (p. 116) include aminoglycosides (amikacin, capreomycin or kanamycin) and fluoroquinolones (moxifloxacin or levofloxacin), discussed above. Other established second-line agents administered orally are cycloserine (which causes neurological side-effects); ethionamide or prothionamide (which are not active with *InhA*-gene-mediated resistance but have reasonable CSF penetration; their side-effect profile includes gastrointestinal disturbance, hepatotoxicity and

neurotoxicity); and paraminosalicylic acid (which causes rashes and gastrointestinal upset). Linezolid may also be used and has good CSF penetration, while meropenem with co-amoxiclav is occasionally chosen. New drugs developed for XDR-TB include delamanid and bedaquiline; their adverse effects include QT prolongation and cardiac arrhythmias. Their co-administration with other agents with a similar side-effect profile (e.g. fluoroquinolones) therefore requires careful risk assessment.

Clofazimine

Clofazimine is used against *M. leprae* and resistant strains of *M. tuberculosis*. Its mode of action may involve induction of oxidative stress and it is weakly bactericidal. Oral absorption is variable and it is excreted in the bile. Side-effects include gastrointestinal upset, dry eyes and skin, and skin pigmentation, especially in those with pigmented skin.

Antifungal agents

See Box 6.24.

i 6.24 Antifungal agents

Agent	Usual route(s) of administration	Clinically relevant antifungal spectrum
Imidazoles		
Miconazole		
Econazole	Topical	*Candida* spp., dermatophytes
Clotrimazole		
Ketoconazole	Topical, oral	*Malassezia* spp., dermatophytes, agents of eumycetoma
Triazoles		
Fluconazole	Oral, IV	Yeasts (*Candida* and *Cryptococcus* spp.)
Itraconazole	Oral, IV	Yeasts, dermatophytes, dimorphic fungi (p. 300), *Aspergillus* spp.
Voriconazole	Oral, IV	Yeasts and most filamentous fungi (excluding mucoraceous moulds)
Posaconazole	Oral, IV	Yeasts and many filamentous fungi (including most mucoraceous moulds)
Isavuconazole	Oral, IV	Yeasts and many filamentous fungi (variable activity against mucoraceous moulds)
Echinocandins		
Anidulafungin		*Candida* spp., *Aspergillus* spp. (no activity against *Cryptococcus* spp. or mucoraceous moulds)
Caspofungin	IV only	
Micafungin		
Polyenes		
Amphotericin B	IV	Yeasts and most dimorphic and filamentous fungi (including mucoraceous moulds)
Nystatin	Topical	
Others		
5-fluorocytosine	Oral, IV	Yeasts
Griseofulvin	Oral	Dermatophytes
Terbinafine	Topical, oral	Dermatophytes

6

Azole antifungals

The azoles (imidazoles and triazoles) inhibit synthesis of ergosterol, a constituent of the fungal cell membrane. Side-effects vary but include gastrointestinal upset, hepatitis and rash. Azoles are inhibitors of cytochrome P450 enzymes, so tend to increase exposure to cytochrome P450-metabolised drugs (p. 24).

Imidazoles

Miconazole, econazole, clotrimazole and ketoconazole are relatively toxic and therefore administered topically. Clotrimazole is used extensively to treat superficial fungal infections. Triazoles are used for systemic treatment because they are less toxic.

Triazoles

Fluconazole is effective against yeasts (*Candida* and *Cryptococcus* spp.) and has a long half-life (approximately 30 hours) and an excellent safety profile. The drug is highly water-soluble and distributes widely to all body sites and tissues, including CSF. Itraconazole is lipophilic and distributes extensively, including to toenails and fingernails. CSF penetration is poor. Because oral absorption is erratic, therapeutic drug monitoring is required. Voriconazole is well absorbed orally but variability in levels requires therapeutic drug monitoring. It is used mainly in aspergillosis (p. 596). Side-effects include photosensitivity, hepatitis and transient retinal toxicity. Posaconazole and isavuconazole are broad-spectrum azoles, with activity against *Candida* spp., *Aspergillus* spp. and some mucoraceous moulds. Isavuconazole is non-inferior to voriconazole in the management of invasive aspergillosis and may be considered as an alternative when voriconazole is not tolerated.

Echinocandins

The echinocandins inhibit β-1,3-glucan synthesis in the fungal cell wall. They have few significant adverse effects. Caspofungin, anidulafungin and micafungin are used to treat systemic candidosis, and caspofungin is also used in aspergillosis.

Polyenes

Amphotericin B (AmB) deoxycholate causes cell death by binding to ergosterol and damaging the fungal cytoplasmic membrane. Its use in resource-rich countries has been largely supplanted by less toxic agents. Its long half-life enables once-daily administration. CSF penetration is poor.

Adverse effects include immediate anaphylaxis, other infusion-related reactions and nephrotoxicity. Nephrotoxicity may be sufficient to require dialysis and occurs in most patients who are adequately dosed. It may be ameliorated by concomitant infusion of normal saline. Irreversible nephrotoxicity occurs with large cumulative doses of AmB.

Nystatin has a similar spectrum of antifungal activity to AmB. Its toxicity limits it to topical use, e.g. in oral and vaginal candidiasis.

Lipid formulations of amphotericin B

Lipid formulations of AmB have been developed to reduce AmB toxicity and have replaced AmB deoxycholate in many regions. They consist of AmB encapsulated in liposomes (liposomal AmB, L-AmB) or complexed with phospholipids (AmB lipid complex, ABLC). The drug becomes active on dissociating from its lipid component. Adverse effects are similar to, but considerably less frequent than, those with AmB deoxycholate, and efficacy is similar. Lipid formulations of AmB are used in invasive fungal disease, as empirical therapy in patients with neutropenic fever (p. 1327), and also in visceral leishmaniasis (p. 282).

Other antifungal agents

Flucytosine

Flucytosine (5-fluorocytosine) has particular activity against yeasts. When it is used as monotherapy, acquired resistance develops rapidly, so it should be given in combination with another antifungal agent. Adverse effects include myelosuppression, gastrointestinal upset and hepatitis.

Griseofulvin

Griseofulvin has been largely superseded by terbinafine and itraconazole for treatment of dermatophyte infections, except in children, for whom these agents remain largely unlicensed. It is deposited in keratin precursor cells, which become resistant to fungal invasion.

Terbinafine

Terbinafine distributes with high concentration to sebum and skin, with a half-life of more than 1 week. It is used topically for dermatophyte skin infections and orally for onychomycosis. The major adverse reaction is hepatic toxicity (approximately 1:50 000 cases). Terbinafine is not recommended for breastfeeding mothers.

Antiviral agents

Most viral infections in immunocompetent individuals resolve without intervention. Antiviral therapy is available for a limited number of infections only (Box 6.25).

Antiretroviral agents

These agents, used predominantly against HIV, are discussed on page 324.

Anti-herpesvirus agents

Aciclovir, valaciclovir, penciclovir and famciclovir

These antivirals are acyclic analogues of guanosine, which inhibit viral DNA polymerase after being phosphorylated by virus-derived thymidine kinase (TK). Aciclovir is poorly absorbed after oral dosing; better levels are achieved intravenously or by use of the prodrug valaciclovir. Famciclovir is the prodrug of penciclovir. Resistance is mediated by viral TK or polymerase mutations.

Ganciclovir

Chemical modification of the aciclovir molecule allows preferential phosphorylation by protein kinases of cytomegalovirus (CMV) and other β-herpesviruses (e.g. human herpesvirus (HHV) 6/7) and hence greater inhibition of the DNA polymerase, but at the expense of increased toxicity. Ganciclovir is administered intravenously or as a prodrug (valganciclovir) orally.

Cidofovir

Cidofovir inhibits viral DNA polymerases with potent activity against CMV, including most ganciclovir-resistant CMV. It also has activity against aciclovir-resistant herpes simplex virus (HSV) and varicella zoster virus (VZV), HHV6 and occasionally adenovirus, poxvirus, papillomavirus or polyoma virus, and may be used to treat these infections in immunocompromised hosts.

i 6.25 Antiviral agents

Drug	Route(s) of administration	Indications	Significant side-effects
Antiretroviral therapy (ART, p. 324)	Oral	HIV infection (including AIDS)	CNS symptoms, anaemia, lipodystrophy
Anti-herpesvirus agents Aciclovir	Topical/oral/IV	Herpes zoster Chickenpox (esp. in immunosuppressed) Herpes simplex infections: encephalitis (IV only), genital tract, oral, ophthalmic	Significant side-effects rare Hepatitis, renal impairment and neurotoxicity reported rarely
Valaciclovir	Oral	Herpes zoster, herpes simplex	As for aciclovir
Famciclovir	Oral	Herpes zoster, herpes simplex (genital)	As for aciclovir
Penciclovir	Topical	Labial herpes simplex	Local irritation
Ganciclovir	IV	Treatment and prevention of CMV infection in immunosuppressed	Gastrointestinal symptoms, liver dysfunction, neurotoxicity, myelosuppression, renal impairment, fever, rash, phlebitis at infusion sites Potential teratogenicity
Valganciclovir	Oral	Treatment and prevention of CMV infection in immunosuppressed	As for ganciclovir but neutropenia is predominant
Cidofovir	IV/topical	HIV-associated CMV infections and occasionally other viruses (see text)	Renal impairment, neutropenia
Foscarnet	IV	CMV and aciclovir-resistant HSV and VZV infections in immunosuppressed	Gastrointestinal symptoms, renal impairment, electrolyte disturbances, genital ulceration, neurotoxicity
Anti-influenza agents Zanamivir	Inhalation	Influenza A and B	Allergic reactions (very rare)
Oseltamivir	Oral	Influenza A and B	Gastrointestinal side-effects, rash, hepatitis (very rare)
Peramivir	IV, IM		
Amantadine, rimantadine	Oral	Influenza A (but see text)	CNS symptoms, nausea
Agents used in other virus infections* Ribavirin	Oral/IV/inhalation	Lassa fever (IV) RSV infection in infants (inhalation)	Haemolytic anaemia, cough, dyspnoea, bronchospasm and ocular irritation (when given by inhalation)

*Antiviral agents used in viral hepatitis are discussed on pages 875 and 878. (AIDS = acquired immunodeficiency syndrome; CMV = cytomegalovirus; CNS = central nervous system; HIV = human immunodeficiency virus; HSV = herpes simplex virus; IM = intramuscular; IV = intravenous; RSV = respiratory syncytial virus; VZV = varicella zoster virus)

Foscarnet

This analogue of inorganic pyrophosphate acts as a non-competitive inhibitor of HSV, VZV, HHV6/7 or CMV DNA polymerase. It does not require significant intracellular phosphorylation and so may be effective when HSV or CMV resistance is due to altered drug phosphorylation. It has variable CSF penetration.

Anti-influenza agents

Zanamivir and oseltamivir

These agents inhibit influenza A and B neuraminidase, which is required for release of virus from infected cells (see Fig. 6.2, p. 101). They are used in the treatment and prophylaxis of influenza. Administration within 48 hours of disease onset reduces the duration of symptoms by approximately 1–1½ days. In the UK, their use is limited mainly to adults with chronic respiratory or renal disease, significant cardiovascular disease, immunosuppression or diabetes mellitus, during known outbreaks. Peramivir has been developed as a distinct chemical structure, which means that it retains activity against some oseltamivir- and zanamivir-resistant strains. It has poor oral bioavailability and has been developed as an intravenous or intramuscular formulation for treatment of severe

cases of influenza, e.g. in intensive care units. It is now approved for use in adults in a number of countries. An intravenous formulation of zanamivir is also in development for critically ill patients. Laninamivir is approved as an intranasal formulation in Japan.

Amantadine and rimantadine

These drugs reduce replication of influenza A by inhibition of viral M2 protein ion channel function, which is required for uncoating (see Fig. 6.2). Resistance develops rapidly and is widespread, and amantadine and rimantadine should be used only if the prevalence of resistance locally is known to be low. They are no longer recommended for treatment or prophylaxis in the UK or USA, having been superseded by zanamivir and oseltamivir. However, they may still be indicated to treat oseltamivir-resistant influenza A in patients unable to take zanamivir (e.g. ventilated patients).

Other agents used to treat viruses

Antiviral agents used to treat hepatitis B and C virus are discussed on pages 875 and 878, and those used against HIV-1 are described on page 324.

Ribavirin

Ribavirin is a guanosine analogue that inhibits nucleic acid synthesis in a variety of viruses. It is used in particular in the treatment of hepatitis C virus but also against certain viral haemorrhagic fevers, e.g. Lassa fever, although it has not been useful against Ebola virus.

Antiparasitic agents

Antimalarial agents

Artemisinin (qinghaosu) derivatives

Artemisinin originates from a herb (sweet wormwood, *Artemisia annua*), which was used in Chinese medicine to treat fever. Its derivatives, artemether and artesunate, were developed for use in malaria in the 1970s. Their mechanism of action is unknown. They are used in the treatment, but not prophylaxis, of malaria, usually in combination with other antimalarials, and are effective against strains of *Plasmodium* spp. that are resistant to other antimalarials. Artemether is lipid-soluble and may be administered via the intramuscular and oral routes. Artesunate is water-soluble and is administered intravenously or orally. Serious adverse effects are uncommon. Current advice for malaria in pregnancy is that the artemisinin derivatives should be used to treat uncomplicated *falciparum* malaria in the second and third trimesters, but should not be prescribed in the first trimester until more information becomes available.

Atovaquone

Atovaquone inhibits mitochondrial function. It is an oral agent, used for treatment and prophylaxis of malaria, in combination with proguanil (see below), without which it is ineffective. It is also employed in the treatment of mild cases of *Pneumocystis jirovecii* pneumonia, where there is intolerance to co-trimoxazole. Significant adverse effects are uncommon.

Folate synthesis inhibitors (proguanil, pyrimethamine–sulfadoxine)

Proguanil inhibits dihydrofolate reductase and is used for malaria prophylaxis. Pyrimethamine–sulfadoxine may be used in the treatment of malaria.

Quinoline-containing compounds

Chloroquine and quinine are believed to act by intraparasitic inhibition of haem polymerisation, resulting in toxic build-up of intracellular haem. The mechanisms of action of other agents in this group (quinidine, amodiaquine, mefloquine, primaquine, etc.) may differ. They are employed in the treatment and prophylaxis of malaria. Primaquine is used for radical cure of malaria due to *Plasmodium vivax* and *P. ovale* (destruction of liver hypnozoites). Chloroquine may also be given for extra-intestinal amoebiasis.

Chloroquine can cause a pruritus sufficient to compromise adherence to therapy. If used in long-term, high-dose regimens, it causes an irreversible retinopathy. Overdosage leads to life-threatening cardiotoxicity. The side-effect profile of mefloquine includes neuropsychiatric effects ranging from mood change, nightmares and agitation to hallucinations and psychosis. Quinine may cause hypoglycaemia and cardiotoxicity, especially when administered parenterally. Primaquine causes haemolysis in people with glucose-6-phosphate dehydrogenase deficiency (p. 948), which should be excluded before therapy. Chloroquine is considered safe in pregnancy but mefloquine should be avoided in the first trimester.

Lumefantrine

Lumefantrine is used in combination with artemether to treat uncomplicated *falciparum* malaria, including chloroquine-resistant strains. Its mechanism of action is unknown. Significant adverse effects are uncommon.

Drugs used in trypanosomiasis

Benznidazole

Benznidazole is an oral agent used to treat South American trypanosomiasis (Chagas' disease, p. 279). Significant and common adverse effects include dose-related peripheral neuropathy, purpuric rash and granulocytopenia.

Eflornithine

Eflornithine inhibits biosynthesis of polyamines by ornithine decarboxylase inhibition, and is used in West African trypanosomiasis (*T. brucei gambiense* infection) of the central nervous system. It is administered as an intravenous infusion 4 times daily, which may be logistically difficult in the geographical areas affected by this disease. Significant adverse effects are common and include convulsions, gastrointestinal upset and bone marrow depression.

Melarsoprol

This is an arsenical agent, used to treat central nervous system infections in East and West African trypanosomiasis (*T. brucei rhodesiense* and *gambiense*). It is administered intravenously. Melarsoprol treatment is associated with peripheral neuropathy and reactive arsenical encephalopathy (RAE), which carries a significant mortality.

Nifurtimox

Nifurtimox is administered orally to treat South American trypanosomiasis (Chagas' disease). Gastrointestinal and neurological adverse effects are common.

Pentamidine isetionate

Pentamidine is an inhibitor of DNA replication used in West African trypanosomiasis (*T. brucei gambiense*) and, to a lesser extent, in visceral and cutaneous leishmaniasis. It is also prescribed in *Pneumocystis jirovecii* pneumonia. It is administered via intravenous or intramuscular routes. It is a relatively toxic drug, commonly causing rash, renal impairment, profound hypotension (especially on rapid infusion), electrolyte disturbances, blood dyscrasias and hypoglycaemia.

Suramin

Suramin is a naphthaline dye derivative, used to treat East African trypanosomiasis (*T. brucei rhodesiense*). It is administered intravenously. Adverse effects are common and include rash, gastrointestinal disturbance, blood dyscrasias, peripheral neuropathies and renal impairment.

Other antiprotozoal agents

Pentavalent antimonials

Sodium stibogluconate and meglumine antimoniate inhibit protozoal glycolysis by phosphofructokinase inhibition. They are used parenterally (intravenous or intramuscular) to treat leishmaniasis. Adverse effects include arthralgia, myalgias, raised hepatic transaminases, pancreatitis and electrocardiogram changes. Severe cardiotoxicity leading to death is not uncommon.

Diloxanide furoate

This oral agent is used to eliminate luminal cysts following treatment of intestinal amoebiasis, or in asymptomatic cyst excreters. The drug is absorbed slowly (enabling luminal persistence) and has no effect in hepatic amoebiasis. It is a relatively non-toxic drug, the most significant adverse effect being flatulence.

Iodoquinol (di-iodohydroxyquinoline)

Iodoquinol is a quinoline derivative (p. 128) with activity against *Entamoeba histolytica* cysts and trophozoites. It is used orally to treat asymptomatic cyst excreters or, in association with another amoebicide (e.g. metronidazole), to treat extra-intestinal amoebiasis. Long-term use of this drug is not recommended, as neurological adverse effects include optic neuritis and peripheral neuropathy.

Nitazoxanide

Nitazoxanide is an inhibitor of pyruvate–ferredoxin oxidoreductase-dependent anaerobic energy metabolism in protozoa. It is a broad-spectrum agent, active against various nematodes, tapeworms, flukes and intestinal protozoa. Nitazoxanide also has activity against some anaerobic bacteria and viruses. It is administered orally in giardiasis and cryptosporidiosis. Adverse effects are usually mild and involve the gastrointestinal tract (e.g. nausea, diarrhoea and abdominal pain).

Paromomycin

Paromomycin is an aminoglycoside (p. 122) that is used to treat visceral leishmaniasis and intestinal amoebiasis. It is not significantly absorbed when administered orally, and is therefore given orally for intestinal amoebiasis and by intramuscular injection for leishmaniasis. It showed early promise in the treatment of HIV-associated cryptosporidiosis but subsequent trials have demonstrated that this effect is marginal at best.

Drugs used against helminths

Benzimidazoles (albendazole, mebendazole)

These agents act by inhibiting both helminth glucose uptake, causing depletion of glycogen stores, and fumarate reductase. Albendazole is used for hookworm, ascariasis, threadworm, *Strongyloides* infection, trichinellosis, *Taenia solium* (cysticercosis) and hydatid disease. Mebendazole is used for hookworm, ascariasis, threadworm and whipworm. The drugs are administered orally. Absorption is relatively poor but is increased by a fatty meal. Significant adverse effects are uncommon.

Bithionol

Bithionol is used to treat fluke infections with *Fasciola hepatica*. It is well absorbed orally. Adverse effects are mild (e.g. nausea, vomiting, diarrhoea, rashes) but relatively common (approximately 30%).

Diethylcarbamazine

Diethylcarbamazine (DEC) is an oral agent used to treat filariasis and loiasis. Treatment of filariasis is often followed by fever, headache, nausea, vomiting, arthralgia and prostration. This is caused by the host response to dying microfilariae, rather than the drug, and may be reduced by pre-treatment with glucocorticoids.

Ivermectin

Ivermectin binds to helminth nerve and muscle cell ion channels, causing increased membrane permeability. It is an oral agent, used in *Strongyloides* infection, filariasis and onchocerciasis. Significant side-effects are uncommon.

Niclosamide

Niclosamide inhibits oxidative phosphorylation, causing paralysis of helminths. It is an oral agent, used in *Taenia saginata* and intestinal *T. solium* infection. Systemic absorption is minimal and it has few significant side-effects.

Piperazine

Piperazine inhibits neurotransmitter function, causing helminth muscle paralysis. It is an oral agent, used in ascariasis and threadworm (*Enterobius vermicularis*) infection. Significant adverse effects are uncommon but include neuropsychological reactions such as vertigo, delirium and convulsions.

Praziquantel

Praziquantel increases membrane permeability to Ca^{2+}, causing violent contraction of worm muscle. It is the drug of choice for schistosomiasis and is also used in *T. saginata*, *T. solium* (cysticercosis) and fluke infections (*Clonorchis*, *Paragonimus*) and in echinococcosis. It is administered orally and is well absorbed. Adverse effects are usually mild and transient, and include nausea and abdominal pain.

Pyrantel pamoate

This agent causes spastic paralysis of helminth muscle through a suxamethonium-like action. It is used orally in ascariasis and threadworm infection. Systemic absorption is poor and adverse effects are uncommon.

Thiabendazole

Thiabendazole inhibits fumarate reductase, which is required for energy production in helminths. It is used orally in *Strongyloides* infection and topically to treat cutaneous larva migrans. Significant adverse effects are uncommon.

Further information

Websites

cdc.gov *Centers for Disease Control and Prevention, Atlanta, USA. Provides information on all aspects of communicable disease, including prophylaxis against malaria.*
dh.gov.uk *UK Department of Health. The publications section provides current UK recommendations for immunisation.*
ecdc.europa.eu *European Centre for Disease Prevention and Control. Includes data on prevalence of antibiotic resistance in Europe.*
gov.uk/government/organisations/public-health-england *Public Health England. Provides information on infectious diseases relating mainly to England, including community infection control.*
idsociety.org *Infectious Diseases Society of America. Publishes up-to-date, evidence-based guidelines.*
who.int *World Health Organization. Provides up-to-date information on global aspects of infectious disease, including outbreak updates. Also has information on the 'World Antibiotic Awareness Week' campaign.*

SHL Thomas

7

Poisoning

Comprehensive evaluation of the poisoned patient 132

General approach to the poisoned patient 134
Triage and resuscitation 134
Clinical assessment and investigations 134
Psychiatric assessment 135
General management 135

Poisoning by specific pharmaceutical agents 137
Analgesics 137
Antidepressants 138
Cardiovascular medications 140
Iron 140
Antipsychotic drugs 141
Antidiabetic agents 141
Pharmaceutical agents less commonly taken in poisoning 141

Drugs of misuse 141
Depressants 141
Stimulants and entactogens 143
Hallucinogens 143
Dissociative drugs 144
Volatile substances 144
Body packers and body stuffers 144

Chemicals and pesticides 144
Carbon monoxide 144
Organophosphorus insecticides and nerve agents 145
Carbamate insecticides 146
Paraquat 147
Methanol and ethylene glycol 147
Corrosive substances 147
Aluminium and zinc phosphide 148
Copper sulphate 148
Chemicals less commonly taken in poisoning 148
Chemical warfare agents 149

Environmental poisoning 149

Food-related poisoning 149

Plant poisoning 150

Comprehensive evaluation of the poisoned patient

1 Airway, breathing, circulation
Respiration rate,
oxygen saturation,
pulse, BP,
dysrhythmias

2 Level of consciousness
Presence of seizures,
delirium, agitation
or psychosis

3 Chest
Evidence of aspiration,
bronchoconstriction

4 Movement and muscles
Tone, fasciculations,
myoclonus, tremor,
paralysis, ataxia

5 Reflexes
Tendon reflexes, plantar
responses, inducible clonus

6 Eyes
Miosis or mydriasis,
diplopia or strabismus,
lacrimation

▲ Pinpoint pupil

▲ Injected conjunctiva

7 Abdomen
Hepatic or epigastric
tenderness, ileus,
palpable bladder

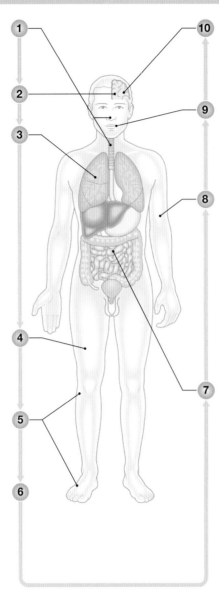

10 Psychiatric evaluation
Features of psychiatric illness,
mental capacity

9 Mouth
Dry mouth, excessive salivation

8 Skin
Temperature, cyanosis,
flushing, sweating,
blisters, pressure areas,
piloerection,
evidence of self-harm

▲ Self-cutting

▲ Chemical burn

▲ Needle tracks

Insets (Self-cutting) From Douglas G, Nicol F, Robertson C (eds). Macleod's Clinical examination, 11th edn. Churchill Livingstone, Elsevier Ltd; 2005. (Chemical burn) www.firewiki.net. (Needle tracks) www.deep6inc.com. (Pinpoint pupil) http://drugrecognition.com/images. (Injected conjunctiva) http:// knol.google.com.

---

i   Taking a history in poisoning

- What toxin(s) have been taken and how much?
- What time were they taken and by what route?
- Has alcohol or any other substance (or substances, including drugs of misuse) been taken as well?
- Obtain details from witnesses (e.g. family, friends, ambulance personnel) of the circumstances of the overdose
- Assess immediate suicide risk in those with apparent self-harm (full psychiatric evaluation when patient has recovered physically)

- Assess capacity to make decisions about accepting or refusing treatment
- Establish past medical history, drug history and allergies, social and family history
- Record all information carefully

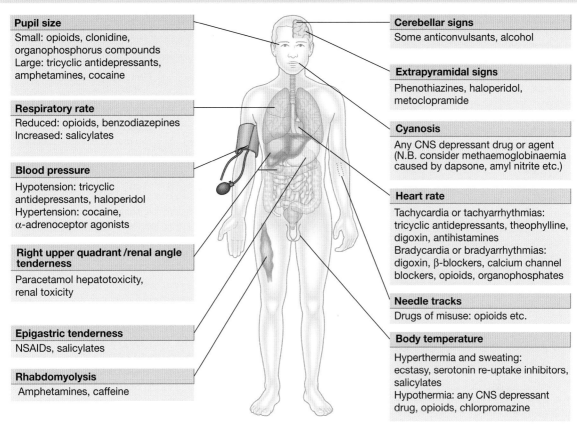

Pupil size
Small: opioids, clonidine, organophosphorus compounds
Large: tricyclic antidepressants, amphetamines, cocaine

Respiratory rate
Reduced: opioids, benzodiazepines
Increased: salicylates

Blood pressure
Hypotension: tricyclic antidepressants, haloperidol
Hypertension: cocaine, α-adrenoceptor agonists

Right upper quadrant /renal angle tenderness
Paracetamol hepatotoxicity, renal toxicity

Epigastric tenderness
NSAIDs, salicylates

Rhabdomyolysis
Amphetamines, caffeine

Cerebellar signs
Some anticonvulsants, alcohol

Extrapyramidal signs
Phenothiazines, haloperidol, metoclopramide

Cyanosis
Any CNS depressant drug or agent (N.B. consider methaemoglobinaemia caused by dapsone, amyl nitrite etc.)

Heart rate
Tachycardia or tachyarrhythmias: tricyclic antidepressants, theophylline, digoxin, antihistamines
Bradycardia or bradyarrhythmias: digoxin, β-blockers, calcium channel blockers, opioids, organophosphates

Needle tracks
Drugs of misuse: opioids etc.

Body temperature
Hyperthermia and sweating: ecstasy, serotonin re-uptake inhibitors, salicylates
Hypothermia: any CNS depressant drug, opioids, chlorpromazine

7

Clinical signs of poisoning by pharmaceutical agents and drugs of misuse.

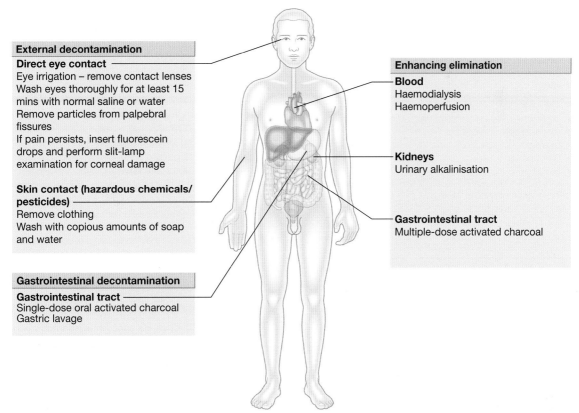

External decontamination
Direct eye contact
Eye irrigation – remove contact lenses
Wash eyes thoroughly for at least 15 mins with normal saline or water
Remove particles from palpebral fissures
If pain persists, insert fluorescein drops and perform slit-lamp examination for corneal damage

Skin contact (hazardous chemicals/ pesticides)
Remove clothing
Wash with copious amounts of soap and water

Gastrointestinal decontamination
Gastrointestinal tract
Single-dose oral activated charcoal
Gastric lavage

Enhancing elimination
Blood
Haemodialysis
Haemoperfusion

Kidneys
Urinary alkalinisation

Gastrointestinal tract
Multiple-dose activated charcoal

Decontamination and enhanced elimination. One of the key aspects in the evaluation of a poisoned patient is deciding if decontamination and/or enhanced elimination is required.

Acute poisoning is common, accounting for about 1% of hospital admissions in the UK. Common or otherwise important substances involved are shown in Box 7.1. In developed countries, the most frequent cause is intentional drug overdose in the context of self-harm, often involving prescribed or 'over-the-counter' medicines. Accidental poisoning is also common, especially in children and the elderly (Box 7.2). Toxicity also results from alcohol or recreational substance use, or following occupational or environmental exposure. Poisoning is a major cause of death in young adults, but most deaths occur before patients reach medical attention, and mortality is low (<1%) in those admitted to hospital.

In developing countries, the frequency of self-harm is more difficult to estimate. Because of their widespread availability and use, household and agricultural products, such as pesticides and herbicides, are common sources of poisoning and have a much higher case fatality. In China and South-east Asia, pesticides account for about 300 000 suicides each year. Snake bite and other forms of envenomation are also important causes of morbidity and mortality internationally and are discussed in Chapter 8.

7.1 Important substances involved in poisoning

In the UK

- Analgesics: paracetamol and non-steroidal anti-inflammatory drugs (NSAIDs)
- Antidepressants: tricyclic antidepressants (TCAs), selective serotonin re-uptake inhibitors (SSRIs) and lithium
- Cardiovascular agents: β-blockers, calcium channel blockers and cardiac glycosides
- Drugs of misuse: depressants (e.g. opiates, benzodiazepines), stimulants and entactogens (e.g. amphetamines, MDMA, mephedrone, cocaine), hallucinogens (e.g. cannabis, synthetic cannabinoid receptor agonists, LSD)
- Carbon monoxide
- Alcohol

In South and South-east Asia

- Organophosphorus and carbamate insecticides
- Aluminium and zinc phosphide
- Oleander
- Corrosives
- Snake venoms (Ch. 8)

(LSD = lysergic acid diethylamide; MDMA = 3,4-methylene-dioxymethamphetamine, ecstasy)

7.2 Poisoning in old age

- **Aetiology**: may result from accidental poisoning (e.g. due to delirium or dementia) or drug toxicity as a consequence of impaired renal or hepatic function or drug interaction. Toxic prescription medicines are more likely to be available.
- **Psychiatric illness**: self-harm is less common than in younger adults but more frequently associated with depression and other psychiatric illness, as well as chronic illness and pain. There is a higher risk of subsequent suicide.
- **Severity of poisoning**: increased morbidity and mortality result from reduced renal and hepatic function, lower functional reserve, increased sensitivity to sedative agents and frequent comorbidity.

General approach to the poisoned patient

A general approach is shown on pages 132–133. In many countries, poisons centres are available to provide advice on management of suspected poisoning with specific substances. Information is also available online (p. 150).

Triage and resuscitation

Patients who are seriously poisoned must be identified early so that appropriate management is not delayed. Triage involves:

- immediately assessing vital signs
- identifying the poison(s) involved and obtaining adequate information about them
- identifying patients at risk of further attempts at self-harm and removing any remaining hazards.

Those with possible external contamination with chemical or environmental toxins should undergo appropriate decontamination (p. 133). Critically ill patients must be resuscitated (p. 174).

The Glasgow Coma Scale (GCS) is commonly employed to assess conscious level, although not specifically validated in poisoning. The AVPU (alert/verbal/painful/unresponsive) scale is also a rapid and simple method. An electrocardiogram (ECG) should be performed and cardiac monitoring instituted in all patients with cardiovascular features or where exposure to potentially cardiotoxic substances is suspected. Patients who may need antidotes should be weighed if possible, so that appropriate weight-related doses can be prescribed.

Substances unlikely to be toxic in humans should be identified so that inappropriate admission and intervention are avoided (Box 7.3).

Clinical assessment and investigations

History and examination are described on page 132. Occasionally, patients may be unaware of or confused about what they have taken, or may exaggerate (or, less commonly, underestimate) the size of the overdose, but rarely mislead medical staff deliberately. In regions of the world where self-poisoning is illegal, patients may be reticent about giving a history.

Toxic causes of abnormal physical signs are shown on page 133. The patient may have a cluster of clinical features ('toxidrome') suggestive of poisoning with a particular drug type, e.g. anticholinergic, serotoninergic (see Box 7.10), stimulant, sedative, opioid (see Box 7.12) or cholinergic (see Box 7.14) feature clusters. Poisoning is a common cause of coma, especially

7.3 Substances of very low toxicity

- Writing/educational materials, e.g. pencil lead, crayons, chalk
- Decorating products, e.g. emulsion paint, wallpaper paste
- Cleaning/bathroom products (except dishwasher tablets and liquid laundry detergent capsules, which can be corrosive)
- Pharmaceuticals: oral contraceptives, most antibiotics (but not tetracyclines or antituberculous drugs), vitamins B, C and E, prednisolone, emollients and other skin creams, baby lotion
- Miscellaneous: plasticine, silica gel, most household plants, plant food, pet food, soil

Causes	Consequences	Treatment
Non-toxic • Congenital methaemoglobinaemias *Toxic (Oxidising agents)* • Organic nitrites • Nitrates • Benzocaine • Dapsone • Chloroquine • Aniline dyes • Chlorobenzene • Naphthalene • Copper sulphate	• Haemoglobin–oxygen dissociation curve is shifted to the left (see Fig. 23.5) • Oxygen delivery to tissues is reduced • There is apparent 'cyanosis' • Breathlessness, fatigue, headache and chest pain occur • Delirium, impaired consciousness and seizures may occur in severe cases	• Methylthioninium chloride ('methylene blue') 1–2 mg/kg (intravenous) is given • Reduces methaemoglobin (see below) • Used for symptomatic patients with severe methaemoglobinaemia (e.g. >30%) • Patients with anaemia or other comorbidities may need treatment at lower concentrations

Fig. 7.1 **Methaemoglobinaemia.**

	7.4 Causes of acidosis in the poisoned patient		
Cause	**Normal lactate***	**High lactate**	
Toxic	Salicylates Methanol Ethylene glycol Paraldehyde	Metformin Iron Cyanide Sodium valproate Carbon monoxide	
Other	Renal failure Ketoacidosis Severe diarrhoea	Shock	

*Unless circulatory shock is present, when it will be high in any case.

	7.5 Anion and osmolar gaps in poisoning	
	Anion gap	**Osmolar gap**
Calculation	$[Na^+ + K^+] - [Cl^- + HCO_3^-]$	[Measured osmolality] − $[(2 \times Na) + Urea + Glucose]$[1]
Reference range	12–16 mmol/L	< 10
Common toxic causes of elevation[2]	Ethanol Ethylene glycol Methanol Salicylates Iron Cyanide	Ethanol Ethylene glycol Methanol

[1]All units should be in mmol/L, except osmolality, which should be in mOsmol/kg. For non-SI units, the corresponding formula is [Measured osmolality (mOsmol/kg)] − [(2 × Na (mEq/L)) + Urea/2.8 (mg/dL) + Glucose/18 (mg/dL)]. [2]Box 14.19 (p. 365) gives non-toxic causes.

in younger people, but it is important to exclude other potential causes (p. 194).

Urea, electrolytes and creatinine should be measured in all patients with suspected systemic poisoning. Arterial blood gases should be checked in those with significant respiratory or circulatory compromise, or after poisoning with substances likely to affect acid–base status (Box 7.4). Calculation of anion and osmolar gaps may help to inform diagnosis and management (Box 7.5). Potent oxidising agents may cause methaemoglobinaemia, with consequent blue discoloration of skin and blood, and reduced oxygen delivery to the tissues (Fig. 7.1).

For some substances, management may be facilitated by measurement of the amount of toxin in the blood. Qualitative urine screens for potential toxins, including near-patient testing kits, have a limited clinical role.

Psychiatric assessment

Patients presenting with drug overdose in the context of self-harm should undergo psychiatric evaluation prior to discharge by a

health professional with appropriate training (p. 1187). This should occur after they have recovered from poisoning, unless there is an urgent issue, such as uncertainty about their capacity to decline medical treatment.

General management

Patients presenting with eye/skin contamination should undergo local decontamination measures. These are described on page 133.

Gastrointestinal decontamination

Patients who have ingested potentially life-threatening quantities of toxins may be considered for gastrointestinal decontamination if poisoning has been recent (p. 133).

Activated charcoal

Given orally as a slurry, activated charcoal absorbs toxins in the bowel as a result of its large surface area. It can prevent absorption of an important proportion of the ingested dose of toxin, but efficacy decreases with time and current guidelines do not encourage use more than 1 hour after overdose, unless a sustained-release preparation has been taken or when gastric emptying may be delayed. Use is ineffective for some toxins that do not bind to activated charcoal (Box 7.6). In patients with impaired swallowing or a reduced level of consciousness, activated charcoal, even via a nasogastric tube, carries a risk of aspiration pneumonitis, which can be reduced (but not eliminated) by protecting the airway with a cuffed endotracheal tube.

Multiple doses of oral activated charcoal (50 g 6 times daily in an adult) may enhance the elimination of some substances at any time after poisoning (Box 7.7). This interrupts enterohepatic circulation or reduces the concentration of free drug in the gut lumen, to the extent that drug diffuses from the blood back into the bowel to be absorbed on to the charcoal ('gastrointestinal dialysis'). A laxative is generally given with the charcoal to reduce the risk of constipation or intestinal obstruction by charcoal 'briquette' formation in the gut lumen.

Evidence suggests that single or multiple doses of activated charcoal do not improve clinical outcomes after poisoning with pesticides or oleander.

Gastric aspiration and lavage

Gastric aspiration and/or lavage is very infrequently indicated in acute poisoning, as it is no more effective than activated charcoal

for most substances and complications are common, especially pulmonary aspiration. It is contraindicated if strong acids, alkalis or petroleum distillates have been ingested. Use may be justified for life-threatening overdoses of those substances that are not absorbed by activated charcoal (see Box 7.6).

Whole bowel irrigation

This involves the administration of large quantities of osmotically balanced polyethylene glycol and electrolyte solution (1–2 L/hr for an adult), usually by a nasogastric tube, until the rectal effluent is clear. It is occasionally indicated to enhance the elimination of ingested packets of illicit drugs or slow-release tablets such as iron and lithium that are not absorbed by activated charcoal. Contraindications include inadequate airway protection, haemodynamic instability, gastrointestinal haemorrhage, obstruction or ileus. Whole bowel irrigation may precipitate nausea and vomiting, abdominal pain and electrolyte disturbances.

Urinary alkalinisation

Urinary excretion of weak acids and bases is affected by urinary pH, which changes the extent to which they are ionised. Highly ionised molecules pass poorly through lipid membranes and therefore little tubular reabsorption occurs and urinary excretion is increased. If the urine is alkalinised (pH>7.5) by the administration of sodium bicarbonate (e.g. 1.5 L of 1.26% sodium bicarbonate over 2 hrs), weak acids (e.g. salicylates, methotrexate) are highly ionised, resulting in enhanced urinary excretion.

Urinary alkalinisation is currently recommended for patients with clinically significant salicylate poisoning when the criteria for haemodialysis are not met (see below). It is also sometimes used for poisoning with methotrexate. Complications include alkalaemia, hypokalaemia and occasionally alkalotic tetany (p. 367). Hypocalcaemia may occur but is rare.

Haemodialysis and haemoperfusion

These techniques can enhance the elimination of poisons that have a small volume of distribution and a long half-life after overdose; use is appropriate when poisoning is sufficiently severe. The toxin must be small enough to cross the dialysis membrane (haemodialysis) or must bind to activated charcoal (haemoperfusion) (see Box 7.7). Haemodialysis can also correct acid–base and metabolic disturbances associated with poisoning (p. 135).

Lipid emulsion therapy

Lipid emulsion therapy is increasingly used for poisoning with lipid-soluble agents, such as local anaesthetics, tricyclic antidepressants, calcium channel blockers and lipid-soluble β-adrenoceptor antagonists (β-blockers) such as propranolol. It involves intravenous infusion of 20% lipid emulsion (e.g. Intralipid, suggested initial dose 1.5 mL/kg, followed by a continued infusion of 0.25 mL/kg/min until there is clinical improvement). It is thought that lipid-soluble toxins partition into the intravenous lipid, reducing target tissue concentrations. The elevated myocardial free fatty acid concentrations may also have beneficial effects on myocardial metabolism and performance by counteracting the inhibition of myocardial fatty acid oxidation produced by some cardiotoxins, enabling increased adenosine triphosphate (ATP) synthesis and energy production. Some animal studies have suggested efficacy and case reports of use in human poisoning have also been

---

i | **7.6 Substances poorly adsorbed by activated charcoal**

Medicines

- Iron
- Lithium

Chemicals

- Acids*
- Mercury
- Alkalis*
- Methanol
- Ethanol
- Petroleum distillates*
- Ethylene glycol

*Gastric lavage contraindicated.

---

i | **7.7 Poisons effectively eliminated by multiple doses of activated charcoal, haemodialysis or haemoperfusion**

Multiple doses of activated charcoal

- Carbamazepine
- Quinine
- Dapsone
- Theophylline
- Phenobarbital

Haemodialysis

- Ethylene glycol
- Salicylates
- Isopropanol
- Sodium valproate
- Methanol
- Lithium

Haemoperfusion

- Theophylline
- Phenobarbital
- Phenytoin
- Amobarbital
- Carbamazepine

i 7.8 Complications of poisoning and their management

Complication	Examples of causative agents	Management
Coma	Sedative agents	Appropriate airway protection and ventilatory support Oxygen saturation and blood gas monitoring Pressure area and bladder care Identification and treatment of aspiration pneumonia
Seizures	NSAIDs Anticonvulsants TCAs Theophylline	Appropriate airway and ventilatory support IV benzodiazepine (e.g. diazepam 10–20 mg, lorazepam 2–4 mg) Correction of hypoxia, acid–base and metabolic abnormalities
Acute dystonias	Typical antipsychotics Metoclopramide	Procyclidine, benzatropine or diazepam
Hypotension Due to vasodilatation	Vasodilator antihypertensives Anticholinergic agents TCAs	IV fluids Vasopressors (rarely indicated; p. 206)
Due to myocardial suppression	β-blockers Calcium channel blockers TCAs	Optimisation of volume status Inotropic agents (p. 206)
Ventricular tachycardia Monomorphic, associated with QRS prolongation	Sodium channel blockers	Correction of electrolyte and acid–base abnormalities and hypoxia Sodium bicarbonate (e.g. 50 mL 8.4% solution, repeated if necessary)
Torsades de pointes, associated with QT_c prolongation	Anti-arrhythmic drugs (quinidine, amiodarone, sotalol) Antimalarials Organophosphate insecticides Antipsychotic agents Antidepressants Antibiotics (erythromycin)	Correction of electrolyte and acid–base abnormalities and hypoxia Magnesium sulphate, 2 g IV over 1–2 mins, repeated if necessary

(NSAID = non-steroidal anti-inflammatory drug; TCA = tricyclic antidepressant)

---

encouraging, with recovery of circulatory collapse reported in cases where other treatment modalities have been unsuccessful. No controlled trials of this technique have been performed, however, and efficacy remains uncertain.

Supportive care

For most poisons, antidotes and methods to accelerate elimination are inappropriate, unavailable or incompletely effective. Outcome is dependent on appropriate nursing and supportive care, and treatment of complications (Box 7.8).

Antidotes

Antidotes are available for some poisons and work by a variety of mechanisms (Box 7.9). The use of some of these in the management of specific poisons is described below.

Poisoning by specific pharmaceutical agents

Analgesics

Paracetamol

Paracetamol (acetaminophen) is the drug most commonly used in overdose in the UK. Toxicity is caused by an intermediate reactive metabolite that binds covalently to cellular proteins,

i 7.9 Specific antidotes used to treat poisoning

Mechanism of action	Examples of antidote	Poisoning treated
Glutathione repleters	Acetylcysteine Methionine	Paracetamol
Receptor antagonists	Naloxone	Opioids
	Flumazenil	Benzodiazepines
	Atropine	Organophosphorus compounds Carbamates
Alcohol dehydrogenase inhibitors	Fomepizole Ethanol	Ethylene glycol Methanol
Chelating agents	Desferrioxamine	Iron
	Hydroxocobalamin Dicobalt edetate	Cyanide
	DMSA Sodium calcium edetate	Lead
Reducing agents	Methylthioninium chloride	Organic nitrites
Cholinesterase reactivators	Pralidoxime	Organophosphorus compounds
Antibody fragments	Digoxin Fab fragments	Digoxin

(DMSA = dimercaptosuccinic acid)

causing cell death. This results in hepatic and occasionally renal failure. In therapeutic doses, the toxic metabolite is detoxified in reactions requiring glutathione, but in overdose, glutathione reserves become exhausted.

Management

Activated charcoal may be used in patients presenting within 1 hour. Antidotes for paracetamol act by replenishing hepatic glutathione and should be administered to all patients with acute poisoning and paracetamol concentrations above a 'treatment line' provided on paracetamol poisoning nomograms (Fig. 7.2). The threshold used for these nomograms varies between countries, however, and local guidance should be followed. Acetylcysteine given intravenously (or orally in some countries) is highly efficacious if administered within 8 hours of the overdose. However, efficacy declines thereafter, so administration should not be delayed in patients presenting after 8 hours to await a paracetamol blood concentration result. The antidote can be stopped if the paracetamol concentration is shown to be below the nomogram treatment line. Liver and renal function, International Normalised Ratio (INR) and a venous bicarbonate should also be measured. Arterial blood gases and lactate should be assessed in patients with reduced bicarbonate or severe liver function abnormalities; metabolic acidosis indicates severe poisoning.

Anaphylactoid reactions are the most important adverse effects of acetylcysteine and are related to dose-related histamine release. Common features are itching and urticaria, and in severe cases, bronchospasm and hypotension. Most cases can be managed by temporary discontinuation of acetylcysteine and administration of an antihistamine.

An alternative antidote is methionine 2.5 g orally (adult dose) every 4 hours to a total of four doses, but this may be less effective, especially after delayed presentation. Liver transplantation should be considered for paracetamol poisoning with life-threatening liver failure (p. 856).

If multiple ingestions of paracetamol have taken place over several hours ('staggered overdose') or days (e.g. chronic therapeutic excess), acetylcysteine may be indicated; specific treatment recommendations vary between countries.

Fig. 7.2 Paracetamol treatment nomogram (UK). Above the treatment line, benefits of treatment outweigh risk. Below it, risks of treatment outweigh benefits.

Salicylates (aspirin)

Clinical features

Salicylate overdose commonly causes nausea, vomiting, sweating, tinnitus and deafness. Direct stimulation of the respiratory centre produces hyperventilation and respiratory alkalosis. Peripheral vasodilatation with bounding pulses and profuse sweating occurs in moderately severe cases. Serious poisoning is associated with metabolic acidosis, hypoprothrombinaemia, hyperglycaemia, hyperpyrexia, renal failure, pulmonary oedema, shock and cerebral oedema. Agitation, delirium, coma and fits may occur, especially in children. Toxicity is enhanced by acidosis, which increases salicylate transfer across the blood–brain barrier.

Management

Activated charcoal should be administered if the patient presents within 1 hour. Multiple doses may enhance salicylate elimination but are not routinely recommended.

The plasma salicylate concentration should be measured at least 2 (symptomatic patients) or 4 hours (asymptomatic patients) after overdose and repeated in suspected serious poisoning, as concentrations may continue to rise for several hours. Clinical status, however, is more important than the salicylate concentration when assessing severity.

Dehydration should be corrected carefully because of the risk of pulmonary oedema. Metabolic acidosis should be treated with intravenous sodium bicarbonate (8.4%), after plasma potassium has been corrected. Urinary alkalinisation is indicated for adults with salicylate concentrations above 500 mg/L.

Haemodialysis is very effective for removing salicylate and correcting associated acid–base and fluid balance abnormalities. It should be considered when serum concentrations are above 700 mg/L in adults with severe toxic features, or in renal failure, pulmonary oedema, coma, convulsions or refractory acidosis.

Non-steroidal anti-inflammatory drugs

Clinical features

Overdose of most non-steroidal anti-inflammatory drugs (NSAIDs) usually causes only minor abdominal discomfort, vomiting and/ or diarrhoea, but convulsions can occur occasionally, especially with mefenamic acid. Coma, prolonged seizures, apnoea, liver dysfunction and renal failure may follow substantial overdose but are rare. Features of toxicity are unlikely to develop in patients who are asymptomatic more than 6 hours after overdose.

Management

Electrolytes, liver function tests and a full blood count should be checked in all but the most trivial cases. Activated charcoal may be given if the patient presents within 1 hour. Symptomatic treatment for nausea and gastrointestinal irritation may be needed.

Antidepressants

Tricyclic antidepressants

Overdose with tricyclic antidepressants (TCAs) carries a high morbidity and mortality because of their sodium channel-blocking, anticholinergic and α-adrenoceptor-blocking effects.

Clinical features

Anticholinergic effects are common (Box 7.10). Severe complications include convulsions, coma and arrhythmias (ventricular

i	**7.10** Anticholinergic and serotonergic feature clusters	
	Anticholinergic	**Serotonin syndrome**
Common causes	Benzodiazepines Antipsychotics TCAs Antihistamines Scopolamine Benzatropine Belladonna Some plants and mushrooms (see Box 7.18)	SSRIs MAOIs TCAs Amphetamines Tryptamines Buspirone Bupropion (especially in combination)
Clinical features		
Cardiovascular	Tachycardia, hypertension	Tachycardia, hyper- or hypotension
Central nervous system	Delirium, hallucinations, sedation	Delirium, hallucinations, sedation, coma
Muscle	Myoclonus	Shivering, tremor, myoclonus, raised creatine kinase
Temperature	Fever	Fever
Eyes	Diplopia, mydriasis	Normal pupil size
Abdomen	Ileus, palpable bladder	Diarrhoea, vomiting
Mouth	Dry	
Skin	Flushing, hot, dry	Flushing, sweating
Complications	Seizures	Seizures Rhabdomyolysis Renal failure Metabolic acidosis Coagulopathies

(MAOI = monoamine oxidase inhibitor; SSRI = selective serotonin re-uptake inhibitor; TCA = tricyclic antidepressant)

Fig. 7.3 ECG in severe tricyclic antidepressant poisoning. This rhythm strip shows a broad QRS complex due to impaired conduction.

tachycardia, ventricular fibrillation and, less commonly, heart block). Hypotension results from inappropriate vasodilatation or impaired myocardial contractility. Serious complications appear more common with dosulepin and amitriptyline.

Management

Activated charcoal should be administered if the patient presents within 1 hour. A 12-lead ECG should be taken and continuous cardiac monitoring maintained for at least 6 hours. Prolongation of the QRS interval (especially if >0.16 secs) indicates severe sodium channel blockade and a high risk of arrhythmia (Fig. 7.3). QT interval prolongation may also occur. Arterial blood gases should be measured in suspected severe poisoning.

In patients with arrhythmias, significant QRS or QT prolongation or acidosis, intravenous sodium bicarbonate (50 mL of 8.4%

solution) should be administered and repeated to correct pH. The correction of the acidosis and the sodium loading that results may bring about rapid improvement in ECG features and arrhythmias. Hypoxia and electrolyte abnormalities should also be corrected. Anti-arrhythmic drugs should only be given on specialist advice. Prolonged seizures should be treated initially with intravenous benzodiazepines (see Box 7.8).

Selective serotonin and noradrenaline re-uptake inhibitors

Selective serotonin re-uptake inhibitor (SSRI) antidepressants (e.g. fluoxetine, paroxetine, fluvoxamine, sertraline, citalopram, escitalopram) are increasingly used to treat depression and are less toxic in overdose than TCAs. The related serotonin–noradrenaline re-uptake inhibitors (SNRIs), such as venlafaxine and duloxetine, are also commonly used but are more toxic than SSRIs in overdose.

Clinical features and management

Overdose of SSRIs may produce nausea and vomiting, tremor, insomnia and sinus tachycardia. Agitation, drowsiness and convulsions occur infrequently and may be delayed for several hours. Serotonin syndrome may occur (see Box 7.10), especially if SSRIs are taken in combination or with other serotonergic agents. Cardiac arrhythmias occur infrequently and most patients require supportive care only. The toxic effects of SNRIs are similar but tachycardia, hypertension or hypotension and ECG changes (QRS and QT prolongation) may be more prominent and hypoglycaemia can also arise.

Lithium

Severe lithium toxicity is uncommon after intentional acute overdose but is more often encountered in patients taking therapeutic doses, frequently as a result of interactions with drugs such as diuretics or NSAIDs. Severe toxicity is more common after acute overdose in patients already taking chronic therapy ('acute on chronic' poisoning).

Clinical features

Nausea, diarrhoea, polyuria, dizziness and tremor may progress to muscular weakness, drowsiness, delirium, myoclonus, fasciculations, choreoathetosis and renal failure. Coma, seizures, ataxia, cardiac dysrhythmias such as heart block, blood pressure disturbances and renal failure may occur in severe poisoning.

Management

Activated charcoal is ineffective. Early gastric lavage is of theoretical benefit, but lithium tablets are likely to remain intact in the stomach and may be too large for aspiration via a lavage tube. Whole bowel irrigation is often used after substantial overdose but efficacy is unproven.

Lithium concentrations should be measured immediately (symptomatic patients) or after at least 6 hours (asymptomatic patients) following acute overdose. The usual therapeutic range is 0.4–1.0 mmol/L. Adequate hydration should be maintained with intravenous fluids. Seizures should be treated as in Box 7.8.

Haemodialysis should be considered for severe toxicity associated with high lithium concentrations (e.g. >4.0 mmol/L after chronic or 'acute on chronic' poisoning, or >7.5 mmol/L after acute poisoning). Lithium concentrations are reduced substantially during dialysis, but rebound increases occur after discontinuation and multiple sessions are usually required.

Cardiovascular medications

Although not common, cardiovascular drug overdose is important because features of toxicity are often severe.

Beta-blockers

Major features of toxicity are bradycardia and hypotension; heart block, pulmonary oedema and cardiogenic shock occur in severe poisoning. Those with additional sodium channel-blocking effects (e.g. propranolol, acebutolol, carvedilol) may cause seizures, delirium and coma, while sotalol, which also blocks potassium channels, may cause QT_c prolongation and torsades de pointes (Box 7.8 and p. 476).

Management

Intravenous fluids may reverse hypotension but care is required to avoid pulmonary oedema. Bradycardia and hypotension may respond to high doses of atropine (up to 3 mg in an adult) or an infusion of isoproterenol. Glucagon (5–10 mg over 10 mins, then 1–5 mg/hr by infusion) counteracts β-blockade by stimulating intracellular cyclic adenosine monophosphate (cAMP) production and is now more commonly used. In severe cases, 'hyperinsulinaemia euglycaemic therapy' has been used, as described under calcium channel blockers below. The efficacy of lipid emulsion therapy in severe poisoning with lipid-soluble β-blockers, such as propranolol, carvedilol and oxprenolol, is uncertain.

Calcium channel blockers

L-type calcium channel blockers are highly toxic in overdose. Dihydropyridines (e.g. nifedipine, amlodipine) cause vasodilatation, whereas diltiazem and verapamil have predominantly cardiac effects, including bradycardia and reduced myocardial contractility.

Clinical features

Hypotension due to vasodilatation or myocardial depression is common and bradycardias and heart block may also occur, especially with verapamil and diltiazem. Gastrointestinal disturbances, delirium, metabolic acidosis, hyperglycaemia and hyperkalaemia may also be present.

Management

Hypotension should be corrected with intravenous fluids, taking care to avoid pulmonary oedema. Persistent hypotension may respond to intravenous calcium gluconate (10 mg IV over 5 mins, repeated as required). Isoproterenol and glucagon may also be useful. Successful use of intravenous insulin with glucose (10–20% dextrose with insulin initially at 0.5–2.0 U/kg/hr, increasing to 5–10 U/kg/hr according to clinical response), so-called 'hyperinsulinaemia euglycaemic therapy', has been reported in patients unresponsive to other strategies. The mechanism of action remains to be fully elucidated, but in states of shock myocardial metabolism switches from use of free fatty acids to glucose. Calcium channel blocker poisoning is also associated with hypoinsulinaemia and insulin resistance, impeding glucose uptake by myocytes. High doses of insulin inhibit lipolysis and increase glucose uptake and the efficiency of glucose utilisation. Cardiac pacing may be needed for severe unresponsive bradycardias or heart block. Lipid emulsion therapy has also been used in severe poisoning with apparent benefit, although evidence is largely anecdotal.

Digoxin and oleander

Poisoning with digoxin is usually accidental, arising from prescription of an excessive dose, impairment of renal function or drug interactions. In South Asia, deliberate self-poisoning with yellow oleander (*Thevetia peruviana*), containing cardiac glycosides, is common.

Clinical features

Cardiac effects include tachyarrhythmias (either atrial or ventricular) and bradycardias, with or without atrioventricular block. Ventricular bigeminy is common and atrial tachycardia with evidence of atrioventricular block is highly suggestive of the diagnosis. Severe poisoning is often associated with hyperkalaemia. Non-cardiac features include delirium, headache, nausea, vomiting, diarrhoea and (rarely) altered colour vision. Digoxin poisoning can be confirmed by elevated plasma concentration (usual therapeutic range 1.3–2.5 mmol/L). After chronic exposure, concentrations >5 mmol/L suggest serious poisoning.

Management

Activated charcoal is commonly administered to patients presenting soon after acute ingestion, although evidence of benefit is lacking. Urea, electrolytes and creatinine should be measured, a 12-lead ECG performed and cardiac monitoring instituted. Hypoxia, hypokalaemia (sometimes caused by concurrent diuretic use), hypomagnesaemia and acidosis increase the risk of arrhythmias and should be corrected. Significant bradycardias may respond to atropine, although temporary pacing is sometimes needed. Ventricular arrhythmias may respond to intravenous magnesium (see Box 7.8). If available, digoxin-specific antibody fragments should be administered when there are severe refractory ventricular arrhythmias or bradycardias. These are effective for both digoxin and yellow oleander poisoning.

Iron

Overdose with iron can cause severe and sometimes fatal poisoning, with toxicity of individual iron preparations related to their elemental iron content.

Clinical features

Early features include gastrointestinal disturbance with the passage of grey or black stools, progressing to hyperglycaemia, leucocytosis, haematemesis, rectal bleeding, drowsiness, convulsions, coma, metabolic acidosis and cardiovascular collapse in severe cases. Early symptoms may improve or resolve within 6–12 hours, but hepatocellular necrosis can develop 12–24 hours after overdose and occasionally progresses to hepatic failure. Gastrointestinal strictures are late complications.

Management

Activated charcoal is ineffective but gastric lavage may be considered in patients presenting soon after substantial overdose, although efficacy is unknown. Serum iron concentration should be measured at least 4 hours after overdose or earlier if there are features of toxicity. Desferrioxamine chelates iron and should be administered immediately in patients with severe features, without waiting for serum iron concentrations, as well as symptomatic patients with high serum iron concentrations (e.g. >5 mg/L). Desferrioxamine may cause hypotension, allergic reactions and occasionally pulmonary oedema. Otherwise, treatment is supportive and directed at complications.

Antipsychotic drugs

Antipsychotic drugs (p. 1198) are often prescribed for patients at high risk of self-harm or suicide and are often taken in overdose.

Clinical features

Anticholinergic features (see Box 7.10) including drowsiness, tachycardia and hypotension, are common and convulsions may occur. Acute dystonias, including oculogyric crisis, torticollis and trismus, may occur after overdose with typical antipsychotics like haloperidol or chlorpromazine. QT interval prolongation and torsades de pointes can occur with some typical (e.g. haloperidol) and atypical (e.g. quetiapine, amisulpride, ziprasidone) agents.

Management

Activated charcoal may be of benefit if given early. Cardiac monitoring should be undertaken for at least 6 hours. Management is largely supportive, with treatment directed at complications (see Box 7.8).

Antidiabetic agents

Overdose is uncommon but toxic effects can be severe.

Clinical features

Sulphonylureas, meglitinides (e.g. nateglinide, repaglinide) and parenteral insulin cause hypoglycaemia when taken in overdose, although insulin is non-toxic if ingested by mouth. The duration of hypoglycaemia depends on the half-life or release characteristics of the preparation and may be prolonged over several days with long-acting agents such as glibenclamide, insulin zinc suspension or insulin glargine.

Features of hypoglycaemia include nausea, agitation, sweating, aggression, delirium, tachycardia, hypothermia, drowsiness, convulsions and coma (p. 738). Permanent neurological damage can occur if hypoglycaemia is prolonged. Hypoglycaemia can be diagnosed using bedside glucose strips but venous blood should also be sent for laboratory confirmation.

Metformin is uncommonly associated with hypoglycaemia. Its major toxic effect is lactic acidosis, which can have a high mortality, and is particularly common in older patients and those with renal or hepatic impairment, or when ethanol has been co-ingested. Other features of metformin overdose are nausea, vomiting, diarrhoea, abdominal pain, drowsiness, coma, hypotension and cardiovascular collapse.

There is limited experience of overdose involving thiazolidinediones (e.g. pioglitazone) and dipeptidyl peptidase 4 (DPP-4) inhibitors (e.g. sitagliptin) but significant hypoglycaemia is unlikely.

Management

Activated charcoal should be considered for recent substantial overdose. Venous blood glucose and urea and electrolytes should be measured and measurement repeated regularly. Hypoglycaemia should be corrected using oral or intravenous glucose (50 mL of 50% dextrose); an infusion of 10–20% dextrose may be required to prevent recurrence. Intramuscular glucagon can be used as an alternative, especially if intravenous access is unavailable. Failure to regain consciousness within a few minutes of normalisation of the blood glucose can indicate that a central nervous system (CNS) depressant has also been ingested, the hypoglycaemia has been prolonged, or there is another cause of coma (e.g. cerebral haemorrhage or oedema).

i 7.11 Clinical features and specific management of drugs less commonly involved in poisoning		
Substance	**Clinical features**	**Management**
Anticonvulsants		
Carbamazepine, phenytoin	Cerebellar signs Convulsions Cardiac arrhythmias Coma	Multiple-dose activated charcoal (carbamazepine)
Sodium valproate	Coma Metabolic acidosis	Haemodialysis for severe poisoning
Isoniazid	Peripheral neuropathy Convulsions	Activated charcoal IV pyridoxine
Theophylline	Cardiac arrhythmias Convulsions Coma	Multiple-dose activated charcoal
Antimalarial drugs		
Chloroquine	Acidosis and hypokalaemia Visual loss Convulsions, coma ECG changes and arrhythmias	Correction of pH (but not potassium) Monitoring and treatment of cardiac rhythm High-dose diazepam with mechanical ventilation
Quinine	Tremor, tinnitus, deafness, ataxia, convulsions, coma Haemolysis ECG changes and arrhythmias Retinal toxicity	Correction of pH (but not potassium) Monitoring and treatment of cardiac rhythm Multiple-dose activated charcoal No effective treatment for visual loss

Arterial blood gases and plasma lactate should be taken after metformin overdose; acidosis should be corrected with intravenous sodium bicarbonate (250 mL 1.26% solution or 50 mL 8.4% solution, repeated as necessary). In severe cases, haemodialysis or haemodiafiltration is used.

Pharmaceutical agents less commonly taken in poisoning

An overview of the clinical features and management for drugs less commonly involved in poisoning is provided in Box 7.11.

Drugs of misuse

Drugs of misuse are common causes of toxicity requiring hospital admission. Management has recently become more complex because of the emergence of 'novel psychoactive substances' (NPS). These are often chemically related to traditional drugs of misuse, but with structural modifications made to evade legal control. The constituents of branded NPS products are often unknown and knowledge about the clinical features and management of NPS toxicity is limited.

Depressants

These produce CNS depression, including drowsiness, ataxia, delirium and coma, sometimes with respiratory depression, airway compromise, aspiration pneumonia and respiratory arrest

	7.12 Stimulant, sedative and opioid feature clusters		
	Stimulant	**Sedative hypnotic**	**Opioid**
Common causes	Amphetamines MDMA ('ecstasy') Ephedrine Pseudoephedrine Cocaine Cannabis Phencyclidine Cathinones (e.g. mephedrone) Benzylpiperazine	Benzodiazepines Barbiturates Ethanol GHB	Heroin Morphine Methadone Fentanyl and derivatives Oxycodone Dihydrocodeine Codeine Pethidine Buprenorphine Dextropropoxyphene Tramadol
Clinical features			
Respiratory	Tachypnoea	Reduced respiratory rate and ventilation[1]	Reduced respiratory rate and ventilation
Cardiovascular	Tachycardia, hypertension	Hypotension[1]	Hypotension, relative bradycardia
Central nervous system	Restlessness, anxiety, anorexia, insomnia Hallucinations	Delirium, hallucinations, slurred speech Sedation, coma[1]	Delirium, hallucinations, slurred speech Sedation, coma[2]
Muscle	Tremor	Ataxia, reduced muscle tone	Ataxia, reduced muscle tone
Temperature	Fever	Hypothermia	Hypothermia
Eyes	Mydriasis	Diplopia, strabismus, nystagmus Normal pupil size	Miosis
Abdomen	Abdominal pain, diarrhoea	–	Ileus
Mouth	Dry	–	–
Skin	Piloerection	Blisters, pressure sores	Needle tracks[2]
Complications	Seizures Myocardial infarction Dysrhythmias Rhabdomyolysis Renal failure Intracerebral haemorrhage or infarction	Respiratory failure[1] Aspiration	Respiratory failure[2] Non-cardiogenic pulmonary oedema Aspiration

[1]Especially barbiturates. [2]IV use.
(GHB = gamma hydroxybutyrate; MDMA = 3,4-methylene-dioxymethamphetamine)

(Box 7.12). Other complications of coma include pressure blisters or sores and rhabdomyolysis. Effects are potentiated by other CNS depressants, including alcohol.

Essential supportive care is detailed in Box 7.8. Antidotes are available for some depressants.

Benzodiazepines

Benzodiazepines (e.g. diazepam) and related substances (e.g. zopiclone) are of low toxicity when taken alone in overdose but can enhance CNS and respiratory depression when taken with other sedative agents, including alcohol. They are more hazardous in the elderly and those with chronic lung or neuromuscular disease (see Box 7.12).

The specific benzodiazepine antagonist flumazenil (0.5 mg IV, repeated if needed) increases conscious level in patients with benzodiazepine overdose, but carries a risk of seizures and is contraindicated in patients co-ingesting pro-convulsants (e.g. TCAs) and those with a history of epilepsy.

Opioids

Toxicity may result from misuse of illicit drugs such as heroin or from intentional or accidental overdose of medicinal opiates. Intravenous or smoked heroin gives a rapid, intensely pleasurable experience, often accompanied by heightened sexual arousal. Physical dependence occurs within a few weeks of regular high-dose use. Withdrawal can start within 12 hours, causing intense craving, rhinorrhoea, lacrimation, yawning, perspiration, shivering, piloerection, vomiting, diarrhoea and abdominal cramps. Examination reveals tachycardia, hypertension, mydriasis and facial flushing.

Commonly encountered opioids and clinical features of poisoning are shown in Box 7.12. Needle tracks may be visible in intravenous users and there may be drug-related paraphernalia. Methadone may also cause QT_c prolongation and torsades de pointes. Features of opioid poisoning can be prolonged for up to 48 hours after use of long-acting agents such as methadone or oxycodone.

Use of the specific opioid antagonist naloxone (0.4–2 mg IV in an adult, repeated if necessary) may obviate the need for intubation, although excessive doses may precipitate acute withdrawal in chronic opiate users and breakthrough pain in those receiving opioids for pain management. Repeated doses or an infusion are often required because the half-life of the antidote is short compared to that of most opiates, especially those with prolonged elimination. Patients should be monitored for at least 6 hours after the last naloxone dose. Rare complications of naloxone therapy include fits, ventricular arrhythmias and pulmonary oedema.

Gamma hydroxybutyrate

Gamma hydroxybutyrate (GHB), and the related compounds gamma butyrolactone (GBL) and 1,4 butanediol are sedative liquids with psychedelic and body-building effects.

As well as sedative hypnotic features (see Box 7.12), toxicity may cause nausea, diarrhoea, vertigo, tremor, myoclonus, extrapyramidal signs, euphoria, bradycardia, convulsions, metabolic acidosis, hypokalaemia and hyperglycaemia. Coma usually resolves abruptly within a few hours but occasionally persists for several days. Dependence may develop in regular users, who experience severe, prolonged withdrawal effects if use is discontinued suddenly.

Management is largely supportive. All patients should be observed for a minimum of 2 hours and until symptoms resolve, with monitoring of blood pressure, heart rate, respiratory rate and oxygenation. Withdrawal symptoms may require treatment with very high doses of benzodiazepine.

Stimulants and entactogens

These are sympathomimetic and serotonergic amines that have overlapping clinical features, depending on the balance of their stimulant (see Box 7.12) and serotonergic (see Box 7.10) effects. As well as traditional drugs such as cocaine, amphetamines and ecstasy, the group includes many more recently emerging novel psychoactive substances, including cathinones (e.g. mephedrone), piperazines (e.g. benzylpiperazine), piperadines (e.g. ethylphenidate), benzofurans (e.g. 5-aminopropylbenzofuran) and NBOMe compounds (e.g. 25I-NBOMe).

Cocaine

Cocaine is available as a water-soluble hydrochloride salt powder suitable for nasal inhalation ('snorting'), or as insoluble free-base ('crack' cocaine) 'rocks' that, unlike the hydrochloride salt, vaporise at high temperature and can be smoked, giving a more rapid and intense effect.

Effects appear rapidly after inhalation and especially after smoking. Sympathomimetic stimulant effects predominate (see Box 7.12). Serious complications usually occur within 3 hours of use and include coronary artery spasm, leading to myocardial ischaemia or infarction, hypotension and ventricular arrhythmias. Cocaine toxicity should be considered in younger adults presenting with ischaemic chest pain. Hyperpyrexia, rhabdomyolysis, acute renal failure and disseminated intravascular coagulation may occur.

A 12-lead ECG and ECG monitoring should be undertaken. ST segment elevation may occur in the absence of myocardial infarction and troponin T estimations are the most sensitive and specific markers of myocardial damage. Benzodiazepines and intravenous nitrates are useful for managing patients with chest pain or hypertension. Acidosis should be corrected and physical cooling measures used for hyperthermia. Beta-blockers may be contraindicated because of the risk of unopposed α-adrenoceptor stimulation, but this is debated. Coronary angiography should be considered in patients with myocardial infarction or acute coronary syndromes.

Amphetamines and cathinones

Amphetamine-related compounds include amphetamine sulphate ('speed'), methylamphetamine ('crystal meth') and 3,4-methylene-dioxymethamphetamine (MDMA, 'ecstasy'). Synthetic cathinones include mephedrone and methylenedioxypyrovalerone. Tolerance is common, leading regular users to seek ever higher doses.

Toxic features usually appear within a few minutes of use and last 4–6 hours, or substantially longer after a large overdose. Sympathomimetic stimulant and serotonergic effects are common (see Boxes 7.10 and 7.12). Some users develop hyponatraemia as a result of excessive water-drinking or inappropriate vasopressin (antidiuretic hormone, ADH) secretion. Muscle rigidity, pain and bruxism (clenching of the jaw), hyperpyrexia, rhabdomyolysis, metabolic acidosis, acute renal failure, disseminated intravascular coagulation, hepatocellular necrosis, acute respiratory distress syndrome (ARDS) and cardiovascular collapse have all been described following MDMA use. Cerebral infarction and haemorrhage have been reported, especially after intravenous amphetamine use.

Management is supportive and directed at complications (see Box 7.8).

Hallucinogens

Cannabis

Derived from the dried leaves and flowers of *Cannabis sativa*, cannabis produces euphoria, perceptual alterations and conjunctival injection, followed by enhanced appetite, relaxation and occasionally hypertension, tachycardia, slurred speech and ataxia. Effects occur 10–30 minutes after smoking or 1–3 hours after ingestion, and last 4–8 hours. High doses may produce anxiety, delirium, hallucinations and psychosis. Psychological dependence is common, but tolerance and withdrawal symptoms are unusual. Long-term use is thought to increase the lifetime risk of psychosis. Serious acute toxicity is uncommon and supportive treatment is all that is required.

Synthetic cannabinoid receptor agonists

Large numbers of synthetic cannabinoid receptor agonists (SCRAs), synthetic compounds sometimes referred to collectively as 'spice', are now used as legal alternatives to cannabis; examples include PB-22, 5F-PB-22, 5F-AKB-48, STS-135, SF-ADB and MDMB-CHMICA. They are usually sprayed on to a herbal smoking mix and packaged as smoking products with appealing brand names. These may contain more than one SCRA and content may change with time.

The toxic effects of SCRAs differ from those of cannabis, being generally more marked and including agitation, panic, delirium, hallucinations, tachycardia, ECG changes, hypertonia, dyspnoea and vomiting. Coma, respiratory acidosis, seizures, hypokalaemia and renal dysfunction are also reported. Treatment of intoxication is supportive.

Tryptamines

These are predominantly 5-hydroxytryptamine (5-HT, serotonin; especially 5-HT2a) agonists with associated stimulant effects. Typical clinical features include hallucinations, agitation, delirium, hypertension, tachycardia, sweating, anxiety and headache. Serotonin syndrome may occur (see Box 7.10), especially if tryptamines are used in combination with other serotonergic agents. Naturally occurring examples are psilocin and psilocybin, found in 'magic mushrooms', and dimethyltryptamine (DMT) in traditional ayahuasca brews. Synthetic tryptamines, such as alpha-methyltryptamine (AMT), have been encountered recently.

d-Lysergic acid diethylamide

d-Lysergic acid diethylamide (LSD) is a synthetic ergoline usually ingested as small squares of impregnated absorbent paper (often printed with a distinctive design) or as 'microdots'. The drug causes perceptual effects, such as heightened visual awareness of colours or distortion of images. Hallucinations may be pleasurable or terrifying ('bad trip'). Other features are delirium, agitation, aggression, dilated pupils, hypertension, pyrexia and metabolic acidosis. Psychosis may sometimes last several days.

Patients with psychotic reactions or CNS depression should be observed in hospital, preferably in a quiet, dimly lit room to minimise external stimulation. A benzodiazepine that can be used for sedation is required, avoiding antipsychotics if possible, as they may precipitate cardiovascular collapse or convulsions.

Dissociative drugs

Ketamine, its *N*-ethyl derivative methoxetamine and phencyclidine (now rarely encountered) produce a sense of dissociation from reality, often associated with visual and auditory distortions. Memory loss, impaired consciousness, agitation, hallucinations, tremors and numbness may also occur. Long-term ketamine (and probably methoxetamine) use can cause severe chronic cystitis with dysuria, frequency, urgency, haematuria and incontinence. Treatment of intoxication is supportive.

Volatile substances

Inhalation of volatile nitrites (e.g. amyl nitrite, isobutyl nitrite), often sold in bottles or vials as 'poppers', is reported to produce a feeling of pleasure and warmth, relax the anal sphincter and prolong orgasm. These potent vasodilators commonly provoke headache, dizziness, hypotension and tachycardia. They also oxidise haemoglobin to produce methaemoglobinaemia, with resulting breathlessness and delirium. Severe cases are treated with methylthioninium chloride ('methylene blue', see Fig 7.1).

Several volatile solvents found in household products, such as propane, butane, toluene and trichloroethylene, have a mild euphoriant effect if inhaled. Serious toxic effects can occur, including reduced level of consciousness, seizures and cardiac arrhythmias; there is also a risk of asphyxia from some methods of inhalation.

Nitrous oxide is an anaesthetic gas, but small canisters of it are sold for the domestic production of whipped cream and the contents of these can be transferred to balloons for inhalation. The gas has euphoriant effects ('laughing gas'), but hazards include asphyxia from inhalation without oxygen, or vitamin B_{12} inactivation from chronic use leading to megaloblastic anaemia, psychosis and other neurological sequelae.

Body packers and body stuffers

Body packers ('mules') attempt to smuggle illicit drugs (usually cocaine, heroin or amphetamines) by ingesting multiple small packages wrapped in several layers of clingfilm or in condoms. Body stuffers are those who have ingested unpackaged or poorly wrapped substances, often to avoid arrest. Both groups are at risk of severe toxicity if the packages rupture. This is more likely for body stuffers, who may develop symptoms of poisoning within 8 hours of ingestion. The risk of poisoning depends on the quality of the wrapping, and the amount and type of drug

Fig. 7.4 Abdominal X-ray of a body packer showing multiple drug-filled condoms.

ingested. Cocaine, for example, presents a much higher risk than heroin because of its high toxicity and lack of a specific antidote.

Patients suspected of body packing or stuffing should be admitted for observation. A careful history taken in private is important, but for obvious reasons patients may withhold details of the drugs involved. The mouth, rectum and vagina should be examined as possible sites for concealed drugs. A urine toxicology screen performed at intervals may provide evidence of leakage, although positive results may reflect earlier drug use. Packages may be visible on plain abdominal films (Fig. 7.4) but ultrasound and computed tomography (CT) are more sensitive. One of these (preferably CT) should be performed in all suspected body packers.

Antimotility agents are often used by body packers to prevent premature passage of packages; it can take several days for packages to pass spontaneously, during which the carrier is at risk from package rupture. Whole bowel irrigation is commonly used to accelerate passage and is continued until all packages have passed. Surgery may be required when there is mechanical bowel obstruction or when evolving clinical features suggest package rupture, especially with cocaine.

Chemicals and pesticides

Carbon monoxide

Carbon monoxide (CO) is a colourless, odourless gas produced by faulty appliances burning organic fuels. It is also present in vehicle exhaust fumes and sometimes in smoke from house fires. It binds with haemoglobin and cytochrome oxidase, reducing tissue oxygen delivery and inhibiting cellular respiration. CO is a common cause of death by poisoning and most patients die before reaching hospital.

Clinical features

Early features include headache, nausea, irritability, weakness and tachypnoea. The cause of these non-specific features may not be obvious if the exposure is occult, such as from a faulty domestic appliance. Subsequently, ataxia, nystagmus, drowsiness and hyper-reflexia may develop, progressing to coma, convulsions, hypotension, respiratory depression, cardiovascular collapse and death. Myocardial ischaemia may result in arrhythmias or myocardial infarction. Cerebral oedema is common and rhabdomyolysis may cause myoglobinuria and renal failure. In those who recover from acute toxicity, longer-term neuropsychiatric effects are common, such as personality change, memory loss and concentration impairment. Extrapyramidal effects, urinary or faecal incontinence, and gait disturbance may also occur. Poisoning during pregnancy may cause fetal hypoxia and intrauterine death.

Management

Patients should be removed from exposure as soon as possible and resuscitated as necessary. A high concentration of oxygen should be administered via a tightly fitting facemask; this reduces the half-life of carboxyhaemoglobin from 4–6 hours to about 40 minutes. Measurement of carboxyhaemoglobin is useful for confirming exposure; levels >20% suggest significant exposure but do not correlate well with the severity of poisoning, partly because concentrations fall rapidly after removal of the patient from exposure, especially if supplemental oxygen has been given.

An ECG should be performed in all patients with acute CO poisoning, especially those with pre-existing heart disease. Arterial blood gas analysis should be checked in those with serious poisoning. Pulse oximetry may provide misleading oxygen saturations because carboxyhaemoglobin and oxyhaemoglobin are both measured. Excessive intravenous fluid administration should be avoided, particularly in the elderly, because of the risk of pulmonary and cerebral oedema. Convulsions should be controlled with diazepam.

Hyperbaric oxygen therapy is controversial. At 2.5 atmospheres, this reduces the half-life of carboxyhaemoglobin to about 20 minutes and increases the amount of oxygen dissolved in plasma 10-fold, but systematic reviews have not consistently shown improved clinical outcomes. The logistical difficulties of transporting sick patients to hyperbaric chambers and managing them therein are substantial.

Organophosphorus insecticides and nerve agents

Organophosphorus (OP) compounds (Box 7.13) are widely used as pesticides, especially in developing countries. Case fatality following deliberate ingestion is high (5–20%).

Nerve agents, developed for chemical warfare, are derived from OP insecticides and are much more toxic. They are commonly classified as G (originally synthesised in Germany) or V ('venomous') agents. The 'G' agents, such as tabun, sarin and soman, are volatile, absorbed by inhalation or via the skin, and dissipate rapidly after use. 'V' agents, such as VX, are contact poisons unless aerosolised, and contaminate ground for weeks or months.

The toxicology and management of nerve agent and pesticide poisoning are similar.

Mechanism of toxicity

OP compounds inactivate acetylcholinesterase (AChE), resulting in the accumulation of acetylcholine (ACh) in cholinergic synapses (Fig. 7.5). Initially, spontaneous hydrolysis of the OP–enzyme

i | **7.13 Organophosphorus compounds**

Nerve agents
- G agents: sarin, tabun, soman
- V agents: VX, VE

Insecticides

Dimethyl compounds
- Dichlorvos
- Fenthion
- Malathion
- Methamidophos

Diethyl compounds
- Chlorpyrifos
- Diazinon
- Parathion-ethyl
- Quinalphos

Fig. 7.5 Mechanism of toxicity of organophosphorus compounds and treatment with oxime.

complex allows reactivation of the enzyme but, subsequently, loss of a chemical group from the OP–enzyme complex prevents further enzyme reactivation. After this process (termed 'ageing') has taken place, new enzyme needs to be synthesised before function can be restored. The rate of 'ageing' is an important determinant of toxicity and is more rapid with dimethyl (3.7 hrs) than diethyl (31 hrs) compounds (Box 7.13) and especially rapid after exposure to nerve agents (soman in particular), which cause 'ageing' within minutes.

Clinical features and management

OP poisoning causes an acute cholinergic phase, which may occasionally be followed by the intermediate syndrome or organophosphate-induced delayed polyneuropathy (OPIDN). The onset, severity and duration of poisoning depend on the route of exposure and agent involved.

i	**7.14 Cholinergic features in poisoning***	
	Muscarinic	**Nicotinic**
Respiratory	Bronchorrhoea, bronchoconstriction	Reduced ventilation
Circulation	Bradycardia, hypotension	Tachycardia, hypertension
Higher mental function	Anxiety, delirium, psychosis	
Muscle	–	Fasciculation, paralysis
Temperature	Fever	–
Eyes	Diplopia, miosis, lacrimation	Mydriasis
Abdomen	Vomiting, profuse diarrhoea	–
Mouth	Salivation	–
Skin	Sweating	–
Complications	Coma, seizures, respiratory depression	

*Both muscarinic and nicotinic features occur in OP poisoning. Nicotinic features occur in nicotine poisoning and black widow spider bites. Cholinergic features are sometimes seen with some mushrooms.

Acute cholinergic syndrome

This usually starts within a few minutes of exposure and nicotinic or muscarinic features may be present (Box 7.14). Vomiting and profuse diarrhoea are typical following ingestion. Bronchoconstriction, bronchorrhoea and salivation may cause severe respiratory compromise. Excess sweating and miosis are characteristic and the presence of muscular fasciculations strongly suggests the diagnosis, although this feature is often absent, even in serious poisoning. Subsequently, generalised flaccid paralysis may develop and affect respiratory and ocular muscles, resulting in respiratory failure. Ataxia, coma, convulsions, cardiac repolarisation abnormalities and torsades de pointes may occur.

Management

The airway should be cleared of excessive secretions, breathing and circulation assessed, high-flow oxygen administered and intravenous access obtained. Appropriate external decontamination is needed (p. 133). Gastric lavage or activated charcoal may be considered if the patient presents sufficiently early. Seizures should be treated as described in Box 7.8. The ECG, oxygen saturation, blood gases, temperature, urea and electrolytes, amylase and glucose should be monitored closely.

Early use of sufficient doses of atropine is potentially life-saving in patients with severe toxicity. Atropine reverses ACh-induced bronchospasm, bronchorrhoea, bradycardia and hypotension. When the diagnosis is uncertain, a marked increase in heart rate associated with skin flushing after a 1 mg intravenous dose makes OP poisoning unlikely. In OP poisoning, atropine (2 mg IV) should be administered and this dose should be doubled every 5–10 minutes until clinical improvement occurs. Further bolus doses should be given until secretions are controlled, the skin is dry, blood pressure is adequate and heart rate is >80 bpm. Large doses may be needed, but excessive doses may cause anticholinergic effects (see Box 7.10).

In severe poisoning requiring atropine, an oxime such as pralidoxime chloride or obidoxime is generally recommended, if available, although efficacy is debated. This may reverse or prevent muscle weakness, convulsions or coma, especially if

given rapidly after exposure. Oximes reactivate AChE that has not undergone 'ageing' and are therefore less effective with dimethyl compounds and nerve agents, especially soman. Oximes may provoke hypotension, especially if administered rapidly.

Intravenous magnesium sulphate has been reported to increase survival in animals and in small human studies of OP poisoning; however, further clinical trial evidence is needed before this can be recommended routinely.

Ventilatory support should be instituted before the patient develops respiratory failure. Benzodiazepines may be used to treat agitation, fasciculations and seizures and for sedation during mechanical ventilation.

Exposure is confirmed by measurement of plasma or red blood cell cholinesterase activity but antidote use should not be delayed pending results. Plasma cholinesterase is reduced more rapidly but is less specific than red cell cholinesterase. Values correlate poorly with the severity of clinical features but are usually <10% in severe poisoning, 20–50% in moderate poisoning and >50% in subclinical poisoning.

The acute cholinergic phase usually lasts 48–72 hours, with most patients requiring intensive cardiorespiratory support and monitoring. Cholinergic features may be prolonged over several weeks with some lipid-soluble agents.

Intermediate syndrome

About 20% of patients with OP poisoning develop weakness that spreads rapidly from the ocular muscles to those of the head and neck, proximal limbs and the muscles of respiration, resulting in ventilatory failure. This 'intermediate syndrome' generally develops 1–4 days after exposure, often after resolution of the acute cholinergic syndrome, and may last 2–3 weeks. There is no specific treatment and supportive care is needed, including maintenance of airway and ventilation.

Organophosphate-induced delayed polyneuropathy

Organophosphate-induced delayed polyneuropathy (OPIDN) is a rare complication that usually occurs 2–3 weeks after acute exposure. It is a mixed sensory/motor polyneuropathy, affecting long myelinated neurons especially, and appears to result from inhibition of enzymes other than AChE. It is a feature of poisoning with some OPs such as triorthocresyl phosphate but is less common with nerve agents. Early clinical features are muscle cramps followed by numbness and paraesthesiae, proceeding to flaccid paralysis of the lower and subsequently the upper limbs, with foot and wrist drop and a high-stepping gait, progressing to paraplegia. Sensory loss may also be present but is variable. Initially, tendon reflexes are reduced or lost but mild spasticity may develop later.

There is no specific therapy for OPIDN. Regular physiotherapy may limit deformity caused by muscle-wasting. Recovery is often incomplete and may be limited to the hands and feet, although substantial functional recovery after 1–2 years may occur, especially in younger patients.

Carbamate insecticides

Carbamate insecticides such as bendiocarb, carbofuran, carbaryl and methomyl inhibit a number of tissue esterases, including AChE. The mechanism, clinical features and management of toxicity are similar to those of OP compounds. However, clinical features are usually less severe and of shorter duration, because the carbamate–AChE complex dissociates quickly, with a half-life of 30–40 minutes, and does not undergo ageing. Also, carbamates penetrate the CNS poorly. Intermediate syndrome and OPIDN are not common features of carbamate poisoning. In spite of this, case fatality can be high for some carbamates, depending on their formulation.

Atropine may be given intravenously as for OP poisoning (p. 146). Diazepam may be used to relieve anxiety. The use of oximes is unnecessary.

Paraquat

Paraquat is a herbicide that is widely used across the world, although it has been banned in the European Union and some other countries for several years. It is highly toxic if ingested, with clinical features including oral burns, vomiting and diarrhoea, progressing to pneumonitis, pulmonary fibrosis and multi-organ failure.

Exposure can be confirmed by a urinary dithionite test, while the plasma paraquat concentration indicates prognosis. There is no specific antidote but activated charcoal is commonly administered. Immunosuppression with glucocorticoids and cyclophosphamide is sometimes used but evidence for benefit is weak. Irrespective of treatment, death is common and may occur within 24 hours with substantial poisoning or after 1–2 weeks with lower doses.

Methanol and ethylene glycol

Ethylene glycol (1,2-ethanediol) is found in antifreeze, brake fluids and, in lower concentrations, windscreen washes. Methanol is present in some antifreeze products and commercially available industrial solvents, and in low concentrations in some screen washes and methylated spirits. It may also be an adulterant of illicitly produced alcohol. Both are rapidly absorbed after ingestion. Methanol and ethylene glycol are not of high intrinsic toxicity but are converted via alcohol dehydrogenase to toxic metabolites that are largely responsible for their clinical effects (Fig. 7.6).

Clinical features

Early features of poisoning with either methanol or ethylene glycol include vomiting, ataxia, drowsiness, dysarthria and nystagmus. As toxic metabolites are formed, metabolic acidosis, tachypnoea, coma and seizures may develop.

Toxic effects of ethylene glycol include ophthalmoplegia, cranial nerve palsies, hyporeflexia and myoclonus. Renal pain

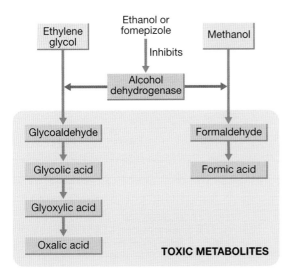

Fig. 7.6 Metabolism of methanol and ethylene glycol.

and acute tubular necrosis occur because of renal calcium oxalate precipitation. Hypocalcaemia, hypomagnesaemia and hyperkalaemia are common.

Methanol poisoning causes headache, delirium and vertigo. Visual impairment and photophobia develop, associated with optic disc and retinal oedema and impaired pupil reflexes. Blindness may be permanent, although some recovery may occur over several months. Pancreatitis and abnormal liver function have also been reported.

Management

Urea and electrolytes, chloride, bicarbonate, glucose, calcium, magnesium, albumin, plasma osmolarity and arterial blood gases should be measured in all patients with suspected methanol or ethylene glycol toxicity. The osmolar and anion gaps should be calculated (see Box 7.5). Initially, poisoning is associated with an increased osmolar gap, but as toxic metabolites are produced, an increased anion gap develops, associated with metabolic acidosis. The diagnosis can be confirmed by measurement of ethylene glycol or methanol concentrations but assays are not widely available.

An antidote, ideally fomepizole but otherwise ethanol, should be administered to all patients with suspected significant exposure while awaiting the results of laboratory investigations. These block alcohol dehydrogenase and delay the formation of toxic metabolites until the parent drug is eliminated in the urine or by dialysis. The antidote should be continued until ethylene glycol or methanol concentrations are undetectable. Metabolic acidosis should be corrected with sodium bicarbonate (e.g. 250 mL of 1.26% solution, repeated as necessary). Convulsions should be treated with an intravenous benzodiazepine. In ethylene glycol poisoning, hypocalcaemia should be corrected only if there are severe ECG features or if seizures occur, as this may increase calcium oxalate crystal formation. In methanol poisoning, folinic acid should be administered to enhance the metabolism of the toxic metabolite, formic acid.

Haemodialysis or haemodiafiltration should be used in severe poisoning, especially if renal failure is present or there is visual loss in the context of methanol poisoning. It should be continued until acute toxic features are no longer present and ethylene glycol/methanol concentrations are undetectable.

Corrosive substances

Products containing strong acids (e.g. hydrochloric or sulphuric acid) or alkalis (e.g. sodium hydroxide, calcium carbonate) may be ingested, accidentally or intentionally, causing gastrointestinal pain, ulceration and necrosis, with risk of perforation.

External decontamination (p. 133), if needed, should be performed after initial resuscitation. Gastric lavage should not be attempted and neutralising chemicals should not be administered after large ingestions because of the risk of tissue damage from heat release. Cardiorespiratory monitoring is necessary and full blood count, renal function, coagulation and acid–base status should be assessed. An erect chest X-ray should be performed if perforation is suspected and may show features of mediastinitis or gas under the diaphragm. Strong analgesics should be administered for pain.

Severe abdominal or chest pain, abdominal distension, shock or acidosis may indicate perforation and should prompt an urgent CT scan of chest and abdomen and surgical review. In the absence of perforation, drooling, dysphagia, stridor or oropharyngeal burns suggest possible severe oesophageal damage and early endoscopy by an experienced operator should be considered. Delayed endoscopy (e.g. after several days) may carry a higher risk of perforation.

Aluminium and zinc phosphide

These rodenticides and fumigants are a common means of self-poisoning in northern India. The mortality rate for aluminium phosphide ingestion has been estimated at 60%; zinc phosphide ingestion appears less toxic, at about 2%. When ingested, both compounds react with gastric acid to form phosphine, a potent pulmonary and gastrointestinal toxicant. Clinical features include severe gastrointestinal disturbances, chest tightness, cough and breathlessness progressing to ARDS and respiratory failure, tremor, paraesthesiae, convulsions, coma, tachycardia, metabolic acidosis, electrolyte disturbances, hypoglycaemia, myocarditis, liver and renal failure, and leucopenia. Ingestion of a few tablets can be fatal.

Treatment is supportive and directed at correcting electrolyte abnormalities and treating complications; there is no specific antidote. Early gastric lavage is sometimes used, often with vegetable oil to reduce the release of toxic phosphine, but the benefit is uncertain.

Copper sulphate

This is used as a fungicide. If it is ingested, clinical features of toxicity include nausea, vomiting, abdominal pain, diarrhoea, discoloured (blue/green) secretions, corrosive effects on the gastrointestinal tract, renal or liver failure, methaemoglobinaemia, haemolysis, rhabdomyolysis, convulsions and coma. Treatment is as for other corrosive substances (see above) and should address complications, including use of methylthioninium chloride for methaemoglobinaemia (see Fig. 7.1). Chelation therapy is unlikely to be beneficial after acute exposure.

Chemicals less commonly taken in poisoning

An overview of the clinical features and management for chemicals less commonly involved in poisoning is provided in Box 7.15.

---

i **7.15 Clinical features and specific management of chemicals less commonly involved in poisoning**

Substance	Clinical features	Management
Lead e.g. Chronic occupational exposure, leaded paint, water contaminated by lead pipes, use of kohl cosmetics	Abdominal pain Microcytic anaemia with basophilic stippling Headache and encephalopathy Motor neuropathy Nephrotoxicity Hypertension Hypocalcaemia	Prevention of further exposure Measurement of blood lead concentration, full blood count and blood film, urea and electrolytes, liver function tests and calcium Abdominal X-ray in children to detect pica Bone X-ray for 'lead lines' Chelation therapy with DMSA or sodium calcium edetate
Petroleum distillates e.g. White spirit, kerosene	Vomiting Aspiration pneumonitis	Gastric lavage contraindicated Activated charcoal ineffective Oxygen and nebulised bronchodilators Chest X-ray to assess pulmonary effects
Organochlorines e.g. DDT, lindane, dieldrin, endosulfan	Nausea, vomiting Agitation Fasciculation Paraesthesiae (face, extremities) Convulsions Coma Respiratory depression Cardiac arrhythmias Hyperthermia Rhabdomyolysis Pulmonary oedema Disseminated intravascular coagulation	Activated charcoal (with nasogastric aspiration for liquid preparations) within 1 hr of ingestion Cardiac monitoring
Pyrethroid insecticides e.g. Cypermethrin, permethrin, imiprothrin	Skin contact: dermatitis, skin paraesthesiae Eye contact: lacrimation, photophobia and oedema of the eyelids Inhalation: dyspnoea, nausea, headaches Ingestion: epigastric pain, nausea, vomiting, headache, coma, convulsions, pulmonary oedema	Symptomatic and supportive care Washing contaminated skin makes irritation worse
Anticoagulant rodenticides e.g. Brodifacoum, bromadialone and warfarin	Abnormal bleeding (prolonged)	Monitor INR/prothrombin time Vitamin K_1 by slow IV injection if there is coagulopathy Fresh frozen plasma or specific clotting factors for bleeding

(DMSA = dimercaptosuccinic acid)

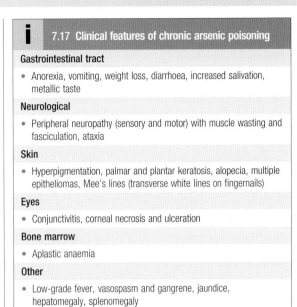

7.16 Chemical warfare agents		
Examples	Clinical effects	Antidotes*
Nerve agents		
Tabun Sarin Soman VX	See page 145 and Box 7.13	Atropine Oximes (p. 145)
Blistering agents		
Nitrogen/sulphur Mustard Lewisite	Eyes: watering, blepharospasm, corneal ulceration Skin: erythema, blistering Respiratory: cough, hoarseness, dyspnoea, pneumonitis	None
Choking agents		
Chlorine Phosgene	Eyes: watering, blepharospasm, corneal ulceration Respiratory: cough, hoarseness, dyspnoea, pneumonitis	None
Blood agents		
Cyanide	Cardiovascular: dizziness, shock Respiratory: dyspnoea, cyanosis CNS: anxiety, headache, delirium, convulsions, coma, fixed dilated pupils Other: vomiting, lactic acidosis	Dicobalt edetate Hydroxocobalamin

*Appropriate resuscitation, decontamination and supportive care are essential after exposure to all chemical warfare agents. Use appropriate personal protective equipment.

Chemical warfare agents

Some toxins have been developed for use as chemical warfare agents. These are summarised in Box 7.16.

Environmental poisoning

Arsenism

Chronic arsenic exposure from drinking water has been reported in many countries, especially India, Bangladesh, Nepal, Thailand, Taiwan, China, Mexico and South America, where a large proportion of the drinking water (ground water) has a high arsenic content, placing large populations at risk. The World Health Organisation (WHO) guideline value for arsenic content in tube well water is 10 µg/L.

Health effects associated with chronic exposure to arsenic in drinking water are shown in Box 7.17. In exposed individuals, high concentrations of arsenic are present in bone, hair and nails. Specific treatments are of no benefit in chronic arsenic toxicity and recovery from the peripheral neuropathy may never be complete, so the emphasis should be on prevention.

Fluorosis

Fluoride poisoning can result from exposure to excessive quantities of fluoride (> 10 ppm) in drinking water, industrial

7.17 Clinical features of chronic arsenic poisoning
Gastrointestinal tract
• Anorexia, vomiting, weight loss, diarrhoea, increased salivation, metallic taste
Neurological
• Peripheral neuropathy (sensory and motor) with muscle wasting and fasciculation, ataxia
Skin
• Hyperpigmentation, palmar and plantar keratosis, alopecia, multiple epitheliomas, Mee's lines (transverse white lines on fingernails)
Eyes
• Conjunctivitis, corneal necrosis and ulceration
Bone marrow
• Aplastic anaemia
Other
• Low-grade fever, vasospasm and gangrene, jaundice, hepatomegaly, splenomegaly
Increased risk of malignancy
• Lung, liver, bladder, kidney, larynx and lymphoid system

exposure to fluoride dust or consumption of brick teas. Clinical features include yellow staining and pitting of permanent teeth, osteosclerosis, soft tissue calcification, deformities (e.g. kyphosis) and joint ankylosis. Changes in the bones of the thoracic cage may lead to rigidity that causes dyspnoea on exertion. Very high doses of fluoride may cause abdominal pain, nausea, vomiting, seizures and muscle spasm. In calcium-deficient children, the toxic effects of fluoride manifest even at marginally high exposures to fluoride.

In endemic areas, such as Jordan, Turkey, Chile, India, Bangladesh, China and Tibet, fluorosis is a major public health problem, especially in communities engaged in physically strenuous agricultural or industrial activities. Dental fluorosis is endemic in East Africa and some West African countries.

Food-related poisoning

Paralytic shellfish poisoning

Paralytic shellfish poisoning is caused by consumption of bivalve molluscs (e.g. mussels, clams, oysters, cockles and scallops) contaminated with saxitoxins, which are concentrated in the shellfish as a result of constant filtration of toxic algae during algal blooms (e.g. 'red tide'). Symptoms develop within 10–120 minutes of eating the contaminated shellfish and include gastrointestinal disturbances, paraesthesia around the mouth or in the extremities, ataxia, mental state changes and dysphagia. In severe cases, paralysis and respiratory failure can develop. There is no specific antidote and treatment is supportive. Most cases resolve over a few days.

Ciguatera poisoning

Ciguatera toxin and related toxins are produced by dinoflagellate plankton that adhere to algae and seaweed. These accumulate in the tropical herbivorous fish that feed on these and in their larger predators (e.g. snapper, barracuda), especially in the

i 7.18 Some poisonous plants and fungi, with their clinical effects

Species (common name)	Toxins	Important features of toxicity
Plants		
Abrus precatorius (jequirity bean)	Abrin	Gastrointestinal effects, drowsiness, delirium, convulsions, multi-organ failure
Ricinus communis (castor oil plant)	Ricin	
Aconitum napellus (aconite, wolf's banc, monkshood)	Aconite	Gastrointestinal effects, paraesthesiae, convulsions, ventricular tachycardia
Aconitum ferox (Indian aconite, bikh)		
Atropa belladonna (deadly nightshade)	Atropine, scopolamine, hyocyamine	Anticholinergic toxidrome (see Box 7.10)
Datura stramonium (Jimson weed, thorn apple)		
Brugmansia spp. (angel's trumpet)		
Colchicum autumnale (autumn crocus)	Colchicine	Gastrointestinal effects, hypotension, cardiogenic shock
Conium maculatum (hemlock)	Toxic nicotinic alkaloids	Hypersalivation, gastrointestinal effects, followed by muscular paralysis
Digitalis purpurea (foxglove)	Cardiac glycosides	Cardiac glycoside toxicity (p. 140)
Nerium oleander (pink oleander)		
Thevetia peruviana (yellow oleander)		
Laburnum anagyroides (laburnum)	Cytosine	Gastrointestinal effects; convulsions in severe cases
Taxus baccata (yew)	Taxane alkaloids	Hypotension, bradycardia, respiratory depression, convulsions, coma, arrhythmias
Fungi		
Amanita phalloides (death cap mushroom)	Amatoxins	Gastrointestinal effects, progressing to liver failure
Cortinarius spp.	Orellanine	Gastrointestinal effects, fever, progressing to renal failure
Psilocybe semilanceata ('magic mushrooms')	Psilocybin, psilocin	Hallucinations

Pacific and Caribbean. Human exposure occurs through eating contaminated fish, even if well cooked. Nausea, vomiting, diarrhoea and abdominal pain develop within a few hours, followed by paraesthesia, ataxia, blurred vision, ataxia and tremor. Convulsions and coma can occur, although death is uncommon. Fatigue and peripheral neuropathy can be long-term effects. There is no specific treatment. In the South Pacific and Caribbean, there are approximately 50 000 cases per year, with a case fatality of 0.1%.

Scombrotoxic fish poisoning

Under poor storage conditions, histidine in scombroid fish (e.g. tuna, mackerel, bonito, skipjack and the canned dark meat of sardines) may be converted by bacteria to histamine and other chemicals. Within minutes of consumption, flushing, burning, sweating, urticaria, pruritus, headache, colic, nausea and vomiting, diarrhoea, bronchospasm and hypotension may occur. Management is with nebulised salbutamol, intravenous antihistamines and, occasionally, intravenous fluid replacement.

Plant poisoning

A substantial number of plants and fungi are potentially toxic if consumed, with patterns of poisoning depending on their geographical distribution. Some toxic examples and the clinical features of toxicity are shown in Box 7.18.

Further information

Books and journal articles

Bateman DN, Jefferson R, Thomas SHL, et al. (eds). Oxford desk reference: toxicology. Oxford: Oxford University Press; 2014.
Benson BE, Hoppu K, Troutman WG, et al. Position paper update: gastric lavage for gastrointestinal decontamination. Clin Toxicol 2013; 51:140–146.
Chyka PA, Seger D, Krenzelok EP, et al. Position paper: single-dose activated charcoal. Clin Toxicol 2005; 43:61–87.
Thompson JP, Watson ID, Thanacoody HK, et al. Guidelines for laboratory analyses for poisoned patients in the United Kingdom. Ann Clin Biochem 2014; 51:312–325.

Websites

curriculum.toxicology.wikispaces.net/ *Free access to educational material related to poisoning.*
toxbase.org *Toxbase, the clinical toxicology database of the UK National Poisons Information Service. Free for UK health professionals but registration is required. Access for overseas users by special arrangement. Low-cost smartphone app available.*
toxnet.nlm.nih.gov *US National Library of Medicine's Toxnet: a hazardous substances databank, including Toxline for references to literature on drugs and other chemicals.*
who.int/gho/phe/chemical_safety/poisons_centres/en/ *World directory of poisons centres held by the WHO, including interactive map and contact details.*

8

J White

Envenomation

Comprehensive evaluation of the envenomed patient 152

Geographical distribution of venomous snakes 153

Bedside tests in the envenomed patient 153

Overview of envenomation 154
Venom 154
Venomous animals 154
Clinical effects 155

General approach to the envenomed patient 156
First aid 156
Assessment and management in hospital 158
Treatment 159
Follow-up 160

Envenomation by specific animals 160
Venomous snakes 160
Scorpions 161
Spiders 161
Paralysis ticks 161
Venomous insects 161
Marine venomous and poisonous animals 162

Comprehensive evaluation of the envenomed patient

1 Airway, breathing, circulation
Blood pressure
Pulse
Respiration rate
Oxygen saturation
Dysrhythmias

2 Level of consciousness
Confusion
Agitation
Seizures

3 Mouth, gums
Evidence of bleeding
Increased salivation
Drooling

4 Cranial nerves
Drooling
Dysarthria
Dysphagia
Upper airway compromise

▲ Bilateral mild ptosis

▲ Ptosis and lateral
ophthalmoplegia

▲ Fixed dilated pupils

5 Chest
Pulmonary oedema
Diminished respiration

Copyright © Julian White.

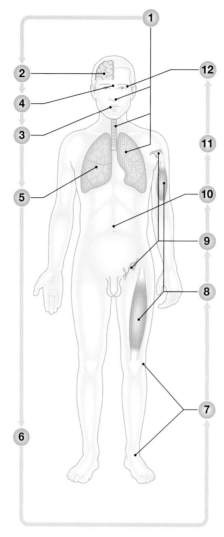

12 Eyes
Miosis or mydriasis
Increased lacrimation
Corneal injury (venom spit injury)

▲ Chemosis – can indicate
capillary leak syndrome

11 Skin
In addition to (6):
Piloerection
Erythema
Blistering
Infection

▲ Local increased sweating

10 Abdomen
Intra-abdominal, retroperitoneal
or renal pathology

9 Lymph nodes
Tender or enlarged nodes
draining bite/sting area

8 Muscles
Weakness
Tenderness
Pain

7 Reflexes
Decreased or absent reflexes

6 Bite/sting site
Pain
Swelling
Bruising
Discoloration
Necrosis

▲ Local bleeding, blistering

▲ Local bleeding

Geographical distribution of venomous snakes

Indian krait
Bungarus caeruleus

European adder
Vipera aspis

Russell's viper
Daboia russelii

Green pit viper
Trimeresurus gramineus

Puff adder
Bitis arietans

Saw-scaled viper
Echis carinatus

South American rattlesnake
Crotalus durissus

Black-necked spitting cobra
Naja nigricollis

Common Indian cobra
Naja naja

Monacled cobra
Naja kaouthia

The geographical location of a snakebite determines the likely animal(s) involved and the nature and risks of the envenomation. *Copyright © Julian White.*

Bedside tests in the envenomed patient

1 Obtain a clean **glass** container (test tube or bottle) that is either new, or has only been washed with water (not detergent/soap)

2 Place 2–3 mL venous blood in the **glass** container

3 Allow to stand undisturbed for 20 mins

4 Gently invert/tip the glass container checking for presence of a blood clot

4a Clot present = negative test (no coagulopathy present)

4b Clot absent = positive test (coagulopathy present)

Examination of urine. Haematuria may indicate a coagulopathy. Dark urine is suggestive of myoglobinuria, which is a sign of extensive rhabdomyolysis. *Copyright © Julian White.*

Twenty-minute whole-blood clotting test (20WBCT). The presence of coagulopathy is a key indicator of major envenoming for some species. While full laboratory coagulation studies may be the ideal, the 20WBCT has emerged as a simple standardised bedside test of coagulopathy, applicable even in areas with limited health facilities. *Copyright © Julian White.*

Overview of envenomation

Envenomation occurs when a venomous animal injects sufficient venom by a bite or a sting into a prey item or perceived predator to cause deleterious local and/or systemic effects. This is defined as a venom-induced disease (VID). Venomous animals generally use their venom to acquire and, in some cases, pre-digest prey, with defensive use a secondary function for many species. Accidental encounters between venomous animals and humans are frequent, particularly in the rural tropics, where millions of cases of venomous bites and stings occur annually. Globally, an increasing number of exotic venomous animals are kept privately, so cases of envenoming may present to hospitals where doctors have insufficient knowledge to manage potentially complex presentations. Doctors everywhere should thus be aware of the basic principles of management of envenomation and how to seek expert support. It is important for doctors to know what types of venomous animal are likely to occur in their geographical area (hospital hinterland; p. 153) and the types of envenoming they may cause.

Venom

Venom is a complex mixture of diverse components (notably toxins), often with several separate toxins that can cause adverse effects in humans, and each is potentially capable of multiple effects (Box 8.1). Venom is produced at considerable metabolic cost, so is used sparingly; thus only some bites/stings by venomous animals result in significant envenoming, the remainder being 'dry bites'. The concept of dry bites is important in understanding approaches to first aid and medical management.

Venomous animals

There are many animal groups that contain venomous species (Box 8.2). The epidemiological estimates reflect the importance of snakes and scorpions as causes of severe or lethal envenomation, but also the fragmentary nature of the data. For snakes, recent studies have proposed widely varying estimates of epidemiological impact, but even the higher estimates may be too low. A recent

i 8.2 Venomous animals and human envenoming

Phyla	Principal venomous animal groups	Estimated number of human cases/year	Estimated number of human deaths/year
Chordata	Snakes	>2.5 million	>100 000
	Spiny fish	? >100 000	Close to zero
	Stingrays	? >100 000	? <10
Arthropoda	Scorpions	>1 million	? <5000
	Spiders	? >100 000	? <100
	Paralysis ticks	? >1000	? <10
	Insects	? >1 million	? >1000*
Mollusca	Cone snails	? <1000	? <10
	Blue-ringed octopus	? <100	? <10
Coelenterata	Jellyfish	? >1 million	? <10

*Social insect stings cause death by anaphylaxis rather than primary venom toxicity, except for massive multiple sting attacks.
Copyright © Julian White.

i 8.1 Key venom effects*

Venom component	Clinical effects	Type of venomous animal
Neurotoxin Paralytic	Flaccid paralysis	Some snakes Paralysis ticks Cone snails Blue-ringed octopus
Excitatory	Neuroexcitation: autonomic storm, cardiotoxicity, pulmonary oedema	Some scorpions, spiders, jellyfish (irukandji)
Myotoxins	Systemic or local myolysis	Some snakes
Cardiotoxins	Direct or indirect cardiotoxicity; cardiac collapse, shock	Some snakes, scorpions, spiders and jellyfish (box jellyfish)
Haemostasis system toxins	Variation from rapid coagulopathy and bleeding to thrombosis, deep venous thrombosis and pulmonary emboli	Many snakes and a few scorpions (*Hemiscorpius*) Brazilian caterpillars (*Lonomia*)
Haemorrhagic toxins	Local vessel damage, fluid extravasation, blistering, ecchymosis, shock	Mainly some snakes
Nephrotoxins	Renal damage	Some snakes, massed bee and wasp stings
Necrotoxins	Local tissue injury/necrosis, shock	Some snakes, a few scorpions (*Hemiscorpius*), spiders (recluse spiders), jellyfish and stingrays
Allergic toxins	Induction of acute allergic response (direct and indirect)	Almost all venoms but particularly those of social insects (i.e. bees, wasps, ants)

*All venom components have lethal potential.
Copyright © Julian White.

comprehensive study in India indicated there are at least 45 000 snakebite-related deaths in that country annually, far above both government figures and previous estimates. In many areas of the poor rural tropics, health resources are limited and few envenoming cases are either seen or recorded within the official hospital system, compared to the actual community burden of disease. While fatal cases may gain most attention, long-term disability from envenomation affects significantly more people and has a major social and economic cost.

Stings by social insects such as bees and wasps may also cause lethal anaphylaxis. Other venomous animals may commonly envenom humans but cause mostly non-lethal effects. A few animals only rarely envenom humans but have a high potential for severe or lethal envenoming. These include box jellyfish, cone snails, blue-ringed octopus, paralysis ticks and Australian funnel web spiders. Within any given group, particularly snakes, there may be a wide range of clinical presentations. Some are described here but for a more detailed discussion of the types of venomous animal, their venoms and their effects on humans, see toxinology.com.

Clinical effects

With the exception of dry bites, where no significant toxin effects occur, venomous bites/stings can result in three broad classes of effect.

Local effects

These vary from trivial to severe (Box 8.3). There may be minimal or no local effects with some snakebites (not even pain), yet lethal systemic envenoming may still be present. For other species,

---

local effects predominate over systemic, and for some, such as certain snakes, both are important (p. 152). Some species commonly cause local necrosis, notably some snakes, brown recluse spiders, an Iranian scorpion (*Hemiscorpius lepturus*) and some stingrays.

General systemic effects

By definition, these are non-specific (Box 8.3). Shock is an important complication of major local envenoming by some snake species and, if inadequately treated, can prove lethal, especially in children.

Specific systemic effects

These are important in both diagnosis and treatment.

- *Neurotoxic flaccid paralysis* can develop very rapidly, progressing from mild weakness to full respiratory paralysis in less than 30 minutes (blue-ringed octopus bite, cone snail sting), or may develop far more slowly, over hours (some snakes) to days (paralysis tick). For neurotoxic snakes, the cranial nerves are usually involved first, with ptosis a common initial sign, often progressing to partial and later complete ophthalmoplegia, fixed dilated pupils, drooling and loss of upper airway protection (p. 152). From this, paralysis may extend to the limbs, with weakness and loss of deep tendon reflexes, the neck ('broken neck' sign), then finally respiratory paralysis affecting the diaphragm.
- *Excitatory neurotoxins* cause an 'autonomic storm', often with profuse sweating (p. 152), variable cardiac effects and cardiac failure, sometimes with pulmonary oedema (notably, Australian funnel web spider bite, some scorpions such as Indian red scorpion). This type of envenomation can be rapidly fatal (many scorpions, funnel web spiders), or may cause distressing symptoms but constitute a lesser risk of death (widow spiders, banana spiders).
- *Myotoxicity* can be localised in the bitten limb, or systemic, affecting mostly skeletal muscles. It can initially be silent, then present with generalised muscle pain, tenderness, myoglobinuria (p. 153) and huge rises in serum creatine kinase (CK). Secondary renal failure can precipitate potentially lethal hyperkalaemic cardiotoxicity.
- *Cardiotoxicity* is often secondary but symptoms and signs are non-specific in most cases. For some scorpions, envenomation can cause direct cardiac effects, including decreased cardiac output, arrhythmias and pulmonary oedema.
- *Haemostasis system toxins* cause a variety of effects, depending on the type of toxin (Fig. 8.1). Coagulopathy may present as bruising and bleeding from the bite site (p. 152), gums and intravenous sites. Surgical interventions are high-risk in such cases. Other venoms cause thrombosis, usually presenting as deep venous thrombosis (DVT), pulmonary embolus or stroke (particularly Caribbean/Martinique vipers).
- *Haemorrhagic toxins* cause vascular damage, especially in the bitten limb, with extravasation of fluid and sometimes hypotensive shock; this is a problem associated with some snakebites. The role of these toxins in causing late-developing capillary leak syndrome (p. 152), again

---

> **i** | **8.3 Local and systemic effects of envenomation**
>
> **Local effects**
>
> | | |
> |---|---|
> | • Pain | • Blistering |
> | • Sweating | • Necrosis |
> | • Erythema | • Swelling |
> | • Major direct tissue trauma (e.g. stingray injuries) | • Bleeding and bruising |
>
> **Non-specific systemic effects**
>
> | | |
> |---|---|
> | • Headache | • Pulmonary oedema |
> | • Nausea | • Dizziness |
> | • Vomiting and diarrhoea | • Collapse |
> | • Abdominal pain | • Convulsions |
> | • Tachycardia or bradycardia | • Shock |
> | • Hypertension or hypotension | • Cardiac arrest |
>
> **Specific systemic effects**
>
> - Neurotoxic flaccid paralysis (descending or ascending)
> - Excitatory neurotoxicity (catecholamine storm-like and similar)
> - Rhabdomyolysis (systemic or local)
> - Coagulopathy (procoagulant/fibrinolytic or anticoagulant or thrombotic or antiplatelet)
> - Cardiotoxicity (decreased/abnormal cardiac function or arrhythmia or arrest)
> - Acute kidney injury (polyuria or oliguria or anuria or isolated elevated creatinine/urea)
>
> *Copyright © Julian White.*

8

1 Haemorrhagic metalloproteinases and disintegrins
Damage blood vessel wall, cause leakage of blood, degrade platelet plug response

2 Procoagulants
Activate specific coagulation factors to activate clotting cascade and promote formation of fibrin clots. Can also activate fibrinolytic system, resulting in defibrination and reduced ability to form protective clots

3 Direct fibrinolytics
Split fibrinogen, often abnormally, resulting in poor clot formation and a bleeding tendency

4 Other haemostasis system toxins
Target various parts of haemostasis, either as activators (e.g. plasminogen activators), or as inhibitors of coagulation (e.g. serpin inactivators, platelet aggregation inhibitors)

Fig. 8.1 Sites of action of venoms on the haemostasis system. *Copyright © Julian White.*

associated with some snakebites (notably Russell's viper), is uncertain.

- *Renal damage* in envenoming is mostly secondary, although some species, such as Russell's vipers, can cause primary renal damage. The presentation is similar in both cases, with changes in urine output (polyuria, oliguria or anuria) or rises in creatinine and urea. In cases with intravascular haemolysis, secondary renal damage is likely. The clinical effects of specific animals in different regions of the world are shown in Boxes 8.4–8.6.

General approach to the envenomed patient

First aid

First aid can be crucial in determining the outcome for envenomed patients, yet throughout much of the world inappropriate and dangerous first aid is often administered.

---

i   8.4 Selected important venomous animals in Asia

Scientific name[1]	Common name	Clinical effects	Antivenom/antidote/treatment
Indian subcontinent			
Bungarus spp. (E)	Kraits	Flaccid paralysis[2,3], myolysis[4], hyponatraemia[5]	Indian PV or specific
Naja spp. (E)	Cobras	Flaccid paralysis[3], local necrosis/blistering, shock	Indian PV or specific
Ophiophagus hannah (E)	King cobra	Flaccid paralysis[3], local necrosis, shock	Indian PV or specific
Echis spp. (Vv)	Saw-scaled vipers	Procoagulant coagulopathy, local necrosis/blistering, renal failure	Indian PV or specific
Daboia russelii (Vv)	Russell's viper	Procoagulant coagulopathy, local necrosis/blistering, myolysis, renal failure, shock, flaccid paralysis[2]	Indian PV or specific
Hypnale spp. (Vc)	Hump-nosed vipers	Procoagulant coagulopathy, shock, renal failure	Try Indian PV
Trimeresurus[6] spp. (Vc)	Green pit vipers	Procoagulant coagulopathy, local necrosis, shock	Indian PV or specific
Hottentotta spp. (Sc)	Indian scorpions	Neuroexcitation, cardiotoxicity	Indian specific AV Prazosin
East Asia			
Bungarus spp. (E)	Kraits	Flaccid paralysis[2,3]	Specific AV from country
Naja spp. (E)	Cobras (some spitters)	Flaccid paralysis[3], local necrosis/blistering, shock	Specific AV from country
Ophiophagus hannah (E)	King cobra	Flaccid paralysis[3], local necrosis, shock	King cobra AV
Calloselasma rhodostoma (Vc)	Malayan pit viper	Procoagulant coagulopathy, local necrosis/blistering, renal failure, shock	Specific AV from country
Daboia siamensis (Vv)	Russell's viper	Procoagulant coagulopathy, local necrosis/blistering, renal failure, shock	Specific AV from country
Gloydius spp. (Vc)	Mamushis, pit vipers	Procoagulant coagulopathy, local necrosis/blistering, shock, renal failure, flaccid paralysis[2]	Specific AV from country
Trimeresurus[6] spp. (Vc)	Green pit vipers, habus	Procoagulant coagulopathy, local necrosis/blistering, shock	Specific AV from country

[1]Family names: C = 'Colubridae' (mostly 'non-venomous'; family subject to major taxonomic revisions); E = Elapidae (all venomous); Sc = Scorpionoidea; Vc = Viperidae Crotalinae (New World and Asian vipers); Vv = Viperidae viperinae (Old World vipers). [2]Pre-synaptic. [3]Post-synaptic. [4]Only reported so far for *B. candidus, B. niger* and *B. caeruleus.* [5]Only reported so far for *B. multicinctus* and *B. candidus.* [6]Genus is subject to major taxonomic change (split into at least eight genera). (AV = antivenom; PV = polyvalent)
More information is available from WHO-SEARO *Guidelines for the management of snake-bites* and from toxinology.com.
Copyright © Julian White.

ℹ	8.5 Selected important venomous animals in the Americas and Australia

Scientific name[1]	Common name	Clinical effects	Antivenom/antidote/treatment
North America			
Crotalus spp. (Vc)	Rattlesnakes	Procoagulant coagulopathy, local necrosis/blistering (flaccid paralysis[2] rare), shock	CroFab AV or Bioclon Antivipmyn AV
Sistrurus spp. (Vc)	Massasaugas	Procoagulant coagulopathy, local necrosis/blistering, shock	CroFab AV or Bioclon Antivipmyn AV
Agkistrodon spp. (Vc)	Copperheads and moccasins	Procoagulant coagulopathy, local necrosis/blistering, shock	CroFab AV or Bioclon Antivipmyn AV
Micrurus spp. (E)	Coral snakes	Flaccid paralysis[3]	Bioclon Coralmyn AV
Latrodectus mactans	Widow spider	Neuroexcitation	MSD Widow spider AV
Centruroides sculpturatus	Arizona bark scorpion	Neuroexcitation	Bioclon Anascorp AV
Central and South America			
Crotalus spp. (Vc)	Rattlesnakes	Flaccid paralysis[2], myolysis, procoagulant coagulopathy, shock, renal failure	Specific AV from country
Bothrops spp. (Vc)	Lancehead vipers	Procoagulant coagulopathy, local necrosis/blistering, shock, renal failure	Specific AV from country
Bothriechis spp. (Vc)	Eyelash pit vipers	Shock, pain and swelling	Specific AV from country
Lachesis spp. (Vc)	Bushmasters	Procoagulant coagulopathy, shock, renal failure, local necrosis/blistering	Specific AV from country
Micrurus spp. (E)	Coral snakes	Flaccid paralysis[2,3], myolysis, renal failure	Specific AV from country
Tityus serrulatus	Brazilian scorpion	Neuroexcitation, shock	Instituto Butantan scorpion AV
Loxosceles spp.	Recluse spiders	Local necrosis	Instituto Butantan spider AV
Phoneutria nigriventer	Banana spider	Neuroexcitation, shock	Instituto Butantan spider AV
Potamotrygon, Dasyatis spp.	Freshwater stingrays	Necrosis of bite area, shock, severe pain and oedema	No available AV; good wound care
Australia			
Pseudonaja spp. (E)	Brown snakes	Procoagulant coagulopathy, renal failure, flaccid paralysis[2] (rare)	CSL brown snake AV or PVAV
Notechis spp. (E)	Tiger snakes	Procoagulant coagulopathy, myolysis, flaccid paralysis[2,3], renal failure	CSL tiger snake AV or PVAV
Oxyuranus spp. (E)	Taipans	Procoagulant coagulopathy, flaccid paralysis[2,3], myolysis, renal failure	CSL taipan or PVAV
Acanthophis spp. (E)	Death adders	Flaccid paralysis[3]	CSL death adder or PVAV
Pseudechis spp.	Black and mulga snakes	Anticoagulant coagulopathy, myolysis, renal failure	CSL black snake AV or PVAV
Enhydrina schistosa	Sea snakes (all species globally)	Flaccid paralysis and/or myolysis	CSL sea snake AV
Atrax, Hadronyche spp.	Funnel web spiders	Neuroexcitation, shock	CSL funnel web spider AV
Latrodectus hasseltii	Red back spider	Neuroexcitation, pain and sweating	CSL red back spider AV
Chironex fleckeri	Box jellyfish	Neuroexcitation, cardiotoxicity, local necrosis	CSL box jellyfish AV
Synanceia spp.	Stonefish	Severe local pain	CSL stonefish AV

[1]For family name, see Box 8.4. [2]Pre-synaptic. [3]Post-synaptic.
(PVAV = polyvalent antivenom)
Copyright © Julian White.

A significant proportion of venom is transported from the bite/sting site via the lymphatic system, particularly for venoms with larger molecular weight toxins, such as many snake venoms. It is recommended that for most forms of envenoming, the patient should be kept still, the bitten limb immobilised with a splint and vital systems supported, where required. A patent upper airway should be specifically ensured and respiratory support provided, if required. For some animals, notably snakes in certain regions, the use of a local pressure pad bandage over the bite site (Myanmar) or a pressure immobilisation bandage (Australia, New Guinea) is recommended.

Ineffective or dangerous first aid, such as suction devices, 'cut and suck', local chemicals, snake stones (stones of some sort placed over the snakebite) and tourniquets, should not be used. Tourniquets, in particular, have the potential to cause catastrophic distal limb injuries in snakebite when applied too narrowly or too tightly, or left on too long.

Transporting patients

Where possible, transport should be brought to the patient. It is also vital to obtain medical assessment and intervention at the earliest opportunity, however, so any delay in transporting the patient to a medical facility should be avoided. Severely envenomed patients may develop life-threatening problems, such as shock or respiratory failure, during transport, so ideally the transport method used should allow for management of these problems en route.

In resource-poor environments, simple solutions for rapid transport have been successfully employed, such as motorbikes or similar with the patient supported between the driver in front and another person behind the patient. However, this method cannot cope with a patient developing airway compromise or respiratory failure, such as from developing neurotoxicity.

i 8.6 Selected important venomous animals in Africa and Europe

Scientific name[1]	Common name	Clinical effects	Antivenom/antidote/treatment
Africa			
Naja spp. (E)	Cobras		
	Non-spitters	Flaccid paralysis[3] ± local necrosis/blistering	South African PV or Sanofi Pasteur FavAfrica AV
	Spitters	Local necrosis/blistering (flaccid paralysis[3] uncommon)	South African PV or Sanofi Pasteur FavAfrica AV
Dendroaspis spp. (E)	Mambas	Mamba neurotoxic flaccid paralysis and muscle fasciculation, shock, necrosis (uncommon)	South African PV or Sanofi Pasteur FavAfrica AV
Hemachatus haemachatus (E)	Rinkhals	Flaccid paralysis[3], local necrosis, shock	South African PV
Atheris spp. (Vv)	Bush vipers	Procoagulant coagulopathy, shock, pain and swelling	No available AV (can try South African AV)
Bitis spp. (Vv)	Puff adders etc.	Procoagulant coagulopathy, shock, cardiotoxicity, local necrosis/blistering	South African PV or Sanofi Pasteur FavAfrica AV
Causus spp. (Vv)	Night adders	Pain and swelling	No available AV
Echis spp. (Vv)	Carpet vipers	Procoagulant coagulopathy, shock, renal failure, local necrosis/blistering	Specific anti-*Echis* AV for species/geographical region or Sanofi Pasteur FavAfrica AV
Cerastes spp. (Vv)	Horned desert vipers	Procoagulant coagulopathy, local necrosis, shock	Specific or polyspecific AV covering *Cerastes* from country of origin
Dispholidus typus (C)	Boomslang	Procoagulant coagulopathy, shock	Boomslang AV
Androctonus spp.	North African scorpions	Neuroexcitation	Specific scorpion AV (Algeria, Tunisia, Sanofi Pasteur Scorpifav)
Lelurus quinquestriatus	Yellow scorpion	Neuroexcitation, shock	Specific scorpion AV (Algeria, Tunisia, Sanofi Pasteur Scorpifav)
Europe			
Vipera spp. (Vv)	Vipers and adders	Shock, local necrosis/blistering, procoagulant coagulopathy (flaccid paralysis[2] rare)	ViperaTab AV or Zagreb AV or SanofiPasteur Viperfav AV

[1]For family name, see Box 8.4. [2]Pre-synaptic. [3]Post-synaptic.
More information is available from WHO *Guidelines for the prevention and clinical management of snakebite in Africa* and from toxinology.com.
Copyright © Julian White.

Assessment and management in hospital

On arrival at a health station or hospital, there are two immediate priorities:

- identifying and treating any life-threatening problems (e.g. circulatory shock, respiratory failure; see Ch. 16)
- determining whether envenoming is present and if that requires urgent treatment.

Assessment and management of life-threatening problems

Patients who are seriously envenomed must be identified early so that appropriate management is not delayed. Critically ill patients must be resuscitated (p. 202) and this takes precedence over administration of any antivenom. Clinicians should look for signs of:

- shock/hypotension
- airway and/or respiratory compromise (likely to be secondary to flaccid paralysis)
- major bleeding, including internal bleeding (especially intracranial)
- impending limb compromise from inappropriate first aid (e.g. a tourniquet) – though beware sudden envenoming on removal of a tourniquet.

In a patient with severe neurotoxic flaccid paralysis, who is still able to maintain sufficient respiratory function for survival, clinical assessment may suggest irretrievable brain injury (fixed dilated pupils, absent reflexes, no withdrawal response to painful stimuli, no movement of limbs, fixed forward gaze with gross ptosis; p. 152) when, in fact, the patient is conscious.

Assessment for evidence of envenoming

As in other areas of medicine, comprehensive assessment of a patient bitten/stung by a venomous animal requires a good history, a careful targeted examination and, where appropriate, 'laboratory' testing (though the latter may just consist of simple bedside tests performed by the doctor; p. 153). Animals that are unlikely to cause serious envenomation in humans should be identified so that inappropriate admission and intervention are avoided. Occasionally, patients may be unaware they have been bitten/stung and thus provide a misleading history. In regions of the world where keeping or handling venomous animals is illegal, patients may be reticent in giving a truthful history. Multiple bites or stings are more likely to cause major envenoming.

The following key questions should be asked:

- When was the patient exposed to the venomous bite/sting?
- Was the organism causing it seen and what did it look like (size, colour)?
- What were the circumstances (on land, in water etc.)?
- Was there more than one bite/sting?
- What first aid was used, when and for how long?
- What symptoms has the patient had (local and systemic)?
- Are there symptoms suggesting systemic envenoming (paralysis, rhabdomyolysis, coagulopathy etc.)?

- Is there any significant past medical history and medication use?
- Is there a past exposure to antivenom/venom and allergies?

If patients state that they have been bitten by a particular species, ensure this information is accurate. Private keepers of venomous animals may not have accurate knowledge of what they are keeping, and misidentification of a snake, scorpion or spider can have dire consequences if the wrong antivenom is used.

An outline of some principal findings on examination of the envenomed patient is shown on page 152. The patient may have a cluster of clinical features suggestive of a particular type of envenoming (see Box 8.1).

Even with dangerously venomous animals, some bites/stings will be dry bites and will not require antivenom. The time to onset of first symptoms and signs of envenomation is variable, depending on both animal and patient factors. It may range from a matter of minutes post-bite/sting to 24 hours later in some cases. Therefore, the initial assessment, if normal, must be repeated multiple times during the first 24 hours. Some types of envenomation will not cause symptoms or signs at all, or they may appear very late, long after the optimum time for treatment has passed. Evidence of envenomation may become apparent only through laboratory testing.

Laboratory investigations

Specific tests for venom are currently commercially available only for Australian snakebites but are likely to be developed for snakebites in other regions. They are not available for other types of envenomation, where venom concentrations are low. For snakebite, a screen for envenoming includes full blood count, coagulation screen, urea and electrolytes, creatinine, CK and electrocardiogram (ECG). Lung function tests, peripheral oximetry or arterial blood gases may be indicated in cases with potential or established respiratory failure. In areas without access to routine laboratory tests, the 20-minute whole-blood clotting test (20WBCT) is useful (p. 153).

Treatment

Once a diagnosis of likely envenoming has been made, the next and urgent decision is whether to give antivenom. Antivenom may not be the only crucial treatment, however. For a snakebite by a potentially lethal species such as Russell's viper, the patient might have local effects with oedema, blistering, necrosis, and resultant fluid shifts causing shock, and at the same time have systemic effects such as intractable vomiting, coagulopathy, paralysis and secondary renal failure. Specific treatment with antivenom will be required to reverse the coagulopathy and may prevent worsening of the paralysis and reduce the vomiting, but will not greatly affect the local tissue damage or the renal failure or shock. The latter will require intravenous fluid therapy, possibly respiratory support, renal dialysis and local wound care, perhaps including antibiotics.

Each venomous animal will cause a particular pattern of envenomation, requiring a tailored response. Listing all of these is beyond the scope of this chapter (see 'Further information' below).

Antivenom

Antivenom, sometimes inappropriately labelled as 'anti-snake venom' (ASV), is the most important tool in treating

i	**8.7 Indications for antivenom**

General indications

- Shock/cardiac collapse
- Respiratory compromise
- Rapidly increasing swelling of the bitten limb
- Active bleeding
- Intractable non-specific symptoms, including recurrent vomiting

Specific indications

- Developing paralytic features (ptosis etc.)
- Developing rhabdomyolysis
- Developing coagulopathy
- Developing renal failure
- Developing neuroexcitatory envenoming

Copyright © Julian White.

8

envenoming. It is made by hyperimmunising an animal, usually horses, to produce antibodies against venom. Once refined, these bind to venom toxins and render them inactive or allow their rapid clearance. Antivenom is available only for certain venomous animals and cannot reverse all types of envenoming. With a few exceptions, it should be given intravenously, with adrenaline (epinephrine) ready in case of anaphylaxis. It should be used only when clearly indicated, and indications will vary between venomous animals (Box 8.7). It is critical that the correct antivenom is used at the appropriate dose. Doses vary widely between antivenoms. In some situations (such as the Indian subcontinent), pre-treatment with subcutaneous adrenaline may reduce the chance of anaphylaxis to antivenom.

Antivenom can sometimes reverse post-synaptic neurotoxic paralysis (α-bungarotoxin-like neurotoxins) but will not usually reverse established pre-synaptic paralysis (β-bungarotoxin-like neurotoxins), so should be given before major paralysis has occurred (Fig. 8.2). Coagulopathy is best reversed by antivenom, but even after all venom is neutralised, there may be a delay of hours before normal coagulation is restored. More antivenom should not be given because coagulopathy has failed to normalise fully in the first 1–3 hours (except in very particular circumstances). Thrombocytopenia may persist for days, despite antivenom. The role of antivenom in reversing established rhabdomyolysis and renal failure is uncertain. Antivenom may help limit local tissue effects or injury in the bitten limb but this is quite variable and time-dependent. Neuroexcitatory envenoming can respond very well to antivenom (Australian funnel web spider bites and Mexican, South American and Indian scorpion stings) but there is controversy about the effectiveness of antivenom for some species (some North African and Middle Eastern scorpions). The role of antivenom in limiting local venom effects, including necrosis, is also controversial; it is most likely to be effective when given early.

All patients receiving antivenom are at risk of both early and late adverse reactions, including anaphylaxis (early; not always related to immunoglobulin E (IgE)) and serum sickness (late).

Non-antivenom treatments

Anticholinesterases are used as an adjunctive treatment for post-synaptic paralysis.

Prazosin (an α-adrenoceptor antagonist) is used in the management of hypertension or pulmonary oedema in scorpion sting cardiotoxicity, particularly for Indian red scorpion stings, though antivenom is now the preferred treatment.

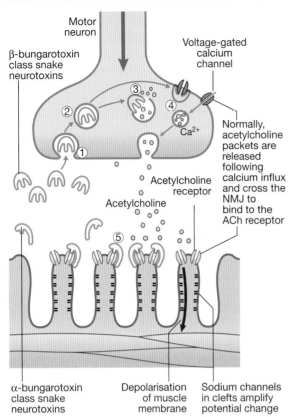

Fig. 8.2 Principal snake venom neurotoxins acting at the neuromuscular junction (NMJ). The pre-synaptic neurotoxins (β-bungarotoxin-like) bind to the cell membrane of the terminal axon (1), form a synaptosome (2) and enter the cell, where they disrupt acetylcholine (ACh) production (3) and damage intracellular structures, including ion channels (4). On initial entry, they cause release of excess ACh, followed by cessation of all ACh release, causing irreversible paralysis until the cell is repaired (days to weeks later). The post-synaptic neurotoxins (α-bungarotoxin-like) bind adjacent to the ACh receptor on the external surface of the muscle end plate and block ACh binding (5), thereby ceasing neurotransmission. Because this action is external to the cell and does not cause cell damage, it is potentially a reversible paralysis. *Copyright © Julian White.*

Antibiotics are not routinely required for most bites/stings, though a few animals, such as some South American pit vipers and stingrays, regularly cause significant wound infection or abscess. Tetanus is a risk in some types of bite or sting, such as snakebite, but intramuscular toxoid should not be given until any coagulopathy is reversed.

Mechanical ventilation (p. 202) is vital for established respiratory paralysis that will not reverse with antivenom and may be required for prolonged periods (up to several months in some cases).

Fasciotomy as a treatment for potential compartment syndrome or severe limb swelling is an overused and often disastrous surgical intervention in snakebite and is associated with poor functional outcomes. It should be reserved as a treatment of last resort and be used only in cases where compartment syndrome is confirmed by intracompartment pressure measurement and after first trying limb elevation and antivenom, and ensuring that any coagulopathy has resolved.

Follow-up

Cases with significant envenomation and those receiving antivenom should be followed up to ensure any complications have resolved and to identify any delayed envenoming.

Envenomation by specific animals

Venomous snakes

Venomous snakes represent the single most important cause of envenomation globally, affecting millions of humans annually and resulting in large numbers of deaths and patients left with long-term disability. Of the 3000-plus snake species, more than 1000 either are venomous or produce oral toxins. The most important venomous snake families are the Viperidae (vipers; includes typical vipers (subfamily Viperinae) and pit-vipers, with heat-sensing pit organs (subfamily Crotalinae)) and the Elapidae (cobras, kraits, mambas, coral snakes, sea snakes, Australian snakes). However, there are also dangerous species among the Atractaspididae (side-fanged burrowing vipers of Africa and the Middle East) and the non-front-fanged colubrids (NFFC snakes; several families, including the 'back-fanged' boomslang and vine snakes of Africa and the keelbacks of Asia).

A selection of important species is included in Boxes 8.4–8.6.

Clinical features and management

As with other forms of envenoming, the management of snakebite follows the standard assessment guidelines described previously (p. 152). The nature of the risks posed will depend on the specific snake fauna in a given region (p. 153). For example, in the Indian subcontinent, the major snakebite risks are claimed to come from the 'big four': cobras, kraits, Russell's viper and saw-scaled vipers. This list is misleading, though, as it omits other important snakes, including the hump-nosed vipers, king cobra and green pit vipers, all of which can cause severe or lethal envenoming and may not be covered by current Indian antivenoms. Even for those snakes recognised as causing envenoming, there may be major geographical variation in venom and features of envenoming. For Russell's viper (*Daboia* spp.), Sri Lankan specimens can cause rhabdomyolysis and flaccid paralysis, in addition to classic severe coagulopathy, haemorrhage, local bite site injury and acute kidney injury (AKI). Indian populations of the same snake are not associated with either rhabdomyolysis or paralysis, but in parts of Southern India may cause anterior pituitary haemorrhage and/or capillary leak syndrome (hypotensive shock plus vascular leakage resulting in pulmonary oedema). Capillary leak syndrome is also encountered with populations of Burmese Russell's viper (Myanmar), where AKI is especially common and severe.

Antivenom raised against venom from one population of these snakes is often poorly effective against bites from snakes from other regions. Similarly, each of the several species of saw-scaled vipers (*Echis* spp.) spread from West Africa across the Middle East to the Indian subcontinent, including Sri Lanka, has specific venoms that may not be neutralised by antivenoms raised against other species in the genus; Indian antivenoms are ineffective against African species. It follows that, in managing snakebite envenomation, it is critically important to choose the appropriate antivenom and to understand that this may not include every antivenom claiming to cover a given species.

It is unwise to assume that everything is known about envenoming by snakes because new clinical information and syndromes are emerging as more detailed studies are carried out. For instance, krait bites (*Bungarus* spp.), long associated with 'painless' bites, later development of devastating flaccid paralysis and a high mortality rate, are now known to have some venom diversity. At least some species can cause rhabdomyolysis and/or severe hyponatraemia, and while bites may be painless, systemic envenomation can cause severe abdominal pain in at least some patients. Among cobra bites, the previous division into 'non-spitting', neurotoxic species and 'spitting', less neurotoxic species that cause local necrosis is less clear. Non-spitters are now known to spit in parts of their range (e.g. *Naja kaouthia* in West Bengal) and may cause local necrosis in addition to paralysis. Previously clear diagnostic indicators for envenomation by particular types of snakes, such as Russell's vipers and saw-scaled vipers causing coagulopathy, have also become less sure, as it is now known that other snakes, such as hump-nosed vipers (*Hypnale* spp.) and green pit vipers (*Trimeresurus* spp.), found in similar regions, can also cause marked coagulopathy and yet are often not covered by available antivenoms. The ability to cause life-threatening coagulopathy, associated with snakes previously considered harmless, such as the keelbacks in Asia (*Rhabdophis* spp.), can further complicate the diagnostic and management process, as antivenom against these snakes is currently available only in Japan.

Scorpions

Scorpions are second only to snakes in their venomous impact on humankind. Most medically important scorpions are in the family Buthidae and have complex neuroexcitatory venoms with highly specific ion-channel toxins. Classically, stings by these scorpions (some key genera listed in Boxes 8.4–8.6) cause moderate to severe local pain and rapid-onset systemic envenoming with development of a catecholamine storm-like syndrome as the toxins target the nervous system. There may be tachycardia or bradycardia, hyper- or hypotension, profuse sweating, salivation, cardiac dysfunction and pulmonary oedema. Cardiac collapse can occur, especially in children. Other clinical features may vary, depending on the scorpion species.

The Iranian scorpion, *Hemiscorpius lepturus* (principally southwest Iran), causes a quite different presentation, with an initial minor sting, followed by progressive development of bite site or limb necrosis and a potentially lethal systemic envenoming, characterised by intravascular haemolysis, disseminated intravascular coagulation (DIC), secondary renal failure and shock.

Clinical features and management

The approach to management varies with species and region. In Latin America, specific antivenoms are routinely used and associated with improved outcomes and dramatic falls in mortality rate. In India, the past reliance on prazosin has been replaced with use of specific antivenom, again with improved outcomes. In contrast, in parts of North Africa, past reliance on antivenom has been replaced with use of cardiac support and arguably poorer outcomes.

In Iran, *H. lepturus* stings are treated with antivenom, though as presentation is often delayed because the sting initially appears to be minor, the role of late antivenom is unclear.

Spiders

There are vast numbers and great species diversity of spiders, with two broad taxonomic groupings: the more 'primitive' Mygalomorphs (several medically important species, especially Australian funnel web spiders (*Atrax*, *Hadronyche* and *Illawarra*)) and the far more diverse Araneomorphs (main clinically important species in the genera *Latrodectus* (widow spiders), *Loxosceles* (brown recluse spiders) and *Phoneutria* (banana or wandering spiders)).

Clinical features and management

While spiders and spider bites are common, only those genera noted above commonly cause medically significant effects. In most cases this is a neuroexcitatory envenoming, sometimes similar to severe scorpion envenoming (notable from Australian funnel web spiders), but the recluse spiders cause an often painless bite that develops into local skin necrosis and sometimes a systemic illness similar to that caused by the Iranian scorpion, *H. lepturus*, and with similar lethal potential.

For most of these spiders, antivenom remains the key treatment and is life-saving in some cases. Recent studies suggesting that anti-*Latrodectus* antivenom is ineffective have not been confirmed by independent studies and are in contrast to decades of positive clinical experience.

Paralysis ticks

Most ticks are vectors for disease but a few species in Australia, North America and parts of Africa can cause flaccid paralysis. Toxins in the saliva act as potent pre-synaptic neurotoxins that can cause gradual-onset ascending flaccid paralysis.

There are no antivenoms for tick paralysis. Treatment is based on removal of all ticks and supportive care, including intubation/ventilation where required. The paralysis usually resolves by about 48 hours following removal of all ticks.

Venomous insects

A number of insects are venomous but very few cause significant envenoming in humans.

Venomous lepidopterans

The *Lonomia* caterpillars of South America, especially Brazil, have numerous protective venomous spines that, on contact with the skin, can discharge a potent procoagulant venom that can cause a progressive and sometimes fatal consumptive coagulopathy, with terminal haemorrhagic and/or organ failure events. Treatment includes use of a Brazilian specific antivenom and supportive care.

Venomous hymenopterans

Many bees, wasps, hornets and some ants have modified ovipositors in the abdomen that act as stings, attached to venom glands. The quantity of venom injected in a single sting is insufficient to cause significant envenomation, but as many of these venoms are potently allergenic, it can cause severe and sometimes fatal anaphylaxis in sensitised persons (p. 75). Massed stings by hundreds of these insects in a swarm, however, can cause life-threatening systemic envenoming, often with intravascular haemolysis, DIC, shock and multi-organ failure. 'Africanised' bees are a particular risk for such attacks in South

America and now in parts of North America. The giant wasps and hornets of Asia can similarly cause systemic envenoming with multiple attacks. Invasive ants, such as *Solenopsis* spp., are colonising new regions and can cause both allergic reactions and unpleasant local reactions.

Marine venomous and poisonous animals

The marine environment is dominated by animal life, and many species utilise toxins, either self-produced or taken up from the environment, to arm themselves for either defence or predation. Many of these animals can cause adverse effects in humans, either as a direct venom effect on bites/stings (venomous spiny fish, sea snakes, stingrays, jellyfish, sea urchins, some starfish, cone snails, selected octopuses etc.), or through poisoning if eaten (fugu, ciguatera, scombroid, several types of shellfish poisoning; p. 149).

For venomous marine animals, there is antivenom available only for sea snakes, which can cause rhabdomyolysis and/paralytic neurotoxicity; box jellyfish, which can cause very rapid cardiac collapse; and stonefish, which cause intense sting-site pain. In general, marine venoms respond to heat; thus a hot water immersion or shower (about 45°C) is effective at reducing local pain, particularly for jellyfish, stinging fish and stingray stings. For stingray stings, the venom may cause local tissue damage both through sting trauma and a venom effect; wounds penetrating the abdomen or chest are potentially lethal and wounds should be adequately explored, cleaned and allowed to heal by secondary intention. For bites by the blue-ringed octopus and stings by cone snails, rapid-acting venom can cause early cardiovascular collapse and flaccid paralysis. Supportive care is crucial in ensuring survival from these potentially lethal and seemingly trivial local wounds. Sea urchin and venomous starfish wounds can result in multiple penetrating spines, which cause pain and act as a nidus for secondary infection, but surgical removal of spines can be difficult and unrewarding.

Further information

Books and journal articles

Meier J, White J. Handbook of clinical toxicology of animal venoms and poisons. Boca Raton: CRC Press; 1995.

World Health Organisation, Regional Office for Africa. Guidelines for the prevention and clinical management of snakebite in Africa; 2010 (afro.who.int).

World Health Organisation, Regional Office for South-East Asia. Guidelines for the management of snake-bites; 2010 (searo .who.int).

Websites

toxinology.com *Clinical toxinology guide from the University of Adelaide.*

M Byers

9

Environmental medicine

Radiation exposure 164

Extremes of temperature 165

High altitude 168

Under water 169

Humanitarian crisis 171

Environmental medicine deals with the interactions between the environment and human health. While previously concerned mainly with controlling infectious diseases, the focus at present is predominantly on the multiple physical, chemical, biological and social factors that pose risks to human health. As the environment continually alters, whether through population growth, economic development or climate change, it plays an important role in disease causation – one that may increase over time. This chapter deals principally with acute effects of environmental hazards on individuals and should be read in conjunction with the chapters on Poisoning (Ch. 7) and Acute Medicine and Critical Illness (Ch. 10). Chapter 5 deals with more general effects of environmental factors on population health.

Radiation exposure

Radiation includes ionising (Fig. 9.1) and non-ionising radiations (ultraviolet (UV), visible light, laser, infrared and microwave). While global industrialisation and the generation of fluorocarbons have raised concerns about loss of the ozone layer, leading to an increased exposure to UV rays, and disasters such as the Chernobyl and Fukushima nuclear power station explosions have demonstrated the harm of ionising radiation, it is important to remember that it can be harnessed for medical benefit. Ionising radiation is used in X-rays, computed tomography (CT), radionuclide scans and radiotherapy, and non-ionising UV for therapy in skin diseases and laser therapy for diabetic retinopathy.

Types of ionising radiation

These include charged subatomic alpha and beta particles, uncharged neutrons or high-energy electromagnetic radiations such as X-rays and gamma rays. When they interact with atoms, energy is released and the resulting ionisation can lead to molecular damage. The clinical effects of different forms of radiation depend on their range in air and tissue penetration (Fig. 9.1).

Dosage and exposure

The dose of radiation is based on the energy absorbed by a unit mass of tissue and is measured in grays (Gy), with 1 Gy representing 1 J/kg. To take account of different types of radiation and variations in the sensitivity of various tissues, weighting factors are used to produce a unit of effective dose, measured in sieverts (Sv). This value reflects the absorbed dose weighted for the damaging effects of a particular form of radiation and is most valuable in evaluating the long-term effects of exposure.

'Background radiation' refers to our exposure to naturally occurring radioactivity (e.g. radon gas and cosmic radiation). This produces an average annual individual dose of approximately 2.6 mSv per year, although this figure varies according to local geology.

Effects of radiation exposure

Effects on the individual are classified as either deterministic or stochastic.

Deterministic effects

Deterministic (threshold) effects occur with increasing severity as the dose of radiation rises above a threshold level. Tissues with actively dividing cells, such as bone marrow and gastrointestinal mucosa, are particularly sensitive to ionising radiation. Lymphocyte depletion is the most sensitive marker of bone marrow injury, and after exposure to a fatal dose, marrow aplasia is a common cause of death. However, gastrointestinal mucosal toxicity may cause earlier death due to profound diarrhoea, vomiting, dehydration and sepsis. The gonads are highly radiosensitive and radiation may result in temporary or permanent sterility. Eye exposure can lead to cataracts and the skin is susceptible to radiation burns. Irradiation of the lung may induce acute inflammatory reactions or pulmonary fibrosis, and irradiation of the central nervous system may cause permanent neurological deficit. Bone necrosis and lymphatic fibrosis are characteristic following regional irradiation, particularly for breast cancer. The thyroid gland is not inherently sensitive but its ability to concentrate iodine makes it susceptible to damage after exposure to relatively low doses of radioactive iodine isotopes, such as those released from Chernobyl.

Stochastic effects

Stochastic (chance) effects occur with increasing probability as the dose of radiation increases. Carcinogenesis represents a stochastic effect. With acute exposures, leukaemias may arise after an interval of around 2–5 years and solid tumours after an

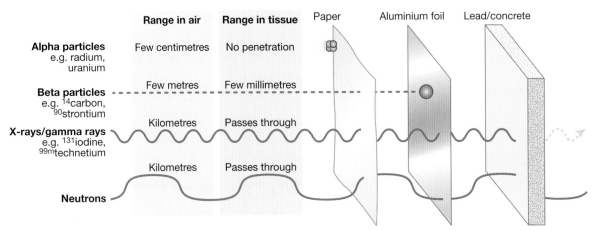

Fig. 9.1 Properties of different ionising radiations.

interval of about 10–20 years. Thereafter the incidence rises with time. An individual's risk of developing cancer depends on the dose received, the time to accumulate the total dose and the interval following exposure.

Management of radiation exposure

Exposed people should be removed from ongoing exposure ('get inside, stay inside'), and should take off affected clothing and shower to stop further contamination. If contamination of food and water supplies may have occurred, only bottled water and food in sealed containers should be consumed. The principal problems after large-dose exposures are maintenance of adequate hydration, control of sepsis and management of marrow aplasia. Associated injuries such as thermal burns need specialist management within 48 hours of active resuscitation. Internal exposure to radioisotopes should be treated with chelating agents (such as Prussian blue used to chelate [137]caesium after ingestion). White-cell colony stimulation and haematopoietic stem cell transplantation may need to be considered for marrow aplasia.

Extremes of temperature

Thermoregulation

Body heat is generated by basal metabolic activity and muscle movement, and lost by conduction (which is more effective in water than in air), convection, evaporation and radiation (most important at lower temperatures when other mechanisms conserve heat) (Box 9.1). Body temperature is controlled in the hypothalamus, which is directly sensitive to changes in core temperature and indirectly responds to temperature-sensitive neurons in the skin. The normal 'set-point' of core temperature is tightly regulated within the range 37±0.5°C, which is necessary to preserve the normal function of many enzymes and other metabolic processes. The temperature set-point is increased in response to infection (p. 218).

i	9.1 Thermoregulation: responses to hot and cold environments		
	Mechanism	**Hot environment**	**Cold environment**
Heat production	Basal metabolic rate	→	↓ in hypothermia
	Muscle activity	↓ by lethargy	↑ by shivering ↓ in severe hypothermia
Heat loss	Conduction*	↑ by vasodilatation	↓ by vasoconstriction ↑↑ in water <31°C
	Convection*	↑ by vasodilatation ↓ by lethargy	↓ by vasoconstriction ↑ by wind and movement
	Evaporation*	↑↑ by sweating ↓ by high humidity	↑ by hyperventilation
	Radiation	↑ by vasodilatation	↓ by vasoconstriction (but is the major heat loss in dry cold)

*These losses are dependent on the relative ambient and skin temperatures.

In a cold environment, protective mechanisms include cutaneous vasoconstriction and shivering; however, any muscle activity that involves movement may promote heat loss by increasing convective loss from the skin, and respiratory heat loss by stimulating ventilation. In a hot environment, sweating is the main mechanism for increasing heat loss. This usually occurs when the ambient temperature rises above 32.5°C or during exercise.

Hypothermia

Hypothermia exists when the body's normal thermal regulatory mechanisms are unable to maintain heat in a cold environment and core temperature falls below 35°C (Fig. 9.2). Moderate hypothermia occurs below 32°C and severe hypothermia below 28°C. Other systems define hypothermia on the basis of symptoms rather than absolute temperature.

While infants are susceptible to hypothermia because of their poor thermoregulation and high body surface area to weight ratio, it is the elderly who are at highest risk (Box 9.2). Hypothyroidism is often a contributory factor in old age, while

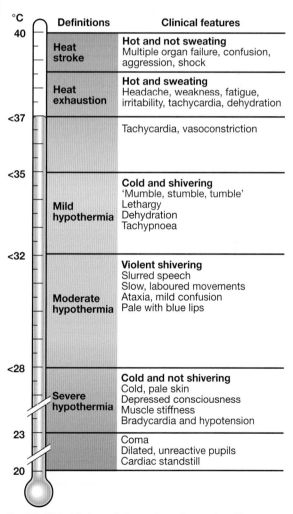

Fig. 9.2 Clinical features of abnormal core temperature. The hypothalamus normally maintains core temperature at 37°C, but this set-point is altered in, for example, fever (pyrexia, p. 218), and may be lost in hypothalamic disease (p. 679). In these circumstances, the clinical picture at a given core temperature may be different.

9.2 Thermoregulation in old age

- **Age-associated changes**: impairments in vasomotor function, skeletal muscle response and sweating mean that older people react more slowly to changes in temperature.
- **Increased comorbidity**: thermoregulatory problems are more likely in the presence of pathology such as atherosclerosis and hypothyroidism, and medication such as sedatives and hypnotics.
- **Hypothermia**: this may arise as a primary event, but more commonly complicates other acute illness, e.g. pneumonia, stroke or fracture.
- **Ambient temperature**: financial pressures and older equipment may result in inadequate heating during cold weather.

Fig. 9.3 Electrocardiogram showing J waves (arrows) in a hypothermic patient.

alcohol and other drugs (e.g. phenothiazines) commonly impede the thermoregulatory response in younger people. More rarely, hypothermia is secondary to hypothyroidism, glucocorticoid insufficiency, stroke, hepatic failure or hypoglycaemia.

Hypothermia also occurs in healthy individuals whose thermoregulatory mechanisms are intact but insufficient to cope with the intensity of the thermal stress. Typical examples include immersion in cold water, when core temperature may fall rapidly (acute hypothermia), exposure to extreme climates such as during hill walking (subacute hypothermia), and slow-onset hypothermia, as develops in an immobilised older individual (subchronic hypothermia). This classification is important, as it determines the method of rewarming.

Clinical features

Diagnosis is dependent on recognition of the environmental circumstances and measurement of core (rectal) body temperature. Clinical features depend on the degree of hypothermia (Fig. 9.2).

In a cold patient, it is very difficult to diagnose death reliably by clinical means. It has been suggested that, in extreme environmental conditions, irreversible hypothermia is probably present if there is asystole (no carotid pulse for 1 min), the chest and abdomen are rigid, the core temperature is <13°C and serum potassium is >12 mmol/L. However, in general, resuscitative measures should continue until the core temperature is normal and only then should a diagnosis of brain death be considered (p. 211).

Investigations

Blood gases, a full blood count, electrolytes, chest X-ray and electrocardiogram (ECG) are all essential investigations. Haemoconcentration and metabolic acidosis are common, and the ECG may show characteristic J waves, which occur at the junction of the QRS complex and the ST segment (Fig. 9.3). Cardiac arrhythmias, including ventricular fibrillation, may occur. Although the arterial oxygen tension may be normal when measured at room temperature, the arterial PO_2 in the blood falls by 7% for each 1°C fall in core temperature. Serum aspartate

aminotransferase and creatine kinase may be elevated secondary to muscle damage and the serum amylase is often high due to subclinical pancreatitis. If the cause of hypothermia is not obvious, additional investigations for thyroid and pituitary–adrenal dysfunction (p. 633), hypoglycaemia (p. 725) and the possibility of drug intoxication (p. 134) should be performed.

Management

Following resuscitation, the objectives of management are to rewarm the patient in a controlled manner while treating associated hypoxia (by oxygenation and ventilation if necessary), fluid and electrolyte disturbance, and cardiovascular abnormalities, particularly arrhythmias. Careful handling is essential to avoid precipitating the latter. The method of rewarming is dependent not on the absolute core temperature, but on haemodynamic stability and the presence or absence of an effective cardiac output.

Mild hypothermia

Outdoors, continued heat loss is prevented by sheltering the patient from the cold, replacing wet clothing, covering the head and insulating him or her from the ground. Once in hospital, even in the presence of profound hypothermia, if there is an effective cardiac output then forced-air rewarming, heat packs placed in axillae and groins and around the abdomen, inhaled warmed air and correction of fluid and electrolyte disturbances are usually sufficient. Rewarming rates of 1–2°C per hour are effective in leading to a gradual and safe return to physiological normality. Underlying conditions should be treated promptly (e.g. hypothyroidism with triiodothyronine 10 μg IV 3 times daily; p. 640).

Severe hypothermia

In the case of severe hypothermia (<28°C), patients with cardiopulmonary arrest (non-perfusing rhythm), or those with cardiac instability (systolic blood pressure <90 mmHg or ventricular arrhythmias), the aim is to restore perfusion, and rapid rewarming at a rate of >2°C per hour is required. This is best achieved by cardiopulmonary bypass or extracorporeal membrane oxygenation (ECMO). If these are unavailable, then veno–veno haemofiltration, and pleural, peritoneal, thoracic or bladder lavage with warmed fluids are alternatives. Direct heat sources, such as hot water or heat pads, should be used with caution, as these can provoke cardiac arrhythmias or cause burns. Monitoring of cardiac rhythm and arterial blood gases, including H+ (pH), is essential. Significant acidosis may require correction (p. 364).

Cold injury

Freezing cold injury (frostbite)

This represents the direct freezing of body tissues and usually affects the extremities: in particular, the fingers, toes, ears and face. Risk factors include smoking, peripheral vascular disease, dehydration and alcohol consumption. The tissues may become anaesthetised before freezing and, as a result, the injury often goes unrecognised at first. Frostbitten tissue is initially pale and doughy to the touch and insensitive to pain (Fig. 9.4). Once frozen, the tissue is hard.

Rewarming should not occur until it can be achieved rapidly in a water bath. Give oxygen and aspirin 300 mg as soon as possible. Frostbitten extremities should be rewarmed in warm water at 37–39°C, with antiseptic added. Adequate analgesia is necessary, as rewarming is very painful. Vasodilators such as

Fig. 9.4 Frostbite in a female Everest sherpa.

pentoxifylline (a phosphodiesterase inhibitor) have been shown to improve tissue survival. Once it has thawed, the injured part must not be re-exposed to the cold, and should be dressed and rested. While wound débridement may be necessary, amputations should be delayed for 60–90 days, as good recovery may occur over an extended period. As yet, the role of hyperbaric oxygen in the treatment of frostbite requires further research.

Non-freezing cold injury (trench or immersion foot)

This results from prolonged exposure to cold, damp conditions. The limb (usually the foot) appears cold, ischaemic and numb, but there is no freezing of the tissue. On rewarming, the limb appears mottled and thereafter becomes hyperaemic, swollen and painful. Recovery may take many months, during which period there may be chronic pain and sensitivity to cold. The pathology remains uncertain but probably involves endothelial injury. Gradual rewarming is associated with less pain than rapid rewarming. The pain and associated paraesthesia are difficult to control with conventional analgesia and may require amitriptyline (50 mg nocte), best instituted early. The patient is at risk of further damage on subsequent exposure to the cold.

Chilblains

Chilblains are tender, red or purplish skin lesions that occur in the cold and wet. They are often seen in horse riders, cyclists and swimmers, and are more common in women than men. They are short-lived and, although painful, not usually serious.

Heat-related illness

When generation of heat exceeds the body's capacity for heat loss, core temperature rises. Non-exertional heat illness (NEHI) occurs with a high environmental temperature in those with attenuated thermoregulatory control mechanisms: the elderly, the young, those with comorbidity or those taking drugs that affect thermoregulation (particularly phenothiazines, diuretics and alcohol). Exertional heat illness (EHI), on the other hand, typically develops in athletes when heat production exceeds the body's ability to dissipate it.

Acclimatisation mechanisms to environmental heat include stimulation of the sweat mechanism with increased sweat volume, reduced sweat sodium content and secondary hyperaldosteronism to maintain body sodium balance. The risk of heat-related illness falls as acclimatisation occurs. Heat illness can be prevented to a

i	**9.3** Differential diagnosis in patients with elevated core body temperature

- Heat illness (heat exhaustion, heat stroke)
- Sepsis, including meningitis
- Malaria
- Drug overdose
- Serotonin syndrome (pp. 139 and 1199)
- Malignant hyperpyrexia
- Thyroid storm (p. 639)

large extent by adequate replacement of salt and water, although excessive water intake alone should be avoided because of the risk of dilutional hyponatraemia (p. 357).

A spectrum of illnesses occurs in the heat (see Fig. 9.2). The cause is usually obvious but the differential diagnosis should be considered (Box 9.3).

Heat cramps

These painful muscle contractions occur following vigorous exercise and profuse sweating in hot weather. There is no elevation of core temperature. The mechanism is considered to be extracellular sodium depletion as a result of persistent sweating, exacerbated by replacement of water but not salt. Symptoms usually respond rapidly to rehydration with oral rehydration salts or intravenous saline.

Heat syncope

This is similar to a vasovagal faint (p. 181) and is related to peripheral vasodilatation in hot weather.

Heat exhaustion

Heat exhaustion occurs with prolonged exertion in hot and humid weather, profuse sweating and inadequate salt and water replacement. There is an elevation in core (rectal) temperature to between 37°C and 40°C, leading to the clinical features shown in Figure 9.2. Blood analyses may show evidence of dehydration with mild elevation of the blood urea, sodium and haematocrit. Treatment involves removal of the patient from the heat, and active evaporative cooling using tepid sprays and fanning ('strip–spray–fan'). Fluid losses are replaced with either oral rehydration mixtures or intravenous isotonic saline. Up to 5 L positive fluid balance may be required in the first 24 hours. Untreated, heat exhaustion may progress to heat stroke.

Heat stroke

Heat stroke occurs when the core body temperature rises above 40°C and is a life-threatening condition. The symptoms of heat exhaustion progress to include headache, nausea and vomiting. Neurological manifestations include a coarse muscle tremor and confusion, aggression or loss of consciousness. The patient's skin feels very hot, and sweating is often absent due to failure of thermoregulatory mechanisms. Complications include hypovolaemic shock, lactic acidosis, disseminated intravascular coagulation, rhabdomyolysis, hepatic and renal failure, and pulmonary and cerebral oedema.

Duration of hyperthermia is key to the outcome and immediate cooling should begin at the scene, before transfer to hospital. The aim should be to reduce core temperature by >0.2°C per minute to approximately 39°C, while avoiding overshooting and hypothermia. The patient should be resuscitated with evaporative or convective cooling. Fluid resuscitation with crystalloid intravenous fluids should be instituted but solutions containing potassium

9

should be avoided. Intravenous dextrose may be necessary, as hypoglycaemia can occur. Appropriate monitoring of fluid balance, including central venous pressure, is important, as over-aggressive fluid replacement may precipitate pulmonary oedema or further metabolic disturbance. Investigations for complications include routine haematology and biochemistry, coagulation screen, hepatic transaminases (aspartate aminotransferase and alanine aminotransferase), creatine kinase and chest X-ray. Once emergency treatment is established, heat stroke patients are best managed in intensive care.

Heat stroke is an emergency with a significant mortality. However, where temperatures can be reduced to <40°C within 30 minutes of collapse, death rates can approach zero. Patients who have had core temperatures of >40°C should be monitored carefully for later onset of rhabdomyolysis, renal damage and other complications before discharge from hospital. Clear advice to avoid heat and heavy exercise during recovery is important.

High altitude

The physiological effects of high altitude are significant. On Everest, the barometric pressure of the atmosphere falls from sea level by approximately 50% at base camp (5400 m) and approximately 70% at the summit (8848 m). The proportions of oxygen, nitrogen and carbon dioxide in air do not change with the fall in pressure but their partial pressure falls in proportion to barometric pressure (Fig. 9.5). Oxygen tension within the pulmonary alveoli is further reduced at altitude because the partial pressure of water vapour is related to body temperature and not barometric pressure, and so is proportionately greater at altitude, accounting for only 6% of barometric pressure at sea level but 19% at 8848 m.

Physiological effects of high altitude

Reduction in oxygen tension results in a fall in arterial oxygen saturation (Fig. 9.5). This varies widely between individuals, depending

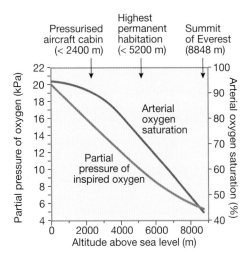

Fig. 9.5 Change in inspired oxygen tension and blood oxygen saturation at altitude. The blue curve shows changes in oxygen availability at altitude and the red curve shows the typical resultant changes in arterial oxygen saturation in a healthy person. Oxygen saturation varies between individuals according to the shape of the oxygen–haemoglobin dissociation curve and the ventilatory response to hypoxaemia. (To convert kPa to mmHg, multiply by 7.5.)

on the shape of the sigmoid oxygen–haemoglobin dissociation curve (see Fig. 23.5, p. 917) and the ventilatory response. Acclimatisation to hypoxaemia at high altitude involves a shift in this dissociation curve (dependent on 2,3-diphosphoglycerate (2,3-DPG)), erythropoiesis, haemoconcentration, and hyperventilation resulting from hypoxic drive, which is then sustained despite hypocapnia by restoration of cerebrospinal fluid pH to normal in prolonged hypoxia. This process takes several days, so travellers need to plan accordingly.

Illnesses at high altitude

Ascent to altitudes up to 2500 m or travel in a pressurised aircraft cabin is harmless to healthy people. Above 2500 m high-altitude illnesses may occur in previously healthy people, and above 3500 m these become common. Sudden ascent to altitudes above 6000 m, as experienced by aviators, balloonists and astronauts, may result in decompression illness with the same clinical features as seen in divers (see below), or even loss of consciousness. However, most altitude illness occurs in travellers and mountaineers.

Acute mountain sickness

Acute mountain sickness (AMS) is a syndrome comprised principally of headache, together with fatigue, anorexia, nausea and vomiting, difficulty sleeping or dizziness. Ataxia and peripheral oedema may be present. The aetiology of AMS is not fully understood but it is thought that hypoxaemia increases cerebral blood flow and hence intracranial pressure. Symptoms occur within 6–12 hours of an ascent and vary in severity from trivial to completely incapacitating. The incidence in travellers to 3000 m may be 40–50%, depending on the rate of ascent.

Treatment of mild cases consists of rest and simple analgesia; symptoms usually resolve after 1–3 days at a stable altitude, but may recur with further ascent. Occasionally, there is progression to cerebral oedema. Persistent symptoms indicate the need to descend but may respond to acetazolamide, a carbonic anhydrase inhibitor that induces a metabolic acidosis and stimulates ventilation; acetazolamide may also be used as prophylaxis if a rapid ascent is planned.

High-altitude cerebral oedema

The cardinal symptoms of high-altitude cerebral oedema (HACE) are ataxia and altered consciousness. HACE is rare, life-threatening and usually preceded by AMS. In addition to features of AMS, the patient suffers confusion, disorientation, visual disturbance, lethargy and ultimately loss of consciousness. Papilloedema and retinal haemorrhages are common and focal neurological signs may be found.

Treatment is directed at improving oxygenation. Descent is essential and dexamethasone (8 mg immediately and 4 mg 4 times daily) should be given. If descent is impossible, oxygen therapy in a portable pressurised bag may be helpful.

High-altitude pulmonary oedema

High-altitude pulmonary oedema (HAPE) is a life-threatening condition that usually occurs in the first 4 days after ascent above 2500 m. Unlike HACE, HAPE may occur de novo without the preceding signs of AMS. Presentation is with symptoms of dry cough, exertional dyspnoea and extreme fatigue. Later, the cough becomes wet and sputum may be blood-stained. Tachycardia and tachypnoea occur at rest and crepitations may often be heard in both lung fields. There may be profound hypoxaemia, pulmonary hypertension and radiological evidence of diffuse alveolar oedema. It is not known whether the alveolar oedema is a result of mechanical stress on the pulmonary capillaries associated with the high pulmonary arterial pressure, or an effect of hypoxia on capillary permeability. Reduced arterial oxygen saturation is not diagnostic but is a marker for disease progression.

Treatment is directed at reversal of hypoxia with immediate descent and oxygen administration. Nifedipine (20 mg 4 times daily) should be given to reduce pulmonary arterial pressure, and oxygen therapy in a portable pressurised bag should be used if descent is delayed.

Chronic mountain sickness (Monge's disease)

This occurs on prolonged exposure to altitude and has been reported in residents of Colorado, South America and Tibet. Patients present with headache, poor concentration and other signs of polycythaemia. The haemoglobin concentration is high (>200 g/L) and the haematocrit raised (>65%). Affected individuals are cyanosed and often have finger clubbing.

High-altitude retinal haemorrhage

This occurs in over 30% of trekkers at 5000 m. The haemorrhages are usually asymptomatic and resolve spontaneously. Visual defects can occur with haemorrhage involving the macula but there is no specific treatment.

Venous thrombosis

This has been reported at altitudes of >6000 m. Risk factors include dehydration, inactivity and the cold. The use of the oral contraceptive pill at high altitude should be considered carefully, as this is an additional risk factor.

Refractory cough

A cough at high altitude is common and usually benign. It may be due to breathing dry, cold air and to increased mouth breathing, with consequent dry oral mucosa. This may be indistinguishable from the early signs of HAPE.

Air travel

Commercial aircraft usually cruise at 10000–12000 m, with the cabin pressurised to an equivalent of around 2400 m. At this altitude, the partial pressure of oxygen is 16 kPa (120 mmHg), leading to a PaO_2 in healthy people of 7.0–8.5 kPa (53–64 mmHg). Oxygen saturation is also reduced but to a lesser degree (see Fig. 9.5). Although well tolerated by healthy people, this degree of hypoxia may be dangerous in patients with respiratory disease.

Advice for patients with respiratory disease

The British Thoracic Society has published guidance on the management of patients with respiratory disease who want to fly. Specialist pre-flight assessment is advised for all patients who have hypoxaemia (oxygen saturation <95%) at sea level, and includes spirometry and a hypoxic challenge test with 15% oxygen (performed in hospital). Air travel may have to be avoided or undertaken only with inspired oxygen therapy during the flight. Asthmatic patients should be advised to carry their inhalers in their hand baggage. Following pneumothorax, flying should be avoided while air remains in the pleural cavity, but can be considered after proven resolution or definitive (surgical) treatment.

Advice for other patients

Other circumstances in which patients are more susceptible to hypoxia require individual assessment. These include cardiac arrhythmia, sickle-cell disease and ischaemic heart disease. Most airlines decline to carry pregnant women after the 36th week of gestation. In complicated pregnancies it may be advisable to avoid air travel at an earlier stage. Patients who have had recent abdominal surgery, including laparoscopy, should avoid flying until all intraperitoneal gas is reabsorbed. Divers should not fly for 24 hours after a dive requiring decompression stops.

Ear and sinus pain due to changes in gas volume are common but usually mild, although patients with chronic sinusitis and otitis media may need specialist assessment. A healthy mobile tympanic membrane visualised during a Valsalva manœuvre usually suggests a patent Eustachian tube.

On long-haul flights, patients with diabetes mellitus may need to adjust their insulin or oral hypoglycaemic dosing according to the timing of in-flight and subsequent meals (p. 750). Advice is available from Diabetes UK and other websites. Patients should be able to provide documentary evidence of the need to carry needles and insulin.

Deep venous thrombosis

Air travellers have an increased risk of venous thrombosis (p. 975), due to a combination of factors, including loss of venous emptying because of prolonged immobilisation (lack of muscular activity) and reduced barometric pressure on the tissues, together with haemoconcentration as a result of oedema and perhaps a degree of hypoxia-induced diuresis.

Venous thrombosis can probably be prevented by avoiding dehydration and excess alcohol, and by exercising muscles during the flight. Without a clear cost–benefit analysis, prophylaxis with aspirin or heparin cannot be recommended routinely, but may be considered in high-risk cases.

Under water

Drowning and near-drowning

Drowning is defined as death due to asphyxiation following immersion in a fluid, while near-drowning is defined as survival for longer than 24 hours after suffocation by immersion. Drowning remains a common cause of accidental death throughout the world and is particularly common in young children (Box 9.4). In about 10% of cases, no water enters the lungs and death follows intense laryngospasm ('dry' drowning). Prolonged immersion in cold water, with or without water inhalation, results in a rapid fall in core body temperature and hypothermia (p. 165).

Following inhalation of water, there is a rapid onset of ventilation–perfusion imbalance with hypoxaemia, and the development

i	9.4 Most common causes of drowning by age	
Infants/young children		
• Domestic baths	• Garden pools	
Adolescents		
• Swimming pools	• Rivers, sea, etc.	
Adults		
• Water sports, boating, fishing	• Occupational	
Older people		
• Domestic baths		

of diffuse pulmonary oedema. Fresh water is hypotonic and, although rapidly absorbed across alveolar membranes, impairs surfactant function, which leads to alveolar collapse and right-to-left shunting of unoxygenated blood. Absorption of large amounts of hypotonic fluid can result in haemolysis. Salt water is hypertonic and inhalation provokes alveolar oedema, but the overall clinical effect is similar to that of freshwater drowning.

Clinical features

Those rescued alive (near-drowning) are often unconscious and not breathing. Hypoxaemia and metabolic acidosis are inevitable features. Acute lung injury usually resolves rapidly over 48–72 hours, unless infection occurs (Fig. 9.6). Complications include dehydration, hypotension, haemoptysis, rhabdomyolysis, renal failure and cardiac arrhythmias. A small number of patients, mainly the more severely ill, progress to develop the acute respiratory distress syndrome (ARDS; p. 198).

Survival is possible after immersion for up to 30 minutes in very cold water, as the rapid development of hypothermia after immersion may be protective, particularly in children. Long-term outcome depends on the severity of the cerebral hypoxic injury and is predicted by the duration of immersion, delay in resuscitation, intensity of acidosis and the presence of cardiac arrest.

Management

Initial management requires cardiopulmonary resuscitation with administration of oxygen and maintenance of the circulation (p. 456). It is important to clear the airway of foreign bodies and protect the cervical spine. Continuous positive airways pressure (CPAP; p. 202) should be considered for spontaneously breathing patients with oxygen saturations of <94%. Observation is required for a minimum of 24 hours. Prophylactic antibiotics are only required if exposure was to obviously contaminated water.

Fig. 9.6 Near-drowning. Chest X-ray of a 39-year-old farmer, 2 weeks after immersion in a polluted freshwater ditch for 5 min before rescue. Airspace consolidation and cavities in the left lower lobe reflect secondary staphylococcal pneumonia and abscess formation.

Diving-related illness

The underwater environment is extremely hostile. Other than drowning, most diving illness is related to changes in barometric pressure and its effect on gas behaviour.

Ambient pressure under water increases by 101 kPa (1 atmosphere, 1 ata) for every 10 metres of seawater (msw) or 33 eet of seawater (fsw) depth. As divers descend, the partial pressures of the gases they are breathing increase (Box 9.5), and the blood and tissue concentrations of dissolved gases rise accordingly. Nitrogen is a weak anaesthetic agent, and if the inspiratory pressure of nitrogen is allowed to increase above 320 kPa (3.2 ata; i.e. a depth of approximately 30 msw), it produces 'narcosis', resulting in impairment of cognitive function and manual dexterity, not unlike alcohol intoxication. For this reason, compressed air can be used only for shallow diving. Oxygen is also toxic at inspired pressures above approximately 40 kPa (0.4 ata; inducing apprehension, muscle twitching, euphoria, sweating, tinnitus, nausea and vertigo), so 100% oxygen cannot be used as an alternative. For dives deeper than approximately 30 msw, mixtures of oxygen with nitrogen and/or helium are used.

While drowning remains the most common diving-related cause of death, another important group of disorders usually present once the diver returns to the surface: decompression illness (DCI) and barotrauma.

Clinical features
Decompression illness

This includes decompression sickness (DCS) and arterial gas embolism (AGE). While the vast majority of symptoms of DCI present within 6 hours of a dive, they can also be provoked by flying (further decompression), and thus patients may present to medical services at sites far removed from the dive.

Exposure of individuals to increased partial pressures of nitrogen results in additional nitrogen being dissolved in body tissues; the amount dissolved depends on the depth/pressure and on the duration of the dive. On ascent, the tissues become supersaturated with nitrogen, and this places the diver at risk of producing a critical quantity of gas (bubbles) in tissues if the ascent is too fast. The gas so formed may cause symptoms locally, peripherally due to bubbles passing through the pulmonary vascular bed (Box 9.6) or by embolisation elsewhere. Arterial embolisation may occur if the gas load in the venous system exceeds the lungs' abilities to excrete nitrogen, or when bubbles pass through a patent foramen ovale (present asymptomatically

i	9.5 Physics of breathing compressed air while diving in sea water			
Depth	Lung volume	Barometric pressure	PiO_2	PiN_2
Surface	100%	101 kPa (1 ata)	21 kPa (0.21 ata)	79 kPa (0.78 ata)
10 m	50%	202 kPa (2 ata)	42 kPa (0.42 ata)	159 kPa (1.58 ata)
20 m	33%	303 kPa (3 ata)	63 kPa (0.63 ata)	239 kPa (2.34 ata)
30 m	25%	404 kPa (4 ata)	84 kPa (0.84 ata)	319 kPa (3.12 ata)

<table>
<tr><td>i</td><td>9.6 Assessment of a patient with decompression illness*</td></tr>
</table>

Evolution

- Progressive
- Static
- Relapsing
- Spontaneously improving

Manifestations

- Pain: often large joints, e.g. shoulder ('the bends')
- Neurological: any deficit is possible
- Audiovestibular: vertigo, tinnitus, nystagmus; may mimic inner ear barotrauma
- Pulmonary: chest pain, cough, haemoptysis, dyspnoea; may be due to arterial gas embolism (AGE)
- Cutaneous: itching, erythematous rash
- Lymphatic: tender lymph nodes, oedema
- Constitutional: headache, fatigue, general malaise

Dive profile

- Depth
- Type of gas used
- Duration of dive

*Information required by diving specialists to decide appropriate treatment. See contact details on page 172.

in 25–30% of adults; p. 531). Although DCS and AGE can be indistinguishable, their early treatment is the same.

Barotrauma

During the ascent phase of a dive, the gas in the diver's lungs expands due to the decreasing pressure. The diver must therefore ascend slowly and breathe regularly; if ascent is rapid or the diver holds his/her breath, the expanding gas may cause lung rupture (pulmonary barotrauma). This can result in pneumomediastinum, pneumothorax or AGE as a result of gas passing directly into the pulmonary venous system. Other air-filled body cavities may be subject to barotrauma, including the ear and sinuses.

Management

The patient is nursed horizontally and airway, breathing and circulation are assessed. Treatment includes the following:

- *High-flow oxygen* is given by a tight-fitting mask using a rebreathing bag. This assists in the washout of excess inert gas (nitrogen) and may reduce the extent of local tissue hypoxia resulting from focal embolic injury.
- *Fluid replacement* (oral or intravenous) corrects the intravascular fluid loss from endothelial bubble injury and dehydration associated with immersion. Maintenance of an adequate peripheral circulation is important for the excretion of excess dissolved gas.
- *Recompression* is the definitive therapy. Transfer to a recompression facility may be by surface or air, provided that the altitude remains low (<300 m) and the patient continues to breathe 100% oxygen. Recompression reduces the volume of gas within tissues (Boyle's law), forces nitrogen back into solution and is followed by slow decompression, allowing the nitrogen load to be excreted.

The majority of patients make a complete recovery with treatment, although a small but significant proportion are left with neurological disability.

Humanitarian crisis

Humanitarian crises are common. If the medical profession is to help, it must understand that the emergency treatment of a few sick and injured people is not always the priority and that there is a set of basic needs that must be addressed in order to do the most for the most.

A humanitarian crisis can take many forms: an environmental disaster, mass emigration due to drought, conflict or famine, a disease outbreak or any number of natural or man-made events. When this event overwhelms the resources of the affected country's government, then the international community will often step in to help. Although a full examination of the subject is beyond the scope of this book, there are a few basic principles for managing a humanitarian crisis.

The response is broken down into four phases:

1. recognition (first week)
2. emergency response (first month)
3. consolidation phase (to crisis resolution or crisis containment)
4. handover and withdrawal.

Recognition

Recognition of a disaster may be obvious in a sudden event such as an earthquake or a tidal wave, but less obvious in a disease outbreak or when it stems from internal conflict. The recognition phase is for the host nation rather than the international community, and requests for support will come from the affected country's government.

Emergency response

During the emergency phase, responders (whether international, governmental or the charity sector) will undertake an initial assessment of need, set objectives, mobilise resources, coordinate with other agencies and deploy to the crisis in order to deliver an initial response.

Consolidation phase

The consolidation phase involves matching resources to need, dealing with the crisis, building resilience, supporting infrastructure (human and physical) and instituting systems to manage the ongoing health needs of the population.

Handover and withdrawal

Once the crisis is under control and the country is able to manage within resources, a phased withdrawal can occur.

Health-care priorities

When the normal infrastructure of a country or area fails, then populations are at risk, whether they shelter in place or flee, leading to mass migration. For health-care teams, rather than logisticians, rescue teams or security forces, there are well-defined priorities, which must be in place (Box 9.7). This must all occur during the emergency phase and is followed by the

9.7 Priorities in a humanitarian crisis

1. Assessment of population need
2. Safe water and sanitation
3. Food and nutrition
4. Shelter and warmth
5. Emergency health care
6. Immunisation of risk groups
7. Control of communicable diseases
8. Ongoing health surveillance and reporting
9. Training and deployment of indigenous health-care workers
10. Handover of responsibility to local authorities

implementation of a public health surveillance and reporting system and the mobilisation of local human resources, and their training and deployment during the consolidation phase in order to prepare for handover to the local competent authority and withdrawal.

Further information

Websites

altitude.org *A website written by doctors with expertise and experience of expedition and altitude medicine and critical care.*

diversalertnetwork.org *Advice on the clinical management of diving illness and emergency assistance services.*

emergency.cdc.gov/radiation/ *The Centers for Disease Control and Prevention provides information and links on all forms of radiation for patients and professionals.*

msf.org *Information and advice about all aspects of responding to humanitarian crises around the world.*

Telephone numbers

Two organisations can offer national and international advice on diving emergencies and recompression facilities:

- Within the UK, the National Diving Accident Helpline on +44 (0)7831 151523 (24 hours).
- Outside the UK, contact the Divers Alert Network International Emergency Hotline +1-919-684-9111.

VR Tallentire
MJ MacMahon

Acute medicine and critical illness

Clinical examination in critical care 174

Monitoring 175

Acute medicine 176
The decision to admit to hospital 176
Ambulatory care 176

Presenting problems in acute medicine 176
Chest pain 176
Acute breathlessness 179
Syncope/presyncope 181
Delirium 183
Headache 185
Unilateral leg swelling 186

Identification and assessment of deterioration 188
Early warning scores and the role of the medical emergency team 188
Immediate assessment of the deteriorating patient 188
Selecting the appropriate location for ongoing management 189

Common presentations of deterioration 190
Tachypnoea 190
Hypoxaemia 190
Tachycardia 191
Hypotension 193
Hypertension 193
Decreased conscious level 194
Decreased urine output/deteriorating renal function 195

Disorders causing critical illness 196
Sepsis and the systemic inflammatory response 196
Acute respiratory distress syndrome 198
Acute circulatory failure (cardiogenic shock) 199
Post cardiac arrest 200
Other causes of multi-organ failure 201

Critical care medicine 201
Decisions around intensive care admission 201

Stabilisation and institution of organ support 202
Respiratory support 202
Cardiovascular support 204
Renal support 208
Neurological support 208

Daily clinical management in intensive care 208
Clinical review 208
Sedation and analgesia 209
Delirium in intensive care 209
Weaning from respiratory support 209
Extubation 210
Tracheostomy 210
Nutrition 210
Other essential components of intensive care 210

Complications and outcomes of critical illness 211
Adverse neurological outcomes 211
Other long-term problems 212
The older patient 212
Withdrawal of active treatment and death in intensive care 213
Discharge from intensive care 213
Critical care scoring systems 213

Clinical examination in critical care

A Airway

Is the airway patent?
Is the end-tidal CO_2 trace normal?
Are there any signs of airway obstruction?

I Infection

What is the temperature?
Review recent infective markers and trend
What antibiotics are being given and what is the duration of treatment?

H Haematology

What are the haemoglobin/platelet levels?
Are there any signs of bleeding?

G Glucose

What is the glucose level?
Is insulin being administered?

F Fluids, electrolytes and renal system

What is the fluid balance?
Urine volume and colour?
Is there any oedema?
Review the renal biochemistry and electrolyte levels

B Breathing

Is the physiology normal (SpO_2, respiratory rate, tidal volume)?
What is the level of support?
Are there any abnormal signs on chest examination?
Review the ventilator settings, arterial blood gases and recent chest X-ray

C Circulation

Is the physiology normal (heart rate, blood pressure, peripheral temperature, lactate, urine output)?
How much support is required (inotrope, vasopressor)?

E Enteral/exposure

Feeding regime
Stool frequency
Abdominal tenderness/bowel sounds present?

D Disability

Level of responsiveness
Delirium screen
Pupillary responses
Doses of sedative drugs

Monitoring

Electrocardiography
Heart rate, rhythm and QRS morphology

Arterial line trace
Size of the area under the curve is proportional to stroke volume
Narrow peaks suggest low stroke volume as shown here

Oxygen saturation
Saturation of haemoglobin measured by plethysmography (SpO_2). Gives an indication of adequacy of oxygenation, and the quality of tissue perfusion can also be inferred – a flat trace suggests poor peripheral perfusion

Central venous pressure trace
A non-specific guide to volume status and right ventricular function. Increased values in fluid overload and right ventricular failure

Capnography
Numerical value of end-tidal CO_2 ($ETCO_2$) is less than arterial PCO_2 ($PaCO_2$) by a variable amount. Shape of trace can signify airway displacement/obstruction, bronchospasm or a low cardiac output (as shown below)

10

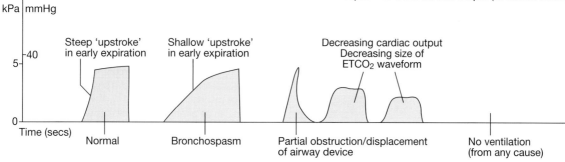

kPa | mmHg

Steep 'upstroke' in early expiration

Shallow 'upstroke' in early expiration

Decreasing cardiac output Decreasing size of $ETCO_2$ waveform

Time (secs)

Normal

Bronchospasm

Partial obstruction/displacement of airway device

No ventilation (from any cause)

Bedside physiological data commonly monitored in an intensive care unit setting.

ℹ **Plethysmography (SpO_2)**

Basic principles

- Uses the different red and infrared absorption profiles of oxyhaemoglobin and deoxyhaemoglobin to estimate arterial oxyhaemoglobin saturation (SaO_2)
- Only pulsatile absorption is measured
- A poor trace correlates with poor perfusion

Sources of error

- Carboxyhaemoglobin – absorption profile is the same as oxyhaemoglobin: falsely elevated SpO_2
- Methaemoglobinaemia – SpO_2 will tend towards 85%
- Ambient light/poor application of probe/ severe tricuspid regurgitation (pulsatile venous flow): falsely depressed SpO_2
- Reduced accuracy below 80% saturation
- Hyperbilirubinaemia does not affect SpO_2

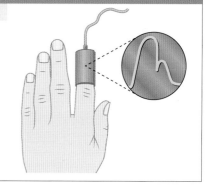

Hospital medicine is becoming ever more specialised and people are living longer while accruing increasing numbers of chronic disease diagnoses. Rather than diminishing the role of the generalist, these factors paradoxically create a need for experts in the undifferentiated presentation. In the UK such physicians are known as 'general physicians', while in the US they are referred to as 'hospitalists'.

Acute illness can present in a large variety of ways, depending on the nature of the illness, the underlying health of the individual, and their cultural and religious background. The skills of prompt diagnosis formation and provision of appropriate treatment rely on the integration of information from all the available sources, along with careful consideration of underlying chronic health problems.

Patients who deteriorate while in hospital make up a small but important cohort. If they are well managed, in-hospital cardiac arrest rates will be low. This can be achieved through the combined effects of prompt resuscitation and appropriate end-of-life decision-making. Early recognition of deterioration by ward teams and initial management by health-care professionals operating within a functioning rapid response system are the central tenets of any system designed to improve the outcomes of deteriorating ward patients.

Intensive care medicine has developed into a prominent specialty, central to the safe functioning of a modern acute hospital. Scientific endeavour has resulted in a much better understanding of the molecular pathophysiology of processes such as sepsis and acute respiratory distress syndrome, which account for much premature death worldwide.

Acute medicine

Acute medicine is the part of general medicine that is concerned with the immediate and early management of medical patients who require urgent care. As a specialty, it is closely aligned with emergency medicine and intensive care medicine, but is firmly rooted within general medicine. Acute physicians manage the adult medical take and lead the development of acute care pathways that aim to reduce variability, improve care and cut down hospital admissions.

The decision to admit to hospital

Every patient presenting to hospital should be assessed by a clinician who is able to determine whether or not admission is required. The requirement for admission is determined by many factors, including the severity of illness, the patient's physiological reserve, the need for urgent investigations, the nature of proposed treatments and the patient's social circumstances. In many cases, it is clear early in the assessment process that a patient requires admission. In such cases, a move into a medical receiving unit – often termed a medical admissions unit (MAU) or acute medical unit (AMU) – should be facilitated as soon as the initial assessment has been completed and urgent investigations and/or treatments have been instigated. In hospitals where such units do not exist, patients will need to be moved to a downstream ward once treatment has been commenced and they have been deemed sufficiently stable. Following the initial assessment, it may be possible to discharge stable patients home with a plan for early follow-up (such as a rapid-access specialist clinic appointment).

Ambulatory care

In some hospitals, it is increasingly possible for patient care to be coordinated in an ambulatory setting, negating the need for a patient to remain in hospital overnight. In the context of acute medicine, ambulatory care can be employed for conditions that are perceived by either the patient or the referring practitioner as requiring prompt clinical assessment by a competent decision-maker with access to appropriate diagnostic resources. The patient may return on several occasions for investigation, observation, consultation or treatment. Some presentations, such as a unilateral swollen leg (p. 186), lend themselves to this type of management (Box 10.1). If indicated, a Doppler ultrasound can be arranged, and patients with confirmed deep vein thromboses can be anticoagulated on an outpatient basis. Successful ambulatory care requires careful patient selection; while many patients may cherish the opportunity to sleep at home, others may find frequent trips to hospital or clinic too difficult due to frailty, poor mobility or transport difficulties.

Presenting problems in acute medicine

Chest pain

Chest pain is a common symptom in patients presenting to hospital. The differential diagnosis is wide (Box 10.2), and a

i 10.1 Groups of patients who are potentially suitable for ambulatory care		
Group	Example(s)	Quality and safety issues
Diagnostic exclusion group	Chest pain – possible myocardial infarction; breathlessness – possible pulmonary embolism	Even when a specific condition has been excluded, there is still a need to explain the patient's symptoms through the diagnostic process
Low-risk stratification group	Non-variceal upper gastrointestinal bleed with low Blatchford score (p. 780); community-acquired pneumonia with low CURB-65 score (p. 583)	Appropriate treatment plans should be in place
Specific procedure group	Replacement of percutaneous endoscopic gastrostomy (PEG) tube; drainage of pleural effusion/ascites	The key to implementation is how ambulatory care for this group of patients can be delivered when they present out of hours
Outpatient group with supporting infrastructure	Deep vein thrombosis (DVT); cellulitis	These are distinct from the conditions listed above because the infrastructure required to manage them is quite different

---

| | **10.2 Differential diagnosis of chest pain** |

Central

Cardiac
- Myocardial ischaemia (angina)
- Myocardial infarction
- Myocarditis
- Pericarditis
- Mitral valve prolapse syndrome

Aortic
- Aortic dissection
- Aortic aneurysm

Oesophageal
- Oesophagitis
- Oesophageal spasm
- Mallory–Weiss syndrome
- Oesophageal perforation (Boerhaave's syndrome)

Pulmonary embolus

Mediastinal
- Malignancy

Anxiety/emotion[1]

Peripheral

Lungs/pleura
- Pulmonary infarct
- Pneumonia
- Pneumothorax
- Malignancy
- Tuberculosis
- Connective tissue disorders

Musculoskeletal[2]
- Osteoarthritis
- Rib fracture/injury
- Acute vertebral fracture
- Costochondritis (Tietze's syndrome)
- Intercostal muscle injury
- Epidemic myalgia (Bornholm disease)

Neurological
- Prolapsed intervertebral disc
- Herpes zoster
- Thoracic outlet syndrome

[1]May also cause peripheral chest pain. [2]Can sometimes cause central chest pain.

detailed history and thorough clinical examination are paramount to ensure that the subsequent investigative pathway is appropriate.

Presentation

Chest 'pain' is clearly a subjective phenomenon and may be described by patients in a variety of different ways. Whether the patient describes 'pain', 'discomfort' or 'pressure' in the chest, there are some key features that must be elicited from the history.

Site and radiation

Pain secondary to myocardial ischaemia is typically located in the centre of the chest. It may radiate to the neck, jaw, and upper or even lower arms. Occasionally, it may be experienced only at the sites of radiation or in the back. The pain of myocarditis or pericarditis is characteristically felt retrosternally, to the left of the sternum, or in the left or right shoulder. The severe pain of aortic dissection is typically central with radiation through to the back. Central chest pain may also occur with tumours affecting the mediastinum, oesophageal disease (p. 791) or disease of the thoracic aorta (p. 505). Pain situated over the left anterior chest and radiating laterally is unlikely to be due to cardiac ischaemia and may have many causes, including pleural or lung disorders, musculoskeletal problems or anxiety. Rarely, sharp, left-sided chest pain that is suggestive of a musculoskeletal problem may be a feature of mitral valve prolapse (p. 520).

Characteristics

Pleurisy, a sharp or 'catching' chest pain aggravated by deep breathing or coughing, is indicative of respiratory pathology, particularly pulmonary infection or infarction. However, the pain associated with myocarditis or pericarditis is often also described as 'sharp' and may 'catch' during inspiration, coughing or lying flat. It typically varies in intensity with movement and the phase of respiration. A malignant tumour invading the chest wall or ribs can cause gnawing, continuous local pain. The pain of myocardial ischaemia is typically dull, constricting, choking or 'heavy', and is usually described as squeezing, crushing, burning or aching. Patients often emphasise that it is a discomfort rather than a pain. Angina occurs during (not after) exertion and is promptly relieved (in less than 5 minutes) by rest. It may also be precipitated or exacerbated by emotion but tends to occur more readily during exertion, after a large meal or in a cold wind. In crescendo or unstable angina, similar pain may be precipitated by minimal exertion or at rest. The increase in venous return or preload induced by lying down may also be sufficient to provoke pain in vulnerable patients (decubitus angina). Patients with reversible airways obstruction, such as asthma, may also describe exertional chest tightness that is relieved by rest. This may be difficult to distinguish from myocardial ischaemia. Bronchospasm may be associated with wheeze, atopy and cough (p. 556). Musculoskeletal chest pain is variable in site and intensity but does not usually fall into any of the patterns described above. The pain may vary with posture or movement of the upper body, or be associated with a specific movement (bending, stretching, turning). Many minor soft tissue injuries are related to everyday activities, such as driving, manual work and sport.

Onset

The pain associated with myocardial infarction (MI) typically takes several minutes or even longer to develop to its maximal intensity; similarly, angina builds up gradually in proportion to the intensity of exertion. Pain that occurs after, rather than during, exertion is usually musculoskeletal or psychological in origin. The pain of aortic dissection (severe and 'tearing'), massive pulmonary embolism (PE) or pneumothorax is usually very sudden in onset. Other causes of chest pain tend to develop more gradually, over hours or even days.

Associated features

The pain of MI, massive PE or aortic dissection is often accompanied by autonomic disturbance, including sweating, nausea and vomiting. Some patients describe a feeling of impending death, referred to as 'angor animi'. Breathlessness, due to pulmonary congestion arising from transient ischaemic left ventricular dysfunction, is often a prominent feature of myocardial ischemia. Breathlessness may also accompany any of the respiratory causes of chest pain and can be associated with cough, wheeze or other respiratory symptoms. Patients with myocarditis or pericarditis may describe a prodromal viral illness. Gastrointestinal disorders, such as gastro-oesophageal reflux or peptic ulceration, may present with chest pain that is hard to distinguish from myocardial ischaemia; it may even be precipitated by exercise and be relieved by nitrates. However, it is usually possible to elicit a history relating chest pain to supine posture or eating, drinking or oesophageal reflux. The pain of gastro-oesophageal reflux often radiates to the interscapular region and dysphagia may be present. Severe chest pain arising after retching or vomiting, or following oesophageal instrumentation, should raise the possibility of oesophageal perforation.

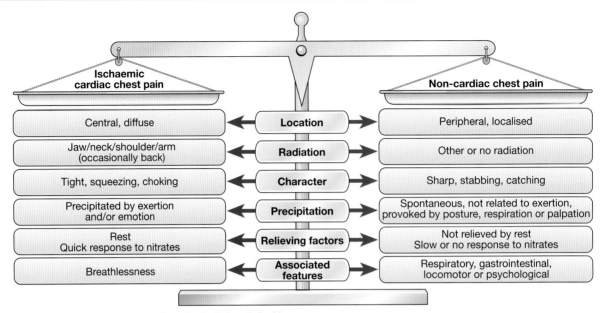

Fig. 10.1 Identifying ischaemic cardiac pain: the 'balance' of evidence.

Anxiety-induced chest pain may be associated with breathlessness (without hypoxaemia), throat tightness, perioral tingling and other evidence of emotional distress. It is important to remember, however, that chest pain itself can be an extremely frightening experience, and so psychological and organic features often coexist. Anxiety may amplify the effects of organic disease and a confusing clinical picture may result.

A detailed and clear history is key to narrowing the differential diagnosis of chest pain. Figure 10.1 shows how certain features of the history, particularly when combined, can tip the balance of evidence towards or away from ischaemic cardiac chest pain.

Clinical assessment

Cardiorespiratory examination may detect clinical signs that help guide ongoing investigation. Patients with a history compatible with myocardial ischaemia should have a 12-lead electrocardiogram (ECG) performed while clinical examination proceeds. Ongoing chest pain with clinical features of shock or pulmonary oedema, or ECG evidence of ventricular arrhythmia or complete heart block should prompt urgent cardiology review and referral to a higher level of care.

Chest pain that is accompanied by clinical evidence of increased intracardiac pressure (especially a raised jugular venous pressure) increases the likelihood of myocardial ischaemia or massive PE. The legs should be examined for clinical evidence of deep vein thrombosis.

A large pneumothorax should be evident on clinical examination, with absent breath sounds and a hyper-resonant percussion note on the affected side. Other unilateral chest signs, such as bronchial breathing or crackles, are most likely to indicate a respiratory tract infection, and a chest X-ray should be expedited.

Pericarditis may be accompanied by a pericardial friction rub. In aortic dissection, syncope or neurological deficit may occur. Examination may reveal asymmetrical pulses, features of undiagnosed Marfan's syndrome (p. 508) or a new early diastolic murmur representing aortic regurgitation.

Any disease process involving the pleura may restrict rib movement and a pleural rub may be audible on the affected side. Local tenderness of the chest wall is likely to indicate musculoskeletal pain but can also be found in pulmonary infarction.

Subdiaphragmatic inflammatory pathology, such as a liver abscess, cholecystitis or ascending cholangitis, can mimic pneumonia by causing fever, pleuritic chest pain and a small sympathetic pleural effusion, usually on the right. Likewise, acute pancreatitis can present with thoracic symptoms, and an amylase or lipase level should be requested where appropriate. It is imperative that the abdomen is examined routinely in all patients presenting with pleuritic chest pain.

Initial investigations

Chest X-ray, ECG and biomarkers (e.g. troponin, D-dimer) play a pivotal role in the evaluation of chest pain. However, indiscriminate ordering of such investigations may result in diagnostic confusion and over-investigation. The choice of investigation(s) is intimately linked to the history and examination findings. A chest X-ray and 12-lead ECG should be performed in the vast majority of patients presenting to hospital with chest pain. Pregnancy is not a contraindication to chest X-ray, but particular consideration should be given to whether the additional diagnostic information justifies breast irradiation.

The chest X-ray may confirm the suspected diagnosis, particularly in the case of pneumonia. Small pneumothoraces are easily missed, as are rib fractures or small metastatic deposits, and all should be considered individually during chest X-ray review. A widened mediastinum suggests acute aortic dissection but a normal chest X-ray does not exclude the diagnosis. Provided it has been more than 1 hour since the onset of pain, chest X-ray in oesophageal rupture may reveal subcutaneous emphysema, pneumomediastinum or a pleural effusion.

Patients with a history compatible with myocardial ischaemia require an urgent 12-lead ECG. Acute chest pain with ECG changes indicating a ST segment elevation myocardial infarction (STEMI) suggests that the patient is likely to benefit from immediate reperfusion therapy. Specific information relating to cocaine or amphetamine use should be sought, particularly in younger

i	10.3 Causes of elevated serum troponin other than acute coronary syndrome

Cardiorespiratory causes

- Pulmonary embolism
- Acute pulmonary oedema
- Tachyarrhythmias
- Myocarditis/myopericarditis
- Aortic dissection
- Cardiac trauma
- Cardiac surgery/ablation

Non-cardiorespiratory causes

- Prolonged hypotension
- Severe sepsis
- Severe burns
- Stroke
- Subarachnoid haemorrhage
- End-stage renal failure

patients. In the context of a compatible history, an ECG showing ischaemic changes that do not meet STEMI criteria should prompt regular repeat ECGs and treatment for non-ST segment elevation myocardial infarction (NSTEMI)/unstable angina. Measurement of serum troponin concentration on admission is often helpful in cases where there is diagnostic doubt, but a negative result should always prompt a repeat sample 6–12 hours after maximal pain. Acute coronary syndrome may be diagnosed with confidence in patients with a convincing history of ischaemic pain (Fig. 10.1) and either ECG evidence of ischaemia or an elevated serum troponin. If an elevated serum troponin is found in a patient who has an atypical history or is at low risk of ischaemic heart disease, then alternative causes of raised troponin should be considered (Box 10.3). Further management of acute coronary syndromes is discussed on page 498.

In the absence of convincing ECG evidence of myocardial ischaemia, other life-threatening causes of chest pain, such as aortic dissection, massive PE and oesophageal rupture, should be considered. Suspicion of aortic dissection (background of hypertension, trauma, pregnancy or previous aortic surgery) should prompt urgent thoracic computed tomography (CT) or transoesophageal echocardiography. An ECG in the context of massive PE most commonly reveals only a sinus tachycardia, but may show new right axis deviation, right bundle branch block or a dominant R wave in V_1. The classical finding of $S_1Q_3T_3$ (a deep S wave in lead I, with a Q wave and T wave inversion in lead III) is rare. If massive PE is suspected and the patient is haemodynamically unstable, a transthoracic echocardiogram, to seek evidence of right heart strain and exclude alternative diagnoses such as tamponade, is extremely useful.

If the patient is deemed to be at low risk of PE, a D-dimer test can be informative, as a negative result effectively excludes the diagnosis. The D-dimer test should be performed only if there is clinical suspicion of PE, as false-positive results can lead to unnecessary investigations. If the D-dimer is positive, there is high clinical suspicion, or there is other convincing evidence of PE (such as features of right heart strain on the ECG), prompt imaging should be arranged (p. 619 and Fig. 17.67).

Acute breathlessness

In acute breathlessness, the history, along with a rapid but careful examination, will usually suggest a diagnosis that can be confirmed by routine investigations including chest X-ray, 12-lead ECG and arterial blood gas (ABG) sampling.

Presentation

A key feature of the history is the speed of onset of breathlessness. Acute severe breathlessness (over minutes or hours) has a distinct

Fig. 10.2 Inhaled foreign body. [A] Chest X-ray showing a tooth lodged in a main bronchus. [B] Bronchoscopic appearance of inhaled foreign body (tooth) with a covering mucous film.

differential diagnosis list to chronic exertional breathlessness. The presence of associated cardiovascular (chest pain, palpitations, sweating and nausea) or respiratory symptoms (cough, wheeze, haemoptysis, stridor) can narrow the differential diagnosis yet further. A previous history of left ventricular dysfunction, asthma or exacerbations of chronic obstructive pulmonary disease (COPD) is important. In the severely ill patient, it may be necessary to obtain the history from accompanying witnesses. In children, the possibility of inhalation of a foreign body (Fig. 10.2) or acute epiglottitis should always be considered. There is often more than one underlying diagnosis; a thorough assessment should continue, even after a possible diagnosis has been reached, particularly if the severity of symptoms does not seem to be adequately explained. The causes of acute severe breathlessness are covered here; chronic exertional dyspnoea is discussed further on page 557.

Clinical assessment

Airway obstruction, anaphylaxis and tension pneumothorax require immediate identification and treatment. If any of these is suspected, treatment should not be delayed while additional investigations are performed, and anaesthetic support is likely to be required. In the absence of an immediately life-threatening cause, the following should be assessed and documented:

- level of consciousness
- degree of central cyanosis
- work of breathing (rate, depth, pattern, use of accessory muscles)
- adequacy of oxygenation (SpO_2)

- ability to speak (in single words or sentences)
- cardiovascular status (heart rate and rhythm, blood pressure (BP) and peripheral perfusion).

Pulmonary oedema is suggested by a raised jugular venous pressure and bi-basal crackles or diffuse wheeze, while asthma or COPD is characterised by wheeze and prolonged expiration. A hyper-resonant hemithorax with absent breath sounds raises the possibility of pneumothorax, while severe breathlessness with normal breath sounds may indicate PE. Leg swelling may suggest cardiac failure or, if asymmetrical, venous thrombosis.

The presence of wheeze is not always indicative of bronchospasm. In acute left heart failure, an increase in the left ventricular diastolic pressure causes the pressure in the left atrium, pulmonary veins and pulmonary capillaries to rise. When the hydrostatic pressure of the pulmonary capillaries exceeds the oncotic pressure of plasma (about 25–30 mmHg), fluid moves from the capillaries into the interstitium. This stimulates respiration through a series of autonomic reflexes, producing rapid, shallow respiration, and congestion of the bronchial mucosa may cause wheeze (sometimes known as cardiac asthma). Sitting upright or standing may provide some relief by helping to reduce congestion at the apices of the lungs. The patient may be unable to speak and is typically distressed, agitated, sweaty and pale. Respiration is rapid, with recruitment of accessory muscles, coughing and wheezing. Sputum may be profuse, frothy and blood-streaked or pink. Extensive crepitations and rhonchi are usually audible in the chest and there may also be signs of right heart failure.

Any arrhythmia may cause breathlessness, but usually does so only if the heart is structurally abnormal, such as with the onset of atrial fibrillation in a patient with mitral stenosis. In such cases, the classic mid-diastolic rumbling murmur with pre-systolic accentuation may be heard. Patients sometimes describe chest tightness as 'breathlessness'. However, myocardial ischaemia may also induce true breathlessness by provoking transient left ventricular dysfunction. When breathlessness is the dominant or sole feature of myocardial ischaemia, it is known as 'angina equivalent'. A history of chest tightness or close correlation with exercise should be sought.

Initial investigations

As shown in Box 10.4, amalgamation of a clear history and thorough clinical examination with chest X-ray, ECG and ABG findings will usually indicate the primary cause of breathlessness. If bronchospasm is suspected, measurement of peak expiratory flow will assist in the assessment of severity and should be performed whenever possible. An ABG will often provide additional information to SpO_2 measurement alone, particularly if there is clinical evidence (drowsiness, delirium, asterixis) or a strong likelihood of hypercapnia. An acute rise in $PaCO_2$ will increase the HCO_3^- by only a small amount, resulting in inadequate buffering and acidaemia. Renal compensation and a large rise in HCO_3^- will take at least 12 hours. In acute type II respiratory failure (p. 565), the rate of rise of $PaCO_2$ is a better indicator of severity than the absolute value.

An ABG is essential in the context of smoke inhalation to measure carboxyhaemoglobin level, and is central to the identification of metabolic acidosis or the diagnosis of psychogenic hyperventilation (Box 10.4). If 'angina equivalent' is suspected,

	10.4 Clinical features in acute breathlessness				
Condition	History	Signs	Chest X-ray	ABG	ECG
Pulmonary oedema	Chest pain, palpitations, orthopnoea, cardiac history*	Central cyanosis, ↑JVP, sweating, cool extremities, basal crackles*	Cardiomegaly, oedema/pleural effusions*	↓PaO_2 ↓$PaCO_2$	Sinus tachycardia, ischaemia*, arrhythmia
Massive pulmonary embolus	Risk factors, chest pain, pleurisy, syncope*, dizziness*	Central cyanosis, ↑JVP*, absence of signs in the lung*, shock (tachycardia, hypotension)	Often normal Prominent hilar vessels, oligaemic lung fields*	↓PaO_2 ↓$PaCO_2$	Sinus tachycardia, RBBB, $S_1Q_3T_3$ pattern ↑T(V_1–V_4)
Acute severe asthma	History of asthma, asthma medications, wheeze*	Tachycardia, pulsus paradoxus, cyanosis (late), →JVP*, ↓peak flow, wheeze*	Hyperinflation only (unless complicated by pneumothorax)*	↓PaO_2 ↓$PaCO_2$ (↑$PaCO_2$ in extremis)	Sinus tachycardia (bradycardia in extremis)
Acute exacerbation of COPD	Previous episodes*, smoker. If in type II respiratory failure, may be drowsy	Cyanosis, hyperinflation*, signs of CO_2 retention (flapping tremor, bounding pulses)*	Hyperinflation*, bullae, complicating pneumothorax	↓ or ↓↓PaO_2 ↑$PaCO_2$ in type II failure ± ↑H^+, ↑HCO_3^- in chronic type II failure	Normal, or signs of right ventricular strain
Pneumonia	Prodromal illness*, fever*, rigors*, pleurisy*	Fever, delirium, pleural rub*, consolidation*, cyanosis (if severe)	Pneumonic consolidation*	↓PaO_2 ↓$PaCO_2$ (↑ in extremis)	Tachycardia
Metabolic acidosis	Evidence of diabetes mellitus or renal disease, aspirin or ethylene glycol overdose	Fetor (ketones), hyperventilation without heart or lung signs*, dehydration*, air hunger	Normal	PaO_2 normal ↓↓$PaCO_2$, ↑H^+ ↓HCO_3^-	
Psychogenic	Previous episodes, digital or perioral dysaesthesia	No cyanosis, no heart or lung signs, carpopedal spasm	Normal	PaO_2 normal* ↓↓$PaCO_2$, ↓H^+**	

*Valuable discriminatory feature.
(ABG = arterial blood gas; COPD = chronic obstructive pulmonary disease; JVP = jugular venous pressure; RBBB = right bundle branch block)

objective evidence of myocardial ischaemia from stress testing may help to establish the diagnosis.

Syncope/presyncope

The term 'syncope' refers to sudden loss of consciousness due to reduced cerebral perfusion. 'Presyncope' refers to lightheadedness, in which the individual thinks he or she may 'black out'. Dizziness and presyncope are particularly common in old age (Box 10.5). Symptoms are disabling, undermine confidence and independence, and can affect a person's ability to work or to drive.

There are three principal mechanisms that underlie recurrent presyncope or syncope:

- *cardiac syncope* due to mechanical cardiac dysfunction or arrhythmia
- *neurocardiogenic syncope (also known as vasovagal or reflex syncope)*, in which an abnormal autonomic reflex causes bradycardia and/or hypotension
- *postural hypotension*, in which physiological peripheral vasoconstriction on standing is impaired, leading to hypotension.

There are, however, other causes of loss of consciousness, and differentiating syncope from seizure is a particular challenge. Psychogenic blackouts (also known as non-epileptic seizures or pseudoseizures) also need to be considered in the differential diagnosis.

| 10.5 Dizziness in old age |

- **Prevalence**: common, affecting up to 30% of people aged >65 years.
- **Symptoms**: most frequently described as a combination of unsteadiness and lightheadedness.
- **Most common causes**: postural hypotension and cardiovascular disease. Many patients have more than one underlying cause.
- **Arrhythmia**: can present with lightheadedness either at rest or on activity.
- **Anxiety**: frequently associated with dizziness but rarely the only cause.
- **Falls**: multidisciplinary workup is required if dizziness is associated with falls.

Presentation

The history from the patient *and* a witness is the key to establishing a diagnosis. The terms used for describing the symptoms associated with syncope vary so much among patients that they should not be taken for granted. Some patients use the term 'blackout' to describe a purely visual symptom, rather than loss of consciousness. Some may understand 'dizziness' to mean an abnormal perception of movement (vertigo), some will consider this a feeling of faintness, and others will regard it as unsteadiness. The clinician thus needs to elucidate the exact nature of the symptoms that the patient experiences. The potential differential diagnoses of syncope and presyncope, on the basis of the symptoms described, is shown in Figure 10.3.

The history should always be supplemented by a direct eye-witness account if available. Careful history with corroboration will usually establish whether there has been full consciousness, altered consciousness, vertigo, transient amnesia or something else. Attention should be paid to potential triggers (e.g. medication, micturition, exertion, prolonged standing), the patient's appearance (e.g. colour, seizure activity), the duration of the episode, and the speed of recovery (Box 10.6). Cardiac syncope is usually sudden but can be associated with premonitory lightheadedness, palpitation or chest discomfort. The blackout is usually brief and recovery rapid. Exercise-induced syncope can be the presenting feature of a number of serious pathologies (such as hypertrophic obstructive cardiomyopathy or exercise-induced arrhythmia) and always requires further investigation. Neurocardiogenic syncope will often be associated with a situational trigger (such as pain or emotion), and the patient may experience flushing, nausea, malaise and clamminess for several minutes afterwards. Recovery is usually quick and without subsequent delirium, provided the patient has assumed a supine position. There is often some brief stiffening and limb-twitching, which requires differentiation from seizure-like movements. It is rare for syncope to cause injury or to cause amnesia after regaining awareness. Patients with seizures do not exhibit pallor, may have abnormal movements, usually take more than 5 minutes to recover and are often confused. Aspects of the history that can help to differentiate seizure from syncope are shown in Box 10.7.

A diagnosis of psychogenic blackout (also known as non-epileptic seizure, pseudoseizure or psychogenic seizure) may be suggested by specific emotional triggers, dramatic movements

i	10.6 Typical features of cardiac syncope, neurocardiogenic syncope and seizures		
	Cardiac syncope	**Neurocardiogenic syncope**	**Seizures**
Premonitory symptoms	Often none Lightheadedness Palpitation Chest pain Breathlessness	Nausea Lightheadedness Sweating	Delirium Hyperexcitability Olfactory hallucinations 'Aura'
Unconscious period	Extreme 'death-like' pallor	Pallor	Prolonged (>1 min) unconsciousness Motor seizure activity* Tongue-biting Urinary incontinence
Recovery	Rapid (<1 min) Flushing	Slow Nausea Lightheadedness	Prolonged delirium (>5 mins) Headache Focal neurological signs

*N.B. Cardiac syncope can also cause convulsions by inducing cerebral anoxia.

Fig. 10.3 The differential diagnosis of syncope and presyncope.

10.7 How to differentiate seizures from syncope	Seizure	Syncope
Aura (e.g. olfactory)	+	−
Cyanosis	+	−
Lateral tongue-biting	+	−/+
Post-ictal delirium	+	−
Post-ictal amnesia	+	−
Post-ictal headache	+	−
Rapid recovery	−	+

or vocalisation, or by very prolonged duration (hours). A history of rotational vertigo is suggestive of a labyrinthine or vestibular disorder (p. 1086). Postural hypotension is normally obvious from the history, with presyncope or, less commonly, syncope occurring within a few seconds of standing. The history should include enquiry about predisposing medications (diuretics, vasodilators, antidepressants) and conditions (such as diabetes mellitus and Parkinson's disease).

Clinical assessment

Examination of the patient may be entirely normal, but may reveal clinical signs that favour one form of syncope. The systolic murmurs of aortic stenosis or hypertrophic obstructive cardiomyopathy are important findings, particularly if paired with a history of lightheadedness or syncope on exertion. BP taken when supine and then after 1 and 3 minutes of standing may, when combined with symptoms, provide robust evidence of symptomatic postural hypotension.

Clinical suspicion of hypersensitive carotid sinus syndrome (sensitivity of carotid baroreceptors to external pressure such as a tight collar) should prompt monitoring of the ECG and BP during carotid sinus pressure, provided there is no carotid bruit or history of cerebrovascular disease. A positive cardio-inhibitory response is defined as a sinus pause of 3 seconds or more; a positive vasodepressor response is defined as a fall in systolic BP of more than 50 mmHg. Carotid sinus pressure will produce positive findings in about 10% of elderly individuals, but fewer than 25% of these experience spontaneous syncope. Symptoms should not, therefore, be attributed to hypersensitive carotid sinus syndrome unless they are reproduced by carotid sinus pressure.

Initial investigations

A 12-lead ECG is essential in all patients presenting with syncope or presyncope. Lightheadedness may occur with many arrhythmias, but blackouts (Stokes–Adams attacks, p. 477) are usually due to profound bradycardia or malignant ventricular tachyarrhythmias. The ECG may show evidence of conducting system disease (e.g. sinus bradycardia, atrioventricular block, bundle branch block), which would predispose a patient to bradycardia, but the key to establishing a diagnosis is to obtain an ECG recording *while symptoms are present*. Since minor rhythm disturbances are common, especially in the elderly, symptoms must occur at the same time as a recorded arrhythmia before a diagnosis can be made. Ambulatory ECG recordings are helpful only if symptoms occur several times per week. Patient-activated ECG recorders are useful for examining the rhythm in patients with recurrent dizziness but are not helpful in assessing sudden blackouts. When these investigations fail to establish a cause in patients with presyncope or syncope, an implantable ECG recorder can be sited subcutaneously over the upper left chest. This device continuously records the cardiac rhythm and will activate automatically if extreme bradycardia or tachycardia occurs. The ECG memory can also be tagged by the patient, using a hand-held activator as a form of 'symptom diary'. Stored ECGs can be accessed by the implanting centre, using a telemetry device in a clinic, or using a home monitoring system via an online link.

Head-up tilt-table testing is a provocation test used to establish the diagnosis of vasovagal syncope. It involves positioning the patient supine on a padded table that is then tilted to an angle of 60–70° for up to 45 minutes, while the ECG and BP responses are monitored. A positive test is characterised by bradycardia (cardio-inhibitory response) and/or hypotension (vasodepressor response), associated with typical symptoms.

Delirium

Delirium is a syndrome of transient, reversible cognitive dysfunction that is more common in old age. It is associated with high rates of mortality, complications and institutionalisation, and with longer lengths of stay. The recognised risk factors for delirium are shown in Box 10.8.

Presentation

Delirium manifests as a disturbance of arousal with global impairment of mental function, causing drowsiness with

---

10.8 Risk factors for delirium

Predisposing factors

- Old age
- Dementia
- Frailty
- Sensory impairment
- Polypharmacy
- Renal impairment

Precipitating factors

- Intercurrent illness
- Surgery
- Change of environment or ward
- Sensory deprivation (e.g. darkness) or overload (e.g. noise)
- Medications (e.g. opioids, psychotropics)
- Dehydration
- Pain
- Constipation
- Urinary catheterisation
- Acute urinary retention
- Hypoxia
- Fever
- Alcohol withdrawal

10.9 How to make a diagnosis of delirium: the 4AT

1. Alertness

This includes patients who may be markedly drowsy (e.g. difficult to rouse and/or obviously sleepy during assessment) or agitated/hyperactive. Observe the patient. If asleep, attempt to wake with speech or gentle touch on shoulder. Ask the patient to state their name and address to assist rating:

- Normal (fully alert, but not agitated, throughout assessment) — 0
- Mild sleepiness for <10 secs after waking, then normal — 0
- Clearly abnormal — 4

2. AMT4

Age, date of birth, place (name of the hospital or building), current year:

- No mistakes — 0
- 1 mistake — 1
- ≥2 mistakes/untestable — 2

3. Attention

Say to the patient: 'Please tell me the months of the year in backwards order, starting at December.' To assist initial understanding, one prompt of 'What is the month before December?' is permitted:

- Achieves ≥7 months correctly — 0
- Starts but scores <7 months/refuses to start — 1
- Untestable (cannot start because unwell, drowsy, inattentive) — 2

4. Acute change or fluctuating course

Evidence of significant change or fluctuation in: alertness, cognition, other mental function (e.g. paranoia, hallucinations) arising over the last 2 weeks and still evident in last 24 hrs:

- No — 0
- Yes — 4

Total 4AT score (maximum possible score 12)

≥4: possible delirium ± cognitive impairment
1–3: possible cognitive impairment
0: delirium or severe cognitive impairment unlikely (but delirium still possible if information in 4 incomplete)

(AMT4 = Abbreviated Mental Test 4)

---

disorientation, perceptual errors and muddled thinking. The three broad subtypes of delirium – hypoactive, hyperactive and mixed – can be differentiated on the basis of psychomotor changes. Patients with hyperactive delirium are often agitated and restless, whereas hypoactive delirium can present as lethargy and sedation, and is frequently misdiagnosed as depression or dementia. Fluctuation is typical and delirium is often worse at

10

night, when delirious patients can present significant management difficulties. Emotional disturbance (anxiety, irritability or depression) is common. History-taking from a delirious patient is frequently impossible, and every effort should be made to obtain a collateral history from a close friend or relative. As delirium is particularly common in patients with dementia, the collateral history should ask specifically about onset and course of delirium, along with any functional consequences in comparison to the patient's norm.

Clinical assessment

In order to manage delirium effectively, the first step is to make a diagnosis. Tools such as the 4AT (Box 10.9) or the Confusion Assessment Method (CAM) can be used to detect delirium and differentiate it from dementia; such screening tools should be applied to all older patients admitted to hospital. Once a diagnosis of delirium has been established, attempts should be made to identify all of the reversible precipitating factors. Symptoms suggestive of a physical illness, such as an infection or stroke, should be elicited. An accurate drug and alcohol history is required, especially to ascertain whether any drugs have been recently stopped or started (see Fig. 10.4 for commonly implicated drugs). Although not always possible in its entirety, a full physical examination of all delirious patients should be attempted, noting in particular:

- pyrexia and any signs of infection in the chest, skin, abdomen or urine (on dipstick testing)
- oxygen saturation and signs of CO_2 retention
- signs of alcohol withdrawal or psychoactive drug use, such as tremor or sweating
- any focal neurological signs.

Certain psychiatric conditions, such as depressive pseudo-dementia and dissociative disorder, can easily be mistaken for delirium. Mental state examination is necessary to seek evidence of associated mood disorder, hallucinations, delusions or behavioural abnormalities. Examination should also include cognitive testing with a tool such as the Mini-Mental State Examination (MMSE) or the Montreal Cognitive Assessment (MoCA) (p. 1181).

Investigations and management

Common causes of delirium, along with appropriate investigative pathways, are shown in Figure 10.4. Alongside investigation and treatment of underlying causes, delirium and disorientation should be minimised by a well-lit and quiet environment, with hearing aids and glasses readily available. Good nursing is needed to preserve orientation, prevent pressure sores and falls, and maintain hydration, nutrition and continence. Sedatives may worsen delirium and should be used as a last resort. Resolution of delirium, particularly in the elderly, may be slow and incomplete. Many patients fail to recover to their pre-morbid level of cognition.

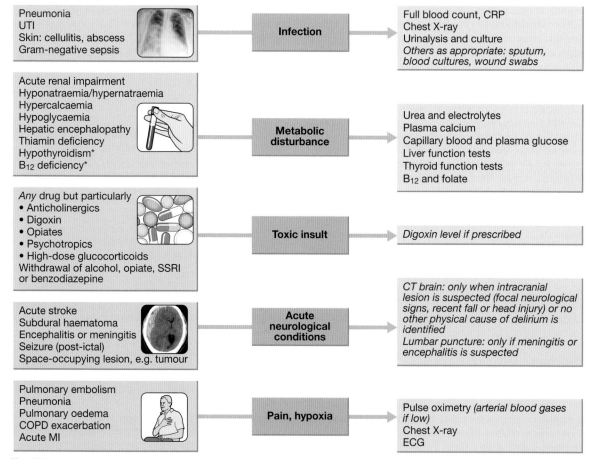

Fig. 10.4 Common causes and investigation of delirium. All investigations are performed routinely, except those in italics. *Tend to present over weeks to months rather than hours to days. The chest X-ray shows right mid- and lower zone consolidation. The CT scan shows a subdural haematoma. (COPD = chronic obstructive pulmonary disease; CRP = C-reactive protein; MI = myocardial infarction; SSRI = selective serotonin re-uptake inhibitor; UTI = urinary tract infection)

Headache

Headache is common and causes considerable worry amongst both patients and clinicians, but rarely represents sinister disease. The causes may be divided into primary or secondary, with primary headache syndromes being vastly more common (Box 10.10).

Presentation

The primary purpose of the history and clinical examination in patients presenting with headache is to identify the small minority of patients with serious underlying pathology. Key features of the history include the temporal evolution of a headache; a headache that reached maximal intensity immediately or within 5 minutes of onset requires rapid assessment for possible subarachnoid haemorrhage. Other 'red flag' symptoms are shown in Box 10.11.

It is important to establish whether the headache comes and goes, with periods of no headache in between (usually migraine), or whether it is present all or almost all of the time. Associated features, such as preceding visual symptoms, nausea/vomiting or photophobia/phonophobia, may support a diagnosis of migraine but others, such as progressive focal symptoms or constitutional upset like weight loss, may suggest a more sinister cause. The headache of cerebral venous thrombosis may be 'throbbing' or 'band-like' and associated with nausea, vomiting or hemiparesis. Raised intracranial pressure (ICP) headache tends to be worse in the morning and when lying flat or coughing, and associated with nausea and/or vomiting.

A description of neck stiffness along with headache and photophobia should raise the suspicion of meningitis (Box 10.12), although this may present in atypical ways in immunosuppressed, alcoholic or pregnant patients. The behaviour of the patient during headache is often instructive; migraine patients typically retire to bed to sleep in a dark room, whereas cluster headache often induces agitated and restless behaviour. The pain of a subarachnoid haemorrhage frequently causes significant distress.

Headache duration is also important to elicit; headaches that have been present for months or years are almost never sinister, whereas new-onset headache, especially in the elderly, is more of a concern. In a patient over 60 years with head pain localised to one or both temples, scalp tenderness or jaw claudication, temporal arteritis (p. 1042) should be considered.

Clinical assessment

An assessment of conscious level (using the Glasgow Coma Scale (GCS); Fig. 10.5) should be performed early and constantly reassessed. A decreased conscious level suggests raised ICP and urgent CT scanning (with airway protection if necessary) is indicated. A full neurological examination may provide clues as to the pathology involved; for example, brainstem signs in the context of acute-onset occipital headache may indicate vertebrobasilar dissection. Neurological signs may, however, be 'falsely localising', as in large subarachnoid haemorrhage or bacterial meningitis. Care should be taken to examine for other evidence of meningitis such as a rash (not always petechial), fever or signs of shock.

Unilateral headache with agitation, ipsilateral lacrimation, facial sweating and conjunctival injection is typical of cluster headache. Conjunctival injection may also be seen in acute glaucoma, accompanied by peri- or retro-orbital pain, clouding of the cornea, decreased visual acuity and, often, systemic upset. Temporal headaches in patients over 60 should prompt examination for enlarged or tender temporal arteries and palpation of temporal pulses (often absent in temporal arteritis). Visual acuity should be assessed promptly, as visual loss is an important complication of temporal arteritis.

Initial investigations

If there is any alteration of conscious level, focal neurological signs, new-onset seizures or a history of head injury, then CT scanning of the head is indicated. The urgency of scanning will depend on the clinical picture and trajectory but in many circumstances

10.10 Primary and secondary headache syndromes

Primary headache syndromes

- Migraine (with or without aura)
- Tension-type headache
- Trigeminal autonomic cephalalgia (including cluster headache)
- Primary stabbing/coughing/exertional/sex-related headache
- Thunderclap headache
- New daily persistent headache syndrome

Secondary causes of headache

- Medication overuse headache (chronic daily headache)
- Intracranial bleeding (subdural haematoma, subarachnoid or intracerebral haemorrhage)
- Raised intracranial pressure (brain tumour, idiopathic intracranial hypertension)
- Infection (meningitis, encephalitis, brain abscess)
- Inflammatory disease (temporal arteritis, other vasculitis, arthritis)
- Referred pain from other structures (orbit, temporomandibular joint, neck)

10.11 'Red flag' symptoms in headache

Symptom	Possible explanation
Sudden onset (maximal immediately or within 5 mins)	Subarachnoid haemorrhage Cerebral venous sinus thrombosis Pituitary apoplexy Meningitis

Focal neurological symptoms (other than for typically migrainous)	Intracranial mass lesion:
	    Vascular
	    Neoplastic
	    Infection

Constitutional symptoms:
    Weight loss
    General malaise
    Pyrexia
    Meningism
    Rash
	Meningitis
	Encephalitis
	Neoplasm (lymphoma or metastases)
	Inflammation (vasculitis)

Raised intracranial pressure (worse on waking/lying down, associated vomiting)	Intracranial mass lesion
New onset aged >60 years	Temporal arteritis

10.12 Identification of bacterial meningitis

In patients presenting with headache, identification of those with bacterial meningitis is a top priority to facilitate rapid antibiotic treatment. In almost all cases there will be one of the following features:
- meningism (neck stiffness, photophobia, positive Kernig's sign)
- fever >38°C
- signs of shock (tachycardia, hypotension, elevated serum lactate)
- rash (not always petechial)

10

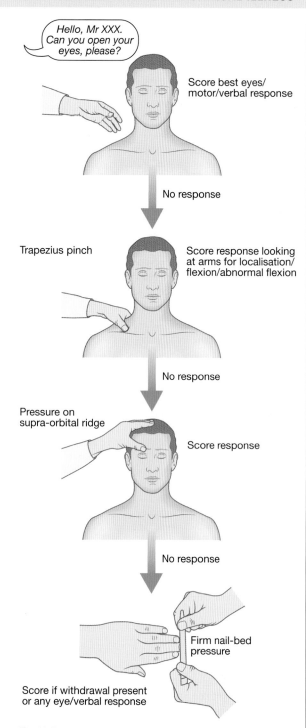

Hello, Mr XXX. Can you open your eyes, please?

Score best eyes/ motor/verbal response

No response

Trapezius pinch

Score response looking at arms for localisation/ flexion/abnormal flexion

No response

Pressure on supra-orbital ridge

Score response

No response

Firm nail-bed pressure

Score if withdrawal present or any eye/verbal response

Fig. 10.5 Assessment of the Glasgow Coma Scale (GCS) score in an obtunded patient. Avoid using a sternal rub, as it causes bruising.

will be immediately required. Intracranial haemorrhage or a space-occupying lesion with mass effect should prompt urgent neurosurgical referral. If bacterial meningitis is suspected (Box 10.12), cerebrospinal fluid (CSF) analysis is required to make a definite diagnosis. Antibiotics should not be delayed for lumbar puncture (LP), which needs to be preceded by CT scanning only if raised ICP is suspected. In cases of thunderclap headache (peak intensity within 5 minutes and lasting over an hour), a normal CT scan should be followed by an LP performed more than 12 hours

after headache onset, to look for evidence of xanthochromia. It is increasingly accepted, however, that a negative CT scan within 6 hours of headache onset has such a high degree of sensitivity for excluding subarachnoid haemorrhage that an LP is not necessary. In such circumstances, a CT angiogram should be considered to exclude other pathology, such as arterial dissection. Many headaches require prompt involvement of specialists. Features of acute glaucoma, for example, require immediate ophthalmological review for measurement of intraocular pressures. Suspected temporal arteritis with an erythrocyte sedimentation rate (ESR) of >50 mm/hr should prompt immediate glucocorticoid therapy and rheumatological referral (see p. 1042 for management). Features of raised ICP in the absence of a mass lesion on neuroimaging may indicate idiopathic intracranial hypertension; CSF opening pressure is likely to be informative.

Unilateral leg swelling

Most leg swelling is caused by oedema, the accumulation of fluid within the interstitial space. There are three explanatory mechanisms for development of oedema that are described in Box 10.13. Unilateral swelling usually indicates a localised pathology in either the venous or the lymphatic system, while bilateral oedema often represents generalised fluid overload combined with the effects of gravity. However, all causes of unilateral leg swelling may present bilaterally, and generalised fluid overload may present with asymmetrical (and therefore apparently unilateral) oedema. Fluid overload may be the result of cardiac failure, pulmonary hypertension (even in the absence of right ventricular failure), renal failure, hypoalbuminaemia or drugs (calcium channel blockers, glucocorticoids, mineralocorticoids, non-steroidal anti-inflammatory drugs (NSAIDs) and others); see Box 16.14 (p. 463) for other causes. The remainder of this section focuses on the causes of 'unilateral' oedema.

Presentation

Any patient who presents with unilateral leg swelling should be assessed with the possibility of deep vein thrombosis (DVT) in mind. The pain and swelling of a DVT is often fairly gradual in onset, over hours or even days. Sudden-onset pain in the posterior aspect of the leg is more consistent with gastrocnemius muscle tear (which may be traumatic or spontaneous) or a ruptured Baker's cyst. Leg swelling and pain associated with paraesthesia or paresis, or in the context of lower limb injury or reduced conscious level, should always prompt concern regarding the possibility of compartment syndrome (Box 10.14).

Clinical assessment

Lower limb DVT characteristically starts in the distal veins, causing an increase in temperature of the limb and dilatation of the superficial veins. Often, however, symptoms and signs are minimal.

i	10.13 Mechanisms of oedema

There are three explanatory mechanisms for the development of oedema that may occur in isolation or combination:
- increased hydrostatic pressure in the venous system due to increased intravascular volume or venous obstruction
- decreased oncotic pressure secondary to a decrease in the plasma proteins that retain fluid within the circulation
- obstruction to lymphatic drainage ('lymphoedema')

✚ 10.14 Identification of compartment syndrome

- Compartment syndrome classically occurs following extrinsic compression of a limb due to trauma or reduced conscious level (especially when caused by drugs or alcohol)
- It usually presents with a tense, firm and exquisitely painful limb
- The pain is characteristically exacerbated by passive muscle stretching or squeezing the compartment
- Altered sensation may be evident distally
- Absent peripheral pulses are a late sign and their presence does not exclude the diagnosis
- Clinical suspicion of compartment syndrome should prompt measurement of creatine kinase and urgent surgical review

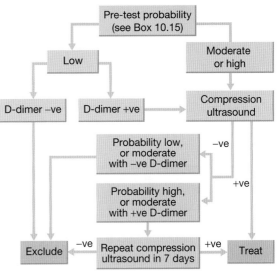

Fig. 10.6 Investigation of suspected deep vein thrombosis. Pre-test probability is calculated in Box 10.15. See also page 11.

Cellulitis is usually characterised by erythema and skin warmth localised to a well-demarcated area of the leg and may be associated with an obvious source of entry of infection (e.g. leg ulcer or insect bite). The patient may be febrile and systemically unwell. Superficial thrombophlebitis is more localised; erythema and tenderness occur along the course of a firm, palpable vein.

Examination of any patient presenting with leg swelling should include assessment for malignancy (evidence of weight loss, a palpable mass or lymphadenopathy). Malignancy is a risk factor for DVT, but pelvic or lower abdominal masses can also produce leg swelling by compressing the pelvic veins or lymphatics. Early lymphoedema is indistinguishable from other causes of oedema. More chronic lymphoedema is firm and non-pitting, often with thickening of the overlying skin, which may develop a 'cobblestone' appearance.

Chronic venous insufficiency is a cause of long-standing oedema that, particularly when combined with another cause of leg swelling, may acutely worsen. Characteristic skin changes (haemosiderin deposition, hair loss, varicose eczema, ulceration) and prominent varicosities are common, and sometimes cause diagnostic confusion with cellulitis. See Box 10.14 for the examination findings associated with compartment syndrome.

Initial investigations

Clinical criteria can be used to rank patients according to their likelihood of DVT, by using scoring systems such as the Wells score (Box 10.15). Figure 10.6 gives an algorithm for investigation of suspected DVT based on initial Wells score. In patients with a low ('unlikely') pre-test probability of DVT, D-dimer levels can be measured; if these are normal, further investigation for DVT is unnecessary. In those with a moderate or high ('likely') probability of DVT or with elevated D-dimer levels, objective diagnosis of DVT should be obtained using appropriate imaging, usually a Doppler ultrasound scan. The investigative pathway for DVT, therefore, differs according to the pre-test probability (p. 11) of DVT. For low-probability DVT, the negative predictive value of the D-dimer test (the most important parameter in this context) is over 99%; if the test is negative, the clinician can discharge the patient with confidence. In patients with a high probability of DVT, the negative predictive value of a D-dimer test falls to somewhere in the region of 97–98%. While this may initially appear to be a high figure, to discharge 2 or 3 patients in every 100 incorrectly would generally be considered an unacceptable error rate. Hence, with the exception of pregnancy (Box 10.16), a combination of clinical probability and blood test results should be used in the diagnosis of venous thromboembolism.

If cellulitis is suspected, serum inflammatory markers, skin swabs and blood cultures should be sent, ideally before antibiotics

ℹ 10.15 Predicting the pre-test probability of deep vein thrombosis (DVT) using the Wells score*

Clinical characteristic	Score
Previous documented DVT	1
Active cancer (patient receiving treatment for cancer within previous 6 months or currently receiving palliative treatment)	1
Paralysis, paresis or recent plaster immobilisation of lower extremities	1
Recently bedridden for ≥3 days, or major surgery within previous 4 weeks	1
Localised tenderness along distribution of deep venous system	1
Entire leg swollen	1
Calf swelling at least 3 cm larger than that on asymptomatic side (measured 10 cm below tibial tuberosity)	1
Pitting oedema confined to symptomatic leg	1
Collateral superficial veins (non-varicose)	1
Alternative diagnosis at least as likely as DVT	−2
Clinical probability	**Total score**
DVT low probability	<1
DVT moderate probability	1–2
DVT high probability	>2

*A dichotomised revised Wells score, which classifies patients as 'unlikely' or 'likely', may also be used.
From Wells PS. Evaluation of D-dimer in the diagnosis of suspected deep-vein thrombosis. N Engl J Med 2003; 349:1227; copyright © 2003 Massachusetts Medical Society.

are given. Ruptured Baker's cyst and calf muscle tear can both be readily diagnosed on ultrasound. If pelvic or lower abdominal malignancy is suspected, a prostate-specific antigen (PSA) level should be measured in males and appropriate imaging with ultrasound (transabdominal or transvaginal) or CT should be undertaken.

10.16 Swollen legs in pregnancy

- **Benign swollen legs**: common in pregnancy; this is usually benign.
- **DVT**: pregnancy is a significant risk factor, however.
- **D-dimer**: should not be measured in pregnancy; it has not been validated in this group.
- **Imaging**: should be arranged on the basis of clinical suspicion alone, and the threshold for undertaking a definite diagnostic test should be low.

Identification and assessment of deterioration

Early warning scores and the role of the medical emergency team

There are many systems that have been developed with the aim of rapidly identifying and managing physiological deterioration. These are referred to as 'rapid response systems'. One popular example of a rapid response system is a medical emergency team (MET). A MET system operates on the basis that when a patient meets certain physiological criteria, the team is alerted. The team is expected to make a rapid assessment and institute immediate management. This may include escalation to critical care or, following liaison with the parent clinical team, ongoing ward-based care.

The trigger for a 'MET' call may be a single parameter – such as a low BP or tachycardia – or may consist of a composite early warning score. Early warning score systems function by the observer allocating a value between 0 and 3 for abnormalities in respiratory rate, SpO_2, temperature, BP, heart rate, neurological response and urine output (Fig. 10.7). The values are summed and the composite score gives an indication of the severity of physiological derangement. Early warning systems can be automated into an electronic format that calculates the score and even alerts the responsible clinician(s) by email or text message.

There are advantages and disadvantages to having a separate MET system, compared with allowing the responsible clinical team to manage deterioration, and to having a composite score or a single parameter detection system. These are outlined in Box 10.17.

Immediate assessment of the deteriorating patient

An approach to assessment of the deteriorating patient can be summarised by the mnemonic 'C-A-B-C-D-E'.

C – Control of obvious problem

For example, if the patient has ventricular tachycardia on the monitor or significant blood loss is apparent, immediate action is required.

A and B – Airway and breathing

If the patient is talking in full sentences, then the airway is clear and breathing is adequate. A rapid history should be obtained while the initial assessment is undertaken. Breathing should be assessed with a focused respiratory examination. Oxygen saturations and ABGs should be checked early (p. 190).

A	NEWS Key 0 1 2 3		Date:							
			Time:							
	Respiratory Rate		≥25							
			21–24							
			12–20							
			9–11							
			≤8							
	SpO2	Chronic Hypoxia	Default							
		≥88	≥91							
			94–95							
	Medical signature required to use scale for patients with Chronic Hypoxia	86–87	92–93							
		≤85	≤91							
	Sign		Unrecordable							
	Inspired 02		% or litres							
	Temperature		≥39°							
			38°							
			37°							
			36°							
			≤35°							
	NEWS SCORE uses Systolic BP		230							
			220							
			210							
			200							
			190							
			180							
			170							
			160							
			150							
			140							
	If manual BP mark as M		130							
			120							
			110							
			100							
			90							
			80							
			70							
			60							
			50							
			Unrecordable							
	Heart Rate		>140							
			130							
			120							
			110							
			100							
			90							
			80							
			70							
			60							
			50							
			40							
			30							
			Regular Y/N							
	Conscious Level		Alert							
			V/P/U							
			New confusion							

Fig. 10.7 Identifying and responding to physiological deterioration.
A An example of an early warning score chart. (NEWS = National Early Warning Score; V/P/U = Verbal/Pain/Unresponsive)

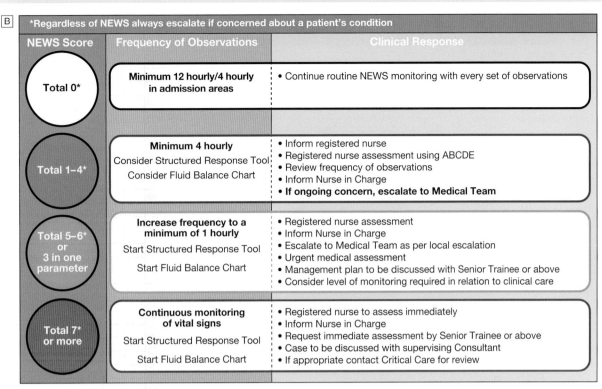

Fig. 10.7, cont'd B Responses to physiological deterioration. *A and B, From Royal College of Physicians. National Early Warning Score (NEWS): standardising the assessment of acute-illness severity in the NHS. Report of a working party. London: RCP, 2012.*

i | 10.17 Advantages and disadvantages of different rapid response systems

System	Advantages	Disadvantages
Single parameter trigger	High sensitivity. Probably picks up subclinical deterioration and allows optimisation	Low specificity. Much time will be spent with patients who are not deteriorating
Composite early warning scoring system, e.g. NEWS or MEWS score	Combines good sensitivity with improved specificity	May miss single parameter deterioration that is still significant, e.g. a drop of 2 GCS points may not trigger an alert
MET system	Brings expertise in deteriorating patients immediately to the bedside	Expensive to have well-trained individuals who are free from other clinical duties. May deskill the ward-based teams in acute care. May not have expertise in highly specific areas of medicine
Clinical team review	Patient is seen by clinicians familiar with the patient and condition	Clinical team may be busy with other urgent duties. There may not be expertise in acute care within the ward-based team

(GCS = Glasgow Coma Scale; MET = Medical Emergency Team; MEWS = Modified Early Warning Score; NEWS = National Early Warning Score)

C – Circulation

A focused cardiovascular examination should include heart rate and rhythm, jugular venous pressure, evidence of bleeding, signs of shock and abnormal heart sounds. The carotid pulse should be palpated in the collapsed or unconscious patient, but peripheral pulses also should be checked in conscious patients. The radial, brachial, foot and femoral pulses may disappear as shock progresses, and this indicates the severity of circulatory compromise.

D – Disability

Conscious level should be assessed using the GCS (see Fig. 10.5 and Box 10.24, pp. 186 and 194). A brief neurological examination looking for focal signs should be performed. Capillary blood glucose should always be measured to exclude hypoglycaemia or severe hyperglycaemia.

E – Exposure and evidence

'Exposure' indicates the need for targeted clinical examination of the remaining body systems, particularly the abdomen and lower limbs. 'Evidence' may be gathered via a collateral history from other health-care professionals or family members, recent investigations, prescriptions or monitoring charts.

Selecting the appropriate location for ongoing management

Any patient who will gain benefit from a critical care area should be admitted. Such patients generally fall into two groups: those with organ dysfunction severe enough to require organ support and those in whom the disease process is clearly setting them on a downward trajectory and in whom early, aggressive management may alter the outcome. Whether an individual patient should be

	10.18 Levels of care and the corresponding admission criteria for intensive care unit (ICU) and high-dependency unit (HDU)	
Level of care	**Criteria**	**Appropriate location**
3	Patients requiring/likely to require endotracheal intubation and invasive mechanical ventilatory support Patients requiring support of two or more organ systems (e.g. inotropes and haemofiltration) Patients with chronic impairment of one or more organ systems (e.g. COPD or severe ischaemic heart disease) who require support for acute reversible failure of another organ	**ICU**

2	Patients requiring detailed observation or monitoring that cannot be provided at ward level:
	   Direct arterial BP monitoring
	   CVP monitoring
	   Fluid balance
	   Neurological observations, regular GCS recording
	Patients requiring support for a single failing organ system, excluding invasive ventilatory support (IPPV):
	   Non-invasive respiratory support (p. 202)
	   Moderate inotropic or vasopressor support
	   Renal replacement therapy in an otherwise stable patient
	Step-down from intensive care requiring additional monitoring or single organ support
		HDU

1	Patients in whom frequent but intermittent observations and medical review are sufficient	**General ward setting**

(BP = blood pressure; COPD = chronic obstructive pulmonary disease; CVP = central venous pressure; GCS = Glasgow Coma Scale; IPPV = intermittent positive pressure ventilation)

admitted to the intensive care or high-dependency unit (ICU/HDU) will depend on local arrangements. A useful tool to assist with the decision regarding location is the 'level of care' required (Box 10.18). Many intensive care units are a mix of level 2 and level 3 beds, which streamlines the admission process.

Common presentations of deterioration

As patients become critically unwell, they usually manifest physiological derangement. The principle underpinning critical care is the simultaneous assessment of illness severity and the stabilisation of life-threatening physiological abnormalities. The goal is to prevent deterioration and effect improvements, as the diagnosis is established and treatment of the underlying disease process is initiated.

It can be useful to consider the physiological changes as a starting point to help delineate urgent investigations and supportive treatment, which should proceed alongside the search for a definitive diagnosis.

Tachypnoea

Pathophysiology

A raised respiratory rate (tachypnoea) is the earliest and most sensitive sign of clinical deterioration. Tachypnoea may be primary (i.e. a problem within the respiratory system) or secondary to pathology elsewhere in the body. Cardiopulmonary causes of tachypnoea have been covered on page 179. Secondary tachypnoea is usually due to a metabolic acidosis, most commonly observed in the context of sepsis, haemorrhage, ketoacidosis or visceral ischaemia. More detailed information on metabolic acidosis can be found on page 364.

Assessment and management

A simple assessment of a patient's clinical status and basic physiology will usually indicate whether urgent intervention is required. In the examination, attention should be paid to the adequacy of chest expansion, air entry and the presence of added sounds such as wheeze.

Analysis of an arterial blood sample is especially helpful in narrowing the differential diagnosis and confirming clinical suspicion of severity. The 'base excess' provides rapid quantification of the component of disease that is metabolic in origin. A base excess lower than −2 mEq/L (or, put another way, a 'base deficit' of more than 2 mEq/L) is likely to represent a metabolic acidosis. A simple rule of thumb is that a lactate of more than 4 mmol/L or a base deficit of more than 10 mEq/L should cause concern and trigger escalation to a higher level of care. In addition to clinical examination, chest radiography and bedside ultrasound can help to distinguish the cause of poor air entry; consolidation and effusion can be readily identified and a significant pneumothorax can be excluded (as shown in Fig. 10.8).

Hypoxaemia

Pathophysiology

Low arterial partial pressure of oxygen (PaO_2) is termed hypoxaemia. It is a common presenting feature of deterioration. Hypoxia is defined as an inadequate amount of oxygen in tissues (or the inability of cells to use the available oxygen for cellular respiration). Hypoxia may be due to hypoxaemia, or may be secondary to impaired cardiac output, the presence of inadequate or dysfunctional haemoglobin, or intracellular dysfunction (such as in cyanide poisoning, where oxygen utilisation at the cellular level is impaired).

Over 97% of oxygen carried in the blood is bound to haemoglobin. The haemoglobin–oxygen dissociation curve delineates the relationship between the percentage saturation of haemoglobin with oxygen (SO_2) and the partial pressure (PO_2) of oxygen in the blood. A shift in the curve will influence the uptake and release of oxygen by the haemoglobin molecule. As capillary PCO_2 rises, the curve moves to the right, increasing the offloading of oxygen in the tissues (the Bohr effect). This increases capillary PO_2 and hence cellular oxygen supply. Shifts of the oxyhaemoglobin dissociation curve can have significant implications in certain disease processes (Fig. 10.9).

Fig. 10.8 Using ultrasound to rule out an anterior pneumothorax. [A] Probe position and orientation. [B] and [C] Two-dimensional (2D) ultrasound images. [D] and [E] M-mode ultrasound images. Key: (1) Intercostal muscle. (2) Rib. (3) Normal bright pleural line –'shimmering appearance' of sliding pleura. (4) Lung. (5) Absent 'shimmering' in pneumothorax and lung not visible. (6) Normal – 'sea shore' sign excludes pneumothorax at that location. The 'sea shore' is represented by the bright granular line with lung (sea) deeper to the bright line. (7) Absent granular pleural line and a repeating linear pattern or 'barcode' sign suggest the presence of pneumothorax.

10

Fig. 10.9 The haemoglobin–oxygen dissociation curve and the effect of CO_2 on oxygen saturations. In pulmonary embolism, compensatory hyperventilation often occurs. $PaCO_2$ decreases, shifting the oxyhaemoglobin saturation curve to the left (green line). Therefore, despite a low PaO_2 (8 kPa/60 mmHg), the saturation reading is 93%.

Due to the shape of the curve, a small drop in arterial PO_2 (PaO_2) below 8 kPa (60 mmHg) will cause a marked fall in SaO_2.

Relative hypoxaemia refers to the comparison between the observed PaO_2 and that which might be expected for a given fraction of inspired oxygen (FiO_2). With the patient breathing air, PaO_2 of 12–14 kPa (90–105 mmHg) would be expected; with the patient breathing 100% oxygen, a PaO_2 of >60 kPa (450 mmHg) would be normal.

Assessment and management

Oxygen therapy should be titrated to avoid hyperoxia (too high a PaO_2; Box 10.19). Hyperoxia is theoretically harmful via a number of mechanisms. This has a clinically significant effect in patients

---

10.19 Prescribing oxygen in critical illness

• Oxygen should be prescribed to achieve a target saturation of 94–98% for most critically unwell patients.
• 88–92% is a more appropriate target range for those at risk of hypercapnic respiratory failure.

---

with acute stroke, those with MI and those who chronically retain CO_2. Adverse effects of hyperoxia include:

• free radical-induced tissue damage
• less efficient buffering of carbon dioxide by oxyhaemoglobin (compared to deoxyhaemoglobin)
• less efficient ventilation–perfusion matching in lung units (due to loss of hypoxic vasoconstriction of under-ventilated lung units)
• decreased hypoxic respiratory drive in individuals with chronic hypercapnia.

When attempting to determine the cause of hypoxaemia, it is useful to consider whether the primary physiological mechanism is a type of shunt, or one of the many causes of ventilation–perfusion mismatch, such as alveolar or central hypoventilation (Fig. 10.10). A classification of common causes of hypoxaemia in hospitalised patients is shown in Box 10.20. In reality, the observed physiological abnormality may represent a combination of inter-related processes, such as severe pulmonary oedema leading to exhaustion, which in turn causes hypoventilation.

Evaluation of risk factors, history and examination will help to differentiate the likely aetiology and guide specific management. Further management of respiratory failure is discussed on page 202.

Tachycardia

Pathophysiology

A heart rate of >110 beats/min in an adult should always be considered abnormal and not attributed to anxiety until other causes have been excluded. Intrinsic cardiac causes (atrial fibrillation (AF), atrial flutter, supraventricular tachycardia and

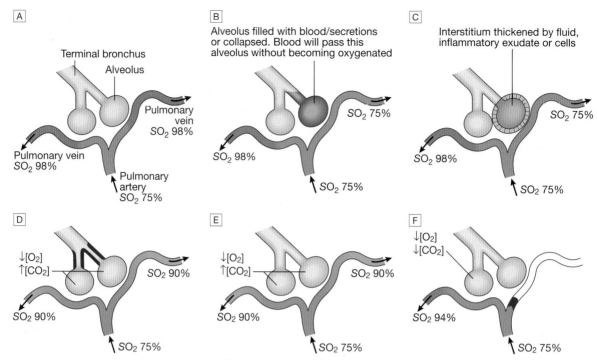

Fig. 10.10 Theoretical mechanisms of hypoxaemia. A Normal physiology. B Shunt caused by alveolar filling, e.g. in pneumonia or alveolar haemorrhage. The mixture of oxygenated and deoxygenated blood causes arterial desaturation. C Shunt caused by interstitial pathology, e.g. pulmonary oedema or fibrosis. Interstitial thickening causes inadequate transfer of oxygen from the alveolus to the blood, leading to shunting and arterial desaturation. Because minute volume is usually maintained, this causes type I respiratory failure. D Ventilation–perfusion ($\dot{V}/\dot{Q}$) mismatch caused by alveolar hypoventilation, e.g. in chronic obstructive pulmonary disease (COPD)/asthma. Alveoli are under-ventilated relative to perfusion. Alveolar PO_2 falls and PCO_2 rises, causing type II respiratory failure. E $\dot{V}/\dot{Q}$ mismatch caused by central hypoventilation, e.g. in neuromuscular disease or narcotic use. The alveoli are relatively over-perfused, causing type II respiratory failure. F $\dot{V}/\dot{Q}$ mismatch caused by a perfusion defect, e.g. a small pulmonary embolism. Pulmonary blood flow is diverted to other alveoli, causing them to be relatively over-perfused and thus reducing alveolar PO_2. Minute volume is increased, so PCO_2 is not elevated.

i **10.20 Common causes of hypoxaemia in hospitalised patients**

Hypoxaemia due to shunt

- Lung collapse
- Consolidation/alveolar haemorrhage
- Interstitial oedema or interstitial infiltration (e.g. fibrosis)
- Silent aspiration of gastric contents

Hypoxaemia due to ventilation–perfusion mismatch

- Pulmonary embolism
- Acute exacerbation of asthma
- COPD (with high minute volume)

Hypoxaemia from hypoventilation

- Effects of opiates
- Severe COPD (with low minute volume)
- Neuromuscular disease/general weakness from other illness

(COPD = chronic obstructive pulmonary disease)

ventricular dysrhythmias) are less common in the general inpatient population than secondary causes of tachycardia.

A cardiac monitor or 12-lead ECG early in the examination will help both determine severity (heart rate >160 beats/min should prompt urgent escalation to a higher level of care) and narrow the differential diagnosis. AF with a rapid ventricular response should usually be regarded as secondary to another insult (mostly commonly, infection) until other diagnoses have been excluded.

Hypovolaemia should not be missed. Concealed bleeding (e.g. into the pleura, gastrointestinal tract or retroperitoneum) may not be apparent initially and assessment of haemoglobin in an acute haemorrhage, when <30 mL/kg of fluid has been administered, can be misleadingly high. Sepsis and other hyper-metabolic conditions may present with a tachycardia that is accompanied by tachypnoea, peripheral vasodilatation and a raised temperature. Other organ dysfunction should be noted from a brief general examination and salient points from the history.

Assessment and management

The management of a tachycardic patient should focus on treating the cause. Treating the rate alone with beta-blockade in an unwell or deteriorating patient should be done only under specialist guidance, in controlled conditions, and when a clear evaluation of the risk–benefit ratio has been undertaken.

The recognition and management of primary cardiac dysrhythmias are discussed on page 468. The most appropriate method of rate control in AF depends primarily on the degree of haemodynamic compromise. An intravenous loading dose of amiodarone is well tolerated and efficacious in the majority of critically ill patients with AF and a very rapid ventricular rate. There are thromboembolic concerns regarding chemical cardioversion of AF of unknown duration. However, in deteriorating patients, the low incidence of embolic events makes this concern of secondary importance to achieving haemodynamic stability.

Digoxin continues to have a role in the treatment of AF in critically unwell but haemodynamically stable patients, when its inotropic properties can be helpful. Electrical cardioversion is reserved for dysrhythmias with extremely high heart rates, following failure of pharmacological management, and/or for those of ventricular origin. It is rarely successful in dysrhythmias secondary to systemic illness.

Hypotension

Pathophysiology

Low BP (hypotension) should always be defined in relation to a patient's usual BP. The calculation of mean arterial pressure (MAP) is shown in Box 10.21; it unifies the systolic and diastolic BPs into a single reference value. A MAP of >65 mmHg will maintain renal perfusion in the majority of patients, although a MAP of up to 80 mmHg may be required in patients with chronic hypertension.

Assessment and management

The first stage of assessment is to decide if the hypotension is physiological or pathological. The MAP is useful as, despite low systolic pressures, it is rare to see a physiological MAP of <65 mmHg. Urine output is particularly useful in the determination of the desirable MAP for an individual patient; oliguria suggests that measures to increase the MAP should be sought (p. 204). If the hypotension is pathological, an assessment of severity should look at whether it is causing physiological harm to the patient (i.e. the patient is shocked).

Shock

Shock means 'circulatory failure'. It can be defined as a level of oxygen delivery (DO_2) that fails to meet the metabolic requirements of the tissues (Box 10.22). Hypotension is a common presentation of shock but the terms are not synonymous. Patients can be hypotensive but not shocked, and oxygen delivery can be critically low in the context of a 'normal' BP. Along with the signs of low cardiac output (Box 10.23), objective markers of inadequate tissue oxygen delivery, such as increasing base deficit, elevated blood lactate and reduced urine output, can aid

10.21 Calculation of mean arterial pressure (MAP)

$$MAP = \text{Diastolic blood pressure} + \frac{(\text{systolic} - \text{diastolic})}{3}$$

At normal heart rates, the heart, on average, spends two-thirds of the cycle in diastole. The MAP reflects this by weighting the value towards the diastolic blood pressure

10.22 Oxygen content and delivery

- Oxygen content of blood = *Haemoglobin level × oxygen saturation × constant
- Cardiac output = Heart rate × stroke volume
- Stroke volume is dependent on cardiac filling (preload) and contractility
- In shock, the most productive measures to improve oxygen delivery are optimising the haemoglobin level and the cardiac output

*Oxygen is almost exclusively bound to haemoglobin; only tiny amounts are dissolved in blood at atmospheric pressure.

10.23 Hypotension in relation to cardiac output: clinical signs and possible causes

	High cardiac output	Low cardiac output
Signs	Warm hands Pulsatile head movement High-volume/strong pulse Low venous pressure	Cold/clammy peripheries Peripheral cyanosis Raised venous pressure
Causes	Sepsis Allergy Drug overdose (e.g. antihypertensive) Acidosis (e.g. diabetic ketoacidosis) Thyrotoxicosis Beri-beri	Bleeding Aortic stenosis and failed compensation Dysrhythmia Obstructive (pulmonary embolism/tamponade/dynamic hyperinflation as in severe asthma) Chronic heart failure

10

early identification. If shock is suspected, resuscitation should be commenced (p. 204).

Hypotensive patients who do not have any evidence of shock are still at significant risk of organ dysfunction. Hypotension should serve as a 'red flag' that there may be serious underlying pathology. Organ failure occurs despite normal or elevated oxygen delivery, so a full assessment of the patient is indicated. A review of the drug chart is essential, as many inpatients will be on antihypertensive medications that are contributing to hypotension. Non-cardiac medications may also have a negative influence on BP; for example, some drugs used for urine outflow tract obstruction, such as tamsulosin, have an α-adrenoceptor-blocking effect.

Hypertension

Pathophysiology

High BP (hypertension) is common and is usually benign in a critical care context. However, it can be the presenting feature of a number of serious disease processes. Furthermore, acute hypertension can result in an acute rise in vascular tone that increases left ventricular end-systolic pressure (afterload). The left ventricle may be unable to eject blood against the increased aortic pressure, and acute pulmonary oedema can result (referred to as 'flash' pulmonary oedema.)

Assessment and management

Before treating an acute rise in BP, it is worth considering a few important diagnoses that may impact on the immediate management:

- *Intracranial event.* Ischaemia of the brainstem (commonly via a pressure effect) will cause acute increases in BP. A neurological examination and CT scan of the head should be considered.
- *Fluid overload.* Once the capacity of the venous blood reservoir becomes saturated, increases in fluid volume will lead to increases in BP. This can occur in younger patients without the onset of peripheral oedema and originate from myocardial dysfunction or impaired renal clearance.
- *Underlying medical problems.* A brief search for a history of renal disease, spinal injury and less common metabolic causes such as phaeochromocytoma can be worthwhile. In women of child-bearing age, pregnancy-induced

hypertension and pre-eclampsia must always be considered.

- *Primary cardiac problems*. Myocardial ischaemia, acute heart failure and aortic dissection can all present with hypertension.
- *Drug-related problems*. Most commonly, these involve a missed antihypertensive medication, but sympathomimetic drugs such as cocaine and amphetamines can be implicated.

The management of hypertension is discussed further on page 510.

Decreased conscious level

Assessment

A reduction in conscious level should prompt an urgent assessment of the patient, a search for the likely cause and an evaluation of the risk of airway loss. The GCS was developed to risk-stratify head injury, but it has become the most widely recognised assessment tool for conscious level (see Box 10.24 for breakdown of GCS assessment, Box 10.25 for how to communicate the findings and Fig. 10.5 for how to assess GCS). While disorders that affect language or limb function (e.g. left hemisphere stroke, locked-in syndrome) may reduce its usefulness, evaluation of the GCS usually provides helpful prognostic information, and serial recordings can plot improvement or deterioration. It is not possible to define a total score below which a patient is unlikely to be able to protect the airway (from aspiration or obstruction), but a motor score of less than 5 would suggest significant risk.

Coma is defined as a persisting state of deep unconsciousness. In practice, this means a sustained GCS of 8 or less. There are many causes of coma (Box 10.26), including neurological (structural or non-structural brain disease) and non-neurological (e.g. type II respiratory failure) ones. The mode of onset of coma and any precipitating event is crucial to establishing the cause, and should be obtained from witnesses. Failure to obtain an adequate history for patients in coma is a common cause of diagnostic delay.

Once the patient is stable from a cardiorespiratory perspective, examination should include accurate assessment of conscious level and a thorough general medical examination, looking for clues such as needle tracks indicating drug abuse, rashes, fever and focal signs of infection, including neck stiffness or evidence of head injury. Focal neurological signs may suggest a structural explanation (stroke or tumour) or may be falsely localising (for example, 6th nerve palsy can occur as a consequence of raised intracerebral pressure). It is vital to exclude non-neurological causes of coma. Sodium and glucose should be measured urgently as part of the initial assessment, as acute hyponatraemia (p. 358) and hypoglycaemia (p. 738) are easily corrected and can cause irreversible brain injury if missed.

🩺 10.25 How to communicate conscious level to other health-care professionals

- It is best to state the physical response along with the numerical score
- For example, 'a patient who doesn't open his eyes, withdraws to pain and makes groaning noises, having a GCS of E1, M4, V2, making a total of 7' is preferable to 'a male with a GCS of 7'

ℹ 10.24 Glasgow Coma Scale (GCS)*

Eye-opening (E)

• Spontaneous	4
• To speech	3
• To pain	2
• Nil	1

Best motor response (M)

• Obeys commands	6
• Localises to painful stimulus	5
• Flexion to painful stimulus or withdraws hand from pain	4
• Abnormal flexion (internal rotation of shoulder, flexion of wrist)	3
• Extensor response (external rotation of shoulder, extension of wrist)	2
• Nil	1

Verbal response (V)

• Orientated	5
• Confused conversation	4
• Inappropriate words	3
• Incomprehensible sounds	2
• Nil	1

Coma score = E + M + V

Always present GCS as breakdown, not a sum score (unless 3 or 15)

• Minimum sum	3
• Maximum sum	15

*Record the best score observed. When the patient is intubated, there can be no verbal response. The suffix 'T' should replace the verbal component of the score, and the remainder of the score is therefore a maximum of 10.

ℹ 10.26 Causes of coma

Metabolic disturbance

- Drug overdose
- Diabetes mellitus:
  Hypoglycaemia
  Ketoacidosis
  Hyperosmolar coma
- Hyponatraemia
- Uraemia
- Hepatic failure (hyperammonaemia)
- Inborn errors of metabolism causing hyperammonaemia
- Hyperammonaemia on refeeding following profound anorexia
- Respiratory failure
- Hypothermia
- Hypothyroidism

Trauma

- Cerebral contusion
- Extradural haematoma
- Subdural haematoma
- Diffuse axonal injury

Vascular disease

- Subarachnoid haemorrhage
- Brainstem infarction/ haemorrhage
- Intracerebral haemorrhage
- Cerebral venous sinus thrombosis

Infections

- Meningitis
- Encephalitis
- Cerebral abscess
- Systemic sepsis

Others

- Epilepsy
- Brain tumour
- Functional ('pseudo-coma')

Fig. 10.11 Hyperacute changes in conscious state are commonly of vascular origin. CT of the brain is unlikely to identify many vascular causes but a CT angiogram of the circle of Willis is a high-yield investigation in this context. [A] Non-contrast CT of the head showing hyperdense thrombus in the basilar artery (arrow). This is a specific, but not sensitive, sign. [B] CT angiogram of the circle of Willis demonstrating thrombosis in the basilar artery (arrow). This has better sensitivity for acute vascular occlusion.

Further investigations should be guided by the clinical presentation and examination findings; a sudden onset suggests a vascular cause. An early CT scan of the brain may demonstrate any gross pathology but if a brainstem stroke is suspected (Fig. 10.11), a CT angiogram of the circle of Willis will provide more useful information, as a non-contrast CT is frequently negative in this context. If there are features suggestive of cerebral venous thrombosis, such as thrombophilia or sinus infection, a CT venogram should be performed. Meningitis or encephalitis may be suggested by the history, signs of infection or subtle radiological findings. If these diagnoses are considered, it is best to commence treatment with broad-spectrum antibiotics and antivirals while awaiting more definitive diagnostic information.

Other drug, metabolic and hepatic causes of reduced conscious level are dealt with in the relevant chapters. An ammonia level (sent on ice) can narrow the differential diagnosis to a metabolic or hepatic cause if there is diagnostic doubt; levels >100 µmol/L (140 µg/dL) are significantly abnormal. Psychiatric conditions such as catatonic depression or neurological conditions such as the autoimmune encephalitides can cause a reduced level of consciousness, but they are diagnoses of exclusion and will require specialist input.

Management

Moving an unconscious patient into the recovery position is best for airway protection while preparations are made for escalation to a higher level of care. The decision regarding intubation for airway protection is always difficult. Length of stay in intensive care is significantly reduced if there is no secondary organ dysfunction. Therefore, early intubation and the prevention of lung injury constitute the safer option if there is any doubt about a patient's ability to protect the airway from obstruction or aspiration.

Decreased urine output/deteriorating renal function

Assessment

A urine output of 0.5 mL/kg/hr is a commonly quoted, though admittedly arbitrary target. Although some patients can produce urine volumes below this level with no change in their renal biochemistry, such low volumes should alert the clinician to the possibility of suboptimal renal perfusion.

Oliguria in association with hypotension or an increase in serum creatinine level (even if small) should prompt examination for the underlying cause. Pre-renal causes predominate in the general inpatient population, so optimising the MAP by administration of intravenous fluids (and possibly vasopressors) is the first priority. In the majority of inpatients there is no role for high volumes (i.e. >30 mL/kg) of intravenous fluid if the MAP is normal. Exceptions to this rule include patients with clinical dehydration or high fluid losses such as in burns, diabetes emergencies (pp. 735 and 738) and diabetes insipidus (p. 687), where fluid management should be guided by local protocols.

Diagnosis and management

Further assessment and management of oliguria are explained on page 391. Two other important causes of renal failure in the inpatient population are abdominal compartment syndrome and rhabdomyolysis.

Abdominal compartment syndrome

Abdominal compartment syndrome occurs when raised pressure within the abdomen reduces perfusion to the abdominal organs. It is most commonly seen in surgical patients, but can occur in medical conditions with extreme fluid retention such as liver cirrhosis. When it is suspected, intra-abdominal pressure can be monitored via a pressure transducer connected to a urinary catheter (following instillation of 25 mL of 0.9% saline into the bladder). Values over 20 mmHg suggest abdominal compartment syndrome is present. Urgent measures should be taken to reduce the pressure, such as decompression of the stomach, bladder and peritoneum if ascites is present. If conservative measures fail, a laparostomy should be considered.

Rhabdomyolysis

Rhabdomyolysis occurs when there is an injury to a large volume of skeletal muscle, usually because a single limb or muscle compartment has been ischaemic for a prolonged period. It can also occur following trauma and crush injury or after over-exertion of muscles. Over-exertion can occur after intense physical exercise or as part of a medical condition that causes widespread muscular activity, such as malignant hyperpyrexia or neuroleptic malignant syndrome. A creatine kinase (CK) level of >1000 U/L is highly suggestive, although it can rise to tens of thousands in severe cases. Management should focus on identification and correction of the underlying cause and support for multi-organ dysfunction. Forced alkaline diuresis (using intravenous bicarbonate infusion and furosemide) can be used to maintain a good flow of less acidic fluid within the renal tubules and reduce myoglobin precipitation.

Disorders causing critical illness

Sepsis and the systemic inflammatory response

Sepsis is one of the most common causes of multi-organ failure. Sepsis requires the presence of infection with a resultant systemic inflammatory state; organ dysfunction occurs from a combination of the two processes. The definition of sepsis has undergone various iterations and there is still a lack of consensus as to the exact wording that best reflects this complex, multisystem process (Box 10.27).

Aetiology and pathogenesis

To understand how an infection can lead to progressive multi-organ failure, it is essential to have a grasp of the pathophysiology.

Initiation of the inflammatory response

The process begins with infection in one part of the body that triggers a localised inflammatory response. Appropriate source control and a competent immune system will, in most cases, contain the infection at this stage. However, if certain factors are present, the infection may become systemic. The causative factors are not fully elucidated but probably include:

- a genetic predisposition to sepsis
- a large microbiological load
- high virulence of the organism
- delay in source control (either surgical or antimicrobial)
- resistance of the organism to treatment
- patient factors (immune status, nutrition, frailty).

Mediators are released from damaged cells (called 'alarmins') and these, coupled with direct stimulation of immune cells by the molecular patterns of the microorganism, trigger the inflammatory response. An example of such direct stimulation is that of lipopolysaccharide, which is found on the surface of Gram-negative bacteria. It strongly stimulates an immune response and is commonly used in research settings to initiate a septic cascade.

Viral and fungal infections can cause a syndrome that is clinically indistinguishable from bacterial sepsis. Likewise, numerous

non-infective processes, such as pancreatitis, burns, trauma, major surgery and drug reactions, can cause alarmins to be released and initiate the process of systemic inflammation.

Propagation of the inflammatory response

Once activated, immune cells such as macrophages release the inflammatory cytokines interleukin-2 (IL-2), IL-6 and tumour necrosis factor alpha, which, in turn, activate neutrophils. Activated neutrophils express adhesion factors and release various other inflammatory and toxic substances; the net effects are vasodilatation (via activation of inducible nitric oxide synthase enzymes) and damage to the endothelium. Neutrophils migrate into the interstitial space; fluid and plasma proteins will also leak through the damaged endothelium, leading to oedema and intravascular fluid depletion.

Activation of the coagulation system

Damaged endothelium triggers the coagulation cascade (via tissue factor, factor VII, and reduced activity of proteins C and S) and thrombus forms within the microvasculature. A vicious circle of endothelial injury, intravascular coagulation and microvascular occlusion develops, causing more tissue damage and further release of inflammatory mediators. In severe sepsis, intravascular coagulation can become widespread. This is referred to as disseminated intravascular coagulation (DIC) and usually heralds the onset of multi-organ failure. Specific aspects of the diagnosis and management of DIC are discussed on page 978.

Organ damage from sepsis

Any and all organs may be injured by severe sepsis. The pathological mechanisms are shown in Figure 10.12.

Lactate physiology

Lactate is an excellent biomarker for the severity of sepsis. Hyperlactataemia (serum lactate >2.4 mmol/L or 22 mg/dL) is used as a marker of severity. Figure 10.13 explains the physiology of hyperlactataemia; it is caused by all types of shock and therefore is not specific to sepsis. A lactate level of >8 mmol/L (>73 mg/dL) is associated with an extremely high mortality and should trigger immediate escalation. Measures to optimise oxygen delivery should be sought, and the adequacy of resuscitation measured by lactate clearance.

The anti-inflammatory cascade

As the inflammatory state develops, a compensatory anti-inflammatory system is activated involving the release of anti-inflammatory cytokines such as IL-4 and IL-10 from immune cells. While such mechanisms are necessary to keep the inflammatory response in check, they may lead to a period of immunosuppression after the initial septic episode. Patients recovering from severe sepsis are prone to developing secondary infections due to a combination of this immunosuppression and the presence of indwelling devices.

Management

The most important action is to consider sepsis as the cause of a patient's deterioration. Aligned to this is the requirement to consider other diagnoses that could be causing the presentation, such as haemorrhage, PE, anaphylaxis or a low cardiac output state.

Resuscitation in sepsis

General resuscitative measures are discussed on page 204. Early resuscitation can be aided by following the requirements of the

---

10.27 Definitions of sepsis and septic shock*

Sepsis

Patients with suspected infection who have 2 or more of:
- *Hypotension* – systolic blood pressure <100 mmHg
- *Altered mental status* – Glasgow Coma Scale score ≤14
- *Tachypnoea* – respiratory rate ≥22 breaths/min

Sepsis can also be diagnosed by suspected infection and an increase of ≥2 points on the Sequential Organ Failure Assessment (SOFA) score (p. 214)

Septic shock

A subset of sepsis with underlying circulatory or cellular/metabolic abnormalities associated with a substantially increased mortality:
- Sepsis and both of (after fluid resuscitation):
  1. Persistent hypotension requiring vasopressors to maintain a MAP >65 mmHg
  2. Serum lactate >2 mmol/L (18 mg/dL)

*From the Third International Consensus Definitions for Sepsis and Septic Shock (Sepsis-3).

'Sepsis Six' (Box 10.28). Red cell transfusion should be used to target a haemoglobin concentration of 70–90 g/L (7–9 g/dL). Albumin 4% can be used as colloid solution and has the theoretical benefit of remaining in the intravascular space for longer than crystalloid. Early intubation is recommended in severe cases to facilitate further management and reduce oxygen demand.

Appropriate antibiotics should be administered as early as possible (Box 10.29). The antibiotic choice will depend on local patterns of resistance, patient risk factors and the likely source of infection. Information on likely organisms and appropriate antibiotics can be found on pages 117 and 226. Microbiological samples (such as blood cultures, urine or CSF) should be taken, but this should not delay antibiotic administration, if obtaining samples is difficult.

Early source control

Source control requires an accurate diagnosis; urgent investigations should be performed as soon as physiological stability has been established. A CT scan of the chest and abdomen with contrast is a high-yield test in this context. Specific points in the history should be reviewed, such as risk factors for human immunodeficiency virus (HIV), contacts with tuberculosis and underlying immune status. Immunocompromised patients will be susceptible to a far broader spectrum of infectious microorganisms (p. 223).

Fig. 10.12 Pathophysiology of organ damage in sepsis. *Macrovascular.* Severe hypovolaemia, vasodilatation or septic cardiomyopathy can reduce oxygen delivery, causing tissue hypoxia. Paradoxically, most patients with sepsis have an increased cardiac output and oxygen delivery. *Microvascular.* Tissue injury can occur from hypoxia secondary to microvascular injury and thrombosis. Damaged epithelium permits neutrophils, proteins and fluid to leak out. *Shunting.* Organs fail in sepsis despite supranormal blood flow. It is likely that arteriovenous shunt pathways exist within vascular beds; these shunts open up in septic shock. *Cellular.* Cells are damaged by a number of mechanisms in sepsis: (1) direct injury by microorganisms; (2) injury from toxins produced by immune cells, e.g. oxygen free radicals; (3) mitochondrial injury causing cytopathic hypoxia – cells are unable to metabolise oxygen; (4) apoptosis – if the cell injury is sufficient, capsase enzymes are activated within the nucleus and programmed cell death occurs; (5) hypoxia from micro- and macrovascular pathology.

✚	10.28 The 'Sepsis Six'*

1. Deliver high-flow oxygen
2. Take blood cultures
3. Administer intravenous antibiotics
4. Measure serum lactate and send full blood count
5. Start intravenous fluid replacement
6. Commence accurate measurement of urine output

*International recommendations for the immediate management of suspected sepsis from the Surviving Sepsis Campaign (all to be delivered within 1 hr of the initial diagnosis of sepsis).

✚	10.29 Early administration of antibiotics in suspected sepsis

• Broad-spectrum antibiotics should be administered as soon as possible after sepsis is suspected
• Every hour of delayed treatment is associated with a 5–10% increase in mortality

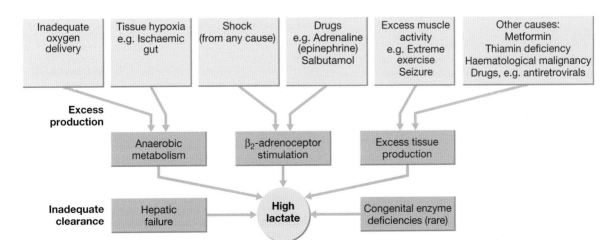

Fig. 10.13 Physiology of hyperlactataemia.

10.30 Central and mixed venous oxygen saturations

- Saturation of venous blood sampled from the right atrium or superior vena cava (central) or pulmonary artery (mixed venous)
- Both values reflect the balance of supply and demand of oxygen to the tissues
- Mixed venous oxygen saturation is a measure of whole-body supply and demand of oxygen; central venous oxygen saturation measures the supply and demand of oxygen from the upper body. Normal mixed venous oxygen saturation is 70%. Lower values than this suggest inadequate oxygen delivery
- Central venous oxygen saturation is more variable, depending on whether the patient is awake or anaesthetised, but a value of 70% is considered normal
- Where cytopathic hypoxia occurs, oxygen extraction is impaired and the central and mixed venous oxygen saturations may be >80%. This is often a poor prognostic sign

Noradrenaline (norepinephrine) for refractory hypotension

Central venous access should be established early in the resuscitation process and a noradrenaline infusion commenced. If there is severe hypotension, it is not necessary to wait until 30 mL/kg of fluid has been administered before commencing noradrenaline; early vasopressor use may improve the outcome from acute kidney injury. Measurement of central and mixed venous oxygen saturations may provide additional prognostic information (Box 10.30).

Other therapies for refractory hypotension

Refractory hypotension is due to either inadequate cardiac output or inadequate systemic vascular resistance (vasoplegia). When vasoplegia is suspected, it may be necessary to add vasopressin (antidiuretic hormone, ADH). This is a potent vasoconstrictor that may be used to augment noradrenaline (norepinephrine) in achieving an acceptable MAP. Intravenous glucocorticoids are also commonly used in refractory hypotension. There is little evidence that they improve the overall outcome, but they do lead to a more rapid reversal of the shocked state. There is a small increased risk of secondary infection following glucocorticoid use.

Septic cardiomyopathy

The myocardium can be affected by the septic process, presenting as either acute left or right ventricular dysfunction. A bedside echocardiogram is particularly useful to confirm the diagnosis, as ECG changes are usually non-specific. Dobutamine or adrenaline (epinephrine) can be used to augment cardiac output, and intravenous calcium should be replaced if ionised calcium is low.

Other interventions such as intravenous bicarbonate in profound metabolic acidosis, high-volume haemofiltration/haemodialysis and extracorporeal support are sometimes used, but currently lack evidence of benefit.

Review of the underlying pathology

While sepsis is the most common cause of acute systemic inflammation, up to 20% of patients initially treated for sepsis will have a non-infectious cause: that is, a sepsis mimic (Box 10.31). These conditions should be considered where the clinical picture is not typical, no source of sepsis can be found, or the inflammatory response seems excessive in the context of local infection. Early reconsideration of the diagnosis of sepsis is crucial, as many of the 'sepsis mimics' offer a finite time window for specific intervention, after which irreversible organ damage will have occurred.

 10.31 Sepsis mimics

- Pancreatitis
- Drug reactions
- Widespread vasculitis – catastrophic antiphospholipid syndrome, Goodpasture's syndrome
- Autoimmune diseases – inflammatory bowel disease, rheumatoid arthritis, systemic lupus erythematosus
- Malignancy – carcinoid syndrome
- Haematological conditions – haemophagocytic syndrome, diffuse lymphoma, thrombotic thrombocytopenic purpura

Acute respiratory distress syndrome

Aetiology and pathogenesis

Acute respiratory distress syndrome (ARDS) is a diffuse neutrophilic alveolitis caused by a range of conditions and characterised by bilateral radiographic infiltrates and hypoxaemia (Box 10.32). Activated neutrophils are sequestered into the lungs and capillary permeability is increased, with damage to cells within the alveoli. The pathophysiology is part of the inflammatory spectrum described in 'Sepsis' above, and the triggers are similar: infective and non-infective inflammatory processes. These processes result in exudation and accumulation of protein-rich cellular fluid within alveoli and the formation of characteristic 'hyaline membranes'. Local release of cytokines and chemokines by activated macrophages and neutrophils results in progressive recruitment of inflammatory cells. Secondary effects include loss of surfactant and impaired surfactant production. The net effect is alveolar collapse and reduced lung compliance, most marked in dependent regions of the lung (mainly dorsal in supine patients). The affected airspaces become fluid-filled and can no longer contribute to ventilation, resulting in hypoxaemia (due to increased pulmonary shunt) and hypercapnia (due to inadequate ventilation in some areas of the lung): that is, ventilation–perfusion mismatch.

Diagnosis and management

ARDS can be difficult to distinguish from fluid overload or cardiac failure. Classic chest X-ray and CT appearances are shown in Figures 10.14 and 10.15, respectively. Occasionally, conditions may present in a similar way to ARDS but respond to alternative treatments; an example of this might be a glucocorticoid-responsive interstitial pneumonia (p. 605). Management of ARDS is supportive, including use of lung-protective mechanical ventilation, inducing a negative fluid balance and treating the underlying cause. Establishing the severity of ARDS (Box 10.33) is useful, as severe disease will require more proactive management such as prone positioning or extracorporeal membrane oxygenation (ECMO; p. 204).

 10.32 Berlin definition of ARDS

- Onset within 1 week of a known clinical insult, or new or worsening respiratory symptoms
- Bilateral opacities on chest X-ray, not fully explained by effusions, lobar/lung collapse or nodules
- Respiratory failure not fully explained by cardiac failure or fluid overload. Objective assessment (e.g. by echocardiography) must exclude hydrostatic oedema if no risk factor is present
- Impaired oxygenation (see Box 10.33)

Fig. 10.14 Chest X-ray in acute respiratory distress syndrome (ARDS). Note bilateral lung infiltrates, pneumomediastinum, pneumothoraces with bilateral chest drains, surgical emphysema, and fractures of the ribs, right clavicle and left scapula.

Fig. 10.15 CT scan of the thorax in a patient with severe ARDS. Note the pathology is mainly in the dorsal (dependent) parts of the lung.

10

 10.33 Determining the severity of ARDS

Severity of hypoxaemia is calculated using a Pa/FiO_2 ratio. This is a number calculated by using the PaO_2 from an arterial blood gas measurement divided by the fraction of inspired oxygen (FiO_2, expressed as a fraction).

For example, a patient with a PaO_2 of 10 kPa (75 mmHg) on 50% oxygen, i.e. FiO_2 of 0.5, would have a Pa/FiO_2 ratio of 20 kPa (150 mmHg). This would be defined as moderately severe ARDS, if the other Berlin criteria were met (see Box 10.32). All measurements should be taken on a minimum of 5 cmH$_2$O of PEEP or CPAP.

- Mild: 40–26.6 kPa (300–200 mmHg)
- Moderate: 26.6–13.3 kPa (200–100 mmHg)
- Severe: ≤13.3 kPa (≤100 mmHg)

(CPAP = continuous positive airway pressure; PEEP = positive end-expiratory pressure)

✚ 10.34 Acute myocardial infarction: haemodynamic subsets

Cardiac output	Pulmonary oedema	
	No	Yes
Normal	Good prognosis and requires no treatment for heart failure	Due to moderate left ventricular dysfunction. Treat with vasodilators and diuretics
Low	Due to right ventricular dysfunction or concomitant hypovolaemia. Give fluid challenge and consider pulmonary artery catheter to guide therapy	Extensive myocardial infarction and poor prognosis. Consider intra-aortic balloon pump, vasodilators, diuretics and inotropes

Acute circulatory failure (cardiogenic shock)

Definition and aetiology

Cardiogenic shock is defined as hypoperfusion due to inadequate cardiac output or, more technically, a cardiac index of <2.2 L/min/m² (see Box 10.42). While cardiogenic shock is the final common pathway of many disease processes (e.g. sepsis, anaphylaxis, haemorrhage), the important primary causes of acute heart failure or cardiogenic shock (Fig. 10.16) are described here.

Myocardial infarction

In the majority of cases, cardiogenic shock following acute MI is due to left ventricular dysfunction. However, it may also be due to infarction of the right ventricle, or a variety of mechanical complications, including tamponade (due to infarction and rupture of the free wall), an acquired ventricular septal defect (due to

infarction and rupture of the septum) and acute mitral regurgitation (due to infarction or rupture of the papillary muscles).

Severe myocardial systolic dysfunction causes a fall in cardiac output, BP and coronary perfusion pressure. Diastolic dysfunction causes a rise in left ventricular end-diastolic pressure, pulmonary congestion and oedema, leading to hypoxaemia that worsens myocardial ischaemia. This is further exacerbated by peripheral vasoconstriction. These factors combine to create the 'downward spiral' of cardiogenic shock (Fig. 10.17). Hypotension, oliguria, delirium and cold, clammy peripheries are the manifestations of a low cardiac output, whereas breathlessness, hypoxaemia, cyanosis and inspiratory crackles at the lung bases are typical features of pulmonary oedema. If necessary, a Swan–Ganz catheter can be used to measure the pulmonary artery pressures and cardiac output (p. 206). These findings can be used to categorise patients with acute MI into four haemodynamic subsets (Box 10.34) and titrate therapy accordingly.

In cardiogenic shock associated with acute MI, immediate percutaneous coronary intervention should be performed (p. 491). The viable myocardium surrounding a fresh infarct may contract poorly for a few days and then recover. This phenomenon is known as myocardial stunning and means that acute heart failure

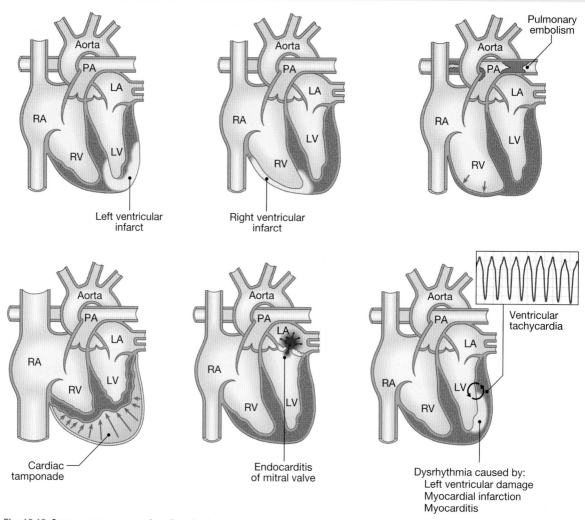

Fig. 10.16 Some common causes of cardiogenic shock.

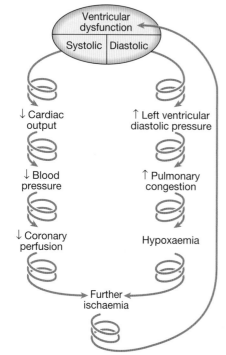

Fig. 10.17 The downward spiral of cardiogenic shock.

should be treated intensively because overall cardiac function may subsequently improve.

Acute massive pulmonary embolism

Massive PE may complicate leg or pelvic vein thrombosis and usually presents with sudden collapse. The clinical features and treatment are discussed on page 619. Bedside echocardiography may demonstrate a small, under-filled, vigorous left ventricle with a dilated right ventricle; it is sometimes possible to see thrombus in the right ventricular outflow tract or main pulmonary artery. In practice, it can be difficult to distinguish massive PE from a right ventricular infarct on transthoracic echocardiogram. CT pulmonary angiography usually provides a definitive diagnosis.

Acute valvular pathology, aortic dissection and cardiac tamponade

These conditions should be considered in an undifferentiated presentation of shock. The diagnosis and management of these conditions is discussed on pages 514, 506 and 544.

Post cardiac arrest

The initial management of cardiac arrest is discussed on page 456. Following the return of spontaneous circulation (ROSC), the majority of cardiac arrest survivors will need a period of time in intensive care to achieve physiological stability, identify and manage the underlying cause of the arrest, and optimise neurological recovery.

Acute management

A MAP of >70 mmHg should be maintained to optimise cerebral perfusion. Shock is common following ROSC and is caused by a combination of the underlying condition leading to the arrest, myocardial stunning and a post-arrest vasodilated state. Support with inotropes, vasopressors and occasionally mechanical support from an intra-aortic balloon pump or venous–arterial ECMO (p. 207) may be required. Specific cardiac interventions and their indications are described in Chapter 16. Other physiological targets are listed in Box 10.35.

Prognosis

Predicting which patients will not recover from the brain injury sustained at the time of cardiac arrest is very difficult. Certain features suggest that the outcome will be poor: for example, the absence of pupillary and corneal reflexes, absence of a motor response and persistent myoclonic jerking.

Tools to assist prognostication following cardiac arrest are shown in Box 10.36. The clinician should, where feasible, delay prognostication until a period of 72 hours of targeted temperature management has been completed. The bilateral absence of the 'N20' spike on the somato-sensory evoked potential is the most specific test to predict irrecoverable brain injury. This test is performed by administering an electrical impulse over a peripheral nerve and recording the electrical impulses measured by the scalp electrodes overlying the part of the brain expected to receive the impulse. Where this is not available, prognostication based on all other available information, along with the perceived wishes relating to the level of disability the individual would be prepared to accept, should allow a decision regarding ongoing treatment to be made. Where there is doubt, more time should be given to allow assessment of neurological recovery.

Other causes of multi-organ failure

As previously discussed, sepsis is the most common cause of multi-organ failure. However, multi-organ failure secondary to single organ dysfunction, such as cardiac failure, liver failure, renal failure or respiratory failure, is also common. The multisystem insult in these disease processes goes beyond the direct biochemical damage and tissue hypoxia caused by the primary organ dysfunction. It probably reflects cellular signalling pathways and the release of other systemic toxins by the failing organ, referred to as organ 'crosstalk'.

Multi-organ failure can also be caused by a physiological insult that damages a wide variety of cells in different organs, including toxins from extrinsic sources such as envenomation and intrinsic sources such as myoglobin in rhabdomyolysis (p. 195). Multi-organ failure can also be caused by profound physical injury to cells from processes such as nuclear radiation, heat exposure or blast trauma.

Critical care medicine

Decisions around intensive care admission

Being a patient in intensive care is seldom a pleasant experience. The interventions are usually painful and the loss of liberties that are normally taken for granted can be devastating. While much of the unpleasant sensory and emotional experience can be modified with high-quality care and analgesia, there is a strong case that it can only be morally 'right' to admit a patient to intensive care if the end justifies the means. There must be a realistic hope that the patient will regain a quality of life that would be worth the pain and suffering that he or she will experience in intensive care. Few patients are able to comprehend fully what it means to be critically ill, so the physician should guide the process of determining who should be admitted to intensive care.

Selecting the appropriate level of intervention for an individual patient can be very difficult. The decision-making process should involve an assessment of the likelihood of reversibility of the disease, the magnitude of the interventions required, the underlying level of frailty, and the personal beliefs and wishes of the patient (commonly expressed through their next of kin).

As technology and science have improved, conditions that were previously regarded as terminal can now be supported and life can be considerably prolonged (Box 10.37). There have been several prominent examples of individuals who have received intensive care, but where an onlooker might have considered treatment to be futile owing to frailty, comorbidity or profound neurological injury. Such cases will, in part, shape the views and expectations of society, and it is unlikely that making decisions in this area will become any easier. Some suggested techniques to aid decision-making are listed in Box 10.38.

10

| **10.35 Physiological targets following a return of spontaneous circulation (ROSC)** |

- *Temperature management.* Facilitate maintenance of temperature at 36°C and avoidance of pyrexia by the use of a cooling blanket. This should be continued for 72 hrs. Muscle relaxants may be required to prevent shivering
- *Blood pressure management.* Aim for a MAP of at least 70 mmHg and a systolic blood pressure of >120 mmHg
- *Glucose control.* Control the glucose to 6–10 mmol/L (108–180 mg/dL)
- *Normal CO_2* (4.5–6 kPa, 33–45 mmHg) *and oxygen saturation* (94–98%). Avoid both hypoxaemia and hyperoxia

---

| **10.36 Prognostication after cardiac arrest: predictors of poor neurological recovery** |

Coexisting problems

- Multi-organ failure
- Significant comorbidities

Clinical

- Persisting and generalised myoclonus
- Absence of pupillary or corneal reflexes
- Poor motor response (absent or extensor response)

Biochemical

- A neuron-specific enolase >33 µg/L

Imaging

- CT showing loss of grey–white differentiation
- Focal cause or consequence of cardiac arrest, e.g. subarachnoid haemorrhage

Electrophysiology

- EEG patterns may suggest brain injury, e.g. burst suppression
- Somato-sensory evoked potentials – bilateral absence of the N20 spike (recorded from scalp electrodes from cutaneous electrical impulse over the median nerve)

10.37 Critical illness in the context of congenital conditions

- **Longer survival**: there are many congenital conditions that would, in the past, have been fatal in childhood, but now patients survive into adulthood. Decision-making can be difficult when the adolescent has impaired decision-making capacity.
- **Parental views**: in such circumstances, the views of the parent or legal guardian become paramount.
- **Goals of care**: often a detailed explanation of what is, and is not, achievable in intensive care allows the direction of care to be switched to palliative when life expectancy is poor and quality of life is severely impaired.
- **Decision-making**: such conversations may require input from experts in the patient's congenital condition(s), and advanced decision-making regarding ICU admission should be encouraged whenever patients and families feel able to discuss such issues.

10.38 Techniques to improve admission decision-making

- *Always act in the best interests of the patient*: external influences are commonly present but these should be of only secondary importance
- *Maximise patient capacity*: wherever possible, the patient should be involved in discussions of escalation and resuscitation status
- *Communicate openly and honestly with the next of kin*: when communicating potential outcomes, it is best to use natural frequencies rather than percentages. For example, 'If we had 100 patients with the same illness as your mother, only 10 would survive' is easier for most people to understand than 'there is a 90% chance of death'
- *Reach mutual agreement with the next of kin*: it is rare for there to be discord between clinicians and family, and in most cases the most appropriate course of action is clear
- *Seek additional opinions*: other clinicians involved in the care of the patient will provide useful input. The premise should be to err on the side of escalation where the most appropriate course of action is unclear. Where there is an unresolvable difference in opinion, a mediation process or court ruling may be required to make the final decision. Thankfully, this is a very infrequent occurrence
- *Plan ahead*: advance planning in chronic, progressive disease can make the decision easier. Some health facilities use an escalation form, which specifies the interventions that should be offered or are acceptable to the patient. This can be useful as the binary decision of for/not for resuscitation fails to account for the array of interventions that can be performed before cardiac arrest occurs

Stabilisation and institution of organ support

In order to stabilise a critically unwell patient, the primary problem should be corrected as quickly as possible: for example, source control in sepsis and control of the bleeding point in haemorrhage. Immediate resuscitation and prioritisation of the safety of the patient are clearly important, but there is only a limited role for 'optimising' the patient if such measures may significantly delay a definitive treatment, such as laparotomy for a perforated viscus. In some cases, the definitive treatment is not readily apparent or treatments take time to have their full effect. In these cases, adequate organ support to stabilise the patient while the treatment is given becomes the main goal of care.

Respiratory support

Non-invasive respiratory support

Non-invasive respiratory support provides a bridge between simple oxygen delivery devices and invasive ventilation. It can be used in patients who are in respiratory distress but do not have an indication for invasive ventilation, or in those who are not suitable for intubation and ventilation for chronic health reasons. Patients must be cooperative, able to protect their airway, and have the strength to breathe spontaneously and cough effectively. Clinicians should avoid using non-invasive respiratory support to prolong the dying process in irreversible conditions such as end-stage lung disease. Likewise, a failure to respond to treatment or further deterioration should trigger a decision regarding intubation, as delayed invasive ventilation in this context is associated with worse outcome.

High-flow nasal cannulae

High-flow nasal cannulae (HFNCs) are devices that provide very high gas flows of fully humidified oxygen and air. They offer distinct advantages over non-invasive ventilation (NIV) in selected patients, mainly those with type I respiratory failure (particularly pneumonia) who have not reached an indication for invasive ventilation. They allow patient comfort and increased expectoration while providing some degree of positive end-expiratory pressure (PEEP) and a high oxygen concentration that can be titrated to the SO_2.

Continuous positive pressure ventilation

Continuous positive pressure ventilation therapy involves the application of a continuous positive airway pressure (CPAP) throughout the patient's breathing cycle, typically 5–10 cmH$_2$O. It helps to recruit collapsed alveoli and can enhance clearance of alveolar fluid. It is particularly effective at treating pulmonary atelectasis (which may be post-operative) and pulmonary oedema. It uses a simpler device than NIV but otherwise offers no direct benefit over it.

Non-invasive ventilation or bi-level ventilation

NIV provides ventilatory support via a tight-fitting nasal or facial mask. It can be delivered by using a simple bi-level ventilation (BiPAP) turbine ventilator, or an intensive care ventilator. These machines can deliver pressure at a higher level (approximately 15–25 cmH$_2$O) for inspiration and a lower pressure (usually 4–10 cmH$_2$O) to allow expiration. Ventilation can be spontaneous (triggered by a patient's breaths) or timed (occurring at a set frequency). Systems that synchronise with a patient's efforts are better tolerated and tend to be more effective in respiratory failure. Timed breaths are used for patients with central apnoea. NIV is the first-line therapy in patients with type II respiratory failure secondary to an acute exacerbation of COPD because it reduces the work of breathing and offloads the diaphragm, allowing it to recover strength. It is also useful in pulmonary oedema, obesity hypoventilation syndromes and some neuromuscular disorders. It should be initiated early, especially when severe respiratory acidosis secondary to hypercapnia is present. NIV can also be used to support selected patients with hypercapnia secondary to pneumonia, or during weaning from invasive ventilation, but its effectiveness in these contexts is less certain; early intubation or re-intubation is probably more beneficial.

Intubation and intermittent positive pressure ventilation

Taking control of the respiratory system in a critically ill patient is one of the most significant and risky periods in a patient's journey. Critical incidents are common because the patient is often deteriorating rapidly and is exhausted. The potential for cardiovascular collapse is further exacerbated by the negatively inotropic and vasodilating drugs used to induce anaesthesia, and the period of apnoea invoked to facilitate intubation (Box 10.39).

The main aims of intermittent positive pressure ventilation (IPPV) are to avoid critical hypoxaemia and hypercapnia while minimising damage to the alveoli and encouraging the patient to

breathe spontaneously once it is safe to do so. The determination of what constitutes *critical* will depend on the status of each patient. For example, a patient with raised ICP will have a strong indication for normocapnia (because hypercapnia increases ICP). Unfortunately, achieving the minute volumes required to maintain normocapnia can, in itself, be harmful to the lungs (p. 204).

Ventilator modes

Following intubation, most patients have a period of paralysis from the muscle relaxation. Mandatory ventilation is, therefore, required for a variable period, depending on the severity of the lung injury, the underlying disease process and the general condition of the patient. Mandatory ventilation means that the ventilator will deliver set parameters (either a set tidal volume or a set inspiratory pressure), regardless of patient effort. A physician can choose to support additional patient effort in between mandatory breaths with pressure support. This requires sufficient patient effort to 'trigger' the ventilator to deliver a synchronised breath, in time with the patient's own ventilation. Other parameters that should be considered when using mechanical ventilation are shown in Figure 10.18.

As a patient's illness resolves, or if the lung injury necessitating intubation is not severe, periods of spontaneous breathing with pressure support are commenced. While spontaneous breathing is preferable to mandatory ventilation modes, the shearing forces of patient effort can exacerbate lung injury in patients with severely damaged lungs. It is, therefore, important that a patient is permitted to breathe in a planned and controlled way.

10.39 Optimising safety during intubation

- Intervene early in the disease process (once it has become clear that the disease trajectory is downward)
- Use a stable anaesthetic technique: low doses of sedative agents and rapidly acting paralytic agents
- Remember that intubation should be performed by the most experienced operator available
- Use techniques to optimise oxygenation and ventilation in the period around intubation, e.g. keeping non-invasive ventilation in situ for pre-oxygenation, leaving high-flow nasal cannulae on for the intubation process, and using a video-laryngoscope in an anticipated difficult intubation

---

Plateau pressure
Airway pressure during an inspiratory hold. Keeping plateau pressure as low as possible above PEEP is the most protective strategy for the lungs

Respiratory rate and minute volume
Depend on the minute volume required to achieve the desired PCO_2, and whether the patient is breathing spontaneously. Rates are commonly 20–30 breaths/min

Ventilator mode
Mandatory, spontaneous, or mandatory with the ability to take spontaneous breaths (as shown here)

FiO_2
Fraction of inspired oxygen. This is usually titrated to oxygen saturations targeting 92–95%

Pressure–time graph

Volume–time graph

Flow–time graph

Tidal volume
Usual target is 6 mL/kg of predicted body weight (PBW)

Positive end-expiratory pressure (PEEP)
The pressure within the respiratory system during expiration, commonly 5–15 cmH$_2$O. Higher levels of PEEP often improve oxygenation but put strain on the right heart (as it makes it harder to pump blood through the pulmonary circulation)

Fig. 10.18 Settings to be considered when commencing mechanical ventilation.

Ventilator-induced lung injury

Every positive-pressure breath causes cyclical inflation of alveoli followed by deflation. The resultant damage to alveoli occurs via several possible mechanisms:

- distending forces from the tidal volume, termed 'volutrauma'
- the pressure used to inflate the lung, referred to as 'barotrauma'
- alveoli collapsing at the end of expiration, called 'atelectotrauma'
- the release of inflammatory cytokines in response to cyclical distension, called 'biotrauma'.

The threshold of injurious ventilation is unique to each patient. Moderate ventilator pressures and volumes used to ventilate healthy lungs may not cause ventilator-induced lung injury (VILI), but the same settings may cause significant VILI if delivered to a patient with lungs that are already damaged from another disease process.

Strategies that may reduce the incidence and severity of VILI include:

- *Permissive hypercapnia.* In the majority of patients who are ventilated for respiratory failure, it is preferable to tolerate moderate degrees of hypercapnia rather than strive for normal blood gases at the expense of VILI. For example, in a patient with isolated respiratory failure, a physician may choose to tolerate a $PaCO_2$ of up to 10 kPa (75 mmHg), provided the H^+ is <63 nmol/L (pH >7.2).
- *'Open lung' ventilation.* Maintaining a positive pressure within the airways at the end of expiration prevents atelectotrauma. Use of low tidal volumes, higher levels of PEEP (Fig. 10.18) and recruitment manœuvres (occasional short periods of sustained high airway pressures to open up alveoli that have collapsed) can reduce the incidence of VILI.
- *Paralysis.* When respiratory failure is severe, patient effort may worsen VILI. An infusion of muscle relaxant can be used to moderate dyssynchrony with the ventilator.

Advanced respiratory support

Airway pressure release ventilation

Airway pressure release ventilation (APRV) is a mode of ventilation that lengthens the inspiratory time to the extreme, with a very short period of time for expiration. It relies on spontaneous movement of the diaphragm from patient effort to facilitate the mixing of gas within the respiratory system during the long period in full inspiration, followed by a very short period of low pressure to allow passive expiration. It has not, however, been demonstrated to be superior to conventional modes of ventilation, but may have a role in moderate to severe ARDS.

Prone positioning

In ARDS, the posterior parts of the lung lose airspaces due to atelectasis and inflammatory exudate. By placing patients on their front, the pattern of fluid distribution within the lung changes, and ventilation–perfusion matching is improved. This is used to enhance oxygenation in moderate to severe ARDS, and may have some disease-modifying effects as the dependent areas of the lung are changed periodically. Although there are risks associated with nursing a patient in the prone position, it is becoming a widespread therapy. Patients are usually placed in the prone position for 12–24 hours and then rotated back to the supine position for a similar period. This cycle continues until there is evidence of resolving lung injury.

Extracorporeal respiratory support

Sometimes, despite optimal invasive ventilation, it is not possible to maintain adequate oxygenation or prevent a profound respiratory acidosis. When a patient has a reversible cause of respiratory failure (or is a potential lung transplant recipient) and facilities are available, extracorporeal respiratory support should be considered.

Venous–venous extracorporeal membrane oxygenation

In venous–venous extracorporeal membrane oxygenation (VV ECMO), large-bore central venous cannulae are inserted into the superior vena cava (SVC) and/or the inferior vena cava (IVC) via the femoral or jugular veins, and advanced under ultrasound or fluoroscopic guidance (Fig. 10.19). Venous blood is then pumped through a membrane oxygenator. This device has thousands of tiny silicone tubes with air/oxygen gas on the other side of the tubes (the membrane). This facilitates the passage of oxygen into the blood and diffusion of carbon dioxide across the membrane, where it is removed by a constant flow of gas (sweep gas). The oxygenated blood is then returned to the right atrium, from where it flows through the lungs as it would in the physiological state. This means that even if the lungs are contributing no oxygenation or carbon dioxide removal, a patient can remain well oxygenated and normocapnic.

Extracorporeal carbon dioxide removal

In some patients it is possible to maintain oxygenation but there is refractory hypercapnia. There are devices available that can remove carbon dioxide using a much lower blood flow rate than VV ECMO. Consequently, smaller venous cannulae, similar to those used in renal dialysis, can be sufficient to have a 'CO_2 dialysis' effect. This can be useful in patients in whom normocapnia is essential (such as those with a raised ICP), or those with refractory hypercapnia and adequate oxygenation. In addition, extracorporeal carbon dioxide removal can be used to reduce the required minute volume, which is a beneficial strategy for protecting the lungs against VILI or facilitating early extubation.

Cardiovascular support

Initial resuscitation

A brief assessment can usually yield enough information to determine whether a patient is at significant risk of an imminent cardiac arrest. If the patient is obtunded and there is no palpable radial or brachial pulse, then treatment should proceed as described on page 457.

In anaphylactic shock, or undifferentiated shock in a peri-arrest situation, a single dose of intramuscular adrenaline (epinephrine) 0.5 mg (0.5 mL of 1:1000) can be life-saving. If expertise is available, a small dose of intravenous adrenaline can delay cardiac arrest long enough to identify the cause of shock and institute other supportive measures; a suggested dose would be 50 µg (0.5 mL of 1:10000). If haemorrhage is considered a possibility, a 'major haemorrhage' alert should be activated, facilitating rapid access to large volumes of blood and blood products. A classification of shock is shown in Box 10.40.

A

Controller console

RPM 4000

Pressures
Saturations
Flow

Centrifugal pump

Gas out

Membrane oxygenator

Gas in

Oxygenated blood returned to vein (V–V) or artery (V–A)

Venous blood from patient (usually inferior vena cava)

B

From ECMO circuit

Venous 'return' cannula
Superior vena cava
Right atrium now full of oxygenated blood
Tricuspid valve
Right ventricle

Venous 'return' cannula

Venous 'access' cannula

Inguinal ligament
Femoral artery
Access ECMO cannula
Skin puncture site in proximal thigh
Femoral vein

To ECMO circuit

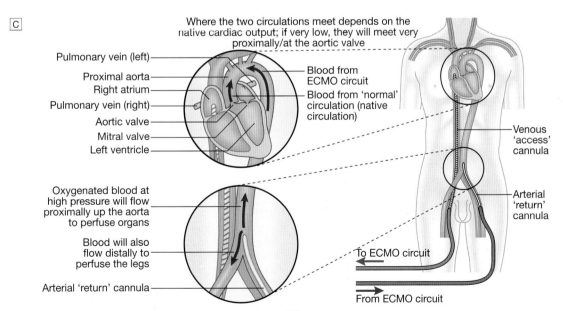

C

Where the two circulations meet depends on the native cardiac output; if very low, they will meet very proximally/at the aortic valve

Pulmonary vein (left)
Proximal aorta
Right atrium
Pulmonary vein (right)
Aortic valve
Mitral valve
Left ventricle

Blood from ECMO circuit
Blood from 'normal' circulation (native circulation)

Venous 'access' cannula

Oxygenated blood at high pressure will flow proximally up the aorta to perfuse organs
Blood will also flow distally to perfuse the legs
Arterial 'return' cannula

Arterial 'return' cannula

To ECMO circuit
From ECMO circuit

Fig. 10.19 Principles of extracorporeal membrane oxygenation (ECMO). A Basic ECMO circuit: venous–arterial (VA) and venous–venous (VV). B Example of a VV ECMO circuit. C Example of a VA ECMO circuit.

i | **10.40 Categories of shock**

Category	Description
Hypovolaemic	Can be haemorrhagic or non-haemorrhagic in conditions such as hyperglycaemic hyperosmolar state (p. 738) and burns
Cardiogenic	See page 199
Obstructive	Obstruction to blood flow around the circulation, e.g. major pulmonary embolism, cardiac tamponade, tension pneumothorax
Septic	See page 196
Anaphylactic	Inappropriate vasodilatation triggered by an allergen (e.g. bee sting), often associated with endothelial disruption and capillary leak (p. 75)
Neurogenic	Caused by major brain or spinal injury, which disrupts brainstem and neurogenic vasomotor control. High cervical cord trauma may result in disruption of the sympathetic outflow tracts, leading to inappropriate bradycardia and hypotension. Guillain–Barré syndrome (p. 1140) can involve the autonomic nervous system, resulting in periods of severe hypo- or hypertension
Others	e.g. Drug-related such as calcium channel blocker overdose; Addisonian crisis

i | **10.41 Actions of commonly used vasoactive agents**

Drug	Action		
	Vasoconstrictor	Inotrope	Chronotrope
Adrenaline (epinephrine)	++	+++	++
Noradrenaline (norepinephrine)	++++	+	+
Dobutamine	–	++++	+++
Vasopressin	+++++	No action	– (reflex bradycardia)

Venous access for the administration of drugs and fluids is vital but often difficult in critically unwell patients. Wide-bore cannulae are required for rapid fluid administration. In extremis, the external jugular vein can be cannulated; it is often prominent in low cardiac output states and readily visible on the lateral aspect of the neck. Occluding the vein distally with finger pressure makes it easier to cannulate, but care must be taken to remain high in the neck to avoid causing a pneumothorax. Intra-osseous or central venous access can be established if there are no visible peripheral veins. Ultrasound can provide assistance for rapid and safe venous cannulation. Rapid infusion devices are widely available and should be used for the delivery of warmed, air-free fluid and blood products.

Fluid and vasopressor use

Resuscitation of the shocked patient should include a 10 mL/kg fluid challenge. Using colloid or crystalloid is acceptable; starch solutions are associated with additional renal dysfunction and should be avoided. The fluid challenge can be repeated if shock persists, to a maximum total of 30 mL/kg of fluid. However, commencing vasopressor therapy early in resuscitation is better than delaying until a large volume of fluid has been given. Amongst other beneficial effects, vasopressors induce venoconstriction, reducing the capacitance of the circulation and effectively mobilising more fluid into the circulation.

If a patient remains shocked after 30 mL/kg of fluid has been administered, a re-evaluation of the likely cause is required, looking particularly for concealed haemorrhage or an obstructive pathology. A bedside echocardiogram is especially useful at this stage to evaluate cardiac output and exclude tamponade. Noradrenaline (norepinephrine) should be commenced as the first-line vasoactive agent in most cases, unless there is a strong indication to use a pure inotropic or chronotropic agent: for example, in cardiogenic shock or shock associated with bradycardia. If there is evidence of low cardiac output, adrenaline (epinephrine) or dobutamine should be commenced. Both agents are equally effective, but dobutamine causes more vasodilatation and additional noradrenaline may be required to maintain an adequate MAP. Vasopressin is added if hypotension persists despite high doses of noradrenaline and cardiac output is thought to be adequate.

In extreme situations it is acceptable to start infusions of inotropes through a well-sited, large-bore peripheral cannula, although central venous access and an arterial line (for monitoring) should be inserted as soon as possible. The actions of commonly used vasoactive drugs are summarised in Box 10.41.

Advanced haemodynamic monitoring

There are many different devices available to estimate cardiac output. Such devices employ a variety of mechanisms, including the Doppler effect of moving blood, changes in electrical impedance of the thorax, or the dilution of either an indicator substance or heat (thermodilution). The information is processed within the equipment, and often integrated with additional data, such as the arterial pressure waveform, to give an estimate of cardiac output and stroke volume.

When the aetiology of shock is straightforward and the patient is responding as predicted to treatment, the value of devices that estimate cardiac output is limited. Portable echocardiography has the advantage of giving qualitative information – for example, demonstrating aortic stenosis or a regional wall motion abnormality – as well as quantitative information on stroke volume, but it requires technical expertise.

Pulmonary artery (PA) catheters, sometimes referred to as Swan–Ganz catheters (Fig. 10.20), are invasive but provide useful information on pulmonary pressures, cardiac output, mixed venous oxygen saturations (see Box 10.30) and, by extrapolation, whether the cause of the shock is vasodilatation or pump failure. They can be helpful in complex cases, such as shock after cardiac surgery, or in patients with suspected pulmonary hypertension (Box 10.42). However, PA catheters are associated with some rare but serious complications, including lung infarction, PA rupture and thrombosis of the catheter itself. Such complications occur infrequently in centres that use PA catheters regularly; it should be stressed that a lack of familiarity within the wider clinical team is a relative contraindication to their use.

Mechanical cardiovascular support

When shock is so severe that it is not possible to maintain sufficient organ perfusion with fluids and inotropic support, it is

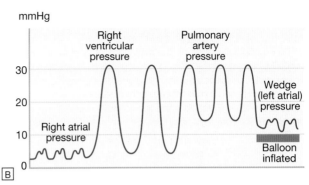

Fig. 10.20 A pulmonary artery (Swan–Ganz) catheter. A There is a small balloon at the tip of the catheter and pressure can be measured through the central lumen. The catheter is inserted via an internal jugular, subclavian or femoral vein and advanced through the right heart until the tip lies in the pulmonary artery. When the balloon is deflated, the pulmonary artery pressure can be recorded. B Advancing the catheter with the balloon inflated will 'wedge' the catheter in the pulmonary artery. Blood cannot then flow past the balloon, so the tip of the catheter will now record the pressure transmitted from the pulmonary veins and left atrium (known as the pulmonary artery capillary wedge pressure), which provides an indirect measure of the left atrial pressure. (LA = left atrium; LV = left ventricle; RA = right atrium; RV = right ventricle)

i	**10.42 Interpreting haemodynamic data**			
Variable	**Units**	**Reference range**	**Interpretation**	
Cardiac output (CO)	litres/minute (L/min)	4–8 L/min	Low cardiac output suggests pump failure	
Cardiac index (CI) Cardiac output referenced to the size of the patient	litres/minute/metre^2 (L/min/m^2)	2.5–4 L/min/m^2	More useful than raw cardiac output alone, especially in smaller patients	
Central venous pressure (CVP)	mmHg	0–6 mmHg	Reflects right atrial pressure – a non-specific measurement of right ventricular (RV) function and volume status Low levels suggest good RV function or hypovolaemia	
Pulmonary artery systolic pressure (PA systolic)	mmHg	15–30 mmHg	Difficult to interpret in isolation Low levels suggest vasodilatation, hypovolaemia or right heart failure High levels are seen in many pathologies, e.g. left heart failure, primary pulmonary arterial hypertension (PAH), fluid overload	
Pulmonary artery diastolic pressure (PA diastolic)	mmHg	5–15 mmHg	As with PA systolic pressure, difficult to interpret in isolation	
Pulmonary artery capillary wedge pressure (PACWP)	mmHg	2–10 mmHg (should be within a few mmHg of PA diastolic)	Reasonable indication of left atrial pressure – raised in left heart failure and fluid overload Measurement is associated with injury to PA so should only be taken occasionally	
Transpulmonary gradient (PA diastolic – PACWP)	mmHg	1–5 mmHg	A high gradient suggests the pathology is in the pulmonary arteries, e.g. primary PAH	

sometimes necessary to use an internal device to augment or replace the inadequate native cardiac output.

Intra-aortic balloon pump

An intra-aortic balloon counter-pulsation device is a long tube that is usually inserted into the femoral artery and fed proximally into the thoracic aorta. The basic principle is that a helium-filled balloon is able to inflate and deflate rapidly in time with the cardiac cycle. It is inflated in diastole, thus augmenting forward flow of blood to the abdominal organs and improving diastolic pressure proximal to the balloon, thereby optimising coronary perfusion. While the principle is appealing, and an intra-aortic balloon pump (IABP) is often effective in achieving predetermined physiological goals, this does not translate into improved survival

in cardiogenic shock. There are risks associated with thrombosis formation on the balloon, mesenteric ischaemia and femoral artery pseudo-aneurysm following removal of the device.

Venous–arterial extracorporeal membrane oxygenation

Venous–arterial extracorporeal membrane oxygenation (VA ECMO) can be life-saving in profound cardiogenic shock and has even been used effectively in refractory cardiac arrest. The circuit and principles are very similar to those described in 'VV ECMO' above (see p. 204 and Fig. 10.19) with one important difference: oxygenated blood is returned to the arterial system (rather than into the right atrium). This means that the pump needs to generate sufficient pressure to allow blood to flow through the systemic circulation. The sites of venous and arterial access can be either central (via a thoracotomy or sternotomy) or peripheral via cannulae in the IVC/SVC and the femoral/subclavian artery. If the return cannula is peripherally sited (e.g. in the femoral artery), blood will flow back up the aorta from distal to proximal and perfuse the organs.

The outcome depends on the avoidance of complications (primarily, bleeding at the cannula site, intracranial haematoma, air embolism, infection and thrombosis) and improvement of the underlying condition. Most causes of profound cardiogenic shock are unlikely to resolve, and the potential availability of a longer-term solution, such as cardiac transplantation or insertion of a ventricular assist device, is a prerequisite for commencing VA ECMO in most centres.

Renal support

Renal replacement therapy (RRT) is explained in detail on page 420. The key points relating to RRT in an intensive care context are:

- Haemodynamic instability is common. Continuous therapies are widely believed to cause less haemodynamic instability than intermittent dialysis. However, many units use intermittent dialysis without significant problems.
- Haemodialysis and haemofiltration are equally good. Although there are theoretical benefits to removing inflammatory cytokines with haemofiltration, this does not translate into improved survival.
- Anticoagulation is usually achieved using citrate or heparin. Citrate has a better profile for anticoagulating the extracorporeal circuit without inducing an increased bleeding risk, but may accumulate in patients with profound multi-organ failure and should be avoided in very unstable individuals.
- Most patients who survive intensive care will regain adequate renal function to live without long-term renal support.
- A thorough investigation for reversible causes of renal dysfunction should always be undertaken in conjunction with instigation of renal support (see Fig. 15.18, p. 411).
- Shock appears to reverse more rapidly when renal support is instituted. Commencing renal support soon after a patient develops renal 'injury' (when serum creatinine is more than two times higher than baseline) is probably beneficial in the context of septic shock.

Neurological support

A diverse range of neurological conditions require management in intensive care. These include the various causes of coma, spinal cord injury, peripheral neuromuscular disease and prolonged seizures.

The goals of care in such cases are to:
- Protect the airway, if necessary by endotracheal intubation.
- Provide respiratory support to correct hypoxaemia and hypercapnia.
- Treat circulatory problems, e.g. neurogenic pulmonary oedema in subarachnoid haemorrhage, autonomic disturbances in Guillain–Barré syndrome, and spinal shock following high spinal cord injuries.
- Manage acute brain injury with control of ICP.

- Manage status epilepticus using antiepileptic agents such as levetiracetam, phenytoin and benzodiazepines. In refractory cases an infusion of sodium thiopental or ketamine may be required.

The aim of management in acute brain injury is to optimise cerebral oxygen delivery by maintaining normal arterial oxygen content and a cerebral perfusion pressure (CPP) of >60 mmHg. Secondary insults to the brain, such as hypoxaemia, hyper-/hypoglycaemia and prolonged seizures, must be avoided. ICP rises in acute brain injury as a result of haematoma, contusions, oedema or ischaemic swelling. Raised ICP causes damage to the brain in two ways: direct damage to the brainstem and motor tracts as a result of downward pressure and herniation through the tentorium cerebelli and foramen magnum, and indirect damage by reducing CPP. Cerebral blood flow is dependent on an adequate CPP. The CPP is determined by the formula:

$$CPP = MAP - ICP$$

ICP can be measured by pressure transducers that are inserted directly into the brain tissue. The normal upper limit for ICP is 15 mmHg and an upper acceptable limit of 20 mmHg is usually adopted in intensive care. Sustained pressures of >30 mmHg are associated with a poor prognosis. Various strategies are used to control ICP: maintaining normocapnia, preventing any impedance to venous drainage from the head, giving osmotic agents such as mannitol and hypertonic saline, and using hypothermia and decompressive craniectomy. No single technique has been shown to improve outcome in severe intracranial hypertension.

CPP should be maintained above 60 mmHg by ensuring adequate fluid replacement and, if necessary, by treating hypotension with a vasopressor such as noradrenaline (norepinephrine). Complex neurological monitoring must be combined with frequent clinical assessment of GCS, pupillary response to light, and focal neurological signs.

Daily clinical management in intensive care

Clinical review

In intensive care, detailed clinical examination should be performed daily to identify changes to a patient's condition and review the latest diagnostic information. Further focused clinical reviews are usually incorporated into twice-daily ward rounds. Each ward round offers an ideal opportunity to monitor and document compliance with relevant care bundles. A care bundle is a group of interventions that, when implemented concurrently, have provided evidence of clinical benefit. The mnemonic 'FAST HUG' provides a useful checklist of interventions that reduce intensive care complications: feeding, analgesia, sedation, thromboprophylaxis, head of bed elevation (to reduce the incidence of passive aspiration), ulcer prophylaxis and glucose control.

Other key aspects of the daily review are outlined on page 174. The overarching aim of the review is to identify the issues that are impeding recovery from critical illness, and make alterations to address them. In addition, specific and realistic goals for each relevant organ system should be defined, facilitating the autonomous titration of therapy by the bedside critical care nurse. An example of daily goals may be: 'Titrate the noradrenaline (norepinephrine) to achieve a MAP of 65 mmHg, aim for a negative fluid balance, titrate FiO_2 to achieve oxygen saturations

i	**10.43 Properties of sedative and analgesic agents used in ICU**		
Drug	**Mode of action**	**Advantages**	**Disadvantages**
Propofol	Intravenous anaesthetic	Rapid onset and offset	Large cumulative doses can cause multi-organ failure, especially in children – the 'propofol infusion syndrome'
Alfentanil	Potent opiate analgesic	Rapid onset and offset	High doses may be required. Agitation may persist
Morphine	Opioid	Analgesia	Active metabolites and accumulation cause slow offset
Midazolam	Benzodiazepine sedative	Can be used in children	Active metabolites and accumulation cause slow offset
Remifentanil	Very potent opiate	Analgesia and tube tolerance	Respiratory depression – extreme caution in non-intubated patients
Dexmedetomidine	α_2-adrenergic agonist	Excellent tube tolerance. Less delirium. Can be used in awake patients	Cost and availability

of 92–95% and titrate sedation to a RASS score of 0 to –1' (Box 10.44).

Sedation and analgesia

Most patients require sedation and analgesia to ensure comfort, relieve anxiety and tolerate mechanical ventilation. Some conditions, such as critically high ICP or critical hypoxaemia, require deep sedation to reduce tissue oxygen requirements and protect the brain from the peaks in ICP associated with coughing or gagging. For the majority of patients, however, optimal sedation is an awake and lucid patient who is comfortable and able to tolerate an endotracheal tube (termed 'tube tolerance').

Over-sedation is associated with longer ICU stays, a higher prevalence of delirium, prolonged requirement for mechanical ventilation, and an increased incidence of ICU-acquired infection. Box 10.43 compares the various agents used for sedation in intensive care. The key principles are that the patient should primarily receive analgesia, rather than anaesthesia, and caution should be used with drugs that accumulate in hepatic and renal dysfunction. Often a combination of drugs is used to achieve the optimal balance of sedation and analgesia.

Sedation is monitored via clinical sedation scales that record responses to voice and physical stimulation. The Richmond Agitation–Sedation Scale (RASS) is the best-recognised tool (see Box 10.44 for details). Regular use of a scoring system to adjust sedation is associated with a shorter ICU stay. Many ICUs also have a daily 'sedation break', when all sedation is stopped in appropriate cases for a short period. This is commonly combined with a trial of spontaneous breathing aiming to shorten the duration of mechanical ventilation.

Delirium in intensive care

Delirium is discussed on page 183. It is extremely common in critically ill patients and often becomes apparent as sedation is reduced. Hypoactive delirium is far more common than hyperactive delirium, but is easily missed unless routine screening is undertaken. A widely used bedside assessment is the CAM-ICU score. The patient is requested to squeeze the examiner's hand in response to instruction and questions, aiming to ascertain whether disordered thought or sensory inattention is present.

Delirium of any type is associated with poorer outcome. Management is focused on non-pharmacological interventions such as early mobilisation, reinstatement of day–night routine,

i	**10.44 Richmond Agitation–Sedation Scale (RASS)**	
Score	**Term**	**Description**
+4	Combative	Overtly combative, violent or immediate danger to staff
+3	Very agitated	Pulls on/removes tubes or catheters, or aggressive to staff
+2	Agitated	Frequent non-purposeful movement or patient–ventilator dyssynchrony
+1	Restless	Anxious or apprehensive but no aggressive or vigorous movements
0	Alert and calm	
–1	Drowsy	Not fully alert but sustained awakening (> 10 secs) with eye opening/contact to voice
–2	Light sedation	Brief awakening (<10 secs) with eye contact to voice
–3	Moderate sedation	Movement but no eye contact to voice
–4	Deep sedation	Movement to physical stimulation but no response to voice
–5	Unrousable	No response to voice or physical stimulation

noise reduction, cessation of drugs known to precipitate delirium, and treatment of potential underlying causes such as thiamin replacement in patients at risk of Wernicke's encephalopathy. Patients with agitated delirium that is refractory to verbal de-escalation should initially be managed with small doses of intramuscular antipsychotics, changed to the enteral route once control is established. Atypical antipsychotics such as olanzapine and quetiapine are more efficacious than traditional drugs such as haloperidol. Pharmacological interventions are not useful as prophylaxis or in hypoactive delirium. Additional information on diagnosis and management of delirium can be found on page 184.

Weaning from respiratory support

As the condition that necessitated ventilation resolves, respiratory support is gradually reduced: the process of 'weaning' from ventilation. Some approaches to weaning are described below.

Spontaneous breathing trials

A spontaneous breathing trial involves the removal of all respiratory support followed by close observation of how long the patient is able to breathe unassisted. The technique is particularly effective when linked to a reduction in sedation. PEEP and pressure support are reduced to low levels, or patients are disconnected from the ventilator and breathe oxygen or humidified air through the endotracheal tube. Signs of failure include rapid shallow breathing, hypoxaemia, rising $PaCO_2$, sweating and agitation. Patients who pass a spontaneous breathing trial are assessed for suitability of extubation (endotracheal tube removal).

Progressive reduction in pressure support ventilation

Progressive reduction in pressure support ventilation (PSV) is applied to each breath over a period of hours or days, according to patient response. Some ICU ventilators have software that allows the facility to wean the support provided automatically.

A useful tool to guide the weaning process is the rapid shallow breathing index (RSBI). This composite score of a patient's spontaneous respiratory rate and tidal volume (respiratory rate divided by tidal volume in litres) gives a numerical indication of how difficult the patient is finding breathing at that particular level of support. A RSBI value of > 100 suggests that a patient is working at a level that would be unsustainable for longer periods.

Extubation

It is not possible to predict whether a patient is ready to be extubated accurately; the timing relies heavily on clinical judgement. There are, however, some simple rules that can aid decision-making. Patients must have stable ABGs with resolution of hypoxaemia and hypercapnia despite minimal ventilator pressure support and a low FiO_2. Conscious level must be adequate to protect the airway, comply with physiotherapy, and cough. Furthermore, an assessment must be made as to whether the patient can sustain the required minute volume without ventilator support. This depends on the condition of patients' lungs, their strength and other factors affecting the $PaCO_2$, such as temperature and metabolic rate. The need for re-intubation following extubation is associated with poorer outcome, but patients who are not given the opportunity to breathe without a ventilator will also be at increased risk of ventilator-associated complications such as pneumonia and myopathy.

Tracheostomy

A tracheostomy is a percutaneous tube passed into the trachea (usually between the first and second, or second and third tracheal rings) to facilitate longer-term ventilation. The advantages and disadvantages of tracheostomy insertion are listed in Box 10.45. When ventilation weaning has been unsuccessful, a tracheostomy provides a bridge between intubation and extubation; the patient can have increasing periods free of ventilator support but easily have support reinstated. A tracheostomy can be inserted percutaneously, using a bronchoscope in the trachea for guidance, or surgically under direct vision. Occasionally, a patient will have a tracheostomy in situ following a laryngectomy. Such

i	**10.45 Advantages and disadvantages of tracheostomy**

Advantages

- Patient comfort
- Improved oral hygiene
- Access for tracheal toilet
- Ability to speak with cuff deflated and a speaking valve attached
- Reduced equipment 'dead space' (the volume of tubing)
- Earlier weaning and ICU discharge
- Reduced sedation requirement
- Reduced vocal cord damage

Disadvantages

- Immediate complications: hypoxaemia, haemorrhage
- Tracheostomy site infection
- Tracheal damage; late stenosis

patients are important to identify, as emergency management in the event of a tracheostomy problem (blockage or displacement) must be through the tracheostomy site; access will not be possible via the upper airway.

Nutrition

It is crucial that critically ill patients receive adequate calories, protein and essential vitamins and minerals. Calculation of exact requirements is complex and requires the expertise of a dietitian. It is, however, useful to make a rough estimation of requirements (p. 705). Under-feeding leads to muscle wasting and delayed recovery, while over-feeding can lead to biliary stasis, jaundice and steatosis. Enteral feeding is preferred where possible because it avoids the infective complications of total parenteral nutrition (TPN) and helps to maintain gut integrity. However, TPN is recommended for patients who are likely to have a sustained period without effective enteral feeding, or who are already malnourished. Caution must be taken to avoid the consequences of refeeding syndrome (p. 706).

Other essential components of intensive care

Survival after critical illness depends, to a large extent, on the prevention of medical complications during recovery from the primary insult.

Thromboprophylaxis

DVT, venous catheter-related thrombosis and PE are common in critically ill patients. Low-molecular-weight heparin (LMWH) should be administered to all patients, unless there is a contraindication. Often patients at highest risk of thrombosis, such as those with hepatic dysfunction or those who have suffered major trauma, have a relative contraindication to heparin. Such cases mandate daily evaluation of the risk–benefit ratio, and LMWH should be administered as soon as it is deemed safe to do so. Mechanical thromboprophylaxis, such as intermittent calf compression devices, are useful adjuvants in high-risk patients.

Glucose control

Hyperglycaemia is harmful in critical illness and may occur in people with pre-existing diabetes or undiagnosed diabetes, following administration of high-dose glucocorticoids, or as a consequence of 'stress hyperglycaemia'. Hyperglycaemia is commonly managed by infusion of intravenous insulin titrated against a 'sliding scale'. Intensive management of hyperglycaemia with insulin can result in hypoglycaemia, which may also be harmful in critical illness. Therefore, a compromise is to titrate insulin to a blood glucose level of 6–10 mmol/L (108–180 mg/dL).

Blood transfusion

Many critically ill patients become anaemic due to reduced red cell production and red cell loss through bleeding and blood sampling. However, red cell transfusion carries inherent risks of immunosuppression, fluid overload, organ dysfunction from microemboli, and transfusion reactions. In stable patients, a haemoglobin level of 70 g/L (7 g/dL) is a safe compromise between optimisation of oxygen delivery and the risks of transfusion. This transfusion threshold should be adjusted upwards for situations where oxygen delivery is critical, such as in patients with active myocardial ischaemia.

Peptic ulcer prophylaxis

Stress ulceration during critical illness is a serious complication. Proton pump inhibitors or histamine-2 receptor antagonists are effective at reducing the incidence of ulceration. There is, however, a suggestion that the use of these agents, particularly in conjunction with antibiotics, may increase the incidence of nosocomial infection, especially with *Clostridium difficile* (p. 264). It is therefore common practice to stop ulcer prophylaxis once consistent absorption of enteral feed is established.

Complications and outcomes of critical illness

The majority of patients will survive their episode of critical illness. While some will return to full, active lives, there are many who have ongoing physical, emotional and psychological problems.

Adverse neurological outcomes

Brain injury

Head injury, hypoxic–ischaemic injury and infective, inflammatory and vascular pathologies can all irreversibly injure the brain. If treatment is unsuccessful, patients will either die or be left with a degree of disability. In the latter situation, the provision of ongoing organ support will depend on the severity of the injury, the prognosis, and the wishes of the patient (usually expressed via relatives). Brain death is a state in which cortical and brainstem function is irreversibly lost. Diagnostic criteria for brain death vary between countries (Box 10.46); if satisfied, these criteria allow physicians to withdraw active treatment and discuss the potential for organ donation. Diagnosing brain death is complex and should be done only by physicians with appropriate expertise, as clinical differentiation from reduced consciousness can be challenging (Box 10.47). Where there is doubt – for example, in patients with coexisting spinal injury or localised brainstem pathology – additional investigations should be performed.

The 'locked-in' syndrome, in which the patient is paralysed except for eye movements, requires preserved hemispheric

---

i | **10.46 UK criteria for the diagnosis of brain death**

Preconditions for considering a diagnosis of brain death

- The patient is deeply comatose:
  - a. There must be no suspicion that coma is due to depressant drugs, such as narcotics, hypnotics, tranquillisers
  - b. Hypothermia has been excluded – rectal temperature must exceed 35°C
  - c. There is no profound abnormality of serum electrolytes, acid–base balance or blood glucose concentrations, and any metabolic or endocrine cause of coma has been excluded
- The patient is maintained on a ventilator because spontaneous respiration has been inadequate or has ceased. Drugs, including neuromuscular blocking agents, must have been excluded as a cause of the respiratory failure
- The diagnosis of the disorder leading to brain death has been firmly established. There must be no doubt that the patient is suffering from irremediable structural brain damage

Tests for confirming brain death

- All brainstem reflexes are absent:
  - a. The pupils are fixed and unreactive to light
  - b. The corneal reflexes are absent
  - c. The vestibulo-ocular reflexes are absent – there is no eye movement following the injection of 20 mL of ice-cold water into each external auditory meatus in turn
  - d. There are no motor responses to adequate stimulation within the cranial nerve distribution
  - e. There is no gag reflex and no reflex response to a suction catheter in the trachea
- No respiratory movement occurs when the patient is disconnected from the ventilator for long enough to allow the carbon dioxide tension to rise above the threshold for stimulating respiration ($PaCO_2$ must reach 6.7 kPa/50 mmHg)

The diagnosis of brain death should be made by two doctors of a specified status and experience. The tests are usually repeated after a short interval to allow blood gases to normalise before brain death is finally confirmed

---

function (and thus consciousness), but a lesion in the ventral pons (usually caused by infarction) results in complete paralysis. The term 'vegetative state' implies some retention of brainstem function and minimal cortical function, with loss of awareness of the environment. In contrast, 'minimally conscious state' implies that there is some degree of awareness and intact brainstem function. Confident distinction between these states is important and requires careful assessment, often over a period of time. Brain death is, by definition, irreversible but other states may offer hope for improvement.

ICU-acquired weakness

Weakness is common among survivors of critical illness. It is usually symmetrical, proximal and most marked in the lower limbs. Critical illness polyneuropathy and myopathy can occur simultaneously and, within the constraints of an altered sensorium, it can be impossible to distinguish the two conditions clinically. Risk factors for both processes include the severity of multi-organ failure, poor glycaemic control and the use of muscle relaxants and glucocorticoids.

Critical illness polyneuropathy

This is due to peripheral nerve axonal loss and characteristically presents as proximal muscle weakness with preserved sensation.

i	10.47 Classification of brain death and reduced conscious states			
Diagnosis	**Features**		**Investigation**	**Prognosis**
Brain death	See Box 10.46		Often not required if cranial imaging shows compatible cause and patient meets clinical criteria In diagnostic doubt: four-vessel angiogram (fluoroscopic or CT) of cerebral vessels or isotope scan of brain to demonstrate absence of cerebral blood flow	Time of confirmed brain death is recorded as time of death Potential to donate organs – donation after brain death (DBD) donor
Vegetative state (VS) 'Persistent VS' >1 month 'Permanent VS' >1 year	No reaction to verbal stimuli Some reaction to noxious stimuli Sleep–wake cycles (periods of eye opening) Maintained respiratory drive Intact brainstem reflexes Occasional automatic movements (yawning, swallowing)		Cranial imaging for primary cause Maintained cortical blood flow	Poor. May be better with traumatic aetiology
Minimally conscious state	Some reaction to verbal stimuli Some reaction to noxious stimuli Spontaneous movements Intact brainstem reflexes		EEG demonstrates reactivity	Variable. Recovery of function more likely than in VS
Locked-in syndrome	Cortex is intact but bilateral motor tracts are damaged Can be partial or complete, i.e. some response to verbal stimuli (e.g. vertical eye movements to communicate) Variable brainstem reflexes No limb movement to noxious stimuli		Imaging for primary cause – commonly MRI or CT will show brainstem or pontine infarction	Variable and depends on cause – progress can continue over months to years

It may also manifest as failure to wean from the ventilator secondary to respiratory muscle weakness. Electrophysiological studies of the affected nerves can be helpful, especially to rule out other potential causes such as Guillain–Barré syndrome. Conduction studies typically show reduced amplitude of transmitted voltage action potential with preserved velocity (compare with findings in Guillain–Barré syndrome; pp. 1076 and 1140). There are no specific treatments aside from resolution of the underlying cause and rehabilitation. Weakness may persist long into the convalescence stage of illness. In some cases, the clinical picture may be more in keeping with individual nerve involvement. This may be due to local pressure effects or part of a generalised picture. Great care must be taken to avoid pressure on high-risk areas such as the neck of the fibula where the common peroneal nerve navigates a superficial course. Nerve palsies such as foot drop can be permanent.

Critical illness myopathy

Although loss of muscle bulk is related to immobility and the catabolic state of critical illness, it is likely that microvascular and intracellular pathophysiological processes are also involved in critical illness myopathy. These processes result in loss of actin myofibrils and muscle weakness. Typically, the CK is normal or only mildly elevated. Like critical illness polyneuropathy, critical illness myopathy is usually a clinical diagnosis. Nerve conduction studies and electromyography may be suggestive of critical illness myopathy, and helpful in ruling out other pathology, but a muscle biopsy is required to confirm the diagnosis (p. 1076). It characteristically shows selective loss of the thick myofibrils and muscle necrosis. Management is conservative and the prognosis is good in ICU survivors.

Other long-term problems

The experience of critical illness and the necessary invasive management can leave patients with profound psychological sequelae akin to the post-traumatic stress syndrome seen in many survivors of conflict. Specialist help is required in managing these issues. Sometimes recovering patients benefit from returning to the ICU to see the environment in a different way and gain a better understanding of the processes and procedures that haunt them.

Long-term physical consequences are also common. Many diseases are not completely cured but follow a relapsing–remitting course; patients who have been critically ill with sepsis are far more likely than others in the general population to suffer from it again. Organ damage often persists and iatrogenic complications are common (e.g. damage to the vocal cords or tracheal stenosis from mucosal pressure caused by the cuff of the endotracheal tube). Intensive care follow-up clinics provide an excellent forum for addressing such issues, and for coordinating care involving a variety of medical specialties.

The older patient

Critically ill older patients present additional challenges following intensive care discharge (Box 10.48). As the ability to make a full recovery depends on frailty rather than chronological age, it can be helpful to use a validated frailty scoring system (p. 1306) to inform admission decision-making.

Rehabilitation medicine has much to offer survivors of critical illness, and an early referral is beneficial when it is clear that a patient is likely to survive with significant morbidity.

10.48 The critically ill older patient

- **ICU demography**: increasing numbers of critically ill older patients are admitted to the ICU; more than 50% of patients in many general ICUs are over 65 years old.
- **Outcome**: affected to some extent by age, as reflected in APACHE II (see Box 10.50), but age should not be used as the sole criterion for withholding or withdrawing ICU support.
- **Cardiopulmonary resuscitation (CPR)**: successful hospital discharge following in-hospital CPR is rare in patients over 70 years old in the presence of significant chronic disease.
- **Functional independence**: tends to be lost during an ICU stay and prolonged rehabilitation may subsequently be necessary.
- **Specific problems**:
  - Skin fragility and ulceration
  - Poor muscle strength: difficulty weaning from ventilator and mobilising
  - Delirium: compounded by sedatives and analgesics
  - High prevalence of underlying nutritional deficiency.

Withdrawal of active treatment and death in intensive care

Futility

The idea of futility is not new: Hippocrates stated that physicians should 'refuse to treat those who are overmastered by their disease, realising that in such cases medicine is powerless'. In intensive care, where the concept of futility is often used as a criterion to limit or withdraw life-sustaining treatment, it is helpful to have a working definition on which families and physicians can agree. It is, therefore, reasonable to define futility in such circumstances as the point at which recovery to a quality of life that the patient would find acceptable has passed. The primary insult may be neurological (irreversible brain injury not meeting criteria for brain death), or multi-organ failure that is refractory to treatment.

Death

Whilst most patients prefer to die at home, many spend their final days in hospital. Chapter 34 details the medical, legal and ethical priorities that should guide patient management once the decision to withdraw active treatment has been made (p. 1354). The decision to shift the focus of care to palliation should not change its intensity; it is the over-arching objective that changes. Only interventions that will improve the quality of a patient's remaining life should be offered. In the ICU, it is often appropriate to continue infusions of sedatives and analgesics, as reducing or stopping them may cause unnecessary pain and agitation. Measures that were instituted to prolong life should be withdrawn (usually including cessation of inotropes and extubation) to allow the patient to die peacefully with their family and friends present.

Organ donation

Donation after brain death

The diagnosis of brain death is discussed on page 211. Once brain death has been confirmed, consideration should be given to organ donation, termed 'donation after brain death' (DBD). Time of death is recorded as the time when the first series of brain death tests are undertaken, although the deceased

patient continues to be ventilated. The practice of organ donation varies throughout the world but the principles remain the same.

Organ donation specialists are contacted and they begin the process of establishing the suitability of any organs for transplantation and matching potential recipients. Many patients will have expressed their wishes through an organ donor registration scheme but agreement of family and next of kin is a moral (and sometimes legal) prerequisite. Once the organ retrieval theatre team have been assembled and all preliminary tests have been completed, the deceased patient is transferred to the operating theatre and the organs are sequentially removed.

Donation after cardiac death

If a patient does not meet brain death criteria but withdrawal of treatment has been agreed, donation of organs with residual function may be appropriate. This is termed 'donation after cardiac death' (DCD). If the patient dies within a short period following the commencement of 'warm ischaemic time' (the time to asystole following the onset of physiological derangement after the withdrawal of active treatment), then DCD can proceed. The deceased patient is transferred to an operating theatre and the agreed organs (often lungs, liver, kidney and pancreas) are retrieved. As heart valves and corneas can be retrieved later (within a longer time frame), tissue retrieval may occur in the mortuary.

Postmortem examination or autopsy

There are several indications to request a postmortem examination. A coroner (or legal equivalent) may initiate the process if a death is unexpected or violent, or has occurred under suspicious circumstances. The treating physician(s) may request one if they are unable to establish a cause of death or there is agreement that it may yield information of interest to the family or clinical team. The postmortem diagnosis is frequently at odds with the antemortem diagnosis and it is a very useful learning exercise to review the results with all those involved in the patient's care.

Discharge from intensive care

Discharge is appropriate when the original indication for admission has resolved and the patient has sufficient physiological reserve to continue to recover without the facilities of intensive care. Many ICUs and HDUs function as combined units, allowing 'step-down' of patients to HDU care without changing the clinical team involved. Discharge from ICU is stressful for patients and families, and clear communication with the clinical team accepting responsibility is vital. Nursing ratios change from 1:1 (one nurse per patient) or 1:2 to much lower staffing levels. Discharges from ICU or HDU to standard wards should take place within normal working hours to ensure adequate medical and nursing support and detailed handover. Discharge outside normal working hours is associated with higher ICU re-admission rates and increased mortality. The receiving team should be provided with a written summary, including the information listed in Box 10.49. The ICU team should remain available for advice; many ICU teams provide an outreach service to supply advice and facilitate continuity of care.

Critical care scoring systems

Admission and discharge criteria vary between ICUs, so it is important to define the characteristics of the patients admitted in

10

10.49 How to write an ICU discharge summary: information to be included

- Summary of diagnosis and progress in intensive care
- Current medications and changes to regular medications with justifications
- Antibiotic regime and suggested review dates
- Results of positive microbiological tests
- Positions of invasive devices and insertion dates
- Escalation plan in the event of deterioration
- Pending investigations and specialty consultations
- If the physiology remains abnormal due to chronic disease, rapid response triggers should be adjusted accordingly

order to assess the effects of the care provided on the outcomes achieved. Two systems are widely used to measure severity of illness (see Box 10.50 for further details):

- *APACHE II*: Acute Physiology Assessment and Chronic Health Evaluation
- *SOFA score*: Sequential Organ Failure Assessment tool.

When combined with the admission diagnosis, scoring systems have been shown to correlate well with the risk of death in hospital. Such outcome predictions are useful at a population level but lack the specificity to be of use in decision-making for individual patients. This is in contrast to well-validated, disease-specific tools, such as the CURB-65 tool for pneumonia, which can be helpful in guiding individual management (see Fig. 17.32, p. 583).

Predicted mortality figures by diagnosis have been calculated from large databases generated from a range of ICUs. These allow a particular unit to evaluate its performance compared to the reference ICUs by calculating standardised mortality ratios (SMRs) for each diagnostic group. A value of unity indicates the same performance as the reference ICUs, while a value below 1 indicates a better than predicted outcome. If a unit has a high SMR in a certain diagnostic category, it should prompt investigation

i 10.50 Comparison of APACHE II and SOFA scores

APACHE II score

- An assessment of admission characteristics (e.g. age and pre-existing organ dysfunction) and the maximum/minimum values of 12 routine physiological measurements during the first 24 hours of admission (e.g. temperature, blood pressure, GCS) that reflect the physiological impact of the illness
- Composite score out of 71
- Higher scores are given to patients with more serious underlying diagnoses, medical history or physiological instability; higher mortality correlates with higher scores

SOFA score

- A score of 1–4 is allocated to six organ systems (respiratory, cardiovascular, liver, renal, coagulation and neurological) to represent the degree of organ dysfunction, e.g. platelet count $>150\times10^9$/L scores 1 point, $<25\times10^9$/L scores 4 points
- Composite score out of 24
- Higher scores are associated with increased mortality

into the management of patients with that diagnosis, in order to identify aspects of care that could be improved.

Further information

Websites

criticalcarereviews.com *Reviews and appraisal of ICU topics.*
emcrit.org *Online podcasts and general information on emergency medicine and critical care.*
esicm.org *European Society of Intensive Care Medicine: guidelines, recommendations, consensus conference reports.*
lifeinthefastlane.com *Information on a range of intensive care and emergency medicine topics.*
survivingsepsis.org *Surviving Sepsis website.*

DH Dockrell
S Sundar
BJ Angus

Infectious disease

Clinical examination of patients with infectious disease 216

Presenting problems in infectious diseases 218
Fever 218
Positive blood culture 225
Sepsis 226
Acute diarrhoea and vomiting 227
Infections acquired in the tropics 230
Infections in adolescence 234
Infections in pregnancy 234

Viral infections 236
Systemic viral infections with exanthem 236
Systemic viral infections without exanthem 240
Viral infections of the skin 247
Gastrointestinal viral infections 249
Respiratory viral infections 249
Viral infections with neurological involvement 249
Viral infections with rheumatological involvement 250

Prion diseases 250

Bacterial infections 250
Bacterial infections of the skin, soft tissues and bones 250
Systemic bacterial infections 254
Gastrointestinal bacterial infections 262
Respiratory bacterial infections 265
Bacterial infections with neurological involvement 267
Mycobacterial infections 267
Rickettsial and related intracellular bacterial infections 270
Chlamydial infections 272

Protozoal infections 273
Systemic protozoal infections 273
Leishmaniasis 281
Gastrointestinal protozoal infections 286

Infections caused by helminths 288
Intestinal human nematodes 288
Tissue-dwelling human nematodes 290
Zoonotic nematodes 293
Trematodes (flukes) 294
Cestodes (tapeworms) 297

Ectoparasites 299

Fungal infections 300
Superficial mycoses 300
Subcutaneous mycoses 300
Systemic mycoses 301

Clinical examination of patients with infectious disease

5 **Eyes**
Conjunctival petechiae
Painful red eye in uveitis
Loss of red reflex in endophthalmitis
Roth's spots in infective endocarditis
Haemorrhages and exudates
of cytomegalovirus retinitis
Choroidal lesions of tuberculosis

Roth's spots in
endocarditis

4 **Head and neck**
Lymphadenopathy
Parotidomegaly
Abnormal tympanic membranes

3 **Oropharynx**
Dental caries
Tonsillar enlargement or exudate
Candidiasis

▲ Streptococcal tonsillitis

2 **Hands and nails**
Finger clubbing
Splinter haemorrhages
Janeway lesions
Signs of chronic liver disease
Vasculitis lesions

▲ Splinter haemorrhages
in endocarditis

1 **Skin**
Generalised erythema
Rash (see opposite)
IV injection track marks
Surgical scars
Prosthetic devices, e.g. central
venous catheters
Tattoos

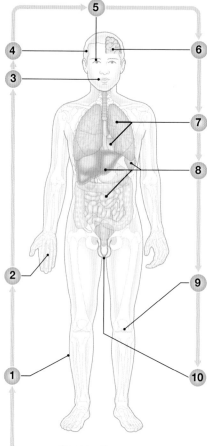

Observation
• Temperature
• Sweating
• Weight loss
• Respiratory distress
• Altered consciousness
• Pallor
• Jaundice

6 **Neurological**
Neck stiffness
Photophobia
Delirium
Focal neurological signs

7 **Heart and lungs**
Tachycardia, hypotension
Murmurs or prosthetic heart
sounds
Pericardial rub
Signs of consolidation
Pleural or pericardial effusion

▲ Chest X-ray consolidation
in pneumonia

8 **Abdomen**
Hepatosplenomegaly
Ascites
Renal angle tenderness
Localised tenderness or
guarding with decreased bowel
sounds, e.g. in left iliac fossa
with diverticulitis
Mass lesions
Surgical drains

9 **Musculoskeletal**
Joint swelling, erythema or
tenderness
Localised tender spine suggestive
of epidural abscesses or discitis
Draining sinus of
chronic osteomyelitis

10 **Genitalia and rectum**
Ulceration or discharge
Testicular swelling or nodules
Inguinal lymphadenopathy
Prostatic tenderness
Rectal fluctuance

▲ Testicular swelling
in adult mumps

Insets (splinter haemorrhages) Courtesy of Dr Nick Beeching, Royal Liverpool University Hospital; (Roth's spots) Courtesy of Prof. Ian Rennie, Royal Hallamshire Hospital, Sheffield.

Figs A–C opposite Courtesy of Dr Ravi Gowda, Royal Hallamshire Hospital, Sheffield.

i Fever

Documentation of fever

- 'Feeling hot' or sweaty does not necessarily signify fever – diagnosed only when a body temperature of over 38.0°C is recorded
- Axillary and aural measurement is less accurate than oral or rectal
- Outpatients may be trained to keep a temperature chart

Rigors

- Shivering (followed by excessive sweating) occurs with a rapid rise in body temperature from any cause

Night sweats

- Associated with particular infections (e.g. TB, infective endocarditis); sweating from any cause is worse at night

Excessive sweating

- Alcohol, anxiety, thyrotoxicosis, diabetes mellitus, acromegaly, lymphoma and excessive environmental heat all cause sweating without temperature elevation

Recurrent fever

- There are various causes, e.g. *Borrelia recurrentis*, bacterial abscess

Accompanying features

- Severe headache and photophobia, although characteristic of meningitis, may accompany other infections.
- Delirium during fever is more common in young children or the elderly
- Myalgia may occur with viral infections, such as influenza, and with sepsis including meningococcal sepsis
- Shock may accompany severe infections and sepsis (p. 196)

i History-taking in suspected infectious disease*

Presenting complaint

- Diverse manifestations of infectious disease make accurate assessment of features and duration critical; e.g. fever and cough lasting 2 days imply an acute respiratory tract infection but suggest TB if they last 2 months

Review of systems

- Must be comprehensive

Past medical history

- Define the 'host' and likelihood of infection(s)
- Include surgical and dental procedures involving prosthetic materials
- Document previous infections

Medication history

- Include non-prescription drugs, use of antimicrobials and immunosuppressants
- Identify medicines that interact with antimicrobials or that may cause fever

Allergy history

- Esp. to antimicrobials, noting allergic manifestation (e.g. rash versus anaphylaxis)

Family and contact history

- Note infections and their duration
- Sensitively explore exposure to key infections, e.g. TB and HIV

Travel history

- Include countries visited and where previously resident (relevant to exposure and likely vaccination history, e.g. likelihood of BCG vaccination in childhood)

Occupation

- e.g. Anthrax in leather tannery workers

Recreational pursuits

- e.g. Leptospirosis in canoeists and windsurfers

Animal exposures

- Include pets, e.g. dogs/hydatid disease

Dietary history

- Consider under-cooked meats, shellfish, unpasteurised dairy products or well water
- Establish who else was exposed, e.g. to food-borne pathogens

History of intravenous drug injection or receipt of blood products

- Risks for blood-borne viruses, e.g. HIV-1, HBV and HCV

Sexual history

- Explore in a confidential manner (Ch. 13); remember that the most common mode of HIV-1 transmission is heterosexual (Ch. 12)

Vaccination history and use of prophylactic medicines

- Consider occupation- or age-related vaccines
- In a traveller or infection-predisposed patient, establish adherence to prophylaxis

*Always consider non-infectious aetiologies in the differential diagnosis. (HBV/HCV = hepatitis B/C virus; HIV-1 = human immunodeficiency virus-1; TB = tuberculosis)

1 Skin lesions in infectious diseases

- Diffuse erythema, e.g. A
- Migrating erythema, e.g. enlarging rash of erythema migrans in Lyme disease (see Fig. 11.21, p. 256)
- Purpuric or petechial rashes, e.g. B
- Macular or papular rashes, e.g. primary infection with HIV (see Box 12.8, p. 312)
- Vesicular or blistering rash, e.g. C
- Erythema multiforme (see Fig. 29.53 and Box 29.32, pp. 1264 and 1265)
- Nodules or plaques, e.g. Kaposi's sarcoma (p. 315)
- Erythema nodosum (D and Box 29.33, p. 1265)

Streptococcal toxic shock syndrome.

Meningococcal sepsis.

Shingles.

Erythema nodosum.

11

The principles of infection and its investigation and therapy are described in Chapter 6. This chapter and the following ones on human immunodeficiency virus/acquired immunodeficiency syndrome (HIV/AIDS) and sexually transmitted infection (STI) describe the approach to patients with potential infectious disease, the individual infections and the resulting syndromes.

Presenting problems in infectious diseases

Infectious diseases present with myriad clinical manifestations. Many of these are described in other chapters or below.

Fever

'Fever' implies an elevated core body temperature of more than 38.0°C (p. 138). Fever is a response to cytokines and acute phase proteins (pp. 65 and 70), and occurs in infections and in non-infectious conditions.

Clinical assessment

The differential diagnosis is very broad so clinical features are used to guide the most appropriate investigations. The systematic approach described on page 216 should be followed. Box 11.1 describes the assessment of elderly patients.

Investigations

If the clinical features do not suggest a specific infection, then initial investigations should include:

- a full blood count (FBC) with differential, including eosinophil count
- urea and electrolytes, liver function tests (LFTs), blood glucose and muscle enzymes
- inflammatory markers, erythrocyte sedimentation rate (ESR) and C-reactive protein (CRP)
- a test for antibodies to HIV-1 (p. 310)
- autoantibodies, including antinuclear antibodies (ANA)
- chest X-ray and electrocardiogram (ECG)
- urinalysis and urine culture
- blood culture (p. 106)
- throat swab for culture or polymerase chain reaction (PCR)

11.1 Fever in old age

- **Temperature measurement**: fever may be missed because oral temperatures are unreliable. Rectal measurement may be needed but core temperature is increasingly measured using eardrum reflectance.
- **Delirium**: common with fever, especially in those with underlying cerebrovascular disease or dementia.
- **Prominent causes of pyrexia of unknown origin**: include tuberculosis and intra-abdominal abscesses, complicated urinary tract infection and infective endocarditis. Non-infective causes include polymyalgia rheumatica/temporal arteritis and tumours. A smaller fraction of cases remain undiagnosed than in young people.
- **Pitfalls in the elderly**: conditions such as stroke or thromboembolic disease can cause fever but every effort must be made to exclude concomitant infection.
- **Common infectious diseases in the very frail** (e.g. nursing home residents): pneumonia, urinary tract infection, soft tissue infection and gastroenteritis.

- other specimens, as indicated by history and examination, e.g. wound swab; sputum culture; stool culture, microscopy for ova and parasites, and *Clostridium difficile* toxin assay
- specific tests and their priority, indicated by geographical location: malaria films on 3 consecutive days or a malaria rapid diagnostic test (antigen detection, p. 276), a test for non-structural protein 1 (NS1) in dengue (antigen detection) and blood cultures for *Salmonella* Typhi, as well as abdominal ultrasound, would be standard initial tests in many regions in Africa, Asia, Oceania, and Central and South America.

Subsequent investigations in patients with HIV-related (p. 313), immune-deficient (p. 223), nosocomial or travel-related (p. 230) pyrexia and in individuals with associated symptoms or signs of involvement of the respiratory, gastrointestinal or neurological systems are described elsewhere.

Management

Fever and its associated systemic symptoms can be treated with paracetamol, and by tepid sponging to cool the skin. Replacement of salt and water is important in patients with drenching sweats. Further management is focused on the underlying cause.

Fever with localising symptoms or signs

In most patients, the site of infection is apparent after clinical evaluation (p. 216), and the likelihood of infection is reinforced by investigation results (e.g. neutrophilia with raised ESR and CRP in bacterial infections). Not all apparently localising symptoms are reliable, however; headache, breathlessness and diarrhoea can occur in sepsis or malaria without localised infection in the central nervous system (CNS), respiratory tract or gastrointestinal tract, and abdominal pain may be a feature of basal pneumonia. Careful interpretation of the clinical features is vital (e.g. severe headache associated with photophobia, rash and neck stiffness suggests meningitis, whereas moderate headache with cough and rhinorrhoea is consistent with a viral upper respiratory tract infection).

Common infections that present with fever are shown in Figure 11.1. Further investigation and management are specific to the cause, but may include empirical antimicrobial therapy (p. 116) pending confirmation of the microbiological diagnosis.

Pyrexia of unknown origin

Pyrexia of unknown origin (PUO) was classically defined as a temperature above 38.0°C on multiple occasions for more than 3 weeks, without diagnosis, despite initial investigation in hospital for 1 week. The definition has been relaxed to allow for investigation over 3 days of inpatient care, three outpatient visits or 1 week of intensive ambulatory investigation. Subsets of PUO are described as HIV-1 related, immune-deficient or nosocomial. Up to one-third of cases of PUO remain undiagnosed.

Clinical assessment

Major causes of PUO are outlined in Box 11.2. Rare causes, such as periodic fever syndromes (p. 81), should be considered in those with a family history. Children and younger adults are more likely to have infectious causes – in particular, viral infections. Older adults are more likely to have certain infectious and non-infectious causes (see Box 11.1). Detailed history and examination should be repeated at regular intervals to detect emerging features (e.g. rashes, signs of infective endocarditis

Fig. 11.1 Common infectious syndromes presenting with fever and localised features. Major causes are grouped by approximate anatomical location and include central nervous system infection; respiratory tract infections; abdominal, pelvic or urinary tract infections; and skin and soft tissue infections (SSTIs) or osteomyelitis. For each site of infection, particular syndromes and their common causes are described elsewhere in the book. The causative organisms vary, depending on host factors, which include whether the patient has lived in or visited a tropical country or particular geographical location, has acquired the infection in a health-care environment or is immunocompromised. *Insets (cellulitis of the leg) Courtesy of Dr Ravi Gowda, Royal Hallamshire Hospital, Sheffield; (pulmonary tuberculosis) Courtesy of Dr Ann Chapman, Royal Hallamshire Hospital, Sheffield; (empyema, pyogenic liver abscess, diverticular abscess, tuberculous osteomyelitis) Courtesy of Dr Robert Peck, Royal Hallamshire Hospital, Sheffield.*

(p. 527) or features of vasculitis). In men, the prostate should be considered as a potential source of infection.

Clinicians should be alert to the possibility of factitious fever, in which high temperature recordings are engineered by the patient (Box 11.3).

Investigations

If initial investigation of fever is negative, further microbiological and non-microbiological investigations should be considered (Boxes 11.4 and 11.5). As with initial investigation of fever described above, the selection and prioritisation of tests will be influenced by the geographical location of potential exposure to pathogens (Box 11.4). These will usually include:

- induced sputum or other specimens for mycobacterial stains and culture
- serological tests, including an HIV test, and ferritin estimation
- imaging of the abdomen by ultrasonography or computed tomography (CT)
- echocardiography.

Lesions identified on imaging should usually be biopsied in order to seek evidence of relevant pathogens by culture, histopathology or nucleic acid detection. Particularly in patients who have received prior antimicrobials, 16S rRNA analysis (Box 6.2, p. 101) may aid diagnosis if a microorganism is not cultured. The chance of a successful diagnosis is greatest if procedures for obtaining

11.2 Aetiology of pyrexia of unknown origin (PUO)

Infections (~30%)

Specific locations
- Abscesses: hepatobiliary, diverticular, urinary tract (including prostate), pulmonary, CNS
- Infections of oral cavity (including dental), head and neck (including sinuses)
- Bone and joint infections
- Infective endocarditis*

Specific organisms
- TB (particularly extrapulmonary)*
- HIV-1 infection
- Other viral infections: cytomegalovirus (CMV), Epstein–Barr virus (EBV)
- Fungal infections (e.g. *Aspergillus* spp., *Candida* spp. or dimorphic fungi)
- Infections with fastidious organisms (e.g. *Bartonella* spp., *Tropheryma whipplei*)

Specific patient groups
- Recently spent time in a region with geographically restricted infection:
  Malaria*, dengue, rickettsial infections, *Brucella* spp., amoebic liver abscess, enteric fevers (Africa, Asia, Oceania, Central and South America), *Leishmania* spp. (southern Europe, India, Africa and Latin America), *Burkholderia pseudomallei* (South-east Asia), Middle East respiratory syndrome coronavirus (MERS-CoV; Arabian Peninsula)
- Residence in or travel to a region with endemic infection:
  TB* (Africa, Asia, Central and South America), extensively drug-resistant TB (XDR-TB; South Africa), *Brucella* spp. (Africa, Asia, Central and South America), HIV-1 (Africa, Asia), *Trypanosoma cruzi* (Central and South America)
- Nosocomial infections:
  Pneumonia*, infections related to prosthetic materials and surgical procedures, urinary tract infections, central venous catheter infections
- HIV-positive individuals:
  Acute retroviral syndrome
  AIDS-defining infections (disseminated *Mycobacterium avium* complex (DMAC), *Pneumocystis jirovecii* pneumonia, CMV and others)

Malignancy (~20%)

Haematological malignancy
- Lymphoma*, leukaemia and myeloma

Solid tumours
- Renal, liver, colon, stomach, pancreas

Connective tissue disorders (~15%)

Older adults
- Temporal arteritis/polymyalgia rheumatica*

Younger adults
- Still's disease (juvenile rheumatoid arthritis)*
- Systemic lupus erythematosus (SLE)
- Vasculitic disorders, including polyarteritis nodosa, rheumatoid disease with vasculitis and granulomatosis with polyangiitis (formerly known as Wegener's granulomatosis)
- Polymyositis
- Behçet's disease
- Rheumatic fever (in regions where still endemic, e.g. Asia, Oceania and parts of Africa)

Miscellaneous (~20%)

Cardiovascular
- Atrial myxoma, aortitis, aortic dissection

Respiratory
- Sarcoidosis, pulmonary embolism and other thromboembolic disease, extrinsic allergic alveolitis

Gastrointestinal
- Inflammatory bowel disease, granulomatous hepatitis, alcoholic liver disease, pancreatitis

Endocrine/metabolic
- Thyrotoxicosis, thyroiditis, hypothalamic lesions, phaeochromocytoma, adrenal insufficiency, hypertriglyceridaemia

Haematological
- Haemolytic anaemia, paroxysmal nocturnal haemoglobinuria, thrombotic thrombocytopenic purpura, myeloproliferative disorders, Castleman's disease, graft-versus-host disease (after allogeneic haematopoietic stem cell transplantation)

Inherited
- Familial Mediterranean fever and periodic fever syndromes

Drug reactions*
- e.g. Antibiotic fever, drug hypersensitivity reactions etc.

Factitious fever

Idiopathic (~15%)

*Most common causes within each group.

 11.3 Clues to the diagnosis of factitious fever

- A patient who looks well
- Bizarre temperature chart with absence of diurnal variation and/or temperature-related changes in pulse rate
- Temperature >41°C
- Absence of sweating during defervescence
- Normal erythrocyte sedimentation rate and C-reactive protein despite high fever
- Evidence of self-injection or self-harm
- Normal temperature during supervised (observed) measurement
- Infection with multiple commensal organisms (e.g. enteric or mouth flora)

and transporting the correct samples in the appropriate media are carefully planned between the clinical team, the radiologist or surgeon performing the procedure, and the local microbiologist and histopathologist. Positron emission tomography (PET) scans may aid diagnosis of vasculitis or help selection of biopsy sites. Liver biopsy may be justified – for example, to identify idiopathic granulomatous hepatitis – if there are biochemical or radiological abnormalities. Bone marrow biopsies have a diagnostic yield of up to 15%, most often revealing haematological malignancy, myelodysplasia or tuberculosis, and also identifying brucellosis, typhoid fever or visceral leishmaniasis. Bone marrow should be sent for culture, as well as microscopy. Laparoscopy is occasionally undertaken with biopsy of abnormal tissues. Splenic aspiration in specialist centres is the diagnostic test of choice for

11.4 Microbiological investigation of pyrexia of unknown origin[1]

Location-independent investigations

Microscopy
- Blood for atypical lymphocytes (EBV, CMV, HIV-1, hepatitis viruses or *Toxoplasma gondii*)
- Respiratory samples for mycobacteria and fungi
- Stool for ova, cysts and parasites
- Biopsy for light microscopy (bacteria, mycobacteria, fungi) and/or electron microscopy (viruses, protozoa (e.g. microsporidia) and other fastidious organisms (e.g. *Tropheryma whipplei*))
- Urine for white or red blood cells and mycobacteria (early morning urine ×3)

Culture
- Aspirates and biopsies (e.g. joint, deep abscess, debrided tissues)
- Blood, including prolonged culture and special media conditions
- Sputum for mycobacteria
- CSF
- Gastric aspirate for mycobacteria
- Stool
- Swabs
- Urine ± prostatic massage in older men

Antigen detection
- Blood, e.g. HIV p24 antigen, cryptococcal antigen, *Aspergillus* galactomannan ELISA and for *Aspergillus* and other causes of invasive, fungal infection (1,3)-β-D-glucan
- CSF for cryptococcal antigen
- Bronchoalveolar lavage fluid for *Aspergillus* galactomannan
- Nasopharyngeal aspirate/throat swab for respiratory viruses, e.g. IAV or RSV
- Urine, e.g. for *Legionella* antigen

Nucleic acid detection
- Blood for *Bartonella* spp. and viruses
- CSF for viruses and key bacteria (meningococcus, pneumococcus, *Listeria monocytogenes*)
- Nasopharyngeal aspirate/throat swab for respiratory viruses

- Sputum for *Mycobacterium tuberculosis* (MTB) and rifampicin (RIF) resistance with geneXpert MTB/RIF cartridge-based nucleic acid amplification test
- Bronchoalveolar lavage fluid, e.g. for respiratory viruses
- Tissue specimens, e.g. for *T. whipplei*
- Urine, e.g. for *Chlamydia trachomatis*, *Neisseria gonorrhoeae*
- Stool, e.g. for norovirus, rotavirus

Immunological tests
- Serology (antibody detection) for viruses, including HIV-1, and some bacteria
- Interferon-gamma release assay for diagnosis of exposure to tuberculosis (but note this will not distinguish latent from active disease and can only be used to trigger further investigations of active disease)

Geographically restricted tests[2]

Microscopy
- Blood for trypanosomiasis, malaria and *Borrelia* spp.
- Stool for geographically restricted ova, cysts and parasites
- Biopsy for light microscopy (dimorphic fungi, *Leishmania* spp. and other parasites)
- Urine for red blood cells and schistosome ova

Antigen detection
- Blood, e.g. dengue virus NS1 antigen, *Histoplasma* antigen (restricted availability) and malaria antigen (e.g. HRP-2 for *Plasmodium falciparum* or parasite-specific LDH for *P. falciparum* and *P. vivax*)

Nucleic acid detection
- Blood for causes of viral haemorrhagic fever
- CSF for geographically restricted viruses, e.g. Japanese encephalitis virus
- Nasopharyngeal aspirate/throat swab or bronchoalveolar lavage fluid for geographically restricted respiratory viruses, e.g. MERS-CoV

Immunological tests
- Serology (antibody detection) for viruses, dimorphic fungi and protozoa

[1]This list does not apply to every patient with a pyrexia of unknown origin. Appropriate tests should be selected in a stepwise manner, according to specific predisposing factors, epidemiological exposures and local availability, and should be discussed with a microbiologist. [2]Addition of these tests should be guided by the location of presentation or travel history.
(CMV = cytomegalovirus; CSF = cerebrospinal fluid; EBV = Epstein–Barr virus; ELISA = enzyme-linked immunosorbent assay; HIV-1 = human immunodeficiency virus-1; HRP-2 = histidine-rich protein 2; IAV = influenza A virus; LDH = lactate dehydrogenase; MERS-CoV = Middle East respiratory syndrome coronavirus; NS1 = non-structural 1; RSV = respiratory syncytial virus)

11

11.5 Additional investigations in PUO

- Serological tests for connective tissue disorders:
  - Autoantibody screen
  - Complement levels
  - Immunoglobulins
  - Cryoglobulins
- Ferritin
- Echocardiography
- Ultrasound of abdomen
- CT/MRI of thorax, abdomen and/or brain
- Imaging of the skeletal system:
  - Plain X-rays
  - CT/MRI spine
  - Isotope bone scan

- Labelled white cell scan
- Positron emission tomography (PET)/single-photon emission computed tomography (SPECT)
- Biopsy:
  - Bronchoscopy and lavage ± transbronchial biopsy
  - Lymph node aspirate or biopsy
  - Biopsy of radiological lesion
  - Biopsy of liver
  - Bone marrow aspirate and biopsy
  - Lumbar puncture
  - Laparoscopy and biopsy
  - Temporal artery biopsy

suspected visceral leishmaniasis. Temporal artery biopsy should be considered in patients over the age of 50 years, even in the absence of physical signs or a raised ESR. 'Blind' biopsy of other structures in the absence of localising signs or laboratory or radiology results is unhelpful.

Prognosis

No cause is found in approximately 10% of PUO cases, but as long as there is no significant weight loss or signs of another disease, the long-term mortality is low.

Fever in the injection drug-user

Intravenous injection of recreational drugs is widespread in many parts of the world (p. 1184). Infective organisms are introduced by non-sterile (often shared) injection equipment (Fig. 11.2). The risks increase with prolonged drug use and injection into large veins of the groin and neck necessitated by progressive thrombosis of superficial peripheral veins. The most common causes of fever are soft tissue or respiratory infections.

Clinical assessment

The history should address the following risk factors:

- *Site of injection.* Femoral vein injection is associated with vascular complications such as deep venous thrombosis (50% of which are septic) and accidental arterial injection with false aneurysm formation or a compartment syndrome due to swelling within the fascial sheath. Local complications include ilio-psoas abscess, and septic arthritis of the hip joint or sacroiliac joint. Injection of the jugular vein can be associated with cerebrovascular complications. Subcutaneous and intramuscular injection has been related to infection by clostridial species, the spores of which contaminate heroin. *Clostridium novyi*

6 Cardiovascular system
Systolic 'V' waves in JVP of tricuspid regurgitation (p. 526)
Regurgitant murmurs in endocarditis

5 Nervous system
Signs of drug intoxication
Encephalopathy
Signs of meningitis
Focal neurological features or seizures in septic embolism/ mycotic aneurysm/abscess
Cranial nerve palsies of botulism
Trismus, muscle rigidity or spasms in tetanus
Localised pain over vertebrae with epidural abscess

4 Optic fundi
Roth's spots
Candidal cotton wool spots

3 Oropharynx
Dental infections
Oropharyngeal candidiasis or other signs of HIV-1 infection

2 Hands and nails
Splinter haemorrhages
Signs of chronic liver disease

1 Skin and soft tissues (any site)
Cellulitis
Purulent drainage
Abscesses
Ulcers
Bullae or extreme pain suggestive of necrotising fasciitis

7 Respiratory system
Consolidation in pneumonia
Upper lobe signs in tuberculosis
Pleural rub with septic pulmonary emboli

8 Abdomen
Jaundice ± tender liver edge with hepatitis
Pain in left upper quadrant with splenic abscess

9 Bone and joints
Osteomyelitis
Septic arthritis

10 Injection sites
Abscesses
Fistula
Haematoma
Pseudoaneurysm

11 Femoral stretch test
Passive extension of the hip joint causes pain and reflex muscle spasm in ilio-psoas abscess

12 Legs
Signs of DVT
Vasculitis or ischaemic signs of septic emboli, endocarditis or vasospasm
Compartment syndrome

Observation

▲ Skin abscesses in an injection drug-user

▲ Sharing injecting equipment may transmit blood-borne viruses

▲ Hip flexor spasm in an injection drug-user with ilio-psoas abscess

Fig. 11.2 Fever in the injection drug-user: key features of clinical examination. Full examination (p. 216) is required but features most common amongst injection drug-users are shown here. (DVT = deep venous thrombosis; JVP = jugular venous pulse)

causes a local lesion with significant toxin production, leading to shock and multi-organ failure. Tetanus, wound botulism, anthrax and gas gangrene also occur.

- *Technical details of injection.* Sharing of needles and other injecting paraphernalia (including spoons and filters) increases the risk of blood-borne virus infection (e.g. HIV-1, hepatitis B or C virus). Some users lubricate their needles by licking them prior to injection, thus introducing mouth organisms (e.g. anaerobic streptococci, *Fusobacterium* spp. and *Prevotella* spp.). Contamination of commercially available lemon juice, used to dissolve heroin before injection, has been associated with blood-stream infection with *Candida* spp.
- *Substances injected.* Injection of cocaine is associated with a variety of vascular complications. Certain formulations of heroin have been linked with particular infections, e.g. wound botulism with black tar heroin. Drugs are often mixed with other substances, e.g. talc.
- *Blood-borne virus status.* Results of previous HIV-1 and hepatitis virus tests or vaccinations for hepatitis viruses should be recorded.
- *Surreptitious use of antimicrobials.* Addicts may use antimicrobials to self-treat infections, masking initial blood culture results.

Key findings on clinical examination are shown in Figure 11.2. It can be difficult to distinguish the effects of infection from the effects of drugs or drug withdrawal (excitement, tachycardia, sweating, marked myalgia, delirium). Stupor and delirium may result from drug administration but may also indicate meningitis or encephalitis. Non-infected venous thromboembolism is also common in this group.

Investigations

The initial investigations are as for any fever (see above), including a chest X-ray and blood cultures. Since blood sampling may be difficult, contamination is often a problem. Echocardiography to detect infective endocarditis should be performed in all injection drug-users with bacteraemia due to *Staphylococcus aureus* or other organisms associated with endocarditis (Fig. 11.3A); thromboembolic phenomena; or a new or previously undocumented murmur. Endovascular infection should also be suspected if lung abscesses or pneumatoceles are detected radiologically. Infected thrombus at injection sites, such as the groin, is common, and may lead to abscess formation. Additional imaging should be focused on sites of injection or of localising symptoms and signs (Fig. 11.3B). Any pathological fluid collections should be sampled.

Urinary toxicology tests may suggest a non-infectious cause of the presenting complaint. While being investigated, all injection drug-users should be offered testing for infection with hepatitis B and C virus and HIV-1.

Injection drug-users may have more than one infection. Skin and soft tissue infections are most often due to *Staph. aureus* or streptococci, and sometimes to *Clostridium* spp. or anaerobes. Pulmonary infections are most often due to the common pathogens causing community-acquired pneumonia, tuberculosis or septic emboli (Fig. 11.3C). Endocarditis with septic emboli commonly involves *Staph. aureus* and viridans streptococci, but *Pseudomonas aeruginosa* and *Candida* spp. are also encountered.

Management

Empirical therapy of fever in the injection drug-user includes an antistaphylococcal penicillin (e.g. flucloxacillin) or, if meticillin-resistant *Staph. aureus* (MRSA) is prevalent in the community, a

Fig. 11.3 Causes of fever in injection drug-users. A Endocarditis: large vegetation on the tricuspid valve (arrow). B Septic arthritis of the left sternoclavicular joint (arrow A) (note the erosion of the bony surfaces at the sternoclavicular joint) with overlying soft tissue collection (arrow B). C Tricuspid valve endocarditis caused by *Staphylococcus aureus*. Thoracic CT scan shows multiple embolic lesions with cavitation (arrows). The patient presented with haemoptysis. *C, Courtesy of Dr Julia Greig, Royal Hallamshire Hospital, Sheffield.*

glycopeptide (e.g. vancomycin) or lipopeptide (e.g.daptomycin). Once microbiological results are available, therapy can be narrowed to focus on the microorganism identified. In injection drug-users, meticillin-sensitive *Staph. aureus* is customarily treated with high-dose intravenous flucloxacillin, with shorter durations for uncomplicated right-sided endocarditis. Right-sided endocarditis caused by MRSA is usually treated with 4 weeks of vancomycin plus gentamicin for the first week. Specialist advice should be sought.

For localised infections of the skin and soft tissues, oral therapy with agents active against staphylococci, streptococci and anaerobes is appropriate (e.g. flucloxacillin plus co-amoxiclav or clindamycin). Non-adherence to prescribed antimicrobial regimens leads to a high rate of complications.

Fever in the immunocompromised host

Immunocompromised hosts include those with congenital immunodeficiency (p. 77), HIV infection (Ch. 12) and iatrogenic immunosuppression induced by chemotherapy (p. 1330), transplantation (p. 88) or immunosuppressant medicines, including high-dose glucocorticoids. Metabolic abnormalities, such as under-nutrition or hyperglycaemia, may also contribute. Multiple elements of the immune system are potentially compromised. A patient may have impaired neutrophil function from chemotherapy, impaired T-cell and/or B-cell responses due to underlying malignancy, T-cell and phagocytosis defects due to glucocorticoids, mucositis from chemotherapy and an impaired skin barrier due to insertion of a central venous catheter.

Fever may result from infectious or non-infectious causes, including drugs, vasculitis, neoplasm, lymphoproliferative disease, graft-versus-host disease (in recipients of haematopoietic stem cell transplants (HSCT; p. 936), organising pneumonitis or Sweet's syndrome (reddish nodules or plaques with fever and leucocytosis, in association with haematological malignancy).

Clinical assessment

The following should be addressed in the history:

- Identification of the immunosuppressant factors and nature of the immune defect.
- Any past infections and their treatment. Infections may recur and antimicrobial resistance may have been acquired in response to prior therapy.
- Exposure to infections, including opportunistic infections that would not cause disease in an immunocompetent host.
- Prophylactic medicines and vaccinations administered.

Examination should include inspection of the normal physical barriers provided by skin and mucosal surfaces and, in particular, central venous catheters, the mouth, sinuses, ears and perianal area (digital rectal examination should be avoided). Disseminated infections can manifest as cutaneous lesions. The areas around fingernails and toenails should also be inspected closely.

Investigations

Initial screening tests are as described above (p. 218). Immunocompromised hosts often have decreased inflammatory responses leading to attenuation of physical signs, such as neck stiffness with meningitis, radiological features and laboratory findings, such as leucocytosis. Chest CT scan should be considered in addition to chest X-ray when respiratory symptoms occur. Abdominal imaging may also be warranted, particularly if there is right lower quadrant pain, which may indicate typhlitis (inflammation of the caecum) in neutropenic patients. Blood cultures from a central venous catheter, urine cultures, and stool cultures if diarrhoea is present are also recommended.

Nasopharyngeal aspirates are sometimes diagnostic, as immunocompromised hosts may shed respiratory viruses for prolonged periods. Skin lesions should be biopsied if nodules are present, and investigation should include fungal stains. Useful molecular techniques include PCR for cytomegalovirus (CMV) and *Aspergillus* spp. DNA, and antigen assays (e.g. cryptococcal antigen (CrAg) for *Cryptococcus neoformans*, galactomannan for *Aspergillus* spp. in blood, and (1,3)-β-D-glucan for *Aspergillus* spp. and other causes of invasive fungal infection (though this will not identify mucoraceous moulds) or *Legionella pneumophila* type 1 in urine). Antibody detection is rarely useful in immunocompromised patients. Patients with respiratory signs or symptoms should be considered for bronchoalveolar lavage to detect *Pneumocystis jirovecii*, other fungi, bacteria and viruses.

Neutropenic fever

Neutropenic fever is defined as a neutrophil count of less than 0.5×10^9/L (p. 925) and a single axillary temperature above 38.5°C or three recordings above 38.0°C over a 12-hour period, although the infection risk increases progressively as the neutrophil count drops below 1.0×10^9/L. Patients with neutropenia are particularly prone to bacterial and fungal infection. Gram-positive organisms are the most common pathogens, particularly in association with in-dwelling catheters.

Empirical broad-spectrum antimicrobial therapy is commenced as soon as neutropenic fever occurs and cultures have been obtained. The most common regimens for neutropenic sepsis are broad-spectrum penicillins, such as piperacillin–tazobactam IV. The routine addition of aminoglycosides to these agents is not supported by trial data. If fever has not resolved after 3–5 days, empirical antifungal therapy (e.g. caspofungin) is added (p. 125). An alternative antifungal strategy is to use azole prophylaxis in high-risk patients and markers of early fungal infection, such as galactomannan and/or fungal PCR, to guide initiation of antifungal treatment (a 'pre-emptive approach').

Post-transplantation fever

Fever in transplant recipients may be due to infection, episodes of graft rejection in solid organ transplant recipients, or graft-versus-host disease following HSCT (p. 936).

Infections in solid organ transplant recipients are grouped according to the time of onset (Box 11.6). Those in the first month are mostly related to the underlying condition or surgical complications. Those occurring 1–6 months after transplantation are characteristic of impaired T-cell function. Risk factors for CMV infection have been identified; patients commonly receive either prophylaxis or intensive monitoring involving regular testing for CMV DNA by PCR and early initiation of anti-CMV therapy using intravenous ganciclovir or oral valganciclovir if tests become positive.

Following HSCT, infections in the first 4 weeks are more common in patients receiving a myeloablative-conditioning

i 11.6 Infections in transplant recipients	
Time post transplantation	Infections
Solid organ transplant recipients	
0–1 month	Bacterial or fungal infections related to the underlying condition or surgical complications
1–6 months	CMV, other opportunistic infections (e.g. *Pneumocystis jirovecii* pneumonia)
>6 months	Bacterial pneumonia, other bacterial community-acquired infections, shingles, cryptococcal infection, PTLD
Myeloablative haematopoietic stem cell transplant recipients	
Pre-engraftment (typically 0–4 weeks) Post-engraftment:	Bacterial and fungal infections, respiratory viruses or HSV reactivation
Early (<100 days)	CMV, *Pneumocystis jirovecii* pneumonia, moulds or other opportunistic infections
Late (>100 days)	Community-acquired bacterial infections, shingles, CMV, PTLD

(CMV = cytomegalovirus; HSV = herpes simplex virus; PTLD = post-transplant lymphoproliferative disorder)

regimen (Box 11.6). Later infections are more common if an allogeneic procedure is performed.

Post-transplant lymphoproliferative disorder (PTLD) is an Epstein–Barr virus (EBV)-associated lymphoma that can complicate transplantation, particularly when primary EBV infection occurs after transplantation.

Positive blood culture

Blood-stream infection (BSI) is a frequent presentation of infection. This can be community-acquired or hospital-acquired ('nosocomial'). The most common causes are shown in Box 11.7. In immunocompromised hosts, a wider range of microorganisms may be isolated, e.g. fungi in neutropenic hosts.

Primary BSI describes the situation in which there is no known extravascular source of infection (e.g. pneumonia or urinary tract infection), and is more common in *Staph. aureus* BSI. In community-acquired *Staph. aureus* bacteraemia, 20–30% of cases are associated with infectious endocarditis and up to 10% are due to osteomyelitis. Peripheral and central venous catheters are an important source of nosocomial BSI.

BSI has an associated mortality of 15–40%, depending on the setting, host and microbial factors.

Clinical assessment

The history should determine the setting in which BSI has occurred. Host factors predisposing to infection include skin disease, diabetes mellitus, injection drug use, the presence of a central venous, urinary or haemodialysis catheter, and surgical procedures, especially those involving the implantation of prosthetic materials (in particular, endovascular prostheses).

Physical examination should focus on signs of endocarditis (p. 527), evidence of bone or joint infection (tenderness or restriction of movement), and abdominal or flank tenderness. Central venous catheters should be examined for erythema or purulence at the exit site. Particularly in cases with *Candida* spp. infection or suspected infectious endocarditis, fundoscopy after pupil dilatation should be performed.

Investigations

Positive blood cultures may be caused by contaminants. When isolated from only one bottle, or from all bottles from one venesection, coagulase-negative staphylococci often represent contamination. Repeated isolation of this organism, however, should raise suspicion of infective endocarditis or, in a patient with any form of prosthetic material, prosthesis infection. Viridans streptococci occasionally cause transient non-significant

bacteraemia or blood culture contamination but, in view of their association with infective endocarditis, significant infection must always be excluded. *Bacillus* spp. ('aerobic spore bearers') and *Clostridium* spp. often represent incidental transient bacteraemia or contamination, but certain species (e.g. *C. septicum*) are more likely to be genuine pathogens.

Further investigations are influenced by the causative organism and setting. Initial screening tests are similar to those for fever (p. 218) and should include chest X-ray, urine culture and, in many cases, ultrasound or other imaging of the abdomen. Imaging should also include any areas of bone or joint pain and any prosthetic material, e.g. a prosthetic joint or an aortic graft.

Echocardiography should be considered for those patients with BSI who have valvular heart disease or clinical features of endocarditis (p. 527), those whose cultures reveal an organism that is a common cause of endocarditis (e.g. *Staph. aureus*, viridans streptococci or enterococci), those in whom multiple blood cultures are positive for the same organism, and those with a rapid positive result on culture. The sensitivities of transthoracic echocardiography (TTE) and transoesophageal echocardiography (TOE) for the detection of vegetations are 50–90% and over 95%, respectively. Therefore, if TTE is negative, TOE should be performed.

Certain rare causes of BSI have specific associations that warrant further investigation. Endocarditis caused by *Streptococcus gallolyticus* subsp. *gallolyticus* (formerly *Strep. bovis* biotype I) and BSI with *C. septicum* are both associated with colonic carcinoma and their isolation is an indication for colonoscopy.

Management

BSI requires antimicrobial therapy and attention to the source of infection, including surgical drainage if appropriate. Two weeks of therapy may be sufficient for *Staph. aureus* BSI from central and peripheral venous catheter infections when the source is identified and removed, for uncomplicated skin and soft tissue infections, and for uncomplicated right-sided infective endocarditis. Other *Staph. aureus* BSIs are usually treated for 4–6 weeks.

Central venous catheter infections

Infections of central venous catheters typically involve the catheter lumen and are associated with fever, positive blood cultures and, in some cases, signs of purulence or exudate at the site of insertion. Infection is more common in temporary catheters inserted into the groin or jugular vein than in those in the subclavian vein. Tunnelled catheters, e.g. Hickman catheters, may also develop tunnel site infections.

Staphylococci account for 70–90% of catheter infections, with coagulase-negative staphylococci more common than *Staph. aureus*. Other causes include enterococci and Gram-negative bacilli. Unusual Gram-negative organisms, such as *Citrobacter freundii* and *Pseudomonas fluorescens*, raise the possibility of non-sterile infusion equipment or infusate. *Candida* spp. are a common cause of line infections, particularly in association with total parenteral nutrition. Non-tuberculous mycobacteria may cause tunnel infections.

Investigations and management

In bacteraemic patients with fever and no other obvious source of infection, a catheter infection is likely. Local evidence of erythema, purulence or thrombophlebitis supports the diagnosis. However, microbiological confirmation is essential (p. 106). Catheter-related infection is suggested by higher colony counts

i	**11.7 Common causes of blood-stream infection**

Community-acquired

• *Escherichia coli*	• *Streptococcus pneumoniae*
• *Staphylococcus aureus*, including MRSA	• Other streptococci

Nosocomial

• *Staph. aureus*, including MRSA	• Enterococci, including VRE
• Coagulase-negative staphylococci	• Gram-negative bacteria
	• *Candida* spp.

(MRSA = meticillin-resistant *Staphylococcus aureus*; VRE = vancomycin-resistant enterococci)

or shorter time to positivity in blood cultures obtained through the catheter than in peripheral blood cultures. If the line is removed, a semi-quantitative culture of the tip may confirm the presence of 15 or more colony-forming units, but this is retrospective and does not detect luminal infection.

For coagulase-negative staphylococcal line infections, the options are to remove the line and provide 5–7 days' therapy or, particularly in the case of tunnelled catheters, to treat empirically with a glycopeptide antibiotic, e.g. vancomycin, with or without the use of antibiotic-containing lock therapy to the catheter for approximately 14 days. For *Staph. aureus* infection, the chance of curing an infection with the catheter in situ is low and the risks from infection are high. Therefore, unless the risks of catheter removal outweigh the benefits, treatment involves catheter removal, followed by 14 days of antimicrobial therapy; the same applies to infections with *Pseudomonas aeruginosa*, *Candida* spp., atypical mycobacteria or *Bacillus* spp. Infections complicated by endocarditis, thrombophlebitis, metastatic infection or tunnel infection also require catheter removal.

Infection prevention is a key component of the management of vascular catheters. Measures include strict attention to hand hygiene, optimal siting, full aseptic technique on insertion and subsequent interventions, skin antisepsis with chlorhexidine and isopropyl alcohol, daily assessment of catheter sites (e.g. with visual infusion phlebitis (VIP) score; see Box 11.37, p. 251), and daily consideration of the continuing requirement for catheterisation. The use of catheters impregnated with antimicrobials, such as chlorhexidine or silver, is advocated in some settings.

Sepsis

Sepsis is discussed on page 196 and there are many causes (Box 11.8). The results of blood cultures and pre-existing host factors guide initial investigations. Patients who are immunocompromised may have a broader range of causal pathogens that may be harder to culture, including mycobacteria and fungi. In many regions, malaria and dengue must also be excluded.

Severe skin and soft tissue infections

Skin and soft tissue infections (SSTIs) are an important cause of sepsis. Cases can be classified as in Box 11.9, according to the clinical features and microbiological findings. In some cases, severe systemic features may be out of keeping with mild local features.

Necrotising fasciitis

In necrotising fasciitis, cutaneous erythema and oedema progress to bullae or areas of necrosis. Unlike in cellulitis, pain may be disproportionately intense in relation to the visible cutaneous features or may spread beyond the zone of erythema. The infection spreads quickly along the fascial plane. Type 1 necrotising fasciitis is a mixed infection with Gram-negative bacteria and anaerobes, often seen post-operatively in diabetic or immunocompromised hosts. Subcutaneous gas may be present. Type 2 necrotising fasciitis is caused by group A or other streptococci. Approximately 60% of cases are associated with streptococcal toxic shock syndrome (p. 253). Type 3 infection

11.8 Causes of sepsis	
Infection	Setting
Bacterial	
Staphylococcus aureus, coagulase-negative staphylococci	Bacteraemia may be associated with endocarditis, intravascular cannula infection, or skin or bone foci
Streptococcus pneumoniae	Invasive pneumococcal disease, usually with pneumonia or meningitis; asplenia
Other streptococci	Invasive streptococcal disease, especially necrotising fasciitis
	Viridans streptococci in neutropenic host with severe mucositis
Staphylococcal or streptococcal toxic shock syndrome	Toxin-mediated, blood cultures negative; clues include erythrodermic rash and epidemiological setting
Enterococci	Most often with abdominal focus
Neisseria meningitidis	Sepsis in children or young adults with petechial rash and/or meningitis
Escherichia coli, other Gram-negative bacteria	Urinary or biliary tract infection, or other abdominal infections
Pseudomonas aeruginosa, multidrug-resistant Gram-negative bacteraemia	Nosocomial infection
Salmonella Typhi or Paratyphi	In countries with a high incidence of enteric fever
Yersinia pestis	In plague
Burkholderia pseudomallei	Endemic in areas of Thailand; more likely to involve patients with diabetes mellitus or immunocompromised
Capnocytophaga canimorsus	Associated with dog bites and asplenic individuals
Clostridium difficile	Severe colitis, particularly in the elderly
Polymicrobial infection with Gram-negatives and anaerobes	Bowel perforation, bowel ischaemia
Mycobacterium tuberculosis, *M. avium* complex (MAC)	HIV-positive or immunocompromised with miliary tuberculosis or disseminated MAC
Fungal	
Candida spp.	Line infection or post-operative complication, nosocomial or immunocompromised host
Histoplasma capsulatum, other dimorphic fungi	Immunocompromised host
Parasitic	
Falciparum malaria	Malaria with high-level parasitaemia and multi-organ failure or as a complication of bacterial superinfection
Babesia microti	Asplenic individual
Strongyloides stercoralis hyperinfection syndrome	Gram-negative infection complicating *Strongyloides* infection in immunocompromised host

11.9 Severe necrotising soft tissue infections

- Necrotising fasciitis (primarily confined to subcutaneous fascia and fat)
- Clostridial anaerobic cellulitis (confined to skin and subcutaneous tissue)
- Non-clostridial anaerobic cellulitis
- Progressive bacterial synergistic gangrene (*Staphylococcus aureus* + micro-aerophilic streptococcus) ('Meleney's gangrene', primarily confined to skin)
- Pyomyositis (discrete abscesses within individual muscle groups)
- Clostridial myonecrosis (gas gangrene)
- Anaerobic streptococcal myonecrosis (non-clostridial infection mimicking gas gangrene)
- Group A streptococcal necrotising myositis

Fig. 11.4 Excision following necrotising fasciitis in an injection drug-user.

involves organisms such as *Aeromonas hydrophila* and *Vibrio vulnificus*, which is found in tropical to subtropical regions and is associated with marine exposure. Type 4 is caused by fungi such as mucoraceous moulds and may also vary geographically in incidence with recent reports of increased cases in India and other regions.

Necrotising fasciitis is a medical emergency, requiring immediate surgical débridement with inspection of the involved muscle groups, in addition to antimicrobial therapy (Fig. 11.4). Empirical treatment is with broad-spectrum agents (e.g. piperacillin–tazobactam plus clindamycin; meropenem with clindamycin). Ceftazidime or ciprofloxacin with doxycycline may be used where marine exposure is a factor, and antifungals for suspected fungal necrotising fasciitis, but it is important to combine these with effective coverage against streptococcal infection. MRSA-associated necrotising fasciitis has emerged in some regions and in these places appropriate therapy for MRSA, such as a glycopeptide or linezolid, should be added to the empirical regimen until microbiological results allow narrowing of the antimicrobial spectrum. Hyperbaric oxygen therapy may be considered for polymicrobial infection. Group A streptococcal infection is treated with benzylpenicillin plus clindamycin, and often immunoglobulin, though to date clinical trials have not provided clear evidence of the benefit of immunoglobulin.

Gas gangrene

Although *Clostridium* spp. may colonise or contaminate wounds, no action is required unless there is evidence of spreading infection. Infection may be limited to tissue that is already damaged (anaerobic cellulitis) or may involve healthy muscle (gas gangrene).

In anaerobic cellulitis, usually due to *C. perfringens* or other clostridia infecting devitalised tissue following a wound, gas forms locally and extends along tissue planes but bacteraemia does not occur. Prompt surgical débridement of devitalised tissue and therapy with penicillin or clindamycin is usually effective.

Gas gangrene (clostridial myonecrosis) is defined as acute invasion of healthy living muscle undamaged by previous trauma, and is most commonly caused by *C. perfringens*. In at least 70% of cases, it follows deep penetrating injury sufficient to create an anaerobic (ischaemic) environment and allow clostridial introduction and proliferation. Severe pain at the site of the injury progresses rapidly over 18–24 hours. Skin colour changes from pallor to bronze/purple discoloration and the skin is tense, swollen, oedematous and exquisitely tender. Gas in tissues may be obvious, with crepitus on clinical examination, or visible on X-ray, CT or ultrasound. Signs of systemic toxicity develop rapidly, with high leucocytosis, multi-organ dysfunction, raised creatine kinase and evidence of disseminated intravascular coagulation and haemolysis. Antibiotic therapy with high-dose intravenous penicillin and clindamycin is recommended, coupled with aggressive surgical débridement of the affected tissues. Alternative agents include cephalosporins and metronidazole. Hyperbaric oxygen has a putative but controversial role.

Other SSTIs

'Synergistic gangrene' is a polymicrobial infection with anaerobes and other bacteria (*Staph. aureus* or Gram-negatives). When this affects the genital/perineal area, it is known as 'Fournier's gangrene'. Severe gangrenous cellulitis in immunocompromised hosts may involve Gram-negative bacteria or fungi. *Entamoeba histolytica* can cause soft tissue necrosis following abdominal surgery in areas of the world where infection is common. Contact with sea water or shellfish consumption in tropical to subtropical regions worldwide, such as the Gulf of Mexico, can lead to infection with *Vibrio vulnificus*. This infection causes soft tissue necrosis and bullae, and may lead to necrotising fasciitis. Patients with chronic liver disease are particularly susceptible to this infection and can develop sepsis.

Acute diarrhoea and vomiting

Acute diarrhoea (p. 783), sometimes with vomiting, is the predominant symptom in infective gastroenteritis (Box 11.10). Acute diarrhoea may also be a symptom of other infectious and non-infectious diseases (Box 11.11). Stress, whether psychological or physical, can also produce loose stools.

The World Health Organisation (WHO) estimates that there are more than 1.7 billion cases of acute diarrhoea annually globally, with 760 000 deaths in children under 5. In developed countries, diarrhoea remains an important problem, with the elderly being most vulnerable (Box 11.12). The majority of episodes are due to infections spread by the faecal–oral route and transmitted either on fomites, on contaminated hands, or in food or water. Measures such as the provision of clean drinking water, appropriate disposal of human and animal sewage, and the application of simple principles of food hygiene can all limit gastroenteritis.

The clinical features of food-borne gastroenteritis vary. Some organisms (*Bacillus cereus*, *Staph. aureus* and *Vibrio cholerae*) elute exotoxins that cause vomiting and/or so-called 'secretory' diarrhoea (watery diarrhoea without blood or faecal leucocytes,

11.10 Causes of infectious gastroenteritis

Toxin in food: <6 hrs incubation

- *Bacillus cereus* (p. 262)
- *Staphylococcus aureus* (p. 262)
- *Clostridium* spp. enterotoxin (p. 262)

Bacterial: 12–72 hrs incubation

- Enterotoxigenic *Escherichia coli* (ETEC, p. 263)
- Shiga toxin-producing *E. coli* (EHEC, p. 263)*
- Enteroinvasive *E. coli* (EIEC, p. 263)*
- *Vibrio cholerae* (p. 264)
- *Salmonella* (p. 262)
- *Shigella** (p. 265)
- *Campylobacter** (p. 262)
- *Clostridium difficile** (p. 264)

Viral: short incubation

- Rotavirus (p. 249)
- Norovirus (p. 249)

Protozoal: long incubation

- Giardiasis (p. 287)
- Cryptosporidiosis (pp. 287 and 317)
- Microsporidiosis (p. 317)
- Amoebic dysentery (p. 286)*
- Cystoisosporiasis (p. 233)

*Associated with bloody diarrhoea.

11.11 Differential diagnosis of acute diarrhoea and vomiting

Infectious causes

- Gastroenteritis
- *Clostridium difficile* infection (p. 264)
- Acute diverticulitis (p. 833)
- Sepsis (p. 196)
- Pelvic inflammatory disease (p. 336)
- Meningococcaemia (p. 1119)
- Pneumonia (especially 'atypical disease', p. 582)
- Malaria (p. 273)

Non-infectious causes

Gastrointestinal

- Inflammatory bowel disease (p. 813)
- Bowel malignancy (p. 827)
- Overflow from constipation (p. 834)
- Enteral tube feeding

Metabolic

- Diabetic ketoacidosis (p. 735)
- Thyrotoxicosis (p. 635)
- Uraemia (p. 414)
- Neuro-endocrine tumours releasing (e.g.) VIP or 5-HT

Drugs and toxins

- NSAIDs
- Cytotoxic agents
- Antibiotics
- Proton pump inhibitors
- Dinoflagellates (p. 149)
- Plant toxins (p. 150)
- Heavy metals
- Ciguatera fish poisoning (p. 149)
- Scombrotoxic fish poisoning (p. 150)

(5-HT = 5-hydroxytryptamine, serotonin; NSAIDs = non-steroidal anti-inflammatory drugs; VIP = vasoactive intestinal peptide)

11.12 Infectious diarrhoea in old age

- **Incidence**: not increased but the impact is greater.
- **Mortality**: most deaths due to gastroenteritis in the developed world are in adults aged over 70. Most are presumed to be caused by dehydration leading to organ failure.
- ***Clostridium difficile* infection (CDI)**: more common, especially in hospital and nursing home settings, usually following antibiotic exposure.

reflecting small bowel dysfunction). In general, the time from ingestion to the onset of symptoms is short and, other than dehydration, little systemic upset occurs. Other organisms, such as *Shigella* spp., *Campylobacter* spp. and enterohaemorrhagic *Escherichia coli* (EHEC), may directly invade the mucosa of the small bowel or produce cytotoxins that cause mucosal ulceration, typically affecting the terminal small bowel and colon. The incubation period is longer and more systemic upset occurs, with prolonged bloody diarrhoea. *Salmonella* spp. are capable of invading enterocytes and of causing both a secretory response and invasive disease with systemic features. This is seen with *Salmonella* Typhi and *Salmonella* Paratyphi (enteric fever), but may occasionally be seen with other non-typhoidal *Salmonella* spp., particularly in the immunocompromised host and the elderly.

Clinical assessment

The history should address foods ingested (Box 11.13), duration and frequency of diarrhoea, presence of blood or steatorrhoea, abdominal pain and tenesmus, and whether other people have been affected. Fever and bloody diarrhoea suggest an invasive, colitic, dysenteric process. An incubation period of less than 18 hours suggests toxin-mediated food poisoning, and longer than 5 days suggests diarrhoea caused by protozoa or helminths. Person-to-person spread suggests certain infections, such as shigellosis or cholera.

Examination includes assessment of the degree of dehydration. Assessment for early signs of hypotension, such as thirst, headache, altered skin turgor, dry mucous membranes and postural hypotension, is important, particularly in tropical regions where dehydration progresses rapidly. Signs of more marked dehydration include supine hypotension and tachycardia, decreased urinary output, delirium and sunken eyes. The blood pressure, pulse rate, urine output and ongoing stool losses should be monitored closely.

11.13 Foods associated with infectious illness, including gastroenteritis

Raw seafood

- Norovirus
- *Vibrio* spp.
- Hepatitis A

Raw eggs

- *Salmonella* serovars

Undercooked meat or poultry

- *Salmonella* serovars
- *Campylobacter* spp.
- EHEC
- Hepatitis E (pork products)
- *Clostridium perfringens*

Unpasteurised milk or juice

- *Salmonella* serovars.
- *Campylobacter* spp.
- EHEC
- *Yersinia enterocolitica*

Unpasteurised soft cheeses

- *Salmonella* serovars
- *Campylobacter* spp.
- ETEC
- *Yersinia enterocolitica*
- *Listeria monocytogenes*

Home-made canned goods

- *Clostridium botulinum*

Raw hot dogs, pâté

- *Listeria monocytogenes*

(EHEC = enterohaemorrhagic *Escherichia coli*; ETEC = enterotoxigenic *E. coli*)

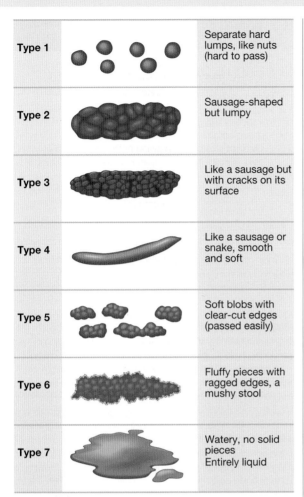

Type 1		Separate hard lumps, like nuts (hard to pass)
Type 2		Sausage-shaped but lumpy
Type 3		Like a sausage but with cracks on its surface
Type 4		Like a sausage or snake, smooth and soft
Type 5		Soft blobs with clear-cut edges (passed easily)
Type 6		Fluffy pieces with ragged edges, a mushy stool
Type 7		Watery, no solid pieces Entirely liquid

Fig. 11.5 Bristol stool chart. The stool is given a 'score' of 1–7 by reference to the verbal and visual description. This is recorded on a chart (usually known as a 'Bristol stool chart') or in a patient monitoring database. *Adapted from Lewis SJ, Heaton KW. Stool form scale as a useful guide to intestinal transit time. Scand J Gastroenterol 1997; 32:920–924.*

The severity of diarrhoea may be assessed by reference to the Bristol stool form scale (Bristol stool chart), which allows an objective assessment of stool consistency by providing a verbal and visual reference scale (Fig. 11.5). The Bristol stool form scale was developed in the 1990s to monitor patients with irritable bowel syndrome, but its main use (at least in UK hospitals) is to monitor hospital inpatients with loose stool to assist in decisions on stool sampling and infection prevention precautions, especially in relation to *C. difficile*.

Investigations

These include stool inspection for blood and microscopy for leucocytes, and also an examination for ova, cysts and parasites if the history indicates residence or travel to areas where these infections are prevalent. Stool culture should be performed and *C. difficile* toxin sought. FBC and serum electrolytes indicate the degree of inflammation and dehydration. Where cholera is prevalent, examination of a wet film with dark-field microscopy for darting motility may provide a diagnosis. In a malarious area, a blood film for malaria parasites should be obtained. Blood and urine cultures and a chest X-ray may identify alternative sites of infection, particularly if the clinical features suggest a syndrome other than gastroenteritis.

Management

All patients with acute, potentially infective diarrhoea should be appropriately isolated to minimise person-to-person spread of infection. If the history suggests a food-borne source, public health measures must be implemented to identify the source and to establish whether other linked cases exist (p. 114).

Fluid replacement

Replacement of fluid losses in diarrhoeal illness is crucial and may be life-saving.

Although normal daily fluid intake in an adult is only 1–2 L, there is considerable additional fluid movement in and out of the gut in secretions (see Fig. 21.7, p. 769). Altered gut resorption with diarrhoea can result in substantial fluid loss; for example, 10–20 L of fluid may be lost in 24 hours in cholera. The fluid lost in diarrhoea is isotonic, so both water and electrolytes need to be replaced. Absorption of electrolytes from the gut is an active process requiring energy. Infected mucosa is capable of very rapid fluid and electrolyte transport if carbohydrate is available as an energy source. Oral rehydration solutions (ORS) therefore contain sugars, as well as water and electrolytes (Box 11.14). ORS can be just as effective as intravenous replacement fluid, even in the management of cholera. In mild to moderate gastroenteritis, adults should be encouraged to drink fluids and, if possible, continue normal dietary food intake. If this is impossible – due to vomiting, for example – intravenous fluid administration will be required. In very sick patients or those with cardiac or renal disease, monitoring of urine output and central venous pressure may be necessary.

The volume of fluid replacement required should be estimated based on the following considerations:

- *Replacement of established deficit*. After 48 hours of moderate diarrhoea (6–10 stools per 24 hrs), the average adult will be 2–4 L depleted from diarrhoea alone. Associated vomiting will compound this. Adults with this symptomatology should therefore be given rapid replacement of 1–1.5 L, either orally (ORS) or by intravenous infusion (normal saline), within the first 2–4 hours of presentation. Longer symptomatology or more persistent/severe diarrhoea rapidly produces fluid losses comparable to diabetic ketoacidosis and is a metabolic emergency requiring active intervention.

i	**11.14 Composition of oral rehydration solution and other replacement fluids***			
Fluid	**Na**	**K**	**Cl**	**Energy**
WHO	90	20	80	54
Dioralyte	60	20	60	71
Pepsi	6.5	0.8	–	400
7UP	7.5	0.2	–	320
Apple juice	0.4	26	–	480
Orange juice	0.2	49	–	400
Breast milk	22	36	28	670

*Values given in mmol/L for electrolyte and kcal/L for energy components.
(WHO = World Health Organisation)

- *Replacement of ongoing losses*. The average adult's diarrhoeal stool accounts for a loss of 200 mL of isotonic fluid. Stool losses should be carefully charted and an estimate of ongoing replacement fluid calculated. Commercially available rehydration sachets are conveniently produced to provide 200 mL of ORS; one sachet per diarrhoea stool is an appropriate estimate of supplementary replacement requirements.
- *Replacement of normal daily requirement*. The average adult has a daily requirement of 1–1.5 L of fluid in addition to the calculations above. This will be increased substantially in fever or a hot environment.

Antimicrobial agents

In non-specific gastroenteritis, routine use of antimicrobials does not improve outcome and may lead to antimicrobial resistance or side-effects. They are usually used where there is systemic involvement, a host with immunocompromise or significant comorbidity.

Evidence suggests that, in EHEC infections, the use of antibiotics may make the complication of haemolytic uraemic syndrome (HUS; p. 408) more likely due to increased toxin release. Antibiotics should therefore not be used in this condition.

Conversely, antibiotics are indicated in *Shigella dysenteriae* infection and in invasive salmonellosis – in particular, typhoid fever. Antibiotics may also be advantageous in cholera epidemics, reducing infectivity and controlling the spread of infection.

Antidiarrhoeal, antimotility and antisecretory agents

These agents are not usually recommended in acute infective diarrhoea. Loperamide, diphenoxylate and opiates are potentially dangerous in dysentery in childhood, causing intussusception. Antisecretory agents, such as bismuth and chlorpromazine, may make the stools appear more bulky but do not reduce stool fluid losses and may cause significant sedation. Adsorbents, such as kaolin or charcoal, have little effect.

Non-infectious causes of food poisoning

While acute food poisoning and gastroenteritis are most frequently caused by infections, non-infectious causes must also be considered in the differential diagnosis. These are discussed on page 149.

Antimicrobial-associated diarrhoea

Antimicrobial-associated diarrhoea (AAD) is a common complication of antimicrobial therapy, especially with broad-spectrum agents. It is most common in the elderly but can occur at all ages. Although the specific mechanism is unknown in most cases of AAD, *C. difficile* (p. 264) is implicated in 20–25% of cases and is the most common cause among patients with evidence of colitis. *C. perfringens* is a rarer cause that usually remains undiagnosed, and *Klebsiella oxytoca* may also cause antibiotic-associated haemorrhagic colitis.

Infections acquired in the tropics

Recent decades have seen unprecedented increases in long-distance business and holiday travel, as well as extensive migration. Although certain diseases retain their relatively fixed geographical distribution, being dependent on specific vectors or weather conditions, many travel with their human hosts and some may then be transmitted to other people. This means

11.15 How to assess health needs in travellers before departure*

- Destination
- Personal details, including previous travel experience
- Dates of trip
- Itinerary and purpose of trip
- Personal medical history, including pregnancy, medication and allergies (e.g. to eggs, vaccines, antibiotics)
- Past vaccinations:
  - Childhood schedule followed? Diphtheria, tetanus, pertussis, polio, *Neisseria meningitidis* types B/C, *Haemophilus influenzae* B (HiB)
  - Travel-related? Typhoid, yellow fever, hepatitis A, hepatitis B, meningococcal ACW135Y, rabies, Japanese B encephalitis, tick-borne encephalitis
- Malaria prophylaxis: questions influencing the choice of antimalarial drugs are destination, past experience with antimalarials, history of epilepsy or psychiatric illness

*Further information is available at fitfortravel.nhs.uk.

that the pattern of infectious diseases seen in each country changes constantly, and travel history and information on countries previously lived in, particularly during childhood, are crucial.

In general, the diversity of infectious diseases is greater in tropical than in temperate countries, and people in temperate countries have immunity to a narrower range of infections, reflecting less exposure in childhood and less ongoing boosting of immunity later in life, so that the most common travel-associated infections are those that are acquired by residents of temperate countries during visits to the tropics. In addition, those who have lived in tropical areas may lose immunity when they move to temperate countries and become susceptible when visiting their homeland.

Most travel-associated infections can be prevented. Pre-travel advice is tailored to the destination and the traveller (Box 11.15). It includes avoidance of insect bites (using at least 20% diethyltoluamide (DEET)), sun protection (sunscreen with a sun protection factor (SPF) of at least 15), food and water hygiene ('Boil it, cook it, peel it or forget it!'), how to respond to travellers' diarrhoea (seek medical advice if bloody or if it lasts more than 48 hrs) and, if relevant, safe sex (condom use).

Fever acquired in the tropics

Presentation with unexplained fever is common in travellers who are visiting or have recently travelled to tropical areas. Fever may also occur in those living in tropical regions if they have not developed immunity to the endemic pathogen or if this immunity is compromised by factors such as pregnancy. Frequent final diagnoses in such patients are malaria, typhoid fever, viral hepatitis and dengue fever. Travellers to affected areas may have viral haemorrhagic fevers (VHFs) such as Ebola, Lassa, Crimean–Congo and Marburg (see Box 11.36, p. 245), avian influenza (H5N1) or Middle East respiratory syndrome (MERS), which require special isolation precautions.

Clinical assessment

The approach to unexplained fever is as described above and key questions relating to infections acquired in tropical regions are listed in Box 11.16. Medicines purchased in some countries may have reduced efficacy, e.g. for malaria prophylaxis. Consult reliable up-to-date sources about resistance to antimalarial drugs in the country visited. Vaccinations against yellow fever and hepatitis A and B are sufficiently effective to virtually exclude these infections. Oral and injectable typhoid vaccinations are 70–90% effective.

The differential diagnosis is guided by the clinical scenario, presence of specific exposures (Box 11.17) and incubation period (Box 11.18). *Falciparum* malaria tends to present between 7 and 28 days after exposure in an endemic area. VHF, dengue and rickettsial infection can usually be excluded if more than 21 days have passed between leaving the area and onset of illness.

11.16 How to obtain a history from travellers to the tropics with fever

Questions	Factors to ascertain
Countries visited and dates of travel	Relate travel to known outbreaks of infection or antimicrobial resistance
Determine the environment visited	Travel to rural environments, forests, rivers or lakes
Clarify where the person slept	Sleeping in huts, use of bed nets, sleeping on the ground
Establish what he/she was doing	Exposure to people with medical illness, animals, soil, lakes and rivers
History of insect bites	Type of insect responsible, circumstances (location, time of day etc.), preventive measures
Dietary history	Ingestion of uncooked foods, salads and vegetables, meats (especially if under-cooked), shellfish, molluscs, unpasteurised dairy products, unbottled water and sites at which food prepared
Sexual history	History of sexual intercourse with commercial sex workers, local population or travellers from other countries
Malaria prophylaxis	Type of prophylaxis
Vaccination history	Receipt of pre-travel vaccines and appropriateness to area visited
History of any treatments received while abroad	Receipt of medicines, local remedies, blood transfusions or surgical procedures

11.17 Specific exposures and causes of fever in the tropics

Exposure	Infection or disease
Mosquito bite	Malaria, dengue fever, Chikungunya, filariasis, tularaemia
Tsetse fly bite	African trypanosomiasis
Tick bite	Rickettsial infections including typhus, Lyme disease, tularaemia, Crimean–Congo haemorrhagic fever, Kyasanur forest disease, babesiosis, tick-borne encephalitis
Louse bite	Typhus
Flea bite	Plague
Sandfly bite	Leishmaniasis, arbovirus infection
Reduviid bug	Chagas' disease
Animal contact	Q fever, brucellosis, anthrax, plague, tularaemia, viral haemorrhagic fevers, rabies
Fresh-water swimming	Schistosomiasis, leptospirosis, *Naegleria fowleri*
Exposure to soil	Inhalation: dimorphic fungi Inhalation or inoculation: *Burkholderia pseudomallei* Inoculation (most often when barefoot): hookworms, *Strongyloides stercoralis*
Raw or under-cooked fruit and vegetables	Enteric bacterial infections, hepatitis A or E virus, *Fasciola hepatica*, *Toxocara* spp., *Echinococcus granulosus* (hydatid disease), *Entamoeba histolytica*
Under-cooked pork	*Taenia solium* (cysticercosis)
Crustaceans or molluscs	Paragonimiasis, gnathostomiasis, *Angiostrongylus cantonensis* infection, hepatitis A virus, cholera
Unpasteurised dairy products	Brucellosis, salmonellosis, abdominal tuberculosis, listeriosis
Untreated water	Enteric bacterial infections, giardiasis, *Cryptosporidium* spp. (chronic in immunocompromised), hepatitis A or E virus

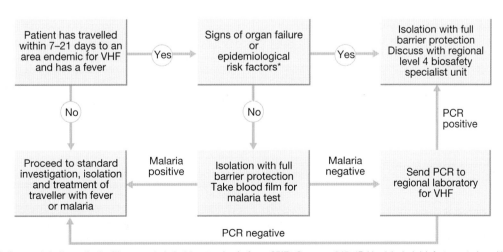

Fig. 11.6 Approach to the patient with suspected viral haemorrhagic fever (VHF). See page 245. *Epidemiological risk factors: staying with a febrile individual, caring for a sick individual, or contact with body fluids from a suspected human or animal case of VHF. (PCR = polymerase chain reaction)

11.18 Incubation times and illnesses in travellers

<2 weeks

Non-specific fever
- Malaria
- Chikungunya
- Dengue
- Scrub typhus
- Spotted group rickettsiae
- Acute HIV
- Acute hepatitis C virus
- *Campylobacter*
- Salmonellosis
- Shigellosis
- East African trypanosomiasis
- Leptospirosis
- Relapsing fever
- Influenza
- Yellow fever

Fever and coagulopathy (usually thrombocytopenia)
- Malaria
- VHF
- Meningococcaemia
- Enteroviruses
- Leptospirosis and other bacterial pathogens associated with coagulopathy

Fever and central nervous system involvement
- Malaria
- Typhoid fever
- Rickettsial typhus (epidemic caused by *Rickettsia prowazekii*)
- Meningococcal meningitis
- Arboviral encephalitis
- East African trypanosomiasis
- Other causes of encephalitis or meningitis
- Angiostrongyliasis
- Rabies

Fever and pulmonary involvement
- Influenza
- Pneumonia, including *Legionella* pneumonia
- Acute histoplasmosis
- Acute coccidioidomycosis
- Q fever
- SARS

Fever and rash
- Viral exanthems (rubella, measles, varicella, mumps, HHV-6, enteroviruses)
- Chikungunya
- Dengue
- Spotted or typhus group rickettsiosis
- Typhoid fever
- Parvovirus B19
- HIV-1

2–6 weeks
- Malaria
- Tuberculosis
- Hepatitis A, B, C and E viruses
- Visceral leishmaniasis
- Acute schistosomiasis
- Amoebic liver abscess
- Leptospirosis
- African trypanosomiasis
- VHF
- Q fever
- Acute American trypanosomiasis
- Viral causes of mononucleosis syndromes

>6 weeks
- Non-*falciparum* malaria
- Tuberculosis
- Hepatitis B and E viruses
- HIV-1
- Visceral leishmaniasis
- Filariasis
- Onchocerciasis
- Schistosomiasis
- Amoebic liver abscess
- Chronic mycoses
- African trypanosomiasis
- Rabies
- Typhoid fever

(HHV-6 = human herpesvirus-6; SARS = severe acute respiratory syndrome; VHF = viral haemorrhagic fever)
Adapted from Traveller's Health Yellow Book, CDC Health Information for International Travel 2008.

11.19 Investigation of tropically acquired acute fever without localising signs

Features on full blood count	Further investigations
Neutrophil leucocytosis	
Bacterial sepsis	Blood culture
Leptospirosis	Culture of blood and urine, serology
Borreliosis (tick- or louse-borne relapsing fever)	Blood film
Amoebic liver abscess	Ultrasound
Normal white cell count and differential	
Malaria (may have low platelets or anaemia)	Blood film, antigen test
Typhoid fever	Blood and stool culture
Typhus	Serology
Lymphocytosis	
Viral fevers, including VHF	Serology, PCR
Infectious mononucleosis	Monospot test, serology
Malaria	Blood film, antigen test
Rickettsial fevers	Serology
Atypical lymphocytes	
Dengue and other VHF	Serology, antigen, PCR
Infectious mononucleosis-like syndromes	Serology, PCR
HIV (acute retroviral syndrome)	Serology, antigen
Hepatitis viruses	Serology, antigen, PCR
Parasitic, malaria, trypanosomiasis	Blood film, antigen test, PCR

(PCR = polymerase chain reaction; VHF = viral haemorrhagic fever)

Investigations and management

Initial investigations should start with blood films for malaria parasites, FBC, urinalysis and chest X-ray if indicated. Box 11.19 lists diagnoses and investigations to consider in unexplained acute fever.

Management is directed at the underlying cause. In patients with suspected VHF (p. 245), strict infection control measures with isolation and barrier nursing are implemented to prevent contact with the patient's body fluids. The risk of VHF should be determined using epidemiological risk factors and clinical signs (Fig. 11.6), and further management undertaken as described on page 246.

Diarrhoea acquired in the tropics

Gastrointestinal illness is the most common infection amongst visitors to the tropics, with *Salmonella* spp., *Campylobacter* spp. and *Cryptosporidium* spp. infections prevalent worldwide (Box 11.20). *Shigella* spp. and *Entamoeba histolytica* (amoebiasis) are usually encountered in visitors to or residents of the Indian subcontinent or sub-Saharan and southern Africa.

The approach to patients with acute diarrhoea is described on page 227. The benefits of treating travellers' diarrhoea with antimicrobials are marginal, with slight reductions in stool

11.20 Most common causes of travellers' diarrhoea

- Enterotoxigenic *E. coli* (ETEC)
- *Shigella* spp.
- *Campylobacter jejuni*
- *Salmonella* serovars
- *Plesiomonas shigelloides*
- Non-cholera *Vibrio* spp.
- *Aeromonas* spp.

Clinical examination is summarised on page 216. Particular attention should be paid to the skin, throat, eyes, nail beds, lymph nodes, abdomen and heart. Patients may be unaware of tick bites or eschars (p. 270). Body temperature should be measured at least twice daily.

frequency and likelihood of cure at 72 hours offset by increased side-effects. The differential diagnosis of diarrhoea persisting for more than 14 days is wide (see Box 21.18, p. 784). Parasitic and bacterial causes, tropical malabsorption, inflammatory bowel disease and neoplasia should all be considered. Box 11.21 lists causes encountered particularly in visitors to or residents of the tropics. The workup should include tests for parasitic causes of chronic diarrhoea, such as examination of stool and duodenal aspirates for ova and parasites, and serological investigation.

Tropical sprue is a malabsorption syndrome (p. 807) with no defined aetiology. It was typically associated with a long period of residence in the tropics or with overland travel but is now rarely seen. *Giardia lamblia* infection may progress to a malabsorption syndrome that mimics tropical sprue. If no cause is found, empirical treatment for *Giardia lamblia* infection with metronidazole is often helpful.

HIV-1 has now emerged as a major cause of chronic diarrhoea. This may be due to HIV enteropathy or infection with agents such as *Cryptosporidium* spp., *Cystoisospora belli* (syn. *Isospora belli*) or microsporidia (p. 316). However, many other causes of chronic AIDS-associated diarrhoea seen in the developed world are less common in tropical settings, e.g. CMV or disseminated *Mycobacterium avium* complex infections.

Eosinophilia acquired in the tropics

Eosinophilia occurs in a variety of haematological, allergic and inflammatory conditions discussed on page 927. It may also arise in HIV-1 and human T-cell lymphotropic virus (HTLV)-1 infection. However, eosinophils are important in the immune response to parasitic infections, in particular those involving parasites with a tissue migration phase. In the context of travel to or residence in the tropics, a patient with an eosinophil count of more than 0.4×10^9/L should be investigated for both non-parasitic (see Box 23.9, p. 926) and parasitic causes (Box 11.22).

The response to parasite infections is often different when travellers to and residents of endemic areas are compared. Travellers often have recent and light infections associated with eosinophilia. Residents have often been infected for a long time, have evidence of chronic pathology and no longer have eosinophilia.

Clinical assessment

A history of travel to known endemic areas for schistosomiasis, onchocerciasis and the filariases will indicate possible causes. Assessment should establish how long patients have spent in endemic areas and the history should address all the elements in Box 11.16.

Physical signs or symptoms that suggest a parasitic cause for eosinophilia include transient rashes (schistosomiasis or strongyloidiasis), fever (Katayama syndrome; p. 295), pruritus (onchocerciasis) or migrating subcutaneous swellings (loiasis, gnathostomiasis) (see Box 11.22). Paragonimiasis can give rise to haemoptysis, and the migratory phase of intestinal nematodes or lymphatic filariasis may cause cough, wheezing and transient pulmonary infiltrates. Schistosomiasis, strongyloidiasis and gnathostomiasis induce transient respiratory symptoms with infiltrates in the acute stages and, when eggs reach the pulmonary vasculature in chronic schistosomiasis infection, can

i | 11.21 Causes of chronic diarrhoea acquired in the tropics

- *Giardia lamblia*
- Strongyloidiasis
- Enteropathic *Escherichia coli*
- HIV enteropathy
- Intestinal flukes
- Tropical sprue
- Chronic intestinal schistosomiasis
- Chronic calcific pancreatitis
- Hypolactasia (primary and secondary)

i | 11.22 Parasite infections that cause eosinophilia

Infestation	Pathogen	Clinical syndrome with eosinophilia
Strongyloidiasis	*Strongyloides stercoralis*	Larva currens
Soil-transmitted helminthiases		
Hookworm	*Necator americanus*	Anaemia
	Ancylostoma duodenale	Anaemia
Ascariasis	*Ascaris lumbricoides*	Löffler's syndrome
Toxocariasis	*Toxocara canis*	Visceral larva migrans
Schistosomiasis	*Schistosoma haematobium*	Katayama fever
	S. mansoni, S. japonicum	Chronic infection
Filariases		
Loiasis	*Loa loa*	Skin nodules
Wuchereria bancrofti	*W. bancrofti*	Lymphangitis, lymphadenopathy, orchitis, intermittent bouts of cellulitis, lymphoedema and elephantiasis
Brugia malayi	*B. malayi*	Brugian elephantiasis similar but typically less severe than that caused by *W. bancrofti*
Mansonella perstans	*M. perstans*	Asymptomatic infection, occasionally subconjunctival nodules
Onchocerciasis	*Onchocerca volvulus*	Visual disturbance, dermatitis
Other nematode infections	*Trichinella spiralis*	Myositis
	Gnathostoma spinigerum	Pruritus, migratory nodules, eosinophilic meningitis
Cestode infections	*Taenia saginata, T. solium*	Usually asymptomatic; eosinophilia associated with migratory phase
	Echinococcus granulosus	Lesions in liver or other organ; eosinophilia associated with leakage from cyst
Liver flukes	*Fasciola hepatica*	Hepatic symptoms; eosinophilia associated with migratory phase
	Clonorchis sinensis	As for fascioliasis
	Opisthorchis felineus	As for fascioliasis
Lung fluke	*Paragonimus westermani*	Lung lesions

i 11.23 Initial investigation of eosinophilia

Investigation	Pathogens sought
Stool microscopy	Ova, cysts and parasites
Terminal urine	Ova of *Schistosoma haematobium*
Duodenal aspirate	Filariform larvae of *Strongyloides*, liver fluke ova
Day bloods	Microfilariae *Brugia malayi*, *Loa loa*
Night bloods	Microfilariae *Wuchereria bancrofti*
Skin snips	*Onchocerca volvulus*
Slit-lamp examination	*Onchocerca volvulus*
Serology	Schistosomiasis, filariasis, strongyloidiasis, hydatid, trichinosis, gnathostomiasis etc.

result in shortness of breath with features of right heart failure due to pulmonary hypertension. Fever and hepatosplenomegaly are seen in schistosomiasis, *Fasciola hepatica* infection and toxocariasis (visceral larva migrans). Intestinal worms, such as *Ascaris lumbricoides* and *Strongyloides stercoralis*, can cause abdominal symptoms, including intestinal obstruction and diarrhoea. In the case of heavy infestation with *Ascaris*, this may be due to fat malabsorption and there may be associated nutritional deficits. *Schistosoma haematobium* can cause haematuria or haematospermia. *Toxocara* spp. can give rise to choroidal lesions with visual field defects. *Angiostrongylus cantonensis* and gnathostomiasis induce eosinophilic meningitis, and the hyperinfection syndrome caused by *S. stercoralis* in immunocompromised hosts induces meningitis due to Gram-negative bacteria. Myositis is a feature of trichinosis (trichinellosis) and cysticercosis, while periorbital oedema is found in trichinosis.

Investigations

The diagnosis of a parasitic infestation requires direct visualisation of adult worms, larvae or ova. Serum antibody detection may not distinguish between active and past infection and is often unhelpful in those born in endemic areas. Radiological investigations may provide circumstantial evidence of parasite infestation. Box 11.23 describes initial investigations for eosinophilia.

Management

A specific diagnosis guides therapy. In the absence of a specific diagnosis, many clinicians will give an empirical course of praziquantel if the individual has potentially been exposed to schistosomiasis, or with albendazole/ivermectin if strongyloidiasis or intestinal nematodes are likely causes.

■ Skin conditions acquired in the tropics

Community-based studies in the tropics consistently show that skin infections (bacterial and fungal), scabies and eczema are the most common skin problems (Box 11.24). Scabies and eczema are discussed on pages 1241 and 1244. Cutaneous leishmaniasis and onchocerciasis have defined geographical distributions (pp. 284 and 292). In travellers, secondarily infected insect bites, pyoderma, cutaneous larva migrans and non-specific dermatitis are common.

During the investigation of skin lesions, enquiry should be made about habitation, activities undertaken and regions visited (see Box 11.16). Examples of skin lesions in tropical disease are shown in Figure 11.7.

i 11.24 Rash in tropical travellers/residents

Maculopapular rash
- Dengue
- HIV-1
- Typhoid
- *Spirillum minus*
- Rickettsial infections
- Measles

Petechial or purpuric rash
- Viral haemorrhagic fevers
- Yellow fever
- Meningococcal sepsis
- Leptospirosis
- Rickettsial spotted fevers
- Malaria

Vesicular rash
- Monkeypox
- Insect bites
- Rickettsial pox

Urticarial rash
- Katayama fever (schistosomiasis)
- *Toxocara* spp.
- *Strongyloides stercoralis*
- Fascioliasis

Ulcers
- Leishmaniasis
- *Mycobacterium ulcerans* (Buruli ulcer)
- Dracunculosis
- Anthrax
- Rickettsial eschar
- Tropical ulcer (*Fusobacterium ulcerans* and *Treponema vincentii*)
- Ecthyma (staphylococci, streptococci)

Papules
- Scabies
- Insect bites
- Prickly heat
- Ringworm
- Onchocerciasis

Nodules or plaques
- Leprosy
- Chromoblastomycosis
- Dimorphic fungi
- Trypanosomiasis
- Onchocerciasis
- Myiasis (larvae of tumbu fly or botfly)
- Tungiasis (*Tunga penetrans*)

Migratory linear rash
- Cutaneous larva migrans (CLM; dog hookworms)
- *Strongyloides stercoralis* (larva currens, more rapid than CLM)

Migratory papules/nodules
- *Loa loa*
- Gnathostomiasis
- Schistosomiasis

Thickened skin
- Mycetoma (actinomycetoma/eumycetoma)
- Elephantiasis (filariasis)

Skin biopsies are helpful in diagnosing aetiology. Culture of biopsy material may be needed to diagnose bacterial, fungal, parasitic and mycobacterial infections.

Infections in adolescence

Particular issues of relevance in adolescent patients are shown in Box 11.25.

Infections in pregnancy

Box 11.26 shows some of the infections encountered in pregnancy.

Fig. 11.7 Examples of skin lesions in patients with fever in the tropics. **A** Subcutaneous nodule due to botfly infection. **B** Emerging larva after treatment with petroleum jelly. **C** Eschar of scrub typhus. **D** Rat bite fever. *A, B and D, Courtesy of Dr Ravi Gowda, Royal Hallamshire Hospital, Sheffield. C, Courtesy of Dr Rattanaphone Phetsouvanh, Mahosot Hospital, Vientiane, PDR Laos.*

11.25 Key issues in infectious diseases in adolescence

- **Common infectious syndromes**: infectious mononucleosis, bacterial pharyngitis, whooping cough, pneumonia, staphylococcal skin/soft tissue infections, urinary tract infections, acute gastroenteritis.
- **Life-threatening infections**: meningococcal infection (sepsis and/ or meningitis).
- **Sexually transmitted infections**: human papillomavirus (HPV), HIV-1, hepatitis B virus and chlamydia. These may reflect either voluntary sexual activity or sexual coercion/abuse.
- **Travel-related infections**: diarrhoea, malaria etc. are relatively common.
- **Infections in susceptible groups**: patients with cystic fibrosis, congenital immunodeficiency, acute leukaemia and other adolescent malignancies are vulnerable to specific groups of infections.
- **Infections requiring prolonged antimicrobial use**: adherence to chronic therapy is challenging, for both oral (antituberculous or antiretroviral) and systemic (osteomyelitis, septic arthritis or post-operative infections) treatments. Outpatient antimicrobial therapy is preferred to minimise hospitalisation.
- **Vaccination**: engagement with age-specific vaccine programmes should be ensured, e.g. HPV, childhood booster vaccines and meningococcal vaccine.
- **Risk reduction**: education relating to sexual health and alcohol and recreational drug usage is important.

11

11.26 Infections in pregnancy

Infection	Consequence	Prevention and management
Rubella	Congenital malformation	Childhood vaccination and vaccination of non-immune mothers post-delivery
Cytomegalovirus	Neonatal infection, congenital malformation	Limited prevention strategies
Zika virus	Congenital malformation	Avoidance of travel, delay in pregnancy if infected
Varicella zoster virus	Neonatal infection, congenital malformation, severe infection in mother	VZ immunoglobulin (see Box 11.31)
Herpes simplex virus (HSV)	Congenital or neonatal infection	Aciclovir and consideration of caesarean section for mothers who shed HSV from genital tract at time of delivery. Aciclovir for infected neonates
Hepatitis B virus	Chronic infection of neonate	Hepatitis B immunoglobulin and active vaccination of newborn
Hepatitis E virus	Fulminant hepatitis, pre-term delivery, fetal loss	Maintenance of standard food hygiene practices
HIV-1	Chronic infection of neonate	Antiretroviral drugs for mother and infant and consideration of caesarean section if HIV-1 viral load detectable. Avoidance of breastfeeding
Parvovirus B19	Congenital infection	Avoidance of individuals with acute infection if pregnant
Measles	More severe infection in mother and neonate, fetal loss	Childhood vaccination, human normal immunoglobulin in non-immune pregnant contacts and vaccination post-delivery
Dengue	Neonatal dengue if mother has infection <5 weeks prior to delivery	Vector (mosquito) control
Syphilis	Congenital malformation	Serological testing in pregnancy with prompt treatment of infected mothers
Neisseria gonorrhoeae and *Chlamydia trachomatis*	Neonatal conjunctivitis (ophthalmia neonatorum, p. 340)	Treatment of infection in mother and neonate
Listeriosis	Neonatal meningitis or bacteraemia, bacteraemia or pyrexia of unknown origin in mother	Avoidance of unpasteurised cheeses and other dietary sources
Brucellosis	Possibly increased incidence of fetal loss	Avoidance of unpasteurised dairy products
Group B streptococcal infection	Neonatal meningitis and sepsis. Sepsis in mother after delivery	Risk- or screening-based antimicrobial prophylaxis in labour (recommendations vary between countries)
Toxoplasmosis	Congenital malformation	Diagnosis and prompt treatment of cases, avoidance of under-cooked meat while pregnant
Malaria	Fetal loss, intrauterine growth retardation, severe malaria in mother	Avoidance of insect bites. Intermittent preventative treatment during pregnancy to decrease incidence in high-risk countries

Viral infections

Systemic viral infections with exanthem

Childhood exanthems are characterised by fever and widespread rash. Maternal antibody usually gives protection for the first 6–12 months of life. Comprehensive immunisation programmes have dramatically reduced the number of paediatric infections but incomplete uptake results in infections in later life.

Measles

The WHO has set the objective of eradicating measles globally using the live attenuated vaccine. However, vaccination of more than 95% of the population is required to prevent outbreaks. Natural illness produces life-long immunity.

Clinical features

Infection is by respiratory droplets with an incubation period of 6–19 days. A prodromal illness occurs, 1–3 days before the rash, with upper respiratory symptoms, conjunctivitis and the presence of the pathognomonic Koplik's spots: small white spots surrounded by erythema on the buccal mucosa (Fig. 11.8A). As natural antibody develops, the maculopapular rash appears, spreading from the face to the extremities (Fig. 11.8B). Generalised lymphadenopathy and diarrhoea are common. Complications are more common in older children and adults, and include otitis media, bacterial pneumonia, transient hepatitis, pancreatitis and clinical encephalitis (approximately 0.1% of cases). A rare late complication is subacute sclerosing panencephalitis (SSPE), which occurs up to 7 years after infection. Diagnosis is clinical (although this has become unreliable in areas where measles is no longer common) and by detection of antibody (serum immunoglobulin M (IgM), seroconversion or salivary IgM).

Measles is a serious disease in the malnourished, vitamin-deficient or immunocompromised, in whom the typical rash may be missing and persistent infection with a giant cell pneumonitis or encephalitis may occur. In tuberculosis infection, measles suppresses cell-mediated immunity and may exacerbate disease; for this reason, measles vaccination should be deferred until after commencing antituberculous treatment. Measles does not cause congenital malformation but may be more severe in pregnant women.

Mortality clusters at the extremes of age, averaging 1:1000 in developed countries and up to 1:4 in developing countries. Death usually results from a bacterial superinfection, occurring as a complication of measles: most often pneumonia, diarrhoeal disease or noma/cancrum oris, a gangrenous stomatitis. Death may also result from complications of measles encephalitis.

Management and prevention

Normal immunoglobulin attenuates the disease in the immunocompromised (regardless of vaccination status) and in non-immune pregnant women, but must be given within 6 days of exposure. Vaccination can be used in outbreaks and vitamin A may improve the outcome in uncomplicated disease. Antibiotic therapy is reserved for bacterial complications. All children aged 12–15 months should receive measles vaccination (as combined measles, mumps and rubella (MMR), a live attenuated vaccine), and a further MMR dose at age 4 years.

Rubella (German measles)

Rubella causes exanthem in the non-immunised.

Clinical features

Rubella is spread by respiratory droplet, with infectivity from up to 10 days before to 2 weeks after the onset of the rash. The incubation period is 15–20 days. In childhood, most cases are subclinical, although clinical features may include fever, maculopapular rash spreading from the face, and lymphadenopathy. Complications are rare but include thrombocytopenia and hepatitis. Encephalitis and haemorrhage are occasionally reported. In adults, arthritis involving hands or knees is relatively common, especially in women.

If transplacental infection takes place in the first trimester or later, persistence of the virus is likely and severe congenital disease may result (Box 11.27). Even if normal at birth, the infant has an increased incidence of other diseases developing later, e.g. diabetes mellitus.

Diagnosis

Laboratory confirmation of rubella is required if there has been contact with a pregnant woman. This is achieved either by detection of rubella IgM in serum or by IgG seroconversion. In the exposed pregnant woman, absence of rubella-specific IgG confirms the potential for congenital infection.

Prevention

All children should be immunised with MMR vaccine. Congenital rubella syndrome may be controlled by testing women of child-bearing age for rubella antibodies and offering vaccination if seronegative. Antenatal rubella screening was offered to pregnant mothers in the UK for many years for this reason. However, this

Fig. 11.8 Measles. A Koplik's spots (arrows) seen on buccal mucosa in the early stages of clinical measles. B Typical measles rash.

11.27 Rubella infection: risk of congenital malformation	
Stage of gestation	Likelihood of malformations
1–2 months	65–85% chance of illness, multiple defects/spontaneous abortion
3 months	30–35% chance of illness, usually a single congenital defect (most frequently deafness, cataract, glaucoma, mental retardation or congenital heart disease, especially pulmonary stenosis or patent ductus arteriosus)
4 months	10% risk of congenital defects, most commonly deafness
>20 weeks	Occasional deafness

practice ceased in 2016 because: rubella is so rare in the UK as to be considered eliminated; pre-pregnancy MMR vaccination is considered to be a more effective method of protecting pregnant women; and the screening test may give inaccurate results, causing unnecessary stress to pregnant women.

Parvovirus B19

Parvovirus B19 causes exanthem and other clinical syndromes. Some 50% of children and 60–90% of adults are seropositive. Most infections are spread by the respiratory route, although spread via contaminated blood is also possible. The virus has particular tropism for red cell precursors.

Clinical features

Many infections are subclinical. Clinical manifestations result after an incubation period of 14–21 days (Box 11.28). The classic exanthem (erythema infectiosum) is preceded by a prodromal fever and coryzal symptoms. A 'slapped cheek' rash is characteristic but the rash is very variable (Fig. 11.9). In adults, polyarthropathy is common. Infected individuals have a transient block in erythropoiesis for a few days, which is of no clinical consequence, except in individuals with increased red cell turnover due to haemoglobinopathy or haemolytic anaemia. These individuals develop an acute anaemia that may be severe (transient aplastic crisis; p. 968). Erythropoiesis usually recovers spontaneously after 10–14 days. Immunocompromised individuals, including those with congenital immunodeficiency or AIDS, can develop a more sustained block in erythropoiesis in response to the chronic viraemia that results from their inability to clear the infection. Infection during the first two trimesters of pregnancy can result in intrauterine infection and impact on fetal bone marrow; it causes 10–15% of non-immune (non-Rhesus-related) hydrops fetalis, a rare complication of pregnancy.

Diagnosis

IgM to parvovirus B19 suggests recent infection but may persist for months and false positives occur. Seroconversion to IgG positivity confirms infection but in isolation a positive IgG is of little diagnostic utility. Detection of parvovirus B19 DNA in blood is particularly useful in immunocompromised patients. Giant pronormoblasts or haemophagocytosis may be demonstrable in the bone marrow.

Management

Infection is usually self-limiting. Symptomatic relief for arthritic symptoms may be required. Severe anaemia requires transfusion.

11.28 Clinical features of parvovirus B19 infection	
Affected age group	Clinical manifestations
Fifth disease (erythema infectiosum) Small children	Three clinical stages: a 'slapped cheek' appearance, followed by a maculopapular rash progressing to a reticulate eruption on the body and limbs, then a final stage of resolution. Often the child is quite well throughout
Gloves and socks syndrome Young adults	Fever and an acral purpuric eruption with a clear margin at the wrists and ankles. Mucosal involvement also occurs
Arthropathies Adults and occasionally children	Symmetrical small-joint polyarthropathy. In children it tends to involve the larger joints in an asymmetrical distribution
Impaired erythropoiesis Adults, those with haematological disease, the immunosuppressed	Mild anaemia; in an individual with an underlying haematological abnormality it can precipitate transient aplastic crisis, or in the immunocompromised a more sustained but often milder pure red cell aplasia
Hydrops fetalis Transplacental fetal infection	Asymptomatic or symptomatic maternal infection that can cause fetal anaemia with an aplastic crisis, leading to non-immune hydrops fetalis and spontaneous abortion

Fig. 11.9 Slapped cheek syndrome. The typical facial rash of parvovirus B19 infection.

Persistent viraemia in immunocompromised hosts may require immunoglobulin therapy to clear the virus.

Pregnant women should avoid contact with cases of parvovirus B19 infection; if they are exposed, serology should be performed to establish whether they are non-immune.

Passive prophylaxis with normal immunoglobulin has been suggested for non-immune pregnant women exposed to infection but there are limited data to support this recommendation. The pregnancy should be closely monitored by ultrasound scanning, so that hydrops fetalis can be treated by fetal transfusion.

Human herpesvirus 6 and 7

Human herpesvirus 6 (HHV-6) is a lymphotropic virus that causes a childhood viral exanthem (exanthem subitum), rare cases of an infectious mononucleosis-like syndrome and infection in the immunocompromised host. Infection is almost universal, with approximately 95% of children acquiring this virus by 2 years of age. Transmission is via saliva.

i	11.29 Herpesvirus infections	
Virus	**Infection**	
Herpes simplex virus (HSV)		
HSV-1 (p. 247)	Herpes labialis ('cold sores') Stomatitis, pharyngitis Corneal ulceration Finger infections ('whitlows') Eczema herpeticum Encephalitis	
HSV-2 (p. 247)	Genital ulceration and neonatal infection (acquired during vaginal delivery) Acute meningitis or transverse myelitis; rarely, encephalitis	
Varicella zoster virus (VZV)	Chickenpox (varicella) Shingles (herpes zoster)	
Cytomegalovirus (CMV) (p. 242)	Congenital infection Infectious mononucleosis (heterophile antibody-negative) Hepatitis Disease in immunocompromised patients: retinitis, encephalitis, pneumonitis, hepatitis, enteritis Fever with abnormalities in haematological parameters	
Epstein–Barr virus (EBV) (p. 241)	Infectious mononucleosis Burkitt's and other lymphomas Nasopharyngeal carcinoma Oral hairy leucoplakia (AIDS patients) Other lymphomas, post-transplant lymphoproliferative disorder (p. 225)	
Human herpesvirus 6 and 7 (HHV-6, HHV-7)	Exanthem subitum Disease in immunocompromised patients	
Human herpesvirus 8 (HHV-8) (p. 248)	Kaposi's sarcoma, primary effusion lymphoma, multicentric Castleman's disease	

HHV-7 is very closely related to HHV-6 and is believed to be responsible for a proportion of cases of exanthem subitum. Like HHV-6, HHV-7 causes an almost universal infection in childhood, with subsequent latent infection and occasional infection in the immunocompromised host.

Clinical features

Exanthem subitum is also known as roseola infantum or sixth disease (Box 11.29). A high fever is followed by a maculopapular rash as the fever resolves. Fever and/or febrile convulsions may also occur without a rash. Rarely, older children or adults may develop an infectious mononucleosis-like illness, hepatitis or rash. In the immunocompromised, infection is rare but can cause fever, rash, hepatitis, pneumonitis, cytopenia or encephalitis.

Diagnosis and management

Exanthem subitum is usually a clinical diagnosis but can be confirmed by antibody and/or DNA detection. The disease is self-limiting. Treatment with ganciclovir or foscarnet is used in immunocompromised hosts infected with HHV-6.

Chickenpox (varicella)

Varicella zoster virus (VZV) is a dermotropic and neurotropic virus that produces primary infection, usually in childhood, which may reactivate in later life. VZV is spread by aerosol and direct contact. It is highly infectious to non-immune individuals. Disease in children is usually well tolerated. Manifestations are more severe in adults, pregnant women and the immunocompromised.

Clinical features

The incubation period is 11–20 days, after which a vesicular eruption begins (Fig. 11.10), often on mucosal surfaces first, followed by rapid dissemination in a centripetal distribution (most dense on trunk and sparse on limbs). New lesions occur every 2–4 days and each crop is associated with fever. The rash progresses from small pink macules to vesicles and pustules within 24 hours. Infectivity lasts from up to 4 days (but usually 48 hours) before the lesions appear until the last vesicles crust over. Due to intense itching, secondary bacterial infection from scratching is the most common complication of primary chickenpox. Self-limiting cerebellar ataxia and encephalitis are rare complications.

Adults, pregnant women and the immunocompromised are at increased risk of visceral involvement, which presents as pneumonitis, hepatitis or encephalitis. Pneumonitis can be fatal and is more likely to occur in smokers. Maternal infection in

Fig. 11.10 Varicella zoster virus infection. A Chickenpox. B Shingles in a thoracic dermatome.

early pregnancy carries a 3% risk of neonatal damage with developmental abnormalities of eyes, CNS and limbs. Chickenpox within 5 days of delivery leads to severe neonatal varicella with visceral involvement and haemorrhage.

Diagnosis

Diagnosis is primarily clinical, by recognition of the rash. If necessary, this can be confirmed by detection of antigen (direct immunofluorescence) or DNA (PCR) of aspirated vesicular fluid. Serology is used to identify seronegative individuals at risk of infection.

Management and prevention

The benefits of antivirals for uncomplicated primary VZV infection in children are marginal, shortening the duration of rash by only 1 day, and treatment is not normally required. Antivirals are, however, used for uncomplicated chickenpox in adults when the patient presents within 24–48 hours of onset of vesicles, in all patients with complications, and in those who are immunocompromised, including pregnant women, regardless of duration of vesicles (Box 11.30). More severe disease, particularly in immunocompromised hosts, requires initial parenteral therapy. Immunocompromised patients may have prolonged viral shedding and may require prolonged treatment until all lesions crust over.

Human VZ immunoglobulin (VZIG) is used to attenuate infection in people who have had significant contact with VZV, are susceptible to infection (i.e. have no history of chickenpox or shingles and are seronegative for VZV IgG) and are at risk of severe disease (e.g. immunocompromised or pregnant) (Box 11.31). Ideally, VZIG should be given within 7 days of exposure, but it may attenuate disease even if given up to 10 days afterwards. Susceptible contacts who develop severe chickenpox after receiving VZIG should be treated with aciclovir.

A live, attenuated VZV vaccine is available and in routine use in the USA and other countries, but in the UK its use has been restricted to non-immune health-care workers and household contacts of immunocompromised individuals. Children receive one dose after 1 year of age and a second dose at 4–6 years of age; seronegative adults receive two doses at least 1 month apart. The vaccine may also be used prior to planned iatrogenic immunosuppression, e.g. before transplant and for the elderly aged over 70 to prevent shingles.

Shingles (herpes zoster)

After initial infection, VZV persists in latent form in the dorsal root ganglion of sensory nerves and can reactivate in later life.

Clinical features

Burning discomfort occurs in the affected dermatome following reactivation and discrete vesicles appear 3–4 days later. This is associated with a brief viraemia, which can produce distant satellite 'chickenpox' lesions. Occasionally, paraesthesia occurs without rash ('zoster sine herpete'). Severe disease, a prolonged duration of rash, multiple dermatomal involvement or recurrence suggests underlying immune deficiency, including HIV. Chickenpox may be contracted from a case of shingles but not vice versa.

Although thoracic dermatomes are most commonly involved (Fig. 11.10B), the ophthalmic division of the trigeminal nerve is also frequently affected; vesicles may appear on the cornea and lead to ulceration. This condition can lead to blindness and urgent ophthalmology review is required. Geniculate ganglion involvement causes the Ramsay Hunt syndrome of facial palsy,

11.30 Therapy for herpes simplex and varicella zoster virus infection	
Disease state	**Treatment options**
Primary genital HSV	Famciclovir 250 mg 3 times daily for 7–10 days Valaciclovir 1 g twice daily for 7–10 days Oral aciclovir 200 mg 5 times daily or 400 mg 3 times daily for 7–10 days
Severe and preventing oral intake	Aciclovir 5 mg/kg 3 times daily IV until patient can tolerate oral therapy
Recurrent genital HSV-1 or 2	Oral aciclovir 200 mg 5 times daily or 400 mg 3 times daily for 5 days Famciclovir 125 mg twice daily for 5 days Valaciclovir 500 mg twice daily for 3–5 days or 2 g twice daily for 1 day. Shorter durations increasingly favoured
Primary or recurrent oral HSV	Usually no treatment If required, usually short duration, e.g. valaciclovir 2 g twice daily for 1 day
Mucocutaneous HSV infection in immunocompromised host	Aciclovir 5 mg/kg 3 times daily IV for 7–10 days Oral aciclovir 400 mg 4 times daily for 7–10 days Famciclovir 500 mg 3 times daily for 7–10 days Valaciclovir 1 g twice daily for 7–10 days
Chickenpox in adult or child	Oral aciclovir 800 mg 5 times daily for 5 days Famciclovir 500 mg 3 times daily for 5 days Valaciclovir 1 g 3 times daily for 5 days
Immunocompromised host/pregnant woman	Aciclovir 5 mg/kg 3 times daily IV until patient is improving, then complete therapy with oral therapy until all lesions are crusting over
Shingles	Treatment and doses as for chickenpox but duration typically 7–10 days
Visceral involvement (non-CNS) in HSV	Aciclovir IV 5 mg/kg 3 times daily for 14 days
Visceral involvement (non-CNS) in VZV	Aciclovir IV 5 mg/kg 3 times daily for 7 days
Severe complications (encephalitis, disseminated infection)	Aciclovir IV 10 mg/kg 3 times daily (up to 20 mg/kg in neonates) for 14–21 days
HSV disease suppression	Aciclovir 400 mg twice daily Famciclovir 250 mg twice daily Valaciclovir 500 mg daily

(CNS = central nervous system; HSV = herpes simplex virus; VZV = varicella zoster virus)

ipsilateral loss of taste and buccal ulceration, plus a rash in the external auditory canal. This may be mistaken for Bell's palsy (p. 1082). Bowel and bladder dysfunction occur with sacral nerve root involvement. The virus occasionally causes cranial nerve palsy, myelitis or encephalitis. Granulomatous cerebral angiitis is a cerebrovascular complication that leads to a stroke-like syndrome in association with shingles, especially in an ophthalmic distribution.

Post-herpetic neuralgia causes troublesome persistence of pain for 1–6 months or longer, following healing of the rash. It is more common with advanced age.

Fig. 11.11 Typical unilateral mumps. [A] Note the loss of angle of the jaw on the affected (right) side. [B] Comparison showing normal (left) side.

Management

Early therapy with aciclovir or related agents has been shown to reduce both early- and late-onset pain, especially in patients over 65 years. Post-herpetic neuralgia requires aggressive analgesia, along with agents such as amitriptyline 25–100 mg daily, gabapentin (commencing at 300 mg daily and building slowly to 300 mg twice daily or more) or pregabalin (commencing at 75 mg twice daily and building up to 100 mg or 200 mg 3 times daily if tolerated). Capsaicin cream (0.075%) may be helpful. Although controversial, glucocorticoids have not been demonstrated to reduce post-herpetic neuralgia to date.

Enteroviral exanthems

Coxsackie or echovirus infections can lead to a maculopapular eruption or roseola-like rash that occurs after fever falls. Enteroviral infections are discussed further under viral infections of the skin (see below).

Systemic viral infections without exanthem

Other systemic viral infections present with features other than a rash suggestive of exanthem. Rashes may occur in these conditions but differ from those seen in exanthems or are not the primary presenting feature.

Mumps

Mumps is a systemic viral infection characterised by swelling of the parotid glands. Infection is endemic worldwide and peaks at 5–9 years of age. Vaccination has reduced the incidence in children but incomplete coverage and waning immunity with time have led to outbreaks in young adults. Infection is spread by respiratory droplets.

Clinical features

The median incubation period is 19 days, with a range of 15–24 days. Classical tender parotid enlargement, which is bilateral in 75%, follows a prodrome of pyrexia and headache (Fig. 11.11). Meningitis complicates up to 10% of cases. The CSF reveals a lymphocytic pleocytosis or, less commonly, neutrophils. Rare complications include encephalitis, transient hearing loss, labyrinthitis, electrocardiographic abnormalities, pancreatitis and arthritis.

Approximately 25% of post-pubertal males with mumps develop epididymo-orchitis but, although testicular atrophy occurs, sterility is unlikely. Oophoritis is less common. Abortion may occur if infection takes place in the first trimester of pregnancy. Complications may occur in the absence of parotitis.

Diagnosis

The diagnosis is usually clinical. In atypical presentations without parotitis, serology for mumps-specific IgM or IgG seroconversion (fourfold rise in IgG convalescent titre) confirms the diagnosis. Virus can also be cultured from urine in the first week of infection or detected by PCR in urine, saliva or CSF.

Management and prevention

Treatment is with analgesia. There is no evidence that glucocorticoids are of value for orchitis. Mumps vaccine is one of the components of the combined MMR vaccine.

Influenza

Influenza is an acute systemic viral infection that primarily affects the respiratory tract and carries a significant mortality. It is caused by influenza A virus or, in milder form, influenza B virus. Infection is seasonal, and variation in the haemagglutinin (H) and neuraminidase (N) glycoproteins on the surface of the virus leads to disease of variable intensity each year. Minor changes in haemagglutinin are known as 'genetic drift', whereas a switch in the haemagglutinin or neuraminidase antigen is termed 'genetic shift'. Nomenclature of influenza strains is based on these glycoproteins, e.g. H1N1, H3N2 etc. Genetic shift results in the circulation of a new influenza strain within a community to which few people are immune, potentially initiating an influenza epidemic or pandemic in which there is a high attack rate and there may be increased disease severity.

Clinical features

After an incubation period of 1–3 days, uncomplicated disease leads to fever, malaise and cough. Viral pneumonia may occur, although pulmonary complications are most often due to superinfection with Strep. pneumoniae, Staph. aureus or other bacteria. Rare extrapulmonary manifestations include myositis, myocarditis, pericarditis and neurological complications (Reye's syndrome in children, encephalitis or transverse myelitis). Mortality is greatest in the elderly, those with medical comorbidities and pregnant women. Polymorphisms in the gene encoding an antiviral protein, interferon-induced transmembrane protein 3 (IFITM3), are associated with more severe influenza.

Diagnosis

Acute infection is diagnosed by viral antigen or RNA detection in a nasopharyngeal sample. The disease may also be diagnosed retrospectively by serology.

Management and prevention

Management involves early microbiological identification of cases and good infection control, with an emphasis on hand hygiene and preventing dissemination of infection by coughing and sneezing. Administration of neuraminidase inhibitor, oral oseltamivir (75 mg twice daily) or inhaled zanamivir (10 mg twice daily) for 5 days, can reduce the severity of symptoms if started within 48 hours of symptom onset (or possibly later in immunocompromised individuals). These agents have superseded routine use of amantadine and rimantadine. Antiviral drugs can also be used as prophylaxis in high-risk individuals during the 'flu' season. Resistance can emerge to all of these agents and so updated local advice should be followed with regard to the sensitivity to antivirals of the circulating strain.

Prevention relies on seasonal vaccination of the elderly, children 2–7 years of age and individuals with chronic medical illnesses that place them at increased risk of the complications of influenza, such as chronic cardiopulmonary diseases or immune compromise, as well as their health-care workers. The vaccine composition changes each year to cover the 'predicted' seasonal strains but vaccination may fail when a new pandemic strain emerges.

Avian influenza

Avian influenza is caused by transmission of avian influenza A viruses to humans. Avian viruses, such as H5N1, possess alternative haemagglutinin antigens to seasonal influenza strains. Most cases have had contact with sick poultry, predominantly in South-east Asia, and person-to-person spread has been limited to date. Infections with H5N1 viruses have been severe, with enteric features and respiratory failure. Treatment depends on the resistance pattern but often involves oseltamivir. Vaccination against seasonal 'flu' does not adequately protect against avian influenza. There is a concern that adaptation of an avian strain to allow effective person-to-person transmission is likely to lead to a global pandemic of life-threatening influenza.

Swine influenza

Re-assortment of swine, avian and human influenza strains can occur in pigs and lead to outbreaks of swine 'flu' in humans, as occurred in 2009, when an outbreak of H1N1pdm2009 influenza spread around the world from Mexico. Cases were still occurring

in the Indian subcontinent in 2014–16. Symptoms included more gastrointestinal symptoms than with seasonal influenza, respiratory failure and seizures or encephalitis. Severe disease was a feature of infants, adults less than 50 years, those with chronic lung or neurological disease, obese patients and pregnant women, but with time the clinical features have become indistinguishable from those of seasonal influenza.

Infectious mononucleosis and Epstein–Barr virus

Infectious mononucleosis (IM) is a clinical syndrome characterised by pharyngitis, cervical lymphadenopathy, fever and lymphocytosis (known colloquially as glandular fever). It is most often caused by Epstein–Barr virus (EBV) but other infections can produce a similar clinical syndrome (Box 11.32).

EBV is a gamma herpesvirus. In developing countries, subclinical infection in childhood is virtually universal. In developed countries, primary infection may be delayed until adolescence or early adult life. Under these circumstances, about 50% of infections result in typical IM. The virus is usually acquired from asymptomatic excreters via saliva, either by droplet infection or environmental contamination in childhood, or by kissing among adolescents and adults. EBV is not highly contagious and isolation of cases is unnecessary.

Clinical features

EBV infection has a prolonged but undetermined incubation period, followed in some cases by a prodrome of fever, headache and malaise. This is followed by IM with severe pharyngitis, which may include tonsillar exudates and non-tender anterior and posterior cervical lymphadenopathy. Palatal petechiae, periorbital oedema, splenomegaly, inguinal or axillary lymphadenopathy, and macular, petechial or erythema multiforme rashes may occur. In most cases, fever resolves over 2 weeks, and fatigue and other abnormalities settle over a further few weeks. Complications are listed in Box 11.33. Death is rare but can occur due to respiratory obstruction, haemorrhage from splenic rupture, thrombocytopenia or encephalitis.

The diagnosis of EBV infection outside the usual age in adolescence and young adulthood is more challenging. In children under 10 years the illness is mild and short-lived, but in adults over 30 years of age it can be severe and prolonged. In both groups, pharyngeal symptoms are often absent. EBV may present with jaundice, as a PUO or with a complication.

Long-term complications of EBV infection

Lymphoma complicates EBV infection in immunocompromised hosts, and some forms of Hodgkin lymphoma are EBV-associated (p. 961). The endemic form of Burkitt's lymphoma complicates EBV infection in areas of sub-Saharan Africa where falciparum malaria is endemic. Nasopharyngeal carcinoma is a geographically restricted tumour seen in China and Alaska that is associated with EBV infection. X-linked lymphoproliferative (Duncan's) syndrome is a familial lymphoproliferative disorder that follows primary EBV infection in boys without any other history of immunodeficiency;

i	**11.32 Causes of infectious mononucleosis syndrome**
• Epstein–Barr virus infection	• HIV-1 primary infection (p. 311)
• Cytomegalovirus	• Toxoplasmosis
• Human herpesvirus-6 or 7	

it is due to mutation of the *SAP* gene, causing failure of T-cell and NK-cell activation and inability to contain EBV infection.

Investigations

Atypical lymphocytes are common in EBV infection but also occur in other causes of IM, acute retroviral syndrome with HIV infection, viral hepatitis, mumps and rubella (Fig. 11.12A). They are also a feature of dengue, malaria and other geographically restricted infections (see Box 11.19). A 'heterophile' antibody is present during the acute illness and convalescence, which is detected by the Paul–Bunnell or 'Monospot' test. (A heterophile antibody is an antibody that has affinity for antigens other than the specific one, in this case animal immunoglobulins; the Paul–Bunnell and Monospot tests exploit this feature by detecting the ability of test serum to agglutinate sheep and horse red blood cells, respectively.). Sometimes antibody production is delayed, so an initially negative test should be repeated. However, many children and 10% of adolescents with IM do not produce heterophile antibody at any stage.

Specific EBV serology confirms the diagnosis. Acute infection is characterised by IgM antibodies against the viral capsid, antibodies to EBV early antigen and the initial absence of antibodies to EBV nuclear antigen (anti-EBNA). Seroconversion of anti-EBNA at approximately 1 month after the initial illness may confirm the diagnosis in retrospect. CNS infections may be diagnosed by detection of viral DNA in CSF.

Management

Treatment is largely symptomatic. If a throat culture yields a β-haemolytic streptococcus, penicillin should be given. Administration of ampicillin or amoxicillin in this condition commonly causes an itchy macular rash and should be avoided (Fig. 11.12B). When pharyngeal oedema is severe, a short course of glucocorticoids, e.g. prednisolone 30 mg daily for 5 days, may help. Current antiviral drugs are not active against EBV.

Return to work or school is governed by physical fitness rather than laboratory tests; contact sports should be avoided until splenomegaly has resolved because of the danger of splenic rupture. Unfortunately, about 10% of patients with IM suffer a chronic relapsing syndrome.

Cytomegalovirus

Cytomegalovirus (CMV), like EBV, circulates readily among children. A second period of virus acquisition occurs among teenagers and young adults, peaking between the ages of 25 and 35 years, rather later than with EBV infection. CMV infection is persistent, and is characterised by subclinical cycles of active virus replication and by persistent low-level virus shedding. Most post-childhood infections are therefore acquired from asymptomatic excreters who shed virus in saliva, urine, semen and genital secretions. Sexual transmission and oral spread are common among adults but infection may also be acquired by women caring for children with asymptomatic infections.

Clinical features

Most post-childhood CMV infections are subclinical, although some young adults develop an IM-like syndrome and some have a prolonged influenza-like illness lasting 2 weeks or more. Physical signs resemble those of IM but in CMV infections hepatomegaly is

---

i	11.33 Complications of Epstein–Barr virus infection

Common

- Severe pharyngeal oedema
- Antibiotic-induced rash (80–90% with ampicillin)
- Hepatitis (80%)
- Prolonged post-viral fatigue (10%)
- Jaundice (<10%)

Uncommon

Neurological
- Cranial nerve palsies
- Polyneuritis
- Transverse myelitis
- Meningoencephalitis

Haematological
- Haemolytic anaemia
- Thrombocytopenia

Renal
- Abnormalities on urinalysis
- Interstitial nephritis

Cardiac
- Myocarditis
- ECG abnormalities
- Pericarditis

Rare
- Ruptured spleen
- Respiratory obstruction
- Agranulocytosis
- X-linked lymphoproliferative syndrome

EBV-associated malignancy
- Nasopharyngeal carcinoma
- Burkitt's lymphoma
- Hodgkin lymphoma (certain subtypes only)
- Primary CNS lymphoma
- Lymphoproliferative disease in immunocompromised

Fig. 11.12 Features of infectious mononucleosis. A Atypical lymphocytes in peripheral blood. B Skin reaction to ampicillin.

more common, while lymphadenopathy, splenomegaly, pharyngitis and tonsillitis occur less often. Jaundice is uncommon and usually mild. Complications include meningoencephalitis, Guillain–Barré syndrome, autoimmune haemolytic anaemia, thrombocytopenia, myocarditis and skin eruptions, such as ampicillin-induced rash. Immunocompromised patients can develop hepatitis, oesophagitis, colitis, pneumonitis, retinitis, encephalitis and polyradiculitis.

Women who develop a primary CMV infection during pregnancy have about a 40% chance of passing CMV to the fetus, causing congenital infection and disease at any stage of gestation. Features include petechial rashes, hepatosplenomegaly and jaundice; 10% of infected infants will have long-term CNS sequelae, such as microcephaly, cerebral calcifications, chorioretinitis and deafness. Infections in the newborn usually are asymptomatic or have features of an IM-like illness, although some studies suggest that subtle sequelae affecting hearing or mental development may occur.

Investigations

Atypical lymphocytosis is not as prominent as in EBV infection and heterophile antibody tests are usually negative. LFTs are often abnormal, with an alkaline phosphatase level raised out of proportion to transaminases. Serological diagnosis depends on the detection of CMV-specific IgM antibody plus a fourfold rise or seroconversion of IgG. In the immunocompromised, antibody detection is unreliable and detection of CMV in an involved organ by PCR, antigen detection, culture or histopathology establishes the diagnosis. Detection of CMV in the blood may be useful in transplant populations but not in HIV-positive individuals, since in HIV infection CMV reactivates at regular intervals, but these episodes do not correlate well with episodes of clinical disease. Detection of CMV in urine is not helpful in diagnosing infection, except in neonates, since CMV is intermittently shed in the urine throughout life following infection.

Management

Only symptomatic treatment is required in the immunocompetent patient. Immunocompromised individuals are treated with ganciclovir 5 mg/kg IV twice daily or with oral valganciclovir 900 mg twice daily for at least 14 days. Foscarnet or cidofovir is also used in CMV treatment of immunocompromised patients who are resistant to or intolerant of ganciclovir-based therapy. They can be given intravitreally if required.

Dengue

Dengue is a febrile illness caused by a flavivirus transmitted by mosquitoes. It is endemic in Asia, the Pacific, Africa and the Americas (Fig. 11.13). Approximately 400 million infections and 100 million clinically apparent infections occur annually, and dengue is the most rapidly spreading mosquito-borne viral illness. The principal vector is the mosquito *Aedes aegypti*, which breeds

in standing water; collections of water in containers, water-based air coolers and tyre dumps are a good environment for the vector in large cities. *Aedes albopictus* is a vector in some South-east Asian countries. There are four serotypes of dengue virus, all producing a similar clinical syndrome; type-specific immunity is life-long but immunity against the other serotypes lasts only a few months. Dengue haemorrhagic fever (DHF) and dengue shock syndrome (DSS) occur in individuals who are immune to one dengue virus serotype and are then infected with another. Prior immunity results in increased uptake of virus by cells expressing the antibody Fc receptor and increased T-cell activation with resultant cytokine release, causing capillary leak and disseminated intravascular coagulation (DIC; p. 978). Previously, dengue was seen in small children and DHF/DSS in children 2–15 years old, but these conditions are now being seen in children less than 2 years old, and most frequently in those 16–45 years of age or older, in whom severe organ dysfunction is more common. Other epidemiological changes include the spread of dengue into rural communities and greater case fatality in women.

Clinical features

Many cases of dengue infection are asymptomatic in children. Clinical disease presents with undifferentiated fever termed dengue-like illness. When dengue infection occurs with characteristic symptoms or signs it is termed 'dengue' (Box 11.34). A rash frequently follows the initial febrile phase as the fever settles. Laboratory features include leucopenia, neutropenia,

i	**11.34 Clinical features of dengue fever**

Incubation period

- 2–7 days

Prodrome

- 2 days of malaise and headache

Acute onset

- Fever, backache, arthralgias, headache, generalised pains ('break-bone fever'), pain on eye movement, lacrimation, scleral injection, anorexia, nausea, vomiting, pharyngitis, upper respiratory tract symptoms, relative bradycardia, prostration, depression, hyperaesthesia, dysgeusia, lymphadenopathy

Fever

- Continuous or 'saddle-back', with break on 4th or 5th day and then recrudescence; usually lasts 7–8 days

Rash

- Initial flushing faint macular rash in first 1–2 days. Maculopapular, scarlet morbilliform blanching rash from days 3–5 on trunk, spreading centrifugally and sparing palms and soles; onset often with fever defervescence. May desquamate on resolution or give rise to petechiae on extensor surfaces

Convalescence

- Slow and may be associated with prolonged fatigue syndrome, arthralgia or depression

Complications

- Dengue haemorrhagic fever and disseminated intravascular coagulation
- Dengue shock syndrome
- Severe organ involvement
- Vertical transmission if infection within 5 weeks of delivery

◻ Dengue   ◻ Yellow fever   ◼ Dengue + yellow fever

Fig. 11.13 Endemic zones of yellow fever and dengue.

thrombocytopenia and elevated alanine aminotransferase (ALT) or aspartate aminotransferase (AST). Many symptomatic infections run an uncomplicated course but complications or a protracted convalescence may ensue. Warning signs justify intense medical management and monitoring for progression to severe dengue. Atypical clinical features of dengue are increasingly common, especially in infants or older patients (Box 11.35). These, along with DHF or DSS, are recognised as features of severe dengue in the 2015 case definition.

The period 3–7 days after onset of fever is termed the 'critical' phase, during which signs of DHF or DSS may develop. In mild forms, petechiae occur in the arm when a blood pressure cuff is inflated to a point between systolic and diastolic blood pressure and left for 5 minutes (the positive 'tourniquet test') – a non-specific test of capillary fragility and thrombocytopenia. As the extent of capillary leak increases, DSS develops, with a raised haematocrit, tachycardia and hypotension, pleural effusions and ascites. This may progress to metabolic acidosis and multi-organ failure, including acute respiratory distress syndrome (ARDS; p. 198). Minor (petechiae, ecchymoses, epistaxis) or major (gastrointestinal or vaginal) haemorrhage, a feature of DHF, may occur. Cerebrovascular bleeding may be a complication of severe dengue.

Diagnosis

In endemic areas, mild dengue must be distinguished from other viral infections. The diagnosis can be confirmed by seroconversion of IgM or a fourfold rise in IgG antibody titres. Serological tests may detect cross-reacting antibodies from infection or vaccination against other flaviviruses, including yellow fever virus, Japanese encephalitis virus and West Nile virus. Isolation of dengue virus or detection of dengue virus RNA by PCR (p. 106) in blood or CSF is available in specialist laboratories. Commercial enzyme-linked immunosorbent assay (ELISA) kits to detect the NS1 viral antigen, although less sensitive than PCR, are available in many endemic areas.

Management and prevention

Treatment is supportive, emphasising fluid replacement and appropriate management of shock and organ dysfunction, which is a major determinant of morbidity and mortality. With intensive care support, mortality rates are 1% or less. Aspirin should be avoided due to bleeding risk. Glucocorticoids have not been shown to help. No existing antivirals are effective.

Breeding places of *Aedes* mosquitoes should be abolished and the adults destroyed by insecticides. A recently licensed vaccine is available.

Yellow fever

Yellow fever is a haemorrhagic fever of the tropics, caused by a flavivirus. It is a zoonosis of monkeys in West and Central African, and South and Central American tropical rainforests, where it may cause devastating epidemics (Fig. 11.13). Transmission is by tree-top mosquitoes, *Aedes africanus* (Africa) and *Haemagogus* spp. (America). The infection is introduced to humans either by infected mosquitoes when trees are felled, or by monkeys raiding human settlements. In towns, yellow fever may be transmitted between humans by *Aedes aegypti*, which breeds efficiently in small collections of water. The distribution of this mosquito is far wider than that of yellow fever, and more widespread infection is a continued threat.

Yellow fever causes approximately 200 000 infections each year, mainly in sub-Saharan Africa, and the number is increasing. Overall mortality is around 15%, although this varies widely. Humans are infectious during the viraemic phase, which starts 3–6 days after the bite of the infected mosquito and lasts for 4–5 days.

Clinical features

After an incubation period of 3–6 days, yellow fever is often a mild febrile illness lasting less than 1 week, with headache, myalgia, conjunctival erythema and bradycardia. This is followed by fever resolution (defervescence) but, in some cases, fever recurs after a few hours to days. In more severe disease, fever recrudescence is associated with lower back pain, abdominal pain and somnolence, prominent nausea and vomiting, bradycardia and jaundice. Liver damage and DIC lead to bleeding with petechiae, mucosal haemorrhages and gastrointestinal bleeding. Shock, hepatic failure, renal failure, seizures and coma may ensue.

11.35 WHO case definitions of dengue, 2015

Probable dengue fever

- Exposure in an endemic area
- Fever
- Two of:
    Nausea/vomiting
    Rash
    Aches/pains
    Positive tourniquet test
    Leucopenia
    Any warning sign

Laboratory confirmation important

Needs regular medical observation and instruction in the warning signs

If there are no warning signs, need for hospitalisation is influenced by age, comorbidities, pregnancy and social factors

Dengue with warning signs

- Probable dengue plus one of:
    Abdominal pain or tenderness
    Persistent vomiting
    Signs of fluid accumulation, e.g. pleural effusion or ascites
    Mucosal bleed
    Hepatomegaly >2 cm
    Rapid increase in haematocrit with fall in platelet count

Needs medical intervention, e.g. intravenous fluid

Severe dengue

- Severe plasma leakage leading to:
    Shock (dengue shock syndrome)
    Fluid accumulation with respiratory distress
- Severe haemorrhagic manifestations, e.g. gastrointestinal haemorrhage
- Severe organ involvement (atypical features):
    Liver AST or ALT ≥1000 U/L
    CNS: impaired consciousness, meningoencephalitis, seizures
    Cardiomyopathy, conduction defects, arrhythmias
    Other organs, e.g. acute kidney injury, pancreatitis, acute lung injury, disseminated intravascular coagulopathy, rhabdomyolysis

Needs emergency medical treatment and specialist care with intensive care input

(ALT = alanine aminotransferase; AST = aspartate aminotransferase)
Adapted from https://wwww.cdc.gov/nndss/conditions/dengue-virus-infections/case-definition/2015/

Diagnosis

The differential diagnosis includes malaria, typhoid, viral hepatitis, leptospirosis, haemorrhagic fevers and aflatoxin poisoning. Diagnosis of yellow fever can be confirmed by detection of virus in the blood in the first 3–4 days of illness (e.g. by culture or reverse transcription polymerase chain reaction (RT-PCR)), the presence of IgM or a fourfold rise in IgG antibody titre. Leucopenia is characteristic. Liver biopsy should be avoided in life due to the risk of fatal bleeding. Postmortem features, such as acute mid-zonal necrosis and Councilman bodies with minimal inflammation in the liver, are suggestive but not specific. Immunohistochemistry for viral antigens improves specificity.

Management and prevention

Treatment is supportive, with meticulous attention to fluid and electrolyte balance, urine output and blood pressure. Blood transfusions, plasma expanders and peritoneal dialysis may be necessary. Patients should be isolated, as their blood and body products may contain virus particles.

A single vaccination with a live attenuated vaccine gives full protection for at least 10 years and many travellers do not require a booster unless specified by individual countries' travel requirements. Potential side-effects include hypersensitivity, encephalitis and systemic features of yellow fever (viscerotropic disease) caused by the attenuated virus. Vaccination is not recommended in people who are significantly immunosuppressed. The risk of vaccine side-effects must be balanced against the risk of infection for less immunocompromised hosts, pregnant women and older patients. An internationally recognised certificate of vaccination is sometimes necessary when crossing borders.

Viral haemorrhagic fevers

Viral haemorrhagic fevers (VHFs) are zoonoses caused by several different viruses (Box 11.36). They are geographically restricted and previously occurred in rural settings or in health-care facilities. The largest outbreak of VHF to date started in 2014, with Ebola

11.36 Viral haemorrhagic fevers

Disease	Reservoir	Transmission	Incubation period	Geography	Mortality rate	Clinical features of severe disease[1]
Lassa fever	Multimammate rats (*Mastomys natalensis*)	Urine from rat Body fluids from patients	6–21 days	West Africa	15%	Haemorrhage, shock, encephalopathy, ARDS (responds to ribavirin), deafness in survivors
Ebola fever	Fruit bats (*Pteropodidae* family) and bush meat	Body fluids from patients Handling infected primates	2–21 days	Central Africa Outbreaks as far north as Sudan	25–90%	Haemorrhage and/or diarrhoea, hepatic failure and acute kidney injury
Marburg fever	Undefined	Body fluids from patients Handling infected primates	3–9 days	Central Africa Outbreak in Angola	25–90%	Haemorrhage, diarrhoea, encephalopathy, orchitis
Yellow fever	Monkeys	Mosquitoes	3–6 days	See Figure 11.13	~15%	Hepatic failure, acute kidney injury, haemorrhage
Dengue	Humans	*Aedes aegypti*	2–7 days	See Figure 11.13	<10%[2]	Haemorrhage, shock
Crimean–Congo haemorrhagic fever	Small vertebrates Domestic and wild animals	*Ixodes* tick Body fluids	1–3 days up to 9 days 3–6 days up to 13 days	Africa, Asia, Eastern Europe	30%	Encephalopathy, early haemorrhage, hepatic failure, acute kidney injury, ARDS
Rift Valley fever	Domestic livestock	Contact with animals, mosquito or other insect bites	2–6 days	Africa, Arabian peninsula	1%	Haemorrhage, blindness, meningoencephalitis (complications only in a minority)
Kyasanur fever	Monkeys	Ticks	3–8 days	Karnataka State, India	5–10%	Haemorrhage, pulmonary oedema, neurological features, iridokeratitis in survivors
Bolivian and Argentinian haemorrhagic fever (Junin and Machupo viruses)	Rodents (*Calomys* spp.)	Urine, aerosols Body fluids from case (rare)	5–19 days (3–6 days for parenteral)	South America	15–30%	Haemorrhage, shock, cerebellar signs (may respond to ribavirin)
Haemorrhagic fever with renal syndrome (Hantaan fever)	Rodents	Aerosols from faeces	5–42 days (typically 14 days)	Northern Asia, northern Europe, Balkans	5%	Acute kidney injury, cerebrovascular accidents, pulmonary oedema, shock (hepatic failure and haemorrhagic features only in some variants)

[1]All potentially have circulatory failure. [2]Mortality of uncomplicated and haemorrhagic dengue fever, respectively.
(ARDS = acute respiratory distress syndrome)

circulating in Guinea, Liberia and Sierra Leone. The outbreak resulted in over 28 000 cases by 2016.

Serological surveys have shown that Lassa fever is widespread in West Africa and may lead to up to 500 000 infections annually. Mortality overall may be low, as 80% of cases are asymptomatic, but in hospitalised cases mortality averages 15%. Ebola outbreaks have occurred at a rate of approximately one per year in Africa, involving up to a few hundred cases prior to the 2014 outbreak. Marburg has been documented less frequently, with outbreaks in the Democratic Republic of Congo and Uganda, but the largest outbreak to date involved 163 cases in Angola in 2005. Mortality rates of Ebola and Marburg are high.

VHFs have extended into Europe, with an outbreak of Congo–Crimean haemorrhagic fever (CCHF) in Turkey in 2006, and cases of haemorrhagic fever with renal syndrome in the Balkans and Russia. An outbreak of CCHF in 2011 in Gujarat, India, involved several health-care workers and emphasised the importance of maintaining a high index of suspicion for VHF and implementing appropriate infection control measures at the first opportunity. Kyasanur forest disease is a tick-borne VHF currently confined to a small focus in Karnataka, India; there are about 500 cases annually. Monkeys are the principal hosts but, with forest felling, there are fears that this disease will increase.

New outbreaks and new agents are identified sporadically. Details on recent disease outbreaks can be found at the WHO website (see 'Further information').

Clinical features

VHFs present with non-specific fever, malaise, body pains, sore throat and headache. On examination, conjunctivitis, throat injection, an erythematous or petechial rash, haemorrhage, lymphadenopathy and bradycardia may be noted. The viruses cause endothelial dysfunction with the development of capillary leak. Bleeding is due to endothelial damage and platelet dysfunction. Hypovolaemic shock and ARDS may develop (p. 198).

Haemorrhage is a late feature of most VHFs and most patients present with earlier features. In Lassa fever, joint and abdominal pain is prominent. A macular blanching rash may be present but bleeding is unusual, occurring in only 20% of hospitalised patients. Encephalopathy may develop and deafness affects 30% of survivors. In CCHF, bleeding, manifest by haematemesis or bleeding per rectum, may be an early feature, accompanied by derangement of LFTs.

The clue to the viral aetiology comes from the travel and exposure history. Travel to an outbreak area, activity in a rural environment and contact with sick individuals or animals within 21 days all increase the risk of VHF. Enquiry should be made about insect bites, hospital visits and attendance at ritual funerals (Ebola virus infection). For Lassa fever, retrosternal pain, pharyngitis and proteinuria have a positive predictive value of 80% in West Africa.

Investigations and management

Non-specific findings include leucopenia, thrombocytopenia and proteinuria. In Lassa fever, an AST of >150 U/L is associated with a 50% mortality. It is important to exclude other causes of fever, especially malaria, typhoid and respiratory tract infections. Most patients suspected of having a VHF in the UK turn out to have malaria.

A febrile patient from an endemic area within the 21-day incubation period, who has specific epidemiological risk factors (see Fig. 11.6) or signs of organ failure or haemorrhage, should be treated as being at high risk of VHF; appropriate infection control measures must be implemented and the patient transferred to a centre with biosafety level (BSL) 4 facilities if testing positive. Individuals with a history of travel within 21 days and fever, but without the relevant epidemiological features or signs of VHF, are classified as medium-risk and should have an initial blood sample tested to exclude malaria. If this is negative, relevant specimens (blood, throat swab, urine and pleural fluid, if available) are collected and sent to an appropriate reference laboratory for nucleic acid detection (PCR), virus isolation and serology. If patients are still felt to be at significant risk of VHF or if infection is confirmed, they should be transferred to a specialised high-security infectious disease unit. All further laboratory tests should be performed at BSL 4. Transport requires an ambulance with BSL 3 facilities.

In addition to general supportive measures, ribavirin is given intravenously (100 mg/kg, then 25 mg/kg daily for 3 days and 12.5 mg/kg daily for 4 days) when Lassa fever or South American haemorrhagic fevers are suspected.

Prevention

Ribavirin has been used as prophylaxis in close contacts in Lassa fever but there are no formal trials of its efficacy.

Ebola virus disease (EVD)

Ebola virus disease (EVD) is thought to spread to human populations from fruit bats, sometimes indirectly via contact with infected primates or other animals. Person-to-person spread, via contact with blood, secretions or body parts, establishes EVD in populations. Family members, health-care workers and people performing traditional burials are at particular risk. The 2014 outbreak involved the Zaire strain of Ebola virus.

Clinical features

The incubation period is 2–21 days but typically 8–10 days. Fever and non-specific signs are accompanied by abdominal pain, diarrhoea, vomiting and hiccups. A maculopapular rash occurs after 5–7 days in some. Although bleeding from the gums or venepuncture sites or in the stool occurs, haemorrhage may be less prominent than in other VHFs and is often a terminal event, as observed in the 2014 epidemic. In contrast, fluid losses from diarrhoea are more marked and reach 10 L a day. Complications include meningoencephalitis, uveitis and miscarriages in pregnant women.

Investigations

Lymphopenia occurs, followed by neutrophilia, atypical lymphocytes, thrombocytopenia and coagulation abnormalities. Elevations of AST/ALT, features of acute kidney injury, electrolyte disturbances and proteinuria are also observed. The virus is detected by a PCR in blood or body fluids, but may need retesting if the duration of symptoms is less than 3 days. Serology provides a retrospective diagnosis.

Management

Treatment is supportive and aimed at fluid replacement. Bacterial super-infections should be promptly treated. A cocktail of monoclonal antibodies against Ebola virus, ZMapp, has been used in a few cases, but efficacy requires further studies. Mortality is approximately 40%. Survivors recover from the second week of illness but experience late sequelae, including arthritis (76%), uveitis (60%) and deafness (24%), while skin sloughing is common. Relapse with meningitis is reported months after recovery.

Prevention

Ebola virus may be detected in the semen months after recovery. Male survivors are therefore encouraged to practise safe sex for 12 months after symptom onset or until semen tests negative on two occasions, but recommendations are evolving. Public health measures are essential for outbreak control and involve contact surveillance and monitoring through the incubation period, separating healthy from sick individuals, practising safe burial methods and ensuring appropriate infection control measures to protect health-care and laboratory workers, including provision of personal protective equipment such as gloves, gowns and full-face protection (face shield or masks combined with goggles). An Ebola glycoprotein vaccine, rVZV-ZEBOV, was shown to be effective in 2016 after a trial in West Africa.

Zika virus

Zika virus is a flavivirus spread from primate hosts by *Aedes aegypti* and *Aedes albopictus*, which bite during the day. Described in Africa and Asia since 2015, it has been epidemic in the Caribbean and Central and South America, where a mosquito–man–mosquito transmission cycle is established. It also can be transmitted in semen.

Clinical features

The incubation period is 3–12 days. Infection is asymptomatic or mild, resembling dengue with fever, arthralgia, conjunctivitis and maculopapular rash. Complications include increased reports of Guillain–Barré syndrome. The major concern has been a marked increase in microcephaly in pregnant women infected with Zika virus, as well as increased rates of cerebral calcification, deafness, visual problems such as chorioretinal scarring, joint contractures (arthrogryposis), hydrops fetalis and growth retardation. Zika virus appears to infect neural progenitor cells.

Investigations

Routine blood tests are usually normal but may show leucopenia, thrombocytopenia or increased transaminases. PCR detects virus in the first week of illness or in urine up to 14 days. Serology provides a retrospective diagnosis but cross-reacts with other flaviviruses. Plaque-reduction neutralisation testing can be used to detect virus-specific neutralising antibodies and distinguish between cross-reacting antibodies in primary flavivirus infections.

Prevention

Prevention focuses on avoiding mosquito bites. Since Zika virus may be found in the semen or genital secretions for prolonged periods, infected individuals should practise safe sex for at least 6 months and planned pregnancy should be postponed for at least 6 months. Individuals who have travelled to an endemic area but are asymptomatic should practise safe sex and avoid pregnancy for at least 2 months. As this is an evolving area, updated guidance should be sought. There is currently no vaccine.

Viral infections of the skin

Herpes simplex virus 1 and 2

Herpes simplex viruses (HSVs) cause recurrent mucocutaneous infection; HSV-1 typically involves the mucocutaneous surfaces of the head and neck (Fig. 11.14), while HSV-2 predominantly involves the genital mucosa (pp. 333 and 336), although there is overlap (see Box 11.29). The seroprevalence of HSV-1 is 30–100%, varying by socioeconomic status, while that of HSV-2 is 20–60%. Infection is acquired by inoculation of viruses shed by an infected individual on to a mucosal surface in a susceptible person. The virus infects sensory and autonomic neurons and establishes latent infection in the nerve ganglia. Primary infection is followed by episodes of reactivation throughout life.

Clinical features

Primary HSV-1 or 2 infection is more likely to be symptomatic later in life, causing gingivostomatitis, pharyngitis or painful genital tract lesions. The primary attack may be associated with fever and regional lymphadenopathy.

Recurrence

Recurrent attacks occur throughout life, most often in association with concomitant medical illness, menstruation, mechanical trauma, immunosuppression, psychological stress or, for oral lesions, ultraviolet light exposure. HSV reactivation in the oral mucosa produces the classical 'cold sore' or 'herpes labialis'. Prodromal hyperaesthesia is followed by rapid vesiculation, pustulation and crusting. Recurrent HSV genital disease is a common cause of recurrent painful ulceration (pp. 333 and 336). An inoculation lesion on the finger gives rise to a paronychia, termed a 'whitlow', in contacts of patients with herpetic lesions (Fig. 11.14B).

Fig. 11.14 Cutaneous manifestations of herpes simplex virus 1 (HSV-1). A Acute HSV-1. There were also vesicles in the mouth – herpetic stomatitis. B Herpetic whitlow. C Eczema herpeticum. HSV-1 infection spreads rapidly in eczematous skin.

Complications

Disseminated cutaneous lesions can occur in individuals with underlying dermatological diseases, such as eczema (eczema herpeticum) (Fig. 11.14C). Herpes keratitis presents with pain and blurring of vision; characteristic dendritic ulcers are visible on slit-lamp examination and may produce corneal scarring and permanent visual impairment.

Primary HSV-2 can cause meningitis or transverse myelitis. HSV is the leading cause of sporadic viral encephalitis (p. 1121); this follows either primary or secondary disease, usually with HSV-1. A haemorrhagic necrotising temporal lobe cerebritis produces temporal lobe epilepsy and altered consciousness/coma. Without treatment, mortality is 80%. HSV is also implicated in the pathogenesis of Bell's palsy with a lower motor neuron 7th nerve palsy, although antivirals have not been demonstrated to improve outcome.

Neonatal HSV disease is usually associated with primary infection of the mother at term (see Box 11.26). In excess of two-thirds of cases develop disseminated disease with cutaneous lesions, hepatitis, pneumonitis and frequently encephalitis.

Immunocompromised hosts can develop visceral disease with oesophagitis, hepatitis, pneumonitis, encephalitis or retinitis.

Diagnosis

Differentiation from other vesicular eruptions is achieved by demonstration of virus in vesicular fluid, usually by direct immunofluorescence or PCR. HSV encephalitis is diagnosed by a positive PCR for HSV in CSF. Serology is of limited value.

Management

Therapy of localised disease must commence in the first 48 hours of clinical disease (primary or recurrent); thereafter it is unlikely to influence clinical outcome. Oral lesions in an immunocompetent individual may be treated with topical aciclovir. All severe manifestations should be treated, regardless of the time of presentation (see Box 11.30). Suspicion of HSV encephalopathy requires immediate empirical antiviral therapy. Aciclovir resistance is encountered occasionally in immunocompromised hosts, in which case foscarnet is the treatment of choice.

Human herpesvirus 8

Human herpesvirus 8 (HHV-8) (see Box 11.29) causes Kaposi's sarcoma in both AIDS-related and endemic non-AIDS-related forms (p. 314). HHV-8 is spread via saliva, and men who have sex with men have an increased incidence of infection. Seroprevalence varies widely, being highest in sub-Saharan Africa. HHV-8 also causes two rare haematological malignancies: primary effusion lymphoma and multicentric Castleman's disease. Current antivirals are not effective.

Enterovirus infections

Hand, foot and mouth disease

This systemic infection is caused by Coxsackie viruses usually, or occasionally by echoviruses. It affects children and occasionally adults, resulting in local or household outbreaks, particularly in the summer months. A relatively mild illness with fever and lymphadenopathy develops after an incubation period of approximately 10 days; 2–3 days later, a painful papular or vesicular rash appears on palmoplantar surfaces of hands and feet, with associated oral lesions on the buccal mucosa and tongue that ulcerate rapidly. A papular erythematous rash may appear on buttocks and thighs. Antiviral treatment is not available and management consists of symptom relief with analgesics.

Herpangina

This infection, caused by Coxsackie viruses, primarily affects children and teenagers in the summer months. It is characterised by a small number of vesicles at the soft/hard palate junction, often associated with high fever, an extremely sore throat and headache. The lesions are short-lived, rupturing after 2–3 days and rarely persisting for more than 1 week. Treatment is with analgesics if required. Culture of the virus from vesicles or DNA detection by PCR differentiates herpangina from HSV.

Poxviruses

These DNA viruses are rare but potentially important pathogens.

Smallpox (variola)

Smallpox, which has high mortality, was eradicated worldwide by a global vaccination programme but interest has re-emerged due to its potential as a bioweapon. The virus is spread by the respiratory route or contact with lesions, and is highly infectious.

The incubation period is 7–17 days. A prodrome with fever, headache and prostration leads, in 1–2 days, to the rash, which develops through macules and papules to vesicles and pustules, worst on the face and distal extremities. Lesions in one area are all at the same stage of development with no cropping (unlike chickenpox). Vaccination can lead to a modified course of disease with milder rash and lower mortality.

If a case of smallpox is suspected, national public health authorities must be contacted. Electron micrography (like Fig. 11.15) and DNA detection tests (PCR) are used to confirm diagnosis.

Monkeypox

Despite the name, the animal reservoirs for this virus are probably small squirrels and rodents. It causes a rare zoonotic infection in communities in the rainforest belt of Central Africa, producing a vesicular rash that is indistinguishable from smallpox, but differentiated by the presence of lymphadenopathy. Little person-to-person transmission occurs. Outbreaks outside

Fig. 11.15 Electron micrograph of molluscum contagiosum, a poxvirus. *Courtesy of Prof. Goura Kudesia, Northern General Hospital, Sheffield.*

Africa have been linked to importation of African animals as exotic pets. Diagnosis is by electron micrography or DNA detection (PCR).

Cowpox

Humans in contact with infected cows develop large vesicles, usually on the hands or arms and associated with fever and regional lymphadenitis. The reservoir is thought to be wild rodents.

Vaccinia virus

This laboratory strain is the basis of the existing vaccine to prevent smallpox. Widespread vaccination is no longer recommended due to the likelihood of local spread from the vaccination site (potentially life-threatening in those with eczema (eczema vaccinatum) or immune deficiency) and of encephalitis. However, vaccination may still be recommended for key medical staff.

Other poxviruses: orf and molluscum contagiosum

See page 1239 and Figure 11.15.

Gastrointestinal viral infections

Norovirus (Norwalk agent)

Norovirus is the most common cause of infectious gastroenteritis in the UK and leads to outbreaks in hospital wards, cruise ships and military camps. Food handlers may transmit this virus, which is relatively resistant to decontamination procedures. The incubation period is 24–48 hours. High attack rates and prominent vomiting are characteristic. Diagnosis may be achieved by electron microscopy, antigen or DNA detection (PCR) in stool samples, although the characteristic clinical and epidemiological features mean that microbiological confirmation is not always necessary. The virus is highly infectious and cases should be isolated and environmental surfaces cleaned with detergents and disinfected with bleach.

Astrovirus

Astroviruses cause diarrhoea in small children and occasionally in immunocompromised adults.

Rotavirus

Rotaviruses infect enterocytes and are a major cause of diarrhoeal illness in young children worldwide. There are winter epidemics in developed countries, particularly in nurseries. Adults in close contact with cases may develop disease. The incubation period is 48 hours and patients present with watery diarrhoea, vomiting, fever and abdominal pain. Dehydration is prominent. Diagnosis is aided by commercially available enzyme immunoassay kits, which require fresh or refrigerated stool samples. Immunity develops to natural infection. Monovalent and multivalent vaccines have been licensed in many countries and have now demonstrated efficacy in large trials in Africa and the Americas.

Hepatitis viruses (A–E)

See Chapter 22.

Other viruses

Adenoviruses are frequently identified from stool culture and implicated as a cause of diarrhoea in children. They have also been linked to cases of intussusception.

Respiratory viral infections

These infections are described on page 581.

Adenoviruses, rhinoviruses and enteroviruses (Coxsackie viruses and echoviruses) often produce non-specific upper respiratory tract symptoms but may cause viral pneumonia. Parainfluenza and respiratory syncytial viruses cause upper respiratory tract disease, croup and bronchiolitis in small children and pneumonia in the immunocompromised. Respiratory syncytial virus also causes pneumonia in nursing home residents and may be associated with nosocomial pneumonia. Metapneumovirus and bocavirus cause upper and occasionally lower respiratory tract infection, especially in immunosuppressed individuals. The severe acute respiratory syndrome (SARS), caused by the SARS coronavirus, emerged as a major respiratory pathogen during an outbreak in 2002–2003, with 8000 cases and 10% mortality (p. 582).

Middle East respiratory syndrome coronavirus (MERS-CoV)

In 2012, a novel coronavirus, distantly related to the SARS coronavirus, caused several deaths connected with pneumonia in patients originating from the Middle East. The Middle East respiratory syndrome coronavirus (MERS-CoV) appears to be a zoonosis, involving transmission from bats to camels and then to humans. Over 20 countries have reported cases, although most cases have a history of travel to Saudi Arabia or other countries in the Arabian Peninsula. By 2016 there had been over 1700 reported cases.

Clinical features

The incubation period in person-to-person transmission is 2–14 (average 5) days. Any age may be infected but the severe form of MERS-CoV mainly occurs in patients over 50 with medical comorbidities. Initial symptoms are fever, chills, headache, myalgia, dry cough and dyspnoea. Abdominal pain and diarrhoea may be prominent. The mean period from symptom onset to hospitalisation is 4 days, and 5 days to intensive care unit admission. Illness is complicated by rapid development of respiratory failure and features of ARDS and multi-organ failure. Mortality is 35%.

Diagnosis and management

Laboratory features include lymphopenia, thrombocytopenia and raised lactate dehydrogenase (LDH). Diagnosis is confirmed by PCR of serum, nasopharyngeal or other respiratory samples. Serology may also be useful. Treatment is supportive. Strict infection control measures should be implemented for anyone with fever, severe respiratory illness and epidemiological risk factors. Patients should be managed in an airborne infection isolation room with contact and airborne infection control measures, including personal protective equipment for health-care workers.

Viral infections with neurological involvement

See also page 1121.

Japanese B encephalitis

This flavivirus is an important cause of endemic encephalitis in Japan, China, Russia, South-east Asia, India and Pakistan; outbreaks also occur elsewhere. There are 10 000–20 000 cases reported to the WHO annually. Pigs and aquatic birds are the virus reservoirs and transmission is by mosquitoes. Exposure to rice paddies is a recognised risk factor.

Clinical features

The incubation period is 4–21 days. Most infections are subclinical in childhood and 1% or less of infections lead to encephalitis. Initial systemic illness with fever, malaise and anorexia is followed by headache, photophobia, vomiting and changes in brainstem function. Other neurological features include meningism, seizures, cranial nerve palsies, flaccid or spastic paralysis and extrapyramidal syndromes. Mortality with neurological disease is 25%. Most children die from respiratory failure. Some 50% of survivors have neurological sequelae.

Investigations, management and prevention

Other infectious causes of encephalitis should be excluded (p. 1121). There is neutrophilia and often hyponatraemia. CSF analysis reveals lymphocytosis and elevated protein. Serological testing of serum and CSF aids diagnosis but may cross-react with dengue and other flaviviruses.

Treatment is supportive. Vaccination is recommended for travellers to endemic areas during the monsoon. Some endemic countries include vaccination in their childhood schedules.

West Nile virus

This flavivirus is an important cause of neurological disease in an area that extends from Australia, India and Russia through Africa and Southern Europe and across to North America. The disease has an avian reservoir and a mosquito vector. Older people are at increased risk of neurological disease.

Clinical features

Most infections are asymptomatic. After 2–6 days' incubation, a mild febrile illness and arthralgia may occur. A prolonged incubation may be seen in immunocompromised individuals. Children may develop a maculopapular rash. Neurological disease is seen in 1% and is characterised by encephalitis, meningitis or asymmetric flaccid paralysis with 10% mortality.

Diagnosis and management

Diagnosis is by serology or detection of viral RNA in blood or CSF. Serological tests may show cross-reactivity with other flaviviruses, including vaccine strains. Treatment is supportive.

Enterovirus 71

Enterovirus 71 has caused outbreaks around the globe of enteroviral disease with hand, foot and mouth disease (p. 248) and aseptic meningitis. Some cases have been complicated by encephalitis with flaccid paralysis or by brainstem involvement and death. The virus can be isolated from vesicle fluid, stool or CSF, and viral RNA can be detected in CSF by RT-PCR.

Nipah virus encephalitis

Nipah virus is a paramyxovirus in the Henipavirus genus, which caused an epidemic of encephalitis amongst Malaysian pig farmers in 1999 and subsequently caused outbreaks in Bangladesh and India. Mortality is around 30%. Diagnosis is by PCR or serology.

Human T-cell lymphotropic virus type I

Human T-cell lymphotropic virus type I (HTLV-1) is a retrovirus that causes chronic infection with development of adult T-cell leukaemia/lymphoma (ATL) or HTLV-1-associated myelopathy (HAM) in a subset of those infected (see Box 23.57, p. 964). It is found mainly in Japan, the Caribbean, Central and South America, and the Seychelles. HAM or tropical spastic paraparesis occurs in less than 5% of those with chronic infection, and presents with gait disturbance, spasticity of the lower extremities, urinary incontinence, impotence and sensory disturbance. Myositis and uveitis may also occur with HTLV-1 infection. Serology, sometimes confirmed with PCR, establishes the diagnosis. Treatment is usually supportive.

Viral infections with rheumatological involvement

Rheumatological syndromes characterise a variety of viral infections ranging from exanthems, such as rubella and parvovirus B19 (p. 237), to blood-borne viruses, such as HBV and HIV-1 and the sequelae of EVD.

Chikungunya virus

Chikungunya is an alphavirus that causes fever, rash and arthropathy. It is found principally in Africa and Asia, including India. Humans and non-human primates are the main reservoir and the main vector is the *Aedes aegypti* mosquito. Cases occur in epidemics on a background of sporadic cases. In 2007, an outbreak extended as far north as Italy.

The incubation period is 2–12 days. A period of fever may be followed by an afebrile phase and then recrudescence of fever. Children may develop a maculopapular rash. Adults are susceptible to arthritis, which causes early morning pain and swelling, most often in the small joints. Arthritis can persist for months and may become chronic in individuals who are positive for human leucocyte antigen (HLA)-B27. Related alphaviruses causing similar syndromes include Sindbis virus (Scandinavia and Africa), O'nyong-nyong virus (Central Africa), Ross River virus (Australia) and Mayaro virus (Caribbean and South America).

Diagnosis is by serology but cross-reactivity between alphaviruses occurs. Treatment is symptomatic.

Prion diseases

Prions cause transmissible spongiform encephalopathies and are discussed on page 1126.

Bacterial infections

Bacterial infections of the skin, soft tissues and bones

Most infections of the skin, soft tissues and bone are caused by either *Staph. aureus* or streptococci (mainly *Strep. pyogenes*) (see pp. 1019 and 1237).

Staphylococcal infections

Staphylococci are usually found colonising the anterior nares and skin. Some staphylococci produce coagulase, an enzyme that converts fibrinogen to fibrin in rabbit plasma, causing it to clot. *Staph. aureus* is coagulase-positive, and most other species are coagulase-negative. In modern laboratory practice, however, the identification of *Staph. aureus* rarely involves the coagulase test.

Staph. aureus is the main cause of staphylococcal infections. *Staph. intermedius* is another coagulase-positive staphylococcus, which causes infection following dog bites. Among coagulase-negative organisms, *Staph. epidermidis* is the predominant commensal organism of the skin, and can cause severe infections in those with central venous catheters or implanted prosthetic materials. *Staph. saprophyticus* is part of the normal vaginal flora and causes urinary tract infections in sexually active young women. Others implicated in human infections include *Staph. lugdunensis*, *Staph. schleiferi*, *Staph. haemolyticus* and *Staph. caprae*. Coagulase-negative staphylococci are not usually identified to species level.

Staphylococci are particularly dangerous if they gain access to the blood stream, having the potential to disseminate widely (Fig. 11.16). In any patient with staphylococcal bacteraemia, especially injection drug-users, the possibility of endocarditis must be considered (p. 527). Growth of *Staph. aureus* in blood cultures should not be dismissed as a 'contaminant' unless all possible underlying sources have been excluded and repeated blood culture is negative. Any evidence of spreading cellulitis indicates the urgent need for an antistaphylococcal antibiotic, such as flucloxacillin (unless there is a likely risk of MRSA). This is particularly true for mid-facial cellulitis, which can result in cavernous sinus thrombophlebitis.

In addition, *Staph. aureus* can cause severe systemic disease due to the effects of toxin produced at superficial sites in the absence of tissue invasion by bacteria.

Skin infections

Staphylococcal infections cause ecthyma, folliculitis, furuncles, carbuncles, bullous impetigo and the scalded skin syndrome (pp. 1235–1237). They may also be involved in necrotising infections of the skin and subcutaneous tissues (p. 226).

Wound infections

Many wound infections are caused by staphylococci, which may significantly prolong post-operative hospital stays

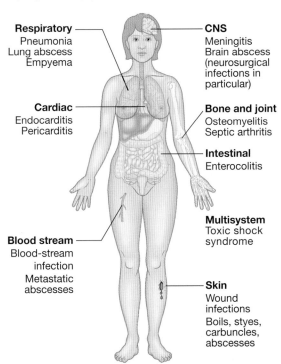

Fig. 11.16 Infections caused by *Staphylococcus aureus*.

Respiratory
Pneumonia
Lung abscess
Empyema

Cardiac
Endocarditis
Pericarditis

Blood stream
Blood-stream infection
Metastatic abscesses

CNS
Meningitis
Brain abscess (neurosurgical infections in particular)

Bone and joint
Osteomyelitis
Septic arthritis

Intestinal
Enterocolitis

Multisystem
Toxic shock syndrome

Skin
Wound infections
Boils, styes, carbuncles, abscesses

(Fig. 11.17A). Prevention involves careful attention to hand hygiene, skin preparation and aseptic technique, and the use of topical and systemic antibiotic prophylaxis.

Treatment is by drainage of any abscesses plus adequate dosage of antistaphylococcal antibiotics, done early, particularly if prosthetic implants have been inserted.

Cannula-related infection

Staphylococcal infection associated with cannula sepsis (Fig. 11.17B and p. 196) and thrombophlebitis is an important and common reason for morbidity following hospital admission. The Visual Infusion Phlebitis (VIP) score aids cannula evaluation (Box 11.37). Staphylococci have a predilection for plastic, rapidly

Fig. 11.17 Manifestations of skin infection with *Staphylococcus aureus*. A Wound infection. B Cannula-related infection.

11.37 How to assess an intravenous cannula using the Visual Infusion Phlebitis (VIP) score		
Clinical features	**Score**	**Assessment and management**
IV site appears healthy	0	**No signs of phlebitis** Observe cannula

One of the following is evident:
   Slight pain near IV site
   Slight redness near IV site
	1	**Possible first signs of phlebitis**
		Observe cannula

Two of the following are evident:
   Pain near IV site
   Erythema
   Swelling
	2	**Early stage of phlebitis**
		Resite cannula

ALL of the following are evident and extensive:
   Pain along path of cannula
   Erythema
   Induration
	3	**Medium stage of phlebitis**
		Resite cannula
		Consider treatment

ALL of the following are evident and extensive:
   Pain along path of cannula
   Erythema
   Induration
   Palpable venous cord
	4	**Advanced stage of phlebitis or start of thrombophlebitis**
		Resite cannula
		Consider treatment

ALL of the following are evident:
   Pain along path of cannula
   Erythema
   Induration
   Palpable venous cord
   Pyrexia
	5	**Advanced stage of thrombophlebitis**
		Initiate treatment
		Resite cannula

Adapted from Jackson A. Nursing Times 1997; 94:68–71.

forming a biofilm on cannulae, which remains as a source of bacteraemia. Local poultice application may relieve symptoms but cannula removal and antibiotic treatment with flucloxacillin (or a glycopeptide if MRSA is suspected) are necessary if there is any suggestion of spreading infection.

Meticillin-resistant Staph. aureus

Resistance to meticillin is due to a penicillin-binding protein mutation in *Staph. aureus*. Resistance to vancomycin/teicoplanin (glycopeptides) in either glycopeptide intermediate *Staph. aureus* (GISA) or, rarely, vancomycin-resistant (VRSA) strains threatens the ability to manage serious infections produced by such organisms. Meticillin-resistant *Staph. aureus* (MRSA) is now a major worldwide health care-acquired pathogen, accounting for up to 40% of staphylococcal bacteraemia in developed countries. Community-acquired MRSA (c-MRSA) currently accounts for 50% of all MRSA infections in the USA. These organisms have also acquired other toxins, such as Panton–Valentine leukocidin (PVL), and cause rapidly fatal infection in young people. Clinicians must be aware of the potential danger of these infections and be prepared to take whatever appropriate infection control measures are locally advised (p. 111).

Treatment options for MRSA are shown in Box 6.16 (p. 117). Treatment should always be based on the results of antimicrobial susceptibility testing, since resistance to all these agents occurs. Milder MRSA infections may be treated with clindamycin, tetracyclines or co-trimoxazole. Glycopeptides, linezolid and daptomycin are reserved for treatment of more severe infections. Toxin-producing MRSA infections should be treated with protein-inhibiting antibiotics (clindamycin, linezolid).

Staphylococcal toxic shock syndrome

Staphylococcal toxic shock syndrome (TSS) is a serious and life-threatening disease associated with infection by *Staph. aureus*, which produces a specific toxin (toxic shock syndrome toxin 1, TSST1). It was formerly seen in young women in association with the use of highly absorbent intravaginal tampons but can occur with any *Staph. aureus* infection involving a relevant toxin-producing strain. The toxin acts as a 'super-antigen', triggering significant T-cell activation and massive cytokine release.

TSS has an abrupt onset with high fever, generalised systemic upset (myalgia, headache, sore throat and vomiting), a widespread erythematous blanching rash resembling scarlet fever, and hypotension. It rapidly progresses over a few hours to multi-organ failure, leading to death in 10–20%. Recovery is accompanied at 7–10 days by desquamation (Fig. 11.18).

The diagnosis is clinical and may be confirmed in menstrual cases by finding a retained tampon with staphylococci on Gram stain. Subsequent culture and demonstration of toxin production are confirmatory.

Management

Treatment is with immediate and aggressive fluid resuscitation and an intravenous antistaphylococcal antimicrobial (flucloxacillin or vancomycin), usually with the addition of a protein synthesis inhibitor (e.g. clindamycin) to inhibit toxin production. Intravenous immunoglobulin is occasionally added in the most severe cases. Women who recover from tampon-associated TSS should avoid tampons for at least 1 year and be advised that the condition can recur.

Fig. 11.18 Full-thickness desquamation after staphylococcal toxic shock syndrome.

Streptococcal infections

Streptococci are oropharyngeal and gut commensals, which appear as Gram-positive cocci in chains (see Fig. 6.3, p. 102). They are classified by the pattern of haemolysis they produce on blood agar (see Fig. 6.4, p. 102), by their 'Lancefield groups' (Box 11.38) and more recently by speciation on matrix-assisted laser desorption/ionisation time-of-flight (MALDI-TOF) mass spectometry. Some streptococci (e.g. *Strep. milleri* group) defy simple classification.

Group A streptococci (GAS) are the leading cause of bacterial pharyngitis. Although the presence of fever, tender anterior lymphadenopathy and purulent tonsillar exudate and the absence of cough make streptococcal pharyngitis more likely than viral infection, clinical features alone are unreliable for diagnosing streptococcal pharyngitis. GAS are also the major cause of cellulitis, erysipelas and impetigo (pp. 1237 and 1235). Groups C and G streptococci cause cellulitis, particularly in elderly, diabetic or immunocompromised patients. Group B streptococci (GBS) colonise the gut and vagina. They cause post-partum and neonatal sepsis, as well as other deep infections (infective endocarditis, septic arthritis, osteomyelitis etc.), especially in the elderly.

Streptococcal scarlet fever

Group A (or occasionally groups C and G) streptococci causing pharyngitis, tonsillitis or other infection may lead to scarlet fever, if the infecting strain produces a streptococcal pyrogenic exotoxin. Scarlet fever is most common in school-age children, but can also occur in young adults who have contact with young children. A diffuse erythematous rash occurs, which blanches on pressure (Fig. 11.19A), classically with circumoral pallor. The tongue, initially coated, becomes red and swollen ('strawberry tongue', Fig. 11.19B). The disease lasts about 7 days, the rash disappearing in 7–10 days, followed by a fine desquamation. Residual petechial lesions in the antecubital fossa may be seen ('Pastia's sign', Fig. 11.19C).

Treatment involves intravenous benzylpenicillin or an oral penicillin plus symptomatic measures.

11.38 Streptococcal and related infections

β-haemolytic group A (*Strep. pyogenes*)

- Skin and soft tissue infection (including erysipelas, impetigo, necrotising fasciitis)
- Streptococcal toxic shock syndrome
- Puerperal sepsis
- Scarlet fever
- Glomerulonephritis
- Rheumatic fever
- Bone and joint infection
- Tonsillitis

β-haemolytic group B (*Strep. agalactiae*)

- Neonatal infections, including meningitis
- Female pelvic infections
- Cellulitis

β-haemolytic group C (various zoonotic streptococci)

- Cellulitis
- Endocarditis
- Pharyngitis
- Septic arthritis

α-, β- or non-haemolytic group D (*Enterococcus faecalis, E. faecium*)

- Endocarditis
- Intra-abdominal infections
- Urinary tract infection

α- or non-haemolytic group D (*Strep. gallolyticus* subsp. *gallolyticus/S. bovis* biotype I)

- Bacteraemia/endocarditis associated with large bowel malignancy

β-haemolytic group G streptococci

- Cellulitis
- Endocarditis
- Liver abscess
- Septic arthritis

α-haemolytic optochin-resistant (viridans streptococci – *Strep. mitis, Strep. sanguis, Strep. mutans, Strep. salivarius*)

- Sepsis in immunosuppressed
- Endocarditis

α-haemolytic optochin-sensitive (*Strep. pneumoniae*)

- Pneumonia
- Meningitis
- Endocarditis
- Otitis media
- Sepsis
- Spontaneous bacterial peritonitis
- Sinusitis

Variable haemolysis (*Strep. milleri* group – *Strep. anginosus, Strep. intermedius, Strep. constellatus*)

- Endocarditis
- Intra-abdominal infections
- Urinary tract infection

Anaerobic streptococci (*Peptostreptococcus* spp.)

- Sepsis in immunosuppressed
- Endocarditis

N.B. All streptococci can cause sepsis.

Streptococcal toxic shock syndrome

Group A (or occasionally group C or G) streptococci can produce one of a variety of toxins, such as pyogenic exotoxin A. Like staphylococcal TSST1 (see above), these act as super-antigens. Initially, an influenza-like illness occurs, with signs of localised infection in 50% of cases, most often involving the skin and soft tissues. A faint erythematous rash, mainly on the chest, rapidly progresses to circulatory shock. Without aggressive management, multi-organ failure will develop.

Fluid resuscitation must be undertaken, along with parenteral antistreptococcal antibiotic therapy, usually with benzylpenicillin and clindamycin, to inhibit toxin production. Intravenous immunoglobulin is often administered. If necrotising fasciitis is present, it should be treated as described on page 227 with urgent débridement.

Treponematoses

Syphilis

This disease is described on page 337.

Endemic treponematoses

Yaws

Yaws is a granulomatous disease, mainly involving the skin and bones; it is caused by *Treponema pertenue*, morphologically and serologically indistinguishable from the causative organisms of syphilis and pinta. It is important to establish the geographical origin and sexual history of patients to exclude false-positive syphilis serology due to endemic treponemal infections. Between 1950 and 1960, WHO campaigns treated over 60 million people and eradicated yaws from many areas, but the disease has persisted patchily throughout the tropics; there was a resurgence in the 1980s and 1990s in West and Central Africa and the South Pacific.

Organisms are transmitted by bodily contact from a patient with infectious yaws through minor abrasions of the skin of another patient, usually a child. After an incubation period of 3–4 weeks, a proliferative granuloma containing numerous treponemes develops at the site of inoculation. This primary lesion is followed by secondary eruptions. In addition, there may be hypertrophic periosteal lesions of many bones, with underlying cortical rarefaction. Lesions of late yaws are characterised

Fig. 11.19 Clinical features of scarlet fever. [A] Characteristic rash with blanching on pressure. [B] 'Strawberry tongue'. [C] Pastia's sign: a petechial rash in the cubital fossa.

11.39 Diagnosis and treatment of yaws, pinta and bejel

Diagnosis of early stages

- Detection of spirochaetes in exudate of lesions by dark ground microscopy

Diagnosis of latent and early stages

- Positive serological tests, as for syphilis (see Box 13.8, p. 339)

Treatment of all stages

- Single intramuscular injection of 1.2 g long-acting penicillin, e.g. benzathine benzylpenicillin

by destructive changes that closely resemble the osteitis and gummas of tertiary syphilis and that heal with scarring and deformity. Investigations and management are outlined in Box 11.39. Improved housing and hygiene, combined with mass chemotherapy programmes, have achieved dramatic success in the control of yaws.

Pinta and bejel

These two treponemal infections occur in poor rural populations with low standards of domestic hygiene but are found in separate parts of the world. They have features in common, notably that they are transmitted by contact, usually within the family and not sexually, and in the case of bejel, through common eating and drinking utensils. Their diagnosis and management are as for yaws (Box 11.39).

- *Pinta.* Pinta is found only in South and Central America, where its incidence is declining. The infection is confined to the skin. The early lesions are scaly papules or dyschromic patches on the skin. The late lesions are often depigmented and disfiguring.
- *Bejel.* Bejel is the Middle Eastern name for non-venereal syphilis, which has a patchy distribution across sub-Saharan Africa, the Middle East, Central Asia and Australia. It has been eradicated from Eastern Europe. Transmission is most commonly from the mouth of the mother or child and the primary mucosal lesion is seldom seen. The early and late lesions resemble those of secondary and tertiary syphilis (p. 337) but cardiovascular and neurological disease is rare.

Tropical ulcer

Tropical ulcer is due to a synergistic bacterial infection caused by a fusobacterium (*F. ulcerans*, an anaerobe) and *Treponema vincentii*. It is common in hot, humid regions. The ulcer is most common on the lower legs and develops as a papule that rapidly breaks down to a sharply defined, painful ulcer. The base of the ulcer has a foul slough. Penicillin and metronidazole are useful in the early stages but rest, elevation and dressings are the mainstays of treatment.

Buruli ulcer

This ulcer is caused by *Mycobacterium ulcerans* and occurs widely in tropical rainforests. In 1999, a survey in Ghana found 6500 cases; there are an estimated 10 000 cases in West Africa as a whole.

The initial lesion is a small subcutaneous nodule on the arm or leg. This breaks down to form a shallow, necrotic ulcer with deeply undermined edges, which extends rapidly. Healing may occur

after 6 months but granuloma formation and the accompanying fibrosis cause contractures and deformity. Clumps of acid-fast bacilli can be detected in the ulcer floor.

A combination of rifampicin and streptomycin can cure the infection. Infected tissue should be removed surgically. Health campaigns in Ghana have successfully focused on early removal of the small, pre-ulcerative nodules.

Systemic bacterial infections

Brucellosis

Brucellosis is an enzootic infection (i.e. endemic in animals) caused by Gram-negative bacilli. The four species causing human disease and their animal hosts are: *Brucella melitensis* (goats, sheep and camels in Europe, especially the Mediterranean basin, the Middle East, Africa, India, Central Asia and South America), *B. abortus* (cattle, mainly in Africa, Asia and South America), *B. suis* (pigs in South Asia) and *B. canis* (dogs). *B. melitensis* causes the most severe disease; *B. suis* is often associated with abscess formation.

Infected animals may excrete *Brucella* spp. in their milk for prolonged periods and human infection is acquired by ingesting contaminated dairy products (especially unpasteurised milk), uncooked meat or offal. Animal urine, faeces, vaginal discharge and uterine products may transmit infection through abraded skin or via splashes and aerosols to the respiratory tract and conjunctiva.

Clinical features

Brucella spp. are intracellular organisms that survive for long periods within the reticulo-endothelial system. This explains the disease chronicity and tendency to relapse, even after antimicrobial therapy.

Acute illness is characterised by a high swinging temperature, rigors, lethargy, headache, joint and muscle pains, and scrotal pain. Occasionally, there is delirium, abdominal pain and constipation. Physical signs are non-specific, e.g. enlarged lymph nodes. Splenomegaly may cause thrombocytopenia.

Localised infection (Fig. 11.20), which occurs in about 30% of patients, is more likely if diagnosis and treatment are delayed.

Diagnosis

Definitive diagnosis depends on culture of the organism. Blood cultures are positive in 75–80% of *B. melitensis* and 50% of *B. abortus* infections. Bone marrow culture is not routine but may increase the diagnostic yield if antibiotics have been used prior to culture. CSF culture in neurobrucellosis is positive in about 30% of cases. The laboratory should be alerted to a suspected diagnosis of brucellosis, as the organism may infect laboratory workers and must be cultured at the appropriate biosafety level.

Serology may also aid diagnosis. In endemic areas, a single high antibody titre of more than 1/320 or a fourfold rise in titre is needed to support a diagnosis of acute infection. The test usually takes several weeks to become positive but should eventually detect 95% of acute infections.

Management

Aminoglycosides show synergistic activity with tetracyclines against brucellae. Treatment regimens for different forms of brucellosis are outlined in Box 11.40.

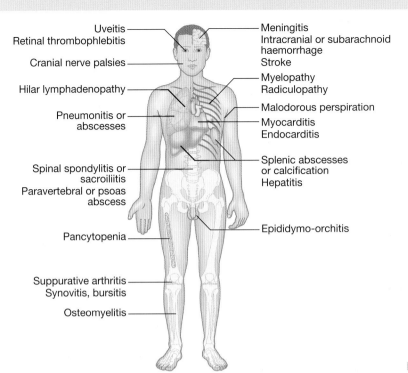

Fig. 11.20 Clinical features of brucellosis.

Uveitis
Retinal thrombophlebitis
Cranial nerve palsies
Hilar lymphadenopathy
Pneumonitis or abscesses
Spinal spondylitis or sacroiliitis
Paravertebral or psoas abscess
Pancytopenia
Suppurative arthritis
Synovitis, bursitis
Osteomyelitis

Meningitis
Intracranial or subarachnoid haemorrhage
Stroke
Myelopathy
Radiculopathy
Malodorous perspiration
Myocarditis
Endocarditis
Splenic abscesses or calcification
Hepatitis
Epididymo-orchitis

 11.40 Treatment of brucellosis

Adults with non-localised disease

- Doxycycline 100 mg twice daily orally for 6 weeks *plus* gentamicin 5 mg/kg IV once daily for 7 days
  or
- Doxycycline 100 mg twice daily *plus* rifampicin 600–900 mg orally once daily for 6 weeks

Bone disease

- Doxycycline 100 mg twice daily *plus* rifampicin 600–900 mg once daily orally for 6 weeks *plus* gentamicin 5 mg/kg IV once daily for 7 days
  or
- Ciprofloxacin 750 mg twice daily orally *plus* rifampicin 600–900 mg orally once daily for 3 months

Neurobrucellosis

- Doxycycline 100 mg twice daily *plus* rifampicin 600–900 mg orally once daily for 6 weeks *plus* ceftriaxone 2vg IV twice daily until the cerebrospinal fluid is clear (though susceptibility should be confirmed because sensitivity to third-generation cephalosporins varies among strains)

Endocarditis

- Almost always needs surgical intervention
  plus
- Doxycycline 100 mg twice daily, rifampicin 600–900 mg orally once daily and co-trimoxazole 5 mg/kg of trimethoprim component for 6 months *plus* gentamicin 5 mg/kg IV once daily for 2–4 weeks

Pregnancy

- Rifampicin 600–900 mg orally once daily and co-trimoxazole 5 mg/kg of trimethoprim component for 4 weeks, but caution in last week of pregnancy due to displacement of bilirubin from albumin by drugs and risk of kernicterus to the fetus

---

Borrelia infections

Borrelia are flagellated spirochaetal bacteria that infect humans after bites from ticks or lice. They cause a variety of human infections worldwide (Box 11.41).

Lyme disease

Lyme disease (named after the town of Old Lyme in Connecticut, USA) is caused by *B. burgdorferi*, which occurs in the USA, Europe, Russia, China, Japan and Australia. In Europe, two additional genospecies are also encountered, *B. afzelii* and *B. garinii*. The reservoir of infection is ixodid (hard) ticks that feed on a variety of large mammals, particularly deer. Birds may spread ticks over a wide area. The organism is transmitted to humans via the bite of infected ticks; larval, nymphal and adult forms are all capable of spreading infection.

Ehrlichiosis is a common co-infection with Lyme disease. Two forms occur: *Anaplasma phagocytophilum*, human granulocytic anaplasmosis (HGA); and *Ehrlichia chaffeensis*, human monocytic ehrlichiosis (HME).

Clinical features

There are three stages of disease. Progression may be arrested at any stage.

- *Early localised disease.* The characteristic feature is a skin reaction around the site of the tick bite, known as erythema migrans (Fig. 11.21). Initially, a red 'bull's eye' macule or papule appears 2–30 days after the bite. It then enlarges peripherally with central clearing and may persist for months. Atypical forms are common. The lesion is not pathognomonic of Lyme disease since similar lesions can occur after tick bites. Acute manifestations, such as fever, headache and regional lymphadenopathy, may develop with or without the rash.

11

Fig. 11.21 Rash of erythema migrans in Lyme disease with metastatic secondary lesions. *Courtesy of Dr Ravi Gowda, Royal Hallamshire Hospital, Sheffield.*

- *Early disseminated disease.* Dissemination occurs via the blood stream and lymphatics. There may be a systemic reaction with malaise, arthralgia and, occasionally, metastatic areas of erythema migrans (Fig. 11.21). Neurological involvement may follow weeks or months after infection. Common features include lymphocytic meningitis, cranial nerve palsies (especially unilateral or bilateral facial nerve palsy) and peripheral neuropathy. Radiculopathy, often painful, may present a year or more after initial infection. Carditis, sometimes accompanied by atrioventricular conduction defects, occurs in the USA but is rare in Europe.

- *Late disease.* Late manifestations include arthritis, polyneuritis and encephalopathy. Prolonged arthritis, particularly affecting large joints, and brain parenchymal involvement, causing neuropsychiatric abnormalities, may occur but are rare in the UK. Acrodermatitis chronica atrophicans is an uncommon late complication seen more frequently in Europe than North America. Doughy, patchy discoloration occurs on the peripheries, eventually leading to shiny atrophic skin. The lesions are easily mistaken for those of peripheral vascular disease. In patients coming from an endemic area or having risk factors, who have facial nerve palsy, Lyme disease should be considered.

Diagnosis

The diagnosis of early Lyme borreliosis is often clinical. Culture from biopsy material is not generally available, has a low yield and may take longer than 6 weeks. Antibody detection is frequently negative early in the course of the disease but sensitivity increases to 90–100% in disseminated or late disease. Immunofluorescence or ELISA can give false-positive reactions in a number of conditions, including other spirochaetal infections, infectious mononucleosis, rheumatoid arthritis and systemic lupus erythematosus (SLE). Immunoblot (Western blot) techniques are more specific and, although technically demanding, should be used to confirm the diagnosis. Microorganism DNA detection by PCR has been applied to blood, urine, CSF and biopsies of skin and synovium.

Management

Recent evidence suggests that asymptomatic patients with positive antibody tests should not be treated. However, erythema migrans always requires therapy because organisms may persist and cause progressive disease, even if the skin lesions resolve. Standard therapy consists of a 14-day course of doxycycline (200 mg daily) or amoxicillin (500 mg 3 times daily). Some 15% of patients with early disease will develop a mild Jarisch–Herxheimer reaction (JHR) during the first 24 hours of therapy (p. 339). In pregnant women and small children with penicillin allergy, or in those allergic to amoxicillin and doxycycline, 14-day treatment with cefuroxime axetil (500 mg twice daily) or erythromycin (250 mg 4 times daily) may be used.

Disseminated disease and arthritis require therapy for a minimum of 28 days. Arthritis may respond poorly and prolonged or repeated courses may be necessary. Neuroborreliosis is treated with parenteral β-lactam antibiotics for 3–4 weeks; third-generation cephalosporins such as ceftriaxone are the preferred therapy.

Prevention

Protective clothing and insect repellents should be used in tick-infested areas. Since the risk of borrelial transmission is lower in the first few hours of a blood feed, prompt removal of ticks is advisable. Unfortunately, larval and nymphal ticks are tiny and may not be noticed. Where risk of transmission is high, a single 200 mg dose of doxycycline, given within 72 hours of exposure, has been shown to prevent erythema migrans.

Louse-borne relapsing fever

The human body louse, *Pediculus humanus*, causes itching. Borreliae (*B. recurrentis*) are liberated from infected lice when they are crushed during scratching, which also inoculates the borreliae into the skin. The disease occurs worldwide, with epidemic relapsing fever most often seen in Central/East Africa and South America.

The borreliae multiply in the blood, where they are abundant in the febrile phases, and invade most tissues, especially the liver, spleen and meninges.

Clinical features

Onset is sudden with fever. The temperature rises to 39.5–40.5°C, accompanied by a tachycardia, headache, generalised aching, injected conjunctivae (Fig. 11.22) and herpes labialis. Thrombocytopenia is associated with a petechial rash and epistaxis. As the disease progresses tender hepatosplenomegaly, accompanied by jaundice and elevated transaminases, is common. There may be severe serosal and intestinal haemorrhage, delirium and meningism. The fever ends in crisis between the fourth and tenth days, often associated with profuse sweating, hypotension and circulatory and cardiac failure. There may be no further fever but, in a proportion of patients, after an afebrile period of about 7 days, there are one or more relapses, which are usually milder and less prolonged. In the absence of specific treatment, the mortality rate is up to 40%, especially among the elderly and malnourished.

Investigations and management

Dark ground microscopy of a wet film or Wright–Giemsa stained thick and thin films demonstrate the organism in blood from a febrile patient.

Treatment aims to eradicate the organism and prevent relapses, while minimising the severe JHR that inevitably follows successful chemotherapy. The safest treatment is procaine penicillin 300 mg IM, followed the next day by 0.5 g tetracycline. Tetracycline alone is effective and prevents relapse, but may give rise to a worse reaction. Doxycycline 200 mg once orally in place of tetracycline has the advantage of also being curative for typhus, which often accompanies epidemics of relapsing fever. JHR is best managed in a high-dependency unit with expert nursing and medical care.

The patient, clothing and all contacts must be freed from lice, as in epidemic typhus.

Fig. 11.22 Louse-borne relapsing fever. Injected conjunctivae.

Tick-borne relapsing fever

Soft ticks (*Ornithodoros* spp.) transmit *B. duttonii* (and other *Borrelia* species) through saliva while feeding on their host. People sleeping in mud houses are at risk, as the tick hides in crevices during the day and feeds on humans during the night. Rodents are the reservoir in all parts of the world except East Africa, where humans are the reservoir. Clinical manifestations are similar to those seen with the louse-borne disease but microorganisms are detected in fewer patients on dark field microscopy. A 7-day course (due to a higher relapse rate than in louse-borne relapsing fever) of treatment with either tetracycline (500 mg 4 times daily) or erythromycin (500 mg 4 times daily) is needed.

Leptospirosis

Microbiology and epidemiology

Leptospirosis is one of the most common zoonotic diseases, favoured by a tropical climate and flooding during the monsoon but occurring worldwide. Leptospires are tightly coiled, thread-like organisms about 5–7 μm in length, which are actively motile; each end is bent into a hook. *Leptospira interrogans* is pathogenic for humans. The genus can be separated into more than 200 serovars (subtypes) belonging to 23 serogroups.

Leptospirosis appears to be ubiquitous in wildlife and in many domestic animals. The organisms persist indefinitely in the convoluted tubules of the kidney and are shed into the urine in massive numbers, but infection is asymptomatic in the host. The most frequent hosts are rodents, especially the common rat (*Rattus norvegicus*). Particular leptospiral serogroups are associated with characteristic animal hosts; for example, *L. ictero-haemorrhagiae* is the classical parasite of rats and *L. canicola* of dogs. There is nevertheless considerable overlap in host–serogroup associations.

Leptospires can enter their human hosts through intact skin or mucous membranes but entry is facilitated by cuts and abrasions. Prolonged immersion in contaminated water will also favour invasion, as the spirochaete can survive in water for months. Leptospirosis is common in the tropics and also in freshwater sports enthusiasts.

Clinical features

After a relatively brief bacteraemia, invading organisms are distributed throughout the body, mainly in kidneys, liver, meninges and brain. The incubation period averages 1–2 weeks. Four main clinical syndromes can be discerned and clinical features can involve multiple different organ systems (Fig. 11.23).

Bacteraemic leptospirosis

Bacteraemia with any serogroup can produce a non-specific illness with high fever, weakness, muscle pain and tenderness (especially of the calf and back), intense headache and photophobia, and sometimes diarrhoea and vomiting. Conjunctival congestion is the only notable physical sign. The illness comes to an end after about 1 week, or else merges into one of the other forms of infection.

Aseptic meningitis

Classically associated with *L. canicola* infection, this illness is very difficult to distinguish from viral meningitis. The conjunctivae may be congested but there are no other differentiating signs. Laboratory clues include a neutrophil leucocytosis, abnormal LFTs, and the occasional presence of albumin and casts in the urine.

11

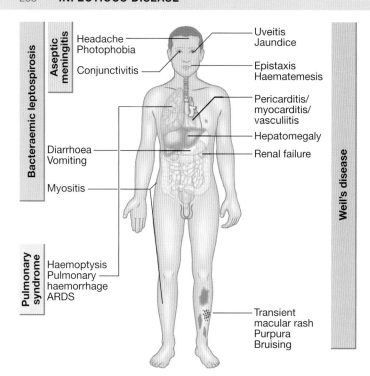

Fig. 11.23 Clinical syndromes of leptospirosis.
(ARDS = acute respiratory distress syndrome)

Icteric leptospirosis (Weil's disease)

Fewer than 10% of symptomatic infections result in severe icteric illness. Weil's disease is a dramatic life-threatening event, characterised by fever, haemorrhages, jaundice and acute kidney injury. Conjunctival hyperaemia is a frequent feature. The patient may have a transient macular erythematous rash but the characteristic skin changes are purpura and large areas of bruising. In severe cases there may be epistaxis, haematemesis and melaena, or bleeding into the pleural, pericardial or subarachnoid spaces. Thrombocytopenia, probably related to activation of endothelial cells with platelet adhesion and aggregation, is present in 50% of cases. Jaundice is deep and the liver is enlarged but there is usually little evidence of hepatic failure or encephalopathy. Acute kidney injury, primarily caused by impaired renal perfusion and acute tubular necrosis, manifests as oliguria or anuria, with the presence of albumin, blood and casts in the urine.

Weil's disease may also be associated with myocarditis, encephalitis and aseptic meningitis. Uveitis and iritis may appear months after apparent clinical recovery.

Pulmonary syndrome

This syndrome has long been recognised in the Far East and has been described during an outbreak of leptospirosis in Nicaragua. It is characterised by haemoptysis, patchy lung infiltrates on chest X-ray, and respiratory failure. Total bilateral lung consolidation and ARDS (p. 324) with multi-organ dysfunction may develop, with a high mortality (over 50%).

Diagnosis

A polymorphonuclear leucocytosis is accompanied in severe infection by thrombocytopenia and elevated blood levels of creatine kinase. In jaundiced patients, there is hepatitis and the prothrombin time may be prolonged. The CSF in leptospiral meningitis shows a variable cellular response, a moderately elevated protein level and normal glucose content. Acute kidney injury due to interstitial nephritis is common.

In the tropics, dengue, malaria, typhoid fever, scrub typhus and hantavirus infection are important differential diagnoses.

Definitive diagnosis of leptospirosis depends on isolation of the organism, serological tests or detection of specific DNA. In general, however, it is probably under-diagnosed.

- Blood cultures are most likely to be positive if taken before the 10th day of illness. Special media are required and cultures may have to be incubated for several weeks.
- Leptospires appear in the urine during the second week of illness, and in untreated patients may be recovered on culture for several months.
- Serological tests are diagnostic if seroconversion or a fourfold increase in titre is demonstrated. The microscopic agglutination test (MAT) is the investigation of choice and can become positive by the end of the first week. IgM ELISA and immunofluorescent techniques are easier to perform, however, while rapid immunochromatographic tests are specific but of only moderate sensitivity in the first week of illness.
- Detection of leptospiral DNA by PCR is possible in blood in early symptomatic disease, and in urine from the eighth day of illness and for many months thereafter.

Management and prevention

The general care of the patient is critically important. Blood transfusion for haemorrhage and careful attention to renal function, the usual cause of death, are especially important. Acute kidney injury is potentially reversible with adequate support, such as dialysis. Most infections are self-limiting. Therapy with either oral doxycycline (100 mg twice daily for 1 week) or intravenous penicillin (900 mg 4 times daily for 1 week) is effective but may not prevent the development of renal failure. Parenteral ceftriaxone (1 g daily) is as effective as penicillin. JHR may occur but is usually mild. Uveitis is treated with a combination of systemic antibiotics and local glucocorticoids. There is no role for the routine use of glucocorticoids in the management of leptospirosis.

Trials in military personnel have shown that infection with *L. interrogans* can be prevented by taking prophylactic doxycycline 200 mg weekly.

Plague

Plague is caused by *Yersinia pestis*, a small Gram-negative bacillus that is spread between rodents by their fleas. If domestic rats become infected, infected fleas may bite humans. Hunters and trappers can contract plague from handling rodents. In the late stages of human plague, *Y. pestis* may be expectorated and spread between humans by droplets, causing 'pneumonic plague'.

Epidemics of plague, such as the 'Black Death', have occurred since ancient times. It is often said that the first sign of plague is the appearance of dead rats. Plague foci are widely distributed throughout the world, including the USA; human cases are reported from about 10 countries per year (Fig. 11.24).

Y. pestis is a potential bioweapon because of the possibility of person-to-person spread and the high fatality rate associated with pneumonic plague.

Clinical features

Organisms inoculated through the skin are transported rapidly to the draining lymph nodes, where they elicit a severe inflammatory response that may be haemorrhagic. If the infection is not contained, sepsis ensues and necrotic, purulent or haemorrhagic lesions develop in many organs. Oliguria and shock follow, and disseminated intravascular coagulation may result in widespread haemorrhage. Inhalation of *Y. pestis* causes alveolitis. The incubation period is 3–6 days but shorter in pneumonic plague.

Bubonic plague

In this, the most common form of the disease, onset is usually sudden, with a rigor, high fever, dry skin and severe headache. Soon, aching and swelling at the site of the affected lymph nodes begin. The groin is the most common site of this 'bubo', made up of the swollen lymph nodes and surrounding tissue. Some infections are relatively mild but, in the majority of patients, toxaemia quickly increases, with a rapid pulse, hypotension and delirium. The spleen is usually palpable.

Septicaemic plague

Those not exhibiting a bubo usually deteriorate rapidly and have a high mortality. The elderly are more prone to this form of illness.

■ Frequent transmission   ▢ Infrequent or suspected transmission

Fig. 11.24 Foci of the transmission of plague. *Reproduced by permission of the World Health Organisation.*

The patient is toxic and may have gastrointestinal symptoms, such as nausea, vomiting, abdominal pain and diarrhoea. DIC may occur, manifested by bleeding from various orifices or puncture sites, along with ecchymoses. Hypotension, shock, renal failure and ARDS may lead to further deterioration. Meningitis, pneumonia and expectoration of blood-stained sputum containing *Y. pestis* may complicate septicaemic, or occasionally bubonic, plague.

Pneumonic plague

Following primary infection in the lung, the onset of disease is very sudden, with cough and dyspnoea. The patient soon expectorates copious blood-stained, frothy, highly infective sputum, becomes cyanosed and dies. Chest radiology reveals bilateral infiltrates, which may be nodular and progress to an ARDS-like picture.

Investigations

The organism may be cultured from blood, sputum and bubo aspirates. For rapid diagnosis, Gram, Giemsa and Wayson's stains (the latter containing methylene blue) are applied to smears from these sites. *Y. pestis* is seen as bipolar staining coccobacilli, sometimes referred to as having a 'safety pin' appearance. Smears are also subjected to antigen detection by immunofluorescence, using *Y. pestis* F1 antigen-specific antibodies. The diagnosis may be confirmed by seroconversion or a single high titre (>128) of anti-F1 antibodies in serum. DNA detection by PCR is under evaluation.

Plague is a notifiable disease under international health regulations (p. 114).

Management

If the diagnosis is suspected on clinical and epidemiological grounds, treatment must be started as soon as, or even before, samples have been collected for laboratory diagnosis. Streptomycin (1 g twice daily) or gentamicin (1 mg/kg 3 times daily) is the drug of choice. Tetracycline (500 mg 4 times daily) and chloramphenicol (12.5 mg/kg 4 times daily) are alternatives. Fluoroquinolones (ciprofloxacin and levofloxacin) may be as effective but there is less clinical experience. Treatment may also be needed for acute circulatory failure, DIC and hypoxia.

Prevention and infection control

Rats and fleas should be controlled. In endemic areas, people should avoid handling and skinning wild animals. The patient should be isolated for the first 48 hours or until clinical improvement begins. Attendants must wear gowns, masks and gloves. Exposed symptomatic or asymptomatic people who have been in close contact with a patient with pneumonic plague should receive post-exposure antibiotic prophylaxis (doxycycline 100 mg or ciprofloxacin 500 mg twice daily) for 7 days.

A recombinant subunit vaccine (protein antigens F1 + V) is in development.

Listeriosis

Listeria monocytogenes is an environmental Gram-positive bacillus that can contaminate food. Outbreaks have been associated with raw vegetables, soft cheeses, under-cooked chicken, fish, meat and pâtés. The bacterium demonstrates 'cold enrichment', outgrowing other contaminating bacteria during refrigeration. Although food-borne outbreaks of gastroenteritis have been reported in immunocompetent individuals, *Listeria* causes more significant invasive infection, especially in pregnant women, older adults (over 55 years) and the immunocompromised.

11

In pregnancy, in addition to systemic symptoms of fever and myalgia, listeriosis causes chorioamnionitis, fetal deaths, abortions and neonatal infection. In other susceptible individuals, it causes systemic illness due to bacteraemia without focal symptoms. Meningitis, similar to other bacterial meningitis but with normal CSF glucose, is the next most common presentation; CSF usually shows increased neutrophils but occasionally only the mononuclear cells are increased (see Box 25.6, p. 1078).

Investigations and management

Diagnosis is made by blood and CSF culture. The organism grows readily in culture media.

The most effective regimen consists of a combination of intravenous amoxicillin or ampicillin plus an aminoglycoside. A sulfamethoxazole/trimethoprim combination can be used in those with penicillin allergy. Cephalosporins are of no use in this infection, as the organism is inherently resistant, an important consideration when treating meningitis empirically.

Proper treatment of foods before eating is the key to preventing listeriosis. Pregnant women are advised to avoid high-risk products, including soft cheeses.

Typhoid and paratyphoid (enteric) fevers

Typhoid and paratyphoid fevers, which are transmitted by the faecal–oral route, are important causes of fever in the Indian subcontinent, sub-Saharan Africa and Latin America. Elsewhere, they are relatively rare. Enteric fevers are caused by infection with *Salmonella* Typhi and *Salmonella* Paratyphi A and B. After a few days of bacteraemia, the bacilli localise, mainly in the lymphoid tissue of the small intestine, resulting in typical lesions in the Peyer's patches and follicles. These swell at first, then ulcerate and usually heal. After clinical recovery, about 5% of patients become chronic carriers (i.e. continue to excrete the bacteria after 1 year); the bacilli may live in the gallbladder for months or years and pass intermittently in the stool and, less commonly, in the urine.

Clinical features

Typhoid fever

Clinical features are outlined in Box 11.42. The incubation period is typically about 10–14 days but can be longer, and the onset may be insidious. The temperature rises in a stepladder fashion for 4 or 5 days with malaise, increasing headache, drowsiness and aching in the limbs. Constipation may be caused by swelling of lymphoid tissue around the ileocaecal junction, although in children diarrhoea and vomiting may be prominent early in the illness. The pulse is often slower than would be expected from the height of the temperature, i.e. a relative bradycardia.

At the end of the first week, a rash may appear on the upper abdomen and on the back as sparse, slightly raised, rose-red spots, which fade on pressure. It is usually visible only on white skin. Cough and epistaxis occur. Around the 7th–10th day, the spleen becomes palpable. Constipation is followed by diarrhoea and abdominal distension with tenderness. Bronchitis and delirium may develop. If untreated, by the end of the second week the patient may be profoundly ill.

Paratyphoid fever

The course tends to be shorter and milder than that of typhoid fever and the onset is often more abrupt with acute enteritis. The rash may be more abundant and the intestinal complications less frequent.

Complications

These are given in Box 11.43. Haemorrhage from, or a perforation of, the ulcerated Peyer's patches may occur at the end of the second week or during the third week of the illness. A drop in temperature to normal or subnormal levels may be falsely reassuring in patients with intestinal haemorrhage. Additional complications may involve almost any viscus or system because of the bacteraemia present during the first week. Bone and joint infection is common in children with sickle-cell disease.

Investigations

In the first week, diagnosis may be difficult because, in this invasive stage with bacteraemia, the symptoms are those of a generalised infection without localising features. Typically, there is a leucopenia. Blood culture establishes the diagnosis and multiple cultures increase the yield. Stool cultures are often positive in the second and third weeks. The Widal test detects antibodies to the O and H antigens but is not specific.

Management

Antibiotic therapy must be guided by in vitro sensitivity testing. Chloramphenicol (500 mg 4 times daily), ampicillin (750 mg 4 times daily) and co-trimoxazole (2 tablets or IV equivalent twice daily) are losing their effect due to resistance in many areas of the world, especially India and South-east Asia. Fluoroquinolones are the drugs of choice (e.g. ciprofloxacin 500 mg twice daily), if nalidixic acid screening predicts susceptibility, but resistance is common, especially in the Indian subcontinent and also in the UK. Extended-spectrum cephalosporins (ceftriaxone and cefotaxime) are useful alternatives but have a slightly increased

---

i	11.42 Clinical features of typhoid fever	
First week		
• Fever	• Constipation	
• Headache	• Diarrhoea and vomiting in	
• Myalgia	children	
• Relative bradycardia		
End of first week		
• Rose spots on trunk	• Abdominal distension	
• Splenomegaly	• Diarrhoea	
• Cough		
End of second week		
• Delirium, complications, then coma and death (if untreated)		

---

i	11.43 Complications of typhoid fever	
Bowel		
• Perforation	• Haemorrhage	
Septic foci		
• Bone and joint infection	• Cholecystitis	
• Meningitis		
Toxic phenomena		
• Myocarditis	• Nephritis	
Chronic carriage		
• Persistent gallbladder carriage		

treatment failure rate. Azithromycin (500 mg once daily) is an alternative when fluoroquinolone resistance is present but has not been validated in severe disease. Treatment should be continued for 14 days. Pyrexia may persist for up to 5 days after the start of specific therapy. Even with effective chemotherapy, there is still a danger of complications, recrudescence of the disease and the development of a carrier state.

Chronic carriers were formerly treated for 4 weeks with ciprofloxacin but may require an alternative agent and duration, as guided by antimicrobial sensitivity testing. Cholecystectomy may be necessary.

Prevention

Improved sanitation and living conditions reduce the incidence of typhoid. Travellers to countries where enteric infections are endemic should be inoculated with one of the three available typhoid vaccines (two inactivated injectable and one oral live attenuated).

Tularaemia

Tularaemia is primarily a zoonotic disease of the northern hemisphere. It is caused by a highly infectious Gram-negative bacillus, *Francisella tularensis*. *F. tularensis* is passed transovarially (ensuring transmission from parent to progeny) in ticks, which allows persistence in nature without the absolute requirement for an infected animal reservoir. It is a potential weapon for bioterrorism. Wild rabbits, rodents and domestic dogs or cats are potential reservoirs, and ticks, mosquitoes or other biting flies are the vectors.

Infection is introduced either through an arthropod or animal bite or via contact with infected animals, soil or water through skin abrasions. The most common 'ulceroglandular' variety of the disease (70–80%) is characterised by skin ulceration with regional lymphadenopathy. There is also a purely 'glandular' form. Alternatively, inhalation of the infected aerosols may result in pulmonary tularaemia, presenting as pneumonia. Rarely, the portal of entry of infection may be the conjunctiva, leading to a nodular, ulcerated conjunctivitis with regional lymphadenopathy (an 'oculoglandular' form). Typhoidal tularaemia is a rare and serious form of tularaemia with vomiting, diarrhoea and hepatosplenomegaly, which may be complicated by pneumonia and meningitis.

Investigations and management

Demonstration of a single high titre (≥1:160) or a fourfold rise in 2–3 weeks in the tularaemia tube agglutination test confirms the diagnosis. Bacterial yield from the lesions is extremely poor. DNA detection methods to enable rapid diagnosis are in development.

Treatment consists of a 10–21-day course of parenteral aminoglycosides, streptomycin (7.5–10 mg/kg twice daily) or gentamicin (1.7 mg/kg 3 times daily), with doxycycline or ciprofloxacin offered as alternatives.

Melioidosis

Melioidosis is caused by *Burkholderia pseudomallei*, a saprophyte found in soil and water (rice paddy fields). Infection is by inoculation or inhalation, leading to bacteraemia, which is followed by the formation of abscesses in the lungs, liver and spleen. Patients with diabetes, renal stones, thalassaemia or severe burns are particularly susceptible. The disease is most common in South-east Asia and northern Australia, and carries a significant mortality. Disease may present years or decades after the initial exposure.

Clinical features

Pneumonia is the most common feature but localised skin nodules and abscesses, or sepsis, especially in diabetics, may occur. Diarrhoea and hepatosplenomegaly may be observed. The chest X-ray can resemble cavitatory tuberculosis. In chronic forms, multiple abscesses occur in subcutaneous tissue, liver, spleen and bone, accompanied by profound weight loss.

Investigations and management

Culture of blood, sputum or pus on selective media, e.g. Ashdown agar, may yield *B. pseudomallei*. Latex agglutination has been developed as a rapid diagnostic test in Thailand and PCR-based tests are also available. Indirect haemagglutination testing can be helpful in travellers; however, most people in endemic areas are seropositive.

In the acute illness, prompt initiation of empirical therapy is life-saving. Ceftazidime 100 mg/kg (2 g 3 times daily) or meropenem (0.5–1 g 3 times daily) is given for 2–3 weeks, followed by maintenance therapy of co-trimoxazole (sulfamethoxazole 1600 mg plus trimethoprim 320 mg twice daily) or doxycycline 200 mg daily for 3–6 months. Abscesses should be drained surgically.

Actinomycete infections

Nocardiosis

Nocardiosis is an uncommon infection caused by aerobic Actinomycetes of the genus *Nocardia*, which are found in the soil. Infection occurs most frequently by direct traumatic inoculation or occasionally via inhalation or ingestion. Nocardiosis can result in localised cutaneous ulcers or nodules, most often in the lower limbs. Chronic destructive infection in tropical countries can result in actinomycetoma, involving soft tissues with occasional penetration to the bone. Actinomycetoma may also be caused by other aerobic Actinomycetes, and a similar clinical syndrome, eumycetoma, is caused by filamentous fungi. Both conditions are discussed on page 301. Systemic *Nocardia* infection, most commonly in immunocompromised individuals, results in suppurative disease with lung and brain abscesses.

On microscopy, *Nocardia* spp. appear as long, filamentous, branching Gram-positive rods, which are also weakly acid-fast. They are easily grown in culture but require prolonged incubation.

Treatment of systemic infection is guided by sensitivity testing and typically requires combinations of imipenem with ceftriaxone, amikacin or co-trimoxazole, often for 6–12 months or longer. Meropenem, tigecycline, linezolid and minocycline may also be used with severe disease or with allergy, or when intolerance prevents use of the preferred agents. Abscesses are drained surgically when this is feasible. Localised cutaneous infection is usually treated with a single agent for 1–3 months. Treatment of actinomycetoma is discussed on page 301.

Actinomyces *spp.*

Actinomyces are anaerobic Actinomycetes, which are predominantly commensals of the oral cavity. They are capable of causing deep, suppurating infection in the head and neck (cervicofacial actinomycosis) and the lungs (thoracic actinomycosis). They also cause suppurating disease in the pelvis, associated with intrauterine contraceptive devices (IUCDs). Modern diagnostic techniques demonstrate that actinomycosis is caused by many different *Actinomyces* species, the most common of which is *Actinomyces israelii*. Treatment of established disease requires prolonged (about 6–12 months) of penicillin or doxycycline. Early disease may respond to shorter antibiotic courses.

Gastrointestinal bacterial infections

The approach to patients presenting with acute gastroenteritis is described on page 227.

Staphylococcal food poisoning

Staph. aureus is transmitted via the hands of food handlers to foodstuffs such as dairy products, including cheese, and cooked meats. Inappropriate storage of these foods allows growth of the organism and production of one or more heat-stable enterotoxins that cause the symptoms.

Nausea and profuse vomiting develop within 1–6 hours. Diarrhoea may not be marked. The toxins that cause the syndrome act as 'super-antigens' and induce a significant neutrophil leucocytosis that may be clinically misleading. Most cases settle rapidly but severe dehydration can occasionally be life-threatening.

Antiemetics and appropriate fluid replacement are the mainstays of treatment. Suspect food should be cultured for staphylococci and demonstration of toxin production. The public health authorities should be notified if food vending is involved.

Bacillus cereus food poisoning

Ingestion of the pre-formed heat-stable exotoxins of *B. cereus* causes rapid onset of vomiting and some diarrhoea within hours of food consumption, which resolves within 24 hours. Fried rice and freshly made sauces are frequent sources; the organism grows and produces enterotoxin during storage (Fig. 11.25). If viable bacteria are ingested and toxin formation takes place within the gut lumen, then the incubation period is longer (12–24 hours) and watery diarrhoea and cramps are the predominant symptoms. The disease is self-limiting but can be quite severe.

Rapid and judicious fluid replacement and appropriate notification of the public health authorities are all that is required.

Clostridium perfringens food poisoning

Spores of *C. perfringens* are widespread in the guts of large animals and in soil. If contaminated meat products are incompletely cooked and stored in anaerobic conditions, *C. perfringens* spores germinate and viable organisms multiply. Subsequent reheating of the food causes release of enterotoxin. Symptoms (diarrhoea and cramps) occur some 6–12 hours following ingestion. The illness is usually self-limiting.

Clostridial enterotoxins are potent and most people who ingest them will be symptomatic. 'Point source' outbreaks, in which a number of cases all become symptomatic following ingestion, classically occur after school or canteen lunches where meat stews are served.

Clostridial necrotising enteritis (CNE) or pigbel is an often-fatal type of food poisoning caused by a β-toxin of *C. perfringens*, type C. The toxin is normally inactivated by certain proteases or by normal cooking. Pigbel is more likely in protein malnutrition or in the presence of trypsin inhibitors, either in foods such as sweet potatoes or during infection with *Ascaris* sp. roundworms.

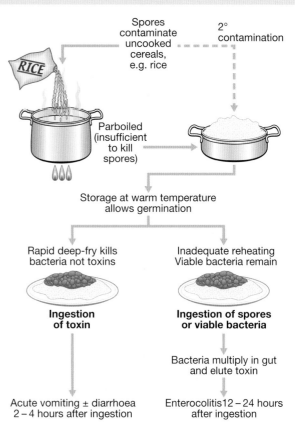

Fig. 11.25 *Bacillus cereus* food poisoning.

Campylobacter jejuni infection

This infection is essentially a zoonosis, although contaminated water may be implicated, as the organism can survive for many weeks in fresh water. The most common sources of the infection are chicken, beef and contaminated milk products. Pet puppies have also been sources. *Campylobacter* infection is now the most common cause of bacterial gastroenteritis in the UK, accounting for some 100 000 cases per annum, most of which are sporadic.

The incubation period is 2–5 days. Colicky abdominal pain may be severe and mimic acute appendicitis or other surgical pathology. Nausea, vomiting and significant diarrhoea, frequently containing blood, are common features. The majority of *Campylobacter* infections affect fit young adults and are self-limiting after 5–7 days. About 10–20% will have prolonged symptomatology, occasionally meriting treatment with a macrolide, most often azithromycin, as many organisms are resistant to ciprofloxacin.

Approximately 1% of cases will develop bacteraemia and possible distant foci of infection. *Campylobacter* spp. have been linked to Guillain–Barré syndrome and post-infectious reactive arthritis (pp. 1140 and 1031).

Salmonella spp. infection

Salmonella enterica serovars other than *Salmonella* Typhi and Paratyphi (p. 260), of which there are more than 2000, can cause gastroenteritis. They are widely distributed throughout the animal kingdom. Two serovars are most important worldwide: *Salmonella* Enteritidis phage type 4 and *Salmonella* Typhimurium dt.104. The latter may be resistant to commonly used antibiotics such as ciprofloxacin. Some strains have a clear relationship to particular animal species, e.g. *Salmonella* Arizonae and pet reptiles. Transmission is by contaminated water or food, particularly poultry, egg products and minced beef, direct person-to-person spread or the handling of exotic pets such as salamanders, lizards or turtles. The incidence of *Salmonella* enteritis is falling in the UK due to an aggressive culling policy in broiler chicken stocks, coupled with vaccination.

The incubation period of *Salmonella* gastroenteritis is 12–72 hours and the predominant feature is diarrhoea, sometimes with passage of blood. Vomiting may be present at the outset. Approximately 5% of cases are bacteraemic and invasive non-typhoidal salmonellosis is a leading cause of bacteraemia in sub-Saharan Africa. Reactive (post-infective) arthritis occurs in approximately 2%.

Antibiotics are not indicated for uncomplicated *Salmonella* gastroenteritis but are prescribed for bacteraemia. Salmonellae are notorious for persistent infection and can seed endothelial surfaces such as an atherosclerotic aorta. Mortality, as with other forms of gastroenteritis, is higher in the elderly (see Box 11.12, p. 228).

Escherichia coli infection

Many serotypes of *E. coli* constitute part of the human gut microbiome. Clinical disease requires either colonisation with a new or previously unrecognised strain, or the acquisition by current colonising bacteria of a particular pathogenicity factor for mucosal attachment or toxin production. Travel to unfamiliar areas of the world allows contact with different strains of endemic *E. coli* and the development of travellers' diarrhoea. Enteropathogenic strains may be found in the gut of healthy individuals and, if these people move to a new environment, close contacts may develop symptoms.

At least five different clinico-pathological patterns of diarrhoea are associated with specific strains of *E. coli* with characteristic virulence factors.

Enterotoxigenic *E. coli*

Enterotoxigenic *E. coli* (ETEC) is the most common cause of travellers' diarrhoea, although there are other causes (see Box 11.20, p. 232). The organisms produce either a heat-labile or a heat-stable enterotoxin, causing marked secretory diarrhoea and vomiting after 1–2 days' incubation. The illness is usually mild and self-limiting after 3–4 days. Antibiotics are of questionable value (p. 232).

Entero-invasive *E. coli*

Illness caused by entero-invasive *E. coli* (EIEC) is very similar to *Shigella* dysentery (p. 265) and is caused by invasion and destruction of colonic mucosal cells. No enterotoxin is produced. Acute watery diarrhoea, abdominal cramps and some scanty blood-staining of the stool are common. The symptoms are rarely severe and are usually self-limiting.

Enteropathogenic *E. coli*

Enteropathogenic *E. coli* (EPEC) organisms are very important in infant diarrhoea. They are able to attach to the gut mucosa, inducing a specific 'attachment and effacement' lesion and causing destruction of microvilli and disruption of normal absorptive capacity. The symptoms vary from mild non-bloody diarrhoea to quite severe illness, but without bacteraemia.

Entero-aggregative *E. coli*

Entero-aggregative *E. coli* (EAEC) strains adhere to the mucosa but also produce a locally active enterotoxin and demonstrate a particular 'stacked brick' aggregation to tissue culture cells when viewed by microscopy. They have been associated with prolonged diarrhoea in children in South America, South-east Asia and India.

Enterohaemorrhagic *E. coli*

A number of distinct 'O' serotypes of *E. coli* possess both the genes necessary for adherence (see 'EPEC' above) and plasmids encoding two distinct enterotoxins (verotoxins), which are identical to the toxins produced by *Shigella* ('shiga toxins 1 and 2'). *E. coli* O157:H7 is perhaps the best known of these verotoxin-producing *E. coli* (VTEC) but others, including types O126 and O11, are also implicated. In 2011, an outbreak of food-borne illness linked to fenugreek seeds occurred in Germany and was due to *E. coli* O104:H4, an EAEC strain that had acquired genes encoding shiga toxin 2a. Although the incidence of enterohaemorrhagic *E. coli* (EHEC) is considerably lower than that of *Campylobacter* and *Salmonella* infection, it is increasing in the developing world.

The reservoir of infection is in the gut of herbivores. The organism has an extremely low infecting dose (10–100 organisms). Runoff water from pasture lands where cattle have grazed, which is used to irrigate vegetable crops, as well as contaminated milk, meat products (especially hamburgers that have been incompletely cooked), lettuce, radish shoots and apple juice have all been implicated as sources (Fig. 11.26).

The incubation period is between 1 and 7 days. Initial watery diarrhoea becomes uniformly blood-stained in 70% of cases and

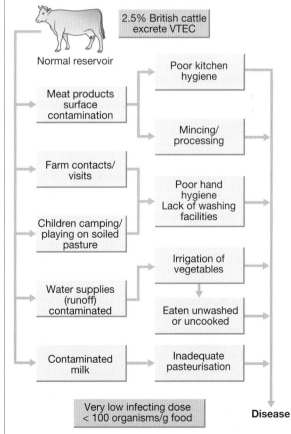

Fig. 11.26 Verocytotoxigenic *Escherichia coli* (VTEC) infections.

is associated with severe abdominal pain. There is little systemic upset, vomiting or fever.

Enterotoxins have both a local effect on the bowel and a distant effect on particular body tissues, such as glomerular apparatus, heart and brain. The potentially life-threatening haemolytic uraemic syndrome (HUS, p. 408) occurs in 10–15% of sufferers from this infection, arising 5–7 days after the onset of symptoms. It is most likely at the extremes of age, is heralded by a high peripheral leucocyte count, and may be induced, particularly in children, by antibiotic therapy.

HUS is treated by dialysis if necessary and may be averted by plasma exchange. Antibiotics should be avoided since they can stimulate toxin release.

Clostridium difficile infection

C. difficile is the most commonly diagnosed cause of antibiotic-associated diarrhoea (p. 230), and is an occasional constituent of the gut microbiome. C. difficile can produce two toxins (A and B). C. difficile infection (CDI) usually follows antimicrobial therapy, which alters the composition of the gastrointestinal flora and may result in colonisation with toxigenic C. difficile, if the patient is exposed to C. difficile spores. The combination of toxin production and the ability to produce environmentally stable spores accounts for the clinical features and transmissibility of CDI. A hypervirulent strain of C. difficile, ribotype 027, has emerged, which produces more toxin and more severe disease than other C. difficile strains.

Clinical features

Disease manifestations range from diarrhoea to life-threatening pseudomembranous colitis. Around 80% of cases occur in people over 65 years of age, many of whom are frail with comorbid diseases. Symptoms usually begin in the first week of antibiotic therapy but can occur at any time up to 6 weeks after treatment has finished. The onset is often insidious, with lower abdominal pain and diarrhoea that may become profuse and watery. The presentation may resemble acute ulcerative colitis with bloody diarrhoea, fever and even toxic dilatation and perforation. Ileus is also seen in pseudomembranous colitis.

Investigations

C. difficile can be isolated from stool culture in 30% of patients with antibiotic-associated diarrhoea and over 90% of those with pseudomembranous colitis, but also from 5% of healthy adults and up to 20% of elderly patients in residential care. The diagnosis of CDI therefore rests on detection of toxins A or B in the stool. Current practice in the UK is to screen stool from patients with a compatible clinical syndrome by detection either of glutamate dehydrogenase (GDH), an enzyme produced by C. difficile, or of C. difficile nucleic acid (e.g. by PCR); if screening is positive, a C. difficile toxin ELISA or a tissue culture cytotoxicity assay is performed.

The rectal appearances at sigmoidoscopy may be characteristic, with erythema, white plaques or an adherent pseudomembrane (Fig. 11.27), or may resemble ulcerative colitis. In some cases, the rectum is spared and abnormalities are observed in the proximal colon. Patients who are ill require abdominal and erect chest X-rays to exclude perforation or toxic dilatation. CT may be useful when the diagnosis is in doubt.

Management

The precipitating antibiotic should be stopped and the patient should be isolated. Supportive therapy includes intravenous

Fig. 11.27 Clostridium difficile infection. Colonoscopic view showing numerous adherent 'pseudomembranes' on the mucosa.

fluids and bowel rest. First-line antimicrobial therapy involves metronidazole (500 mg orally 3 times daily for 10 days) or vancomycin (125 mg orally 4 times daily for 7–10 days). Although vancomycin is more effective than metronidazole against hypervirulent C. difficile strains (e.g. ribotype 027), it is more expensive and may drive the emergence of vancomycin resistance in other organisms (e.g. enterococci, Staph. aureus). For these reasons, some authorities reserve its use for relapse (15–30% of patients), failure of initial response or severe infection. Fidaxomicin is associated with a lower relapse rate than vancomycin but is more expensive. Intravenous immunoglobulin and/or glucocorticoids are sometimes given in the most severe or refractory cases, and faecal transplantation from a healthy donor is increasingly used to manage relapses by restoring a more advantageous gut microbiome profile. Surgical intervention needs to be considered early in severe cases.

Yersinia enterocolitica infection

Yersinia enterocolitica, commonly found in pork, causes mild to moderate gastroenteritis and can produce significant mesenteric adenitis after an incubation period of 3–7 days. It predominantly causes disease in children but adults may also be affected. The illness resolves slowly. Complications include reactive arthritis (p. 1031; 10–13% of cases), which may be persistent, and anterior uveitis.

Cholera

Cholera, caused by Vibrio cholerae serotype O1, is the archetypal toxin-mediated bacterial cause of acute watery diarrhoea. The enterotoxin activates adenylate cyclase in the intestinal epithelium, inducing net secretion of chloride and water. V. cholerae O1 has two biotypes, classical and El Tor, and each of these has two distinct serotypes, Inaba and Ogawa. Following its origin in the Ganges valley, devastating epidemics have occurred, often in association with large religious festivals, and pandemics have spread worldwide. The seventh pandemic, due to the El Tor biotype, began in 1961 and spread via the Middle East to become endemic in Africa, subsequently spreading throughout South and Central America. Numbers of cases of cholera have been increasing, with outbreaks in Ghana in 2014 and Tanzania in 2015. El Tor is more resistant to commonly used antimicrobials than classical Vibrio, and causes prolonged carriage in 5% of infections. An atypical serotype, O139, has been responsible for localised outbreaks in Bangladesh.

Infection spreads via the stools or vomit of symptomatic patients or of the much larger number of subclinical cases. Organisms survive for up to 2 weeks in fresh water and 8 weeks in salt water. Transmission is normally through infected drinking water, shellfish and food contaminated by flies, or on the hands of carriers.

Clinical features

Severe diarrhoea without pain or colic begins suddenly and is followed by vomiting. Following the evacuation of normal gut faecal contents, typical 'rice water' material is passed, consisting of clear fluid with flecks of mucus. Classical cholera produces enormous loss of fluid and electrolytes, leading to intense dehydration with muscular cramps. Shock and oliguria develop but mental clarity remains. Death from acute circulatory failure may occur rapidly unless fluid and electrolytes are replaced. Improvement is rapid with proper treatment.

The majority of infections, however, cause mild illness with slight diarrhoea. Occasionally, a very intense illness, 'cholera sicca', occurs, with loss of fluid into dilated bowel, killing the patient before typical gastrointestinal symptoms appear. The disease is more dangerous in children.

Diagnosis and management

Clinical diagnosis is easy during an epidemic. Otherwise, the diagnosis should be confirmed bacteriologically. Stool dark-field microscopy shows the typical 'shooting star' motility of *V. cholerae*. Rectal swab or stool cultures allow identification. Cholera is notifiable under international health regulations.

Maintenance of circulation by replacement of water and electrolytes is paramount (p. 229). Ringer-Lactate is the best fluid for intravenous replacement. Vomiting usually stops once the patient is rehydrated, and fluid should then be given orally up to 500 mL hourly. Early intervention with oral rehydration solutions that include resistant starch, based on either rice or cereal, shortens the duration of diarrhoea and improves prognosis. Severe dehydration, as indicated by altered consciousness, skin tenting, very dry tongue, decreased pulses, low blood pressure or minimal urine output, mandates intravenous replacement. Total fluid requirements may exceed 50 L over a period of 2–5 days. Accurate records are greatly facilitated by the use of a 'cholera cot', which has a reinforced hole under the patient's buttocks, beneath which a graded bucket is placed.

Three days' treatment with tetracycline 250 mg 4 times daily, a single dose of doxycycline 300 mg or ciprofloxacin 1 g in adults reduces the duration of excretion of *V. cholerae* and the total volume of fluid needed for replacement.

Prevention

Strict personal hygiene is vital and drinking water should come from a clean piped supply or be boiled. Flies must be denied access to food. Oral vaccines containing killed *V. cholerae* with or without the B subunit of cholera toxin are used in specific settings.

In epidemics, improvements in sanitation and access to clean water, public education and control of population movement are vital. Mass single-dose vaccination and treatment with tetracycline are valuable. Disinfection of discharges and soiled clothing, and scrupulous hand-washing by medical attendants reduce spread.

▌*Vibrio parahaemolyticus* infection

This marine organism produces a disease similar to enterotoxigenic *E. coli* (see above). It is very common where ingestion of raw seafood is widespread (e.g. Japan). After an incubation period of approximately 20 hours, explosive diarrhoea, abdominal cramps and vomiting occur. Systemic symptoms of headache and fever are frequent but the illness is self-limiting after 4–7 days. Rarely, a severe septic illness arises; in this case, *V. parahaemolyticus* can be isolated using specific halophilic culture.

▌Bacillary dysentery (shigellosis)

Shigellae are Gram-negative rods, closely related to *E. coli*, that invade the colonic mucosa. There are four main groups: *Sh. dysenteriae*, *flexneri*, *boydii* and *sonnei*. In the tropics, bacillary dysentery is usually caused by *Sh. flexneri*, while in the UK most cases are caused by *Sh. sonnei*. Shigellae are often resistant to multiple antibiotics, especially in tropical countries. The organism only infects humans and its spread is facilitated by its low infecting dose of around 10 organisms.

Spread may occur via contaminated food or flies, but person-to-person transmission by unwashed hands after defaecation is the most important factor. Outbreaks occur in psychiatric hospitals, residential schools and other closed institutions, and dysentery is a constant accompaniment of wars and natural catastrophes, which bring crowding and poor sanitation in their wake. *Shigella* infection may spread rapidly among men who have sex with men.

Clinical features

Disease severity varies from mild *Sh. sonnei* infections that may escape detection to more severe *Sh. flexneri* infections, while those due to *Sh. dysenteriae* may be fulminating and cause death within 48 hours.

In a moderately severe illness, the patient complains of diarrhoea, colicky abdominal pain and tenesmus. Stools are small, and after a few evacuations contain blood and purulent exudate with little faecal material. Fever, dehydration and weakness occur, with tenderness over the colon. Reactive arthritis or iritis may occasionally complicate bacillary dysentery (p. 1031).

Management and prevention

Oral rehydration therapy or, if diarrhoea is severe, intravenous replacement of water and electrolyte loss is necessary. Antibiotic therapy is with ciprofloxacin (500 mg twice daily for 3 days) Azithromycin and ceftriaxone are alternatives but resistance occurs to all agents, especially in Asia. The use of antidiarrhoeal medication should be avoided.

The prevention of faecal contamination of food and milk and the isolation of cases may be difficult, except in limited outbreaks. Hand-washing is very important.

Respiratory bacterial infections

Most of these infections are described in Chapter 17.

▌Diphtheria

Infection with *Corynebacterium diphtheriae* occurs most commonly in the upper respiratory tract and is usually spread by droplet infection. Infection may also complicate skin lesions, especially in alcoholics. The organisms remain localised at the site of infection but release of a soluble exotoxin damages the heart muscle and the nervous system.

Diphtheria has been eradicated from many parts of the world by mass vaccination using a modified exotoxin but remains

11

11.44 Clinical features of diphtheria

Acute infection

- Membranous tonsillitis
- *or* Nasal infection
- *or* Laryngeal infection
- *or* Skin/wound/conjunctival infection (rare)

Complications

- Laryngeal obstruction or paralysis
- Myocarditis
- Peripheral neuropathy

important in areas where vaccination has been incomplete, e.g. in Russia and South-east Asia. The disease is notifiable in all countries of Europe and North America, and international guidelines have been issued by the WHO for the management of infection.

Clinical features

The average incubation period is 2–4 days. The disease begins insidiously with a sore throat (Box 11.44). Despite modest fever, there is usually marked tachycardia. The diagnostic feature is the 'wash-leather' elevated, greyish-green membrane on the tonsils. It has a well-defined edge, is firm and adherent, and is surrounded by a zone of inflammation. There may be swelling of the neck ('bull neck') and tender enlargement of the lymph nodes. In the mildest infections, especially where there is a high degree of immunity, a membrane may not appear and inflammation is minimal.

With anterior nasal infection there is nasal discharge, frequently blood-stained. In laryngeal diphtheria, a husky voice and high-pitched cough signal potential respiratory obstruction requiring urgent tracheostomy. If infection spreads to the uvula, fauces and nasopharynx, the patient is gravely ill.

Death from acute circulatory failure may occur within the first 10 days. Late complications arise as a result of toxin action on the heart or nervous system. About 25% of survivors of the early toxaemia may later develop myocarditis with arrhythmias or cardiac failure. These are usually reversible, with no permanent damage other than heart block in survivors.

Neurological involvement occurs in 75% of cases. After tonsillar or pharyngeal diphtheria, it usually starts after 10 days with palatal palsy. Paralysis of accommodation often follows, manifest by difficulty in reading small print. Generalised polyneuritis with weakness and paraesthesia may follow in the next 10–14 days. Recovery from such neuritis is always ultimately complete.

Management

A clinical diagnosis of diphtheria must be notified to the public health authorities and the patient sent urgently to a specialist infectious diseases unit. Empirical treatment should commence after collection of appropriate swabs.

Diphtheria antitoxin is produced from hyperimmune horse serum. It neutralises circulating toxin but has no effect on toxin already fixed to tissues, so it must be injected intramuscularly without awaiting the result of a throat swab. However, reactions to this foreign protein include a potentially lethal immediate anaphylactic reaction (p. 75) and a 'serum sickness' with fever, urticaria and joint pains, which occurs 7–12 days after injection. A careful history of previous horse serum injections or allergic reactions should be taken and a small test injection of serum

should be given half an hour before the full dose in every patient. Adrenaline (epinephrine) solution must be available to deal with any immediate type of reaction (0.5–1.0 mL of 1/1000 solution IM). An antihistamine is also given. In a severely ill patient, the risk of anaphylactic shock is outweighed by the mortal danger of diphtheritic toxaemia. A dose of up to 100 000 IU of antitoxin is injected intravenously if the test dose is tolerated. For disease of moderate severity, 16 000–40 000 IU IM will suffice, and for mild cases 4000–8000 IU.

Penicillin (1200 mg 4 times daily IV) or amoxicillin (500 mg 3 times daily) should be administered for 2 weeks to eliminate *C. diphtheriae*. Patients allergic to penicillin can be given erythromycin. Due to poor immunogenicity of primary infection, all sufferers should be immunised with diphtheria toxoid following recovery.

Patients must be managed in strict isolation and attended by staff with a clearly documented immunisation history until three swabs 24 hours apart are culture-negative.

Prevention

Active immunisation should be given to all children. If diphtheria occurs in a closed community, contacts should be given erythromycin, which is more effective than penicillin in eradicating the organism in carriers.

All contacts should also be immunised or given a booster dose of toxoid. Booster doses are required every 10 years to maintain immunity.

Pneumococcal infection

Strep. pneumoniae (the pneumococcus) is the leading cause of community-acquired pneumonia globally (p. 582) and one of the leading causes of infection-related mortality. Otitis media, meningitis and sinusitis are also frequently caused by *Strep. pneumoniae*. Occasional patients present with bacteraemia without obvious focus. Asplenic individuals are at risk of fulminant pneumococcal disease with purpuric rash.

Increasing rates of penicillin resistance have been reported around the world for *Strep. pneumoniae*, although they remain low in the UK. Strains with cephalosporin resistance causing meningitis require treatment with a combination of cephalosporins, glycopeptides and rifampicin. Macrolide resistance is also increasing. Newer quinolones are also used (e.g. levofloxacin) but rates of resistance are rising.

Vaccination of infants with the protein conjugate pneumococcal vaccine decreases *Strep. pneumoniae* infection in infants and in their relatives. The polysaccharide pneumococcal vaccine is used in individuals predisposed to *Strep. pneumoniae* infection and the elderly, but only modestly reduces pneumococcal bacteraemia and does not prevent pneumonia. All asplenic individuals should receive vaccination against *Strep. pneumoniae*.

Anthrax

Anthrax is an endemic zoonosis in many countries; it causes human disease following inoculation of the spores of *Bacillus anthracis*. *B. anthracis* was the first bacterial pathogen described by Koch and the model pathogen for 'Koch's postulates' (see Box 6.1, p. 100). It is a Gram-positive organism with a central spore. The spores can survive for years in soil. Infection is commonly acquired from contact with animals, particularly herbivores. The ease of production of *B. anthracis* spores makes this infection a candidate for biological warfare or bioterrorism. *B. anthracis* produces a number of toxins that mediate the clinical features of disease.

Clinical features

These depend on the route of entry of the anthrax spores.

Cutaneous anthrax

This skin lesion is associated with occupational exposure to anthrax spores during processing of hides and bone products. It accounts for the vast majority of clinical cases. Animal infection is a serious problem in Africa, India, Pakistan and the Middle East.

Spores are inoculated into exposed skin. A single lesion develops as an irritable papule on an oedematous haemorrhagic base. This progresses to a depressed black eschar. Despite extensive oedema, pain is infrequent.

Gastrointestinal anthrax

This is associated with the ingestion of contaminated meat. The caecum becomes infected, which produces nausea, vomiting, anorexia and fever, followed in 2–3 days by severe abdominal pain and bloody diarrhoea. Toxaemia and death can develop rapidly thereafter.

Inhalational anthrax

This form of the disease is extremely rare but has been associated with bioterrorism. Without rapid and aggressive therapy at the onset of symptoms, the mortality is 50–90%. Fever, dyspnoea, cough, headache and sepsis develop 3–14 days following exposure. Typically, the chest X-ray shows only widening of the mediastinum and pleural effusions, which are haemorrhagic. Meningitis may occur.

Management

B. anthracis can be cultured from skin swabs from lesions. Skin lesions are readily curable with early antibiotic therapy. Treatment is with ciprofloxacin (500 mg twice daily) until penicillin susceptibility is confirmed; the regimen can then be changed to benzylpenicillin with doses up to 2.4 g IV given 6 times daily or phenoxymethylpenicillin 500–1000 mg 4 times daily administered for 10 days. The addition of an aminoglycoside may improve the outlook in severe disease. In view of concerns about concomitant inhalational exposure, particularly in the era of bioterrorism, a further 2-month course of ciprofloxacin 500 mg twice daily or doxycycline 100 mg twice daily orally is added to eradicate inhaled spores. Inhalational anthrax is treated with ciprofloxacin and clindamycin for at least 14 days, followed by therapy to eradicate spores. Monoclonal antibodies against *B. anthracis* protective antigen can be added for systemic infection. Prophylaxis with ciprofloxacin (500 mg twice daily for 2 months) is recommended for anyone at high risk of inhalational exposure to anthrax spores and should be combined with three doses of anthrax vaccine adsorbed (AVA).

Bacterial infections with neurological involvement

Infections affecting the CNS, including bacterial meningitis, botulism and tetanus, are described on page 1117.

Mycobacterial infections

Tuberculosis

Tuberculosis is predominantly, although by no means exclusively, a respiratory disease and is described on page 588.

Leprosy

Leprosy (Hansen's disease) is a chronic granulomatous disease affecting skin and nerves and caused by *Mycobacterium leprae*, a slow-growing mycobacterium that cannot be cultured in vitro. The clinical manifestations are determined by the degree of the patient's cell-mediated immunity (CMI; p. 69) towards *M. leprae* (Fig. 11.28). High levels of CMI with elimination of leprosy bacilli produces tuberculoid leprosy, whereas absent CMI results in lepromatous leprosy. Complications arise due to nerve damage, immunological reactions and bacillary infiltration. People with leprosy are frequently stigmatised and using the word 'leper' is inappropriate.

Epidemiology and transmission

Some 4 million people have leprosy and around 750 000 new cases are detected annually. About 70% of the world's leprosy patients live in India, with the disease endemic in Brazil, Indonesia, Mozambique, Madagascar, Tanzania and Nepal.

Untreated lepromatous patients discharge bacilli from the nose. Infection occurs through the nose, followed by haematogenous spread to skin and nerve. The incubation period is 2–5 years for tuberculoid cases and 8–12 years for lepromatous cases. Leprosy incidence peaks at 10–14 years, and is more common in males and in household contacts of leprosy cases.

Pathogenesis

M. leprae has tropism for Schwann cells and skin macrophages. In tuberculoid leprosy, effective CMI controls bacillary multiplication ('paucibacillary') and organised epithelioid granulomata form. In lepromatous leprosy, there is abundant bacillary multiplication ('multibacillary'), e.g. in Schwann cells and perineurium. Between these two extremes is a continuum, varying from patients with

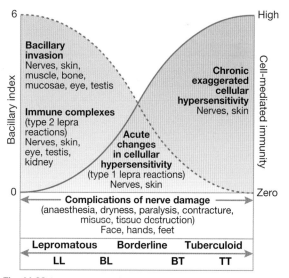

Fig. 11.28 Leprosy: mechanisms of damage and tissue affected. Mechanisms under the broken line are characteristic of disease near the lepromatous end of the spectrum, and those under the solid line are characteristic of the tuberculoid end. They overlap in the centre where, in addition, instability predisposes to type 1 lepra reactions. At the peak in the centre, neither bacillary growth nor cell-mediated immunity has the upper hand. (BL = borderline lepromatous; BT = borderline tuberculoid) *Adapted from Bryceson ADM, Pfaltzgraff RE. Leprosy, 3rd edn. Churchill Livingstone, Elsevier Ltd; 1990.*

moderate CMI (borderline tuberculoid) to patients with little cellular response (borderline lepromatous).

Immunological reactions evolve as the immune response develops and the bacillary antigenic stimulus varies, particularly in borderline patients. Delayed hypersensitivity reactions produce type 1 (reversal) reactions, while immune complexes contribute to type 2 (erythema nodosum leprosum) reactions.

HIV/leprosy co-infected patients have typical lepromatous and tuberculoid leprosy skin lesions and typical leprosy histology and granuloma formation. Surprisingly, even with low circulating CD4 counts, tuberculoid leprosy may be observed and there is not an obvious shift to lepromatous leprosy.

Clinical features

Box 11.45 gives the cardinal features of leprosy. Types of leprosy are compared in Box 11.46.

- *Skin.* The most common skin lesions are macules or plaques. Tuberculoid patients have few, hypopigmented lesions (Fig. 11.29A). In lepromatous leprosy, papules, nodules or diffuse infiltration of the skin occur. The earliest lesions are ill defined; gradually, the skin becomes infiltrated and thickened. Facial skin thickening leads to the characteristic leonine facies (Fig. 11.29B).

11.45 Cardinal features of leprosy

- Skin lesions, typically anaesthetic at tuberculoid end of spectrum
- Thickened peripheral nerves
- Acid-fast bacilli on skin smears or biopsy

11.46 Clinical characteristics of the polar forms of leprosy

Clinical and tissue-specific features	Lepromatous	Tuberculoid
Skin and nerves Number and distribution	Widely disseminated	One or a few sites, asymmetrical
Skin lesions Definition:		
Clarity of margin	Poor	Good
Elevation of margin	Never	Common
Colour:		
Dark skin	Slight hypopigmentation	Marked hypopigmentation
Light skin	Slight erythema	Coppery or red
Surface	Smooth, shiny	Dry, scaly
Central healing	None	Common
Sweat and hair growth	Impaired late	Impaired early
Loss of sensation	Late	Early and marked
Nerve enlargement and damage	Late	Early and marked
Bacilli (bacterial index)	Many (5 or 6+)	Absent (0)
Natural history	Progressive	Self-healing
Other tissues	Upper respiratory mucosa, eye, testes, bones, muscle	None
Reactions	Immune complexes (type 2)	Cell-mediated (type 1)

- *Anaesthesia.* In skin lesions, the small dermal sensory and autonomic nerve fibres are damaged, causing localised sensory loss and loss of sweating. Anaesthesia can occur in the distribution of a damaged large peripheral nerve. A 'glove and stocking' sensory neuropathy is also common in lepromatous leprosy.
- *Nerve damage.* Peripheral nerve trunks are affected at 'sites of predilection'. These are the ulnar (elbow), median (wrist), radial (humerus), radial cutaneous (wrist), common peroneal (knee), posterior tibial and sural nerves (ankle), facial nerve (zygomatic arch) and great auricular nerve (posterior triangle of the neck). Damage to peripheral nerve trunks produces characteristic signs with regional sensory loss and muscle dysfunction (Fig. 11.29C). All these nerves should be examined for enlargement and tenderness, and tested for motor and sensory function. The CNS is not affected.
- *Eye involvement.* Blindness is a devastating complication for a patient with anaesthetic hands and feet. Eyelid closure is impaired when the facial nerve is affected. Damage to the trigeminal nerve causes anaesthesia of the cornea and conjunctiva. The cornea is then susceptible to trauma and ulceration.
- *Other features.* Many organs can be affected. Nasal collapse occurs secondary to bacillary destruction of the nasal cartilage and bone. Diffuse infiltration of the testes causes testicular atrophy and the acute orchitis that occurs with type 2 reactions. This results in azoospermia and hypogonadism.

Leprosy reactions

Leprosy reactions (Box 11.47) are events superimposed on the cardinal features shown in Box 11.45.

- *Type 1 (reversal) reactions.* These occur in 30% of borderline patients (BT, BB or BL – see below) and are delayed hypersensitivity reactions. Skin lesions become

---

11.47 Reactions in leprosy

	Lepra reaction type 1 (reversal)	Lepra reaction type 2 (erythema nodosum leprosum)
Mechanism	Cell-mediated hypersensitivity	Immune complexes
Clinical features	Painful tender nerves, loss of function Swollen skin lesions New skin lesions	Tender papules and nodules; may ulcerate Painful tender nerves, loss of function Iritis, orchitis, myositis, lymphadenitis Fever, oedema
Management	Prednisolone 40 mg, reducing over 3–6 months[1]	Moderate: prednisolone 40 mg daily Severe: thalidomide[2] or prednisolone 40–80 mg daily, reducing over 1–6 months; local if eye involved[3]

[1]Indicated for any new impairment of nerve or eye function. [2]Contraindicated in women who may become pregnant. [3]1% hydrocortisone drops or ointment and 1% atropine drops.

Fig. 11.29 Clinical features of leprosy.
A Tuberculoid leprosy. Single lesion with a well-defined active edge and anaesthesia within the lesion. B Lepromatous leprosy. Widespread nodules and infiltration, with loss of the eyebrows. This man also has early collapse of the nose. C Borderline tuberculoid leprosy with severe nerve damage. This boy has several well-defined, hypopigmented, macular, anaesthetic lesions. He has severe nerve damage affecting both ulnar and median nerves bilaterally and has sustained severe burns to his hands. D Reversal (type 1) reactions. Erythematous, oedematous lesions.

11

erythematous (Fig. 11.29D). Peripheral nerves become tender and painful, with sudden loss of nerve function. These reactions may occur spontaneously, after starting treatment and also after completion of multidrug therapy (MDT).

- *Type 2 (erythema nodosum leprosum, ENL) reactions.* These are partly due to immune complex deposition and occur in BL and LL patients who produce antibodies and have a high antigen load. They manifest with malaise, fever and crops of small pink nodules on the face and limbs. Iritis and episcleritis are common. Other signs are acute neuritis, lymphadenitis, orchitis, bone pain, dactylitis, arthritis and proteinuria. ENL may continue intermittently for several years.

Borderline cases

In borderline tuberculoid (BT) cases, skin lesions are more numerous than in tuberculoid (TT) cases, and there is more severe nerve damage and a risk of type 1 reactions. In borderline leprosy (BB) cases, skin lesions are numerous and vary in size, shape and distribution; annular lesions are characteristic and nerve damage is variable. In borderline lepromatous (BL) cases, there are widespread small macules in the skin and widespread nerve involvement; both type 1 and type 2 reactions occur.

Pure neural leprosy (i.e. without skin lesions) occurs principally in India and accounts for 10% of patients. There is asymmetrical involvement of peripheral nerve trunks and no visible skin lesions. On nerve biopsy, all types of leprosy have been found.

Investigations

The diagnosis is clinical, made by finding a cardinal sign of leprosy and supported by detecting acid-fast bacilli in slit-skin smears or typical histology in a skin biopsy. Slit-skin smears

---

i | **11.48 Principles of leprosy treatment**

- Stop the infection with chemotherapy
- Treat reactions
- Educate the patient about leprosy
- Prevent disability
- Support the patient socially and psychologically

---

are obtained by scraping dermal material on to a glass slide. The smears are then stained for acid-fast bacilli, the number counted per high-power field and a score derived on a logarithmic scale (0–6): the bacterial index (BI). Smears are useful for confirming the diagnosis and monitoring response to treatment. Neither serology nor PCR is sensitive or specific enough for diagnosis.

Management

The principles of treatment are outlined in Box 11.48. All leprosy patients require MDT with an approved first-line regimen (Box 11.49).

Rifampicin is a potent bactericidal for *M. leprae* but should always be given in combination with other antileprotics, since a single-step mutation can confer resistance. Dapsone is bacteriostatic. It commonly causes mild haemolysis and rarely anaemia. Clofazimine is a red, fat-soluble crystalline dye, weakly bactericidal for *M. leprae*. Skin discoloration (red to purple–black) and ichthyosis are troublesome side-effects, particularly on pale skins. New bactericidal drugs against *M. leprae* have been identified, notably fluoroquinolones (pefloxacin and ofloxacin). Minocycline and clarithromycin may also be used. These agents are now established second-line drugs. Minocycline causes a grey pigmentation of skin lesions.

i	11.49 Modified WHO-recommended multidrug therapy (MDT) regimens in leprosy			
Type of leprosy[1]	Monthly supervised treatment	Daily self-administered treatment	Duration of treatment[2]
Paucibacillary	Rifampicin 600 mg	Dapsone 100 mg	6 months
Multibacillary	Rifampicin 600 mg Clofazimine 300 mg	Clofazimine 50 mg Dapsone 100 mg	12 months
Paucibacillary single-lesion	Ofloxacin 400 mg Rifampicin 600 mg Minocycline 100 mg		Single dose

[1]Classification uses the bacillary index (BI) in slit-skin smears or, if BI is not available, the number of skin lesions:
- paucibacillary single-lesion leprosy (1 skin lesion)
- paucibacillary (2–5 skin lesions)
- multibacillary (>5 skin lesions).

[2]Studies from India have shown that multibacillary patients with an initial BI of >4 need longer treatment, for at least 24 months.

Although single-dose treatment is less effective than the conventional 6-month treatment for paucibacillary leprosy, it is an operationally attractive field regimen recommended by the WHO.

Lepra reactions are treated as shown in Box 11.47. Chloroquine can also be used.

Patient education

This is essential and should patients should be informed that, after 3 days of chemotherapy, they are not infectious and can lead a normal social life. It should emphasise that gross deformities are not inevitable.

Patients with anaesthetic hands or feet need to avoid and treat burns or other minor injuries. Good footwear is important. Physiotherapy helps maintain range of movement of affected muscles and neighbouring joints.

Prognosis

Untreated, tuberculoid leprosy has a good prognosis; it may self-heal and peripheral nerve damage is limited. Lepromatous leprosy (LL) is a progressive condition with high morbidity if untreated.

After treatment, the majority of patients, especially those who have no nerve damage at the time of diagnosis, do well, with resolution of skin lesions. Borderline patients are at risk of developing type 1 reactions, which may result in devastating nerve damage.

Prevention and control

The previous strategy of centralised leprosy control campaigns has been superseded by integrated programmes, with primary health-care workers in many countries now responsible for case detection and provision of MDT. It is not yet clear how successful this will be, especially in the time-consuming area of disability prevention.

BCG vaccination has been shown to give good but variable protection against leprosy; adding killed M. leprae to BCG does not enhance protection.

Rickettsial and related intracellular bacterial infections

Rickettsial fevers

The rickettsial fevers are the most common tick-borne infections. It is important to ask potentially infected patients about contact with ticks, lice or fleas. There are two main groups of rickettsial fevers: spotted fevers and typhus (Box 11.50).

Pathogenesis

The rickettsiae are intracellular Gram-negative organisms that parasitise the intestinal canal of arthropods. Infection of humans through the skin occurs from the excreta of arthropods, but the saliva of some biting vectors is infected. The organisms multiply in capillary endothelial cells, producing lesions in the skin, CNS, heart, lungs, liver, kidneys and skeletal muscles. Endothelial proliferation, associated with a perivascular reaction, may cause thrombosis and purpura. In epidemic typhus, the brain is the target organ; in scrub typhus, the cardiovascular system and lungs in particular are attacked. An eschar, a black necrotic crusted sore, is often found in tick- and mite-borne typhus (see Fig. 11.7C, p. 235). This is due to vasculitis following immunological recognition of the inoculated organism. Regional lymph nodes often enlarge.

Spotted fever group

Rocky Mountain spotted fever

Rickettsia rickettsii is transmitted by tick bites. It is widely distributed and increasing in western and south-eastern states of the USA and also in Central and South America. The incubation period is about 7 days. The rash appears on about the third or fourth day of illness, looking at first like measles, but in a few hours a typical maculopapular eruption develops. The rash spreads in 24–48 hours from wrists, forearms and ankles to the back, limbs and chest, and then to the abdomen, where it is least pronounced. Larger cutaneous and subcutaneous haemorrhages may appear in severe cases. The liver and spleen become palpable. At the extremes of life, the mortality is 2–12%.

Other spotted fevers

R. conorii (boutonneuse fever) and *R. africae* (African tick bite fever) cause Mediterranean and African tick typhus, which also occurs on the Indian subcontinent. The incubation period is approximately 7 days. Infected ticks may be picked up by walking on grasslands, or dogs may bring ticks into the house. Careful examination might reveal a diagnostic eschar, and the maculopapular rash on the trunk, limbs, palms and soles. There may be delirium and meningeal signs in severe infections but recovery is usual. *R. africae* can be associated with multiple eschars. Some cases, particularly those with *R. africae*, present without rash ('spotless spotted fever'). Other spotted fevers are shown in Box 11.50.

Typhus group

Scrub typhus fever

Scrub typhus is caused by *Orientia tsutsugamushi* (formerly *Rickettsia tsutsugamushi*), transmitted by mites. It occurs in the Far East, Myanmar, Pakistan, Bangladesh, India, Indonesia, the South Pacific islands and Queensland, particularly where patches of forest cleared for plantations have attracted rats and mites.

In many patients, one eschar or more develops, surrounded by an area of cellulitis (see Fig. 11.7C, p. 235) and

i 11.50 Features of rickettsial infections

Disease	Organism	Reservoir	Vector	Geographical area	Rash	Gangrene	Target organs	Mortality
Spotted fever group								
Rocky Mountain spotted fever	*R. rickettsii*	Rodents, dogs, ticks	*Ixodes* tick	North, Central and South America	Morbilliform Haemorrhagic	Often	Bronchi, myocardium, brain, skin	2–12%[2]
Boutonneuse fever	*R. conorii*	Rodents, dogs, ticks	*Ixodes* tick	Mediterranean, Africa, South-west Asia, India	Maculopapular	–	Skin, meninges	2.5%[3]
Siberian tick typhus	*R. sibirica*	Rodents, birds, domestic animals, ticks	Various ticks	Siberia, Mongolia, northern China	Maculopapular	–	Skin, meninges	Rare[3]
Australian tick typhus	*R. australis*	Rodents, ticks	Ticks	Australia	Maculopapular	–	Skin, meninges	Rare[3]
Oriental spotted fever	*R. japonica*	Rodents, dogs, ticks	Ticks	Japan	Maculopapular	–	Skin, meninges	Rare[3]
African tick bite fever[1]	*R. africae*	Cattle, game, ticks	*Ixodes* tick	South Africa	Can be spotless	–	Skin, meninges	Rare[3]
Typhus group								
Scrub typhus	*Orientia tsutsugamushi*	Rodents	*Trombicula* mite	South-east Asia	Maculopapular	Unusual	Bronchi, myocardium, brain, skin	Rare[3]
Epidemic typhus	*R. prowazekii*	Humans	Louse	Worldwide	Morbilliform Haemorrhagic	Often	Brain, skin, bronchi, myocardium	Up to 40%
Endemic typhus	*R. typhi*	Rats	Flea	Worldwide	Slight	–	–	Rare[3]

[1]Eschar at bite site and local lymphadenopathy. [2]Highest in adult males. [3]Except in infants, older people and the debilitated.

enlargement of regional lymph nodes. The incubation period is about 9 days.

Mild or subclinical cases are common. The onset of symptoms is usually sudden, with headache (often retro-orbital), fever, malaise, weakness and cough. In severe illness, the general symptoms increase, with apathy and prostration. An erythematous maculopapular rash often appears on about the 5th–7th day and spreads to the trunk, face and limbs, including the palms and soles, with generalised painless lymphadenopathy. The rash fades by the 14th day. The temperature rises rapidly and continues as a remittent fever (i.e. the difference between maximum and minimum temperature exceeds 1°C), remaining above normal with sweating until it falls on the 12th–18th day. In severe infection, the patient is prostrate with cough, pneumonia, delirium and deafness. Cardiac failure, renal failure and haemorrhage may develop. Convalescence is often slow and tachycardia may persist for some weeks.

Epidemic (louse-borne) typhus

Epidemic typhus is caused by *R. prowazekii* and is transmitted by infected faeces of the human body louse, usually through scratching the skin. Patients suffering from epidemic typhus infect lice, which leave when the patient is febrile. In conditions of overcrowding, the disease spreads rapidly. It is prevalent in parts of Africa, especially Ethiopia and Rwanda, and in the South American Andes and Afghanistan. Large epidemics have occurred in Europe, usually as a sequel to war. The incubation period is usually 12–14 days.

There may be a few days of malaise but the onset is more often sudden, with rigors, fever, frontal headaches, pains in the back and limbs, constipation and bronchitis. The face is flushed and cyanotic, the eyes are congested and the patient becomes confused. The rash appears on the 4th–6th day. In its early stages, it disappears on pressure but soon becomes petechial with subcutaneous mottling. It appears first on the anterior folds of the axillae, sides of the abdomen or backs of hands, then on the trunk and forearms. The neck and face are seldom affected. During the second week, symptoms increase in severity. Sores develop on the lips. The tongue becomes dry, brown, shrunken and tremulous. The spleen is palpable, the pulse feeble and the patient stuporous and delirious. The temperature falls rapidly at the end of the second week and the patient recovers gradually. In fatal cases, the patient usually dies in the second week from toxaemia, cardiac or renal failure, or pneumonia.

Endemic (flea-borne) typhus

Flea-borne or 'endemic' typhus caused by *R. typhi* is endemic worldwide. Humans are infected when the faeces or contents of a crushed flea, which has fed on an infected rat, are introduced into the skin. The incubation period is 8–14 days. The symptoms resemble those of a mild louse-borne typhus. The rash may be scanty and transient.

Investigation of rickettsial infection

Routine blood investigations are not diagnostic. There is usually hepatitis and thrombocytopenia. Diagnosis is made on clinical grounds and response to treatment, and may be confirmed by antibody detection or PCR in specialised laboratories. Differential diagnoses include malaria, which should be excluded, typhoid, meningococcal sepsis and leptospirosis.

Management of rickettsial fevers

The different rickettsial fevers vary in severity but all respond to tetracycline 500 mg 4 times daily, doxycycline 200 mg daily or chloramphenicol 500 mg 4 times daily for 7 days. Louse-borne typhus and scrub typhus can be treated with a single dose of 200 mg doxycycline, repeated for 2–3 days to prevent relapse. Chloramphenicol- and doxycycline-resistant strains of *O. tsutsugamushi* have been reported from Thailand and patients here may need treatment with rifampicin.

Nursing care is important, especially in epidemic typhus. Sedation may be required for delirium and blood transfusion for haemorrhage. Relapsing fever and typhoid are common intercurrent infections in epidemic typhus, and pneumonia in scrub typhus, which require diagnosis and treatment. Convalescence is usually protracted, especially in older people.

To prevent rickettsial infection, lice, fleas, ticks and mites need to be controlled with insecticides.

Q fever

Q fever occurs worldwide and is caused by the rickettsia-like organism *Coxiella burnetii*, an obligate intracellular organism that survives in the extracellular environment. Cattle, sheep and goats are important reservoirs and the organism is transmitted by inhalation of aerosolised particles. An important characteristic of *C. burnetii* is its antigenic variation, called phase variation, due to a change of lipopolysaccharide (LPS). When isolated from animals or humans, *C. burnetii* expresses phase I antigen and is very infectious (a single bacterium is sufficient to infect a human). In culture, there is an antigenic shift to the phase II form, which is not infectious. Measurement of antigenic shift helps differentiate acute and chronic Q fever.

Clinical features

The incubation period is 3–4 weeks. The initial symptoms are non-specific with fever, headache and chills; in 20% of cases, a maculopapular rash occurs. Other presentations include pneumonia and hepatitis. Chronic Q fever may present with osteomyelitis, encephalitis and endocarditis.

Investigations and management

Diagnosis is usually serological and the stage of the infection can be distinguished by isotype tests and phase-specific antigens. Phase I and II IgM titres peak at 4–6 weeks. In chronic infections, IgG titres to phase I and II antigens may be raised.

Prompt treatment of acute Q fever with doxycycline reduces fever duration. Treatment of Q fever endocarditis is problematic, requiring prolonged therapy with doxycycline and rifampicin or ciprofloxacin with hydroxychloroquine; even then, organisms are not always eradicated. Valve surgery is often required (p. 526).

Bartonellosis

This group of diseases is caused by intracellular Gram-negative bacilli closely related to the rickettsiae, which have been discovered to be important causes of 'culture-negative' endocarditis. They are found in many domestic pets, such as cats, although for several the host is undefined (Box 11.51). The principal human pathogens are *Bartonella quintana*, *B. henselae* and *B. bacilliformis*. *Bartonella* infections are associated with the following:

- *Trench fever*. This is a relapsing fever with severe leg pain and is caused by *B. quintana*. The disease is not fatal but is very debilitating.
- *Bacteraemia and endocarditis in the homeless*. Endocarditis due to *B. quintana* or *B. henselae* is associated with severe damage to the heart valves.

i 11.51 Clinical diseases caused by *Bartonella* spp.			
Reservoir	Vector	Organism	Disease
Cats	Flea	*B. henselae*	Cat scratch disease, bacillary angiomatosis, endocarditis
Undefined	Lice	*B. quintana*	Trench fever, bacillary angiomatosis, endocarditis
Undefined	Sandfly	*B. bacilliformis*	Carrion's disease: Oroya fever and verruga peruana
Undefined	Flea	*B. rochalimae*	Fever, rash, anaemia, splenomegaly

- *Cat scratch disease*. *B. henselae* causes this common benign lymphadenopathy in children and young adults. A vesicle or papule develops on the head, neck or arms after a cat scratch. The lesion resolves spontaneously but there may be regional lymphadenopathy that persists for up to 4 months before also resolving spontaneously. Rare complications include retinitis and encephalopathy.
- *Bacillary angiomatosis*. This is an HIV-associated disease caused by *B. quintana* or *B. henselae* (p. 316).
- *Oroya fever and verruga peruana* (*Carrion's disease*). This is endemic in areas of Peru. It is a biphasic disease caused by *B. bacilliformis*, transmitted by sandflies of the genus *Phlebotomus*. Fever, haemolytic anaemia and microvascular thrombosis with end-organ ischaemia are features. It is frequently fatal if untreated.

Investigations and management

Bartonellae can be cultured in specialised laboratories but PCR is often used to diagnose infection. Serum antibody detection is possible but cross-reactions occur with *Chlamydia* and *Coxiella* spp.

Bartonella spp. are typically treated with macrolides or tetracyclines. Antibiotic use is guided by clinical need. Cat scratch disease usually resolves spontaneously but *Bartonella* endocarditis requires valve replacement and combination antibiotic therapy with doxycycline and gentamicin.

Chlamydial infections

These are listed in Box 11.52 and are also described on pages 340 and 582.

i 11.52 Chlamydial infections	
Organism	Disease caused
Chlamydia trachomatis	Trachoma Lymphogranuloma venereum (see Box 13.12, p. 341) Cervicitis, urethritis, proctitis (p. 334)
Chlamydia psittaci	Psittacosis (see Box 17.36, p. 582)
Chlamydophila (Chlamydia) pneumoniae	Atypical pneumonia (see Box 17.36, p. 582) Acute/chronic sinusitis

Trachoma

Trachoma is a chronic keratoconjunctivitis caused by *Chlamydia trachomatis* and is the most common cause of avoidable blindness. The classic trachoma environment is dry and dirty, causing children to have eye and nose discharges. Transmission occurs through flies, on fingers and within families. In endemic areas, the disease is most common in children.

Pathology and clinical features

The onset is usually insidious. Infection may be asymptomatic, lasts for years, may be latent over long periods and may recrudesce. The conjunctiva of the upper lid is first affected with vascularisation and cellular infiltration. Early symptoms include conjunctival irritation and blepharospasm. The early follicles are characteristic (Fig. 11.30) but clinical differentiation from conjunctivitis due to other causes may be difficult. Scarring causes inversion of the lids (entropion) so that the lashes rub against the cornea (trichiasis). The cornea becomes vascularised and opaque. The problem may not be detected until vision begins to fail.

Investigations and management

Intracellular inclusions may be demonstrated in conjunctival scrapings by staining with iodine or immunofluorescence. Although chlamydiae may, in theory, be isolated in chick embryo or cell culture or detected by nucleic acid amplification tests, these methods are rarely available in the areas where trachoma is encountered, and in any case their sensitivity and specificity are poorly established. Diagnosis of trachoma is therefore based on clinical and epidemiological features.

A single dose of azithromycin (20 mg/kg) has been shown to be superior to 6 weeks of tetracycline eye ointment twice daily for individuals in mass treatment programmes. Deformity and scarring of the lids, and corneal opacities, ulceration and scarring require surgical treatment after control of local infection.

Prevention

Personal and family hygiene should be improved. Proper care of the eyes of newborn and young children is essential. Family contacts should be examined. The WHO is promoting the SAFE strategy for trachoma control (surgery, antibiotics, facial cleanliness and environmental improvement).

Fig. 11.30 Trachoma. Trachoma is characterised by hyperaemia and numerous pale follicles. *Courtesy of Institute of Ophthalmology, Moorfields Eye Hospital, London.*

Protozoal infections

Protozoa are responsible for many important infectious diseases. They can be categorised according to whether they cause systemic or local infection. Trichomoniasis is described on page 335.

Systemic protozoal infections

Malaria

Malaria in humans is caused by *Plasmodium falciparum*, *P. vivax*, *P. ovale* (subspecies *curtisi* and *wallikeri*), *P. malariae* and the predominantly simian parasite *P. knowlesi*. It is transmitted by the bite of female anopheline mosquitoes and occurs throughout the tropics and subtropics at altitudes below 1500 metres (Fig. 11.31). The WHO estimates that 214 million cases of clinical malaria occurred in 2015, 88% of these in Africa, especially among children and pregnant women. WHO prevention and treatment campaigns reduced the incidence of malaria between 1950 and 1960, but since 1970 there has been resurgence. Furthermore, *P. falciparum* has now become resistant to chloroquine and sulfadoxine-pyrimethamine, initially in South-east Asia and now throughout Africa. The WHO's Millennium Development Goal malaria target aimed to halt the spread of the disease by 2015 and this has been achieved. The 'Roll Back Malaria' campaign was designed to halve mortality by 2010 by utilising the 'best evidence' vector and disease control methods, such as artemisinin combination therapy (ACT).

Travellers are susceptible to malaria (p. 230). Most cases are due to *P. falciparum*, usually from Africa, and of these 1% die because of late diagnosis. Migrants from endemic countries who spend long periods of time in non-endemic countries are particularly at risk if they visit friends and family in their country of origin. They have lost their partial immunity and frequently do not take malaria prophylaxis. A few people living near airports in Europe have acquired malaria from accidentally imported mosquitoes.

Pathogenesis

Life cycle of the malarial parasite

The female anopheline mosquito becomes infected when it feeds on human blood containing gametocytes, the sexual forms of the malarial parasite (Figs 11.32 and 11.33). Development in the mosquito takes 7–20 days, and results in sporozoites accumulating in the salivary glands and being inoculated into the human blood stream. Sporozoites disappear from human blood within half an hour and enter the liver. After some days, merozoites leave the liver and invade red blood cells, where further asexual cycles of multiplication take place, producing schizonts.

Fig. 11.31 Distribution of malaria. (For up-to-date information see the Malaria Atlas Project (MAP): map.ox.ac.uk.)

Rupture of the schizont releases more merozoites into the blood and causes fever, the periodicity of which depends on the species of parasite.

P. vivax and *P. ovale* may persist in liver cells as dormant forms, hypnozoites, capable of developing into merozoites months or years later. Thus the first attack of clinical malaria may occur long after the patient has left the endemic area, and the disease may relapse after treatment with drugs that only kill the erythrocytic stage of the parasite.

P. falciparum, *P. knowlesi* and *P. malariae* have no persistent exo-erythrocytic phase but recrudescence of fever may result from multiplication of parasites in red cells that have not been eliminated by treatment and immune processes (Box 11.53).

Pathology

Red cells infected with malaria are prone to haemolysis. This is most severe with *P. falciparum*, which invades red cells of all ages but especially young cells; *P. vivax* and *P. ovale* invade reticulocytes, and *P. malariae* normoblasts, so that infections

Fig. 11.32 Scanning electron micrograph of *Plasmodium falciparum* oöcysts lining an anopheline mosquito's stomach.

i	11.53 Relationships between life cycle of parasite and clinical features of malaria		
Cycle/ feature	*Plasmodium vivax*, *P. ovale*	*P. malariae*	*P. falciparum*
Pre-patent period (minimum incubation)	8–25 days	15–30 days	8–25 days
Exo-erythrocytic cycle	Persistent as hypnozoites	Pre-erythrocytic only	Pre-erythrocytic only
Asexual cycle	48 hrs synchronous	72 hrs synchronous	<48 hrs asynchronous
Fever periodicity	Alternate days	Every third day	None
Delayed onset	Common	Rare	Rare
Relapses	Common up to 2 years	Recrudescence many years later	Recrudescence up to 1 year

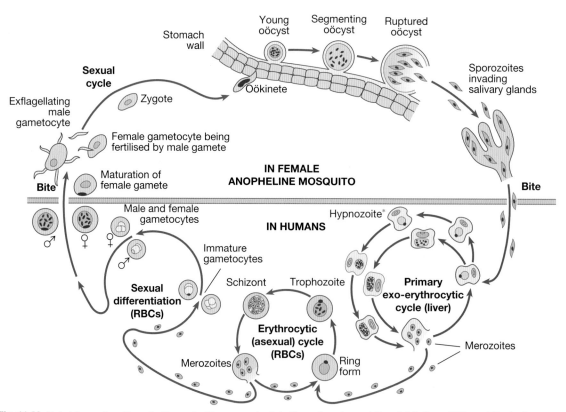

Fig. 11.33 **Malarial parasites: life cycle.** Hypnozoites(*) are present only in *Plasmodium vivax* and *P. ovale* infections. (RBC = red blood cell)

remain lighter. Anaemia may be profound and is worsened by dyserythropoiesis, splenomegaly and depletion of folate stores.

In *P. falciparum* malaria, red cells containing trophozoites adhere to vascular endothelium in post-capillary venules in brain, kidney, liver, lungs and gut by the formation of 'knob' proteins. They also form 'rosettes' and rouleaux with uninfected red cells. Vessel congestion results in organ damage, which is exacerbated by rupture of schizonts, liberating toxic and antigenic substances (Fig. 11.33).

P. falciparum has influenced human evolution, with the appearance of protective mutations such as sickle-cell (HbS; p. 951), thalassaemia (p. 953), glucose-6-phosphate dehydrogenase (G6PD) deficiency (p. 948) and HLA-B53. *P. falciparum* does not grow well in red cells that contain haemoglobin F, C or especially S. Haemoglobin S heterozygotes (AS) are protected against the lethal complications of malaria. *P. vivax* cannot enter red cells that lack the Duffy blood group; therefore many West Africans and African Americans are protected.

Clinical features

The clinical features of malaria are non-specific and the diagnosis must be suspected in anyone returning from an endemic area who has features of infection.

P. falciparum infection

This is the most dangerous of the malarias. The onset is often insidious, with malaise, headache and vomiting. Cough and mild diarrhoea are also common. The fever has no particular pattern. Jaundice is common due to haemolysis and hepatic dysfunction. The liver and spleen enlarge and may become tender. Anaemia develops rapidly, as does thrombocytopenia.

A patient with *falciparum* malaria, apparently not seriously ill, may rapidly develop dangerous complications (Fig. 11.34 and Box 11.54). Cerebral malaria is manifested by delirium, seizures or coma, usually without localising signs. Children die rapidly without any specific symptoms other than fever. Immunity is impaired in pregnancy and the parasite can preferentially bind to the placental protein chondroitin sulphate A. Abortion and intrauterine growth retardation from parasitisation of the maternal side of the placenta are frequent. Previous splenectomy increases the risk of severe malaria.

P. vivax and *P. ovale* infection

In many cases, the illness starts with several days of continued fever before the development of classical bouts of fever on alternate days. Fever starts with a rigor. The patient feels cold and the temperature rises to about 40°C. After half an hour to

11

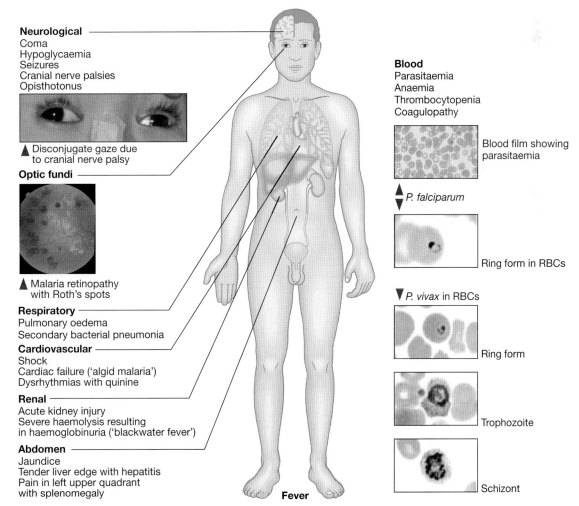

Neurological
Coma
Hypoglycaemia
Seizures
Cranial nerve palsies
Opisthotonus

▲ Disconjugate gaze due to cranial nerve palsy

Optic fundi

▲ Malaria retinopathy with Roth's spots

Respiratory
Pulmonary oedema
Secondary bacterial pneumonia

Cardiovascular
Shock
Cardiac failure ('algid malaria')
Dysrhythmias with quinine

Renal
Acute kidney injury
Severe haemolysis resulting in haemoglobinuria ('blackwater fever')

Abdomen
Jaundice
Tender liver edge with hepatitis
Pain in left upper quadrant with splenomegaly

Blood
Parasitaemia
Anaemia
Thrombocytopenia
Coagulopathy

Blood film showing parasitaemia

▲▼ *P. falciparum*

Ring form in RBCs

▼ *P. vivax* in RBCs

Ring form

Trophozoite

Schizont

Fever

Fig. 11.34 Features of *Plasmodium falciparum* infection. (RBC = red blood cell) *Insets (malaria retinopathy) Courtesy of Dr Nicholas Beare, Royal Liverpool University Hospital; (blood films of* P. vivax *and* P. falciparum) *Courtesy of Dr Kamolrat Silamut, Mahidol Oxford Research Unit, Bangkok, Thailand.*

11.54 Severe manifestations/complications of *falciparum* malaria and their immediate management

Coma (cerebral malaria)

- Maintain airway
- Nurse on side
- Exclude other treatable causes of coma (e.g. hypoglycaemia, bacterial meningitis)
- Avoid harmful ancillary treatments such as glucocorticoids, heparin and adrenaline (epinephrine)
- Intubate if necessary

Hyperpyrexia

- Tepid sponging, fanning, cooling blanket
- Antipyretic drug (paracetamol)

Convulsions

- Maintain airway
- Treat promptly with diazepam or paraldehyde injection

Hypoglycaemia

- Measure blood glucose
- Give 50% dextrose injection followed by 10% dextrose infusion (glucagon may be ineffective)

Severe anaemia (packed cell volume <15%)

- Transfuse fresh whole blood or packed cells if pathogen screening of donor blood is available

Acute pulmonary oedema

- Nurse at 45°, give oxygen, venesect 250 mL of blood, give diuretic, stop intravenous fluids
- Intubate and add PEEP/CPAP (p. 202) in life-threatening hypoxaemia
- Haemofilter

Acute kidney injury

- Exclude pre-renal causes
- Fluid resuscitation if appropriate
- Peritoneal dialysis (haemofiltration or haemodialysis if available)

Spontaneous bleeding and coagulopathy

- Transfuse screened fresh whole blood (cryoprecipitate/fresh frozen plasma and platelets if available)
- Vitamin K injection

Metabolic acidosis

- Exclude or treat hypoglycaemia, hypovolaemia and Gram-negative sepsis
- Fluid resuscitation
- Give oxygen

Shock ('algid malaria')

- Suspect Gram-negative sepsis
- Take blood cultures
- Give parenteral antimicrobials
- Correct haemodynamic disturbances

Aspiration pneumonia

- Give parenteral antimicrobial drugs
- Change position
- Physiotherapy
- Give oxygen

Hyperparasitaemia

- Consider exchange transfusion (e.g. >10% of circulating erythrocytes parasitised in non-immune patient with severe disease)

Specific therapy

- Intravenous artesunate
- Mefloquine should be avoided due to increased risk of post-malaria neurological syndrome

(CPAP = continuous positive airway pressure; PEEP = positive end-expiratory pressure)
From WHO. Severe falciparum malaria. In: Severe and complicated malaria, 3rd edn. Trans Roy Soc Trop Med Hyg 2000; 94 (suppl. 1):S1–41.

---

an hour, the hot or flush phase begins. It lasts several hours and gives way to profuse perspiration and a gradual fall in temperature. The cycle is repeated 48 hours later. Gradually, the spleen and liver enlarge and may become tender. Anaemia develops slowly. Relapses are frequent in the first 2 years after leaving the malarious area and infection may be acquired from blood transfusion.

P. malariae and P. knowlesi infection

This is usually associated with mild symptoms and bouts of fever every third day. Parasitaemia may persist for many years, with the occasional recrudescence of fever or without producing any symptoms. Chronic *P. malariae* infection causes glomerulonephritis and long-term nephrotic syndrome in children. *P. knowlesi* is usually mild but can deteriorate rapidly.

Investigations

Giemsa-stained thick and thin blood films should be examined whenever malaria is suspected. In the thick film, erythrocytes are lysed, releasing all blood stages of the parasite. This, as well as the fact that more blood is used in thick films, facilitates the diagnosis of low-level parasitaemia. A thin film is essential to confirm the diagnosis, species and, in *P. falciparum* infections,

to quantify the parasite load (by counting the percentage of infected erythrocytes). *P. falciparum* parasites may be very scanty, especially in patients who have been partially treated. With *P. falciparum*, only ring forms are normally seen in the early stages (Fig. 11.34); with the other species, all stages of the erythrocytic cycle may be found. Gametocytes appear after about 2 weeks, persist after treatment and are harmless, except that they are the source by which more mosquitoes become infected.

Immunochromatographic rapid diagnostic tests (RDTs) for malaria antigens, such as OptiMAL (which detects the *Plasmodium* LDH of *P. falciparum* and *vivax*) and Parasight-F (which detects the *P. falciparum* histidine-rich protein 2), are extremely sensitive and specific for *falciparum* malaria but less so for other species. They should be used in parallel with blood film examination but are especially useful where the microscopist is less experienced in examining blood films (e.g. in the UK). They are less sensitive for low-level parasitaemia and positivity may persist for a month or more in some individuals. The QBC Malaria Test is a fluorescence microscopy-based malaria diagnostic test that is also widely used.

DNA detection (PCR) is used mainly in research and is useful for determining whether a patient has a recrudescence of the same malaria parasite or a reinfection with a new parasite.

Management

Mild *P. falciparum* malaria

Since *P. falciparum* is now resistant to chloroquine and sulfadoxine-pyrimethamine (Fansidar) almost worldwide, an artemisinin-based treatment is recommended (Box 11.55) and WHO policy in Africa recommends always using ACT, e.g. co-artemether or artesunate–amodiaquine. Unfortunately, artemisinin resistance has now been reported in South-east Asia.

11.55 Malaria treatment

Mild malaria

Preferred therapy
- Co-artemether (CoArtem or Riamet); contains artemether and lumefantrine (4 tablets orally at 0, 8, 24, 36, 48 and 60 hrs)

Alternative therapy
- Quinine (600 mg of quinine salt 3 times daily orally for 5–7 days), together with or followed by doxycycline (200 mg once daily orally for 7 days)
    Use clindamycin not doxycycline if the patient is a pregnant woman or young child
    or
- Atovaquone–proguanil (Malarone, 4 tablets orally once daily for 3 days)

Pregnancy
- Co-artemether but avoid in early pregnancy.
- If not using co-artemether, use quinine plus clindamycin (450 mg 3 times daily orally for 7 days)

Other regimens
- Artesunate (200 mg orally daily for 3 days) and mefloquine (1 g orally on day 2 and 500 mg orally on day 3)

Severe malaria

Preferred therapy
- Artesunate 2.4 mg/kg IV at 0, 12 and 24 hrs and then once daily for 7 days. Once the patient is able to recommence oral intake, switch to 2 mg/kg orally once daily, to complete a total cumulative dose of 17–18 mg/kg

Alternative therapy
- Quinine, loading dose 20 mg/kg IV over 4 hrs, up to a maximum of 1.4 g, then maintenance doses of 10 mg/kg quinine salt given as 4-hr infusions 3 times daily for the first 48 hrs then twice a day, up to a maximum of 700 mg per dose or until the patient can take drugs orally. Combine with doxycycline (or clindamycin if there are contraindications to doxycycline)
- Note the loading dose should not be given if quinine, quinidine or mefloquine has been administered in the previous 24 hrs
- Patients should be monitored by ECG while receiving quinine, with special attention to QRS duration and QT interval

Non-*falciparum* malaria

Preferred therapy
- Chloroquine: 600 mg chloroquine base orally, followed by 300 mg base in 6 hrs, then 150 mg base twice daily for 2 more days plus primaquine (30 mg orally daily (for *P. vivax*) or 15 mg orally daily (for *P. ovale*) for 14 days) after confirming G6PD-negative

Patients with mild to moderate G6PD deficiency and *P. vivax* or *P. ovale*
- Chloroquine plus primaquine 0.75 mg/kg weekly orally for 8 weeks

Chloroquine-resistant *P. vivax*
- Co-artemether as for *P. falciparum*

(G6PD = glucose-6-phosphate dehydrogenase)

Complicated *P. falciparum* malaria

Severe malaria should be considered in any non-immune patient with a parasite count greater than 2% or with complications, and is a medical emergency (see Box 11.54). Management includes early and appropriate antimalarial chemotherapy, active treatment of complications, correction of fluid, electrolyte and acid–base balance, and avoidance of harmful ancillary treatments.

The treatment of choice is intravenous artesunate. Late haemolysis is a treatment side-effect in some patients. Rectal administration of artesunate is also being developed to allow administration in remote rural areas. Quinine salt is the alternative.

Exchange transfusion has not been tested in randomised controlled trials but may be beneficial for non-immune patients with persisting high parasitaemias (>10% circulating erythrocytes).

Non-*falciparum* malaria

P. vivax, *P. ovale*, *P. knowlesi* and *P. malariae* infections should be treated with oral chloroquine but some chloroquine resistance has been reported from Indonesia. 'Radical cure' is achieved in patients with *P. vivax* or *P. ovale* malaria using a course of primaquine, which destroys the hypnozoite phase in the liver. Haemolysis may develop in those who are G6PD-deficient. Cyanosis due to the formation of methaemoglobin in the red cells is more common but not dangerous (see Fig. 7.1, p. 135). All are sensitive to ACTs.

Prevention

Clinical attacks of malaria may be preventable with chemoprophylaxis using chloroquine, atovaquone plus proguanil (Malarone), doxycycline or mefloquine. Box 11.56 gives the recommended doses for protection of the non-immune. The risk of malaria in the area to be visited and the degree of chloroquine resistance guide the recommendations for prophylaxis. Updated recommendations are summarised at fitfortravel.nhs.uk. Fansidar should not be used for chemoprophylaxis, as deaths have occurred from agranulocytosis or Stevens–Johnson syndrome (pp. 1224 and 1254). Mefloquine is useful in areas of multiple drug resistance, such as East and Central Africa and Papua New Guinea. Experience shows it to be safe for at least 2 years but there are several contraindications to its use (Box 11.56).

Expert advice is required for individuals unable to tolerate the first-line agents listed or in whom they are contraindicated. Mefloquine should be started 2–3 weeks before travel to give time for assessment of side-effects. Chloroquine should not be taken continuously as a prophylactic for more than 5 years without regular ophthalmic examination, as it may cause irreversible retinopathy. Pregnant and lactating women may take proguanil or chloroquine safely.

Prevention also involves advice about the use of high-percentage diethyltoluamide (DEET), covering up extremities when out after dark, and sleeping under permethrin-impregnated mosquito nets.

Malaria control in endemic areas

There are major initiatives to reduce and eliminate malaria in endemic areas. Successful programmes combine vector control, including indoor residual spraying, use of long-lasting insecticide-treated bed nets (ITNs) and intermittent preventative therapy (IPT; repeated dose of prophylactic drugs in high-risk groups, such as children and pregnant women, which reduces malaria and anaemia).

Research to produce a fully protective malaria vaccine is ongoing.

Antimalarial tablets	Adult prophylactic dose	Regimen
Chloroquine resistance high		
Mefloquine[2]	250 mg weekly	Started 2–3 weeks before travel and continued until 4 weeks after
or Doxycycline[3,4]	100 mg daily	Started 1 week before and continued until 4 weeks after travel
or Malarone[4]	1 tablet daily	From 1–2 days before travel until 1 week after return
Chloroquine resistance absent		
Chloroquine[5] and proguanil	300 mg base weekly ⎫ 100–200 mg daily ⎭	Started 1 week before and continued until 4 weeks after travel

[1]Choice of regimen is determined by area to be visited, length of stay, level of malaria transmission, level of drug resistance, presence of underlying disease in the traveller and concomitant medication taken. [2]Contraindicated in the first trimester of pregnancy, lactation, cardiac conduction disorders, epilepsy, psychiatric disorders; may cause neuropsychiatric disorders. [3]Causes photosensitisation and sunburn if high-protection sunblock is not used. [4]Avoid in pregnancy. [5]British preparations of chloroquine usually contain 150 mg base, French preparations 100 mg base and American preparations 300 mg base.

Babesiosis

Babesiosis is a tick-borne intra-erythrocytic protozoon parasite. There are more than 100 species of *Babesia*, all of which have an animal reservoir, typically either rodents or cattle, and are transmitted to humans via the tick vector *Ixodes scapularis*. Most American cases of babesiosis are due to *B. microti* and most European cases to *B. divergens*. Patients present with fever and malaise 1–4 weeks after a tick bite. Illness may be complicated by haemolytic anaemia. Severe illness is seen in splenectomised patients. The diagnosis is made by blood-film examination. Treatment is with quinine and clindamycin.

African trypanosomiasis (sleeping sickness)

African sleeping sickness is caused by trypanosomes (Fig. 11.35) conveyed to humans by the bites of infected tsetse flies, and is unique to sub-Saharan Africa (Fig. 11.36). The incidence of sleeping sickness across Africa has declined by over 60% since 1990 due to better control measures. *Trypanosoma brucei gambiense* trypanosomiasis has a wide distribution in West and Central Africa and accounts for 90% of human African trypanosomiasis (HAT). *T. brucei rhodesiense* trypanosomiasis is found in parts of East and Central Africa. In West Africa, transmission is mainly at the riverside, where the fly rests in the shade of trees; no animal reservoir has been identified for *T. gambiense*. *T. rhodesiense* has a large reservoir in numerous wild animals and transmission takes place in the shade of woods bordering grasslands. Rural populations employed in agriculture, fishing and animal husbandry are susceptible. Local people and tourists visiting forests infested with tsetse flies and animal reservoirs may become infected.

Clinical features

A bite by a tsetse fly is painful and commonly becomes inflamed; if trypanosomes are introduced, the site may again become painful and swollen about 10 days later ('trypanosomal chancre'), associated with regional lymphadenopathy. Within 2–3 weeks of infection, the trypanosomes invade the blood stream. The disease is characterised by an early haematolymphatic (stage 1) and a late encephalitic phase (stage 2), in which the parasite crosses the blood–brain barrier and chronic encephalopathy develops.

Rhodesiense infections

In these infections, the disease is more acute and severe than in *gambiense* infections, so that, within days or a few weeks,

Fig. 11.35 Trypanosomiasis. Scanning electron micrograph showing trypanosomes swimming among erythrocytes.

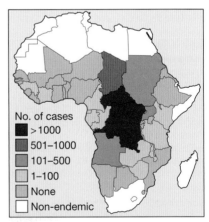

No. of cases
- >1000
- 501–1000
- 101–500
- 1–100
- None
- Non-endemic

Fig. 11.36 Distribution of human African trypanosomiasis. Data are from 2009. *From Simarro PP, Diarra A, Ruiz Postigo JA, et al. The human African trypanosomiasis control and surveillance programme of the World Health Organization 2000–2009: the way forward. PLoS Negl Trop Dis 2011; 5(2):e1007.*

the patient is usually severely ill and may have developed pleural effusions and signs of myocarditis or hepatitis. There may be a petechial rash. The patient may die before there are signs of involvement of the CNS. If the illness is less acute, drowsiness, tremors and coma develop.

Gambiense infections

The distinction between early and late stages may not be apparent in *gambiense* infections. The disease usually runs a slow course over months or years, with irregular bouts of fever and enlargement of lymph nodes. These are characteristically firm, discrete, rubbery and painless, and are particularly prominent in the posterior triangle of the neck ('Winterbottom's sign'). The spleen and liver may become palpable. After some months without treatment, the CNS is invaded. Patients develop headache, altered behaviour, blunting of higher mental functions, insomnia by night and sleepiness by day, delirium and eventually tremors, pareses, wasting, coma and death.

Investigations

Trypanosomiasis should be considered in any febrile patient from an endemic area. In *rhodesiense* infections, thick and thin malaria blood films will reveal trypanosomes. The trypanosomes may be seen in the blood or from puncture of the primary lesion in the earliest stages of *gambiense* infections, but it is usually easier to demonstrate them by aspiration of a lymph node. Concentration methods include buffy coat microscopy and miniature anion exchange chromatography.

Due to the cyclical nature of parasitaemia, the diagnosis is often made by demonstration of antibodies using a simple, rapid screening card agglutination trypanosomiasis test (CATT) for *gambiense* HAT, followed by parasitological confirmation. No reliable serological test is available for *rhodesiense* HAT. PCR diagnosis is available, although technical requirements limit its availability in endemic regions. If the CNS is affected, the cell count ($>20 \times 10^9$ leucocytes/L) and protein content of the CSF are increased and the glucose is diminished. A very high level of serum IgM or the presence of IgM in the CSF is suggestive of trypanosomiasis. Recognition of CNS involvement is critical, as failure to treat it might be fatal.

Management

Therapeutic options for African trypanosomiasis are limited and most antitrypanosomal drugs are toxic and expensive. The prognosis is good if treatment is begun early, before the brain has been invaded. At this stage, intravenous suramin, after a test dose of 100–200 mg, should be given for *rhodesiense* infections, followed by five injections of 20 mg/kg every 7 days. For *gambiense* infections, deep intramuscular or intravenous pentamidine 4 mg/kg for 7 days is given.

For the treatment of stage 2 (nervous system) infection caused by *gambiense* HAT, patients were previously treated with melarsoprol (an arsenical). Treatment-related mortality with melarsoprol is 4–12% due to reactive encephalopathy. Now eflornithine (DFMO), an irreversible inhibitor of ornithine decarboxylase (100 and 150 mg/kg IV 4 times daily for 14 days for adults and children, respectively), is a safer and cost-effective option. Combinations of eflornithine (400 mg daily for 7 days) with oral nifurtimox (15 mg/kg daily for 15 days) have been shown to decrease relapses, deaths and drug toxicity. Stage 2 *rhodesiense* infection is treated with melarsoprol 2.2 mg/kg IV for 10 days.

Prevention

In endemic *gambiense* areas, various measures are taken against tsetse flies, and field teams help detect and treat early HAT. In *rhodesiense* endemic areas, control is difficult.

█ American trypanosomiasis (Chagas' disease)

Chagas' disease occurs widely in South and Central America. The cause is *Trypanosoma cruzi*, transmitted to humans from the faeces of a reduviid (triatomine) bug, in which the trypanosomes develop before infecting humans. These bugs live in wild forests in crevices, burrows and palm trees. The *Triatoma infestans* bug has become domesticated in the Southern Cone countries (Argentina, Brazil, Chile, Paraguay and Uruguay). It lives in the mud and wattle walls and thatched roofs of simple rural houses and emerges at night to feed and defaecate on the sleeping occupants. Infected faeces are rubbed in through the conjunctiva, mucosa of mouth or nose, or abrasions of the skin. Over 100 species of mammal – domestic, peridomestic and wild – may serve as reservoirs of infection. In some areas, blood transfusion accounts for about 5% of cases. Congenital transmission occasionally occurs.

Pathology

The trypanosomes migrate via the blood stream, develop into amastigote forms in the tissues and multiply intracellularly by binary fission. In the acute phase (primarily cell-mediated), inflammation of parasitised, as well as non-parasitised, cardiac muscles and capillaries occurs, resulting in acute myocarditis. In the chronic phase, focal myocardial atrophy, signs of chronic passive congestion and thromboembolic phenomena, cardiomegaly and apical cardiac aneurysm are salient findings. In the digestive form of disease, focal myositis and discontinuous lesions of the intramural myenteric plexus are seen, predominantly in the oesophagus and colon.

Clinical features

Acute phase

Clinical manifestations of the acute phase are seen in only 1–2% of individuals infected before the age of 15 years. Young children (1–5 years) are most commonly affected. The entrance of *T. cruzi* through an abrasion produces a dusky-red, firm swelling and enlargement of regional lymph nodes. A conjunctival lesion, although less common, is characteristic; the unilateral firm, reddish swelling of the lids may close the eye and constitutes 'Romaña's sign'. In a few patients, an acute generalised infection soon appears, with a transient morbilliform or urticarial rash, fever, lymphadenopathy and enlargement of the spleen and liver. In a small minority of patients, acute myocarditis and heart failure or neurological features, including personality changes and signs of meningoencephalitis, may be seen. The acute infection may be fatal to infants.

Chronic phase

About 50–70% of infected patients become seropositive and develop an indeterminate form when no parasitaemia is detectable. They have a normal lifespan with no symptoms but are a natural reservoir for the disease and maintain the life cycle of parasites. After a latent period of several years, 10–30% of chronic cases develop low-grade myocarditis and damage to conducting fibres, which causes cardiomyopathy characterised by cardiac dilatation, arrhythmias, partial or complete heart block and sudden death. In nearly 10% of patients, damage to Auerbach's plexus results in dilatation of various parts of the alimentary canal, especially the colon and oesophagus, so-called 'mega' disease. Dilatation of the bile ducts and bronchi are also recognised sequelae. Autoimmune processes may be responsible for much of the damage. There are geographical variations of the basic pattern

11

of disease. Reactivation of Chagas' disease can occur in patients with HIV if the CD4 count falls lower than 200 cells/mm[3]; this can cause space-occupying lesions with a presentation similar to *Toxoplasma gondii*, encephalitis, encephalitis, meningoencephalitis or myocarditis.

Investigations

T. cruzi is easily detectable in a blood film in the acute illness. In chronic disease, it may be recovered in up to 50% of cases by xenodiagnosis, in which infection-free, laboratory-bred reduviid bugs feed on the patient; subsequently, the hindgut or faeces of the bug are examined for parasites. Parasite DNA detection by PCR in the patient's blood is a highly sensitive method for documentation of infection and, in addition, can be employed in faeces of bugs used in xenodiagnosis tests to improve sensitivity. Antibody detection is also highly sensitive.

Management and prevention

Parasiticidal agents are used to treat the acute phase, congenital disease and early chronic phase (within 10 years of infection). Nifurtimox is given orally. The dose, which has to be carefully supervised to minimise toxicity while preserving parasiticidal activity, is 10 mg/kg daily orally, divided into three equal doses for 90 days. The paediatric dose is 15 mg/kg daily. Cure rates of 80% in acute disease are obtained. Benznidazole is an alternative, given at a dose of 5 mg/kg daily orally, in two divided doses for 60 days; children receive 10 mg/kg daily. Both nifurtimox and benznidazole are toxic, with adverse reaction rates of 30–55%. Parasiticidal treatment of the chronic phase is usually performed but, in the cardiac or digestive 'mega' diseases, does not reverse tissue damage. Surgery may be needed.

Preventative measures include improvement of housing and destruction of reduviid bugs by spraying of houses with insecticides. Blood and organ donors should be screened.

Toxoplasmosis

Toxoplasma gondii is an intracellular parasite. The sexual phase of the parasite's life cycle (Fig. 11.37) occurs in the small intestinal epithelium of the domestic cat. Oöcysts are shed in cat faeces and are spread to intermediate hosts (pigs, sheep and also humans) through widespread contamination of soil. Oöcysts may survive in moist conditions for weeks or months. Once they are ingested, the parasite transforms into rapidly dividing tachyzoites through cycles of asexual multiplication. Microscopic tissue cysts develop containing bradyzoites, which persist for the lifetime of the host. Cats become infected or reinfected by ingesting tissue cysts in prey such as rodents and birds.

Human infection occurs via oöcyst-contaminated soil, salads and vegetables, or by ingestion of raw or under-cooked meats containing tissue cysts. Sheep, pigs and rabbits are the most common meat sources. Outbreaks of toxoplasmosis have been linked to the consumption of unfiltered water. In developed countries, toxoplasmosis is the most common protozoal infection; around 22% of adults in the UK are seropositive. Most primary infections are subclinical; however, toxoplasmosis is thought to account for about 15% of heterophile antibody-negative infectious mononucleosis (p. 241). In India or Brazil, approximately 40–60% of pregnant females are seropositive for *T. gondii*. In HIV-1 infection (p. 320), toxoplasmosis is an important opportunistic infection with considerable morbidity and mortality. Generalised toxoplasmosis has been described after accidental laboratory infection with highly virulent strains.

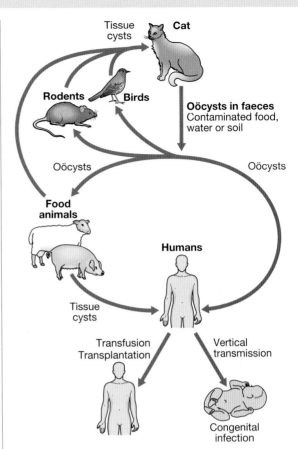

Fig. 11.37 Life cycle of *Toxoplasma gondii*.

Clinical features

In most immunocompetent individuals, including children and pregnant women, the infection goes unnoticed. In approximately 10% of patients, it causes a self-limiting illness, most common in adults aged 25–35 years. The presenting feature is usually localised or generalised painless lymphadenopathy. The cervical nodes are primarily involved but mediastinal, mesenteric or retroperitoneal groups may be affected. The spleen is seldom palpable. Most patients have no systemic symptoms but some complain of malaise, fever, fatigue, muscle pain, sore throat and headache. Complete resolution usually occurs within a few months, although symptoms and lymphadenopathy tend to fluctuate unpredictably and some patients do not recover completely for a year or more. Encephalitis, myocarditis, polymyositis, pneumonitis or hepatitis occasionally occur in immunocompetent patients but are more frequent in immunocompromised hosts. Retinochoroiditis (Fig. 11.38) is usually the result of congenital infection but has also been reported in acquired disease.

Congenital toxoplasmosis

Acute toxoplasmosis, mostly subclinical, affects 0.3–1% of pregnant women, with an approximately 60% transmission rate to the fetus, which rises with increasing gestation. Seropositive females infected 6 months before conception have no risk of fetal transmission. Congenital disease affects approximately 40% of infected fetuses, and is more likely and more severe with infection early in gestation (see Box 11.26, p. 235). Many fetal infections are subclinical at birth but long-term sequelae include retinochoroiditis, microcephaly and hydrocephalus.

Fig. 11.38 Retinochoroiditis due to toxoplasmosis.

Investigations

In contrast to immunocompromised patients, in whom the diagnosis often requires direct detection of parasites, serology is often used in immunocompetent individuals. The Sabin–Feldman dye test (indirect fluorescent antibody test), which detects IgG antibody, is most commonly used. Recent infection induces a fourfold or greater increase in titre when paired sera are tested in parallel. Peak titres of 1/1000 or more are reached within 1–2 months of the onset of infection, and serology then becomes an unreliable indicator of recent infection. The detection of significant levels of *Toxoplasma*-specific IgM antibody may be useful in confirming acute infection. A false-positive result or persistence of IgM antibodies for years after infection makes interpretation difficult; however, negative IgM antibodies virtually rule out acute infection.

During pregnancy, it is critical to differentiate recent from past infection; the presence of high-avidity IgG antibodies excludes infection acquired in the preceding 3–4 months.

If necessary, the presence of *Toxoplasma* organisms in a lymph node biopsy or other tissue can be detected histochemically with *T. gondii* antiserum, or by the use of PCR to detect *Toxoplasma*-specific DNA.

Management

In immunocompetent subjects, uncomplicated toxoplasmosis is self-limiting and responds poorly to antimicrobial therapy. Treatment with sulfadiazine, pyrimethamine and folinic acid is usually reserved for severe or progressive disease, and for infection in immunocompromised patients.

In pregnant women with established recent infection, spiramycin (3 g daily in divided doses) is given until term. Once fetal infection is established, treatment with sulfadiazine and pyrimethamine plus calcium folinate is recommended (spiramycin does not cross the placental barrier). The cost/benefit of routine *Toxoplasma* screening and treatment in pregnancy is being debated in many countries. There is insufficient evidence to determine the effects on mother or baby of current antiparasitic treatment for women who seroconvert in pregnancy.

Leishmaniasis

Leishmaniasis is caused by unicellular, flagellate, intracellular protozoa belonging to the genus *Leishmania* (order Kineto-

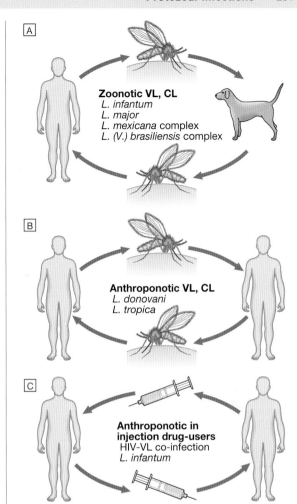

Fig. 11.39 Transmission of leishmaniasis. [A] Zoonotic transmission. [B] Anthroponotic transmission. [C] Anthroponotic transmission in the injection drug-user. (CL = cutaneous leishmaniasis; VL = visceral leishmaniasis)

plastidae). There are 21 leishmanial species that cause diverse clinical syndromes, which can be placed into three broad groups:

- visceral leishmaniasis (VL, kala-azar)
- cutaneous leishmaniasis (CL)
- mucosal leishmaniasis (ML).

Epidemiology and transmission

Although most clinical syndromes are caused by zoonotic transmission of parasites from animals (chiefly canine and rodent reservoirs) to humans through phlebotomine sandfly vectors (Fig. 11.39A), humans are the only known reservoir (anthroponotic person-to-person transmission) in major VL foci in the Indian subcontinent and in injection drug-users (Fig. 11.39B and C). Leishmaniasis occurs in approximately 100 countries around the world, with an estimated annual incidence of 0.9–1.3 million new cases (25% VL).

The life cycle of *Leishmania* is shown in Figure 11.40. Flagellar promastigotes (10–20 μm) are introduced by the feeding female sandfly. The promastigotes are taken up by neutrophils, which undergo apoptosis and are then engulfed by macrophages, in which the parasites transform into amastigotes (2–4 μm; Leishman–Donovan body). These multiply, causing macrophage

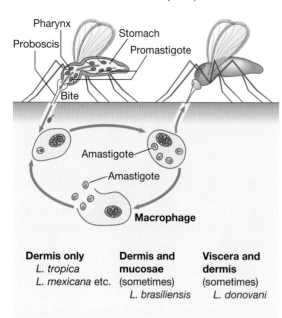

Sandfly
(*Phlebotomus* in eastern hemisphere,
Lutzomyia and *Psychodopygus*
in western hemisphere)

Pharynx
Proboscis
Stomach
Promastigote
Bite
Amastigote
Amastigote
Macrophage

Dermis only	**Dermis and mucosae** (sometimes)	**Viscera and dermis** (sometimes)
L. tropica *L. mexicana* etc.	*L. brasiliensis*	*L. donovani*

Fig. 11.40 Life cycle of *Leishmania*. *From Knight R. Parasitic disease in man. Churchill Livingstone, Elsevier Ltd; 1982.*

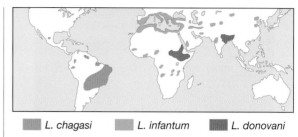

L. chagasi   L. infantum   L. donovani

Fig. 11.41 World distribution of visceral leishmaniasis.

Fig. 11.42 Splenic smear showing numerous intracellular, and a few extracellular, amastigotes. *Courtesy of Dr S. Sundar and Dr H.W. Murray.*

lysis and infection of other cells. Sandflies pick up amastigotes when feeding on infected patients or animal reservoirs. In the sandfly, the parasite transforms into a flagellar promastigote, which multiplies by binary fission in the gut of the vector and migrates to the proboscis to infect a new host.

Sandflies live in hot and humid climates in the cracks and crevices of mud or straw houses and lay eggs in organic matter. People living in such conditions are more prone to leishmaniasis. Female sandflies bite during the night and preferentially feed on animals; humans are incidental hosts.

Visceral leishmaniasis (kala-azar)

VL is caused by the protozoon *Leishmania donovani* complex (comprising *L. donovani*, *L. infantum* and *L. chagasi*). India, Sudan, Bangladesh and Brazil account for 90% of cases of VL. Other affected regions include the Mediterranean, East Africa, China, Arabia, Israel and other South American countries (Fig. 11.41). In addition to sandfly transmission, VL has also been reported to follow blood transfusion, and disease can present unexpectedly in immunosuppressed patients – for example, after renal transplantation and in HIV infection.

The majority of people infected remain asymptomatic. In visceral disease, the spleen, liver, bone marrow and lymph nodes are primarily involved.

Clinical features

In the Indian subcontinent, adults and children are equally affected; elsewhere, VL is mainly a disease of small children and infants, except in adults with HIV co-infection. The incubation period ranges from weeks to months (occasionally, several years).

The first sign of infection is high fever, usually accompanied by rigor and chills. Fever intensity decreases over time and patients may become afebrile for intervening periods ranging from weeks to months. This is followed by a relapse of fever, often of lesser intensity. Splenomegaly develops quickly in the first few weeks and becomes massive as the disease progresses. Moderate hepatomegaly occurs later. Lymphadenopathy is common in Africa, the Mediterranean and South America but is rare in the Indian subcontinent. Blackish discoloration of the skin, from which the disease derived its name, kala-azar (the Hindi word for 'black fever'), is a feature of advanced illness but is now rarely seen. Pancytopenia is common. Moderate to severe anaemia develops rapidly and can cause cardiac failure. Thrombocytopenia, often compounded by hepatic dysfunction, may result in bleeding from the retina, gastrointestinal tract and nose. In advanced illness, hypoalbuminaemia may manifest as pedal oedema, ascites and anasarca (gross generalised oedema and swelling).

As disease progresses, there is profound immunosuppression and secondary infections are very common. These include tuberculosis, pneumonia, gastroenteritis, severe amoebic or bacillary dysentery, boils, cellulitis, chickenpox, shingles and scabies. Without adequate treatment, most patients with clinical VL die.

Investigations

Pancytopenia is the dominant feature, with granulocytopenia and monocytosis. Polyclonal hypergammaglobulinaemia, chiefly IgG followed by IgM, and hypoalbuminaemia are seen later.

Demonstration of amastigotes (Leishman–Donovan bodies) in splenic smears is the most efficient means of diagnosis, with 98% sensitivity (Fig. 11.42); however, it carries a risk of serious haemorrhage in inexperienced hands. Safer methods, such as bone marrow or lymph node smears, are not as sensitive but are frequently employed. Parasites may be demonstrated in buffy coat smears, especially in immunosuppressed patients. Sensitivity is improved by culturing the aspirate material or by using PCR for DNA detection and species identification, but these tests can only be performed in specialised laboratories.

Serodiagnosis, by ELISA or immunofluorescence antibody test, is employed in developed countries. In endemic regions, a highly sensitive direct agglutination test using stained promastigotes and an equally efficient rapid immunochromatographic k39 strip test have become popular. These tests remain positive for several months after cure has been achieved, so do not predict response to treatment or relapse. The vast majority of people exposed to the parasite do not develop clinical illness but may have positive serological tests thereafter. Formal gel (aldehyde) or other similar tests based on the detection of raised globulin have limited value and should not be employed for the diagnosis of VL.

Differential diagnosis

This includes malaria, typhoid, tuberculosis, schistosomiasis and many other infectious and neoplastic conditions, some of which may coexist with VL. Fever, splenomegaly, pancytopenia and non-response to antimalarial therapy may provide clues before specific laboratory diagnosis is made.

Management

Pentavalent antimonials

Antimony (Sb) compounds were the first drugs to be used for the treatment of leishmaniasis and remain the mainstay of treatment in most parts of the world. The exception is the Indian subcontinent, especially Bihar state, where almost two-thirds of cases are refractory to Sb treatment. Traditionally, pentavalent antimony is available as sodium stibogluconate (100 mg/mL) in English-speaking countries and meglumine antimoniate (85 mg/mL) in French-speaking ones. The daily dose is 20 mg/kg body weight, intravenously or intramuscularly, for 28–30 days. Side-effects are common and include arthralgia, myalgia, raised hepatic transaminases, pancreatitis (especially in patients co-infected with HIV) and ECG changes (T-wave inversion and reduced amplitude). Severe cardiotoxicity, manifest by concave ST segment elevation, prolongation of QT_c greater than 0.5 msec and ventricular dysrhythmias, is not uncommon. The incidence of cardiotoxicity and death is particularly high with improperly manufactured Sb.

Amphotericin B

Amphotericin B deoxycholate, given once daily or on alternate days at a dose of 0.75–1.00 mg/kg for 15–20 doses, is used as the first-line drug in many regions where there is a significant level of Sb unresponsiveness. It has a cure rate of nearly 100%. Infusion-related side-effects, such as high fever with rigor, thrombophlebitis, diarrhoea and vomiting, are extremely common. Serious side-effects, including renal or hepatic toxicity, hypokalaemia and thrombocytopenia, are observed frequently.

Lipid formulations of amphotericin B (p. 126) are less toxic. AmBisome is first-line therapy in Europe for VL. Dosing recommendations vary according to geographical region. In the Indian subcontinent, a total dose of 10 or 15 mg/kg, administered in a single dose or as multiple doses over several days, respectively, is considered adequate, whereas in Africa 14–18 mg/kg, and in South America and Europe 21–24 mg/kg, in divided doses, typically spread over 10 days, is recommended for immunocompetent patients. High daily doses of the lipid formulations are well tolerated, and in one study a single dose of 10 mg/kg of AmBisome cured 96% of Indian patients. The manufacturer of AmBisome has donated a large quantity of the drug for use in the Kala-azar Elimination Programme in India, Nepal and Bangladesh, leading to its adoption as the first-line drug in treatment.

Other drugs

The oral drug miltefosine, an alkyl phospholipid, has been approved in several countries for the treatment of VL. A daily dose of 50 mg (patient's body weight <25 kg) to 100 mg (≥25 kg), or 2.5 mg/kg for children, for 28 days cures over 90% of patients. Side-effects include mild to moderate vomiting and diarrhoea, and rarely skin allergy or renal or liver toxicity. Since it is a teratogenic drug, it cannot be used in pregnancy; female patients are advised not to become pregnant for the duration of treatment and 3 months thereafter because of its half-life of nearly 1 week.

Paromomycin is an aminoglycoside that has undergone trials in India and Africa, and is highly effective if given intramuscularly at 11 mg/kg of paromomycin base, daily for 3 weeks. No significant auditory or renal toxicity is seen. The drug is approved in India for VL treatment.

Pentamidine isethionate was used to treat Sb-refractory patients with VL. However, declining efficacy and serious side-effects, such as type 1 diabetes mellitus, hypoglycaemia and hypotension, have led to it being abandoned.

Multidrug therapy of VL is likely to be used increasingly to prevent emergence of drug resistance, and in India short-course combinations (a single dose of AmBisome 5 mg/kg with either 7 days of miltefosine or 10 days of paromomycin, or 10 days each of miltefosine and paromomycin) were as effective as standard therapy. In India, in treatment centres where the cold chain (a temperature-controlled supply chain) is not maintained, 10 days of paromomycin combined with miltefosine is an alternative treatment regimen.

Response to treatment

A good response results in fever resolution, improved well-being, reduction in splenomegaly, weight gain and recovery of blood counts. Patients should be followed regularly for 6–12 months, as some may experience relapse irrespective of the treatment regimen.

HIV–visceral leishmaniasis co-infection

HIV-induced immunosuppression (Ch. 12) increases the risk of contracting VL 100–1000 times. Most cases of HIV–VL co-infection have been reported from Spain, France, Italy and Portugal. Antiretroviral therapy (ART) has led to a remarkable decline in the incidence of VL co-infection in Europe. However, numbers are increasing in Africa (mainly Ethiopia), Brazil and the Indian subcontinent.

Although the clinical triad of fever, splenomegaly and hepatomegaly is found in the majority of co-infected patients, those with low CD4 count may have atypical clinical presentations. VL may present with gastrointestinal involvement (stomach, duodenum or colon), ascites, pleural or pericardial effusion, or involvement of lungs, tonsil, oral mucosa or skin. Diagnostic principles remain the same as those in non-HIV patients. Parasites are numerous and easily demonstrable, even in buffy coat preparations. Sometimes amastigotes are found in unusual sites, such as bronchoalveolar lavage fluid, pleural fluid or biopsies of the gastrointestinal tract. Serological tests have low sensitivity. DNA detection by PCR of the blood or its buffy coat is at least 95% sensitive and accurately tracks recovery and relapse.

11

Treatment of VL with HIV co-infection is essentially the same as in immunocompetent patients but there are some differences in outcome. Conventional amphotericin B (0.7 mg/kg/day for 28 days) may be more effective in achieving initial cure than Sb (20 mg/kg/day for 28 days). Using high-dose liposomal amphotericin B (4 mg/kg on days 1–5, 10, 17, 24, 31 and 38), a high cure rate is possible. However, co-infected patients have a tendency to relapse within 1 year and maintenance chemotherapy with monthly liposomal amphotericin B is useful.

Post-kala-azar dermal leishmaniasis

After treatment and apparent recovery from VL in India and Sudan, some patients develop dermatological manifestations due to local parasitic infection.

Clinical features

In India, dermatological changes occur in a small minority of patients 6 months to at least 3 years after the initial infection. They are seen as macules, papules, nodules (most frequently) and plaques, which have a predilection for the face, especially the area around the chin. The face often appears erythematous (Fig. 11.43A). Hypopigmented macules can occur over all parts of the body and are highly variable in extent. There are no systemic symptoms and little spontaneous healing occurs.

In Sudan, approximately 50% of patients with VL develop post-kala-azar dermal leishmaniasis (PKDL), experiencing skin manifestations concurrently with VL or within the following 6 months. In addition to the dermatological features, a measles-like micropapular rash (Fig. 11.43B) may be seen all over the body. In Sudan, children are more frequently affected than in India. Spontaneous healing occurs in about three-quarters of cases within 1 year.

Investigations and management

The diagnosis is clinical, supported by demonstration of scanty parasites in lesions by slit-skin smear and culture. Immunofluorescence and immunohistochemistry may demonstrate the parasite in skin tissues. In the majority of patients, serological tests (direct agglutination test or k39 strip tests) are positive.

Treatment of PKDL is difficult. In India, Sb for 120 days, several courses of amphotericin B infusions, or miltefosine for 12 weeks is required. In Sudan, Sb for 2 months is considered adequate. In the absence of a physical handicap, most patients are reluctant to complete the treatment. PKDL patients are a human reservoir, and focal outbreaks have been linked to patients with PKDL in areas previously free of VL.

Prevention and control

Sandfly control through insecticide spray is very important. Mosquito nets or curtains treated with insecticides will keep out the tiny sandflies. In endemic areas with zoonotic transmission, infected or stray dogs should be destroyed.

In areas with anthroponotic transmission, early diagnosis and treatment of human infections, to reduce the reservoir and control epidemics of VL, is extremely important. Serology is useful in diagnosis of suspected cases in the field. No vaccine is currently available.

Cutaneous and mucosal leishmaniasis

Cutaneous leishmaniasis

CL (oriental sore) occurs in both the Old World (Asia, Africa and Europe) and the New World (the Americas). Transmission is described on page 281.

In the Old World, CL is mild. It is found around the Mediterranean basin, throughout the Middle East and Central Asia as far as Pakistan, and in sub-Saharan West Africa and Sudan (Fig. 11.44). The causative organisms for Old World zoonotic CL are *L. major*, *L. tropica* and *L. aethiopica* (Box 11.57). Anthroponotic CL is caused by *L. tropica*, and is confined to urban or suburban areas of the Old World. Afghanistan is currently the biggest focus but infection is endemic in Pakistan, the western deserts of India, Iran, Iraq, Syria and other areas of the Middle East. In recent years, there has been an increase in the incidence of zoonotic CL in both the Old and the New Worlds due to urbanisation and deforestation, which led to peridomestic transmission (in and around human dwellings).

Fig. 11.43 Post-kala-azar dermal leishmaniasis. A In India, with macules, papules, nodules and plaques. B In Sudan, with micronodular rash. *A, From Sundar S, Kumar K, Chakravarty J, et al. Cure of antimony-unresponsive Indian post-kala-azar dermal leishmaniasis with oral miltefosine. Trans R Soc Trop Med Hyg 2006; 100(7):698–700. B, Courtesy of Dr E.E. Zijlstra.*

New World CL is a more significant disease, which may disfigure the nose, ears and mouth, and is caused by the *L. mexicana* complex (comprising *L. mexicana*, *L. amazonensis* and *L. venezuelensis*) and by the *Viannia* subgenus *L. (V.) brasiliensis* complex (comprising *L. (V.) guyanensis*, *L. (V.) panamensis*, *L. (V.) brasiliensis* and *L. (V.) peruviana*).

CL is commonly imported and should be considered in the differential diagnosis of an ulcerating skin lesion, especially in travellers who have visited endemic areas of the Old World or forests in Central and South America.

Pathogenesis

Inoculated parasites are taken up by dermal macrophages, in which they multiply and form a focus for lymphocytes, epithelioid cells and plasma cells. Self-healing may occur with necrosis of infected macrophages, or the lesion may become chronic with ulceration of the overlying epidermis, depending on the aetiological pathogen.

Clinical features

The incubation period is typically 2–3 months (range 2 weeks to 5 years). In all types of CL a papule develops at the site of

i	**11.57 Types of Old World cutaneous leishmaniasis**	
Leishmania spp.	**Host**	**Clinical features**
L. tropica	Dogs	Slow evolution, less severe
L. major	Gerbils, desert rodents	Rapid necrosis, wet sores
L. aethiopica	Hyraxes	Solitary facial lesions with satellites

| ■ *L. mexicana* | ■ *L. infantum* | ■ *L. major* |
| ■ *L. brasiliensis* | ■ *L. tropica* | ■ *L. aethiopica* |

Fig. 11.44 World distribution of cutaneous leishmaniasis.

the vector bite. The small, red papules may be single or multiple and increase gradually in size, reaching 2–10 cm in diameter. A crust forms, overlying an ulcer with a granular base and with raised borders (Fig. 11.45). These ulcers develop a few weeks or months after the bite. There can be satellite lesions, especially in *L. major* and occasionally in *L. tropica* infections. Regional lymphadenopathy, pain, pruritus and secondary bacterial infections may occur.

Lesions of *L. mexicana* and *L. peruviana* closely resemble those seen in the Old World, but lesions on the pinna of the ear are common and are chronic and destructive. *L. mexicana* is responsible for chiclero ulcers, the self-healing sores of Mexico.

If immunity is effective, there is usually spontaneous healing in *L. tropica*, *L. major* and *L. mexicana* lesions. In some patients with anergy to *Leishmania*, the skin lesions of *L. aethiopica*, *L. mexicana* and *L. amazonensis* infections progress to the development of diffuse CL; this is characterised by spread of the infection from the initial ulcer, usually on the face, to involve the whole body in the form of non-ulcerative nodules. Occasionally, in *L. tropica* infections, sores that have apparently healed relapse persistently (recidivans or lupoid leishmaniasis).

Mucosal leishmaniasis

The *Viannia* subgenus extends widely from the Amazon basin as far as Paraguay and Costa Rica, and is responsible for deep sores and ML. In *L. (V.) brasiliensis* complex infections, cutaneous lesions may be followed by mucosal spread of the disease simultaneously or even years later. Young men with chronic lesions are particularly at risk, and 2–40% of infected persons develop 'espundia', metastatic lesions in the mucosa of the nose or mouth. This is characterised by thickening and erythema of the nasal mucosa, typically starting at the junction of the nose and upper lip. Later, ulceration develops. The lips, soft palate, fauces and larynx may also be invaded and destroyed, leading to considerable suffering and deformity. There is no spontaneous healing, and death may result from severe respiratory tract infections due to massive destruction of the pharynx.

Investigations in CL and ML

CL is often diagnosed on the basis of the lesions' clinical characteristics. Parasitological confirmation is important, however, because clinical manifestations may be mimicked by other infections. Amastigotes can be demonstrated on a slit-skin smear with Giemsa staining; alternatively, they can be cultured from the sores early during the infection. Parasites seem to be particularly

11

Fig. 11.45 Cutaneous leishmaniasis. [A] Papule. [B] Ulcer. *B, Courtesy of Dr Ravi Gowda, Royal Hallamshire Hospital, Sheffield.*

difficult to isolate from sores caused by *L. brasiliensis*, responsible for the vast majority of cases in Brazil. Touch preparations from biopsies and histopathology usually have a low sensitivity. Culture of fine needle aspiration material has been reported to be the most sensitive method.

ML is more difficult to diagnose parasitologically. The leishmanin skin test measures delayed-type hypersensitivity to killed *Leishmania* organisms. A positive test is defined as induration of more than 5 mm, 48 hours after intradermal injection. The test is positive, except in diffuse CL and during active VL. PCR is used increasingly for diagnosis and speciation, which is useful in selecting therapy.

Management of CL and ML

Small lesions may self-heal or are treated by freezing with liquid nitrogen or curettage. There is no ideal antimicrobial therapy. Treatment should be individualised on the basis of the causative organism, severity of the lesions, availability of drugs, tolerance of the patient for toxicity, and local resistance patterns.

In CL, topical application of paromomycin 15% plus methylbenzethonium chloride 12% is beneficial. Intralesional antimony (Sb 0.2–0.8 mL/lesion) up to 2 g seems to be rapidly effective in suitable cases; it is well tolerated and economic, and is safe in patients with cardiac, liver or renal diseases.

In ML, and in CL when the lesions are multiple or in a disfiguring site, it is better to treat with parenteral Sb in a dose of 20 mg/kg/day (usually given for 20 days for CL and 28 days for ML), or with conventional or liposomal amphotericin B (see treatment of VL above). Sb is also indicated to prevent the development of mucosal disease, if there is any chance that a lesion acquired in South America is due to an *L. brasiliensis* strain. Refractory CL or ML should be treated with an amphotericin B preparation.

Other regimens may be effective. Two to four doses of pentamidine (2–4 mg/kg), administered on alternate days, are effective in New World CL caused by *L. guyanensis*. In ML, 8 injections of pentamidine (4 mg/kg on alternate days) cure the majority of patients. Ketoconazole (600 mg daily for 4 weeks) has shown some potential against *L. mexicana* infection. In Saudi Arabia, fluconazole (200 mg daily for 6 weeks) reduced healing times and cured 79% of patients with CL caused by *L. major*. In India, itraconazole (200 mg daily for 6 weeks) produced good results in CL.

Prevention of CL and ML

Personal protection against sandfly bites is important. No effective vaccine is yet available.

Gastrointestinal protozoal infections

Amoebiasis

Amoebiasis is caused by *Entamoeba histolytica*, which is spread between humans by its cysts. It is one of the leading parasitic causes of morbidity and mortality in the tropics and is occasionally acquired in non-tropical countries. Two non-pathogenic *Entamoeba* species (*E. dispar* and *E. moshkovskii*) are morphologically identical to *E. histolytica*, and are distinguishable only by molecular techniques, isoenzyme studies or monoclonal antibody typing. However, only *E. histolytica* causes amoebic dysentery or liver abscess. The life cycle of the amoeba is shown in Figure 11.46A.

Pathology

Cysts of *E. histolytica* are ingested in water or uncooked foods contaminated by human faeces. Infection may also be acquired through anal/oral sexual practices. In the colon, trophozoite forms emerge from the cysts. The parasite invades the mucous membrane of the large bowel, producing lesions that are maximal

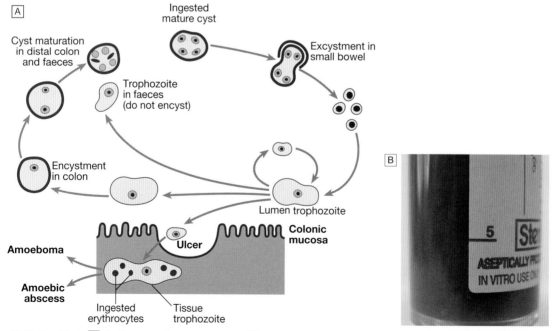

Fig. 11.46 Amoebiasis. **A** The life cycle of *Entamoeba histolytica*. **B** The chocolate-brown appearance of aspirated material from an amoebic liver abscess. *A, From Knight R. Parasitic disease in man. Churchill Livingstone, Elsevier Ltd; 1982. B, Courtesy of Dr Ravi Gowda, Royal Hallamshire Hospital, Sheffield.*

in the caecum but extend to the anal canal. These are flask-shaped ulcers, varying greatly in size and surrounded by healthy mucosa. A localised granuloma (amoeboma), presenting as a palpable mass in the rectum or a filling defect in the colon on radiography, is a rare complication that should be differentiated from carcinoma. Amoebic ulcers may cause severe haemorrhage but rarely perforate the bowel wall.

Amoebic trophozoites can emerge from the vegetative cyst from the bowel and be carried to the liver in a portal venule. They can multiply rapidly and destroy the liver parenchyma, causing an abscess (see also p. 879). The liquid contents at first have a characteristic pinkish colour, which may later change to chocolate-brown (said to resemble anchovy sauce).

Cutaneous amoebiasis, though rare, causes progressive genital, perianal or peri-abdominal surgical wound ulceration.

Clinical features

Intestinal amoebiasis – amoebic dysentery

Most amoebic infections are asymptomatic. The incubation period of amoebiasis ranges from 2 weeks to many years, followed by a chronic course with abdominal pains and two or more unformed stools a day. Offensive diarrhoea, alternating with constipation, and blood or mucus in the stool are common. There may be abdominal pain, especially in the right lower quadrant (which may mimic acute appendicitis). A dysenteric presentation with passage of blood, simulating bacillary dysentery or ulcerative colitis, occurs particularly in older people, in the puerperium and with super-added pyogenic infection of the ulcers.

Amoebic liver abscess

The abscess is usually found in the right hepatic lobe. There may not be associated diarrhoea. Early symptoms may be only local discomfort and malaise; later, a swinging temperature and sweating may develop, usually without marked systemic symptoms or signs. An enlarged, tender liver, cough and pain in the right shoulder are characteristic but symptoms may remain vague and signs minimal. A large abscess may penetrate the diaphragm, rupturing into the lung, and may be coughed up through a hepatobronchial fistula. Rupture into the pleural or peritoneal cavity, or rupture of a left lobe abscess in the pericardial sac, is less common but more serious.

Investigations

The stool and any exudate should undergo prompt microscopic examination for motile trophozoites containing red blood cells. Movements cease rapidly as the stool preparation cools. Several stools may need to be examined in chronic amoebiasis before cysts are found. Sigmoidoscopy may reveal typical flask-shaped ulcers, which should be scraped and examined immediately for E. histolytica. In endemic areas, one-third of the population are symptomless passers of amoebic cysts.

An amoebic abscess of the liver is suspected on clinical grounds; there is often a neutrophil leucocytosis and a raised right hemidiaphragm on chest X-ray. Confirmation is by ultrasonic scanning. Aspirated pus from an amoebic abscess has the characteristic chocolate-brown appearance but only rarely contains free amoebae (Fig. 11.46B).

Serum antibodies are detectable by immunofluorescence in over 95% of patients with hepatic amoebiasis and intestinal amoeboma, but in only about 60% of dysenteric amoebiasis. DNA detection by PCR has been shown to be useful in diagnosis of E. histolytica infections but is not generally available.

Management

Intestinal and early hepatic amoebiasis responds quickly to oral metronidazole (800 mg 3 times daily for 5–10 days) or other long-acting nitroimidazoles like tinidazole or ornidazole (both in doses of 2 g daily for 3 days). Nitazoxanide (500 mg twice daily for 3 days) is an alternative drug. Either diloxanide furoate or paromomycin, in doses of 500 mg orally 3 times daily for 10 days after treatment, should be given to eliminate luminal cysts.

If a liver abscess is large or threatens to burst, or if the response to chemotherapy is not prompt, aspiration is required and is repeated if necessary. Rupture of an abscess into the pleural cavity, pericardial sac or peritoneal cavity necessitates immediate aspiration or surgical drainage. Small serous effusions resolve without drainage.

Prevention

Personal precautions against contracting amoebiasis include not eating fresh, uncooked vegetables or drinking unclean water.

Giardiasis

Infection with Giardia lamblia is found worldwide and is common in the tropics. It particularly affects children, tourists and immunosuppressed individuals, and is the parasite most commonly imported into the UK. In cystic form, it remains viable in water for up to 3 months and infection usually occurs by ingesting contaminated water. Its flagellar trophozoite form attaches to the duodenal and jejunal mucosa, causing inflammation.

Clinical features and investigations

After an incubation period of 1–3 weeks, there is diarrhoea, abdominal pain, weakness, anorexia, nausea and vomiting. On examination, there may be abdominal distension and tenderness. Chronic diarrhoea and malabsorption may occur, with bulky stools that float.

Stools obtained at 2–3-day intervals should be examined for cysts. Duodenal or jejunal aspiration by endoscopy gives a higher diagnostic yield. The 'string test' may be used, in which one end of a piece of string is passed into the duodenum by swallowing and retrieved after an overnight fast; expressed fluid is then examined for the presence of G. lamblia trophozoites. A number of stool antigen detection tests are available. Jejunal biopsy specimens may show G. lamblia on the epithelial surface.

Management

Treatment is with a single dose of tinidazole 2 g, metronidazole 400 mg 3 times daily for 10 days, or nitazoxanide 500 mg orally twice daily for 3 days.

Cryptosporidiosis

Cryptosporidium spp. are coccidian protozoal parasites of humans and domestic animals. Infection is acquired by the faecal–oral route through contaminated water supplies. The incubation period is approximately 7–10 days and is followed by watery diarrhoea and abdominal cramps. The illness is usually self-limiting but in immunocompromised patients, especially those with HIV, the illness can be devastating, with persistent severe diarrhoea and substantial weight loss (p. 317).

Cyclosporiasis

Cyclospora cayetanensis is a globally distributed coccidian protozoal parasite of humans. Infection is acquired by ingestion of contaminated water and recent food-borne outbreaks have been associated with raspberries and coriander (cilantro). The incubation period of approximately 2–11 days is followed by diarrhoea with abdominal cramps, which may remit and relapse. Although usually self-limiting, the illness may last as long as 6 weeks, with significant weight loss and malabsorption, and is more severe in immunocompromised individuals. Diagnosis is by detection of oöcysts on faecal microscopy or PCR of stool. Treatment may be necessary in a few cases, using co-trimoxazole 960 mg twice daily for 7 days.

Infections caused by helminths

Helminths (from the Greek *helmins*, meaning worm) include three groups of parasitic worm (Box 11.58), large multicellular organisms with complex tissues and organs.

Intestinal human nematodes

Adult nematodes living in the human gut can cause disease. There are two types:

- the hookworms, which have a soil stage in which they develop into larvae that then penetrate the host
- a group of nematodes that survive in the soil merely as eggs, which have to be ingested for their life cycle to continue.

The geographical distribution of hookworms is limited by the larval requirement for warmth and humidity. Soil-transmitted nematode infections can be prevented by avoidance of faecal soil contamination (adequate sewerage disposal) or skin contact (wearing shoes), and by strict personal hygiene.

Ancylostomiasis (hookworm)

Ancylostomiasis is caused by *Ancylostoma duodenale* or *Necator americanus*. The complex life cycle is shown in Figure 11.47. The adult hookworm is 1 cm long and lives in the duodenum and upper jejunum. Eggs are passed in the faeces. In warm, moist, shady soil, the larvae develop into rhabditiform and then the infective filariform stages; they then penetrate human skin and are carried to the lungs. After entering the alveoli, they ascend the bronchi, are swallowed and mature in the small intestine, reaching maturity 4–7 weeks after infection. The worms attach to the mucosa of the small intestine by their buccal capsule (Fig. 11.48) and withdraw blood. The mean daily blood loss from one *A. duodenale* is 0.15 mL and that from *N. americanus* 0.03 mL.

Hookworm infection is a leading cause of anaemia in the tropics and subtropics. *A. duodenale* is endemic in the Far East and Mediterranean coastal regions, and is also present in Africa, while *N. americanus* is endemic in West, East and Central Africa, and Central and South America, as well as in the Far East.

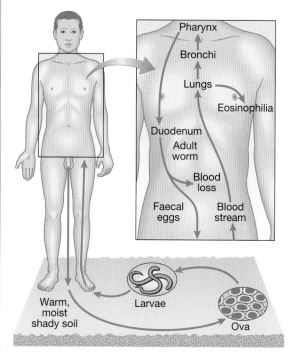

Fig. 11.47 Ancylostomiasis. Life cycle of *Ancylostoma*.

Fig. 11.48 *Ancylostoma duodenale.* Electron micrograph showing the ventral teeth. *From Gibbons LM. SEM guide to the morphology of nematode parasites of vertebrates. Farnham Royal, Slough: Commonwealth Agricultural Bureau International; 1986.*

---

i **11.58 Classes of helminth that parasitise humans**

Nematodes or roundworms

- Intestinal human nematodes: *Ancylostoma duodenale, Necator americanus, Strongyloides stercoralis, Ascaris lumbricoides, Enterobius vermicularis, Trichuris trichiura*
- Tissue-dwelling human nematodes: *Wuchereria bancrofti, Brugia malayi, Loa loa, Onchocerca volvulus, Dracunculus medinensis, Mansonella perstans, Dirofilaria immitis*
- Zoonotic nematodes: *Trichinella spiralis*

Trematodes or flukes

- Blood flukes: *Schistosoma haematobium, S. mansoni, S. japonicum, S. mekongi, S. intercalatum*
- Lung flukes: *Paragonimus* spp.
- Hepatobiliary flukes: *Clonorchis sinensis, Fasciola hepatica, Opisthorchis felineus*
- Intestinal flukes: *Fasciolopsis buski*

Cestodes or tapeworms

- Intestinal tapeworms: *Taenia saginata, T. solium, Diphyllobothrium latum, Hymenolepis nana*
- Tissue-dwelling cysts or worms: *Taenia solium, Echinococcus granulosus*

Clinical features

An allergic dermatitis, usually on the feet (ground itch), may be experienced at the time of infection. The passage of the larvae through the lungs in a heavy infection causes a paroxysmal cough with blood-stained sputum, associated with patchy pulmonary consolidation and eosinophilia. When the worms reach the small intestine, vomiting and epigastric pain resembling peptic ulcer disease may occur. Sometimes, frequent loose stools are passed. The degree of iron and protein deficiency depends not only on the worm burden but also on patient nutrition and iron stores. Anaemia with high-output cardiac failure may result. The mental and physical development of children may be delayed in severe infection.

Investigations

There is eosinophilia. The characteristic ovum can be recognised in the stool. If hookworms are present in numbers sufficient to cause anaemia, faecal occult blood testing will be positive.

Management

A single dose of albendazole (400 mg) is the treatment of choice. Alternatively, mebendazole 100 mg twice daily for 3 days may be used. Anaemia and heart failure associated with hookworm infection respond well to oral iron, even when severe; blood transfusion is rarely required.

Strongyloidiasis (threadworm)

Strongyloides stercoralis is a small nematode (2 mm×0.4 mm) that parasitises the mucosa of the upper part of the small intestine, often in large numbers, causing persistent eosinophilia. The eggs hatch in the bowel but only larvae are passed in the faeces. In moist soil, they moult and become the infective filariform larvae. After penetrating human skin, they undergo a development cycle similar to that of hookworms, except that the female worms burrow into the intestinal mucosa and submucosa. Some larvae in the intestine may develop into filariform larvae, which may then penetrate the mucosa or the perianal skin and lead to autoinfection and persistent infection. Patients with *Strongyloides* infection persisting for more than 35 years have been described. Strongyloidiasis occurs in the tropics and subtropics, and is especially prevalent in the Far East.

Clinical features

These are shown in Box 11.59. The classic triad of symptoms consists of abdominal pain, diarrhoea and urticaria. Cutaneous

11.59 Clinical features of strongyloidiasis
Penetration of skin by infective larvae
• Itchy rash
Presence of worms in gut
• Abdominal pain, diarrhoea, steatorrhoea, weight loss
Allergic phenomena
• Urticarial plaques and papules, wheezing, arthralgia
Autoinfection
• Transient itchy, linear, urticarial weals across abdomen and buttocks (larva currens)
Systemic (super-)infection
• Diarrhoea, pneumonia, meningoencephalitis, death

manifestations, either urticaria or larva currens (a highly characteristic pruritic, elevated, erythematous lesion, rapidly advancing along the course of larval migration), are characteristic and occur in 66% of patients.

Systemic strongyloidiasis (the *Strongyloides* hyperinfection syndrome), with dissemination of larvae throughout the body, occurs with immune suppression (HIV or HTLV-1 infection, immunosuppressant treatment). Patients present with severe, generalised abdominal pain, abdominal distension and shock. Massive larval invasion of the lungs causes cough, wheeze and dyspnoea; cerebral involvement has manifestations ranging from subtle neurological signs to coma. Gram-negative sepsis frequently complicates the picture.

Investigations

There is eosinophilia. Serology (ELISA) is helpful but definitive diagnosis depends on finding the larvae. The faeces should be examined microscopically for motile larvae; excretion is intermittent and so repeated examinations are necessary. Larvae may be found in jejunal aspirates or detected using the string test (p. 287). Larvae may also be cultured from faeces.

Management

A course of two doses of ivermectin (200 µg/kg), administered on successive days, is effective. Alternatively, albendazole is given orally (15 mg/kg twice daily for 3 days). A second course may be required. For the *Strongyloides* hyperinfection syndrome, ivermectin is given at 200 µg/kg for 5–7 days.

Ascaris lumbricoides (roundworm)

This pale yellow nematode is 20–35 cm long. Humans are infected by eating food contaminated with mature ova. *Ascaris* larvae hatch in the duodenum, migrate through the lungs, ascend the bronchial tree, are swallowed and mature in the small intestine. This tissue migration can provoke both local and general hypersensitivity reactions, with pneumonitis, eosinophilic granulomas, wheezing and urticaria.

Clinical features

Intestinal ascariasis causes symptoms ranging from vague abdominal pain to malnutrition. The large size of the adult worm and its tendency to aggregate and migrate cause obstructive complications. Tropical and subtropical areas are endemic for ascariasis, and here it causes up to 35% of all intestinal obstructions, most commonly in the terminal ileum. Obstruction can be complicated further by intussusception, volvulus, haemorrhagic infarction and perforation. Other complications include blockage of the bile or pancreatic duct and obstruction of the appendix by adult worms. Ascariasis in non-endemic areas has been associated with pig husbandry and may be caused by *Ascaris suum*, which is indistinguishable from (and possibly the same species as) *Ascaris lumbricoides*.

Investigations

The diagnosis is made microscopically by finding ova in the faeces. Adult worms are frequently expelled rectally or orally. Occasionally, the worms are demonstrated radiographically by a barium examination. There is eosinophilia.

Management

A single dose of albendazole (400 mg), pyrantel pamoate (11 mg/kg; maximum 1 g), or ivermectin (150–200 µg/kg), or alternatively mebendazole (100 mg twice daily for 3 days) treats intestinal ascariasis. Patients should be warned that they might expel numerous whole, large worms. Obstruction due to ascariasis should be treated with nasogastric suction, piperazine and intravenous fluids. Complete intestinal obstruction and its complications require urgent surgical intervention.

Prevention

Community chemotherapy programmes reduce *Ascaris* infection. The whole community can be treated every 3 months for several years. Alternatively, schoolchildren are targeted; treating them lowers the prevalence of ascariasis in the community.

Enterobius vermicularis (threadworm)

This helminth is common worldwide and affects mainly children. After the ova are swallowed, development takes place in the small intestine but the adult worms are found chiefly in the colon.

Clinical features

The female lays ova around the anus, causing intense itching, especially at night. The ova are often carried to the mouth on the fingers and so reinfection or human-to-human infection occurs (Fig. 11.49). In females, the genitalia may be involved. The adult worms may be seen moving on the buttocks or in the stool.

Investigations

Ova are detected in stool samples or by applying the adhesive surface of cellophane tape to the perianal skin in the morning. This is then examined on a glass slide under the microscope. A perianal swab, moistened with saline, also allows diagnosis.

Management

A single dose of mebendazole (100 mg), albendazole (400 mg), pyrantel pamoate (11 mg/kg) or piperazine (4 g) treats infection and is repeated after 2 weeks to control auto-reinfection. If infection recurs in a family, each member should be treated. All nightclothes and bed linen are laundered during treatment. Fingernails must be kept short and hands washed carefully before meals. Subsequent therapy is reserved for family members with recurrent infection.

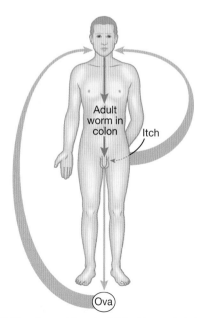

Fig. 11.49 Threadworm. Life cycle of *Enterobius vermicularis*.

Trichuris trichiura (whipworm)

Whipworm infections are common worldwide with poor hygiene. Infection follows ingestion of earth or food contaminated with ova, which have become infective after lying for 3 weeks or more in moist soil. The adult worm is 3–5 cm long and has a coiled anterior end resembling a whip. Whipworms inhabit the caecum, lower ileum, appendix, colon and anal canal. There are usually no symptoms, but intense infections in children may cause persistent diarrhoea or rectal prolapse, and growth retardation. The diagnosis is readily made by identifying ova in faeces. Treatment is with mebendazole in doses of 100 mg twice daily or albendazole 400 mg daily for 3 days for patients with light infections, and for 5–7 days for those with heavy infections.

Tissue-dwelling human nematodes

Filarial worms are tissue-dwelling nematodes. The larval stages are inoculated by biting mosquitoes or flies, each specific to a particular filarial species. The larvae develop into adult worms (2–50 cm long), which, after mating, produce millions of microfilariae (170–320 μm long) that migrate in blood or skin. The life cycle is completed when the vector takes up microfilariae by biting humans. In the insect, ingested microfilariae develop into infective larvae for inoculation in humans, normally the only host.

Disease is due to the host's immune response to the worms (both adult and microfilariae), particularly dying worms, and its pattern and severity vary with the site and stage of each species (Box 11.60). The worms are long-lived: microfilariae survive 2–3 years and adult worms 10–15 years. The infections are chronic and worst in individuals constantly reinfected.

Lymphatic filariasis

The filarial worms *Wuchereria bancrofti* and *Brugia malayi* infect approximately 120 million people globally and cause clinical outcomes ranging from subclinical infection to hydrocele and elephantiasis.

W. bancrofti is usually transmitted by night-biting culicine or anopheline mosquitoes (Fig. 11.50). The adult worms, 4–10 cm in length, live in the lymphatics, and the females produce microfilariae that circulate in large numbers in the peripheral blood, usually at night. The infection is widespread in tropical Africa, on the North African coast, in coastal areas of Asia, Indonesia and northern Australia, the South Pacific islands, the West Indies and also in North and South America.

i	**11.60 Pathogenicity of filarial infections depending on site and stage of worms**	
Worm species	**Adult worm**	**Microfilariae**
Wuchereria bancrofti and *Brugia malayi*	Lymphatic vessels+++	Blood− Pulmonary capillaries++
Loa loa	Subcutaneous+	Blood+
Onchocerca volvulus	Subcutaneous+	Skin+++ Eye+++
Mansonella perstans	Retroperitoneal−	Blood−
Mansonella streptocerca	Skin+	Skin++
(+++ severe; ++ moderate; + mild; − rarely pathogenic)		

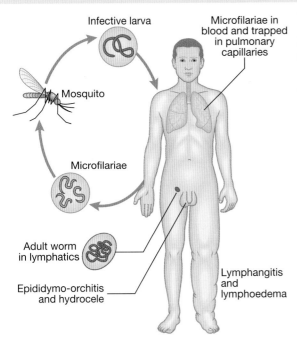

Fig. 11.50 *Wuchereria bancrofti* and *Brugia malayi*. Life cycle of organisms and pathogenesis of lymphatic filariasis.

B. malayi usually causes less severe disease than *W. bancrofti* and is transmitted by *Mansonia* or *Anopheles* mosquitoes in Indonesia, Borneo, Malaysia, Vietnam, South China, South India and Sri Lanka.

Pathology

Several factors contribute to the pathogenesis of lymphatic filariasis. Toxins released by adult worms cause lymphangiectasia; this dilatation of the lymphatic vessels leads to lymphatic dysfunction and the chronic clinical manifestations of lymphatic filariasis, lymphoedema and hydrocele. Death of the adult worm results in acute filarial lymphangitis. The filariae are symbiotically infected with rickettsia-like bacteria (*Wolbachia* spp.), and lipopolysaccharide released from *Wolbachia* triggers inflammation. Lymphatic obstruction persists after death of the adult worm. Secondary bacterial infections cause tissue destruction. The host response to microfilariae is central to the pathogenesis of tropical pulmonary eosinophilia.

Clinical features

Acute filarial lymphangitis presents with fever, pain, tenderness and erythema along the course of inflamed lymphatic vessels. Inflammation of the spermatic cord, epididymis and testis is common. Episodes last a few days but may recur several times a year. Temporary oedema becomes more persistent and regional lymph nodes enlarge. Progressive enlargement, coarsening, corrugation, fissuring and bacterial infection of the skin and subcutaneous tissue develop gradually, causing irreversible 'elephantiasis'. The scrotum may reach an enormous size. Chyluria and chylous effusions are milky and opalescent; on standing, fat globules rise to the top.

Acute lymphatic manifestations of filariasis must be differentiated from thrombophlebitis and infection. Oedema and lymphatic obstructive changes must be distinguished from congestive cardiac failure, malignancy, trauma and idiopathic abnormalities of the lymphatic system. Silicates absorbed from volcanic soil can also cause non-filarial elephantiasis.

Tropical pulmonary eosinophilia is a complication, seen mainly in India, due to microfilariae trapped in the pulmonary capillaries that are destroyed by allergic inflammation. Patients present with paroxysmal cough, wheeze and fever. If untreated, this may progress to debilitating chronic interstitial lung disease.

Investigations

In the earliest stages of lymphangitis, the diagnosis is made on clinical grounds, supported by eosinophilia and sometimes by positive filarial serology. Filarial infections cause the highest eosinophil counts of all helminthic infections.

Microfilariae can be found in the peripheral blood at night, and either are seen moving in a wet blood film or are detected by microfiltration of a sample of lysed blood. They are usually present in hydrocele fluid, which may occasionally yield an adult filaria. By the time elephantiasis develops, microfilariae become difficult to find. Calcified filariae may sometimes be demonstrable by radiography. Movement of adult worms can be seen on scrotal ultrasound. PCR-based tests for detection of *W. bancrofti* and *B. malayi* DNA from blood have been developed.

Indirect fluorescence and ELISA detect antibodies in over 95% of active cases and 70% of established elephantiasis. The test becomes negative 1–2 years after cure. Serological tests cannot distinguish the different filarial infections. Highly sensitive and specific, commercially available, immunochromatographic card tests detect circulating *W. bancrofti* antigen using fingerprick blood samples taken at any time of the day.

In tropical pulmonary eosinophilia, serology is strongly positive and IgE levels are massively elevated but circulating microfilariae are not found. The chest X-ray shows miliary changes or mottled opacities. Pulmonary function tests show a restrictive picture.

Management

Treatment is aimed at halting and reversing disease progression. Diethylcarbamazine (DEC, 2 mg/kg orally 3 times daily for 12 days, or 6 mg/kg as a single dose) kills microfilariae and adult worms. Most adverse effects seen with DEC treatment are due to the host response to dying microfilariae, which is directly proportional to the microfilarial load. The main symptoms are fever, headache, nausea, vomiting, arthralgia and prostration. These usually occur within 24–36 hours of the first dose of DEC. Antihistamines or glucocorticoids treat these allergic phenomena. Combining albendazole (400 mg) with ivermectin (200 μg/kg) in a single dose, with or without DEC (300 mg), is also highly effective in clearing the parasites. Treatment of *Wolbachia* with doxycycline (200 mg/day) for 4–8 weeks provides additional benefit by eliminating the bacteria; this leads to interruption of parasite embryogenesis. For tropical pulmonary eosinophilia, DEC for 14 days is the treatment of choice.

Chronic lymphatic pathology

Experience in India and Brazil shows that active management of chronic lymphatic pathology can alleviate symptoms. Patients should be taught meticulous skin care of their lymphoedematous limbs to prevent secondary bacterial and fungal infections. Tight bandaging, massage and bed rest with elevation of the affected limb help to control the lymphoedema. Prompt diagnosis and antibiotic therapy of bacterial cellulitis prevent further lymphatic damage and worsening of existing elephantiasis. Plastic surgery may be indicated in established elephantiasis. Relief can be obtained by removal of excess tissue but recurrences are probable

11

unless new lymphatic drainage is established. Hydroceles and chyluria can be repaired surgically.

Prevention

Treatment of the whole population in endemic areas with annual single-dose DEC (6 mg/kg), either alone or in combination with albendazole or ivermectin, can reduce filarial transmission. Mass treatment should be combined with mosquito control programmes.

Loiasis

Loiasis is caused by infection with the filaria *Loa loa*. The disease is endemic in forested and swampy parts of Western and Central Africa. The adult worms, 3–7 cm×4 mm, chiefly parasitise the subcutaneous tissue of humans, releasing larval microfilariae into the peripheral blood in the daytime. The vector is *Chrysops*, a forest-dwelling, day-biting fly.

The host response to *Loa loa* is usually absent or mild, so that the infection may be harmless. From time to time a short-lived, inflammatory, oedematous swelling (a Calabar swelling) is produced around an adult worm. Heavy infections, especially when treated, may cause encephalitis.

Clinical features

The infection is often symptomless. The incubation period is commonly over a year but may be just 3 months. The first sign is usually a Calabar swelling: an irritating, tense, localised swelling that may be painful, especially if it is near a joint. The swelling is generally on a limb; it measures a few centimetres in diameter but may be diffuse and extensive. It usually disappears after a few days but may persist for 2–3 weeks. Several swellings may appear at irregular intervals, often in adjacent sites. Sometimes, there is urticaria and pruritus elsewhere. Occasionally, a worm may be seen wriggling under the skin, especially that of an eyelid, and may cross the eye under the conjunctiva, taking many minutes to do so.

Investigations

Diagnosis is by demonstrating microfilariae in blood taken during the day, but they may not always be found in patients with Calabar swellings. Antifilarial antibodies are positive in 95% of patients and there is massive eosinophilia. Occasionally, a calcified worm may be seen on X-ray.

Management

DEC (see above) is curative, in a dose of 9–12 mg/kg daily, continued for 21 days. Treatment may precipitate a severe reaction in patients with a heavy microfilaraemia, characterised by fever, joint and muscle pain, and encephalitis; microfilaraemic patients should be given glucocorticoid cover.

Prevention

Building houses away from trees and having dwellings wire-screened reduce infections. Protective clothing and insect repellents are also useful. DEC in a dose of 5 mg/kg daily for 3 days each month is partially protective.

Onchocerciasis (river blindness)

Onchocerciasis results from infection by the filarial *Onchocerca volvulus*. The infection is conveyed by flies of the genus *Simulium*, which breed in rapidly flowing, well-aerated water. Adult flies inflict painful bites during the day, both inside and outside houses. While

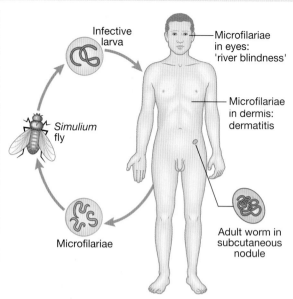

Fig. 11.51 *Onchocerca volvulus.* Life cycle of organism and pathogenesis of onchocerciasis.

feeding, they pick up the microfilariae, which mature into the infective larva and are transmitted to a new host in subsequent bites. Humans are the only known hosts (Fig. 11.51).

Onchocerciasis is endemic in sub-Saharan Africa, Yemen and a few foci in Central and South America. It is estimated that 26 million people are infected, of whom 500 000 are visually impaired and 270 000 blind. Due to onchocerciasis, huge tracts of fertile land lie virtually untilled and individuals and communities are impoverished.

Pathology

After inoculation of larvae by a bite, the worms mature in 2–4 months and live for up to 17 years in subcutaneous and connective tissues. At sites of trauma, over bony prominences and around joints, fibrosis may form nodules around adult worms, which otherwise cause no direct damage. Innumerable microfilariae, discharged by the female *O. volvulus*, move actively in these nodules and in the adjacent tissues. The microfilariae are widely distributed in the skin and may invade the eye. Live microfilariae elicit little tissue reaction but dead ones may cause severe allergic inflammation, leading to hyaline necrosis and loss of collagen and elastin. Death of microfilariae in the eye causes inflammation and may lead to blindness.

Clinical features

The infection may remain symptomless for months or years. The first symptom is usually itching, localised to one quadrant of the body and later becoming generalised and involving the eyes. Transient oedema of part or all of a limb is an early sign, followed by papular urticaria spreading gradually from the site of infection. This is difficult to see on dark skins, in which the most common signs are papules excoriated by scratching, spotty hyperpigmentation from resolving inflammation, and chronic changes of a rough, thickened or inelastic, wrinkled skin. Both infected and uninfected superficial lymph nodes enlarge and may hang down in folds of loose skin in the groin. Hydrocele, femoral hernias and scrotal elephantiasis can occur. Firm subcutaneous nodules of more than 1 cm in diameter (onchocercomas) occur in chronic infection.

Eye disease is most common in highly endemic areas and is associated with chronic heavy infections and nodules on the head. Early manifestations include itching, lacrimation and conjunctival injection. These cause conjunctivitis; sclerosing keratitis with pannus formation; uveitis, which may lead to glaucoma and cataract; and, less commonly, choroiditis and optic neuritis. Classically, 'snowflake' deposits are seen in the edges of the cornea.

Investigations

The finding of nodules or characteristic lesions of the skin or eyes in a patient from an endemic area, associated with eosinophilia, is suggestive. Skin snips or shavings, taken with a corneoscleral punch or scalpel blade from calf, buttock and shoulder, are placed in saline under a cover slip on a microscope slide and examined after 4 hours. Microfilariae are seen wriggling free in all but the lightest infections. Slit-lamp examination may reveal microfilariae moving in the anterior chamber of the eye or trapped in the cornea. A nodule may be removed and incised, showing the coiled, thread-like adult worm.

Filarial antibodies are positive in up to 95% of patients. Rapid strip tests to detect antibody or antigen are under clinical evaluation. When there is a strong suspicion of onchocerciasis but tests are negative, a provocative Mazzotti test, in which administration of 0.5–1.0 mg/kg of DEC exacerbates pruritus or dermatitis, strongly suggests onchocerciasis.

Management

Ivermectin is recommended, in a single dose of 100–200 μg/kg, repeated several times at 3-monthly intervals to prevent relapses. It kills microfilariae and has minimal toxicity. In the rare event of a severe reaction causing oedema or postural hypotension, prednisolone 20–30 mg may be given daily for 2 or 3 days. Ivermectin has little macrofilaricidal effect so that, 1 year after ivermectin treatment, skin microfilarial densities regain at least 20% of pre-treatment levels; repeated treatments are required for the lifespan of the adult worm. Eradication of *Wolbachia* with doxycycline (100 mg daily for 6 weeks) prevents worm reproduction.

Prevention

Mass treatment with ivermectin reduces community morbidity and slows the progression of eye disease but it does not clear worm infection. *Simulium* can be destroyed in its larval stage by the application of insecticide to streams. Long trousers, skirts and sleeves discourage the fly from biting.

Dracunculiasis (Guinea worm)

Infestation with the Guinea worm *Dracunculus medinensis* manifests when the female worm, over a metre long, emerges from the skin. Humans are infected by ingesting a small crustacean, *Cyclops*, which inhabits wells and ponds, and contains the infective larval stage of the worm. The worm was widely distributed across Africa and the Middle East but successful global eradication programmes have limited the infection to a few countries in sub-Saharan Africa. However, recent findings of dog dracunculiasis in Chad and Ethiopia pose a new threat to eradication efforts.

Management and prevention

Traditionally, the protruding worm is extracted by winding it out gently over several days on a matchstick. The worm must never be broken. Antibiotics for secondary infection and prophylaxis of tetanus are also required.

A global eradication campaign aims to provide clean drinking water and eradicate water fleas from drinking water by simple filtration of water through a plastic mesh filter and chemical treatment of water supplies.

Other filariases

Mansonella perstans

This filarial worm is transmitted by the midges *Culicoides austeni* and *C. grahami*. It is common throughout equatorial Africa, as far south as Zambia, and also in Trinidad and parts of northern and eastern South America.

M. perstans has never been proven to cause disease but it may be responsible for a persistent eosinophilia and occasional allergic manifestations. *M. perstans* is resistant to ivermectin and DEC, and the infection may persist for many years.

Dirofilaria immitis

This dog heartworm infects humans, causing skin and lung lesions. It is not uncommon in the USA, Japan and Australia.

Zoonotic nematodes

Trichinosis (trichinellosis)

Trichinella spiralis is a nematode that parasitises rats and pigs, and is transmitted to humans by ingestion of partially cooked infected pork, particularly sausage or ham, or occasionally by bear meat. Symptoms result from invasion of intestinal submucosa by ingested larvae, which develop into adult worms, and the secondary invasion of striated muscle by fresh larvae produced by these adult worms. Outbreaks have occurred in countries where pork is eaten.

Clinical features

The clinical features of trichinosis are determined by the larval numbers. A light infection with a few worms may be asymptomatic; a heavy infection causes nausea and diarrhoea 24–48 hours after the infected meal. A few days later, the symptoms associated with larval invasion predominate: there is fever and oedema of the face, eyelids and conjunctivae; invasion of the diaphragm may cause pain, cough and dyspnoea; and involvement of the muscles of the limbs, chest and mouth causes stiffness, pain and tenderness in affected muscles. Larval migration may cause acute myocarditis and encephalitis. Eosinophilia is observed after the second week. An intense infection may prove fatal but those who survive recover completely.

Investigations

Frequently, people who have eaten infected pork from a common source develop symptoms at about the same time. Biopsy from the deltoid or gastrocnemius muscle after the third week of symptoms may reveal encysted larvae. Serological tests are also helpful.

Management

Treatment is with albendazole (400 mg twice daily for 8–14 days) or mebendazole (200–400 mg three times daily for 3 days, followed by 400–500 mg three times daily for 10 days). Treatment commenced early in infection kills newly formed adult worms in the submucosa and reduces the number of larvae reaching the

11

muscles. Glucocorticoids are necessary to control the serious effects of acute inflammation.

Anisakiasis (herring worm)

This infection is caused by the larvae of a fish nematode (*Anisakis simplex* or *Pseudoterranova decipiens*) and is associated with consumption of under-cooked fish or squid. The parasite cannot complete its life cycle in humans but larval ingestion is associated with pharyngeal tingling, abdominal pain, diarrhoea and vomiting. Diagnosis is made by identification of the larva by patients or endoscopists, and albendazole (400 mg twice a day for 5 days) can be used in treatment if larvae are not removed.

Cutaneous larva migrans

Cutaneous larva migrans (CLM) is the most common linear lesion seen in travellers (Fig. 11.52). Intensely pruritic, linear, serpiginous lesions result from the larval migration of the dog hookworm (*Ancylostoma caninum*). The track moves across the skin at a rate of 2–3 cm/day. This contrasts with the fast-moving transient rash of *Strongyloides* (p. 289). Although the larvae of dog hookworms frequently infect humans, they do not usually develop into the adult form. The most common site for CLM is the foot but elbows, breasts and buttocks may be affected. Most patients with CLM have recently visited a beach where the affected part was exposed. The diagnosis is clinical. Treatment may be local with 12-hourly application of 15% thiabendazole cream, or systemic with a single dose of albendazole (400 mg) or ivermectin (150–200 µg/kg).

Angiostrongylus cantonensis

The rat lungworm infects humans in Asia and the Pacific basin, via infected snails or contaminated water. It causes eosinophilic meningitis. The role of combination therapy with glucocorticoids and albendazole remains controversial.

Fig. 11.52 Cutaneous larva migrans. *Courtesy of Dr Ravi Gowda, Royal Hallamshire Hospital, Sheffield.*

Gnathostomiasis

Gnathostomiasis is a nematode infection that occurs predominantly in South-east Asia and is due to *Gnathostoma spinigerum*. It also occurs in other parts of Asia, Central and South America, and Africa. Humans are infected by the larvae from intermediate hosts (raw or under-cooked freshwater fish, shrimps and frogs) and are not definitive hosts, so the life cycle is incomplete. Pruritic, painful, migratory nodules appear 3–4 weeks after ingestion due to larval migration. Complications include cough, visual disturbance, eosinophilic meningitis or encephalitis. Serology confirms diagnosis and the preferred treatment is albendazole (400 mg twice daily) for 21 days, but its role in visual or neurological disease is uncertain as it may increase larval migration.

Trematodes (flukes)

These leaf-shaped worms are parasitic to humans and animals. Their complex life cycles may involve one or more intermediate hosts, often freshwater molluscs.

Schistosomiasis

Schistosomiasis is a major cause of morbidity in the tropics. The species commonly causing disease in humans are: *Schistosoma haematobium*, *S. mansoni*, *S. japonicum*, *S. mekongi* and *S. intercalatum*. *S. haematobium* is sometimes called bilharzia or bilharziasis. Schistosome eggs have been found in Egyptian mummies.

The life cycle is shown in Figure 11.53A. The ovum is passed in the urine or faeces of infected individuals and gains access to fresh water, where the ciliated miracidium inside it is liberated; it enters its intermediate host, a species of freshwater snail, and multiplies. Large numbers of fork-tailed cercariae are then liberated into the water, where they may survive for 2–3 days. Cercariae can penetrate the skin or the mucous membrane of the mouth of humans. They transform into schistosomulae and moult as they pass through the lungs; then they are carried by the blood stream to the liver, and so to the portal vein, where they mature. The male worm is up to 20 mm in length and the more slender cylindrical female, usually enfolded longitudinally by the male, is longer (Fig. 11.53B). Within 4–6 weeks of infection, they migrate to the venules draining the pelvic viscera, where the females deposit ova.

Pathology

Disease is usually due to passage of eggs through mucosa and to the granulomatous reaction to eggs deposited in tissues. The eggs of *S. haematobium* pass mainly through the bladder wall but may also involve the rectum, seminal vesicles, vagina, cervix and uterine tubes. *S. mansoni* and *S. japonicum* eggs pass mainly through the wall of the lower bowel or are carried to the liver. The most serious, although rare, site of ectopic egg deposition is the CNS. Granulomas are composed of macrophages, eosinophils, and epithelioid and giant cells around an ovum. Later, there is fibrosis and eggs calcify, which is often visible radiologically. Eggs of *S. haematobium* may leave the vesical plexus and be carried directly to the lung. Those of *S. mansoni* and *S. japonicum* may also reach the lungs after the development of portal hypertension and consequent portasystemic collateral circulation. Egg deposition in the pulmonary vasculature, and the resultant host response, can lead to pulmonary hypertension.

Fig. 11.53 *Schistosoma*. A Life cycle. B Scanning electron micrograph of adult schistosome worms, showing the larger male worm embracing the thinner female.

Clinical features

Recent travellers, especially those overlanding through Africa, may present with allergic manifestations and eosinophilia; residents of schistosomiasis-endemic areas are more likely to present with chronic urinary tract pathology or portal hypertension.

During the early stages of infection, there may be itching lasting 1–2 days at the site of cercarial penetration ('swimmer's itch'). After a symptom-free period of 3–5 weeks, acute schistosomiasis (Katayama syndrome) may present with allergic manifestations, such as urticaria, fever, muscle aches, abdominal pain, headaches, cough and sweating. On examination, hepatomegaly, splenomegaly, lymphadenopathy and pneumonia may be present. These allergic phenomena may be severe in infections with *S. mansoni* and *S. japonicum*, but are rare with *S. haematobium*. The features subside after 1–2 weeks.

Chronic schistosomiasis is due to egg deposition and occurs months to years after infection. The symptoms and signs depend on the intensity of infection and the species of infecting schistosome (Box 11.61).

Schistosoma haematobium

Humans are the only natural hosts of *S. haematobium*, which is highly endemic in Egypt and East Africa, and occurs throughout Africa and the Middle East (Fig. 11.54). Infection can be acquired after a brief exposure, such as swimming in freshwater lakes in Africa.

Painless terminal haematuria is usually the first and most common symptom. Frequency of micturition follows, due to bladder neck obstruction. Later, frequent urinary tract infections, bladder or ureteric stones, hydronephrosis, and ultimately renal failure with a contracted calcified bladder may occur. Pain is often felt in the iliac fossa or in the loin, and radiates to the groin. In several endemic areas, there is a strong epidemiological

i	**11.61 Pathogenesis of schistosomiasis**	
Time	***Schistosoma haematobium***	***S. mansoni* and *S. japonicum***
Cercarial penetration		
Days	Papular dermatitis at site of penetration	As for *S. haematobium*
Larval migration and maturation		
Weeks	Pneumonitis, myositis, hepatitis, fever, 'serum sickness', eosinophilia, seroconversion	As for *S. haematobium*
Early egg deposition		
Months	Cystitis, haematuria	Colitis, granulomatous hepatitis, acute portal hypertension
	Ectopic granulomatous lesions: skin, CNS etc. Immune complex glomerulonephritis	As for *S. haematobium*
Late egg deposition		
Years	Fibrosis and calcification of ureters, bladder: bacterial infection, calculi, hydronephrosis, carcinoma Pulmonary granulomas and pulmonary hypertension	Colonic polyposis and strictures, periportal fibrosis, portal hypertension As for *S. haematobium*

association of *S. haematobium* infection with squamous cell carcinoma of the bladder. Disease of the seminal vesicles may lead to haematospermia. Females may develop schistosomal papillomas of the vulva, and schistosomal lesions of the cervix may be mistaken for cancer. Intestinal symptoms may follow

11

S. mansoni   S. intercalatum

S. haematobium   S. japonicum   S. mekongi

Fig. 11.54 Geographical distribution of schistosomiasis. *From Cook GC, ed. Manson's tropical diseases, 20th edn. Saunders, Elsevier Inc.; 1995.*

Fig. 11.55 Ova of *Schistosoma haematobium* in urine. Note the terminal spike.

involvement of the bowel wall. Ectopic worms cause skin or spinal cord lesions.

The severity of *S. haematobium* infection varies greatly and many with a light infection are asymptomatic. However, as adult worms can live for 20 years or more and lesions may progress, these patients should always be treated.

Schistosoma mansoni

S. mansoni is endemic throughout Africa, the Middle East, Venezuela, Brazil and the Caribbean (Fig. 11.54).

Characteristic symptoms begin 2 months or more after infection. They may be slight – no more than malaise – or consist of abdominal pain and frequent stools that contain blood-stained mucus. With severe advanced disease, increased discomfort from rectal polyps may be experienced. The early hepatomegaly is reversible but portal hypertension may cause massive splenomegaly, fatal haematemesis from oesophageal varices, or progressive ascites (p. 868). Liver function is initially preserved because the pathology is fibrotic rather than cirrhotic. *S. mansoni* and other schistosome infections predispose to the carriage of *Salmonella*, in part because *Salmonella* may attach to the schistosomes and in part because shared antigens on schistosomes may induce immunological tolerance to *Salmonella*.

Schistosoma japonicum, S. mekongi and S. intercalatum

In addition to humans, the adult worm of *S. japonicum* infects the dog, rat, field mouse, water buffalo, ox, cat, pig, horse and sheep. Although other *Schistosoma* spp. can infect species other than humans, the non-human reservoir seems to be particularly important only in transmission for *S. japonicum*. *S. japonicum* is prevalent in the Yellow River and Yangtze–Jiang basins in China, where the infection is a major public health problem. It also has a focal distribution in the Philippines, Indonesia and Thailand (Fig. 11.54). The related *S. mekongi* occurs in Laos, Thailand and Myanmar, and *S. intercalatum* in West and Central Africa.

The pathology of *S. japonicum* is similar to that of *S. mansoni*, but as this worm produces more eggs, the lesions tend to be more extensive and widespread. The clinical features resemble those of severe infection with *S. mansoni*, with added neurological features. The small and large bowel may be affected, and hepatic fibrosis with splenic enlargement is usual. Deposition of eggs or worms in the CNS, especially in the brain or spinal cord, causes symptoms in about 5% of infections, notably epilepsy, blindness, hemiplegia or paraplegia.

Investigations

There is marked eosinophilia. Serological tests (ELISA) are useful as screening tests but remain positive after treatment.

In *S. haematobium* infection, dipstick urine testing shows blood and albumin. The eggs can be found by microscopic examination of the centrifuged deposit of terminal stream urine (Fig. 11.55). Ultrasound assesses the urinary tract; bladder wall thickening, hydronephrosis and bladder calcification can be detected. Cystoscopy reveals 'sandy' patches, bleeding mucosa and later distortion.

In a heavy infection with *S. mansoni* or *S. japonicum*, the characteristic egg with its lateral spine can usually be found in the stool. When the infection is light or of long duration, a rectal biopsy can be examined. Sigmoidoscopy may show inflammation or bleeding. Biopsies should be examined for ova.

Management

The object of therapy is to kill the adult schistosomes and stop egg-laying. Praziquantel (20 mg/kg orally twice daily for 1 day) is the drug of choice for all forms of schistosomiasis except *S. japonicum* and *S. mekongi*, for which 60 mg/kg (20 mg for 3 doses) is recommended. The drug produces parasitological cure in 80% of treated individuals and over 90% reduction in egg counts in the remainder. Side-effects are uncommon but include nausea and abdominal pain. Praziquantel therapy in early infection reverses hepatomegaly, bladder wall thickening and granulomas.

Surgery may be required to deal with residual lesions such as ureteric stricture, small fibrotic urinary bladders, or granulomatous masses in the brain or spinal cord. Removal of rectal papillomas by diathermy or by other means may provide symptomatic relief.

Prevention

No single means of controlling schistosomiasis has been established to date. The life cycle is terminated if fresh water containing the snail host is not contaminated by ova-containing urine or faeces. The provision of latrines and of a safe water supply, however, remains a major problem in rural areas throughout the

i | **11.62 Diseases caused by flukes in the bile duct**

	Clonorchiasis	Opisthorchiasis	Fascioliasis
Parasite	*Clonorchis sinensis*	*Opisthorchis felineus*	*Fasciola hepatica*
Other mammalian hosts	Dogs, cats, pigs	Dogs, cats, foxes, pigs	Sheep, cattle
Mode of spread	Ova in faeces, water	As for *C. sinensis*	Ova in faeces on to wet pasture
1st intermediate host	Snails	Snails	Snails
2nd intermediate host	Freshwater fish	Freshwater fish	Encysts on vegetation
Geographical distribution	Far East, especially South China	Far East, especially North-east Thailand	Cosmopolitan, including UK
Pathology	*Escherichia coli* cholangitis, abscesses, biliary carcinoma	As for *C. sinensis*	Toxaemia, cholangitis, eosinophilia
Symptoms	Often symptom-free, recurrent jaundice	As for *C. sinensis*	Unexplained fever, tender liver, may be ectopic, e.g. subcutaneous fluke
Diagnosis	Ova in stool or duodenal aspirate	As for *C. sinensis*	As for *C. sinensis*, also serology
Prevention	Cook fish	Cook fish	Avoid contaminated watercress
Treatment	Praziquantel 25 mg/kg 3 times daily for 2 days	As for *C. sinensis* but for 1 day only	Triclabendazole 10 mg/kg single dose; repeat treatment may be required*

*In the UK, available from the Hospital for Tropical Diseases, London.

11

tropics. Furthermore, *S. japonicum* has so many hosts besides humans that latrines would have little impact. Population mass treatment annually helps prevent *S. haematobium* and *S. mansoni* infection but so far has had little success with *S. japonicum*. Targeting the intermediate host, the snail, is problematic and has not, on its own, proved successful. For personal protection, contact with infected water must be avoided.

Liver flukes

Liver flukes infect at least 20 million people and remain an important public health problem in endemic areas. They are associated with abdominal pain, hepatomegaly and relapsing cholangitis. *Clonorchis sinensis* and *Opisthorchis felineus* are major aetiological agents of bile duct cancer. The three major liver flukes have similar life cycles and pathologies, as outlined in Box 11.62.

Other flukes of medical importance include lung and intestinal flukes (see Box 11.58).

Cestodes (tapeworms)

Cestodes are ribbon-shaped worms that inhabit the intestinal tract. They have no alimentary system and absorb nutrients through the tegumental surface. The anterior end, or scolex, has suckers for attaching to the host. From the scolex, a series of progressively developing segments arise, the proglottides, which may continue to show active movements when shed. Cross-fertilisation takes place between segments. Ova, present in large numbers in mature proglottides, remain viable for weeks, and during this period they may be consumed by the intermediate host. Larvae liberated from the ingested ova pass into the tissues of the intermediate host, forming larval cysticerci.

Tapeworms cause two distinct patterns of disease: either intestinal infection or systemic cysticercosis (Fig. 11.56). *Taenia saginata* (beef tapeworm), *Taenia asiatica* and *Diphyllobothrium latum* (fish tapeworm) cause only intestinal infection in humans, following ingestion of intermediate hosts. *Taenia solium* causes intestinal infection if a cysticerci-containing intermediate host

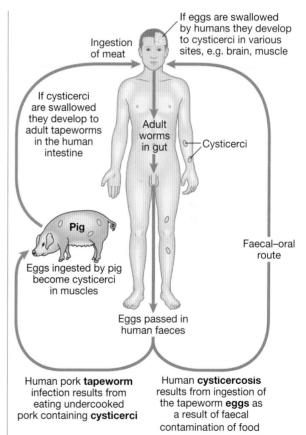

Human pork **tapeworm** infection results from eating undercooked pork containing **cysticerci**

Human **cysticercosis** results from ingestion of the tapeworm **eggs** as a result of faecal contamination of food

Fig. 11.56 Cysticercosis. Life cycle of *Taenia solium*.

is ingested, and cysticercosis (systemic infection from larval migration) if ova are ingested. *Echinococcus granulosus* (dog tapeworm) does not cause human intestinal infection, but causes hydatid disease (which is analogous to cysticercosis) following ingestion of ova and subsequent larval migration.

Intestinal tapeworm

Humans acquire tapeworm by eating under-cooked beef infected with the larval stage of *T. saginata*, under-cooked pork containing the larval stage of *T. solium* or *T. asiatica*, or under-cooked freshwater fish containing larvae of *D. latum*. Usually, only one adult tapeworm is present in the gut but up to 10 have been reported. The ova of all the three *Taenia* are indistinguishable microscopically. However, examination of scolex and proglottides can differentiate them: *T. solium* has a rostellum and two rows of hooklets on the scolex, and discharges multiple proglottides (3–5) attached together with lower degrees of uterine branching (approximately 10); *T. saginata* has only four suckers in its scolex, and discharges single proglottids with greater uterine branching (up to 30); *T. asiatica* has a rostellum without hooks on its scolex and is difficult to differentiate from *T. saginata*, except that there are fewer uterine branches (16–21).

Taenia solium

T. solium, the pork tapeworm, is common in central Europe, South Africa, South America and parts of Asia. It is not as large as *T. saginata*. The adult worm is found only in humans following the ingestion of pork containing cysticerci. Intestinal infection is treated with praziquantel (5–10 mg/kg) or niclosamide (2 g), both as a single dose, or alternatively with nitazoxanide (500 mg twice daily for 3 days). These are followed by a mild laxative (after 1–2 hours) to prevent retrograde intestinal autoinfection. Cooking pork well prevents intestinal infection. Great care must be taken while attending a patient harbouring an adult worm to avoid ingestion of ova or segments.

Taenia saginata

Infection with *T. saginata* occurs in all parts of the world. The adult worm may be several metres long and produces little or no intestinal upset in human beings, but identification of segments in the faeces or on underclothing may distress the patient. Ova may be found in the stool. Praziquantel is the drug of choice; niclosamide or nitazoxanide is an alternative. Prevention depends on efficient meat inspection and the thorough cooking of beef.

Taenia asiatica

T. asiatica is a newly recognised species of *Taenia*, restricted to Asia. It is acquired by eating uncooked meat or viscera of pigs. Clinical features and treatment are similar to those of *T. saginata*.

Cysticercosis

Human cysticercosis is acquired by ingesting *T. solium* tapeworm ova, from either contaminated fingers or food (Fig. 11.56). The larvae are liberated from eggs in the stomach, penetrate the intestinal mucosa and are carried to many parts of the body, where they develop and form cysticerci, 0.5–1 cm cysts that contain the head of a young worm. They do not grow further or migrate. Common locations are the subcutaneous tissue, skeletal muscles and brain (Fig. 11.57).

Clinical features

Superficial cysts can be palpated under the skin or mucosa as pea-like ovoid bodies, but cause few or no symptoms and will eventually die and become calcified.

Fig. 11.57 Neurocysticercosis. T2-weighted axial image of the brain showing multiple lesions of neurocysticercosis (large arrows show the largest lesions).

Heavy brain infections, especially in children, may cause features of encephalitis. More commonly, however, cerebral signs do not occur until the larvae die, 5–20 years later. Epilepsy, including new-onset focal seizures, personality changes, staggering gait and signs of hydrocephalus are the most common features.

Investigations

Calcified cysts in muscles can be recognised radiologically. In the brain, however, less calcification takes place and larvae are only occasionally visible by plain X-ray; CT or magnetic resonance imaging (MRI) will usually show them. Epileptic fits starting in adult life suggest the possibility of cysticercosis if the patient has lived in or travelled to an endemic area. The subcutaneous tissue should be palpated and any nodule excised for histology. Radiological examination of the skeletal muscles may be helpful. Antibody detection is available for serodiagnosis.

Management and prevention

Albendazole (15 mg/kg daily for a minimum of 8 days) has now become the drug of choice for parenchymal neurocysticercosis. Praziquantel (50 mg/kg in 3 divided doses daily for 10 days) is another option. Prednisolone (10 mg 3 times daily) is also given for 14 days, starting 1 day before the albendazole or praziquantel. In addition, antiepileptic drugs should be given until the reaction in the brain has subsided. Operative intervention is indicated for hydrocephalus. Studies from India and Peru suggest that most small, solitary cerebral cysts will resolve without treatment.

Echinococcus granulosus (*Taenia echinococcus*) and hydatid disease

Dogs are the definitive hosts of the tiny tapeworm *E. granulosus*. The larval stage, a hydatid cyst, normally occurs in sheep, cattle,

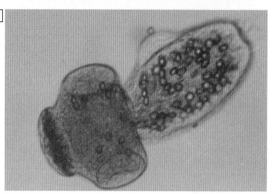

Fig. 11.58 Hydatid disease. A Life cycle of *Echinococcus granulosus*. B Daughter cysts removed at surgery. C Within the daughter cysts are the protoscolices.

camels and other animals that are infected from contaminated pastures or water. By handling a dog or drinking contaminated water, humans may ingest eggs (Fig. 11.58). The embryo is liberated from the ovum in the small intestine and invades the blood stream, spreading to the liver. The resultant cyst grows very slowly, sometimes intermittently. It is composed of an enveloping fibrous pericyst, laminated hyaline membrane (ectocyst) and inner germinal layers (endocyst) that give rise to daughter cysts, or a germinating cystic brood capsule in which larvae (protoscolices) develop. Over time, some cysts calcify and become non-viable. The disease is common in the Middle East, North and East Africa, Australia and Argentina. Foci of infection persist in the UK in rural Wales and Scotland. *E. multilocularis*, which has a cycle between foxes and voles, causes a similar but more severe infection, 'alveolar hydatid disease', which invades the liver like cancer.

Clinical features

A hydatid cyst is typically acquired in childhood and, after growing for years, may cause pressure symptoms. These vary, depending on the site involved. In nearly 75% of patients with hydatid disease, the right lobe of the liver is invaded and contains a single cyst. In others, a cyst may be found in lung, bone, brain or elsewhere.

Investigations

The diagnosis depends on the clinical, radiological and ultrasound findings in a patient that has close contact with dogs in an endemic area. Complement fixation and ELISA are positive in 70–90% of patients.

Management and prevention

Hydatid cysts should be excised wherever possible. Great care is taken to avoid spillage and cavities are sterilised with 0.5% silver nitrate or 2.7% sodium chloride. Albendazole (400 mg twice daily for 3 months) should also be used and is often combined with PAIR (percutaneous puncture, aspiration, injection of scolicidal agent and re-aspiration). Praziquantel (20 mg/kg twice daily for 14 days) also kills protoscolices perioperatively.

Prevention is difficult when there is a close association with dogs. Personal hygiene, satisfactory disposal of carcasses, meat inspection and deworming of dogs reduces the prevalence of disease.

Other tapeworms

Other cestodes' adult or larval stages may infect humans. Sparganosis is a condition in which an immature worm develops in humans, usually subcutaneously, as a result of eating or applying to the skin the secondary or tertiary intermediate host, such as frogs or snakes.

Ectoparasites

Ectoparasites only interact with the outermost surfaces of the host; see also page 1241.

Jiggers (tungiasis)

This is widespread in tropical America and Africa, and is caused by the sand flea *Tunga penetrans*. The pregnant flea burrows into the skin around toes and produces large numbers of eggs.

The burrows are intensely irritating and the whole inflammatory nodule should be removed with a sterile needle. Secondary infection of lesions is common.

Myiasis

Myiasis is due to skin infestation with larvae of the South American botfly, *Dermatobia hominis*, or the African tumbu fly, *Cordylobia anthropophaga*. The larvae develop in a subcutaneous space with a central sinus. This orifice is the air source for the larvae, and periodically the larval respiratory spiracles protrude through the sinus. Patients with myiasis feel movement within the larval burrow and can experience intermittent sharp, lancinating pains. Myiasis is diagnosed clinically and should be suspected with any furuncular lesion accompanied by pain and a crawling sensation in the skin. The larva may be suffocated by blocking the respiratory orifice with petroleum jelly and gently removing it with tweezers. Secondary infection of myiasis is rare and rapid healing follows removal of intact larvae.

Fungal infections

Fungal infections, or mycoses, are classified as superficial, subcutaneous or systemic (deep), depending on the degree of tissue invasion. They are caused by filamentous fungi (moulds), by yeasts or by fungi that vary between these two forms, depending on environmental conditions (dimorphic fungi; Fig. 11.59).

Superficial mycoses

Superficial cutaneous fungal infections caused by dermatophyte fungi are described in Chapter 29.

Candidiasis (thrush)

Superficial candidiasis is caused by *Candida* spp., mainly *C. albicans*. Manifestations include oropharyngeal (pp. 790 and 1240) and vaginal candidiasis ('thrush'), intertrigo and chronic paronychia. Superficial candidiasis often follows antibiotic therapy. Intertrigo is characterised by inflammation in skin folds with surrounding 'satellite lesions'. Chronic paronychia is associated with frequent wetting of the hands. Superficial candidiasis is treated mainly with topical azoles (p. 126), oral azoles being reserved for refractory or recurrent disease. Severe oropharyngeal and oesophageal candidiasis is a consequence of CD4[+] T-lymphocyte depletion/dysfunction, as in HIV infection (p. 316). Recurrent vaginal or penile candidiasis may be a manifestation of diabetes mellitus. Rarely, mutations in the autoimmune regulator gene (*AIRE*) or signal transducer and activator of transcription 1 (*STAT1*) cause a syndrome of chronic mucocutaneous candidiasis (p. 689). This is characterised by *Candida* infections of skin, mucosa and nails, with hyperkeratotic nails and erythematous periungual skin. Patients have cell-mediated immune defects against *Candida* and may have polyendocrinopathy and autoimmune features.

Subcutaneous mycoses

Chromoblastomycosis

Chromoblastomycosis is a predominantly tropical or subtropical disease caused by environmental dematiaceous (dark-pigmented) fungi, most commonly *Fonsecaea pedrosoi*. Other causes include *F. compacta*, *Cladophialophora carrionii* and *Phialophora verrucosa*. The disease is a cutaneous/subcutaneous mycosis acquired by traumatic inoculation. Commonly affected areas

Filamentous fungi (moulds)	Dimorphic fungi	Yeasts
Characterised by the production of elongated, cylindrical, often septate cells (hyphae) and conidia (spores)	Exist in filamentous (top) or yeast (bottom) form, depending on environmental conditions	Characterised by the production of oval or round cells, which reproduce by binary fission (budding)
Examples: • *Aspergillus* spp. (*A. fumigatus* shown here) • *Fusarium* spp. • Dermatophyte fungi (*Tricophyton* spp., *Microsporum* spp. etc.) • Mucorales	Examples: • *Histoplasma capsulatum*, *Coccidioides immitis*, *Paracoccidioides brasiliensis* (shown here), *Blastomyces dermatidis* • *Sporothrix schenkii* • *Talaromyces marneffei* • *Malassezia* spp.	Examples: • *Candida* spp.* • *Cryptococcus* spp. (*C. neoformans* shown here)

Fig. 11.59 Classification of medically important fungi. Fungal classification is based on simple morphological characteristics. *Pneumocystis jirovecii* is morphologically distinct from other fungi and does not fit into this classification. *Although *Candida albicans* exists in a number of forms, including filamentous (hyphae and pseudohyphae), it is generally encountered in its yeast form so is classified in this category. *Insets (dimorphic fungi) Courtesy of Beatriz Gomez and Angela Restrepo, CIB, Medellín, Colombia.*

include the foot, ankle and lower leg. Lesions may start several months after the initial injury, and medical attention is often sought several years later. The initial lesion is a papule. Further papules develop and coalesce to form irregular plaques. Nodular lesions may produce a characteristic 'cauliflower' appearance.

Diagnosis is by histopathological examination of infected material, which shows dematiaceous, rounded, thick-walled 'sclerotic bodies' with septa at right angles to each other. The aetiological agent is confirmed by culture. Therapeutic approaches include antifungal agents, cryosurgery and surgical excision, alone or in combination, but the optimal therapy is unknown. Itraconazole and terbinafine are the most effective antifungal agents. However, posaconazole has also been used with a good outcome.

Mycetoma (eumycetoma and actinomycetoma)

Mycetoma is a chronic suppurative infection of the deep soft tissues and bones, most commonly of the limbs but also of the abdominal or chest wall or head. It is caused by either filamentous fungi, Eumyces (eumycetoma – 40%) or aerobic Actinomycetes (actinomycetoma – 60%). Many fungi cause eumycetomas, the most common being *Madurella mycetomatis*, *M. grisea*, *Leptosphaeria senegalensis* and *Scedosporium apiospermum*; causes of actinomycetoma include *Nocardia, Streptomyces* and *Actinomadura* spp. Both groups produce characteristically coloured 'grains' (microcolonies), the colour depending on the organism (black grains – eumycetoma, red and yellow grains – actinomycetoma, white grains – either). The disease occurs mostly in the tropics and subtropics.

Clinical features

The disease is acquired by inoculation (e.g. from a thorn) and most commonly affects the foot (Madura foot). Mycetoma begins as a painless swelling at the implantation site, which becomes chronic and progressive, grows and spreads steadily within the soft tissues, eventually extending into bone. Nodules develop under the epidermis and these rupture, revealing sinuses through which grains may be discharged. Sinuses heal with scarring, while fresh sinuses appear elsewhere. Deeper tissue invasion and bone involvement are less rapid and extensive in eumycetoma than actinomycetoma. There is little pain and usually no fever or lymphadenopathy, but there is progressive disability.

Investigations

Diagnosis of mycetoma involves identification of grains in pus, and/or histopathological examination of tissue. Culture is necessary for species identification and susceptibility testing. Serological tests are not available.

Management

Eumycetoma is usually treated with a combination of surgery and antifungal therapy. Antifungal susceptibility testing, if available, is recommended, although clinical outcome does not necessarily correspond to in vitro test results. Itraconazole and ketoconazole (both 200–400 mg/day) are used most commonly. Success has also been reported with terbinafine monotherapy, and refractory cases have responded to voriconazole or posaconazole. Amphotericin B is not usually effective. Therapy is continued for 6–12 months or longer. In extreme cases, amputation may be required. Actinomycetoma is treated with prolonged antibiotic combinations, most commonly streptomycin and dapsone. Dapsone is replaced by co-trimoxazole in intolerance or refractory

disease. Success has also been reported wth co-trimoxazole plus amikacin, with rifampicin added in difficult cases and to prevent recurrence.

Phaeohyphomycosis

Phaeohyphomycoses are a heterogeneous group of fungal diseases caused by a large number (more than 70) of dematiaceous fungi. In phaeohyphomycosis, the tissue form of the fungus is predominantly mycelial (filamentous), as opposed to eumycetoma (grain) or chromoblastomycosis (sclerotic body). Disease may be superficial, subcutaneous or deep. The most serious manifestation is cerebral phaeohyphomycosis, which presents with a ring-enhancing, space-occupying cerebral lesion. Optimal therapy for this condition has not been established but usually consists of neurosurgical intervention and antifungal (usually triazole) therapy. Causative agents are *Cladophialophora bantiana*, *Fonsecaea* spp. and *Rhinocladiella mackenziei*, which occurs mainly in the Middle East and is usually fatal.

Sporotrichosis

Sporotrichosis is caused by *Sporothrix schenckii*, a dimorphic fungal saprophyte of plants in tropical and subtropical regions. Disease is caused by dermal inoculation of the fungus, usually from a thorn (occasionally from a cat scratch). In fixed cutaneous sporotrichosis, a subcutaneous nodule develops at the site of infection and subsequently ulcerates, with a purulent discharge. The disease may then spread along the cutaneous lymphatic channels, resulting in multiple cutaneous nodules that ulcerate and discharge (lymphocutaneous sporotrichosis). Rarer forms include cutaneous disease presenting with arthritis. Later, draining sinuses may form. Pulmonary sporotrichosis occurs as a result of inhalation of the conidia (spores) and causes chronic cavitary fibronodular disease with haemoptysis and constitutional symptoms. Disseminated disease may occur, especially in patients with HIV.

Investigations

Typical yeast forms detected on histology confirm diagnosis but are rarely seen; the fungus can also be cultured from biopsy specimen. A latex agglutination test detects *S. schenckii* antibodies in serum.

Management

Cutaneous and lymphocutaneous disease is treated with itraconazole (200–400 mg daily, prescribed as the oral solution, which has better bioavailability than the capsule formulation) for 3–6 months. Alternative agents include a saturated solution of potassium iodide (SSKI, given orally), initiated with 5 drops and increased to 40–50 drops 3 times daily, or terbinafine (500 mg twice daily). Localised hyperthermia may be used in pregnancy (to avoid azole use). Osteoarticular disease requires a longer course of therapy (at least 12 months). Severe or life-threatening disease is treated with amphotericin B (lipid formulation preferred).

Systemic mycoses

Aspergillosis

Aspergillosis is an opportunistic systemic mycosis, which affects the respiratory tract predominantly. It is described on page 596.

11

Candidiasis

Systemic candidiasis is an opportunistic mycosis caused by *Candida* spp. The most common cause is *C. albicans*. Other agents include *C. dubliniensis*, *C. glabrata*, *C. krusei*, *C. parapsilosis* and *C. tropicalis*. *Candida* species identification often predicts susceptibility to fluconazole: *C. krusei* is universally resistant, many *C. glabrata* isolates have reduced susceptibility or are resistant, and other species are mostly susceptible. Candidiasis is usually an endogenous disease that originates from oropharyngeal, genitourinary or skin colonisation, although nosocomial spread occurs. *C. auris* is an emerging species, which has a particular propensity for nosocomial transmission.

Syndromes of systemic candidiasis

Acute disseminated candidiasis

This usually presents as candidaemia (isolation of *Candida* spp. from the blood). The main predisposing factor is the presence of a central venous catheter. Other major factors include recent abdominal surgery, total parenteral nutrition (TPN), recent antimicrobial therapy and localised *Candida* colonisation. Up to 40% of cases will have ophthalmic involvement, with characteristic retinal 'cotton wool' exudates. As this is a sight-threatening condition, candidaemic patients should have a full ophthalmoscopy review. Skin lesions (non-tender pink/red nodules) may be seen. Although predominantly a disease of intensive care and surgical patients, acute disseminated candidiasis and/or *Candida* endophthalmitis is seen occasionally in injection drug-users, due to candidal contamination of citric acid or lemon juice used to dissolve heroin.

Chronic disseminated candidiasis (hepatosplenic candidiasis)

Persistent fever in a neutropenic patient, despite antibacterial therapy and neutrophil recovery, associated with the development of abdominal pain, raised alkaline phosphatase and multiple lesions in abdominal organs (e.g. liver, spleen and/or kidneys) on radiological imaging, suggests a diagnosis of hepatosplenic candidiasis. This represents a form of immune reconstitution syndrome (p. 104) in patients recovering from neutropenia and usually lasts for several months, despite appropriate therapy.

Other manifestations

Renal tract candidiasis, osteomyelitis, septic arthritis, peritonitis, meningitis and endocarditis are all well recognised and are usually sequelae of acute disseminated disease. Diagnosis and treatment of these conditions require specialist mycological advice.

Management

Blood cultures positive for *Candida* spp. must never be ignored. Acute disseminated candidiasis is treated with antifungal therapy, removal of any in-dwelling central venous catheter (whether known to be the source of infection or not) and removal of any documented source. Candidaemia should be treated initially with an echinocandin (p. 126), with subsequent adjustment (usually to intravenous or oral fluconazole) guided by clinical response, species identification and susceptibility testing. Treatment should continue for a minimum of 14 days. Alternative therapies include voriconazole and amphotericin B formulations.

Chronic disseminated candidiasis requires prolonged treatment over several months with fluconazole or other agents, depending on species and clinical response. The duration of the condition may be reduced by adjuvant therapy with systemic glucocorticoids.

Fig. 11.60 Cryptococcal disease. A 23-year-old HIV-positive male developed headache and left-sided weakness. **A** MRI scan of the brain showed a space-occupying lesion (arrow) with surrounding oedema. **B** Histopathological examination of the lesion stained with Grocott's silver stain showed encapsulated yeasts. *Cryptococcus neoformans* was cultured.

Cryptococcosis

Cryptococcosis is a systemic mycosis caused by two environmental yeast species, *Cr. neoformans* and *Cr. gattii*. *Cr. neoformans* is distributed worldwide and is primarily an opportunistic pathogen, most commonly associated with HIV infection (p. 321). *Cr. gattii* is a primary pathogen with a widespread distribution that includes Australasia, Africa, Canada (Vancouver Island) and the north-western USA.

Cryptococcosis is acquired by inhalation of yeasts. These may disseminate to any organ, most commonly the CNS and skin. The manifestations of *Cr. neoformans* are most severe in immunocompromised individuals. Conversely, *Cr. gattii* causes severe disease in immunocompetent hosts. Disseminated cryptococcosis (sepsis with cryptococci present in the blood stream or at multiple sites) is largely restricted to immunocompromised patients. CNS manifestations of cryptococcosis include meningitis (p. 321) and cryptococcoma (Fig. 11.60), the latter more likely with *Cr. gattii* infection. Manifestations of pulmonary cryptococcosis range from severe pneumonia (in more immunocompromised patients) to asymptomatic disease with single or multiple pulmonary nodules, sometimes exhibiting cavitation (in patients with lesser immunosuppression). Cryptococcal nodules may mimic other causes of lung pathology, such as tuberculosis or malignancy, and diagnosis requires histopathology and/or culture.

Treatment of severe cryptococcosis is the same as for cryptococcal meningitis, initially with liposomal amphotericin B (p. 321). Mild pulmonary disease is usually treated with fluconazole, although for asymptomatic nodules resection of the lesions is likely to be sufficient.

Fusariosis

Fusarium spp. cause disseminated disease in patients with prolonged neutropenia. The disease presents with

Fig. 11.61 *Fusarium* infection. A patient presented with fever and skin nodules after developing neutropenia secondary to haematopoietic stem cell transplantation and chemotherapy for relapsed leukaemia. *Fusarium solani* was cultured from skin lesions and blood cultures. **A** Tender, erythematous papules/nodules on upper arm. **B** Gram stain of *Fusarium* in blood culture medium.

antibiotic-resistant fever and evidence of dissemination (e.g. skin nodules, endophthalmitis, septic arthritis, pulmonary disease; Fig. 11.61). In contrast to *Aspergillus* spp., *Fusarium* spp. is often recovered from blood cultures. Treatment is challenging because of resistance to antifungal agents; voriconazole, posaconazole or lipid-formulated amphotericin B is most often prescribed.

Mucormycosis

Mucormycosis is a severe but uncommon opportunistic systemic mycosis caused by a number of 'mucoraceous' moulds, most commonly *Lichtheimia* (formerly *Absidia*) spp., *Rhizomucor* spp., *Mucor* spp. and *Rhizopus* spp. Disease patterns include rhinocerebral/craniofacial, pulmonary, cutaneous and systemic disease. All are characterised by the rapid development of severe tissue necrosis, which is almost always fatal if left untreated. The most common predisposing factors are profound immunosuppression from neutropenia and/or haematopoietic stem cell transplantation, uncontrolled diabetes mellitus, iron chelation therapy with desferrioxamine and severe burns.

Definitive diagnosis is by culture but histopathological confirmation is required, as the fungi may be environmental contaminants. Treatment requires a combination of antifungal therapy and surgical débridement, with correction of predisposing factor(s) if possible. High-dose lipid-formulated amphotericin B is most commonly used. Posaconazole is active against many mucoraceous moulds in vitro and may be used as a second-line agent or as oral 'step-down' therapy.

Talaromyces (formerly *Penicillium*) *marneffei* infection

T. marneffei is a thermally dimorphic pathogen (filamentous in environmental conditions and yeast at body temperature), which causes disease in South-east Asia, mainly in association with HIV infection (although immunocompetent patients may also be infected). Acquisition is usually by inhalation of environmental spores, with primary lung infection followed by haematogenous dissemination. A generalised papular rash, which progresses to widespread necrosis and ulceration, is a characteristic feature. Skin lesions may resemble molluscum contagiosum. Diagnosis is by histopathology and/or culture of respiratory secretions, blood or any infected clinical material (e.g. skin lesions, bone marrow, biopsies). Treatment involves an amphotericin B formulation followed by itraconazole (in severe infection), or itraconazole alone.

Histoplasmosis

Histoplasmosis is a primary systemic mycosis caused by the dimorphic fungus *Histoplasma capsulatum*. *H. capsulatum* var. *capsulatum* is endemic to east-central USA (especially the Mississippi and Ohio river valleys), parts of Canada, Latin America, the Caribbean, East and South-east Asia, and Africa. It occurs sporadically in Australia and India, and is very rare in Europe. *H. capsulatum* var. *duboisii* is found in West Africa and Madagascar.

The primary reservoir of *H. capsulatum* is soil enriched by bird and bat droppings, in which the fungus remains viable for many years. Infection is by inhalation of infected dust. Natural infections are found in bats, which represent a secondary reservoir of infection. Histoplasmosis is a specific hazard for explorers of caves and people who clear out bird (including chicken) roosts.

Pathology

The organism is inhaled in the form of conidia or hyphal fragments and transforms to the yeast phase during infection. Conidia or yeasts are phagocytosed by alveolar macrophages and neutrophils, and this may be followed by haematogenous dissemination to any organ. Subsequent development of a T-lymphocyte response brings the infection under control, resulting in a latent state in most exposed individuals.

Clinical features

Disease severity depends on the quantity of spores inhaled and the immune status of the host. In most cases, infection is asymptomatic. Pulmonary symptoms are the most common presentation, with fever, non-productive cough and an influenza-like illness. Erythema nodosum, myalgia and joint pain frequently occur, and chest radiography may reveal a pneumonitis with hilar or mediastinal lymphadenopathy.

Patients with pre-existing lung disease, such as chronic obstructive pulmonary disease (COPD) or emphysema, may develop chronic pulmonary histoplasmosis (CPH). The predominant features of this condition, which may easily be mistaken for tuberculosis, are fever, cough, dyspnoea, weight loss and night sweats. Radiological findings include fibrosis, nodules, cavitation and hilar/mediastinal lymphadenopathy.

Disease caused by *H. capsulatum* var. *duboisii* presents more commonly with papulonodular and ulcerating lesions of the skin and underlying subcutaneous tissue and bone (sometimes referred to as 'African histoplasmosis'). Multiple lesions of the ribs are common and the bones of the limbs may be affected. Lung involvement is relatively rare. Radiological examination may show rounded foci of bone destruction, sometimes associated

11

with abscess formation. Other disease patterns include a visceral form with liver and splenic invasion, and disseminated disease.

Acute disseminated histoplasmosis is seen with immuno-compromise, including HIV infection. Features include fever, pancytopenia, hepatosplenomegaly, lymphadenopathy and often a papular skin eruption. Chronic disseminated disease presents with fever, anorexia and weight loss. Cutaneous and mucosal lesions, lymphadenopathy, hepatosplenomegaly and meningitis may develop. *Emergomyces africanus* (formerly *Emmonsia* sp.) is a dimorphic fungus recently described in South Africa, which causes a disseminated histoplasmosis-like illness, mainly associated with HIV infection. Histopathologically, yeast forms appear similar to histoplasmosis and can be distinguished only by PCR.

Investigations

Histoplasmosis should be suspected in endemic areas with every undiagnosed infection in which there are pulmonary signs, enlarged lymph nodes, hepatosplenomegaly or characteristic cutaneous/bony lesions. Radiological examination in long-standing cases may show calcified lesions in the lungs, spleen or other organs. In the more acute phases of the disease, single or multiple soft pulmonary shadows with enlarged tracheobronchial nodes are seen on chest X-ray.

Laboratory diagnosis is by direct detection (histopathology or antigen detection), culture and serology; although antigen detection is the most effective method, it is not widely available. Serology utilises complement fixation testing or immunodiffusion; interpretation is complex and requires a specialist. *Histoplasma* antigen may be detectable in blood or urine. Culture is definitive but slow (up to 12 weeks). Histopathology may show characteristic intracellular yeasts. Diagnosis of subcutaneous or bony infection is mainly by histopathological examination and/or culture.

Management

Mild pulmonary disease does not require treatment. However, if prolonged, it may be treated with itraconazole. More severe pulmonary disease is treated with an amphotericin B formulation for 2 weeks, followed by itraconazole for 12 weeks, with methylprednisolone added for the first 2 weeks of therapy if there is hypoxia or ARDS. CPH is treated with itraconazole oral solution for 12–24 months, and disseminated histoplasmosis with an amphotericin B formulation followed by itraconazole. Lipid formulations of amphotericin B are preferred but their use is subject to availability. In subcutaneous and bone infection, patterns of remission and relapse are more common than cure. A solitary bony lesion may require local surgical treatment only.

Coccidioidomycosis

This is a primary systemic mycosis caused by the dimorphic fungi *Coccidioides immitis* and *C. posadasii*, found in the south-western USA and Central and South America. The disease is acquired by inhalation of conidia (arthrospores). In 60% of cases it is asymptomatic but in the remainder it affects the lungs, lymph nodes and skin. Rarely (in approximately 0.5%), it may spread haematogenously to bones, adrenal glands, meninges and other organs, particularly in those with immunocompromise.

Pulmonary coccidioidomycosis has two forms: primary and progressive. If symptomatic, primary coccidioidomycosis presents with cough, fever, chest pain, dyspnoea and (commonly) arthritis and a rash (erythema multiforme). Progressive disease presents with systemic upset (e.g. fever, weight loss, anorexia) and features of lobar pneumonia, and may resemble tuberculosis.

Coccidioides meningitis (which may be associated with CSF eosinophils) is the most severe disease manifestation; it is fatal if untreated and requires life-long suppressive therapy with antifungal azoles.

Investigations and management

Diagnosis is by direct histopathological detection in specimens, culture of infected tissue or fluids, or antibody detection. IgM may be detected after 1–3 weeks of disease by precipitin tests. IgG appears later and is detected with the complement fixation test. Change in IgG titre may be used to monitor clinical progress.

Treatment depends on specific disease manifestations and ranges from regular clinical reassessment without antifungal therapy (in mild pulmonary, asymptomatic cavitary or single nodular disease) to high-dose treatment with an antifungal azole, which may be continued indefinitely (e.g. in meningitis). Amphotericin B is used in diffuse pneumonia, disseminated disease and, intrathecally, in meningitis. Posaconazole has been used successfully in refractory disease.

Paracoccidioidomycosis

This is a primary systemic mycosis caused by inhalation of the dimorphic fungus *Paracoccidioides brasiliensis*, which is restricted to South America. The disease affects the lungs, mucous membranes (painful destructive ulceration in 50% of cases), skin, lymph nodes and adrenal glands (hypoadrenalism). Diagnosis is by microscopy and culture of lesions, and antibody detection. Oral itraconazole solution (200 mg/day) has demonstrated 98% efficacy and is currently the treatment of choice (mean duration 6 months). Ketoconazole, fluconazole, voriconazole and 2–3-year courses of sulphonamides are alternatives. Amphotericin B is used in severe or refractory disease, followed by an azole or sulphonamide.

Blastomycosis

Blastomyces dermatitidis is a dimorphic fungus endemic to restricted parts of North America, mainly around the Mississippi and Ohio rivers. Very occasionally, it is reported from Africa. The disease usually presents as a chronic pneumonia similar to pulmonary tuberculosis. Bones, skin and the genitourinary tract may also be affected. Diagnosis is by culture of the organism or identification of the characteristic yeast form in a clinical specimen. Antibody detection is rarely helpful. Treatment is with amphotericin B (severe disease) or itraconazole.

Further information

Websites

britishinfection.org *British Infection Association; source of general information on communicable diseases.*

cdc.gov *Centers for Disease Control, USA; source of general information about infectious diseases.*

fitfortravel.nhs.uk *Scottish site with valuable information for travellers.*

https://www.gov.uk/government/organisations/public-health-england *Public Health England; information on infectious diseases in the UK.*

idsociety.org *Infectious Diseases Society of America; source of general information relating to infectious diseases and of authoritative practice guidelines.*

who.int. *especially* www.who.int/csr/don *World Health Organisation; invaluable links on travel medicine with updates on outbreaks of infections, changing resistance patterns and vaccination requirements.*

G Maartens

HIV infection and AIDS

Clinical examination in HIV disease 306

Epidemiology 308
Global and regional epidemics 308
Modes of transmission 308

Virology and immunology 309

Diagnosis and investigations 310
Diagnosing HIV infection 310
Viral load and CD4 counts 311

Clinical manifestations of HIV 311

Presenting problems in HIV infection 312
Lymphadenopathy 313
Weight loss 313
Fever 313
Mucocutaneous disease 314
Gastrointestinal disease 316
Hepatobiliary disease 317
Respiratory disease 318
Nervous system and eye disease 319
Rheumatological disease 321
Haematological abnormalities 322
Renal disease 322
Cardiac disease 322
HIV-related cancers 322

Prevention of opportunistic infections 323
Preventing exposure 323
Chemoprophylaxis 323
Immunisation 324

Antiretroviral therapy 324
ART complications 325
ART in special situations 326
Prevention of HIV 327

Clinical examination in HIV disease

2 Oropharynx
Mucous membranes

▲ Oropharyngeal candidiasis

▲ Oral hairy leucoplakia

Herpes simplex
Aphthous ulcers
Kaposi's sarcoma

Teeth

▲ Gingivitis/periodontitis

1 Skin
Papular pruritic eruption

▲ Kaposi's sarcoma

▲ Molluscum contagiosum

Herpes zoster
Seborrhoeic dermatitis

3 Neck
Lymph node enlargement
  Tuberculosis
  Lymphoma
  Kaposi's sarcoma
  Persistent generalised
  lymphadenopathy
Parotidomegaly

▲ Cervical lymphadenopathy

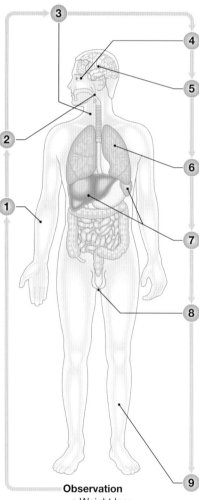

Observation
• Weight loss
• Tachypnoea
• Fevers and sweats

4 Eyes
Retina
  Toxoplasmosis
  HIV retinopathy
  Progressive outer retinal
  necrosis

▲ Cytomegalovirus retinitis

5 Central nervous system
Higher mental function
  HIV dementia
  Progressive multifocal
  leucoencephalopathy
Focal signs
  Toxoplasmosis
  Primary CNS lymphoma
Neck stiffness
  Cryptococcal meningitis
  Tuberculous meningitis
  Pneumococcal meningitis

6 Chest
Lungs
  Pleural effusion
  Tuberculosis
  Kaposi's sarcoma
  Parapneumonic

7 Abdomen
Hepatosplenomegaly

8 Anogenital region
Rashes

▲ Anal cancer

Condylomas
Herpes simplex
Ulcers

9 Legs
Peripheral nerve examination
  Spastic paraparesis
  Peripheral neuropathy

Inset (oral hairy leucoplakia) Courtesy of Audiovisual Dept, St Mary's Hospital, London.

i **HIV clinical staging classifications**

World Health Organisation (WHO) clinical stage (used in low- and middle-income countries)	Centers for Disease Control (CDC) clinical categories (used in high-income countries)
Stage 1 Asymptomatic Persistent generalised lymphadenopathy	**Category A** Primary HIV infection Asymptomatic Persistent generalised lymphadenopathy
Stage 2 Unexplained moderate weight loss (<10% of body weight) Recurrent upper respiratory tract infections Herpes zoster Angular cheilitis Recurrent oral ulceration Papular pruritic eruptions Seborrhoeic dermatitis Fungal nail infections	**Category B** Bacillary angiomatosis Candidiasis, oropharyngeal (thrush) Candidiasis, vulvovaginal; persistent, frequent or poorly responsive to therapy Cervical dysplasia (moderate or severe)/cervical carcinoma in situ Constitutional symptoms, such as fever (38.5°C) or diarrhoea lasting >1 month Oral hairy leucoplakia Herpes zoster, involving two distinct episodes or more than one dermatome Idiopathic thrombocytopenic purpura Listeriosis Pelvic inflammatory disease, particularly if complicated by tubo-ovarian abscess Peripheral neuropathy
Stage 3 Unexplained severe weight loss (>10% of body weight) Unexplained chronic diarrhoea for >1 month Unexplained persistent fever (>37.5°C for >1 month) Persistent oral candidiasis Oral hairy leucoplakia Pulmonary tuberculosis Severe bacterial infections Acute necrotising ulcerative stomatitis, gingivitis or periodontitis Unexplained anaemia (<80 g/L (8 g/dL)), neutropenia (<0.5×10^9/L) and/or chronic thrombocytopenia (<50×10^9/L)	
Stage 4	**Category C**

Candidiasis of oesophagus, trachea, bronchi or lungs
Cervical carcinoma – invasive
Cryptococcosis – extrapulmonary
Cryptosporidiosis, chronic (>1 month)
Cytomegalovirus disease (outside liver, spleen and nodes)
Herpes simplex chronic (>1 month) ulcers or visceral
HIV encephalopathy
HIV wasting syndrome
Cystoisosporiasis (formerly known as isosporiasis), chronic (>1 month)
Kaposi's sarcoma
Lymphoma (cerebral or B-cell non-Hodgkin)
Mycobacterial infection, non-tuberculous, extrapulmonary or disseminated
Mycosis – disseminated endemic (e.g. coccidioidomycosis, talaromycosis (formerly penicilliosis), histoplasmosis)
Pneumocystis pneumonia
Pneumonia, recurrent bacterial
Progressive multifocal leucoencephalopathy
Toxoplasmosis – cerebral
Tuberculosis – extrapulmonary (CDC includes pulmonary)
Sepsis, recurrent (including non-typhoidal *Salmonella*) (CDC only includes *Salmonella*)

Symptomatic HIV-associated nephropathy*
Symptomatic HIV-associated cardiomyopathy*
Leishmaniasis, atypical disseminated*

*These conditions are in WHO stage 4 but not in CDC category C.

12

Epidemiology

The acquired immunodeficiency syndrome (AIDS) was first recognised in 1981, although the earliest documented case of HIV infection has been traced to a blood sample from the Democratic Republic of Congo in 1959. AIDS is caused by the human immunodeficiency virus (HIV), which progressively impairs cellular immunity. The origin of HIV is a zoonotic infection with simian immunodeficiency viruses (SIV) from African primates, probably first infecting local hunters. SIVs do not cause disease in their natural primate hosts. HIV-1 was transmitted from chimpanzees and HIV-2 from sooty mangabey monkeys. HIV-1 is the cause of the global HIV pandemic, while HIV-2, which causes a similar illness to HIV-1 but progresses more slowly and is less transmissible, is restricted mainly to western Africa. It has been estimated that both HIV-1 and HIV-2 first infected humans about 100 years ago. HIV-2 will not be discussed further in this chapter.

There are three groups of HIV-1, representing three separate transmission events from chimpanzees: M ('major', worldwide distribution), O ('outlier') and N ('non-major and non-outlier'). Groups O and N are restricted to West Africa. Group M consists of nine subtypes: A–D, F–H, J and K (subtypes E and I were subsequently shown to be recombinants of other subtypes). Globally, subtype C (which predominates in sub-Saharan Africa and India) accounts for half of infections and appears to be more readily transmitted. Subtype B predominates in Western Europe, the Americas and Australia. In Europe, the prevalence of non-B subtypes is increasing because of migration. Subtypes A and D are associated with slower and faster disease progression, respectively.

Global and regional epidemics

In 2015 it was estimated that there were 36.7 million people living with HIV/AIDS, 2.1 million new infections and 1.1 million AIDS-related deaths. The global epidemiology of HIV has been changed by expanding access to combination antiretroviral therapy (ART), which reached 17 million people in 2015: the annual number of AIDS-related deaths has almost halved since the peak in 2005, the number of new infections has decreased by 40% since the peak in 1997, and the number of people living with HIV has increased. Regions have marked differences in HIV prevalence, incidence and dominant modes of transmission (Box 12.1). HIV has had a devastating impact in sub-Saharan Africa,

particularly in southern Africa, where average life expectancy of the general population fell to below 40 years before the introduction of ART.

Modes of transmission

HIV is transmitted by sexual contact, by exposure to blood (e.g. injection drug use, occupational exposure in health-care workers) and blood products, or to infants of HIV-infected mothers (who may be infected in utero, perinatally or via breastfeeding). Worldwide, the major route of transmission is heterosexual. The risk of contracting HIV after exposure to infected body fluid is dependent on the integrity of the exposed site, the type and volume of fluid, and the level of viraemia in the source person. The approximate transmission risk after exposure is given in Box 12.2. Factors that increase the risk of transmission are listed in Box 12.3.

A high proportion of patients with haemophilia in high-income countries had been infected through contaminated blood products by the time HIV antibody screening was adopted in 1985. Routine screening of blood and blood products for HIV infection has virtually eliminated this as a mode of transmission. However, the World Health Organisation (WHO) estimates that, because of the lack of adequate screening facilities in resource-poor countries, 5–10% of blood transfusions globally are with HIV-infected blood.

i | 12.2 Risk of HIV transmission after single exposure to an HIV-infected source

HIV exposure	Approximate risk
Sexual	
Vaginal intercourse: female to male	0.05%
Vaginal intercourse: male to female	0.1%
Anal intercourse: insertive	0.05%
Anal intercourse: receptive	0.5%
Oral intercourse: insertive	0.005%
Oral intercourse: receptive	0.01%
Blood exposure	
Blood transfusion	90%
Intravenous drug-users sharing needles	0.67%
Percutaneous needlestick injury	0.3%
Mucous membrane splash	0.09%
Mother to child	
Vaginal delivery	15%
Breastfeeding (per month)	0.5%

i | 12.1 Regional HIV prevalence in 2015, incidence trend and dominant mode of transmission

Region	People living with HIV (millions)	HIV incidence trend (2011–2015)	Dominant transmission
Sub-Saharan Africa	25.5	Decreasing	Heterosexual
Asia and Pacific	5.1	Stable	IDU, heterosexual
Latin America and Caribbean	2	Stable	MSM, heterosexual
Western and Central Europe, and North America	2.4	Stable	MSM
Eastern Europe and Central Asia	1.5	Increasing	IDU
Middle East and North Africa	0.23	Stable	IDU, MSM

(IDU = injection drug-users; MSM = men who have sex with men)

i	**12.3 Factors increasing the risk of transmission of HIV**

Common to all transmission categories

- High viral load

Sexual transmission

• STIs, especially genital ulcers	• Receptive anal intercourse
• Cervical ectopy	• Depot intramuscular progesterone contraceptive use
• Rectal or vaginal lacerations	
• Menstruation	
• Uncircumcised male partner	

Injection drug use transmission

• Sharing equipment	• Concomitant cocaine use
• Linked commercial sex	• Incarceration
• Intravenous use	

Occupational transmission

• Deep injury	• Needle was in a blood vessel
• Visible blood on device	

Vertical transmission

• Prolonged rupture of membranes	• Older gestational age

(STIs = sexually transmitted infections)

Virology and immunology

HIV is an enveloped ribonucleic acid (RNA) retrovirus from the lentivirus family. After mucosal exposure, HIV is transported via dendritic cells to the lymph nodes, where infection becomes established. This is followed by viraemia and dissemination to lymphoid organs, which are the main sites of viral replication.

Each mature virion has a lipid membrane lined by a matrix protein that is studded with glycoprotein (gp) 120 and gp41 spikes. The inner cone-shaped protein core (p24) houses two copies of the single-stranded RNA genome and viral enzymes. The HIV genome consists of three characteristic retroviral genes – *gag* (encodes a polyprotein that is processed into structural proteins, including p24), *pol* (codes for the enzymes reverse transcriptase, integrase and protease) and *env* (codes for envelope proteins gp120 and gp41) – as well as six regulatory genes.

HIV infects cells bearing the CD4 receptor; these are T-helper lymphocytes, monocyte–macrophages, dendritic cells, and microglial cells in the central nervous system (CNS). Entry into the cell commences with binding of gp120 to the CD4 receptor (Fig. 12.1), which results in a conformational change in gp120 that permits binding to one of two chemokine co-receptors (CXCR4 or CCR5). The chemokine co-receptor CCR5 is utilised during initial infection, but later on the virus may adapt to use CXCR4. Individuals who are homozygous for the CCR5 delta

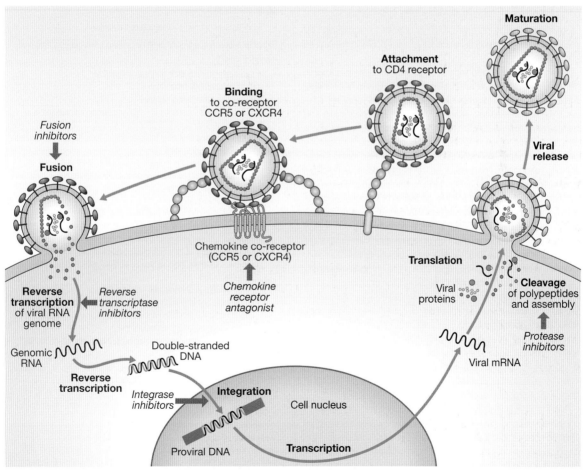

Fig. 12.1 Life cycle of HIV. Red arrows indicate sites of action of antiretroviral drugs.

32 mutation do not express CCR5 on CD4 cells and are immune to HIV infection. Chemokine co-receptor binding is followed by membrane fusion and cellular entry involving gp41. After penetrating the cell and uncoating, a deoxyribonucleic acid (DNA) copy is transcribed from the RNA genome by the reverse transcriptase enzyme, which is carried by the infecting virion. Reverse transcription is an error-prone process and multiple mutations arise with ongoing replication, which results in considerable viral genetic heterogeneity. Viral DNA is transported into the nucleus and integrated within the host cell genome by the integrase enzyme. Integrated virus is known as proviral DNA and persists for the life of the cell. Cells infected with proviral HIV DNA produce new virions only if they undergo cellular activation, resulting in the transcription of viral messenger RNA (mRNA) copies, which are then translated into viral peptide chains. The precursor polyproteins are then cleaved by the viral protease enzyme to form new viral structural proteins and enzymes that migrate to the cell surface and are assembled using the host cellular apparatus to produce infectious viral particles; these bud from the cell surface, incorporating the host cell membrane into the viral envelope. The mature virion then infects other CD4 cells and the process is repeated. CD4 lymphocytes that are replicating HIV have a very short survival time of about 1 day. It has been estimated that in asymptomatic HIV-infected people, more than 10^{10} virions are produced and 10^9 CD4 lymphocytes destroyed each day. The CD4 lymphocytes are destroyed primarily by the host immune response rather than by cytopathic effects of HIV.

A small percentage of T-helper lymphocytes enter a post-integration latent phase. Latently infected cells are important as sanctuary sites from antiretroviral drugs, which act only on replicating virus. Current ART is unable to eradicate HIV infection due to the persistence of proviral DNA in long-lived latent CD4 cells.

The host immune response to HIV infection is both humoral, with the development of antibodies to a wide range of antigens, and cellular, with a dramatic expansion of HIV-specific CD8 cytotoxic T lymphocytes, resulting in a CD8 lymphocytosis and reversal of the usual CD4:CD8 ratio. CD8 cytotoxic T lymphocytes kill activated CD4 cells that are replicating HIV, but not latently infected CD4 cells. HIV evades destruction despite this vigorous immune response, in part because the highly conserved regions of gp120 and gp41 that are necessary for viral attachment and entry are covered by highly variable glycoprotein loops that change over time as a result of mutations selected for by the immune response. The initial peak of viraemia in primary infection settles to a plateau phase of persistent chronic viraemia. With time, there is gradual attrition of the T-helper lymphocyte population and, as these cells are pivotal in orchestrating the immune response, the patient becomes susceptible to opportunistic diseases. The predominant opportunist infections in HIV-infected people are the consequences of impaired cell-mediated rather than antibody-mediated immunity (e.g. mycobacteria, herpesviruses). However, there is also a B-lymphocyte defect with impaired antibody production to new antigens and dysregulated antibody production with a polyclonal increase in gamma globulins, resulting in an increased risk of infection with encapsulated bacteria, notably *Streptococcus pneumoniae*.

The immune activation in response to HIV infection does not completely resolve on effective ART. This residual inflammatory state has been implicated in the pathogenesis of several non-AIDS morbidities that occur at a higher rate in HIV-infected people on ART than in the general population: cardiovascular, neurological and liver disease, chronic kidney disease and non-AIDS cancers.

Diagnosis and investigations

Diagnosing HIV infection

Globally, the trend is towards universal HIV testing, rather than testing only those patients at high risk or those with manifestations of HIV infection. However, in the UK, testing is still targeted to high-risk groups (Box 12.4). HIV is diagnosed by detecting host antibodies either with rapid point-of-care tests or in the laboratory, where enzyme-linked immunosorbent assay (ELISA) tests are usually done. Most tests detect antibodies to both HIV-1 and HIV-2. A positive antibody test from two different immunoassays is sufficient to confirm infection. Western blot assays can also be used to confirm infection but they are expensive and sometimes yield indeterminate results. Screening tests often include an assay for p24 antigen in addition to antibodies, in order to detect patients with primary infection before the antibody response occurs. Nucleic acid amplification tests (usually polymerase chain reaction, PCR) to detect HIV RNA are used to diagnose infections in infants of HIV-infected mothers, who carry maternal antibodies to HIV for up to 15 months irrespective of whether they are infected, and to diagnose primary infection before

 12.4 Patients who should be offered and recommended HIV testing in the UK[1]

Patients accessing specialist sexual health services (including genitourinary medicine)

- All patients who attend for testing or treatment

Patients accessing primary care (including emergency care) and secondary care

- All patients attending their first appointment at:
  Drug dependency programmes
  Pregnancy termination services
  Services treating hepatitis B or C, lymphoma or tuberculosis
- All patients who:
  Have symptoms that may indicate HIV or for which HIV is part of the differential diagnosis
  Are from a country or group with high rate of HIV infection
  Are male, or trans women, who have sex with men
  Report sexual contact with someone from a country with high rate of HIV infection
  Disclose high-risk sexual practices, e.g. 'chemsex' (p. 332)
  Are diagnosed with, or request testing for, a sexually transmitted infection
  Report a history of injecting drug use
  Are the sexual partners of people known to be HIV-positive or at high risk of HIV
- In areas of high[2] and extremely high[3] prevalence:
  All patients not previously diagnosed with HIV who register with a general practice or undergo blood testing for any reason
- In areas of extremely high prevalence[3]:
  All emergency care and secondary care patients not previously diagnosed with HIV
  At each general practice consultation consider offering opportunistic HIV testing

Prison inmates

- All new inmates not previously diagnosed with HIV

[1]Adapted from *National Institute for Health and Care Excellence NG60 – HIV testing: increasing uptake among people who may have undiagnosed HIV NICE guideline* (Dec. 2016). [2]Prevalence of diagnosed HIV is 2–5 per 1000 people aged 15–59. [3]Prevalence of diagnosed HIV is ≥ 5 per 1000 people aged 15–59.

12.5 How to carry out pre-test counselling

- Discuss meaning of positive and negative test results
- Realise importance of maintaining confidentiality
- Identify person to whom positive result could be disclosed
- Explore knowledge and explain natural history of HIV
- Discuss transmission and risk reduction
- Assess coping strategy
- Explain test procedure
- Obtain informed consent

12.6 How to carry out post-test counselling

Test result negative

- Discuss transmission and need for behaviour modification
- Advise second test 3 months after last exposure

Test result positive

- Explain meaning of result
- Organise medical follow-up
- Assess coping strategy
- Stress importance of disclosure
- Explain value of antiretroviral therapy
- Provide written information and useful Internet resources
- Discuss confidentiality issues
- Organise emotional and practical support (names/phone numbers)
- Facilitate notification of sexual partners

12.7 Baseline investigations

- CD4 count
- Viral load
- Hepatitis B surface antigen
- Hepatitis C antibody
- Liver function tests
- Full blood count
- Urinalysis, serum creatinine
- Syphilis serology
- Cervical smear in women
- Serum cryptococcal antigen (if CD4 <100)
- Tuberculin skin test
- Sexually transmitted infection screen

antibodies have developed. PCR is more sensitive than p24 antigen detection for diagnosing primary infection.

The purpose of HIV testing is not simply to identify infected individuals, but also to educate people about prevention and transmission of the virus. Counselling in the client's home language is essential both before testing and after the result is obtained (Boxes 12.5 and 12.6). There are major advantages to using rapid point-of-care HIV tests in that pre- and post-test counselling can be done at the same visit.

A number of baseline investigations should be done at the initial medical evaluation (Box 12.7). The extent of these investigations will depend on the resources available.

Viral load and CD4 counts

CD4 counts

CD4 lymphocyte counts are usually determined by flow cytometry but cheaper methods have been developed for low-income countries. The CD4 count is the most clinically useful laboratory indicator of the degree of immune suppression; it is used, together with clinical staging, in decisions to start prophylaxis against opportunistic infections, and is of great value in the differential diagnosis of clinical problems.

The CD4 count varies by up to 20% from day to day and is also transiently reduced by intercurrent infections. Due to this variability, major therapeutic decisions should not be taken on the basis of a single count. The percentage of lymphocytes that are CD4$^+$, rather than the absolute count, is routinely used in paediatrics, as the normal CD4 counts in infants and young children are much higher than in adults. In adults, the CD4 percentage is occasionally useful when evaluating significant reductions in an individual's CD4 count, which may be associated with transient lymphopenia due to intercurrent infection or pregnancy. In this case, the CD4 percentage will be unchanged.

The normal CD4 count is over 500 cells/mm^3. The rate of decline in CD4 count is highly variable. People with CD4 counts between 200 and 500 cells/mm^3 have a low risk of developing major opportunistic infections. Morbidity due to inflammatory dermatoses, herpes zoster, oral candidiasis, tuberculosis, bacterial pneumonia and HIV-related immune disorders (e.g. immune thrombocytopenia) becomes increasingly common as CD4 counts decline. Once the count is below 200 cells/mm^3, there is severe immune suppression and a high risk of AIDS-defining conditions. It is important to note that patients can be asymptomatic despite very low CD4 counts and that major opportunistic diseases occasionally present with high CD4 counts.

The CD4 count should be performed every 3–6 months in patients on ART, together with measurement of the viral load.

Viral load

The level of viraemia is measured by quantitative PCR of HIV RNA, known as the viral load. Determining the viral load is crucial for monitoring responses to ART (p. 324). People with high viral loads (e.g. >100 000 copies/mL) experience more rapid declines in CD4 count, while those with low viral loads (<1000 copies/mL) usually have slow or even no decline in CD4 counts.

Transient increases in viral load occur with intercurrent infections and immunisations, so the test should be done at least 2 weeks afterwards. Viral loads are variable; only changes in viral load of more than 0.5 log$_{10}$ copies/mL are considered clinically significant.

Clinical manifestations of HIV

Clinical staging of patients should be done at the initial medical examination, as it provides prognostic information and is a key criterion for initiating prophylaxis against opportunistic infections. Two clinical staging systems are used internationally (p. 307). In both, patients are staged according to the most severe manifestation and do not improve their classification. For example, a patient who is asymptomatic following a major opportunistic disease (AIDS) remains at stage 4 or category C of the WHO and CDC systems, respectively, and never reverts to earlier stages. Finally, patients do not always progress steadily through all stages and may present with AIDS, having been asymptomatic.

Primary HIV infection

Primary infection is symptomatic in more than 50% of cases but the diagnosis is often missed. The incubation period is usually 2–4 weeks after exposure. The duration of symptoms is variable but is seldom longer than 2 weeks. The clinical manifestations (Box 12.8) resemble those of infectious mononucleosis/glandular fever (p. 241), but the presence of maculopapular rash or mucosal ulceration strongly suggests primary HIV infection

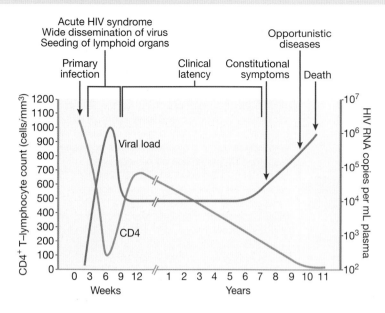

Fig. 12.2 Virological and immunological progression of untreated HIV infection.

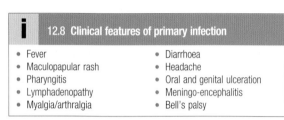

12.8 Clinical features of primary infection

- Fever
- Maculopapular rash
- Pharyngitis
- Lymphadenopathy
- Myalgia/arthralgia
- Diarrhoea
- Headache
- Oral and genital ulceration
- Meningo-encephalitis
- Bell's palsy

rather than the other viral causes of infectious mononucleosis. In infectious mononucleosis due to Epstein–Barr virus (EBV) or in cytomegalovirus (CMV), rashes generally occur only if aminopenicillins are given. Atypical lymphocytosis occurs less frequently than in EBV infection. Transient lymphopenia, including CD4 lymphocytes, is found in most cases (Fig. 12.2), which may result in opportunistic infections, notably oropharyngeal candidiasis. Major opportunistic infections like *Pneumocystis jirovecii* pneumonia (PJP) may rarely occur. Thrombocytopenia and moderate elevation of liver enzymes are commonly present. The differential diagnosis of primary HIV includes acute EBV, primary CMV infection, rubella, primary toxoplasmosis and secondary syphilis.

Early diagnosis is made by detecting HIV RNA by PCR or p24 antigenaemia. The appearance of specific anti-HIV antibodies in serum (seroconversion) occurs 2–12 weeks after the development of symptoms. The window period during which antibody tests may be false negative is prolonged when post-exposure prophylaxis has been used.

Asymptomatic infection

A prolonged period of clinical latency follows primary infection, during which infected individuals are asymptomatic. Persistent generalised lymphadenopathy with nodes typically <2 cm diameter is a common finding. Eventually, the lymph nodes regress, with destruction of node architecture as disease advances.

Viraemia peaks during primary infection and then drops as the immune response develops, to reach a plateau about 3 months later. The level of viraemia post seroconversion is a predictor of the rate of decline in CD4 counts, which is highly variable and explained in part by genetic factors affecting the immune

response. The median time from infection to the development of AIDS in adults is about 9 years (see Fig. 12.2). A small proportion of untreated HIV-infected people are long-term non-progressors, with CD4 counts in the reference range for 10 years or more. Some long-term non-progressors have undetectable viral loads and are known as 'elite controllers'.

Minor HIV-associated disorders

A wide range of disorders indicating some impairment of cellular immunity occur in most patients before they develop AIDS (CDC category B or WHO stages 2 and 3). Careful examination of the mouth is important when patients are being followed up, as oral candidiasis and oral hairy leucoplakia are common conditions that require initiation of prophylaxis against opportunistic infections, irrespective of the CD4 count.

Acquired immunodeficiency syndrome

AIDS is defined by the development of specified opportunistic infections, cancers and severe manifestations of HIV itself (p. 307). CDC category C is the most widely used definition of AIDS. WHO updated its classification more recently and added a few conditions of similar prognosis to its stage 4 disease.

Presenting problems in HIV infection

HIV itself is associated with a wide variety of clinical manifestations, and opportunistic diseases add many more. All body systems can be affected by HIV. The CD4 count is useful in differential diagnosis (Box 12.9): opportunistic diseases that may present at higher CD4 counts become increasingly common as CD4 counts decline, so the CD4 count helps to rule out certain disorders. For example, in a patient with a pulmonary infiltrate and a CD4 count of 350 cells/mm³, pulmonary tuberculosis is a likely diagnosis and PJP is very unlikely, but if the patient's CD4 count is 50 cells/mm³, both PJP and tuberculosis are likely.

Globally, tuberculosis is the most common cause of morbidity and mortality in HIV-infected patients. Tuberculosis should be considered in the differential diagnosis of most presenting problems in patients from communities where tuberculosis is common.

i	12.9 CD4 count and risk of common HIV-associated diseases

<500 cells/mm³

- Tuberculosis
- Bacterial pneumonia
- Herpes zoster
- Oropharyngeal candidiasis
- Non-typhoid salmonellosis
- Kaposi's sarcoma
- Non-Hodgkin lymphoma
- HIV-associated idiopathic thrombocytopenic purpura

<200 cells/mm³

- *Pneumocystis jirovecii* pneumonia
- Chronic herpes simplex ulcers
- Oesophageal candidiasis
- *Cystoisospora belli* (syn. *Isospora belli*) diarrhoea
- HIV wasting syndrome
- HIV-associated dementia
- Peripheral neuropathy
- Endemic mycoses

<100 cells/mm

- Cerebral toxoplasmosis
- Cryptococcal meningitis
- Cryptosporidiosis and microsporidiosis
- Primary CNS lymphoma
- Cytomegalovirus
- Disseminated *Mycobacterium avium* complex (MAC)
- Progressive multifocal leucoencephalopathy

Lymphadenopathy

Persistent generalised lymphadenopathy due to HIV is described above under asymptomatic infection. Lymphadenopathy may also be due to malignancy (Kaposi's sarcoma or lymphoma) or infections, especially tuberculosis, which is an extremely common cause in low- and middle-income countries. Tuberculous lymph nodes are often matted and may become fluctuant due to extensive caseous necrosis; inexperienced clinicians often perform incision and drainage inappropriately when simple aspiration is all that is required. Symmetrical generalised lymphadenopathy may occur in disseminated tuberculosis. Lymphoma typically presents with large, firm, asymmetric nodes. Rapid enlargement of a node, asymmetric enlargement or lymphadenopathy associated with constitutional symptoms (even if the nodes are symmetrical)

warrants further investigation. Lymph node needle aspiration (using a wide-bore needle such as 19G if tuberculosis is suspected) should be performed. One slide should be air-dried and sent for staining for acid-fast bacilli, which has about a 70% yield in tuberculosis. The other slide should be fixed and sent for cytology. If caseous liquid is aspirated, this should be sent for mycobacterial culture or PCR. If needle aspiration is unhelpful, or if lymphoma or Kaposi's sarcoma is suspected, excision biopsy should be performed.

Weight loss

Weight loss is a very common finding in advanced HIV infection. The HIV wasting syndrome is an AIDS-defining condition and is defined as weight loss of more than 10% of body weight, plus either unexplained chronic diarrhoea (lasting over 1 month) or chronic weakness and unexplained prolonged fever (lasting over 1 month). This is a diagnosis of exclusion. If the weight loss is rapid (more than 1 kg a month), then major opportunistic infections or cancers become more likely. Painful oral conditions and nausea from drugs contribute by limiting intake. Depression is very common and can cause significant weight loss. Measurement of C-reactive protein is helpful in the work-up of weight loss, as this is markedly raised with most opportunistic diseases but not with HIV itself. Erythrocyte sedimentation rate (ESR) is elevated by HIV infection and is therefore not useful. The presence of fever or diarrhoea is helpful in the differential diagnosis of weight loss (Fig. 12.3).

Fever

Fever is a very common presenting feature. Common causes of prolonged fever with weight loss are listed in Figure 12.3. Non-typhoid *Salmonella* bacteraemia, which commonly presents with fever in low-income countries, is accompanied by diarrhoea in only about 50% of patients. Pyrexia of unknown origin (PUO) in HIV infection is defined as temperature over 38°C with no cause found after 4 weeks in outpatients or 3 days in inpatients, and initial investigations such as chest X-rays, urinalysis and

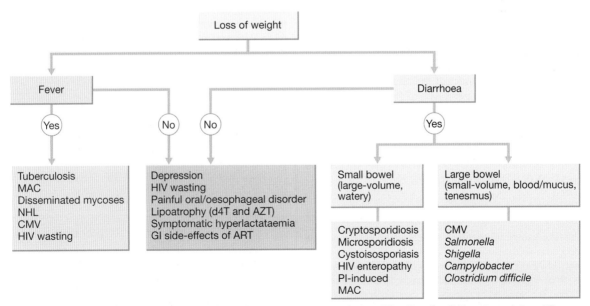

Fig. 12.3 Presentation and differential diagnosis of weight loss. (ART = antiretroviral therapy; AZT = zidovudine; CMV = cytomegalovirus; d4T = stavudine; KS = Kaposi's sarcoma; MAC = *Mycobacterium avium* complex; NHL = non-Hodgkin lymphoma; PI = protease inhibitor)

Fig. 12.4. Disseminated histoplasmosis presenting with diffuse papular rash and fever. Skin biopsy was diagnostic. *Courtesy of Professor Graeme Meintjes.*

blood cultures have failed to identify the cause. HIV itself can present with prolonged fever but this is a diagnosis of exclusion, as a treatable cause will be found in most patients. Abdominal imaging, preferably by computed tomography (CT), should be requested. Abdominal nodes (especially if they are hypodense in the centre) or splenic microabscesses strongly suggest tuberculosis. Mycobacterial blood cultures, which can also detect fungi, should be performed. Bone marrow aspirate and trephine biopsy are helpful if the full blood count shows cytopenias. Liver biopsy may be helpful if the liver enzymes are elevated but is invasive and seldom necessary. Mycobacterial and fungal stains and cultures should be done on all biopsies. Chest X-rays should be repeated after about a week, as micronodular or interstitial infiltrates may have become apparent (see p. 319 for differential diagnosis).

Tuberculosis is by far the most common cause of PUO in low- and middle-income countries, and in these settings a trial of empirical therapy is warranted after cultures have been sent. In high-income countries, disseminated *Mycobacterium avium* complex (MAC) infection is an important cause of PUO, often also presenting with diarrhoea and splenomegaly. Disseminated endemic mycoses (e.g. histoplasmosis, coccidioidomycosis, talaromycosis) present with PUO, often with papular skin eruptions or mucosal ulcerations (Fig. 12.4). Skin biopsy for histology and fungal culture is often diagnostic.

Mucocutaneous disease

The skin and mouth must be carefully examined, as mucocutaneous manifestations are extremely common in HIV and many prognostically important conditions can be diagnosed by simple inspection. The differential diagnosis of dermatological conditions is simplified by categorising disorders according to the lesion type (Box 12.10). Some common dermatological diseases, notably psoriasis, are exacerbated by HIV. The risk of many drug rashes is increased in HIV-infected patients. Skin biopsy should

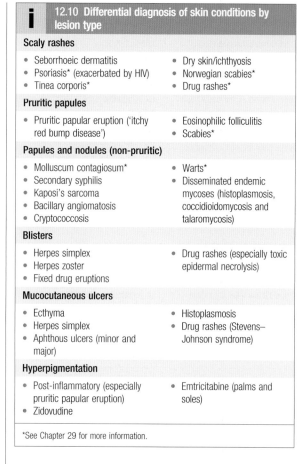

i	12.10 Differential diagnosis of skin conditions by lesion type

Scaly rashes

- Seborrhoeic dermatitis
- Psoriasis* (exacerbated by HIV)
- Tinea corporis*
- Dry skin/ichthyosis
- Norwegian scabies*
- Drug rashes*

Pruritic papules

- Pruritic papular eruption ('itchy red bump disease')
- Eosinophilic folliculitis
- Scabies*

Papules and nodules (non-pruritic)

- Molluscum contagiosum*
- Secondary syphilis
- Kaposi's sarcoma
- Bacillary angiomatosis
- Cryptococcosis
- Warts*
- Disseminated endemic mycoses (histoplasmosis, coccidioidomycosis and talaromycosis)

Blisters

- Herpes simplex
- Herpes zoster
- Fixed drug eruptions
- Drug rashes (especially toxic epidermal necrolysis)

Mucocutaneous ulcers

- Ecthyma
- Herpes simplex
- Aphthous ulcers (minor and major)
- Histoplasmosis
- Drug rashes (Stevens–Johnson syndrome)

Hyperpigmentation

- Post-inflammatory (especially pruritic papular eruption)
- Zidovudine
- Emtricitabine (palms and soles)

*See Chapter 29 for more information.

be taken, and sent for histology and culture for mycobacteria and fungi, in patients with papular rashes or if there are constitutional symptoms coinciding with the development of the rash.

Seborrhoeic dermatitis

Seborrhoeic dermatitis is very common in HIV. The severity increases as the CD4 count falls. It presents as scaly red patches, typically in the nasolabial folds and in hairy areas. Fungal infections are thought to play a role in the pathogenesis of this condition. It responds well to a combined topical antifungal and glucocorticoid. Selenium sulphide shampoo is helpful for scalp involvement.

Fig. 12.5 Severe mucocutaneous herpes simplex. Chronic anogenital or perioral ulcers are very common in advanced HIV infection.

i	12.11 Treatment of common opportunistic infections in adults with AIDS		
Opportunistic infection	**Treatment**	**Alternative treatment**	**Secondary prophylaxis***
Pneumocystis jirovecii pneumonia	Co-trimoxazole 20/100 mg/kg/day (in 4 divided doses) for 21 days; maximum per dose 320/1600 mg Early adjunctive prednisone 40 mg twice daily, if hypoxic	Clindamycin 900 mg 3 times daily IV (switch to 600 mg 3 times daily PO once improving) plus primaquine 30 mg daily for 21 days	Co-trimoxazole 160/800 mg daily
Cerebral toxoplasmosis	Sulfadiazine 15 mg/kg 4 times daily plus pyrimethamine 200 mg stat, then 75 mg daily plus folinic acid 15–25 mg daily for 6 weeks	Co-trimoxazole 320/1600 mg twice daily for 4 weeks, then 160/800 mg twice daily for 3 months	Co-trimoxazole 160/800 mg daily
Cryptococcosis	Liposomal amphotericin B 4 mg/kg/day IV plus flucytosine 25 mg/kg 4 times daily for 14 days, followed by fluconazole 400 mg daily for 8 weeks	Amphotericin B 1 mg/kg/day IV plus fluconazole 800 mg daily for 14 days, followed by fluconazole 400 mg daily for 8 weeks	Fluconazole 200 mg daily (for minimum of 1 year)
Oesophageal candidiasis	Fluconazole 200 mg daily for 14 days	Itraconazole 200 mg daily for 14–21 days	Not usually recommended
Disseminated *Mycobacterium avium* complex	Clarithromycin 500 mg twice daily plus ethambutol 15 mg/kg daily	Azithromycin 500 mg daily plus ethambutol 15 mg/kg daily	Continue treatment for minimum of 1 year
Herpes simplex ulcers	Aciclovir 400 mg 3 times daily for 5–10 days	Valaciclovir 500 mg or famciclovir 125 mg twice daily for 5–10 days	Aciclovir 400 mg twice daily only if recurrences are frequent/severe
Cystoisospora belli diarrhoea	Co-trimoxazole 160/800 mg 4 times daily for 10 days	Ciprofloxacin 500 mg twice daily for 10 days	Co-trimoxazole 160/800 mg daily

*Secondary prophylaxis may be discontinued once CD4 counts have increased to >200 cells/mm³ on antiretroviral therapy for at least 3 months.

Herpes simplex infections

Recurrences of herpes simplex infection are very common and primarily affect the nasolabial and anogenital areas (Fig. 12.5). As immune suppression worsens, the ulcers take longer to heal and become more extensive. Ulcers that persist for more than 4 weeks are AIDS-defining. The diagnosis is clinical, but PCR of vesicle fluid or from ulcer swabs may be diagnostic with unusual presentations. Response to a course of antiviral drug such as aciclovir is good but relapses are common. Frequent relapses that persist despite ART should be treated with aciclovir 400 mg twice daily for 6–12 months (Box 12.11).

Herpes zoster

This usually presents with a pathognomonic vesicular rash on an erythematous base in a dermatomal distribution (p. 239). The median CD4 count at the first episode of zoster is 350 cells/mm³. In patients with advanced HIV disease, the rash may be multidermatomal and recurrent episodes may occur. Disseminated zoster is rare. In HIV-infected patients, zoster is generally more extensive and has a longer duration, and there is a higher risk of developing post-herpetic neuralgia. High doses of aciclovir or its congeners should be given for all cases with active disease, irrespective of the time since the onset of the rash. Post-herpetic neuralgia is difficult to manage. Analgesic adjuvants, e.g. amitriptyline and pregabalin, should be commenced in all patients with prolonged pain. Topical capsaicin has modest efficacy.

Kaposi's sarcoma

Kaposi's sarcoma (KS) is a spindle-cell tumour of lympho-endothelial origin. All forms of KS are due to sexually transmitted human herpesvirus 8, also known as KS-associated herpesvirus. KS occurs in four patterns:

- *classic KS*: rare, indolent and restricted largely to elderly Mediterranean or Jewish men
- *endemic KS*: occurs in sub-Saharan Africa, is more aggressive, presents at earlier ages than classic KS, and affects men more than women
- *KS in patients on immunosuppressant drugs*: usually transplant recipients, who experience disseminated disease
- *AIDS-associated KS*.

In Africa, the male-to-female ratio of AIDS-associated KS is much lower than is seen with endemic KS, but men are still more affected than women, despite the fact that the seroprevalence of human herpesvirus 8 is the same in both sexes.

AIDS-associated KS is always a multicentric disease. Early mucocutaneous lesions are macular and may be difficult to diagnose. Subsequently, lesions become papular or nodular, and may ulcerate. KS lesions typically have a red–purple colour (Fig. 12.6 and p. 306) but may become hyperpigmented, especially in dark-skinned patients. As the disease progresses, the skin lesions become more numerous and larger. Lymphoedema is common, as lymphatic vessels are infiltrated. KS also commonly spreads to lymph nodes and viscerally, especially to the lungs and gastrointestinal tract. Visceral disease occasionally occurs in the absence of mucocutaneous involvement. B symptoms of fever, night sweats and weight loss may occur.

KS may respond to ART. Chemotherapy should be reserved for those patients who fail to remit on ART, or be given together with ART if there are poor prognostic features such as visceral involvement, oedema, ulcerated lesions and B symptoms.

Bacillary angiomatosis

Bacillary angiomatosis is a bacterial infection caused by *Bartonella henselae* or *B. quintana*. Skin lesions range from solitary superficial red–purple lesions resembling KS or pyogenic granuloma, to

Fig. 12.6 Oral Kaposi's sarcoma. A full examination is important to detect disease that may affect the palate, gums, fauces or tongue.

multiple subcutaneous nodules or plaques. Lesions are painful and may bleed or ulcerate. The infection may become disseminated with fevers, lymphadenopathy and hepatosplenomegaly. Diagnosis is made by biopsy of a lesion and Warthin–Starry silver staining, which reveals aggregates of bacilli. Treatment with doxycycline or azithromycin is effective.

Papular pruritic eruption

Papular pruritic eruption ('itchy red bump disease') is an intensely itchy, symmetrical rash affecting the trunk and extremities. It is thought to be due to an allergic reaction to insect bites. In sub-Saharan Africa, it is the most common skin manifestation of HIV. Post-inflammatory hyperpigmentation is common. Topical glucocorticoids, emollients and antihistamines are useful but response is variable. Measures to reduce insect bites are logical but difficult to implement in low-income settings.

Drug rashes

Cutaneous hypersensitivity to drugs is said to occur 100 times more frequently in HIV infection. The most common type is an erythematous maculopapular rash, which may be scaly. The drugs most commonly associated with rashes are sulphonamides and non-nucleoside reverse transcriptase inhibitors (NNRTIs – see below). Severe, life-threatening features of drug rashes include blistering (when this affects more than 30% of surface area it is known as toxic epidermal necrolysis), involvement of mucous membranes (Stevens–Johnson syndrome, pp. 1224 and 1254), or systemic involvement with fever or organ dysfunction (especially hepatitis, which is often delayed for a week or two after the rash develops). Because sulphonamides are important in the treatment and prophylaxis of opportunistic infections, rechallenge or desensitisation is often attempted in patients who have previously experienced rashes, provided the reaction was not life-threatening. Details of rashes caused by ART are given below.

Oral conditions

Oropharyngeal candidiasis is very common. It is nearly always caused by *C. albicans* (p. 300), but azole-resistant *Candida* species may be selected for if there have been repeated courses of azole drugs. Pseudomembranous candidiasis is the most common manifestation, with white patches on the buccal mucosa

(p. 306) that can be scraped off to reveal a red raw surface. Erythematous candidiasis is more difficult to diagnose and presents with a reddened mucosa and a smooth shiny tongue. Angular cheilitis due to *Candida* is a common manifestation. Topical antifungals are usually effective. Antifungal lozenges are more effective than antifungal solutions. Systemic azole therapy, usually fluconazole, should be given if topical therapy fails or if there are oesophageal symptoms.

Oral hairy leucoplakia (p. 306) appears as corrugated white plaques running vertically on the side of the tongue and is virtually pathognomonic of HIV disease. It is usually asymptomatic and is due to EBV.

Oral ulcers are common. Herpetiform oral ulcers occur in primary infection. Herpes simplex typically affects the nasolabial area but may cause oral ulcers. In early disease, minor aphthous ulcers are common. In advanced disease, giant aphthous ulcers occur. These destroy tissue, are painful and need to be differentiated from herpes simplex and CMV ulcers by biopsy. They respond to systemic glucocorticoids and ART. A number of disseminated endemic mycoses, notably histoplasmosis (p. 303), may cause oral ulcers, usually associated with constitutional symptoms. Finally, superficial oral ulcers may occur as part of the Stevens–Johnson syndrome, usually caused by sulphonamides or NNRTIs.

KS often involves the mouth, especially the hard palate (see above and Fig. 12.6). Nodular oral lesions are associated with a worse prognosis.

Gingivitis is very common. Good oral hygiene and regular dental check-ups are important. Acute necrotising ulcerative gingivitis and periostitis (p. 306) can result in loss of teeth; they should be treated with a course of metronidazole and a dental referral should be made.

Nail disorders

Fungal infections (onychomycosis, p. 1240) are very common and often involve multiple nails. Blue–black discoloration of nails is common and may be due to HIV or to the antiretroviral drug zidovudine.

Gastrointestinal disease

Oesophageal diseases

Oesophageal candidiasis (Fig. 12.7) is the most common cause of pain on swallowing (odynophagia), dysphagia and regurgitation. Concomitant oral candidiasis is present in about 70% of patients. Systemic azole therapy, e.g. fluconazole 200 mg daily for 14 days, is usually curative but relapses are common (Box 12.11). Patients whose oesophageal symptoms fail to respond to azoles should be investigated with oesophagoscopy. Major aphthous ulceration and CMV ulcers are the most likely causes and need to be differentiated by biopsy. Occasionally, herpes simplex oesophagitis or KS is responsible.

Diarrhoea

Chronic diarrhoea is a very common presenting problem in patients with advanced HIV, especially in areas where there is no access to safe water. It is a major cause of wasting. The differential diagnosis of diarrhoea depends on whether the presentation is with large- or small-bowel symptoms (see Fig. 12.3). The presentation and aetiology of acute diarrhoea are similar to those in HIV-uninfected patients.

i | **12.12 Common causes of chronic watery diarrhoea**

	Cryptosporidiosis	Microsporidiosis	Cystoisosporiasis (formerly isosporiasis)
Organism	Protozoan	Fungus	Protozoan
Species	*Cryptosporidium parvum* *C. hominis*	*Enterozoon bieneusi* *Encephalitozoon intestinalis* etc.	*Cystoisospora belli*
Animal host	Multiple	Multiple	No
Distribution	Global	Global	Tropics
Stool examination	Acid-fast stain	Trichrome stain Polymerase chain reaction	Acid-fast stain
Specific treatment	No established therapy	Albendazole (some species)	Co-trimoxazole

Fig. 12.7 Oesophageal candidiasis. Endoscopy showing typical pseudomembranous candidiasis.

Fig. 12.8 Cryptosporidiosis. Duodenal biopsy may be necessary to confirm cryptosporidiosis or microsporidiosis. The arrow indicates an oöcyst.

Large-bowel diarrhoea

Acute diarrhoea caused by the bacterial enteric pathogens *Campylobacter*, *Shigella* and *Salmonella* occurs more frequently than in HIV-uninfected people and the illness is more severe. Bacteraemia is much more common, notably due to non-typhoid *Salmonella* (p. 262). Diarrhoea caused by *Clostridium difficile* should be considered if there has been prior exposure to antibiotics, as is often the case in patients with symptomatic HIV.

CMV colitis presents with chronic large-bowel symptoms and fever in patients with CD4 counts below 100 cells/mm³. On colonoscopy, ulcers are seen, mostly involving the left side of the colon. Biopsy of ulcers shows typical 'owl's-eye' inclusion bodies.

Small-bowel diarrhoea

Chronic small-bowel diarrhoea may be due to HIV enteropathy but this is a diagnosis of exclusion. It typically presents with chronic watery diarrhoea and wasting without fever. Infection with one of three unicellular organisms is responsible for most cases: cryptosporidiosis, microsporidiosis and cystoisosporiasis (formerly known as isosporiasis) (Box 12.12). All three organisms are intracellular parasites that invade enterocytes. If the diagnosis is not made by stool microscopy on at least two specimens, a duodenal biopsy should be performed (Fig. 12.8). Electron microscopy is essential for speciation of microsporidia.

About 40% of patients with disseminated MAC infections have watery diarrhoea. Fever is a prominent feature of MAC infection, which helps differentiate it from cryptosporidiosis, microsporidiosis and cystoisosporiasis. Intestinal tuberculosis typically involves the ileocaecal area and may present with fever, weight loss and diarrhoea, but the diarrhoea is seldom profuse.

Hepatobiliary disease

Chronic viral hepatitis

Hepatitis B and/or C (HBV and HCV) co-infection is common in HIV-infected people due to shared risk factors for transmission. The natural history of both HBV and HCV is altered by HIV co-infection. In the ART era, chronic liver disease from viral hepatitis has emerged as a major cause of morbidity and mortality. HBV and HCV are further described on pages 873 and 877.

Hepatitis B

HBV infection is common in several groups of people at risk of HIV infection: residents of low- and middle-income countries, injection drug-users, haemophiliacs and MSM. HIV co-infection increases HBV viraemia, is associated with less elevation of transaminase (presumably due to immune suppression), and increases the risk of liver fibrosis and hepatocellular carcinoma. Several nucleoside reverse transcriptase inhibitors (NRTIs; lamivudine, emtricitabine and tenofovir) are also effective against HBV. HBV status should be checked at baseline in all HIV-infected patients. Treatment with anti-HBV drugs should be considered for all patients who have active HBV replication (HBeAg-positive or HBV DNA >2000 IU/mL) and/or evidence of inflammation or fibrosis on liver biopsy (see also p. 876). A flare of hepatitis may be associated with improved immune function after starting ART or discontinuing

12

antiretrovirals that have anti-HBV activity. HBV co-infection increases the risk of antiretroviral hepatotoxicity.

Hepatitis C

HCV infection is extremely common in injection drug-users and haemophiliacs. HIV co-infection increases HCV viraemia and increases the risk of liver fibrosis and hepatocellular carcinoma. Treatment for HCV should preferably be deferred in patients with CD4 counts <200 cells/mm³ until they are stable on ART. As with HBV co-infection, a flare of hepatitis may be associated with improved immune function after starting ART, and there is an increased risk of antiretroviral hepatotoxicity. Response to anti-HCV therapy is similar to that seen in HIV-uninfected people, but there are important drug–drug interactions between several antiretrovirals and the newer HCV protease inhibitors.

HIV cholangiopathy

HIV cholangiopathy, a form of secondary sclerosing cholangitis (p. 888), may occur in patients with severe immune suppression. In some patients, coexisting intestinal infection with CMV, cryptosporidiosis or microsporidiosis is present, but it is uncertain if these organisms play an aetiological role. Papillary stenosis is common and is amenable to cautery via endoscopic retrograde cholangiopancreatography (ERCP), which provides symptomatic relief. Acalculous cholecystitis is a common complication of cholangiopathy. ART may improve the condition.

Respiratory disease

Pulmonary disease is very common and is the major reason for hospital admission. Most patients who are admitted for respiratory diseases will have either bacterial pneumonia, pulmonary tuberculosis or PJP. PJP is more common in high-income countries, while tuberculosis is more common in low- and middle-income countries. An approach to the differential diagnosis of all three conditions is given in Box 12.13.

Pneumocystis jirovecii pneumonia

The key presenting feature of *Pneumocystis jirovecii* pneumonia (PJP) is progressive dyspnoea with a duration of less than 12 weeks. Dry cough and fever are common. The chest X-ray typically shows a bilateral interstitial infiltrate spreading out from the hilar

Fig. 12.9 *Pneumocystis* pneumonia: typical chest X-ray appearance. Note the interstitial bilateral infiltrate.

regions (Fig. 12.9) but may be normal initially. High-resolution CT scan is more sensitive than chest X-ray, usually showing typical 'ground-glass' interstitial infiltrates. Pneumatoceles may occur and may rupture, resulting in a pneumothorax. The diagnosis is made with silver stains, PCR or immunofluorescence of broncho-alveolar lavage or induced sputum (note that spontaneously produced sputum should not be sent, as the yield is low). Treatment is with high-dose co-trimoxazole, together with adjunctive systemic glucocorticoids if the patient is hypoxic (see Box 12.11).

Pulmonary tuberculosis

Tuberculosis is the most common cause of admission in countries with a high tuberculosis incidence. Pulmonary tuberculosis in patients with mild immune suppression typically presents as in HIV-uninfected patients, with a chronic illness and apical pulmonary cavities (p. 588). However, in patients with CD4 counts below 200 cells/mm³, there are four important differences in the clinical presentation of pulmonary tuberculosis:

- Tuberculosis progresses more rapidly, with a subacute or even acute presentation. The diagnosis therefore needs to be made and therapy commenced promptly. A trial of empirical therapy is often started while awaiting the results of mycobacterial cultures.
- The chest X-ray appearance alters: cavities are rarely seen, pulmonary infiltrates are no longer predominantly in apical areas, and pleural effusions and hilar or mediastinal lymphadenopathy are common (Fig. 12.10). A normal chest X-ray is not unusual in symptomatic patients with tuberculosis confirmed on sputum culture. These atypical findings can result in a delayed or missed diagnosis.
- Sputum smears, which are positive in most HIV-uninfected adults with pulmonary tuberculosis, are negative in more than half of patients. The main reason for this is the absence of pulmonary cavities.
- Many patients have disseminated tuberculosis, sometimes with a classic miliary pattern on chest X-ray, but more

i	12.13 Comparative features of bacterial pneumonia, *Pneumocystis jirovecii* pneumonia and pulmonary tuberculosis		
	Bacterial pneumonia	**Pneumocystis jirovecii pneumonia**	**Pulmonary tuberculosis**
Duration	Acute	Subacute	Variable
Dyspnoea	Common	Prominent	Occasional
White cell count	Increased	Normal	Variable
Chest X-ray			
Infiltrate	Consolidation	Interstitial	Variable
Bilateral infiltrate	Occasional	Usual	Common
Effusion	Occasional	No	Common
Nodes	Rare	No	Common
C-reactive protein	Markedly increased	Variable	Increased

Fig. 12.10 Chest X-ray of pulmonary tuberculosis in advanced HIV infection. Lower-zone infiltrates and hilar or mediastinal nodes in a patient with a CD4 count of <200 cells/mm³.

commonly presenting with pulmonary infiltrates together with extrapulmonary tuberculosis. The most common sites of concomitant extrapulmonary tuberculosis are the pleura and lymph nodes. Acid-fast bacilli are more often found on wide-needle aspirate of nodes than on sputum (p. 313). Pleural aspirate showing a lymphocytic exudate suggests tuberculosis as a likely cause and pleural biopsy will usually confirm the diagnosis.

Tuberculosis in HIV-infected patients responds well to standard short-course therapy (p. 592).

Bacterial pneumonia

The incidence of bacterial pneumonia is increased about 100-fold by HIV infection. The severity, likelihood of bacteraemia, risk of recurrent pneumonia, and mortality are all increased compared with HIV-uninfected patients. The aetiology is similar to that of community-acquired pneumonia in HIV-uninfected patients with co-morbidity: *S. pneumoniae* is the most common cause, followed by *Haemophilus influenzae*, Enterobacteriaceae (e.g. *Klebsiella pneumoniae*) and *Staphylococcus aureus*. The prevalence of atypical bacteria in HIV-infected patients with pneumonia is similar to that in the general population. Treatment is with a broad-spectrum β-lactam (e.g. ceftriaxone, amoxicillin–clavulanate), with the addition of a macrolide if the pneumonia is severe.

Uncommon bacteria causing pneumonia include *Pseudomonas aeruginosa*, *Nocardia* (which mimics tuberculosis) and *Rhodococcus equi* (which can cause pulmonary cavities).

Miscellaneous causes of pulmonary infiltrates

Pulmonary cryptococcosis may present as a component of disseminated disease or be limited to the lungs. The chest X-ray appearances are variable. Cryptococcomas occur less commonly than in HIV-uninfected people. The most common radiographic pattern seen in HIV infection is patchy consolidation, often with small areas of cavitation resembling tuberculosis. Pleural involvement is rare. The disseminated endemic mycoses (histoplasmosis, coccidioidomycosis and talaromycosis) often cause diffuse pulmonary infiltrates, mimicking miliary tuberculosis.

Lymphoid interstitial pneumonitis is a slowly progressive disorder causing a diffuse reticulonodular infiltrate. It is caused by a benign polyclonal lymphocytic interstitial infiltrate and is part of the diffuse infiltrative lymphocytosis syndrome (DILS – see p. 321). Patients may have other features of DILS, notably parotidomegaly.

KS often spreads to the lungs. Typical chest X-ray appearances are large, irregular nodules, linear reticular patterns and pleural effusions. Bronchoscopy is diagnostic.

Nervous system and eye disease

The central and peripheral nervous systems are commonly involved in HIV, either as a direct consequence of HIV infection or due to opportunistic diseases. An approach to common presentations is outlined in Figure 12.11.

Cognitive impairment

HIV-associated neurocognitive disorders

HIV is a neurotropic virus and invades the CNS early during infection. Meningo-encephalitis may occur at seroconversion. About 50% of HIV-infected people have abnormal neuropsychiatric testing. The term HIV-associated neurocognitive disorder (HAND) describes a spectrum of disorders: asymptomatic neurocognitive impairment (which is the most common), minor neurocognitive disorder and HIV-associated dementia (also called HIV encephalopathy). The proportion of patients with symptomatic HAND increases with declining CD4 counts. HIV-associated dementia is a subcortical dementia characterised by impairment of executive function, psychomotor retardation and impaired memory. There is no diagnostic test for HIV-associated dementia. CT or magnetic resonance imaging (MRI) shows diffuse cerebral atrophy out of keeping with age. It is important to exclude depression, cryptococcal meningitis and neurosyphilis. ART usually improves HIV-associated dementia but milder forms of HAND often persist.

Progressive multifocal leucoencephalopathy

Progressive multifocal leucoencephalopathy (PML) is a progressive disease that presents with stroke-like episodes and cognitive

Fig. 12.11 Presentation and differential diagnosis of HIV-related neurological disorders. (CMV = cytomegalovirus; HAND = HIV-associated neurocognitive disorder; PCNSL = primary CNS lymphoma; PML = progressive multifocal leucoencephalopathy)

Fig. 12.12 Progressive multifocal leucoencephalopathy. Non-enhancing white-matter lesions without surrounding oedema are seen.

Fig. 12.13 Cerebral toxoplasmosis. Multiple ring-enhancing lesions with surrounding oedema are characteristic.

impairment. Vision is often impaired due to involvement of the occipital cortex. PML is caused by the JC virus. A combination of characteristic appearances on MRI (Fig. 12.12) and detection of JC virus DNA in the cerebrospinal fluid (CSF) by PCR is diagnostic. No specific treatment exists and prognosis remains poor despite ART.

CMV encephalitis

This presents with behavioural disturbance, cognitive impairment and a reduced level of consciousness. Focal signs may also occur. Detection of CMV DNA in the CSF supports the diagnosis. Response to anti-CMV therapy is usually poor.

Space-occupying lesions

Space-occupying lesions in AIDS patients typically present over days to weeks. The most common cause is toxoplasmosis. As toxoplasmosis responds rapidly to therapy, a trial of anti-toxoplasmosis therapy should be given to all patients presenting with space-occupying lesions while the results of diagnostic tests are being awaited.

Cerebral toxoplasmosis

Cerebral toxoplasmosis is caused by reactivation of residual *Toxoplasma gondii* cysts from past infection, which results in the development of space-occupying lesions. The characteristic findings on imaging are multiple space-occupying lesions with ring enhancement on contrast and surrounding oedema (Fig. 12.13). *Toxoplasma* serology shows evidence of previous exposure (positive immunoglobulin (Ig)G antibodies); a negative serological test effectively rules out toxoplasmosis but a positive test is not specific. The standard therapy for toxoplasmosis is sulfadiazine with pyrimethamine, together with folinic acid, to reduce the risk of bone marrow suppression (see Box 12.11). However, co-trimoxazole has been shown to be as effective and less toxic, and is also more widely available. Response to a trial of therapy is usually diagnostic, with clinical improvement in 1–2 weeks and shrinkage of lesions on imaging in 2–4 weeks. Definitive diagnosis is by brain biopsy but this is seldom necessary.

Fig. 12.14 Primary CNS lymphoma. A single enhancing periventricular lesion with moderate oedema is typical.

Primary CNS lymphoma

Primary CNS lymphomas (PCNSLs) are high-grade B-cell lymphomas associated with EBV infection. Characteristically, imaging demonstrates a single homogeneously enhancing, periventricular lesion with surrounding oedema (Fig. 12.14). If it is considered safe to perform a lumbar puncture, PCR for EBV DNA in the CSF has a high sensitivity and specificity for PCNSL. Brain biopsy is definitive but carries a risk of morbidity and may be non-diagnostic in up to one-third. The prognosis is poor.

Tuberculoma

Lesions resemble toxoplasmosis on imaging, except that oedema tends to be less marked and single lesions occur more commonly.

There may be evidence of tuberculosis elsewhere. The CSF may show features consistent with tuberculous meningitis. Response to antituberculosis therapy is slow and paradoxical expansion of lesions despite therapy is not uncommon.

Stroke

There is a higher incidence of stroke in patients with HIV disease. Atherosclerosis is accelerated by the presence of inflammation due to the immune response to HIV, which is not completely suppressed by ART, and by dyslipidaemia caused by some antiretroviral drugs. HIV vasculopathy, which is thought to be a vasculitis, can also cause a stroke. It is important to exclude tuberculous meningitis and meningovascular syphilis in all patients who present with a stroke.

Meningitis

Cryptococcal meningitis

Cryptococcus neoformans is the most common cause of meningitis in AIDS patients. Patients usually present subacutely with headache, vomiting and decreased level of consciousness. Neck stiffness is present in less than half. CSF pleocytosis is often mild or even absent, and protein and glucose concentrations are variable. It is important to request CSF cryptococcal antigen tests in all HIV-infected patients undergoing lumbar puncture, as this test has a high sensitivity and specificity. Treatment is with amphotericin B (plus flucytosine if available) for 2 weeks, followed by fluconazole (see Box 12.11). Raised intracranial pressure is common and should be treated with repeated therapeutic lumbar punctures, removing sufficient CSF to reduce pressure to less than 20 cmH$_2$O. (Most experts are reluctant to withdraw more than 30 mL at a time.)

Tuberculous meningitis

The presentation and CSF findings of tuberculous meningitis are similar to those in HIV-uninfected patients (p. 1120), except that concomitant tuberculosis at other sites is more common in HIV infection.

Peripheral nerve disease

HIV infection causes axonal degeneration, resulting in a sensorimotor peripheral neuropathy in about one-third of AIDS patients. The incidence increases with lower CD4 counts, older age and increased height. Sensory symptoms predominate. Treatment involves foot care, analgesia and analgesic adjuvants. ART has minimal effect on halting or reversing the process. The NRTIs stavudine and didanosine, now largely abandoned due to their toxicity, can cause drug-induced peripheral neuropathy, which is typically more painful and more rapidly progressive than HIV neuropathy.

Acute inflammatory demyelinating polyneuropathy is an uncommon manifestation, usually occurring in primary infection. It resembles Guillain–Barré syndrome (p. 1140), except that CSF pleocytosis is more prominent. Mononeuritis may also occur, commonly involving the facial nerve.

Myelopathy and radiculopathy

The most common cause of myelopathy in HIV infection is cord compression from tuberculous spondylitis. Vacuolar myelopathy is seen in advanced disease and is due to HIV. It typically presents with a slowly progressive paraparesis with no sensory level. MRI of the spine is normal but is an important investigation to exclude other causes. Most patients have concomitant HIV-associated dementia.

CMV polyradiculitis presents with painful legs, progressive flaccid paraparesis, saddle anaesthesia, absent reflexes and sphincter dysfunction. CSF shows a neutrophil pleocytosis (which is unusual for a viral infection), and the detection of CMV DNA by PCR confirms the diagnosis. Functional recovery is poor despite treatment with ganciclovir or valganciclovir.

Psychiatric disease

Significant psychiatric morbidity is very common and is a major risk factor for poor adherence. Reactive depression is the most common disorder. Diagnosis is often difficult, as many patients have concomitant HAND. Substance misuse is common in many groups of people at risk of HIV. Some antiretroviral drugs can cause psychiatric adverse effects and these are detailed on page 326.

Retinopathy

CMV retinitis presents with painless, progressive visual loss in patients with severe immune suppression. On fundoscopy, the vitreous is clear. Haemorrhages and exudates are seen in the retina (p. 306), often with sheathing of vessels ('frosted branch angiitis'). The disease usually starts unilaterally but progressive bilateral involvement occurs in most untreated patients. Diagnosis is usually clinical, but if there is doubt, demonstrating CMV DNA by PCR of vitreous fluid is diagnostic. Treatment with ganciclovir or valganciclovir stops progression of the disease but lost vision does not recover. Some patients may develop immune recovery uveitis in response to ART, with intraocular inflammation, macular oedema and cataract formation that require prompt treatment with oral and intraocular glucocorticoids to prevent further visual loss.

Three other conditions may mimic CMV retinitis: ocular toxoplasmosis, which typically presents with a vitritis and retinitis without retinal haemorrhages; HIV retinopathy, a microangiopathy that causes cotton wool spots, which are not sight-threatening; and varicella zoster virus, which can cause rapidly progressive outer retinal necrosis.

Rheumatological disease

The immune dysregulation associated with HIV infection may result in autoantibody formation, usually in low titres. Mild arthralgias and a fibromyalgia-like syndrome are common in HIV-infected people.

Arthritis

HIV can cause a seronegative arthritis, which resembles rheumatoid arthritis. A more benign oligoarthritis may also occur. Reactive arthritis is more severe in HIV infection (p. 1031).

Diffuse infiltrative lymphocytosis syndrome

Diffuse infiltrative lymphocytosis syndrome (DILS) is a benign disorder involving polyclonal CD8 lymphocytic infiltration of tissues, which has some features in common with Sjögren's syndrome (p. 1038). It is linked to human leucocyte antigen (HLA)-DRB1. Most patients have a marked CD8 lymphocytosis. DILS usually presents in patients with mild immune suppression. The most common manifestation is bilateral parotid gland enlargement; the glands are often massive, with lymphoepithelial cysts

Fig. 12.15 CT scan of parotid glands showing multiple cysts (arrows) in a patient with the diffuse infiltrative lymphocytosis syndrome.

on histology (Fig. 12.15). Sicca symptoms are common but usually mild. Lymphocytic interstitial pneumonitis is the most common manifestation outside the salivary glands. Generalised lymphadenopathy may occur, with nodes larger than those seen with persistent generalised lymphadenopathy of HIV. Hepatitis, mononeuritis, polyarthritis and polymyositis may also occur. The manifestations outside the salivary glands usually respond to systemic glucocorticoids. Parotid gland enlargement may be treated by aspiration of parotid cysts and instillation of a sclerosant for cosmetic reasons, and surgery is best avoided. DILS may regress on ART but response is variable.

Haematological abnormalities

Disorders of all three major cell lines may occur in HIV. In advanced disease, haematopoiesis is impaired due to the direct effect of HIV and by cytokines. Pancytopenia may occur as a consequence of HIV but it is important to exclude a disorder infiltrating the bone marrow, such as mycobacterial or fungal infections, or lymphoma.

Anaemia

Normochromic, normocytic anaemia is very common in advanced HIV disease. Opportunistic diseases may cause anaemia of chronic disease (e.g. tuberculosis) or marrow infiltration (e.g. MAC, tuberculosis, lymphoma, fungi). Anaemia is a common adverse effect of zidovudine, which also causes a macrocytosis. Red cell aplasia is rare and may be caused either by parvovirus B19 infection or by lamivudine.

Neutropenia

Isolated neutropenia is occasionally due to HIV but is nearly always caused by drug toxicity (e.g. zidovudine, co-trimoxazole, ganciclovir).

Thrombocytopenia

Mild thrombocytopenia is common in HIV-infected people. Transient thrombocytopenia is frequently found in primary infection. The most common disorder causing severe thrombocytopenia is immune-mediated platelet destruction resembling idiopathic thrombocytopenic purpura (p. 971). This responds to glucocorticoids or intravenous immunoglobulin, together with ART. Splenectomy should be avoided if possible because it further increases the risk of infection with encapsulated bacteria. Severe thrombocytopenia with a microangiopathic anaemia also occurs in a thrombotic thrombocytopenic purpura-like illness (p. 979), which has a better prognosis and fewer relapses than the classical disease.

Renal disease

Acute kidney injury is common, usually due to acute infection or nephrotoxicity of drugs (e.g. tenofovir (p. 412), amphotericin B (p. 126)) HIV-associated nephropathy (HIVAN) is the most important cause of chronic kidney disease (CKD) and is seen most frequently in patients of African descent and those with low CD4 counts. Progression to end-stage disease is more rapid than with most other causes of CKD, and renal size is usually preserved. HIVAN presents with nephrotic syndrome, CKD or a combination of both. ART has some effect in slowing progression of HIVAN. Other important HIV-associated renal diseases include HIV immune complex kidney diseases and thrombotic microangiopathy. With the overall improvement in life expectancy from ART, conditions such as diabetes mellitus, hypertension and vascular disease add to the burden of CKD. Outcomes of renal transplantation are good in patients on ART.

Cardiac disease

HIV-associated cardiomyopathy resembles idiopathic dilated cardiomyopathy (p. 539) but progresses more rapidly. ART may improve cardiac failure but does not reverse established cardiomyopathy. Pericardial disease due to opportunistic diseases is not uncommon. Globally, the most common cause is tuberculous pericardial effusions. Tuberculous constrictive pericarditis is less common than in HIV-uninfected people. KS and lymphoma may cause pericardial effusions. Septic pericarditis, usually due to *S. pneumoniae*, is uncommon.

HIV is associated with an increased risk of myocardial infarction due to accelerated atherogenesis caused by the inflammatory state, which is not completely suppressed by ART, and by dyslipidaemia caused by some antiretroviral drugs.

HIV-related cancers

The AIDS-defining cancers are KS (see above), cervical cancer and non-Hodgkin lymphoma (NHL, p. 964). NHL may occur at any CD4 count but is more commonly seen with counts below 200 cells/mm^3. Almost all NHLs are B-cell tumours and most are stage 3 or 4. Long-term remission rates similar to those in patients without HIV can be achieved with NHL in AIDS patients using ART and chemotherapy (including the anti-B-cell monoclonal antibody rituximab if it is a B-cell tumour).

The incidence of a number of other cancers induced by viruses is also increased in HIV-infected people (Box 12.14). Regular cytological examination of the cervix, and of the anus in people who practise anal sex, should be performed to detect pre-malignant lesions, which are easier to treat. In general, the incidence of cancers that are not induced by viruses is similar to that in the general population.

i	12.14 Approximate incidence ratio of virus-related cancers compared to the general population	
Viral cancers		**Incidence ratio**
Human herpesvirus 8-related		
Kaposi's sarcoma		3600
Epstein–Barr virus-related		
Non-Hodgkin lymphoma		80
Hodgkin lymphoma		10
Human papillomavirus-related		
Cervical cancer		6
Vulval cancer		6
Anal cancer		30
Penile cancer		4
Hepatitis B/C virus-related		
Hepatocellular carcinoma		5

Prevention of opportunistic infections

The best way to prevent opportunistic infections is to improve the CD4 count with ART. However, infections continue to occur in the ART era as CD4 counts take time to improve if ART is initiated in patients with profound immune suppression, immune reconstitution on ART is often suboptimal, and CD4 counts may decline because antiretroviral resistance develops.

Preventing exposure

The best method for avoiding infection is to prevent exposure to the infectious agent. This is possible only for a few opportunistic infections, however. Furthermore, many opportunistic infections occur after reactivation of latent/dormant infection after prior exposure; examples include herpes simplex virus, zoster (shingles), CMV, toxoplasmosis, cryptococcosis and the endemic mycoses.

Safe water and food

Cryptosporidiosis, microsporidiosis and cystoisosporiasis may be water-borne. If there is no access to safe water, then water should be boiled before drinking. Food-borne illnesses are also important in HIV infection, notably *Salmonella* species. *Toxoplasma* exposure is related to eating raw or undercooked meat. People living with HIV infection need to be informed about food hygiene and the importance of adequately cooked meat.

Tuberculosis

Preventing exposure to tuberculosis is important when there is an infectious case in the household, in clinics and in hospitals. Adequate ventilation, masks and safe coughing procedures reduce the risk of exposure.

Malaria vector control

All HIV-infected individuals living in malarious areas should practise vector control, as malaria occurs more frequently and is more severe in HIV-infected people. The most cost-effective way to achieve this is by using insecticide-impregnated bed nets. Other modalities of vector control that are of benefit to the community, such as reducing standing water and spraying with residual insecticides and larvicides, should also be implemented.

Safer sex

HIV-infected individuals should practise safer sex in order to reduce the transmission of HIV. Even if their partners are HIV-infected, condoms should be used, as HIV mutants that have developed antiretroviral drug resistance can be transmitted. Safer sex will also lower the risk of acquiring herpes simplex virus and human herpesvirus 8.

Pets

Toxoplasma gondii can be acquired from kittens or cat litter, and people living with HIV infection should avoid handling either. Cryptosporidiosis can be transmitted from animals, and patients should be advised to wash their hands after handling animals.

Chemoprophylaxis

Chemoprophylaxis is the use of antimicrobial agents to prevent infections. Primary prophylaxis is used to prevent opportunistic infections that have not yet occurred. Secondary prophylaxis is used to prevent recurrence of opportunistic infections because many may recur after an initial response to therapy (see Box 12.11). Secondary prophylaxis can be discontinued when ART results in immune reconstitution, with CD4 counts increasing to over 200 cells/mm^3, but for CMV and MAC, prophylaxis can be stopped if CD4 counts increase to more than 100 cells/mm^3.

Co-trimoxazole primary prophylaxis

Co-trimoxazole reduces the incidence of a number of opportunistic infections (Box 12.15), resulting in lower hospitalisation and mortality rates. The indications for initiating co-trimoxazole are either clinical evidence of immune suppression (WHO clinical stages 3 or 4) or laboratory evidence of immune suppression (CD4 count <200 cells/mm^3). In low-income countries where malaria and/or severe bacterial infections are highly prevalent, the WHO recommends initiating co-trimoxazole regardless of CD4 counts or clinical stage. The recommended dose of co-trimoxazole is 960 mg daily, but trials have shown that half this dose is as effective and may be associated with less toxicity. Co-trimoxazole prophylaxis can be discontinued when CD4 counts increase to more than 200 cells/mm^3 on ART, except in low-income countries where it should be continued life-long.

Co-trimoxazole prophylaxis is well tolerated. The most common side-effect is hypersensitivity, causing a maculo-papular rash. If therapy is discontinued, desensitisation or rechallenge under antihistamine cover should be attempted, unless the rash was accompanied by systemic symptoms or mucosal involvement. Prophylactic doses of co-trimoxazole can also cause neutropenia, but this is very uncommon and routine monitoring of blood counts is not necessary. If co-trimoxazole cannot be tolerated, then

i	12.15 Opportunistic infections reduced by co-trimoxazole

- *Pneumocystis jirovecii* pneumonia
- Cerebral toxoplasmosis
- Bacterial pneumonia
- Bacteraemia
- Cystoisosporiasis
- Malaria

dapsone 100 mg daily should be substituted. Dapsone is equally effective at reducing the incidence of *P. jirovecii* pneumonia, but has little or no effect on reducing the other opportunistic infections prevented by co-trimoxazole.

Tuberculosis preventive therapy

Trials in patients not on ART showed that preventive therapy, either with isoniazid or combinations of rifamycins with isoniazid, reduces the risk of tuberculosis only in HIV-infected patients with a positive tuberculin skin test. In HIV infection, induration of 5 mm or more on a Mantoux test is regarded as positive. Recent evidence indicates that tuberculin skin tests do not predict benefit in patients starting ART or established on ART in high tuberculosis prevalence settings.

There is no CD4 count or clinical threshold for starting or stopping tuberculosis preventive therapy. It is important to rule out active tuberculosis before starting preventive therapy, and symptom screening has been shown to be adequate to achieve this (Box 12.16). The usual duration of isoniazid preventive therapy is 6 months but this does not provide long-term reduction in the risk of tuberculosis. Isoniazid for 36 months has been shown to be much more effective in people with a positive tuberculin skin test. Rifampicin or rifapentine combined with isoniazid for 12 weeks has been shown to be at least as effective as 6–12 months of isoniazid.

Mycobacterium avium complex prophylaxis

In high-income countries, a macrolide (azithromycin or clarithromycin) is recommended to prevent MAC in patients with a CD4 count below 50 cells/mm³, which can be discontinued once the CD4 count has risen to over 100 cells/mm³ on ART. MAC is uncommon in low- and middle-income countries and primary prophylaxis is thus not warranted.

Preventing cryptococcosis

Serum cryptococcal antigen test should be done in patients with a CD4 count below 100 cells/mm³. If this is positive, pre-emptive therapy with fluconazole should be commenced.

Immunisation

There are significant problems associated with vaccination in HIV infection. Firstly, vaccination with live organisms is contraindicated in patients with severe immune suppression, as this may result in disease from the attenuated organisms. Secondly, immune responses to vaccination are impaired in HIV-infected patients. If the CD4 count is below 200 cells/mm³, then immune responses to immunisation are very poor. Therefore it is preferable to wait until the CD4 count has increased to more than 200 cells/mm³ on ART before immunisation is given, and essential if live virus vaccines are used. All patients should be given a conjugate pneumococcal vaccine and annual influenza vaccination. Hepatitis B vaccination should be given to those who are not immune. In the UK, the following additional vaccines are also recommended:

- *hepatitis A*: in those at risk
- *human papillomavirus*: in people <40 years old
- *measles, mumps and rubella (MMR)*: in those with negative measles serology
- *meningococcus*: in people <25 years old, those with asplenia or complement deficiency, during outbreaks
- *diphtheria/tetanus/acellular pertussis (dTaP)/inactivated poliovirus vaccine (IPV)*: meeting general indications
- *chickenpox*: if seronegative; those who are seropositive should receive the shingles vaccine.

Bacille Calmette–Guérin (BCG) is contraindicated in all HIV-infected people.

Antiretroviral therapy

ART has transformed HIV from a progressive illness with a fatal outcome into a chronic manageable disease with a near-normal life expectancy.

The goals of ART are to:

- reduce the viral load to an undetectable level for as long as possible
- improve the CD4 count to over 200 cells/mm³ so that severe HIV-related disease is unlikely
- improve the quantity and quality of life without unacceptable drug toxicity
- reduce HIV transmission.

Many of the antiretroviral drugs that were initially used have largely been abandoned because of toxicity or poor efficacy. The drugs that are currently recommended are shown in Box 12.17, and their targets in the HIV life cycle in Figure 12.1.

Selecting antiretroviral regimens

The standard combination antiretroviral regimens are two NRTIs together with an NNRTI, protease inhibitor (PI) or integrase inhibitor. Dual NRTI combinations are usually emtricitabine or lamivudine (they have the same mechanism of action and so are never combined), together with one of abacavir, tenofovir or zidovudine. It is possible to construct effective regimens without NRTIs if there is intolerance or resistance to the NRTIs. Currently used PIs should always be administered with ritonavir, which

---

i | 12.16 Symptom screen for tuberculosis before isoniazid preventive therapy

All of the following must be absent:
- Active cough
- Weight loss
- Night sweats
- Fever

---

i | 12.17 Commonly used antiretroviral drugs

Classes	Drugs
Nucleoside reverse transcriptase inhibitors (NRTIs)	Abacavir, emtricitabine, lamivudine, tenofovir, zidovudine*
Non-nucleoside reverse transcriptase inhibitors (NNRTIs)	Efavirenz*, rilpivirine (only if viral load <100 000)
Protease inhibitors (PIs)	Atazanavir, darunavir, lopinavir*
Integrase inhibitors	Raltegravir, dolutegravir, elvitegravir
Chemokine receptor inhibitor	Maraviroc

*These drugs are no longer recommended as first-line options in high-income countries due to their toxicity.

itself is a PI that is toxic in therapeutic doses. Low doses of ritonavir dramatically increase the concentrations and elimination half-lives of other PIs by inhibiting the efflux pump P-glycoprotein and the cytochrome P450 isoenzyme CYP3A.

Most guidelines from high-income countries, including the UK, allow clinicians to choose a starting regimen of dual NRTIs combined with an NNRTI, or a PI or an integrase inhibitor, as these three regimens have similar efficacy. Subsequent ART regimen switches for virological failure are guided by the results of resistance testing (see below). For low- and middle-income countries, the WHO recommends a public health approach to using ART with standardised first-line (NNRTI plus dual NRTIs) and second-line (ritonavir-boosted PI plus dual NRTIs) regimens. NNRTIs are preferred by the WHO in first-line regimens, as they are cheaper than PIs and better tolerated. Furthermore, NNRTIs need to be given with two fully active NRTIs because they have a low genetic barrier to resistance (see below), whereas PI-containing regimens are effective even when there are some mutations conferring resistance to the NRTIs. PIs in second-line regimens are therefore preferable in settings where resistance testing is not widely available. The public health approach to using ART can be implemented by nurses and has been successfully applied in resource-poor settings.

Criteria for starting ART

Guidelines now recommend starting ART in all people with confirmed HIV infection, irrespective of CD4 count or clinical status. Early initiation of ART, compared with the previous strategy of deferring ART until CD4 thresholds or clinical disease occurs, has been shown to reduce morbidity and mortality, and has the additional benefit of reducing the risk of transmission.

It is seldom necessary to start ART urgently. Several consultations are required to give patients insight into the need for life-long ART, to stress the importance of adherence and to formulate a personal treatment plan. Disclosure of HIV status, joining support groups and using patient-nominated treatment supporters should be encouraged, as these have been shown to improve adherence. Recognition and management of depression and substance abuse is also important.

In patients with major opportunistic infections, ART should generally be started within 2 weeks, with two important exceptions: in cryptococcal meningitis, ART should be deferred for 5 weeks, as earlier initiation increases the risk of death; and in tuberculosis, ART should be deferred until 8 weeks (except if the CD4 count is <50 cells/mm^3), as earlier initiation increases the risk of the immune reconstitution inflammatory syndrome (see below).

Monitoring efficacy

The most important measure of ART efficacy is the viral load. A baseline viral load should be measured prior to initiating treatment. Viral load measurement should be repeated 4 weeks after starting ART, when there should be at least a 10-fold decrease. The viral load should be suppressed after 6 months. Once the viral load is suppressed, measurement should be repeated 6-monthly. Failure of ART is defined by the viral load becoming detectable after suppression. In most guidelines, a viral load threshold is used to define virological failure, e.g. more than 200 (UK) or more than 1000 (WHO) copies/mL. Adherence support should be enhanced if virological failure is detected, and measurement of the viral load repeated to confirm failure before switching to a new ART regimen.

CD4 counts are generally monitored every 6 months together with the viral load, but there is little point in repeating the CD4 count in patients who maintain virological suppression and whose CD4 count is >350 cells/mm^3. The CD4 count increases rapidly in the first month, followed by a more gradual increase. In the first year, the CD4 count typically increases by 100–150 cells/mm^3, and about 80 cells/mm^3 per annum thereafter until the reference range is reached, provided the viral load is suppressed. However, CD4 responses are highly variable: in about 15–30% of patients the CD4 count does not increase despite virological suppression, and in a similar proportion of patients the CD4 response is good despite the presence of virological failure. If ART is stopped, the CD4 count rapidly falls to the baseline value before ART was commenced.

Antiretroviral resistance

Reverse transcription is error-prone, generating a large number of mutations. If the viral load is suppressed on ART, viral replication is suppressed and resistance mutations will not be selected. If ART is taken and there is ongoing replication, due to either resistant mutations or suboptimal adherence, mutations conferring resistance to antiretroviral drugs will be selected. Antiretroviral drugs differ in their ability to select for resistant mutations. Some drugs (e.g. emtricitabine, lamivudine, efavirenz) have a low genetic barrier to resistance, rapidly selecting for a single mutation conferring high-level resistance. PIs and some NRTIs (e.g. zidovudine) select for resistance mutations slowly, and multiple resistant mutations often need to accumulate before the drug's efficacy is lost. Patients who develop antiretroviral resistance may transmit resistant virus to others and will eventually develop clinical failure.

Antiretroviral resistance is assessed by sequencing the relevant viral genes to detect mutations that are known to confer resistance. The patient must be taking ART when the test is performed, as otherwise the wild-type virus will predominate and resistant mutations will not be detected. The resistant proviral DNA is archived in latent CD4 cells and will re-emerge rapidly on re-exposure to the antiretroviral. In regions where resistance testing is affordable, it is recommended at baseline (to detect primary resistance) and at every confirmed virological failure, in order to select the most appropriate antiretrovirals in a new regimen.

ART complications

Immune reconstitution inflammatory syndrome

Immune reconstitution inflammatory syndrome (IRIS) is a common early complication of ART, especially in patients who start ART with CD4 counts below 50 cells/mm^3. IRIS presents either with paradoxical deterioration of an existing opportunistic disease (including infections that are responding to appropriate therapy) or with the unmasking of a new infection. The clinical presentation of IRIS events is often characterised by an exaggerated immune response, with pronounced inflammatory features. For example, patients with CMV retinitis developing IRIS on ART develop a uveitis; inflammatory haloes occur around KS lesions. Paradoxical tuberculosis IRIS events are common but it is important to exclude multidrug resistance, which could be responsible for the deterioration. IRIS is associated with a mortality of around 5% but this is higher when it complicates CNS infections.

The management of IRIS is to continue ART and to ensure that the opportunistic disease is adequately treated. Symptomatic treatments are helpful. Glucocorticoids are often used for more severe IRIS manifestations but they should not be given to patients with KS, as this can result in rapid progression of KS lesions.

Lipodystrophy

Long-term use of ART is associated with changes in body fat distribution called lipodystrophy, which can present either with fat accumulation (e.g. visceral fat, 'buffalo hump') or with subcutaneous fat loss ('lipoatrophy', Fig. 12.16), or with both fat loss and accumulation. The thymidine analogue NRTIs (stavudine and, to a lesser extent, zidovudine) are associated with fat loss. Switching to the non-thymidine NRTIs, abacavir or tenofovir, will result in very gradual improvement of lipoatrophy.

Previously, PIs were thought to be the cause of fat accumulation. However, recent studies have shown that all classes of antiretrovirals are associated with fat gain to a similar extent, and visceral adiposity is similar to that seen in the general population. Although not yet fully resolved, the current weight of evidence is that fat gain on ART is a return to normal by treating HIV infection.

Hypersensitivity rashes

These are common but must be differentiated from the other causes described on page 314. The NRTI abacavir typically causes a systemic hypersensitivity reaction, which is limited to people with HLA-B*5701, about 50% of whom will develop a hypersensitivity reaction. HLA testing should be done before abacavir is given and the drug should not be prescribed for people who are HLA-B*5701-positive, which is rare in people of African descent. Rechallenge must never be attempted after abacavir hypersensitivity, as fatal reactions may occur.

Drug rashes are very common with NNRTIs. When the NNRTI rash is mild and not accompanied by systemic involvement, the suspected drug is often continued and antihistamines are administered. The rash usually resolves. If it worsens or if systemic features develop, the NNRTI should be discontinued.

Other adverse effects

The NNRTI efavirenz causes insomnia, agitation, euphoria or dysphoria in many patients but tolerance to its neuropsychiatric effects develops in a few weeks in most patients. The NRTI zidovudine can cause anaemia and neutropenia, and tenofovir may cause nephrotoxicity and loss of bone mineral density. Some PIs are associated with dyslipidaemias and may increase the risk of myocardial infarction.

ART in special situations

Pregnancy

All pregnant women should have HIV testing at an early stage in pregnancy. The CD4 count falls by about 25% during pregnancy due to haemodilution. The course of HIV disease progression is not altered by pregnancy. In the pre-ART era, the rate of mother-to-child transmission was 15–40%, with rates being influenced by several factors (see Box 12.3).

ART has dramatically reduced the risk of mother-to-child transmission of HIV to less than 1%. All pregnant women should start ART at the beginning of the second trimester, unless they have advanced disease, when ART should be started in the first trimester.

Caesarean section is associated with a lower risk of mother-to-child transmission than vaginal delivery, but the mode of delivery does not affect transmission risk if the viral load is suppressed on ART.

HIV is also transmitted by breastfeeding. In high-income countries, exclusive formula feeding is generally recommended. In resource-poor settings, however, formula feeding is associated with a risk of infant morbidity and mortality, which may negate the benefit of not transmitting HIV to the infant. There is minimal risk of transmitting HIV by breastfeeding in women with a suppressed viral load on ART. Furthermore, providing antiretrovirals to infants (usually nevirapine monotherapy) while they are breastfeeding has been shown to reduce the risk of transmission. Breastfeeding is therefore now encouraged in resource-poor settings. Infants should be exclusively breastfed for the first 6 months, as mixed

---

12.18 HIV infection in old age

- **Epidemiology**: the HIV-infected population is ageing due to the life-prolonging effects of ART.
- **Immunity**: age-related decline increases the risk of infections. CD4 counts decline more rapidly as age extends beyond 40 years, resulting in faster disease progression. CD4 responses to ART decrease with increasing age.
- **Dementia**: HIV causes cerebral atrophy and neurocognitive disorders; dementia is therefore more common and more severe than in the HIV-uninfected elderly.
- **Vascular disease**: HIV is associated with an increased risk, exacerbated by some antiretrovirals that increase the risk of vascular disease by causing dyslipidaemia or insulin resistance.
- **Polypharmacy**: treatment of co-morbidities is complex due to the many drug interactions with antiretrovirals.

Fig. 12.16 Fat loss complicating long-term use of the thymidine analogue NRTIs stavudine and zidovudine.

feeding (with formula or solids) is associated with a higher risk of transmission.

Diagnosis of HIV in infancy requires the detection of HIV RNA by PCR, as maternal antibodies to HIV, which persist for up to 15 months, will give a false-positive result on antibody assays. PCR should ideally be carried out within 6 weeks of birth to facilitate early ART initiation. If the baby is breastfed, the PCR should be repeated 2 weeks after weaning.

Prevention of HIV

An effective HIV vaccine remains elusive due to the extensive genetic diversity of HIV and the lack of a safe attenuated virus. Measures for the prevention of HIV transmission are shown in Box 12.19.

Pre-exposure prophylaxis

Pre-exposure prophylaxis (PrEP) with daily tenofovir plus emtricitabine has been shown to reduce the risk of HIV acquisition in people at ongoing high risk (e.g. from sex or injecting drug use) and is well tolerated. Regular HIV testing should be done in people on PrEP.

Post-exposure prophylaxis

Post-exposure prophylaxis (PEP) is recommended when the risk is deemed to be significant after a careful risk assessment, in both occupational and non-occupational settings. The first dose should be given as soon as possible, preferably within 6–8 hours. There is no point in starting PEP after 72 hours. Tenofovir together with emtricitabine is the most widely used dual NRTI combination, together with either a PI or an integrase inhibitor. PEP should not be given if the exposed person is HIV-infected. HIV antibody testing should be performed at 3 months after exposure.

 12.19 Prevention measures for HIV transmission

Sexual

- Sex education programmes in schools
- Easily accessible voluntary counselling and testing centres
- Promotion of safer sex practices (delaying sexual debut, condom use, fewer sexual partners)
- Effective ART for HIV-infected individuals
- Pre-exposure prophylaxis for high-risk groups
- Male circumcision
- Post-exposure prophylaxis

Parenteral

- Blood product transmission: donor questionnaire, routine screening of donated blood
- Injection drug use: education, needle/syringe exchange, avoidance of 'shooting galleries', methadone maintenance programmes

Perinatal

- Routine 'opt-out' antenatal HIV antibody testing
- Measures to reduce vertical transmission (see text)

Occupational

- Education/training: universal precautions, needlestick injury avoidance
- Post-exposure prophylaxis

12

Further information

Websites with updated clinical guidelines

aidsinfo.nih.gov *AIDSinfo, a service of the US Department of Health and Human Services (HHS).*
bhiva.org *British HIV Association.*
who.int/hiv/pub *World Health Organisation.*

Sexually transmitted infections

Clinical examination in men 330

Clinical examination in women 331

Approach to patients with a suspected STI 332

Presenting problems in men 333
Urethral discharge 333
Genital itch and/or rash 333
Genital ulceration 333
Genital lumps 334
Proctitis in men who have sex with men 334

Presenting problems in women 335
Vaginal discharge 335
Lower abdominal pain 336
Genital ulceration 336
Genital lumps 336
Chronic vulval pain and/or itch 336

Prevention of STI 336

Sexually transmitted bacterial infections 337
Syphilis 337
Gonorrhoea 339
Chlamydial infection 340
Other sexually transmitted bacterial infections 341

Sexually transmitted viral infections 341
Genital herpes simplex 341
Human papillomavirus and anogenital warts 342
Molluscum contagiosum 343
Viral hepatitis 343

Clinical examination in men

5 Skin of penis
(Retract prepuce if present)
Genital warts
Ulcers
Be aware of normal anatomical features such as coronal papillae, or prominent sebaceous or parafrenal glands

▲ Coronal papillae

4 Scrotal contents
Abnormal masses or tenderness (epididymo-orchitis)

3 Pubic area
Pthirus pubis (crab louse)

2 Skin around groin and scrotum
Warts
Tinea cruris

1 Inguinal glands
Significant enlargement

6 Urethral meatus

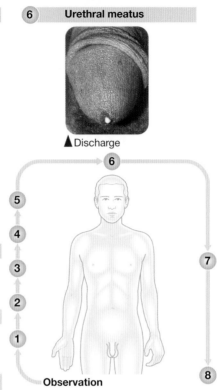

▲ Discharge

Observation
• Mouth
• Eyes
• Joints
• Skin:
  Rash of secondary syphilis
  Scabies
  Manifestations of HIV infection (Ch. 12)

7 Perianal area
(Men who have sex with men, and heterosexual men)

▲ Warts

8 Rectum
(Men who have sex with men practising receptive anal intercourse)

▲ Proctoscope

▲ Proctitis

Insets (Perianal warts) From McMillan A, Scott GR. Sexually transmitted infections: a colour guide. Churchill Livingstone, Elsevier Ltd; 2000. (Coronal papillae, mucopus) From McMillan A, Young H, Ogilvie MM, Scott GR. Clinical practice in sexually transmissible infections. Saunders, Elsevier Inc.; 2002.

---

i Investigations for STIs in heterosexual males

• First-void urine (FVU)* is the specimen of choice for the combined nucleic acid amplification test (NAAT) for gonorrhoea and chlamydia
• Alternatively, for gonorrhoea, a urethral swab plated directly on a selective medium such as modified New York City (MNYC), or sent in an appropriate transport medium, can be cultured to allow for assessment of antimicrobial sensitivities
• Serological test for syphilis (STS), e.g. enzyme immunoassay (EIA) for antitreponemal immunoglobulin G (IgG) antibody
• Human immunodeficiency virus (HIV) test (see note)

*A urethral swab can be submitted if the patient is unable to pass urine.

i Investigations for STIs in men who have sex with men

• FVU*, and pharyngeal and rectal swabs for combined NAAT for gonorrhoea and chlamydia
• STS (repeat testing may be necessary in the event of negative test results in the first few weeks following exposure)
• Serological tests for hepatitis A/B (with a view to vaccination if seronegative)
• HIV test (see note)

*A urethral swab can be submitted if the patient is unable to pass urine.

HIV testing

It should always be standard practice to offer HIV testing as part of screening for sexually transmitted infection (STI) because the benefits of early diagnosis outweigh other considerations. Extensive pre-test counselling is not required in most instances, but it is important to establish efficient pathways for referral of patients at high risk for whom the clinician wishes specialist support, and for those diagnosed as HIV-positive.

Clinical examination in women

4 Labia majora and minora
Ulcers
Vulvitis

▲ Warts

3 Pubic area

▲ *Pthirus pubis* (crab louse)

2 Inguinal glands
Significant enlargement

1 Abdomen
Abnormal masses or tenderness

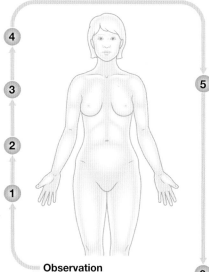

Observation
- Mouth
- Eyes
- Joints
- Skin:
  Rash of secondary syphilis
  Scabies
  Manifestations of HIV
  infection (Ch. 12)

5 Perineum and perianal skin
Warts
Ulcers

▲ Inflammation

6 Vagina and cervix
Abnormal discharge
Warts
Ulcers
Inflammation
In women with lower abdominal
pain, bimanual examination for
adnexal tenderness
(pelvic inflammatory disease)

▲ Speculum

13

Inset (Inflammation) From McMillan A, Young H, Ogilvie MM, Scott GR. Clinical practice in sexually transmissible infections. Saunders, Elsevier Inc.; 2002.

i Investigations for STIs in women	**i** Management goals in suspected STI	**i** Those at particular risk from STIs*
• Self-taken vaginal swab, or clinician-obtained cervical or vaginal swab, for combined NAAT for gonorrhoea and chlamydia • Alternatively, for gonorrhoea, cervical and urethral swabs plated directly on a selective medium such as MNYC, or sent in appropriate transport medium, can be cultured to allow for assessment of antimicrobial sensitivities • Wet mount for microscopy or high vaginal swab (HVS) for culture of *Trichomonas* • STS, e.g. EIA for antitreponemal IgG antibody • HIV test (see note)	• Relief of any symptoms • Screening for treatable STI that may not be causing symptoms • Tracing and treatment of sexual contacts who may also be infected • Advice to reduce risk of infection in the future	• Sex workers, male and female • Clients of sex workers • Men who have sex with men • Injecting drug users (sex for money or drugs) and their partners • Frequent travellers *Adapted from WHO/UNAIDS, 1997.

Sexually transmitted infections (STIs) are a group of contagious conditions whose principal mode of transmission is by intimate sexual activity involving the moist mucous membranes of the penis, vulva, vagina, cervix, anus, rectum, mouth and pharynx, along with their adjacent skin surfaces. A wide range of infections may be sexually transmitted, including syphilis, gonorrhoea, human immunodeficiency virus (HIV), genital herpes, genital warts, chlamydia and trichomoniasis. Bacterial vaginosis and genital candidiasis are not regarded as STIs, although they are common causes of vaginal discharge in sexually active women. Chancroid, lymphogranuloma venereum (LGV) and granuloma inguinale are usually seen in tropical countries. Hepatitis viruses A, B, C and D (p. 871) may be acquired sexually, as well as by other routes. Although primarily transmitted by mosquito bite, cases of male-to-female sexual transmission of Zika virus have been described and the virus is known to persist in semen for several months (p. 247).

The World Health Organization (WHO) estimates that 357 million curable STIs (*Trichomonas vaginalis*, *Chlamydia trachomatis*, gonorrhoea and syphilis) occur worldwide each year. In the UK in 2014, the most common treatable STIs diagnosed were chlamydia (220 000 cases) and gonorrhoea (nearly 40 000 cases). Genital warts are the second most common complaint seen in genitourinary medicine (GUM) departments. In addition to causing morbidity themselves, STIs may increase the risk of transmitting or acquiring HIV infection (Ch. 12).

As coincident infection with more than one STI is seen frequently, GUM clinics routinely offer a full set of investigations at the patient's first visit (pp. 330–331), regardless of the reason for attendance. In other settings, less comprehensive investigation may be appropriate.

The extent of the examination largely reflects the likelihood of HIV infection or syphilis. Most heterosexuals in the UK are at such low risk of these infections that routine extragenital examination is unnecessary. This is not the case in parts of the world where HIV is endemic, or for men who have sex with men (MSM) in the UK. In other words, the extent of the examination is determined by the sexual history (Box 13.1).

Approach to patients with a suspected STI

Patients concerned about the possible acquisition of an STI are often anxious. Staff must be friendly, sympathetic and reassuring; they should have the ability to put patients at ease, while emphasising that clinic attendance is confidential. The history focuses on genital symptoms, with reference to genital ulceration, rash, irritation, pain, swelling and urinary symptoms, especially dysuria. In men, the clinician should ask about urethral discharge, and in women, vaginal discharge, pelvic pain or dyspareunia. Enquiry about general health should include menstrual and obstetric history, cervical cytology, recent medication, especially with antimicrobial or antiviral agents, previous STI and allergy. Immunisation status for hepatitis A and B should be noted, as should information about alcohol intake and recreational drug use. Some MSM use new psychoactive substances (NPS), formerly referred to in the UK as 'legal highs', to enhance their sexual experience. Often described as 'chemsex', this has been associated with outbreaks of infections including syphilis, LGV and hepatitis C.

A detailed sexual history is imperative (Box 13.1), as this informs the clinician of the degree of risk for certain infections, as well as specific sites that should be sampled; for example, rectal samples should be taken from men who have had unprotected anal sex with other men. Sexual partners, whether male or female, and casual or regular, should be recorded. Sexual practices – insertive or receptive vaginal, anal, orogenital or oroanal – should be noted, as should choice of contraception for women, and condom use for both sexes.

STI during pregnancy

Many STIs can be transmitted from mother to child in pregnancy, either transplacentally or during delivery. Possible outcomes are highlighted in Box 13.2.

STI in children

The presence of an STI in a child may be indicative of sexual abuse, although vertical transmission may explain some presentations in the first 2 years. In an older child and in adolescents, STI may

---

13.1 How to take a sexual history

- In your lifetime, have your sexual partners been male, female or both?
- Do you have a regular sexual partner at present?
- If yes:
    How long have you been together?
    When did you last have sex with anyone else?
- If no:
    When did you last have sex?
    Was this a regular or a casual partner?
- Do/did you use a condom?

13.2 Possible outcomes of STI in pregnancy

Organism	Mode of transmission	Outcome for fetus/neonate	Outcome for mother
Treponema pallidum	Transplacental	Ranges from no effect to severe stigmata or miscarriage/stillbirth	None directly relating to the pregnancy
Neisseria gonorrhoeae	Intrapartum	Severe conjunctivitis	Possibility of ascending infection postpartum
Chlamydia trachomatis	Intrapartum	Conjunctivitis, pneumonia	Possibility of ascending infection postpartum
Herpes simplex	Usually intrapartum, but transplacental infection may occur rarely	Ranges from no effect to severe disseminated infection	Rarely, primary infection during 2nd/3rd trimesters becomes disseminated, with high maternal mortality
Human papillomaviruses	Intrapartum	Anogenital warts or laryngeal papillomas are very rare	Warts may become more florid during pregnancy, but usually regress postpartum

be the result of voluntary sexual activity. Specific issues regarding the management of STI and other infections in adolescence are discussed in Box 11.25 (p. 235).

Presenting problems in men

Urethral discharge

In the UK the most important causes of urethral discharge are gonorrhoea and chlamydia. In a significant minority of cases, tests for both of these infections are negative, a scenario often referred to as non-specific urethritis (NSU). Some of these cases may be caused by *Trichomonas vaginalis*, herpes simplex virus (HSV), mycoplasmas, ureaplasmas or adenoviruses. A small minority seem not to have an infectious aetiology.

Gonococcal urethritis usually causes symptoms within 7 days of exposure. The discharge is typically profuse and purulent. Chlamydial urethritis has an incubation period of 1–4 weeks, and tends to result in milder symptoms than gonorrhoea; there is overlap, however, and microbiological confirmation should always be sought.

Investigations

A presumptive diagnosis of urethritis can be made from a Gram-stained smear of the urethral exudate (Fig. 13.1), which will demonstrate significant numbers of polymorphonuclear leucocytes (≥5 per high-power field). A working diagnosis of gonococcal urethritis is made if Gram-negative intracellular diplococci (GNDC) are seen; if no GNDC are seen, a label of NSU is applied.

If microscopy is not available, urine samples and/or swabs should be taken and empirical antimicrobials prescribed. A first-void urine (FVU) sample should be submitted for a combined nucleic acid amplification test (NAAT) for gonorrhoea and chlamydia; a urethral swab is an alternative if the patient cannot pass urine. When gonorrhoea is suspected, a urethral swab should be sent for culture and antimicrobial sensitivities of *Neisseria gonorrhoeae*. Tests for other potential causes of urethritis are not performed routinely.

A swab should also be taken from the pharynx because gonococcal infection here is not reliably eradicated by single-dose therapy. In MSM, swabs for gonorrhoea and chlamydia should be taken from the rectum.

Fig. 13.1 A Gram-stained urethral smear from a man with gonococcal urethritis. Gram-negative diplococci are seen within polymorphonuclear leucocytes.

Management

This depends on local epidemiology and the availability of diagnostic resources. Treatment is often presumptive, with prescription of multiple antimicrobials to cover the possibility of gonorrhoea and/or chlamydia. This is likely to include a single-dose treatment for gonorrhoea, which is desirable because it eliminates the risk of non-adherence. The recommended agents for treating gonorrhoea vary according to local antimicrobial resistance patterns (p. 340). Appropriate treatment for chlamydia (p. 340) should also be prescribed because concurrent infection is present in up to 50% of men with gonorrhoea. Non-gonococcal, non-chlamydial urethritis is treated as for chlamydia.

Patients should be advised to avoid sexual contact until it is confirmed that any infection has resolved and, whenever possible, recent sexual contacts should be traced. The task of contact tracing – also called partner notification – is best performed by trained nurses based in GUM clinics; it is standard practice in the UK to treat current sexual partners of men with gonococcal or non-specific urethritis without waiting for microbiological confirmation.

If symptoms clear, a routine test of cure is not necessary, but patients should be re-interviewed to confirm that there was no immediate vomiting or diarrhoea after treatment, that there has been no risk of reinfection, and that traceable partners have sought medical advice.

Genital itch and/or rash

Patients may present with many combinations of penile/genital symptoms, which may be acute or chronic, and infectious or non-infectious. Box 13.3 provides a guide to diagnosis.

Balanitis refers to inflammation of the glans penis, often extending to the under-surface of the prepuce, in which case it is called balanoposthitis. Tight prepuce and poor hygiene may be aggravating factors. Candidiasis is sometimes associated with immune deficiency, diabetes mellitus, and the use of broad-spectrum antimicrobials, glucocorticoids or antimitotic drugs. Local saline bathing is usually helpful, especially when no cause is found.

Genital ulceration

The most common cause of ulceration is genital herpes. Classically, multiple painful ulcers affect the glans, coronal sulcus or shaft of penis (Fig. 13.2), but solitary lesions occur rarely. Perianal ulcers may be seen in MSM. The diagnosis is made by gently scraping material from lesions and sending this in an appropriate transport medium for culture or detection of HSV DNA by polymerase chain reaction (PCR). Increasingly, laboratories will also test for *Treponema pallidum* by PCR.

In the UK, the possibility of syphilis or any other ulcerating STI is much less likely unless the patient is an MSM and/or has had a sexual partner from a region where tropical STIs are more common. The classic lesion of primary syphilis (chancre) is single, painless and indurated; however, multiple lesions are seen rarely and anal chancres are often painful. Diagnosis is made in GUM clinics by dark-ground microscopy and/or PCR on a swab from a chancre, but in other settings by serological tests for syphilis (p. 338). Other rare infective causes seen in the UK include varicella zoster virus (p. 238) and trauma with secondary infection. Tropical STIs, such as chancroid,

13

i 13.3 Differential diagnosis of genital itch and/or rash in men

Likely diagnosis	Acute or chronic	Itch	Pain	Discharge (non-urethral)	Specific characteristics	Diagnostic test	Treatment
Subclinical urethritis	Either	±	–	±	Often intermittent	Gram stain and urethral swabs	As for urethral discharge
Candidiasis	Acute	✓	–	White	Post-coital	Microscopy	Antifungal cream, e.g. clotrimazole
Anaerobic (erosive) balanitis	Acute	±	–	Yellow	Offensive	Clinical	Saline bathing ± metronidazole
Pthirus pubis ('crab lice') infection	Either	✓	–	–	Lice and nits seen attached to pubic hairs	Can be by microscopy but usually visual	According to local policy – often permethrin
Lichen planus (p. 1252)	Either	±	–	–	Violaceous papules ± Wickham's striae	Clinical	None or mild topical glucocorticoid, e.g. hydrocortisone
Lichen sclerosus	Chronic	±	–	–	Ivory–white plaques, scarring	Clinical or biopsy	Strong topical glucocorticoid, e.g. clobetasol
Plasma cell balanitis of Zoon	Chronic	✓	–	±	Shiny, inflamed circumscribed areas	Clinical or biopsy	Strong topical glucocorticoid, e.g. clobetasol
Dermatoses, e.g. eczema or psoriasis	Either	✓	–	–	Similar to lesions elsewhere on skin	Clinical	Mild topical glucocorticoid, e.g. hydrocortisone
Genital herpes	Acute	±	✓	–	Atypical ulcers are not uncommon	Swab for HSV PCR	Oral antiviral, e.g. aciclovir
Circinate balanitis	Either	–	–	–	Painless erosions with raised edges; usually as part of sexually acquired reactive arthritis (SARA, p. 1031)	Clinical	Mild topical glucocorticoid, e.g. hydrocortisone

(HSV PCR = herpes simplex virus polymerase chain reaction)

Fig. 13.2 Penile herpes simplex (HSV-2) infection.

LGV and granuloma inguinale, are described in Box 13.12 (p. 341). Inflammatory causes include Stevens–Johnson syndrome (pp. 1224 and 1254), Behçet's disease (p. 1043) and fixed drug reactions. In older patients, malignant and pre-malignant conditions, such as squamous cell carcinoma and erythroplasia of Queyrat (intra-epidermal carcinoma), should be considered.

Genital lumps

The most common cause of genital 'lumps' is warts (p. 342). These are classically found in areas of friction during sex, such as the parafrenal skin and prepuce of the penis. Warts may also be seen in the urethral meatus, and less commonly on the shaft or around the base of the penis. Perianal warts are surprisingly common in men who do not have anal sex.

The differential diagnosis includes molluscum contagiosum and skin tags. Adolescent boys may confuse normal anatomical features such as coronal papillae (p. 330), parafrenal glands or sebaceous glands (Fordyce spots) with warts.

Proctitis in men who have sex with men

STIs that may cause proctitis in MSM include gonorrhoea, chlamydia, herpes and syphilis. The substrains of *Chlamydia trachomatis* that cause LGV (L1–3) have been associated with outbreaks of severe proctitis in Northern Europe, including the UK. Symptoms include mucopurulent anal discharge, rectal bleeding, pain and tenesmus.

Examination may show mucopus and erythema with contact bleeding (p. 330). In addition to the diagnostic tests listed on page 330, a PCR test for HSV and a request for identification of the LGV substrain should be arranged if chlamydial infection is detected. Treatment is directed at the individual infections.

MSM may also present with gastrointestinal symptoms from infection with organisms such as *Entamoeba histolytica* (p. 286), *Shigella* spp. (p. 265), *Campylobacter* spp. (p. 262) and *Cryptosporidium* spp. (pp. 287 and 317).

Presenting problems in women

Vaginal discharge

The natural vaginal discharge may vary considerably, especially under differing hormonal influences such as puberty, pregnancy or prescribed contraception. A sudden or recent change in discharge, especially if associated with alteration of colour and/or smell, or vulval itch/irritation, is more likely than a gradual or long-standing change to indicate an infective cause.

Local epidemiology is particularly important when assessing possible causes. In the UK, most cases of vaginal discharge are not sexually transmitted, being due to either candidal infection or bacterial vaginosis (BV). Worldwide, the most common treatable STI causing vaginal discharge is trichomoniasis; other possibilities include gonorrhoea and chlamydia. HSV may cause increased discharge, although vulval pain and dysuria are usually the predominant symptoms. Non-infective causes include retained tampons, malignancy and/or fistulae.

Speculum examination often allows a relatively accurate diagnosis, with appropriate treatment to follow (Box 13.4). If the discharge is homogeneous and off-white in colour, vaginal pH is greater than 4.5, and Gram stain microscopy reveals scanty or absent lactobacilli with significant numbers of Gram-variable organisms, some of which may be coating vaginal squamous cells (so-called Clue cells, Fig. 13.3), the likely diagnosis is BV. If there is vulval and vaginal erythema, the discharge is curdy in nature, vaginal pH is less than 4.5, and Gram stain microscopy reveals fungal spores and pseudohyphae, the diagnosis is candidiasis. Trichomoniasis tends to cause a profuse yellow or green discharge and is usually associated with significant

vulvovaginal inflammation. Diagnosis is made by observing motile flagellate protozoa on a wet-mount microscopy slide of vaginal material and/or by culture.

If examination reveals the discharge to be cervical in origin, the possibility of chlamydial or gonococcal infection is increased and appropriate cervical or vaginal swabs should be taken (p. 331). In addition, Gram stain of cervical and urethral material may reveal GNDC, allowing presumptive treatment for gonorrhoea to be given. If gonococcal cervicitis is suspected, swabs should also be taken from the pharynx and rectum; infections at these sites are not reliably eradicated by single-dose therapy and a test of cure will therefore be required.

GUM clinics in the UK may offer sexually active women presenting with vaginal discharge an STI screen (p. 331). In other settings, such as primary care or gynaecology, testing for chlamydia and gonorrhoea may be considered in young women (<25 years old), those who have changed partner recently, and those not using a barrier method of contraception, even if a non-STI cause of discharge is suspected clinically.

Treatment of infections causing vaginal discharge is shown in Box 13.4.

Fig. 13.3 Gram stain of a Clue cell from a patient with bacterial vaginosis. The margin of this vaginal epithelial cell is obscured by a coating of anaerobic organisms. *From McMillan A, Young H, Ogilvie MM, Scott GR. Clinical practice in sexually transmissible infections. Saunders, Elsevier Inc.; 2002.*

i	**13.4 Infections that cause vaginal discharge**	
Cause	**Clinical features**	**Treatment (in pregnancy seek specialist advice)**
Candidiasis	Vulval and vaginal inflammation Curdy white discharge adherent to walls of vagina Low vaginal pH	Clotrimazole[1] 500 mg pessary once at night and clotrimazole cream twice daily *or* Econazole[1] pessary 150 mg for 3 nights and econazole cream twice daily (topical creams for 7 days) *or* Fluconazole[2] 150 mg orally stat
Trichomoniasis	Vulval and vaginal inflammation Frothy yellow/green discharge	Metronidazole[3] 400 mg twice daily orally for 5–7 days *or* Metronidazole[3] 2 g orally as a single dose
Bacterial vaginosis	No inflammation White homogeneous discharge High vaginal pH	Metronidazole[3] 2 g stat or 400 mg twice daily orally for 5–7 days Metronidazole[3] vaginal gel 0.75% daily for 5 days Clindamycin[1,4] vaginal cream 2% daily for 7 days
Streptococcal/staphylococcal infection	Purulent vaginal discharge	Choice of antibiotic depends on sensitivity tests

[1]Clotrimazole, econazole and clindamycin damage latex condoms and diaphragms. [2]Avoid in pregnancy and breastfeeding. [3]Avoid alcoholic drinks until 48 hours after finishing treatment. Avoid high-dose regimens in pregnancy or breastfeeding. [4]*Clostridium difficile* colitis has been reported with the use of clindamycin cream.

13

Lower abdominal pain

Pelvic inflammatory disease (PID, infection or inflammation of the Fallopian tubes and surrounding structures) is part of the extensive differential diagnosis of lower abdominal pain in women, especially those who are sexually active. The possibility of PID is increased if, in addition to acute/subacute pain, there is dyspareunia, abnormal vaginal discharge and/or bleeding. There may also be systemic features, such as fever and malaise. On examination, lower abdominal pain is usually bilateral, and vaginal examination reveals adnexal tenderness with or without cervical excitation. Unfortunately, a definitive diagnosis can only be made by laparoscopy. A pregnancy test should be performed (as well as the diagnostic tests on p. 331) because the differential diagnosis includes ectopic pregnancy.

Broad-spectrum antibiotics, including those active against gonorrhoea and chlamydia, such as ofloxacin and metronidazole, should be prescribed if PID is suspected, along with appropriate analgesia. Delaying treatment increases the likelihood of adverse sequelae, such as abscess formation, and tubal scarring that may lead to ectopic pregnancy or infertility. Hospital admission may be indicated for severe symptoms.

Genital ulceration

The most common cause of ulceration is genital herpes. Classically, multiple painful ulcers affect the introitus, labia and perineum, but solitary lesions occur rarely. Inguinal lymphadenopathy and systemic features, such as fever and malaise, are more common than in men. Diagnosis is made by gently scraping material from lesions and sending this in an appropriate transport medium for culture or detection of HSV DNA by PCR. Increasingly, laboratories will also test such samples for *Treponema pallidum* by PCR. In the UK, the possibility of any other ulcerating STI is unlikely unless the patient has had a sexual partner from a region where tropical STIs are more common (see Box 13.12).

Inflammatory causes include lichen sclerosus, Stevens–Johnson syndrome (pp. 1224 and 1254), Behçet's disease (p. 1043) and fixed drug reactions. In older patients, malignant and pre-malignant conditions, such as squamous cell carcinoma, should be considered.

Genital lumps

The most common cause of genital 'lumps' is warts. These are classically found in areas of friction during sex, such as the fourchette and perineum. Perianal warts are surprisingly common in women who do not have anal sex.

The differential diagnosis includes molluscum contagiosum, skin tags, and normal papillae or sebaceous glands.

Chronic vulval pain and/or itch

Women may present with a range of chronic symptoms that may be intermittent or continuous (Box 13.5).

Recurrent candidiasis may lead to hypersensitivity to candidal antigens, with itch and erythema becoming more prominent than increased discharge. Effective treatment may require regular oral antifungals, e.g. fluconazole 150 g once a week, plus a combined antifungal/glucocorticoid cream.

Prevention of STI

Case-finding

Early diagnosis and treatment facilitated by active case-finding will help to reduce the spread of infection by limiting the period of infectivity; tracing and treating sexual partners will also reduce the risk of reinfection. Unfortunately, the majority of individuals with an STI are asymptomatic and therefore unlikely to seek medical attention. Improving access to diagnosis in primary care or non-medical settings, especially through opportunistic testing, may help. However, the impact of medical intervention through improved access alone is likely to be small.

Changing behaviour

The prevalence of STIs is driven largely by sexual behaviour. Primary prevention encompasses efforts to delay the onset of sexual activity and limit the number of sexual partners thereafter. Encouraging the use of barrier methods of contraception will also help to reduce the risk of transmitting or acquiring STIs. This

i 13.5 Chronic vulval pain and/or itch					
Likely diagnosis	Itch	Pain	Specific characteristics	Diagnostic test	Treatment
Candidiasis	✓	±	Usually cyclical	Microscopy (culture for yeasts other than *Candida albicans* in recurrent/refractory disease)	Oral antifungal, e.g. fluconazole 150 mg
Lichen planus	±	–	Violaceous papules ± Wickham's striae	Clinical	No treatment, or mild topical glucocorticoid, e.g. hydrocortisone
Lichen sclerosus	±	–	Ivory–white plaques, scarring ± labial resorption	Clinical or biopsy	Strong topical glucocorticoid, e.g. clobetasol
Vestibulitis	–	✓	Dyspareunia common, pain on touching erythematous area	Clinical	Refer to specialist vulva clinic
Vulvodynia	–	✓	Pain usually neuropathic in nature	Clinical	Refer to specialist vulva clinic
Dermatoses, e.g. eczema or psoriasis	✓	–	Similar to lesions elsewhere on skin	Clinical	Mild topical glucocorticoid, e.g. hydrocortisone
Genital herpes	±	✓	Atypical ulcers are not uncommon	Swab for HSV PCR	Oral antiviral, e.g. aciclovir

(HSV PCR = herpes simplex virus polymerase chain reaction)

is especially important in the setting of 'sexual concurrency', where sexual relationships overlap.

Unfortunately, there is contradictory evidence as to which (if any) interventions can reduce sexual activity. Knowledge alone does not translate into behaviour change, and broader issues, such as poor parental role modelling, low self-esteem, peer group pressure in the context of the increased sexualisation of our societies, gender power imbalance and homophobia, all need to be addressed. Throughout the world there is a critical need to enable women to protect themselves from undisciplined and coercive male sexual activity. Economic collapse and the turmoil of war regularly lead to situations where women are raped or must turn to prostitution to feed themselves and their children, and an inability to negotiate safe sex increases their risk of acquiring STI, including HIV.

Sexually transmitted bacterial infections

Syphilis

Syphilis is caused by infection, through abrasions in the skin or mucous membranes, with the spirochaete *Treponema pallidum*. In adults the infection is usually sexually acquired; however, transmission by kissing, blood transfusion and percutaneous injury has been reported. Transplacental infection of the fetus can occur.

The natural history of untreated syphilis is variable. Infection may remain latent throughout, or clinical features may develop at any time. The classification of syphilis is shown in Box 13.6. All infected patients should be treated. Penicillin remains the drug of choice for all stages of infection.

Acquired syphilis

Early syphilis

Primary syphilis

The incubation period is usually between 14 and 28 days, with a range of 9–90 days. The primary lesion or chancre (Fig. 13.4) develops at the site of infection, usually in the genital area. A dull red macule develops, becomes papular and then erodes to form an indurated ulcer (chancre). The draining inguinal lymph nodes may become moderately enlarged, mobile, discrete and rubbery. The chancre and the lymph nodes are both painless and non-tender, unless there is concurrent or secondary infection. Without treatment, the chancre will resolve within 2–6 weeks to leave a thin atrophic scar.

i	**13.6 Classification of syphilis**	
Stage	**Acquired**	**Congenital**
Early	Primary Secondary Latent	Clinical and latent
Late	Latent Benign tertiary Cardiovascular Neurosyphilis	Clinical and latent

Fig. 13.4 Primary syphilis. A painless ulcer (chancre) is shown in the coronal sulcus of the penis. This is usually associated with inguinal lymphadenopathy. *Courtesy of Dr P. Hay, St George's Hospital, London.*

Chancres may develop on the vaginal wall and on the cervix. Extragenital chancres are found in about 10% of patients, affecting sites such as the finger, lip, tongue, tonsil, nipple, anus or rectum. Anal chancres often resemble fissures and may be painful.

Secondary syphilis

This occurs 6–8 weeks after the development of the chancre, when treponemes disseminate to produce a multisystem disease. Constitutional features, such as mild fever, malaise and headache, are common. Over 75% of patients present with a rash on the trunk and limbs that may later involve the palms and soles; this is initially macular but evolves to maculopapular or papular forms, which are generalised, symmetrical and non-irritable. Scales may form on the papules later. Lesions are red, changing to a 'gun-metal' grey as they resolve. Without treatment, the rash may last for up to 12 weeks. Condylomata lata (papules coalescing to plaques) may develop in warm, moist sites such as the vulva or perianal area. Generalised non-tender lymphadenopathy is present in over 50% of patients. Mucosal lesions, known as mucous patches, may affect the genitalia, mouth, pharynx or larynx and are essentially modified papules, which become eroded. Rarely, confluence produces characteristic 'snail track ulcers' in the mouth.

Other features, such as meningitis, cranial nerve palsies, anterior or posterior uveitis, hepatitis, gastritis, glomerulonephritis or periostitis, are sometimes seen. Neurological involvement may be more common in HIV-positive patients.

The differential diagnosis of secondary syphilis can be extensive, but in the context of a suspected STI, primary HIV infection is the most important alternative condition to consider (Ch. 12). Non-STI conditions that mimic the rash include psoriasis, pityriasis rosea, scabies, allergic drug reaction, erythema multiforme and pityriasis (tinea) versicolor.

The clinical manifestations of secondary syphilis will resolve without treatment but relapse may occur, usually within the first year of infection. Thereafter, the disease enters the phase of latency.

Latent syphilis

This phase is characterised by the presence of positive syphilis serology or the diagnostic cerebrospinal fluid (CSF) abnormalities of neurosyphilis in an untreated patient with no evidence of clinical disease. It is divided into early latency (within 2 years of infection), when syphilis may be transmitted sexually, and late latency, when the patient is no longer sexually infectious.

13

Transmission of syphilis from a pregnant woman to her fetus, and rarely by blood transfusion, is possible for several years following infection.

Late syphilis

Late latent syphilis

This may persist for many years or for life. Without treatment, over 60% of patients might be expected to suffer little or no ill health. Coincidental prescription of antibiotics for other illnesses, such as respiratory tract or skin infections, may treat latent syphilis serendipitously and make the interpretation of serological test results difficult (see below).

Benign tertiary syphilis

This may develop between 3 and 10 years after infection but is now rarely seen in the UK. Skin, mucous membranes, bone, muscle or viscera can be involved. The characteristic feature is a chronic granulomatous lesion called a gumma, which may be single or multiple. Healing with scar formation may impair the function of the structure affected. Skin lesions may take the form of nodules or ulcers, while subcutaneous lesions may ulcerate with a gummy discharge. Healing occurs slowly, with the formation of characteristic tissue-paper scars. Mucosal lesions may occur in the mouth, pharynx, larynx or nasal septum, appearing as punched-out ulcers. Of particular importance is gummatous involvement of the tongue, healing of which may lead to leucoplakia with the attendant risk of malignant change. Gummas of the tibia, skull, clavicle and sternum have been described, as has involvement of the brain, spinal cord, liver, testis and, rarely, other organs. Resolution of active disease should follow treatment, though some tissue damage may be permanent. Paroxysmal cold haemoglobinuria (p. 950) may be seen.

Cardiovascular syphilis

This may present many years after initial infection. Aortitis, which may involve the aortic valve and/or the coronary ostia, is the key feature. Clinical features include aortic incompetence, angina and aortic aneurysm (p. 505). The condition typically affects the ascending aorta and sometimes the aortic arch; aneurysm of the descending aorta is rare. Treatment with penicillin will not correct anatomical damage and surgical intervention may be required.

Neurosyphilis

This may also take years to develop. Asymptomatic infection is associated with CSF abnormalities in the absence of clinical signs. Meningovascular disease, tabes dorsalis and general paralysis of the insane constitute the symptomatic forms (p. 1125). Neurosyphilis and cardiovascular syphilis may coexist and are sometimes referred to as quaternary syphilis.

Congenital syphilis

Congenital syphilis is rare where antenatal serological screening is practised. Antisyphilitic treatment in pregnancy treats the fetus, if infected, as well as the mother.

Treponemal infection may give rise to a variety of outcomes after 4 months of gestation, when the fetus becomes immunocompetent:

- miscarriage or stillbirth, prematurely or at term
- birth of a syphilitic baby (a very sick baby with hepatosplenomegaly, bullous rash and perhaps pneumonia)

---

i | 13.7 Clinical features of congenital syphilis

Early congenital syphilis (neonatal period)

- Maculopapular rash
- Condylomata lata
- Mucous patches
- Fissures around mouth, nose and anus
- Rhinitis with nasal discharge (snuffles)

- Hepatosplenomegaly
- Osteochondritis/periostitis
- Generalised lymphadenopathy
- Choroiditis
- Meningitis
- Anaemia/thrombocytopenia

Late congenital syphilis

- Benign tertiary syphilis
- Periostitis
- Paroxysmal cold haemoglobinuria
- Neurosyphilis

- 8th nerve deafness
- Interstitial keratitis
- Clutton's joints (painless effusion into knee joints)

Stigmata

- Hutchinson's incisors (anterior–posterior thickening with notch on narrowed cutting edge)
- Mulberry molars (imperfectly formed cusps/deficient dental enamel)
- High arched palate
- Maxillary hypoplasia
- Saddle nose (following snuffles)

- Rhagades (radiating scars around mouth, nose and anus following rash)
- Salt and pepper scars on retina (from choroiditis)
- Corneal scars (from interstitial keratitis)
- Sabre tibia (from periostitis)
- Bossing of frontal and parietal bones (healed periosteal nodes)

- birth of a baby who develops signs of early congenital syphilis during the first few weeks of life (Box 13.7)
- birth of a baby with latent infection who either remains well or develops congenital syphilis/stigmata later in life (see Box 13.7).

Investigations in adult cases

Treponema pallidum may be identified in serum collected from chancres, or from moist or eroded lesions in secondary syphilis using a dark-field microscope, a direct fluorescent antibody test or PCR.

The serological tests for syphilis (STS) are listed in Box 13.8. These are antibody tests that almost always remain positive, even after successful treatment. Prolonged untreated infection results in higher titres that may not decline at all. Interpretation of results requires knowledge of any treatment, which may include antibiotics given coincidentally, e.g. for skin or respiratory tract infections.

Many centres use treponemal enzyme immunoassays (EIAs) for IgG and IgM antibodies to screen for syphilis. EIA for antitreponemal IgM becomes positive at approximately 2 weeks, while non-treponemal tests become positive about 4 weeks after primary syphilis. All positive results in asymptomatic patients must be confirmed by repeat tests.

Biological false-positive reactions occur occasionally; these are most commonly seen with Venereal Diseases Research Laboratory (VDRL) or rapid plasma reagin (RPR) tests (when treponemal tests will be negative). Acute false-positive reactions may be associated with infections, such as infectious mononucleosis, chickenpox and malaria, and may also occur in pregnancy. Chronic false-positive reactions may be associated with autoimmune diseases. False-negative results for non-treponemal tests may be found in secondary syphilis because extremely high antibody levels can

13.8 Serological tests for syphilis

Non-treponemal (non-specific) tests

- Venereal Diseases Research Laboratory (VDRL) test
- Rapid plasma reagin (RPR) test

Treponemal (specific) antibody tests

- Treponemal antigen-based enzyme immunoassay (EIA) for IgG and IgM
- *Treponema pallidum* haemagglutination assay (TPHA)
- *T. pallidum* particle agglutination assay (TPPA)
- Fluorescent treponemal antibody-absorbed (FTA-ABS) test

prevent the formation of the antibody–antigen lattice necessary for the visualisation of the flocculation reaction (the prozone phenomenon).

In benign tertiary and cardiovascular syphilis, examination of CSF should be considered because asymptomatic neurological disease may coexist. The CSF should also be examined in patients with clinical signs of neurosyphilis (p. 1125) and in both early and late congenital syphilis. Positive STS may be found in patients who are being investigated for neurological disease, especially dementia. In many instances, the serology reflects previous infection unrelated to the presenting complaint, especially when titres are low. Examination of CSF is occasionally necessary.

Chest X-ray, electrocardiogram (ECG) and echocardiogram are useful in the investigation of cardiovascular syphilis. Biopsy may be required to diagnose gumma.

Endemic treponematoses, such as yaws, endemic (non-venereal) syphilis (bejel) and pinta (pp. 253 and 254), are caused by treponemes that are morphologically indistinguishable from *T. pallidum* and cannot be differentiated by serological tests. A VDRL or RPR test may help to elucidate the correct diagnosis because adults with late yaws usually have low titres.

Investigations in suspected congenital syphilis

Passively transferred maternal antibodies from an adequately treated mother may give rise to positive serological tests in her baby. In this situation, non-treponemal tests should become negative within 3–6 months of birth. A positive EIA test for antitreponemal IgM suggests early congenital syphilis. A diagnosis of congenital syphilis mandates investigation of the mother, her partner and any siblings.

Management

Penicillin is the drug of choice. Currently, a single dose of 2.4 megaunits of intramuscular benzathine benzylpenicillin is recommended for early syphilis (<2 years' duration), with three doses at weekly intervals being recommended in late syphilis. A 14-day course of procaine penicillin is recommended for the treatment of neurosyphilis, supplemented by a 3-day course of prednisolone (see below). Doxycycline is indicated for patients allergic to penicillin, except in pregnancy (see below). Azithromycin is less favoured due to the potential for resistance. All patients must be followed up to ensure cure, and partner notification is of particular importance. Resolution of clinical signs in early syphilis with declining titres for non-treponemal tests, usually to undetectable levels within 6 months for primary syphilis and 12–18 months for secondary syphilis, is an indicator of successful treatment. Specific treponemal antibody tests may remain positive for life. In patients who have had syphilis for many years there may be little serological response following treatment.

Pregnancy

Penicillin is the treatment of choice in pregnancy. Erythromycin stearate can be given if there is penicillin hypersensitivity, but it crosses the placenta poorly; the newborn baby must therefore be treated with a course of penicillin and consideration given to retreating the mother. Some specialists recommend penicillin desensitisation for pregnant mothers so that penicillin can be given during temporary tolerance. A 10-day course of ceftriaxone is a further alternative. Babies should be treated in hospital with the help of a paediatrician.

Treatment reactions

- *Anaphylaxis*. Penicillin is a common cause; on-site facilities should be available for management (p. 75).
- *Jarisch–Herxheimer reaction*. This is an acute febrile reaction that follows treatment and is characterised by headache, malaise and myalgia; it resolves within 24 hours. It is common in early syphilis and rare in late syphilis. Fetal distress or premature labour can occur in pregnancy.
  The reaction may also cause worsening of neurological (cerebral artery occlusion) or ophthalmic (uveitis, optic neuritis) disease, myocardial ischaemia (inflammation of the coronary ostia) and laryngeal stenosis (swelling of a gumma). Prednisolone 40–60 mg daily for 3 days is recommended to prevent the reaction in patients with these forms of the disease; antisyphilitic treatment can be started 24 hours after introducing glucocorticoids. In high-risk situations it is wise to initiate therapy in hospital.
- *Procaine reaction*. Fear of impending death occurs immediately after the accidental intravenous injection of procaine penicillin and may be associated with hallucinations or fits. Symptoms are short-lived, but verbal assurance and sometimes physical restraint are needed. The reaction can be prevented by aspiration before intramuscular injection to ensure the needle is not in a blood vessel.

Gonorrhoea

Gonorrhoea is caused by infection with *Neisseria gonorrhoeae* and may involve columnar epithelium in the lower genital tract, rectum, pharynx and eyes. Transmission is usually the result of vaginal, anal or oral sex. Gonococcal conjunctivitis may be caused by accidental infection from contaminated fingers. Untreated mothers may infect babies during delivery, resulting in ophthalmia neonatorum (Fig. 13.5). Infection of children beyond the neonatal period usually indicates sexual abuse.

Clinical features

The incubation period is usually 2–10 days. In men the anterior urethra is commonly infected, causing urethral discharge and dysuria, but symptoms are absent in about 10% of cases. Examination will usually show a mucopurulent or purulent urethral discharge. Rectal infection in MSM is usually asymptomatic but may present with anal discomfort, discharge or rectal bleeding. Proctoscopy may reveal either no abnormality, or clinical evidence of proctitis (p. 334) such as inflamed rectal mucosa and mucopus.

In women, the urethra, paraurethral glands/ducts, Bartholin's glands/ducts or endocervical canal may be infected. The rectum may also be involved either due to contamination from a urogenital site or as a result of anal sex. Occasionally, the rectum is the

13

Fig. 13.5 Gonococcal ophthalmia neonatorum. *From McMillan A, Scott GR. Sexually transmitted infections: a colour guide. Churchill Livingstone, Elsevier Ltd; 2000.*

	13.9 Treatment of uncomplicated anogenital gonorrhoea

Uncomplicated infection

- Ceftriaxone 500 mg IM plus azithromycin 1 g orally *or*
- Cefixime 400 mg stat *or*
- Ciprofloxacin 500 mg orally stat[1,2] *or*
- Ofloxacin 400 mg orally stat[1,2]

Pregnancy and breastfeeding

- Ceftriaxone 500 mg plus azithromycin 1 g IM stat *or*
- Spectinomycin 2 g IM stat[3]

Pharyngeal gonorrhoea

- Ceftriaxone 500 mg IM plus azithromycin 1 g stat *or*
- Ciprofloxacin 500 mg[1,2] orally stat *or*
- Ofloxacin 400 mg[1,2] orally stat

[1]Contraindicated in pregnancy and breastfeeding. [2]If prevalence of quinolone resistance for *Neisseria gonorrhoeae* is <5%. [3]May be available only in specialist clinics.

	13.10 Complications of delayed therapy in gonorrhoea

- Acute prostatitis
- Epididymo-orchitis
- Bartholin's gland abscess
- Pelvic inflammatory disease (may lead to infertility or ectopic pregnancy)
- Disseminated gonococcal infection

only site infected. About 80% of women who have gonorrhoea are asymptomatic. There may be vaginal discharge or dysuria but these symptoms are often due to additional infections, such as chlamydia (see below), trichomoniasis or candidiasis, making full investigation essential (p. 331). Lower abdominal pain, dyspareunia and intermenstrual bleeding may be indicative of PID. Clinical examination may show no abnormality, or pus may be expressed from urethra, paraurethral ducts or Bartholin's ducts. The cervix may be inflamed, with mucopurulent discharge and contact bleeding.

Pharyngeal gonorrhoea is the result of receptive orogenital sex and is usually symptomless. Gonococcal conjunctivitis is an uncommon complication, presenting with purulent discharge from the eye(s), severe inflammation of the conjunctivae and oedema of the eyelids, pain and photophobia. Gonococcal ophthalmia neonatorum presents similarly with purulent conjunctivitis and oedema of the eyelids. Conjunctivitis must be treated urgently to prevent corneal damage.

Disseminated gonococcal infection (DGI) is seen rarely, and typically affects women with asymptomatic genital infection. Symptoms include arthritis of one or more joints, pustular skin lesions, tenosynovitis and fever. Gonococcal endocarditis has been described.

Investigations

Gram-negative diplococci may be seen on microscopy of smears from infected sites (see Fig. 13.1). Pharyngeal smears are difficult to analyse due to the presence of other diplococci, so the diagnosis must be confirmed by culture or NAAT.

Management of adults

Emerging resistance is making it increasingly difficult to cure gonorrhoea with a single oral dose of antimicrobials, and recommended treatment in the UK has changed to intramuscular ceftriaxone 500 mg given with an oral dose of azithromycin 1 g, in the hope that combination therapy will slow down the development of cephalosporin resistance. The alternatives listed in Box 13.9 are less likely to be effective.

Longer courses of antibiotics are required for complicated infection. The partner(s) of patients with gonorrhoea should be seen as soon as possible. Delay in treatment may lead to complications (Box 13.10).

Chlamydial infection

Chlamydial infection in men

Chlamydia is transmitted and presents in a similar way to gonorrhoea; however, urethral symptoms are usually milder and may be absent in over 50% of cases. Conjunctivitis is also milder than in gonorrhoea; pharyngitis does not occur. The incubation period varies from 1 week to a few months. Without treatment, symptoms may resolve but the patient remains infectious for several months. Complications, such as epididymo-orchitis and sexually acquired reactive arthritis (SARA, p. 1031), are rare. Sexually transmitted pathogens, such as chlamydia or gonococci, are usually responsible for epididymo-orchitis in men aged less than 35 years, whereas bacteria such as Gram-negative enteric organisms are more commonly implicated in older men.

Treatments for chlamydia are listed in Box 13.11. NSU is treated identically. The partner(s) of men with chlamydia should be treated, even if laboratory tests for chlamydia are negative. Investigation is not mandatory but serves a useful epidemiological purpose; moreover, positive results encourage further attempts at contact-tracing.

Chlamydial infection in women

The cervix and urethra are commonly involved. Infection is asymptomatic in about 80% of patients but may cause intermenstrual and/or post-coital bleeding, dysuria or vaginal discharge. Lower abdominal pain and dyspareunia are features of PID. Examination may reveal mucopurulent cervicitis, contact

13.11 Treatment of chlamydial infection

Standard regimens

- Azithromycin 1 g orally as a single dose[1] *or*
- Doxycycline 100 mg twice daily orally for 7 days[2]

Alternative regimens

- Erythromycin 500 mg four times daily orally for 7 days *or* 500 mg twice daily for 2 weeks *or*
- Ofloxacin 200 mg twice daily orally for 7 days[2]

[1]Safety in pregnancy and breastfeeding has not been fully established.
[2]Contraindicated in pregnancy and breastfeeding.

bleeding from the cervix, evidence of PID or no obvious clinical signs. Treatment options are listed in Box 13.11. The patient's male partner(s) should be investigated and treated.

Many infections clear spontaneously but others persist. PID, with the risk of tubal damage and subsequent infertility or ectopic pregnancy, is a rare but important long-term complication. Other complications include perihepatitis, chronic pelvic pain, conjunctivitis and SARA (p. 1031). Perinatal transmission may lead to ophthalmia neonatorum and/or pneumonia in the neonate.

Other sexually transmitted bacterial infections

Chancroid, granuloma inguinale and LGV as causes of genital ulcers in the tropics are described in Box 13.12. LGV is also a cause of proctitis in MSM (p. 334).

Sexually transmitted viral infections

Genital herpes simplex

Infection with herpes simplex virus type 1 (HSV-1) or type 2 (HSV-2) produces a wide spectrum of clinical problems (p. 247), and may facilitate HIV transmission. Infection is usually acquired sexually (vaginal, anal, orogenital or oroanal), but perinatal transmission to the neonate may also occur. Primary infection at the site of HSV entry, which may be symptomatic or asymptomatic, establishes latency in local sensory ganglia. Recurrences, either symptomatic or asymptomatic viral shedding, are a consequence of HSV reactivation. The first symptomatic episode is usually the most severe. Although HSV-1 is classically associated with orolabial herpes and HSV-2 with anogenital herpes, HSV-1 now accounts for more than 50% of anogenital infections in the UK.

Clinical features

The first symptomatic episode presents with irritable vesicles that soon rupture to form small, tender ulcers on the external genitalia (Fig. 13.6 and see Fig. 13.2). Lesions at other sites (e.g. urethra, vagina, cervix, perianal area, anus or rectum) may cause dysuria, urethral or vaginal discharge, or anal, perianal or rectal pain. Constitutional symptoms, such as fever, headache and malaise, are common. Inguinal lymph nodes become enlarged and tender, and there may be nerve root pain in the 2nd and 3rd sacral dermatomes.

Extragenital lesions may develop at other sites, such as the buttock, finger or eye, due to auto-inoculation. Oropharyngeal infection may result from orogenital sex. Complications, such

13

13.12 Salient features of lymphogranuloma venereum, chancroid and granuloma inguinale (Donovanosis)

Infection and distribution	Organism	Incubation period	Genital lesion	Lymph nodes	Diagnosis	Management
Lymphogranuloma venereum (LGV) E/W Africa, India, SE Asia, S America, Caribbean	*Chlamydia trachomatis* types L1, 2, 3	3–30 days	Small, transient, painless ulcer, vesicle, papule; often unnoticed	Tender, usually unilateral, matted, suppurative bubo; inguinal/femoral nodes involved[1]	Serological tests for L1–3 serotypes; swab from ulcer or bubo pus for *Chlamydia*	Doxycycline[2] twice daily orally for 21 days *or* Erythromycin 500 mg four times daily orally
Chancroid Africa, Asia, Central and S America	*Haemophilus ducreyi* (short Gram-negative bacillus)	3–10 days	Single or multiple painful ulcers with ragged undermined edges	As above but unilocular, suppurative bubo; inguinal nodes involved in ~50%	Microscopy and culture of scrapings from ulcer or pus from bubo	Azithromycin[3] 1 g orally once *or* Ceftriaxone 250 mg IM once *or* Ciprofloxacin[2] 500 mg twice daily orally for 3 days
Granuloma inguinale Australia, India, Caribbean, S Africa, S America, Papua New Guinea	*Klebsiella granulomatis* (Donovan bodies)	3–40 days	Ulcers or hypertrophic granulomatous lesions; usually painless[4]	Initial swelling of inguinal nodes, then spread of infection to form abscess or ulceration through adjacent skin	Microscopy of cellular material for intracellular bipolar-staining Donovan bodies	Azithromycin[3] 1 g weekly orally or 500 mg daily orally *or* Doxycycline[2] 100 mg twice daily orally *or* Ceftriaxone 1 g IM daily

N.B. Partners of patients with LGV, chancroid and granuloma inguinale should be investigated and treated, even if asymptomatic.
[1]The genito-ano-rectal syndrome is a late manifestation of LGV. [2]Doxycycline and ciprofloxacin are contraindicated in pregnancy and breastfeeding. [3]The safety of azithromycin in pregnancy and breastfeeding has not been fully assessed. [4]Mother-to-baby transmission of granuloma inguinale may rarely occur.

Fig. 13.6 Herpetic ulceration of the vulva. *From McMillan A, Scott GR. Sexually transmitted infections: a colour guide. Churchill Livingstone, Elsevier Ltd; 2000.*

as urinary retention due to autonomic neuropathy, and aseptic meningitis, are occasionally seen.

First episodes usually heal within 2–4 weeks without treatment; recurrences are usually milder and of shorter duration than the initial attack. They occur more often in HSV-2 infection and their frequency tends to decrease with time. Prodromal symptoms, such as irritation or burning at the subsequent site of recurrence, or neuralgic pain affecting buttocks, legs or hips are commonly seen. The first symptomatic episode may be a recurrence of a previously undiagnosed primary infection. Recurrent episodes of asymptomatic viral shedding are important in the transmission of HSV.

Diagnosis

Swabs are taken from vesicular fluid or ulcers for detection of DNA by PCR, or tissue culture and typing as either HSV-1 or 2. Electron microscopy of such material will give only a presumptive diagnosis, as herpes group viruses appear similar. Type-specific antibody tests are available but are not sufficiently accurate for general use.

Management

First episode

The following 5-day oral regimens should be started within 5 days of the beginning of the episode, or while lesions are still forming:

- aciclovir 400 mg three times daily
- valaciclovir 500 mg twice daily.

Famciclovir 250 mg three times daily or aciclovir 200 mg five times daily is an alternative.

Analgesia may be required and saline bathing can be soothing. Treatment may be continued for longer than 5 days if new lesions develop. Occasionally, intravenous therapy may be indicated if oral therapy is poorly tolerated or aseptic meningitis occurs.

Catheterisation via the suprapubic route is advisable for urinary retention due to autonomic neuropathy because the transurethral route may introduce HSV into the bladder.

Recurrent genital herpes

Symptomatic recurrences are usually mild and may require no specific treatment other than saline bathing. For more severe episodes, patient-initiated treatment at onset, with one of the following 5-day oral regimens, should reduce the duration of the recurrence:

- aciclovir 200 mg five times daily
- famciclovir 125–250 mg twice daily
- valaciclovir 500 mg twice daily.

In a few patients, treatment started at the onset of prodromal symptoms may abort recurrence.

Suppressive therapy may be required for patients with frequent recurrences, especially if these are experienced at intervals of less than 4 weeks. Treatment should be given for a minimum of 1 year before stopping to assess recurrence rate. About 20% of patients will experience reduced attack rates thereafter, but for those whose recurrences remain unchanged, resumption of suppressive therapy is justified. Aciclovir 400 mg twice daily is most commonly prescribed.

Management in pregnancy

If her partner is known to be infected with HSV, a pregnant woman with no previous anogenital herpes should be advised to protect herself during sexual intercourse because the risk of disseminated infection is increased in pregnancy. Consistent condom use during pregnancy may reduce transmission of HSV. Genital herpes acquired during the first or second trimester of pregnancy is treated with aciclovir as clinically indicated. Although aciclovir is not licensed for use in pregnancy in the UK, there is considerable clinical evidence to support its safety. Third-trimester acquisition of infection has been associated with life-threatening haematogenous dissemination and should be treated with aciclovir.

Vaginal delivery should be routine in women who are symptomless in late pregnancy. Caesarean section is sometimes considered if there is a recurrence at the beginning of labour, although the risk of neonatal herpes through vaginal transmission is very low. Caesarean section is often recommended if primary infection occurs after 34 weeks because the risk of viral shedding is very high in labour.

Human papillomavirus and anogenital warts

Human papillomavirus (HPV) DNA typing has demonstrated over 90 genotypes (p. 1238), of which HPV-6, HPV-11, HPV-16 and HPV-18 most commonly infect the genital tract through sexual transmission. It is important to differentiate between the benign genotypes (HPV-6 and 11) that cause anogenital warts, and genotypes such as 16 and 18 that are associated with dysplastic conditions and cancers of the genital tract but are not a cause of benign warts. All genotypes usually result in subclinical infection of the genital tract rather than clinically obvious lesions affecting penis, vulva, vagina, cervix, perineum or anus.

Clinical features

Anogenital warts caused by HPV may be single or multiple, exophytic, papular or flat. Perianal warts (p. 330), while being more common in MSM, are also found in heterosexual men and in women. Rarely, a giant condyloma (Buschke–Löwenstein tumour) develops, with local tissue destruction. Atypical warts should be biopsied. In pregnancy, warts may dramatically increase in size and number, making treatment difficult. Rarely, they are large enough to obstruct labour and, in this case, delivery by caesarean section will be required. Uncommonly, perinatal transmission of HPV leads to anogenital warts, or possibly laryngeal papillomas, in the neonate.

Management

The use of condoms can help prevent the transmission of HPV to non-infected partners, but HPV may affect parts of the genital area not protected by condoms. Vaccination against HPV infection has been introduced and is in routine use in many countries. There are three types of vaccine:

- *A bivalent vaccine* offers protection against HPV types 16 and 18, which account for approximately 75% of cervical cancers in the UK.
- *A quadrivalent vaccine* offers additional protection against HPV types 6 and 11, which account for over 90% of genital warts.
- *A nonovalent vaccine* protects against five additional high-risk types (31, 33, 45, 52 and 58).

All vaccines have been shown to be highly effective in the prevention of cervical intra-epithelial neoplasia in young women, and the quadrivalent and nonovalent vaccines have also been demonstrated to be highly effective in protecting against HPV-associated genital warts. It is currently recommended that HPV vaccination should be administered prior to the onset of sexual activity, typically at age 11–13, in a course of three injections. In the UK, only girls are offered vaccination, but it is possible that vaccination will be extended to MSM in whom HPV transmission is associated with an increased risk of anal cancer. As no vaccine protects against all oncogenic types of HPV, cervical screening programmes will still be necessary.

A variety of treatments are available for established disease, including the following:

- *Podophyllotoxin, 0.5% solution or 0.15% cream* (contraindicated in pregnancy), applied twice daily for 3 days, followed by 4 days' rest, for up to 4 weeks, is suitable for home treatment of external warts.
- *Imiquimod cream* (contraindicated in pregnancy), applied 3 times weekly (and washed off after 6–10 hours) for up to 16 weeks, is also suitable for home treatment of external warts.
- *Catephen* (an extract of the green tea plant, *Camellia sinensis*) is applied by the patient three times daily for up to 16 weeks.
- *Cryotherapy* using liquid nitrogen to freeze warty tissue is suitable for external and internal warts but often requires repeated clinic visits.
- *Hyfrecation* – electrofulguration that causes superficial charring – is suitable for external and internal warts. Hyfrecation results in smoke plume, which contains HPV DNA and has the potential to cause respiratory infection in the operator/patient. Masks should be worn during the procedure and adequate extraction of fumes should be provided.

- *Surgical removal* may be used to excise refractory warts, especially pedunculated perianal lesions, under local or general anaesthesia.

Molluscum contagiosum

Infection by molluscum contagiosum virus, both sexual and non-sexual, produces flesh-coloured, umbilicated, hemispherical papules usually up to 5 mm in diameter after an incubation period of 3–12 weeks (Fig. 13.7). Larger lesions may be seen in HIV infection (p. 306). Lesions are often multiple and, once established in an individual, may spread by auto-inoculation. They are found on the genitalia, lower abdomen and upper thighs when sexually acquired. Facial lesions are highly suggestive of underlying HIV infection. Diagnosis is made clinically or very rarely by electron microscopy. Typically, lesions persist for several months before spontaneous resolution occurs. Treatment regimens are therefore cosmetic; they include cryotherapy, hyfrecation, topical applications of 0.15% podophyllotoxin cream (contraindicated in pregnancy) or expression of the central core.

Fig. 13.7 Molluscum contagiosum of the shaft of the penis.
From McMillan A, Scott GR. Sexually transmitted infections: a colour guide. Churchill Livingstone, Elsevier Ltd; 2000.

13

Viral hepatitis

The hepatitis viruses A–D (p. 871) may be sexually transmitted:

- *Hepatitis A (HAV).* Insertive oroanal sex, insertive digital sex, insertive anal sex and multiple sexual partners have been linked with HAV transmission in MSM. HAV transmission in heterosexual men and women is also possible through oroanal sex.
- *Hepatitis B (HBV).* Insertive oroanal sex, anal sex and multiple sexual partners are linked with HBV infection in MSM. Heterosexual transmission of HBV is well documented and commercial sex workers are at particular risk. Hepatitis D (HDV) may also be sexually transmitted.
- *Hepatitis C (HCV).* Sexual transmission of HCV is well documented in MSM but less so in heterosexuals. Sexual transmission is less efficient than for HBV.

The sexual partner(s) of patients with HAV and HBV should be seen as soon as possible and offered immunisation where appropriate. Patients with HAV should abstain from all forms of unprotected sex until non-infectious. Those with HBV should likewise abstain from unprotected sex until they are non-infectious or until their partners have been vaccinated successfully. No active or passive immunisation is available for protection against HCV but the consistent use of condoms is likely to protect susceptible partners. Active immunisation against HAV and HBV should be offered to susceptible people at risk of infection. Many STI clinics offer HAV immunisation to MSM along with routine HBV immunisation; a combined HAV and HBV vaccine is available.

Further information

Books and journal articles

Pattman R, Sankar N, Elawad B, et al. (eds). Oxford handbook of genitourinary medicine, HIV, and sexual health. Oxford: Oxford University Press; 2010.
Rogstad KE (ed.). ABC of sexually transmitted infections, 6th edn. Oxford: Wiley–Blackwell; 2011.

Website

bashh.org/guidelines British Association for Sexual Health and HIV; updates on treatment of all STIs.

A Mather
L Burnett
DR Sullivan
P Stewart

14

Clinical biochemistry and metabolic medicine

Clinical examination in biochemical and metabolic disorders 346

Biochemical investigations 348

Water and electrolyte homeostasis 349

Sodium homeostasis 349
Functional anatomy and physiology 349
Presenting problems in sodium and water balance 352
  Hypovolaemia 352
  Hypervolaemia 353

Water homeostasis 355
Functional anatomy and physiology 355
Presenting problems in regulation of osmolality 356
  Hyponatraemia 357
  Hypernatraemia 358

Potassium homeostasis 360
Functional anatomy and physiology 360
Presenting problems in potassium homeostasis 361
  Hypokalaemia 361
  Hyperkalaemia 362

Acid–base homeostasis 363
Functional anatomy and physiology 363
Presenting problems in acid–base balance 364
  Metabolic acidosis 364
  Metabolic alkalosis 366
  Respiratory acidosis 367
  Respiratory alkalosis 367
  Mixed acid–base disorders 367

Calcium homeostasis 367

Magnesium homeostasis 367
Functional anatomy and physiology 367
Presenting problems in magnesium homeostasis 367
  Hypomagnesaemia 368
  Hypermagnesaemia 368

Phosphate homeostasis 368
Functional anatomy and physiology 368
Presenting problems in phosphate homeostasis 368
  Hypophosphataemia 368
  Hyperphosphataemia 369

Disorders of amino acid metabolism 369

Disorders of carbohydrate metabolism 370

Disorders of complex lipid metabolism 370

Lipids and lipoprotein metabolism 370
Functional anatomy and physiology 371
Lipids and cardiovascular disease 373
Investigations 373
Presenting problems in lipid metabolism 373
  Hypercholesterolaemia 373
  Hypertriglyceridaemia 374
  Mixed hyperlipidaemia 375
  Rare dyslipidaemias 375
Principles of management 375

The porphyrias 378

Clinical examination in biochemical and metabolic disorders

Many biochemical and metabolic disorders are clinically silent or present with non-specific manifestations, and are first detected by laboratory testing. Several abnormalities can be picked up by history and physical examination, however, as summarised below.

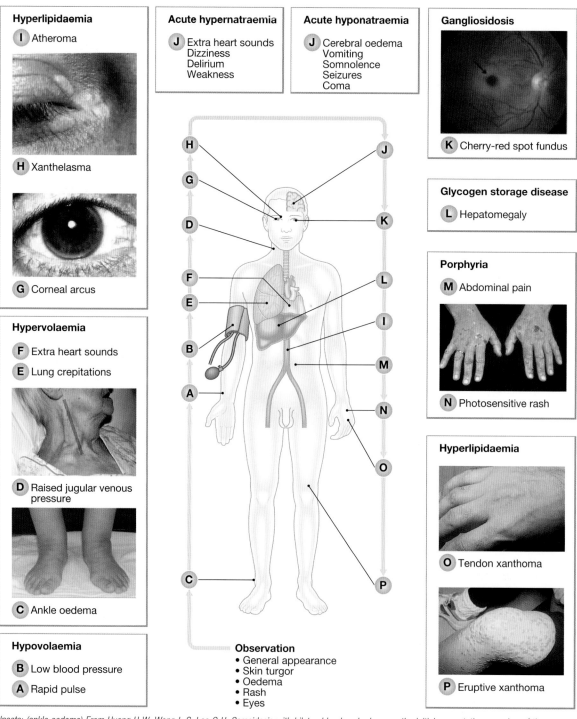

Hyperlipidaemia

I Atheroma

H Xanthelasma

G Corneal arcus

Hypervolaemia

F Extra heart sounds

E Lung crepitations

D Raised jugular venous pressure

C Ankle oedema

Hypovolaemia

B Low blood pressure

A Rapid pulse

Acute hypernatraemia

J Extra heart sounds
Dizziness
Delirium
Weakness

Acute hyponatraemia

J Cerebral oedema
Vomiting
Somnolence
Seizures
Coma

Observation
• General appearance
• Skin turgor
• Oedema
• Rash
• Eyes

Gangliosidosis

K Cherry-red spot fundus

Glycogen storage disease

L Hepatomegaly

Porphyria

M Abdominal pain

N Photosensitive rash

Hyperlipidaemia

O Tendon xanthoma

P Eruptive xanthoma

Insets: (ankle oedema) From Huang H-W, Wong L-S, Lee C-H. Sarcoidosis with bilateral leg lymphedema as the initial presentation: a review of the literature. Dermatologica Sinica 2016; 34:29–32; (raised jugular venous pressure) Newby D, Grubb N. Cardiology: an illustrated colour text. Edinburgh: Churchill Livingstone, Elsevier Ltd; 2005; (cherry-red spots) Vieira de Rezende Pinto WB, Sgobbi de Souza PV, Pedroso JL, et al. Variable phenotype and severity of sialidosis expressed in two siblings presenting with ataxia and macular cherry-red spots. J Clin Neurosci 2013; 20:1327–1328; (photosensitive rash) Ferri FF. Ferri's Color atlas and text of clinical medicine. Philadelphia: Saunders, Elsevier Inc.; 2009; courtesy of the Institute of Dermatology, London.

Assessment of volume status and electrolyte disturbances

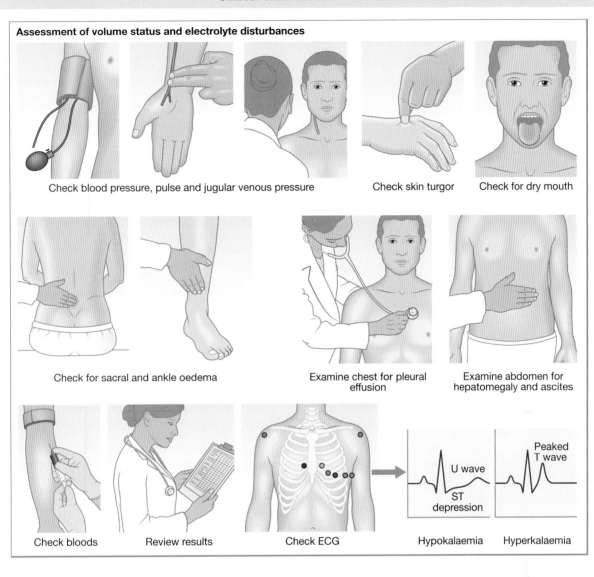

Check blood pressure, pulse and jugular venous pressure

Check skin turgor

Check for dry mouth

Check for sacral and ankle oedema

Examine chest for pleural effusion

Examine abdomen for hepatomegaly and ascites

Check bloods

Review results

Check ECG

U wave

ST depression

Peaked T wave

Hypokalaemia

Hyperkalaemia

14

Check for signs of hyperlipidaemia

Check skin and tendons for xanthomas

Check eyes for arcus and xanthelasma

There is a worldwide trend towards increased use of laboratory-based diagnostic investigations, and biochemical investigations in particular. In the health-care systems of developed countries, it has been estimated that 60–70% of all critical decisions taken in regard to patients, and over 90% of data stored in electronic medical records systems, involve a laboratory service or result.

This chapter covers a diverse group of disorders affecting adults that are not considered elsewhere in this book, whose primary manifestation is in abnormalities of biochemistry laboratory results, or whose underlying pathophysiology involves disturbance in specific biochemical pathways.

Biochemical investigations

There are three broad reasons why a clinician may request a biochemical laboratory investigation:

- to screen an asymptomatic subject for the presence of disease
- to assist in diagnosis of a patient's presenting complaint
- to monitor changes in test results, as a marker of disease progression or response to treatment.

Contemporary medical practice has become increasingly reliant on laboratory investigation and, in particular, on biochemical investigation. This has been associated with extraordinary improvements in the analytical capacity and speed of laboratory instrumentation and the following operational trends:

- Large central biochemistry laboratories feature extensive use of automation and information technology. Specimens are transported from clinical areas to the laboratory using high-speed transport systems (such as pneumatic tubes) and identified with machine-readable labels (such as bar codes). Laboratory instruments have been miniaturised and integrated with robot transport systems to enable multiple rapid analyses of a single sample. Statistical process control techniques are used to assure the quality of analytical results, and increasingly to monitor other aspects of the laboratory, such as the time taken to complete the analysis ('turn-around time').

- Point-of-care testing (POCT) brings selected laboratory analytical systems into clinical areas, to the patient's bedside or even connected to an individual patient. These systems allow the clinician to receive results almost instantaneously for immediate treatment of the patient, although often with lesser precision or at greater cost than using a central laboratory.

- The diversity of analyses has widened considerably with the introduction of many techniques borrowed from the chemical or other industries (Box 14.1).

Good medical practice involves the appropriate ordering of laboratory investigations and correct interpretation of test results (Box 14.2). The key principles, including the concepts of sensitivity and specificity, are described on page 4. Reference intervals for laboratory results are provided in Chapter 35. Many laboratory investigations can be subject to variability arising from whether the sample is being taken in the fed or fasted state; the timing of sample collection, in relation to diurnal variation of analytes; dosage intervals for therapeutic drug monitoring; sample type, such as serum plasma; use of anticoagulants, such as EDTA, which can interfere with some assays; or artefacts, such as

14.1 Range of analytical modalities used in the clinical biochemistry laboratory

Analytical modality	Analyte	Typical applications
Ion-selective electrodes	Blood gases, electrolytes (Na, K, Cl)	Point-of-care testing (POCT) High-throughput analysers
Colorimetric chemical reaction or coupled enzymatic reaction	Simple mass or concentration measurement (creatinine, phosphate) Simple enzyme activity	High-throughput analysers
Ligand assay (usually immunoassay)	Specific proteins Hormones Drugs	Increasingly available for POCT or high-throughput analysers
Chromatography: gas chromatography (GC), high-performance liquid chromatography (HPLC), thin-layer chromatography (TLC)	Organic compounds	Therapeutic drug monitoring (TDM)
Mass spectroscopy (MS)		Drug screening (drugs of misuse) Vitamins Biochemical metabolites
Spectrophotometry, turbidimetry, nephelometry, fluorimetry	Haemoglobin derivatives Specific proteins Immunoglobulins	Xanthochromia Lipoproteins Paraproteins
Electrophoresis	Proteins Some enzymes	Paraproteins Isoenzyme analysis
Atomic absorption (AA) Inductively coupled plasma/mass spectroscopy (ICP-MS)	Trace elements and metals	Quantitation of heavy metals
Molecular diagnostics	Nucleic acid quantification and/or sequence	Inherited and somatic cell mutations (Ch. 3) Genetic polymorphisms (Ch. 3) Variations in rates of drug metabolism (Ch. 2) Microbial diagnosis (Ch. 6)

14.2 How to interpret urea and electrolytes results*

Sodium

- Largely reflects changes in sodium and water balance
- See 'Hypernatraemia' and 'Hyponatraemia' (pp. 358 and 357)

Potassium

- May reflect K shifts in and out of cells
- Low levels usually mean excessive losses (gastrointestinal or renal)
- High levels usually mean renal dysfunction
- See 'Hypokalaemia' and 'Hyperkalaemia' (pp. 361 and 362)

Chloride

- Generally changes in parallel with plasma Na
- Low in metabolic alkalosis
- High in some forms of metabolic acidosis

Bicarbonate

- Abnormal in acid–base disorders
- See Box 14.18 (p. 365)

Urea

- Increased with a fall in glomerular filtration rate (GFR), reduced renal perfusion or urine flow rate, and in high protein intake or catabolic states
- See page 386

Creatinine

- Increased with a fall in GFR, in individuals with high muscle mass, and with some drugs
- See Fig. 15.2 (p. 387)

*The term urea and electrolytes (U&Es) refers to urea, electrolyes and creatinine. In some countries this is abbreviated to EUC (electrolytes/urea/creatinine).

Fig. 14.1 Normal distribution of body water and electrolytes. Schematic representation of volume (L = litres) and composition (dominant ionic species only shown) of the intracellular fluid (ICF) and extracellular fluid (ECF) in a 70 kg male. The main difference in composition between the plasma and interstitial fluid (ISF) is the presence of appreciable concentrations of protein in the plasma but not the ISF. The Na/K differential is maintained by the Na,K-adenosine triphosphatase (ATPase) pump.

taking a venous sample proximal to the site of an intravenous infusion. It is therefore important for clinical and laboratory staff to communicate effectively and for clinicians to follow local recommendations concerning collection and transport of samples in the appropriate container and with appropriate labelling.

Water and electrolyte homeostasis

Total body water (TBW) is approximately 60% of body weight in an adult male, although the proportion is somewhat more for infants and less for women. In a 70 kg man TBW is therefore about 40 L. Approximately 25 L is located inside cells (the intracellular fluid or ICF), while the remaining 15 L is in the extracellular fluid (ECF) compartment (Fig. 14.1). Most of the ECF (approximately 12 L) is interstitial fluid, which is within the tissues but outside cells, whereas the remainder (about 3 L) is in the plasma compartment.

The ion composition between the main body fluid compartments intracellularly and extracellularly is illustrated in Figure 14.1. The dominant positively charged ion (cation) within cells is potassium, whereas phosphates and negatively charged proteins constitute the major intracellular negatively charged ions (anions). In the ECF the dominant cation is sodium, while chloride and, to a lesser extent, bicarbonate are the most important ECF anions. An important difference between the intravascular (plasma) and interstitial compartments of the ECF is that only plasma contains significant concentrations of protein.

The major force maintaining the difference in cation concentrations between the ICF and ECF is the sodium–potassium

pump (Na,K-activated adenosine triphosphatase (ATPase)), which is present in all cell membranes. Maintenance of these gradients is essential for many cell processes, including the excitability of conducting tissues such as nerve and muscle. The difference in protein content between the plasma and the interstitial fluid compartment is maintained by the impermeability of the capillary wall to protein. This protein concentration gradient (the colloid osmotic, or oncotic, pressure of the plasma) contributes to the balance of forces across the capillary wall that favour fluid retention within the plasma compartment.

The concentration of sodium in the ECF plays a pivotal role in determining plasma osmolality and thereby controlling intracellular volume through changes in water balance between the intracellular and extracellular space. In contrast, plasma volume is largely controlled by total body sodium, which determines volume change. Therefore, disturbances in water homeostasis typically present with biochemical abnormalities such as hyponatraemia or hypernatraemia, whereas disturbances in sodium homeostasis present with hypervolaemia or hypovolaemia as the result of expansion or contraction of ECF volume, respectively.

Sodium homeostasis

Most of the body's sodium is located in the ECF, where it is by far the most abundant cation. Accordingly, total body sodium is the principal determinant of ECF volume. Sodium intake varies widely between individuals, ranging between 50 and 250 mmol/24 hrs. The kidneys can compensate for these wide variations in sodium intake by increasing excretion of sodium when there is sodium overload, and retaining sodium in the presence of sodium depletion, to maintain normal ECF volume and plasma volume.

Functional anatomy and physiology

The functional unit for renal excretion is the nephron (Fig. 14.2). Blood undergoes ultrafiltration in the glomerulus, generating a fluid that is free from cells and protein and which resembles plasma in its electrolyte composition. This is delivered into the renal tubules, where reabsorption of water and various electrolytes occurs. (More detail on the structure and function of the glomerulus is given in Ch. 15.) The glomerular filtration rate (GFR) is approximately 125 mL/min (equivalent to 180 L/24 hrs) in a normal adult. Over 99% of the filtered fluid is reabsorbed into the blood in the peritubular capillaries during its passage through successive segments of the nephron, largely as a result of tubular reabsorption of sodium. The processes mediating sodium reabsorption, and the factors that regulate it, are key to understanding clinical disturbances and pharmacological interventions of sodium and fluid balance.

The nephron can be divided into at least four different functional segments in terms of sodium reabsorption (Fig. 14.3).

Proximal renal tubule

About 65% of the filtered sodium load is reabsorbed in the proximal renal tubule. The cellular mechanisms are complex but some of the key features are shown in Figure 14.3A. Filtered sodium in the luminal fluid enters the proximal tubular cell through transporters in the apical membrane that couple sodium transport to the entry of glucose, amino acid, phosphate and other organic molecules. Entry of sodium into the tubular cells at this site is also linked to secretion of H+ ions, through the sodium–hydrogen exchanger (NHE-3). Intracellular H+ ions are generated within tubular cells from the breakdown of carbonic acid, which is produced from carbon dioxide and water under the influence of carbonic anhydrase. Large numbers of Na,K-ATPase pumps

are present on the basolateral membrane of tubular cells, which transport sodium from the cells into the blood. In addition, a large component of the transepithelial flux of sodium, water and other dissolved solutes occurs through gaps *between* the cells (the 'shunt' pathway). Overall, fluid and electrolyte reabsorption is almost isotonic in this segment, as water reabsorption is matched very closely to sodium fluxes, such that the osmolality of fluid passing into the loop of Henle is very similar to that of plasma. A component of this water flow also passes *through* the cells, via aquaporin-1 (AQP-1) water channels, which are not sensitive to hormonal regulation.

Loop of Henle

The thick ascending limb of the loop of Henle (Fig. 14.3B) reabsorbs a further 25% of the filtered sodium but is impermeable to water, resulting in dilution of the luminal fluid. The primary driving force is the Na,K-ATPase on the basolateral cell membrane, but in this segment sodium enters the cell from the lumen through a specific carrier molecule, the Na,K,2Cl co-transporter ('triple co-transporter', or NKCC2), which allows electroneutral entry of these ions into the renal tubular cell by balancing transport of anions (Na+/K+) with cations (Cl-). Some of the potassium accumulated inside the cell recirculates across the apical membrane back into the lumen through a specific potassium channel (ROMK), providing a continuing supply of potassium to match the high concentrations of sodium and chloride in the lumen. A small positive transepithelial potential difference exists in the lumen of this segment relative to the interstitium, and this serves to drive cations such as sodium, potassium, calcium and magnesium between the cells, forming a reabsorptive shunt pathway.

Early distal renal tubule

About 6% of filtered sodium is reabsorbed in the early distal tubule (also called distal convoluted tubule) (Fig. 14.3C), again driven by the activity of the basolateral Na,K-ATPase. In this segment, entry of sodium into the cell from the luminal fluid occurs through a sodium–chloride co-transport carrier (NCCT). This segment is also impermeable to water, resulting in further dilution of the luminal fluid. There is no significant transepithelial flux of potassium in this segment, but calcium is reabsorbed through the mechanism shown in Figure 14.3C: a basolateral sodium–calcium exchanger leads to low intracellular concentrations of calcium, promoting calcium entry from the luminal fluid through a calcium channel.

Late distal renal tubule and collecting ducts

The late distal tubule and cortical collecting duct are anatomically and functionally continuous (Fig. 14.3D). Here, sodium entry from the luminal fluid occurs through the epithelial sodium channel (ENaC), generating a substantial lumen-negative transepithelial potential difference. This sodium flux into the tubular cells is balanced by secretion of potassium and hydrogen ions into the lumen and by reabsorption of chloride ions. Potassium is accumulated in the cell by the basolateral Na,K-ATPase, and passes into the luminal fluid down its electrochemical gradient, through an apical potassium channel (ROMK). Chloride ions pass largely between cells. Hydrogen ion secretion is mediated by an H+-ATPase located on the luminal membrane of the intercalated cells, which constitute approximately one-third of the epithelial cells in this segment of the nephron. The distal tubule and collecting duct have a variable permeability to water, depending on circulating levels of vasopressin (antidiuretic hormone, ADH).

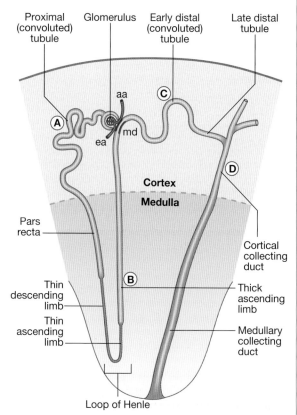

Fig. 14.2 The nephron. Letters A–D refer to tubular segments shown in more detail in Figure 14.3. (aa = afferent arteriole; ea = efferent arteriole; md = macula densa)

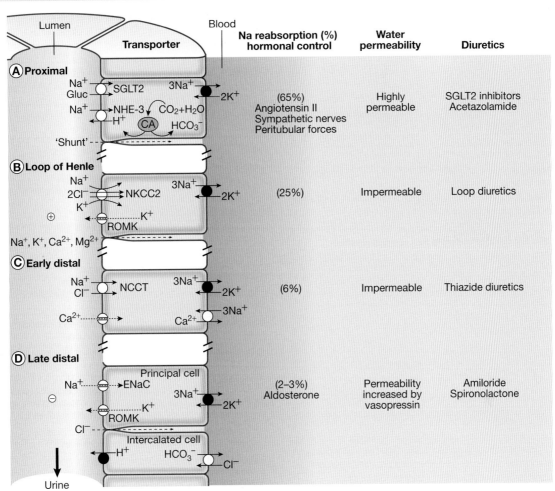

Fig. 14.3 Principal transport mechanisms in segments of the nephron. The apical membrane of tubular cells is the side facing the lumen and the basolateral membrane is the side facing the blood. Black circles indicate active transport pumps linked to ATP hydrolysis and white symbols indicate ion channels and transporter molecules. Details of the proportion of sodium reabsorbed, influence of regulatory factors, water permeability and sites of action for different classes of diuretics are shown. The SGLT2 inhibitors are primarily used for the treatment of diabetes but have diuretic properties by blocking SGLT2 in the proximal tubule. At the same site, acetazolamide inhibits carbonic anhydrase (CA), which, by reducing production of hydrogen ions by proximal tubular cells, inhibits sodium–hydrogen exchange through the NHE-3 transporter. Loop diuretics block the NKCC2 transporter in the loop of Henle, whereas thiazide diuretics block the NCCT channel in the early distal tubule. Amiloride and spironolactone block the ENaC channel in the late distal tubule and collecting ducts. See text for further details and abbreviations.

All ion transport processes in this segment are stimulated by the steroid hormone aldosterone, which can increase sodium reabsorption in this segment to a maximum of 2–3% of the filtered sodium load.

Less than 1% of sodium reabsorption occurs in the medullary collecting duct, where it is inhibited by atrial natriuretic peptide (ANP) and brain natriuretic peptide (BNP).

Regulation of sodium transport

The amount of sodium excreted by the kidney is dependent on the filtered load of sodium (which is largely determined by GFR) and the control of tubular sodium reabsorption. A number of interrelated mechanisms serve to maintain whole-body sodium balance, and hence ECF volume, by matching urinary sodium excretion to sodium intake (Fig. 14.4), and controlling those two processes.

Important sensing mechanisms include volume receptors in the cardiac atria and the intrathoracic veins, as well as pressure receptors located in the central arterial tree (aortic arch and carotid

sinus) and the afferent arterioles within the kidney. A further afferent signal is generated within the kidney itself: the enzyme renin is released from specialised smooth muscle cells in the walls of the afferent and efferent arterioles, at the point where they make contact with the early distal tubule (at the macula densa; see Fig. 14.2) to form the juxtaglomerular apparatus. Renin release is stimulated by:

- reduced perfusion pressure in the afferent arteriole
- increased sympathetic nerve activity
- decreased sodium chloride concentration in the distal tubular fluid.

Renin acts on the peptide substrate, angiotensinogen (which is produced by the liver), to produce angiotensin I, which is cleaved by angiotensin-converting enzyme (ACE), largely in the pulmonary capillary bed, to produce angiotensin II (see Fig. 18.18, p. 666). Angiotensin II has multiple actions: it stimulates proximal tubular sodium reabsorption and release of aldosterone from the zona glomerulosa of the adrenal cortex, and causes vasoconstriction of small arterioles. Aldosterone amplifies sodium

Fig. 14.4 Mechanisms involved in the regulation of sodium transport. (ANP = atrial natriuretic peptide; BNP = brain natriuretic peptide; ECF = extracellular fluid; GFR = glomerular filtration rate; RAA = renin–angiotensin–aldosterone system; SNS = sympathetic nervous system. ⊕ indicates an effect to stimulate Na reabsorption and hence reduce Na excretion, while ⊖ indicates an effect to inhibit Na reabsorption and hence increase Na excretion)

retention by its action on the cortical collecting duct. The net effect of activation of the renin–angiotensin system is to raise blood pressure and cause sodium and water retention, thereby correcting hypovolaemia.

Changes in GFR alter peritubular hydrostatic pressure and oncotic pressure in opposite directions, resulting in a change in sodium reabsorption. In particular, with hypovolaemia, and a reduction in hydrostatic pressure and an increase in oncotic pressure, there is an increase in sodium reabsorption.

The sympathetic nervous system also acts to increase sodium retention, both through haemodynamic mechanisms (afferent arteriolar vasoconstriction and GFR reduction) and by direct stimulation of proximal tubular sodium reabsorption. In contrast, other humoral mediators, such as the natriuretic peptides, which inhibit sodium reabsorption, contribute to natriuresis during periods of sodium and volume excess.

Increases in sodium intake cause hypervolaemia, which increases renal perfusion and GFR and suppresses renin production through increased delivery of sodium into the macula densa. This sets in motion a train of events opposite to those that occur in hypovolaemia, to cause an increase in sodium excretion.

Presenting problems in sodium and water balance

When the balance of sodium intake and excretion is disturbed, any tendency for plasma sodium concentration to change is usually corrected by the osmotic mechanisms controlling water balance (p. 349). As a result, disorders in sodium balance present chiefly as alterations in the ECF volume, resulting in hypovolaemia or hypervolaemia, rather than as an alteration in plasma sodium concentration. Clinical manifestations of altered ECF volume are illustrated in Box 14.3.

Hypovolaemia

Hypovolaemia is defined as a reduction in circulating blood volume. The most common causes are loss or sequestration

14.3 Clinical features of hypovolaemia and hypervolaemia

	Hypovolaemia	Hypervolaemia
Symptoms	Thirst Dizziness on standing Weakness	Ankle swelling Abdominal swelling Breathlessness
Signs	Postural hypotension Tachycardia Dry mouth Reduced skin turgor Reduced urine output Weight loss Delirium, stupor	Peripheral oedema Raised JVP Pulmonary crepitations Pleural effusion Ascites Weight gain Hypertension (sometimes)

(JVP = jugular venous pressure)

14.4 Causes of hypovolaemia

Mechanism	Examples
Inadequate sodium intake	Environmental deprivation, inadequate therapeutic replacement
Gastrointestinal sodium loss	Vomiting, diarrhoea, nasogastric suction, external fistula
Skin sodium loss	Excessive sweating, burns
Renal sodium loss	Diuretic therapy, mineralocorticoid deficiency, tubulointerstitial disease
Internal sequestration*	Bowel obstruction, peritonitis, pancreatitis, crush injury
Reduced blood volume	Acute blood loss

*A cause of circulatory volume depletion, although total body sodium and water may be normal or increased.

of sodium-containing fluids or acute blood loss, as summarised in Box 14.4.

Pathogenesis

Loss of sodium-containing fluid triggers the changes in renal sodium handling and activation of the renin–angiotensin system that were described on page 349. Loss of whole blood, as in acute haemorrhage, is another cause of hypovolaemia, and elicits the same mechanisms for the conservation of sodium and water as loss of sodium-containing fluid.

Clinical features

Hypovolaemia is primarily a clinical diagnosis, based on characteristic symptoms such as thirst, dizziness and weakness along with characteristic clinical signs (see Box 14.3) in the context of a relevant precipitating illness.

Investigations

Serum sodium concentrations are usually normal in hypovolaemia. The GFR is usually maintained unless the hypovolaemia is very severe or prolonged, but urinary flow rate is reduced as a consequence of activation of sodium- and water-retaining mechanisms in the nephron. Serum creatinine, which reflects GFR, is usually normal, but serum urea concentration is typically elevated due to a low urine flow rate, which is accompanied by increased tubular reabsorption of urea. Similarly, serum uric acid may also rise, reflecting increased reabsorption in the proximal renal tubule. The urine osmolality increases due to increased reabsorption of sodium and water, while the urine sodium concentration falls and sodium excretion may fall to less than 0.1% of the filtered sodium load.

Management

Management of sodium and water depletion has two main components:

- treat the cause where possible, to stop ongoing salt and water losses
- replace the salt and water deficits, and provide ongoing maintenance requirements, usually by intravenous fluid replacement when depletion is severe.

Intravenous fluid therapy

Intravenous fluid therapy can be used to maintain water, sodium and potassium intake when the patient is fasting, such as during an acute illness or post-operatively. If any deficits or continuing pathological losses are identified, additional fluid and electrolytes will be required. In prolonged periods of fasting (more than a few days), attention also needs to be given to providing sufficient caloric and nutritional intake to prevent excessive catabolism of body energy stores (p. 704). The daily maintenance requirements for water and electrolytes in a typical adult are shown in Box 14.5 and the composition of some widely available intravenous fluids are given in Box 14.6. The choice of fluid and the rate of administration depend on the clinical circumstances, as assessed at the bedside and from laboratory data, as described in Box 14.7.

The choice of intravenous fluid therapy in the treatment of significant hypovolaemia relates to the concepts in Figure 14.1. If fluid containing neither sodium nor protein is given, it will distribute in the body fluid compartments in proportion to the normal distribution of total body water. For example, administration of 1 L of 5% dextrose contributes little (approximately 3/40 of the infused volume) towards expansion of the plasma volume, which makes this fluid unsuitable for restoring the circulation and perfusion of vital organs. Intravenous infusion of an isotonic (normal) saline solution, on the other hand, is more effective at expanding the ECF, although only a small proportion (about 3/15) of the infused volume actually contributes to plasma volume.

You would expect that solutions containing plasma proteins (colloids) would be better retained within the vascular space and to be more effective at correcting hypovolaemia than protein-free fluids (crystalloids). However, recent clinical studies have not shown any advantage of giving albumin-containing infusions in the treatment of acute hypovolaemia. Furthermore, synthetic colloids such as dextrans have been shown to be associated with an increased risk of acute kidney injury and mortality in the critically ill. Therefore, crystalloids are the fluid of choice for resuscitation in acute hypovolaemia. More studies, however, are required to clarify the most appropriate crystalloid in this situation, given that normal saline can cause a mild metabolic acidosis, perhaps related to excessive chloride loading, whereas 'balanced solutions', such as Hartmann's, may cause a mild hyponatraemia, as its composition is slightly hypotonic.

Hypervolaemia

Hypervolaemia is the result of sodium and water excess and is rare in patients with normal cardiac and renal function, since

---

14.7 How to assess fluid and electrolyte balance in hospitalised patients

Step 1: assess clinical volume status

- Examine patient for signs of hypovolaemia or hypervolaemia (see Box 14.3)
- Check daily weight change

Step 2: review fluid balance chart

- Check total volumes IN and OUT on previous day (IN–OUT is positive by ~400 mL in normal balance, reflecting insensible fluid losses of ~800 mL and metabolic water generation of ~400 mL)
- Check cumulative change in daily fluid balance over previous 3–5 days
- Correlate chart figures with weight change and clinical volume status to estimate net fluid balance

Step 3: assess ongoing pathological process

- Check losses from gastrointestinal tract and surgical drains
- Estimate increased insensible losses (e.g. in fever) and internal sequestration ('third space')

Step 4: check plasma U&Es (see Box 14.2)

- Check plasma Na as marker of relative water balance
- Check plasma K as a guide to extracellular K balance
- Check HCO_3^- as a clue to acid–base disorder
- Check urea and creatinine to monitor renal function

Step 5: prescribe appropriate intravenous fluid replacement therapy

- Replace basic water and electrolytes each day (see Box 14.5)
- Allow for anticipated oral intake and pathological fluid loss
- Adjust amounts of water (if IV, usually given as isotonic 5% dextrose), sodium and potassium according to plasma electrolyte results

---

14.5 Basic daily water and electrolyte requirements

	Requirement per kg	Typical 70 kg adult
Water	35–45 mL/kg	2.45–3.15 L/24 hrs
Sodium	1.5–2 mmol/kg	105–140 mmol/24 hrs
Potassium	1.0–1.5 mmol/kg	70–105 mmol/24 hrs

14.6 Composition of some isotonic intravenous fluids

Fluid	D-glucose	Calories	Na⁺ (mmol/L)	Cl⁻ (mmol/L)	Other (mmol/L)
5% dextrose	50 g	200	0	0	0
Normal (0.9%) saline	0	0	154	154	0
Hartmann's solution	0	0	131	111	K⁺ 5 Ca²⁺ 2 Lactate⁻ 29

14

the kidney has a large capacity to increase renal excretion of sodium and water via the homeostatic mechanisms described on page 349.

Pathogenesis

The most common systemic disorders responsible for hypervolaemia are outlined in Box 14.8. In cardiac failure, cirrhosis and nephrotic syndrome, sodium retention occurs in response to circulatory insufficiency caused by the primary disorder, as illustrated in Figure 14.5. The pathophysiology is different in renal failure, when the primary cause of volume expansion is the profound reduction in GFR impairing sodium and water excretion, while secondary tubular mechanisms are of lesser importance. In Conn's syndrome (p. 674), the pathophysiology also differs, in that increased secretion of aldosterone directly stimulates sodium reabsorption.

Clinical features

Peripheral oedema is the most common physical sign of hypervolaemia since the excess fluid leaks out of the capillaries to expand the interstitial compartment of the ECF. This is particularly the case in nephrotic syndrome and chronic liver disease, in which hypoalbuminaemia is a prominent feature. The main exception is primary hyperaldosteronism (Conn's syndrome), which presents with hypertension and often hypokalaemia, but in which peripheral oedema is not commonly seen.

Investigations

Although hypervolaemia is accompanied by an excess of total body sodium, serum sodium concentrations are normal due to the accompanying water retention. Serum concentrations of potassium are normal except in Conn's syndrome, where there is hypokalaemia due to the increased aldosterone production (p. 674). Creatinine, GFR and urea are usually normal, unless the underlying cause of hypervolaemia is renal failure. General investigations may reveal evidence of cardiac, renal or liver disease.

Management

The management of hypervolaemia involves a number of components:

- specific treatment directed at the underlying cause, such as ACE inhibitors in heart failure and glucocorticoids in minimal change nephropathy
- restriction of dietary sodium (to 50–80 mmol/24 hrs) to match the diminished excretory capacity
- treatment with diuretics.

Diuretic therapy

Diuretics play a pivotal role in the treatment of hypervolaemia due to salt and water retention and in hypertension (p. 513). They act by inhibiting sodium reabsorption at various locations along the nephron (see Fig. 14.3). Their potency and adverse effects relate to their mechanism and site of action.

Carbonic anhydrase inhibitors Acetazolamide is a carbonic anhydrase inhibitor that inhibits intracellular production of H^+ ions in the proximal tubule, reducing the fraction of sodium reabsorption that is exchanged for H^+ by the apical membrane sodium–hydrogen exchanger. It is a weak diuretic but is seldom used clinically for this purpose, since only a small fraction of proximal sodium reabsorption uses this mechanism, and much of the sodium that is not reabsorbed in the proximal tubule can be reabsorbed by downstream segments of the nephron.

Sodium-dependent glucose transporter inhibitors Inhibitors of the sodium-dependent glucose transporter 2 (SGLT2), such as dapagliflozin and canagliflozin, simultaneously block glucose and sodium reabsorption in the proximal tubule. They have mild diuretic properties but are principally used to lower blood glucose in the treatment of diabetes (p. 745).

Loop diuretics Loop diuretics, such as furosemide, inhibit sodium reabsorption in the thick ascending limb of the loop of Henle, by blocking the action of the apical membrane NKCC2 co-transporter. Because this segment reabsorbs a large fraction

14.8 Causes of sodium and water excess	
Mechanism	**Examples**
Impaired renal function	Primary renal disease
Primary hyperaldosteronism*	Conn's syndrome
Secondary hyperaldosteronism (see Fig. 14.5)	Congestive cardiac failure Cirrhotic liver disease Nephrotic syndrome Protein-losing enteropathy Malnutrition Idiopathic/cyclical oedema Renal artery stenosis*

*Conditions in this box *other than* primary hyperaldosteronism and renal artery stenosis are typically associated with generalised oedema.

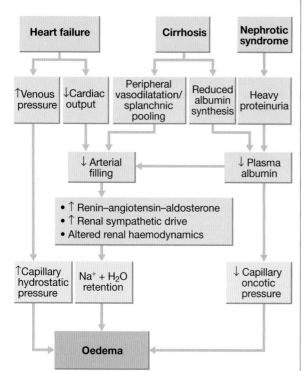

Fig. 14.5 Secondary mechanisms causing sodium excess and oedema in cardiac failure, cirrhosis and nephrotic syndrome. Primary renal retention of Na and water may also contribute to oedema formation when glomerular filtration rate is significantly reduced (see Box 14.8 and p. 395).

of the filtered sodium, these drugs are potent diuretics, and are commonly used in diseases associated with significant oedema. Loop diuretics cause excretion not only of sodium (and with it water) but also of potassium. This occurs largely as a result of delivery of increased amounts of sodium to the late distal tubule and cortical collecting ducts, where sodium reabsorption is associated with excretion of potassium, and is amplified if circulating aldosterone levels are high.

Thiazide diuretics Thiazide diuretics inhibit sodium reabsorption in the early distal tubule, by blocking the NCCT co-transporter in the apical membrane. Since this segment reabsorbs a much smaller fraction of the filtered sodium, these are less potent than loop diuretics, but are widely used in the treatment of hypertension and less severe oedema. Like loop diuretics, thiazides increase excretion of potassium through delivery of increased amounts of sodium to the late distal tubule and collecting duct. They are the diuretics that are most likely to be complicated by the development of hyponatraemia, as outlined on page 357.

Potassium-sparing diuretics Potassium-sparing diuretics act on the late distal renal tubule and cortical collecting duct segment to inhibit sodium reabsorption. Since sodium reabsorption and potassium secretion are linked at this site, the reduced sodium reabsorption is accompanied by reduced potassium secretion. The apical sodium channel (see Fig. 14.3) is blocked by amiloride and triamterene, while spironolactone and eplerenone also act at this site by blocking binding of aldosterone to the mineralocorticoid receptor.

Osmotic diuretics These act independently of a specific transport mechanism. As they are freely filtered at the glomerulus but not reabsorbed by any part of the tubular system, they retain fluid osmotically within the tubular lumen and limit the extent of sodium reabsorption in multiple segments. Mannitol is the most commonly used osmotic diuretic. It is given by intravenous infusion to achieve short-term diuresis in conditions such as cerebral oedema.

Clinical use of diuretics

The following principles should be observed when using diuretics:

- Use the minimum effective dose.
- Use for as short a period of time as necessary.
- Monitor regularly for adverse effects.

The choice of diuretic is determined by the potency required, the presence of coexistent conditions, and the side-effect profile.

Adverse effects encountered with the most frequently used classes of diuretic (loop drugs and thiazide drugs) are summarised in Box 14.9. Volume depletion and electrolyte disorders are the most common, as predicted from their mechanism of action. The metabolic side-effects listed are rarely of clinical significance and may reflect effects on K$^+$ channels that influence insulin secretion (p. 723). Since most drugs from these classes are sulphonamides, there is a relatively high incidence of hypersensitivity reactions, and occasional idiosyncratic side-effects in a variety of organ systems.

The side-effect profile of the potassium-sparing diuretics differs in a number of important respects from that of other diuretics. The disturbances in potassium, magnesium and acid–base balance are in the opposite direction, so that normal or increased levels of potassium and magnesium are found in the blood, and there is a tendency to metabolic acidosis, especially when renal function is impaired.

---

i | **14.9 Adverse effects of loop-acting and thiazide diuretics**

Renal side-effects

- Hypovolaemia
- Hyponatraemia
- Hypokalaemia
- Metabolic alkalosis
- Hyperuricaemia
- Hypomagnesaemia
- Hypercalciuria (loop)
- Hypocalciuria (thiazide)

Metabolic side-effects

- Glucose intolerance/ hyperglycaemia
- Hyperlipidaemia

Miscellaneous side-effects

- Hypersensitivity reactions
- Erectile dysfunction
- Acute pancreatitis/cholecystitis (thiazides)

An important feature of the most commonly used diuretic drugs (furosemide, thiazides and amiloride) is that they act on their target molecules from the luminal side of the tubular epithelium. Since they are highly protein-bound in the plasma, very little reaches the urinary fluid by glomerular filtration, but there are active transport mechanisms for secreting organic acids and bases, including these drugs, across the proximal tubular wall into the lumen, resulting in adequate drug concentrations being delivered to later tubular segments. This secretory process may be impaired by certain other drugs, and also by accumulated organic anions as occurs in chronic kidney disease and chronic liver failure, leading to resistance to diuretics.

Diuretic resistance is encountered under a variety of circumstances, including impaired renal function, activation of sodium-retaining mechanisms, impaired oral bioavailability (such as in patients with gastrointestinal disease) and decreased renal blood flow. In these circumstances, short-term intravenous therapy with a loop-acting agent such as furosemide may be useful. Combinations of diuretics administered orally may also increase potency. Either a loop or a thiazide drug can be combined with a potassium-sparing drug, and all three classes can be used together for short periods, with carefully supervised clinical and laboratory monitoring.

Water homeostasis

Daily water intake can vary from about 500 mL to several litres a day. About 800 mL of water is lost daily through the stool, sweat and the respiratory tract (insensible losses) and about 400 mL is generated daily through oxidative metabolism (metabolic water). The kidneys are chiefly responsible for adjusting water excretion to balance intake, endogenous production and losses so as to maintain total body water content and serum osmolality within the reference range of 280–296 mOsmol/kg.

Functional anatomy and physiology

While regulation of total ECF volume is largely achieved through renal control of sodium excretion, mechanisms exist to allow for the excretion of urine that is hypertonic or hypotonic in relation to plasma to maintain constant plasma osmolality.

These functions are largely achieved by the loop of Henle and the collecting ducts (see Fig. 14.2). The countercurrent configuration of flow in adjacent limbs of the loop (Fig. 14.6) involves osmotic movement of water from the descending limbs and reabsorption of

14

— Passive diffusion of H$_2$O ═══ Portions of tubule impermeable to H$_2$O
←σ Active transport of NaCl * Permeability to H$_2$O increased by vasopressin

Fig. 14.6 Mechanisms of renal water handling. (1) Filtrate from the proximal tubule is isosmotic to plasma and cortical interstitial fluid. (2) Water moves down its osmotic gradient, concentrating the filtrate but not diluting the interstitium, as the vasa recta carries away the water. (3) The filtrate is at its highest concentration at the bend of the loop and therefore the surrounding medulla is also concentrated. (4) NaCl is pumped out of the filtrate in the thick ascending limb and early distal tubule, increasing the interstitial fluid osmolality. (5) The filtrate has a concentration of 100 mOsmol/kg as it leaves the early distal tubule. **A** In the face of water deficit, vasopressin causes water permeability of the collecting ducts, resulting in osmotic reabsorption of water. **B** In the situation of water overload, vasopressin secretion is suppressed and urine remains dilute.

solute from neighbouring ascending limbs, to set up a gradient of osmolality from isotonic (like plasma) in the renal cortex to hypertonic (around 1200 mOsmol/kg) in the inner part of the medulla. At the same time, the fluid emerging from the thick ascending limb is hypotonic compared to plasma because it has been diluted by the reabsorption of sodium, but not water, from the thick ascending limb and is further diluted in the early distal tubule. As this dilute fluid passes from the cortex through the collecting duct system to the renal pelvis, it traverses the medullary interstitial gradient of osmolality set up by the operation of the loop of Henle, and water is able to be reabsorbed.

Further changes in the urine osmolality on passage through the collecting ducts depend on the circulating level of vasopressin, which is released by the posterior pituitary gland under conditions of increased plasma osmolality or hypovolaemia (p. 688).

• When water intake is high and plasma osmolality is normal or low–normal (Fig. 14.6B), vasopressin levels are suppressed and the collecting ducts remain impermeable to water. The luminal fluid osmolality remains low, resulting in the excretion of a dilute urine (minimum osmolality approximately 50 mOsmol/kg in a healthy young person).

• When water intake is restricted and plasma osmolality is high (Fig. 14.6A), or in the presence of plasma volume depletion, vasopressin levels rise. This causes water permeability of the collecting ducts to increase through binding of vasopressin to the V2 receptor, which enhances collecting duct water permeability through the insertion of AQP-2 channels into the luminal cell membrane. This results in osmotic reabsorption of water along the entire length of the collecting duct, with maximum urine

osmolality approaching that in the medullary tip (up to 1200 mOsmol/kg).

Parallel to these changes in vasopressin release are changes in water-seeking behaviour triggered by the sensation of thirst, which also becomes activated as plasma osmolality rises.

In summary, for adequate dilution of the urine there must be:

• adequate solute delivery to the loop of Henle and early distal tubule
• normal function of the loop of Henle and early distal tubule
• absence of vasopressin in the circulation.

If any of these processes is faulty, water retention and hyponatraemia may result.

Conversely, to achieve concentration of the urine there must be:

• adequate solute delivery to the loop of Henle
• normal function of the loop of Henle
• vasopressin release into the circulation
• vasopressin action on the collecting ducts.

Failure of any of these steps may result in inappropriate water loss and hypernatraemia.

Presenting problems in regulation of osmolality

Changes in plasma osmolality are largely determined by changes in serum sodium concentration and its associated anions. Changes in sodium concentration usually occur because of disturbances in water balance either because there is a relative excess of body water compared to total body sodium (hyponatraemia) or a relative lack of body water compared to total body sodium (hypernatraemia). Abnormalities of water balance can result from disturbances in urinary concentration or dilution.

If extracellular osmolality falls abruptly, water flows rapidly across cell membranes, causing cell swelling, whereas cell shrinkage occurs when osmolality rises. Cerebral function is particularly sensitive to such volume changes, particularly brain swelling during hypo-osmolality, which can lead to an increase in intracerebral pressure and reduced cerebral perfusion.

Hyponatraemia

Hyponatraemia is defined as a serum Na <135 mmol/L. It is a common electrolyte abnormality with many potential underlying causes, as summarised in Box 14.10.

Pathophysiology

In all cases, hyponatraemia is caused by greater retention of water relative to sodium. The causes are best categorised according to associated changes in the ECF volume (Box 14.10).

Hyponatraemia with hypovolaemia

In this situation there is depletion of sodium and water but the sodium deficit exceeds the water deficit, causing hypovolaemia and hyponatraemia (see Box 14.3). The cause of sodium loss is usually apparent and common examples are shown in Box 14.10.

Hyponatraemia with euvolaemia

In this situation there are no major disturbances of body sodium content and the patient is clinically euvolaemic. Excess body water may be the result of abnormally high intake, either orally (primary polydipsia) or as a result of medically infused fluids (as intravenous dextrose solutions, or by absorption of sodium-free bladder irrigation fluid after prostatectomy).

Water retention also occurs in the syndrome of inappropriate secretion of antidiuretic hormone, or vasopressin (SIADH). In this condition, an endogenous source of vasopressin (either cerebral or tumour-derived) promotes water retention by the kidney in the absence of an appropriate physiological stimulus (Box 14.11). The clinical diagnosis requires the patient to be euvolaemic, with no evidence of cardiac, renal or hepatic disease potentially associated with hyponatraemia. Other non-osmotic stimuli that cause release of vasopressin (pain, stress, nausea) should also be excluded. Supportive laboratory findings are shown in Box 14.11.

Hyponatraemia with hypervolaemia

In this situation, excess water retention is associated with sodium retention and volume expansion, as in heart failure, liver disease or kidney disease.

Clinical features

Hyponatraemia is often asymptomatic but can also be associated with profound disturbances of cerebral function, manifesting as anorexia, nausea, vomiting, delirium, lethargy, seizures and coma. The likelihood of symptoms occurring is related to the speed at which hyponatraemia develops rather than the severity of hyponatraemia. This is because water rapidly flows into cerebral cells when plasma osmolality falls acutely, causing them to become swollen and ischaemic. However, when hyponatraemia develops gradually, cerebral neurons have time to respond by reducing intracellular osmolality, through excreting potassium and reducing synthesis of intracellular organic osmolytes (Fig. 14.7). The osmotic gradient favouring water movement into the cells is thus reduced and symptoms are avoided. This process takes about 24–48 hours and hyponatraemia is therefore classified as acute (<48 hours) and chronic (>48 hours). Hyponatraemia can also be defined as mild (130–135 mmol/L), moderate (125–129 mmol/L) or severe (<124 mmol/L), based on biochemical findings or on the degree of severity of symptoms (Box 14.12).

Investigations

An algorithm for the clinical assessment of patients with hyponatraemia is shown in Figure 14.8. Artefactual causes of hyponatraemia should be considered in all cases. These include severe hyperlipidaemia or hyperproteinaemia, when the aqueous fraction of the serum specimen is reduced because of the volume occupied by the macromolecules (although this artefact is dependent on the assay technology). Transient hyponatraemia

14

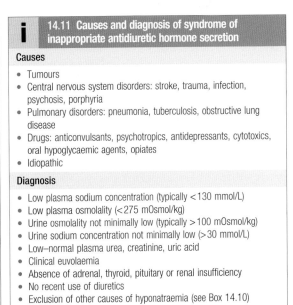

i	14.10 Causes of hyponatraemia	
Volume status	**Examples**	

Hypovolaemic	Renal sodium losses:
	    Diuretic therapy (especially thiazides)
	    Adrenocortical failure
	Gastrointestinal sodium losses:
	    Vomiting
	    Diarrhoea
	Skin sodium losses:
	    Burns	

Euvolaemic	Primary polydipsia Excessive electrolyte-free water infusion SIADH Hypothyroidism	
Hypervolaemic	Congestive cardiac failure Cirrhosis Nephrotic syndrome Chronic kidney disease (during free water intake)	

(SIADH = syndrome of inappropriate antidiuretic hormone (vasopressin) secretion; see Box 14.11).

14.11 Causes and diagnosis of syndrome of inappropriate antidiuretic hormone secretion

Causes

- Tumours
- Central nervous system disorders: stroke, trauma, infection, psychosis, porphyria
- Pulmonary disorders: pneumonia, tuberculosis, obstructive lung disease
- Drugs: anticonvulsants, psychotropics, antidepressants, cytotoxics, oral hypoglycaemic agents, opiates
- Idiopathic

Diagnosis

- Low plasma sodium concentration (typically <130 mmol/L)
- Low plasma osmolality (<275 mOsmol/kg)
- Urine osmolality not minimally low (typically >100 mOsmol/kg)
- Urine sodium concentration not minimally low (>30 mmol/L)
- Low–normal plasma urea, creatinine, uric acid
- Clinical euvolaemia
- Absence of adrenal, thyroid, pituitary or renal insufficiency
- No recent use of diuretics
- Exclusion of other causes of hyponatraemia (see Box 14.10)
- Appropriate clinical context (above)

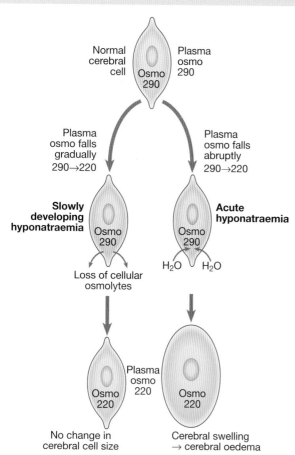

Fig. 14.7 Hyponatraemia and the brain. Numbers represent osmolality (osmo) in mOsmol/kg.

	14.12 Symptoms and severity of hyponatraemia	
Severity	**Serum sodium**	**Symptoms**
Mild	130–135 mmol/L	None
Moderate	125–129 mmol/L	Nausea Delirium Headache
Severe	<124 mmol/L	Vomiting Somnolence Seizures Coma Cardiorespiratory arrest

may also occur due to osmotic shifts of water out of cells during hyperosmolar states caused by acute hyperglycaemia or by mannitol infusion, but in these cases plasma osmolality is normal.

When these conditions have been excluded, serum and urine electrolytes and osmolality (Fig. 14.8) are usually the only tests required to clarify the underlying cause. Hypovolaemic hyponatraemia is characterised by a low urinary sodium concentration (<30 mmol/L) when there are extrarenal causes of sodium loss and high urinary sodium concentration (>30 mmol/L) in patients with excessive renal sodium loss.

Measurement of vasopressin is not generally helpful in distinguishing between different categories of hyponatraemia. This is because concentrations of vasopressin are raised both in

hypovolaemic states and in most chronic hypervolaemic states, as the impaired circulation in those disorders activates vasopressin release through non-osmotic mechanisms. Indeed, patients with these disorders may have higher circulating vasopressin (ADH) levels than patients with SIADH. The only disorders listed in Box 14.10 in which vasopressin is suppressed are primary polydipsia and iatrogenic water intoxication, where the hypo-osmolar state inhibits vasopressin release from the pituitary.

Management

The treatment of hyponatraemia is critically dependent on its rate of development, severity, presence of symptoms and underlying cause. If hyponatraemia has developed rapidly (<48 hours) and there are signs of cerebral oedema, such as obtundation or convulsions, sodium levels should be restored rapidly to normal by infusion of hypertonic (3%) sodium chloride. A common approach is to give an initial bolus of 150 mL over 20 minutes, which may be repeated once or twice over the initial hours of observation, depending on the neurological response and rise in plasma sodium.

Rapid correction of hyponatraemia that has developed more slowly (>48 hours) can be hazardous, since brain cells adapt to slowly developing hypo-osmolality by reducing the intracellular osmolality, thus maintaining normal cell volume (see Fig. 14.7). Under these conditions, an abrupt increase in extracellular osmolality can lead to water shifting out of neurons, abruptly reducing their volume and causing them to detach from their myelin sheaths. The resulting 'myelinolysis' can produce permanent structural and functional damage to mid-brain structures, and is generally fatal. The rate of correction of the plasma Na concentration in chronic asymptomatic hyponatraemia should not exceed 10 mmol/L/24 hrs, and an even slower rate is generally safer.

The underlying cause should also be treated. For hypovolaemic patients, this involves controlling the source of sodium loss, and administering intravenous saline if clinically warranted. Patients with euvolaemic hyponatraemia generally respond to fluid restriction in the range of 600–1000 mL/24 hrs, accompanied where possible by withdrawal of the precipitating stimulus (such as drugs causing SIADH). In patients with persistent hyponatraemia due to prolonged SIADH, oral urea therapy (30–45 g/day) can be used, which provides a solute load to promote water excretion. Oral vasopressin receptor antagonists such as tolvaptan may also be used to block the vasopressin-mediated component of water retention in a range of hyponatraemic conditions, but concerns exist with regard to the risk of overly rapid correction of hyponatraemia with these agents. Hypervolaemic patients with hyponatraemia need treatment of the underlying condition, accompanied by cautious use of diuretics in conjunction with strict fluid restriction. Potassium-sparing diuretics may be particularly useful in this context when there is significant secondary hyperaldosteronism.

Hypernatraemia

Hypernatraemia is defined as existing when the serum Na is >145 mmol/L. The causes are summarised in Box 14.13, grouped according to any associated disturbance in total body sodium content.

Pathophysiology

Hypernatraemia occurs due to inadequate concentration of the urine in the face of restricted water intake. This can arise because

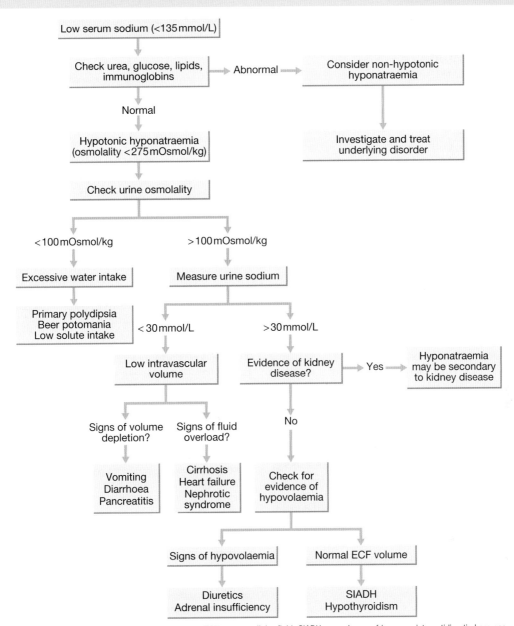

Fig. 14.8 Algorithm for the diagnosis of hyponatraemia. (ECF = extracellular fluid; SIADH = syndrome of inappropriate antidiuretic hormone (vasopressin) secretion)

14.13 Causes of hypernatraemia	
Volume status	**Examples**

Hypovolaemic	Renal sodium losses:
	  Diuretic therapy (especially osmotic diuretic, or
	  loop diuretic during water restriction)
	  Glycosuria (hyperglycaemic hyperosmolar
	  state, p. 738)
	Gastrointestinal sodium losses:
	  Colonic diarrhoea
	Skin sodium losses:
	  Excessive sweating

Euvolaemic	Diabetes insipidus (central or nephrogenic) (p. 687)
Hypervolaemic	Enteral or parenteral feeding Intravenous or oral salt administration Chronic kidney disease (during water restriction)

of failure to generate an adequate medullary concentration gradient in the kidney due to low GFR or loop diuretic therapy, but more commonly is caused by failure of the vasopressin system. This can occur because of pituitary damage (cranial diabetes insipidus, p. 687) or because the collecting duct cells are unable to respond to circulating vasopressin concentrations in the face of restricted water intake (nephrogenic diabetes insipidus). Whatever the underlying cause, sustained or severe hypernatraemia generally reflects an impaired thirst mechanism or responsiveness to thirst.

Clinical features

Patients with hypernatraemia generally have reduced cerebral function, either as a primary problem or as a consequence of the hypernatraemia itself, which results in dehydration of neurons and brain shrinkage. In the presence of an intact thirst mechanism and preserved capacity to obtain and ingest water,

14.14 Hyponatraemia and hypernatraemia in old age

- **Decline in GFR**: older patients are predisposed to both hyponatraemia and hypernatraemia, mainly because, as glomerular filtration rate declines with age, the capacity of the kidney to dilute or concentrate the urine is impaired.
- **Hyponatraemia**: occurs when free water intake continues in the presence of a low dietary salt intake and/or diuretic drugs (particularly thiazides).
- **Vasopressin release**: water retention is aggravated by any condition that stimulates vasopressin release, especially heart failure. Moreover, the vasopressin response to non-osmotic stimuli may be brisker in older subjects. Appropriate water restriction may be a key part of management.
- **Hypernatraemia**: occurs when water intake is inadequate, due to physical restrictions preventing access to drinks and/or blunted thirst. Both are frequently present in patients with advanced dementia or following a severe stroke.
- **Dietary salt**: hypernatraemia is aggravated if dietary supplements or medications with a high sodium content (especially effervescent preparations) are administered. Appropriate prescription of fluids is a key part of management.

Fig. 14.9 Feedback control of plasma potassium concentration.

hypernatraemia may not progress very far. If adequate water is not obtained, dizziness, delirium, weakness and, ultimately, coma and death can result.

Management

Treatment of hypernatraemia depends on both the rate of development and the underlying cause. If there is reason to think that the condition has developed rapidly, neuronal shrinkage may be acute and relatively rapid correction may be attempted. This can be achieved by infusing an appropriate volume of intravenous fluid (isotonic 5% dextrose or hypotonic 0.45% saline) at an initial rate of 50–70 mL/hr. In older, institutionalised patients, however, it is more likely that the disorder has developed slowly, and extreme caution should be exercised in lowering plasma sodium to avoid the risk of cerebral oedema. Where possible, the underlying cause should also be addressed (Box 14.13).

Elderly patients are predisposed, in different circumstances, to both hyponatraemia and hypernatraemia, and a high index of suspicion of these electrolyte disturbances is appropriate in elderly patients with recent alterations in behaviour (Box 14.14).

Potassium homeostasis

Potassium is the major intracellular cation (see Fig. 14.1), and the steep concentration gradient for potassium across the cell membrane of excitable cells plays an important part in generating the resting membrane potential and allowing the propagation of the action potential that is crucial to normal functioning of nerve, muscle and cardiac tissues. Control of body potassium balance is described below.

Functional anatomy and physiology

The kidneys normally excrete some 90% of the daily intake of potassium, typically 80–100 mmol/24 hrs. Potassium is freely filtered at the glomerulus; around 65% is reabsorbed in the proximal tubule and a further 25% in the thick ascending limb of the loop of Henle. Little potassium is transported in the early distal tubule but a significant secretory flux of potassium into

the urine occurs in the late distal tubule and cortical collecting duct to ensure that the amount removed from the blood is proportional to the ingested load.

The mechanism for potassium secretion in the distal parts of the nephron is shown in Figure 14.3D. Movement of potassium from blood to lumen is dependent on active uptake across the basal cell membrane by the Na,K-ATPase, followed by diffusion of potassium through the ROMK channel into the tubular fluid. The electrochemical gradient for potassium movement into the lumen is contributed to both by the high intracellular potassium concentration and by the negative luminal potential difference relative to the blood.

A number of factors influence the rate of potassium secretion. Luminal influences include the rate of sodium delivery and fluid flow through the late distal tubule and cortical collecting ducts. This is a major factor responsible for the increased potassium loss that accompanies diuretic treatment. Agents interfering with the generation of the negative luminal potential also impair potassium secretion, and this is the basis of reduced potassium secretion associated with potassium-sparing diuretics such as amiloride. Factors acting on the blood side of this tubular segment include plasma potassium and pH, such that hyperkalaemia and alkalosis both enhance potassium secretion directly. However, the most important factor in the acute and chronic adjustment of potassium secretion to match metabolic potassium load is aldosterone.

As shown in Figure 14.9, a negative feedback relationship exists between the plasma potassium concentration and aldosterone. In addition to its regulation by the renin–angiotensin system (see Fig. 18.18, p. 666), aldosterone is released from the adrenal cortex in direct response to an elevated plasma potassium. Aldosterone then acts on the kidney to enhance potassium secretion, hydrogen secretion and sodium reabsorption, in the late distal tubule and cortical collecting ducts. The resulting increased excretion of potassium maintains plasma potassium within a narrow range (3.6–5.0 mmol/L). Factors that reduce angiotensin II levels may indirectly affect potassium balance by blunting the rise in aldosterone that would otherwise be provoked by hyperkalaemia. This accounts for the increased risk of hyperkalaemia during therapy with ACE inhibitors and related drugs.

Presenting problems in potassium homeostasis

Changes in the distribution of potassium between the ICF and ECF compartments can alter plasma potassium concentration, without any overall change in total body potassium content. Potassium is driven into the cells by extracellular alkalosis and by a number of hormones, including insulin, catecholamines (through the β_2-receptor) and aldosterone. Any of these factors can produce hypokalaemia, whereas extracellular acidosis, lack of insulin, and insufficiency or blockade of catecholamines or aldosterone can cause hyperkalaemia due to efflux of potassium from the intracellular compartment.

Hypokalaemia

Hypokalaemia is a common electrolyte disturbance and is defined as existing when serum K^+ falls below 3.5 mmol/L. The main causes of hypokalaemia are shown in Box 14.15.

i 14.15 Causes of hypokalaemia	
Cause	**Other features and comment**
Reduced intake Dietary deficiency Potassium-free intravenous fluids	Urine K^+ > 20–30 mmol/24 hrs
Redistribution into cells Alkalosis Insulin Catecholamines β-adrenergic agonists Hypokalaemic periodic paralysis	Caused by flux of K^+ into cells
Increased urinary excretion Activation of mineralocorticoid receptor:	Urine K^+ > 20–30 mmol/24 hrs

Conn's syndrome
   Cushing's syndrome
   Glucocorticoid excess
   Carbenoxelone/liquorice
	Associated with hypertension and alkalosis

Genetic disorders: Liddle's syndrome	Associated with hypertension and alkalosis
Bartter's syndrome Gitelman's syndrome	Associated with hypertension, alkalosis and hypomagnesaemia
Renal tubular acidosis Type 1 (distal) Type 2 (proximal)	Inherited and acquired forms; associated with high serum chloride. Type 2 associated with glycosuria, aminoaciduria and phosphaturia
Acetazolamide	Associated with acidosis

Diuresis:
   Loop diuretics
   Thiazides
   Recovery from acute tubular necrosis
   Recovery from renal obstruction
	Increased sodium delivery to distal tubule

Increased gastrointestinal loss	Urine K^+ < 20–30 mmol/L

Upper gastrointestinal tract:
   Vomiting
   Nasogastric aspiration
	Loss of gastric acid
	 Associated with metabolic alkalosis

Lower gastrointestinal tract:
   Diarrhoea
   Laxative abuse
   Villous adenoma
   Bowel obstruction/fistula
   Ureterosigmoidostomy
	Associated with metabolic acidosis

Pathophysiology

Hypokalaemia is generally indicative of abnormal potassium loss from the body, through either the kidney or the gastrointestinal tract. Renal causes of hypokalaemia can be divided into those with and those without hypertension. Hypokalaemia in the presence of hypertension may be due to increased aldosterone secretion in Conn's syndrome (p. 674) or a genetic defect affecting sodium channels in the distal nephron (Liddle's syndrome). Excessive intake of liquorice or treatment with carbenoxolone may result in a similar clinical picture, due to inhibition of the renal 11βHSD2 enzyme, which inactivates cortisol in peripheral tissues.

If blood pressure is normal or low, hypokalaemia can be classified according to the associated change in acid–base balance. Inherited defects in tubular transport should be suspected when hypokalaemia occurs in association with hypotension and alkalosis, provided that diuretic use has been excluded. One such disease is Bartter's syndrome, in which sodium reabsorption in the thick ascending limb of Henle is defective, usually due to a loss-of-function mutation of the NKCC2 transporter. The clinical and biochemical features are similar to those in chronic treatment with furosemide. In Gitelman's syndrome there is a loss-of-function mutation affecting the NCCT transporter in the early distal tubule. The clinical and biochemical features are similar to chronic thiazide treatment. Note that while both Bartter's and Gitelman's syndromes are characterised by hypokalaemia and hypomagnesaemia, urinary calcium excretion is increased in Bartter's syndrome but decreased in Gitelman's syndrome, analogous to the effects of the loop and thiazide diuretics, respectively, on calcium transport (see Box 14.9).

If hypokalaemia occurs in the presence of a normal blood pressure and metabolic acidosis, renal tubular acidosis (proximal or 'classical' distal) should be suspected (p. 364).

When hypokalaemia is due to potassium wasting through the gastrointestinal tract, the cause is usually obvious clinically. In some cases, when there is occult induction of vomiting, the hypokalaemia is characteristically associated with metabolic alkalosis, due to loss of gastric acid. If, however, potassium loss has occurred through the surreptitious use of aperients, the hypokalaemia is generally associated with metabolic acidosis. In both cases, urinary potassium excretion is low unless there is significant extracellular volume depletion, which can raise urinary potassium levels by stimulating aldosterone production.

Hypokalaemia can also be caused by redistribution of potassium into cells as the result of insulin, β-adrenoceptor agonists and alkalosis, or as the result of K^+ flux into muscle in hypokalaemic periodic paralysis, which is associated with mutations in several genes that regulate transmembrane ion flow into muscle cells. Finally, reduced dietary intake of potassium can contribute to hypokalaemia but is seldom the only cause, except in extreme cases.

Clinical features

Patients with mild hypokalaemia (plasma K^+ 3.0–3.3 mmol/L) are generally asymptomatic, but more profound reductions in plasma potassium often lead to muscular weakness and associated tiredness. Ventricular ectopic beats or more serious arrhythmias may occur and the arrhythmogenic effects of digoxin may be potentiated. Typical electrocardiogram (ECG) changes occur, affecting the T wave in particular (p. 347). Functional bowel obstruction may occur due to paralytic ileus. Long-standing hypokalaemia may cause renal tubular damage (hypokalaemic nephropathy) and can interfere with the tubular response to vasopressin (acquired nephrogenic diabetes insipidus), resulting in polyuria and polydipsia.

14

Investigations

Measurement of plasma electrolytes, bicarbonate, urine potassium and sometimes of plasma calcium and magnesium is usually sufficient to establish the diagnosis. If the diagnosis remains unclear, plasma renin should be measured. Levels are low in patients with primary hyperaldosteronism (p. 674) and other forms of mineralocorticoid excess, but raised in other causes of hypokalaemia. When there is no obvious clinical clue to which pathway is involved, measurement of urinary potassium may be helpful; if the kidney is the route of potassium loss, the urine potassium is high (>30 mmol/24 hrs), whereas if potassium is being lost through the gastrointestinal tract, the kidney retains potassium, resulting in a lower urinary potassium (generally <20 mmol/24 hrs). It should be noted, however, that if gastrointestinal fluid loss is also associated with hypovolaemia, activation of the renin–angiotensin–aldosterone system may occur, causing increased loss of potassium in the urine.

The cause of hypokalaemia may remain unclear despite the above investigations when urinary potassium measurements are inconclusive and the history is incomplete or unreliable. Many such cases are associated with metabolic alkalosis, and in this setting the measurement of urine chloride concentration can be helpful. A low urine chloride (<30 mmol/L) is characteristic of vomiting (spontaneous or self-induced, in which chloride is lost in HCl in the vomit), while a urine chloride >40 mmol/L suggests diuretic therapy (acute phase) or a tubular disorder such as Bartter's or Gitelman's syndrome. Differentiation between occult diuretic use and primary tubular disorders can be achieved by performing a screen of urine for diuretic drugs.

Management

Treatment of hypokalaemia involves first determining the cause and correcting this where possible. If the problem is mainly one of redistribution of potassium into cells, reversal of the process responsible may be sufficient to restore plasma potassium without providing supplements. In most cases, however, some form of potassium replacement will be required. This can generally be achieved with slow-release potassium chloride tablets, but in more acute circumstances intravenous potassium chloride may be necessary. The rate of administration depends on the severity of hypokalaemia and the presence of cardiac or neuromuscular complications, but should generally not exceed 10 mmol of potassium per hour. In patients with severe, life-threatening hypokalaemia, the concentration of potassium in the infused fluid may be increased to 40 mmol/L if a peripheral vein is used, but higher concentrations must be infused into a large 'central' vein with continuous cardiac monitoring.

In the less common situation where hypokalaemia occurs in the presence of systemic acidosis, alkaline salts of potassium, such as potassium bicarbonate, can be given by mouth. If magnesium depletion is also present, replacement of magnesium may also be required, since low cell magnesium can promote tubular potassium secretion, causing ongoing urinary losses. In some circumstances, potassium-sparing diuretics, such as amiloride, can assist in the correction of hypokalaemia, hypomagnesaemia and metabolic alkalosis, especially when renal loss of potassium is the underlying cause.

▌Hyperkalaemia

Hyperkalaemia is a common electrolyte disorder, which is defined as existing when serum K^+ is >5 mmol/L. The causes of hyperkalaemia are summarised in Box 14.16.

ℹ 14.16 Causes of hyperkalaemia

Cause	Other features and comment
Artefactual	
Haemolysis during venepuncture	Release of intracellular K^+ during sample collection, transit or clotting
Haemolysis in vitro	
Thrombocytosis/leucocytosis	
Increased intake	
Dietary potassium	
Potassium-containing intravenous fluids	
Redistribution from cells	
Acidosis	
Insulin deficiency	
Severe hyperglycaemia	
β-adrenergic blockers (β-blockers)	Caused by flux of intracellular K^+ into plasma
Hyperkalaemic periodic paralysis	
Rhabdomyolysis	
Severe haemolysis	
Tumour lysis syndrome	
Reduced urinary excretion	
Reduced glomerular filtration:	
Acute kidney injury	Plasma creatinine typically
Chronic kidney disease	>500 μmol/L (5.67 mg/dL)
Reduced mineralocorticoid receptor activation:	
Addison's disease	
Congenital adrenal hyperplasia	
Isolated aldosterone deficiency	
Angiotensin-converting enzyme (ACE) inhibitors	ACE inhibitors and ARBs reduce aldosterone levels
Angiotensin-receptor blockers (ARBs)	
Calcineurin inhibitors	All block the mineralocorticoid receptor
Spironolactone	
Eplerenone	
Heparin	Heparin inhibits aldosterone production
Inhibitors of renin production:	
Non-steroidal anti-inflammatory drugs (NSAIDs)	
β-blockers	
Tubulointerstitial disease:	
Interstitial nephritis	
Diabetic nephropathy	
Obstructive uropathy	
Other:	
Amiloride	Blocks K^+ exchange in distal tubule
Gordon's syndrome	Direct effect on K^+ transport in renal tubule

Pathophysiology

It is important to remember that hyperkalaemia can be artefactual due to haemolysis of blood specimens during collection or in vitro, or due to release of potassium from platelets in patients with thrombocytosis.

True hyperkalaemia, however, can occur either because of redistribution of potassium between the ICF and ECF, or because potassium intake exceeds excretion. Redistribution of potassium from the ICF to the ECF may take place in the presence of systemic acidosis, or when the circulating levels of insulin, catecholamines and aldosterone are reduced, or when the effects of these hormones are blocked (p. 361).

High dietary potassium intake may contribute to hyperkalaemia, but is seldom the only explanation unless renal excretion mechanisms are impaired. The mechanism of hyperkalaemia in acute kidney injury and chronic kidney disease is impaired excretion of potassium into the urine as the result of a reduced GFR. In addition, acute kidney injury can be associated with severe hyperkalaemia when there is an increased potassium load, such as in rhabdomyolysis or in sepsis, particularly when acidosis is present. In chronic kidney disease, adaptation to moderately elevated plasma potassium levels commonly occurs. However, acute rises in potassium triggered by excessive dietary intake, hypovolaemia or drugs (see below) may occur and destabilise the situation.

Hyperkalaemia can also develop when tubular potassium secretory processes are impaired, even if the GFR is normal. This can arise in association with low levels of aldosterone, as is found in Addison's disease, hyporeninaemic hypoaldosteronism or inherited disorders such as congenital isolated hypoaldosteronism, in which there is a defect in aldosterone biosynthesis, and pseudohypoaldosteronism type 2 (Gordon's syndrome), caused by mutations in the *WNK2* and *WNK4* genes, which causes decreased potassium secretion in the renal tubules.

Drug-induced causes include ACE inhibitors, angiotensin-receptor blockers (ARBs), non-steroidal anti-inflammatory drugs (NSAIDs) and β-adrenoceptor antagonists (β-blockers).

In another group of conditions, tubular potassium secretion is impaired as the result of aldosterone resistance. This can occur in a variety of diseases in which there is inflammation of the tubulointerstitium, such as systemic lupus erythematosus; following renal transplantation; during treatment with potassium-sparing diuretics; and in a number of inherited disorders of tubular transport.

In aldosterone deficiency or aldosterone resistance, hyperkalaemia may be associated with acid retention, giving rise to the pattern of hyperkalaemic distal ('type 4') renal tubular acidosis (p. 364).

Clinical features

Mild to moderate hyperkalaemia (<6.5 mmol/L) is usually asymptomatic. More severe hyperkalaemia can present with progressive muscular weakness, but sometimes there are no symptoms until cardiac arrest occurs. The typical ECG changes are shown on page 347. Peaking of the T wave is an early ECG sign, but widening of the QRS complex presages a dangerous cardiac arrhythmia. However, these characteristic ECG findings are not always present, even in severe hyperkalaemia.

Investigations

Measurement of electrolytes, creatinine and bicarbonate, when combined with clinical assessment, usually provides the explanation for hyperkalaemia. In aldosterone deficiency, plasma sodium concentration is characteristically low, although this can occur with many causes of hyperkalaemia. Addison's disease should be excluded unless there is an obvious alternative diagnosis, as described on page 671.

Management

Treatment of hyperkalaemia depends on its severity and the rate of development, but opinions vary as to what level of

14.17 Treatment of severe hyperkalaemia	
Objective	**Therapy**
Stabilise cell membrane potential[1]	IV calcium gluconate (10 mL of 10% solution)
Shift K⁺ into cells	Inhaled β_2-adrenoceptor agonist IV glucose (50 mL of 50% solution) and insulin (5 IU Actrapid) IV sodium bicarbonate[2]
Remove K⁺ from body	IV furosemide and normal saline[3] Ion-exchange resin (e.g. Resonium) orally or rectally Dialysis

[1]If severe hyperkalaemia (K⁺ typically >6.5 mmol/L). [2]If acidosis present. [3]If adequate residual renal function.

serum potassium constitutes severe hyperkalaemia and requires urgent treatment. Patients who have potassium concentrations <6.5 mmol/L in the absence of neuromuscular symptoms or ECG changes can be treated with a reduction of potassium intake and correction of predisposing factors. However, in acute and/or severe hyperkalaemia (plasma potassium >6.5–7.0 mmol/L), more urgent measures must be taken (Box 14.17). The first step should be infusion of 10 mL 10% calcium gluconate to stabilise conductive tissue membranes (calcium has the opposite effect to potassium on conduction of an action potential). Measures to shift potassium from the ECF to the ICF should also be applied, as they generally have a rapid effect and may avert arrhythmias. Ultimately, a means of removing potassium from the body is generally necessary. When renal function is reasonably preserved, loop diuretics (accompanied by intravenous saline if hypovolaemia is present) may be effective. In renal failure, dialysis may be required. Oral ion exchange resins, such as sodium polystyrene sulfonate (SPS), have traditionally been used to bind and excrete gastrointestinal potassium. There are concerns, however, with regard to SPS's lack of proven efficacy and safety, with a number of reports of intestinal necrosis associated with its use. Alternative cation exchanges have been developed and are currently being trialled, with the aim of providing more effective and safer alternatives for the treatment of hyperkalaemia.

Acid–base homeostasis

The pH of arterial plasma is normally 7.40, corresponding to an H⁺ concentration of 40 nmol/L, and under normal circumstances H⁺ concentrations do not vary outside the range of 37–45 nmol/L (pH 7.43–7.35). Abnormalities of acid–base balance can occur in a wide range of diseases. Increases in H⁺ concentration cause acidosis with a decrease in pH, whereas decreases in H⁺ concentration cause alkalosis with a rise in pH.

Functional anatomy and physiology

A variety of physiological mechanisms maintain pH of the ECF within narrow limits. The first is the action of blood and tissue buffers, of which the most important involves reaction of H⁺ ions with bicarbonate to form carbonic acid, which, under the

14

influence of the enzyme carbonic anhydrase (CA), dissociates to form CO_2 and water:

$$CO_2 + H_2O \underset{CA}{\longleftrightarrow} H_2CO_3 \rightleftharpoons H^+ + HCO_3^-$$

This buffer system is important because bicarbonate is present at a relatively high concentration in ECF (21–29 mmol/L), and two of its key components are under physiological control: CO_2 by the lungs, and bicarbonate by the kidneys. These relationships are illustrated in Figure 14.10 (a form of the Henderson–Hasselbalch equation).

Respiratory compensation for acid–base disturbances can occur quickly. In response to acid accumulation, pH changes in the brainstem stimulate ventilatory drive, reduce PCO_2 and increase pH (p. 555). Conversely, systemic alkalosis leads to inhibition of ventilation, causing a rise in PCO_2 and reduction in pH, although it should be noted that this mechanism has limited capacity to change pH because hypoxia provides an alternative stimulus to drive ventilation.

The kidneys provide a third line of defence against disturbances of arterial pH. When acid accumulates due to chronic respiratory or metabolic (non-renal) causes, the kidneys have the long-term capacity to enhance urinary excretion of acid, effectively increasing the plasma bicarbonate.

Renal control of acid–base balance

Regulation of acid–base balance occurs at several sites in the kidney. The proximal tubule reabsorbs about 85% of the filtered bicarbonate ions, through the mechanism for H^+ secretion illustrated in Figure 14.3A. This is dependent on the enzyme carbonic anhydrase, both in the cytoplasm of the proximal tubular cells and on the luminal surface of the brush border membranes. The system has a high capacity and is required to rescue filtered bicarbonate, but does not lead to significant acidification of the luminal fluid.

Distal nephron segments also have an important role in acid excretion. Hydrogen ions are secreted into the lumen by an H^+-ATPase in the intercalated cells of the cortical collecting duct and the outer medullary collecting duct cells. The H^+ ions

$$pH = 6.1 + \log \frac{[HCO_3^-]}{0.03 \times PCO_2}$$

Fig. 14.10 Relationship between pH, PCO_2 (in mmHg) and plasma bicarbonate concentration (in mmol/L). *Note that changes in HCO_3^- concentration are also part of the renal correction for sustained metabolic acid–base disturbances as long as the kidney itself is not the cause of the primary disturbance.

are generated in the tubular cell from the hydration of CO_2 to form carbonic acid, which dissociates into an H^+ ion secreted luminally, and a bicarbonate ion that passes across the basolateral membrane into the blood. The secreted H^+ ions contribute to the reabsorption of any residual bicarbonate present in the luminal fluid, by generating intracellular OH^- that reacts with CO_2 to form HCO_3^-, which exits across the basolateral membrane. However, H^+ secretion also contributes net acid for removal from the body, bound to a variety of urinary buffers, of which phosphate and ammonia are the most important. Urinary buffers are required to prevent a reduction in urinary pH, which would create an unfavourable gradient that would prevent further H^+ secretion. Filtered phosphate (HPO_4^{2-}) combines with H^+ in the distal tubular lumen to form dihydrogen phosphate ($H_2PO_4^-$), which is excreted in the urine with sodium. Ammonia (NH_3) is generated within tubular cells by deamination of the amino acid glutamine by the enzyme glutaminase. The NH_3 then reacts with secreted H^+ in the tubular lumen to form ammonium (NH_4^+), which becomes trapped in the luminal fluid and is excreted with chloride ions.

These two mechanisms remove approximately 1 mmol/kg of hydrogen ions from the body per day, which equates to the non-volatile acid load arising from the metabolism of dietary protein. The slightly alkaline plasma pH of 7.4 (H^+ 40 nmol/L) that is maintained during health can be accounted for by the kidney's ability to generate an acidic urine (typically pH 5–6 (H^+ 1000–10 000 nmol/L), in which the net daily excess of metabolic acid produced by the body can be excreted.

Presenting problems in acid–base balance

Patients with disturbances of acid–base balance may present clinically either with the effects of tissue malfunction due to disturbed pH (such as altered cardiac and central nervous system function), or with secondary changes in respiration that occur as a response to the underlying metabolic change (such as Kussmaul respiration during metabolic acidosis). The clinical picture is often dominated by the underlying cause rather than the acid–base abnormality itself. Frequently, acid–base disturbances only become evident when the venous plasma bicarbonate concentration is measured and found to be abnormal, or when blood gas analysis shows abnormalities in pH, PCO_2 or bicarbonate.

The most common patterns of abnormality in blood gas parameters are shown in Box 14.18. Note that the terms acidosis and alkalosis strictly refer to the underlying direction of the acid–base change, while acidaemia and alkalaemia more correctly refer to the net change present in the blood. Interpretation of arterial blood gases is also described on page 555.

In metabolic disturbances, respiratory compensation is almost immediate, so that the predicted compensatory change in PCO_2 is achieved soon after the onset of the metabolic disturbance. In respiratory disorders, on the other hand, a small initial change in bicarbonate occurs as a result of chemical buffering of CO_2, largely within red blood cells, but over days and weeks the kidney achieves further compensatory changes in bicarbonate concentration as a result of long-term adjustments in acid secretory capacity. When the clinically obtained acid–base parameters do not accord with the predicted compensation shown, a mixed acid–base disturbance should be suspected (p. 367).

Metabolic acidosis

Metabolic acidosis occurs when an acid other than carbonic acid (due to CO_2 retention) accumulates in the body, resulting in a

14.18 Principal patterns of acid–base disturbance

Disturbance	Blood H^+	Primary change	Compensatory response	Predicted compensation
Metabolic acidosis	>40[1]	$HCO_3^- < 24$ mmol/L	$PCO_2 < 5.33$ kPa[2]	PCO_2 fall in kPa = 0.16 × HCO_3^- fall in mmol/L
Metabolic alkalosis	<40[1]	$HCO_3^- > 24$ mmol/L	$PCO_2 > 5.33$ kPa[2,3]	PCO_2 rise in kPa = 0.08 × HCO_3^- rise in mmol/L
Respiratory acidosis	>40[1]	$PCO_2 > 5.33$ kPa[2]	$HCO_3^- > 24$ mmol/L	Acute: HCO_3^- rise in mmol/L = 0.75 × PCO_2 rise in kPa Chronic: HCO_3^- rise in mmol/L = 2.62 × PCO_2 rise in kPa
Respiratory alkalosis	<40[1]	$PCO_2 < 5.33$ kPa[2]	$HCO_3^- < 24$ mmol/L	Acute: HCO_3^- fall in mmol/L = 1.50 × PCO_2 fall in kPa Chronic: HCO_3^- fall in mmol/L = 3.75 × PCO_2 fall in kPa

[1]H^+ of 40 nmol/L = pH of 7.40. [2]PCO_2 of 5.33 kPa = 40 mmHg. [3]PCO_2 does not rise above 7.33 kPa (55 mmHg) because hypoxia then intervenes to drive respiration.

14.19 Causes of metabolic acidosis

Disorder	Mechanism
Normal anion gap	
Ingestion or infusion of inorganic acid	Therapeutic infusion of or poisoning with NH_4Cl, HCl
Gastrointestinal HCO_3^- loss	Loss of HCO_3^- in diarrhoea, small bowel fistula, urinary diversion procedure
Renal tubular acidosis (RTA)	Urinary loss of HCO_3^- in proximal RTA; impaired tubular acid secretion in distal RTA
Increased anion gap **Endogenous acid load**	
Diabetic ketoacidosis	Accumulation of ketones[1] with hyperglycaemia (p. 735)
Starvation ketosis Alcoholic ketoacidosis	Accumulation of ketones without hyperglycaemia (p. 725)
Lactic acidosis	Shock, liver disease, drugs
Kidney disease	Accumulation of organic acids
Exogenous acid load	
Aspirin poisoning	Accumulation of salicylate[2]
Methanol poisoning	Accumulation of formate
Ethylene glycol poisoning	Accumulation of glycolate, oxalate

[1]Ketones include acid anions acetoacetate and β-hydroxybutyrate (p. 725).
[2]Salicylate poisoning is also associated with respiratory alkalosis due to direct ventilatory stimulation.

14.20 Causes of renal tubular acidosis

Proximal renal tubular acidosis (type II RTA)
- Inherited:
  - Fanconi's syndrome
  - Cystinosis
  - Wilson's disease
- Paraproteinaemia:
  - Myeloma
- Amyloidosis
- Hyperparathyroidism
- Heavy metal toxicity:
  - Lead, cadmium and mercury poisoning
- Drugs:
  - Carbonic anhydrase inhibitors
  - Ifosfamide

Classical distal renal tubular acidosis (type I RTA)
- Inherited
- Autoimmune diseases:
  - Systemic lupus erythematosus
  - Sjögren's syndrome
- Hyperglobulinaemia
- Toxins and drugs:
  - Toluene
  - Lithium
  - Amphotericin

Hyperkalaemic distal renal tubular acidosis (type IV RTA)
- Hypoaldosteronism (primary or secondary)
- Obstructive nephropathy
- Renal transplant rejection
- Drugs:
  - Amiloride
  - Spironolactone

14

fall in the plasma bicarbonate. The causes of metabolic acidosis are summarised in Box 14.19, subdivided into two categories, depending on whether the anion gap is normal or raised.

Pathophysiology

Metabolic acidosis with a normal anion gap occurs when there is a primary loss of bicarbonate from the ECF, or when there is poisoning with or therapeutic infusion of a mineral acid such as hydrochloric acid or ammonium chloride. Renal tubular acidosis (RTA) is an important cause of metabolic acidosis with a normal anion gap. It can be caused by a defect in one of three processes:

- impaired bicarbonate reabsorption in the proximal tubule (proximal RTA)
- impaired acid secretion in the late distal tubule or cortical collecting duct intercalated cells (classical distal RTA)
- impaired sodium reabsorption in the late distal tubule or cortical collecting duct, which is associated with reduced secretion of both potassium and H^+ ions (hyperkalaemic distal RTA).

Various subtypes of RTA are recognised and the most common causes are shown in Box 14.20. The inherited forms of RTA are due to mutations in the genes that regulate acid or bicarbonate transport in the renal tubules (see Fig. 14.3).

Acidosis with an increased anion gap is most commonly seen in ketoacidosis, renal failure and lactic acidosis, where there is endogenous production of anions distinct from Cl^- and HCO_3^-. Ketoacidosis is caused by insulin deficiency and is exacerbated by catecholamine and stress hormone excess, which combine to cause lipolysis and the formation of acidic ketones (acetoacetate, 3-hydroxybutyrate and acetone). The most common cause of ketoacidosis is diabetic ketoacidosis (DKA); its aetiology and management are discussed on page 735. Starvation ketoacidosis occurs when there is reduced food intake in situations of high glucose demand, such as in neonates, and in pregnant or breastfeeding women. In alcoholic ketoacidosis, there is usually a background of chronic malnutrition and a recent alcohol binge. Two subtypes of lactic acidosis have been defined:

- type 1, due to tissue hypoxia and peripheral generation of lactate, as in patients with circulatory failure and shock
- type 2, due to impaired metabolism of lactate, as in liver disease or by a number of drugs and toxins, including metformin, which inhibit lactate metabolism (p. 746).

Metabolic acidosis with an increased anion gap may also be a consequence of exogenous acid loads from poisoning with aspirin, methanol or ethylene glycol.

Clinical features

Normal anion gap metabolic acidosis is usually due either to bicarbonate loss in diarrhoea, where the clinical diagnosis is generally obvious, or to RTA. Although some forms of RTA are inherited, it may also be an acquired disorder, and in these circumstances the discovery of metabolic acidosis may serve as an early clue to the underlying diagnosis. The presentation of increased anion gap acidosis is usually dominated by clinical features of the underlying disease, such as uncontrolled diabetes mellitus, kidney failure or shock, or may be suggested by the clinical history of starvation, alcoholism or associated symptoms, such as visual complaints in methanol poisoning (p. 147).

Investigations

The different types of metabolic acidosis can be distinguished by blood gas measurements, along with measurements of creatinine, electrolytes and bicarbonate. Under normal circumstances, the anion gap, defined as the numerical difference between the main measured cations ($Na^+ + K^+$) and the anions ($Cl^- + HCO_3^-$) is about 5–11 mmol/L. This gap is normally made up of anions, such as phosphate and sulphate, as well as albumin. RTA should be suspected when there is a hyperchloraemic acidosis with a normal anion gap in the absence of gastrointestinal disturbance. The diagnosis can be confirmed by finding an inappropriately high urine pH (>5.5) in the presence of systemic acidosis. Sometimes, distal RTA may be incomplete, such that the plasma bicarbonate concentration may be normal under resting conditions. In this case, an acid challenge test can be performed by administration of an acid load in the form of ammonium chloride to reduce plasma bicarbonate. The diagnosis of incomplete distal RTA can be confirmed if the urine pH fails to fall below 5.3 in the presence of a low bicarbonate.

The different subtypes of RTA can be differentiated by various biochemical features. Patients with proximal and distal RTA often present with features of profound hypokalaemia, while type IV RTA is associated with hyperkalaemia. Proximal RTA is frequently associated with urinary wasting of amino acids, phosphate and glucose (Fanconi's syndrome), as well as bicarbonate and potassium. Patients with this disorder can lower the urine pH when the acidosis is severe and plasma bicarbonate levels have fallen below 16 mmol/L, since distal H^+ secretion mechanisms are intact. In the classical form of distal RTA, however, acid accumulation is relentless and progressive, resulting in mobilisation of calcium from bone and osteomalacia with hypercalciuria, renal stone formation and nephrocalcinosis. Potassium is also lost in classical distal RTA, while it is retained in hyperkalaemic distal RTA.

Investigations in patients with raised anion gap metabolic acidosis show features of the underlying cause, such as reduced GFR in renal failure and raised urine or blood ketones in ketoacidosis. In DKA, blood glucose is raised, while in starvation and alcoholic acidosis blood glucose is not elevated and may be low. Measurement of plasma lactate is helpful in the diagnosis of lactic acidosis when values are increased over the normal maximal level of 2 mmol/L.

Management

The first step in management of metabolic acidosis is to identify and correct the underlying cause when possible (see Box 14.19). This may involve controlling diarrhoea, treating diabetes mellitus, correcting shock, stopping drugs that might cause the condition, or using dialysis to remove toxins. Since metabolic acidosis is frequently associated with sodium and water depletion, resuscitation with intravenous fluids is often needed. In alcoholism and starvation ketosis, intravenous glucose is indicated. By stimulating endogenous insulin secretion, this will reverse hepatic ketone production. Malnourished patients may also require thiamin, potassium, magnesium and phosphate supplements (p. 706). Use of intravenous bicarbonate in metabolic acidosis is controversial. Because rapid correction of acidosis can induce hypokalaemia or a fall in plasma ionised calcium, the use of bicarbonate infusions is best reserved for situations where the underlying disorder cannot be readily corrected and acidosis is severe (H^+ >100 nmol/L, pH <7.00) or associated with evidence of tissue dysfunction.

The acidosis in RTA can sometimes be controlled by treating the underlying cause (see Box 14.20), but usually supplements of sodium and potassium bicarbonate are also necessary in types I and II RTA to achieve a target plasma bicarbonate level of >18 mmol/L and normokalaemia. In type IV RTA, loop diuretics, thiazides or fludrocortisone (as appropriate to the underlying diagnosis) may be effective in correcting the acidosis and the hyperkalaemia.

Metabolic alkalosis

Metabolic alkalosis is characterised by an increase in the plasma bicarbonate concentration and the plasma pH (see Box 14.18). There is a compensatory rise in PCO_2 due to hypoventilation but this is limited by the need to avoid hypoxia. Classical causes include primary hyperaldosteronism (Conn's syndrome, p. 674), Cushing's syndrome (p. 666) and glucocorticoid therapy (p. 670). Occasionally, overuse of antacid salts for treatment of dyspepsia produces a similar pattern.

Pathophysiology

Metabolic alkalosis is best classified according to the accompanying changes in ECF volume. Hypovolaemic metabolic alkalosis is the most common pattern. This can be caused by sustained vomiting, in which acid-rich fluid is lost directly from the body, or by treatment with loop diuretics or thiazides. In the case of sustained vomiting, loss of gastric acid is the immediate cause of the alkalosis, but several factors act to sustain or amplify this in the context of volume depletion (Fig. 14.11). Loss of sodium and fluid leads to hypovolaemia and secondary hyperaldosteronism, triggering proximal sodium bicarbonate reabsorption and additional acid secretion by the distal tubule. Hypokalaemia occurs due to potassium loss in the vomitus and by the kidney as the result of secondary hyperaldosteronism, and itself is a stimulus to acid secretion. Additionally, the compensatory rise in PCO_2 further enhances tubular acid secretion. The net result is sustained metabolic alkalosis with an inappropriately acid urine, which cannot be corrected until the deficit in circulating volume has been replaced.

Normovolaemic (or hypervolaemic) metabolic alkalosis occurs when bicarbonate retention and volume expansion occur simultaneously.

Clinical features

Clinically, apart from manifestations of the underlying cause, there may be few symptoms or signs related to alkalosis itself. When the rise in systemic pH is abrupt, however, plasma ionised calcium falls and signs of increased neuromuscular irritability, such as tetany, may develop (p. 663).

Investigations

The diagnosis can be confirmed by measurement of electrolytes and arterial blood gases.

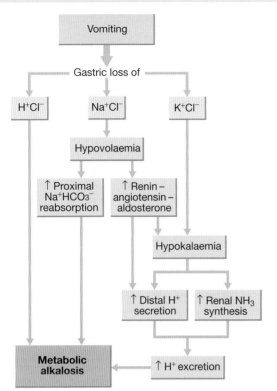

Fig. 14.11 Generation and maintenance of metabolic alkalosis during prolonged vomiting. Loss of H⁺Cl⁻ generates metabolic alkalosis, which is maintained by renal changes.

Diagram labels: Vomiting → Gastric loss of → H⁺Cl⁻, Na⁺Cl⁻, K⁺Cl⁻; Na⁺Cl⁻ → Hypovolaemia → ↑ Proximal Na⁺HCO₃⁻ reabsorption, ↑ Renin–angiotensin–aldosterone → Hypokalaemia → ↑ Distal H⁺ secretion, ↑ Renal NH₃ synthesis → ↑ H⁺ excretion → Metabolic alkalosis

Management

Metabolic alkalosis with hypovolaemia can be corrected by intravenous infusions of 0.9% saline with potassium supplements. This reverses the secondary hyperaldosteronism and allows the kidney to excrete the excess alkali in the urine. In metabolic alkalosis with normal or increased volume, treatment should focus on management of the underlying endocrine cause (Ch. 18).

Respiratory acidosis

Respiratory acidosis occurs when there is accumulation of CO_2 due to type II respiratory failure (p. 565). This results in a rise in the PCO_2, with a compensatory increase in plasma bicarbonate concentration, particularly when the disorder is of long duration and the kidney has fully developed its capacity for increased acid excretion.

This acid–base disturbance can arise from lesions anywhere along the neuromuscular pathways from the brain to the respiratory muscles that result in impaired ventilation. It can also arise during intrinsic lung disease if there is significant mismatching of ventilation and perfusion.

Clinical features are primarily those of the underlying cause of the respiratory disorder, such as paralysis, chest wall injury or chronic obstructive lung disease, but the CO_2 accumulation may itself lead to drowsiness that further depresses respiratory drive.

Management involves correction of causative factors where possible, but ultimately ventilatory support may be necessary.

Respiratory alkalosis

Respiratory alkalosis develops when there is a period of sustained hyperventilation, resulting in a reduction of PCO_2 and increase in plasma pH. If the condition is sustained, renal compensation occurs, such that tubular acid secretion is reduced and the plasma bicarbonate falls.

Respiratory alkalosis is usually of short duration, occurring in anxiety states or as the result of over-vigorous assisted ventilation. It can be prolonged in the context of pregnancy, pulmonary embolism, chronic liver disease, and ingestion of certain drugs such as salicylates that directly stimulate the respiratory centre in the brainstem.

Clinical features are those of the underlying cause but agitation associated with perioral and digital tingling may also occur, as alkalosis promotes the binding of calcium to albumin, resulting in a reduction in ionised calcium concentrations. In severe cases, Trousseau's sign and Chvostek's sign may be positive, and tetany or seizures may develop (p. 663).

Management involves correction of identifiable causes, reduction of anxiety, and a period of rebreathing into a closed bag to allow CO_2 levels to rise.

Mixed acid–base disorders

It is not uncommon for more than one disturbance of acid–base metabolism to be present at the same time in the same patient: for example, a respiratory acidosis due to narcotic overdose with metabolic alkalosis due to vomiting. In these situations, the arterial pH will represent the net effect of all primary and compensatory changes. Indeed, the pH may be normal, but the presence of underlying acid–base disturbances can be gauged from concomitant abnormalities in the PCO_2 and bicarbonate concentration.

In assessing these disorders, all clinical influences on the patient's acid–base status should be identified, and reference should be made to the table of predicted compensation given in Box 14.18. If the compensatory change is discrepant from the rules of thumb provided, more than one disturbance of acid–base metabolism may be suspected.

Calcium homeostasis

Disorders of calcium homeostasis are discussed in Chapter 18 and bone disease is discussed in Chapter 24.

Magnesium homeostasis

Magnesium is mainly an intracellular cation. It is important to the function of many enzymes, including the Na,K-ATPase, and can regulate both potassium and calcium channels. Its overall effect is to stabilise excitable cell membranes.

Functional anatomy and physiology

Renal handling of magnesium involves filtration of free plasma magnesium at the glomerulus (about 70% of the total), with extensive reabsorption (50–70%) in the loop of Henle and other parts of the proximal and distal renal tubule. Magnesium reabsorption is also enhanced by parathyroid hormone (PTH).

Presenting problems in magnesium homeostasis

Disturbances in magnesium homeostasis usually occur because of increased loss of magnesium through the gut or kidney or

14

inability to excrete magnesium normally in patients with renal impairment.

Hypomagnesaemia

Hypomagnesaemia is defined as existing when plasma magnesium concentrations are below the reference range of 0.75–1.0 mmol/L (1.5–2.0 mEq/L).

Pathophysiology

Hypomagnesaemia usually is a reflection of magnesium depletion (Box 14.21), which can be caused by excessive magnesium loss from the gastrointestinal tract (notably in chronic diarrhoea) or the kidney (during prolonged use of loop diuretics). Excessive alcohol ingestion can cause magnesium depletion through both gut and renal losses. Some inherited tubular transport disorders, such as Gitelman's and Bartter's syndromes, can also result in urinary magnesium wasting (p. 361). Magnesium depletion has important effects on calcium homeostasis because magnesium is required for the normal secretion of PTH in response to a fall in serum calcium, and because hypomagnesaemia causes end-organ resistance to PTH.

Clinical features

Mild degrees of hypomagnesaemia may be asymptomatic but more severe hypomagnesaemia may be associated with symptoms of hypocalcaemia, such as tetany, cardiac arrhythmias (notably torsades de pointes, p. 476), central nervous excitation and seizures, vasoconstriction and hypertension. Hypomagnesaemia and magnesium depletion are also associated (through uncertain mechanisms) with hyponatraemia and hypokalaemia, which may contribute to some of the clinical manifestations.

i	14.21 Causes of hypomagnesaemia	
Mechanism	**Examples**	
Inadequate intake	Starvation	
	Malnutrition	
	Alcoholism	
	Parenteral alimentation	
Excessive losses		
Gastrointestinal	Prolonged vomiting/nasogastric aspiration	
	Chronic diarrhoea/laxative abuse	
	Malabsorption	
	Small bowel bypass surgery	
	Fistulae	
Urinary	Diuretic therapy	
	Alcohol	
	Tubulotoxic drugs:	
	Gentamicin	
	Cisplatin	
	Volume expansion	
	Diabetic ketoacidosis	
	Post-obstructive diuresis	
	Recovery from acute tubular necrosis	
	Inherited tubular transport defect:	
	Bartter's syndrome	
	Gitelman's syndrome	
	Primary renal magnesium wasting	
Miscellaneous	Acute pancreatitis	
	Foscarnet therapy	
	Proton pump inhibitor therapy	
	Hungry bone syndrome	
	Diabetes mellitus	

Management

The underlying cause should be identified and treated where possible. When symptoms are present, the treatment of choice is intravenous magnesium chloride at a rate not exceeding 0.5 mmol/kg in the first 24 hours. If intravenous access is not feasible, magnesium sulphate can be given intramuscularly. Oral magnesium salts have limited effectiveness due to poor absorption and may cause diarrhoea. If hypomagnesaemia is caused by diuretic treatment, adjunctive use of a potassium-sparing agent can also help by reducing magnesium loss into the urine.

Hypermagnesaemia

This is a much less common abnormality than hypomagnesaemia. Predisposing conditions include acute kidney injury, chronic kidney disease and adrenocortical insufficiency. The condition is generally precipitated in patients at risk from an increased intake of magnesium, or from the use of magnesium-containing medications, such as antacids, laxatives and enemas.

Clinical features include bradycardia, hypotension, reduced consciousness and respiratory depression.

Management involves ceasing all magnesium-containing drugs and reducing dietary magnesium intake, improving renal function if possible, and promoting urinary magnesium excretion using a loop diuretic with intravenous hydration, if residual renal function allows. Calcium gluconate may be given intravenously to ameliorate cardiac effects. Dialysis may be necessary in patients with poor renal function.

Phosphate homeostasis

Inorganic phosphate (mainly present as HPO_4^{2-}) is intimately involved in cell energy metabolism, intracellular signalling and bone and mineral homeostasis (Ch. 24). The normal plasma concentration is 0.8–1.4 mmol/L (2.48–4.34 mg/dL).

Functional anatomy and physiology

Phosphate is freely filtered at the glomerulus and approximately 65% is reabsorbed by the proximal tubule, through an apical sodium–phosphate co-transport carrier. A further 10–20% is reabsorbed in the distal tubules, leaving a fractional excretion of some 10% to pass into the urine, usually as $H_2PO_4^-$. Proximal reabsorption is decreased by PTH, fibroblast growth factor 23 (FGF23), volume expansion, osmotic diuretics and glucose infusion.

Presenting problems in phosphate homeostasis

The following section deals primarily with conditions that cause acute disturbances in serum phosphate concentrations. Chronic disorders that are accompanied by phosphate depletion, such as osteomalacia and hypophosphataemic rickets, are discussed in Chapter 24. Acute kidney injury and chronic kidney disease, which are associated with hyperphosphataemia, are discussed below and also in Chapter 15.

Hypophosphataemia

Hypophosphataemia is defined as existing when serum phosphate values fall below 0.8 mmol/L (2.48 mg/dL). The causes are shown in Box 14.22, subdivided into the underlying pathogenic mechanisms.

i	14.22 Causes of hypophosphataemia	
Mechanism	**Examples**	
Redistribution into cells	Refeeding after starvation	
	Respiratory alkalosis	
	Treatment for diabetic ketoacidosis	
Inadequate intake or absorption	Malnutrition	
	Malabsorption	
	Chronic diarrhoea	
	Phosphate binders	
	Antacids	
	Vitamin D deficiency or resistance	
Increased renal excretion	Hyperparathyroidism	
	Extracellular fluid volume expansion with diuresis	
	Osmotic diuretics	
	Fanconi's syndrome	
	Familial hypophosphataemic rickets	
	Tumour-induced hypophosphataemic rickets	

Pathophysiology

Phosphate may redistribute into cells during periods of increased energy utilisation (such as refeeding after a period of starvation) and during systemic alkalosis. However, severe hypophosphataemia usually represents an overall body deficit due to either inadequate intake or absorption through the gut, or excessive renal losses, most notably in primary hyperparathyroidism (p. 663) or as the result of acute plasma volume expansion, osmotic diuresis and diuretics acting on the proximal renal tubule. Less common causes include inherited defects of proximal sodium–phosphate co-transport and tumour-induced osteomalacia due to ectopic production of the hormone FGF23 (p. 1053).

Clinical features

The clinical features of phosphate depletion are wide-ranging, reflecting the involvement of phosphate in many aspects of metabolism. Defects appear in the blood (impaired function and survival of all cell lineages), skeletal muscle (weakness, respiratory failure), cardiac muscle (congestive cardiac failure), smooth muscle (ileus), central nervous system (decreased consciousness, seizures and coma) and bone (osteomalacia in severe prolonged hypophosphataemia, p. 1053).

Investigations

Measurement of creatinine, electrolytes, phosphate, albumin, calcium and alkaline phosphatase should be performed. In selected cases, measurement of PTH and 25(OH)D may be helpful to exclude osteomalacia or hypophosphataemic rickets. The combination of hypophosphataemia and hypercalcaemia suggests primary hyperparathyroidism, which should be further investigated by measurements of PTH, as described on page 663. The presence of hypocalcaemia suggests hypophosphataemic rickets, which should be further investigated as described on page 1053.

Management

Management of hypophosphataemia due to decreased dietary intake or excessive losses involves administering oral phosphate supplements and high-protein/high-dairy dietary supplements that are rich in naturally occurring phosphate. Intravenous treatment with sodium or potassium phosphate salts can be used in critical situations, but there is a risk of precipitating hypocalcaemia and metastatic calcification. Management of primary hyperparathyroidism and hypophosphataemic rickets are described in more detail on pages 664 and 1053.

Hyperphosphataemia

Hyperphosphataemia is most commonly caused by acute kidney injury or chronic kidney disease (pp. 413 and 419).

Pathophysiology

In acute kidney injury and chronic kidney disease, the primary cause is reduced phosphate excretion as the result of a low GFR. In contrast, the hyperphosphataemia in hypoparathyroidism and pseudohypoparathyroidism is due to increased tubular phosphate reabsorption. Redistribution of phosphate from cells into the plasma can also be a contributing factor in the tumour lysis syndromes and other catabolic states. Phosphate accumulation can be aggravated in any of these conditions if the patient takes phosphate-containing preparations or inappropriate vitamin D therapy.

Clinical features

The clinical features relate to hypocalcaemia and metastatic calcification, particularly in chronic kidney disease with tertiary hyperparathyroidism (when a high calcium–phosphate product occurs).

Management

Hyperphosphataemia in patients with kidney disease should be treated with dietary phosphate restriction and the use of oral phosphate binders (p. 418). Hyperphosphataemia in hypoparathyroidism and pseudohypoparathyroidism does not usually require treatment. Hyperphosphataemia associated with tumour lysis syndromes and catabolic states can be treated with intravenous normal saline, which is given to promote phosphate excretion.

Disorders of amino acid metabolism

Congenital disorders of amino acid metabolism usually present in the neonatal period and may involve life-long treatment regimens. However, some disorders, particularly those involved in amino acid transport, may not present until later in life.

Phenylketonuria

Phenylketonuria (PKU) is inherited as an autosomal recessive disorder caused by loss-of-function mutations in the *PAH* gene, which encodes phenylalanine hydroxylase, an enzyme required for degradation of phenylalanine. As a result, phenylalanine accumulates at high levels in the neonate's blood, causing intellectual disability.

The diagnosis of PKU is almost always made by routine neonatal screening (p. 56). Treatment involves life-long adherence to a low-phenylalanine diet. Early and adequate dietary treatment prevents major intellectual disability, although there may still be a slight reduction in IQ.

Homocystinuria

Homocystinuria is an autosomal recessive disorder caused by loss-of-function mutations in the *CBS* gene, which encodes cystathionine β-synthase. The enzyme deficiency causes accumulation of homocysteine and methionine in the blood. Many cases of homocystinuria are diagnosed through newborn screening programmes.

14

Clinical manifestations are wide-ranging and involve the eyes (ectopia lentis – displacement of the lens), central nervous system (intellectual disability, delayed developmental milestones, seizures, psychiatric disturbances), skeleton (resembling Marfan's syndrome, and also with generalised osteoporosis), vascular system (thrombotic lesions of arteries and veins) and skin (hypopigmentation).

Treatment is dietary, involving a methionine-restricted, cystine-supplemented diet, as well as large doses of pyridoxine.

Disorders of carbohydrate metabolism

The most common disorder of carbohydrate metabolism is diabetes mellitus, which is discussed in Chapter 20. There are also some rare inherited defects, discussed below.

Galactosaemia

Galactosaemia is caused by loss-of-function mutations in the *GALT* gene, which encodes galactose-1-phosphate uridyl transferase. It is usually inherited in an autosomal recessive manner. The neonate is unable to metabolise galactose, one of the hexose sugars contained in lactose. Vomiting or diarrhoea usually begins within a few days of ingestion of milk, and the neonate may become jaundiced. Failure to thrive is the most common clinical presentation. The classic form of the disease results in hepatomegaly, cataracts and intellectual disability. Fulminant infection with *Escherichia coli* is a frequent complication. Treatment involves life-long avoidance of galactose- and lactose-containing foods.

The widespread inclusion of galactosaemia in newborn screening programmes has resulted in the identification of a number of milder ('Duarte') variants.

Glycogen storage diseases

Glycogen storage diseases (GSDs, or glycogenoses) result from inherited defects in one of the many enzymes responsible for the formation or breakdown of glycogen, a complex carbohydrate that can be broken down quickly to release glucose during exercise or between meals.

There are several major types of GSD, which are classified by a number, by the name of the defective enzyme, or eponymously

after the physician who first described the condition (Box 14.23). Most forms of GSD are inherited in an autosomal recessive manner.

The diagnosis of GSD is made on the basis of the symptoms, physical examination and results of biochemical tests. Occasionally, a muscle or liver biopsy is required to confirm the enzyme defect. Different types of GSD present at different ages, and some may require life-long modifications of diet and lifestyle.

Disorders of complex lipid metabolism

Complex lipids are key components of the cell membrane that are normally catabolised in organelles called lysosomes. The lysosomal storage diseases are a heterogeneous group of disorders caused by loss-of-function mutations in various lysosomal enzymes (Box 14.24), resulting in an inability to break down complex glycolipids or other intracellular macromolecules. These disorders have diverse clinical manifestations, typically including intellectual disability. Some can be treated with enzyme replacement therapy, while others (such as Tay–Sachs disease) can be prevented through community participation in genetic carrier screening programmes.

Lipids and lipoprotein metabolism

The three main biological classes of lipid are:

- cholesterol, which is composed of hydrocarbon rings
- triglycerides (TGs), which are esters composed of glycerol linked to three long-chain fatty acids
- phospholipids, which are composed of a hydrophobic 'tail' consisting of two long-chain fatty acids linked through glycerol to a hydrophilic head containing a phosphate group.

Phospholipids are present in cell membranes and are important signalling molecules.

Despite their poor water solubility, lipids need to be absorbed from the gastrointestinal tract and transported throughout the body. This is achieved by incorporating lipids within lipoproteins. Plasma cholesterol and TGs are clinically important because they are major treatable risk factors for cardiovascular disease, while severe hypertriglyceridaemia also predisposes to acute pancreatitis.

i	14.23 Glycogen storage diseases			
Type	**Eponym**	**Enzyme deficiency**	**Clinical features and complications**
I	Von Gierke	Glucose-6-phosphatase	Childhood presentation, hypoglycaemia, hepatomegaly
II	Pompe	α-glucosidase (acid maltase)	Classical presentation in infancy, muscle weakness (may be severe)
III	Cori	Glycogen debrancher enzyme	Childhood presentation, hepatomegaly, mild hypoglycaemia
IV	Andersen	Brancher enzyme	Presentation in infancy, severe muscle weakness (may affect heart), cirrhosis
V	McArdle	Muscle glycogen phosphorylase	Exercise-induced fatigue and myalgia
VI	Hers	Liver phosphorylase	Mild hepatomegaly
VII	Tarui	Muscle phosphofructokinase	Exercise-induced fatigue and myalgia
IX[1]		Liver phosphorylase kinase	Mild hepatomegaly
0		Hepatic glycogen synthase	Fasting hypoglycaemia, post-prandial hyperglycaemia
X[2]		Muscle phosphoglycerate mutase	Exercise-induced myoglobinuria

[1]Note that type VIII has been merged into type IX and no longer exists as a separate entity. [2]Recent progress in molecular genetics has recognised a number of additional, rarer types of glycogen storage disease. These are not shown in this table, which stops at type X.

i 14.24 Lysosomal storage diseases

Lysosomal storage disease	Enzyme deficiency	Clinical features	Human enzyme replacement therapy
Fabry's disease	α-galactosidase A	Variable age of onset Neurological (pain in extremities) Dermatological (hypohidrosis, angiokeratomas) Cerebrovascular (renal, cardiac, central nervous system)	Available for clinical use
Gaucher's disease (various types)	Glucocerebrosidase	Splenic and liver enlargement, with variable severity of disease Some types also have neurological involvement	Available for clinical use in some types
Mucopolysaccharidosis Hurler's syndrome Hunter's syndrome Sanfilippo's syndrome Morquio's syndrome + several other types	Several enzymes involved in breakdown of glycosaminoglycans	Vary with syndrome: can cause intellectual disability, skeletal and joint abnormalities, abnormal facies, obstructive respiratory diseases and recurrent respiratory infections	Available for clinical use in some types; clinical trials under way for other types
Niemann–Pick disease	Acid sphingomyelinase	Most common presentation is as a progressive neurological disorder, accompanied by organomegaly Some variants do not have neurological symptoms	Clinical trials planned for some types
GM2-gangliosidosis Tay–Sachs disease Hexosaminidase activator deficiency Sandhoff's disease	Hexosaminidase A Hexosaminidase activator Hexosaminidase A and B	Severe progressive neurological disorder Cherry-red spot in macula Organomegaly in Sandhoff's disease	

14

Functional anatomy and physiology

Lipids are transported and metabolised by apolipoproteins, which combine with lipids to form spherical or disc-shaped lipoproteins, consisting of a hydrophobic core and a less hydrophobic coat (Fig. 14.12). The structure of some apolipoproteins also enables them to act as enzyme co-factors or cell receptor ligands. Variations in lipid and apolipoprotein composition result in distinct classes of lipoprotein that perform specific metabolic functions.

Processing of dietary lipid

The intestinal absorption of dietary lipid is described on page 768 (see also Fig. 14.13). Enterocytes lining the gut extract monoglyceride and free fatty acids from micelles and re-esterify them into TGs, which are combined with a truncated form of apolipoprotein B (Apo B48) as it is synthesised. Intestinal cholesterol derived from dietary and biliary sources is also absorbed through a specific intestinal membrane transporter termed NPC1L1. This produces chylomicrons containing TG and cholesterol ester that are secreted basolaterally into lymphatic lacteals and carried to the circulation through the thoracic duct. On entering the blood stream, nascent chylomicrons are modified by further addition of apolipoproteins. Chylomicron TGs are hydrolysed by lipoprotein lipase located on the endothelium of tissue capillary beds. This releases fatty acids that are used locally for energy production or stored as TG in muscle or fat. The residual 'remnant' chylomicron particle is avidly cleared by low-density lipoprotein receptors (LDLRs) in the liver, which recognise Apo E on the remnant lipoproteins. Complete absorption of dietary lipids takes about 6–10 hours, so chylomicrons are usually undetectable in the plasma after a 12-hour fast.

The main dietary determinants of plasma cholesterol concentrations are the intake of saturated and *trans*-unsaturated fatty acids, which reduce LDLR levels (see below), whereas dietary cholesterol has surprisingly little effect on fasting cholesterol levels. Plant sterols and drugs that inhibit cholesterol absorption are effective because they also reduce the re-utilisation of biliary cholesterol. The dietary determinants of plasma TG concentrations are complex since excessive intake of carbohydrate, fat or alcohol may all contribute to increased plasma TG by different mechanisms.

Endogenous lipid synthesis

In the fasting state, the liver is the major source of plasma lipids (Fig. 14.13). The liver may acquire lipids by uptake, synthesis or conversion from other macronutrients. These lipids are transported to other tissues by secretion of very low-density lipoproteins (VLDLs), which are rich in TG but differ from chylomicrons in that they are less massive and contain full-length Apo B100. Following secretion into the circulation, VLDLs undergo metabolic processing similar to that of chylomicrons. Hydrolysis of VLDL TG releases fatty acids to tissues and converts VLDLs into 'remnant' particles, referred to as intermediate-density lipoproteins (IDLs). Most IDLs are rapidly cleared by LDLRs in the liver but some are

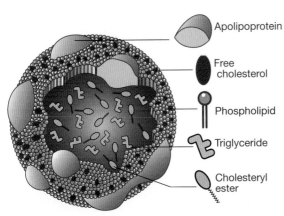

Fig. 14.12 Structure of lipoproteins.

- Apolipoprotein
- Free cholesterol
- Phospholipid
- Triglyceride
- Cholesteryl ester

Fig. 14.13 Absorption, transport and storage of lipids. Pathways of lipid transport are shown; in addition, cholesterol ester transfer protein exchanges triglyceride and cholesterol ester between very low-density lipoprotein/chylomicrons and high-/low-density lipoprotein, and free fatty acids released from peripheral lipolysis can be taken up in the liver. (ABCA1/ABCG1 = adenosine triphosphate-binding cassette A1/G1; Apo = apolipoprotein; BA = bile acids; C = cholesterol; CE = cholesterol ester; FFA = free fatty acids; HDL = mature high-density lipoprotein; HL = hepatic lipase; HMGCoAR = hydroxy-methyl-glutaryl-co-enzyme A reductase; IDL = intermediate-density lipoprotein; iHDL = immature high-density lipoprotein; LCAT = lecithin cholesterol acyl transferase; LDL = low-density lipoprotein; LDLR = low-density lipoprotein receptor (Apo B100 receptor); LPL = lipoprotein lipase; PCSK9 = proprotein convertase subtilisin kexin 9; SRB1 = scavenger receptor B1; TG = triglyceride; VLDL = very low-density lipoprotein)

processed by hepatic lipase, which converts the particle to an LDL by removing TG and most materials other than Apo B100, and free and esterified cholesterol. The catabolism of TG-rich chylomicrons and VLDL by lipoprotein lipase is modulated by Apos C2 and C3 on the surface of these particles.

The LDL particles act as a source of cholesterol for cells and tissues (Fig. 14.13). LDL cholesterol is internalised by receptor-mediated endocytosis through the LDLR. Delivery of cholesterol via this pathway down-regulates expression of LDLR and reduces the synthesis and activity of the rate-limiting enzyme for cholesterol synthesis, hydroxy-methyl-glutaryl-co-enzyme A (HMGCoA) reductase. Another important regulator of LDLR levels is the sterol-sensitive protease proprotein convertase subtilisin kexin 9 (PCSK9), which degrades the LDLR. Intracellular free cholesterol concentrations are maintained within a narrow range by the inhibitory effects of LDL on expression of LRLR, fine-tuning

of the half-life of LDLR through PCSK9, and modulation of cholesterol esterification.

Cholesterol transport

Peripheral tissues are further guarded against excessive cholesterol accumulation by high-density lipoproteins (HDLs; Fig. 14.13). Lipid-poor Apo A1 (derived from the liver, intestine and th e outer layer of chylomicrons and VLDL) accepts cellular cholesterol and phospholipid from a specific membrane transporter known as the ATP-binding cassette A1 (ABCA1). This produces small HDLs that are able to accept more free cholesterol from cholesterol-rich regions of the cell membrane known as 'rafts' via another membrane transporter (ABCG1). The cholesterol that has been accepted by these small HDLs is esterified by lecithin cholesterol acyl transferase (LCAT), thus maintaining an uptake gradient and remodelling the particle into a mature spherical HDL. These HDLs release their cholesterol to the liver and other cholesterol-requiring tissues via the scavenger receptor B1 (SRB1).

The cholesterol ester transfer protein (CETP) in plasma allows transfer of cholesterol from HDLs or LDLs to VLDLs or chylomicrons in exchange for TG. When TG is elevated, the action of CETP may reduce HDL cholesterol and remodel LDLs into 'small, dense' LDL particles that may be more atherogenic in the blood-vessel wall. Animal species that lack CETP are resistant to atherosclerosis.

Lipids and cardiovascular disease

Plasma lipoprotein levels are major modifiable risk factors for cardiovascular disease. Increased levels of atherogenic lipoproteins (especially LDL, but also IDL, and possibly chylomicron remnants) contribute to the development of atherosclerosis (p. 484). A sub-population of LDL particles bears an additional protein known as apolipoprotein (a), which shares homology with plasminogen. The combination of LDL and apolipoprotein (a) is known as lipoprotein (a) (Lp(a)). It transports oxidised phospholipid and is regarded as atherogenic because its plasma concentration is an independent risk factor for cardiovascular disease. Following chemical modifications such as oxidation, Apo B-containing lipoproteins are no longer cleared by normal mechanisms. They trigger a self-perpetuating inflammatory response, during which they are taken up by macrophages to form foam cells, a hallmark of atherosclerotic lesions. These processes also have an adverse effect on endothelial function.

Conversely, HDL removes cholesterol from the tissues to the liver, where it is metabolised and excreted in bile. HDL may also counteract some components of the inflammatory response, such as the expression of vascular adhesion molecules by the endothelium. Consequently, low HDL cholesterol levels, which are often associated with TG elevation, are also associated with atherosclerosis.

Investigations

Lipid measurements are usually performed for the following reasons:

- screening for primary or secondary prevention of cardiovascular disease
- investigation of patients with clinical features of lipid disorders (p. 347) and their relatives
- monitoring of response to diet, weight control and medication.

Abnormalities of lipid metabolism most commonly come to light following these tests. Non-fasting measurements of total cholesterol (TC) and HDL cholesterol (HDL-C) allow estimation of non-HDL cholesterol (non-HDLC, calculated as TC – HDL-C), but a 12-hour fasting sample is required to standardise TG measurement and allow calculation of LDL cholesterol (LDL-C) according to the Friedewald formula:

$$LDL\text{-}C = TC - HDL\text{-}C - (TG/2.2)\,mmol/L$$

or

$$LDL\text{-}C = TC - HDL\text{-}C - (TG/5)\,mg/dL$$

The formula becomes unreliable when TG levels exceed 4 mmol/L (350 mg/dL). Measurements of non-HDLC or Apo B100 may assess risk of cardiovascular disease more accurately than LDL-C, particularly when TG levels are increased. The use of non-fasting samples is increasing because non-fasting TG is a more sensitive marker of the risk of cardiovascular disease. Nevertheless, a 12-hour fast is required for formal diagnosis of the presence of hypertriglyceridaemia or use of the Friedewald equation. Consideration must be given to confounding factors, such as recent illness, after which cholesterol, LDL and HDL levels temporarily decrease in proportion to severity. Results that will affect major decisions, such as initiation of drug therapy, should be confirmed with a repeat measurement.

Elevated levels of TG are common in obesity, diabetes and insulin resistance (Chs 19 and 20), and are frequently associated with low HDL and increased 'small, dense' LDL. Under these circumstances, LDL-C may under-estimate risk. This is one situation in which measurement of non-HDLC or Apo B may provide more accurate risk assessment.

Presenting problems in lipid metabolism

Hyperlipidaemia can occur in association with various diseases and drugs, as summarised in Box 14.25. Overt or subclinical hypothyroidism (p. 639) may cause hypercholesterolaemia, and so measurement of thyroid function is warranted in most cases, even in the absence of typical symptoms and signs.

Once secondary causes are excluded, primary lipid abnormalities may be diagnosed. Primary lipid abnormalities can be classified according to the predominant lipid problem: hypercholesterolaemia, hypertriglyceridaemia or mixed hyperlipidaemia (Box 14.26). Although single-gene disorders are encountered in all three categories, most cases are due to multiple-gene (polygenic) loci interacting with environmental factors. Clinical consequences of dyslipidaemia vary somewhat between these causes (pp. 346–347).

Hypercholesterolaemia

Hypercholesterolaemia is a polygenic disorder that is the most common cause of a mild to moderate increase in

i 14.25 Causes of secondary hyperlipidaemia

Secondary hypercholesterolaemia

Moderately common
- Drugs:
  Diuretics
  Ciclosporin
  Glucocorticoids
  Androgens
  Antiretroviral agents
- Hypothyroidism
- Pregnancy
- Cholestatic liver disease

Less common
- Nephrotic syndrome
- Anorexia nervosa
- Porphyria
- Hyperparathyroidism

Secondary hypertriglyceridaemia

Common
- Type 2 diabetes mellitus
- Chronic renal disease
- Abdominal obesity
- Excess alcohol
- Hepatocellular disease
- Drugs:
  β-blockers
  Retinoids
  Glucocorticoids
  Antiretroviral agents

14

i 14.26 Classification of hyperlipidaemia

Disease	Elevated lipid results	Elevated lipoprotein	CHD risk	Pancreatitis risk
Predominant hypercholesterolaemia				
Polygenic (majority)	TC ± TG	LDL ± VLDL	+	–
Familial hypercholesterolaemia (LDLR defect, defective Apo B100, increased function of *PCSK9*)	TC ± TG	LDL ± VLDL	+++	–
Hyperalphalipoproteinaemia	TC ± TG	HDL	–	–
Predominant hypertriglyceridaemia				
Polygenic (majority)	TG	VLDL ± LDL	Variable	+
Lipoprotein lipase deficiency	TG ≫ TC	Chylo	?	+++
Familial hypertriglyceridaemia	TG > TC	VLDL ± Chylo	?	++
Mixed hyperlipidaemia				
Polygenic (majority)	TC + TG	VLDL + LDL	Variable	+
Familial combined hyperlipidaemia*	TC and/or TG	LDL and/or VLDL	++	+
Dysbetalipoproteinaemia*	TC and/or TG	IDL	+++	+

+ = slightly increased risk; ++ = increased risk; +++ = greatly increased risk; ? = risk unclear

*Familial combined hyperlipidaemia and dysbetalipoproteinaemia may also present as predominant hypercholesterolaemia or predominant hypertriglyceridaemia.

(Apo B100 = apolipoprotein B100; CHD = coronary heart disease; Chylo = chylomicrons; HDL = high-density lipoprotein; IDL = intermediate-density lipoprotein; LDL = low-density lipoprotein; LDLR = low-density lipoprotein receptor; TC = total cholesterol; TG = triglycerides; VLDL = very low-density lipoprotein)

 14.27 Familial hypercholesterolaemia in adolescence

- **Statin treatment**: may be required from the age of about 10. It does not compromise normal growth and maturation.
- **Smoking**: patients should be strongly advised not to smoke.
- **Adherence to medication:** critically important to the success of treatment. Simple regimens should be used and education and support provided.

LDL-C (Box 14.26). Physical signs, such as corneal arcus and xanthelasma, may be found in this as well as other forms of lipid disturbance (p. 346). The risk of cardiovascular disease is proportional to the degree of LDL-C (or Apo B) elevation, but is modified by other major risk factors, including low HDL-C and high Lp(a).

Familial hypercholesterolaemia (FH) is a more severe disorder with a prevalence of at least 0.4% in most populations. It is usually caused by loss-of-function mutations affecting the *LDLR* gene, which results in an autosomal dominant pattern of inheritance. A similar syndrome can arise with loss-of-function mutations in the ligand-binding domain of Apo B100 or gain-of-function mutations in *PCSK9*, which promote LDLR degradation. Causative mutations can be detected in one of these three genes by genetic testing in about 70% of patients with FH. Most patients with these types of FH have LDL-C levels that are approximately twice as high as in normal subjects of the same age and gender. Affected patients suffer from severe hypercholesterolaemia and premature cardiovascular disease. FH may be accompanied by xanthomas of the Achilles or extensor digitorum tendons (p. 346), which are strongly suggestive of FH. The onset of corneal arcus before age 40 is also suggestive of this condition. Identification of an index case of FH (the first case of FH in a family) should trigger genetic and biochemical screening of other family members, which is a cost-effective method for case detection. Affected individuals should be managed from childhood (Box 14.27).

Homozygous FH may occur sporadically, especially in populations in which there is a 'founder' gene effect or consanguineous marriage. Homozygosity results in more extensive xanthomas and precocious cardiovascular disease, often in childhood. Hyperalphalipoproteinaemia refers to increased levels of HDL-C. In the absence of an increase in LDL-C, this condition rarely causes cardiovascular disease, but exceptions can occur so it should not be regarded as universally benign.

Familial combined hyperlipidaemia, and dysbetalipoproteinaemia, may present with the pattern of predominant hypercholesterolaemia (see 'Mixed hyperlipidaemia' below).

Hypertriglyceridaemia

Hypertriglyceridaemia also usually involves polygenic factors (see Box 14.26). Other common causes include excess alcohol intake, medications (such as β-blockers and retinoids), type 2 diabetes, impaired glucose tolerance, central obesity or other manifestations of insulin resistance (p. 728) and impaired absorption of bile acids. It is often accompanied by post-prandial hyperlipidaemia and reduced HDL-C, both of which may contribute to cardiovascular risk. Excessive intake of alcohol or dietary fat, or other exacerbating factors, may precipitate a massive increase in TG levels, which, if they exceed 10 mmol/L (880 mg/dL), may pose a risk of acute pancreatitis.

Monogenic forms of hypertriglyceridaemia also occur due to loss-of-function mutations in the genes encoding lipoprotein lipase, Apo C2 or *ANGPTL4*, which coordinate the lipolytic breakdown of TG-rich lipoproteins. These cause recessively inherited forms of severe hypertriglyceridaemia that is not readily amenable to drug treatment. They can present in childhood and may be associated with episodes of acute abdominal pain and pancreatitis. In common with other causes of severe hypertriglyceridaemia, hepatomegaly, lipaemia retinalis and eruptive xanthomas may occur (p. 346). Familial hypertriglyceridaemia may also be inherited in a dominant manner due to mutations in the *APOA5* gene, which encodes Apo A5 – a co-factor that is essential for lipoprotein lipase activity. These disorders may also be associated with increased risk of cardiovascular disease.

Familial combined hyperlipidaemia, and dysbetalipoproteinaemia, may present with the pattern of predominant hypertriglyceridaemia (see 'Mixed hyperlipidaemia', below).

Mixed hyperlipidaemia

It is difficult to define quantitatively the distinction between predominant hyperlipidaemias and mixed hyperlipidaemia. The term 'mixed' usually implies the presence of hypertriglyceridaemia, as well as an increase in LDL-C or IDL. Treatment of massive hypertriglyceridaemia may improve TG faster than cholesterol, thus temporarily mimicking mixed hyperlipidaemia.

Primary mixed hyperlipidaemia is usually polygenic and, like predominant hypertriglyceridaemia, often occurs in association with type 2 diabetes, impaired glucose tolerance, central obesity or other manifestations of insulin resistance (p. 728). Both components of mixed hyperlipidaemia may contribute to the risk of cardiovascular disease.

Familial combined hyperlipidaemia is a term used to identify an inherited tendency towards the over-production of atherogenic Apo B-containing lipoproteins. It results in elevation of cholesterol, TG or both in different family members at different times. It is associated with an increased risk of cardiovascular disease but it does not produce any pathognomonic physical signs. In practice, this relatively common condition is substantially modified by factors such as age and weight. It may not be a monogenic condition, but rather one end of a heterogeneous spectrum that overlaps insulin resistance.

Dysbetalipoproteinaemia (also referred to as type 3 hyperlipidaemia, broad-beta dyslipoproteinaemia or remnant hyperlipidaemia) involves accumulation of roughly equimolar levels of cholesterol and TG. It is caused by homozygous inheritance of the Apo E2 allele, which is the isoform least avidly recognised by the LDLR. In conjunction with other exacerbating factors, such as obesity or diabetes, it leads to accumulation of atherogenic IDL and chylomicron remnants. Premature cardiovascular disease is common, as is peripheral vascular disease. It may also result in the formation of palmar xanthomas, tuberous xanthomas or tendon xanthomas.

Rare dyslipidaemias

Several rare disturbances of lipid metabolism have been described (Box 14.28). They provide important insights into lipid metabolism and its impact on risk of cardiovascular disease.

14.28 Miscellaneous and rare forms of hyperlipidaemia

Condition	Lipoprotein pattern	CVD risk
Tangier disease	Very low HDL, low TC	+
Apo A1 deficiency	Very low HDL	++
Apo A1 Milano	Very low HDL	–
Fish eye disease	Very low HDL, high TG	–
LCAT deficiency	Very low HDL, high TG	?
Autosomal recessive FH	Very high LDL	++
Sitosterolaemia	High plant sterols including sitosterol	+
Cerebrotendinous xanthomatosis	Bile acid defect (cholestanol accumulation)	+

+ = slightly increased risk; ++ = increased risk.
(CVD = cardiovascular disease; FH = familial hypercholesterolaemia; HDL = high-density lipoprotein; LCAT = lecithin cholesterol acyl transferase; LDL = low-density lipoprotein; TC = total cholesterol; TG = triglycerides)

Fish eye disease, Apo A1 Milano and lecithin cholesterol acyl transferase (LCAT) deficiency demonstrate that very low HDL-C levels do not necessarily cause cardiovascular disease, but Apo A1 deficiency, and possibly Tangier disease, demonstrate that low HDL-C can be atherogenic under some circumstances. Autosomal recessive *FH* and *PCSK9* gain-of-function mutations reveal the importance of proteins that chaperone the LDLR. Sitosterolaemia and cerebrotendinous xanthomatosis demonstrate that sterols other than cholesterol can cause xanthomas and cardiovascular disease, while *PCSK9* loss-of-function mutations, abetalipoproteinaemia and hypobetalipoproteinaemia suggest that low levels of Apo B-containing lipoproteins reduce the risk of cardiovascular disease. The only adverse health outcomes associated with extremely low plasma lipid levels in the latter two conditions are attributable to fat-soluble vitamin deficiency, or impaired transport of lipid from intestine or liver.

Principles of management

Lipid-lowering therapies have a key role in the secondary and primary prevention of cardiovascular diseases (p. 487). Assessment of absolute risk of cardiovascular disease, treatment of all modifiable risk factors and optimisation of lifestyle, especially diet and exercise, are central to management in all cases. Patients with the greatest absolute risk of cardiovascular disease derive the greatest absolute benefit from treatment. Public health organisations recommend thresholds for the introduction of lipid-lowering therapy based on the identification of patients in very high-risk categories, or those calculated to be at high absolute risk according to algorithms or tables such as the Joint British Societies Coronary Risk Prediction Chart (see Fig. 16.77, p. 511). These tables, which are based on large epidemiological studies, should be recalibrated for the local population, if possible. In general, patients who have cardiovascular disease, diabetes mellitus, chronic renal impairment, familial hypercholesterolaemia or an absolute risk of cardiovascular disease of more than 20% in the ensuing 10 years are arbitrarily regarded as having sufficient risk to justify drug treatment. Age is such an overwhelming determinant of absolute cardiovascular risk that some recent recommendations consider 'lifetime' risk. This diminishes the pressure to treat very elderly patients and supports earlier intervention in non-elderly patients.

Public health organisations also recommend target levels for patients receiving drug treatment. High-risk patients should aim for HDL-C >1 mmol/L (38 mg/dL) and fasting TG <2 mmol/L (approximately 180 mg/dL), while target levels for LDL-C have been reduced to 1.8 mmol/L (76 mg/dL) or less. In general, total cholesterol should be <5 mmol/L (190 mg/dL) during treatment, and <4 mmol/L (approximately 150 mg/dL) in high-risk patients and in secondary prevention of cardiovascular disease. Recent trials have demonstrated continuous benefit of LDL-C reduction to a level of 1.4 mmol/L (54 mg/dL), so further reduction in treatment targets may be anticipated.

Non-pharmacological management

Patients with lipid abnormalities should receive medical advice and, if necessary, dietary counselling to:
• reduce intake of saturated and *trans*-unsaturated fat to less than 7–10% of total energy
• reduce intake of cholesterol to <250 mg/day
• replace sources of saturated fat and cholesterol with alternative foods, such as lean meat, low-fat dairy

14

products, polyunsaturated spreads and low-glycaemic-index carbohydrates
- reduce energy-dense foods such as fats and soft drinks, while increasing activity and exercise to maintain or lose weight
- increase consumption of cardioprotective and nutrient-dense foods, such as vegetables, unrefined carbohydrates, fish, pulses, nuts, legumes, and fruit
- adjust alcohol consumption, reducing intake if excessive or if associated with hypertension, hypertriglyceridaemia or central obesity
- achieve additional benefits with preferential intake of foods containing lipid-lowering nutrients such as n-3 fatty acids, dietary fibre and plant sterols.

The response to diet is usually apparent within 3–4 weeks but dietary adjustment may need to be introduced gradually. Although hyperlipidaemia in general, and hypertriglyceridaemia in particular, can be very responsive to these measures, LDL-C reductions are often only modest in routine clinical practice. Explanation, encouragement and persistence are often required to assist patient adherence. Even minor weight loss can substantially reduce cardiovascular risk, especially in centrally obese patients (p. 700).

All other modifiable cardiovascular risk factors should be assessed and treated. If possible, intercurrent drug treatments that adversely affect the lipid profile should be replaced.

Pharmacological management

The main diagnostic categories provide a useful framework for management and the selection of first-line pharmacological treatment (Fig. 14.14).

Hypercholesterolaemia

Hypercholesterolaemia can be treated with one or more of the cholesterol-lowering drugs as described below.

Statins

These reduce cholesterol synthesis by inhibiting the HMGCoA reductase enzyme. The reduction in cholesterol synthesis up-regulates production of the LDLR, which increases clearance of LDL and its precursor, IDL, resulting in a secondary reduction in LDL synthesis. Statins reduce LDL-C by up to 60%, reduce TG by up to 40% and increase HDL-C by up to 10%. They also reduce the concentration of intermediate metabolites such as isoprenes, which may lead to other effects such as suppression of the inflammatory response. There is clear evidence of protection against total and coronary mortality, stroke and cardiovascular events across the spectrum of cardiovascular disease risk.

Statins are generally well tolerated and serious side-effects are rare (well below 2%). Liver function test abnormalities and muscle problems, such as myalgia, asymptomatic increase in creatine kinase (CK), myositis and, infrequently, rhabdomyolysis, are the most common. Side-effects are more likely in patients who are elderly, debilitated or receiving other drugs that interfere with statin degradation, which usually involves cytochrome P450 3A4 or glucuronidation.

Ezetimibe

Ezetimibe inhibits activity of the intestinal mucosal transporter NPC1L1, which is responsible for absorption of dietary and biliary cholesterol. The resulting depletion of hepatic cholesterol up-regulates hepatic LDLR production. This mechanism of action is synergistic with the effect of statins. Monotherapy in a 10 mg/day dose reduces LDL-C by 15–20%. Slightly greater (17–25%) incremental LDL-C reduction occurs when ezetimibe is added to statins. Ezetimibe is well tolerated, and evidence of a beneficial effect on cardiovascular disease endpoints is now available. Plant sterol-supplemented foods, which also reduce cholesterol absorption, lower LDL-C by 7–15%.

Bile acid-sequestering resins

Drugs in this class include colestyramine, colestipol and colesevelam. These prevent the reabsorption of bile acids, thereby increasing de novo bile acid synthesis from hepatic cholesterol. As with ezetimibe, the resultant depletion of hepatic cholesterol up-regulates LDL receptor activity and reduces LDL-C in a manner that is synergistic with the action of statins. Resins reduce LDL-C and modestly increase HDL-C, but may increase TG. They are safe but may interfere with bioavailability of other drugs. Colesevelam has fewer gastrointestinal effects than older

Fig. 14.14 **Flow chart for the drug treatment of hyperlipidaemia.** *Interrupt treatment if creatine kinase is more than 5–10 times the upper limit of normal, or if elevated with muscle symptoms, or if alanine aminotransferase is more than 2–3 times the upper limit. To convert triglyceride (TG) in mmol/L to mg/dL, multiply by 88. To convert low-density lipoprotein (LDL)-C in mmol/L to mg/dL, multiply by 38.

preparations that are less well tolerated. The depletion of bile acids is sensed via the farnesyl X receptor and the response may also improve glucose metabolism.

PCSK9 inhibitors

Monoclonal antibodies have been developed that neutralise PCSK9, an enzyme that degrades the LDLR. This causes levels of LDLR to increase, which markedly reduces LDL-C. The PCSK9 inhibitors currently available are evolocumab and alirocumab, which are administered by subcutaneous injection every 2–4 weeks. These drugs are well tolerated and highly effective. Reductions in LDL-C of about 50–60% have been observed in patients who have not responded adequately to standard lipid-lowering therapy and this has been accompanied by a reduction in the risk of cardiovascular events of about 15%. The PCSK9 inhibitors do not deplete intracellular concentrations and, because of that, do not trigger compensatory mechanisms that blunt the effect of other cholesterol-lowering medications.

Nicotinic acid

Pharmacological doses reduce peripheral fatty acid release, with the result that VLDL and LDL decline while HDL-C increases. Recent randomised clinical trials have been disappointing regarding effects on atherosclerosis and cardiovascular events. The same may be said of novel agents that inhibit cholesterol ester transfer protein. Neither of these HDL-C-raising drugs is indicated in current lipid management.

Combination therapy

In many patients, treatment of predominant hypercholesterolaemia can be achieved by diet plus the use of a statin in sufficient doses to achieve target LDL-C levels. Patients who do not reach LDL targets on the highest tolerated statin dose, or who are intolerant of statins, may receive ezetimibe, plant sterols, or resins. Ezetimibe and resins are safe and effective in combination with a statin because the mechanisms of action of individual therapies complement each other while blunting each other's compensatory mechanisms.

Hypertriglyceridaemia

Predominant hypertriglyceridaemia can be treated with one of the TG-lowering drugs described below (see Fig. 14.14).

Fibrates

These stimulate peroxisome proliferator-activated receptor (PPAR) alpha, which controls the expression of gene products that mediate the metabolism of TG and HDL. As a result, synthesis of fatty acids, TG and VLDL is reduced, while that of lipoprotein lipase, which catabolises TG, is enhanced. In addition, production of Apo A1 and ABC A1 is up-regulated, leading to increased reverse cholesterol transport via HDL. Consequently, fibrates reduce TG by up to 50% and increase HDL-C by up to 20%, but LDL-C changes are variable.

Fewer large-scale trials have been conducted with fibrates than with statins. The results are less conclusive, but reduced rates of cardiovascular disease have been reported with fibrate therapy in the subgroup of patients with low HDL-C levels and elevated TG (TG >2.3 mmol/L (200 mg/dL)). Fibrates are usually well tolerated but share a similar side-effect profile to statins. In addition, they may increase the risk of cholelithiasis and prolong the action of anticoagulants. Accumulating evidence suggests that they may also have a protective effect against diabetic microvascular complications.

Highly polyunsaturated long-chain n-3 fatty acids

These include eicosapentaenoic acid (EPA) and docosahexaenoic acid (DHA), which comprise approximately 30% of the fatty acids in fish oil. EPA and DHA are potent inhibitors of VLDL TG formation. Intakes of more than 2 g n-3 fatty acid (equivalent to 6 g of most forms of fish oil) per day lower TG in a dose-dependent fashion. Up to 50% reduction in TG may be achieved with 15 g fish oil per day. Changes in HDL-C are variable but fish oils do not routinely reduce LDL-C. Fish oil fatty acids have also been shown to inhibit platelet aggregation and improve cardiac arrhythmia in animal models. Dietary and pharmacological trials suggested that n-3 fatty acids may reduce mortality from coronary heart disease, but the benefit of fish oil supplements has been less conclusive in recent trials. Fish oils appear to be safe and well tolerated but dietary fish consumption is the preferred source.

Patients with predominant hypertriglyceridaemia who do not respond to lifestyle intervention can be treated with fibrates or fish oil, depending on individual response and tolerance. If target levels are not achieved, the fibrates, fish oil and possibly nicotinic acid can be combined. Massive hypertriglyceridaemia may require more aggressive limitation of dietary fat intake (< 10–20% energy as fat). Any degree of insulin deficiency should be corrected because insulin is required for optimal activity of lipoprotein lipase. The initial target for patients with massive hypertriglyceridaemia is TG < 10 mmol/L (880 mg/dL), to reduce the risk of acute pancreatitis.

Mixed hyperlipidaemia

Mixed hyperlipidaemia can be difficult to treat. First-line therapy with statins alone is unlikely to achieve target levels once fasting TGs exceed approximately 4 mmol/L (350 mg/dL). Fibrates

14.29 Management of hyperlipidaemia in old age

- **Prevalence of atherosclerotic cardiovascular disease**: greatest in old age.
- **Associated cardiovascular risk**: lipid levels become less predictive, as do other risk factors apart from age itself.
- **Benefit of statin therapy**: maintained up to the age of 80 years but evidence is lacking beyond this.
- **Life expectancy and statin therapy**: lives saved by intervention are associated with shorter life expectancy than in younger patients, and so the impact of statins on quality-adjusted life years is smaller in old age.

14.30 Dyslipidaemia in pregnancy

- **Lipid metabolism**: lipid and lipoprotein levels increase during pregnancy. This includes an increase in low-density lipoprotein cholesterol, which resolves post-partum. Remnant dyslipidaemia and hypertriglyceridaemia may be exacerbated during pregnancy.
- **Treatment**: dyslipidaemia is rarely thought to warrant urgent treatment so pharmacological therapy is usually contraindicated when conception or pregnancy is anticipated. Teratogenicity has been reported with systemically absorbed agents, and non-absorbed agents may interfere with nutrient bioavailability.
- **Monitoring**: while still uncommon among women of child-bearing age, cardiovascular disease is increasing in prevalence. Pre-conception cardiovascular review should be considered for women at high risk to optimise medications for pregnancy and to ensure that the patient will be able to withstand the demands of pregnancy and labour.

14

are first-line therapy for dysbetalipoproteinaemia, but they may not control the cholesterol component in other forms of mixed hyperlipidaemia. Combination therapy is often required. Effective combinations include:

- statin plus fenofibrate (recognising that the risk of myopathy is increased with gemfibrozil, but fenofibrate is relatively safe in this regard)
- statin plus fish oil when TG is not too high
- fibrate plus ezetimibe when cholesterol is not too high.

Monitoring of therapy

The effects of lipid-lowering therapy should be assessed after 6 weeks (12 weeks for fibrates). At this point, it is prudent to review side-effects, lipid response (see target levels above), CK and liver function tests. During longer-term follow-up, adherence to treatment, diet and exercise should be assessed, with monitoring of weight, blood pressure and lipid levels. The presence of cardiovascular symptoms or signs should be noted and absolute cardiovascular risk assessed periodically. Effective statin therapy may be associated with a paradoxical and as yet unexplained increase in coronary calcium score.

It is not necessary to perform routine checks of CK and liver function unless symptoms occur, or if statins are used in combination with fibrates, or other drugs that may interfere with their clearance. If myalgia or weakness occurs in association with CK elevation over 5–10 times the upper limit of normal, or if sustained alanine aminotransferase (ALT) elevation more than 2–3 times the upper limit of normal occurs that is not accounted for by fatty liver (p. 882), treatment should be discontinued and alternative therapy sought.

The principles of the management of dyslipidaemia can be applied broadly, but the objectives of treatment in the elderly (Box 14.29) and the safety of pharmacological therapy in pregnancy (Box 14.30) warrant special consideration.

The porphyrias

This group of disorders is caused by inherited abnormalities in the haem biosynthetic pathway (Fig. 14.15). Most of the described forms are due to partial enzyme deficiencies with a dominant mode of inheritance. They are commonly classified as hepatic or erythropoietic, depending on whether the major site of excess porphyrin production is in the liver or red cell.

The porphyrias have a penetrance in the order of 25%, emphasising the importance of environmental factors in disease expression. In porphyria cutanea tarda (PCT), which is the most

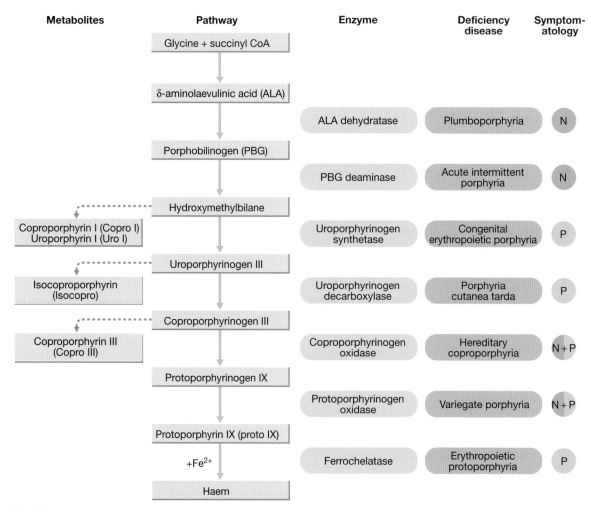

Fig. 14.15 Haem biosynthetic pathway and enzyme defects responsible for the porphyrias. (ALA = δ-aminolaevulinic acid; CoA = co-enzyme A; N = neurovisceral; P = photosensitive; PBG = porphobilinogen)

| i | 14.31 Diagnostic biochemical findings in the porphyrias[1] | | | |

| Condition | Elevated porphyrins and precursors | | |
	Blood	Urine	Faeces
ALA dehydratase deficiency (plumboporphyria)	Proto IX[2]	ALA, Copro III[2]	
Acute intermittent porphyria (AIP)		ALA, PBG	
Congenital erythropoietic porphyria (CEP)	Uro I	Uro I	Copro I
Porphyria cutanea tarda (PCT)		Uro I	Isocopro
Hereditary coproporphyria (HCP)		ALA, PBG, Copro III	Copro III
Variegate porphyria (VP)		ALA, PBG, Copro III	Proto IX
Erythropoietic protoporphyria (EPP)	Proto IX		Proto IX

[1]Refer to Figure 14.15 for metabolic pathways. [2]The paradoxical rise in coproporphyrin III (Copro III) and protoporphyrin (Proto) in this very rare condition is poorly understood. (ALA = δ-aminolaevulinic acid; Isocopro = isocoproporphyrin; PBG = porphobilinogen; Uro = uroporphyrin)

common cause of porphyria, environmental triggers include alcohol, iron accumulation, exogenous oestrogens and exposure to various chemicals. Many cases are associated with hepatitis C infection and this should always be screened for on presentation.

Clinical features

The clinical features of porphyria fall into two broad categories: photosensitivity and acute neurovisceral syndrome. The enzyme defects responsible for the diseases are shown in Figure 14.15.

Photosensitive skin manifestations, attributable to excess production and accumulation of porphyrins in the skin, cause pain, erythema, bullae, skin erosions, hirsutism and hyperpigmentation, and occur predominantly on areas of the skin that are exposed to sunlight (p. 1220). The skin also becomes sensitised to damage from minimal trauma.

The other pattern of presentation is with an acute neurological syndrome. This almost always presents with acute abdominal pain together with features of autonomic dysfunction, such as tachycardia, hypertension and constipation. Neuropsychiatric manifestations, hyponatraemia due to inappropriate ADH release (p. 357), and an acute neuropathy may also occur (p. 1138). The neuropathy is predominantly motor and may, in severe cases, progress to respiratory failure.

There is no proven explanation for the episodic nature of the attacks in porphyria, which can relapse and remit or follow a prolonged and unremitting course. Sometimes, specific triggers can be identified, such as alcohol, fasting, or drugs such as anticonvulsants, sulphonamides, oestrogen and progesterone. The oral contraceptive pill is a common precipitating factor. In a significant number, no precipitant can be identified.

Investigations

The diagnosis of porphyria and classification into the various forms have traditionally relied on measurements of porphyrins and porphyrin precursors found in blood, urine and faeces (Box 14.31). The diagnosis is straightforward when the metabolites are significantly elevated, but this is not always the case in asymptomatic individuals who may have normal porphyrin studies.

More recently, measurement of the enzymes that are deficient in the various porphyrias has provided further diagnostic information. An example is measurement of porphobilinogen deaminase activity in red blood cells to diagnose acute intermittent porphyria. There is often considerable overlap between enzyme activities in affected and normal subjects, however. Furthermore, some of the enzymes occur in the mitochondria, for which it is more

difficult to obtain suitable specimens for analysis. All the genes of the haem biosynthetic pathway have now been characterised. This has made it possible to identify affected individuals in families by genetic testing, a significant advance considering that penetrance of porphyria is low.

Metabolite excretory patterns are always grossly abnormal during an acute attack or with cutaneous manifestations of porphyria, and are diagnostic of the particular porphyria. A normal metabolite profile under these circumstances effectively excludes porphyria. Metabolites usually remain abnormal for long periods after an acute attack, and in some individuals never return to normal. The diagnosis is not so straightforward in patients who are in remission, or in asymptomatic individuals with a positive family history. Neurological porphyria rarely manifests before puberty, nor can it be readily diagnosed after the menopause as porphyrin excretion may be normal. Genetic testing for disease-specific mutations can clarify the situation.

Management

For patients predisposed to neurovisceral attacks, general management includes avoidance of any agents known to precipitate acute porphyria. Specific management includes intravenous glucose, as provision of 5000 kilojoules per day can, in some cases, terminate acute attacks through a reduction in δ-aminolaevulinic acid (ALA) synthetase activity, leading to reduced ALA and porphyrin synthesis. More recently, administration of haem (in various forms such as haematin or haem arginate) has been shown to reduce metabolite excretory rates, relieve pain and accelerate recovery. Cyclical acute attacks in women sometimes respond to suppression of the menstrual cycle using gonadotrophin-releasing hormone analogues. In rare cases with frequent prolonged attacks or attacks intractable to treatment, liver transplantation has been effective.

There are few specific or effective measures to treat the photosensitive manifestations. The primary goal is to avoid sun exposure and skin trauma. Barrier sun creams containing zinc or titanium oxide are the most effective products. New colourless creams containing nanoparticle formulations have improved patient acceptance. Beta-carotene is used in some patients with erythropoietic porphyria with some efficacy. Afamelanotide, a synthetic analogue of alpha-melanocyte stimulating hormone (α-MSH), has also been shown to provide protection in erythropoietic protoporphyria, and is now undergoing approval in many countries. In porphyria cutanea tarda, a course of venesections to remove iron can result in long-lasting clinical and biochemical remission,

14

especially if exposure to identified precipitants, such as alcohol or oestrogens, is reduced. Alternatively, a prolonged course of low-dose chloroquine therapy is effective.

Further information

Journal articles

Spasovski G, Vanholder R, Allolio B, et al. Clinical practice guideline on diagnosis and treatment of hyponatraemia. Eur J Endocrinol 2014; 170:G1–G47.

Walsh S, Unwin R. Renal tubular disorders. Clin Med 2012; 12(5):476–479.

Websites

emedicine.medscape.com *The Nephrology link on this site contains a useful compendium of articles.*

lipidsonline.org *Summarises management strategies for dyslipidaemia.*

ncbi.nlm.nih.gov *The link to OMIM (Online Mendelian Inheritance in Man) provides updated information on the genetic basis of metabolic disorders.*

porphyria-europe.com and drugs-porphyria.org *Excellent resources on drug safety in porphyria.*

B Conway
PJ Phelan
GD Stewart

15

Nephrology and urology

Clinical examination of the kidney and urinary tract 382

Functional anatomy and physiology 384

Investigation of renal and urinary tract disease 386
Glomerular filtration rate 386
Urine investigations 387
Blood tests 388
Imaging 389
Renal biopsy 391

Presenting problems in renal and urinary tract disease 391
Oliguria/anuria 391
Haematuria 391
Proteinuria 392
Oedema 395
Hypertension 396
Loin pain 396
Dysuria 396
Frequency 396
Polyuria 396
Nocturia 397
Urinary incontinence 397

Glomerular diseases 397
Glomerulonephritis 397

Tubulo-interstitial diseases 401

Genetic renal diseases 403
Inherited glomerular diseases 403
Inherited tubulo-interstitial diseases 404
Isolated defects of tubular function 405
Cystic diseases of the kidney 405

Renal vascular diseases 406
Renal artery stenosis 406
Acute renal infarction 408
Diseases of small intrarenal vessels 408

Renal involvement in systemic conditions 409

Acute kidney injury 411

Chronic kidney disease 415

Renal replacement therapy 420
Conservative treatment 421
Haemodialysis 421
Haemofiltration 423
Haemodiafiltration 423
Peritoneal dialysis 424
Renal transplantation 424

Renal disease in pregnancy 426

Renal disease in adolescence 426

Drugs and the kidney 426
Drug-induced renal disease 426
Prescribing in renal disease 426

Infections of the urinary tract 426

Urolithiasis 431

Diseases of the collecting system and ureters 433
Congenital abnormalities 433
Retroperitoneal fibrosis 434

Tumours of the kidney and urinary tract 434

Urinary incontinence 436

Prostate disease 437

Testicular tumours 439

Erectile dysfunction 440

Clinical examination of the kidney and urinary tract

Many diseases of the kidney and urinary tract are clinically silent, at least in the early stages. Accordingly, it is common for these conditions to be detected first by routine blood tests or on dipstick testing of the urine. Several important abnormalities can also be picked up on physical examination, however, and these are summarised below.

5 Fundoscopy

▲ Hypertensive changes

4 Jugular venous pressure

Elevated in fluid overload

3 Blood pressure

Often elevated

2 Skin

Yellow complexion*
Bruising*
Excoriation of pruritus*
Reduced skin turgor in fluid depletion

1 Hands

▲ Splinter haemorrhages

▲ 'Brown line' pigmentation of nails

6 Lungs

Crepitations in fluid overload

Observation

- Tiredness
- Respiratory rate and depth increased in metabolic acidosis
- Pallor*

*Features of advanced chronic kidney disease (see also Fig. 15.22)

7 Heart

Extra heart sounds in fluid overload
Pericardial friction rub*

8 Abdomen

Renal mass
Local tenderness
Renal or other arterial bruits in renal vascular disease
Rectal examination — prostate

9 Genitalia

Scrotal swellings

▲ Phimosis

10 Sacral oedema

11 Ankle oedema

12 Peripheral neuropathy*

13 Urinalysis for blood and protein

14 Urine microscopy

See Fig. 15.3

Blood pressure measurements

Blood tests for abnormal creatinine and electrolytes

Urinalysis for protein, blood, nitrites and leucocytes

Abdominal examination for palpable kidneys

Percussing for tenderness in renal angle

Digital rectal examination for prostate enlargement

Checking sacrum and ankles for pitting oedema

Clinical examination techniques to evaluate urological and renal abnormalities. *Inset (Dipstick): From Pitkin J, Peattie AB, Magowan BA. Obstetrics and gynaecology: An lilustrated colour text. Edinburgh: Churchill Livingstone, Elsevier Ltd; 2003.*

15

Male lower urinary tract demonstrating the relationship of the bladder, urethra, vas deferens and testes.

This chapter describes the disorders of the kidneys and urinary tract that are commonly encountered in routine practice, as well as giving an overview of the highly specialised field of renal replacement therapy. Disorders of renal tubular function, which may cause alterations in electrolyte and acid–base balance, are described in Chapter 14.

Functional anatomy and physiology

The kidneys

The kidneys play a central role in excretion of many metabolic breakdown products, including ammonia and urea from protein, creatinine from muscle, uric acid from nucleic acids, drugs and toxins. They achieve this by making large volumes of an ultrafiltrate of plasma (120 mL/min, 170 L/24 hrs) at the glomerulus, and selectively reabsorbing components of this ultrafiltrate at points along the nephron. The rates of filtration and reabsorption are controlled by many hormonal and haemodynamic signals to regulate fluid and electrolyte balance (p. 349), blood pressure (p. 447), and acid–base (p. 363) and calcium–phosphate homeostasis (pp. 367 and 368). In addition, the kidneys activate vitamin D and control the synthesis of red blood cells by producing erythropoietin. Strategies to replace each of these important functions are required when managing patients with kidney failure.

Each kidney is approximately 11–14 cm in length in healthy adults; they are located retroperitoneally on either side of the aorta and inferior vena cava between the 12th thoracic and 3rd lumbar vertebrae (Fig. 15.1A). The right kidney is usually a few centimetres lower because the liver lies above it. Both kidneys rise and descend several centimetres with respiration.

The kidneys have a rich blood supply and receive approximately 20–25% of cardiac output through the renal arteries, which arise from the abdominal aorta. The renal arteries undergo various subdivisions within the kidney, eventually forming interlobular arteries that run through the renal cortex. These eventually give rise to afferent glomerular arterioles that supply the glomeruli. The efferent arteriole, leading from the glomerulus, supplies the distal nephron and medulla in a 'portal' circulation (Fig. 15.1B). This highly unusual arrangement of two serial capillary beds reflects the role of the afferent and efferent arterioles in autoregulation of glomerular filtration.

The nephron

Each kidney contains approximately 1 million individual functional units, called nephrons. Each nephron consists of a glomerulus, which is responsible for ultrafiltration of blood, a proximal renal tubule, a loop of Henle, a distal renal tubule and a collecting duct, which together are responsible for selective reabsorption of water and electrolytes that have been filtered at the glomerulus (see Fig. 14.2, p. 350, and Fig. 15.1B). Under normal circumstances, more than 99% of the 170 L of glomerular filtrate that is produced each day is reabsorbed in the tubules. The remainder passes through the collecting ducts of multiple nephrons and drains into the renal pelvis and ureters.

The glomerulus

The glomerulus comprises a tightly packed loop of capillaries supplied by an afferent arteriole and drained by an efferent arteriole. It is surrounded by a cup-shaped extension of the proximal tubule termed Bowman's capsule, which is composed of epithelial cells. The glomerular capillary endothelial cells contain pores (fenestrae), through which circulating molecules can pass to reach the underlying glomerular basement membrane (GBM), which is formed by fusion of the basement membranes of tubular epithelial and vascular endothelial cells (Fig. 15.1C and D). Glomerular epithelial cells (podocytes) have multiple long foot processes that interdigitate with those of the adjacent epithelial cells, thereby maintaining a selective barrier to filtration (Fig. 15.1E). Mesangial cells lie in the central region of the glomerulus. They have contractile properties similar to those of vascular smooth muscle cells and play a role in regulating glomerular filtration rate.

Under normal circumstances, the glomerulus is impermeable to proteins the size of albumin (67 kDa) or larger, while proteins of 20 kDa or smaller are filtered freely. The ability of molecules between 20 and 67 kDa to pass through the GBM is variable and depends on the size (smaller molecules are filtered more easily) and charge (positively charged molecules are filtered more easily). Very little lipid is filtered by the glomerulus.

Filtration pressure at the glomerulus is normally maintained at a constant level, in the face of wide variations in systemic blood pressure and cardiac output, by alterations in muscle tone within the afferent and efferent arterioles and mesangial cells. This is known as autoregulation. Reduced renal perfusion pressure increases local production of prostaglandins that mediate vasodilatation of the afferent arteriole, thereby increasing the intraglomerular pressure (Fig. 15.1D). In addition, renin is released by specialised smooth muscle cells in the juxtaglomerular apparatus in response to reduced perfusion pressure, stimulation of sympathetic nerves or low sodium concentration of fluid in the distal convoluted tubule at the macula densa. Renin cleaves angiotensinogen to release angiotensin I, which is further cleaved by angiotensin-converting enzyme (ACE) to produce angiotensin II. This restores glomerular perfusion pressure in the short term by causing vasoconstriction of the efferent arterioles within the kidney to raise intraglomerular pressure selectively (Fig. 15.1D), and by inducing systemic vasoconstriction to increase blood pressure and thus renal perfusion pressure. In the longer term, angiotensin II increases plasma volume by stimulating aldosterone release, which enhances sodium reabsorption by the renal tubules (see Fig. 18.18, p. 666). Consumption of non-steroidal anti-inflammatory preparations and renin–angiotensin system inhibitors in the context of volume depletion may impair the ability of the kidney to maintain glomerular filtration and exacerbate pre-renal failure (see Fig. 15.19, p. 413).

Renal tubules, loop of Henle and collecting ducts

The proximal renal tubule, loop of Henle, distal renal tubule and collecting ducts are responsible for reabsorption of water, electrolytes and other solutes, as well as regulating acid–base balance, as described in detail on page 350 and in Figure 14.3. They also play a key role in regulating calcium homeostasis by converting 25-hydroxyvitamin D to the active metabolite 1,25-dihydroxyvitamin D (p. 1049). Failure of this process contributes to the pathogenesis of hypocalcaemia and bone disease that occurs in chronic kidney disease (CKD, p. 415). Fibroblast-like cells that lie in the interstitium of the renal cortex are responsible for production of erythropoietin, which in turn is required for production of red blood cells. Erythropoietin synthesis is regulated by oxygen tension; anaemia and hypoxia increase production, whereas polycythaemia and hyperoxia inhibit it.

15

Fig. 15.1 Functional anatomy of the kidney. [A] Anatomical relationships of the kidney. [B] A single nephron. For the functions of different segments, see Figures 14.2 and 14.3 (pp. 350 and 351). [C] Histology of a normal glomerulus. [D] Schematic cross-section of a glomerulus, showing five capillary loops, to illustrate structure and show cell types. [E] Electron micrograph of the filtration barrier. (GBM = glomerular basement membrane) *(C) Courtesy of Dr J.G. Simpson, Aberdeen Royal Infirmary.*

Failure of erythropoietin production plays an important role in the pathogenesis of anaemia in CKD.

The ureters and bladder

The ureters drain urine from the renal pelvis (Fig. 15.1A) and deliver it to the bladder, a muscular organ that lies anteriorly in the lower part of the pelvis, just behind the pubic bone. The function of the bladder is to store and then release urine during micturition. The bladder is richly innervated. Sympathetic nerves arising from T10–L2 relay in the pelvic ganglia to cause relaxation of the detrusor muscle and contraction of the bladder neck (both via α-adrenoceptors), thereby preventing release of urine from the bladder. The distal sphincter mechanism is innervated by somatic motor fibres from sacral segments S2–4, which reach the sphincter either by the pelvic plexus or via the pudendal nerves. Afferent sensory impulses pass to the cerebral cortex, from where reflex-increased sphincter tone and suppression of detrusor contraction inhibit micturition until it is appropriate. Conversely, parasympathetic nerves arising from S2–4 stimulate detrusor contraction, promoting micturition.

The micturition cycle has a storage (filling) phase and a voiding (micturition) phase. During the filling phase, the high compliance of the detrusor muscle allows the bladder to fill steadily without a rise in intravesical pressure. As bladder volume increases, stretch receptors in its wall cause reflex bladder relaxation and increased sphincter tone. The act of micturition is initiated first by voluntary and then by reflex relaxation of the pelvic floor and distal sphincter mechanism, followed by reflex detrusor contraction. These actions are coordinated by the pontine micturition centre. Intravesical pressure remains greater than urethral pressure until the bladder is empty.

The prostate gland

The prostate gland is situated at the base of the bladder, surrounding the proximal urethra (p. 383). Exocrine glands within the prostate produce fluid, which comprises about 20% of the volume of ejaculated seminal fluid and is rich in zinc and proteolytic enzymes. The remainder of the ejaculate is formed in the seminal vesicles and bulbo-urethral glands, with spermatozoa arising from the testes.

Smooth muscle fibres within the prostate, which are under sympathetic control, play a role in controlling urine flow through the bulbar urethra, and also contract at orgasm to move seminal fluid through ejaculatory ducts into the bulbar urethra (emission). Contraction of the bulbocavernosus muscle (via a spinal muscle reflex) then ejaculates the semen out of the urethra.

The penis

Blood flow into the corpus cavernosum of the penis is controlled by sympathetic nerves from the thoracolumbar plexus, which maintain smooth muscle contraction (p. 383). In response to afferent input from the glans penis and from higher centres, pelvic splanchnic parasympathetic nerves actively relax the cavernosal smooth muscle via neurotransmitters such as nitric oxide, acetylcholine, vasoactive intestinal polypeptide (VIP) and prostacyclin, with consequent dilatation of the lacunar space. At the same time, draining venules are compressed, trapping blood in the lacunar space with consequent elevation of pressure and erection (tumescence) of the penis.

Investigation of renal and urinary tract disease

Glomerular filtration rate

The glomerular filtration rate (GFR) is the sum of the ultrafiltration rates from plasma into the Bowman's space in each nephron and is a measure of renal excretory function. It is proportionate to body size and the reference value is usually expressed after correction for body surface area as 120±25 mL/min/1.73 m². The GFR may be measured directly by injecting and measuring the clearance of compounds such as inulin or radiolabelled ethylenediamine-tetra-acetic acid (EDTA), which are completely filtered at the glomerulus and are not secreted or reabsorbed by the renal tubules (Box 15.1). This is not performed routinely, however, and is usually reserved for special circumstances, such as the assessment of renal function in potential live kidney donors. Instead, GFR is usually assessed indirectly in clinical

---

 15.1 How to estimate glomerular filtration rate (GFR)

Measuring GFR

- Direct measurement using labelled ethylenediamine-tetra-acetic acid (EDTA) or inulin
- Creatinine clearance (CrCl):
  Minor tubular secretion of creatinine causes CrCl to exaggerate GFR when renal function is poor; can be affected by drugs (e.g. trimethoprim, cimetidine)
  Needs 24-hr urine collection (inconvenient and often unreliable)

$$CrCl\,(mL/min) = \frac{urine\ creatinine\ concentration\ (\mu mol/L) \times volume\ (mL)}{plasma\ creatinine\ concentration\ (\mu mol/L) \times time\ (min)}$$

Estimating GFR with equations

- The Modification of Diet in Renal Disease (MDRD) study equation (see www.renal.org/eGFR):
  Requires knowledge of age and sex only; it can therefore be reported automatically by laboratories
  For limitations, see Box 15.2

$$eGFR = 175^* \times (creatinine\ in\ \mu mol/L/88.4)^{-1.154} \times (age\ in\ yrs)^{-0.203} \times (0.742\ if\ female) \times (1.21\ if\ black)$$

- The Chronic Kidney Disease Epidemiology Collaboration (CKD-EPI) equation:
  More accurately estimates the actual GFR than the MDRD eGFR in those with relatively preserved renal function

$$eGFR = 141 \times min\,(SCr/\kappa,\ 1)^{\alpha} \times max\,(SCr/\kappa,\ 1)^{-1.209} \times 0.993^{Age} \times 1.018\ (if\ female) \times 1.159\ (if\ black)$$

  Where SCr = serum creatinine in μmol/L
  κ=61.9 if female and 79.6 if male
  α=−0.329 if female and −0.411 if male
  min = whichever is the minimum of serum creatinine/κ or 1
  max = whichever is the maximum of serum creatinine/κ or 1
- No equations perform well in unusual circumstances, such as extremes of body (and muscle) mass or in acutely unwell patients (see Box 15.2)

*A correction factor of 175 is used for isotope dilution mass spectrometry traceable creatinine measurements. To convert creatinine in mg/dL to μmol/L, multiply by 88.4.

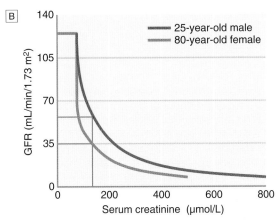

Fig. 15.2 Serum creatinine and the glomerular filtration rate (GFR).
A The relationship between serum creatinine and estimated GFR (eGFR) is non-linear; small increases above the normal range (e.g. 80–100 μmol/L; green lines) can therefore indicate a substantial decline in renal function (e.g. 105–80 mL/min/1.73 m²; conversely, in the high range, large changes in creatinine (e.g. 400–600 μmol/L; blue lines) can occur with only small declines in renal function (e.g. 20–15 mL/min/1.73m²). **B** Creatinine is dependent on muscle mass; the same creatinine value may therefore reflect very different levels of renal function depending on the age and sex of the individual. To convert creatinine in mg/dL to μmol/L, multiply by 88.4.

practice by measuring serum levels of endogenously produced compounds that are excreted by the kidney. The most widely used is serum creatinine, which is produced by muscle at a constant rate, is almost completely filtered at the glomerulus, and is not reabsorbed. Although creatinine is secreted to a small degree by the proximal tubule, this is only usually significant in terms of GFR estimation in severe renal impairment, where it accounts for a larger proportion of the creatinine excreted. Accordingly, provided muscle mass remains constant, changes in serum creatinine concentrations closely reflect changes in GFR. The relationship between serum creatinine and GFR is not linear, however, and a modest elevation in serum creatinine above the normal range may therefore reflect a substantial decline in GFR (Fig. 15.2). For this reason, several methods have been developed to estimate GFR from serum creatinine measurements (see Box 15.1) but the most widely used is the Modification of Diet in Renal Disease (MDRD) equation. Routine reporting by laboratories of estimated GFR (eGFR) has increased recognition of moderate kidney damage and encouraged early deployment

of protective therapies; however, some limitations remain (Boxes 15.2 and 15.3). In particular, the MDRD formula is based on the serum creatinine value and so is heavily influenced by muscle mass; eGFR may therefore be misleading in individuals whose muscle bulk is outside the normal range for their sex and age. Measurement of other endogenous metabolites, such as cystatin C, may provide a more accurate estimate of GFR in this setting; this test, however, is not yet widely available in routine clinical practice.

Direct measurement of creatinine clearance by collecting a 24-hour urine sample and relating serum creatinine levels to urinary creatinine excretion (see Box 15.1) is now less commonly performed due to the difficulty in obtaining accurate 24-hour urine collections. It may still have a role in assessing renal function in patients at extremes of muscle mass, where the creatinine-based equations perform poorly.

Urine investigations

Screening for the presence of blood (p. 391), protein (p. 392), glucose, ketones, nitrates and leucocytes, and assessment of urinary pH and osmolality can be achieved by dipstick testing. The presence of leucocytes and nitrites in urine is indicative of renal tract infection. Urine pH can provide diagnostic information in the assessment of renal tubular acidosis (p. 365).

Urine microscopy (Fig. 15.3) may detect dysmorphic erythrocytes, which suggest the presence of nephritis or red cell casts, indicative of glomerular disease. White cell casts are strongly suggestive of pyelonephritis. Microscopy may also detect the presence of bacteria in those with urinary infection and crystals in patients with renal stone disease. It should be noted that calcium oxalate and urate crystals can sometimes be found in normal urine that has been left to stand, due to crystal formation ex vivo.

15

i | 15.3 Stages of chronic kidney disease (CKD)

Stage[1]	Definition[2]	Description	Prevalence[4]	Clinical presentation[5]
1	Kidney damage[3] with normal or high GFR (>90)	Normal function	3.5%	Asymptomatic
2	Kidney damage and GFR 60 89	Mild CKD	3.9%	Asymptomatic
3A 3B	GFR 45–59 GFR 30–44	Mild to moderate CKD Moderate to severe CKD	7.6% (3A and 3B combined)	Usually asymptomatic Anaemia in some patients at 3B Most are non-progressive or progress very slowly
4	GFR 15–29	Severe CKD	0.4%	First symptoms often at GFR <20 Electrolyte problems likely as GFR falls
5	GFR <15 or on dialysis	Kidney failure	0.1%	Significant symptoms and complications usually present Dialysis initiation varies but usually at GFR <10

[1]Stages of CKD 1–5 were originally defined by the US National Kidney Foundation Kidney Disease Quality Outcomes Initiative 2002. In the 2013 Kidney Disease Outcomes Quality Initiative (K/DOQI) CKD guideline update, the suffices A1, A2 and A3 are recommended, indicating the presence of albuminuria of <30, 30–300 and >300 mg/24 hrs respectively, in view of the prognostic importance of albuminuria. [2]Two GFR values 3 months apart are required to assign a stage. All GFR values are in mL/min/1.73 m². [3]Kidney damage means pathological abnormalities or markers of damage, including abnormalities in urine tests or imaging studies. [4]From Hill NR, Fatoba ST, Oke JL et al. Global prevalence of chronic kidney disease – a systematic review and meta-analysis. PLoS One 2016; 11:e0158765. [5]For further information, see page 415.

Fig. 15.3 Urine microscopy. [A] Erythrocytes due to bleeding from lower in the urinary tract (×400). [B] Dysmorphic erythrocytes due to glomerular inflammation (×400). [C] Hyaline casts in normal urine. [D] Erythrocytes and a red cell cast in glomerulonephritis (×100). Panels A–C are phase contrast images; D is a bright field image. *(A, B) Courtesy of Dr G.M. Iadorola and Dr F. Quarello, B. Bosco Hospital, Turin (from www.sin-italia.org/imago/sediment/sed.htm).*

Urine collection over a 24-hour period may be performed to measure excretion of solutes, such as calcium, oxalate and urate, in patients with recurrent renal stone disease (p. 431). Proteinuria can also be measured on 24-hour collections but is usually now quantified by protein/creatinine ratio on spot urine samples.

Other dynamic tests of tubular function, including concentrating ability (p. 688), ability to excrete a water load (p. 357) and ability to excrete acid (p. 415), and calculation of fractional calcium, phosphate or sodium excretion, are valuable in some circumstances but are usually performed in very specific contexts.

The fractional excretion of these ions can be calculated by the general formula: 100×(urine concentration of analyte×serum creatinine) / (serum concentration of analyte×urinary creatinine). Calculation of fractional excretion of sodium (FENa) can help in the setting of acute kidney injury (AKI) to differentiate volume depletion, when the tubules are avidly conserving sodium (FENa typically <1.0%), from acute tubular necrosis, when the tubules are damaged and are less able to conserve sodium (FENa typically >1.0%). In clinical practice this is seldom required.

Blood tests

Haematology

A normochromic normocytic anaemia is common in CKD and is due in part to deficiency of erythropoietin and bone marrow suppression secondary to toxins retained in CKD. Other causes of anaemia include iron deficiency from urinary tract bleeding, and haemolytic anaemia secondary to disorders such as haemolytic uraemic syndrome (HUS) and thrombotic thrombocytopenic purpura (TTP). Other abnormalities may be observed that reflect underlying disease processes, such as neutrophilia and raised erythrocyte sedimentation rate (ESR) in vasculitis or sepsis, and lymphopenia and raised ESR in systemic lupus erythematosus (SLE). Fragmented red cells on blood film and low platelets may be observed in thrombotic microangiopathies such as HUS/TTP and malignant hypertension. Pancytopenia may occur in SLE or bone marrow suppression due to myeloma.

Biochemistry

Abnormalities of routine biochemistry are common in renal disease. Serum levels of creatinine may be raised, reflecting reduced GFR (see above), as may serum potassium. Serum levels of urea are often increased in kidney disease but this analyte has limited value as a measure of GFR since levels increase with protein intake, following gastrointestinal haemorrhage and in catabolic states. Conversely, urea levels may be reduced in patients with chronic liver disease or anorexia and in malnourished patients, independently of changes in renal function. In the absence of the other causes mentioned above, an elevated urea:creatinine ratio is indicative of volume depletion and pre-renal failure. Serum calcium tends to be reduced and phosphate increased in CKD, in association with high parathyroid hormone (PTH) levels caused by reduced production of 1,25-dihydroxyvitamin D (1,25(OH)$_2$D) by the kidney (secondary hyperparathyroidism). In some patients, this may be accompanied by raised serum alkaline phosphatase levels, which are indicative of renal osteodystrophy. Serum bicarbonate may be low in renal failure and in renal tubular acidosis. Serum albumin may be low in liver disease, as a negative acute phase response or due to malnutrition/malabsorption, but if it is a new finding it should prompt urinalysis to exclude nephrotic syndrome. Other biochemical abnormalities may be observed that reflect underlying disease processes, such as raised glucose and HbA$_{1c}$ levels in diabetes mellitus (p. 726) and raised levels of C-reactive protein (CRP) in sepsis and vasculitis.

Immunology

Antinuclear antibodies, antibodies to extractable nuclear antigens and anti-double-stranded DNA antibodies may be detected in patients with renal disease secondary to SLE (p. 1034). Antineutrophil cytoplasmic antibodies (ANCAs) may be detected in patients with glomerulonephritis secondary to systemic vasculitis (p. 1040), as may antibodies to GBM in patients with Goodpasture's syndrome (p. 401), and low levels of complement may be observed in a number of kidney diseases (see Box 15.17, p. 401).

Imaging

Ultrasound

Renal ultrasound is a valuable non-invasive technique that may be performed to assess renal size and to investigate patients who are suspected of having obstruction of the urinary tract (Fig. 15.4), renal tumours, cysts or stones. Ultrasound can also be used to provide images of the prostate gland and bladder, and to estimate the completeness of emptying in patients with suspected bladder outflow obstruction. In addition, it can reveal other abdominal, pelvic and retroperitoneal pathology. Ultrasonography may show increased signal in the renal cortex with loss of distinction between cortex and medulla, which is characteristic of CKD. Doppler imaging can be used to study blood flow in extrarenal and larger intrarenal vessels, and to assess the resistivity index (peak systolic velocity – end-diastolic velocity/peak systolic velocity in the intrarenal arteries), which may be elevated (>0.7) in various diseases, including acute tubular necrosis and rejection of a renal transplant. However, renal ultrasound is operator-dependent and the results are often less clear in obese patients.

Computed tomography

Computed tomography urography (CTU) is used to evaluate cysts and mass lesions in the kidney or filling defects within the collecting systems. It usually entails an initial scan without contrast medium, and subsequent scans following injection of contrast to obtain a nephrogram image and images during the excretory phases. CTU has largely replaced the previous gold-standard investigation of intravenous urography (IVU) for investigation of the upper urinary tract, having the advantage of providing complete staging information and details of surrounding organs. Contrast enhancement is particularly useful for characterising mass lesions within the kidney and differentiating benign from malignant lesions (see Fig. 15.32A, p. 435). CT without contrast gives clear definition of retroperitoneal anatomy regardless of obesity and is superior to ultrasound in this respect. Non-contrast CT of kidneys, ureters and bladder (CTKUB) is the method of choice for demonstrating stones within the kidney or ureter (see Fig. 15.29, p. 432). For investigation of patients with renal trauma, a triple-phase CT scan with a delayed phase, to assess the integrity of the collecting system, is performed. Drawbacks of contrast-enhanced CT scans include the fact that relatively large doses of contrast medium are required, which can cause renal dysfunction, and that the radiation dose is significant (Box 15.4).

Magnetic resonance imaging

Magnetic resonance imaging (MRI) offers excellent resolution and gives good distinction between different tissue types (see Fig. 15.15, p. 406). It is very useful for local staging of prostate, bladder and penile cancers. Magnetic resonance angiography (MRA) provides an alternative to CT for imaging renal vessels but involves administration of gadolinium-based contrast media, which may carry risks for patients with impaired renal function (Box 15.4). Whilst MRA gives good images of the main renal vessels, stenosis of small branch arteries may be missed.

Renal arteriography

Renal arteriography involves taking X-rays following an injection of contrast medium directly into the renal artery. The main indication is to investigate renal artery stenosis (p. 406) or haemorrhage following renal trauma. Renal angiography can often be combined with therapeutic balloon dilatation or stenting of the renal artery. It can be used to occlude bleeding vessels and arteriovenous fistulae by the insertion of thin platinum wires (coils). These curl up within the vessel and promote thrombosis, thereby securing haemostasis.

15

| A Normal kidney | B Simple renal cyst | C Hydronephrosis | D Renal stone | E Renal tumour T1b |

Fig. 15.4 Renal ultrasound. [A] Normal kidney. The normal cortex is less echo-dense (blacker) than the adjacent liver. (RC = renal cortex; RS = renal sinus – calyx, renal pelvis, blood vessels, sinus fat) [B] Typical simple renal cyst: round, echo-free content, no septa, posterior acoustic enhancement. (C = calyx; P = thinned parenchyma; RP = renal pelvis; U = ureter) [C] The renal pelvis and calyces are dilated due to obstruction. The thinness of the parenchyma indicates chronic obstruction. [D] A typical renal stone with posterior shadowing. (AS = posterior acoustic shadow) [E] A T1b renal tumour. (K = kidney; L = liver; T = tumour) *(A–E) Courtesy of Dr Tobias Klatte, Addenbrooke's Hospital, Cambridge.*

i | **15.4 Renal complications of radiological investigations**

Contrast nephrotoxicity

- Acute deterioration in renal function commencing <48 hrs after administration of IV radiographic contrast media

Risk factors

- Pre-existing renal impairment
- Use of high-osmolality, ionic contrast media and repetitive dosing in short time periods
- Diabetes mellitus
- Myeloma

Prevention

- Provide hydration with free oral fluids plus IV isotonic saline 500 mL, then 250 mL/hr during procedure
- Avoid nephrotoxic drugs; withhold non-steroidal anti-inflammatory drugs (NSAIDs). Omit metformin for 48 hrs after the procedure, in case renal impairment occurs
- N-acetylcysteine may provide some protection but data are conflicting
- If the risks are high, consider alternative methods of imaging

Cholesterol atheroembolism

- Typically follows days to weeks after intra-arterial investigations or interventions (p. 409)

Nephrogenic sclerosing fibrosis after MRI contrast agents

- Chronic progressive sclerosis of skin, deeper tissues and other organs, associated with gadolinium-based contrast agents
- Only reported in patients with renal impairment, typically on dialysis or with GFR <15 mL/min/1.73 m^2, but caution is advised in patients with GFR <30 mL/min/1.73 m^2

Pyelography

Pyelography involves direct injection of contrast medium into the collecting system from above (antegrade) or below (retrograde). It offers the best views of the collecting system and upper tract, and is often used to identify the cause of urinary tract obstruction (p. 391). Antegrade pyelography requires the insertion of a fine needle into the pelvicalyceal system under ultrasound or radiographic control. In addition to visualising the cause of obstruction, percutaneous nephrostomy drainage can be established and often stents can be passed through any obstruction. Retrograde pyelography can be performed by inserting a ureteric catheter into the ureteric orifice at cystoscopy (Fig. 15.5) and again a stent can be inserted to bypass any obstruction.

Radionuclide studies

These are functional studies requiring the injection of gamma ray-emitting radiopharmaceuticals that are taken up and excreted by the kidney, a process that can be monitored by an external gamma camera.

Dynamic radionuclide studies are performed with mercaptoacetyltriglycine labelled with technetium (^{99m}Tc-MAG3), which is filtered by the glomerulus and excreted into the urine. Imaging following ^{99m}Tc-MAG3 injection can provide valuable information about the perfusion of each kidney but is not a reliable method for identifying renal artery stenosis. In patients with significant obstruction of the outflow tract, ^{99m}Tc-MAG3 persists in the renal pelvis and a loop diuretic fails to accelerate its disappearance. This can be useful in determining the functional significance of an equivocally obstructed collecting system without undertaking pyelography.

Fig. 15.5 Retrograde pyelography. The best views of the normal collecting system are shown by pyelography. A catheter has been passed into the left renal pelvis at cystoscopy. The anemone-like calyces are sharp-edged and normal. *Courtesy of Dr A.P. Bayliss and Dr P. Thorpe, Aberdeen Royal Infirmary.*

Formal measurements of GFR can be made by radionuclide studies following the injection of diethylenetriamine penta-acetic acid (^{99m}Tc-DPTA).

Static radionuclide studies are performed with dimercaptosuccinic acid labelled with technetium (^{99m}Tc-DMSA), which is taken up by proximal tubular cells. Following intravenous injection, images of the renal cortex are obtained that show the shape, size and relative function of each kidney (Fig. 15.6). This is a sensitive method for demonstrating cortical scarring in reflux nephropathy and a way of assessing the individual function of each kidney.

Radionuclide bone scanning following the injection of methylene diphosphonate (^{99m}Tc-MDP) is indicated to assess the presence and extent of bone metastases in men with advanced prostate cancer (p. 438).

Fig. 15.6 DMSA radionuclide scan. A posterior view is shown of a normal left kidney and a small right kidney (with evidence of cortical scarring at upper and lower poles) that contributes only 39% of total renal function.

Indications

- Acute kidney injury and chronic kidney disease of uncertain aetiology
- Nephrotic syndrome or glomerular proteinuria (protein:creatinine ratio >100 mg/mol) in adults
- Nephrotic syndrome in children that has atypical features or is not responding to treatment
- Nephritic syndrome
- Renal transplant dysfunction
- Rarely performed for isolated haematuria or isolated low-grade proteinuria in the absence of impaired renal function or evidence of a multisystem disorder

Contraindications

- Disordered coagulation or thrombocytopenia. Aspirin and other antiplatelet agents increase bleeding risk
- Uncontrolled hypertension
- Kidneys <60% predicted size
- Solitary kidney* (except transplants)

Complications

- Pain, usually mild
- Bleeding into urine, usually minor but may produce clot colic and obstruction
- Bleeding around the kidney, occasionally massive and requiring angiography with intervention, or surgery
- Arteriovenous fistula, rarely significant clinically

*Relative contraindication.

Renal biopsy

Renal biopsy is used to establish the diagnosis and severity of renal disease in order to judge the prognosis and need for treatment (Box 15.5). The procedure is performed transcutaneously under local anaesthetic with ultrasound or contrast radiography guidance to ensure accurate needle placement into a renal pole. Light microscopy, electron microscopy and immunohistological assessment of the specimen may all be required.

Presenting problems in renal and urinary tract disease

Oliguria/anuria

Oliguria is defined as being present when less than 400 mL of urine is passed per day, whereas anuria is deemed to exist when less than 100 mL of urine is passed per day.

The volume of urine produced represents a balance between the amount of fluid that is filtered at the glomerulus and that reabsorbed by the renal tubules. When GFR is low, urine volumes may still be normal if tubular reabsorption is also reduced; hence urine volume alone is a poor indicator of the severity of kidney disease. Oliguria and anuria may be caused by a reduction in urine production, as in pre-renal AKI, when GFR is reduced and tubular homeostatic mechanisms increase reabsorption to conserve salt and water. A high solute load or associated tubular dysfunction may, however, produce normal or high urine volumes in such cases until the pre-renal insult becomes severe and GFR is markedly reduced, such as occurs in diabetic ketoacidosis

Condition	Examples
Urinary obstruction (complete)	Urinary retention due to prostatic enlargement, urethral stenosis, bladder tumour Bilateral ureteric obstruction due to retroperitoneal fibrosis, cancer, radiation injury Bilateral renal stones (usually staghorn calculi) Massive crystalluria obstruction of tubules (rare)
Lack of renal perfusion (bilateral)	Aortic dissection involving renal arteries Severe acute tubular necrosis Severe functional hypoperfusion (cardiorenal, hepatorenal)
Rapidly progressive glomerulonephritis	Anti-glomerular basement membrane disease, severe antineutrophil cytoplasmic antibody (ANCA) vasculitis (100% glomerular crescents on biopsy)

with marked glycosuria. Urine volumes are variable in AKI due to intrinsic renal disease, but a rapid decline in urine volume may be observed. Anuria should prompt a differential including complete urinary obstruction, severe vascular compromise or rapidly progressive glomerulonephritis (Box 15.6).

Obstruction of the renal tract can produce oliguria and anuria, but to do so, obstruction must be complete and occur distal to the bladder neck, be bilateral, or be unilateral on the side of a single functioning kidney. Unilateral ureteric obstruction may not lead to any noticeable reduction in urine output. The presence of pain that is exacerbated by a fluid load suggests an acute obstruction of the renal tract, and its characteristics may be of value in reaching a diagnosis. Obstruction at the bladder neck is associated with lower midline abdominal discomfort, whereas ureteric obstruction typically presents as loin pain radiating to the groin and at the level of the renal pelvis may present as flank pain. Chronic obstruction rarely produces pain but may give rise to a dull ache. Urethral strictures should be considered as a possible cause, especially in patients with a history of instrumentation of the renal tract.

The presence of bladder enlargement in a middle-aged or elderly man suggests benign or malignant enlargement of the prostate gland as a potential cause of oliguria or anuria (pp. 437 and 438). It is important to note that many cases of acute urinary retention are observed after general anaesthesia, particularly in patients with pre-existing prostatic enlargement. Partial obstruction can be associated with a normal or even high urine volume due to chronic tubular injury, which causes loss of tubular concentrating ability. Management of oliguria and anuria should be directed at the underlying cause and is outlined later in the chapter (p. 413).

Haematuria

Healthy individuals may have occasional red blood cells in the urine (up to 12 500 cells/mL), but the presence of visible (macroscopic) haematuria or non-visible haematuria (microscopic, only detectable on dipstick testing) is indicative of significant bleeding from somewhere in the urinary tract (Fig. 15.7). Once infection, menstruation and causes of a positive urinary dipstick in the absence of red cells (haemoglobinuria/myoglobinuria) have

15

i 15.7 Interpretation of non-visible haematuria

Dipstick test positive	Urine microscopy	Suggested cause
Haematuria	White blood cells	Infection
	Abnormal epithelial cells	Tumour
	Red cell casts	
	Dysmorphic erythrocytes (phase contrast microscopy)	Glomerular bleeding*
Haemoglobinuria	No red cells	Intravascular haemolysis
Myoglobinuria (brown urine)	No red cells	Rhabdomyolysis

*Glomerular bleeding implies that the GBM is ruptured. It can occur physiologically following very strenuous exertion but usually indicates intrinsic renal disease and is an important feature of the nephritic syndrome.

i 15.8 Investigation of nephritic syndrome

Cause	Investigations
Rapidly progressive glomerulonephritis (RPGN)	
Post-infectious glomerulonephritis	ASOT, C3, C4
Anti-GBM disease	Anti-GBM antibody
Small-vessel vasculitis	p-ANCA, c-ANCA
Lupus nephritis	ANA, dsDNA, C3, C4
Mild glomerulonephritic presentation	
IgA nephropathy	Serum IgA (polyclonal rise in 50% of patients)
Mesangioproliferative glomerulonephritis	C3, C4, hepatitis B,C + HIV serology, ANA, dsDNA, immunoglobulins, PPE
Alport's syndrome*	Genetic screening, hearing test

*Not a glomerulonephritis but may present in a similar manner with haematuria, variable proteinuria, hypertension and slowly declining renal function.
(ANA = antinuclear antibody; ANCA = antineutrophil cytoplasmic antibody; ASOT = anti-streptolysin O titre; C3, C4 = complement proteins 3, 4; dsDNA = double-stranded DNA; GBM = glomerular basement membrane; HIV = human immunodeficiency virus; IgA = immunoglobulin A; PPE = plasma protein electrophoresis)

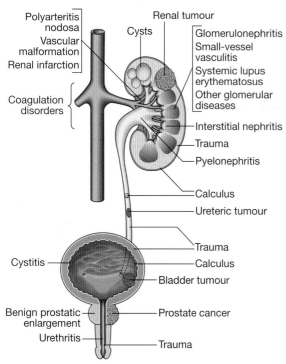

Fig. 15.7 Causes of haematuria.

been excluded (Box 15.7), both visible and persistent non-visible haematuria require investigation, as they may be caused by malignancy or indicate glomerulonephritis.

Visible haematuria is most likely to be caused by tumour, which can affect any part of the urogenital tract (Fig. 15.7), and patients with visible haematuria must therefore be referred to urology for imaging (ultrasound or CT scan) and cystoscopy (Fig. 15.8). Other common causes of visible haematuria are urine infection and stones. Visible haematuria may also be encountered in patients with IgA nephropathy, typically following an upper respiratory tract infection.

Non-visible haematuria may also indicate an underlying tumour, and all patients over 40 years old with persistent (detected on at least 2 of 3 consecutive dipstick tests) non-visible haematuria should therefore undergo imaging and cystoscopy. In younger patients, an underlying tumour is much less likely, and if a

glomerular cause is not suspected (see below), it may be appropriate to manage them by periodic observation in primary care, although occasionally these individuals develop significant overt renal disease during follow-up.

Glomerular bleeding occurs when inflammatory, destructive or degenerative processes disrupt the GBM, permitting passage of red blood cells into the urine. A characteristic feature of glomerular bleeding is an 'active urinary sediment' (the presence of dysmorphic red blood cells or red cell casts on microscopy); this is not always present, however. Patients with visible and non-visible haematuria should also be assessed for hypertension, proteinuria, reduced/declining renal function, family history of renal disease or features of systemic disease (Fig. 15.8). The presence of any of these features raises the possibility of intrinsic renal pathology and warrants referral to nephrology for further investigation, including consideration of renal biopsy.

Nephritic syndrome

The nephritic syndrome is characterised by the presence of haematuria in association with hypertension, oliguria, fluid retention and reduced/declining renal function. Many patients with glomerulonephritis, particularly those with milder disease, do not exhibit all of these features; their combined presence, however, is typical of a rapidly progressive glomerulonephritis and warrants urgent investigation. In many cases, investigation will include a renal biopsy to confirm diagnosis and guide management, but less invasive investigations may also be useful (Box 15.8).

Patients with nephritic syndrome may also exhibit varying degrees of proteinuria, including nephrotic-range proteinuria; the prominence of haematuria on dipstick should, however, alert the physician to the possibility of a glomerulonephritis. Indeed, it is important to recognise that the characteristic features of nephritic syndrome and nephrotic syndrome do not always present in isolation, but should be considered to be the extreme phenotypes at either end of a spectrum of presentations (Fig. 15.9).

Proteinuria

While very small amounts of high-molecular-weight proteins and moderate amounts of low-molecular-weight proteins pass

Fig. 15.8 Investigation of haematuria. *Symptomatic: lower urinary tract voiding symptoms such as hesitancy, frequency, urgency and dysuria. (ACR = albumin:creatinine ratio; BP = blood pressure; CT = computed tomography; eGFR = estimated glomerular filtration rate; NVH = non-visible haematuria; UTI = urinary tract infection)

15

Fig. 15.9 Nephritic and nephrotic syndrome. At one extreme, specific injury to podocytes causes proteinuria and nephrotic syndrome. The histology to the left shows diabetic nephropathy. At the other end of the spectrum, inflammation leads to cell damage and proliferation, breaks form in the glomerular basement membrane (GBM) and blood leaks into urine. In its extreme form, with acute sodium retention and hypertension, such disease is labelled nephritic syndrome. The histology to the right shows a glomerulus with many extra nuclei from proliferating intrinsic cells, and influx of inflammatory cells leading to crescent formation (arrows) in response to severe post-infectious glomerulonephritis. (FSGS = focal and segmental glomerulosclerosis; IgA = immunoglobulin A; MCGN = mesangiocapillary glomerulonephritis; SLE = systemic lupus erythematosus)

through the healthy GBM, these proteins normally are completely reabsorbed by receptors on tubular cells. Hence, in healthy individuals, less than 150 mg of protein is excreted in the urine each day, much of which is derived from tubular cells. This includes Tamm–Horsfall protein (uromodulin), encoded by the *UMOD* gene that has recently been linked to tubulo-interstitial

disease (see Box 15.20, p. 405). The presence of larger amounts of protein is usually indicative of significant renal disease.

Proteinuria is usually asymptomatic and is often picked up by urinalysis, although large amounts of protein may make the urine frothy. Transient proteinuria can occur after vigorous exercise, during fever, in heart failure and in people with urinary

15.9 Quantifying proteinuria in random urine samples

ACR[1]	PCR[2]	Typical dipstick results[3]	Significance
<3.5 (female) <2.5 (male)	<25	–	Normal
3.5–30	25–50	–	Moderately elevated albuminuria
30–70	50–100	+ to ++	Dipstick positive
70–300	100–350	++ to +++	Glomerular disease more likely; equivalent to >1 g/24 hrs
>300	>350	+++ to ++++	Nephrotic range: almost always glomerular disease, equivalent to > 3.5 g/24 hrs

[1]Urinary albumin (mg/L)/urine creatinine (mmol/L). [2]Urine protein (mg/L)/urine creatinine (mmol/L). (If urine creatinine is measured in mg/dL, reference values for PCR and ACR can be derived by dividing by 11.31.) [3]Dipstick results are affected by urine concentration and are occasionally weakly positive on normal samples.

tract infection. Patients should be assessed for the presence of these conditions and urine testing repeated once the potential trigger has been treated or resolved.

Testing for proteinuria is best done on an early morning sample, as some individuals exhibit orthostatic proteinuria. In these patients, typically less than 1 g/24 hrs of protein is excreted only in association with an upright posture, the first morning sample being negative. Orthostatic proteinuria is regarded as a benign disorder that does not require treatment.

Moderately elevated albuminuria (microalbuminuria)

In healthy individuals, there is virtually no urinary excretion of large-molecular-weight serum proteins, such as albumin, in contrast to modest urinary excretion of tubule-derived proteins. The presence of even moderate amounts of albuminuria (previously referred to as microalbuminuria) is therefore abnormal, and may indicate early glomerular pathology, at a time when the standard dipstick test remains negative (Box 15.9). Screening for moderately elevated albuminuria should be performed regularly in patients with diabetes, as persistently elevated levels warrant therapy with inhibitors of the renin–angiotensin–aldosterone system, even in normotensive individuals, to reduce the rate of loss of renal function (see Box 20.39, p. 758). Persistent moderately increased albuminuria has also been associated with cardiovascular mortality in patients with and without diabetes, but an explanation for this association has not yet been established.

Overt (dipstick-positive) proteinuria

Urinary dipstick testing is a valuable screening tool for the detection of proteinuria; it is only semi-quantitative, however, as it is highly dependent on the concentration of the urine. Typically, standard dipsticks test positive for protein once the urinary protein exceeds approximately 0.5 g/24 hrs; however, trace to 1+ on dipstick may be observed in very concentrated urine from individuals with no evidence of renal pathology. Hence all patients with persistent proteinuria on dipstick should have the amount of protein quantified to guide further investigations (Fig. 15.10). When more than 1 g of protein per day is being excreted, glomerular disease is likely and this is an indication for renal biopsy. Since quantification by 24-hour urine collection is often inaccurate, the protein:creatinine ratio (PCR) in a spot sample of urine is preferred. This makes an allowance for the variable degree of urinary dilution and can be used to extrapolate to 24-hour values (Box 15.9). Changes in PCR also give valuable information about the progression of renal disease and response to therapy in CKD.

Fig. 15.10 Investigation of proteinuria. (ACR = albumin:creatinine ratio; PCR = protein:creatinine ratio.)

It is possible to measure albumin:creatinine ratio (ACR), but this requires a more expensive immunoassay and is usually reserved for situations when high sensitivity is required, such as detection of the early stages of diabetic nephropathy (p. 757).

It is sometimes helpful to identify the type of protein in the urine. Large amounts of low-molecular-weight proteins, such as β_2-microglobulin (molecular weight 12 kDa), in the urine suggest renal tubular damage and are referred to as tubular proteinuria. This rarely exceeds 1.5–2 g/24 hrs (maximum PCR 150–200 mg/mmol; see Box 15.9 for conversion of mg/mmol to mg/dL).

Free immunoglobulin light chains (molecular weight 25 kDa) are filtered freely at the glomerulus but are poorly identified by dipstick tests. Hence, electrophoresis of the urine and specific immunodetection methods are required to detect immunoglobulin light chains, known as 'Bence Jones protein'. This may occur in AL amyloidosis (p. 81) and in B-cell dyscrasias but is particularly important as a marker for myeloma (p. 966).

Nephrotic syndrome

Nephrotic syndrome is characterised by very heavy proteinuria (>3.5 g/24 hrs), hypoalbuminaemia and oedema (see below). Blood volume may be normal, reduced or increased. Renal sodium retention is an early and universal feature; the mechanisms of this are shown in Figure 14.5 (p. 354). The diseases that cause nephrotic syndrome all affect the glomerulus (see Fig. 15.9), either directly, by damaging podocytes, or indirectly, by causing scarring or deposition of exogenous material such as amyloid into the glomerulus.

Investigation of nephrotic syndrome usually involves renal biopsy, although non-invasive tests may also be helpful in suggesting the underlying cause (Box 15.10). In children, minimal change disease is by far the most common cause of nephrotic syndrome and therefore renal biopsy is not usually required unless the patient fails to respond to high-dose glucocorticoid therapy. Similarly, most patients with diabetes presenting with nephrotic syndrome will have diabetic nephropathy, and so renal biopsy is usually not performed unless the course of the disease is atypical (rapidly increasing proteinuria or rapid decline in renal function; p. 757).

Management of nephrotic syndrome should be directed at the underlying cause. In addition, nephrotic syndrome is associated with a number of complications (Box 15.11), which may require supportive management unless the nephrosis is expected to resolve rapidly, such as in glucocorticoid-responsive minimal change disease.

Oedema

Oedema is caused by an excessive accumulation of fluid within the interstitial space. Clinically, this can be detected by persistence of an indentation in tissue following pressure on the affected area (pitting oedema). Pitting oedema tends to accumulate in the ankles during the day and improves overnight as the interstitial fluid is reabsorbed. Non-pitting oedema is typical of lymphatic obstruction and may also occur as the result of excessive matrix deposition in tissues: for example, in hypothyroidism (p. 639) or systemic sclerosis (p. 1037).

Clinical assessment

Dependent areas, such as the ankles and lower legs, are typically affected first but oedema can be restricted to the sacrum in bed-bound patients. With increasing severity, oedema spreads to affect the upper parts of the legs, the genitalia and abdomen. Ascites is common and often an earlier feature in children or young adults, and in liver disease. Pleural effusions are common but frank pulmonary oedema is rare. Facial oedema on waking is common. Features of intravascular volume depletion (tachycardia, postural hypotension) may occur when oedema is due to decreased

15

---

i · 15.10 Investigation of nephrotic syndrome

Cause	Typical age group	Investigations
Fulminant presentation		
Minimal change disease	Children, young adults, occasionally seen in older patients	None specific
Primary focal segmental glomerulosclerosis	Young adults	None specific
Subacute presentation		
Membranous nephropathy	Middle-aged to older patients	Hepatitis B, C + HIV serology, ANA, dsDNA
Amyloid	Older patients	Immunoglobulins, PPE, Bence Jones protein, serum free light chains
Gradual progression		
Diabetic nephropathy	Any age, but rarely <10 years from diagnosis of type 1 diabetes	Glucose, glycosylated haemoglobin

(ANA = antinuclear antibody; dsDNA = double-stranded DNA; HIV = human immunodeficiency virus; PPE = plasma protein electrophoresis)

---

i · 15.11 Consequences of the nephrotic syndrome and their management

Feature	Mechanism	Consequence	Management
Hypoalbuminaemia	Urinary protein losses exceed synthetic capacity of liver	Reduced oncotic pressure Oedema	Treatment of underlying cause
Avid sodium retention	Secondary hyperaldosteronism Additional poorly characterised intrarenal mechanisms	Oedema	Diuretics and a low-sodium diet*
Hypercholesterolaemia	Non-specific increase in lipoprotein synthesis by liver in response to low oncotic pressure	High rate of atherosclerosis	Statins, ezetimibe
Hypercoagulability	Relative loss of inhibitors of coagulation (antithrombin III, protein C and S) and increase in liver synthesis of procoagulant factors	Venous thromboembolism	Consideration of prophylaxis in chronic or severe nephrotic syndrome
Infection	Hypogammaglobulinaemia due to urinary loss of immunoglobulins	Pneumococcal and meningococcal infection	Consideration of vaccination

*Severe nephrotic syndrome may need very large doses of combinations of diuretics acting on different parts of the nephron (e.g. loop diuretic plus thiazide plus amiloride). In occasional patients with hypovolaemia, intravenous salt-poor albumin infusions may help to establish a diuresis, although efficacy is controversial. Over-diuresis risks secondary impairment of renal function through hypovolaemia.

15.12 Causes of oedema

Increased total extracellular fluid

- Congestive heart failure
- Renal failure
- Liver disease

High local venous pressure

- Deep venous thrombosis or venous insufficiency
- Pregnancy
- Pelvic tumour

Low plasma oncotic pressure/serum albumin

- Nephrotic syndrome
- Liver failure
- Malnutrition/malabsorption

Increased capillary permeability

- Leakage of proteins into the interstitium, reducing the osmotic pressure gradient that draws fluid into the lymphatics and blood
- Infection/inflammation
- Severe sepsis
- Calcium channel blockers

Lymphatic obstruction

- Infection: filariasis, lymphogranuloma venereum (pp. 290 and 341)
- Malignancy
- Radiation injury
- Congenital abnormality

oncotic pressure or increased capillary permeability. If oedema is localised – for example, to one ankle but not the other – then venous thrombosis, inflammation or lymphatic disease should be suspected.

Investigations

Oedema may be due to a number of causes (Box 15.12), which are usually apparent from the history and examination of the cardiovascular system and abdomen. Blood should be taken for measurement of urea and electrolytes, liver function and serum albumin, and the urine tested for protein. Further imaging of the liver, heart or kidneys may be indicated, based on history and clinical examination. Where ascites or pleural effusions occur in isolation, aspiration of fluid with measurement of protein and glucose, and microscopy for cells, will usually help to clarify the diagnosis in differentiating a transudate (typical of oedema) from an exudate (more suggestive of local pathology, p. 564).

Management

Mild oedema usually responds to elevation of the legs, compression stockings, or a thiazide or a low dose of a loop diuretic, such as furosemide or bumetanide. In nephrotic syndrome, renal failure and severe cardiac failure, very large doses of diuretics, sometimes in combination, may be required to achieve a negative sodium and fluid balance. Restriction of sodium intake and fluid intake may be required. Diuretics are not helpful in the treatment of oedema caused by venous or lymphatic obstruction or by increased capillary permeability. Specific causes of oedema, such as venous thrombosis, should be treated.

Hypertension

Hypertension is a very common feature of renal disease. Additionally, the presence of hypertension identifies a population at risk of developing CKD and current recommendations are that hypertensive patients should have renal function checked annually. Control of hypertension is very important in patients with renal impairment because of its close relationship with further decline of renal function (p. 420) and because of the exaggerated cardiovascular risk associated with CKD. Pathophysiology and management are discussed on pages 509 and 510.

Loin pain

Loin pain is often caused by musculoskeletal disease but can be a manifestation of renal tract disease; in the latter case, it may arise from renal stones, ureteric stones, renal tumours, acute pyelonephritis and urinary tract obstruction. Acute loin pain radiating anteriorly and often to the groin is termed renal colic. When combined with haematuria, this is typical of ureteric obstruction due to calculi (p. 431). Precipitation of loin pain by a large fluid intake (Dietl's crisis) suggests upper urinary tract obstruction caused by a congenital abnormality of the pelvi-ureteric junction (p. 433).

Dysuria

Dysuria refers to painful urination, often described as burning, scalding or stinging, and commonly accompanied by suprapubic pain. It is often associated with frequency of micturition and a feeling of incomplete emptying of the bladder. By far the most common cause is urinary tract infection, as described on page 426. Other diagnoses that need to be considered in patients with dysuria include sexually transmitted infections (p. 329) and bladder stones (p. 431).

Frequency

Frequency describes daytime micturition more often than a patient would expect. It may be a consequence of polyuria, when urine volume is normal or high, but is also found in patients with dysuria and prostatic diseases, when the urine volume is normal.

Polyuria

Polyuria is defined as a urine volume in excess of 3 L/24 hrs. Various underlying conditions, both renal and extrarenal, may be responsible, as outlined in Box 15.13.

Investigation of polyuria includes measurement of urea, creatinine and electrolytes, glucose, calcium and albumin. A 24-hour urine collection may be helpful to confirm the severity of polyuria. The presence of nocturnal polyuria suggests a

15.13 Causes of polyuria

- Excess fluid intake
- Osmotic diuresis: hyperglycaemia, hypercalcaemia
- Cranial diabetes insipidus
- Nephrogenic diabetes insipidus:
    Rare inherited mutations in vasopressin receptor or aquaporin 2 genes
    Lithium
    Diuretics
    Interstitial nephritis
    Hypokalaemia
    Hypercalcaemia

pathological cause. Investigation and management of suspected diabetes insipidus are described on page 688.

Nocturia

Nocturia is defined as waking up at night to void urine. It may be a consequence of polyuria but may also result from increased fluid intake or diuretic use in the late evening (including caffeine). Nocturia also occurs in CKD, and in prostatic enlargement when it is associated with poor stream, hesitancy, incomplete bladder emptying, terminal dribbling and urinary frequency due to partial urethral obstruction (p. 437). Nocturia may also occur due to sleep disturbance without any functional abnormalities of the urinary tract.

Urinary incontinence

Urinary incontinence is defined as any involuntary leakage of urine. It may occur in patients with a normal urinary tract, as the result of dementia or poor mobility, or transiently during an acute illness or hospitalisation, especially in older people (see Box 15.54, p. 436). The pathophysiology, investigation and management of urinary incontinence are discussed in detail later in the chapter (p. 436).

Glomerular diseases

Glomerular diseases account for a significant proportion of acute and chronic kidney disease. Most patients with glomerular disease do not present acutely and are asymptomatic until abnormalities are detected on routine screening of blood or urine samples.

There are many causes of glomerular damage, including immunological injury, inherited diseases such as Alport's syndrome (p. 403), metabolic diseases such as diabetes mellitus (p. 757), and deposition of abnormal proteins such as amyloid in the glomeruli (p. 81). The glomerular cell types that may be the target of injury are shown in Figure 15.11. Proteinuria is the hallmark of glomerular disease; however, the response of the glomerulus to injury and hence the predominant clinical features vary according to the nature of the insult, ranging from fulminant nephrotic syndrome to rapidly progressive glomerulonephritis (see Fig. 15.9). Several prognostic indicators are common to all causes of glomerulonephritis (Box 15.14) and may be helpful in assessing the need for immunosuppressive therapy.

Glomerulonephritis

While glomerulonephritis literally means 'inflammation of glomeruli', the term is often used more broadly to describe all types of glomerular disease, even though some of these (e.g. minimal change nephropathy) are not associated with inflammation.

	15.14 Poor prognostic indicators in glomerular disease

- Male sex
- Hypertension
- Persistent and severe proteinuria
- Elevated creatinine at time of presentation
- Rapid rate of decline in renal function
- Tubulo-interstitial fibrosis observed on renal biopsy

Most types of glomerulonephritis are immunologically mediated and several respond to immunosuppressive drugs. Deposition of antibody occurs in many types of glomerulonephritis and testing for circulating or glomerular deposition of antibodies may aid diagnosis (see Fig. 15.11 and Boxes 15.8 and 15.10). In small-vessel vasculitis, no glomerular antibody deposition is observed (pauci-immune), but the antibodies may be indirectly pathogenic by activating neutrophils to promote endothelial injury (Fig. 15.11).

Glomerulonephritis is generally classified in terms of the histopathological appearances, as summarised in Box 15.15 and Figure 15.12. Many non-specialists find the terminology used in describing glomerulonephritis to be confusing; some definitions are provided in Box 15.16. It is important to stress that the histological appearance rarely confirms a specific renal disease but rather suggests a limited range of diagnoses, which may be confirmed by further investigation. Conversely, some diseases, such as lupus, are associated with more than one histological pattern of injury. The most common histological subtypes may be categorised according to their typical clinical presentation, as discussed below. Genetic disorders associated with glomerular disease are described later (p. 403).

Circulating immune complexes
Cryoglobulinaemia *(Cryoglobulins in serum)*
Serum sickness
Endocarditis

Endothelium (indirectly)
Small-vessel vasculitis
ANCA (serum)

GBM
Goodpasture's disease
Anti-GBM antibody (serum + IF on biopsy; see Fig.15.12H)

Mesangium
IgA nephropathy *(polyclonal rise in serum IgA in 50% patients; IF on biopsy; see Fig.15.12G)*

Podocyte
Membranous nephropathy
Anti-phosphilipase A2 receptor 1 (serum + IF on biopsy; experimental at present; see Fig.15.12F)

Planted antigens
SLE – *ANA, anti-dsDNA (serum)*
Post-infectious glomerulonephritis

Fig. 15.11 Glomerulonephritis associated with antibody production. Antibodies and antigen–antibody (immune) complexes may target or be deposited in specific components of the glomerulus, resulting in different patterns of histological injury and clinical presentation. Testing for antibody deposition in the glomerulus by immunofluorescence (IF) on renal biopsy tissue or for antibodies in the serum may aid diagnosis. Diagnostic tests are shown in italics. (ANA = antinuclear antibody; ANCA = antineutrophil cytoplasmic antibody; dsDNA = double-stranded DNA; GBM = glomerular basement membrane; IgA = immunoglobulin A; SLE = systemic lupus erythematosus)

Diseases typically presenting with nephrotic syndrome

In these diseases, the injury is focused on the podocyte and there is little histological evidence of inflammation or cell proliferation in the glomerulus (non-proliferative, Fig. 15.12). Minimal change and primary focal segmental glomerulosclerosis (FSGS) typically present with fulminant nephrotic syndrome, whereas in membranous nephropathy and secondary FSGS, the nephrosis tends to be more indolent in nature. Other causes of nephrotic syndrome due to systemic disease are discussed elsewhere, including diabetic nephropathy (p. 757) and amyloid (p. 81).

Minimal change nephropathy

Minimal change disease occurs at all ages but accounts for most cases of nephrotic syndrome (see Box 15.15) in children and about one-quarter of adult cases. It is caused by reversible dysfunction of podocytes. On light microscopy, the glomeruli appear normal (Fig. 15.12A), but fusion of podocyte foot processes is observed on electron microscopy. The presentation is with nephrotic syndrome, which typically is severe; it remits

---

i | **15.15 Glomerulonephritis categorised by clinical presentation and histological classification**

Histology	Immune deposits	Pathogenesis	Associations	Comments
Nephrotic presentation				
Minimal change				
Normal, except on electron microscopy, where fusion of podocyte foot processes is observed (non-specific finding)	None	Unknown; probable circulating factor promoting podocyte injury Some cases are genetic (p. 403)	Atopy Drugs, most commonly NSAIDs Haematological malignancies	Acute and often severe nephrotic syndrome Good response to glucocorticoids Dominant cause of idiopathic nephrotic syndrome in childhood
Focal segmental glomerulosclerosis (FSGS)				
Segmental scars in some glomeruli No acute inflammation Podocyte foot process fusion seen in primary FSGS	Non-specific trapping in focal scars	Unknown; circulating factors may increase glomerular permeability Injury to podocytes may be common feature Some cases are genetic (p. 403)	*APOL1* variant in people of West African descent Causes of secondary FSGS include: Healing of previous local glomerular injury HIV infection Heroin misuse Morbid obesity Chronic hypertension	*Primary FSGS* presents as idiopathic nephrotic syndrome but is less responsive to treatment than minimal change; may progress to renal impairment, and can recur after transplantation *Secondary FSGS* presents with variable proteinuria and outcome
Membranous nephropathy				
Thickening of GBM Progressing to increased matrix deposition and glomerulosclerosis	Granular subepithelial IgG	Antibodies to a podocyte surface antigen (commonly phospholipase A_2 receptor 1), with complement-dependent podocyte injury	*HLA-DQA1* (for idiopathic) Drugs: Penicillamine, NSAIDs, heavy metals Hepatitis B virus Malignancy Lupus[1]	Common cause of adult idiopathic nephrotic syndrome One-third progress, one-third spontaneously remit and one-third remain stable; may respond to glucocorticoids and immunosuppressants
Mild glomerulonephritic presentation				
IgA nephropathy				
Increased mesangial matrix and cells Focal segmental nephritis in acute disease	Mesangial IgA (and C3)	Unknown Mucosal infections (e.g. helminths) may be involved	Usually idiopathic, flares triggered by upper respiratory infection Liver disease Coeliac disease	Common disease with range of presentations, usually including haematuria and hypertension Henoch–Schönlein purpura is an acute IgA variant common in children
Mesangiocapillary glomerulonephritis				
Immunoglobulin type	Immunoglobulins	Deposition of circulating immune complexes or 'planted' antigens	Infections, autoimmunity or monoclonal gammopathies	Most common pattern found in association with subacute bacterial infection, but also with cryoglobulinaemia ± hepatitis C virus, and others
Complement type	Complement components	Complement abnormalities, inherited or acquired Dense deposit disease is associated with abnormal activation of alternative complement pathway	Complement gene mutations C3 nephritic factor and partial lipodystrophy	In dense deposit disease, intramembranous deposits No proven treatments

Continued

i 15.15 Glomerulonephritis categorised by clinical presentation and histological classification – continued

Histology	Immune deposits	Pathogenesis	Associations	Comments
Rapidly progressive glomerulonephritis presentation				
Focal necrotising glomerulonephritis				
Segmental inflammation and/or necrosis in some glomeruli ± crescent formation	Variable according to cause but typically negative (or 'pauci-immune')	Small-vessel vasculitis, often ANCA-mediated	Primary or secondary small-vessel vasculitis	Often occurs in systemic disease Responds to treatment with glucocorticoids and immunosuppressants
***Diffuse proliferative glomerulonephritis*[2]**				
Infection-related diffuse proliferative glomerulonephritis[3]				
Diffuse proliferation of endothelial and mesangial cells Infiltration by neutrophils and macrophages ± crescent formation	Subendothelial and subepithelial	Immune complex-mediated (e.g. to streptococcal infection with presumed cross-reactive epitopes)	Post-streptococcal Concurrent infection with staphylococci, endocarditis	Presents with severe sodium and fluid retention, hypertension, haematuria, oliguria Usually resolves spontaneously
Anti-glomerular basement membrane disease				
Usually crescentic nephritis	Linear IgG along GBM	Autoantibodies to α3 chain of type IV collagen in GBM	*HLA-DR15* (previously known as *DR2*)	Associated with lung haemorrhage but renal or lung disease may occur alone Treat with glucocorticoids, cyclophosphamide and plasma exchange

[1]Systemic lupus erythematosus can cause almost any histological injury pattern, most commonly membranous nephropathy or diffuse proliferative glomerulonephritis.
[2]In addition to the association with infection and anti-GBM disease, a diffuse proliferative glomerulonephritis picture may also be seen with lupus and occasionally IgA nephropathy. [3]Infection may also present with mesangioproliferative glomerulonephritis and membranous nephropathy (HIV).
(ANA = antinuclear antibody; ANCA = antineutrophil cytoplasmic antibody; *APOL1* = apolipoprotein L1; GBM = glomerular basement membrane; HLA = human leucocyte antigen; IgA = immunoglobulin A; NSAIDs = non-steroidal anti-inflammatory drugs)

15

A Normal glomerulus **B** Focal segmental GS **C** Focal necrotising GN **D** Membranous GN

E Crescentic GN **F** Membranous GN **G** IgA nephropathy **H** Anti-GBM disease

Fig. 15.12 Histopathology of glomerular disease. (**A**–**E** *Light microscopy*) **A** A normal glomerulus. Note the open capillary loops and thinness of their walls. **B** Focal segmental glomerulosclerosis (GS). The portion of the glomerulus arrowed shows loss of capillary loops and cells, which are replaced by matrix. **C** Focal necrotising glomerulonephritis (GN). A portion of the glomerulus (N = focal necrotising lesion) is replaced by bright pink material with some 'nuclear dust'. Neutrophils may be seen elsewhere in the glomerulus. There is surrounding interstitial inflammation (I). This is most commonly associated with small-vessel vasculitis and may progress to crescentic nephritis (see **E**). **D** Membranous glomerulonephritis. The capillary loops (C) are thickened (compare with the normal glomerulus) and there is expansion of the mesangial regions by matrix deposition (M). However, there is no gross cellular proliferation or excess of inflammatory cells. **E** Crescentic glomerulonephritis. The lower part of Bowman's space is occupied by a semicircular formation ('crescent', Cr) of large pale cells, compressing the glomerular tuft. This is seen in aggressive inflammatory glomerulonephritis. *Antibody deposition in the glomerulus.* (**F**–**H** *Direct immunofluorescence*) **F** Granular deposits of IgG along the basement membrane in a subepithelial pattern, typical of membranous GN. **G** Immunoglobulin A (IgA) deposits in the mesangium, as seen in IgA nephropathy. **H** Ribbon-like linear deposits of anti-GBM antibodies along the glomerular basement membrane in Goodpasture's disease. The glomerular structure is well preserved in all of these examples. *(A, C, D, E) Courtesy of Dr J.G. Simpson, Aberdeen Royal Infirmary. (F, G, H) Courtesy of Dr R. Herriot.*

15.16 Terminology used in glomerulonephritis

Light microscopy

- *Focal*: affecting some but not all glomeruli
- *Diffuse*: affecting >50% of glomeruli
- *Segmental*: affecting a portion of a glomerulus
- *Global*: affecting all of the glomerulus
- *Necrotising*: severe injury leading to an area of necrosis, usually associated with vasculitis
- *Crescentic*: a crescent-shaped area of inflammatory cells responding to severe glomerular injury

Electron microscopy

- *Subendothelial immune deposits*: found between the endothelial cell and the GBM – often found in nephritic presentations
- *Intramembranous immune deposits*: found within the GBM – found in the dense deposit variant of mesangiocapillary glomerulonephritis
- *Subepithelial immune deposits*: found between the epithelial cell and the GBM – often found in nephrotic presentations, including membranous presentation of lupus

(GBM = glomerular basement membrane)

with high-dose glucocorticoid therapy (1 mg/kg prednisolone for 6 weeks), though the response to therapy is often less satisfactory in older patients. Some patients who respond incompletely (glucocorticoid-resistant) or relapse frequently need maintenance glucocorticoids (glucocorticoid dependence), cytotoxic therapy or other agents. Glucocorticoid resistance in children warrants a biopsy to exclude an alternative diagnosis, but if minimal change is confirmed, a genetic cause should be considered (p. 403). Minimal change disease typically does not progress to CKD but can present with problems related to the nephrotic syndrome (see Box 15.11) and complications of treatment.

Focal segmental glomerulosclerosis

Primary focal segmental glomerulosclerosis (FSGS) (Fig. 15.12B) can occur in all age groups but is particularly common in people of West African descent, who, compared with other ethnicities, have a much higher carriage rate of an apolipoprotein L1 (*APOL1*) gene variant that is associated with increased risk of FSGS. Histological analysis shows sclerosis initially limited to segments of the glomeruli, which may also show positive staining for deposits of C3 and IgM on immunofluorescence. Since FSGS is a focal process, abnormal glomeruli may not be seen on renal biopsy if only a few are sampled, leading to an initial diagnosis of minimal change nephropathy. In most cases the underlying cause is unknown (primary FSGS) and these patients typically present with abrupt onset of severe nephrotic syndrome. Primary FSGS may respond to high-dose glucocorticoid therapy (0.5–2.0 mg/kg/day) but the response is rarely as rapid or complete as for minimal change disease. Immunosuppressive drugs, such as ciclosporin, cyclophosphamide and mycophenolate mofetil, have also been used but their efficacy is uncertain. Progression to CKD is common in patients who do not respond to glucocorticoids and the disease frequently recurs after renal transplantation.

FSGS may also be secondary to other diseases such as human immunodeficiency virus (HIV) renal disease (particularly in African Americans), morbid obesity or chronic hypertension. In addition, it may reflect scarring from previous focal glomerular injury resulting from HUS, cholesterol embolism or vasculitis. Patients with secondary FSGS typically present with more modest proteinuria than those with primary disease and rarely exhibit full-blown nephrotic syndrome. Management of secondary FSGS is focused on treating the underlying cause and reducing proteinuria by inhibiting the renin–angiotensin system (p. 417).

Membranous nephropathy

Membranous nephropathy is the most common cause of nephrotic syndrome in Caucasian adults. It is caused by antibodies (usually autoantibodies) directed at antigen(s) expressed on the surface of podocytes, including the M-type phospholipase A_2 receptor 1. While most cases are idiopathic, a proportion are associated with other causes, such as heavy metal poisoning, drugs, infections, lupus and tumours (see Box 15.15 and Fig. 15.12D and F). Approximately one-third of patients with idiopathic membranous nephropathy undergo spontaneous remission, one-third remain in a nephrotic state, and one-third develop progressive CKD. High doses of glucocorticoids and cyclophosphamide may improve both the nephrotic syndrome and the long-term prognosis. However, because of the toxicity of these regimens, many nephrologists reserve such treatment for those with severe nephrotic syndrome or deteriorating renal function. Treatment of secondary membranous nephropathy is directed at the underlying cause.

Diseases typically presenting with mild nephritic syndrome

Patients with mild glomerulonephritis typically present with non-visible haematuria and modest proteinuria, and their renal disease tends to follow a slowly progressive course. IgA nephropathy and mesangiocapillary glomerulonephritis (MCGN) typically fall in this category. Their presentation is highly variable, however; IgA nephropathy occasionally presents with rapidly progressive glomerulonephritis while MCGN may present with nephrotic syndrome. Other diseases that present with haematuria, modest proteinuria and slow progression include Alport's syndrome (p. 403).

IgA nephropathy

This is one of the most common types of glomerulonephritis and can present in many ways. Haematuria is the earliest sign and non-visible haematuria is almost universal, while hypertension is also very common. These are often detected during routine screening: for example, at occupational medical examinations. Proteinuria can also occur but is usually a later feature. In many cases, there is slowly progressive loss of renal function leading to end-stage renal disease (ESRD). A particular hallmark of IgA nephropathy in young adults is the occurrence of acute self-limiting exacerbations, often with visible haematuria, in association with minor respiratory infections. This may be so acute as to resemble acute post-infectious glomerulonephritis, with fluid retention, hypertension and oliguria with dark or red urine. Characteristically, the latency from clinical infection to nephritis is short: a few days or less. Asymptomatic presentations dominate in older adults, with non-visible haematuria, hypertension and reduction in GFR. Occasionally, IgA nephropathy progresses rapidly in association with crescent formation on biopsy. Management is largely directed towards the control of blood pressure, with renin–angiotensin system inhibitors preferable in those with proteinuria. There is some evidence for additional benefit from several months of high-dose glucocorticoid treatment in those at high-risk of progressive disease (see Box 15.14), but no strong evidence for other immunosuppressive agents. A role for other therapies, such as fish oil, remains uncertain.

Henoch–Schönlein purpura

This condition most commonly occurs in children but can also be observed in adults. It is a systemic vasculitis that often arises in response to an infectious trigger. It presents with a tetrad of features:

- a characteristic petechial rash typically affecting buttocks and lower legs
- abdominal pain due to vasculitis involving the gastrointestinal tract
- arthralgia
- renal disease characterised by visible or non-visible haematuria, with or without proteinuria.

Renal biopsy shows mesangial IgA deposition and appearances that are indistinguishable from acute IgA nephropathy (Fig. 15.12G). Treatment is supportive in nature; in most patients, the prognosis is good, with spontaneous resolution, though relapses are common. Some patients, particularly adults and those with severe or persistent proteinuria, progress to develop ESRD.

Mesangiocapillary glomerulonephritis

Mesangiocapillary glomerulonephritis (MCGN), also known as membranoproliferative glomerulonephritis, is a pattern of injury seen on renal biopsy that is characterised by an increase in mesangial cellularity with thickening of glomerular capillary walls. The typical presentation is with proteinuria and haematuria. Several underlying causes have been identified, as summarised in Box 15.15. It can be classified into two main subtypes. The first is characterised by deposition of immunoglobulins within the glomeruli. This subtype is associated with chronic infections, autoimmune diseases and monoclonal gammopathy. The second is characterised by deposition of complement in the glomeruli and is associated with inherited or acquired abnormalities in the complement pathway. This category comprises 'dense deposit disease', which is typified by electron-dense deposits within the GBM, and C3 glomerulonephritis that shows deposits similar to immunoglobulin-type MCGN.

Treatment of MCGN associated with immunoglobulin deposits consists of the identification and treatment of the underlying disease, if possible, and the use of immunosuppressive drugs such as mycophenolate mofetil or cyclophosphamide. There are few specific treatments for MCGN associated with complement dysregulation, although eculizumab, the anti-C5 inhibitor that prevents formation of the membrane attack complex, has shown promise.

Diseases typically presenting with rapidly progressive glomerulonephritis

Rapidly progressive glomerulonephritis (RPGN) is characterised by rapid loss of renal function over days to weeks, usually in association with hypertension and oedema. Non-visible haematuria is almost always present with variable amounts of proteinuria, while characteristic red cell casts and dysmorphic red cells may be observed on urine microscopy (see Fig. 15.3). Renal biopsy typically shows crescentic lesions (see Fig. 15.12E), often associated with necrotising lesions within the glomerulus (Fig. 15.12C), particularly in small-vessel vasculitides.

This pattern of presentation is typical of post-infectious glomerulonephritis, anti-GBM disease and small-vessel vasculitides (p. 1040). It can also be observed in SLE (p. 1034) and occasionally in IgA and other nephropathies (see Fig. 15.9).

i	**15.17 Causes of glomerulonephritis associated with low serum complement**

- Post-infectious glomerulonephritis
- Subacute bacterial infection, especially endocarditis
- Systemic lupus erythematosus
- Cryoglobulinaemia
- Mesangiocapillary glomerulonephritis, usually complement type

Anti-glomerular basement membrane disease

Anti-GBM disease is a rare autoimmune disease in which antibodies develop against the α3 chain of type 4 collagen GBM. Expression of the α3 chain is largely restricted to the basement membranes of glomeruli and lungs, and hence the disease may present with rapidly progressive glomerulonephritis, lung haemorrhage, or disease of both organs, when it is known as Goodpasture's disease. Goodpasture's disease is more common in younger patients, while elderly patients often present with renal-limited disease. Patients with anti-GBM disease should be treated with plasma exchange combined with glucocorticoids and immunosuppressants, but early diagnosis is essential, as renal function is rarely recoverable in those requiring dialysis at presentation.

The combination of glomerulonephritis and pulmonary haemorrhage (Goodpasture's syndrome) may also be observed with small-vessel vasculitis (particularly granulomatosis with polyangiitis, previously known as Wegener's granulomatosis) and lupus.

Infection-related glomerulonephritis

RPGN may occur either during or following an infection. In both cases, circulating immune complexes are present and activation of the complement system promotes consumption of complement factors, resulting in low serum C3 and C4 concentration, as observed in many causes of glomerulonephritis (Box 15.17).

Post-infectious glomerulonephritis is observed most commonly in children and young adults, and typically presents 10 days *after* a streptococcal throat infection or longer after a skin infection. The clinical presentation ranges from mild abnormalities on urinalysis to RPGN with severe AKI. The anti-streptolysin (ASO) test is positive in up to 95% of patients with streptococcal throat infections. Treatment is supportive, with control of blood pressure and fluid overload with salt restriction, diuretics and dialysis if required. Antibiotic therapy is rarely needed, as the renal disease occurs after the infection has subsided. The medium-term prognosis for children and most adults is good, with recovery of renal function typical even in those requiring dialysis therapy. Some patients may develop CKD 20–30 years after the original presentation, however.

An immune complex-mediated disease may also be observed *during* an infection, typically a staphylococcal infection such as endocarditis, skin infection or pneumonia, but also with subacute endocarditis due to *Streptococcus viridans*. This occurs more commonly in older adults and the presentation tends not to be as fulminant as with post-streptococcal disease. In addition to supportive measures, antibiotic therapy is required, as infection is usually concurrent with renal disease.

Tubulo-interstitial diseases

These diseases primarily affect the renal tubules and interstitial components of the renal parenchyma. They are characterised

15

by tubular dysfunction with electrolyte abnormalities, moderate levels of proteinuria and varying degrees of renal impairment. Often the urinary output may be relatively preserved for any given GFR, and indeed there may be polyuria and nocturia.

Acute interstitial nephritis

Acute interstitial nephritis (AIN) is an immune-mediated disorder, characterised by acute inflammation affecting the tubulo-interstitium of the kidney. It is commonly drug-induced, with proton pump inhibitors (PPIs) fast becoming the most common cause, but can be caused by other toxins, and can complicate a variety of systemic diseases and infections (Box 15.18).

Clinical features

The clinical presentation is typically with renal impairment but, in some patients with drug-induced AIN, there may be signs of a generalised drug hypersensitivity reaction with fever, rash and eosinophilia. Proteinuria is generally modest (PCR < 100 mg/mmol) and tubular in type (see Box 15.25, p. 412). The urine may contain white blood cells and white cell casts but is sterile on culture. Eosinophils are present in up to 70% of patients but this is a non-specific finding. AIN should always be considered in patients with non-oliguric AKI. There may be a rapid deterioration of renal function in some cases of drug-induced AIN, causing the condition to be mistaken for RPGN.

Investigations

Renal biopsy is usually required to confirm the diagnosis (Fig. 15.13D). This typically shows evidence of intense inflammation, with infiltration of the tubules and interstitium by polymorphonuclear leucocytes and lymphocytes. Eosinophils may also be observed, especially in drug-induced AIN. Often granulomas may be evident, especially in drug-induced AIN or sarcoidosis (p. 608). The degree of chronic inflammation in a biopsy is a useful predictor of long-term renal function. Eosinophiluria may be present but is not a good discriminator for AIN.

Management

Some patients with drug-induced AIN recover following withdrawal of the drug alone, but high-dose glucocorticoids (prednisolone 1 mg/kg/day) may accelerate recovery and prevent long-term scarring. Other specific causes (see Box 15.18) should be treated, if possible.

Chronic interstitial nephritis

Chronic interstitial nephritis (CIN) is characterised by renal dysfunction with fibrosis and infiltration of the renal parenchyma by lymphocytes, plasma cells and macrophages, in association with tubular damage.

> **i** | **15.18 Causes of acute interstitial nephritis**
>
> **Allergic**
>
> Many drugs but particularly:
> - Penicillins
> - Non-steroidal anti-inflammatory drugs (NSAIDs)
> - Proton pump inhibitors
> - Mesalazine (delayed)
>
> **Immune**
> - Autoimmune nephritis ± uveitis
> - Transplant rejection
>
> **Infections**
> - Acute bacterial pyelonephritis
> - Leptospirosis
> - Tuberculosis
> - Hantavirus
>
> **Toxic**
> - Myeloma light chains
> - Mushrooms (*Cortinarius*)

A Normal tubular histology

B Acute tubular necrosis

C Acute pyelonephritis

D Acute interstitial nephritis

Fig. 15.13 Tubular histopathology. A Normal tubular histology. The tubules are back to back. Brush borders can be seen on the luminal borders of cells in the proximal tubule. B Acute tubular necrosis. There are scattered breaks (B) in tubular basement membranes, swelling and vacuolation of tubular cells, and, in places, apoptosis and necrosis of tubular cells with shedding of cells into the lumen. During the regenerative phase, there is increased tubular mitotic activity. The interstitium (I) is oedematous and infiltrated by inflammatory cells. The glomeruli (not shown) are relatively normal, although there may be endothelial cell swelling and fibrin deposition. C Acute bacterial pyelonephritis. A widespread inflammatory infiltrate that includes many neutrophils is seen. Granulocyte casts (G) are forming within some dilated tubules (T). Other tubules are scarcely visible because of the extent of the inflammation and damage. D Acute (allergic) interstitial nephritis. In this patient who received a non-steroidal anti-inflammatory drug (NSAID), an extensive mononuclear cell infiltrate (no neutrophils) involving tubules (T) is seen. This inflammation does not involve the glomeruli (not shown). Sometimes eosinophils are prominent. Transplant rejection looks similar to this.

Pathophysiology

This disease may follow on from AIN that does not resolve, or may be associated with ingestion of various toxins and drugs, or with metabolic and chronic inflammatory diseases, as summarised in Box 15.19. In many patients, CIN presents at a late stage and no underlying cause can be identified. Genetic causes may underlie many of these cases (p. 404). Toxins that have been associated with CIN include those contained within the plant *Aristolochia clematitis* (birthwort). These are probably responsible for the severe nephrotoxicity that can be associated with treatment with herbal medicines in Asia and for Balkan nephropathy, which affects isolated rural communities in Bosnia, Bulgaria, Croatia, Romania and Serbia, possibly through contaminated flour. The nephropathy is commonly linked with tumours of the collecting system and is probably due to the mutagenic effects of the plant toxin on the urothelial epithelium. Ingestion of mushrooms within the *Cortinarius* genus can cause a devastating and irreversible renal tubular toxicity. It is encountered occasionally in Scandinavia and Scotland.

15.19 Causes of chronic interstitial nephritis

Acute interstitial nephritis

- Any of the causes of acute interstitial nephritis, if persistent (see Box 15.18)

Glomerulonephritis

- Varying degrees of interstitial inflammation occur in association with most types of inflammatory glomerulonephritis

Immune/inflammatory

- Sarcoidosis
- Sjögren's syndrome
- Chronic transplant rejection
- Systemic lupus erythematosus, primary autoimmune

Toxic

- *Aristolochia* in herbal medicines
- Lead
- Balkan nephropathy
- Mushrooms (*Cortinarius*)

Drugs

- All drugs causing acute interstitial nephritis
- Tenofovir
- Lithium toxicity
- Analgesic nephropathy
- Ciclosporin, tacrolimus

Infection

- Consequence of severe pyelonephritis

Congenital/developmental

- Vesico-ureteric reflux: associated but causation not clear
- Renal dysplasias: often associated with reflux
- Inherited: now well recognised but mechanisms unclear
- Other: Wilson's disease, sickle-cell nephropathy, medullary sponge kidney (nephrocalcinosis)

Metabolic and systemic diseases

- Calcium phosphate crystallisation after excessive phosphate administration (e.g. phosphate enemas in patients with chronic kidney disease)
- Hypokalaemia
- Hyperoxaluria

Clinical features

Most patients with CIN present in adult life with CKD, hypertension and small kidneys. Urinalysis abnormalities are non-specific. A minority present with salt-losing nephropathy, characterised by hypotension, polyuria and features of sodium and water depletion. People with CIN have an impairment of urine-concentrating ability and sodium conservation, which puts them at risk of AKI due to salt and water depletion during an acute illness. Renal tubular acidosis (p. 365) may complicate CIN but is seen most often in myeloma, sarcoidosis, cystinosis, amyloidosis and Sjögren's syndrome.

Management

Management is supportive in nature, with correction of acidosis and hyperkalaemia; replacement of fluid and electrolytes, as required; and renal replacement therapy if irreversible renal damage has occurred.

Papillary necrosis

The renal papillae lie within a hypertonic environment in the renal medulla, at the end of the vasa recta. They are susceptible to ischaemic damage because of this and can undergo necrosis when their vascular supply is impaired as the result of diabetes mellitus, sickle-cell disease or long-term ingestion of NSAIDs. The condition may occasionally occur in other diseases. There is an association with pyelonephritis but it is difficult to determine whether this is a cause of papillary necrosis or a complication. The clinical presentation is variable. Some patients are asymptomatic and clinically silent, whereas others present with renal colic and renal impairment as necrosed papillae slough off and cause ureteric obstruction. Urinalysis may be normal but more frequently haematuria and sterile pyuria are present. Significant proteinuria is unusual, unless there is renal failure. The imaging method of choice to make the diagnosis is CTU or intravenous pyelography. Management is based on relieving obstruction, where present, and withdrawal of the offending drugs.

Genetic renal diseases

The advent of modern genetic techniques such as next-generation sequencing has allowed us to understand the breadth of inherited renal diseases on a much deeper level than before.

Inherited glomerular diseases

Alport's syndrome

A number of uncommon diseases may involve the glomerulus in childhood but the most important one affecting adults is Alport's syndrome. Most cases arise from a mutation or deletion of the *COL4A5* gene on the X chromosome, which encodes type IV collagen, resulting in inheritance as an X-linked recessive disorder (p. 48). Mutations in *COL4A3* or *COL4A4* genes are less common and cause autosomal recessive disease. The accumulation of abnormal collagen results in a progressive degeneration of the GBM (Fig. 15.14). Affected patients progress from haematuria to ESRD in their late teens or twenties. Female carriers of *COL4A5* mutations usually have haematuria but less commonly develop significant renal disease. Some other basement membranes containing the same collagen isoforms are similarly involved, notably in the cochlea, so that Alport's syndrome is associated with sensorineural deafness and ocular abnormalities.

15

Fig. 15.14 Alport's syndrome. [A] Diagrammatic structure of the normal glomerular basement membrane (GBM). [B] The normal GBM (electron micrograph) contains mostly the tissue-specific (α3, α4 and α5) chains of type IV collagen. [C] In Alport's syndrome, this network is disrupted and replaced by α1 and α2 chains. Although the GBM appears structurally normal in early life, in time thinning appears, progressing to thickening, splitting and degeneration. *(B, C) Courtesy of Dr J. Collar, St Mary's Hospital, London.*

Angiotensin-converting enzyme (ACE) inhibitors may slow but not prevent loss of kidney function. Patients with Alport's syndrome are good candidates for renal replacement therapy (RRT), as they are young and usually otherwise healthy. They can develop an immune response to the normal collagen antigens present in the GBM of the donor kidney and, in a small minority, anti-GBM disease develops and destroys the allograft.

Thin glomerular basement membrane disease

In thin glomerular basement membrane disease there is glomerular bleeding, which is usually non-visible, without associated hypertension, proteinuria or a reduction in GFR. The glomeruli appear normal by light microscopy but, on electron microscopy, the GBM is abnormally thin. The condition may be familial and some patients are carriers of Alport mutations. This does not appear to account for all cases, and in many patients the cause is unclear. Monitoring of these patients is advisable, as proteinuria may develop in some and there appears to be an increased rate of progressive CKD in the long term.

Hereditary nephrotic syndrome

Many genes have been discovered that cause early-onset nephrotic syndrome, often with an FSGS pattern of injury. Inheritance may be autosomal dominant or recessive, the former conditions having a less severe and later-onset phenotype and often exhibiting incomplete penetrance. The involved genes almost all code for podocyte proteins, including nephrin ('Finnish-type' nephropathy) and podocin, which both cause early congenital nephrotic syndrome. Autosomal dominant mutations in various genes may cause FSGS as part of systemic syndromes; the genes include *INF2* (Charcot–Marie–Tooth disease), *LMX1B* (nail–patella syndrome) and *WT1* (abnormal genitalia, Wilms' tumour, mental retardation).

Inheriting variants in the *APOL1* gene, which is observed predominantly in people of West African ancestry, leads to a greatly increased risk of kidney disease including FSGS (p. 400).

Inherited tubulo-interstitial diseases

It has become evident in recent years that a significant number of cases of CKD with low or absent proteinuria have genetic causes, which may be inherited in an autosomal dominant or recessive pattern (Box 15.20). The histological pattern of injury is identical to other forms of CIN (p. 402). This is a heterogeneous group of inherited disorders. Small cysts are sometimes evident, explaining the previous name of medullary cystic kidney disease, but tubulo-interstitial nephritis is the predominant pattern of injury. Many of these conditions, especially those formerly known as nephronophthisis, are associated with retinal dystrophies and brain or other abnormalities, and some may be associated with hyperuricaemia or gout (*UMOD* or *HNF1-beta* mutations). Modern genetics have brought clarity to a disease spectrum comprising many different conditions with inexact previous names.

---

i **15.20 Hereditary tubulo-interstitial kidney diseases**

Inheritance	Gene(s)	Other name(s)	Clinical features
Autosomal dominant	*UMOD*	MCKD type 2 Juvenile hyperuricaemic nephropathy	Gout
	MUC1	MCKD type 1	Progressive CKD without other manifestations
	HNF1-beta	Juvenile hyperuricaemic nephropathy	Cystic kidneys, solitary kidney; gout; MODY; abnormal LFTs; pancreatic atrophy; hypomagnesaemia
	REN (codes for renin)	Juvenile hyperuricaemic nephropathy	Gout; hyperkalaemia; salt-losing nephropathy
Autosomal recessive	*NPHP* genes (17 discovered so far)	Nephronophthisis Part of many syndromes (Bardet–Biedl)	Common cause of paediatric ESRD Occurs earlier than AD interstitial nephritis Extrarenal manifestation common (learning difficulty, eye/limb problems)

(AD = autosomal dominant; CKD = chronic kidney disease; ESRD = end-stage renal disease; LFTs = liver function tests; MCKD = medullary cystic kidney disease; MODY = maturity-onset diabetes of the young)

Isolated defects of tubular function

An increasing number of disorders have been identified that are caused by specific defects in transporter molecules expressed in renal tubular cells. Only the most common are mentioned here. Renal glycosuria is a benign autosomal recessive defect of tubular reabsorption of glucose, caused by mutations of the sodium/glucose co-transporter *SGLT2*. Glucose appears in the urine in the presence of a normal blood glucose concentration. It is notable that *SGLT2* inhibitors have been developed as a treatment for diabetes mellitus and evidence suggests they may improve renal and cardiovascular outcomes.

Cystinuria is a rare condition, in which reabsorption of filtered cystine, ornithine, arginine and lysine is defective. It is caused by mutations in the *SLC3A1* amino acid transporter gene. The high concentration of cystine in urine leads to cystine stone formation (p. 431).

Other uncommon tubular disorders include hereditary hypophosphataemic rickets (p. 1052), in which reabsorption of filtered phosphate is reduced; nephrogenic diabetes insipidus (p. 687), in which the tubules are resistant to the effects of vasopressin (antidiuretic hormone, ADH); and Bartter's and Gitelman's syndromes, in which there is sodium-wasting and hypokalaemia (p. 361).

The term 'Fanconi's syndrome' is used to describe generalised proximal tubular dysfunction. The condition typically presents with low blood phosphate and uric acid concentrations, glycosuria, aminoaciduria and proximal renal tubular acidosis. In addition to the causes of interstitial nephritis described above, some congenital metabolic disorders are associated with Fanconi's syndrome, notably Wilson's disease, cystinosis and hereditary fructose intolerance.

Renal tubular acidosis describes the common end-point of a variety of diseases affecting distal (classical or type 1) or proximal (type 2) renal tubular function. These syndromes are described on page 365.

Cystic diseases of the kidney

It is common to encounter patients with a single renal cyst or even multiple cysts as an incidental finding, especially in those aged 50 years and over. Usually, these cysts are of no clinical consequence and are asymptomatic, but occasionally they can cause pain or haematuria. In addition, several specific diseases are recognised as being caused by the formation of multiple renal cysts. These are discussed in more detail below.

Adult polycystic kidney disease

Adult polycystic kidney disease (PKD) is a common condition, with a prevalence of approximately 1:1000, and is inherited as an autosomal dominant trait. Small cysts lined by tubular epithelium develop from infancy or childhood and enlarge slowly and irregularly. The surrounding normal kidney tissue is compressed and progressively damaged. Mutations in the *PKD1* gene account for 85% of cases and those in *PKD2* for about 15% (coding for polycystin 1 and 2, respectively). ESRD occurs in approximately 50% of patients with *PKD1* mutations, with a mean age of onset of 52 years, but in a minority of patients with *PKD2* mutations, with a mean age of onset of 69 years. It has been estimated that between 5% and 10% of patients on RRT have PKD.

> **15.21 Adult polycystic kidney disease: common clinical features**
>
> - Vague discomfort in loin or abdomen due to increasing mass of renal tissue
> - Acute loin pain or renal colic due to haemorrhage into a cyst
> - Hypertension
> - Haematuria (with little or no proteinuria)
> - Urinary tract or cyst infections
> - Renal failure

Clinical features

Common clinical features are shown in Box 15.21. Affected people are usually asymptomatic until later life but hypertension usually occurs from the age of 20 onwards. One or both kidneys may be palpable and the surface may feel nodular. About 30% of patients with PKD also have hepatic cysts (see Fig. 22.39, p. 893) but disturbance of liver function is rare. Sometimes (almost always in women) this causes massive and symptomatic hepatomegaly, usually concurrent with renal enlargement but occasionally with only minor renal involvement. Berry aneurysms of cerebral vessels are an associated feature in about 5% of patients with PKD. This feature appears to be largely restricted to certain families (and presumably specific mutations). Mitral and aortic regurgitation is frequent but rarely severe, and colonic diverticula and abdominal wall hernias may occur.

Investigations

The diagnosis is usually based on family history, clinical findings and ultrasound examination. Ultrasound demonstrates cysts in approximately 95% of affected patients over the age of 20 and is the screening method of choice, but may not detect small developing cysts in younger subjects. Cysts may also be identified by other imaging modalities, such as MRI (Fig. 15.15). Simple renal cysts may occur in normal individuals but are uncommon below the age of 30. The following criteria exist for an ultrasound diagnosis of PKD in patients with a family history but unknown genotype:

- 15–39 years of age: at least three unilateral or bilateral kidney cysts
- 40–59 years of age: at least two cysts in each kidney
- 60 years or older: at least four cysts in each kidney.

It is now possible to make a molecular diagnosis by mutation screening of *PDK1* or *PDK2* but this is seldom used in routine clinical practice because the genes are so large and have many possible mutations. Next-generation sequencing allows faster and simpler genetic screening for *PKD1* and *PKD2*. This is likely to be used in cases with an uncertain diagnosis (young patients, few cysts, lack of family history), for workup of living kidney donors, or for screening for mutations associated with a worse prognosis (see below). Screening for intracranial aneurysms is not generally indicated but can be done by MR angiography in families with a history of subarachnoid haemorrhage. The yield of screening is low, however, and the risk:benefit ratio of intervention in asymptomatic aneurysms in this disease is not clear.

Management

Blood pressure control is important because cardiovascular morbidity and mortality are so common in renal disease, but evidence is lacking that controlling blood pressure to generally recommended CKD targets (e.g. <130/80 mmHg) influences renal outcomes. There are data suggesting that targeting a very low blood pressure (<110/75 mmHg) with ACE inhibitors or angiotensin II

15

Fig. 15.15 MRI images of the kidneys. [A] Normal kidneys.
[B] Polycystic kidneys; although the kidney enlargement is extreme, this patient had only slightly reduced GFR.

receptor blocker (ARBs) leads to slower increases in kidney volume, but no improvements in eGFR decline were observed and these targets are often not tolerated. This tight blood pressure target did lead to a greater decline in left ventricular mass index, which may have implications for improved cardiovascular risk later in life.

The vasopressin V2 receptor antagonist tolvaptan may retard kidney volume increase and slow the rate of GFR decline. It has now been licensed in many countries for patients at high risk of progression. Risk factors for progression include large kidneys (more specifically height-adjusted kidney volume), truncating *PKD1* mutations, and family history of early progression, as well as male sex, hypertension, proteinuria and development of early symptomatic cysts.

Patients with PKD are usually good candidates for dialysis and transplantation. Sometimes kidneys are so large that one or both have to be removed to make space for a renal transplant. Otherwise, they are usually left in situ unless they are a source of pain or infection.

Other cystic diseases

Renal cysts and diabetes syndrome is caused by *HNF1-beta* mutations (see above); it has a varying renal phenotype that often causes cysts but also may cause a tubulo-interstitial pattern of injury or congenital absence of a kidney. It also causes a form of MODY (p. 733).

Autosomal recessive PKD is caused by mutations in the *PKHD1* gene, encoding fibrocystin. It is less common than autosomal dominant PKD (about 1:20 000 live births). Patients often present in infancy or young childhood with renal cysts and congenital hepatic fibrosis.

Some uncommon autosomal dominantly inherited conditions are associated with multiple renal cysts and tumours in adult life. In tuberous sclerosis (p. 1264), replacement of renal tissue by multiple angiomyolipomas may occasionally cause renal failure in adults. Patients may also develop renal cysts and have a higher risk of renal cell carcinoma. Other organs affected include the skin (adenoma sebaceum on the face) and brain (causing seizures and mental retardation). The von Hippel–Lindau syndrome (p. 1132) is associated with multiple renal cysts, renal adenomas and renal adenocarcinoma. Other involved organs include the central nervous system (haemangioblastomas), pancreas (serous cystadenomas) and adrenals (phaeochromocytoma).

A number of other rarer inherited cystic diseases are recognised that have some similarities to PKD but distinct genetic causes. Multicystic dysplastic kidneys are often unilateral and are a developmental abnormality found in children. Most of these seem to involute during growth, leaving a solitary kidney in adults.

Acquired cystic kidney disease can develop in patients with a very long history of renal failure, so it is not an inherited cystic disease. It is associated with increased erythropoietin production and sometimes with the development of renal cell carcinoma.

Renal vascular diseases

Diseases that affect renal blood vessels may cause renal ischaemia, leading to acute or chronic kidney disease or secondary hypertension. The rising prevalence of atherosclerosis and diabetes mellitus in ageing populations has made renovascular disease an important cause of ESRD.

Renal artery stenosis

A stenosis of more than 50% may be observed on imaging of the renal arteries in up to 20% of older patients with advanced kidney disease; however, a haemodynamically significant effect will be present in only a relatively small proportion. Renal artery stenosis is the most common cause of secondary hypertension, with an estimated prevalence of about 2% in unselected patients, but this may increase to 4% in older patients who have evidence of atherosclerotic disease elsewhere. Most cases of renal artery stenosis are caused by atherosclerosis but fibromuscular dysplasia involving the vessel wall may be responsible in younger patients. Rare causes include vasculitis, thromboembolism and aneurysms of the renal artery.

Pathophysiology

Renal artery stenosis results in a reduction in renal perfusion pressure, which activates the renin–angiotensin system, leading to increased circulating levels of angiotensin II. This results in hypertension by provoking vasoconstriction and increasing aldosterone production by the adrenal, causing sodium retention by the renal tubules (p. 351). Significant reduction of renal blood flow occurs when there is more than 70% narrowing of the artery, and this is commonly associated with distal, post-stenotic dilatation. Atherosclerotic lesions are typically ostial and are associated with more widespread atherosclerosis within the aorta and other vessels, particularly the iliac vessels. There is often concurrent small-vessel disease in affected kidneys, due to subclinical atheroemboli. As the stenosis becomes more severe, global renal ischaemia leads to shrinkage of the affected kidney and may cause renal failure if bilateral, or if unilateral in the presence of a single kidney (ischaemic nephropathy).

In younger patients, fibromuscular dysplasia is a more likely cause of renal artery stenosis. This is an uncommon disorder of unknown cause. It is characterised by hypertrophy of the media (medial fibroplasia), which narrows the artery but rarely leads to total occlusion. It may be associated with disease in other arteries; for example, those who have carotid artery dissections are more likely to have renal arteries with this appearance. It most commonly presents with hypertension in patients aged 15–30 years, and women are affected more frequently than men. Irregular narrowing (beading) may occur in the distal renal artery and this sometimes extends into the intrarenal branches of the vessel. Rarely, renal artery stenosis may occur as a complication of large-vessel vasculitis, such as Takayasu's arteritis and polyarteritis nodosa (pp. 1041 and 1042).

Untreated, atheromatous renal artery stenosis is thought to progress to complete arterial occlusion in about 15% of cases. This figure increases with more severe degrees of stenosis. If the progression is gradual, collateral vessels may develop and some function may be preserved, preventing infarction and loss of kidney structure. Conversely, at least 85% of patients with renal artery stenosis will not develop progressive renal impairment, and many patients die from coronary, cerebral or other vascular disease rather than renal failure. Unfortunately, methods of predicting which patients are at risk of progression or who will respond to treatment are still imperfect.

Clinical features

Renal artery stenosis can present in various ways including hypertension, acute pulmonary oedema, progressive renal failure (with bilateral disease) or a deterioration in renal function when ACE inhibitors or ARBs are administered. Although many patients experience a slight drop in GFR when commencing these drugs, an increase in serum creatinine of 30% or more raises the possibility of renal artery stenosis. Acute pulmonary oedema is particularly characteristic of bilateral renovascular disease. It typically occurs at night and is associated with severe hypertension, often in the context of normal or only mildly impaired renal and cardiac function. Clinical evidence of generalised vascular disease may be observed, particularly in the legs and in older patients with atherosclerotic renal artery stenosis. Clinical features associated with an increased risk of renal artery stenosis in hypertensive patients are summarised in Box 15.22. However, given the risk of imaging and angiography in patients with renal disease (see Box 15.4, p. 390), further investigation should only be performed if intervention is being contemplated (see below).

Investigations

When appropriate, imaging of the renal vasculature with either CT angiography or MR angiography should be performed to confirm the diagnosis (Fig. 15.16). Both give good views of the main renal arteries, the vessels predominantly involved and the most amenable to intervention. Biochemical testing may reveal impaired renal function and an elevated plasma renin activity, sometimes with hypokalaemia due to hyperaldosteronism. Ultrasound may also reveal a discrepancy in size between the two kidneys,

although this is insufficiently sensitive or specific to be of value in diagnosis of renovascular disease in hypertensive patients.

Management

The first-line management in patients with renal artery stenosis is medical therapy with antihypertensive drugs, supplemented, where appropriate, by statins and low-dose aspirin in those with atherosclerotic disease. Interventions to correct the vessel narrowing should be considered in:

* young patients (age below 40) suspected of having renal artery stenosis
* those whose blood pressure cannot easily be controlled with antihypertensive agents
* those who have a history of 'flash' pulmonary oedema
* those with accelerated phase (malignant) hypertension
* those whose renal function is deteriorating.

The most commonly used technique is angioplasty. The best results are obtained in non-atheromatous fibromuscular dysplasia, where correction of the stenosis has a high chance of success in improving blood pressure and protecting renal function. Beyond the indications above, angioplasty and stenting is now rarely

15.22 Presentation and clinical features of renal artery stenosis

Renal artery stenosis is more likely if:

* hypertension is severe, of recent onset or difficult to control
* kidneys are asymmetrical in size
* flash pulmonary oedema occurs repeatedly*
* there is peripheral vascular disease of the lower limbs
* there is renal impairment*
* renal function has deteriorated on angiotensin-converting enzyme inhibitors or angiotensin II receptor blockers

*Particularly with bilateral disease.

Fig. 15.16 Renal artery stenosis. A magnetic resonance angiogram following injection of contrast. The abdominal aorta is severely irregular and atheromatous. The left renal artery is stenosed (arrow).

15

performed in atherosclerotic disease, as randomised trials such as ASTRAL and CORAL have produced no convincing evidence for overall benefit in terms of renal function, blood pressure control or cardiovascular outcomes. The risks of angioplasty and stenting include renal artery occlusion, renal infarction and atheroemboli (p. 409) from manipulations in a severely diseased aorta. Small-vessel disease distal to the stenosis may preclude substantial functional recovery.

Acute renal infarction

This is an uncommon condition that occurs as the result of sudden occlusion of the renal arteries. The presentation is typically with loin pain of acute onset, usually in association with non-visible haematuria, but pain may be absent in some cases. Severe hypertension is common but not universal. Blood levels of lactate dehydrogenase (LDH) and CRP are commonly raised. The condition may be caused by thrombosis of a renal artery or by thromboemboli from a distant source, when occlusion may occur in branch arteries distal to the main renal artery. This can cause multiple infarcts within the renal parenchyma of both kidneys, which may be visualised by CT scanning. If occlusion of the main renal arteries is bilateral or if there is occlusion in a single functioning kidney, the presentation is with AKI and the patient is typically anuric. Patients with bilateral occlusion usually have evidence of widespread vascular disease and may show evidence of aortic occlusion, with absent femoral pulses and reduced lower limb perfusion. Management is largely supportive, and includes anticoagulation if a source of thromboembolism is identified. It is sometimes possible to perform stenting of an acutely blocked main renal artery to try to restore renal blood flow; in most cases, however, presentation is too late to salvage renal function.

Diseases of small intrarenal vessels

Thrombotic microangiopathies

A number of conditions are associated with acute damage and occlusion of small blood vessels (arterioles and capillaries) in the kidney (Box 15.23) and other organs. A common feature of these syndromes is microangiopathic haemolytic anaemia (MAHA), in which haemolysis and red cell fragmentation arise as consequences of damage incurred to red blood cells during passage through the abnormal vessels. The red blood cell fragments (schistocytes) may be observed on blood films, together with laboratory features of intravascular haemolysis (p. 947), including an elevated unconjugated bilirubin level, raised serum LDH concentration and decreased circulating levels of haptoglobin. A reticulocytosis is often seen. Endothelial injury is pronounced, leading to increased platelet adherence and a marked reduction in the platelet count. These abnormal blood parameters should alert the physician to the possibility of a thrombotic microangiopathy and may also be useful in monitoring response to treatment. The key is to distinguish between the various aetiologies, as the management differs according to the primary cause (Box 15.23).

Haemolytic uraemic syndrome

Haemolytic uraemic syndrome (HUS) is characterised by thrombotic microangiopathy that predominantly affects the renal microcirculation, with involvement of other organs (including the brain) observed in more severe cases.

The most common cause of HUS is infection with organisms that produce enterotoxins called Shiga-like toxin or verotoxins. The organisms most commonly implicated are enterohaemorrhagic *Escherichia coli* (p. 263) and *Shigella dysenteriae* (p. 265). The

i | 15.23 Thrombotic microangiopathies associated with acute renal damage

Condition	Typical features	Management
Primary thrombotic microangiopathies		
Haemolytic uraemic syndrome:	Renal failure prominent in all causes	
Shiga toxin +ve HUS	Bloody diarrhoea; check stool for *Escherichia coli* O157:H7	Supportive therapy
Complement-mediated	Positive family history; screen for complement factor mutations	Plasma exchange, eculizumab
Drug-induced: quinine, calcineurin and VEGF-A inhibitors	Drug exposure, fever with quinine	Cessation of offending drug
Thrombotic thrombocytopenic purpura	Neurological manifestations prominent; check ADAMTS-13 activity	Plasma exchange (p. 979)
Thrombotic microangiopathy associated with systemic disorders		
Disseminated intravascular coagulation (DIC)	Clotting system involvement: elevated D-dimers, low fibrinogen, prolonged PT and APTT	Treatment of primary cause (p. 979)
Malignancy	May occur with breast, prostate, lung, pancreas and GI tumours	Treatment of tumour where possible
Systemic sclerosis	Cutaneous features of systemic sclerosis	Blood pressure control with ACE inhibitors (p. 1037)
Pre-eclampsia and HELLP syndrome	Typically in third trimester; abnormal LFTs	Resolution with delivery (p. 1276)
Malignant hypertension	Blood pressure typically very high; evidence of hypertensive retinopathy including papilloedema	Blood pressure control

(ACE = angiotensin-converting enzyme; ADAMTS-13 = a disintegrin and metalloproteinase with a thrombospondin type 1 motif, member 13; APTT = activated partial thromboplastin time; GI = gastrointestinal; HELLP = haemolysis, elevated liver enzymes and low platelets; HUS = haemolytic uraemic syndrome; LFTs = liver function tests; PT = prothrombin time; VEGF = vascular endothelial growth factor)

E. coli O157:H7 serotype is the best known but other serotypes that produce verotoxins may also be responsible. Although these bacteria live as commensals in the gut of cattle and other livestock, they can cause haemorrhagic diarrhoea in humans when the infection is contracted from contaminated food products, water or other infected individuals. In a proportion of cases, verotoxin produced by the organisms enters the circulation and binds to specific glycolipid receptors that are expressed on the surface of microvascular endothelial cells. Most cases are sporadic but large outbreaks related to poor sanitation may occur. In developed countries, Shiga-like toxin-associated HUS is now the most common cause of AKI in children. Recovery is good in most patients but sometimes RRT may be required for up to 14 days. No other specific treatments have been shown to accelerate renal recovery.

In the absence of bloody diarrhoea, other (atypical) causes of HUS should be considered: in particular, abnormalities of the complement system. Familial forms are due to mutations in various genes that encode components or regulators of the complement cascade, including factor H (*CFH*), factor B (*CFB*), membrane co-factor protein (*MCP*) and complement component 3 (*C3*). The penetrance of familial HUS is incomplete, indicating that environmental triggers are also involved: often infection, including diarrhoea. Sporadic cases may be associated with the development of autoantibodies to complement factor H. In addition to supportive care, including RRT if necessary, management of complement-mediated HUS includes plasma exchange to replace complement component and remove pathogenic autoantibodies. Recently, impressive results have been reported with the anti-C5 monoclonal antibody, eculizumab, which binds to C5, thereby preventing activation of the terminal complement cascade.

Thrombotic thrombocytopenic purpura

Like HUS, thrombotic thrombocytopenic purpura (TTP) is characterised by microangiopathic haemolytic anaemia and thrombocytopenia; in contrast, however, the brain is more commonly affected in TTP and involvement of the kidney is usually less prominent. TTP is an autoimmune disorder caused by antibodies against ADAMTS-13, which is involved in regulating platelet aggregation, and a low (< 10%) serum ADAMTS-13 activity level may be useful in distinguishing TTP from HUS. This distinction is important, as early therapy with plasma exchange is crucial in TTP. More details are provided on page 979.

Cholesterol emboli

These present with renal impairment, haematuria, proteinuria and sometimes eosinophilia with inflammatory features that can mimic a small-vessel vasculitis. The symptoms are provoked by showers of cholesterol-containing microemboli, arising in atheromatous plaques in major arteries. The diagnosis should be suspected when these clinical features occur in patients with widespread atheromatous disease, who have undergone interventions such as surgery or arteriography. They may also be precipitated by anticoagulants and thrombolytic agents. On clinical examination, signs of large-vessel disease and microvascular occlusion in the lower limbs (ischaemic toes, livedo reticularis) are common but not invariable (Fig. 15.17). There is no specific treatment.

Small-vessel vasculitis

Renal disease caused by small-vessel vasculitis usually presents with a clinical picture typical of a glomerulonephritis (see Figs 15.9 and 15.12C, pp. 393 and 399). More information is given on page 410.

Fig. 15.17 The foot of a patient who suffered extensive atheroembolism following coronary artery stenting.

Renal involvement in systemic conditions

The kidneys may be directly involved in a number of multisystem diseases or secondarily affected by diseases of other organs. Involvement may be at a pre-renal, renal (glomerular or interstitial) or post-renal level. Many of the diseases are described in other sections of this chapter or in other chapters of the book.

Diabetes mellitus

Diabetic nephropathy is the most common cause of CKD in developed countries. In patients with diabetes, there is a steady advance from moderately elevated albuminuria (microalbuminuria) to dipstick-positive proteinuria, in association with evolving hypertensive and progressive renal failure, as described on page 757. Few patients require renal biopsy to establish the diagnosis, but atypical features such as very rapid progression of proteinuria/decline in renal function or the absence of other microvascular damage, including retinopathy, should lead to suspicion that an alternative condition could be present.

Management with ACE inhibitors and ARBs to slow progression is described on page 757. In some patients, proteinuria may be eradicated and progression completely halted, even if renal function is abnormal, although most still have progressive disease, albeit at a slower rate. Emerging evidence suggests that SGLT2 inhibitors, such as empagliflozin, a new agent for diabetes that causes glycosuria (p. 748), may lead to improved cardiovascular and renal outcomes, at the expense of increased genital infections.

Multiple myeloma

In myeloma, a malignant clone of plasma cells produces a paraprotein, often a monoclonal light chain (p. 966). Renal manifestations are dominated by these toxic light chains, which may cause a variety of insults (Box 15.24). Hypercalcaemia may also occur due to bony metastases.

Hepatic–renal disease

Severe hepatic dysfunction may cause a haemodynamically mediated type of renal failure, hepatorenal syndrome (HRS), described on page 864. Patients with chronic liver disease are also predisposed to develop AKI (acute tubular necrosis) in response to relatively minor insults, including bleeding, diuretic therapy and infection. Differentiating true HRS from AKI can be difficult. Patients with true HRS are often difficult to treat

15

i	15.24 Renal manifestations of multiple myeloma		
Condition	**Presentation**	**Pathogenesis**	
Cast nephropathy ('myeloma kidney')	AKI Little/no proteinuria	Light chains combine with Tamm–Horsfall protein precipitating in tubules	
Fanconi's syndrome	Aminoaciduria, phosphaturia, glycosuria Proximal (type II) RTA	Proximal tubular injury due to light chain deposition in tubular epithelium	
AL (primary) amyloidosis*	Proteinuria/nephrotic syndrome Renal impairment	Misfolded lights chains (usually lambda) form amyloid, which is deposited in glomeruli	
Monoclonal immunoglobulin deposition disease*	Proteinuria (may be in nephrotic range) Renal impairment	Usually light chains (frequently kappa) are deposited in glomeruli, causing a nodular glomerulosclerosis	
Hypercalcaemia	Thirst, polyuria, bony and abdominal pain, headache	Bony destruction from metastases	

*These may also occur as primary conditions without myeloma being present.
(AKI = acute kidney injury; RTA = renal tubular acidosis)

by dialysis and have a poor prognosis. Where treatment is justified – for example, if there is a good chance of recovery or of a liver transplant – slow or continuous treatments are less likely to precipitate or exacerbate hepatic encephalopathy. IgA nephropathy (p. 400) is more common in patients with chronic liver disease.

Sarcoidosis

The most common renal manifestation of sarcoidosis is hypercalcaemia from 1-α-vitamin D formation in granulomas. Less commonly, it may lead to a granulomatous interstitial nephritis, sometimes presenting acutely, where renal function may improve with glucocorticoid therapy. Postmortem examinations reveal a chronic interstitial nephritis in 15–30% of patients with sarcoidosis but clinically relevant disease appears to be much less common.

Systemic vasculitis

Small-vessel vasculitis (p. 1040) commonly affects the kidneys, with rapid and profound impairment of glomerular function. Histologically, there is a focal inflammatory glomerulonephritis, usually with focal necrosis (see Box 15.15, p. 398, and Fig. 15.12C, p. 399) and often with crescentic changes (see Fig. 15.12C). Typically, the patient is systemically unwell with an acute phase response, weight loss and arthralgia. In some patients, it presents as a kidney-limited disorder, with rapidly deteriorating renal function and crescentic nephritis (a rapidly progressive glomerulonephritis). In others, pulmonary haemorrhage may occur, which can be life-threatening.

The most important cause is ANCA vasculitis (p. 1041). Two subtypes are recognised, microscopic polyangiitis (MPA) and granulomatosis with polyangiitis. Both may present with glomerulonephritis and pulmonary haemorrhage, along with constitutional symptoms. Gastrointestinal involvement and neuropathy may also occur. Serological testing for antibodies to myeloperoxidase (MPO) and proteinase 3 (PR3) is usually positive but these are not specific and a biopsy of affected tissue should be obtained, if possible, to confirm the diagnosis.

The standard treatment of glomerulonephritis associated with systemic vasculitis is high-dose glucocorticoids combined with cyclophosphamide, or mycophenolate mofetil (p. 1041). Recent studies indicate that rituximab (p. 1006), when combined with high-dose glucocorticoids, is as effective as oral cyclophosphamide and high-dose glucocorticoids in the treatment of ANCA-associated vasculitis. Plasma exchange can offer additional benefit in patients with progressive renal damage who are not responding adequately to immunosuppressive therapy.

Glomerulonephritis secondary to vasculitis may rarely be seen in rheumatoid arthritis, SLE and cryoglobulinaemia, although SLE usually involves the kidney in different ways (see below).

Medium- to large-vessel vasculitis, such as polyarteritis nodosa (p. 1042), does not cause glomerulonephritis but can cause hypertension, renal aneurysms and infarction if the renal vessels are involved.

Systemic sclerosis

Renal involvement is a serious complication of systemic sclerosis, which is more likely to occur in diffuse cutaneous systemic sclerosis (DCSS) than in limited cutaneous systemic sclerosis (LCSS) (p. 1037). The renal lesion is caused by intimal cell proliferation and luminal narrowing of intrarenal arteries and arterioles. There is intense intrarenal vasospasm and plasma renin activity is markedly elevated. Renal involvement usually presents clinically with severe hypertension, microangiopathic features and progressive oliguric renal failure ('scleroderma renal crisis'). Use of ACE inhibitors to control the hypertension has improved the 1-year survival from 20% to 75% but about 50% of patients continue to require RRT. Onset or acceleration of the syndrome after glucocorticoid use or cessation of ACE inhibitors is well described.

Systemic lupus erythematosus

Subclinical renal involvement, with non-visible haematuria and proteinuria but minimally impaired or normal renal function, is common in systemic lupus erythematosus (SLE). Usually, this is due to glomerular disease, although interstitial nephritis may also occur, particularly in patients with overlap syndromes such as mixed connective tissue disease and Sjögren's syndrome (p. 1038).

Almost any histological pattern of glomerular disease can be observed in SLE and the clinical presentation ranges from florid, rapidly progressive glomerulonephritis to nephrotic syndrome. The most common presentation is with subacute disease and inflammatory features (haematuria, hypertension, variable renal impairment), accompanied by heavy proteinuria that often reaches nephrotic levels. In severely affected patients, the most common histological pattern is a proliferative glomerulonephritis with substantial deposits of immunoglobulins on immunofluorescence. Randomised controlled trials have shown that the risk of ESRD in lupus nephritis is significantly reduced by high-dose glucocorticoids administered in combination with cyclophosphamide, usually given as regular intravenous pulses. Subsequently, it has been shown that the combination of glucocorticoids and mycophenolate mofetil is equally as effective, for both induction and maintenance treatment.

Many patients with SLE who develop ESRD go into remission, possibly because of immunosuppression related to the ESRD.

Patients with ESRD caused by SLE are usually good candidates for dialysis and transplantation. Although it may recur in renal allografts, the immunosuppression required to prevent allograft rejection usually controls SLE.

Sickle-cell nephropathy

Improved survival of patients with sickle-cell disease (p. 951) means that a high proportion now live to develop chronic complications of microvascular occlusion. In the kidney, these changes are most pronounced in the medulla, where the vasa recta are the site of sickling because of hypoxia and hypertonicity. Loss of urinary concentrating ability and polyuria are the earliest changes; distal renal tubular acidosis and impaired potassium excretion are typical. Papillary necrosis may also occur (p. 403). A minority of patients develop ESRD. This is managed according to the usual principles, but response to recombinant erythropoietin is poor because of the haemoglobinopathy. Patients with sickle trait have an increased incidence of unexplained non-visible haematuria.

Acute kidney injury

Acute kidney injury (AKI), previously referred to as acute renal failure, is not a diagnosis; rather it describes the situation where there is a sudden and often reversible loss of renal function, which develops over days or weeks and is often accompanied by a reduction in urine volume. Approximately 7% of all hospitalised patients and 20% of acutely ill patients develop AKI. In uncomplicated AKI mortality is low, even when RRT is required. In AKI associated with sepsis and multiple organ failure, mortality is 50–70% and the outcome is usually determined by the severity of the underlying disorder and other complications, rather than by kidney injury itself. Elderly patients are at higher risk of developing AKI and have a worse outcome (Box 15.25).

Pathophysiology

There are many causes of AKI and it is frequently multifactorial. It is helpful to classify it into three subtypes:
- 'pre-renal', when perfusion to the kidney is reduced
- 'renal', when the primary insult affects the kidney itself
- 'post-renal', when there is obstruction to urine flow at any point from the tubule to the urethra (Fig. 15.18).

In pre-renal AKI, a reduction in perfusion reduces GFR. If the insult is not corrected, this may lead to 'renal' injury: namely, acute tubular necrosis (ATN). Histologically, the kidney shows inflammatory changes, focal breaks in the tubular basement membrane and interstitial oedema (see Fig. 15.13B, p. 402). Dead tubular cells may also be shed into the tubular lumen, leading to tubular obstruction. Although tubular cell damage is the dominant feature under the microscope, there may also be profound alterations in the renal microcirculation. Renal AKI may be caused by nephrotoxic drugs (p. 426), which can cause ATN or allergic interstitial nephritis. The other common 'renal' cause is glomerulonephritis, in which there is direct inflammatory damage to the glomeruli (p. 416).

Post-renal AKI occurs as the result of obstruction to the renal tract. This leads to elevation of intraluminal ureteral pressure transmitted to the nephrons after prolonged obstruction, with a subsequent fall in GFR. If the obstruction is not relieved, the low GFR is maintained by a drop in renal blood flow rate via thromboxane A_2 and angiotensin II. This leads to chronic

Fig. 15.18 Causes of acute kidney injury.

PRE-RENAL

Impaired perfusion:
- Cardiac failure
- Sepsis
- Blood loss
- Dehydration
- Vascular occlusion

RENAL

Glomerulonephritis
Small-vessel vasculitis
Acute tubular necrosis
- Drugs
- Toxins
- Prolonged hypotension
Interstitial nephritis
- Drugs
- Toxins
- Inflammatory disease
- Infection

POST-RENAL

Urinary calculi (bilateral)
Retroperitoneal fibrosis
Benign prostatic enlargement
Bladder cancer
Prostate cancer
Cervical cancer
Urethral stricture/valves
Meatal stenosis/phimosis

renal injury over time (several weeks). Recovery of renal function depends on the duration of obstruction and also the pre-morbid GFR.

Clinical features

Early recognition and intervention is important in AKI; all emergency admissions to hospital should have renal function, blood pressure, temperature and pulse checked on arrival and should undergo a risk assessment for the likelihood of developing AKI. This includes looking at coexisting diseases such as diabetes and vascular and liver disease, which make AKI more likely, as well as gathering information on drug treatments such as ACE inhibitors and NSAIDs, which may be associated with renal dysfunction. If a patient is found to have a high serum creatinine, it is important to establish whether this is an acute or acute-on-chronic phenomenon, or a sign of CKD (see Fig. 15.22, p. 416). Previous measurements of renal function can be of great value in differentiating these possibilities. Patients with AKI need to be assessed quickly to determine the likely underlying cause. Clinical features and pertinent investigations for the different causes of AKI are shown in Box 15.25. Various criteria have been proposed to classify AKI and to help identify high-risk patients, guide treatment and provide information regarding prognosis but are mostly used in a research setting to standardise diagnosis. The most commonly used are the KDIGO, AKIN and RIFLE criteria.

Pre-renal AKI

Patients with pre-renal AKI are typically hypotensive and tachycardic with signs of poor peripheral perfusion, such as delayed capillary return. Tachycardia and postural hypotension (a fall in blood pressure of >20/10 mmHg from lying to standing) are valuable signs of early hypovolaemia. Many patients with sepsis

15

i	**15.25 Categorising acute kidney injury based on history, examination and investigations**		
Type of AKI	**History**	**Examination**	**Investigations**
Pre-renal	Volume depletion (vomiting, diarrhoea, burns, haemorrhage) Drugs (diuretics, ACE inhibitors, ARBs, NSAIDs, calcineurin inhibitors, iodinated contrast) Liver disease Cardiac failure	Low BP (including postural drop) Tachycardia Weight decrease Dry mucous membranes and increased skin turgor JVP not visible even when lying down	Urine Na <20 mmol/L Fractional excretion Na <1% High urea:creatinine ratio Urinalysis bland
Renal ATN	Prolonged pre-renal state Sepsis Toxic ATN: drugs (aminoglycosides, cisplatin, tenofovir, methotrexate, iodinated contrast) Other (rhabdomyolysis, snake bite, *Amanita* mushrooms)	Vital signs Fluid assessment Limbs for compartment syndrome	Urine Na >40 mmol/L Fractional excretion Na ≥1% Dense granular ('muddy brown') casts Creatine kinase
Glomerular	Rash, weight loss, arthralgia Chest symptoms (pulmonary renal syndromes) IV drug use	Hypertension Oedema Purpuric rash, uveitis, arthritis	Proteinuria, haematuria Red cell casts, dysmorphic red cells ANCA, anti-GBM, ANA, C3 and C4 Viral hepatitis screen, HIV Renal biopsy
Tubulo-interstitial	Interstitial nephritis: drugs (PPIs, penicillins, NSAIDs) Sarcoidosis Tubular obstruction: 1. Myeloma (cast nephropathy) 2. Tubular crystal nephropathy: Drugs (aciclovir, indinavir, triamterene, methotrexate) Oxalate (fat malabsorption, ethylene glycol) Urate (tumour lysis)	Fever Rash	Leucocyturia Eosinophiluria (and a peripheral eosinophilia) White cell casts Minimal proteinuria Paraprotein Calcium (myeloma, sarcoidosis) Urine microscopy for crystals Serum urate Urine collection for oxalate
Vascular (including renal infarction, renal vein thrombosis, cholesterol emboli, malignant hypertension)	Flank pain, trauma Anticoagulation Recent angiography (cholesterol emboli) Nephrotic syndrome (renal vein thrombosis) Systemic sclerosis (renal crisis) Diarrhoea (HUS)	BP (malignant hypertension) Fundoscopy Livedo reticularis (cholesterol emboli) Sclerodactyly	Normal urinalysis or some haematuria C3 and C4 (cholesterol emboli, TMA) Doppler renal ultrasound CT angiography Platelets, haemolytic screen, LDH Consider ADAMTS13 and complement genetics (if TMA)
Post-renal	Prostate cancer history Neurogenic bladder Cervical carcinoma Retroperitoneal fibrosis Bladder outlet symptoms	Rectal examination (prostate and anal tone) Distended bladder Pelvic mass	Urinalysis frequently normal (may reveal haematuria depending on cause) Renal ultrasound (hydronephrosis) Isotope renogram (delayed excretion) if ultrasound inconclusive

(ACE = angiotensin-converting enzyme; ANA = antinuclear antibody; ANCA = antineutrophil cytoplasmic antibody; ARBs = angiotensin receptor blockers; BP = blood pressure; GBM = glomerular basement membrane; HIV = human immunodeficiency virus; HUS = haemolytic uraemic syndrome; JVP = jugular venous pulse; LDH = lactate dehydrogenase; Na = sodium; NSAIDs = non-steroidal anti-inflammatory drugs; PPIs = proton pump inhibitors; TMA = thrombotic microangiopathy)

initially present with poor peripheral perfusion, as mentioned above, but then show evidence of peripheral vasodilatation once they have undergone initial resuscitation with intravenous fluids. However, this is accompanied by relative underfilling of the arterial tree and the kidney responds as it would to absolute hypovolaemia, with renal vasoconstriction. It is important to note that pre-renal AKI may also occur without systemic hypotension, particularly in patients taking NSAIDs or ACE inhibitors (Fig. 15.19). The cause of hypotension is often obvious, but concealed blood loss can occur into the gastrointestinal tract, retroperitoneum, following trauma (particularly with pelvic and femoral fractures), and into the pregnant uterus. Large volumes of intravascular fluid may also be lost into tissues after crush injuries or burns, and in severe inflammatory skin diseases or sepsis. Uncorrected renal hypoperfusion causing pre-renal azotaemia may progress to ATN.

Renal AKI

Factors that can help differentiate the various causes of intrinsic renal AKI are summarised in Box 15.25. Patients with

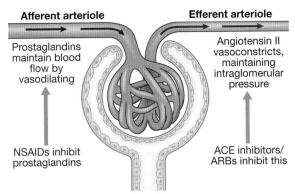

Afferent arteriole

Efferent arteriole

Prostaglandins maintain blood flow by vasodilating

Angiotensin II vasoconstricts, maintaining intraglomerular pressure

NSAIDs inhibit prostaglandins

ACE inhibitors/ ARBs inhibit this

Fig. 15.19 Renal haemodynamics and autoregulation of glomerular filtration rate (GFR). It is evident from this figure how angiotensin-converting enzyme (ACE) inhibitors/angiotensin receptor blockers (ARBs) may be associated with profound drops in GFR in the context of bilateral renal artery stenosis or intravascular volume depletion (which decrease perfusion to afferent arterioles). (NSAIDs = non-steroidal anti-inflammatory drugs)

glomerulonephritis demonstrate haematuria and proteinuria, and may have clinical manifestations of an underlying disease, such as SLE or systemic vasculitis. Although blood tests, including an immunological screen, should be performed to clarify the diagnosis in glomerulonephritis, a renal biopsy is usually required. Drug-induced acute interstitial nephritis is harder to spot but should be suspected in a previously well patient if there is an acute deterioration of renal function coinciding with introduction of a new drug treatment. Drugs that are commonly implicated include PPIs, NSAIDs and many antibiotics.

Post-renal AKI

Patients should be examined clinically to look for evidence of a distended bladder and should also undergo imaging with ultrasound to detect evidence of obstruction above the level of the bladder. Post-renal AKI is usually accompanied by hydronephrosis.

Management

Management options common to all forms of AKI are discussed in more detail below and summarised in Box 15.26.

Haemodynamic status

If hypovolaemia is present, it should be corrected by replacement of intravenous fluid or blood; excessive administration of fluid should be avoided, since this can provoke pulmonary oedema and worsen outcome in AKI. Monitoring of central venous pressure may be of value in determining the rate of administration of fluid in these circumstances. Balanced crystalloid solutions, such as Plasma-Lyte, Hartmann's or Ringer's lactate, may be preferable to isotonic saline (0.9% NaCl) when large volumes of fluid resuscitation are required, in order to avoid hyperchloraemic acidosis, but whether this substantially influences outcome remains unclear. Administration of hydroxyethyl starch solutions should be avoided, since they have been associated with higher rates of established AKI. Critically ill patients may require inotropic drugs to restore an effective blood pressure but clinical trials do not support a specific role for low-dose dopamine.

Hyperkalaemia and acidosis

Hyperkalaemia is common, particularly in patients with rhabdomyolysis, burns, haemolysis or metabolic acidosis

(p. 362). If serum K$^+$ concentration is >6.5 mmol/L, this should be treated immediately, as described in Box 14.17 (p. 363), to prevent life-threatening cardiac arrhythmias. Metabolic acidosis develops unless prevented by loss of hydrogen ions through vomiting. Severe acidosis can be ameliorated with sodium bicarbonate if volume status allows. Restoration of blood volume will correct acidosis by restoring kidney function. Infusions of isotonic sodium bicarbonate may also be used, if acidosis is severe, to reduce life-threatening hyperkalaemia (Box 15.26).

Cardiopulmonary complications

Pulmonary oedema (Fig. 15.20) may be caused by the administration of excessive amounts of fluids relative to urine

---

i | **15.26 Management of acute kidney injury**

- Assess fluid status as this will determine fluid prescription:
  If hypovolaemic: optimise systemic haemodynamic status with fluid challenge and inotropic drugs if necessary
  Once euvolaemic, match fluid intake to urine output plus an additional 500 mL to cover insensible losses
  If fluid-overloaded, prescribe diuretics (loop diuretics at high dose will often be required); if the response is unsatisfactory, dialysis may be required
- Administer calcium resonium to stabilise myocardium and glucose and insulin to correct hyperkalaemia if K$^+$ >6.5 mmol/L (see Box 14.17, p. 363) as a holding measure until a definitive method of removing potassium is achieved (dialysis or restoration of renal function)
- Consider administering sodium bicarbonate (100 mmol) to correct acidosis if H$^+$ is >100 nmol/L (pH <7.0)
- Discontinue potentially nephrotoxic drugs and reduce doses of therapeutic drugs according to level of renal function
- Ensure adequate nutritional support
- Consider proton pump inhibitors to reduce the risk of upper gastrointestinal bleeding
- Screen for intercurrent infections and treat promptly if present
- In case of urinary tract obstruction, drain lower or upper urinary tract as necessary

Fig. 15.20 Pulmonary oedema in acute kidney injury. The appearances are indistinguishable from left ventricular failure but the heart size is usually normal. Blood pressure is often high.

output and by increased pulmonary capillary permeability. If pulmonary oedema is present and urine output cannot be rapidly restored, treatment with dialysis may be required to remove excess fluid. Temporary respiratory support may also be necessary using non-invasive ventilation. Once initial resuscitation has been performed, fluid intake should be matched to urine output plus 500 mL per day to cover insensible losses, unless diarrhoea is present, in which case additional fluids may be required.

Electrolyte disturbances

Electrolyte disturbances, such as dilutional hyponatraemia, may occur if the patient has continued to drink freely despite oliguria or has received inappropriate amounts of intravenous dextrose. They can be avoided by paying careful attention to fluid balance and by giving intravenous fluids slowly. Modest hypocalcaemia is common but rarely requires treatment. Serum phosphate levels are usually high but may fall in patients on daily or continuous renal replacement therapy (CRRT), necessitating phosphate replacement.

Dietary measures

Adequate nutritional support should be ensured and it is important to give sufficient amounts of energy and adequate amounts of protein; high protein intake should be avoided. This is particularly important in patients with sepsis and burns who are hypercatabolic. Enteral or parenteral nutrition may be required (p. 707).

Infection

Patients with AKI are at substantial risk of intercurrent infection because humoral and cellular immune mechanisms are depressed. Regular clinical examination, supplemented by microbiological investigation where appropriate, is required to diagnose infection. If infection is discovered, it should be treated promptly according to standard principles (Ch. 6).

Medications

Patients with drug-induced kidney injury (p. 402) should have the offending drug withdrawn. Additionally, vasoactive medications, such as NSAIDs and ACE inhibitors, should be discontinued, as they may prolong AKI (see Fig 15.19). H_2-receptor antagonists or PPIs should be given to prevent gastrointestinal bleeding. Other drug treatments should be reviewed and the doses adjusted if necessary, to take account of renal function. Non-essential drug treatments should be stopped.

Renal tract obstruction

In post-renal AKI, the obstruction should be relieved as soon as possible. This may involve urinary catheterisation for bladder outflow obstruction, or correction of ureteric obstruction with a ureteric stent or percutaneous nephrostomy.

Renal replacement therapy

Conservative management can be successful in AKI with meticulous attention to fluid balance, electrolytes and nutrition, but RRT may be required in patients who are not showing signs of recovery with these measures (Box 15.26). No specific cut-off values for serum urea or creatinine have been identified at which RRT should be commenced, and clinical trials of earlier versus later RRT in unselected patients with AKI have not shown differences in outcome. Furthermore, RRT can be a risky intervention, since it requires the placement of central venous catheters that may become infected and it may represent a major haemodynamic

Fig. 15.21 **Recovery from acute kidney injury (AKI).** Many patients make a full recovery of renal function (1). If the insult is prolonged or prior renal function not normal, however, patients may develop progressive chronic kidney disease (2) or, rarely, irreversible, complete loss of renal function (3). (ESRD = end-stage renal disease)

challenge in unstable patients. Accordingly, the decision to institute RRT should be made on an individual basis, taking account of the potential risks and benefits, comorbidity and an assessment of whether early or delayed recovery is likely. Severe uraemia with pericarditis and neurological signs (uraemic encephalopathy) is uncommon in AKI but, when present, is a strong indication for RRT; other indications are given in Box 15.35 (p. 422). The two main options for RRT in AKI are intermittent haemodialysis and CRRT (see Box 15.38, p. 424). Peritoneal dialysis is also an option if haemodialysis is not available (p. 424).

Recovery from AKI

Most cases of AKI will recover after the insult resolves but recovery may be impaired in pre-existing CKD or a prolonged severe insult (Fig. 15.21). Recovery is heralded by a gradual return of urine output and a steady improvement in plasma biochemistry. Initially, there is often a diuretic phase in which urine output increases rapidly and remains excessive for several days before returning to normal. This may be due in part to tubular damage and to temporary loss of the medullary concentration gradient. After a few days, urine volume falls to normal as the concentrating

15.27 Acute kidney injury in old age

- **Physiological change**: nephrons decline in number with age and average GFR falls progressively, so many elderly patients will have established CKD and less functional reserve. Small acute declines in renal function may therefore have a significant impact.
- **Creatinine**: as muscle mass falls with age, less creatinine is produced each day. Serum creatinine can be misleading as a guide to renal function.
- **Renal tubular function**: declines with age, leading to loss of urinary concentrating ability.
- **Drugs**: increased drug prescription in older people (diuretics, ACE inhibitors and NSAIDs) may contribute to the risk of AKI.
- **Causes**: infection, renal vascular disease, prostatic obstruction, hypovolaemia and severe cardiac dysfunction are common.
- **Mortality**: rises with age, primarily because of comorbid conditions.

mechanism and tubular reabsorption are restored. During the recovery phase of AKI, it may be necessary to provide temporary supplementation of bicarbonate, potassium and sometimes calcium, phosphate and magnesium.

AKI in old age is described in Box 15.27.

Chronic kidney disease

Chronic kidney disease (CKD) refers to an irreversible deterioration in renal function that usually develops over a period of years (see Box 15.3, p. 388). Initially, it manifests only as a biochemical abnormality but, eventually, loss of the excretory, metabolic and endocrine functions of the kidney leads to the clinical symptoms and signs of renal failure, collectively referred to as uraemia. When death is likely without RRT (CKD stage 5), it is called end-stage renal disease (ESRD).

Epidemiology

The social and economic consequences of CKD are considerable. In many countries, estimates of the prevalence of CKD stages 3–5 (eGFR <60 mL/min/1.73 m^2) are around 5–7%, mostly affecting people aged 65 years and above (see Box 15.3). The prevalence of CKD in patients with hypertension, diabetes and vascular disease is substantially higher, and targeted screening for CKD should be considered in these and other high-risk groups. More than 25% of the population aged over 75 years have an eGFR of <60 mL/min/1.73 m^2, mostly stage 3A CKD, which in this context typically reflects an increased cardiovascular risk burden. In these patients, investigation and management should be focused on cardiovascular risk prevention, as very few will ever develop ESRD. Many primary renal diseases, however, are more common in the elderly, so investigation is warranted for those with declining renal function or with haematuria/proteinuria on dipstick.

Pathophysiology

Common causes of CKD are shown in Box 15.28. In many cases, the underlying diagnosis is unclear, especially among the large number of elderly patients with stage 3 CKD (see Box 15.3).

15.28 Common causes of chronic kidney disease

Disease	Proportion	Comments
Diabetes mellitus	20–40%	Large racial and geographical differences
Interstitial diseases	20–30%	Often drug-induced
Glomerular diseases	10–20%	IgA nephropathy is most common
Hypertension	5–20%	Causality controversial, much may be secondary to another primary renal disease
Systemic inflammatory diseases	5–10%	Systemic lupus erythematosus, vasculitis
Renovascular disease	5%	Mostly atheromatous, may be more common
Congenital and inherited	5%	Polycystic kidney disease, Alport's syndrome
Unknown	5–20%	

Many patients diagnosed at a late stage have bilateral small kidneys; renal biopsy is rarely undertaken in this group since it is more risky, less likely to provide a histological diagnosis because of the severity of damage, and unlikely to alter management.

Clinical features

The typical presentation is for a raised urea and creatinine to be found incidentally during routine blood tests, often during screening of high-risk patients, such as those with diabetes or hypertension. Most patients with slowly progressive disease are asymptomatic until GFR falls below 30 mL/min/1.73 m^2 and some can remain asymptomatic with much lower GFR values than this. An early symptom is nocturia, due to the loss of concentrating ability and increased osmotic load per nephron, but this is non-specific. When GFR falls below 15–20 mL/min/1.73 m^2, symptoms and signs are common and can affect almost all body systems (Fig. 15.22). They typically include tiredness or breathlessness, which may, in part, be related to renal anaemia or fluid overload. With further deterioration in renal function, patients may suffer pruritus, anorexia, weight loss, nausea, vomiting and hiccups. In very advanced renal failure, respiration may be particularly deep (Kussmaul breathing) due to profound metabolic acidosis, and patients may develop muscular twitching, fits, drowsiness and coma.

Investigations

The recommended investigations in patients with CKD are shown in Box 15.29. Their main aims are:

- to exclude AKI requiring rapid investigation; in patients with unexpectedly high urea and creatinine (when there is an increase from previous results or no prior results are available), renal function should be retested within 2 weeks to avoid missing AKI
- to identify the underlying cause where possible, since this may influence the treatment
- to identify reversible factors that may worsen renal function, such as hypertension or urinary tract obstruction
- to screen for complications of CKD, such as anaemia and renal osteodystrophy
- to screen for cardiovascular risk factors.

Referral to a nephrologist is appropriate for patients with potentially treatable underlying disease and those who are likely to progress to ESRD. Suggested referral criteria are listed in Box 15.30.

Management

The aims of management in CKD are to:

- monitor renal function
- prevent or slow further renal damage
- limit complications of renal failure
- treat risk factors for cardiovascular disease
- prepare for RRT, if appropriate (p. 420).

Monitoring of renal function

The rate of change in renal function varies between patients and may vary over time in each individual. Renal function should therefore be monitored every 6 months in patients with stage 3 CKD, but more frequently in patients who are deteriorating rapidly or have stage 4 or 5 CKD. A plot of GFR against time (Fig. 15.23) can demonstrate whether therapy has been successful in slowing progression, detect any unexpected increase in the rate of decline that may warrant further investigation, and help

Fig. 15.22 **Physical signs in advanced chronic kidney disease.** (*Features of renal replacement therapy)

Labels in figure:
- Yellow complexion
- Pallor
- Jugular venous pressure raised in fluid overload or pericardial tamponade
- Dual-lumen central venous catheter for dialysis access (right or left)*
- Pericardial friction rub
- Pulsus paradoxus in pericardial tamponade
- Arteriovenous fistulae for dialysis access*
- Transplanted kidney (right or left) with overlying scar*
- Tenckhoff catheter for peritoneal dialysis (right or left)*
- 'Brown line' pigmentation of nails
- Excoriation of pruritus
- Increased respiratory rate and depth in metabolic acidosis
- Bruising easily
- Peripheral neuropathy
  Absent reflexes
  Reduced sensation
  Paraesthesia
  'Restless legs'

i	**15.29 Suggested investigations in chronic kidney disease**	
Initial tests	**Interpretation**
Urea and creatinine	To assess stability/progression: compare to previous results
Urinalysis and quantification of proteinuria	Haematuria and proteinuria may indicate glomerular disease and need for biopsy (p. 391). Proteinuria indicates risk of progressive CKD requiring preventive ACE inhibitor or ARB therapy
Electrolytes	To identify hyperkalaemia and acidosis
Calcium, phosphate, parathyroid hormone and 25(OH)D	Assessment of renal osteodystrophy
Albumin	Low albumin: consider malnutrition, inflammation, nephrotic syndrome
Full blood count (±Fe, ferritin, folate, B$_{12}$)	If anaemic, exclude common non-renal explanations, then manage as renal anaemia
Lipids, glucose ±HbA$_{1c}$	Cardiovascular risk high in CKD: treat risk factors aggressively
Renal ultrasound	Only if there are obstructive urinary symptoms, persistent haematuria, family history of polycystic kidney disease or progressive CKD. Small kidneys suggest chronicity. Asymmetric renal size suggests renovascular or developmental disease
Hepatitis and HIV serology	If dialysis or transplant is planned. Hepatitis B vaccination recommended if seronegative
Other tests	Consider relevant tests from Box 15.25, especially if the cause of CKD is unknown

(ACE = angiotensin-converting enzyme; ARB = angiotensin II receptor blocker; 25(OH)D = 25-hydroxyvitamin D)

predict when ESRF will be reached to facilitate timely planning for RRT.

Reduction of rate of progression

Slowing the rate of progression of CKD may reduce complications and delay symptom onset and the need for RRT (Fig. 15.23). Therapies directed towards the primary cause of CKD should be employed where possible; tight blood pressure control is applicable to CKD regardless of cause, however, and reducing proteinuria is a key target in those with glomerular disease.

Antihypertensive therapy Lowering of blood pressure slows the rate at which renal function declines in CKD, independently of the agent used (apart from those with proteinuria; see below) and

Fig. 15.23 **Plot of estimated glomerular filtration rate (eGFR) against time in a patient with type 1 diabetes mellitus.** After approximately 6 years of monitoring (blue arrow), this patient entered an aggressive treatment programme aimed at optimising blood pressure (BP) and glycaemic control. The reduction in BP was accompanied by a fall in proteinuria (protein:creatinine ratio, PCR; shown in mg/mmol). At the previous rate of decline in renal function (dashed line), he was likely to reach the level of renal function at which dialysis therapy is typically required (eGFR=10 mL/min/1.73 m²) within 18 months; however, the relative stabilisation in his renal function (dotted line) means that this has been deferred, potentially for several years.

ℹ 15.30 Criteria for referral of chronic kidney disease patients to a nephrologist

- eGFR <30 mL/min/1.73 m²
- Rapid deterioration in renal function (>25% from previous or >15 mL/min/1.73 m²/year)
- Significant proteinuria (PCR >100 mg/mmol or ACR >70 mg/mmol), unless known to be due to diabetes and patient is already on appropriate medications
- ACR >30 mg/mmol with non-visible haematuria
- Hypertension that remains poorly controlled despite at least four antihypertensive medications
- Suspicion of renal involvement in multisystem disease

---

has additional benefits in lowering the risk of hypertensive heart failure, stroke and peripheral vascular disease. No threshold for beneficial effects has been identified and any reduction of blood pressure appears to be beneficial. Various targets have been suggested, such as 140/90 mmHg for patients with CKD and no albuminuria (ACR <3 mg/mmol). A lower target of 130/80 mmHg should be considered for those who have moderately elevated albuminuria (ACR 3–3 mg/mmol), and is recommended for those with an ACR of more than 30 mg/mmol. Even lower targets, such as 125/75 mmHg, may be prudent in patients with CKD and heavy proteinuria (PCR >100 mg/mmol or ACR >70 mg/mmol). Achieving these blood pressure targets often requires multiple drugs, and therapeutic success may be limited by adverse effects and poor adherence.

Reduction of proteinuria Patients with proteinuria are at higher risk of progression of renal disease, and there is strong evidence that reducing proteinuria reduces the risk of progression. ACE inhibitors and ARBs reduce proteinuria and retard the progression of CKD. These effects are partly due to the reduction in blood pressure but there is evidence for a specific beneficial effect in patients with proteinuria (PCR >50 mg/mmol or ACR >30 mg/mmol) through a reduction in glomerular perfusion pressure. In addition, ACE inhibitors have been shown to reduce the risk of cardiovascular events and all-cause mortality in CKD. Accordingly, ACE inhibitors and/or ARBs should be prescribed to all patients with diabetic nephropathy and patients with CKD and proteinuria, irrespective of whether or not hypertension is present.

While ACE inhibitors and ARBs are excellent drugs for patients with diabetes or CKD and proteinuria, they need to be prescribed with care in certain circumstances. Initiation of treatment with ACE inhibitors and ARBs may be accompanied by an immediate reduction in GFR; patients should therefore have their renal function checked within 7–10 days of initiating or increasing the dose of an ACE inhibitor or ARB. Treatment can be continued so long as the reduction in GFR is not greater than 25% and is not progressive. Angiotensin II is critical for autoregulation of GFR in the context of low renal perfusion (see Fig. 15.1D, p. 385), and so ACE inhibitors or ARBs may exacerbate pre-renal failure (see Fig. 15.19). Patients on ACE inhibitors/ARBs should therefore be warned to stop taking the medication if they become unwell, such as with fever, vomiting or diarrhoea, restarting once they are better. This also applies to other common medications used in patients with CKD, such as diuretics, metformin and NSAIDs, and this advice may be reinforced by providing written information such as 'sick-day rule' cards (Box 15.31). ACE inhibitors and ARBs increase serum potassium and should not be commenced in patients with baseline potassium >5.5 mmol/L. In patients with serum potassium >6.0 mmol/L, the dose of ACE inhibitors or ARBs should be reduced or discontinued entirely, but only after all other measures to reduce potassium have been considered (see below). Combination therapy with ACE inhibitors and ARBs or direct renin inhibitors has not been shown to reduce progression of kidney disease but is associated with higher rates of hyperkalaemia and AKI, and is therefore to be avoided.

15

15.31 Exemplar medicine sick-day card

When you are unwell with vomiting, diarrhoea or fever, stop taking the following medications:
- ACE inhibitors: medicines ending in '-pril', e.g. lisinopril, ramipril
- Angiotensin receptor blockers: medicines ending in '-sartan', e.g. irbesartan, losartan, candesartan
- Non-steroidal anti-inflammatory painkillers: e.g. ibuprofen (Brufen), diclofenac (Voltarol)
- Diuretics: e.g. furosemide, bendroflumethiazide, indapamide, spironolactone
- Metformin: a medicine for diabetes.

Restart when you are well again (after 24–48 hours of eating and drinking normally).

15.32 Foods high in potassium

- Fruit: bananas, avocados, figs, rhubarb
- Vegetables: tomatoes, spinach, parsnips, courgettes, sprouts, potatoes (including baked, fries, wedges; boiling vegetables reduces potassium content)
- Sweets/snacks: crisps, chocolate, toffee, nuts (including peanut butter)
- Drinks: beer, cider, wine (spirits contain less potassium), hot chocolate, fruit juice, milk, yoghurt
- Salt substitutes, such as Lo-Salt: sodium chloride is substituted with potassium chloride

Treatment of complications

The kidneys have many functions in addition to excretion of waste (p. 384). Treatments that substitute for all of the normal roles of the kidneys must therefore be instigated to maintain normal body homeostasis and prevent complications.

Maintenance of fluid and electrolyte balance The kidneys excrete waste and regulate many electrolytes, and so patients with CKD may accumulate waste products and develop electrolyte abnormalities.

Urea is a key product of protein degradation and accumulates with progressive CKD. All patients with stages 4 and 5 CKD should be given dietetic advice aimed at preventing excessive consumption of protein. Severe protein restriction is not recommended, however; there is no evidence that this reduces the rate of decline in renal function but may lead to malnutrition.

Potassium often accumulates in patients with advanced CKD, who should be provided with dietary advice to reduce daily potassium intake to below 70 mmol (Box 15.32). Potassium-binding compounds limit absorption of potassium from the gut and may be a useful adjunctive therapy. Calcium resonium is not recommended other than as a very short-term measure, as it can be associated with bowel necrosis; however, newer agents, such as zirconium cyclosilicate and patiromer, appear promising for chronic use. Other measures that may help regulate potassium include diuretic therapy and control of acidosis with sodium bicarbonate (see below). Consideration should be given to stopping or reducing drugs that elevate potassium, such as potassium-sparing diuretics and ACE inhibitors/ARBs; however, this has to be balanced against the potential benefit that such drugs may have on retarding progression of renal and cardiovascular disease, and hence withdrawal should be reserved for when other measures have failed.

The inability of the failing kidney to excrete sodium and water loads commonly leads to their accumulation, which may manifest as oedema and may drive hypertension. Patients with evidence of volume expansion should be instructed to consume a low-sodium diet (< 100 mmol/24 hrs), and in severe cases fluid intake should also be restricted. Diuretics are commonly required, and as renal function deteriorates, increasing doses of potent loop diuretics or synergistic combinations of loop, thiazide and potassium-sparing diuretics may be necessary.

Occasionally, some patients with tubulo-interstitial disease can develop 'salt-wasting' disease and may require a high sodium and water intake, including supplements of sodium salts, to prevent fluid depletion and worsening of renal function.

Acid–base balance Reduced ability to excrete organic acids in patients with CKD may lead to an anion-gap metabolic acidosis. In addition, in patients with tubulo-interstitial disease or diabetic nephropathy, there may be specific defects in acid–base regulation within the kidney, causing a non-anion-gap renal tubular acidosis (p. 365). Although acidosis is usually asymptomatic, it may be associated with increased tissue catabolism and decreased protein synthesis, and may exacerbate bone disease and the rate of decline in renal function. Hence, plasma bicarbonate concentrations should be maintained above 22 mmol/L by prescribing sodium bicarbonate supplements (starting dose of 1 g 8-hourly, increasing as required). There is some evidence that correcting acidosis may reduce the rate of decline in renal function.

Renal bone disease Disturbances of calcium and phosphate metabolism are almost universal in advanced CKD (Fig. 15.24). The sequence of events that leads to renal bone disease is complex, but two primary factors are impaired excretion of phosphate and failure of the renal tubular cells to convert 25-hydroxyvitamin D to its active metabolite, 1,25-dihydroxyvitamin D. A rise in serum phosphate levels promotes production of the hormone fibroblast growth factor 23 (FGF23) from osteocytes (Fig. 24.3, p. 986) and stimulates parathyroid hormone (PTH) release and hyperplasia of the parathyroid glands. The FGF23 and PTH promote tubular phosphate excretion, thereby partly compensating for the reduced glomerular filtration of phosphate. The reduced 1,25-dihydroxyvitamin D levels impair intestinal absorption of calcium. In addition, raised levels of serum phosphate complex with calcium in the extracellular space, leading to calcium phosphate deposition. Both the reduced absorption and increased deposition of calcium cause hypocalcaemia, which also stimulates PTH production by the parathyroid glands. Hence in many patients with CKD, compensatory responses initially maintain phosphate and calcium levels at the upper and lower ends of their respective normal ranges, at the expense of an elevated PTH level (secondary hyperparathyroidism). This is associated with a gradual transfer of calcium and phosphate from the bone to other tissues, leading to bone resorption (osteitis fibrosa cystica), and in severe cases this may result in bony pain and increased risk of fractures. Conversely there is increased deposition of calcium phosphate in many tissues, most notably blood vessels and heart valves, which may contribute to the increased risk of cardiovascular disease in patients with CKD (p. 420). In some cases, tertiary hyperparathyroidism supervenes, due to autonomous production of PTH by the enlarged parathyroid glands; this presents with hypercalcaemia. Additional problems in bone metabolism include low bone turnover (adynamic bone disease) in patients who have been over-treated with vitamin D metabolites, osteomalacia with over-treatment of

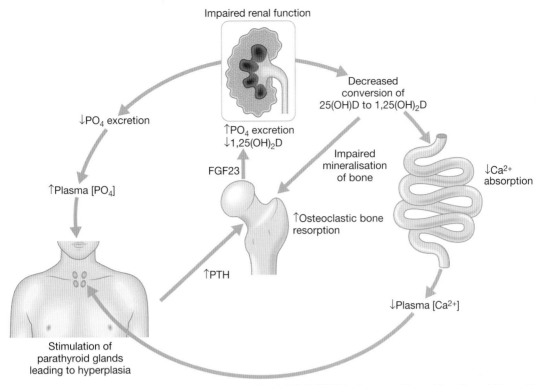

Fig. 15.24 **Pathogenesis of renal osteodystrophy.** Low 1,25-dihydroxyvitamin D (1,25(OH)$_2$D) levels cause calcium malabsorption and this, combined with high phosphate levels, causes hypocalcaemia, which increases parathyroid hormone (PTH) production by the parathyroid glands. The raised level of PTH increases osteoclastic bone resorption. Although production of fibroblast growth factor 23 (FGF23) from osteocytes also increases, promoting phosphate excretion, this is insufficient to prevent hyperphosphataemia in advanced chronic kidney disease.

hyperphosphataemia (p. 369), and osteoporosis in patients with poor nutritional intake.

The key focus in the management of renal bone disease should be directed towards the two main driving factors, hyperphosphataemia and inadequate activation of vitamin D. Hyperphosphataemia should be treated by dietary restriction of foods with high phosphate content (milk, cheese, eggs and protein-rich foods) and by the use of phosphate-binding drugs. Various drugs are available, including calcium carbonate, aluminium hydroxide, lanthanum carbonate and polymer-based phosphate binders such as sevelamer. The aim is to maintain serum phosphate values at or below 1.5 mmol/L (4.6 mg/dL) if possible, but many of these drugs are difficult to take and adherence can be a problem. Active vitamin D metabolites (either 1-α-hydroxyvitamin D or 1,25-dihydroxyvitamin D) should be administered in patients who are hypocalcaemic or have serum PTH levels more than twice the upper limit of normal. The dose should be adjusted to try to reduce PTH levels to between 2 and 4 times the upper limit of normal to limit hyperparathyroidism while avoiding over-suppression of bone turnover and adynamic bone disease, but care must be exercised in order to avoid hypercalcaemia. In patients with persistent hypercalcaemia (tertiary hyperparathyroidism), parathyroidectomy may be required. If parathyroidectomy is unsuccessful or not possible, calcimimetic agents, such as cinacalcet, may be used. These bind to the calcium-sensing receptor in the parathyroid glands and reduce PTH secretion.

Anaemia Anaemia is common in patients with CKD and contributes to many of the non-specific symptoms, including fatigue and

15.33 Causes of anaemia in chronic kidney disease

- Deficiency of erythropoietin
- Toxic effects of uraemia on marrow precursor cells
- Reduced red cell survival
- Blood loss due to capillary fragility and poor platelet function
- Reduced intake, absorption and utilisation of dietary iron

shortness of breath. Haemoglobin can be as low as 50–70 g/L in CKD stage 5, although it is often less severe or absent in patients with polycystic kidney disease. Several mechanisms are implicated, as summarised in Box 15.33. Iron deficiency is common in patients with CKD, and even more prevalent in those on haemodialysis as a result of haemolysis in the dialysis circuit. Hence many patients require iron supplements, which may be given intravenously for those with iron intolerance or in situations where adherence may be difficult. Once iron deficiency and other causes of anaemia have been excluded or corrected, recombinant human erythropoietin is very effective in correcting the anaemia of CKD and improving symptoms. Erythropoietin treatment does not influence mortality, however, and correcting haemoglobin to normal levels may carry some extra risk, including hypertension and thrombosis. The target haemoglobin is usually between 100 and 120 g/L. Erythropoietin is less effective in the presence of iron deficiency, active inflammation or malignancy, in particular myeloma.

Treatment of risk factors for cardiovascular disease

The risk of cardiovascular disease is substantially increased in patients with a GFR below 60 mL/min/1.73 m^2 and in those with proteinuria, the combination of reduced eGFR and proteinuria being particularly unfavourable. Patients with CKD have a higher prevalence of traditional risk factors for atherosclerosis, such as hypertension, hyperlipidaemia and diabetes; however, additional mechanisms of cardiovascular disease may also be implicated. Left ventricular hypertrophy is commonly found in patients with CKD, secondary to hypertension or anaemia. Calcification of the media of blood vessels, heart valves, myocardium and the conduction system of the heart is also common and may be due, in part, to the high serum phosphate levels. Reflecting this fact, serum FGF23 levels, which increase in response to serum phosphate, are an independent predictor of mortality in CKD. Both left ventricular hypertrophy and cardiac calcification may increase the risk of arrhythmias and sudden cardiac death, which is a much more common mode of death in patients with CKD than in the general population, particularly in those with more advanced disease and those on dialysis.

To reduce vascular risk, patients with CKD should be encouraged to adopt a healthy lifestyle, including regular exercise, and weight loss and smoking cessation where appropriate. Lipid-lowering drugs reduce cardiovascular events in patients with CKD, although their efficacy may be less once patients require dialysis.

Preparing for renal replacement therapy

It is crucial for patients who are known to have progressive CKD to be prepared well in advance for the institution of RRT. This involves ensuring that they are referred to a nephrologist in a timely manner, as those who are referred late, when they are either at the stage of or very close to requiring dialysis, tend to have poorer outcomes.

Several decisions need to be taken in discussion with the patient and family. The first is to decide whether RRT is an appropriate choice or whether conservative treatment might be preferable (p. 421). This is especially relevant in patients with significant comorbidity. For those who decide to go ahead with RRT, there are further choices between haemodialysis and peritoneal dialysis (Box 15.34), between hospital and home treatment, and on referral for renal transplantation.

Since there is no evidence that early initiation of RRT improves outcome, the overall aim is to commence RRT when symptoms of CKD begin to impact on quality of life but before serious complications have occurred. While there is wide variation between patients, this typically occurs when the eGFR approaches 10 mL/min/1.73 m^2. This may be a useful marker to predict the timing of initiation of RRT by extrapolating from a plot of serial eGFR measurements over time (see Fig. 15.23).

Preparations for starting RRT should begin at least 12 months before the predicted start date. This involves providing the patient with psychological and social support, assessing home circumstances and discussing the various choices of treatment (Fig. 15.25). Depression is common in patients who are on or approaching RRT, and support from the renal multidisciplinary team should be provided both for them and for their relatives, to explain and help them adapt to the changes to lifestyle that may be necessary once RRT starts; this may help to reduce their anxieties about these changes. Physical preparations include establishment of timely access for haemodialysis or peritoneal dialysis and vaccination against hepatitis B.

15.34 Comparison of haemodialysis and peritoneal dialysis

Haemodialysis	Peritoneal dialysis
Efficient; 4 hrs three times per week is usually adequate	Less efficient; four exchanges per day are usually required, each taking 30–60 mins (continuous ambulatory peritoneal dialysis) or 8–10 hrs each night (automated peritoneal dialysis)
2–3 days between treatments	A few hours between treatments
Requires visits to hospital (although home treatment is possible for some patients)	Performed at home
Requires adequate venous circulation for vascular access	Requires an intact peritoneal cavity without major scarring from previous surgery
Careful adherence to diet and fluid restrictions required between treatments	Diet and fluid less restricted
Fluid removal compressed into treatment periods; may cause symptoms and haemodynamic instability	Slow continuous fluid removal, usually asymptomatic
Infections related to vascular access may occur	Peritonitis and catheter-related infections may occur
Patients are usually dependent on others	Patients can take full responsibility for their treatment

Renal replacement therapy

Renal replacement therapy (RRT) may be required on a temporary basis in patients with AKI or on a permanent basis for those with advanced CKD. Since the advent of long-term RRT in the 1960s, the numbers of patients with ESRD who are kept alive by dialysis and transplantation have increased considerably. By the end of 2014, almost 59 000 patients were on RRT in the UK, with a median age of 65 years. After a long period of expansion, the number of patients on dialysis in the UK and USA has begun to stabilise; however, the total number of patients on RRT continues to expand, due to an increasing proportion (53%) of patients with a functional transplant. The remaining patients were on haemodialysis (41%) and peritoneal dialysis (6%).

There are variations in the numbers of patients receiving RRT in different countries because of differences in the incidence of predisposing disease, as well as differences in medical practice. For example, the incidence rate for RRT in the USA was about three times higher than in the UK (363 versus 115 patients per million population), and the prevalence rate was more than twice as high (2034 versus 913 per million population). Diabetic kidney disease is the most common cause of ESRD in many countries, accounting for 26% of all ESRD in the UK and almost 50% in the USA. The large increase in the prevalence of type 2 diabetes in developing countries is resulting in a predictable rise in cases of ESRD, which is challenging already stretched health-care resources.

Survival on dialysis is strongly influenced by age and presence of complications such as diabetes (Fig. 15.26). For this reason, conservative care rather than RRT may be a more appropriate option for older patients or those with extensive comorbidities. Although many young patients without extrarenal disease lead

A **Haemodialysis**

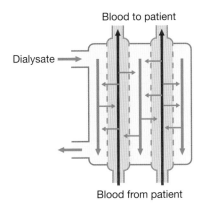

Blood to patient

Dialysate →

Blood from patient

B **Haemofiltration**

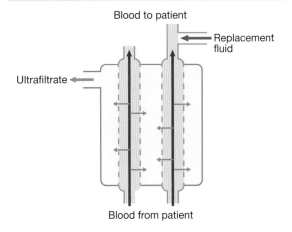

Blood to patient

← Replacement fluid

Ultrafiltrate ←

Blood from patient

C **Peritoneal dialysis**

— Peritoneal cavity

— Peritoneal membrane

— PD fluid

— Catheter

D **Transplantation**

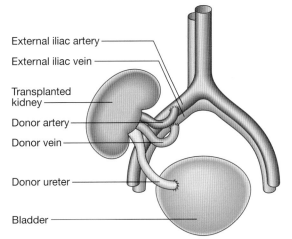

External iliac artery ———

External iliac vein ———

Transplanted kidney ———

Donor artery ———

Donor vein ———

Donor ureter ———

Bladder ———

Fig. 15.25 Options for renal replacement therapy. A In haemodialysis, there is diffusion of solutes from blood to dialysate across a semipermeable membrane down a concentration gradient. B In haemofiltration, both water and solutes are filtered across a porous semipermeable membrane by a pressure gradient. Replacement fluid is added to the filtered blood before it is returned to the patient. C In peritoneal dialysis (PD), fluid is introduced into the abdominal cavity using a catheter. Solutes diffuse from blood across the peritoneal membrane to PD fluid down a concentration gradient, and water diffuses through osmosis (see text for details). D In transplantation, the blood supply of the transplanted kidney is generally anastomosed to the external iliac vessels and the ureter to the bladder. The transplanted kidney replaces all functions of the failed kidney.

normal and active lives on RRT, those aged 30–34 have a mortality rate 25 times higher than that of age-matched controls.

The aim of RRT is to replace the excretory functions of the kidney and to maintain normal electrolyte concentrations and fluid balance. Various options are available, including haemodialysis, haemofiltration, haemodiafiltration, peritoneal dialysis and renal transplantation, and each of these is discussed in more detail below. Indications for starting RRT in both AKI and CKD may be found in Box 15.35.

Conservative treatment

In older patients with multiple comorbidities, conservative treatment of stage 5 CKD, aimed at limiting the adverse symptoms of ESRD without commencing RRT, is increasingly viewed as a positive choice (Box 15.36). Current evidence suggests that survival of these patients without dialysis can be similar or only

slightly shorter than that of patients who undergo RRT, but they avoid the hospitalisation and interventions associated with dialysis. Patients are offered full medical, psychological and social support to optimise and sustain their existing renal function and to treat complications, such as anaemia, for as long as possible, with appropriate palliative care in the terminal phase of their disease. Many of these patients enjoy a good quality of life for several years. When quality of life on dialysis is poor, it is appropriate to consider discontinuing it, following discussion with the patient and family, and to offer palliative care.

Haemodialysis

Haemodialysis is the most common form of RRT in ESRD and is also used in AKI. Haemodialysis involves gaining access to the circulation, either through a central venous catheter or an arteriovenous fistula or graft. The patient's blood is pumped through a haemodialyser, which allows bidirectional diffusion of

i **15.35 Indications for dialysis with examples for AKI and CKD**

Indication*	Acute examples	Chronic examples
Fluid overload	Acute pulmonary oedema	Intractable dependent oedema resistant to diuretics Pulmonary oedema Severe hypertension
Hyperkalaemia	High potassium (generally >6.5 mmol/L) with ECG changes (especially broad QRS)	Potassium resistant to dietary control and medical intervention
Uraemia	Pericarditis Encephalopathy	Uraemic syndrome including anorexia, nausea, lethargy etc. (generally not until eGFR <10 mL/min/1.73 m²)
Metabolic acidosis	Severe acidosis (H⁺ >79 nmol/L; pH <7.1)	Chronic acidosis resistant to bicarbonate therapy
Other (often relative indications)	Bleeding diathesis considered due to uraemia-induced platelet dysfunction	Intractable anaemia despite erythropoietin and iron Hyperphosphataemia despite binders

*The presence of anuria in AKI will modify the above indications, as these complications will not resolve if the patient is persistently anuric. Most indications to commence chronic dialysis are relative indications; a holistic approach is taken to making this decision.
(ECG = electrocardiogram; eGFR = estimated glomerular filtration rate)

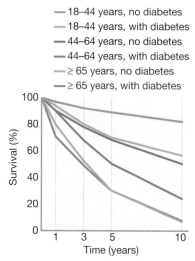

— 18–44 years, no diabetes
— 18–44 years, with diabetes
— 44–64 years, no diabetes
— 44–64 years, with diabetes
— ≥ 65 years, no diabetes
— ≥ 65 years, with diabetes

Fig. 15.26 Percentage survival after commencing renal replacement therapy according to age group and presence of diabetes.

15.36 Renal replacement therapy in old age

- **Quality of life**: age itself is not a barrier to good quality of life on RRT.
- **Coexisting cardiovascular disease**: older people are more sensitive to fluid balance changes, predisposing to hypotension during dialysis with rebound hypertension between dialysis sessions. A failing heart cannot cope with fluid overload, and pulmonary oedema develops easily.
- **Provision of treatment**: often only hospital-provided haemodialysis is suitable and older patients require more medical and nursing time.
- **Survival on dialysis**: difficult to predict for an individual patient, but old age plus substantial comorbidity are associated with poor median survival. Similar survival may be achieved through conservative care, without the complications associated with dialysis.
- **Withdrawal from dialysis**: may be appropriate whenever quality of life deteriorates irreversibly, usually in the context of severe comorbidity.
- **Transplantation**: relative risks of surgery and immunosuppression exclude most older people from transplantation.
- **Conservative therapy**: without dialysis but with adequate support. This is an appropriate option for patients at high risk of complications from dialysis, who have a limited prognosis and little hope of functional recovery.

solutes between blood and the dialysate across a semipermeable membrane down a concentration gradient (Fig. 15.25A). The composition of the dialysate can be varied to achieve the desired gradient, and fluid can be removed by applying negative pressure to the dialysate side.

Haemodialysis in AKI

Haemodialysis offers the best rate of small solute clearance in AKI, compared with other techniques such as haemofiltration, but should be started gradually because of the risk of delirium and convulsions due to cerebral oedema (dialysis disequilibrium). Typically, 1–2 hours of dialysis is prescribed initially but, subsequently, patients with AKI who are haemodynamically stable can be treated by 4–5 hours of haemodialysis on alternate days, or 2–3 hours every day. During dialysis, it is standard practice to anticoagulate patients with heparin but the dose may be reduced if there is a bleeding risk. Epoprostenol can be used as an alternative but carries a risk of hypotension. In patients undergoing short treatments and in those with abnormal clotting, it may be possible to avoid anticoagulation altogether.

In AKI, dialysis is performed through a large-bore, dual-lumen catheter inserted into the femoral or internal jugular vein (Fig. 15.27A). Subclavian lines are avoided where possible, largely due to bleeding risk. Also, thromboses or stenoses here will compromise the ability to form a functioning fistula in the arm if the patient fails to recover renal function and needs chronic dialysis.

Haemodialysis in CKD

In CKD, vascular access for haemodialysis is gained by formation of an arteriovenous fistula (AVF), usually in the forearm, up to a year before dialysis is contemplated (Fig. 15.27B). After 4–6 weeks, increased pressure transmitted from the artery to the vein leading from the fistula causes distension and thickening of the vessel wall (arterialisation). Large-bore needles can then be

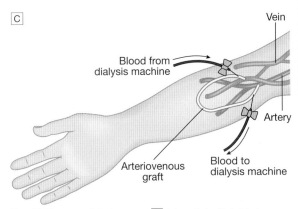

Fig. 15.27 Haemodialysis access. [A] A tunnelled cuffed dialysis catheter. [B] An arteriovenous fistula. [C] An arteriovenous graft.

inserted into the vein to provide access for each haemodialysis treatment.

Preservation of arm veins is thus very important in patients with progressive renal disease who may require haemodialysis in the future. If creation of an AVF is not possible, synthetic polytetrafluoroethylene (PTFE) grafts may be fashioned between an artery and a vein, or central venous catheters may be used for short-term access (Fig. 15.27C). These are tunnelled under the skin to reduce infection risk. All patients must be screened

in advance for hepatitis B, hepatitis C and HIV, and vaccinated against hepatitis B if they are not immune. All dialysis units should have segregation facilities for hepatitis B-positive patients, given its easy transmissibility. Patients with hepatitis C and HIV are less infectious and can be treated satisfactorily using machine segregation and standard infection control measures.

Haemodialysis is usually carried out for 3–5 hours three times weekly, either at home or in an outpatient dialysis unit. The intensity and frequency of dialysis should be adjusted to achieve a reduction in urea during dialysis (urea reduction ratio) of over 65%; below this level there is an associated increase in mortality. Most patients notice an improvement in symptoms during the first 6 weeks of treatment. The intensity of dialysis can be increased by:

- escalating the number of standard sessions to four or more per week
- performing short, frequent dialysis sessions of 2–3 hours 5–7 times per week
- performing nocturnal haemodialysis, when low blood-pump speeds and single-needle dialysis are used for approximately 8 hours overnight 5–6 times per week.

More frequent dialysis and nocturnal dialysis can achieve better fluid balance and phosphate control, improve left ventricular mass and possibly improve mortality, although the latter has not yet been robustly demonstrated. Box 15.37 summarises some of the problems related to haemodialysis.

Haemofiltration

This technique is principally used in the treatment of AKI as CRRT (Box 15.38). Large volumes of water are filtered from blood across a porous semipermeable membrane under a pressure gradient. Solutes are removed via 'solvent drag'. Replacement fluid of a suitable electrolyte composition is added to the blood after it exits the haemofilter. If removal of fluid is required, then less fluid is added back than is removed (see Fig. 15.25B). Haemofiltration may be either intermittent or continuous, and typically 1–2 L of filtrate is replaced per hour (equivalent to a GFR of 15–30 mL/min/1.73 m^2); higher rates of filtration may be of benefit in patients with sepsis and multi-organ failure. In continuous arteriovenous haemofiltration (CAVH), the extracorporeal blood circuit is driven by the arteriovenous pressure difference, but poor filtration rates and clotting of the filter are common and this treatment has fallen out of favour. Continuous venovenous haemofiltration (CVVH) is pump-driven, providing a reliable extracorporeal circulation. Issues concerning anticoagulation are similar to those for haemodialysis, but may be more problematic because longer or continuous anticoagulation is necessary.

Haemodiafiltration

This technique combines haemodialysis with approximately 20–30 L of ultrafiltration (with replacement of filtrate) over a 3–5-hour treatment. It uses a large-pore membrane and combines the improved clearance of medium-sized molecules observed in haemofiltration with the higher small-solute clearance of haemodialysis. It is sometimes used in the treatment of AKI, often as continuous therapy (Box 15.38). It is increasingly favoured in the treatment of CKD but is more expensive than haemodialysis and the long-term benefits are not yet established.

15

i 15.37 Problems with haemodialysis

Problem	Clinical features	Cause	Treatment
During treatments			
Hypotension	Sudden ↓BP; often leg cramps; sometimes chest pain	Fluid removal and hypovolaemia	Saline infusion; exclude cardiac ischaemia; quinine may help cramp
Cardiac arrhythmias	Hypotension; sometimes chest pain	Potassium and acid base shifts	Check K^+ and arterial blood gases; review dialysis prescription; stop dialysis
Haemorrhage	Blood loss (overt or occult); hypotension	Anticoagulation Venous needle disconnection	Stop dialysis; seek source; consider heparin-free treatment
Air embolism	Circulatory collapse; cardiac arrest	Disconnected or faulty lines and equipment malfunction	Stop dialysis
Dialyser hypersensitivity	Acute circulatory collapse	Allergic reaction to dialysis membrane or sterilisant	Stop dialysis; change to different artificial kidney
Between treatments			
Pulmonary oedema	Breathlessness	Fluid overload	Ultrafiltration ± dialysis
Systemic sepsis	Rigors; fever; ↓BP	Usually involves vascular access devices (catheter or fistula)	Blood cultures; antibiotics

(BP = blood pressure)

i 15.38 Types of continuous renal replacement therapy (CRRT) used in AKI management*

- CVVH: continuous venovenous haemofiltration
- CVVHD: continuous venovenous haemodialysis
- CVVHDF: continuous venovenous haemodiafiltration

*Most CRRT machines may perform all of these treatments. Continuous arteriovenous treatments (i.e. continuous arteriovenous haemofiltration) have fallen out of favour.

Peritoneal dialysis

Peritoneal dialysis is principally used in the treatment of CKD, though it may occasionally be employed in AKI. It requires the insertion of a permanent Silastic catheter into the peritoneal cavity (see Fig. 15.25C). Two types are in common use. In continuous ambulatory peritoneal dialysis (CAPD), about 2 L of sterile, isotonic dialysis fluid are introduced and left in place for approximately 4–6 hours. Metabolic waste products diffuse from peritoneal capillaries into the dialysis fluid down a concentration gradient. The fluid is then drained and fresh dialysis fluid introduced, in a continuous four-times-daily cycle. The inflow fluid is rendered hyperosmolar by the addition of glucose or glucose polymer; this results in net removal of fluid from the patient during each cycle, due to diffusion of water from the blood through the peritoneal membrane down an osmotic gradient (ultrafiltration). The patient is mobile and able to undertake normal daily activities. Automated peritoneal dialysis (APD) is similar to CAPD but uses a mechanical device to perform the fluid exchanges during the night, leaving the patient free, or with only a single exchange to perform, during the day.

CAPD is particularly useful in children, as a first treatment in adults with residual renal function, and as a treatment for elderly patients with cardiovascular instability. The long-term use of peritoneal dialysis may be limited by episodes of bacterial peritonitis and damage to the peritoneal membrane, including encapsulating peritoneal sclerosis, but some patients have been treated successfully for more than 10 years. Box 15.39 summarises some of the problems related to CAPD treatment.

Renal transplantation

Renal transplantation offers the best chance of long-term survival in ESRD and is the most cost-effective treatment. All patients with ESRD should be considered for transplantation but many are not suitable due to a combination of comorbidity and advanced age (although no absolute age limit applies). Active malignancy, vasculitis, cardiovascular disease and a high risk of recurrence of renal disease (generally glomerulonephritides) are common contraindications to transplantation.

Kidney grafts may be taken from a deceased donor in the UK after brain death (40%) or circulatory death (24%), or from a living donor (36%). As described on page 88, matching of a donor to a specific recipient is strongly influenced by immunological factors, since graft rejection is the major cause of transplant failure. Compatibility of ABO blood group between donor and recipient is usually required and the degree of matching for major histocompatibility (MHC) antigens, particularly human leucocyte antigen DR (HLA-DR), influences the incidence of rejection. Immediately prior to transplantation, cross-matching should be performed for anti-HLA antibodies (traditionally mixing of recipient serum with donor lymphocytes) (p. 88). Positive tests predict early rejection and worse graft survival. Although some ABO- and HLA-incompatible transplants are now possible, this involves appropriate preparation with pre-transplant plasma exchange and/or immunosuppression, so that recipient antibodies to the donor's tissue are reduced to acceptably low levels. This option is generally only available for living donor transplants because of the preparation required. Paired exchanges, in which a donor–recipient pair who are incompatible, either in blood group or HLA, are computer-matched with another pair to overcome the mismatch, are also used to help increase the number of successful transplants that can be performed.

During the transplant operation, the kidney is placed in the pelvis; the donor vessels are usually anastomosed to the recipient's external iliac artery and vein, and the donor ureter to the bladder (see Fig. 15.25D). The native kidneys are usually left in place but may be removed pre-transplant if they are a source of repeated sepsis or to make room for a transplant in patients with very large kidneys due to adult polycystic kidney disease.

i 15.39 Problems with continuous ambulatory peritoneal dialysis

Problem	Clinical features	Cause	Treatment
Peritonitis	Cloudy drainage fluid; abdominal pain and systemic sepsis are variable	Usually entry of skin contaminants via catheter; bowel organisms less common	Culture of peritoneal dialysis fluid Intraperitoneal antibiotics, tobramycin, vancomycin Catheter removal sometimes required
Catheter exit site infection	Erythema and pus around exit site	Usually skin organisms	Antibiotics; sometimes surgical drainage
Ultrafiltration failure	Fluid overload	Damage to peritoneal membrane, leading to rapid transport of glucose and loss of osmotic gradient	Replacement of glucose with synthetic, poorly absorbed polymers for some exchanges (icodextrin)
Peritoneal membrane failure	Inadequate clearance of urea etc.	Scarring/damage to peritoneal membrane	Increase in exchange volumes; consideration of automated peritoneal dialysis or switch to haemodialysis
Sclerosing peritonitis	Intermittent bowel obstruction Malnutrition	Unknown; typically occurs after many years	Switch to haemodialysis (may still progress) Surgery and tamoxifen may be used

i 15.40 Common causes of renal allograft dysfunction

Time post transplant	Cause	Risk factors
Hours to days	Renal artery/vein thrombosis	Technically difficult surgery Thrombophilia/SLE
	Ureteric leak Delayed graft function (i.e. transplant does not start working immediately)	Small bladder/anuria pre-transplant Prolonged cold ischaemia time* Donation after circulatory death Older, hypertensive donor with stroke as cause of death, high tacrolimus level
	Hyperacute rejection	Pre-formed anti-HLA antibodies HLA mismatch Previous transplant
Weeks	Acute rejection (especially <3 months; can occur later with non-adherence/insufficient immunosuppression)	Pre-formed anti-HLA antibodies HLA mismatch Previous transplant
Months	BK virus nephropathy	Intensive immunosuppression Ureteric stent use
	Renal artery stenosis	Donor disease Injury at organ retrieval
Years	Chronic allograft injury (often antibody-mediated)	Previous acute rejections Non-adherence/insufficient immunosuppression
Any time	Tacrolimus/ciclosporin toxicity	High doses/serum levels Concurrent use of drugs that inhibit cytochrome P450 system
	Sepsis (opportunistic and conventional) Recurrence of disease: Early (FSGS/MCGN) Later (IgA nephropathy/membranous glomerulonephritis)	Primary FSGS and MCGN Previous transplant recurrence

*Time from organ retrieval in the donor, with cold perfusion occurring ex vivo, until implantation into the recipient. (FSGS = focal segmental glomerulosclerosis; HLA = human leucocyte antigen; IgA = immunoglobulin A; MCGN = mesangiocapillary glomerulonephritis; SLE = systemic lupus erythematosus)

All transplant patients require regular life-long follow-up to monitor renal function and complications of immunosuppression. Allograft dysfunction is often asymptomatic and picked up during routine surveillance blood tests. The common causes at different time points post transplant are summarised in Box 15.40. Immunosuppressive therapy (see Box 4.26, p. 89) is required to prevent rejection and is more intensive in the early post-transplantation period, when rejection risk is highest. A common regimen is triple therapy with prednisolone; ciclosporin or tacrolimus; and azathioprine or mycophenolate mofetil. Sirolimus is an alternative that can be introduced later but is generally not used initially due to impaired wound healing. Antibodies to deplete or modulate specific lymphocyte populations are increasingly used for induction and for treatment of glucocorticoid-resistant acute rejection. Basiliximab, an interleukin (IL)-2 receptor antagonist, is frequently used at induction to lower rates of rejection. Acute cellular rejection is usually treated, in the first instance, by short courses of high-dose glucocorticoids, such as intravenous methylprednisolone on three consecutive days. Anti-lymphocyte preparations (e.g. anti-thymocyte globulin, ATG) are used for glucocorticoid-resistant rejection. Antibody-mediated rejection is more difficult to treat and usually requires plasma exchange and intravenous immunoglobulin (p. 89). Complications of immunosuppression include infections and malignancy (p. 89). Approximately 50% of white patients develop skin malignancy by 15 years after transplantation.

The prognosis after kidney transplantation is good. Recent UK statistics for transplants from cadaver donors indicate 96% patient survival and 93% graft survival at 1 year, and 88% patient survival and 84% graft survival at 5 years. Even better figures are obtained with living donor transplantation (91% graft survival at 5 years).

Renal disease in pregnancy

Pregnancy has important physiological effects on the renal system. Some diseases are more common in pregnancy (Box 15.41), the manifestations of others are modified during pregnancy, and a few diseases, such as pre-eclampsia (see Box 30.8, p. 1276), are unique to pregnancy. These are discussed in detail in Chapter 30.

 15.41 Renal diseases in pregnancy

- **Eclampsia**: severe hypertension, encephalopathy and fits
- **Disseminated intravascular coagulation**
- **Thrombotic microangiopathy**: may also occur post-partum (post-partum thrombotic thrombocytopenic purpura/haemolytic uraemic syndrome)
- **Acute fatty liver of pregnancy**
- **'HELLP' syndrome**: haemolysis, elevated liver enzymes, low platelets (thrombotic microangiopathy with abnormal liver function)

Renal disease in adolescence

Many causes of renal failure present during infancy or childhood, such as congenital urological malformations and inherited disorders like cystinosis and autosomal recessive polycystic kidney disease. The consequences continue throughout the patient's life and the situation often arises whereby patients transition from paediatric to adult nephrology services. Some of the issues and challenges surrounding this transition are summarised in Box 15.42.

 15.42 Kidney disease in adolescence

- **Adherence**: young adults moving from parental supervision may become disengaged. There may also be reduced adherence to prophylactic and therapeutic treatment.
- **Adverse events**: there is an increased risk of transplant loss and other adverse events in young adults on renal replacement therapy.
- **Management**: joint transition clinics should be established with the paediatric team to facilitate transfer to adult specialist clinics.

Drugs and the kidney

Drug-induced renal disease

The kidney is susceptible to damage by drugs because it is the route of excretion of many water-soluble compounds, including drugs and their metabolites. Some may reach high concentrations in the renal cortex as a result of proximal tubular transport mechanisms. Others are concentrated in the medulla by the operation of the countercurrent system. The same applies to certain toxins.

Toxic renal damage may occur by a variety of mechanisms (Box 15.43). Very commonly, drugs contribute to the development of acute tubular necrosis as one of multiple insults. Numerically, reactions to NSAIDs and ACE inhibitors are the most important. Haemodynamic renal impairment, acute tubular necrosis and allergic reactions are usually reversible if recognised early enough. Other types, however, especially those associated with extensive fibrosis, are less likely to be reversible.

Non-steroidal anti-inflammatory drugs

Impairment of renal function may develop in patients on NSAIDs, since prostaglandins play an important role in regulating renal blood flow by vasodilating afferent arterioles (see Fig. 15.19, p. 413). This is particularly likely in patients with other disorders, such as volume depletion, heart failure, cirrhosis, sepsis and pre-existing renal impairment. In addition, idiosyncratic immune reactions may occur, causing minimal change nephrotic syndrome, membranous nephropathy (p. 400) and acute interstitial nephritis (p. 402). Analgesic nephropathy (p. 403) is now a rare complication of long-term use.

ACE inhibitors

These abolish the compensatory angiotensin II-mediated vasoconstriction of the glomerular efferent arteriole that takes place in order to maintain glomerular perfusion pressure distal to a renal artery stenosis and in renal hypoperfusion (see Figs 15.1 and 15.19, pp. 385 and 413). Monitoring of renal function before and after initiation of therapy is essential and an expected rise in creatinine of about 20% is frequently observed.

Prescribing in renal disease

Many drugs and drug metabolites are excreted by the kidney and so the presence of renal impairment alters the required dose and frequency (p. 31).

Infections of the urinary tract

In health, bacterial colonisation is confined to the lower end of the urethra and the remainder of the urinary tract is sterile (see Ch. 6). The urinary tract can become infected with various bacteria but the most common is *E. coli* derived from the gastrointestinal tract. The most common presenting problem is cystitis with urethritis (generally referred to as urinary tract infection).

Urinary tract infection

Urinary tract infection (UTI) is the term used to describe acute urethritis and cystitis caused by a microorganism. It is a common disorder, accounting for 1–3% of consultations in general medical practice. The prevalence of UTI in women is about 3% at the age of 20, increasing by about 1% in each subsequent decade. In males, UTI is uncommon, except in the first year of life and in men over 60, when it may complicate bladder outflow obstruction.

i   15.43 Mechanisms and examples of drug-induced renal disease/dysfunction

Mechanism	Drug or toxin	Comments
Haemodynamic	NSAIDs	Reduce renal blood flow due to inhibition of prostaglandin synthesis causing afferent arteriolar vasoconstriction
	ACE inhibitors	Reduce efferent glomerular arteriolar tone, so especially problematic in the presence of renal artery stenosis and other causes of renal hypoperfusion (e.g. NSAIDs)
	Radiographic contrast media	Multifactorial aetiology may include intense vasoconstriction
Acute tubular necrosis	Aminoglycosides, amphotericin	In most examples there is evidence of direct tubular toxicity but haemodynamic and other factors probably contribute
	Paracetamol overdose	May occur with or without serious hepatotoxicity
	Radiographic contrast media	Directly toxic to proximal tubular cells
Loss of tubular/collecting duct function	Lithium	Dose-related, partially reversible loss of concentrating ability
	Cisplatin	Occurs at lower exposures than cause acute tubular necrosis
	Aminoglycosides, amphotericin	
Glomerulonephritis (immune-mediated)	Penicillamine, gold	Membranous nephropathy
	Penicillamine, propylthiouracil, hydralazine	Crescentic or focal necrotising glomerulonephritis in association with ANCA and systemic small-vessel vasculitis
	NSAIDs	Minimal change nephropathy, membranous nephropathy
Interstitial nephritis (immune-mediated)	NSAIDs, penicillins, proton pump inhibitors, many others	Acute interstitial nephritis
Interstitial nephritis (toxicity)	Lithium	As a consequence of acute toxicity
	Ciclosporin, tacrolimus	Chronic interstitial nephritis
Interstitial nephritis (with papillary necrosis)	Various NSAIDs (p. 403)	Ischaemic damage secondary to NSAID effects on renal blood flow
Tubular obstruction (crystal formation)	Aciclovir	Crystals of the drug form in tubules. Aciclovir is now more common than the original example of sulphonamides
	Chemotherapy	Uric acid crystals form as a consequence of tumour lysis (typically, a first-dose effect in haematological malignancy)
Nephrocalcinosis	Oral sodium phosphate-containing bowel cleansing agents	Precipitation of calcium phosphate occurring in 1–4% and exacerbated by volume depletion. Usually mild but damage can be irreversible
Retroperitoneal fibrosis	Ergolinic dopamine agonists (cabergoline), methysergide*, practolol*	Idiopathic retroperitoneal fibrosis is more common (p. 434)

*These drugs are no longer in use in the UK.
(ACE = angiotensin-converting enzyme; ANCA = antineutrophil cytoplasmic antibody; NSAIDs = non-steroidal anti-inflammatory drugs)

15

Pathophysiology

Urine is an excellent culture medium for bacteria; in addition, the urothelium of susceptible persons may have more receptors, to which virulent strains of *E. coli* become adherent. In women, the ascent of organisms into the bladder is easier than in men; the urethra is shorter and the absence of bactericidal prostatic secretions may be relevant. Sexual intercourse may cause minor urethral trauma and transfer bacteria from the perineum into the bladder. Instrumentation of the bladder may also introduce organisms. Multiplication of organisms then depends on a number of factors, including the size of the inoculum and virulence of the bacteria. Conditions that predispose to UTI are shown in Box 15.44.

Clinical features

Typical features of cystitis and urethritis include:
- abrupt onset of frequency of micturition and urgency
- burning pain in the urethra during micturition (dysuria)
- suprapubic pain during and after voiding

- intense desire to pass more urine after micturition, due to spasm of the inflamed bladder wall (strangury)
- urine that may appear cloudy and have an unpleasant odour
- non-visible or visible haematuria.

Systemic symptoms are usually slight or absent. However, infection in the lower urinary tract can spread to cause acute pyelonephritis. This is suggested by prominent systemic symptoms with fever, rigors, vomiting, hypotension and loin pain, guarding or tenderness, and may be an indication for hospitalisation. Only about 30% of patients with acute pyelonephritis have associated symptoms of cystitis or urethritis. Prostatitis is suggested by perineal or suprapubic pain, pain on ejaculation and prostatic tenderness on rectal examination.

The differential diagnosis of lower urinary tract symptoms includes urethritis due to sexually transmitted disease, notably chlamydia (p. 340) and urethritis associated with reactive arthritis (p. 1031). Some patients, usually female, have symptoms suggestive of urethritis and cystitis but no bacteria are cultured from the urine (the 'urethral syndrome'). Possible explanations include infection with organisms not readily cultured by ordinary

15.44 Risk factors for urinary tract infection

Bladder outflow obstruction

- Benign prostatic enlargement
- Prostate cancer
- Urethral stricture

Anatomical abnormalities

- Vesico-ureteric reflux
- Uterine prolapse
- Bladder fistula

Neurological problems

- Multiple sclerosis
- Spina bifida
- Diabetic neuropathy

Foreign bodies

- Urethral suprapubic catheter
- Ureteric stent
- Nephrostomy tube
- Urolithiasis

Loss of host defences

- Atrophic urethritis and vaginitis in post-menopausal women
- Diabetes mellitus

15.45 Investigation of patients with urinary tract infection

All patients

- Dipstick* estimation of nitrite, leucocyte esterase and glucose
- Microscopy/cytometry of urine for white blood cells, organisms
- Urine culture

Infants, children, and anyone with fever or complicated infection

- Full blood count; urea, electrolytes, creatinine
- Blood cultures

Pyelonephritis: men; children; women with recurrent infections

- Renal tract ultrasound or CT
- Pelvic examination in women, rectal examination in men

Continuing haematuria or other suspicion of bladder lesion

- Cystoscopy

*May substitute for microscopy and culture in simple uncomplicated infection.

15.46 Urinary infection in old age

- **Prevalence of asymptomatic bacteriuria**: rises with age. Among the most frail in institutional care it rises to 40% in women and 30% in men.
- **Decision to treat**: treating asymptomatic bacteriuria does not improve chronic incontinence or decrease mortality or morbidity from symptomatic urinary infection. It risks adverse effects from the antibiotic and promotion of the emergence of resistant organisms. Bacteriuria should not be treated in the absence of urinary symptoms.
- **Source of infection**: the urinary tract is the most frequent source of bacteraemia in older patients admitted to hospital.
- **Incontinence**: new or increased incontinence is a common presentation of UTI in older women.
- **Treatment**: post-menopausal women with acute lower urinary tract symptoms may require longer than 3 days' therapy.

of typical clinical features and abnormalities on urinalysis. Most urinary pathogens can reduce nitrate to nitrite, and neutrophils and nitrites can usually be detected in symptomatic infections by urine dipstick tests for leucocyte esterase and nitrite, respectively. The absence of both nitrites and leucocyte esterase in the urine makes UTI unlikely. Interpretation of bacterial counts in the urine, and of what is a 'significant' culture result, is based on probabilities. Urine taken by suprapubic aspiration should be sterile, so the presence of any organisms is significant. If the patient has symptoms and there are neutrophils in the urine, a small number of organisms is significant. In asymptomatic patients, more than 10^5 organisms/mL is usually regarded as significant (asymptomatic bacteriuria; see below).

Typical organisms causing UTI in the community include *E. coli* derived from the gastrointestinal tract (about 75% of infections), *Proteus* spp., *Pseudomonas* spp., streptococci and *Staphylococcus epidermidis*. In hospital, *E. coli* still predominates but *Klebsiella* and streptococci are becoming more common. Certain strains of *E. coli* have a particular propensity to invade the urinary tract.

Investigations to detect underlying predisposing factors for UTI are used selectively, most commonly in children, men or patients with recurrent infections (see Box 15.45).

Management

Antibiotics are recommended in all cases of proven UTI (Box 15.47). If urine culture has been performed, treatment may be started while awaiting the result. For infection of the lower urinary tract, treatment for 3 days is the norm and is less likely to induce significant alterations in bowel flora than more prolonged therapy. Trimethoprim or nitrofurantoin is the usual first choice of drug for initial treatment; however, between 10% and 40% of organisms causing UTI are resistant to trimethoprim, the lower rates being seen in community-based practice. Trimethoprim and nitrofurantoin are not recommended if eGFR is <30 mL/min/1.73m² due to reduced efficacy/increased risk of toxicity. In addition, trimethoprim may increase serum potassium and creatinine levels and lead to artefactual reductions in eGFR, which resolve once the drug is discontinued. Quinolone antibiotics such as ciprofloxacin and norfloxacin, and cefalexin are also generally effective. Co-amoxiclav and amoxicillin are no longer recommended as blind therapy, as up to 30% of organisms are resistant. They may be used once cultures confirm that the organism is sensitive. Penicillins and cephalosporins are safe to use in pregnancy but trimethoprim, sulphonamides, quinolones and tetracyclines should be avoided.

methods (such as *Chlamydia* and certain anaerobes), intermittent or low-count bacteriuria, reaction to toiletries or disinfectants, symptoms related to sexual intercourse, or post-menopausal atrophic vaginitis.

The differential diagnosis of acute pyelonephritis includes pyelonephrosis, acute appendicitis, diverticulitis, cholecystitis, salpingitis, ruptured ovarian cyst or ectopic pregnancy. In pyelonephrosis due to upper urinary tract obstruction, patients may become extremely ill, with fever, leucocytosis and positive blood cultures. With a perinephric abscess, there is marked pain and tenderness, and often bulging of the loin on the affected side. Urinary symptoms may be absent in this situation and urine testing negative, containing neither pus cells nor organisms.

Investigations

An approach to investigation is shown in Box 15.45. In an otherwise healthy woman with a single lower urinary tract infection, urine culture prior to treatment is not mandatory. Investigation is necessary, however, in patients with recurrent infection or after failure of initial treatment, during pregnancy, or in patients susceptible to serious infection, such as the immunocompromised, those with diabetes or an indwelling catheter, and older people (Box 15.46). The diagnosis can be made from the combination

i	15.47 Antibiotic regimens for urinary tract infection in adults[1]				
Scenario	**Drug**	**Regimen**		**Duration**	**Comment**
Cystitis					
First choices	Trimethoprim	200 mg twice daily			
	Nitrofurantoin	50 mg 4 times daily			7–10 days in men
Second choices[1]	Cefalexin	250 mg 4 times daily	}	3 days	
	Ciprofloxacin	250 mg twice daily			
	Pivmecillinam	400 mg 3 times daily			
In pregnancy	Nitrofurantoin	50 mg 4 times daily	}	7 days	Avoid trimethoprim and quinolones during pregnancy; avoid nitrofurantoin at term
	Cefalexin	250 mg 4 times daily			
Prophylactic therapy					
First choice	Trimethoprim	100 mg at night	}	Continuous	
Second choice[1]	Nitrofurantoin	50 mg at night			
Pyelonephritis					
First choice	Cefalexin	1 g 4 times daily		14 days	} Admit to hospital if no response within 24 hrs
	Ciprofloxacin	500 mg twice daily		7 days	
Second choice	Gentamicin[2]	Adjust dose according to renal function and serum levels	}	14 days	Switch to appropriate oral agent as soon as possible
	Cefuroxime	750–1500 mg 3 times daily			
Epididymo-orchitis					
First choice	Ciprofloxacin	500 mg twice daily			
Young men	Doxycycline	100 mg twice daily	}	14 days	Refer young men to genito-urinary department to check for *Neisseria gonorrhoeae*, which requires addition of a single dose of ceftriaxone 500 mg IM
Older men	Ciprofloxacin	500 mg twice daily			
Acute prostatitis					
First choice	Trimethoprim	200 mg twice daily	}	28 days	
Second choice	Ciprofloxacin	500 mg twice daily			

[1]In all cases, the choice of drug should take locally determined antibiotic resistance patterns into account. [2]See Hartford nomogram (Fig. 6.18, p. 122). (IM = intramuscular)

In more severe infection, antibiotics should be continued for 7–14 days. Seriously ill patients may require intravenous therapy with gentamicin for a few days (Box 15.47), later switching to an oral agent.

A fluid intake of at least 2 L/day is usually recommended, although this is not based on evidence and may make symptoms of dysuria worse.

Persistent or recurrent UTI

If the causative organism persists on repeat culture despite treatment, or if there is reinfection with any organism after an interval, then an underlying cause is more likely to be present (see Box 15.44) and more detailed investigation is justified (see Box 15.45). In women, recurrent infections are common and investigation is justified only if infections are frequent (three or more per year) or unusually severe. Recurrent UTI, particularly in the presence of an underlying cause, may result in permanent renal damage, whereas uncomplicated infections rarely (if ever) do so (see chronic reflux nephropathy, p. 430).

If an underlying cause cannot be treated, suppressive antibiotic therapy (see Box 15.47) can be used to prevent recurrence and reduce the risk of sepsis and renal damage. Urine should be cultured at regular intervals; a regimen of two or three antibiotics in sequence, rotating every 6 months, is often used in an attempt to reduce the emergence of resistant organisms. Other simple measures may help to prevent recurrence (Box 15.48). Trimethoprim or nitrofurantion is recommended for prophylaxis. Alternative antibiotics include cefalexin, co-amoxiclav

i	15.48 Prophylactic measures to be adopted by women with recurrent urinary infections

- Fluid intake of at least 2 L/day
- Regular complete emptying of bladder
- Good personal hygiene
- Emptying of bladder before and after sexual intercourse
- Cranberry juice/tablets may be effective

and ciprofloxacin, but these should be avoided if possible because of adverse effects and the generation of resistance.

Asymptomatic bacteriuria

This is defined as more than 10^5 organisms/mL in the urine of apparently healthy asymptomatic patients. Approximately 1% of children under the age of 1 year, 1% of schoolgirls, 0.03% of schoolboys and men, 3% of non-pregnant adult women and 5% of pregnant women have asymptomatic bacteriuria. It is increasingly common in those aged over 65. There is no evidence that this condition causes renal scarring in adults who are not pregnant and have a normal urinary tract, and, in general, treatment is not indicated. Up to 30% will develop symptomatic infection within 1 year, however. Treatment is required in infants, pregnant women and those with urinary tract abnormalities.

Catheter-related bacteriuria

In patients with a urinary catheter, bacteriuria increases the risk of Gram-negative bacteraemia five-fold. Bacteriuria is common,

15

however, and almost universal during long-term catheterisation. Treatment is usually avoided in asymptomatic patients, as this may promote antibiotic resistance. Careful sterile insertion technique is important and the catheter should be removed as soon as it is not required.

Acute pyelonephritis

The kidneys are infected in a minority of patients with UTI. Acute renal infection (pyelonephritis) presents as a classic triad of loin pain, fever and tenderness over the kidneys. The renal pelvis is inflamed and small abscesses are often evident in the renal parenchyma (see Fig. 15.13C, p. 402).

Renal infection is almost always caused by organisms ascending from the bladder, and the bacterial profile is the same as for lower urinary tract infection (p. 428). Rarely, bacteraemia may give rise to renal or perinephric abscesses, most commonly due to staphylococci. Predisposing factors, such as cysts or renal scarring, facilitate infection.

Rarely, acute pyelonephritis is associated with papillary necrosis. Fragments of renal papillary tissue are passed per urethra and can be identified histologically. They may cause ureteric obstruction and, if this occurs bilaterally or in a single kidney, it may lead to AKI. Predisposing factors include diabetes mellitus, chronic urinary obstruction, analgesic nephropathy and sickle-cell disease. A necrotising form of pyelonephritis with gas formation, 'emphysematous pyelonephritis', is occasionally seen in patients with diabetes mellitus. Xanthogranulomatous pyelonephritis is a chronic infection that can resemble renal cell cancer. It is usually associated with obstruction, is characterised by accumulation of foamy macrophages and generally requires nephrectomy. Infection of cysts in polycystic kidney disease (p. 405) calls for prolonged antibiotic treatment.

Appropriate investigations are shown in Box 15.45 and management is described above and in Box 15.47. Intravenous rehydration may be needed in severe cases. If complicated infection is suspected or response to treatment is not prompt, urine should be re-cultured and renal tract ultrasound performed to exclude urinary tract obstruction or a perinephric collection. If obstruction is present, drainage by a percutaneous nephrostomy or ureteric stent should be considered.

Tuberculosis

Tuberculosis of the kidney and renal tract is secondary to tuberculosis elsewhere (p. 588) and is the result of blood-borne infection. Initially, lesions develop in the renal cortex; these may ulcerate into the renal pelvis and involve the ureters, bladder, epididymis, seminal vesicles and prostate. Calcification in the kidney and stricture formation in the ureter are typical.

Clinical features may include symptoms of bladder involvement (frequency, dysuria); haematuria (sometimes macroscopic); malaise, fever, night sweats, lassitude and weight loss; loin pain; associated genital disease; and chronic renal failure as a result of urinary tract obstruction or destruction of kidney tissue.

Neutrophils are present in the urine but routine urine culture may be negative ('sterile pyuria'). Special techniques of microscopy and culture may be required to identify tubercle bacilli and are most usefully performed on early morning urine specimens. Bladder involvement should be assessed by cystoscopy. Radiology of the urinary tract and a chest X-ray to look for pulmonary tuberculosis are mandatory. Anti-tuberculous chemotherapy follows standard regimens (p. 592). Surgery to relieve urinary

tract obstruction or to remove a very severely infected kidney may be required.

Reflux nephropathy

This condition, which was previously known as chronic pyelonephritis, is a specific type of chronic interstitial nephritis associated with vesico-ureteric reflux (VUR) in early life and with the appearance of scars in the kidney, as demonstrated by various imaging techniques. About 12% of patients in Europe requiring treatment for ESRD may have this disorder but diagnostic criteria are imprecise.

Pathophysiology

Reflux nephropathy is thought to be due to chronic reflux of urine from the bladder into the ureters, in association with recurrent UTI in childhood. It was previously assumed that ascending infection was necessary for progressive renal damage in patients with VUR but there is evidence to suggest that renal scars can occur, even in the absence of infection. Furthermore, epidemiological surveys and controlled trials have found that efforts to correct VUR by using surgical or other means are ineffective in halting progression of the disease.

Susceptibility to VUR has a genetic component and may be associated with renal dysplasia and other congenital abnormalities of the urinary tract. It can be connected with outflow obstruction, usually caused by urethral valves, but usually occurs with an apparently normal bladder.

Clinical features

Usually, the renal scarring and dilatation are asymptomatic and the patient may present at any age with hypertension (sometimes severe), proteinuria or features of CKD. There may be no history of overt UTI. However, symptoms arising from the urinary tract may be present and include frequency of micturition, dysuria and aching lumbar pain. VUR may occur in children but diminishes as the child grows, and usually has disappeared by adulthood. Urinalysis often shows the presence of leucocytes and moderate proteinuria (usually <1 g/24 hrs) but these are not invariable. The risk of renal stone formation is increased. A number of women first present with hypertension and/or proteinuria in pregnancy. Children and adults with small or unilateral renal scars have a good prognosis, provided renal growth is normal. With significant unilateral scars there is usually compensatory hypertrophy of the contralateral kidney. In patients with more severe bilateral disease, prognosis is related to the severity of renal dysfunction, hypertension and proteinuria. If the serum creatinine is normal and hypertension and proteinuria are absent, then the long-term prognosis is usually good.

Investigations

Renal scarring can be detected by ultrasound but it has poor sensitivity and is only capable of detecting major defects and excluding significant obstruction. Radionuclide DMSA scans are more sensitive (see Fig. 15.6, p. 390), and serial imaging by MRI or CT may be useful in assessing progression. Abnormalities may be unilateral or bilateral and of any grade of severity. Gross scarring of the kidneys, commonly at the poles, is seen, with reduced kidney size and narrowing of the cortex and medulla. Renal scars may be juxtaposed to dilated calyces. In patients who develop heavy proteinuria and hypertension, renal biopsies show glomerulomegaly and focal glomerulosclerosis, probably as a secondary response to reduced nephron numbers. Radionuclide

Fig. 15.28 Vesico-ureteric reflux (grade IV) shown by micturating cystogram. The bladder has been filled with contrast medium through a urinary catheter. After micturition, there was gross vesico-ureteric reflux into widely distended ureters and pelvicalyceal systems. *Courtesy of Dr A.P. Bayliss and Dr P. Thorpe, Aberdeen Royal Infirmary.*

i 15.49 Composition of renal stones	
Composition	**Percentage**
Calcium oxalate[1]	60%
Calcium phosphate	15%
Uric acid	10%
Magnesium ammonium phosphate (struvite)[2]	15%
Cystine and others	1%

[1]Stones often contain small amounts of calcium phosphate. [2]Associated with urine infection.

i 15.50 Predisposing factors for kidney stones

Environmental and dietary causes
- Low urine volumes: high ambient temperatures, low fluid intake
- Diet: high protein, high sodium, low calcium
- High sodium excretion
- High oxalate excretion
- High urate excretion
- Low citrate excretion

Acquired causes
- Hypercalcaemia of any cause (p. 661)
- Ileal disease or resection (increases oxalate absorption and urinary excretion)
- Renal tubular acidosis type I (distal, p. 365)

Congenital and inherited causes
- Familial hypercalciuria
- Medullary sponge kidney
- Cystinuria
- Renal tubular acidosis type I (distal)
- Primary hyperoxaluria

techniques can also be used to demonstrate VUR as a non-invasive alternative to micturating cystourethrography (MCUG; the bladder is filled with contrast media through a urinary catheter and images are taken during and after micturition; Fig. 15.28). As surgical intervention for VUR has declined in popularity (see below), however, this type of imaging is used less often.

Management

Infection, if present, should be treated; if recurrent, it should be prevented with prophylactic therapy, as described for UTI (p. 429). If recurrent pyelonephritis occurs in an abnormal kidney with minimal function, nephrectomy may be indicated. Occasionally, hypertension is cured by the removal of a diseased kidney when the disease is predominantly or entirely unilateral.

As most childhood reflux tends to disappear spontaneously and trials have shown small or no benefits from anti-reflux surgery, such intervention is now less common. Severe reflux may be managed by ureteric reimplantation or subtrigonal injection of Teflon or polysaccharide (STING) beneath the ureteric orifice.

Urolithiasis

Renal stone disease is common, affecting people of all countries and ethnic groups. In the UK, the prevalence is about 1.2%, with a lifetime risk of developing a renal stone by age 60–70 of approximately 7% in men. In some regions, the risk is higher, most notably in countries such as Saudi Arabia, where the lifetime risk of developing a renal stone in men aged 60–70 is just over 20%.

Pathophysiology

Urinary calculi consist of aggregates of crystals, usually containing calcium or phosphate in combination with small amounts of proteins and glycoproteins. The most common types are summarised in Box 15.49. A number of risk factors have been identified for renal stone formation (Box 15.50). In developed countries, however, most calculi occur in healthy young men, in whom investigations reveal no clear predisposing cause. Renal stones vary greatly in size, from sand-like particles anywhere in the urinary tract to large, round stones in the bladder. In developing countries, bladder stones are common, particularly in children. In developed countries, the incidence of childhood bladder stones is low; renal stones in adults are more common. Staghorn calculi fill the whole renal pelvis and branch into the calyces (Fig. 15.29); they are usually associated with infection and composed largely of struvite. Deposits of calcium may be present throughout the renal parenchyma, giving rise to fine calcification within it (nephrocalcinosis), especially in patients with renal tubular acidosis, hyperparathyroidism, vitamin D intoxication and healed renal tuberculosis. Cortical nephrocalcinosis may occur in areas of cortical necrosis, typically after AKI in pregnancy or other severe AKI.

Clinical features

The clinical presentation is highly variable. Many patients with renal stone disease are asymptomatic, whereas others present with pain, haematuria, UTI or urinary tract obstruction. A common presentation is with acute loin pain radiating to the anterior

15

Fig. 15.29 Computed tomogram of the kidneys, ureters and bladder (CTKUB): coronal view showing a staghorn calculus in the left kidney. *Courtesy of Dr I. Mendichovszky, University of Cambridge.*

	15.51 Investigations for renal stones		
Sample	Test	First stone	Recurrent stone
Stone	Chemical composition[1]		✓
Blood	Calcium	✓	✓
	Phosphate	✓	✓
	Uric acid	✓	✓
	Urea and electrolytes	✓	✓
	Bicarbonate	✓	✓
	Parathyroid hormone[2]		(✓)
Urine	Dipstick test for protein, blood, glucose	✓	✓
	Amino acids		✓
24-hr urine	Urea		✓
	Creatinine clearance		✓
	Sodium		✓
	Calcium		✓
	Oxalate		✓
	Uric acid		✓

[1]The most valuable test if a stone can be obtained. [2]Only if serum calcium or urinary calcium excretion is high.

abdominal wall, together with haematuria: a symptom complex termed renal or ureteric colic. This is most commonly caused by ureteric obstruction by a calculus but the same symptoms can occur in association with a sloughed renal papilla, tumour or blood clot. The patient is suddenly aware of pain in the loin, which radiates round the flank to the groin and often into the testis or labium, in the sensory distribution of the first lumbar nerve. The pain steadily increases in intensity to reach a peak in a few minutes. The patient is restless and generally tries unsuccessfully to obtain relief by changing position or pacing the room. There is pallor, sweating and often vomiting. Frequency, dysuria and haematuria may occur. The intense pain usually subsides within 2 hours but may continue unabated for hours or days. It is usually constant during attacks, although slight fluctuations in severity may be seen. Subsequent to an attack of renal colic, intermittent dull pain in the loin or back may persist for several hours.

Investigations

Patients with symptoms of renal colic should be investigated to determine whether or not a stone is present, to identify its location and to assess whether it is causing obstruction. About 90% of stones contain calcium and these can be visualised on plain abdominal X-ray (radio-opaque stones) but non-contrast CTKUB (Fig. 15.29) is the gold standard for diagnosing a stone within the kidney or ureter, as 99% are visible using this method. Ultrasound can show stones within the kidney and dilatation of the renal pelvis and ureter if the stone is obstructing urine flow; it is useful in unstable patients or young women, in whom exposure to ionising radiation is undesirable.

A minimum set of investigations (Box 15.51) should be performed in patients with a first renal stone. The yield of more detailed investigation is low, and hence usually reserved for young patients, those with recurrent or multiple stones, or those with complicated or unexpected presentations. Chemical analysis of stones is often helpful in defining the underlying cause. Since most stones pass spontaneously through the urinary tract, ideally the urine should be sieved for a few days after an episode of colic in order to collect the calculus for analysis.

Management

The immediate treatment of renal colic is with analgesia and antiemetics. Renal colic is often unbearably painful and demands powerful analgesia; diclofenac orally or as a suppository (100 mg) is often very effective, followed by morphine (10–20 mg) or pethidine (100 mg) intramuscularly. Around 90% of stones of less than 4 mm diameter pass spontaneously, but this applies to only 10% of stones bigger than 6 mm, and these may require intervention (see below). Patients with renal or ureteric stones are at high risk of infection; if surgery is contemplated, the patient should be covered with appropriate antibiotics. Immediate action is required if infection occurs in the stagnant urine proximal to the stone (pyonephrosis), and in patients with a solitary kidney who develop anuria in association with a stone in the ureter.

Stones that do not pass spontaneously through the urinary tract may need to be removed surgically, using ureteroscopy and stone fragmentation usually with a laser, or percutaneous nephrolithotomy (PCNL) and fragmentation with an ultrasonic disaggregator. Alternatively, stones can be fragmented by extracorporeal shock wave lithotripsy (ESWL), in which shock waves generated outside the body are focused on the stone, breaking it into small pieces that can pass easily down the ureter. The indications for intervention to manage or remove stones from the renal tract are summarised in Box 15.52. Procedures vary, depending on the site (Fig. 15.30).

Measures to prevent further stone formation are guided by the investigations in Box 15.51. Some general principles apply to almost every patient with calcium-containing stones (Box 15.53). More specific measures apply to some types. Urate stones can be prevented by allopurinol but its role in patients with calcium

i | **15.52 Indications for intervention to manage and remove stones from the urinary tract**

Clinical presentation	Procedure
Obstruction and/or anuria	Emergency nephrostomy or stent
Pyonephrosis associated with stone	Emergency nephrostomy or stent
Stone in a patient with solitary kidney	Urgent PCNL, stent, ESWL or ureteroscopy*
Severe pain and persistence of stone in renal tract	Urgent PCNL, stent, ESWL or ureteroscopy*
Pain and persistence of stone in renal tract	Elective PCNL, ESWL or ureteroscopy*

*Procedure depends on site of stone; see Fig. 15.30.
(ESWL = extracorporeal shock wave lithotripsy; PCNL = percutaneous nephrolithotomy)

i | **15.53 Measures to prevent calcium stone formation**

Diet

Fluid
- At least 2 L output per day (intake 3–4 L): check with 24-hr urine collections
- Intake distributed throughout the day (especially before bed)

Sodium
- Restrict intake

Protein
- Moderate, not high

Calcium
- Maintain good calcium intake (calcium forms an insoluble salt with dietary oxalate, lowering oxalate absorption and excretion)
- Avoid calcium supplements separate from meals (increase calcium excretion without reducing oxalate excretion)

Oxalate
- Avoid foods that are rich in oxalate (spinach, rhubarb)

Drugs

Thiazide diuretics
- Reduce calcium excretion
- Valuable in recurrent stone-formers and hypercalciuria

Allopurinol
- If urate excretion high (unproven except for urate stones)

Avoid
- Vitamin D supplements (increase calcium absorption and excretion)
- Vitamin C supplementation (increases oxalate excretion)

15

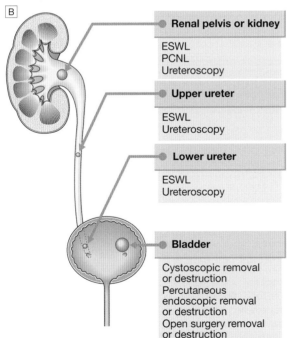

Fig. 15.30 Options for removal of urinary stones. |A| A patient undergoing extracorporeal shock wave lithotripsy (ESWL). |B| The procedures that are used for removal of stones in the urinary tract, shown in relation to the site of the stone. (PCNL = percutaneous nephrolithotomy)

Renal pelvis or kidney
ESWL
PCNL
Ureteroscopy

Upper ureter
ESWL
Ureteroscopy

Lower ureter
ESWL
Ureteroscopy

Bladder
Cystoscopic removal or destruction
Percutaneous endoscopic removal or destruction
Open surgery removal or destruction

stones and high urate excretion is uncertain. Stones formed in cystinuria can be reduced by penicillamine therapy. It may also be helpful to attempt to alkalinise the urine with sodium bicarbonate, as a high pH discourages urate and cystine stone formation.

Diseases of the collecting system and ureters

Congenital abnormalities

Various congenital anomalies of the urinary tract can occur (Fig. 15.31); they affect more than 10% of infants. If not immediately lethal, they can lead to complications in later life, including obstructive nephropathy and CKD.

Single kidneys

About 1 in 500 infants is born with only one kidney. Although this is usually compatible with normal life, it may be associated with other abnormalities.

Medullary sponge kidney disease

Medullary sponge kidney is a congenital disorder characterised by malformation of the papillary collecting ducts in the pericalyceal region of the renal pyramids. This leads to the formation of microscopic and large medullary cysts. Patients often present as adults with renal stones but the prognosis is generally good. The diagnosis is made by ultrasound, CT or intravenous urography, where contrast medium is seen to fill dilated or cystic tubules, which are sometimes calcified.

Fig. 15.31 Congenital abnormalities of the urinary tract. (PUJ = pelvi-ureteric junction)

Ureterocele

A ureterocele occurs behind a pin-hole ureteric orifice when the intramural part of the ureter dilates and bulges into the bladder. It can become very large and cause lower urinary tract obstruction. Incision of the pin-hole opening relieves the obstruction.

Ectopic ureters and duplex kidneys

Ectopic ureters occur with congenital duplication of one or both kidneys (duplex kidneys). Developmentally, the ureter has two main branches and, if this arrangement persists, the two ureters of the duplex kidneys may drain separately into the bladder. The lower pole moiety enters the bladder superiorly and laterally, while the upper pole moiety enters the bladder inferomedially to the lower pole moiety ureter or, more rarely, enters the vagina or seminal vesicle. The lower pole moiety has an ineffective valve mechanism, so that urine passes up the ureter on voiding (vesico-ureteric reflux, p. 430), whereas the upper pole moiety is often associated with a ureterocele.

Megaureter

A megaureter is a ureter dilated to more than 5 mm in diameter. It may be obstructed or non-obstructed and refluxing or non-refluxing. Some 50% of cases are asymptomatic but patients may present with pain, haematuria or infection. Radiographic and pressure/flow studies may be needed to determine whether there is obstruction to urine flow. Patients with symptoms or reduced renal function are treated. Ideally, treatment is expectant with antibiotic prophylaxis. Surgery (narrowing of the ureter and/or reimplantation) may, however, be needed for recurrent symptoms, reduction of more than 10% in renal function or complications (i.e. stones).

Pelvi-ureteric junction obstruction

Pelvi-ureteric junction obstruction (PUJO) causes idiopathic hydronephrosis and results from a functional obstruction at the junction of the ureter and renal pelvis. The abnormality is likely to be congenital and is often bilateral. It can be seen in very young children but gross hydronephrosis may present at any age. The common presentation is ill-defined renal pain or ache, exacerbated by drinking large volumes of liquid (Dietl's crisis). Rarely, it is asymptomatic. The diagnosis is often suspected after ultrasound or CT scan, and can be confirmed with a ^{99m}Tc-MAG3 renogram followed by diuretic. In a PUJO, the MAG3 renogram shows a pathognomonic 'rising curve' as the radioisotope accumulates in the renal pelvis and still does not drain following the diuretic injection. Treatment is surgical excision of the pelvi-ureteric junction and reanastomosis (pyeloplasty), which can now be performed laparoscopically. Less invasive alternatives are also possible, including balloon dilatation and endoscopic pyelotomy, but are generally less effective.

Retroperitoneal fibrosis

Fibrosis of the retroperitoneal connective tissues may encircle and compress the ureter(s), causing obstruction. The fibrosis is most commonly idiopathic but can represent a reaction to infection, radiation or aortic aneurysm, or be caused by metastatic cancer. It is recognised as part of the spectrum of disorders associated with elevated IgG4 levels (p. 890). Rarely, it can be associated with inflammatory bowel disease. Patients usually present with ill-defined symptoms of ureteric obstruction. Typically, there is an acute phase response (high CRP and ESR, and polyclonal hypergammaglobulinaemia). Imaging with CT or IVU shows ureteric obstruction with medial deviation of the ureters. Idiopathic retroperitoneal fibrosis may respond well to glucocorticoids (with a reduction in inflammatory marker levels) but ureteric stenting is often necessary to relieve obstruction and preserve renal function. Failure to improve indicates the need for surgery (ureterolysis), both to relieve obstruction and to exclude malignancy.

Tumours of the kidney and urinary tract

Several malignant tumours can affect the kidney and urinary tract, including renal cell cancer, upper urinary tract urothelial cancers, bladder carcinoma, prostate carcinoma, and cancers of the testis and penis. The urogenital tract can also be affected by benign tumours and secondary tumour deposits, which can cause obstructive uropathy. Renal cell cancer and bladder carcinoma are described here, while prostate cancer (p. 438) and testicular tumours (p. 439) are covered later in this chapter.

Renal cell cancer

Renal cell cancer (RCC) is by far the most common malignant tumour of the kidney in adults, making up 2.5% of all adult cancers, with a prevalence of 16 cases per 100 000 population. It is twice as common in males. The peak incidence is between 65 and 75 years of age and it is uncommon before 40. The tumour arises from renal tubular cells. Haemorrhage and necrosis give the cut surface a characteristic mixed golden-yellow and red appearance (Fig. 15.32B). Microscopically, clear cell RCCs are the most common histological subtype (85%), with papillary,

Fig. 15.32 Renal cell cancer. A In this CT, the right kidney is expanded by a low-density tumour, which fails to take up contrast material. Tumour is shown extending into the renal vein and inferior vena cava (arrow). B Pathology specimen showing typical necrosis of a renal cell cancer. *(A, B) Courtesy of Dr A.P. Bayliss and Dr P. Thorpe, Aberdeen Royal Infirmary.*

chromophobe and collecting duct tumours comprising the remainder. In RCC, there is potentially spread along the renal vein and the inferior vena cava. Direct invasion of perinephric tissues is common. Lymphatic spread occurs to para-aortic nodes, while blood-borne metastases (which may be solitary) most commonly develop in the lungs, bone and brain.

Clinical features

In 50% of patients, asymptomatic renal tumours are identified as an incidental finding during imaging investigations carried out for other reasons. Among symptomatic patients, about 60% present with haematuria, 40% with loin pain and 25% with a palpable mass. About 10% present with a triad of pain, haematuria and a mass; this usually represents advanced disease. A remarkable range of systemic effects may be present, including fever, raised ESR, polycythaemia, disorders of coagulation, hypercalcaemia, and abnormalities of plasma proteins and liver function tests. The patient may present with pyrexia of unknown origin (PUO) or, rarely, with neuropathy. Some of these systemic effects are caused by secretion of products by the tumour, such as renin, erythropoietin, parathyroid hormone-related protein (PTHrP) and gonadotrophins. The effects disappear when the tumour is removed but may reappear when metastases develop.

Investigations

Ultrasound is often the initial investigation and allows differentiation between solid tumour and simple renal cysts. If the results are suggestive of a tumour, contrast-enhanced CT of the abdomen and chest should be performed for staging (Fig. 15.32A). For tumours with no evidence of metastatic spread and when the nature of the lesion is uncertain, ultrasound or CT-guided biopsy may be used to avoid nephrectomy for benign disease.

Management

Radical nephrectomy that includes the perirenal fascial envelope is the treatment of choice. Nephrectomy is commonly performed laparoscopically, with equivalent outcomes to open surgery. Partial nephrectomy, which may be carried out by open or minimally invasive surgery, is recommended for tumours of 4 cm or less, as there is a lower incidence of long-term cardiac- and

renal-related morbidity. Patients at high operative risk who have small tumours may also be treated percutaneously by cryotherapy or radiofrequency ablation. There is an evolving role for active surveillance with serial imaging in selected patients with small renal masses of less than 4 cm. Surgery may also play a role in the treatment of solitary metastases, since these can remain single for long periods and excision may be curative.

RCC is resistant to most chemotherapeutic agents. For many years, cytokine therapy with interferon and interleukin-2 was used in metastatic renal cancer but, in recent years, two new classes of targeted drugs have been introduced and are now the mainstay of therapy. These are the tyrosine kinase inhibitors sunitinib and pazopanib, and the mammalian target of rapamycin (mTOR) inhibitors temsirolimus and everolimus.

In previous years, patients who presented with distant metastases were treated with cytoreductive nephrectomy, in which nephrectomy was coupled with systemic cytokine treatment, since this was shown to improve survival as compared with either treatment in isolation. It is, at present, unclear whether this survival benefit still prevails with the newer agents mentioned above.

Studies that antedate the introduction of these new agents show that, if the tumour is confined to the kidney, 5-year survival is 75%, but this falls to 5% when there are distant metastases.

Urothelial tumours

Tumours arising from the transitional epithelium of the renal tract can affect the renal pelvis, ureter, bladder or urethra. They are rare under the age of 40, affect men 3–4 times more often than women, and account for about 3% of all malignant tumours. The bladder is by far the most frequently affected site. Although almost all tumours are transitional cell carcinomas (otherwise known as urothelial cancers), squamous carcinoma may occur in urothelium that has undergone metaplasia, usually following chronic inflammation due to stones or schistosomiasis. The appearance of a transitional cell tumour ranges from a delicate papillary structure with a relatively good prognosis to a solid ulcerating mass in more aggressive disease.

15

Pathophysiology

Risk factors include cigarette smoking and exposure to industrial carcinogens such as aromatic amines, aniline dyes and aldehydes.

Clinical features

More than 80% of patients present with painless, visible haematuria. It should be assumed that such bleeding is from a tumour until proven otherwise (p. 391). Tumours of the ureter or bladder may also cause symptoms of obstruction, depending on the site of involvement, and tumours of the bladder present with dysuria or storage symptoms. Physical examination is usually unremarkable, except in patients with very advanced disease, when bimanual examination may reveal a palpable mass.

Investigations

Cystoscopy (usually flexible cystoscopy under a local anaesthetic) is mandatory to evaluate the bladder in cases of haematuria or suspected bladder cancer. Imaging of the upper urinary tract (CT urogram is the gold standard but IVU combined with renal ultrasound is also acceptable) is also important to rule out abnormalities of the kidney, ureters and renal pelvis in patients with haematuria. If a suspicious defect is seen on CT urography or IVU in the ureter or renal pelvis, a retrograde ureteropyelogram, ureteroscopy and biopsy are required. If evidence of a solid invasive urothelial tumour is found, CT of the abdomen, pelvis and chest should be performed to define tumour stage.

Management

Most bladder tumours are low-grade superficial lesions that can be successfully treated endoscopically by transurethral resection of the tumour. Intravesical chemotherapy with mitomycin C is usually administered as a one-off treatment post resection to prevent tumour recurrence, or may be given as a prolonged course to treat multiple low-grade bladder tumours. Patients with carcinoma in situ have a high risk of progression to invasive cancer. These patients often respond well to intravesical bacille Calmette–Guérin (BCG) treatment but more radical treatment may also be needed if this is unsuccessful. Following initial treatment and endoscopic clearance of bladder tumours, regular check cystoscopies are required to look for evidence of recurrence. Patients with recurrences of superficial disease can usually be treated by further resection and diathermy, but if this is unsuccessful, a cystectomy may be needed.

The management of invasive bladder tumours involves radical cystectomy with urinary diversion into an incontinent ileal conduit or a continent catheterisable bowel pouch; the latter is usually reserved for patients under the age of 70 years.

The prognosis of bladder tumours depends on tumour stage and grade. About 5% of patients with low-grade superficial bladder cancer progress to develop invasion of the bladder muscle, compared with about 50% of those with high-grade superficial bladder cancers. Overall, the 5-year survival for patients with muscle-invasive bladder cancer of either grade is 50–70%.

Urothelial cell carcinoma of the renal pelvis and ureter is usually treated by open or laparoscopic nephro-ureterectomy, but if the tumour is solitary and low-grade, it can be treated endoscopically.

Inherited tumour syndromes affecting the renal tract

Some uncommon autosomal dominantly inherited conditions are associated with multiple renal tumours in adult life. In tuberous sclerosis (p. 1264), replacement of renal tissue by multiple angiomyolipomas (tubers) may occasionally cause renal failure in adults; they may also bleed, requiring embolisation. The von Hippel–Lindau syndrome (p. 1132) is associated with multiple renal cysts, renal adenomas and clear cell renal cell cancers. Other organs affected include the central nervous system (haemangioblastomas), pancreas and adrenals (phaeochromocytoma).

Urinary incontinence

Urinary incontinence is defined as any involuntary leakage of urine. It may occur in patients with a normal urinary tract, as the result of dementia or poor mobility, or transiently during an acute illness or hospitalisation, especially in older people (Box 15.54). The prevalence of any form of incontinence in all females is 25–45%, with a concomitant socioeconomic burden. Childbirth, hysterectomy, obesity, recurrent UTI, smoking, caffeine and constipation are risk factors for incontinence.

Pathophysiology

As urine accumulates in the bladder during the storage phase, the sphincter tone gradually increases, but there are no significant changes in vesical pressure, detrusor pressure or intra-abdominal pressure. During voiding, intravesical pressure increases as a result of detrusor contraction and the sphincter relaxes, allowing urine to flow from the bladder until it is empty. Clinical disorders associated with incontinence are connected with various abnormalities in this cycle and these are discussed in more detail below.

Stress incontinence

This occurs because passive bladder pressure exceeds the urethral pressure, due either to poor pelvic floor support or a weak urethral sphincter. Usually there is an element of both these factors. Stress incontinence is very common in women and seen most frequently following childbirth. It is rare in men and usually follows surgery to the prostate. The presentation is with incontinence during coughing, sneezing or exertion. In women, perineal inspection may reveal leakage of urine when the patient coughs.

Urge incontinence

This usually occurs because of detrusor over-activity, which produces an increased bladder pressure that overcomes the urethral sphincter. Urgency with or without incontinence may also be driven by a hypersensitive bladder resulting from UTI or a bladder stone. Detrusor over-activity is usually idiopathic,

15.54 Incontinence in old age

- **Prevalence**: urinary incontinence affects 15% of women and 10% of men aged over 65 years.
- **Cause**: incontinence may be transient and due to delirium, urinary infection, medication (such as diuretics), faecal impaction or restricted mobility, and these should be treated before embarking on further specific investigation.
- **Detrusor over-activity**: established incontinence in old age is most commonly due to detrusor over-activity, which may be caused by damage to central inhibitory centres or local detrusor muscle abnormalities.
- **Catheterisation**: poor manual dexterity or cognitive impairment may necessitate the help of a carer to assist with intermittent catheterisation.

other than in patients with neurological conditions such as spina bifida or multiple sclerosis, in whom it is neurogenic (p. 1093). The incidence of urge incontinence increases with age, occurring in 10–15% of the population aged over 65 years and in approximately 50% of patients requiring nursing home care. It is also seen in men with lower urinary tract obstruction and most often remits after the obstruction is relieved.

Continual incontinence

This is suggestive of a fistula, usually between the bladder and vagina (vesicovaginal), or the ureter and vagina (ureterovaginal). It is most common following gynaecological surgery but is also seen in patients with gynaecological malignancy or post radiotherapy. In parts of the world where obstetric services are scarce, prolonged obstructed labour can be a common cause of vesicovaginal fistulae. Continual incontinence may also be seen in infants with congenital ectopic ureters. Occasionally, stress incontinence is so severe that the patient leaks continuously.

Overflow incontinence

This occurs when the bladder becomes chronically over-distended and may lead to AKI (high-pressure chronic urinary retention). It is most commonly seen in men with benign prostatic enlargement or bladder neck obstruction (see below) but may arise in either sex as a result of failure of the detrusor muscle (atonic bladder). The latter may be idiopathic but more commonly is the result of damage to the pelvic nerves, either from surgery (commonly, hysterectomy or rectal excision), trauma or infection, or from compression of the cauda equina by disc prolapse, trauma or tumour. Incontinence due to prostatic enlargement can be regarded as a type of overflow incontinence.

Post-micturition dribble

This is very common in men, even in the relatively young. It is due to a small amount of urine becoming trapped in the U-bend of the bulbar urethra, which leaks out when the patient moves. Post-micturition dribble is more pronounced if associated with a urethral diverticulum or urethral stricture. It may occur in women with a urethral diverticulum and may mimic stress incontinence.

Clinical features

Patients should be encouraged to keep a voiding diary, including the measured volume voided, frequency of voiding, a note of incontinence pad usage, precipitating factors and associated features, such as urgency, since this can be of diagnostic value. Structured questionnaires may help objectively quantify symptoms. The patient should be assessed for evidence of cognitive impairment and impaired mobility. A neurological assessment should be performed to detect disorders such as multiple sclerosis that may affect the nervous supply of the bladder, and the lumbar spine should be inspected for features of spina bifida occulta. Perineal sensation and anal sphincter tone should be assessed. Rectal examination is needed to assess the prostate in men and to exclude faecal impaction as a cause of incontinence. Genital examination should be done to identify phimosis or paraphimosis in men, and vaginal mucosal atrophy, cystoceles or rectoceles in women.

Investigations

Urinalysis and culture should be performed in all patients. Ultrasound examination can be helpful in identifying patients with overflow incontinence who have incomplete bladder emptying, as they may reveal a significant amount of fluid in the bladder (>100 mL) post micturition. Urine flow rates and full urodynamic assessment by cystometrography may be required to diagnose the type of incontinence and are indicated in selected cases when the diagnosis is unclear on clinical grounds. A CT scan and cystoscopy should be performed in patients with continual incontinence who are suspected of having a fistula. Imaging with MRI is indicated when a urethral diverticulum is suspected.

Management

Weight reduction in obese patients will aid resolution of incontinence. Women with stress incontinence respond well to physiotherapy. The mainstay of treatment for urge incontinence is bladder retraining, which involves teaching patients to hold more urine voluntarily in their bladder, assisted by anticholinergic medication. Surgery may be required in patients who have severe daytime incontinence despite conservative treatment. The treatment of incontinence secondary to fistula formation is surgical. Patients with overflow incontinence due to bladder obstruction should be treated surgically or with long-term catheterisation (intermittent or continuous). Incontinence secondary to neurological diseases can be managed by intermittent self-catheterisation.

Prostate disease

Prostatitis

This results from inflammation of the prostate gland. Acute or chronic bacterial prostatitis can be caused by infection with the same bacteria that are associated with UTI (p. 426) but prostatitis can also be 'non-bacterial', in which case no organism can be cultured from the urine. This is also known as chronic pelvic pain syndrome. Clinical features of prostatitis include frequency, dysuria, painful ejaculation, perineal or groin pain, difficulty passing urine and, in acute disease, considerable systemic disturbance. The prostate is enlarged and tender. Bacterial prostatitis is confirmed by a positive culture from urine or from urethral discharge obtained after prostatic massage, and the treatment of choice is a quinolone antibiotic. A 4–6-week course of antibiotics is required (see Box 15.47, p. 429). Treatment of chronic pelvic pain syndrome is challenging but some patients respond to a combination of α-blockers, NSAIDs and amitriptyline.

Benign prostatic enlargement

Benign prostatic enlargement (BPE) is extremely common. It has been estimated that about half of all men aged 80 years and over will have lower urinary tract symptoms associated with bladder outlet obstruction (BOO) due to BPE. Benign prostatic hyperplasia (BPH) is the histological abnormality that underlies BPE.

Pathophysiology

The prostate gland increases in volume by 2.4 cm^3 per year on average from 40 years of age. The process begins in the periurethral (transitional) zone and involves both glandular and stromal tissue to a variable degree. The cause is unknown, although BPE does not occur in patients with hypogonadism, suggesting that hormonal factors may be important.

Clinical features

The primary symptoms of BPE arise because of difficulty in voiding urine due to obstruction of the urethra by the prostate; these voiding symptoms consist of hesitancy, poor urinary flow and a sensation of incomplete emptying. Other storage

15

Symptom	Question	Example score
Straining	How often have you had to push or strain to begin urination?	1
Urgency	How often have you found it difficult to postpone urination?	2
Hesitancy	How often have you found that you stopped and started again several times when you urinated?	1
Incomplete emptying	How often have you had a sensation of not emptying your bladder completely after you finished urinating?	3
Frequency	How often have you had to urinate again less than 2 hours after you finished urinating?	1
Weak stream	How often have you had a weak urinary stream?	2
Nocturia	How many times did you most typically get up to urinate from the time you went to bed at night until the time you got up in the morning?	1
Total score		11

0 = not at all; 1 = less than one-fifth of the time; 2 = less than half the time; 3 = about half of the time; 4 = more than half of the time; 5 = almost always.
A score of 0–7 indicates mild symptoms, 8–19 moderate symptoms and 20–35 severe symptoms. In the example shown, the patient had moderate symptoms.

15.56 Treatment for benign prostatic enlargement

Medical
- Prostate < 30 g: α-adrenoceptor blockers
- Prostate > 30 g: 5α-reductase inhibitors ± α-adrenoceptor blockers

Surgical
- Transurethral resection of the prostate (TURP)
- Laser enucleation
- Laser vaporisation
- Open prostatectomy

post-void residual volume of urine assessed with ultrasound, and prostate volume by transrectal ultrasound scan (TRUS). Objective assessment of obstruction is possible by urodynamics but this is seldom required. If symptoms or signs, such as a palpable bladder, nocturnal enuresis, recurrent UTI or a history of renal stones, are present, renal function should be assessed; if it is abnormal, screening should be conducted for evidence of obstructive uropathy by ultrasound examination.

Management

Patients who present with acute retention require urgent treatment and should undergo immediate catheterisation to relieve the obstruction. Those with mild to moderate symptoms can be treated by medication (Box 15.56). The first-line treatments are α_{1A}-adrenoceptor blockers such as tamsulosin, which reduce the tone of smooth muscle cells in the prostate and bladder neck, thereby reducing the obstruction. The 5α-reductase inhibitors finasteride and dutasteride inhibit conversion of testosterone to the nine times more potent dihydrotestosterone in the prostate and so cause the prostate to reduce in size. This class of drugs is indicated in patients with an estimated prostate size of more than 30 g or a prostate-specific antigen (PSA) level of more than 1.4 ng/mL. Patients who fail to respond to a single drug may be treated with a combination of α-blockers and 5α-reductase inhibitors, since this is more efficacious than either agent alone. Symptoms that are resistant to medical therapy require surgical treatment to remove some of the prostate tissue that is causing urethral obstruction. This is usually achieved by transurethral resection of the prostate (TURP) but enucleation of the prostate by holmium laser or vaporisation by potassium-titanyl-phosphate (KTP) laser (Greenlight laser) is equally effective and has potentially fewer complications. Open surgery is rarely needed, unless the gland is very large.

Prostate cancer

Prostate cancer is the most common malignancy in men in the UK, with a prevalence of 105 per 100 000 population. It is also common in northern Europe and the USA (particularly in the African American population) but is rare in China and Japan. It is uncommon in India but the incidence is increasing. Prostate cancer rarely occurs before the age of 50 and has a mean age at presentation of 70 years.

Pathophysiology

Prostate cancers tend to arise within the peripheral zone of the prostate and almost all are adenocarcinomas. Metastatic spread to pelvic lymph nodes occurs early and metastases to bone, mainly the lumbar spine and pelvis, are common. Genetic factors are known to play an important role in pathogenesis,

symptoms include urinary frequency, urgency of micturition and urge incontinence, although these are not specific to BPE. Some patients present suddenly with acute urinary retention, when they are unable to micturate and develop a painful, distended bladder. This is often precipitated by excessive alcohol intake, constipation or prostatic infection. Severity of symptoms can be ascertained by using the International Prostate Symptom Score (IPSS) questionnaire (Box 15.55), which serves as a valuable starting point for assessment of the patient. Once a baseline value is established, any improvement or deterioration may be monitored on subsequent visits. The IPSS may be combined with a quality-of-life score, in which patients are asked the following question: 'If you were to spend the rest of your life with your urinary condition the way it is now, how would you feel about that?' Responses range from 0 (delighted) to 6 (terrible).

Patients may also present with chronic urinary retention. Here, the bladder slowly distends due to inadequate emptying over a long period of time. Patients with chronic retention can also develop acute retention: so-called acute-on-chronic retention. This condition is characterised by pain-free bladder distension, which may result in hydroureter, hydronephrosis and renal failure (high-pressure chronic retention, of which nocturnal incontinence is a pathognomonic symptom). On digital rectal examination (DRE), patients with BPE have evidence of prostatic enlargement with a smooth prostate gland. Abdominal examination may also reveal evidence of bladder enlargement in patients with urinary retention.

Investigations

The diagnosis of BOO secondary to BPE is a clinical one but flow rates can be accurately measured with a flow meter, and multiple genetic loci have been found to predispose to the disease in genome-wide association studies. A family history of prostate cancer greatly increases a man's chances of developing the disease.

Clinical features

Most patients either are asymptomatic or present with lower urinary tract symptoms indistinguishable from BPE. On DRE the prostate may feel nodular and stony-hard, and the median sulcus may be lost, but up to 45% of tumours are impalpable. Symptoms and signs due to metastases are much less common at the initial presentation but may include back pain, weight loss, anaemia and obstruction of the ureters.

Investigations

Measurement of PSA levels in a peripheral blood sample, together with DRE, is the cornerstone of diagnosis. Prior to a PSA test, men should be given careful counselling about the limitations of the test: namely, a normal level does not exclude prostate cancer, while a high value does not confirm the diagnosis but will open a discussion about biopsy and possible future treatments with potential side-effects (Box 15.57). The need for radical treatment of localised prostate cancer is still not established; radical treatments have significant potential morbidity and mortality, yet early identification and treatment of prostate cancer may save lives. Current evidence suggests that population-based screening for prostate cancer with PSA is of limited value, due in part to the fact that over 700 patients would need to be screened to cure 1 man of prostate cancer. Individuals suspected of having prostate cancer, based on an elevated PSA and/or abnormal DRE, should undergo transrectal ultrasound-guided prostate biopsies. About 40% of patients with a serum PSA of 4.0–10 ng/mL or more will have prostate cancer on biopsy, although 25% of patients with a PSA of less than 4 ng/mL may also have prostate cancer. Occasionally, a small focus of tumour is found incidentally in patients undergoing TURP for benign hyperplasia. If the diagnosis of prostate cancer is confirmed, staging should be performed by pelvic MRI to assess the presence and extent of local involvement. An isotope bone scan should be carried out if distant metastases are suspected (rare if the PSA is below 20 ng/mL); very high levels of serum PSA (>100 ng/mL) almost always indicate distant bone metastases. Following diagnosis, serial assessment of PSA levels is useful for monitoring response to treatment and disease progression.

Management

Tumour confined to the prostate is potentially curable by radical prostatectomy, radical radiotherapy or brachytherapy (implantation of small radioactive particles into the prostate). These options should be considered only in patients with more than 10 years' life expectancy. Patients who are found to have small-volume, low-grade disease do not appear to require specific treatment but should be followed up periodically with PSA testing, DRE and a schedule of biopsies; this is known as active surveillance. Prostatic cancer, like breast cancer, is sensitive to steroid hormones; metastatic prostate cancer is treated by androgen depletion, involving either surgery (orchidectomy) or, more commonly, androgen-suppressing drugs. Androgen receptor blockers, such as bicalutamide or cyproterone acetate, may also prevent tumour cell growth. Gonadotrophin-releasing hormone (GnRH) analogues, such as goserelin, continuously occupy pituitary receptors, preventing them from responding to the GnRH pulses that normally stimulate luteinising hormone (LH) and follicle-stimulating hormone (FSH) release. This initially causes an increase in testosterone before producing a prolonged reduction, and for this reason the initial dose must be covered with an androgen receptor blocker to prevent a tumour flare.

A small proportion of patients fail to respond to endocrine treatment. A larger number respond for a year or two but then the disease progresses. Chemotherapy with docetaxel can then be effective and provide a modest (around 3 months) survival advantage. Radiotherapy is useful for localised bone pain but the basis of treatment remains pain control by analgesia (p. 1331). Provided that patients do not die of another cause, the 10-year survival rate of patients with tumours localised to the prostate is 95%, but if metastases are present, this falls to 10%. Life expectancy is not reduced in patients with small foci of tumour.

i	**15.57 Advantages and disadvantages of prostate-specific antigen (PSA) testing in order to identify men with prostate cancer**

Advantages
- Identification of prostate cancer at a treatable stage, which otherwise may not have been identified*

Disadvantages
- High false-positive rate: 50–60% of men with an elevated PSA will not have prostate cancer
- High false-negative rate: 25% of men with a normal PSA have prostate cancer
- Leads to further invasive tests (biopsy) with morbidity (e.g. sepsis or bleeding)
- May lead to diagnosis of prostate cancer, which is often over-treated by surgery or radiotherapy with associated side-effects (e.g. impotence or incontinence)
- If PSA is elevated but biopsy is normal, there is a potential need for further testing and associated anxiety

*The advantages of identifying prostate cancer earlier than would be the case if the man developed symptomatic disease must be considered against the limitations of PSA testing.

Testicular tumours

Testicular tumours are uncommon, with a prevalence of 5 cases per 100 000 population. They occur mainly in young men aged between 20 and 40 years. They often secrete α-fetoprotein (AFP) and β-human chorionic gonadotrophin (β-hCG), which are useful biochemical markers for both diagnosis and prognosis. Seminoma and teratoma account for 85% of all tumours of the testis. Leydig cell tumours are less common.

Seminomas arise from seminiferous tubules and represent a relatively low-grade malignancy. Metastases can occur through lymphatic spread, however, and typically involve the lungs.

Teratomas arise from primitive germinal cells and tend to occur at a younger age than seminomas. They may contain cartilage, bone, muscle, fat and a variety of other tissues, and are classified according to the degree of differentiation. Well-differentiated tumours are the least aggressive; at the other extreme, trophoblastic teratoma is highly malignant. Occasionally, teratoma and seminoma occur together.

Leydig cell tumours are usually small and benign but secrete oestrogens, leading to presentation with gynaecomastia (p. 657).

Clinical features and investigations

The common presentation is incidental discovery of a painless testicular lump, although some patients complain of a testicular ache.

All suspicious scrotal lumps should be imaged by ultrasound. Serum levels of AFP and β-hCG are elevated in extensive disease. Oestradiol may be elevated, suppressing LH, FSH and testosterone. Accurate staging is based on CT of the lungs, liver and retroperitoneal area.

Management and prognosis

The primary treatment is surgical orchidectomy. Subsequent treatment depends on the histological type and stage. Radiotherapy is the treatment of choice for early-stage seminoma. Teratoma confined to the testes may be managed conservatively, but more advanced cancers are treated with chemotherapy, usually the combination of bleomycin, etoposide and cisplatin. Follow-up is by CT and assessment of AFP and β-hCG. Retroperitoneal lymph node dissection is now performed only for residual or recurrent nodal masses.

The 5-year survival rate for patients with seminoma is 90–95%. For teratomas, the 5-year survival varies between 60% and 95%, depending on tumour type, stage and volume.

Erectile dysfunction

Causes of erectile failure are shown in Box 15.58. Vascular, neuropathic and psychological causes are most common. Exclusion of previously unrecognised cardiovascular disease is important in men presenting with erectile dysfunction. With the exception of diabetes mellitus, endocrine causes are relatively uncommon and are characterised by loss of libido, as well as erectile dysfunction. Erectile dysfunction and reduced libido occur in over 50% of men with advanced CKD or those on dialysis, and is a markedly under-diagnosed problem. It is important to discuss matters frankly with the patient, and to establish whether there are associated features of hypogonadism (p. 655) and if erections occur at any other time. If the patient has erections on wakening, vascular and neuropathic causes are much less likely and a psychological cause should be suspected.

Investigations

Blood should be taken for glucose, lipids, thyroid function tests, prolactin, testosterone, LH and FSH. A number of further tests are available but are rarely employed because they do not usually influence management. These include nocturnal tumescence monitoring (using a plethysmograph placed around the shaft of the penis overnight) to establish whether blood supply and nerve function are sufficient to allow erections to occur during sleep; intracavernosal injection of prostaglandin E_1 to test the adequacy of blood supply; internal pudendal artery angiography; and tests of autonomic and peripheral sensory nerve conduction.

Management

First-line therapy is usually with oral phosphodiesterase type 5 inhibitors, such as sildenafil, which elevate cyclic guanosine monophosphate (cGMP) levels in vascular smooth muscle cells of the corpus cavernosum, causing vasodilatation and penile erection. Co-administration of these drugs with nitric oxide donors, such as glycerol trinitrate, is contraindicated because of the risk of severe hypotension. Other treatments for impotence include self-administered intracavernosal injection or urethral administration of prostaglandin E1; vacuum devices that achieve an erection maintained by a tourniquet around the base of the penis; and prosthetic implants, either of a fixed rod or an inflatable reservoir. Psychotherapy involving the patient and sexual partner may be helpful for psychological problems. Erectile dysfunction associated with peripheral neuropathy and vascular disease is difficult to treat. If hypogonadism is detected, it should be managed as described on page 655.

Further information

Websites

edren.org *Renal Unit, Royal Infirmary of Edinburgh; information about individual diseases, protocols for immediate in-hospital management and more.*
edrep.org/resources *Educational resources.*
nephron.com *The links under 'Physicians' include useful urology pages, eGFR and other calculators, and other resources.*
renal.org/ckd *UK Renal Association; current UK guidelines on the detection, referral and management of CKD.*
renalfellow.blogspot.co.uk/ *Educational blog written by renal trainees for trainees.*
uroweb.org/guidelines *European Association of Urology guidelines; current European guidelines on the management of all common urological conditions.*

 15.58 Causes of erectile dysfunction

With reduced libido

- Hypogonadism
- Depression

With intact libido

- Psychological problems, including anxiety
- Vascular insufficiency (atheroma)
- Neuropathic causes (diabetes mellitus, alcohol excess, multiple sclerosis)
- Drugs (β-blockers, thiazide diuretics)

DE Newby
NR Grubb

16

Cardiology

Clinical examination of the cardiovascular system 442

Functional anatomy and physiology 444
Anatomy 444
Physiology 446

Investigation of cardiovascular disease 448
Electrocardiogram 448
Cardiac biomarkers 450
Chest X-ray 450
Echocardiography 451
Computed tomography 452
Magnetic resonance imaging 452
Cardiac catheterisation 453
Electrophysiology 454
Radionuclide imaging 454

Presenting problems in cardiovascular disease 454
Chest pain on exertion 454
Severe prolonged chest pain 455
Breathlessness 455
Syncope 455
Palpitation 455
Cardiac arrest 456
Abnormal heart sounds 457
Heart failure 461

Cardiac arrhythmias 468

Principles of management of cardiac arrhythmias 479
Anti-arrhythmic drugs 479
Non-pharmacological treatments 482

Coronary artery disease 484
Angina pectoris 487
Acute coronary syndrome 493
Non-cardiac surgery in patients with heart disease 501

Peripheral arterial disease 502

Diseases of the aorta 505
Aortic aneurysm 505
Aortic dissection 506
Aortitis 508
Marfan's syndrome 508
Coarctation of the aorta 508
Hypertension 508

Diseases of the heart valves 514
Rheumatic heart disease 515
Mitral valve disease 517
Aortic valve disease 521
Tricuspid valve disease 525
Pulmonary valve disease 526
Prosthetic valves 526
Infective endocarditis 527

Congenital heart disease 531

Diseases of the myocardium 538
Myocarditis 538
Cardiomyopathy 538
Cardiac tumours 541

Diseases of the pericardium 542

Clinical examination of the cardiovascular system

6 Face, mouth and eyes
Pallor
Central cyanosis
Dental caries
Fundi (retinopathy)
Stigmata of
hyperlipidaemia
and thyroid disease

▲ Malar flush

▲ Poor oral hygiene in a patient with infective endocarditis

▲ Xanthelasma

5 Jugular venous pulse
(see opposite)
Height
Waveform

▲ Jugular venous pulse

4 Carotid pulses
Volume
Character
Bruits
(see opposite)

3 Blood pressure

2 Radial pulse
Rate
Rhythm

1 Hands
Clubbing
Splinter haemorrhages
and other stigmata of
infective endocarditis

▲ Splinter haemorrhage

▲ Cyanosis and clubbing in a patient with complex cyanotic congenital heart disease

7 Precordium
Inspect
Palpate
(see opposite)

8 Auscultation
(see opposite)

9 Back
Lung crepitations
Sacral oedema

10 Abdomen
Hepatomegaly
Ascites
Aortic aneurysm
Bruits

11 Tendon xanthomas
(hyperlipidaemia)

12 Femoral pulses
Radio-femoral delay
Bruits

13 Legs
Peripheral pulses
Oedema

▲ Vasculitis in a patient with infective endocarditis

▲ Peripheral oedema in a patient with congestive cardiac failure

Observation
Symptoms and well-being
• Breathlessness
• Distress etc.
Body habitus
• Body mass (obesity, cachexia)
• Marfan's and other syndromes
Tissue perfusion
• Skin temperature
• Sweating
• Urine output

Insets (Splinter haemorrhage, jugular venous pulse, malar flush, tendon xanthomas) From Newby D, Grubb N. Cardiology: an illustrated colour text. Edinburgh: Churchill Livingstone, Elsevier Ltd; 2005.

4 Examination of the arterial pulse

- The character of the pulse is determined by stroke volume and arterial compliance, and is best assessed by palpating a major artery, such as the carotid or brachial artery.
- Aortic regurgitation, anaemia, sepsis and other causes of a large stroke volume typically produce a bounding pulse with a high amplitude and wide pulse pressure (panel A).
- Aortic stenosis impedes ventricular emptying. If severe, it causes a slow-rising, weak and delayed pulse (panel A).
- Sinus rhythm produces a pulse that is regular in time and force. Arrhythmias may cause irregularity. Atrial fibrillation produces a pulse that is irregular in time and volume (panel B).

A

B

5 Examination of the jugular venous pulse

The internal jugular vein, superior vena cava and right atrium are in continuity, so the height of the jugular venous pulsation reflects right atrial pressure. When the patient is placed at 45°, with the head supported and turned to the left, the jugular venous pulse is visible along the line of the sternocleidomastoid muscle (see opposite). In health it is normally just visible above the clavicle.

- The height of the jugular venous pulse is determined by right atrial pressure and is therefore elevated in right heart failure and reduced in hypovolaemia.
- If the jugular venous pulse is not easily seen, it may be exposed by applying firm pressure over the abdomen.
- In sinus rhythm, the two venous peaks, the a and v waves, approximate to atrial and ventricular systole, respectively.
- The x descent reflects atrial relaxation and apical displacement of the tricuspid valve ring. The y descent reflects atrial emptying early in diastole. These signs are subtle.
- Tricuspid regurgitation produces giant v waves that coincide with ventricular systole.

i Distinguishing venous/arterial pulsation in the neck

- The venous pulse has two peaks in each cardiac cycle; the arterial pulse has one peak.
- The height of the venous pulse varies with respiration (falls on inspiration) and position.
- Abdominal compression causes the venous pulse to rise.
- The venous pulse is not easily palpable and can be occluded with light pressure.

7 Palpation of the precordium

Technique

- Place fingertips over apex (1) to assess for position and character. Place heel of hand over left sternal edge (2) for a parasternal heave or 'lift'. Assess for thrills in all areas, including the aortic and pulmonary areas (3). Normal position is the 5th or 6th intercostal space, at the mid-clavicular line.

Common abnormalities of the apex beat

- Volume overload, such as mitral or aortic regurgitation: displaced, thrusting
- Pressure overload, such as aortic stenosis, hypertension: discrete, heaving
- Dyskinetic, such as left ventricular aneurysm: displaced, incoordinate

Other abnormalities

- Palpable S1 (tapping apex beat: mitral stenosis)
- Palpable P2 (severe pulmonary hypertension)
- Left parasternal heave or 'lift' felt by heel of hand (right ventricular hypertrophy)
- Palpable thrill (aortic stenosis)

8 Auscultation of the heart

- Use the diaphragm to examine at the apex, lower left sternal edge (tricuspid area) and upper left (pulmonary area) and right (aortic area) sternal edges.
- Use the bell to examine low-pitched noises, particularly at the apex for the mid-diastolic murmur of mitral stenosis.
- Time the sounds and murmurs by feeling the carotid pulse; the first heart sound (S1) just precedes the upstroke of the pulse and the second heart sound (S2) is out of step with it. If present, a third heart sound (S3) immediately follows S2, and a fourth heart sound (S4) just precedes S1. Systolic murmurs are synchronous with the pulse.
- Listen for radiation of systolic murmurs, over the base of the neck (aortic stenosis) and in the axilla (mitral incompetence).
- Listen over the left sternal border with the patient sitting forward (aortic incompetence), then at the apex with the patient rolled on to the left side (mitral stenosis).

16

The haemodynamic effects of respiration are discussed on page 447, and the analysis and interpretation of heart sounds and murmurs on page 457.

Cardiovascular disease is the most frequent cause of adult death in the Western world. In the UK, one-third of men and one-quarter of women will die as a result of ischaemic heart disease. In many developed countries, the incidence of ischaemic heart disease has been falling for the last two or three decades, but it is rising in Eastern Europe and Asia. Cardiovascular disease will soon become the leading cause of death on all continents. Strategies for the treatment and prevention of heart disease can be highly effective and have been subjected to rigorous evaluation. The evidence base for the treatment of cardiovascular disease is stronger than for almost any other disease group.

Valvular heart disease is common but the aetiology varies in different parts of the world. On the Indian subcontinent and in Africa, it is predominantly due to rheumatic fever, whereas calcific aortic valve disease is the most common problem in developed countries.

Prompt recognition of the development of heart disease is limited by two key factors. Firstly, it is often latent; coronary artery disease can proceed to an advanced stage before the patient notices any symptoms. Secondly, the diversity of symptoms attributable to heart disease is limited, so different pathologies may frequently present with the same symptoms.

Functional anatomy and physiology

Anatomy

The heart acts as two serial pumps that share several electrical and mechanical components. The right heart circulates blood to the lungs where it is oxygenated, and the left heart circulates it to the rest of the body (Fig. 16.1). The atria are thin-walled structures that act as priming pumps for the ventricles, which provide most of the energy required to maintain the circulation. The atria are situated posteriorly within the mediastinum where the left atrium (LA) sits anterior to the oesophagus and descending aorta. The right atrium (RA) receives blood from the superior and inferior venae cavae and the coronary sinus. The LA receives blood from four pulmonary veins, two from each of the left and right lungs. The ventricles are thick-walled structures, adapted to circulating blood through large vascular beds under pressure. The atria and ventricles are separated by the annulus fibrosus, which forms the skeleton for the atrioventricular (AV) valves and electrically insulates the atria from the ventricles. The right ventricle (RV) is about 2–3 mm thick and triangular in shape. It extends from the annulus fibrosus to near the cardiac apex and sits anterior and to the right of the left ventricle (LV). The anterosuperior surface of the RV is rounded and convex, and its posterior extent is bounded by the interventricular septum, which bulges into the chamber. Its upper extent is conical, forming the conus arteriosus or outflow tract, from which the pulmonary artery arises. The LV is more conical in shape and in cross-section is nearly circular. It extends from the LA to the apex of the heart. The LV myocardium is normally around 10 mm thick because it pumps blood at a higher pressure than the RV.

Normally, the heart occupies less than 50% of the transthoracic diameter in the frontal plane, as seen on a chest X-ray. On the patient's left, the cardiac silhouette is formed by the aortic arch, the pulmonary trunk, the left atrial appendage and the LV. On the right, the silhouette is formed by the RA and the superior and inferior venae cavae, and the lower right border is formed by the RV (Fig. 16.2). In disease states or congenital cardiac abnormalities, the silhouette may change as a result of hypertrophy or dilatation.

Coronary circulation

The left main and right coronary arteries arise from the left and right sinuses of the aortic root, distal to the aortic valve (Fig. 16.3). Within 2.5 cm of its origin, the left main coronary artery divides into the left anterior descending artery (LAD), which runs in the anterior interventricular groove, and the left circumflex artery (CX), which runs posteriorly in the atrioventricular groove.

Fig. 16.1 Direction of blood flow through the heart. The blue arrows show deoxygenated blood moving through the right heart to the lungs. The red arrows show oxygenated blood moving from the lungs to the systemic circulation. The normal pressures are shown for each chamber in mmHg.

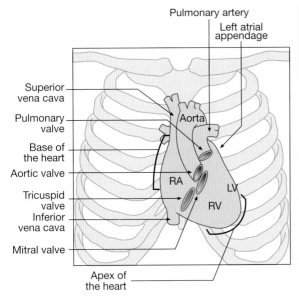

Fig. 16.2 **Surface anatomy of the heart.** The positions of the major cardiac chambers and heart valves are shown. (LV = left ventricle; RA = right atrium; RV = right ventricle)

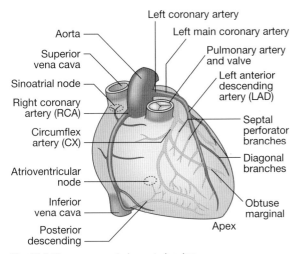

Fig. 16.3 **The coronary arteries: anterior view.**

The LAD gives branches to supply the anterior part of the septum (septal perforators) and the anterior, lateral and apical walls of the LV. The CX gives marginal branches that supply the lateral, posterior and inferior segments of the LV. The right coronary artery (RCA) runs in the right atrioventricular groove, giving branches that supply the RA, RV and inferoposterior aspects of the LV. The posterior descending artery runs in the posterior interventricular groove and supplies the inferior part of the interventricular septum. This vessel is a branch of the RCA in approximately 90% of people (dominant right system) and is supplied by the CX in the remainder (dominant left system). The coronary anatomy varies greatly from person to person and there are many normal variants.

The RCA supplies the sinoatrial (SA) node in about 60% of individuals and the AV node in about 90%. Proximal occlusion of the RCA therefore often results in sinus bradycardia and may also cause AV nodal block. Abrupt occlusion of the RCA, due

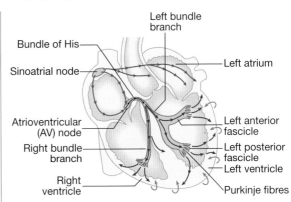

Fig. 16.4 **The cardiac conduction system.** Depolarisation starts in the sinoatrial node and spreads through the atria (blue arrows), and then through the atrioventricular node (black arrows). Depolarisation then spreads through the bundle of His and the bundle branches to reach the ventricular muscle (red arrows). Repolarisation spreads from epicardium to endocardium (green arrows).

to coronary thrombosis, results in infarction of the inferior part of the LV and often the RV. Abrupt occlusion of the LAD or CX causes infarction in the corresponding territory of the LV, and occlusion of the left main coronary artery is usually fatal.

The venous system follows the coronary arteries but drains into the coronary sinus in the atrioventricular groove, and then to the RA. An extensive lymphatic system drains into vessels that travel with the coronary vessels and then into the thoracic duct.

Conduction system

The SA node is situated at the junction of the superior vena cava and RA (Fig. 16.4). It comprises specialised atrial cells that depolarise at a rate influenced by the autonomic nervous system and by circulating catecholamines. During normal (sinus) rhythm, this depolarisation wave propagates through both atria via sheets of atrial myocytes. The annulus fibrosus forms a conduction barrier between atria and ventricles, and the only pathway through it is the AV node. This is a midline structure, extending from the right side of the interatrial septum, penetrating the annulus fibrosus anteriorly. The AV node conducts relatively slowly, producing a necessary time delay between atrial and ventricular contraction. The His–Purkinje system is composed of the bundle of His extending from the AV node into the interventricular septum, the right and left bundle branches passing along the ventricular septum and into the respective ventricles, the anterior and posterior fascicles of the left bundle branch, and the smaller Purkinje fibres that ramify through the ventricular myocardium. The tissues of the His–Purkinje system conduct very rapidly and allow near-simultaneous depolarisation of the entire ventricular myocardium.

Nerve supply of the heart

The heart is innervated by both sympathetic and parasympathetic fibres. Adrenergic nerves from the cervical sympathetic chain supply muscle fibres in the atria and ventricles, and the electrical conducting system. Activation of β_1-adrenoceptors in the heart results in positive inotropic and chronotropic effects, whereas activation of β_2-adrenoceptors in vascular smooth muscle causes vasodilatation. Parasympathetic pre-ganglionic fibres and sensory fibres reach the heart through the vagus nerves. Cholinergic nerves supply the AV and SA nodes via muscarinic (M2) receptors.

16

Under resting conditions, vagal inhibitory activity predominates and the heart rate is slow. Adrenergic stimulation, associated with exercise, emotional stress, fever and so on, causes the heart rate to increase. In disease states, the nerve supply to the heart may be affected. For example, in heart failure the sympathetic system may be up-regulated, and in diabetes mellitus the nerves themselves may be damaged by autonomic neuropathy (p. 758) so that there is little variation in heart rate.

Physiology

Myocardial contraction

Myocardial cells (myocytes) are about 50–100 µm long; each cell branches and interdigitates with adjacent cells. An intercalated disc permits electrical conduction via gap junctions, and mechanical conduction via the fascia adherens, to adjacent cells (Fig. 16.5A). The basic unit of contraction is the sarcomere (2 µm long), which is aligned to those of adjacent myofibrils, giving a striated appearance due to the Z-lines (Fig. 16.5B and C). Actin filaments are attached at right angles to the Z-lines and interdigitate with thicker parallel myosin filaments. The cross-links between actin and myosin molecules contain myofibrillar adenosine triphosphatase (ATPase), which breaks down adenosine triphosphate (ATP) to provide the energy for contraction (Fig. 16.5E). Two chains of actin molecules form a helical structure, with a second molecule, tropomyosin, in the grooves of the actin helix, and a further molecule complex, troponin, attached to every seventh actin molecule (Fig. 16.5D).

During the plateau phase of the action potential, calcium ions enter the cell and are mobilised from the sarcoplasmic reticulum. They bind to troponin and thereby precipitate contraction by shortening of the sarcomere through the interdigitation of the actin and myosin molecules. The force of cardiac muscle contraction, or inotropic state, is regulated by the influx of calcium ions through 'slow calcium channels'. The extent to which the sarcomere can shorten determines stroke volume of the ventricle. It is maximally shortened in response to powerful inotropic drugs or marked exercise. However, the enlargement of the heart seen in heart failure is due to slippage of the myofibrils and adjacent cells rather than lengthening of the sarcomere.

Cardiac peptides

Cardiomyocytes secrete peptides that have humoral effects on the vasculature and kidneys. Atrial natriuretic peptide (ANP) is a

Fig. 16.5 **Schematic of myocytes and the contraction process within a muscle fibre.** [A] Myocytes are joined together through intercalated discs. [B] Within the myocytes, myofibrils are composed of longitudinal and transverse tubules extending from the sarcoplasmic reticulum. [C] The expanded section shows a schematic of an individual sarcomere with thick filaments composed of myosin and thin filaments composed primarily of actin. [D] Actin filaments are composed of troponin, tropomyosin and actin subunits. [E] The three stages of contraction, resulting in shortening of the sarcomere. (1) The actin-binding site is blocked by tropomyosin. (2) ATP-dependent release of calcium ions, which bind to troponin, displacing tropomyosin. The binding site is exposed. (3) Tilting of the angle of attachment of the myosin head, resulting in fibre shortening. (ADP = adenosine diphosphate; ATP = adenosine triphosphate)

28-amino acid peptide, which includes an amino acid ring that acts as a vasodilator, thereby reducing blood pressure (BP), and acts as a diuretic by promoting renal excretion of water and sodium. It is released by atrial myocytes in response to stretch. Brain natriuretic peptide (BNP), which was originally identified in extracts of porcine brain, is a 32-amino acid polypeptide produced by ventricular cardiomyocytes in response to stretch, as occurs in heart failure. Like ANP, it has diuretic properties. Neprilysin is an enzyme present in the circulation that is produced by the kidney and other tissues. It breaks down ANP, BNP and other proteins and, in so doing, acts as a vasoconstrictor. It forms a therapeutic target in patients with heart failure (p. 466).

Circulation

The RA receives deoxygenated blood from the superior and inferior venae cavae and discharges blood to the RV, which in turn pumps it into the pulmonary artery. Blood passes through the pulmonary arterial and alveolar capillary bed, where it is oxygenated, then drains through the pulmonary veins into the LA. Blood then passes into the LV, which pumps it into the aorta (see Fig. 16.1). During ventricular contraction (systole), the tricuspid valve in the right heart and the mitral valve in the left heart close, and the pulmonary and aortic valves open. In diastole, the pulmonary and aortic valves close, and the two AV valves open. Collectively, these atrial and ventricular events constitute the cardiac cycle of filling and ejection of blood from one heart beat to the next. Blood passes from the heart through the large central elastic arteries into muscular arteries before encountering the resistance vessels, and ultimately the capillary bed, where there is exchange of nutrients, oxygen and waste products of metabolism. The central arteries, such as the aorta, are predominantly composed of elastic tissue with little or no vascular smooth muscle cells. When blood is ejected from the heart, the compliant aorta expands to accommodate the volume of blood before the elastic recoil sustains BP and flow following cessation of cardiac contraction. This is called the Windkessel effect and it prevents excessive rises in systolic BP while sustaining diastolic BP, thereby reducing cardiac afterload and maintaining coronary perfusion. These benefits are lost with progressive arterial stiffening, which occurs with ageing and advanced renal disease. Passing down the arterial tree, vascular smooth muscle cells progressively play a greater role until the resistance arterioles are encountered. Although all vessels contribute, the resistance vessels (diameter 50–200 μm) provide the greatest contribution to systemic vascular resistance, with small changes in radius having a marked influence on blood flow; resistance is inversely proportional to the fourth power of the radius (Poiseuille's Law). The tone of these resistance vessels is tightly regulated by humoral, neuronal and mechanical factors. Neurogenic constriction operates via α-adrenoceptors on vascular smooth muscle, and dilatation via muscarinic and β$_2$-adrenoceptors. In addition, systemic and locally released vasoactive substances influence tone; vasoconstrictors include noradrenaline (norepinephrine), angiotensin II and endothelin-1, whereas adenosine, bradykinin, prostaglandins and nitric oxide are vasodilators. Resistance to blood flow rises with viscosity and is mainly influenced by the haematocrit.

Coronary blood vessels receive sympathetic and parasympathetic innervation. While stimulation of α-adrenoceptors causes vasoconstriction and stimulation of β$_2$-adrenoceptors causes vasodilatation, the predominant effect of sympathetic stimulation in coronary arteries is vasodilatation. Parasympathetic stimulation also causes modest dilatation of normal coronary arteries. Because of these homeostatic mechanisms that regulate vessel tone, narrowing or stenosis in a coronary artery does not limit flow, even during exercise, until the cross-sectional area of the vessel is reduced by at least 70%.

Endothelium

The endothelium plays a vital role in the control of vascular homeostasis. It synthesises and releases many vasoactive mediators that cause vasodilatation, including nitric oxide, prostacyclin and endothelium-derived hyperpolarising factor, and vasoconstriction, including endothelin-1 and angiotensin II. A balance exists whereby the release of such factors contributes to the maintenance and regulation of vascular tone and BP. Damage to the endothelium may disrupt this balance and lead to vascular dysfunction, tissue ischaemia and hypertension.

The endothelium has a major influence on key regulatory steps in the recruitment of inflammatory cells and on the formation and dissolution of thrombus. Once activated, the endothelium expresses surface receptors such as E-selectin, intercellular adhesion molecule type 1 (ICAM-1) and platelet–endothelial cell adhesion molecule type 1 (PECAM-1), which mediate rolling, adhesion and migration of inflammatory leucocytes into the subintima. The endothelium also stores and releases the multimeric glycoprotein von Willebrand factor, which promotes thrombus formation by linking platelet adhesion to denuded surfaces, especially in the arterial vasculature. In contrast, once intravascular thrombus forms, tissue plasminogen activator is rapidly released from a dynamic storage pool within the endothelium to induce fibrinolysis and thrombus dissolution. These processes are critically involved in the development and progression of atherosclerosis, and endothelial function and injury are seen as central to the pathogenesis of many cardiovascular disease states.

Respiration

Cardiac output, BP and pulse rate change with respiration as the result of changes in blood flow to the right and left heart, as summarised in Box 16.1. During inspiration the fall in intrathoracic pressure causes increased return of venous blood into the chest and right side of the heart, which increases cardiac output from the RV. A substantial amount of blood is sequestered in the lungs, however, due to increased capacitance of the pulmonary vascular bed, which causes a reduction in blood flow to the left side of the heart. This causes a reduction in cardiac output from the LV and a slight fall in BP. With expiration the opposite sequence of events occurs; there is a fall in venous return to the right heart with a reduction in RV output, and a rise in the venous return to the left side of the heart with an increase in LV output. As the result of these changes, BP normally falls during inspiration

16

i 16.1 Haemodynamic effects of respiration		
	Inspiration	**Expiration**
Jugular venous pressure	Falls	Rises
Blood pressure	Falls (up to 10 mmHg)	Rises
Heart rate	Accelerates	Slows
Second heart sound	Splits*	Fuses*

*Inspiration prolongs right ventricular ejection, delaying P$_2$, and shortens left ventricular ejection, bringing forward A$_2$; expiration produces the opposite effects.

but rises during expiration. These changes are exaggerated in patients with severe airways obstruction secondary to asthma or chronic obstructive pulmonary disease (COPD) leading to pulsus paradoxus, which describes an exaggerated fall in BP during inspiration. As well as being found in airways obstruction, pulsus paradoxus is also characteristic of cardiac tamponade (p. 544). Here, cardiac filling is constrained by external pressure, and on inspiration compression of the RV impedes the normal increase in flow through it on inspiration. The interventricular septum then moves to the left, impeding left ventricular filling and cardiac output. This produces a marked fall in BP (>10 mmHg fall during inspiration).

Investigation of cardiovascular disease

Several investigations may be required in the diagnosis of cardiac disease and assessment of its severity. Basic tests, such as electrocardiography, chest X-ray and echocardiography, can be performed in an outpatient clinic or at the bedside, whereas more complex procedures such as cardiac catheterisation, radionuclide imaging, computed tomography (CT) and magnetic resonance imaging (MRI) require specialised facilities.

Electrocardiogram

The electrocardiogram (ECG) is used to assess cardiac rhythm and conduction, and is the main test used in the diagnosis of myocardial ischaemia and infarction.

The physiological basis of an ECG recording is the fact that electrical depolarisation of myocardial tissue produces a small dipole current, which can be detected by electrode pairs on the body surface. These signals are amplified and either printed or displayed on a monitor (Fig. 16.6). During sinus rhythm, the SA node triggers atrial depolarisation, producing a P wave. Depolarisation proceeds slowly through the AV node, which is too small to produce a depolarisation wave detectable from the body surface. The bundle of His, bundle branches and Purkinje system are then activated, initiating ventricular myocardial depolarisation, which produces the QRS complex. The muscle mass of the ventricles is much larger than that of the atria, so

the QRS complex is larger than the P wave. The interval between the onset of the P wave and the onset of the QRS complex is termed the 'PR interval' and largely reflects the duration of AV nodal conduction. Injury to the left or right bundle branch delays ventricular depolarisation, widening the QRS complex. Selective injury of one of the left fascicles (hemiblock, p. 479) affects the electrical axis. Repolarisation is slower and spreads from the epicardium to the endocardium. Atrial repolarisation does not cause a detectable signal but ventricular repolarisation produces the T wave. The QT interval represents the total duration of ventricular depolarisation and repolarisation.

The 12-lead ECG

The 12-lead ECG (Box 16.2) is generated from 10 electrodes that are attached to the skin. One electrode is attached to each limb and six electrodes are attached to the chest. In addition, the left arm, right arm and left leg electrodes are attached to a central terminal acting as an additional virtual electrode in the centre of the chest (the right leg electrode acts as an earthing electrode). The 12 'leads' of the ECG refer to recordings made from pairs or sets of these electrodes. They comprise three groups: three dipole limb leads, three augmented voltage limb leads and six unipole chest leads.

Leads I, II and III are the dipole limb leads and refer to recordings obtained from pairs of limb electrodes. Lead I records

16.2 How to read a 12-lead electrocardiogram: examination sequence	
Rhythm strip (lead II)	To determine heart rate and rhythm
Cardiac axis	Normal if QRS complexes +ve in leads I/II
P-wave shape	Tall P waves denote right atrial enlargement (P pulmonale) and notched P waves denote left atrial enlargement (P mitrale)
PR interval	Normal = 0.12–0.20 sec. Prolongation denotes impaired atrioventricular nodal conduction. A short PR interval occurs in Wolff–Parkinson–White syndrome (p. 474)
QRS duration	If >0.12 sec, ventricular conduction is abnormal (left or right bundle branch block)
QRS amplitude	Large QRS complexes occur in slim young patients and in patients with left ventricular hypertrophy
Q waves	May signify previous myocardial infarction
ST segment	ST elevation may signify myocardial infarction, pericarditis or left ventricular aneurysm; ST depression may signify ischaemia or infarction
T waves	T-wave inversion has many causes, including myocardial ischaemia or infarction, and electrolyte disturbances
QT interval	Normal <0.42 sec. QT prolongation may occur with congenital long QT syndrome, low K^+, Mg^{2+} or Ca^{2+}, and some drugs (see Box 16.26, p. 476)
ECG conventions	Depolarisation towards electrode: +ve deflection Depolarisation away from electrode: −ve deflection Sensitivity: 10 mm = 1 mV Paper speed: 25 mm per sec Each large (5 mm) square = 0.2 sec Each small (1 mm) square = 0.04 sec Heart rate = 1500/RR interval (mm) (i.e. 300 ÷ number of large squares between beats)

Fig. 16.6 **The electrocardiogram.** The components correspond to depolarisation and repolarisation, as depicted in Figure 16.4. The upper limit of the normal range for each interval is given in brackets.

the signal between the right (negative) and left (positive) arms. Lead II records the signal between the right arm (negative) and left leg (positive). Lead III records the signal between the left arm (negative) and left leg (positive). These three leads thus record electrical activity along three different axes in the frontal plane. Leads aVR, aVL and aVF are the augmented voltage limb leads. These record electrical activity between a limb electrode and a modified central terminal. For example, lead aVL records the signal between the left arm (positive) and a central (negative) terminal, formed by connecting the right arm and left leg electrodes (Fig. 16.7). Similarly augmented signals are obtained from the right arm (aVR) and left leg (aVF). These leads also record electrical activity in the frontal plane, with each lead 120° apart. Lead aVF thus examines activity along the axis +90°, and lead aVL along the axis −30°, and so on.

When depolarisation moves towards a positive electrode, it produces a positive deflection in the ECG; depolarisation in the opposite direction produces a negative deflection. The

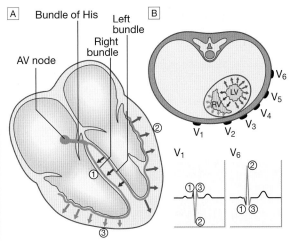

Fig. 16.8 **The sequence of activation of the ventricles.** [A] Activation of the septum occurs first (red arrows), followed by spreading of the impulse through the left ventricle (LV, blue arrows) and then the right ventricle (RV, green arrows). [B] Normal electrocardiographic complexes from leads V_1 and V_6.

average vector of ventricular depolarisation is known as the frontal cardiac axis. When the vector is at right angles to a lead, the depolarisation in that lead is equally negative and positive (isoelectric). In Figure 16.7A, the QRS complex is isoelectric in aVL, negative in aVR and most strongly positive in lead II; the main vector or axis of depolarisation is therefore 60°. The normal cardiac axis lies between −30° and +90°. Examples of left and right axis deviation are shown in Figures 16.7B and C.

There are six chest leads, V_1–V_6, derived from electrodes placed on the anterior and lateral left side of the chest, over the heart. Each lead records the signal between the corresponding chest electrode (positive) and the central terminal (negative). Leads V_1 and V_2 lie approximately over the RV, V_3 and V_4 over the interventricular septum, and V_5 and V_6 over the LV (Fig. 16.8). The LV has the greater muscle mass and contributes the major component of the QRS complex.

The shape of the QRS complex varies across the chest leads. Depolarisation of the interventricular septum occurs first and moves from left to right; this generates a small initial negative deflection in lead V_6 (Q wave) and an initial positive deflection in lead V_1 (R wave). The second phase of depolarisation is activation of the body of the LV, which creates a large positive deflection or R wave in V_6 (with reciprocal changes in V_1). The third and final phase involves the RV and produces a small negative deflection or S wave in V_6.

Exercise ECG

In exercise or stress electrocardiography a 12-lead ECG is recorded during exercise on a treadmill or bicycle ergometer. It is similar to a resting ECG, except that the limb electrodes are placed on the shoulders and hips rather than the wrists and ankles. The Bruce Protocol is the most commonly used. During an exercise ECG, BP is recorded and symptoms are assessed. Common indications for exercise testing are shown in Box 16.3. The test is considered positive if angina occurs, BP falls or fails to increase, or if there are ST segment shifts of more than 1 mm (see Fig. 16.57, p. 490). Exercise testing is useful in confirming the diagnosis of coronary artery disease in patients with suspected angina, and under these circumstances has good sensitivity and specificity (Box 16.3). False-negative

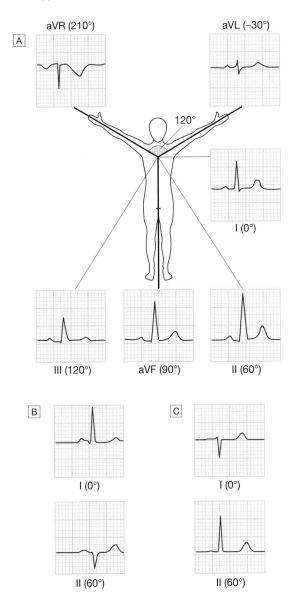

Fig. 16.7 **The appearance of the ECG from different leads in the frontal plane.** [A] Normal. [B] Left axis deviation, with negative deflection in lead II and positive in lead I. [C] Right axis deviation, with negative deflection in lead I and positive in lead II.

results can, however, occur in patients with coronary artery disease, and not all patients with a positive test have coronary disease. This is especially true in low-risk individuals, such as asymptomatic young or middle-aged women, in whom an abnormal response is more likely to represent a false-positive than a true-positive test. Stress testing is contraindicated in the presence of acute coronary syndrome, decompensated heart failure and severe hypertension.

Ambulatory ECG

Ambulatory ECG recordings can be obtained using a portable digital recorder. These devices usually provide limb lead ECG recordings only, on a continuous basis for periods of between 1 and 7 days. The main indication for ambulatory ECG is in the investigation of patients with suspected arrhythmia, such as those with intermittent palpitation, dizziness or syncope. In this situation a standard ECG provides only a snapshot of the cardiac rhythm and is unlikely to detect an intermittent arrhythmia, so a longer period of recording is required (see Fig. 16.32, p. 469). Ambulatory ECG can also be used to assess rate control in patients with atrial fibrillation, and to detect transient myocardial ischaemia using ST segment analysis. If symptoms are infrequent, special recorders can be issued that can be activated by the patient when a symptom episode occurs and placed on the chest wall to record the cardiac rhythm at that point in time. With some devices, the recording can be transmitted to hospital electronically. If the symptoms are very infrequent but potentially serious, such as syncope, implantable 'loop recorders' resembling a leadless pacemaker can be used and implanted subcutaneously to record cardiac rhythm for prolonged periods of between 1 and 3 years.

Cardiac biomarkers

Several biomarkers are available that can be measured in peripheral blood to assess myocardial dysfunction and ischaemia.

Brain natriuretic peptide

Brain natriuretic peptide (BNP) is a peptide hormone of 32 amino acids with diuretic properties. It is secreted by the LV as a 108-amino acid prohormone, which is cleaved to produce active BNP, and an inactive 76-amino acid N-terminal fragment (NT-proBNP). Circulating levels are elevated in conditions associated with LV systolic dysfunction. Generally, NT-proBNP is measured in preference to BNP since it has a longer half-life. Measurements of NT-proBNP are indicated for the diagnosis of LV dysfunction and to assess prognosis and response to therapy in patients with heart failure (p. 461).

Cardiac troponins

Troponin I and troponin T are structural cardiac muscle proteins (see Fig. 16.5) that are released during myocyte damage and necrosis, and represent the cornerstone of the diagnosis of acute myocardial infarction (MI, Box 16.47, p. 493). Modern assays are extremely sensitive, however, and can detect minor degrees of myocardial damage, so that elevated plasma troponin concentrations may be observed in conditions other than acute MI, such as pulmonary embolus, septic shock and pulmonary oedema.

Chest X-ray

This is useful for determining the size and shape of the heart, and the state of the pulmonary blood vessels and lung fields. Most information is given by a postero-anterior (PA) projection taken in full inspiration. Anteroposterior (AP) projections can be performed when patient movement is restricted but result in magnification of the cardiac shadow.

An estimate of overall heart size can be made by comparing the maximum width of the cardiac outline with the maximum internal transverse diameter of the thoracic cavity. The term cardiomegaly is used to describe an enlarged cardiac silhouette when the ratio of cardiac width to the width of the lung fields is greater than 0.5. Cardiomegaly can be caused by chamber dilatation, especially left ventricular dilatation, or by a pericardial effusion, but may also be due to a mediastinal mass or pectus excavatum (p. 628). Cardiomegaly is not a sensitive indicator of left ventricular systolic dysfunction since the cardiothoracic ratio is normal in many patients with poor left ventricular function and is not specific, since many patients with cardiomegaly on chest X-ray have normal echocardiograms.

Dilatation of individual cardiac chambers can be recognised by the characteristic alterations to the cardiac silhouette (Fig. 16.9):

- Left atrial dilatation results in prominence of the left atrial appendage, creating the appearance of a straight left heart border, a double cardiac shadow to the right of the sternum, and widening of the angle of the carina (bifurcation of the trachea) as the left main bronchus is pushed upwards.
- Right atrial enlargement projects from the right heart border towards the right lower lung field.
- Left ventricular dilatation causes prominence of the left heart border and enlargement of the cardiac silhouette. Left ventricular hypertrophy produces rounding of the left heart border (Fig. 16.10).
- Right ventricular dilatation increases heart size, displaces the apex upwards and straightens the left heart border.

Lateral or oblique projections may be useful for detecting pericardial calcification in patients with constrictive pericarditis (p. 543) or a calcified thoracic aortic aneurysm, as these abnormalities may be obscured by the spine on the PA view.

The lung fields on the chest X-ray may show congestion and oedema in patients with heart failure (see Fig. 16.27, p. 464), and an increase in pulmonary blood flow ('pulmonary plethora') in those with left-to-right shunt. Pleural effusions may also occur in heart failure.

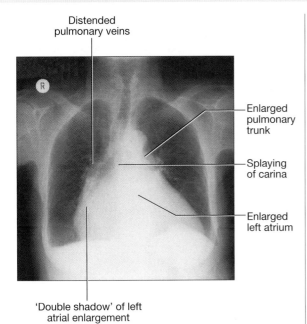

Distended pulmonary veins

Enlarged pulmonary trunk

Splaying of carina

Enlarged left atrium

'Double shadow' of left atrial enlargement

Fig. 16.9 Chest X-ray of a patient with mitral stenosis and regurgitation indicating enlargement of the LA and prominence of the pulmonary artery trunk.

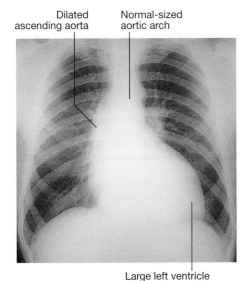

Dilated ascending aorta

Normal-sized aortic arch

Large left ventricle

Fig. 16.10 Chest X-ray of a patient with aortic regurgitation, left ventricular enlargement and dilatation of the ascending aorta.

Echocardiography

Transthoracic echocardiography

Transthoracic echocardiography, commonly referred to as 'echo', is obtained by placing an ultrasound transducer on the chest wall to image the heart structures as a real-time two-dimensional 'slice'. This can be used for rapid evaluation of various aspects of cardiac structure and function. Common indications for echocardiography are shown in Box 16.4.

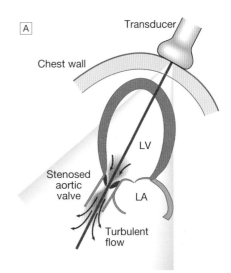

A

Transducer

Chest wall

LV

Stenosed aortic valve

LA

Turbulent flow

B

1 AV Vmax	2.98 m/s
AV Vmean	1.94 m/s
AV maxPG	35.52 mmHg
AV meanPG	18.19 mmHg
AV VTI	52.98 cm
AV Env.Ti	273.57 ms
HR	219.32 BPM

Fig. 16.11 Doppler echocardiography in aortic stenosis. A The aortic valve is imaged and a Doppler beam passed directly through the left ventricular outflow tract and the aorta into the turbulent flow beyond the stenosed valve. B The velocity of the blood cells is recorded to determine the maximum velocity and hence the pressure gradient across the valve. In this example, the peak velocity is approximately 450 cm/sec (4.5 m/sec), indicating severe aortic stenosis (peak gradient of 81 mmHg).

Doppler echocardiography

Doppler echocardiography provides information on blood flow within the heart and the great vessels. It is based on the Doppler principle that sound waves reflected from moving objects, such as red blood cells, undergo a frequency shift. Doppler echocardiography can therefore detect the speed and direction of blood flow in the heart chambers and great vessels. The greater the frequency shift, the faster the blood is moving. The information can be presented either as a plot of blood velocity against time for a particular point in the heart (Fig. 16.11) or as

16

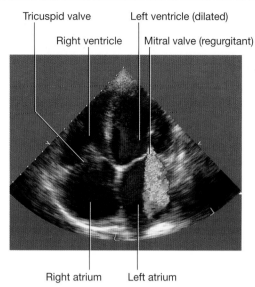

Tricuspid valve   Left ventricle (dilated)

Right ventricle   Mitral valve (regurgitant)

Right atrium   Left atrium

Fig. 16.12 Echocardiographic illustration of the principal cardiac structures in the 'four-chamber' view. Colour-flow Doppler has been used to demonstrate mitral regurgitation: a flame-shaped (yellow/blue) turbulent jet into the left atrium.

a colour overlay on a two-dimensional real-time echo picture (colour-flow Doppler, Fig. 16.12). Doppler echocardiography is useful in the detection of valvular regurgitation, where the direction of blood flow is reversed and turbulence is seen, and is also used to detect pressure gradients across stenosed valves. For example, the normal resting systolic flow velocity across the aortic valve is approximately 1 m/sec; in the presence of aortic stenosis, this is increased as blood accelerates through the narrow orifice. In severe aortic stenosis, the peak aortic velocity may be increased to 5 m/sec (see Fig. 16.11). An estimate of the pressure gradient across a valve or lesion is given by the modified Bernoulli equation:

$$\text{Pressure gradient (mmHg)} = 4 \times (\text{peak velocity in m/sec})^2$$

Advanced techniques include three-dimensional echocardiography, intravascular ultrasound (defines vessel wall abnormalities and guides coronary intervention), intracardiac ultrasound (provides high-resolution images), tissue Doppler imaging (quantifies myocardial contractility and diastolic function) and speckle tracking (assesses myocardial motion and strain).

Transoesophageal echocardiography

Transoesophageal echocardiography (TOE) involves passing an endoscope-like ultrasound probe into the oesophagus and upper stomach under light sedation and positioning it behind the LA. It is particularly useful for imaging structures such as the left atrial appendage, pulmonary veins, thoracic aorta and interatrial septum, which may be poorly visualised by transthoracic echocardiography, especially if the patient is overweight or has obstructive airway disease. The high-resolution images that can be obtained makes TOE particularly valuable for investigating patients with prosthetic (especially mitral) valve dysfunction, congenital abnormalities such as atrial septal defects, aortic dissection, infective endocarditis (vegetations that are too small to be detected by transthoracic echocardiography) and systemic embolism (intracardiac thrombus or masses).

Fig. 16.13 Computed tomography coronary angiography, demonstrating normal coronary arteries (arrows). A Three-dimensional image. B Two-dimensional image.

Stress echocardiography

Stress echocardiography is used to investigate patients with suspected coronary artery disease who are unsuitable for exercise stress testing, such as those with mobility problems or pre-existing bundle branch block. A two-dimensional echo is performed before and after infusion of a moderate to high dose of an inotrope, such as dobutamine. Myocardial segments with poor perfusion become ischaemic and contract poorly under stress, manifesting as a wall motion abnormality on the scan. Stress echocardiography is sometimes used to examine myocardial viability in patients with impaired left ventricular function. Low-dose dobutamine can induce contraction in 'hibernating' myocardium; such patients may benefit from bypass surgery or percutaneous coronary intervention.

Computed tomography

Computed tomography (CT) is useful for imaging the cardiac chambers, great vessels, pericardium, and mediastinal structures and masses. Multidetector scanners can acquire up to 320 slices per rotation, allowing very high-resolution imaging in a single heart beat. CT is often performed using a timed injection of X-ray contrast to produce clear images of blood vessels and associated pathologies. Contrast scans are very useful for imaging the aorta in suspected aortic dissection (see Fig. 16.74, p. 507), and the pulmonary arteries and branches in suspected pulmonary embolism (p. 619).

Some centres use cardiac CT scans for quantification of coronary artery calcification, which may serve as an index of cardiovascular risk. However, modern multidetector scanning allows non-invasive coronary angiography (Fig. 16.13) with a spatial resolution approaching that of conventional coronary arteriography and at a lower radiation dose. CT coronary angiography is particularly useful in the initial assessment of patients with chest pain and a low or intermediate likelihood of disease, since it has a high negative predictive value in excluding coronary artery disease. Modern volume scanners are also able to assess myocardial perfusion, often at the same sitting.

Magnetic resonance imaging

Magnetic resonance imaging (MRI) can be used to generate cross-sectional images of the heart, lungs and mediastinal structures. It provides better differentiation of soft tissue structures than CT but is poor at demonstrating calcification. MRI scans need to be 'gated' to the ECG, allowing the scanner to produce moving images of the heart and mediastinal structures throughout the cardiac cycle. MRI is very useful for imaging the aorta, including suspected dissection (see Fig. 16.73, p. 507), and can define the anatomy of the heart and great vessels in patients with congenital heart disease. It is also useful for detecting infiltrative conditions affecting the heart and for evaluation of the RV that is difficult to image by echocardiography.

Physiological data can be obtained from the signal returned from moving blood, which allows quantification of blood flow across regurgitant or stenotic valves. It is also possible to analyse regional wall motion in patients with suspected coronary disease or cardiomyopathy.

Myocardial perfusion and viability can also be readily assessed by MRI. When enhanced by gadolinium-based contrast media, areas of myocardial hypoperfusion can be identified with better spatial resolution than nuclear medicine techniques. Later redistribution of this contrast, so-called delayed enhancement, can be used to identify myocardial scarring and fibrosis: this is a particular strength of cardiac MRI (Fig. 16.14). This can help in selecting patients for revascularisation procedures, or in identifying those with myocardial infiltration, such as that seen with sarcoid heart disease and arrhythmogenic right ventricular cardiomyopathy.

Cardiac catheterisation

This involves passing a specialised catheter through a peripheral vein or artery into the heart under X-ray guidance. Cardiac catheterisation allows BP and oxygen saturation to be measured in the cardiac chambers and great vessels, and is used to perform angiograms by injecting contrast media into a chamber or blood vessel.

Left heart catheterisation involves accessing the arterial circulation, usually through the radial artery, to allow catheterisation of the aorta, LV and coronary arteries. Coronary angiography is the most widely performed procedure, in which the left and right coronary arteries are selectively imaged, providing information about the extent and severity of coronary stenoses, thrombus and calcification (Fig. 16.15). Additional anatomical

Fig. 16.14 **Cardiac magnetic resonance imaging.** [A] Recent inferior myocardial infarction with black area of microvascular obstruction (arrow). [B] Old anterior myocardial infarction with large area of subendocardial delayed gadolinium enhancement (white area, arrows).

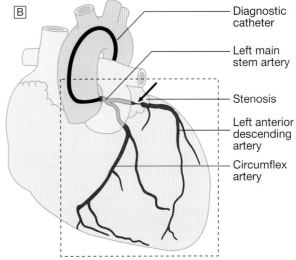

Fig. 16.15 **The left anterior descending and circumflex coronary arteries with a stenosis (arrow) in the left anterior descending vessel.** [A] Coronary artery angiogram. [B] Schematic of the vessels and branches.

(intravascular ultrasound, optical coherence tomography) or functional (pressure wire) assessments are sometimes used to define plaque characteristics and severity more precisely. This permits planning of percutaneous coronary intervention and coronary artery bypass graft surgery. Left ventriculography can be performed during the procedure to determine the size and function of the LV and to demonstrate mitral regurgitation. Aortography defines the size of the aortic root and thoracic aorta, and can help quantify aortic regurgitation. Left heart catheterisation is a day-case procedure and is relatively safe, with serious complications occurring in only approximately 1 in 1000 cases.

Right heart catheterisation is used to assess right heart and pulmonary artery pressures, and to detect intracardiac shunts by measuring oxygen saturations in different chambers. For example, a step up in oxygen saturation from 65% in the RA to 80% in the pulmonary artery is indicative of a large left-to-right shunt that might be due to a ventricular septal defect. Cardiac output can also be measured using thermodilution techniques. Left atrial pressure can be measured directly by puncturing the interatrial septum from the RA with a special catheter. For most purposes, however, a satisfactory approximation to left atrial pressure can be obtained by 'wedging' an end-hole or balloon catheter in a branch of the pulmonary artery. Swan–Ganz balloon catheters are often used to monitor pulmonary 'wedge' pressure as a guide to left heart filling pressure in critically ill patients (p. 206).

Electrophysiology

Patients with known or suspected arrhythmia are investigated by percutaneous placement of electrode catheters into the heart via the femoral and neck veins. An electrophysiology study (EPS) is most commonly performed to evaluate patients for catheter ablation and is normally done at the same time as the ablation procedure. EPS is occasionally used for risk stratification of patients suspected of being at risk of ventricular arrhythmias.

Radionuclide imaging

Radionuclide imaging can be used to evaluate cardiac function but is declining in popularity due to the availability of MRI, which does not involve exposure to radiation and provides equivalent or superior quality data to radionuclide imaging.

▌ Blood pool imaging

The patient is given an intravenous injection of radioisotope-labelled blood cells, and after 4–5 minutes the distribution of isotope in the heart is evaluated by a gamma camera at different phases of the cardiac cycle, thereby permitting the calculation of ventricular ejection fractions. It also allows the assessment of the size and 'shape' of the cardiac chambers.

▌ Myocardial perfusion scanning

The patient is given an intravenous injection of a radioactive isotope, such as ^{99}technetium tetrofosmin, and scintiscans of the myocardium are subsequently obtained by gamma camera at rest and during stress (see Fig. 16.58, p. 490). Either exercise stress or pharmacological stress (using the inotrope dobutamine or the vasodilator dipyridamole) can be used. More sophisticated quantitative information can be obtained with positron emission tomography (PET), which can also be used to assess myocardial metabolism, but this is available in only a few centres.

Presenting problems in cardiovascular disease

Cardiovascular disease gives rise to a relatively limited range of symptoms. Making the correct diagnosis depends on careful analysis of the factors that provoke symptoms, the subtle differences in how they are described by the patient, the clinical findings and the results of investigations. A close relationship between symptoms and exercise is the hallmark of heart disease. The New York Heart Association (NYHA) functional classification is used to grade disability (Box 16.5).

Chest pain on exertion

There are many other non-cardiac causes of chest pain, as discussed in Chapter 10. This section will focus on exertional chest pain, which is a typical presenting symptom of coronary artery disease.

Clinical assessment

A careful history is crucial in determining whether chest pain is cardiac or not. Chest pain on effort is the hallmark of angina pectoris (Fig. 16.16). The reproducibility, predictability and relationship to physical exertion (and occasionally emotion) of the chest pain are the most important features. The duration of symptoms should be noted because patients with recent-onset angina are at greater risk than those with long-standing and unchanged symptoms. Physical examination is often normal but

---

i | **16.5 New York Heart Association (NYHA) functional classification**

Class I
• No limitation during ordinary activity

Class II
• Slight limitation during ordinary activity

Class III
• Marked limitation of normal activities without symptoms at rest

Class IV
• Unable to undertake physical activity without symptoms; symptoms may be present at rest

Fig. 16.16 Typical ischaemic cardiac pain. Characteristic hand gestures used to describe cardiac pain. Typical radiation of pain is shown in the schematic.

may reveal evidence of risk factors for cardiovascular disease, such as xanthoma or xanthelasma indicating hyperlipidaemia (p. 373). Signs of anaemia (p. 923) or thyrotoxicosis (p. 635) may be identified, both of which can exacerbate angina. Cardiovascular examination may reveal evidence of left ventricular dysfunction (p. 442) or cardiac murmurs in patients with aortic valve disease and hypertrophic cardiomyopathy. Other manifestations of arterial disease, such as bruits and loss of peripheral pulses, may also be observed.

Investigations

A full blood count, fasting blood glucose, lipids, thyroid function tests and a 12-lead ECG are the most important baseline investigations. An exercise ECG is helpful in identifying high-risk patients who require further investigation and treatment but cannot reliably exclude the presence of coronary artery disease (p. 449). In patients with chest pain where the exercise ECG is normal but where there is a suspicion of coronary artery disease, CT coronary angiography should be performed. If a murmur is found, echocardiography should be performed to check for valve disease or hypertrophic cardiomyopathy.

Severe prolonged chest pain

Severe prolonged cardiac chest pain may be due to acute myocardial infarction or to unstable angina (p. 493). These are known collectively as the acute coronary syndromes.

Clinical assessment

Acute coronary syndrome is suggested by a previous history of stable angina but an episode of acute severe chest pain at rest can be the first presentation of coronary artery disease. Making the correct diagnosis depends on analysing the character of the pain and its associated features. Physical examination may reveal signs of risk factors for coronary artery disease as described for exertional chest pain, and pallor or sweating, which is indicative of autonomic disturbance and typical of acute coronary syndrome. Other features, such as arrhythmia, hypotension and heart failure, may occur. Patients presenting with symptoms consistent with an acute coronary syndrome require admission to hospital and urgent investigation because there is a high risk of avoidable complications.

Investigations

A 12-lead ECG is mandatory and is the most useful method of initial triage, along with measurement of serum troponin I or T. The diagnosis of an acute coronary syndrome is supported by ST segment elevation or depression on ECG and an elevated level of troponin I or T, which demonstrates that there has been myocardial damage.

If the diagnosis remains unclear after initial investigation, repeat ECG recordings should be performed and are particularly useful if they can be obtained during an episode of pain. If the plasma troponin concentrations are normal at baseline, repeat measurements should be made 6–12 hours after the onset of symptoms or admission to hospital. New ECG changes or an elevated plasma troponin concentration confirm the diagnosis of an acute coronary syndrome. If the pain settles and does not recur, there are no new ECG changes and troponin concentrations remain normal, the patient can be discharged from hospital but further investigations may be indicated to look for evidence of coronary artery disease, as discussed on page 484.

Management

The differential diagnosis and management of acute coronary syndrome are described in more detail on pages 494 and 498.

Breathlessness

Cardiac causes of breathlessness include cardiac arrhythmias, acute and chronic heart failure, acute coronary syndrome, valvular disease, cardiomyopathy and constrictive pericarditis, all discussed later in this chapter. The differential diagnosis of breathlessness is wide, however, and has many other non-cardiac causes. These are discussed in more detail on pages 179 and 557.

Syncope

The term 'syncope' refers to loss of consciousness due to reduced cerebral perfusion. The differential diagnosis, investigation and management of syncope are discussed on page 181.

Palpitation

Palpitation is a common and sometimes frightening symptom that is usually due to a disorder of cardiac rhythm. Patients use the term to describe many sensations, including an unusually erratic, fast, slow or forceful heart beat, or even chest pain or breathlessness.

Clinical assessment

Initial evaluation should concentrate on determining the likely mechanism of palpitation and whether or not there is significant underlying heart disease. A detailed description of the sensation is essential and patients should be asked to describe their symptoms clearly, or to demonstrate the sensation of rhythm by tapping with their hand. A provisional diagnosis can usually be made on the basis of a thorough history (Box 16.6 and Fig. 16.17). Recurrent but short-lived bouts of an irregular heart beat are usually due to atrial or ventricular extrasystoles (ectopic beats). Some patients will describe the experience as a 'flip' or a 'jolt' in the chest, while others report dropped or missed beats. Extrasystoles are often more frequent during periods of stress or debility; they can be triggered by alcohol or nicotine.

Episodes of a pounding, forceful and relatively fast (90–120/min) heart beat are a common manifestation of anxiety. These may also reflect a hyperdynamic circulation, such as anaemia, pregnancy and thyrotoxicosis, and can occur in some forms of valve disease such as aortic regurgitation. Discrete bouts of a

16.6 How to evaluate palpitation

- Is the palpitation continuous or intermittent?
- Is the heart beat regular or irregular?
- What is the approximate heart rate?
- Do symptoms occur in discrete attacks?
  - Is the onset abrupt? How do attacks terminate?
- Are there any associated symptoms?
  - Chest pain, lightheadedness, polyuria (a feature of supraventricular tachycardia, p. 473)
- Are there any precipitating factors, such as exercise or alcohol excess?
- Is there a history of structural heart disease, such as coronary artery disease or valvular heart disease?

16

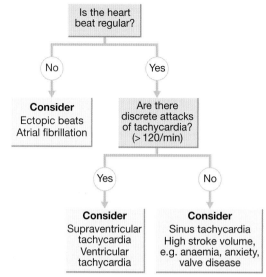

Fig. 16.17 A simple approach to the diagnosis of palpitation.

Fig. 16.18 Ventricular fibrillation. A bizarre chaotic rhythm, initiated in this case by two ventricular ectopic beats in rapid succession.

i	16.7 Causes of sudden arrhythmic death

Coronary artery disease (85%)

- Myocardial ischaemia
- Acute myocardial infarction
- Prior myocardial infarction with myocardial scarring

Structural heart disease (10%)

- Aortic stenosis (p. 521)
- Hypertrophic cardiomyopathy (p. 539)
- Dilated cardiomyopathy (p. 539)
- Arrhythmogenic right ventricular dysplasia (p. 540)
- Congenital heart disease (p. 531)

No structural heart disease (5%)

- Long QT syndrome (p. 476)
- Brugada syndrome (p. 477)
- Wolff–Parkinson–White syndrome (p. 474)
- Adverse drug reactions (torsades de pointes, p. 476)
- Severe electrolyte abnormalities

very rapid (over 120/min) heart beat are more likely to be due to a paroxysmal supraventricular or ventricular tachycardia. In contrast, episodes of atrial fibrillation typically present with irregular and usually rapid palpitation.

Investigation

If initial assessment suggests that the palpitation is due to an arrhythmia, the diagnosis should be confirmed by an ECG recording during an episode using an ambulatory ECG monitor or a patient-activated ECG recorder. Additional investigations may be required depending on the nature of the arrhythmia, as discussed on page 468.

Management

Palpitation is usually benign and even if the patient's symptoms are due to an arrhythmia, the outlook is good if there is no underlying structural heart disease. Most cases are due to an awareness of the normal heart beat, a sinus tachycardia or benign extrasystoles, in which case an explanation and reassurance may be all that is required. Palpitation associated with pre-syncope or syncope (p. 181) may reflect more serious structural or electrical disease and should be investigated without delay. Other arrhythmias may require treatment, as discussed in more detail on page 479.

Cardiac arrest

Cardiac arrest describes the sudden and complete loss of cardiac output due to asystole, ventricular tachycardia or fibrillation, or loss of mechanical cardiac contraction (pulseless electrical activity). The clinical diagnosis is based on the victim being unconscious and pulseless; breathing may take some time to stop completely after cardiac arrest. Death is virtually inevitable, unless effective treatment is given promptly. Sudden cardiac death is usually caused by a catastrophic arrhythmia and accounts for 25–30% of deaths from cardiovascular disease, claiming an estimated 70 000 to 90 000 lives each year in the UK. Many of these deaths are potentially preventable.

Pathogenesis

Coronary artery disease is the most common cause of cardiac arrest. Ventricular fibrillation or ventricular tachycardia is common in the first few hours of MI and many victims die before medical help is sought. Up to one-third of people developing MI die before reaching hospital, emphasising the importance of educating the public to recognise symptoms and to seek medical help quickly. Acute myocardial ischaemia in the absence of infarction can also cause these arrhythmias, but less commonly. Patients with a history of previous MI are at increased risk of sudden arrhythmic death, especially if there is extensive left ventricular scarring and impairment, or if there is ongoing myocardial ischaemia. Cardiac arrest may be caused by ventricular fibrillation (Fig. 16.18), pulseless ventricular tachycardia (p. 457), asystole or pulseless electrical activity. These can complicate many types of heart disease, including cardiomyopathies, and sometimes can occur in the absence of recognised structural abnormalities. The causes are listed in Box 16.7. Sudden death less often occurs because of an acute mechanical catastrophe such as cardiac rupture or aortic dissection (pp. 496 and 506).

Clinical assessment and management

Basic life support

When a patient with suspected cardiac arrest is encountered, the ABCDE approach to management should be followed; this involves prompt assessment and restoration of the **A**irway, maintenance of ventilation using rescue **B**reathing ('mouth-to-mouth' breathing), and maintenance of the **C**irculation using chest compressions; **D**isability, in resuscitated patients, refers to assessment of neurological status, and **E**xposure entails removal of clothes to enable defibrillation, auscultation of the chest, and assessment for a rash caused by anaphylaxis, for injuries and so on (Fig. 16.19). The term basic life support (BLS)

In-hospital resuscitation

Collapsed / sick patient

↓

Shout for HELP and assess patient

↓

Signs of life?

NO ← → **YES**

NO branch:

Call resuscitation team

↓

CPR 30:2 with oxygen and airway adjuncts

↓

Apply pads/monitor Attempt defibrillation if appropriate

↓

Advanced life support when resuscitation team arrives

YES branch:

Assess ABCDE Recognise and treat Oxygen, monitoring, IV access

↓

Call resuscitation team if appropriate

↓

Handover to resuscitation team

Fig. 16.19 Algorithm for adult basic life support. For further information, see www.resus.org.uk. (CPR = cardiopulmonary resuscitation) *From Resuscitation Council (UK) guidelines: https://www.resus.org.uk/ resuscitation-guidelines/in-hospital-resuscitation/.*

encompasses manœuvres that aim to maintain a low level of circulation until more definitive treatment with advanced life support can be given. Chest compression-only ('hands-only') cardiopulmonary resuscitation (CPR) is easier for members of the public to learn and administer, and is now advocated in public education campaigns.

Advanced life support

Advanced life support (ALS) (Fig. 16.20) aims to restore normal cardiac rhythm by defibrillation when the cause of cardiac arrest is a tachyarrhythmia, or to restore cardiac output by correcting other reversible causes of cardiac arrest. The initial priority is to assess the patient's cardiac rhythm by attaching a defibrillator or monitor. Once that this has been done, treatment should be instituted based on the clinical findings.

Ventricular fibrillation or pulseless ventricular tachycardia should be treated with immediate defibrillation. Defibrillation is more likely to be effective if a biphasic shock defibrillator is used, where the polarity of the shock is reversed midway through its delivery. Defibrillation is usually administered using a 150-joule biphasic shock, and CPR resumed immediately for 2 minutes without attempting to confirm restoration of a pulse because restoration of mechanical cardiac output rarely occurs immediately after successful defibrillation. If, after 2 minutes, a pulse is not restored, a further biphasic shock of 150–200 joules should be given. Thereafter, additional biphasic shocks of 150–200 joules are given every 2 minutes after each cycle of CPR. During resuscitation, adrenaline (epinephrine, 1 mg IV) should be given every 3–5 minutes and consideration given to the use

of intravenous amiodarone, especially if ventricular fibrillation or ventricular tachycardia re-initiates after successful defibrillation.

Ventricular fibrillation of low amplitude, or 'fine VF', may mimic asystole. If asystole cannot be confidently diagnosed, the patient should be treated for VF and defibrillated. If an electrical rhythm is observed that would be expected to produce a cardiac output, 'pulseless electrical activity' is present. Pulseless electrical activity should be treated by continuing CPR and adrenaline (epinephrine) administration while seeking such causes. Asystole should be treated similarly, with the additional support of atropine and sometimes external or transvenous pacing in an attempt to generate an electrical rhythm. There are many potentially reversible causes of cardiac arrest; the main ones can be easily remembered as a list of four Hs and four Ts (Fig. 16.20).

The Chain of Survival

This term refers to the sequence of events that is necessary to maximise the chances of a cardiac arrest victim surviving (Fig. 16.21). Survival is most likely if all links in the chain are strong: that is, if the arrest is witnessed, help is called immediately, basic life support is administered by a trained individual, the emergency medical services respond promptly, and defibrillation is achieved within a few minutes. Good training in both basic and advanced life support is essential and should be maintained by regular refresher courses. In recent years, public access defibrillation has been introduced in places of high population density, particularly where traffic congestion may impede the response of emergency services, such as railway stations, airports and sports stadia. Designated individuals can respond to a cardiac arrest using BLS and an automated external defibrillator.

Survivors of cardiac arrest

Patients who survive a cardiac arrest caused by acute MI need no specific treatment beyond that given to those recovering from an uncomplicated infarct, since their prognosis is similar (p. 498). Those with reversible causes, such as exercise-induced ischaemia or aortic stenosis, should have the underlying cause treated if possible. Survivors of ventricular tachycardia or ventricular fibrillation arrest in whom no reversible cause can be identified may be at risk of another episode, and should be considered for an implantable cardiac defibrillator (p. 483) and anti-arrhythmic drug therapy. In these patients, the risk is reduced by treatment of heart failure with β-adrenoceptor antagonists (β-blockers) and angiotensin-converting enzyme (ACE) inhibitors, and by coronary revascularisation.

Abnormal heart sounds

The first indication of heart disease may be the discovery of an abnormal sound on auscultation (Box 16.8). This may be incidental – for example, during a routine childhood examination – or may be prompted by symptoms of heart disease.

Clinical assessment

The aims of clinical assessment are, firstly, to determine if the abnormal sound is cardiac; secondly, to determine if it is pathological; and thirdly, to try to determine its cause.

Is the sound cardiac?

Additional heart sounds and murmurs demonstrate a consistent relationship to a specific part of the cardiac cycle, whereas extracardiac sounds, such as a pleural rub or venous hum,

16

Advanced life support

Unresponsive and
not breathing normally?

Call resuscitation team

CPR 30:2
Attach defibrillator/monitor
Minimise interruptions

Assess rhythm

**Shockable
(VF/Pulseless VT)**

**Non-shockable
(PEA/Asystole)**

1 shock
Minimise
interruptions

Return of spontaneous
circulation

Immediately resume
CPR for 2 mins
Minimise interruptions

**Immediate post-cardiac
arrest treatment**
• Use ABCDE approach
• Aim for SaO_2 of 94–98%
• Aim for normal $PaCO_2$
• 12-lead ECG
• Treat precipitating cause
• Targeted temperature
  management

Immediately resume
CPR for 2 mins
Minimise interruptions

During CPR
• Ensure high-quality chest compressions
• Minimise interruptions to compressions
• Give oxygen
• Use waveform capnography
• Perform continuous compressions when
  advanced airway in place
• Gain vascular access (intravenous or
  interosseous)
• Give adrenaline (epinephrine) every
  3–5 min
• Give amiodarone after 3 shocks

Treat reversible causes

Hypoxia   Thrombosis – coronary or pulmonary
Hypovolaemia   Tension pneumothorax
Hypo-/hyperkalaemia/metabolic   Tamponade – cardiac
Hypothermia/hyperthermia   Toxins

Consider
• Ultrasound imaging
• Mechanical chest compressions to facilitate transfer/treatment
• Coronary angiography and percutaneous coronary intervention
• Extracorporeal CPR

Fig. 16.20 Algorithm for adult advanced life support. For further information, see www.resus.org.uk. (CPR = cardiopulmonary resuscitation:
PEA = pulseless electrical activity; VF = ventricular fibrillation; VT = ventricular tachycardia) *From Resuscitation Council (UK) guidelines:
https://www.resus.org.uk/resuscitation-guidelines/adult-advanced-life-support/.*

Fig. 16.21 The Chain of Survival in cardiac arrest. (ALS = advanced life support; CPR = cardiopulmonary resuscitation)

16.8 Normal and abnormal heart sounds

Sound	Timing	Characteristics	Mechanisms	Variable features
First heart sound (S1)	Onset of systole	Usually single or narrowly split	Closure of mitral and tricuspid valves	Loud: hyperdynamic circulation (anaemia, pregnancy, thyrotoxicosis); mitral stenosis Soft: heart failure; mitral regurgitation
Second heart sound (S2)	End of systole	Split on inspiration Single on expiration (p. 447)	Closure of aortic and pulmonary valve A_2 first P_2 second	Fixed wide splitting with atrial septal defect Wide but variable splitting with delayed right heart emptying (right bundle branch block) Reversed splitting due to delayed left heart emptying (left bundle branch block)
Third heart sound (S3)	Early in diastole, just after S2	Low pitch, often heard as 'gallop'	From ventricular wall due to abrupt cessation of rapid filling	Physiological: young people, pregnancy Pathological: heart failure, mitral regurgitation
Fourth heart sound (S4)	End of diastole, just before S1	Low pitch	Ventricular origin (stiff ventricle and augmented atrial contraction) related to atrial filling	Absent in atrial fibrillation A feature of severe left ventricular hypertrophy
Systolic clicks	Early or mid-systole	Brief, high-intensity sound	Valvular aortic stenosis Valvular pulmonary stenosis Floppy mitral valve Prosthetic heart sounds from opening and closing of normally functioning mechanical valves	Click may be lost when stenotic valve becomes thickened or calcified Prosthetic clicks lost when valve obstructed by thrombus or vegetations
Opening snap (OS)	Early in diastole	High pitch, brief duration	Opening of stenosed leaflets of mitral valve Prosthetic heart sounds	Moves closer to S2 as mitral stenosis becomes more severe. May be absent in calcific mitral stenosis

16.9 Features of a benign or innocent heart murmur

- Soft
- Mid-systolic
- Heard at left sternal edge
- No radiation
- No other cardiac abnormalities

16.10 How to assess a heart murmur

When does it occur?

- Time the murmur using heart sounds, carotid pulse and the apex beat. Is it systolic or diastolic?
- Does the murmur extend throughout systole or diastole or is it confined to a shorter part of the cardiac cycle?

How loud is it? (intensity)

- Grade 1: very soft (audible only in ideal conditions)
- Grade 2: soft
- Grade 3: moderate
- Grade 4: loud with associated thrill
- Grade 5: very loud
- Grade 6: heard without stethoscope

  Note: Diastolic murmurs are very rarely above grade 4

Where is it heard best? (location)

- Listen over the apex and base of the heart, including the aortic and pulmonary areas

Where does it radiate?

- Listen at the neck, axilla or back

What does it sound like? (pitch and quality)

- Pitch is determined by flow (high pitch indicates high-velocity flow)
- Is the intensity constant or variable?

do not. Pericardial friction produces a characteristic scratching noise termed a pericardial rub, which may have two components corresponding to atrial and ventricular systole, and may vary with posture and respiration.

Is the sound pathological?

Pathological sounds and murmurs are the product of turbulent blood flow or rapid ventricular filling due to abnormal loading conditions. Some added sounds are physiological but may also occur in pathological conditions; for example, a third sound is common in young people and in pregnancy but is also a feature of heart failure (Box 16.8). Similarly, a systolic murmur due to turbulence across the right ventricular outflow tract may occur in hyperdynamic states such as anaemia or pregnancy, but may also be due to pulmonary stenosis or an intracardiac shunt leading to volume overload of the RV, such as an atrial septal defect. Benign murmurs do not occur in diastole (Box 16.9), and systolic murmurs that radiate or are associated with a thrill are almost always pathological.

What is the origin of the sound?

Timing, intensity, location, radiation and quality are all useful clues to the origin and nature of an additional sound or murmur (Box 16.10). Radiation of a murmur is determined by the direction of turbulent blood flow and is detectable only when there is a high-velocity jet, such as in mitral regurgitation (radiation from apex to axilla) or aortic stenosis (radiation from base to neck). Similarly, the pitch and quality of the sound can help to distinguish

the murmur, such as the 'blowing' murmur of mitral regurgitation or the 'rasping' murmur of aortic stenosis. The position of a murmur in relation to the cardiac cycle is crucial and should be assessed by timing it with the heart sounds, carotid pulse and apex beat (Figs 16.22 and 16.23).

Systolic murmurs

Ejection systolic murmurs are associated with ventricular outflow tract obstruction and occur in mid-systole with a

16.11 Features of some common systolic murmurs				
Condition	Timing and duration	Quality	Location and radiation	Associated features
Aortic stenosis	Mid-systolic	Loud, rasping	Base and left sternal edge, radiating to suprasternal notch and carotids	Single second heart sound Ejection click (in young patients) Slow rising pulse Left ventricular hypertrophy (pressure overload)
Mitral regurgitation	Pansystolic	Blowing	Apex, radiating to axilla	Soft first heart sound Third heart sound Left ventricular hypertrophy (volume overload)
Ventricular septal defect	Pansystolic	Harsh	Lower left sternal edge, radiating to whole precordium	Thrill Biventricular hypertrophy
Benign	Mid-systolic	Soft	Left sternal edge, no radiation	No other signs of heart disease

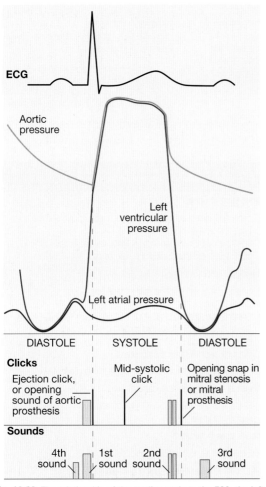

Fig. 16.22 The relationship of the cardiac cycle to the ECG, the left ventricular pressure wave and the position of heart sounds.

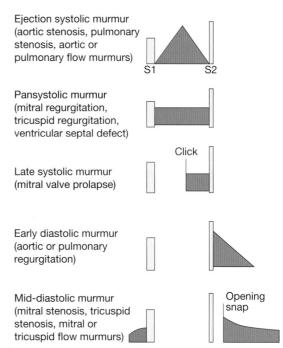

Fig. 16.23 The timing and pattern of cardiac murmurs.

crescendo–decrescendo pattern, reflecting the changing velocity of blood flow (Box 16.11). Pansystolic murmurs maintain a constant intensity and extend from the first heart sound throughout systole to the second heart sound, sometimes obscuring it. They occur when blood leaks from a ventricle into a low-pressure chamber at an even or constant velocity. Mitral regurgitation, tricuspid regurgitation and ventricular septal defect are the only causes of a pansystolic murmur. Late systolic murmurs are unusual but may

occur in mitral valve prolapse, if the mitral regurgitation is confined to late systole, and hypertrophic obstructive cardiomyopathy, if dynamic obstruction occurs late in systole.

Diastolic murmurs

These are due to accelerated or turbulent flow across the mitral or tricuspid valves. They are low-pitched noises that are often difficult to hear and should be evaluated with the bell of the stethoscope. A mid-diastolic murmur may be due to mitral stenosis (located at the apex and axilla), tricuspid stenosis (located at the left sternal edge), increased flow across the mitral valve (for example, the to-and-fro murmur of severe mitral regurgitation) or increased flow across the tricuspid valve (for example, a left-to-right shunt through a large atrial septal defect). Early diastolic murmurs have a soft, blowing quality with a decrescendo pattern and should be evaluated with the diaphragm of the stethoscope. They are due to regurgitation across the aortic or pulmonary valves and are best heard at the left sternal edge, with the patient sitting forwards in held expiration.

Continuous murmurs

These result from a combination of systolic and diastolic flow, such as occurs with a persistent ductus arteriosus, and must be distinguished from extracardiac noises such as bruits from arterial shunts, venous hums (high rates of venous flow in children) and pericardial friction rubs.

Investigations

If clinical evaluation suggests that the additional sound is cardiac and likely to be pathological, then echocardiography is indicated to determine the underlying cause.

Management

Management of patients with additional cardiac sounds depends on the underlying cause. More details are provided in the sections on specific valve defects and congenital anomalies later in this chapter (pp. 514 and 531).

Heart failure

Heart failure describes the clinical syndrome that develops when the heart cannot maintain adequate output, or can do so only at the expense of elevated ventricular filling pressure. In mild to moderate forms of heart failure, symptoms occur only when the metabolic demand increases during exercise or some other form of stress. In severe heart failure, symptoms may be present at rest. In clinical practice, heart failure may be diagnosed when a patient with significant heart disease develops the signs or symptoms of a low cardiac output, pulmonary congestion or systemic venous congestion at rest or on exercise. Three types of heart failure are recognised.

Left heart failure

This is characterised by a reduction in left ventricular output and an increase in left atrial and pulmonary venous pressure. If left heart failure occurs suddenly – for example, as the result of an acute MI – the rapid increase in left atrial pressure causes pulmonary oedema. If the rise in atrial pressure is more gradual, as occurs with mitral stenosis, there is reflex pulmonary vasoconstriction, which protects the patient from pulmonary oedema. However, the resulting increase in pulmonary vascular resistance causes pulmonary hypertension, which in turn impairs right ventricular function.

Right heart failure

This is characterised by a reduction in right ventricular output and an increase in right atrial and systemic venous pressure. The most common causes are chronic lung disease, pulmonary embolism and pulmonary valvular stenosis. The term 'cor pulmonale' is used to describe right heart failure that is secondary to chronic lung disease.

Biventricular heart failure

In biventricular failure, both sides of the heart are affected. This may occur because the disease process, such as dilated cardiomyopathy or ischaemic heart disease, affects both ventricles or because disease of the left heart leads to chronic elevation of the left atrial pressure, pulmonary hypertension and right heart failure.

Epidemiology

Heart failure predominantly affects the elderly; the prevalence rises from 1% in those aged 50–59 years to over 10% in those aged 80–89 years. In the UK, most patients admitted to hospital with heart failure are more than 70 years old; they typically remain hospitalised for a week or more and may be left with chronic disability. Although the outlook depends, to some extent, on the underlying cause of the problem, untreated heart failure generally carries a poor prognosis; approximately 50% of patients with severe heart failure due to left ventricular dysfunction will die within 2 years because of either pump failure or malignant ventricular arrhythmias. The most common causes are coronary artery disease and myocardial infarction but almost all forms of heart disease can lead to heart failure, as summarised in Box 16.12. An accurate diagnosis is important because treatment of the underlying cause may reverse heart failure or prevent its progression.

Pathogenesis

Heart failure occurs when cardiac output fails to meet the demands of the circulation. Cardiac output is determined by preload (the volume and pressure of blood in the ventricles at the end of diastole), afterload (the volume and pressure of blood in the ventricles during systole) and myocardial contractility, forming the basis of Starling's Law (Fig. 16.24). The causes of heart failure are discussed below.

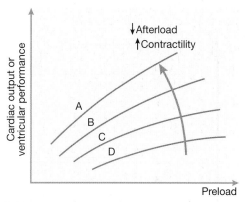

Fig. 16.24 Starling's Law. Normal (A), mild (B), moderate (C) and severe (D) heart failure. Ventricular performance is related to the degree of myocardial stretching. An increase in preload (end-diastolic volume, end-diastolic pressure, filling pressure or atrial pressure) will therefore enhance function; however, overstretching causes marked deterioration. In heart failure, the curve moves to the right and becomes flatter. An increase in myocardial contractility or a reduction in afterload will shift the curve upwards and to the left (green arrow).

Ventricular dysfunction

Ventricular dysfunction is the most common cause of heart failure. This can occur because of impaired systolic contraction due to myocardial disease, or diastolic dysfunction where there is abnormal ventricular relaxation due to a stiff, non-compliant ventricle. This is most commonly found in patients with left ventricular hypertrophy. Systolic dysfunction and diastolic dysfunction often coexist, particularly in patients with coronary artery disease. Ventricular dysfunction reduces cardiac output, which, in turn, activates the sympathetic nervous system (SNS) and renin–angiotensin–aldosterone system (RAAS). Under normal circumstances, activation of the SNS and RAAS supports cardiac function but, in the setting of impaired ventricular function, the consequences are negative and lead to an increase in both afterload and preload (Fig. 16.25). A vicious circle may then be

i	16.12 Mechanisms of heart failure	
Cause	**Examples**	**Features**
Reduced ventricular contractility	Myocardial infarction (segmental dysfunction) Myocarditis/cardiomyopathy (global dysfunction)	In coronary artery disease, 'akinetic' or 'dyskinetic' segments contract poorly and may impede the function of normal segments by distorting their contraction and relaxation patterns Progressive ventricular dilatation
Ventricular outflow obstruction (pressure overload)	Hypertension, aortic stenosis (left heart failure) Pulmonary hypertension, pulmonary valve stenosis (right heart failure)	Initially, concentric ventricular hypertrophy allows the ventricle to maintain a normal output by generating a high systolic pressure. Later, secondary changes in the myocardium and increasing obstruction lead to failure with ventricular dilatation and rapid clinical deterioration
Ventricular inflow obstruction	Mitral stenosis, tricuspid stenosis	Small, vigorous ventricle; dilated, hypertrophied atrium. Atrial fibrillation is common and often causes marked deterioration because ventricular filling depends heavily on atrial contraction
Ventricular volume overload	Left ventricular volume overload (mitral or aortic regurgitation) Ventricular septal defect Right ventricular volume overload (atrial septal defect) Increased metabolic demand (high output)	Dilatation and hypertrophy allow the ventricle to generate a high stroke volume and help to maintain a normal cardiac output. However, secondary changes in the myocardium lead to impaired contractility and worsening heart failure
Arrhythmia	Atrial fibrillation Tachycardia Complete heart block	Tachycardia does not allow for adequate filling of the heart, resulting in reduced cardiac output and back pressure Prolonged tachycardia causes myocardial fatigue Bradycardia limits cardiac output, even if stroke volume is normal
Diastolic dysfunction	Constrictive pericarditis Restrictive cardiomyopathy Left ventricular hypertrophy and fibrosis Cardiac tamponade	Marked fluid retention and peripheral oedema, ascites, pleural effusions and elevated jugular veins Bi-atrial enlargement (restrictive filling pattern and high atrial pressures). Atrial fibrillation may cause deterioration Good systolic function but poor diastolic filling Hypotension, elevated jugular veins, pulsus paradoxus, poor urine output

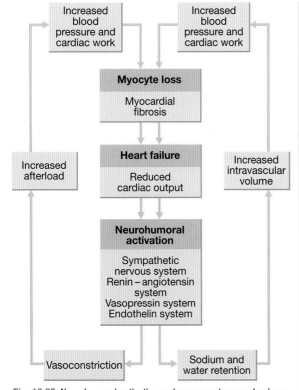

Fig. 16.25 Neurohumoral activation and compensatory mechanisms in heart failure. There is a vicious circle in progressive heart failure.

established because any additional fall in cardiac output causes further activation of the SNS and RAAS, and an additional increase in peripheral vascular resistance.

Activation of the RAAS causes vasoconstriction and sodium and water retention. This is primarily mediated by angiotensin II, a potent constrictor of arterioles, in both the kidney and the systemic circulation (Fig. 16.25). Activation of the SNS also occurs and can initially sustain cardiac output through increased myocardial contractility and heart rate. Prolonged sympathetic stimulation has negative effects, however, causing cardiac myocyte apoptosis, cardiac hypertrophy and focal myocardial necrosis. Sympathetic stimulation also contributes to vasoconstriction and predisposes to arrhythmias. Sodium and water retention is further enhanced by the release of aldosterone, endothelin-1 (a potent vasoconstrictor peptide with marked effects on the renal vasculature) and, in severe heart failure, vasopressin (antidiuretic hormone, ADH). Natriuretic peptides are released from the atria in response to atrial dilatation and compensate to an extent for the sodium-conserving effect of aldosterone, but this mechanism is overwhelmed in heart failure. Pulmonary and peripheral oedema occurs because of high left and right atrial pressures, and is compounded by sodium and water retention, caused by impairment of renal perfusion and by secondary hyperaldosteronism. If the underlying cause is a myocardial infarction, cardiac contractility is impaired and SNS and RAAS activation causes hypertrophy of non-infarcted segments, with thinning, dilatation and expansion of the infarcted segment (see Fig. 16.64, p. 496). This leads to further deterioration in ventricular function and worsening heart failure.

High-output failure

Sometimes cardiac failure can occur in patients without heart disease due to a large arteriovenous shunt, or where there is an excessively high cardiac output due to beri-beri (p. 714), severe anaemia or thyrotoxicosis.

Valvular disease

Heart failure can also be caused by valvular disease in which there is impaired filling of the ventricles due to mitral or tricuspid stenosis; where there is obstruction to ventricular outflow, as occurs in aortic and tricuspid stenosis and hypertrophic cardiomyopathy; or as the result of ventricular overload secondary to valvular regurgitation.

Clinical assessment

Heart failure may develop suddenly, as in MI, or gradually, as in valvular heart disease. When there is gradual impairment of cardiac function, several compensatory changes take place. The term compensated heart failure is sometimes used to describe the condition of those with impaired cardiac function, in whom adaptive changes have prevented the development of overt heart failure. However, a minor event, such as an intercurrent infection or development of atrial fibrillation, may precipitate acute heart failure in these circumstances (Box 16.13). Similarly, acute heart failure sometimes supervenes as the result of a decompensating episode, on a background of chronic heart failure; this is called acute-on-chronic heart failure.

Acute left heart failure

Acute left heart failure presents with a sudden onset of dyspnoea at rest that rapidly progresses to acute respiratory distress, orthopnoea and prostration. Often there is a clear precipitating factor, such as an acute MI, which may be apparent from the history. The patient appears agitated, pale and clammy. The peripheries are cool to the touch and the pulse is rapid, but in some cases there may be an inappropriate bradycardia that may contribute to the acute episode of heart failure. The BP is usually high because of SNS activation, but may be normal or low if the patient is in cardiogenic shock.

The jugular venous pressure (JVP) is usually elevated, particularly with associated fluid overload or right heart failure. In acute heart failure, there has been no time for ventricular dilatation and the apex is not displaced. A 'gallop' rhythm, with a third heart sound, is heard quite early in the development of acute left-sided heart failure. A new systolic murmur may signify acute mitral regurgitation or ventricular septal rupture. Chest examination may reveal crepitations at the lung bases if there is pulmonary oedema, or crepitations throughout the lungs if this

is severe. There may be an expiratory wheeze. Patients with acute-on-chronic heart failure may have additional features of chronic heart failure (see below). Potential precipitants, such as an upper respiratory tract infection or inappropriate cessation of diuretic medication, may be identified on clinical examination or history-taking.

Chronic heart failure

Patients with chronic heart failure commonly follow a relapsing and remitting course, with periods of stability and episodes of decompensation, leading to worsening symptoms that may necessitate hospitalisation. The clinical picture depends on the nature of the underlying heart disease, the type of heart failure that it has evoked, and the changes in the SNS and RAAS that have developed (see Box 16.12 and Fig. 16.26).

Low cardiac output causes fatigue, listlessness and a poor effort tolerance; the peripheries are cold and the BP is low. To maintain perfusion of vital organs, blood flow is diverted away from skeletal muscle and this may contribute to fatigue and weakness. Poor renal perfusion leads to oliguria and uraemia.

Pulmonary oedema due to left heart failure presents with dyspnoea and inspiratory crepitations over the lung bases. In contrast, right heart failure produces a high JVP with hepatic congestion and dependent peripheral oedema. In ambulant patients the oedema affects the ankles, whereas in bed-bound patients it collects around the thighs and sacrum. Ascites or pleural effusion may occur (Fig. 16.26). Heart failure is not the only cause of oedema (Box 16.14).

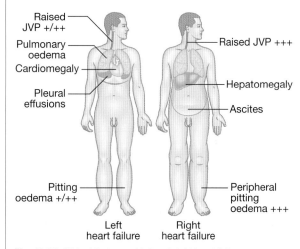

Fig. 16.26 Clinical features of left and right heart failure.
(JVP = jugular venous pressure)

	16.13 Factors that may precipitate or aggravate heart failure in pre-existing heart disease

- Myocardial ischaemia or infarction
- Intercurrent illness
- Arrhythmia
- Inappropriate reduction of therapy
- Administration of a drug with negative inotropic (β-blocker) or fluid-retaining properties (non-steroidal anti-inflammatory drugs, glucocorticoids)
- Pulmonary embolism
- Conditions associated with increased metabolic demand (pregnancy, thyrotoxicosis, anaemia)
- Intravenous fluid overload

	16.14 Differential diagnosis of peripheral oedema

- Cardiac failure: right or combined left and right heart failure, pericardial constriction, cardiomyopathy
- Chronic venous insufficiency: varicose veins
- Hypoalbuminaemia: nephrotic syndrome, liver disease, protein-losing enteropathy; often widespread, can affect arms and face
- Drugs:
    Sodium retention: fludrocortisone, non-steroidal anti-inflammatory drugs
    Increasing capillary permeability: nifedipine, amlodipine
- Idiopathic: women > men
- Chronic lymphatic obstruction

Chronic heart failure is sometimes associated with marked weight loss (cardiac cachexia), caused by a combination of anorexia and impaired absorption due to gastrointestinal congestion, poor tissue perfusion due to a low cardiac output, and skeletal muscle atrophy due to immobility.

Complications of heart failure

Several complications may occur in advanced heart failure, as described below.

- *Renal failure* is caused by poor renal perfusion due to low cardiac output and may be exacerbated by diuretic therapy, ACE inhibitors and angiotensin receptor blockers (ARBs).
- *Hypokalaemia* may be the result of treatment with potassium-losing diuretics or hyperaldosteronism caused by activation of the renin–angiotensin system and impaired aldosterone metabolism due to hepatic congestion. Most of the body's potassium is intracellular and there may be substantial depletion of potassium stores, even when the plasma concentration is in the reference range.
- *Hyperkalaemia* may be due to the effects of drugs that promote renal resorption of potassium, in particular the combination of ACE inhibitors, ARBs and mineralocorticoid receptor antagonists. These effects are amplified if there is renal dysfunction due to low cardiac output or atherosclerotic renal vascular disease.
- *Hyponatraemia* is a feature of severe heart failure and is a poor prognostic sign. It may be caused by diuretic therapy, inappropriate water retention due to high vasopressin secretion, or failure of the cell membrane ion pump.
- *Impaired liver function* is caused by hepatic venous congestion and poor arterial perfusion, which frequently cause mild jaundice and abnormal liver function tests; reduced synthesis of clotting factors can make anticoagulant control difficult.
- *Thromboembolism*. Deep vein thrombosis and pulmonary embolism may occur due to the effects of a low cardiac output and enforced immobility. Systemic emboli occur in patients with atrial fibrillation or flutter, or with intracardiac thrombus complicating conditions such as mitral stenosis, MI or left ventricular aneurysm.
- *Atrial and ventricular arrhythmias* are very common and may be related to electrolyte changes such as hypokalaemia and hypomagnesaemia, the underlying cardiac disease, and the pro-arrhythmic effects of sympathetic activation. Atrial fibrillation occurs in approximately 20% of patients with heart failure and causes further impairment of cardiac function. Ventricular ectopic beats and runs of non-sustained ventricular tachycardia are common findings in patients with heart failure and are associated with an adverse prognosis.
- *Sudden death* occurs in up to 50% of patients with heart failure and is most probably due to ventricular fibrillation.

Investigations

A chest X-ray should be performed in all cases. This may show abnormal distension of the upper lobe pulmonary veins with the patient in the erect position (Fig. 16.27). Vascularity of the lung fields becomes more prominent and the right and left pulmonary arteries dilate. Subsequently, interstitial oedema causes thickened interlobular septa and dilated lymphatics. These are evident as horizontal lines in the costophrenic angles (septal or 'Kerley

Reticular shadowing of alveolar oedema · **Prominence of upper lobe blood vessels** · **Enlarged hilar vessels**

Septal or 'Kerley B' lines · **Enlarged cardiac silhouette; usually with coexisting chronic heart failure**

Fig. 16.27 Radiological features of heart failure. A Chest X-ray of a patient with pulmonary oedema. B Enlargement of lung base showing septal or 'Kerley B' lines (arrow).

B' lines). More advanced changes due to alveolar oedema cause a hazy opacification spreading from the hilar regions, and pleural effusions. Echocardiography is very useful and should be considered in all patients with heart failure in order to:

- determine the aetiology
- detect hitherto unsuspected valvular heart disease, such as occult mitral stenosis, and other conditions that may be amenable to specific remedies
- identify patients who will benefit from long-term drug therapy.

Serum urea, creatinine and electrolytes, haemoglobin and thyroid function may help to establish the nature and severity of the underlying heart disease and detect any complications. BNP is elevated in heart failure and is a prognostic marker, as well as being useful in differentiating heart failure from other causes of breathlessness or peripheral oedema.

Management of acute heart failure

Acute heart failure with pulmonary oedema is a medical emergency that should be treated urgently. The patient should initially be kept rested, with continuous monitoring of cardiac rhythm, BP and

16.15 Management of acute pulmonary oedema	
Action	**Effect**
Sit the patient up	Reduces preload
Give high-flow oxygen	Corrects hypoxia
Ensure continuous positive airway pressure (CPAP) of 5–10 mmHg by tight-fitting mask	Reduces preload and pulmonary capillary hydraulic gradient
Administer nitrates:* IV glyceryl trinitrate (10–200 µg/min) Buccal glyceryl trinitrate 2–5 mg	Reduces preload and afterload
Administer a loop diuretic: Furosemide (50–100 mg IV)	Combats fluid overload

*The dose of nitrate should be titrated upwards every 10 mins until there is an improvement or systolic blood pressure is <110 mmHg.

i 16.16 General measures for the management of heart failure

Education
- Explanation of nature of disease, treatment and self-help strategies

Diet
- Good general nutrition and weight reduction for the obese
- Avoidance of high-salt foods and added salt, especially for patients with severe congestive heart failure

Alcohol
- Moderation or elimination of alcohol consumption; alcohol-induced cardiomyopathy requires abstinence

Smoking
- Cessation

Exercise
- Regular moderate aerobic exercise within limits of symptoms

Vaccination
- Consideration of influenza and pneumococcal vaccination

pulse oximetry. Intravenous opiates can be of value in distressed patients but must be used sparingly, as they may cause respiratory depression and exacerbation of hypoxaemia and hypercapnia. The key elements of management are summarised in Box 16.15.

If these measures prove ineffective, inotropic agents such as dobutamine (2.5–10 µg/kg/min) may be required to augment cardiac output, particularly in hypotensive patients. Insertion of an intra-aortic balloon pump may be beneficial in patients with acute cardiogenic pulmonary oedema and shock. Following management of the acute episode, additional measures must be instituted to control heart failure in the longer term, as discussed below.

Management of chronic heart failure

The aims of treatment in chronic heart failure are to improve cardiac function by increasing contractility, optimising preload or decreasing afterload, and controlling cardiac rate and rhythm (see Fig. 16.25). This can be achieved by a combination of drug treatment or non-drug treatments, as discussed below.

Education

Education of patients and their relatives about the causes and treatment of heart failure can improve adherence to a management plan (Box 16.16). Some patients may need to weigh themselves daily, as a measure of fluid load, and adjust their diuretic therapy accordingly.

Drug treatment

A wide variety of drug treatments are now available for the treatment of heart failure. Drugs that reduce preload are appropriate in patients with high end-diastolic filling pressures and evidence of pulmonary or systemic venous congestion, whereas those that reduce afterload or increase myocardial contractility are more useful in patients with signs and symptoms of a low cardiac output.

Diuretics Diuretics promote urinary sodium and water excretion, leading to a reduction in blood plasma volume (p. 354), which in turn reduces preload and improves pulmonary and systemic venous congestion. They may also reduce afterload and ventricular volume, leading to a fall in ventricular wall tension and increased cardiac efficiency. Although a fall in preload (ventricular filling pressure) normally reduces cardiac output, patients with heart failure are beyond the apex of the Starling curve, so there may

Fig. 16.28 The effect of treatment on ventricular performance curves in heart failure. Diuretics and venodilators (A), angiotensin-converting enzyme (ACE) inhibitors and mixed vasodilators (B), and positive inotropic agents (C).

be a substantial and beneficial fall in filling pressure with either no change or an improvement in cardiac output (see Figs 16.24 and 16.28). Nevertheless, the dose of diuretics needs to be titrated carefully so as to avoid excessive volume depletion, which can cause a fall in cardiac output with hypotension, lethargy and renal failure. This is especially likely in patients with a marked diastolic component to their heart failure.

Oedema may persist, despite oral loop diuretic therapy, in some patients with severe chronic heart failure, particularly if there is renal impairment. Under these circumstances an intravenous infusion of furosemide (5–10 mg/hr) may initiate a diuresis. Combining a loop diuretic with a thiazide diuretic such as bendroflumethiazide (5 mg daily) may also prove effective but care must be taken to avoid an excessive diuresis.

Mineralocorticoid receptor antagonists, such as spironolactone and eplerenone, are potassium-sparing diuretics that are of particular benefit in patients with heart failure with severe left ventricular systolic dysfunction. They have been shown to improve long-term clinical outcome in individuals with severe heart failure or heart failure following acute MI but may cause hyperkalaemia, particularly when used with an ACE inhibitor.

16

Angiotensin-converting enzyme inhibitors ACE inhibitors play a central role in the management of heart failure since they interrupt the vicious circle of neurohumoral activation that is characteristic of the disease by preventing the conversion of angiotensin I to angiotensin II. This, in turn, reduces peripheral vasoconstriction, activation of the sympathetic nervous system (Fig. 16.29), and salt and water retention due to aldosterone release, as well as preventing the activation of the renin–angiotensin system caused by diuretic therapy.

In moderate and severe heart failure, ACE inhibitors can produce a substantial improvement in effort tolerance and in mortality. They can also improve outcome and prevent the onset of overt heart failure in patients with poor residual left ventricular function following MI.

Adverse effects of ACE inhibitors include symptomatic hypotension and impairment of renal function, especially in patients with bilateral renal artery stenosis or those with pre-existing renal disease. An increase in serum potassium concentration may also occur, which can be beneficial in offsetting the hypokalaemia associated with loop diuretic therapy. Short-acting ACE inhibitors can cause marked falls in BP, particularly in the elderly or when started in the presence of hypotension, hypovolaemia or hyponatraemia. In stable patients without hypotension (systolic BP over 100 mmHg), ACE inhibitors can usually be safely started in the community. In other patients, however, it is usually advisable to withhold diuretics for 24 hours before starting treatment with a small dose of a long-acting agent, preferably given at night (Box 16.18). Renal function and serum potassium must be monitored and should be checked 1–2 weeks after starting therapy.

Angiotensin receptor blockers ARBs act by blocking the action of angiotensin II on the heart, peripheral vasculature and kidney. In heart failure, they produce beneficial haemodynamic changes that are similar to the effects of ACE inhibitors (Fig. 16.29) but are generally better tolerated. They have comparable effects on mortality and are a useful alternative for patients who cannot tolerate ACE inhibitors. Like ACE inhibitors they should be started at a low dose and titrated upwards, depending on response (Box 16.18). Unfortunately, they share all the more serious adverse effects of ACE inhibitors, including renal dysfunction and hyperkalaemia. ARBs are normally used as an alternative to ACE inhibitors, but the two can be combined in patients with resistant or recurrent heart failure.

Neprilysin inhibitors The only drug currently in this class is sacubitril, a small-molecule inhibitor of neprilysin, which is

---

16.17 Congestive cardiac failure in old age

- **Incidence**: rises with age and affects 5–10% of those in their eighties.
- **Common causes**: coronary artery disease, hypertension and calcific degenerative valvular disease.
- **Diastolic dysfunction**: often prominent, particularly in those with a history of hypertension.
- **ACE inhibitors**: improve symptoms and mortality but are more frequently associated with postural hypotension and renal impairment than in younger patients.
- **Loop diuretics**: usually required but may be poorly tolerated in those with urinary incontinence and men with prostate enlargement.

---

i 16.18 Dosages of ACE inhibitors, β-blockers and angiotensin receptor blockers in heart failure

	Starting dose	Target dose
ACE inhibitors		
Enalapril	2.5 mg twice daily	10 mg twice daily
Lisinopril	2.5 mg daily	20 mg daily
Ramipril	1.25 mg daily	10 mg daily
Angiotensin receptor blockers		
Losartan	25 mg daily	100 mg daily
Candesartan	4 mg daily	32 mg daily
Valsartan	40 mg daily	160 mg daily
β-blockers		
Bisoprolol	1.25 mg daily	10 mg daily
Metoprolol	25 mg twice daily	100 mg twice daily
Carvedilol	3.125 mg twice daily	25 mg twice daily

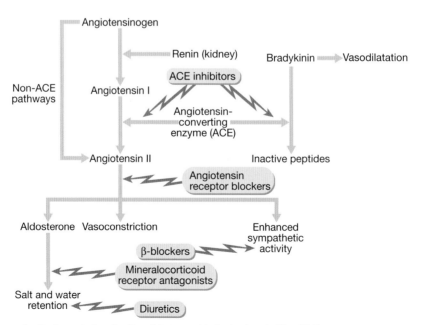

Fig. 16.29 Neurohumoral activation and sites of action of drugs used in the treatment of heart failure.

responsible for the breakdown of the endogenous diuretics ANP and BNP. Used in combination with the ARB valsartan (sacubitril–valsartan), it has been shown to produce additional symptomatic and mortality benefit over ACE inhibition and is now recommended in the management of resistant heart failure.

Vasodilators These drugs are valuable in chronic heart failure, when ACE inhibitors or ARBs are contraindicated. Venodilators, such as nitrates, reduce preload, and arterial dilators, such as hydralazine, reduce afterload (see Fig. 16.28). Their use is limited by pharmacological tolerance and hypotension.

Beta-adrenoceptor blockers Beta-blockade helps to counteract the deleterious effects of enhanced sympathetic stimulation and reduces the risk of arrhythmias and sudden death. When initiated in standard doses β-blockers may precipitate acute-on-chronic heart failure, but when given in small incremental doses they can increase ejection fraction, improve symptoms, reduce the frequency of hospitalisation and reduce mortality in patients with chronic heart failure. A typical regimen is bisoprolol, starting at a dose of 1.25 mg daily and increased gradually over a 12-week period to a target maintenance dose of 10 mg daily. Beta-blockers are more effective at reducing mortality than ACE inhibitors, with a relative risk reduction of 33% versus 20%, respectively.

Ivabradine Ivabradine acts on the I_f inward current in the SA node, resulting in reduction of heart rate. It reduces hospital admission and mortality rates in patients with heart failure due to moderate or severe left ventricular systolic impairment. In trials, its effects were most marked in patients with a relatively high heart rate (over 77/min), so ivabradine is best suited to patients who cannot take β-blockers or whose heart rate remains high despite β-blockade. It is ineffective in patients with atrial fibrillation.

Digoxin Digoxin (p. 482) can be used to provide rate control in patients with heart failure and atrial fibrillation. In patients with severe heart failure (NYHA class III–IV, see Box 16.5), digoxin reduces the likelihood of hospitalisation for heart failure, although it has no effect on long-term survival.

Amiodarone This is a potent anti-arrhythmic drug (p. 481) that has little negative inotropic effect and may be valuable in patients with poor left ventricular function. It is effective only in the treatment of symptomatic arrhythmias and should not be used as a preventative agent in asymptomatic patients. Amiodarone is used for prevention of symptomatic atrial arrhythmias and of ventricular arrhythmias when other pharmacological options have been exhausted.

Non-pharmacological treatments

Implantable cardiac defibrillators These devices are indicated in patients with symptomatic ventricular arrhythmias and heart failure, since they improve prognosis and survival (p. 483).

Resynchronisation devices In patients with marked intraventricular conduction delay, prolonged depolarisation may lead to uncoordinated left ventricular contraction. When this is associated with severe symptomatic heart failure, cardiac resynchronisation devices may be helpful. Here, both the LV and RV are paced simultaneously (Fig. 16.30) to generate a more coordinated left ventricular contraction and improve cardiac output. This is associated with improved symptoms and survival.

Coronary revascularisation Coronary artery bypass surgery or percutaneous coronary intervention may improve function in

Fig. 16.30 Chest X-ray of a biventricular pacemaker and defibrillator (cardiac resynchronisation therapy). The right ventricular lead (RV) is in position in the ventricular apex and is used for both pacing and defibrillation. The left ventricular lead (LV) is placed via the coronary sinus, and the right atrial lead (RA) is placed in the right atrial appendage; both are used for pacing only.

areas of the myocardium that are 'hibernating' because of inadequate blood supply, and can be used to treat carefully selected patients with heart failure and coronary artery disease. If necessary, 'hibernating' myocardium can be identified by stress echocardiography and specialised nuclear or magnetic resonance imaging.

Cardiac transplantation Cardiac transplantation is an established and successful treatment for patients with intractable heart failure. Coronary artery disease and dilated cardiomyopathy are the most common indications. The use of transplantation is limited by the efficacy of modern drug and device therapies, as well as the availability of donor hearts, so it is generally reserved for young patients with severe symptoms despite optimal therapy.

Conventional heart transplantation is contraindicated in patients with pulmonary vascular disease due to long-standing left heart failure, complex congenital heart disease such as Eisenmenger's syndrome, or primary pulmonary hypertension because the RV of the donor heart may fail in the face of high pulmonary vascular resistance. However, heart–lung transplantation can be successful in patients with Eisenmenger's syndrome, and lung transplantation has been used for primary pulmonary hypertension.

Although cardiac transplantation usually produces a dramatic improvement in the recipient's quality of life, serious complications may occur:

- *Rejection*. In spite of routine therapy with ciclosporin A, azathioprine and glucocorticoids, episodes of rejection are common and may present with heart failure, arrhythmias or subtle ECG changes. Cardiac biopsy is often used to confirm the diagnosis before starting treatment with high-dose glucocorticoids.
- *Accelerated atherosclerosis*. Recurrent heart failure is often due to progressive atherosclerosis in the coronary arteries of the donor heart. This is not confined to patients who underwent transplantation for coronary artery disease and is probably a manifestation of chronic rejection. Angina is rare because the heart has been denervated.

16

- *Infection*. Opportunistic infection with organisms such as cytomegalovirus or *Aspergillus* remains a major cause of death in transplant recipients.

Ventricular assist devices Because of the limited supply of donor organs, ventricular assist devices (VAD) may be employed as a bridge to cardiac transplantation and as short-term restoration therapy following a potentially reversible insult such as viral myocarditis. In some patients, VADs may be used as a long-term therapy if no other options exist.

These devices assist cardiac output by using a roller, centrifugal or pulsatile pump that, in some cases, is implantable and portable. They withdraw blood through cannulae inserted in the atria or ventricular apex and pump it into the pulmonary artery or aorta. They are designed not only to unload the ventricles but also to provide support to the pulmonary and systemic circulations. Their more widespread application is limited by high complication rates (haemorrhage, systemic embolism, infection, neurological and renal sequelae), although some improvements in survival and quality of life have been demonstrated in patients with severe heart failure.

Cardiac arrhythmias

A cardiac arrhythmia is defined as a disturbance of the electrical rhythm of the heart. Cardiac arrhythmias are often a manifestation of structural heart disease but may also occur because of abnormal conduction or depolarisation in an otherwise healthy heart. There are many types of cardiac arrhythmia, as discussed later in this section. By convention, however, a heart rate of more than 100/min is called a tachycardia, and a heart rate of less than 60/min is called a bradycardia.

Pathogenesis

Cardiac arrhythmias usually occur as the result of pathology affecting the conduction system of the heart. The cardiac cycle is normally initiated by an electrical discharge from the SA node. The atria and ventricles then activate sequentially as electrical depolarisation passes through specialised conducting tissues (see Fig. 16.4, p. 445). The sinus node acts as a pacemaker and its intrinsic rate is regulated by the autonomic nervous system; vagal activity decreases the heart rate and sympathetic activity increases heart rate through cardiac sympathetic nerves and circulating catecholamines.

There are three main mechanisms of tachycardia:

- *Increased automaticity*. The tachycardia is produced by spontaneous depolarisation of an ectopic focus in the atria, atrioventricular junction or ventricles, often in response to catecholamines. Single depolarisations lead to atrial, junctional or ventricular premature (ectopic) beats. Repeated depolarisation leads to atrial, junctional or ventricular tachycardia.
- *Re-entry*. The tachycardia is initiated by an ectopic beat and sustained by a re-entry circuit (Fig. 16.31). Most tachyarrhythmias are caused by re-entry.
- *Triggered activity*. This can cause ventricular arrhythmias in patients with coronary artery disease. It is a form of secondary depolarisation arising from an incompletely repolarised cell membrane. Arrhythmias may be supraventricular (sinus, atrial or junctional) or ventricular in origin.

Supraventricular rhythms usually produce narrow QRS complexes because the ventricles are depolarised in their normal sequence via the AV node, the bundle of His and associated Purkinje fibres. In contrast, ventricular rhythms produce broad, bizarre QRS complexes because the ventricles are activated in an abnormal sequence. Occasionally, supraventricular tachycardia can mimic ventricular tachycardia and present as a broad-complex tachycardia due to coexisting bundle branch block or the presence of an additional atrioventricular connection (accessory pathway, see below).

Bradycardia may be due to reduced automaticity of the SA node or abnormalities of conduction through the AV node. If the sinus rate becomes unduly slow, another, more distal part of the conducting system may assume the role of pacemaker. This is known as an escape rhythm and may arise in the AV node or His bundle (junctional rhythm) or in the ventricles (idioventricular rhythm).

Clinical features

Many arrhythmias are asymptomatic but sustained tachycardias typically present with rapid palpitation, dizziness, chest discomfort or breathlessness. Extreme tachycardias can also cause syncope because the heart is unable to contract or relax properly at extreme rates. Bradycardias tend to cause symptoms that reflect low cardiac output, including fatigue, lightheadedness and syncope. Extreme bradycardias or tachycardias can precipitate sudden death or cardiac arrest.

Investigations

The first-line investigation is a standard 12-lead ECG, which can be diagnostic in many cases. If arrhythmias are intermittent and the resting ECG is normal, an attempt should be made to capture the abnormal rhythm using an ambulatory ECG or a patient-activated ECG.

Fig. 16.31 **The mechanism of re-entry.** Re-entry can occur when there are two alternative pathways with different conducting properties, such as the atrioventricular node and an accessory pathway, or an area of normal and an area of ischaemic tissue. Here, pathway A conducts slowly and recovers quickly, while pathway B conducts rapidly and recovers slowly. (1) In sinus rhythm, each impulse passes down both pathways before entering a common distal pathway. (2) As the pathways recover at different rates, a premature impulse may find pathway A open and B closed. (3) Pathway B may recover while the premature impulse is travelling selectively down pathway A. The impulse can then travel retrogradely up pathway B, setting up a closed loop or re-entry circuit. (4) This may initiate a tachycardia that continues until the circuit is interrupted by a change in conduction rates or electrical depolarisation.

Management

Features of individual arrhythmias are discussed below. Management depends on the nature of the arrhythmia and the general principles of medical management are discussed on page 479.

Sinus arrhythmia

This is defined as a cyclical alteration of the heart rate during respiration, with an increase during inspiration and a decrease during expiration. Sinus arrhythmia is a normal phenomenon and can be quite pronounced in children. Absence of this normal variation in heart rate with breathing or with changes in posture may be a feature of diabetic neuropathy (p. 758), autonomic involvement in patients with diseases of peripheral nerves (p. 1138) or increased sympathetic drive. Sinus arrhythmia does not require treatment.

Sinus bradycardia

This may occur in healthy people at rest and is a common finding in athletes. Some pathological causes are listed in Box 16.19. If sinus bradycardia is asymptomatic, then no treatment is required. Symptomatic sinus bradycardia may occur acutely during an MI and can be treated with intravenous atropine (0.6–1.2 mg). Patients with recurrent or persistent symptomatic sinus bradycardia should be considered for pacemaker implantation.

Sinus tachycardia

Sinus tachycardia is usually due to an increase in sympathetic activity associated with exercise, emotion and pregnancy. Healthy young adults can produce a rapid sinus rate, up to 200/min, during intense exercise. Sinus tachycardia does not require treatment but sometimes may reflect an underlying disease, as summarised in Box 16.19.

Sick sinus syndrome

Sick sinus syndrome can occur at any age but is most common in older people. It is caused by fibrosis, degenerative changes or ischaemia of the SA node and is characterised by a variety of arrhythmias (Box 16.20). The typical presentation is with

| **i** | **16.19 Some pathological causes of sinus bradycardia and tachycardia** |

Sinus bradycardia
- Myocardial infarction
- Sinus node disease (sick sinus syndrome)
- Hypothermia
- Hypothyroidism

- Cholestatic jaundice
- Raised intracranial pressure
- Drugs (β-blockers, digoxin, verapamil)

Sinus tachycardia
- Anxiety
- Fever
- Anaemia
- Heart failure

- Thyrotoxicosis
- Phaeochromocytoma
- Drugs (β-agonists)

| **i** | **16.20 Common features of sinoatrial disease** |

- Sinus bradycardia
- Sinoatrial block (sinus arrest)
- Paroxysmal atrial fibrillation

- Paroxysmal atrial tachycardia
- Atrioventricular block

palpitation, dizzy spells or syncope, due to intermittent tachycardia, bradycardia, or pauses with no atrial or ventricular activity (SA block or sinus arrest) (Fig. 16.32).

A permanent pacemaker may benefit patients with troublesome symptoms due to spontaneous bradycardias, or those with symptomatic bradycardias induced by drugs required to prevent tachyarrhythmias. Atrial pacing may prevent episodes of atrial fibrillation. Pacing improves symptoms but not prognosis, and is not indicated in patients who are asymptomatic.

Atrial ectopic beats

Atrial ectopic beats usually cause no symptoms but can give the sensation of a missed beat or an abnormally strong beat. The ECG (Fig. 16.33) shows a premature but otherwise normal QRS complex; if visible, the preceding P wave has a different morphology because the atria activate from an abnormal site. In most cases these are of no consequence, although very frequent atrial ectopic beats may herald the onset of atrial fibrillation.

16

Fig. 16.32 Sinoatrial disease (sick sinus syndrome). A continuous rhythm strip from a 24-hour ECG tape recording illustrating periods of sinus rhythm, atrial ectopics, junctional beats, sinus bradycardia, sinus arrest and paroxysmal atrial fibrillation.

Fig. 16.33 Atrial ectopic beats. The first, second and fifth complexes are normal sinus beats. The third, fourth and sixth complexes are atrial ectopic beats with identical QRS complexes and abnormal (sometimes barely visible) P waves.

Treatment is rarely necessary but β-blockers can be used if symptoms are intrusive.

Atrial tachycardia

Atrial tachycardia may be a manifestation of increased atrial automaticity, sinoatrial disease or digoxin toxicity. It produces a narrow-complex tachycardia with abnormal P-wave morphology, sometimes associated with AV block if the atrial rate is rapid. It may respond to β-blockers, which reduce automaticity, or class I or III anti-arrhythmic drugs (see Box 16.30 below). The ventricular response in rapid atrial tachycardias may be controlled by AV node-blocking drugs. Catheter ablation (p. 484) can be used to target the ectopic site and should be offered as an alternative to anti-arrhythmic drugs in patients with recurrent atrial tachycardia.

Atrial flutter

Atrial flutter is characterised by a large (macro) re-entry circuit, usually within the right atrium encircling the tricuspid annulus. The atrial rate is approximately 300/min, and is usually associated with 2:1, 3:1 or 4:1 AV block (with corresponding heart rates of 150, 100 or 75/min). Rarely, in young patients, every flutter wave is conducted, producing a rate of 300/min and, potentially, haemodynamic compromise. The ECG shows saw-tooth flutter waves (Fig. 16.34). When there is regular 2:1 AV block, it may be difficult to identify flutter waves that are buried in QRS complexes and T waves. Atrial flutter should always be suspected when there is a narrow-complex tachycardia of 150/min. Carotid sinus pressure or intravenous adenosine may help to establish the diagnosis by temporarily increasing the degree of AV block and revealing flutter waves (Fig. 16.35).

Management

Medical management with digoxin, β-blockers or verapamil is often successful in controlling the ventricular rate (p. 479). In many cases, however, it may be preferable to try to restore sinus rhythm by direct current (DC) cardioversion. Following cardioversion, β-blockers or amiodarone can be used to prevent recurrent episodes of atrial flutter. Class Ic anti-arrhythmic drugs such as flecainide are contraindicated because there is a risk of slowing the flutter circuit, facilitating 1:1 AV nodal conduction and producing a paradoxical extreme tachycardia and haemodynamic compromise. Catheter ablation is a highly effective treatment, offering a greater than 90% chance of complete cure, and is the treatment of choice for patients with persistent symptoms. Anticoagulant management in patients with atrial flutter, including management around cardioversion, is identical to that of patients with atrial fibrillation (p. 471).

Fig. 16.34 Atrial flutter. Simultaneous recording showing atrial flutter with 4:1 atrioventricular block. Flutter waves are visible only in leads II and III.

Fig. 16.35 Carotid sinus pressure in atrial flutter: continuous trace. The diagnosis of atrial flutter with 2:1 block was established when carotid sinus pressure produced temporary atrioventricular block, revealing the flutter waves.

Atrial fibrillation

Atrial fibrillation (AF) is the most common sustained cardiac arrhythmia, with an overall prevalence of 0.5% in the adult population of the UK. The prevalence rises with age, affecting 1% of those aged 60–64 years, increasing to 9% of those aged over 80 years. It is associated with significant morbidity and a twofold increase in mortality. This is mainly because of its association with underlying heart disease but also because of its association with systemic embolism and stroke.

Pathogenesis

AF is a complex arrhythmia characterised by both abnormal automatic firing and the presence of multiple interacting re-entry circuits looping around the atria. Episodes of AF are initiated by rapid bursts of ectopic beats arising from conducting tissue in the pulmonary veins or from diseased atrial tissue. It becomes sustained because of re-entrant conduction within the atria or sometimes because of continuous ectopic firing (Fig. 16.36). Re-entry is more likely to occur in atria that are enlarged or in which conduction is slow, as is the case in many forms of heart disease. During episodes of AF, the atria beat rapidly but in an uncoordinated and ineffective manner. The ventricles are activated irregularly at a rate determined by conduction through the AV node. This produces the characteristic 'irregularly irregular' pulse. The ECG (Fig. 16.37) shows normal but irregular QRS complexes; there are no P waves but the baseline may show irregular fibrillation waves. Commonly, AF is classified as paroxysmal (intermittent episodes that self-terminate within 7 days), persistent

Fig. 16.36 Mechanisms initiating atrial fibrillation. (1) Ectopic beats, often arising from the pulmonary veins, trigger atrial fibrillation. (2) Re-entry within the atria maintains atrial fibrillation, with multiple interacting re-entry circuits operating simultaneously.

Fig. 16.37 Two examples of atrial fibrillation. The QRS complexes are irregular and there are no P waves. **A** There is usually a fast ventricular rate, between 120 and 160/min, at the onset of atrial fibrillation. **B** In chronic atrial fibrillation, the ventricular rate may be much slower, due to the effects of medication and AV nodal fatigue.

i	**16.21 Common causes of atrial fibrillation**
• Coronary artery disease (including acute MI) • Valvular heart disease, especially rheumatic mitral valve disease • Hypertension • Sinoatrial disease • Hyperthyroidism	• Alcohol • Cardiomyopathy • Congenital heart disease • Chest infection • Pulmonary embolism • Pericardial disease • Idiopathic (lone atrial fibrillation)

of loss of atrial function and heart rate control. A fall in BP may cause lightheadedness, and chest pain may occur with underlying coronary artery disease. In older patients, AF may not be associated with a rapid ventricular rate and may be asymptomatic, only to be discovered as a result of a routine examination or an ECG. Asymptomatic AF may also present with systemic embolism and is a major cause of stroke in the elderly.

Investigations

Assessment of patients with newly diagnosed AF should include a full history, physical examination, a 12-lead ECG, echocardiogram and thyroid function tests to exclude thyrotoxicosis. This is an unusual but potentially treatable cause of AF. Additional investigations may be needed to determine the nature and extent of any underlying heart disease. In particular echocardiographic assessment is useful to identify any structural heart disease, particularly mitral valve disease.

Management

Management depends on whether the AF is transient or persistent and whether there is a clear precipitating factor. When AF complicates an acute illness such as a chest infection or pulmonary embolism, treatment of the underlying disorder will often restore sinus rhythm. Where AF does not resolve, the main objectives are to control heart rate during periods of AF, restore sinus rhythm, prevent recurrence of AF and reduce the risk of thromboembolism. Management of paroxysmal and persistent AF is discussed below.

Paroxysmal atrial fibrillation

Occasional attacks of AF that are well tolerated do not necessarily require treatment. Beta-blockers are normally used as first-line therapy if symptoms are troublesome, since they reduce the ectopic firing that normally initiates the arrhythmia. They are particularly useful for treating patients with AF associated with coronary artery disease, hypertension and cardiac failure. Class Ic drugs (see Box 16.30), such as propafenone or flecainide, are also effective at preventing episodes but should not be given to patients with coronary artery disease or left ventricular dysfunction. Flecainide is seldom used alone, since it can precipitate atrial flutter, and is usually prescribed with a rate-limiting β-blocker. Class III drugs can also be used; amiodarone is the most effective agent for preventing AF but side-effects restrict its use to when other measures fail. Dronedarone is an effective alternative but is contraindicated in patients with heart failure or significant left ventricular impairment. Digoxin and verapamil are not effective for the prevention of AF but can help with rate control by slowing conduction through the AV node. Catheter ablation can be considered where anti-arrhythmic drug therapy is ineffective or causes side-effects. Ablation can disconnect the pulmonary veins from the LA electrically, preventing ectopic triggering of AF. In addition, lines of conduction block can be created

16

(prolonged episodes that can be terminated by electrical or pharmacological cardioversion) or permanent. It can be difficult to identify what type of AF patients have at first presentation but this usually becomes clearer as time progresses. Unfortunately for many patients, paroxysmal AF becomes permanent as the underlying disease process progresses. This is partly because of electrophysiological changes that occur in the atria within a few hours of the onset of AF and which tend to maintain fibrillation: a process called electrical remodelling. When AF persists for a period of months, structural remodelling also occurs, leading to atrial fibrosis and dilatation that predispose to chronicity of the AF. Early treatment of AF can sometimes prevent the arrhythmia from becoming persistent.

Many forms of heart disease can present with AF (Box 16.21), particularly those that are associated with enlargement or dilatation of the atria. Alcohol excess, hyperthyroidism and chronic lung disease are also common causes of AF, although multiple predisposing factors may coexist, such as the combination of alcohol, hypertension and coronary artery disease. About 50% of all patients with paroxysmal AF and 20% of patients with persistent or permanent AF have structurally normal hearts; this is known as 'lone atrial fibrillation'.

Clinical features

The typical presentation is with palpitation, breathlessness and fatigue. In patients with poor ventricular function or valve disease, AF may precipitate or aggravate cardiac failure because within the atria to prevent re-entry. Ablation prevents AF in approximately 75% of patients with prior drug-resistant episodes, although a repeat procedure is sometimes required before this is achieved. Ablation for AF is an attractive treatment when drugs are ineffective or poorly tolerated but may be complicated by cardiac tamponade, stroke, phrenic nerve injury and, rarely, pulmonary vein stenosis.

Persistent atrial fibrillation

There are two options for treating persistent AF. One is to attempt to restore and maintain sinus rhythm and the second is to accept the presence of AF and to try to control the ventricular rate. With both options prophylaxis against thromboembolism is required on either a short-term or long-term basis.

Rhythm control An attempt to restore sinus rhythm is particularly appropriate if the arrhythmia causes troublesome symptoms and if there is a modifiable or treatable underlying cause. Electrical DC cardioversion (p. 482) or pharmacological cardioversion may be used. Cardioversion is initially successful in most patients but relapse is frequent (25–50% at 1 month and 70–90% at 1 year). Attempts to restore and maintain sinus rhythm are most successful if AF has been present for less than 3 months, the patient is young and there is no important structural heart disease.

Immediate cardioversion is appropriate if AF has been present for less than 48 hours. In stable patients with no history of structural heart disease, intravenous flecainide (2 mg/kg over 30 mins, maximum dose 150 mg) can be used for pharmacological cardioversion and will restore sinus rhythm in 75% of patients within 8 hours. In patients with structural or ischaemic heart disease, intravenous amiodarone can be given through a central venous catheter. Cardioversion is an alternative treatment and is often effective when drugs fail. If AF has been present for 48 hours or longer, or if there is doubt about its duration, DC cardioversion should be deferred until the patient has been established on effective oral anticoagulation for a minimum of 4 weeks and any underlying problems, such as hypertension or alcohol excess, have been corrected. Consideration should be given to prophylactic treatment with amiodarone to reduce the risk of recurrence. Catheter ablation is sometimes used to restore and maintain sinus rhythm in resistant cases but is a less effective treatment than for paroxysmal AF.

Rate control If sinus rhythm cannot be restored, treatment should be directed at maintaining an appropriate heart rate. Digoxin, β-blockers and rate-limiting calcium antagonists, such as verapamil or diltiazem (p. 479), reduce the ventricular rate by slowing AV conduction. This alone may produce a striking improvement in cardiac function, particularly in patients with mitral stenosis. Beta-blockers and rate-limiting calcium antagonists are more effective than digoxin at controlling the heart rate during exercise and have additional benefits in patients with hypertension or structural heart disease. Combination therapy with digoxin and a β-blocker can help with rate control but calcium channel antagonists should not be used with β-blockers because of the risk of bradycardia.

In exceptional cases, poorly controlled and symptomatic AF can be treated by implanting a permanent pacemaker and then deliberately inducing complete AV nodal block with catheter ablation. This is known as the 'pace and ablate' strategy.

Thromboprophylaxis Loss of atrial contraction and left atrial dilatation cause stasis of blood in the LA and may lead to thrombus formation in the left atrial appendage. This predisposes patients to stroke and other forms of systemic embolism.

16.22 Atrial fibrillation in old age

- **Prevalence**: rises with age, reaching 9% in those over 80 years.
- **Symptoms**: sometimes asymptomatic but often accompanied by diastolic heart failure.
- **Hyperthyroidism**: atrial fibrillation may emerge as the dominant feature of otherwise silent or occult hyperthyroidism.
- **Cardioversion**: followed by high rates (~70% at 1 year) of recurrent atrial fibrillation.
- **Stroke**: atrial fibrillation is an important cause of cerebral embolism, found in 15% of all stroke patients and 2–8% of those with transient ischaemic attacks (TIAs).
- **Anticoagulation**: although the risk of thromboembolism rises, the hazards of anticoagulation also become greater with age because of increased comorbidity, particularly cognitive impairment and falls.
- **Target INR**: if anticoagulation is recommended in those over 75 years, care should be taken to maintain an INR below 3.0 because of the increased risk of intracranial haemorrhage.
- **Directly acting oral anticoagulants**: alternatives to warfarin. No blood monitoring is required, there are fewer drug interactions, and fixed dosing may aid adherence. Dabigatran dose is reduced from 150 mg twice daily to 110 mg twice daily in those over 80 or if creatinine clearance is less than 30 mL/min. Rivaroxaban dose is reduced from 20 mg once daily to 15 mg once daily if creatinine clearance is 30–49 mL/min, and is contraindicated below 30 mL/min.

Patients undergoing cardioversion to restore sinus rhythm require temporary anticoagulation to reduce the risk of systemic embolus. This can be achieved with warfarin, aiming for an international normalised ratio (INR) target of 2.0–3.0. Increasingly, direct-acting oral anticoagulant drugs (see below) are used as an alternative. Anticoagulation should be started for at least 4 weeks before cardioversion and should be maintained for at least 3 months following successful cardioversion.

In patients with chronic AF, the annual risk of stroke is influenced by many factors and a decision has to be made in which the risk of stroke is balanced against the risk of bleeding with anticoagulation. Patients with AF secondary to mitral valve disease should always be anticoagulated because the risk is so high. In other patients, clinical scoring systems can be used to assess the risk of stroke and bleeding. The risk of stroke is usually assessed by the CHA$_2$DS$_2$-VASc score (Box 16.23), whereas the HAS-BLED score can be used to estimate the bleeding risk (Box 16.24). Patients with a HAS-BLED score of 3 or more points may require more careful monitoring if anticoagulated.

In patients with intermittent AF, stroke risk is similar to that in patients with persistent AF when adjusted for CHA$_2$DS$_2$-VASc score. The risk of embolism is only weakly related to the frequency and duration of AF episodes, so stroke prevention guidelines do not distinguish between those with paroxysmal, persistent and permanent AF.

Several agents can be used to reduce stroke risk in AF. Warfarin therapy adjusted to a target INR of 2.0–3.0 reduces the risk of stroke by about two-thirds at the cost of an annual risk of bleeding of 1–1.5% and is indicated for patients with a CHA$_2$D$_S$-VASc score of 2 or more, unless there are coexisting clinical risk factors that increase the risk of bleeding. These include peptic ulcer, uncontrolled hypertension, alcohol misuse, frequent falls, poor adherence and the use of other drugs that might interact with warfarin. If bleeding does occur in warfarin-treated patients, anticoagulation can be reversed by administering vitamin K or clotting factors.

The factor Xa inhibitors rivaroxaban, apixaban and edoxaban, and the direct thrombin inhibitor dabigatran (collectively referred

16.23 CHA₂DS₂-VASc stroke risk scoring system for non-valvular atrial fibrillation

	Parameter	Score
C	Congestive heart failure	1 point
H	Hypertension history	1 point
A₂	Age ≥75 years	2 points
D	Diabetes mellitus	1 point
S₂	Previous stroke or transient ischemic attack (TIA)	2 points
V	Vascular disease	1 point
A	Age 65–74 years	1 point
Sc	Sex category female	1 point
	Maximum total score	9 points

Annual stroke risk
0 points = 0% (no prophylaxis required)
1 point = 1.3% (oral anticoagulant recommended in males only)
2+ points = > 2.2% (oral anticoagulant recommended)

From European Society of Cardiology Clinical practice guidelines: atrial fibrillation (management of) 2010 and focused update (2012). Eur Heart J 2012; 33:2719–2747.

16.24 HAS-BLED bleeding risk scoring system for patients receiving oral anticoagulation

	Parameter	Score
H	Hypertension; current systolic blood pressure >160 mmHg	1 point
A	Abnormal liver function (cirrhosis OR bilirubin > twice upper limit of reference range or transaminases > three times upper limit of reference range	1 point
	Abnormal renal function (creatinine >200 μmol/L (2.26 mg/dL)	1 point
S	Stroke history	1 point
B	Bleeding: prior major event	1 point
L	Labile INR on warfarin	1 point
E	Elderly: age ≥65 years	1 point
D	Drugs:	
	Use of antiplatelet drugs	1 point
	High alcohol consumption	1 point
	Maximum total score	9 points
	HAS-BLED score of ≥3 points requires close patient monitoring	

to as directly acting oral anticoagulants, or DOACs), can be used as an alternative. They are at least as effective as warfarin at preventing thrombotic stroke and are associated with a lower risk of intracranial haemorrhage. Other advantages include the lack of requirement for monitoring and the fact that they have fewer drug interactions. Agents that reverse the effects of DOACs have been developed. These include idarucizumab, which binds to dabigatran and allows acute bleeding complications to be managed more effectively.

Aspirin should not be used since it has little or no effect on embolic stroke and is associated with significant bleeding risk.

Supraventricular tachycardia

The term supraventricular tachycardia (SVT) describes the occurrence of a group of regular tachycardias that have a

Fig. 16.38 Supraventricular tachycardia. The rate is 180/min and the QRS complexes are normal.

similar appearance on ECG. These are usually narrow-complex tachycardias and are characterised by a re-entry circuit or automatic focus involving the atria. The three principal types are atrioventricular nodal re-entrant tachycardia (AVNRT), atrioventricular re-entrant tachycardia (AVRT) and atrial tachycardia. The term SVT is technically incorrect as, in many cases, the ventricles also form part of the re-entry circuit.

Atrioventricular nodal re-entrant tachycardia

AVNRT is a type of SVT caused by re-entry in a circuit involving the AV node and its two right atrial input pathways: a superior 'fast' pathway and an inferior 'slow' pathway (see Fig. 16.39A below). This produces a regular tachycardia with a rate of 120–240/min. It tends to occur in the absence of structural heart disease and episodes may last from a few seconds to many hours. The patient is usually aware of a rapid, very forceful, regular heart beat and may experience chest discomfort, lightheadedness or breathlessness. Polyuria, mainly due to the release of ANP, is sometimes a feature. The ECG (Fig. 16.38) usually shows a tachycardia with normal QRS complexes but occasionally there may be rate-dependent bundle branch block.

Management

Treatment is not always necessary. However, an acute episode may be terminated by carotid sinus pressure or by the Valsalva manœuvre. Adenosine (3–12 mg rapidly IV in incremental doses until tachycardia stops) or verapamil (5 mg IV over 1 min) will restore sinus rhythm in most cases. Intravenous β-blocker or flecainide can also be used. In rare cases, when there is severe haemodynamic compromise, the tachycardia should be terminated by DC cardioversion (p. 482).

In patients with recurrent SVT, catheter ablation (p. 484) is the most effective therapy and will permanently prevent SVT in more than 90% of cases. Alternatively, prophylaxis with oral β-blocker, verapamil or flecainide may be used but commits predominantly young patients to long-term drug therapy and can create difficulty in female patients, as these drugs are normally avoided during pregnancy.

Atrioventricular re-entrant tachycardia

In this condition there is an abnormal band of conducting tissue that connects the atria and ventricles. This so-called accessory pathway comprises rapidly conducting fibres that resemble Purkinje tissue, in that they conduct very rapidly and are rich in sodium channels. In about 50% of cases, this pathway conducts only in the retrograde direction (from ventricles to atria) and thus does not alter the appearance of the ECG in sinus rhythm. This is known as a concealed accessory pathway. In the rest, the pathway also conducts in an antegrade direction (from atria to ventricles), so AV conduction in sinus rhythm is mediated via both the AV node and the accessory pathway, distorting the QRS complex. Premature ventricular activation via the pathway shortens the PR interval and produces a 'slurred' initial deflection

16

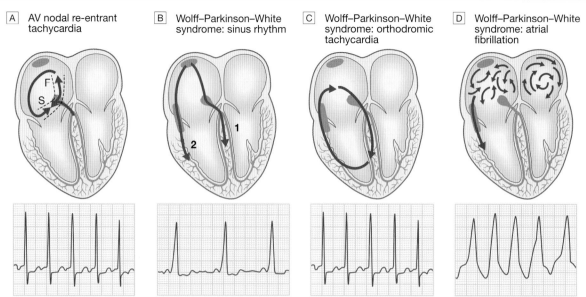

Fig. 16.39 **Atrioventricular nodal re-entrant tachycardia (AVNRT) and Wolff–Parkinson–White (WPW) syndrome.** A AV node re-entrant tachycardia. The mechanism of AVNRT occurs via two right atrial AV nodal input pathways: the slow (S) and fast (F) pathways. Antegrade conduction occurs via the slow pathway; the wavefront enters the AV node and passes into the ventricles, at the same time re-entering the atria via the fast pathway. In WPW syndrome, there is a strip of accessory conducting tissue that allows electricity to bypass the AV node and spread from the atria to the ventricles rapidly and without delay. When the ventricles are depolarised through the AV node the ECG is normal, but when the ventricles are depolarised through the accessory conducting tissue the ECG shows a very short PR interval and a broad QRS complex. B Sinus rhythm. In sinus rhythm, the ventricles are depolarised through (1) the AV node and (2) the accessory pathway, producing an ECG with a short PR interval and broadened QRS complexes; the characteristic slurring of the upstroke of the QRS complex is known as a delta wave. The degree of pre-excitation (the proportion of activation passing down the accessory pathway) and therefore the ECG appearances may vary a lot, and at times the ECG can look normal. C Orthodromic tachycardia. This is the most common form of tachycardia in WPW. The re-entry circuit passes antegradely through the AV node and retrogradely through the accessory pathway. The ventricles are therefore depolarised in the normal way, producing a narrow-complex tachycardia that is indistinguishable from other forms of supraventricular tachycardia. D Atrial fibrillation. In this rhythm, the ventricles are largely depolarised through the accessory pathway, producing an irregular broad-complex tachycardia that is often more rapid than the example shown.

of the QRS complex, called a delta wave (Fig. 16.39B). This is known as a manifest accessory pathway. As the AV node and accessory pathway have different conduction speeds and refractory periods, a re-entry circuit can develop, causing tachycardia (Fig. 16.39C); when associated with symptoms, the condition is known as Wolff–Parkinson–White syndrome. The ECG during this tachycardia is almost indistinguishable from that of AVNRT (Fig. 16.39A).

Management

Carotid sinus pressure or intravenous adenosine can terminate the tachycardia. If AF occurs, it may produce a dangerously rapid ventricular rate because the accessory pathway lacks the rate-limiting properties of the AV node (Fig. 16.39D). This is known as pre-excited atrial fibrillation and may cause collapse, syncope and even death. It should be treated as an emergency, usually with DC cardioversion.

Catheter ablation is first-line treatment in symptomatic patients and is nearly always curative. Alternatively, prophylactic anti-arrhythmic drugs, such as flecainide or propafenone (p. 481), can be used to slow conduction in, and prolong the refractory period of, the accessory pathway. Long-term drug therapy is not the preferred treatment for most patients and amiodarone should not be used, as its side-effect profile cannot be justified and ablation is safer and more effective. Digoxin and verapamil shorten the refractory period of the accessory pathway and should not be used.

Ventricular premature beats

Ventricular premature beats (VPBs) are frequently found in healthy people and their prevalence increases with age. Ectopic beats in patients with otherwise normal hearts are more prominent at rest and disappear with exercise. Sometimes VPBs are a manifestation of subclinical coronary artery disease or cardiomyopathy but also may occur in patients with established heart disease following an MI. Most patients with VPBs are asymptomatic but some present with an irregular heart beat, missed beats or abnormally strong beats, due to increased cardiac output of the post-ectopic sinus beat. On examination the pulse is irregular, with weak or missed beats as a result of the fact that the stroke volume is low because left ventricular contraction occurs before filling is complete (Fig. 16.40). The ECG shows broad and bizarre complexes because the ventricles are activated sequentially rather than simultaneously. The complexes may be unifocal (identical beats arising from a single ectopic focus) or multifocal (varying morphology with multiple foci, Fig. 16.40). 'Couplet' and 'triplet' are the terms used to describe two or three successive ectopic beats. A run of alternating sinus and ventricular ectopic beats is known as ventricular 'bigeminy'. The significance depends on the presence or absence of underlying heart disease.

Management

Treatment may not be necessary, unless the patient is highly symptomatic, in which case β-blockers or, in some situations,

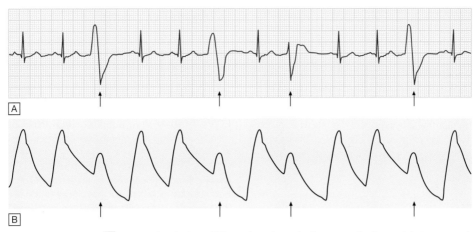

Fig. 16.40 Ventricular ectopic beats. A There are broad, bizarre QRS complexes (arrows) with no preceding P wave in between normal sinus beats. Their configuration varies, so these are multifocal ectopics. B A simultaneous arterial pressure trace is shown. The ectopic beats result in a weaker pulse (arrows), which may be perceived as a 'dropped beat'.

catheter ablation can be used. There is no evidence that anti-arrhythmic therapy improves prognosis but the discovery of very frequent VPBs in a patient not known to have heart disease should prompt further investigations with echocardiography and an exercise ECG to screen for structural heart disease and ischaemic heart disease. It is common for VPBs to occur during the course of an acute MI. Persistent, frequent VPBs (over 10/hr) in patients who have survived the acute phase of MI indicate a poorer long-term outcome. In this situation, anti-arrhythmic drugs do not improve and may even worsen prognosis. The exception is β-blockers, which should be prescribed for other reasons (p. 500). Similarly, heart failure of any cause is associated with VPBs. While they indicate an adverse prognosis, this is not improved by anti-arrhythmic drugs. Effective treatment of the heart failure may suppress the ectopic beats. VPBs are also a feature of digoxin toxicity.

Ventricular tachycardia

Ventricular tachycardia (VT) occurs most commonly in the settings of acute MI, chronic coronary artery disease and cardiomyopathy. It is associated with extensive ventricular disease, impaired left ventricular function and ventricular aneurysm. In these settings, VT may cause haemodynamic compromise or degenerate into ventricular fibrillation (p. 456). VT is caused by abnormal automaticity or triggered activity in ischaemic tissue, or by re-entry within scarred ventricular tissue. Patients may complain of palpitation or symptoms of low cardiac output, including dyspnoea, lightheadedness and syncope. The ECG shows tachycardia and broad, abnormal QRS complexes with a rate of more than 120/min (Fig. 16.41). It may be difficult to distinguish VT from SVT with bundle branch block or pre-excitation (WPW syndrome) on ECG but features in favour of VT are listed in Box 16.25. A 12-lead ECG (Fig. 16.42) or electrophysiology study (p. 454) may help establish the diagnosis. When there is doubt, it is safer to manage the problem as VT.

Patients recovering from MI sometimes have periods of idioventricular rhythm ('slow' VT) at a rate only slightly above the preceding sinus rate and below 120/min. These episodes often reflect reperfusion of the infarct territory and may be a good sign. They are usually self-limiting and asymptomatic, and do not require treatment. Other forms of sustained VT require treatment, often as an emergency.

Fig. 16.41 Ventricular tachycardia: fusion beat (arrow). In ventricular tachycardia, there is independent atrial and ventricular activity. Occasionally, a P wave is conducted to the ventricles through the AV node, producing a normal sinus beat in the middle of the tachycardia (a capture beat); more commonly, however, the conducted impulse fuses with an impulse from the tachycardia (a fusion beat). This can occur only when there is atrioventricular dissociation and is therefore diagnostic of ventricular tachycardia.

16.25 Features more in keeping with ventricular tachycardia
• History of myocardial infarction
• Atrioventricular dissociation (pathognomonic)
• Capture/fusion beats (pathognomonic; see Fig. 16.41)
• Extreme left axis deviation
• Very broad QRS complexes (>140 msecs)
• No response to carotid sinus massage or intravenous adenosine

Occasionally, VT occurs in patients with otherwise healthy hearts ('normal heart VT'), usually because of abnormal automaticity in the right ventricular outflow tract or one of the fascicles of the left bundle branch.

Management

Prompt action to restore sinus rhythm is required and should usually be followed by prophylactic therapy. Synchronised DC cardioversion is the treatment of choice if systolic BP is less than 90 mmHg. If the arrhythmia is well tolerated, intravenous amiodarone may be given as a bolus, followed by a continuous infusion (p. 481). Intravenous lidocaine can be used but may depress left ventricular function, causing hypotension or acute heart failure. Hypokalaemia, hypomagnesaemia, acidosis and hypoxia should be corrected if present.

Beta-blockers are effective at preventing VT by reducing ventricular automaticity. Amiodarone can be added if additional control is needed. Class Ic anti-arrhythmic drugs should not be used for prevention of VT in patients with coronary artery disease or heart failure because they depress myocardial function and can increase the likelihood of a dangerous arrhythmia. In patients with poor left ventricular function or where VT is associated with haemodynamic compromise, the use of an implantable cardiac defibrillator is recommended (p. 483). Rarely, surgery with resection of a ventricular aneurysm or catheter ablation can be used to interrupt the arrhythmia focus or circuit in patients with VT associated with a myocardial infarct scar. The treatment of choice for VT occurring in a normal heart is catheter ablation, which often can be curative.

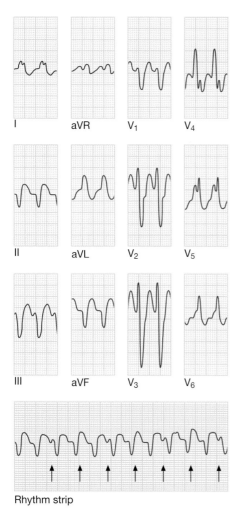

Rhythm strip

Fig. 16.42 Ventricular tachycardia: 12-lead ECG. There are typically very broad QRS complexes and marked left axis deviation. There is also atrioventricular dissociation; some P waves are visible and others are buried in the QRS complexes (arrows).

Torsades de pointes

This form of polymorphic VT is a complication of prolonged ventricular repolarisation (prolonged QT interval). The ECG shows rapid irregular complexes that seem to twist around the baseline as the mean QRS axis changes (Fig. 16.43). The arrhythmia is usually non-sustained and repetitive, but may degenerate into ventricular fibrillation. During periods of sinus rhythm, the ECG will usually show a prolonged QT interval (>0.44 sec in men, >0.46 sec in women when corrected to a heart rate of 60/min).

Some of the common causes are listed in Box 16.26. The arrhythmia is more common in women and is often triggered by a combination of factors, such as administration of QT-prolonging medications and hypokalaemia. The congenital long QT syndromes are a family of genetic disorders that are characterised by mutations in genes that code for cardiac sodium or potassium channels. Long QT syndrome subtypes have different triggers, which are important when counselling patients. Adrenergic stimulation through vigorous exercise is a common trigger in long QT type 1, and a sudden noise may trigger arrhythmias in long QT type 2. Arrhythmias are more common during sleep in type 3.

Management

Intravenous magnesium (8 mmol over 15 mins, then 72 mmol over 24 hrs) should be given in all cases. If this is ineffective,

i	16.26 Causes of long QT interval and torsades de pointes

Bradycardia

- Bradycardia compounds other factors that cause torsades de pointes

Electrolyte disturbance

- Hypokalaemia
- Hypomagnesaemia
- Hypocalcaemia

Drugs*

- Disopyramide, flecainide and other class Ia, Ic anti-arrhythmic drugs (p. 479)
- Sotalol, amiodarone and other class III anti-arrhythmic drugs
- Amitriptyline and other tricyclic antidepressants
- Chlorpromazine and other phenothiazines
- Erythromycin and other macrolides

Congenital syndromes

- Long QT1: gene affected *KCNQI*: K+ channel, 30–35%
- Long QT2: gene affected *HERG*: K+ channel, 25–30%
- Long QT3: gene affected *SCN5A*: Na+ channel, 5–10%
- Long QT4–12: rare; various genes implicated

*Many other drugs that are not shown can be associated with prolongation of the QT interval. See www.crediblemeds.org for a complete list.

Fig. 16.43 Torsades de pointes. A bradycardia with a long QT interval is followed by polymorphic ventricular tachycardia that is triggered by an R on T ectopic.

atrial pacing should be tried, since it can suppress the arrhythmia through rate-dependent shortening of the QT interval. Intravenous isoprenaline is a reasonable alternative to pacing but should be avoided in patients with the congenital long QT syndromes. Once initial control has been achieved, efforts should be made to identify and treat the underlying cause or stop medications that predispose to the arrhythmia. If the underlying cause cannot be corrected or the arrhythmia is the result of an inherited syndrome, then long-term pharmacological therapy may be necessary. Beta-blockers are effective at preventing syncope in patients with congenital long QT syndrome. Some patients, particularly those with extreme QT interval prolongation (>500 msecs) or certain high-risk genotypes, should be considered for an implantable defibrillator. Left stellate ganglion block may be of value in patients with resistant arrhythmias.

Brugada syndrome is a related genetic disorder that may present with polymorphic VT or sudden death. It is characterised by a defect in sodium channel function and an abnormal ECG (right bundle branch block and ST elevation in V_1 and V_2 but not usually prolongation of the QT interval). The only known effective treatment is an implantable defibrillator.

Atrioventricular block

This usually occurs as the result of disease affecting the AV node. AV block can be intermittent, however, and may become evident only when the conducting tissue is stressed by a rapid atrial rate. Reflecting this fact, atrial tachyarrhythmias are often associated with AV block (see Fig. 16.37). Episodes of ventricular asystole may also complicate complete heart block or Mobitz type II second-degree AV block. Several types of AV block are recognised.

First-degree atrioventricular block

In this condition, AV conduction is delayed and so the PR interval is prolonged (>0.20 sec; Fig. 16.44). It rarely causes symptoms and does not usually require treatment.

Second-degree atrioventricular block

Here dropped beats occur because some impulses from the atria fail to conduct to the ventricles. Two subtypes are recognised. In Mobitz type I second-degree AV block (Fig. 16.45), there is

progressive lengthening of successive PR intervals, culminating in a dropped beat. The cycle then repeats itself. This is known as the Wenckebach phenomenon and is usually due to impaired conduction in the AV node itself. The phenomenon may be physiological and is sometimes observed at rest or during sleep in athletic young adults with high vagal tone.

In Mobitz type II second-degree AV block (Fig. 16.46), the PR interval of the conducted impulses remains constant but some P waves are not conducted. This is usually caused by disease of the His–Purkinje system and carries a risk of asystole.

In 2:1 AV block (Fig. 16.47), alternate P waves are conducted, so it is impossible to distinguish between Mobitz type I and type II block.

Third-degree atrioventricular block

In third-degree AV block, conduction fails completely and the atria and ventricles beat independently. This is known as AV dissociation, as shown in Fig. 16.48. Ventricular activity is maintained by an escape rhythm arising in the AV node or bundle of His (narrow QRS complexes) or the distal Purkinje tissues (broad QRS complexes). Distal escape rhythms tend to be slower and less reliable. Complete AV block (Box 16.27) produces a slow (25–50/min), regular pulse that does not vary with exercise, except in the case of congenital complete AV block. There is usually a compensatory increase in stroke volume, producing a large-volume pulse. Cannon waves may be visible in the neck and the intensity of the first heart sound varies due to the loss of AV synchrony.

Clinical features

The typical presentation is with recurrent syncope or 'Stokes–Adams' attacks. These episodes are characterised by sudden

Fig. 16.44 First-degree atrioventricular block. The PR interval is prolonged and measures 0.26 sec.

Fig. 16.45 Second-degree atrioventricular block (Mobitz type I – the Wenckebach phenomenon). The PR interval progressively increases until a P wave is not conducted. The cycle then repeats itself. In this example, conduction is at a ratio of 4:3, leading to groupings of three ventricular complexes in a row.

Fig. 16.46 Second-degree atrioventricular block (Mobitz type II). The PR interval of conducted beats is normal but some P waves are not conducted. The constant PR interval distinguishes this from the Wenckebach phenomenon.

Fig. 16.47 Second-degree atrioventricular block with fixed 2:1 block. Alternate P waves are not conducted. This may be due to Mobitz type I or II block.

Fig. 16.48 Complete (third-degree) atrioventricular block. There is complete dissociation of atrial and ventricular complexes. The atrial rate is 80/min and the ventricular rate is 38/min.

i	**16.27 Causes of complete atrioventricular block**

Congenital

Acquired

- Idiopathic fibrosis
- Myocardial infarction/ischaemia
- Inflammation:
  Infective endocarditis
  Sarcoidosis
  Chagas' disease
- Trauma
- Drugs:
  Digoxin
  β-blockers
  Calcium antagonists

loss of consciousness that occurs without warning and results in collapse. A brief anoxic seizure (due to cerebral ischaemia) may occur if there is prolonged asystole. There is pallor and a death-like appearance during the attack, but when the heart starts beating again there is a characteristic flush. In distinction to epilepsy, recovery is rapid. Sinoatrial disease and neurocardiogenic syncope (p. 181) may cause similar symptoms.

Management

This depends on the clinical circumstances. Acute inferior MI is often complicated by transient AV block because the right coronary artery (RCA) supplies the AV node. There is usually a reliable escape rhythm and, if the patient remains well, no treatment is required. Symptomatic second- or third-degree AV block may respond to atropine (0.6 mg IV, repeated as necessary) or, if this fails, a temporary pacemaker. In most cases, the AV block will resolve within 7–10 days.

Second- or third-degree AV heart block complicating acute anterior MI indicates extensive ventricular damage involving both bundle branches and carries a poor prognosis. Asystole may ensue and a temporary pacemaker should be inserted promptly. If the patient presents with asystole, intravenous atropine (3 mg) or intravenous isoprenaline (2 mg in 500 mL 5% dextrose, infused at 10–60 mL/hr) may help to maintain the circulation until a temporary pacing electrode can be inserted. Temporary pacing can provide effective rhythm support in the short term.

Patients with symptomatic bradyarrhythmias associated with AV block should be treated with a permanent pacemaker. Asymptomatic first-degree or Mobitz type I second-degree AV block (Wenckebach phenomenon) does not require treatment but may be an indication of underlying heart disease. A permanent pacemaker is usually indicated in patients with asymptomatic Mobitz type II second-degree AV block or third-degree AV heart block because of the risk of asystole and sudden death. Pacing improves prognosis.

Bundle branch block

Damage to the right or left bundle branch of the conducting system can occur as a result of many pathologies, including ischaemic heart disease, hypertensive heart disease and cardiomyopathy. However, right bundle branch block (RBBB) can occur as a normal variant in healthy individuals (Box 16.28). In left bundle branch block (LBBB) and RBBB, depolarisation proceeds through a slow myocardial route in the affected ventricle rather than through the rapidly conducting Purkinje tissues that constitute the bundle branches. This causes delayed conduction into the LV or RV, broadens the QRS complex (≥ 0.12 sec) and produces characteristic alterations in QRS morphology (Figs 16.49 and

i	**16.28 Common causes of bundle branch block**

Right bundle branch block

- Normal variant
- Right ventricular hypertrophy or strain, e.g. pulmonary embolism
- Congenital heart disease, e.g. atrial septal defect
- Coronary artery disease

Left bundle branch block

- Coronary artery disease
- Hypertension
- Aortic valve disease
- Cardiomyopathy

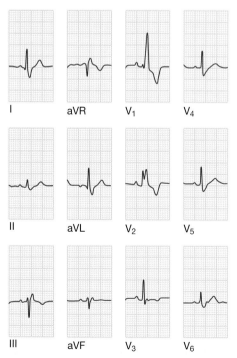

Fig. 16.49 Right bundle branch block. Note the wide QRS complexes with 'M'-shaped configuration in leads V_1 and V_2 and a wide S wave in lead I.

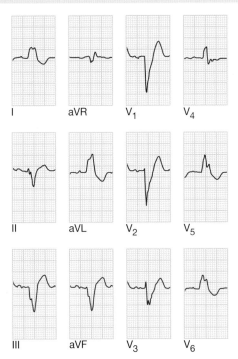

Fig. 16.50 Left bundle branch block. Note the wide QRS complexes with loss of the Q wave or septal vector in lead I and 'M'-shaped QRS complexes in V_5 and V_6.

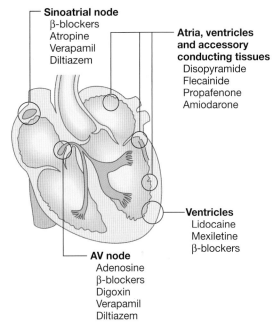

Fig. 16.51 Classification of anti-arrhythmic drugs by site of action.

i	**16.29 Classification of anti-arrhythmic drugs by effect on the intracellular action potential***

Class I: membrane-stabilising agents (sodium channel blockers)

(a) Block Na⁺ channel and prolong action potential
- Quinidine, disopyramide

(b) Block Na⁺ channel and shorten action potential
- Lidocaine, mexiletine

(c) Block Na⁺ channel with no effect on action potential
- Flecainide, propafenone

Class II: β-adrenoceptor antagonists (β-blockers)
- Atenolol, bisoprolol, metoprolol

Class III: drugs whose main effect is to prolong the action potential
- Amiodarone, dronedarone, sotalol

Class IV: slow calcium channel blockers
- Verapamil, diltiazem

*Some drugs such as digoxin, ivabradine and adenosine have no place in this classification, while others such as amiodarone have properties in more than one class.

16.50). Damage to the left bundle can also occur after it divides into anterior and posterior fascicles, when it is called hemiblock. In this case, the QRS complex is not broadened but the direction of ventricular depolarisation is changed, causing left axis deviation in left anterior hemiblock and right axis deviation in left posterior hemiblock (see Fig. 16.7, p. 449). The combination of RBBB and left anterior or posterior hemiblock is known as bifascicular block. LBBB usually signifies important underlying heart disease and also causes ventricular incoordination, which may aggravate symptoms in patients with heart failure. This can be treated in selected patients by cardiac resynchronisation therapy (p. 484).

Principles of management of cardiac arrhythmias

Cardiac arrhythmias can be managed with either anti-arrhythmic drug therapy or external devices that depolarise the heart by passing an electric current through it. These strategies are relevant across a range of indications and are discussed in more detail here.

Anti-arrhythmic drugs

Traditionally, the Vaughan Williams system has been used to categorise anti-arrhythmic drugs based on their effects on the action potential. More recently, increased understanding of the mechanisms of action has allowed further subclassification, based on the cardiac ion channels and receptors on which they act (Box 16.29 and Fig. 16.51). The individual agents, dosages and most common side-effects are summarised in Box 16.30 and the general principles of use are summarised in Box 16.31.

Class I drugs

Class I drugs act principally by suppressing excitability and slowing conduction in atrial or ventricular muscle. They block sodium channels, of which there are several types in cardiac tissue. These drugs should generally be avoided in patients with heart failure because they depress myocardial function, and class Ia and Ic drugs are often pro-arrhythmic.

Class Ia drugs

These prolong cardiac action potential duration and increase the tissue refractory period. They are used to prevent both atrial and ventricular arrhythmias.

Disopyramide

This is an effective drug but causes anticholinergic side-effects, such as urinary retention, and can precipitate glaucoma. It can

16

16.30 Uses, dosages and side-effects of anti-arrhythmic drugs

Drug	Main uses	Route	Dose (adult)	Important side-effects
Class I				
Disopyramide	Prevention and treatment of atrial and ventricular tachyarrhythmias	IV / Oral	2 mg/kg at 30 mg/min, then 0.4 mg/kg/hr (max 800 mg/day) / 300–800 mg daily in divided dosage	Myocardial depression, hypotension, dry mouth, urinary retention
Lidocaine	Treatment and short-term prevention of VT and VF	IV	Bolus 50–100 mg, 4 mg/min for 30 mins, then 2 mg/min for 2 hrs, then 1 mg/min for 24 hrs	Myocardial depression, delirium, convulsions
Mexiletine	Prevention and treatment of ventricular tachyarrhythmias	IV / Oral	Loading dose: 100–250 mg at 25 mg/min, then 250 mg in 1 hr, then 250 mg in 2 hrs Maintenance therapy: 0.5 mg/min / 200–250 mg 3 times daily	Myocardial depression, gastrointestinal irritation, delirium, dizziness, tremor, nystagmus, ataxia
Flecainide	Prevention and treatment of atrial and ventricular tachyarrhythmias	IV / Oral	2 mg/kg over 10 mins, then if required 1.5 mg/kg/hr for 1 hr, then 0.1 mg/kg/hr / 50–100 mg twice daily	Myocardial depression, dizziness
Propafenone	Prevention and treatment of atrial and ventricular tachyarrhythmias	Oral	150 mg 3 times daily for 1 week, then 300 mg twice daily	Myocardial depression, dizziness
Class II				
Atenolol	Treatment and prevention of SVT and AF, prevention of VEs and exercise-induced VF	IV	2.5 mg at 1 mg/min, repeated at 5-min intervals (max 10 mg)	Myocardial depression, bradycardia, bronchospasm, fatigue, depression, nightmares, cold peripheries
		Oral	25–100 mg daily	
Bisoprolol		Oral	2.5–10 mg daily	
Metoprolol		IV	5 mg over 2 mins to a maximum of 15 mg	
Class III				
Amiodarone	Serious or resistant atrial and ventricular tachyarrhythmias	IV / Oral	5 mg/kg over 20–120 mins, then up to 15 mg/kg/24 hrs / Initially 600–1200 mg/day, then 100–400 mg daily	Photosensitivity skin discoloration, corneal deposits, thyroid dysfunction, alveolitis, nausea and vomiting, hepatotoxicity, peripheral neuropathy, torsades de pointes; potentiates digoxin and warfarin
Dronedarone	Paroxysmal atrial fibrillation	Oral	400 mg twice daily	Renal and hepatic dysfunction requiring regular blood monitoring
Sotalol*	AF, rarely ventricular tachyarrhythmias	IV / Oral	10–20 mg slowly / 40–160 mg twice daily	Can cause torsades de pointes
Class IV				
Verapamil	Teatment of SVT, control of AF	IV / Oral	5–10 mg over 30 secs / 40–120 mg 3 times daily or 240 mg SR daily	Myocardial depression, hypotension, bradycardia, constipation
Other				
Atropine	Treatment of bradycardia and/or hypotension due to vagal overactivity	IV	0.6–3 mg	Dry mouth, thirst, blurred vision, atrial and ventricular extrasystoles
Adenosine	Teatment of SVT, aid to diagnosis in unidentified tachycardia	IV	3 mg over 2 secs, followed if necessary by 6 mg, then 12 mg at intervals of 1–2 mins	Flushing, dyspnoea, chest pain Avoid in asthma
Digoxin	Treatment and prevention of SVT, rate control of AF	IV / Oral	Loading dose: 0.5–1 mg (total), 0.5 mg over 30 mins, then 0.25–0.5 mg after 4–6 hrs / 0.5 mg repeated after 6 hrs, then 0.0625–0.25 mg daily	Gastrointestinal disturbance, xanthopsia, arrhythmias See Box 16.33

*Sotalol also has class II activity as a β-blocker.
(AF = atrial fibrillation; IV = intravenous; SR = sustained-release formulation; SVT = supraventricular tachycardia; VE = ventricular ectopic; VF = ventricular fibrillation; VT = ventricular tachycardia)

depress myocardial function and should be avoided in cardiac failure.

Quinidine
Now rarely used, quinidine increases mortality and causes gastrointestinal upset.

Class Ib drugs
These shorten the action potential and tissue refractory period. They act on channels found predominantly in ventricular myocardium and so are used to treat or prevent VT and VF.

Lidocaine
This must be given intravenously and has a very short plasma half-life.

Mexiletine
This can be given intravenously or orally but has many side-effects.

Class Ic drugs
These affect the slope of the action potential without altering its duration or refractory period. They are used mainly for prophylaxis of AF but are effective in prophylaxis and treatment

16.31 Anti-arrhythmic drugs: principles of use

Anti-arrhythmic drugs are potentially toxic and should be used carefully according to the following principles:
- Many arrhythmias are benign and do not require specific treatment
- Precipitating or causal factors should be corrected if possible:
  Alcohol excess
  Caffeine consumption
  Myocardial ischaemia
  Hyperthyroidism
  Acidosis
  Hypokalaemia
  Hypomagnesaemia
- If drug therapy is required, it is best to use as few drugs as possible
- In difficult cases, programmed electrical stimulation (electrophysiological study) may help to identify the optimum therapy
- When managing life-threatening arrhythmias, it is essential to ensure that prophylactic treatment is effective. Ambulatory monitoring and exercise testing may be of value
- Patients on long-term anti-arrhythmic drugs should be reviewed regularly and attempts made to withdraw therapy if the factors that precipitated the arrhythmias are no longer operative
- For patients with recurrent supraventricular tachycardia, radiofrequency ablation is often preferable to long-term drug therapy

of supraventricular or ventricular arrhythmias. They are useful for WPW syndrome because they block conduction in accessory pathways. They should not be used in patients with previous MI because they increase the risk of arrhythmia in this setting.

Flecainide

This is effective for prevention of AF, and an intravenous infusion may be used for pharmacological cardioversion of AF of less than 24 hours' duration. *Since flecainide can cause slow atrial flutter with a paradoxically rapid ventricular rate, it should be prescribed along with an AV node-blocking drug such as a β-blocker to control the ventricular rate.*

Propafenone

This also has some β-blocker (class II) properties. Important interactions with digoxin, warfarin and cimetidine have been described.

Class II drugs

This group comprises the β-adrenoceptor antagonists (β-blockers). These agents reduce the rate of SA node depolarisation and cause relative block in the AV node, making them useful for rate control in atrial flutter and AF. They can be used to prevent VT and SVT. They reduce myocardial excitability and the risk of arrhythmic death in patients with coronary artery disease and heart failure.

Non-selective β-blockers

These act on both β_1 and β_2 receptors. Beta$_2$-blockade causes side-effects, such as bronchospasm and peripheral vasoconstriction. Propranolol is non-selective and is subject to extensive first-pass metabolism in the liver. The effective oral dose is therefore unpredictable and must be titrated after treatment is started with a small dose. Other non-selective drugs include nadolol and carvedilol.

Cardioselective β-blockers

These act mainly on myocardial β_1 receptors and are relatively well tolerated. Bisoprolol and metoprolol are examples of cardioselective β-blockers.

Sotalol

This is a racemic mixture of two isomers with non-selective β-blocker (mainly l-sotalol) and class III (mainly d-sotalol) activity. It may cause torsades de pointes.

Class III drugs

Class III drugs act by prolonging the plateau phase of the action potential, thus lengthening the refractory period. These drugs are very effective at preventing atrial and ventricular tachyarrhythmias. They cause QT interval prolongation and can predispose to torsades de pointes and VT, especially in patients with other predisposing risk factors (see Box 16.26). Disopyramide and sotalol have some class III activity but the main drug in this class is amiodarone, as discussed below.

Amiodarone

While amiodarone is primarily considered a class III drug, it also has class I, II and IV activity. It is probably the most effective drug currently available for controlling paroxysmal AF. It is also used to prevent episodes of recurrent VT, particularly in patients with poor left ventricular function or those with implantable defibrillators (to prevent unnecessary DC shocks). Amiodarone has a very long tissue half-life (25–110 days). An intravenous or oral loading regime is often used to achieve therapeutic tissue concentrations rapidly. The drug's effects may last for weeks or months after treatment has been stopped. Side-effects are common (up to one-third of patients), numerous and potentially serious. Drug interactions are also common (see Box 16.30).

Dronedarone

Dronedarone is related to amiodarone but has a short tissue half-life and fewer side-effects. It has recently been shown to be effective at preventing episodes of atrial flutter and AF. It is contraindicated in patients with permanent AF, or if there is heart failure or left ventricular impairment, because it increases mortality. Regular liver function test monitoring is required.

Class IV drugs

These block the 'slow calcium channel', which is important for impulse generation and conduction in atrial and nodal tissue, although it is also present in ventricular muscle. Their main indications are prevention of SVT (by blocking the AV node) and rate control in patients with AF.

Verapamil

This is the most widely used drug in this class. Intravenous verapamil may cause profound bradycardia or hypotension, and should not be used in conjunction with β-blockers.

Diltiazem

This has similar properties to verapamil.

Other anti-arrhythmic drugs

Atropine sulphate

Atropine is a muscarinic receptor antagonist that increases the sinus rate and SA and AV conduction. It is the treatment of choice for severe bradycardia or hypotension due to vagal over-activity. It is used for initial management of symptomatic bradyarrhythmias complicating inferior MI, and in cardiac arrest due to asystole. The usual dose is 0.6 mg IV, repeated if necessary

16

i | **16.32 Response to intravenous adenosine**

Arrhythmia	Response
Supraventricular tachycardia	Termination
Atrial fibrillation, atrial flutter, atrial tachycardia	Transient atrioventricular block
Ventricular tachycardia	No effect

i | **16.33 Digoxin toxicity**

Extracardiac manifestations

- Anorexia, nausea, vomiting
- Diarrhoea
- Altered colour vision (xanthopsia)

Cardiac manifestations

- Bradycardia
- Multiple ventricular ectopics
- Ventricular bigeminy (alternate ventricular ectopics)
- Atrial tachycardia (with variable block)
- Ventricular tachycardia
- Ventricular fibrillation

to a maximum of 3 mg. Repeat dosing may be necessary because the drug disappears rapidly from the circulation after parenteral administration. Side-effects are listed in Box 16.30.

Adenosine

This works by binding to A1 receptors in conducting tissue, producing a transient AV block lasting a few seconds. It is used to terminate SVTs when the AV node is part of the re-entry circuit, or to help establish the diagnosis in difficult arrhythmias, such as atrial flutter with 2:1 AV block (see Fig. 16.35) or broad-complex tachycardia (Boxes 16.30 and 16.32). Adenosine is given as an intravenous bolus, initially 3 mg over 2 secs (see Box 16.30). If there is no response after 1–2 minutes, 6 mg should be given; if necessary, after another 1–2 minutes the maximum dose of 12 mg may be given. Patients should be warned to expect short-lived and sometimes distressing flushing, breathlessness and chest pain. Adenosine can cause bronchospasm and should be avoided in patients with asthma; its effects are greatly potentiated by dipyridamole and inhibited by theophylline and other xanthines.

Digoxin

Digoxin is a glycoside purified from the European foxglove, *Digitalis lanata*, which slows conduction and prolongs the refractory period in the AV node. This effect helps to control the ventricular rate in AF and may interrupt SVTs involving the AV node. Digoxin also shortens refractory periods and enhances excitability and conduction in other parts of the heart, including accessory conduction pathways. It may therefore increase atrial and ventricular ectopic activity and can lead to more complex atrial and ventricular tachyarrhythmias. Digoxin is largely excreted by the kidneys, and the maintenance dose (see Box 16.30) should be reduced in children, older people and those with renal impairment. It is widely distributed and has a long tissue half-life (36 hours), so that effects may persist for several days. Measurement of plasma digoxin concentration helps identify digoxin toxicity or under-treatment (Box 16.33).

Non-pharmacological treatments

A variety of non-pharmacological treatments are available for the treatment of arrhythmias. These include the use of electrical devices that work by passing an electric current through the heart, and catheter-based strategies that disrupt abnormal conduction tissues responsible for the generation of arrhythmias.

Electrical cardioversion

Electrical cardioversion, also known as direct current (DC) cardioversion, is useful for terminating an organised rhythm, such as AF or VT. The electric current interrupts the arrhythmia and produces a brief period of asystole, which is usually followed by the resumption of sinus rhythm. Cardioversion is usually carried out as an elective procedure under general anaesthesia. The electric shock is delivered immediately after the R wave because, if it is applied during ventricular repolarisation (on the T wave), it may provoke VF. High-energy shocks may cause chest wall pain post-procedure, so, if there is no urgency, it is appropriate to begin with a lower-amplitude shock of about 50 joules initially, going on to larger shocks if necessary.

Defibrillation

Defibrillators deliver a DC, high-energy, short-duration shock via two large electrodes or paddles coated with conducting jelly or a gel pad, positioned over the upper right sternal edge and the apex. Defibrillators are primarily used in the management of cardiac arrest due to VF and deliver an unsynchronised shock, since the precise timing of the discharge is not important in this situation. Modern units deliver a biphasic shock, during which the shock polarity is reversed mid-shock. This reduces the total shock energy required to depolarise the heart. In VF and other emergencies, the energy of the first and second shocks should be 150 joules and thereafter up to 200 joules; there is no need for an anaesthetic, as the patient is unconscious.

Temporary pacemakers

Temporary pacing involves delivery of an electrical impulse into the heart to initiate tissue depolarisation and to trigger cardiac contraction. This is achieved by inserting a bipolar pacing electrode through the internal jugular, subclavian or femoral vein and positioning it at the apex of the RV, using fluoroscopic imaging. The electrode is connected to an external pacemaker with an adjustable energy output and pacing rate. The ECG of right ventricular pacing is characterised by regular broad QRS complexes with a left bundle branch block pattern. Each complex is immediately preceded by a 'pacing spike' (Fig. 16.52). Nearly all pulse generators are used in the 'demand' mode, so that the pacemaker will operate only if the heart rate falls below a preset level. Occasionally, temporary atrial or dual-chamber pacing (see below) is used.

Temporary pacing is indicated in the management of transient AV block and other arrhythmias complicating acute MI or cardiac surgery, to maintain the rhythm in other situations of reversible bradycardia (such as metabolic disturbance or drug overdose), or as a bridge to permanent pacing. Complications include pneumothorax, brachial plexus or subclavian artery injury, local infection or sepsis (usually with *Staphylococcus aureus*), and pericarditis. Failure of the system may be due to lead displacement or a progressive increase in the threshold (exit block) caused by tissue oedema. Complication rates increase with time and so a temporary pacing system should ideally not be used for more than 7 days.

Transcutaneous pacing is administered by delivering an electrical stimulus through two large adhesive gel pad electrodes

Fig. 16.52 Dual-chamber pacing. The first three beats show atrial and ventricular pacing with narrow pacing spikes in front of each P wave and QRS complex. The last four beats show spontaneous P waves with a different morphology and no pacing spike; the pacemaker senses or tracks these P waves and maintains atrioventricular synchrony by pacing the ventricle after an appropriate interval.

placed over the apex and upper right sternal edge, or over the anterior and posterior chest. It is easy and quick to set up, but causes discomfort because it induces forceful pectoral and intercostal muscle contraction. Modern external cardiac defibrillators often incorporate a transcutaneous pacing system that can be used during an emergency until transvenous pacing is established.

Permanent pacemakers

Permanent pacemakers are small, flat, metal devices that are implanted under the skin, usually in the pectoral area. They contain a battery, a pulse generator, and programmable electronics that allow adjustment of pacing and memory functions. Pacing electrodes (leads) can be placed via the subclavian or cephalic veins into the RV (usually at the apex), the right atrial appendage or, to maintain AV synchrony, both.

Permanent pacemakers are controlled using an external programmer through a wireless telemetry system, allowing rate, output, timing and other parameters to be adjusted. This allows the device settings to be tailored to the patient's needs. Aside from their therapeutic role, pacemakers store useful diagnostic data about the patient's heart rate trends and the occurrence of tachyarrhythmias, such as VT.

Single-chamber atrial pacing is indicated in patients with SA disease without AV block and also in patients with continuous AF and bradycardia. Here the pacemaker acts as an external sinus node. Dual-chamber pacing is most often used in patients with second- or third-degree AV block. Here, the atrial electrode is used to detect spontaneous atrial activity and trigger ventricular pacing (Fig. 16.52), thereby preserving AV synchrony and allowing the ventricular rate to increase, together with the sinus node rate, during exercise and other forms of stress. Dual-chamber pacing has many advantages over ventricular pacing, including superior haemodynamics and better effort tolerance; a lower prevalence of atrial arrhythmias in patients with SA disease; and avoidance of 'pacemaker syndrome', in which a fall in BP and dizziness occur due to loss of AV synchrony.

A code is used to signify the pacing mode (Box 16.34). For example, a system that paces the atrium, senses the atrium and is inhibited if it senses spontaneous activity is designated AAI. Most dual-chamber pacemakers are programmed to a mode termed DDD; in this case, ventricular pacing is triggered by a sensed sinus P wave and inhibited by a sensed spontaneous QRS complex. A fourth letter, 'R', is added if the pacemaker has a rate response function. For example, the letters AAIR indicate an atrial demand pacemaker with a rate response function. Rate-responsive pacemakers are used in patients with chronotropic incompetence, who are unable to increase their heart

i 16.34 International generic pacemaker code		
Chamber paced	**Chamber sensed**	**Response to sensing**
O = none	O = none	O = none
A = atrium	A = atrium	T = triggered
V = ventricle	V = ventricle	I = inhibited
D = both	D = both	D = both

rate during exercise. These devices have a sensor that triggers an increase in heart rate in response to movement or increased respiratory rate. The sensitivity of the sensor is programmable, as is the maximum paced heart rate.

Early complications of permanent pacing include pneumothorax, cardiac tamponade, infection and lead displacement. Late complications include infection (which usually necessitates removing the pacing system), erosion of the generator or lead, chronic pain related to the implant site, and lead fracture due to mechanical fatigue.

Implantable cardiac defibrillators

In addition to the functions of a permanent pacemaker, implantable cardiac defibrillators (ICDs) can also detect and terminate life-threatening ventricular tachyarrhythmias. ICDs are larger than pacemakers mainly because of the need for a large battery and capacitor to enable cardioversion or defibrillation. ICD leads are similar to pacing leads but have one or two shock coils along the length of the lead, used for delivering defibrillation. ICDs treat ventricular tachyarrhythmias using overdrive pacing, cardioversion or defibrillation. They are implanted in a similar manner to pacemakers and carry a similar risk of complications. In addition, patients can be prone to psychological problems and anxiety, particularly if they have experienced repeated shocks from their device.

The evidence-based indications for ICD implantation are shown in Box 16.35. These can be divided into secondary prevention indications, when patients have already had a potentially life-threatening ventricular arrhythmia, and primary prevention indications, when patients are considered to be at significant future risk of arrhythmic death. A common primary prevention indication is in patients with inherited conditions associated with a high risk of sudden cardiac death, such as long QT syndrome (p. 476), hypertrophic cardiomyopathy (p. 539) and arrhythmogenic right ventricular dysplasia (p. 540). Treatment with ICDs is expensive

i 16.35 Key indications for implantable cardiac defibrillator therapy
Primary prevention
• After myocardial infarction, if the left ventricular ejection fraction is <30%
• Mild to moderate symptomatic heart failure on optimal drug therapy, with left ventricular ejection fraction <35%
• Some patients with inherited cardiac conditions (long QT syndrome, cardiomyopathy)
Secondary prevention
• Survivors of ventricular fibrillation or ventricular tachycardia cardiac arrest not having a transient or reversible cause
• Ventricular tachycardia with haemodynamic compromise or significant left ventricular impairment (left ventricular ejection fraction <35%)

16

and so the indications for which the devices are routinely implanted depend on the health-care resources available.

Cardiac resynchronisation therapy

Cardiac resynchronisation therapy (CRT) is a useful treatment for selected patients with heart failure, in whom cardiac function is impaired by the presence of left bundle branch block. This conduction defect is associated with poorly coordinated left ventricular contraction that can aggravate heart failure in susceptible patients. The systems used to deliver CRT comprise a right atrial lead, a right ventricular lead, and a third lead that is placed via the coronary sinus into one of the veins on the epicardial surface of the LV (see Fig. 16.30, p. 467). Simultaneous septal and left ventricular epicardial pacing resynchronises left ventricular contraction.

CRT improves symptoms and quality of life, and reduces mortality in patients with moderate to severe (NYHA class III–IV) heart failure who are in sinus rhythm, with left bundle branch block and left ventricular ejection fraction of 35% or less. CRT also prevents heart failure progression in similar patients with mild (NYHA class I–II) heart failure symptoms. These devices are more effective in patients in sinus rhythm than in those with AF. Most devices are also defibrillators (CRT-D) because many patients with heart failure are predisposed to ventricular arrhythmias. CRT pacemakers (CRT-P) are used when the focus is palliation of symptoms rather than prolonging life.

Catheter ablation therapy

Catheter ablation therapy is the treatment of choice for patients with SVT or atrial flutter, and is a useful treatment for some patients with AF or ventricular arrhythmias (Fig. 16.53). It involves inserting a series of catheter electrodes into the heart through the venous system. These are used to record the activation sequence of the heart in sinus rhythm, during tachycardia and after pacing manœuvres. Once the arrhythmia focus or circuit, such as an accessory pathway in WPW syndrome, has been identified, a catheter is used to ablate the culprit tissue. This can be done either by using heat, which is termed radiofrequency ablation, or by freezing, which is termed cryoablation. The procedure takes approximately 1–4 hours and does not require a general anaesthetic, although the patient may experience some discomfort

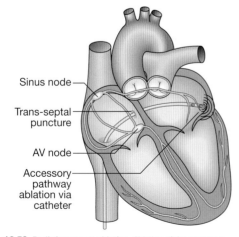

Fig. 16.53 Radiofrequency ablation. Ablation of the accessory conducting pathway in Wolff–Parkinson–White syndrome (see text for details). (AV = atrioventricular node)

during the ablation procedure. Serious complications are rare (<1%) but include complete heart block requiring pacemaker implantation, and cardiac tamponade. For many arrhythmias, radiofrequency ablation is very attractive because it offers the prospect of a lifetime cure, thereby eliminating the need for long-term drug therapy.

The technique has revolutionised the management of many arrhythmias and is now the treatment of choice for AVNRT and AV re-entrant (accessory pathway) tachycardias, when it is curative in over 90% of cases. Focal atrial tachycardias and atrial flutter can also be treated by radiofrequency ablation, although some patients subsequently experience episodes of AF. The applications of the technique are expanding and it can now be used to treat some forms of VT. Catheter ablation techniques are also employed to prevent AF. This involves ablation at two sites: the ostia of the pulmonary veins, from which ectopic beats may trigger paroxysms of arrhythmia, and in the LA itself, where re-entry circuits maintain AF, once established. This is effective at reducing episodes of AF in around 70–80% of younger patients with structurally normal hearts, and tends to be reserved for patients with drug-resistant AF because the procedure carries a risk of cardiac tamponade, and rarely stroke or death.

In patients with permanent AF and poor rate control, in whom drugs are ineffective or are not tolerated, rate control can be achieved by implantation of a permanent pacemaker, followed by ablation of the AV node to induce complete AV block and bradycardia, thus allowing the pacemaker to assume control of the heart rate.

Coronary artery disease

Coronary artery disease (CAD) is the most common cause of angina and acute coronary syndrome and the most common cause of death worldwide. The World Health Organisation (WHO) has estimated that 3.8 million men and 3.4 million women die from cardiovascular disease (CVD) each year, and since 1990, more people have died from CVD than any other cause. It also has a devastating effect on quality of life. Disability-adjusted life years, a measure of healthy years of life lost, can be used to indicate the burden of disease rather than the resulting deaths. It has been estimated that CAD is responsible for 10% of disability-adjusted life years in low-income countries and 18% in high-income ones. In the UK, 1 in 3 men and 1 in 4 women die from CAD, an estimated 188 000 people have a myocardial infarct each year, and approximately 2.3 million people are living with CAD. The death rates from CAD in the UK are among the highest in Western Europe (more than 70 000 people) but are falling, particularly in younger age groups; over the last 50 years, CAD mortality has more than halved. In Eastern Europe and much of Asia, however, the rates of CAD are rapidly rising. Occult CAD is common in those who present with other forms of atherosclerotic vascular disease, such as intermittent claudication or stroke, and is an important cause of morbidity and mortality in these patients.

Pathogenesis

In the vast majority of patients, CAD is caused by atherosclerosis (Box 16.36) but rarely it can occur as the result of aortitis (p. 508), vasculitis (p. 1040) and autoimmune connective tissue diseases (p. 1034). Atherosclerosis is a progressive inflammatory disorder of the arterial wall that is characterised by focal lipid-rich deposits of atheroma that remain clinically silent until they become large enough to impair tissue perfusion, or until ulceration and disruption of the lesion result in thrombotic occlusion or distal embolisation of the vessel. Atherosclerosis begins early in life with deposits of lipids in the vessel wall, which tend to occur at sites of altered arterial shear stress, such as bifurcations, and are associated with abnormalities of endothelial function at that site. Abnormalities of arterial function have been detected among high-risk children and adolescents, such as cigarette smokers and those with familial hyperlipidaemia or hypertension. Early lesions have been found in the arteries of victims of accidental death in the second and third decades of life but clinical manifestations often do not appear until the sixth, seventh or eighth decade. During evolution of an atherosclerotic plaque, monocytes and other inflammatory cells bind to receptors expressed by endothelial cells. Subsequently, they migrate into the intima, and take up oxidised low-density lipoprotein (LDL) particles by phagocytosis to become lipid-laden macrophages or foam cells. Extracellular lipid pools appear in the intimal space when foam cells die and release their contents (Fig. 16.54). In response to cytokines and growth factors produced by activated macrophages, smooth muscle cells migrate from the media of the arterial wall into the intima, and change from a contractile to a fibroblastic phenotype, which can stabilise the atherosclerotic lesion. If this is successful, the lipid core will be covered by smooth muscle cells and matrix, producing a stable atherosclerotic plaque that will remain asymptomatic until it becomes large enough to obstruct arterial flow.

In an established atherosclerotic plaque, macrophages mediate inflammation and smooth muscle cells promote repair. If inflammation predominates, the plaque becomes active or unstable and may be complicated by ulceration and thrombosis. Cytokines, such as interleukin-1, tumour necrosis factor-alpha, interferon-gamma, platelet-derived growth factors and matrix metalloproteinases, are released by activated macrophages. They cause the intimal smooth muscle cells overlying the plaque to become senescent and the collagen cross-links within the plaque to degrade. This results in thinning of the protective fibrous cap, making the lesion vulnerable to mechanical stress that ultimately causes erosion, fissuring or rupture of the plaque surface (Fig. 16.54). Any breach in the integrity of the plaque will expose its contents to blood and will trigger platelet aggregation and

16.36 Coronary artery disease: clinical manifestations and pathology	
Clinical problem	**Pathology**
Stable angina	Ischaemia due to fixed atheromatous stenosis of one or more coronary arteries
Unstable angina	Ischaemia caused by dynamic obstruction of a coronary artery due to plaque rupture or erosion with superimposed thrombosis
Myocardial infarction	Myocardial necrosis caused by acute occlusion of a coronary artery due to plaque rupture or erosion with superimposed thrombosis
Heart failure	Myocardial dysfunction due to infarction or ischaemia
Arrhythmia	Altered conduction due to ischaemia or infarction
Sudden death	Ventricular arrhythmia, asystole or massive myocardial infarction

16

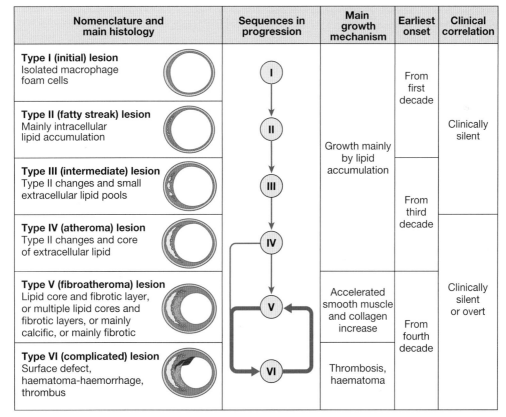

Nomenclature and main histology	Sequences in progression	Main growth mechanism	Earliest onset	Clinical correlation
Type I (initial) lesion Isolated macrophage foam cells	I	Growth mainly by lipid accumulation	From first decade	Clinically silent
Type II (fatty streak) lesion Mainly intracellular lipid accumulation	II			
Type III (intermediate) lesion Type II changes and small extracellular lipid pools	III		From third decade	
Type IV (atheroma) lesion Type II changes and core of extracellular lipid	IV			Clinically silent or overt
Type V (fibroatheroma) lesion Lipid core and fibrotic layer, or multiple lipid cores and fibrotic layers, or mainly calcific, or mainly fibrotic	V	Accelerated smooth muscle and collagen increase	From fourth decade	
Type VI (complicated) lesion Surface defect, haematoma-haemorrhage, thrombus	VI	Thrombosis, haematoma		

Fig. 16.54 The six stages of atherosclerosis. American Heart Association classification. *From Stary HC, Chandler B, Dinsmore RE et al. A definition of advanced types of atherosclerotic lesions and a histological classification of atherosclerosis. Circulation 1995; 92:1355–1374. © 1995 American Heart Association.*

thrombosis that extend into the atheromatous plaque and the arterial lumen. This may cause partial or complete obstruction at the site of the lesion or distal embolisation, resulting in infarction or ischaemia of the affected organ. This common mechanism underlies acute coronary syndromes, as well as other manifestations of atherosclerotic disease such as lower limb ischaemia (p. 502) and stroke (Ch. 26).

The number and complexity of arterial plaques increase with age and risk factors (see below) but the rate of progression of individual plaques is variable. There is a complex and dynamic interaction between mechanical wall stress and atherosclerotic lesions. Vulnerable plaques are characterised by a lipid-rich core, a thin fibrocellular cap, speckled calcification and an increase in inflammatory cells that release specific enzymes to degrade matrix proteins. In contrast, stable plaques are typified by a small lipid pool, a thick fibrous cap, heavy calcification and plentiful collagenous cross-links. Fissuring or rupture tends to occur at sites of maximal mechanical stress, particularly the margins of an eccentric plaque, and may be triggered by a surge in BP, such as during exercise or emotional stress. Surprisingly, most plaque events are subclinical and heal spontaneously, although this may allow thrombus to be incorporated into the lesion, producing plaque growth and further obstruction to flow.

Atherosclerosis may induce complex changes in the media that lead to arterial remodelling. Some arterial segments may slowly constrict (negative remodelling), while others may gradually enlarge (positive remodelling). These changes are important because they may amplify or minimise the degree to which atheroma encroaches into the arterial lumen.

Many risk factors have been identified for atherosclerosis but the causes are incompletely understood, since unknown factors account for up to 40% of the variation in risk from one person to the next.

Age and sex

Age is the most powerful independent risk factor for atherosclerosis and gender also plays a role. Pre-menopausal women have lower rates of disease than men, although the gender difference disappears after the menopause. Hormone replacement therapy (HRT) is not effective in the prevention of CAD, and HRT in post-menopausal women is associated with an increased risk of cardiovascular events.

Genetics

Atherosclerotic CAD often runs in families and a positive family history is common in patients with early-onset disease (age <50 in men and <55 in women). Twin studies have shown that a monozygotic twin of an affected individual has an eightfold increased risk and a dizygotic twin a fourfold increased risk of dying from CAD, compared to the general population due to a combination of shared genetic, environmental and lifestyle factors. The most common risk factors, such as hypertension, hyperlipidaemia and diabetes mellitus, are inherited in a polygenic manner.

Smoking

There is a strong relationship between cigarette smoking and CAD, especially in younger (<70 years) individuals, and this is probably the most important modifiable risk factor.

Hypertension

The incidence of atherosclerosis increases as BP rises, and this is related to systolic and diastolic BP, as well as pulse pressure. Antihypertensive therapy reduces cardiovascular mortality, stroke and heart failure.

Hypercholesterolaemia

The risk of atherosclerosis rises with serum cholesterol concentrations and lowering serum total and LDL cholesterol concentrations reduces the risk of cardiovascular events.

Diabetes mellitus

This is a potent risk factor for all forms of atherosclerosis, especially type 2 diabetes mellitus. It is often associated with diffuse disease that is difficult to treat. Insulin resistance (normal glucose homeostasis with high levels of insulin) is associated with obesity and physical inactivity, and is also a risk factor for CAD (p. 730). Glucose intolerance makes a major contribution to the high incidence of ischaemic heart disease in people from the Indian subcontinent and some other ethnic groups.

Haemostatic factors

Platelet activation and high plasma fibrinogen concentrations are associated with an increased risk of coronary thrombosis, whereas antiphospholipid antibodies are associated with recurrent arterial thromboses (p. 977).

Physical activity

Regular exercise (brisk walking, cycling or swimming for 20 minutes two or three times a week) has a protective effect, whereas inactivity roughly doubles the risk of CAD and is a major risk factor for stroke.

Obesity

Obesity, particularly if central or truncal, is an independent risk factor, although it is often associated with other adverse factors such as hypertension, diabetes mellitus and physical inactivity.

Alcohol

Excess alcohol consumption is associated with hypertension and cerebrovascular disease.

Diet

Diets deficient in fresh fruit, vegetables and polyunsaturated fatty acids are associated with an increased risk of cardiovascular disease. The introduction of a Mediterranean-style diet reduces cardiovascular events. However, dietary supplements, such as vitamins C and E, beta-carotene, folate and fish oils, do not reduce cardiovascular events and, in some cases, have been associated with harm.

Personality

While certain personality traits are associated with an increased risk of coronary disease there is no evidence to support the popular belief that stress is a major cause of CAD.

Social deprivation

Social deprivation is strongly related to cardiovascular disease. This may be partly due to associations with lifestyle risk factors, such as smoking and alcohol excess, which are more common in socially deprived individuals. Social deprivation does appear to be an independent risk factor for cardiovascular disease, however. Current guidelines recommend that treatment thresholds should be lowered for patients from socially deprived areas.

The effect of risk factors can be multiplicative rather than additive. People with a combination of risk factors are at greatest risk and so assessment should take account of all identifiable risk factors. It is important to distinguish between relative risk (the proportional increase in risk) and absolute risk (the actual chance of an event). For example, a man of 35 years with a plasma cholesterol of 7 mmol/L (approximately 170 mg/dL), who smokes 40 cigarettes a day, is much more likely to die from coronary disease within the next decade than a non-smoking man of the same age with a normal cholesterol, but the absolute likelihood of his dying during this time is still small (high relative risk, low absolute risk).

Management

Two approaches can be employed. Primary prevention aims to introduce lifestyle changes or therapeutic interventions to prevent CAD and other forms of atherosclerosis in the whole population or in healthy individuals with an elevated risk of disease. Secondary prevention involves initiating treatment in patients who already have had an event, with the aim of reducing the risk of subsequent events.

Primary prevention

The population-based strategy aims to modify the risk factors of the whole population through diet and lifestyle advice, on the basis that even a small reduction in smoking or average cholesterol, or modification of exercise and diet will produce worthwhile benefits (Box 16.37). Some risk factors, such as obesity and smoking, are also associated with a higher risk of other diseases and should be actively discouraged through public health measures. The effectiveness of this approach has been demonstrated by introduction of legislation to restrict smoking in public places, which has been associated with reductions in rates of MI.

The targeted strategy aims to identify and treat high-risk individuals, who usually have a combination of risk factors that can be quantified by composite scoring systems. It is important to consider the absolute risk of atheromatous cardiovascular disease that an individual is facing before initiating treatment, since this will help to determine whether the potential benefits of intervention are likely to outweigh the expense, inconvenience and possible side-effects of treatment. For example, a 65-year-old man with an average BP of 150/90 mmHg, who smokes and has diabetes mellitus with a total:high-density lipoprotein (HDL) cholesterol ratio of 8, has a 10-year risk of MI or stroke of 56%. Conversely, a 55-year-old woman who has an identical BP, is a non-smoker, does not have diabetes mellitus, and has a total:HDL cholesterol ratio of 6 has a much better outlook, with a 10-year coronary MI or stroke risk of 5.7%. Lowering cholesterol will reduce the risk in both of these individuals by 30% and lowering BP will produce a further 20% reduction. In combination, both strategies would reduce the risk of an event from 56% to 25% in the male patient and from 5.7% to 2.5% in the female patient. Thresholds for treatment vary

in different countries. In the UK and North America, current guidelines recommend initiation of cholesterol and BP-lowering therapies in individuals with a 10-year cardiovascular risk of 7.5–10%.

Secondary prevention

This involves targeting interventions at individuals who already have evidence of cardiovascular disease. Patients who recover from a clinical event such as an MI are usually keen to help themselves and are particularly receptive to lifestyle advice, such as dietary modification and smoking cessation. Additional interventions that should be introduced in patients with angina pectoris or an acute coronary syndrome are discussed in more detail below.

Angina pectoris

Angina pectoris is a symptom complex caused by transient myocardial ischaemia, which occurs whenever there is an imbalance between myocardial oxygen supply and demand (Box 16.38).

Pathogenesis

Atherosclerosis is by far the most common cause of angina pectoris. Angina may also occur in aortic valve disease and hypertrophic cardiomyopathy, and when the coronary arteries are involved with vasculitis or aortitis. The underlying mechanisms and risk factors for atherosclerosis have already been discussed. Approximately 10% of patients who report stable angina on effort have normal coronary arteries on angiography. The main causes are discussed in more detail below.

16

Coronary artery spasm

Angina may result from vasospasm of the coronary arteries. This may coexist with atherosclerosis, especially in unstable angina (see below), but may occur as an isolated phenomenon in less than 1% of cases, in patients with normal coronary arteries on angiography. This is sometimes known as variant angina; when it is accompanied by transient ST elevation on the ECG, it is termed Prinzmetal's angina.

Syndrome X

The constellation of typical angina on effort, objective evidence of myocardial ischaemia on stress testing, and normal coronary arteries on angiography is sometimes known as syndrome X. Many of these patients are women and the mechanism of their

	16.37 Population-based strategies to prevent coronary disease

- Do not smoke
- Take regular exercise (minimum of 20 mins, three times per week)
- Maintain an 'ideal' body weight
- Eat a mixed diet rich in fresh fruit and vegetables
- Aim to get no more than 10% of energy intake from saturated fat

	16.38 Factors influencing myocardial oxygen supply and demand

Oxygen demand: cardiac work

- Heart rate
- Blood pressure
- Myocardial contractility
- Left ventricular hypertrophy
- Valve disease

Oxygen supply: coronary blood flow*

- Duration of diastole
- Coronary perfusion pressure (aortic diastolic minus coronary sinus or right atrial diastolic pressure)
- Coronary vasomotor tone
- Oxygenation:
  Haemoglobin
  Oxygen saturation

*Coronary blood flow occurs mainly in diastole.

---

i   **16.39 Activities precipitating angina**

Common

- Physical exertion
- Cold exposure
- Heavy meals
- Intense emotion

Uncommon

- Vivid dreams (nocturnal angina)
- Lying flat (decubitus angina)

---

i   **16.40 Canadian Cardiovascular Society (CCS) angina score**

Class I

- Angina only during strenuous or prolonged physical activity

Class II

- Slight limitation, with angina only during vigorous physical activity

Class III

- Moderate limitation where symptoms occur with everyday activities

Class IV

- Inability to perform any activity without angina or angina at rest, i.e. severe limitation

---

i   **16.41 Risk stratification in stable angina***

High risk	Low risk
Post-infarct angina	Predictable exertional angina
Poor effort tolerance	Good effort tolerance
Ischaemia at low workload	Ischaemia only at high workload
Left main or three-vessel disease	Single-vessel or two-vessel disease
Poor left ventricular function	Good left ventricular function

*Patients may fall between these two categories.

---

symptoms is often unclear. This disorder is poorly understood; it carries a good prognosis but may respond to anti-anginal therapy.

Other causes

Angina can occur in association with aortic stenosis, hypertrophic obstructive cardiomyopathy and aortitis, all of which are discussed in more detail later in this chapter. It may also rarely be found in association with vasculitis (p. 1040).

Clinical features

The history is the most important factor in making the diagnosis (p. 454). Stable angina is characterised by central chest pain, discomfort or breathlessness that is predictably precipitated by exertion or other forms of stress (Box 16.39), and is promptly relieved by rest (see Fig. 10.1, p. 178). Some patients find the discomfort comes when they start walking and that later it does not return despite greater effort ('warm-up angina'). The Canadian Cardiovascular Society (CCS) scoring system is commonly used to grade the severity of angina (Box 16.40). This is of clinical value, not only in documenting the severity of angina but also in assessing prognosis (p. 493).

Physical examination is frequently unremarkable but should include a careful search for evidence of valve disease (particularly aortic), important risk factors (hypertension, diabetes mellitus), left ventricular dysfunction (cardiomegaly, gallop rhythm), other manifestations of arterial disease (carotid bruits, peripheral arterial disease), and unrelated conditions that may exacerbate angina (anaemia, thyrotoxicosis).

Investigations

Symptoms are a poor guide to the extent of CAD. Because of this, stress testing and non-invasive imaging are advisable in patients who are potential candidates for revascularisation. An algorithm for the investigation and treatment of patients with stable angina is shown in Figure 16.55. The first-line investigation is an exercise ECG, which should be performed using a standard treadmill or bicycle ergometer protocol (p. 449) while monitoring the patient's pulse, BP and general condition. Planar or down-sloping ST segment depression of 1 mm or more is indicative of ischaemia (Fig. 16.56). Up-sloping ST depression is less specific; it often occurs in normal individuals and false-positive results can occur with digoxin therapy, left ventricular hypertrophy, bundle branch block and WPW syndrome. The amount of exercise that can be tolerated and the extent of ST segment change (Fig. 16.57) that occurs can be of value in identifying high-risk individuals with severe coronary disease in combination with other clinical features (Box 16.41). However, exercise testing may be normal in a significant proportion of patients with CAD or may be inconclusive because an adequate heart rate cannot be achieved due to reduced mobility or other non-cardiac problems. Accordingly, if clinical suspicion is high and the exercise ECG is normal or inconclusive, further imaging with myocardial perfusion scanning or stress echocardiography is indicated. A perfusion defect present during stress but not at rest provides evidence of reversible myocardial ischaemia (Fig. 16.58), whereas a persistent perfusion defect seen during both phases of the study is usually indicative of previous MI. Increasingly, CT coronary arteriography is being used to document the presence or absence of CAD in patients with suspected angina. It can clarify the diagnosis, help to guide optimal treatment and avoid the need for cardiac catheterisation in patients who do not have CAD or who have mild disease only (see Fig. 16.55).

Coronary angiography provides detailed anatomical information about the extent and nature of CAD (see Fig. 16.15, p. 453). It is usually performed when coronary artery bypass graft surgery or percutaneous coronary intervention is being considered (p. 491).

Management

This should begin with a careful explanation of the problem and a discussion of the lifestyle and medical interventions that can be deployed to relieve symptoms and improve prognosis (Box 16.42). Anxiety and misconceptions often contribute to disability; for example, some patients avoid all forms of exertion because they believe that each attack of angina is a 'mini-heart attack' that results in permanent damage. Education and reassurance can dispel these misconceptions and make a huge difference to the patient's quality of life.

The principles of management involve:

- a careful assessment of the extent and severity of arterial disease
- identification and treatment of risk factors
- advice on smoking cessation
- introduction of drug treatment for symptom control
- identification of high-risk patients for treatment to improve life expectancy.

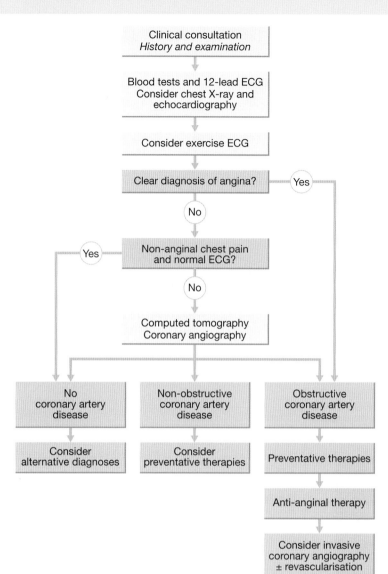

Fig. 16.55 **A scheme for the investigation and treatment of stable angina on effort.** This scheme is best adopted for patients without prior known coronary artery disease. For patients with known coronary artery disease, further stress imaging (echocardiography, radionuclide perfusion or magnetic resonance perfusion) rather than computed tomography coronary angiography is recommended.

Fig. 16.56 **Forms of exercise-induced ST depression.** A Planar ST depression is usually indicative of myocardial ischaemia. B Down-sloping depression also usually indicates myocardial ischaemia. C Up-sloping depression may be a normal finding.

16.42 Advice to patients with stable angina

- Do not smoke
- Aim for an ideal body weight
- Take regular exercise (exercise up to, but not beyond, the point of chest discomfort is beneficial and may promote collateral vessels)
- Avoid severe unaccustomed exertion, and vigorous exercise after a heavy meal or in very cold weather
- Take sublingual nitrate before undertaking exertion that may induce angina

All patients with angina secondary to CAD should receive antiplatelet therapy. Low-dose (75 mg) aspirin should be prescribed for all patients and continued indefinitely since it reduces the risk of MI. Clopidogrel (75 mg daily) is an equally effective alternative if aspirin causes dyspepsia or other side-effects. Similarly, all patients should be prescribed a statin, even if cholesterol is normal.

Anti-anginal drug therapy

The goal of anti-anginal therapy is to control symptoms using a regimen that is as simple as possible and does not cause side-effects. Five groups of drug can be used in the prevention and treatment of angina but there is little evidence that one group is more effective than another. It is conventional to start therapy with sublingual glyceryl trinitrate (GTN) and a β-blocker, and then add a calcium channel antagonist or a long-acting nitrate if needed. If the combination of two drugs fails to achieve an acceptable symptomatic response, revascularisation should be considered

Nitrates

Nitrates act directly on vascular smooth muscle to produce venous and arteriolar dilatation. Several preparations are available,

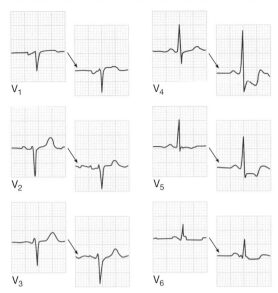

Fig. 16.57 A positive exercise test (chest leads only). The resting 12-lead ECG shows some minor T-wave changes in the inferolateral leads but is otherwise normal. After 3 minutes' exercise on a treadmill, there is marked planar ST depression in leads V_4 and V_5 (right-hand offset). Subsequent coronary angiography revealed critical three-vessel coronary artery disease.

Fig. 16.58 A myocardial perfusion scan showing reversible anterior myocardial ischaemia. The images are cross-sectional tomograms of the left ventricle. The resting scans (left) show even uptake of the [99]technetium-labelled tetrofosmin and look like doughnuts. During stress there is reduced uptake of technetium, particularly along the anterior wall (arrows), and the scans look like crescents (right).

i 16.43 Duration of action of some nitrate preparations		
Preparation	**Peak action**	**Duration of action**
Sublingual GTN	4–8 mins	10–30 mins
Buccal GTN	4–10 mins	30–300 mins
Transdermal GTN	1–3 hrs	Up to 24 hrs
Oral isosorbide dinitrate	45–120 mins	2–6 hrs
Oral isosorbide mononitrate	45–120 mins	6–10 hrs
(GTN = glyceryl trinitrate)		

as shown in Box 16.43. They help angina by lowering preload and afterload, which reduces myocardial oxygen demand, and by increasing myocardial oxygen supply through coronary vasodilatation. Sublingual GTN, administered from a metered-dose aerosol (400 μg per spray) or as a tablet (300 or 500 μg), is indicated for acute attacks and will usually relieve an attack in 2–3 minutes. Patients should also be encouraged to use the drug prophylactically before taking exercise that is liable to provoke symptoms. Sublingual GTN has a short duration of action and side-effects include headache, symptomatic hypotension and, rarely, syncope. A more prolonged therapeutic effect can be achieved by giving GTN transcutaneously as a patch (5–10 mg daily) or as a slow-release buccal tablet (1–5 mg 4 times daily). Isosorbide dinitrate (10–20 mg 3 times daily) and isosorbide mononitrate (20–60 mg once or twice daily) can be given by mouth, unlike GTN, which undergoes extensive metabolism in the liver. Headache is common with oral nitrates but tends to diminish if the patient perseveres with the treatment. Continuous nitrate therapy can cause pharmacological tolerance but this can be avoided by a 6–8-hour nitrate-free period, best achieved at night when the patient is inactive. If nocturnal angina is a predominant symptom, long-acting nitrates can be given at the end of the day.

Beta-blockers

These lower myocardial oxygen demand by reducing heart rate, BP and myocardial contractility, but they may provoke bronchospasm in patients with asthma. The properties and side-effects of β-blockers are discussed on page 500. In theory, non-selective β-blockers may aggravate coronary vasospasm by blocking coronary artery $β_2$-adrenoceptors, and so a once-daily cardioselective preparation such as slow-release metoprolol (50–200 mg daily) or bisoprolol (5–15 mg daily) is preferable. Beta-blockers should not be withdrawn abruptly, as rebound effects may precipitate dangerous arrhythmias, worsening angina or MI. This is known as the β-blocker withdrawal syndrome.

Calcium channel antagonists

These drugs lower myocardial oxygen demand by reducing BP and myocardial contractility. Since dihydropyridine calcium antagonists, such as nifedipine and amlodipine, may cause a reflex tachycardia, it is best to use them in combination with a β-blocker. In contrast, verapamil and diltiazem can be used as monotherapy because they slow SA node firing, inhibit conduction through the AV node and tend to cause bradycardia. They are particularly useful when β-blockers are contraindicated. Calcium channel antagonists reduce myocardial contractility and must be used with care in patients with poor LV function, since they can

16.44 Calcium channel antagonists used for the treatment of angina		
Drug	**Dose**	**Feature**
Nifedipine	5–20 mg 3 times daily*	May cause marked tachycardia
Nicardipine	20–40 mg 3 times daily	May cause less myocardial depression than the other calcium antagonists
Amlodipine	2.5–10 mg daily	Ultra-long-acting
Verapamil	40–80 mg 3 times daily*	Commonly causes constipation; useful anti-arrhythmic properties (p. 481)
Diltiazem	60–120 mg 3 times daily*	Similar anti-arrhythmic properties to verapamil

*Once- or twice-daily slow-release preparations are available.

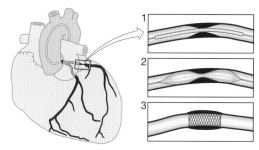

Fig. 16.59 Percutaneous coronary intervention. A guidewire is advanced from the radial (or femoral) artery to the coronary artery under radiographic control (1). A fine balloon catheter is then advanced over the guidewire to the stenotic coronary artery and the balloon is inflated to dilate the stenosis (2). When this has been achieved, a stent is usually placed at the site of the stenosis to maintain patency of the artery (3) (see text for more details).

aggravate or precipitate heart failure. Other unwanted effects include peripheral oedema, flushing, headache and dizziness (Box 16.44).

Potassium channel activators

Nicorandil (10–30 mg twice daily orally) is the only drug in this class that is currently available for clinical use. It acts as a vasodilator with effects on the arterial and venous systems, and has the advantage that it does not exhibit the tolerance seen with nitrates.

I_f channel antagonist

Ivabradine is the first of this class of drug. It induces bradycardia by modulating ion channels in the sinus node. It does not inhibit myocardial contractility and appears to be safe in patients with heart failure.

Ranolazine

This drug inhibits the late inward sodium current in coronary artery smooth muscle cells, with a secondary effect on calcium flux and vascular tone, reducing angina symptoms.

Non-pharmacological treatments

Percutaneous coronary intervention

Percutaneous coronary intervention (PCI) involves passing a fine guidewire across a coronary stenosis under radiographic control and using it to position a balloon, which is then inflated to dilate the stenosis (Fig. 16.59). This can be combined with deployment of a coronary stent, which is a piece of metallic 'scaffolding' that can be impregnated with drugs with antiproliferative properties and that helps to maximise and maintain dilatation of a stenosed vessel. The routine use of stents in appropriate vessels reduces both acute complications and the incidence of clinically important restenosis (Fig. 16.60).

Treatment with PCI often provides excellent symptom control but it does not improve survival in patients with chronic stable angina. It is mainly used in single- or two-vessel disease. Stenoses in bypass grafts can be dilated, as well as those in the native coronary arteries. The technique is often used to provide palliative therapy for patients with recurrent angina after coronary artery bypass grafting.

The main acute complications of PCI are occlusion of the target vessel or a side branch by thrombus or a loose flap of intima (coronary artery dissection), and consequent myocardial

damage. This occurs in about 2–5% of procedures and can often be corrected by deploying a stent, although emergency coronary artery bypass grafting may occasionally be required if stenting is unsuccessful. Minor myocardial damage, as indicated by elevation of sensitive intracellular markers (p. 497), occurs in up to 10% of cases. The main long-term complication of PCI is restenosis, in up to one-third of cases. This is due to a combination of elastic recoil and smooth muscle proliferation and tends to occur within 3 months. Stenting substantially reduces the risk of restenosis, probably because it allows the operator to achieve more complete dilatation. Drug-eluting stents reduce this risk further by allowing an antiproliferative drug, such as sirolimus or paclitaxel, to elute slowly from the coating and prevent neo-intimal hyperplasia and in-stent restenosis. These are especially indicated in diabetic patients, or in patients with long or calcific lesions, or small target-vessel diameter. Recurrent angina (affecting up to 5–10% of patients receiving an intracoronary stent at 6 months) may require further PCI or bypass grafting.

The risk of complications and the likely success of the procedure are closely related to the morphology of the stenoses, the experience of the operator and the presence of important comorbidity, such as diabetes and peripheral arterial disease. A good outcome is less likely if the target lesion is complex, long, eccentric or calcified, lies on a bend or within a tortuous vessel, involves a branch or contains thrombus.

Adjunctive therapy with a potent platelet inhibitor such as the P2Y12 receptor antagonists (clopidogrel, prasugrel or ticagrelor) in combination with aspirin and heparin improves the outcome following PCI.

Coronary artery bypass grafting

The internal mammary arteries, radial arteries or reversed segments of the patient's own saphenous vein can be used to bypass coronary artery stenoses (Fig. 16.61). This usually involves major surgery under cardiopulmonary bypass but, in some cases, grafts can be applied to the beating heart: 'off-pump' surgery. The operative mortality is approximately 1.5% but risks are higher in elderly patients, those with poor left ventricular function and those with significant comorbidity, such as renal failure.

Approximately 90% of patients are free of angina 1 year after coronary artery bypass grafting (CABG), but fewer than 60% of patients are asymptomatic after 5 or more years. Early post-operative angina is usually due to graft failure arising from technical problems during the operation, or poor 'run-off' due

Fig. 16.60 Primary percutaneous coronary intervention. A Acute right coronary artery occlusion. B Initial angioplasty demonstrates a large thrombus filling defect (arrows). C Complete restoration of normal flow following intracoronary stenting.

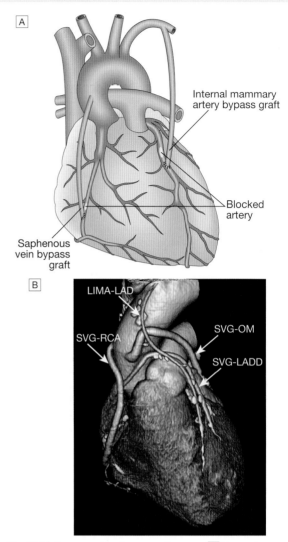

Fig. 16.61 Coronary artery bypass graft surgery. A Narrowed or stenosed arteries are bypassed using saphenous vein grafts connected to the aorta or by utilising the internal mammary artery. B Three-dimensional reconstruction of multidetector CT of the heart. The image shows the patent saphenous vein grafts (SVG) to the right coronary artery (RCA), obtuse marginal branch (OM) and diagonal branch (LADD), and left internal mammary artery graft (LIMA) to the left anterior descending (LAD) coronary artery.

to disease in the distal native coronary vessels. Late recurrence of angina may be caused by progressive disease in the native coronary arteries or graft degeneration. Fewer than 50% of vein grafts are patent 10 years after surgery. Arterial grafts have a much better long-term patency rate, however, with more than 80% of internal mammary artery grafts patent at 10 years. This has led many surgeons to consider total arterial revascularisation during CABG surgery. Aspirin (75–150 mg daily) and clopidogrel (75 mg daily) both improve graft patency, and one or the other

should be prescribed indefinitely. Intensive lipid-lowering therapy slows the progression of disease in the native coronary arteries and bypass grafts, and reduces clinical cardiovascular events. There is substantial excess cardiovascular morbidity and mortality in patients who continue to smoke after bypass grafting. Persistent smokers are twice as likely to die in the 10 years following surgery than those who give up at surgery.

Survival is improved by CABG in symptomatic patients with left main stem stenosis or three-vessel coronary disease when the LAD, CX and right coronary arteries are involved, or two-vessel disease involving the proximal LAD coronary artery. Improvement in survival is most marked in those with impaired left ventricular function or positive stress testing prior to surgery and in those who have undergone left internal mammary artery grafting.

Neurological complications are common, with a 1–5% risk of perioperative stroke. Between 30% and 80% of patients develop short-term cognitive impairment that typically resolves within 6 months. There are also reports of long-term cognitive decline that may be evident in more than 30% of patients at 5 years. PCI and CABG are compared in Box 16.45.

Prognosis

The prognosis of CAD is related to the number of diseased vessels and the degree of left ventricular dysfunction. A patient with single-vessel disease and good left ventricular function has a 5-year survival of more than 90%. In contrast, a patient with severe left ventricular dysfunction and extensive three-vessel disease has a 5-year survival of less than 30% unless revascularisation is performed. Symptoms are a poor guide to prognosis, since spontaneous improvement in angina due to the development of collateral vessels is common. Nevertheless, the 5-year mortality of patients with severe angina (CCS angina scale III or IV, see Box 16.40) is nearly double that of patients with mild symptoms.

i	16.45 Comparison of percutaneous coronary intervention (PCI) and coronary artery bypass grafting (CABG)		
		PCI	**CABG**
Death		<0.5%	<1.5%
Myocardial infarction*		2%	10%
Hospital stay		12–36 hrs	5–8 days
Return to work		2–5 days	6–12 weeks
Recurrent angina		15–20% at 6 months	10% at 1 year
Repeat revascularisation		10–20% at 2 years	2% at 2 years
Neurological complications		Rare	Common (see text)
Other complications		Emergency CABG Vascular damage related to access site	Diffuse myocardial damage Infection (chest, wound) Wound pain

*Defined as CK-MB >2× normal (p. 497).

16.46 Angina in old age

- **Incidence**: coronary artery disease increases in old age and affects women almost as often as men.
- **Comorbid conditions**: anaemia and thyroid disease are common and may worsen angina.
- **Calcific aortic stenosis**: common and should be sought in all older people with angina.
- **Atypical presentations**: when myocardial ischaemia occurs, age-related changes in myocardial compliance and diastolic relaxation can cause the presentation to be with symptoms of heart failure, such as breathlessness, rather than with chest discomfort.
- **Angioplasty and coronary artery bypass surgery**: provide symptomatic relief, although with increased procedure-related morbidity and mortality. Outcome is determined by the number of diseased vessels, severity of cardiac dysfunction and the number of concomitant diseases, as much as by age itself.

Acute coronary syndrome

Acute coronary syndrome is a term that encompasses both unstable angina and myocardial infarction. Unstable angina is characterised by new-onset or rapidly worsening angina (crescendo angina), angina on minimal exertion or angina at rest in the absence of myocardial damage. Myocardial infarction differs from unstable angina, since there is evidence of myocardial necrosis. The term acute myocardial infarction (MI) should be used when there is evidence of myocardial necrosis in a clinical setting consistent with acute myocardial ischaemia. Under these conditions, any one of the criteria shown in Box 16.47 fulfils the criteria for the diagnosis of an acute MI. The diagnosis of a previous MI can be made when any one of the features shown in Box 16.48 is present.

Acute coronary syndrome may present as a new phenomenon in patients with no previous history of heart disease or against a background of chronic stable angina. Approximately 12% of patients with acute coronary syndrome die within 1 month and 20% within 6 months of the index event. The risk markers that are indicative of an adverse prognosis include recurrent ischaemia, extensive ECG changes at rest or during pain, raised troponin I or T levels, arrhythmias and haemodynamic complications

i	16.47 Criteria for diagnosis of an acute myocardial infarction (MI)

- Detection of a rise and/or fall of cardiac biomarker values (preferably cardiac troponin (cTn)), with at least one value above the 99th centile upper reference limit (URL) and with at least one of the following:
  1. Symptoms of ischaemia
  2. New or presumed new significant ST segment–T wave (ST–T) changes or new left bundle branch block (LBBB)
  3. Development of pathological Q waves in the ECG
  4. Imaging evidence of new loss of viable myocardium or new regional wall motion abnormality
  5. Identification of an intracoronary thrombus by angiography or postmortem
- Cardiac death with symptoms suggestive of myocardial ischaemia and presumed new ischaemic ECG changes or new LBBB, but death occurred before cardiac biomarkers were obtained, or before cardiac biomarker values would be increased
- Percutaneous coronary intervention (PCI)-related MI is arbitrarily defined by elevation of cTn values (>5×99th centile URL) in patients with normal baseline values (≤99th centile URL) or a rise of cTn values >20% if the baseline values are elevated and are stable or falling. In addition, either (i) symptoms suggestive of myocardial ischaemia, or (ii) new ischaemic ECG changes, or (iii) angiographic findings consistent with a procedural complication, or (iv) imaging demonstration of new loss of viable myocardium or new regional wall motion abnormality are required
- Stent thrombosis associated with MI when detected by coronary angiography or postmortem in the setting of myocardial ischaemia and with a rise and/or fall of cardiac biomarker values with at least one value above the 99th centile URL
- Coronary artery bypass grafting (CABG)-related MI is arbitrarily defined by elevation of cardiac biomarker values (>10×99th centile URL) in patients with normal baseline cTn values (≤99th centile URL). In addition, either (i) new pathological Q waves or new LBBB, or (ii) angiographic documented new graft or new native coronary artery occlusion, or (iii) imaging evidence of new loss of viable myocardium or new regional wall motion abnormality is required

Adapted from Thygesen K, Alpert JS, Jaffe AS et al. Third universal definition of myocardial infarction. Eur Heart J 2012; 33:2551–2267.

16

(hypotension, mitral regurgitation) during episodes of ischaemia. Careful assessment and risk stratification are important because these guide the use of more complex pharmacological and interventional treatments (Figs 16.62 and 16.70), which can improve outcome (p. 501).

Pathogenesis

Acute coronary syndrome almost always occurs in patients who have atherosclerosis. The culprit lesion that precipitates the acute

	16.48 Criteria for diagnosis of a prior myocardial infarction

- Pathological Q waves with or without symptoms in the absence of non-ischaemic causes
- Imaging evidence of a region of loss of viable myocardium that is thinned and fails to contract, in the absence of a non-ischaemic cause
- Pathological findings of a prior myocardial infarction

Adapted from Thygesen K, Alpert JS, Jaffe AS et al. Third universal definition of myocardial infarction. Eur Heart J 2012; 33:2551–2267.

event is usually a complex ulcerated or fissured atheromatous plaque with adherent platelet-rich thrombus and local coronary artery spasm (see Fig. 16.54). These vascular changes during an acute coronary syndrome are dynamic, such that the degree of obstruction may either increase, leading to complete vessel occlusion, or regress due to the effects of platelet disaggregation and endogenous fibrinolysis. In acute MI, occlusive thrombus is almost always present at the site of rupture or erosion of an atheromatous plaque. The thrombus may undergo spontaneous lysis over the course of the next few days, although, by this time, irreversible myocardial damage has occurred. Without treatment, the artery responsible for the MI remains permanently occluded in 20–30% of patients. Since the process of infarction progresses over several hours (Fig. 16.63), most patients present when it is still possible to salvage myocardium and improve outcome.

Clinical features

The differential diagnosis of acute coronary syndrome is wide and includes most causes of central chest pain or collapse (p. 176). Chest pain at rest is the cardinal symptom but breathlessness, vomiting and collapse are also common features (Box 16.49).

1. Find points for each predictive factor

Killip class	Points	SBP (mmHg)	Points	Heart rate (beats/min)	Points	Age (years)	Points	Serum creatinine level (μmol/L)	Points	Other risk factors	Points
I	0	≤ 80	58	≤ 50	0	≤ 30	0	0–34	1		
II	20	80–99	53	50–69	3	30–39	8	35–70	4	Cardiac arrest at admission	39
III	39	100–119	43	70–89	9	40–49	25	71–105	7		
IV	59	120–139	34	90–109	15	50–59	41	106–140	10	ST-segment deviation	28
		140–159	24	110–149	24	60–69	58	141–176	13		
		160–199	10	150–199	38	70–79	75	177–353	21	Elevated cardiac enzyme levels	14
		≥ 200	0	≥ 200	46	80–89	91	≥ 353	28		
						≥ 90	100				

2. Sum points for all predictive factors

Killip class	+	SBP	+	Heart rate	+	Age	+	Creatinine level	+	Cardiac arrest at admission	+	ST-segment deviation	+	Elevated cardiac enzyme levels	=	Total points

3. Look up risk corresponding to total points

Total points	≤ 60	70	80	90	100	110	120	130	140	150	160	170	180	190	200	210	220	230	240	≥ 250
Probability of in-hospital death (%)	≤ 0.2	0.3	0.4	0.6	0.8	1.1	1.6	2.1	2.9	3.9	5.4	7.3	9.8	13	18	23	29	36	44	≥ 52

Examples

A patient has Killip class II, SBP of 99 mmHg, heart rate of 100 beats/min, is 65 years of age, has a serum creatinine level of 76 μmol/L, did not have a cardiac arrest at admission but did have ST-segment deviation and elevated enzyme levels. His score would be: 20 + 53 + 15 + 58 + 7 + 0 + 28 + 14 = 195. This gives about a 16% risk of having an in-hospital death.

Similarly, a patient with Killip class I, SBP of 80 mmHg, heart rate of 60 beats/min, who is 55 years of age, has a serum creatinine level of 30 μmol/L, and no risk factors would have the following score: 0 + 58 + 3 + 41 + 1 = 103. This gives about a 0.9% risk of having an in-hospital death.

Fig. 16.62 Risk stratification in the acute coronary syndrome: the GRACE score. Killip class refers to a categorisation of the severity of heart failure based on easily obtained clinical signs. The main clinical features are as follows: class I = no heart failure; class II = crackles audible halfway up the chest; class III = crackles heard in all the lung fields; class IV = cardiogenic shock. To convert creatinine in μmol/L to mg/dL, divide by 88.4. (SBP = systolic blood pressure) *From Scottish Intercollegiate Guidelines Network (SIGN) Guideline no. 93 – Acute coronary syndromes; February 2007.*

1 hour   4 hours   8 hours

■ Infarction   ■ Ischaemia

Fig. 16.63 The time course of myocardial infarction. The relative proportion of ischaemic, infarcting and infarcted tissue slowly changes over a period of 12 hours. In the early stages of myocardial infarction, a significant proportion of the myocardium in jeopardy is potentially salvageable.

✚ 16.49 Clinical features of acute coronary syndromes	
Symptoms	
• Prolonged cardiac pain: chest, throat, arms, epigastrium or back	• Nausea and vomiting
	• Breathlessness
• Anxiety and fear of impending death	• Collapse/syncope
Physical signs	
Signs of sympathetic activation	
• Pallor	• Tachycardia
• Sweating	
Signs of vagal activation	
• Vomiting	• Bradycardia
Signs of impaired myocardial function	
• Hypotension, oliguria, cold peripheries	• Third heart sound
	• Quiet first heart sound
• Narrow pulse pressure	• Diffuse apical impulse
• Raised jugular venous pressure	• Lung crepitations
Low-grade fever	
Complications	
• Mitral regurgitation	• Pericarditis

The pain occurs in the same sites as angina but is usually more severe and lasts longer; it is often described as a tightness, heaviness or constriction in the chest. In acute MI the pain can be excruciating, and the patient's expression and pallor may vividly convey the seriousness of the situation. Most patients are breathless and, in some, this is the only symptom. Painless or 'silent' MI may also occur and is particularly common in older patients or those with diabetes mellitus. If syncope occurs, it is usually caused by an arrhythmia or profound hypotension. Vomiting and sinus bradycardia are often due to vagal stimulation and are particularly common in patients with inferior MI. Nausea and vomiting may also be caused or aggravated by opiates given for pain relief. Sometimes infarction occurs in the absence of physical signs. Sudden death, from ventricular fibrillation or asystole, may occur immediately and often within the first hour. If the patient survives this most critical stage, the liability to dangerous arrhythmias remains, but diminishes as each hour goes by. It is vital that patients know not to delay calling for help if symptoms occur. Complications may occur in all forms of acute coronary syndrome but have become less frequent in the modern era of immediate or early coronary revascularisation. Specific complications of acute coronary syndromes and their management are discussed below.

ℹ 16.50 Common arrhythmias in acute coronary syndrome	
• Ventricular fibrillation	• Atrial tachycardia
• Ventricular tachycardia	• Sinus bradycardia (particularly
• Accelerated idioventricular	after inferior myocardial
rhythm	infarction)
• Ventricular ectopics	• Atrioventricular block
• Atrial fibrillation	

Arrhythmias

Arrhythmias are common in patients with acute coronary syndrome (Box 16.50) but are often transient and of no haemodynamic or prognostic importance. The risk of arrhythmia can be minimised by adequate pain relief, rest and the correction of hypokalaemia. VF occurs in 5–10% of patients who reach hospital and is thought to be the major cause of death in those who die before receiving medical attention. Prompt defibrillation restores sinus rhythm and is life-saving. The prognosis of patients with early VF (within the first 48 hours) who are successfully and promptly resuscitated is identical to that of patients who do not suffer VF. The presence of ventricular arrhythmias during the convalescent phase of acute coronary syndrome may be a marker of poor ventricular function and may herald sudden death. Selected patients may benefit from electrophysiological testing and specific anti-arrhythmic therapy (including ICDs, p. 483). AF is a common but frequently transient arrhythmia, and usually does not require emergency treatment. However, if it causes a rapid ventricular rate with hypotension or circulatory collapse, prompt cardioversion is essential. In other situations, digoxin or a β-blocker is usually the treatment of choice. AF may be a feature of impending or overt left ventricular failure, and therapy may be ineffective if heart failure is not recognised and treated appropriately. Anticoagulation is required if AF persists. Bradycardia may occur but does not require treatment unless there is hypotension or haemodynamic deterioration, in which case atropine (0.6–1.2 mg IV) may be given. Inferior MI may be complicated by AV block, which is usually temporary and often resolves following reperfusion therapy. If there is clinical deterioration due to second-degree or complete AV block, a temporary pacemaker should be considered. AV block complicating anterior infarction is more serious because asystole may suddenly supervene. A prophylactic temporary pacemaker should be inserted in these patients (p. 482).

Recurrent angina

Patients who develop recurrent angina at rest or on minimal exertion following an acute coronary syndrome are at high risk and should be considered for prompt coronary angiography with a view to revascularisation. Patients with dynamic ECG changes and ongoing pain should be treated with intravenous glycoprotein IIb/IIIa receptor antagonists. Patients with resistant pain or marked haemodynamic changes should be considered for intra-aortic balloon counterpulsation and emergency coronary revascularisation. Post-infarct angina occurs in up to 50% of patients treated with thrombolysis. Most patients have a residual stenosis in the infarct-related vessel, despite successful thrombolysis, and this may cause angina if there is still viable myocardium downstream. For this reason, all patients who have received successful thrombolysis should be considered for early (within the first 6–24 hours) coronary angiography with a view to coronary revascularisation.

16

Acute heart failure

Acute heart failure usually reflects extensive myocardial damage and is associated with a poor prognosis. All the other complications of MI are more likely to occur when acute heart failure is present. The assessment and management of heart failure is discussed in more detail on pages 463 and 465.

Pericarditis

This only occurs following infarction and is particularly common on the second and third days. The patient may recognise that a different pain has developed, even though it is at the same site, and that it is positional and tends to be worse or sometimes present only on inspiration. A pericardial rub may be audible. Opiate-based analgesia should be used. Non-steroidal (NSAIDs) and steroidal anti-inflammatory drugs may increase the risk of aneurysm formation and myocardial rupture in the early recovery period, and should be avoided.

Dressler's syndrome

This syndrome is characterised by persistent fever, pericarditis and pleurisy, and is probably due to autoimmunity. The symptoms tend to occur a few weeks or even months after MI and often subside after a few days. If the symptoms are prolonged or severe, treatment with high-dose aspirin, NSAIDs or even glucocorticoids may be required.

Papillary muscle rupture

This typically presents with acute pulmonary oedema and shock due to the sudden onset of severe mitral regurgitation. Examination usually reveals a pansystolic murmur and third heart sound but the murmur may be quiet or absent in patients with severe mitral regurgitation. The diagnosis is confirmed by echocardiography, and emergency valve replacement may be necessary. Lesser degrees of mitral regurgitation due to papillary muscle dysfunction are common and may be transient.

Ventricular septum rupture

This usually presents with sudden haemodynamic deterioration accompanied by a new and loud pansystolic murmur radiating to the right sternal border, which may be difficult to distinguish from acute mitral regurgitation. Rupture of the intraventricular septum causes left-to-right shunting through a ventricular septal defect, which tends to cause acute right heart failure rather than pulmonary oedema. Doppler echocardiography and right heart catheterisation will confirm the diagnosis. Treatment is by emergency surgical repair; without this, the condition is usually fatal.

Ventricular rupture

Rupture of the ventricle may lead to cardiac tamponade and is usually fatal (p. 544), although it is occasionally possible to support a patient with an incomplete rupture until emergency surgery can be performed.

Embolism

Thrombus often forms on the endocardial surface of freshly infarcted myocardium. This can lead to systemic embolism and occasionally causes a stroke or ischaemic limb. Venous thrombosis and pulmonary embolism may occur but have become less common with the use of prophylactic anticoagulants and early mobilisation.

Ventricular remodelling

This is a potential complication of an acute transmural MI due to thinning and stretching of the infarcted segment. This leads

Fig. 16.64 Infarct expansion and ventricular remodelling. Full-thickness myocardial infarction causes thinning and stretching of the infarcted segment (infarct expansion), which leads to increased wall stress with progressive dilatation and hypertrophy of the remaining ventricle (ventricular remodelling).

to an increase in wall stress with progressive dilatation and hypertrophy of the remaining ventricle (ventricular remodelling, Fig. 16.64). As the ventricle dilates, it becomes less efficient and heart failure may supervene. Infarct expansion occurs over a few days and weeks but ventricular remodelling can take years. ACE inhibitor and mineralocorticoid receptor antagonist therapies reduce late ventricular remodelling and can prevent the onset of heart failure (p. 465).

Ventricular aneurysm

Ventricular aneurysm develops in approximately 10% of patients with MI and is particularly common when there is persistent occlusion of the infarct-related vessel. Heart failure, ventricular arrhythmias, mural thrombus and systemic embolism are all recognised complications of aneurysm formation. Other features include a paradoxical impulse on the chest wall, persistent ST elevation on the ECG, and sometimes an unusual bulge from the cardiac silhouette on the chest X-ray. Echocardiography is diagnostic. Surgical removal of a left ventricular aneurysm carries a high morbidity and mortality but is sometimes necessary.

Investigations

Electrocardiogram

The standard 12-lead ECG is central to confirming the diagnosis but may be difficult to interpret if there is bundle branch block or previous MI. The initial ECG may be normal or non-diagnostic in one-third of cases. Repeated ECGs are important, especially where the diagnosis is uncertain or the patient has recurrent or persistent symptoms. The earliest ECG change is usually ST-segment deviation. With proximal occlusion of a major coronary artery, ST-segment elevation (or new bundle branch block) is seen initially, with later diminution in the size of the R wave and, in transmural (full-thickness) infarction, development of a Q wave. Subsequently, the T wave becomes inverted because of a change in ventricular repolarisation; this change persists after the ST segment has returned to normal. These sequential features (Fig. 16.65) are sufficiently reliable for the approximate age of the infarct to be deduced.

In non-ST segment elevation acute coronary syndrome, there is partial occlusion of a major vessel or complete occlusion of

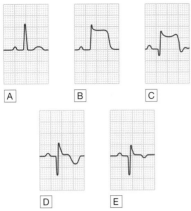

Fig. 16.65 The serial evolution of ECG changes in transmural myocardial infarction. [A] Normal ECG complex. [B] Acute ST elevation ('the current of injury'). [C] Progressive loss of the R wave, developing Q wave, resolution of the ST elevation and terminal T-wave inversion. [D] Deep Q wave and T-wave inversion. [E] Old or established infarct pattern; the Q wave tends to persist but the T-wave changes become less marked. The rate of evolution is very variable but, in general, stage B appears within minutes, stage C within hours, stage D within days and stage E after several weeks or months. This should be compared with the 12-lead ECGs in Figures 16.66–16.68.

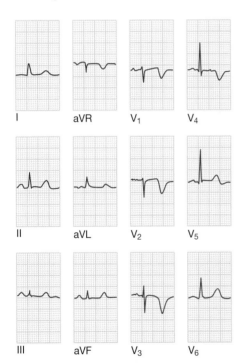

Fig. 16.66 Recent anterior non-ST elevation (subendocardial) myocardial infarction. This ECG demonstrates deep symmetrical T-wave inversion, together with a reduction in the height of the R wave in leads V_1, V_2, V_3 and V_4.

a minor vessel, causing unstable angina or partial-thickness (subendocardial) MI. This is usually associated with ST-segment depression and T-wave changes. In the presence of infarction, this may be accompanied by some loss of R waves in the absence of Q waves (Fig. 16.66).

The ECG changes are best seen in the leads that 'face' the ischaemic or infarcted area. When there has been anteroseptal infarction, abnormalities are found in one or more leads from

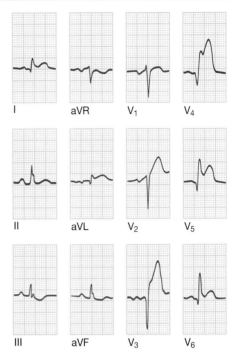

Fig. 16.67 Acute transmural anterior myocardial infarction. This ECG was recorded from a patient who had developed severe chest pain 6 hours earlier. There is ST elevation in leads I, aVL, V_2, V_3, V_4, V_5 and V_6, and there are Q waves in leads V_3, V_4 and V_5. Anterior infarcts with prominent changes in leads V_2, V_3 and V_4 are sometimes called 'anteroseptal' infarcts, as opposed to 'anterolateral' infarcts, in which the ECG changes are predominantly found in V_4, V_5 and V_6.

V_1 to V_4, while anterolateral infarction produces changes from V_4 to V_6, in aVL and in lead I. Inferior infarction is best shown in leads II, III and aVF, while, at the same time, leads I, aVL and the anterior chest leads may show 'reciprocal' changes of ST depression (Figs 16.67 and 16.68). Infarction of the posterior wall of the LV does not cause ST elevation or Q waves in the standard leads, but can be diagnosed by the presence of reciprocal changes (ST depression and a tall R wave in leads V_1–V_4). Some infarctions (especially inferior) also involve the RV. This may be identified by recording from additional leads placed over the right precordium.

Cardiac biomarkers

Serial measurements of serum troponin should be taken. In unstable angina, there is no detectable rise in troponin and the diagnosis is made on the basis of the clinical history and ECG changes. In contrast, MI causes a rise in plasma troponin T and I concentrations and other cardiac muscle enzymes (p. 450; Fig. 16.69 and see Box 16.47). Levels of troponins T and I increase within 3–6 hours, peak at about 36 hours and remain elevated for up to 2 weeks. A full blood count may reveal the presence of a leucocytosis, which reaches a peak on the first day. The erythrocyte sedimentation rate (ESR) and C-reactive protein (CRP) are also elevated. Lipids should be measured within 24 hours of presentation because there is often a transient fall in cholesterol in the 3 months following infarction.

Radiography

A chest X-ray should be performed since this may demonstrate pulmonary oedema that is not evident on clinical examination (see Fig. 16.27, p. 464). The heart size is often normal but

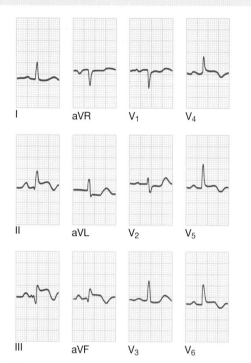

Fig. 16.68 Acute transmural inferolateral myocardial infarction. This ECG was recorded from a patient who had developed severe chest pain 4 hours earlier. There is ST elevation in inferior leads II, III and aVF and lateral leads V_4, V_5 and V_6. There is also 'reciprocal' ST depression in leads aVL and V_2.

Fig. 16.69 Changes in plasma cardiac biomarker concentrations after myocardial infarction. Creatine kinase (CK) and troponins T (Tn-T) and I (Tn-I) are the first to rise, followed by aspartate aminotransferase (AST) and then lactate (hydroxybutyrate) dehydrogenase (LDH). In patients treated with reperfusion therapy, a rapid rise in plasma creatine kinase (curve CK(R)) occurs, due to a washout effect.

there may be cardiomegaly due to pre-existing myocardial damage.

Echocardiography

Echocardiography is normally performed before discharge from hospital and is useful for assessing ventricular function and for detecting important complications, such as mural thrombus, cardiac rupture, ventricular septal defect, mitral regurgitation and pericardial effusion.

Coronary angiography

Coronary arteriography should be considered with a view to revascularisation in all patients at moderate or high risk of a further

16.51 Late management of myocardial infarction

Risk stratification and further investigation (see text)

Lifestyle modification
- Diet (weight control, lipid-lowering, 'Mediterranean diet')
- Cessation of smoking
- Regular exercise

Secondary prevention drug therapy
- Antiplatelet therapy (aspirin and/or clopidogrel)
- β-blocker
- ACE inhibitor/ARB
- Statin
- Additional therapy for control of diabetes and hypertension
- Mineralocorticoid receptor antagonist

Rehabilitation

Devices
- Implantable cardiac defibrillator (high-risk patients)

(ACE = angiotensin-converting enzyme; ARB = angiotensin receptor blocker)

event, including those who fail to settle on medical therapy, those with extensive ECG changes, those with an elevated plasma troponin and those with severe pre-existing stable angina (Fig. 16.70). This often reveals disease that is amenable to PCI or urgent CABG (see below).

Management

All patients with suspected acute coronary syndrome should be admitted urgently to hospital because there is a significant risk of death or recurrent myocardial ischaemia during the early unstable phase. Appropriate medical therapy can reduce the incidence of these complications by at least 60%. The key elements of immediate in-hospital management are shown in Figure 16.70. Patients should ideally be managed in a dedicated cardiac unit, where the necessary expertise, monitoring and resuscitation facilities are available. Clinical risk factor analysis using tools such as the GRACE score (see Fig. 16.62) should be performed to identify patients that should be selected for intensive therapy, and specifically early inpatient coronary angiography (thresholds vary, but a score of 140 points or more indicates early intervention). If there are no complications and risk factor analysis shows that angiography is not required, the patient can be mobilised from the second day and discharged after 2–3 days. Low-risk patients without spontaneous angina should undergo an exercise tolerance test approximately 4 weeks after the acute coronary syndrome. This will help to identify those individuals with residual myocardial ischaemia who require further investigation, and may help to boost the confidence of the remainder. Management of the acute event is discussed below and the principles of long-term management are summarised in Box 16.51.

Analgesia

Adequate analgesia is essential, not only to relieve distress but also to lower adrenergic drive and thereby reduce vascular resistance, BP, infarct size and susceptibility to ventricular arrhythmias. Intravenous opiates (initially, morphine sulphate 5–10 mg or diamorphine 2.5–5 mg) and antiemetics (initially, metoclopramide 10 mg) should be administered, and titrated by giving repeated small aliquots until the patient is comfortable. Intramuscular injections should be avoided because the clinical effect may be delayed by poor skeletal muscle perfusion, and a painful haematoma may form following thrombolytic or antithrombotic therapy.

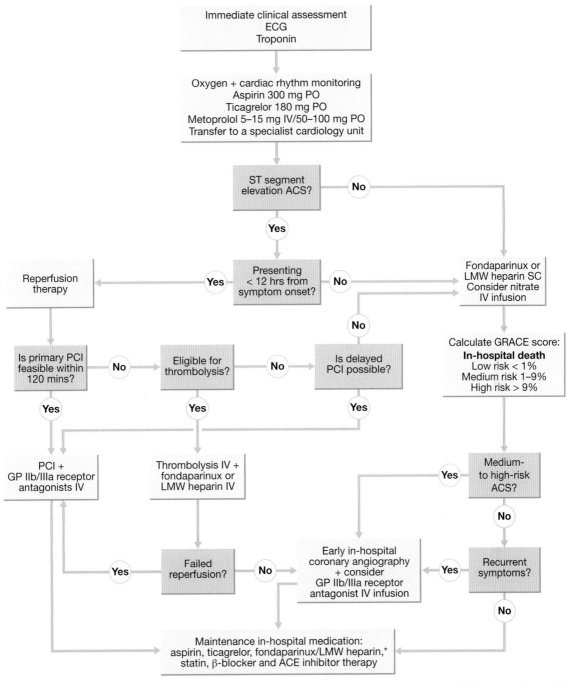

Fig. 16.70 Summary of treatment for acute coronary syndrome (ACS). *Not required following PCI. For details of the GRACE score, see Figure 16.62. (ACE = angiotensin-converting enzyme; ECG = electrocardiogram; GP = glycoprotein; IV = intravenous; LMW = low-molecular-weight; PCI = percutaneous coronary intervention; PO = by mouth; SC = subcutaneous) *Adapted from SIGN 93, Feb 2007, and updated in SIGN 148, April 2016.*

Reperfusion therapy

Immediate reperfusion therapy with PCI (see Fig. 16.60) is indicated when the ECG shows new bundle branch block or characteristic ST-segment elevation in two contiguous leads of 1 mm or more in the limb leads or 2 mm or more in the chest leads. This procedure has revolutionised the outcomes for these patients and is the treatment of choice for those presenting within 12 hours of symptom onset (Fig. 16.70). If PCI cannot be performed within 120 minutes for any reason, and thrombolysis is contraindicated, the procedure should be performed as soon as practically possible. Patients should be considered for PCI within the first 24 hours, even if they have reperfused spontaneously or with thrombolytic therapy. Coronary artery patency is restored in over 95% of patients undergoing PCI. The procedure preserves left ventricular function with a marked reduction in the progression to heart failure, more than halves rates of recurrent MI and dramatically improves mortality with more than 95% 1-year survival rates in clinical trials. Successful therapy is also associated with rapid pain relief, resolution of acute ST elevation and occasional transient arrhythmias.

Selected medium- to high-risk patients do benefit from in-hospital coronary angiography and coronary revascularisation but this does not need to take place in the first 12 hours unless there are high-risk features, such as ongoing chest pain or ECG changes. Reperfusion therapy with PCI confers no immediate mortality benefit in patients with non-ST segment elevation acute coronary syndrome.

Thrombolytic therapy

If primary PCI cannot be achieved in a timely manner (see Fig. 16.70), thrombolytic therapy should be administered. Although the survival advantage is not as good as primary PCI, mortality is reduced and this is maintained for at least 10 years. The benefit of thrombolytic therapy is greatest in those patients who receive treatment within the first 12 hours and especially the first 2 hours. Modern thrombolytic agents, such as tenecteplase (TNK) and reteplase (rPA), are analogues of human tissue plasminogen activator and can be given as an intravenous bolus, assisting prompt treatment in the emergency department or in the pre-hospital setting. The major hazard of thrombolytic therapy is bleeding. Cerebral haemorrhage causes 4 extra strokes per 1000 patients treated, and the incidence of other major bleeds is between 0.5% and 1%. Accordingly, the treatment should be withheld if there is a significant risk of serious bleeding (Box 16.52). For some patients, thrombolytic therapy is contraindicated or fails to achieve coronary arterial reperfusion (Fig. 16.70). Emergency PCI may then be considered, particularly where there is evidence of cardiogenic shock. Even where thrombolysis successfully achieves reperfusion, PCI should be considered within 24 hours to prevent recurrent infarction and improve outcome.

Antithrombotic therapy

Oral administration of 75–325 mg aspirin daily improves survival, with a 25% relative risk reduction in mortality. The first tablet (300 mg) should be given orally within the first 12 hours and therapy should be continued indefinitely if there are no side-effects. A P2Y12 receptor antagonist should be given in combination with aspirin for up to 12 months. The strongest evidence is for ticagrelor (180 mg, followed by 90 mg twice daily) but prasugrel (60 mg, followed by 10 mg daily) is an alternative. If the patient is intolerant of aspirin, clopidogrel is a suitable alternative (300 mg, followed by 75 mg daily). Glycoprotein IIb/IIIa receptor antagonists, such as tirofiban and abciximab, block the final common pathway of platelet aggregation and are potent inhibitors of platelet-rich thrombus formation. They are of particular benefit in high-risk patients with acute coronary syndromes who undergo PCI, especially those with a high thrombus burden at angiography or who have received inadequate prior antiplatelet therapy. These intravenous agents are administered in addition to oral aspirin and a P2Y12 inhibitor such as clopidogrel. Anticoagulation further reduces the risk of thromboembolic complications, and prevents re-infarction in the absence of reperfusion therapy or after

successful thrombolysis. Anticoagulation can be achieved using unfractionated heparin, fractioned (low-molecular-weight) heparin or a pentasaccharide such as subcutaneous fondaparinux (2.5 mg daily). Comparative clinical trials show that the pentasaccharides have the best safety and efficacy profile but low-molecular-weight heparin, such as subcutaneous enoxaparin (1 mg/kg twice daily), is a reasonable alternative. Anticoagulation should be continued for 8 days or until discharge from hospital or coronary revascularisation has been completed. A period of treatment with warfarin should be considered if there is persistent AF or evidence of extensive anterior infarction with mural thrombus because these patients are at increased risk of systemic thromboembolism.

Anti-anginal therapy

Sublingual glyceryl trinitrate (300–500 µg) is a valuable first-aid measure in unstable angina or threatened infarction, and intravenous nitrates (glyceryl trinitrate 0.6–1.2 mg/hr or isosorbide dinitrate 1–2 mg/hr) are useful for the treatment of left ventricular failure and the relief of recurrent or persistent ischaemic pain. Intravenous β-blockers (atenolol 5–10 mg or metoprolol 5–15 mg given over 5 mins) relieve pain, reduce arrhythmias and improve short-term mortality in patients who present within 12 hours of the onset of symptoms (Fig. 16.70). However, they should be avoided if there is heart failure (pulmonary oedema), hypotension (systolic BP < 105 mmHg) or bradycardia (heart rate < 65/min). Nifedipine or amlodipine can be added to the β-blocker if there is persistent chest discomfort but these drugs may cause tachycardia if used alone. Verapamil and diltiazem should be used if a β-blocker is contraindicated. In the longer term, treatment with an oral β-blocker reduces long-term mortality by approximately 25% among the survivors of an acute MI. Patients with heart failure, irreversible COPD or peripheral arterial disease derive similar, if not greater, secondary preventative benefits from β-blocker therapy and should receive maintenance therapy unless it is poorly tolerated. Unfortunately, a minority of patients do not tolerate β-blockers because of bradycardia, AV block, hypotension or asthma.

Renin–angiotensin blockade

Long-term treatment with ACE inhibitors such as enalapril (10 mg twice daily) or ramipril (2.5–5 mg twice daily) can counteract ventricular remodelling, prevent the onset of heart failure, improve survival, reduce recurrent MI and avoid rehospitalisation. The

---

16.52 Relative contraindications to thrombolytic therapy

- Active internal bleeding
- Previous subarachnoid or intracerebral haemorrhage
- Uncontrolled hypertension
- Recent surgery (within 1 month)
- Recent trauma (including traumatic resuscitation)
- High probability of active peptic ulcer
- Pregnancy

16.53 Myocardial infarction in old age

- **Atypical presentation**: often with anorexia, fatigue, weakness, delirium or falls rather than chest pain.
- **Case fatality**: rises steeply. Hospital mortality exceeds 25% in those over 75 years old, which is five times greater than that seen in those aged less than 55 years.
- **Survival benefit of treatments**: not influenced by age. The absolute benefit of evidence-based treatments may therefore be greatest in older people.
- **Hazards of treatments**: rise with age (for example, increased risk of intracerebral bleeding after thrombolysis) and are due partly to increased comorbidity.
- **Quality of evidence**: older patients, particularly those with significant comorbidity, were under-represented in many of the randomised controlled clinical trials that helped to establish the treatment of myocardial infarction. The balance of risk and benefit for many treatments, such as thrombolysis and primary percutaneous transluminal coronary angiography, in frail older people is uncertain.

benefits are greatest in those with overt heart failure (clinical or radiological) but extend to patients with asymptomatic left ventricular dysfunction and those with preserved left ventricular function. They should therefore be considered in all patients with acute coronary syndrome. Caution must be exercised in hypovolaemic or hypotensive patients because ACE inhibition may exacerbate hypotension and impair coronary perfusion. In patients intolerant of ACE inhibitors, ARBs such as valsartan (40–160 mg twice daily) or candesartan (4–16 mg daily) are alternatives and are better tolerated.

Mineralocorticoid receptor antagonists

Patients with acute MI and left ventricular dysfunction (ejection fraction <35%) and either pulmonary oedema or diabetes mellitus further benefit from additional mineralocorticoid receptor antagonism (eplerenone 25–50 mg daily, or spironolactone 25–50 mg daily).

Lipid-lowering therapy

The benefits of lowering serum cholesterol following acute coronary syndrome have been demonstrated in several large-scale randomised trials. All patients should receive therapy with HMG CoA reductase enzyme inhibitors (statins) after acute coronary syndrome, irrespective of serum cholesterol concentrations. Patients with serum LDL cholesterol concentrations above 3.2 mmol/L (approximately 120 mg/dL) benefit from more intensive therapy, such as atorvastatin (80 mg daily). Other agents, such as ezetimibe, fibrates, anion exchange resins and injectable PCSK9 inhibitors, may be used in cases where total cholesterol or LDL cholesterol cannot be lowered adequately using statins alone.

Smoking cessation

The 5-year mortality of patients who continue to smoke cigarettes is double that of those who quit smoking at the time of their acute coronary syndrome. Giving up smoking is the single most effective contribution a patient can make to his or her future. The success of smoking cessation can be increased by supportive advice and pharmacological therapy (p. 94).

Diet and exercise

Maintaining an ideal body weight, eating a Mediterranean-style diet, taking regular exercise, and achieving good control of hypertension and diabetes mellitus may all improve the long-term outlook.

Rehabilitation

The necrotic muscle of an acute myocardial infarct takes 4–6 weeks to be replaced with fibrous tissue and it is conventional to restrict physical activities during this period. When there are no complications, the patient can mobilise on the second day, return home in 2–3 days and gradually increase activity, with the aim of returning to work in 4 weeks. The majority of patients may resume driving after 1–4 weeks, although, in most countries, drivers of heavy goods and public service vehicles require special assessment before returning to work. Emotional problems, such as denial, anxiety and depression, are common and must be addressed. Some patients are severely and even permanently incapacitated as a result of the psychological effects of acute coronary syndrome rather than the physical ones, and all benefit from thoughtful explanation, counselling and reassurance. Many patients mistakenly believe that stress was the cause of their heart attack and may restrict their activity inappropriately. The patient's spouse or partner will also require emotional support,

information and counselling. Formal rehabilitation programmes, based on graded exercise protocols with individual and group counselling, are often very successful and, in some cases, have been shown to improve the long-term outcome.

Implantable defibrillators

ICDs are of benefit in preventing sudden cardiac death in patients who have severe left ventricular impairment (ejection fraction ≤30%) after MI (p. 483).

Prognosis

The prognosis of patients who have survived an acute coronary syndrome is related to the extent of residual myocardial ischaemia, the degree of myocardial damage and the presence of ventricular arrhythmias. In almost one-quarter of all cases of MI, death occurs within a few minutes without medical care. Half the deaths occur within 24 hours of the onset of symptoms and about 40% of all affected patients die within the first month. The prognosis of those who survive to reach hospital is much better, with a 28-day survival of more than 85%. Patients with unstable angina have a mortality of approximately half that of patients with MI. Early death is usually due to an arrhythmia and is independent of the extent of MI. However, late outcomes are determined by the extent of myocardial damage, and unfavourable features include poor left ventricular function, AV block and persistent ventricular arrhythmias. The prognosis is worse for anterior than for inferior infarcts. Bundle branch block and high cardiac marker levels both indicate extensive myocardial damage. Old age, depression and social isolation are also associated with a higher mortality. Of those who survive an acute attack, more than 80% live for a further year, about 75% for 5 years, 50% for 10 years and 25% for 20 years.

Non-cardiac surgery in patients with heart disease

Non-cardiac surgery, particularly major vascular, abdominal or thoracic surgery, can precipitate serious perioperative cardiac complications, such as MI and death, in patients with CAD and other forms of heart disease. Careful pre-operative cardiac assessment may help to determine the balance of benefit versus risk on an individual basis, and identify measures that minimise the operative risk (Box 16.54).

A hypercoagulable state is part of the normal physiological response to surgery, and may promote coronary thrombosis leading to an acute coronary syndrome in the early post-operative period. Patients with a history of recent PCI or acute coronary syndrome are at greatest risk and, whenever possible, elective non-cardiac surgery should be avoided for 3 months after such an event. Where possible, antiplatelet agents, statins and β-blocker therapies should be continued throughout the perioperative period.

| **i** | **16.54 Major risk factors for cardiac complications of non-cardiac surgery** |

- Recent (< 6 months) myocardial infarction or unstable angina
- Severe coronary artery disease: left main stem or three-vessel disease
- Severe stable angina on effort
- Severe left ventricular dysfunction
- Severe valvular heart disease (especially aortic stenosis)

Careful attention to fluid balance during and after surgery is particularly important in patients with impaired left ventricular function and valvular heart disease because vasopressin is released as part of the normal physiological response to surgery and, in these circumstances, the over-zealous administration of intravenous fluids can easily precipitate heart failure. Patients with severe valvular heart disease, particularly aortic stenosis and mitral stenosis, are also at increased risk because they may not be able to increase their cardiac output in response to the stress of surgery.

AF may be triggered by hypoxia, myocardial ischaemia or heart failure, and is a common post-operative complication in patients with pre-existing heart disease. It usually terminates spontaneously when the precipitating factors have been eliminated, but digoxin or β-blockers can be prescribed to control the heart rate.

Peripheral arterial disease

Peripheral arterial disease (PAD) has been estimated to affect about 20% of individuals aged 55–75 years in the UK. Only 25% of patients present with symptoms, the most common of which is intermittent claudication (IC). About 1–2% of patients with IC per year progress to a point where amputation and/or revascularisation are required. However, the annual mortality rate of people with IC is about 5%, which is 2–3 times higher than the general population of the same age and gender. The cause of death is typically an MI or stroke, reflecting the fact that IC nearly always occurs in association with widespread atherosclerosis.

Pathogenesis

In developed countries, almost all PAD is due to atherosclerosis and the risk factors are the same as described in patients with CAD. As with CAD, plaque rupture is responsible for the most serious manifestations of PAD, and not infrequently occurs in a plaque that hitherto has been asymptomatic. The clinical manifestations depend on the anatomical site, the presence or absence of a collateral supply, the speed of onset and the mechanism of injury (Box 16.55). Approximately 5–10% of patients with PAD have diabetes but this proportion increases to 30–40% in those with severe limb ischaemia. The mechanism of PAD in diabetes is atheroma affecting the medium-sized to large arteries rather than obstructive microangiopathy and so diabetes is not a contraindication to lower limb revascularisation. Nevertheless, diabetic patients with PAD pose a number of particular problems (Box 16.56).

Clinical features

Symptomatic PAD affects the legs about eight times more commonly than the arms. Several locations may be affected, including the aortoiliac vessels, the femoropopliteal vessels and the infrapopliteal vessels. One or more of these segments may be affected in a variable and asymmetric manner. In the arm, the subclavian artery is the most common site of disease. Peripheral artery disease can present clinically in a variety of ways, as detailed below.

Intermittent claudication

This is the most common presentation of PAD affecting the lower limbs. It is characterised by ischaemic pain affecting the muscles of the leg. The pain is usually felt in the calf because

	16.55 Factors influencing the clinical manifestations of peripheral arterial disease (PAD)

Anatomical site

Cerebral circulation
- TIA, amaurosis fugax, vertebrobasilar insufficiency

Renal arteries
- Hypertension and renal failure

Mesenteric arteries
- Mesenteric angina, acute intestinal ischaemia

Limbs (legs ≫ arms)
- Intermittent claudication, critical limb ischaemia, acute limb ischaemia

Collateral supply

- In a patient with a complete circle of Willis, occlusion of one carotid artery may be asymptomatic
- In a patient without cross-circulation, stroke is likely

Speed of onset

- Where PAD develops slowly, a collateral supply will develop
- Sudden occlusion of a previously normal artery is likely to cause severe distal ischaemia

Mechanism of injury

Haemodynamic
- Plaque must reduce arterial diameter by 70% ('critical stenosis') to reduce flow and pressure at rest. On exertion a moderate stenosis may become 'critical'. This mechanism tends to have a relatively benign course due to collateralisation

Thrombotic
- Occlusion of a long-standing critical stenosis may be asymptomatic due to collateralisation. However, acute rupture and thrombosis of a non-haemodynamically significant plaque usually has severe consequences

Atheroembolic
- Symptoms depend on embolic load and size
- Carotid (TIA, amaurosis fugax or stroke) and peripheral arterial (blue toe/finger syndrome) plaque are common examples

Thromboembolic
- Usually secondary to atrial fibrillation
- The consequences are usually dramatic, as the thrombus load is often large and occludes a major, previously healthy, non-collateralised artery suddenly and completely

(TIA = transient ischaemic attack)

the disease most commonly affects the superficial femoral artery, but it may be felt in the thigh or buttock if the iliac arteries are involved. Typically, the pain comes on after walking, often once a specific distance has been covered, and rapidly subsides on resting. Resumption of walking leads to a return of the pain. Most patients describe a cyclical pattern of exacerbation and resolution due to the progression of disease and the subsequent development of collaterals. When PAD affects the upper limbs, arm claudication may occur, although this is uncommon.

Critical limb ischaemia

Critical limb ischaemia (CLI) is defined as rest pain requiring opiate analgesia, and/or ulceration or gangrene that has been present for more than 2 weeks, in the presence of an ankle BP of less than 50 mmHg. The typical progression of symptoms in CLI is summarised in Figure 16.71. Rest pain only, with ankle pressures above 50 mmHg, is known as subcritical limb ischaemia (SCLI). The term severe limb ischaemia (SLI) is used to describe

i	16.56 Peripheral vascular disease in diabetes	
Feature	**Difficulty**	
Arterial calcification	Spuriously high ABPI due to incompressible ankle vessels. Inability to clamp arteries for the purposes of bypass surgery. Resistant to angioplasty	
Immunocompromise	Prone to rapidly spreading cellulitis, gangrene and osteomyelitis	
Multisystem arterial disease	Coronary and cerebral arterial disease increase the risks of intervention	
Distal disease	Diabetic vascular disease has a predilection for the calf vessels. Although vessels in the foot are often spared, performing a satisfactory bypass or angioplasty to these small vessels is a technical challenge	
Sensory neuropathy	Even severe ischaemia and/or tissue loss may be completely painless. Diabetic patients often present late with extensive destruction of the foot. Loss of proprioception leads to abnormal pressure loads and worsens joint destruction (Charcot joints)	
Motor neuropathy	Weakness of the long and short flexors and extensors leads to abnormal foot architecture, abnormal pressure loads, callus formation and ulceration	
Autonomic neuropathy	Leads to a dry foot deficient in sweat that normally lubricates the skin and is antibacterial. Scaling and fissuring create a portal of entry for bacteria. Abnormal blood flow in the bones of the ankle and foot may also contribute to osteopenia and bony collapse	

(ABPI = ankle–brachial pressure index)

✚	16.57 Symptoms AND signs of acute limb ischaemia	
Symptoms/signs	**Comment**	
Pain, Pallor, Pulselessness	May be absent in complete acute ischaemia, and can be present in chronic ischaemia	
Perishing cold	Unreliable, as the ischaemic limb takes on the ambient tempetature	
Paraesthesia, Paralysis	Important features of impending irreversible ischaemia	

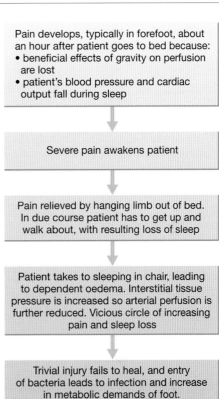

Fig. 16.71 Progressive night pain and the development of tissue loss.

16

the situation where either CLI and SCLI occurs. Whereas IC is usually due to single-segment plaque, SLI is always due to multilevel disease. Many patients with SLI have not previously sought medical advice, principally because they have other comorbidity that prevents them from walking to a point where IC develops. Patients with SLI are at high risk of losing their limb, and sometimes their life, in a matter of weeks or months without surgical bypass or endovascular revascularisation by angioplasty or stenting. Treatment of these patients is difficult, however, because most are elderly with extensive and severe disease and significant multisystem comorbidities.

Acute limb ischaemia

This is most frequently caused by acute thrombotic occlusion of a pre-existing stenotic arterial segment, thromboembolism, and trauma that may be iatrogenic. The typical presentation is with paralysis (inability to wiggle toes/fingers) and paraesthesia (loss of light touch over the dorsum of the foot/hand), the so-called 'Ps of acute ischaemia' (Box 16.57). These features are non-specific, however, and inconsistently related to its severity. Pain on squeezing the calf indicates muscle infarction and impending irreversible ischaemia. All patients with suspected acutely ischaemic limbs must be discussed immediately with a vascular surgeon; a few hours can make the difference between death/amputation and complete recovery of limb function. If there are no contraindications (acute aortic dissection or

trauma, particularly head injury), an intravenous bolus of heparin (3000–5000 U) should be administered to limit propagation of thrombus and protect the collateral circulation. Distinguishing thrombosis from embolism is frequently difficult but is important because treatment and prognosis are different (Box 16.58). Acute limb ischaemia due to thrombosis in situ can usually be treated medically in the first instance with intravenous heparin (target activated partial thromboplastin time (APTT) 2.0–3.0), antiplatelet agents, high-dose statins, intravenous fluids to avoid dehydration, correction of anaemia, oxygen and sometimes prostaglandins, such as iloprost. Embolism will normally result in extensive tissue necrosis within 6 hours unless the limb is revascularised. The indications for thrombolysis, if any, remain controversial. Irreversible ischaemia mandates early amputation or palliative care.

Atheroembolism

This may be a presenting feature of PAD affecting the subclavian arteries. The presentation is with blue fingers, which are due to

16.58 Distinguishing features of embolism and thrombosis in peripheral arteries		
Clinical features	**Embolism**	**Thrombosis**
Severity	Complete (no collaterals)	Incomplete (collaterals)
Onset	Seconds or minutes	Hours or days
Limb	Leg 3:1 arm	Leg 10:1 arm
Multiple sites	Up to 15%	Rare
Embolic source	Present (usually atrial fibrillation)	Absent
Previous claudication	Absent	Present
Palpation of artery	Soft, tender	Hard, calcified
Bruits	Absent	Present
Contralateral leg pulses	Present	Absent
Diagnosis	Clinical	Angiography
Treatment	Embolectomy, warfarin	Medical, bypass, thrombolysis
Prognosis	Loss of life > loss of limb	Loss of limb > loss of life

16.59 Clinical features of chronic lower limb ischaemia
• Pulses: diminished or absent • Bruits: denote turbulent flow but bear no relationship to the severity of the underlying disease • Reduced skin temperature • Pallor on elevation and rubor on dependency (Buerger's sign) • Superficial veins that fill sluggishly and empty ('gutter') on minimal elevation • Muscle-wasting • Skin and nails: dry, thin and brittle • Loss of hair

small emboli lodging in digital arteries. This may be confused with Raynaud's phenomenon (p. 1035) but the symptoms of atheroembolism are typically unilateral rather than bilateral as in Raynaud's.

Subclavian steal

This can be a feature of PAD affecting the upper limbs. The presentation is with dizziness, cortical blindness and/or collapse, which occurs when the arm is used and is thought to be caused by diversion (or steal) of blood from the brain to the limbs via the vertebral artery.

Investigations

The presence and severity of ischaemia can usually be determined by clinical examination (Box 16.59) and measurement of the ankle–brachial pressure index (ABPI), which is the ratio between the highest systolic ankle and brachial blood pressures. In health, the ABPI is over 1.0, in IC typically 0.5–0.9 and in CLI usually less than 0.5. Further investigation with duplex ultrasonography, MRI or CT with intravenous injection of contrast agents may be used to characterise the sites of involvement further. Intra-arterial digital subtraction angiography (IA-DSA) is usually reserved for those undergoing endovascular revascularisation. Other investigations should include a full blood count to look for evidence of treatable secondary causes, such as thrombocythaemia; measurement of

16.60 Medical therapy for peripheral arterial disease

• Smoking cessation
• Regular exercise (30 mins of walking, three times per week)
• Antiplatelet agent (aspirin 75 mg or clopidogrel 75 mg daily)
• Reduction of cholesterol:
    Statins
    Diet
    Weight loss
• Diagnosis and treatment of diabetes mellitus
• Diagnosis and treatment of associated conditions:
    Hypertension
    Anaemia
    Heart failure

lipids to check for evidence of hyperlipidaemia; and measurement of blood glucose to check for evidence of diabetes.

Management

Key elements of medical management are summarised in Box 16.60. This consists of smoking cessation (if applicable), taking regular exercise, antiplatelet therapy with low-dose aspirin or clopidogrel, therapy with a statin, and treatment of coexisting disease such as diabetes, hypertension or polycythaemia. Recently, the antiplatelet drug vorapaxar, a selective antagonist of the protease-activated receptor 1 (PAR-1) that regulates platelet activation, has been licensed in combination with either aspirin or clopidogrel in patients with PAD. The peripheral vasodilator cilostazol has been shown to improve walking distance and should be considered in patients who do not respond adequately to best medical therapy. Intervention with angioplasty, stenting, endarterectomy or bypass is usually considered only after medical therapy has been given at least 6 months to effect symptomatic improvement, and then just in patients who are severely disabled or whose livelihood is threatened by their disability. Subclavian artery disease is usually treated by means of angioplasty and stenting, as carotid–subclavian bypass surgery can be technically difficult.

Buerger's disease

Buerger's disease or thromboangiitis obliterans is an inflammatory disease of the arteries that is distinct from atherosclerosis and usually presents in young (20–30 years) male smokers. It is most common in those from the Mediterranean and North Africa. It characteristically affects distal arteries, giving rise to claudication in the feet or rest pain in the fingers or toes. Wrist and ankle pulses are absent but brachial and popliteal pulses are present. It may also affect the veins, giving rise to superficial thrombophlebitis. It often remits if the patient stops smoking. Symptomatic therapy with vasodilators such as prostacyclin and calcium antagonists or sympathectomy may also be helpful. Major limb amputation is the most frequent outcome if patients continue to smoke.

Raynaud's syndrome

This common disorder affects 5–10% of young women aged 15–30 years in temperate climates. It does not progress to ulceration or infarction, and significant pain is unusual. The underlying cause is unclear and no investigation is necessary. The patient should be reassured and advised to avoid exposure to cold. Usually, no other treatment is required, although

16.61 Atherosclerotic vascular disease in old age

- **Prevalence**: related almost exponentially to age in developed countries, although atherosclerosis is not considered part of the normal ageing process.
- **Statin therapy**: no role in the primary prevention of atherosclerotic disease in those over 75 years but reduces cardiovascular events in those with established vascular disease, albeit with no reduction in overall mortality.
- **Presentation in the frail**: frequently with advanced multisystem arterial disease, along with a host of other comorbidities.
- **Intervention in the frail**: in those with extensive disease and limited life expectancy, the risks of surgery may outweigh the benefits, and symptomatic care is all that should be offered.

16.62 Abdominal aortic aneurysm (AAA): common presentations

Incidental

- On physical examination, plain X-ray or, most commonly, abdominal ultrasound
- Even large AAAs can be difficult to feel, so many remain undetected until they rupture
- Studies are currently under way to determine whether screening will reduce the number of deaths from rupture

Pain

- In the central abdomen, back, loin, iliac fossa or groin

Thromboembolic complications

- Thrombus within the aneurysm sac may be a source of emboli to the lower limbs
- Less commonly, the aorta may undergo thrombotic occlusion

Compression

- Surrounding structures such as the duodenum (obstruction and vomiting) and the inferior vena cava (oedema and deep vein thrombosis)

Rupture

- Into the retroperitoneum, the peritoneal cavity or surrounding structures (most commonly the inferior vena cava, leading to an aortocaval fistula)

vasodilators such as nifedipine can may be helpful if symptoms are troublesome. More severe Raynaud's syndrome can also occur in association with digital ulceration in patients with connective tissue disease. This is discussed in more detail on page 1035.

Diseases of the aorta

Aortic aneurysm

Aortic aneurysm is defined to exist when there is an abnormal dilatation of the aortic lumen. The most common site is the infrarenal abdominal aorta. The suprarenal abdominal aorta and a variable length of the descending thoracic aorta may be affected in 10–20% of patients but the ascending aorta is usually spared. Abdominal aortic aneurysms (AAAs) affect men three times more commonly than women and are estimated to occur in about 5% of men over the age of 60 years.

Pathogenesis

The most common cause of aortic aneurysm is atherosclerosis, the risk factors for which have previously been described (p. 484). Genetic factors that predispose to hypertension, hyperlipidaemia and diabetes all play a role in the pathogenesis of aortic aneurysm but there appears to be an additional and specific genetic component since aortic aneurysm tends to run in families. This may explain in part why only some patients with risk factors for atheroma develop aneurysmal disease. Marfan's syndrome is an inherited disorder of connective tissue that is associated with aortic aneurysm and aortic dissection (p. 508). The features and management of this disorder are discussed on page 508.

Clinical features

The clinical presentation is dependent on the site of the aneurysm. Thoracic aneurysms may typically present with acute severe chest pain (p. 176) but other features, including aortic regurgitation, compressive symptoms such as stridor (trachea, bronchus), hoarseness (recurrent laryngeal nerve) and superior vena cava syndrome, may occur (Fig. 16.72A). If the aneurysm erodes into an adjacent structure, such as the oesophagus or bronchus, the presentation may be with massive bleeding. AAAs affect the infrarenal segment of the aorta. They can present in a number of ways, as summarised in Box 16.62. The usual age at presentation is 65–75 years for elective presentations and 75–85 years for emergency presentations.

Investigations

Ultrasound is the best way of establishing the diagnosis of an abdominal aneurysm and of following up patients with asymptomatic aneurysms that are not yet large enough to warrant surgical repair. In the UK, a national screening programme for men over 65 years of age has been introduced using ultrasound scanning. For every 10 000 men scanned, 65 ruptures are prevented and 52 lives saved. CT provides more accurate information about the size and extent of the aneurysm, the surrounding structures and the presence of any other intra-abdominal pathology. It is the standard pre-operative investigation but is not suitable for surveillance because of the high cost and radiation dose.

Management

The risks of surgery generally outweigh the risks of rupture until an asymptomatic AAA has reached a maximum of 5.5 cm in diameter. All symptomatic AAAs should be considered for repair, not only to rid the patient of symptoms but also because pain often predates rupture. Distal embolisation is a strong indication for repair, regardless of size, because otherwise limb loss is common. Most patients with a ruptured AAA do not survive to reach hospital, but if they do and surgery is thought to be appropriate, there must be no delay in getting them to the operating theatre to clamp the aorta.

Open AAA repair has been the treatment of choice in both the elective and the emergency settings, and entails replacing the aneurysmal segment with a prosthetic (usually Dacron) graft. The 30-day mortality for this procedure is approximately 5–8% for elective asymptomatic AAA, 10–20% for emergency symptomatic AAA and 50% for ruptured AAA. However, patients who survive the operation to leave hospital have a long-term survival approaching that of the normal population. Increasingly, endovascular aneurysm repair (EVAR), using a stent graft introduced via the femoral arteries in the groin, is

16

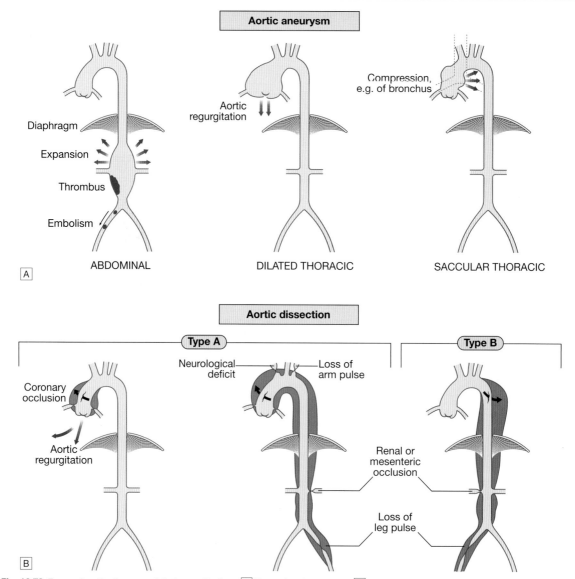

Fig. 16.72 Types of aortic disease and their complications. [A] Types of aortic aneurysm. [B] Types of aortic dissection.

replacing open surgery. It is cost-effective and likely to become the treatment of choice for infrarenal AAA. It is possible to treat many suprarenal and thoraco-abdominal aneurysms by EVAR too. If the aneurysm is secondary to Marfan's syndrome, treatment with β-blockers reduces the rate of aortic dilatation and the risk of rupture. Elective replacement of the ascending aorta may also be considered in patients with evidence of progressive aortic dilatation but carries a mortality of 5–10%.

Aortic dissection

Aortic dissection occurs when a breach in the integrity of the aortic wall allows arterial blood to enter the media, which is then split into two layers, creating a false lumen alongside the existing or true lumen (Fig. 16.72B). The aortic valve may be damaged and the branches of the aorta may be compromised. Typically, the false lumen eventually re-enters the true lumen, creating a double-barrelled aorta, but it may also rupture into

the left pleural space or pericardium with fatal consequences. The peak incidence is in the sixth and seventh decades but dissection can occur in younger patients, usually in association with Marfan's syndrome, pregnancy or trauma; men are affected twice as frequently as women.

Pathogenesis

The primary event is often a spontaneous or iatrogenic tear in the intima of the aorta; multiple tears or entry points are common. Other dissections are triggered by primary haemorrhage in the media of the aorta, which then ruptures through the intima into the true lumen. This form of spontaneous bleeding from the vasa vasorum is sometimes confined to the aortic wall, when it may present as a painful intramural haematoma. Aortic disease and hypertension are the most important aetiological factors but other conditions may also be implicated (Box 16.63). Chronic dissections may lead to aneurysmal dilatation of the aorta, and thoracic aneurysms may be complicated by dissection. It can therefore be difficult to identify the primary pathology.

Aortic dissection is classified anatomically and for management purposes into type A and type B (see Fig. 16.72B), involving or sparing the ascending aorta, respectively. Type A dissections account for two-thirds of cases and frequently also extend into the descending aorta.

Clinical features

Involvement of the ascending aorta typically gives rise to anterior chest pain, and involvement of the descending aorta to intrascapular back pain. The pain is typically described as 'tearing' and very abrupt in onset; collapse is common. Unless there is major haemorrhage, the patient is invariably hypertensive. There may be asymmetry of the brachial, carotid or femoral pulses and signs of aortic regurgitation. Occlusion of aortic branches may cause MI (coronary), stroke (carotid), paraplegia (spinal), mesenteric infarction with an acute abdomen (coeliac and superior mesenteric), renal failure (renal) and acute limb (usually leg) ischaemia.

i	16.63 Risk factors for aortic dissection

- Hypertension (in 80%)
- Atherosclerosis
- Coarctation
- Genetic:
  Marfan's syndrome
  Ehlers–Danlos syndrome
- Fibromuscular dysplasia
- Previous cardiac surgery:
  CABG
  Aortic valve replacement

- Pregnancy (usually third trimester)
- Trauma
- Iatrogenic:
  Cardiac catheterisation
  Intra-aortic balloon pumping

(CABG = coronary artery bypass grafting)

Investigations

The investigations of choice are CT or MR angiography (Figs 16.73 and 16.74), both of which are highly specific and sensitive. A chest X-ray should be performed. It characteristically shows broadening of the upper mediastinum and distortion of the aortic 'knuckle' but these findings are absent in 10% of cases. A left-sided pleural effusion is common. The ECG may show left ventricular hypertrophy in patients with hypertension or, rarely, changes

Fig. 16.73 Sagittal view of an MRI scan from a patient with long-standing aortic dissection, illustrating a biluminal aorta. There is sluggish flow in the false lumen (FL), accounting for its grey appearance. (TL = true lumen)

16

Fig. 16.74 Images from a patient with an acute type B aortic dissection that had ruptured into the left pleural space and was repaired by deploying an endoluminal stent graft. A CT scan illustrating an intimal flap (arrow) in the descending aorta and a large pleural effusion. B Aortogram illustrating aneurysmal dilatation; a stent graft has been introduced from the right femoral artery and is about to be deployed. C CT scan after endoluminal repair. The pleural effusion has been drained but there is a haematoma around the descending aorta. D Aortogram illustrating the stent graft. E Three-dimensional reconstruction of an aortic stent graft. E, Courtesy of Dr T. Lawton.

Fig. 16.75 Echocardiograms from a patient with a chronic aortic dissection. Colour flow Doppler shows flow from the larger false lumen (FL) into the true lumen (TL), characteristic of chronic disease.

of acute MI (usually inferior). Doppler echocardiography may show aortic regurgitation, a dilated aortic root and, occasionally, the flap of the dissection. TOE is particularly helpful because transthoracic echocardiography can provide images of the first 3–4 cm of the ascending aorta only (Fig. 16.75).

Management

The early mortality of acute dissection is approximately 1–5% per hour and so treatment is urgently required. Initial management comprises pain control and antihypertensive treatment. Type A dissections require emergency surgery to replace the ascending aorta. Type B aneurysms are treated medically unless there is actual or impending external rupture, or vital organ (gut, kidneys) or limb ischaemia, as the morbidity and mortality associated with surgery are very high. The aim of medical management is to maintain a mean arterial pressure (MAP) of 60–75 mmHg to reduce the force of the ejection of blood from the LV. First-line therapy is with β-blockers; the additional α-blocking properties of labetalol make it especially useful. Rate-limiting calcium channel blockers, such as verapamil or diltiazem, are used if β-blockers are contraindicated. Sodium nitroprusside may be considered if these fail to control BP adequately.

Percutaneous or minimal access endoluminal repair is sometimes possible and involves either 'fenestrating' (perforating) the intimal flap so that blood can return from the false to the true lumen (so decompressing the former), or implanting a stent graft placed from the femoral artery (see Fig. 16.74).

Aortitis

Syphilis is a rare cause of aortitis that characteristically produces saccular aneurysms of the ascending aorta containing calcification. Other rare conditions associated with aortitis include Takayasu's disease (p. 1041), reactive arthritis (p. 1031), giant cell arteritis (p. 1042) and ankylosing spondylitis (p. 1028).

Marfan's syndrome

Marfan's syndrome is an inherited disorder of connective tissue that is associated with a high risk of aortic aneurysm and dissection. It is inherited in an autosomal dominant manner but some cases are due to new mutations. It is a rare disorder that is estimated to affect about 0.02% of the population.

Marfan's syndrome is caused by protein-coding mutations affecting the *FBN1* gene, which encodes fibrillin, an extracellular matrix protein. The causal mutations disrupt the mechanical integrity of connective tissue, giving rise to a wide range of clinical features.

Clinical features

Aortic dissection and aneurysm are the most serious complications of Marfan's syndrome but many other clinical manifestations may be observed. These include aortic and mitral valve regurgitation; skin laxity and joint hypermobility; abnormalities of body habitus, including long arms, legs and fingers (arachnodactyly), scoliosis, pectus excavatum and a high-arched palate; ocular abnormalities, such as lens dislocation and retinal detachment; and an increased risk of pneumothorax.

Investigations

The diagnosis is usually suspected on the basis of the characteristic clinical features and can be confirmed by genetic testing. Imaging by chest X-ray may reveal evidence of aortic dilatation but echocardiography is more sensitive and can also demonstrate valvular disease, if present. Patients with Marfan's syndrome should undergo serial monitoring of the aortic root by echocardiography; if evidence of dilatation is observed, then elective surgery should be considered.

Management

Treatment with β-blockers reduces the risk of aortic dilatation and should be given in all patients with Marfan's syndrome. Activities that are associated with increases in cardiac output are best avoided. Surgery to replace the aortic root can be performed in patients with progressive aortic dilatation.

Coarctation of the aorta

Coarctation of the aorta is the term used to describe a narrowing distal to the origin of the left subclavian artery. It is most commonly due to congenital heart disease (p. 531), but narrowing of the aorta leading to similar symptoms can occur in other conditions such as Takayasu's arteritis (p. 1041) and trauma. Diagnosis and management of coarctation are discussed on page 534.

Hypertension

The risk of cardiovascular diseases such as stroke and CAD is closely related to levels of BP. BP follows a normal distribution in the general population and there is no specific cut-off above which the risk of cardiovascular risk suddenly increases. The diagnosis of hypertension is therefore made when systolic and diastolic values rise above a specific threshold that corresponds to the level of BP at which the risk of cardiovascular complications and benefits of treatment outweigh the treatment costs and potential side-effects of therapy. The British Hypertension Society classification, provided in Box 16.64, defines mild hypertension as existing when the BP is above 140/90 mmHg. Similar thresholds have been published by the European Society of Hypertension and the WHO–International Society of Hypertension. The cardiovascular risks associated with high BP depend on the combination of risk factors in an individual, such as age, gender, weight, physical activity, smoking, family history, serum cholesterol, diabetes mellitus and pre-existing vascular disease.

16.64 Definition of hypertension

Category	Systolic blood pressure (mmHg)	Diastolic blood pressure (mmHg)
Blood pressure		
Optimal	<120	<80
Normal	<130	85
High normal	130–139	85–89
Hypertension		
Grade 1 (mild)	140–159	90–99
Grade 2 (moderate)	160–179	100–109
Grade 3 (severe)	≥180	>110
Isolated systolic hypertension		
Grade 1	140–159	<90
Grade 2	≥160	<90

16.65 Causes of secondary hypertension

Alcohol

Obesity

Pregnancy

Renal disease
- Parenchymal renal disease, particularly glomerulonephritis
- Renal vascular disease
- Polycystic kidney disease

Endocrine disease
- Phaeochromocytoma
- Cushing's syndrome
- Primary hyperaldosteronism (Conn's syndrome)
- Glucocorticoid-suppressible hyperaldosteronism
- Hyperparathyroidism
- Acromegaly
- Primary hypothyroidism
- Thyrotoxicosis
- Congenital adrenal hyperplasia due to 11β-hydroxylase or 17α-hydroxylase deficiency
- Liddle's syndrome (p. 361)
- 11β-hydroxysteroid dehydrogenase deficiency

Drugs

Coarctation of the aorta

Pathogenesis

Many factors may contribute to the regulation of BP and the development of hypertension, including renal dysfunction, peripheral resistance, vessel tone, endothelial dysfunction, autonomic tone, insulin resistance and neurohumoral factors. In more than 95% of cases, however, no specific underlying cause of hypertension can be found. Such patients are said to have essential hypertension. Hypertension is more common in some ethnic groups, particularly African Americans and Japanese, and approximately 40–60% is explained by genetic factors. Age is a strong risk factor in all ethnic groups. Important environmental factors include a high salt intake, heavy consumption of alcohol, obesity and lack of exercise. Impaired intrauterine growth and low birth weight are associated with an increased risk of hypertension later in life. In about 5% of cases, hypertension is secondary to a specific disease, as summarised in Box 16.65.

Hypertension has a number of adverse effects on the cardiovascular system. In larger arteries (>1 mm in diameter), the internal elastic lamina is thickened, smooth muscle is hypertrophied and fibrous tissue is deposited. The vessels dilate and become tortuous, and their walls become less compliant. In smaller arteries (<1 mm), hyaline arteriosclerosis occurs in the wall, the lumen narrows and aneurysms may develop. Widespread atheroma develops and may lead to coronary

Fig. 16.76 Retinal changes in hypertension. **A** Grade 4 hypertensive retinopathy showing swollen optic disc, retinal haemorrhages and multiple cotton wool spots (infarcts). **B** Central retinal vein thrombosis showing swollen optic disc and widespread fundal haemorrhage, commonly associated with systemic hypertension. *A and B, Courtesy of Dr B. Cullen.*

and cerebrovascular disease, particularly if other risk factors are present. These structural changes in the vasculature often perpetuate and aggravate hypertension by increasing peripheral vascular resistance and reducing renal blood flow, thereby activating the renin–angiotensin–aldosterone axis (p. 461).

Clinical features

Hypertension is usually asymptomatic until the diagnosis is made at a routine physical examination or when a complication arises. Reflecting this fact, a BP check is advisable every 5 years in adults over 40 years of age to pick up occult hypertension. Sometimes clinical features may be observed that can give a clue to the underlying cause of hypertension. These include radio-femoral delay in patients with coarctation of the aorta (see Fig. 16.93, p. 534), enlarged kidneys in patients with polycystic kidney disease (p. 405), abdominal bruits that may suggest renal artery stenosis (p. 406), and the characteristic facies and habitus of Cushing's syndrome (Box 16.65). Examination may also reveal evidence of risk factors for hypertension, such as central obesity and hyperlipidaemia. Other signs may be observed that are due to the complications of hypertension. These include signs of left ventricular hypertrophy, accentuation of the aortic component of the second heart sound, and a fourth heart sound. AF is common and may be due to diastolic dysfunction caused by left ventricular hypertrophy or the effects of CAD.

Severe hypertension can cause left ventricular failure in the absence of CAD, particularly when there is an impairment of renal function. The optic fundi are often abnormal (see Fig. 16.76 below) and there may be evidence of generalised atheroma or

16

16.66 Hypertensive retinopathy

Grade 1

- Arteriolar thickening, tortuosity and increased reflectiveness ('silver wiring')

Grade 2

- Grade 1 plus constriction of veins at arterial crossings ('arteriovenous nipping')

Grade 3

- Grade 2 plus evidence of retinal ischaemia (flame-shaped or blot haemorrhages and 'cotton wool' exudates)

Grade 4

- Grade 3 plus papilloedema

16.67 How to measure blood pressure

- Use a machine that has been validated, well maintained and properly calibrated
- Measure sitting BP routinely, with additional standing BP in elderly and diabetic patients and those with possible postural hypotension; rest the patient for 2 minutes
- Remove tight clothing from the arm
- Support the arm at the level of the heart
- Use a cuff of appropriate size (the bladder must encompass more than two-thirds of the arm)
- Lower the pressure slowly (2 mmHg per second)
- Read the BP to the nearest 2 mmHg
- Use phase V (disappearance of sounds) to measure diastolic BP
- Take two measurements at each visit

specific complications, such as aortic aneurysm, PAD or stroke. Examination of the optic fundi reveals a gradation of changes linked to the severity of hypertension; fundoscopy can, therefore, provide an indication of the arteriolar damage occurring elsewhere (Box 16.66). 'Cotton wool' exudates are associated with retinal ischaemia or infarction, and fade in a few weeks (Fig. 16.76A). 'Hard' exudates (small, white, dense deposits of lipid) and microaneurysms ('dot' haemorrhages) are more characteristic of diabetic retinopathy (see Fig. 27.8, p. 1176). Hypertension is also associated with central retinal vein thrombosis (Fig. 16.76B).

Investigations

A decision to embark on antihypertensive therapy effectively commits the patient to life-long treatment, so readings must be as accurate as possible. The objectives are to:

- confirm the diagnosis by obtaining accurate, representative BP measurements
- identify contributory factors and any underlying causes
- assess other risk factors and quantify cardiovascular risk
- detect any complications that are already present
- identify comorbidity that may influence the choice of antihypertensive therapy.

Blood pressure measurements

BP measurements should be made to the nearest 2 mmHg, in the sitting position with the arm supported, and repeated after 5 minutes' rest if the first recording is high (Box 16.67). To avoid spuriously high readings in obese subjects, the cuff should contain a bladder that encompasses at least two-thirds of the arm circumference. Exercise, anxiety, discomfort and unfamiliar surroundings can all lead to a transient rise in BP. Sphygmomanometry, particularly when performed by a doctor, can cause a transient elevation in BP, which has been termed 'white coat' hypertension. It has been estimated that up to 20% of patients who are found to have raised BP at outpatient clinics have a normal BP when it is recorded by automated devices used at home. The risk of cardiovascular disease in these patients is less than that in patients with sustained hypertension but greater than that in normotensive subjects. If clinic BP measurements show borderline levels of BP or if white coat hypertension is suspected, then ambulatory measurement or home-based measurements may be of value in confirming the diagnosis.

Ambulatory blood pressure measurements

A series of automated ambulatory BP measurements obtained over 24 hours or longer provide a better profile than a limited

16.68 Investigation of hypertension

- Urinalysis for blood, protein and glucose
- Blood urea, electrolytes and creatinine
    Hypokalaemic alkalosis may indicate primary hyperaldosteronism but is usually due to diuretic therapy
- Blood glucose
- Serum total and HDL cholesterol
- Thyroid function tests
- 12-lead ECG (left ventricular hypertrophy, coronary artery disease)

(HDL = high-density lipoprotein)

number of clinic readings and correlate more closely with evidence of target organ damage than casual BP measurements. Treatment thresholds and targets (see Box 16.71 below) must be adjusted downwards, however, because ambulatory BP readings are systematically lower (approximately 12/7 mmHg) than clinic measurements. The average ambulatory daytime (not 24-hour or night-time) BP should be used to guide management decisions.

Home blood pressure measurements

Patients can measure their own BP at home using a range of commercially available semi-automatic devices. The value of such measurements is less well established and is dependent on the environment and timing of the readings measured. Home or ambulatory BP measurements are particularly helpful in patients with unusually labile BP, those with refractory hypertension, those who may have symptomatic hypotension, and those in whom white coat hypertension is suspected.

Other investigations

All hypertensive patients should undergo a limited number of investigations (Box 16.68) but additional investigations are appropriate in patients younger than 40 years of age or those with resistant hypertension (Box 16.69). Family history, lifestyle (exercise, salt intake, smoking habit) and other risk factors should also be recorded. A careful history will identify those patients with drug- or alcohol-induced hypertension and may elicit the symptoms of other causes of secondary hypertension, such as phaeochromocytoma (paroxysmal headache, palpitation and sweating, p. 675) or complications such as CAD.

Management

The objective of antihypertensive therapy is to reduce the incidence of adverse cardiovascular events, particularly CAD, stroke and heart failure. Randomised controlled trials have demonstrated that antihypertensive therapy can reduce the incidence of stroke and, to a lesser extent, CAD. The relative benefits (approximately 30% reduction in risk of stroke and 20% reduction in risk of CAD) are similar in all patient groups, so the absolute benefit of treatment (total number of events prevented)

---

i   16.69 Specialised investigation of hypertension

- Chest X-ray: to detect cardiomegaly, heart failure, coarctation of the aorta
- Ambulatory BP recording: to assess borderline or 'white coat' hypertension
- Echocardiogram: to detect or quantify left ventricular hypertrophy
- Renal ultrasound: to detect possible renal disease
- Renal angiography: to detect or confirm the presence of renal artery stenosis
- Urinary catecholamines: to detect possible phaeochromocytoma (p. 675)
- Urinary cortisol and dexamethasone suppression test: to detect possible Cushing's syndrome (p. 666)
- Plasma renin activity and aldosterone: to detect possible primary aldosteronism (p. 674)

---

is greatest in those at highest risk. For example, to extrapolate from the Medical Research Council (MRC) Mild Hypertension Trial (1985), 566 young patients would have to be treated with bendroflumethiazide for 1 year to prevent 1 stroke, while in the MRC trial of antihypertensive treatment in the elderly (1992), 1 stroke was prevented for every 286 patients treated for 1 year.

A formal estimate of absolute cardiovascular risk, which takes account of all the relevant risk factors, may help to determine whether the likely benefits of therapy will outweigh its costs and hazards. A variety of risk algorithms are available for this purpose, such as the Joint British Societies risk calculator (Fig. 16.77 and see 'Further information'). Most of the excess morbidity and mortality associated with hypertension are attributable to CAD and many treatment guidelines are therefore based on estimates of the 10-year CAD risk. Total cardiovascular risk can be estimated by multiplying CAD risk by 4/3 (i.e. if CAD risk is 30%, cardiovascular risk is 40%). The value of this approach can be illustrated by comparing the two hypothetical cases on page 487.

Intervention thresholds

Systolic BP and diastolic BP are both powerful predictors of cardiovascular risk. The British Hypertension Society management

Fig. 16.77 Example of cardiovascular risk prediction chart for non-diabetic men. Cardiovascular risk is predicted from the patient's age, sex, smoking habit, BP and cholesterol ratio. The ratio of total to high-density lipoprotein (HDL) cholesterol can be determined in a non-fasting blood sample. Where HDL cholesterol concentration is unknown, it should be assumed to be 1 mmol/L; the lipid scale should be used as total serum cholesterol. Current guidelines suggest initiation of primary prevention in individuals with a 10-year cardiovascular risk ≥20%. Patients with diabetes mellitus should be assumed to have a 10-year cardiovascular risk of ≥20% and receive secondary prevention therapy. Modified charts exist for women. For further details, see www.who.int/cardiovascular_diseases/guidelines/Pocket_GL_information.

- To estimate an individual's absolute 10-year risk of developing cardiovascular disease (CVD), choose the panel for the appropriate gender, smoking status and age. Within this, define the level of risk from the point where the coordinates for systolic blood pressure (SBP) and ratio of the total to HDL-cholesterol cross.
- Highest-risk individuals (red areas) are those whose 10-year CVD risk exceeds 20%, which is approximately equivalent to a 10-year coronary artery disease risk of >15%. As a minimum, those with CVD risk >30% (shown by the line within the red area) should be targeted and treated now. When resources allow, others with a CVD risk >20% should be targeted progressively.
- The chart also assists in identification of individuals with a moderately high 10-year CVD risk, in the range of 10–20% (orange area) and those in whom it is <10% (green area).
- Smoking status should reflect lifetime exposure to tobacco. For further information, see www.bhf.org.uk.

From Joint British Societies Cardiovascular Risk Prediction Chart, reproduced with permission from the University of Manchester.

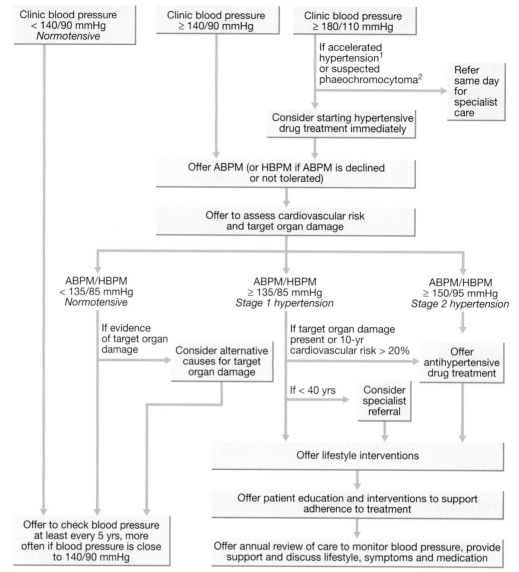

Fig. 16.78 Management of hypertension: British Hypertension Society guidelines. [1]Signs of papilloedema or retinal haemorrhage. [2]Labile or postural hypotension, headache, palpitations, pallor and diaphoresis. (ABPM = ambulatory blood pressure monitoring; HBPM = home blood pressure monitoring) *From NICE Clinical Guideline 127 – Hypertension in adults; August 2011.*

guidelines therefore utilise both readings, and treatment should be initiated if they exceed the given threshold (Fig. 16.78).

Patients with diabetes or cardiovascular disease are at particularly high risk and the threshold for initiating antihypertensive therapy is therefore lower (≥140/90 mmHg) in these patient groups. The thresholds for treatment in the elderly are the same as for younger patients (Box 16.70).

Treatment targets

The optimum BP for reduction of major cardiovascular events has been found to be 139/83 mmHg, and even lower in patients with diabetes mellitus. Moreover, reducing BP below this level causes no harm. The targets suggested by the British Hypertension Society (Box 16.71) are ambitious. Primary care strategies have been devised to improve screening and detection of hypertension that, in the past, remained undetected in up to half

16.70 Hypertension in old age

- **Prevalence**: hypertension affects more than half of all people over the age of 60 years (including isolated systolic hypertension).
- **Risks**: hypertension is the most important risk factor for myocardial infarction, heart failure and stroke in older people.
- **Benefit of treatment**: absolute benefit from therapy is greatest in older people (at least up to age 80 years).
- **Target blood pressure**: targets be relaxed in older people to 150/90 mmHg.
- **Tolerance of treatment**: antihypertensives are tolerated as well as in younger patients.
- **Drug of choice**: low-dose thiazides but, in the presence of coexistent disease such as gout or diabetes, other agents may be more appropriate.

Age	Clinic BP (mmHg)	Ambulatory or home BP (mmHg)[2]
<80 years	<140/90	<135/85
≥80 years	<150/90	<140/85

[1]Both systolic and diastolic values should be attained. [2]Average BP during waking hours.

of affected individuals. Application of new guidelines should help establish patients on appropriate treatment, and allow step-up if lifestyle modification and first-line drug therapy fail to control hypertension.

Patients taking antihypertensive therapy require follow-up at regular intervals to monitor BP, minimise side-effects and reinforce lifestyle advice.

Non-drug therapy

Appropriate lifestyle measures may obviate the need for drug therapy in patients with borderline hypertension, reduce the dose and/or the number of drugs required in patients with established hypertension, and directly reduce cardiovascular risk.

Correcting obesity, reducing alcohol intake, restricting salt intake, taking regular physical exercise and increasing consumption of fruit and vegetables can all lower BP. Moreover, stopping smoking, eating oily fish and adopting a diet that is low in saturated fat may produce further reductions in cardiovascular risk that are independent of changes in BP.

Drug therapy

Thiazides The mechanism of action of these drugs is incompletely understood and it may take up to a month for the maximum effect to be observed. An appropriate daily dose is 2.5 mg bendroflumethiazide or 0.5 mg cyclopenthiazide. More potent loop diuretics, such as furosemide (40 mg daily) or bumetanide (1 mg daily), have few advantages over thiazides in the treatment of hypertension, unless there is substantial renal impairment or they are used in conjunction with an ACE inhibitor.

ACE inhibitors ACE inhibitors (enalapril 20 mg daily, ramipril 5–10 mg daily or lisinopril 10–40 mg daily) are effective and usually well tolerated. They should be used with care in patients with impaired renal function or renal artery stenosis because they can reduce glomerular filtration rate and precipitate renal failure. Electrolytes and creatinine should be checked before and 1–2 weeks after commencing therapy. Side-effects include first-dose hypotension, cough, rash, hyperkalaemia and renal dysfunction.

Angiotensin receptor blockers ARBs (irbesartan 150–300 mg daily, valsartan 40–160 mg daily) have similar efficacy to ACE inhibitors but they do not cause cough and are better tolerated.

Calcium channel antagonists Amlodipine (5–10 mg daily) and nifedipine (30–90 mg daily) are effective and usually well-tolerated antihypertensive drugs that are particularly useful in older people. Side-effects include flushing, palpitations and fluid retention. The rate-limiting calcium channel antagonists (diltiazem 200–300 mg daily, verapamil 240 mg daily) can be useful when hypertension coexists with angina but may cause bradycardia. The main side-effect of verapamil is constipation.

Beta-blockers These are no longer used as first-line antihypertensive therapy, except in patients with another indication for the drug such as angina. Metoprolol (100–200 mg daily), atenolol (50–100 mg daily) and bisoprolol (5–10 mg daily), which preferentially block cardiac β_1-adrenoceptors, should be used rather than non-selective agents that also block β_2-adrenoceptors, which mediate vasodilatation and bronchodilatation.

Combined β- and α-blockers Labetalol (200 mg–2.4 g daily in divided doses) and carvedilol (6.25–25 mg twice daily) are combined β- and α-adrenoceptor antagonists that are sometimes more effective than pure β-blockers. Labetalol can be used as an infusion in malignant phase hypertension (see below).

Other vasodilators A variety of other vasodilators may be used. These include the α_1-adrenoceptor antagonists prazosin (0.5–20 mg daily in divided doses), indoramin (25–100 mg twice daily) and doxazosin (1–16 mg daily), and drugs that act directly on vascular smooth muscle, such as hydralazine (25–100 mg twice daily) and minoxidil (10–50 mg daily). Side-effects include first-dose and postural hypotension, headache, tachycardia and fluid retention. Minoxidil also causes increased facial hair and is therefore unsuitable for female patients.

Aspirin Antiplatelet therapy is a powerful means of reducing cardiovascular risk but may cause bleeding, particularly intracerebral haemorrhage, in a small number of patients. The benefits are thought to outweigh the risks in hypertensive patients aged 50 years or over who have well-controlled BP and either target organ damage or diabetes or a 10-year CAD risk of at least 15% (or 10-year cardiovascular disease risk of at least 20%).

Statins Treating hyperlipidaemia can produce a substantial reduction in cardiovascular risk. These drugs are strongly indicated in patients who have established vascular disease, or hypertension with a high (at least 10% in 10 years) risk of developing cardiovascular disease (p. 376).

Choice of antihypertensive drug

Trials that have compared thiazides, calcium antagonists, ACE inhibitors and ARBs have not shown consistent differences in outcome, efficacy, side-effects or quality of life. Beta-blockers, which previously featured as first-line therapy in guidelines, have a weaker evidence base. The choice of antihypertensive therapy is initially dictated by the patient's age and ethnic background, although cost and convenience will influence the exact drug and preparation used. Response to initial therapy and side-effects guide subsequent treatment. Comorbid conditions also have an influence on initial drug selection (Box 16.72); for example, a β-blocker might be the most appropriate treatment for a patient with angina. Thiazide diuretics and dihydropyridine calcium channel antagonists are the most suitable drugs for treatment in older people.

Combination therapy

Although some patients can be treated with a single antihypertensive drug, a combination of drugs is often required to achieve optimal control (Fig. 16.79). Combination therapy may be desirable for other reasons; for example, low-dose therapy with two drugs may produce fewer unwanted effects than treatment with the maximum dose of a single drug. Some drug combinations have complementary or synergistic actions; for example, thiazides increase activity of the renin–angiotensin system, while ACE inhibitors block it.

16

i 16.72 The influence of comorbidity on choice of antihypertensive drug therapy

Class of drug	Compelling indications	Possible indications	Caution	Compelling contraindications
α-blockers	Benign prostatic hypertrophy	–	Postural hypotension, heart failure[1]	Urinary incontinence
ACE inhibitors	Heart failure Left ventricular dysfunction, post-MI or established CAD Type 1 diabetic nephropathy Secondary stroke prevention[4]	Chronic renal disease[2] Type 2 diabetic nephropathy	Renal impairment[2] PAD[3]	Pregnancy Renovascular disease[2]
Angiotensin II receptor blockers	ACE inhibitor intolerance Type 2 diabetic nephropathy Hypertension with left ventricular hypertrophy Heart failure in ACE-intolerant patients, after MI	Left ventricular dysfunction after MI Intolerance of other antihypertensive drugs Proteinuric or chronic renal disease[2] Heart failure	Renal impairment[2] PAD[3]	Pregnancy
β-blockers	MI, angina Heart failure[5]	–	Heart failure[5] PAD Diabetes (except with CAD)	Asthma or chronic obstructive pulmonary disease Heart block
Calcium channel blockers (dihydropyridine)	Older patients, isolated systolic hypertension	Angina	–	–
Calcium channel blockers (rate-limiting)	Angina	Older patients	Combination with β-blockade	Atrioventricular block, heart failure
Thiazides or thiazide-like diuretics	Older patients, isolated systolic hypertension, heart failure, secondary stroke prevention	–	–	Gout[6]

[1]In heart failure when used as monotherapy. [2]ACE inhibitors or ARBs may be beneficial in chronic renal failure and renovascular disease but should be used with caution, close supervision and specialist advice when there is established and significant renal impairment. [3]Caution with ACE inhibitors and ARBs in PAD because of association with renovascular disease. [4]In combination with a thiazide or thiazide-like diuretic. [5]β-blockers are used increasingly to treat stable heart failure but may worsen acute heart failure. [6]Thiazides or thiazide-like diuretics may sometimes be necessary to control BP in people with a history of gout, ideally used in combination with allopurinol.
(ACE = angiotensin-converting enzyme; ARBs = angiotensin II receptor blockers; CAD = coronary artery disease; MI = myocardial infarction; PAD = peripheral arterial disease)

Refractory hypertension

Refractory hypertension refers to the situation where multiple drug treatments do not give adequate control of BP. Although this may be due to genuine resistance to therapy in some cases, a more common cause of treatment failure is non-adherence to drug therapy. Resistant hypertension can also be caused by failure to recognise an underlying cause, such as renal artery stenosis or phaeochromocytoma. There is no easy solution to problems with adherence but simple treatment regimens, attempts to improve rapport with the patient and careful supervision can all help. Spironolactone is a particularly useful addition in patients with treatment-resistant hypertension.

Accelerated hypertension

Accelerated or malignant hypertension is a rare condition that can complicate hypertension of any aetiology. It is characterised by accelerated microvascular damage with necrosis in the walls of small arteries and arterioles (fibrinoid necrosis) and by intravascular thrombosis. The diagnosis is based on evidence of high BP and rapidly progressive end-organ damage, such as retinopathy (grade 3 or 4), renal dysfunction (especially proteinuria) and/or hypertensive encephalopathy (see above). Left ventricular failure may occur and, if this is untreated, death occurs within months.

Management

In accelerated phase hypertension, lowering BP too quickly may compromise tissue perfusion due to altered autoregulation and can cause cerebral damage, including occipital blindness, and precipitate coronary or renal insufficiency. Even in the presence of cardiac failure or hypertensive encephalopathy, a controlled reduction to a level of about 150/90 mmHg over a period of 24–48 hours is ideal.

In most patients, it is possible to avoid parenteral therapy and bring BP under control with bed rest and oral drug therapy. Intravenous or intramuscular labetalol (2 mg/min to a maximum of 200 mg), intravenous GTN (0.6–1.2 mg/hr), intramuscular hydralazine (5 or 10 mg aliquots repeated at half-hourly intervals) and intravenous sodium nitroprusside (0.3–1.0 μg/kg body weight/min) are all effective but require careful supervision, preferably in a high-dependency unit.

Diseases of the heart valves

The heart valves allow forward movement of blood through the cardiac chambers when they are open and prevent backward flow when they are closed. Diseased valve may become narrowed, obstructing forward flow, or become leaky, causing backward flow or regurgitation. Breathlessness is a common symptom of valve disease, and acute severe breathlessness may be a presenting symptom of valve failure. The causes of this are shown in Box 16.73. Predisposition to valvular disease may be genetically determined, can arise as the result of rheumatic fever or infections, or can occur in association with dilatation of

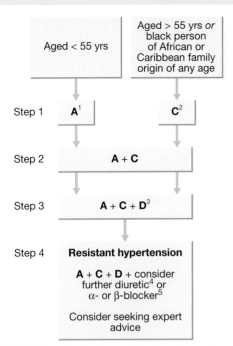

Fig. 16.79 **Antihypertensive drug combinations.** Black patients are those of African or Caribbean descent and not mixed-race, Asian or Chinese patients. [1]A = Angiotensin-converting enzyme (ACE) inhibitor or consider angiotensin II receptor blocker (ARB); choose a low-cost ARB. [2]C = calcium channel blocker (CCB); a CCB is preferred but consider a thiazide-like diuretic if a CCB is not tolerated or the person has oedema, evidence of heart failure or a high risk of heart failure. [3]D = thiazide-type diuretic. [4]Consider a low dose of spironolactone or higher doses of a thiazide-like diuretic. At the time of publication by NICE (August 2011), spironolactone did not have a UK marketing authorisation for this indication. Informed consent should be obtained and documented. [5]Consider an α- or β-blocker if further diuretic therapy is not tolerated, or is contraindicated or ineffective. *From NICE Clinical Guideline 127 – Hypertension in adults; August 2011.*

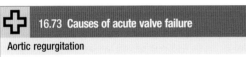

16.73 Causes of acute valve failure

Aortic regurgitation

- Aortic dissection
- Infective endocarditis

Mitral regurgitation

- Papillary muscle rupture due to acute myocardial infarction
- Infective endocarditis
- Rupture of chordae due to myxomatous degeneration

Prosthetic valve failure

- Mechanical valves: fracture, jamming, thrombosis, dehiscence
- Biological valves: degeneration with cusp tear

---

the cardiac chambers in heart failure. The principal causes of valvular disease are summarised in Box 16.74.

Rheumatic heart disease

Acute rheumatic fever

Acute rheumatic fever usually affects children and young adults between the ages of 5 and 15 years. It is now rare in high-income countries in Western Europe and North America, where the

16.74 Principal causes of valve disease

Valve regurgitation

- Congenital
- Acute rheumatic carditis
- Chronic rheumatic carditis
- Infective endocarditis
- Cardiac failure*

- Syphilitic aortitis
- Traumatic valve rupture
- Senile degeneration
- Damage to chordae and papillary muscles

Valve stenosis

- Congenital
- Rheumatic carditis

- Senile degeneration

*Causes dilatation of the valve ring.

---

incidence is about 0.5 cases per 100 000, but remains endemic in the Indian subcontinent, Africa and South America. Recent studies indicate that the current incidence of rheumatic heart disease in India ranges between 13 and 150 cases per 100 000 population per year and it is by far the most common cause of acquired heart disease in childhood and adolescence in that country.

Pathogenesis

The condition is triggered by an immune-mediated delayed response to infection with specific strains of group A streptococci, which have antigens that cross-react with cardiac myosin and sarcolemmal membrane proteins. Antibodies produced against the streptococcal antigens cause inflammation in the endocardium, myocardium and pericardium, as well as the joints and skin. Histologically, fibrinoid degeneration is seen in the collagen of connective tissues. Aschoff nodules are pathognomonic and occur only in the heart. They are composed of multinucleated giant cells surrounded by macrophages and T lymphocytes, and are not seen until the subacute or chronic phases of rheumatic carditis.

Clinical features

Acute rheumatic fever is a multisystem disorder that usually presents with fever, anorexia, lethargy and joint pain, 2–3 weeks after an episode of streptococcal pharyngitis. There may be no history of sore throat, however. Arthritis occurs in approximately 75% of patients. Other features include rashes, subcutaneous nodules, carditis and neurological changes (Fig. 16.80). The diagnosis, made using the revised Jones criteria (Box 16.75), is based on two or more major manifestations, or one major and two or more minor manifestations, along with evidence of preceding streptococcal infection. A presumptive diagnosis of acute rheumatic fever can be made without evidence of preceding streptococcal infection in cases of isolated chorea or pancarditis, if other causes of these have been excluded. In cases of established rheumatic heart disease or prior rheumatic fever, a diagnosis of acute rheumatic fever can be made based only on the presence of multiple minor criteria and evidence of preceding group A streptococcal pharyngitis.

Carditis

Rheumatic fever causes a pancarditis involving the endocardium, myocardium and pericardium to varying degrees. Its incidence declines with increasing age, ranging from 90% at 3 years to around 30% in adolescence. It may manifest as breathlessness (due to heart failure or pericardial effusion), palpitations or chest pain (usually due to pericarditis or pancarditis). Other features include tachycardia, cardiac enlargement and new or changed

Sydenham's chorea
St Vitus dance

Prior sore throat

Carditis
Dyspnoea (CCF)
Syncope
Pericarditis (pain, rub)
Carey Coombs murmur
Aortic or mitral
regurgitation
Heart block

**Subcutaneous
nodules** (over bones
or tendons)

Fever
39° C
38° C
37° C

**Flitting
polyarthritis**
+ arthralgia

Oedema
(heart failure)

Erythema marginatum

Fig. 16.80 Clinical features of rheumatic fever. Bold labels indicate Jones major criteria. (CCF = congestive cardiac failure) *Inset (Erythema marginatum) From Savin JA, Hunter JAA, Hepburn NC. Skin signs in clinical medicine. London: Mosby–Wolfe, Elsevier; 1997.*

---

i | 16.75 Jones criteria for the diagnosis of rheumatic fever

Major manifestations

- Carditis
- Polyarthritis
- Chorea
- Erythema marginatum
- Subcutaneous nodules

Minor manifestations

- Fever
- Arthralgia
- Raised erythrocyte sedimentation rate or C-reactive protein
- Previous rheumatic fever
- Leucocytosis
- First-degree atrioventricular block

Plus

- Supporting evidence of preceding streptococcal infection: recent scarlet fever, raised antistreptolysin O or other streptococcal antibody titre, positive throat culture*

*Evidence of recent streptococcal infection is particularly important if there is only one major manifestation.

---

murmurs. A soft systolic murmur due to mitral regurgitation is very common. A soft mid-diastolic murmur (the Carey Coombs murmur) is typically due to valvulitis, with nodules forming on the mitral valve leaflets. Aortic regurgitation occurs in 50% of cases but the tricuspid and pulmonary valves are rarely involved. Pericarditis may cause chest pain, a pericardial friction rub and precordial tenderness. Cardiac failure may be due to myocardial dysfunction or valvular regurgitation. ECG evidence commonly includes ST and T wave changes. Conduction defects, including AV block, sometimes occur and may cause syncope.

Arthritis

This is the most common major manifestation and occurs early when streptococcal antibody titres are high. An acute painful, asymmetric and migratory inflammation of the large joints typically affects the knees, ankles, elbows and wrists. The joints are involved in quick succession and are usually red, swollen and tender for between a day and 4 weeks.

Skin lesions

Erythema marginatum occurs in less than 5% of patients. The lesions start as red macules that fade in the centre but remain red at the edges, and occur mainly on the trunk and proximal extremities but not the face. The resulting red rings or 'margins' may coalesce or overlap (Fig. 16.80). Subcutaneous nodules occur in 5–7% of patients. They are small (0.5–2.0 cm), firm and painless, and are best felt over extensor surfaces of bone or tendons. They typically appear more than 3 weeks after the onset of other manifestations and therefore help to confirm rather than make the diagnosis.

Sydenham's chorea

Sydenham's chorea, also known as St Vitus dance, is a late neurological manifestation that appears at least 3 months after the episode of acute rheumatic fever, when all the other signs may have disappeared. It occurs in up to one-third of cases and is more common in females. Emotional lability may be the first feature and is typically followed by purposeless, involuntary, choreiform movements of the hands, feet or face. Speech may be explosive and halting. Spontaneous recovery usually occurs within a few months. Approximately one-quarter of affected patients will go on to develop chronic rheumatic valve disease.

Other features

Other systemic manifestations, such as pleurisy, pleural effusion and pneumonia, may occur but are rare.

Investigations

Blood should be taken for measurement of ESR and CRP since these are useful for monitoring progress of the disease (Box 16.76). Throat cultures should be taken but positive results are obtained in only 10–25% of cases since the infection has often resolved by the time of presentation. Serology for antistreptolysin O antibodies (ASO) should be performed. Raised levels provide supportive evidence for the diagnosis but are normal in one-fifth of adult cases of rheumatic fever and most cases of chorea. Echocardiography should be carried out and typically shows mitral regurgitation with dilatation of the mitral annulus and prolapse of the anterior mitral leaflet; it may also demonstrate aortic regurgitation and pericardial effusion.

Management

The aims of management are to limit cardiac damage and relieve symptoms.

Bed rest

Bed rest is important, as it lessens joint pain and reduces cardiac workload. The duration should be guided by symptoms, along with temperature, leucocyte count and ESR, and should be continued until these have settled. Patients can then return to normal physical activity but strenuous exercise should be avoided in those who have had carditis.

Treatment of cardiac failure

Cardiac failure should be treated as necessary. Some patients, particularly those in early adolescence, can develop a fulminant form of the disease with severe mitral regurgitation and, sometimes, concomitant aortic regurgitation. If heart failure in these cases

16.76 Investigations in acute rheumatic fever

Evidence of a systemic illness

- Leucocytosis, raised erythrocyte sedimentation rate and C-reactive protein

Evidence of preceding streptococcal infection

- Throat swab culture: group A β-haemolytic streptococci (also from family members and contacts)
- Antistreptolysin O antibodies (ASO titres): rising titres, or levels of >200 U (adults) or >300 U (children)

Evidence of carditis

- Chest X-ray: cardiomegaly; pulmonary congestion
- ECG: first- and, rarely, second-degree atrioventricular block; features of pericarditis; T-wave inversion; reduction in QRS voltages
- Echocardiography: cardiac dilatation and valve abnormalities

does not respond to medical treatment, valve replacement may be necessary and is often associated with a dramatic decline in rheumatic activity. Occasionally, AV block may occur but is seldom progressive and usually resolves spontaneously. Rarely, pacemaker insertion may be required.

Antibiotics

A single dose of benzathine benzylpenicillin (1.2 million U IM) or oral phenoxymethylpenicillin (250 mg 4 times daily for 10 days) should be given on diagnosis to eliminate any residual streptococcal infection. If the patient is penicillin-allergic, erythromycin or a cephalosporin can be used. Patients are susceptible to further attacks of rheumatic fever if another streptococcal infection occurs, and long-term prophylaxis with penicillin should be given with oral phenoxymethylpenicillin (250 mg twice daily) or as benzathine benzylpenicillin (1.2 million U IM monthly), if adherence is in doubt. Sulfadiazine or erythromycin may be used if the patient is allergic to penicillin; sulphonamides prevent infection but are not effective in the eradication of group A streptococci. Further attacks of rheumatic fever are unusual after the age of 21, when antibiotic treatment can usually be stopped. The duration of prophylaxis should be extended if an attack has occurred in the last 5 years, or if the patient lives in an area of high prevalence and has an occupation (such as teaching) with a high risk of exposure to streptococcal infection. In those with residual heart disease, prophylaxis should continue until 10 years after the last episode or 40 years of age, whichever is later. While long-term antibiotic prophylaxis prevents further attacks of acute rheumatic fever, it does not protect against infective endocarditis.

Aspirin

This usually relieves the symptoms of arthritis rapidly and a response within 24 hours helps confirm the diagnosis. A reasonable starting dose is 60 mg/kg body weight/day, divided into six doses. In adults, 100 mg/kg per day may be needed up to the limits of tolerance or a maximum of 8 g per day. Mild toxicity includes nausea, tinnitus and deafness; vomiting, tachypnoea and acidosis are more serious. Aspirin should be continued until the ESR has fallen and then gradually tailed off.

Glucocorticoids

These produce more rapid symptomatic relief than aspirin and are indicated in cases with carditis or severe arthritis. There is no evidence that long-term steroids are beneficial. Prednisolone

(1.0–2.0 mg/kg per day in divided doses) should be continued until the ESR is normal and then tailed off.

Chronic rheumatic heart disease

Chronic valvular heart disease develops in at least half of those affected by rheumatic fever with carditis. Two-thirds of cases occur in women. Some episodes of rheumatic fever pass unrecognised and it is possible to elicit a history of rheumatic fever or chorea in only about half of all patients with chronic rheumatic heart disease.

The mitral valve is affected in more than 90% of cases; the aortic valve is the next most frequently involved, followed by the tricuspid and then the pulmonary valve. Isolated mitral stenosis accounts for about 25% of all cases, and an additional 40% have mixed mitral stenosis and regurgitation.

Pathogenesis

The main pathological process in chronic rheumatic heart disease is progressive fibrosis. The heart valves are predominantly affected but involvement of the pericardium and myocardium also occurs and may contribute to heart failure and conduction disorders. Fusion of the mitral valve commissures and shortening of the chordae tendineae may lead to mitral stenosis with or without regurgitation. Similar changes in the aortic and tricuspid valves produce distortion and rigidity of the cusps, leading to stenosis and regurgitation. Once a valve has been damaged, the altered haemodynamic stresses perpetuate and extend the damage, even in the absence of a continuing rheumatic process.

Mitral valve disease

Mitral stenosis

Mitral stenosis is almost always rheumatic in origin, although in older people it can be caused by heavy calcification of the mitral valve. There is also a rare form of congenital mitral stenosis.

Pathogenesis

In rheumatic mitral stenosis, the mitral valve orifice is slowly diminished by progressive fibrosis, calcification of the valve leaflets, and fusion of the cusps and subvalvular apparatus. The mitral valve orifice is normally about 5 cm^2 in diastole but can be reduced to <1 cm^2 in severe mitral stenosis. The patient is usually asymptomatic until the orifice is <2 cm^2. As stenosis progresses, left ventricular filling becomes more dependent on left atrial contraction. There is dilatation and hypertrophy of the LA and left atrial pressure rises, leading to pulmonary venous congestion and breathlessness. Any increase in heart rate shortens diastole when the mitral valve is open and produces a further rise in left atrial pressure. Situations that demand an increase in cardiac output, such as pregnancy and exercise, also increase left atrial pressure and are poorly tolerated.

Atrial fibrillation is very common due to progressive dilatation of the LA. Its onset often precipitates pulmonary oedema because the accompanying tachycardia and loss of atrial contraction lead to marked haemodynamic deterioration and a rapid rise in left atrial pressure. In the absence of AF, a more gradual rise in left atrial pressure may occur. In the presence or absence of AF, pulmonary hypertension may occur, which can protect the patient from pulmonary oedema. Pulmonary hypertension leads to right ventricular hypertrophy and dilatation, tricuspid regurgitation and right heart failure. Fewer than 20% of patients

16

remain in sinus rhythm but many of these have a small fibrotic LA and severe pulmonary hypertension.

Clinical features

Effort-related dyspnoea is usually the dominant symptom (Box 16.77). Typically, exercise tolerance diminishes very slowly over many years until symptoms eventually occur at rest. Patients frequently do not appreciate the extent of their disability until the diagnosis is made and their valve disease is treated. Acute pulmonary oedema or pulmonary hypertension can lead to haemoptysis. Fatigue is a common symptom due to a low cardiac output. Thromboembolism is a common complication, especially in patients with AF. Prior to the advent of anticoagulant therapy, emboli caused one-quarter of all deaths.

The physical signs of mitral stenosis are often found before symptoms develop and their recognition is of particular importance in pregnancy. The forces that open and close the mitral valve increase as left atrial pressure rises. The first heart sound (S1) is therefore loud and can be palpable (tapping apex beat). An opening snap may be audible and moves closer to the second sound (S2) as the stenosis becomes more severe and left atrial pressure rises. However, the first heart sound and opening snap may be inaudible if the valve is heavily calcified.

Turbulent flow produces the characteristic low-pitched mid-diastolic murmur and sometimes a thrill (Fig. 16.81). The murmur is accentuated by exercise and during atrial systole (pre-systolic accentuation). Early in the disease, a pre-systolic murmur may be

i	16.77 Clinical features of mitral stenosis	
Clinical feature		**Cause**
Symptoms		
Breathlessness		Pulmonary congestion, low cardiac output
Fatigue		Low cardiac output
Oedema, ascites		Right heart failure
Palpitation		Atrial fibrillation
Haemoptysis		Pulmonary congestion, pulmonary embolism
Cough		Pulmonary congestion
Chest pain		Pulmonary hypertension
Thromboembolism		Atrial stasis and atrial fibrillation
Signs		
Atrial fibrillation		Atrial dilatation
Mitral facies		Low cardiac output
Auscultation:		
Loud first heart sound, opening snap		Pressure gradient across the valve
Mid-diastolic murmur		
Crepitations		Left heart failure
Pulmonary oedema		
Pleural effusions		
Right ventricular heave, loud P_2		Pulmonary hypertension

Fig. 16.81 Mitral stenosis: murmur and the diastolic pressure gradient between left atrium (LA) and left ventricle (LV). (Mean gradient is reflected by the area between LA and LV in diastole.) The first heart sound is loud, and there is an opening snap (OS) and mid-diastolic murmur (MDM) with pre-systolic accentuation. **A** Echocardiogram showing reduced opening of the mitral valve in diastole. **B** Colour Doppler showing turbulent flow.

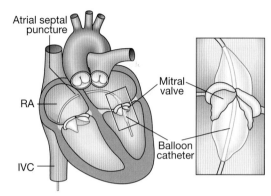

Fig. 16.82 Mitral valvuloplasty. A guidewire is introduced into the right atrium (RA) from the femoral vein and the inferior vena cava (IVC). The inter-atrial septum is punctured, providing access to the left atrium and mitral valve. A balloon catheter is then advanced over the guidewire across the mitral valve and the balloon dilated to stretch the valve and reduce the degree of stenosis.

the only auscultatory abnormality, but in patients with symptoms, the murmur extends from the opening snap to the first heart sound. Coexisting mitral regurgitation causes a pansystolic murmur that radiates towards the axilla.

Pulmonary hypertension may ultimately lead to right ventricular hypertrophy and dilatation with secondary tricuspid regurgitation, which causes a systolic murmur and giant '*v* waves' in the venous pulse.

Investigations

Doppler echocardiography is the investigation of choice for evaluation of suspected mitral stenosis (Fig. 16.81). Cardiac catheterisation may also be required if surgery or valvuloplasty is being considered, to screen for coexisting conditions such as CAD. The ECG may show either AF or bifid P waves (P mitrale) associated with left atrial hypertrophy (Box 16.78). A typical chest X-ray is shown in Figure 16.9 (p. 451).

Management

Patients with mild symptoms can be treated medically but intervention by balloon valvuloplasty, mitral valvotomy or mitral valve replacement should be considered if the patient remains symptomatic despite medical treatment or if pulmonary hypertension develops.

Medical management

This consists of anticoagulation to reduce the risk of systemic embolism, ventricular rate control with digoxin, β-blockers or rate-limiting calcium antagonists in AF, and diuretic to control pulmonary congestion. Antibiotic prophylaxis against infective endocarditis is no longer routinely recommended.

Mitral balloon valvuloplasty and valve replacement

Valvuloplasty is the treatment of choice if specific criteria are fulfilled (Box 16.79 and Fig. 16.82), although surgical closed or open mitral valvotomy is an acceptable alternative. Patients who have undergone mitral valvuloplasty or valvotomy should be followed up at 1–2-yearly intervals because restenosis may occur. Clinical symptoms and signs are a guide to the severity

of mitral restenosis but Doppler echocardiography provides a more accurate assessment.

Valve replacement is indicated if there is substantial mitral reflux or if the valve is rigid and calcified (p. 526).

Mitral regurgitation

Rheumatic disease is the principal cause in countries where rheumatic fever is common but elsewhere, including in the UK, other causes are more important (Box 16.80). Mitral regurgitation may also follow mitral valvotomy or valvuloplasty.

Pathogenesis

Chronic mitral regurgitation causes gradual dilatation of the LA with little increase in pressure and therefore relatively few symptoms. Nevertheless, the LV dilates slowly and the left ventricular diastolic and left atrial pressures gradually increase as a result of chronic volume overload of the LV. In contrast, acute mitral regurgitation causes a rapid rise in left atrial pressure (because left atrial compliance is normal) and marked symptomatic deterioration.

Fig. 16.83 Mitral regurgitation: murmur and systolic wave in left atrial pressure. The first sound is normal or soft and merges with a pansystolic murmur (PSM) extending to the second heart sound. A third heart sound occurs with severe regurgitation. **A** A transoesophageal echocardiogram shows mitral valve prolapse, with one leaflet bulging towards the left atrium (LA, arrow). **B** This results in a jet of mitral regurgitation on colour Doppler (arrow).

Mitral valve prolapse

This is also known as 'floppy' mitral valve and is a common cause of mild mitral regurgitation (Fig. 16.83). Some cases are thought to be due to a developmental abnormality of the mitral valve and others due to degenerative myxomatous change in a normal mitral valve. Rarely, mitral valve prolapse may occur in association with Marfan's syndrome (p. 508).

In its mildest forms, the valve remains competent but bulges back into the atrium during systole, causing a mid-systolic click but no murmur. In the presence of a regurgitant valve, the click is followed by a late systolic murmur, which lengthens as the regurgitation becomes more severe. A click is not always audible and the physical signs may vary with both posture and respiration. Progressive elongation of the chordae tendineae leads to increasing mitral regurgitation, and if chordal rupture occurs, regurgitation suddenly becomes severe. This is rare before the fifth or sixth decade of life.

Mitral valve prolapse is associated with a variety of typically benign arrhythmias, atypical chest pain and a very small risk of embolic stroke or transient ischaemic attack (TIA). Nevertheless, the overall long-term prognosis is good.

Other causes of mitral regurgitation

Mitral valve function depends on the chordae tendineae and their papillary muscles; dilatation of the LV distorts the geometry of these and may cause mitral regurgitation (Box 16.80). Dilated cardiomyopathy and heart failure from CAD are common causes of so-called 'functional' mitral regurgitation. Endocarditis is an important cause of acute mitral regurgitation.

Clinical features

Symptoms and signs depend on the underlying cause and how suddenly the regurgitation develops (Box 16.81). Chronic mitral regurgitation produces a symptom complex that is similar to that of mitral stenosis but sudden-onset mitral regurgitation usually presents with acute pulmonary oedema.

The regurgitant jet causes an apical systolic murmur (Fig. 16.83), which radiates into the axilla and may be accompanied by a thrill. Increased forward flow through the mitral valve causes a loud third heart sound and even a short mid-diastolic murmur. The apex beat feels active and rocking due to left ventricular volume overload and is usually displaced to the left as a result of left ventricular dilatation.

Investigations

Echocardiography is a pivotal investigation. The severity of regurgitation can be assessed by Doppler and information may also be gained on papillary muscle function and valve prolapse. An ECG should be performed and commonly shows AF, as a consequence of atrial dilatation. Cardiac catheterisation is

---

i 16.81 Clinical features of mitral regurgitation

Clinical feature	Cause
Symptoms	
Breathlessness	Pulmonary congestion
Fatigue	Low cardiac output
Oedema, ascites	Right heart failure
Palpitation	Atrial fibrillation
Signs	
Atrial fibrillation	Atrial dilatation
Displaced apex beat	Cardiomegaly
Auscultation:	
Apical pansystolic murmur	Regurgitation of blood from left ventricle to left atrium
Soft S1	Valve does not close properly
Apical S3	Rapid flow of blood into left ventricle
Crepitations	
Pulmonary oedema	Left heart failure
Pleural effusions	
Right ventricular heave	Pulmonary hypertension
Raised jugular venous pressure	Right heart failure
Oedema	Right heart failure

---

i 16.82 Investigations in mitral regurgitation

ECG

- Left atrial hypertrophy
- Atrial fibrillation

Chest X-ray

- Enlarged left atrium
- Enlarged left ventricle
- Pulmonary venous congestion
- Pulmonary oedema (if acute)

Echo

- Dilated left atrium, left ventricle
- Dynamic left ventricle (unless myocardial dysfunction predominates)
- Structural abnormalities of mitral valve

Doppler

- Detects and quantifies regurgitation

Cardiac catheterisation

- Dilated left atrium, dilated left ventricle, mitral regurgitation
- Pulmonary hypertension
- Coexisting coronary artery disease

---

indicated when surgery is being considered (Box 16.82). During catheterisation, the severity of mitral regurgitation can be assessed by left ventriculography and by the size of the *v* (systolic) waves in the left atrial or pulmonary artery wedge pressure trace.

Management

Mitral regurgitation of moderate severity can be treated medically with diuretics and vasodilators. Digoxin and anticoagulants should be given if AF is present (Box 16.83). If systemic hypertension is present, it should be treated with vasodilators such as ACE inhibitors or ARBs, since high afterload may worsen the degree of regurgitation. All patients should be reviewed at regular intervals, both clinically and by echocardiography. Worsening symptoms, progressive cardiomegaly or echocardiographic evidence of deteriorating left ventricular function are indications for mitral valve replacement or repair. Mitral valve repair is now the treatment of choice for severe mitral regurgitation, even in asymptomatic

---

i 16.83 Medical management of mitral regurgitation

- Diuretics
- Vasodilators if hypertension is present
- Digoxin if atrial fibrillation is present
- Anticoagulants if atrial fibrillation is present

---

patients, because results are excellent and early repair prevents irreversible left ventricular damage. Mitral regurgitation often accompanies left ventricular failure associated with CAD. If such patients are to undergo CABG surgery, it is common practice to repair the valve and restore mitral valve function by inserting an annuloplasty ring to overcome annular dilatation and to bring the valve leaflets closer together. Unfortunately, it can be difficult to determine whether it is the ventricular dilatation or the mitral regurgitation that is the predominant problem. If ventricular dilatation is the underlying cause of mitral regurgitation, then mitral valve repair or replacement may actually worsen ventricular function, as the ventricle can no longer empty into the low-pressure LA.

Aortic valve disease

Aortic stenosis

There are several causes of aortic stenosis but the age at which patients present can give a clue to the most likely diagnosis (Box 16.84). In congenital aortic stenosis, obstruction is present from birth or becomes apparent during infancy. With bicuspid aortic valves, obstruction may take years to develop as the valve becomes fibrotic and calcified, and these patients present as young to middle-aged adults. Rheumatic disease of the aortic valve presents at a similar age but is usually accompanied by mitral valve disease. In older people, structurally normal aortic valves may become stenotic as the result of fibrosis and calcification. Haemodynamically significant stenosis develops slowly, typically occurring at 30–60 years in those with rheumatic disease, 50–60 years in those with bicuspid aortic valves and 70–90 years in those with calcific tricuspid disease.

Pathogenesis

Cardiac output is initially maintained in patients with aortic stenosis at the cost of a steadily increasing pressure gradient across the aortic valve. With progression of the stenosis the LV becomes increasingly hypertrophied and coronary blood flow may be inadequate to supply the myocardium, such that

---

i 16.84 Causes of aortic stenosis

Infants, children, adolescents

- Congenital aortic stenosis
- Congenital subvalvular aortic stenosis
- Congenital supravalvular aortic stenosis

Young adults to middle-aged

- Calcification and fibrosis of congenitally bicuspid aortic valve
- Rheumatic aortic stenosis

Middle-aged to elderly

- Senile degenerative aortic stenosis
- Calcification of bicuspid valve
- Rheumatic aortic stenosis

16

angina can develop even in the absence of coexisting CAD. The fixed outflow obstruction limits the increase in cardiac output required on exercise. Eventually, the LV can no longer overcome the outflow tract obstruction and LV failure results, leading to pulmonary oedema.

Clinical features

Aortic stenosis is commonly picked up in asymptomatic patients at routine clinical examination but the three cardinal symptoms are angina, breathlessness and syncope (Box 16.85). Angina arises either because of the increased demands of the hypertrophied LV working against the high-pressure outflow tract obstruction, or the presence of coexisting CAD, which affects over 50% of patients. Exertional breathlessness suggests cardiac decompensation as a consequence of the excessive pressure overload placed on the LV. Syncope usually occurs on exertion when cardiac

output fails to rise to meet demand, leading to a fall in BP. Sometimes patients with severe aortic stenosis do not complain of symptoms. If, on clinical evaluation, this appears to be due to a sedentary lifestyle, a careful exercise test may reveal symptoms on modest exertion.

The characteristic clinical signs of severe aortic stenosis are shown in Box 16.85. A harsh ejection systolic murmur radiates to the neck, with a soft second heart sound, particularly in those with calcific valves. The murmur is often likened to a saw cutting wood and may (especially in older patients) have a musical quality like the 'mew' of a seagull (Fig. 16.84). The severity of aortic stenosis may be difficult to gauge clinically, as older patients with a non-compliant 'stiff' arterial system may have an apparently normal carotid upstroke in the presence of severe aortic stenosis. Milder degrees of stenosis may be difficult to distinguish from aortic sclerosis, in which the valve is thickened or calcified but not obstructed. A careful examination should be made for other valve lesions, particularly in rheumatic heart disease, when there is frequently concomitant mitral valve disease. In contrast to patients with mitral stenosis, which tends to progress very slowly, patients with aortic stenosis typically remain asymptomatic for many years but deteriorate rapidly when symptoms develop; if otherwise untreated, they usually die within 3–5 years of presentation.

Investigations

Echocardiography is a pivotal investigation in patients suspected of having aortic stenosis. It can demonstrate restricted valve opening (Fig. 16.85) and Doppler assessment permits calculation of the systolic gradient across the aortic valve, from which the severity of stenosis can be assessed (see Fig. 16.11, p. 451). In

---

i 16.85 Clinical features of aortic stenosis

Symptoms

- Mild or moderate stenosis: usually asymptomatic
- Exertional dyspnoea
- Angina
- Exertional syncope
- Sudden death
- Episodes of acute pulmonary oedema

Signs

- Ejection systolic murmur
- Slow-rising carotid pulse
- Thrusting apex beat (left ventricular pressure overload)
- Narrow pulse pressure
- Signs of pulmonary venous congestion

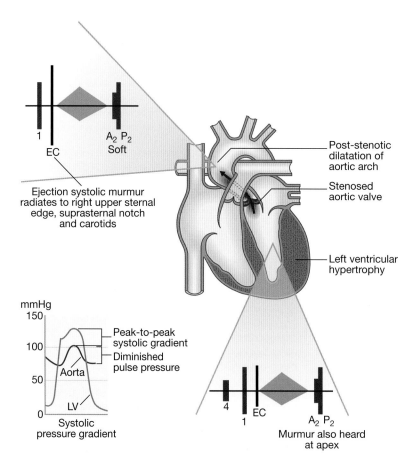

Fig. 16.84 Aortic stenosis. Pressure traces show the systolic gradient between left ventricle (LV) and aorta. The 'diamond-shaped' murmur is heard best with the diaphragm in the aortic outflow and also at the apex. An ejection click (EC) may be present in young patients with a bicuspid aortic valve but not in older patients with calcified valves. Aortic stenosis may lead to left ventricular hypertrophy with a fourth sound at the apex and post-stenotic dilatation of the aortic arch. Figure 16.11 (p. 451) shows the typical Doppler signal with aortic stenosis.

Fig. 16.85 Two-dimensional echocardiogram comparing a normal individual and a patient with calcific aortic stenosis. A Normal individual in diastole; the aortic leaflets are closed and thin, and a point of coaptation is seen (arrow). B Calcific aortic stenosis in diastole; the aortic leaflets are thick and calcified (arrow). C Normal in systole; the aortic leaflets are open (arrows). D Calcific aortic stenosis in systole; the thickened leaflets have barely moved (arrows). *From Newby D, Grubb N. Cardiology: an illustrated colour text. Edinburgh: Churchill Livingstone, Elsevier Ltd; 2005.*

i | **16.86 Investigations in aortic stenosis**

ECG

- Left ventricular hypertrophy
- Left bundle branch block

Chest X-ray

- May be normal; sometimes enlarged left ventricle and dilated ascending aorta on postero-anterior view, calcified valve on lateral view

Echo

- Calcified valve with restricted opening, hypertrophied left ventricle

Doppler

- Measurement of severity of stenosis
- Detection of associated aortic regurgitation

Cardiac catheterisation

- Mainly to identify associated coronary artery disease
- May be used to measure gradient between left ventricle and aorta

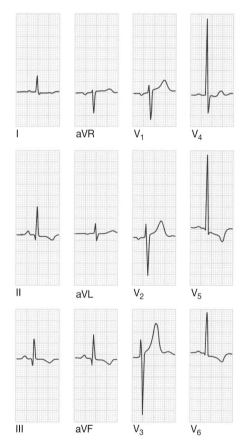

Fig. 16.86 Left ventricular hypertrophy. QRS complexes in limb leads have increased amplitude with a very large R wave in V_6 and S wave in V_2. There is ST depression and T-wave inversion in leads II, III, aVF, V_5 and V_6: a 'left ventricular strain' pattern.

patients with impaired left ventricular function, velocities across the aortic valve may be diminished because of a reduced stroke volume; this is called low-flow aortic stenosis. When marked aortic regurgitation or elevated cardiac output is present, velocities are increased because of an increased stroke volume and this may overestimate stenosis severity on Doppler echocardiography. In advanced cases, ECG features of hypertrophy (Box 16.86) are often pronounced (Fig. 16.86), and down-sloping ST segments

16.87 Aortic stenosis in old age

- **Incidence**: the most common form of valve disease affecting the very old.
- **Symptoms**: a common cause of syncope, angina and heart failure in the very old.
- **Signs**: because of increasing stiffening in the central arteries, low pulse pressure and a slow rising pulse may not be present.
- **Trans-catheter aortic valve implantation (TAVI)**: a good option in older individuals because less invasive than surgery.
- **Surgery**: can be successful in those aged 80 years or more in the absence of comorbidity, but with a higher operative mortality. The prognosis without surgery is poor once symptoms have developed.
- **Valve replacement type**: a biological valve is often preferable to a mechanical one because this obviates the need for anticoagulation, and the durability of biological valves usually exceeds the patient's anticipated life expectancy.

 16.88 Causes of aortic regurgitation

Congenital

- Bicuspid valve or disproportionate cusps

Acquired

- Rheumatic disease
- Infective endocarditis
- Trauma
- Causes of aortic dilatation:
  - Marfan's syndrome
  - Aneurysm
  - Aortic dissection
  - Syphilis
  - Ankylosing spondylitis

 16.89 Clinical features of aortic regurgitation

Symptoms

Mild to moderate aortic regurgitation

- Often asymptomatic
- Palpitations

Severe aortic regurgitation

- Breathlessness
- Angina

Signs

Pulses

- Large-volume or 'collapsing' pulse
- Low diastolic and increased pulse pressure
- Bounding peripheral pulses
- Capillary pulsation in nail beds: Quincke's sign
- Femoral bruit ('pistol shot'): Duroziez's sign
- Head nodding with pulse: de Musset's sign

Murmurs

- Early diastolic murmur
- Systolic murmur (increased stroke volume)
- Austin Flint murmur (soft mid-diastolic)

Other signs

- Displaced, heaving apex beat (volume overload)
- Pre-systolic impulse
- Fourth heart sound
- Crepitations (pulmonary venous congestion)

and T inversion ('strain pattern') are seen in the lateral leads, reflecting left ventricular fibrosis. Nevertheless, the ECG can be normal, despite severe stenosis. Imaging with CT and MRI may be useful in assessing the degree of valve calcification and stenosis, respectively, and may help where there is uncertainty.

Management

Irrespective of the severity of valve stenosis, patients with asymptomatic aortic stenosis have a good immediate prognosis and conservative management is appropriate. Such patients should be kept under review, as the development of angina, syncope, symptoms of low cardiac output or heart failure has a poor prognosis and is an indication for prompt surgery. In practice, patients with moderate or severe stenosis should be evaluated every 1–2 years with Doppler echocardiography to detect evidence of progression in severity. The intervals between reviews should be more frequent (typically 3–6-monthly) in older patients with heavily calcified valves.

Patients with symptomatic severe aortic stenosis should have prompt aortic valve replacement. Delay exposes the patient to the risk of sudden death or irreversible deterioration in ventricular function. Old age is not a contraindication to valve replacement and results are very good in experienced centres, even for those in their eighties (Box 16.87). This is especially the case with transcatheter aortic valve implantation (TAVI, p. 527). Aortic balloon valvuloplasty is useful in congenital aortic stenosis but has limited value in older patients with calcific aortic stenosis.

Anticoagulants are required only in patients who have AF or those who have had a valve replacement with a mechanical prosthesis.

Aortic regurgitation

This condition can result from either disease of the aortic valve cusps, infection, trauma or dilatation of the aortic root. The causes are summarised in Box 16.88.

Pathogenesis

Regurgitation of blood through the aortic valve causes the LV to dilate as cardiac output increases to maintain the demands of the circulation. The stroke volume of the LV may eventually be doubled and the major arteries are then conspicuously pulsatile. As the disease progresses, left ventricular failure develops, leading to a rise in left ventricular end-diastolic pressure and pulmonary oedema.

Clinical features

Until the onset of breathlessness, the only symptom may be an awareness of the heart beat (Box 16.89), particularly when lying on the left side, which results from the increased stroke volume. Paroxysmal nocturnal dyspnoea is sometimes the first symptom, and peripheral oedema or angina may occur. The characteristic murmur is best heard to the left of the sternum during held expiration (Fig. 16.87); a thrill is rare. A systolic murmur due to the increased stroke volume is common and does not necessarily indicate stenosis. The regurgitant jet causes fluttering of the mitral valve and, if severe, causes partial closure of the anterior mitral leaflet, leading to functional mitral stenosis and a soft mid-diastolic (Austin Flint) murmur.

Acute severe regurgitation may occur as the result of perforation of an aortic cusp in endocarditis. In this circumstance, there may be no time for compensatory left ventricular hypertrophy and dilatation to develop and the features of heart failure may predominate. The classical signs of aortic regurgitation in such patients may be masked by tachycardia and an abrupt rise in

Fig. 16.87 **Aortic regurgitation.** The early diastolic murmur is best heard at the left sternal edge and may be accompanied by an ejection systolic ('to and fro') murmur. The aortic arch and left ventricle (LV) may become dilated. The inset shows a Doppler echocardiogram with the regurgitant jet (arrows). *Inset (Colour Doppler echo) From Newby D, Grubb N. Cardiology: an illustrated colour text. Edinburgh: Churchill Livingstone, Elsevier Ltd; 2005.*

i	**16.90 Investigations in aortic regurgitation**

ECG

• Initially normal, later left ventricular hypertrophy and T-wave inversion

Chest X-ray

• Cardiac dilatation, maybe aortic dilatation
• Features of left heart failure

Echo

• Dilated left ventricle	• Doppler detects reflux
• Hyperdynamic left ventricle	• Fluttering anterior mitral leaflet

Cardiac catheterisation*

• Dilated left ventricle	• Dilated aortic root
• Aortic regurgitation	

*Not always required.

left ventricular end-diastolic pressure. The pulse pressure may also be normal or near-normal and the diastolic murmur may be short or even absent.

Investigations

Doppler echocardiography is the investigation of first choice for detecting regurgitation (Box 16.90). In severe acute aortic regurgitation, the rapid rise in left ventricular diastolic pressure may cause premature mitral valve closure. Cardiac catheterisation and aortography are usually performed to assess the severity of regurgitation, to determine if there is dilatation of the aorta and to screen for the presence of coexisting CAD. MRI can also be useful in assessing the degree and extent of aortic dilatation if this is suspected on chest X-ray or echocardiography.

Management

Treatment may be required for underlying conditions, such as endocarditis or syphilis. Aortic valve replacement is indicated if aortic regurgitation causes symptoms, and this may need to be combined with aortic root replacement and coronary bypass surgery. Those with chronic aortic regurgitation can remain asymptomatic for many years because compensatory ventricular dilatation and hypertrophy occur, but should be advised to report the development of any symptoms of breathlessness or angina. Asymptomatic patients should also be followed up annually with echocardiography for evidence of increasing ventricular size. If this occurs or if the end-systolic dimension increases to 55 mm or more, then aortic valve replacement should be undertaken. If systemic hypertension is present, vasodilators should be used to control systolic BP. There is conflicting evidence regarding the need for aortic valve replacement in asymptomatic patients with severe aortic regurgitation. When aortic root dilatation is the cause of aortic regurgitation, as can occur in Marfan's syndrome, aortic root replacement is usually necessary.

Tricuspid valve disease

Tricuspid stenosis

Tricuspid stenosis is usually rheumatic in origin and is rare in developed countries. Tricuspid disease occurs in fewer than 5% of patients with rheumatic heart disease and then nearly always occurs in association with mitral and aortic valve disease. Tricuspid stenosis and regurgitation may also occur in the carcinoid syndrome (p. 678).

Clinical features and investigations

Although the symptoms of mitral and aortic valve disease predominate, tricuspid stenosis may cause symptoms of right heart failure, including hepatic discomfort and peripheral oedema.

The main clinical feature is a raised JVP with a prominent *a* wave, and a slow *y* descent due to the loss of normal rapid right ventricular filling (p. 443). There is also a mid-diastolic murmur, best heard at the lower left or right sternal edge. This is generally higher-pitched than the murmur of mitral stenosis and is increased by inspiration. Right heart failure causes hepatomegaly with pre-systolic pulsation (large *a* wave), ascites and peripheral oedema. The diagnosis can be confirmed by Doppler echocardiography, which shows similar appearances to those of rheumatic mitral stenosis.

Management

In patients who require surgery to other valves, either the tricuspid valve can also be replaced or treated with valvotomy. Balloon valvuloplasty can be used to treat rare cases of isolated tricuspid stenosis.

Tricuspid regurgitation

Tricuspid regurgitation is common, and is most frequently functional, occurring as a result of right ventricular dilatation due to right heart failure or biventricular failure. It may also be the result of other conditions, as summarised in Box 16.91.

Clinical features

Symptoms are usually non-specific, with tiredness related to reduced cardiac output, and oedema and hepatic enlargement due to venous congestion. The most prominent sign is a 'giant' *v* wave in the jugular venous pulse (a *cv* wave replaces the normal *x* descent). Other features include a pansystolic murmur at the left sternal edge and a pulsatile liver. Echocardiography may reveal dilatation of the RV. If the valve has been affected by rheumatic disease, the leaflets will appear thickened and, in endocarditis, vegetations may be seen.

Management

Tricuspid regurgitation due to right ventricular dilatation often improves when the cardiac failure is treated. Patients with a normal pulmonary artery pressure tolerate isolated tricuspid reflux well, and valves damaged by endocarditis do not usually need to be replaced. Patients undergoing mitral valve replacement, who have tricuspid regurgitation due to marked dilatation of the tricuspid annulus, benefit from valve repair with an annuloplasty ring to bring the leaflets closer together. Those with rheumatic damage may require tricuspid valve replacement.

16.91 Causes of tricuspid regurgitation

Primary

- Rheumatic heart disease
- Endocarditis, particularly in intravenous drug-users
- Ebstein's congenital anomaly (see Box 16.102)

Secondary

- Right ventricular failure
- Right ventricular infarction
- Pulmonary hypertension

Pulmonary valve disease

Pulmonary stenosis

This can occur in the carcinoid syndrome but is usually congenital, in which case it may be isolated or associated with other abnormalities, such as Fallot's tetralogy (p. 536).

Clinical features

The principal finding on examination is an ejection systolic murmur, loudest at the left upper sternum and radiating towards the left shoulder. There may be a thrill, best felt when the patient leans forwards and breathes out. The murmur is often preceded by an ejection sound (click). Delay in right ventricular ejection may cause wide splitting of the second heart sound. Severe pulmonary stenosis is characterised by a loud, harsh murmur, an inaudible pulmonary closure sound (P_2), an increased right ventricular heave, and prominent *a* waves in the jugular pulse.

Investigations

Doppler echocardiography is the definitive investigation. ECG may show evidence of right ventricular hypertrophy, and post-stenotic dilatation in the pulmonary artery may be observed on the chest X-ray.

Management

Mild to moderate isolated pulmonary stenosis is relatively common and does not usually progress or require treatment. Severe pulmonary stenosis (resting gradient >50 mmHg with a normal cardiac output) can be treated by percutaneous pulmonary balloon valvuloplasty or, if this is not available, by surgical valvotomy. Long-term results are very good. Post-operative pulmonary regurgitation is common but benign.

Pulmonary regurgitation

This is rare in isolation and is usually associated with pulmonary artery dilatation due to pulmonary hypertension. It may complicate mitral stenosis, producing an early diastolic decrescendo murmur at the left sternal edge that is difficult to distinguish from aortic regurgitation (Graham Steell murmur). The pulmonary hypertension may be secondary to other disease of the left side of the heart, primary pulmonary vascular disease or Eisenmenger's syndrome (p. 532). Trivial pulmonary regurgitation is a frequent finding in normal individuals and has no clinical significance.

Prosthetic valves

Diseased heart valves can be replaced with mechanical or biological prostheses. The three most commonly used types of mechanical prosthesis are the ball and cage, tilting single disc and tilting bi-leaflet valves. All generate prosthetic sounds or clicks on auscultation. Pig or allograft valves mounted on a supporting stent are the most commonly used biological valves. They generate normal heart sounds. All prosthetic valves used in the aortic position produce a systolic flow murmur.

All mechanical valves require long-term anticoagulation because they can cause systemic thromboembolism or may develop valve thrombosis or obstruction (Box 16.92); the prosthetic clicks may become inaudible if the valve malfunctions. Biological valves have the advantage of not requiring anticoagulants to maintain proper function; however, many patients undergoing valve replacement surgery, especially mitral valve replacement, will have AF that

16.92 Anticoagulation targets and prosthetic heart valves	
Mechanical valves	**Target INR**
Ball and cage (e.g. Starr–Edwards) **Tilting disc** (e.g. Bjork–Shiley)	3.0–4.0
Bi-leaflet (e.g. St Jude)	2.5–3.0
Biological valves with atrial fibrillation	2.0–3.0
(INR = international normalised ratio)	

Fig. 16.88 Transcatheter aortic valve implantation (TAVI): bioprosthetic valve.

requires anticoagulation anyway. Biological valves are less durable than mechanical valves and may degenerate 7 or more years after implantation, particularly when used in the mitral position. They are more durable in the aortic position and in older patients, so are particularly appropriate for patients over 65 undergoing aortic valve replacement.

Transcatheter aortic valve implantation

For patients being considered for aortic valve surgery, especially due to aortic stenosis, transcatheter aortic valve implantation (TAVI) is an emerging alternative to surgical aortic valve replacement. The native valve is not removed but is compressed by the new bioprosthetic valve, which is implanted within it. The bioprosthetic valve is mounted on a large stent-like structure and is implanted through a catheter inserted in the femoral artery (Fig. 16.88). TAVI has several major advantages. It avoids the need for a sternotomy, is associated with a short recovery period, can be used in high-risk and otherwise inoperable patients, and is much better tolerated by elderly patients. Complications include stroke (2%) and heart block necessitating pacemaker implantation (5–15%).

Prosthetic valve dysfunction

Symptoms or signs of unexplained heart failure in a patient with a prosthetic heart valve may be due to valve dysfunction, and urgent assessment is required. Metallic valves can suffer strut fracture and fail, causing catastrophic regurgitation. Alternatively, they may thrombose and cause systemic thromboembolism or valve obstruction, especially in the presence of inadequate anticoagulation. Biological valve dysfunction is usually associated with the development of a regurgitant murmur and may begin to develop 8–10 years after implantation.

Infective endocarditis

This is caused by microbial infection of a heart valve, the lining of a cardiac chamber or blood vessel, or by a congenital anomaly. Both native and prosthetic valves can be affected. The most common causes of infective endocarditis are streptococci and staphylococci but other organisms may also be involved.

Epidemiology

The incidence of infective endocarditis in community-based studies ranges from 5 to 15 cases per 100 000 per annum. More than 50% of patients are over 60 years of age (Box 16.93). In a large British study, the underlying condition was rheumatic heart disease in 24% of patients, congenital heart disease in 19%, and other cardiac abnormalities such as calcified aortic valve or floppy mitral valve in 25%. The remaining 32% were not thought to have a pre-existing cardiac abnormality. Bacterial endocarditis is a serious illness; the case fatality is approximately 20% even with treatment, and is even higher in those with prosthetic valve endocarditis and those infected with antibiotic-resistant organisms.

Pathophysiology

Infective endocarditis typically occurs at sites of pre-existing endocardial damage, but infection with particularly virulent or aggressive organisms such as *Staphylococcus aureus* can cause endocarditis in a previously normal heart. Staphylococcal endocarditis of the tricuspid valve is a common complication of intravenous drug use. Many acquired and congenital cardiac lesions are vulnerable, particularly areas of endocardial damage caused by a high-pressure jet of blood, such as ventricular septal defect, mitral regurgitation and aortic regurgitation, many of which are haemodynamically insignificant. In contrast, the risk of endocarditis at the site of haemodynamically important low-pressure lesions, such as a large atrial septal defect, is minimal.

Infection tends to occur at sites of endothelial damage because they attract deposits of platelets and fibrin that are vulnerable to colonisation by blood-borne organisms. The avascular valve tissue and presence of fibrin and platelet aggregates help to protect proliferating organisms from host defence mechanisms. When the infection is established, vegetations composed of organisms, fibrin and platelets grow and may become large enough to cause obstruction or embolism. Adjacent tissues are destroyed and abscesses may form. Valve regurgitation may develop or increase if the affected valve is damaged by tissue distortion, cusp perforation or disruption of chordae. Extracardiac manifestations, such as vasculitis and skin lesions, may occur as the result of either emboli or immune complex deposition. Mycotic aneurysms may develop in arteries at the site of infected emboli. In fatal cases, infarction of the spleen and kidneys and, sometimes, an immune glomerulonephritis may be found at postmortem.

16

	16.93 Endocarditis in old age

- **Symptoms and signs**: may be non-specific, with delirium, weight loss, malaise and weakness, and the diagnosis may not be suspected.
- **Common causative organisms**: often enterococci (from the urinary tract) and *Streptococcus gallolyticus* subsp. *gallolyticus* (from a colonic source).
- **Morbidity and mortality**: much higher.

i 16.94 Microbiology of infective endocarditis

Pathogen	Of native valve (n = 280)	In injection drug users (n = 87)	Of prosthetic valve	
			Early (n = 15)	Late (n = 72)
Staphylococci	124 (44%)	60 (69%)	10 (67%)	33 (46%)
Staph. aureus	106 (38%)	60 (69%)	3 (20%)	15 (21%)
Coagulase-negative	18 (6%)	0	7 (47%)	18 (25%)
Streptococci	86 (31%)	7 (8%)	0	25 (35%)
Oral	59 (21%)	3 (3%)	0	19 (26%)
Others (non-enterococcal)	27 (10%)	4 (5%)	0	6 (8%)
Enterococcus spp.	21 (8%)	2 (2%)	1 (7%)	5 (7%)
HACEK	12 (4%)	0	0	1 (1%)
Polymicrobial	6 (2%)	8 (9%)	0	1 (1%)
Other bacteria	12 (4%)	4 (5%)	0	2 (3%)
Fungi	3 (1%)	2 (2%)	0	0
Negative blood culture	16 (6%)	4 (5%)	4 (27%)	5 (7%)

(HACEK = **H**aemophilus aphrophilus – now known as *Aggregatibacter aphrophilus*–**A**ggregatibacter actinomycetemcomitans; **C**ardiobacterium hominis; **E**ikenella corrodens; and **K**ingella kingae)
Adapted from Moreillon P, Que YA. Infective endocarditis. Lancet 2004; 363:139–149.

Microbiology

Over three-quarters of cases are caused by streptococci or staphylococci. Viridans streptococci, such as *Streptococcus mitis* and *Strep. sanguis*, which are commensals in the oral cavity, can enter the blood stream on chewing or tooth-brushing, or at the time of dental treatment, and are common causes of subacute endocarditis (Box 16.94). Other organisms, including *Enterococcus faecalis*, *E. faecium* and *Strep. gallolyticus* subsp. *gallolyticus* (previously known as *Strep. bovis*), may enter the blood from the bowel or urinary tract. Patients who are found to have endocarditis caused by *Strep. gallolyticus* should undergo colonoscopy, since this organism is associated with large-bowel malignancy.

Staph. aureus has now overtaken streptococci as the most common cause of acute endocarditis. It originates from skin infections, abscesses or vascular access sites such as intravenous and central lines, or from intravenous drug use. It is highly virulent and invasive, usually producing florid vegetations, rapid valve destruction and abscess formation. Other causes of acute endocarditis include *Strep. pneumoniae* and *Strep. pyogenes*.

Post-operative endocarditis after cardiac surgery may affect native or prosthetic heart valves or other prosthetic materials. The most common organisms are coagulase-negative staphylococci such as *Staph. epidermidis*, which are part of the normal skin flora. There is frequently a history of wound infection with the same organism. Coagulase-negative staphylococci cause native valve endocarditis in approximately 5% of cases and this possibility should always be considered before they are dismissed as blood culture contaminants. Another coagulase-negative staphylococcus, *Staph. lugdenensis*, causes a rapidly destructive acute endocarditis that is associated with previously normal valves and multiple emboli. Unless accurately identified, it may also be overlooked as a contaminant.

In Q fever endocarditis due to *Coxiella burnetii*, the patient often has a history of contact with farm animals. The aortic valve is usually affected and there may also be hepatitis, pneumonia and purpura. Life-long antibiotic therapy may be required.

In about 3–4% of cases, endocarditis may be caused by Gram-negative bacteria of the so-called HACEK group (**H**aemophilus aphrophilus – now known as *Aggregatibacter aphrophilus*–**A**ggregatibacter actinomycetemcomitans; **C**ardiobacterium hominis; **E**ikenella corrodens; and **K**ingella kingae). These are slow-growing, fastidious Gram-negative organisms that are oropharyngeal commensals. The diagnosis may be revealed only after prolonged culture and the organisms may be resistant to penicillin.

Brucella endocarditis is associated with a history of contact with goats or cattle and often affects the aortic valve.

Yeasts and fungi, such as *Candida* and *Aspergillus*, may attack previously normal or prosthetic valves, particularly in immunocompromised patients or those with in-dwelling intravenous catheters. Abscesses and emboli are common, therapy is difficult, surgery is often required and mortality is high. Concomitant bacterial infection may be present.

Clinical features

Endocarditis can take either an acute or a more insidious 'subacute' form. There is considerable overlap, however, because the clinical pattern is influenced not only by the organism but also by the site of infection, prior antibiotic therapy and the presence of a valve or shunt prosthesis. The subacute form may abruptly develop acute life-threatening complications, such as valve disruption or emboli. The Duke criteria for diagnosis of infective endocarditis are shown in Box 16.95.

Subacute endocarditis

This should be suspected when a patient with congenital or valvular heart disease develops a persistent fever, complains of unusual tiredness, night sweats or weight loss, or develops new signs of valve dysfunction or heart failure. Less often, it presents as an embolic stroke or peripheral arterial embolism. Other features (Fig. 16.89) include purpura and petechial haemorrhages in the skin and mucous membranes, and splinter haemorrhages under the fingernails or toenails. Osler's nodes are painful, tender swellings at the fingertips that are probably the product of vasculitis; they are rare. Digital clubbing is a late sign. The spleen is frequently palpable; in *Coxiella* infections, the spleen and the

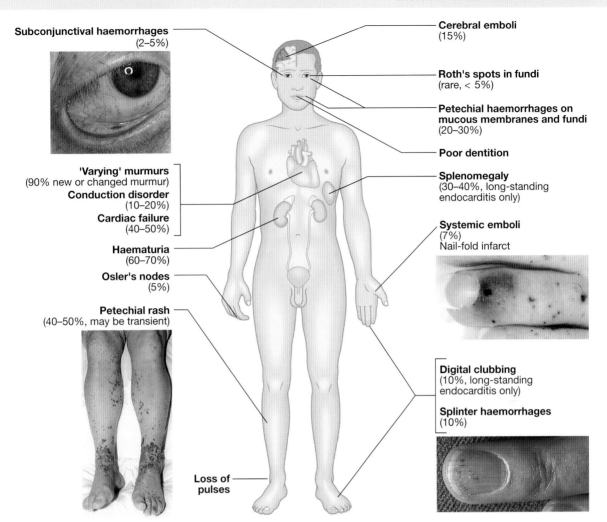

Subconjunctival haemorrhages
(2–5%)

Cerebral emboli
(15%)

Roth's spots in fundi
(rare, < 5%)

Petechial haemorrhages on mucous membranes and fundi
(20–30%)

Poor dentition

'Varying' murmurs
(90% new or changed murmur)
Conduction disorder
(10–20%)
Cardiac failure
(40–50%)

Splenomegaly
(30–40%, long-standing endocarditis only)

Haematuria
(60–70%)

Systemic emboli
(7%)
Nail-fold infarct

Osler's nodes
(5%)

Petechial rash
(40–50%, may be transient)

Digital clubbing
(10%, long-standing endocarditis only)

Splinter haemorrhages
(10%)

Loss of pulses

16

Fig. 16.89 **Clinical features that may be present in endocarditis.** *Insets (Petechial rash, nail-fold infarct) From Newby D, Grubb N. Cardiology: an illustrated colour text. Edinburgh: Churchill Livingstone, Elsevier Ltd; 2005.*

---

i **16.95 Diagnosis of infective endocarditis***

Major criteria

Positive blood culture
- Typical organism from two cultures
- Persistent positive blood cultures taken >12 hrs apart
- Three or more positive cultures taken over >1 hr

Endocardial involvement
- Positive echocardiographic findings of vegetations
- New valvular regurgitation

Minor criteria
- Predisposing valvular or cardiac abnormality
- Intravenous drug misuse
- Pyrexia ≥38°C
- Embolic phenomenon
- Vasculitic phenomenon
- Blood cultures suggestive: organism grown but not achieving major criteria
- Suggestive echocardiographic findings

*Modified Duke criteria. Patients with two major, or one major and three minor, or five minor have definite endocarditis. Patients with one major and one minor, or three minor have possible endocarditis.

liver may be considerably enlarged. Non-visible haematuria is common. The finding of any of these features in a patient with persistent fever or malaise is an indication for re-examination to detect hitherto unrecognised heart disease.

Acute endocarditis

This presents as a severe febrile illness with prominent and changing heart murmurs and petechiae. Clinical stigmata of chronic endocarditis are usually absent. Embolic events are common, and cardiac or renal failure may develop rapidly. Abscesses may be detected on echocardiography. Partially treated acute endocarditis behaves like subacute endocarditis.

Post-operative endocarditis

This may present as an unexplained fever in a patient who has had heart valve surgery. The infection usually involves the valve ring and may resemble subacute or acute endocarditis, depending on the virulence of the organism. Morbidity and mortality are high and revision surgery is often required. The range of organisms is similar to that seen in native valve disease, but when endocarditis occurs during the first few weeks after surgery it is usually due to infection with a coagulase-negative staphylococcus that was introduced during the perioperative period.

Investigations

Blood culture (see Fig. 6.6, p. 107) is the pivotal investigation to identify the organism that is the cause of the infection and to guide antibiotic therapy. Three to six sets of blood cultures should bo takon prior to commoncing thorapy and should not wait for episodes of pyrexia. The first two specimens will detect bacteraemia in 90% of culture-positive cases. A meticulous aseptic technique is essential. Taking discrete sets of blood cultures from peripheral sites at intervals of ≥ 6 hours reduces the risk of misdiagnosis due to contamination with skin commensals. Isolation of a typical organism in more than one culture provides strong evidence in favour of the diagnosis (Box 16.95). An in-dwelling line should not be used to take cultures. Both aerobic and anaerobic cultures are required.

Echocardiography is key for detecting and following the progress of vegetations, for assessing valve damage and for detecting abscess formation. Vegetations as small as 2–4 mm can be detected by transthoracic echocardiography, and even smaller ones (1–1.5 mm) can be visualised by trans-oesophageal echocardiography (TOE), which is particularly valuable for identifying abscess formation and investigating patients with prosthetic heart valves. Vegetations may be difficult to distinguish in the presence of an abnormal valve; the sensitivity of transthoracic echo is approximately 65% but that of TOE is more than 90%. Failure to detect vegetations does not exclude the diagnosis.

Elevation of the ESR, a normocytic normochromic anaemia, and leucocytosis are common but not invariable. Measurement of serum CRP is more reliable than the ESR in monitoring progress. Proteinuria may occur and non-visible haematuria is usually present.

The ECG may show the development of AV block (due to aortic root abscess formation) and occasionally infarction due to emboli. The chest X-ray may show evidence of cardiac failure and cardiomegaly.

Management

A multidisciplinary approach, with cooperation between the physician, surgeon and microbiologist, increases the chance of a successful outcome. Any source of infection should be removed as soon as possible; for example, a tooth with an apical abscess should be extracted.

Empirical treatment depends on the mode of presentation, the suspected organism and the presence of a prosthetic valve or penicillin allergy. If the presentation is subacute, antibiotic treatment should ideally be withheld until the results of blood cultures are available. However, if empirical antibiotic treatment is considered necessary, amoxicillin (2 g 6 times daily IV) should be considered (with or without gentamicin). If the presentation is acute, empirical therapy should be started with vancomycin (1 g twice daily IV) and gentamicin (1 mg/kg twice daily IV), with dose adjustment based on antibiotic levels. The same regimen is used in true penicillin allergy. Patients with suspected prosthetic valve endocarditis should be treated with vancomycin and gentamicin at the above-mentioned doses, plus rifampicin orally in a dose of 300–600 mg twice daily. Following identification of the causal organism, determination of the minimum inhibitory concentration (MIC) for the organism helps guide antibiotic therapy. Recommended regimens for some of the most common scenarios are shown in Box 16.96. More detailed information

16.96 Antimicrobial treatment of common causative organisms in infective endocarditis

Antimicrobial susceptibility	Antimicrobial	Dose	Native valve	Prosthetic valve
Streptococci				
Penicillin MIC ≤0.125 mg/L	Benzylpenicillin IV	1.2 g 6 times daily	4 weeks[1]	6 weeks
Penicillin MIC >0.125, ≤0.5 mg/L	Benzylpenicillin IV and gentamicin IV	2.4 g 6 times daily / 1 mg/kg twice daily[2]	4 weeks / 2 weeks	6 weeks / 2 weeks
Penicillin MIC >0.5 mg/L	Vancomycin IV and gentamicin IV	1 g twice daily[3] / 1 mg/kg twice daily[2]	4 weeks / 4 weeks	6 weeks / 6 weeks
Enterococci				
Amoxicillin MIC ≤4 mg/L and gentamicin MIC ≤128 mg/L	Amoxicillin IV and gentamicin IV[2]	2 g 6 times daily / 1 mg/kg twice daily[2]	4 weeks / 4 weeks	6 weeks / 6 weeks
Amoxicillin MIC >4 mg/L and gentamicin MIC ≤128 mg/L	Vancomycin IV and gentamicin IV[2]	1 g twice daily[3] / 1 mg/kg twice daily[2]	4 weeks / 4 weeks	6 weeks / 6 weeks
Staphylococci – native valve				
Meticillin-sensitive	Flucloxacillin IV	2 g 4–6 times daily[4]	4 weeks	–
Meticillin-resistant, vancomycin MIC ≤2 mg/L, rifampicin-sensitive	Vancomycin IV / Rifampicin orally	1 g twice daily[3] / 300–600 mg twice daily	4 weeks / 4 weeks	– / –
Staphylococci – prosthetic valve				
Meticillin-sensitive	Flucloxacillin IV and gentamicin IV and rifampicin orally	2 g 4–6 times daily / 1 mg/kg twice daily[2] / 300–600 mg twice daily	– / – / –	6 weeks / 6 weeks / 6 weeks
Meticillin-resistant, vancomycin MIC ≤2 mg/L, rifampicin-sensitive	Vancomycin IV and rifampicin orally	1 g twice daily[3] / 300–600 mg twice daily	– / –	6 weeks / 6 weeks

[1]When conditions in Box 16.97 are met, 2 weeks of benzylpenicillin and gentamicin (1 mg/kg twice daily) may be sufficient. Ceftriaxone 2 g once daily IV/IM can be used instead of benzylpenicillin for those with non-severe penicillin allergy. [2]Pre-dose gentamicin level should be ≤1 mg/L, post-dose 3–5 mg/L. Adjust dose according to levels and renal function. [3]Pre-dose vancomycin level should be 15–20 mg/L. Adjust dose according to levels and renal function. [4]Use 6 times daily if weight >85 kg.
(IV = intravenous; MIC = minimum inhibitory concentration)
Adapted from Gould FK, Denning DW, Elliott TS, et al. Guidelines for the diagnosis and antibiotic treatment of endocarditis in adults: a report of the working party of the British Society for Antimicrobial Chemotherapy. J Antimicrob Chemother 2012; 67:269–289.

16.97 Conditions for the short-course treatment of endocarditis caused by fully sensitive streptococci

- Native valve infection
- Minimum inhibitory concentration (MIC) ≤0.125 mg/L
- No adverse prognostic factors (heart failure, aortic regurgitation, conduction defect)
- No evidence of thromboembolic disease
- No vegetations >5 mm diameter
- Clinical response within 7 days

16.98 Indications for cardiac surgery in infective endocarditis*

- Heart failure due to valve damage
- Failure of antibiotic therapy (persistent/uncontrolled infection)
- Large vegetations on left-sided heart valves with echo appearance suggesting high risk of emboli
- Previous evidence of systemic emboli
- Abscess formation

*Patients with prosthetic valve endocarditis or fungal endocarditis often require cardiac surgery.

16.99 Incidence and relative frequency of congenital cardiac malformations

Lesion	% of all congenital heart defects
Ventricular septal defect	30
Atrial septal defect	10
Persistent ductus arteriosus	10
Pulmonary stenosis	7
Coarctation of aorta	7
Aortic stenosis	6
Tetralogy of Fallot	6
Complete transposition of great arteries	4
Others	20

16.100 Presentation of congenital heart disease throughout life

Birth and neonatal period

- Cyanosis
- Heart failure

Infancy and childhood

- Cyanosis
- Heart failure
- Arrhythmia
- Murmur
- Failure to thrive

Adolescence and adulthood

- Heart failure
- Murmur
- Arrhythmia
- Eisenmenger's syndrome
- Hypertension (coarctation)
- Complications of previous cardiac surgery:
  Arrhythmia related to scarring
  Heart failure secondary to scarring

16

can be found in the 2012 British Society for Antimicrobial Chemotherapy guidelines (see 'Further reading').

A 2-week treatment regimen may be sufficient for fully sensitive strains of streptococci, provided specific conditions are met (Box 16.97).

Cardiac surgery with débridement of infected material and valve replacement may be required in a substantial proportion of patients, particularly those with *Staph. aureus* and fungal infections (Box 16.98). Antimicrobial therapy must be started before surgery.

Prevention

Until recently, antibiotic prophylaxis was routinely given to people at risk of infective endocarditis undergoing interventional procedures. However, as this has not been proven to be effective and the link between episodes of infective endocarditis and interventional procedures has not been demonstrated, antibiotic prophylaxis is no longer offered routinely.

Congenital heart disease

Congenital heart disease can be the result of defects in the formation of the heart or great vessels or can arise because the anatomical changes that occur during transition between the fetus and the newborn child fail to proceed normally. Congenital heart disease usually presents in childhood but some patients do not present until adult life. It has been estimated that the incidence of haemodynamically significant congenital cardiac abnormalities is about 0.8% of live births (Box 16.99). Defects that are well tolerated, such as atrial septal defect, may cause no symptoms until adult life or may be detected incidentally on routine examination or chest X-ray. Congenital defects that were previously fatal in childhood can now be corrected, or at least partially, so that survival to adult life is the norm. Such patients remain well for many years but subsequently re-present in later

life with related problems such as arrhythmia or heart failure (Box 16.100).

Pathophysiology

Understanding the fetal circulation helps clarify how some forms of congenital heart disease occur. Figure 16.90 shows the fetal circulation and the changes that normally occur immediately after birth. In the fetus there is little blood flow through the lungs, which are collapsed because they are not required for gas exchange. Instead, oxygenated blood from the placenta passes directly from the right atrium to the left side of the heart through the foramen ovale without having to flow through the lungs, and also from the pulmonary artery into the aorta via the ductus arteriosus.

During early embryonic life, the heart develops as a single tube that folds back on itself and then divides into two separate circulations. Failure of septation can cause some forms of atrial and ventricular septal defect, whereas failure of alignment of the great vessels with the ventricles contributes to transposition of the great arteries, tetralogy of Fallot and truncus arteriosus. Atrial septal defects occur because the foramen ovale fails to close at birth, as is normal. Similarly, a persistent ductus arteriosus will remain persistent if it fails to close after birth. Failure of the aorta to develop at the point of the aortic isthmus and where the ductus arteriosus attaches can lead to coarctation of the aorta. Maternal infection and exposure to drugs or toxins are important causes of congenital heart disease. Maternal rubella infection is associated with persistent ductus arteriosus, pulmonary valvular

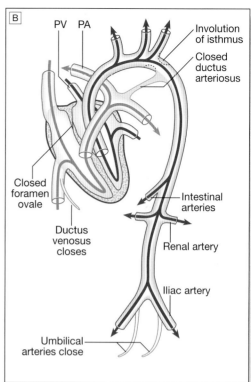

Fig. 16.90 Changes in the circulation at birth. [A] In the fetus, oxygenated blood comes through the umbilical vein where it enters the inferior vena cava (IVC) via the ductus venosus (red). The oxygenated blood streams from the right atrium (RA) through the open foramen ovale to the left atrium (LA) and via the left ventricle (LV) into the aorta. Venous blood from the superior vena cava (SVC, blue) crosses under the main blood stream into the RA and then, partly mixed with oxygenated blood (purple), into the right ventricle (RV) and pulmonary artery (PA). The pulmonary vasculature has a high resistance and so little blood passes to the lungs; most blood passes through the ductus arteriosus to the descending aorta. The aortic isthmus is a constriction in the aorta that lies in the aortic arch before the junction with the ductus arteriosus and limits the flow of oxygen-rich blood to the descending aorta. This configuration means that less oxygen-rich blood is supplied to organ systems that take up their function mainly after birth, e.g. the kidneys and intestinal tract. [B] At birth, the lungs expand with air and pulmonary vascular resistance falls, so that blood now flows to the lungs and back to the LA. The left atrial pressure rises above right atrial pressure and the flap valve of the foramen ovale closes. The umbilical arteries and the ductus venosus close. In the next few days, the ductus arteriosus closes under the influence of hormonal changes (particularly prostaglandins) and the aortic isthmus expands. (PV = pulmonary vein) *Adapted from Drews U. Colour atlas of embryology. Stuttgart: Georg Thieme; 1995.*

and/or artery stenosis, and atrial septal defect. Maternal alcohol misuse is associated with septal defects, and maternal lupus erythematosus with congenital complete heart block. Genetic or chromosomal abnormalities, such as Down's syndrome, may cause septal defects, and gene defects have also been identified as leading to specific abnormalities, such as Marfan's syndrome (p. 508) and DiGeorge's syndrome (deletion in chromosome 22q).

Clinical features

Symptoms may be absent, or the child may be breathless or fail to attain normal growth and development. Some defects are not compatible with extrauterine life and lead to neonatal death. Clinical signs vary with the anatomical lesion. Murmurs, thrills or signs of cardiomegaly may be present. In coarctation of the aorta, radio-femoral delay may be noted (Fig. 16.91) and some female patients have the features of Turner's syndrome (p. 659). Features of other congenital conditions, such as Marfan's syndrome or Down's syndrome, may also be apparent. Cerebrovascular events and cerebral abscesses may complicate severe cyanotic congenital disease.

Early diagnosis is important because many types of congenital heart disease are amenable to surgery, but this opportunity is lost if secondary changes, such as irreversible pulmonary hypertension, occur.

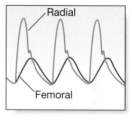

Fig. 16.91 Radio-femoral delay. The difference in pulse pressures is shown.

Central cyanosis and digital clubbing

Central cyanosis of cardiac origin occurs when desaturated blood enters the systemic circulation without passing through the lungs (right-to-left shunting). In the neonate, the most common cause is transposition of the great arteries, in which the aorta arises from the RV and the pulmonary artery from the LV in association with a ventricular septal defect. In older children, cyanosis is usually the consequence of a ventricular septal defect combined with severe pulmonary stenosis (as in tetralogy of Fallot) or with pulmonary vascular disease (Eisenmenger's syndrome). Prolonged cyanosis is associated with finger and toe clubbing (p. 442).

Growth retardation and learning difficulties

These may occur with large left-to-right shunts at ventricular or great arterial level, and also with other defects, especially if they form part of a genetic syndrome. Major intellectual impairment is uncommon in children with isolated congenital heart disease; minor learning difficulties can occur, however. Cerebral function can also be affected after cardiac surgery if cerebral perfusion is compromised.

Syncope

In the presence of increased pulmonary vascular resistance or severe left or right ventricular outflow obstruction, exercise may provoke syncope as systemic vascular resistance falls but pulmonary vascular resistance rises, worsening right-to-left shunting and cerebral oxygenation. Syncope can also occur because of associated arrhythmias.

Pulmonary hypertension

Persistently raised pulmonary flow with a left-to-right shunt causes increased pulmonary vascular resistance followed by pulmonary hypertension. Progressive changes, including obliteration of distal arterioles, take place and are irreversible. At this stage, central cyanosis occurs and digital clubbing develops. The chest X-ray shows enlarged central pulmonary arteries and peripheral 'pruning' of the pulmonary vessels. The ECG shows features of right ventricular hypertrophy.

Eisenmenger's syndrome

In patients with severe and prolonged pulmonary hypertension the left-to-right shunt may reverse, resulting in right-to-left shunt and marked cyanosis. This is termed Eisenmenger's syndrome. The cyanosis in Eisenmenger's syndrome may be more apparent in the feet and toes than in the upper part of the body, resulting in so-called differential cyanosis. Eisenmenger's syndrome is more common with large ventricular septal defects or persistent ductus arteriosus than with atrial septal defects. Patients with Eisenmenger's syndrome are at particular risk from abrupt changes in afterload that exacerbate right-to-left shunting, such as vasodilatation, anaesthesia and pregnancy.

Congenital heart disease in pregnancy

During pregnancy, there is a 50% increase in plasma volume, a 40% increase in whole blood volume and a similar increase in cardiac output, so problems may arise in women with congenital heart disease (Box 16.101). Many with palliated or untreated disease will tolerate pregnancy well, however. Pregnancy is particularly hazardous in the presence of conditions associated with cyanosis or severe pulmonary hypertension; maternal mortality in patients with Eisenmenger's syndrome is more than 50%.

16.101 Pregnancy in women with congenital heart disease

- **Obstructive lesions**: poorly tolerated and associated with significant maternal morbidity and mortality.
- **Cyanotic conditions**: especially poorly tolerated. Specialised pre-conception counselling should explain the increased risks.
- **Surgically corrected disease**: patients often tolerate pregnancy well.
- **Children of patients with congenital heart disease**: 2–5% will be born with cardiac abnormalities, especially if the mother is affected. The risk may be up to 20% in babies born of women with left-sided lesions.

Persistent ductus arteriosus

Normally, the ductus arteriosus closes soon after birth but in this anomaly it fails to do so. Persistence of the ductus is often associated with other abnormalities and is more common in females.

Pathophysiology

During fetal life, before the lungs begin to function, most of the blood from the pulmonary artery passes through the ductus arteriosus into the aorta (see Fig. 16.90). Persistence of the ductus causes a continuous AV shunt from the aorta to the pulmonary artery since pressure in the aorta is higher than that in the pulmonary circulation. The volume of the shunt depends on the size of the ductus but as much as 50% of the left ventricular output may be recirculated through the lungs, with a consequent increase in the work of the heart (Fig. 16.92). A large left-to-right shunt in infancy may cause a considerable rise in pulmonary artery pressure and sometimes this leads to progressive pulmonary vascular damage.

Clinical features

With small shunts there may be no symptoms for years, but when the ductus is large, growth and development may be retarded. Usually, there is no disability in infancy but cardiac failure may eventually ensue, dyspnoea being the first symptom. A continuous 'machinery' murmur is heard with late systolic accentuation, maximal in the second left intercostal space below the clavicle (Fig. 16.92). It is frequently accompanied by a thrill. Pulses are increased in volume.

Enlargement of the pulmonary artery may be detected radiologically. The ECG is usually normal. If pulmonary vascular resistance increases, pulmonary artery pressure may rise until it equals or exceeds aortic pressure. The shunt through the defect

16

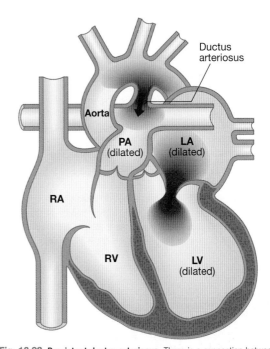

Fig. 16.92 Persistent ductus arteriosus. There is a connection between the aorta and the pulmonary artery with left-to-right shunting. (LA = left atrium; LV = left ventricle; PA = pulmonary artery; RA = right atrium; RV = right ventricle)

may then reverse, causing Eisenmenger's syndrome. The murmur becomes quieter, may be confined to systole or may disappear.

Investigations

Echocardiography is the investigation of choice although the persistent ductus requires specific echocardiographic views, such as from the suprasternal notch, to reveal it. The ECG shows evidence of right ventricular hypertrophy

Management

A persistent ductus can be closed at cardiac catheterisation with an implantable occlusive device. Closure should be undertaken in infancy if the shunt is significant and pulmonary resistance not elevated, but this may be delayed until later childhood in those with smaller shunts, for whom closure remains advisable to reduce the risk of endocarditis. When the ductus is structurally intact, a prostaglandin synthetase inhibitor (indometacin or ibuprofen) may be used in the first week of life to induce closure. However, in the presence of a congenital defect with impaired lung perfusion, such as occurs in severe pulmonary stenosis and left-to-right shunt through the ductus, it may be advisable to improve oxygenation by keeping the ductus open with prostaglandin treatment. Unfortunately, these treatments do not work if the ductus is intrinsically abnormal.

Coarctation of the aorta

This condition is twice as common in males and occurs in 1 in 4000 children. It is associated with other abnormalities, most frequently bicuspid aortic valve and 'berry' aneurysms of the cerebral circulation (p. 1160). Acquired coarctation of the aorta is rare but may follow trauma or occur as a complication of a progressive arteritis (Takayasu's disease, p. 1041).

Pathogenesis

Narrowing of the aorta occurs in the region where the ductus arteriosus joins the aorta, at the isthmus just below the origin of the left subclavian artery (see Fig. 16.90). This causes raised BP affecting vessels of the head and neck proximal to the coarctation, and reduced BP and impaired circulation distally.

Clinical features

Aortic coarctation is an important cause of cardiac failure in the newborn but symptoms are often absent in older children or adults. Headaches may occur from hypertension proximal to the coarctation, and occasionally weakness or cramps in the legs may result from decreased circulation in the lower part of the body. The BP is raised in the upper body but normal or low in the legs. The femoral pulses are weak and delayed in comparison with the radial pulse (see Fig. 16.91). A systolic murmur is usually heard posteriorly, over the coarctation. There may also be an ejection click and systolic murmur in the aortic area due to a bicuspid aortic valve. As a result of the aortic narrowing, collaterals form; they mainly involve the periscapular, internal mammary and intercostal arteries, and may result in localised bruits.

Investigations

Imaging by MRI is the investigation of choice (Fig. 16.93). The chest X-ray in early childhood is often normal but later may show changes in the contour of the aorta (indentation of the descending aorta, '3 sign') and notching of the under-surfaces of the ribs from collaterals. The ECG may show evidence of left ventricular hypertrophy, which can be confirmed by echocardiography.

Fig. 16.93 MRI scan of coarctation of the aorta. The aorta is severely narrowed just beyond the arch at the start of the descending aorta (arrow A). Extensive collaterals have developed; a large internal mammary artery (arrow B) and several intercostal arteries (arrows C) are shown. Unusually, in this case, there is also a coarctation of the abdominal aorta (arrow D).

Management

In untreated cases, death may occur from left ventricular failure, dissection of the aorta or cerebral haemorrhage. Surgical correction is advisable in all but the mildest cases. If this is carried out sufficiently early in childhood, persistent hypertension can be avoided. Patients repaired in late childhood or adult life often remain hypertensive or develop recurrent hypertension later on. Recurrence of stenosis may occur as the child grows and this may be managed by balloon dilatation and sometimes stenting. The latter may be used as the primary treatment. Coexistent bicuspid aortic valve, which occurs in over 50% of cases, may lead to progressive aortic stenosis or regurgitation, and also requires long-term follow-up.

Atrial septal defect

Atrial septal defect is one of the most common congenital heart defects and occurs twice as frequently in females. Most are 'ostium secundum' defects, involving the fossa ovalis that, in utero, was the foramen ovale (see Fig. 16.90). 'Ostium primum' defects result from a defect in the atrioventricular septum and are associated with a 'cleft mitral valve' (split anterior leaflet).

Pathogenesis

Since the normal RV is more compliant than the LV, a patent foramen ovale is associated with shunting of blood from the LA to the RA, and then to the RV and pulmonary arteries (Fig. 16.94). As a result, there is gradual enlargement of the right side of the heart and of the pulmonary arteries. Pulmonary hypertension and shunt reversal sometimes complicate atrial septal defect, but are less common and tend to occur later in life than with other types of left-to-right shunt.

Clinical features

Most children are asymptomatic for many years and the condition is often detected at routine clinical examination or following a chest X-ray. Symptoms that can occur include dyspnoea, chest infections,

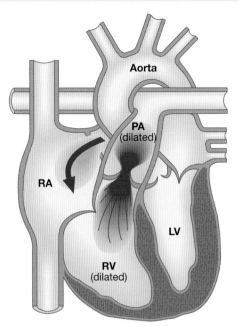

Fig. 16.94 Atrial septal defect. Blood flows across the atrial septum (arrow) from left to right. The murmur is produced by increased flow velocity across the pulmonary valve, as a result of left-to-right shunting and a large stroke volume. The density of shading is proportional to velocity of blood flow. (LV = left ventricle; PA = pulmonary artery; RA = right atrium; RV = right ventricle)

Fig. 16.95 Transoesophageal echocardiogram of an atrial septal defect. The defect is clearly seen (arrow) between the left atrium above and right atrium below. Doppler colour-flow imaging shows flow (blue) across the defect.

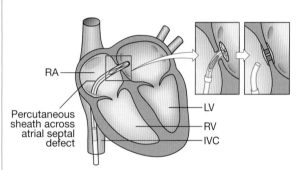

Fig. 16.96 Percutaneous closure of atrial septal defect. The closure device is delivered across the interatrial septum and a disc deployed on either side to seal the defect. (IVC = inferior vena cava; LV = left ventricle; PA = pulmonary artery; RA = right atrium; RV = right ventricle)

cardiac failure and arrhythmias, especially AF. The characteristic physical signs are the result of the volume overload of the RV:

- wide, fixed splitting of the second heart sound: wide because of delay in right ventricular ejection (increased stroke volume and RBBB), and fixed because the septal defect equalises left and right atrial pressures throughout the respiratory cycle
- a systolic flow murmur over the pulmonary valve.

In children with a large shunt, there may be a diastolic flow murmur over the tricuspid valve. Unlike a mitral flow murmur, this is usually high-pitched.

Investigations

Echocardiography is diagnostic. It directly demonstrates the defect and typically shows right ventricular dilatation, right ventricular hypertrophy and pulmonary artery dilatation. The precise size and location of the defect are best defined by TOE (Fig. 16.95). The chest X-ray typically shows enlargement of the heart and the pulmonary artery, as well as pulmonary plethora. The ECG usually demonstrates incomplete RBBB because right ventricular depolarisation is delayed as a result of ventricular dilatation (with a 'primum' defect, there is also left axis deviation).

Management

Atrial septal defects in which pulmonary flow is increased 50% above systemic flow (i.e. a flow ratio of 1.5:1) are often large enough to be clinically recognisable and should be closed surgically. (Smaller defects may be managed conservatively and patients are monitored with echocardiography.) Closure can also be accomplished at cardiac catheterisation using implantable closure devices (Fig. 16.96). The long-term prognosis thereafter is excellent, unless pulmonary hypertension has developed.

Severe pulmonary hypertension and shunt reversal are both contraindications to surgery.

Ventricular septal defect

Ventricular septal defect is the most common congenital cardiac defect, occurring once in 500 live births. The defect may be isolated or part of complex congenital heart disease.

Pathogenesis

Congenital ventricular septal defect occurs as a result of incomplete septation of the ventricles. Embryologically, the interventricular septum has a membranous and a muscular portion, and the latter is further divided into inflow, trabecular and outflow portions. Most congenital defects are 'perimembranous', occurring at the junction of the membranous and muscular portions of the septum.

Clinical features

Flow from the high-pressure LV to the low-pressure RV during systole produces a pansystolic murmur, usually heard best at the left sternal edge but radiating all over the precordium (Fig. 16.97). A small defect often produces a loud murmur (maladie de Roger) in the absence of other haemodynamic disturbance. Conversely, a large defect produces a softer murmur,

16

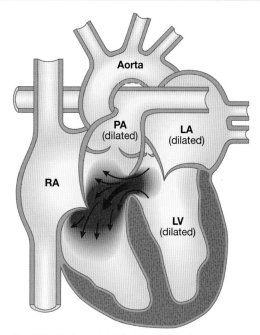

Fig. 16.97 Ventricular septal defect. In this example, a large left-to-right shunt (arrows) has resulted in chamber enlargement. (LA = left atrium; LV = left ventricle; PA = pulmonary artery; RA = right atrium)

particularly if pressure in the RV is elevated. This may be found immediately after birth, while pulmonary vascular resistance remains high, or when the shunt is reversed in Eisenmenger's syndrome. Congenital ventricular septal defect may present as cardiac failure in infants, as a murmur with only minor haemodynamic disturbance in older children or adults, or, rarely, as Eisenmenger's syndrome. In a proportion of infants, the murmur becomes quieter or disappears due to spontaneous closure of the defect.

If cardiac failure complicates a large defect, it is usually absent in the immediate postnatal period and becomes apparent only in the first 4–6 weeks of life. In addition to the murmur, there is prominent parasternal pulsation, tachypnoea and indrawing of the lower ribs on inspiration.

Investigations

Doppler echocardiography should be performed since it helps to identify the small septal defects that are not haemodynamically significant and are likely to close spontaneously. Patients with larger defects should be monitored by serial ECG and echocardiography to screen for signs of pulmonary hypertension. With larger defects, the chest X-ray shows pulmonary congestion and the ECG shows bilateral ventricular hypertrophy.

Management

Small ventricular septal defects require no specific treatment. If there is cardiac failure in infancy, this should initially be treated medically with digoxin and diuretics. Persisting failure is an indication for surgical repair of the defect. Percutaneous closure devices are under development.

If serial ECG and echocardiography suggest that pulmonary hypertension is developing, surgical repair should be performed. Surgical closure is contraindicated in fully developed Eisenmenger's

syndrome, in which case heart–lung transplantation is the only effective treatment. The long-term prognosis is generally very good. An exception is in Eisenmenger's syndrome, when death normally occurs in the second or third decade of life, but a few individuals survive to the fifth decade without transplantation.

Tetralogy of Fallot

This is complex defect consisting of right ventricular outflow tract obstruction and right ventricular hypertrophy, a large ventricular septal defect and an over-riding aorta that, when combined with the septal defect, allows blood to be pumped directly from the RV into the aorta. It occurs in about 1 in 2000 births and is the most common cause of cyanosis in infancy after the first year of life.

Pathogenesis

Tetralogy of Fallot occurs as the result of abnormal development of the bulbar septum that separates the ascending aorta from the pulmonary artery, and which normally aligns and fuses with the outflow part of the interventricular septum. The right ventricular outflow obstruction is most often subvalvular (infundibular) but may be valvular, supravalvular or a combination of these (Fig. 16.98). The subvalvular component of the right ventricular outflow obstruction is dynamic and may increase suddenly under adrenergic stimulation. The ventricular septal defect is usually large and similar in aperture to the aortic orifice. The combination results in elevated right ventricular pressure and right-to-left shunting of cyanotic blood across the ventricular septal defect into the aorta.

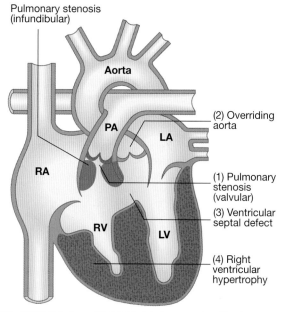

Fig. 16.98 Tetralogy of Fallot. The tetralogy comprises (1) pulmonary stenosis, (2) overriding of the ventricular septal defect by the aorta, (3) a ventricular septal defect and (4) right ventricular hypertrophy. (LA = left atrium; LV = left ventricle; PA = pulmonary artery; RA = right atrium; RV = right ventricle)

Clinical features

Children are usually cyanosed but this may not be the case in the neonate because it is only when right ventricular pressure rises to equal or exceed left ventricular pressure that a large right-to-left shunt develops. The affected child may suddenly become increasingly cyanosed, often after feeding or a crying attack, and may become apnoeic and unconscious. These attacks are called 'Fallot's spells'. In older children, Fallot's spells are uncommon but cyanosis becomes increasingly apparent, with stunting of growth, digital clubbing and polycythaemia. Some children characteristically obtain relief by squatting after exertion, which increases the afterload of the left heart and reduces the right-to-left shunting. This is called Fallot's sign. The natural history before the development of surgical correction was variable but most patients died in infancy or childhood.

On examination, the most characteristic feature is the combination of cyanosis with a loud ejection systolic murmur in the pulmonary area (as for pulmonary stenosis). Cyanosis may be absent in the newborn or in patients with only mild right ventricular outflow obstruction, however. This is called acyanotic tetralogy of Fallot.

Investigations

Echocardiography is diagnostic and demonstrates that the aorta is not continuous with the anterior ventricular septum. The ECG shows right ventricular hypertrophy and the chest X-ray shows an abnormally small pulmonary artery and a 'boot-shaped' heart.

Management

The definitive management is total correction of the defect by surgical relief of the pulmonary stenosis and closure of the ventricular septal defect. Primary surgical correction may be undertaken prior to the age of 5 years. If the pulmonary arteries are too hypoplastic, then palliation in the form of a Blalock–Taussig shunt may be performed, with an anastomosis created between the pulmonary artery and subclavian artery. This improves pulmonary blood flow and pulmonary artery development, and may facilitate later definitive correction.

The prognosis after total correction is good, especially if the operation is performed in childhood. Follow-up is needed to identify residual shunting, recurrent pulmonary stenosis and arrhythmias. An implantable defibrillator is sometimes recommended in adulthood.

Other causes of cyanotic congenital heart disease

There are other causes of cyanotic congenital heart disease, as summarised in Box 16.102. Echocardiography is usually the definitive diagnostic procedure, supplemented, if necessary, by cardiac catheterisation.

Adult congenital heart disease

There are increasing numbers of children who have had surgical correction of congenital defects and who may have further problems as adults. The transition period between paediatric and adult care needs to be managed in a carefully planned manner, addressing many diverse aspects of care (Box 16.103). Those who have undergone correction of coarctation of the aorta may develop hypertension in adult life. Those with transposition of the great arteries who have had a 'Mustard' repair, in which

16.102 Other causes of cyanotic congenital heart disease

Defect	Features
Tricuspid atresia	Absent tricuspid orifice, hypoplastic RV, RA-to-LA shunt, ventricular septal defect shunt, other anomalies Surgical correction may be possible
Transposition of the great vessels	Aorta arises from the morphological RV, pulmonary artery from LV Shunt via atria, ductus and possibly ventricular septal defect Palliation by balloon atrial septostomy/enlargement Surgical correction possible
Pulmonary atresia	Pulmonary valve atretic and pulmonary artery hypoplastic RA-to-LA shunt, pulmonary flow via ductus Palliation by balloon atrial septostomy Surgical correction may be possible
Ebstein's anomaly	Tricuspid valve is dysplastic and displaced into RV, RV 'atrialised' Tricuspid regurgitation and RA-to-LA shunt Wide spectrum of severity Arrhythmias Surgical repair possible but significant risk

(LA = left atrium; LV = left ventricle; RA = right atrium; RV = right ventricle)

16.103 Congenital heart disease in adolescence

- **Patients**: a heterogeneous population with residual disease and sequelae that vary according to the underlying lesion and in severity; each patient must be assessed individually.
- **Management plan**: should be agreed with the patient and include short- and long-term goals and timing of transition to adult care.
- **Risks of surgery**: non-cardiac surgery for associated congenital abnormalities carries increased risks and needs to be planned, with careful pre-operative assessment. Risks include thrombosis, embolism from synthetic shunts or patches, and volume overload from fluid shifts. Operative approaches should address cosmetic concerns, such as site of implantation of abdominal generator.
- **Exercise**: patients with mild or repaired defects can undertake moderately vigorous exercise but those with complex defects, cyanosis, ventricular dysfunction or arrhythmias require specialist evaluation and individualised advice regarding exercise.
- **Genetics**: Between 10% and 15% have a genetic basis and this should be assessed to understand the impact it may have for the patient's own future children. A family history, genetic evaluation of syndromic versus non-syndromic disorders and, sometimes, cytogenetics are required.
- **Education and employment**: may be adversely affected and occupational activity levels need to be assessed.
- **End of life**: some adolescents with complex disorders may misperceive and think they have been cured; transition to adult services may be the first time they receive information about mortality. Expectations on life expectancy need to be managed and adolescents are often willing to engage with this and play a role in decision-making.

blood is redirected at atrial level leaving the RV connected to the aorta, may develop right ventricular failure in adult life. This is because the RV is unsuited for function at systemic pressures and may begin to dilate and fail when patients are in their twenties or thirties.

16

Those who have had surgery involving the atria may develop atrial arrhythmias, and those who have ventricular scars may develop ventricular arrhythmias and need consideration for placement of an ICD. Such patients require careful follow-up from the teenage years throughout adult life, so that problems can be identified early and appropriate medical or surgical treatment instituted. The management of patients with grown-up congenital heart disease (GUCH) is complex and has developed as a cardiological subspecialty.

Diseases of the myocardium

Although the myocardium is involved as the result of ischaemia in CAD and in valvular heart disease, this section focus on conditions that primarily affect the heart muscle.

Myocarditis

This is an acute inflammatory condition that can have an infectious, toxic or autoimmune aetiology (Box 16.104). Myocarditis can complicate many infections in which inflammation may be due directly to infection of the myocardium or the effects of circulating toxins. Viral infections are the most common causes, such as Coxsackie (35 cases per 1000 infections) and influenza A and B (25 cases per 1000 infections) viruses. Myocarditis may occur several weeks after the initial viral symptoms, and susceptibility is increased by glucocorticoid treatment, immunosuppression, radiation, previous myocardial damage and exercise. Some bacterial and protozoal infections may be complicated by myocarditis; for example, approximately 5% of patients with Lyme disease (*Borrelia burgdorferi*, p. 255) develop myopericarditis, which is often associated with AV block. Toxins such as alcohol and drugs such as cocaine, lithium and doxorubicin may directly injure the myocardium. Other drugs, including penicillins and sulphonamides, and poisons such as lead and carbon monoxide may cause a hypersensitivity reaction and associated myocarditis. Occasionally, autoimmune conditions, such as systemic lupus erythematosus and rheumatoid arthritis, are associated with myocarditis.

Clinical features

Myocarditis may present in one of four ways:

- *Fulminant myocarditis* follows a viral prodrome or influenza-like illness and results in severe heart failure or cardiogenic shock.
- *Acute myocarditis* presents over a longer period with heart failure; it can lead to dilated cardiomyopathy.
- *Chronic active myocarditis* is rare and associated with chronic myocardial inflammation.
- *Chronic persistent myocarditis* is characterised by focal myocardial infiltrates and can cause chest pain and arrhythmia without necessarily causing ventricular dysfunction.

Myocarditis is self-limiting in most patients and the immediate prognosis is good. Death may, however, occur due to a ventricular arrhythmia or rapidly progressive heart failure. Myocarditis has been reported as a cause of sudden and unexpected death in young athletes. Some forms of myocarditis may lead to chronic low-grade myocarditis or dilated cardiomyopathy (see below). For example, in Chagas' disease (p. 279), the patient frequently recovers from the acute infection but goes on to develop a chronic dilated cardiomyopathy 10 or 20 years later.

Investigations

The diagnosis of myocarditis is often made after other more common causes of cardiac dysfunction have been excluded. Echocardiography should be performed and may reveal left ventricular dysfunction that is sometimes regional (due to focal myocarditis). Cardiac MRI is also useful since it may show diagnostic patterns of myocardial inflammation or infiltration. The ECG is frequently abnormal but the changes are non-specific. Blood should be taken for analysis of troponin I and T, and creatine kinase. Levels may be elevated in the early phases. Occasionally, endomyocardial biopsy may be required to confirm the diagnosis.

Management

Treatment of myocarditis is primarily supportive. Treatment for cardiac failure or arrhythmias should be given and patients should be advised to avoid intense physical exertion because there is some evidence that this can induce potentially fatal ventricular arrhythmias. There is no evidence of benefit from treatment with glucocorticoids and immunosuppressive agents.

Specific antimicrobial therapy may be used if a causative organism has been identified but this is rare. Patients who do not respond adequately to medical treatment may temporarily require circulatory support with a mechanical ventricular assist device. Rarely, cardiac transplantation may be required.

Cardiomyopathy

Cardiomyopathies are primary diseases of the myocardium, which are classified according to their effects on cardiac structure and function (Fig. 16.99). They can be inherited or be caused by infections or exposure to toxins. In some cases no cause is identified.

---

i 16.104 Some causes of myocarditis

Infections

Viral
- Coxsackie
- Adenovirus
- Influenza A
- Human immunodeficiency virus (HIV)
- Influenza B

Bacterial
- *Borrelia burgdorferi* (Lyme disease)
- *Mycoplasma pneumoniae*

Protozoal
- *Trypanosoma cruzi* (Chagas' disease)
- *Toxoplasma gondii*

Fungal
- *Aspergillus*

Parasitic
- *Shistosoma*

Drugs/Toxins
- Alcohol
- Anthracyclines
- Clozapine
- Cocaine
- Lithium

Autoimmune
- Systemic lupus erythematosus
- Systemic sclerosis
- Rheumatoid arthritis
- Sarcoidosis
- Hypersensitivity reaction to penicillins, sulphonamides, lead, carbon monoxide

Fig. 16.99 Types of cardiomyopathy. A Normal heart. B Hypertrophic cardiomyopathy: asymmetric septal hypertrophy (ASH) with systolic anterior motion of the mitral valve (SAM), causing mitral reflux and dynamic left ventricular outflow tract obstruction. C Hypertrophic cardiomyopathy: concentric hypertrophy. D Hypertrophic cardiomyopathy: apical hypertrophy. E Dilated cardiomyopathy. F Arrhythmogenic right ventricular cardiomyopathy. G Obliterative cardiomyopathy. H Restrictive cardiomyopathy.

16

Dilated cardiomyopathy

In North America and Europe, symptomatic dilated cardiomyopathy has an incidence of 20 per 100 000 and a prevalence of 38 per 100 000. Men are affected more than twice as often as women.

Pathogenesis

Cardiomyopathy is characterised by dilatation and impaired contraction of the LV and often the RV. Left ventricular mass is increased but wall thickness is normal or reduced (Fig. 16.99). Dilatation of the valve rings can lead to functional mitral and tricuspid incompetence. Histological changes are variable but include myofibrillary loss, interstitial fibrosis and T-cell infiltrates. The term 'dilated cardiomyopathy' encompasses a heterogeneous group of conditions. Alcohol may be an important cause in some patients. At least 25% of cases are inherited as an autosomal dominant trait and a variety of single-gene mutations have been identified. Most of these mutations affect proteins in the cytoskeleton of the myocytes, such as dystrophin, lamin A and C, emerin and metavinculin. Many are also associated with abnormalities of skeletal muscle. Conversely, most of the X-linked inherited skeletal muscular dystrophies, such as Becker and Duchenne (p. 1143), are associated with cardiomyopathy. Finally, a late autoimmune reaction to viral myocarditis is thought to be the cause in a substantial subgroup of patients with dilated cardiomyopathy; a similar mechanism is believed to be responsible for the myocardial involvement that occurs in up to 10% of patients with advanced human immunodeficiency virus (HIV) infection.

Clinical features

Most patients present with heart failure or are found to have the condition during routine investigation. Arrhythmia, thromboembolism and sudden death may occur at any stage; sporadic chest pain is a surprisingly frequent symptom. The differential diagnosis includes ventricular dysfunction due to CAD, and a diagnosis of dilated cardiomyopathy should be made only when this has been excluded.

Investigations

Echocardiography and cardiac MRI are the most useful investigations. Although ECG changes are common, they are non-specific. Genetic testing is indicated if more than one family member is diagnosed with the condition.

Management

The focus of management is to control heart failure using the strategies described earlier in this chapter (p. 464). Although some patients remain well for many years, the prognosis is variable and cardiac transplantation may be indicated. Patients with dilated cardiomyopathy and moderate or severe heart failure are at risk of sudden arrhythmic death and this can be reduced by rigorous medical therapy with β-blockers and either ACE inhibitors or ARBs. Some patients may be considered for implantation of a cardiac defibrillator and/or cardiac resynchronisation therapy (pp. 483 and 484).

Hypertrophic cardiomyopathy

This is the most common form of cardiomyopathy, with a prevalence of approximately 100 per 100 000. It is characterised by inappropriate and elaborate left ventricular hypertrophy with malalignment of the myocardial fibres and myocardial fibrosis. The hypertrophy may be generalised or confined largely to the interventricular septum (asymmetric septal hypertrophy, Fig. 16.99) or other regions of the heart. A specific variant termed apical hypertrophic cardiomyopathy is common in the Far East.

Pathogenesis

Hypertrophic cardiomyopathy is a genetic disorder, usually with autosomal dominant transmission, a high degree of penetrance and variable expression. In most patients, it is due to a single-point mutation in one of the genes that encode sarcomeric contractile proteins. There are three common groups of mutation with different phenotypes. Beta-myosin heavy-chain mutations are associated with elaborate ventricular hypertrophy. Troponin mutations are associated with little, and sometimes even no, hypertrophy but marked myocardial fibre disarray, exercise-induced hypotension and a high risk of sudden death. Myosin-binding protein C mutations tend to present late in life and are often associated with hypertension and arrhythmia. In all subtypes, heart failure may develop because the stiff, non-compliant LV impedes diastolic filling. Septal hypertrophy may also cause dynamic left ventricular outflow tract obstruction (hypertrophic obstructive cardiomyopathy, HOCM) and mitral regurgitation due to abnormal systolic anterior motion of the anterior mitral valve leaflet.

Clinical features

Effort-related symptoms, such as angina, breathlessness, arrhythmia and sudden death, are the dominant clinical presentations. The symptoms and signs are similar to those of aortic stenosis, except that, in hypertrophic cardiomyopathy, the character of the arterial pulse is jerky (Box 16.105). The annual mortality from sudden death is 2–3% among adults and 4–6% in children and adolescents (Box 16.106). Sudden death typically occurs during or just after vigorous physical activity and is thought to be due to ventricular arrhythmias. Hypertrophic cardiomyopathy is the most common cause of sudden death in young athletes. In patients who do not suffer fatal arrhythmias, the natural history is variable but clinical deterioration is often slow.

	16.105 Clinical features of hypertrophic cardiomyopathy

Symptoms

- Angina on effort
- Syncope on effort
- Dyspnoea on effort
- Sudden death

Signs

- Jerky pulse*
- Palpable left ventricular hypertrophy
- Double impulse at the apex (palpable fourth heart sound due to left atrial hypertrophy)
- Mid-systolic murmur at the base*
- Pansystolic murmur (due to mitral regurgitation) at the apex

*Signs of left ventricular outflow tract obstruction may be augmented by standing up (reduced venous return), inotropes and vasodilators (e.g. sublingual nitrate).

	16.106 Risk factors for sudden death in hypertrophic cardiomyopathy

- A history of previous cardiac arrest or sustained ventricular tachycardia
- Recurrent syncope
- An adverse genotype and/or family history
- Exercise-induced hypotension
- Non-sustained ventricular tachycardia on ambulatory ECG monitoring
- Marked increase in left ventricular wall thickness

Investigations

Echocardiography is the investigation of choice and is usually diagnostic. Sometimes the diagnosis is more difficult when another cause of left ventricular hypertrophy is present but the degree of hypertrophy in hypertrophic cardiomyopathy is usually greater than in physiological hypertrophy and the pattern is asymmetrical. The ECG is abnormal and shows features of left ventricular hypertrophy with a wide variety of often bizarre abnormalities, including deep T-wave inversion. Genetic testing can be performed and is helpful in screening relatives of affected individuals.

Management

Beta-blockers, rate-limiting calcium antagonists and disopyramide can help to relieve symptoms and prevent syncopal attacks. Arrhythmias often respond to treatment with amiodarone. No pharmacological treatment has been identified that can improve prognosis, however. Outflow tract obstruction can be improved by partial surgical resection (myectomy) or by iatrogenic infarction of the basal septum (septal ablation) using a catheter-delivered alcohol solution. An ICD should be considered in patients with clinical risk factors for sudden death (Box 16.106). Digoxin and vasodilators may increase outflow tract obstruction and should be avoided.

Arrhythmogenic ventricular cardiomyopathy

Arrhythmogenic ventricular cardiomyopathy (AVC) predominantly affects the myocardium of the right ventricle. It is inherited in an autosomal dominant manner and has a prevalence of approximately 10 per 100 000. The genetic defect involves desmosomal protein genes, most commonly plakophilin 2 (*PKP-2*), although current genetic testing protocols will not identify the culprit gene in many cases. It is characterised by replacement of patches of the right ventricular myocardium with fibrous and fatty tissue (see Fig. 16.99). In some cases, the LV is also involved and this is associated with a poorer prognosis. The diagnosis is based on a complex set of criteria that take account of the ECG, structural assessment, genetics and arrhythmias. The dominant clinical problems are ventricular arrhythmias, sudden death and right-sided cardiac failure. The ECG typically shows a slightly broadened QRS complex and inverted T waves in the right precordial leads. MRI is a helpful diagnostic tool and is used, along with the 12-lead ECG and ambulatory ECG monitoring, to screen the first-degree relatives of affected individuals. Management is based on treating right-sided cardiac failure with diuretics and cardiac arrhythmias with β-blockers or, in patients at high risk of sudden death, an implantable defibrillator can be offered.

Restrictive cardiomyopathy

In this rare condition, ventricular filling is impaired because the ventricles are 'stiff' (see Fig. 16.99). This leads to high atrial pressures with atrial hypertrophy, dilatation and, later, AF. Amyloidosis is the most common cause in the UK, although other forms of infiltration due to glycogen storage diseases, idiopathic perimyocyte fibrosis and a familial form of restrictive cardiomyopathy can also occur. The diagnosis can be difficult and requires assessment with Doppler echocardiography, CT or MRI, and endomyocardial biopsy. Treatment is symptomatic but the prognosis is usually poor and transplantation may be indicated.

Obliterative cardiomyopathy

This is a rare form of restrictive cardiomyopathy, involving the endocardium of one or both ventricles; it is characterised by thrombosis and fibrosis, with gradual obliteration of the ventricular cavities by fibrous tissue (see Fig. 16.99). The mitral and tricuspid valves become regurgitant. Heart failure and pulmonary and systemic embolism are prominent features. It can sometimes be associated with eosinophilia and can occur in eosinophilic leukaemia and eosinophilic granulomatosis with polyangiitis (formerly known as Churg–Strauss syndrome, p. 1043). In tropical countries, the disease can be responsible for up to 10% of cardiac deaths. Mortality is high: 50% at 2 years. Anticoagulation and antiplatelet therapy are used, and diuretics may help symptoms of heart failure. Surgery (tricuspid and/or mitral valve replacement with decortication of the endocardium) may be helpful in selected cases.

Takotsubo cardiomyopathy

Takotsubo cardiomyopathy (Takotsubo syndrome) is a form of acute left ventricular dysfunction characterised by dilatation of the left ventricular apex and adjacent myocardium, with associated left ventricular impairment. The mechanism is poorly understood but may involve noradrenergic coronary vasoconstriction and acute left ventricular outflow obstruction. It is often associated with acute environmental or emotional stress (such as a bereavement) and presents with chest pain, breathlessness and sometimes cardiac failure. It occurs more frequently in women than in men. In terms of both symptoms and the ECG, the condition mimics acute ST elevation acute coronary syndrome. The diagnosis is usually made at coronary angiography, when CAD is found to be absent or minimal. Echocardiography then shows characteristic 'apical ballooning' of the LV. The dilated apex and narrow outflow of the LV resemble a Japanese octopus trap, or takotsubo (Fig. 16.100).

Fig. 16.100 Takotsubo cardiomyopathy. Left ventriculogram following injection of contrast in a patient with Takotsubo cardiomyopathy. The outline of the dilated left ventricle is indicated by arrows.

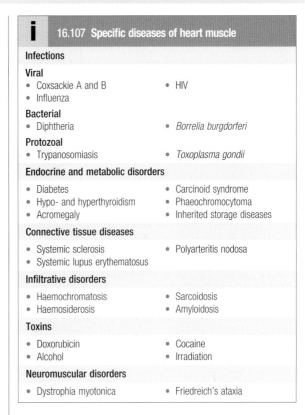

i	**16.107 Specific diseases of heart muscle**

Infections

Viral
- Coxsackie A and B
- Influenza
- HIV

Bacterial
- Diphtheria
- *Borrelia burgdorferi*

Protozoal
- Trypanosomiasis
- *Toxoplasma gondii*

Endocrine and metabolic disorders
- Diabetes
- Hypo- and hyperthyroidism
- Acromegaly
- Carcinoid syndrome
- Phaeochromocytoma
- Inherited storage diseases

Connective tissue diseases
- Systemic sclerosis
- Systemic lupus erythematosus
- Polyarteritis nodosa

Infiltrative disorders
- Haemochromatosis
- Haemosiderosis
- Sarcoidosis
- Amyloidosis

Toxins
- Doxorubicin
- Alcohol
- Cocaine
- Irradiation

Neuromuscular disorders
- Dystrophia myotonica
- Friedreich's ataxia

16

Left ventricular dysfunction usually recovers within 4–5 days, although this can take weeks in some cases. Treatment is with a β-blocker, to prevent arrhythmia, and an ACE inhibitor, to treat left ventricular dysfunction. These drugs are continued only until cardiac function has recovered.

Secondary causes of cardiomyopathy

Many systemic conditions can produce a picture that is indistinguishable from dilated cardiomyopathy, including connective tissue disorders, sarcoidosis, haemochromatosis and alcoholic heart muscle disease (Box 16.107). In contrast, amyloidosis and eosinophilic heart disease produce symptoms and signs similar to those found in restrictive or obliterative cardiomyopathy, whereas the heart disease associated with Friedreich's ataxia (p. 1116) can mimic hypertrophic cardiomyopathy.

Treatment and prognosis are determined by the underlying disorder. Abstention from alcohol may lead to a dramatic improvement in patients with alcoholic heart muscle disease.

Cardiac tumours

Primary cardiac tumours are rare (<0.2% of autopsies) but the heart and mediastinum may be the sites of metastases. Most primary tumours are benign (75%) and, of these, the majority are myxomas. The remainder are fibromas, lipomas, fibroelastomas and haemangiomas.

Atrial myxoma

Myxomas most commonly arise in the LA as single or multiple polypoid tumours, attached by a pedicle to the interatrial septum.

They are usually gelatinous but may be solid and even calcified, with superimposed thrombus.

On examination, the first heart sound is usually loud, and there may be a murmur of mitral regurgitation with a variable diastolic sound (tumour 'plop') due to prolapse of the mass through the mitral valve. The tumour can be detected incidentally on echocardiography, or following investigation of pyrexia, syncope, arrhythmias or emboli. Occasionally, the condition presents with malaise and features suggestive of a connective tissue disorder, including a raised ESR.

Treatment is by surgical excision. If the pedicle is removed, fewer than 5% of tumours recur.

Diseases of the pericardium

The normal pericardial sac contains about 50 mL of fluid, similar to lymph, which lubricates the surface of the heart. The pericardium limits distension of the heart, contributes to the haemodynamic interdependence of the ventricles, and acts as a barrier to infection. Nevertheless, congenital absence of the pericardium does not result in significant clinical or functional limitations.

Acute pericarditis

This is due to an acute inflammatory process affecting the pericardium, which may coexist with myocarditis.

Pathogenesis

A number of causes are recognised (Box 16.108), but in some cases the cause is unclear. All forms of pericarditis may produce a pericardial effusion that, depending on the aetiology, may be fibrinous, serous, haemorrhagic or purulent. A fibrinous exudate may eventually lead to varying degrees of adhesion formation, whereas serous pericarditis often produces a large effusion of turbid, straw-coloured fluid with a high protein content. A haemorrhagic effusion is often due to malignant disease, particularly carcinoma of the breast or bronchus, and lymphoma. Purulent pericarditis is rare and may occur as a complication of sepsis, by direct spread from an intrathoracic infection, or from a penetrating injury.

Clinical features

The typical presentation is with chest pain that is retrosternal, radiates to the shoulders and neck, and is typically aggravated by deep breathing, movement, a change of position, exercise and swallowing. A low-grade fever is common. A pericardial

i	16.108 Causes of acute pericarditis and pericardial effusion
Infection	
• Viral	• Tuberculosis
• Bacterial	
Inflammatory	
• Rheumatoid arthritis	• Rheumatic fever
• Systemic lupus erythematosus	
Other	
• Post-myocardial infarction	• Malignancy
• Uraemia	• Trauma

friction rub is a high-pitched, superficial scratching or crunching noise, produced by movement of the inflamed pericardium, and is diagnostic of pericarditis; it is usually heard in systole but may also be audible in diastole and frequently has a 'to-and-fro' quality.

Investigations

The diagnosis can often be made on the basis of clinical features and the ECG; the latter shows ST elevation with upward concavity (Fig. 16.101) over the affected area, which may be widespread. PR interval depression is a very specific indicator of acute pericarditis. Later, there may be T-wave inversion, particularly if there is a degree of myocarditis. Echocardiography may be normal or may reveal pericardial effusion, in which case regular echocardiographic monitoring is recommended.

Management

The pain usually responds to aspirin (600 mg 6 times daily) but a more potent anti-inflammatory agent, such as indometacin (50 mg 3 times daily), may be required. Colchicine or glucocorticoids can also suppress symptoms but there is no evidence that they accelerate cure. In viral pericarditis, recovery usually occurs within a few days or weeks but there may be recurrences (chronic relapsing pericarditis). Purulent pericarditis requires treatment with antimicrobial therapy, pericardiocentesis and, if necessary, surgical drainage.

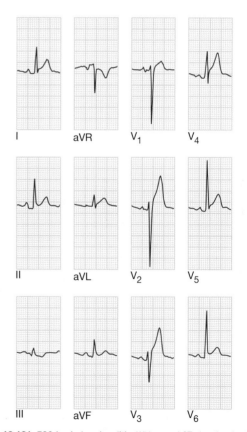

Fig. 16.101 ECG in viral pericarditis. Widespread ST elevation (leads I, II, aVL and V₁–V₆) is shown. The upward concave shape of the ST segments (see leads II and V₆) and the unusual distribution of changes (involving anterior and inferior leads) help to distinguish pericarditis from acute myocardial infarction.

Pericardial effusion

Pericardial effusion often accompanies pericarditis and can have a number of causes, as shown in Box 16.108.

Clinical features

With the onset of an effusion the heart sounds may become quieter, and a friction rub, if present, may diminish in intensity but is not always abolished. Larger effusions may be accompanied by a sensation of retrosternal oppression. While most effusions do not have significant haemodynamic effects, large or rapidly developing effusions may cause cardiac tamponade. This term is used to describe acute heart failure due to compression of the heart and is described in detail below. Typical physical findings are a markedly raised JVP, hypotension, pulsus paradoxus (p. 448) and oliguria. Atypical presentations may occur when the effusion is loculated as a result of previous pericarditis or cardiac surgery.

Investigations

Echocardiography is the definitive investigation and is helpful in monitoring the size of the effusion and its effect on cardiac function (Fig. 16.102). The QRS voltages on the ECG are often reduced in the presence of a large effusion. The QRS complexes may alternate in amplitude due to a to-and-fro motion of the heart within the fluid-filled pericardial sac (electrical alternans). The chest X-ray may show an increase in the size of the cardiac silhouette and, when there is a large effusion, this has a globular appearance. Aspiration of the effusion may be required for diagnostic purposes and, if necessary, for treatment of large effusions, as described below.

Management

Patients with large effusions that are causing haemodynamic compromise or cardiac tamponade should undergo aspiration of the effusion. This involves inserting a needle under echocardiographic guidance medial to the cardiac apex or below the xiphoid process, directed upwards towards the left shoulder. The route of choice will depend on the experience of the operator, the shape of the patient and the position of the effusion. A pericardial drain may be placed to provide symptomatic relief. Complications of pericardiocentesis include arrhythmias, damage to a coronary artery and bleeding, with exacerbation of tamponade as a result of injury to the RV. When tamponade is due to cardiac rupture or aortic dissection, pericardial aspiration may precipitate further potentially fatal bleeding and, in these situations, emergency surgery is the treatment of choice. A viscous, loculated or recurrent effusion may also require formal surgical drainage.

Tuberculous pericarditis

Tuberculous pericarditis may complicate pulmonary tuberculosis but may also be the first manifestation of the infection. In Africa, a tuberculous pericardial effusion is a common feature of AIDS (p. 322). The condition typically presents with chronic malaise, weight loss and a low-grade fever. An effusion usually develops and the pericardium may become thick and unyielding, leading to pericardial constriction or tamponade. An associated pleural effusion is often present.

The diagnosis may be confirmed by aspiration of the fluid and direct examination or culture for tubercle bacilli. Treatment requires specific antituberculous chemotherapy (p. 592); in addition, a 3-month course of prednisolone (initial dose 60 mg a day, tapering down rapidly) improves outcome.

Chronic constrictive pericarditis

Constrictive pericarditis is due to progressive thickening, fibrosis and calcification of the pericardium. In effect, the heart is encased in a solid shell and cannot fill properly. The calcification may extend into the myocardium, so there may also be impaired myocardial contraction. The condition often follows an attack of tuberculous pericarditis but can also complicate haemopericardium, viral pericarditis, rheumatoid arthritis and purulent pericarditis. It is often impossible to identify the original insult.

Clinical features

The symptoms and signs of systemic venous congestion are the hallmarks of constrictive pericarditis. AF is common and there is often dramatic ascites and hepatomegaly (Box 16.109). Breathlessness is not a prominent symptom because the lungs are seldom congested. The condition is sometimes overlooked but should be suspected in any patient with unexplained right heart failure and a small heart.

Investigations

A chest X-ray, which may show pericardial calcification (Fig. 16.103), and echocardiography often help to establish the diagnosis. CT scanning is useful for imaging the pericardial calcification. Constrictive pericarditis is often difficult to distinguish

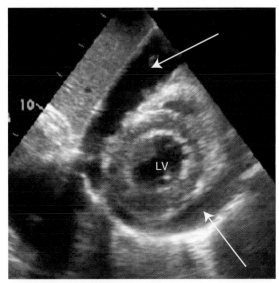

Fig. 16.102 Pericardial effusion: echocardiogram (apical view). Short-axis view of the heart showing a large circumferential pericardial effusion (arrows). (LV = left ventricle)

i	16.109 Clinical features of constrictive pericarditis

- Fatigue
- Rapid, low-volume pulse
- Elevated JVP with a rapid *y* descent
- Loud early third heart sound or 'pericardial knock'
- Kussmaul's sign
- Hepatomegaly
- Ascites
- Peripheral oedema
- Pulsus paradoxus

(JVP = jugular venous pressure)

Fig. 16.103 Lateral chest X-ray from a patient with severe heart failure due to chronic constrictive pericarditis. There is heavy calcification of the pericardium.

from restrictive cardiomyopathy and in such cases complex echo–Doppler studies and cardiac catheterisation may be required.

Management

The resulting diastolic heart failure is treated using loop diuretics and aldosterone antagonists, such as spironolactone. Surgical resection of the diseased pericardium can lead to a dramatic improvement but carries a high morbidity, with disappointing results in up to 50% of patients.

Cardiac tamponade

This term is used to describe acute heart failure due to compression of the heart as the result of a large pericardial effusion. Tamponade may complicate any form of pericarditis but can be caused by malignant disease, by blood in the pericardial space following trauma, or by rupture of the free wall of the myocardium following MI.

Clinical features

Patients with tamponade are unwell, with hypotension, tachycardia and a markedly raised JVP. Other clinical features are summarised in Box 16.110.

Investigations

The pivotal investigation is echocardiography, which can confirm the diagnosis and also helps to identify the optimum site for

 16.110 Clinical features of cardiac tamponade

- Dyspnoea
- Collapse
- Tachycardia
- Hypotension
- Gross elevation of the JVP
- Soft heart sounds with an early third heart sound
- Pulsus paradoxus (a large fall in BP during inspiration, when the pulse may be impalpable)
- Kussmaul's sign (a paradoxical rise in JVP during inspiration)

(JVP = jugular venous pressure)

aspiration of the fluid. The ECG may show features of the underlying disease, such as pericarditis or acute MI. When there is a large pericardial effusion, the ECG complexes are small and there may be electrical alternans: a changing axis with alternate beats caused by the heart swinging from side to side in the pericardial fluid. A chest X-ray shows an enlarged globular heart but can look normal.

Management

Cardiac tamponade is a medical emergency. When the diagnosis is confirmed, percutaneous pericardiocentesis should be performed as soon as possible, which usually results in a dramatic improvement. In some cases, surgical drainage may be required.

Further information

Websites

acc.org *American College of Cardiology (ACC): free access to guidelines for the evaluation and management of many cardiac conditions.*

americanheart.org *American Heart Association (AHA): free access to all the ACC/AHA/ESC guidelines, AHA scientific statements and fact sheets for patients.*

escardio.org *European Society of Cardiology (ESC): free access to guidelines for the diagnosis and management of many cardiac conditions, and to educational modules.*

jbs3risk.com *Joint British Societies for the Prevention of Cardiovascular Disease: risk calculator.*

Journal articles

Gould FK, Denning DW, Elliott TS, et al. Guidelines for the diagnosis and antibiotic treatment of endocarditis in adults: a report of the working party of the British Society for Antimicrobial Chemotherapy. J Antimicrob Chemother 2012; 67:269–289.

PT Reid
JA Innes

17

Respiratory medicine

Clinical examination of the respiratory system 546

Functional anatomy and physiology 548

Investigation of respiratory disease 550
Imaging 551
Endoscopic examination 553
Immunological and serological tests 554
Microbiological investigations 554
Respiratory function testing 554

Presenting problems in respiratory disease 556
Cough 556
Breathlessness 557
Chest pain 558
Finger clubbing 559
Haemoptysis 559
The incidental pulmonary nodule 560
Pleural effusion 562
Respiratory failure 565

Obstructive pulmonary diseases 567
Asthma 567
Chronic obstructive pulmonary disease 573
Bronchiectasis 578
Cystic fibrosis 580

Infections of the respiratory system 581
Upper respiratory tract infection 581
Pneumonia 582
Tuberculosis 588
Respiratory diseases caused by fungi 596

Tumours of the bronchus and lung 598
Primary tumours of the lung 599
Secondary tumours of the lung 603
Tumours of the mediastinum 603

Interstitial and infiltrative pulmonary diseases 605
Diffuse parenchymal lung disease 605
Lung diseases due to systemic inflammatory disease 610
Pulmonary eosinophilia and vasculitides 611
Lung diseases due to irradiation and drugs 612
Rare interstitial lung diseases 613

Occupational and environmental lung disease 613
Occupational airway disease 613
Pneumoconiosis 614
Lung diseases due to organic dusts 616
Asbestos-related lung and pleural diseases 617
Occupational lung cancer 618
Occupational pneumonia 618

Pulmonary vascular disease 619
Pulmonary embolism 619
Pulmonary hypertension 621

Diseases of the upper airway 622
Diseases of the nasopharynx 622
Sleep-disordered breathing 622
Laryngeal disorders 624
Tracheal disorders 625

Pleural disease 625

Diseases of the diaphragm and chest wall 627
Disorders of the diaphragm 627
Deformities of the chest wall 628

Clinical examination of the respiratory system

6 — 9 Thorax
(see opposite)

5 Face, mouth and eyes
Pursed lips
Central cyanosis
Anaemia
Horner's syndrome
(Ch. 25)

4 Jugular venous pulse
Elevated
Pulsatile

3 Blood pressure
Arterial paradox

2 Radial pulse
Rate
Rhythm

1 Hands
Digital clubbing
Tar staining
Peripheral cyanosis
Signs of occupation
CO_2 retention flap

▲ Finger clubbing

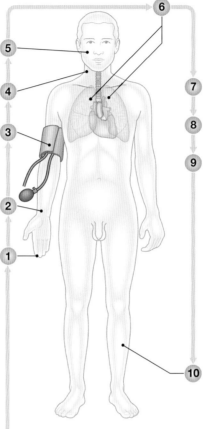

6 Inspection
Deformity
(e.g. pectus excavatum)
Scars
Intercostal indrawing
Symmetry of expansion
Hyperinflation
Paradoxical rib movement
(low flat diaphragm)

▲ Idiopathic kyphoscoliosis

7 Palpation
From the front:
Trachea central
Cricosternal distance
Cardiac apex displaced
Expansion
From behind:
Cervical lymphadenopathy
Expansion

8 Percussion
Resonant or dull
'Stony dull' (effusion)

9 Auscultation
Breath sounds:
normal, bronchial, louder or softer
Added sounds:
wheezes, crackles, rubs
Spoken voice (vocal resonance):
absent (effusion), increased
(consolidation)
Whispered voice:
whispering pectoriloquy

10 Leg oedema
Salt and water retention
Cor pulmonale
Venous thrombosis

Observation
- Respiratory rate
- Cachexia, fever, rash
- Sputum (see below)
- Fetor
- Locale:
 Oxygen delivery
 (mask, cannulae)
 Nebulisers
 Inhalers

Sputum

▲ Serous/frothy/pink
Pulmonary oedema

▲ Mucopurulent
Bronchial or pneumonic
infection

▲ Purulent
Bronchial or pneumonic
infection

▲ Blood-stained
Cancer, tuberculosis,
bronchiectasis,
pulmonary embolism

Insets (idiopathic kyphoscoliosis) Courtesy of Dr I. Smith, Papworth Hospital, Cambridge; (serous, mucopurulent and purulent sputum) Courtesy of Dr J. Foweraker, Papworth Hospital, Cambridge.

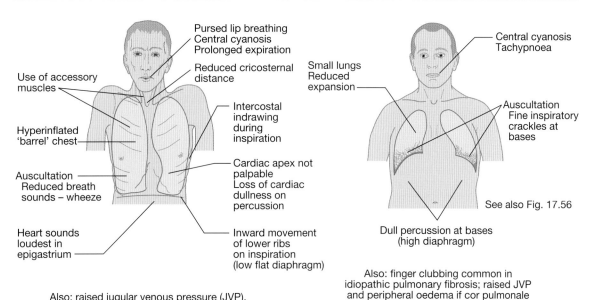

Chronic obstructive pulmonary disease

- Pursed lip breathing
- Central cyanosis
- Prolonged expiration
- Reduced cricosternal distance
- Use of accessory muscles
- Intercostal indrawing during inspiration
- Hyperinflated 'barrel' chest
- Auscultation — Reduced breath sounds – wheeze
- Cardiac apex not palpable
- Loss of cardiac dullness on percussion
- Heart sounds loudest in epigastrium
- Inward movement of lower ribs on inspiration (low flat diaphragm)

Also: raised jugular venous pressure (JVP), peripheral oedema from salt and water retention and/or cor pulmonale

Pulmonary fibrosis

- Central cyanosis
- Tachypnoea
- Small lungs
- Reduced expansion
- Auscultation — Fine inspiratory crackles at bases
- Dull percussion at bases (high diaphragm)

See also Fig. 17.56

Also: finger clubbing common in idiopathic pulmonary fibrosis; raised JVP and peripheral oedema if cor pulmonale

Right middle lobe pneumonia

Obscures R heart border on X-ray

Inspection
   Tachypnoea
   Central cyanosis (if severe)
Palpation
   ↓Expansion on R
Percussion
   Dull R mid-zone and axilla
Auscultation
   Bronchial breath sounds and ↑vocal resonance over consolidation and whispering pectoriloquy
   Pleural rub if pleurisy

Right upper lobe collapse

X-ray
   Deviated trachea (to R)
   Elevated horizontal fissure
   ↓Volume R hemithorax
   Central (hilar) mass may be seen

Inspection
   ↓Volume R upper zone
Palpation
   Trachea deviated to R
   ↓Expansion R upper zone
Percussion
   Dull R upper zone
Auscultation
   ↓Breath sounds with central obstruction

Right pneumothorax

Inspection
   Tachypnoea (pain, deflation reflex)
Palpation
   ↓Expansion R side
Percussion
   Resonant or hyper-resonant on R
Auscultation
   Absent breath sounds on R

Tension pneumothorax also causes
   Deviation of trachea to opposite side
   Tachycardia and hypotension

Large right pleural effusion

Inspection
   Tachypnoea
Palpation
   ↓Expansion on R
   Trachea and apex may be moved to L
Percussion
   Stony dull
   R mid- and lower zones
Auscultation
   Absent breath sounds and vocal resonance R base
   Bronchial breathing or crackles above effusion

17

Insets (upper lobe collapse) From http://3.bp.blogspot.com; (pneumothorax) http://chestatlas.com; (pleural effusion) www.ispub.com.

Respiratory disease is responsible for a major burden of morbidity and untimely death, with conditions such as tuberculosis, pandemic influenza and pneumonia the most important in world health terms. The increasing prevalence of allergy, asthma and chronic obstructive pulmonary disease (COPD) contributes to the overall burden of chronic disease in the community. By 2025, the number of cigarette smokers worldwide is anticipated to increase to 1.5 billion, ensuring a growing burden of tobacco-related respiratory conditions.

Respiratory disease covers a breadth of pathologies, including infectious, inflammatory, neoplastic and degenerative processes. The practice of respiratory medicine thus requires collaboration with a range of disciplines. Recent advances have improved the lives of many patients with obstructive lung disease, cystic fibrosis, obstructive sleep apnoea and pulmonary hypertension, but the outlook remains poor for lung and other respiratory cancers and for some of the fibrosing lung conditions.

Functional anatomy and physiology

The lungs occupy the upper two-thirds of the bony thorax, bounded medially by the spine, the heart and the mediastinum and inferiorly by the diaphragm. During breathing, free movement of the lung surface relative to the chest wall is facilitated by sliding contact between the parietal and visceral pleura, which cover the inner surface of the chest wall and the lung, respectively, and are normally in close apposition. Inspiration involves downward contraction of the dome-shaped diaphragm (innervated by the phrenic nerves originating from C3, 4 and 5) and upward,

outward movement of the ribs on the costovertebral joints, caused by contraction of the external intercostal muscles (innervated by intercostal nerves originating from the thoracic spinal cord). Expiration is largely passive, driven by elastic recoil of the lungs.

The conducting airways from the nose to the alveoli connect the external environment with the extensive, thin and vulnerable alveolar surface. As air is inhaled through the upper airways, it is filtered in the nose, heated to body temperature and fully saturated with water vapour; partial recovery of this heat and moisture occurs on expiration. Total airway cross-section is smallest in the glottis and trachea, making the central airway particularly vulnerable to obstruction by foreign bodies and tumours. Normal breath sounds originate mainly from the rapid turbulent airflow in the larynx, trachea and main bronchi.

The multitude of small airways within the lung parenchyma has a very large combined cross-sectional area (over 300 cm^2 in the third-generation respiratory bronchioles), resulting in very slow flow rates. Airflow is virtually silent here and gas transport occurs largely by diffusion in the final generations. Major bronchial and pulmonary divisions are shown in Figure 17.1.

The acinus (Fig. 17.2) is the gas exchange unit of the lung and comprises branching respiratory bronchioles and clusters of alveoli. Here the air makes close contact with the blood in the pulmonary capillaries (gas-to-blood distance <0.4 μm), and oxygen uptake and CO_2 excretion occur. The alveoli are lined with flattened epithelial cells (type I pneumocytes) and a few, more cuboidal, type II pneumocytes. The latter produce surfactant, which is a mixture of phospholipids that reduces surface tension and counteracts the tendency of alveoli to collapse under surface

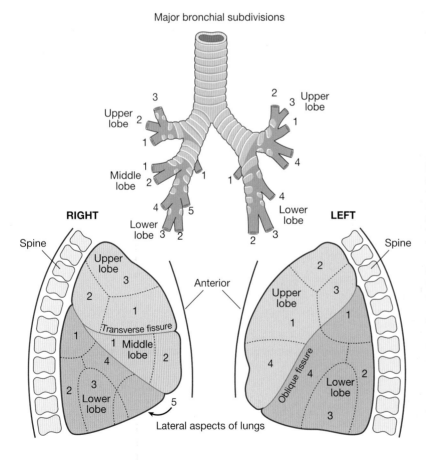

Major bronchial subdivisions

Fig. 17.1 The major bronchial divisions and the fissures, lobes and segments of the lungs. The angle of the oblique fissure means that the left upper lobe is largely anterior to the lower lobe. On the right, the transverse fissure separates the upper from the anteriorly placed middle lobe, which is matched by the lingular segment on the left side. The site of a lobe determines whether physical signs are mainly anterior or posterior. Each lobe is composed of two or more bronchopulmonary segments that are supplied by the main branches of each lobar bronchus. *Bronchopulmonary segments:* **Right** *Upper lobe:* (1) Anterior, (2) Posterior, (3) Apical. *Middle lobe:* (1) Lateral, (2) Medial. *Lower lobe:* (1) Apical, (2) Posterior basal, (3) Lateral basal, (4) Anterior basal, (5) Medial basal. **Left** *Upper lobe:* (1) Anterior, (2) Apical, (3) Posterior, (4) Lingular. *Lower lobe:* (1) Apical, (2) Posterior basal, (3) Lateral basal, (4) Anterior basal.

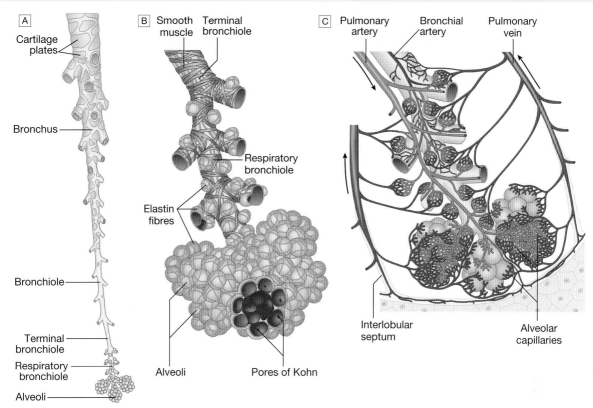

Fig. 17.2 Functional anatomy of the lung. [A] The tapering, branching bronchus is armoured against compression by plates of cartilage. The more distal bronchioles are collapsible, but held patent by surrounding elastic tissue. [B] The unit of lung supplied by a terminal bronchiole is called an acinus. The bronchiolar wall contains smooth muscle and elastin fibres. The latter also run through the alveolar walls. Gas exchange occurs in the alveoli, which are connected to each other by the pores of Kohn. [C] Vascular anatomy of an acinus. Both the pulmonary artery (carrying desaturated blood) and the bronchial artery (systemic supply to airway tissue) run along the bronchus. The venous drainage to the left atrium follows the interlobular septa. *From www.Netter.com: Illustrations 155 (bronchus, acinus) and 191 (circulation), Elsevier.*

tension. Type II pneumocytes can divide to reconstitute type I pneumocytes after lung injury.

Lung mechanics

Healthy alveolar walls contain a fine network of elastin and collagen fibres (Fig. 17.2). The volume of the lungs at the end of a tidal ('normal') breath out is called the functional residual capacity (FRC). At this volume, the inward elastic recoil of the lungs (resulting from elastin fibres and surface tension in the alveolar lining fluid) is balanced by the resistance of the chest wall to inward distortion from its resting shape, causing negative pressure in the pleural space. Elastin fibres allow the lung to be easily distended at physiological lung volumes, but collagen fibres cause increasing stiffness as full inflation is approached, so that, in health, the maximum inspiratory volume is limited by the lung (rather than the chest wall). Within the lung, the weight of tissue compresses the dependent regions and distends the uppermost parts, so a greater portion of an inhaled breath passes to the basal regions, which also receive the greatest blood flow as a result of gravity. Elastin fibres in alveolar walls maintain small airway patency by radial traction on the airway walls. Even in health, however, these small airways narrow during expiration because they are surrounded by alveoli at higher pressure, but are prevented from collapsing by radial elastic traction. The volume that can be exhaled is thus limited purely by the capacity of the expiratory muscles to distort the chest wall inwards. In emphysema, loss of alveolar walls leaves the small airways unsupported, and their collapse on expiration causes air trapping and limits expiration at a high end-expiratory volume (p. 575).

Control of breathing

The respiratory motor neurons in the posterior medulla oblongata are the origin of the respiratory cycle. Their activity is modulated by multiple external inputs in health and in disease (see Fig. 17.9):

- Central chemoreceptors in the ventrolateral medulla sense the pH of the cerebrospinal fluid (CSF) and are indirectly stimulated by a rise in arterial PCO_2.
- The carotid bodies sense hypoxaemia but are mainly activated by arterial PO_2 values below 8 kPa (60 mmHg). They are also sensitised to hypoxia by raised arterial PCO_2.
- Muscle spindles in the respiratory muscles sense changes in mechanical load.
- Vagal sensory fibres in the lung may be stimulated by stretch, by inhaled toxins or by disease processes in the interstitium.
- Cortical (volitional) and limbic (emotional) influences can override the automatic control of breathing.

Ventilation/perfusion matching and the pulmonary circulation

To achieve optimal gas exchange within the lungs, the regional distribution of ventilation and perfusion must be matched. At

17.1 Respiratory function in old age

- **Reserve capacity**: a significant reduction in function can occur with ageing with only minimal effect on normal breathing, but the ability to combat acute disease is reduced.
- **Decline in FEV$_1$**: the FEV$_1$/FVC (forced expiratory volume/forced vital capacity, p. 55) ratio falls by around 0.2% per year from 70% at the age of 40–45 years, due to a decline in elastic recoil in the small airways with age. Smoking accelerates this decline threefold on average. Symptoms usually occur only when FEV$_1$ drops below 50% of predicted.
- **Increasing ventilation–perfusion mismatch**: the reduction in elastic recoil causes a tendency for the small airways to collapse during expiration, particularly in dependent areas of the lungs, thus reducing ventilation.
- **Reduced ventilatory responses to hypoxia and hypercapnia**: older people may be less tachypnoeic for any given fall in PaO_2 or rise in $PaCO_2$.
- **Impaired defences against infection**: due to reduced numbers of glandular epithelial cells, which lead to a reduction in protective mucus.
- **Decline in maximum oxygen uptake**: due to a combination of impairments in muscle, and the respiratory and cardiovascular systems. This leads to a reduction in cardiorespiratory reserve and exercise capacity.
- **Loss of chest wall compliance**: due to reduced intervertebral disc spaces and ossification of the costal cartilages; respiratory muscle strength and endurance also decline. These changes become important only in the presence of other respiratory disease.

Fig. 17.3 The mucociliary escalator. Scanning electron micrograph of the respiratory epithelium showing large numbers of cilia (C) overlaid by the mucus 'raft' (M).

segmental and subsegmental level, hypoxia constricts pulmonary arterioles and airway CO_2 dilates bronchi, helping to maintain good regional matching of ventilation and perfusion. Lung disease may create regions of relative under-ventilation or under-perfusion, which disturb this regional matching, causing respiratory failure (p. 565). In addition to causing ventilation–perfusion mismatch, diseases that destroy capillaries or thicken the alveolar capillary membrane (e.g. emphysema or fibrosis) can impair gas diffusion directly.

The pulmonary circulation in health operates at low pressure (approximately 24/9 mmHg) and can accommodate large increases in flow with minimal rise in pressure, e.g. during exercise. Pulmonary hypertension occurs when vessels are destroyed by emphysema, obstructed by thrombus, involved in interstitial inflammation or thickened by pulmonary vascular disease. The right ventricle responds by hypertrophy, with right axis deviation and P pulmonale (tall, peaked p waves) on the electrocardiogram (ECG), and clinical features of right heart failure; the term 'cor pulmonale' is often used for these findings.

Lung defences

Upper airway defences

Large airborne particles are trapped by nasal hairs, and smaller particles settling on the mucosa are cleared towards the oropharynx by the columnar ciliated epithelium that covers the turbinates and septum (Fig. 17.3). During cough, expiratory muscle effort against a closed glottis results in high intrathoracic pressure, which is then released explosively. The flexible posterior tracheal wall is pushed inwards by the high surrounding pressure, which reduces tracheal cross-section and thus maximises the airspeed to achieve effective expectoration. The larynx also acts

as a sphincter, closing to protect the airway during swallowing and vomiting.

Lower airway defences

The sterility, structure and function of the lower airways are maintained by close cooperation between the innate and adaptive immune responses (pp. 62 and 67).

The innate response in the lungs is characterised by a number of non-specific defence mechanisms. Inhaled particulate matter is trapped in airway mucus and cleared by the mucociliary escalator. Cigarette smoke increases mucus secretion but reduces mucociliary clearance and predisposes towards lower respiratory tract infections, including pneumonia. Defective mucociliary transport is also a feature of several rare diseases, including Kartagener's syndrome, Young's syndrome and ciliary dysmotility syndrome, which are characterised by repeated sino-pulmonary infections and bronchiectasis.

Airway secretions contain an array of antimicrobial peptides (such as defensins, immunoglobulin A (IgA) and lysozyme), antiproteinases and antioxidants. Many assist with the opsonisation and killing of bacteria and the regulation of the powerful proteolytic enzymes secreted by inflammatory cells. In particular, α_1-antitrypsin regulates neutrophil elastase, and deficiency of this may be associated with premature emphysema.

Macrophages engulf microbes, organic dusts and other particulate matter. They are unable to digest inorganic agents, such as asbestos or silica, which cause their death and lead to the release of powerful proteolytic enzymes that damage the lung. Neutrophil numbers in the airway are low but the pulmonary circulation contains a marginated pool that may be recruited rapidly in response to bacterial infection. This may explain the prominence of lung injury in sepsis syndromes and trauma.

Adaptive immunity is characterised by the specificity of the response and the development of memory. Lung dendritic cells facilitate antigen presentation to T and B lymphocytes.

Investigation of respiratory disease

A detailed history, thorough examination and basic haematological and biochemical tests usually indicate the likely diagnosis and differential. A number of other investigations are normally required to confirm the diagnosis and/or monitor disease activity.

Imaging

The 'plain' chest X-ray

This is performed on the majority of patients suspected of having chest disease. A posteroanterior (PA) film provides information on the lung fields, heart, mediastinum, vascular structures and thoracic cage (Fig. 17.4). Additional information may be obtained from a lateral film, particularly if pathology is suspected behind the heart shadow or deep in the diaphragmatic sulci. An approach to interpreting the chest X-ray is given in Box 17.2 and common abnormalities are listed in Box 17.3.

Increased shadowing may represent accumulation of fluid, lobar collapse or consolidation. Uncomplicated consolidation should not change the position of the mediastinum and the presence of an air bronchogram means that proximal bronchi are patent. Collapse (implying obstruction of the lobar bronchus) is accompanied by loss of volume and displacement of the mediastinum towards the affected side (Fig. 17.5).

The presence of ring shadows (thickened bronchi seen end-on), tramline shadows (thickened bronchi side-on) or tubular shadows (bronchi filled with secretions) suggests bronchiectasis, but computed tomography is a much more sensitive test than plain X-ray in bronchiectasis. The presence of pleural fluid is suggested by a dense basal shadow, which, in the erect patient, ascends towards the axilla (p. 547). In large pulmonary embolism, relative oligaemia may cause a lung field to appear abnormally dark.

17.2 How to interpret a chest X-ray	
Name, date, orientation	Films are posteroanterior (PA) unless marked AP to denote that they are anteroposterior
Lung fields	Equal translucency? Check horizontal fissure from right hilum to sixth rib at the anterior axillary line Masses? Consolidation? Cavitation?
Lung apices	Check behind the clavicles. Masses? Consolidation? Cavitation?
Trachea	Central (midway between the clavicular heads)? Paratracheal mass? Goitre?
Heart	Normal shape? Cardiothoracic ratio (should be < half the intrathoracic diameter) Retrocardiac mass?
Hila	Left should be higher than right Shape (should be concave laterally; if convex, consider mass or lymphadenopathy)? Density?
Diaphragm	Right should be higher than left Hyperinflation (no more than 10 ribs should be visible posteriorly above the diaphragm)?
Costophrenic angles	Acute and well defined (pleural fluid or thickening, if not)?
Soft tissues	Breast shadows in females Chest wall for masses or subcutaneous emphysema
Bones	Ribs, vertebrae, scapulae and clavicles Any fracture visible at bone margins or lucencies?

17

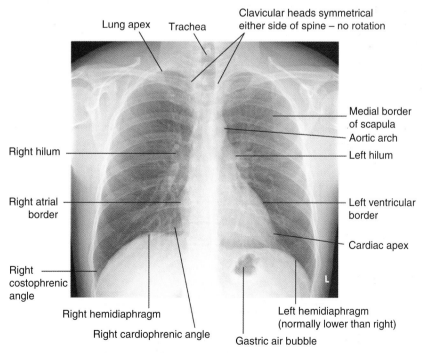

Fig. 17.4 The normal chest X-ray. The lung markings consist of branching and tapering lines radiating out from the hila. Where airways and vessels turn towards the film, they can appear as open or filled circles (see upper pole of right hilum). The scapulae may overlie the lung fields; trace the edge of bony structures to avoid mistaking them for pleural or pulmonary shadows. To check for hyperinflation, count the ribs; if more than 10 are visible posteriorly above the diaphragm, the lungs are hyperinflated. *From Innes JA. Davidson's Essentials of medicine. Edinburgh: Churchill Livingstone, Elsevier Ltd; 2009.*

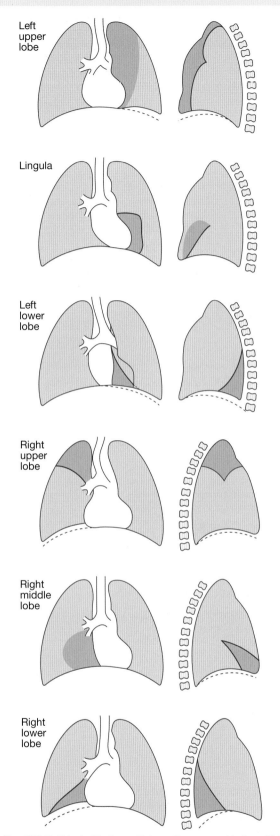

Fig. 17.5 Radiological features of lobar collapse caused by bronchial obstruction. The dotted line in the drawings represents the normal position of the diaphragm. The dark pink area represents the extent of shadowing seen on the X-ray.

Left upper lobe

Lingula

Left lower lobe

Right upper lobe

Right middle lobe

Right lower lobe

> **i** **17.3 Common chest X-ray abnormalities**
>
> **Pulmonary and pleural shadowing**
>
> - Consolidation: infection, infarction, inflammation and, rarely, bronchoalveolar cell carcinoma
> - Lobar collapse: mucus plugging, tumour, compression by lymph nodes
> - Solitary nodule: see page 560
> - Multiple nodules: miliary tuberculosis (TB), dust inhalation, metastatic malignancy, healed varicella pneumonia, rheumatoid disease
> - Ring shadows, tramlines and tubular shadows: bronchiectasis
> - Cavitating lesions: tumour, abscess, infarct, pneumonia (*Staphylococcus/Klebsiella*), granulomatosis with polyangiitis (formerly known as Wegener's granulomatosis)
> - Reticular, nodular and reticulonodular shadows: diffuse parenchymal lung disease, infection
> - Pleural abnormalities: fluid, plaques, tumour
>
> **Increased translucency**
>
> - Bullae
> - Pneumothorax
> - Oligaemia
>
> **Hilar abnormalities**
>
> - Unilateral hilar enlargement: TB, lung cancer, lymphoma
> - Bilateral hilar enlargement: sarcoid, lymphoma, TB, silicosis
>
> **Other abnormalities**
>
> - Hiatus hernia
> - Surgical emphysema

Computed tomography

Computed tomography (CT) provides detailed images of the pulmonary parenchyma, mediastinum, pleura and bony structures. The displayed range of densities can be adjusted to highlight different structures, such as the lung parenchyma, the mediastinal vascular structures or bone. Cross-sectional formatting allows recognition of the axial distribution of the disease, while coronal reformation displays the craniocaudal distribution. In cases of suspected lung cancer, CT is central to both diagnosis and staging, and facilitates percutaneous needle biopsy. CT identifies the extent and appearance of pleural thickening (see Fig. 17.65) and reliably differentiates pleural and pericardial fat from other pathologies. High-resolution thin-section scanning provides detailed images of the pulmonary parenchyma and is particularly useful in assessing diffuse parenchymal lung disease (see Fig. 17.56), identifying airway thickening, bronchiectasis (see Fig. 17.29) and emphysema (see Fig. 17.27). The relative contribution of competing pathologies to a breathless patient may be assessed. Prone imaging may be used to differentiate the gravity-induced posterobasal attenuation seen in supine scans. CT pulmonary angiography (CTPA) has become the investigation of choice in the diagnosis of pulmonary thromboembolism (see Fig. 17.68), when it may either confirm the suspected embolism or highlight an alternative diagnosis. It has largely replaced the radioisotope-based ventilation–perfusion scan, although the latter continues to provide useful information in the pre-operative assessment of patients being considered for lung resection and in the assessment of pulmonary hypertension. CT may assist in identifying the cavitation of tuberculosis, fungal infection (p. 300) and other signs of infection (halo – air crescent). Finally, CT may be used to assess disease progression, thereby predicting prognosis, and in screening to detect the earliest signs of disease.

Fig. 17.6 Computed tomography and positron emission tomography combined to reveal intrathoracic metastases. [A] In a patient with lung cancer, CT shows some posterior pleural thickening. [B] PET scanning reveals FDG uptake in two pleural lesions (arrows). [C] The lesions are highlighted in yellow in the combined PET/CT image. *A–C, From http://radiology.rsnajnls.org.*

Positron emission tomography

Positron emission tomography (PET) scanners employ the radiotracer ^{18}F-fluorodeoxyglucose (FDG) to quantify the rate of glucose metabolism by cells. The [18]FDG is rapidly taken up by metabolically active tissue, where it is phosphorylated and 'trapped' in the cell. The assessment of [18]FDG uptake may be qualitative (visual analysis) or semi-quantitative, using the standardised uptake value (SUV) (Fig. 17.6). PET is useful in the staging of mediastinal lymph nodes and distal metastatic disease in patients with lung cancer and in the investigation of pulmonary nodules. Co-registration of PET and CT (PET-CT) enhances localisation and characterisation of metabolically active deposits (Fig. 17.6). PET may also differentiate benign from malignant pleural disease and can be used to assess the extent of extrapulmonary disease in sarcoidosis. However, [18]FDG uptake by a lesion is affected by a large number of parameters, including equipment used, the physics, and biological factors such as amount of body fat and brown fat uptake and the level of fasting blood glucose.

Magnetic resonance imaging

Conventional magnetic resonance imaging (MRI) of the lung parenchyma is seldom useful, although the technique is increasingly finding a role in the differentiation of benign from malignant pleural disease, and in delineating invasion of the chest wall or diaphragm by tumour.

Ultrasound

Transthoracic ultrasound has evolved into a point-of-care investigation to assess the pleural space (see Fig. 17.15). In the hands of an experienced operator it can distinguish pleural fluid from pleural thickening, identify a pneumothorax and, by directly visualising the diaphragm and solid organs such as the liver, spleen and kidneys, may be used to guide pleural aspiration, biopsy and intercostal chest drain insertion safely. It is also used to guide needle biopsy of superficial lymph node or chest wall masses and provides useful information on the shape and movement of the diaphragm.

Endoscopic examination

Laryngoscopy

The larynx may be inspected directly with a fibreoptic laryngoscope and this is useful in cases of suspected vocal cord dysfunction, when paradoxical movement of the vocal cords may mimic asthma. Left-sided lung tumours may involve the left recurrent laryngeal nerve, paralysing the left vocal cord and leading to a hoarse voice and a 'bovine' cough. Continuous laryngoscopy during exercise tests allows the identification of exercise-induced laryngeal obstruction.

Bronchoscopy

The trachea and the first 3–4 generations of bronchi may be inspected using a flexible bronchoscope. Flexible bronchoscopy is usually performed under local anaesthesia with sedation, on an outpatient basis. Abnormal tissue in the bronchial lumen or wall can be biopsied, and bronchial brushings, washings or aspirates can be taken for cytological or bacteriological examination. Small biopsy specimens of lung tissue, taken by forceps passed through the bronchial wall (transbronchial biopsies), may be helpful in the diagnosis of bronchocentric disorders such as sarcoidosis and diffuse malignancy but are generally too small to be of diagnostic value in other diffuse parenchymal pulmonary disease (p. 605).

Rigid bronchoscopy requires general anaesthesia and is reserved for specific situations, such as massive haemoptysis or removal of a foreign body (see Fig. 10.2, p. 179), and can facilitate endobronchial laser therapy and stenting.

Endobronchial ultrasound

Endobronchial ultrasound (EBUS) allows directed needle aspiration from peribronchial nodes and is used increasingly to stage lung cancer. It may also be useful in non-malignant conditions, such as tuberculosis of the mediastinal lymph nodes or sarcoid. Lymph nodes down to the main carina can also be sampled using a mediastinoscope passed through a small incision at the suprasternal notch under general anaesthetic. Lymph nodes in the lower mediastinum may be biopsied via the oesophagus using endoscopic ultrasound (EUS), an oesophageal endoscope equipped with an ultrasound transducer and biopsy needle.

Thoracoscopy

Thoracoscopy, which involves the insertion of an endoscope through the chest wall, facilitates biopsy under direct vision and is performed by surgeons and an increasing number of physicians. This modality is the gold standard for the evaluation of the pleural interface, characterisation of complex pleural effusion, and identification of exudate and haemorrhage, as well as the analysis of superior sulcus tumours, as it enables more accurate staging.

17

Immunological and serological tests

The diagnosis of asthma may be supported by demonstrating an elevated level of immunoglobulin E (IgE), and the measurement of IgE directed against specific antigens can be useful in assessing the contribution of specific allergens to the presentation. Many autoimmune diseases present with pulmonary involvement and autoantibodies may be identified in the serum. Serum precipitins are antibodies that form visible lines of precipitated glycoprotein when they encounter their specific antigen in an agarose gel or on an acetate cellulose sheet. They may identify a reaction to fungi such as *Aspergillus* (p. 596) or to antigens involved in hypersensitivity pneumonitis, such as farmer's lung (p. 616). IgG enzyme immunoassay may be used interchangeably. The presence of pneumococcal antigen in sputum, blood or urine may be of diagnostic importance in pneumonia. Respiratory viruses can be detected in nose/throat swabs by immunofluorescence and *Legionella* infection may diagnosed by detection of the urinary antigen. The detection of galactomannan, a component of the cell wall of *Aspergillus*, may assist in the diagnosis of invasive aspergillosis, and interferon-gamma release assays are useful in the detection of latent tuberculosis.

Microbiological investigations

Sputum, pleural fluid, throat swabs, blood, and bronchial washings and aspirates can be examined for bacteria, fungi and viruses. The use of hypertonic saline to induce expectoration of sputum may obviate the need for more invasive procedures, such as

bronchoscopy. Molecular tests are increasingly being used to provide rapid and accurate identification of many infective organisms. Nucleic acid amplification tests (NAATs) identify common respiratory viruses, such as influenza, adenovirus and respiratory syncytial virus, and have largely replaced paired serology for *Mycoplasma*, *Legionella* and other organisms. NAATs are increasingly adopted as the first-line investigation for identification of tuberculosis and rapid identification of drug resistance.

Cytology and histopathology

Cytological examination of exfoliated cells in pleural fluid or bronchial brushings and washings, or of fine needle aspirates from lymph nodes or pulmonary lesions, can support a diagnosis of malignancy but a larger tissue biopsy is often necessary, particularly as this allows immunohistochemistry using a panel of antibodies to characterise the tumour. Histopathology may also allow identification of infective agents such as *Mycobacterium tuberculosis*, *Pneumocystis jirovecii* or fungi. Differential cell counts in bronchial lavage fluid may help to distinguish pulmonary changes due to sarcoidosis (p. 608) from those caused by idiopathic pulmonary fibrosis (p. 605) or hypersensitivity pneumonitis (p. 616).

Respiratory function testing

Respiratory function tests are used to aid diagnosis, quantify functional impairment, and monitor treatment or progression of disease. Airway narrowing, lung volume and gas exchange capacity are quantified and compared with normal values

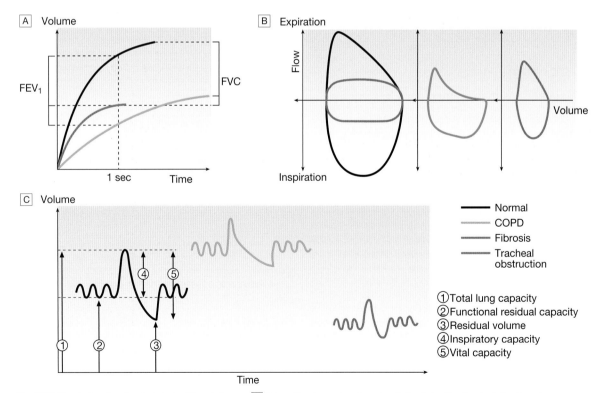

Fig. 17.7 Respiratory function tests in health and disease. **A** Volume/time traces from forced expiration in health, chronic obstructive pulmonary disease (COPD) and fibrosis. COPD causes slow, prolonged and limited exhalation. In fibrosis, forced expiration results in rapid expulsion of a reduced forced vital capacity (FVC). Forced expiratory volume (FEV_1) is reduced in both diseases but disproportionately so, compared to FVC, in COPD. **B** The same data plotted as flow/volume loops. In COPD, collapse of intrathoracic airways limits flow, particularly during mid- and late expiration. The blue trace illustrates large airway obstruction, which particularly limits peak flow rates. **C** Lung volume measurement. Volume/time graphs during quiet breathing with a single maximal breath in and out. COPD causes hyperinflation with increased residual volume. Fibrosis causes a proportional reduction in all lung volumes.

adjusted for age, gender, height and ethnic origin. In diseases characterised by airway narrowing (e.g. asthma, bronchitis and emphysema), maximum expiratory flow is limited by dynamic compression of small intrathoracic airways, some of which may close completely during expiration, limiting the volume that can be expired ('obstructive' defect). Hyperinflation of the chest results and can become extreme if elastic recoil is also lost due to parenchymal destruction, as in emphysema. In contrast, diseases that cause interstitial inflammation and/or fibrosis lead to progressive loss of lung volume ('restrictive' defect) with normal expiratory flow rates. Typical laboratory traces are illustrated in Figure 17.7.

Measurement of airway obstruction

Airway narrowing is assessed by asking patients to breathe in fully, then blow out as hard and fast as they can into a peak flow meter or a spirometer. Peak flow meters are cheap and convenient for home monitoring of peak expiratory flow (PEF) in the detection and monitoring of asthma but results are effort-dependent. More accurate and reproducible measures are obtained by maximum forced expiration into a spirometer. The forced expired volume in 1 second (FEV_1) is the volume exhaled in the first second, and the forced vital capacity (FVC) is the total volume exhaled. FEV_1 is disproportionately reduced in airflow obstruction, resulting in FEV_1/FVC ratios of less than 70%. In this situation, spirometry should be repeated following inhaled short-acting β_2-adrenoceptor agonists (e.g. salbutamol); an increase of >12% and >200 mL in FEV_1 or FVC indicates significant reversibility. A large improvement in FEV_1 (>400 mL) and variability in peak flow over time are features of asthma (p. 567).

To distinguish large airway narrowing (e.g. tracheal stenosis or compression; see Fig. 18.12, p. 648) from small airway narrowing, spirometry data are plotted as flow/volume loops. These display flow in relation to lung volume (rather than time) during maximum expiration and inspiration, and the pattern of flow reveals the site of airflow obstruction (Fig. 17.7B).

Lung volumes

Spirometry can measure only the volume of gas that can be exhaled; it cannot measure the gas remaining in the lungs after a maximal expiration. All the gas in the lungs can be measured by rebreathing an inert non-absorbed gas (usually helium) and recording how much the test gas is diluted by lung gas at equilibrium. This measures the volume of intrathoracic gas that mixes freely with tidal breaths. Alternatively, lung volume may be measured by body plethysmography (p. 175), which determines the pressure/volume relationship of the thorax. This method measures total intrathoracic gas volume, including poorly ventilated areas such as bullae. The terms used to describe lung volume are shown in Figure 17.7C.

Transfer factor

To measure the capacity of the lungs to exchange gas, patients inhale a test mixture of 0.3% carbon monoxide, which is taken up avidly by haemoglobin in pulmonary capillaries. After a short breath-hold, the rate of disappearance of CO into the circulation is calculated from a sample of expirate, and expressed as the TL_{CO} or carbon monoxide transfer factor. Helium is also included in the test breath to allow calculation of the volume of lung examined by the test breath. Transfer factor expressed per unit lung volume is termed K_{CO}. Common respiratory function abnormalities are summarised in Box 17.4.

17.4 How to interpret respiratory function abnormalities

	Asthma	Chronic bronchitis	Emphysema	Pulmonary fibrosis
FEV_1	↓↓	↓↓	↓↓	↓
FVC	↓	↓	↓	↓↓
FEV_1/FVC	↓	↓	↓	→/↑
TL_{CO}	→	→	↓↓	↓↓
K_{CO}	→/↑	→	↓	→/↓
TLC	→/↑	↑	↑↑	↓
RV	→/↑	↑	↑↑	↓

(RV = residual volume; TLC = total lung capacity; see text for other abbreviations)

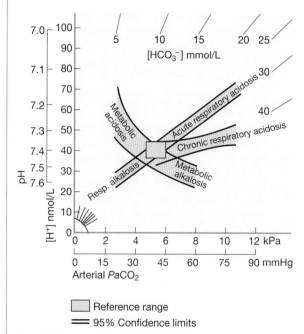

Fig. 17.8 Changes in blood [H+], $PaCO_2$ and plasma [HCO_3^-] in acid–base disorders. The rectangle indicates normal limits for [H+] and $PaCO_2$. The bands represent 95% confidence limits of single disturbances in human blood. To determine the likely cause of an acid–base disorder, plot the values of [H+] and $PaCO_2$ from an arterial blood gas measurement. The diagram indicates whether any acidosis or alkalosis results primarily from a respiratory disorder of $PaCO_2$ or from a metabolic derangement. *Reprinted with permission from Elsevier (Flenley D. Lancet 1971; 1:1921).*

Arterial blood gases and oximetry

The measurement of hydrogen ion concentration, PaO_2 and $PaCO_2$, and derived bicarbonate concentration in an arterial blood sample is essential for assessing the degree and type of respiratory failure and for measuring acid–base status. This is discussed in detail on pages 363 and 565. Interpretation of results is made easier by blood gas diagrams (Fig. 17.8), which indicate whether any acidosis or alkalosis is due to acute or chronic respiratory derangements of $PaCO_2$ or to metabolic causes.

Pulse oximeters with finger or ear probes measure the difference in absorbance of light by oxygenated and deoxygenated blood and calculate the percentage of haemoglobin that is oxygenated (the oxygen saturation). This allows non-invasive continuous

17

assessment of oxygen saturation in patients and its response to oxygen therapy.

Exercise tests

Resting measurements may be unhelpful in early disease or in patients complaining only of exercise-induced symptoms. Exercise testing with spirometry before and after can help to reveal exercise-induced asthma. Walk tests include the self-paced 6-minute walk and the externally paced incremental 'shuttle' test, where patients walk at increasing pace between two cones 10 m apart. These provide simple, repeatable assessments of disability and response to treatment. Cardiopulmonary bicycle exercise testing, with measurement of metabolic gas exchange, ventilation and ECG changes, is useful for quantifying exercise limitation and detecting occult cardiovascular or respiratory limitation in a breathless patient.

Presenting problems in respiratory disease

Cough

Cough is the most frequent symptom of respiratory disease and is caused by stimulation of sensory nerves in the mucosa of the pharynx, larynx, trachea and bronchi. Acute sensitisation of the normal cough reflex occurs in a number of conditions and it is typically induced by changes in air temperature or exposure to irritants, such as cigarette smoke or perfumes. Distinguishing characteristics of various causes of cough are detailed in Box 17.5.

The explosive quality of a normal cough is lost in patients with respiratory muscle paralysis or vocal cord palsy. Paralysis of a single vocal cord gives rise to a prolonged, low-pitched, inefficient 'bovine' cough accompanied by hoarseness. Coexistence of an inspiratory noise (stridor) indicates partial obstruction of a major airway (e.g. laryngeal oedema, tracheal tumour, scarring, compression or inhaled foreign body) and requires urgent investigation and treatment. Sputum production is common in patients with acute or chronic cough, and its nature and appearance can provide clues to the aetiology (p. 546).

Aetiology

Acute transient cough is most commonly caused by viral tracheo-bronchial infection, post-nasal drip resulting from rhinitis or sinusitis, aspiration of a foreign body, or throat-clearing secondary to laryngitis or pharyngitis. When cough occurs in the context of more serious diseases, such as pneumonia, aspiration, congestive heart failure or pulmonary embolism, it is usually easy to diagnose from other clinical features.

Patients with chronic cough present more of a challenge, especially when physical examination, chest X-ray and lung function studies are normal. In this context, it is most often explained by cough-variant asthma (where cough may be the principal or exclusive clinical manifestation), post-nasal drip secondary to nasal or sinus disease, or gastro-oesophageal reflux disease (GORD) with aspiration. Diagnosis of the latter may require oesophageal pH monitoring or a prolonged trial of anti-reflux therapy (p. 793). Between 10% and 15% of patients (particularly women) taking angiotensin-converting enzyme (ACE) inhibitors develop a drug-induced chronic cough. *Bordetella pertussis* infection in adults (p. 582) can result in cough lasting up to 3 months. While most patients with lung cancer have an abnormal chest X-ray on presentation, fibreoptic bronchos-copy or thoracic CT is advisable in most adults (especially smokers) with otherwise unexplained cough of recent onset, as this may reveal a small endobronchial tumour or unexpected foreign body (see Fig. 10.2, p. 179). In a small percentage of patients, dry cough may be the presenting feature of interstitial lung disease.

i	**17.5 Cough**		
Origin	**Common causes**	**Clinical features**
Pharynx	Post-nasal drip	History of chronic rhinitis
Larynx	Laryngitis, tumour, whooping cough, croup	Voice or swallowing altered, harsh or painful cough Paroxysms of cough, often associated with stridor
Trachea	Tracheitis	Raw retrosternal pain with cough
Bronchi	Bronchitis (acute) and chronic obstructive pulmonary disease (COPD)	Dry or productive, worse in mornings
	Asthma	Usually dry, worse at night
	Eosinophilic bronchitis	Features similar to asthma but airway hyper-reactivity absent
	Lung cancer	Persistent (often with haemoptysis)
Lung parenchyma	Tuberculosis	Productive (often with haemoptysis)
	Pneumonia	Dry initially, productive later
	Bronchiectasis	Productive, changes in posture induce sputum production
	Pulmonary oedema	Often at night (may be productive of pink, frothy sputum)
	Interstitial fibrosis	Dry and distressing
Drug side-effect	Angiotensin-converting enzyme (ACE) inhibitors	Dry cough
Aspiration	Gastro-oesophageal reflux disease (GORD)	History of acid reflux, heartburn, hiatus hernia Obesity

Adapted from Munro JF, Campbell IW. Macleod's Clinical examination, 10th edn. Edinburgh: Churchill Livingstone, Elsevier Ltd; 2000.

Breathlessness

Breathlessness or dyspnoea can be defined as the feeling of an uncomfortable need to breathe. It is unusual among sensations, as it has no defined receptors, no localised representation in the brain, and multiple causes both in health (e.g. exercise) and in diseases of the lungs, heart or muscles.

Pathophysiology

Stimuli to breathing resulting from disease processes are shown in Figure 17.9. Respiratory diseases can stimulate breathing and dyspnoea by:

- stimulating intrapulmonary sensory nerves (e.g. pneumothorax, interstitial inflammation and pulmonary embolus)
- increasing the mechanical load on the respiratory muscles (e.g. airflow obstruction or pulmonary fibrosis)
- causing hypoxia, hypercapnia or acidosis, which stimulate chemoreceptors.

In cardiac failure, pulmonary congestion reduces lung compliance and can also obstruct the small airways. Reduced cardiac output also limits oxygen supply to the skeletal muscles during exercise, causing early lactic acidaemia and further stimulating breathing via the central chemoreceptors.

Breathlessness and the effects of treatment can be quantified using a symptom scale. Patients tend to report breathlessness in proportion to the sum of the above stimuli to breathing.

Individual patients differ greatly in the intensity of breathlessness reported for a given set of circumstances, but breathlessness scores during exercise within individuals are reproducible and can be used to monitor the effects of therapy.

Differential diagnosis

Patients with breathlessness present either with chronic exertional symptoms or as an emergency with acute breathlessness, when symptoms are prominent even at rest. The causes can be classified accordingly (Box 17.6).

Chronic exertional breathlessness

The cause of breathlessness is often apparent from a careful clinical history. Key questions are detailed below.

How is your breathing at rest and overnight?

In COPD, there is a fixed, structural limit to maximum ventilation, and a tendency for progressive hyperinflation during exercise. Breathlessness is apparent mainly when walking and patients usually report minimal symptoms at rest and overnight. In contrast, patients with significant asthma are often woken from their sleep by breathlessness with chest tightness and wheeze.

Orthopnoea is common in COPD, as well as in heart disease, because airflow obstruction is made worse by cranial displacement of the diaphragm by the abdominal contents when recumbent, so many patients choose to sleep propped up. Thus it is not a useful differentiating symptom unless there is a clear history of previous angina or infarction to suggest cardiac disease.

17

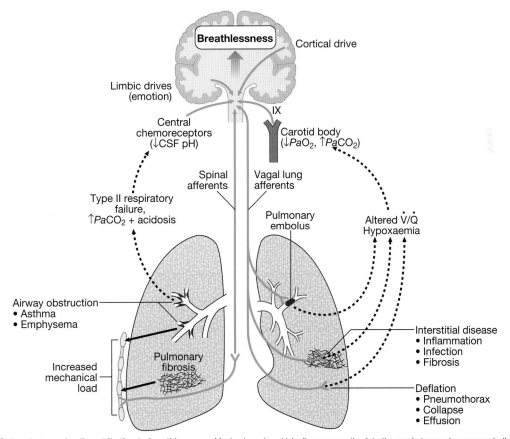

Fig. 17.9 Respiratory stimuli contributing to breathlessness. Mechanisms by which disease can stimulate the respiratory motor neurons in the medulla. Breathlessness is usually felt in proportion to the sum of these stimuli. Further explanation is given on page 179. (CSF = cerebrospinal fluid; $\dot{V}/\dot{Q}$ = ventilation/perfusion match)

i 17.6 Causes of breathlessness

System	Acute dyspnoea	Chronic exertional dyspnoea
Cardiovascular	*Acute pulmonary oedema (p. 463)	Chronic heart failure (p. 463) Myocardial ischaemia (angina equivalent) (p. 180)
Respiratory	*Acute severe asthma *Acute exacerbation of COPD *Pneumothorax *Pneumonia *Pulmonary embolus ARDS Inhaled foreign body (especially in children) Lobar collapse Laryngeal oedema (e.g. anaphylaxis)	*COPD *Chronic asthma Lung cancer Interstitial lung disease (sarcoidosis, fibrosing alveolitis, extrinsic allergic alveolitis, pneumoconiosis) Chronic pulmonary thromboembolism Lymphangitis carcinomatosis (may cause intolerable breathlessness) Large pleural effusion(s)
Others	Metabolic acidosis (e.g. diabetic ketoacidosis, lactic acidosis, uraemia, overdose of salicylates, ethylene glycol poisoning) Psychogenic hyperventilation (anxiety- or panic-related)	Severe anaemia Obesity Deconditioning

*Denotes a common cause.
(ARDS = acute respiratory distress syndrome; COPD = chronic obstructive pulmonary disease)

How much can you do on a good day?

Noting 'breathless on exertion' is not enough; the approximate distance the patient can walk on the level should be documented, along with capacity to climb inclines or stairs. Variability within and between days is a hallmark of asthma; in mild asthma, the patient may be free of symptoms and signs when well. Gradual, progressive loss of exercise capacity over months and years, with consistent disability over days, is typical of COPD. When asthma is suspected, the degree of variability is best documented by home peak flow monitoring.

Relentless, progressive breathlessness that is also present at rest, often accompanied by a dry cough, suggests interstitial fibrosis. Impaired left ventricular function can also cause chronic exertional breathlessness, cough and wheeze. A history of angina, hypertension or myocardial infarction raises the possibility of a cardiac cause. This may be confirmed by a displaced apex beat, a raised JVP and cardiac murmurs (although these signs can occur in severe hypoxic lung disease with fluid retention). The chest X-ray may show cardiomegaly and an ECG and echocardiogram may provide evidence of left ventricular disease. Measurement of arterial blood gases may help, as, in the absence of an intracardiac shunt or pulmonary oedema, the PaO_2 in cardiac disease is normal and the $PaCO_2$ is low or normal.

Did you have breathing problems in childhood or at school?

When present, a history of childhood wheeze increases the likelihood of asthma, although this history may be absent in late-onset asthma. A history of atopic allergy also increases the likelihood of asthma.

Do you have other symptoms along with your breathlessness?

Digital or perioral paraesthesiae and a feeling that 'I cannot get a deep enough breath in' are typical features of psychogenic hyperventilation but this cannot be diagnosed until investigations have excluded other potential causes. Additional symptoms include lightheadedness, central chest discomfort or even carpopedal spasm due to acute respiratory alkalosis. These alarming symptoms may provoke further anxiety and exacerbate hyperventilation. Psychogenic breathlessness rarely disturbs sleep, frequently occurs at rest, may be provoked by stressful situations and may even be relieved by exercise. The Nijmegen

i 17.7 Factors suggesting psychogenic hyperventilation

- 'Inability to take a deep breath'
- Frequent sighing/erratic ventilation at rest
- Short breath-holding time in the absence of severe respiratory disease
- Difficulty in performing and/or inconsistent spirometry measures
- High score (over 26) on Nijmegen questionnaire
- Induction of symptoms during submaximal hyperventilation
- Resting end-tidal CO_2 <4.5%
- Associated digital and/or perioral paraesthesiae

questionnaire can be used to score some of the typical symptoms of hyperventilation (Box 17.7). Arterial blood gases show normal PO_2, low PCO_2 and alkalosis.

Pleuritic chest pain in a patient with chronic breathlessness, particularly if it occurs in more than one site over time, should raise suspicion of thromboembolic disease. Thromboembolism may occasionally present as chronic breathlessness with no other specific features and should always be considered before a diagnosis of psychogenic hyperventilation is made.

Morning headache is an important symptom in patients with breathlessness, as it may signal the onset of carbon dioxide retention and respiratory failure. This is particularly significant in patients with musculoskeletal disease impairing respiratory function (e.g. kyphoscoliosis or muscular dystrophy).

Acute severe breathlessness

This is one of the most common and dramatic medical emergencies. Although respiratory causes are common, it can result from cardiac disease, metabolic disease or poisoning causing acidosis, or from psychogenic causes. The approach to patients with acute severe breathlessness is covered on page 179.

Chest pain

Chest pain can result from cardiac, respiratory, oesophageal or musculoskeletal disorders. The approach to this common symptom is covered on page 176.

Finger clubbing

Finger clubbing describes painless swelling of the soft tissues of the terminal phalanges, causing increased longitudinal and lateral convexity of the nail (Fig. 17.10). Upward displacement of the proximal nail margin causes the anteroposterior diameter of the finger at that point to exceed that at the distal interphalangeal joint. It also removes the normal hyponychial angle between the proximal part of the nail and the adjoining skin. Clubbing usually affects the fingers symmetrically and commonly also involves the toes, but can be unilateral if caused by a proximal vascular condition, e.g. arteriovenous shunts for dialysis. It is sometimes congenital but in over 90% of patients it indicates a serious underlying disorder. The most common underlying causes are suppurative or malignant lung disease but a variety of other conditions can cause clubbing (Box 17.8). Clubbing may recede if the underlying condition resolves, e.g. following lung transplantation for cystic fibrosis.

Haemoptysis

Coughing up blood, irrespective of the amount, is an alarming symptom and patients nearly always seek medical advice. Care should be taken to establish that it is true haemoptysis and not haematemesis, or gum or nose bleeding. Haemoptysis must always be assumed to have a serious cause until this is excluded (Box 17.9).

Many episodes of haemoptysis remain unexplained, even after full investigation, and are likely to be due to simple bronchial infection. A history of repeated small haemoptysis, or blood-streaking of sputum, is highly suggestive of lung cancer. Fever, night sweats and weight loss suggest tuberculosis. Pneumococcal pneumonia often causes 'rusty'-coloured sputum but can cause frank haemoptysis, as can all suppurative pneumonic infections, including lung abscess (p. 586). Bronchiectasis (p. 578) and intracavitary mycetoma (p. 597) can cause catastrophic bronchial haemorrhage, and in these patients there may be a history of previous tuberculosis or pneumonia in early life. Finally, pulmonary thromboembolism is a common cause of haemoptysis and should always be considered.

Physical examination may reveal additional clues. Finger clubbing suggests lung cancer or bronchiectasis; other signs of malignancy, such as cachexia, hepatomegaly and lymphadenopathy, should also be sought. Fever, pleural rub and signs of consolidation occur in pneumonia or pulmonary infarction; a minority of patients with pulmonary infarction also have unilateral leg swelling or pain suggestive of deep venous

Fig. 17.10 Finger clubbing. [A] Anterior view. [B] Lateral view. *From Douglas G, Nicol F, Robertson C. Macleod's Clinical examination, 13th edn. Edinburgh: Churchill Livingstone, Elsevier Ltd; 2013.*

i 17.8 Differential diagnosis of finger clubbing
Congenital or familial (5–10%)
Acquired
Thoracic (~80%)

• Chronic suppurative conditions:	• Tumours:
Pulmonary tuberculosis	Lung cancer
Bronchiectasis	Mesothelioma
Lung abscess	Fibroma
Empyema	• Pulmonary fibrosis
Cystic fibrosis	
Cardiovascular	
• Cyanotic congenital heart disease	• Arteriovenous shunts and aneurysms
• Infective endocarditis	
Gastrointestinal	
• Cirrhosis	• Coeliac disease
• Inflammatory bowel disease	
Others	
• Thyrotoxicosis (thyroid acropachy)	• Primary hypertrophic osteoarthropathy

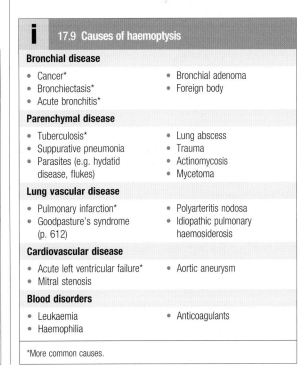

i 17.9 Causes of haemoptysis
Bronchial disease

• Cancer*	• Bronchial adenoma
• Bronchiectasis*	• Foreign body
• Acute bronchitis*	
Parenchymal disease	
• Tuberculosis*	• Lung abscess
• Suppurative pneumonia	• Trauma
• Parasites (e.g. hydatid disease, flukes)	• Actinomycosis
	• Mycetoma
Lung vascular disease	
• Pulmonary infarction*	• Polyarteritis nodosa
• Goodpasture's syndrome (p. 612)	• Idiopathic pulmonary haemosiderosis
Cardiovascular disease	
• Acute left ventricular failure*	• Aortic aneurysm
• Mitral stenosis	
Blood disorders	
• Leukaemia	• Anticoagulants
• Haemophilia	

*More common causes.

17

thrombosis. Rashes, haematuria and digital infarcts point to an underlying systemic disease, such as a vasculitis, which may be associated with haemoptysis.

Management

In severe acute haemoptysis, the patient should be nursed upright (or on the side of the bleeding, if this is known), given high-flow oxygen and resuscitated as required. Bronchoscopy in the acute phase is difficult and often merely shows blood throughout the bronchial tree. Infusions of the antifibrinolytic agent tranexamic acid or the vasopressin precursor terlipressin may help to limit bleeding but evidence of efficacy is limited. If radiology shows an obvious central cause, then rigid bronchoscopy under general anaesthesia may allow intervention to stop bleeding; however, the source often cannot be visualised. Intubation with a divided endotracheal tube may allow protected ventilation of the unaffected lung to stabilise the patient. Bronchial arteriography and embolisation (Fig. 17.11), or even emergency surgery, can be life-saving in the acute situation.

In the vast majority of cases, however, the haemoptysis itself is not life-threatening and a logical sequence of investigations can be followed:

- chest X-ray, which may provide evidence of a localised lesion, including tumour (malignant or benign), pneumonia, mycetoma or tuberculosis
- full blood count (FBC) and clotting screen
- bronchoscopy after acute bleeding has settled, which may reveal a central lung cancer (not visible on the chest X-ray) and permit biopsy and tissue diagnosis
- CTPA, which may show underlying pulmonary thromboembolic disease or alternative causes not seen on the chest X-ray (e.g. pulmonary arteriovenous malformation or small or hidden tumours).

Fig. 17.11 Bronchial artery angiography. An angiography catheter has been passed via the femoral artery and aorta into an abnormally dilated right bronchial artery (arrows). Contrast is seen flowing into the lung. This patient had post-tuberculous bronchiectasis and presented with massive haemoptysis. Bronchial artery embolisation was successfully performed.

The 'incidental' pulmonary nodule

A pulmonary nodule may be defined as a well or poorly circumscribed, approximately rounded structure that appears on imaging as a focal opacity less than 3 cm in diameter that is surrounded by aerated lung. The increased use of helical multi-detector CT (Fig 17.12) has been accompanied by an epidemic of 'incidental' pulmonary nodules. Nodules must not be dismissed as 'incidental', however, until an important and treatable infective or malignant condition in its earliest stage is excluded or stability over at least 2 years has been demonstrated.

The list of potential causes of pulmonary nodules is extensive and most are benign (Box 17.10). Features on a CT scan consistent with a benign lesion include being less than 5 mm in diameter or less than 80 mm^3 in volume; diffuse, central, laminated or popcorn calcification; or the presence of macroscopic fat. In addition, perifissural lymph nodes and subpleural nodules with a lentiform or triangular shape do not require any further investigation.

In cases where a benign lesion cannot be confidently assumed, further assessment depends on both the appearance of the nodule and the clinical context. These assessments may be aided by the use of computer prediction models (Box 17.11).

Fig. 17.12 Thoracic CT scan showing a solitary pulmonary nodule identified in the right upper lobe (arrow).

i | 17.10 Causes of pulmonary nodules

Common causes

- Lung cancer
- Single metastasis
- Localised pneumonia
- Lung abscess
- Tuberculoma
- Pulmonary infarct

Uncommon causes

- Benign tumour
- Lymphoma
- Arteriovenous malformation
- Hydatid cyst (p. 298)
- Bronchogenic cyst
- Rheumatoid nodule
- Granulomatosis with polyangiitis (Wegener's granulomatosis)
- Pulmonary sequestration
- Pulmonary haematoma
- 'Pseudotumour' – fluid collection in a fissure
- Aspergilloma (usually surrounded by air crescent)
- *Cryptococcus*
- *Aspergillus* nodule

i	17.11 Clinical and radiographic features distinguishing benign from malignant nodules*		
Feature	**Risk of malignancy**	**Feature**	**Risk of malignancy**
Characteristics of nodule		**Characteristics of patient**	
Size	Nearly all >3 cm but fewer than 1% <4 mm are malignant	Age	Increases with age and is uncommon below age of 40
Margin	Usually smooth in benign lesions	Smoking history	Increases in proportion to duration and amount smoked
	Spiculated suggests malignancy	Other	Increased by history of lung cancer in first-degree
Calcification or fat	Laminated or central deposition of calcification suggests granuloma		relative and by exposure to asbestos, silica, uranium and radon
	'Popcorn' pattern suggests hamartoma		
	Fat may suggest hamartoma or lipoid granuloma		
Location	70% of lung cancers occur in upper lobes		
	Benign lesions are equally distributed throughout upper and lower lobes		

*Linear or sheet-like lung opacities are unlikely to represent neoplasms and do not require follow-up. Some nodular opacities may be sufficiently typical of scarring for follow-up not to be warranted.
Adapted from MacMahon H, Austin JH, Gamsu G, et al. Guidelines for management of small pulmonary nodules detected on CT scans: a statement from the Fleischner Society. Radiology 2005; 237:395–400.

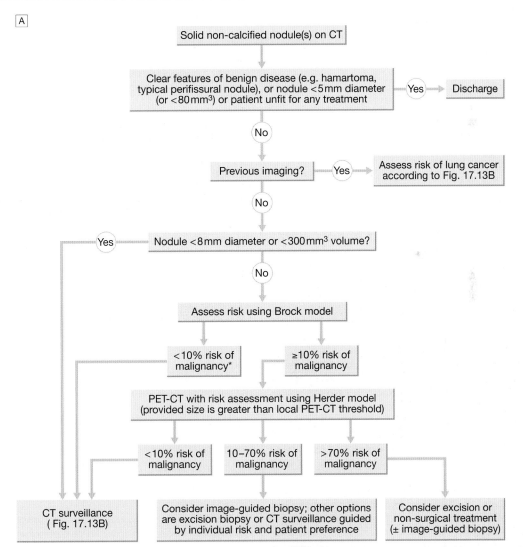

Fig. 17.13 Recommendations on the assessment of a solid pulmonary nodule. [A] Initial approach to solid pulmonary nodules. The Brock model is an online calculator that can also be downloaded as an app (https://brocku.ca/lung-cancer-risk-calculator). The model integrates data on age, sex, family history of cancer, the presence of emphysema, nodule size, nodule type, nodule position, nodule count and speculation, and calculates the probability that a nodule will become malignant within a 2- to 4-year follow-up period. Herder is a similar model. *Consider positron emission tomography–computed tomography (PET-CT) for larger nodules in young patients with low risk by Brock score, as this score was developed in a screening cohort (50–75 years) and so performance in younger patients is unproven. *Continues overleaf.*

B

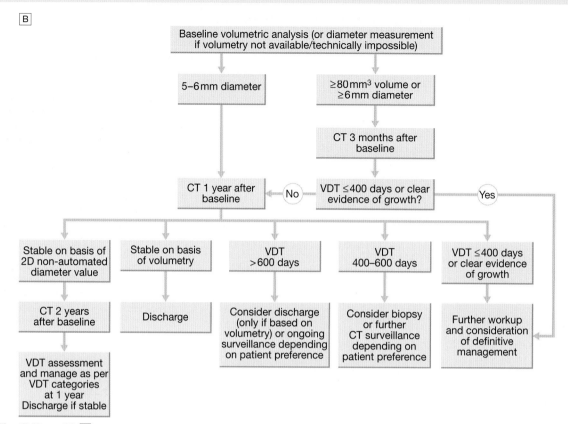

Fig. 17.13, cont'd [B] Solid pulmonary nodule surveillance algorithm. (VDT = volume doubling time) *From Callister ME, Baldwin DR, Akram AR, et al. British Thoracic Society Guidelines on the investigation and management of pulmonary nodules. Thorax 2015; Suppl. 2:ii1–ii54.*

A variety of diagnostic approaches may be considered, including bronchoscopy, percutaneous needle biopsy, PET, interval CT scanning or even surgical resection of the lesion. Pulmonary nodules are invariably beyond the vision of the bronchoscope and, with the notable exception of pulmonary infection (e.g. tuberculosis), the yield from blind washings is low, although this may improve as advances in endobronchial imaging are adopted. If the nodule is favourably located and of sufficient size, percutaneous needle biopsy under ultrasound or CT guidance may be employed. The risk of pneumothorax is approximately 15% and around 7% require intercostal drainage, so this should be contemplated only in individuals with an FEV$_1$ of more than 35% predicted. Haemorrhage into the lung or pleural space, air embolism and tumour seeding are rare but recognised complications.

Where clinical suspicion remains high despite a benign or indeterminate biopsy or where a nodule is considered to be of sufficiently high risk for malignancy to merit proceeding straight to surgery, then surgical resection may be the best management, as surgery remains the best chance of curing lung cancer. It is important for the logic underlying this approach to be discussed with the patient and the consequences of resection of a benign lesion explained.

PET scanning provides useful information about nodules of at least 1 cm in diameter. The presence of high metabolic activity is strongly suggestive of malignancy, while an inactive 'cold' nodule is consistent with benign disease. However, a high SUV is a marker of glucose metabolism, not malignancy, and PET has significant limitations in regions with high endemic rates of infectious or granulomatous disease. False-negative results may occur with neuro-endocrine tumours and minimally invasive lepidic adenocarcinoma. Detection of neuro-endocrine tumours may be improved by the use of ^{68}Ga-Dotatoc in place of FDG.

If the nodule is small and inaccessible, interval CT scanning may be employed. A repeat CT scan at 3 months will reliably detect growth in larger nodules and may also demonstrate resolution. Further interval scans may be arranged, depending on the clinical context (Fig. 17.13).

Particular care must be taken with subsolid nodules, particularly if further imaging demonstrates the development of a new solid component, as these may represent a pre-malignant or an early invasive form of adenocarcinoma.

In cases where the probability of cancer is low, the potential risk of further scanning must be considered. Subsequent scans often detect further nodules, increase the risk of false-positive findings and lead to unnecessary patient anxiety while exposing the individual to increased radiation.

Pleural effusion

The accumulation of serous fluid within the pleural space is termed pleural effusion. The accumulation of frank pus is termed empyema (p. 564), that of blood is haemothorax, and that of chyle is a chylothorax. In general, pleural fluid accumulates as a result of either increased hydrostatic pressure or decreased osmotic pressure ('transudative' effusion, as seen in cardiac, liver or renal failure), or from increased microvascular pressure due to disease of the pleura or injury in the adjacent lung ('exudative' effusion). The causes of the majority of pleural effusions (Boxes 17.12 and 17.13) are identified by a thorough history, examination and relevant investigations.

Clinical assessment

Symptoms (pain on inspiration and coughing) and signs of pleurisy (a pleural rub) often precede the development of an effusion, especially in patients with underlying pneumonia, pulmonary infarction or connective tissue disease. When breathlessness is the only symptom, however, the onset may be insidious, depending on the size and rate of accumulation. The physical signs are detailed on page 547.

17.12 Causes of pleural effusion

Common causes

- Pneumonia ('parapneumonic effusion')
- Tuberculosis
- Pulmonary infarction*
- Malignant disease
- Cardiac failure*
- Subdiaphragmatic disorders (subphrenic abscess, pancreatitis etc.)

Uncommon causes

- Hypoproteinaemia* (nephrotic syndrome, liver failure, malnutrition)
- Connective tissue diseases* (particularly systemic lupus erythematosus and rheumatoid arthritis)
- Post-myocardial infarction syndrome
- Acute rheumatic fever
- Meigs' syndrome (ovarian tumour plus pleural effusion)
- Myxoedema*
- Uraemia*
- Asbestos-related benign pleural effusion

*May cause bilateral effusions.

Investigations

Radiological investigations

The classical appearance of pleural fluid on the erect PA chest film is of a curved shadow at the lung base, blunting the costophrenic angle and ascending towards the axilla (p. 547). Fluid appears to track up the lateral chest wall. In fact, fluid surrounds the whole lung at this level but casts a radiological shadow only where the X-ray beam passes tangentially across the fluid against the lateral chest wall. Around 200 mL of fluid is required in order for it to be detectable on a PA chest X-ray. Previous scarring or adhesions in the pleural space can cause localised effusions. Pleural fluid localised below the lower lobe ('subpulmonary effusion') simulates an elevated hemidiaphragm. Pleural fluid localised within an oblique fissure may produce a rounded opacity that may be mistaken for a tumour.

Ultrasound is more accurate than plain chest X-ray for determining the presence of fluid. A clear hypoechoic space is consistent with a transudate and the presence of moving, floating densities suggests an exudate. The presence of septation most likely indicates an evolving empyema or resolving haemothorax. CT scanning is indicated where malignant disease is suspected.

Pleural aspiration and biopsy

In some conditions (e.g. left ventricular failure), it should not be necessary to sample fluid unless atypical features are present; appropriate treatment should be administered and the effusion re-evaluated. In most other circumstances, however, diagnostic sampling is required. Simple aspiration provides information on the colour and texture of fluid and these alone may immediately suggest an empyema or chylothorax. The presence of blood is consistent with pulmonary infarction or malignancy but may result from a traumatic tap. Biochemical analysis allows classification into

17.13 Pleural effusion: main causes and features

Cause	Appearance of fluid	Type of fluid	Predominant cells in fluid	Other diagnostic features
Tuberculosis	Serous, usually amber-coloured	Exudate	Lymphocytes (occasionally polymorphs)	Positive tuberculin test Isolation of *Mycobacterium tuberculosis* from pleural fluid (20%) Positive pleural biopsy (80%) Raised adenosine deaminase
Malignant disease	Serous, often blood-stained	Exudate	Serosal cells and lymphocytes Often clumps of malignant cells	Positive pleural biopsy (40%) Evidence of malignancy elsewhere
Cardiac failure	Serous, straw-coloured	Transudate	Few serosal cells	Other signs of cardiac failure Response to diuretics
Pulmonary infarction	Serous or blood-stained	Exudate (rarely transudate)	Red blood cells Eosinophils	Evidence of pulmonary infarction Obvious source of embolism Factors predisposing to venous thrombosis
Rheumatoid disease	Serous Turbid if chronic	Exudate	Lymphocytes (occasionally polymorphs)	Rheumatoid arthritis: rheumatoid factor and anti-cyclic citrullinated peptide (anti-CCP) antibodies Cholesterol in chronic effusion; very low glucose in pleural fluid
Systemic lupus erythematosus (SLE)	Serous	Exudate	Lymphocytes and serosal cells	Other signs of SLE Antinuclear factor or anti-DNA positive
Acute pancreatitis	Serous or blood-stained	Exudate	No cells predominate	Higher amylase in pleural fluid than in serum
Obstruction of thoracic duct	Milky	Chyle	None	Chylomicrons

17

17.14 Light's criteria for distinguishing pleural transudate from exudate

Exudate is likely if one or more of the following criteria are met:
• Pleural fluid protein:serum protein ratio >0.5
• Pleural fluid LDH:serum LDH ratio >0.6
• Pleural fluid LDH > two-thirds of the upper limit of normal serum LDH

(LDH = lactate dehydrogenase)

17.15 Clinical features of empyema

Systemic features

• Pyrexia, usually high and remittent
• Rigors, sweating, malaise and weight loss
• Polymorphonuclear leucocytosis, high C-reactive protein

Local features

• Pleural pain; breathlessness; cough and sputum, usually because of underlying lung disease; copious purulent sputum if empyema ruptures into a bronchus (bronchopleural fistula)
• Clinical signs of pleural effusion

transudate and exudate (Box 17.14) and Gram stain may suggest parapneumonic effusion. The predominant cell type provides useful information and cytological examination is essential. A low pH suggests infection but may also be seen in rheumatoid arthritis, ruptured oesophagus or advanced malignancy.

Ultrasound- or CT-guided pleural biopsy provides tissue for pathological and microbiological analysis. Where necessary, video-assisted thoracoscopy allows visualisation of the pleura and direct guidance of a biopsy.

Management

Therapeutic aspiration may be required to palliate breathlessness but removing more than 1.5 L at a time is associated with a small risk of re-expansion pulmonary oedema. An effusion should never be drained to dryness before establishing a diagnosis, as biopsy may be precluded until further fluid accumulates. Treatment of the underlying cause – e.g. heart failure, pneumonia, pulmonary embolism or subphrenic abscess – will often be followed by resolution of the effusion. The management of pleural effusion in pneumonia, tuberculosis and malignancy is dealt with below.

Empyema

This is a collection of pus in the pleural space, which may be as thin as serous fluid or so thick that it is impossible to aspirate, even through a wide-bore needle. Microscopically, neutrophil leucocytes are present in large numbers. An empyema may involve the whole pleural space or only part of it ('loculated' or 'encysted' empyema) and is usually unilateral. It is always secondary to infection in a neighbouring structure, usually the lung, most commonly due to the bacterial pneumonias and tuberculosis. Over 40% of patients with community-acquired pneumonia develop an associated pleural effusion ('parapneumonic' effusion) and about 15% of these become secondarily infected. Other causes are infection of a haemothorax following trauma or surgery, oesophageal rupture, and rupture of a subphrenic abscess through the diaphragm.

Both pleural surfaces are covered with a thick, shaggy, inflammatory exudate. The pus in the pleural space is often under considerable pressure, and if the condition is not adequately treated, pus may rupture into a bronchus, causing a bronchopleural fistula and pyopneumothorax, or track through the chest wall with the formation of a subcutaneous abscess or sinus, so-called empyema necessitans.

Clinical assessment

An empyema should be suspected in patients with pulmonary infection if there is severe pleuritic chest pain or persisting or recurrent pyrexia, despite appropriate antibiotic treatment. In other cases, the primary infection may be so mild that it passes unrecognised and the first definite clinical features are due to the

Fig. 17.14 Chest X-ray showing a 'D'-shaped shadow in the left mid-zone, consistent with an empyema. In this case, an intercostal chest drain has been inserted but the loculated collection of pus remains.

empyema itself. Once an empyema has developed, systemic features are prominent (Box 17.15).

Investigations

Chest X-ray appearances may be indistinguishable from those of pleural effusion, although pleural adhesions may confine the empyema to form a 'D'-shaped shadow against the inside of the chest wall (Fig. 17.14). When air is present as well as pus (pyopneumothorax), a horizontal 'fluid level' marks the air/liquid interface. Ultrasound shows the position of the fluid, the extent of pleural thickening and whether fluid is in a single collection or multiloculated, containing fibrin and debris (Fig. 17.15). CT provides information on the pleura, underlying lung parenchyma and patency of the major bronchi.

Ultrasound or CT is used to identify the optimal site for aspiration, which is best performed using a wide-bore needle. If the fluid is thick and turbid pus, empyema is confirmed. Other features suggesting empyema are a fluid glucose of less than 3.3 mmol/L (60 mg/dL), lactate dehydrogenase (LDH) of more than 1000 IU/L, or a fluid pH of less than 7.0 (H⁺ >100 nmol/L). However, pH measurement should be avoided if pus is thick, as it damages blood gas machines. The pus is frequently sterile on culture if antibiotics have already been given. The distinction between tuberculous and non-tuberculous disease can be difficult and may require pleural biopsy, histology, culture and/or a NAAT.

Fig. 17.15 Pleural ultrasound showing septation. *Courtesy of Dr P. Sivasothy, Department of Respiratory Medicine, Addenbrooke's Hospital, Cambridge.*

Management

An empyema will heal only if infection is eradicated and the empyema space is obliterated, allowing apposition of the visceral and parietal pleural layers. This can only occur if re-expansion of the compressed lung is secured at an early stage by removal of all the pus from the pleural space. When the pus is sufficiently thin, this is most easily achieved by the insertion of a wide-bore intercostal tube into the most dependent part of the empyema space. If the initial aspirate reveals turbid fluid or frank pus, or if loculations are seen on ultrasound, the tube should be put on suction (−5 to −10 cmH$_2$O) and flushed regularly with 20 mL normal saline. If the organism causing the empyema can be identified, the appropriate antibiotic should be given for 2–4 weeks. Empirical antibiotic treatment (e.g. intravenous co-amoxiclav or cefuroxime with metronidazole) should be used if the organism is unknown. Intrapleural fibrinolytic therapy is of no benefit.

An empyema can often be aborted if these measures are started early, but if the intercostal tube is not providing adequate drainage – e.g. when the pus is thick or loculated – surgical intervention is required to clear the empyema cavity of pus and break down any adhesions. Surgical 'decortication' of the lung may also be required if gross thickening of the visceral pleura is preventing re-expansion of the lung. Surgery is also necessary if a bronchopleural fistula develops.

Despite the widespread availability of antibiotics that are effective against pneumonia, empyema remains a significant cause of morbidity and mortality.

Respiratory failure

The term 'respiratory failure' is used when pulmonary gas exchange fails to maintain normal arterial oxygen and carbon dioxide levels. Its classification into types I and II is defined by the absence or presence of hypercapnia (raised $PaCO_2$).

Pathophysiology

When disease impairs ventilation of part of a lung (e.g. in asthma or pneumonia), perfusion of that region results in hypoxic and CO_2-laden blood entering the pulmonary veins. Increased ventilation of neighbouring regions of normal lung can increase CO_2 excretion, correcting arterial CO_2 to normal, but cannot augment oxygen uptake because the haemoglobin flowing through these normal regions is already fully saturated. Admixture of blood from the under-ventilated and normal regions thus results in hypoxia with normocapnia, which is called 'type I respiratory failure'. Diseases causing this include all those that impair ventilation locally with sparing of other regions (Box 17.16).

Arterial hypoxia with hypercapnia (type II respiratory failure) is seen in conditions that cause generalised, severe ventilation–perfusion mismatch, leaving insufficient normal lung to correct $PaCO_2$, or any disease that reduces total ventilation. The latter includes not just diseases of the lung but also disorders affecting any part of the neuromuscular mechanism of ventilation (Box 17.16).

Management of acute respiratory failure

Prompt diagnosis and management of the underlying cause is crucial. In type I respiratory failure, high concentrations of oxygen (40–60% by mask) will usually relieve hypoxia by increasing the alveolar PO_2 in poorly ventilated lung units. Occasionally, however (e.g. severe pneumonia affecting several lobes), mechanical ventilation may be needed to relieve hypoxia. Patients who need high concentrations of oxygen for more than a few hours should receive humidified oxygen.

17

17.16 How to interpret blood gas abnormalities in respiratory failure

	Type I		Type II	
	Hypoxia (PaO_2 <8.0 kPa (60 mmHg)) Normal or low $PaCO_2$ (≤6 kPa (45 mmHg))		Hypoxia (PaO_2 <8.0 kPa (60 mmHg)) Raised $PaCO_2$ (>6 kPa (45 mmHg))	
	Acute	Chronic	Acute	Chronic
H$^+$	→	→	↑	→ or ↑
Bicarbonate	→	→	→	↑
Causes	Acute asthma Pulmonary oedema Pneumonia Lobar collapse Pneumothorax Pulmonary embolus ARDS	COPD Lung fibrosis Lymphangitic carcinomatosis Right-to-left shunts	Acute severe asthma Acute exacerbation of COPD Upper airway obstruction Acute neuropathies/paralysis Narcotic drugs Primary alveolar hypoventilation Flail chest injury	COPD Sleep apnoea Kyphoscoliosis Myopathies/muscular dystrophy Ankylosing spondylitis

(ARDS = acute respiratory distress syndrome; COPD = chronic obstructive pulmonary disease)

Acute type II respiratory failure is an emergency requiring immediate intervention. It is useful to distinguish between patients with high ventilatory drive (rapid respiratory rate and accessory muscle recruitment) who cannot move sufficient air, and those with reduced or inadequate respiratory effort. In the former, particularly if inspiratory stridor is present, acute upper airway obstruction from foreign body inhalation or laryngeal obstruction (angioedema, carcinoma or vocal cord paralysis) must be considered, as the Heimlich manœuvre (p. 625), immediate intubation or emergency tracheostomy may be life-saving.

More commonly, the problem is in the lungs, with severe generalised bronchial obstruction from COPD or asthma, acute respiratory distress syndrome (ARDS) arising from a variety of insults (p. 198), or occasionally tension pneumothorax (p. 625). In all such cases, high-concentration (e.g. 60%) oxygen should be administered, pending a rapid examination of the respiratory system and measurement of arterial blood gases. Patients with the trachea deviated away from a silent and resonant hemithorax are likely to have tension pneumothorax, and air should be aspirated from the pleural space and a chest drain inserted as soon as possible. Patients with generalised wheeze, scanty breath sounds bilaterally or a history of asthma or COPD should be treated with salbutamol 2.5 mg nebulised with oxygen, repeated until bronchospasm is relieved. Failure to respond to initial treatment, declining conscious level and worsening respiratory acidosis (H^+ >50 nmol/L (pH <7.3), $PaCO_2$ >6.6 kPa (50 mmHg)) on blood gases are all indications that supported ventilation is required (p. 202).

A small percentage of patients with severe chronic COPD and type II respiratory failure develop abnormal tolerance to raised $PaCO_2$ and may become dependent on hypoxic drive to breathe. In these patients only, lower concentrations of oxygen (24–28% by Venturi mask) should be used to avoid precipitating worsening respiratory depression (see below). In all cases, regular monitoring of arterial blood gases is important to assess progress.

Patients with acute type II respiratory failure who have reduced drive or conscious level may be suffering from sedative poisoning, CO_2 narcosis or a primary failure of neurological drive (e.g. following intracerebral haemorrhage or head injury). History from a witness may be invaluable, and reversal of specific drugs with (for example) opiate antagonists is occasionally successful, but should not delay intubation and supported mechanical ventilation in appropriate cases.

Chronic and 'acute on chronic' type II respiratory failure

The most common cause of chronic type II respiratory failure is severe COPD. Although $PaCO_2$ may be persistently raised, there is no persisting acidaemia because the kidneys retain bicarbonate, correcting arterial pH to normal. This 'compensated' pattern, which may also occur in chronic neuromuscular disease or kyphoscoliosis, is maintained until there is a further acute illness (Box 17.16), such as an exacerbation of COPD that precipitates an episode of 'acute on chronic' respiratory failure, with acidaemia and initial respiratory distress followed by drowsiness and eventually coma. These patients have lost their chemosensitivity to elevated $PaCO_2$, and so they may paradoxically depend on hypoxia for respiratory drive and are at risk of respiratory depression if given high concentrations of oxygen, e.g. during ambulance transfers or in emergency departments. Moreover, in contrast to acute severe asthma, some patients with 'acute on chronic' type II respiratory failure

due to COPD may not appear distressed, despite being critically ill with severe hypoxaemia, hypercapnia and acidaemia. While the physical signs of CO_2 retention (delirium, flapping tremor, bounding pulses and so on) can be helpful if present, they may not be, so measurement of arterial blood gases is mandatory in the assessment of initial severity and response to treatment.

Management

The principal aims of treatment in acute on chronic type II respiratory failure are to achieve a safe PaO_2 (>7.0 kPa (52 mmHg)) without increasing $PaCO_2$ and acidosis, while identifying and treating the precipitating condition. In these patients, it is not necessary to achieve a normal PaO_2; even a small increase will greatly improve tissue oxygen delivery, since their PaO_2 values are often on the steep part of the oxygen dissociation curve (see Fig. 10.9, p. 191). The risks of worsening hypercapnia and coma must be balanced against those of severe hypoxaemia, which include potentially fatal arrhythmias and hypoxic brain damage. Immediate treatment is shown in Box 17.17. Patients who are conscious and have adequate respiratory drive may benefit from non-invasive ventilation (NIV), which has been shown to reduce the need for intubation and shorten hospital stay in acidotic exacerbations of COPD. Patients who are drowsy and have low respiratory drive require an urgent decision regarding intubation and ventilation, as this is likely to be the only effective treatment, even though weaning off the ventilator may be difficult in severe disease. The decision is challenging, and important factors to consider include patient and family wishes, presence of a potentially remediable precipitating condition, prior functional

---

17.17 Assessment and management of 'acute on chronic' type II respiratory failure

Initial assessment

Patient may not appear distressed, despite being critically ill
- Conscious level (response to commands, ability to cough)
- CO_2 retention (warm periphery, bounding pulses, flapping tremor)
- Airways obstruction (wheeze, prolonged expiration, hyperinflation, intercostal indrawing, pursed lips)
- Cor pulmonale (peripheral oedema, raised jugular venous pressure, hepatomegaly, ascites)
- Background functional status and quality of life
- Signs of precipitating cause (see Box 17.16)

Investigations

- Arterial blood gases (severity of hypoxaemia, hypercapnia, acidaemia, bicarbonate)
- Chest X-ray

Management

- Maintenance of airway
- Treatment of specific precipitating cause
- Frequent physiotherapy ± pharyngeal suction
- Nebulised bronchodilators
- Controlled oxygen therapy:
  Start with 24% Venturi mask
  Aim for a PaO_2 > 7 kPa (52 mmHg) (a PaO_2 < 5 (37 mmHg) is dangerous)
- Antibiotics if evidence of infection
- Diuretics if evidence of fluid overload

Progress

- If $PaCO_2$ continues to rise or a safe PaO_2 cannot be achieved without severe hypercapnia and acidaemia, mechanical ventilatory support may be required capacity and quality of life. The various types of non-invasive (via a face or nasal mask) or invasive (via an endotracheal tube) ventilation are detailed on page 202.

Respiratory stimulant drugs, such as doxapram, have been superseded by intubation and mechanical ventilation in patients with CO_2 narcosis.

Home ventilation for chronic respiratory failure

NIV is of great value in the long-term treatment of respiratory failure due to spinal deformity, neuromuscular disease and central alveolar hypoventilation. Some patients with advanced lung disease, e.g. cystic fibrosis, also benefit from NIV for respiratory failure. In these conditions, type II respiratory failure can develop slowly and insidiously. Morning headache (due to elevated $PaCO_2$) and fatigue are common symptoms but, in many cases, the diagnosis is revealed only by sleep studies or morning blood gas analysis. In the initial stages, ventilation is insufficient for metabolic needs only during sleep, when there is a physiological decline in ventilatory drive. Over time, however, CO_2 retention becomes chronic, with renal compensation of acidosis. Treatment by home-based NIV overnight is often sufficient to restore the daytime PCO_2 to normal, and to relieve fatigue and headache. In advanced disease (e.g. muscular dystrophies or cystic fibrosis), daytime NIV may also be required.

Lung transplantation

Lung transplantation is an established treatment for carefully selected patients with advanced lung disease unresponsive to medical treatment (Box 17.18). Single-lung transplantation may be used for selected patients with advanced emphysema or lung fibrosis. This is contraindicated in patients with chronic bilateral pulmonary infection, such as cystic fibrosis and bronchiectasis, because the transplanted lung is vulnerable to cross-infection in the context of post-transplant immunosuppression, and for these individuals bilateral lung transplantation is the standard procedure. Combined heart–lung transplantation is still occasionally needed for patients with advanced congenital heart disease, such as Eisenmenger's syndrome, and is preferred by some surgeons for the treatment of primary pulmonary hypertension unresponsive to medical therapy.

The prognosis following lung transplantation is improving steadily with modern immunosuppressive drugs: over 50% 10-year survival in some UK centres. Chronic rejection with obliterative bronchiolitis continues to afflict some recipients, however. Glucocorticoids are used to manage acute rejection, but drugs that inhibit cell-mediated immunity specifically, such as ciclosporin, mycophenolate and tacrolimus (p. 89), are used to prevent chronic rejection. Azithromycin, statins and total lymphoid

irradiation are employed to treat obliterative bronchiolitis but late organ failure remains a significant problem.

The major factor limiting the availability of lung transplantation is the shortage of donor lungs. To improve organ availability, techniques to recondition the lungs in vitro after removal from the donor are being developed.

Obstructive pulmonary diseases

Asthma

Asthma is a chronic inflammatory disorder of the airways, in which many cells and cellular elements play a role. Chronic inflammation is associated with airway hyper-responsiveness that leads to recurrent episodes of wheezing, breathlessness, chest tightness and coughing, particularly at night and in the early morning. These episodes are usually associated with widespread but variable airflow obstruction within the lung that is often reversible, either spontaneously or with treatment.

The prevalence of asthma increased steadily over the latter part of last century. As asthma affects all age groups, it is one of the most common and important long-term respiratory conditions in terms of global years lived with disability (Fig. 17.16).

The development and course of asthma and the response to treatment are influenced by genetic determinants, while the rapid rise in prevalence implies that environmental factors are critically important in the development and expression of the disease. The potential role of indoor and outdoor allergens, microbial exposure, diet, vitamins, breastfeeding, tobacco smoke, air pollution and obesity have been explored but no clear consensus has emerged.

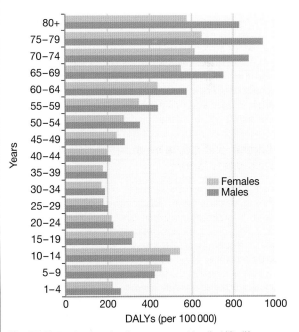

Fig. 17.16 The burden of asthma, measured by disability life years (DALYs) per 100 000 population. The burden of asthma is greatest in children approaching adolescence and the elderly. The burden is similar in males and females at ages below 30–34 but at older ages the burden is higher in males. *From The Global Asthma Report 2014. Copyright 2014 The Global Asthma Network.*

i	**17.18 Indications for lung transplantation**

Parenchymal lung disease

- Cystic fibrosis
- Emphysema
- Pulmonary fibrosis
- Obliterative bronchiolitis
- Langerhans cell histiocytosis (p. 613)
- Lymphangioleiomyomatosis (p. 613)

Pulmonary vascular disease

- Primary pulmonary hypertension
- Thromboembolic pulmonary hypertension
- Veno-occlusive disease
- Eisenmenger's syndrome (p. 532)

Fig. 17.17 Airway hyper-reactivity in asthma. This is demonstrated by bronchial challenge tests with sequentially increasing concentrations of either histamine, or methacholine or mannitol. The reactivity of the airways is expressed as the concentration or dose of either chemical required to produce a specific decrease (usually 20%) in the forced expired volume in 1 second (FEV_1) (PC_{20} or PD_{20}, respectively).

Fig. 17.18 Changes in peak flow following allergen challenge. A similar biphasic response is observed following a variety of different challenges. Occasionally, an isolated late response is seen with no early reaction.

Pathophysiology

Airway hyper-reactivity (AHR) – the tendency for airways to narrow excessively in response to triggers that have little or no effect in normal individuals – is integral to the diagnosis of asthma and appears to be related, although not exclusively, to airway inflammation (Fig. 17.17). Other factors likely to be important in the behaviour of airway smooth muscle include the degree of airway narrowing and neurogenic mechanisms.

The relationship between atopy (the propensity to produce IgE) and asthma is well established and in many individuals there is a clear relationship between sensitisation and allergen exposure, as demonstrated by skin-prick reactivity or elevated serum-specific IgE. Common examples of allergens include house dust mites, pets such as cats and dogs, pests such as cockroaches, and fungi. Inhalation of an allergen into the airway is followed by an early and late-phase bronchoconstrictor response (Fig. 17.18). Allergic mechanisms are also implicated in some cases of occupational asthma (p. 613).

In cases of aspirin-sensitive asthma, the ingestion of salicylates results in inhibition of the cyclo-oxygenase enzymes, preferentially shunting the metabolism of arachidonic acid through the lipoxygenase pathway with resultant production of the asthmogenic cysteinyl leukotrienes. In exercise-induced asthma, hyperventilation results in water loss from the pericellular lining fluid of the respiratory mucosa, which, in turn, triggers mediator release. Heat loss from the respiratory mucosa may also be important.

In persistent asthma, a chronic and complex inflammatory response ensues, characterised by an influx of numerous inflammatory cells, the transformation and participation of airway structural cells, and the secretion of an array of cytokines, chemokines and growth factors. Examination of the inflammatory cell profile in induced sputum samples demonstrates that, although asthma is predominantly characterised by airway eosinophilia, neutrophilic inflammation predominates in some patients while in others scant inflammation is observed: so-called 'pauci-granulocytic' asthma.

With increasing severity and chronicity of the disease, remodelling of the airway may occur, leading to fibrosis of the airway wall, fixed narrowing of the airway and a reduced response to bronchodilator medication.

Clinical features

Typical symptoms include recurrent episodes of wheezing, chest tightness, breathlessness and cough. Asthma is commonly mistaken for a cold or a persistent chest infection (e.g. longer than 10 days). Classical precipitants include exercise, particularly in cold weather, exposure to airborne allergens or pollutants, and viral upper respiratory tract infections. Wheeze apart, there is often very little to find on examination. An inspection for nasal polyps and eczema should be performed. Rarely, a vasculitic rash may suggest eosinophilic granulomatosis with polyangiitis (formerly known as Churg–Strauss syndrome; p. 1043).

Patients with mild intermittent asthma are usually asymptomatic between exacerbations. Individuals with persistent asthma report ongoing breathlessness and wheeze but these are variable, with symptoms fluctuating over the course of one day, or from day to day or month to month.

Asthma characteristically displays a diurnal pattern, with symptoms and lung function being worse in the early morning. Particularly when poorly controlled, symptoms such as cough and wheeze disturb sleep. Cough may be the dominant symptom in some patients, and the lack of wheeze or breathlessness may lead to a delay in reaching the diagnosis of so-called 'cough-variant asthma'.

Some patients with asthma have a similar inflammatory response in the upper airway. Careful enquiry should be made as to a history of sinusitis, sinus headache, a blocked or runny nose and loss of sense of smell.

Although the aetiology of asthma is often elusive, an attempt should be made to identify any agents that may contribute to the appearance or aggravation of the condition. Particular enquiry should be made about potential allergens, such as exposure to a pet cat, guinea pig, rabbit or horse, pest infestation, exposure to moulds following water damage to a home or building, and any potential occupational agents (p. 613).

In some circumstances, the appearance of asthma is triggered by medications. Beta-blockers, even when administered topically as eye drops, may induce bronchospasm, as may aspirin and other non-steroidal anti-inflammatory drugs (NSAIDs). The classical aspirin-sensitive patient is female and presents in middle age with asthma, rhinosinusitis and nasal polyps. Aspirin-sensitive patients may also report symptoms following alcohol and foods containing salicylates. Other medications implicated include the oral contraceptive pill, cholinergic agents and prostaglandin $F_{2\alpha}$. Betel nuts contain arecoline, which is structurally similar to methacholine and can aggravate asthma. An important minority of patients develop a particularly severe form of asthma and this appears to be more common in women. Allergic triggers are less important and airway neutrophilia predominates.

Diagnosis

The diagnosis of asthma is predominantly clinical and is based on the combination of the history, lung function and 'other' tests, which allows high, intermediate or low probability of asthma to emerge. The approach may vary from patient to patient and may need to be re-evaluated following the introduction of treatment.

Supportive evidence is provided by the demonstration of variable airflow obstruction, preferably by using spirometry (Box 17.19) to measure FEV_1 and FVC. This identifies the obstructive defect, defines its severity, and provides a baseline for bronchodilator reversibility (Fig. 17.19). If spirometry is not available, a peak flow meter may be used. Symptomatic patients should be instructed to record peak flow readings after rising in the morning and before retiring in the evening. A diurnal variation in PEF of more than 20% (the lowest values typically being recorded in the morning) is considered diagnostic, and the magnitude of variability provides some indication of disease severity (Fig. 17.20). A trial of glucocorticoids (e.g. 30 mg daily for 2 weeks) may be useful in establishing the diagnosis, by demonstrating an improvement in either FEV_1 or PEF.

It is not uncommon for patients whose symptoms are suggestive of asthma to have normal lung function. In these circumstances, the demonstration of AHR by challenge tests may be useful to confirm the diagnosis (see Fig. 17.17). AHR has a high negative predictive value but positive results may be seen in other conditions, such as COPD, bronchiectasis and cystic fibrosis. The use of exercise tests is useful when symptoms are predominantly related to exercise (Fig. 17.21).

The diagnosis may be supported by the presence of atopy demonstrated by skin-prick tests or measurement of total and allergen-specific IgE, an FE_{NO} (a surrogate of eosinophilic airway inflammation) of ≥40 parts per billion in a glucocorticoid-naïve adult, or a peripheral blood eosinophilia. Chest X-ray appearances are often normal but lobar collapse may be seen if mucus occludes a large bronchus and, if accompanied by the presence of flitting infiltrates, may suggest that asthma has been complicated by allergic bronchopulmonary aspergillosis (p. 596). A high-resolution CT scan (HRCT) may be useful to detect bronchiectasis.

Management

Setting goals

Asthma is a chronic condition but may be controlled with appropriate treatment in the majority of patients. The goal of treatment should be to obtain and maintain complete control (Box 17.20) but aims may be modified according to the circumstances

17.19 How to make a diagnosis of asthma

Compatible clinical history *plus either/or*:
- FEV_1 ≥12% (and 200 mL) increase following administration of a bronchodilator/trial of glucocorticoids. Greater confidence is gained if the increase is >15% and >400 mL
- >20% diurnal variation on ≥ 3 days in a week for 2 weeks on PEF diary
- FEV_1 ≥15% decrease after 6 mins of exercise

(FEV_1 = forced expiratory volume in 1 sec; PEF = peak expiratory flow)

17

Fig. 17.19 **Reversibility test.** Forced expiratory manœuvres before and 20 minutes after inhalation of a β_2-adrenoceptor agonist. Note the increase in forced expiratory volume in 1 second (FEV_1) from 1.0 to 2.5 L.

Fig. 17.20 **Serial recordings of peak expiratory flow (PEF) in a patient with asthma.** Note the sharp overnight fall (morning dip) and subsequent rise during the day. Following the introduction of glucocorticoids, there is an improvement in PEF rate and reduction of morning dipping.

i 17.20 Levels of asthma control

Characteristic	Controlled	Partly controlled (any present in any week)	Uncontrolled
Daytime symptoms	None (≤ twice/week)	> twice/week	
Limitations of activities	None	Any	
Nocturnal symptoms/awakening	None	Any	≥ 3 features of partly controlled asthma present in any week
Need for rescue/'reliever' treatment	None (≤ twice/week)	> twice/week	
Lung function (PEF or FEV$_1$)	Normal	< 80% predicted or personal best (if known) on any day	
Exacerbation	None	≥ 1/year	1 in any week

(FEV1 = forced expiratory volume in 1 sec; PEF = peak expiratory flow)

Fig. 17.21 **Exercise-induced asthma.** Serial recordings of forced expiratory volume in 1 second (FEV$_1$) in a patient with bronchial asthma before and after 6 minutes of strenuous exercise. Note initial rise on completion of exercise, followed by sudden fall and gradual recovery. Adequate warm-up exercise or pre-treatment with a β$_2$-adrenoceptor agonist, nedocromil sodium or a leukotriene antagonist can protect against exercise-induced symptoms.

 17.21 Asthma in pregnancy

- **Clinical course**: women with well-controlled asthma usually have good pregnancy outcomes. Pregnancy in women with more severe asthma can precipitate worsening control and lead to increased maternal and neonatal morbidity.
- **Labour and delivery**: 90% have no symptoms.
- **Safety data**: good for β$_2$-agonists, inhaled glucocorticoids, theophyllines, oral prednisolone, and chromones.
- **Oral leukotriene receptor antagonists**: no evidence that these harm the fetus and they should not be stopped in women who have previously demonstrated significant improvement in asthma control prior to pregnancy.
- **Glucocorticoids**: women on maintenance prednisolone >7.5 mg/day should receive hydrocortisone 100 mg 3–4 times daily during labour.
- **Prostaglandin F$_{2\alpha}$**: may induce bronchospasm and should be used with extreme caution.
- **Breastfeeding**: use medications as normal.
- **Uncontrolled asthma**: associated with maternal (hyperemesis, hypertension, pre-eclampsia, vaginal haemorrhage, complicated labour) and fetal (intrauterine growth restriction and low birth weight, preterm birth, increased perinatal mortality, neonatal hypoxia) complications.

and the patient. Unfortunately, surveys consistently demonstrate that the majority of individuals with asthma report suboptimal control, perhaps reflecting the poor expectations of patients and their clinicians.

Whenever possible, patients should be encouraged to take responsibility for managing their own disease. A full explanation of the nature of the condition, the relationship between symptoms and inflammation, the importance of key symptoms such as nocturnal waking, the different types of medication and, if appropriate, the use of PEF to guide management decisions should be given. A variety of tools/questionnaires have been validated to assist in assessing asthma control. Written action plans can be helpful in developing self-management skills.

Avoidance of aggravating factors

This is particularly important in the management of occupational asthma (p. 613) but may also be relevant in atopic patients, when removing or reducing exposure to relevant antigens, such as a

pet, may effect improvement. House dust mite exposure may be minimised by replacing carpets with floorboards and using mite-impermeable bedding. So far, improvements in asthma control following such measures have been difficult to demonstrate. Many patients are sensitised to several ubiquitous aeroallergens, making avoidance strategies largely impractical. Measures to reduce fungal exposure may be applicable in specific circumstances and medications known to precipitate or aggravate asthma should be avoided. Smoking cessation (p. 94) is particularly important, as smoking not only encourages sensitisation but also induces a relative glucocorticoid resistance in the airway.

The stepwise approach to the management of asthma

See Figure 17.22.

Step 1: Occasional use of inhaled short-acting β$_2$-adrenoreceptor agonist bronchodilators

A variety of different inhaled devices are available and the choice of device should be guided by patient preference and competence

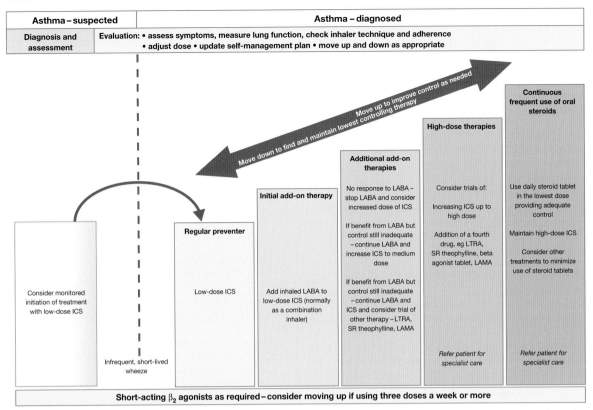

Asthma – suspected	Asthma – diagnosed
Diagnosis and assessment	**Evaluation:** • assess symptoms, measure lung function, check inhaler technique and adherence • adjust dose • update self-management plan • move up and down as appropriate

Move up to improve control as needed

Move down to find and maintain lowest controlling therapy

Continuous frequent use of oral steroids

High-dose therapies

Additional add-on therapies

Initial add-on therapy

Regular preventer

Consider monitored initiation of treatment with low-dose ICS

Infrequent, short-lived wheeze

Low-dose ICS

Add inhaled LABA to low-dose ICS (normally as a combination inhaler)

No response to LABA – stop LABA and consider increased dose of ICS

If benefit from LABA but control still inadequate – continue LABA and increase ICS to medium dose

If benefit from LABA but control still inadequate – continue LABA and ICS and consider trial of other therapy – LTRA, SR theophylline, LAMA

Consider trials of:

Increasing ICS up to high dose

Addition of a fourth drug, eg LTRA, SR theophylline, beta agonist tablet, LAMA

Refer patient for specialist care

Use daily steroid tablet in the lowest dose providing adequate control

Maintain high-dose ICS

Consider other treatments to minimize use of steroid tablets

Refer patient for specialist care

Short-acting β₂ agonists as required – consider moving up if using three doses a week or more

Fig. 17.22 Management approach in adults based on asthma control. (ICS = inhaled corticosteroids (glucocorticoids); LABA = long-acting β$_2$-agonist; LAMA = long-acting muscarinic antagonist; LTRA = leukotriene receptor antagonist; SR = sustained-release) *From British Thoracic Society and SIGN guideline 153: British guideline on the management of asthma (2016).*

17

- Remove the cap and shake the inhaler
- Breathe out gently and place the mouthpiece into the mouth
- Incline the head backwards to minimise oropharyngeal deposition
- Simultaneously, begin a slow deep inspiration, depress the canister and continue to inhale
- Hold the breath for 10 seconds

Fig. 17.23 How to use a metered-dose inhaler.

in its use. The metered-dose inhaler remains the most widely prescribed (Fig. 17.23).

For patients with mild intermittent asthma (symptoms less than once a week for 3 months and fewer than two nocturnal episodes per month), it is usually sufficient to prescribe an inhaled short-acting β$_2$-agonist, such as salbutamol or terbutaline, to be used as required. However, many patients (and their physicians) under-estimate the severity of asthma. A history of a severe exacerbation should lead to a step-up in treatment.

Step 2: Introduction of regular preventer therapy

Regular anti-inflammatory therapy (preferably inhaled glucocorticoids (ICS), such as beclometasone, budesonide (BUD), fluticasone, mometasone or ciclesonide) should be started in addition to inhaled β$_2$-agonists taken on an as-required basis for any patient who:

- has experienced an exacerbation of asthma in the last 2 years
- uses inhaled β$_2$-agonists three times a week or more
- reports symptoms three times a week or more
- is awakened by asthma one night per week.

For adults, a reasonable starting dose is 400 µg beclometasone dipropionate (BDP) or equivalent per day in adults, although higher doses may be required in smokers. Alternative but much less effective preventive agents include chromones, leukotriene receptor antagonists and theophyllines.

Step 3: Add-on therapy

If a patient remains poorly controlled despite regular use of an inhaled glucocorticoid, a thorough review should be undertaken of adherence, inhaler technique and ongoing exposure to modifiable aggravating factors. A further increase in the dose of inhaled glucocorticoid may benefit some patients but, in general, add-on therapy should be considered in adults taking 800 µg/day BDP (or equivalent).

The addition of a long-acting β$_2$-agonist (LABA) to an inhaled glucocorticoid provides more effective asthma control compared with increasing the dose of inhaled glucocorticoid alone. Fixed-combination inhalers of glucocorticoids and LABAs have been developed; these are more convenient, increase adherence and prevent patients using a LABA as monotherapy – the latter may be accompanied by an increased risk of life-threatening attacks or asthma death. The onset of action of formoterol is similar to that of salbutamol such that, in carefully selected patients, a fixed combination of budesonide and formoterol may be used as both rescue and maintenance therapy.

Oral leukotriene receptor antagonists (e.g. montelukast 10 mg daily) are generally less effective than LABAs as add-on therapy but may facilitate a reduction in the dose of inhaled glucocorticoid and control exacerbations.

Step 4: Poor control on moderate dose of inhaled glucocorticoid and add-on therapy: addition of a fourth drug

In adults, the dose of inhaled glucocorticoid may be increased to 2000 μg BDP/BUD (or equivalent) daily. A nasal glucocorticoid preparation should be used in patients with prominent upper airway symptoms. Leukotriene receptor antagonists, long-acting antimuscarinic agents, theophyllines or a slow-release β₂-agonist may be considered. If the trial of add-on therapy is ineffective, it should be discontinued.

Step 5: Continuous or frequent use of oral glucocorticoids

At this stage, prednisolone therapy (usually administered as a single daily dose in the morning) should be prescribed in the lowest amount necessary to control symptoms. Patients who are on long-term glucocorticoid tablets (>3 months) or are receiving more than three or four courses per year will be at risk of systemic side-effects (p. 670). The risk of osteoporosis in this group can be reduced by giving bisphosphonates (p. 1047). In patients who continue to experience symptoms and asthma exacerbation and demonstrate impaired lung function despite step 5 treatment, omalizumab, a monoclonal antibody directed against IgE, should be considered for those with a prominent atopic phenotype, and mepolizumab, a monoclonal antibody that blocks the binding of IL-5 to its receptor on eosinophils, should be considered in those with eosinophilic-mediated disease. The use of immunosuppressants, such as methotrexate, ciclosporin or oral gold, is less common nowadays, as the response is variable and the limited benefits may be easily offset by side-effects.

Step-down therapy

Once asthma control is established, the dose of inhaled (or oral) glucocorticoid should be titrated to the lowest dose at which effective control of asthma is maintained. Decreasing the dose of glucocorticoid by around 25–50% every 3 months is a reasonable strategy for most patients.

Exacerbations of asthma

The course of asthma may be punctuated by exacerbations with increased symptoms, deterioration in lung function, and an increase in airway inflammation. Exacerbations are most commonly precipitated by viral infections but moulds (*Alternaria* and *Cladosporium*), pollens (particularly following thunderstorms) and air pollution are also implicated. Most attacks are characterised by a gradual deterioration over several hours to days but some appear to occur with little or no warning: so-called brittle asthma. An important minority of patients appear to have a blunted perception of airway narrowing and fail to appreciate the early signs of deterioration.

Management of mild to moderate exacerbations

Doubling the dose of inhaled glucocorticoids does not prevent an impending exacerbation. Short courses of 'rescue' glucocorticoids (prednisolone 30–60 mg daily) are therefore often required to regain control. Tapering of the dose to withdraw treatment is

not necessary, unless glucocorticoid has been given for more than 3 weeks.

Indications for 'rescue' courses include:

- symptoms and PEF progressively worsening day by day, with a fall of PEF below 60% of the patient's personal best recording
- onset or worsening of sleep disturbance by asthma
- persistence of morning symptoms until midday
- progressively diminishing response to an inhaled bronchodilator
- symptoms that are sufficiently severe to require treatment with nebulised or injected bronchodilators.

Management of acute severe asthma

Box 17.22 highlights the immediate assessment requirements in acute asthma. Measurement of PEF is mandatory, unless the patient is too ill to cooperate, and is most easily interpreted when expressed as a percentage of the predicted normal or of the previous best value obtained on optimal treatment (Fig. 17.24). Arterial blood gas analysis is essential to determine the $PaCO_2$, a normal or elevated level being particularly dangerous. A chest X-ray is not immediately necessary, unless pneumothorax is suspected.

Treatment includes the following measures:

- *Oxygen.* High concentrations (humidified if possible) should be administered to maintain the oxygen saturation above 92% in adults. The presence of a high $PaCO_2$ should not be taken as an indication to reduce oxygen concentration but as a warning sign of a severe or life-threatening attack. Failure to achieve appropriate oxygenation is an indication for assisted ventilation.
- *High doses of inhaled bronchodilators.* Short-acting β₂-agonists are the agent of choice. In hospital, they are most conveniently given via a nebuliser driven by oxygen, but delivery of multiple doses of salbutamol via a metered-dose inhaler through a spacer device provides equivalent bronchodilatation and can be used in primary care. Ipratropium bromide provides further bronchodilator therapy and should be added to salbutamol in acute severe or life-threatening attacks.

✚ 17.22 Immediate assessment of acute severe asthma

Acute severe asthma

- PEF 33–50% predicted (<200 L/min)
- Heart rate ≥110 beats/min
- Respiratory rate ≥25 breaths/min
- Inability to complete sentences in 1 breath

Life-threatening features

- PEF <33% predicted (<100 L/min)
- SpO_2 <92% or PaO_2 <8 kPa (60 mmHg) (especially if being treated with oxygen)
- Normal or raised $PaCO_2$
- Silent chest
- Cyanosis
- Feeble respiratory effort
- Bradycardia or arrhythmias
- Hypotension
- Exhaustion
- Delirium
- Coma

Near-fatal asthma

- Raised $PaCO_2$ and/or requiring mechanical ventilation with raised inflation pressures

(PEF = peak expiratory flow)

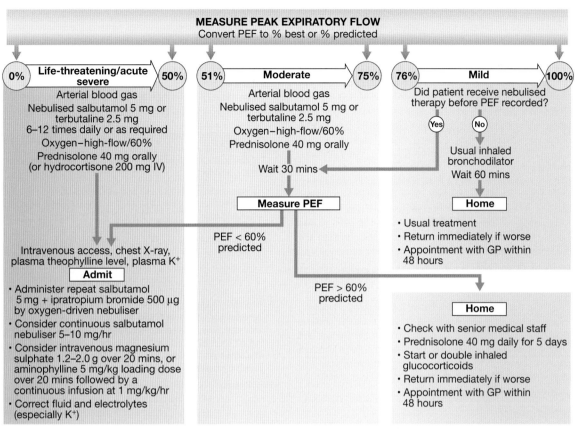

MEASURE PEAK EXPIRATORY FLOW
Convert PEF to % best or % predicted

0% — **Life-threatening/acute severe** — **50%**
Arterial blood gas
Nebulised salbutamol 5 mg or terbutaline 2.5 mg 6–12 times daily or as required
Oxygen–high-flow/60%
Prednisolone 40 mg orally (or hydrocortisone 200 mg IV)

51% — **Moderate** — **75%**
Arterial blood gas
Nebulised salbutamol 5 mg or terbutaline 2.5 mg
Oxygen–high-flow/60%
Prednisolone 40 mg orally
Wait 30 mins

76% — **Mild** — **100%**
Did patient receive nebulised therapy before PEF recorded?
Yes / No
Usual inhaled bronchodilator
Wait 60 mins

Measure PEF

Home (mild)
• Usual treatment
• Return immediately if worse
• Appointment with GP within 48 hours

Intravenous access, chest X-ray, plasma theophylline level, plasma K⁺
Admit
• Administer repeat salbutamol 5 mg + ipratropium bromide 500 µg by oxygen-driven nebuliser
• Consider continuous salbutamol nebuliser 5–10 mg/hr
• Consider intravenous magnesium sulphate 1.2–2.0 g over 20 mins, or aminophylline 5 mg/kg loading dose over 20 mins followed by a continuous infusion at 1 mg/kg/hr
• Correct fluid and electrolytes (especially K⁺)

PEF < 60% predicted

PEF > 60% predicted

Home
• Check with senior medical staff
• Prednisolone 40 mg daily for 5 days
• Start or double inhaled glucocorticoids
• Return immediately if worse
• Appointment with GP within 48 hours

Fig. 17.24 Immediate treatment of patients with acute severe asthma.

17

• *Systemic glucocorticoids.* These reduce the inflammatory response and hasten the resolution of an exacerbation. They should be administered to all patients with an acute severe attack. They can usually be administered orally as prednisolone but intravenous hydrocortisone may be used in patients who are vomiting or unable to swallow.

There is no evidence base for the use of intravenous fluids but many patients are dehydrated due to high insensible water loss and will probably benefit. Potassium supplements may be necessary, as repeated doses of salbutamol can lower serum potassium.

If patients fail to improve, a number of further options may be considered. Intravenous magnesium may provide additional bronchodilatation in patients whose presenting PEF is below 30% predicted. Some patients appear to benefit from the use of intravenous aminophylline but cardiac monitoring is recommended.

PEF should be recorded every 15–30 minutes and then every 4–6 hours. Pulse oximetry should ensure that SaO_2 remains above 92%, but repeat arterial blood gases are necessary if the initial $PaCO_2$ measurements were normal or raised, the PaO_2 was below 8 kPa (60 mmHg) or the patient deteriorates. Box 17.23 lists the indications for endotracheal intubation and intermittent positive pressure ventilation (IPPV).

Prognosis

The outcome from acute severe asthma is generally good but a considerable number of deaths occur in young people and many are preventable. Failure to recognise the severity of an attack, on the part of either the assessing physician or the

17.23 Indications for assisted ventilation in acute severe asthma

• Coma
• Respiratory arrest
• Deterioration of arterial blood gas tensions despite optimal therapy:
  PaO_2 <8 kPa (60 mmHg) and falling
  $PaCO_2$ >6 kPa (45 mmHg) and rising
  pH low and falling (H⁺ high and rising)
• Exhaustion, delirium, drowsiness

patient, contributes to delay in delivering appropriate therapy and to under-treatment.

Prior to discharge, patients should be stable on discharge medication (nebulised therapy should have been discontinued for at least 24 hours) and the PEF should have reached 75% of predicted or personal best. The acute attack should prompt a look for and avoidance of any trigger factors, the delivery of asthma education and the provision of a written self-management plan. The patient should be offered an appointment with a GP or asthma nurse within 2 working days of discharge, and follow-up at a specialist hospital clinic within a month.

Chronic obstructive pulmonary disease

Chronic obstructive pulmonary disease (COPD) is defined as a preventable and treatable disease characterised by persistent airflow limitation that is usually progressive and associated with an enhanced chronic inflammatory response in the airways and the lung to noxious particles or gases. Exacerbations and co-morbidities contribute to the overall severity in individual patients. Related diagnoses include chronic bronchitis (cough and sputum for at least 3 consecutive months in each of 2 consecutive years) and emphysema (abnormal permanent enlargement of the airspaces distal to the terminal bronchioles, accompanied by destruction of their walls and without obvious fibrosis). Extrapulmonary effects include weight loss and skeletal muscle dysfunction (Fig. 17.25). Commonly associated co-morbid conditions include cardiovascular disease, cerebrovascular disease, the metabolic syndrome (p. 730), osteoporosis, depression and lung cancer.

The prevalence of COPD is directly related to the prevalence of risk factors in the community, such as tobacco smoking, coal dust exposure or the use of biomass fuels, and to the age of the population being studied. Those with the most severe disease bear the greatest personal impact of the condition and contribute to its significant social and economic consequences on society. It is predicted that, by 2030, COPD will represent the seventh leading cause of disability and fourth most common cause of death worldwide.

Risk factors are shown in Box 17.24. Cigarette smoking represents the most significant risk factor for COPD and the risk of developing the condition relates to both the amount and duration of smoking. It is unusual to develop COPD with less than 10 pack years (1 pack year = 20 cigarettes/day/year) and not all smokers develop the condition, suggesting that individual susceptibility factors are important.

Pathophysiology

COPD has both pulmonary and systemic components (Fig. 17.25). The presence of airflow limitation combined with premature airway closure leads to gas trapping and hyperinflation, adversely affecting pulmonary and chest wall compliance. Pulmonary hyperinflation also results, which flattens the diaphragmatic muscles and leads to an increasingly horizontal alignment of the intercostal muscles, placing the respiratory muscles at a mechanical disadvantage. The work of breathing is therefore markedly increased – first on exercise, when the time for expiration is further shortened, but then, as the disease advances, at rest.

17.24 Risk factors for development of chronic obstructive pulmonary disease

Environmental factors
- Tobacco smoke: accounts for 95% of cases in the UK
- Indoor air pollution: cooking with biomass fuels in confined areas in developing countries
- Occupational exposures, such as coal dust, silica and cadmium
- Low birth weight: may reduce maximally attained lung function in young adult life
- Lung growth: childhood infections or maternal smoking may affect growth of lung during childhood, resulting in a lower maximally attained lung function in adult life
- Infections: recurrent infection may accelerate decline in FEV_1; persistence of adenovirus in lung tissue may alter local inflammatory response, predisposing to lung damage; HIV infection is associated with emphysema
- Low socioeconomic status
- Cannabis smoking

Host factors
- Genetic factors: α_1-antitrypsin deficiency; other COPD susceptibility genes are likely to be identified
- Airway hyper-reactivity

(FEV_1 = forced expiratory volume in 1 sec)

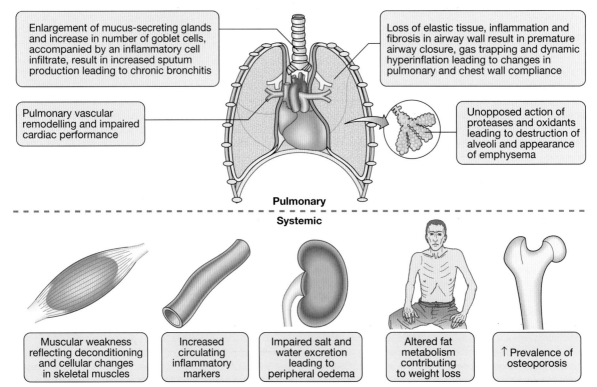

Enlargement of mucus-secreting glands and increase in number of goblet cells, accompanied by an inflammatory cell infiltrate, result in increased sputum production leading to chronic bronchitis

Loss of elastic tissue, inflammation and fibrosis in airway wall result in premature airway closure, gas trapping and dynamic hyperinflation leading to changes in pulmonary and chest wall compliance

Pulmonary vascular remodelling and impaired cardiac performance

Unopposed action of proteases and oxidants leading to destruction of alveoli and appearance of emphysema

Pulmonary

Systemic

Muscular weakness reflecting deconditioning and cellular changes in skeletal muscles

Increased circulating inflammatory markers

Impaired salt and water excretion leading to peripheral oedema

Altered fat metabolism contributing to weight loss

↑ Prevalence of osteoporosis

Fig. 17.25 The pulmonary and systemic features of chronic obstructive pulmonary disease.

Fig. 17.26 The pathology of emphysema. A Normal lung.
B Emphysematous lung, showing gross loss of the normal surface area available for gas exchange. *B, Courtesy of the British Lung Foundation.*

Emphysema (Fig. 17.26) may be classified by the pattern of the enlarged airspaces: centriacinar, panacinar and paraseptal. Bullae form in some individuals. This results in impaired gas exchange and respiratory failure.

Clinical features

COPD should be suspected in any patient over the age of 40 years who presents with symptoms of chronic bronchitis and/or breathlessness. Depending on the presentation, important differential diagnoses include chronic asthma, tuberculosis, bronchiectasis and congestive cardiac failure.

Cough and associated sputum production are usually the first symptoms, and are often referred to as a 'smoker's cough'. Haemoptysis may complicate exacerbations of COPD but should not be attributed to COPD without thorough investigation.

Breathlessness usually prompts presentation to a health professional. The level should be quantified for future reference, often by documenting what the patient can manage before stopping; scales such as the modified Medical Research Council (MRC) dyspnoea scale may be useful (Box 17.25). In advanced disease, enquiry should be made as to the presence of oedema (which may be seen for the first time during an exacerbation) and morning headaches (which may suggest hypercapnia).

Physical signs (p. 546) are non-specific, correlate poorly with lung function, and are seldom obvious until the disease is advanced. Breath sounds are typically quiet; crackles may accompany infection but, if persistent, raise the possibility of bronchiectasis. Finger clubbing is not a feature of COPD and should trigger further investigation for lung cancer or fibrosis. Right heart failure may develop in patients with advanced COPD,

i	17.25 Modified Medical Research Council (MRC) dyspnoea scale	
Grade	**Degree of breathlessness related to activities**	
0	No breathlessness, except with strenuous exercise	
1	Breathlessness when hurrying on the level or walking up a slight hill	
2	Walks slower than contemporaries on level ground because of breathlessness or has to stop for breath when walking at own pace	
3	Stops for breath after walking about 100 m or after a few minutes on level ground	
4	Too breathless to leave the house, or breathless when dressing or undressing	

particularly if there is coexisting sleep apnoea or thromboembolic disease ('cor pulmonale'). However, even in the absence of heart failure, COPD patients often have pitting oedema from salt and water retention caused by renal hypoxia and hypercapnia. The term 'cor pulmonale' is a misnomer in such patients, as they do not have heart failure. Fatigue, anorexia and weight loss may point to the development of lung cancer or tuberculosis, but are common in patients with severe COPD and the body mass index (BMI) is of prognostic significance. Depression and anxiety are also common and contribute to morbidity.

Two classical phenotypes have been described: 'pink puffers' and 'blue bloaters'. The former are typically thin and breathless, and maintain a normal $PaCO_2$ until the late stage of disease. The latter develop (or tolerate) hypercapnia earlier and may develop oedema and secondary polycythaemia. In practice, these phenotypes often overlap.

Investigations

Although there are no reliable radiographic signs that correlate with the severity of airflow limitation, a chest X-ray is essential to identify alternative diagnoses such as cardiac failure, other complications of smoking such as lung cancer, and the presence of bullae. A blood count is useful to exclude anaemia or document polycythaemia, and in younger patients with predominantly basal emphysema α_1-antitrypsin should be assayed.

The diagnosis requires objective demonstration of airflow obstruction by spirometry and is established when the post-bronchodilator FEV_1/FVC is <70%. The severity of COPD may be defined in relation to the post-bronchodilator FEV_1 (Box 17.26).

Measurement of lung volumes provides an assessment of hyperinflation. This is generally performed by helium dilution technique (p. 515); however, in patients with severe COPD, and in particular large bullae, body plethysmography is preferred because the use of helium may under-estimate lung volumes. The presence of emphysema is suggested by a low gas transfer (p. 515). Exercise tests provide an objective assessment of exercise tolerance and provide a baseline on which to judge the response to bronchodilator therapy or rehabilitation programmes; they may also be valuable when assessing prognosis. Pulse oximetry may prompt referral for a domiciliary oxygen assessment if less than 93%.

The assessment of health status by the St George's Respiratory Questionnaire (SGRQ) is commonly used for research. In practice, the COPD Assessment Test and the COPD Control Questionnaire are easier to administer. HRCT is likely to play an increasing role in the assessment of COPD, as it allows the detection,

17

i	17.26 Spirometric classification of COPD severity based on post-bronchodilator FEV$_1$				
		Severity of airflow obstruction post-bronchodilator			
PD FEV$_1$/ FVC	FEV$_1$% predicted	ATS/ERS (2004)	GOLD (2008)	NICE Clinical Guideline 101 (2010)	
<0.7	≥80%	Mild	Stage I – mild	Stage I – mild[1]	
<0.7	50–79%	Moderate	Stage II – moderate	Stage II – moderate	
<0.7	30–49%	Severe	Stage III – severe	Stage III – severe	
<0.7	<30%	Very severe	Stage IV – very severe[2]	Stage IV – very severe[2]	

[1]Mild COPD should not be diagnosed on lung function alone if the patient is asymptomatic. [2]Or FEV$_1$ <50% with respiratory failure.
(ATS/ERS = American Thoracic Society/European Respiratory Journal; FEV$_1$ = forced expiratory volume in 1 sec; GOLD = Global Initiative for Chronic Obstructive Lung Disease; PD = post-bronchodilator)
Adapted from National Institute for Health and Care Excellence (NICE) CG101 – Chronic obstructive pulmonary disease in over 16s: diagnosis and management; 2010.

Fig. 17.27 Gross emphysema. High-resolution computed tomogram showing emphysema, most evident in the right lower lobe.

characterisation and quantification of emphysema (Fig. 17.27) and is more sensitive than the chest X-ray at detecting bullae. It is also used to guide lung volume reduction surgery.

Assessment of severity

The severity of COPD has traditionally been defined in relation to the FEV% predicted. However, assessing the impact of COPD on individual patients in terms of the symptoms and limitations in activity that they experience and whether they suffer frequent or significant exacerbations may provide a more clinically relevant assessment and help guide management.

Management

The management of COPD focuses on improving breathlessness, reducing the frequency and severity of exacerbations, and improving health status and prognosis.

Reducing exposure to noxious particles and gases

Sustained smoking cessation in mild to moderate COPD is accompanied by a reduced decline in FEV$_1$ compared to persistent

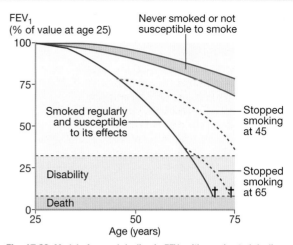

Fig. 17.28 Model of annual decline in FEV$_1$ with accelerated decline in susceptible smokers. When smoking is stopped, subsequent loss is similar to that in healthy non-smokers. (FEV$_1$ = forced expiratory volume in 1 second)

smokers, and cessation (p. 94) remains the only strategy that impacts favourably on the natural history of COPD. Complete cessation is accompanied by an improvement in lung function and deceleration in the rate of FEV$_1$ decline (Fig. 17.28). In regions where the indoor burning of biomass fuels is important, the introduction of non-smoking cooking devices or alternative fuels should be encouraged.

Bronchodilators

Bronchodilator therapy is central to the management of breathlessness. The inhaled route is preferred and a number of different agents delivered by a variety of devices are available. Choice should be informed by patient preference and inhaler assessment. Short-acting bronchodilators may be used for patients with mild disease but longer-acting bronchodilators are usually more appropriate for those with moderate to severe disease. Significant improvements in breathlessness may be reported despite minimal changes in FEV$_1$, probably reflecting improvements in lung emptying that reduce dynamic hyperinflation and ease the work of breathing. Oral bronchodilator therapy, such as theophylline preparations, may be contemplated in patients who cannot use inhaled devices efficiently but their use may be limited by side-effects, unpredictable metabolism and drug interactions; hence the requirement to monitor plasma levels. Orally active, highly selective phosphodiesterase inhibitors remain under appraisal.

Combined inhaled glucocorticoids and bronchodilators

The fixed combination of an inhaled glucocorticoid and a LABA improves lung function, reduces the frequency and severity of exacerbations and improves quality of life. These advantages may be accompanied by an increased risk of pneumonia, particularly in the elderly. LABA/inhaled glucocorticoid combinations are frequently given with a long-acting muscarinic antagonist (LAMA). LAMAs should be used with caution in patients with significant heart disease or a history of urinary retention.

Oral glucocorticoids

Oral glucocorticoids are useful during exacerbations but maintenance therapy contributes to osteoporosis and impaired skeletal muscle function, and should be avoided. Oral glucocorticoid trials assist in the diagnosis of asthma but do not predict response to inhaled glucocorticoids in COPD.

Pulmonary rehabilitation

Exercise should be encouraged at all stages and patients reassured that breathlessness, while distressing, is not dangerous. Multidisciplinary programmes that incorporate physical training, disease education and nutritional counselling reduce symptoms, improve health status and enhance confidence. Most programmes include two to three sessions per week, last between 6 and 12 weeks, and are accompanied by demonstrable and sustained improvements in exercise tolerance and health status.

Oxygen therapy

Long-term domiciliary oxygen therapy (LTOT) improves survival in selected patients with COPD complicated by severe hypoxaemia (arterial PaO_2 <7.3 kPa (55 mmHg); Box 17.27). It is most conveniently provided by an oxygen concentrator and patients should be instructed to use oxygen for a minimum of 15 hours/day; greater benefits are seen in those who use it for more than 20 hours/day. The aim of therapy is to increase the PaO_2 to at least 8 kPa (60 mmHg) or SaO_2 to at least 90%. Ambulatory oxygen therapy should be considered in patients who desaturate on exercise and show objective improvement in exercise capacity and/or dyspnoea with oxygen. Oxygen flow rates should be adjusted to maintain SaO_2 above 90%.

Surgical intervention

Bullectomy may be considered when large bullae compress surrounding normal lung tissue. Patients with predominantly upper lobe emphysema, preserved gas transfer and no evidence of pulmonary hypertension may benefit from lung volume reduction surgery (LVRS), in which peripheral emphysematous lung tissue is resected with the aim of reducing hyperinflation and decreasing the work of breathing. Both bullectomy and LVRS can be performed thorascopically, minimising morbidity. Lung transplantation may benefit carefully selected patients with advanced disease (p. 567).

Other measures

Patients with COPD should be offered an annual influenza vaccination and, as appropriate, pneumococcal vaccination. Obesity, poor nutrition, depression and social isolation should be identified and, if possible, improved. Mucolytic agents are occasionally used but evidence of benefit is limited.

Palliative care

Addressing end-of-life needs is an important, yet often ignored, aspect of care in advanced disease. Morphine preparations may be used for palliation of breathlessness in advanced disease and benzodiazepines in low dose may reduce anxiety. Decisions regarding resuscitation should be addressed in advance of critical illness.

17.27 Prescription of long-term oxygen therapy in COPD

Arterial blood gases are measured in clinically stable patients on optimal medical therapy on at least two occasions 3 weeks apart:
- PaO_2 <7.3 kPa (55 mmHg) irrespective of $PaCO_2$ and FEV_1 <1.5 L
- PaO_2 7.3–8 kPa (55–60 mmHg) plus pulmonary hypertension, peripheral oedema or nocturnal hypoxaemia
- the patient has stopped smoking

Use at least 15 hrs/day at 2–4 L/min to achieve a PaO_2 >8 kPa (60 mmHg) without unacceptable rise in $PaCO_2$

17.28 Calculation of the BODE index

Variable	Points on BODE index			
	0	1	2	3
FEV_1	≥65	50–64	36–49	≤35
Distance walked in 6 mins (m)	≥350	250–349	150–249	≤149
MRC dyspnoea scale*	0–1	2	3	4
Body mass index	>21	≤21		

A patient with a BODE score of 0–2 has a mortality rate of around 10% at 52 months, whereas a patient with a BODE score of 7–10 has a mortality rate of around 80% at 52 months.

*See Box 17.25.
(BODE – see text; FEV_1 = forced expiratory volume in 1 sec)

Prognosis

COPD has a variable natural history but is usually progressive. The prognosis is inversely related to age and directly related to the post-bronchodilator FEV_1. Additional poor prognostic indicators include weight loss and pulmonary hypertension. A composite score (BODE), comprising the body mass index (B), the degree of airflow obstruction (O), a measurement of dyspnoea (D) and exercise capacity (E) may assist in predicting death from respiratory and other causes (Box 17.28). Respiratory failure, cardiac disease and lung cancer represent common modes of death.

Acute exacerbations of COPD

Acute exacerbations of COPD are characterised by an increase in symptoms and deterioration in lung function and health status. They become more frequent as the disease progresses and are usually triggered by bacteria, viruses or a change in air quality. They may be accompanied by the development of respiratory failure and/or fluid retention and represent an important cause of death.

Many patients can be managed at home with the use of increased bronchodilator therapy, a short course of oral glucocorticoids and, if appropriate, antibiotics. The presence of cyanosis, peripheral oedema or an alteration in consciousness should prompt referral to hospital. In other patients, consideration of comorbidity and social circumstances may influence decisions regarding hospital admission.

Oxygen therapy

In patients with an exacerbation of severe COPD, high concentrations of oxygen may cause respiratory depression and worsening acidosis (p. 566). Controlled oxygen at 24% or 28% should be used with the aim of maintaining a PaO_2 of more than 8 kPa (60 mmHg) (or an SaO_2 of more than 90%) without worsening acidosis.

Bronchodilators

Nebulised short-acting β_2-agonists combined with an anticholinergic agent (e.g. salbutamol and ipratropium) should be administered. With careful supervision it is usually safe to drive nebulisers with oxygen, but if concern exists regarding oxygen sensitivity, they may be driven by compressed air and supplemental oxygen delivered by nasal cannula.

17

Glucocorticoids

Oral prednisolone reduces symptoms and improves lung function. Doses of 30 mg for 10 days are currently recommended but shorter courses may be acceptable. Prophylaxis against osteoporosis should be considered in patients who receive repeated courses of glucocorticoids (p. 670).

Antibiotic therapy

The role of bacteria in exacerbations remains controversial and there is little evidence for the routine administration of antibiotics. They are currently recommended for patients reporting an increase in sputum purulence, sputum volume or breathlessness. In most cases simple regimens are advised, such as an aminopenicillin, a tetracycline or a macrolide. Co-amoxiclav is only required in regions where β-lactamase-producing organisms are known to be common.

Non-invasive ventilation

Non-invasive ventilation is safe and effective in patients with an acute exacerbation of COPD complicated by mild to moderate respiratory acidosis (H^+ ≥45 nmol/L, pH <7.35), and should be considered early in the course of respiratory failure to reduce the need for endotracheal intubation, treatment failure and mortality. It is not useful in patients who cannot protect their airway. Mechanical ventilation may be contemplated when there is a reversible cause for deterioration (e.g. pneumonia) or when no prior history of respiratory failure has been noted.

Additional therapy

Exacerbations may be accompanied by the development of peripheral oedema; this usually responds to diuretics. There has been a vogue for using an infusion of intravenous aminophylline but evidence for benefit is limited and attention must be paid to the risk of inducing arrhythmias and drug interactions. The use of the respiratory stimulant doxapram has been largely superseded by the development of NIV but it may be useful for a limited period in selected patients with a low respiratory rate.

17.29 Obstructive pulmonary disease in old age

- **Asthma**: may appear de novo in old age, so airflow obstruction should not always be assumed to be due to COPD.
- **Peak expiratory flow recordings**: older people with poor vision have difficulty reading PEF meters.
- **Perception of bronchoconstriction**: impaired by age, so an older patient's description of symptoms may not be a reliable indicator of severity.
- **Stopping smoking**: the benefits on the rate of loss of lung function decline with age but remain valuable up to the age of 80.
- **Metered-dose inhalers**: many older people cannot use these because of difficulty coordinating and triggering the device. Even mild cognitive impairment virtually precludes their use. Frequent demonstration and re-instruction in the use of all devices are required.
- **Mortality rates for acute asthma**: higher in old age, partly because patients under-estimate the severity of bronchoconstriction and also develop a lower degree of tachycardia and pulsus paradoxus for the same degree of bronchoconstriction.
- **Treatment decisions**: advanced age in itself is not a barrier to intensive care or mechanical ventilation in an acute episode of asthma or COPD, but this decision may be difficult and should be shared with the patient (if possible), the relatives and the GP.

Discharge

Discharge from hospital may be contemplated once patients are clinically stable on their usual maintenance medication. Hospital at-home teams may provide short-term nebuliser loan, improving discharge rates and providing additional support for the patient.

Bronchiectasis

Bronchiectasis means abnormal dilatation of the bronchi. Chronic suppurative airway infection with sputum production, progressive scarring and lung damage occur, whatever the cause.

Aetiology and pathology

Bronchiectasis may result from a congenital defect affecting airway ion transport or ciliary function, such as cystic fibrosis (see below), or may be acquired secondary to damage to the airways by a destructive infection, inhaled toxin or foreign body. The result is chronic inflammation and infection in the airways. Box 17.30 shows the common causes, of which tuberculosis is the most common worldwide.

Localised bronchiectasis may occur due to the accumulation of pus beyond an obstructing bronchial lesion, such as enlarged tuberculous hilar lymph nodes, a bronchial tumour or an inhaled foreign body (e.g. an aspirated peanut).

The bronchiectatic cavities may be lined by granulation tissue, squamous epithelium or normal ciliated epithelium. There may also be inflammatory changes in the deeper layers of the bronchial wall and hypertrophy of the bronchial arteries. Chronic inflammatory and fibrotic changes are usually found in the surrounding lung tissue, resulting in progressive destruction of the normal lung architecture in advanced cases.

Clinical features

The symptoms are shown in Box 17.31.

Physical signs in the chest may be unilateral or bilateral. If the bronchiectatic airways do not contain secretions and there is no associated lobar collapse, there are no abnormal physical signs. When there are large amounts of sputum in the bronchiectatic spaces, numerous coarse crackles may be heard over the affected areas. Collapse with retained secretions blocking a proximal bronchus may lead to locally diminished breath sounds, while advanced disease may cause scarring and overlying bronchial

---

17.30 Causes of bronchiectasis

Congenital

- Cystic fibrosis
- Ciliary dysfunction syndromes:
  Primary ciliary dyskinesia (immotile cilia syndrome)
  Kartagener's syndrome (sinusitis and transposition of the viscera)
- Primary hypogammaglobulinaemia (p. 79)

Acquired: children

- Severe infections in infancy (especially whooping cough, measles)
- Primary tuberculosis
- Inhaled foreign body

Acquired: adults

- Suppurative pneumonia
- Pulmonary tuberculosis
- Allergic bronchopulmonary aspergillosis complicating asthma (p. 596)
- Bronchial tumours

Fig. 17.29 Computed tomogram of bronchiectasis. Extensive dilatation of the bronchi, with thickened walls (arrows) in both lower lobes.

breathing. Acute haemoptysis is an important complication of bronchiectasis; management is described on page 560.

Investigations

In addition to common respiratory pathogens, sputum culture may reveal *Pseudomonas aeruginosa* and *Staphylococcus aureus*, fungi such as *Aspergillus* and various mycobacteria. Frequent cultures are necessary to ensure appropriate treatment of resistant organisms.

Bronchiectasis, unless very gross, is not usually apparent on a chest X-ray. In advanced disease, thickened airway walls, cystic bronchiectatic spaces and associated areas of pneumonic consolidation or collapse may be visible. CT is much more sensitive and shows thickened, dilated airways (Fig. 17.29).

A screening test can be performed in patients suspected of having a ciliary dysfunction syndrome by measuring the time taken for a small pellet of saccharin placed in the anterior chamber of the nose to reach the pharynx, at which point the patient can taste it. This time should not exceed 20 minutes but is greatly prolonged in patients with ciliary dysfunction. Ciliary beat frequency may also be assessed from biopsies taken from the nose. Structural abnormalities of cilia can be detected by electron microscopy.

Management

In patients with airflow obstruction, inhaled bronchodilators and glucocorticoids should be used to enhance airway patency.

Physiotherapy

Patients should be shown how to perform regular daily physiotherapy to assist the drainage of excess bronchial secretions. Efficiently executed, this is of great value both in reducing the amount of cough and sputum, and in preventing recurrent episodes of bronchopulmonary infection. Patients should lie in a position in which the lobe to be drained is uppermost. Deep breathing, followed by forced expiratory manœuvres (the 'active cycle of breathing' technique), helps to move secretions in the dilated bronchi towards the trachea, from which they can be cleared by vigorous coughing. Devices that increase airway pressure either by a constant amount (positive expiratory pressure mask) or in an oscillatory manner (flutter valve) aid sputum clearance in some patients and a variety of techniques should be tried to find the one that suits the individual. The optimum duration and frequency of physiotherapy depend on the amount of sputum but 5–10 minutes twice daily is a minimum for most patients.

Antibiotic therapy

For most patients with bronchiectasis, the appropriate antibiotics are the same as those used in COPD (p. 578) but larger doses and longer courses are required, and resolution of symptoms is often incomplete. When secondary infection occurs with staphylococci and Gram-negative bacilli, in particular *Pseudomonas* species, antibiotic therapy becomes more challenging and should be guided by the microbiological sensitivities. For *Pseudomonas*, oral ciprofloxacin (500–750 mg twice daily) or an intravenous anti-pseudomonal β-lactam (e.g. piperacillin–tazobactam or ceftazidime) will be required. Haemoptysis in bronchiectasis often responds to treatment of the underlying infection, although percutaneous embolisation of the bronchial circulation by an interventional radiologist may be necessary in severe cases.

Surgical treatment

Excision of bronchiectatic areas is indicated in only a small proportion of cases. These are usually patients in whom the bronchiectasis is confined to a single lobe or segment on CT. Unfortunately, many of those in whom medical treatment proves unsuccessful are also unsuitable for surgery because of either extensive bilateral bronchiectasis or coexisting severe airflow obstruction. In progressive forms of bronchiectasis, resection of destroyed areas of lung that are acting as a reservoir of infection should be considered only as a last resort.

Prognosis

The disease is progressive when associated with ciliary dysfunction and cystic fibrosis, and eventually causes respiratory failure. In other patients, the prognosis can be relatively good if physiotherapy is performed regularly and antibiotics are used aggressively.

Prevention

As bronchiectasis commonly starts in childhood following measles, whooping cough or a primary tuberculous infection, adequate prophylaxis for and treatment of these conditions are essential. Early recognition and treatment of bronchial obstruction are also important.

17

Cystic fibrosis

Genetics, pathogenesis and epidemiology

Cystic fibrosis (CF) is the most common fatal genetic disease in Caucasians, with autosomal recessive inheritance, a carrier rate of 1 in 25, and an incidence of about 1 in 2500 live births (pp. 40 and 48). It is much less common in people of African descent and rarer still in Asians. CF is the result of mutations affecting a gene on the long arm of chromosome 7, which codes for a chloride channel known as cystic fibrosis transmembrane conductance regulator (*CFTR*); this influences salt and water movement across epithelial cell membranes. The most common *CFTR* mutation in northern European and American populations is ΔF508 but over 2000 mutations of this gene have now been identified. The genetic defect causes increased sodium and chloride content in sweat and increased resorption of sodium and water from respiratory epithelium (Fig. 17.30). Relative dehydration of the airway epithelium is thought to predispose to chronic bacterial infection and ciliary dysfunction, leading to bronchiectasis. The gene defect also causes disorders in the gut epithelium, pancreas, liver and reproductive tract (see below).

In the 1960s, few patients with CF survived childhood, yet with aggressive treatment of airway infection and nutritional support, life expectancy has improved dramatically, so that there are now more adults than children with CF in many developed countries. Until recently, the diagnosis was most commonly made from the clinical picture (bowel obstruction, failure to thrive, steatorrhoea and/or chest symptoms in a young child), supported by sweat electrolyte testing and genotyping. Patients with unusual phenotypes were commonly missed, however, and late diagnosis led to poorer outcomes. Neonatal screening for CF using immunoreactive trypsin and genetic testing of newborn blood samples is now routine in the UK and should reduce delayed diagnosis and improve outcomes. Pre-implantation and/or prenatal testing may be offered to those known to be at high risk (p. 56).

Clinical features

The lungs are macroscopically normal at birth, but bronchiolar inflammation and infections usually lead to bronchiectasis in childhood. At this stage, the lungs are most commonly infected with *Staph. aureus*; however, in adulthood, many patients become colonised with *P. aeruginosa, Stenotrophomonas maltophilia* or other Gram-negative bacilli. Recurrent exacerbations of bronchiectasis, initially in the upper lobes but subsequently throughout both lungs, cause progressive lung damage, resulting ultimately in death from respiratory failure. Other clinical manifestations are shown in Box 17.32. Most men with CF are infertile due to failure of development of the vas deferens, but microsurgical sperm aspiration and in vitro fertilisation are possible. Genotype is a poor predictor of disease severity in individuals; even siblings with matching genotypes may have different phenotypes. This suggests that other 'modifier genes', as yet unidentified, influence clinical outcome.

Management

Treatment of CF lung disease

The management of CF lung disease is that of severe bronchiectasis. All patients with CF who produce sputum should perform chest physiotherapy daily, and more frequently during exacerbations. While infections with *Staph. aureus* can often be managed with oral antibiotics, intravenous treatment (frequently self-administered at home through an implanted subcutaneous vascular access device) is usually needed for *Pseudomonas* infections.

Unfortunately, the bronchi of many patients with CF eventually become colonised with pathogens that are resistant to most antibiotics. Resistant strains of *P. aeruginosa*, *Stenotrophomonas maltophilia* and *Burkholderia cepacia* are the main culprits and may require prolonged treatment with unusual combinations of antibiotics. *Aspergillus* and non-tuberculous mycobacteria are also frequently found in the sputum of patients with CF but in most cases these behave as benign 'colonisers' of the bronchiectatic airways and do not require specific therapy. An

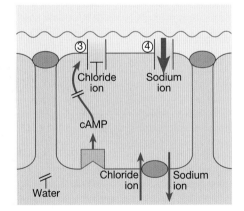

A Normal   **B** Cystic fibrosis

Airway lumen
Apical surface
Chloride ion   Sodium ion
EPITHELIAL CELL
cAMP
Basal surface   Chloride ion   Sodium ion
Water

Chloride ion   Sodium ion
cAMP
Chloride ion   Sodium ion
Water

β₂-adrenoceptor

Fig. 17.30 Cystic fibrosis: basic defect in the pulmonary epithelium. **A** The cystic fibrosis gene (*CFTR*) codes for a chloride channel (1) in the apical (luminal) membrane of epithelial cells in the conducting airways. This is normally controlled by cyclic adenosine monophosphate (cAMP) and indirectly by β-adrenoceptor stimulation, and is one of several apical ion channels that control the quantity and solute content of airway-lining fluid. Normal channels appear to inhibit the adjacent epithelial sodium channels (2). **B** In cystic fibrosis, one of many cystic fibrosis gene defects causes absence or defective function of this chloride channel (3). This leads to reduced chloride secretion and loss of inhibition of sodium channels, with excessive sodium resorption (4) and dehydration of the airway lining. The resulting abnormal airway-lining fluid predisposes to infection by mechanisms still to be fully explained.

17.32 Complications of cystic fibrosis

Respiratory

- Progressive airway obstruction
- Infective exacerbations of bronchiectasis
- Respiratory failure
- Spontaneous pneumothorax
- Haemoptysis
- Lobar collapse due to secretions
- Pulmonary hypertension
- Nasal polyps

Gastrointestinal and hepatic

- Malabsorption and steatorrhoea
- Distal intestinal obstruction syndrome
- Biliary cirrhosis
- Portal hypertension, varices and splenomegaly
- Gallstones

Others

- Diabetes (25% of adults)
- Delayed puberty
- Male infertility
- Stress incontinence due to repeated forced cough
- Psychosocial problems
- Osteoporosis
- Arthropathy
- Cutaneous vasculitis

17.34 Cystic fibrosis in adolescence

Issues for the patient

- Move to adult CF centre – loss of trusted paediatric team
- Feelings of being different from peers due to chronic illness
- Demanding treatments that conflict with social and school life
- Pressure to take responsibility for self-care
- Relationship/fertility concerns

Issues for the patient's parents

- Loss of control over patient's treatment – feeling excluded
- Loss of trusted paediatric team
- Need to develop trust in adult team
- Feelings of helplessness when adolescent rebels or will not take treatment

Issues for the CF team

- Reluctance or refusal by patient to engage with transition
- Management of deterioration due to non-adherence
- Motivation of adolescents to self-care
- Provision of adolescent-friendly health-care environment

17.33 Treatments that reduce chest exacerbations and/or improve lung function in cystic fibrosis

Therapy	Patients treated
Nebulised recombinant human DNase 2.5 mg daily	Age ≥ 5, FVC $> 40\%$ predicted
Nebulised tobramycin 300 mg twice daily, given in alternate months	Patients colonised with *Pseudomonas aeruginosa*
Regular oral azithromycin 500 mg 3 times a week	Patients colonised with *P. aeruginosa*
Nebulised hypertonic saline 4 mL 7%, twice daily	Age ≥ 6, FEV$_1$ > 40% predicted

(FEV$_1$ = forced expiratory volume in 1 sec; FVC = forced vital capacity)

exception is *Mycobacterium abscessus*, which is multi-resistant, may be transmissible between patients with CF and can cause progressive lung destruction that is hard to treat.

Some patients have coexistent asthma, which is treated with inhaled bronchodilators and glucocorticoids; allergic bronchopulmonary aspergillosis (p. 596) also occurs occasionally in CF.

Four maintenance treatments have been shown to cause modest rises in lung function and/or to reduce the frequency of chest exacerbations in patients with CF (Box 17.33). Individual responses are variable and should be carefully monitored to avoid burdening patients with treatments that prove ineffective.

For advanced CF lung disease, home oxygen and NIV may be necessary to treat respiratory failure. Ultimately, lung transplantation can produce dramatic improvements but is limited by donor organ availability.

Treatment of non-respiratory manifestations of CF

There is a clear link between good nutrition and prognosis in CF. Malabsorption occurs in 85% of patients due to exocrine pancreatic failure and is treated with oral pancreatic enzymes and vitamin supplements. The increased calorie requirements of patients with CF are met by supplemental feeding, including nasogastric or gastrostomy tube feeding if required. Diabetes

eventually develops in over 25% of patients and often requires insulin therapy. Osteoporosis secondary to malabsorption and chronic ill health should be sought and treated.

Novel therapies for cystic fibrosis

Small molecules designed to correct the function of particular *CFTR* defects are being developed. One such drug, ivacaftor (a *CFTR* 'potentiator'), is now an established oral treatment for the 5% of patients with the G551D mutation, causing sustained improvements in FEV$_1$ and weight, and normalising the sweat test. The combination of ivacaftor and lumacaftor (a *CFTR* 'corrector') has been found to have modest short-term benefit in patients with DF508 mutations. Improved versions of these treatments may soon offer similar benefits for these patients. Somatic gene therapy for CF is also under development. Manufactured normal copies of the CF gene are 'packaged' in liposomes or virus vectors and administered to the airways by aerosol inhalation. Trials are under way but more efficient gene delivery methods are needed to make this practical.

Infections of the respiratory system

Infections of the upper and lower respiratory tract are a major cause of morbidity and mortality, particularly in patients at the extremes of age and those with pre-existing lung disease or immune suppression.

Upper respiratory tract infection

Upper respiratory tract infections (URTIs), such as coryza (the common cold), acute pharyngitis and acute tracheobronchitis, are the most common of all communicable diseases and represent the most frequent cause of short-term absenteeism from work and school. The vast majority are caused by viruses (p. 249) and, in adults, are usually short-lived and rarely serious.

Acute coryza is the most common URTI and is usually the result of rhinovirus infection. In addition to general malaise, acute coryza typically causes nasal discharge, sneezing and cough. Involvement of the pharynx results in a sore throat, and that of

17

the larynx a hoarse or lost voice. If complicated by a tracheitis or bronchitis, chest tightness and wheeze typical of asthma occur. Specific investigation is rarely warranted and treatment with simple analgesics, antipyretics and decongestants is all that is required. Symptoms usually resolve quickly, but if repeated URTIs 'go to the chest', a more formal diagnosis of asthma ought to be considered. A variety of viruses causing URTI may also trigger exacerbations of asthma or COPD and aggravate other lung diseases.

Bordetella pertussis, the cause of whooping cough, is an important source of URTI. It is highly contagious and is notifiable in the UK. Vaccination confers protection and is usually offered in infancy, but its efficacy wanes in adult life and the infection is easily spread. Adults usually experience a mild illness similar to acute coryza but some individuals develop paroxysms of coughing that can persist for weeks to months, earning whooping cough the designation of 'the cough of 100 days'. The diagnosis may be confirmed by bacterial culture, polymerase chain reaction (PCR) from a nasopharyngeal swab or serological testing. If the illness is recognised early in the clinical course, macrolide antibiotics may ameliorate the course.

Rhinosinusitis typically causes a combination of nasal congestion, blockage or discharge and may be accompanied by facial pain/pressure or loss of smell. Examination usually confirms erythematous swollen nasal mucosa and pus may be evident. Nasal polyps should be sought and dental infection excluded. Treatment with topical glucocorticoids, nasal decongestants and regular nasal douching is usually sufficient and, although bacterial infection is often present, antibiotics are indicated only if symptoms persist for more than 5 days. Persistent symptoms or recurrent episodes should prompt a referral to an ear, nose and throat specialist.

Influenza is discussed on page 240.

Pneumonia

Pneumonia is as an acute respiratory illness associated with recently developed radiological pulmonary shadowing that may be segmental, lobar or multilobar. The context in which pneumonia develops is highly suggestive of the likely organism(s) involved; therefore, pneumonias are usually classified as community- or hospital-acquired, or those occurring in immunocompromised hosts. 'Lobar pneumonia' is a radiological and pathological term referring to homogeneous consolidation of one or more lung lobes, often with associated pleural inflammation; bronchopneumonia refers to more patchy alveolar consolidation associated with bronchial and bronchiolar inflammation, often affecting both lower lobes.

Community-acquired pneumonia

Figures from the UK suggest that an estimated 5–11/1000 adults suffer from community-acquired pneumonia (CAP) each year, accounting for around 5–12% of all lower respiratory tract infections. CAP may affect all age groups but is particularly common at the extremes of age; for example, worldwide, CAP continues to kill more children than any other illness and the propensity to ease the passing of the debilitated and the elderly led to designation of pneumonia as the 'old man's friend'.

Most cases are spread by droplet infection, and while CAP may occur in previously healthy individuals, several factors may impair the effectiveness of local defences and predispose to CAP (Box 17.35). *Streptococcus pneumoniae* (Fig. 17.31) remains the

Fig. 17.31 Gram stain of sputum showing Gram-positive diplococci characteristic of *Streptococcus pneumoniae* (arrows).

i	**17.35 Factors that predispose to pneumonia**

- Cigarette smoking
- Upper respiratory tract infections
- Alcohol
- Glucocorticoid therapy
- Old age
- Recent influenza infection
- Pre-existing lung disease
- HIV
- Indoor air pollution

i	**17.36 Organisms causing community-acquired pneumonia**

Bacteria

- *Streptococcus pneumoniae*
- *Mycoplasma pneumoniae*
- *Legionella pneumophila*
- *Chlamydia pneumoniae*
- *Haemophilus influenzae*
- *Staphylococcus aureus*
- *Chlamydia psittaci*
- *Coxiella burnetii* (Q fever)
- *Klebsiella pneumoniae* (Freidländer's bacillus)

Viruses

- Influenza, parainfluenza
- Measles
- Herpes simplex
- Varicella
- Adenovirus
- Cytomegalovirus
- Coronaviruses (SARS-CoV and MERS-CoV)

(MERS = Middle East respiratory syndrome; SARS = severe acute respiratory syndrome)

most common infecting agent, and thereafter the likelihood that other organisms may be involved depends on the age of the patient and the clinical context. Viral infections are recognised as important causes of CAP in children and their contribution to adult CAP is increasingly recognised. The common causative organisms are shown in Box 17.36.

Clinical features

Pneumonia, particularly lobar pneumonia, usually presents as an acute illness. Systemic features, such as fever, rigors, shivering and malaise, predominate and delirium may be present. The appetite is invariably lost and headache frequently reported.

Pulmonary symptoms include cough, which at first is characteristically short, painful and dry, but later is accompanied by the expectoration of mucopurulent sputum. Rust-coloured sputum may be produced by patients with *Strep. pneumoniae* infection and the occasional patient may report haemoptysis.

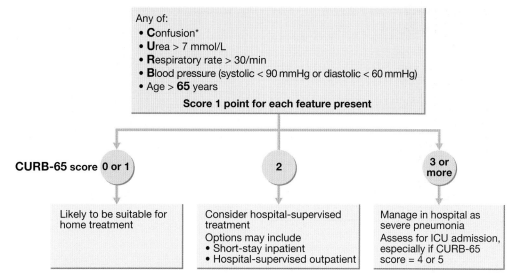

Fig. 17.32 Hospital CURB-65. *Defined as a mental test score of 8 or less, or new disorientation in person, place or time. (ICU = intensive care unit; urea of 7 mmol/L ≅ 20 mg/dL)

Pleuritic chest pain may be a presenting feature and on occasion may be referred to the shoulder or anterior abdominal wall. Upper abdominal tenderness is sometimes apparent in patients with lower lobe pneumonia or those with associated hepatitis. Less typical presentations may be seen in the very young and the elderly.

While different organisms often give rise to a similar clinical and radiological picture, it may be possible to infer the likely agent from the clinical context. *Mycoplasma pneumoniae* is more common in young people and rare in the elderly, whereas *Haemophilus influenzae* is more common in the elderly, particularly if underlying lung disease is present. *Legionella pneumophila* occurs in local outbreaks centred on contaminated cooling towers in hotels, hospitals and other industries. *Staph. aureus* is more common following an episode of influenza. *Klebsiella* pneumonia has a specific association with alcohol abuse and often presents with a particularly severe bacteraemic illness. Recent foreign travel raises the possibility of infections that may otherwise be unusual in the UK, e.g. MERS-coronavirus (Middle East; p. 249), melioidosis caused by *Burkholderia pseudomallei* (South-east Asia and northern Australia; p. 261) and endemic fungal infection (North, Central or South America; p. 301). Certain occupations may be associated with exposure to specific bacteria (p. 618).

Clinical examination should first focus on the respiratory and pulse rates, blood pressure and an assessment of the mental state, as these are important in forming a judgement as to severity of the illness (Fig. 17.32). Chest signs (p. 547) vary, depending on the inflammatory response, which proceeds through stages of acute exudation, red and then grey hepatisation, and finally resolution. When consolidated, the lung is typically dull to percussion and, as conduction of sound is enhanced, auscultation reveals bronchial breathing and whispering pectoriloquy; crackles are heard throughout. An assessment of the state of nutrition is important, particularly in the elderly. The presence of herpes labialis may point to streptococcal infection, as may the finding of 'rusty' sputum.

The differential diagnosis of pneumonia is shown in Box 17.37.

Investigations

The object of investigations, which are summarised in Box 17.38, is to confirm the diagnosis, assess the severity and

---

> **i** | **17.37 Differential diagnosis of pneumonia**
>
> - Pulmonary infarction
> - Pulmonary/pleural tuberculosis
> - Pulmonary oedema (can be unilateral)
> - Pulmonary eosinophilia (p. 611)
> - Malignancy: bronchoalveolar cell carcinoma
> - Cryptogenic organising pneumonia/bronchiolitis obliterans organising pneumonia (COP/BOOP) (p. 606)

17

identify the development of complications. While many cases of mild to moderate CAP can be successfully managed without identification of the organism, a range of microbiological tests should be performed on patients with severe CAP.

Management

The most important aspects of management include oxygenation, fluid balance and antibiotic therapy. In severe or prolonged illness, nutritional support may be required.

Oxygen

Oxygen should be administered to all patients with tachypnoea, hypoxaemia, hypotension or acidosis with the aim of maintaining the PaO_2 ≥8 kPa (60 mmHg) or SaO_2 ≥92%. High concentrations (≥35%), preferably humidified, should be used in all patients who do not have hypercapnia associated with COPD. Continuous positive airway pressure (CPAP) should be considered in those who remain hypoxic despite high-concentration oxygen therapy, and these patients should be managed in a high-dependency or intensive care environment where mechanical ventilation may be rapidly employed. Indications for ITU referral are summarised in Box 17.39.

Fluid balance

Intravenous fluids should be considered in those with severe illness, in older patients and those with vomiting. It may be appropriate to discontinue hypertensive agents temporarily. Otherwise, an adequate oral intake of fluid should be encouraged. Inotropic support may be required in patients with shock (p. 204).

17.38 Investigations in community-acquired pneumonia

Blood

Full blood count
- Very high (>20×10⁹/L) or low (<4×10⁹/L) white cell count: marker of severity
- Neutrophil leucocytosis >15×10⁹/L: suggests bacterial aetiology
- Haemolytic anaemia: occasional complication of *Mycoplasma*

Urea and electrolytes
- Urea >7 mmol/L (~20 mg/dL): marker of severity
- Hyponatraemia: marker of severity

Liver function tests
- Abnormal if basal pneumonia inflames liver
- Hypoalbuminaemia: marker of severity

Erythrocyte sedimentation rate/C-reactive protein
- Non-specifically elevated

Blood culture
- Bacteraemia: marker of severity

Cold agglutinins
- Positive in 50% of patients with *Mycoplasma*

Arterial blood gases
- Measure when SaO_2 <93% or when clinical features are severe, to assess ventilatory failure or acidosis

Sputum

Sputum samples
- Gram stain (see Fig. 17.31), culture and antimicrobial sensitivity testing

Oropharynx swab
- Polymerase chain reaction for *Mycoplasma pneumoniae* and other atypical pathogens

Urine
- Pneumococcal and/or *Legionella* antigen

Chest X-ray

Lobar pneumonia
- Patchy opacification evolves into homogeneous consolidation of affected lobe
- Air bronchogram (air-filled bronchi appear lucent against consolidated lung tissue) may be present (Fig. 17.33)

Bronchopneumonia
- Typically patchy and segmental shadowing

Complications
- Para-pneumonic effusion, intrapulmonary abscess or empyema

Staphylococcus aureus
- Suggested by multilobar shadowing, cavitation, pneumatoceles and abscesses

Pleural fluid
- Always aspirate and culture when present in more than trivial amounts, preferably with ultrasound guidance

Fig. 17.33 Pneumonia of the right middle lobe. **A** Posteroanterior view: consolidation in the right middle lobe with characteristic opacification beneath the horizontal fissure and loss of normal contrast between the right heart border and lung. **B** Lateral view: consolidation confined to the anteriorly situated middle lobe.

17.39 Indications for referral to ITU

- CURB score of 4–5 (see Fig. 17.32), failing to respond rapidly to initial management
- Persisting hypoxia (PaO_2 <8 kPa (60 mmHg)), despite high concentrations of oxygen
- Progressive hypercapnia
- Severe acidosis
- Circulatory shock
- Reduced conscious level

Antibiotic treatment

Prompt administration of antibiotics improves the outcome. The initial choice of antibiotic is guided by clinical context, severity assessment, local knowledge of antibiotic resistance patterns and, at times, epidemiological information. Current regimens are detailed in Box 17.40. In most patients with uncomplicated pneumonia a 5-day course is adequate, although treatment is usually required for longer in patients with *Legionella*, staphylococcal or *Klebsiella* pneumonia. Oral antibiotics are usually adequate unless the patient has a severe illness, impaired consciousness, loss of swallowing reflex or functional or anatomical reasons for malabsorption.

Treatment of pleural pain

It is important to relieve pleural pain in order to allow the patient to breathe normally and cough efficiently. For the majority, simple analgesia with paracetamol, co-codamol or NSAIDs is sufficient. In some patients, opiates may be required but must be used with extreme caution in individuals with poor respiratory function.

Physiotherapy

Physiotherapy is not usually indicated in patients with CAP, although it may be helpful to assist expectoration in patients who suppress cough because of pleural pain.

17.40 Antibiotic treatment for community-acquired pneumonia*

Low severity CAP (CURB-65 score 0-1)

- Amoxicillin 500 mg 3 times daily orally (or IV if necessary)

If patient is allergic to penicillin

- Doxycycline 200 mg loading dose then 100 mg/day orally *or* Clarithromycin 500 mg twice daily orally

Moderate severity CAP (CURB-65 score 2)

- Amoxicillin 500 mg–1 g 3 times daily orally (or IV if oral medication not possible) *or* Benzylpenicillin 1.2 g 4 times daily IV
- *plus* Clarithromycin 500 mg twice daily orally/IV

If patient is allergic to penicillin

- Doxycycline 200 mg loading dose then 100 mg/day orally *or* Levofloxacin 500 mg/day orally

Severe CAP (CURB-65 score 3-5)

- Co-amoxiclav 1.2 g 3 times daily IV or Cefuroxime 1.5 g 3 times daily IV *or* Ceftriaxone 1–2 g daily IV
- *plus* Clarithromycin 500 mg twice daily IV
- *or* Benzylpenicillin 1.2 g 4 times daily IV *plus* Levofloxacin 500 mg twice daily IV

If *Legionella* is strongly suspected

- Consider adding Levofloxacin 500 mg twice daily IV

---

*Antibiotic use in individual patients should take into account local guidance and antibiotic sensitivity patterns.
Adapted from British Thoracic Society Guidelines.

 17.41 Complications of pneumonia

- Para-pneumonic effusion – common
- Empyema (p. 564)
- Retention of sputum causing lobar collapse
- Deep vein thrombosis and pulmonary embolism
- Pneumothorax, particularly with *Staphylococcus aureus*
- Suppurative pneumonia/lung abscess
- ARDS, renal failure, multi-organ failure (p. 198)
- Ectopic abscess formation (*Staph. aureus*)
- Hepatitis, pericarditis, myocarditis, meningoencephalitis
- Arrhythmias (e.g. atrial fibrillation)
- Pyrexia due to drug hypersensitivity

(ARDS = acute respiratory distress syndrome)

Prognosis

Most patients respond promptly to antibiotic therapy. Fever may persist for several days, however, and the chest X-ray often takes several weeks or even months to resolve, especially in old age. Delayed recovery suggests either that a complication has occurred (Box 17.41) or that the diagnosis is incorrect (see Box 17.37). Alternatively, the pneumonia may be secondary to a proximal bronchial obstruction or recurrent aspiration. The mortality rate of adults with non-severe pneumonia is very low (<1%); hospital death rates are typically between 5% and 10% but may be as high as 50% in severe illness.

Discharge and follow-up

The decision to discharge a hospitalised patient depends on the home circumstances and the likelihood of complications. A chest X-ray need not be repeated before discharge in patients making a satisfactory clinical recovery. Clinical review by GP or hospital should be arranged around 6 weeks later and a chest X-ray obtained if there are persistent symptoms, physical signs or reasons to suspect underlying malignancy.

Prevention

Current smokers should be advised to stop. Influenza and pneumococcal vaccination should be considered in patients at highest risk of pneumonia (e.g. those over 65 or with chronic lung, heart, liver or kidney disease, diabetes or immunosuppression). Because of the mode of spread, *Legionella pneumophila* has important public health implications and usually requires notification to the appropriate health authority for investigation of potential sources. In resource-poor settings, tackling malnourishment and indoor air pollution, and encouraging immunisation against measles, pertussis and *Haemophilus influenzae* type b are particularly important in children.

Hospital-acquired pneumonia

Hospital-acquired pneumonia (HAP) or nosocomial pneumonia refers to a new episode of pneumonia occurring at least 2 days after admission to hospital. It is the second most common hospital-acquired infection (HAI) and the leading cause of HAI-associated death. The elderly are particularly at risk, as are patients in intensive care units, especially when mechanically ventilated; here, the term ventilator-associated pneumonia (VAP) is applied. Health-care-associated pneumonia (HCAP) refers to the development of pneumonia in a person who has spent at least 2 days in hospital within the last 90 days, or has attended a haemodialysis unit, or received intravenous antibiotics, or been resident in a nursing home or other long-term care facility. The factors predisposing to the development of pneumonia in a hospitalised patient are listed in Box 17.42.

Clinical features and investigation

The diagnosis should be considered in any hospitalised or ventilated patient who develops purulent sputum (or endotracheal secretions), new radiological infiltrates, an otherwise unexplained increase in oxygen requirement, a core temperature >38.3°C, and a leucocytosis or leucopenia. The clinical features and radiographic signs are variable and non-specific, however, raising a broad differential diagnosis that includes pulmonary embolism, ARDS, pulmonary oedema, pulmonary haemorrhage and drug toxicity. Therefore, in contrast to CAP, microbiological confirmation should

17

 17.42 Factors predisposing to hospital-acquired pneumonia

Reduced host defences against bacteria

- Reduced immune defences (e.g. glucocorticoid treatment, diabetes, malignancy)
- Reduced cough reflex (e.g. post-operative)
- Disordered mucociliary clearance (e.g. anaesthetic agents)
- Bulbar or vocal cord palsy

Aspiration of nasopharyngeal or gastric secretions

- Immobility or reduced conscious level
- Vomiting, dysphagia (N.B. stroke disease), achalasia or severe reflux
- Nasogastric intubation

Bacteria introduced into lower respiratory tract

- Endotracheal intubation/tracheostomy
- Infected ventilators/nebulisers/bronchoscopes
- Dental or sinus infection

Bacteraemia

- Abdominal sepsis
- Intravenous cannula infection
- Infected emboli

be sought whenever possible. Adequate sputum samples may be difficult to obtain in the frail elderly person and physiotherapy should be considered to aid expectoration. In patients who are mechanically ventilated, bronchoscopy-directed protected brush specimens, bronchoalveolar lavage (BAL) or endotracheal aspirates may be obtained.

Management

The principles of management are similar to those of CAP, focusing on adequate oxygenation, appropriate fluid balance and antibiotics. The choice of empirical antibiotic therapy is considerably more challenging, however, given the diversity of pathogens and the potential for drug resistance.

The organisms implicated in early-onset HAP (occurring within 4–5 days of admission) are similar to those involved in CAP. In patients who have received no previous antibiotics, co-amoxiclav or cefuroxime represents a sensible choice. If the patient has received a course of recent antibiotics, then piperacillin/tazobactam or a third-generation cephalosporin should be considered.

Late-onset HAP is more often attributable to Gram-negative bacteria (e.g. *Escherichia coli*, *Pseudomonas aeruginosa*, *Klebsiella* spp. and *Acinetobacter baumannii*), *Staph. aureus* (including meticillin-resistant *Staph. aureus* (MRSA)) and anaerobes, and the choice of antibiotics ought to cover these possibilities. Antipseudomonal cover may be provided by a carbapenem (meropenem), an anti-pseudomonal cephalosporin or piperacillin–tazobactam. MRSA cover may be provided by glycopeptides such as vancomycin or linezolid. *A. baumannii* is usually sensitive to carbapenems but resistant cases may require nebulised and/or intravenous colistin. The choice of agents is most appropriately guided by knowledge of local patterns of microbiology and antibiotic resistance. It is sensible to commence broad-based cover, discontinuing less appropriate antibiotics as culture results become available. In the absence of good evidence, the duration of antibiotic therapy remains a matter for clinical judgement. Physiotherapy is important to aid expectoration in the immobile and elderly, and adequate nutritional support is often required.

Prevention

Despite appropriate management, the mortality from HAP is high (approximately 30%), mandating prevention whenever possible. Good hygiene is paramount, particularly with regard to hand-washing and any equipment used. Steps should be taken to minimise the chances of aspiration and to limit the use of stress ulcer prophylaxis with proton pump inhibitors. Oral antiseptic (chlorhexidine 2%) may be used to decontaminate the upper airway and some intensive care units employ selective decontamination of the digestive tract when the anticipated requirement for ventilation will exceed 48 hours.

Suppurative pneumonia, aspiration pneumonia and pulmonary abscess

These conditions are considered together, as their aetiology and clinical features overlap. Suppurative pneumonia is characterised by destruction of the lung parenchyma by the inflammatory process. Although microabscess formation is a characteristic histological feature, 'pulmonary abscess' is usually taken to refer to lesions in which there is a large localised collection of pus, or a cavity lined by chronic inflammatory tissue, from which pus has escaped by rupture into a bronchus.

Suppurative pneumonia and pulmonary abscess often develop after the inhalation of septic material during operations on the nose, mouth or throat, under general anaesthesia, or of vomitus during anaesthesia or coma, particularly if oral hygiene is poor. Additional risk factors for aspiration pneumonia include bulbar or vocal cord palsy, achalasia or oesophageal reflux, and alcoholism. Aspiration tends to localise to dependent areas of the lung, such as the apical segment of the lower lobe in a supine patient. These conditions may also complicate local bronchial obstruction from a neoplasm or foreign body.

Infections are usually due to a mixture of anaerobes and aerobes in common with the typical flora encountered in the mouth and upper respiratory tract. Isolates of *Prevotella melaninogenica*, *Fusobacterium necrophorum*, anaerobic or microaerophilic cocci, and *Bacteroides fragilis* may be identified. When suppurative pneumonia or a pulmonary abscess occurs in a previously healthy lung, the most likely infecting organisms are *Staph. aureus* or *K. pneumoniae*. *Actinomyces* infections (mostly *A. israelii*) cause chronic suppurative pulmonary infections, which may be associated with poor dental hygiene. Actinomycosis presents a particular diagnostic challenge because of the slow growth of actinomycetes.

Bacterial infection of a pulmonary infarct or a collapsed lobe may also produce a suppurative pneumonia or lung abscess. The organism(s) isolated from the sputum include *Strep. pneumoniae*, *Staph. aureus*, *Streptococcus pyogenes*, *H. influenzae* and, in some cases, anaerobic bacteria. In many cases, however, no pathogen can be isolated, particularly when antibiotics have been given.

Some strains of community-acquired MRSA (CA-MRSA) produce the cytotoxin Panton–Valentine leukocidin. The organism is mainly responsible for suppurative skin infection but may be associated with rapidly progressive severe necrotising pneumonia.

Lemierre's syndrome is a rare cause of pulmonary abscesses. The usual causative agent is the anaerobe *Fusobacterium necrophorum*. The illness typically commences as a sore throat,

17.43 Respiratory infection in old age

- **Increased risk of and from respiratory infection**: because of reduced immune responses, increased closing volumes, reduced respiratory muscle strength and endurance, altered mucus layer, poor nutritional status and the increased prevalence of chronic lung disease.
- **Predisposing factors**: other medical conditions may predispose to infection, e.g. swallowing difficulties due to stroke increase the risk of aspiration pneumonia.
- **Atypical presentation**: older patients often present with delirium, rather than breathlessness or cough.
- **Mortality**: the vast majority of deaths from pneumonia in developed countries occur in older people.
- **Influenza**: has a much higher complication rate, and morbidity and mortality. Vaccination significantly reduces morbidity and mortality in old age but uptake is poor.
- **Tuberculosis**: most cases in old age represent reactivation of previous, often unrecognised, disease and may be precipitated by glucocorticoid therapy, diabetes mellitus and the factors above. Cryptic miliary tuberculosis is an occasional alternative presentation. Older people more commonly suffer adverse effects from antituberculous chemotherapy and require close monitoring.

| **i** | **17.44 Clinical features of suppurative pneumonia** |

Symptoms

- Cough with large amounts of sputum, sometimes fetid and blood-stained
- Pleural pain common
- Sudden expectoration of copious amounts of foul sputum if abscess ruptures into a bronchus

Clinical signs

- High remittent pyrexia
- Profound systemic upset
- Digital clubbing may develop quickly (10–14 days)
- Consolidation on chest examination; signs of cavitation rarely found
- Pleural rub common
- Rapid deterioration in general health, with marked weight loss if not adequately treated

painful swollen neck, fever, rigor, haemoptysis and dyspnoea; spread into the jugular veins leads to thrombosis and metastatic dispersal of the organisms.

Injecting drug-users are at particular risk of developing haematogenous lung abscess, often in association with endocarditis affecting the pulmonary and tricuspid valves.

A non-infective form of aspiration pneumonia – exogenous lipid pneumonia – may follow the aspiration of animal, vegetable or mineral oils.

The clinical features of suppurative pneumonia are summarised in Box 17.44.

Investigations

Radiological features of suppurative pneumonia include homogeneous lobar or segmental opacity consistent with consolidation or collapse. Abscesses are characterised by cavitation and a fluid level. Occasionally, a pre-existing emphysematous bulla becomes infected and appears as a cavity containing an air–fluid level.

Management

Aspiration pneumonia can usually be treated with amoxicillin and metronidazole. Co-amoxiclav also has a suitable antibiotic spectrum but increases the risk of *Clostridium difficile* infection. Further modification of antibiotics should be informed by clinical response and microbiological results. CA-MRSA is usually susceptible to a variety of oral non-β-lactam antibiotics, such as trimethoprim/sulfamethoxazole, clindamycin, tetracyclines and linezolid. Parenteral therapy with vancomycin or linezolid can also be considered. *Fusobacterium necrophorum* is highly susceptible to β-lactam antibiotics and to metronidazole, clindamycin and third-generation cephalosporins. Prolonged treatment for 4–6 weeks may be required in some patients with lung abscess. Established pulmonary actinomycosis requires 6–12 months' treatment with intravenous or oral penicillin, or with a tetracycline in penicillin-allergic patients.

Physiotherapy is of great value, especially when suppuration is present in the lower lobes or when a large abscess cavity has formed. In most patients there is a good response to treatment, and although residual fibrosis and bronchiectasis are common sequelae, these seldom give rise to serious morbidity. Surgery should be contemplated if no improvement occurs despite optimal medical therapy. Removal or treatment of any obstructing endobronchial lesion is essential.

Pneumonia in the immunocompromised patient

Patients immunocompromised by drugs or disease (particularly human immunodeficiency virus (HIV) infection; p. 318) are at increased risk of pulmonary infection and pneumonia is the most common cause of death in this group. The majority of infections are caused by the same pathogens that cause pneumonia in immunocompetent individuals, but in patients with more profound immunosuppression less common organisms, or those normally considered to be of low virulence or non-pathogenic, may become 'opportunistic' pathogens. Depending on the clinical context, clinicians should consider the possibility of Gram-negative bacteria, especially *P. aeruginosa*, viruses, fungi, mycobacteria, and less common organisms such as *Nocardia* spp. Infection is often due to more than one organism.

Clinical features

These typically include fever, cough and breathlessness but are influenced by the degree of immunosuppression, and the presentation may be less specific in the more profoundly immunosuppressed. The onset of symptoms tends to be swift in those with a bacterial infection but more gradual in patients with opportunistic organisms such as *Pneumocystis jirovecii* and mycobacterial infections (p. 318). In *P. jirovecii* pneumonia, symptoms of cough and breathlessness can be present several days or weeks before the onset of systemic symptoms or the appearance of radiographic abnormality. The clinical features of invasive pulmonary aspergillosis are dealt with on page 597.

Investigations

The approach is informed by the clinical context and severity of the illness. Invasive investigations, such as bronchoscopy, BAL, transbronchial biopsy or surgical lung biopsy, are often impractical, as many patients are too ill to undergo these safely; however, 'induced sputum' (p. 554) offers a relatively safe method of obtaining microbiological samples. HRCT can be helpful:

- focal unilateral airspace opacification favours bacterial infection, mycobacteria or *Nocardia*
- bilateral opacification favours *P. jirovecii* pneumonia, fungi, viruses and unusual bacteria, e.g. *Nocardia*
- cavitation may be seen with *N. asteroides*, mycobacteria and fungi
- the presence of a 'halo sign' (a zone of intermediate attenuation between the nodule and the lung parenchyma) may suggest aspergillosis (p. 596)
- pleural effusions suggest pyogenic bacterial infections and are uncommon in *P. jirovecii* pneumonia.

Management

In theory, treatment should be based on an established aetiological diagnosis; in practice, however, the causative agent is frequently unknown. Factors that favour a bacterial aetiology include neutropenia, rapid onset and deterioration. In these circumstances, broad-spectrum antibiotic therapy should be commenced immediately, e.g. a third-generation cephalosporin, or a quinolone, plus an antistaphylococcal antibiotic, or an antipseudomonal penicillin plus an aminoglycoside. Thereafter, treatment may be tailored according to the results of investigations and the clinical response. Depending on the clinical context and response to treatment, antifungal or antiviral therapies may be added. The management of *P. jirovecii* infection is detailed on page 318 and that of invasive aspergillosis on page 596.

17

Fig. 17.34 Worldwide incidence of tuberculosis (2014). Estimated new cases (all forms) per 100 000 population. *From World Health Organisation. Global tuberculosis report, 20th edn. Geneva: WHO; 2015.*

Tuberculosis

Epidemiology

Tuberculosis (TB) is caused by infection with *Mycobacterium tuberculosis* (MTB), which is part of a complex of organisms including *M. bovis* (reservoir cattle) and *M. africanum* (reservoir humans). The resurgence in TB in the UK observed over the latter part of the last century has finally halted and notification of TB has fallen by around 1.5% per year since 2000. None the less, its impact on world health remains significant. An estimated 9.6 million new cases were recorded in 2014, with the majority presenting in the world's poorest nations, which struggle to cover the costs associated with management and control programmes (Fig. 17.34). In the same year, 1.5 million men, women and children died of TB, and TB continues to rank alongside HIV as a leading cause of death worldwide.

Pathology and pathogenesis

M. bovis infection arises mainly drinking non-sterilised milk from infected cows. *M. tuberculosis* is spread by the inhalation of aerosolised droplet nuclei from other infected patients. Once inhaled, the organisms lodge in the alveoli and initiate the recruitment of macrophages and lymphocytes. Macrophages undergo transformation into epithelioid and Langhans cells, which aggregate with the lymphocytes to form the classical tuberculous granuloma (Fig. 17.35). Numerous granulomas aggregate to form a primary lesion or 'Ghon focus' (a pale yellow, caseous nodule, usually a few millimetres to 1–2 cm in diameter), which is characteristically situated in the periphery of the lung. Spread of organisms to the hilar lymph nodes is followed by a similar pathological reaction, and the combination of the primary lesion and regional lymph nodes is referred to as the 'primary complex of Ranke'. Reparative processes encase the primary complex in a fibrous capsule, limiting the spread of bacilli. If no further complications ensue, this lesion eventually calcifies and is clearly seen on a chest X-ray. Lymphatic or haematogenous spread may occur before immunity is established, however, seeding secondary foci in other organs, including lymph nodes, serous membranes, meninges, bones, liver, kidneys and lungs, which may lie dormant for years. The only clue that infection has occurred may be the appearance of a cell-mediated, delayed-type hypersensitivity reaction to tuberculin, demonstrated by tuberculin skin testing or an interferon gamma release assay (IGRA): so-called latent TB

Fig. 17.35 Tuberculous granuloma. Normal lung tissue is lost and replaced by a mass of fibrous tissue with granulomatous inflammation characterised by large numbers of macrophages and multinucleate giant cells (white arrow). The central area of this focus shows caseous degeneration (black arrow). *Courtesy of Dr William Wallace, Department of Pathology, Royal Infirmary of Edinburgh.*

(p. 594). If these reparative processes fail, primary progressive disease ensues (Fig. 17.36). The estimated lifetime risk of developing disease after primary infection is 10%, with roughly half of this risk occurring in the first 2 years after infection. Factors predisposing to TB are summarised in Box 17.45 and the natural history of infection with TB is summarised in Box 17.46.

Clinical features: pulmonary disease

Primary pulmonary TB

Primary TB refers to the infection of a previously uninfected (tuberculin-negative) individual. A few patients develop a self-limiting febrile illness but clinical disease occurs only if there is a hypersensitivity reaction or progressive infection (Box 17.47). Progressive primary disease may appear during the course of the initial illness or after a latent period of weeks or months.

Miliary TB

Blood-borne dissemination gives rise to miliary TB, which may present acutely but more frequently is characterised by 2–3 weeks of fever, night sweats, anorexia, weight loss and a

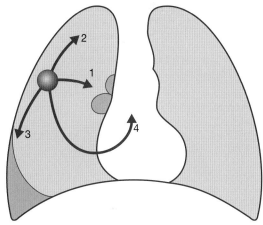

Fig. 17.36 Primary pulmonary tuberculosis. (1) Spread from the primary focus to hilar and mediastinal lymph glands to form the 'primary complex', which heals spontaneously in most cases. (2) Direct extension of the primary focus – progressive pulmonary tuberculosis. (3) Spread to the pleura – tuberculous pleurisy and pleural effusion. (4) Blood-borne spread: *few bacilli* – pulmonary, skeletal, renal, genitourinary infection, often months or years later; *massive spread* – miliary pulmonary tuberculosis and meningitis.

 17.45 Factors increasing the risk of tuberculosis

Patient-related

- Age (children > young adults < elderly)
- First-generation immigrants from high-prevalence countries
- Close contacts of patients with smear-positive pulmonary TB
- Overcrowding (prisons, collective dormitories); homelessness (doss houses and hostels)
- Chest X-ray evidence of self-healed TB
- Primary infection <1 year previously
- Smoking: cigarettes, bidis (Indian cigarettes made of tobacco wrapped in temburini leaves) and cannabis

Associated diseases

- Immunosuppression: HIV, anti-tumour necrosis factor (TNF) and other biologic therapies, high-dose glucocorticoids, cytotoxic agents
- Malignancy (especially lymphoma and leukaemia)
- Diabetes mellitus
- Chronic kidney disease
- Silicosis
- Gastrointestinal disease associated with malnutrition (gastrectomy, jejuno-ileal bypass, cancer of the pancreas, malabsorption)
- Deficiency of vitamin D or A
- Recent measles in children

17.46 Natural history of untreated primary tuberculosis

Time from infection	Manifestations
3–8 weeks	Primary complex, positive tuberculin skin test
3–6 months	Meningeal, miliary and pleural disease
Up to 3 years	Gastrointestinal, bone and joint, and lymph node disease
Around 8 years	Renal tract disease
From 3 years onwards	Post-primary disease due to reactivation or re-infection

Adapted from Davies PDO, ed. Clinical tuberculosis. London: Hodder Arnold; 1998.

 17.47 Features of primary tuberculosis

Infection (4–8 weeks)

- Influenza-like illness
- Skin test conversion
- Primary complex

Disease

- Lymphadenopathy: hilar (often unilateral), paratracheal or mediastinal
- Collapse (especially right middle lobe)
- Consolidation (especially right middle lobe)
- Obstructive emphysema
- Cavitation (rare)
- Pleural effusion
- Miliary
- Meningitis
- Pericarditis

Hypersensitivity

- Erythema nodosum
- Phlyctenular conjunctivitis
- Dactylitis

17.48 Cryptic tuberculosis

- Age over 60 years
- Intermittent low-grade pyrexia of unknown origin
- Unexplained weight loss, general debility (hepatosplenomegaly in 25–50%)
- Normal chest X-ray
- Blood dyscrasias; leukaemoid reaction, pancytopenia
- Negative tuberculin skin test
- Confirmation by biopsy with granulomas and/or acid-fast bacilli in liver or bone marrow

17

dry cough. Hepatosplenomegaly may develop and the presence of a headache may indicate coexistent tuberculous meningitis. Auscultation of the chest is frequently normal but in more advanced disease widespread crackles are evident. Fundoscopy may show choroidal tubercles. The classical appearances on chest X-ray are of fine 1–2 mm lesions ('millet seed') distributed throughout the lung fields, although occasionally the appearances are coarser. Anaemia and leucopenia reflect bone marrow involvement. 'Cryptic' miliary TB is an unusual presentation sometimes seen in old age (Box 17.48).

Post-primary pulmonary TB

Post-primary disease refers to exogenous ('new' infection) or endogenous (reactivation of a dormant primary lesion) infection in a person who has been sensitised by earlier exposure. It is most frequently pulmonary and characteristically occurs in the apex of an upper lobe, where the oxygen tension favours survival of the strictly aerobic organism. The onset is usually insidious, developing slowly over several weeks. Systemic symptoms include fever, night sweats, malaise and loss of appetite and weight, and are accompanied by progressive pulmonary symptoms (Box 17.49). Very occasionally, this form of TB may present with one of the complications listed in Box 17.50. Radiological changes include ill-defined opacification in one or both of the upper lobes, and as progression occurs, consolidation, collapse and cavitation develop to varying degrees (Fig. 17.37). It is often difficult to distinguish active from quiescent disease on radiological criteria alone but the presence of a miliary pattern or cavitation favours active disease. In extensive disease, collapse may be marked and results in significant displacement of the trachea and mediastinum. Occasionally, a caseous lymph node may drain into an adjoining bronchus, leading to tuberculous pneumonia.

Clinical features: extrapulmonary disease

Extrapulmonary TB accounts for 20% of cases in those who are HIV-negative but is more common in HIV-positive patients.

Lymphadenitis

Lymph nodes are the most common extrapulmonary site of disease. Cervical and mediastinal glands are affected most frequently, followed by axillary and inguinal, and more than one region may be involved. Disease may represent primary infection, spread from contiguous sites or reactivation. Supraclavicular lymphadenopathy is often the result of spread from mediastinal disease. The nodes are usually painless and initially mobile but become matted together with time. When caseation and liquefaction occur, the swelling becomes fluctuant and may discharge through the skin with the formation of a 'collar-stud' abscess and sinus formation. Approximately half of cases fail to show any constitutional features, such as fevers or night sweats. The tuberculin test is usually strongly positive. During or after treatment, paradoxical enlargement, development of new nodes and suppuration may all occur but without evidence of continued infection; surgical excision is rarely necessary. In non-immigrant children in the UK, most mycobacterial lymphadenitis is caused by opportunistic mycobacteria, especially of the *M. avium* complex.

Gastrointestinal tuberculosis

TB can affect any part of the bowel and patients may present with a wide range of symptoms and signs (Fig. 17.38). Upper gastrointestinal tract involvement is rare and is usually an unexpected histological finding in an endoscopic or laparotomy specimen. Ileocaecal disease accounts for approximately half of abdominal TB cases. Fever, night sweats, anorexia and weight loss are usually prominent and a right iliac fossa mass may be palpable. Up to 30% of cases present with an acute abdomen. Ultrasound or CT may reveal thickened bowel wall, abdominal lymphadenopathy, mesenteric thickening or ascites. Barium enema and small bowel enema reveal narrowing, shortening and

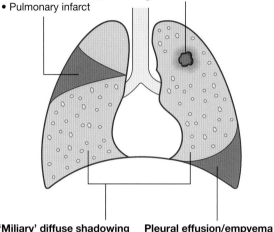

Cavitation
Differential diagnosis
- Pneumonia/lung abscess
- Lung cancer
- Pulmonary infarct
- Granulomatosis with polyangiitis (Wegener's granulomatosis)
- Progressive massive fibrosis

Consolidation/collapse
Differential diagnosis
- Pneumonia
- Bronchial carcinoma
- Pulmonary infarct

'Miliary' diffuse shadowing
Differential diagnosis
- Sarcoidosis
- Malignancy
- Pneumoconiosis
- Infection (e.g. histoplasmosis)

Pleural effusion/empyema
Differential diagnosis
- Bacterial pneumonia
- Pulmonary infarction
- Carcinoma
- Connective tissue disorder

Fig. 17.37 Chest X-ray: major manifestations and differential diagnosis of pulmonary tuberculosis. Less common manifestations include pneumothorax, acute respiratory distress syndrome (ARDS; p. 198), cor pulmonale and localised emphysema.

distortion of the bowel, with caecal involvement predominating. Diagnosis rests on obtaining histology by either colonoscopy or mini-laparotomy. The main differential diagnosis is Crohn's disease (p. 813). Tuberculous peritonitis is characterised by abdominal distension, pain and constitutional symptoms. The ascitic fluid is exudative and cellular, with a predominance of lymphocytes. Laparoscopy reveals multiple white 'tubercles' over the peritoneal and omental surfaces. Low-grade hepatic dysfunction is common in miliary disease, in which biopsy reveals granulomas. Occasionally, patients may be frankly icteric, with a mixed hepatic/cholestatic picture.

Pericardial disease

Disease occurs in two forms (see Fig. 17.38 and p. 542): pericardial effusion and constrictive pericarditis. Fever and night sweats are rarely prominent and the presentation is usually insidious, with breathlessness and abdominal swelling. Coexistent pulmonary disease is very rare, with the exception of pleural effusion. Pulsus paradoxus, a raised JVP, hepatomegaly, prominent ascites and peripheral oedema are common to both types. Pericardial effusion is associated with increased pericardial dullness and a globular enlarged heart on chest X-ray, and pericardial calcification occurs in around 25% of cases. Constriction is associated with an early third heart sound and, occasionally, atrial fibrillation. Diagnosis is based on the clinical, radiological and echocardiographic findings (p. 542). The effusion is frequently blood-stained. Open pericardial biopsy can be performed where there is diagnostic uncertainty. The addition of glucocorticoids to antituberculosis treatment has been shown to help both forms of pericardial disease.

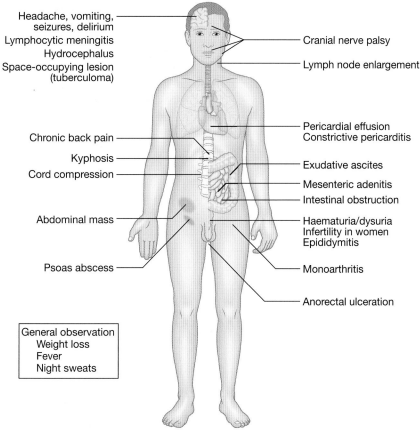

Headache, vomiting, seizures, delirium
Lymphocytic meningitis
Hydrocephalus
Space-occupying lesion (tuberculoma)

Cranial nerve palsy

Lymph node enlargement

Chronic back pain

Kyphosis

Cord compression

Pericardial effusion
Constrictive pericarditis

Exudative ascites

Mesenteric adenitis

Intestinal obstruction

Abdominal mass

Haematuria/dysuria
Infertility in women
Epididymitis

Psoas abscess

Monoarthritis

Anorectal ulceration

General observation
Weight loss
Fever
Night sweats

Fig. 17.38 Systemic presentations of extrapulmonary tuberculosis.

17

Central nervous system disease

Meningeal disease represents the most important form of central nervous system TB. Unrecognised and untreated, it is rapidly fatal. Even when appropriate treatment is prescribed, mortality rates of 30% have been reported, while survivors may be left with neurological sequelae. Clinical features, investigations and management are described on page 1120.

Bone and joint disease

The spine is the most common site for bony TB (Pott's disease), which usually presents with chronic back pain and typically involves the lower thoracic and lumbar spine (see Fig. 17.38). The infection starts as a discitis and then spreads along the spinal ligaments to involve the adjacent anterior vertebral bodies, causing angulation of the vertebrae with subsequent kyphosis. Paravertebral and psoas abscess formation is common and the disease may present with a large (cold) abscess in the inguinal region. CT or MRI is valuable in gauging the extent of disease, the amount of cord compression, and the site for needle biopsy or open exploration, if required. The major differential diagnosis is malignancy, which tends to affect the vertebral body and leave the disc intact. Important complications include spinal instability or cord compression.

TB can affect any joint but most frequently involves the hip or knee. Presentation is usually insidious, with pain and swelling; fever and night sweats are uncommon. Radiological changes are often non-specific but, as disease progresses, reduction in joint space and erosions appear. Poncet's arthropathy is an immunologically mediated polyarthritis that usually resolves within 2 months of starting treatment.

Genitourinary disease

Fever and night sweats are rare with renal tract TB and patients are often only mildly symptomatic for many years. Haematuria, frequency and dysuria are often present, with sterile pyuria found on urine microscopy and culture. In women, infertility from endometritis, or pelvic pain and swelling from salpingitis or a tubo-ovarian abscess occurs occasionally. In men, genitourinary TB may present as epididymitis or prostatitis.

Investigations

The presence of an otherwise unexplained cough for more than 2–3 weeks, particularly in regions where TB is prevalent, or typical chest X-ray or CT changes (Fig. 17.39) should prompt further investigation (Box 17.51). Direct microscopy of a sputum smear remains the most important first step. At least two sputum samples (including at least one obtained in the early morning) from a spontaneously produced deep cough should be obtained. Induced sputum may be used in those unable to expectorate. In selected cases, bronchoscopy and lavage or aspiration of a lymph node by EBUS may be used.

Light-emitting diode fluorescent microscopy with auramine staining is increasingly replacing the more traditional standard light microscopy and Ziehl–Neelsen stain (Fig. 17.40) or the use of mercury-vapour fluorescent microscopy. A positive smear is sufficient for the presumptive diagnosis of TB but definitive

Fig. 17.39 Typical changes of tuberculosis. The chest X-ray shows bilateral upper lobe airspace shadowing with cavitation.

Fig. 17.40 Positive Ziehl–Neelsen stain. Mycobacteria (arrow) retain the red carbol fuchsin stain, despite washing with acid and alcohol. *Courtesy of Adam Hill.*

ℹ 17.51 Diagnosis of tuberculosis

Specimens required

Pulmonary
- Sputum* (induced with nebulised hypertonic saline if patient not expectorating)
- Bronchoscopy with washings or BAL
- Gastric washing* (mainly used for children)

Extrapulmonary
- Fluid examination (cerebrospinal, ascitic, pleural, pericardial, joint): yield classically very low
- Tissue biopsy (from affected site): bone marrow/liver may be diagnostic in disseminated disease

Diagnostic tests
- Tuberculin skin test: low sensitivity/specificity; useful only in primary or deep-seated infection
- Stain
  Ziehl–Neelsen
  Auramine fluorescence
- Nucleic acid amplification
- Culture
  Solid media (Löwenstein–Jensen, Middlebrook)
  Liquid media (e.g. MGIT)
- Pleural fluid: adenosine deaminase
- Response to empirical antituberculous drugs (usually seen after 5–10 days)

Baseline blood tests
- Full blood count, C-reactive protein, erythrocyte sedimentation rate, urea and electrolytes, liver function tests

*At least two but preferably three, including an early morning sample.
(BAL = bronchoalveolar lavage; MGIT = mycobacteria growth indicator tube)

---

diagnosis requires culture. The probability of detecting acid-fast bacilli is proportional to the bacillary burden in the sputum. Smear-negative sputum should also be cultured, as only 10–100 viable organisms are required for sputum to be culture-positive. A diagnosis of smear-negative TB may be made in advance of culture if the chest X-ray appearances are typical of TB.

The slow growth of MTB on solid (typically between 4 and 6 weeks) and automated and semi-automated liquid (typically around 2 weeks) culture media has prompted the development of rapid NAATs (p. 106). For example, Xpert MTB/RIF (a DNA detection-based NAAT) has the capacity to detect MTB (and rifampicin resistance) in less than 2 hours. However, while it is specific to MTB, it is not sufficiently sensitive to have replaced culture.

The diagnosis of extrapulmonary TB can be more challenging. There are generally fewer organisms (particularly in meningeal or pleural fluid), so culture, histopathological examination of tissue and/or NAAT may be required. Stimulation of T cells by mycobacterial antigens leads to increased levels of adenosine deaminase in pleural, pericardial, cerebrospinal and ascitic fluid, and so may assist in confirming suspected TB.

In the presence of HIV, examination of sputum may still be useful, as subclinical pulmonary disease is common. Lateral flow urinary lipoarabinomannan assay (LF-LAM) may be useful in the severely ill patient with a CD4 count of 100 cells/µL or less.

Drug sensitivity testing

The rapid detection of drug resistance is central both to the management of the individual with TB and to control of the disease in the population. The gold standard remains culture, in either solid or liquid media, but the use of other phenotypic tests, such as microscopically observed drug susceptibility (MODS), colorimetric redox indicator (CRI) methods and nitrate reductase assay, offer low-cost alternatives, depending on the resource and expertise available. The potential for molecular tests to provide rapid drug sensitivity testing (DST) is improving, particularly with regard to the detection of rifampicin resistance, which is important because rifampicin forms the cornerstone of 6-month chemotherapy. Rapid identification of rifampicin resistance is provided by Xpert MTB/RIF. Line probe assays (LPAs) use PCR and reverse hybridisation to detect genetic sequences linked to resistance to both rifampicin and isoniazid, and increasingly to resistance to pyrazinamide, ethambutol and other second-line agents.

Management

Chemotherapy

The treatment of TB is based on the principle of an initial intensive phase to reduce the bacterial population rapidly, followed by a continuation phase to destroy any remaining bacteria (Box 17.52). Standard treatment involves 6 months' treatment with isoniazid and rifampicin, supplemented in the first 2 months with

i 17.52 Treatment of new tuberculosis patients (World Health Organisation recommendations)

Intensive phase	Continuation phase	Comments
Standard regimen		
2 months of HRZE	4 months of HR	
2 months of HRZE	4 months of HRE	Applies only in countries with high levels of isoniazid resistance in new TB patients, and where isoniazid drug susceptibility testing in new patients is not done (or results are unavailable) before the continuation phase begins
Dosing frequency		
Daily*	Daily	Optimal
Daily*	3 times/week	Acceptable alternative for any new patient receiving directly observed therapy
3 times/week	3 times/week	Acceptable alternative, provided that the patient is receiving directly observed therapy and is NOT living with HIV or living in an HIV-prevalent setting

*Daily (rather than 3 times weekly) intensive-phase dosing may help to prevent acquired drug resistance in TB patients starting treatment with isoniazid resistance.
(H = isoniazid; R = rifampicin; Z = pyrazinamide; E = ethambutol)
Adapted from World Health Organisation. Treatment of tuberculosis guidelines, 4th edn; 2010.

i 17.53 Main adverse reactions of first-line antituberculous drugs

	Isoniazid	Rifampicin	Pyrazinamide	Streptomycin	Ethambutol
Mode of action	Cell wall synthesis	DNA transcription	Unknown	Protein synthesis	Cell wall synthesis
Major adverse reactions	Peripheral neuropathy[1] Hepatitis[2] Rash	Febrile reactions Hepatitis Rash Gastrointestinal disturbance	Hepatitis Gastrointestinal disturbance Hyperuricaemia	8th nerve damage Rash	Retrobulbar neuritis[3] Arthralgia
Less common adverse reactions	Lupoid reactions Seizures Psychoses	Interstitial nephritis Thrombocytopenia Haemolytic anaemia	Rash Photosensitisation Gout	Nephrotoxicity Agranulocytosis	Peripheral neuropathy Rash

[1]The risk may be reduced by prescribing pyridoxine. [2]More common in patients with a slow acetylator status and in alcoholics. [3]Reduced visual acuity and colour vision may be reported with higher doses and are usually reversible.

17

pyrazinamide and ethambutol. Fixed-dose tablets combining two or three drugs are preferred. Treatment should be commenced immediately in any patient who is smear-positive, and in those who are smear-negative but with typical chest X-ray changes and no response to standard antibiotics.

Six months of therapy is appropriate for all patients with new-onset pulmonary TB and most cases of extrapulmonary TB. However, 12 months of therapy is recommended for meningeal TB, including involvement of the spinal cord in cases of spinal TB; in these cases, ethambutol may be replaced by streptomycin. Pyridoxine should be prescribed in pregnant women and malnourished patients to reduce the risk of peripheral neuropathy with isoniazid. Where drug resistance is not anticipated, patients can be assumed to be non-infectious after 2 weeks of appropriate therapy.

Most patients can be treated at home. Admission to a hospital unit with appropriate isolation facilities should be considered where there is uncertainty about the diagnosis, intolerance of medication, questionable treatment adherence, adverse social conditions or a significant risk of multidrug-resistant TB (culture-positive after 2 months on treatment, or contact with known multidrug-resistant TB).

Patients treated with rifampicin should be advised that their urine, tears and other secretions will develop a bright, orange/red coloration, and women taking the oral contraceptive pill must be warned that its efficacy will be reduced and alternative contraception may be necessary. Ethambutol and streptomycin should be used with caution in renal impairment, with appropriate

dose reduction and monitoring of drug levels. Adverse drug reactions occur in about 10% of patients but are significantly more common with HIV co-infection (Box 17.53).

Baseline liver function and regular monitoring are important for patients treated with standard therapy. Rifampicin may cause asymptomatic hyperbilirubinaemia but, along with isoniazid and pyrazinamide, may also cause hepatitis. Mild asymptomatic increases in transaminases are common but significant hepatotoxicity only occurs in 2–5%. It is appropriate to stop treatment and allow any symptoms to subside and the liver function tests to recover before commencing a stepwise re-introduction of the individual drugs. Less hepatotoxic regimens may be considered, including streptomycin, ethambutol and fluoroquinolones.

Glucocorticoids reduce inflammation and limit tissue damage; they are currently recommended when treating pericardial or meningeal disease, and in children with endobronchial disease. They may confer benefit in TB of the ureter, pleural effusions and extensive pulmonary disease, and can suppress hypersensitivity drug reactions. Surgery should be considered in cases complicated by massive haemoptysis, loculated empyema, constrictive pericarditis, lymph node suppuration, and spinal disease with cord compression, but usually only after a full course of antituberculosis treatment.

The effectiveness of therapy for pulmonary TB is assessed by further sputum smear at 2 months and at 5 months. Treatment failure is defined as a positive sputum smear or culture at 5 months or any patient with a multidrug-resistant strain, regardless of whether they are smear-positive or negative. Extrapulmonary TB must be assessed clinically or radiographically, as appropriate.

Control and prevention

TB is preventable, particularly so in those with latent TB. Supporting the development of laboratory and health-care services to improve detection and treatment of active and latent TB is an important component of this goal.

Detection of latent TB

The majority of individuals exposed to MTB harbour the bacteria, which remain dormant. They do not develop any signs of active disease and are non-infectious. They are however, at risk of developing active TB disease and becoming infectious. The lifetime risk of TB disease for a person with documented latent TB infection is estimated at 5–15%, with the majority of cases occurring within the first 5 years after initial infection.

Latent TB may be identified by the presence of immune responses to *M. tuberculosis* antigens. Contact tracing is a legal requirement in many countries. It has the potential to identify the probable index case, other cases infected by the same index patient (with or without evidence of disease), and close contacts who should receive BCG vaccination (see below) or chemotherapy. Approximately 10–20% of close contacts of patients with smear-positive pulmonary TB and 2–5% of those with smear-negative, culture-positive disease have evidence of TB infection.

Cases are commonly identified using the tuberculin skin test (TST; Fig. 17.41) or an IGRA (Fig. 17.42). An otherwise asymptomatic contact who tests positive but has a normal chest X-ray may be treated with chemoprophylaxis to prevent infection from progressing to clinical disease. Chemoprophylaxis should be offered to adults up to the age of 65 (although age-specific cut-off varies by country). It should also be considered for HIV-infected close contacts of a patient with smear-positive disease. A course of rifampicin and isoniazid for 3 months or isoniazid for 6 months is effective.

Tuberculin skin testing may be associated with false-positive reactions in those who have had a BCG vaccination and in areas where exposure to non-tuberculous mycobacteria is high. The skin tests may also be falsely negative in the setting of immunosuppression or overwhelming TB infection.

IGRAs detect the release of interferon-gamma (IFN-γ) from sensitised T cells in response to antigens, such as early secretory antigenic target (ESAT)-6 or culture filtrate protein (CFP)-10, which are encoded by genes specific to *Mycobacterium tuberculosis* and are not shared with BCG or opportunistic mycobacteria (Fig. 17.42). IGRAs are more specific than skin testing and logistically more convenient, as they require a single blood test rather than two clinic visits. In the UK, a dual strategy of TST followed by IGRA is recommended. TST remains the first choice in children, while IGRA represents the first choice for individuals with HIV.

Directly observed therapy

Poor adherence to therapy is a major factor in prolonged illness, risk of relapse, and the emergence of drug resistance. Directly observed therapy (DOT) involves the supervised administration of therapy 3 times weekly to improve adherence. DOT has become an important control strategy in resource-poor nations. In the UK, it is currently recommended for patients thought unlikely to be adherent to therapy: homeless people and drifters, alcohol or

Fig. 17.41 The tuberculin skin test. [A] The reaction to the intradermal injection of tuberculin purified protein derivative (PPD) on the inner surface of the forearm is read between 48 and 72 hours. [B] The diameter of the indurated area should be measured across the forearm and is positive when ≥5 mm.

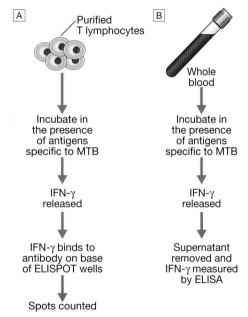

Fig. 17.42 The principles of interferon-gamma release assays (IGRAs). A sample of either (A) purified T cells (T-SPOT.TB test) or (B) whole blood (QuantiFERON–TB Gold test) is incubated in the presence of antigens specific to *Mycobacterium tuberculosis* (MTB). The release of interferon-gamma (IFN-γ) by the cells is measured by enzyme-linked immunosorbent assay (ELISA). (ELISPOT = enzyme-linked immunosorbent spot assay)

drug users, patients with serious mental illness and those with a history of non-adherence.

TB and HIV/AIDS

The close links between HIV and TB, particularly in sub-Saharan Africa, and the potential for both diseases to overwhelm health-care funding in resource-poor nations have been recognised, with the promotion of programmes that link detection and treatment of TB with detection and treatment of HIV. It is recommended that all patients with TB should be tested for HIV infection. Mortality is high and TB is a leading cause of death in HIV patients. Full discussion of its presentation and management is given on page 318.

Drug-resistant TB

Drug-resistant TB is defined by the presence of resistance to any first-line agent. Multidrug-resistant tuberculosis (MDR-TB) is defined by resistance to at least rifampicin and isoniazid, with or without other drug resistance. Globally, an estimated 3.3% of new TB cases and 20% of previously treated cases have MDR-TB. In 2014, an estimated 190 000 people died of MDR-TB. Extensively drug-resistant tuberculosis (XDR-TB) is defined as resistance to at least rifampicin and isoniazid, in addition to any quinolone and at least one injectable second-line agent. An estimated 9.7% of people with MDR-TB have XDR-TB. The prevalence of MDR-TB is rising, particularly in the former Soviet Union, Central Asia and Africa. It is more common in individuals with a prior history of TB, particularly if treatment has been inadequate, and those with HIV infection. Box 17.54 lists the factors contributing to the emergence of drug-resistant TB. Diagnosis is challenging, especially in resource-poor settings, and although cure may be possible, it requires prolonged treatment with less effective, more toxic and more expensive therapies. The mortality rate from MDR-TB is high and that from XDR-TB higher still.

Vaccines

BCG (the Calmette–Guérin bacillus), a live attenuated vaccine derived from *M. bovis*, is the most established TB vaccine. It is administered by intradermal injection and is highly immunogenic. BCG appears to be effective in preventing disseminated disease, including tuberculous meningitis, in children, but its efficacy in adults is inconsistent and new vaccines are urgently needed. Current vaccination policies vary worldwide according to incidence and health-care resources, but usually target children and other high-risk individuals. BCG is very safe, with the occasional complication of local abscess formation. It should not be administered to those who are immunocompromised (e.g. by HIV) or pregnant.

Prognosis

Following successful completion of chemotherapy, cure should be anticipated in the majority of patients. There is a small (<5%) and unavoidable risk of relapse. Most relapses occur within

5 months and usually have the same drug susceptibility. In the absence of treatment, a patient with smear-positive TB will remain infectious for an average of 2 years; in 1 year, 25% of untreated cases will die. Death is more likely in those who are smear-positive and those who smoke. A few patients die unexpectedly soon after commencing therapy and it is possible that some have subclinical hypoadrenalism that is unmasked by a rifampicin-induced increase in glucocorticoid metabolism. HIV-positive patients have higher mortality rates and a modestly increased risk of relapse.

Opportunistic mycobacterial infection

Other species of environmental mycobacteria (often termed 'atypical') may cause human disease (Box 17.55). The sites commonly involved are the lungs, lymph nodes, skin and soft tissues. The most widely recognised of these mycobacteria, *M. avium* complex (MAC), is well described in severe HIV disease (CD4 count <50 cells/mL – p. 324). However, several others (including MAC) colonise and/or infect apparently immunocompetent patients with chronic lung diseases such as COPD, bronchiectasis, pneumoconiosis, old TB, or cystic fibrosis. The clinical presentation varies from a relatively indolent course in some to an aggressive course characterised by cavitatory or nodular disease in others. Radiological appearances may be similar to classical TB, but in patients with bronchiectasis, opportunistic infection may present with lower-zone nodules. The most commonly reported organisms include *M. kansasii*, *M. malmoense*, *M. xenopi* and *M. abscessus* but geographical variation is marked. *M. abscessus* and *M. fortuitum* grow rapidly but the majority grow slowly. More rapid diagnostic systems are under development, including DNA probes, high-performance liquid chromatography (HPLC), PCR restriction enzyme analysis (PRA) and 16S rRNA gene sequence analysis. With the exception of *M. kansasii*, drug sensitivity testing is usually unhelpful in predicting treatment response. In the UK, these organisms are not notifiable to local public health departments as they are not normally communicable, although there is some evidence of patient-to-patient transmission of *M. abscessus* in cystic fibrosis.

17

i	17.54 Factors contributing to the emergence of drug-resistant tuberculosis

- Drug shortages
- Poor-quality drugs
- Lack of appropriate supervision
- Transmission of drug-resistant strains
- Prior antituberculosis treatment
- Treatment failure (smear-positive at 5 months)

i	17.55 Site-specific opportunistic mycobacterial disease

Pulmonary

- *M. xenopi*
- *M. kansasii*
- *M. malmoense*
- MAC
- *M. abscessus* (in cystic fibrosis)

Lymph node

- MAC
- *M. malmoense*
- *M. fortuitum*
- *M. chelonei*

Soft tissue/skin

- *M. leprae*
- *M. ulcerans* (prevalent in Africa, northern Australia and South-east Asia)
- *M. marinum*
- *M. fortuitum*
- *M. chelonae*

Disseminated

- MAC (HIV-associated)
- *M. haemophilum*
- *M. genavense*
- *M. fortuitum*
- *M. chelonae*
- BCG

(BCG = bacille Calmette–Guérin; MAC = *Mycobacterium avium* complex – *M. scrofulaceum*, *M. intracellulare* and *M. avium*)

Respiratory diseases caused by fungi

The majority of fungi encountered by humans are harmless saprophytes but in certain circumstances (Box 17.56) some species may cause disease by infecting human tissue, promoting damaging allergic reactions or producing toxins. 'Mycosis' is the term applied to disease caused by fungal infection. The conditions associated with *Aspergillus* species are listed in Box 17.57.

Allergic bronchopulmonary aspergillosis

Allergic bronchopulmonary aspergillosis (ABPA) occurs as a result of a hypersensitivity reaction to germinating fungal spores in the airway wall. The condition may complicate the course of asthma and cystic fibrosis, and is a recognised cause of pulmonary eosinophilia (p. 611). The prevalence of ABPA is approximately 1–2% in asthma and 5–10% in CF. A variety of human leucocyte antigens (HLAs) convey both an increased and a decreased risk of developing the condition, suggesting that genetic susceptibility is important.

Clinical features

Clinical features depend on the stage of the disease. Common manifestations in the early phases include fever, breathlessness, cough productive of bronchial casts and worsening of asthmatic symptoms. The appearance of radiographic infiltrates may cause ABPA to be mistaken for pneumonia but the diagnosis may also be suggested by segmental or lobar collapse on chest X-rays of patients whose asthma symptoms are stable. Diagnostic features are shown in Box 17.58 and the typical *Aspergillus* hyphae in Figure 17.43. If bronchiectasis develops, the symptoms and complications of that disease often overshadow those of asthma.

Management

ABPA is generally considered an indication for regular therapy with low-dose oral glucocorticoids (prednisolone 7.5–10 mg daily) with the aim of suppressing the immunopathological responses and preventing progressive tissue damage. In some patients, itraconazole (400 mg/day) facilitates a reduction in oral

17.56 Factors predisposing to pulmonary fungal disease

Systemic factors

- Haematological malignancy
- HIV
- Diabetes mellitus
- Chronic alcoholism
- Radiotherapy
- Glucocorticoids, cytotoxic chemotherapy, biologic therapies and other immunosuppressant medication

Local factors

- Tissue damage by suppuration or necrosis
- Alteration of normal bacterial flora by antibiotic therapy

17.57 Classification of bronchopulmonary aspergillosis

- Allergic bronchopulmonary aspergillosis (asthmatic pulmonary eosinophilia)
- Extrinsic allergic alveolitis (*Aspergillus clavatus*)
- Intracavitary aspergilloma
- Invasive pulmonary aspergillosis
- Chronic and subacute pulmonary aspergillosis

17.58 Features of allergic bronchopulmonary aspergillosis

- Asthma (in the majority of cases)
- Proximal bronchiectasis (inner two-thirds of chest CT field)
- Positive skin test to an extract of *Aspergillus fumigatus*
- Elevated total serum immunoglobulin E (IgE) >417 kU/L (1000 ng/mL)
- Elevated *A. fumigatus*-specific IgE or IgG
- Peripheral blood eosinophilia >0.5×10⁹/L
- Presence or history of chest X-ray abnormalities
- Fungal hyphae of *A. fumigatus* on microscopic examination of sputum

Fig. 17.43 Branching *Aspergillus* hyphae seen in allergic bronchopulmonary aspergillosis. The figure shows the use of calcofluor white, a non-specific fluorochrome stain that binds to fungi and fluoresces when exposed to light of the appropriate wavelength. *Aspergillus fumigatus* was subsequently grown on culture. *Courtesy of Mr T. Russell and Dr M. Hanson, Department of Microbiology, NHS Lothian.*

glucocorticoids; a 4-month trial is usually recommended to assess its efficacy. The use of specific anti-IgE monoclonal antibodies is under consideration. Exacerbations, particularly when associated with new chest X-ray changes, should be treated promptly with prednisolone (40–60 mg daily) and physiotherapy. If persistent lobar collapse occurs, bronchoscopy (usually under general anaesthetic) should be performed to remove impacted mucus and ensure prompt re-inflation.

Chronic pulmonary aspergillosis

The term chronic pulmonary aspergillosis (CPA) encompasses simple aspergilloma, chronic cavitary pulmonary aspergillosis, chronic fibrosing pulmonary aspergillosis, *Aspergillus* nodule and semi-invasive aspergillosis. They are uncommon conditions and challenging to diagnose and treat.

Simple aspergilloma

Cavities left by diseases such as TB or by damaged bronchi provide favourable conditions in which inhaled *Aspergillus* may lodge and germinate. At the earliest stage, CT scanning may identify an irregular mucosal wall and, as fungal growth progresses, this finally collapses into the cavity, forming a fungal ball that may be identified on imaging (Fig. 17.44).

Simple aspergillomas are often asymptomatic. They can, however, give rise to a variety of non-specific symptoms, such as lethargy and weight loss, and may cause recurrent haemoptysis, which may be life-threatening.

Fig. 17.44 Computed tomogram of aspergilloma in the left upper lobe. The rounded fungal ball is separated from the wall of the cavity by an 'air crescent' (arrow).

The typical radiological picture is invariably accompanied by elevated serum precipitins/IgG to *A. fumigatus*. Sputum microscopy typically demonstrates scanty hyphal fragments and is usually positive on culture. Less than half exhibit skin hypersensitivity to extracts of *A. fumigatus*. Rarely, other filamentous fungi can cause intracavity mycetoma and are identified by culture.

Asymptomatic cases do not require treatment but haemoptysis should be controlled by surgery. Tranexamic acid or bronchial artery embolisation may provide a bridge to surgery or palliate haemoptysis when surgery is not possible. Instillation of antifungal agents, such as amphotericin B, via a catheter placed into the cavity has been reported but is rarely used in the UK.

Chronic cavitary pulmonary aspergillosis and chronic fibrosing pulmonary aspergillosis

The features of chronic cavitary pulmonary aspergillosis (CCPA) include cough (with or without haemoptysis), weight loss, anorexia and fatigue over months or years, with associated fever, night sweats and elevated inflammatory markers. Radiological features include thick-walled cavities (predominantly apical), pulmonary infiltrates and pleural thickening (Fig. 17.45). Once again, diagnosis rests on a combination of radiological examination, histopathology, isolation of fungus from the respiratory tract and detection of *Aspergillus* IgG in serum. Treatment usually involves prolonged courses of itraconazole or voriconazole. Cure is unusual and the most frequent pattern is chronic relapse/remission with gradual deterioration. Surgical intervention is fraught with complications and should be avoided. Many patients are malnourished and require nutritional support. Glucocorticoids should be avoided. As CCPA progresses, fibrotic destruction of the lung results and the condition may then be referred to as chronic fibrosing pulmonary aspergillosis (CFPA).

Aspergillus *nodule*

The formation of one or more nodules is a less common manifestation of *Aspergillus* infection. In addition to lung cancer, the *Aspergillus* nodule may mimic TB but cavitation is unusual. Cryptococcosis or coccidioidomycosis should be considered in areas where these conditions are endemic.

Subacute invasive aspergillosis

Subacute invasive aspergillosis (SIA) was previously referred to as chronic necrotising or semi-invasive pulmonary aspergillosis.

Fig. 17.45 Chronic pulmonary aspergillosis. [A] The chest X-ray shows pleural thickening with loss of lung volume at the left apex (arrow). [B] High-resolution computed tomography reveals multiple small cavities and pleural thickening with an aspergilloma and surrounding air crescent (arrow) in one of the cavities. *Courtesy of Professor David Denning, National Aspergillosis Centre, Manchester, UK.*

The clinical and radiological picture is similar to CCPA but lung biopsy demonstrates invasion of lung tissue by hyphae. The development of SIA is favoured by mild immunocompromise and should be suspected in patients with diabetes mellitus, malnutrition or alcoholism, or with advanced age and in prolonged glucocorticoid use. It is also seen in the presence of COPD, non-tuberculous mycobacteria or HIV infection. SIA should be treated in a similar manner to invasive pulmonary aspergillosis.

Invasive pulmonary aspergillosis

Invasive pulmonary aspergillosis (IPA) is most commonly a complication of profound neutropenia caused by drugs (especially immunosuppressive agents) and/or disease (Box 17.59).

Clinical features

Acute IPA causes a severe necrotising pneumonia and must be considered in any immunocompromised patient who develops fever, new respiratory symptoms (particularly pleural pain or haemoptysis) or a pleural rub. Invasion of pulmonary vessels causes thrombosis and infarction, and systemic spread may occur

17

17.59 Risk factors for invasive aspergillosis

- Neutropenia: risk related to duration and degree
- Solid organ or allogeneic stem cell transplantation
- Prolonged high-dose glucocorticoid therapy
- Leukaemia and other haematological malignancies
- Cytotoxic chemotherapy
- Advanced HIV disease
- Severe chronic obstructive pulmonary disease
- Critically ill patients on intensive care units
- Chronic granulomatous disease

17.60 Criteria for the diagnosis of probable invasive pulmonary aspergillosis

Host factors

- Recent history of neutropenia ($<0.5\times10^9$/L for ≥10 days) temporally related to the onset of fungal disease
- Recipient of allogeneic stem cell transplant
- Prolonged use of glucocorticoids (average minimum 0.3 mg/kg/day prednisolone or equivalent) for >3 weeks (excludes allergic bronchopulmonary aspergillosis)
- Treatment with other recognised T-cell immune suppressants, such as ciclosporin, tumour necrosis factor, alpha-blockers, specific monoclonal antibodies (e.g. alemtuzumab) or nucleoside analogues during the last 90 days
- Inherited severe immune deficiency, e.g. chronic granulomatous disease or severe combined immune deficiency (p. 79)

Clinical criteria[1]

- The presence of one of the following on CT:
  Dense, well-circumscribed lesion(s) with or without a halo sign
  Air crescent sign
  Cavity

Tracheobronchitis

- Tracheobronchial ulceration, nodule, pseudomembrane, plaque or eschar seen on bronchoscopy

Mycological criteria

- Mould in sputum, BAL fluid or bronchial brush, indicated by one of the following:
  Recovery of fungal elements indicating a mould of *Aspergillus*
  Recovery by culture of a mould of *Aspergillus*
- Indirect tests (detection of antigen or cell wall constituents)
  Galactomannan antigen in plasma, serum or BAL fluid
  β-1,3-glucan detected in serum (detects other species of fungi, as well as *Aspergillus*)[2]

[1]Must be consistent with the mycological findings and temporally related to current episode. [2]May be useful as a preliminary screening tool for invasive aspergillosis.
(BAL = bronchoalveolar lavage)
Adapted from De Pauw B, Walsh TJ, Donnelly JP, et al. Revised definitions of invasive fungal disease from the European Organisation for Research and Treatment of Cancer/Mycoses Study Group. Clin Infect Dis 2008; 46:1813–1821.

to the brain, heart, kidneys and others organs. Tracheobronchial aspergillosis involvement is characterised by the formation of fungal plaques and ulceration.

HRCT characteristically shows macronodules (usually ≥1 cm), which may be surrounded by a 'halo' of intermediate attenuation if captured early (<5 days). Culture or histopathological evidence of *Aspergillus* in diseased tissues provides a definitive diagnosis

but the majority of patients are too ill for invasive tests, such as bronchoscopy or lung biopsy. Other investigations include detection of *Aspergillus* cell-wall components (galactomannan and β-1,3-glucan) in blood or BAL fluid and *Aspergillus* DNA by PCR. Diagnosis is often inferred from a combination of features (Box 17.60).

Management and prevention

IPA carries a high mortality rate, especially if treatment is delayed. The drug of choice is voriconazole. Second-line agents include liposomal amphotericin, caspofungin, posaconazole and isavuconazole. Response may be assessed clinically, radiologically and serologically (by estimation of the circulating galactomannan level). Recovery is dependent on immune reconstitution, which may be accompanied by enlargement and/or cavitation of pulmonary nodules.

Patients at risk of *Aspergillus* (and other fungal infections) should be managed in rooms with high-efficiency particulate air (HEPA) filters and laminar airflow. In areas with high spore counts, patients are advised to wear a mask if venturing outside their hospital room. Posaconazole (200 mg 3 times daily) or itraconazole (200 mg/day) may be prescribed for primary prophylaxis, and patients with a history of definite or probable IPA should be considered for secondary prophylaxis before further immunosuppression.

Other fungal infections

Mucormycosis (p. 303) may present with a pulmonary syndrome that is clinically indistinguishable from acute IPA. Diagnosis relies on histopathology (where available) and/or culture of the organism from diseased tissue. The principles of treatment are as for other forms of mucormycosis: correction of predisposing factors, antifungal therapy with high-dose lipid amphotericin B or posaconazole (second line), and surgical débridement.

The endemic mycoses (histoplasmosis, coccidioidomycosis, blastomycosis and *Emergomyces* infection) and cryptococcosis are discussed on pages 302–304. *Pneumocystis jirovecii* pneumonia is described on page 318.

Tumours of the bronchus and lung

Lung cancer is the most common cause of death from cancer worldwide, causing 1.59 million deaths per year (Box 17.61). Tobacco use is the major preventable cause. Just as tobacco use and cancer rates are falling in some developed countries, both smoking and lung cancer are rising in Eastern Europe and in many developing countries. The great majority of tumours in the lung are primary lung cancers and, in contrast to many other tumours, the prognosis remains poor, with fewer than 30% of patients surviving at 1 year and 6–8% at 5 years.

17.61 The burden of lung cancer

- 1.8 million new cases worldwide each year
- Most common cancer in men
- Rates rising in women:
  Female lung cancer deaths outnumber male in some Nordic countries
  Has overtaken breast cancer in several countries
- More than a threefold increase in deaths since 1950
- More than 50% of cases have metastatic disease at diagnosis

Primary tumours of the lung

Aetiology

Cigarette smoking is by far the most important cause of lung cancer. It is thought to be directly responsible for at least 90% of cases, the risk being proportional to the amount smoked and to the tar content of cigarettes. The death rate from the disease in heavy smokers is 40 times that in non-smokers. Risk falls slowly after smoking cessation but remains above that in non-smokers for many years. It is estimated that 1 in 2 smokers dies from a smoking-related disease, about half in middle age. The effect of 'passive' smoking is more difficult to quantify but is currently thought to be a factor in 5% of all lung cancer deaths. Exposure to naturally occurring radon is another risk. The incidence of lung cancer is slightly higher in urban than in rural dwellers, which may reflect differences in atmospheric pollution (including tobacco smoke) or occupation, since a number of industrial materials are associated with lung cancer (p. 1320). In recent years, the strong link between smoking and ill health has led many governments to legislate against smoking in public places, and smoking prevalence and some smoking-related diseases are already declining in these countries (p. 94).

Lung cancer

The incidence of lung cancer increased dramatically during the 20th century as a direct result of the tobacco epidemic (Fig. 17.46).

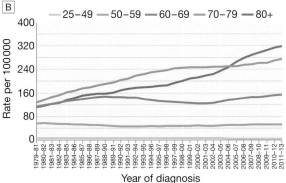

Fig. 17.46 Mortality trends from lung cancer in UK, 1979–2013, by age and year of death. A Males. B Females. Note the decline in mortality from lung cancer in men and increase in mortality in older women towards the end of this period, reflecting changes in smoking habits. *From Cancer Research UK: http://www.cancerresearchuk.org/health-professional/cancer-statistics/statistics-by-cancer-type/lung-cancer/mortality. Accessed January 2017.*

In women, smoking prevalence and deaths from lung cancer continue to increase, and more women now die of lung cancer than breast cancer in the USA and the UK.

Pathology

Lung cancers arise from the bronchial epithelium or mucous glands. The common cell types are listed in Box 17.62. When the tumour occurs in a large bronchus, symptoms arise early but tumours originating in a peripheral bronchus can grow very large without producing symptoms, resulting in delayed diagnosis. Peripheral squamous tumours may undergo central necrosis and cavitation and may resemble a lung abscess on X-ray (Fig. 17.47). Lung cancer may involve the pleura directly or by lymphatic spread and may extend into the chest wall, invading the intercostal nerves or the brachial plexus and causing pain. Lymphatic spread to mediastinal and supraclavicular lymph nodes often occurs before diagnosis. Blood-borne metastases occur most commonly in liver, bone, brain, adrenals and skin. Even a small primary tumour may cause widespread metastatic deposits and this is a particular characteristic of small-cell lung cancers.

Clinical features

Lung cancer presents in many different ways, reflecting local, metastatic or paraneoplastic tumour effects.

Cough This is the most common early symptom. It is often dry but secondary infection may cause purulent sputum. A change in the character of a smoker's cough, particularly if associated with other new symptoms, should always raise suspicion of lung cancer.

Haemoptysis Haemoptysis is common, especially with central bronchial tumours. Although it may be caused by bronchitic

17

i	**17.62 Common cell types in lung cancer**
Cell type	**%**
Adenocarcinoma	35–40
Squamous	25–30
Small-cell	15
Large-cell	10–15

Fig. 17.47 Large cavitated lung cancer in left lower lobe.

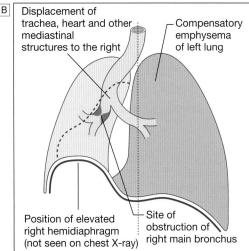

Fig. 17.48 Collapse of the right lung: effects on neighbouring structures. A Chest X-ray. B The typical abnormalities are highlighted.

infection, haemoptysis in a smoker should always be investigated to exclude a lung cancer. Occasionally, central tumours invade large vessels, causing sudden massive haemoptysis that may be fatal.

Bronchial obstruction This is another common presentation. The clinical and radiological manifestations (Figs 17.48 and 17.5, p. 552; Box 17.63) depend on the site and extent of the obstruction, any secondary infection and the extent of coexisting lung disease. Complete obstruction causes collapse of a lobe or lung, with breathlessness, mediastinal displacement and dullness to percussion with reduced breath sounds. Partial bronchial obstruction may cause a monophonic, unilateral wheeze that fails to clear with coughing, and may also impair the drainage of secretions to cause pneumonia or lung abscess as a presenting problem. Pneumonia that recurs at the same site or responds slowly to treatment, particularly in a smoker, should always suggest an underlying lung cancer. Stridor (a harsh inspiratory noise) occurs when the larynx, trachea or a main bronchus is narrowed by the primary tumour or by compression from malignant enlargement of the subcarinal and paratracheal lymph nodes.

17.63 Causes of large bronchus obstruction

Common

- Lung cancer or adenoma
- Enlarged tracheobronchial lymph nodes (malignant or tuberculous)
- Inhaled foreign bodies (especially right lung)
- Bronchial casts or plugs consisting of inspissated mucus or blood clot (especially asthma, cystic fibrosis, haemoptysis, debility)
- Collections of mucus or mucopus retained in the bronchi as a result of ineffective expectoration (especially postoperative following abdominal surgery)

Rare

- Aortic aneurysm
- Giant left atrium
- Pericardial effusion
- Congenital bronchial atresia
- Fibrous bronchial stricture (e.g. following tuberculosis or bronchial surgery/lung transplant)

Breathlessness Breathlessness may be caused by collapse or pneumonia, or by tumour causing a large pleural effusion or compressing a phrenic nerve and leading to diaphragmatic paralysis.

Pain and nerve entrapment Pleural pain may indicate malignant pleural invasion, although it can occur with distal infection. Intercostal nerve involvement causes pain in the distribution of a thoracic dermatome. Cancer in the lung apex may cause Horner's syndrome (ipsilateral partial ptosis, enophthalmos, miosis and hypohidrosis of the face; p. 1091) due to involvement of the sympathetic nerves to the eye at or above the stellate ganglion. Pancoast's syndrome (pain in the inner aspect of the arm, sometimes with small muscle wasting in the hand) indicates malignant destruction of the T1 and C8 roots in the lower part of the brachial plexus by an apical lung tumour.

Mediastinal spread Involvement of the oesophagus may cause dysphagia. If the pericardium is invaded, arrhythmia or pericardial effusion may occur. Superior vena cava obstruction by malignant nodes causes suffusion and swelling of the neck and face, conjunctival oedema, headache and dilated veins on the chest wall and is most commonly due to lung cancer. Involvement of the left recurrent laryngeal nerve by tumours at the left hilum causes vocal cord paralysis, voice alteration and a 'bovine' cough (lacking the normal explosive character). Supraclavicular lymph nodes may be palpably enlarged or identified using ultrasound; if so, a needle aspirate may provide a simple means of cytological diagnosis.

Metastatic spread This may lead to focal neurological defects, epileptic seizures, personality change, jaundice, bone pain or skin nodules. Lassitude, anorexia and weight loss usually indicate metastatic spread.

Finger clubbing Overgrowth of the soft tissue of the terminal phalanx, leading to increased nail curvature and nail bed fluctuation, is often seen (p. 546).

Hypertrophic pulmonary osteoarthropathy (HPOA) This is a painful periostitis of the distal tibia, fibula, radius and ulna, with local tenderness and sometimes pitting oedema over the anterior shin. X-rays reveal subperiosteal new bone formation. While

---

i 17.64 Non-metastatic extrapulmonary manifestations of lung cancer

Endocrine (Ch. 18)

- Inappropriate antidiuretic hormone (ADH, vasopressin) secretion, causing hyponatraemia
- Ectopic adrenocorticotrophic hormone secretion
- Hypercalcaemia due to secretion of parathyroid hormone-related peptides
- Carcinoid syndrome (p. 678)
- Gynaecomastia

Neurological (Ch. 25)

- Polyneuropathy
- Myelopathy
- Cerebellar degeneration
- Myasthenia (Lambert–Eaton syndrome, p. 1142)

Other

- Digital clubbing
- Hypertrophic pulmonary osteoarthropathy
- Nephrotic syndrome
- Polymyositis and dermatomyositis
- Eosinophilia

---

most frequently associated with lung cancer, HPOA can occur with other tumours.

Non-metastatic extrapulmonary effects (Box 17.64) The syndrome of inappropriate antidiuretic hormone secretion (SIADH, p. 357) and ectopic adrenocorticotrophic hormone secretion (p. 670) are usually associated with small-cell lung cancer. Hypercalcaemia may indicate malignant bone destruction or production of hormone-like peptides by a tumour. Associated neurological syndromes may occur with any type of lung cancer.

Investigations

The main aims of investigation are to confirm the diagnosis, establish the histological cell type and define the extent of the disease.

Imaging

Lung cancer produces a range of appearances on chest X-ray, from lobar collapse (see Fig. 17.5, p. 552) to mass lesions, effusion or malignant rib destruction (Fig. 17.49). CT should be performed early, as it may reveal mediastinal or metastatic spread and is helpful for planning biopsy procedures, e.g. in establishing whether a tumour is accessible by bronchoscopy or percutaneous CT-guided biopsy.

Biopsy and histopathology

Over half of primary lung tumours can be visualised and sampled directly by biopsy and brushing using a flexible bronchoscope. Bronchoscopy also allows an assessment of operability, from the proximity of central tumours to the main carina (Fig. 17.50).

For tumours that are too peripheral to be accessible by bronchoscope, the yield of 'blind' bronchoscopic washings and brushings from the radiologically affected area is low and percutaneous needle biopsy under CT or ultrasound guidance is a more reliable way to obtain a histological diagnosis. There is a small risk of iatrogenic pneumothorax, which may preclude the procedure if there is extensive coexisting COPD. In patients with a peripheral tumour and enlarged hilar or paratracheal lymph nodes on CT, bronchoscopy with EBUS-guided node sampling may allow both diagnosis and staging. In those who are unfit

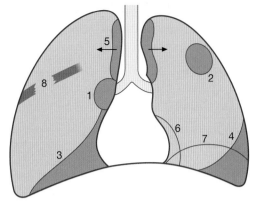

Fig. 17.49 Common radiological presentations of lung cancer.
(1) Unilateral hilar enlargement suggests a central tumour or hilar glandular involvement. However, a peripheral tumour in the apex of a lower lobe can look like an enlarged hilar shadow on the posteroanterior X-ray. (2) Peripheral pulmonary opacity (p. 560) is usually irregular but well circumscribed, and may contain irregular cavitation. It can be very large. (3) Lung, lobe or segmental collapse is usually caused by tumour occluding a proximal bronchus. Collapse may also be due to compression of a bronchus by enlarged lymph glands. (4) Pleural effusion usually indicates tumour invasion of the pleural space or, very rarely, infection in collapsed lung tissue distal to a lung cancer. (5) Paratracheal lymphadenopathy may cause widening of the upper mediastinum. (6) A malignant pericardial effusion may cause enlargement of the cardiac shadow. (7) A raised hemidiaphragm may be caused by phrenic nerve palsy. Screening will show paradoxical upward movement when the patient sniffs. (8) Osteolytic rib destruction indicates direct invasion of the chest wall or metastatic spread.

17

Fig. 17.50 Bronchoscopic view of a lung cancer. There is distortion of mucosal folds, partial occlusion of the airway lumen and abnormal tumour tissue.

for invasive investigation, sputum cytology may reveal malignant cells, although the yield is low.

In patients with pleural effusions, pleural aspiration and biopsy is the preferred investigation. Where facilities exist, thoracoscopy increases yield by allowing targeted biopsies under direct vision. In patients with metastatic disease, the diagnosis can often be confirmed by needle aspiration or biopsy of affected lymph nodes, skin lesions, liver or bone marrow.

Tumour stage	Lymph node spread			
	N0 (None)	N1 (Ipsilateral hilar)	N2 (Ipsilateral mediastinal or subcarinal)	N3 (Contralateral or supraclavicular)
T1a (≤1 cm)	IA1 (92%)	IIB (53%)	IIIA (36%)	IIIB (26%)
T1b (>1 to ≤2 cm)	IA2 (83%)			
T1c (>2 to ≤3 cm)	IA3 (77%)			
T2a (>3 to ≤4 cm)	IB (68%)			
T2b (>4 cm to ≤5 cm)	IIA (60%)			
T3 (>5 cm)	IIB (53%)			
T4 (>7 cm or invading heart, vessels, oesophagus, carina etc.)	IIIA (36%)		IIIB (26%)	IIIC (13%)
M1a Lung metastasis/effusion	IVA (10%)			
M1b Single extrathoracic metastasis				
M1c Multiple extrathoracic metastases	IVB (0%)			

Fig. 17.51 Tumour stage and 5-year survival in non-small-cell lung cancer. The figure shows the relationship between tumour extent (size, lymph node status and metastases) and prognosis (% survival at 5 years for each clinical stage). *Based on data from Detterbeck FC, Boffa DJ, Kim AW, Tanoue T. The eighth edition lung cancer stage classification. Chest 2017; 151:193–203.*

Staging to guide treatment

The propensity of small-cell lung cancer to metastasise early means these patients are usually not suitable for surgical intervention. In non-small-cell lung cancer (NSCLC), treatment and prognosis are determined by disease extent, so careful staging is required. CT is used early to detect obvious local or distant spread. Enlarged upper mediastinal nodes may be sampled using an EBUS-equipped bronchoscope or by mediastinoscopy. Nodes in the lower mediastinum can be sampled through the oesophageal wall using endoscopic ultrasound. Combined CT and whole-body PET (see Fig. 17.6, p. 553) is commonly used to detect occult but metabolically active metastases. Head CT, radionuclide bone scanning, liver ultrasound and bone marrow biopsy are generally reserved for patients with clinical, haematological or biochemical evidence of tumour spread to these sites. Information on tumour size and nodal and metastatic spread is then collated to assign the patient to one of seven staging groups that determine optimal management and prognosis (Fig. 17.51). Detailed physiological testing is required to assess whether respiratory and cardiac function is sufficient to allow aggressive treatment.

Management

Surgical resection carries the best hope of long-term survival but some patients treated with radical radiotherapy and chemotherapy also achieve prolonged remission or cure. In over 75% of cases, treatment with the aim of cure is not possible or is inappropriate due to extensive spread or comorbidity. Such patients are offered palliative therapy and best supportive care. Radiotherapy and, in some cases, chemotherapy can relieve symptoms.

Surgical treatment

Accurate pre-operative staging, coupled with improvements in surgical and post-operative care, now offers 5-year survival rates of over 75% in stage I disease (N0, tumour confined within visceral pleura) and 55% in stage II disease, which includes resection in patients with ipsilateral peribronchial or hilar node involvement.

Radiotherapy

While much less effective than surgery, radical radiotherapy can offer long-term survival in selected patients with localised disease in whom comorbidity precludes surgery. Radical radiotherapy is usually combined with chemotherapy when lymph nodes are involved (stage III). Highly targeted (stereotactic) radiotherapy may be given in 3–5 treatments for small lesions.

The greatest value of radiotherapy, however, is in the palliation of distressing complications, such as superior vena cava obstruction, recurrent haemoptysis, and pain caused by chest wall invasion or by skeletal metastatic deposits. Obstruction of the trachea and main bronchi can also be relieved temporarily. Radiotherapy can be used in conjunction with chemotherapy in the treatment of small-cell carcinoma and is particularly efficient at preventing the development of brain metastases in patients who have had a complete response to chemotherapy (p. 1331).

Chemotherapy

The treatment of small-cell carcinoma with combinations of cytotoxic drugs, sometimes with radiotherapy, can increase median survival from 3 months to well over a year. The use of combinations of chemotherapeutic drugs requires considerable skill and should be overseen by multidisciplinary teams of clinical oncologists and specialist nurses. Combination chemotherapy leads to better outcomes than single-agent treatment. Regular cycles of therapy, including combinations of intravenous cyclophosphamide, doxorubicin and vincristine or intravenous cisplatin and etoposide, are commonly used.

In NSCLC chemotherapy is less effective, though platinum-based chemotherapy regimens offer 30% response rates and a modest increase in survival, and are widely used. Some non-small-cell lung tumours, particularly adenocarcinomas in non-smokers, carry detectable mutations, e.g. in the epidermal growth factor receptor (*EGFR*) gene. Tyrosine kinase inhibitors, such as erlotinib and monoclonal antibodies to EGFR (e.g. bevacizumab), show improved treatment responses in metastatic

NSCLC and *EGFR* mutations, and similar approaches are being developed to target other known genetic abnormalities.

In NSCLC there is some evidence that chemotherapy given before surgery may increase survival and can effectively 'down-stage' disease with limited nodal spread. Post-operative chemotherapy is now proven to enhance survival rates when operative samples show nodal involvement by tumour.

Nausea and vomiting are common side-effects of chemotherapy and are best treated with 5-HT$_3$ receptor antagonists (p. 1353).

Laser therapy and stenting

Palliation of symptoms caused by major airway obstruction can be achieved in selected patients using bronchoscopic laser treatment to clear tumour tissue and allow re-aeration of collapsed lung. The best results are achieved in tumours of the main bronchi. Endobronchial stents can be used to maintain airway patency in the face of extrinsic compression by malignant nodes.

General aspects of management

The best outcomes are obtained when lung cancer is managed in specialist centres by multidisciplinary teams, including oncologists, thoracic surgeons, respiratory physicians and specialist nurses. Effective communication, pain relief and attention to diet are important. Lung tumours can cause clinically significant depression and anxiety, and these may need specific therapy. The management of non-metastatic endocrine manifestations is described in Chapter 18. When a malignant pleural effusion is present, an attempt should be made to drain the pleural cavity using an intercostal drain; provided that the lung fully re-expands, pleurodesis with a sclerosing agent, such as talc, should be performed to prevent recurrent effusion.

Prognosis

The overall prognosis in lung cancer is very poor, 70% of patients dying within a year of diagnosis and only 6–8% surviving 5 years after diagnosis. The best prognosis is with well-differentiated squamous cell tumours that have not metastasised and are amenable to surgical resection. The clinical features and prognosis of some less common tumours are given in Box 17.65.

Secondary tumours of the lung

Blood-borne metastatic deposits in the lungs may be derived from many primary carcinomas, in particular breast, kidney, uterus, ovary, testes and thyroid, and also from osteogenic and other sarcomas. These secondary deposits are usually multiple and bilateral. Often there are no respiratory symptoms and the diagnosis is incidental on X-ray. Breathlessness may occur if a considerable amount of lung tissue has been replaced by metastatic tumour. Endobronchial deposits are uncommon but can cause haemoptysis and lobar collapse.

Lymphatic infiltration may develop in carcinoma of the breast, stomach, bowel, pancreas or bronchus. 'Lymphangitic carcinomatosis' causes severe, rapidly progressive breathlessness with marked hypoxaemia. The chest X-ray shows diffuse pulmonary shadowing radiating from the hilar regions, often with septal lines, and CT shows characteristic polygonal thickened interlobular septa. Palliation of breathlessness with opiates may help (p. 1353).

Tumours of the mediastinum

Figure 17.52 shows the major compartments of the mediastinum and Box 17.66 lists likely causes of a mediastinal mass.

i 17.66 Causes of a mediastinal mass

Superior mediastinum

- Retrosternal goitre
- Persistent left superior vena cava
- Prominent left subclavian artery
- Thymic tumour
- Dermoid cyst
- Lymphoma
- Aortic aneurysm

Anterior mediastinum

- Retrosternal goitre
- Dermoid cyst
- Thymic tumour
- Lymphoma
- Aortic aneurysm
- Germ cell tumour
- Pericardial cyst
- Hiatus hernia through the diaphragmatic foramen of Morgagni

Posterior mediastinum

- Neurogenic tumour
- Paravertebral abscess
- Oesophageal lesion
- Aortic aneurysm
- Foregut duplication

Middle mediastinum

- Lung cancer
- Lymphoma
- Sarcoidosis
- Bronchogenic cyst
- Hiatus hernia

i 17.65 Rare types of lung tumour				
Tumour	**Status**	**Histology**	**Typical presentation**	**Prognosis**
Adenosquamous carcinoma	Malignant	Tumours with areas of unequivocal squamous and adeno-differentiation	Peripheral or central lung mass	Stage-dependent
Neuro-endocrine (carcinoid) tumour (p. 678)	Low-grade malignant	Neuro-endocrine differentiation	Bronchial obstruction, cough	95% 5-year survival with resection
Bronchial gland adenoma	Benign	Salivary gland differentiation	Tracheobronchial irritation/obstruction	Local resection curative
Bronchial gland carcinoma	Low-grade malignant	Salivary gland differentiation	Tracheobronchial irritation/obstruction	Local recurrence
Hamartoma	Benign	Mesenchymal cells, cartilage	Peripheral lung nodule	Local resection curative
Bronchoalveolar carcinoma	Malignant	Tumour cells line alveolar spaces	Alveolar shadowing, productive cough	Variable, worse if multifocal

Fig. 17.52 The divisions of the mediastinum. (1) Superior mediastinum. (2) Anterior mediastinum. (3) Middle mediastinum. (4) Posterior mediastinum. Sites of the more common mediastinal tumours are also illustrated. *From Johnson N McL. Respiratory medicine. Oxford: Blackwell Science; 1986.*

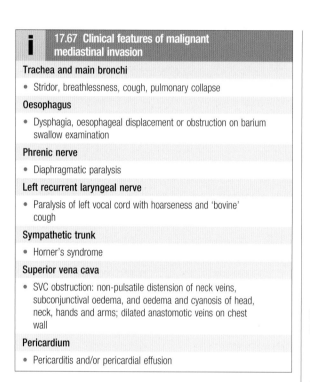

i 17.67 Clinical features of malignant mediastinal invasion

Trachea and main bronchi

• Stridor, breathlessness, cough, pulmonary collapse

Oesophagus

• Dysphagia, oesophageal displacement or obstruction on barium swallow examination

Phrenic nerve

• Diaphragmatic paralysis

Left recurrent laryngeal nerve

• Paralysis of left vocal cord with hoarseness and 'bovine' cough

Sympathetic trunk

• Horner's syndrome

Superior vena cava

• SVC obstruction: non-pulsatile distension of neck veins, subconjunctival oedema, and oedema and cyanosis of head, neck, hands and arms; dilated anastomotic veins on chest wall

Pericardium

• Pericarditis and/or pericardial effusion

Fig. 17.53 Intrathoracic goitre (arrows) extending from right upper mediastinum.

Benign tumours and cysts in the mediastinum are often diagnosed when a chest X-ray is undertaken for some other reason. In general, they do not invade vital structures but may cause symptoms by compressing the trachea or the superior vena cava. A dermoid cyst may very occasionally rupture into a bronchus.

Malignant mediastinal tumours are distinguished by their power to invade, as well as compress, surrounding structures. As a result, even a small malignant tumour can produce symptoms, although, more commonly, the tumour has attained a considerable size before this happens (Box 17.67). The most common cause is mediastinal lymph node metastasis from lung cancer but lymphomas, leukaemia, malignant thymic tumours and germ-cell tumours can cause similar features. Aortic and innominate aneurysms have destructive features resembling those of malignant mediastinal tumours.

Investigations

A benign mediastinal tumour generally appears on chest X-ray as a sharply circumscribed mediastinal opacity encroaching on one or both lung fields (Fig. 17.53). CT (or MRI) is the investigation of choice for mediastinal tumours (e.g. see Fig. 18.12, p. 648). A malignant mediastinal tumour seldom has a clearly defined margin and often presents as a general broadening of the mediastinum.

Bronchoscopy may reveal a primary lung cancer causing mediastinal lymphadenopathy. EBUS may be used to guide sampling of peribronchial masses. The posterior mediastinum can be imaged and biopsied via the oesophagus using endoscopic ultrasound (p. 553).

Mediastinoscopy under general anaesthetic can be used to visualise and biopsy masses in the superior and anterior mediastinum but surgical exploration of the chest, with removal of part or all of the tumour, is often required to obtain a histological diagnosis.

Management

Benign mediastinal tumours should be removed surgically because most produce symptoms sooner or later. Cysts may become infected, while neural tumours have the potential to undergo malignant transformation. The operative mortality is low in the absence of coexisting cardiovascular disease, COPD or extreme age.

Interstitial and infiltrative pulmonary diseases

Diffuse parenchymal lung disease

The diffuse parenchymal lung diseases (DPLDs) are a heterogeneous group of conditions affecting the pulmonary parenchyma (interstitium) and/or alveolar lumen, which are frequently considered collectively as they share a sufficient number of clinical physiological and radiographic similarities (Box 17.68).

17.68 Features common to the diffuse parenchymal lung diseases

Clinical presentation

- Cough: usually dry, persistent and distressing
- Breathlessness: usually slowly progressive; insidious onset; acute in some cases

Examination findings

- Crackles: typically bilateral and basal
- Clubbing: common in idiopathic pulmonary fibrosis but also seen in other types, e.g. asbestosis
- Central cyanosis and signs of right heart failure in advanced disease

Radiology

- Chest X-ray: typically small lung volumes with reticulonodular shadowing but may be normal in early or limited disease
- High-resolution computed tomography: combinations of ground glass changes, reticulonodular shadowing, honeycomb cysts and traction bronchiectasis, depending on stage of disease

Pulmonary function

- Typically restrictive ventilatory defect with reduced lung volumes and impaired gas transfer; exercise tests assess exercise tolerance and exercise-related fall in SaO_2

They often present with cough, which is typically dry and distressing, and breathlessness, which is often insidious in onset but thereafter relentlessly progressive. Physical examination reveals the presence of inspiratory crackles and in many cases digital clubbing develops. Pulmonary function tests typically show a restrictive ventilatory defect in the presence of small lung volumes and reduced gas transfer. The typical radiographic findings include, in the earliest stages, ground glass and reticulonodular shadowing, with progression to honeycomb cysts and traction bronchiectasis. While these appearances may be seen on a 'plain' chest X-ray, they are most easily appreciated on HRCT, which has assumed a central role in the evaluation of DPLD (Fig. 17.54). The current classification is shown in Figure 17.55 and the potential differential diagnoses in Box 17.69.

Idiopathic interstitial pneumonias

The idiopathic interstitial pneumonias represent a major subgroup of DPLD that are grouped together as a result of their unknown aetiology (Box 17.70). They are often distinguished by the predominant histological pattern on tissue biopsy; hence they are frequently referred to by their pathological description, e.g. usual interstitial pneumonia (UIP) or non-specific interstitial pneumonia (NSIP). The most important of these is idiopathic pulmonary fibrosis.

Idiopathic pulmonary fibrosis

Idiopathic pulmonary fibrosis is defined as a progressive fibrosing interstitial pneumonia of unknown cause, occurring in adults and associated with the histological or radiological pattern of UIP. Important differentials include fibrosing diseases caused

17.69 Conditions that mimic diffuse parenchymal lung disease	
Infection	
• Viral pneumonia	• Tuberculosis
• *Pneumocystis jirovecii*	• Parasite, e.g. filariasis
• *Mycoplasma pneumoniae*	• Fungal infection
Malignancy	
• Leukaemia and lymphoma	• Multiple metastases
• Lymphangitic carcinomatosis	• Bronchoalveolar carcinoma
Pulmonary oedema	
Aspiration pneumonitis	

17

Fig. 17.54 Algorithm for the investigation of patients with interstitial lung disease following initial clinical and chest X-ray examination.

Fig. 17.55 Classification of diffuse parenchymal lung disease.

i	**17.70 Idiopathic interstitial pneumonias**
Clinical diagnosis	**Notes**
Usual interstitial pneumonia (UIP)	Idiopathic pulmonary fibrosis – see text
Non-specific interstitial pneumonia (NSIP)	See page 608
Respiratory bronchiolitis–interstitial lung disease	More common in men and smokers. Usually presents at age 40–60 years. Smoking cessation may lead to improvement. Natural history unclear
Acute interstitial pneumonia	Often preceded by viral upper respiratory tract infection. Severe exertional dyspnoea, widespread pneumonic consolidation and diffuse alveolar damage on biopsy. Prognosis often poor
Desquamative interstitial pneumonia (DIP)	More common in men and smokers. Presents at age 40–60 years. Insidious onset of dyspnoea. Clubbing in 50%. Biopsy shows increased macrophages in alveolar space, septal thickening and type II pneumocyte hyperplasia. Prognosis generally good
Cryptogenic organising pneumonia ('bronchiolitis obliterans organising pneumonia' – BOOP)	Presents as clinical and radiological pneumonia. Systemic features and markedly raised erythrocyte sedimentation rate common. Finger clubbing absent. Biopsy shows florid proliferation of immature collagen (Masson bodies) and fibrous tissue. Response to glucocorticoids classically excellent
Lymphocytic interstitial pneumonia (LIP)	More common in women, slow onset over years. Investigate for associations with connective tissue disease or HIV. Unclear whether glucocorticoids are helpful

by occupational exposure, medication or connective tissue diseases, which must be excluded by careful history, examination and investigation.

The histological features of the condition are suggestive of repeated episodes of focal damage to the alveolar epithelium consistent with an autoimmune process but the aetiology remains elusive: speculation has included exposure to viruses (e.g. Epstein–Barr virus), occupational dusts (metal or wood), drugs (antidepressants) or chronic gastro-oesophageal reflux. Familial cases are rare but genetic factors that control the inflammatory and fibrotic response are likely to be important. There is a strong association with cigarette smoking.

Clinical features

IPF usually presents in the older adult and is uncommon before the age of 50 years. With the advent of widespread CT scanning it may present as an incidental finding in an otherwise asymptomatic individual but more typically presents with progressive breathlessness (which may have been insidious) and a non-productive cough. Constitutional symptoms are unusual. Clinical findings include finger clubbing and the presence of bi-basal fine late inspiratory crackles likened to the unfastening of Velcro.

Investigations

These are summarised in Box 17.71. Established IPF will be apparent on chest X-ray as a bilateral lower lobe and subpleural reticular shadowing. The chest X-ray may be normal in individuals with early or limited disease, however. HRCT typically demonstrates a patchy, predominantly peripheral, subpleural and basal reticular pattern and, in more advanced disease, the presence of honeycombing cysts and traction bronchiectasis

17.71 Investigations in diffuse parenchymal lung disease

Laboratory investigations

- Full blood count: lymphopenia in sarcoid; eosinophilia in pulmonary eosinophilias and drug reactions; neutrophilia in hypersensitivity pneumonitis
- Ca^{2+}: may be elevated in sarcoid
- Lactate dehydrogenase: may be elevated in active alveolitis
- Serum angiotensin-converting enzyme: non-specific indicator of disease activity in sarcoid
- Erythrocyte sedimentation rate and C-reactive protein: non-specifically raised
- Autoimmune screen: anti-cyclic citrullinated peptide (anti-CCP) and other autoantibodies may suggest connective tissue disease

Radiology

- See Box 17.68

Pulmonary function

- See Box 17.68

Bronchoscopy

- Bronchoalveolar lavage: differential cell counts may point to sarcoid and drug-induced pneumonitis, pulmonary eosinophilias, hypersensitivity pneumonitis or cryptogenic organising pneumonia; useful to exclude infection
- Transbronchial biopsy: useful in sarcoid and differential of malignancy or infection
- Bronchial biopsy: occasionally useful in sarcoid

Video-assisted thoracoscopic lung biopsy (in selected cases)

- Allows pathological classification: presence of asbestos bodies may suggest asbestosis; silica in occupational fibrosing lung disease

Others

- Liver biopsy: may be useful in sarcoidosis
- Urinary calcium excretion: may be useful in sarcoidosis

Fig. 17.56 Idiopathic pulmonary fibrosis. Typical high-resolution CT images demonstrate the bilateral, predominantly basal and peripheral reticular opacities, accompanied by honeycombing in the later stages. A Anteroposterior view. B Transverse section. *Courtesy of Dr Andrew Baird, Consultant Radiologist, NHS Lothian, Edinburgh, UK.*

(Fig. 17.56). When these features are present, HRCT has a high positive predictive value for the diagnosis of IPF and recourse to biopsy is seldom necessary. HRCT appearances may also be sufficiently characteristic to suggest an alternative diagnosis such as hypersensitivity pneumonitis (p. 616) or sarcoidosis (p. 608). The presence of pleural plaques may suggest asbestosis (p. 618).

Pulmonary function tests classically show a restrictive defect with reduced lung volumes and gas transfer. However, lung volumes may be preserved in patients with concomitant emphysema. Dynamic tests are useful to document exercise tolerance and demonstrate exercise-induced arterial hypoxaemia, but as IPF advances, arterial hypoxaemia and hypocapnia are present at rest.

Bronchoscopy is seldom indicated unless there is serious consideration of differential diagnoses of infection or a malignant process; lymphocytosis may suggest chronic hypersensitivity pneumonitis. The tissue samples obtained by transbronchial lung biopsy are invariably insufficient to be of value, and if tissue is required, a surgical lung biopsy should be sought. Lung biopsy should be considered in cases of diagnostic uncertainty or with atypical features. UIP is the histological pattern predominantly encountered in IPF (Fig. 17.57); however, it is also found in asbestosis, hypersensitivity pneumonitis, connective tissue diseases and drug reactions.

It is not uncommon to identify a mildly positive antinuclear antibody (ANA) or anti-cyclic citrullinated peptide 2 (anti-CCP2) and repeat serological testing may be performed, as lung disease may precede the appearance of connective tissue disease.

Management

The management options for IPF are improving. If the vital capacity is between 50% and 80% predicted, patients may be offered either pirfenidone (an antifibrotic agent) or nintedanib (a tyrosine kinase inhibitor). Both of these agents have been shown to reduce the rate of decline in lung function. Patients taking pirfenidone should be advised to avoid direct exposure to sunlight and use photoprotective clothing and high-protection sunscreens. Nintedanib may be accompanied by diarrhoea. Neither drug improves cough or breathlessness and treatment should be discontinued if lung function declines by more than 10% over the first year of treatment. Medication to control gastro-oesophageal reflux may improve the cough. Current smokers should be apprised of the increased risk of lung cancer and advised to stop. Influenza and pneumococcal vaccination should be recommended. Patients should be encouraged to exercise and participate in pulmonary rehabilitation using ambulatory oxygen if appropriate. Domiciliary oxygen should be considered for palliation of breathlessness in severe cases. Where appropriate, lung transplantation should be considered. The optimum treatment for acute exacerbations is unknown. Treatment is largely supportive. Broad-spectrum antibiotics may

Fig. 17.57 Pathology of usual interstitial pneumonia. [A] Lung tissue showing subpleural scarring, most prominently down the posterior edge of the lower lobe. This distribution of fibrosis is typical of usual interstitial pneumonitis. The fibrosis may be associated with prominent cystic change known as 'honeycomb lung'. [B] Histology showing severe interstitial fibrosis with loss of the normal alveolar architecture and the development of 'honeycomb' cysts. *Courtesy of Dr William Wallace, Department of Pathology, Royal Infirmary of Edinburgh.*

be combined with glucocorticoids and sometimes additional immunosuppression but there are few data to support this approach.

Prognosis

The natural history is usually one of steady decline; however, some patients are prone to exacerbations accompanied by an acute deterioration in breathlessness, disturbed gas exchange, and new ground glass changes or consolidation on HRCT. In advanced disease, central cyanosis is detectable and patients may develop pulmonary hypertension and features of right heart failure. A median survival of 3 years is widely quoted; the rate of disease progression varies considerably, however, from death within a few months to survival with minimal symptoms for many years. Serial lung function testing may provide useful prognostic information, relative preservation of lung function suggesting longer survival and significantly impaired gas transfer and/or desaturation on exercise heralding a poorer prognosis. The finding of high numbers of fibroblastic foci on biopsy suggests a more rapid deterioration.

Non-specific interstitial pneumonia

The clinical picture of fibrotic NSIP is similar to that of IPF, although patients tend to be women and younger in age. As with UIP, the condition may present as an isolated idiopathic pulmonary condition, but an NSIP pattern is often associated with connective tissue disease, certain drugs, chronic hypersensitivity pneumonitis or HIV infection and care must be taken to exclude these possibilities. As with UIP, the pulmonary condition may precede the appearance of connective tissue disease. HRCT findings are less specific than with IPF and lung biopsy may be required. The prognosis is significantly better than that of IPF, particularly in the cellular form of the condition, and the 5-year mortality rate is typically less than 15%.

Sarcoidosis

Sarcoidosis is a multisystem granulomatous disorder of unknown aetiology that is characterised by the presence of non-caseating granulomas (Fig. 17.58). The condition is more frequently described in colder parts of northern Europe. It also appears to be more common and more severe in those from a West Indian or Asian background; Eskimos, Arabs and Chinese are

Fig. 17.58 Sarcoidosis of the lung. Histology showing non-caseating granulomas (arrows). *Courtesy of Dr William Wallace, Department of Pathology, Royal Infirmary of Edinburgh.*

rarely affected. The tendency for sarcoid to present in the spring and summer has led to speculation about the role of infective agents, including mycobacteria, propionibacteria and viruses, but the cause remains elusive. Genetic susceptibility is supported by familial clustering; a range of class II HLA alleles confer protection from, or susceptibility to, the condition. Sarcoidosis occurs less frequently in smokers. It may be associated with common variable immunodeficiency (p. 79).

Clinical features

Sarcoidosis is considered with other DPLDs, as over 90% of cases affect the lungs, but the condition can involve almost any organ (Fig. 17.59 and Box 17.72). Löfgren's syndrome – an acute illness characterised by erythema nodosum, peripheral arthropathy, uveitis, bilateral hilar lymphadenopathy (BHL), lethargy and occasionally fever – is often seen in young women. Alternatively, BHL may be detected in an otherwise asymptomatic individual undergoing a chest X-ray for other purposes. Pulmonary disease may also present in a more insidious manner with cough, exertional breathlessness and radiographic infiltrates; chest auscultation is often surprisingly unremarkable. Fibrosis

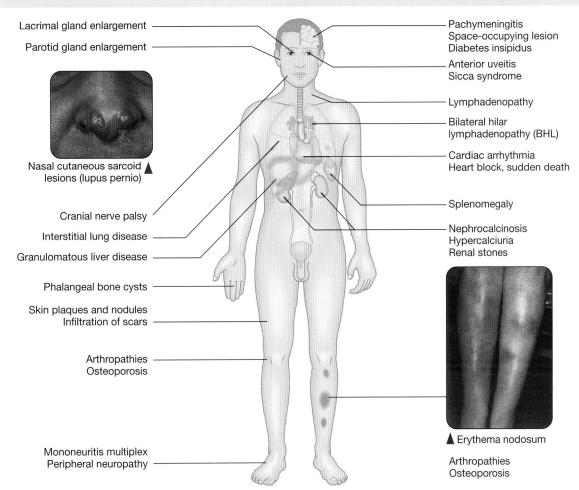

Lacrimal gland enlargement

Parotid gland enlargement

Nasal cutaneous sarcoid ▲
lesions (lupus pernio)

Cranial nerve palsy

Interstitial lung disease

Granulomatous liver disease

Phalangeal bone cysts

Skin plaques and nodules
Infiltration of scars

Arthropathies
Osteoporosis

Mononeuritis multiplex
Peripheral neuropathy

Pachymeningitis
Space-occupying lesion
Diabetes insipidus

Anterior uveitis
Sicca syndrome

Lymphadenopathy

Bilateral hilar
lymphadenopathy (BHL)

Cardiac arrhythmia
Heart block, sudden death

Splenomegaly

Nephrocalcinosis
Hypercalciuria
Renal stones

▲ Erythema nodosum

Arthropathies
Osteoporosis

17

Fig. 17.59 Possible systemic involvement in sarcoidosis. *Inset (Erythema nodosum): From Savin JA, Hunter JAA, Hepburn NC. Skin signs in clinical medicine. London: Mosby–Wolfe; 1997.*

17.72 Presentation of sarcoidosis

- Asymptomatic: abnormal routine chest X-ray (~30%) or abnormal liver function tests
- Respiratory and constitutional symptoms (20–30%)
- Erythema nodosum and arthralgia (20–30%)
- Ocular symptoms (5–10%)
- Skin sarcoid (including lupus pernio) (5%)
- Superficial lymphadenopathy (5%)
- Other (1%), e.g. hypercalcaemia, diabetes insipidus, cranial nerve palsies, cardiac arrhythmias, nephrocalcinosis

17.73 Chest X-ray changes in sarcoidosis

Stage I: BHL (usually symmetrical); paratracheal nodes often enlarged
- Often asymptomatic but may be associated with erythema nodosum and arthralgia. The majority of cases resolve spontaneously within 1 year

Stage II: BHL and parenchymal infiltrates
- Patients may present with breathlessness or cough. The majority of cases resolve spontaneously

Stage III: parenchymal infiltrates without BHL
- Disease less likely to resolve spontaneously

Stage IV: pulmonary fibrosis
- Can cause progression to ventilatory failure, pulmonary hypertension and cor pulmonale

(BHL = bilateral hilar lymphadenopathy)

occurs in around 20% of cases of pulmonary sarcoidosis and may cause a silent loss of lung function. Pleural disease is uncommon and finger clubbing is not a feature. Complications such as bronchiectasis, aspergilloma, pneumothorax, pulmonary hypertension and cor pulmonale have been reported but are rare.

Investigations

Lymphopenia is characteristic and liver function tests may be mildly deranged. Hypercalcaemia may be present (reflecting increased formation of calcitriol – 1,25-dihydroxyvitamin D – by alveolar macrophages), particularly if the patient has been exposed to strong sunlight. Hypercalciuria may also be seen and may lead to nephrocalcinosis. Serum angiotensin-converting enzyme (ACE)

may provide a non-specific marker of disease activity and can assist in monitoring the clinical course. Chest radiography has been used to stage sarcoid (Box 17.73). In patients with pulmonary infiltrates, pulmonary function testing may show a restrictive defect accompanied by impaired gas exchange. Exercise tests may reveal oxygen desaturation. Bronchoscopy may demonstrate a 'cobblestone' appearance of the mucosa, and bronchial and transbronchial biopsies usually show non-caseating granulomas, as may samples from the mediastinal nodes obtained by EBUS. Bronchoalveolar lavage fluid typically contains an increased CD4:CD8 T-cell ratio. Characteristic HRCT appearances include reticulonodular opacities that follow a perilymphatic distribution centred on bronchovascular bundles and the subpleural areas. PET scanning can detect extrapulmonary disease.

The occurrence of erythema nodosum with BHL on chest X-ray is often sufficient for a confident diagnosis, without recourse to a tissue biopsy. Similarly, a typical presentation with classical HRCT features may also be accepted. In other instances, however, the diagnosis should be confirmed by histological examination of the involved organ. The presence of anergy (e.g. to tuberculin skin tests) may support the diagnosis.

Management

Patients who present with acute illness and erythema nodosum should receive NSAIDs and, on occasion, a short course of glucocorticoids. The majority of patients enjoy spontaneous remission and so, if there is no evidence of organ damage, systemic glucocorticoid therapy can be withheld for 6 months. However, prednisolone (at a starting dose of 20–40 mg/day) should be commenced immediately in the presence of hypercalcaemia, pulmonary impairment, renal impairment and uveitis. Topical glucocorticoids may be useful in cases of mild uveitis, and inhaled glucocorticoids have been used to shorten the duration of systemic glucocorticoid use in asymptomatic parenchymal sarcoid. Patients should be warned that strong sunlight may precipitate hypercalcaemia and endanger renal function.

Features suggesting a less favourable outlook include age over 40, Afro-Caribbean ethnicity, persistent symptoms for more than 6 months, the involvement of more than three organs, lupus pernio (see Fig. 17.59) and a stage III/IV chest X-ray. In patients with severe disease, methotrexate (10–20 mg/week), azathioprine (50–150 mg/day) and specific tumour necrosis factor alpha (TNF-α) inhibitors (p. 1006) have been effective. Chloroquine, hydroxychloroquine and low-dose thalidomide may be useful in cutaneous sarcoid with limited pulmonary involvement. Selected patients may be referred for consideration of single lung transplantation. The overall mortality is low (1–5%) and usually reflects cardiac involvement or pulmonary fibrosis.

Lung diseases due to systemic inflammatory disease

The acute respiratory distress syndrome

See page 198.

Respiratory involvement in connective tissue disorders

Pulmonary complications of connective tissue disease are common, affecting the airways, alveoli, pulmonary vasculature, diaphragm and chest wall muscles, and the chest wall itself. In some instances, pulmonary disease may precede the appearance of the connective tissue disorder (Box 17.74). Indirect associations between connective tissue disorders and respiratory complications include those due to disease in other organs, e.g. thrombocytopenia causing haemoptysis; pulmonary toxic effects of drugs used to treat the connective tissue disorder (e.g. gold and methotrexate); and secondary infection due to the disease itself, neutropenia or immunosuppressive drug regimens.

Rheumatoid disease

Pulmonary involvement in rheumatoid disease is important, accounting for around 10–20% of the mortality associated with the condition (p. 1021). The majority of cases occur within 5 years of the rheumatological diagnosis but pulmonary manifestations may precede joint involvement in 10–20%. Pulmonary fibrosis is the most common pulmonary manifestation. All forms of interstitial disease have been described but NSIP is probably the most common. A rare variant of localised upper lobe fibrosis and cavitation is occasionally seen.

Pleural effusion is common, especially in men with seropositive disease. Effusions are usually small and unilateral, but can be large and bilateral. Most resolve spontaneously. Biochemical testing shows an exudate with markedly reduced glucose levels and raised lactate dehydrogenase (LDH). Effusions that fail to resolve spontaneously may respond to a short course of oral prednisolone (30–40 mg daily) but some become chronic.

Rheumatoid pulmonary nodules are usually asymptomatic and detected incidentally on imaging. They are most often multiple and subpleural in site (Fig. 17.60). Solitary nodules can mimic primary lung cancer; when multiple, the differential

i	**17.74 Respiratory complications of connective tissue disorders**				
Disorder	**Airways**	**Parenchyma**	**Pleura**	**Diaphragm and chest wall**
Rheumatoid arthritis	Bronchitis, obliterative bronchiolitis, bronchiectasis, crico-arytenoid arthritis, stridor	Pulmonary fibrosis, nodules, upper lobe fibrosis, infections	Pleurisy, effusion, pneumothorax	Poor healing of intercostal drain sites
Systemic lupus erythematosus	–	Pulmonary fibrosis, 'vasculitic' infarcts	Pleurisy, effusion	Diaphragmatic weakness (shrinking lungs)
Systemic sclerosis	Bronchiectasis	Pulmonary fibrosis, aspiration pneumonia	–	Cutaneous thoracic restriction (hidebound chest)
Dermatomyositis/polymyositis	Lung cancer	Pulmonary fibrosis	–	Intercostal and diaphragmatic myopathy
Granulomatosis with polyangiitis	Epistaxis, nasal discharge crusting, subglottic stenosis	Pulmonary nodules that may cavitate	Pleurisy, effusion	–

Fig. 17.60 Rheumatoid (necrobiotic) nodules. Thoracic CT just below the level of the main carina, showing the typical appearance of peripheral pleural-based nodules (arrows). The nodule in the left lower lobe shows characteristic cavitation.

diagnoses include pulmonary metastatic disease. Cavitation raises the possibility of TB and predisposes to pneumothorax. The combination of rheumatoid nodules and pneumoconiosis is known as Caplan's syndrome (p. 615).

Bronchitis and bronchiectasis are both more common in rheumatoid patients. Rarely, the potentially fatal condition called obliterative bronchiolitis may develop. Bacterial lower respiratory tract infections are frequent. Treatments given for rheumatoid arthritis may also be relevant: glucocorticoid therapy predisposes to infections, methotrexate may cause pulmonary fibrosis, and anti-TNF therapy has been associated with the reactivation of TB.

Systemic lupus erythematosus

Pleuropulmonary involvement is more common in lupus than in any other connective tissue disorder and may be a presenting problem, when it is sometimes attributed incorrectly to infection or pulmonary embolism. Up to two-thirds of patients have repeated episodes of pleurisy, with or without effusions. Effusions may be bilateral and may also involve the pericardium.

The most serious manifestation of lupus is an acute alveolitis that may be associated with diffuse alveolar haemorrhage. This condition is life-threatening and requires either immediate immunosuppression with glucocorticoids or a step-up in immunosuppressive treatment, if already started.

Pulmonary fibrosis is a relatively uncommon manifestation of systemic lupus erythematosus (SLE). Some patients with SLE present with exertional dyspnoea and orthopnoea but without overt signs of pulmonary fibrosis. The chest X-ray reveals elevated diaphragms and pulmonary function testing shows reduced lung volumes. This condition has been described as 'shrinking lungs' and has been attributed to diaphragmatic myopathy.

SLE patients with antiphospholipid antibodies are at increased risk of venous and pulmonary thromboembolism and require life-long anticoagulation.

Systemic sclerosis

Most patients with systemic sclerosis (p. 1037) eventually develop diffuse pulmonary fibrosis; at necropsy more than 90% have evidence of lung fibrosis. In some patients it is indolent, but when progressive, as in IPF, the median survival time is around 4 years. Pulmonary fibrosis is rare in the CREST variant of progressive systemic sclerosis but isolated pulmonary hypertension may develop.

Other pulmonary complications include recurrent aspiration pneumonias secondary to oesophageal disease. Rarely, sclerosis of the skin of the chest wall may be so extensive and cicatrising as to restrict chest wall movement – the so-called 'hidebound chest'.

Pulmonary eosinophilia and vasculitides

Pulmonary eosinophilia refers to the association of radiographic (usually pneumonic) abnormalities and peripheral blood eosinophilia. The term encompasses a group of disorders of different aetiology (Box 17.75). Eosinophils are the predominant cell recovered in sputum or BAL, and eosinophil products are likely to the prime mediators of tissue damage.

Acute eosinophilic pneumonia

Acute eosinophilic pneumonia is an acute febrile illness (of less than 5 days' duration), characterised by diffuse pulmonary infiltrates and hypoxic respiratory failure. The pathology is usually that of diffuse alveolar damage. Diagnosis is confirmed by BAL, which characteristically demonstrates >25% eosinophils. The condition is usually idiopathic but drug reactions should be considered. Glucocorticoids invariably induce prompt and complete resolution.

Chronic eosinophilic pneumonia

Chronic eosinophilic pneumonia typically presents in an insidious manner with malaise, fever, weight loss, breathlessness and unproductive cough. It is more common in middle-aged females. The classical chest X-ray appearance has been likened to the photographic negative of pulmonary oedema with bilateral, peripheral and predominantly upper lobe parenchymal shadowing. The peripheral blood eosinophil count is almost always very high, and the erythrocyte sedimentation rate (ESR) and total serum IgE are elevated. BAL reveals a high proportion of eosinophils

17.75 Pulmonary eosinophilia

Extrinsic (cause known)
- Helminths: e.g. *Ascaris, Toxocara, Filaria*
- Drugs: nitrofurantoin, para-aminosalicylic acid (PAS), sulfasalazine, imipramine, chlorpropamide, phenylbutazone
- Fungi: e.g. *Aspergillus fumigatus* causing allergic bronchopulmonary aspergillosis (p. 596)

Intrinsic (cause unknown)
- Cryptogenic eosinophilic pneumonia
- Eosinophilic granulomatosis with polyangiitis (formerly Churg–Strauss syndrome), diagnosed on the basis of four or more of the following features:
  - Asthma
  - Peripheral blood eosinophilia >1.5×10^9/L (or >10% of a total white cell count)
  - Mononeuropathy or polyneuropathy
  - Pulmonary infiltrates
  - Paranasal sinus disease
  - Eosinophilic vasculitis on biopsy of an affected site
- Hypereosinophilic syndrome
- Polyarteritis nodosa (p. 1042; rare)

in the lavage fluid. Response to prednisolone (20–40 mg daily) is usually dramatic. Prednisolone can usually be withdrawn after a few weeks without relapse but long-term, low-dose therapy is occasionally necessary.

Tropical pulmonary eosinophilia

Tropical pulmonary eosinophilia occurs as a result of a mosquito-borne filarial infection with *Wuchereria bancrofti* or *Brugia malayi* (p. 290). The condition presents with fever, weight loss, dyspnoea and asthma-like symptoms. The peripheral blood eosinophilia is marked, as is the elevation of total IgE. High antifilarial antibody titres are seen. The diagnosis may be confirmed by a response to treatment with diethylcarbamazine (6 mg/kg/day for 3 weeks). Tropical pulmonary eosinophilia must be distinguished from infection with *Strongyloides stercoralis* (p. 289) as, in strongyloidiasis, glucocorticoids may cause a life-threatening hyperinfection syndrome. Ascariasis ('larva migrans') and other hookworm infestation are covered in Chapter 11.

Granulomatosis with polyangiitis

Granulomatosis with polyangiitis (formerly referred to as Wegener's granulomatosis) is a rare vasculitic and granulomatous condition (p. 1041). The lung is commonly involved in systemic forms of the disease but a limited pulmonary form may also occur. Respiratory symptoms include cough, haemoptysis and chest pain. Associated upper respiratory tract manifestations include nasal discharge and crusting, and otitis media. Fever, weight loss and anaemia are common. Radiological features include multiple nodules and cavitation that may resemble primary or metastatic carcinoma, or a pulmonary abscess. Tissue biopsy confirms the distinctive pattern of necrotising granulomas and necrotising vasculitis. Other respiratory complications include tracheal subglottic stenosis and saddle nose deformity. The differential diagnoses include mycobacterial and fungal infection and other forms of pulmonary vasculitis, including polyarteritis nodosa (pulmonary infarction), microscopic polyangiitis, eosinophilic granulomatosis with polyangiitis (formerly Churg–Strauss syndrome: marked tissue eosinophilia and association with asthma), necrotising sarcoid, bronchocentric granulomatosis and lymphomatoid granulomatosis.

Goodpasture's disease

This describes the association of pulmonary haemorrhage and glomerulonephritis, in which IgG antibodies bind to the glomerular or alveolar basement membranes (p. 401). Pulmonary disease usually precedes renal involvement and includes radiographic infiltrates and hypoxia with or without haemoptysis. It occurs more commonly in men and almost exclusively in smokers.

Lung diseases due to irradiation and drugs

Radiotherapy

Targeting radiotherapy to certain tumours is inevitably accompanied by irradiation of normal lung tissue. Although delivered in divided doses, the effects are cumulative. Acute radiation pneumonitis is typically seen within 6–12 weeks and presents with cough and dyspnoea. This may resolve spontaneously but responds to glucocorticoid treatment. Chronic interstitial fibrosis may present several months later with symptoms of exertional dyspnoea and cough. Changes are often confined to the area irradiated but may be bilateral. Established post-irradiation fibrosis does not usually

respond to glucocorticoid treatment. The pulmonary effects of radiation (p. 1332) are exacerbated by treatment with cytotoxic drugs, and the phenomenon of 'recall pneumonitis' describes the appearance of radiation injury in a previously irradiated area when chemotherapy follows radiotherapy. If the patient survives, there are long-term risks of lung cancer.

Drugs

Drugs may cause a variety of pulmonary conditions (Box 17.76). Pulmonary fibrosis may occur in response to a variety of drugs but is seen most frequently with bleomycin, methotrexate, amiodarone and nitrofurantoin. Eosinophilic pulmonary reactions can also be caused by drugs. The pathogenesis may be an immune reaction similar to that in hypersensitivity pneumonitis, which specifically attracts large numbers of eosinophils into the lungs. This type of reaction is well described as a rare reaction to a variety of antineoplastic agents (e.g. bleomycin), antibiotics (e.g. sulphonamides), sulfasalazine and the anticonvulsants phenytoin and carbamazepine. Patients usually present with breathlessness, cough and fever. The chest X-ray characteristically shows patchy shadowing. Most cases resolve completely on withdrawal of the drug, but if the reaction is severe, rapid resolution can be obtained with glucocorticoids.

Drugs may also cause other lung diseases, such as asthma, pulmonary haemorrhage, pleural effusion and, rarely, pleural thickening. An ARDS-like syndrome of acute non-cardiogenic pulmonary oedema may present with dramatic onset of breathlessness, severe hypoxaemia and signs of alveolar oedema

i 17.76 Drug-induced respiratory disease

Non-cardiogenic pulmonary oedema (ARDS)
- Hydrochlorothiazide
- Thrombolytics (streptokinase)
- Intravenous β-adrenoceptor agonists (e.g. for premature labour)
- Aspirin and opiates (in overdose)

Non-eosinophilic alveolitis
- Amiodarone, flecainide, gold, nitrofurantoin, cytotoxic agents – especially bleomycin, busulfan, mitomycin C, methotrexate, sulfasalazine

Pulmonary eosinophilia
- Antimicrobials (nitrofurantoin, penicillin, tetracyclines, sulphonamides, nalidixic acid)
- Drugs used in joint disease (gold, aspirin, penicillamine, naproxen)
- Cytotoxic drugs (bleomycin, methotrexate, procarbazine)
- Psychotropic drugs (chlorpromazine, dosulepin, imipramine)
- Anticonvulsants (carbamazepine, phenytoin)
- Others (sulfasalazine, nadolol)

Pleural disease
- Bromocriptine, amiodarone, methotrexate, methysergide
- Induction of systemic lupus erythematosus – phenytoin, hydralazine, isoniazid

Asthma
- Pharmacological mechanisms (β-blockers, cholinergic agonists, aspirin and NSAIDs)
- Idiosyncratic reactions (tamoxifen, dipyridamole)

(ARDS = acute respiratory distress syndrome; NSAIDs = non-steroidal anti-inflammatory drugs)

on the chest X-ray. This syndrome has been reported most frequently in cases of opiate overdose in drug addicts (p. 142) but also after salicylate overdose, and there are occasional reports of its occurrence after therapeutic doses of drugs, including hydrochlorothiazides and some cytotoxic agents.

17.77 Interstitial lung disease in old age

- **Idiopathic pulmonary fibrosis**: the most common interstitial lung disease, with a poor prognosis.
- **Chronic aspiration pneumonitis**: must always be considered in elderly patients presenting with bilateral basal shadowing on a chest X-ray.
- **Granulomatosis with polyangiitis (Wegener's granulomatosis)**: a rare condition but more common in old age. Renal involvement is more common at presentation and upper respiratory problems are fewer.
- **Asbestosis**: symptoms may appear only in old age because of the prolonged latent period between exposure and disease.
- **Drug-induced interstitial lung disease**: more common, presumably because of the increased chance of exposure to multiple drugs.
- **Rarer interstitial disease**: sarcoidosis, idiopathic pulmonary haemosiderosis, alveolar proteinosis and eosinophilic pneumonia rarely present.
- **Increased dyspnoea**: coexistent muscle weakness, chest wall deformity (e.g. thoracic kyphosis) and deconditioning may all exacerbate dyspnoea associated with interstitial lung disease.
- **Surgical lung biopsy**: often inappropriate in the very frail. A diagnosis therefore frequently depends on clinical and high-resolution computed tomography findings alone.

Rare interstitial lung diseases

See Box 17.78.

Occupational and environmental lung disease

The role of occupation and environmental exposure in lung disease is a particularly important area of respiratory medicine. Occupational lung disease is common and, in addition to the challenges of its diagnosis and management, often involves discussions about the workplace and, in some circumstances, litigation. Many countries encourage the registration of cases of occupational lung disease.

Occupational airway disease

Occupational asthma

Occupational asthma should be considered in any individual of working age who develops new-onset asthma, particularly if the individual reports improvement in asthma symptoms during periods away from work, e.g. at weekends and on holidays. Workers in certain occupations appear to be at particularly high risk (Box 17.79) and the condition is more common in smokers and atopic individuals. Depending on the intensity of exposure, asthmatic symptoms usually develop within the first few years of employment but are classically preceded by a latent period. Symptoms of rhinoconjunctivitis often precede

17

17.78 Rare interstitial lung diseases

Disease	Presentation	Chest X-ray	Course
Idiopathic pulmonary haemosiderosis	Haemoptysis, breathlessness, anaemia	Bilateral infiltrates, often perihilar Diffuse pulmonary fibrosis	Rapidly progressive in children Slow progression or remission in adults Death from massive pulmonary haemorrhage or cor pulmonale and respiratory failure
Alveolar proteinosis	Breathlessness and cough Occasionally fever, chest pain and haemoptysis	Diffuse bilateral shadowing, often more pronounced in the hilar regions Air bronchogram	Spontaneous remission in one-third Whole-lung lavage or granulocyte–macrophage colony-stimulating factor (GM–CSF) therapy may be effective
Langerhans cell histiocytosis (histiocytosis X)	Breathlessness, cough, pneumothorax	Diffuse interstitial shadowing progressing to honeycombing	Course unpredictable but may progress to respiratory failure Smoking cessation may be followed by significant improvement Poor response to immunosuppressive treatment
Neurofibromatosis	Breathlessness and cough in a patient with multiple organ involvement with neurofibromas, including skin	Bilateral reticulonodular shadowing of diffuse interstitial fibrosis	Slow progression to death from respiratory failure Poor response to glucocorticoid therapy
Alveolar microlithiasis	May be asymptomatic Breathlessness and cough	Diffuse calcified micronodular shadowing more pronounced in the lower zones	Slowly progressive to cor pulmonale and respiratory failure May stabilise in some
Lymphangioleiomyomatosis	Haemoptysis, breathlessness, pneumothorax and chylous effusion in females	Diffuse bilateral shadowing CT shows characteristic thin-walled cysts with well-defined walls throughout both lungs	Progressive to death within 10 years Oestrogen ablation and progesterone therapy of doubtful value Consider lung transplantation
Pulmonary tuberous sclerosis	Very similar to lymphangioleiomyomatosis, except occasionally occurs in men		

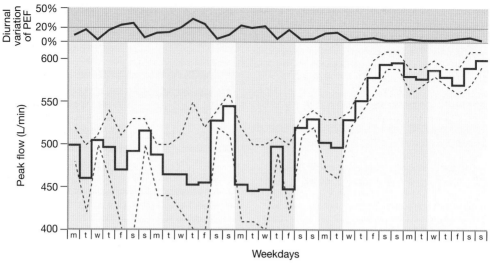

Fig. 17.61 Peak flow readings in occupational asthma. In this example, an individual with suspected occupational asthma has performed serial peak flow recording both at and away from work. The maximum, mean and minimum values are plotted daily. Days at work are indicated by the shaded areas. The diurnal variation is displayed at the top. Here, a period away from work is followed by a marked improvement in peak flow readings and a reduction in diurnal variation. (PEF = peak expiratory flow)

i   17.79 Occupational asthma

Most frequently reported causative agents

- Isocyanates
- Flour and grain dust
- Colophony and fluxes
- Latex
- Animals
- Aldehydes
- Wood dust

Workers most commonly reported to occupational asthma schemes

- Paint sprayers
- Bakers and pastry-makers
- Nurses
- Chemical workers

the development of asthma. When occupational asthma follows exposure to high-molecular-weight proteins, sensitisation may be demonstrated by skin testing or measurement of specific IgE to the agent in question. Confirmation of occupational asthma should be sought from lung function tests. This usually involves serial recording of peak flow at work at least four times per day for a minimum of 3 weeks and, if possible, including a period away from work (Fig. 17.61). In certain circumstances, specific challenge tests are required to confirm the diagnosis.

It may be possible to remove the worker from the implicated agent, but when this cannot be done, consideration of personal protective equipment and workplace hygiene may allow the worker to retain their job and livelihood. Specialist follow-up in such situations is highly advisable. A favourable prognosis is indicated by a short history of symptoms and normal lung function at diagnosis. Where reduction or avoidance of exposure fails to bring about resolution, the management is identical to that of any patient with asthma (p. 569).

Reactive airways dysfunction syndrome

Reactive airways dysfunction syndrome or acute irritant-induced asthma refers to the development of a persistent asthma-like syndrome following the inhalation of an airway irritant: typically, a single, specific exposure to a gas, smoke, fume or vapour in very high concentrations. Pulmonary function tests show airflow obstruction and airway hyper-reactivity, and the management is similar to that of asthma. Once developed, the condition often persists but it is common for symptoms to improve over years.

Chronic obstructive pulmonary disease

While tobacco smoking remains the most important preventable cause of COPD, there is increasing recognition that other noxious particles and gases can cause, or aggravate, the condition. Occupational COPD is recognised in workers exposed to coal dust, crystalline silica and cadmium. In many parts of the developing world, indoor air pollution from the burning of biomass fuels in confined spaces used for cooking contributes to the development of COPD.

Byssinosis

Byssinosis occurs in workers of cotton and flax mills exposed to cotton brack (dried leaf and plant debris). An acute form of the disease may occur, but more typically, byssinosis develops after 20–30 years' exposure. Typical symptoms include chest tightness or breathlessness accompanied by a drop in lung function; classically, these are most severe on the first day of the working week ('Monday fever') or on return to work following a period away. As the week progresses, symptoms improve and the fall in lung function becomes less dramatic. Continued exposure leads to the development of persistent symptoms and a progressive decline in FEV_1, similar to that observed in COPD.

Pneumoconiosis

Pneumoconiosis may be defined as a permanent alteration of lung structure due to the inhalation of mineral dust and the tissue reactions of the lung to its presence, excluding bronchitis and emphysema (Box 17.80). Not all dusts are pathogenic. For example, silica is highly fibrogenic, whereas iron (siderosis), tin (stannosis) and barium (baritosis) are almost inert. Beryllium causes an interstitial granulomatous disease similar to sarcoidosis. In

	17.80 Lung diseases caused by exposure to inorganic dusts		
Cause	**Occupation**	**Description**	**Characteristic pathological features**
Coal dust Silica	Coal mining Mining, quarrying, stone dressing, metal grinding, pottery, boiler scaling	Coal worker's pneumoconiosis Silicosis	Focal and interstitial fibrosis, centrilobular emphysema, progressive massive fibrosis
Asbestos	Demolition, ship breaking, manufacture of fireproof insulating materials, pipe and boiler lagging	Asbestos-related disease	Pleural plaques, diffuse pleural thickening, acute benign pleurisy, carcinoma of lung, interstitial fibrosis, mesothelioma
Iron oxide	Arc welding	Siderosis	Mineral deposition only
Tin oxide	Tin mining	Stannosis	Tin-laden macrophages
Beryllium	Aircraft, atomic energy and electronics industries	Berylliosis	Granulomas, interstitial fibrosis

many types of pneumoconiosis, a long period of dust exposure is required before radiological changes appear and these may precede clinical symptoms. The most important pneumoconioses include coal worker's pneumoconiosis, silicosis and asbestosis.

Coal worker's pneumoconiosis

Coal worker's pneumoconiosis (CWP) follows prolonged inhalation of coal dust. Dust-laden alveolar macrophages aggregate to form macules in or near the centre of the secondary pulmonary lobule and a fibrotic reaction ensues, resulting in the appearance of scattered discrete fibrotic lesions. Classification is based on the size and extent of radiographic nodularity. Simple coal worker's pneumoconiosis (SCWP) refers to the appearance of small radiographic nodules in an otherwise asymptomatic individual. SCWP does not impair lung function and, once exposure ceases, will seldom progress. Progressive massive fibrosis (PMF) refers to the formation of conglomerate masses (mainly in the upper lobes), which may cavitate. The development of PMF is usually associated with cough, sputum that may be black (melanoptysis) and breathlessness. The chest X-ray appearances may be confused with lung cancer, TB and granulomatosis with polyangiitis. PMF may progress, even after coal dust exposure ceases, and in extreme cases leads to respiratory failure and right ventricular failure.

Caplan's syndrome describes the coexistence of rheumatoid arthritis and rounded fibrotic nodules 0.5–5 cm in diameter. They show pathological features similar to a rheumatoid nodule, including central necrosis, palisading histiocytes, and a peripheral rim of lymphocytes and plasma cells. This syndrome may also occur in other types of pneumoconiosis.

Silicosis

Silicosis results from the inhalation of crystalline silica, usually in the form of quartz, by workers cutting, grinding and polishing stone. Classic silicosis is most common and usually manifests after 10–20 years of continuous silica exposure, during which time the patient remains asymptomatic. Accelerated silicosis is associated with a much shorter duration of dust exposure (typically 5–10 years), may present as early as after 1 year of exposure and, as the name suggests, follows a more aggressive course. Intense exposure to very fine crystalline silica dust can cause a more acute disease: silicoproteinosis, similar to alveolar proteinosis (see Box 17.78).

Radiological features are similar to those of CWP, with multiple well-circumscribed 3–5 mm nodular opacities predominantly in the mid- and upper zones. As the disease progresses, PMF

Fig. 17.62 Silicosis. [A] A chest X-ray from a patient with silicosis, showing the presence of small rounded nodules, predominantly seen in the upper zones. [B] High-resolution computed tomogram from the same patient, demonstrating conglomeration of nodules with posterior bias.

may develop (Fig. 17.62). Enlargement of the hilar glands with an 'egg-shell' pattern of calcification is said to be characteristic but is non-specific. Silica is highly fibrogenic and the disease is usually progressive, even when exposure ceases; hence the affected worker should invariably be removed from further exposure. Individuals with silicosis are at increased risk of TB

17

(silicotuberculosis), lung cancer and COPD; associations with renal and connective tissue disease have also been described.

Berylliosis

Exposure to beryllium is encountered in the aerospace, engineering, telecommunications and biomedical industries. The presence of cough, progressive breathlessness, night sweats and arthralgia in a worker exposed to dusts, fumes or vapours containing beryllium should raise suspicion of berylliosis. The radiographic appearances are similar in type and distribution to those of sarcoid and biopsy shows sarcoid-like granulomas. The diagnosis may be confirmed by specialised tests of lymphocyte function.

Less common pneumoconioses

Siderosis refers to the development of a benign iron oxide pneumoconiosis in welders and other iron foundry workers. Baritosis may be seen in barium process workers and stannosis in tin refining. Haematite lung occurs in iron ore miners and resembles silicosis but stains the lung red. Diamond polishers may develop hard metal disease, which is similar to UIP but the pathology shows a giant-cell interstitial pneumonia. Workers exposed to aluminium oxide develop bauxite pneumoconiosis, sometimes referred to as shaver's disease. Popcorn worker's lung is a form of obliterative bronchiolitis following ingestion of diacetyl used in butter flavouring.

Lung diseases due to organic dusts

A wide range of organic agents may cause respiratory disorders (Box 17.81). Disease results from a local immune response to animal proteins or fungal antigens in mouldy vegetable matter. Hypersensitivity pneumonitis is the most common of these conditions.

i	17.81 Examples of lung diseases caused by organic dusts		
Disorder	**Source**	**Antigen/agent**	
Farmer's lung*	Mouldy hay, straw, grain	*Saccharopolyspora rectivirgula* (formerly *Micropolyspora faeni*) *Aspergillus fumigatus*	
Bird fancier's lung*	Avian excreta, proteins and feathers	Avian serum proteins	
Malt worker's lung*	Mouldy maltings	*Aspergillus clavatus*	
Cheese worker's lung*	Mouldy cheese	*Aspergillus clavatus* *Penicillium casei*	
Maple bark stripper's lung*	Bark from stored maple	*Cryptostroma corticale*	
Saxophone player's lung*	Reed of any wind instrument	*Fusarium* spp. *Penicillium* spp. *Cladosporium* spp.	
Byssinosis	Textile industries	Cotton, flax, hemp dust	
Inhalation ('humidifier') fever	Contamination of air conditioning	Thermophilic actinomycetes	

*Presents as hypersensitivity pneumonitis.

Hypersensitivity pneumonitis

Hypersensitivity pneumonitis (HP; also called extrinsic allergic alveolitis) results from the inhalation of a wide variety of organic antigens that give rise to a diffuse immune complex reaction in the walls of alveoli and bronchioles. Common causes include farmer's lung and bird fancier's lung. Other examples are shown in Box 17.81. HP is not exclusively occupational or environmental and other important causes include medications (see Box 17.76).

The pathology of HP is consistent with both type III and type IV immunological mechanisms (p. 83). Precipitating IgG antibodies may be detected in the serum and a type III Arthus reaction is believed to occur in the lung, where the precipitation of immune complexes results in activation of complement and an inflammatory response in the alveolar walls, characterised by the influx of mononuclear cells and foamy histiocytes. The presence of poorly formed non-caseating granulomas in the alveolar walls suggests that type IV responses are also important. The distribution of the inflammatory infiltrate is predominantly peribronchiolar. Chronic forms of the disease may be accompanied by fibrosis. For reasons that remain uncertain, there is a lower incidence of HP in smokers compared to non-smokers.

Clinical features

The presentation of HP varies from an acute form to a more indolent pattern in accordance with the antigen load. For example, the farmer exposed to mouldy hay, as occurs when the hay is gathered and stored damp during a wet summer, or the pigeon fancier cleaning a large pigeon loft will, within a few hours, report influenza-like symptoms accompanied by cough, breathlessness and wheeze. The individual with low-level antigen exposure, however, such as the owner of an indoor pet bird, will typically present in a more indolent fashion with slowly progressive breathlessness; in some cases, established fibrosis may be present by the time the disease is recognised. Chest auscultation typically reveals widespread end-inspiratory crackles and squeaks.

Investigations

In cases of acute HP, the chest X-ray typically shows ill-defined patchy airspace shadowing, which, given the systemic features, may be confused with pneumonia. HRCT is more likely to show bilateral ground-glass shadowing and areas of consolidation superimposed on small centrilobar nodular opacities with an upper and middle lobe predominance (Fig. 17.63). In more chronic disease, features of fibrosis, such as volume loss, linear opacities and architectural distortion, appear. In common with other fibrotic diseases, pulmonary function tests show a restrictive ventilatory defect with reduced lung volumes and impaired gas transfer, dynamic tests may detect oxygen desaturation and, in more advanced disease, type I respiratory failure is present at rest.

Diagnosis

The diagnosis of HP is usually based on the characteristic clinical and radiological features, together with the identification of a potential source of antigen at the patient's home or place of work (Box 17.82). It may be supported by a positive serum precipitin test or by more sensitive serological investigations. It is important, however, to be aware that the presence of precipitins in the absence of other features does not make the diagnosis; the great majority of farmers with positive precipitins do not have farmer's lung, and up to 15% of pigeon breeders may have positive serum precipitins yet remain healthy.

Fig. 17.63 Hypersensitivity pneumonitis. [A] High-resolution computed tomogram showing typical patchy ground-glass opacification. [B] Histology shows evidence of an interstitial inflammatory infiltrate in the lung, and expanding alveolar walls, with a peribronchial distribution. Within the infiltrate, there are foci of small, poorly defined non-caseating granulomas (inset), which often lie adjacent to the airways. In this case, there is little in the way of established lung fibrosis but this can be marked. *A, Courtesy of Dr S. Jackson, Western General Hospital, Edinburgh. B, Courtesy of Dr William Wallace, Dept of Pathology, Royal Infirmary of Edinburgh.*

---

i | **17.82 Predictive factors in the identification of hypersensitivity pneumonitis**

- Exposure to a known offending antigen
- Positive precipitating antibodies to offending antigen
- Recurrent episodes of symptoms
- Inspiratory crackles on examination
- Symptoms occurring 4–8 hours after exposure
- Weight loss

Where HP is suspected but the cause is not readily apparent, a visit to the patient's home or workplace should be arranged. Occasionally, such as when an agent previously unrecognised as causing HP is suspected, provocation testing may be necessary to prove the diagnosis; if positive, inhalation of the relevant antigen is followed after 3–6 hours by pyrexia and a reduction in vital capacity and gas transfer factor. BAL fluid usually shows an increase in the number of CD8$^+$ T lymphocytes and transbronchial biopsy can occasionally provide sufficient tissue for a confident diagnosis; however, open lung biopsy may be necessary.

Management

If it is practical, the patient should cease exposure to the inciting agent. In some cases this may be difficult, however, because of either implications for livelihood (e.g. farmers) or addiction to

hobbies (e.g. pigeon breeders). Dust masks with appropriate filters may minimise exposure and may be combined with methods of reducing levels of antigen (e.g. drying hay before storage). In acute cases, prednisolone should be given for 3–4 weeks, starting with an oral dose of 40 mg per day. Severely hypoxaemic patients may require high-concentration oxygen therapy initially. Most patients recover completely, but if unchecked, fibrosis may progress to cause severe respiratory disability, hypoxaemia, pulmonary hypertension, cor pulmonale and eventually death.

Inhalation ('humidifier') fever

Inhalation fever shares similarities with HP. It occurs as a result of contaminated humidifiers or air-conditioning units that release a fine spray of microorganisms into the atmosphere. The illness is characterised by self-limiting fever and breathlessness; permanent sequelae are unusual. An identical syndrome can also develop after disturbing an accumulation of mouldy hay, compost or mulch. So-called 'hot tub lung' appears to be attributable to *Mycobacterium avium*. Outbreaks of HP in workers using metalworking fluids appear to be linked to *Acinetobacter* or *Ochrobactrum*.

Asbestos-related lung and pleural diseases

Asbestos is a naturally occurring silicate. Asbestos fibres may be classified as either chrysotile (white asbestos), which accounts for 90% of the world's production, or serpentine (crocidolite or blue asbestos, and amosite or brown asbestos). The favourable thermal and chemical insulation properties led to its extensive use by the shipbuilding and construction industries throughout the latter part of the 20th century. Exposure to asbestos may be followed, after a lengthy latent period, by the development of both pleural and pulmonary disease.

Pleural plaques

Pleural plaques are the most common manifestation of past asbestos exposure, being discrete circumscribed areas of hyaline fibrosis situated on the parietal pleura of the chest wall,

Fig. 17.64 Asbestos-related benign pleural plaques. Chest X-ray showing extensive calcified pleural plaques ('candle wax' appearance – arrows), particularly marked on the diaphragm and lateral pleural surfaces.

17

diaphragm, pericardium or mediastinum. They are virtually always asymptomatic, usually being identified as an incidental finding on a chest X-ray (Fig. 17.64) or thoracic CT scan, particularly when partially calcified. They do not cause impairment of lung function and are benign.

Acute benign asbestos pleurisy

Benign asbestos pleurisy is estimated to occur in around 20% of asbestos workers but many episodes are subclinical and pass unreported. When symptomatic, patients present with features of pleurisy, including mild fever and systemic disturbance. The diagnosis therefore necessitates the exclusion of other known causes of pleurisy and pleural effusion. Repeated episodes may be followed by the development of diffuse (visceral) pleural thickening.

Diffuse pleural thickening

Diffuse pleural thickening (DPT) refers to thickening of the visceral pleura. In contrast to pleural plaques, if this is sufficiently extensive, it may cause restrictive lung function impairment, exertional breathlessness and, occasionally, persistent chest pain. The typical appearances of DPT on chest X-ray include thickening of the pleura along the chest wall and obliteration of the costophrenic angles. Earlier manifestations detected by CT scanning include parenchymal bands (Fig. 17.65) and 'round atelectasis'. There is no treatment and the condition may be progressive in around one-third of individuals. In exceptionally severe cases, surgical decortication may be considered. A pleural biopsy may be required to exclude mesothelioma.

Fig. 17.65 Thoracic CT scan showing right-sided pleural thickening and an associated parenchymal band.

Asbestosis

Fibrosis of the lung following asbestos exposure generally requires substantial exposure over several years and is rarely associated with low-level or bystander exposure. In common with other fibrosing lung diseases, asbestosis usually presents with exertional breathlessness and fine, late inspiratory crackles over the lower zones. Finger clubbing may be present. Pulmonary function tests and HRCT appearances are similar to those of UIP. These features, accompanied by a history of substantial asbestos exposure, are generally sufficient to establish the diagnosis and lung biopsy is rarely necessary. When biopsy is

performed, asbestosis may be diagnosed when alveolar septal fibrosis is accompanied by an average of at least two asbestos bodies per square centimetre of lung tissue. In some cases, asbestos fibre counts may be performed on lung biopsy material to establish the diagnosis.

Asbestosis is usually slowly progressive and has a better prognosis than IPF, but in advanced cases respiratory failure, pulmonary hypertension and cor pulmonale may still develop. About 40% of patients (who usually smoke) develop lung cancer and 10% may develop mesothelioma.

Mesothelioma

Mesothelioma is a malignant tumour affecting the pleura or, less commonly, the peritoneum. Its occurrence almost invariably suggests past asbestos exposure, which may be low-level. There is typically a long latent interval between first exposure and the onset of clinical manifestations, and this accounts for the continued increasing incidence many years after control measures have been implemented. Around 1 in 170 of all British men born in the 1940s will die of mesothelioma.

Pleural mesothelioma typically presents with increasing breathlessness resulting from pleural effusion or unremitting chest pain, reflecting involvement of the chest wall. As the tumour progresses, it encases the underlying lung and may invade the parenchyma, the mediastinum and the pericardium. Metastatic disease, although not often clinically detectable in life, is a common finding on postmortem.

Mesothelioma is almost invariably fatal. Highly selected patients may be considered for radical surgery but, in the majority of patients, therapy is invariably directed towards palliation of symptoms. The use of chemotherapy may improve quality of life and is accompanied by a small survival benefit, typically regarded as being around 3 months. Radiotherapy can be used to control pain and limit the risk of tumour seeding at biopsy sites. Pleural effusions are managed with drainage and pleurodesis. Typical figures for survival from onset of symptoms are around 16 months for epithelioid tumours, 10 months for sarcomatoid tumours and 15 months for biphasic tumours, with only a minority of patients surviving for longer periods.

Occupational lung cancer

Individuals exposed to substantial quantities of asbestos are at increased risk of lung cancer, particularly if they smoke tobacco. Increased risks of lung cancer have also been reported in workers who develop silicosis and those exposed to radon gas, beryllium, diesel exhaust fumes, cadmium, chromium, and dust and fumes from coke plants.

Occupational pneumonia

Occupational and environmental exposures may be linked to the development of pneumonia. Pneumococcal vaccine is recommended for welders. Farm workers, abattoir workers and hide factory workers may be exposed to *Coxiella burnetii*, the causative agent of Q fever. The organisms are excreted from milk, urine, faeces and amniotic fluid; they may be transmitted by cattle ticks or contaminated dust from the milking floor, or by drinking milk that is inadequately pasteurised. Birds (often parrots) or budgerigars infected with *Chlamydia psittaci* can cause psittacosis. Sewage workers, farmers, animal handlers and vets run an increased risk of leptospiral pneumonia, and contact with rabbits, hares, muskrats and ground squirrels is associated with tularaemic pneumonia, caused by *Francisella tularensis*. Anthrax (wool-sorter's disease) may occur in workers exposed to infected hides, hair, bristle, bonemeal and animal carcases.

Pulmonary vascular disease

Pulmonary embolism

The majority of pulmonary emboli arise from the propagation of lower limb deep vein thrombosis (p. 186). Rare causes include septic emboli (from endocarditis affecting the tricuspid or pulmonary valves), tumour (especially choriocarcinoma), fat following fracture of long bones such as the femur, air, and amniotic fluid, which may enter the mother's circulation following delivery.

Clinical features

The diagnosis of pulmonary embolism (PE) may be aided by asking three questions:

- Is the clinical presentation consistent with PE?
- Does the patient have risk factors for PE?
- Are there any alternative diagnoses that can explain the patient's presentation?

Clinical presentation varies, depending on number, size and distribution of emboli and on underlying cardiorespiratory reserve (Box 17.83). A recognised risk factor is present in 80–90% (see Box 23.65, p. 975). The presence of one or more risk factors increases the risk further still.

Investigations

A variety of non-specific radiographic appearances have been described (Fig. 17.66) but the chest X-ray is most useful in

i 17.83 Features of pulmonary thromboemboli			
	Acute massive PE	Acute small/medium PE	Chronic PE
Pathophysiology	Major haemodynamic effects: ↓cardiac output; acute right heart failure	Occlusion of segmental pulmonary artery → infarction ± effusion	Chronic occlusion of pulmonary microvasculature, right heart failure
Symptoms	Faintness or collapse, crushing central chest pain, apprehension, severe dyspnoea	Pleuritic chest pain, restricted breathing, haemoptysis	Exertional dyspnoea Late: symptoms of pulmonary hypertension or right heart failure
Signs	Major circulatory collapse: tachycardia, hypotension, ↑JVP, RV gallop rhythm, loud P₂, severe cyanosis, ↓urinary output	Tachycardia, pleural rub, raised hemidiaphragm, crackles, effusion (often blood-stained), low-grade fever	Early: may be minimal Later: RV heave, loud P₂ Terminal: signs of right heart failure
Chest X-ray	Usually normal; may be subtle oligaemia	Pleuropulmonary opacities, pleural effusion, linear shadows, raised hemidiaphragm	Enlarged pulmonary artery trunk, enlarged heart, prominent right ventricle
Electrocardiogram	$S_1Q_3T_3$ anterior T-wave inversion, RBBB	Sinus tachycardia	RV hypertrophy and strain
Arterial blood gases	Markedly abnormal with ↓PaO_2 and ↓$PaCO_2$, metabolic acidosis	May be normal or ↓PaO_2 or ↓$PaCO_2$	Exertional ↓PaO_2 or desaturation on formal exercise testing
Alternative diagnoses	Myocardial infarction, pericardial tamponade, aortic dissection	Pneumonia, pneumothorax, musculoskeletal chest pain	Other causes of pulmonary hypertension

(JVP = jugular venous pressure; PE = pulmonary embolism; RBBB = right bundle branch block; RV = right ventricular)

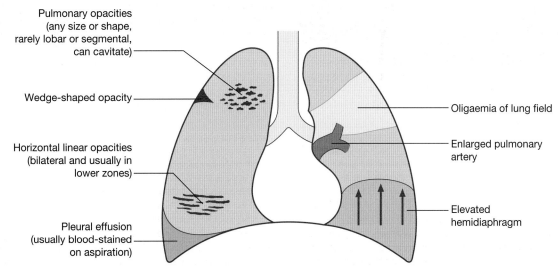

Fig. 17.66 Features of pulmonary thromboembolism/infarction on chest X-ray.

Pulmonary opacities (any size or shape, rarely lobar or segmental, can cavitate)

Wedge-shaped opacity

Horizontal linear opacities (bilateral and usually in lower zones)

Pleural effusion (usually blood-stained on aspiration)

Oligaemia of lung field

Enlarged pulmonary artery

Elevated hemidiaphragm

17

excluding key differential diagnoses, e.g. pneumonia or pneumothorax. Normal appearances in an acutely breathless and hypoxaemic patient should raise the suspicion of PE, as should bilateral changes in anyone presenting with unilateral pleuritic chest pain.

The ECG is often normal but is useful in excluding other important differential diagnoses, such as acute myocardial infarction and pericarditis. The most common findings in PE include sinus tachycardia and anterior T-wave inversion but these are non-specific; larger emboli may cause right heart strain revealed by an $S_1Q_3T_3$ pattern, ST-segment and T-wave changes, or the appearance of right bundle branch block.

Arterial blood gases typically show a reduced PaO_2 and a normal or low $PaCO_2$, and an increased alveolar–arterial oxygen gradient, but may be normal in a significant minority. A metabolic acidosis may be seen in acute massive PE with cardiovascular collapse.

An elevated D-dimer (see Fig. 10.6, p. 187) is of limited value, as it may be raised in a variety of other conditions, including myocardial infarction, pneumonia and sepsis. However, low levels, particularly in the context of a low clinical risk, have a high negative predictive value and further investigation is usually unnecessary (Fig. 17.67). The result of the D-dimer assay should be disregarded in high-risk patients, as further investigation is mandatory even when normal. The serum troponin I (see Box 10.3, p. 179) may be elevated, reflecting right heart strain.

CTPA is the first-line diagnostic test (Fig. 17.68). It has the advantage of visualising the distribution and extent of the emboli or highlighting an alternative diagnosis, such as consolidation, pneumothorax or aortic dissection. The sensitivity of CT scanning may be increased by simultaneous visualisation of the femoral and popliteal veins, although this is not widely practised. As the contrast media may be nephrotoxic, care should be taken in patients with renal impairment, and CTPA avoided in those with a history of allergy to iodinated contrast media. In these cases, either V̇/Q̇ scanning or ventilation/perfusion single photon emission computed tomography (V̇/Q̇ SPECT) may be considered.

Colour Doppler ultrasound of the leg veins may be used in patients with suspected PE, particularly if there are clinical signs in a limb, as many will have identifiable proximal thrombus in the leg veins.

Bedside echocardiography is extremely helpful in the differential diagnosis and assessment of acute circulatory collapse (p. 199). Acute dilatation of the right heart is usually present in massive PE, and thrombus (embolism in transit) may be visible. Important differential diagnoses, including left ventricular failure, aortic dissection and pericardial tamponade, can also be identified.

Conventional pulmonary angiography is still useful in selected settings or for the delivery of catheter-based therapies.

Management
General measures

Prompt recognition and treatment are potentially life-saving. Sufficient oxygen should be given to hypoxaemic patients to maintain arterial oxygen saturation above 90%. Circulatory shock should be treated with intravenous fluids or plasma expander, but inotropic agents are of limited value as the hypoxic dilated right ventricle is already close to maximally stimulated by endogenous catecholamines. Diuretics and vasodilators should also be avoided, as they will reduce cardiac output. Opiates may be necessary to relieve pain and distress but should be used with caution

Fig. 17.68 CT pulmonary angiogram. The arrow points to a saddle embolism in the bifurcation of the pulmonary artery.

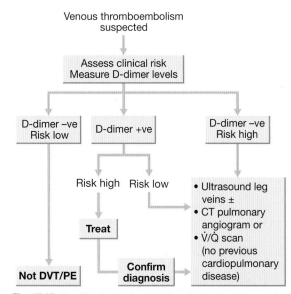

Fig. 17.67 Algorithm for the investigation of patients with suspected pulmonary thromboembolism. Clinical risk is based on the presence of risk factors for venous thromboembolism and the probability of another diagnosis. (DVT = deep vein thrombosis; PE = pulmonary embolism)

17.84 Pulmonary embolism in pregnancy

- **Maternal mortality**: venous thromboembolism is the leading direct cause in the UK.
- **CT pulmonary angiography**: may be performed safely (0.01–0.06 mGy). It is important to consider the risk of radiation to breast tissue (particularly if there is a family history of breast carcinoma).
- **V̇/Q̇ scanning**: greater radiation dose to fetus (0.11–0.22 mGy) but significantly less to maternal breast tissue.
- **In utero radiation exposure**: estimated incidence of childhood malignancy is about 1 in 16 000 per mGy.
- **Warfarin**: teratogenic, so pulmonary embolism should be treated with low-molecular-weight heparin during pregnancy.

in the hypotensive patient. External cardiac massage may be successful in the moribund patient by dislodging and breaking up a large central embolus.

Anticoagulation

The main principle of treatment for PE is anticoagulation, which is discussed for PE and other forms of VTE on page 975.

Thrombolytic and surgical therapy

Thrombolysis is indicated in any patient presenting with acute massive PE accompanied by cardiogenic shock. In the absence of shock, the benefits are less clear but thrombolysis may be considered in those presenting with right ventricular dilatation and hypokinesis or severe hypoxaemia. Patients must be screened carefully for haemorrhagic risk, as there is a high risk of intracranial haemorrhage. Surgical pulmonary embolectomy may be considered in selected patients but carries a high mortality.

Caval filters

A patient in whom anticoagulation is contraindicated, who has suffered massive haemorrhage on anticoagulation, or recurrent VTE despite anticoagulation, should be considered for an inferior vena caval filter. Retrievable caval filters are particularly useful in individuals with temporary risk factors. The caval filter should be used only until anticoagulation can be safely initiated, at which time the filter should be removed if possible.

Prognosis

Immediate mortality is greatest in those with echocardiographic evidence of right ventricular dysfunction or cardiogenic shock. Once anticoagulation is commenced, however, the risk of mortality rapidly falls. The risk of recurrence is highest in the first 6–12 months after the initial event, and at 10 years around one-third of individuals will have suffered a further event.

Pulmonary hypertension

Pulmonary hypertension (PH) is defined as a mean pulmonary artery pressure (PAP) of at least 25 mmHg at rest, as measured by right heart catheterisation. The definition may be further refined by consideration of the pulmonary wedge pressure (PWP), the cardiac output and the transpulmonary pressure gradient (mean PAP – mean PWP). The clinical classification of PH is shown in Box 17.85. Further classification is based on the degree of functional disturbance, assessed using the New York Heart Association (NYHA) grades I–IV. Although respiratory failure due to intrinsic pulmonary disease is the most common cause of PH, severe PH may occur as a primary disorder, as a complication of connective tissue disease (e.g. systemic sclerosis), or as a result of chronic thromboembolic events.

Primary pulmonary hypertension (PPH) is a rare but important disease that predominantly affects women aged between 20 and 30 years. Familial disease is rarer still but is known to be associated with mutations in the gene encoding type II bone morphogenetic protein receptor (*BMPR2*), a member of the transforming growth factor beta (TGF-β) superfamily. Mutations in this gene have been identified in some patients with sporadic PH. Pathological features include hypertrophy of both the media and the intima of the vessel wall and a clonal expansion of endothelial cells, which take on the appearance of plexiform lesions. There is marked narrowing of the vessel lumen and this, together with the frequently observed in situ thrombosis, leads to an increase in pulmonary vascular resistance and PH.

---

i 17.85 Classification of pulmonary hypertension

Pulmonary arterial hypertension

- Primary pulmonary hypertension: sporadic and familial
- Secondary to: connective tissue disease (limited cutaneous systemic sclerosis), congenital systemic to pulmonary shunts, portal hypertension, HIV infection, exposure to various drugs or toxins, and persistent pulmonary hypertension of the newborn

Pulmonary venous hypertension

- Left-sided atrial or ventricular heart disease
- Left-sided valvular heart disease
- Pulmonary veno-occlusive disease
- Pulmonary capillary haemangiomatosis

Pulmonary hypertension associated with disorders of the respiratory system and/or hypoxaemia

- Chronic obstructive pulmonary disease
- Diffuse parenchymal lung disease
- Sleep-disordered breathing
- Alveolar hypoventilation disorders
- Chronic exposure to high altitude
- Neonatal lung disease
- Alveolar capillary dysplasia
- Severe kyphoscoliosis

Pulmonary hypertension caused by chronic thromboembolic disease

- Thromboembolic obstruction of the proximal pulmonary arteries
- In situ thrombosis
- Sickle-cell disease

Miscellaneous

- Inflammatory conditions
- Extrinsic compression of central pulmonary veins

Adapted from Dana Point 2008. Simonneau G, Robbins IM, Beghetti M, et al. Updated clinical classification of pulmonary hypertension. J Am Coll Cardiol 2009; 54:S43–S54.

Clinical features

PH presents insidiously and is often diagnosed late. Typical symptoms include breathlessness, chest pain, fatigue, palpitation and syncope. Important signs include elevation of the JVP (with a prominent 'a' wave if in sinus rhythm), a parasternal heave (right ventricular hypertrophy), accentuation of the pulmonary component of the second heart sound and a right ventricular third heart sound. Signs of interstitial lung disease or cardiac, liver or connective tissue disease may suggest the underlying cause.

Investigations

PH is suspected if an ECG shows a right ventricular 'strain' pattern or a chest X-ray shows enlarged pulmonary arteries, peripheral pruning and right ventricle enlargement (Fig. 17.69). Doppler assessment of the tricuspid regurgitant jet by transthoracic echocardiography provides a non-invasive estimate of the PAP, which is equal to $4 \times$(tricuspid regurgitation velocity)^2. Further assessment should be by right heart catheterisation to assess pulmonary haemodynamics, measure vasodilator responsiveness and thus guide further therapy.

Management

Specialist centres should direct the management of PH. Diuretic therapy should be prescribed for patients with right heart failure. Supplemental oxygen should be given to maintain resting PaO_2

Fig. 17.69 Chest X-ray showing the typical appearance in pulmonary hypertension.

above 8 kPa (60 mmHg). Anticoagulation should be considered unless there is an increased risk of bleeding. Digoxin may be useful in patients who develop atrial tachyarrhythmias. Pregnancy carries a very high risk of death and women of child-bearing age should be counselled appropriately. Excessive physical activity that leads to distressing symptoms should be avoided but otherwise patients should be encouraged to remain active. Pneumococcal and influenza vaccination should be recommended. Nitrates should be avoided owing to the risk of hypotension, and β-blockers are poorly tolerated. Cyclizine can aggravate PH and should also be avoided.

Disease-targeted strategies have focused on replacing endogenous prostacyclins with infusions of epoprostenol or treprostinil or nebulised iloprost; blocking endothelin-mediated vasoconstriction with agents such as bosentan, ambrisentan or macitentan; or enhancing endogenous nitric oxide-mediated vasodilatation with phosphodiesterase V inhibitors, such as sildenafil or tadalafil, or the guanylate cyclase stimulator riociguat. High-dose calcium channel blockers may be appropriate in those with an acute vasodilator response.

Selected patients are referred for double-lung transplantation, and pulmonary thrombo-endarterectomy may be contemplated in those with chronic proximal pulmonary thromboembolic disease. Atrial septostomy (the creation of a right-to-left shunt) decompresses the right ventricle and improves haemodynamic performance; it may be used as a bridge to transplantation or as a palliative measure.

Diseases of the upper airway

Diseases of the nasopharynx

▎ Allergic rhinitis

This is a disorder in which there are episodes of nasal congestion, watery nasal discharge and sneezing. It may be seasonal or perennial, and is due to an immediate hypersensitivity reaction in the nasal mucosa. Seasonal antigens include pollens from grasses, flowers, weeds or trees. Grass pollen is responsible for hay fever, the most common type of seasonal allergic rhinitis in northern Europe, which is at its peak between May and July.

This is a worldwide problem, however, which may be aggravated during harvest seasons.

Perennial allergic rhinitis may be a specific reaction to antigens derived from house dust, fungal spores or animal dander, but similar symptoms can be caused by physical or chemical irritants, e.g. pungent odours or fumes, including strong perfumes, cold air and dry atmospheres. The phrase 'vasomotor rhinitis' is often used in this context, as the term 'allergic' is a misnomer.

Clinical features

In the seasonal type, there are frequent sudden attacks of sneezing, with profuse watery nasal discharge and nasal obstruction. These attacks last for a few hours and are often accompanied by smarting and watering of the eyes and conjunctival irritation. In perennial rhinitis, the symptoms are similar but more continuous and usually less severe. Skin hypersensitivity tests with the relevant antigen are usually positive in seasonal allergic rhinitis but are less useful in perennial rhinitis.

Management

In those sensitised to house dust, simple measures, such as thorough dust removal from the bed area, leaving a window open and renewing old pillows, are often helpful. Avoidance of pollen and antigens from domestic pets, however desirable and beneficial, is usually impractical.

The following medications, singly or in combination, are usually effective in both seasonal and perennial allergic rhinitis:

- an antihistamine such as loratadine
- sodium cromoglicate nasal spray
- glucocorticoid nasal spray, e.g. beclometasone dipropionate, fluticasone, mometasone or budesonide.

When symptoms are very severe, resistant to usual treatments and seriously interfering with school, business or social activities, immunotherapy (desensitisation) is also used but carries the risk of serious reactions and must be managed in specialist centres. Vasomotor rhinitis is often difficult to treat but may respond to ipratropium bromide, administered into each nostril 3 times daily.

Sleep-disordered breathing

A variety of respiratory disorders affect sleep or are affected by sleep. Cough and wheeze disturbing sleep are characteristic of asthma, while the hypoventilation that accompanies normal sleep can precipitate respiratory failure in patients with disordered ventilation due to kyphoscoliosis, diaphragmatic paralysis or muscle disease (e.g. muscular dystrophy).

In contrast, a small but important group of disorders cause problems only during sleep. Patients may have normal lungs and daytime respiratory function, but during sleep have either abnormalities of ventilatory drive (central sleep apnoea) or upper airway obstruction (obstructive sleep apnoea). Of these, the obstructive sleep apnoea/hypopnoea syndrome is by far the most common and important. When this coexists with COPD, severe respiratory failure can result, even if the COPD is mild.

▎ The sleep apnoea/hypopnoea syndrome

Recurrent upper airway obstruction during sleep, sufficient to cause sleep fragmentation and daytime sleepiness, is thought to affect 2% of women and 4% of men aged 30–60 in Caucasian populations. Daytime sleepiness, especially in monotonous situations, results in a threefold increased risk of road traffic accidents and a ninefold increased risk of single-vehicle accidents.

Aetiology

Sleep apnoea results from recurrent occlusion of the pharynx during sleep, usually at the level of the soft palate. Inspiration results in negative pressure within the pharynx. During wakefulness, upper airway dilating muscles, including palatoglossus and genioglossus, contract actively during inspiration to preserve airway patency. During sleep, muscle tone declines, impairing the ability of these muscles to maintain pharyngeal patency. In a minority of people, a combination of an anatomically narrow palatopharynx and under-activity of the dilating muscles during sleep results in inspiratory airway obstruction. Incomplete obstruction causes turbulent flow, resulting in snoring (44% of men and 28% of women aged 30–60 snore). More severe obstruction triggers increased inspiratory effort and transiently wakes the patient, allowing the dilating muscles to re-open the airway. These awakenings are so brief that patients have no recollection of them. After a series of loud deep breaths that may wake their bed partner, the patient rapidly returns to sleep, snores and becomes apnoeic once more. This cycle of apnoea and awakening may repeat itself many hundreds of times per night and results in severe sleep fragmentation and secondary variations in blood pressure, which may predispose over time to cardiovascular disease.

Predisposing factors to the sleep apnoea/hypopnoea syndrome include male gender, which doubles the risk, and obesity, which is found in about 50% because parapharyngeal fat deposits tend to narrow the pharynx. Nasal obstruction or a recessed mandible can further exacerbate the problem. Acromegaly and hypothyroidism also predispose by causing submucosal infiltration and narrowing of the upper airway. Sleep apnoea is often familial, where the maxilla and mandible are back-set, narrowing the upper airway. Alcohol and sedatives predispose to snoring and apnoea by relaxing the upper airway dilating muscles. As a result of marked sympathetic activation during apnoea, sleep-disordered breathing is associated over time with sustained hypertension and an increased risk of coronary events and stroke. Associations have also been described with insulin resistance, the metabolic syndrome and type 2 diabetes. Treatment of sleep apnoea reduces sympathetic drive and blood pressure, and may also improve these associated metabolic disorders.

Clinical features

Excessive daytime sleepiness is the principal symptom and snoring is virtually universal. The patient usually feels that he or she has been asleep all night but wakes unrefreshed. Bed partners report loud snoring in all body positions and often have noticed multiple breathing pauses (apnoeas). Difficulty with concentration, impaired cognitive function and work performance, depression, irritability and nocturia are other features.

Investigations

Provided that the sleepiness does not result from inadequate time in bed or from shift work, anyone who repeatedly falls asleep during the day when not in bed, who complains that his or her work is impaired by sleepiness, or who is a habitual snorer with multiple witnessed apnoeas should be referred for a sleep assessment. A more quantitative assessment of daytime sleepiness can be obtained by questionnaire (Box 17.86).

Overnight studies of breathing, oxygenation and sleep quality are diagnostic (Fig. 17.70) but the level of investigation depends on local resources and the probability of the diagnosis. The current

i | **17.86 Epworth sleepiness scale**

How likely are you to doze off or fall asleep in the situations described below? Choose the most appropriate number for each situation from the following scale:

0 = would never doze
1 = slight chance of dozing
2 = moderate chance of dozing
3 = high chance of dozing

- Sitting and reading
- Watching TV
- Sitting inactive in a public place (e.g. a theatre or a meeting)
- As a passenger in a car for an hour without a break
- Lying down to rest in the afternoon when circumstances permit
- Sitting and talking to someone
- Sitting quietly after a lunch without alcohol
- In a car, while stopped for a few minutes in the traffic

Normal subjects average 5.9 (SD 2.2) and patients with severe obstructive sleep apnoea average 16.0 (SD 4.4).

Fig. 17.70 Sleep apnoea/hypopnoea syndrome: overnight oxygen saturation trace. The left-hand panel shows the trace of a patient who had 53 apnoeas plus hypopnoeas/hour, 55 brief awakenings/hour and marked oxygen desaturation. The right-hand panel shows the effect of continuous positive airway pressure (CPAP) of 10 cmH$_2$O delivered through a tight-fitting nasal mask: it abolished his breathing irregularity and awakenings, and improved oxygenation. *Courtesy of Professor N.J. Douglas.*

threshold for diagnosing moderate sleep apnoea/hypopnoea syndrome is 15 or more apnoeas/hypopnoeas per hour of sleep, where an apnoea is defined as a 10-second or longer breathing pause and a hypopnoea a 10-second or longer 50% reduction in breathing.

Several other conditions can cause daytime sleepiness but can usually be excluded by a careful history (Box 17.87). Narcolepsy is a rare cause of sudden-onset sleepiness, occurring in 0.05% of the population (p. 1105). Idiopathic hypersomnolence occurs in younger individuals and is characterised by long nocturnal sleeps.

Management

The major hazard to patients and those around them is traffic accidents, so drivers must be strongly advised not to drive until treatment has relieved their sleepiness. In a minority, relief of nasal obstruction or the avoidance of alcohol may prevent obstruction. Advice to obese patients to lose weight is often unheeded and the majority of patients need to use continuous

17

17.87 Differential diagnosis of persistent sleepiness

Lack of sleep

- Inadequate time in bed
- Extraneous sleep disruption (e.g. babies/children)
- Shift work
- Excessive caffeine intake
- Physical illness (e.g. pain)

Sleep disruption

- Sleep apnoea/hypopnoea syndrome
- Periodic limb movement disorder (recurrent limb movements during non-REM sleep, frequent nocturnal awakenings; p. 1106)

Sleepiness with relatively normal sleep

- Narcolepsy
- Idiopathic hypersomnolence (rare)
- Neurological lesions (e.g. hypothalamic or upper brainstem infarcts or tumours)
- Drugs

Psychological/psychiatric

- Depression

17.88 Causes of chronic laryngitis

- Repeated attacks of acute laryngitis
- Excessive use of the voice, especially in dusty atmospheres
- Heavy tobacco smoking
- Mouth-breathing from nasal obstruction
- Chronic infection of nasal sinuses

17.89 Causes of laryngeal obstruction

- Inflammatory or allergic oedema, or exudate
- Spasm of laryngeal muscles
- Inhaled foreign body
- Inhaled blood clot or vomitus in an unconscious patient
- Tumours of the larynx
- Bilateral vocal cord paralysis
- Fixation of both cords in rheumatoid disease

positive airway pressure (CPAP) delivered by a nasal mask every night to splint the upper airway open. When CPAP is tolerated, the effect is often dramatic (Fig. 17.70), with relief of somnolence and improved daytime performance, quality of life and survival. Unfortunately, 30–50% of patients do not tolerate CPAP. Mandibular advancement devices that fit over the teeth and hold the mandible forward, thus opening the pharynx, are an alternative that is effective in some patients. There is no evidence that palatal surgery is of benefit.

Laryngeal disorders

The larynx is commonly affected by acute self-limiting infections (p. 581). Other disorders include chronic laryngitis, laryngeal tuberculosis, laryngeal paralysis and laryngeal obstruction. Tumours of the larynx are relatively common, particularly in smokers. For further details, the reader should refer to an otolaryngology text.

Chronic laryngitis

The common causes are listed in Box 17.88. The chief symptoms are hoarseness or loss of voice (aphonia). There is irritation of the throat and a spasmodic cough. The disease pursues a chronic course, frequently uninfluenced by treatment, and the voice may become permanently impaired. Other causes of chronic hoarseness include use of inhaled glucocorticoid treatment, tuberculosis, laryngeal paralysis or tumour.

In some patients, a chest X-ray may reveal an unsuspected lung cancer or pulmonary tuberculosis. If these are not found, laryngoscopy should be performed to exclude a local structural cause.

When no specific treatable cause is found, the voice must be rested completely. This is particularly important in public speakers and singers. Smoking should be avoided. Some benefit may be obtained from frequent inhalations of medicated steam.

Laryngeal paralysis

Interruption of the motor nerve supply of the larynx is nearly always unilateral and, because of the intrathoracic course of the left recurrent laryngeal nerve, usually left-sided. One or both recurrent laryngeal nerves may be damaged by thyroidectomy, carcinoma of the thyroid or anterior neck injury. Rarely, the vagal trunk itself is involved by tumour, aneurysm or trauma.

Clinical features and management

Hoarseness always accompanies laryngeal paralysis, whatever its cause. Paralysis of organic origin is seldom reversible, but when only one vocal cord is affected, hoarseness may improve or even disappear after a few weeks, as the normal cord compensates by crossing the midline to approximate with the paralysed cord on phonation.

'Bovine cough' is a characteristic feature of organic laryngeal paralysis, and lacks the explosive quality of normal coughing because the cords fail to close the glottis. Sputum clearance may also be impaired. A normal cough in patients with partial loss of voice or aphonia virtually excludes laryngeal paralysis. Stridor is occasionally present but seldom severe, except when laryngeal paralysis is bilateral.

Laryngoscopy is required to establish the diagnosis of laryngeal paralysis. The paralysed cord lies in the so-called 'cadaveric' position, midway between abduction and adduction.

The cause should be treated, if possible. In unilateral paralysis, persistent dysphonia may be improved by the injection of Teflon into the affected vocal cord. In bilateral organic paralysis, tracheal intubation, tracheostomy or plastic surgery on the larynx may be necessary.

Psychogenic hoarseness and aphonia

Psychogenic causes of hoarseness or aphonia may be suggested by associated symptoms in the history (p. 1187). Laryngoscopy may be necessary, however, to exclude a physical cause. In psychogenic aphonia, only the voluntary movement of adduction of the vocal cords is seen to be impaired. Speech therapy may be helpful.

Laryngeal obstruction

Laryngeal obstruction is more liable to occur in children than in adults because of the smaller size of the glottis. Important causes are given in Box 17.89. Sudden complete laryngeal obstruction by a foreign body produces the clinical picture of acute asphyxia:

violent but ineffective inspiratory efforts with indrawing of the intercostal spaces and the unsupported lower ribs, accompanied by cyanosis. Unrelieved, the condition progresses to coma and death within a few minutes. When, as in most cases, the obstruction is incomplete at first, the main clinical features are progressive breathlessness accompanied by stridor and cyanosis. Urgent treatment to prevent complete obstruction is needed.

Management

Transient laryngeal obstruction due to exudate and spasm, which may occur with acute pharyngitis in children and with whooping cough, is potentially dangerous but can usually be relieved by steam inhalation. Laryngeal obstruction from all other causes carries a high mortality and demands prompt treatment.

When a foreign body causes laryngeal obstruction in children, it can often be dislodged by turning the patient head downwards and squeezing the chest vigorously. In adults, a sudden forceful compression of the upper abdomen (Heimlich manœuvre) may be effective. Otherwise, the cause of the obstruction should be investigated by direct laryngoscopy, which may also permit the removal of an unsuspected foreign body or the insertion of a tube past the obstruction into the trachea. Tracheostomy must be performed without delay if these procedures fail to relieve obstruction but, except in dire emergencies, this should be performed in theatre by a surgeon.

In diphtheria, antitoxin should be administered, and for other infections the appropriate antibiotic should be given. In angioedema, complete laryngeal occlusion can usually be prevented by treatment with adrenaline (epinephrine; 0.5–1 mg (0.5–1 mL of 1 : 1000) IM), chlorphenamine maleate (10–20 mg by slow intravenous injection) and intravenous hydrocortisone sodium succinate (200 mg).

Tracheal disorders

Tracheal obstruction

External compression by lymph nodes containing metastases, usually from a lung cancer, is a more frequent cause of tracheal obstruction than primary benign or malignant tumours. The trachea may also be compressed by a retrosternal goitre (see Fig. 18.12, p. 648). Rare causes include an aneurysm of the aortic arch and (in children) tuberculous mediastinal lymph nodes. Tracheal stenosis is an occasional complication of tracheostomy, prolonged intubation, granulomatosis with polyangiitis (Wegener's granulomatosis; p. 1041) or trauma.

Clinical features and management

Stridor can be detected in every patient with severe tracheal narrowing. Bronchoscopic examination of the trachea should be undertaken without delay to determine the site, degree and nature of the obstruction.

Localised tumours of the trachea can be resected but reconstruction after resection may be technically difficult. Endobronchial laser therapy, bronchoscopically placed tracheal stents, chemotherapy and radiotherapy are alternatives to surgery. The choice of treatment depends on the nature of the tumour and the general health of the patient. Benign tracheal strictures can sometimes be dilated but may require resection.

Tracheo-oesophageal fistula

This may be present in newborn infants as a congenital abnormality. In adults, it is usually due to malignant lesions in the mediastinum, such as carcinoma or lymphoma, eroding both the trachea and oesophagus to produce a communication between them. Swallowed liquids enter the trachea and bronchi through the fistula and provoke coughing.

Surgical closure of a congenital fistula, if undertaken promptly, is usually successful. There is usually no curative treatment for malignant fistulae, and death from overwhelming pulmonary infection rapidly supervenes.

Pleural disease

Pleurisy, pleural effusion, empyema and asbestos-associated pleural disease have been described above.

Pneumothorax

Pneumothorax is the presence of air in the pleural space, which can either occur spontaneously, or result from iatrogenic injury or trauma to the lung or chest wall (Box 17.90). Primary spontaneous pneumothorax occurs in patients with no history of lung disease. Smoking, tall stature and the presence of apical subpleural blebs are risk factors. Secondary pneumothorax affects patients with pre-existing lung disease and is associated with higher mortality rates (Fig. 17.71).

Where the communication between the airway and the pleural space seals off as the lung deflates and does not re-open, the

i 17.90 Classification of pneumothorax
Spontaneous
Primary
• No evidence of overt lung disease; air escapes from the lung into the pleural space through rupture of a small pleural bleb, or the pulmonary end of a pleural adhesion
Secondary
• Underlying lung disease, most commonly chronic obstructive pulmonary disease and tuberculosis; also seen in asthma, lung abscess, pulmonary infarcts, lung cancer and all forms of fibrotic and cystic lung disease
Traumatic
• Iatrogenic (e.g. following thoracic surgery or biopsy) or chest wall injury

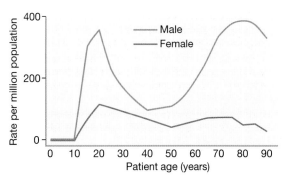

Fig. 17.71 Bimodal age distribution for hospital admissions for pneumothorax in England. The incidence of primary spontaneous pneumothorax peaks in males aged 15–30 years. Secondary spontaneous pneumothorax occurs mainly in males over 55 years.

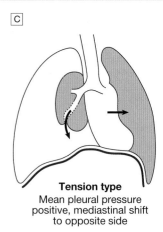

Closed type
Mean pleural pressure negative

Open type
Mean pleural pressure atmospheric

Tension type
Mean pleural pressure positive, mediastinal shift to opposite side

Fig. 17.72 Types of spontaneous pneumothorax. A Closed type. B Open type. C Tension (valvular) type.

pneumothorax is referred to as 'closed' (Fig. 17.72A). The mean pleural pressure remains negative, spontaneous reabsorption of air and re-expansion of the lung occur over a few days or weeks, and infection is uncommon. This contrasts with an 'open' pneumothorax, where the communication fails to seal and air continues to pass freely between the bronchial tree and pleural space (Fig. 17.72B). An example of the latter is a bronchopleural fistula, which can facilitate the transmission of infection from the airways into the pleural space, leading to empyema. An open pneumothorax is commonly seen following rupture of an emphysematous bulla, tuberculous cavity or lung abscess into the pleural space.

Occasionally, the communication between the airway and the pleural space acts as a one-way valve, allowing air to enter the pleural space during inspiration but not to escape on expiration. This is a tension pneumothorax. Large amounts of trapped air accumulate progressively in the pleural space and the intrapleural pressure rises to well above atmospheric levels. This causes mediastinal displacement towards the opposite side, with compression of the opposite normal lung and impairment of systemic venous return, causing cardiovascular compromise (Fig. 17.72C).

Clinical features

The most common symptoms are sudden-onset unilateral pleuritic chest pain or breathlessness. In those individuals with underlying lung disease, breathlessness can be severe and may not resolve spontaneously. In patients with a small pneumothorax, physical examination may be normal. A larger pneumothorax (>15% of the hemithorax) results in decreased or absent breath sounds (p. 547). The combination of absent breath sounds and a resonant percussion note is diagnostic of pneumothorax.

By contrast, in tension pneumothorax there is rapidly progressive breathlessness associated with a marked tachycardia, hypotension, cyanosis and tracheal displacement away from the side of the silent hemithorax. Occasionally, tension pneumothorax may occur without mediastinal shift, if malignant disease or scarring has splinted the mediastinum.

Investigations

The chest X-ray shows the sharply defined edge of the deflated lung with complete translucency (no lung markings) between this and the chest wall (p. 547). Care must be taken to differentiate between a large pre-existing emphysematous bulla and a

---

17.91 Pleural disease in old age

- **Spontaneous pneumothorax**: invariably associated with underlying lung disease in old age and has a significant mortality. Surgical or chemical pleurodesis is advised in all such patients.
- **Rib fracture**: common cause of pleural-type pain; may be spontaneous (due to coughing), traumatic or pathological. Underlying osteomalacia may contribute to poor healing, especially in the housebound with no exposure to sunlight.
- **Tuberculosis**: should always be considered and actively excluded in any elderly patient presenting with a unilateral pleural effusion.
- **Mesothelioma**: more common in older individuals than younger people due to a long latency period between asbestos exposure (often more than 20 years) and the development of disease.
- **Analgesia**: frail older people are particularly sensitive to the respiratory depressant effects of opiate-based analgesia and careful monitoring is required when using these agents for pleural pain.

---

pneumothorax. CT is used in difficult cases to avoid misdirected attempts at aspiration. X-rays may also show the extent of any mediastinal displacement and reveal any pleural fluid or underlying pulmonary disease.

Management

Primary pneumothorax, in which the lung edge is less than 2 cm from the chest wall and the patient is not breathless, normally resolves without intervention. In young patients presenting with a moderate or large spontaneous primary pneumothorax, percutaneous needle aspiration of air is a simple and well-tolerated alternative to intercostal tube drainage, with a 60–80% chance of avoiding the need for a chest drain (Fig. 17.73). In patients with significant underlying chronic lung disease, however, secondary pneumothorax may cause respiratory distress. In these individuals, the success rate of aspiration is much lower, and intercostal tube drainage and inpatient observation are usually required, particularly in those over 50 years old and those with respiratory compromise. If there is a tension pneumothorax, immediate release of the positive pressure by insertion of a blunt cannula into the pleural space may be beneficial, allowing time to prepare for chest drain insertion.

When needed, intercostal drains are inserted in the fourth, fifth or sixth intercostal space in the mid-axillary line, connected to an underwater seal or one-way Heimlich valve, and secured firmly

Fig. 17.73 Management of spontaneous pneumothorax. (1) Immediate decompression prior to insertion of the intercostal drain. (2) Aspirate in the second intercostal space anteriorly in the mid-clavicular line using a 16F cannula; discontinue if resistance is felt, the patient coughs excessively, or more than 2.5 L of air are removed. (3) The post-aspiration chest X-ray is not a reliable indicator of whether a pleural leak remains, and all patients should be told to attend again immediately in the event of deterioration.

to the chest wall. Clamping of an intercostal drain is potentially dangerous and rarely indicated. The drain should be removed the morning after the lung has fully re-inflated and bubbling has stopped. Continued bubbling after 5–7 days is an indication for surgery. If bubbling in the drainage bottle stops before full re-inflation, the tube is either blocked or kinked or displaced. Supplemental oxygen may speed resolution, as it accelerates the rate at which nitrogen is reabsorbed by the pleura.

Patients with a closed pneumothorax should be advised not to fly, as the trapped gas expands at altitude. After complete resolution, there is no clear evidence to indicate how long patients should avoid flying for, although British Thoracic Society guidelines suggest that waiting 1–2 weeks, with confirmation of full inflation prior to flight, is prudent. Patients should also be advised to stop smoking and informed about the risks of a recurrent pneumothorax. Diving is potentially dangerous after pneumothorax, unless a surgical pleurodesis has sealed the lung to the chest wall.

Recurrent spontaneous pneumothorax

After primary spontaneous pneumothorax, recurrence occurs within a year of either aspiration or tube drainage in approximately 25% of patients and should prompt definitive treatment. Surgical pleurodesis is recommended in all patients following a second pneumothorax and should be considered following the first episode of secondary pneumothorax if low respiratory reserve makes recurrence hazardous. Pleurodesis can be achieved

by pleural abrasion or parietal pleurectomy at thoracotomy or thoracoscopy.

Diseases of the diaphragm and chest wall

Disorders of the diaphragm

Congenital disorders

Diaphragmatic hernias

Congenital defects of the diaphragm can allow herniation of abdominal viscera. Posteriorly situated hernias through the foramen of Bochdalek are more common than anterior hernias through the foramen of Morgagni.

Eventration of the diaphragm

Abnormal elevation or bulging of one hemidiaphragm, more often the left, results from total or partial absence of muscular development of the septum transversum. Most eventrations are asymptomatic and are detected by chance on X-ray in adult life but severe respiratory distress can be caused in infancy if the diaphragmatic muscular defect is extensive.

Acquired disorders

Elevation of a hemidiaphragm may result from paralysis or other structural causes (Box 17.92). The phrenic nerve may be damaged by lung cancer, disease of cervical vertebrae, tumours of the cervical cord, shingles, trauma (including road traffic and birth injuries), surgery, and stretching of the nerve by mediastinal masses and aortic aneurysms. Idiopathic diaphragmatic paralysis occasionally occurs in otherwise fit patients. Paralysis of one hemidiaphragm results in loss of around 20% of ventilatory capacity but may not be noticed by otherwise healthy individuals. Ultrasound screening can be used to demonstrate paradoxical upward movement of the paralysed hemidiaphragm on sniffing. CT of the chest and neck is the best way to exclude occult disease affecting the phrenic nerve.

Bilateral diaphragmatic weakness occurs in peripheral neuropathies of any type, including Guillain–Barré syndrome (p. 1140); in disorders affecting the anterior horn cells, e.g. poliomyelitis (p. 1123); in muscular dystrophies; and in connective tissue disorders, such as SLE and polymyositis (pp. 1034 and 1039).

Hiatus hernia is common (p. 791). Diaphragmatic rupture is usually caused by a crush injury and may not be detected until years later. Respiratory disorders that cause pulmonary hyperinflation, e.g. emphysema, and those that result in small stiff lungs, e.g. diffuse pulmonary fibrosis, compromise diaphragmatic function and predispose to fatigue.

17

i	**17.92 Causes of elevation of a hemidiaphragm**
• Phrenic nerve paralysis • Eventration of the diaphragm • Decrease in volume of one lung (e.g. lobectomy, unilateral pulmonary fibrosis) • Severe pleuritic pain	• Pulmonary infarction • Subphrenic abscess • Large volume of gas in the stomach or colon • Large tumours or cysts of the liver

Deformities of the chest wall

Thoracic kyphoscoliosis

Abnormalities of alignment of the dorsal spine and their consequent effects on thoracic shape may be caused by:

- congenital abnormality
- vertebral disease, including tuberculosis, osteoporosis and ankylosing spondylitis
- trauma
- neuromuscular disease, such as poliomyelitis.

Simple kyphosis (increased anterior curvature of the thoracic spine) causes less pulmonary embarrassment than kyphoscoliosis (anteroposterior and lateral curvature). Kyphoscoliosis, if severe, restricts and distorts expansion of the chest wall and impairs diaphragmatic function, causing ventilation–perfusion mismatch in the lungs. Patients with severe deformity may develop type II respiratory failure (initially manifest during sleep), pulmonary hypertension and right ventricular failure. They can often be successfully treated with non-invasive ventilatory support (p. 202).

Pectus excavatum

Pectus excavatum (funnel chest) is an idiopathic condition in which the body of the sternum, usually only the lower end, is curved inwards. The heart is displaced to the left and may be compressed between the sternum and the vertebral column but only rarely is there associated disturbance of cardiac function. The deformity may restrict chest expansion and reduce vital capacity. Operative correction is rarely performed, and then only for cosmetic reasons.

Pectus carinatum

Pectus carinatum (pigeon chest) is frequently caused by severe asthma during childhood. Very occasionally, this deformity can be produced by rickets or be idiopathic.

Further information

Websites

brit-thoracic.org.uk *British Thoracic Society: access to guidelines on a range of respiratory conditions.*

ersnet.org *European Respiratory Society: provides information on education and research, and patient information.*

ginasthma.com *Global Initiative for Asthma: comprehensive overview of asthma.*

goldcopd.org *Global Initiative for Chronic Obstructive Lung Disease: comprehensive overview of COPD.*

thoracic.org *American Thoracic Society: provides information on education and research, and patient information.*

MWJ Strachan
JDC Newell-Price

18

Endocrinology

Clinical examination in endocrine disease 630

An overview of endocrinology 632
Functional anatomy and physiology 632
Endocrine pathology 632
Investigation of endocrine disease 633
Presenting problems in endocrine disease 633

The thyroid gland 634
Functional anatomy, physiology and investigations 634
Presenting problems in thyroid disease 635
  Thyrotoxicosis 635
  Hypothyroidism 639
  Asymptomatic abnormal thyroid function tests 642
  Thyroid lump or swelling 642
Autoimmune thyroid disease 643
Transient thyroiditis 646
Iodine-associated thyroid disease 647
Simple and multinodular goitre 648
Thyroid neoplasia 649
Congenital thyroid disease 650

The reproductive system 651
Functional anatomy, physiology and investigations 651
Presenting problems in reproductive disease 653
  Delayed puberty 653
  Precocious puberty 654
  Amenorrhoea 654
  Male hypogonadism 655
  Infertility 656
  Gynaecomastia 657
  Hirsutism 657
Polycystic ovarian syndrome 658
Turner's syndrome 659
Klinefelter's syndrome 660

The parathyroid glands 661
Functional anatomy, physiology and investigations 661
Presenting problems in parathyroid disease 661
  Hypercalcaemia 661
  Hypocalcaemia 662
Primary hyperparathyroidism 663
Familial hypocalciuric hypercalcaemia 664
Hypoparathyroidism 664

The adrenal glands 665
Functional anatomy and physiology 665
Presenting problems in adrenal disease 666
  Cushing's syndrome 666
  Therapeutic use of glucocorticoids 670
  Adrenal insufficiency 671
  Incidental adrenal mass 673
Primary hyperaldosteronism 674
Phaeochromocytoma and paraganglioma 675
Congenital adrenal hyperplasia 676

The endocrine pancreas and gastrointestinal tract 676
Presenting problems in endocrine pancreas disease 676
  Spontaneous hypoglycaemia 676
Gastroenteropancreatic neuro-endocrine tumours 678

The hypothalamus and the pituitary gland 679
Functional anatomy, physiology and investigations 679
Presenting problems in hypothalamic and pituitary disease 681
  Hypopituitarism 681
  Pituitary tumour 683
  Hyperprolactinaemia/galactorrhoea 684
Prolactinoma 684
Acromegaly 685
Craniopharyngioma 687
Diabetes insipidus 687

Disorders affecting multiple endocrine glands 688
Multiple endocrine neoplasia 688
Autoimmune polyendocrine syndromes 689
Late effects of childhood cancer therapy 689

Clinical examination in endocrine disease

Endocrine disease causes clinical syndromes with symptoms and signs involving many organ systems. The emphasis of the clinical examination depends on the gland or hormone that is thought to be abnormal.

Diabetes mellitus (described in detail in Ch. 20) and thyroid disease are the most common endocrine disorders.

5 Blood pressure
Hypertension in Cushing's and Conn's syndromes, phaeochromocytoma
Hypotension in adrenal insufficiency

4 Pulse
Atrial fibrillation
Sinus tachycardia
Bradycardia

3 Skin
Hair distribution
Dry/greasy
Pigmentation/pallor
Bruising
Vitiligo
Striae
Thickness

▲ Vitiligo in organ-specific autoimmune disease

2 Hands
Palmar erythema
Tremor
Acromegaly
Carpal tunnel syndrome

▲ Pigmentation of creases due to high ACTH levels in Addison's disease

▲ Acromegalic hands. Note soft tissue enlargement causing 'spade-like' changes

1 Height and weight

6 Head

▲ Prognathism in acromegaly

Eyes
  Graves' disease (see opposite)
  Diplopia
  Visual field defect (see opposite)
Hair
  Alopecia
  Frontal balding

Facial features
  Hypothyroid
  Hirsutism
  Acromegaly
  Cushing's

Mental state
  Lethargy
  Depression
  Delirium
  Libido

7 Neck
Voice
  Hoarse, e.g. hypothyroid
  Virilised
Thyroid gland (see opposite)
  Goitre
  Nodules

Multinodular goitre ◀

8 Breasts
Galactorrhoea
Gynaecomastia

9 Body fat
Central obesity in Cushing's syndrome and growth hormone deficiency

10 Bones
Fragility fractures (e.g. of vertebrae, neck of femur or distal radius)

11 Genitalia
Virilisation
Pubertal development
Testicular volume

12 Legs
Proximal myopathy
Myxoedema

▲ Pretibial myxoedema in Graves' disease

Observation
• Most examination in endocrinology is by observation
• Astute observation can often yield 'spot' diagnosis of endocrine disorders
• The emphasis of examination varies depending on which gland or hormone is thought to be involved

6 Examination of the visual fields by confrontation

- Sit opposite patient
- You and patient cover opposite eyes
- Bring red pin (or wiggling finger) slowly into view from extreme of your vision, as shown
- Ask patient to say 'now' when it comes into view
- Continue to move pin into centre of vision and ask patient to tell you if it disappears
- Repeat in each of four quadrants
- Repeat in other eye

A bitemporal hemianopia is the classical finding in pituitary macroadenomas (p. 683)

6 Examination in Graves' ophthalmopathy

- **Inspect** from front and side
  Periorbital oedema (Fig. 18.8)
  Conjunctival inflammation (chemosis)
  Corneal ulceration
  Proptosis (exophthalmos)*
  Lid retraction*

- **Range of eye movements**
  Lid lag on descending gaze*
  Diplopia on lateral gaze

- **Pupillary reflexes**
  Afferent defect (pupils constrict further on swinging light to unaffected eye, Box 25.22)

- **Vision**
  Visual acuity impaired
  Loss of colour vision
  Visual field defects

Right proptosis and afferent pupillary defect

- **Ophthalmoscopy**
  Optic disc pallor
  Papilloedema

*Note position of eyelids relative to iris.

18

7 Examination of the thyroid gland

- **Inspect** from front to side

- **Palpate** from behind
  Thyroid moves on swallowing
  Check if lower margin is palpable
  Cervical lymph nodes
  Tracheal deviation

- **Auscultate** for bruit
  Ask patient to hold breath
  If present, check for radiating murmur

- **Percuss** for retrosternal thyroid

- Consider systemic signs of thyroid dysfunction (Box 18.7) incl. tremor, palmar erythema, warm peripheries, tachycardia, lid lag

- Consider signs of Graves' disease incl. ophthalmopathy, pretibial myxoedema

- Check for Pemberton's sign, i.e. facial engorgement when arms raised above head

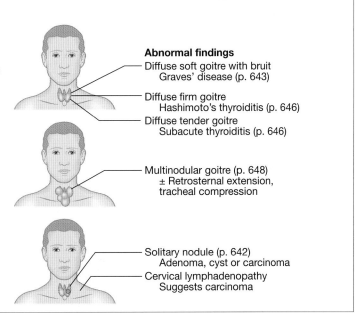

Abnormal findings
Diffuse soft goitre with bruit
  Graves' disease (p. 643)

Diffuse firm goitre
  Hashimoto's thyroiditis (p. 646)
Diffuse tender goitre
  Subacute thyroiditis (p. 646)

Multinodular goitre (p. 648)
  ± Retrosternal extension, tracheal compression

Solitary nodule (p. 642)
  Adenoma, cyst or carcinoma
Cervical lymphadenopathy
  Suggests carcinoma

Endocrinology concerns the synthesis, secretion and action of hormones. These are chemical messengers released from endocrine glands that coordinate the activities of many different cells. Endocrine diseases can therefore affect multiple organs and systems. This chapter describes the principles of endocrinology before dealing with the function and diseases of each gland in turn.

Some endocrine disorders are common, particularly those of the thyroid, parathyroid glands, reproductive system and β cells of the pancreas (Ch. 20). For example, thyroid dysfunction occurs in more than 10% of the population in areas with iodine deficiency, such as the Himalayas, and 4% of women aged 20–50 years in the UK. Less common endocrine syndromes are described later in the chapter.

Few endocrine therapies have been evaluated by randomised controlled trials, in part because hormone replacement therapy (e.g. with levothyroxine) has obvious clinical benefits and placebo-controlled trials would be unethical. Where trials have been performed, they relate mainly to use of therapy that is 'optional' and/or more recently available, such as oestrogen replacement in post-menopausal women, androgen therapy in older men and growth hormone replacement.

An overview of endocrinology

Functional anatomy and physiology

Some endocrine glands, such as the parathyroids and pancreas, respond directly to metabolic signals, but most are controlled by hormones released from the pituitary gland. Anterior pituitary hormone secretion is controlled in turn by substances produced in the hypothalamus and released into portal blood, which drains directly down the pituitary stalk (Fig. 18.1). Posterior pituitary hormones are synthesised in the hypothalamus and transported down nerve axons, to be released from the posterior pituitary. Hormone release in the hypothalamus and pituitary is regulated by numerous stimuli and through feedback control by hormones produced by the target glands (thyroid, adrenal cortex and gonads). These integrated endocrine systems are called 'axes' and are listed in Figure 18.2.

A wide variety of molecules can act as hormones, including peptides such as insulin and growth hormone, glycoproteins such as thyroid-stimulating hormone, and amines such as noradrenaline (norepinephrine). The biological effects of hormones are mediated by binding to receptors. Many receptors are located on the cell surface. These interact with various intracellular signalling molecules on the cytosolic side of the plasma membrane to affect cell function, usually through changes in gene expression. Some hormones, most notably steroids, triiodothyronine (T_3) and vitamin D, bind to specific intracellular receptors. The hormone/receptor complex forms a ligand-activated transcription factor, which regulates gene expression directly (p. 39).

The classical model of endocrine function involves hormones synthesised in endocrine glands, which are released into the circulation and act at sites distant from those of secretion (as in Fig. 18.1). However, additional levels of regulation are now recognised. Many other organs secrete hormones or contribute to the peripheral metabolism and activation of prohormones. A notable example is the production of oestrogens from adrenal androgens in adipose tissue by the enzyme aromatase. Some hormones, such as neurotransmitters, act in a paracrine fashion

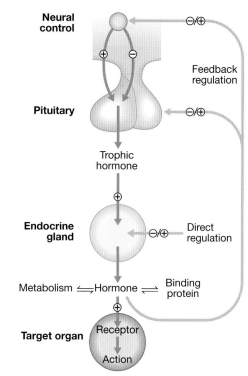

Fig. 18.1 An archetypal endocrine axis. Regulation by negative feedback and direct control is shown, along with the equilibrium between active circulating free hormone and bound or metabolised hormone.

to affect adjacent cells, or act in an autocrine way to affect behaviour of the cell that produces the hormone.

Endocrine pathology

For each endocrine axis or major gland, diseases can be classified as shown in Box 18.1. Pathology arising within the gland is often called 'primary' disease (e.g. primary hypothyroidism in Hashimoto's thyroiditis), while abnormal stimulation of the gland is often called 'secondary' disease (e.g. secondary hypothyroidism in patients with a pituitary tumour and thyroid-stimulating hormone

---

i | **18.1 Classification of endocrine disease**

Hormone excess

• Primary gland over-production
• Secondary to excess trophic substance

Hormone deficiency

• Primary gland failure
• Secondary to deficient trophic hormone

Hormone hypersensitivity

• Failure of inactivation of hormone
• Target organ over-activity/hypersensitivity

Hormone resistance

• Failure of activation by hormone
• Target organ resistance

Non-functioning tumours

• Benign
• Malignant

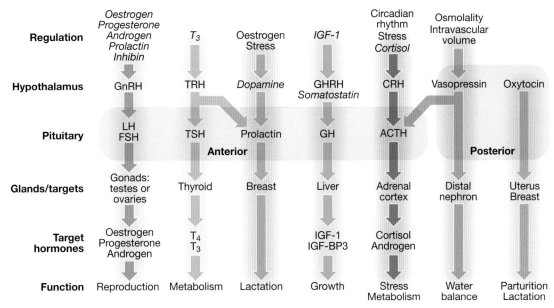

Fig. 18.2 The principal endocrine 'axes'. Some major endocrine glands are not controlled by the pituitary. These include the parathyroid glands (regulated by calcium concentrations, p. 661), the adrenal zona glomerulosa (regulated by the renin–angiotensin system, p. 665) and the endocrine pancreas (Ch. 20). Italics show negative regulation. (ACTH = adrenocorticotrophic hormone; CRH = corticotrophin-releasing hormone; FSH = follicle-stimulating hormone; GH = growth hormone; GHRH = growth hormone-releasing hormone; GnRH = gonadotrophin-releasing hormone; IGF-1 = insulin-like growth factor-1; IGF-BP3 = IGF-binding protein-3; LH = luteinising hormone: T_3 = triiodothyronine; T_4 = thyroxine; TRH = thyrotrophin-releasing hormone; TSH = thyroid-stimulating hormone; vasopressin = antidiuretic hormone (ADH))

deficiency). Some pathological processes can affect multiple endocrine glands (p. 688); these may have a genetic basis (such as organ-specific autoimmune endocrine disorders and the multiple endocrine neoplasia (MEN) syndromes) or be a consequence of therapy for another disease (e.g. following treatment of childhood cancer with chemotherapy and/or radiotherapy).

Investigation of endocrine disease

Biochemical investigations play a central role in endocrinology. Most hormones can be measured in blood but the circumstances in which the sample is taken are often crucial, especially for hormones with pulsatile secretion, such as growth hormone; those that show diurnal variation, such as cortisol; or those that demonstrate monthly variation, such as oestrogen or progesterone. Some hormones are labile and need special collection, handling and processing requirements, e.g. collection in a special tube and/or rapid transportation to the laboratory on ice. Local protocols for hormone measurement should be carefully followed. Other investigations, such as imaging and biopsy, are more frequently reserved for patients who present with a tumour. The principles of investigation are shown in Box 18.2. The choice of test is often pragmatic, taking local access to reliable sampling facilities and laboratory measurements into account.

Presenting problems in endocrine disease

Endocrine diseases present in many different ways and to clinicians in many different disciplines. Classical syndromes are described in relation to individual glands in the following sections. Often, however, the presentation is with non-specific symptoms (Box 18.3) or with asymptomatic biochemical abnormalities. In

i | **18.2 Principles of endocrine investigation**

Timing of measurement

- Release of many hormones is rhythmical (pulsatile, circadian or monthly), so random measurement may be invalid and sequential or dynamic tests may be required

Choice of dynamic biochemical test

- Abnormalities are often characterised by loss of normal regulation of hormone secretion
- If hormone deficiency is suspected, choose a stimulation test
- If hormone excess is suspected, choose a suppression test
- The more tests there are to choose from, the less likely it is that any single test is infallible, so avoid interpreting one result in isolation

Imaging

- 'Functional' as well as conventional 'structural' imaging can be performed as secretory endocrine cells can also take up labelled substrates, e.g. radio-labelled iodine or octreotide
- Most endocrine glands have a high prevalence of 'incidentalomas', so do not scan unless the biochemistry confirms endocrine dysfunction or the primary problem is a tumour

Biopsy

- Many endocrine tumours are difficult to classify histologically (e.g. adrenal carcinoma and adenoma)

addition, endocrine diseases are encountered in the differential diagnosis of common complaints discussed in other chapters of this book, including electrolyte abnormalities (Ch. 14), hypertension (Ch. 16), obesity (Ch. 19) and osteoporosis (Ch. 24). Although diseases of the adrenal glands, hypothalamus and pituitary are relatively rare, their diagnosis often relies on astute clinical observation in a patient with non-specific complaints, so it is important that clinicians are familiar with their key features.

18

18.3 Examples of non-specific presentations of endocrine disease

Symptom	Most likely endocrine disorder(s)
Lethargy and depression	Hypothyroidism, diabetes mellitus, hyperparathyroidism, hypogonadism, adrenal insufficiency, Cushing's syndrome
Weight gain	Hypothyroidism, Cushing's syndrome
Weight loss	Thyrotoxicosis, adrenal insufficiency, diabetes mellitus
Polyuria and polydipsia	Diabetes mellitus, diabetes insipidus, hyperparathyroidism, hypokalaemia (Conn's syndrome)
Heat intolerance	Thyrotoxicosis, menopause
Palpitation	Thyrotoxicosis, phaeochromocytoma
Headache	Acromegaly, pituitary tumour, phaeochromocytoma
Muscle weakness (usually proximal)	Thyrotoxicosis, Cushing's syndrome, hypokalaemia (e.g. Conn's syndrome), hyperparathyroidism, hypogonadism
Coarsening of features	Acromegaly, hypothyroidism

18.4 Classification of thyroid disease

	Primary	Secondary
Hormone excess	Graves' disease Multinodular goitre Adenoma Subacute thyroiditis	TSHoma
Hormone deficiency	Hashimoto's thyroiditis Atrophic hypothyroidism	Hypopituitarism
Hormone hypersensitivity	–	
Hormone resistance	Thyroid hormone resistance syndrome 5'-monodeiodinase deficiency	
Non-functioning tumours	Differentiated carcinoma Medullary carcinoma Lymphoma	

The thyroid gland

Diseases of the thyroid, summarised in Box 18.4, predominantly affect females and are common, occurring in about 5% of the population. The thyroid axis is involved in the regulation of cellular differentiation and metabolism in virtually all nucleated cells, so that disorders of thyroid function have diverse manifestations. Structural diseases of the thyroid gland, such as goitre, commonly occur in patients with normal thyroid function.

Functional anatomy, physiology and investigations

Thyroid physiology is illustrated in Figure 18.3. The parafollicular C cells secrete calcitonin, which is of no apparent physiological significance in humans. The follicular epithelial cells synthesise thyroid hormones by incorporating iodine into the amino acid tyrosine on the surface of thyroglobulin (Tg), a protein secreted into the colloid of the follicle. Iodide is a key substrate for thyroid hormone synthesis; a dietary intake in excess of 100 μg/day is required to maintain thyroid function in adults. The thyroid secretes predominantly thyroxine (T_4) and only a small amount of triiodothyronine (T_3); approximately 85% of T_3 in blood is produced from T_4 by a family of monodeiodinase enzymes that are active in many tissues, including liver, muscle, heart and kidney. Selenium is an integral component of these monodeiodinases. T_4 can be regarded as a prohormone, since it has a longer half-life in blood than T_3 (approximately 1 week compared with approximately 18 hours), and binds and activates thyroid hormone receptors less effectively than T_3. T_4 can also be converted to the inactive metabolite, reverse T_3.

T_3 and T_4 circulate in plasma almost entirely (>99%) bound to transport proteins, mainly thyroxine-binding globulin (TBG). It is the unbound or free hormones that diffuse into tissues and exert diverse metabolic actions. Some laboratories use assays that measure total T_4 and T_3 in plasma but it is increasingly common to measure free T_4 and free T_3. The theoretical advantage of the

free hormone measurements is that they are not influenced by changes in the concentration of binding proteins. For example, TBG levels are increased by oestrogen (such as in the combined oral contraceptive pill) and this will result in raised total T_3 and T_4, although free thyroid hormone levels are normal.

Production of T_3 and T_4 in the thyroid is stimulated by thyrotrophin (thyroid-stimulating hormone, TSH), a glycoprotein released from the thyrotroph cells of the anterior pituitary in response to the hypothalamic tripeptide, thyrotrophin-releasing hormone (TRH). A circadian rhythm of TSH secretion can be demonstrated with a peak at 0100 hrs and trough at 1100 hrs, but the variation is small so that thyroid function can be assessed reliably from a single blood sample taken at any time of day and does not usually require any dynamic stimulation or suppression tests. There is a negative feedback of thyroid hormones on the hypothalamus and pituitary such that in thyrotoxicosis, when plasma concentrations of T_3 and T_4 are raised, TSH secretion is suppressed. Conversely, in hypothyroidism due to disease of the thyroid gland, low T_3 and T_4 are associated with high circulating TSH levels. The relationship between TSH and T_4 is classically described as inverse log-linear (Fig. 18.4). The anterior pituitary is, though, very sensitive to minor changes in thyroid hormone levels within the reference range. For example, in an individual whose free T_4 level is usually 15 pmol/L (1.17 ng/dL), a rise or fall of 5 pmol/L (0.39 ng/dL) would be associated on the one hand with undetectable TSH, and on the other hand with a raised TSH. For this reason, TSH is usually regarded as the most useful investigation of thyroid function. However, interpretation of TSH values without considering thyroid hormone levels may be misleading in patients with pituitary disease; for example, TSH is inappropriately low or 'normal' in secondary hypothyroidism (see Box 18.5 and Box 18.53, p. 680). Moreover, TSH may take several weeks to 'catch up' with T_4 and T_3 levels; for example, levothyroxine therapy will raise T_4 and T_3 levels within approximately 2 weeks but it may take 4–6 weeks for the TSH to reach a steady state. Heterophilic antibodies (host antibodies with affinity to the animal antibodies used in biological assays, p. 242) can also interfere with the TSH assay and cause a spurious high or low measurement. Common patterns of abnormal thyroid function test results and their interpretation are shown in Box 18.5.

Other modalities commonly employed in the investigation of thyroid disease include measurement of antibodies against

Fig. 18.3 Structure and function of the thyroid gland. (1) Thyroglobulin (Tg) is synthesised and secreted into the colloid of the follicle. (2) Inorganic iodide (I⁻) is actively transported into the follicular cell ('trapping'). (3) Iodide is transported on to the colloidal surface by a transporter (pendrin, defective in Pendred's syndrome, p. 650) and 'organified' by the thyroid peroxidase enzyme, which incorporates it into the amino acid tyrosine on the surface of Tg to form monoiodotyrosine (MIT) and diiodotyrosine (DIT). (4) Iodinated tyrosines couple to form T_3 and T_4. (5) Tg is endocytosed. (6) Tg is cleaved by proteolysis to free the iodinated tyrosine and thyroid hormones. (7) Iodinated tyrosine is dehalogenated to recycle the iodide. (8) T_4 is converted to T_3 by 5'-monodeiodinase.

Fig. 18.4 The relationship between serum thyroid-stimulating hormone (TSH) and free T_4. Due to the classic negative feedback loop between T_4 and TSH, there is an inverse relationship between serum free T_4 and the log of serum TSH. To convert pmol/L to ng/dL, divide by 12.87.

the TSH receptor or other thyroid antigens (see Box 18.8), radioisotope imaging, fine needle aspiration biopsy and ultrasound. Their use is described below.

Presenting problems in thyroid disease

The most common presentations are hyperthyroidism (thyrotoxicosis), hypothyroidism and enlargement of the thyroid (goitre or thyroid nodule). Widespread availability of thyroid function tests has led to the increasingly frequent identification of patients with abnormal results who either are asymptomatic or have non-specific complaints such as tiredness and weight gain.

Thyrotoxicosis

Thyrotoxicosis describes a constellation of clinical features arising from elevated circulating levels of thyroid hormone. The most common causes are Graves' disease, multinodular goitre and autonomously functioning thyroid nodules (toxic adenoma) (Box 18.6). Thyroiditis is more common in parts of the world where relevant viral infections occur, such as North America.

Clinical assessment

The clinical manifestations of thyrotoxicosis are shown in Box 18.7 and an approach to differential diagnosis is given in

18.5 How to interpret thyroid function test results

TSH	T$_4$	T$_3$	Most likely interpretation(s)
U.D.	Raised	Raised	Primary thyrotoxicosis
U.D. or low	Raised	Normal	Over-treatment of hypothyroidism with levothyroxine Factitious thyrotoxicosis
U.D.	Normal[1]	Raised	Primary T$_3$ toxicosis
U.D.	Normal[1]	Normal[1]	Subclinical thyrotoxicosis
U.D. or low	Raised	Low or normal	Non-thyroidal illness Amiodarone therapy
U.D. or low	Low	Raised	Over-treatment of hypothyroidism with liothyronine (T$_3$)
U.D.	Low	Low	Secondary hypothyroidism[4] Transient thyroiditis in evolution
Normal	Low	Low[2]	Secondary hypothyroidism[4]
Mildly elevated 5–20 mIU/L	Low	Low[2]	Primary hypothyroidism Secondary hypothyroidism[4]
Elevated > 20 mIU/L	Low	Low[2]	Primary hypothyroidism
Mildly elevated 5–20 mIU/L	Normal[3]	Normal[2]	Subclinical hypothyroidism
Elevated 20–500 mIU/L	Normal	Normal	Artefact Heterophilic antibodies (host antibodies with affinity to the animal antibodies used in TSH assays)
Elevated	Raised	Raised	Non-adherence to levothyroxine replacement – recent 'loading' dose Secondary thyrotoxicosis[4] Thyroid hormone resistance

[1]Usually upper part of reference range. [2]T$_3$ is not a sensitive indicator of hypothyroidism and should not be requested. [3]Usually lower part of reference range. [4]i.e. Secondary to pituitary or hypothalamic disease. Note that TSH assays may report detectable TSH.
(TSH = thyroid-stimulating hormone; U.D. = undetectable)

18.6 Causes of thyrotoxicosis and their relative frequencies

Cause	Frequency[1] (%)
Graves' disease	76
Multinodular goitre	14
Solitary thyroid adenoma	5
Thyroiditis Subacute (de Quervain's)[2] Post-partum[2]	3 0.5
Iodide-induced Drugs (amiodarone)[2] Radiographic contrast media[2] Iodine supplementation programme[2]	1 – –
Extrathyroidal source of thyroid hormone Factitious thyrotoxicosis[2] Struma ovarii[2,3]	0.2 –
TSH-induced TSH-secreting pituitary adenoma Choriocarcinoma and hydatidiform mole[4]	0.2 –
Follicular carcinoma ± metastases	0.1

[1]In a series of 2087 patients presenting to the Royal Infirmary of Edinburgh over a 10-year period. [2]Characterised by negligible radioisotope uptake. [3]i.e. Ovarian teratoma containing thyroid tissue. [4]Human chorionic gonadotrophin has thyroid-stimulating activity.
(TSH = thyroid-stimulating hormone)

Figure 18.5. The most common symptoms are weight loss with a normal or increased appetite, heat intolerance, palpitations, tremor and irritability. Tachycardia, palmar erythema and lid lag are common signs. Not all patients have a palpable goitre, but experienced clinicians can discriminate the diffuse soft goitre of Graves' disease from the irregular enlargement of a multinodular goitre. All causes of thyrotoxicosis can cause lid retraction and lid lag, due to potentiation of sympathetic innervation of the levator palpebrae muscles, but only Graves' disease causes other features of ophthalmopathy, including periorbital oedema, conjunctival irritation, exophthalmos and diplopia. Pretibial myxoedema (p. 646) and the rare thyroid acropachy (a periosteal hypertrophy, indistinguishable from finger clubbing) are also specific to Graves' disease.

Investigations

The first-line investigations are serum T$_3$, T$_4$ and TSH. If abnormal values are found, the tests should be repeated and the abnormality confirmed in view of the likely need for prolonged medical treatment or destructive therapy. In most patients, serum T$_3$ and T$_4$ are both elevated, but T$_4$ is in the upper part of the reference range and T$_3$ is raised (T$_3$ toxicosis) in about 5%. Serum TSH is undetectable in primary thyrotoxicosis, but values can be raised in the very rare syndrome of secondary thyrotoxicosis caused by a TSH-producing pituitary adenoma. When biochemical thyrotoxicosis has been confirmed, further investigations should be undertaken to determine the underlying cause, including measurement of TSH receptor antibodies (TRAb, elevated in Graves' disease; Box 18.8) and radioisotope scanning, as shown in Figure 18.5. Other non-specific abnormalities are common

18.7 Clinical features of thyroid dysfunction

Thyrotoxicosis		Hypothyroidism	
Symptoms	Signs	Symptoms	Signs
Common			
Weight loss despite normal or increased appetite	Weight loss	Weight gain	Weight gain
Heat intolerance, sweating	Tremor	Cold intolerance	
Palpitations, tremor	Palmar erythema	Fatigue, somnolence	
Dyspnoea, fatigue	Sinus tachycardia	Dry skin	
Irritability, emotional lability	Lid retraction, lid lag	Dry hair	
		Menorrhagia	
Less common			
Osteoporosis (fracture, loss of height)	Goitre with bruit[1]	Constipation	Hoarse voice
Diarrhoea, steatorrhoea	Atrial fibrillation[2]	Hoarseness	Facial features:
Angina	Systolic hypertension/increased pulse pressure	Carpal tunnel syndrome	Purplish lips
Ankle swelling	Cardiac failure[2]	Alopecia	Malar flush
Anxiety, psychosis	Hyper-reflexia	Aches and pains	Periorbital oedema
Muscle weakness	Ill-sustained clonus	Muscle stiffness	Loss of lateral eyebrows
Periodic paralysis (predominantly in Chinese and other Asian groups)	Proximal myopathy	Deafness	Anaemia
	Bulbar myopathy[2]	Depression	Carotenaemia
Pruritus, alopecia		Infertility	Erythema ab igne
Amenorrhoea/oligomenorrhoea			Bradycardia hypertension
Infertility, spontaneous abortion			Delayed relaxation of reflexes
Loss of libido, impotence			Dermal myxoedema
Excessive lacrimation			
Rare			
Vomiting	Gynaecomastia	Psychosis (myxoedema madness)	Ileus, ascites
Apathy	Spider naevi	Galactorrhoea	Pericardial and pleural effusions
Anorexia	Onycholysis	Impotence	Cerebellar ataxia
Exacerbation of asthma	Pigmentation		Myotonia

[1]In Graves' disease only. [2]Features found particularly in elderly patients.

18

18.8 Prevalence of thyroid autoantibodies (%)

	Antibodies to:		
	Thyroid peroxidase[1]	Thyroglobulin	TSH receptor[2]
Normal population	8–27	5–20	0
Graves' disease	50–80	50–70	80–95
Autoimmune hypothyroidism	90–100	80–90	10–20
Multinodular goitre	~30–40	~30–40	0
Transient thyroiditis	~30–40	~30–40	0

[1]Thyroid peroxidase (TPO) antibodies are the principal component of what was previously measured as thyroid 'microsomal' antibodies. [2]Thyroid-stimulating hormone receptor antibodies (TRAb) can be agonists (stimulatory, causing Graves' thyrotoxicosis) or antagonists ('blocking', causing hypothyroidism).

(Box 18.9). An electrocardiogram (ECG) may demonstrate sinus tachycardia or atrial fibrillation.

Radio-iodine uptake tests measure the proportion of isotope that is trapped in the whole gland but have been largely superseded by ^{99m}technetium scintigraphy scans, which also indicate trapping, are quicker to perform with a lower dose of radioactivity, and provide a higher-resolution image. In low-uptake thyrotoxicosis, the cause is usually a transient thyroiditis (p. 646). Occasionally, patients induce 'factitious thyrotoxicosis' by consuming excessive amounts of a thyroid hormone preparation, most often levothyroxine. The exogenous levothyroxine suppresses pituitary TSH secretion and hence iodine uptake, serum thyroglobulin and release of endogenous thyroid hormones. The T_4:T_3 ratio (typically 30 : 1 in conventional thyrotoxicosis) is increased to above 70 : 1 because circulating T_3 in factitious thyrotoxicosis is derived exclusively from the peripheral monodeiodination of T_4 and not from thyroid secretion. The combination of negligible iodine uptake, high T_4:T_3 ratio and a low or undetectable thyroglobulin is diagnostic.

Management

Definitive treatment of thyrotoxicosis depends on the underlying cause and may include antithyroid drugs, radioactive iodine or surgery. A non-selective β-adrenoceptor antagonist (β-blocker), such as propranolol (160 mg daily) or nadolol (40–80 mg daily), will alleviate but not abolish symptoms in most patients within 24–48 hours. Beta-blockers should not be used for long-term

Fig. 18.5 Establishing the differential diagnosis in thyrotoxicosis. [1]Graves' ophthalmopathy refers to clinical features of exophthalmos and periorbital and conjunctival oedema, not simply the lid lag and lid retraction that can occur in all forms of thyrotoxicosis. [2]Thyroid-stimulating hormone (TSH) receptor antibodies are very rare in patients without autoimmune thyroid disease but occur in only 80–95% of patients with Graves' disease; a positive test is therefore confirmatory but a negative test does not exclude Graves' disease. Other thyroid antibodies (e.g. anti-peroxidase and anti-thyroglobulin antibodies) are unhelpful in the differential diagnosis since they occur frequently in the population and are found with several of the disorders that cause thyrotoxicosis. [3]Scintigraphy is not necessary in most cases of drug-induced thyrotoxicosis. [4] [99m]Technetium pertechnetate scans of patients with thyrotoxicosis. In low-uptake thyrotoxicosis, most commonly due to a viral, post-partum or iodine-induced thyroiditis, there is negligible isotope detected in the region of the thyroid, although uptake is apparent in nearby salivary glands (not shown here). In a toxic adenoma there is lack of uptake of isotope by the rest of the thyroid gland due to suppression of serum TSH. In multinodular goitre there is relatively low, patchy uptake within the nodules; such an appearance is not always associated with a palpable thyroid. In Graves' disease there is diffuse uptake of isotope.

i	**18.9 Non-specific laboratory abnormalities in thyroid dysfunction***

Thyrotoxicosis

- Serum enzymes: raised alanine aminotransferase, γ-glutamyl transferase (GGT), and alkaline phosphatase from liver and bone
- Raised bilirubin
- Mild hypercalcaemia
- Glycosuria: associated diabetes mellitus, 'lag storage' glycosuria

Hypothyroidism

- Serum enzymes: raised creatine kinase, aspartate aminotransferase, lactate dehydrogenase (LDH)
- Hypercholesterolaemia
- Anaemia: normochromic normocytic or macrocytic
- Hyponatraemia

*These abnormalities are not useful in differential diagnosis, so the tests should be avoided and any further investigation undertaken only if abnormalities persist when the patient is euthyroid.

treatment of thyrotoxicosis but are extremely useful in the short term, while patients are awaiting hospital consultation or following ^{131}I therapy. Verapamil may be used as an alternative to β-blockers, e.g. in patients with asthma, but usually is only effective in improving tachycardia and has little effect on the other systemic manifestations of thyrotoxicosis.

Atrial fibrillation in thyrotoxicosis

Atrial fibrillation occurs in about 10% of patients with thyrotoxicosis. The incidence increases with age, so that almost half of all males with thyrotoxicosis over the age of 60 are affected. Moreover, subclinical thyrotoxicosis (p. 642) is a risk factor for atrial fibrillation. Characteristically, the ventricular rate is little influenced by digoxin but responds to the addition of a β-blocker. Thromboembolic vascular complications are particularly common in thyrotoxic atrial fibrillation so that anticoagulation is required, unless contraindicated. Once thyroid hormone and TSH concentrations have been returned to normal, atrial fibrillation will spontaneously revert to sinus rhythm in about 50% of patients but cardioversion may be required in the remainder.

i	18.10 The Burch–Wartofsky scoring system for thyrotoxic crisis	
Diagnostic parameters		**Score**
Temperature (°C)		
≤ 37.1		0
37.2–37.7		5
37.8–38.2		10
38.3–38.8		15
38.9–39.2		20
39.3–39.9		25
≥ 40.0		30
Central nervous system		
Absent		0
Mild (agitation)		10
Moderate (delirium, psychosis, extreme lethargy)		20
Severe (seizures, coma)		30
Gastrointestinal system		
Absent		0
Moderate (diarrhoea, nausea, vomiting, abdominal pain)		10
Severe (unexplained jaundice)		20
Cardiovascular system: pulse rate (beats/min)		
≤89		0
90–109		5
110–119		10
120–129		15
130–139		20
≥140		25
Atrial fibrillation		
Absent		0
Present		10
Congestive heart failure		
Absent		0
Mild (peripheral oedema)		5
Moderate (bi-basal crepitations)		10
Severe (pulmonary oedema)		20
Precipitant history		
Absent		0
Present		10

Scores should be totalled.

Score ≥45 = likely thyrotoxic crisis; 25–44 = impending thyrotoxic crisis; <25 = unlikely to represent thyroid crisis.

Adapted from Burch HB, Wartofsky L. Life-threatening thyrotoxicosis. Thyroid storm. Endocrinol Metab Clin N Am 1993; 22:263–277.

Thyrotoxic crisis ('thyroid storm')

This is a rare but life-threatening complication of thyrotoxicosis. The most prominent signs are fever, agitation, delirium, tachycardia or atrial fibrillation and, in the older patient, cardiac failure. The Burch–Wartofsky system may be used to help establish the diagnosis (Box 18.10). Thyrotoxic crisis is a medical emergency and has a mortality of 10% despite early recognition and treatment. It is most commonly precipitated by infection in a patient with previously unrecognised or inadequately treated thyrotoxicosis. It may also develop in known thyrotoxicosis shortly after thyroidectomy in an ill-prepared patient or within a few days of ^{131}I therapy, when acute radiation damage may lead to a transient rise in serum thyroid hormone levels.

Patients should be rehydrated and given propranolol, either orally (80 mg 4 times daily) or intravenously (1–5 mg 4 times daily). Sodium ipodate (500 mg per day orally) will restore serum T_3 levels to normal in 48–72 hours. This is a radiographic contrast medium that not only inhibits the release of thyroid hormones but also reduces the conversion of T_4 to T_3, and is therefore more effective than potassium iodide or Lugol's solution. Dexamethasone (2 mg 4 times daily) and amiodarone have similar effects. Oral carbimazole 40–60 mg daily (p. 644) should be given to inhibit the synthesis of new thyroid hormone. If the patient is unconscious or uncooperative, carbimazole can be administered rectally with good effect but no preparation is available for parenteral use. After 10–14 days the patient can usually be maintained on carbimazole alone.

Hypothyroidism

Hypothyroidism is a common condition with various causes (Box 18.11), but autoimmune disease (Hashimoto's thyroiditis) and thyroid failure following ^{131}I or surgical treatment of thyrotoxicosis account for over 90% of cases, except in areas where iodine deficiency is endemic. Women are affected approximately six times more frequently than men.

Clinical assessment

The clinical presentation depends on the duration and severity of the hypothyroidism. Those in whom complete thyroid failure has developed insidiously over months or years may present with many of the clinical features listed in Box 18.7. A consequence of prolonged hypothyroidism is the infiltration of many body tissues by the mucopolysaccharides hyaluronic acid and chondroitin

i	18.11 Causes of hypothyroidism		
Causes		**Anti-TPO antibodies[1]**	**Goitre[2]**
Autoimmune			
Hashimoto's thyroiditis		++	±
Spontaneous atrophic hypothyroidism		–	–
Graves' disease with TSH receptor-blocking antibodies		+	±
Iatrogenic			
Radioactive iodine ablation		+	±
Thyroidectomy		+	–
Drugs:			
Carbimazole, methimazole, propylthiouracil		+	±
Amiodarone		+	±
Lithium		–	±
Transient thyroiditis			
Subacute (de Quervain's) thyroiditis		+	±
Post-partum thyroiditis		+	±
Iodine deficiency			
e.g. In mountainous regions		–	++
Congenital			
Dyshormonogenesis		–	++
Thyroid aplasia		–	–
Infiltrative			
Amyloidosis, Riedel's thyroiditis, sarcoidosis etc.		+	++
Secondary hypothyroidism			
TSH deficiency		–	–

[1]As shown in Box 18.8, thyroid autoantibodies are common in the healthy population, so might be present in anyone. ++ high titre; + more likely to be detected than in the healthy population; – not especially likely. [2]Goitre: – absent; ± may be present; ++ characteristic.
(TPO = thyroid peroxidase; TSH = thyroid-stimulating hormone)

18

Fig. 18.6 An approach to adults with suspected primary hypothyroidism. This scheme ignores congenital causes of hypothyroidism (see Box 18.11), such as thyroid aplasia and dyshormonogenesis (associated with nerve deafness in Pendred's syndrome, p. 650), which are usually diagnosed in childhood. [1]Immunoreactive thyroid-stimulating hormone (TSH) may be detected at normal or even modestly elevated levels in patients with pituitary failure; unless T_4 is only marginally low, TSH should be >20 mIU/L to confirm the diagnosis of primary hypothyroidism. [2]The usual abnormality in sick euthyroidism is a low TSH but any pattern can occur. [3]Thyroid peroxidase (TPO) antibodies are highly sensitive but not very specific for autoimmune thyroid disease (see Boxes 18.8 and 18.11). [4]Specialist advice is most appropriate where indicated. Secondary hypothyroidism is rare, but is suggested by deficiency of pituitary hormones or by clinical features of pituitary tumour such as headache or visual field defect (p. 683). Rare causes of hypothyroidism with goitre include dyshormonogenesis and infiltration of the thyroid (see Box 18.11).

sulphate, resulting in a low-pitched voice, poor hearing, slurred speech due to a large tongue, and compression of the median nerve at the wrist (carpal tunnel syndrome). Infiltration of the dermis gives rise to non-pitting oedema (myxoedema), which is most marked in the skin of the hands, feet and eyelids. The resultant periorbital puffiness is often striking and may be combined with facial pallor due to vasoconstriction and anaemia, or a lemon-yellow tint to the skin caused by carotenaemia, along with purplish lips and malar flush. Most cases of hypothyroidism are not clinically obvious, however, and a high index of suspicion needs to be maintained so that the diagnosis is not overlooked in individuals complaining of non-specific symptoms such as tiredness, weight gain, depression or carpal tunnel syndrome.

The key discriminatory features in the history and examination are highlighted in Figure 18.6. Care must be taken to identify patients with transient hypothyroidism, in whom life-long levothyroxine therapy is inappropriate. This is often observed during the first 6 months after thyroidectomy or ^{131}I treatment of Graves' disease, in the post-thyrotoxic phase of subacute thyroiditis and in post-partum thyroiditis. In these conditions, levothyroxine treatment is not always necessary, as the patient may be asymptomatic during the short period of thyroid failure.

Investigations

In the vast majority of cases, hypothyroidism results from an intrinsic disorder of the thyroid gland (primary hypothyroidism). In this situation, serum T_4 is low and TSH is elevated, usually in excess of 20 mIU/L. Measurements of serum T_3 are unhelpful since they do not discriminate reliably between euthyroidism and hypothyroidism. Secondary hypothyroidism is rare and is caused

by failure of TSH secretion in an individual with hypothalamic or anterior pituitary disease. Other non-specific abnormalities are shown in Box 18.9. In severe, prolonged hypothyroidism, the ECG classically demonstrates sinus bradycardia with low-voltage complexes and ST-segment and T-wave abnormalities. Measurement of thyroid peroxidase antibodies is helpful but further investigations are rarely required (Fig. 18.6).

Management

Treatment is with levothyroxine replacement. It is customary to start with a low dose of 50 μg per day for 3 weeks, increasing thereafter to 100 μg per day for a further 3 weeks and finally to a maintenance dose of 100–150 μg per day. In younger patients, it is safe to initiate levothyroxine at a higher dose (e.g. 100 μg per day), to allow a more rapid normalisation of thyroid hormone levels. Levothyroxine has a half-life of 7 days so it should always be taken as a single daily dose and at least 6 weeks should pass before repeating thyroid function tests (as TSH takes several weeks to reach a steady state) and adjusting the dose. Patients feel better within 2–3 weeks. Reduction in weight and periorbital puffiness occurs quickly but the restoration of skin and hair texture and resolution of any effusions may take 3–6 months. As illustrated in Figure 18.6, most patients do not require specialist review but will need life-long levothyroxine therapy.

The dose of levothyroxine should be adjusted to maintain serum TSH within the reference range. To achieve this, serum T_4 often needs to be in the upper part of the reference range because the T_3 required for receptor activation is derived exclusively from conversion of T_4 within the target tissues, without the usual contribution from thyroid secretion. Some physicians advocate

18.12 Situations in which an adjustment of the dose of levothyroxine may be necessary

Increased dose required

Use of other medication
- Increase T_4 clearance: phenobarbital, phenytoin, carbamazepine, rifampicin, sertraline*, chloroquine*
- Interfere with intestinal T_4 absorption: colestyramine, sucralfate, aluminium hydroxide, ferrous sulphate, dietary fibre supplements, calcium carbonate

Pregnancy or oestrogen therapy
- Increases concentration of serum thyroxine-binding globulin

After surgical or ^{131}I ablation of Graves' disease
- Reduces thyroidal secretion with time

Malabsorption

Decreased dose required

Ageing
- Decreases T_4 clearance

Graves' disease developing in patient with long-standing primary hypothyroidism
- Switch from production of blocking to stimulating TSH receptor antibodies

*Mechanism not fully established.

combined replacement with T_4 (levothyroxine) and T_3 (liothyronine) or preparations of animal thyroid extract but this approach remains controversial and is not supported by robust evidence. Some patients remain symptomatic despite normalisation of TSH and may wish to take extra levothyroxine, which suppresses TSH. However, suppressed TSH is a risk factor for osteoporosis and atrial fibrillation (see below; subclinical thyrotoxicosis), so this approach cannot be recommended.

It is important to measure thyroid function every 1–2 years once the dose of levothyroxine is stabilised. This encourages adherence to therapy and allows adjustment for variable underlying thyroid activity and other changes in levothyroxine requirements (Box 18.12). Some patients have a persistent elevation of serum TSH despite an ostensibly adequate replacement dose of levothyroxine; most commonly, this is a consequence of suboptimal adherence to therapy. There may be differences in bioavailability between the numerous generic preparations of levothyroxine and so, if an individual is experiencing marked changes in serum TSH despite optimal adherence, the prescription of a branded preparation of levothyroxine could be considered. There is some limited evidence that suggests levothyroxine absorption may be better when the drug is taken before bed and can be further optimised by adding a vitamin C supplement; such strategies may be considered in patients with malabsorption. In some poorly compliant patients, levothyroxine is taken diligently or even in excess for a few days prior to a clinic visit, resulting in the seemingly anomalous combination of a high serum T_4 and high TSH (see Box 18.5).

Levothyroxine replacement in ischaemic heart disease

Hypothyroidism and ischaemic heart disease are common conditions that often occur together. Although angina may remain unchanged in severity or paradoxically disappear with restoration of metabolic rate, exacerbation of myocardial ischaemia, infarction and sudden death are recognised complications of levothyroxine replacement, even using doses as low as 25 µg per day. In patients with known ischaemic heart disease, thyroid hormone

replacement should be introduced at low dose and increased very slowly under specialist supervision. It has been suggested that T_3 has an advantage over T_4, since T_3 has a shorter half-life and any adverse effect will reverse more quickly, but the more distinct peak in hormone levels after each dose of T_3 is a disadvantage. Coronary intervention may be required if angina is exacerbated by levothyroxine replacement therapy.

Hypothyroidism in pregnancy

Women with hypothyroidism usually require an increased dose of levothyroxine in pregnancy; inadequately treated hypothyroidism in pregnancy has been associated with impaired cognitive development in the fetus. This is discussed in more detail on page 1279 (see also Box 18.18).

Myxoedema coma

This is a very rare presentation of hypothyroidism in which there is a depressed level of consciousness, usually in an elderly patient who appears myxoedematous. Body temperature may be as low as 25°C, convulsions are not uncommon, and cerebrospinal fluid (CSF) pressure and protein content are raised. The mortality rate is 50% and survival depends on early recognition and treatment of hypothyroidism and other factors contributing to the altered consciousness level, such as medication, cardiac failure, pneumonia, dilutional hyponatraemia and respiratory failure.

Myxoedema coma is a medical emergency and treatment must begin before biochemical confirmation of the diagnosis. Suspected cases should be treated with an intravenous injection of 20 µg liothyronine, followed by further injections of 20 µg 3 times daily until there is sustained clinical improvement. In survivors, there is a rise in body temperature within 24 hours and, after 48–72 hours, it is usually possible to switch patients to oral levothyroxine in a dose of 50 µg daily. Unless it is apparent that the patient has primary hypothyroidism, the thyroid failure should also be assumed to be secondary to hypothalamic or pituitary disease and treatment given with hydrocortisone 100 mg IM 3 times daily, pending the results of T_4, TSH and cortisol measurement (p. 680). Other measures include slow rewarming (p. 166), cautious use of intravenous fluids, broad-spectrum antibiotics and high-flow oxygen.

Symptoms of hypothyroidism with normal thyroid function tests

The classic symptoms of hypothyroidism are, by their very nature, non-specific (see Box 18.3). There is a wide differential diagnosis for symptoms such as 'fatigue', 'weight gain' and 'low mood'. As has been noted, outside the context of pituitary and hypothalamic disease, serum TSH is an excellent measure of an individual's thyroid hormone status. However, some individuals believe that they have hypothyroidism despite normal serum TSH concentrations. There are a large number of websites that claim that serum TSH is not a good measure of thyroid hormone status and suggest that other factors, such as abnormalities of T_4 to T_3 conversion, may lead to low tissue levels of active thyroid hormones. Such websites often advocate a variety of tests of thyroid function of dubious scientific validity, including measurement of serum reverse T_3, 24-hour urine T_3, basal body temperature, skin iodine absorption, and levels of selenium in blood and urine. Individuals who believe they have hypothyroidism, despite normal conventional tests of thyroid function, can be difficult to manage. They require reassurance that their symptoms are being taken seriously and that organic disease has been carefully considered; if their symptoms persist, referral to a

18

team specialising in medically unexplained symptoms should be considered.

Asymptomatic abnormal thyroid function tests

One of the most common problems in medical practice is how to manage patients with abnormal thyroid function tests who have no obvious signs or symptoms of thyroid disease. These can be divided into three categories.

Subclinical thyrotoxicosis

Serum TSH is undetectable and serum T_3 and T_4 are at the upper end of the reference range. This combination is most often found in older patients with multinodular goitre. These patients are at increased risk of atrial fibrillation and osteoporosis, and hence the consensus view is that they have mild thyrotoxicosis and require therapy, usually with ^{131}I. Otherwise, annual review is essential, as the conversion rate to overt thyrotoxicosis with elevated T_4 and/or T_3 concentrations is 5% each year.

Subclinical hypothyroidism

Serum TSH is raised and serum T_3 and T_4 concentrations are at the lower end of the reference range. This may persist for many years, although there is a risk of progression to overt thyroid failure, particularly if antibodies to thyroid peroxidase are present or if the TSH rises above 10 mIU/L. In patients with non-specific symptoms, a trial of levothyroxine therapy may be appropriate. In those with positive autoantibodies or a TSH greater than 10 mIU/L, it is better to treat the thyroid failure early rather than risk loss to follow-up and subsequent presentation with profound hypothyroidism. Levothyroxine should be given in a dose sufficient to restore the serum TSH concentration to normal.

Non-thyroidal illness ('sick euthyroidism')

This typically presents with a low serum TSH, raised T_4 and normal or low T_3 in a patient with systemic illness who does not have clinical evidence of thyroid disease. These abnormalities are caused by decreased peripheral conversion of T_4 to T_3 (with conversion instead to reverse T_3), altered levels of binding proteins and their affinity for thyroid hormones, and often reduced secretion of TSH. During convalescence, serum TSH concentrations may increase to levels found in primary hypothyroidism. As thyroid function tests are difficult to interpret in patients with non-thyroidal illness, it is wise to avoid performing thyroid function tests unless there is clinical evidence of concomitant thyroid disease. If an abnormal result is found, treatment should only be given with specialist advice and the diagnosis should be re-evaluated after recovery.

Thyroid lump or swelling

A lump or swelling in the thyroid gland can be a source of considerable anxiety for patients. There are numerous causes but, broadly speaking, a thyroid swelling is either a solitary nodule, a multinodular goitre or a diffuse goitre (Box 18.13). Nodular thyroid disease is more common in women and occurs in approximately 30% of the adult female population. The majority of thyroid nodules are impalpable but may be identified when imaging of the neck is performed for another reason, such as during Doppler ultrasonography of the carotid arteries or computed tomographic pulmonary angiography. Increasingly, thyroid nodules are identified during staging of patients with cancer with computed tomography (CT), magnetic resonance

18.13 Causes of thyroid enlargement

Diffuse goitre
- Simple goitre
- Hashimoto's thyroiditis[1]
- Graves' disease
- Drugs: iodine, amiodarone, lithium
- Iodine deficiency (endemic goitre)[1]
- Suppurative thyroiditis[2]
- Transient thyroiditis[2]
- Dyshormonogenesis[1]
- Infiltrative: amyloidosis, sarcoidosis etc.
- Riedel's thyroiditis[2]

Multinodular goitre

Solitary nodule
- Colloid cyst
- Hyperplastic nodule
- Follicular adenoma
- Papillary carcinoma
- Follicular carcinoma
- Medullary cell carcinoma
- Anaplastic carcinoma
- Lymphoma
- Metastasis

[1]Goitre likely to shrink with levothyroxine therapy. [2]Usually tender.

imaging (MRI) or positron emission tomography (PET) scans. Palpable thyroid nodules occur in 4–8% of adult women and 1–2% of adult men, and classically present when the individual (or a friend or relative) notices a lump in the neck. Multinodular goitre and solitary nodules sometimes present with acute painful enlargement due to haemorrhage into a nodule.

Patients with thyroid nodules often worry that they have cancer but the reality is that only 5–10% of thyroid nodules are malignant. A nodule presenting in childhood or adolescence, particularly if there is a past history of head and neck irradiation, or one presenting in an elderly patient should heighten suspicion of a primary thyroid malignancy (p. 649). The presence of cervical lymphadenopathy also increases the likelihood of malignancy. Rarely, a secondary deposit from a renal, breast or lung carcinoma presents as a painful, rapidly growing, solitary thyroid nodule. Thyroid nodules identified on PET scanning have an approximately 33% chance of being malignant.

Clinical assessment and investigations

Swellings in the anterior part of the neck most commonly originate in the thyroid and this can be confirmed by demonstrating that the swelling moves on swallowing (p. 631). It is often possible to distinguish clinically between the three main causes of thyroid swelling. There is a broad differential diagnosis of anterior neck swellings, which includes lymphadenopathy, branchial cysts, dermoid cysts and thyroglossal duct cysts (the latter are classically located in the midline and move on protrusion of the tongue). An ultrasound scan should be performed urgently, if there is any doubt as to the aetiology of an anterior neck swelling.

Serum T_3, T_4 and TSH should be measured in all patients with a goitre or solitary thyroid nodule. The finding of biochemical thyrotoxicosis or hypothyroidism (both of which may be subclinical) should lead to investigations, as already described on pages 636 and 640.

Thyroid scintigraphy

Thyroid scintigraphy with ^{99m}technetium should be performed in an individual with a low serum TSH and a nodular thyroid to confirm the presence of an autonomously functioning ('hot') nodule (see Fig. 18.5). In such circumstances, further evaluation is not necessary. 'Cold' nodules on scintigraphy have a much higher likelihood of malignancy, but the majority are benign and so scintigraphy is not routinely used in the evaluation of thyroid nodules when TSH is normal.

Thyroid ultrasound

If thyroid function tests are normal, an ultrasound scan will often determine the nature of the thyroid swelling. Ultrasound can establish whether there is generalised or localised swelling of the thyroid. Inflammatory disorders causing a diffuse goitre, such as Graves' disease and Hashimoto's thyroiditis, demonstrate a diffuse pattern of hypoechogenicity and, in the case of Graves' disease, increased thyroid blood flow may be seen on colour-flow Doppler. The presence of thyroid autoantibodies will support the diagnosis of Graves' disease or Hashimoto's thyroiditis, while their absence in a younger patient with a diffuse goitre and normal thyroid function suggests a diagnosis of 'simple goitre' (p. 648).

Ultrasound can readily determine the size and number of nodules within the thyroid and can distinguish solid nodules from those with a cystic element. Ultrasound is used increasingly as the key investigation in defining the risk of malignancy in a nodule. Size of the nodule is not a predictor of the risk of malignancy but there are other ultrasound characteristics that are associated with a higher likelihood of malignancy. These include hypoechoicity, intranodular vascularity, the presence of microcalcification and irregular or lobulated margins. A purely cystic nodule is highly unlikely to be malignant and a 'spongiform' appearance is also highly predictive of a benign aetiology. Individual nodules within a multinodular goitre have the same risk of malignancy as a solitary nodule. Thyroid ultrasonography is a highly specialised investigation and the accurate stratification of risk of malignancy of a thyroid nodule requires skill and expertise.

Fine needle aspiration cytology

Fine needle aspiration cytology is recommended for thyroid nodules that are suspicious for malignancy or are radiologically indeterminate. Fine needle aspiration of a thyroid nodule can be performed in the outpatient clinic, usually under ultrasound guidance. Aspiration may be therapeutic for a cyst, although recurrence on more than one occasion is an indication for surgery. Fine needle aspiration cytology cannot differentiate between a follicular adenoma and a follicular carcinoma, and in 10–20% of cases an inadequate specimen is obtained.

Management

Nodules with a benign appearance on ultrasound may be observed in an ultrasound surveillance programme; when the suspicion of malignancy is very low, the patient may be reassured and discharged. In parts of the world with borderline low iodine intake, there is evidence that levothyroxine therapy, in doses that suppress serum TSH, may reduce the size of some nodules. This should not be routine practice in iodine-sufficient populations.

Nodules that are suspicious for malignancy are treated by surgical excision, by either lobectomy or thyroidectomy. Nodules that are radiologically and/or cytologically indeterminate are more of a management challenge and often end up being surgically excised. Molecular techniques may, in the future, improve the diagnostic accuracy of thyroid cytology and allow a more conservative strategy for individuals with an indeterminate biopsy. Nodules in which malignancy is confirmed by formal histology are treated as described on page 649.

A diffuse or multinodular goitre may also require surgical treatment for cosmetic reasons or if there is compression of local structures (resulting in stridor or dysphagia). [131]I therapy may also cause some reduction in size of a multinodular goitre. Levothyroxine therapy may shrink the goitre of Hashimoto's disease, particularly if serum TSH is elevated.

Autoimmune thyroid disease

Thyroid diseases are amongst the most prevalent antibody-mediated autoimmune diseases and are associated with other organ-specific autoimmunity (Ch. 4 and p. 689). Autoantibodies may produce inflammation and destruction of thyroid tissue, resulting in hypothyroidism, goitre (in Hashimoto's thyroiditis) or sometimes even transient thyrotoxicosis ('Hashitoxicosis'), or they may stimulate the TSH receptor to cause thyrotoxicosis (in Graves' disease). There is overlap between these conditions, since some patients have multiple autoantibodies.

Graves' disease

Graves' disease can occur at any age but is unusual before puberty and most commonly affects women aged 30–50 years. The most common manifestation is thyrotoxicosis with or without a diffuse goitre. The clinical features and differential diagnosis are described on page 635. Graves' disease also causes ophthalmopathy and, rarely, pretibial myxoedema (p. 646). These extrathyroidal features usually occur in thyrotoxic patients but can arise in the absence of thyroid dysfunction.

Graves' thyrotoxicosis

Pathophysiology

The thyrotoxicosis results from the production of immunoglobulin G (IgG) antibodies directed against the TSH receptor on the thyroid follicular cell, which stimulate thyroid hormone production and proliferation of follicular cells, leading to goitre in the majority of patients. These antibodies are termed thyroid-stimulating immunoglobulins or TSH receptor antibodies (TRAb) and can be detected in the serum of 80–95% of patients with Graves' disease. The concentration of TRAb in the serum is presumed to fluctuate to account for the natural history of Graves' thyrotoxicosis (Fig. 18.7). Thyroid failure seen in some patients may result from the presence of blocking antibodies against the TSH receptor, and from tissue destruction by cytotoxic antibodies and cell-mediated immunity.

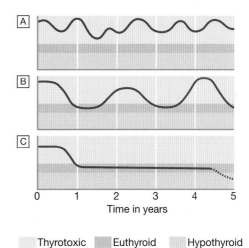

Thyrotoxic   Euthyroid   Hypothyroid

Fig. 18.7 Natural history of the thyrotoxicosis of Graves' disease.
[A] and [B] The majority (60%) of patients have either prolonged periods of thyrotoxicosis of fluctuating severity, or periods of alternating relapse and remission. [C] It is the minority who experience a single short-lived episode followed by prolonged remission and, in some cases, by the eventual onset of hypothyroidism.

Graves' disease has a strong genetic component. There is 50% concordance for thyrotoxicosis between monozygotic twins but only 5% concordance between dizygotic twins. Genomewide association studies have identified polymorphisms at the MHC, CTLA4, PTPN22, TSHR1 and FCRL3 loci as predisposing genetic variants. Many of these loci have been implicated in the pathogenesis of other autoimmune diseases.

A suggested trigger for the development of thyrotoxicosis in genetically susceptible individuals may be infection with viruses or bacteria. Certain strains of the gut organisms Escherichia coli and Yersinia enterocolitica possess cell membrane TSH receptors and it has been suggested that antibodies to these microbial antigens may cross-react with the TSH receptors on the host thyroid follicular cell. In regions of iodine deficiency (p. 647), iodine supplementation can precipitate thyrotoxicosis, but only in those with pre-existing subclinical Graves' disease. Smoking is weakly associated with Graves' thyrotoxicosis but strongly linked with the development of ophthalmopathy.

Management

Symptoms of thyrotoxicosis respond to β-blockade (p. 637) but definitive treatment requires control of thyroid hormone secretion. The different options are compared in Box 18.14. Some clinicians adopt an empirical approach of prescribing a course of antithyroid drug therapy and then recommending ^{131}I or surgery if relapse occurs. In many centres, however, ^{131}I is used extensively as a first-line therapy, given the high risk of relapse following a course of antithyroid drugs. A number of observational studies have linked therapeutic ^{131}I with increased incidence of some malignancies, particularly of the thyroid and gastrointestinal tract, but the results have been inconsistent; the association may be with Graves' disease rather than its therapy, and the magnitude of the effect, if any, is small. Experience from the disaster at the Chernobyl nuclear power plant in 1986 suggests that younger people are more sensitive to radiation-induced thyroid cancer.

Antithyroid drugs The most commonly used are carbimazole and its active metabolite, methimazole (not available in the UK). Propylthiouracil is equally effective. These drugs reduce the synthesis of new thyroid hormones by inhibiting the iodination of tyrosine (see Fig. 18.3). Carbimazole also has an immunosuppressive action, leading to a reduction in serum TRAb concentrations, but this is not enough to influence the natural history of the thyrotoxicosis significantly.

Antithyroid drugs should be introduced at high doses (carbimazole 40–60 mg daily or propylthiouracil 400–600 mg daily). Usually, this results in subjective improvement within 10–14 days and renders the patient clinically and biochemically euthyroid at 6–8 weeks. At this point, the dose can be reduced and titrated to maintain T_4 and TSH within their reference range. In most patients, carbimazole is continued at 5–20 mg per day for 12–18 months in the hope that remission will occur. Between 50% and 70% of patients with Graves's disease will subsequently relapse, usually within 2 years of stopping treatment. Risk factors for relapse include younger age, male sex, presence of a goitre, and higher TRAb titres at both diagnosis and cessation of antithyroid therapy. Rarely, T_4 and TSH levels fluctuate between those of thyrotoxicosis and hypothyroidism at successive review appointments, despite good drug adherence, presumably due to rapidly changing concentrations of TRAb. In these patients, satisfactory control can be achieved by blocking thyroid hormone synthesis with carbimazole 30–40 mg daily and adding levothyroxine 100–150 µg daily as replacement therapy (a 'block and replace' regime).

Antithyroid drugs can have adverse effects. The most common is a rash. Agranulocytosis is a rare but potentially serious complication that cannot be predicted by routine measurement of white blood cell count but which is reversible on stopping treatment. Patients should be warned to stop the drug and seek medical advice immediately, should a severe sore throat or fever develop while on treatment. Propylthiouracil is associated with a small but definite risk of hepatotoxicity, which, in some instances, has resulted in liver failure requiring liver transplantation, and even in death. It should therefore be considered second-line therapy to carbimazole and be used only during pregnancy or breastfeeding (p. 1279), or if an adverse reaction to carbimazole has occurred.

i	18.14 Comparison of treatments for the thyrotoxicosis of Graves' disease		
Management	**Common indications**	**Contraindications**	**Disadvantages/complications**
Antithyroid drugs (carbimazole, propylthiouracil)	First episode in patients <40 years	Breastfeeding (propylthiouracil suitable)	Hypersensitivity rash 2% Agranulocytosis 0.2% Hepatotoxicity (with propylthiouracil) – very rare but potentially fatal >50% relapse rate usually within 2 years of stopping drug
Subtotal thyroidectomy[1]	Large goitre Poor drug adherence, especially in young patients Recurrent thyrotoxicosis after course of antithyroid drugs in young patients	Previous thyroid surgery Dependence on voice, e.g. opera singer, lecturer[2]	Hypothyroidism (~25%) Transient hypocalcaemia (10%) Permanent hypoparathyroidism (1%) Recurrent laryngeal nerve palsy[2] (1%)
Radio-iodine	Patients >40 years[3] Recurrence following surgery irrespective of age Other serious comorbidity	Pregnancy or planned pregnancy within 6 months of treatment Active Graves' ophthalmopathy[4]	Hypothyroidism: ~40% in first year, 80% after 15 years Most likely treatment to result in exacerbation of ophthalmopathy[4]

[1]A near-total thyroidectomy is now the favoured operation for Graves' thyrotoxicosis in many institutions and is associated with a higher risk of some complications, including hypothyroidism (nearly 100%), but a reduced risk of persistent or recurrent thyrotoxicosis. [2]It is not only vocal cord palsy due to recurrent laryngeal nerve damage that alters the voice following thyroid surgery; the superior laryngeal nerves are frequently transected and this results in minor changes in voice quality. [3]In many institutions, ^{131}I is used more liberally and is prescribed for much younger patients. [4]The extent to which radio-iodine exacerbates ophthalmopathy is controversial and practice varies; some use prednisolone to reduce this risk.

Thyroid surgery Patients should be rendered euthyroid with antithyroid drugs before operation. Oral potassium iodide, 60 mg three times daily, is often added for 10 days before surgery to inhibit thyroid hormone release and reduce the size and vascularity of the gland, making surgery technically easier. Traditionally, a 'subtotal' thyroidectomy is performed, in which a portion of one lobe of the thyroid is left in situ, with the aim of rendering the patient euthyroid. While complications of surgery are rare and 80% of patients are euthyroid, 15% are permanently hypothyroid and 5% remain thyrotoxic. As a consequence, many endocrine surgeons now opt to perform a 'near-total' thyroidectomy, leaving behind only a small portion of gland adjacent to the recurrent laryngeal nerves. This strategy invariably results in permanent hypothyroidism and is probably associated with a higher risk of hypoparathyroidism, but maximises the potential for cure of thyrotoxicosis.

Radioactive iodine ^{131}I is administered orally as a single dose and is trapped and organified in the thyroid (see Fig. 18.3). [131]I emits both β and γ radiation and, although it decays within a few weeks, it has long-lasting inhibitory effects on survival and replication of follicular cells. The variable radio-iodine uptake and radiosensitivity of the gland means that the choice of dose is empirical; in most centres, approximately 400–600 MBq (approximately 10–15 mCi) is administered. This regimen is effective in 75% of patients within 4–12 weeks. During the lag period, symptoms can be controlled by a β-blocker or, in more severe cases, by carbimazole. However, carbimazole reduces the efficacy of ^{131}I therapy because it prevents organification of ^{131}I in the gland, and so should be avoided until 48 hours after radio-iodine administration. If thyrotoxicosis persists after 6 months, a further dose of ^{131}I can be given. The disadvantage of ^{131}I treatment is that the majority of patients eventually develop hypothyroidism. [131]I is usually avoided in patients with Graves' ophthalmopathy and evidence of significant active orbital inflammation. It can be administered with caution in those with mild or 'burnt-out' eye disease, when it is customary to cover the treatment with a 6-week tapering course of oral prednisolone. In women of reproductive age, pregnancy must be excluded before administration of ^{131}I and avoided for 6 months thereafter; men are also advised against fathering children for 6 months after receiving [131]I.

Thyrotoxicosis in pregnancy

Thyrotoxicosis in pregnancy may be associated with significant maternal and fetal morbidity. Management is very specialised and is discussed on page 1279 (see also Box 18.18).

Thyrotoxicosis in adolescence

Thyrotoxicosis can occasionally occur in adolescence and is almost always due to Graves' disease. The presentation may be atypical and management challenging, as summarised in Box 18.15.

Graves' ophthalmopathy

This condition is immunologically mediated but the autoantigen has not been identified. Within the orbit (and the dermis) there is cytokine-mediated proliferation of fibroblasts that secrete hydrophilic glycosaminoglycans. The resulting increase in interstitial fluid content, combined with a chronic inflammatory cell infiltrate, causes marked swelling and ultimately fibrosis of the extraocular muscles (Fig. 18.8) and a rise in retrobulbar pressure. The eye is displaced forwards (proptosis, exophthalmos, p. 631) and in severe cases there is optic nerve compression.

18.15 Thyrotoxicosis in adolescence

- **Presentation**: may present with a deterioration in school performance or symptoms suggestive of attention deficit hyperactivity disorder.
- **Antithyroid drug therapy**: prolonged courses may be required because remission rates following an 18-month course of therapy are much lower than in adults.
- **Adherence**: adherence to antithyroid drug therapy is often suboptimal, resulting in poor disease control that may adversely affect performance at school.
- **Radio-iodine therapy**: usually avoided in adolescents because of concerns about risk of future malignancy.

Fig. 18.8 Graves' disease. **A** Bilateral ophthalmopathy in a 42-year-old man. The main symptoms were diplopia in all directions of gaze and reduced visual acuity in the left eye. The periorbital swelling is due to retrobulbar fat prolapsing into the eyelids, and increased interstitial fluid as a result of raised intraorbital pressure. **B** Transverse CT of the orbits, showing the enlarged extraocular muscles. This is most obvious at the apex of the left orbit (arrow), where compression of the optic nerve caused reduced visual acuity.

Ophthalmopathy, like thyrotoxicosis (see Fig. 18.7), typically follows an episodic course and it is helpful to distinguish patients with active inflammation (periorbital oedema and conjunctival inflammation with changing orbital signs) from those in whom the inflammation has 'burnt out'. Eye disease is detectable in up to 50% of thyrotoxic patients at presentation, but active ocular inflammation may occur before or after thyrotoxic episodes (exophthalmic Graves' disease). It is more common in cigarette smokers and is exacerbated by poor control of thyroid function, especially hypothyroidism. The most frequent presenting symptoms are related to increased exposure of the cornea, resulting from proptosis and lid retraction. There may be excessive lacrimation made worse by wind and bright light, a 'gritty' sensation in the eye, and pain due to conjunctivitis or corneal ulceration. In addition, there may be reduction of visual acuity and/or visual fields as a consequence of corneal oedema or optic nerve compression. Other signs of optic nerve compression include reduced colour vision and a relative afferent pupillary defect (pp. 631 and 1088). If the extraocular muscles are involved and do not act in concert, diplopia results.

The majority of patients require no treatment other than reassurance. Smoking cessation should be actively encouraged. Methylcellulose eye drops and gel counter the gritty discomfort of dry eyes, and tinted glasses or side shields attached to spectacle frames reduce the excessive lacrimation triggered by sun or wind. In patients with mild Graves' ophthalmopathy, oral selenium (100 µg twice daily for 6 months) improves quality of life, reduces ocular involvement and slows progression of disease; the mechanism of action is not known but may relate to an antioxidant effect. More severe inflammatory episodes are treated with glucocorticoids (e.g. pulsed intravenous methylprednisolone) and sometimes orbital radiotherapy. There is also an increasing trend to use alternative immunosuppressive therapies, such as rituximab and ciclosporin. Loss of visual acuity is an indication for urgent surgical decompression of the orbit. In 'burnt-out' disease, surgery to the extraocular muscles, and later the eyelids, may improve diplopia, conjunctival exposure and cosmetic appearance.

Pretibial myxoedema

This infiltrative dermopathy occurs in fewer than 5% of patients with Graves' disease and has similar pathological features as occur in the orbit. It takes the form of raised pink-coloured or purplish plaques on the anterior aspect of the leg, extending on to the dorsum of the foot (p. 630). The lesions may be itchy and the skin may have a 'peau d'orange' appearance with growth of coarse hair; less commonly, the face and arms are affected. Treatment is rarely required but in severe cases topical glucocorticoids may be helpful.

Hashimoto's thyroiditis

Hashimoto's thyroiditis is characterised by destructive lymphoid infiltration of the thyroid, ultimately leading to a varying degree of fibrosis and thyroid enlargement. There is an increased risk of thyroid lymphoma (p. 650), although this is exceedingly rare. The nomenclature of autoimmune hypothyroidism is confusing. Some authorities reserve the term 'Hashimoto's thyroiditis' for the condition of patients with positive antithyroid peroxidase autoantibodies and a firm goitre who may or may not be hypothyroid, and use the term 'spontaneous atrophic hypothyroidism' for the condition of hypothyroid patients without a goitre in whom TSH receptor-blocking antibodies may be more important than antithyroid peroxidase antibodies. However, these syndromes can both be considered as variants of the same underlying disease process.

Hashimoto's thyroiditis increases in incidence with age and affects approximately 3.5 per 1000 women and 0.8 per 1000 men each year. Many present with a small or moderately sized diffuse goitre, which is characteristically firm or rubbery in consistency. Around 25% of patients are hypothyroid at presentation. In the remainder, serum T_4 is normal and TSH normal or raised, but these patients are at risk of developing overt hypothyroidism in future years. Antithyroid peroxidase antibodies are present in the serum in more than 90% of patients with Hashimoto's thyroiditis. In those under the age of 20 years, antinuclear factor (ANF) may also be positive.

Levothyroxine therapy is indicated as treatment for hypothyroidism (p. 640) and also to shrink an associated goitre.

In this context, the dose of levothyroxine should be sufficient to suppress serum TSH to low but detectable levels.

Transient thyroiditis

Subacute (de Quervain's) thyroiditis

In its classical painful form, subacute thyroiditis is a transient inflammation of the thyroid gland occurring after infection with Coxsackie, mumps or adenoviruses. There is pain in the region of the thyroid that may radiate to the angle of the jaw and the ears, and is made worse by swallowing, coughing and movement of the neck. The thyroid is usually palpably enlarged and tender. Systemic upset is common. Affected patients are usually females aged 20–40 years. Painless transient thyroiditis can also occur after viral infection and in patients with underlying autoimmune disease. The condition can also be precipitated by drugs, including interferon-α and lithium.

Irrespective of the clinical presentation, inflammation in the thyroid gland occurs and is associated with release of colloid and stored thyroid hormones, but also with damage to follicular cells and impaired synthesis of new thyroid hormones. As a result, T_4 and T_3 levels are raised for 4–6 weeks until the pre-formed colloid is depleted. Thereafter, there is usually a period of hypothyroidism of variable severity before the follicular cells recover and normal thyroid function is restored within 4–6 months (Fig. 18.9). In the thyrotoxic phase, the iodine uptake is low because the damaged follicular cells are unable to trap iodine and because TSH secretion is suppressed. Low-titre thyroid autoantibodies appear transiently in the serum, and the erythrocyte sedimentation rate (ESR) is usually raised. High-titre autoantibodies suggest an underlying autoimmune pathology and greater risk of recurrence and ultimate progression to hypothyroidism.

The pain and systemic upset usually respond to simple measures such as non-steroidal anti-inflammatory drugs (NSAIDs). Occasionally, however, it may be necessary to prescribe prednisolone 40 mg daily for 3–4 weeks. The thyrotoxicosis is mild and treatment with a β-blocker is usually adequate. Antithyroid drugs are of no benefit because thyroid hormone synthesis is impaired rather than enhanced. Careful monitoring of thyroid function and symptoms is required so that levothyroxine can be prescribed temporarily in the hypothyroid phase. Care must be taken to identify patients presenting with hypothyroidism who

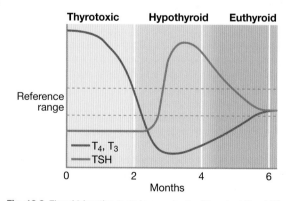

Fig. 18.9 Thyroid function tests in an episode of transient thyroiditis. This pattern might be observed in classical subacute (de Quervain's) thyroiditis, painless thyroiditis or post-partum thyroiditis. The duration of each phase varies between patients.

are in the later stages of a transient thyroiditis, since they are unlikely to require life-long levothyroxine therapy (see Fig. 18.6).

Post-partum thyroiditis

The maternal immune response, which is modified during pregnancy to allow survival of the fetus, is enhanced after delivery and may unmask previously unrecognised subclinical autoimmune thyroid disease. Surveys have shown that transient biochemical disturbances of thyroid function occur in 5–10% of women within 6 months of delivery (see Box 18.18). Those affected are likely to have antithyroid peroxidase antibodies in the serum in early pregnancy. Symptoms of thyroid dysfunction are rare and there is no association between postnatal depression and abnormal thyroid function tests. However, symptomatic thyrotoxicosis presenting for the first time within 12 months of childbirth is likely to be due to post-partum thyroiditis and the diagnosis is confirmed by a negligible radio-isotope uptake. The clinical course and treatment are similar to those of painless subacute thyroiditis (see above). Post-partum thyroiditis tends to recur after subsequent pregnancies, and eventually patients progress over a period of years to permanent hypothyroidism.

Iodine-associated thyroid disease

Iodine deficiency

Iodine is an essential micronutrient and is a key component of T_4 and T_3. The World Health Organisation (WHO) recommends a daily intake of iodine of 150 µg/day for adult men and women; higher levels are recommended for pregnant women (p. 1279). Dietary sources of iodine include seafood, dairy products, eggs and grains. Dietary iodine deficiency is a major worldwide public health issue, with an estimated one-third of the world population living in areas of iodine insufficiency. Iodine deficiency is particularly common in Central Africa, South-east Asia and the Western Pacific. It is associated with the development of thyroid nodules and goitre (endemic goitre); the reduced substrate available for thyroid hormone production increases thyroid activity to maximise iodine uptake and recycling, and this acts as a potent stimulus for enlargement of the thyroid and nodule formation. Most affected patients are euthyroid with normal or raised TSH levels, although hypothyroidism can occur with severe iodine deficiency. Suspected iodine deficiency can be assessed by measuring iodine in urine (either a 24-hour collection or a spot sample). Endemic goitre can be treated by iodine supplementation, and a reduction in nodule and goitre size can be seen, particularly if it is commenced in childhood. Iodine deficiency is not associated with an increased risk of Graves' disease or thyroid cancer, but the high prevalence of nodular autonomy does result in an increased risk of thyrotoxicosis and this risk may be further increased by iodine supplementation. Conversely, iodine supplementation may also increase the prevalence of subclinical hypothyroidism and autoimmune hypothyroidism. These complex effects of iodine supplementation are further discussed below.

In pregnancy, iodine deficiency is associated with impaired brain development, and severe deficiency can cause cretinism. Worldwide, iodine deficiency is the most common cause of preventable impaired cognitive development in children (p. 1279). The WHO and other international organisations have made reversal of iodine deficiency a priority and have helped organise national supplementation programmes. These have mainly involved the iodisation of table salt, but have also included schemes to administer oral or intramuscular iodised oil to at-risk populations and the addition of iodine to wells supplying water to local communities. These schemes have been extremely effective in reducing the prevalence of iodine deficiency, but lower consumption of table salt has actually led to an increase in iodine deficiency in some developed countries like Australia and New Zealand.

Iodine-induced thyroid dysfunction

Iodine has complex effects on thyroid function. Very high concentrations of iodine inhibit thyroid hormone synthesis and release (known as the Wolff–Chaikoff effect) and this forms the rationale for iodine treatment in thyroid crisis (p. 637) and prior to thyroid surgery for thyrotoxicosis (p. 645). This is an autoregulatory response to protect the body from the sudden release of large amounts of thyroid hormone in response to the ingestion of a substantial load of iodine. This effect only lasts for about 10 days, after which it is followed by an 'escape phenomenon': essentially, the return to normal organification of iodine and thyroid peroxidase action (see Fig. 18.3). Therefore, if iodine is given to prepare an individual with Graves' disease for surgery, the operation must happen within 10–14 days; otherwise, a significant relapse of the thyrotoxicosis could occur.

Iodine deficiency and underlying thyroid disease can both moderate the effects of iodine on thyroid function. In iodine-deficient parts of the world, transient thyrotoxicosis may be precipitated by prophylactic iodinisation programmes. In iodine-sufficient areas, thyrotoxicosis can be precipitated by iodine-containing radiographic contrast medium or expectorants in individuals who have underlying thyroid disease predisposing to thyrotoxicosis, such as multinodular goitre or Graves' disease in remission. Induction of thyrotoxicosis by iodine is called the Jod–Basedow effect. Chronic excess iodine administration can also result in hypothyroidism; this is, in effect, a failure to escape from the Wolff–Chaikoff effect and usually occurs in the context of prior insult to the thyroid by, for example, autoimmune disease, thyroiditis, lithium, antithyroid drugs or surgery.

Amiodarone

The anti-arrhythmic agent amiodarone has a structure that is analogous to that of T_4 (Fig. 18.10) and contains huge amounts of iodine; a 200 mg dose contains 75 mg iodine. Amiodarone also has a cytotoxic effect on thyroid follicular cells and inhibits conversion of T_4 to T_3 (increasing the ratio of T_4:T_3). Most patients receiving amiodarone have normal thyroid function but up to 20% develop hypothyroidism or thyrotoxicosis, and so thyroid function should be monitored regularly. TSH provides the best indicator of thyroid function.

The thyrotoxicosis can be classified as either:

- *type I*: iodine-induced excess thyroid hormone synthesis in patients with an underlying thyroid disorder, such as

Fig. 18.10 **The structure of amiodarone.** Note the similarities to T_4 (see Fig. 18.3).

nodular goitre or latent Graves' disease (an example of the Jod–Basedow effect).

- *type II*: thyroiditis due to a direct cytotoxic effect of amiodarone administration.

These patterns can overlap and may be difficult to distinguish clinically, as iodine uptake is low in both. There is no widely accepted management algorithm, although the iodine excess renders the gland resistant to [131]I. Antithyroid drugs may be effective in patients with the type I form but are ineffective in type II thyrotoxicosis. Prednisolone is beneficial in the type II form. A pragmatic approach is to commence combination therapy with an antithyroid drug and glucocorticoid in patients with significant thyrotoxicosis. A rapid response (within 1–2 weeks) usually indicates a type II picture and permits withdrawal of the antithyroid therapy; a slower response suggests a type I picture, in which case antithyroid drugs may be continued and prednisolone withdrawn. Potassium perchlorate can also be used to inhibit iodine trapping in the thyroid. If the cardiac state allows, amiodarone should be discontinued, but it has a long half-life (50–60 days) and so its effects are long-lasting. To minimise the risk of type I thyrotoxicosis, thyroid function should be measured in all patients prior to commencement of amiodarone therapy, and amiodarone should be avoided if TSH is suppressed.

Hypothyroidism should be treated with levothyroxine, which can be given while amiodarone is continued.

Simple and multinodular goitre

These terms describe diffuse or multinodular enlargement of the thyroid, which occurs sporadically and is of unknown aetiology.

Simple diffuse goitre

This form of goitre usually presents between the ages of 15 and 25 years, often during pregnancy, and tends to be noticed by friends and relatives rather than the patient. Occasionally, there is a tight sensation in the neck, particularly when swallowing. The goitre is soft and symmetrical, and the thyroid enlarged to two or three times normal. There is no tenderness, lymphadenopathy or overlying bruit. Concentrations of T_3, T_4 and TSH are normal and no thyroid autoantibodies are detected in the serum. No treatment is necessary and the goitre usually regresses. In some, however, the unknown stimulus to thyroid enlargement persists and, as a result of recurrent episodes of hyperplasia and involution during the following 10–20 years, the gland becomes multinodular with areas of autonomous function.

Multinodular goitre

The natural history is shown in Figure 18.11. Patients with thyroid enlargement in the absence of thyroid dysfunction or positive autoantibodies (i.e. with 'simple goitre'; see above) as young adults may progress to develop nodules. These nodules grow at varying rates and secrete thyroid hormone 'autonomously', thereby suppressing TSH-dependent growth and function in the rest of the gland. Ultimately, complete suppression of TSH occurs in about 25% of cases, with T_4 and T_3 levels often within the reference range (subclinical thyrotoxicosis, p. 642), but sometimes elevated (toxic multinodular goitre; see Fig. 18.5).

Clinical features and investigations

Multinodular goitre is usually diagnosed in patients presenting with thyrotoxicosis, a large goitre with or without tracheal compression,

Age (in years)	15–25	26–55	> 55
Goitre	Diffuse	Nodular	Nodular
Tracheal compression/ deviation	No	Minimal	Yes
T_3, T_4	Normal	Normal	Raised
TSH	Normal	Normal or undetectable	Undetectable

Fig. 18.11 Natural history of simple goitre.

Fig. 18.12 Computed tomogram showing retrosternal multinodular goitre (black arrow). This is causing acute severe breathlessness and stridor due to tracheal compression (white arrow).

or sudden painful swelling caused by haemorrhage into a nodule or cyst. The goitre is nodular or lobulated on palpation and may extend retrosternally; however, not all multinodular goitres causing thyrotoxicosis are easily palpable. Very large goitres can cause mediastinal compression with stridor (Fig. 18.12), dysphagia and obstruction of the superior vena cava. Hoarseness due to recurrent laryngeal nerve palsy can occur but is far more suggestive of thyroid carcinoma.

The diagnosis can be confirmed by ultrasonography and/or thyroid scintigraphy (see Fig. 18.5). In patients with large goitres, a flow-volume loop is a good screening test for significant tracheal compression (see Fig. 17.7, p. 554). If intervention is contemplated, a CT or MRI of the thoracic inlet should be performed to quantify the degree of tracheal displacement or compression and the extent of retrosternal extension. Nodules should be evaluated for the possibility of thyroid neoplasia, as described on page 649.

Management

If the goitre is small, no treatment is necessary but annual thyroid function testing should be arranged, as the natural history is progression to a toxic multinodular goitre. Thyroid surgery is indicated for large goitres that cause mediastinal compression or that are cosmetically unattractive. [131]I can result in a significant reduction in thyroid size and may be of value in elderly patients. Levothyroxine therapy is of no benefit in shrinking multinodular goitres in iodine-sufficient countries and may simply aggravate any associated thyrotoxicosis.

In toxic multinodular goitre, treatment is usually with [131]I. The iodine uptake is lower than in Graves' disease, so a higher dose may be administered (up to 800 Mbq (approximately 20 mCi)) and hypothyroidism is less common. In thyrotoxic patients with a large goitre, thyroid surgery may be indicated. Long-term treatment with antithyroid drugs is not usually employed, as relapse is invariable after drug withdrawal; drug therapy is normally reserved for frail older patients in whom surgery or ^{131}I is not an appropriate option.

Asymptomatic patients with subclinical thyrotoxicosis (p. 642) are increasingly being treated with ^{131}I on the grounds that a suppressed TSH is a risk factor for atrial fibrillation and, particularly in post-menopausal women, osteoporosis.

Thyroid neoplasia

Patients with thyroid tumours usually present with a solitary nodule (p. 642). Most are benign and a few of these, called 'toxic adenomas', secrete excess thyroid hormones. Primary thyroid malignancy is rare, accounting for less than 1% of all carcinomas, and has an incidence of 25 per million per annum. As shown in Box 18.16, it can be classified according to the cell type of origin. With the exception of medullary carcinoma, thyroid cancer is more common in females.

Toxic adenoma

A solitary toxic nodule is the cause of less than 5% of all cases of thyrotoxicosis. The nodule is a follicular adenoma, which autonomously secretes excess thyroid hormones and inhibits endogenous TSH secretion, with subsequent atrophy of the rest of the thyroid gland. The adenoma is usually greater than 3 cm in diameter.

Most patients are female and over 40 years of age. Although many nodules are palpable, the diagnosis can be made with certainty only by thyroid scintigraphy (see Fig. 18.5). The

thyrotoxicosis is usually mild and in almost 50% of patients the plasma T_3 alone is elevated (T_3 thyrotoxicosis). [131]I (400–800 MBq (10–20 mCi)) is highly effective and is an ideal treatment since the atrophic cells surrounding the nodule do not take up iodine and so receive little or no radiation. For this reason, permanent hypothyroidism is unusual. Hemithyroidectomy is an alternative management option.

Differentiated carcinoma

Papillary carcinoma

This is the most common of the malignant thyroid tumours and accounts for 90% of radiation-induced thyroid cancer. It may be multifocal and spread is initially to regional lymph nodes. Some patients present with cervical lymphadenopathy and no apparent thyroid enlargement; in such instances, the primary lesion may be less than 10 mm in diameter.

Follicular carcinoma

This is usually a single encapsulated lesion. Spread to cervical lymph nodes is rare. Metastases are blood-borne and are most often found in bone, lungs and brain.

Management

The management of thyroid cancers should be individualised and planned in multidisciplinary team meetings that include all specialists involved in the service; this should include thyroid surgeons, endocrinologists, oncologists, pathologists, radiologists and nurse specialists. Large tumours, those with adverse histological features and/or tumours with metastatic disease at presentation are usually managed by total thyroidectomy followed by a large dose of [131]I (1100 or 3700 MBq (approximately 30 or 100 mCi)) to ablate any remaining normal or malignant thyroid tissue. Thereafter, long-term treatment with levothyroxine in a dose sufficient to suppress TSH (usually 150–200 μg daily) is given, as there is evidence that growth of differentiated thyroid carcinomas is TSH-dependent. Smaller tumours with no adverse histological features may require only thyroid lobectomy.

Follow-up involves measurement of serum thyroglobulin, which should be undetectable in patients whose normal thyroid has been ablated and who are taking a suppressive dose of levothyroxine. Thyroglobulin antibodies may interfere with the assay and, depending on the method employed, may result in a falsely low or high result. Detectable thyroglobulin, in the absence of assay interference, is suggestive of tumour recurrence or metastases, particularly if the thyroglobulin titre is rising across serial measurements. Local recurrence or metastatic disease may be localised by ultrasound, CT, MRI and/or whole-body scanning with ^{131}I, and may be treated with further surgery and/or ^{131}I therapy. [131]I treatment in thyroid cancer and isotope scanning both require serum TSH concentrations to be elevated (>20 mIU/L). This may be achieved by stopping levothyroxine for 4–6 weeks, inducing symptomatic hypothyroidism, or by administering intramuscular injections of recombinant human TSH. Patients usually find the latter approach preferable but it is more expensive. Those with locally advanced or metastatic papillary and follicular carcinoma that is refractory to ^{131}I may be considered for therapy with sorafenib or lenvatinib. These drugs are multi-targeted tyrosine kinase inhibitors and have been shown in trials to prolong progression-free survival by between 5 and 14 months. They have multiple toxicities, however, including poor appetite, weight loss, fatigue, diarrhoea, mucositis, rashes, hypertension and blood dyscrasias. The potential benefits of

18

i 18.16 Malignant thyroid tumours			
Type of tumour	Frequency (%)	Age at presentation (years)	10-year survival (%)
Follicular cells			
Differentiated carcinoma:			
Papillary	75–85	20–40	98
Follicular	10–20	40–60	94
Anaplastic	<5	>60	9
Parafollicular C cells			
Medullary carcinoma	5–8	>40*	78
Lymphocytes			
Lymphoma	<5	>60	45
*Patients with medullary carcinoma as part of multiple endocrine neoplasia (MEN) types 2 and 3 (p. 688) may present in childhood.			

therapy therefore have to be carefully weighed against side-effects that can significantly impair quality of life.

Prognosis

Most patients with papillary and follicular thyroid cancer will be cured with appropriate treatment. Adverse prognostic factors include older age at presentation, the presence of distant metastases, male sex and certain histological subtypes. However, ^{131}I therapy can be effective in treating those with distant metastases, particularly small-volume disease in the lungs, and so prolonged survival is quite common.

Anaplastic carcinoma and lymphoma

These two conditions are difficult to distinguish clinically but are distinct cytologically and histologically. Patients are usually over 60 years of age and present with rapid thyroid enlargement over 2–3 months. The goitre is hard and there may be stridor due to tracheal compression and hoarseness due to recurrent laryngeal nerve palsy. There is no effective treatment for anaplastic carcinoma, although surgery and radiotherapy may be considered in some circumstances. In older patients, median survival is only 7 months.

The prognosis for lymphoma, which may arise from pre-existing Hashimoto's thyroiditis, is better (p. 961), with a median survival of 9 years. Some 98% of tumours are non-Hodgkin's lymphomas, usually the diffuse large B-cell subtype. Treatment is with combination chemotherapy and external beam radiotherapy (p. 965).

Medullary carcinoma

This tumour arises from the parafollicular C cells of the thyroid. In addition to calcitonin, the tumour may secrete 5-hydroxytryptamine (5-HT, serotonin), various peptides of the tachykinin family, adrenocorticotrophic hormone (ACTH) and prostaglandins. As a consequence, carcinoid syndrome (p. 678) and Cushing's syndrome (p. 666) may occur.

Patients usually present in middle age with a firm thyroid mass. Cervical lymph node involvement is common but distant metastases are rare initially. Serum calcitonin levels are raised and are useful in monitoring response to treatment. Despite the very high levels of calcitonin found in some patients, hypocalcaemia is extremely rare; however, hypercalcitoninaemia can be associated with severe, watery diarrhoea.

Treatment is by total thyroidectomy with removal of regional cervical lymph nodes. Since the C cells do not concentrate iodine and are not responsive to TSH, there is no role for ^{131}I therapy or TSH suppression with levothyroxine. External beam radiotherapy may be considered in some patients at high risk of local recurrence. Vandetanib and cabozantinib are tyrosine kinase inhibitors licensed for patients with progressive advanced medullary cancer. The prognosis is less good than for papillary and follicular carcinoma, but individuals can live for many decades with persistent disease that behaves in an indolent fashion.

Medullary carcinoma of the thyroid occurs sporadically in 70–90% cases; in 10–30% of cases, there is a genetic predisposition that is inherited in an autosomal dominant fashion and is due to an activating mutation in the *RET* gene. This inherited tendency normally forms part of one of the MEN syndromes (MEN 2 (also known as MEN 2a) or MEN 3 (also known as MEN 2b), p. 688) but, occasionally, susceptibility to medullary carcinoma is the only inherited trait (familial medullary thyroid cancer).

18.17 The thyroid gland in old age

Thyrotoxicosis

- **Causes**: commonly due to multinodular goitre.
- **Clinical features**: apathy, anorexia, proximal myopathy, atrial fibrillation and cardiac failure predominate.
- **Non-thyroidal illness**: thyroid function tests are performed more frequently in the elderly but interpretation may be altered by intercurrent illness.

Hypothyroidism

- **Clinical features**: non-specific features, such as physical and mental slowing, are often attributed to increasing age and the diagnosis is delayed.
- **Myxoedema coma** (p. 641): more likely in the elderly.
- **Levothyroxine dose**: to avoid exacerbating latent or established heart disease, the starting dose should be 25 µg daily. Levothyroxine requirements fall with increasing age and few patients need more than 100 µg daily.
- **Other medication** (see Box 18.12): may interfere with absorption or metabolism of levothyroxine, necessitating an increase in dose.

Riedel's thyroiditis

This is not a form of thyroid cancer but the presentation is similar and the differentiation can usually be made only by thyroid biopsy. It is an exceptionally rare condition of unknown aetiology, in which there is extensive infiltration of the thyroid and surrounding structures with fibrous tissue. There may be associated mediastinal and retroperitoneal fibrosis. Presentation is with a slow-growing goitre that is irregular and stony-hard. There is usually tracheal and oesophageal compression necessitating partial thyroidectomy. Other recognised complications include recurrent laryngeal nerve palsy, hypoparathyroidism and eventually hypothyroidism.

Congenital thyroid disease

Early treatment with levothyroxine is essential to prevent irreversible brain damage in children (cretinism) with congenital hypothyroidism. Routine screening of TSH levels in heel-prick blood samples obtained 5–7 days after birth (as part of the Guthrie test) has revealed an incidence of approximately 1 in 3000, resulting from thyroid agenesis, ectopic or hypoplastic glands, or dyshormonogenesis. Congenital hypothyroidism is thus six times more common than phenylketonuria. It is now possible to start levothyroxine replacement therapy within 2 weeks of birth. Developmental assessment of infants treated at this early stage has revealed no differences between cases and controls in most children.

Dyshormonogenesis

Several autosomal recessive defects in thyroid hormone synthesis have been described; the most common results from deficiency of the intrathyroidal peroxidase enzyme. Homozygous individuals present with congenital hypothyroidism; heterozygotes present in the first two decades of life with goitre, normal thyroid hormone levels and a raised TSH. The combination of dyshormonogenetic goitre and nerve deafness is known as Pendred's syndrome and is due to mutations in pendrin, the protein that transports iodide to the luminal surface of the follicular cell (see Fig. 18.3).

18.18 Thyroid disease in pregnancy

Normal pregnancy

- **Trimester-specific reference ranges**: should be used to interpret thyroid function test results in pregnancy.

Iodine deficiency

- **Iodine requirements**: increased in pregnancy. The World Health Organisation (WHO) recommends a minimum intake of 250 µg/day.
- **Iodine deficiency**: the major cause of preventable impaired cognitive development in children worldwide.

Hypothyroidism

- **Impaired cognitive development in the offspring**: may be associated with hypothyroidism that is not adequately treated.
- **Levothyroxine replacement therapy dose requirements**: increase by 30–50% from early in pregnancy. Monitoring to maintain TSH results within the trimester-specific reference range is recommended in early pregnancy and at least once in each trimester.

Thyrotoxicosis

- **Gestational thyrotoxicosis**: associated with multiple pregnancies and hyperemesis gravidarum. Transient and usually does not require antithyroid drug treatment.
- **Graves' disease**: the most common cause of sustained thyrotoxicosis in pregnancy
- **Antithyroid drugs**: propylthiouracil should be used in the first trimester, with carbimazole substituted in the second and third trimesters.

Post-partum thyroiditis

- **Screening**: not recommended for every woman, but thyroid function should be tested 4–6 weeks post-partum in those with a personal history of thyroid disease, goitre or other autoimmune disease including type 1 diabetes, in those known to have positive antithyroid peroxidase antibodies, or when there is clinical suspicion of thyroid dysfunction.

Thyroid hormone resistance

This is a rare disorder in which the pituitary and hypothalamus are resistant to feedback suppression of TSH by T_3, sometimes due to mutations in the thyroid hormone receptor β or because of defects in monodeiodinase activity. The result is high levels of TSH, T_4 and T_3, often with a moderate goitre that may not be noted until adulthood. Thyroid hormone signalling is highly complex and involves different isozymes of both monodeiodinases and thyroid hormone receptors in different tissues. For that reason, other tissues may or may not share the resistance to thyroid hormone and there may be features of thyrotoxicosis (e.g. tachycardia). This condition can be difficult to distinguish from an equally rare TSH-producing pituitary tumour (TSHoma; see Box 18.5, p. 636); administration of TRH results in elevation of TSH in thyroid hormone resistance and not in TSHoma, but an MRI scan of the pituitary may be necessary to exclude a macroadenoma.

The reproductive system

Clinical practice in reproductive medicine is shared between several specialties, including gynaecology, urology, paediatrics, psychiatry and endocrinology. The following section is focused on disorders managed by endocrinologists.

Fig. 18.13 Male reproductive physiology. (FSH = follicle-stimulating hormone; LH = luteinising hormone)

Functional anatomy, physiology and investigations

The physiology of male and female reproductive function is illustrated in Figures 18.13 and 18.14, respectively. Pathways for synthesis of sex steroids are shown in Figure 18.19 (p. 667).

The male

In the male, the testis serves two principal functions: synthesis of testosterone by the interstitial Leydig cells under the control of luteinising hormone (LH), and spermatogenesis by Sertoli cells under the control of follicle-stimulating hormone (FSH) (but also requiring adequate testosterone). Negative feedback suppression of LH is mediated principally by testosterone, while secretion of another hormone by the testis, inhibin, suppresses FSH. The axis can be assessed easily by a random blood sample for testosterone, LH and FSH. Testosterone levels are higher in the morning and therefore, if testosterone is marginally low, sampling should be repeated with the patient fasted at 0900 hrs. Testosterone is largely bound in plasma to sex hormone-binding globulin and this can also be measured to calculate the 'free androgen index' or the 'bioavailable' testosterone. Testicular function can also be tested by semen analysis.

There is no equivalent of the menopause in men, although testosterone concentrations decline slowly from the fourth decade onwards.

Fig. 18.14 Female reproductive physiology and the normal menstrual cycle. (FSH = follicle-stimulating hormone; LH = luteinising hormone)

The female

In the female, physiology varies during the normal menstrual cycle. FSH stimulates growth and development of ovarian follicles during the first 14 days after the menses. This leads to a gradual increase in oestradiol production from granulosa cells, which initially suppresses FSH secretion (negative feedback) but then, above a certain level, stimulates an increase in both the frequency and amplitude of gonadotrophin-releasing hormone (GnRH) pulses, resulting in a marked increase in LH secretion (positive feedback). The mid-cycle 'surge' of LH induces ovulation. After release of the ovum, the follicle differentiates into a corpus luteum, which secretes progesterone. Unless pregnancy occurs during the cycle, the corpus luteum regresses and the fall in progesterone levels results in menstrual bleeding. Circulating levels of oestrogen and progesterone in pre-menopausal women are, therefore, critically dependent on the time of the cycle. The most useful 'test' of ovarian function is a careful menstrual history: if menses are regular, measurement of gonadotrophins and oestrogen is not necessary. In addition, ovulation can be confirmed by measuring plasma progesterone levels during the luteal phase ('day 21 progesterone').

Cessation of menstruation (the menopause) occurs at an average age of approximately 50 years in developed countries. In the 5 years before, there is a gradual increase in the number of anovulatory cycles and this is referred to as the climacteric. Oestrogen and inhibin secretion falls and negative feedback results in increased pituitary secretion of LH and FSH (both typically to levels above 30 IU/L (3.3 μg/L)).

The pathophysiology of male and female reproductive dysfunction is summarised in Box 18.19.

i 18.19 Classification of diseases of the reproductive system		
	Primary	**Secondary**
Hormone excess	Polycystic ovarian syndrome Granulosa cell tumour Leydig cell tumour Teratoma	Pituitary gonadotrophinoma
Hormone deficiency	Menopause Hypogonadism (see Box 18.20) Turner's syndrome Klinefelter's syndrome	Hypopituitarism Kallmann's syndrome (isolated GnRH deficiency) Severe systemic illness, including anorexia nervosa
Hormone hypersensitivity	Idiopathic hirsutism	
Hormone resistance	Androgen resistance syndromes Complete ('testicular feminisation') Partial (Reifenstein's syndrome) 5α-reductase type 2 deficiency	
Non-functioning tumours	Ovarian cysts Carcinoma Teratoma Seminoma	

(GnRH = gonadotrophin-releasing hormone)

Presenting problems in reproductive disease

Delayed puberty

Normal pubertal development is discussed on page 1290. Puberty is considered to be delayed if the onset of the physical features of sexual maturation has not occurred by a chronological age that is 2.5 standard deviations (SD) above the national average. In the UK, this is by the age of 14 in boys and 13 in girls. Genetic factors have a major influence in determining the timing of the onset of puberty, such that the age of menarche (the onset of menstruation) is often comparable within sibling and mother–daughter pairs and within ethnic groups. However, because there is also a threshold for body weight that acts as a trigger for normal puberty, the onset of puberty can be influenced by other factors including nutritional status and chronic illness (p. 694).

Clinical assessment

The differential diagnosis is shown in Box 18.20. The key issue is to determine whether the delay in puberty is simply because the 'clock is running slow' (constitutional delay of puberty) or because there is pathology in the hypothalamus/pituitary (hypogonadotrophic hypogonadism) or the gonads (hypergonadotrophic hypogonadism). A general history and physical examination should be performed with particular reference to previous or current medical disorders, social circumstances and family history. Body proportions, sense of smell and pubertal stage should be carefully documented and, in boys, the presence or absence of testes in the scrotum noted. Current weight and height may be plotted on centile charts, along with parental heights. Previous growth measurements in childhood, which can usually be obtained from health records, are extremely useful. Healthy growth usually follows a centile. Usually, children with constitutional delay have always been small but have maintained a normal growth velocity that is appropriate for bone age. Poor linear growth, with 'crossing of the centiles', is more likely to be associated with acquired disease. Issues that are commonly encountered in the management of adolescents with delayed puberty are summarised in Box 18.21.

Constitutional delay of puberty

This is the most common cause of delayed puberty, but is a much more frequent explanation for lack of pubertal development in boys than in girls. Affected children are healthy and have usually been more than 2 SD below the mean height for their age throughout childhood. There is often a history of delayed puberty in siblings or parents. Since sex steroids are essential for fusion of the epiphyses, 'bone age' can be estimated by X-rays of epiphyses, usually in the wrist and hand; in constitutional delay, bone age is lower than chronological age. Constitutional delay of puberty should be considered as a normal variant, as puberty will commence spontaneously. However, affected children can experience significant psychological distress because of their lack of physical development, particularly when compared with their peers.

Hypogonadotrophic hypogonadism

This may be due to structural, inflammatory or infiltrative disorders of the pituitary and/or hypothalamus (see Box 18.54, p. 681). In such circumstances, other pituitary hormones, such as growth hormone, are also likely to be deficient.

'Functional' gonadotrophin deficiency is caused by a variety of factors, including low body weight, chronic systemic illness (as a consequence of the disease itself or secondary malnutrition), endocrine disorders and profound psychosocial stress.

Isolated gonadotrophin deficiency is usually due to a genetic abnormality that affects the synthesis of either GnRH or gonadotrophins. The most common form is Kallmann's syndrome, in which there is primary GnRH deficiency and, in most affected individuals, agenesis or hypoplasia of the olfactory bulbs, resulting in anosmia or hyposmia. If isolated gonadotrophin deficiency is left untreated, the epiphyses fail to fuse, resulting in tall stature with disproportionately long arms and legs relative to trunk height (eunuchoid habitus).

Cryptorchidism (undescended testes) and gynaecomastia are commonly observed in all forms of hypogonadotrophic hypogonadism.

18.20 Causes of delayed puberty and hypogonadism

Constitutional delay

Hypogonadotrophic hypogonadism
- Structural hypothalamic/pituitary disease (see Box 18.54, p. 681)
- Functional gonadotrophin deficiency:
  - Chronic systemic illness (e.g. asthma, malabsorption, coeliac disease, cystic fibrosis, renal failure)
  - Psychological stress
  - Anorexia nervosa
  - Excessive physical exercise
  - Hyperprolactinaemia
  - Other endocrine disease (e.g. Cushing's syndrome, primary hypothyroidism)
- Isolated gonadotrophin deficiency (Kallmann's syndrome)

Hypergonadotrophic hypogonadism
- Acquired gonadal damage:
  - Chemotherapy/radiotherapy to gonads
  - Trauma/surgery to gonads
  - Autoimmune gonadal failure
  - Mumps orchitis
  - Tuberculosis
  - Haemochromatosis
- Developmental/congenital gonadal disorders:
  - Steroid biosynthetic defects
  - Anorchidism/cryptorchidism in males
  - Klinefelter's syndrome (47XXY, male phenotype)
  - Turner's syndrome (45XO, female phenotype)

18.21 Delayed puberty

- **Aetiology**: in boys the most common cause is constitutional delay, whereas in girls there is inevitably a structural hypothalamic/pituitary abnormality or a factor that affects their function.
- **Psychological effects**: whatever the underlying cause, delayed puberty is often associated with substantial psychological distress.
- **Investigations**: a karyotype should be performed in all adolescents with hypergonadotrophic hypogonadism, to exclude Turner's and Klinefelter's syndromes, unless there is an obvious precipitating cause.
- **Medical induction of puberty**: if this is being considered, it needs to be managed carefully and carried out in a controlled fashion, to avoid premature fusion of the epiphyses.

18

Hypergonadotrophic hypogonadism

Hypergonadotrophic hypogonadism associated with delayed puberty is usually due to Klinefelter's syndrome in boys and Turner's syndrome in girls (pp. 659 and 660). Other causes of primary gonadal failure are shown in Box 18.20.

Investigations

Key measurements are LH and FSH, testosterone (in boys) and oestradiol (in girls). Chromosome analysis should be performed if gonadotrophin concentrations are elevated. If gonadotrophin concentrations are low, then the differential diagnosis lies between constitutional delay and hypogonadotrophic hypogonadism. A plain X-ray of the wrist and hand may be compared with a set of standard films to obtain a bone age. Full blood count, renal function, liver function, thyroid function and coeliac disease autoantibodies (p. 806) should be measured, but further tests may be unnecessary if the blood tests are normal and the child has all the clinical features of constitutional delay. If hypogonadotrophic hypogonadism is suspected, neuroimaging and further investigations are required (p. 680).

Management

Puberty can be induced using low doses of oral oestrogen in girls (e.g. ethinylestradiol 2 µg daily) or testosterone in boys (testosterone gel or depot testosterone esters). Higher doses carry a risk of early fusion of epiphyses. This therapy should be given in a specialist clinic where the progress of puberty and growth can be carefully monitored. In children with constitutional delay, this 'priming' therapy can be discontinued when endogenous puberty is established, usually in less than a year. In children with hypogonadism, the underlying cause should be treated and reversed if possible. If hypogonadism is permanent, sex hormone doses are gradually increased during puberty and full adult replacement doses given when development is complete.

Precocious puberty

Precocious puberty (PP) is the early development of any secondary sexual characteristics before the age of 9 years in a boy and 6–8 years of age in a girl. Central PP is due to the early maturation of the hypothalamic–pituitary–gonadal axis and thus is gonadotrophin-dependent. It is more common in girls than boys and often no structural cause is identified, i.e. 'the physiological clock is running fast'. Structural causes are found more commonly in younger children and in boys and include:

- central nervous system (CNS) tumours such as astrocytomas, germ-cell tumours secreting human chorionic gonadotrophin (hCG) and hypothalamic harmartomas
- CNS injury caused by infection, inflammation or trauma/surgery
- congenital CNS structural abnormalities.

Pseudo (or peripheral) PP is much less common, and is due to excess sex steroids in the absence of pituitary gonadotrophins, with causes including congenital adrenal hyperplasia and McCune–Albright syndrome (p. 1055).

Investigations

Measurement of basal and GnRH-stimulated gonadotrophin levels will allow categorisation into central or peripheral PP, with gonadotrophin levels rising in central PP. Imaging of the CNS is required in cases of central PP, while adrenal and ovarian imaging is indicated in peripheral PP.

Management

Social and psychological difficulties may accompany the onset of PP and the premature closure of the epiphyses can result in reduced final height. In central PP, development can be arrested with long-acting GnRH analogues. In both central and peripheral PP, treatment of any underlying cause is indicated.

Amenorrhoea

Primary amenorrhoea may be diagnosed in a female who has never menstruated; this usually occurs as a manifestation of delayed puberty but may also be a consequence of anatomical defects of the female reproductive system, such as endometrial hypoplasia or vaginal agenesis. Secondary amenorrhoea describes the cessation of menstruation in a female who has previously had periods. The causes of this common presentation are shown in Box 18.22. In non-pregnant women, secondary amenorrhoea is almost invariably a consequence of either ovarian or hypothalamic/pituitary dysfunction. Premature ovarian failure (premature menopause) is defined, arbitrarily, as occurring before 40 years of age. Rarely, endometrial adhesions (Asherman's syndrome) can form after uterine curettage, surgery or infection with tuberculosis or schistosomiasis, preventing endometrial proliferation and shedding.

Clinical assessment

The underlying cause can often be suspected from associated clinical features and the patient's age. Hypothalamic/pituitary disease and premature ovarian failure result in oestrogen deficiency, which causes a variety of symptoms usually associated with the menopause (Box 18.23). A history of galactorrhoea should be sought. Significant weight loss of any cause can cause amenorrhoea by suppression of gonadotrophins. Weight gain may suggest hypothyroidism, Cushing's syndrome or, very rarely, a hypothalamic lesion. Hirsutism, obesity and long-standing irregular periods suggest polycystic ovarian

i	18.22 Causes of secondary amenorrhoea

Physiological
- Pregnancy
- Menopause

Hypogonadotrophic hypogonadism (see Box 18.20)

Ovarian dysfunction
- Hypergonadotrophic hypogonadism (see Box 18.20)
- Polycystic ovarian syndrome
- Androgen-secreting tumours

Uterine dysfunction
- Asherman's syndrome

i	18.23 Symptoms of oestrogen deficiency

Vasomotor effects
- Hot flushes
- Sweating

Psychological
- Anxiety
- Irritability
- Emotional lability

Genitourinary
- Dyspareunia
- Urgency of micturition
- Vaginal infections

syndrome (PCOS, p. 658). The presence of other autoimmune disease raises the possibility of autoimmune premature ovarian failure.

Investigations

Pregnancy should be excluded in women of reproductive age by measuring urine or serum hCG. Serum LH, FSH, oestradiol, prolactin, testosterone, T_4 and TSH should be measured and, in the absence of a menstrual cycle, can be taken at any time. Investigation of hyperprolactinaemia is described on page 684. High concentrations of LH and FSH with low or low-normal oestradiol suggest primary ovarian failure. Ovarian autoantibodies may be positive when there is an underlying autoimmune aetiology, and a karyotype should be performed in younger women to exclude mosaic Turner's syndrome. Elevated LH, prolactin and testosterone levels with normal oestradiol are common in PCOS. Low levels of LH, FSH and oestradiol suggest hypothalamic or pituitary disease and a pituitary MRI is indicated.

There is some overlap in gonadotrophin and oestrogen concentrations between women with hypogonadotrophic hypogonadism and PCOS. If there is doubt as to the underlying cause of secondary amenorrhoea, then the response to 5 days of treatment with an oral progestogen (e.g. medroxyprogesterone acetate 10 mg twice daily) can be assessed. In women with PCOS, the progestogen will cause maturation of the endometrium and menstruation will occur a few days after the progestogen is stopped. In women with hypogonadotrophic hypogonadism, menstruation does not occur following progestogen withdrawal because the endometrium is atrophic as a result of oestrogen deficiency. If doubt persists in distinguishing oestrogen deficiency from a uterine abnormality, the capacity for menstruation can be tested with 1 month of treatment with cyclical oestrogen and progestogen (usually administered as a combined oral contraceptive pill).

Assessment of bone mineral density by dual X-ray absorptiometry (DXA, p. 989) may be appropriate in patients with low androgen and oestrogen levels.

Management

Where possible, the underlying cause should be treated. For example, women with functional amenorrhoea due to excessive exercise and low weight should be encouraged to reduce their exercise and regain some weight. The management of structural pituitary and hypothalamic disease is described on page 684 and that of PCOS on page 658.

In oestrogen-deficient women, replacement therapy may be necessary to treat symptoms and/or to prevent osteoporosis. Women who have had a hysterectomy can be treated with oestrogen alone but those with a uterus should be treated with combined oestrogen/progestogen therapy, since unopposed oestrogen increases the risk of endometrial cancer. Cyclical hormone replacement therapy (HRT) regimens typically involve giving oestrogen on days 1–21 and progestogen on days 14–21 of the cycle, and this can be conveniently administered as the oral contraceptive pill. If oestrogenic side-effects (fluid retention, weight gain, hypertension and thrombosis) are a concern, then lower-dose oral or transdermal HRT may be more appropriate.

The timing of the discontinuation of oestrogen replacement therapy is still a matter of debate. In post-menopausal women, HRT has been shown to relieve menopausal symptoms and to prevent osteoporotic fractures but is associated with adverse effects, which are related to the duration of therapy and to the patient's age. In patients with premature menopause, HRT should be continued up to the age of around 50 years, but continued beyond this age only if there are continued symptoms of oestrogen deficiency on discontinuation.

Management of infertility in oestrogen-deficient women is described on page 656.

Male hypogonadism

The clinical features of both hypo- and hypergonadotrophic hypogonadism include loss of libido, lethargy with muscle weakness, and decreased frequency of shaving. Patients may also present with gynaecomastia, infertility, delayed puberty, osteoporosis or anaemia of chronic disease. The causes of hypogonadism are listed in Box 18.20. Mild hypogonadism may also occur in older men, particularly in the context of central adiposity and the metabolic syndrome (p. 730). Postulated mechanisms are complex and include reduction in sex hormone-binding globulin by insulin resistance and reduction in GnRH and gonadotrophin secretion by cytokines or oestrogen released by adipose tissue. Testosterone levels also fall gradually with age in men (see Box 18.30) and this is associated with gonadotrophin levels that are low or inappropriately within the 'normal' range. There is an increasing trend to measure testosterone in older men, typically as part of an assessment of erectile dysfunction and lack of libido.

Investigations

Male hypogonadism is confirmed by demonstrating a low fasting 0900-hr serum testosterone level. The distinction between hypo- and hypergonadotrophic hypogonadism is by measurement of random LH and FSH. Patients with hypogonadotrophic hypogonadism should be investigated as described for pituitary disease on page 680. Patients with hypergonadotrophic hypogonadism should have the testes examined for cryptorchidism or atrophy, and a karyotype should be performed (to identify Klinefelter's syndrome).

Management

Testosterone replacement is clearly indicated in younger men with significant hypogonadism to prevent osteoporosis and to restore muscle power and libido. Debate exists as to whether replacement therapy is of benefit in mild hypogonadism associated with ageing and central adiposity, particularly in the absence of structural pituitary/hypothalamic disease or other pituitary hormone deficiency. In such instances, a therapeutic trial of testosterone therapy may be considered if symptoms are present (e.g. low libido and erectile dysfunction), but the benefits of therapy must be carefully weighed against the potential for harm.

Routes of testosterone administration are shown in Box 18.24. First-pass hepatic metabolism of testosterone is highly efficient, so bioavailability of ingested preparations is poor. Doses of systemic testosterone can be titrated against symptoms; circulating testosterone levels may provide only a rough guide to dosage because they may be highly variable (Box 18.24). Testosterone therapy can aggravate prostatic carcinoma; prostate-specific antigen (PSA) should be measured before commencing testosterone therapy in men older than 50 years and monitored annually thereafter. Haemoglobin concentration should also be monitored in older men, as androgen replacement can cause polycythaemia. Testosterone replacement inhibits spermatogenesis; treatment for fertility is described below.

18

18.24 Options for androgen replacement therapy

Route of administration	Preparation	Dose	Frequency	Comments
Intramuscular	Testosterone enantate	50–250 mg	Every 3–4 weeks	Produces peaks and troughs of testosterone levels that are outside the physiological range and may be symptomatic
	Testosterone undecanoate	1000 mg	Every 3 months	Smoother profile than testosterone enantate, with less frequent injections
Subcutaneous	Testosterone pellets	600–800 mg	Every 4–6 months	Smoother profile than testosterone enantate but implantation causes scarring and infection
Transdermal	Testosterone patch	5–10 mg	Daily	Stable testosterone levels but high incidence of skin hypersensitivity
	Testosterone gel	50–100 mg	Daily	Stable testosterone levels; transfer of gel can occur following skin-to-skin contact with another person
Oral	Testosterone undecanoate	40–120 mg	Twice daily	Very variable testosterone levels; risk of hepatotoxicity

Infertility

Infertility affects around 1 in 7 couples of reproductive age, often causing psychological distress. The main causes are listed in Box 18.25. In women, it may result from anovulation or abnormalities of the reproductive tract that prevent fertilisation or embryonic implantation, often damaged Fallopian tubes from previous infection. In men, infertility may result from impaired sperm quality (e.g. reduced motility) or reduced sperm number. Azoospermia or oligospermia is usually idiopathic but may be a consequence of hypogonadism (see Box 18.20). Microdeletions of the Y chromosome are increasingly recognised as a cause of severely abnormal spermatogenesis. In many couples, more than one factor causing subfertility is present, and in a large proportion no cause can be identified.

18.25 Causes of infertility

Female factor (35–40%)
- Ovulatory dysfunction:
  Polycystic ovarian syndrome
  Hypogonadotrophic hypogonadism (see Box 18.20)
  Hypergonadotrophic hypogonadism (see Box 18.20)
- Tubular dysfunction:
  Pelvic inflammatory disease (chlamydia, gonorrhoea)
  Endometriosis
  Previous sterilisation
  Previous pelvic or abdominal surgery
- Cervical and/or uterine dysfunction:
  Congenital abnormalities
  Fibroids
  Treatment for cervical carcinoma
  Asherman's syndrome

Male factor (35–40%)
- Reduced sperm quality or production:
  Y chromosome microdeletions
  Varicocele
  Hypergonadotrophic hypogonadism (see Box 18.20)
  Hypogonadotrophic hypogonadism (see Box 18.20)
- Tubular dysfunction:
  Varicocele
  Congenital abnormality of vas deferens/epididymis
  Previous sexually transmitted infection (chlamydia, gonorrhoea)
  Previous vasectomy

Unexplained or mixed factor (20–35%)

Clinical assessment

A history of previous pregnancies, relevant infections and surgery is important in both men and women. A sexual history must be explored sensitively, as some couples have intercourse infrequently or only when they consider the woman to be ovulating, and psychosexual difficulties are common. Irregular and/or infrequent menstrual periods are an indicator of anovulatory cycles in the woman, in which case causes such as PCOS should be considered. In men, the testes should be examined to confirm that both are in the scrotum and to identify any structural abnormality, such as small size, absent vas deferens or the presence of a varicocele.

Investigations

Investigations should generally be performed after a couple has failed to conceive despite unprotected intercourse for 12 months, unless there is an obvious abnormality like amenorrhoea. Both partners need to be investigated. The male partner needs a semen analysis to assess sperm count and quality. Home testing for ovulation (by commercial urine dipstick kits, temperature measurement, or assessment of cervical mucus) is not recommended, as the information is often counterbalanced by increased anxiety if interpretation is inconclusive. In women with regular periods, ovulation can be confirmed by an elevated serum progesterone concentration on day 21 of the menstrual cycle. Transvaginal ultrasound can be used to assess uterine and ovarian anatomy. Tubal patency may be examined at laparoscopy or by hysterosalpingography (HSG; a radio-opaque medium is injected into the uterus and should normally outline the Fallopian tubes). In vitro assessments of sperm survival in cervical mucus may be done in cases of unexplained infertility but are rarely helpful.

Management

Couples should be advised to have regular sexual intercourse, ideally every 2–3 days throughout the menstrual cycle. It is not uncommon for 'spontaneous' pregnancies to occur in couples undergoing investigations for infertility or with identified causes of male or female subfertility.

In women with anovulatory cycles secondary to PCOS (p. 658), clomifene, which has partial anti-oestrogen action, blocks negative feedback of oestrogen on the hypothalamus/pituitary, causing gonadotrophin secretion and thus ovulation. In women with gonadotrophin deficiency or in whom anti-oestrogen therapy is unsuccessful, ovulation may be induced by direct stimulation of the ovary by daily injection of FSH and an injection of hCG to induce follicular rupture at the appropriate time. In hypothalamic disease, pulsatile GnRH therapy with a portable infusion pump can be used to stimulate pituitary gonadotrophin secretion (note that non-pulsatile administration of GnRH or its analogues paradoxically suppresses LH and FSH secretion). Whatever method of ovulation induction is employed, monitoring of response is essential to avoid multiple ovulation. For clomifene, ultrasound monitoring is recommended for at least the first cycle. During gonadotrophin therapy, closer monitoring of follicular growth by transvaginal ultrasonography and blood oestradiol levels is mandatory. 'Ovarian hyperstimulation syndrome' is characterised by grossly enlarged ovaries and capillary leak with circulatory shock, pleural effusions and ascites. Anovulatory women who fail to respond to ovulation induction or who have primary ovarian failure may wish to consider using donated eggs or embryos, surrogacy and adoption.

Surgery to restore Fallopian tube patency can be effective but in vitro fertilisation (IVF) is normally recommended. IVF is widely used for many causes of infertility and in unexplained cases of prolonged (>3 years) infertility. The success of IVF depends on age, with low success rates in women over 40 years.

Men with hypogonadotrophic hypogonadism who wish fertility are usually given injections of hCG several times a week (recombinant FSH may also be required in men with hypogonadism of pre-pubertal origin); it may take up to 2 years to achieve satisfactory sperm counts. Surgery is rarely an option in primary testicular disease but removal of a varicocele can improve semen quality. Extraction of sperm from the epididymis for IVF, and intracytoplasmic sperm injection (ICSI, when single spermatozoa are injected into each oöcyte) are being used increasingly in men with oligospermia or poor sperm quality who have primary testicular disease. Azoospermic men may opt to use donated sperm but this may be in short supply.

Gynaecomastia

Gynaecomastia is the presence of glandular breast tissue in males. Normal breast development in women is oestrogen-dependent, while androgens oppose this effect. Gynaecomastia results from an imbalance between androgen and oestrogen activity, which may reflect androgen deficiency or oestrogen excess. Causes are listed in Box 18.26. The most common are physiological: for example, in the newborn baby (due to maternal and placental oestrogens), in pubertal boys (in whom oestradiol concentrations

---

18.26 Causes of gynaecomastia

Idiopathic

Physiological

Drug-induced
- Cimetidine
- Digoxin
- Anti-androgens (cyproterone acetate, spironolactone)
- Some exogenous anabolic steroids (diethylstilbestrol)
- Cannabis

Hypogonadism (see Box 18.20)

Androgen resistance syndromes

Oestrogen excess
- Liver failure (impaired steroid metabolism)
- Oestrogen-secreting tumour (e.g. of testis)
- Human chorionic gonadotrophin-secreting tumour (e.g. of testis or lung)

---

reach adult levels before testosterone) and in elderly men (due to decreasing testosterone concentrations). Prolactin excess alone does not cause gynaecomastia (p. 684).

Clinical assessment

A drug history is important. Gynaecomastia is often asymmetrical and palpation may allow breast tissue to be distinguished from the prominent adipose tissue (lipomastia) around the nipple that is often observed in obesity. Features of hypogonadism should be sought (see above) and the testes examined for evidence of cryptorchidism, atrophy or a tumour.

Investigations

If a clinical distinction between gynaecomastia and adipose tissue cannot be made, then ultrasonography or mammography is required. A random blood sample should be taken for testosterone, LH, FSH, oestradiol, prolactin and hCG. Elevated oestrogen concentrations are found in testicular tumours and hCG-producing neoplasms.

Management

An adolescent with gynaecomastia who is progressing normally through puberty may be reassured that the gynaecomastia will usually resolve once development is complete. If puberty does not proceed normally, then there may be an underlying abnormality that requires investigation (p. 653). Gynaecomastia may cause significant psychological distress, especially in adolescent boys, and surgical excision may be justified for cosmetic reasons. Androgen replacement will usually improve gynaecomastia in hypogonadal males and any other identifiable underlying cause should be addressed if possible. The anti-oestrogen tamoxifen may also be effective in reducing the size of the breast tissue.

Hirsutism

Hirsutism refers to the excessive growth of terminal hair (the thick, pigmented hair usually associated with the adult male chest) in an androgen-dependent distribution in women (upper lip, chin, chest, back, lower abdomen, thigh, forearm) and is one of the most common presentations of endocrine disease. It should be distinguished from hypertrichosis, which is generalised excessive growth of vellus hair (the thin, non-pigmented hair that is typically found all over the body from childhood onwards). The aetiology of androgen excess is shown in Box 18.27.

Clinical assessment

The severity of hirsutism is subjective. Some women suffer profound embarrassment from a degree of hair growth that others would not consider remarkable. Important observations are a drug and menstrual history, calculation of body mass index, measurement of blood pressure, and examination for virilisation (clitoromegaly, deep voice, male-pattern balding, breast atrophy) and associated features, including acne vulgaris or Cushing's syndrome (p. 666). Hirsutism of recent onset associated with virilisation is suggestive of an androgen-secreting tumour but this is rare.

Investigations

A random blood sample should be taken for testosterone, prolactin, LH and FSH. If there are clinical features of Cushing's syndrome, further investigations should be performed (p. 667).

If testosterone levels are more than twice the upper limit of normal for females, idiopathic hirsutism and PCOS are less likely, especially if LH and FSH levels are low. Under these

18

i **18.27 Causes of hirsutism**

Cause	Clinical features	Investigation findings	Treatment
Idiopathic	Often familial Mediterranean or Asian background	Normal	Cosmetic measures Anti-androgens
Polycystic ovarian syndrome	Obesity Oligomenorrhoea or secondary amenorrhoea Infertility	LH:FSH ratio > 2.5:1 Minor elevation of androgens* Mild hyperprolactinaemia	Weight loss Cosmetic measures Anti-androgens (Metformin, glitazones may be useful)
Congenital adrenal hyperplasia (95% 21-hydroxylase deficiency)	Pigmentation History of salt-wasting in childhood, ambiguous genitalia, or adrenal crisis when stressed Jewish background	Elevated androgens* that suppress with dexamethasone Abnormal rise in 17-OH-progesterone with ACTH	Glucocorticoid replacement administered in reverse rhythm to suppress early morning ACTH
Exogenous androgen administration	Athletes Virilisation	Low LH and FSH Analysis of urinary androgens may detect drug of misuse	Stop steroid misuse
Androgen-secreting tumour of ovary or adrenal cortex	Rapid onset Virilisation: clitoromegaly, deep voice, balding, breast atrophy	High androgens* that do not suppress with dexamethasone Low LH and FSH CT or MRI usually demonstrates a tumour	Surgical excision
Cushing's syndrome	Clinical features of Cushing's syndrome (p. 667)	Normal or mild elevation of adrenal androgens* See investigations (p. 667)	Treat the cause (p. 667)

*e.g. Serum testosterone levels in women: <2 nmol/L (<58 ng/dL) is normal; 2–5 nmol/L (58–144 ng/dL) is minor elevation; >5 nmol/L (>144 ng/dL) is high and requires further investigation.
(ACTH = adrenocorticotrophic hormone; CT = computed tomography; FH = follicle-stimulating hormone; LH = luteinising hormone; MRI = magnetic resonance imaging)

circumstances, other causes of androgen excess should be sought. Congenital adrenal hyperplasia due to 21-hydroxylase deficiency is diagnosed by a short ACTH stimulation test with measurement of 17-OH-progesterone (p. 676). In patients with androgen-secreting tumours, serum testosterone does not suppress following a 48-hour low-dose dexamethasone suppression test. The tumour should then be sought by CT or MRI of the adrenals and ovaries.

Management

This depends on the cause (Box 18.27). Options for the treatment of PCOS and idiopathic hirsutism are similar and are described below.

Polycystic ovarian syndrome

Polycystic ovarian syndrome (PCOS) affects up to 10% of women of reproductive age. It is a heterogeneous disorder (Box 18.28), often associated with obesity, for which the primary cause remains uncertain. Genetic factors probably play a role, since PCOS often affects several family members. The severity and clinical features of PCOS vary markedly between individual patients but diagnosis is usually made during the investigation of hirsutism (p. 657) or amenorrhoea/oligomenorrhoea (p. 655). Infertility may also be present (p. 656). There is no universally accepted definition but it has been recommended that a diagnosis of PCOS requires the presence of two of the following three features:

• menstrual irregularity
• clinical or biochemical androgen excess
• multiple cysts in the ovaries (most readily detected by transvaginal ultrasound; Fig. 18.15).

i **18.28 Features of polycystic ovarian syndrome**

Mechanisms*	Manifestations
Pituitary dysfunction	High serum LH High serum prolactin
Anovulatory menstrual cycles	Oligomenorrhoea Secondary amenorrhoea Cystic ovaries Infertility
Androgen excess	Hirsutism Acne
Obesity	Hyperglycaemia Elevated oestrogens
Insulin resistance	Dyslipidaemia Hypertension

*These mechanisms are interrelated; it is not known which, if any, is primary. PCOS probably represents the common endpoint of several different pathologies.
(LH = luteinising hormone)

Women with PCOS are at increased risk of glucose intolerance and some authorities recommend screening for type 2 diabetes and other cardiovascular risk factors associated with the metabolic syndrome (p. 730).

Management

This should be directed at the presenting complaint but all PCOS patients who are overweight should be encouraged to lose weight, as this can improve several symptoms, including menstrual irregularity, and reduces the risk of type 2 diabetes.

18.29 Anti-androgen therapy

Mechanism of action	Drug	Dose	Hazards
Androgen receptor antagonism	Cyproterone acetate	2, 50 or 100 mg on days 1–11 of 28-day cycle with ethinylestradiol 30 μg on days 1–21	Hepatic dysfunction Feminisation of male fetus Progesterone receptor agonist Dysfunctional uterine bleeding
	Spironolactone	100–200 mg daily	Electrolyte disturbance
	Flutamide	Not recommended	Hepatic dysfunction
5α-reductase inhibition (prevent conversion of testosterone to active dihydrotestosterone)	Finasteride	5 mg daily	Limited clinical experience; possibly less efficacious than other treatments
Suppression of ovarian steroid production and elevation of sex hormone-binding globulin	Oestrogen	See combination with cyproterone acetate above *or* Conventional oestrogen-containing contraceptive	Venous thromboembolism Hypertension Weight gain Dyslipidaemia Increased breast and endometrial carcinoma

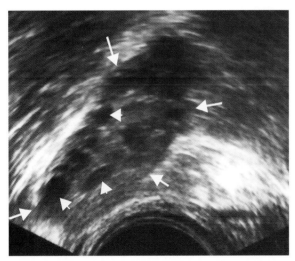

Fig. 18.15 Polycystic ovary. A transvaginal ultrasound scan showing multiple cysts (some indicated by small arrows) in the ovary (highlighted by bigger arrows) of a woman with polycystic ovarian syndrome.

Menstrual irregularity and infertility

Most women with PCOS have oligomenorrhoea, with irregular, heavy menstrual periods. This may not require treatment unless fertility is desired. Metformin (p. 746), by reducing insulin resistance, may restore regular ovulatory cycles in overweight women, although it is less effective than clomifene (p. 656) at restoring fertility as measured by successful pregnancy. Thiazolidinediones (p. 747) also enhance insulin sensitivity and restore menstrual regularity in PCOS but are contraindicated in women planning pregnancy.

In women who have very few periods each year or are amenorrhoeic, the high oestrogen concentrations associated with PCOS can cause endometrial hyperplasia. Progestogens can be administered on a cyclical basis to induce regular shedding of the endometrium and a withdrawal bleed, or a progestogen-impregnated intrauterine coil can be fitted.

Hirsutism

For hirsutism, most patients will have used cosmetic measures, such as shaving, bleaching and waxing, before consulting a

doctor. Electrolysis and laser treatment are effective for small areas like the upper lip and for chest hair but are expensive. Eflornithine cream inhibits ornithine decarboxylase in hair follicles and may reduce hair growth when applied daily to affected areas of the face.

If conservative measures are unsuccessful, anti-androgen therapy is given (Box 18.29). The life cycle of a hair follicle is at least 3 months and no improvement is likely before this time, when follicles have shed their hair and replacement hair growth has been suppressed. Metformin and thiazolidinediones are less effective at treating hirsutism than at restoring menstrual regularity. Unless weight is lost, hirsutism will return if therapy is discontinued. The patient should know that prolonged exposure to some agents may not be desirable and they should be stopped before pregnancy.

Turner's syndrome

Turner's syndrome affects around 1 in 2500 females. It is classically associated with a 45XO karyotype but other cytogenetic abnormalities may be responsible, including mosaic forms (e.g. 45XO/46XX or 45XO/46XY) and partial deletions of an X chromosome.

Clinical features

These are shown in Figure 18.16.

Individuals with Turner's syndrome invariably have short stature from an early age and this is often the initial presenting symptom. It is probably due to haploinsufficiency of the *SHOX* gene, one copy of which is found on both the X and Y chromosomes, which encodes a protein that is predominantly found in bone fibroblasts.

The genital tract and external genitalia in Turner's syndrome are female in character, since this is the default developmental outcome in the absence of testes. Ovarian tissue develops normally until the third month of gestation, but thereafter there is gonadal dysgenesis with accelerated degeneration of oöcytes and increased ovarian stromal fibrosis, resulting in 'streak ovaries'. The inability of ovarian tissue to produce oestrogen results in loss of negative feedback and elevation of FSH and LH concentrations.

There is a wide variation in the spectrum of associated somatic abnormalities. The severity of the phenotype is, in part, related to

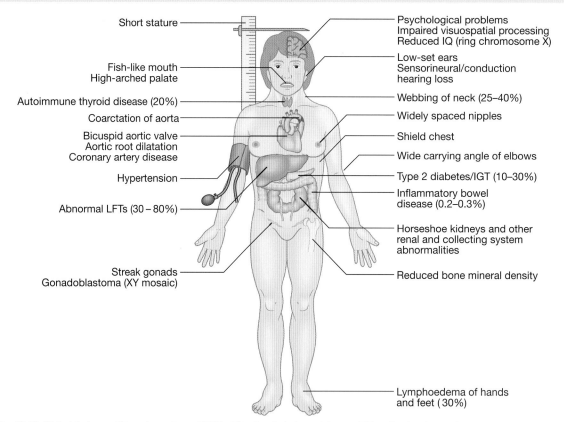

Short stature

Fish-like mouth
High-arched palate

Autoimmune thyroid disease (20%)

Coarctation of aorta

Bicuspid aortic valve
Aortic root dilatation
Coronary artery disease

Hypertension

Abnormal LFTs (30 – 80%)

Streak gonads
Gonadoblastoma (XY mosaic)

Psychological problems
Impaired visuospatial processing
Reduced IQ (ring chromosome X)

Low-set ears
Sensorineural/conduction
hearing loss

Webbing of neck (25–40%)

Widely spaced nipples

Shield chest

Wide carrying angle of elbows

Type 2 diabetes/IGT (10–30%)

Inflammatory bowel
disease (0.2–0.3%)

Horseshoe kidneys and other
renal and collecting system
abnormalities

Reduced bone mineral density

Lymphoedema of hands
and feet (30%)

Fig. 18.16 Clinical features of Turner's syndrome (45XO). (IGT = impaired glucose tolerance; LFTs = liver function tests)

the underlying cytogenetic abnormality. Mosaic individuals may have only mild short stature and may enter puberty spontaneously before developing gonadal failure.

Diagnosis and management

The diagnosis of Turner's syndrome can be confirmed by karyotype analysis. Short stature, although not directly due to growth hormone deficiency, responds to high doses of growth hormone. Prophylactic gonadectomy is recommended for individuals with 45XO/46XY mosaicism because there is an increased risk of gonadoblastoma. Pubertal development can be induced with oestrogen therapy but causes fusion of the epiphyses and cessation of growth. The timing of pubertal induction therefore needs to be carefully planned. Adults with Turner's syndrome require long-term oestrogen replacement therapy and should be monitored periodically for the development of aortic root dilatation, hearing loss and other somatic complications.

Klinefelter's syndrome

Klinefelter's syndrome affects approximately 1 in 1000 males and is usually associated with a 47XXY karyotype. However, other cytogenetic variants may be responsible, especially 46XY/47XXY mosaicism. The principal pathological abnormality is dysgenesis of the seminiferous tubules. This is evident from infancy (and possibly even in utero) and progresses with age. By adolescence, hyalinisation and fibrosis are present within the seminiferous tubules and Leydig cell function is impaired, resulting in hypogonadism.

18.30 Gonadal function in old age

- **Post-menopausal osteoporosis**: a major public health issue due to the high incidence of associated fragility fractures, especially of hip.
- **Hormone replacement therapy**: should be prescribed only above the age of 50 for the short-term relief of symptoms of oestrogen deficiency.
- **Sexual activity**: many older people remain sexually active.
- **'Male menopause'**: does not occur, although testosterone concentrations do fall with age. Testosterone therapy in mildly hypogonadal men may be of benefit for body composition, muscle and bone. Large randomised trials are required to determine whether benefits outweigh potentially harmful effects on the prostate and cardiovascular system.
- **Androgens in older women**: hirsutism and balding occur. In those rare patients with elevated androgen levels, this may be pathological, e.g. from an ovarian tumour.

Clinical features

The diagnosis is typically made in adolescents who have presented with gynaecomastia and failure to progress normally through puberty. Affected individuals usually have small, firm testes. Tall stature is apparent from early childhood, reflecting characteristically long leg length associated with 47XXY, and may be exacerbated by androgen deficiency with lack of epiphyseal closure in puberty. Other clinical features may include learning difficulties and behavioural disorders, as well as an increased risk of breast cancer and type 2 diabetes in later life. The spectrum of clinical features is wide and some individuals, especially those with 46XY/47XXY mosaicism, may pass through puberty normally and be identified only during investigation for infertility.

Diagnosis and management

Klinefelter's syndrome is suggested by the typical phenotype in a patient with hypergonadotrophic hypogonadism and can be confirmed by karyotype analysis. Individuals with clinical and biochemical evidence of androgen deficiency require androgen replacement (see Box 18.24). There are reports of successful pregnancy occurring following ICSI therapy where spermatocytes have been retrieved from the gonads of men with Klinefelter's syndrome.

The parathyroid glands

Parathyroid hormone (PTH) plays a key role in the regulation of calcium and phosphate homeostasis and vitamin D metabolism, as shown in Figure 24.61 (p. 1051). The consequences of altered function of this axis in gut and renal disease are covered on pages 783 and 418, respectively. Other metabolic bone diseases are explored on page 1044. Here, the investigation of hypercalcaemia and hypocalcaemia and disorders of the parathyroid glands are discussed.

Functional anatomy, physiology and investigations

The four parathyroid glands lie behind the lobes of the thyroid and weigh between 25 and 40 mg. The parathyroid chief cells respond directly to changes in calcium concentrations via a G protein-coupled cell surface receptor (the calcium-sensing receptor) located on the cell surface (see Fig. 25.55). When serum ionised calcium levels fall, PTH secretion rises. PTH is a single-chain polypeptide of 84 amino acids. It acts on the renal tubules to promote reabsorption of calcium and reduce reabsorption of phosphate, and on the skeleton to increase osteoclastic bone resorption and bone formation. PTH also promotes the conversion of 25-hydroxyvitamin D to the active metabolite, 1,25-dihydroxyvitamin D; the 1,25-dihydroxyvitamin D, in turn, enhances calcium absorption from the gut.

More than 99% of total body calcium is in bone. Prolonged exposure of bone to high levels of PTH is associated with increased osteoclastic activity and new bone formation, but the net effect is to cause bone loss with mobilisation of calcium into the extracellular fluid. In contrast, pulsatile release of PTH causes net bone gain, an effect that is exploited therapeutically in the treatment of osteoporosis (p. 1048).

The differential diagnosis of disorders of calcium metabolism requires measurement of calcium phosphate, alkaline phosphatase, renal function, PTH and 25-hydroxyvitamin D. Although the parathyroid glands detect and respond to ionised calcium levels, most clinical laboratories measure only total serum calcium levels. About 50% of total calcium is bound to organic ions, such as citrate or phosphate, and to proteins, especially albumin. Accordingly, if the serum albumin level is reduced, total calcium concentrations should be 'corrected' by adjusting the value for calcium upwards by 0.02 mmol/L (0.08 mg/dL) for each 1 g/L reduction in albumin below 40 g/L. If albumin concentrations are significantly low, as in severe acute illness and other chronic illness such as liver cirrhosis, this correction is less accurate and measurement of ionised calcium is needed.

Calcitonin is secreted from the parafollicular C cells of the thyroid gland. Although it is a useful tumour marker in medullary carcinoma of thyroid (p. 650) and can be given therapeutically in Paget's disease of bone (p. 1053), its release from the thyroid is of no clinical relevance to calcium homeostasis in humans.

Disorders of the parathyroid glands are summarised in Box 18.31.

Presenting problems in parathyroid disease

Hypercalcaemia

Hypercalcaemia is one of the most common biochemical abnormalities and is often detected during routine biochemical analysis in asymptomatic patients. However, it can present with chronic symptoms, as described below, and occasionally as an acute emergency with severe hypercalcaemia and dehydration.

i | 18.31 Classification of diseases of the parathyroid glands

	Primary	Secondary
Hormone excess	Primary hyperparathyroidism Parathyroid adenoma Parathyroid carcinoma[1] Parathyroid hyperplasia[2] Tertiary hyperparathyroidism Following prolonged secondary hyperparathyroidism	Secondary hyperparathyroidism Chronic kidney disease Malabsorption Vitamin D deficiency
Hormone deficiency	Hypoparathyroidism Post-surgical Autoimmune Inherited	
Hormone hypersensitivity	Autosomal dominant hypercalciuric hypocalcaemic (CASR-activating mutation)	
Hormone resistance	Pseudohypoparathyroidism Familial hypocalciuric hypercalcaemia	
Non-functioning tumours	Parathyroid carcinoma[1]	

[1]Parathyroid carcinomas may or may not produce parathyroid hormone. [2]In multiple endocrine neoplasia (MEN) syndromes (p. 688).
(CASR = calcium-sensing receptor)

Causes of hypercalcaemia are listed in Box 18.32. Of these, primary hyperparathyroidism and malignant hypercalcaemia are by far the most common. Familial hypocalciuric hypercalcaemia (FHH) is a rare but important cause that needs differentiation from primary hyperparathyroidism (HPT). Lithium may cause hyperparathyroidism by reducing the sensitivity of the calcium-sensing receptor.

Clinical assessment

Symptoms and signs of hypercalcaemia include polyuria and polydipsia, renal colic, lethargy, anorexia, nausea, dyspepsia and peptic ulceration, constipation, depression, drowsiness and impaired cognition. Patients with malignant hypercalcaemia can have a rapid onset of symptoms and may have clinical features that help to localise the tumour.

The classic symptoms of primary hyperparathyroidism are described by the adage 'bones, stones and abdominal groans', but few patients present in this way nowadays and the disorder is most often picked up as an incidental finding on biochemical testing. About 50% of patients with primary hyperparathyroidism are asymptomatic while others have non-specific symptoms such as fatigue, depression and generalised aches and pains. Some present with renal calculi and it has been estimated that 5% of first stone formers and 15% of recurrent stone formers have primary hyperparathyroidism (p. 663). Hypertension is a common feature of hyperparathyroidism. Parathyroid tumours are almost never palpable.

A family history of hypercalcaemia raises the possibility of FHH or MEN (p. 688).

Investigations

The most discriminatory investigation is measurement of PTH. If PTH levels are detectable or elevated in the presence of hypercalcaemia, then primary hyperparathyroidism is the most likely diagnosis. High plasma phosphate and alkaline phosphatase accompanied by renal impairment suggest tertiary hyperparathyroidism. Hypercalcaemia may cause nephrocalcinosis and renal tubular impairment, resulting in hyperuricaemia and hyperchloraemia.

Patients with FHH can present with a similar biochemical picture to primary hyperparathyroidism but typically have low urinary calcium excretion (a ratio of urinary calcium clearance to creatinine clearance of <0.01). The diagnosis of FHH can be confirmed by screening family members for hypercalcaemia and/or identifying an inactivating mutation in the gene encoding the calcium-sensing receptor.

If PTH is low and no other cause is apparent, then malignancy with or without bony metastases is likely. PTH-related peptide, which is often responsible for the hypercalcaemia associated with malignancy, is not detected by PTH assays, but can be measured by a specific assay (although this is not usually necessary). Unless the source is obvious, the patient should be screened for malignancy with a chest X-ray, myeloma screen (p. 967) and CT as appropriate.

Management

Treatment of severe hypercalcaemia and primary hyper-parathyroidism is described on pages 663 and 1327, respectively. FHH does not require any specific intervention.

Hypocalcaemia

Aetiology

Hypocalcaemia is much less common than hypercalcaemia. The differential diagnosis is shown in Box 18.33. The most common

---

 18.32 Causes of hypercalcaemia

With normal or elevated parathyroid hormone (PTH) levels

- Primary or tertiary hyperparathyroidism
- Lithium-induced hyperparathyroidism
- Familial hypocalciuric hypercalcaemia

With low PTH levels

- Malignancy (lung, breast, myeloma, renal, lymphoma, thyroid)
- Elevated 1,25-dihydroxyvitamin D (vitamin D intoxication, sarcoidosis, human immunodeficiency virus, other granulomatous disease)
- Thyrotoxicosis
- Paget's disease with immobilisation
- Milk-alkali syndrome
- Thiazide diuretics
- Glucocorticoid deficiency

---

i 18.33 Differential diagnosis of hypocalcaemia

	Total serum calcium	Ionised serum calcium	Serum phosphate	Serum PTH	Comments
Hypoalbuminaemia	↓	↔	↔	↔	Adjust calcium upwards by 0.02 mmol/L (0.1 mg/dL) for every 1 g/L reduction in albumin below 40 g/L
Alkalosis	↔	↓	↔	↔ or ↑	p. 366
Vitamin D deficiency	↓	↓	↓	↑	p. 1049
Chronic renal failure	↓	↓	↑	↑	Due to impaired vitamin D hydroxylation Serum creatinine ↑
Hypoparathyroidism	↓	↓	↑	↓	See text
Pseudohypoparathyroidism	↓	↓	↑	↑	Characteristic phenotype (see text)
Acute pancreatitis	↓	↓	↔ or ↓	↑	Usually clinically obvious Serum amylase ↑
Hypomagnesaemia	↓	↓	Variable	↓ or ↔	Treatment of hypomagnesaemia may correct hypocalcaemia

(↑ = levels increased; ↓ = levels reduced; ↔ = levels normal) cause of hypocalcaemia is a low serum albumin with normal ionised calcium concentration. Conversely, ionised calcium may be low in the face of normal total serum calcium in patients with alkalosis: for example, as a result of hyperventilation.

Hypocalcaemia may also develop as a result of magnesium depletion and should be considered in patients with malabsorption, those on diuretic or proton pump inhibitor therapy, and/or those with a history of alcohol excess. Magnesium deficiency causes hypocalcaemia by impairing the ability of the parathyroid glands to secrete PTH (resulting in PTH concentrations that are low or inappropriately in the reference range) and may also impair the actions of PTH on bone and kidney.

Clinical assessment

Mild hypocalcaemia is often asymptomatic but, with more profound reductions in serum calcium, tetany can occur. This is characterised by muscle spasms due to increased excitability of peripheral nerves.

Children are more liable to develop tetany than adults and present with a characteristic triad of carpopedal spasm, stridor and convulsions, although one or more of these may be found independently of the others. In carpopedal spasm, the hands adopt a characteristic position with flexion of the metacarpophalangeal joints of the fingers and adduction of the thumb ('main d'accoucheur'). Pedal spasm can also occur but is less frequent. Stridor is caused by spasm of the glottis. Adults can also develop carpopedal spasm in association with tingling of the hands and feet and around the mouth, but stridor and fits are rare.

Latent tetany may be detected by eliciting Trousseau's sign: inflation of a sphygmomanometer cuff on the upper arm to more than the systolic blood pressure is followed by carpal spasm within 3 minutes. Less specific is Chvostek's sign, in which tapping over the branches of the facial nerve as they emerge from the parotid gland produces twitching of the facial muscles.

Hypocalcaemia can cause papilloedema and prolongation of the ECG QT interval, which may predispose to ventricular arrhythmias. Prolonged hypocalcaemia and hyperphosphataemia (as in hypoparathyroidism) may cause calcification of the basal ganglia, grand mal epilepsy, psychosis and cataracts. Hypocalcaemia associated with hypophosphataemia, as in vitamin D deficiency, causes rickets in children and osteomalacia in adults (p. 1049).

Management

Emergency management of hypocalcaemia associated with tetany is given in Box 18.34. Treatment of chronic hypocalcaemia is described on page 1051.

Primary hyperparathyroidism

Primary hyperparathyroidism is caused by autonomous secretion of PTH, usually by a single parathyroid adenoma, which can vary in diameter from a few millimetres to several centimetres. It should be distinguished from secondary hyperparathyroidism, in which there is a physiological increase in PTH secretion to compensate for prolonged hypocalcaemia (such as in vitamin D deficiency, p. 1049), and from tertiary hyperparathyroidism, in which continuous stimulation of the parathyroids over a prolonged period of time results in adenoma formation and autonomous PTH secretion (Box 18.35). This is most commonly seen in individuals with advanced chronic kidney disease (p. 418).

The prevalence of primary hyperparathyroidism is about 1 in 800 and it is 2–3 times more common in women than men; 90% of patients are over 50 years of age. It also occurs in the familial MEN syndromes (p. 688), in which case hyperplasia or multiple adenomas of all four parathyroid glands are more likely than a solitary adenoma.

Clinical and radiological features

The clinical presentation of primary hyperparathyroidism is described on page 667. Parathyroid bone disease is now rare due to earlier diagnosis and treatment. Osteitis fibrosa results from increased bone resorption by osteoclasts with fibrous replacement in the lacunae. This may present as bone pain and tenderness, fracture and deformity. Chondrocalcinosis can occur due to deposition of calcium pyrophosphate crystals within articular cartilage. It typically affects the menisci at the knees and can result in secondary degenerative arthritis or predispose to attacks of acute pseudogout (p. 1016). Skeletal X-rays are usually normal in mild primary hyperparathyroidism, but in patients with advanced disease characteristic changes are observed. In the early stages there is demineralisation, with subperiosteal erosions and terminal resorption in the phalanges. A 'pepper-pot' appearance may be seen on lateral X-rays of the skull. Reduced bone mineral density, resulting in either osteopenia or osteoporosis, is now the most common skeletal manifestation of hyperparathyroidism. This is usually not evident radiographically and requires assessment by DXA (p. 989).

In nephrocalcinosis, scattered opacities may be visible within the renal outline. There may be soft tissue calcification in arterial walls and hands and in the cornea.

Investigations

The diagnosis can be confirmed by finding a raised PTH level in the presence of hypercalcaemia, provided that FHH is excluded

---

✚ 18.34 Management of severe hypocalcaemia

Immediate management

- 10–20 mL 10% calcium gluconate IV over 10–20 mins
- Continuous IV infusion may be required for several hours (equivalent of 10 mL 10% calcium gluconate/hr)
- Cardiac monitoring is recommended

If associated with hypomagnesaemia

- 50 mmol (1.23 g) magnesium chloride IV over 24 hrs
- Most parenteral magnesium will be excreted in the urine, so further doses may be required to replenish body stores

---

i 18.35 Hyperparathyroidism

Type	Serum calcium	PTH
Primary Single adenoma (90%) Multiple adenomas (4%) Nodular hyperplasia (5%) Carcinoma (1%)	Raised	Not suppressed
Secondary Chronic renal failure Malabsorption Osteomalacia and rickets	Low	Raised
Tertiary	Raised	Not suppressed

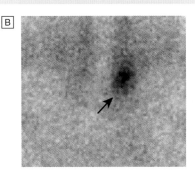

Fig. 18.17 ^{99m}Tc-sestamibi scan of a patient with primary hyperparathyroidism secondary to a parathyroid adenoma. **A** After 1 hour, there is uptake in the thyroid gland (thick arrow) and the enlarged left inferior parathyroid gland (thin arrow). **B** After 3 hours, uptake is evident only in the parathyroid (thin arrow).

(p. 664). Parathyroid scanning by ^{99m}Tc-sestamibi scintigraphy (MIBI; Fig. 18.17) and an ultrasound examination can be performed prior to surgery, in an attempt to localise an adenoma; a concordant finding of tissue consistent with a parathyroid gland and uptake on the MIBI scan allows a targeted resection. Negative imaging does not exclude the diagnosis, however, and four-gland exploration may be needed.

Management

The treatment of choice for primary hyperparathyroidism is surgery, with excision of a solitary parathyroid adenoma or hyperplastic glands. Experienced surgeons will identify solitary tumours in more than 90% of cases. Patients with parathyroid bone disease run a significant risk of developing hypocalcaemia post-operatively but the risk of this can be reduced by correcting vitamin D deficiency pre-operatively.

Surgery is usually indicated for individuals aged less than 50 years, with clear-cut symptoms or documented complications (such as renal stones, renal impairment or osteoporosis), and (in asymptomatic patients) significant hypercalcaemia (corrected serum calcium >2.85 mmol/L (>11.4 mg/dL)). Patients who are treated conservatively without surgery should have calcium biochemistry and renal function checked annually and bone density monitored periodically. They should be encouraged to maintain a high oral fluid intake to avoid renal stones.

Occasionally, primary hyperparathyroidism presents with severe life-threatening hypercalcaemia. This is often due to dehydration and should be managed medically with intravenous fluids and bisphosphonates, as described on page 1327. If this is not effective, then urgent parathyroidectomy should be considered.

Cinacalcet (p. 419) is a calcimimetic that enhances the sensitivity of the calcium-sensing receptor, so reducing PTH levels, and is licensed for tertiary hyperparathyroidism and as a treatment for patients with primary hyperparathyroidism who are unwilling to have surgery or are medically unfit.

Familial hypocalciuric hypercalcaemia

This autosomal dominant disorder is caused by an inactivating mutation in one of the alleles of the calcium-sensing receptor gene, which reduces the ability of the parathyroid gland to 'sense' ionised calcium concentrations. As a result, higher than normal calcium levels are required to suppress PTH secretion. The typical presentation is with mild hypercalcaemia with PTH concentrations that are 'inappropriately' at the upper end of the reference range or are slightly elevated. Calcium-sensing receptors in the renal tubules are also affected and this leads to increased renal tubular reabsorption of calcium and hypocalciuria (as measured in the vitamin D-replete individual by a fractional calcium excretion or 24-hour calcium excretion). The hypercalcaemia of FHH is always asymptomatic and complications do not occur. The main risk of FHH is that of the patient being subjected to an unnecessary (and ineffective) parathyroidectomy if misdiagnosed as having primary hyperparathyroidism. Testing of family members for hypercalcaemia is helpful in confirming the diagnosis and it is also possible to perform genetic testing. No treatment is necessary.

Hypoparathyroidism

The most common cause of hypoparathyroidism is damage to the parathyroid glands (or their blood supply) during thyroid surgery. Rarely, hypoparathyroidism can occur as a result of infiltration of the glands with iron in haemochromatosis (p. 895) or copper in Wilson's disease (p. 896).

There are a number of rare congenital or inherited forms of hypoparathyroidism. One form is associated with autoimmune polyendocrine syndrome type 1 (p. 689) and another with DiGeorge syndrome (p. 79). Autosomal dominant hypoparathyroidism is the mirror image of FHH (see above), in that an activating mutation in the calcium-sensing receptor reduces PTH levels, resulting in hypocalcaemia and hypercalciuria.

Pseudohypoparathyroidism

In this disorder, the individual is functionally hypoparathyroid but, instead of PTH deficiency, there is tissue resistance to the effects of PTH, such that PTH concentrations are markedly elevated. The PTH receptor itself is normal but the downstream signalling pathways are defective due to mutations that affect *GNAS1*, which encodes the Gsα protein, a molecule involved in signal transduction downstream of the PTH receptor and other G protein-coupled receptors. There are several subtypes but the most common (pseudohypoparathyroidism type 1a) is characterised by hypocalcaemia and hyperphosphataemia, in association with short stature, short fourth metacarpals and metatarsals, rounded face, obesity and subcutaneous calcification; these features are collectively referred to as Albright's hereditary osteodystrophy (AHO). Type 1a pseudohypoparathyroidism occurs only when the *GNAS1* mutation is inherited on the maternal chromosome (maternal imprinting, p. 49).

The term pseudopseudohypoparathyroidism is used to describe patients who have clinical features of AHO but normal serum calcium and PTH concentrations; it occurs when the *GNAS1* mutation is inherited on the paternal chromosome. The inheritance of these disorders is an example of genetic imprinting (p. 49). The difference in clinical features occurs as a result of the fact that renal cells exclusively express the maternal *GNAS1* allele, whereas both maternal and paternal alleles are expressed in other cell types; this explains why maternal inheritance is associated with hypocalcaemia and resistance to PTH (which regulates serum calcium and phosphate levels largely by an effect on the renal tubule), and why paternal inheritance is associated with skeletal and other abnormalities in the absence of hypocalcaemia and raised PTH values.

Management of hypoparathyroidism

Persistent hypoparathyroidism and pseudohypoparathyroidism are treated with oral calcium salts and vitamin D analogues, either 1α-hydroxycholecalciferol (alfacalcidol) or 1,25-dihydroxycholecalciferol (calcitriol). This therapy needs careful monitoring because of the risks of iatrogenic hypercalcaemia, hypercalciuria and nephrocalcinosis. Recombinant PTH is available as subcutaneous injection therapy for osteoporosis (p. 1048) and, although not currently licensed, has been used in hypoparathyroidism (but not in pseudohypoparathyroidism). It is much more expensive than calcium and vitamin D analogue therapy but has the advantage that it is less likely to cause hypercalciuria. There is no specific treatment for AHO other than to try to maintain calcium levels within the reference range using active vitamin D metabolites.

> **18.36 The parathyroid glands in old age**
>
> - **Osteoporosis**: always exclude osteomalacia and hyperparathyroidism by checking vitamin D and calcium concentrations.
> - **Primary hyperparathyroidism**: more common with ageing. Older people can often be observed without surgical intervention.
> - **Hypercalcaemia**: may cause delirium.
> - **Vitamin D deficiency**: common because of limited exposure to the sun and reduced ability of older skin to synthesise cholecalciferol.

The adrenal glands

The adrenals comprise several separate endocrine glands within a single anatomical structure. The adrenal medulla is an extension of the sympathetic nervous system that secretes catecholamines into capillaries rather than synapses. Most of the adrenal cortex is made up of cells that secrete cortisol and adrenal androgens, and form part of the hypothalamic–pituitary–adrenal (HPA) axis. The small outer glomerulosa of the cortex secretes aldosterone under the control of the renin–angiotensin system. These functions are important in the integrated control of cardiovascular, metabolic and immune responses to stress.

There is increasing evidence that subtle alterations in adrenal function contribute to the pathogenesis of common diseases such as hypertension, obesity and type 2 diabetes mellitus. However, classical syndromes of adrenal hormone deficiency and excess are relatively rare.

Functional anatomy and physiology

Adrenal anatomy and function are shown in Figure 18.18. Histologically, the cortex is divided into three zones, but these function as two units (zona glomerulosa and zonae fasciculata/reticularis) that produce corticosteroids in response to humoral stimuli. Pathways for the biosynthesis of corticosteroids are shown in Figure 18.19. Investigation of adrenal function is described under specific diseases below. The different types of adrenal disease are shown in Box 18.37.

Glucocorticoids

Cortisol is the major glucocorticoid in humans. Levels are highest in the morning on waking and lowest in the middle of the night. Cortisol rises dramatically during stress, including any illness. This elevation protects key metabolic functions (such as the maintenance of cerebral glucose supply during starvation) and inhibits potentially damaging inflammatory responses to infection and injury. The clinical importance of cortisol deficiency is, therefore, most obvious at times of stress.

More than 95% of circulating cortisol is bound to protein, principally cortisol-binding globulin, which is increased by oestrogens. It is the free fraction that is biologically active. Cortisol regulates cell function by binding to glucocorticoid receptors that regulate the transcription of many genes. Cortisol can also activate mineralocorticoid receptors, but it does not normally do so because most cells containing mineralocorticoid receptors also express an enzyme called 11β-hydroxysteroid dehydrogenase type 2 (11β-HSD2), which inactivates cortisol by converting it to cortisone. Inhibitors of 11β-HSD2 (such as liquorice) or mutations in the gene that encodes 11β-HSD2 cause cortisol to act as a mineralocorticoid, resulting in sodium retention and hypertension (see Box 18.46).

18

	Primary	Secondary
18.37 Classification of diseases of the adrenal glands		
Hormone excess	Non-ACTH-dependent Cushing's syndrome Primary hyperaldosteronism Phaeochromocytoma	ACTH-dependent Cushing's syndrome Secondary hyperaldosteronism
Hormone deficiency	Addison's disease Congenital adrenal hyperplasia	Hypopituitarism
Hormone hypersensitivity	11β-hydroxysteroid dehydrogenase type 2 deficiency Liddle's syndrome	
Hormone resistance	Pseudohypoaldosteronism Glucocorticoid resistance syndrome	
Non-functioning tumours	Adenoma Carcinoma (usually functioning) Metastatic tumours	

(ACTH = adrenocorticotrophic hormone)

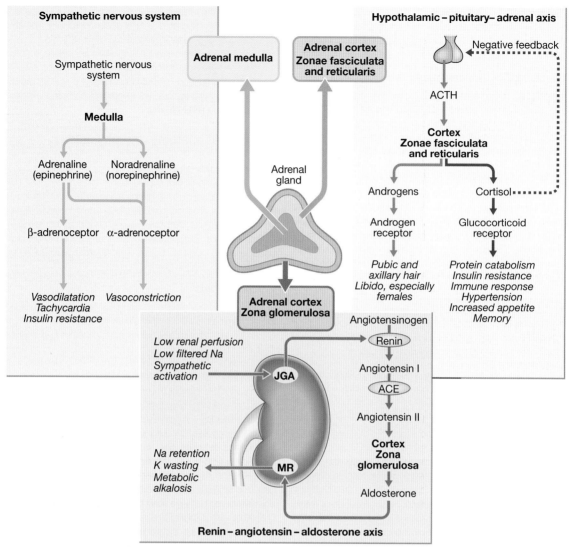

Fig. 18.18 Structure and function of the adrenal glands. (ACE = angiotensin-converting enzyme; ACTH = adrenocorticotrophic hormone; JGA = juxtaglomerular apparatus; MR = mineralocorticoid receptor)

Mineralocorticoids

Aldosterone is the most important mineralocorticoid. It binds to mineralocorticoid receptors in the kidney and causes sodium retention and increased excretion of potassium and protons (p. 351). The principal stimulus to aldosterone secretion is angiotensin II, a peptide produced by activation of the renin–angiotensin system (see Fig. 18.18). Renin activity in the juxtaglomerular apparatus of the kidney is stimulated by low perfusion pressure in the afferent arteriole, low sodium filtration leading to low sodium concentrations at the macula densa, or increased sympathetic nerve activity. As a result, renin activity is increased in hypovolaemia and renal artery stenosis, and is approximately doubled when standing up from a recumbent position.

Catecholamines

In humans, only a small proportion of circulating noradrenaline (norepinephrine) is derived from the adrenal medulla; much more is released from sympathetic nerve endings. Conversion of noradrenaline to adrenaline (epinephrine) is catalysed by catechol O-methyltransferase (COMT), which is induced by glucocorticoids.

Blood flow in the adrenal is centripetal, so that the medulla is bathed in high concentrations of cortisol and is the major source of circulating adrenaline. However, after surgical removal of the adrenal medullae, there appear to be no clinical consequences attributable to deficiency of circulating catecholamines.

Adrenal androgens

Adrenal androgens are secreted in response to ACTH and are the most abundant steroids in the blood stream. They are probably important in the initiation of puberty (adrenarche). The adrenals are also the major source of androgens in adult females and may be important in female libido.

Presenting problems in adrenal disease

Cushing's syndrome

Cushing's syndrome is caused by excessive activation of glucocorticoid receptors. It is most commonly iatrogenic, due to prolonged administration of synthetic glucocorticoids such as

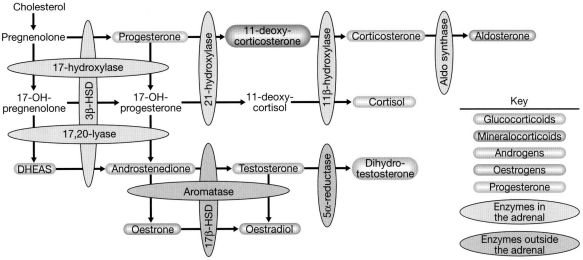

Fig. 18.19 The major pathways of synthesis of steroid hormones. (DHEAS = dehydroepiandrosterone sulphate; HSD = hydroxysteroid dehydrogenase)

prednisolone. Endogenous Cushing's syndrome is uncommon but is caused by chronic over-production of cortisol by the adrenal glands, either as the result of an adrenal tumour or because of excessive production of ACTH by a pituitary tumour or ectopic ACTH production by other tumours.

Aetiology

The causes are shown in Box 18.38. Amongst endogenous causes, pituitary-dependent cortisol excess (by convention, called Cushing's disease) accounts for approximately 80% of cases. Both Cushing's disease and cortisol-secreting adrenal tumours are four times more common in women than men. In contrast, ectopic ACTH syndrome (often due to a small-cell carcinoma of the bronchus) is more common in men.

Clinical assessment

The diverse manifestations of glucocorticoid excess are shown in Figure 18.20. Many of these are not specific to Cushing's syndrome and, because spontaneous Cushing's syndrome is rare, the positive predictive value of any single clinical feature alone is low. Moreover, some common disorders can be confused with Cushing's syndrome because they are associated with alterations in cortisol secretion, e.g. obesity and depression (Box 18.38). Features that favour Cushing's syndrome in an obese patient are bruising, myopathy and thin skin. Any clinical suspicion of cortisol excess is best resolved by further investigation.

It is vital to exclude iatrogenic causes in all patients with Cushing's syndrome since even inhaled or topical glucocorticoids can induce the syndrome in susceptible individuals. A careful drug history must therefore be taken before embarking on complex investigations. An 0800–0900-hr serum cortisol of < 100 nmol/L (3.6 μg/dL) in a patient with a normal sleep–wake pattern and Cushingoid appearance is consistent with exogenous synthetic glucocorticoid use (common) or cyclical secretion of cortisol from endogenous Cushing's (uncommon).

Some clinical features are more common in ectopic ACTH syndrome. While ACTH-secreting pituitary tumours retain some negative feedback sensitivity to cortisol, this is absent in tumours that produce ectopic ACTH, typically resulting in higher levels of both ACTH and cortisol than are observed in pituitary-driven disease. The high ACTH levels are associated with marked

> ### i 18.38 Classification of endogenous Cushing's syndrome
>
> **ACTH-dependent – 80%**
>
> - Pituitary adenoma secreting ACTH (Cushing's disease) – 70%
> - Ectopic ACTH syndrome (bronchial carcinoid, small-cell lung carcinoma, other neuro-endocrine tumour) – 10%
>
> **Non-ACTH-dependent – 20%**
>
> - Adrenal adenoma – 15%
> - Adrenal carcinoma – 5%
> - ACTH-independent macronodular hyperplasia; primary pigmented nodular adrenal disease; McCune–Albright syndrome (together < 1%)
>
> **Hypercortisolism due to other causes (also referred to as pseudo-Cushing's syndrome)**
>
> - Alcohol excess (biochemical and clinical features)
> - Major depressive illness (biochemical features only, some clinical overlap)
> - Primary obesity (mild biochemical features, some clinical overlap)
>
> (ACTH = adrenocorticotrophic hormone)

pigmentation because of binding to melanocortin 1 receptors on melanocytes in the skin. The high cortisol levels also overcome the capacity of 11β-HSD2 to inactivate cortisol in the kidney (p. 665), causing hypokalaemic alkalosis that aggravates myopathy and hyperglycaemia (by inhibiting insulin secretion). When the tumour that is secreting ACTH is malignant, then the onset is usually rapid and may be associated with cachexia. For these reasons, the classical features of Cushing's syndrome are less common in ectopic ACTH syndrome; if present, they suggest that a less aggressive tumour, such as a bronchial carcinoid, is responsible.

In Cushing's disease, the pituitary tumour is usually a microadenoma (< 10 mm in diameter); hence other features of a pituitary macroadenoma (hypopituitarism, visual failure or disconnection hyperprolactinaemia, p. 684) are rare.

Investigations

The large number of tests available for Cushing's syndrome reflects the fact that each one has limited specificity and sensitivity

18

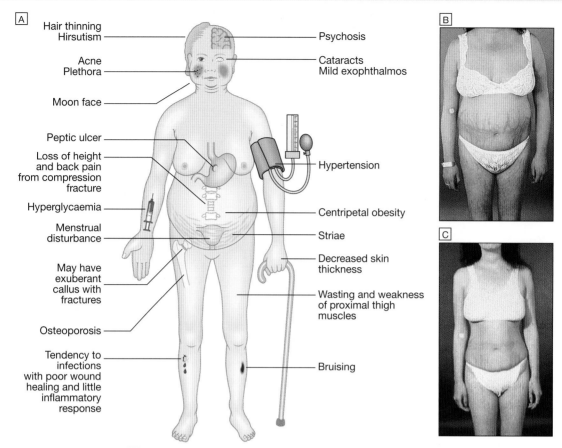

Hair thinning
Hirsutism

Acne
Plethora

Moon face

Peptic ulcer

Loss of height
and back pain
from compression
fracture

Hyperglycaemia

Menstrual
disturbance

May have
exuberant
callus with
fractures

Osteoporosis

Tendency to
infections
with poor wound
healing and little
inflammatory
response

Psychosis

Cataracts
Mild exophthalmos

Hypertension

Centripetal obesity

Striae

Decreased skin
thickness

Wasting and weakness
of proximal thigh
muscles

Bruising

Fig. 18.20 Cushing's syndrome. A Clinical features common to all causes. B A patient with Cushing's disease before treatment. C The same patient 1 year after the successful removal of an ACTH-secreting pituitary microadenoma by trans-sphenoidal surgery.

in isolation. Accordingly, several tests are usually combined to establish the diagnosis. Testing for Cushing's syndrome should be avoided under conditions of stress, such as an acute illness, because this activates the HPA axis, causing potentially spurious results. The diagnosis of Cushing's is a two-step process:

1. to establish whether the patient has Cushing's syndrome (Fig. 18.21)
2. to define its cause (Fig. 18.22).

Some additional tests are useful in all cases of Cushing's syndrome, including plasma electrolytes, glucose, glycosylated haemoglobin and bone mineral density measurement.

Establishing the presence of Cushing's syndrome

In patients where there is appropriate clinical suspicion, Cushing's syndrome is confirmed by using two of three main tests:

1. failure to suppress serum cortisol with low doses of oral dexamethasone
2. loss of the normal circadian rhythm of cortisol, with inappropriately elevated late-night serum or salivary cortisol
3. increased 24-hour urine free cortisol (see Fig. 18.21).

Dexamethasone is used for suppression testing because it does not cross-react in immunoassays for cortisol. An overnight dexamethasone suppression test (ONDST) involves administration of 1 mg dexamethasone at 2300 hrs and measurement of serum cortisol at 0900 hrs the following day. In a low-dose dexamethasone suppression test (LDDST), serum cortisol is measured following administration of 0.5 mg dexamethasone 4 times daily for 48 hours. For either test, a normal response is a serum cortisol of <50 nmol/L (1.8 µg/dL). It is important for any oestrogens to be stopped for 6 weeks prior to investigation to allow corticosteroid-binding globulin (CBG) levels to return to normal and to avoid false-positive responses, as most cortisol assays measure total cortisol, including that bound to CBG. Cyclicity of cortisol secretion is a feature of all types of Cushing's syndrome and, if very variable, can confuse diagnosis. Use of multiple salivary cortisol samples over weeks or months can be helpful in diagnosis but an elevated salivary cortisol alone should not be taken as proof of diagnosis. In iatrogenic Cushing's syndrome, cortisol levels are low unless the patient is taking a glucocorticoid (such as prednisolone) that cross-reacts in immunoassays with cortisol.

Determining the underlying cause

Once the presence of Cushing's syndrome is confirmed, measurement of plasma ACTH is the key to establishing the differential diagnosis; it is best measured in the morning around 0900 hrs. In the presence of excess cortisol secretion, an undetectable ACTH (<1.1 pmol/L (5 ng/L)) indicates an adrenal cause, while ACTH levels of >3.3 pmol/L (15 ng/L) suggest a pituitary cause or ectopic ACTH. ACTH levels between these values represent a 'grey area' and further evaluation by a specialist is required. Tests to discriminate pituitary from ectopic sources of ACTH rely on the fact that pituitary tumours, but not ectopic tumours, retain some features of normal regulation of

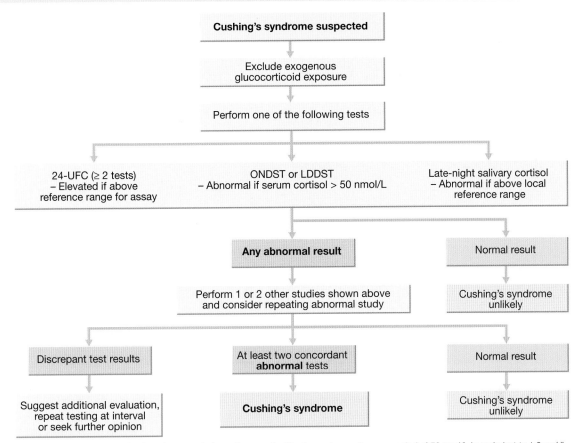

Fig. 18.21 Sequence of investigations in suspected spontaneous Cushing's syndrome. A serum cortisol of 50 nmol/L is equivalent to 1.8 μg/dL. (LDDST = low-dose dexamethasone suppression test; ONDST = overnight dexamethasone suppression test; UFC = urinary free cortisol)

18

ACTH secretion. Thus, in pituitary-dependent Cushing's disease, ACTH secretion is suppressed by high-dose dexamethasone and ACTH is stimulated by corticotrophin-releasing hormone (CRH). In a high-dose dexamethasone suppression test (HDDST), serum cortisol is measured before and after administration of 2 mg of dexamethasone 4 times daily for 48 hours.

Techniques for localisation of tumours secreting ACTH or cortisol are listed in Figure 18.22. MRI detects around 60% of pituitary microadenomas secreting ACTH. If available, bilateral inferior petrosal sinus sampling (BIPSS) with measurement of ACTH is the best means of confirming Cushing's disease, unless MRI shows a tumour bigger than 6 mm, in which case it may not be needed. CT or MRI detects most adrenal tumours; adrenal carcinomas are usually large (>5 cm) and have other features of malignancy (p. 673).

Management

Untreated severe Cushing's syndrome has a 50% 5-year mortality. Most patients are treated surgically, but medical therapy may be given in severe cases for a few weeks prior to operation to improve the clinical state. A number of drugs are available that inhibit glucocorticoid biosynthesis, including metyrapone and ketoconazole. The dose of these agents is best titrated against serum cortisol levels or 24-hour urine free cortisol.

Cushing's disease

Trans-sphenoidal surgery carried out by an experienced surgeon with selective removal of the adenoma is the treatment of choice,

with approximately 70% of patients going into immediate remission. Around 20% of patients suffer a recurrence, often years later, emphasising the need for life-long follow-up.

Laparoscopic bilateral adrenalectomy performed by an expert surgeon effectively cures ACTH-dependent Cushing's syndrome, but in patients with pituitary-dependent Cushing's syndrome this can result in Nelson's syndrome. In Nelson's syndrome, the loss of negative feedback from endogenous cortisol results in growth of the pituitary tumour, often leading to an invasive pituitary macroadenoma (which causes local mass effects) and very high ACTH levels (which cause pigmentation). The risk of Nelson's syndrome is reported as being reduced by pituitary irradiation in some series, but not all.

The somatostatin analogue pasireotide is also licensed for the treatment of Cushing's disease and works by suppressing ACTH secretion by the tumour. It may cause tumour shrinkage but cortisol levels are likely to return to pre-treatment levels following cessation of therapy. Pasireotide has to be administered by twice-daily subcutaneous injection and is relatively expensive. It is an alternative to drugs that inhibit glucocorticoid biosynthesis in patients who are not suitable for a surgical approach.

Adrenal tumours

Laparoscopic adrenal surgery is the treatment of choice for adrenal adenomas. Surgery offers the only prospect of cure for adrenocortical carcinomas but, in general, prognosis is poor with high rates of recurrence, even in patients with localised disease at presentation. Radiotherapy to the tumour bed reduces

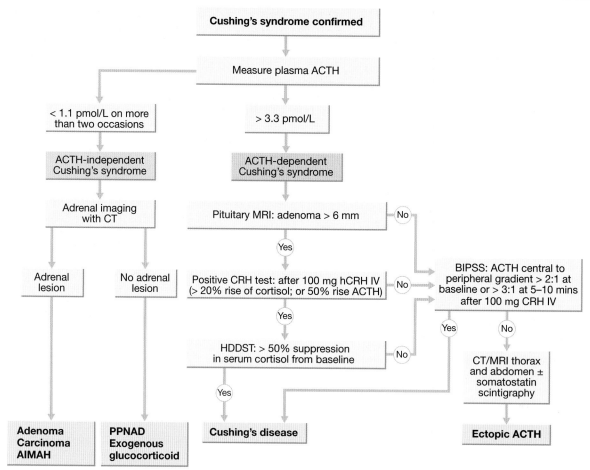

Fig. 18.22 Determining the cause of confirmed Cushing's syndrome. To convert pmol/L to ng/L, multiply by 4.541. (ACTH = adrenocorticotrophic hormone; AIMAH = ACTH-independent macronodular adrenal hyperplasia; BIPSS = bilateral inferior petrosal sinus sampling; hCRH = human corticotrophin-releasing hormone; HDDST = high-dose dexamethasone suppression test; PPNAD = primary pigmented nodular adrenal disease)

the risk of local recurrence; systemic therapy consists of the adrenolytic drug mitotane and chemotherapy, but responses are often poor.

Ectopic ACTH syndrome

Localised tumours, such as bronchial carcinoid, should be removed surgically. In patients with incurable malignancy, it is important to reduce the severity of the Cushing's syndrome using medical therapy (see above) or, if appropriate, bilateral adrenalectomy.

Therapeutic use of glucocorticoids

The remarkable anti-inflammatory properties of glucocorticoids have led to their use in a wide variety of clinical conditions but the hazards are significant. Equivalent doses of commonly used glucocorticoids are listed in Box 18.39. Topical preparations (dermal, rectal and inhaled) can also be absorbed into the systemic circulation, and although this rarely occurs to a sufficient degree to produce clinical features of Cushing's syndrome, it can result in significant suppression of endogenous ACTH and cortisol secretion. Severe Cushing's syndrome can result if there is concomitant administration of inhaled glucocorticoids and strong inhibitors of the liver enzyme CYP450 3A4, such as the antiretroviral drug ritonavir (p. 324).

18.39 Approximate equivalent doses of glucocorticoids

- Hydrocortisone: 20 mg
- Cortisone acetate: 25 mg
- Prednisolone: 5 mg
- Dexamethasone: 0.5 mg

Adverse effects of glucocorticoids

The clinical features of glucocorticoid excess are illustrated in Figure 18.20. Adverse effects are related to dose, duration of therapy, and pre-existing conditions that might be worsened by glucocorticoid therapy, such as diabetes mellitus or osteoporosis. Osteoporosis is a particularly important problem because, for a given bone mineral density, the fracture risk is greater in glucocorticoid-treated patients than in post-menopausal osteoporosis. Therefore, when systemic glucocorticoids are prescribed and the anticipated duration of steroid therapy is more than 3 months, bone-protective therapy should be considered, as detailed on page 1005. Rapid changes in glucocorticoid levels can also lead to marked mood disturbances, including depression, mania and insomnia. Glucocorticoid use also increases the white blood cell count (predominantly neutrophils), which must be taken into account when assessing patients with possible infection.

The anti-inflammatory effect of glucocorticoids may mask signs of disease. For example, perforation of a viscus may be masked and the patient may show no febrile response to an infection. Although there is debate about whether or not glucocorticoids increase the risk of peptic ulcer when used alone, they act synergistically with NSAIDs, including aspirin, to increase the risk of serious gastrointestinal adverse effects. Latent tuberculosis may be reactivated and patients on glucocorticoids are at risk of severe varicella zoster virus infection, so should avoid contact with chickenpox or shingles if they are non-immune.

Management of glucocorticoid withdrawal

All glucocorticoid therapy, even if inhaled or applied topically, can suppress the HPA axis. In practice, this is likely to result in a crisis due to adrenal insufficiency on withdrawal of treatment only if glucocorticoids have been administered orally or systemically for longer than 3 weeks, if repeated courses have been prescribed within the previous year, or if the dose is higher than the equivalent of 7.5 mg prednisolone per day. In these circumstances, the drug, when it is no longer required for the underlying condition, must be withdrawn slowly at a rate dictated by the duration of treatment. If glucocorticoid therapy has been prolonged, then it may take many months for the HPA axis to recover. All patients must be advised to avoid sudden drug withdrawal. They should be issued with a steroid card and/or wear an engraved bracelet (Box 18.40).

Recovery of the HPA axis is aided if there is no exogenous glucocorticoid present during the nocturnal surge in ACTH secretion. This can be achieved by giving glucocorticoid in the morning. Giving ACTH to stimulate adrenal recovery is of no value, as the pituitary remains suppressed.

In patients who have received glucocorticoids for longer than a few weeks, especially if the period is months to years, it is often valuable to confirm that the HPA axis is recovering during glucocorticoid withdrawal. Withdrawal has to be very slow, usually by a dose reduction equivalent of prednisolone 1 mg per month or slower. Once the dose of glucocorticoid is reduced to a minimum (e.g. 5 mg prednisolone or 0.5 mg

dexamethasone per day), then serum cortisol can be measured at 0900 hrs before the next dose. If this is <100 nmol/L (3.6 µg/dL), slow reduction should be continued with a repeat 0900 hrs serum cortisol when the dose of prednisolone is 3 mg per day. Once 0900 hrs serum cortisol is >100 nmol/L, then an ACTH stimulation test should be performed (see Box 18.43) to confirm if glucocorticoids can be withdrawn completely. Even when glucocorticoids have been successfully withdrawn, short-term replacement therapy is often advised during significant intercurrent illness occurring in subsequent months, as the HPA axis may not be able to respond fully to severe stress.

Adrenal insufficiency

Adrenal insufficiency results from inadequate secretion of cortisol and/or aldosterone. It is potentially fatal and notoriously variable in its presentation. A high index of suspicion is therefore required in patients with unexplained fatigue, hyponatraemia or hypotension. Causes are shown in Box 18.41. The most common is ACTH deficiency (secondary adrenocortical failure), usually because of inappropriate withdrawal of chronic glucocorticoid therapy or a pituitary tumour (p. 683). Congenital adrenal hyperplasia and Addison's disease (primary adrenocortical failure) are rare causes.

Clinical assessment

The clinical features of adrenal insufficiency are shown in Box 18.42. In Addison's disease, either glucocorticoid or mineralocorticoid deficiency may come first, but eventually all patients fail to secrete both classes of corticosteroid.

Patients may present with chronic features and/or in acute circulatory shock. With a chronic presentation, initial symptoms are often misdiagnosed as chronic fatigue syndrome or depression. In primary adrenal insufficiency, weight loss is a uniform presenting feature. Adrenocortical insufficiency should also be considered in patients with hyponatraemia, even in the absence of symptoms (p. 357).

Features of an acute adrenal crisis include circulatory shock with severe hypotension, hyponatraemia, hyperkalaemia and, in some instances, hypoglycaemia and hypercalcaemia. Muscle cramps, nausea, vomiting, diarrhoea and unexplained fever

18.40 Advice to patients on glucocorticoid replacement therapy

Intercurrent stress

- Febrile illness: double dose of hydrocortisone

Surgery

- Minor operation: hydrocortisone 100 mg IM with pre-medication
- Major operation: hydrocortisone 100 mg 4 times daily for 24 hrs, then 50 mg IM 4 times daily until ready to take tablets

Vomiting

- Patients must have parenteral hydrocortisone if unable to take it by mouth

Steroid card

- Patient should carry this at all times; it should give information regarding diagnosis, steroid, dose and doctor

Bracelet and emergency pack

- Patients should be encouraged to buy a bracelet and have it engraved with the diagnosis, current treatment and a reference number for a central database
- Patients should be given a hydrocortisone emergency pack and trained in the self-administration of hydrocortisone 100 mg IM; they should be advised to take the pack on holidays/trips abroad

18.41 Causes of adrenocortical insufficiency

Secondary (↓ACTH)

- Withdrawal of suppressive glucocorticoid therapy
- Hypothalamic or pituitary disease

Primary (↑ACTH)

Addison's disease

Common causes
- Autoimmune:
  Sporadic
  Polyglandular
  syndromes (p. 688)
- Tuberculosis
- HIV/AIDS
- Metastatic carcinoma
- Bilateral adrenalectomy

Rare causes
- Lymphoma
- Intra-adrenal haemorrhage (Waterhouse–Friderichsen syndrome following meningococcal sepsis)
- Amyloidosis
- Haemochromatosis

Corticosteroid biosynthetic enzyme defects
- Congenital adrenal hyperplasias
- Drugs: metyrapone, ketoconazole, etomidate

(ACTH = adrenocorticotrophic hormone)

18

i | **18.42 Clinical and biochemical features of adrenal insufficiency**

	Glucocorticoid insufficiency	Mineralocorticoid insufficiency	ACTH excess	Adrenal androgen insufficiency
Withdrawal of exogenous glucocorticoid	+	−	−	+
Hypopituitarism	+	−	−	+
Addison's disease	+	+	+	+
Congenital adrenal hyperplasia (21-hydroxylase deficiency)	+	+	+	−
Clinical features	Weight loss, anorexia Malaise, weakness Nausea, vomiting Diarrhoea or constipation Postural hypotension Shock Hypoglycaemia Hyponatraemia (dilutional) Hypercalcaemia	Hypotension Shock Hyponatraemia (depletional) Hyperkalaemia	Pigmentation of: Sun-exposed areas Pressure areas (e.g. elbows, knees) Palmar creases, knuckles Mucous membranes Conjunctivae Recent scars	Decreased body hair and loss of libido, especially in females

(ACTH = adrenocorticotrophic hormone)

 18.43 How and when to do an ACTH stimulation test

Use

- Diagnosis of primary or secondary adrenal insufficiency
- Assessment of HPA axis in patients taking suppressive glucocorticoid therapy
- Relies on ACTH-dependent adrenal atrophy in secondary adrenal insufficiency, so may not detect acute ACTH deficiency (e.g. in pituitary apoplexy, p. 683)

Dose

- 250 μg ACTH$_{1-24}$ (Synacthen) by IM injection at any time of day

Blood samples

- 0 and 30 mins for plasma cortisol
- 0 mins also for ACTH (on ice) if Addison's disease is being considered (patient not known to have pituitary disease or to be taking exogenous glucocorticoids)

Results

- Normal subjects: plasma cortisol > 500 nmol/L (approximately 18 μg/dL)* either at baseline or at 30 mins
- Incremental change in cortisol is not a criterion

*The exact cortisol concentration depends on the cortisol assay being used.
(ACTH = adrenocorticotrophic hormone; HPA = hypothalamic–pituitary–adrenal)

---

may be present. The crisis is often precipitated by intercurrent disease, surgery or infection.

Vitiligo occurs in 10–20% of patients with autoimmune Addison's disease (p. 630).

Investigations

Treatment should not be delayed to wait for results in patients with suspected acute adrenal crisis. Here, a random blood sample should be stored for subsequent measurement of serum cortisol and, if possible, plasma ACTH; if the patient's clinical condition permits, it may be appropriate to spend 30 minutes performing a short ACTH stimulation test (Box 18.43) before administering hydrocortisone, but delays must be avoided if there

is circulatory compromise. Investigations should be performed before treatment is given in patients who present with features suggestive of chronic adrenal insufficiency.

Assessment of glucocorticoids

Random plasma cortisol is usually low in patients with adrenal insufficiency but it may be within the reference range, yet inappropriately low, for a seriously ill patient. Random measurement of normal levels of plasma cortisol cannot therefore be used to confirm or refute the diagnosis, unless the value is above 500 nmol/L (> 18 μg/dL), which effectively excludes adrenal insufficiency.

More useful is the short ACTH stimulation test (also called the tetracosactrin or short Synacthen test) described in Box 18.43. Cortisol levels fail to increase in response to exogenous ACTH in patients with primary or secondary adrenal insufficiency. These can be distinguished by measurement of ACTH (which is low in ACTH deficiency and high in Addison's disease).

Assessment of mineralocorticoids

Mineralocorticoid secretion in patients with suspected Addison's disease cannot be adequately assessed by electrolyte measurements since hyponatraemia occurs in both aldosterone and cortisol deficiency (see Box 18.42 and p. 357). Hyperkalaemia is common, but not universal, in aldosterone deficiency. Plasma renin and aldosterone should be measured in the supine position. In mineralocorticoid deficiency, plasma renin activity is high, with plasma aldosterone being either low or in the lower part of the reference range.

Assessment of adrenal androgens

This is not necessary in men because testosterone from the testes is the principal androgen. In women, dehydroepiandrosterone sulphate (DHEAS) and androstenedione may be measured in a random specimen of blood, though levels are highest in the morning.

Other tests to establish the cause

Patients with unexplained secondary adrenocortical insufficiency should be investigated as described on page 680. In patients with elevated ACTH, further tests are required to establish the cause of Addison's disease. Adrenal autoantibodies are frequently positive in autoimmune adrenal failure. If antibody tests are negative, imaging of the adrenal glands with CT or MRI is indicated. Tuberculosis causes adrenal calcification, visible on plain X-ray or ultrasound scan. A human immunodeficiency virus (HIV) test should be performed if risk factors for infection are present (p. 310). Adrenal metastases are a rare cause of adrenal insufficiency. Patients with evidence of autoimmune adrenal failure should be screened for other organ-specific autoimmune diseases, such as thyroid disease, pernicious anaemia and type 1 diabetes.

Management

Patients with adrenocortical insufficiency always need glucocorticoid replacement therapy and usually, but not always, mineralocorticoid therapy. There is some evidence that adrenal androgen replacement may also be beneficial in women. Other treatments depend on the underlying cause. The emergency management of adrenal crisis is described in Box 18.44.

Glucocorticoid replacement

Adrenal replacement therapy consists of oral hydrocortisone (cortisol) 15–20 mg daily in divided doses, typically 10 mg on waking and 5 mg at around 1500 hrs. These are physiological replacement doses that should not cause Cushingoid side-effects. The dose may need to be adjusted for the individual patient but this is subjective. Excess weight gain usually indicates over-replacement, while persistent lethargy or hyperpigmentation may be due to an inadequate dose or lack of absorption. Measurement of serum cortisol levels is not usually helpful. Advice to patients dependent on glucocorticoid replacement is given in Box 18.40.

Mineralocorticoid replacement

Fludrocortisone (9α-fluoro-hydrocortisone) is administered at the usual dose of 0.05–0.15 mg daily, and adequacy of replacement may be assessed by measurement of blood pressure, plasma electrolytes and plasma renin. It is indicated for virtually every patient with primary adrenal insufficiency but is not needed in secondary adrenal insufficiency.

18.44 Management of adrenal crisis

Correct volume depletion

- IV saline as required to normalise blood pressure and pulse
- In severe hyponatraemia (<125 mmol/L) avoid increases of plasma Na >10 mmol/L/day to prevent pontine demyelination (p. 358)
- Fludrocortisone is not required during the acute phase of treatment

Replace glucocorticoids

- IV hydrocortisone succinate 100 mg stat, and 100 mg 4 times daily for first 12–24 hrs
- Continue parenteral hydrocortisone (50–100 mg IM 4 times daily) until patient is well enough for reliable oral therapy

Correct other metabolic abnormalities

- Acute hypoglycaemia: IV 10% glucose
- Hyperkalaemia: should respond to volume replacement but occasionally requires specific therapy (see Box 14.17, p. 363)

Identify and treat underlying cause

- Consider acute precipitant, such as infection
- Consider adrenal or pituitary pathology (see Box 18.41)

18.45 Glucocorticoids in old age

- **Adrenocortical insufficiency**: often insidious and may present with tiredness, drowsiness, delirium, falls, immobility and orthostatic hypotension.
- **Glucocorticoid therapy**: especially hazardous in older people, who are already relatively immunocompromised and susceptible to osteoporosis, diabetes, hypertension and other complications.
- **'Physiological' glucocorticoid replacement therapy**: increased risk of adrenal crisis because adherence may be poor and there is a greater incidence of intercurrent illness. Patient and carer education, with regular reinforcement of the principles described in Box 18.40, is crucial.

Androgen replacement

Androgen replacement with DHEAS (50 mg/day) is occasionally given to women with primary adrenal insufficiency who have symptoms of reduced libido and fatigue, but the evidence in support of this is not robust and treatment may be associated with side-effects such as acne and hirsutism.

Incidental adrenal mass

It is not uncommon for a mass in the adrenal gland to be identified on a CT or MRI scan of the abdomen that has been performed for another indication. Such lesions are known as adrenal 'incidentalomas'. The prevalence increases with age and they are present in up to 10% of adults aged 70 years and older.

Eighty-five per cent of adrenal incidentalomas are non-functioning adrenal adenomas. The remainder includes functional tumours of the adrenal cortex (secreting cortisol, aldosterone or androgens), phaeochromocytomas, primary and secondary carcinomas, hamartomas and other rare disorders, including granulomatous infiltrations.

Clinical assessment and investigations

There are two key questions to be resolved: is the lesion secreting hormones, and is it benign or malignant?

Patients with an adrenal incidentaloma are usually asymptomatic. However, clinical signs and symptoms of excess glucocorticoids (p. 665), mineralocorticoids (see below), catecholamines (p. 666) and, in women, androgens (p. 666) should be sought. Investigations should include a dexamethasone suppression test, urine or plasma metanephrines and, in virilised women, measurement of serum testosterone, DHEAS and androstenedione. Patients with hypertension should be investigated for mineralocorticoid excess, as described below. In bilateral masses consistent with adrenocortical lesions, 17-OH-progesterone should also be measured.

CT and MRI are equally effective in assessing the malignant potential of an adrenal mass, using the following parameters:

- *Size.* The larger the lesion, the greater the malignant potential. Around 90% of adrenocortical carcinomas are over 4 cm in diameter, but specificity is poor since only approximately 25% of such lesions are malignant.
- *Configuration.* Homogeneous and smooth lesions are more likely to be benign. The presence of metastatic lesions elsewhere increases the risk of malignancy, but as many as two-thirds of adrenal incidentalomas in patients with cancer are benign.
- *Presence of lipid.* Adenomas are usually lipid-rich, resulting in an attenuation of below 10 Hounsfield units (HU) on

18

an unenhanced CT, and in signal dropout on chemical shift MRI.

• *Enhancement.* Benign lesions demonstrate rapid washout of contrast, whereas malignant lesions tend to retain contrast.

Histology in a sample obtained by CT-guided biopsy is rarely indicated, and is not useful in distinguishing an adrenal adenoma from an adrenocortical carcinoma. Biopsy is occasionally helpful in confirming adrenal metastases from other cancers, but should be avoided if either phaeochromocytoma or primary adrenal cancer is suspected in order to avoid precipitation of a hypertensive crisis or seeding of tumour cells, respectively.

Management

In patients with radiologically benign, non-functioning lesions of less than 4 cm in diameter, surgery is required only if serial imaging suggests tumour growth. Functional lesions and tumours of more than 4 cm in diameter should be considered for surgery, though many centres will not operate on tumours of more than 4 cm if all other characteristics suggest benign disease. Optimal management of patients with low-grade cortisol secretion, as demonstrated by the dexamethasone suppression test, remains to be established.

Primary hyperaldosteronism

Estimates of the prevalence of primary hyperaldosteronism vary according to the screening tests employed, but it may occur in as many as 10% of people with hypertension. Indications to test for mineralocorticoid excess in hypertensive patients include hypokalaemia (including hypokalaemia induced by thiazide diuretics), poor control of blood pressure with conventional therapy, a family history of early-onset hypertension, or presentation at a young age.

Causes of excessive activation of mineralocorticoid receptors are shown in Box 18.46. It is important to differentiate primary hyperaldosteronism, caused by an intrinsic abnormality of the adrenal glands resulting in aldosterone excess, from secondary

hyperaldosteronism, which is usually a consequence of enhanced activity of renin in response to inadequate renal perfusion and hypotension. Most individuals with primary hyperaldosteronism have bilateral adrenal hyperplasia (idiopathic hyperaldosteronism), while only a minority have an aldosterone-producing adenoma (APA; Conn's syndrome). Glucocorticoid-suppressible hyperaldosteronism is a rare autosomal dominant condition in which aldosterone is secreted 'ectopically' from the adrenal zonae fasciculata/reticularis in response to ACTH. Rarely, the mineralocorticoid receptor pathway in the distal nephron is activated, even though aldosterone concentrations are low.

Clinical features

Individuals with primary hyperaldosteronism are usually asymptomatic but may have features of sodium retention or potassium loss. Sodium retention may cause oedema, while hypokalaemia may cause muscle weakness (or even paralysis, especially in South-east Asian populations), polyuria (secondary to renal tubular damage, which produces nephrogenic diabetes insipidus) and occasionally tetany (because of associated metabolic alkalosis and low ionised calcium). Blood pressure is elevated but accelerated phase hypertension is rare.

Investigations

Biochemical

Routine blood tests may show a hypokalaemic alkalosis. Sodium is usually at the upper end of the reference range in primary hyperaldosteronism, but is characteristically low in secondary hyperaldosteronism (because low plasma volume stimulates vasopressin (antidiuretic hormone, ADH) release and high angiotensin II levels stimulate thirst). The key measurements are plasma renin and aldosterone (Box 18.46), and in many centres the aldosterone : renin ratio (ARR) is employed as a screening test for primary hyperaldosteronism in hypertensive patients. Almost all antihypertensive drugs interfere with this ratio (β-blockers inhibit while diuretics stimulate renin secretion). Thus, individuals with an elevated ARR require further testing after stopping antihypertensive drugs for at least 4 weeks. If necessary, antihypertensive agents that have minimal effects on the renin–angiotensin system, such as calcium antagonists and α-blockers, may be substituted. Oral potassium supplementation may also be required, as hypokalaemia itself suppresses renin activity. If, on repeat testing, plasma renin is low and aldosterone concentrations are elevated, then further investigation under specialist supervision may include suppression tests (sodium loading) and/or stimulation tests (captopril or furosemide administration) to differentiate angiotensin II-dependent aldosterone secretion in idiopathic hyperplasia from autonomous aldosterone secretion typical of an APA.

Imaging and localisation

Imaging with CT or MRI will identify most APAs (Fig. 18.23) but it is important to recognise the risk of false positives (non-functioning adrenal adenomas are common) and false negatives (imaging may have insufficient resolution to identify adenomas with a diameter of less than 0.5 cm). If the imaging is inconclusive and there is an intention to proceed with surgery on the basis of strong biochemical evidence of an APA, then adrenal vein catheterisation with measurement of aldosterone (and cortisol to confirm positioning of the catheters) is required. In some centres, this is performed even in the presence of a unilateral 'adenoma', to avoid inadvertent removal of an incidental non-functioning adenoma contralateral to a radiologically inapparent cause of aldosterone excess.

 18.46 Causes of mineralocorticoid excess

With renin high and aldosterone high (secondary hyperaldosteronism)

• Inadequate renal perfusion (diuretic therapy, cardiac failure, liver failure, nephrotic syndrome, renal artery stenosis)
• Renin-secreting renal tumour (very rare)

With renin low and aldosterone high (primary hyperaldosteronism)

• Adrenal adenoma secreting aldosterone (Conn's syndrome)
• Idiopathic bilateral adrenal hyperplasia
• Glucocorticoid-suppressible hyperaldosteronism (rare)

With renin low and aldosterone low (non-aldosterone-dependent activation of mineralocorticoid pathway)

• Ectopic ACTH syndrome
• Liquorice misuse (inhibition of 11β-HSD2)
• Liddle's syndrome
• 11-deoxycorticosterone-secreting adrenal tumour
• Rare forms of congenital adrenal hyperplasia and 11β-HSD2 deficiency

(11β-HSD2 = 11β-hydroxysteroid dehydrogenase type 2; ACTH = adrenocorticotrophic hormone)

Fig. 18.23 Aldosterone-producing adenoma causing Conn's syndrome. [A] CT scan of left adrenal adenoma (arrow). [B] The tumour is 'canary yellow' because of intracellular lipid accumulation.

Management

Mineralocorticoid receptor antagonists (spironolactone and eplerenone) are valuable in treating both hypokalaemia and hypertension in all forms of mineralocorticoid excess. Up to 20% of males develop gynaecomastia on spironolactone. Amiloride (10–40 mg/day), which blocks the epithelial sodium channel regulated by aldosterone, is an alternative.

In patients with an APA, medical therapy is usually given for a few weeks to normalise whole-body electrolyte balance before unilateral adrenalectomy. Laparoscopic surgery cures the biochemical abnormality but, depending on the pre-operative duration, hypertension remains in as many as 70% of cases, probably because of irreversible damage to the systemic microcirculation.

Phaeochromocytoma and paraganglioma

These are rare neuro-endocrine tumours that may secrete catecholamines (adrenaline/epinephrine, noradrenaline/norepinephrine). Approximately 80% of these tumours occur in the adrenal medulla (phaeochromocytomas), while 20% arise elsewhere in the body in sympathetic ganglia (paragangliomas). Most are benign but approximately 15% show malignant features. Around 40% are associated with inherited disorders, including neurofibromatosis (p. 1131), von Hippel–Lindau syndrome (p. 1132), MEN 2 and MEN 3 (p. 688). Paragangliomas are particularly associated with mutations in the succinate

dehydrogenase B, C and D genes. Other genetic causes include mutations in *SDHA*, *SDHAF2*, *TMEN127* and *MAX*.

Clinical features

These depend on the pattern of catecholamine secretion and are listed in Box 18.47.

Some patients present with hypertension, although it has been estimated that phaeochromocytoma accounts for less than 0.1% of cases of hypertension. The presentation may be with a complication of hypertension, such as stroke, myocardial infarction, left ventricular failure, hypertensive retinopathy or accelerated phase hypertension. The apparent paradox of postural hypotension between episodes is explained by 'pressure natriuresis' during hypertensive episodes so that intravascular volume is reduced. There may also be features of the familial syndromes associated with phaeochromocytoma. Paragangliomas are often non-functioning.

Investigations

Excessive secretion of catecholamines can be confirmed by measuring metabolites in plasma and/or urine (metanephrine and normetanephrine). There is a high 'false-positive' rate, as misleading metanephrine concentrations may be seen in stressed patients (during acute illness, following vigorous exercise or severe pain) and following ingestion of some drugs such as tricyclic antidepressants. For this reason, a repeat sample should usually be requested if elevated levels are found, although, as a rule, the higher the concentration of metanephrines, the more likely the diagnosis of phaeochromocytoma/paraganglioma. Serum chromogranin A is often elevated and may be a useful tumour marker in patients with non-secretory tumours and/or metastatic disease. Genetic testing should be considered in individuals with other features of a genetic syndrome, in those with a family history of phaeochromocytoma/paraganglioma, and in those presenting under the age of 50 years.

Localisation

Phaeochromocytomas are usually identified by abdominal CT or MRI (Fig. 18.24). Localisation of paragangliomas may be more difficult. Scintigraphy using meta-iodobenzyl guanidine (MIBG) can be useful, particularly if combined with CT, for adrenal phaeochromocytoma but is often negative in paraganglioma. ^{18}F-deoxyglucose PET is especially useful for detection of malignant disease and for confirming an imaging abnormality as a paraganglioma in an individual with underlying risk due to genetic mutation. Less widely available, [68]gallium dotatate PET/CT imaging has high sensitivity for paraganglioma.

Management

In functioning tumours, medical therapy is required to prepare the patient for surgery, preferably for a minimum of 6 weeks,

Fig. 18.24 CT scan of abdomen showing large left adrenal phaeochromocytoma. The normal right adrenal (white arrow) contrasts with the large heterogeneous phaeochromocytoma arising from the left adrenal gland (black arrow).

to allow restoration of normal plasma volume. The most useful drug in the face of very high circulating catecholamines is the α-blocker phenoxybenzamine (10–20 mg orally 3–4 times daily) because it is a non-competitive antagonist, unlike prazosin or doxazosin. If α-blockade produces a marked tachycardia, then a β-blocker such as propranolol can be added. On no account should a β-blocker be given before an α-blocker, as this may cause a paradoxical rise in blood pressure due to unopposed α-mediated vasoconstriction.

During surgery, sodium nitroprusside and the short-acting α-antagonist phentolamine are useful in controlling hypertensive episodes, which may result from anaesthetic induction or tumour mobilisation. Post-operative hypotension may occur and require volume expansion and, very occasionally, noradrenaline (norepinephrine) infusion, but is uncommon if the patient has been prepared with phenoxybenzamine.

Metastatic tumours may behave in an aggressive or a very indolent fashion. Management options include debulking surgery, radionuclide therapy with ^{131}I-MIBG, chemotherapy and (chemo) embolisation of hepatic metastases; some may respond to tyrosine kinase and angiogenesis inhibitors.

Congenital adrenal hyperplasia

Pathophysiology and clinical features

Inherited defects in enzymes of the cortisol biosynthetic pathway (see Fig. 18.19) result in insufficiency of hormones downstream of the block, with impaired negative feedback and increased ACTH secretion. ACTH then stimulates the production of steroids upstream of the enzyme block. This produces adrenal hyperplasia and a combination of clinical features that depend on the severity and site of the defect in biosynthesis. All of these enzyme abnormalities are inherited as autosomal recessive traits.

The most common enzyme defect is 21-hydroxylase deficiency. This results in impaired synthesis of cortisol and aldosterone, and accumulation of 17-OH-progesterone, which is then diverted to form adrenal androgens. In about one-third of cases, this defect is severe and presents in infancy with features of glucocorticoid and mineralocorticoid deficiency (see Box 18.42) and androgen excess,

such as ambiguous genitalia in girls. In the other two-thirds, mineralocorticoid secretion is adequate but there may be features of cortisol insufficiency and/or ACTH and androgen excess, including precocious pseudo-puberty, which is distinguished from 'true' precocious puberty by low gonadotrophins. Sometimes the mildest enzyme defects are not apparent until adult life, when females may present with amenorrhoea and/or hirsutism (pp. 762 and 763). This is called 'non-classical' or 'late-onset' congenital adrenal hyperplasia.

Defects of all the other enzymes in Figure 18.19 are rare. Both 17-hydroxylase and 11β-hydroxylase deficiency may produce hypertension due to excess production of 11-deoxycorticosterone, which has mineralocorticoid activity.

Investigations

Circulating 17-OH-progesterone levels are raised in 21-hydroxylase deficiency but this may be demonstrated only after ACTH administration in late-onset cases. To avoid salt-wasting crises in infancy, 17-OH-progesterone can be routinely measured in heelprick blood spot samples taken from all infants in the first week of life. Assessment is otherwise as described for adrenal insufficiency on page 672.

In siblings of affected children, antenatal genetic diagnosis can be made by amniocentesis or chorionic villus sampling. This allows prevention of virilisation of affected female fetuses by administration of dexamethasone to the mother to suppress ACTH levels.

Management

The aim is to replace deficient corticosteroids and to suppress ACTH-driven adrenal androgen production. A careful balance is required between adequate suppression of adrenal androgen excess and excessive glucocorticoid replacement resulting in features of Cushing's syndrome. In children, growth velocity is an important measurement, since either under- or over-replacement with glucocorticoids suppresses growth. In adults, there is no uniformly agreed adrenal replacement regime, and clinical features (menstrual cycle, hirsutism, weight gain, blood pressure) and biochemical profiles (plasma renin, 17-OH-progesterone and testosterone levels) provide a guide.

Women with late-onset 21-hydroxylase deficiency may not require corticosteroid replacement. If hirsutism is the main problem, anti-androgen therapy may be just as effective (p. 659).

The endocrine pancreas and gastrointestinal tract

A series of hormones are secreted from cells distributed throughout the gastrointestinal tract and pancreas. Functional anatomy and physiology are described on pages 723 and 848. Diseases associated with abnormalities of these hormones are listed in Box 18.48. Most are rare, with the exception of diabetes mellitus (Ch. 20).

Presenting problems in endocrine pancreas disease

Spontaneous hypoglycaemia

Hypoglycaemia most commonly occurs as a side-effect of treatment with insulin or sulphonylurea drugs in people with

18.48 Classification of endocrine diseases of the pancreas and gastrointestinal tract		
	Primary	Secondary
Hormone excess	Insulinoma Gastrinoma (Zollinger–Ellison syndrome, p. 802) Carcinoid syndrome (secretion of 5-HT) Glucagonoma VIPoma Somatostatinoma	Hypergastrinaemia of achlorhydria Hyperinsulinaemia after bariatric surgery
Hormone deficiency	Diabetes mellitus	
Hormone resistance	Insulin resistance syndromes (e.g. type 2 diabetes mellitus, lipodystrophy, Donohue's syndrome)	
Non-functioning tumours	Pancreatic carcinoma Pancreatic neuro-endocrine tumour	

(5-HT = 5-hydroxytryptamine, serotonin)

Fig. 18.25 Differential diagnosis of spontaneous hypoglycaemia. Measurement of insulin and C-peptide concentrations during an episode is helpful in determining the underlying cause.

diabetes mellitus. In non-diabetic individuals, symptomatic hypoglycaemia is rare, but it is not uncommon to detect venous blood glucose concentrations below 3.0 mmol/L (54 mg/dL) in asymptomatic patients. For this reason, and because the symptoms of hypoglycaemia are non-specific, a hypoglycaemic disorder should be diagnosed only if all three conditions of Whipple's triad are met (Fig. 18.25). There is no specific blood glucose concentration at which spontaneous hypoglycaemia can be said to occur, although the lower the blood glucose concentration, the more likely it is to have pathological significance. Investigations are unlikely to be needed unless glucose concentrations below 3.0 mmol/L are observed, many patients with true hypoglycaemia demonstrating glucose levels below 2.2 mmol/L (40 mg/dL).

Clinical assessment

The clinical features of hypoglycaemia are described in the section on insulin-induced hypoglycaemia on page 738. Individuals with chronic spontaneous hypoglycaemia often have attenuated autonomic responses and 'hypoglycaemia unawareness', and may present with a wide variety of features of neuroglycopenia, including odd behaviour and convulsions. The symptoms are usually episodic and relieved by consumption of carbohydrate. Symptoms occurring while fasting (such as before breakfast) or following exercise are much more likely to be representative of pathological hypoglycaemia than those that develop after food (post-prandial or 'reactive' symptoms). Hypoglycaemia should be considered in all comatose patients, even if there is an apparently obvious cause, such as hemiplegic stroke or alcohol intoxication.

Investigations

Does the patient have a hypoglycaemic disorder?

Patients who present acutely with delirium, coma or convulsions should be tested for hypoglycaemia at the bedside with a capillary blood sample and an automated meter. While this is sufficient to exclude hypoglycaemia, blood glucose meters are relatively inaccurate in the hypoglycaemic range and the diagnosis should

always be confirmed by a laboratory-based glucose measurement. At the same time, a sample should be taken for later measurement of alcohol, insulin, C-peptide, cortisol and sulphonylurea levels, if hypoglycaemia is confirmed. Taking these samples during an acute presentation prevents subsequent unnecessary dynamic tests and is of medico-legal importance in cases where poisoning is suspected.

Patients who attend the outpatient clinic with episodic symptoms suggestive of hypoglycaemia present a more challenging problem. The main diagnostic test is the prolonged (72-hour) fast. If symptoms of hypoglycaemia develop during the fast, then blood samples should be taken to confirm hypoglycaemia and for later measurement of insulin and C-peptide. Hypoglycaemia is then corrected with oral or intravenous glucose and Whipple's triad completed by confirmation of the resolution of symptoms. The absence of clinical and biochemical evidence of hypoglycaemia during a prolonged fast effectively excludes the diagnosis of a hypoglycaemic disorder.

What is the cause of the hypoglycaemia?

In the acute setting, the underlying diagnosis is often obvious. In non-diabetic individuals, alcohol excess is the most common cause of hypoglycaemia in the UK but other drugs – e.g. salicylates, quinine and pentamidine – may also be implicated. Hypoglycaemia is one of many metabolic derangements that occur in patients with hepatic failure, renal failure, adrenal insufficiency, sepsis or malaria.

Hypoglycaemia in the absence of insulin, or any insulin-like factor, in the blood indicates impaired gluconeogenesis and/or availability of glucose from glycogen in the liver. Hypoglycaemia associated with high insulin and low C-peptide concentrations is indicative of administration of exogenous insulin, either factitiously or feloniously. Adults with high insulin and C-peptide concentrations during an episode of hypoglycaemia are most likely to have an insulinoma but sulphonylurea ingestion should also be considered (particularly in individuals with access to such medication, such as health-care professionals or family members of someone with type 2 diabetes). Suppressed plasma β-hydroxybutyrate helps confirm inappropriate insulin secretion during fasting. Usually, insulinomas in the pancreas

18.49 Spontaneous hypoglycaemia in old age

- **Presentation**: may present with focal neurological abnormality. Blood glucose should be checked in all patients with acute neurological symptoms and signs, especially stroke, as these will reverse with early treatment of hypoglycaemia.

are small (<5 mm diameter) but can be identified by CT, MRI or ultrasound (endoscopic or laparoscopic). Imaging should include the liver since around 10% of insulinomas are malignant and may metastasise to the liver. Rarely, large non-pancreatic tumours, such as sarcomas, may cause recurrent hypoglycaemia because of their ability to produce excess pro-insulin-like growth factor-2 (pro-IGF-2), which has considerable structural homology to insulin.

Management

Treatment of acute hypoglycaemia should be initiated as soon as laboratory blood samples have been taken and should *not* be deferred until formal laboratory confirmation has been obtained. Intravenous dextrose (5% or 10%) is effective in the short term in the obtunded patient and should be followed on recovery with oral unrefined carbohydrate (starch). Continuous dextrose infusion may be necessary, especially in sulphonylurea poisoning. Intramuscular glucagon (1 mg) stimulates hepatic glucose release but is ineffective in patients with depleted glycogen reserves, such as in alcohol excess or liver disease.

Chronic recurrent hypoglycaemia in insulin-secreting tumours can be treated by regular consumption of oral carbohydrate combined with agents that inhibit insulin secretion (diazoxide or somatostatin analogues). Insulinomas are resected when benign, providing the individual is fit enough to undergo surgery. Metastatic malignant insulinomas may be incurable and are managed along the same lines as other metastatic neuro-endocrine tumours (see below).

Gastroenteropancreatic neuro-endocrine tumours

Neuro-endocrine tumours (NETs) are a heterogeneous group derived from neuro-endocrine cells in many organs, including the gastrointestinal tract, lung, adrenals (phaeochromocytoma, p. 675) and thyroid (medullary carcinoma, p. 650). Most NETs occur sporadically but a proportion are associated with genetic cancer syndromes, such as MEN 1, 2 and 3 and neurofibromatosis type 1 (pp. 688 and 1131). NETs may secrete hormones into the circulation.

Gastroenteropancreatic NETs arise in organs that are derived embryologically from the gastrointestinal tract. Most commonly, they occur in the small bowel but they can also arise elsewhere in the bowel, pancreas, thymus and bronchi. The term 'carcinoid' is often used when referring to non-pancreatic gastroenteropancreatic NETs because, when initially described, they were thought to behave in an indolent fashion compared with conventional cancers. It is now recognised that there is a wide spectrum of malignant potential for all NETs; some are benign (most insulinomas and appendiceal carcinoid tumours), while others have an aggressive clinical course with widespread metastases (small-cell carcinoma of the lung). The majority of gastroenteropancreatic NETs behave in an intermediate manner, with relatively slow growth but a propensity to invade and metastasise to remote organs, especially the liver.

18.50 Pancreatic neuro-endocrine tumours

Tumour	Hormone	Effects
Gastrinoma	Gastrin	Peptic ulcer and steatorrhoea (Zollinger–Ellison syndrome, p. 802)
Insulinoma	Insulin	Recurrent hypoglycaemia (see above)
VIPoma	Vasoactive intestinal peptide (VIP)	Watery diarrhoea and hypokalaemia
Glucagonoma	Glucagon	Diabetes mellitus, necrolytic migratory erythema
Somatostatinoma	Somatostatin	Diabetes mellitus and steatorrhoea

18.51 Clinical features of the carcinoid syndrome

- Episodic flushing, wheezing and diarrhoea
- Facial telangiectasia
- Cardiac involvement (tricuspid regurgitation, pulmonary stenosis, right ventricular endocardial plaques) leading to heart failure

Clinical features

Patients with gastroenteropancreatic NETs often have a history of abdominal pain over many years prior to diagnosis and usually present with local mass effects, such as small-bowel obstruction, appendicitis, and pain from hepatic metastases. Thymic and bronchial carcinoids occasionally present with ectopic ACTH syndrome (p. 667). Pancreatic NETs can also cause hormone excess (Box 18.50) but most are non-functional. The classic 'carcinoid syndrome' (Box 18.51) occurs when vasoactive hormones reach the systemic circulation. In the case of gastrointestinal carcinoids, this invariably means that the tumour has metastasised to the liver or there are peritoneal deposits, which allow secreted hormones to gain access to the systemic circulation; hormones secreted by the primary tumour into the portal vein are metabolised and inactivated in the liver. The features of Zollinger–Ellison syndrome are described on page 802.

Investigations

A combination of imaging with ultrasound, CT, MRI and/or radio-labelled somatostatin analogue (Fig. 18.26) will usually identify the primary tumour and allow staging, which is crucial for determining prognosis. Biopsy of the primary tumour or a metastatic deposit is required to confirm the histological type. NETs demonstrate immunohistochemical staining for the proteins chromogranin A and synaptophysin, and the histological grade provides important prognostic information: the higher the Ki67 proliferation index, the worse the prognosis.

Carcinoid syndrome is confirmed by measuring elevated concentrations of 5-hydroxyindoleacetic acid (5-HIAA), a metabolite of serotonin, in a 24-hour urine collection. False positives can occur, particularly if the individual has been eating certain foods, such as avocado and pineapple. Plasma chromogranin A can be measured in a fasting blood sample, along with the hormones listed in Box 18.50. All of these can be useful as tumour markers.

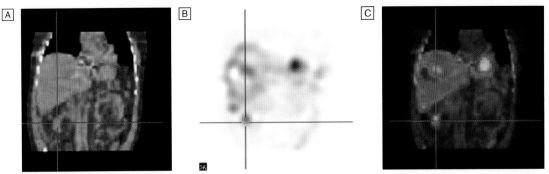

Fig. 18.26 Octreotide scintigraphy in a metastatic neuro-endocrine tumour. [A] Coronal CT scan showing hepatomegaly and a mass inferior to the liver (at the intersection of the horizontal and vertical red lines). [B] Octreotide scintogram showing patches of increased uptake in the upper abdomen. [C] When the octreotide and CT scans are superimposed, it shows that the areas of increased uptake are in hepatic metastases and in the tissue mass, which may be lymph nodes or a primary tumour.

Management

Treatment of solitary tumours is by surgical resection. If metastatic or multifocal primary disease is present, then surgery is usually not indicated, unless there is a complication such as gastrointestinal obstruction. Diazoxide can reduce insulin secretion in insulinomas, and high doses of proton pump inhibitors suppress acid production in gastrinomas. Somatostatin analogues are effective in reducing the symptoms of carcinoid syndrome and of excess glucagon and vasoactive intestinal peptide (VIP) production. The slow-growing nature of NETs means that conventional cancer therapies, such as chemotherapy and radiotherapy, have limited efficacy, but use of somatostatin analogues is associated with improved progression-free survival. Other treatments, such as interferon, targeted radionuclide therapy with ^{131}I-MIBG and radio-labelled somatostatin analogues (which may be taken up by NET metastases), and resection/embolisation/ablation of hepatic metastases, may have a role in the palliation of symptoms but debate exists as to whether this prolongs life. The tyrosine kinase inhibitor sunitinib and the mammalian target of rapamycin (mTOR) inhibitor everolimus have shown significant improvements in progression-free survival in patients with advanced and progressive pancreatic and lung NETS that are not poorly differentiated, and should be considered as part of standard therapy.

The hypothalamus and the pituitary gland

Diseases of the hypothalamus and pituitary have an annual incidence of approximately 3:100 000 and a prevalence of 30–70 per 100 000. The pituitary plays a central role in several major endocrine axes, so that investigation and treatment invariably involve several other endocrine glands.

Functional anatomy, physiology and investigations

The anatomical relationships of the pituitary are shown in Figure 18.27 and its numerous functions are shown in Figure 18.2 (p. 633). The pituitary gland is enclosed in the sella turcica and bridged over by a fold of dura mater called the diaphragma sellae, with the sphenoidal air sinuses below and the optic chiasm above. The cavernous sinuses are lateral to the pituitary fossa and contain the 3rd, 4th and 6th cranial nerves and the internal

Fig. 18.27 Anatomical relationships of the normal pituitary gland and hypothalamus. See also Figure 18.2 (p. 633). [A] Sagittal MRI. [B] Coronal MRI. (AP = anterior pituitary; CS = cavernous sinus; H = hypothalamus; IC = internal carotid artery; OC = optic chiasm; PP = posterior pituitary; PS = pituitary stalk; SS = sphenoid sinus; TV = third ventricle)

carotid arteries. The gland is composed of two lobes, anterior and posterior, and is connected to the hypothalamus by the infundibular stalk, which has portal vessels carrying blood from the median eminence of the hypothalamus to the anterior lobe and nerve fibres to the posterior lobe.

	Primary	Secondary
i 18.52 Classification of diseases of the pituitary and hypothalamus		
Non-functioning tumours	Pituitary adenoma Craniopharyngioma Metastatic tumours	
Hormone excess Anterior pituitary	Prolactinoma Acromegaly Cushing's disease Rare TSH-, LH- and FSH-secreting adenomas	Disconnection hyperprolactinaemia
Hypothalamus and posterior pituitary	Syndrome of inappropriate antidiuretic hormone (SIADH, p. 357)	
Hormone deficiency Anterior pituitary	Hypopituitarism	GnRH deficiency
Hypothalamus and posterior pituitary	Cranial diabetes insipidus	(Kallmann's syndrome)
Hormone resistance	Growth hormone resistance (Laron dwarfism) Nephrogenic diabetes insipidus	

(FSH = follicle-stimulating hormone; GnRH = gonadotrophin-releasing hormone; LH = luteinising hormone; TSH = thyroid-stimulating hormone)

Diseases of the hypothalamus and pituitary are classified in Box 18.52. By far the most common disorder is an adenoma of the anterior pituitary gland.

Investigation of patients with pituitary disease

Although pituitary disease presents with diverse clinical manifestations (see below), the approach to investigation is similar in all cases (Box 18.53).

The approach to testing for hormone deficiency is outlined in Box 18.53. Details are given in the sections on individual glands elsewhere in this chapter. Tests for hormone excess vary according to the hormone in question. For example, prolactin is not secreted in pulsatile fashion, although it rises with significant psychological stress. Assuming that the patient was not distressed by venepuncture, a random measurement of serum prolactin is sufficient to diagnose hyperprolactinaemia. In contrast, growth hormone is secreted in a pulsatile fashion. A high random level does not confirm acromegaly; the diagnosis is confirmed only by failure of growth hormone to be suppressed during an oral glucose tolerance test, and a high serum insulin-like growth factor-1 (IGF-1). Similarly, in suspected ACTH-dependent Cushing's disease (p. 666), random measurement of plasma cortisol is unreliable and the diagnosis is usually made by a dexamethasone suppression test.

The most common local complication of a large pituitary tumour is compression of the optic pathway. The resulting visual field defect can be documented using a Goldman's perimetry chart.

MRI reveals 'abnormalities' of the pituitary gland in as many as 10% of 'healthy' middle-aged people. It should therefore be performed only if there is a clear biochemical abnormality or if a patient presents with clinical features of pituitary tumour (see below). A pituitary tumour may be classified as either a macroadenoma (>10 mm diameter) or a microadenoma (<10 mm diameter).

Surgical biopsy is usually only performed as part of a therapeutic operation. Conventional histology identifies tumours as chromophobe (usually non-functioning), acidophil (typically prolactin- or growth hormone-secreting) or basophil (typically ACTH-secreting); immunohistochemistry may confirm their secretory capacity but is poorly predictive of growth potential of the tumour.

 18.53 How to investigate patients with suspected pituitary hypothalamic disease

Identify pituitary hormone deficiency

ACTH deficiency
- Short ACTH stimulation test (see Box 18.43)
- Insulin tolerance test (see Box 18.56): only if there is uncertainty in interpretation of short ACTH stimulation test (e.g. acute presentation)

LH/FSH deficiency
- In the male, measure random serum testosterone, LH and FSH
- In the pre-menopausal female, ask if the menses are regular
- In the post-menopausal female, measure random serum LH and FSH (FSH normally >30 IU/L and LH >20 IU/L)

TSH deficiency
- Measure random serum T_4
- Note that TSH is often detectable in secondary hypothyroidism

Growth hormone deficiency
Only investigate if growth hormone replacement therapy is being contemplated (p. 682)
- Measure immediately after exercise
- Consider other stimulatory tests (see Box 18.55)

Cranial diabetes insipidus
Only investigate if patient complains of polyuria/polydipsia, which may be masked by ACTH or TSH deficiency
- Exclude other causes of polyuria with blood glucose, potassium and calcium measurements
- Water deprivation test (see Box 18.61) or 5% saline infusion test

Identify hormone excess

- Measure random serum prolactin
- Investigate for acromegaly (glucose tolerance test) or Cushing's syndrome (p. 667) if there are clinical features

Establish the anatomy and diagnosis

- Consider visual field testing
- Image the pituitary and hypothalamus by MRI or CT

(ACTH = adrenocorticotrophic hormone; FSH = follicle-stimulating hormone; LH = luteinising hormone; TSH = thyroid-stimulating hormone)

Presenting problems in hypothalamic and pituitary disease

The clinical features of pituitary disease are shown in Figure 18.28. Younger women with pituitary disease most commonly present with secondary amenorrhoea (p. 654) or galactorrhoea (in hyperprolactinaemia). Post-menopausal women and men of any age are less likely to report symptoms of hypogonadism and so are more likely to present late with larger tumours causing visual field defects. Nowadays, many patients present with the incidental finding of a pituitary tumour on a CT or MRI scan.

Hypopituitarism

Hypopituitarism describes combined deficiency of any of the anterior pituitary hormones. The clinical presentation is variable and depends on the underlying lesion and the pattern of resulting hormone deficiency. The most common cause is a pituitary macroadenoma but other causes are listed in Box 18.54.

Clinical assessment

The presentation is highly variable. For example, following radiotherapy to the pituitary region, there is a characteristic sequence of loss of pituitary hormone secretion. Growth hormone secretion is often the earliest to be lost. In adults, this produces lethargy, muscle weakness and increased fat mass but these features are not obvious in isolation. Next, gonadotrophin (LH and FSH) secretion becomes impaired with loss of libido in the male and oligomenorrhoea or amenorrhoea in the female. Later, in the male there may be gynaecomastia and decreased frequency of shaving. In both sexes, axillary and pubic hair eventually become

i 18.54 Causes of anterior pituitary hormone deficiency	
Structural	
• Primary pituitary tumour	• Chordoma
• Adenoma*	• Germinoma (pinealoma)
• Carcinoma (exceptionally rare)	• Arachnoid cyst
• Craniopharyngioma*	• Rathke's cleft cyst
• Meningioma*	• Haemorrhage (apoplexy)
• Secondary tumour (including leukaemia and lymphoma)	
Inflammatory/infiltrative	
• Sarcoidosis	• Lymphocytic hypophysitis
• Infections, e.g. pituitary abscess, tuberculosis, syphilis, encephalitis	• Haemochromatosis
	• Langerhans cell histiocytosis
Congenital deficiencies	
• GnRH (Kallmann's syndrome)*	• TRH
• GHRH*	• CRH
Functional*	
• Chronic systemic illness	• Excessive exercise
• Anorexia nervosa	
Other	
• Head injury*	• Post-partum necrosis (Sheehan's syndrome)
• (Para)sellar surgery*	
• (Para)sellar radiotherapy*	• Opiate analgesia

*The most common causes of pituitary hormone deficiency.
(CRH = corticotrophin-releasing hormone; GHRH = growth hormone-releasing hormone; GnRH = gonadotrophin-releasing hormone; TRH = thyrotrophin-releasing hormone)

18

Local complications
• Headache
• Visual field defect
• Disconnection hyperprolactinaemia
• Diplopia (cavernous sinus involvement)
• Acute infarction/expansion (pituitary apoplexy)

Hormone excess

Hyperprolactinaemia
• Galactorrhoea
• Amenorrhoea
• Hypogonadism

Acromegaly
• Headache
• Sweating
• Change in shoe and ring size

Cushing's disease
• Weight gain
• Bruising
• Myopathy
• Hypertension
• Striae
• Depression

Macroadenoma (arrows) > 10 mm diameter

Microadenoma (arrow) < 10 mm diameter

Hypopituitarism

Growth hormone
• Lethargy

Gonadotrophins
• Lethargy
• Loss of libido
• Hair loss
• Amenorrhoea

ACTH
• Lethargy
• Postural hypotension
• Pallor
• Hair loss

TSH
• Lethargy

Vasopressin (usually post-surgical)
• Thirst and polyuria

Fig. 18.28 Common symptoms and signs to consider in a patient with suspected pituitary disease. (ACTH = adrenocorticotrophic hormone; TSH = thyroid-stimulating hormone)

18.55 Tests of growth hormone secretion

GH levels are commonly undetectable, so a choice from the range of 'stimulation' tests is required:
- Insulin-induced hypoglycaemia
- Arginine (may be combined with GHRH)
- Glucagon
- Clonidine (in children)

(GH = growth hormone; GHRH = growth hormone-releasing hormone)

18.56 How and when to do an insulin tolerance test

Use
- Assessment of the HPA axis
- Assessment of GH deficiency
- Indicated when there is doubt after the other tests in Box 18.53
- Usually performed in specialist centres, especially in children
- IV glucose and hydrocortisone must be available for resuscitation

Contraindications
- Ischaemic heart disease
- Epilepsy
- Severe hypopituitarism (0800 hrs plasma cortisol <180 nmol/L (6.6 µg/dL))

Dose
- 0.15 U/kg body weight soluble insulin IV

Aim
- To produce adequate hypoglycaemia (tachycardia and sweating with blood glucose <2.2 mmol/L (40 mg/dL))

Blood samples
- 0, 30, 45, 60, 90, 120 mins for blood glucose, plasma cortisol and growth hormone

Results
- Normal subjects: GH > 6.7 µg/L (20 mIU/L)*
- Normal subjects: cortisol >550 nmol/L (approximately 20.2 µg/dL)*

*The precise cut-off figure for a satisfactory cortisol and GH response depends on the assay used and so varies between centres.
(GH = growth hormone; HPA = hypothalamic–pituitary–adrenal)

sparse or even absent and the skin becomes characteristically finer and wrinkled. Chronic anaemia may also occur. The next hormone to be lost is usually ACTH, resulting in symptoms of cortisol insufficiency (including postural hypotension and a *dilutional* hyponatraemia). In contrast to primary adrenal insufficiency (p. 671), angiotensin II-dependent zona glomerulosa function is not lost and hence aldosterone secretion maintains normal plasma potassium. In contrast to the pigmentation of Addison's disease due to high levels of circulating ACTH acting on the skin melanocytes, a striking degree of pallor is usually present. Finally, TSH secretion is lost with consequent secondary hypothyroidism. This contributes further to apathy and cold intolerance. In contrast to primary hypothyroidism, frank myxoedema is rare, presumably because the thyroid retains some autonomous function. The onset of all of the above symptoms is notoriously insidious. However, patients sometimes present acutely unwell with glucocorticoid deficiency. This may be precipitated by a mild infection or injury, or may occur secondary to pituitary apoplexy (p. 683).

Other features of pituitary disease may be present (Fig. 18.28).

Investigations

The strategy for investigation of pituitary disease is described in Box 18.53. In acutely unwell patients, the priority is to diagnose and treat cortisol deficiency (p. 672). Other tests can be undertaken later. Specific dynamic tests for diagnosing hormone deficiency are described in Boxes 18.43 and 18.55. More specialised biochemical tests, such as insulin tolerance tests (Box 18.56), GnRH and TRH tests, are rarely required. All patients with biochemical evidence of pituitary hormone deficiency should have an MRI or CT scan to identify pituitary or hypothalamic tumours. If a tumour is not identified, then further investigations are indicated to exclude infectious or infiltrative causes.

Management

Treatment of acutely ill patients is similar to that described for adrenocortical insufficiency on page 673, except that sodium depletion is not an important component to correct. Chronic hormone replacement therapies are described below. Once the cause of hypopituitarism is established, specific treatment – of a pituitary macroadenoma, for example (see below) – may be required.

Cortisol replacement

Hydrocortisone should be given if there is ACTH deficiency. Suitable doses are described in the section on adrenal disease on page 672. Mineralocorticoid replacement is not required.

Thyroid hormone replacement

Levothyroxine 50–150 µg once daily should be given as described on page 640. Unlike in primary hypothyroidism, measuring

TSH is not helpful in adjusting the replacement dose because patients with hypopituitarism often secrete glycoproteins that are measured in the TSH assays but are not bioactive. The aim is to maintain serum T_4 in the upper part of the reference range. It is dangerous to give thyroid replacement in adrenal insufficiency without first giving glucocorticoid therapy, since this may precipitate adrenal crisis.

Sex hormone replacement

This is indicated if there is gonadotrophin deficiency in women under the age of 50 and in men to restore normal sexual function and to prevent osteoporosis (p. 1044).

Growth hormone replacement

Growth hormone (GH) is administered by daily subcutaneous self-injection to children and adolescents with GH deficiency and, until recently, was discontinued once the epiphyses had fused. However, although hypopituitary adults receiving 'full' replacement with hydrocortisone, levothyroxine and sex steroids are usually much improved by these therapies, some individuals remain lethargic and unwell compared with a healthy population. Some of these patients feel better, and have objective improvements in their fat:muscle mass ratio and other metabolic parameters, if they are also given GH replacement. Treatment with GH may also help young adults to achieve a higher peak bone mineral density. The principal side-effect is sodium retention, manifest as peripheral oedema or carpal tunnel syndrome if given in excess. For this reason, GH replacement should be started at a low dose, with monitoring of the response by measurement of serum IGF-1.

Pituitary tumour

Pituitary tumours produce a variety of mass effects, depending on their size and location, but also present as incidental findings on CT or MRI, or with hypopituitarism, as described above. A wide variety of disorders can present as mass lesions in or around the pituitary gland (see Box 18.54). Most intrasellar tumours are pituitary macroadenomas (most commonly non-functioning adenomas; see Fig. 18.28), whereas suprasellar masses may be craniopharyngiomas (see Fig. 18.31). The most common cause of a parasellar mass is a meningioma.

Clinical assessment

Clinical features are shown in Figure 18.28. A common but non-specific presentation is with headache, which may be the consequence of stretching of the diaphragma sellae. Although the classical abnormalities associated with compression of the optic chiasm are bitemporal hemianopia (see Fig. 18.29) or upper quadrantanopia, any type of visual field defect can result from suprasellar extension of a tumour because it may compress the optic nerve (unilateral loss of acuity or scotoma) or the optic tract (homonymous hemianopia). Optic atrophy may be apparent on ophthalmoscopy. Lateral extension of a sellar mass into the cavernous sinus with subsequent compression of the 3rd, 4th or 6th cranial nerve may cause diplopia and strabismus, but in anterior pituitary tumours this is an unusual presentation.

Occasionally, pituitary tumours infarct or there is bleeding into cystic lesions. This is termed 'pituitary apoplexy' and may result in sudden expansion with local compression symptoms and acute-onset hypopituitarism. Non-haemorrhagic infarction can also occur in a normal pituitary gland; predisposing factors include catastrophic obstetric haemorrhage (Sheehan's syndrome), diabetes mellitus and raised intracranial pressure.

Investigations

Patients suspected of having a pituitary tumour should undergo MRI or CT. While some lesions have distinctive neuro-radiological features, the definitive diagnosis is made on histology after surgery. All patients with (para)sellar space-occupying lesions should have pituitary function assessed as described in Box 18.53.

Management

Modalities of treatment of common pituitary and hypothalamic tumours are shown in Box 18.57. Associated hypopituitarism should be treated as described above.

Urgent treatment is required if there is evidence of pressure on visual pathways. The chances of recovery of a visual field defect are proportional to the duration of symptoms, with full recovery unlikely if the defect has been present for longer than 4 months. In the presence of a sellar mass lesion, it is crucial that serum prolactin is measured before emergency surgery is performed. If the prolactin is over 5000 mIU/L (236 ng/mL), then the lesion is likely to be a macroprolactinoma and should respond to a dopamine agonist with shrinkage of the lesion, making surgery unnecessary (see Fig. 18.29).

Most operations on the pituitary are performed using the trans-sphenoidal approach via the nostrils, while transfrontal surgery via a craniotomy is reserved for suprasellar tumours and is much less frequently needed. It is uncommon to be able to resect lateral extensions into the cavernous sinuses, although with modern endoscopic techniques this is more feasible. All operations on the pituitary carry a risk of damaging normal endocrine function; this risk increases with the size of the primary lesion.

Pituitary function (see Box 18.53) should be retested 4–6 weeks following surgery, primarily to detect the development of any new hormone deficits. Rarely, the surgical treatment of a sellar lesion can result in recovery of hormone secretion that was deficient pre-operatively.

Following surgery, usually after 3–6 months, imaging should be repeated. If there is a significant residual mass and the histology confirms an anterior pituitary tumour, external radiotherapy may be given to reduce the risk of recurrence but the risk:benefit ratio needs careful individualised discussion. Radiotherapy is not useful in patients requiring urgent therapy because it takes many months or years to be effective and there is a risk of acute swelling of the mass. Fractionated radiotherapy carries a life-long risk of hypopituitarism (50–70% in the first 10 years) and annual pituitary function tests are obligatory. There is also concern that radiotherapy might impair cognitive function, cause vascular changes and even induce primary brain tumours, but these side-effects have not been quantified reliably and are likely

18

i 18.57 Therapeutic modalities for functioning and non-functioning hypothalamic and pituitary tumours				
	Surgery	Radiotherapy	Medical	Comment
Non-functioning pituitary macroadenoma	1st line	2nd line	–	
Prolactinoma	2nd line	2nd line	1st line Dopamine agonists	Dopamine agonists usually cause macroadenomas to shrink
Acromegaly	1st line	2nd line	2nd line Somatostatin analogues Dopamine agonists GH receptor antagonists	Medical therapy does not reliably cause macroadenomas to shrink Radiotherapy and medical therapy are used in combination for inoperable tumours
Cushing's disease	1st line	2nd line	2nd line Steroidogenesis inhibitors Pasireotide	Radiotherapy may take many years to reduce ACTH excess and medical therapies may be used as a bridge. Bilateral adrenalectomy may also be considered if the pituitary tumour is not completely resectable
Craniopharyngioma	1st line	2nd line	–	
(ACTH = adrenocorticotrophic hormone; GH = growth hormone)				

to be rare. Stereotactic radiosurgery allows specific targeting of residual disease in a more focused fashion.

Non-functioning tumours should be followed up by repeated imaging at intervals that depend on the size of the lesion and on whether or not radiotherapy has been administered. For smaller lesions that are not causing mass effects, therapeutic surgery may not be indicated and the lesion may simply be monitored by serial neuroimaging without a clear-cut diagnosis having been established.

Hyperprolactinaemia/galactorrhoea

Hyperprolactinaemia is a common abnormality that usually presents with hypogonadism and/or galactorrhoea (lactation in the absence of breastfeeding). Since prolactin stimulates milk secretion but not breast development, galactorrhoea rarely occurs in men and only does so if gynaecomastia has been induced by hypogonadism (p. 655). The differential diagnosis of hyperprolactinaemia is shown in Box 18.58. Many drugs, especially dopamine antagonists, elevate prolactin concentrations. Pituitary tumours can cause hyperprolactinaemia by directly secreting prolactin (prolactinomas, see below), or by compressing the infundibular stalk and thus interrupting the tonic inhibitory effect of hypothalamic dopamine on prolactin secretion ('disconnection' hyperprolactinaemia).

Prolactin usually circulates as a free (monomeric) hormone in plasma but, in some individuals, prolactin becomes bound to an IgG antibody. This complex is known as macroprolactin and such patients have macroprolactinaemia (not to be confused with macroprolactinoma, a prolactin-secreting pituitary tumour of more than 1 cm in diameter). Since macroprolactin cannot cross blood-vessel walls to reach prolactin receptors in target tissues, it is of no pathological significance. Some commercial prolactin assays do not distinguish prolactin from macroprolactin and so macroprolactinaemia is a cause of spurious hyperprolactinaemia. Identification of macroprolactin requires gel filtration chromatography or polyethylene glycol precipitation techniques, and one of these tests should be performed in all patients with hyperprolactinaemia if the prolactin assay is known to cross-react.

Clinical assessment

In women, in addition to galactorrhoea, hypogonadism associated with hyperprolactinaemia causes secondary amenorrhoea and anovulation with infertility (p. 654). Important points in the history include drug use, recent pregnancy and menstrual history. The quantity of milk produced is variable and it may be observed only by manual expression. In men there is decreased libido, reduced shaving frequency and lethargy (p. 655). Unilateral galactorrhoea may be confused with nipple discharge, and breast examination to exclude malignancy or fibrocystic disease is important. Further assessment should address the features in Figure 18.28.

Investigations

Pregnancy should first be excluded before further investigations are performed in women of child-bearing potential. The upper limit of normal for many assays of serum prolactin is approximately 500 mIU/L (24 ng/mL). In non-pregnant and non-lactating patients, monomeric prolactin concentrations of 500–1000 mIU/L (24–47 ng/mL) are likely to be induced by stress or drugs, and a repeat measurement is indicated. Levels between 1000 and 5000 mIU/L (47–236 ng/mL) are likely to be due to either drugs, a microprolactinoma or 'disconnection' hyperprolactinaemia. Levels above 5000 mIU/L (236 ng/mL) are highly suggestive of a macroprolactinoma.

Patients with prolactin excess should have tests of gonadal function (p. 651), and T_4 and TSH should be measured to exclude primary hypothyroidism causing TRH-induced prolactin excess. Unless the prolactin falls after withdrawal of relevant drug therapy, a serum prolactin consistently above the reference range is an indication for MRI or CT scan of the hypothalamus and pituitary. Patients with a macroadenoma also need tests for hypopituitarism (see Box 18.53).

Management

If possible, the underlying cause should be corrected (e.g. cessation of offending drugs and giving levothyroxine replacement in primary hypothyroidism). If dopamine antagonists are the cause, then dopamine agonist therapy is contraindicated; if gonadal dysfunction is the primary concern, sex steroid replacement therapy may be indicated. Troublesome physiological galactorrhoea can also be treated with dopamine agonists (see Box 18.59). Management of prolactinomas is described below.

Prolactinoma

Most prolactinomas in pre-menopausal women are microadenomas because the symptoms of prolactin excess usually result in early presentation. Prolactin-secreting cells of the anterior pituitary share a common lineage with GH-secreting cells, so occasionally prolactinomas can secrete excess GH and cause acromegaly. In prolactinomas there is a relationship between prolactin concentration and tumour size: the higher the level, the bigger the tumour. Some macroprolactinomas can elevate prolactin concentrations above 100 000 mIU/L

---

i | 18.58 Causes of hyperprolactinaemia

Physiological

- Stress (e.g. post-seizure)
- Pregnancy
- Lactation
- Nipple stimulation
- Sleep
- Coitus
- Exercise
- Baby crying

Drug-induced

Dopamine antagonists
- Antipsychotics (phenothiazines and butyrophenones)
- Antidepressants
- Antiemetics (e.g. metoclopramide, domperidone)

Dopamine-depleting drugs
- Reserpine
- Methyldopa

Oestrogens
- Oral contraceptive pill

Pathological

Common
- Disconnection hyperprolactinaemia (e.g. non-functioning pituitary macroadenoma)
- Prolactinoma (usually microadenoma)
- Primary hypothyroidism
- Polycystic ovarian syndrome
- Macroprolactinaemia

Uncommon
- Pituitary tumour secreting prolactin and growth hormone
- Hypothalamic disease
- Renal failure

Rare
- Chest wall reflex (e.g. post herpes zoster)

(4700 ng/mL). The investigation of prolactinomas is the same as for other pituitary tumours (see above).

Management

As shown in Box 18.57, several therapeutic modalities can be employed in the management of prolactinomas.

Medical

Dopamine agonist drugs are first-line therapy for the majority of patients (Box 18.59). They usually reduce serum prolactin concentrations and cause significant tumour shrinkage after several months of therapy (Fig. 18.29), but visual field defects, if present, may improve within days of first administration. It is possible to withdraw dopamine agonist therapy without recurrence of hyperprolactinaemia after a few years of treatment in some

Fig. 18.29 Shrinkage of a macroprolactinoma following treatment with a dopamine agonist. A MRI scan showing a pituitary macroadenoma (T) compressing the optic chiasm (C). B MRI scan of the same tumour following treatment with a dopamine agonist. The macroadenoma, which was a prolactinoma, has decreased in size substantially and is no longer compressing the optic chiasm.

patients with a microadenoma. Also, after the menopause, suppression of prolactin is required in microadenomas only if galactorrhoea is troublesome, since hypogonadism is then physiological and tumour growth unlikely. In patients with macroadenomas, drugs can be withdrawn only after curative surgery or radiotherapy and under close supervision.

Ergot-derived dopamine agonists (bromocriptine and cabergoline) can bind to 5-HT$_{2B}$ receptors in the heart and elsewhere and have been associated with fibrotic reactions, particularly tricuspid valve regurgitation, when used in high doses in patients with Parkinson's disease. At the relatively low doses used in prolactinomas most data suggest that systematic screening for cardiac fibrosis is unnecessary, but if dopamine agonist therapy is prolonged, periodic screening by echocardiography or use of non-ergot agents (quinagolide) may be indicated.

Surgery and radiotherapy

Surgical decompression is usually necessary only when a macroprolactinoma has failed to shrink sufficiently with dopamine agonist therapy, and this may be because the tumour has a significant cystic component. Surgery may also be performed in patients who are intolerant of dopamine agonists. Microadenomas can be removed selectively by trans-sphenoidal surgery with a cure rate of about 80%, but recurrence is possible; the cure rate for surgery in macroadenomas is substantially lower.

External irradiation may be required for some macroadenomas to prevent regrowth if dopamine agonists are stopped.

Pregnancy

Hyperprolactinaemia often presents with infertility, so dopamine agonist therapy may be followed by pregnancy. Patients with microadenomas should be advised to withdraw dopamine agonist therapy as soon as pregnancy is confirmed. In contrast, macroprolactinomas may enlarge rapidly under oestrogen stimulation and these patients should continue dopamine agonist therapy and need measurement of prolactin levels and visual fields during pregnancy. All patients should be advised to report headache or visual disturbance promptly.

Acromegaly

Acromegaly is caused by growth hormone (GH) secretion from a pituitary tumour, usually a macroadenoma, and carries an approximate twofold excess mortality when untreated.

i	18.59 Dopamine agonist therapy: drugs used to treat prolactinomas		
Drug	**Oral dose***	**Advantages**	**Disadvantages**
Bromocriptine	2.5–15 mg/day 2–3 times daily	Available for parenteral use Short half-life; useful in treating infertility Proven long-term efficacy	Ergotamine-like side-effects (nausea, headache, postural hypotension, constipation) Frequent dosing so poor adherence Rare reports of fibrotic reactions in various tissues
Cabergoline	250–1000 µg/week 2 doses/week	Long-acting, so missed doses less important Reported to have fewer ergotamine-like side-effects	Limited data on safety in pregnancy Associated with cardiac valvular fibrosis in Parkinson's disease
Quinagolide	50–150 µg/day Once daily	A non-ergot with few side-effects in patients intolerant of the above	Limited data on safety in pregnancy

*Tolerance develops for the side-effects. All of these agents, especially bromocriptine, must be introduced at low dose and increased slowly. If several doses of bromocriptine are missed, the process must start again.

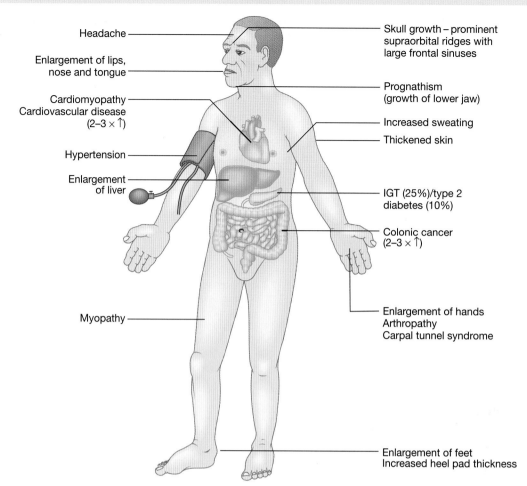

Headache

Enlargement of lips,
nose and tongue

Cardiomyopathy
Cardiovascular disease
(2–3 × ↑)

Hypertension

Enlargement
of liver

Myopathy

Skull growth – prominent
supraorbital ridges with
large frontal sinuses

Prognathism
(growth of lower jaw)

Increased sweating

Thickened skin

IGT (25%)/type 2
diabetes (10%)

Colonic cancer
(2–3 × ↑)

Enlargement of hands
Arthropathy
Carpal tunnel syndrome

Enlargement of feet
Increased heel pad thickness

Fig. 18.30 Clinical features of acromegaly. (IGT = impaired glucose tolerance)

Clinical features

If GH hypersecretion occurs before puberty, then the presentation is with gigantism. More commonly, GH excess occurs in adult life and presents with acromegaly. If hypersecretion starts in adolescence and persists into adult life, then the two conditions may be combined. The clinical features are shown in Figure 18.30. The most common complaints are headache and sweating. Additional features include those of any pituitary tumour (see Fig. 18.28).

Investigations

The clinical diagnosis must be confirmed by measuring GH levels during an oral glucose tolerance test and measuring serum IGF-1. In normal subjects, plasma GH suppresses to below 0.5 μg/L (approximately 2 mIU/L). In acromegaly, GH does not suppress and in about 30% of patients there is a paradoxical rise; IGF-1 is also elevated. The rest of pituitary function should be investigated as described in Box 18.53. Prolactin concentrations are elevated in about 30% of patients due to co-secretion of prolactin from the tumour. Additional tests in acromegaly may include screening for colonic neoplasms with colonoscopy.

Management

The main aims are to improve symptoms and to normalise serum GH and IGF-1 to reduce morbidity and mortality. Treatment is summarised in Box 18.57.

Surgical

Trans-sphenoidal surgery is usually the first line of treatment and may result in cure of GH excess, especially in patients with microadenomas. More often, surgery serves to debulk the tumour and further second-line therapy is required, according to post-operative imaging and glucose tolerance test results.

Radiotherapy

External radiotherapy is usually employed as second-line treatment if acromegaly persists after surgery, to stop tumour growth and lower GH levels. However, GH levels fall slowly (over many years) and there is a risk of hypopituitarism.

Medical

If acromegaly persists after surgery, medical therapy is usually employed to lower GH levels to below 1.0 μg/L (approximately 3 mIU/L) and to normalise IGF-1 concentrations. Medical therapy may be discontinued after several years in patients who have received radiotherapy. Somatostatin analogues (such as octreotide, lanreotide or pasireotide) can be administered as slow-release injections every few weeks. Somatostatin analogues can also be used as primary therapy for acromegaly either as an alternative or in advance of surgery, given evidence that they can induce modest tumour shrinkage in some patients. Dopamine agonists are less effective at lowering GH but may sometimes be helpful, especially with associated prolactin excess.

Pegvisomant is a peptide GH receptor antagonist administered by daily self-injection and may be indicated in some patients whose GH and IGF-1 concentrations fail to suppress sufficiently following somatostatin analogue therapy.

Craniopharyngioma

Craniopharyngiomas are benign tumours that develop in cell rests of Rathke's pouch, and may be located within the sella turcica, or commonly in the suprasellar space. They are often cystic, with a solid component that may or may not be calcified (Fig. 18.31). In young people, they are diagnosed more commonly than pituitary adenomas. They may present with pressure effects on adjacent structures, hypopituitarism and/or cranial diabetes insipidus. Other clinical features directly related to hypothalamic damage may also occur. These include hyperphagia and obesity, loss of the sensation of thirst and disturbance of temperature regulation, and these features can be significant clinical challenges to manage.

Craniopharyngiomas can be treated by the trans-sphenoidal route but surgery may also involve a craniotomy, with a relatively high risk of hypothalamic damage and other complications. If the

Fig. 18.31 Craniopharyngioma. [A] This developmental tumour characteristically presents in younger patients; it is often cystic and calcified, as shown in this MRI scan (arrows). [B] Pathology specimen.

tumour has a large cystic component, it may be safer to place in the cyst cavity a drain that is attached to a subcutaneous access device, rather than attempt a resection. Whatever form it takes, surgery is unlikely to be curative and radiotherapy may often be given to reduce the risk of relapse. Unfortunately, craniopharyngiomas often recur, requiring repeated surgery. They often cause considerable morbidity, usually from hypothalamic obesity, water balance problems and/or visual failure.

Diabetes insipidus

This uncommon disorder is characterised by the persistent excretion of excessive quantities of dilute urine and by thirst. It is classified into two types:

- cranial diabetes insipidus, in which there is deficient production of vasopressin by the hypothalamus
- nephrogenic diabetes insipidus, in which the renal tubules are unresponsive to vasopressin.

The underlying causes are listed in Box 18.60.

Clinical features

The most marked symptoms are polyuria and polydipsia. The patient may pass 5–20 L or more of urine in 24 hours. This is of low specific gravity and osmolality. If the patient has an intact thirst mechanism, is conscious and has access to oral fluids, then he or she can maintain adequate fluid intake. However, in an unconscious patient or a patient with damage to the hypothalamic thirst centre, diabetes insipidus is potentially lethal. If there is associated cortisol deficiency, then diabetes insipidus may not be manifest until glucocorticoid replacement therapy is given. The most common differential diagnosis is primary polydipsia, caused by drinking excessive amounts of fluid in the absence of a defect in vasopressin or thirst control.

18

i	**18.60 Causes of diabetes insipidus**

Cranial

Structural hypothalamic or high stalk lesion
- See Box 18.54

Idiopathic

Genetic defect
- Dominant (*AVP* gene mutation)
- Recessive (DIDMOAD syndrome – association of diabetes insipidus with diabetes mellitus, optic atrophy, deafness)

Nephrogenic

Genetic defect
- V2 receptor mutation
- Aquaporin-2 mutation
- Cystinosis

Metabolic abnormality
- Hypokalaemia
- Hypercalcaemia

Drug therapy
- Lithium
- Demeclocycline

Poisoning
- Heavy metals

Chronic kidney disease
- Polycystic kidney disease
- Sickle-cell anaemia
- Infiltrative disease

18.61 How and when to do a water deprivation test

Use

- To establish a diagnosis of diabetes insipidus and to differentiate cranial from nephrogenic causes

Protocol

- No coffee, tea or smoking on the test day
- Free fluids until 0730 hrs on the morning of the test, but discourage patients from 'stocking up' with extra fluid in anticipation of fluid deprivation
- No fluids from 0730 hrs
- Attend at 0830 hrs for measurement of body weight and plasma and urine osmolality
- Record body weight, urine volume, urine and plasma osmolality and thirst score on a visual analogue scale every 2 hrs for up to 8 hrs
- Stop the test if the patient loses 3% of body weight
- If plasma osmolality reaches >300 mOsmol/kg and urine osmolality <600 mOsmol/kg, then administer DDAVP (see text) 2 μg IM

Interpretation

- Diabetes insipidus is confirmed by a plasma osmolality >300 mOsmol/kg with a urine osmolality <600 mOsmol/kg
- Cranial diabetes insipidus is confirmed if urine osmolality rises by at least 50% after DDAVP
- Nephrogenic diabetes insipidus is confirmed if DDAVP does not concentrate the urine
- Primary polydipsia is suggested by low plasma osmolality at the start of the test

Investigations

Diabetes insipidus can be confirmed if serum vasopressin is undetectable (although the assay for this is not widely available) or the urine is not maximally concentrated (i.e. <600 mmol/kg) in the presence of increased plasma osmolality (i.e. >300 mOsmol/kg). Sometimes, the diagnosis can be confirmed or refuted by random simultaneous samples of blood and urine, but more often a dynamic test is required. The water deprivation test described in Box 18.61 is widely used, but an alternative is to infuse hypertonic (5%) saline and measure vasopressin secretion in response to increasing plasma osmolality. Thirst can also be assessed during these tests on a visual analogue scale. Anterior pituitary function and suprasellar anatomy should be assessed in patients with cranial diabetes insipidus (see Box 18.53).

In primary polydipsia, the urine may be excessively dilute because of chronic diuresis, which 'washes out' the solute gradient across the loop of Henle, but plasma osmolality is low rather than high. DDAVP (see below) should not be administered to patients with primary polydipsia, since it will prevent excretion of water and there is a risk of severe water intoxication if the patient continues to drink fluid to excess.

In nephrogenic diabetes insipidus, appropriate further tests may include plasma electrolytes, calcium, ultrasound of the kidneys and urinalysis.

Management

Treatment of cranial diabetes insipidus is with des-amino-des-aspartate-arginine vasopressin (desmopressin, DDAVP), an analogue of vasopressin that has a longer half-life. For chronic replacement therapy DDAVP may be administered intranasally and orally, although the latter formulation has variable bioavailability. In sick patients, DDAVP should be given by intramuscular injection. The dose of DDAVP should be adjusted on the basis

18.62 The pituitary and hypothalamus in old age

- **Late presentation**: often with large tumours causing visual disturbance, because early symptoms such as amenorrhoea and sexual dysfunction do not occur or are not recognised.
- **Coincidentally discovered pituitary tumours**: may not require surgical intervention if the visual apparatus is not involved, because of slow growth.
- **Hyperprolactinaemia**: less impact in post-menopausal women who are already 'physiologically' hypogonadal. Macroprolactinomas, however, require treatment because of their potential to cause mass effects.

of serum sodium concentrations and/or osmolality. The principal hazard is excessive treatment, resulting in water intoxication and hyponatraemia. Conversely, inadequate treatment results in thirst and polyuria. The ideal dose prevents nocturia but allows a degree of polyuria from time to time before the next dose (e.g. DDAVP nasal dose 5 μg in the morning and 10 μg at night).

The polyuria in nephrogenic diabetes insipidus is improved by thiazide diuretics (e.g. bendroflumethiazide 5–10 mg/day), amiloride (5–10 mg/day) and NSAIDs (e.g. indometacin 15 mg 3 times daily), although the last of these carries a risk of reducing glomerular filtration rate.

Disorders affecting multiple endocrine glands

Multiple endocrine neoplasia

Multiple endocrine neoplasias (MEN) are rare autosomal dominant syndromes characterised by hyperplasia and formation of adenomas or malignant tumours in multiple glands. They fall into four groups, as shown in Box 18.63. Some other genetic diseases also have an increased risk of endocrine tumours; for example, phaeochromocytoma is associated with von Hippel–Lindau syndrome (p. 1132) and neurofibromatosis type 1 (p. 1131).

The MEN syndromes should be considered in all patients with two or more endocrine tumours and in patients with solitary tumours who report other endocrine tumours in their family. Inactivating mutations in MEN 1 (MENIN), a tumour suppressor gene on chromosome 11, cause MEN 1, whereas MEN 2 and 3 (also known as MEN 2a and 2b, respectively) are caused by gain-of-function mutations in the RET proto-oncogene on chromosome 10. These cause constitutive activation of the membrane-associated tyrosine kinase RET, which controls the development of cells that migrate from the neural crest. In contrast, loss-of-function mutations of the RET kinase cause Hirschsprung's disease (p. 834). MEN 4 is extremely rare and is associated with loss-of-function mutations in the CDNK1B gene on chromosome 12; this gene codes for the protein p27, which has putative tumour suppressor activity. Predictive genetic testing can be performed on relatives of individuals with MEN syndromes, after appropriate counselling (p. 59).

Individuals who carry mutations associated with MEN should be entered into a surveillance programme. In MEN 1, this typically involves annual history, examination and measurements of serum calcium and prolactin, and MRI of the pituitary and pancreas every 2 years; some centres also perform regular CT or MRI scans

18.63 Multiple endocrine neoplasia (MEN) syndromes

MEN 1 (Wermer's syndrome)

- Primary hyperparathyroidism
- Pituitary tumours
- Pancreatic neuro-endocrine tumours (e.g. non-functioning, insulinoma, gastrinoma)
- Bronchial and thymic carcinoids
- Adrenal tumours
- Cutaneous lesions (e.g. lipomas, collagenomas, angiofibromas)

MEN 2 (also known as MEN 2a or Sipple's syndrome)

- Primary hyperparathyroidism
- Medullary carcinoma of thyroid
- Phaeochromocytoma

MEN 3 (also known as MEN 2b)

- As for MEN 2 above (though medullary thyroid cancer occurs earlier, even within the first year of life)
- Marfanoid habitus
- Skeletal abnormalities (e.g. craniosynostosis)
- Abnormal dental enamel
- Multiple mucosal neuromas

MEN 4

- Primary hyperparathyroidism
- Pituitary tumours
- Possible tumours in the adrenals, reproductive organs, kidneys
- Possible pancreatic, gastric, bronchial and cervical neuro-endocrine tumours

18.64 Autoimmune polyendocrine syndromes (APS)*

Type 1 (APECED)

- Addison's disease
- Hypoparathyroidism
- Type 1 diabetes
- Primary hypothyroidism
- Chronic mucocutaneous candidiasis
- Nail dystrophy
- Dental enamel hypoplasia

Type 2 (Schmidt's syndrome)

- Addison's disease
- Primary hypothyroidism
- Graves' disease
- Pernicious anaemia
- Primary hypogonadism
- Type 1 diabetes
- Vitiligo
- Coeliac disease
- Myasthenia gravis

*In both types of APS, the precise pattern of disease varies between affected individuals.
(APECED = autoimmune poly-endocrinopathy-candidiasis-ectodermal dystrophy)

of the chest. In individuals with MEN 2 and 3, annual history, examination and measurement of serum calcium, calcitonin and urinary or plasma catecholamine metabolites should be performed. Because the penetrance of medullary carcinoma of the thyroid approaches 100% in individuals with a *RET* mutation, prophylactic thyroidectomy should be performed in early childhood in most patients. The precise timing of surgery in childhood should be guided by the specific mutation in the *RET* gene.

Autoimmune polyendocrine syndromes

Two distinct autoimmune polyendocrine syndromes are known: APS types 1 and 2.

The most common is APS type 2 (Schmidt's syndrome), which typically presents in women between the ages of 20 and 60. It is usually defined as the occurrence in the same individual of two or more autoimmune endocrine disorders, some of which are listed in Box 18.64. The mode of inheritance is autosomal dominant with incomplete penetrance and there is a strong association with HLA-DR3 and CTLA-4.

Much less common is APS type 1, which is also termed autoimmune poly-endocrinopathy-candidiasis-ectodermal dystrophy (APECED). This is inherited in an autosomal recessive fashion and is caused by loss-of-function mutations in the autoimmune regulator gene *AIRE*, which is responsible for the presentation of self-antigens to thymocytes in utero. This is essential for the deletion of thymocyte clones that react against self-antigens and hence for the development of immune tolerance (p. 82). The most common clinical features are described in Box 18.64, although the pattern of presentation is variable and other autoimmune disorders are often observed.

Late effects of childhood cancer therapy

The therapies used to treat cancers in children and adolescents, including radiotherapy and chemotherapy, may cause long-term endocrine dysfunction (p. 1298).

18

Further information

Websites

british-thyroid-association.org *British Thyroid Association: provider of guidelines, e.g. treatment of hypothyroidism and the investigation and management of thyroid cancer.*

btf-thyroid.org *British Thyroid Foundation: a resource for patient leaflets and support for patients with thyroid disorders.*

endocrinology.org *British Society for Endocrinology: useful online education resources and links to patient support group.*

endo-society.org *American Endocrine Society: provider of clinical practice guidelines.*

pituitary.org.uk *Pituitary Foundation: a resource for patient and general practitioner leaflets and further information.*

thyroid.org *American Thyroid Association: provider of clinical practice guidelines.*

AG Shand
JPH Wilding

19

Nutritional factors in disease

Clinical examination in nutritional disorders 692

Clinical assessment and investigation of nutritional status 693

Nutritional factors and disease 694
Physiology of nutrition 694

Disorders of altered energy balance 698
Obesity 698
Under-nutrition 704

Micronutrients, minerals and their diseases 711
Vitamins 711
Inorganic micronutrients 716

Clinical examination in nutritional disorders

3 Hands
Muscle wasting (dorsal interossei, thenar eminences)
Finger clubbing
Leukonychia (low albumin)
Koilonychia (iron deficiency)

▲ Koilonychia

2 Simple anthropometrics (see right)
Body mass index
Triceps skin fold thickness
Waist circumference

1 Observation
Signs of weight loss:
  Prominent ribs
  Muscle wasting
  ↓Skin turgor

▲ Scaphoid abdomen

▲ Clinical effects of short bowel syndrome after multiple resection in Crohn's disease

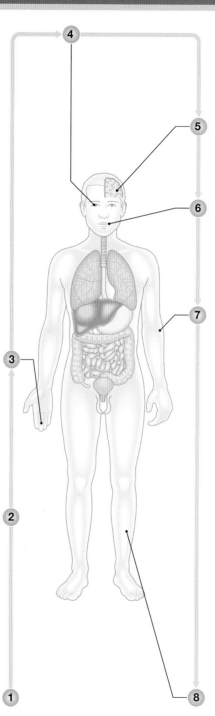

4 Eyes
Sunken eyes
Pallor
Jaundice
Bitot spots (↓vitamin A; see Fig. 19.12)

5 Affect
Fatigue
Depression
Dementia

6 Mouth
Pallor
Angular stomatitis (↓B$_{12}$, folate, iron)
Glossitis (↓B$_{12}$, folate, iron)
Gingivitis, bleeding gums (↓vitamin C; see Fig. 19.14)
Poorly fitting dentures

▲ Gingivitis

7 Skin
Dry, flaky skin or dermatitis (see Fig. 19.13)
Hair loss
Specific abnormalities:
  Petechiae, corkscrew hairs (↓vitamin C)
  Dermatitis of pellegra (↓niacin)

▲ Corkscrew hairs

8 Legs
Pitting oedema
Ulcers

Insets (Scaphoid abdomen) From Chandra A, Quinones-Baldrich WJ. Chronic mesenteric ischemia: How to select patients for invasive treatment. Sem Vasc Surg 2010; 23:21–28; (Koilonychia) Habif TP. Clinical Dermatology, 6th edn. Philadelphia: Saunders, Elsevier Inc.; 2016; (Gingivitis) Newman MG, Takei H, Klokkevold PR, et al. Carranza's Clinical Periodontology, 12th edn. Philadelphia: Saunders, Elsevier Inc.; 2015; (Corkscrew hairs) Bolognia JL, Jorizzo JL, Schaffer JV, et al. Dermatology, 3rd edn. Philadelphia: Saunders, Elsevier Inc.; 2012.

Clinical assessment and investigation of nutritional status

Under-nutrition can go unnoticed in patients with multiple comorbidities. It is vital to be aware of under-nutrition as a potential reason for any acute medical presentation or as a modifier of it. Early nutritional assessment is crucial and a dietary history provides useful information (especially when taken by a dietitian). Points to note include past medical and surgical history (e.g. abdominal or intestinal surgery), a drug history and a specific diet history. Evidence of recent weight loss and muscle wasting should be sought. Simple, validated tools are available to screen patients for nutritional problems. Body composition reflects energy balance and is assessed by clinical anthropomorphic measurements. More sophisticated techniques may be used to assess body composition or functional capacity if required.

i Important elements of the diet history

Ask about weight

- Current weight
- Weight 2 weeks, 1 month and 6 months ago
- Assessment of degree of change

Ask about current food intake

- Quantity of food and if any change
- Quality of food taken
- Whether normal food is being eaten
- Avoidance of specific food types (e.g. solids)
- Any nutritional supplements
- Reliance on supplements/tube feeding
- Any change in appetite or interest in food
- Any taste disturbance

Ask about symptoms that interfere with eating

- Oral ulcers or oral pain
- Difficulties swallowing
- Nausea/vomiting
- Early satiety
- Alteration in bowel habit
- Abdominal (or other) pain

Ask about activity levels/performance status

- Normal activity
- Slightly reduced activity
- Inactive < 50% of the time
- Inactive most of the time

2 Body mass index (BMI)

$$BMI = \frac{wt\ (kg)}{ht\ (m)^2}$$

Example: an adult of 70 kg with a height of 1.75 m has a BMI of $70/1.75^2 = 22.9$ kg/m^2

- BMI is a useful way of identifying under- or over-nutrition but cannot discriminate between lean body or muscle mass and fat mass
- Fat mass is also subject to ethnic variation; for the same BMI, Asians tend to have more body fat than Europeans
- If height cannot be determined (e.g. in older people or those unable to stand), measurement of the femoral length or 'knee height' is a good surrogate

Measurement of knee height.

2 Measures of body composition and nutritional status

Body composition

- Anthropometry (see below)
- Bioelectrical impedance
- Dual X-ray absorptiometry (DXA)

Muscle function and global nutritional status

- Hand grip strength (dynamometer test) – poor grip associated with increased mortality

Obesity and fat distribution (android vs gynoid)

- Waist:hip ratio (circumferences measured midway between superior iliac crest and lower border of rib cage, and at greater trochanters, respectively)

Body fat content and muscle mass

- Triceps skinfold thickness (when combined with mid-/upper arm circumference estimates muscle mass)

Triceps skinfold thickness. Lean patients 6–12 mm; obese patients 40–50 mm.

19

BMI score	Weight loss score	Acute disease score
> 20 = 0	Unplanned loss in 6 months	Acute illness with no nutritional intake for 5 days = 2
18.5 – 20 = 1	< 5% = 0	
< 18.5 = 2	5 – 10% = 1	
	> 10% = 2	

Total score

Total = 0 – Low risk	Total = 1 – Medium risk	Total ≥ 2 – High risk
• Routine clinical care	• Document dietary intake for 3 days	• Refer to dietitian/nutrition support team
• Repeat screen weekly	• Repeat screen weekly	• Review plan weekly

Screening hospitalised patients for risk of malnutrition. Acute illnesses include decompensated liver disease, cancer cachexia or being kept 'nil by mouth'. *Adapted from the British Association of Parenteral and Enteral Nutrition Malnutrition Universal Screening Tool (www.bapen.org.uk).*

Nutritional factors and disease

Obtaining adequate nutrition is a fundamental requirement for the survival of every individual and species. The politics of food provision for humans are complex and constitute a prominent factor in wars, natural disasters and the global economy. In recent decades, economic success has been rewarded by plentiful nutrition unknown to previous generations, which has led to a pandemic of obesity and its consequences for health, yet in many parts of the world, famine and under-nutrition still represent a huge burden. Quality, as well as quantity, of food influences health, with governmental advice on healthy diets maximising fruit and vegetable intakes (Fig. 19.1). Inappropriate diets have been linked to diseases such as coronary heart disease and cancer. Deficiencies of vitamins or minerals lead to avoidable conditions, such as anaemia due to iron deficiency or blindness due to severe vitamin A deficiency. A proper understanding of nutrition is therefore essential in dealing with the needs of individual patients and in informing the planning of public policy.

Physiology of nutrition

Nutrients in the diet can be classified into 'macronutrients', which are eaten in relatively large amounts to provide fuel for energy, and 'micronutrients' (e.g. vitamins and minerals), which do not contribute to energy balance but are required in small amounts because they are not synthesised in the body.

Energy balance

The laws of thermodynamics dictate that energy balance is achieved when energy intake = energy expenditure (Fig. 19.2). Energy expenditure has several components. The basal metabolic rate (BMR) describes the obligatory energy expenditure required to maintain metabolic functions in tissues and hence sustain life. It is most closely predicted by fat-free mass (i.e. total body mass minus fat mass), which is lower in females and older people (Fig. 19.2B). Extra metabolic energy is consumed during growth, pregnancy and lactation, and when febrile. Metabolic

energy is also required for thermal regulation, and expenditure is higher in cold or hot environments. The energy required for digestion of food (diet-induced thermogenesis; Fig. 19.2D) accounts for approximately 10% of total energy expenditure, with protein requiring more energy than other macronutrients. Another component of energy expenditure is governed by the level of muscular activity, which can vary considerably with occupation and lifestyle (Fig. 19.2C). Physical activity levels are usually defined as multiples of BMR.

Energy intake is determined by the 'macronutrient' content of food. Carbohydrates, fat, protein and alcohol provide fuel for oxidation in the mitochondria to generate energy (as adenosine triphosphate (ATP); p. 49). The energy provided by each of these elements differs:

- carbohydrates (16 kJ/g)
- fat (37 kJ/g)
- protein (17 kJ/g)
- alcohol (29 kJ/g).

Regulation of energy balance

Energy intake and expenditure are highly regulated (Fig. 19.3). A link with reproductive function ensures that pregnancy is most likely to occur during times of nutritional plenty, when both mother and baby have a better chance of survival. Improved nutrition is thought to be the reason for the increasingly early onset of puberty in many societies. At the other extreme, anorexia nervosa and excessive exercise can lead to amenorrhoea (p. 654).

Regulation of energy balance is coordinated in the hypothalamus, which receives afferent signals that indicate nutritional status in the short term (e.g. the stomach hormone ghrelin, which falls immediately after eating and rises gradually thereafter, to suppress satiety and signal that it is time for the next meal) and the long term (e.g. the adipose hormone leptin, which increases with growing fat mass and may also link fat mass to reproductive function). The hypothalamus responds with changes in many local neurotransmitters that alter activity in a number of pathways that influence energy balance (Fig. 19.3), including hormones acting on the pituitary gland (see Fig. 18.2, p. 633), and neural control circuits that connect with the cerebral cortex and autonomic nervous system.

Responses to under- and over-nutrition

These complex regulatory pathways allow adaptation to variations in nutrition. In response to starvation, reproductive function is suppressed, BMR is reduced, and there are profound psychological effects, including energy conservation through lethargy. These adjustments can 'defend' body weight within certain limits. In the low-insulin state of starvation (see Fig. 20.5, p. 725), however, fuels are liberated from stores initially in glycogen (in liver and muscle), then in triglyceride (lipolysis in adipose tissue, with excess free fatty acid supply to the liver leading to ketosis) and finally in protein (proteolysis in muscle). In those with a high glucose requirement, such as neonates and women who are pregnant or breastfeeding, starvation can result in ketoacidosis associated with normal or low blood glucose (p. 365).

In response to over-nutrition, BMR is increased, and extra energy is consumed in the work of carrying increased fat stores, so that body weight is again 'defended' within certain limits. In the high-insulin state of over-nutrition, excess energy is invested in fatty acids and stored as triglycerides; these are deposited principally in adipose tissue but they may also accumulate in the liver (non-alcoholic fatty liver disease; p. 882) and skeletal muscle. If hypothalamic function is abnormal (e.g. in those with

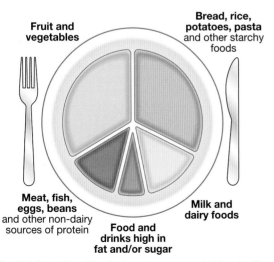

Fig. 19.1 Proportion of key food groups recommended for a healthy, well-balanced diet. *Crown copyright. Department of Health in association with the Welsh Government, the Scottish Government and the Food Standards Agency in Northern Ireland.*

Fruit and vegetables

Bread, rice, potatoes, pasta and other starchy foods

Meat, fish, eggs, beans and other non-dairy sources of protein

Food and drinks high in fat and/or sugar

Milk and dairy foods

Fig. 19.2 Determinants of energy balance. **A** Energy intake is shown as national averages, highlighting the differences in sources of energy in different countries (but obscuring substantial regional variations). The targets are recommendations as a percentage of food energy only (Source: Dept of Health 1991). For WHO targets, see Box 19.4. In the UK, it is assumed that 5% of energy intake will be derived from alcohol. **B** Data for normal basal metabolic rate (BMR) were obtained from healthy men and women in various countries. BMR declines from middle age and is lower in women, even after adjustment for body size because of differences in fat-free mass. **C** Energy is required for movement and activity. Physical activity level (PAL) is the multiple of BMR by which total energy expenditure is increased by activity. **D** Energy is consumed in order to digest food. *Leisure or sport activity increases PAL by ~0.3 for each 30–60 minutes of moderate exercise performed 4–5 times per week. The UK population median for PAL is 1.6, with estimates of 1.5 for the 'less active' and 1.8 for the 'more active'.

craniopharyngioma; see Fig. 18.31, p. 687) or in rare patients with mutations in relevant genes (e.g. in leptin or melanocortin-4 receptors), loss of response to satiety signals, together with loss of adaptive changes in energy expenditure, result in relentless weight gain.

Macronutrients (energy-yielding nutrients)

Carbohydrates

Types of carbohydrate and their dietary sources are listed in Box 19.1. The 'available' carbohydrates (starches and sugars)
are broken down to monosaccharides before absorption from the gut (p. 768), and supply over half the energy in a normal, well-balanced diet (see Fig. 19.2A). No individual carbohydrate is an essential nutrient, as carbohydrates can be synthesised de novo from glycerol or protein. If the available carbohydrate intake is less than 100 g per day, however, increased lipolysis leads to ketosis (see Fig. 20.7, p. 730).

Dietary guidelines do not restrict the intake of intrinsic sugars in fruit and vegetables or the sugars in milk. However, intake of non-milk extrinsic sugars (sucrose, maltose, fructose), which increase the risk of dental caries and diabetes mellitus, should

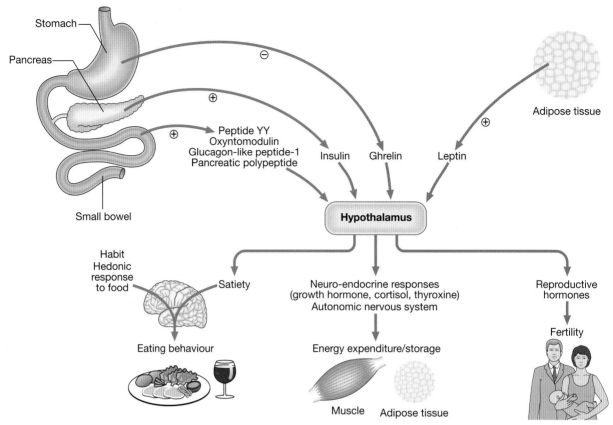

Fig. 19.3 Regulation of energy balance and its link with reproduction. ⊕ indicates factors that are stimulated by eating and induce satiety. ⊖ indicates factors that are suppressed by eating and inhibit satiety.

i	**19.1 Dietary carbohydrates**			
Class	**Components**	**Examples**	**Source**	
Free sugars	Monosaccharides Disaccharides	Glucose, fructose Sucrose, lactose, maltose	Intrinsic: fruits, milks, vegetables Extrinsic (extracted, refined): beet or cane sucrose, high-fructose corn syrup	
Short-chain carbohydrates	Oligosaccharides	Maltodextrins, fructo-oligosaccharides		
Starch polysaccharides	Rapidly digestible Slowly digestible Resistant		Cereals (wheat, rice), root vegetables (potato), legumes (lentils, beans, peas)	
Non-starch polysaccharides (NSPs; dietary fibre)	Fibrous Viscous	Cellulose Hemicellulose Pectins Gums	Plants	
Sugar alcohols		Sorbitol, xylitol	Sorbitol: stone fruits (apples, peaches, prunes) Xylitol: maize, berry fruits Both used as low-calorie sugar alternatives	

be limited. Individuals who do not produce lactase ('lactose-intolerant') are advised to avoid or limit dairy products and foods with added lactose. Starches in cereal foods, root foods and legumes provide the largest proportion of energy in most diets around the world. All starches are polymers of glucose, linked by the same 1–4 glycosidic linkages. Some starches are digested promptly by salivary and then pancreatic amylase, however, producing rapid delivery of glucose to the blood. Other starches are digested more slowly, either because they are protected in the structure of the food, or because of their crystal structure, or because the molecule is unbranched (amylose). These differences are the basis for the 'glycaemic index' of foods. This is the area under the curve of the rise in blood glucose concentration in the 2 hours following ingestion of 50 g carbohydrate, expressed as a percentage of the response to 50 g anhydrous glucose. There is evidence linking high glycaemic index foods, particularly foods containing large amounts of sugars such as glucose, sucrose or fructose (e.g. in soft drinks) with obesity and type 2 diabetes

(p. 932). Sugar alcohols (e.g. sorbitol) that are not absorbed form the gut and are used as replacement sweeteners can cause diarrhoea if eaten in large amounts.

Dietary fibre

Dietary fibre is plant food that is not digested by human enzymes in the gastrointestinal tract. Most dietary fibre is known as 'non-starch polysaccharides' (NSPs) (see Box 19.1). A small percentage of 'resistant' dietary starch may also pass unchanged into the large intestine. Dietary fibre can be broken down by the resident bacteria in the colon to produce short-chain fatty acids. This is essential fuel for the enterocytes and contributes to bowel health. The extent of flatus formed is dependent on the food source.

Some types of NSP, notably the hemicellulose of wheat, increase the water-holding capacity of colonic contents and the bulk of faeces. They relieve simple constipation, appear to prevent diverticulosis and may reduce the risk of cancer of the colon. Other viscous, indigestible polysaccharides like pectin and guar gum are important in the upper gastrointestinal tract, where they slow gastric emptying, contribute to satiety, and reduce bile salt absorption and hence plasma cholesterol concentration.

Fats

Fat has the highest energy density of the macronutrients (37 kJ/g) and excessive consumption may be an insidious cause of obesity (see Fig. 19.2A). Free fatty acids are absorbed in chylomicrons (pp. 371 and 372; see Fig. 21.5, p. 768), allowing access of complex molecules into the circulation. Fatty acid structures are shown in Figure 19.4. The principal polyunsaturated fatty acid (PUFA) in plant seed oils is linoleic acid ($18:2\ \omega6$). This and α-linolenic acid ($18:3\ \omega3$) are the 'essential' fatty acids, which humans cannot synthesise de novo. They undergo further desaturation and elongation, to produce, for example, γ-linolenic acid ($18:3\ \omega6$) and arachidonic acid ($20:4\ \omega6$). These are precursors of prostaglandins and eicosanoids, and form part of the structure of lipid membranes in all cells. Fish oils are rich in $\omega3$ PUFA (e.g. eicosapentaenoic ($20:5\ \omega3$) and docosahexaenoic ($22:6\ \omega3$), which promote the anti-inflammatory cascade of prostaglandin production and occur in the lipids of the human brain and retina. They inhibit thrombosis by competitively antagonising thromboxane A_2 formation. Replacing saturated

fat (i.e. from animal sources: butter, ghee or lard) with PUFA in the diet can lower the concentration of circulating low-density lipoprotein (LDL) cholesterol and may help prevent coronary heart disease. High intakes of *trans* fatty acids (TFAs; isomers of the natural *cis* fatty acids) reflect the use of oils that have been partially hydrogenated in the food industry. It is recommended that TFAs are limited to less than 2% of the dietary fat intake, as they are associated with cardiovascular disease. Changes in industrial practice in the UK and US have meant that TFA intake is now below 1%, with the residual amounts coming from milk as a result of ruminant digestion.

Cholesterol is also absorbed directly from food in chylomicrons and is an important substrate for steroid and sterol synthesis, but not an important source of energy.

Proteins

Proteins are made up of some 20 different amino acids, of which nine are 'essential' (Box 19.2), i.e. they cannot be synthesised in humans but are required for synthesis of important proteins. Another group of five amino acids are termed 'conditionally essential', meaning that they can be synthesised from other amino acids, provided there is an adequate dietary supply. The remaining amino acids can be synthesised in the body by transamination, provided there is a sufficient supply of amino groups.

The nutritive or 'biological' value of different proteins depends on the relative proportions of essential amino acids they contain. Proteins of animal origin, particularly from eggs, milk and meat, are generally of higher biological value than proteins of vegetable origin, which are low in one or more of the essential amino acids. When two different vegetable proteins are eaten together (e.g. a cereal and a legume), however, their amino acid contents are complementary and produce an adequate mix, an important principle in vegan diets.

Dietary recommendations for macronutrients

Recommendations for energy intake (Box 19.3) and proportions of macronutrients (Box 19.4) have been calculated to provide a balance of essential nutrients and minimise the risks of excessive refined sugar (dental caries, high glycaemic index/diabetes mellitus), saturated fat or *trans* fat (obesity, coronary heart disease). Recommended dietary fibre intake is based on avoiding risks of colonic disease. The usual recommended protein intake for a healthy man doing light work is 65–100 g/day. The minimum requirement is around 40 g of protein with a high proportion of essential amino acids or a high biological value.

19

1   14
CH_3 –□–□–□–□–□–□–□–□–□–□–□–□–□– COOH

□ CH_2
■ CH

Saturated fatty acid, e.g. myristic acid (14:0)

18
CH_3 –□–□–□–□–□–□–□–■–■–□–□–□–□–□–□–□– COOH

Monounsaturated fatty acid, e.g. oleic acid (18:1 $\omega9$)

CH_3 –□–□–□–□–■–■–□–■–■–□–□–□–□–□–□– COOH

Polyunsaturated fatty acid, e.g. linoleic acid (18:2 $\omega6$)

Fig. 19.4 Schematic representation of fatty acids. Standard nomenclature specifies the number of carbon atoms and indicates the number and position of the double bond(s) relative to the methyl ($-CH_3$, ω) end of the molecule after a colon.

i | **19.2 Amino acids**

Essential amino acids

- Tryptophan
- Histidine
- Methionine
- Threonine
- Isoleucine
- Valine
- Phenylalanine
- Lysine
- Leucine

Conditionally essential amino acids and their precursors

- Cysteine: methionine, serine
- Tyrosine: phenylalanine
- Arginine: glutamine/glutamate, aspartate
- Proline: glutamate
- Glycine: serine, choline

19.3 Daily adult energy requirements in health

Circumstances	Daily requirements*	
	Females	Males
At rest (basal metabolic rate)	5.4 MJ (1300 kcal)	6.7 MJ (1600 kcal)
Less active	8.0 MJ (1900 kcal)	9.9 MJ (2400 kcal)
Population median	8.8 MJ (2100 kcal)	10.8 MJ (2600 kcal)
More active	9.6 MJ (2300 kcal)	11.8 MJ (2800 kcal)

*These are based on a healthy target body mass index (BMI) of 22.5 kg/m². For a female, height is 162 cm and weight 59.0 kg; for a male, height is 175 cm and weight 68.8 kg. Previous average recommendations of 8.1 MJ (1950 kcal, usually rounded up to 2000 kcal) for females and 10.7 MJ (2500 kcal) for males should continue to be used, as these fall within experimental error.

19.4 WHO recommended population macronutrient goals

Nutrient (% of total energy unless indicated)	Target limits for average population intakes	
	Lower	Upper
Total fat	15	30
Saturated fatty acids	0	10
Polyunsaturated fatty acids	6	10
Trans fatty acids	0	2
Dietary cholesterol (mg/day)	0	300
Total carbohydrate	55	75
Free sugars	0	10
Complex carbohydrate	50	70
Dietary fibre (g/day):		
As non-starch polysaccharides	16	24
As total dietary fibre	27	40
Protein	10	15

Disorders of altered energy balance

Obesity

Obesity is regarded as a pandemic, with potentially disastrous consequences for human health. Over 25% of adults in the UK were obese (i.e. BMI ≥ 30 kg/m²) in 2015, compared with 7% in 1980 and 16% in 1995. Moreover, almost 66% of the UK adult population are overweight (BMI ≥ 25 kg/m²), although there is considerable regional and age group variation. In developing countries, average national rates of obesity are low, but these figures may disguise high rates of obesity in urban communities; for example, nearly 25% of women in urban India are overweight.

There is increasing public awareness of the health implications of obesity. Many will seek medical help for their obesity, others will present with complications of obesity, and increasing numbers are being identified during health screening examinations.

Complications

Obesity has adverse effects on both mortality and morbidity (Fig. 19.5). Changes in mortality are difficult to analyse due to the confounding effects of lower body weight in cigarette smokers and those with other illnesses (such as cancer). It is clear, however, that the lowest mortality rates are seen in Europeans in the BMI range 18.5–24 kg/m² (and at lower BMI in Asians). It is suggested that obesity at age 40 years can reduce life expectancy by up to 7 years for non-smokers and by 13 years for smokers. Coronary heart disease (Fig. 19.6) is the major cause of death but cancer rates are also increased in the overweight, especially colorectal cancer in males and cancer of the gallbladder, biliary tract, breast, endometrium and cervix in females. Obesity has little effect on life expectancy above 70 years of age, but the obese do spend a greater proportion of their active life disabled. The

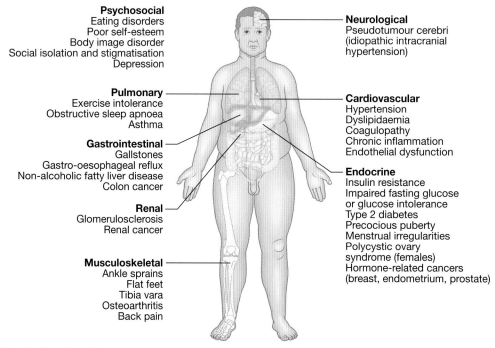

Psychosocial
Eating disorders
Poor self-esteem
Body image disorder
Social isolation and stigmatisation
Depression

Pulmonary
Exercise intolerance
Obstructive sleep apnoea
Asthma

Gastrointestinal
Gallstones
Gastro-oesophageal reflux
Non-alcoholic fatty liver disease
Colon cancer

Renal
Glomerulosclerosis
Renal cancer

Musculoskeletal
Ankle sprains
Flat feet
Tibia vara
Osteoarthritis
Back pain

Neurological
Pseudotumour cerebri
(idiopathic intracranial
hypertension)

Cardiovascular
Hypertension
Dyslipidaemia
Coagulopathy
Chronic inflammation
Endothelial dysfunction

Endocrine
Insulin resistance
Impaired fasting glucose
or glucose intolerance
Type 2 diabetes
Precocious puberty
Menstrual irregularities
Polycystic ovary
syndrome (females)
Hormone-related cancers
(breast, endometrium, prostate)

Fig. 19.5 Complications of obesity.

Fig. 19.6 **Risks of diabetes and cardiovascular disease in overweight and obese women.** Data are from the Nurses' Health Study in the USA, and mostly relate to Caucasian women. In some ethnic groups (e.g. South Asians, Native Americans) and in people with higher waist circumference, the metabolic complications are even more severe at a given level of body mass index.

19.5 Some reasons for the increasing prevalence of obesity – the 'obesogenic' environment

Increasing energy intake

- ↑ Portion sizes
- ↑ Snacking and loss of regular meals
- ↑ Energy-dense food (fat and sugars)
- ↑ Affluence

Decreasing energy expenditure

- ↑ Car ownership
- ↓ Walking to school/work
- ↑ Automation; ↓ manual labour
- ↓ Sports in schools
- ↑ Time spent on computer games and watching TV
- ↑ Central heating

in the liver and muscle, and hence induce insulin resistance and promote type 2 diabetes. Recent research has also highlighted the importance of fat deposition within specific organs, especially the liver, as an important determinant of metabolic risk in the obese.

Aetiology

Accumulation of fat results from a discrepancy between energy consumption and energy expenditure that is too large to be defended by the hypothalamic regulation of BMR. A continuous small daily positive energy balance of only 0.2–0.8 MJ (50–200 kcal; < 10% of intake) would lead to weight gain of 2–20 kg over a period of 4–10 years. Given the cumulative effects of subtle energy excess, body fat content shows 'tracking' with age, such that obese children usually become obese adults. Weight tends to increase throughout adult life, as BMR and physical activity decrease (see Fig. 19.2).

The pandemic of obesity reflects changes in both energy intake and expenditure (Box 19.5), although both are difficult to measure reliably. The estimated average global daily supply of food energy per person increased from approximately 9.8 MJ (2350 kcal) in the 1960s to approximately 11.7 MJ (2800 kcal) in the 1990s, but its delivery is unequal. For example, in India it is estimated that 5% of the population receives 40% of the available food energy, leading to obesity in the urban population in parallel with under-nutrition in some rural communities. In affluent societies, a significant proportion of this food supply is discarded. In the USA, men's average daily energy intake reportedly rose from 10.2 MJ (2450 kcal) in 1971 to 11.0 MJ (2618 kcal) in 2000. Portion sizes, particularly of energy-dense foods such as drinks with highly refined sugar content and salty snacks, have increased. However, UK data suggest that energy intakes have declined (which may in part be due to deliberate restriction or 'dieting'), but this is apparently insufficient to compensate for the decrease in physical activity in recent years. Obesity is correlated positively with the number of hours spent watching television, and inversely with levels of physical activity (e.g. stair climbing). It is suggested that minor activities such as fidgeting, also termed non-exercise activity thermogenesis (NEAT), may contribute to energy expenditure and protect against obesity.

Susceptibility to obesity

Susceptibility to obesity and its adverse consequences undoubtedly varies between individuals. It is not true that obese subjects have a 'slow metabolism', since their BMR is higher than that of lean subjects. Twin and adoption studies confirm a genetic influence on obesity. The pattern of inheritance suggests a polygenic disorder, with small contributions from a number of different genes, together accounting for 25–70% of variation in weight. Recent results from 'genome-wide' association studies of polymorphisms in large numbers of people (p. 45) have

rise in obesity has been accompanied by an epidemic of type 2 diabetes (p. 732) and osteoarthritis, particularly of the knee. Although an increased body size results in greater bone density through increased mechanical stress, it is not certain whether this translates to a lower incidence of osteoporotic fractures (p. 1044). Obesity may have profound psychological consequences, compounded by stigmatisation of the obese in many societies.

Body fat distribution

For some complications of obesity, the distribution rather than the absolute amount of excess adipose tissue appears to be important. Increased intra-abdominal fat causes 'central' ('abdominal', 'visceral', 'android' or 'apple-shaped') obesity, which contrasts with subcutaneous fat accumulation causing 'generalised' ('gynoid' or 'pear-shaped') obesity; the former is more common in men and is more closely associated with type 2 diabetes, the metabolic syndrome and cardiovascular disease (see Fig. 19.5). The key difference between these depots of fat may lie in their vascular anatomy, with intra-abdominal fat draining into the portal vein and thence directly to the liver. Thus many factors that are released from adipose tissue (including free fatty acids; 'adipokines', such as tumour necrosis factor alpha, adiponectin and resistin) may be at higher concentration

19

identified a handful of genes that influence obesity, some of which encode proteins known to be involved in the control of appetite or metabolism and some of which have an unknown function. These genes account for less than 5% of the variation in body weight, however. Genes also influence fat distribution and therefore the risk of the metabolic consequences of obesity, such as type 2 diabetes and fatty liver disease.

A few rare single-gene disorders have been identified that lead to severe childhood obesity. These include mutations of the melanocortin-4 receptor (*MC4R*), which account for approximately 5% of severe early-onset obesity; defects in the enzymes processing propiomelanocortin (*POMC*, the precursor for adrenocorticotrophic hormone (ACTH)) in the hypothalamus; and mutations in the leptin gene (see Fig. 19.3). The latter can be treated by leptin injections. Additional genetic conditions in which obesity is a feature include Prader–Willi (see Box 3.8, p. 51) and Lawrence–Moon–Biedl syndromes.

Reversible causes of obesity and weight gain

In a small minority of patients presenting with obesity, specific causal factors can be identified and treated (Box 19.6). These patients are distinguished from those with idiopathic obesity by their short history, with a recent marked change in the trajectory of their adult weight gain.

Clinical features and investigations

In assessing an individual presenting with obesity, the aims are to:

- quantify the problem
- exclude an underlying cause
- identify complications
- reach a management plan.

i	**19.6 Potentially reversible causes of weight gain**

Endocrine factors

- Hypothyroidism
- Cushing's syndrome
- Insulinoma
- Hypothalamic tumours or injury

Drug treatments

- Atypical antipsychotics (e.g. olanzapine)
- Sulphonylureas, thiazolidinediones, insulin
- Pizotifen
- Glucocorticoids
- Sodium valproate
- β-blockers

Severity of obesity can be quantified using the BMI and waist circumference. The risk of metabolic and cardiovascular complications of obesity is higher in those with a high waist circumference; lower levels of BMI and waist circumference indicate higher risk in Asian populations (Box 19.7).

A dietary history may be helpful in guiding dietary advice (p. 693) but is notoriously susceptible to under-reporting of food consumption. It is important to consider 'pathological' eating behaviour (such as binge eating, nocturnal eating or bulimia; p. 1204), which may be the most important issue to address in some patients. Alcohol is an important source of energy intake and should be considered in detail.

The history of weight gain may help diagnose underlying causes. A patient who has recently gained substantial weight or has gained weight at a faster rate than previously, and is not taking relevant drugs (see Box 19.6), is more likely to have an underlying disorder such as hypothyroidism (p. 639) or Cushing's syndrome (p. 666). All obese patients should have thyroid function tests performed on one occasion, and an overnight dexamethasone suppression test or 24-hour urine free cortisol if Cushing's syndrome is suspected. Monogenic and 'syndromic' causes of obesity are usually relevant only in children presenting with severe obesity.

Assessment of the diverse complications of obesity (see Fig. 19.5) requires a thorough history, examination and screening investigations. The impact of obesity on the patient's life and work is a major consideration. Assessment of other cardiovascular risk factors is important. Blood pressure should be measured with a large cuff, if required (p. 510). Associated type 2 diabetes and dyslipidaemia are detected by measurement of blood glucose or HbA$_{1c}$ and a serum lipid profile, ideally in a fasting morning sample. Elevated serum transaminases occur in patients with non-alcoholic fatty liver disease (p. 884).

Management

The health risks of obesity are largely reversible if identified and treated early. Interventions proven to reduce weight in obese patients also ameliorate cardiovascular risk factors. Lifestyle advice that lowers body weight and increases physical exercise reduces the incidence of type 2 diabetes (p. 743). Given the high prevalence of obesity and the large magnitude of its risks, population strategies to prevent and reverse obesity are high on the public health priority list for many countries. Initiatives include promoting healthy eating in schools, enhancing walking

i	**19.7 Quantifying obesity with BMI and waist circumference for risk of type 2 diabetes and cardiovascular disease**		
		Waist circumference[2]	
BMI (weight in kg/height in m²)	**Classification[1]**	**Men <94 cm** **Women <80 cm**	**Men 94–102 cm** **Women 80–88 cm**	**Men >102 cm** **Women >88 cm**
18.5–24.9	Reference range	Negligible	Mildly increased	Moderate
25.0–29.9	Overweight	Negligible	Moderate	Severe
>30.0	**Obese**			
30.0–34.9	Class I	Moderate	Severe	Very severe
35.0–39.9	Class II	–	Very severe	Very severe
>40.0	Class III	–	Very severe	Very severe

[1]Classification of the World Health Organisation (WHO) and International Obesity Task Force. The Western Pacific Region Office of WHO recommends that, among Asians, BMI >23.0 is overweight and >25.0 is obese. Lower cut-offs for waist circumference have also been proposed for Asians but have not been validated. [2]When BMI is >35 kg/m², waist circumference does not add to the increased risk.

and cycling options for commuters, and liaising with the food industry to reduce energy, sugar and fat content and to label foods appropriately; taxes on high-sugar drinks have also been introduced in some countries. Unfortunately, 'low-fat' foods are often still energy-dense, and current lifestyles with labour-saving devices, sedentary work and passive leisure activities have much lower energy requirements than the manual labour and household duties of previous generations.

Most patients seeking assistance with obesity are motivated to lose weight but have attempted to do so previously without long-term success. Often weight will have oscillated between periods of successful weight loss and then regain of weight. These patients may hold misconceptions that they have an underlying disease, inaccurate perceptions of their energy intake and expenditure, and an unrealistic view of the target weight that they would regard as a 'success'. An empathetic explanation of energy balance, which recognises that some individuals are more susceptible to obesity than others and may find it more difficult to lose body weight and sustain this loss, is important. Exclusion of underlying 'hormone imbalance' with simple tests is reassuring and shifts the focus on to consideration of energy balance. Appropriate goals for weight loss should be agreed, recognising that the slope of the relationship between obesity and many of its complications becomes steeper with increasing BMI, so that a given amount of weight loss achieves greater risk reduction at higher levels of BMI. A reasonable goal for most patients is to lose 5–10% of body weight.

The management plan will vary according to the severity of the obesity (see Box 19.7) and the associated risk factors and complications. It will also be influenced by availability of resources; health-care providers and regulators have generally been careful not to recommend expensive interventions (especially long-term drug therapy and surgery) for everyone who is overweight. Instead, most guidelines focus resources on short-term interventions in those who have high health risks and comorbidities associated with their obesity, and who have demonstrated their capacity to alter their lifestyle to achieve weight loss (Fig. 19.7).

Lifestyle advice

Behavioural modification to avoid some of the effects of the 'obesogenic' environment (see Box 19.5) is the cornerstone of long-term control of weight. Adopting regular eating patterns and maximising physical activity are advised, with reference to the modest extra activity required to increase physical activity level (PAL) ratios (see Fig. 19.2C). Where possible, this should be incorporated in the daily routine (e.g. walking rather than driving to work), as this is more likely to be sustained. Alternative exercise (e.g. swimming) may be considered if musculoskeletal complications prevent walking. Changes in eating behaviour (including food selection, portion size control, avoidance of snacking, regular meals to encourage satiety, and substitution of sugar with artificial sweeteners) should be discussed. Regular support from a dietitian or attendance at a weight loss group may be helpful.

Weight loss diets

In overweight people, adherence to the lifestyle advice given above may gradually induce weight loss. In obese patients, more active intervention is usually required to lose weight before conversion to the 'weight maintenance' advice given above. A significant industry has developed in marketing diets for weight loss. These vary substantially in their balance of macronutrients (Box 19.8) but there is little evidence that they vary in their medium-term (1-year) efficacy. Most involve recommending a reduction of daily total energy intake of −2.5 MJ (600 kcal) from the patient's normal consumption. Modelling data that take into account the reduced energy expenditure as weight is lost suggest that a reduction of energy intake of 100 kJ per day will lead to an eventual body weight change of about 1 kg, with half of the weight change being achieved in about 1 year and 95% of the weight change in about 3 years. Weight loss is highly variable and patient adherence is the major determinant of success. There is some evidence that weight loss diets are most effective in their early weeks and that adherence is improved by novelty of the diet; this provides some justification for switching to a different dietary regimen when weight loss slows on the first diet. Vitamin

Fig. 19.7 Therapeutic options for obesity. Relevant comorbidities include type 2 diabetes, hypertension, cardiovascular disease, sleep apnoea, and waist circumference of >102 cm in men or 88 cm in women. This is an approximate consensus of the numerous national guidelines, which vary slightly in their recommendations and are revised every few years.

i	19.8 Low-calorie diet therapy for obesity				
Diet	**% Carbohydrate**	**% Fat**	**% Protein**	**Comments**	
Normal (typical developed country)	50	30	15		
Moderate fat (e.g. Weight Watchers)	60	25	15	Maintains balance in macronutrients and micronutrients while reducing energy-dense fats	
Low carbohydrate (e.g. Atkins)	10	60	30	Induction of ketosis may suppress hunger	
High protein (e.g. Zone)	43	30	27	Protein has greater satiety effect than other macronutrients	
Low fat (e.g. Ornish)	70	13	17		

supplementation is wise in those diets in which macronutrient balance is markedly disturbed.

In some patients, more rapid weight loss is required, e.g. in preparation for surgery. There is no role for starvation diets, which risk profound loss of muscle mass and the development of arrhythmias (and even sudden death) secondary to elevated free fatty acids, ketosis and deranged electrolytes. Very-low-calorie diets (VLCDs) can be considered for short-term rapid weight loss, producing losses of 1.5–2.5 kg/week, compared to 0.5 kg/week on conventional regimens, but require the supervision of an experienced physician and nutritionist. The composition of the diet should ensure a minimum of 50 g of protein each day for men and 40 g for women to minimise muscle degradation. Energy content should be a minimum of 1.65 MJ (400 kcal) for women of height <1.73 m, and 2.1 MJ (500 kcal) for all men and for women taller than 1.73 m. Side-effects are a problem in the early stages and include orthostatic hypotension, headache, diarrhoea and nausea.

Drugs

A huge investment has been made by the pharmaceutical industry in finding drugs for obesity. The side-effect profile has limited the use of many agents, with notable withdrawals from clinical use of sibutramine (increased cardiovascular events) and rimonabant (psychiatric side-effects) in recent years. Orlistat has been available for many years, and four drugs or drug combinations have recently been approved in the USA and two of these in Europe. There is no role for diuretics, or for thyroxine therapy without biochemical evidence of hypothyroidism. Drug therapy should always be used as an adjunct to lifestyle advice and support, which should be continued throughout treatment.

Orlistat inhibits pancreatic and gastric lipases and thereby decreases the hydrolysis of ingested triglycerides, reducing dietary fat absorption by approximately 30%. The drug is not absorbed and adverse side-effects relate to the effect of the resultant fat malabsorption on the gut: namely, loose stools, oily spotting, faecal urgency, flatus and the potential for malabsorption of fat-soluble vitamins. Orlistat at the standard dose of 120 mg is taken with each of the three main meals of the day; a lower dose (60 mg) is available without prescription in some countries. Its efficacy is shown in Figure 19.8; these effects may be explained because patients taking orlistat adhere better to low-fat diets in order to avoid unpleasant gastrointestinal side-effects.

The combination of low-dose phentermine and topiramate extended release has been approved in the USA; this results in weight loss of approximately 6% greater than placebo and benefits lipids and glucose concentrations. Concerns over teratogenicity of topiramate and cardiovascular effects of phentermine have so far

Fig. 19.8 Effects of orlistat (A), liraglutide (B) and bariatric surgery (C) on weight loss. For the bariatric surgery data, each obese subject undergoing surgery was matched with a control subject whose obesity was managed according to the standard of care for non-operative interventions. Note that the maximum weight loss achieved with orlistat and liraglutide was approximately 10 kg, and that the follow-up period is relatively short; surgery achieves much more substantial and prolonged weight loss. *A, Data from Torgerson JS Hauptman J, Boldrin MS, et al. A randomized study of orlistat as an adjunct to lifestyle changes for the prevention of type 2 diabetes in obese patients. Diabetes Care 2004; 27:155–161. B, Data from le Roux CW, Astrup A, Fujioka K, et al. 3 years of liraglutide versus placebo for type 2 diabetes risk reduction and weight management in individuals with prediabetes: a randomised, double-blind trial. Lancet; published online 22 Feb 2017. C, Data from Sjöström L, Narbro K, Sjöström D, et al. Effects of bariatric surgery on mortality in Swedish obese subjects. N Engl J Med 2007; 357:741–752.*

precluded its approval in Europe. The 5-HT$_{2c}$ inhibitor lorcaserin is also approved in the USA; it is moderately effective and has a relatively low rate of adverse effects. The combination of the opioid antagonist naltrexone and the noradrenaline (norepinephrine)/dopamine re-uptake inhibitor bupropion is also effective. The main adverse effects are dry mouth and constipation. Finally, a higher dose of the injectable glucagon-like peptide-1 (GLP-1) receptor agonist liraglutide (3 mg) is also approved for use and has been shown to reduce the risk of diabetes in patients with pre-diabetes.

Drug therapy is usually reserved for patients with high risk of complications from obesity (see Fig. 19.7), and its optimum timing and duration are controversial. There is evidence that those patients who demonstrate early weight loss (usually defined as 5% after 12 weeks on the optimum dose) achieve greater and longer-term weight loss, and this is reflected in most guidelines for the use of drugs for obesity. Treatment can be stopped in non-responders at this point and an alternative treatment considered. Although life-long therapy is advocated for many drugs that reduce risk on the basis of relatively short-term research trials (e.g. drugs for hypertension and osteoporosis), some patients who continue to take anti-obesity drugs tend to regain weight with time; this may partly reflect age-related weight gain, but significant weight gain should prompt reinforcement of lifestyle advice and, if this is unsuccessful, drug therapy should be discontinued (see Fig. 19.8).

Surgery

'Bariatric' surgery is by far the most effective long-term treatment for obesity (see Fig. 19.8 and Box 19.9) and is the only anti-obesity intervention that has been associated with reduced mortality. Bariatric surgery should be contemplated in motivated patients who have very high risks of complications of obesity (see Fig. 19.7), when extensive dietary and drug therapy has been insufficiently effective. It is usually reserved for those with severe obesity (BMI >40 kg/m^2), or those with a BMI >35 kg/m^2 and significant complications, such as type 2 diabetes or obstructive sleep apnoea, although some evidence-based guidelines now suggest surgery can be considered at a lower weight in people with recent-onset diabetes and a BMI >30 kg/m^2. Only experienced specialist surgeons should undertake these procedures, in collaboration with a multidisciplinary team. Several approaches are used (Fig. 19.9) and all can be performed laparoscopically. The mechanism of weight loss may not simply relate to limiting the stomach or absorptive capacity, but rather in disrupting the release of ghrelin from the stomach or promoting the release of other peptides from the small bowel, thereby enhancing satiety signalling in the hypothalamus. Diabetes may improve rapidly

i **19.9 Effectiveness and adverse effects of laparoscopic bariatric surgical procedures**

Procedure	Expected weight loss (% excess weight)	Adverse effects
Gastric banding	50–60%	Band slippage, erosion, stricture Port site infection Mortality <0.2% in experienced centres
Sleeve gastrectomy	50–60%	Iron deficiency Vitamin B$_{12}$ deficiency Mortality <0.2% in experienced centres
Roux-en-Y gastric bypass	70–80%	Internal hernia Stomal ulcer Dumping syndrome Hypoglycaemia Iron deficiency Vitamin B$_{12}$ deficiency Vitamin D deficiency Mortality 0.5%
Duodenal switch	Up to 100%	Steatorrhoea Protein-calorie malnutrition Iron deficiency Vitamin B$_{12}$ deficiency Calcium, zinc, copper deficiency Mortality 1%

19

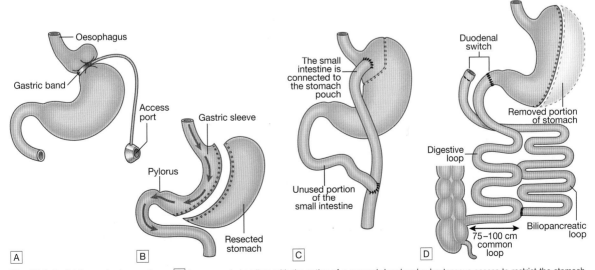

Fig. 19.9 Bariatric surgical procedures. **A** Laparoscopic banding, with the option of a reservoir band and subcutaneous access to restrict the stomach further after compensatory expansion has occurred. **B** Sleeve gastrectomy. **C** Roux-en-Y gastric bypass. **D** Biliopancreatic diversion with duodenal switch.

after surgery, particularly after gastric bypass, and although this may be attributed to severe energy restriction in the perioperative period, it is possible that increased release of incretin hormones such as GLP-1 may contribute to the improvement in glucose control. Complications depend on the approach. Mortality is low in experienced centres but post-operative respiratory problems, wound infection and dehiscence, staple leaks, stomal stenosis, marginal ulcers and venous thrombosis may occur. Additional problems may arise at a later stage, such as pouch and distal oesophageal dilatation, persistent vomiting, 'dumping' (p. 801), hypoglycaemia and micronutrient deficiencies, particularly of folate, vitamin B_{12} and iron, which are of special concern to women contemplating pregnancy; this should be delayed for at least 2 years following surgery.

Cosmetic surgical procedures may be considered in obese patients after successful weight loss. Apronectomy is usually advocated to remove an overhang of abdominal skin, especially if infected or ulcerated. This operation is of no value for long-term weight reduction if food intake remains unrestricted.

Treatment of additional risk factors

Obesity must not be treated in isolation and other risk factors must be addressed, including smoking, excess alcohol consumption, diabetes mellitus, hyperlipidaemia, hypertension and obstructive sleep apnoea. Treatment of these is discussed in the relevant chapters.

Under-nutrition

Starvation and famine

There remain regions of the world, particularly rural Africa, where under-nutrition due to famine is endemic, the prevalence of BMI of less than 18.5 kg/m^2 (Box 19.10) in adults is as high as 20%, and growth retardation due to under-nutrition affects 50% of children. The World Health Organisation (WHO) reports that chronic under-nutrition is responsible for more than half of all childhood deaths worldwide. Starvation is manifest as marasmus (malnutrition with marked muscle wasting) or, when additive complications such as oxidative stress come into play, malnourished children can develop kwashiorkor (malnutrition with oedema). Growth retardation is due to deficiencies of key nutrients (protein, zinc, potassium, phosphate and sulphur). Treatment of these childhood conditions is not discussed in this adult medical textbook. In adults, starvation is the result of chronic sustained negative energy (calorie) balance. Causes are shown in Box 19.11. Causes of weight loss are considered further on page 785.

Clinical features

In starvation, the severity of malnutrition can be assessed by anthropometric measurements, such as BMI (see p. 693 and Box 19.10). Demispan and mid-arm circumference measurements are most useful in monitoring progress during treatment. The clinical features of severe under-nutrition in adults are listed in Box 19.12.

Under-nutrition often leads to vitamin deficiencies, especially of thiamin, folate and vitamin C (see below). Diarrhoea can lead to depletion of sodium, potassium and magnesium. The high mortality rate in famine situations is often due to outbreaks of infection, such as typhus or cholera, but the usual signs of infection may not be apparent. In advanced starvation, patients become completely inactive and may assume a flexed, fetal position. In the last stage of starvation, death comes quietly and often quite suddenly. The very old are most vulnerable. All organs are atrophied at necropsy, except the brain, which tends to maintain its weight.

Investigations

In a famine, laboratory investigations may be impractical but will show that plasma free fatty acids are increased and there is ketosis and a mild metabolic acidosis. Plasma glucose is low

19.11 Causes of under-nutrition and weight loss in adults

Decreased energy intake

- Famine
- Persistent regurgitation or vomiting
- Anorexia, including depression and anorexia nervosa
- Malabsorption (e.g. small intestinal disease)
- Maldigestion (e.g. pancreatic exocrine insufficiency)

Increased energy expenditure

- Increased basal metabolic rate (thyrotoxicosis, trauma, fever, cancer, cachexia)
- Excessive physical activity (e.g. marathon runners)
- Energy loss (e.g. glycosuria in diabetes)
- Impaired energy storage (e.g. Addison's disease, phaeochromocytoma)

19.12 Clinical features of severe under-nutrition in adults

- Weight loss
- Thirst, craving for food, weakness and feeling cold
- Nocturia, amenorrhoea or impotence
- Lax, pale, dry skin with loss of turgor and, occasionally, pigmented patches
- Cold and cyanosed extremities, pressure sores
- Hair thinning or loss (except in adolescents)
- Muscle-wasting, best demonstrated by the loss of the temporalis and periscapular muscles and reduced mid-arm circumference
- Loss of subcutaneous fat, reflected in reduced skinfold thickness and mid-arm circumference
- Hypothermia, bradycardia, hypotension and small heart
- Oedema, which may be present without hypoalbuminaemia ('famine oedema')
- Distended abdomen with diarrhoea
- Diminished tendon jerks
- Apathy, loss of initiative, depression, introversion, aggression if food is nearby
- Susceptibility to infections (Box 19.13)

19.10 Classification of under-nutrition in adults by body mass index (weight/height^2)

BMI (kg/m^2)	Classification
>20	Adequate nutrition
18.5–20	Marginal
<18.5	**Under-nutrition**
17–18.4	Mild
16–17	Moderate
<16	Severe

- Gastroenteritis and Gram-negative sepsis
- Respiratory infections, especially bronchopneumonia
- Certain viral diseases, especially measles and herpes simplex
- Tuberculosis
- Streptococcal and staphylococcal skin infections
- Helminthic infestations

i 19.14 WHO recommended diets for refeeding

Nutrient (per 100 mL)	F-75 diet[1]	F-100 diet[2]
Energy	315 kJ (75 kcal)	420 kJ (100 kcal)
Protein (g)	0.9	2.9
Lactose (g)	1.3	4.2
Potassium (mmol)	3.6	5.9
Sodium (mmol)	0.9	1.9
Magnesium (mmol)	0.43	0.73
Zinc (mg)	2.0	2.3
Copper (mg)	0.25	0.25
Percentage of energy from: Protein Fat	5 32	12 53
Osmolality (mOsmol/kg)	333	419
Dose	170 kJ/kg (40 kcal/kg)	630–920 kJ/kg (150–220 kcal/kg)
Rate of feeding by mouth	2.2 (mL/kg/hr)	Gradual increase in volume, 6 times daily

[1]F-75 is prepared from milk powder (25 g), sugar (70 g), cereal flour (35 g), vegetable oil (27 g) and vitamin and mineral supplements, made up to 1 L with water. [2]F-100 (1 L) contains milk powder (80 g), sugar (50 g), vegetable oil (60 g) and vitamin and mineral supplements (no cereal).

but albumin concentration is often maintained because the liver still functions normally. Insulin secretion is diminished, glucagon and cortisol tend to increase, and reverse T_3 replaces normal triiodothyronine (p. 634). The resting metabolic rate falls, partly because of reduced lean body mass and partly because of hypothalamic compensation (see Fig. 19.2). The urine has a fixed specific gravity and creatinine excretion becomes low. There may be mild anaemia, leucopenia and thrombocytopenia. The erythrocyte sedimentation rate is normal unless there is infection. Tests of delayed skin hypersensitivity, e.g. to tuberculin, are falsely negative. The electrocardiogram shows sinus bradycardia and low voltage.

Management

Whether in a famine or in wasting secondary to disease, the severity of under-nutrition is graded according to BMI (see Box 19.10). People with mild starvation are in no danger; those with moderate starvation need extra feeding; and those who are severely underweight need hospital care.

In severe starvation, there is atrophy of the intestinal epithelium and of the exocrine pancreas, and the bile is dilute. It is critical for the condition to be managed by experts. When food becomes available, it should be given by mouth in small, frequent amounts at first, using a suitable formula preparation (Box 19.14). Individual energy requirements can vary by 30%. During rehabilitation, more concentrated formula can be given with additional food that is palatable and similar to the usual staple meal. Salt should be restricted and micronutrient supplements (e.g. potassium, magnesium, zinc and multivitamins) may be essential. Between 6.3 and 8.4 MJ/day (1500–2000 kcal/day) will arrest progressive under-nutrition but additional energy may be required for regain of weight. During refeeding, a weight gain of 5% body weight per month indicates satisfactory progress. Other care is supportive and includes attention to the skin, adequate hydration, treatment of infections and careful monitoring of body temperature, since thermoregulation may be impaired.

Circumstances and resources are different in every famine but many problems are non-medical and concern organisation, infrastructure, liaison, politics, procurement, security and ensuring that food is distributed on the basis of need. Lastly, plans must be made for the future for prevention and/or earlier intervention if similar circumstances prevail.

Under-nutrition in hospital

It is a paradox that, in spite of record levels of access to food in the developed economies of the world, under-nutrition remains a serious issue in many sectors of society, particularly the elderly and less independent. While the scale of the problem does not match that seen in the developing world, the issues pertaining to poor or impaired health are similar. In the general UK population, 30% of those requiring acute admission to hospital show evidence of serious under-nutrition and 65% of those admitted will lose an

average of 5% of their total body weight during that admission. In the older population, levels of under-nutrition and vitamin deficiencies parallel levels of independent living. In Scotland, 33% of those aged over 65 who are living in their own home are deficient in folic acid and 10% are deficient in vitamin C. The prevalence of vitamin deficiencies rises further in less independent groups in residential or nursing homes.

Under-nutrition is poorly recognised in hospitals and has serious consequences. Physical effects include impaired immunity and muscle weakness, which in turn affect cardiac and respiratory function, and delayed wound healing after surgery with increased risks of post-operative infection. The under-nourished patient is often withdrawn and this may be mistaken for depressive illness. Engagement with treatment and rehabilitation can be adversely affected. Much of this can be avoided through better awareness of the prevalence of under-nutrition, prompt nutritional assessment and monitoring with appropriate intervention. Scoring systems, such as the MUST tool (p. 693), raise awareness across multidisciplinary teams, and encourage staff to assess and monitor food intake and weigh patients regularly.

Causes are often complex (see Box 19.11). Social issues impact on food choices and may cause or exacerbate disease. Social isolation, low levels of disposable income and a lack of knowledge or interest in healthy eating may increase reliance on calorie-dense convenience foods of poor nutritional quality. In turn, the non-specific effects of chronic inflammation, infection or malignancy, as well as specific gastrointestinal disorders, may adversely affect appetite, reducing food intake. Patients may report avoidance of certain foods that exacerbate their symptoms (often fibre-rich, otherwise healthy foods).

A loss of appetite is not specific to gastrointestinal disease and may be seen as a non-specific response to myriad other conditions or their treatments. The most common reported side-effects

19

19.15 Factors affecting adequacy of nutritional intake in hospitalised patients

Factors affecting appetite
- Altered taste
- Nausea and/or vomiting
- Non-specific effects of illness and/or drugs

Issues of quantity
- Is there enough food on the plate?
- Social, cultural, financial, general and mental health issues may all be relevant, individually or in combination

Getting the food from the plate to the mouth
- Generalised reduced mobility
- Reduced manual dexterity
- Loss of limb function

Difficulties chewing the food
- Poorly fitting dentures
- Pain in the oral cavity

Specific problems with the gastrointestinal tract
- Obstruction
- Ischaemia
- Inflammation
- Malabsorption

Cultural issues
- Is the food provided appropriate to the patient's beliefs?

More general evidence of self-neglect
- Evidence of chronic coexisting illness
- Evidence of mental health problems – low mood may be 'cause' or 'effect' in under-nutrition

of many prescription drugs are nausea and gastrointestinal disturbance. Surgical resection of the gastrointestinal tract can have major nutritional sequelae in the years following, ranging from intolerance of normal volumes of food to intestinal failure (where there is partial or complete failure of the intestine to perform its vital functions). There may be no single problem impacting on the intake of adequate nutrition but it helps to consider systematically where the problem(s) might lie (Box 19.15).

Specific issues arising after intestinal surgery

Gastrectomy or partial gastrectomy

There may be a loss of gastric capacity, leading to intolerance of larger volumes of food and early satiety or vomiting. Vagotomy and gastroenterostomy may cause symptoms of dumping syndrome (p. 801), which can lead to food avoidance and weight loss. Many patients who have had gastric surgery will develop iron deficiency (and, less commonly, vitamin D and vitamin B$_{12}$ deficiency) unless adequately supplemented post-operatively.

Proximal small bowel surgery

Those who have had roux-en-Y reconstruction or have blind-ending or excluded loops of small bowel are prone to small intestinal bacterial overgrowth. This may impair absorption of iron, folic acid and vitamin B$_{12}$. Very rarely, it can cause hyperammonaemia and metabolic coma, in which bacterial metabolism of amino acids leads to a lack of citrulline and impairment of the urea cycle.

Pancreatic resection/Whipple's operation

Without adequate post-operative supplementation, this can be a very serious insult to the digestive tract. There is loss of pancreatic exocrine function (causing steatorrhoea and malabsorption of protein, fats and fat-soluble vitamins), as well as the potential for small intestinal bacterial overgrowth (malabsorption of iron, folic acid and vitamin B$_{12}$).

Ileal resection

Ileal resection (p. 810) may give rise to vitamin B$_{12}$ deficiency and, rarely, to steatorrhoea and malabsorption of fat-soluble vitamins.

Massive small bowel resection

This may cause short bowel syndrome and intestinal failure, with impaired ability to absorb fluids, electrolytes and macronutrients adequately without parenteral support.

An approach to assisted nutrition in hospital patients

Once the problems leading to under-nutrition have been recognised, it is important to make an individualised plan to address these issues specifically. In most cases, this means a decision to intervene to tackle and reverse nutritional difficulties. This may involve simply ensuring that adequate supplies of food are delivered and prepared regularly or that dentures fit properly, but may require an assessment of a patient's ability to swallow or of the intestine's ability to digest foods. This must include consideration of the potential for disruption of the normal physiology of absorption and digestion in the context of the patient's medical and surgical history. Whenever possible, it is best to use the most physiological means of feeding, reserving more invasive interventions for when normal physiological mechanisms of swallowing and digestion are impaired or absent. Enteral feeding is preferred to parenteral, provided the intestine is accessible and functioning.

Refeeding syndrome

In severely malnourished individuals, attempts at rapid correction of malnutrition switch the body from a reliance on fat to carbohydrate metabolism. Release of insulin is triggered, shifting potassium, phosphate and magnesium into cells (with water following the osmotic gradient) and causing potentially fatal shifts of fluids and electrolytes from the extracellular to the intracellular compartment. Rapid depletion of (already low) thiamin exacerbates the condition. Clinical features include nausea, vomiting, muscle weakness, seizures, respiratory depression, cardiac arrest and sudden death. The risks of refeeding are greatest in those who are most malnourished (especially chronic alcoholics), but even those who have gone without food for 5 days can be at risk and restitution of feeding should always be done slowly, with careful monitoring of serum potassium, phosphate and magnesium in the first 3–5 days.

Oral nutritional supplements

Poor appetite, immobility, poor dentition or even being kept 'nil by mouth' for hospital procedures all contribute to weight loss. As a first step, patients should be encouraged and helped to eat an adequate amount of normal food. Where swallow and intestinal function remain intact, the simplest form of assisted nutrition is the use of oral nutritional supplements. Most branded products are nutritionally complete (fortified with the daily requirements of vitamins, minerals and trace elements). They most often come in the form of liquid drinks but various formulations and textures exist, including 'shakes' and 'puddings' with a thicker consistency. They are cost-effective and very useful for people who may require just a small number of additional calories each day to maintain or gain weight in the short or longer term. However, in spite of their nutritional value, small volume and range of flavours, many people find them unpalatable or difficult to tolerate.

Enteral feeding

Where swallowing or food ingestion is impaired but intestinal function remains intact, more invasive forms of assisted feeding may be necessary. Enteral tube feeding is usually the intervention of choice. In enteral feeding, nutrition is delivered to and absorbed by the functioning intestine. Delivery usually means bypassing the mouth and oesophagus (or sometimes the stomach and proximal small bowel) by means of a feeding tube (naso-enteral, gastrostomy or jejunostomy feeding). There are a number of theoretical advantages to enteral, as opposed to parenteral, feeding, which have achieved almost mythical status. These include:

- preservation of intestinal mucosal architecture, gut-associated lymphoid tissue, and hepatic and pulmonary immune function
- reduced levels of systemic inflammation and hyperglycaemia
- interference with pathogenicity of gut micro-organisms.

However, the areas in which advantage has been consistently *proven* are:

- fewer episodes of infection
- reduced cost
- earlier return to intestinal function
- reduced length of hospital stay.

Complications

The risks of enteral feeding are those related to tube insertion (Box 19.16) and diarrhoea (Box 19.17).

Route of access

Nasogastric tube feeding This is simple, readily available, comparatively low-cost and most suitable for short-term feeding (up to 4 weeks). Insertion of a nasogastric tube requires care and training (see Box 21.41, p. 805), as potentially serious complications can arise (Box 19.16). Patients with reduced conscious level may pull at tubes and displace them. This can be minimised in the short term by the use of a nasal 'bridle'

device, which fixes the tube around the nasal septum. Although these devices are very effective, there is a risk of damage to the nasal septum (especially bleeding) if a patient persists in pulling forcibly on the tube.

Gastrostomy feeding Gastrostomy is a more invasive insertion technique with higher costs initially. It is most suitable for when longer-term feeding (more than 4 weeks) is required. Gastrostomies are less liable to displacement than nasogastric tubes and the presence of the gastrostomy in the stomach allows for fewer feed interruptions, meaning that more of the prescribed feeds can be administered. Tubes were placed at the time of open surgery until the 1980s, when an endoscopic, minimally invasive technique was developed. A variety of techniques for radiological insertion have also been introduced subsequently. Both endoscopic and radiological gastrostomy insertion involve inflating the stomach, thus apposing it to the anterior abdominal wall. The stomach is then punctured percutaneously and a suitable tube placed (Fig. 19.10). Tubes vary in design but each has an internal retainer device (plastic 'bumper' or balloon) that sits snugly against the gastric mucosa, and an external retainer that limits movement. These retainers hold the gastric wall against the abdominal wall, effectively creating a controlled gastrocutaneous fistula that matures over 2–4 weeks. Radiological gastrostomy placement also utilises percutaneous 'stay sutures', which provide further temporary anchorage and assist in placement. There is no evidence to recommend one technique over another, although the radiological method has advantages in patients with cancers of the head and neck undergoing potentially curative therapy (less chance of tumour 'seeding') and in those with poor respiratory reserve (such as motor neuron disease) since there is no endoscope to compress the upper airways. Reported outcomes are broadly similar for both and the choice of technique should be based on indications and contraindications, operator experience and facilities available. Most important is rigorous patient assessment and selection prior to gastrostomy placement, which should be done by a multidisciplinary nutrition support team, and avoided when the procedure may be too hazardous or the benefits are outweighed by the risks (see Boxes 19.18 and Box 19.27 below).

Post-pyloric feeding In patients with a high risk of pulmonary aspiration or gastroparesis, it may be preferable to feed into the jejunum (via a nasojejunal tube, gastrostomy with jejunal extension or direct placement into jejunum by radiological, endoscopic or laparoscopic means).

Parenteral nutrition

This is usually reserved for clinical situations where the absorptive functioning of the intestine is severely impaired. In parenteral feeding, nutrition is delivered directly into a large-diameter systemic vein, completely bypassing the intestine and portal venous system. As well as being more invasive, more expensive and

19

 19.16 Complications of nasogastric tube feeding

- Tube misplacement, e.g. tracheal or bronchial placement (*rarely*, intracranial placement)
- Reflux of gastric contents and pulmonary aspiration
- Interrupted feeding or inadequate feed volumes
- Refeeding syndrome

 19.17 Diarrhoea related to enteral feeding

Factors contributing to diarrhoea

- Fibre-free feed may reduce short-chain fatty acid production in colon
- Fat malabsorption
- Inappropriate osmotic load
- Pre-existing primary gut problem (e.g. lactose intolerance)
- Infection

Management

- Often responds well to a fibre-containing feed or a switch to an alternative feed
- Simple antidiarrhoeal agents (e.g. loperamide) can be very effective

---

 19.18 Complications of gastrostomy tube feeding

- Reflux of gastric contents and pulmonary aspiration (same as nasogastric tube)
- Risks of insertion (pain, damage to intra-abdominal structures, intestinal perforation, pulmonary aspiration, infection, death)
- Risk of tumour 'seeding' if an endoscopic 'pull-through' technique is used in head and neck or oesophageal cancer patients
- Refeeding syndrome

Fig. 19.10 Percutaneous endoscopic gastrostomy (PEG) placement. A Finger pressure on the anterior abdominal wall is noted by the endoscopist. B Following insertion of a cannula through the anterior abdominal wall into the stomach, a guidewire is threaded through the cannula and grasped by the endoscopic forceps or snare. C The endoscope is withdrawn with the guidewire. The gastrostomy tube is then attached to the guidewire. D The guidewire and tube are pulled back through the mouth, oesophagus and stomach to exit on the anterior abdominal wall, and the endoscope is repassed to confirm the site of placement of the retention device. The latter closely abuts the gastric mucosa; its position is maintained by an external fixation device (see inset). It is also possible to place PEG tubes using fluoroscopic guidance when endoscopy is difficult (radiologically inserted gastrostomy).

---

i 19.19 Complications of parenteral nutrition

Intravenous catheter complications

- Insertion (pneumothorax, haemothorax, arterial puncture)
- Catheter infection (sepsis, discitis, pulmonary or cerebral abscess)
- Central venous thrombosis

Metabolic complications

- Refeeding syndrome
- Electrolyte imbalance
- Hyperglycaemia
- Hyperalimentation
- Fluid overload
- Hepatic steatosis/fibrosis/cirrhosis

---

i 19.20 Parameters for monitoring parenteral nutrition in hospital

Parameter	Monitoring requirement
Electrolytes (sodium, potassium, magnesium) **Bone profile** (calcium, phosphate) **Liver function tests** (bilirubin, alanine aminotransferase, alkaline phosphatase, γ-glutamyl transferase) **Markers of inflammation** (C-reactive protein, leucocyte count)	Daily until stable and then 2–3 times per week
Blood glucose	At least twice daily until stable and then daily
Cholesterol and triglycerides	Weekly initially, reducing to every 3 months when stable

---

less physiological than the enteral route, parenteral nutrition is associated with many more complications (Box 19.19), mainly infective and metabolic (disturbances of electrolytes, hyperglycaemia). Strict adherence to aseptic practice in handling catheters and careful monitoring of clinical (pulse, blood pressure and temperature) and biochemical (urea, electrolytes, glucose and liver function tests) parameters are necessary to minimise risk to the patient (Box 19.20).

The parenteral route may be indicated for patients who are malnourished or at risk of becoming so, and who have an inadequate or unsafe oral intake and a poorly functioning or non-functioning or perforated intestine or an intestine that cannot be accessed by tube feeding. In practice, it is most often required in acutely ill patients with multi-organ failure or in severely under-nourished patients undergoing surgery. It may offer a benefit over oral or enteral feeding prior to surgery in those who are severely malnourished when other routes of feeding have been inadequate. Parenteral nutrition following surgery should be reserved for when enteral nutrition is not tolerated or feasible or where complications (especially sepsis

impair gastrointestinal function, such that oral or enteral feeding is not possible for at least 7 days.

Intestinal failure ('short bowel syndrome')

Intestinal failure (IF) is defined as a reduction in the function of the gut below the minimum necessary for the absorption of macronutrients and/or water and electrolytes such that intravenous supplementation is required to support health and/or growth. The term can be used only when there is both:

- a major reduction in absorptive capacity *and*
- an absolute need for intravenous fluid support.

IF can be further classified according to its onset, metabolic consequences and expected outcome.

- *Type 1 IF*: an acute-onset, usually self-limiting condition with few long-term sequelae. It is most often seen following abdominal surgery or in the context of critical illness. Intravenous support may be required for a few days to weeks.

- *Type 2 IF*: far less common. The onset is also usually acute, following some intra-abdominal catastrophic event (ischaemia, volvulus, trauma or perioperative complication). Septic and metabolic problems are seen, along with complex nutritional issues. It requires multidisciplinary input (nursing, dietetic, medical, biochemical, surgical, radiological and microbiological) and support may be necessary for weeks to months.
- *Type 3 IF*: a chronic condition in which patients are metabolically stable but intravenous support is required over months to years. It may or may not be reversible.

Management

IF is a complex clinical problem with profound and wide-ranging physiological and psychological effects, which is best cared for by a dedicated multidisciplinary team. The majority of IF results from short bowel syndrome (Box 19.21), with chronic intestinal dysmotility and chronic intestinal pseudo-obstruction accounting for most of the remainder. The severity of the physiological upset correlates well with how much functioning intestine remains (rather than how much has been removed). Measurement of the remaining small bowel (from the duodeno-jejunal flexure) at the time of surgery is essential for planning future therapy (Box 19.22). The aims of treatment are to:

- provide nutrition, water and electrolytes to maintain health with normal body weight (and allow normal growth in affected children)
- utilise the enteral or oral routes as much as possible
- minimise the burden of complications of the underlying disease, as well as the IF and its treatment
- allow a good quality of life.

If the ileum and especially the ileum and colon remain intact, long-term nutritional support can usually be avoided. Unlike the jejunum, the ileum can adapt to increase absorption of water and electrolytes over time. The presence of the colon (part or wholly intact) further improves fluid absorption and can generate energy through production of short-chain fatty acids. It is therefore useful to classify patients with a short gut according to whether or not they have any residual colon.

Jejunum–colon patients

Those with an anastomosis between jejunum and residual colon (jejunum–colon patients) may look well in the days or initial weeks

following the acute insult but develop protein-energy malnutrition and significant weight loss, becoming seriously under-nourished over weeks to months.

Stool volume is determined by oral intake, with higher intakes causing more diarrhoea and the potential for dehydration, sodium and magnesium depletion and acute renal failure. The absence of the ileum leads to deficiencies of vitamin B_{12} and fat-soluble vitamins. The absorption of various drugs, including thyroxine, digoxin and warfarin, can be reduced. Approximately 45% of patients will develop gallstones due to disruption of the enterohepatic circulation of bile acids, and 25% may develop calcium oxalate renal stones due to increased colonic absorption of oxalate (see Fig. 21.43, p. 810).

Jejunostomy patients

Patients left with a stoma (usually a jejunostomy) behave very differently, although stool volumes are again determined by oral intake. The jejunum is intrinsically highly permeable, and in the absence of the ileum and its net absorptive role, high losses of fluid, sodium and magnesium dominate the clinical picture from the outset. Dehydration, hyponatraemia, hypomagnesaemia and acute renal failure are the most immediate problems but protein-energy malnutrition will also develop. The jejunum has no real potential for adaptation in terms of absorption, so it is essential to recognise and address the issues of dehydration and electrolyte disturbance early and not expect the problems to improve with time (Box 19.23).

19.23 Management of short bowel patients (and 'high-output' stoma)
Accurate charting of fluid intake and losses
• Vital: oral intake determines stool volume and should be *restricted* rather than encouraged
Dehydration and hyponatraemia
• Must first be corrected intravenously to restore circulating volume and reduce thirst
• Stool volume should be minimised and any ongoing fluid imbalance between oral intake and stool losses replenished intravenously
Measures to reduce stool volume losses
• *Restrict* oral fluid intake to ≤500 mL/24 hrs
• Give a further 1000 mL oral fluid as oral rehydration solution containing 90–120 mmol Na/L (St Mark's solution or Glucodrate, Nestlé)
• Slow intestinal transit (to maximise opportunities for absorption): Loperamide, codeine phosphate
• Reduce volume of intestinal secretions: Gastric acid: omeprazole 20 mg/day orally Other secretions: octreotide 50–100 µg 3 times daily by subcutaneous injection
Measures to increase absorption
• Teduglutide (a recombinant glucagon-like peptide 2) significantly reduces requirements for intravenous fluid and nutritional support

19

19.21 Causes of short bowel syndrome in adults
• Mesenteric ischaemia
• Post-operative complications
• Crohn's disease
• Trauma
• Neoplasia
• Radiation enteritis

19.22 Likely requirements for support according to length of intact residual small bowel					
Residual length of jejunum (cm)	**Oral fluid restriction**	**Oral glucose/electrolyte solution**	**Intravenous fluids**	**Parenteral nutrition**
<200	Yes	Yes	May avoid	May avoid
<100	Yes	Yes	Yes	May avoid
<75	Yes	Yes	Yes	Yes

Small bowel and multivisceral transplantation

Long-term intravenous nutritional support remains the mainstay of therapy for chronic IF but has its own morbidity and mortality. The 10-year survival for patients on long-term home parenteral nutrition is approximately 90%. The majority of deaths are due to the underlying disease process but 5–11% will die from direct complications of parenteral nutrition itself (especially catheter-related sepsis). A minority of patients with chronic IF, for whom the safe administration of parenteral nutrition has become difficult or impossible, may benefit from small bowel transplantation (Box 19.24). The first successful small bowel transplant was carried out in 1988. The introduction of tacrolimus allowed a satisfactory balance of immunosuppression, avoiding rejection while minimising sepsis. Since then, over 2000 transplants have been performed worldwide. Survival rates continue to improve, for both isolated small bowel and multivisceral transplantation (small bowel along with a combination of liver and/or kidney and/or pancreas), although major complications are still frequent (Box 19.25). Current 5-year survival rates are 50–80%, with better outcomes for younger patients and those receiving isolated small bowel procedures.

Further developments in treatment of intestinal failure

Teduglutide is a long-acting recombinant human GLP-2. It enhances intestinal absorption by:

- increasing intestinal blood flow to the intestine
- increasing portal blood flow away from the intestine
- slowing intestinal transit times
- reducing gastric acid secretion.

In patients with short bowel syndrome and IF, the increased intestinal absorptive function induced by teduglutide can significantly reduce the volumes of parenteral fluids and nutrition required, and may allow some patients to regain independence of parenteral support. Recognised side-effects include abdominal cramps and distension (seen in 50%), peristomal swelling, pain, nausea, vomiting and local injection site reactions. Since teduglutide stimulates proliferation of the intestinal epithelium, it should be avoided in those with a history of gastrointestinal malignancy in the past 5 years or a current malignancy. In those patients with a colon, a pre-treatment screening colonoscopy should be undertaken to detect and remove any polyps. Use of teduglutide is currently limited by high costs.

Artificial nutrition at the end of life

Rarely, assisted nutrition may not result in the expected outcomes of reversal of weight loss or improved quality and duration of life. It very seldom reverses other underlying health issues, although it may be used as a short term 'bridge' to help through a patient through a particular crisis.

Such scenarios may present when someone is approaching the end of life, or in the face of weight loss due to advanced

---

19.26 Energy balance in old age

- **Body composition**: muscle mass is decreased and percentage of body fat increased.
- **Energy expenditure**: with the fall in lean body mass, basal metabolic rate is decreased and energy requirements are reduced.
- **Weight loss**: after weight gain throughout adult life, weight often falls beyond the age of 80 years. This may reflect decreased appetite, loss of smell and taste, and decreased interest in and financial resources for food preparation, especially after loss of a partner.
- **BMI**: less reliable in old age as height is lost (due to kyphosis, osteoporotic crush fractures, loss of intervertebral disc spaces). Alternative measurements include arm demispan and knee height (p. 693), which can be extrapolated to estimate height.

---

i **19.24 Potential indications for small bowel transplantation**

Complications of central venous catheters

- Central venous thrombosis leading to loss of two or more intravenous access points
- Severe or recurrent line sepsis
- Recurrent severe acute kidney injury related to dehydration

Metabolic complications of parenteral nutrition

- Parenteral nutrition-related liver fibrosis, cirrhosis and liver failure

---

i **19.27 Ethical and legal considerations in the management of artificial nutritional support**

- Care of the sick involves the duty of providing adequate fluid and nutrients
- Food and fluid should not be withheld from a patient who expresses a desire to eat and drink, unless there is a medical contraindication (e.g. risk of aspiration)
- A treatment plan should include consideration of nutritional issues and should be agreed by all members of the health-care team
- In the situation of palliative care, tube feeding should be instituted only if it is needed to relieve symptoms
- Tube feeding is usually regarded in law as a medical treatment. Like other treatments, the need for such support should be reviewed on a regular basis and changes made in the light of clinical circumstances
- A competent adult patient must give consent for any invasive procedures, including passage of a nasogastric tube or insertion of a central venous cannula
- If a patient is unable to give consent, the health-care team should act in that person's best interests, taking into account any wishes previously expressed by the patient and the views of family
- Under certain specified circumstances (e.g. anorexia nervosa), it is appropriate to provide artificial nutritional support to the unwilling patient

Adapted from British Association for Parenteral and Enteral Nutrition guidelines (www.bapen.org.uk).

---

i **19.25 Complications of small bowel/multivisceral transplantation**

- Sepsis:
  - Enteric bacterial species
  - Staphylococci
  - Fungal species
- Cytomegalovirus infection
- Post-transplantation lymphoproliferative disease (PTLD)
- Graft-versus-host disease
- Acute and chronic rejection
- Chronic renal impairment

respiratory or cardiac failure, malignancy or dementia. In selected cases, a decision not to intervene may be appropriate. An intervention that merely prolongs life without preserving or adding to its quality is seldom justified, particularly if the intervention is not without risk itself. Such decisions are not taken lightly and careful scrutiny of each case is necessary. There should be a thoughtful and sensitive discussion explaining what artificial nutrition can and cannot achieve involving the multidisciplinary team looking after the patient as well as next of kin and, in some cases, legal representatives (Box 19.27).

Nutrition and dementia

Weight loss is seen commonly in people with dementia, and nutritional and eating problems are a significant source of concern for those caring for them. It is appropriate to:

- screen for malnutrition (e.g. MUST, see above)
- assess specific eating difficulties (e.g. Edinburgh Feeding Evaluation in Dementia questionnaire)
- monitor and document body weight
- encourage adequate intake of food
- use oral nutritional supplements.

However, the evidence that artificial nutritional support beyond oral supplementation improves overall functioning or prolongs life in dementia is absent or weak. There may be specific circumstances where a trial of such feeding can be justified (see Box 19.27). Success is more likely in those with mild to moderate dementia, when a temporary and reversible crisis has been precipitated by some acute event. It is important to remember that there is strong evidence to avoid tube feeding in those with advanced dementia because this improves neither the quality nor the duration of life (Fig. 19.11).

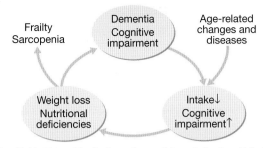

Fig. 19.11 Malnutrition in dementia – a vicious circle. *From Volkert D, Chourdakis M, Faxen-Irving G, et al. ESPEN guidelines on nutrition in dementia. Clin Nutr 2015; 34:1052–1073.*

Micronutrients, minerals and their diseases

Vitamins

Vitamins are organic substances with key roles in certain metabolic pathways, and are categorised into those that are fat-soluble (vitamins A, D, E and K) and those that are water-soluble (vitamins of the B complex group and vitamin C).

Recommended daily intakes of micronutrients (Box 19.28) vary between countries and the nomenclature has become potentially confusing. In the UK, the 'reference nutrient intake' (RNI) has been calculated as the mean plus two standard deviations (SD) of daily intake in the population, which therefore describes normal intake for 97.5% of the population. The lower reference

19

i	19.28 Summary of clinically important vitamins			
		Sources*		
Vitamin	**Rich**	**Important**	**Reference nutrient intake (RNI)**	
Fat-soluble				
A (retinol)	Liver	Milk and milk products, eggs, fish oils	700 µg men 600 µg women	
D (cholecalciferol)	Fish oils	Ultraviolet exposure to skin Egg yolks, margarine, fortified cereals	10 µg if >65 years or no sunlight exposure	
E (tocopherol)	Sunflower oil	Vegetables, nuts, seed oils	No RNI. Safe intake: 4 mg men 3 mg women	
K (phylloquinone, menaquinone)	Soya oil, menaquinones produced by intestinal bacteria	Green vegetables	No RNI. Safe intake: 1 µg/kg	
Water-soluble				
B$_1$ (thiamin)	Pork	Cereals, grains, beans	0.8 mg per 9.68 MJ (2000 kcal) energy intake	
B$_2$ (riboflavin)	Milk	Milk and milk products, breakfast cereals, bread	1.3 mg men 1.1 mg women	
B$_3$ (niacin, nicotinic acid, nicotinamide)	Meat, cereals		17 mg men 13 mg women	
B$_6$ (pyridoxine)	Meat, fish, potatoes, bananas	Vegetables, intestinal microflora synthesis	1.4 mg men 1.2 mg women	
Folate	Liver	Green leafy vegetables, fortified breakfast cereals	200 µg	
B$_{12}$ (cobalamin)	Animal products	Bacterial colonisation	1.5 µg	
Biotin	Egg yolk	Intestinal flora	No RNI. Safe intake: 10–200 µg	
C (ascorbic acid)	Citrus fruit	Fresh fruit, fresh and frozen vegetables	40 mg	

*Rich sources contain the nutrient in high concentration but are not generally eaten in large amounts; important sources contain less but contribute most because larger amounts are eaten.

19.29 Nutrition in pregnancy and lactation

- **Energy requirements**: increased in both mother and fetus but can be met through reduced maternal energy expenditure.
- **Micronutrient requirements**: adaptive mechanisms ensure increased uptake of minerals in pregnancy, but extra increments of some are required during lactation (see Box 19.32). Additional increments of some vitamins are recommended during pregnancy and lactation:

    Vitamin A: for growth and maintenance of the fetus, and to provide some reserve (important in some countries to prevent blindness associated with vitamin A deficiency). Teratogenic in excessive amounts.

    Vitamin D: to ensure bone and dental development in the infant. Higher incidences of hypocalcaemia, hypoparathyroidisim and defective dental enamel have been seen in infants of women not taking vitamin D supplements at >50° latitude.

    Folate: taken pre-conceptually and during the first trimester, reduces the incidence of neural tube defects by 70%.

    Vitamin B$_{12}$: in lactation only.

    Thiamin: to meet increased fetal energy demands.

    Riboflavin: to meet extra demands.

    Niacin: in lactation only.

    Vitamin C: for the last trimester to maintain maternal stores as fetal demands increase.

    Iodine: in countries with high consumption of staple foods (e.g. brassicas, maize, bamboo shoots) that contain goitrogens (thiocyanates or perchlorates) that interfere with iodine uptake, supplements prevent infants being born with cretinism.

 19.30 Vitamin deficiency in old age

- **Requirements**: although requirements for energy fall with age, those for micronutrients do not. If dietary intake falls, a vitamin-rich diet is required to compensate.
- **Vitamin D**: levels are commonly low due to reduced dietary intake, decreased sun exposure and less efficient skin conversion. This leads to bone loss and fractures. Supplements should be given to those at risk of falls in institutional care – the group at highest risk and most likely to benefit.
- **Vitamin B$_{12}$ deficiency**: a causal relationship with dementia has not been identified, but it does produce neuropsychiatric effects and should be checked in all those with declining cognitive function.

nutrient intake (LRNI) is the mean minus 2 SD, below which would be considered deficient in most of the population. These dietary reference values (DRV) have superseded the terms RDI (recommended daily intake) and RDA (recommended daily amount). Other countries use different terminology. Additional amounts of some micronutrients may be required in pregnancy and lactation (Box 19.29).

Vitamin deficiency diseases are most prevalent in developing countries but still occur in developed countries. Older people (Box 19.30) and alcoholics are at risk of deficiencies in B vitamins and in vitamins D and C. Nutritional deficiencies in pregnancy can affect either the mother or the developing fetus, and extra increments of vitamins are recommended in the UK (see Box 19.29). Darker-skinned individuals living at higher latitude, and those who cover up or do not go outside are at increased risk of vitamin D deficiency due to inadequate sunlight exposure. Dietary supplements are recommended for these 'at-risk' groups. Some nutrient deficiencies are induced by diseases or drugs. Deficiencies of fat-soluble vitamins are seen in conditions of fat malabsorption (Box 19.31).

 19.31 Gastrointestinal disorders that may be associated with malabsorption of fat-soluble vitamins

- Biliary obstruction
- Pancreatic exocrine insufficiency
- Coeliac disease
- Ileal inflammation or resection

19.32 Biochemical assessment of vitamin status

Nutrient	Biochemical assessments of deficiency or excess
Vitamin A	Serum retinol may be low in deficiency Serum retinyl esters: when vitamin A toxicity is suspected
Vitamin D	Plasma/serum 25-hydroxyvitamin D (25(OH)D): reflects body stores (liver and adipose tissue) Plasma/serum 1,25(OH)$_2$D: difficult to interpret
Vitamin E	Serum tocopherol:cholesterol ratio
Vitamin K	Coagulation assays (e.g. prothrombin time) Plasma vitamin K
Vitamin B$_1$ (thiamin)	Red blood cell transketolase activity or whole-blood vitamin B$_1$
Vitamin B$_2$ (riboflavin)	Red blood cell glutathione reductase activity or whole-blood vitamin B$_2$
Vitamin B$_3$ (niacin)	Urinary metabolites: 1-methyl-2-pyridone-5-carboxamide, 1-methylnicotinamide
Vitamin B$_6$	Plasma pyridoxal phosphate or erythrocyte transaminase activation coefficient
Vitamin B$_{12}$	Plasma B$_{12}$: poor measure of overall vitamin B$_{12}$ status but will detect severe deficiency Alternatives (methylmalonic acid and holotranscobalamin) are not used routinely
Folate	Red blood cell folate Plasma folate: reflects recent intake but also detects unmetabolised folic acid from foods and supplements
Vitamin C	Leucocyte ascorbic acid: assesses vitamin C tissue stores Plasma ascorbic acid: reflects recent (daily) intake

Some vitamins also have pharmacological actions when given at supraphysiological doses, such as the use of vitamin A for acne (p. 1242). Taking vitamin supplements is fashionable in many countries, although there is no evidence of benefit. Toxic effects are most serious with high dosages of vitamins A, B$_6$ and D.

Investigation of suspected vitamin deficiency or excess may involve biochemical assessment of body stores (Box 19.32). Measurements in blood should be interpreted carefully, however, in conjunction with the clinical presentation.

Fat-soluble vitamins

Vitamin A (retinol)

Pre-formed retinol is found only in foods of animal origin. Vitamin A can also be derived from carotenes, which are present in green and coloured vegetables and some fruits. Carotenes provide most of the total vitamin A in the UK and constitute the only supply in vegans. Retinol is converted to several other important molecules:

- *11-cis-retinaldehyde* is part of the photoreceptor complex in rods of the retina.

- *Retinoic acid* induces differentiation of epithelial cells by binding to specific nuclear receptors, which induce responsive genes. In vitamin A deficiency, mucus-secreting cells are replaced by keratin-producing cells.
- *Retinoids* are necessary for normal growth, fetal development, fertility, haematopoiesis and immune function.

Globally, the most important consequence of vitamin A deficiency is irreversible blindness in young children. Asia is most notably affected and the problem is being addressed through widespread vitamin A supplementation programmes. Adults are not usually at risk because liver stores can supply vitamin A when foods containing vitamin A are unavailable.

Early deficiency causes impaired adaptation to the dark (night blindness). Keratinisation of the cornea (xerophthalmia) gives rise to characteristic Bitot's spots and progresses to keratomalacia, with corneal ulceration, scarring and irreversible blindness (Fig. 19.12). In countries where vitamin A deficiency is endemic, pregnant women should be advised to eat dark green, leafy vegetables and yellow fruits (to build up stores of retinol in the fetal liver), and infants should be fed the same. The WHO

Fig. 19.12 Eye signs of vitamin A deficiency. [A] Bitot's spots in xerophthalmia, showing the white triangular plaques (arrows). [B] Keratomalacia in a 14-month-old child. There is liquefactive necrosis affecting the greater part of the cornea, with typical sparing of the superior aspect. *A, Courtesy of Institute of Ophthalmology, Moorfields Eye Hospital, London. B, From WHO. Report of a joint WHO/USAID meeting, vitamin A deficiency and xerophthalmia (WHO technical report series no. 5 W); 1976.*

is according high priority to prevention in communities where xerophthalmia occurs, giving single prophylactic oral doses of 60 mg retinyl palmitate (providing 200 000 U retinol) to pre-school children. This also reduces mortality from gastroenteritis and respiratory infections.

Repeated moderate or high doses of retinol can cause liver damage, hyperostosis and teratogenicity. Women in countries where deficiency is not endemic are therefore advised not to take vitamin A supplements in pregnancy. Retinol intake may also be restricted in those at risk of osteoporosis. Acute overdose leads to nausea and headache, increased intracranial pressure and skin desquamation. Excessive intake of carotene can cause pigmentation of the skin (hypercarotenosis); this gradually fades when intake is reduced.

Vitamin D

The natural form of vitamin D, cholecalciferol or vitamin D_3, is formed in the skin by the action of ultraviolet (UV) light on 7-dehydrocholesterol, a metabolite of cholesterol. Few foods contain vitamin D naturally and skin exposure to sunlight is the main source. Moving away from the equator, the intensity of UV light decreases, so that at a latitude above 50° (including northern Europe) vitamin D is not synthesised in winter, and even above 30° there is seasonal variation. The body store accumulated during the summer is consumed during the winter. Vitamin D is converted in the liver to 25-hydroxyvitamin D (25(OH)D), which is further hydroxylated in the kidneys to 1,25-dihydroxyvitamin D (1,25(OH)$_2$D), the active form of the vitamin (see Fig. 24.61, p. 1051). This 1,25(OH)$_2$D activates specific intracellular receptors that influence calcium metabolism, bone mineralisation and tissue differentiation. The synthetic form, ergocalciferol or vitamin D_2, is considered to be less potent than endogenous D_3.

Recommended dietary intakes aim to improve musculoskeletal health, preventing rickets and osteomalacia, enhancing muscle strength and reducing the risks of falls in the elderly. Adequate levels of vitamin D may also be important in non-musculoskeletal conditions and may improve immune function (p. 1309). Margarines are fortified with vitamin D in the UK, and milk is fortified in some parts of Europe and in North America. However, the combination of low dietary intake and limited sunlight exposure in the UK has led to recommendations that everyone over the age of 5 should take 10 μg of vitamin D daily. The individuals at highest risk of vitamin D deficiency are those who have limited exposure to sunshine. People who are confined indoors, those who habitually cover up their skin when outdoors and those with darker skins should take 10 μg of vitamin D per day all year round. Other groups may require such supplementation only in the winter months of October to March.

The effects of vitamin D deficiency (calcium deficiency, rickets and osteomalacia) are described on page 1049. An analogue of vitamin D (calcipotriol) is used for treatment of skin conditions such as psoriasis. Excessive doses of cholecalciferol, ergocalciferol or the hydroxylated metabolites cause hypercalcaemia (p. 661).

Vitamin E

There are eight related fat-soluble substances with vitamin E activity. The most important dietary form is α-tocopherol. Vitamin E has many direct metabolic actions:

- It prevents oxidation of polyunsaturated fatty acids in cell membranes by free radicals.
- It helps maintain cell membrane structure.
- It affects DNA synthesis and cell signalling.
- It is involved in the anti-inflammatory and immune systems.

19

Human deficiency is rare and has been described only in premature infants and in malabsorption. It can cause a mild haemolytic anaemia, ataxia and visual scotomas. Vitamin E intakes of up to 3200 mg/day (1000-fold greater than recommended intakes) are considered safe. Diets rich in vitamin E are consumed in countries with lower rates of coronary heart disease, although randomised controlled trials have not demonstrated cardioprotective effects of vitamin E or other antioxidants.

Vitamin K

Vitamin K is supplied in the diet mainly as vitamin K_1 (phylloquinone) in the UK, or as vitamin K_2 (menaquinone) from fermented products in parts of Asia. Vitamin K_2 is also synthesised by bacteria in the colon. Vitamin K is a co-factor for carboxylation reactions: in particular, the production of γ-carboxyglutamate (gla). Gla residues are found in four of the coagulation factor proteins (II, VII, IX and X; p. 918), conferring their capacity to bind to phospholipid surfaces in the presence of calcium. Other important gla proteins are osteocalcin and matrix gla protein, which are important in bone mineralisation.

Vitamin K deficiency leads to delayed coagulation and bleeding. In obstructive jaundice, dietary vitamin K is not absorbed and it is essential to administer the vitamin in parenteral form before surgery. Warfarin and related anticoagulants (p. 939) act by antagonising vitamin K. Vitamin K is given routinely to newborn babies to prevent haemorrhagic disease. Symptoms of excess have been reported only in infants, with synthetic preparations linked to haemolysis and liver damage.

Water-soluble vitamins

Thiamin (vitamin B_1)

Thiamin is widely distributed in foods of both vegetable and animal origin. Thiamin pyrophosphate (TPP) is a co-factor for enzyme reactions involved in the metabolism of macronutrients (carbohydrate, fat and alcohol), including:

- decarboxylation of pyruvate to acetyl-co-enzyme A, which bridges between glycolysis and the tricarboxylic acid (Krebs) cycle
- transketolase activity in the hexose monophosphate shunt pathway
- decarboxylation of α-ketoglutarate to succinate in the Krebs cycle.

In thiamin deficiency, cells cannot metabolise glucose aerobically to generate energy as ATP. Neuronal cells are most vulnerable because they depend almost exclusively on glucose for energy requirements. Impaired glucose oxidation also causes an accumulation of pyruvic and lactic acids, which produce vasodilatation and increased cardiac output.

Deficiency – beri-beri

In the developed world, thiamin deficiency is mainly encountered in chronic alcoholics. Poor diet, impaired absorption, storage and phosphorylation of thiamin in the liver, and the increased requirements for thiamin to metabolise ethanol all contribute. In the developing world, deficiency usually arises as a consequence of a diet based on polished rice. The body has very limited stores of thiamin, so deficiency is manifest after only 1 month on a thiamin-free diet. There are two forms of the disease in adults:

- *Dry (or neurological) beri-beri* manifests with chronic peripheral neuropathy and with wrist and/or foot drop, and may cause Korsakoff's psychosis and Wernicke's encephalopathy (p. 1195).

- *Wet (or cardiac) beri-beri* causes generalised oedema due to biventricular heart failure with pulmonary congestion.

In dry beri-beri, response to thiamin administration is not uniformly good. Multivitamin therapy seems to produce some improvement, however, suggesting that other vitamin deficiencies may be involved. Wernicke's encephalopathy and wet beri-beri should be treated without delay with intravenous vitamin B and C mixture (Pabrinex, p. 1195). Korsakoff's psychosis is irreversible and does not respond to thiamin treatment.

Riboflavin (vitamin B_2)

Riboflavin is required for the flavin co-factors involved in oxidation–reduction reactions. It is widely distributed in animal and vegetable foods. Levels are low in staple cereals but germination increases its content. It is destroyed under alkaline conditions by heat and by exposure to sunlight. Deficiency is rare in developed countries. It mainly affects the tongue and lips and manifests as glossitis, angular stomatitis and cheilosis. The genitals may be involved, as well as the skin areas rich in sebaceous glands, causing nasolabial or facial dyssebacea. Rapid recovery usually follows administration of riboflavin 10 mg daily by mouth.

Niacin (vitamin B_3)

Niacin encompasses nicotinic acid and nicotinamide. Nicotinamide is an essential part of the two pyridine nucleotides, nicotinamide adenine dinucleotide (NAD) and nicotinamide adenine dinucleotide phosphate (NADP), which play a key role as hydrogen acceptors and donors for many enzymes. Niacin can be synthesised in the body in limited amounts from the amino acid tryptophan.

Deficiency – pellagra

Pellagra was formerly endemic among poor people who subsisted chiefly on maize, which contains niacytin, a form of niacin that the body is unable to utilise. Pellagra can develop in only 8 weeks in individuals eating diets that are very deficient in niacin and tryptophan. It remains a problem in parts of Africa, and is occasionally seen in alcoholics and in patients with chronic small intestinal disease in developed countries. Pellagra can occur in Hartnup's disease, a genetic disorder characterised by impaired absorption of several amino acids, including tryptophan. It is also seen occasionally in carcinoid syndrome (p. 678), when tryptophan is consumed in the excessive production of 5-hydroxytryptamine (5-HT, serotonin). Pellagra has been called the disease of the three Ds:

- *Dermatitis*. Characteristically, there is erythema resembling severe sunburn, appearing symmetrically over the parts of the body exposed to sunlight, particularly the limbs and especially on the neck but not the face (Casal's necklace, Fig. 19.13). The skin lesions may progress to vesiculation, cracking, exudation and secondary infection.
- *Diarrhoea*. This is often associated with anorexia, nausea, glossitis and dysphagia, reflecting the presence of a non-infective inflammation that extends throughout the gastrointestinal tract.
- *Dementia*. In severe deficiency, delirium occurs acutely and dementia develops in chronic cases.

Treatment is with nicotinamide, given in a dose of 100 mg 3 times daily orally or parenterally. The response is usually rapid. Within 24 hours the erythema diminishes, the diarrhoea ceases and a striking improvement occurs in the patient's mental state.

Fig. 19.13 Dermatitis due to pellagra (niacin deficiency). The lesions appear on those parts of the body exposed to sunlight. The classic 'Casal's necklace' can be seen around the neck and upper chest. *From Karthikeyan K, Thappa DM. Pellagra and skin. Int J Dermatol 2002; 41:476–481.*

Toxicity

Excessive intakes of niacin may lead to reversible hepatotoxicity. Nicotinic acid is a lipid-lowering agent but at doses above 200 mg a day gives rise to vasodilatory symptoms ('flushing' and/or hypotension).

Pyridoxine (vitamin B$_6$)

Pyridoxine, pyridoxal and pyridoxamine are different forms of vitamin B$_6$ that undergo phosphorylation to produce pyridoxal 5-phosphate (PLP). PLP is the co-factor for a large number of enzymes involved in the metabolism of amino acids. Vitamin B$_6$ is available in most foods.

Deficiency is rare, although certain drugs, such as isoniazid and penicillamine, act as chemical antagonists to pyridoxine. Pyridoxine administration is effective in isoniazid-induced peripheral neuropathy and some cases of sideroblastic anaemia. Large doses of vitamin B$_6$ have an antiemetic effect in radiotherapy-induced nausea. Although vitamin B$_6$ supplements have become popular in the treatment of nausea in pregnancy, carpal tunnel syndrome and pre-menstrual syndrome, there is no convincing evidence of benefit. Very high doses of vitamin B$_6$ taken for several months can cause a sensory polyneuropathy.

Biotin

Biotin is a co-enzyme in the synthesis of fatty acids, isoleucine and valine, and is also involved in gluconeogenesis. Deficiency results from consuming very large quantities of raw egg whites (>30% energy intake) because the avidin they contain binds to and inactivates biotin in the intestine. It may also be seen after long periods of total parenteral nutrition. The clinical features of deficiency include scaly dermatitis, alopecia and paraesthesia.

Folate (folic acid)

Folates exist in many forms. The main circulating form is 5-methyltetrahydrofolate. The natural forms are prone to oxidation. Folic acid is the stable synthetic form. Folate works as a methyl donor for cellular methylation and protein synthesis. It is directly involved in DNA and RNA synthesis, and requirements increase during embryonic development.

Folate deficiency may cause three major birth defects (spina bifida, anencephaly and encephalocele) resulting from imperfect closure of the neural tube, which takes place 3–4 weeks after conception. The UK Department of Health advises that women who have experienced a pregnancy affected by a neural tube defect should take 5 mg of folic acid daily from before conception and throughout the first trimester; this reduces the incidence of these defects by 70%. All women planning a pregnancy are advised to include good sources of folate in their diet, and to take folate supplements throughout the first trimester. Liver is the richest source of folate but an alternative source (e.g. leafy vegetables) is advised in early pregnancy because of the high vitamin A content of liver (p. 712). Folate deficiency has also been associated with heart disease, dementia and cancer. There is mandatory fortification of flour with folic acid in the USA and voluntary fortification of many foods across Europe. There are now concerns that this may contribute to the increased incidence of colon cancer through promotion of the growth of polyps.

Hydroxycobalamin (vitamin B$_{12}$)

Vitamin B$_{12}$ is a co-factor in folate co-enzyme recycling and nerve myelination. Vitamin B$_{12}$ and folate are particularly important in DNA synthesis in red blood cells (p. 943). The haematological disorders (macrocytic or megaloblastic anaemias) caused by their deficiency are discussed on pages 943–945. Vitamin B$_{12}$, but not folate, is needed for the integrity of myelin, so that vitamin B$_{12}$ deficiency is also associated with neurological disease (see Box 23.33, p. 944).

Neurological consequences of vitamin B$_{12}$ deficiency

In older people and chronic alcoholics, vitamin B$_{12}$ deficiency arises from insufficient intake and/or from malabsorption. Several drugs, including neomycin, can render vitamin B$_{12}$ inactive. Adequate intake of folate maintains erythropoiesis and there is a concern that fortification of foods with folate may mask underlying vitamin B$_{12}$ deficiency. In severe deficiency there is insidious, diffuse and uneven demyelination. It may be clinically manifest as peripheral neuropathy or spinal cord degeneration affecting both posterior and lateral columns ('subacute combined degeneration of the spinal cord'; p. 1138), or there may be cerebral manifestations (resembling dementia) or optic atrophy. Vitamin B$_{12}$ therapy improves symptoms in most cases.

Vitamin C (ascorbic acid)

Ascorbic acid is the most active reducing agent in the aqueous phase of living tissues and is involved in intracellular electron transfer. It takes part in the hydroxylation of proline and lysine in protocollagen to hydroxyproline and hydroxylysine in mature collagen. It is very easily destroyed by heat, increased pH and light, and is very soluble in water; hence many traditional cooking methods reduce or eliminate it. Claims that high-dose vitamin C improves immune function (including resistance to the common cold) and cholesterol turnover remain unsubstantiated.

Deficiency – scurvy

Vitamin C deficiency causes defective formation of collagen with impaired healing of wounds, capillary haemorrhage and reduced platelet adhesiveness (normal platelets are rich in ascorbate) (Fig. 19.14). Precipitants and clinical features of scurvy are shown

19

Fig. 19.14 Scurvy. [A] Gingival swelling and bleeding. [B] Perifollicular hyperkeratosis. *A and B, From Ho V, Prinsloo P, Ombiga J. Persistent anaemia due to scurvy. J New Zeal Med Assoc 2007; 120:62. Reproduced with permission.*

---

i 19.33 Scurvy – vitamin C deficiency

Precipitants

Increased requirement
- Trauma, surgery, burns, infections
- Smoking
- Drugs (glucocorticoids, aspirin, indometacin, tetracycline)

Dietary deficiency
- Lack of dietary fruit and vegetables for >2 months
- Infants fed exclusively on boiled milk

Clinical features

- Swollen gums that bleed easily
- Perifollicular and petechial haemorrhages
- Ecchymoses

- Haemarthrosis
- Gastrointestinal bleeding
- Anaemia
- Poor wound healing

---

in Box 19.33. A dose of 250 mg vitamin C 3 times daily by mouth should saturate the tissues quickly. The deficiencies of the patient's diet also need to be corrected and other vitamin supplements given if necessary. Daily intakes of more than 1 g/day have been reported to cause diarrhoea and the formation of renal oxalate stones.

Other dietary organic compounds

There are a number of non-essential organic compounds with purported health benefits, such as reducing risk of heart disease or cancer. Groups of compounds such as the flavonoids and phytoestrogens show bioactivity through their respective antioxidant and oestrogenic or anti-oestrogenic activities. Flavonoids (of which there are a number of different classes of compound) are found in fruit and vegetables, tea and wine; phytoestrogens are found in soy products (with higher intakes in parts of Asia compared to Europe and the USA) and pulses. Caffeine from tea and coffee and carbonated beverages affects the nervous system and can improve mental performance in the short term, with adverse effects seen at higher intakes. Intake of non-carbonic organic acids (which are not metabolised to carbon dioxide), e.g. oxalates, may be restricted in individuals prone to kidney stones.

Inorganic micronutrients

A number of inorganic elements are essential dietary constituents for humans (Box 19.34). Deficiency is seen when there is

inadequate dietary intake of minerals or excessive loss from the body. Toxic effects have also been observed from self-medication and disordered absorption or excretion. Examples of clinical toxicity include excess of iron (haemochromatosis or haemosiderosis), fluoride (fluorosis; p. 149), copper (Wilson's disease) and selenium (selenosis, seen in parts of China). For most minerals, the available biochemical markers do not accurately reflect dietary intake and dietary assessment is required.

Calcium and phosphorus

Calcium is the most abundant cation in the body and powerful homeostatic mechanisms control circulating ionised calcium levels (pp. 661 and 1050). The WHO's dietary guidelines for calcium differ between countries, with higher intakes usually recommended in places with higher fracture prevalence. Between 20% and 30% of calcium in the diet is absorbed, depending on vitamin D status and food source. Calcium requirements depend on phosphorus intakes, with an optimum molar ratio (Ca:P) of 1:1. Excessive phosphorus intakes (e.g. 1–1.5 g/day) with a Ca:P of 1:3 have been shown to cause hypocalcaemia and secondary hyperparathyroidism (p. 662).

Calcium absorption may be impaired in vitamin D deficiency (pp. 661 and 1050) and in malabsorption secondary to small intestinal disease. Calcium deficiency causes impaired bone mineralisation and can lead to osteomalacia in adults. The potential benefits of high calcium intake in osteoporosis are discussed on page 1048. Too much calcium can lead to constipation, and toxicity has been observed in 'milk-alkali syndrome' (p. 662).

Dietary deficiency of phosphorus is rare (except in older people with limited diets) because it is present in nearly all foods and phosphates are added to a number of processed foods. Phosphate deficiency in adults occurs:

- in patients with renal tubular phosphate loss (p. 405)
- in patients receiving a prolonged high dosage of aluminium hydroxide (p. 419)
- in alcoholics sometimes when they are fed with high-carbohydrate foods
- in patients receiving parenteral nutrition if inadequate phosphate is provided.

Deficiency causes hypophosphataemia (p. 368) and muscle weakness secondary to ATP deficiency.

Iron

Iron is involved in the synthesis of haemoglobin and is required for the transport of electrons within cells and for a number of enzyme reactions. Non-haem iron in cereals and vegetables is

	i	**19.34 Summary of clinically important minerals**		

	Sources[1]		**Reference nutrient intake (RNI)**
Mineral	**Rich**	**Important**	
Calcium	Milk and milk products, tofu	Milk, boned fish, green vegetables, beans	700 mg[2]
Phosphorus	Most foods contain phosphorus		550 mg[2]
	Marmite and dry-roasted peanuts	Milk, cereal products, bread and meat	
Magnesium	Whole grains, nuts	Unprocessed and wholegrain foods	300 mg men 270 mg women[2]
Iron	Liver, red meat (haem iron)	Non-haem iron from vegetables, wholemeal bread	8.7 mg 14.8 mg women <50 years
Zinc	Red meat, seafood	Dairy produce, wholemeal bread	9.5 mg men 7 mg women[2]
Iodine	Edible seaweeds	Milk and dairy products	140 μg
Selenium	Fish, wheat grown in selenium-rich soils	Fish	75 μg men 60 μg women[2]
Copper	Shellfish, liver	Bread, cereal products, vegetables	1.2 mg[2]
Fluoride		Drinking water, tea	No RNI. Safe intake: 0.5 mg/kg
Potassium	Dried fruit, potatoes, coffee	Fresh fruit, vegetables, milk	3500 mg
Sodium	Table salt, anchovies	Processed foods, bread, bacon	1600 mg

[1]Rich sources contain the nutrient in high concentration but are not generally eaten in large amounts; important sources contain less but contribute most because larger amounts are eaten. [2]Increased amounts are required in women during lactation.

poorly absorbed but makes the greater contribution to overall intake, compared to the well-absorbed haem iron from animal products. Fruits and vegetables containing vitamin C enhance iron absorption, while the tannins in tea reduce it. Dietary calcium reduces iron uptake from the same meal, which may precipitate iron deficiency in those with borderline iron stores. There is no physiological mechanism for excretion of iron, so homeostasis depends on the regulation of iron absorption (see Fig. 23.18, p. 942). This is regulated at the level of duodenal enterocytes by hepcidin (a peptide secreted by hepatocytes in the duodenum). The expression of hepcidin is suppressed when body iron is low, leading to enhanced efflux of iron into the circulation. The normal daily loss of iron is 1 mg, arising from desquamated surface cells and intestinal losses. A regular loss of only 2 mL of blood per day doubles the iron requirement. On average, an additional 20 mg of iron is lost during menstruation, so pre-menopausal women require about twice as much iron as men (and more if menstrual losses are heavy).

The major consequence of iron deficiency is anaemia (p. 940). This is one of the most important nutritional causes of ill health in all parts of the world. In the UK, it is estimated that 10% women are iron-deficient. Dietary iron overload is occasionally observed and results in iron accumulation in the liver and, rarely, cirrhosis. Haemochromatosis results from an inherited increase in iron absorption (p. 895).

Iodine

Iodine is required for synthesis of thyroid hormones (p. 634). It is present in sea fish, seaweed and most plant foods grown near the sea. The amount of iodine in soil and water influences the iodine content of most foods. Iodine is lacking in the highest mountainous areas of the world (e.g. the Alps and the Himalayas) and in the soil of frequently flooded plains (e.g. Bangladesh).

About a billion people in the world are estimated to have an inadequate iodine intake and hence are at risk of iodine deficiency disorder. Goitre is the most common manifestation, affecting about 200 million people (p. 648).

In those areas where most women have endemic goitre, 1% or more of babies are born with cretinism (characterised by mental and physical retardation). There is a higher than usual prevalence of deafness, slowed reflexes and poor learning in the remaining population. The best way of preventing neonatal cretinism is to ensure adequate levels of iodine during pregnancy. This can be achieved by intramuscular injections with 1–2 mL of iodised poppy seed oil (475–950 mg iodine) to women of child-bearing age every 3–5 years, by administration of iodised oil orally at 6-monthly or yearly intervals to adults and children, or by provision of iodised salt for cooking.

Zinc

Zinc is present in most foods of vegetable and animal origin. It is an essential component of many enzymes, including carbonic anhydrase, alcohol dehydrogenase and alkaline phosphatase.

Acute zinc deficiency has been reported in patients receiving prolonged zinc-free parenteral nutrition and causes diarrhoea, mental apathy, a moist, eczematoid dermatitis, especially around the mouth, and loss of hair. Chronic zinc deficiency occurs in dietary deficiency, malabsorption syndromes, alcoholism and its associated hepatic cirrhosis. It causes the clinical features seen in the very rare congenital disorder known as acrodermatitis enteropathica (growth retardation, hair loss and chronic diarrhoea). Zinc deficiency is thought to be responsible for one-third of the world's population not reaching their optimal height. In the Middle East, chronic deficiency has been associated with dwarfism and hypogonadism. In starvation, zinc deficiency causes thymic atrophy; zinc supplements may accelerate the healing of skin lesions, promote general well-being, improve appetite and reduce the morbidity associated with the under-nourished state, and lower the mortality associated with diarrhoea and pneumonia in children.

19

Selenium

The family of seleno-enzymes includes glutathione peroxidase, which helps prevent free radical damage to cells, and mono-deiodinase, which converts thyroxine to triiodothyronine (p. 634). North American soil has a higher selenium content than European and Asian soil, and the decreasing reliance of Europe on imported American food in recent decades has resulted in a decline in dietary selenium intake.

Selenium deficiency can cause hypothyroidism, cardiomyopathy in children (Keshan's disease) and myopathy in adults. Excess selenium can cause heart disease.

Fluoride

Fluoride helps prevent dental caries because it increases the resistance of the enamel to acid attack. It is a component of bone mineral and some studies have shown anti-fracture effects at low doses, but excessive intakes may compromise bone structure.

If the local water supply contains more than 1 part per million (ppm) of fluoride, the incidence of dental caries is low. Soft waters usually contain no fluoride, while very hard waters may contain over 10 ppm. The benefit of fluoride is greatest when it is taken before the permanent teeth erupt, while their enamel is being laid down. The addition of traces of fluoride (at 1 ppm) to public water supplies is now a widespread practice. Chronic fluoride poisoning is occasionally seen where the water supply contains >10 ppm fluoride. It can also occur in workers handling cryolite (aluminium sodium fluoride), used in smelting aluminium. Fluoride poisoning is described on page 149. Pitting of teeth is a result of too much fluoride as a child.

Sodium, potassium and magnesium

Western diets are high in sodium due to the sodium chloride (salt) that is added to processed food. In the UK, it is suggested that daily salt intakes are kept well below 6 g. The roles of sodium, potassium and magnesium, along with the disease states associated with abnormal intakes or disordered metabolism, are discussed in Chapter 14.

Other essential inorganic nutrients

These include chloride (a counter-ion to sodium and potassium), cobalt (required for vitamin B_{12}), sulphur (a constituent of methionine and cysteine), manganese (needed for or activates many enzymes) and chromium (necessary for insulin action). Deficiency of chromium presents as hyperglycaemia and has been reported in adults as a rare complication of prolonged parenteral nutrition.

Copper metabolism is abnormal in Wilson's disease (p. 896). Deficiency occasionally occurs but only in young children, causing microcytic hypochromic anaemia, neutropenia, retarded growth, skeletal rarefaction and dermatosis.

Further information

Websites

bapen.org.uk *British Society for Parenteral and Enteral Nutrition; includes the MUST tool.*

bsg.org.uk *British Society of Gastroenterology: guidelines on management of patients with a short bowel, enteral feeding for adult hospital patients and the provision of a percutaneously placed enteral tube feeding service.*

espen.org *European Society for Parenteral and Enteral Nutrition: guidelines for adult parenteral nutrition; perioperative care in elective colonic and rectal/pelvic surgery; nutrition in dementia; acute and chronic intestinal failure in adults; and nutrition in cancer patients.*

nice.org.uk *National Institute for Health and Care Excellence: guidance for nutritional support in adults.*

20

ER Pearson
RJ McCrimmon

Diabetes mellitus

Clinical examination of the patient with diabetes 720

Functional anatomy and physiology 723

Investigations 725
Establishing the diagnosis of diabetes 727

Aetiology and pathogenesis of diabetes 728

Presenting problems in diabetes mellitus 734
Hyperglycaemia 734
Presentation with the complications of diabetes 735
Diabetes emergencies 735
    Diabetic ketoacidosis 735
    Hyperglycaemic hyperosmolar state 738
    Hypoglycaemia 738

Management of diabetes 741
Patient education, diet and lifestyle 743
Drugs to reduce hyperglycaemia 745
Insulin therapy 748
Transplantation 752
Management of diabetes in special situations 752

Complications of diabetes 755
Diabetic retinopathy 757
Diabetic nephropathy 757
Diabetic neuropathy 758
The diabetic foot 761

Clinical examination of the patient with diabetes

6 Head
Xanthelasma
Cranial nerve palsy/eye
movements/ptosis

5 Neck
Carotid pulse
Bruits
Thyroid enlargement

4 Axillae

▲ Acanthosis nigricans
in insulin resistance

3 Blood pressure

2 Skin
Bullae
Pigmentation
Granuloma annulare
Vitiligo

1 Hands
(see opposite)

▲ 'Prayer sign'

7 Eyes (see opposite)
Visual acuity
Cataract/lens opacity
Fundoscopy

▲ Exudative maculopathy

Observation
• Weight loss in insulin deficiency
• Obesity in type 2 diabetes
• Mucosal candidiasis
• Dehydration– dry mouth,
  ↓tissue turgor
• Air hunger– Kussmaul breathing
  in ketoacidosis

8 Insulin injection sites
(see opposite)

9 Abdomen
Hepatomegaly
(fatty infiltration of liver)

10 Legs
Muscle-wasting
Sensory abnormality
Hair loss
Tendon reflexes

▲ Necrobiosis lipoidica

11 Feet (see opposite)
Inspection
Peripheral pulses
Sensation

▲ Neuropathic foot ulcer

▲ Charcot neuroarthropathy

Insets (Acanthosis nigricans) From Lim E (ed.). Medicine and surgery: an integrated textbook. Edinburgh: Elsevier Ltd; 2007. (Exudative maculopathy) Courtesy of Dr A.W. Patrick and Dr I.W. Campbell.

Diabetes can affect every system in the body. In routine clinical practice, examination of the patient with diabetes is focused on hands, blood pressure, axillae, neck, eyes, insulin injection sites and feet.

7 Examination of the eyes

Visual acuity

- Check distance vision using Snellen chart at 6 m
- Check near vision using standard reading chart
- Note that visual acuity can alter reversibly with acute hyperglycaemia due to osmotic changes affecting the lens. Most patients with retinopathy do not have altered visual acuity, except after a vitreous haemorrhage or in some cases of maculopathy

Lens opacification

- Look for the red reflex using the ophthalmoscope held 30 cm from the eye

Fundal examination

- Either use a three-field retinal camera or dilate pupils with a mydriatic (e.g. tropicamide) and examine with an ophthalmoscope in a darkened room
- Note features of diabetic retinopathy (p. 1174), including photocoagulation scars from previous laser treatment

Background retinopathy. *Courtesy of Dr A.W. Patrick and Dr I.W. Campbell.*

Proliferative retinopathy. *Courtesy of Dr A.W. Patrick and Dr I.W. Campbell.*

1 Examination of the hands

Several abnormalities are more common in diabetes:

- Limited joint mobility ('cheiroarthropathy') causes painless stiffness. The inability to extend (to 180°) the metacarpophalangeal or interphalangeal joints of at least one finger bilaterally can be demonstrated in the 'prayer sign'
- Dupuytren's contracture (p. 1059) causes nodules or thickening of the skin and knuckle pads
- Carpal tunnel syndrome (p. 1139) presents with wrist pain radiating into the hand
- Trigger finger (flexor tenosynovitis) may be present
- Muscle-wasting/sensory changes may be present in peripheral sensorimotor neuropathy, although this is more common in the lower limbs

8 Insulin injection sites

Main areas used

- Anterior abdominal wall
- Upper thighs/buttocks
- Upper outer arms

Inspection

- Bruising
- Subcutaneous fat deposition (lipohypertrophy)
- Subcutaneous fat loss (lipoatrophy; associated with injection of unpurified animal insulins – now rare)
- Erythema, infection (rare)

Lipohypertrophy of the upper arm.

11 Examination of the feet

Inspection

- Look for evidence of callus formation on weight-bearing areas, clawing of the toes (in neuropathy), loss of the plantar arch, discoloration of the skin (ischaemia), localised infection and ulcers
- Deformity may be present, especially in Charcot neuroarthropathy
- Fungal infection may affect skin between toes, and nails

Circulation

- Peripheral pulses, skin temperature and capillary refill may be abnormal

Sensation

- This is abnormal in stocking distribution in typical peripheral sensorimotor neuropathy
- Testing light touch with monofilaments is sufficient for risk assessment; test other sensation modalities (vibration, pain, proprioception) only when neuropathy is being evaluated

Reflexes

- Ankle reflexes are lost in typical sensorimotor neuropathy
- Test plantar and ankle reflexes

Monofilaments. The monofilament is applied gently until slightly deformed at five points on each foot. Callus should be avoided as sensation is reduced. If the patient feels fewer than 8 out of 10 touches, the risk of foot ulceration is increased 5–10-fold.

20

Diabetes mellitus is a clinical syndrome characterised by an increase in plasma blood glucose (hyperglycaemia). It has many causes (see Box 20.9), most commonly type 1 or type 2 diabetes. Type 1 diabetes is generally considered to result from autoimmune destruction of insulin-producing cells (β cells) in the pancreas, leading to marked insulin deficiency, whereas type 2 diabetes is characterised by reduced sensitivity to the action of insulin and an inability to produce sufficient insulin to overcome this 'insulin resistance'. Hyperglycaemia causes both acute and long-term problems. Acutely, high glucose and lack of insulin can result in marked symptoms, metabolic decompensation and hospitalisation. Chronic hyperglycaemia is responsible for diabetes-specific 'microvascular' complications affecting the eyes (retinopathy), kidneys (nephropathy) and feet (neuropathy).

There is a continuous distribution of blood glucose in the population, with no clear division between people with normal values and those with abnormal ones. The diagnostic criteria for diabetes (a fasting plasma glucose of ≥7.0 mmol/L (126 mg/dL) or glucose 2 hours after an oral glucose challenge of ≥11.1 mmol/L (200 mg/dL); p. 726) have been selected to identify a degree of hyperglycaemia that, if untreated, carries a significant risk of microvascular disease, and in particular diabetic retinopathy. Less severe hyperglycaemia is called 'impaired glucose tolerance'. This is not associated with a substantial risk of microvascular disease, but is connected with an increased risk of large-vessel disease (e.g. atheroma leading to myocardial infarction) and with a greater risk of developing diabetes in future.

The incidence of diabetes is rising. Globally, it is estimated that 415 million people had diabetes in 2015 (10% of the world adult population), and this figure is expected to reach 642 million by 2040. This global pandemic principally involves type 2 diabetes; prevalence varies considerably around the world (Fig. 20.1), being associated with differences in genetic factors, as well as environmental ones such as greater longevity, obesity, unsatisfactory diet, sedentary lifestyle, increasing urbanisation and economic development. A pronounced rise in the prevalence of type 2 diabetes occurs in migrant populations to industrialised countries, as in Asian and Afro-Caribbean immigrants to the UK or USA. Type 2 diabetes is now seen in children and adolescents, particularly in some ethnic groups such as Hispanics, non-Hispanic blacks and Asian Indians.

The incidence of type 1 diabetes is also increasing: between 1960 and 1996, 3% more children were diagnosed worldwide each year. It is generally more common in countries closer to the polar regions. Finland, for instance, has the highest rate of type 1 diagnosis per year at >60 per 100 000 of the population, whereas in China, India and Venezuela the incidence is only 0.1 per 100 000. Type 1 diabetes is most common in Caucasians, and more people are diagnosed in the winter months.

Diabetes is a major burden on health-care facilities in all countries. Globally, in 2015, diabetes caused 5 million deaths in those aged 20–79 years, and health-care expenditure attributed to diabetes was estimated to be at least 673 billion US dollars, or 12% of total health-care expenditure.

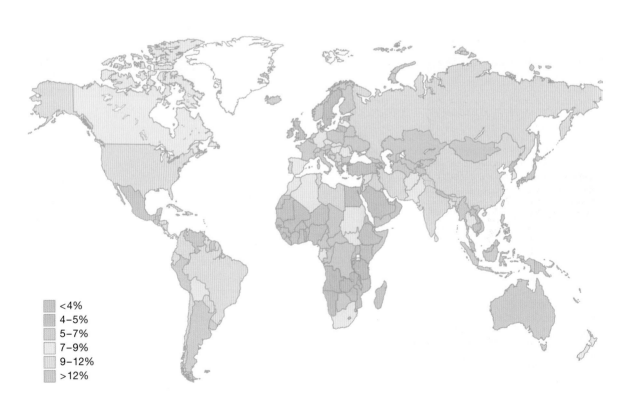

Fig. 20.1 Prevalence (%) of diabetes in those aged 20–79 years, 2015. *Based on estimates from the International Diabetes Federation. IDF Diabetes Atlas, 7th edn. Brussels, Belgium: International Diabetes Federation, 2015. http://www.diabetesatlas.org.*

Functional anatomy and physiology

Regulation of insulin secretion

Insulin is the primary regulator of glucose metabolism and storage (Box 20.1), and is secreted from pancreatic β cells into the portal circulation (Fig. 20.2). The pancreatic β cell is designed to regulate blood glucose concentrations tightly by coupling glucose and other nutrient stimulus with insulin secretion (Fig. 20.2). Entry of glucose into the pancreatic β cell is by facilitated diffusion down its concentration gradient through cell membrane glucose transporters (GLUTs). Glucose is then metabolised by glycolysis and oxidative phosphorylation. The first step of the glycolytic pathway, the conversion of glucose to glucose-6-phosphate, is catalysed by the enzyme glucokinase (GK). Glucokinase has a low affinity for glucose and so its activity under normal physiological conditions varies markedly, according to the concentration of glucose. This makes it a very effective glucose sensor in the β cell. In what is considered a classical direct or triggering pathway, glucose metabolism results in increased intracellular adenosine triphosphate (ATP) and reduced adenosine diphosphate

20.1 Metabolic actions of insulin	
Increase	**Decrease**
Carbohydrate metabolism	
Glucose transport (muscle, adipose tissue)	Gluconeogenesis
Glucose phosphorylation	Glycogenolysis
Glycogen synthesis	
Glycolysis	
Pyruvate dehydrogenase activity	
Pentose phosphate shunt	
Lipid metabolism	
Triglyceride synthesis	Lipolysis
Fatty acid synthesis (liver)	Lipoprotein lipase (muscle)
Lipoprotein lipase activity (adipose tissue)	Ketogenesis
	Fatty acid oxidation (liver)
Protein metabolism	
Amino acid transport	Protein degradation
Protein synthesis	

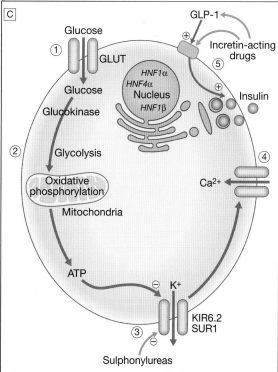

Fig. 20.2 Pancreatic structure and endocrine function. **A** The normal adult pancreas contains about 1 million islets, which are scattered throughout the exocrine parenchyma. Histology is shown in Figure 20.6. **B** The core of each islet consists of β cells that produce insulin, and is surrounded by a cortex of endocrine cells that produce other hormones, including glucagon (α cells), somatostatin (δ cells) and pancreatic polypeptide (PP cells). **C** Schematic representation of the pancreatic β cell. (1) Glucose enters the cell via a glucose transporter (GLUT1 or GLUT2). (2) Glucose then enters glycolysis, and subsequent oxidative phosphorylation in the mitochondria results in a rise in intracellular adenosine triphosphate (ATP). (3) This ATP acts to close the K_{ATP} channel (which consists of four KIR6.2 subunits and four SUR1 subunits). This leads to membrane depolarisation. (4) The rise in membrane potential results in calcium influx due to opening of a voltage-gated calcium channel. This rise in intracellular calcium causes insulin secretory vesicles to fuse with the cell membrane, leading to insulin secretion. (5) Other stimuli, such as glucagon-like peptide-1 (GLP-1) or gastric inhibitory polypeptide (GIP), act on G-protein-coupled receptors to increase cyclic adenosine monophosphate (cAMP) and amplify the insulin secretion. Genetic defects in the β cell result in diabetes. The primary genes are glucokinase (the initial step in glycolysis) and *HNF1α*, *HNF4α* and *HNF1β* (nuclear transcription factors). Two groups of drugs act on the β cell to promote insulin secretion. Sulphonylureas act to close the K_{ATP} channel, causing membrane depolarisation, calcium influx and insulin secretion. Incretin-acting drugs either increase the concentration of endogenous GLP-1 and GIP (the dipeptidyl peptidase 4, or DPP-4, inhibitors) or act as directly on the GLP-1 receptor (GLP-1 receptor agonists). Both of these drug groups act to augment insulin secretion but only following an initial stimulus to insulin secretion through closure of β cell K_{ATP} channels by glucose (or sulphonylureas).

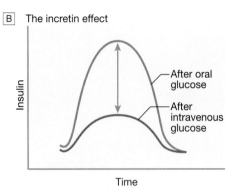

Fig. 20.3 Insulin secretion in response to intravenous or oral glucose. A An acute first phase of insulin secretion occurs in response to an elevated blood glucose, followed by a sustained second phase. B The incretin effect describes the observation that insulin secretion is greater when glucose is given by mouth than when glucose is administered intravenously to achieve the same rise in blood glucose concentrations. The additional stimulus to insulin secretion is mediated by release of peptides from the gut and these actions are exploited in incretin-based therapies (p. 747).

(ADP), which causes closure of an ATP-sensitive potassium channel (K_{ATP}). The resulting membrane depolarisation of the β cell results in insulin secretion due to triggering of calcium release by voltage-sensitive calcium channels. In addition to this pathway, the amount of insulin released can be amplified or potentiated by the background blood glucose, other nutrients and peptides, and by neuronal control via the sympathetic and parasympathetic nervous system. A good example of this potentiation of insulin release is seen with the secretion of two gut peptides following ingestion of food. Glucagon-like peptide-1 (GLP-1) and gastric inhibitory polypeptide (GIP) are released from gastrointestinal L cells and K cells, respectively, following a meal, and act via receptors on the pancreatic β cells to augment insulin secretion. Thus, for a given glucose stimulus to the β cell, there is greater insulin secretion with oral glucose administration (where the gut peptides are released) compared to intravenous glucose administration (which does not stimulate gut peptide release). This enhanced insulin secretion following oral administration of glucose is termed the 'incretin' effect (Fig. 20.3), and GLP-1 and GIP are known as incretin hormones.

Insulin is synthesised as a pro-hormone (pro-insulin) that consists of an α and a β chain, which are linked by C-peptide (Fig. 20.4). The C-peptide is cleaved by β-cell peptidases to create insulin (which now consists of the α and β chains) and free C-peptide. Insulin secretion in response to a glucose stimulus

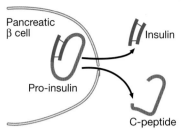

Fig. 20.4 Processing of pro-insulin into insulin and C-peptide. Pro-insulin in the pancreatic β cell is cleaved to release insulin and equimolar amounts of inert C-peptide (connecting peptide). Measurement of C-peptide can be used to assess endogenous insulin secretory capacity.

classically occurs in two phases (see Fig. 20.3). The rapid first phase represents the secretion of pre-formed insulin from granules within the β cells, while the more prolonged second phase is a consequence of newly synthesised insulin.

Regulation of glucagon secretion

Pancreatic islets also contain other endocrine cells such as α cells that secrete the peptide hormone glucagon, and δ cells that produce somatostatin (see Fig. 20.2B). Alpha cells make up about 20% of the human islet cell population. Glucagon has opposite effects to insulin and acts on the liver (and kidney) to stimulate glycogenolysis, leading to increased hepatic glucose production. Regulation of glucagon secretion by the α cell is complex, but β-cell insulin secretion, co-secreted zinc and γ-aminobutyric acid (GABA), as well as somatostatin from δ cells, are thought to have major regulatory roles. This means that insulin and glucagon are tightly, and reciprocally, regulated, such that the ratio of insulin to glucagon in the portal vein is a major determinant of hepatic glucose production. Glucagon is also critically important to the body's defence against hypoglycaemia (p. 738).

Blood glucose homeostasis

Blood glucose is tightly regulated and maintained within a narrow range. This is essential for ensuring a continuous supply of glucose to the central nervous system. The brain has little capacity to store energy in the form of glycogen or triglyceride, and the blood–brain barrier is largely impermeable to fatty acids, so the brain depends on the liver for a constant supply of glucose for oxidation and hence generation of ATP. Glucose homeostasis is achieved through the coordinated actions of multiple organs, but mainly reflects a balance between the entry of glucose into the circulation from the liver, supplemented by intestinal absorption of glucose after meals, and the uptake of glucose by peripheral tissues, particularly skeletal muscle and brain.

After ingestion of a meal containing carbohydrate, normal blood glucose levels are maintained by:

- suppression of hepatic glucose production
- stimulation of hepatic glucose uptake
- stimulation of glucose uptake by peripheral tissues (Fig. 20.5).

The post-prandial rise in portal vein insulin and glucose, together with a fall in portal glucagon concentrations, suppresses hepatic glucose production and results in net hepatic glucose uptake. Depending on the size of the carbohydrate load, around one-quarter to one-third of ingested glucose is taken up in the liver. In addition, insulin stimulates glucose uptake in skeletal muscle and fat, mediated by the glucose transporter GLUT4.

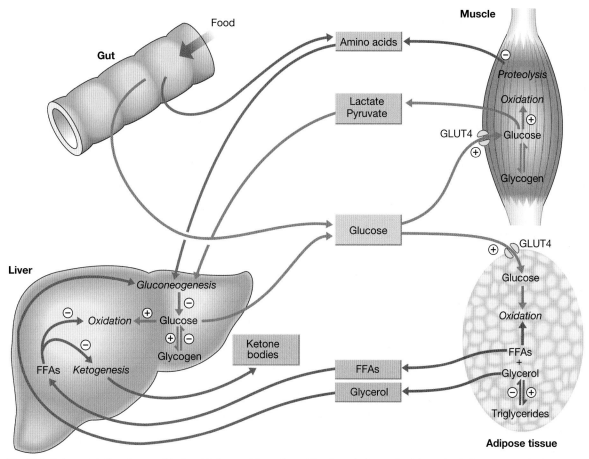

Fig. 20.5 Major metabolic pathways of fuel metabolism and the actions of insulin. ⊕ indicates stimulation and ⊖ indicates suppression by insulin. In response to a rise in blood glucose, e.g. after a meal, insulin is released, suppressing gluconeogenesis and promoting glycogen synthesis and storage. Insulin promotes the peripheral uptake of glucose, particularly in skeletal muscle, and encourages storage (as muscle glycogen). It also promotes protein synthesis and lipogenesis, and suppresses lipolysis. The release of intermediate metabolites, including amino acids (glutamine, alanine), 3-carbon intermediates in oxidation (lactate, pyruvate) and free fatty acids (FFAs), is controlled by insulin. In the absence of insulin, e.g. during fasting, these processes are reversed and favour gluconeogenesis in liver from glycogen, glycerol, amino acids and other 3-carbon precursors.

20

When intestinal glucose absorption declines between meals, portal vein insulin and glucose concentrations fall while glucagon levels rise. This leads to increased hepatic glucose output via gluconeogenesis and glycogen breakdown. The liver now resumes net glucose production and glucose homeostasis is maintained. The main substrates for gluconeogenesis are glycerol and amino acids, as shown in Figure 20.5.

Fat metabolism

Adipocytes (and the liver) synthesise triglyceride from non-esterified ('free') fatty acids (FFAs) and glycerol. Insulin is the major regulator not only of glucose metabolism but also of fatty acid metabolism. High insulin levels after meals promote triglyceride accumulation. In contrast, in the fasting state, low insulin levels permit lipolysis and the release into the circulation of FFAs (and glycerol), which can be oxidised by many tissues. Their partial oxidation in the liver provides energy to drive gluconeogenesis and also produces ketone bodies (acetoacetate, which can be reduced to 3-hydroxybutyrate or decarboxylated to acetone), which are generated in hepatocyte mitochondria. Ketone bodies are organic acids that, when formed in small amounts, are oxidised and utilised as metabolic fuel. However, the rate of

utilisation of ketone bodies by peripheral tissues is limited, and when the rate of production by the liver exceeds their removal, hyperketonaemia results. This occurs physiologically during starvation, when low insulin levels and high catecholamine levels increase lipolysis and delivery of FFAs to the liver.

Investigations

Urine glucose

Testing the urine for glucose with dipsticks is a common screening procedure for detecting diabetes. If possible, testing should be performed on urine passed 1–2 hours after a meal to maximise sensitivity. Glycosuria always warrants further assessment by blood testing (see below). The greatest disadvantage of urine glucose measurement is the individual variation in renal threshold for glucose. The most frequent cause of glycosuria is a low renal threshold, which is common during pregnancy and in young people; the resulting 'renal glycosuria' is a benign condition unrelated to diabetes. Another disadvantage is that some drugs (such as β-lactam antibiotics, levodopa and salicylates) may interfere with urine glucose tests.

Blood glucose

Laboratory glucose testing in blood relies on an enzymatic reaction (glucose oxidase) and is cheap, usually automated and highly reliable. However, blood glucose levels depend on whether the patient has eaten recently, so it is important to consider the circumstances in which the blood sample was taken.

Blood glucose can also be measured with testing sticks that are read with a portable electronic meter. These are used for capillary (fingerprick) testing to monitor diabetes treatment (p. 742). There is some debate as to whether self-monitoring in people with type 2 diabetes improves glycaemic control. Many countries now offer self-monitoring only to people with type 2 diabetes taking sulphonylurea or insulin therapy because of the risk of hypoglycaemia. To make the diagnosis of diabetes, the blood glucose concentration should be estimated using an accurate laboratory method rather than a portable technique.

Glucose concentrations are lower in venous than arterial or capillary (fingerprick) blood. Whole-blood glucose concentrations are lower than plasma concentrations because red blood cells contain relatively little glucose. Venous plasma values are usually the most reliable for diagnostic purposes (Boxes 20.2 and 20.3).

 20.2 Diagnosis of diabetes and pre-diabetes

Diabetes is confirmed by:

- *either* plasma glucose in random sample or 2 hrs after a 75 g glucose load ≥11.1 mmol/L (200 mg/dL) *or*
- fasting plasma glucose ≥7.0 mmol/L (126 mg/dL) *or*
- HbA$_{1c}$ ≥48 mmol/mol

In asymptomatic patients, two diagnostic tests are required to confirm diabetes; the second test should be the same as the first test to avoid confusion

'Pre-diabetes' is classified as:

- impaired fasting glucose = fasting plasma glucose ≥6.1 mmol/L (110 mg/dL) and <7.0 mmol/L (126 mg/dL)
- impaired glucose tolerance = fasting plasma glucose <7.0 mmol/L (126 mg/dL) *and* 2-hr glucose after 75 g oral glucose drink 7.8–11.1 mmol/L (140–200 mg/dL)

HbA$_{1c}$ criteria for pre-diabetes vary. The National Institute for Health and Care Excellence (NICE) guidelines (UK) recommend considering an HbA$_{1c}$ range of 42–47 mmol/mol to be indicative of pre-diabetes; the American Diabetes Association (ADA) guidelines suggest a range of 39–47 mmol/mol. The ADA also suggests a lower fasting plasma glucose limit of ≥ 5.6 mmol/L (100 mg/dL) for impaired fasting glucose.

 20.3 How to perform an oral glucose tolerance test (OGTT)

Preparation before the test

- Unrestricted carbohydrate diet for 3 days
- Fasted overnight for at least 8 hrs
- Rest for 30 mins
- Remain seated for the duration of the test, with no smoking

Sampling

- Measure plasma glucose before and 2 hrs after a 75 g oral glucose drink

---

Interstitial glucose

A relatively new approach to measuring glucose levels in diabetes is through the use of interstitial continuous glucose monitoring (CGM). CGM systems use a tiny sensor inserted under the skin to check glucose levels in interstitial fluid. The sensor can stay in place for up to 2 weeks before being replaced and provides real-time measurements of glucose levels every 1 or 5 minutes (see Fig. 20.16, p. 751). These devices are not as accurate as blood glucose testing, particularly when levels are low or changing rapidly, so users must still check blood glucose with a glucose meter before driving or changing therapy. CGM provides useful information on daily glucose profiles and, in particular, night-time glucose levels. In addition, alarms can be incorporated into the CGM device to warn individuals about hypoglycaemia.

Urine and blood ketones

Acetoacetate can be identified in urine by the nitroprusside reaction, using either tablets or dipsticks. Ketonuria may be found in normal people who have been fasting or exercising strenuously for long periods, vomiting repeatedly, or eating a diet high in fat and low in carbohydrate. Ketonuria is therefore not pathognomonic of diabetes but, if it is associated with glycosuria, the diagnosis of diabetes is highly likely. Urine ketone measurements are semi-quantitative, awkward to perform and retrospective (i.e. the urine has accumulated over several hours). Also, they do not measure the major ketone found in blood during diabetic ketoacidosis (DKA), beta-hydroxybutyrate (β-OHB). Beta-OHB can be measured in blood in the laboratory and also in a fingerprick specimen of capillary blood with a test stick and electronic meter. Whole-blood β-OHB monitoring is useful in assisting with insulin adjustment during intercurrent illness or sustained hyperglycaemia to prevent or detect DKA. Blood β-OHB monitoring is also useful in monitoring resolution of DKA in hospitalised patients (Box 20.4).

Glycated haemoglobin

Glycated haemoglobin provides an accurate and objective measure of glycaemic control over a period of weeks to months.

In diabetes, the slow non-enzymatic covalent attachment of glucose to haemoglobin (glycation) increases the amount in the HbA$_1$ (HbA$_{1c}$) fraction relative to non-glycated adult haemoglobin (HbA$_0$). These fractions can be separated by chromatography;

---

i 20.4 Interpretation of capillary blood ketone measurements

Measurement*	Interpretation
<0.6 mmol/L	Normal; no action required
0.6–1.5 mmol/L	Suggests metabolic control may be deteriorating; the patient should continue to monitor and seek medical advice if sustained/progressive
1.5–3.0 mmol/L	With high blood glucose (>10 mmol/L), there is a high risk of diabetic ketoacidosis; seek medical advice
>3.0 mmol/L	Severe ketosis; in the presence of high glucose (>10 mmol/L) suggests presence of diabetic ketoacidosis; seek urgent medical help

*To convert to mg/dL, multiply values by 18.

i	20.5 Conversion between DCCT and IFCC units for HbA$_{1c}$	
DCCT units (%)		IFCC units (mmol/mol)
4		20
5		31
6		42
7		53
8		64
9		75
10		86
IFCC HbA$_{1c}$ (mmol/mol) = [DCCT HbA$_{1c}$(%)–2.15] × 10.929		

(DCCT = Diabetes Control and Complications Trial; IFCC = International Federation of Clinical Chemistry and Laboratory Medicine)

laboratories may report glycated haemoglobin as total glycated haemoglobin (GHb), HbA$_1$ or HbA$_{1c}$. In most countries, HbA$_{1c}$ is the preferred measurement. The rate of formation of HbA$_{1c}$ is directly proportional to the ambient blood glucose concentration; a rise of 11 mmol/mol in HbA$_{1c}$ corresponds to an approximate average increase of 2 mmol/L (36 mg/dL) in blood glucose. Although HbA$_{1c}$ concentration reflects the integrated blood glucose control over the lifespan of erythrocytes (120 days), HbA$_{1c}$ is most sensitive to changes in glycaemic control occurring in the month before measurement.

Various assay methods are used to measure HbA$_{1c}$, but most laboratories have been reporting HbA$_{1c}$ values (as %) aligned with the reference range that was used in the Diabetes Control and Complications Trial (DCCT). To allow worldwide comparisons of HbA$_{1c}$ values, the International Federation of Clinical Chemistry and Laboratory Medicine (IFCC) has developed a standard method; IFCC-standardised HbA$_{1c}$ values are reported in mmol/mol. In 2011, many countries adopted the IFCC reference method (Box 20.5) and this is used throughout this textbook.

HbA$_{1c}$ estimates may be erroneously diminished in anaemia or during pregnancy, and may be difficult to interpret with some assay methods in patients who have uraemia or a haemoglobinopathy. It is particularly important to be aware of this in some developing countries where nutritional deficiency is common, especially when an absolute cut-off point is used, e.g. in the diagnosis of diabetes.

Islet autoantibodies

As type 1 diabetes is a characterised by autoimmune destruction of the pancreatic β cells, it can be useful in the differential diagnosis of diabetes (see below) to establish evidence of such an autoimmune process. If islet autoantibodies are present at high titre, this can be supportive of a diagnosis of type 1 diabetes. The antibodies that are measured are directed against components of the islet and consist of antibodies to insulin, glutamic acid decarboxylase (GAD), protein tyrosine phosphatase-related proteins (IA-2) and the zinc transporter ZnT8. These antibodies can be detected in the general population; the level at which they are called positive does vary by laboratory but is usually at concentrations greater than the 95th centile or 97.5th centile of the general population. This means that pancreatic autoantibodies can be weakly positive in people who do not have type 1 diabetes. However, if anti-GAD and anti-IA-2 antibodies are measured together, they will be 'positive' (alone or in combination) in approximately 85% of newly diagnosed type 1 diabetes. Some laboratories now include anti-ZnT8 antibodies in their panel of tests, which increases sensitivity for type 1 diabetes to 92%.

C-peptide

C-peptide is the connecting peptide that is cleaved in the production of insulin from pro-insulin (see Fig. 20.4). It can be readily measured in blood and urine by sensitive immunoassays. Serum C-peptide is a marker of endogenous insulin secretion (a synthetic insulin does not contain C-peptide) and is particularly useful if a patient is on exogenous (injected) insulin treatment, when insulin assays would simply detect the injected insulin. Serum C-peptide can help clarify the differential diagnosis of diabetes, as it is usually very low in long-standing type 1 diabetes and very high in severe insulin resistance. It is also useful in the diagnosis of spontaneous hypoglycaemia (p. 676).

Urine protein

Standard urine dipstick testing for albumin detects urinary albumin at concentrations above 300 mg/L, but smaller amounts (microalbuminuria; see Box 15.9, p. 394) can only be measured using specific albumin dipsticks or quantitative biochemical laboratory tests. Microalbuminuria or proteinuria, in the absence of urinary tract infection, is an important indicator of diabetic nephropathy and/or increased risk of macrovascular disease (p. 757).

Establishing the diagnosis of diabetes

Glycaemia can be classified into three categories: normal, impaired (pre-diabetes) and diabetes (see Box 20.2). The glycaemia cut-off that defines diabetes is based on the level above which there is a significant risk of microvascular complications (retinopathy, nephropathy and neuropathy). People categorised as having pre-diabetes have blood glucose levels that carry a negligible risk of microvascular complications but are at increased risk of developing diabetes. Also, because there is a continuous risk of macrovascular disease (atheroma of large conduit blood vessels) with increasing glycaemia in the population, people with pre-diabetes have an increased risk of cardiovascular disease (myocardial infarction, stroke and peripheral vascular disease).

The traditional way to diagnose diabetes or pre-diabetes has been by using random or fasting plasma glucose and/or an oral glucose tolerance test (OGTT). In 2011, the World Health Organisation (WHO) advocated the use of glycated haemoglobin (HbA$_{1c}$, see above) to diagnose diabetes and this has been adopted in some regions. When a person has symptoms of diabetes, the diagnosis can be confirmed with either a fasting glucose of ≥7.0 mmol/L (126 mg/dL) or a random glucose of ≥11.1 mmol/L (200 mg/dL) (see Box 20.2). Asymptomatic individuals should have a second confirmatory test. Diabetes should not be diagnosed on capillary blood glucose results. Alternatively, an HbA$_{1c}$ of ≥48 mmol/mol is also diagnostic of diabetes. As HbA$_{1c}$ reflects the last 2–3 months of glycaemia, it should not be used to diagnose diabetes where the duration of onset is short, i.e. in someone with suspected type 1 diabetes or severe symptomatic hyperglycaemia (p. 734). If there is a high clinical suspicion of diabetes with an HbA$_{1c}$ of less than 48 mmol/mol, then a fasting glucose measurement is required to rule out diabetes. It should be noted that the two populations identified using blood glucose and using HbA$_{1c}$ will not be identical, some

20

being diagnosed with diabetes using one criterion but not the other. When a person is asymptomatic and repeat testing is required, the same method should be used for the confirmatory test to avoid diagnostic confusion.

Pre-diabetes can be subclassified as 'impaired fasting glucose' (IFG), based on a fasting plasma glucose result, or 'impaired glucose tolerance' (IGT), based on the fasting and 2-hour OGTT results (see Box 20.3). Patients with pre-diabetes should be advised of their risk of progression to diabetes, given advice about lifestyle modification to reduce this risk (as for type 2 diabetes, p. 743), and have aggressive management of cardiovascular risk factors such as hypertension and dyslipidaemia. The HbA$_{1c}$ criteria for pre-diabetes are less clear. The NICE guidelines (UK) suggest a range of 42–47 mmol/mol, whereas the American Diabetes Association guidelines recommend a range of 39–47 mmol/mol.

In some people (especially those with pre-existing insulin resistance or low β-cell mass/function), an abnormal blood glucose result is observed during acute severe illness, such as infection or myocardial infarction. This 'stress hyperglycaemia' is a consequence of hormones, such as cortisol and catecholamines, antagonising the action of insulin and thereby increasing insulin resistance. It usually disappears after the acute illness has resolved, but affected individuals have a significantly increased risk of type 2 diabetes in subsequent years. A similar mechanism explains the occurrence of diabetes in some people treated with glucocorticoids (steroid-induced diabetes).

The diagnostic criteria recommended for diabetes in pregnancy are more stringent than those for non-pregnant patients (see Box 20.31). Pregnant women with abnormal glucose tolerance should be referred urgently to a specialist unit for full evaluation. Due to the increased red cell turnover that occurs in pregnancy, an HbA$_{1c}$ test should not be used to diagnose diabetes in pregnancy.

When a diagnosis of diabetes is confirmed, other investigations should include plasma urea, creatinine and electrolytes, lipids, liver and thyroid function tests, blood or urine ketones, and urine protein.

Aetiology and pathogenesis of diabetes

In both of the common types of diabetes, environmental factors interact with genetic susceptibility to determine which people develop the clinical syndrome, and the timing of its onset. However, the underlying genes, precipitating environmental factors and pathophysiology differ substantially between type 1 and type 2 diabetes. Type 1 diabetes was previously termed 'insulin-dependent diabetes mellitus' (IDDM) and is invariably associated with insulin deficiency requiring replacement therapy. Type 2 diabetes was previously termed 'non-insulin-dependent diabetes mellitus' (NIDDM) because patients retain the capacity to secrete insulin, and measured insulin levels are often higher than those seen in people without diabetes. In type 2 diabetes, though, there is an impaired sensitivity to insulin (insulin resistance) and, initially, affected individuals can usually be treated without insulin replacement therapy. However, 20% or more of patients with type 2 diabetes will ultimately develop insulin deficiency requiring replacement therapy, so IDDM and NIDDM were misnomers.

Type 1 diabetes

Pathology

Type 1 diabetes is generally considered a T-cell-mediated autoimmune disease (p. 81) involving destruction of the insulin-secreting β cells in the pancreatic islets. The natural history of type 1 diabetes is based on the model proposed by Eisenbarth in 1986, which proposed that genetically susceptible individuals with a given β-cell mass who were subsequently exposed to an environmental trigger then developed β-cell autoimmunity that led to progressive loss of β cells. This process was seen to take place over a prolonged period (months to years). Marked hyperglycaemia, accompanied by the classical symptoms of diabetes, occurs only when 80–90% of the functional capacity of β cells has been lost. More recent data have led to modifications of this model. For example, it is now recognised that pancreatic β cells can persist in some individuals with very long-standing diabetes and may never reach zero. On the contrary, some individuals present with much higher levels of β-cell viability (40–50%) and that may reflect lower levels of physical activity or increased body mass. Despite this uncertainty, in the natural history of type 1 diabetes there is initially a loss of first-phase insulin secretion, followed by a period of glucose intolerance and clinically undiagnosed diabetes.

The pathology in the pre-diabetic pancreas is characterised by an inflammatory lesion within islets, 'insulitis' (Fig. 20.6), with infiltration of the islets by mononuclear cells containing activated macrophages, helper cytotoxic and suppressor T lymphocytes, natural killer cells and B lymphocytes. Initially, these lesions are patchy and, until a very late stage, lobules containing heavily infiltrated islets are seen adjacent to unaffected lobules. The destructive process is β-cell-specific. It is unclear why other hormone-secreting cells in the islets, such as α and δ cells, remain intact. In addition, while a number of theories such as molecular mimicry, oxidative stress and viral infections have been proposed, the specific mechanisms for inducing autoimmunity in type 1 diabetes are unknown.

Autoimmunity in type 1 diabetes is identified by the presence of autoantibodies to islet and/or β-cell antigens. Islet cell antibodies can be present long before the clinical presentation of type 1 diabetes, and their detection can be useful in confirming a diagnosis of type 1 diabetes, but they are poorly predictive of disease progression and disappear over time (Fig. 20.6). Autoantibodies are typically present in 70–80% of newly diagnosed type 1 diabetes, but this can vary depending on age, gender and ethnicity, as well as quality of the assay employed. Autoantibodies can also be used to predict disease with a 5-year risk of type 1 diabetes of about 20–25% in people with a single positive autoantibody, 50–60% in those with two positive autoantibodies, and 70% in those with three autoantibodies. Type 1 diabetes is associated with other autoimmune disorders (Ch. 4), including thyroid disease (p. 638), coeliac disease (p. 805), Addison's disease (p. 671), pernicious anaemia (p. 944) and vitiligo (p. 1257). The association between type 1 diabetes and coeliac disease is particularly strong; it is estimated that around 1 in 20 people with type 1 diabetes (especially when diagnosed in childhood) will have biopsy-proven coeliac disease and so many countries advocate routine screening for this condition.

Genetic predisposition

Although not showing a simple pattern of inheritance, type 1 diabetes is strongly influenced by genetic factors. The relationship is complex and, as indicated, multifactorial. Monozygotic twins have a disease concordance rate of 30–50%, while dizygotic twins have a concordance of 6–10%. In the USA, the risk of developing type 1 diabetes is 1:20 for those with a first-degree relative, compared with a 1:300 risk in the general population. Children of mothers with type 1 diabetes have a 1–4% risk of

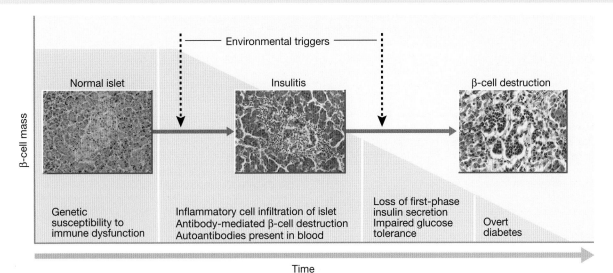

Fig. 20.6 Pathogenesis of type 1 diabetes. Proposed sequence of events in the development of type 1 diabetes. Environmental triggers are described in the text. *Insets (normal islet, β-cell destruction) Courtesy of Dr A. Foulis, Dept of Pathology, University of Glasgow.*

i 20.6 Risk of type 1 diabetes among first-degree relatives of patients with type 1 diabetes	
Relative with type 1 diabetes	**% overall risk**
Identical twin	30–50
Non-identical twin	6–10
HLA-identical sibling	16
Non-HLA-identical sibling	5
Father	10
Mother	1–4
Both parents	Up to 30

developing type 1 diabetes, but children of fathers with type 1 diabetes have a 10% risk. Despite this genetic influence, 80–85% of new cases present in individuals with no known family history of the disease.

The inheritance of type 1 diabetes is polygenic (Box 20.6), with over 20 different regions of the human genome showing an association with type 1 diabetes risk. Most interest has focused on the human leucocyte antigen (HLA) region within the major histocompatibility complex on the short arm of chromosome 6. The HLA haplotypes *DR3* and/or *DR4* are associated with increased susceptibility to type 1 diabetes in Caucasians and are in 'linkage disequilibrium', i.e. they tend to be transmitted together, with the neighbouring alleles of the *HLA-DQA1* and *DQB1* genes. The latter may be the main determinants of genetic susceptibility, since these HLA class II genes code for proteins on the surface of cells that present foreign and self-antigens to T lymphocytes (p. 82). Candidate gene and genome-wide association studies have also implicated other genes in type 1 diabetes, e.g. *CD25*, *PTPN22*, SH2B3, *IL2RA* and *IL-10*. Interestingly, the majority of these disease risk loci are involved in immune responsiveness, such as recognition of pancreatic islet antigens, T-cell development and immune regulation. The genes associated with type 1 diabetes overlap with those for other autoimmune disorders, such as coeliac disease and thyroid disease, consistent with clustering of these conditions in individuals or families.

Environmental predisposition

The wide geographical and seasonal variations in incidence, and the rapid acquisition of local disease incidence rates in migrants from low- to high-incidence countries suggest that environmental factors have an important role in precipitating disease.

Although hypotheses abound, the nature of these environmental factors is unknown. They may trigger type 1 diabetes through direct toxicity to β cells or by stimulating an autoimmune reaction directed against β cells. Potential candidates fall into three main categories: viruses, specific drugs or chemicals, and dietary constituents. Viruses implicated in the aetiology of type 1 diabetes include mumps, Coxsackie B4, retroviruses, rubella (in utero), cytomegalovirus and Epstein–Barr virus. Various dietary nitrosamines (found in smoked and cured meats) and coffee have been proposed as potentially diabetogenic toxins. Bovine serum albumin (BSA), a major constituent of cow's milk, has been implicated, since children who are given cow's milk early in infancy are more likely to develop type 1 diabetes than those who are breastfed. BSA may cross the neonatal gut and raise antibodies that cross-react with a heat-shock protein expressed by β cells. It has also been proposed that reduced exposure to microorganisms in early childhood limits maturation of the immune system and increases susceptibility to autoimmune disease (the 'hygiene hypothesis'). In addition, the high incidence rates in northern Europe have led to the suggestion that low levels of vitamin D may be important, but to date no clear cause–effect relationship has been identified.

Metabolic disturbances in type 1 diabetes

Patients with type 1 diabetes present when progressive β-cell destruction has crossed a threshold at which adequate insulin secretion and normal blood glucose levels can no longer be sustained. Above a certain level, high glucose levels may be toxic to the remaining β cells, so that profound insulin deficiency rapidly ensues, causing the metabolic sequelae shown in Figure 20.7. Hyperglycaemia leads to glycosuria and dehydration, causing fatigue, polyuria, nocturia, thirst and polydipsia, susceptibility to urinary and genital tract infections, and later tachycardia and hypotension. Unrestrained lipolysis and proteolysis result in

20

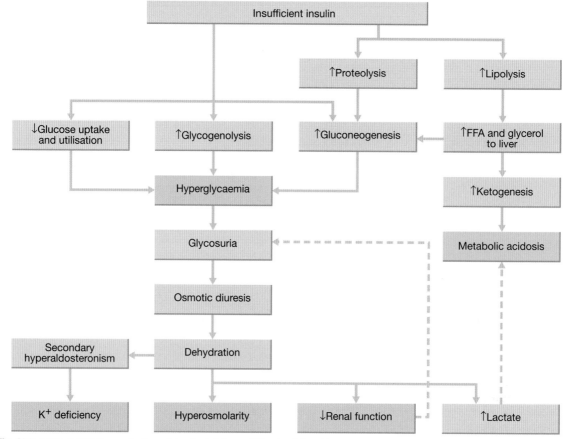

Fig. 20.7 **Acute metabolic complications of insulin deficiency.** (FFA = free fatty acid)

weight loss. Ketoacidosis occurs when generation of ketones exceeds the capacity for their metabolism. Elevated blood H^+ ions drive K^+ out of the intracellular compartment, while secondary hyperaldosteronism encourages urinary loss of K^+. Thus patients usually present with a short history (typically a few weeks) of hyperglycaemic symptoms (thirst, polyuria, nocturia and fatigue), infections and weight loss, and may have developed ketoacidosis (p. 735).

Type 1 diabetes in adults

While type 1 diabetes is classically thought of as a disease of children and young adults (most commonly presenting between 5 and 7 years of age and at or near puberty), it can manifest at any age, with as much as half of cases thought to develop in adults. It is also possible for patients who have a more insidious onset of diabetes to have an autoimmune aetiology; these people are sometimes described as having slow-onset type 1 diabetes or latent autoimmune diabetes of adulthood (LADA). LADA is defined as the presence of islet autoantibodies in high titre (usually GAD antibodies), without rapid progression to insulin therapy (which would usually signify type 1 diabetes). Patients with LADA can often present and be managed similarly to those with type 2 diabetes, but they do progress more rapidly to requiring insulin treatment for glucose control. Not all expert committees recognise LADA as a diagnostic category, however, and consider LADA to be just a subset of autoimmune type 1 diabetes developing in adulthood.

Type 2 diabetes

Pathology

Type 2 diabetes is a diagnosis of exclusion, i.e. it is made when type 1 diabetes and other types of diabetes (see Box 20.9) are ruled out; it is highly heterogeneous. The natural history of typical type 2 diabetes is shown in Figure 20.8. Initially, insulin resistance leads to elevated insulin secretion in order to maintain normal blood glucose levels. However, in susceptible individuals, the pancreatic β cells are unable to sustain the increased demand for insulin and a slowly progressive insulin deficiency develops. Some patients develop diabetes at a young age, usually driven by insulin resistance due to obesity and ethnicity; others, particularly older patients, develop diabetes despite being non-obese and may have more pronounced β-cell failure. The key feature is a 'relative' insulin deficiency, such that there is insufficient insulin production to overcome the resistance to insulin action. This contrasts with type 1 diabetes, in which there is rapid loss of insulin production, resulting in ketoacidosis and death if the insulin is not replaced.

Insulin resistance and the metabolic syndrome

Type 2 diabetes and its pre-diabetes antecedents belong to a cluster of conditions thought to be caused by resistance to insulin action. Thus, people with type 2 diabetes often have associated disorders including hypertension, dyslipidaemia (characterised by elevated levels of small dense low-density lipoprotein (LDL)

Fig. 20.8 Natural history of type 2 diabetes. **A** In the early stage of the disorder, the response to progressive insulin resistance is an increase in insulin secretion by the pancreatic cells, causing hyperinsulinaemia. Eventually, the β cells are unable to compensate adequately and blood glucose rises, producing hyperglycaemia. With further β-cell failure, glycaemic control deteriorates and treatment requirements escalate. **B** Progressive pancreatic β-cell failure in patients with type 2 diabetes in the United Kingdom Prospective Diabetes Study (UKPDS). Beta-cell function was estimated using the homeostasis model assessment (HOMA) and was already below 50% at the time of diagnosis. Thereafter, long-term incremental increases in fasting plasma glucose were accompanied by progressive β-cell dysfunction. If the slope of this progression is extrapolated, it appears that pancreatic dysfunction may have been developing for many years before diagnosis of diabetes. *B, Adapted from Holman RR. Diabetes Res Clin Pract 1998; 40 (Suppl.):S21–S25.*

cholesterol and triglycerides, and a low level of high-density lipoprotein (HDL) cholesterol), non-alcoholic fatty liver disease (p. 882) and, in women, polycystic ovarian syndrome. This cluster has been termed the 'insulin resistance syndrome' or 'metabolic syndrome', and is much more common in individuals who are obese.

The primary cause of insulin resistance remains unclear; it is likely that there are multiple defects in insulin signalling, affecting several tissues. One theory is centred around the adipocyte; this is particularly appealing, as obesity is a major cause of increased insulin resistance. Intra-abdominal 'central' adipose tissue is metabolically active and releases large quantities of FFAs, which may induce insulin resistance because they compete with glucose as a fuel supply for oxidation in peripheral tissues such as muscle. In addition, adipose tissue releases a number of hormones (including a variety of peptides, called 'adipokines' because they are structurally similar to immunological 'cytokines') that act on specific receptors to influence sensitivity to insulin in other tissues. Because the venous drainage of visceral adipose tissue is into the portal vein, central obesity may have a particularly potent influence on insulin sensitivity in the liver, and thereby adversely affect gluconeogenesis and hepatic lipid metabolism.

Physical activity is another important determinant of insulin sensitivity. Inactivity is associated with down-regulation of insulin-sensitive kinases and may promote accumulation of FFAs within skeletal muscle. Sedentary people are therefore more insulin-resistant than active people with the same degree of obesity. Moreover, physical activity allows non-insulin-dependent glucose uptake into muscle, reducing the 'demand' on the pancreatic β cells to produce insulin.

Deposition of fat in the liver is a common association with central obesity and is exacerbated by insulin resistance and/or deficiency. Many people with type 2 diabetes have evidence of fatty infiltration of the liver (non-alcoholic fatty liver disease, NAFLD). This condition may improve with effective

i	**20.7 Risk of developing type 2 diabetes for siblings of individuals with type 2 diabetes**	
Age at onset of type 2 diabetes in proband (years)	**Age-corrected risk of type 2 diabetes for siblings (%)**	
25–44	53	
45–54	37	
55–64	38	
65–80	31	

treatment of the diabetes but, despite this, some patients progress to non-alcoholic steatohepatitis (NASH, p. 882) and cirrhosis.

Pancreatic β-cell failure

In the early stages of type 2 diabetes, reduction in the total mass of pancreatic islet tissue is modest. At the time of diagnosis, around 50% of β-cell function has been lost and this declines progressively (Fig. 20.8B). Some pathological changes are typical of type 2 diabetes, the most consistent of which is deposition of amyloid in the islets. In addition, elevated plasma glucose and FFAs exert toxic effects on pancreatic β cells to impair insulin secretion. However, while β-cell numbers are reduced, β-cell mass is unchanged and glucagon secretion is increased, which may contribute to hyperglycaemia.

Genetic predisposition

Genetic factors are important in type 2 diabetes, as shown by marked differences in susceptibility in different ethnic groups and by studies in monozygotic twins where concordance rates for type 2 diabetes approach 100%. However, many genes are involved and the chance of developing diabetes is also influenced very powerfully by environmental factors (Box 20.7). Genome-wide association studies have identified over 70 genes

20

or gene regions that are associated with type 2 diabetes, each exerting a small effect. Most of the genes known to contribute to risk of type 2 diabetes are involved in β-cell function or in regulation of cell cycling and turnover, suggesting that altered regulation of β-cell mass is a key factor. The largest population genetic effect described to date is seen with variation in *TCF7L2*; the 10% of the population with two copies of the risk variant for this gene have a nearly twofold increase in risk of developing type 2 diabetes. In general, other common variants explain much lower risk than this, many explaining less than a 10% increase in risk only; as only about 10% of the genetic variance in type 2 diabetes is explained by these common genetic variants, this has led some to question the relevance of finding diabetes genes. However, it should be noted that, within a population, the distribution of risk variants will vary, with some patients having inherited a high genetic burden (e.g. more than 40 risk variants) and others having inherited very few. When studies compare those in the top 20% of this risk band with the lowest 20%, those at highest risk are over 2.5 times more likely to develop diabetes. More recent insights into the genetics of type 2 diabetes have highlighted how some genetic variants may be rare and therefore affect only a small proportion of the population, but have large clinical effects. For example, in a Greenlandic population, 3% of people carry a homozygous variant in an insulin signalling gene, *TBC1D4*, that results in muscle insulin resistance; these individuals are over 10 times more likely to develop type 2 diabetes.

Environmental and other risk factors

Diet and obesity

Epidemiological studies show that type 2 diabetes is associated with overeating, especially when combined with obesity and under-activity. Middle-aged people with diabetes eat significantly more and are fatter and less active than their non-diabetic siblings. The risk of developing type 2 diabetes increases 10-fold in people with a body mass index (BMI) of more than 30 kg/m^2 (p. 698). However, although the majority of individuals with type 2 diabetes are obese, only a minority of obese people develop diabetes, as most obese people are able to increase insulin secretion to compensate for the increased demand resulting from obesity and insulin resistance. Those who develop diabetes may have genetically impaired β-cell function, reduced β-cell mass, or a susceptibility of β cells to attack by toxic substances such as FFAs or inflammatory cytokines.

Age

Type 2 diabetes is more common in middle-aged and older individuals (Box 20.8). In the UK, it affects 10% of the population over 65, and over 70% of all cases of diabetes occur after the age of 50 years.

20.8 Diagnosis of diabetes mellitus in old age

- **Prevalence**: increases with age, affecting ~10% of people over 65 years. Half of these are undiagnosed. Impaired β-cell function and exaggerated insulin resistance with ageing both contribute.
- **Glycosuria**: the renal threshold for glucose rises with age, so glycosuria may not develop until the blood glucose concentration is markedly raised.
- **Pancreatic carcinoma**: may present in old age with the development of diabetes, in association with weight loss and diminished appetite.

Ethnicity

Ethnic origin is a major risk factor for development of diabetes. For example, within the USA, the prevalence of diabetes is lowest in Alaskan Natives at 5.5%, moderate for non-Hispanic whites at 7.1%, high for non-Hispanic blacks at 13% and highest in Native Americans at 33%. This considerable variation in prevalence reflects a number of different factors, including a higher BMI and lower socioeconomic class in high-risk groups in the USA; differences in health behaviour, e.g. decreased physical activity and increased smoking; and differences in genetic risk. Studies in high-risk ethnic groups largely demonstrate increased insulin resistance and more central/visceral adiposity than in the lower-risk groups.

Metabolic disturbances in type 2 diabetes

Patients with type 2 diabetes have a slow onset of 'relative' insulin deficiency. Relatively small amounts of insulin are required to suppress lipolysis, and some glucose uptake is maintained in muscle so that, in contrast to type 1 diabetes, lipolysis and proteolysis are not unrestrained and weight loss and ketoacidosis seldom occur. In type 2 diabetes, hyperglycaemia tends to develop slowly over months or years; because of this insidious onset many cases of type 2 diabetes are discovered coincidentally and a large number are undetected. At diagnosis, patients are often asymptomatic or give a long history (typically many months) of fatigue, with or without 'osmotic symptoms' (thirst and polyuria). However, there are some people with type 2 diabetes who present acutely with marked osmotic symptoms and weight loss. These may be presenting late, such that they have already developed β-cell failure, but more usually this decompensation reflects a vicious spiral of decline. As hyperglycaemia worsens, patients often crave sugar and will consume large volumes of sugary drinks to try to quench their thirst; worsening hyperglycaemia is also associated with increasing lipolysis, and the high circulating glucose and FFAs are toxic to the β cell, resulting in 'glucolipotoxicity' and reduced β-cell function. In these patients, ketosis and even DKA can occur; this is classically described in the African American population, where up to half of patients who present with DKA have type 2 diabetes and not type 1 diabetes. The presentation of DKA in type 2 diabetes is referred to as 'ketosis-prone' diabetes or 'Flatbush syndrome', named after the Flatbush neighbourhood of New York, which had a large Caribbean population and where presentation with DKA was common. Importantly in these patients, insulin treatment is required initially but, as the glucose and lipids are controlled, the β cells recover, and they can usually transfer off insulin and on to oral treatments such as metformin after 3 months of insulin treatment.

Intercurrent illness, e.g. with infections, increases the production of stress hormones that oppose insulin action, such as cortisol, growth hormone and catecholamines. This can precipitate an acute exacerbation of insulin resistance and insulin deficiency, and result in more severe hyperglycaemia and dehydration (p. 738).

Other forms of diabetes

Other causes of diabetes are shown in Box 20.9. These can broadly be broken down into genetic disorders including monogenic diabetes (diabetes due to a mutation in or deletion of a single gene) or diabetes as part of a genetic syndrome; endocrine disorders due to excess in hormones that oppose

20.9 Aetiological classification of diabetes mellitus

Type 1 diabetes
- Immune-mediated
- Idiopathic

Type 2 diabetes

Other specific types
- Genetic defects of β-cell function (see Box 20.10)
- Genetic defects of insulin action (e.g. leprechaunism, lipodystrophies)
- Pancreatic disease (e.g. pancreatitis, pancreatectomy, neoplastic disease, cystic fibrosis, haemochromatosis, fibrocalculous pancreatopathy)
- Excess endogenous production of hormonal antagonists to insulin, e.g.:
  - Growth hormone – acromegaly
  - Glucocorticoids – Cushing's syndrome
  - Glucagon – glucagonoma
  - Catecholamines – phaeochromocytoma
  - Thyroid hormones – thyrotoxicosis
- Drug-induced (e.g. glucocorticoids, thiazide diuretics, phenytoin)
- Uncommon forms of immune-mediated diabetes (e.g. IPEX syndrome)
- Associated with genetic syndromes (e.g. Down's syndrome, Klinefelter's syndrome, Turner's syndrome, DIDMOAD (Wolfram's syndrome), Friedreich's ataxia, myotonic dystrophy)

Gestational diabetes

(DIDMOAD = diabetes insipidus, diabetes mellitus, optic atrophy, nerve deafness; IPEX = immunodysregulation polyendocrinopathy X)

20.10 Monogenic diabetes mellitus: maturity-onset diabetes of the young (MODY)

Functional defect	Main type*	Gene mutated*
β-cell glucose sensing	MODY2	*GCK*

The set point for basal insulin release is altered, causing a high fasting glucose, but sufficient insulin is released after meals. As a result, the HbA$_{1c}$ is often normal and microvascular complications are rare. Treatment is rarely required

Functional defect	Main type*	Gene mutated*
β-cell transcriptional regulation	MODY3	*HNF1α*
	MODY5	*HNF1β*
	MODY1	*HNF4α*

Diabetes develops during adolescence/early adulthood and can be managed with diet and tablets for many years, but ultimately, insulin treatment is required. The HNF1α and 4α forms respond particularly well to sulphonylurea drugs. All types are associated with microvascular complications. *HNF1β* mutations also cause renal cysts and renal failure

*Other gene mutations have been found in rare cases. For further information, see diabetesgenes.org.

---

the effects of insulin (Ch. 18); and more generalised diseases of the pancreas.

Pancreatic disease

Pancreatic disease is a relatively common but often unrecognised cause of diabetes, largely related to alcohol excess. Alcohol excess can cause recurrent bouts of acute pancreatitis, with progressive destruction of the pancreas and subsequent diabetes. However, more commonly, chronic alcohol excess can be linked to chronic pancreatitis, which is then termed alcoholic chronic pancreatitis. Although this is associated with recurrent abdominal pain, it is asymptomatic in many patients, resulting in both pancreatic exocrine failure and endocrine failure. While diabetes due to pancreatic insufficiency secondary to alcohol excess can be managed with oral therapy, the insulin deficiency usually requires insulin replacement therapy.

In some geographical regions, there is a form of chronic calcific pancreatitis that is not caused by alcohol excess and causes diabetes to present in adolescence or early adulthood; this condition is called fibrocalculous pancreatic diabetes (FCPD). It is characteristically a disease of the tropics, with variable prevalence across these regions. The aetiology of FCPD is poorly understood. While there is thought to be a genetic predisposition, with mutations in *SPINK1* being described, it is usually seen in malnourished individuals, but it is not clear whether this is a cause or consequence of the disease. FCPD usually presents with recurrent severe abdominal pain in childhood, diabetes developing 10–20 years later; there is a 100-fold increased risk of pancreatic cancer in later life. Insulin treatment is usually required at or soon after diagnosis.

Monogenic diabetes

Monogenic diabetes accounts for approximately 4% of diabetes in those diagnosed under the age of 30 in the UK. While there are a number of monogenic disorders of insulin action, the most common monogenic forms of diabetes are caused by defects in insulin secretion, in part because insulin resistance alone is not sufficient to cause diabetes. Monogenic disorders of the β cell cause two diabetes subtypes: maturity-onset diabetes of the young (MODY; Box 20.10) and neonatal diabetes. The common genes involved in MODY and neonatal diabetes are shown in Figure 20.2C.

MODY is defined as non-insulin-requiring diabetes that develops under the age of 25 years in one family member. MODY is dominantly inherited (p. 46), which means that the diabetes runs in families, many having a family history of diabetes spanning three generations or more. MODY itself is a heterogeneous condition, with multiple subtypes. One form is caused by mutations in glucokinase (see Fig. 20.2B); this is the pancreatic glucose sensor and patients with glucokinase mutations have an altered set-point for glucose. This results in a high fasting glucose (usually >5.5 mmol/L (99 mg/dL)) but a normal post-prandial response. As a result, patients with glucokinase MODY have stable, mild hyperglycaemia, with only a slightly elevated HbA$_{1c}$; they do not require treatment and do not develop diabetes complications. It is therefore important to identify these patients, to avoid unnecessary diabetes treatment and monitoring. The other forms of MODY are mostly caused by defective transcription factors that play a key role in pancreatic β-cell development and function (hepatocyte nuclear factor (HNF) 1α, 1β and 4α). Patients with transcription factor MODY develop diabetes in adolescence or early adulthood and the diabetes is progressive, requiring oral diabetes treatment before eventually needing insulin. Patients with HNF1α and 4α MODY are extremely sensitive to sulphonylureas and this is the treatment of choice for these individuals. HNF1β is a critical transcription factor not only in pancreatic development but also in renal and genital tract development in utero. Patients with *HNF1β* mutations usually have renal abnormalities, including renal cystic disease and genital tract malformation, such as absent or bicornuate uterus or hypospadias and infertility; about 50% of individuals with the gene mutation have young-onset diabetes.

20

Neonatal diabetes is variably defined as diabetes that presents in the neonatal period, although this is usually extended to the first 6 months of life. The presentation is usually that of profound insulin deficiency with marked hyperglycaemia and DKA. Approximately half of patients with neonatal diabetes have a transient form that remits by about 1 year of age, with diabetes recurring in adolescence or early adulthood; the remaining patients have permanent neonatal diabetes. In recent years, the genetics of neonatal diabetes have been unravelled, having a major positive impact for people with this condition. Approximately two-thirds of patients with permanent neonatal diabetes have an activating mutation in the genes encoding the KIR6.2 and SUR1 subunits of the K_{ATP} channel (see Fig. 20.2C). These mutations cause the K_{ATP} channel to be insensitive to the glucose-mediated rise in intracellular ATP; as a result, the pancreatic β cells do not secrete insulin and patients require insulin treatment from soon after birth. It has been shown, however, that these individuals do respond to sulphonylureas; this finding has transformed their care, over 90% being managed with oral sulphonylurea treatment.

Presenting problems in diabetes mellitus

Hyperglycaemia

The diagnosis of diabetes is simple: it is based on confirmation of hyperglycaemia using either fasting or random glucose, an OGTT or HbA_{1c} (p. 727). Diabetes, however, results from a variety of pathological processes, meaning that within this broad category are many aetiological subtypes. Following the identification of hyperglycaemia and subsequent diagnosis of diabetes, the initial management involves a careful clinical assessment of the patient to decide whether immediate treatment is required and, with appropriate investigation, to establish the aetiology of the diabetes, as this will determine subsequent diabetes treatment (Fig. 20.9). The main differential diagnosis to consider is that of type 1 or type 2 diabetes; making a diagnosis of type 1 diabetes is important, as a failure to initiate insulin treatment can result in

Fig. 20.9 New-onset hyperglycaemia. (DKA = diabetic ketoacidosis; GAD = glutamic acid decarboxylase; HHS = hyperosmotic hyperglycaemic state; IA-2 = islet antigen 2; IV = intravenous; SC = subcutaneous)

the development of DKA and death. If the aetiological diagnosis is in doubt, it is important not to delay insulin treatment, which can be withdrawn subsequently if necessary.

Hyperglycaemia causes a wide variety of symptoms (Box 20.11). The classical clinical features of type 1 and type 2 diabetes are compared in Box 20.12. Symptoms of polydipsia, polyuria, nocturia and rapid weight loss are prominent in type 1 diabetes but are often absent in patients with type 2 diabetes, many of whom are asymptomatic or have non-specific complaints such as chronic fatigue and malaise. Uncontrolled diabetes is associated with an increased susceptibility to infection and patients may present with skin sepsis (boils) or genital candidiasis, and complain of pruritus vulvae or balanitis.

While the distinction between type 1 and type 2 diabetes is usually obvious, overlap occurs, particularly in age at onset, duration of symptoms and family history. There are many patients in whom the type of diabetes is not immediately apparent. For example, patients with type 2 diabetes may present with marked and rapid weight loss and even DKA (10–15% of all cases of DKA), and type 2 diabetes is increasingly diagnosed in children and young adults. Type 1 diabetes can occur at any age, not just in younger people, and may develop more insidiously; the presence of pancreatic autoantibodies confirms the diagnosis of slow-onset type 1 diabetes or LADA. Islet autoantibodies are detectable at high titre in many patients with type 1 diabetes, so a negative result should prompt consideration of other aetiologies. Other causes of diabetes (see Box 20.9), such as MODY, should not be forgotten, particularly in those presenting in childhood or as young adults. A history of pancreatic disease, particularly in patients with a history of alcohol excess, makes insulin deficiency more likely.

20.11 Symptoms of hyperglycaemia

- Thirst, dry mouth
- Polyuria
- Nocturia
- Tiredness, fatigue, lethargy
- Change in weight (usually weight loss)
- Blurring of vision
- Pruritus vulvae, balanitis (genital candidiasis)
- Nausea
- Headache
- Hyperphagia; predilection for sweet foods
- Mood change, irritability, difficulty in concentrating, apathy

20.12 Classical features of type 1 and type 2 diabetes

	Type 1	Type 2
Typical age at onset	<40 years	>50 years
Duration of symptoms	Weeks	Months to years
Body weight	Normal or low	Obese
Ketonuria	Yes	No
Rapid death without treatment with insulin	Yes	No
Autoantibodies	Positive in 80–90%	Negative
Diabetic complications at diagnosis	No	25%
Family history of diabetes	Uncommon	Common
Other autoimmune disease	Common	Uncommon

Sometimes the definitive classification of the type of diabetes is only made later, once the natural history or responsiveness to different therapies becomes apparent.

Physical signs in patients with type 2 diabetes at diagnosis depend on the mode of presentation. In Western populations, more than 80% are overweight and the obesity is often central (truncal or abdominal). Obesity is much less evident in Asians. Hypertension is present in at least 50% of patients with type 2 diabetes. Although dyslipidaemia is also common, skin lesions such as xanthelasma and eruptive xanthomas are rare.

Presentation with the complications of diabetes

Patients with long-standing diabetes are at risk of developing a variety of complications (see Box 20.35, p. 756) and as many as 25% of people with type 2 diabetes have evidence of diabetic complications at the time of diagnosis. Thus, diabetes may be first suspected when a patient visits an optometrist or podiatrist, or presents with hypertension or a vascular event such as an acute myocardial infarction or stroke. Blood glucose should therefore be checked in all patients presenting with such pathology. The detailed investigation and management of diabetic complications are described on page 755.

Diabetes emergencies

Diabetic ketoacidosis

Diabetic ketoacidosis (DKA) is a medical emergency and remains a serious cause of morbidity, principally in people with type 1 diabetes. Mortality is low in the UK (approximately 2%) but remains high in developing countries and among non-hospitalised patients. Mortality in DKA is most commonly caused in children and adolescents by cerebral oedema, and in adults by hypokalaemia, acute respiratory distress syndrome and comorbid conditions such as acute myocardial infarction, sepsis or pneumonia.

DKA is characteristic of type 1 diabetes (see Box 20.12) and is often the presenting problem in newly diagnosed patients. However, an increasing number of patients presenting with DKA have underlying type 2 diabetes. This appears to be particularly prevalent in black and non-Hispanic populations. In established type 1 diabetes, DKA may be precipitated by an intercurrent illness because of failure to increase insulin dose appropriately to compensate for the stress response. Sometimes, there is no evidence of a precipitating infection and DKA develops because of errors in self-management. In young patients with recurrent episodes of DKA, up to 20% may have psychological problems complicated by eating disorders.

Pathogenesis

A clear understanding of the biochemical basis and pathophysiology of DKA is essential for its efficient treatment (see Fig. 20.7). The cardinal biochemical features are:

- hyperketonaemia ($\geq$3.0 mmol/L) or ketonuria (more than 2+ on standard urine sticks)
- hyperglycaemia (blood glucose $\geq$11 mmol/L (approximately 200 mg/dL))
- metabolic acidosis (venous bicarbonate <15 mmol/L and/or venous pH <7.3 (H^+>50 nmol/L)).

The hyperglycaemia causes a profound osmotic diuresis leading to dehydration and electrolyte loss, particularly of

20

sodium and potassium. Potassium loss is exacerbated by secondary hyperaldosteronism as a result of reduced renal perfusion. Ketosis stems from insulin deficiency, exacerbated by elevated catecholamines and other stress hormones, leading to unrestrained lipolysis and supply of FFAs for hepatic ketogenesis. When this exceeds the capacity to metabolise acidic ketones, these accumulate in blood. The resulting metabolic acidosis forces hydrogen ions into cells, displacing potassium ions.

The average loss of fluid and electrolytes in moderately severe DKA in an adult is shown in Box 20.13. About half the deficit of total body water is derived from the intracellular compartment and occurs comparatively early in the development of acidosis with relatively few clinical features; the remainder represents loss of extracellular fluid sustained largely in the later stages, when marked contraction of extracellular fluid volume occurs, with haemoconcentration, a decreased blood volume, and finally a fall in blood pressure with associated renal ischaemia and oliguria.

Every patient in DKA is potassium-depleted but the plasma concentration of potassium gives very little indication of the total body deficit. Plasma potassium may even be raised initially due to disproportionate loss of water, catabolism of protein and glycogen, and displacement of potassium from the intracellular compartment by H^+ ions. However, soon after treatment is started, there is likely to be a precipitous fall in the plasma potassium due to dilution of extracellular potassium by administration of intravenous fluids, the movement of potassium into cells induced by insulin, and the continuing renal loss of potassium.

The magnitude of the hyperglycaemia does not correlate with the severity of the metabolic acidosis; moderate elevation of blood glucose may be associated with life-threatening ketoacidosis. Type 1 diabetes in pregnancy is one situation where DKA can occur with blood glucose levels that are not especially high. Conversely, in other situations, hyperglycaemia predominates and acidosis is minimal, with patients presenting in a hyperosmolar state (p. 738).

Clinical assessment

The clinical features of ketoacidosis are listed in Box 20.14. In the fulminating case, the striking features are those of salt and water depletion, with loss of skin turgor, furred tongue and cracked lips, tachycardia, hypotension and reduced intra-ocular pressure. Breathing may be deep and sighing (Kussmaul's sign), the breath is usually fetid, and the sickly-sweet smell of acetone may be apparent. Mental apathy, delirium or a reduced conscious level may be present, although coma is uncommon. Indeed, a patient with dangerous ketoacidosis requiring urgent treatment may walk into the consulting room. For this reason, the term 'diabetic ketoacidosis' is to be preferred to 'diabetic coma', which implies that there is no urgency until unconsciousness supervenes. In fact, it is imperative that energetic treatment is started at the earliest possible stage.

Abdominal pain is sometimes a feature of DKA, particularly in children, and vomiting is common. Serum amylase may be elevated but rarely indicates coexisting pancreatitis. In infected patients, pyrexia may not be present initially because of vasodilatation secondary to acidosis.

Investigations

The following investigations are important but should not delay the institution of intravenous fluid and insulin replacement:

- *Venous blood*: for urea and electrolytes, glucose, bicarbonate and acid–base status (venous blood can be used in portable and fixed blood gas analysers, and differences between venous and arterial pH and bicarbonate are minor).
- *Urine or blood analysis for ketones* (p. 726).
- *Electrocardiogram (ECG).*
- *Infection screen*: full blood count, blood and urine culture, C-reactive protein, chest X-ray. Although leucocytosis invariably occurs in DKA, this represents a stress response and does not necessarily indicate infection.

Assessment of severity

The presence of one or more of the features listed in Box 20.15 is indicative of severe DKA.

Management

DKA is a medical emergency that should be treated in hospital, preferably in a high-dependency area. If available, the diabetes specialist team should be involved. Regular clinical and biochemical review is essential, particularly during the first 24 hours of treatment. Guidelines for the management of DKA are shown in Box 20.16. Early specialist involvement is recommended for high-risk groups such as older people, young adults (18–25 years), pregnant women, and those with heart or kidney failure or other serious comorbidities.

20.13 Average loss of fluid and electrolytes in adult diabetic ketoacidosis of moderate severity

- Water: 6 L
- Sodium: 500 mmol
- Chloride: 400 mmol
- Potassium: 350 mmol

} 3 L extracellular – replace with saline; 3 L intracellular – replace with dextrose

20.14 Clinical features of diabetic ketoacidosis

Symptoms

- Polyuria, thirst
- Weight loss
- Weakness
- Nausea, vomiting
- Leg cramps
- Blurred vision
- Abdominal pain

Signs

- Dehydration
- Hypotension (postural or supine)
- Cold extremities/peripheral cyanosis
- Tachycardia
- Air hunger (Kussmaul breathing)
- Smell of acetone
- Hypothermia
- Delirium, drowsiness, coma (10%)

20.15 Indicators of severe diabetic ketoacidosis

- Blood ketones >6 mmol/L
- Bicarbonate <5 mmol/L
- Venous/arterial pH <7.0 (H^+ >100 nmol/L)
- Hypokalaemia on admission (<3.5 mmol/L)
- Glasgow Coma Scale score <12 (p. 194) or abnormal AVPU scale score (p. 188)
- O_2 saturation <92% on air
- Systolic blood pressure <90 mmHg
- Heart rate >100 or <60 beats per minute
- Anion gap >16 mmol/L

20.16 Emergency management of diabetic ketoacidosis

Time: 0–60 mins

- Establish IV access, assess patient and perform initial investigations
- Commence 0.9% sodium chloride:
  - If systolic BP >90 mmHg, give 1 L over 60 mins
  - If systolic BP <90 mmHg, give 500 mL over 10–15 mins, then re-assess; if BP remains <90 mmHg, repeat and seek senior review
- Commence insulin treatment:
  - 50 U human soluble insulin in 50 mL 0.9% sodium chloride infused intravenously at 0.1 U/kg body weight/hr
  - Continue with SC basal insulin analogue if usually taken by patient
- Perform further investigations: see text
- Establish monitoring schedule:
  - Hourly capillary blood glucose and ketone testing
  - Venous bicarbonate and potassium after 1 and 2 hrs, then every 2 hrs for first 6 hrs
  - Plasma electrolytes every 4 hrs
  - Clinical monitoring of O_2 saturation, pulse, BP, respiratory rate and urine output every hour
- Treat any precipitating cause

Time: 60 mins to 6 hrs

- IV infusion of 0.9% sodium chloride with potassium chloride added as indicated below:
  - 1 L over 2 hrs
  - 1 L over 2 hrs
  - 1 L over 4 hrs
  - 1 L over 4 hrs
  - 1 L over 6 hrs
- Add 10% glucose 125 mL/hr IV when glucose <14 mmol/L (252 mg/dL)
- Be more cautious with fluid replacement in older or young people, pregnant patients and those with renal or heart failure; if plasma sodium is >155 mmol/L, 0.45% sodium chloride may be used

- Adjust potassium chloride infusion:

Plasma potassium (mmol/L)	Potassium replacement (mmol/L of infusion)
>5.5	Nil
3.5–5.5	40
<3.5	Senior review – additional potassium required

Time: 6–12 hrs

- Clinical status, glucose, ketonaemia and acidosis should be improving; request senior review if not
- Continue IV fluid replacement
- Continue insulin administration
- Assess for complications of treatment (fluid overload, cerebral oedema)
- Avoid hypoglycaemia

Time: 12–24 hrs

- By 24 hrs, ketonaemia and acidosis should have resolved (blood ketones <0.3 mmol/L, venous bicarbonate >18 mmol/L)
- If patient is not eating and drinking:
  - Continue IV insulin infusion at lower rate of 2–3 U/hr
  - Continue IV fluid replacement and biochemical monitoring
- If ketoacidosis has resolved and patient is able to eat and drink:
  - Re-initiate SC insulin with advice from diabetes team; do not discontinue IV insulin until 30 mins after SC short-acting insulin injection

Additional procedures

- Consider urinary catheterisation if anuric after 3 hrs or incontinent
- Insert nasogastric tube if obtunded or there is persistent vomiting
- Insert central venous line if cardiovascular system is compromised, to allow fluid replacement to be adjusted accurately; also consider in older patients, pregnant women, renal or cardiac failure, other serious comorbidities and severe DKA
- Measure arterial blood gases; repeat chest X-ray if O_2 saturation <92%
- Institute ECG monitoring in severe cases
- Give thromboprophylaxis with low-molecular-weight heparin

(BP = blood pressure; ECG = electrocardiogram; IV = intravenous; SC = subcutaneous)
Adapted from Joint British Diabetes Societies Inpatient Care Group. The Management of Diabetic Ketoacidosis in Adults, 2nd edn; September 2013; abcd.care.

20

Insulin

A fixed-rate intravenous insulin infusion of 0.1 U/kg body weight/hr is recommended (Box 20.16). Exceptionally, if intravenous administration is not feasible, soluble insulin can be given by intramuscular injection (loading dose of 10–20 U, followed by 5 U hourly), or a fast-acting insulin analogue can be given hourly by subcutaneous injection (initially 0.3 U/kg body weight, then 0.1 U/kg hourly). The blood glucose concentration should fall by 3–6 mmol/L (approximately 55–110 mg/dL) per hour, or blood ketone concentrations fall by at least 0.5 mmol/L/hr. A more rapid decrease in blood glucose should be avoided, as this might precipitate hypoglycaemia and the serious complication of cerebral oedema, particularly in children. Failure of blood glucose to fall within 1 hour of commencing insulin infusion should lead to a re-assessment of insulin dose. Ketosis, dehydration, acidaemia, infection and stress combine to produce severe insulin resistance in some cases, but most will respond to a low-dose insulin regimen. When the blood glucose has fallen, 10% dextrose infusion is introduced and insulin infusion continued to encourage glucose uptake into cells and restoration of normal metabolism. In recent years, it has also become increasingly common to continue with the use of long-acting insulin analogues administered subcutaneously during the initial management of DKA; this provides background insulin for when the intravenous insulin is discontinued, to reduce the risk of in-hospital DKA.

Restoration of the usual insulin regimen, by subcutaneous injection, should not be instituted until the patient is both biochemically stable and able to eat and drink normally.

Fluid replacement

In adults, rapid fluid replacement in the first few hours is usually recommended (Box 20.16). Caution is advised in children and young adults because of the risk of cerebral oedema. Most guidelines favour correction of the extracellular fluid deficit with isotonic saline (0.9% sodium chloride). If the plasma sodium is greater than 155 mmol/L, 0.45% saline may be used initially. Introduction of 10% glucose is recommended when the blood glucose falls below 14 mmol/L (252 mg/dL). The 0.9% saline infusion should be continued to correct circulating volume so both glucose and saline infusions are used concurrently.

Potassium

Careful monitoring of potassium is essential to the management of DKA because both hypo- and hyperkalaemia can occur and are potentially life-threatening. Potassium replacement is not usually recommended with the initial litre of fluid because pre-renal failure may be present secondary to dehydration. Treatment with 0.9% sodium chloride with potassium chloride 40 mmol/L is recommended if the serum potassium is below 5.5 mmol/L and the patient is passing urine (Box 20.16). If the potassium falls below 3.5 mmol/L, the potassium replacement regimen needs to be reviewed. Aim to maintain potassium between 4.0 and 5.5 mmol/L. Cardiac rhythm should be monitored in severe DKA because of the risk of electrolyte-induced cardiac arrhythmia.

Bicarbonate

Adequate fluid and insulin replacement should resolve the acidosis. The use of intravenous bicarbonate therapy is not recommended. Acidosis may reflect an adaptive response, improving oxygen delivery to the tissues, and so excessive bicarbonate may induce a paradoxical increase in cerebrospinal fluid acidosis and has been implicated in the pathogenesis of cerebral oedema in children and young adults.

Phosphate

There is no evidence of benefit with phosphate replacement unless low levels are detected in the presence of respiratory or muscle weakness.

Ongoing management

Where possible, refer the patient to the diabetes specialist team within 24 hours of admission. It is important to review the precipitating factors that led to DKA, glycaemic control and insulin injection technique, as well as to discuss prevention of recurrence and to provide blood ketone meters where available. There is a significant mortality associated with recurrent DKA and so early educational assessment and treatment review are critical.

Hyperglycaemic hyperosmolar state

Hyperglycaemic hyperosmolar state (HHS) is a medical emergency that is different from DKA and so treatment requires a different approach. There is no precise definition of HHS but it is characterised by hypovolaemia, severe hyperglycaemia (>30 mmol/L (600 mg/dL)) and hyperosmolality (serum osmolality >320 mOsmol/kg), without significant ketonaemia (<3 mmol/L) or acidosis (pH >7.3 (H+ <50 nmol/L), bicarbonate >15 mmol/L).

As with DKA, there is glycosuria, leading to an osmotic diuresis with loss of water, sodium, potassium and other electrolytes. However, in HHS, hyperglycaemia usually develops over a longer period (a few days to weeks), causing more profound hyperglycaemia and dehydration (fluid loss may be 10–12 L in a person weighing 100 kg). The reason that patients with HHS do not develop significant ketoacidosis is unclear, although it has been speculated that insulin levels may be too low to stimulate glucose uptake in insulin-sensitive tissues, but are still sufficient to prevent lipolysis and subsequent ketogenesis. A mixed picture of HHS and DKA can occur.

Although typically occurring in older patients, HHS is increasingly seen in younger adults. Common precipitating factors include infection, myocardial infarction, cerebrovascular events or drug therapy (e.g. glucocorticoids). Poor prognostic signs include hypothermia, hypotension (systolic blood pressure <90 mmHg), tachy- or bradycardia, severe hypernatraemia (sodium >160 mmol/L), serum osmolality >360 mOsmol/kg, and the presence of other serious comorbidities. Mortality rates are higher than in DKA – up to 20% in the USA – reflecting the age and frailty of the population and the more frequent presence of comorbidities.

The principles of therapy are shown in Box 20.17. The aims are to normalise osmolality, replace fluid and electrolyte losses, and normalise blood glucose, at the same time as preventing complications such as arterial or venous thrombosis, cerebral oedema and central pontine demyelinosis (Ch. 14). Comorbidities also need to be taken into account; for example, rapid fluid replacement may precipitate cardiac failure in patients with coronary artery disease. Historically, management of HHS has followed DKA guidelines, but increasing recognition of the differences between HHS and DKA has led to new approaches in HHS. In particular, rapid shifts in osmolality should be avoided through more measured fluid replacement regimens that are guided by serial calculations of serum osmolality. Key recommendations are that 0.9% sodium chloride solution alone is used for initial treatment, and that insulin is introduced only when the rate of fall in blood glucose has plateaued.

If osmolality cannot be measured frequently, osmolarity can be calculated as follows and used as a surrogate (based on plasma values in mmol/L):

$$Plasma\ osmolarity = 2[Na^+] + [glucose] + [urea]$$

The normal value is 280–296 mOsmol/L and consciousness is impaired when it is high (>340 mOsmol/L), as commonly occurs in HHS. A limitation of this approach is that hyperglycaemia, by increasing serum osmolality, causes the movement of water out of cells, therefore reducing measured Na+ levels by dilution. In hyperglycaemic patients, the corrected [Na+] should be taken into account. This is calculated by adding 1.6 mmol/L to the measured [Na+] for every 5.55 mmol/L (100 mg/dL) increment of serum glucose above normal.

Hypoglycaemia

Hypoglycaemia is uncommon in people without diabetes but relatively frequent in people with diabetes, mainly due to insulin therapy, and less frequently to use of oral insulin secretagogues such as sulphonylurea drugs, and rarely with other antidiabetic drugs. In people with diabetes, hypoglycaemia is defined as a blood glucose of less than 3.9 mmol/L (70 mg/dL). Severe hypoglycaemia – the need for external assistance to provide glucose, glucagon or other corrective action actively – is greatly feared by people with diabetes and has a major impact on their willingness and ability to achieve target glucose levels. When hypoglycaemia develops in non-diabetic people, it is called 'spontaneous' hypoglycaemia; its definition, causes and investigation are described on page 676.

The critical importance of glucose as a fuel source for the brain means that, in health, a number of mechanisms are in place to ensure that glucose homeostasis is maintained. If blood glucose falls, three primary physiological defence mechanisms operate:

- endogenous insulin release from pancreatic β cells is suppressed
- release of glucagon from pancreatic α cells is increased
- the autonomic nervous system is activated, with release of catecholamines both systemically and within the tissues.

20.17 Emergency management of hyperglycaemic hyperosmolar state

Time 0–60 mins

- Commence IV 0.9% sodium chloride 1 L over 1 hr
- Commence insulin infusion (0.05 U/kg/hr) only if there is significant ketonaemia (3-hydroxybutyrate >1.0 mmol/L)
- Perform initial investigations
- Perform clinical assessment to assess degree of dehydration, mental status and any source of potential sepsis
- Assess foot risk score
- Establish monitoring regimen – generally hourly glucose and calculated osmolality (2Na$^+$ + glucose + urea) for first 6 hrs then 2-hourly if responding
- Insert urinary catheter to monitor hourly urine output and calculate fluid balance
- Commence LMWH in a prophylactic dose
- Consider antibiotic therapy if sepsis suspected

Time 60 mins to 6 hrs

- Continue with 0.9% sodium chloride infusion 0.5–1.0 L/hr, depending on clinical assessment and response (target positive balance of 2–3 L by 6 hrs)
- Calculate osmolality hourly and aim for gradual decline (3–8 mOsmol/kg/hr); if osmolality is increasing and fluid balance adequate, consider 0.45% sodium chloride
- If blood glucose is falling at less than 5 mmol/L/hr, check fluid balance and, if adequate, commence low-dose IV insulin (0.05 U/kg/hr); if insulin is already running, increase rate to 0.1 U/kg/hr
- Maintain potassium in the reference range (3.6–5.0 mmol/L), as with DKA (see Box 20.16)
- Avoid hypoglycaemia – aim to keep blood glucose at 10–15 mmol/L (180–270 mg/dL) in the first 24 hrs. If blood glucose falls below 14 mmol/L (252 mg/dL), commence 5% or 10% glucose infusion in addition to 0.9% saline
- Monitor fluid balance

Time 6–12 hrs

- Ensure clinical and biochemical parameters are improving
- Assess for complications of treatment
- Continue IV fluid replacement to target 3–6 L positive balance by 12 hrs
- Continue treatment of underlying precipitant
- Avoid hypoglycaemia

Time 12–24 hrs

- Ensure clinical and biochemical parameters are improving; measurement can be reduced to 4-hourly; biochemistry does not usually normalise by 24 hrs
- Assess for complications of treatment
- Continue IV fluid replacement to target remaining estimated fluid loss by 24 hrs
- Continue IV insulin with or without 5% or 10% glucose to maintain blood glucose at 10–15 mmol/L (180–270 mg/dL)
- Continue treatment of underlying precipitant
- Avoid hypoglycaemia

Time 24 hrs to day 3

- Ensure clinical and biochemical parameters are improving or normalised; continue IV fluids until eating and drinking; variable-rate insulin and fluids may be required if not
- Convert to appropriate SC insulin regimen when stable
- Assess for signs of fluid overload
- Encourage early mobilisation
- Carry out daily foot checks
- Continue LMWH until discharge
- Ensure review by diabetes team

(DKA = diabetic ketoacidosis; IV = intravenous; LMWH = low-molecular-weight heparin; SC = subcutaneous)
Adapted from Joint British Diabetes Societies Inpatient Care Group. The Management of the Hyperosmolar Hyperglycaemic State (HHS) in Adults with Diabetes; 2012; abcd.care.

20

In addition, stress hormones, such as cortisol and growth hormone, are increased in the blood. These actions reduce whole-body glucose uptake and increase hepatic glucose production, maintaining a glucose supply to the brain. People with type 1 diabetes cannot regulate insulin once it is injected subcutaneously, and so it continues to act, despite the development of hypoglycaemia. In addition, within 5 years of diagnosis, most patients will have lost their ability to release glucagon specifically during hypoglycaemia. The reasons for this are unknown, but may result from loss of α-cell regulation by insulin or other products of the β cell. These two primary defects mean that hypoglycaemia occurs much more frequently in people with type 1 and longer-duration type 2 diabetes.

Clinical assessment

Symptoms of hypoglycaemia (Box 20.18) comprise two main groups: those related to acute activation of the autonomic nervous system and those secondary to glucose deprivation of the brain (neuroglycopenia). Symptoms of hypoglycaemia are idiosyncratic, differing with age and duration of diabetes, and also depending on the circumstances in which hypoglycaemia occurs. Hypoglycaemia also affects mood, inducing a state of increased tension and low energy. Learning to recognise the early onset of hypoglycaemia is an important aspect of the education of people with diabetes treated with insulin.

ⓘ 20.18 Most common symptoms of hypoglycaemia

Autonomic

- Sweating
- Trembling
- Pounding heart
- Hunger
- Anxiety

Neuroglycopenic

- Delirium
- Drowsiness
- Speech difficulty
- Inability to concentrate
- Incoordination
- Irritability, anger

Non-specific

- Nausea
- Tiredness
- Headache

N.B. Symptoms differ with age; children exhibit behavioural changes (such as naughtiness or irritability), while older people experience more prominent neurological symptoms (such as visual disturbance and ataxia).

Circumstances of hypoglycaemia

Risk factors and causes of hypoglycaemia in patients taking insulin or sulphonylurea drugs are listed in Box 20.19. Severe hypoglycaemia can have serious morbidity (e.g. convulsions, coma, focal neurological lesions) and has a mortality of up to

20.19 Hypoglycaemia in diabetes: common causes and risk factors

Medical issues

- Rapid improvement in and/or strict glycaemic control
- Previous severe hypoglycaemia
- Impaired awareness of hypoglycaemia
- Long-duration type 1 diabetes
- Duration of insulin therapy in type 2 diabetes
- Lipohypertrophy at injection sites causing variable insulin absorption
- Severe hepatic dysfunction
- Impaired renal function
- Inadequate treatment of previous hypoglycaemia
- Terminal illness
- Bariatric surgery involving bowel resection
- Unrecognised other endocrine disorder, e.g. Addison's disease

Reduced carbohydrate intake

- Gastroparesis due to autonomic neuropathy causing variable carbohydrate absorption
- Malabsorption, e.g. coeliac disease
- Eating disorder

Lifestyle issues

- Exercise
- Irregular lifestyle
- Increasing age
- Alcohol
- Early pregnancy
- Breastfeeding
- No or inadequate glucose monitoring
- Factitious (deliberately induced)

4% in insulin-treated patients. Rarely, sudden death during sleep occurs in otherwise healthy young patients with type 1 diabetes ('dead-in-bed syndrome') and may result from hypoglycaemia-induced cardiac arrhythmia. Severe hypoglycaemia is very disruptive and impinges on many aspects of the patient's life, including employment, driving (see Box 20.24), travel, sport and personal relationships.

Nocturnal hypoglycaemia in patients with type 1 diabetes is common but often undetected, as hypoglycaemia does not usually waken a person from sleep. Patients may describe poor quality of sleep, morning headaches and vivid dreams or nightmares, or a partner may observe profuse sweating, restlessness, twitching or even seizures. The only reliable way to identify this problem is to measure blood glucose during the night. High glucose levels in the morning are not, as commonly perceived, an indicator of nocturnal hypoglycaemia.

Exercise-induced hypoglycaemia occurs in people with well-controlled, insulin-treated diabetes because of hyperinsulinaemia. Suppression of endogenous insulin secretion to allow increased hepatic glucose production to meet the increased metabolic demand is key to the normal physiological response to exercise. In insulin-treated diabetes, insulin levels may actually increase with exercise because of improved blood flow at the site of injection, and this increases the risk of hypoglycaemia. This means that both insulin and muscle contraction will increase glucose uptake, causing a fall in blood glucose. This occurs most commonly with prolonged and/or aerobic exercise. In addition, the 'double hit' of hypoglycaemia with exercise reflects the additional increased risk of nocturnal hypoglycaemia that can occur after exercise, possibly as a result of glycogen depletion. In contrast, high-intensity exercise because of the marked stimulation to adrenaline (epinephrine) production may actually cause blood glucose to rise significantly. Education is key to preventing exercise-induced hypoglycaemia.

Hypoglycaemia may also occur within the hospital setting. This may result from errors in insulin dose or type of insulin prescribed, infusion of IV insulin without glucose, changes in meal timings or content and failure to provide usual snacks, reduced carbohydrate intake because of vomiting or reduced appetite, or factors related to the hospital admission, e.g. concurrent illness or discontinuation of long-term glucocorticoid therapy.

Awareness of hypoglycaemia

For most individuals, the glucose level (threshold) at which they first become aware of hypoglycaemia is not constant but varies according to the circumstances in which hypoglycaemia arises (e.g. during the night or during exercise). In addition, with longer duration of disease, and particularly in response to frequent hypoglycaemia, the threshold for generation of symptom responses to hypoglycaemia shifts to a lower glucose concentration. This cerebral adaptation has a similar effect on the counter-regulatory hormonal response to hypoglycaemia. Taken together, this means that individuals with type 1 diabetes may have reduced (impaired) awareness of hypoglycaemia. Symptoms can be experienced less intensely, or even be absent, despite blood glucose concentrations below 3.0 mmol/L (55 mg/dL). Such individuals are at an especially high risk of severe hypoglycaemia. The prevalence of impaired awareness of hypoglycaemia increases with time; overall, it affects around 20–25% of people with type 1 diabetes and under 10% with insulin-treated type 2 diabetes.

Management

Acute treatment of hypoglycaemia

Treatment of hypoglycaemia depends on its severity and on whether the patient is conscious and able to swallow (Box 20.20). Oral carbohydrate usually suffices if hypoglycaemia is recognised early. If parenteral therapy is required, then as soon as the patient is able to swallow, glucose should be given orally. Full recovery may not occur immediately and reversal of cognitive impairment may not be complete until 60 minutes after normoglycaemia is restored. When hypoglycaemia has occurred in a patient treated with a long- or intermediate-acting insulin or a long-acting sulphonylurea, such as glibenclamide, the possibility of recurrence should be anticipated; to prevent this, infusion of 10% dextrose, titrated to the patient's blood glucose, or provision of additional carbohydrate may be necessary.

If the patient fails to regain consciousness after blood glucose is restored to normal, then cerebral oedema and other causes of impaired consciousness – such as alcohol intoxication, a post-ictal state or cerebral haemorrhage – should be considered. Cerebral oedema has a high mortality and morbidity.

Following recovery, it is important to try to identify a cause and make appropriate adjustments to the patient's therapy. Unless the reason for a hypoglycaemic episode is clear, the patient should reduce the next dose of insulin by 10–20% and seek medical advice about further adjustments in dose.

The management of self-poisoning with oral antidiabetic agents is described on page 141.

Prevention of hypoglycaemia

Patient education is fundamental to the prevention of hypoglycaemia. Risk factors for, and treatment of, hypoglycaemia should be discussed. The importance of regular blood glucose monitoring and the need to have glucose (and glucagon) readily available should be stressed. A review of insulin and carbohydrate

20.20 Emergency treatment of hypoglycaemia

Biochemical or symptomatic hypoglycaemia (self-treated)

In the UK, it is recommended that all glucose levels <4.0 mmol/L (72 mg/dL) are treated ('4 is the floor'). People with diabetes who recognise developing hypoglycaemia are encouraged to treat immediately. Options available include:

- Oral fast-acting carbohydrate (10–15 g) is taken as glucose drink or tablets or confectionery, e.g. 5–7 Dextrosol tablets (or 4–5 Glucotabs), 90–120 mL *original* Lucozade, 150–200 mL pure fruit juice, 3–4 heaped teaspoons of sugar dissolved in water)
- Repeat capillary glucose measurement 1–15 mins later. If still <4.0 mmol/L, repeat above treatment
- If blood glucose remains <4.0 mmol/L after three cycles (30–45 mins), contact a doctor. Consider glucagon 1 mg IM or 150–200 mL 10% glucose over 15 mins IV
- Once blood glucose is >4.0 mmol/L, take additional long-acting carbohydrate of choice
- Do not omit insulin injection if due but review regimen

Severe (external help required)

This means individuals are either unconscious or unable to treat hypoglycaemia themselves. Treatment is usually by a relative or by paramedical or medical staff. Immediate treatment as below is needed.

- If patient is semiconscious or unconscious, parenteral treatment is required:

  IV 75–100 mL 20% dextrose over 15 mins (=15 g; give 0.2 g/kg in children)*

  Or

  IV 150–200 mL 10% dextrose over 15 mins

  Or

  IM glucagon (1 mg; 0.5 mg in children) – may be less effective in patients on sulphonylurea/under the influence of alcohol
- If patient is conscious and able to swallow:

  Give oral refined glucose as drink or sweets (= 25 g) or 1.5–2 tubes of Glucogel/Dextrogel

  Or

  Apply glucose gel or jam or honey to buccal mucosa
- Repeat blood glucose measurement after 10–15 mins and manage as per biochemical hypoglycaemia

*Use of 50% dextrose is no longer recommended.
Adapted from Joint British Diabetes Societies. The hospital management of hypoglycaemia in adults with diabetes mellitus (2013). Available at: abcd.care.

20.21 Avoidance and treatment of hypoglycaemia during travel

- Carry a supply of fast-acting carbohydrate (non-perishable, in suitable containers):

  Screwtop plastic bottles for glucose drinks
  Packets of powdered glucose (for use in hot, humid climates)
  Confectionery (foil-wrapped in hot climates)
- Ask companions to carry additional oral carbohydrate, and glucagon
- Perform frequent blood glucose testing (carry spare meter and/or visually read strips)
- Use fast-acting insulin analogues for long-distance air travel

be deferred until bedtime (after 2300 hrs), shifting its peak action period to 0500–0700 hrs. It is also a sensible precaution for patients to measure their blood glucose before they retire to bed and to have a carbohydrate snack if the reading is less than 6.0 mmol/L (approximately 110 mg/dL).

Management of diabetes

The aims are to improve symptoms of hyperglycaemia and minimise the risks of long-term microvascular and macrovascular complications. Treatment methods for diabetes include dietary/lifestyle modification, oral antidiabetic drugs and injected therapies. Initial investigation and management is outlined in Figure 20.10. In patients with suspected type 1 diabetes, urgent treatment with insulin is required and prompt referral to a specialist is usually needed. In patients with suspected type 2 diabetes, the first approach to management involves advice about dietary and lifestyle modification. Oral antidiabetic drugs are usually added in those who do not achieve glycaemic targets, or who have symptomatic hyperglycaemia at diagnosis and a high HbA$_{1c}$. However, the guidelines in some countries are to introduce medication immediately on diagnosis of diabetes without waiting to assess the impact of diet and lifestyle changes. Patients with type 2 diabetes who present with marked symptomatic hyperglycaemia or DKA will require initial management with insulin treatment.

For most people, types 1 and 2 diabetes are chronic conditions that will impact on their day-to-day activities and require sustained changes to lifestyle. Education is key to achieving and maintaining a healthy lifestyle and to managing diabetes. Early educational intervention at diagnosis and repeated education are essential if these goals are to be successfully achieved. Management of people with diabetes should be individualised where possible, taking into account personal and cultural beliefs, individual circumstances, comorbidities and other factors.

Diabetes is a complex disorder that progresses in severity with time, so people with diabetes should be seen at regular intervals for the remainder of their lives, either at a specialist diabetic clinic or in primary care where facilities are available and staff are trained in diabetes care. A checklist for follow-up visits is given in Box 20.22. The frequency of visits is variable, ranging from weekly during pregnancy to annually in the case of patients with well-controlled type 2 diabetes.

In parallel with treatment of hyperglycaemia, other risk factors for complications of diabetes need to be addressed, including treatment of hypertension (p. 510) and dyslipidaemia (p. 373), and advice on smoking cessation (p. 94).

management during exercise is particularly useful. Advice for patients when travelling is summarised in Box 20.21.

Relatives and friends also need to be familiar with the symptoms and signs of hypoglycaemia and should be instructed in how to help (including how to inject glucagon).

It is important to recognise that all current insulin replacement regimens are suboptimal and do not accurately replicate normal physiological insulin profiles. Understanding the pharmacokinetics and pharmacodynamics of the insulin regimen in use by the patient will help prevent further hypoglycaemia (p. 748). For example, an individual experiencing regular nocturnal hypoglycaemia between midnight and 0200 hrs may be found to be taking twice-daily soluble and intermediate-acting insulins before breakfast and before the main evening meal between 1700 and 1900 hrs. In this case, the peak action of the isophane insulin will coincide with the period of maximum sensitivity to insulin – namely, 2300–0200 hrs – and increase the risk of nocturnal hypoglycaemia. To address this, the evening dose of depot intermediate-acting insulin should

20

Fig. 20.10 The recommended approach for the management of type 2 diabetes. First-line drug treatment should be metformin. Second- and third-line treatment should be chosen based on the efficacy, hypoglycaemia risk, weight effects and other side-effects, and costs of the therapy in discussion with the patient. (DPP-4-i = dipeptidyl peptidase 4 inhibitor; fxs = fractures; GI = gastrointestinal; GLP-1-RA = glucagon-like peptide 1 receptor agonist; GU = genitourinary; HF, heart failure; SGLT2-i = sodium and glucose transporter 2 inhibitor; SU, sulphonylurea; TZD = thiazolidinedione) *Adapted from the American Diabetes Association/European Association for the Study of Diabetes joint position statement, 2015. Diabetes Care 2015; 38:140–149.*

Self-assessment of glycaemic control

In people with type 2 diabetes, there is not usually a need for regular self-assessment of blood glucose, unless they are treated with insulin, or at risk of hypoglycaemia while taking sulphonylureas. Blood glucose testing can be used for self-education (i.e. demonstrating how different food and exercise regimes affect blood glucose) and may be useful in acute illness. Blood glucose targets vary according to individual circumstances but, in general, fasting glucose levels of 5–7 mmol/L (90–126 mg/dL), pre-meal values of 4–7 mmol/L (72–126 mg/dL) and 2-hour post-meal values of 4–8 mmol/L (72–144 mg/dL) represent optimal control.

Insulin-treated patients should be taught how to monitor their own blood glucose using capillary blood glucose meters. Immediate knowledge of blood glucose levels can be used by patients to guide their insulin dosing and to manage exercise and illness. This can be supplemented with blood testing for ketones when blood glucose is high and/or during intercurrent illness. More recently, continuous glucose monitoring systems (CGMS)

have been developed that allow for a more detailed examination of daily glucose profiles. These can be used continuously as part of day-to-day diabetes management or intermittently as an educational tool.

Urine testing for glucose is not recommended because variability in renal threshold means that some patients with inadequate glycaemic control will not find glucose in their urine.

Therapeutic goals

The target HbA₁c depends on the individual patient. Early on in diabetes (i.e. patients managed by diet or one or two oral agents), a target of 48 mmol/mol or less may be appropriate. However, a higher target of 58 mmol/mol may be more appropriate in older patients with pre-existing cardiovascular disease, or those treated with insulin and therefore at risk of hypoglycaemia. In general, the benefits of lower target HbA₁c (primarily, a lower risk of microvascular disease) need to be weighed against any increased risks (primarily, hypoglycaemia in insulin-treated patients). Type 2 diabetes is usually a progressive condition

20.22 How to review a patient in the diabetes clinic

Lifestyle issues
- General health
- Work or school
- Smoking
- Alcohol intake
- Stress or depression
- Sexual health
- Exercise

Body weight and BMI

Blood pressure
- Individualised target of 130–140/70–80 mmHg, depending on risk factors and presence of nephropathy

Urinalysis
- Analyse fasting specimen for glucose, ketones, albumin (both macro- and micro-albuminuria)

Biochemistry
- Renal, liver and thyroid function
- Lipid profile and estimated 10-year cardiovascular risk to guide need for lipid-lowering therapy (p. 487)

Glycaemic control
- Glycated haemoglobin (HbA_{1c}); individualised target between 48 and 58 mmol/mol
- Inspection of home blood glucose monitoring record (if carried out by patient)

Hypoglycaemic episodes
- Number and cause of severe (requiring assistance for treatment) events and frequency of mild (self-treated) episodes and biochemical hypoglycaemia
- Awareness of hypoglycaemia
- Driving advice

Assessment of injection sites if insulin-treated

Eye examination
- Visual acuities (near and distance)
- Ophthalmoscopy (with pupils dilated) or digital photography

Examination of lower limbs and feet
- Assessment of foot risk (p. 721)

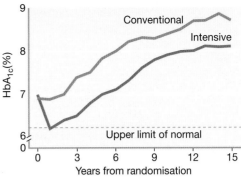

Fig. 20.11 Time course of changes in HbA_{1c} during the United Kingdom Prospective Diabetes Study (UKPDS). In the UKPDS there was loss of glycaemic control with time in patients receiving monotherapy, independently of their randomisation to conventional or intensive glycaemic control, consistent with progressive decline in β-cell function (see Fig. 20.8). *Adapted from UK Prospective Diabetes Study Group. UKPDS 33. Lancet 1998; 352:837–853.*

(Fig. 20.11) unless there are major diet and lifestyle changes, so that there is usually a need to increase diabetes medication over time to achieve the individualised target HbA_{1c}.

In people with type 2 diabetes, treatment of coexisting hypertension and dyslipidaemia is usually required. This can be decided by assessing absolute risk of a cardiovascular disease event (p. 510) and adjusting targets to individual circumstances. The target for blood pressure is usually below 140/80 mmHg, although some guidelines suggest 130/80 mmHg. For lipid-lowering, there is a reduction in cardiovascular risk even with normal cholesterol levels, but statin therapy is usually recommended when the 10-year cardiovascular event risk is at least 20%. As a rule, anyone with type 2 diabetes who is over the age of 40 years should receive a statin, irrespective of baseline cholesterol levels. Some guidelines do not propose a target level once the patient is started on a statin but others suggest a total cholesterol of less than 4.0 mmol/L (approximately 150 mg/dL) and an LDL cholesterol of less than 2.0 mmol/L (approximately 75 mg/dL). Similar targets are appropriate in type 1 diabetes, although there is a shortage of data from clinical trials.

Patient education, diet and lifestyle

The importance of lifestyle changes, such as undertaking regular physical activity, observing a healthy diet and reducing alcohol consumption, should not be under-estimated in improving glycaemic control for people with both type 1 and type 2 diabetes. Many people find this difficult to sustain and constant reinforcement of the benefits of lifestyle change will usually be required. Patients should be encouraged to stop smoking.

Healthy eating

All people with diabetes need to pay special attention to their diet (Box 20.23; see also p. 694). They should have access to a dietitian at diagnosis, at review and at times of treatment change. Nutritional advice should be tailored to individuals and take account of their age, lifestyle, culture and personal circumstances. Structured education programmes are available for both common types of diabetes and, if possible, a clear referral mechanism for diabetes education should be in place.

Between 80% and 90% of people with type 2 diabetes are overweight and so the majority require dietary advice for achieving weight loss, to include caloric restriction. There is, however, limited evidence for the ideal macronutrient composition of the diet in type 2 diabetes. In general, high fat intake (especially saturated fats) is associated with a raised HbA_{1c}, but it is unclear how the type and amount of fat influence post-prandial glucose control. Reduction of caloric intake and weight loss should be the major goals. Some evidence for the Mediterranean diet, low-carbohydrate diets and meal replacements is emerging. Whichever approach is taken, weight loss in overweight and obese individuals with diabetes markedly improves glycaemic control and slows diabetes progression.

Carbohydrate

While it is recognised that the total amount of carbohydrate is the major determinant of post-prandial glucose (p. 694), there is little evidence to support specific strategies for carbohydrate intake in type 2 diabetes or to identify the ideal amount of carbohydrate in their diet. Current UK government Food Standards Agency recommendations are that the total carbohydrate intake should be no more than 50% of energy, and of this non-milk extrinsic sugars (e.g. table sugar, honey,

20

20.23 Dietary management of diabetes

Aims of dietary management

- Achieve good glycaemic control
- Reduce hyperglycaemia and avoid hypoglycaemia
- Assist with weight management:
    Weight maintenance for type 1 diabetes and non-obese type 2 diabetes
    Weight loss for overweight and obese type 2 diabetes
- Reduce the risk of micro- and macrovascular complications
- Ensure adequate nutritional intake
- Avoid 'atherogenic' diets or those that aggravate complications, e.g. high protein intake in nephropathy

Dietary constituents and recommended % of energy intake

- Carbohydrate: 50%:
    Sucrose: up to 10%
- Fat (total): <35%:
    n-6 Polyunsaturated: <10%
    n-3 Polyunsaturated: eat 1 portion (140 g) oily fish once or twice weekly
    Monounsaturated: 10–20%
    Saturated: <10%
- Protein: 10–15% (do not exceed 1 g/kg body weight/day)
- Fruit/vegetables: 5 portions daily

---

glucose and fructose sugars) should not be more than 11%. Low glycaemic index (GI) diets have, in some short-term trials, been shown to improve HbA$_{1c}$, but the literature concerning GI and glycaemic control is mixed. The GI of a carbohydrate-containing food is a measure of the change in blood glucose following its ingestion relative to the rise in blood glucose observed following a liquid OGTT. Different foods can be ranked by their effect on post-prandial glycaemia. Low-GI foods, such as starchy foods (e.g. basmati rice, spaghetti, porridge, noodles, granary bread, and beans and lentils), may reduce post-prandial glucose excursions. However, different methods of food processing and preparation can influence the GI of foods, and this may limit their benefit.

Low-carbohydrate diets may lead to significant reductions in body weight and improved glycaemic control in the short term, although high dropout rates and poor adherence have limited widespread application of this approach. Increased consumption of whole grains has not been shown to improve glycaemic control.

Fat

There is limited evidence on the ideal fat content in the diet of people with diabetes. Current UK government Food Standards Agency recommendations are that intake of total fat should be not more than 35% of energy intake, of which not more than 11% should consist of polyunsaturated fats. The type of fatty acids consumed may be more important when looking at glycaemic targets and risk of cardiovascular disease. Mediterranean diets rich in monounsaturated fats appear more beneficial (Box 20.23). The influence of dietary fats on plasma lipid profile and cardiovascular disease is discussed on page 697.

Salt

People with diabetes should follow the advice given to the general population: namely, adults should limit their sodium intake to no more than 6 g daily.

Weight management

In patients with diabetes, weight management is important, as a high percentage of people with type 2 diabetes are overweight or obese, and many antidiabetic drugs, including insulin, encourage weight gain. Obesity, particularly central obesity with increased waist circumference, also predicts insulin resistance and cardiovascular risk.

Management of obesity is described on page 700. Weight loss can be achieved through a reduction in energy intake and an increase in energy expenditure through physical activity. Lifestyle interventions or pharmacotherapy for obesity, when associated with weight reduction, have beneficial effects on HbA$_{1c}$, but long-term benefits in terms of glycaemic control and microvascular disease have not been adequately assessed. More recently, bariatric surgery (p. 703) has been shown to induce marked weight loss in obese individuals with type 2 diabetes and this is often associated with significant improvements in HbA$_{1c}$ and withdrawal of or reduction in diabetes medications.

Exercise

All patients with diabetes should be advised to achieve a significant level of physical activity and to maintain this in the long term. This can include activities such as walking, gardening, swimming or cycling. Supervised and structured exercise programmes may be of particular benefit in type 2 diabetes. Various guidelines exist for physical activity in the general population. The American Diabetes Association recommends that all adults with diabetes are encouraged to reduce sedentary time, and suggest that adults over 18 years of age should do either 150 minutes per week of moderate-intensity exercise or 75 minutes per week of vigorous-intensity exercise, or a combination thereof. Muscle-strengthening (resistance) exercise is recommended on 2 or more days of the week. Adults over 65 years or those with disabilities should follow the recommended guidelines if possible or be as physically active as they are able. Recent evidence also indicates that extended sedentary time (>90 mins) should be avoided.

People with type 1 diabetes appear to exercise less frequently than the general population, perhaps because of perceived concerns about hypoglycaemia and difficulties in insulin management around exercise. However, the health benefits of exercise are equally important in type 1 diabetes, so this should be addressed in the clinic and specialist advice sought on insulin and carbohydrate management before, during and after exercise.

Alcohol

Alcohol is recognised as having both beneficial and harmful effects on cardiovascular disease and this also appears to apply in patients with diabetes. Alcohol can therefore be taken in moderation in diabetes, with the aim of keeping within national guidelines relating to recommendations for people without diabetes (e.g. in the UK, the weekly recommended maximum is 14 units for women and men). However, alcohol can reduce hypoglycaemia awareness and, by suppressing gluconeogenesis, increase hypoglycaemia risk. The latter occurs when individuals are in the fasted state and so people with diabetes who drink should be advised to eat at the same time. In addition, all patients with diabetes should be made aware of the high calorie content of some alcohols and the implications for body weight management, which are often overlooked.

Driving

European legislation on driving has had a major impact on people with diabetes. Legislation will vary from country to country and so individuals should contact their nurse or doctor to find out if their treatment means they need to inform the licensing authority (Box 20.24). To drive a car or ride a motorcycle in the UK, people with diabetes who take insulin replacement therapy must notify the Driver and Vehicle Licensing Agency (DVLA). They must have adequate awareness of hypoglycaemia, have had no more than one episode of severe hypoglycaemia in the preceding 12 months, meet the standards for visual acuity and visual fields, and not be regarded as a likely risk to the public while driving. In addition, blood glucose testing is required to be performed no more than 2 hours before the start of a journey and every 2 hours while driving. Blood glucose levels should be over 5 mmol/L (90 mg/dL) before driving; if they are below 4.0 mmol/L (72 mg/dL) or there are symptoms of hypoglycaemia, the person should not drive. Legislative requirements for people on insulin therapy who drive larger vehicles such as buses or lorries require, in addition, an annual examination by a diabetes specialist, along with review of 3 months of glucose meter readings. Legislation differs between countries and patients and health-care specialists need to be aware of current requirements.

20.24 Diabetes and driving

- Licensing regulations vary considerably between countries. In the UK, diabetes requiring insulin therapy or any complication that could affect driving should be declared to the Driver and Vehicle Licensing Agency; ordinary driving licences are 'period-restricted' for insulin-treated drivers; and vocational licences (large goods vehicles and public service vehicles) may be granted but require very strict criteria to be met
- The main risk to driving performance is hypoglycaemia. Visual impairment and other complications may occasionally cause problems
- Insulin-treated diabetic drivers should:
    Check blood glucose before driving and 2-hourly during long journeys
    Keep an accessible supply of fast-acting carbohydrate in the vehicle
    Take regular snacks or meals during long journeys
    Stop driving if hypoglycaemia develops
    Refrain from driving until at least 45 mins after treatment of hypoglycaemia (delayed recovery of cognitive function)
    Carry identification in case of injury

Ramadan

The Qur'an requires Muslims to fast during the month of Ramadan from sunrise to sunset. While people with diabetes are a recognised exception to this and are not required to fast, many will choose to do so. In this context, patient education, regular glucose monitoring and adjustment of treatment regimens are essential and should occur weeks prior to Ramadan. The highest risk of hypoglycaemia is in patients treated with

20.25 Recommendations for management of diabetes during Ramadan

- Monitor blood glucose: depending on treatment regimen, glucose levels should be checked daily or several times a day. Patients treated with insulin and insulin secretagogues should measure glucose before, during and after fasting (2–4 times daily)
- Consult diabetes team for medication adjustment at least 1 month prior to Ramadan. Treatment should be evaluated and modified according to risk of hypoglycaemia. Avoid or reduce sulphonylureas and/or insulin daily dosage
- Avoid skipping pre-dawn meals
- Avoid strenuous physical activity during fasting period
- Adjust medication dose and eat a snack in the presence of hypoglycaemia. Break the fast if there is severe or recurrent hypoglycaemia

sulphonylureas and insulin (particularly older people or those with renal failure); such individuals need careful blood glucose monitoring and, if necessary their treatment regimens may need to be adjusted (Box 20.25). Diabetes therapies that do not cause hypoglycaemia may prove safest during Ramadan if glycaemic control permits. DPP-4 inhibitors or GLP-1 receptor agonists may be especially useful because their effect on insulin secretion is glucose-dependent.

Drugs to reduce hyperglycaemia

Patients whose glycaemic control deteriorates after a period of satisfactory control need their therapy to be adjusted. However, this is not a homogeneous group; it includes some patients with late-onset type 1 diabetes who develop an absolute deficiency of insulin, some with type 2 diabetes whose β-cell failure is advanced, and others who are not adhering to the recommended lifestyle changes or medication. Weight loss suggests worsening β-cell function. During continuing follow-up, the majority of patients will require combinations of antidiabetic drugs, often with additional insulin replacement, to obtain satisfactory glycaemic control.

For many years, only a few choices of drug were available for type 2 diabetes – the biguanide metformin, the sulphonylureas and insulin. Insulin is the only treatment for type 1 diabetes, although sometimes metformin is used with insulin in type 1 diabetes. Acarbose is also available but is little used in most countries. Since the late 1990s, however, several new classes of agent have been approved for use in type 2 diabetes, with more in development. These include thiazolidinediones, dipeptidyl peptidase 4 (DPP-4) inhibitors, glucagon-like peptide 1 (GLP-1) receptor agonists, and sodium and glucose transporter 2 (SGLT2) inhibitors. The effects of these drugs are compared in Box 20.26. This makes for an exciting time in diabetes pharmacotherapy but exactly how, when and in what order these agents should be used remains uncertain. The older drugs are cheaper and have established benefits for reducing microvascular disease; they are therefore usually recommended as first-line therapy. Use of the newer drugs is not supported by evidence for reduction in microvascular disease (because the trials have not yet been done) and they are much more expensive, so are often reserved for later therapy after failure of metformin and sulphonylureas. The American Diabetes Association/European Association for the Study of Diabetes (ADA/EASD) consensus

20

		20.26 Effects of drugs used in the treatment of type 2 diabetes							
	Insulin	Sulphonylureas and meglitinides	Metformin	Alpha-glucosidase inhibitors	Thiazolidinediones (glitazones)	DPP-4 inhibitors (gliptins)	GLP-1 receptor agonists	SGLT2 inhibitors
Fasting blood glucose	↓	↓	↓	↘	↓	↓	↓	↓
Post-prandial blood glucose	↓	↓	↓	↓	↓	↓	↓	↓
Plasma insulin	↑	↑	↓	↓	↓	↑	↑	↓
Body weight	↑	↑	→	→	↑	→	↓	↓
Cardiovascular benefit?	No	No	Possible	No	Probable (pioglitazone)	No	Yes	Yes
Risk of hypoglycaemia	++	+	−	−	−	−	−	−
Tolerability	Good	Good	Moderate	Moderate	Moderate	Good	Moderate	Limited experience

(↘ = small reduction; DPP-4 = dipeptidyl peptidase 4; GLP-1 = glucagon-like peptide 1; SGLT2 = sodium and glucose transporter 2)

guidelines are shown in Figure 20.10. These position metformin in the first line, and then aim to encourage choice of second-line treatment to be personalised for each patient. This personalisation is largely based on the adverse risk profile of the drug – in particular, risk of hypoglycaemia (avoid where hypoglycaemia would be a problem, e.g. in drivers of heavy goods vehicles) and weight gain. There is little evidence to guide the clinician and patient in choosing the second- or third-line treatment, and until biomarkers are identified that predict who will respond best and/or experience the fewest side-effects with one drug rather than another, this individualisation of treatment needs to be largely empirical. A trial-and-error approach may be best: stop a drug that does not work or that causes side-effects and trial the next drug. At the time of writing, the ADA/EASD guidelines were already out of date; in 2015/16, the SGLT2 inhibitor empagliflozin and the GLP-1 receptor agonist liraglutide were shown to reduce adverse cardiovascular outcomes and mortality. It is likely that the guidelines will change to take these exciting results into account and we will probably see these newer, more expensive drugs used earlier in the diabetes trajectory.

Biguanides

Metformin is the only biguanide available. Its long-term benefits were shown in the UK Prospective Diabetes Study (UKPDS, p. 756) and it is now widely used as first-line therapy for type 2 diabetes, irrespective of body weight. It is also given as an adjunct to insulin therapy in obese patients with type 1 diabetes. Approximately 25% of patients develop mild gastrointestinal side-effects with metformin, but only 5% are unable to tolerate it even at low dose. The main side-effects are diarrhoea, abdominal cramps, bloating and nausea.

Mechanism of action

The mechanism of action of metformin has not been precisely defined. While classically considered an 'insulin sensitiser' because it lowers insulin levels, its main effects are on fasting glucose and are insulin-independent. Metformin reduces hepatic glucose production, may also increase insulin-mediated glucose uptake, and has effects on gut glucose uptake and utilisation.

At the molecular level, metformin acts as a weak inhibitor of mitochondrial respiration, which increases intracellular adenosine monophosphate (AMP) and reduces adenosine triphosphate (ATP). This has direct effects on the flux through gluconeogenesis, and activates the intracellular energy sensor, AMP-activated protein kinase (AMPK), leading to multiple beneficial metabolic effects. However, metformin is still effective in mice lacking AMPK, and a number of AMPK-independent mechanisms have been proposed.

Clinical use

Metformin is a potent blood glucose-lowering treatment that is weight-neutral or causes weight loss, does not cause hypoglycaemia and has established benefits in microvascular disease. It is employed as first-line therapy in all patients who tolerate it, and its use is maintained when additional agents are added as glycaemia deteriorates (see Fig. 20.10). Metformin is usually introduced at low dose (500 mg twice daily) to minimise the risk of gastrointestinal side-effects. The usual maintenance dose is 1 g twice daily. There is a modified-release formulation of metformin, which may be better tolerated by patients with gastrointestinal side-effects.

Metformin can increase susceptibility to lactic acidosis, although this is much less common than was previously thought. As metformin is cleared by the kidneys, it can accumulate in renal impairment, so the dose should be halved when estimated glomerular filtration rate (eGFR) is 30–45 mL/min/1.73 m², and it should not be used below an eGFR of 30 mL/min/1.73 m². It should be omitted temporarily during any acute illness where acute kidney injury is possible, as this greatly increases the risk of lactic acidosis; insulin treatment may be required while metformin is withheld. Its use is also contraindicated in patients with significantly impaired hepatic function and in those who drink alcohol in excess, in whom the risk of lactic acidosis is significantly increased.

Sulphonylureas

Sulphonylureas are 'insulin secretagogues', i.e. they promote pancreatic β-cell insulin secretion. Similar to metformin, the long-term benefits of sulphonylureas in lowering microvascular complications of diabetes were established in the UKPDS (p. 756).

Mechanism of action

Sulphonylureas act by closing the pancreatic β-cell ATP-sensitive potassium (K_{ATP}) channel, decreasing K^+ efflux, which ultimately triggers insulin secretion (see Fig. 20.2C). Meglitinides (e.g. repaglinide and nateglinide) also work in this way and, although short-acting, are essentially sulphonylurea-like drugs.

Clinical use

Sulphonylureas are an effective therapy for lowering blood glucose and are often used as an add-on to metformin, if glycaemia is inadequately controlled on metformin alone (see Fig. 20.10). The main adverse effects of sulphonylureas are weight gain and hypoglycaemia. The weight gain is not ideal in patients with diabetes who are already overweight or obese, although sulphonylureas are effective treatments in this group. Hypoglycaemia occurs because the closure of K_{ATP} channels brings about unregulated insulin secretion, even with normal or low blood glucose levels.

There are a number of sulphonylureas. In the UK, gliclazide is the most commonly used; in contrast, in the USA, glibenclamide (also known as glyburide) is widely used. Glibenclamide, however, is long-acting and prone to inducing hypoglycaemia, so should be avoided in older patients. Other sulphonylureas include glimepiride and glipizide. The dose–response of all sulphonylureas is steepest at low doses; little additional benefit is obtained when the dose is increased above half-maximal doses.

Alpha-glucosidase inhibitors

The α-glucosidase inhibitors delay carbohydrate absorption in the gut by inhibiting disaccharidases. Acarbose and miglitol are available and are taken with each meal. Both lower post-prandial blood glucose and modestly improve overall glycaemic control. They can be combined with a sulphonylurea. The main side-effects are flatulence, abdominal bloating and diarrhoea. They are used widely in the Far East but infrequently in the UK.

Thiazolidinediones

Mechanism of action

These drugs (also called TZDs, 'glitazones' or PPARγ agonists) bind and activate peroxisome proliferator-activated receptor-γ, a nuclear receptor present mainly in adipose tissue, which regulates the expression of several genes involved in metabolism. TZDs enhance the actions of endogenous insulin, both directly (in the adipose cells) and indirectly (by altering release of 'adipokines', such as adiponectin, which alter insulin sensitivity in the liver). Plasma insulin concentrations are not increased and hypoglycaemia does not occur. TZDs increase pre-adipocyte differentiation, resulting in an increase in fat mass and body weight.

Clinical use

TZDs have been prescribed widely since the late 1990s but a number of adverse effects have become apparent and their use has declined. One popular TZD, rosiglitazone, was reported to increase the risk of myocardial infarction and was withdrawn in 2010. The other TZD in common use, pioglitazone, does not appear to increase the risk of myocardial infarction but may exacerbate cardiac failure by causing fluid retention, and recent data show that it increases the risk of bone fracture and possibly bladder cancer. These observations have led to a dramatic reduction in the use of pioglitazone.

Pioglitazone can be very effective at lowering blood glucose in some patients and appears more effective in insulin-resistant patients. In addition, it has a beneficial effect in reducing fatty liver and NASH (p. 882). Pioglitazone is usually added to metformin with or without sulphonylurea therapy (see Fig. 20.10). It may be given with insulin therapy, when it can be very effective, but the combination of insulin and TZDs markedly increases fluid retention and risk of cardiac failure, so should be used with caution.

Incretin-based therapies: DPP-4 inhibitors and GLP-1 receptor agonists

The incretin effect is the augmentation of insulin secretion seen when a glucose stimulus is given orally rather than intravenously, and reflects the release of incretin peptides from the gut (see Fig. 20.3). The incretin hormones are primarily glucagon-like peptide 1 (GLP-1) and gastric inhibitory polypeptide (GIP), which act to potentiate insulin secretion (see Fig. 20.2). These are rapidly broken down by dipeptidyl peptidase 4 (DPP-4). The incretin effect is diminished in type 2 diabetes, and this has stimulated the development of two incretin-based therapeutic approaches.

The 'gliptins', or DPP-4 inhibitors, prevent breakdown and therefore enhance concentrations of endogenous GLP-1 and GIP. The first DPP-4 inhibitor to market was sitagliptin; others now available include vildagliptin, saxagliptin, linagliptin and alogliptin. These drugs are very well tolerated and are weight-neutral (see Box 20.26). Recent cardiovascular outcome studies have shown mixed results with the DPP-4 inhibitors. The Trial to Evaluate Cardiovascular Outcomes after Treatment with Sitagliptin (TECOS) study reported no adverse cardiovascular outcomes for sitagliptin, but the Saxagliptin Assessment of Vascular Outcomes Recorded in Patients with Diabetes Mellitus – Thrombolysis in Myocardial Infarction (SAVOR-TIMI) study found an increased risk of heart failure in patients treated with saxagliptin.

The GLP-1 receptor agonists have a similar structure to GLP-1 but have been modified to resist breakdown by DPP-4. These agents are not orally active and have to be given by subcutaneous injection. However, they have a key advantage over the DPP-4 inhibitors: because the GLP-1 activity achieved is supra-physiological, it delays gastric emptying and, at the level of the hypothalamus, decreases appetite. Thus, injectable GLP-1 receptor agonists lower blood glucose and result in weight loss – an appealing therapy, as the majority of patients with type 2 diabetes are obese. Currently available GLP-1 receptor agonists include exenatide (twice daily), exenatide modified-release (once weekly), liraglutide (once daily), lixisenatide (once daily) and albiglutide (once weekly). Recently, GLP-1 receptor agonists and long-acting insulin analogue have been combined, enabling co-administration of insulin and GLP-1 receptor agonists with one injection. The GLP-1 receptor agonists vary in their side-effect profile, depending on whether they are administered daily or weekly, but the main side-effect that often limits use is nausea. The Liraglutide Effect and Action in Diabetes: Evaluation of Cardiovascular Outcome Results (LEADER) study has recently demonstrated that liraglutide, when added to usual therapy, results in improved cardiovascular outcomes over placebo in patients at high risk for cardiovascular disease; this contrasts with the Evaluation of Lixisenatide in Acute Coronary Syndrome (ELIXA) study, which showed that lixisenatide was neutral with respect to cardiovascular disease.

20

All the incretin-acting drugs have been reported to be associated with an increased risk of pancreatitis, although this risk is small: between 1 and 10 cases per 1000 patients treated.

Unlike sulphonylureas, both incretin-based therapies promote insulin secretion only when there is a glucose 'trigger' for it. Thus, when the blood glucose is normal, the insulin secretion is not augmented and so these agents do not cause hypoglycaemia when used as monotherapy or with other drugs that do not cause hypoglycaemia.

SGLT2 inhibitors

The sodium and glucose transporter 2 (SGLT2) inhibitor, dapagliflozin, was licensed for use in 2012. Subsequently, canagliflozin and empagliflozin have also been licensed. Glucose is filtered freely in the renal glomeruli and reabsorbed in the proximal tubules. SGLT2 is involved in reabsorption of glucose (Fig. 20.12). Inhibition results in approximately 25% of the filtered glucose not being reabsorbed, with consequent glycosuria. Although this helps to lower blood glucose and results in calorie loss and subsequent weight loss, the glycosuria does also lead to genital fungal infections. There has been increasing use of these agents over the last few years; however, the recent announcement of the Empagliflozin, Cardiovascular Outcomes, and Mortality in Type 2 Diabetes (EMPA-REG Outcomes) trial has the potential to change dramatically the way these drugs are now used. Empagliflozin therapy resulted in a 35% reduction in cardiovascular mortality and a similar reduction in admissions to hospital with heart failure. This result was much greater than anticipated and the mechanism behind it is still being investigated, but this landmark study was the first to show such striking benefits in mortality reduction from a glucose-lowering agent; as such, these drugs should now, at the very least, be used in all patients who fulfil the inclusion criteria of the trial – prior myocardial infarction, coronary artery disease, stroke, unstable angina or occlusive peripheral arterial disease. Euglycaemic diabetic ketoacidosis (i.e. DKA not associated with marked hyperglycaemia) has been recognised as a rare complication of this class of drugs.

Insulin therapy

Manufacture and formulation

Insulin was discovered in 1921 and transformed the management of type 1 diabetes, which was a fatal disorder until then. Up to the 1980s, insulin was obtained by extraction and purification from pancreases of cows and pigs (bovine and porcine insulins), and some patients still prefer to use animal insulins. Recombinant DNA technology enabled large-scale production of human insulin. Unmodified ('soluble' or 'regular') insulin aggregates into hexamers in subcutaneous tissues; these must dissociate before systemic absorption can occur and this process helps extend the duration of action to nearly 8 hours. The amino acid sequence of insulin can be altered to produce analogues of insulin, which differ in their rate of absorption from the site of injection. For example, in insulin lispro, the penultimate lysine and proline residues on the C-terminal end of the β chain are reversed (Fig. 20.13). This prevents the insulin molecules from aggregating as hexamers in subcutaneous tissues after injection and so speeds absorption, leading to a more rapid onset and shorter duration of action than soluble insulin (Box 20.27). The onset of action of insulin analogues may be further hastened by the addition of excipients to the formulation (e.g. nicotinamide and arginine to insulin aspart). Conversely, in insulin glargine, a substitution of glycine for asparagine in the α chain and the addition of two additional arginine residues to the C-terminal end of the β chain serves to prolong the duration of action of the insulin to over 24 hours. The amino acid modifications shift the isoelectric point from a pH of 5.4 to 6.7, making the molecule less soluble at a physiological pH (see Fig. 20.13). Duration of action can also be extended by adding chemicals to soluble insulin solution or by adding other molecules to the insulin structure. Chemical additives include protamine and zinc at neutral pH (isophane or NPH insulin) or excess zinc ions (lente insulins). In insulin detemir and degludec, the duration of action is extended by adding fatty acids to a slightly truncated C-terminal end of the β chain (Fig. 20.13). Following subcutaneous injection, these bind to albumin in the

Fig. 20.12 Glucose filtration and reabsorption by the nephron. Some 90% of filtered glucose is reabsorbed by sodium and glucose transporter 2 (SGLT2) and 10% by SGLT1. SGLT2 inhibitors reduce net reabsorbed glucose by 25%. For a mean plasma glucose of 8 mmol/L (144 mg/dL), this results in a glucose loss of approximately 80 g per day in the urine, which in turn reduces plasma glucose. This equates to 320 kcal per day and subsequent weight loss.

Fast-acting analogues

Lispro   Aspart   Glulisine

Long-acting analogues

Glargine   Detemir/Degludec

Fig. 20.13 Amino acid structure of insulin and insulin analogues. The areas in the shaded colours show the modifications made to the normal structure of insulin. These are important in altering the pharmocokinetic properties of the analogues.

20.27 Duration of action (in hours) of insulin preparations

Insulin	Onset	Peak	Duration
Rapid-acting (insulin analogues: lispro, aspart, glulisine)	<0.5	0.5–2.5	3–4.5
Short-acting (soluble (regular))	0.5–1	1–4	4–8
Intermediate-acting (isophane (NPH), lente)	1–3	3–8	7–14
Long-acting (bovine ultralente)	2–4	6–12	12–30
Long-acting (insulin analogues: glargine, detemir, degludec)	1–2	None	18–26

20.28 How to inject insulin subcutaneously

- Needle sited at right angle to the skin
- Subcutaneous (not intramuscular) injection
- Delivery devices: glass syringe (requires resterilisation), plastic syringe (disposable), pen device (reusable, some disposable), infusion pump

discomfort of injecting bigger volumes and also to reduce variability in insulin delivery from the subcutaneous depot. Therefore, U 200, U 300 and U 500 formulations of insulin are available, which are, respectively, two, three and five times more concentrated than standard insulin. Expert advice should be sought before using concentrated insulin because errors in prescribing can cause severe hypoglycaemia.

Subcutaneous multiple dose insulin therapy

In most patients, insulin is injected subcutaneously several times a day into the anterior abdominal wall, upper arms, outer thighs and buttocks (Box 20.28). Accidental intramuscular injection often occurs in children and thin adults. The rate of absorption of insulin may be influenced by many factors other than the insulin formulation, including the site, depth and volume of injection, skin temperature (warming), local massage and exercise. Absorption is delayed from areas of lipohypertrophy at injection sites (p. 721), which results from the local trophic action of insulin, so repeated injection at the same site should be avoided. Other routes of administration (intravenous and intraperitoneal) are reserved for specific circumstances.

Once absorbed into the blood, insulin has a half-life of just a few minutes. It is removed mainly by the liver and also the kidneys, so plasma insulin concentrations are elevated in patients with liver disease or renal failure. Rarely, the rate of clearance can be affected by binding to insulin antibodies.

blood, from which the insulin slowly disassociates. The duration of action of insulin degludec may also be extended as the fatty acid moiety promotes the formation of multi-hexamers of insulin in the subcutaneous tissues (Box 20.27).

Isophane and lente insulins are cloudy preparations and have to be resuspended prior to injection to ensure adequate mixing of the components. The more modern, structurally modified, long-acting insulins (e.g. glargine, detemir and degludec) are clear and do not require resuspension. Pre-mixed formulations containing short-acting and isophane insulins in various proportions are available.

In most countries, the insulin concentration in available formulations has been standardised at 100 U/mL. Increasing levels of obesity, which are associated with increased daily insulin requirements, have stimulated pharmaceutical companies to develop more concentrated insulin formulations to reduce the

20

- Hypoglycaemia
- Weight gain
- Peripheral oedema (insulin treatment causes salt and water retention in the short term)
- Insulin antibodies
- Local allergy (rare)
- Lipohypertrophy or lipoatrophy at injection sites

Insulin can be administered using a disposable plastic syringe with a fine needle (which can be re-used several times), but this has largely been replaced by pen injectors containing insulin in cartridges sufficient for multiple dosing. These are also available as pre-loaded disposable pens.

For the most part, insulin analogues have replaced soluble and isophane insulins, especially for people with type 1 diabetes, because they allow greater flexibility and convenience and reduce risk of hypoglycaemia (see Box 20.26). Unlike soluble insulin, which should be injected 30–60 minutes before eating, rapid-acting insulin analogues can be administered immediately before, during or even after meals, although are better injected 15 minutes before eating. Long-acting insulin analogues are also better able than isophane insulin to maintain 'basal' insulin levels for up to 24 hours.

Despite these pharmacokinetic benefits, the impact of insulin analogues on overall glycaemic control is minor, but studies consistently show a significant reduction in frequency of hypoglycaemia, particularly overnight.

The complications of insulin therapy are listed in Box 20.29; the most important of these is hypoglycaemia (p. 738). A common problem is fasting hyperglycaemia ('the dawn phenomenon'), which arises through a combination of the normal circadian rhythm and release of hormones such as growth hormone and cortisol during the later part of the night, as well as diminishing levels of overnight isophane insulin. The dawn phenomenon is not a consequence of prior nocturnal hypoglycaemia.

Insulin dosing regimens

The choice of regimen depends on the desired degree of glycaemic control, the severity of underlying insulin deficiency, the patient's lifestyle, and his or her ability to adjust the insulin dose. The time–action profile of different insulin regimens, compared to the secretory pattern of insulin in the non-diabetic state, is shown in Figure 20.14. People with type 1 diabetes are best managed by multiple daily insulin injections or an insulin pump. In type 2 diabetes, insulin is usually initiated as a once-daily long-acting insulin, either alone or in combination with oral antidiabetic agents. However, in time, more frequent insulin injections are usually required.

Twice-daily administration of a short-acting and intermediate-acting insulin (usually soluble and isophane insulins), given in combination before breakfast and the evening meal, is the simplest regimen and is still commonly used in many countries. Initially, two-thirds of the total daily requirement of insulin is given in the morning in a ratio of short-acting to intermediate-acting of 1:2, and the remaining third is given in the evening. Pre-mixed formulations are available that contain different proportions of soluble and isophane insulins (e.g. 30:70 and 50:50). These are useful as they avoid the need for directly mixing insulins, but are inflexible as the individual components cannot be adjusted independently. They need to be resuspended by shaking the

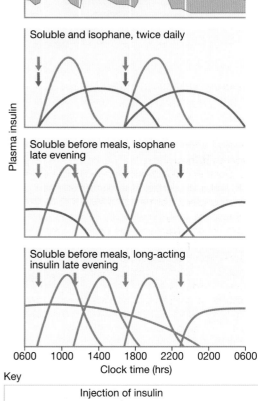

Fig. 20.14 Profiles of plasma insulin associated with different insulin regimens. The schematic profiles are compared with the insulin responses (mean ± 1 standard deviation) observed in non-diabetic adults shown in the top panel (shaded area). These are theoretical patterns of plasma insulin and may differ considerably in magnitude and duration of action between individuals.

vial several times before administration. Fixed-mixture insulins also have altered pharmacodynamic profiles, such that the peak insulin action and time to peak effect are significantly reduced compared with separately injecting the same insulins. This increases the risk of hypoglycaemia.

Multiple injection regimens (intensive insulin therapy) are popular, with short-acting insulin being taken before each meal, and intermediate- or long-acting insulin being injected once or twice daily (basal-bolus regimen, Box 20.30). This type of regimen is more physiological and allows greater freedom with regard to meal timing, as well more variable day-to-day physical activity.

Fig. 20.15 **Insulin pump.** An insulin pump is an alternative means of delivering insulin in type 1 diabetes. Different types are available and include the pump device itself (with controls, processing module and batteries), a disposable reservoir for insulin (inside the pump) and a disposable infusion set (with tubing and a cannula for subcutaneous insertion). Alternative configurations include disposable or semi-disposable pumps, and pumps without infusion tubing. Insulin pumps deliver rapid-acting insulin continuously, and can be adjusted by the user, based on regular glucose monitoring and carbohydrate counting.

---

i | **20.30 Example of a meal bolus calculation**

RL has type 1 diabetes treated with an insulin pump. His pre-breakfast glucose (G) is 12 mmol/L (216 mg/dL). He is having a breakfast meal of cereal with milk containing 30 g of carbohydrate (CHO) in total. His insulin:carbohydrate ratio (ICR) is 10 (1 U of insulin for every 10 g of CHO) and his insulin sensitivity factor (ISF) is 2 (1 U of insulin to bring down blood glucose by 2 mmol/L (36 mg/dL)). He wants to achieve a glucose target (G_T) of 8 mmol/L (144 mg/dL) after eating.

Calculation of estimated bolus dose:

$$Bolus\ dose = (CHO \div ICR) + ((G - G_T) \div ISF)$$
$$= (30 \div 10) + ((12 - 8) \div 2)$$
$$= 5\ U\ of\ insulin$$

Subcutaneous continuous insulin therapy

Subcutaneous continuous insulin therapy, commonly know as the insulin pump, is a system of insulin delivery that uses a battery-operated medical device to deliver insulin continuously to the individual with type 1 diabetes. Device configurations vary between manufacturers but will include the pump with controls, processing module and batteries, a disposable insulin reservoir, and a disposable insulin set including cannula for subcutaneous insertion and a tubing system to deliver insulin from the reservoir to the cannula. Some recent versions are disposable or semi-disposable and eliminate tubing from the infusion set (patch pumps).

Insulin pumps allow the individual more flexibility with bolus insulin injections in both timing and shape (e.g. using an extended bolus when covering high-fat/protein meals such as steak, or when diabetes is complicated by gastroparesis), and also in changing basal insulin infusion rates. This is especially useful overnight when basal rates can be reduced to prevent low glucose, but increased pre-dawn to prevent high glucose. In addition, the temporary basal rates can be used to lessen the risk of hypoglycaemia with exercise. Determining an individual's basal rate on the pump requires help from a specialist, but in essence is determined by fasting for periods of at least 4 hours while periodically evaluating the blood glucose levels and adjusting the pump infusion rate to maintain glucose in the normal range. Basal rates will change and can be influenced by factors such as increasing duration of disease, puberty, weight gain or loss, drugs that affect insulin sensitivity (e.g. glucocorticoids), and a change in fitness levels with exercise on overall glycaemic control. An example of an insulin pump is shown in Figure 20.15.

Closed loop insulin therapy

A further iteration in insulin pump therapy in recent years is the development of a 'closed loop' system, also known as the artificial pancreas (Fig. 20.16). These systems aim to integrate insulin pumps with continuous glucose monitoring systems (CGMS). In a closed loop system, the CGMS device communicates with the insulin pump via a computerised program. This means that real-time glucose data obtained through the CGMS can be used to calculate an insulin dosage to be dispensed through the insulin pump (Fig. 20.17). Features might include a 'low-glucose suspend' function, where detection of hypoglycaemia or a glucose level falling below a pre-set threshold (e.g. 4.0 mmol/L (72 mg/dL)) signals the pump to stop dispensing insulin until the wearer can treat the hypoglycaemia with food or glucose tabs. Current

Fig. 20.16 **Artificial pancreas.** The artificial pancreas (AP) can vary in its set up and the different components employed in its delivery but core to an AP system are: (1) a continuous glucose monitor (CGM) measuring interstitial glucose levels every 5–15 minutes; (2) a smartphone (or personal glucose monitor) with an app that uses the glucose information from the CGM along with modifications inserted by the user to calculate how much insulin should be delivered. This is communicated wirelessly to (3) the insulin pump that delivers insulin subcutaneously as directed.

20

clinical trials in children and adults in the hospital or free-living setting aim to determine how effective this approach will be in optimising management of type 1 diabetes. Widespread use may, however, be limited by cost.

Alternative routes of insulin delivery have also been investigated. Clinical trials with intrapulmonary (inhalation), transdermal and oral insulins are ongoing but as yet none has proven commercially viable. Inhaled insulin has been approved for use in the USA as a mealtime insulin, but experience with this is very limited.

Fig. 20.17 Continuous glucose monitoring (CGM) profiles: sensor data. **A** CGM profile from an individual without diabetes. **B** CGM profile from an individual with type 1 diabetes. The green box shows the reference range. CGM devices may be worn for 7–14 days and the glucose profile of each day illustrated by a different colour. Based on this, the person with diabetes and their health-care team can review overall profiles and adjust treatment as necessary to improve control and avoid hypoglycaemia.

Transplantation

Whole-pancreas transplantation is carried out in a small number of patients with diabetes each year, but it presents problems relating to exocrine pancreatic secretions and long-term immunosuppression is necessary.

There are currently four main types of whole-pancreas transplantation:

- pancreas transplant alone
- simultaneous pancreas–kidney (SPK) transplant, when pancreas and kidney are transplanted simultaneously from the same deceased donor
- pancreas-after-kidney (PAK) transplant, when a cadaveric, or deceased, donor pancreas transplant is performed after a previous, and different, living or deceased donor kidney transplant
- simultaneous deceased donor pancreas and live donor kidney (SPLK) transplant.

The principal complications occurring immediately after surgery include thrombosis, pancreatitis, infection, bleeding and rejection. Prognosis is improving: 1 year after transplantation more than 95% of all patients are still alive and 80–85% of all pancreases are still functional. After transplantation, patients will need life-long immunosuppression, which carries with it an increased risk of infection and cancer.

An alternative form of transplantation is allogenic islet transplantation, which involves the transplantation of islets from a donor pancreas into a person with type 1 diabetes. The isolated pancreatic islets are usually infused into the patient's liver via the portal vein. This approach has now been successfully adopted in a number of centres around the world (Fig. 20.18). At present, islet transplantation is usually suitable only for patients with unstable glycaemic control characterised by recurrent severe hypoglycaemia that cannot be corrected by standard conventional and intensive insulin therapies. Progress is being made towards meeting the needs of supply, purification and storage of islets, but problems remain relating to transplant rejection, and destruction by the patient's autoantibodies against β cells. Nevertheless, the development of methods of inducing tolerance to transplanted islets and the potential use of stem cells (p. 58) mean that this may still prove the most promising approach in the long term. Adoption of newer immunosuppressive protocols has resulted in far better outcomes and now nearly 50% of transplanted patients will be insulin-independent at 3 years post transplantation.

Management of diabetes in special situations

Diabetes in pregnancy

The management of women with pre-existing diabetes who are pregnant or who have developed diabetes in pregnancy (gestational diabetes) is discussed in detail on page 1278 and summarised in Box 20.31. This is a highly specialised area and requires careful and attentive management, as elevated maternal

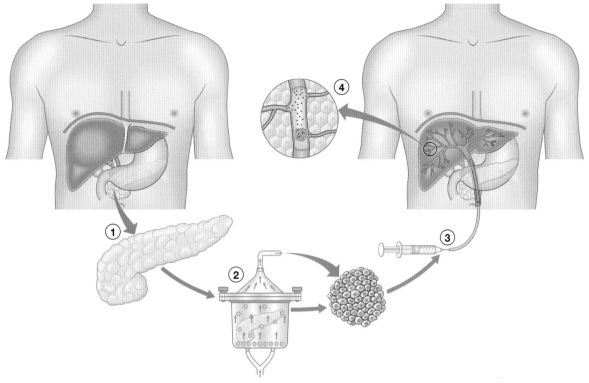

Fig. 20.18 Transplanting islet cells. (1) Pancreas obtained from suitable human donor. (2) Pancreatic islets containing insulin-producing β cells are isolated first in a Ricordi chamber. (3) Islets, once separated and purified, are infused into the hepatic portal vein. (4) Once embedded in the liver, pancreatic islets secrete insulin in response to changes in portal vein glucose.

 Box 20.31 Diabetes in pregnancy

- **Control of established diabetes before and during pregnancy**: must be meticulous, to reduce the risk of complications such as pre-eclampsia, congenital malformations and stillbirth.
- **Gestational diabetes**: most commonly an inability to increase insulin secretion adequately to compensate for pregnancy-induced insulin resistance.
- **Screening for gestational diabetes**: all women at high risk should have an oral glucose tolerance test at 24–28 weeks. Measurement of HbA$_{1c}$ and/or blood glucose at booking visit is usually recommended.
- **Management of gestational diabetes**: reduce intake of refined carbohydrate, and add metformin, glibenclamide and/or insulin if necessary to optimise glycaemic control.
- **Self-monitoring of glucose**: targets are a pre-prandial level of <5.3 mmol/L (95 mg/dL) and a 1-hour or 2-hour post-prandial level of <7.8 mmol/L (140 mg/dL) and <6.4 mmol/L (114 mg/dL), respectively.

 20.32 Diabetes in adolescence

- **Type of diabetes**: type 1 diabetes is predominant in children and adolescents, but type 2 diabetes is now presenting in unprecedented numbers of obese, inactive teenagers. Monogenic diabetes (MODY) should also be considered (see Box 20.10, p. 733).
- **Physiological changes**: hormonal, physical and lifestyle changes in puberty affect dietary intake, exercise patterns and sensitivity to insulin, necessitating alterations in insulin regimen.
- **Emotional changes**: adolescence is a phase of transition into independence (principally from parental care). Periods of rebellion against parental control, experimentation (e.g. with alcohol) and a more chaotic lifestyle are common, and often impact adversely on control of diabetes.
- **Glycaemic control**: a temporary deterioration in control is common, although not universal. It is sometimes more important to maintain contact and engagement with a young person than to insist on tight glycaemic control.
- **Diabetic ketoacidosis**: a few adolescents and young adults present with frequent episodes of DKA, often because of non-adherence to insulin therapy. This is more common in females. Motivating factors may include weight loss, rebellion, and manipulation of family or schooling circumstances.
- **Adolescent diabetes clinics**: these challenges are best tackled with support from a specialised multidisciplinary team, including paediatricians, physicians, nurses and psychologists. Support is required for the patient and parents.

---

blood glucose in pregnancy is associated with significant maternal and fetal morbidity.

Children, adolescents and young adults with diabetes

Most type 1 diabetes is diagnosed in children below 18 years of age, with peak incidence rates between 5 and 7 years of age and at puberty. The management of diabetes in children and adolescents presents particular challenges, which should be addressed in specialised clinics with multidisciplinary input (Box 20.32). Some of the unique aspects of childhood type 1

diabetes management include changing insulin sensitivity related to sexual maturity and physical growth, unique vulnerability to hypoglycaemia (especially in children below 6 years of age) and possibly hyperglycaemia, as well as DKA. In addition, family dynamics, child care and schooling, developmental stages and

20

20.33 Recommended therapeutic targets in childhood and adolescence

Plasma glucose levels

- Before meals 4.0–7.0 mmol/L (72–126 mg/dL)
- After meals 5.0–9.0 mmol/L (90–160 mg/dL)

HbA$_{1c}$

- <53 mmol/mol (7.0%) with a target of 48 mmol/L

Recommended screening

- HbA$_{1c}$ up to four times per year
- Thyroid disease at diagnosis and annually thereafter
- Diabetic retinopathy annually from 12 years
- Albuminuria (albumin:creatinine ratio (ACR) 3–30 mg/mmol; 'microalbuminuria') to detect diabetic kidney disease, annually from 12 years
- Hypertension annually from 12 years

Adapted from National Institute for Health and Care Excellence NG18 – Diabetes (type 1 and type 2) in children and young people: diagnosis and management; 2015.

20.34 How to carry out pre-operative assessment of patients with diabetes

- Assess glycaemic control:
  Consider delaying surgery and refer to the diabetes team if HbA$_{1c}$ >75 mmol/mol; this should be weighed against the need for surgery
- Assess cardiovascular status
  Optimise blood pressure
  Perform an ECG for evidence of (possibly silent) ischaemic heart disease and to assess QTc (p. 448)
- Assess foot risk (p. 761)
  Patients with high-risk feet should have suitable pressure relief provided during post-operative nursing
- For minor/moderate operations where only one meal will be omitted, plan for the patient to be first on the list

ability to self-care all have to be considered in the management plan, as well as, in older children and adolescents, issues of body image, eating disorders and recreational drug and alcohol use. It is also notable that there is very limited clinical research in children with diabetes and so most recommendations are based on expert opinion. The prevalence of type 2 diabetes in those below 20 years has been increasing and is estimated to increase fourfold in the next 40 years. Management of these children and young adults is difficult.

Coeliac disease and thyroid disease are much more common in children with type 1 diabetes than in the general population and so it is currently recommended that these conditions are screened for. Current recommendations for screening in type 1 diabetes are shown in Box 20.33.

Hyperglycaemia in acute medical illness

Hyperglycaemia is often found in patients who are admitted to hospital as an emergency. In most people this occurs in the context of a known diagnosis of diabetes; in some individuals, however, it is a consequence of stress hyperglycaemia (p. 728), while in others it is due to undiagnosed diabetes. Hyperglycaemia on admission to hospital is associated with increased length of stay and increased mortality in a wide variety of acute medical emergencies, including acute coronary syndrome and acute stroke. Intuitively, intensive glycaemic control with intravenous insulin should improve outcomes during acute illness. However, recent studies have shown that strategies aiming for near-normal blood glucose levels in acutely ill patients are associated with either increased mortality or no overall benefit. The reasons for the adverse outcomes are not established, but intensive glycaemic control is inevitably associated with an increased risk of hypoglycaemia because of the inherent limitations of modern insulins, the restricted frequency of glucose monitoring in a ward environment and the relative imprecision of near-patient blood glucose meters. The activation of the sympathetic nervous system and release of counter-regulatory hormones during acute hypoglycaemia could have deleterious consequences for the acutely ill patient.

There is no consensus on the optimum glucose targets in acutely ill patients but extremes of blood glucose should be avoided, and so a target of between 6 and 12 mmol/L (105

and 180 mg/dL) seems appropriate. Achieving such a target may require the use of intravenous insulin and dextrose in some individuals.

Surgery and diabetes

Patients with diabetes are reported to have up to 50% higher perioperative mortality than patients without diabetes. Surgery causes catabolic stress and secretion of counter-regulatory hormones (including catecholamines and cortisol) in both normal and diabetic individuals. This results in increased glycogenolysis, gluconeogenesis, lipolysis, proteolysis and insulin resistance. Starvation exacerbates this process by increasing lipolysis. In the non-diabetic person, these metabolic effects lead to a secondary increase in the secretion of insulin, which exerts a controlling influence. In diabetic patients, either there is absolute deficiency of insulin (type 1 diabetes) or insulin secretion is delayed and impaired (type 2 diabetes), so that in untreated or poorly controlled diabetes, the uptake of metabolic substrate into tissues is significantly reduced, catabolism is increased and, ultimately, metabolic decompensation in the form of DKA may develop in both types of diabetes. In addition, hyperglycaemia impairs wound healing and innate immunity, leading to increased risk of infection. Patients with diabetes are also more likely to have underlying pre-operative morbidity, especially cardiovascular disease. Finally, management errors in diabetes may cause dangerous hyperglycaemia or hypoglycaemia. Careful pre-operative assessment and perioperative management are therefore essential, ideally with support from the diabetes specialist team.

Pre-operative assessment

Unless a surgical intervention is an emergency, patients with diabetes should be assessed well in advance of surgery so that poor glycaemic control and other risk factors can be addressed (Box 20.34). There is good evidence that a higher HbA$_{1c}$ is associated with adverse perioperative outcome. In general, an upper limit for an acceptable HbA$_{1c}$ should be between 64 and 75 mmol/mol (8% and 9%). However, since optimisation of care may take weeks or months to achieve, the benefits need to be weighed against the need for early surgical intervention.

Perioperative management

Figure 20.19 outlines a general approach to perioperative management of diabetes, although this may need to be adapted according to the patient, the surgical procedure and local guidelines. Patients with diabetes who are considered low-risk can attend as day cases or be admitted on the day of surgery.

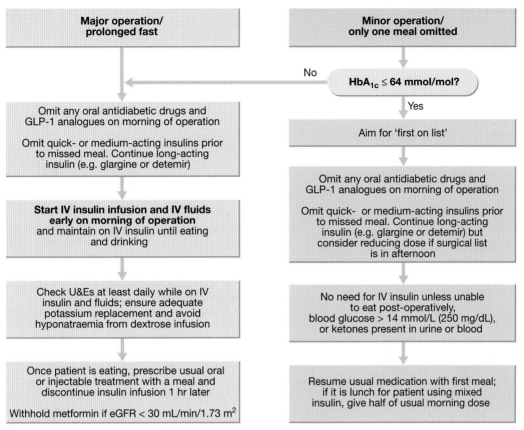

Fig. 20.19 Management of diabetic patients undergoing surgery and general anaesthesia. (eGFR = estimated glomerular filtration rate; GLP-1 = glucagon-like peptide 1; IV = intravenous; U&Es = urea and electrolytes)

Occasionally, patients may be admitted the night before to ensure optimal management.

Post-operative management

Patients who need to continue fasting after surgery should be maintained on intravenous insulin and fluids until they are able to eat and drink (Fig. 20.19). During this time, care must be taken with fluid balance and electrolyte levels. Insulin infusion necessitates dextrose infusion to maintain a supply of glucose but this combination drives down plasma potassium (p. 360) and can result in hyponatraemia. Intravenous fluids during prolonged insulin infusion should therefore include saline and potassium supplementation. UK guidelines recommend the use of dextrose/saline (0.45% saline with 5% dextrose and 0.15% potassium chloride).

Once a patient's usual treatment has been reinstated, care must be taken to continue to control the blood glucose, ideally between 6 and 10 mmol/L (105–180 mg/dL), in order to optimise wound healing and recovery. Patients normally controlled on tablets may require temporary subcutaneous insulin treatment until the increased 'stress' of surgery, wound healing or infection has resolved.

Complications of diabetes

Despite all the treatments now available, the outcome for patients with diabetes remains disappointing. Long-term complications of diabetes still cause significant morbidity and mortality (Boxes 20.35 and 20.36).

Excess mortality in diabetes is caused mainly by large blood vessel disease, particularly myocardial infarction and stroke. Macrovascular disease also causes substantial morbidity from myocardial infarction, stroke, angina, cardiac failure and intermittent claudication. The pathological changes of atherosclerosis in diabetic patients are similar to those in the non-diabetic population but occur earlier in life and are more extensive and severe. Diabetes amplifies the effects of the other major cardiovascular risk factors: smoking, hypertension and dyslipidaemia (Fig. 20.20). Moreover, patients with type 2 diabetes are more likely to have additional cardiovascular risk factors, which co-segregate with insulin resistance in the metabolic syndrome (p. 730). Mortality statistics from the USA indicate that cardiovascular death rates are 1.7 times higher in adults with diabetes aged 20 years or older compared to adults in the same age group who do not have diabetes, while similar figures for myocardial infarction show a 1.8 times greater rate. Hospitalisation rates for stroke were 1.5 times higher in adults with diabetes than in those without diabetes. In addition, 60% of non-traumatic amputations among people aged 20 years or older were reported to be in people with diabetes. Type 1 diabetes is also associated with increased cardiovascular risk. Recent data from Scotland show that the age-adjusted incidence rate ratio for first cardiovascular event was 3 times higher in women and 2.3 times higher in men with type 1 diabetes compared to those without diabetes.

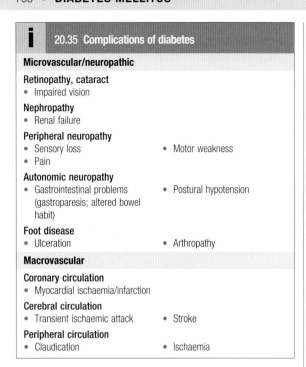

i 20.35 Complications of diabetes

Microvascular/neuropathic

Retinopathy, cataract
- Impaired vision

Nephropathy
- Renal failure

Peripheral neuropathy
- Sensory loss
- Pain
- Motor weakness

Autonomic neuropathy
- Gastrointestinal problems (gastroparesis; altered bowel habit)
- Postural hypotension

Foot disease
- Ulceration
- Arthropathy

Macrovascular

Coronary circulation
- Myocardial ischaemia/infarction

Cerebral circulation
- Transient ischaemic attack
- Stroke

Peripheral circulation
- Claudication
- Ischaemia

Fig. 20.20 Association between HbA$_{1c}$ and risk of microvascular and macrovascular diabetes complications. These data were obtained amongst participants in the UK Prospective Diabetes Study and were adjusted for effects of age, sex and ethnicity; the incidences show what could be expected amongst white men aged 50–54 years at diagnosis of type 2 diabetes, followed up for 10 years. Microvascular disease included retinopathy requiring photocoagulation, vitreous haemorrhage and renal failure. Macrovascular disease included fatal and non-fatal myocardial infarction and sudden death. A 1% change in HbA$_{1c}$ is equivalent to a reduction of 11 mmol/mol.

i 20.36 Mortality in diabetes

Risk versus non-diabetic controls (mortality ratio)

- Overall — 2.6
- Coronary heart disease, Cerebrovascular disease, Peripheral vascular disease — 2.8
- All other causes, including renal failure — 2.7

Causes of death in diabetes (approximate proportion)

- Cardiovascular disease — 70%
- Renal failure — 10%
- Cancer — 10%
- Infections — 6%
- Diabetic ketoacidosis — 1%
- Other — 3%

Risk factors for increased morbidity and mortality in diabetes

- Duration of diabetes
- Early age at onset of disease
- High glycated haemoglobin (HbA$_{1c}$)
- Raised blood pressure
- Proteinuria; microalbuminuria
- Dyslipidaemia
- Obesity

Disease of small blood vessels is a specific complication of diabetes and is termed diabetic microangiopathy. It contributes to mortality through renal failure caused by diabetic nephropathy, and is responsible for substantial morbidity and disability: for example, blindness from diabetic retinopathy, difficulty in walking, chronic ulceration of the feet from peripheral neuropathy, and bowel and bladder dysfunction from autonomic neuropathy. The risk of microvascular disease is positively correlated with the duration and degree of sustained hyperglycaemia, however it is caused and at whatever age it develops.

Pathophysiology

The histopathological hallmark of diabetic microangiopathy is thickening of the capillary basement membrane, with associated increased vascular permeability, which occurs throughout the body. The development of the characteristic clinical syndromes of diabetic retinopathy, nephropathy, neuropathy and accelerated atherosclerosis is thought to result from the local response to generalised vascular injury. For example, in the wall of large vessels, increased permeability of arterial endothelium, particularly when combined with hyperinsulinaemia and hypertension, may increase the deposition of atherogenic lipoproteins. The mechanisms linking hyperglycaemia to these pathological changes are, however, poorly characterised.

Preventing diabetes complications

Glycaemic control

The evidence that improved glycaemic control decreases the risk of developing microvascular complications of diabetes was established by the DCCT in type 1 diabetes and the UKPDS in type 2 diabetes. The DCCT was a large study that lasted 9 years; it randomised patients with type 1 diabetes to intensive treatment (mean HbA$_{1c}$ 53 mmol/mol) and conventional treatment (mean HbA$_{1c}$ 75 mmol/mol). There was a 60% overall reduction in the risk of developing diabetic complications in patients with type 1 diabetes on intensive therapy with strict glycaemic control, compared with those on conventional therapy. No single factor other than glycaemic control had a significant effect on outcome. However, the group that was intensively treated to lower blood glucose had three times the rate of severe hypoglycaemia. The UKPDS randomised patients to intensive treatment (mean HbA$_{1c}$ 53 mmol/mol) versus conventional treatment (mean HbA$_{1c}$ 64 mmol/mol). This study showed that, in type 2 diabetes, the frequency of diabetic complications is lower and progression is slower with good glycaemic control and effective treatment of hypertension, irrespective of the type of therapy used. Extrapolation from the UKPDS suggests that, for every 11 mmol/mol

20.37 Diabetes management in old age

- **Glycaemic control**: the optimal target for glycaemic control in older people has yet to be determined. Strict glycaemic control should be avoided in frail patients with comorbidities and in older patients with long duration of diabetes.
- **Cognitive function and affect**: may benefit from improved glycaemic control but it is important to avoid hypoglycaemia.
- **Hypoglycaemia**: older people have reduced symptomatic awareness of hypoglycaemia and limited knowledge of symptoms, and are at greater risk of, and from, hypoglycaemia.
- **Mortality**: the mortality rate of older people with diabetes is more than double that of age-matched non-diabetic people, largely because of increased deaths from cardiovascular disease.

20.38 Risk factors for diabetic nephropathy

- Poor glycaemic control
- Long duration of diabetes
- Presence of other microvascular complications
- Ethnicity (e.g. Asians, Pima Indians)
- Pre-existing hypertension
- Family history of diabetic nephropathy
- Family history of hypertension

reduction in HbA$_{1c}$, there is a 21% reduction in death related to diabetes, a 14% reduction in myocardial infarction and 30–40% reduction in risk of microvascular complications (Fig. 20.20).

These landmark trials demonstrated that diabetic complications are preventable and that the aim of treatment should be 'near-normal' glycaemia. More recent studies, however, such as the Action to Control Cardiovascular Risk in Diabetes (ACCORD), showed increased mortality in a subgroup of patients who were aggressively treated to lower HbA$_{1c}$ to a target of less than 48 mmol/mol. The patients in this study had poor glycaemic control at baseline, a long duration of diabetes and a high prevalence of cardiovascular disease. It appears that, while a low target HbA$_{1c}$ is appropriate in younger patients with earlier diabetes who do not have underlying cardiovascular disease, aggressive glucose-lowering is not beneficial in older patients with long duration of diabetes and multiple comorbidities (Box 20.37).

Control of other risk factors

Randomised controlled trials have shown that aggressive management of blood pressure minimises the microvascular and macrovascular complications of diabetes. Angiotensin-converting enzyme (ACE) inhibitors are valuable in improving outcome in heart disease and in treating diabetic nephropathy (see below). The management of dyslipidaemia with a statin limits macrovascular disease in people with diabetes (p. 375). This often results in the necessary use of multiple medications, which exacerbates the problem of adherence to therapy by patients; it is not unusual for a patient to be taking two or more diabetes therapies, two or more blood pressure drugs and a statin.

Diabetic retinopathy

Diabetic retinopathy (DR) is one of the most common causes of blindness in adults between 30 and 65 years of age in developed countries. The prevalence of DR increases with duration of diabetes, and almost all individuals with type 1 diabetes and the majority of those with type 2 diabetes will have some degree of DR after 20 years. The pathogenesis, clinical features and management of diabetic retinopathy, as well as screening and prevention, are described on page 1174. Other causes of visual loss in type 2 diabetes are also covered in Chapter 27.

Diabetic nephropathy

Diabetic nephropathy is an important cause of morbidity and mortality in both type 1 and type 2 diabetes. It is now the most common cause of end-stage renal failure in developed countries and accounts for between 20% and 50% of patients starting renal replacement therapy.

About 30% of patients with type 1 diabetes have developed diabetic nephropathy 20 years after diagnosis, but the risk after this time falls to less than 1% per year, and from the outset the risk is not equal in all patients (Box 20.38). The risk of nephropathy in Caucasian populations with type 2 diabetes is similar to those with type 1 diabetes but the rate of progression may be exacerbated by concomitant obesity and other risk factors. The risk of nephropathy is much greater in some ethnic groups, with epigenetic and genetic factors thought to influence this increased risk. Some patients do not develop nephropathy, however, despite having long-standing, poorly controlled diabetes, suggesting that they do not have a genetic predisposition. While variants in a few genes have been implicated in diabetic nephropathy, the major differences in individual risk remain unexplained. With improved standards of care focusing on glycaemic control and blood pressure lowering, the proportion of patients with overt nephropathy is reducing; however, due to the global rise in the incidence of type 2 diabetes, the prevalent number of people with diabetes and end-stage renal failure continues to rise.

The pathophysiology is not fully understood and there are several postulated mechanisms by which hyperglycaemia causes the pathological changes seen in diabetic nephropathy. The central features are activation of the renin–angiotensin system, leading to both intrarenal and systemic effects, as well as direct toxic effects of prolonged hyperglycaemia, leading to renal inflammation and fibrosis. The pattern of progression of renal abnormalities in diabetes is shown schematically in Figure 20.21. Pathologically, the first changes coincide with the onset of microalbuminuria and include thickening of the glomerular basement membrane and accumulation of matrix material in the mesangium. Subsequently, nodular deposits (Fig. 20.22) are characteristic, and glomerulosclerosis worsens as heavy proteinuria develops, until glomeruli are progressively lost and renal function deteriorates.

Diagnosis and screening

Microalbuminuria (Box 20.39) is the presence in the urine of small amounts of albumin, at a concentration below that detectable using a standard urine dipstick. Overt nephropathy is defined as the presence of macroalbuminuria (urinary albumin >300 mg/24 hrs, detectable on urine dipstick). Microalbuminuria is a good predictor of progression to nephropathy in type 1 diabetes. It is a less reliable predictor of nephropathy in older patients with type 2 diabetes, in whom it may be accounted for by other diseases (p. 394), although it is a potentially useful marker of an increased risk of macrovascular disease.

Management

The presence of established microalbuminuria or overt nephropathy should prompt vigorous efforts to reduce the

20

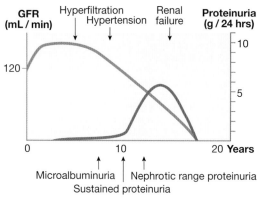

Fig. 20.21 Natural history of diabetic nephropathy. In the first few years of type 1 diabetes mellitus, there is hyperfiltration, which declines fairly steadily to return to a normal value at approximately 10 years (blue line). In susceptible patients (about 30%), after about 10 years, there is sustained proteinuria, and by approximately 14 years it has reached the nephrotic range (red line). Renal function continues to decline, with the end stage being reached at approximately 16 years.

Fig. 20.22 Nodular diabetic glomerulosclerosis. There is thickening of basement membranes, mesangial expansion and a Kimmelstiel–Wilson nodule (arrow), which is pathognomonic of diabetic kidney disease.

---

i | **20.39 Screening for microalbuminuria**

- Screening identifies incipient nephropathy in type 1 and type 2 diabetes; is an independent predictor of macrovascular disease in type 2 diabetes
- Risk factors include high blood pressure, poor glycaemic control and smoking
- Early morning urine is measured for the albumin:creatinine ratio (ACR). Microalbuminuria is present if:
  Male ACR 2.5–30 mg/mmol creatinine
  Female ACR 3.5–30 mg/mmol creatinine
- An elevated ACR should be followed by a repeat test:
  There is established microalbuminuria if 2 out of 3 tests are positive
  An ACR >30 mg/mmol creatinine is consistent with overt nephropathy

---

risk of progression of nephropathy and of cardiovascular disease by:

- aggressive reduction of blood pressure
- aggressive reduction of cardiovascular risk factors
- optimisation of glycaemic control

Blockade of the renin–angiotensin system using either ACE inhibitors or angiotensin 2 receptor blockers (ARBs) has been shown to have an additional benefit over similar levels of blood pressure control achieved with other antihypertensive agents and is recommended as first-line therapy. The addition of a diuretic and/or salt restriction increase both the anti-proteinuric and antihypertensive effect of angiotensin blockade and therefore constitute an ideal second-line treatment. The benefit from blockade of the renin–angiotensin system arises from a reduction in the angiotensin II-mediated vasoconstriction of efferent arterioles in glomeruli (see Fig. 15.1D, p. 385). The resulting dilatation of these vessels decreases glomerular filtration pressure and, therefore, the hyperfiltration and protein leak. Both ACE inhibitors and ARBs increase risk of hyperkalaemia (p. 362) and, in the presence of renal artery stenosis (p. 406), may induce marked deterioration in renal function. Therefore, electrolytes and renal function should be checked after initiation or each dose increase. If blockade of the renin–angiotensin system is not possible, blood pressure should managed with standard treatment, such as calcium channel blockers and diuretics. There may be a role for spironolactone (an aldosterone antagonist) but this is limited by hyperkalaemia.

Halving the amount of albuminuria with an ACE inhibitor or ARB results in a nearly 50% reduction in long-term risk of progression to end-stage renal disease. Some patients do progress, however, with worsening renal function. Renal replacement therapy (p. 420) is often required at a higher eGFR than in other causes of renal failure, due to fluid overload or symptomatic uraemia.

Renal transplantation dramatically improves the life of many, and any recurrence of diabetic nephropathy in the allograft is usually too slow to be a serious problem; associated macrovascular and microvascular disease elsewhere may still progress, however. Pancreatic transplantation (generally carried out at the same time as renal transplantation) can produce insulin independence and delay or reverse microvascular disease, but the supply of organs is limited and this option is available to few. For further information on management, see Chapter 15.

Diabetic neuropathy

Diabetic neuropathy causes substantial morbidity and increases mortality. It is diagnosed on the basis of symptoms and signs, after the exclusion of other causes of neuropathy (p. 1138). Depending on the criteria used for diagnosis, it affects between 50% and 90% of patients with diabetes, and of these, 15–30% will have painful diabetic neuropathy (PDN). Like retinopathy, neuropathy occurs secondary to metabolic disturbance, and prevalence is related to the duration of diabetes and the degree of metabolic control.

Pathological features can occur in any peripheral nerves. They include axonal degeneration of both myelinated and unmyelinated fibres, with thickening of the Schwann cell basal lamina, patchy segmental demyelination and abnormal intraneural capillaries (with basement membrane thickening and microthrombi).

Various classifications of diabetic neuropathy have been proposed. One is shown in Box 20.40 but motor, sensory and autonomic nerves may be involved in varying combinations, so that clinically mixed syndromes usually occur.

Clinical features

Symmetrical sensory polyneuropathy

This is frequently asymptomatic. The most common clinical signs are diminished perception of vibration sensation distally, 'glove

Peripheral neuropathy

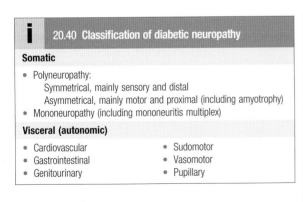

▲ Charcot foot

▲ Neuropathic ulcer

▲ Clawing of toes

Glove and stocking neuropathy

Dry, cracked skin
Callus

Peripheral vascular disease

▲ Proximal arterial occlusion

Loss of leg hair

Absent pulses
Cold feet

▲ Digital gangrene

Fig. 20.23 Diabetic foot disease. Patients with diabetes can have neuropathy, peripheral vascular disease or both. Clawing of the toes is thought to be caused by intrinsic muscle atrophy and subsequent imbalance of muscle function, and causes greater pressure on the metatarsal heads and pressure on flexed toes, leading to increased callus and risk of ulceration. A Charcot foot occurs only in the presence of neuropathy, and results in bony destruction and ultimately deformity (this X-ray shows a resulting 'rocker bottom foot'). The angiogram reveals disease of the superficial femoral arteries (occlusion of the left and stenosis of the right). *Insets (Proximal arterial occlusion) From http://emedicine.medscape.com/article/460178-overview#a0104; (Toe clawing) Bowker JH, Pfeifer MA. Levin and O'Neal's The diabetic foot, 7th edn. Philadelphia: Mosby, Elsevier Inc.; 2008; (Neuropathic foot ulcer) Levy MJ, Valabhji J. Vascular II: The diabetic foot. Surgery 2008; 26:25–28; (Digital gangrene) Swartz MH. Textbook of physical diagnosis, 5th edn. Philadelphia: WB Saunders, Elsevier Inc.; 2006.*

20

> **i 20.40 Classification of diabetic neuropathy**
>
> **Somatic**
>
> - Polyneuropathy:
>   Symmetrical, mainly sensory and distal
>   Asymmetrical, mainly motor and proximal (including amyotrophy)
> - Mononeuropathy (including mononeuritis multiplex)
>
> **Visceral (autonomic)**
>
> - Cardiovascular
> - Gastrointestinal
> - Genitourinary
> - Sudomotor
> - Vasomotor
> - Pupillary

and stocking' impairment of all other modalities of sensation (Fig. 20.23), and loss of tendon reflexes in the lower limbs. In symptomatic patients, sensory abnormalities are predominant. Symptoms include paraesthesiae in the feet (and, rarely, in the hands), pain in the lower limbs (dull, aching and/or lancinating, worse at night, and felt mainly on the anterior aspect of the legs), burning sensations in the soles of the feet, cutaneous hyperaesthesia and, when severe, an abnormal gait (commonly wide-based), often associated with a sense of numbness in the feet. Weakness and atrophy, in particular of the interosseous muscles, develops, leading to structural changes in the foot with loss of lateral and transverse arches, clawing of the toes and exposure of the metatarsal heads. This results in increased

pressure on the plantar aspects of the metatarsal heads, with the development of callus skin at these and other pressure points. Electrophysiological tests (p. 1074) demonstrate slowing of both motor and sensory conduction, and tests of vibration sensitivity and thermal thresholds are abnormal.

A diffuse small-fibre neuropathy causes altered perception of pain and temperature, and is associated with symptomatic autonomic neuropathy; characteristic features include foot ulcers and Charcot neuroarthropathy.

Asymmetrical motor diabetic neuropathy

Sometimes called diabetic amyotrophy, this presents as severe and progressive weakness and wasting of the proximal muscles of the lower (and occasionally the upper) limbs. It is commonly accompanied by severe pain, felt mainly on the anterior aspect of the leg, and hyperaesthesia and paraesthesiae. Sometimes there may also be marked loss of weight ('neuropathic cachexia'). The patient may look extremely ill and be unable to get out of bed. Tendon reflexes may be absent on the affected side(s). Sometimes there are extensor plantar responses and the cerebrospinal fluid protein is often raised. This condition is thought to involve acute infarction of the lower motor neurons of the lumbosacral plexus. Other lesions involving this plexus, such as neoplasms and lumbar disc disease, must be excluded. Although recovery usually occurs within 12 months, some deficits are permanent. Management is mainly supportive.

<table>
<tr><td>i</td><td>20.41 Clinical features of autonomic neuropathy</td></tr>
</table>

Cardiovascular

- Postural hypotension
- Resting tachycardia
- Fixed heart rate

Gastrointestinal

- Dysphagia, due to oesophageal atony
- Abdominal fullness, nausea and vomiting, unstable glycaemia, due to delayed gastric emptying ('gastroparesis')
- Nocturnal diarrhoea ± faecal incontinence
- Constipation, due to colonic atony

Genitourinary

- Difficulty in micturition, urinary incontinence, recurrent infection, due to atonic bladder
- Erectile dysfunction and retrograde ejaculation

Sudomotor

- Nocturnal sweats without hypoglycaemia
- Gustatory sweating
- Anhidrosis; fissures in the feet

Vasomotor

- Feet feel cold, due to loss of skin vasomotor responses
- Dependent oedema, due to loss of vasomotor tone and increased vascular permeability
- Bulla formation

Pupillary

- Decreased pupil size
- Resistance to mydriatics
- Delayed or absent reflexes to light

20.42 How to test cardiovascular autonomic function

Simple reflex tests	Normal	Borderline	Abnormal
Heart rate responses			
To Valsalva manœuvre (15 secs)[1]: ratio of longest to shortest R–R interval	≥1.21		≤1.20
To deep breathing (6 breaths over 1 min): maximum–minimum heart rate	≥15	11–14	≤10
To standing after lying: ratio of R–R interval of 30th to 15th beats	≥1.04	1.01–1.03	≤1.00
Blood pressure response[2]			
To standing: systolic blood pressure fall (mmHg)	≤10	11–29	≥30

Specialised tests

- Heart rate and blood pressure responses to sustained handgrip
- Heart rate variability using power spectral analysis of ECG monitoring
- Heart rate and blood pressure variability using time–domain analysis of ambulatory monitoring
- MIBG (meta-iodobenzylguanidine) scan of the heart

[1]Omit in patients with previous laser therapy for proliferative retinopathy. [2]Avoid arm with arteriovenous fistula in dialysed patients.

Mononeuropathy

Either motor or sensory function can be affected within a single peripheral or cranial nerve. Unlike the gradual progression of distal symmetrical and autonomic neuropathies, mononeuropathies are severe and of rapid onset, but they eventually recover. The nerves most commonly affected are the 3rd and 6th cranial nerves (resulting in diplopia), and the femoral and sciatic nerves. Rarely, involvement of other single nerves results in paresis and paraesthesiae in the thorax and trunk (truncal radiculopathies).

Nerve compression palsies are more common in diabetes, frequently affecting the median nerve and giving the clinical picture of carpal tunnel syndrome, and less commonly the ulnar nerve. Lateral popliteal nerve compression occasionally causes foot drop. Compression palsies may be more common because of glycosylation and thickening of connective tissue and/or because of increased susceptibility of nerves affected by diabetic microangiopathy.

Autonomic neuropathy

This is not necessarily associated with peripheral somatic neuropathy. Parasympathetic or sympathetic nerves may be predominantly affected in one or more visceral systems. The resulting symptoms and signs are listed in Box 20.41 and tests of autonomic function in Box 20.42. The development of autonomic neuropathy is related to poor metabolic control less clearly than to somatic neuropathy, and improved control rarely results in improved symptoms. Within 10 years of developing overt symptoms of autonomic neuropathy, 30–50% of patients are dead, many from sudden cardiorespiratory arrest. Patients with postural hypotension (a drop in systolic pressure of 30 mmHg or more on standing from the supine position) have the highest subsequent mortality.

Gastroparesis

Gastroparesis is diagnosed when there is an objectively measured delay in gastric emptying in the absence of mechanical obstruction. It is most commonly a manifestation of autonomic neuropathy in diabetes, but can occur with eating disorders such as anorexia nervosa or bulimia that are also associated with diabetes. Prevalence rates are estimated to be approximately 5% in type 1 diabetes and 1% in type 2 diabetes. The main symptoms are chronic nausea, vomiting (especially of undigested food), abdominal pain and a feeling of fullness/early satiety. Diagnosis is most commonly made by [99m]-technetium scintigraphy following a solid-phase meal with standard imaging over 4 hours. In this test it is important to recognise that high glucose levels can delay gastric emptying and so every attempt should be made to conduct the test when glucose levels are below 15 mmol/L (270 mg/dL). Other tests include upper gastrointestinal endoscopy, wireless motility capsules and breath testing (pp. 774, 776 and 777). Management is difficult, with glucose levels directly impacting on gastric motility and, conversely, gastroparesis affecting absorption of ingested carbohydrate. Insulin pump therapy may be especially useful in this context; patients on conventional injection therapy may benefit from injecting rapid-acting insulin after a meal rather than before. Recommended dietary changes include following low-fibre and low-residue diets, as well as eating smaller amounts more frequently. Enteral nutrition is rarely required unless gastroparesis is very severe. Recommended pharmacological and interventional therapy is shown in Box 20.43.

Erectile dysfunction

Erectile failure (impotence) affects 30% of diabetic males and is often multifactorial. Although neuropathy and vascular causes are common, psychological factors, including depression, anxiety and reduced libido, may be partly responsible. Alcohol and antihypertensive drugs, such as thiazide diuretics and β-adrenoceptor antagonists (β-blockers), may cause sexual dysfunction and in some patients there may be an endocrine

20.43 Management options for peripheral sensorimotor and autonomic neuropathies

Pain and paraesthesiae from peripheral somatic neuropathies

- Intensive insulin therapy (strict glycaemic control)
- Anticonvulsants (gabapentin, pregabalin, carbamazepine, phenytoin)
- Tricyclic antidepressants (amitriptyline, imipramine)
- Other antidepressants (duloxetine)
- Substance P depleter (capsaicin – topical)
- Opiates (tramadol, oxycodone)
- Membrane stabilisers (mexiletine, IV lidocaine)
- Antioxidant (α-lipoic acid)

Postural hypotension

- Support stockings
- Fludrocortisone
- NSAIDs
- α-adrenoceptor agonist (midodrine)

Gastroparesis

- Dopamine antagonists (metoclopramide, domperidone)
- Erythromycin
- Botulinum toxin
- Gastric pacemaker; percutaneous enteral (jejunal) feeding (see Fig. 19.10, p. 708)

Diarrhoea (p. 783)

- Loperamide
- Broad-spectrum antibiotics
- Clonidine
- Octreotide

Constipation

- Stimulant laxatives (senna)

Atonic bladder

- Intermittent self-catheterisation (p. 1093)

Excessive sweating

- Anticholinergic drugs (propantheline, poldine, oxybutinin)
- Clonidine
- Topical antimuscarinic agent (glycopyrrolate cream)

Erectile dysfunction (p. 440)

- Phosphodiesterase type 5 inhibitors (sildenafil, vardenafil, tadalafil) – oral
- Dopamine agonist (apomorphine) – sublingual
- Prostaglandin E_1 (alprostadil) – injected into corpus cavernosum or intra-urethral administration of pellets
- Vacuum tumescence devices
- Implanted penile prosthesis
- Psychological counselling; psychosexual therapy

(NSAIDs = non-steroidal anti-inflammatory drugs)

20.44 Clinical features of the diabetic foot

	Neuropathy	Ischaemia
Symptoms	None Paraesthesiae Pain Numbness	None Claudication Rest pain
Structural damage	Ulcer Sepsis Abscess Osteomyelitis Digital gangrene Charcot joint	Ulcer Sepsis Gangrene

(p. 502 and Fig. 20.23); with infection is a secondary phenomenon following disruption of the protective epidermis. Most ulcers develop at the site of a plaque of callus skin, beneath which tissue necrosis occurs and eventually breaks through to the surface. In many cases, multiple components are involved but sometimes neuropathy or ischaemia predominates (Box 20.44). Ischaemia alone accounts for a minority of foot ulcers in diabetic patients, with most being either neuropathic or neuro-ischaemic.

Charcot neuroarthropathy is a progressive condition affecting the bones and joints of the foot; it is characterised by early inflammation and then joint dislocation, subluxation and pathological fractures of the foot of neuropathic patients, often resulting in debilitating deformity (Fig. 20.23 and p. 720). Charcot neuroarthropathy can arise in any condition that causes neuropathy (including syphilis, spinal cord injury, syringomyelia etc.) but diabetes is the most common cause. The pathophysiological mechanisms remain poorly understood but may involve unperceived trauma, leading to progressive destruction (the 'neurotraumatic' theory) and/or increased blood flow that results in a mismatch of bone destruction and synthesis (the 'neurovascular' theory). More recent evidence points to disordered inflammation mediated via the nuclear factor kappa B (NFκB)/receptor activator of NFκB ligand (RANKL) pathway, opening the way for trials of the RANKL inhibitor denosumab (p. 1048).

Management

Management can be divided into primary prevention and treatment of an active problem. All patients should be educated in preventative measures (Box 20.45). The feet of people with diabetes should be screened annually, following the steps listed on page 721. Two simple tests are required to grade risk: a 10 g monofilament should be used to assess sensation at five points on each foot, and foot pulses should be palpated (dorsalis pedis and/or posterior tibial). Combined with the clinical scenario, these tests guide appropriate referral and monitoring (Fig. 20.24). Removal of callus skin with a scalpel is best done by a podiatrist who has specialist training and experience in diabetic foot problems.

Foot ulcer

Once a foot ulcer develops, patients should ideally be referred to a multidisciplinary foot team, involving a diabetes specialist, a podiatrist, a vascular surgeon and an orthotist. Treatment involves: débridement of dead tissue; prompt, often prolonged, treatment with antibiotics if required, as infection can accelerate tissue necrosis and lead to gangrene; and pressure relief using customised insoles, specialised orthotic footwear and sometimes total contact plaster cast or an irremovable aircast boot. If an ulcer

cause, such as testosterone deficiency or hyperprolactinaemia. For further information, see page 440.

Management

Management of neuropathies is outlined in Box 20.43.

The diabetic foot

The foot is a frequent site of complications in patients with diabetes and for this reason foot care is particularly important. Tissue necrosis in the feet is a common reason for hospital admission in diabetic patients. Treatment of the foot complications of diabetes accounts for more inpatient days than any other diabetes-related complication.

Aetiology

Foot ulceration occurs as a result of trauma (often trivial) in the presence of neuropathy and/or peripheral vascular disease

20

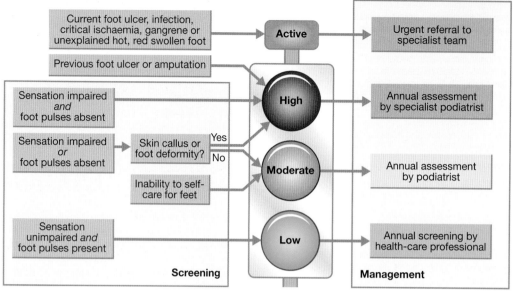

Fig. 20.24 Risk assessment and management of foot problems in diabetes. *Adapted from Scottish Intercollegiate Guidelines Network (SIGN) guideline number 116.*

> **i** | **20.45 Care of the feet in patients with diabetes**
>
> **Preventative advice**
>
> **All diabetic patients**
> - Inspect feet every day
> - Wash feet every day
> - Moisturise skin if dry
> - Cut or file toenails regularly
> - Change socks or stockings every day
> - Avoid walking barefoot
> - Check footwear for foreign bodies
> - Wear suitable, well-fitting shoes
> - Cover minor cuts with sterile dressings
> - Do not burst blisters
> - Avoid over-the-counter corn/callus remedies
>
> **Moderate- and high-risk patients**
> As above plus:
> - Do not attempt corn removal
> - Avoid high and low temperatures
>
> **Podiatric care**
> - A podiatrist is an integral part of the diabetes team to ensure regular and effective podiatry and to educate patients in care of the feet
>
> **Orthotic footwear**
> - Specially manufactured and fitted orthotic footwear is required to prevent recurrence of ulceration and to protect the feet of patients with Charcot neuroarthropathy

is neuro-ischaemic, a vascular assessment is often carried out, by ultrasound or angiography, as revascularisation by angioplasty or surgery may be required to allow the ulcer to heal. In cases of severe secondary infection or gangrene, an amputation may be required. This can be limited to the affected toe or involve more extensive limb amputation.

Charcot neuroarthropathy

Acute Charcot neuroarthropathy almost always presents with signs of inflammation – a hot, red, swollen foot. The initial X-ray may show bony destruction but is often normal. As about 40% of patients with a Charcot joint also have a foot ulcer, it can be difficult to differentiate from osteomyelitis. Magnetic resonance imaging (MRI) of the foot is often helpful. The mainstay of treatment for an active Charcot foot is immobilisation and, ideally, avoidance

of weight-bearing on the affected foot. The rationale is that if no pressure is applied through the foot, the destructive process involving the bones will not result in significant deformity when the acute inflammatory process subsides. Immobilisation is often achieved by a total contact plaster cast or 'aircast' boot. The acute phase frequently lasts 3–6 months and sometimes longer. In the post-acute phase, there is consolidation and remodelling of fracture fragments, eventually resulting in a stable foot.

Further information

Books and journal articles

Diabetes Control and Complications Trial Research Group. The effect of intensive treatment of diabetes on the development and progression of long-term complications in insulin-dependent diabetes mellitus. N Engl J Med 1993; 329:977–986.

Nathan DM, Cleary PA, Backlud JY, et al. Diabetes Control and Complications Trial/Epidemiology of Diabetes Interventions and Complications (DCCT/EDIC) Study Research Group. Intensive diabetes treatment and cardiovascular disease in patients with type 1 diabetes. N Engl J Med 2005; 353:2643–2653.

UK Prospective Diabetes Study (UKPDS) Group. Intensive blood-glucose control with sulphonylureas or insulin compared with conventional treatment and risk of complications in patients with type 2 diabetes (UKPDS 33). Lancet 1998; 352:837–853, 854–865.

Websites

cdc.gov/diabetes/ *Diabetes Public Health Resource. Useful American site with resources for patients and health-care professionals.*

diabetes.org *American Diabetes Association. Includes information on research and advocacy issues.*

diabetes.org.uk *Diabetes UK. Includes information for patients and leaflets.*

idf.org *International Diabetes Federation. Useful information on international aspects of care and education.*

joslin.org *Joslin Diabetes Center. Well-written resource for patients and health-care professionals, and information on diabetes research.*

mydiabetesmyway.scot.nhs.uk *An interactive diabetes website for patients with diabetes and their carers.*

ndei.org *National Diabetes Education Initiative. Web-based education for health-care professionals, including case studies and slides.*

E El-Omar
MH McLean

Gastroenterology

Clinical examination of the gastrointestinal tract 764

Functional anatomy and physiology 766
Oesophagus, stomach and duodenum 766
Small intestine 767
Pancreas 770
Colon 770
Intestinal microbiota 771
Control of gastrointestinal function 771
Gut hormones 772

Investigation of gastrointestinal disease 772
Imaging 772
Tests of infection 777
Tests of function 777
Radioisotope tests 778
Gut hormone testing 778

Presenting problems in gastrointestinal disease 778
Dysphagia 778
Dyspepsia 779
Heartburn and regurgitation 779
Vomiting 780
Gastrointestinal bleeding 780
Diarrhoea 783
Malabsorption 783
Weight loss 785
Constipation 786
Abdominal pain 787

Diseases of the mouth and salivary glands 790

Diseases of the oesophagus 791
Gastro-oesophageal reflux disease 791
Motility disorders 794
Tumours of the oesophagus 796
Perforation of the oesophagus 797

Diseases of the stomach and duodenum 797
Gastritis 797
Peptic ulcer disease 798
Functional disorders 802
Tumours of the stomach 803

Diseases of the small intestine 805
Disorders causing malabsorption 805
Motility disorders 810
Miscellaneous disorders of the small intestine 811
Adverse food reactions 812
Infections of the small intestine 812
Tumours of the small intestine 813

Inflammatory bowel disease 813

Irritable bowel syndrome 824

HIV/AIDS and the gastrointestinal tract 826

Ischaemic gut injury 827

Disorders of the colon and rectum 827
Tumours of the colon and rectum 827
Diverticulosis 833
Constipation and disorders of defecation 834
Anorectal disorders 835

Diseases of the peritoneal cavity 836

Other disorders 837

Diseases of the pancreas 837
Acute pancreatitis 837
Chronic pancreatitis 839
Congenital abnormalities affecting the pancreas 842
Tumours of the pancreas 842

Clinical examination of the gastrointestinal tract

3 Head and neck
Pallor
Jaundice
Angular stomatitis
Glossitis
Parotid enlargement
Mouth ulcers
Dentition
Lymphadenopathy

▲ Virchow's gland in gastric cancer

▲ Atrophic glossitis and angular stomatitis in vitamin B$_{12}$ deficiency

2 Hands
Clubbing
Koilonychia
Signs of liver disease (Ch. 22)

▲ Clubbing in patient with malabsorption

1 Skin and nutritional status
Muscle bulk
Signs of weight loss

▲ Pyoderma gangrenosum in ulcerative colitis

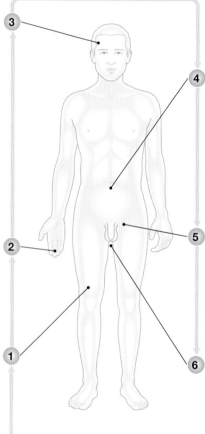

Observation
• Distressed/in pain?
• Fever?
• Dehydrated?
• Habitus
• Skin

4 Abdominal examination
(see opposite)

Observe
Distension
Respiratory movements
Scars
Colour

▲ Multiple surgical scars, a prolapsing ileostomy and enterocutaneous fistulae in a patient with Crohn's disease

Palpate
Tender/guarding
Masses
Viscera
   Liver (Ch. 22)
   Kidneys (Ch. 15)
   Spleen

Percuss
Ascites
Viscera

Auscultate
Bowel sounds
Bruits

5 Groin
Herniae
Lymph nodes

6 Perineum/rectal
(see opposite)
Fistulae
Skin tags
Haemorrhoids
Masses

4 Abdominal examination: possible findings

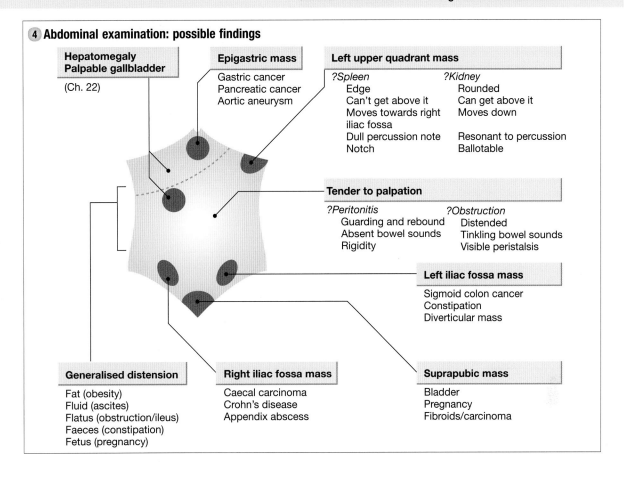

Hepatomegaly
Palpable gallbladder

(Ch. 22)

Epigastric mass

Gastric cancer
Pancreatic cancer
Aortic aneurysm

Left upper quadrant mass

?Spleen	?Kidney
Edge	Rounded
Can't get above it	Can get above it
Moves towards right iliac fossa	Moves down
Dull percussion note	Resonant to percussion
Notch	Ballotable

Tender to palpation

?Peritonitis	?Obstruction
Guarding and rebound	Distended
Absent bowel sounds	Tinkling bowel sounds
Rigidity	Visible peristalsis

Left iliac fossa mass

Sigmoid colon cancer
Constipation
Diverticular mass

Generalised distension

Fat (obesity)
Fluid (ascites)
Flatus (obstruction/ileus)
Faeces (constipation)
Fetus (pregnancy)

Right iliac fossa mass

Caecal carcinoma
Crohn's disease
Appendix abscess

Suprapubic mass

Bladder
Pregnancy
Fibroids/carcinoma

6 Rectal examination: common findings

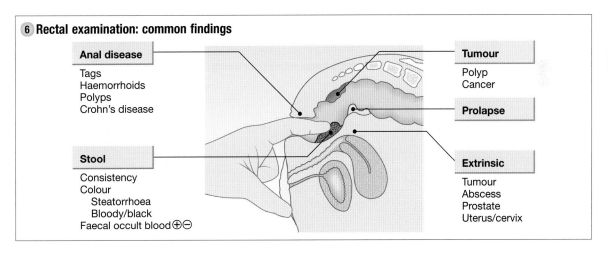

Anal disease

Tags
Haemorrhoids
Polyps
Crohn's disease

Tumour

Polyp
Cancer

Prolapse

Stool

Consistency
Colour
  Steatorrhoea
  Bloody/black
Faecal occult blood ⊕⊖

Extrinsic

Tumour
Abscess
Prostate
Uterus/cervix

21

Diseases of the gastrointestinal tract are a major cause of morbidity and mortality. Approximately 10% of all GP consultations in the UK are for indigestion and 1 in 14 is for diarrhoea. Infective diarrhoea and malabsorption are responsible for much ill health and many deaths in the developing world. The gastrointestinal tract is the most common site for cancer development. Colorectal cancer is the third most common cancer in men and women and population-based screening programmes exist in many countries. Functional bowel disorders affect up to 10–15% of the population and consume considerable health-care resources. The inflammatory bowel diseases, Crohn's disease and ulcerative colitis, together affect 1 in 250 people in the Western world, with substantial associated morbidity.

Functional anatomy and physiology

Oesophagus, stomach and duodenum

The oesophagus is a muscular tube that extends 25 cm from the cricoid cartilage to the cardiac orifice of the stomach. It has an upper and a lower sphincter. A peristaltic swallowing wave propels the food bolus into the stomach (Fig. 21.1).

The stomach acts as a 'hopper', retaining and grinding food, and then actively propelling it into the upper small bowel (Fig. 21.2).

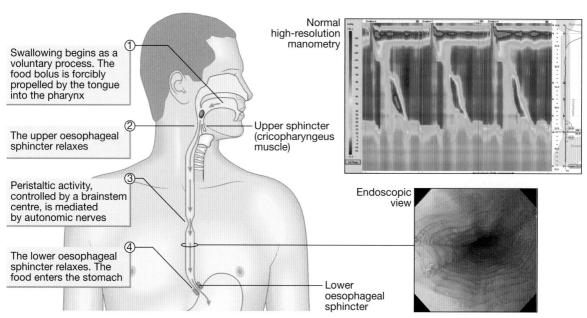

Swallowing begins as a voluntary process. The food bolus is forcibly propelled by the tongue into the pharynx

The upper oesophageal sphincter relaxes

Peristaltic activity, controlled by a brainstem centre, is mediated by autonomic nerves

The lower oesophageal sphincter relaxes. The food enters the stomach

Upper sphincter (cricopharyngeus muscle)

Lower oesophageal sphincter

Normal high-resolution manometry

Endoscopic view

Fig. 21.1 The oesophagus: anatomy and function. The swallowing wave.

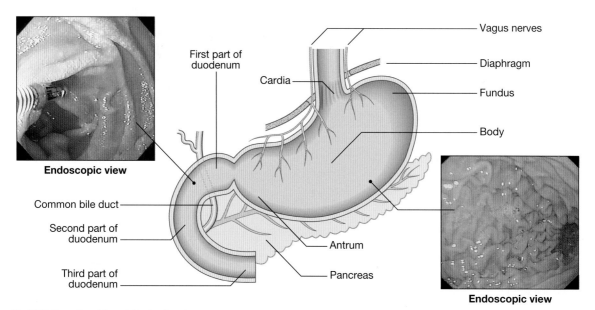

Endoscopic view

First part of duodenum

Cardia

Common bile duct

Second part of duodenum

Third part of duodenum

Vagus nerves

Diaphragm

Fundus

Body

Antrum

Pancreas

Endoscopic view

Fig. 21.2 Normal gastric and duodenal anatomy.

Gastric secretion

Gastrin, histamine and acetylcholine are the key stimulants of acid secretion. Hydrogen and chloride ions are secreted from the apical membrane of gastric parietal cells into the lumen of the stomach by a hydrogen–potassium adenosine triphosphatase (ATPase) ('proton pump') (Fig. 21.3). The hydrochloric acid sterilises the upper gastrointestinal tract and converts pepsinogen, which is secreted by chief cells, to pepsin. The glycoprotein intrinsic factor, secreted in parallel with acid, is necessary for vitamin B_{12} absorption.

Gastrin, somatostatin and ghrelin

The hormone gastrin is produced by G cells in the antrum, whereas somatostatin is secreted from D cells throughout the stomach. Gastrin stimulates acid secretion and mucosal growth while somatostatin suppresses it. Ghrelin, secreted from oxyntic glands, stimulates acid secretion but also appetite and gastric emptying.

Protective factors

Bicarbonate ions, stimulated by prostaglandins, mucins and trefoil factor family (TFF) peptides, together protect the gastro-duodenal mucosa from the ulcerative properties of acid and pepsin.

Small intestine

The small bowel extends from the ligament of Treitz to the ileocaecal valve (Fig. 21.4). During fasting, a wave of peristaltic activity passes down the small bowel every 1–2 hours. Entry of food into the gastrointestinal tract stimulates small bowel peristaltic activity. Functions of the small intestine are:

- digestion (mechanical, enzymatic and peristaltic)
- absorption – the products of digestion, water, electrolytes and vitamins
- protection against ingested toxins
- immune regulation.

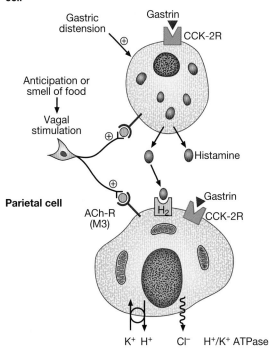

Fig. 21.3 **Control of acid secretion.** Gastrin released from antral G cells in response to food (protein) binds to cholecystokinin receptors (CCK-2R) on the surface of enterochromaffin-like (ECL) cells, which in turn release histamine. The histamine binds to H_2 receptors on parietal cells and this leads to secretion of hydrogen ions in exchange for potassium ions at the apical membrane. Parietal cells also express CCK-2R and it is thought that activation of these receptors by gastrin is involved in regulatory proliferation of parietal cells. Cholinergic (vagal) activity and gastric distension also stimulate acid secretion; somatostatin, vasoactive intestinal polypeptide (VIP) and gastric inhibitory polypeptide (GIP) may inhibit it. (ACh-R = acetylcholine receptor; ATPase = adenosine triphosphatase)

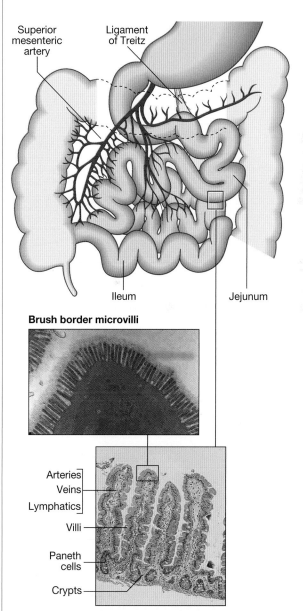

Fig. 21.4 **Small intestine: anatomy.** Epithelial cells are formed in crypts and differentiate as they migrate to the tip of the villi to form enterocytes (absorptive cells) and goblet cells.

Digestion and absorption

Fat

Dietary lipids comprise long-chain triglycerides, cholesterol esters and lecithin. Lipids are insoluble in water and undergo lipolysis and incorporation into mixed micelles before they can be absorbed into enterocytes along with the fat-soluble vitamins A, D, E and K. The lipids are processed within enterocytes and pass via lymphatics into the systemic circulation. Fat absorption and digestion can be considered as a stepwise process, as outlined in Figure 21.5.

Carbohydrates

Starch is hydrolysed by salivary and pancreatic amylases to:

- α-limit dextrins containing 4–8 glucose molecules
- the disaccharide maltose
- the trisaccharide maltotriose.

Disaccharides are digested by enzymes fixed to the microvillous membrane to form the monosaccharides glucose, galactose and fructose. Glucose and galactose enter the cell by an energy-requiring process involving a carrier protein, and fructose enters by simple diffusion.

Protein

The steps involved in protein digestion are shown in Figure 21.6. Intragastric digestion by pepsin is quantitatively modest but important because the resulting polypeptides and amino acids stimulate cholecystokinin (CCK) release from the mucosa of the proximal jejunum, which in turn stimulates release of pancreatic proteases, including trypsinogen, chymotrypsinogen, pro-elastases and procarboxypeptidases, from the pancreas. On exposure to brush border enterokinase, inert trypsinogen is converted to the active proteolytic enzyme trypsin, which activates the other pancreatic pro-enzymes. Trypsin digests proteins to produce oligopeptides, peptides and amino acids. Oligopeptides are further hydrolysed by brush border enzymes to yield dipeptides, tripeptides and amino acids. These small peptides and the amino acids are actively transported into the enterocytes, where intracellular peptidases further digest peptides to amino acids. Amino acids are then actively transported across the basal cell membrane of the enterocyte into the portal circulation and the liver.

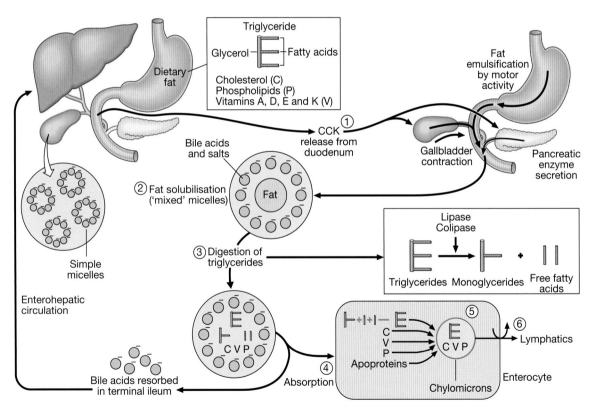

Fig. 21.5 Fat digestion. *Step 1: Luminal phase.* Fatty acids stimulate cholecystokinin (CCK) release from the duodenum and upper jejunum. The CCK stimulates release of amylase, lipase, colipase and proteases from the pancreas, causes gallbladder contraction and relaxes the sphincter of Oddi, allowing bile to flow into the intestine. *Step 2: Fat solubilisation.* Bile acids and salts combine with dietary fat to form mixed micelles, which also contain cholesterol and fat-soluble vitamins. *Step 3: Digestion.* Pancreatic lipase, in the presence of its co-factor, colipase, cleaves long-chain triglycerides, yielding fatty acids and monoglycerides. *Step 4: Absorption.* Mixed micelles diffuse to the brush border of the enterocytes. Within the brush border, long-chain fatty acids bind to proteins, which transport the fatty acids into the cell, whereas cholesterol, short-chain fatty acids, phospholipids and fat-soluble vitamins enter the cell directly. The bile salts remain in the small intestinal lumen and are actively transported from the terminal ileum into the portal circulation and returned to the liver (the enterohepatic circulation). *Step 5: Re-esterification.* Within the enterocyte, fatty acids are re-esterified to form triglycerides. Triglycerides combine with cholesterol ester, fat-soluble vitamins, phospholipids and apoproteins to form chylomicrons. *Step 6: Transport.* Chylomicrons leave the enterocytes by exocytosis, enter mesenteric lymphatics, pass into the thoracic duct and eventually reach the systemic circulation.

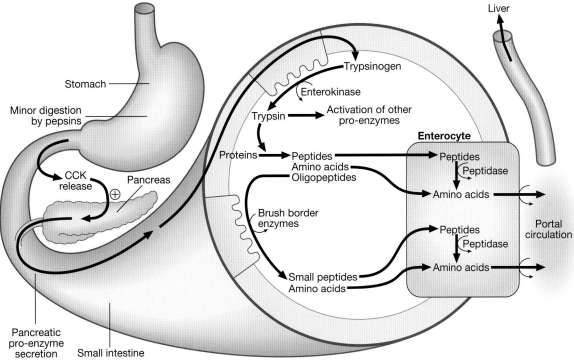

Fig. 21.6 Protein digestion. (CCK = cholecystokinin)

Water and electrolytes

Absorption and secretion of electrolytes and water occur throughout the intestine. Electrolytes and water are transported by two pathways:

- *the paracellular route*, in which passive flow through tight junctions between cells is a consequence of osmotic, electrical or hydrostatic gradients
- *the transcellular route* across apical and basolateral membranes by energy-requiring specific active transport carriers (pumps).

In healthy individuals, fluid balance is tightly controlled, such that only 100 mL of the 8 litres of fluid entering the gastrointestinal tract daily is excreted in stools (Fig. 21.7).

Vitamins and trace elements

Water-soluble vitamins are absorbed throughout the intestine. The absorption of folic acid, vitamin B_{12}, calcium and iron is described on page 943.

Protective function of the small intestine

Physical defence mechanisms

There are several levels of defence in the small bowel (Fig. 21.8). Firstly, the gut lumen contains host bacteria (see below), mucins and secreted antibacterial products, including defensins and immunoglobulins that help combat pathogenic infections. Secondly, epithelial cells have relatively impermeable brush border membranes and passage between cells is prevented by tight and adherens junctions. These cells can react to foreign peptides ('innate immunity') using pattern recognition receptors found on cell surfaces (Toll receptors) or intracellularly. Lastly, in the subepithelial layer, immune responses occur under control of the adaptive immune system in response to pathogenic compounds.

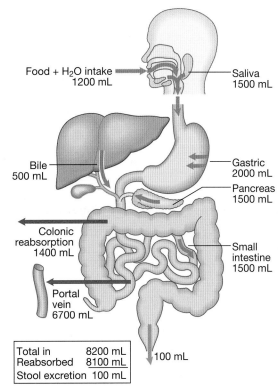

Food + H₂O intake 1200 mL
Saliva 1500 mL
Bile 500 mL
Gastric 2000 mL
Pancreas 1500 mL
Colonic reabsorption 1400 mL
Small intestine 1500 mL
Portal vein 6700 mL
100 mL

Total in	8200 mL
Reabsorbed	8100 mL
Stool excretion	100 mL

Fig. 21.7 Fluid homeostasis in the gastrointestinal tract.

Immunological defence mechanisms

Gastrointestinal mucosa-associated lymphoid tissue (MALT) constitutes 25% of the total lymphatic tissue of the body and is at the heart of adaptive immunity. Within Peyer's patches,

21

Fig. 21.8 Intestinal defence mechanisms. See text for details.

① Lumen
② Epithelium
③ Subepithelial layer

i	21.1 Pancreatic enzymes		
Enzyme	**Substrate**	**Product**
Amylase	Starch and glycogen	Limit dextrans Maltose Maltriose
Lipase **Colipase**	Triglycerides	Monoglycerides and free fatty acids
Proteolytic enzymes Trypsinogen Chymotrypsinogen Pro-elastase Pro-carboxypeptidases	Proteins and polypeptides	Short polypeptides

B lymphocytes differentiate to plasma cells following exposure to antigens and these migrate to mesenteric lymph nodes to enter the blood stream via the thoracic duct. The plasma cells return to the lamina propria of the gut through the circulation and release immunoglobulin A (IgA), which is transported into the lumen of the intestine. Intestinal T lymphocytes help localise plasma cells to the site of antigen exposure, as well as producing inflammatory mediators. Macrophages in the gut phagocytose foreign materials and secrete a range of cytokines, which mediate inflammation. Similarly, activation of mast-cell surface IgE receptors leads to degranulation and release of other molecules involved in inflammation.

Pancreas

The exocrine pancreas (Box 21.1) is necessary for the digestion of fat, protein and carbohydrate. Pro-enzymes are secreted from pancreatic acinar cells in response to circulating gastrointestinal hormones (Fig. 21.9) and are activated by trypsin. Bicarbonate-rich fluid is secreted from ductular cells to produce an optimum alkaline pH for enzyme activity. The endocrine pancreas is discussed in Chapters 18 and 20.

Colon

The colon (Fig. 21.10) absorbs water and electrolytes. It also acts as a storage organ and has contractile activity. Two types of contraction occur. The first of these is segmentation (ring contraction), which leads to mixing but not propulsion; this promotes absorption of water and electrolytes. Propulsive (peristaltic contraction) waves occur several times a day and propel faeces to the rectum. All activity is stimulated after meals through the gastrocolic reflex in response to release of hormones such as 5-hydroxytryptamine (5-HT, serotonin), motilin and CCK. Faecal continence depends on maintenance of the anorectal angle and tonic contraction of the external anal sphincters. On defecation, there is relaxation of the anorectal muscles, increased intra-abdominal pressure from the Valsalva manœuvre and contraction of abdominal muscles, and relaxation of the anal sphincters.

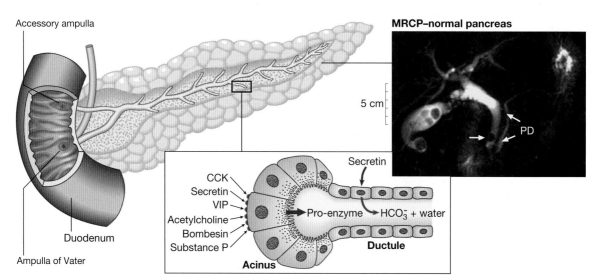

Fig. 21.9 Pancreatic structure and function. Ductular cells secrete alkaline fluid in response to secretin. Acinar cells secrete digestive enzymes from zymogen granules in response to a range of secretagogues. The photograph shows a normal pancreatic duct (PD) and side branches, as defined at magnetic resonance cholangiopancreatography (MRCP). Note the incidental calculi in the gallbladder and common bile duct (arrow). (CCK = cholecystokinin; VIP = vasoactive intestinal polypeptide)

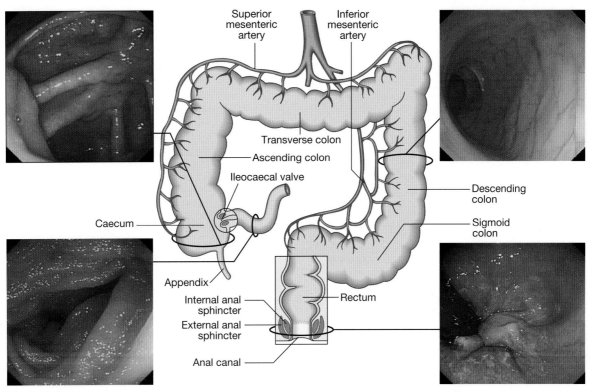

Fig. 21.10 The normal colon, rectum and anal canal.

Intestinal microbiota

The human microbiota comprises 10^{14} microbial residents in the human body, vastly outnumbering host cells. Indeed, the number of bacterial genes in the microbiota genome exceeds that of the host by 100-fold or more. This represents a vast ecosystem that is central to health and homeostasis, and is disordered in disease. In terms of nomenclature, 'microbiota' refers to the microorganisms that live in a particular niche, while 'microbiome' refers to the collective genomes of these microbiota. The metabolic capacity of the gut microbiota is equivalent to that of the liver. The Human Microbiome Project revealed that there are unique communities at different body sites and in the gut particular phyla predominate: namely, Firmicutes, Bacteriodetes, Proteobacteria and Actinobacteria. There is a degree of heritability of this microbiota, as shown in twin studies, but it is clear that there are many environmental factors that can impact, including diet, drugs, physical activity, smoking, stress and natural ageing. Generally, we acquire our adult intestinal microbiota by the age of 2 years. A dysbiosis or imbalance between the different components of the intestinal microbiota has been associated with diseases of the gastrointestinal tract, such as inflammatory bowel disease and colorectal cancer; liver disease, including hepatocellular carcinoma; and pathologies outside the gastrointestinal tract, such as diabetes, obesity, cardiovascular disorders, cerebrovascular disorders, asthma and psychiatric disorders, such as depression. Many challenges remain in understanding the intestinal microbiota and how it impacts on health and disease. It is not clear what constitutes a 'healthy' phenotype; there are questions over best sampling practice from either the faecal stream or the mucosa; and there are technical considerations to ensure consistency in methodologies and data analysis.

Control of gastrointestinal function

Secretion, absorption, motor activity, growth and differentiation of the gut are all modulated by a combination of neuronal and hormonal factors.

The nervous system and gastrointestinal function

The central nervous system (CNS), the autonomic system (ANS) and the enteric nervous system (ENS) interact to regulate gut function. The ANS comprises:

- *parasympathetic pathways* (vagal and sacral efferent), which are cholinergic, and increase smooth muscle tone and promote sphincter relaxation
- *sympathetic pathways*, which release noradrenaline (norepinephrine), reduce smooth muscle tone and stimulate sphincter contraction.

The enteric nervous system

In conjunction with the ANS, the ENS senses gut contents and conditions, and regulates motility, fluid exchange, secretion, blood flow and other key gut functions. It comprises two major networks intrinsic to the gut wall. The myenteric (Auerbach's) plexus in the smooth muscle layer regulates motor control; and the submucosal (Meissner's) plexus exerts secretory control over the epithelium, entero-endocrine cells and submucosal vessels. Together, these plexuses form a two-layered neuronal mesh along the length of

i	21.2 Gut hormones and peptides		
Hormone	**Origin**	**Stimulus**	**Action**
Gastrin	Stomach (G cell)	Products of protein digestion Suppressed by acid and somatostatin	Stimulates gastric acid secretion Stimulates growth of gastrointestinal mucosa
Somatostatin	Throughout gastrointestinal tract (D cell)	Fat ingestion	Inhibits gastrin and insulin secretion Decreases acid secretion Decreases absorption Inhibits pancreatic secretion
Cholecystokinin (CCK)	Duodenum and jejunum (I cells); also ileal and colonic nerve endings	Products of protein digestion Fat and fatty acids Suppressed by trypsin	Stimulates pancreatic enzyme secretion Stimulates gallbladder contraction Relaxes sphincter of Oddi Modulates satiety Decreases gastric acid secretion Reduces gastric emptying Regulates pancreatic growth
Secretin	Duodenum and jejunum (S cells)	Duodenal acid Fatty acids	Stimulates pancreatic fluid and bicarbonate secretion Decreases acid secretion Reduces gastric emptying
Motilin	Duodenum, small intestine and colon (Mo cells)	Fasting Dietary fat	Regulates peristaltic activity, including migrating motor complexes (MMCs)
Gastric inhibitory polypeptide (GIP)	Duodenum (K cells) and jejunum	Glucose and fat	Stimulates insulin release (also known as glucose-dependent insulinotrophic polypeptide) Inhibits acid secretion Enhances satiety
Glucagon-like peptide-1 (GLP-1)	Ileum and colon (L cells)	Carbohydrates, protein and fat	Stimulates insulin release Inhibits acid secretion and gastric emptying Enhances satiety
Vasoactive intestinal peptide (VIP)	Nerve fibres throughout gastrointestinal tract	Unknown	Has vasodilator action Relaxes smooth muscle Stimulates water and electrolyte secretion
Ghrelin	Stomach	Fasting Inhibited by eating	Stimulates appetite, acid secretion and gastric emptying
Peptide YY	Ileum and colon	Feeding	Modulates satiety

the gut. Although connected centrally via the ANS, the ENS can function autonomously using a variety of transmitters, including acetylcholine, noradrenaline (norepinephrine), 5-HT, nitric oxide, substance P and calcitonin gene-related peptide (CGRP). There are local reflex loops within the ENS but also loops involving the coeliac and mesenteric ganglia and the paravertebral ganglia. The parasympathetic system generally stimulates motility and secretion, while the sympathetic system generally acts in an inhibitory manner.

Peristalsis

Peristalsis is a reflex triggered by gut wall distension, which consists of a wave of circular muscle contraction to propel contents from the oesophagus to the rectum. It can be influenced by innervation but functions independently. It results from a basic electrical rhythm originating from the interstitial cells of Cajal in the circular layer of intestinal smooth muscle. These are stellate cells of mesenchymal origin with smooth muscle features, which act as the 'pacemaker' of the gut.

Migrating motor complexes

Migrating motor complexes (MMCs) are waves of contraction spreading from the stomach to the ileum, occurring at a frequency of about 5 per minute every 90 minutes or so, between meals and during fasting. They may serve to sweep intestinal contents distally in preparation for the next meal and are inhibited by eating.

Gut hormones

The origin, action and control of the major gut hormones, peptides and non-peptide signalling transmitters are summarised in Box 21.2.

Investigation of gastrointestinal disease

A wide range of tests is available for the investigation of patients with gastrointestinal symptoms. These can be classified broadly into tests of structure, tests for infection and tests of function.

Imaging

Plain X-rays

Plain X-rays of the abdomen are useful in the diagnosis of intestinal obstruction or paralytic ileus, where dilated loops of bowel and (in the erect position) fluid levels may be seen (Fig. 21.11). Calcified lymph nodes, gallstones and renal stones can also be detected. Chest X-ray (performed with the patient in erect position) is useful in the diagnosis of suspected perforation, as it shows subdiaphragmatic free air (Fig. 21.11).

Fig. 21.11 Examples of plain X-rays. **A** Abdominal X-ray showing dilatation of loops of small bowel (arrows), which are indicative of obstruction (in this case due to adhesions from previous surgery). **B** Chest X-ray showing free air under both hemi-diaphragms (arrows), which is indicative of acute perforation of an abdominal viscus.

i	**21.3 Contrast radiology in the investigation of gastrointestinal disease**		
	Barium swallow/meal	**Barium follow-through**	**Barium enema**
Indications and major uses	Motility disorders (achalasia and gastroparesis) Perforation or fistula (non-ionic contrast)	Diarrhoea and abdominal pain of small bowel origin Possible obstruction by strictures Suspected malabsorption Assessment of Crohn's disease	Altered bowel habit Evaluation of strictures or diverticular disease Megacolon Chronic constipation
Limitations	Risk of aspiration Poor mucosal detail Low sensitivity for early cancer Inability to biopsy	Time-consuming nature Radiation exposure Relative insensitivity	Difficulty in frail or incontinent patients Sigmoidoscopy needed to see rectum Low sensitivity for lesions <1 cm

Fig. 21.12 Examples of contrast radiology. **A** Barium swallow showing a large pharyngeal pouch (P) with retained contrast creating an air–fluid level. **B** Barium follow-through. There are multiple diverticula (arrows) in this patient with jejunal diverticulosis. **C** Barium enema showing severe diverticular disease. There is tortuosity and narrowing of the sigmoid colon with multiple diverticula (arrows).

Contrast studies

X-rays with contrast medium are usually performed to assess not only anatomical abnormalities but also motility. Barium sulphate provides good mucosal coating and excellent opacification but can precipitate impaction proximal to an obstructive lesion. Water-soluble contrast is used to opacify bowel prior to abdominal computed tomography and in cases of suspected perforation.

The double contrast technique improves mucosal visualisation by using gas to distend the barium-coated intestinal surface. Contrast studies are useful for detecting filling defects, such as tumours, strictures, ulcers and motility disorders, but are inferior to endoscopic procedures and more sophisticated cross-sectional imaging techniques, such as computed tomography and magnetic resonance imaging. The major uses and limitations of various contrast studies are shown in Box 21.3 and Figure 21.12.

21

Fig. 21.13 Examples of ultrasound, CT and MRI. [A] Ultrasound showing large gallstone (arrow) with acoustic shadowing. [B] Multidetector coronal CT showing large solid and cystic malignant tumour in the pancreatic tail (arrow). (PV = portal vein; L = liver) [C] Pelvic MRI showing large pelvic abscess (arrow) posterior to the rectum in a patient with Crohn's disease. [D] Fused CT-PET image showing two liver metastases (arrows).

Ultrasound, computed tomography and magnetic resonance imaging

Ultrasound, computed tomography (CT) and magnetic resonance imaging (MRI) are key tests in the evaluation of intra-abdominal disease. They are non-invasive and offer detailed images of the abdominal contents. Fluorodeoxyglucose–positron emission tomography (FDG-PET) is increasingly used in the staging of malignancies and images may be fused with CT to enhance localisation. Their main applications are summarised in Box 21.4 and Figure 21.13.

Endoscopy

Videoendoscopes provide high-definition imaging and accessories can be passed down the endoscope to allow both diagnostic and therapeutic procedures, some of which are illustrated in Figure 21.14. Endoscopes with magnifying lenses allow almost microscopic detail to be observed, and imaging modalities, such as confocal endomicroscopy, autofluorescence and 'narrow-band imaging', are increasingly used to detect subtle abnormalities not visible by standard 'white light' endoscopy.

Upper gastrointestinal endoscopy

This is performed under light intravenous benzodiazepine sedation, or using only local anaesthetic throat spray after the patient has fasted for at least 4 hours. With the patient in the left lateral position, the entire oesophagus (excluding pharynx), stomach and first two parts of duodenum can be seen.

Indications, contraindications and complications are given in Box 21.5.

Endoscopic ultrasound

Endoscopic ultrasound (EUS) combines endoscopy with intraluminal ultrasonography using a high-frequency transducer to produce high-resolution ultrasound images. This allows visualisation through the wall of the gastrointestinal tract and into surrounding tissues, e.g. the pancreas or lymph nodes. It can therefore be used to perform fine needle aspiration or biopsy of mass lesions. EUS is helpful in the diagnosis of pancreatic tumours, chronic pancreatitis, pancreatic cysts, cholangiocarcinoma, common bile duct stones, ampullary lesions and submucosal tumours. It also plays an important role in the staging of certain cancers, e.g. those of oesophagus and pancreas. EUS can also be therapeutic, as in drainage of pancreatic fluid collections and coeliac plexus block for pain management. Possible complications of EUS include bleeding, infection, cardiopulmonary events and perforation.

Capsule endoscopy

Capsule endoscopy (Fig. 21.15) uses a capsule containing an imaging device, battery, transmitter and antenna; as it traverses the small intestine, it transmits images to a battery-powered recorder worn on a belt round the patient's waist. After approximately 8 hours, the capsule is excreted. Images from the capsule are analysed as a video sequence and it is usually possible to localise the segment of small bowel in which lesions are seen. Abnormalities detected usually require enteroscopy

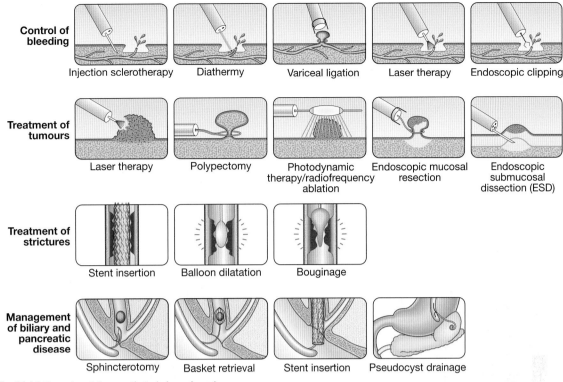

Fig. 21.14 Examples of therapeutic techniques in endoscopy.

i 21.5 Upper gastrointestinal endoscopy

Indications

- Dyspepsia in patients >55 years of age or with alarm symptoms
- Atypical chest pain
- Dysphagia
- Vomiting
- Weight loss
- Acute or chronic gastrointestinal bleeding
- Screening for oesophageal varices in chronic liver disease
- Abnormal CT scan or barium meal
- Duodenal biopsies in the investigation of malabsorption and confirmation of a diagnosis of coeliac disease prior to commencement of gluten-free diet
- Therapy, including treatment of bleeding lesions, banding/injection of varices, dilatation of strictures, insertion of stents, placement of percutaneous gastrostomies, ablation of Barrett's oesophagus and resection of high-grade dysplastic lesions and early neoplasia in the upper gastrointestinal tract

Contraindications

- Severe shock
- Recent myocardial infarction, unstable angina, cardiac arrhythmia*
- Severe respiratory disease*
- Atlantoaxial subluxation*
- Possible visceral perforation

Complications

- Cardiorespiratory depression due to sedation
- Aspiration pneumonia
- Perforation

*These are 'relative' contraindications; in experienced hands, endoscopy can be safely performed.

Fig. 21.15 Wireless capsule endoscopy. A Examples of capsules. B Capsule endoscopy image of bleeding jejunal vascular malformation. *A, Courtesy of Given Imaging.*

21.6 Wireless capsule endoscopy

Indications

- Obscure gastrointestinal bleeding
- Small bowel Crohn's disease
- Assessment of coeliac disease and its complications
- Screening and surveillance in familial polyposis syndromes

Contraindications

- Known or suspected small bowel stricture (risk of capsule retention)
- Caution in people with pacemakers or implantable defibrillators

Complications

- Capsule retention (<1%)

 21.7 Double balloon enteroscopy

Indications

Diagnostic
- Obscure gastrointestinal bleeding
- Malabsorption or unexplained diarrhoea
- Suspicious radiological findings
- Suspected small bowel tumour
- Surveillance of polyposis syndromes

Therapeutic
- Coagulation/diathermy of bleeding lesions
- Jejunostomy placement

Contraindications

- As for upper gastrointestinal endoscopy

Complications

- As for upper gastrointestinal endoscopy
- Post-procedure abdominal pain (≤20%)
- Pancreatitis (1–3%)
- Perforation (especially after resection of large polyps)

 21.8 Colonoscopy

Indications*

- Suspected inflammatory bowel disease
- Chronic diarrhoea
- Altered bowel habit
- Rectal bleeding or iron deficiency anaemia
- Assessment of abnormal CT colonogram or barium enema
- Colorectal cancer screening
- Colorectal adenoma and carcinoma follow-up
- Therapeutic procedures, including endoscopic resection, dilatation of strictures, laser, stent insertion and argon plasma coagulation

Contraindications

- Acute severe ulcerative colitis (unprepared flexible sigmoidoscopy is preferred)
- As for upper gastrointestinal endoscopy

Complications

- Cardiorespiratory depression due to sedation
- Perforation
- Bleeding following polypectomy

*Colonoscopy is not useful in the investigation of constipation.

 21.9 Endoscopy in old age

- **Tolerance**: endoscopic procedures are generally well tolerated, even in very old people.
- **Side-effects from sedation**: older people are more sensitive, and respiratory depression, hypotension and prolonged recovery times are more common.
- **Bowel preparation for colonoscopy**: can be difficult in frail, immobile people. Sodium phosphate-based preparations can cause dehydration or hypotension and should be avoided in those with underlying cardiac or renal failure. Minimal-preparation CT colonograms provide an excellent alternative in these individuals.
- **Antiperistaltic agents**: hyoscine should be avoided in those with glaucoma and can also cause tachyarrhythmias. Glucagon is preferred if an antiperistaltic agent is needed.

for confirmation and therapy. Indications, contraindications and complications are listed in Box 21.6.

Double balloon enteroscopy

While endoscopy can reach the proximal small intestine in most patients, a technique called double balloon enteroscopy is also available, which uses a long endoscope with a flexible overtube. Sequential and repeated inflation and deflation of balloons on the tip of the overtube and enteroscope allow the operator to push and pull along the entire length of the small intestine to the terminal ileum, in order to diagnose or treat small bowel lesions detected by capsule endoscopy or other imaging modalities. Indications, contraindications and complications are listed in Box 21.7.

Sigmoidoscopy and colonoscopy

Sigmoidoscopy can be carried out either in the outpatient clinic using a 20 cm rigid plastic sigmoidoscope or in the endoscopy suite using a 60 cm flexible colonoscope following bowel preparation. When sigmoidoscopy is combined with proctoscopy, accurate detection of haemorrhoids, ulcerative colitis and distal colorectal neoplasia is possible. After full bowel cleansing, it is possible to examine the entire colon and the terminal ileum using a longer colonoscope. Indications, contraindications and complications of colonoscopy are listed in Box 21.8.

Magnetic resonance cholangiopancreatography

Magnetic resonance cholangiopancreatography (MRCP) has largely replaced endoscopic retrograde cholangiopancreatography (ERCP) in the evaluation of obstructive jaundice since it produces comparable images of the biliary tree and pancreas, providing information that complements that obtained from CT and endoscopic ultrasound examination (EUS).

Endoscopic retrograde cholangiopancreatography

Using a side-viewing duodenoscope, it is possible to cannulate the main pancreatic duct and common bile duct. Nowadays, ERCP is used mainly in the treatment of a range of biliary and pancreatic diseases that have been identified by other imaging techniques such as MRCP, EUS and CT. Indications for and risks of ERCP are listed in Box 21.10.

Histology

Biopsy material obtained endoscopically or percutaneously can provide useful information (Box 21.11).

21.10 Endoscopic retrograde cholangiopancreatography

Indications

Diagnostic
- Biliary or pancreatic disease where other imaging is equivocal or contraindicated
- Ampullary biopsy or biliary cytology

Therapeutic
- Biliary disease:
  Removal of common bile duct calculi*
  Palliation of malignant biliary obstruction
  Management of biliary leaks/damage complicating surgery
  Dilatation of benign strictures
  Primary sclerosing cholangitis
- Pancreatic disease:
  Drainage of pancreatic pseudocysts and fistulae
  Removal of pancreatic calculi (selected cases)

Contraindications

- Severe cardiopulmonary comorbidity
- Coagulopathy

Complications

- Occur in 5–10% with a 30-day mortality of 0.5–1%

General
- As for upper endoscopy

Specific
- Biliary disease:
  Bleeding following sphincterotomy
  Cholangitis (if biliary obstruction is not relieved by ERCP)
  Gallstone impaction
- Pancreatic disease:
  Acute pancreatitis
  Infection of pseudocyst

*Laparoscopic surgery is preferred in fit individuals who also require cholecystectomy.

21.11 Reasons for biopsy or cytological examination

- Suspected malignant lesions
- Assessment of mucosal abnormalities
- Diagnosis of infection (*Candida*, *Helicobacter pylori*, *Giardia lamblia*)
- Analysis of genetic mutations

Tests of infection

Bacterial cultures

Stool cultures are essential in the investigation of diarrhoea, especially when it is acute or bloody, in order to identify pathogenic organisms (Ch. 11).

Serology

Detection of antibodies plays a limited role in the diagnosis of gastrointestinal infection caused by organisms such as *Helicobacter pylori*, *Salmonella* species and *Entamoeba histolytica*.

Breath tests

Non-invasive breath tests for *H. pylori* infection are discussed on page 800 and breath tests for suspected small intestinal bacterial overgrowth on page 808.

Tests of function

A number of dynamic tests can be used to investigate aspects of gut function, including digestion, absorption, inflammation and epithelial permeability. Some of the more common ones are listed in Box 21.12. In the assessment of suspected malabsorption, blood tests (full blood count, erythrocyte sedimentation rate (ESR), and measurement of C-reactive protein (CRP), folate, vitamin B_{12},

21.12 Tests of gastrointestinal function

Process	Test	Principle	Comments
Absorption			
Lactose	Lactose H_2 breath test	Measurement of breath H_2 content after 50 g oral lactose. Undigested sugar is metabolised by colonic bacteria in hypolactasia and expired hydrogen is measured	Non-invasive and accurate. May provoke pain and diarrhoea in sufferers
Bile acids	^{75}SeHCAT test	Isotopic quantification of 7-day whole-body retention of oral dose ^{75}Se-labelled homocholyltaurine (>15% = normal, 5–15% = borderline, <5% = abnormal)	Accurate and specific but requires two visits and involves radiation. Results can be equivocal. Serum 7α-hydroxycholestenone is almost as sensitive and specific
	Serum 7α-hydroxycholestenone	Intermediate metabolite of the bile acid synthetic pathway. Serum levels indicate activity of the pathway and are elevated in bile acid diarrhoea	Simple test to perform and only marginally less sensitive and specific than ^{75}SeHCAT test
Pancreatic exocrine function	Pancreolauryl test	Pancreatic esterases cleave fluorescein dilaurate after oral ingestion. Fluorescein is absorbed and quantified in urine	Accurate and avoids duodenal intubation Takes 2 days. Accurate urine collection essential. Rarely performed
	Faecal elastase	Immunoassay of pancreatic enzymes on stool sample	Simple, quick and avoids urine collection. Does not detect mild disease
Mucosal inflammation/ permeability	Faecal calprotectin	A protein secreted non-specifically by neutrophils into the colon in response to inflammation or neoplasia	Useful screening test for gastrointestinal inflammation and for monitoring patients with Crohn's disease and ulcerative colitis. Poor sensitivity for cancer

(^{75}SeHCAT = ^{75}Se-homocholic acid taurine)

21

iron status, albumin, calcium and phosphate) are essential, and endoscopy is undertaken to obtain mucosal biopsies. Faecal calprotectin is very sensitive at detecting mucosal inflammation.

Oesophageal motility

A barium swallow can give useful information about oesophageal motility. Videofluoroscopy, with joint assessment by a speech and language therapist and a radiologist, may be necessary in difficult cases. Oesophageal manometry (see Fig. 21.1), often in conjunction with 24-hour pH measurements, is of value in diagnosing cases of refractory gastro-oesophageal reflux, achalasia and non-cardiac chest pain. Oesophageal impedance testing is useful for detecting non-acid or gas reflux events, especially in patients with atypical symptoms or those who respond poorly to acid suppression.

Gastric emptying

This involves administering a test meal containing solids and liquids labelled with different radioisotopes and measuring the amount retained in the stomach afterwards (Box 21.13). It is useful in the investigation of suspected delayed gastric emptying (gastroparesis) when other studies are normal.

Colonic and anorectal motility

A plain abdominal X-ray taken on day 5 after ingestion of different-shaped inert plastic pellets on days 1–3 gives an estimate of whole-gut transit time. The test is useful in the evaluation of chronic constipation, when the position of any retained pellets can be observed, and helps to differentiate cases of slow transit from those due to obstructed defecation. The mechanism of defecation and anorectal function can be assessed by anorectal manometry, electrophysiological tests and defecating proctography.

Radioisotope tests

Many different radioisotope tests are used (Box 21.13). In some, structural information is obtained, such as the localisation of a Meckel's diverticulum. Others provide functional information, such as the rate of gastric emptying or ability to reabsorb bile acids. Yet others are tests of infection and rely on the presence of bacteria to hydrolyse a radio-labelled test substance followed by detection of the radioisotope in expired air, such as the urea breath test for *H. pylori*.

Gut hormone testing

Excess gut hormone secretion by some gastrointestinal and pancreatic neuro-endocrine tumours can be assessed by measuring levels in blood. Commonly measured hormones include gastrin, somatostatin, vasoactive intestinal polypeptide (VIP) and pancreatic polypeptide.

Presenting problems in gastrointestinal disease

Dysphagia

Dysphagia is defined as difficulty in swallowing. It may coexist with heartburn or vomiting but should be distinguished from both globus sensation (in which anxious people feel a lump in the throat without organic cause) and odynophagia (pain during swallowing, usually from gastro-oesophageal reflux or candidiasis).

Dysphagia can occur due to problems in the oropharynx or oesophagus (Fig. 21.16). Oropharyngeal disorders affect the initiation of swallowing at the pharynx and upper oesophageal sphincter. The patient has difficulty initiating swallowing and complains of choking, nasal regurgitation or tracheal aspiration. Drooling, dysarthria, hoarseness and cranial nerve or other neurological signs may be present. Oesophageal disorders cause dysphagia by obstructing the lumen or by affecting motility. Patients with oesophageal disease complain of food 'sticking' after swallowing, although the level at which this is felt correlates poorly with the true site of obstruction. Swallowing of liquids is normal until strictures become extreme.

Investigations

Dysphagia should always be investigated urgently. Endoscopy is the investigation of choice because it allows biopsy and dilatation of strictures. Even if the appearances are normal, biopsies should be taken to look for eosinophilic oesophagitis. If no abnormality is found, then barium swallow with videofluoroscopic swallowing assessment is indicated to detect major motility disorders. In some cases, oesophageal manometry is required. High-resolution manometry allows accurate classification of abnormalities. Figure 21.16 summarises a diagnostic approach to dysphagia and lists the major causes.

i	21.13 Commonly used radioisotope tests in gastroenterology	
Test	**Isotope**	**Major uses and principle of test**
Gastric emptying study	^{99m}Tc-sulphur ^{111}In-DTPA	Assessment of gastric emptying, particularly for possible gastroparesis
Urea breath test	^{13}C-urea	Non-invasive diagnosis of *Helicobacter pylori*. Bacterial urease enzyme splits urea to ammonia and CO_2, which is detected in expired air
Meckel's scan	^{99m}Tc-pertechnate	Diagnosis of Meckel's diverticulum in cases of obscure gastrointestinal bleeding. Isotope is injected intravenously and localises in ectopic parietal mucosa within diverticulum
Somatostatin receptor scintigraphy (SRS)	^{111}In-DTPA-octreotide	Labelled somatostatin analogue binds to cell surface somatostatin receptors on pancreatic neuro-endocrine tumours
Positron emission tomography (PET)	^{18}F-fluorodeoxyglucose (FDG)	Staging high-grade cancers
	^{68}Gallium-labelled somatostatin analogue	More sensitive and specific than SRS for staging neuro-endocrine tumours

Fig. 21.16 Investigation of dysphagia.

Dyspepsia

Dyspepsia describes symptoms such as discomfort, bloating and nausea, which are thought to originate from the upper gastrointestinal tract. There are many causes (Box 21.14), including some arising outside the digestive system. Heartburn and other 'reflux' symptoms are separate entities and are considered elsewhere. Although symptoms often correlate poorly with the underlying diagnosis, a careful history is important to detect

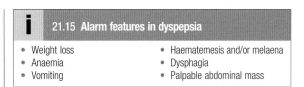

i 21.15 **Alarm features in dyspepsia**	
• Weight loss	• Haematemesis and/or melaena
• Anaemia	• Dysphagia
• Vomiting	• Palpable abdominal mass

'alarm' features requiring urgent investigation (Box 21.15) and to detect atypical symptoms that might be due to problems outside the gastrointestinal tract.

Dyspepsia affects up to 80% of the population at some time in life and most patients have no serious underlying disease. People who present with new dyspepsia at an age of more than 55 years and younger patients unresponsive to empirical treatment require investigation to exclude serious disease. An algorithm for the investigation of dyspepsia is outlined in Figure 21.17.

Heartburn and regurgitation

Heartburn describes retrosternal, burning discomfort, often rising up into the chest and sometimes accompanied by regurgitation of acidic or bitter fluid into the throat. These symptoms often occur after meals, on lying down or with bending, straining or heavy lifting. They are classical symptoms of gastro-oesophageal reflux but up to 50% of patients present with other symptoms, such as chest pain, belching, halitosis, chronic cough or sore throats. In young patients with typical symptoms and a good response to dietary changes, antacids or acid suppression investigation is not required, but in patients over 55 years of age and those with alarm symptoms or atypical features urgent endoscopy is necessary.

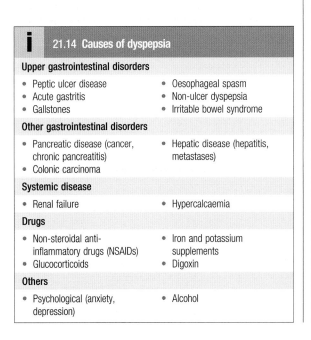

i 21.14 **Causes of dyspepsia**	
Upper gastrointestinal disorders	
• Peptic ulcer disease	• Oesophageal spasm
• Acute gastritis	• Non-ulcer dyspepsia
• Gallstones	• Irritable bowel syndrome
Other gastrointestinal disorders	
• Pancreatic disease (cancer, chronic pancreatitis)	• Hepatic disease (hepatitis, metastases)
• Colonic carcinoma	
Systemic disease	
• Renal failure	• Hypercalcaemia
Drugs	
• Non-steroidal anti-inflammatory drugs (NSAIDs)	• Iron and potassium supplements
• Glucocorticoids	• Digoxin
Others	
• Psychological (anxiety, depression)	• Alcohol

21

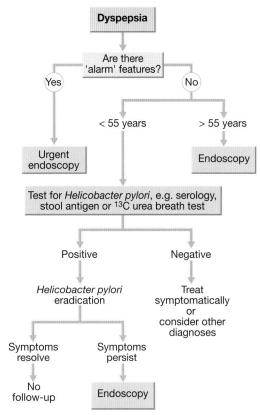

Fig. 21.17 Investigation of dyspepsia.

Vomiting

Vomiting is a complex reflex involving both autonomic and somatic neural pathways. Synchronous contraction of the diaphragm, intercostal muscles and abdominal muscles raises intra-abdominal pressure and, combined with relaxation of the lower oesophageal sphincter, results in forcible ejection of gastric contents. It is important to distinguish true vomiting from regurgitation and to elicit whether the vomiting is acute or chronic (recurrent), as the underlying causes may differ. The major causes are shown in Figure 21.18.

Gastrointestinal bleeding

Acute upper gastrointestinal haemorrhage

This is the most common gastrointestinal emergency, accounting for 50–170 admissions to hospital per 100 000 of the population each year in the UK. The mortality of patients admitted to hospital is about 10% but there is some evidence that outcome is better when individuals are treated in specialised units. Risk scoring systems have been developed to stratify the risk of needing endoscopic therapy or of having a poor outcome (Box 21.16). The advantage of the Blatchford score is that it may be used before endoscopy to predict the need for intervention to treat bleeding. Low scores (2 or less) are associated with a very low risk of adverse outcome. The common causes are shown in Figure 21.19.

Clinical assessment

Haematemesis is red with clots when bleeding is rapid and profuse, or black ('coffee grounds') when less severe. Syncope may occur and is caused by hypotension from intravascular volume depletion. Symptoms of anaemia suggest chronic bleeding. Melaena is the passage of black, tarry stools containing altered blood; it is usually caused by bleeding from the upper gastrointestinal tract, although haemorrhage from the right side of the colon is occasionally responsible. The characteristic colour and smell are the result of the action of digestive enzymes and of bacteria on haemoglobin. Severe acute upper gastrointestinal bleeding can sometimes cause maroon or bright red stool.

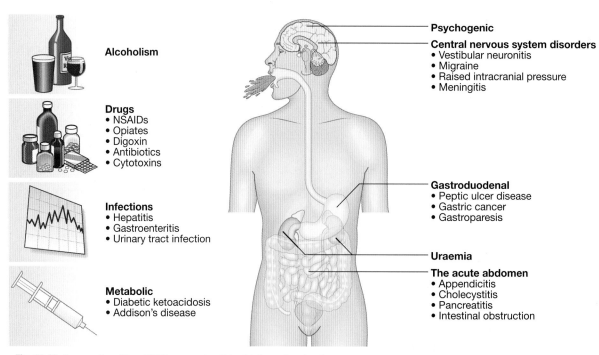

Fig. 21.18 Causes of vomiting. (NSAIDs = non-steroidal anti-inflammatory drugs)

Management

The principles of emergency management of non-variceal bleeding are discussed in detail below. Management of variceal bleeding is discussed on page 869.

i	**21.16 Modified Blatchford score: risk stratification in acute upper gastrointestinal bleeding**

Admission risk marker	Score component value
Blood urea	
≥25 mmol/L (70 mg/dL)	6
10–25 mmol/L (28–70 mg/dL)	4
8–10 mmol/L (22.4–28 mg/dL)	3
6.5–8 mmol/L (18.2–22.4 mg/dL)	2
<6.5 mmol/L (18.2 mg/dL)	0
Haemoglobin for men	
<100 g/L (10 g/dL)	6
100–119 g/L (10–11.9 g/dL)	3
120–129 g/L (12–12.9 g/dL)	1
≥130 g/L (13 g/dL)	0
Haemoglobin for women	
<100 g/L (10 g/dL)	6
100–119 g/L (10–11.9 g/dL)	1
≥120 g/L (12 g/dL)	0
Systolic blood pressure	
<90 mmHg	3
90–99 mmHg	2
100–109 mmHg	1
>109 mmHg	0
Other markers	
Presentation with syncope	2
Hepatic disease	2
Cardiac failure	2
Pulse ≥100 beats/min	1
Presentation with melaena	1
None of the above	0

1. Intravenous access

The first step is to gain intravenous access using at least one large-bore cannula.

2. Initial clinical assessment

- *Define circulatory status.* Severe bleeding causes tachycardia, hypotension and oliguria. The patient is cold and sweating, and may be agitated.
- *Seek evidence of liver disease* (p. 846). Jaundice, cutaneous stigmata, hepatosplenomegaly and ascites may be present in decompensated cirrhosis.
- *Identify comorbidity.* The presence of cardiorespiratory, cerebrovascular or renal disease is important, both because these may be worsened by acute bleeding and because they increase the hazards of endoscopy and surgical operations.

These factors can be combined using the Blatchford score (Box 21.16), which can be calculated at the bedside. A score of 2 or less is associated with a good prognosis, while progressively higher scores are associated with poorer outcomes.

3. Basic investigations

- *Full blood count.* Chronic or subacute bleeding leads to anaemia but the haemoglobin concentration may be normal after sudden, major bleeding until haemodilution occurs. Thrombocytopenia may be a clue to the presence of hypersplenism in chronic liver disease.
- *Urea and electrolytes.* This test may show evidence of renal failure. The blood urea rises as the absorbed products of luminal blood are metabolised by the liver; an elevated blood urea with normal creatinine concentration implies severe bleeding.
- *Liver function tests.* These may show evidence of chronic liver disease.
- *Prothrombin time.* Check when there is a clinical suggestion of liver disease or patients are anticoagulated.
- *Cross-matching.* At least 2 units of blood should be cross-matched if a significant bleed is suspected.

21

Fig. 21.19 Causes of acute upper gastrointestinal haemorrhage. Frequency is given in parentheses. (NSAIDs = non-steroidal anti-inflammatory drugs)

4. Resuscitation

Intravenous crystalloid fluids should be given to raise the blood pressure, and blood should be transfused when the patient is actively bleeding with low blood pressure and tachycardia. Comorbidities should be managed as appropriate. Patients with suspected chronic liver disease should receive broad-spectrum antibiotics.

5. Oxygen

This should be given to all patients in shock.

6. Endoscopy

This should be carried out after adequate resuscitation, ideally within 24 hours, and will yield a diagnosis in 80% of cases. Patients who are found to have major endoscopic stigmata of recent haemorrhage (Fig. 21.20) can be treated endoscopically using a thermal or mechanical modality, such as a 'heater probe' or endoscopic clips, combined with injection of dilute adrenaline (epinephrine) into the bleeding point ('dual therapy'). A biologically inert haemostatic mineral powder (TC325, 'haemospray') can be used as rescue therapy when standard therapy fails. This may stop active bleeding and, combined with intravenous proton pump inhibitor (PPI) therapy, may prevent rebleeding, thus avoiding the need for surgery. Patients found to have bled from varices should be treated by band ligation (p. 870); if this fails, balloon tamponade is another option, while arrangements are made for a transjugular intrahepatic portosystemic shunt (TIPSS).

7. Monitoring

Patients should be closely observed, with hourly measurements of pulse, blood pressure and urine output.

8. Surgery

Surgery is indicated when endoscopic haemostasis fails to stop active bleeding and if rebleeding occurs on one occasion in an elderly or frail patient, or twice in a younger, fitter patient. If available, angiographic embolisation is an effective alternative to surgery in frail patients.

The choice of operation depends on the site and diagnosis of the bleeding lesion. Duodenal ulcers are treated by under-running, with or without pyloroplasty. Under-running for gastric ulcers can also be carried out (a biopsy must be taken to exclude carcinoma). Local excision may be performed, but when neither is possible, partial gastrectomy is required.

9. Eradication

Following treatment for ulcer bleeding, all patients should avoid non-steroidal anti-inflammatory drugs (NSAIDs) and those who test positive for *H. pylori* infection should receive eradication therapy (p. 800). Successful eradication should be confirmed by urea breath or faecal antigen testing.

Lower gastrointestinal bleeding

This may be caused by haemorrhage from the colon, anal canal or small bowel. It is useful to distinguish those patients who present with profuse, acute bleeding from those who present with chronic or subacute bleeding of lesser severity (Box 21.17).

Severe acute lower gastrointestinal bleeding

This presents with profuse red or maroon diarrhoea and with shock. Diverticular disease is the most common cause and is often due to erosion of an artery within the mouth of a diverticulum. Bleeding almost always stops spontaneously, but if it does not, the diseased segment of colon should be resected after confirmation of the site by angiography or colonoscopy. Angiodysplasia is a disease of the elderly, in which vascular malformations develop in the proximal colon. Bleeding can be acute and profuse; it usually

i	**21.17 Causes of lower gastrointestinal bleeding**
Severe acute	
• Diverticular disease	• Meckel's diverticulum
• Angiodysplasia	• Inflammatory bowel disease
• Ischaemia	(rarely)
Moderate, chronic/subacute	
• Fissure	• Large polyps
• Haemorrhoids	• Angiodysplasia
• Inflammatory bowel disease	• Radiation enteritis
• Carcinoma	• Solitary rectal ulcer

Fig. 21.20 Major stigmata of recent haemorrhage and endoscopic treatment. A Active bleeding from a duodenal ulcer. B Haemostasis is achieved after endoscopic injection of adrenaline (epinephrine) and application of a heater probe.

stops spontaneously but commonly recurs. Diagnosis is often difficult. Colonoscopy may reveal characteristic vascular spots and, in the acute phase, visceral angiography can show bleeding into the intestinal lumen and an abnormal large, draining vein. In some patients, diagnosis is achieved only by laparotomy with on-table colonoscopy. The treatment of choice is endoscopic thermal ablation but resection of the affected bowel may be required if bleeding continues. Bowel ischaemia due to occlusion of the inferior mesenteric artery can present with abdominal colic and rectal bleeding. It should be considered in patients (particularly the elderly) who have evidence of generalised atherosclerosis. The diagnosis is made at colonoscopy. Resection is required only in the presence of peritonitis. Meckel's diverticulum with ectopic gastric epithelium may ulcerate and erode into a major artery. The diagnosis should be considered in children or adolescents who present with profuse or recurrent lower gastrointestinal bleeding. A Meckel's ^{99m}Tc-pertechnetate scan is sometimes positive but the diagnosis is commonly made only by laparotomy, at which time the diverticulum is excised.

Subacute or chronic lower gastrointestinal bleeding

This can occur at all ages and is usually due to haemorrhoids or anal fissure. Haemorrhoidal bleeding is bright red and occurs during or after defecation. Proctoscopy can be used to make the diagnosis, but subjects who have altered bowel habit and those who present over the age of 40 years should undergo colonoscopy to exclude coexisting colorectal cancer. Anal fissure should be suspected when fresh rectal bleeding and anal pain occur during defecation.

Major gastrointestinal bleeding of unknown cause

In some patients who present with major gastrointestinal bleeding, upper endoscopy and colonoscopy fail to reveal a diagnosis. When severe life-threatening bleeding continues, urgent CT mesenteric angiography is indicated. This will usually identify the site if the bleeding rate exceeds 1 mL/min and then formal angiographic embolisation can often stop the bleeding. If angiography is negative or bleeding is less severe, push or double balloon enteroscopy can visualise the small intestine (Fig. 21.21) and treat the bleeding source. Wireless capsule endoscopy is often

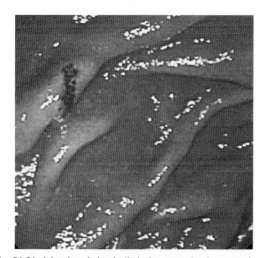

Fig. 21.21 Jejunal angiodysplastic lesion seen at enteroscopy in a patient with recurrent obscure bleeding.

used to define a source of bleeding prior to enteroscopy. When all else fails, laparotomy with on-table endoscopy is indicated.

Chronic occult gastrointestinal bleeding

In this context, occult means that blood or its breakdown products are present in the stool but cannot be seen by the naked eye. Occult bleeding may reach 200 mL per day and cause iron deficiency anaemia. Any cause of gastrointestinal bleeding may be responsible but the most important is colorectal cancer, particularly carcinoma of the caecum, which may produce no gastrointestinal symptoms. In clinical practice, investigation of the upper and lower gastrointestinal tract should be considered whenever a patient presents with unexplained iron deficiency anaemia. Testing the stool for the presence of blood is unnecessary and should not influence whether or not the gastrointestinal tract is imaged because bleeding from tumours is often intermittent and a negative faecal occult blood (FOB) test does not exclude the diagnosis. The only value of FOB testing is as a means of population screening for colonic neoplasia in asymptomatic individuals (p. 832).

Diarrhoea

Diarrhoea is defined as the passage of more than 200 g of stool daily and measurement of stool volume is helpful in confirming this. The most severe symptom in many patients is urgency of defecation, and faecal incontinence is a common event in acute and chronic diarrhoeal illnesses.

Acute diarrhoea

This is extremely common and is usually caused by faecal–oral transmission of bacteria or their toxins, viruses or parasites (Ch. 11). Infective diarrhoea is usually short-lived and patients who present with a history of diarrhoea lasting more than 10 days rarely have an infective cause. A variety of drugs, including antibiotics, cytotoxic drugs, PPIs and NSAIDs, may be responsible.

Chronic or relapsing diarrhoea

The most common cause is irritable bowel syndrome (p. 824), which can present with increased frequency of defecation and loose, watery or pellety stools. Diarrhoea rarely occurs at night and is most severe before and after breakfast. At other times, the patient is constipated and there are other characteristic symptoms of irritable bowel syndrome. The stool often contains mucus but never blood, and 24-hour stool volume is less than 200 g. Chronic diarrhoea can be categorised as being caused by disease of the colon or small bowel, or to malabsorption (Box 21.18). Clinical presentation, examination of the stool, routine blood tests and imaging reveal a diagnosis in many cases. A series of negative investigations usually implies irritable bowel syndrome but some patients clearly have organic disease and need more extensive investigations.

Malabsorption

Diarrhoea and weight loss in patients with a normal diet are likely to be caused by malabsorption. The symptoms are diverse in nature and variable in severity. A few patients have apparently normal bowel habit but diarrhoea is usual and may be watery and voluminous. Bulky, pale and offensive stools that float in the toilet (steatorrhoea) signify fat malabsorption. Abdominal

21

i	21.18 Chronic or relapsing diarrhoea		
	Colonic	**Malabsorption**	**Small bowel**
Clinical features	Blood and mucus in stool Cramping lower abdominal pain	Steatorrhoea Undigested food in the stool Weight loss and nutritional disturbances	Large-volume, watery stool Abdominal bloating Cramping mid-abdominal pain

Some causes	Inflammatory bowel disease
	Microscopic colitis
	Neoplasia
	Ischaemia
	Irritable bowel syndrome
		Pancreatic:
		  Chronic pancreatitis
		  Cancer of pancreas
		  Cystic fibrosis
		Enteropathy:
		  Coeliac disease
		  Tropical sprue
		  Lymphoma
		  Lymphangiectasia
			Crohn's disease
			VIPoma
			Drug-induced:
			  NSAIDs
			  Aminosalicylates
			  SSRIs

Investigations	Faecal calprotectin Ileocolonoscopy with biopsies	Faecal elastase Ultrasound, CT and MRCP Small-bowel biopsy Barium follow-through or small-bowel MRI	Faecal calprotectin Stool volume Gut hormone profile Barium follow-through or small-bowel MRI

(CT = computed tomography; MRCP = magnetic resonance cholangiopancreatography; MRI = magnetic resonance imaging; NSAIDs = non-steroidal anti-inflammatory drugs; SSRIs = selective serotonin re-uptake inhibitors; VIP = vasoactive intestinal polypeptide)

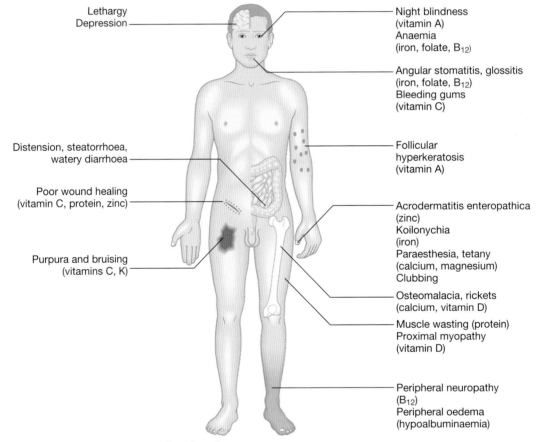

Fig. 21.22 Possible physical consequences of malabsorption.

distension, borborygmi, cramps, weight loss and undigested food in the stool may be present. Some patients complain only of malaise and lethargy. In others, symptoms related to deficiencies of specific vitamins, trace elements and minerals may occur (Fig. 21.22).

Pathophysiology

Malabsorption results from abnormalities of the three processes that are essential to normal digestion:

- *Intraluminal maldigestion* occurs when deficiency of bile or pancreatic enzymes results in inadequate solubilisation and hydrolysis of nutrients. Fat and protein malabsorption results. This may also occur with small bowel bacterial overgrowth.

- *Mucosal malabsorption* results from small bowel resection or conditions that damage the small intestinal epithelium, thereby diminishing the surface area for absorption and depleting brush border enzyme activity.
- *'Post-mucosal' lymphatic obstruction* prevents the uptake and transport of absorbed lipids into lymphatic vessels. Increased pressure in these vessels results in leakage into the intestinal lumen, leading to protein-losing enteropathy.

Investigations

Investigations should be performed both to confirm the presence of malabsorption and to determine the underlying cause. Routine blood tests may show one or more of the abnormalities listed in Box 21.19. Tests to confirm fat and protein malabsorption should be performed, as described on page 777. An approach to the investigation of malabsorption is shown in Figure 21.23.

21.19 Routine blood test abnormalities in malabsorption

Haematology

- Microcytic anaemia (iron deficiency)
- Macrocytic anaemia (folate or B_{12} deficiency)
- Increased prothrombin time (vitamin K deficiency)

Biochemistry

- Hypoalbuminaemia
- Hypocalcaemia
- Hypomagnesaemia
- Hypophosphataemia
- Low serum zinc

Suspected malabsorption

↓

Clinical features of steatorrhoea
- Blood tests (urea and electrolytes, immunoglobulins, Ca^{2+}, Mg^{2+}, full blood count, clotting, albumin, folate, B_{12}, coeliac antibodies)

↓

Investigate small intestine
- Duodenal biopsy
- Barium studies or small bowel MRI
- Faecal calprotectin
- Lactulose/glucose hydrogen breath test

↓ Normal

Investigate pancreas
- Pancreatic function tests, e.g. faecal elastase
- Ultrasound scan/CT
- MRCP

↓ Normal

Consider bile salt malabsorption
- SeHCAT scan
- Serum 7α-hydroxycholestenone

Fig. 21.23 Investigation for suspected malabsorption. (CT = computed tomography; MRCP = magnetic resonance cholangiopancreatography; MRI = magnetic resonance imaging; ^{75}SeHCAT = ^{75}Se-homocholic acid taurine)

Weight loss

Weight loss may be physiological, due to dieting, exercise, starvation, or the decreased nutritional intake that accompanies old age. Weight loss of more than 3 kg over 6 months is significant and often indicates the presence of an underlying disease. Hospital and general practice weight records may be valuable in confirming that weight loss has occurred, as may reweighing patients at intervals; sometimes weight is regained or stabilises in those with no obvious cause. Pathological weight loss can be due to psychiatric illness, systemic disease, gastrointestinal causes or advanced disease of many organ systems (Fig. 21.24).

Physiological causes

Weight loss can occur in the absence of serious disease in healthy individuals who have changes in physical activity or social circumstances. It may be difficult to be sure of this diagnosis in older patients, when the dietary history may be unreliable, and professional help from a dietitian is often valuable under these circumstances.

Psychiatric illness

Features of anorexia nervosa (p. 1203), bulimia (p. 1204) and affective disorders (p. 1198) may be apparent only after formal psychiatric input. Alcoholic patients lose weight as a consequence of self-neglect and poor dietary intake. Depression may cause weight loss.

Systemic disease

Chronic infections, including tuberculosis (p. 588), recurrent urinary or chest infections, and a range of parasitic and protozoan infections (Ch. 11), should be considered. A history of foreign travel, high-risk activities and specific features, such as fever, night sweats, rigors, productive cough and dysuria, must be sought. Promiscuous sexual activity and drug misuse suggest HIV-related illness (Ch. 12). Weight loss is a late feature of disseminated malignancy, but by the time the patient presents, other features of cancer are often present. Chronic inflammatory diseases, such as rheumatoid arthritis (p. 1021) and polymyalgia rheumatica (p. 1042), are often associated with weight loss.

Gastrointestinal disease

Almost any disease of the gastrointestinal tract can cause weight loss. Dysphagia and gastric outflow obstruction (pp. 778 and 801) cause weight loss by reducing food intake. Malignancy at any site may cause weight loss by mechanical obstruction, anorexia or cytokine-mediated systemic effects. Malabsorption from pancreatic diseases (p. 837) or small bowel causes may lead to profound weight loss with specific nutritional deficiencies (p. 704). Inflammatory diseases, such as Crohn's disease or ulcerative colitis (p. 813), cause anorexia, fear of eating and loss of protein, blood and nutrients from the gut.

Metabolic disorders and miscellaneous causes

Weight loss may occur in association with metabolic disorders, as well as end-stage respiratory and cardiac disease.

21

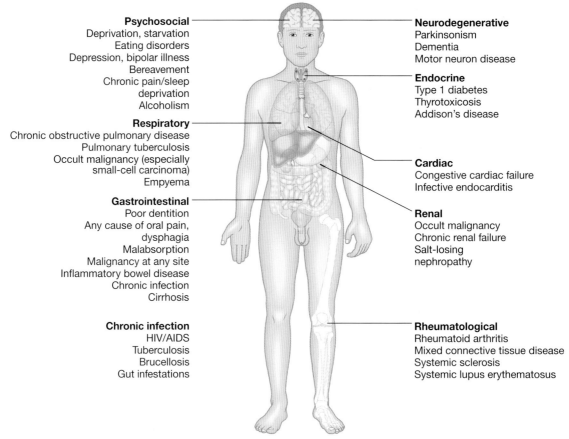

Psychosocial
Deprivation, starvation
Eating disorders
Depression, bipolar illness
Bereavement
Chronic pain/sleep
deprivation
Alcoholism

Respiratory
Chronic obstructive pulmonary disease
Pulmonary tuberculosis
Occult malignancy (especially
small-cell carcinoma)
Empyema

Gastrointestinal
Poor dentition
Any cause of oral pain,
dysphagia
Malabsorption
Malignancy at any site
Inflammatory bowel disease
Chronic infection
Cirrhosis

Chronic infection
HIV/AIDS
Tuberculosis
Brucellosis
Gut infestations

Neurodegenerative
Parkinsonism
Dementia
Motor neuron disease

Endocrine
Type 1 diabetes
Thyrotoxicosis
Addison's disease

Cardiac
Congestive cardiac failure
Infective endocarditis

Renal
Occult malignancy
Chronic renal failure
Salt-losing
nephropathy

Rheumatological
Rheumatoid arthritis
Mixed connective tissue disease
Systemic sclerosis
Systemic lupus erythematosus

Fig. 21.24 Some important causes of weight loss.

Investigations

In cases where the cause of weight loss is not obvious after thorough history taking and physical examination, or where an existing condition is considered unlikely, the following investigations are indicated: urinalysis for glucose, protein and blood; blood tests, including liver function tests, random blood glucose and thyroid function tests; CRP and ESR (may be raised in unsuspected infections, such as tuberculosis, connective tissue disorders and malignancy); and faecal calprotectin. Sometimes invasive tests, such as bone marrow aspiration or liver biopsy, may be necessary to identify conditions like cryptic miliary tuberculosis (p. 588). Rarely, abdominal and pelvic imaging by CT may be required, but before embarking on invasive or very costly investigations it is always worth revisiting the patient's history and reweighing at intervals.

Constipation

Constipation is defined as infrequent passage of hard stools. Patients may also complain of straining, a sensation of incomplete evacuation and either perianal or abdominal discomfort. Constipation may occur in many gastrointestinal and other medical disorders (Box 21.20).

Clinical assessment and management

The onset, duration and characteristics are important; for example, a neonatal onset suggests Hirschsprung's disease, while a recent change in bowel activity in middle age should raise the suspicion of an organic disorder, such as colonic carcinoma. The presence of rectal bleeding, pain and weight loss is important, as are excessive

---

i 21.20 Causes of constipation

Gastrointestinal causes

Dietary
- Lack of fibre and/or fluid intake

Motility
- Slow-transit constipation
- Irritable bowel syndrome
- Drugs (see below)
- Chronic intestinal pseudo-obstruction

Structural
- Colonic carcinoma
- Diverticular disease
- Hirschsprung's disease

Defecation
- Anorectal disease (Crohn's, fissures, haemorrhoids)
- Obstructed defecation

Non-gastrointestinal causes

Drugs
- Opiates
- Anticholinergics
- Calcium antagonists
- Iron supplements
- Aluminium-containing antacids

Neurological
- Multiple sclerosis
- Spinal cord lesions
- Cerebrovascular accidents
- Parkinsonism

Metabolic/endocrine
- Diabetes mellitus
- Hypercalcaemia
- Hypothyroidism
- Pregnancy

Others
- Any serious illness with immobility, especially in the elderly
- Depression

straining, symptoms suggestive of irritable bowel syndrome, a history of childhood constipation and emotional distress.

Careful examination contributes more to the diagnosis than extensive investigation. A search should be made for general medical disorders, as well as signs of intestinal obstruction. Neurological disorders, especially spinal cord lesions, should be sought. Perineal inspection and rectal examination are essential and may reveal abnormalities of the pelvic floor (abnormal descent, impaired sensation), anal canal or rectum (masses, faecal impaction, prolapse).

It is neither possible nor appropriate to investigate every person with constipation. Most respond to increased fluid intake, dietary fibre supplementation, exercise and the judicious use of laxatives. Middle-aged or elderly patients with a short history or worrying symptoms (rectal bleeding, pain or weight loss) must be investigated promptly, by either barium enema or colonoscopy. For those with simple constipation, investigation will usually proceed along the lines described below.

Initial visit

Digital rectal examination, proctoscopy and sigmoidoscopy (to detect anorectal disease), routine biochemistry, including serum calcium and thyroid function tests, and a full blood count should be carried out. If these are normal, a 1-month trial of dietary fibre and/or laxatives is justified.

Next visit

If symptoms persist, then examination of the colon by barium enema or CT colonography is indicated to look for structural disease.

Further investigation

If no cause is found and disabling symptoms are present, then specialist referral for investigation of possible dysmotility may be necessary. The problem may be one of infrequent desire to defecate ('slow transit') or else may result from neuromuscular incoordination and excessive straining ('functional obstructive defecation', p. 803). Intestinal marker studies, anorectal manometry, electrophysiological studies and magnetic resonance proctography can all be used to define the problem.

Abdominal pain

There are four types of abdominal pain:

- *Visceral*. Gut organs are insensitive to stimuli such as burning and cutting but are sensitive to distension, contraction, twisting and stretching. Pain from unpaired structures is usually, but not always, felt in the midline.
- *Parietal*. The parietal peritoneum is innervated by somatic nerves and its involvement by inflammation, infection or neoplasia causes sharp, well-localised and lateralised pain.
- *Referred pain*. Gallbladder pain, for example, may be referred to the back or shoulder tip.
- *Psychogenic*. Cultural, emotional and psychosocial factors influence everyone's experience of pain. In some patients, no organic cause can be found despite investigation, and psychogenic causes (depression or somatisation disorder) may be responsible (pp. 1198 and 1202).

The acute abdomen

This accounts for approximately 50% of all urgent admissions to general surgical units. The acute abdomen is a consequence of one or more pathological processes (Box 21.21):

- *Inflammation*. Pain develops gradually, usually over several hours. It is initially rather diffuse until the parietal

21.21 Causes of acute abdominal pain

Inflammation

- Appendicitis
- Diverticulitis
- Cholecystitis
- Pelvic inflammatory disease
- Pancreatitis
- Pyelonephritis
- Intra-abdominal abscess

Perforation/rupture

- Peptic ulcer
- Diverticular disease
- Ovarian cyst
- Aortic aneurysm

Obstruction

- Intestinal obstruction
- Biliary colic
- Ureteric colic

Other (rare)

- See Box 21.23

peritoneum is involved, when it becomes localised. Movement exacerbates the pain; abdominal rigidity and guarding occur.
- *Perforation*. When a viscus perforates, pain starts abruptly; it is severe and leads to generalised peritonitis.
- *Obstruction*. Pain is colicky, with spasms that cause the patient to writhe around and double up. Colicky pain that does not disappear between spasms suggests complicating inflammation.

Initial clinical assessment

If there are signs of peritonitis (guarding and rebound tenderness with rigidity), the patient should be resuscitated with oxygen, intravenous fluids and antibiotics. In other circumstances, further investigations are required (Fig. 21.25).

Investigations

Patients should have a full blood count, urea and electrolytes, glucose and amylase taken to look for evidence of dehydration, leucocytosis and pancreatitis. Urinalysis is useful in suspected renal colic and pyelonephritis. An erect chest X-ray may show air under the diaphragm, suggestive of perforation, and a plain abdominal film may show evidence of obstruction or ileus (see Fig. 21.11). An abdominal ultrasound may help if gallstones or renal stones are suspected. Ultrasonography is also useful in the detection of free fluid and any possible intra-abdominal abscess. Contrast studies, by either mouth or anus, are useful in the further evaluation of intestinal obstruction, and essential in the differentiation of pseudo-obstruction from mechanical large-bowel obstruction. Other investigations commonly used include CT (seeking evidence of pancreatitis, retroperitoneal collections or masses, including an aortic aneurysm or renal calculi) and angiography (mesenteric ischaemia).

Diagnostic laparotomy should be considered when the diagnosis has not been revealed by other investigations. All patients must be carefully and regularly re-assessed (every 2–4 hours) so that any change in condition that might alter both the suspected diagnosis and clinical decision can be observed and acted on early.

Management

The general approach is to close perforations, treat inflammatory conditions with antibiotics or resection, and relieve obstructions. The speed of intervention and the necessity for surgery depend on the organ that is involved and on a number of other factors,

21

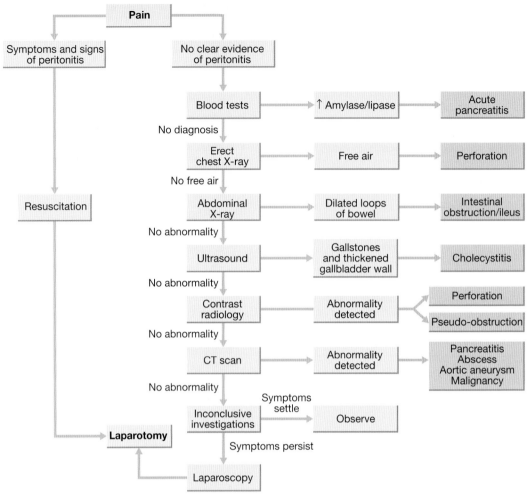

Fig. 21.25 Management of acute abdominal pain: an algorithm.

21.22 Acute abdominal pain in old age

- **Presentation**: severity and localisation may blunt with age. Presentation may be atypical, e.g. with delirium, collapse and/or immobility.
- **Cancer**: a more common cause of acute pain in those over 70 years of age than in those under 50 years. Older people with vague abdominal symptoms should therefore be carefully assessed.
- **Non-specific symptoms**: intra-abdominal inflammatory conditions, such as diverticulitis, may present with non-specific symptoms, such as delirium or anorexia and relatively little abdominal tenderness. The reasons for this are not clear but may stem from altered sensory perception.
- **Outcome of abdominal surgery**: determined by how frail the patient is and whether surgery is elective or emergency, rather than by chronological age.

of which the presence or absence of peritonitis is the most important. A treatment summary of some of the more common surgical conditions follows.

Acute appendicitis

This should be treated by early surgery, since there is a risk of perforation and recurrent attacks with non-operative treatment. The appendix can be removed through a conventional right iliac fossa skin crease incision or by laparoscopic techniques.

Acute cholecystitis

This can be successfully treated non-operatively but the high risk of recurrent attacks and the low morbidity of surgery have made early laparoscopic cholecystectomy the treatment of choice.

Acute diverticulitis

Conservative therapy is standard but if perforation has occurred, resection is advisable. Depending on peritoneal contamination and the state of the patient, primary anastomosis is preferable to a Hartmann's procedure (oversew of rectal stump and end-colostomy).

Small bowel obstruction

If the cause is obvious and surgery inevitable (such as with a strangulated hernia), an early operation is appropriate. If the suspected cause is adhesions from previous surgery, only those patients who do not resolve within the first 48 hours or who develop signs of strangulation (colicky pain becoming constant, peritonitis, tachycardia, fever, leucocytosis) should have surgery.

Large bowel obstruction

Pseudo-obstruction should be treated non-operatively. Some patients benefit from colonoscopic decompression but mechanical obstruction merits resection, usually with a primary anastomosis. Differentiation between the two is made by water-soluble contrast enema.

Perforated peptic ulcer

Surgical closure of the perforation is standard practice but some patients without generalised peritonitis can be treated non-operatively once a water-soluble contrast meal has confirmed spontaneous sealing of the perforation. Adequate and aggressive resuscitation with intravenous fluids, antibiotics and analgesia is mandatory before surgery.

For a more detailed discussion of acute abdominal pain, the reader is referred to the sister volume of this text, *Principles and Practice of Surgery*.

Chronic or recurrent abdominal pain

It is essential to take a detailed history, paying particular attention to features of the pain and any associated symptoms (Boxes 21.23 and 21.24).

i	**21.23 Extra-intestinal causes of chronic or recurrent abdominal pain**

Retroperitoneal

- Aortic aneurysm
- Malignancy
- Lymphadenopathy
- Abscess

Psychogenic

- Depression
- Anxiety
- Hypochondriasis
- Somatisation

Locomotor

- Vertebral compression/fracture
- Abdominal muscle strain

Metabolic/endocrine

- Diabetes mellitus
- Acute intermittent porphyria
- Hypercalcaemia

Drugs/toxins

- Glucocorticoids
- Azathioprine
- Lead
- Alcohol

Haematological

- Sickle-cell disease
- Haemolytic disorders

Neurological

- Spinal cord lesions
- Tabes dorsalis
- Radiculopathy

21.24 How to assess abdominal pain

- Duration
- Site and radiation
- Severity
- Precipitating and relieving factors (food, drugs, alcohol, posture, movement, defecation)
- Nature (colicky, constant, sharp or dull, wakes patient at night)
- Pattern (intermittent or continuous)
- Associated features (vomiting, dyspepsia, altered bowel habit)

Note should be made of the patient's general demeanour, mood and emotional state, signs of weight loss, fever, jaundice or anaemia. If a thorough abdominal and rectal examination is normal, a careful search should be made for evidence of disease affecting other structures, particularly the vertebral column, spinal cord, lungs and cardiovascular system.

Investigations will depend on the clinical features elicited during the history and examination:

- Endoscopy and ultrasound are indicated for epigastric pain, and for dyspepsia and symptoms suggestive of gallbladder disease.
- Colonoscopy is indicated for patients with altered bowel habit, rectal bleeding or features of obstruction suggesting colonic disease.
- CT or MR angiography should be considered when pain is provoked by food in a patient with widespread atherosclerosis, since this may indicate mesenteric ischaemia.
- Persistent symptoms require exclusion of colonic or small bowel disease. However, young patients with pain relieved by defecation, bloating and alternating bowel habit are likely to have irritable bowel syndrome (p. 824). Simple investigations (blood tests, faecal calprotectin and sigmoidoscopy) are sufficient in the absence of rectal bleeding, weight loss and abnormal physical findings.
- Ultrasound, CT and faecal elastase are required for patients with upper abdominal pain radiating to the back. A history of alcohol misuse, weight loss and diarrhoea suggests chronic pancreatitis or pancreatic cancer.
- Recurrent attacks of pain in the loins radiating to the flanks with urinary symptoms should prompt investigation for renal or ureteric stones by abdominal X-ray, ultrasound and computed tomography of the kidneys, ureters and bladder (CT KUB).
- A past history of psychiatric disturbance, repeated negative investigations or vague symptoms that do not fit any disease or organ pattern suggest a psychological origin for the pain. Careful review of case notes and previous investigations, along with open and honest discussion with the patient, reduces the need for further cycles of unnecessary and invasive tests. Care must always be taken, however, not to miss rare pathology, such as acute intermittent porphyria (p. 378), or atypical presentations of common diseases.

Constant abdominal pain

Patients with chronic pain that is constant or nearly always present usually have features to suggest the underlying diagnosis. No cause will be found in a minority, despite thorough investigation, leading to the diagnosis of 'chronic functional abdominal pain'. In these patients, there appears to be abnormal CNS processing of normal visceral afferent sensory input and psychosocial factors are often operative (p. 1186); the most important tasks are to provide symptom control, if not relief, and to minimise the effects of the pain on social, personal and occupational life. Patients are best managed in specialised pain clinics where, in addition to psychological support, appropriate use of drugs, including tricyclic antidepressants, gabapentin or pregabalin, ketamine and opioids, may be necessary.

21

Diseases of the mouth and salivary glands

Aphthous ulceration

Aphthous ulcers are superficial and painful; they occur in any part of the mouth. Recurrent ulcers afflict up to 30% of the population and are particularly common in women prior to menstruation. The cause is unknown, but in severe cases other causes of oral ulceration must be considered (Box 21.25). Biopsy is occasionally necessary for diagnosis.

Management is with topical glucocorticoids (such as 0.1% triamcinolone in Orabase) or choline salicylate (8.7%) gel. Symptomatic relief is achieved using local anaesthetic mouthwashes. Rarely, patients with very severe, recurrent aphthous ulcers may need oral glucocorticoids.

21.25 Causes of oral ulceration	
Aphthous	
• Idiopathic	• Premenstrual
Infection	
• Fungal (candidiasis)	• Bacterial, including syphilis, tuberculosis
• Viral (herpes simplex, HIV)	
Gastrointestinal diseases	
• Crohn's disease	• Coeliac disease
Dermatological conditions	
• Lichen planus	• Dermatitis herpetiformis
• Immunobullous disorders (p. 1255)	• Erythema multiforme
Drugs	
• Nicorandil, NSAIDs, methotrexate, penicillamine, losartan, ACE inhibitors	• Stevens–Johnson syndrome (pp. 1254 and 1264)
	• Cytotoxic drugs
Systemic diseases	
• Systemic lupus erythematosus (p. 1034)	• Behçet's disease (p. 1043)
Neoplasia	
• Carcinoma	• Kaposi's sarcoma
• Leukaemia	

(ACE = angiotensin-converting enzyme; NSAIDs = non-steroidal anti-inflammatory drugs)

Oral cancer

Squamous carcinoma of the oral cavity is common worldwide and the incidence has increased by 25% in the last decade in the UK. The mortality rate is around 50%, largely as a result of late diagnosis. Poor diet, alcohol excess and smoking or tobacco chewing are the traditional risk factors but high-risk, oncogenic strains of human papillomavirus (HPV-16 and HPV-18) have been identified as being responsible for much of the recent increase in incidence, especially in cases affecting the base of tongue, soft palate and tonsils. In parts of Asia, the disease is common among people who chew areca nuts wrapped in leaves of the betel plant ('betel nuts').

i 21.26 Symptoms and signs of oral cancer
• Solitary ulcer without precipitant, e.g. local trauma
• Solitary white patch ('leukoplakia') that fails to wipe off
• Solitary red patch
• Fixed lump
• Lip numbness in absence of trauma or infection
• Trismus (pain/difficulty in opening the mouth)
• Cervical lymphadenopathy

Oral cancer may present in many ways (Box 21.26) and a high index of suspicion is required. All possible sources of local trauma or infection should be treated in patients with suspicious lesions and they should be reviewed after 2 weeks, with biopsy if the lesion persists. Small cancers can be resected but extensive surgery, with neck dissection to remove involved lymph nodes, may be necessary. Some patients can be treated with radical radiotherapy alone, and sometimes radiotherapy is also given after surgery to treat microscopic residual disease. Some tumours may be amenable to photodynamic therapy (PDT), avoiding the need for surgery.

Candidiasis

The yeast *Candida albicans* is a normal mouth commensal but it may proliferate to cause thrush. This occurs in babies, debilitated patients, people receiving glucocorticoid or antibiotic therapy, individuals with diabetes and immunosuppressed patients, especially those receiving cytotoxic therapy and those with HIV infection. White patches are seen on the tongue and buccal mucosa. Odynophagia or dysphagia suggests pharyngeal and oesophageal candidiasis. A clinical diagnosis is sufficient to instigate therapy, although brushings or biopsies can be obtained for mycological examination. Oral thrush is treated using nystatin or amphotericin suspensions or lozenges. Resistant cases or immunosuppressed patients may require oral fluconazole.

Parotitis

Parotitis is caused by viral or bacterial infection. Mumps causes a self-limiting acute parotitis (p. 240). Bacterial parotitis usually occurs as a complication of major surgery. It is a consequence of dehydration and poor oral hygiene, and can be avoided by good post-operative care. Patients present with painful parotid swelling and this can be complicated by abscess formation. Broad-spectrum antibiotics are required, while surgical drainage is necessary for abscesses. Other causes of salivary gland enlargement are listed in Box 21.27.

i 21.27 Causes of salivary gland swelling	
• Infection:	• Tumours:
Mumps	Benign: pleomorphic
Bacterial (post-operative)	adenoma (95% of cases)
• Calculi	Intermediate:
• Sjögren's syndrome (p. 1038)	mucoepidermoid tumour
• Sarcoidosis	Malignant: carcinoma

21.28 Oral health in old age

- **Dry mouth**: affects around 40% of healthy older people.
- **Gustatory and olfactory sensation**: declines and chewing power is diminished.
- **Salivation**: baseline salivary flow falls but stimulated salivation is unchanged.
- **Root caries and periodontal disease**: common partly because oral hygiene deteriorates with increasing frailty.
- **Bacteraemia and sepsis**: may complicate Gram-negative anaerobic infection in the periodontal pockets of the very frail.

Diseases of the oesophagus

Gastro-oesophageal reflux disease

Gastro-oesophageal reflux resulting in heartburn affects approximately 30% of the general population.

Pathophysiology

Occasional episodes of gastro-oesophageal reflux are common in healthy individuals. Reflux is normally followed by oesophageal peristaltic waves that efficiently clear the gullet, alkaline saliva neutralises residual acid and symptoms do not occur. Gastro-oesophageal reflux disease develops when the oesophageal mucosa is exposed to gastroduodenal contents for prolonged periods of time, resulting in symptoms and, in a proportion of cases, oesophagitis. Several factors are known to be involved in the development of gastro-oesophageal reflux disease and these are shown in Figure 21.26.

Abnormalities of the lower oesophageal sphincter

The lower oesophageal sphincter is tonically contracted under normal circumstances, relaxing only during swallowing (p. 766).

Some patients with gastro-oesophageal reflux disease have reduced lower oesophageal sphincter tone, permitting reflux when intra-abdominal pressure rises. In others, basal sphincter tone is normal but reflux occurs in response to frequent episodes of inappropriate sphincter relaxation.

Hiatus hernia

Hiatus hernia (Box 21.29 and Fig. 21.27) causes reflux because the pressure gradient is lost between the abdominal and thoracic cavities, which normally pinches the hiatus. In addition, the oblique angle between the cardia and oesophagus disappears. Many patients who have large hiatus hernias develop reflux symptoms but the relationship between the presence of a hernia and symptoms is poor. Hiatus hernia is very common in individuals who have no symptoms, and some symptomatic patients have only a very small or no hernia. Nevertheless, almost all patients who develop oesophagitis, Barrett's oesophagus or peptic strictures have a hiatus hernia.

Delayed oesophageal clearance

Defective oesophageal peristaltic activity is commonly found in patients who have oesophagitis. It is a primary abnormality, since it persists after oesophagitis has been healed by acid-suppressing drug therapy. Poor oesophageal clearance leads to increased acid exposure time.

Fig. 21.26 Factors associated with the development of gastro-oesophageal reflux disease.

---

i **21.29 Important features of hiatus hernia**

- Herniation of the stomach through the diaphragm into the chest
- Occurs in 30% of the population over the age of 50 years
- Often asymptomatic
- Heartburn and regurgitation can occur
- Gastric volvulus may complicate large hernias

Gastric contents

Gastric acid is the most important oesophageal irritant and there is a close relationship between acid exposure time and symptoms. Pepsin and bile also contribute to mucosal injury.

Defective gastric emptying

Gastric emptying is delayed in patients with gastro-oesophageal reflux disease. The reason is unknown.

Increased intra-abdominal pressure

Pregnancy and obesity are established predisposing causes. Weight loss may improve symptoms.

Dietary and environmental factors

Dietary fat, chocolate, alcohol, tea and coffee relax the lower oesophageal sphincter and may provoke symptoms. The foods that trigger symptoms vary widely between affected individuals.

Patient factors

Visceral sensitivity and patient vigilance play a role in determining symptom severity and consulting behaviour in individual patients.

Clinical features

The major symptoms are heartburn and regurgitation, often provoked by bending, straining or lying down. 'Waterbrash', which is salivation due to reflex salivary gland stimulation as acid enters the gullet, is often present. The patient is often overweight. Some patients are woken at night by choking as refluxed fluid

21

Fig. 21.27 Types of hiatus hernia. **A** Rolling or para-oesophageal. Inset: Barium meal showing a large para-oesophageal hernia with intrathoracic stomach. **B** Sliding. Inset: Barium meal showing a gastric volvulus (small arrows) complicating a sliding hiatus hernia (large arrow).

irritates the larynx. Others develop odynophagia or dysphagia. A variety of other features have been described, such as atypical chest pain that may be severe and can mimic angina; it may be due to reflux-induced oesophageal spasm. Others include hoarseness ('acid laryngitis'), recurrent chest infections, chronic cough and asthma. The true relationship of these features to gastro-oesophageal reflux disease remains unclear.

Complications

Oesophagitis

A range of endoscopic findings is recognised, from mild redness to severe bleeding ulceration with stricture formation, although appearances may be completely normal (Fig. 21.28). There is a poor correlation between symptoms and histological and endoscopic findings.

Barrett's oesophagus

Barrett's oesophagus is a pre-malignant condition, in which the normal squamous lining of the lower oesophagus is replaced by columnar mucosa (columnar lined oesophagus; CLO) that may contain areas of intestinal metaplasia (Fig. 21.29). It is an adaptive response to chronic gastro-oesophageal reflux and is found in 10% of patients undergoing gastroscopy for reflux symptoms. Community-based epidemiological studies suggest that the true prevalence may be up to 1.5–5% of the population, as the condition is often asymptomatic until discovered when the patient presents with oesophageal cancer. The relative risk of oesophageal cancer is increased 40–120-fold but the absolute risk is low (0.1–0.5% per year). The epidemiology and aetiology of Barrett's oesophagus are poorly understood. The prevalence is increasing, and it is more common in men (especially white), the obese and those over 50 years of age. It is weakly associated with smoking but not alcohol intake. The risk of cancer seems to relate to the severity and duration of reflux rather than the presence of Barrett's oesophagus per se, and it has been suggested that duodenogastro-oesophageal reflux of bile, pancreatic enzymes and pepsin, as well as gastric acid,

Fig. 21.28 Severe reflux oesophagitis. There is near-circumferential superficial ulceration and inflammation extending up the gullet.

may be important in the pathogenesis. The molecular events underlying progression of Barrett's oesophagus to dysplasia and cancer are incompletely understood but inactivation of the tumour suppression protein p16 by loss of heterozygosity or promoter hypermethylation is a key event, followed by somatic inactivation of *TP53*, which promotes aneuploidy and tumour progression. Studies are in progress to develop biomarkers that will allow detection of those at higher cancer risk.

Diagnosis This requires multiple systematic biopsies to maximise the chance of detecting intestinal metaplasia and/or dysplasia.

Management Neither potent acid suppression nor anti-reflux surgery stops progression or induces regression of Barrett's

Fig. 21.29 Barrett's oesophagus. Tongues of pink columnar mucosa are seen extending upwards above the oesophago-gastric junction.

oesophagus, and treatment is indicated only for symptoms of reflux or complications, such as stricture. Endoscopic therapies, such as radiofrequency ablation or photodynamic therapy, can induce regression but at present are used only for those with dysplasia or intramucosal cancer. Regular endoscopic surveillance can detect dysplasia at an early stage and may improve survival but, because most Barrett's oesophagus is undetected until cancer develops, surveillance strategies are unlikely to influence the overall mortality rate of oesophageal cancer. Surveillance is expensive and cost-effectiveness studies have been conflicting. It is currently recommended that patients with Barrett's oesophagus with intestinal metaplasia, but without dysplasia, should undergo endoscopy at 3–5-yearly intervals if the length of the Barrettic segment is less than 3 cm and at 2–3-yearly intervals if the length is greater than 3 cm. Those with low-grade dysplasia should be endoscoped at 6-monthly intervals.

For those with high-grade dysplasia or intramucosal carcinoma, the treatment options are either oesophagectomy or endoscopic therapy, with a combination of endoscopic resection of any visibly abnormal areas and radiofrequency ablation of the remaining Barrett's mucosa, as an 'organ-preserving' alternative to surgery. These cases should be discussed in a multidisciplinary team meeting and managed in specialist centres.

Anaemia

Iron deficiency anaemia can occur as a consequence of occult blood loss from long-standing oesophagitis. Most patients have a large hiatus hernia and bleeding can stem from subtle erosions in the neck of the sac ('Cameron lesions'). Nevertheless, hiatus hernia is very common and other causes of blood loss, particularly colorectal cancer, must be considered in anaemic patients, even when endoscopy reveals oesophagitis.

Benign oesophageal stricture

Fibrous strictures can develop as a consequence of long-standing oesophagitis, especially in the elderly and those with poor oesophageal peristaltic activity. The typical presentation is with dysphagia that is worse for solids than for liquids. Bolus obstruction following ingestion of meat causes absolute dysphagia. A history of heartburn is common but not invariable; many elderly patients presenting with strictures have no preceding heartburn.

Diagnosis is by endoscopy, when biopsies of the stricture can be taken to exclude malignancy. Endoscopic balloon dilatation or bouginage is helpful. Subsequently, long-term therapy with a PPI drug at full dose should be started to reduce the risk of recurrent oesophagitis and stricture formation. The patient should be advised to chew food thoroughly and it is important to ensure adequate dentition.

Gastric volvulus

Occasionally, a massive intrathoracic hiatus hernia may twist on itself, leading to a gastric volvulus. This gives rise to complete oesophageal or gastric obstruction and the patient presents with severe chest pain, vomiting and dysphagia. The diagnosis is made by chest X-ray (air bubble in the chest) and barium swallow (see Fig. 21.27B). Most cases spontaneously resolve but recurrence is common, and surgery is usually advised after the acute episode has been treated by nasogastric decompression.

Investigations

Young patients who present with typical symptoms of gastro-oesophageal reflux, without worrying features such as dysphagia, weight loss or anaemia, can be treated empirically without investigation. Investigation is advisable if patients present over the age of 50–55 years, if symptoms are atypical or if a complication is suspected. Endoscopy is the investigation of choice. This is performed to exclude other upper gastrointestinal diseases that can mimic gastro-oesophageal reflux and to identify complications. A normal endoscopy in a patient with compatible symptoms should not preclude treatment for gastro-oesophageal reflux disease.

Twenty-four-hour pH monitoring is indicated if the diagnosis is unclear or surgical intervention is under consideration. This involves tethering a slim catheter with a terminal radiotelemetry pH-sensitive probe above the gastro-oesophageal junction. The intraluminal pH is recorded while the patient undergoes normal activities, and episodes of symptoms are noted and related to pH. A pH of less than 4 for more than 6–7% of the study time is diagnostic of reflux disease. In a few patients with difficult reflux, impedance testing can detect weakly acidic or alkaline reflux that is not revealed by standard pH testing.

Management

A treatment algorithm for gastro-oesophageal reflux is outlined in Figure 21.30. Lifestyle advice should be given, including weight loss, avoidance of dietary items that the patient finds worsen symptoms, elevation of the bed head in those who experience nocturnal symptoms, avoidance of late meals and cessation of smoking. Patients who fail to respond to these measures should be offered PPIs, which are usually effective in resolving symptoms and healing oesophagitis. Recurrence of symptoms is common when therapy is stopped and some patients require life-long treatment at the lowest acceptable dose. When dysmotility features are prominent, domperidone can be helpful. There is no evidence that *H. pylori* eradication has any therapeutic value. Proprietary antacids and alginates can also provide symptomatic benefit. H_2-receptor antagonist drugs relieve symptoms without healing oesophagitis.

Long-term PPI therapy is associated with reduced absorption of iron, B_{12} and magnesium, and a small but increased risk of osteoporosis and fractures (odds ratio 1.2–1.5). The drugs also predispose to enteric infections with *Salmonella*, *Campylobacter* and possibly *Clostridium difficile*, and have recently been shown to have an undesirable impact on the composition of the gut

21

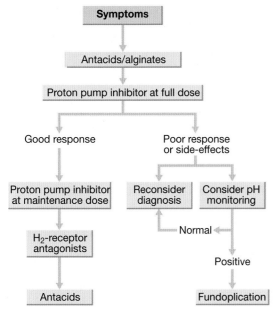

Fig. 21.30 Treatment of gastro-oesophageal reflux disease: a 'step-down' approach.

21.30 Gastro-oesophageal reflux disease in old age

- **Prevalence**: higher.
- **Severity of symptoms**: does not correlate with the degree of mucosal inflammation.
- **Complications**: late complications, such as peptic strictures or bleeding from oesophagitis, are more common.
- **Recurrent pneumonia**: consider aspiration from occult gastro-oesophageal reflux disease.

microbiota. Long-term therapy increases the risk of *Helicobacter*-associated progression of gastric mucosal atrophy (see below) and *H. pylori* eradication is advised in patients requiring PPIs for more than 1 year.

Patients who fail to respond to medical therapy, those who are unwilling to take long-term PPIs and those whose major symptom is severe regurgitation should be considered for laparoscopic anti-reflux surgery (see *Principles and Practice of Surgery*). Although heartburn and regurgitation are alleviated in most patients, a small minority develop complications, such as inability to vomit and abdominal bloating ('gas-bloat' syndrome').

Other causes of oesophagitis

Infection

Oesophageal candidiasis occurs in debilitated patients and those taking broad-spectrum antibiotics or cytotoxic drugs. It is a particular problem in patients with HIV/AIDS, who are also susceptible to a spectrum of other oesophageal infections (p. 316).

Corrosives

Suicide attempt by ingestion of strong household bleach or battery acid is followed by painful burns of the mouth and pharynx and by extensive erosive oesophagitis (p. 147). This may be complicated by oesophageal perforation with mediastinitis and by stricture formation. At the time of presentation, treatment is conservative, based on analgesia and nutritional support; vomiting and endoscopy should be avoided because of the high risk of oesophageal perforation. After the acute phase, a barium swallow should be performed to demonstrate the extent of stricture formation. Endoscopic dilatation is usually necessary but it is difficult and hazardous because strictures are often long, tortuous and easily perforated.

Drugs

Potassium supplements and NSAIDs may cause oesophageal ulcers when the tablets are trapped above an oesophageal stricture. Liquid preparations of these drugs should be used in such patients. Bisphosphonates cause oesophageal ulceration and should be used with caution in patients with known oesophageal disorders.

Eosinophilic oesophagitis

This is more common in children but increasingly recognised in young adults. It occurs more often in atopic individuals and is characterised by eosinophilic infiltration of the oesophageal mucosa. Patients present with dysphagia or food bolus obstruction more often than heartburn, and other symptoms, such as chest pain and vomiting, may be present. Endoscopy is usually normal but mucosal rings (that sometimes need endoscopic dilatation), strictures or a narrow-calibre oesophagus can occur. Children may respond to elimination diets but these are less successful in adults, who should first be treated with PPIs. The condition can be treated with 8–12 weeks of therapy with topical glucocorticoids, such as fluticasone or betamethasone. The usual approach is to prescribe a metered-dose inhaler but to tell the patient to spray this into the mouth and swallow it rather than inhale it. Refractory symptoms sometimes respond to montelukast, a leukotriene inhibitor.

Motility disorders

Pharyngeal pouch

This occurs because of incoordination of swallowing within the pharynx, which leads to herniation through the cricopharyngeus muscle and formation of a pouch. It is rare, affecting 1 in 100 000 people; it usually develops in middle life but can arise at any age. Many patients have no symptoms but regurgitation, halitosis and dysphagia can be present. Some notice gurgling in the throat after swallowing. The investigation of choice is a barium swallow (see Fig. 21.12A), which demonstrates the pouch and reveals incoordination of swallowing, often with pulmonary aspiration. Endoscopy may be hazardous, since the instrument may enter and perforate the pouch. Surgical myotomy ('diverticulotomy'), with or without resection of the pouch, is indicated in symptomatic patients.

Achalasia of the oesophagus

Pathophysiology

Achalasia is characterised by:

- a hypertonic lower oesophageal sphincter, which fails to relax in response to the swallowing wave
- failure of propagated oesophageal contraction, leading to progressive dilatation of the gullet.

The cause is unknown. Defective release of nitric oxide by inhibitory neurons in the lower oesophageal sphincter has been reported, and there is degeneration of ganglion cells within the sphincter and the body of the oesophagus. Loss of the dorsal vagal nuclei within the brainstem can be demonstrated in later stages. Infection with *Trypanosoma cruzi* in Chagas' disease (p. 279) causes a syndrome that is clinically indistinguishable from achalasia.

Clinical features

The presentation is with dysphagia. This develops slowly, is initially intermittent, and is worse for solids and eased by drinking liquids and by standing and moving around after eating. Heartburn does not occur because the closed oesophageal sphincter prevents gastro-oesophageal reflux. Some patients experience episodes of chest pain due to oesophageal spasm. As the disease progresses, dysphagia worsens, the oesophagus empties poorly and nocturnal pulmonary aspiration develops. Achalasia predisposes to squamous carcinoma of the oesophagus.

Investigations

Endoscopy should always be carried out because carcinoma of the cardia can mimic the presentation and radiological and manometric features of achalasia ('pseudo-achalasia'). A barium swallow shows tapered narrowing of the lower oesophagus and, in late disease, the oesophageal body is dilated, aperistaltic and food-filled (Fig. 21.31A). Manometry confirms the high-pressure, non-relaxing lower oesophageal sphincter with poor contractility of the oesophageal body (Fig. 21.31B).

Management

Endoscopic

Forceful pneumatic dilatation using a 30–35-mm-diameter, fluoroscopically positioned balloon disrupts the oesophageal sphincter and improves symptoms in 80% of patients. Some patients require more than one dilatation but those needing frequent dilatation are best treated surgically. Endoscopically directed injection of botulinum toxin into the lower oesophageal sphincter induces clinical remission but relapse is common. Recently, a complex endoscopic technique has been developed in specialist centres (peroral endoscopic myotomy, POEM).

Surgical

Surgical myotomy (Heller's operation), performed either laparoscopically or as an open operation, is effective but is more invasive than endoscopic dilatation. Both pneumatic dilatation and myotomy may be complicated by gastro-oesophageal reflux, and this can lead to severe oesophagitis because oesophageal clearance is so poor. For this reason, Heller's myotomy is accompanied by a partial fundoplication anti-reflux procedure. PPI therapy is often necessary after surgery.

Other oesophageal motility disorders

Diffuse oesophageal spasm presents in late middle age with episodic chest pain that may mimic angina but is sometimes accompanied by transient dysphagia. Some cases occur in response to gastro-oesophageal reflux. Treatment is based on the use of PPI drugs when gastro-oesophageal reflux is present. Oral or sublingual nitrates or nifedipine may relieve attacks of pain. The results of drug therapy are often disappointing, as are the alternatives: pneumatic dilatation and surgical myotomy. 'Nutcracker' oesophagus is a condition in which extremely forceful peristaltic activity leads to episodic chest pain and dysphagia. Treatment is with nitrates or nifedipine. Some patients present with oesophageal motility disorders that do not fit into a specific disease entity. The patients are usually elderly and present with dysphagia and chest pain. Manometric abnormalities, ranging from poor peristalsis to spasm, occur. Treatment is with dilatation and/or vasodilators for chest pain.

Secondary causes of oesophageal dysmotility

In systemic sclerosis or CREST syndrome (p. 1037), the muscle of the oesophagus is replaced by fibrous tissue, which causes failure of peristalsis leading to heartburn and dysphagia. Oesophagitis is often severe and benign fibrous strictures occur. These patients require long-term therapy with PPIs. Dermatomyositis, rheumatoid arthritis and myasthenia gravis may also cause dysphagia.

Benign oesophageal stricture

Benign oesophageal stricture is usually a consequence of gastro-oesophageal reflux disease (Box 21.31) and occurs most often in elderly patients who have poor oesophageal clearance. Rings, caused by submucosal fibrosis, are found at the oesophago-gastric junction ('Schatzki ring') and cause intermittent

21

Fig. 21.31 Achalasia. **A** X-ray showing a dilated, barium-filled oesophagus (O) with fluid level and distal tapering, and a closed lower oesophageal sphincter (LOS). (D = diaphragm) **B** High-resolution manometry in achalasia showing absence of peristaltic swallowing wave in oesophageal body (black arrows) and raised LOS pressure with failure of relaxation on swallowing (white arrow). Compare with normal appearances in Figure 21.1 (p. 766).

dysphagia, often starting in middle age. A post-cricoid web is a rare complication of iron deficiency anaemia (Paterson–Kelly or Plummer–Vinson syndrome), and may be complicated by the development of squamous carcinoma. Benign strictures can be treated by endoscopic dilatation, in which wire-guided bougies or balloons are used to disrupt the fibrous tissue of the stricture.

Tumours of the oesophagus

Benign tumours

The most common is a leiomyoma. This is usually asymptomatic but may cause bleeding or dysphagia.

Carcinoma of the oesophagus

Squamous oesophageal cancer (Box 21.32) is relatively rare in Caucasians (4 : 100 000) but is more common in Iran, parts of Africa and China (200 : 100 000). Squamous cancer can occur in any part of the oesophagus and almost all tumours in the upper oesophagus are squamous cancers. Adenocarcinomas typically arise in the lower third of the oesophagus from Barrett's oesophagus or from the cardia of the stomach. The incidence is increasing and is now approximately 5 : 100 000 in the UK; this is possibly because of the high prevalence of gastro-oesophageal reflux and Barrett's oesophagus in Western populations. Despite modern treatment, the overall 5-year survival of patients presenting with oesophageal cancer is only 13%.

Clinical features

Most patients have a history of progressive, painless dysphagia for solid foods. Others present acutely because of food bolus obstruction. In the late stages, weight loss is often extreme; chest pain or hoarseness suggests mediastinal invasion. Fistulation between the oesophagus and the trachea or bronchial tree leads to coughing after swallowing, pneumonia and pleural effusion. Physical signs may be absent but, even at initial presentation, cachexia, cervical lymphadenopathy or other evidence of metastatic spread is common.

Investigations

The investigation of choice is upper gastrointestinal endoscopy (Fig. 21.32) with biopsy. A barium swallow demonstrates the site and length of the stricture but adds little useful information. Once a diagnosis has been made, investigations should be performed to stage the tumour and define operability. Thoracic and abdominal CT, often combined with positron emission tomography (PET-CT), should be carried out to identify metastatic

Fig. 21.32 Adenocarcinoma of the lower oesophagus. A polypoidal adenocarcinoma in association with Barrett's oesophagus.

Fig. 21.33 Positron emission tomography–computed tomography (PET-CT) staging of oesophageal carcinoma. Whole-body PET scan showing avid uptake in the primary tumour (thick arrow) but also in distant paratracheal (superior thin arrow) and gastro-oesophageal (inferior thin arrow) lymph nodes.

spread and local invasion (Fig. 21.33). Invasion of the aorta, major airways or coeliac axis usually precludes surgery, but patients with resectable disease on imaging should undergo EUS to determine the depth of penetration of the tumour into the oesophageal wall and to detect locoregional lymph node

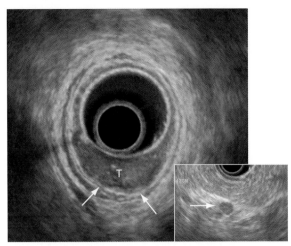

Fig. 21.34 Endoscopic ultrasound staging of oesophageal carcinoma. There is a superficial adenocarcinoma of the oesophagus (T). The submucosa (white band, white arrows) is not involved but there is a small involved local lymph node (white arrow, inset). The tumour is therefore staged T1a, N1.

involvement (Fig. 21.34). These investigations will define the TNM stage of the disease (p. 1322).

Management

The treatment of choice is surgery if the patient presents at a point at which resection is possible. For very early superficial tumours, endoscopic submucosal dissection may offer an alternative to surgery but is not widely used outside of Japan and Korea. Patients with tumours that have extended beyond the wall of the oesophagus (T3) or that have lymph node involvement (N1) carry a 5-year survival of around 10%. This figure improves significantly, however, if the tumour is confined to the oesophageal wall and there is no spread to lymph nodes. Overall survival following 'potentially curative' surgery (all macroscopic tumour removed) is about 30% at 5 years but recent studies have suggested that this can be improved by neoadjuvant chemotherapy. Although squamous carcinomas are radiosensitive, radiotherapy alone is associated with a 5-year survival of only 5% but combined chemoradiotherapy for these tumours can achieve 5-year survival rates of 25–30%.

Approximately 70% of patients have extensive disease at presentation; in these, treatment is palliative and should focus on relief of dysphagia and pain. Endoscopic laser therapy or self-expanding metallic stents can be used to improve swallowing. Palliative radiotherapy may induce shrinkage of both squamous cancers and adenocarcinomas but symptomatic response may be slow. Quality of life can be improved by nutritional support and appropriate analgesia.

Perforation of the oesophagus

The most common cause is endoscopic perforation complicating dilatation or intubation. Malignant, corrosive or post-radiotherapy strictures are more likely to be perforated than peptic strictures. A perforated peptic stricture is managed conservatively using broad-spectrum antibiotics and parenteral nutrition; most cases heal within days. Malignant, caustic and radiotherapy stricture perforations require resection or stenting.

Spontaneous oesophageal perforation ('Boerhaave's syndrome') results from forceful vomiting and retching. Severe chest pain and shock occur as oesophago-gastric contents enter the mediastinum and thoracic cavity. Subcutaneous emphysema, pleural effusions and pneumothorax develop. The diagnosis can be made using a water-soluble contrast swallow but, in difficult cases, both CT and careful endoscopy (usually in an intubated patient) may be required. Treatment is surgical. Delay in diagnosis is a key factor in the high mortality associated with this condition.

Diseases of the stomach and duodenum

Gastritis

Gastritis is a histological diagnosis, although it can also be recognised at endoscopy.

Acute gastritis

Acute gastritis is often erosive and haemorrhagic. Neutrophils are the predominant inflammatory cell in the superficial epithelium. Many cases result from alcohol, aspirin or NSAID ingestion (Box 21.33). Acute gastritis often produces no symptoms but may cause dyspepsia, anorexia, nausea or vomiting, and haematemesis or melaena. Many cases resolve quickly and do not merit investigation; in others, endoscopy and biopsy may be necessary to exclude peptic ulcer or cancer. Treatment should be directed at the underlying cause. Short-term symptomatic therapy with antacids, and acid suppression using PPIs, prokinetics (domperidone) or antiemetics (metoclopramide) may be necessary.

Chronic gastritis due to *Helicobacter pylori* infection

This is the most common cause of chronic gastritis (Box 21.33). The predominant inflammatory cells are lymphocytes and plasma cells. Correlation between symptoms and endoscopic or pathological findings is poor. Most patients are asymptomatic and do not require treatment but patients with dyspepsia may benefit from *H. pylori* eradication.

Autoimmune chronic gastritis

This involves the body of the stomach but spares the antrum; it results from autoimmune damage to parietal cells. The histological features are diffuse chronic inflammation, atrophy and loss of fundic glands, intestinal metaplasia and sometimes hyperplasia of enterochromaffin-like (ECL) cells. Circulating antibodies to parietal cell and intrinsic factor may be present. In some patients, the degree of gastric atrophy is severe and loss of intrinsic factor secretion leads to pernicious anaemia (p. 944). The gastritis itself is usually asymptomatic. Some patients have evidence of other organ-specific autoimmunity, particularly thyroid disease. In the long term, there is a two- to threefold increase in the risk of gastric cancer (see also p. 803).

Ménétrier's disease

In this rare condition, the gastric pits are elongated and tortuous, with replacement of the parietal and chief cells by mucus-secreting cells. The cause is unknown but there is excessive production of transforming growth factor alpha (TGF-α). As a result, the

21

i 21.33 Common causes of gastritis

Acute gastritis (often erosive and haemorrhagic)

- Aspirin, NSAIDs
- *Helicobacter pylori* (initial infection)
- Alcohol
- Other drugs, e.g. iron preparations
- Severe physiological stress, e.g. burns, multi-organ failure, central nervous system trauma
- Bile reflux, e.g. following gastric surgery
- Viral infections, e.g. CMV, herpes simplex virus in HIV/AIDS (p. 316)

Chronic non-specific gastritis

- *H. pylori* infection
- Autoimmune (pernicious anaemia)
- Post-gastrectomy

Chronic 'specific' forms (rare)

- Infections, e.g. CMV, tuberculosis
- Gastrointestinal diseases, e.g. Crohn's disease
- Systemic diseases, e.g. sarcoidosis, graft-versus-host disease
- Idiopathic, e.g. granulomatous gastritis

(CMV = cytomegalovirus; NSAIDs = non-steroidal anti-inflammatory drugs)

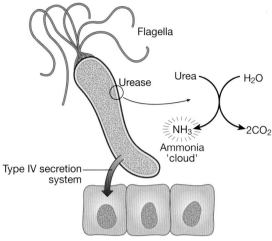

Other factors
- Vacuolating cytotoxin (vacA)
- Cytotoxin-associated gene (cagA)
- Adhesins (babA)
- Outer inflammatory protein A (oipA)

Fig. 21.35 Factors that influence the virulence of *Helicobacter pylori*.

mucosal folds of the body and fundus are greatly enlarged. Most patients are hypochlorhydric. While some patients have upper gastrointestinal symptoms, the majority present in middle or old age with protein-losing enteropathy (p. 811) due to exudation from the gastric mucosa. Endoscopy shows enlarged, nodular and coarse folds, although biopsies may not be deep enough to show all the histological features. Treatment with antisecretory drugs, such as PPIs with or without octreotide, may reduce protein loss and *H. pylori* eradication may be effective, but unresponsive patients require partial gastrectomy.

Peptic ulcer disease

The term 'peptic ulcer' refers to an ulcer in the lower oesophagus, stomach or duodenum, in the jejunum after surgical anastomosis to the stomach or, rarely, in the ileum adjacent to a Meckel's diverticulum. Ulcers in the stomach or duodenum may be acute or chronic; both penetrate the muscularis mucosae but the acute ulcer shows no evidence of fibrosis. Erosions do not penetrate the muscularis mucosae.

Gastric and duodenal ulcer

The prevalence of peptic ulcer (0.1–0.2%) is decreasing in many Western communities as a result of widespread use of *Helicobacter pylori* eradication therapy but it remains high in developing countries. The male-to-female ratio for duodenal ulcer varies from 5:1 to 2:1, while that for gastric ulcer is 2:1 or less. Chronic gastric ulcer is usually single; 90% are situated on the lesser curve within the antrum or at the junction between body and antral mucosa. Chronic duodenal ulcer usually occurs in the first part of the duodenum and 50% are on the anterior wall. Gastric and duodenal ulcers coexist in 10% of patients and more than one peptic ulcer is found in 10–15% of patients.

Pathophysiology

H. pylori

Peptic ulceration is strongly associated with *H. pylori* infection. The prevalence of the infection in developed nations rises with age and

in the UK approximately 50% of people over the age of 50 years are infected. In the developing world infection is more common, affecting up to 90% of adults. These infections are probably acquired in childhood by person-to-person contact. The vast majority of colonised people remain healthy and asymptomatic, and only a minority develop clinical disease. Around 90% of duodenal ulcer patients and 70% of gastric ulcer patients are infected with *H. pylori*. The remaining 30% of gastric ulcers are caused by NSAIDs and this proportion is increasing in Western countries as a result of *H. pylori* eradication strategies.

H. pylori is Gram-negative and spiral, and has multiple flagella at one end, which make it motile, allowing it to burrow and live beneath the mucus layer adherent to the epithelial surface. It uses an adhesin molecule (BabA) to bind to the Lewis b antigen on epithelial cells. Here the surface pH is close to neutral and any acidity is buffered by the organism's production of the enzyme urease. This produces ammonia from urea and raises the pH around the bacterium and between its two cell membrane layers. *H. pylori* exclusively colonises gastric-type epithelium and is found in the duodenum only in association with patches of gastric metaplasia. It causes chronic gastritis by provoking a local inflammatory response in the underlying epithelium (Fig. 21.35). This depends on numerous factors, notably expression of bacterial *cagA* and *vacA* genes. The CagA gene product is injected into epithelial cells, interacting with numerous cell-signalling pathways involved in cell replication and apoptosis. *H. pylori* strains expressing CagA (CagA+) are more often associated with disease than CagA– strains. Most strains also secrete a large pore-forming protein called VacA, which causes increased cell permeability, efflux of micronutrients from the epithelium, induction of apoptosis and suppression of local immune cell activity. Several forms of VacA exist and pathology is most strongly associated with the s1/m1 form of the toxin.

The distribution and severity of *H. pylori*–induced gastritis determine the clinical outcome. In most people, *H. pylori* causes a mild pangastritis with little effect on acid secretion and the majority develop no significant clinical outcomes. In a minority (up to 10% in the West), the infection causes an antral-predominant pattern of gastritis characterised by hypergastrinaemia and a very exaggerated acid production by parietal cells, which could lead to duodenal ulceration (Fig. 21.36). In a much smaller number of infected people, *H. pylori* causes a corpus-predominant pattern of gastritis leading to gastric atrophy and hypochlorhydria. This phenotype is much more common in Asian countries, particularly Japan, China and Korea. The hypochlorhydria allows other bacteria to proliferate within the stomach; these other bacteria continue to drive the chronic inflammation and produce mutagenic nitrites from dietary nitrates, predisposing to the development of gastric cancer (Fig. 21.37). The effects of *H. pylori* are more complex in gastric ulcer patients compared to those with duodenal ulcers. The ulcer probably arises because of impaired mucosal defence resulting from a combination of *H. pylori* infection, NSAIDs and smoking, rather than excess acid.

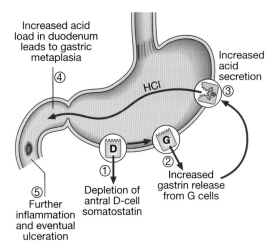

Fig. 21.36 Sequence of events in the pathophysiology of duodenal ulceration.

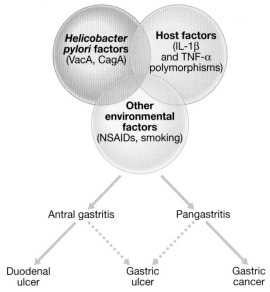

Fig. 21.37 Consequences of *Helicobacter pylori* infection. (CagA = cytotoxin-associated gene; IL-1β = interleukin-1 beta; NSAIDs = non-steroidal anti-inflammatory drugs; TNF-α = tumour necrosis factor alpha; VacA = vacuolating cytotoxin)

NSAIDs

Treatment with NSAIDs is associated with peptic ulcers due to impairment of mucosal defences, as discussed on page 1002.

Smoking

Smoking confers an increased risk of gastric ulcer and, to a lesser extent, duodenal ulcer. Once the ulcer has formed, it is more likely to cause complications and less likely to heal if the patient continues to smoke.

Clinical features

Peptic ulcer disease is a chronic condition with spontaneous relapses and remissions lasting for decades, if not for life. The most common presentation is with recurrent abdominal pain that has three notable characteristics: localisation to the epigastrium, relationship to food and episodic occurrence. Occasional vomiting occurs in about 40% of ulcer subjects; persistent daily vomiting suggests gastric outlet obstruction. In one-third, the history is less characteristic, especially in elderly people or those taking NSAIDs. In this situation, pain may be absent or so slight that it is experienced only as a vague sense of epigastric unease. Occasionally, the only symptoms are anorexia and nausea, or early satiety after meals. In some patients, the ulcer is completely 'silent', presenting for the first time with anaemia from chronic undetected blood loss, as abrupt haematemesis or as acute perforation; in others, there is recurrent acute bleeding without ulcer pain. The diagnostic value of individual symptoms for peptic ulcer disease is poor; the history is therefore a poor predictor of the presence of an ulcer.

Investigations

Endoscopy is the preferred investigation (Fig. 21.38). Gastric ulcers may occasionally be malignant and therefore must always be biopsied and followed up to ensure healing. Patients should be tested for *H. pylori* infection. The current options available are listed in Box 21.34. Some are invasive and require endoscopy; others are non-invasive. They vary in sensitivity and specificity. Breath tests or faecal antigen tests are best because of accuracy, simplicity and non-invasiveness.

21

Fig. 21.38 Endoscopic identification of a duodenal ulcer. The ulcer has a clean base and there are no stigmata of recent haemorrhage.

21.34 Methods for the diagnosis of *Helicobacter pylori* infection		
Test	Advantages	Disadvantages
Non-invasive		
Serology	Rapid office kits available	Lacks specificity
	Good for population studies	Cannot differentiate current from past infection
^{13}C-urea breath test	High sensitivity and specificity	Requires expensive mass spectrometer
Faecal antigen test	Cheap, specific (>95%)	Acceptability
Invasive (antral biopsy)		
Histology	Specificity	False negatives
		Takes several days to process
Rapid urease test	Cheap, quick, specific (>95%)	Sensitivity 85%
Microbiological culture	'Gold standard'	Slow and laborious
	Defines antibiotic sensitivity	Lacks sensitivity

21.36 Indications for *Helicobacter pylori* eradication

Definite

- Peptic ulcer
- Extranodal marginal-zone lymphomas of MALT type
- Family history of gastric cancer
- Previous resection for gastric cancer
- *H. pylori*-positive dyspepsia
- Long-term NSAID or low-dose aspirin users
- Chronic (>1 year) PPI users
- Extragastric disorders:
    Unexplained vitamin B_{12} deficiency*
    Idiopathic thrombocytopenic purpura*
    Iron deficiency anaemia* (see text)

Not indicated

- Gastro-oesophageal reflux disease
- Asymptomatic people without gastric cancer risk factors

*If *H. pylori*-positive on testing.
(MALT = mucosa-associated lymphoid tissue; NSAID = non-steroidal anti-inflammatory drug; PPI = proton pump inhibitor)

21.35 Common side-effects of *Helicobacter pylori* eradication therapy

- Diarrhoea: 30–50% of patients; usually mild but *Clostridium difficile*-associated diarrhoea can occur
- Flushing and vomiting when taken with alcohol (metronidazole)
- Nausea, vomiting
- Abdominal cramps
- Headache
- Rash

21.37 Indications for surgery in peptic ulcer

Emergency

- Perforation
- Haemorrhage

Elective

- Gastric outflow obstruction
- Persistent ulceration despite adequate medical therapy
- Recurrent ulcer following gastric surgery

Management

The aims of management are to relieve symptoms, induce healing and prevent recurrence. *H. pylori* eradication is the cornerstone of therapy for peptic ulcers, as this will successfully prevent relapse and eliminate the need for long-term therapy in the majority of patients.

H. pylori eradication

All patients with proven ulcers who are *H. pylori*-positive should be offered eradication as primary therapy. Treatment is based on a PPI taken simultaneously with two antibiotics (from amoxicillin, clarithromycin and metronidazole) for at least 7 days. High-dose, twice-daily PPI therapy increases efficacy of treatment, as does extending treatment to 10–14 days. Success is achieved in 80–90% of patients, although adherence, side-effects (Box 21.35) and antibiotic resistance influence this. Resistance to amoxicillin is rare but rates of metronidazole resistance reach more than 50% in some countries and rates of clarithromycin resistance of 20–40% have recently become common. Where the latter exceed 15%, a quadruple therapy regimen, consisting of omeprazole (or another PPI), bismuth subcitrate, metronidazole and tetracycline (OBMT) for 10–14 days, is recommended. In areas of low clarithromycin resistance, this regimen should also be offered as second-line therapy to those who remain infected after initial therapy, once adherence has been checked. For those who are still colonised after two treatments, the choice lies between a third attempt guided by antimicrobial sensitivity testing, rescue therapy (levofloxacin, PPI and clarithromycin) or long-term acid suppression.

H. pylori and NSAIDs are independent risk factors for ulcer disease and patients requiring long-term NSAID therapy should first undergo eradication therapy to reduce ulcer risk. Subsequent co-prescription of a PPI along with the NSAID is advised but is not always necessary for patients being given low-dose aspirin, in whom the risk of ulcer complications is lower.

Other indications for *H. pylori* eradication are shown in Box 21.36. Eradication of the infection has proven benefits in several extragastric disorders, including unexplained B_{12} deficiency and iron deficiency anaemia, once sources of gastrointestinal bleeding have been looked for and excluded. Platelet counts improve and may normalise after eradication therapy in patients with idiopathic thrombocytopenic purpura (p. 979); the mechanism for this is unclear.

General measures

Cigarette smoking, aspirin and NSAIDs should be avoided. Alcohol in moderation is not harmful and no special dietary advice is required.

Maintenance treatment

Continuous maintenance treatment should not be necessary after successful *H. pylori* eradication. For the minority who do require it, the lowest effective dose of PPI should be used.

Surgical treatment

Surgery is now rarely required for peptic ulcer disease but it is needed in some cases (Box 21.37).

The operation of choice for a chronic non-healing gastric ulcer is partial gastrectomy, preferably with a Billroth I anastomosis, in which the ulcer itself and the ulcer-bearing area of the stomach are resected. The reason for this is to exclude an underlying cancer. In an emergency, 'under-running' the ulcer for bleeding or 'oversewing' (patch repair) for perforation is all that is required, in addition to taking a biopsy. For giant duodenal ulcers, partial gastrectomy using a 'Polya' or Billroth II reconstruction may be required.

Complications of gastric resection or vagotomy

Up to 50% of patients who undergo gastric surgery for peptic ulcer surgery experience long-term adverse effects. In most cases these are minor but in 10% they significantly impair quality of life.

Dumping Rapid gastric emptying leads to distension of the proximal small intestine as the hypertonic contents draw fluid into the lumen. This leads to abdominal discomfort and diarrhoea after eating. Autonomic reflexes release a range of gastrointestinal hormones that provoke vasomotor features, such as flushing, palpitations, sweating, tachycardia and hypotension. Patients should therefore avoid large meals with high carbohydrate content.

Chemical (bile reflux) gastropathy Duodenogastric bile reflux leads to chronic gastropathy. Treatment with aluminium-containing antacids or sucralfate may be effective. A few patients require revisional surgery with creation of a Roux en Y loop to prevent bile reflux.

Diarrhoea and maldigestion Diarrhoea may develop after any peptic ulcer operation and usually occurs 1–2 hours after eating. Poor mixing of food in the stomach, with rapid emptying, inadequate mixing with pancreaticobiliary secretions, rapid transit and bacterial overgrowth, may lead to malabsorption. Diarrhoea often responds to small, dry meals with a reduced intake of refined carbohydrates. Antidiarrhoeal drugs, such as codeine phosphate (15–30 mg 4–6 times daily) or loperamide (2 mg after each loose stool), are helpful.

Weight loss Most patients lose weight shortly after surgery and 30–40% are unable to regain all the weight that is lost. The usual cause is reduced intake because of a small gastric remnant but diarrhoea and mild steatorrhoea also contribute.

Anaemia Anaemia is common many years after subtotal gastrectomy. Iron deficiency is the most common cause; folic acid and B_{12} deficiency are much less frequent. Inadequate dietary intake of iron and folate, lack of acid and intrinsic factor secretion, mild chronic low-grade blood loss from the gastric remnant and recurrent ulceration are responsible.

Metabolic bone disease Both osteoporosis and osteomalacia can occur as a consequence of calcium and vitamin D malabsorption.

Gastric cancer An increased risk of gastric cancer has been reported from several epidemiological studies. Surgery itself is an independent risk factor for late development of malignancy in the gastric remnant but the risk is higher in those with hypochlorhydria, duodenogastric reflux of bile, smoking and *H. pylori* infection. Although the relative risk is increased, the absolute risk of cancer remains low and endoscopic surveillance is not indicated following gastric surgery.

Complications of peptic ulcer disease

Perforation

When perforation occurs, the contents of the stomach escape into the peritoneal cavity, leading to peritonitis. This is more common in duodenal than in gastric ulcers and is usually found with ulcers on the anterior wall. About one-quarter of all perforations occur in acute ulcers and NSAIDs are often incriminated. Perforation can be the first sign of ulcer and a history of recurrent epigastric pain is uncommon. The most striking symptom is sudden, severe pain; its distribution follows the spread of the gastric contents over the peritoneum. The pain initially develops in the upper abdomen and rapidly becomes generalised; shoulder tip pain is caused by irritation of the diaphragm. The pain is accompanied by shallow respiration, due to limitation of diaphragmatic movements, and by shock. The abdomen is held immobile and there is generalised 'board-like' rigidity. Bowel sounds are absent and liver dullness to percussion decreases due to the presence of gas under the diaphragm. After some hours, symptoms may improve, although abdominal rigidity remains. Later, the patient's condition deteriorates as general peritonitis develops. In at least 50% of cases, an erect chest X-ray shows free air beneath the diaphragm (see Fig. 21.11B, p. 773). If not, a water-soluble contrast swallow will confirm leakage of gastroduodenal contents. After resuscitation, the acute perforation should be treated surgically, either by simple closure or by conversion of the perforation into a pyloroplasty if it is large. On rare occasions, a 'Polya' partial gastrectomy is required. Following surgery, *H. pylori* should be treated (if present) and NSAIDs avoided. Perforation carries a mortality of 25%, reflecting the advanced age and significant comorbidity of the population that are affected.

Gastric outlet obstruction

The causes are shown in Box 21.39. The most common is an ulcer in the region of the pylorus. The presentation is with nausea, vomiting and abdominal distension. Large quantities of gastric content are often vomited and food eaten 24 hours or more previously may be recognised. Physical examination may show evidence of wasting and dehydration. A succussion splash may be elicited 4 hours or more after the last meal or drink. Visible gastric peristalsis is diagnostic of gastric outlet obstruction. Loss of acidic gastric contents leads to alkalosis and dehydration with low serum chloride and potassium and raised serum bicarbonate and urea concentrations (hypochloraemic metabolic alkalosis).

21

> ### 21.38 Peptic ulcer disease in old age
>
> - **Gastroduodenal ulcers**: have a greater incidence, admission rate and mortality.
> - **Causes**: high prevalence of *H. pylori*, use of non-steroidal anti-inflammatory drugs and impaired defence mechanisms.
> - **Atypical presentations**: pain and dyspepsia are frequently absent or atypical. Older people often develop complications, such as bleeding or perforation, without a dyspeptic history.
> - **Bleeding**: older patients require more intensive management because they have more limited reserve to withstand hypovolaemia.

> ### i 21.39 Differential diagnosis and management of gastric outlet obstruction
>
> | Cause | Management |
> | --- | --- |
> | Fibrotic stricture from duodenal ulcer (pyloric stenosis) | Balloon dilatation or surgery |
> | Oedema from pyloric channel or duodenal ulcer | Proton pump inhibitor therapy |
> | Carcinoma of antrum | Surgery |
> | Adult hypertrophic pyloric stenosis | Surgery |

Paradoxical aciduria occurs because of enhanced renal absorption of Na^+ in exchange for H^+. Endoscopy should be performed after the stomach has been emptied using a wide-bore nasogastric tube. Intravenous correction of dehydration is undertaken and, in severe cases, at least 4 L of isotonic saline and 80 mmol of potassium may be necessary during the first 24 hours. In some patients, PPI drugs heal ulcers, relieve pyloric oedema and overcome the need for surgery. Endoscopic balloon dilatation of benign stenoses may be possible in some patients but in others partial gastrectomy is necessary; this is best done after a 7-day period of nasogastric aspiration, which enables the stomach to return to normal size. A gastroenterostomy is an alternative operation but, unless this is accompanied by vagotomy, patients will require long-term PPI therapy to prevent stomal ulceration.

Bleeding

See page 780.

Zollinger–Ellison syndrome

This is a rare disorder characterised by the triad of severe peptic ulceration, gastric acid hypersecretion and a neuro-endocrine tumour (p. 678) of the pancreas or duodenum ('gastrinoma'). It probably accounts for about 0.1% of all cases of duodenal ulceration. The syndrome occurs in either sex at any age, although it is most common between 30 and 50 years of age.

Pathophysiology

The tumour secretes gastrin, which stimulates acid secretion to its maximal capacity and increases the parietal cell mass three- to sixfold. The acid output may be so great that it reaches the upper small intestine, reducing the luminal pH to 2 or less. Pancreatic lipase is inactivated and bile acids are precipitated. Diarrhoea and steatorrhoea result. Around 90% of tumours occur in the pancreatic head or proximal duodenal wall. At least half are multiple and tumour size can vary from 1 mm to 20 cm. Approximately one-half to two-thirds are malignant but are often slow-growing. Between 20% and 60% of patients have multiple endocrine neoplasia (MEN) type 1 (p. 688).

Clinical features

The presentation is with severe and often multiple peptic ulcers in unusual sites, such as the post-bulbar duodenum, jejunum or oesophagus. There is a poor response to standard ulcer therapy. The history is usually short, and bleeding and perforations are common. Diarrhoea is seen in one-third or more of patients and can be the presenting feature.

Investigations

Hypersecretion of acid under basal conditions, with little increase following pentagastrin, may be confirmed by gastric aspiration. Serum gastrin levels are grossly elevated (10- to 1000-fold). Injection of the hormone secretin normally causes no change or a slight decrease in circulating gastrin concentrations, but in Zollinger–Ellison syndrome it produces a paradoxical and dramatic increase in gastrin. Tumour localisation (and staging) is best achieved by a combination of CT and EUS; radio-labelled somatostatin receptor scintigraphy and [68]gallium DOTATATE PET scanning may also be used for tumour detection and staging.

Management

Some 30% of small and single tumours can be localised and resected but many tumours are multifocal (especially in the context of MEN 1). Some patients present with metastatic disease and, in these circumstances, surgery is inappropriate. In the majority of these individuals, continuous therapy with omeprazole or other PPIs can be successful in healing ulcers and alleviating diarrhoea, although double the normal dose is required. The synthetic somatostatin analogue, octreotide, given by subcutaneous injection, reduces gastrin secretion and may be of value. Other treatment options for pancreatic neuro-endocrine tumours are discussed on page 678. Overall 5-year survival is 60–75% and all patients should undergo genetic screening for MEN 1.

Functional disorders

Functional dyspepsia

This is defined as chronic dyspepsia in the absence of organic disease. Other commonly reported symptoms include early satiety, fullness, bloating and nausea. 'Ulcer-like' and 'dysmotility-type' subgroups are often reported but there is overlap between these and with irritable bowel syndrome.

Pathophysiology

The cause is poorly understood but probably covers a spectrum of mucosal, motility and psychiatric disorders.

Clinical features

Patients are usually young (<40 years) and women are affected twice as commonly as men. Abdominal discomfort is associated with a combination of other 'dyspeptic' symptoms, the most common being nausea, satiety and bloating after meals. Morning symptoms are characteristic and pain or nausea may occur on waking. Direct enquiry may elicit symptoms suggestive of irritable bowel syndrome. Peptic ulcer disease must be considered, while in older people intra-abdominal malignancy is a prime concern. There are no diagnostic signs, apart from inappropriate tenderness on abdominal palpation, perhaps. Symptoms may appear disproportionate to clinical well-being and there is no weight loss. Patients often appear anxious. A drug history should be taken and the possibility of a depressive illness should be considered. Pregnancy should be ruled out in young women before radiological studies are undertaken. Alcohol misuse should be suspected when early-morning nausea and retching are prominent.

Investigations

The history will often suggest the diagnosis. All patients should be checked for *H. pylori* infection and patients over the age of 55 years should undergo endoscopy to exclude mucosal disease. While an ultrasound scan may detect gallstones, these are rarely responsible for dyspeptic symptoms.

Management

The most important elements are explanation and reassurance. Possible psychological factors should be explored and the concept of psychological influences on gut function should be explained. Idiosyncratic and restrictive diets are of little benefit but smaller portions and fat restriction may help.

Up to 10% of patients benefit from *H. pylori* eradication therapy and this should be offered to infected individuals. Eradication also removes a major risk factor for peptic ulcers and gastric cancer but at the cost of a small risk of side-effects and worsening symptoms of underlying gastro-oesophageal reflux disease. Drug treatment is not especially successful but merits trial. Antacids, such as hydrotalcite, are sometimes helpful. Prokinetic drugs, such as metoclopramide (10 mg 3 times daily) or domperidone (10–20 mg 3 times daily), may be given before meals if nausea, vomiting or bloating is prominent. Metoclopramide may induce extrapyramidal side-effects, including tardive dyskinesia in young patients. H_2-receptor antagonist drugs may be tried if night pain or heartburn is troublesome. Low-dose tricyclic agents, such as amitriptyline, are of value in up to two-thirds.

Symptoms that can be associated with an identifiable cause of stress resolve with appropriate counselling. Some patients have major psychological disorders that result in persistent or recurrent symptoms and need behavioural or other formal psychotherapy (p. 1190).

Functional causes of vomiting

Psychogenic retching or vomiting may arise in anxiety. It typically occurs on wakening or immediately after breakfast, and only rarely later in the day. The disorder is probably a reaction to facing up to the worries of everyday life; in the young, it can be due to school phobia. Early morning vomiting also occurs in pregnancy, alcohol misuse and depression. Although functional vomiting may occur regularly over long periods, there is little or no weight loss. Children, and less often adults, sometimes suffer from acute and recurrent disabling bouts of vomiting for days at a time. The cause of this cyclical vomiting syndrome is unknown but in some adults it is associated with cannabis use.

In all patients it is essential to exclude other common causes (p. 780). Tranquillisers and antiemetic drugs (metoclopramide 10 mg 3 times daily, domperidone 10 mg 3 times daily, prochlorperazine 5–10 mg 3 times daily) have only a secondary place in management. Antidepressants in full dose may be effective (p. 1199).

Gastroparesis

Defective gastric emptying without mechanical obstruction of the stomach or duodenum can occur as a primary event, due to inherited or acquired disorders of the gastric pacemaker, or can be secondary to disorders of autonomic nerves (particularly diabetic neuropathy) or the gastroduodenal musculature (systemic sclerosis, myotonic dystrophies and amyloidosis). Drugs such as opiates, calcium channel antagonists and those with anticholinergic activity (tricyclics, phenothiazines) can also cause gastroparesis. Early satiety and recurrent vomiting are the major symptoms; abdominal fullness and a succussion splash may be present on examination. Treatment is based on small, frequent, low-fat meals and the use of metoclopramide and domperidone. In severe cases, nutritional failure can occur and long-term jejunostomy feeding or total parenteral nutrition is required. Surgical insertion of a gastric neurostimulator has been successful in some cases, especially those complicating diabetic autonomic neuropathy.

Tumours of the stomach

Gastric carcinoma

Gastric carcinoma is the third leading cause of cancer death worldwide but there is marked geographical variation in incidence. It is most common in China, Japan, Korea (incidence 40/100 000 males), Eastern Europe and parts of South America (20/100 000). Rates in the UK are 12/100 000 for men. In most countries, the incidence is 50% lower in women. In both sexes, it rises sharply

after 50 years of age. Studies of Japanese migrants to the USA have revealed a much lower incidence in the second generation, confirming the importance of environmental factors. The overall prognosis is poor, with less than 30% surviving 5 years, and the best hope for improved survival lies in more efficient detection of tumours at an earlier stage.

Pathophysiology

Infection with *H. pylori* plays a key pathogenic role and the infection has been classified by the International Agency for Research on Cancer (IARC) as a definite human carcinogen. It is associated with chronic atrophic gastritis, gastric mucosal atrophy and gastric cancer (Fig. 21.39). It has been estimated that *H. pylori* infection may contribute to the occurrence of gastric cancer in 70% of cases. Although the majority of *H. pylori*-infected individuals have normal or increased acid secretion, a few become hypo- or achlorhydric and these people are thought to be at greatest risk. *H. pylori*-induced chronic inflammation with generation of reactive oxygen species and depletion of the normally abundant antioxidant ascorbic acid are also important. There is strong evidence that *H. pylori* eradication, especially if achieved before irreversible pre-neoplastic changes (atrophy and intestinal metaplasia) have developed, reduces the risk of cancer development in high-risk populations and is cost-effective.

Diets rich in salted, smoked or pickled foods and the consumption of nitrites and nitrates may increase cancer risk. Carcinogenic *N*-nitroso-compounds are formed from nitrates by the action of nitrite-reducing bacteria that colonise the achlorhydric stomach. Diets lacking in fresh fruit and vegetables, as well as vitamins C and A, may also contribute. Other risk factors are listed in Box 21.40. No predominant genetic abnormality has been identified, although cancer risk is increased two- to threefold in first-degree relatives of patients, and links with blood group A have been reported. Some host genetic factors related to inflammatory genes and prostate stem cell antigen have recently been associated with increased risk of gastric caner. Rarely, gastric cancer may be inherited in an autosomal dominant manner in association with mutations of the *E-cadherin* (*CDH1*) gene.

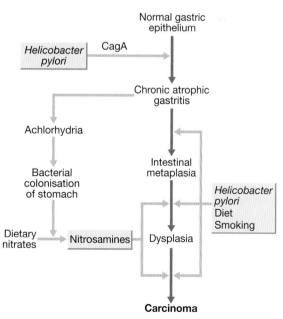

Fig. 21.39 **Gastric carcinogenesis: a possible mechanism.** (CagA = cytotoxin-associated gene)

i 21.40 Risk factors for gastric cancer

- *Helicobacter pylori*
- Smoking
- Alcohol
- Dietary associations (see text)
- Autoimmune gastritis (pernicious anaemia)
- Adenomatous gastric polyps
- Previous partial gastrectomy (>20 years)
- Ménétrier's disease
- Hereditary diffuse gastric cancer families (*CDH1* mutations)
- Familial adenomatous polyposis (p. 828)

Fig. 21.40 Gastric carcinoma. Endoscopic finding of a large polypoidal mass arising from the wall of the stomach.

Virtually all tumours are adenocarcinomas arising from mucus-secreting cells in the base of the gastric crypts. Most develop on a background of chronic atrophic gastritis with intestinal metaplasia and dysplasia. Cancers are either 'intestinal', arising from areas of intestinal metaplasia with histological features reminiscent of intestinal epithelium, or 'diffuse', arising from normal gastric mucosa. Intestinal carcinomas are more common and arise against a background of chronic mucosal injury. Diffuse cancers tend to be poorly differentiated and occur in younger patients. In the developing world, 50% of gastric cancers develop in the antrum; 20–30% occur in the gastric body, often on the greater curve; and 20% are found in the cardia. In Western populations, however, proximal gastric tumours are becoming more common than those arising in the body and distal stomach. This change in disease pattern may be a reflection of changes in lifestyle or the decreasing prevalence of *H. pylori* in the West. Diffuse submucosal infiltration by a scirrhous cancer (linitis plastica) is uncommon. Early gastric cancer is defined as cancer confined to the mucosa or submucosa. It is more often recognised in Japan, where widespread screening is practised. Some cases can be cured by endoscopic mucosal or submucosal resection. The majority of patients (>80%) in the West, however, present with advanced gastric cancer.

Clinical features

Early gastric cancer is usually asymptomatic but may be discovered during endoscopy for investigation of dyspepsia. Two-thirds of patients with advanced cancers have weight loss and 50% have ulcer-like pain. Anorexia and nausea occur in one-third, while early satiety, haematemesis, melaena and dyspepsia alone are less common. Dysphagia occurs in tumours of the gastric cardia that obstruct the gastro-oesophageal junction. Anaemia from occult bleeding is also common. Examination may reveal no abnormalities but signs of weight loss, anaemia and a palpable epigastric mass are not infrequent. Jaundice or ascites signifies metastatic spread. Occasionally, tumour spread occurs to the supraclavicular lymph nodes (Troisier's sign), umbilicus (Sister Joseph's nodule) or ovaries (Krukenberg tumour). Paraneoplastic phenomena, such as acanthosis nigricans, thrombophlebitis (Trousseau's sign) and dermatomyositis, occur rarely. Metastases arise most commonly in the liver, lungs, peritoneum and bone marrow.

Investigations

Upper gastrointestinal endoscopy is the investigation of choice (Fig. 21.40) and should be performed promptly in any dyspeptic patient with 'alarm features' (see Box 21.15, p. 779). Multiple biopsies from the edge and base of a gastric ulcer are required. Barium meal is a poor alternative, since any abnormalities must be followed by endoscopy and biopsy. Once the diagnosis is made, further imaging is necessary for staging and assessment of resectability. CT will provide evidence of intra-abdominal spread or liver metastases. Even with these techniques, laparoscopy with peritoneal washings is required to determine whether the tumour is resectable, as it is the only modality that will reliably detect peritoneal spread.

Management

Surgery

Resection offers the only hope of cure and this can be achieved in about 90% of patients with early gastric cancer. For the majority of patients with locally advanced disease, total gastrectomy with lymphadenectomy is the operation of choice, preserving the spleen if possible. Proximal tumours involving the oesophago-gastric junction also require a distal oesophagectomy. Small, distally sited tumours can be managed by a partial gastrectomy with lymphadenectomy and either a Billroth I or a Roux en Y reconstruction. More extensive lymph node resection may increase survival rates but carries greater morbidity. Even for those who cannot be cured, palliative resection may be necessary when patients present with bleeding or gastric outflow obstruction. Following surgery, recurrence is much more likely if serosal penetration has occurred, although complete removal of all macroscopic tumour combined with lymphadenectomy will achieve a 50–60% 5-year survival. Perioperative chemotherapy with epirubicin, cisplatin and fluorouracil (ECF) improves survival rates.

Palliative treatment

In patients with inoperable tumours, survival can be improved and palliation of symptoms achieved with chemotherapy using 5-fluorouracil and cisplatin, ECF or other platinum- and taxane-based regimens. The biological agent trastuzumab may benefit some patients whose tumours over-express HER2 (p. 1322). Endoscopic laser ablation for control of dysphagia or recurrent bleeding benefits some patients. Carcinomas at the cardia or pylorus may require endoscopic dilatation or insertion of expandable metallic stents for relief of dysphagia or vomiting. A nasogastric tube may offer temporary relief of vomiting due to gastric outlet obstruction (Box 21.41).

21.41 How to insert a nasogastric tube

Equipment

- 8–9F 'fine-bore' tube for feeding or 16–18F 'wide-bore' tube for drainage
- Lubricant jelly
- Cup of water and straw for sipping
- Adhesive tape
- pH (not litmus) paper
- Sickness bowl and tissues
- Catheter drainage bag and clamp (for drainage)

Technique

- A clear explanation and a calm patient are essential
- Establish a 'stop signal' for the patient to use, if needed
- Ask the patient to sit semi-upright
- Examine the nose for deformity or blockage to determine which side to use
- Measure the distance from ear to xiphoid process via the nose and mark the position on the tube
- Advance the lubricated tube tip slowly along the floor of the nasal passage to the oropharynx
- Ask the patient to sip water and advance the tube 2–3 cm with each swallow
- Stop, withdraw and retry if the patient is distressed or coughing, as the tube may have entered the larynx
- Advance until the mark on the tube reaches the tip of the nose and secure with tape
- Aspirate the contents and check pH (gastric acid confirmed if pH <5). If in doubt, perform a chest X-ray to confirm tube position (usually necessary with feeding tubes)
- Attach the catheter drainage bag, if necessary, and clamp

Aftercare

- Flush the tube daily after feeding or drug dosing
- Check position regularly and look for signs of displacement
- Check with the pharmacist what drugs, if any, can be safely given via the tube

Gastric lymphoma

This is a rare tumour, accounting for less than 5% of all gastric malignancies. The stomach is, however, the most common site for extranodal non-Hodgkin lymphoma and 60% of all primary gastrointestinal lymphomas occur at this site. Lymphoid tissue is not found in the normal stomach but lymphoid aggregates develop in the presence of *H. pylori* infection. Indeed, *H. pylori* infection is closely associated with the development of a low-grade lymphoma (classified as extranodal marginal-zone lymphomas of MALT type). EUS plays an important role in staging these lesions by accurately defining the depth of invasion into the gastric wall.

The clinical presentation is similar to that of gastric cancer and endoscopically the tumour appears as a polypoid or ulcerating mass. While initial treatment of low-grade lesions confined to the superficial layers of the gastric wall consists of *H. pylori* eradication and close observation, 25% contain t(11:18) chromosomal translocations. In these cases, additional radiotherapy or chemotherapy is usually necessary. High-grade B-cell lymphomas should be treated by a combination of rituximab, chemotherapy (p. 962), surgery and radiotherapy. The choice depends on the site and extent of tumour, the presence of comorbid illnesses, and other factors, such as symptoms of bleeding and gastric outflow obstruction. The prognosis depends on the stage at diagnosis. Features predicting a favourable prognosis are stage I or II disease, small resectable tumours, tumours with low-grade histology, and age below 60 years.

Other tumours of the stomach

Gastrointestinal stromal cell tumours (GISTs), arising from the interstitial cells of Cajal, are occasionally found at upper gastrointestinal endoscopy. They are differentiated from other mesenchymal tumours by expression of the *c-kit* proto-oncogene, which encodes a tyrosine kinase receptor. These tumours, particularly the smaller lesions of less than 2 cm, are usually benign and asymptomatic, but the larger ones may have malignant potential and may occasionally be responsible for dyspepsia, ulceration and gastrointestinal bleeding. Small lesions (<2 cm) are usually followed by endoscopy, while larger ones require surgical resection. Very large lesions should be treated pre-operatively with imatinib (a tyrosine kinase inhibitor) to reduce their size and make surgery easier. Imatinib can also provide prolonged control of metastatic GISTs.

A variety of polyps occur. Hyperplastic polyps and fundic cystic gland polyps are common and of no consequence. Adenomatous polyps are rare but have malignant potential and should be removed endoscopically.

Occasionally, gastric carcinoid tumours are seen in the fundus and body in patients with long-standing pernicious anaemia. These benign tumours arise from ECL or other endocrine cells, and are often multiple but rarely invasive. Unlike carcinoid tumours arising elsewhere in the gastrointestinal tract, they usually run a benign and favourable course. Large (>2 cm) carcinoids may, however, metastasise and should be removed. Rarely, small nodules of ectopic pancreatic exocrine tissue are found. These 'pancreatic rests' may be mistaken for gastric neoplasms and usually cause no symptoms. EUS is the most useful investigation.

Diseases of the small intestine

Disorders causing malabsorption

Coeliac disease

Coeliac disease is an inflammatory disorder of the small bowel occurring in genetically susceptible individuals, which results from intolerance to wheat gluten and similar proteins found in rye, barley and, to a lesser extent, oats. It can result in malabsorption and responds to a gluten-free diet. The condition occurs worldwide but is more common in northern Europe. The prevalence in the UK is approximately 1%, although 50% of these people are asymptomatic. These include both undiagnosed 'silent' cases of the disease and cases of 'latent' coeliac disease – genetically susceptible people who may later develop clinical coeliac disease.

Pathophysiology

The precise mechanism of mucosal damage is unclear but immunological responses to gluten play a key role (Fig. 21.41). There is a strong genetic component, with around 10% of first-degree relatives of an index case affected, and there is strong (approximately 75%) concordance in monozygotic twins. There is a strong association with human leukocyte antigen (HLA)-DQ2/DQ8. Dysbiosis of the intestinal microbiota has been identified but it is unclear if this is pathological or a response to the underlying mucosal changes.

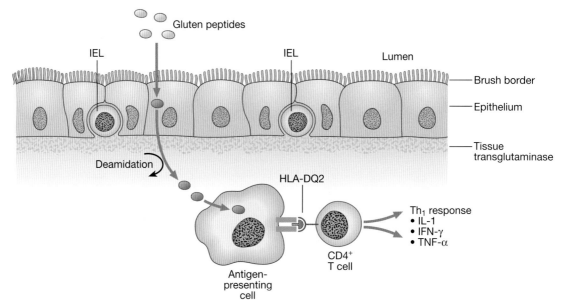

Fig. 21.41 Pathophysiology of coeliac disease. After being taken up by epithelial cells, gluten peptides are deamidated by the enzyme tissue transglutaminase in the subepithelial layer. They are then able to fit the antigen-binding motif on human leucocyte antigen (HLA)-DQ2-positive antigen-presenting cells. Recognition by CD4+ T cells triggers a Th1 immune response with generation of pro-inflammatory cytokines: interleukin-1 (IL-1), interferon gamma (IFN-γ) and tumour necrosis factor alpha (TNF-α). Lymphocytes infiltrate the lamina propria and an increase in intra-epithelial lymphocytes (IELs), crypt hyperplasia and villous atrophy ensue.

Clinical features

Coeliac disease can present at any age. In infancy, it occurs after weaning on to cereals and typically presents with diarrhoea, malabsorption and failure to thrive. In older children, it may present with non-specific features, such as delayed growth. Features of malnutrition are found on examination and mild abdominal distension may be present. Affected children have growth and pubertal delay, leading to short stature in adulthood.

In adults, the disease usually presents during the third or fourth decade and females are affected twice as often as males. The presentation is highly variable, depending on the severity and extent of small bowel involvement. Some have florid malabsorption, while others develop non-specific symptoms, such as tiredness, weight loss, folate deficiency or iron deficiency anaemia. Other presentations include oral ulceration, dyspepsia and bloating. Unrecognised coeliac disease is associated with mild under-nutrition and osteoporosis.

Coeliac disease is associated with other HLA-linked autoimmune disorders and with certain other diseases (Box 21.42). In some centres, people at higher risk of developing coeliac disease, such as those with type 1 diabetes, may undergo periodic antibody screening. Such screening may identify people with asymptomatic or minimally symptomatic disease; there is controversy about the optimum management strategy for such individuals.

Investigations

These are performed to confirm the diagnosis and to look for consequences of malabsorption.

Duodenal biopsy

Endoscopic small bowel biopsy is the gold standard. Endoscopic appearances should not preclude biopsy, as the mucosa usually looks normal. As the histological changes can be patchy, an adequate number of biopsies – currently, more than four biopsies from the second part of the duodenum plus one from the duodenal bulb – should be retrieved. The histological features are

21.42 Disease associations of coeliac disease

- Type 1 diabetes mellitus (2–8%)
- Thyroid disease (5%)
- Primary biliary cirrhosis (3%)
- Sjögren's syndrome (3%)
- Immunoglobulin A deficiency (2%)
- Pernicious anaemia
- Sarcoidosis
- Neurological complications:
  Encephalopathy
  Cerebellar atrophy
  Peripheral neuropathy
  Epilepsy

- Myasthenia gravis
- Dermatitis herpetiformis
- Down's syndrome
- Enteropathy-associated T-cell lymphoma
- Small bowel carcinoma
- Squamous carcinoma of oesophagus
- Ulcerative jejunitis
- Pancreatic insufficiency
- Microscopic colitis
- Splenic atrophy

21.43 Important causes of subtotal villous atrophy

- Coeliac disease
- Tropical sprue
- Dermatitis herpetiformis
- Lymphoma
- HIV-related enteropathy

- Giardiasis
- Hypogammaglobulinaemia
- Radiation
- Whipple's disease
- Zollinger–Ellison syndrome

usually characteristic but other causes of villous atrophy should be considered (Box 21.43 and Fig. 21.42). Sometimes the villi appear normal but there are excess numbers of intra-epithelial lymphocytes (lymphocytic duodenosis).

Antibodies

Antibody tests constitute a valuable screening tool in patients with diarrhoea or other suggestive symptoms but are not a diagnostic substitute for small bowel biopsy at present. Tissue transglutaminase (tTG) is now recognised as the autoantigen for

Fig. 21.42 Jejunal mucosa. [A] Normal. [B] Subtotal villous atrophy in coeliac disease. There is blunting of villi (B), crypt hyperplasia (H) and inflammatory infiltration of the lamina propria (I).

anti-endomysial antibodies. If the antibody screen is positive, adult patients should remain on a gluten-containing diet until duodenal biopsies are taken. High-titre serology in children can be diagnostic without the need for endoscopy and biopsy. Antibody titres usually become negative with successful treatment.

Anti-endomysial antibodies of the IgA class are detectable by immunofluorescence in most untreated cases. They are sensitive (85–95%) and specific (approximately 99%) for the diagnosis, except in very young infants. IgG antibodies, however, must be analysed in patients with coexisting IgA deficiency. The tTG assay has become the serological test of choice in many countries, as it is easier to perform, is semi-quantitative, has more than 95% sensitivity and specificity, and is more accurate in patients with IgA deficiency.

Haematology and biochemistry

A full blood count may show microcytic or macrocytic anaemia from iron or folate deficiency and features of hyposplenism (target cells, spherocytes and Howell–Jolly bodies). Biochemical tests may reveal reduced concentrations of calcium, magnesium, total protein, albumin or vitamin D. Serum IgA measurement is required to ensure an appropriate IgA response and to allow analysis of serological testing.

Other investigations

Measurement of bone density should be considered to look for evidence of osteoporosis, especially in older patients and post-menopausal women.

Management

The aims are to correct existing deficiencies of micronutrients, such as iron, folate, calcium and/or vitamin D, and to achieve mucosal healing through a life-long gluten-free diet. This requires the exclusion of wheat, rye, barley and initially oats, although oats may be re-introduced safely in most patients after 6–12 months. Initially, frequent dietary counselling is required to make sure the diet is being observed, as the most common reason for failure to improve with dietary treatment is accidental or unrecognised gluten ingestion. Mineral and vitamin supplements are also given when indicated but are seldom necessary when a strict gluten-free diet is adhered to. Booklets produced by coeliac societies in many countries, containing diet sheets and recipes for the use of gluten-free flour, are of great value. Dietetic follow-up is key to management. Patients should be followed up after initiation of a gluten-free diet, with assessment of symptoms, weight and nutritional status, and blood should be taken for measurement of tTG or anti-endomysial antibodies. There are currently no additional non-invasive tests to assess small bowel mucosal healing. Repeat small bowel biopsies are not required routinely but should be considered in patients whose symptoms fail to improve and those in whom antibody levels remain high. In these

circumstances, if the diet is satisfactory, then other conditions, such as pancreatic insufficiency or microscopic colitis, should be sought, as should complications of coeliac disease, such as ulcerative jejunitis or enteropathy-associated T-cell lymphoma. There remain a small number of patients who fail to respond adequately to a gluten-free diet and they require therapy with glucocorticoids or immunosuppressive drugs.

Complications

A twofold-increased risk of malignancy, particularly of enteropathy-associated T-cell lymphoma, small bowel carcinoma and squamous carcinoma of the oesophagus, has been reported.

A few patients develop ulcerative jejuno-ileitis. This may present with fever, pain, obstruction or perforation. This diagnosis can be made by barium studies or enteroscopy but laparotomy and full-thickness biopsy may be required. Treatment is difficult. Glucocorticoids are used with mixed success and some patients require surgical resection and parenteral nutrition. The course is often progressive.

Osteoporosis and osteomalacia may occur in patients with long-standing, poorly controlled coeliac disease. These complications are less common in those who adhere strictly to a gluten-free diet.

Dermatitis herpetiformis

This is characterised by crops of intensely itchy blisters over the elbows, knees, back and buttocks (p. 1256). Immunofluorescence shows granular or linear IgA deposition at the dermo-epidermal junction. Almost all patients have partial villous atrophy on duodenal biopsy, identical to that seen in coeliac disease, even though they usually have no gastrointestinal symptoms. In contrast, fewer than 10% of coeliac patients have evidence of dermatitis herpetiformis, although both disorders are associated with the same histocompatibility antigen groups. The rash usually responds to a gluten-free diet but some patients require additional treatment with dapsone (100–150 mg daily).

Tropical sprue

Tropical sprue is defined as chronic, progressive malabsorption in a patient in or from the tropics, associated with abnormalities of small intestinal structure and function. The disease occurs mainly in the West Indies and in southern India, Malaysia and Indonesia.

Pathophysiology

The epidemiological pattern and occasional epidemics suggest that an infective agent may be involved. Although no single bacterium has been isolated, the condition often begins after an acute diarrhoeal illness. Small bowel bacterial overgrowth with *Escherichia coli*, *Enterobacter* and *Klebsiella* is frequently seen. The changes closely resemble those of coeliac disease.

21

Clinical features

There is diarrhoea, abdominal distension, anorexia, fatigue and weight loss. In visitors to the tropics, the onset of severe diarrhoea may be sudden and accompanied by fever. When the disorder becomes chronic, the features of megaloblastic anaemia (vitamin B_{12} and folic acid malabsorption) and other deficiencies, including ankle oedema, glossitis and stomatitis, are common. Remissions and relapses may occur. The differential diagnosis in the indigenous tropical population is an infective cause of diarrhoea. The important differential diagnosis in visitors to the tropics is giardiasis (p. 287).

Management

Tetracycline (250 mg 4 times daily for 28 days) is the treatment of choice and brings about long-term remission or cure. In most patients, pharmacological doses of folic acid (5 mg daily) improve symptoms and jejunal morphology. In some cases, treatment must be prolonged before improvement occurs and occasionally patients must leave the tropics.

Small bowel bacterial overgrowth ('blind loop syndrome')

The normal duodenum and jejunum contain fewer than 10^4/mL organisms, which are usually derived from saliva. The count of coliform organisms never exceeds 10^3/mL. In bacterial overgrowth, there may be 10^8–10^{10}/mL organisms, most of which are normally found only in the colon. Disorders that impair the normal physiological mechanisms controlling bacterial proliferation in the intestine predispose to bacterial overgrowth (Box 21.44). The most important are loss of gastric acidity, impaired intestinal motility and structural abnormalities that allow colonic bacteria to gain access to the small intestine or provide a secluded haven from the peristaltic stream.

Pathophysiology

Bacterial overgrowth can occur in patients with small bowel diverticuli. Another cause is diabetic autonomic neuropathy (p. 760), which reduces small bowel motility and affects enterocyte secretion. In systemic sclerosis, bacterial overgrowth arises because the circular and longitudinal layers of the intestinal muscle are fibrosed and motility is abnormal. In idiopathic

21.44 Causes of small bowel bacterial overgrowth

Mechanism	Examples
Hypo- or achlorhydria	Pernicious anaemia Partial gastrectomy Long-term proton pump inhibitor therapy
Impaired intestinal motility	Systemic sclerosis Diabetic autonomic neuropathy Chronic intestinal pseudo-obstruction
Structural abnormalities	Gastric surgery (blind loop after Billroth II operation) Jejunal diverticulosis Enterocolic fistulae* Extensive small bowel resection Strictures*
Impaired immune function	Hypogammaglobulinaemia

*Most commonly caused by Crohn's disease.

hypogammaglobulinaemia (p. 78), bacterial overgrowth occurs because the IgA and IgM levels in serum and jejunal secretions are reduced. Chronic diarrhoea and malabsorption occur because of bacterial overgrowth and recurrent gastrointestinal infections (particularly giardiasis, p. 287).

Clinical features

The patient presents with watery diarrhoea and/or steatorrhoea, and with anaemia due to B_{12} deficiency. These arise because of deconjugation of bile acids, which impairs micelle formation, and because of bacterial utilisation of vitamin B_{12}. There may also be symptoms from the underlying intestinal cause.

Investigations

The diagnosis of blind loops or fistulae can often be made by barium small bowel meal and follow-through or small bowel MRI enterography. Endoscopic duodenal biopsies are useful in excluding coeliac disease. Jejunal contents for bacteriological examination can also be aspirated at endoscopy but laboratory analysis requires anaerobic and aerobic culture techniques. Bacterial overgrowth can also be diagnosed non-invasively using hydrogen breath tests, although they lack sensitivity. These simple, non-radioactive tests involve serial measurement of breath samples for hydrogen after oral ingestion of 50 g of glucose or lactulose. If bacteria are present within the small bowel, they rapidly metabolise the glucose, causing an early rise in exhaled hydrogen, in advance of that normally resulting from metabolism by colonic flora. Biochemical analysis may reveal low serum levels of vitamin B_{12}, with normal or elevated folate levels because the bacteria produce folic acid. Hypogammaglobulinaemia can be diagnosed by measurement of serum immunoglobulins and by intestinal biopsy, which shows reduced or absent plasma cells and nodular lymphoid hyperplasia.

Management

The underlying cause of small bowel bacterial overgrowth should be addressed, where possible. A course of broad-spectrum antibiotic for 2 weeks is the first-line treatment, although there is no consensus on agent or dose. Examples include tetracycline (250 mg 4 times daily), metronidazole (400 mg 3 times daily), amoxicillin (250 mg 3 times daily) or ciprofloxacin (250 mg twice daily). If breath testing reveals high methane production, addition of neomycin (500 mg twice daily) may be beneficial. Up to 50% of patients do not respond adequately and relapse rates are high. Some patients require up to 4 weeks of treatment and, in a few, continuous rotating courses of antibiotics are necessary. Consideration should be given to the risk of emerging antimicrobial resistance. Intramuscular vitamin B_{12} supplementation may be needed in chronic cases, as the bacteria utilise vitamin B_{12}. Patients with motility disorders, such as diabetes and systemic sclerosis, can sometimes benefit from antidiarrhoeal drugs (diphenoxylate (5 mg 3 times daily orally) or loperamide (2 mg 4–6 times daily) orally). Giardiasis should

21.45 Malabsorption in old age

- **Coeliac disease**: symptoms such as dyspepsia tend to be vague; only 25% present classically with diarrhoea and weight loss. Metabolic bone disease, folate or iron deficiency, coagulopathy and small bowel lymphoma are more common.
- **Small bowel bacterial overgrowth**: more common due to atrophic gastritis, resulting in hypo- or achlorhydria, increased prevalence of jejunal diverticulosis and long-term adverse effects of gastric surgery for ulcer disease.

be controlled in patients with hypogammaglobulinaemia using metronidazole or tinidazole, but if symptoms fail to respond adequately, immunoglobulin infusions may be required.

Whipple's disease

This rare condition is characterised by infiltration of small intestinal mucosa by 'foamy' macrophages, which stain positive with periodic acid–Schiff (PAS) reagent. The disease is a multisystem one and almost any organ can be affected, sometimes long before gastrointestinal involvement becomes apparent (Box 21.46).

Pathophysiology

Whipple's disease is caused by infection with the Gram-positive bacillus *Tropheryma whipplei*, which becomes resident within macrophages in the bowel mucosa. Villi are widened and flattened, containing densely packed macrophages in the lamina propria, which obstruct lymphatic drainage and cause fat malabsorption.

Clinical features

Middle-aged Caucasian men are most frequently affected and presentation depends on the pattern of organ involvement. Low-grade fever is common and most patients have joint symptoms to some degree, often as the first manifestation. Occasionally, neurological manifestations may predominate and CNS involvement is the most serious consequence.

Investigations

Diagnosis is made by the characteristic features on small bowel biopsy, with characterisation of the bacillus by polymerase chain reaction (PCR).

Management

Whipple's disease is often fatal if untreated but responds well, at least initially, to intravenous ceftriaxone (2 g daily for 2 weeks), followed by oral co-trimoxazole for at least 1 year. Symptoms

usually resolve quickly and biopsy changes revert to normal in a few weeks. Long-term follow-up is essential, as clinical relapse occurs in up to one-third of patients, often within the CNS; in this case, the same therapy is repeated or else treatment with doxycycline and hydroxychloroquine is necessary.

Bile acid diarrhoea

Bile acid diarrhoea can occur idiopathically (type 1), as a complication of small bowel resection, post cholecystectomy (type 2) or in association with other conditions such as microscopic colitis, chronic pancreatitis, coeliac disease, small intestinal bacterial overgrowth or diabetes mellitus. The population prevalence is estimated at around 1% and the disease is often under-diagnosed. It is now appreciated that many patients diagnosed with diarrhoea-predominant irritable bowel syndrome have evidence of bile acid diarrhoea. The most common scenario is in patients with Crohn's disease who have undergone ileal resection, which can also lead to other malabsorptive manifestations (Fig. 21.43). Unabsorbed bile salts pass into the colon, stimulating water and electrolyte secretion and causing diarrhoea. If hepatic synthesis of new bile acids cannot keep pace with faecal losses, fat malabsorption occurs. Another consequence is the formation of lithogenic bile, leading to gallstones. Renal calculi, rich in oxalate, develop. Normally, oxalate in the colon is bound to and precipitated by calcium. Unabsorbed bile salts preferentially bind calcium, leaving oxalate to be absorbed, with development of urinary oxalate calculi.

Patients have urgent watery diarrhoea or mild steatorrhoea. Contrast studies and tests of B$_{12}$ and bile acid absorption, such as the ^{75}Se-homocholic acid taurine (SeHCAT) test (p. 777), are useful investigations but are not available throughout the world due to use of synthetic radio-labelled compound. An elevated serum 7α-hydroxycholestenone is a useful non-invasive marker of bile acid diarrhoea. Diarrhoea usually responds well to bile acid sequestrants, such as colestyramine or colesevelam, which bind bile salts in the intestinal lumen. Aluminium hydroxide can be used as an alternative.

Short bowel syndrome

This is discussed in detail on page 708.

Radiation enteritis and proctocolitis

Intestinal damage occurs in 10–15% of patients undergoing radiotherapy for abdominal or pelvic malignancy. The risk varies with total dose, dosing schedule and the use of concomitant chemotherapy.

Pathophysiology

The rectum, sigmoid colon and terminal ileum are most frequently involved. Radiation causes acute inflammation, shortening of villi, oedema and crypt abscess formation. These usually resolve completely but some patients develop an obliterative endarteritis affecting the endothelium of submucosal arterioles over 2–12 months. In the longer term, this can provoke a fibrotic reaction, leading to adhesions, ulceration, strictures, obstruction or fistula to adjacent organs.

Clinical features

In the acute phase, there is nausea, vomiting, cramping abdominal pain and diarrhoea. When the rectum and colon are involved, rectal mucus, bleeding and tenesmus occur. The chronic phase develops after 5–10 years in some patients and produces one or more of the problems listed in Box 21.47.

21

i	**21.46 Clinical features of Whipple's disease**	
Gastrointestinal (>70%)		
• Diarrhoea (75%)	• Protein-losing enteropathy	
• Steatorrhoea	• Ascites	
• Weight loss (90%)	• Hepatosplenomegaly (<5%)	
Musculoskeletal (65%)		
• Seronegative large joint arthropathy	• Sacroiliitis	
Cardiac (10%)		
• Pericarditis	• Endocarditis	
• Myocarditis	• Coronary arteritis	
Neurological (10–40%)		
• Apathy	• Myoclonus	
• Fits	• Meningitis	
• Dementia	• Cranial nerve lesions	
Pulmonary (10–20%)		
• Chronic cough	• Pulmonary infiltrates	
• Pleurisy		
Haematological (60%)		
• Anaemia	• Lymphadenopathy	
Other (40%)		
• Fever	• Pigmentation	

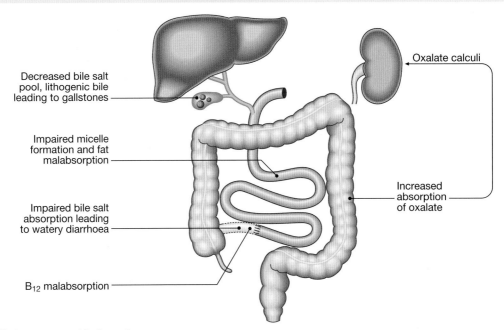

Fig. 21.43 Consequences of ileal resection.

Labels:
- Decreased bile salt pool, lithogenic bile leading to gallstones
- Impaired micelle formation and fat malabsorption
- Impaired bile salt absorption leading to watery diarrhoea
- B$_{12}$ malabsorption
- Oxalate calculi
- Increased absorption of oxalate

---

i	21.47 Chronic complications of intestinal irradiation

- Proctocolitis
- Bleeding from telangiectasia
- Small bowel strictures
- Fistulae: rectovaginal, colovesical, enterocolic
- Adhesions
- Malabsorption: bacterial overgrowth, bile acid diarrhoea (ileal damage)

Investigations

In the acute phase, the rectal changes at sigmoidoscopy resemble ulcerative proctitis (see Fig. 21.53, p. 819). An endoscopic biopsy from the rectal wall is associated with a 2% risk of fistula formation. The extent of the lesion can be assessed by colonoscopy. Barium follow-through or MRI enterography can be of diagnostic value in showing small bowel strictures, ulcers and fistulae.

Management

Diarrhoea in the acute phase should be treated with codeine phosphate, diphenoxylate or loperamide. Antibiotics may be required for bacterial overgrowth. Nutritional supplements are necessary when malabsorption is present. Colestyramine or colesevelam is useful for bile acid diarrhoea. Surgery should be avoided, if possible, because the injured intestine is difficult to resect and anastomose, but may be necessary for obstruction, perforation or fistula.

In radiation proctitis, the underlying pathophysiology is tissue ischaemia rather than inflammation; glucocorticoid enemas are therefore not effective. Traditionally, endoscopic argon plasma coagulation therapy was used but this is of limited benefit and can induce fistula, stricture or perforation. Effective treatments include sucralfate enema and hyperbaric oxygen.

Abetalipoproteinaemia

This rare autosomal recessive disorder is caused by deficiency of apolipoprotein B, which results in failure of chylomicron formation.

It leads to fat malabsorption and deficiency of fat-soluble vitamins. Jejunal biopsy reveals enterocytes distended with resynthesised triglyceride and normal villous morphology. Serum cholesterol and triglyceride levels are low. A number of other abnormalities occur in this syndrome, including acanthocytosis, retinitis pigmentosa and a progressive neurological disorder with cerebellar and dorsal column signs. Symptoms may be improved by a low-fat diet supplemented with medium-chain triglycerides and vitamins A, D, E and K.

Motility disorders

Chronic intestinal pseudo-obstruction

Small intestinal motility is disordered in conditions that affect the smooth muscle or nerves of the intestine. Many cases are 'primary' (idiopathic), while others are 'secondary' to a variety of disorders or drugs (Box 21.48).

Clinical features

There are recurrent episodes of nausea, vomiting, abdominal discomfort and distension, often worse after food. Alternating constipation and diarrhoea occur and weight loss results from malabsorption (due to bacterial overgrowth) and fear of eating. There may also be symptoms of dysmotility affecting other parts of the gastrointestinal tract, such as dysphagia, and features of bladder dysfunction in primary cases. Some patients develop severe abdominal pain for reasons that are poorly understood and this can be difficult to manage.

Investigations

The diagnosis is often delayed and a high index of suspicion is needed. Plain X-rays show distended loops of bowel and air–fluid levels but barium studies demonstrate no mechanical obstruction. Laparotomy is sometimes required to exclude obstruction and to obtain full-thickness biopsies of the intestine. Examination of biopsy material using specialised techniques, such as electron microscopy, and immunohistochemistry can diagnose the many

21.48 Causes of chronic intestinal pseudo-obstruction

Primary or idiopathic

- Rare familial visceral myopathies or neuropathies
- Congenital aganglionosis

Secondary

- Drugs (opiates, tricyclic antidepressants, phenothiazines)
- Smooth muscle disorders (systemic sclerosis, amyloidosis, mitochondrial myopathies)
- Myenteric plexus disorders, e.g. paraneoplastic syndrome in small-cell lung cancer
- Central nervous system disorders (Parkinson's disease, autonomic neuropathy)
- Endocrine and metabolic disorders (hypothyroidism, phaeochromocytoma, acute intermittent porphyria)

rare diseases of enteric smooth muscle and nerves that can cause this syndrome.

Management

This is often difficult. Underlying causes should be addressed and further surgery avoided. Metoclopramide or domperidone may enhance motility and antibiotics are given for bacterial overgrowth. Nutritional and psychological support is also necessary.

Miscellaneous disorders of the small intestine

Protein-losing enteropathy

This term is used when there is excessive loss of protein into the gut lumen, sufficient to cause hypoproteinaemia. Protein-losing enteropathy occurs in many gut disorders but is most common in those in which ulceration occurs (Box 21.49). In other disorders, protein loss can result from increased mucosal permeability or obstruction of intestinal lymphatic vessels. Patients present with peripheral oedema and hypoproteinaemia in the presence of normal liver function, low albumin and globulin, and without proteinuria. The diagnosis can be confirmed by measurement of faecal clearance of α_1-antitrypsin or ^{51}Cr-labelled albumin after intravenous injection. Other investigations should be performed to determine the underlying cause. Treatment is that of the underlying disorder, with nutritional support and measures to control peripheral oedema.

21.49 Causes of protein-losing enteropathy

With mucosal erosions or ulceration

- Crohn's disease
- Ulcerative colitis
- Radiation damage
- Oesophageal, gastric or colonic cancer
- Lymphoma

Without mucosal erosions or ulceration

- Ménétrier's disease
- Bacterial overgrowth
- Coeliac disease
- Tropical sprue
- Eosinophilic gastroenteritis
- Systemic lupus erythematosus

With lymphatic obstruction

- Intestinal lymphangiectasia
- Constrictive pericarditis
- Lymphoma
- Whipple's disease

Intestinal lymphangiectasia

This may be primary, resulting from congenital malunion of lymphatics, or secondary to lymphatic obstruction due to lymphoma, filariasis or constrictive pericarditis. Impaired drainage of intestinal lymphatic vessels leads to discharge of protein and fat-rich lymph into the gastrointestinal lumen. The condition presents with peripheral lymphoedema, pleural effusions or chylous ascites, and steatorrhoea. Investigations reveal hypoalbuminaemia, lymphopenia and reduced serum immunoglobulin concentrations. The diagnosis can be made by CT scanning and by enteroscopy with jejunal biopsy, which shows greatly dilated lacteals. Treatment consists of a low-fat diet with medium-chain triglyceride supplements.

Ulceration of the small intestine

Small bowel ulcers are uncommon and are either idiopathic or secondary to underlying intestinal disorders (Box 21.50). Ulcers are more common in the ileum and cause bleeding, perforation, stricture formation or obstruction. Barium studies and enteroscopy confirm the diagnosis.

21.50 Causes of small intestinal ulcers

- Idiopathic
- Inflammatory bowel disease
- Non-steroidal anti-inflammatory drugs
- Ulcerative jejuno-ileitis
- Lymphoma and carcinoma
- Infections (tuberculosis, typhoid, *Yersinia enterocolitica*)
- Others (radiation, vasculitis)

NSAID-associated small intestinal toxicity

These drugs cause a spectrum of small intestinal lesions ranging from erosions and ulcers to mucosal webs, strictures and, rarely, a condition known as 'diaphragm disease', in which intense submucosal fibrosis results in circumferential stricturing. The condition can present with pain, obstruction, bleeding or anaemia, and may mimic Crohn's disease, carcinoma or lymphoma. Enteroscopy or capsule endoscopy can reveal the diagnosis but sometimes this is discovered only at laparotomy.

Eosinophilic gastroenteritis

This disorder of unknown aetiology can affect any part of the gastrointestinal tract; it is characterised by eosinophil infiltration involving the gut wall, in the absence of parasitic infection or eosinophilia of other tissues. It may be mucosal, muscular or subserosal. Peripheral blood eosinophilia is present in 80% of cases.

Clinical features

There are features of obstruction and inflammation, such as colicky pain, nausea and vomiting, diarrhoea and weight loss. Protein-losing enteropathy occurs and up to 50% of patients have a history of other allergic disorders. Serosal involvement may produce eosinophilic ascites.

Investigations and management

The diagnosis is made by histological assessment of multiple endoscopic biopsies, although full-thickness biopsies are occasionally required. Other investigations should be performed

21

to exclude parasitic infection and other causes of eosinophilia. The serum IgE concentration is often raised. Dietary manipulations are rarely effective, although elimination diets, especially of milk, may benefit a few patients. Severe symptoms are treated with prednisolone (20–40 mg daily) and/or sodium cromoglicate, which stabilises mast cell membranes. The prognosis is good in the majority of patients.

Meckel's diverticulum

This is the most common congenital anomaly of the gastrointestinal tract and occurs in 0.3–3% of people, but the vast majority of affected individuals are asymptomatic throughout life. The diverticulum results from failure of closure of the vitelline duct, with persistence of a blind-ending sac arising from the anti-mesenteric border of the ileum; it usually occurs within 100 cm of the ileocaecal valve and is up to 5 cm long. Approximately 50% contain ectopic gastric mucosa; rarely, colonic, pancreatic or endometrial tissue is present. Complications most commonly occur in the first 2 years of life but are occasionally seen in young adults. Bleeding can result from ulceration of ileal mucosa adjacent to the ectopic parietal cells and presents as recurrent melaena or altered blood per rectum. The diagnosis can be made by scanning the abdomen using a gamma counter following an intravenous injection of ^{99m}Tc-pertechnetate, which is concentrated by ectopic parietal cells. Other complications include intestinal obstruction, diverticulitis, intussusception and perforation. Intervention is unnecessary unless complications occur.

Adverse food reactions

Adverse food reactions are common and are subdivided into food intolerance and food allergy, the former being much more common. In food intolerance, there is an adverse reaction to food that is not immune-mediated and results from pharmacological (histamine, tyramine or monosodium glutamate), metabolic (lactase deficiency) or other mechanisms (toxins or chemical contaminants in food).

Lactose intolerance

Human milk contains around 200 mmol/L (68 g/L) of lactose, which is normally digested to glucose and galactose by the brush border enzyme lactase prior to absorption. In most populations, enterocyte lactase activity declines throughout childhood. The enzyme is deficient in up to 90% of adult Africans, Asians and South Americans but only 5% of northern Europeans.

In cases of genetically determined (primary) lactase deficiency, jejunal morphology is normal. 'Secondary' lactase deficiency occurs as a consequence of disorders that damage the jejunal mucosa, such as coeliac disease and viral gastroenteritis. Unhydrolysed lactose enters the colon, where bacterial fermentation produces volatile short-chain fatty acids, hydrogen and carbon dioxide.

Clinical features

In most people, lactase deficiency is completely asymptomatic. However, some complain of colicky pain, abdominal distension, increased flatus, borborygmi and diarrhoea after ingesting milk or milk products. Irritable bowel syndrome may be suspected but the correct diagnosis is suggested by clinical improvement on lactose withdrawal. The lactose hydrogen breath test is a useful non-invasive investigation.

Dietary exclusion of lactose is recommended, although most sufferers are able to tolerate small amounts of milk without

symptoms. Addition of commercial lactase preparations to milk has been effective in some studies but is costly.

Intolerance of other sugars

'Osmotic' diarrhoea can be caused by sorbitol, an unabsorbable carbohydrate that is used as an artificial sweetener. Fructose contained within fruit juices may also cause diarrhoea if it is consumed in greater quantities than can be absorbed.

Food allergy

Food allergies are immune-mediated disorders, most commonly due to type I hypersensitivity reactions with production of IgE antibodies, although type IV delayed hypersensitivity reactions are also seen (p. 83). Up to 20% of the population perceive themselves as suffering from food allergy but only 1–2% of adults and 5–7% of children have genuine food allergies. The most common culprits are peanuts, milk, eggs, soya and shellfish.

Clinical manifestations occur immediately on exposure and range from trivial to life-threatening or even fatal anaphylaxis. The common oral allergy syndrome results from contact with benzoic acid in certain fresh fruit juices, leading to urticaria and angioedema of the lips and oropharynx. This is not, however, an immune-mediated reaction. 'Allergic gastroenteropathy' has features similar to eosinophilic gastroenteritis, while 'gastro-intestinal anaphylaxis' consists of nausea, vomiting, diarrhoea and sometimes cardiovascular and respiratory collapse. Fatal reactions to trace amounts of peanuts are well documented.

The diagnosis of food allergy is difficult to prove or refute. Skin-prick tests and measurements of antigen-specific IgE antibodies in serum have limited predictive value. Double-blind placebo-controlled food challenges are the gold standard but are laborious and are not readily available. In many cases, clinical suspicion and trials of elimination diets are used.

Treatment of proven food allergy consists of detailed patient education and awareness, strict elimination of the offending antigen, and, in some cases, antihistamines or sodium cromoglicate. Anaphylaxis should be treated as a medical emergency with resuscitation, airway support and intravenous adrenaline (epinephrine). Teachers and other carers of affected children should be trained to deal with this. Patients should wear an information bracelet and be taught to carry and use a preloaded adrenaline syringe.

Infections of the small intestine

Travellers' diarrhoea, giardiasis and amoebiasis

See pages 232, 287 and 286.

Abdominal tuberculosis

Mycobacterium tuberculosis is a rare cause of abdominal disease in Caucasians but must be considered in people in and from the developing world and in AIDS patients. Gut infection usually results from human *M. tuberculosis*, which is swallowed after coughing. Many patients have no pulmonary symptoms and a normal chest X-ray.

The area most commonly affected is the ileocaecal region. The presentation and radiological findings may be very similar to those of Crohn's disease. Abdominal pain can be acute or of several months' duration but diarrhoea is less common in tuberculosis than in Crohn's disease. Low-grade fever is common but not invariable. Like Crohn's disease, tuberculosis can affect any part of the gastrointestinal tract and perianal disease with fistula is recognised. Peritoneal tuberculosis may result in peritonitis with exudative ascites, associated with abdominal pain and fever. Granulomatous hepatitis occurs.

Investigations

Abdominal tuberculosis causes an elevated ESR; a raised serum alkaline phosphatase concentration suggests hepatic involvement. Histological confirmation should be sought by endoscopy, laparoscopy or liver biopsy. Caseation of granulomas is not always seen and acid- and alcohol-fast bacteria are often scanty. Culture may be helpful but identification of the organism may take 6 weeks and diagnosis is now possible on biopsy specimens using PCR-based techniques.

Management

When the presentation is very suggestive of abdominal tuberculosis, chemotherapy with multiple anti-tuberculous drugs should be commenced, even if bacteriological or histological proof is lacking. Isoniazid, pyrazinamide and ethambutol is a common standard regime (p. 590), though the precise choice will be dependent on local drug resistance patterns.

Cryptosporidiosis

Cryptosporidiosis and other protozoal infections, including cystoisosporiasis (Cystoisospora belli) and microsporidiosis, are dealt with on pages 287 and 317.

Tumours of the small intestine

The small intestine is rarely affected by neoplasia and fewer than 5% of all gastrointestinal tumours occur at this site.

Benign tumours

The most common are adenomas, GISTs, lipomas and hamartomas. Adenomas are most often found in the periampullary region and are usually asymptomatic, although occult bleeding or obstruction due to intussusception may occur. Transformation to adenocarcinoma is rare. Multiple adenomas are common in the duodenum of patients with familial adenomatous polyposis (FAP), who merit regular endoscopic surveillance. Hamartomatous polyps with almost no malignant potential occur in Peutz–Jeghers syndrome (p. 829).

Malignant tumours

These are rare and include, in decreasing order of frequency, adenocarcinoma, neuro-endocrine tumours, malignant GIST and lymphoma. The majority occur in middle age or later. Kaposi's sarcoma of the small bowel may arise in patients with AIDS.

Adenocarcinomas

Adenocarcinomas occur with increased frequency in patients with FAP, coeliac disease, small bowel Crohn's disease and Peutz–Jeghers syndrome. This is a rare cancer, accounting for less than 5% of all gastrointestinal malignancies. The non-specific presentation and rarity of these lesions often lead to a delay in diagnosis. Despite advances in imaging and endoscopic techniques, early diagnosis is difficult. Barium follow-through examination or small bowel enterography studies demonstrate most lesions of this type. Enteroscopy, capsule endoscopy, mesenteric angiography and CT also play a role in investigation. Treatment is by surgical resection.

Neuro-endocrine tumours

These are discussed in detail on page 678.

Lymphoma

Non-Hodgkin lymphoma (p. 964) may involve the gastrointestinal tract as part of more generalised disease or may rarely arise in the gut, the small intestine being most commonly affected. Lymphomas occur with increased frequency in patients with coeliac disease, HIV/AIDS and other immunodeficiency states. Most are of B-cell origin, although lymphoma associated with coeliac disease is derived from T cells (enteropathy-associated T-cell lymphoma).

Colicky abdominal pain, obstruction and weight loss are the presenting features and perforation is also seen occasionally. Malabsorption is a feature of diffuse bowel involvement and hepatosplenomegaly is rare.

The diagnosis is made by small bowel biopsy, radiological contrast studies and CT. Staging investigations should be performed as for lymphomas occurring elsewhere (p. 962). Surgical resection, where possible, is the treatment of choice, with radiotherapy and combination chemotherapy reserved for those with advanced disease. The prognosis depends largely on the stage at diagnosis, cell type, patient age and the presence of 'B' symptoms (fever, weight loss, night sweats).

Immunoproliferative small intestinal disease

Immunoproliferative small intestinal disease (IPSID), also known as alpha heavy chain disease, is a rare condition occurring mainly in Mediterranean countries, the Middle East, India, Pakistan and North America. It is a variant of B-cell lymphoma of MALT type and often associated with Campylobacter jejuni infection. The condition varies in severity from relatively benign to frankly malignant.

The small intestinal mucosa is diffusely affected, especially proximally, by a dense lymphoplasmacytic infiltrate. Enlarged mesenteric lymph nodes are also common. Most patients are young adults who present with malabsorption, anorexia and fever. Serum electrophoresis confirms the presence of alpha heavy chains (from the F_c portion of IgA). Prolonged remissions can be obtained with long-term antibiotic therapy but chemotherapy is required for those who fail to respond or who have aggressive disease.

Inflammatory bowel disease

Ulcerative colitis and Crohn's disease are chronic inflammatory bowel diseases that pursue a protracted relapsing and remitting course, usually extending over years. The diseases have many similarities and it is sometimes impossible to differentiate between them. One crucial distinction is that ulcerative colitis involves only the colon, while Crohn's disease can involve any part of the gastrointestinal tract from mouth to anus. A summary of the main features of ulcerative colitis and Crohn's disease is provided in Box 21.51.

The incidence of inflammatory bowel disease (IBD) varies widely between populations. There was a dramatic increase in the incidence of both ulcerative colitis and Crohn's disease in the Western world, starting in the second half of the last century and

21

i 21.51 Comparison of ulcerative colitis and Crohn's disease		
	Ulcerative colitis	Crohn's disease
Age group	Any	Any
Gender	M = F	Slight female preponderance
Incidence	Stable	Increasing
Ethnic group	Any	Any; more common in Ashkenazi Jews
Genetic factors	*HLA-DR*103*; colonic epithelial barrier function (*HNF4α, LAMB1, CDH1*)	Defective innate immunity and autophagy (*NOD2, ATG16L1, IRGM*)
Risk factors	More common in non-/ex-smokers Appendicectomy protects	More common in smokers
Anatomical distribution	Colon only; begins at anorectal margin with variable proximal extension	Any part of gastrointestinal tract; perianal disease common; patchy distribution, skip lesions
Extra-intestinal manifestations	Common	Common
Presentation	Bloody diarrhoea	Variable; pain, diarrhoea, weight loss all common
Histology	Inflammation limited to mucosa; crypt distortion, cryptitis, crypt abscesses, loss of goblet cells	Submucosal or transmural inflammation common; deep fissuring ulcers, fistulae; patchy changes; granulomas
Management	5-ASA; glucocorticoids; azathioprine; biological therapy (anti-TNF, anti-α4β7 integrin); colectomy is curative	Glucocorticoids; azathioprine; methotrexate; biological therapy (anti-TNF, anti-α4β7 integrin); nutritional therapy; smoking cessation; surgery for complications is not curative; 5-ASA is not effective

(5-ASA = 5-aminosalicylic acid; TNF = tumour necrosis factor)

coinciding with the introduction of a more 'hygienic' environment with the advent of domestic refrigeration and the widespread use of antibiotics. The developing world has seen similar patterns, as these countries adopt an increasingly Westernised lifestyle.

In the West, the incidence of ulcerative colitis is stable at 10–20 per 100 000, with a prevalence of 100–200 per 100 000, while the incidence of Crohn's disease is increasing and is now 5–10 per 100 000, with a prevalence of 50–100 per 100 000. Both diseases most commonly start in the second and third decades of life, with a second smaller incidence peak in the seventh decade. Approximately 240 000 people are affected by IBD in the UK (approximately 1.4 million in the USA), equating to a prevalence of about 1 in 250. Life expectancy in patients with IBD is similar to that of the general population. Although many patients require surgery and admission to hospital for other reasons, with substantial associated morbidity, the majority have an excellent work record and pursue a normal life.

Pathophysiology

IBD has both environmental and genetic components, and evidence from genome-wide association studies suggests that genetic variants that predispose to Crohn's disease may have undergone positive selection by protecting against infectious diseases, including tuberculosis (Box 21.52). It is thought that IBD develops because these genetically susceptible individuals mount an abnormal inflammatory response to environmental triggers, such as intestinal bacteria. This leads to inflammation of the intestine with involvement of a wide array of innate and adaptive immune cell responses, with release of inflammatory mediators, including TNF-α, IL-12 and IL-23, which cause tissue damage (Fig. 21.44). There is an association between microbial dysbiosis and IBD. For example, there is a reduced diversity, primarily of Firmicutes and in particular, *Faecalibacterium prausnitzii*. Functional changes in the bacteria are important and include a reduction of anti-inflammatory metabolites, such as

21.52 Factors associated with the development of inflammatory bowel disease

Genetic

- Both CD and UC are common in Ashkenazi Jews
- 10% have first-degree relative/1 or more close relative with IBD
- High concordance in identical twins (40–50% CD; 20–25% UC)
- 163 susceptibility loci identified at genome-wide levels of significance; most confer susceptibility to both CD and UC; many are also susceptibility loci for other inflammatory conditions (especially ankylosing spondylosis and psoriasis)
- UC and CD are both associated with genetic variants at HLA locus, and with multiple genes involved with immune signalling (especially IL-23 and IL-10 pathways)
- CD is associated with genetic defects in innate immunity and autophagy (*NOD2, ATG16L1* and *IRGM* genes)
- UC is associated with genetic defects in barrier function
- *NOD2* is associated with ileal and stricturing disease, and hence a need for resectional surgery
- *HLA-DR*103* is associated with severe UC

Environmental

- UC is more common in non-smokers and ex-smokers
- CD is more common in smokers (relative risk = 3)
- CD is associated with a low-residue, high-refined-sugar diet
- Commensal gut microbiota are altered (dysbiosis) in CD and UC
- Appendicectomy protects against UC

(CD = Crohn's disease; HLA = human leucocyte antigen; IBD = inflammatory bowel disease; IL = interleukin; UC = ulcerative colitis)

butyrate and other short-chain fatty acids. There is emerging evidence that the virome and mycobiome (fungal species) may be important in the development of IBD. In both diseases, the intestinal wall is infiltrated with acute and chronic inflammatory cells, but there are important differences between the conditions in the distribution of lesions and in histological features (Fig. 21.45).

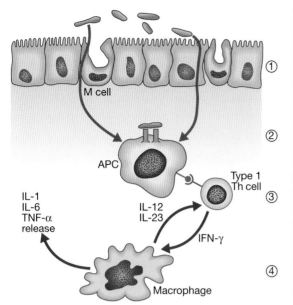

Fig. 21.44 Pathogenesis of inflammatory bowel disease. (1) Bacterial antigens are taken up by specialised M cells, pass between leaky epithelial cells or enter the lamina propria through ulcerated mucosa. (2) After processing, they are presented to type 1 T-helper cells by antigen-presenting cells (APCs) in the lamina propria. (3) T-cell activation and differentiation results in a Th_1 T cell-mediated cytokine response (4) with secretion of cytokines, including interferon gamma (IFN-γ). Further amplification of T cells perpetuates the inflammatory process with activation of non-immune cells and release of other important cytokines, including interleukin 12 (IL-12), IL-23, IL-1, IL-6 and tumour necrosis factor alpha (TNF-α). These pathways occur in all normal individuals exposed to an inflammatory insult and this is self-limiting in healthy subjects. In genetically predisposed persons, dysregulation of innate immunity may trigger inflammatory bowel disease.

Ulcerative colitis

Inflammation invariably involves the rectum (proctitis) and spreads proximally in a continuous manner to involve the entire colon in some cases (pancolitis). In long-standing pancolitis, the bowel can become shortened and post-inflammatory 'pseudopolyps' develop; these are normal or hypertrophied residual mucosa within areas of atrophy (Fig. 21.46). The inflammatory process is limited to the mucosa and spares the deeper layers of the bowel wall (Fig. 21.47). Both acute and chronic inflammatory cells infiltrate the lamina propria and the crypts ('cryptitis'). Crypt abscesses are typical. Goblet cells lose their mucus and, in long-standing

Fig. 21.46 Pseudopolyposis in ulcerative colitis.

21

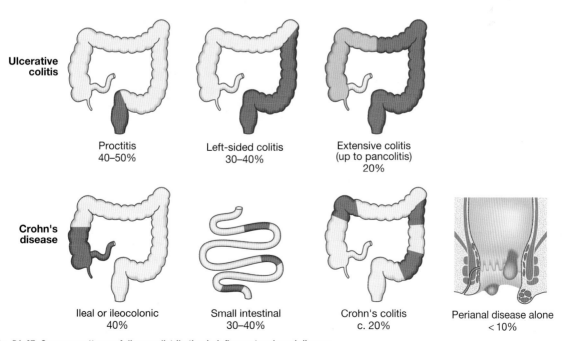

Fig. 21.45 Common patterns of disease distribution in inflammatory bowel disease.

Fig. 21.47 Histology of ulcerative colitis. There is surface ulceration and inflammation is confined to the mucosa with excess inflammatory cells in the lamina propria, loss of goblet cells, and crypt abscesses (arrows). (SM = submucosa)

cases, glands become distorted. Dysplasia, characterised by heaping of cells within crypts, nuclear atypia and increased mitotic rate, may herald the development of colon cancer.

Crohn's disease

The sites most commonly involved are, in order of frequency, the terminal ileum and right side of colon, colon alone, terminal ileum alone, ileum and jejunum. The entire wall of the bowel is oedematous and thickened, and there are deep ulcers that often appear as linear fissures; thus the mucosa between them is described as 'cobblestone'. These may penetrate through the bowel wall to initiate abscesses or fistulae involving the bowel, bladder, uterus, vagina and skin of the perineum. The mesenteric lymph nodes are enlarged and the mesentery is thickened. Crohn's disease has a patchy distribution and the inflammatory process is interrupted by islands of normal mucosa. On histological examination, the bowel wall is thickened with a chronic inflammatory infiltrate throughout all layers (Fig. 21.48).

Clinical features

Ulcerative colitis

The cardinal symptoms are rectal bleeding with passage of mucus and bloody diarrhoea. The presentation varies, depending on the site and severity of the disease (see Fig. 21.45), as well as the presence of extra-intestinal manifestations. The first attack is usually the most severe and is followed by relapses and remissions. Emotional stress, intercurrent infection, gastroenteritis, antibiotics or NSAID therapy may all provoke a relapse. Proctitis causes rectal bleeding and mucus discharge, accompanied by tenesmus. Some patients pass frequent, small-volume fluid stools, while others pass pellety stools due to constipation upstream of the inflamed rectum. Constitutional symptoms do not occur. Left-sided and extensive colitis causes bloody diarrhoea with mucus, often with abdominal cramps. In severe cases, anorexia, malaise, weight loss and abdominal pain occur and the patient is toxic, with fever, tachycardia and signs of peritoneal inflammation (Box 21.53).

Crohn's disease

The major symptoms are abdominal pain, diarrhoea and weight loss. Ileal Crohn's disease (Figs 21.49 and 21.50) may cause

Fig. 21.48 Histology of Crohn's disease. [A] Inflammation is 'transmural'; there is fissuring ulceration (arrow), with inflammation extending into the submucosa (SM). [B] At higher power, a characteristic non-caseating granuloma is seen.

Fig. 21.49 Ileal Crohn's disease. Small bowel magnetic resonance image showing a terminal ileum that is thickened, narrowed and enhancing (arrow), with dilatation immediately proximal to this.

subacute or even acute intestinal obstruction. The pain is often associated with diarrhoea, which is usually watery and does not contain blood or mucus. Almost all patients lose weight because they avoid food, since eating provokes pain. Weight loss may also be due to malabsorption and some patients present with features of fat, protein or vitamin deficiencies. Crohn's colitis presents in an identical manner to ulcerative colitis but rectal

---

i | **21.53 Assessment of disease severity in ulcerative colitis**

	Mild	Moderate	Severe
Daily bowel frequency	<4	4–6	≥6*
Blood in stools	+/–	+/++	+++
Stool volume	<200 g/24 hrs	200–400 g/24 hrs	>400 g/24 hrs
Pulse	<90 beats/min	<90 beats/min	≥90 beats/min*
Temperature	Normal	Normal	≥ 37.8°C*
Haemoglobin	Normal	Normal	<100 g/L (<10 g/dL)*
Erythrocyte sedimentation rate	Normal	Normal	>30 mm/hr* (or equivalent C-reactive protein)
Serum albumin	>35 g/L (>3.5 g/dL)		<30 g/L (<3 g/dL)
Abdominal X-ray	Normal	Normal	Dilated bowel, mucosal islands, thumb-printing of mucosa, or absence of features
Sigmoidoscopy	Normal or erythema/granular mucosa		Severe mucosal inflammatory changes; ulceration; blood in lumen

*The Truelove–Witts criteria for acute severe ulcerative colitis are ≥6 bloody stools/24 hrs plus one or more of: anaemia, fever, tachycardia and high inflammatory markers.

Fig. 21.50 Barium follow-through showing terminal ileal Crohn's disease. A long stricture is present (arrow A), and more proximally there is ulceration with characteristic 'rose thorn' ulcers (arrow B).

i | **21.54 Conditions that can mimic ulcerative or Crohn's colitis**

Infective

Bacterial
- Salmonella
- Shigella
- Campylobacter jejuni
- Escherichia coli O157
- Gonococcal proctitis
- Pseudomembranous colitis
- Chlamydia proctitis

Viral
- Herpes simplex proctitis
- Cytomegalovirus

Protozoal
- Amoebiasis

Non-infective
- Ischaemic colitis
- Collagenous colitis
- Non-steroidal anti-inflammatory drugs
- Diverticulitis
- Radiation proctitis
- Behçet's disease
- Colonic carcinoma

i | **21.55 Differential diagnosis of small bowel Crohn's disease**

- Other causes of right iliac fossa mass:
  - Caecal carcinoma*
  - Appendix abscess*
- Infection (tuberculosis, Yersinia, actinomycosis)
- Mesenteric adenitis
- Pelvic inflammatory disease
- Lymphoma

*Common; other causes are rare.

21

sparing and the presence of perianal disease are features that favour a diagnosis of Crohn's disease. Many patients present with symptoms of both small bowel and colonic disease. A few patients present with isolated perianal disease, vomiting from jejunal strictures or severe oral ulceration.

Physical examination often reveals evidence of weight loss, anaemia with glossitis and angular stomatitis. There is abdominal tenderness, most marked over the inflamed area. An abdominal mass may be palpable and is due to matted loops of thickened bowel or an intra-abdominal abscess. Perianal skin tags, fissures or fistulae are found in at least 50% of patients.

Differential diagnosis

The differential diagnosis is summarised in Box 21.54. The most important issue is to distinguish the first attack of acute colitis from infection. In general, diarrhoea lasting longer than 10 days in Western countries is unlikely to be the result of infection, whereas a history of foreign travel, antibiotic exposure (Clostridium difficile/pseudomembranous colitis) or homosexual contact increases the possibility of infection, which should be excluded by the appropriate investigations (see below). The diagnosis of Crohn's disease is usually more straightforward and is made on the basis of imaging and clinical presentation, but in atypical cases biopsy or surgical resection is necessary to exclude other diseases (Box 21.55).

Complications

Life-threatening colonic inflammation

This can occur in both ulcerative colitis and Crohn's colitis. In the most extreme cases, the colon dilates (toxic megacolon) and bacterial toxins pass freely across the diseased mucosa into the portal and then systemic circulation. This complication arises most commonly during the first attack of colitis and is recognised by the features described in Box 21.53. An abdominal X-ray should be taken daily because, when the transverse colon is dilated to more than 6 cm (Fig. 21.51), there is a high risk of colonic perforation, although this complication can also occur in the absence of toxic megacolon. Severe colonic inflammation with toxic dilatation is a surgical emergency and most often requires colectomy.

Haemorrhage

Haemorrhage due to erosion of a major artery is rare but can occur in both conditions.

Fistulae

These are specific to Crohn's disease. Enteroenteric fistulae can cause diarrhoea and malabsorption due to blind loop syndrome. Enterovesical fistulation causes recurrent urinary infections and pneumaturia. An enterovaginal fistula causes a faeculent vaginal discharge. Fistulation from the bowel may also cause perianal or ischiorectal abscesses, fissures and fistulae.

Cancer

The risk of dysplasia and cancer increases with the duration and extent of uncontrolled colonic inflammation. Thus patients who have long-standing, extensive colitis are at highest risk. Oral mesalazine therapy reduces the risk of dysplasia and neoplasia in ulcerative colitis. Azathioprine also seems to reduce the risk of colorectal cancer in ulcerative colitis and Crohn's colitis. This protective effect probably extends to any medical treatment that results in sustained healing of the colonic mucosa. The

cumulative risk for dysplasia in ulcerative colitis may be as high as 20% after 30 years but is probably lower for Crohn's colitis. The risk is particularly high in patients who have concomitant primary sclerosing cholangitis for unknown reasons. Tumours develop in areas of dysplasia and may be multiple. Patients with long-standing colitis are therefore entered into surveillance programmes beginning 10 years after diagnosis. Targeted biopsies of areas that show abnormalities on staining with indigo carmine or methylene blue increase the chance of detecting dysplasia and this technique (termed pancolonic chromo-endoscopy) has replaced colonoscopy with random biopsies taken every 10 cm in screening for malignancy. The procedure allows patients to be stratified into high-, medium- or low-risk groups to determine the interval between surveillance procedures. Family history of colon cancer is also an important factor to consider. If high-grade dysplasia is found, panproctocolectomy is usually recommended because of the high risk of colon cancer.

Extra-intestinal complications

Extra-intestinal complications are common in IBD and may dominate the clinical picture. Some of these occur during relapse of intestinal disease; others appear to be unrelated to intestinal disease activity (Fig. 21.52).

Investigations

Investigations are necessary to confirm the diagnosis, define disease distribution and activity, and identify complications. Full blood count may show anaemia resulting from bleeding or malabsorption of iron, folic acid or vitamin B_{12}. Platelet count can also be high as a marker of chronic inflammation. Serum albumin concentration falls as a consequence of protein-losing enteropathy, inflammatory disease or poor nutrition. ESR and CRP are elevated in exacerbations and in response to abscess formation. Faecal calprotectin has a high sensitivity for detecting gastrointestinal inflammation and may be elevated, even when the CRP is normal. It is particularly useful for distinguishing inflammatory bowel disease from irritable bowel syndrome at diagnosis, and for subsequent monitoring of disease activity.

Bacteriology

At initial presentation, stool microscopy, culture and examination for *Clostridium difficile* toxin or for ova and cysts, blood cultures and serological tests should be performed. These investigations should be repeated in established disease to exclude superimposed enteric infection in patients who present with exacerbations of IBD. During acute flares necessitating hospital admission, three separate stool samples should be sent for bacteriology to maximise sensitivity.

Endoscopy

Patients who present with diarrhoea plus raised inflammatory markers or alarm features, such as weight loss, rectal bleeding and anaemia, should undergo ileocolonoscopy. Flexible sigmoidoscopy is occasionally performed to make a diagnosis, especially during acute severe presentations when ileocolonoscopy may confer an unacceptable risk; ileocolonoscopy should still be performed at a later date, however, in order to evaluate disease extent. In ulcerative colitis, there is loss of vascular pattern, granularity, friability and contact bleeding, with or without ulceration (Fig. 21.53). In Crohn's disease, patchy inflammation, with discrete, deep ulcers, strictures and perianal disease (fissures, fistulae and skin tags), is typically observed, often with rectal sparing. In established disease, colonoscopy may show active inflammation

Fig. 21.51 Plain abdominal X-ray showing a grossly dilated colon due to severe ulcerative colitis. There is also marked mucosal oedema and 'thumb-printing' (arrows).

Occur during the active phase of inflammatory bowel disease	Unrelated to inflammatory bowel disease activity

Conjunctivitis
Iritis
Episcleritis
Mouth ulcers

Autoimmune hepatitis

Primary sclerosing cholangitis and cholangiocarcinoma (ulcerative colitis)

Fatty liver

Gallstones

Liver abscess/portal pyaemia

Amyloidosis and oxalate calculi

Mesenteric or portal vein thrombosis

Sacroiliitis/ankylosing spondylitis (Crohn's with HLA-B27)

Venous thrombosis

Metabolic bone disease

Large-joint arthritis

Erythema nodosum

Pyoderma gangrenosum

Fig. 21.52 Systemic complications of inflammatory bowel disease. See also Chapters 17 and 18. (HLA = human leukocyte antigen)

Fig. 21.53 Sigmoidoscopic view of moderately active ulcerative colitis. Mucosa is erythematous and friable with contact bleeding. Submucosal blood vessels are no longer visible.

with pseudopolyps or a complicating carcinoma. Biopsies should be taken from each anatomical segment (terminal ileum, right colon, transverse colon, left colon and rectum) to confirm the diagnosis and define disease extent, and also to seek dysplasia in patients with long-standing colitis guided by pancolonic chromo-endoscopy. In Crohn's disease, wireless capsule endoscopy is

useful in the identification of small bowel inflammation but should be avoided in the presence of strictures. Enteroscopy may be required to make a histological diagnosis of small bowel Crohn's disease, when the inflamed segment is out of reach of standard endoscopes. All children and most adults with Crohn's disease should have upper gastrointestinal endoscopy and biopsy to complete their staging. Not only is upper gastrointestinal Crohn's disease relatively common in this group, but also it may help to make a definitive diagnosis in patients who otherwise appear to have non-specific colonic inflammation.

Radiology

Barium enema is a less sensitive investigation than colonoscopy in patients with colitis and, where colonoscopy is incomplete, a CT colonogram is preferred. Small bowel imaging is essential to complete staging of Crohn's disease. Traditional contrast imaging by barium follow-through demonstrates affected areas of the bowel as narrowed and ulcerated, often with multiple strictures (see Fig. 21.50). This has largely been replaced now by MRI enterography, which does not involve exposure to radiation and is a sensitive way of detecting extra-intestinal manifestations and of assessing pelvic and perineal involvement. These studies use an orally administered small bowel-distending agent and intravenous contrast to provide transmural imaging that can usefully distinguish between predominantly inflammatory strictures (that should respond to anti-inflammatory medical strategies)

21

and fibrotic strictures (that require a mechanical solution, such as surgical resection, strictureplasty or endoscopic balloon dilatation). A plain abdominal X-ray is essential in the management of patients who present with severe active disease. Dilatation of the colon (see Fig. 21.51), mucosal oedema (thumb-printing) or evidence of perforation may be found. Patients with proctitis may have features of proximal faecal loading. In small bowel Crohn's disease, there may be evidence of intestinal obstruction or displacement of bowel loops by a mass. Ultrasound is a very powerful tool to detect small bowel inflammation and stricture formation but it is operator-dependent. The role of CT is limited to screening for complications, such as perforation or abscess formation, in the acutely unwell.

Management

Drugs that are used in the treatment of IBD are listed in Box 21.56. Although medical therapy plays an important role, optimal management depends on establishing a multidisciplinary team-based approach involving physicians, surgeons, radiologists, nurse specialists and dietitians. Both ulcerative colitis and Crohn's disease are life-long conditions and have important psychosocial implications; specialist nurses, counsellors and patient support groups have key roles in education, reassurance and coping. The key aims of medical therapy are to:

- treat acute attacks (induce remission)
- prevent relapses (maintain remission)
- prevent bowel damage
- detect dysplasia and prevent carcinoma
- select appropriate patients for surgery.

Ulcerative colitis

Active proctitis Most patients with ulcerative proctitis respond to a 1 g mesalazine suppository but some will additionally require oral 5-aminosalicylate (5-ASA) therapy. Topical glucocorticoids are less effective and are reserved for patients who are intolerant of topical mesalazine. Patients with resistant disease may require treatment with systemic glucocorticoids and immunosuppressants. A stool softener may be required to treat proximal constipation.

Active left-sided or extensive ulcerative colitis In mild to moderately active cases, the combination of a once-daily oral and a topical 5-ASA preparation ('top and tail approach') is usually effective. The topical preparation (1 g foam or liquid enema) is typically withdrawn after 1 month. The oral 5-ASA is continued long-term to prevent relapse and minimise the risk of dysplasia. In patients who do not respond to this approach within 2–4 weeks, oral prednisolone (40 mg daily, tapered by 5 mg/week over an 8-week total course) is indicated. Glucocorticoids should never be used for maintenance therapy. At the first signs of glucocorticoid resistance (lack of efficacy) or in patients who require recurrent glucocorticoid doses to maintain control, immunosuppressive therapy with a thiopurine should be introduced. Simultaneous calcium and vitamin D supplementation should be given along with glucocorticoids for bone protection.

Severe ulcerative colitis Patients who fail to respond to maximal oral therapy and those who present with acute severe colitis (meeting the Truelove–Witts criteria; see Box 21.53) are best managed in hospital and should be monitored jointly by a physician and surgeon:

- *clinically*: for the presence of abdominal pain, temperature, pulse rate, stool blood and frequency

- *by laboratory testing*: haemoglobin, white cell count, albumin, electrolytes, ESR and CRP, stool culture
- *radiologically*: for colonic dilatation on plain abdominal X-rays.

All patients should be given supportive treatment with intravenous fluids to correct dehydration and enteral nutritional support should be provided for malnourished patients (Box 21.57). Intravenous glucocorticoids (methylprednisolone 60 mg or hydrocortisone 400 mg/day) should be given by intravenous infusion or bolus injection. Topical and oral aminosalicylates have no role to play in the acute severe attack. Response to therapy is judged over the first 3 days. Patients who do not respond promptly to glucocorticoids should be considered for medical rescue therapy with ciclosporin (intravenous infusion or oral) or infliximab (5 mg/kg), which can avoid the need for urgent colectomy in approximately 60% of cases.

Patients who develop colonic dilatation (>6 cm), those whose clinical and laboratory measurements deteriorate and those who do not respond after 7–10 days' maximal medical treatment usually require urgent colectomy. Subtotal colectomy can also be performed laparoscopically, given sufficient local expertise. The surgical and medical teams should liaise early in the disease course and, if possible, the patient should have the opportunity to speak with the stoma nurse prior to colectomy.

Maintenance of remission Life-long maintenance therapy is recommended for all patients with left-sided or extensive disease but is not necessary in those with proctitis (although 20% of these patients will develop proximal 'extension' over the lifetime of their disease). Once-daily oral 5-aminosalicylates are the preferred first-line agents. Sulfasalazine has a higher incidence of side-effects but is equally effective and can be considered in patients with coexistent arthropathy. Patients who frequently relapse despite aminosalicylate drugs should be treated with thiopurines (azathioprine or 6-mercaptopurine). Biologic therapy with anti-TNF antibodies (infliximab or adalimumab) or anti-$\alpha 4\beta 7$ integrin antibodies (vedolizumab) can also be considered for maintenance treatment in patients with moderate to severe ulcerative colitis who are intolerant of or non-responsive to thiopurine immunosuppression.

Crohn's disease

Principles of treatment Crohn's disease is a progressive condition that may result in stricture or fistula formation if suboptimally treated. It is therefore important to agree long-term treatment goals with the patient; these are to induce remission and then maintain glucocorticoid-free remission with a normal quality of life. Treatment should focus on monitoring the patient carefully for evidence of disease activity and complications (Box 21.58), and ensuring that mucosal healing is achieved.

Induction of remission Glucocorticoids remain the mainstay of treatment for active Crohn's disease. The drug of first choice in patents with ileal disease is budesonide, since it undergoes 90% first-pass metabolism in the liver and has very little systemic toxicity. A typical regimen is 9 mg once daily for 6 weeks, with a gradual reduction in dose over the subsequent 2 weeks when therapy is stopped. If there is no response to budesonide within 2 weeks, the patient should be switched to prednisolone, which has greater potency. This is typically given in a dose of 40 mg daily, reducing by 5 mg/week over 8 weeks, at which point treatment is stopped. Oral prednisolone in the dose regimen described above is the treatment of choice for inducing remission

i 21.56 Drugs used in the treatment of inflammatory bowel disease

Class	Mechanism of action	Notes

Aminosalicylates (mesalazine (Asacol, Salofalk, Pentasa, Mezavant), olsalazine, sulfasalazine, balsalazide)	Modulate cytokine release from mucosa
	Different means of delivery to colon:
	  pH-dependent (Asacol, Salofalk)
	  time-dependent (Pentasa)
	  bacterial breakdown by colonic bacteria from a carrier molecule (sulfasalazine, balsalazide)
		No proven value in CD
		Available as oral or topical (enema/suppository)
		Sulfasalazine causes side-effects in 10–45%: headache, nausea, diarrhoea, blood dyscrasias
		Other aminosalicylates better tolerated; diarrhoea, headache in 2–5%
		Rarely, renal impairment (check urea and electrolytes 6-monthly)

Glucocorticoids (prednisolone, hydrocortisone, budesonide)	Anti-inflammatory Budesonide is a potent glucocorticoid efficiently cleared from circulation by liver, thereby minimising adrenocortical suppression and steroid side-effects	Topical, oral or IV, according to disease severity Budesonide considered for active ileitis and ileocolitis High vigilance for complications Never used for maintenance therapy Calcium/vitamin D supplements
Thiopurines (azathioprine, mercaptopurine)	Immunomodulation by inducing T-cell apoptosis Azathioprine is metabolised in liver to mercaptopurine, then by TPMT to thioguanine nucleotides	Effective 12 weeks after starting therapy Complications leading to drug withdrawal in approximately 20%: influenza-like syndrome with myalgia, nausea and vomiting; leucopenia in 3%, particularly in inherited TPMT deficiency; hepatotoxicity; pancreatitis 60% of those intolerant of azathioprine will tolerate mercaptopurine Increase in lymphoma (approximately 2–3-fold) and non-melanoma skin cancer (life-long sun protection advised) Check TPMT levels prior to starting treatment and avoid if deficient/ very low due to risk of toxicity Metabolite levels can be measured to tailor therapy Use with caution for patients presenting over the age of 60 years due to risk of malignancy
Methotrexate	Anti-inflammatory	Intolerance in 10–18% Maximal efficacy when given by SC injection once weekly Nausea, stomatitis, diarrhoea, hepatotoxicity and pneumonitis Co-prescription of folic acid and antiemetics. Teratogenic; robust contraception required for males and females
Ciclosporin	Inhibits T-cell activation	Rescue therapy to prevent surgery in UC responding poorly to glucocorticoids. No value in CD Major side-effects in 0–17%: nephrotoxicity, infections, neurotoxicity (including fits) Minor complications in up to 50%: tremor, paraesthesiae, abnormal liver function tests, hirsutism
Anti-TNF antibodies (infliximab and adalimumab)	Suppress inflammation and induce apoptosis of inflammatory cells	Moderate to severe CD, including fistulating disease Moderate to severe UC and acute severe UC as rescue therapy Acute (anaphylactic) and delayed (serum sickness) infusion reactions after multiple infusions; anti-drug antibody titres and drug levels can be measured Contraindicated in infection; reactivation of latent tuberculosis and moderate to severe cardiac failure Increased risk of infections and possibly of malignancy Rarely, neurological adverse events Requires assessment for latent tuberculosis and hepatitis B and C prior to commencement Continue until treatment failure or 12 months and reassess
Anti-α4β7 integrin (vedolizumab)	Blocks integrin expressed on leukocytes and inhibits interaction with gut-specific receptor on endothelium, reducing leukocyte migration to gut mucosa	Moderate to severe CD or moderate to severe UC where treatment with anti-TNF has failed or is not tolerated Side-effects include nasopharyngitis, arthralgia, headache Progressive multifocal leukoencephalopathy risk is reduced due to gut specificity Induction with 300 mg infusion at weeks 0, 2 and 6; maintenance 8-weekly infusions thereafter Discontinue if no improvement after 14 weeks Continue until treatment failure or 12 months and reassess
Antibiotics	Antibacterial	Useful in perianal CD and pouchitis Major concern is peripheral neuropathy with long-term metronidazole
Antidiarrhoeal agents (loperamide, co-phenoxylate)	Reduce gut motility and small bowel secretion Loperamide improves anal function	Avoided in acute flare-ups of disease May precipitate colonic dilatation

(CD = Crohn's disease; IV = intravenous; SC = subcutaneous; TNF = tumour necrosis factor; TPMT = thiopurine methyltransferase; UC = ulcerative colitis)

21

21.57 Medical management of fulminant ulcerative colitis

- Admit to hospital for intensive therapy and monitoring
- Give IV fluids and correct electrolyte imbalance
- Consider transfusion if haemoglobin is <100 g/L (<10 g/dL)
- Give IV methylprednisolone (60 mg daily) or hydrocortisone (400 mg daily)
- Give antibiotics until enteric infection is excluded
- Arrange nutritional support
- Give subcutaneous low-molecular-weight heparin for prophylaxis of venous thromboembolism
- Avoid opiates and antidiarrhoeal agents
- Consider infliximab (5 mg/kg) or ciclosporin (2 mg/kg) in stable patients not responding to 3–5 days of glucocorticoids

21.58 Monitoring of inflammatory bowel disease (IBD)

- Assess symptoms, including extra-intestinal manifestations
- Examine for abdominal mass or perianal disease
- Perform full blood count, urea and electrolytes, liver function tests, albumin, C-reactive protein (CRP)
- Check haematinics (vitamin B_{12}, folate, iron studies) at least annually
- Check faecal calprotectin (to monitor each disease flare/change in therapy and assess response)
- Perform stool cultures (at each flare to exclude infection)
- Assess mucosal healing: surrogate markers (CRP/calprotectin), ileocolonoscopy and/or small bowel magnetic resonance imaging
- Enrol patient in a dedicated IBD clinic (monitoring of stable, uncomplicated patients may be carried out by a nurse or phone clinic)
- Arrange IBD multidisciplinary meeting for acutely ill or complex patients
- Check vaccinations are up to date; ensure surveillance colonoscopy is scheduled where appropriate

21.59 How to give anti-tumour necrosis factor (TNF) therapy in inflammatory bowel disease

- Infliximab (5 mg/kg IV infusion) is given as three loading doses (at 0, 2 and 6 weeks), with 8-weekly maintenance thereafter
- Adalimumab is given as SC injections, which patients can be trained to give themselves. Loading dose is 160 mg, followed by 80 mg 2 weeks later and 40 mg every second week thereafter; some patients require dose escalation to 40 mg once weekly
- Concomitant immunosuppression with a thiopurine or methotrexate may be more efficacious than monotherapy but has more side-effects
- Anti-TNF therapy is contraindicated in the presence of active infection and latent tuberculosis without appropriate prophylaxis; it carries an increased risk of opportunistic infections and a possible increased risk of malignancy; rarely, multiple sclerosis may be unmasked in susceptible individuals. Counselling about the balance of risk and benefit for each patient is important
- Prior to therapy, latent tuberculosis must be excluded
- Live vaccines should not be given
- Certolizumab is effective for luminal Crohn's disease but is not licensed in Europe
- Etanercept is not effective in Crohn's disease

in colonic Crohn's disease. Calcium and vitamin D supplements should be co-prescribed in patients who are on glucocorticoids, to try to compensate for their inhibitory effect on intestinal calcium absorption.

As an alternative to glucocorticoid therapy, enteral nutrition with either an elemental (constituent amino acids) or polymeric (liquid protein) diet may induce remission. Both types of diet are equally effective but the polymeric one is more palatable when taken by mouth. It is particularly effective in children, in whom equal efficacy to glucocorticoids has been demonstrated, and in extensive ileal disease in adults. As well as resting the gut and providing excellent nutritional support, it also has a direct anti-inflammatory effect. It is an effective bridge to urgent staging investigations at first presentation and can be given by mouth or by nasogastric tube. With sufficient explanation, encouragement and motivation, most patients will tolerate it well.

Some individuals with severe colonic disease require admission to hospital for intravenous glucocorticoids. In severe ileal or panenteric disease, induction therapy with an anti-TNF agent is appropriate, provided that acute perforating complications, such as abscess, have not arisen. Both infliximab and adalimumab are licensed for use in the UK. Randomised trials have demonstrated that combination therapy with an anti-TNF antibody and a thiopurine is the most effective strategy for inducing and maintaining remission in luminal Crohn's patients. This strategy is more effective than anti-TNF monotherapy, which, in turn, is more effective than thiopurine monotherapy. Following induction

of remission, a substantial proportion of patients (20–30%) remain well without the requirement for maintenance therapy. Patients with evidence of persistently active disease require further treatment (see below).

Maintenance therapy Immunosuppressive treatment with thiopurines (azathioprine and mercaptopurine) forms the core of maintenance therapy but methotrexate is also effective and can be given once weekly, either orally or by subcutaneous injection. Women and men of child-bearing potential who are prescribed methotrexate must use a robust contraceptive method, and should be counselled to plan pregnancy with a 3-month methotrexate-free period prior to conception since it is teratogenic. Combination therapy with an immunosuppressant and an anti-TNF antibody is the most effective strategy but costs are high and there is an increased risk of serious adverse effects. In the UK, the use of anti-TNF therapy is limited to specific patient subgroups with severe disease (Box 21.59). Vedolizumab is a possible option in patients who have not responded to anti-TNF therapy. It is a humanised monoclonal antibody against anti-$\alpha4\beta7$ integrin. The $\alpha4\beta7$ is expressed on a specific subset of $CD4^+$ leucocytes; vedolizumab binds to this integrin and blocks interaction with MAdCAM-1, expressed on gut endothelial cells, resulting in a reduced influx of immune cells to the inflamed gut mucosa. Serious systemic adverse effects, including progressive multifocal leukoencephalopathy, have been seen with other anti-integrin drugs (such as natalizumab) but this has not emerged with vedolizumab due to its gut specificity. Emerging novel medical therapies for Crohn's disease are currently in phase III clinical trials and are likely to be available for clinical use in the near future. These include ustekinumab (anti-p40, inhibiting both IL-12 and IL-23) and tofacitinib (a Janus kinase inhibitor that blocks pro-inflammatory cytokine signalling).

Cigarette smokers with Crohn's disease should be strongly counselled to stop smoking at every possible opportunity. Those that do not manage to stop smoking fare much worse, with increased rates of relapse and surgical intervention. Careful monitoring of disease activity (see Box 21.58) is the key to maintaining sustained remission and preventing the accumulation of bowel damage in Crohn's disease.

Fistulae and perianal disease Fistulae may develop in relation to active Crohn's disease and are often associated with sepsis. The first step is to define the site by imaging (usually MRI of the pelvis). Surgical exploration by an examination under anaesthetic is usually then required, to delineate the anatomy and drain abscesses. Seton sutures can be inserted through fistula tracts to ensure adequate drainage and to prevent future sepsis. Glucocorticoids are ineffective. Use of antibiotics, such as metronidazole and/or ciprofloxacin, can aid healing as an adjunctive treatment. Thiopurines can be used in chronic disease but do not usually result in fistula healing. Infliximab and adalimumab can heal fistulae and perianal disease in many patients and are indicated when the measures described above have been ineffective. Other options for refractory perianal disease are proctectomy or diverting colostomy.

Surgical treatment

Ulcerative colitis

Up to 60% of patients with extensive ulcerative colitis eventually require surgery. The indications are listed in Box 21.60. Impaired quality of life, with its impact on occupation and social and family life, is the most important of these. Surgery involves removal of the entire colon and rectum, and cures the patient. One-third of those with pancolitis undergo colectomy within 5 years of diagnosis. Before surgery, patients must be counselled by doctors, stoma nurses and patients who have undergone similar surgery. The choice of procedure is either panproctocolectomy with ileostomy, or proctocolectomy with ileal–anal pouch anastomosis. The sister text to this book, *Principles and Practice of Surgery*, should be consulted for further details.

Crohn's disease

The indications for surgery are similar to those for ulcerative colitis. Operations are often necessary to deal with fistulae, abscesses and perianal disease, and may also be required to relieve small or large bowel obstruction. In contrast to ulcerative colitis, surgery is not curative and disease recurrence is the rule. The only method that has consistently been shown to reduce post-operative recurrence is smoking cessation. Antibiotics are effective in the short term only. Use of thiopurines post-surgery is suggested if there are indicators of a high chance of recurrence, i.e. more than one resection or evidence of penetrating disease, such as fistulae or abscess. Otherwise, it is common to undertake colonoscopy 6 months after surgery to inspect and biopsy the anastomosis and neo-terminal ileum. Patients with endoscopic recurrence are then prescribed thiopurines.

Surgery should be as conservative as possible in order to minimise the loss of viable intestine and to avoid the creation of a short bowel syndrome (p. 708). Obstructing or fistulating small bowel disease may require resection of affected tissue. Patients who have localised segments of Crohn's colitis may be managed by segmental resection and/or multiple stricturoplasties, in which the stricture is not resected but instead incised in its longitudinal axis and sutured transversely. Others who have extensive colitis require total colectomy but ileal–anal pouch formation should be avoided because of the high risk of recurrence within the pouch and subsequent fistulae, abscess formation and pouch failure.

Historical datasets show that around 80% of Crohn's patients undergo surgery at some stage and 70% of these require more than one operation during their lifetime. Clinical recurrence following resectional surgery is present in 50% of all cases at 10 years. Emerging data demonstrate that aggressive medical therapy, coupled with intense monitoring, probably reduces the requirement for surgery substantially.

IBD in special circumstances

Childhood

Chronic ill health in childhood or adolescent IBD may result in growth failure, metabolic bone disease and delayed puberty. Loss of schooling and social contact, as well as frequent hospitalisation, can have important psychosocial consequences. Treatment is similar to that described for adults and may require glucocorticoids, immunosuppressive drugs, biological agents and surgery. Monitoring of height, weight and sexual development is crucial. Children with IBD should be managed by specialised paediatric gastroenterologists and transitioned to adult care in dedicated clinics (Box 21.61).

Pregnancy

A women's ability to become pregnant is adversely affected by active IBD. Pre-conceptual counselling should focus on optimising disease control. During pregnancy, the rule of thirds applies: roughly one-third of women improve, one-third get worse and one-third remain stable with active disease. In the post-partum period, these changes sometimes reverse spontaneously. Drug therapy, including aminosalicylates, glucocorticoids and

21

---

i | **21.60 Indications for surgery in ulcerative colitis**

Impaired quality of life
- Loss of occupation or education
- Disruption of family life

Failure of medical therapy
- Dependence on oral glucocorticoids
- Complications of drug therapy

Fulminant colitis

Disease complications unresponsive to medical therapy
- Arthritis
- Pyoderma gangrenosum

Colon cancer or severe dysplasia

21.61 Inflammatory bowel disease in adolescence

- **Delayed growth and pubertal development**: chronic active inflammation, malabsorption, malnutrition and long-term glucocorticoids contribute to short stature and delayed development, with physical and psychological consequences.
- **Metabolic bone disease**: more common with chronic disease beginning in childhood, resulting from chronic inflammation, dietary deficiency and malabsorption of calcium and vitamin D.
- **Drug side-effects and adherence issues**: young people are more likely to require azathioprine or biological therapy than adults. Poor adherence to therapy is more common than with adults, as younger patients may feel well, lack self-motivation to adhere and believe that drugs are ineffective or cause side-effects.
- **Loss of time from education**: physical illness, surgery, fatigue in chronic inflammatory bowel disease, privacy and dignity issues, and social isolation may all contribute.
- **Emotional difficulties**: may result from challenges in coping with illness, problems with forming interpersonal relationships, and issues relating to body image or sexual function.

21.62 Pregnancy and inflammatory bowel disease (IBD)

Pre-conception

- Outcomes are best when pregnancy is carefully planned and disease is in remission
- Methotrexate must be stopped 3 months prior to conception; other IBD drugs should be continued until discussed with a specialist
- Aminosalicylates and azathioprine are safe in pregnancy
- Glucocorticoids are probably safe
- Anti-tumour necrosis factor biological therapy in pregnancy can continue if established pre-pregnancy but should be withheld in the third trimester due to placental transfer of antibody
- No data are available for the use of vedolizumab in pregnancy
- Daily high-dose (>2 mg) folic acid supplements are recommended

Pregnancy

- Two-thirds of patients in remission will remain so in pregnancy
- Active disease is likely to remain active
- Severe active disease carries an increased risk of premature delivery and low birth weight
- Gentle flexible sigmoidoscopy is safe after the first trimester
- X-rays can be performed if clinically indicated but discuss with the radiologist first
- Colonoscopy can be performed safely if the potential benefits outweigh the risks

Labour

- This needs careful discussion between patient, gastroenterologist and obstetrician
- Normal labour and vaginal delivery are possible for most
- Caesarean section may be preferred for patients with perianal Crohn's or an ileo-anal pouch to reduce risks of pelvic floor damage, fistulation and late incontinence

Breastfeeding

- This is safe and does not exacerbate IBD
- Data on the risk to babies from drugs excreted in breast milk are limited; most of these drugs are probably safe
- Patients should discuss breastfeeding and drug therapy with their doctor

azathioprine, can be safely continued throughout pregnancy but methotrexate must be avoided, both during pregnancy and if the patient is trying to conceive (Box 21.62). Anti-TNF agents are transmitted through the placenta (but not breast milk) and are omitted during the last trimester.

Metabolic bone disease

Patients with IBD are prone to developing osteoporosis due to the effects of chronic inflammation, glucocorticoids, weight loss, malnutrition and malabsorption. Osteomalacia can also occur in Crohn's disease that is complicated by malabsorption, but is less common than osteoporosis. The risk of osteoporosis increases with age and with the dose and duration of glucocorticoid therapy.

Refractory Crohn's disease

Crohn's disease can be progressive despite maximal medical therapy and extensive surgery. There are several other immunomodulatory drugs in the clinical trial pipeline (see above).

Microscopic colitis

Microscopic colitis, which comprises two related conditions called lymphocytic colitis and collagenous colitis, has no known cause. The presentation is with watery diarrhoea. The colonoscopic appearances are normal but histological examination of biopsies shows a range of abnormalities. It is therefore recommended that biopsies of the right and left colon plus the terminal ileum should be undertaken in all patients undergoing colonoscopy for diarrhoea. Collagenous colitis is characterised by the presence of a submucosal band of collagen, often with a chronic inflammatory infiltrate. The disease is more common in women and may be associated with rheumatoid arthritis, diabetes, coeliac disease and some drug therapies, such as NSAIDs or PPIs. Treatment with budesonide or 5-aminosalicylates is usually effective but the condition will recur in some patients on discontinuation of therapy.

Irritable bowel syndrome

Irritable bowel syndrome (IBS) is characterised by recurrent abdominal pain in association with abnormal defecation in the absence of a structural abnormality of the gut. About 10–15% of the population are affected at some time but only 10% of these consult their doctors because of symptoms. Nevertheless, IBS is the most common cause of gastrointestinal referral and accounts for frequent absenteeism from work and impaired quality of life. Young women are affected 2–3 times more often than men. Coexisting conditions, such as non-ulcer dyspepsia, chronic fatigue syndrome, dysmenorrhoea and fibromyalgia, are common. IBS is sometimes associated with a history of physical or sexual abuse and this is an important aspect of the history as these patients benefit from psychologically based therapy.

Pathophysiology

The cause of IBS is incompletely understood but biopsychosocial factors are thought to play an important role, along with luminal factors, such as diet and the gut microbiota, as discussed below.

Behavioural and psychosocial factors

Most patients seen in general practice do not have psychological problems but about 50% of patients referred to hospital have a psychiatric illness, such as anxiety, depression, somatisation and neurosis. Panic attacks are also common. Acute psychological stress and overt psychiatric disease are known to alter visceral perception and gastrointestinal motility. There is an increased prevalence of abnormal illness behaviour, with frequent consultations for minor symptoms and reduced coping ability (p. 1202). These factors contribute to but do not cause IBS.

Physiological factors

There is some evidence that IBS may be a serotoninergic (5-HT) disorder, as evidenced by relatively excessive release of 5-HT in diarrhoea-predominant IBS (D-IBS) and relative deficiency with constipation-predominant IBS (C-IBS). Accordingly, 5-HT$_3$ receptor antagonists are effective in D-IBS, while 5-HT$_4$ agonists improve bowel function in C-IBS. There is some evidence that IBS may represent a state of low-grade gut inflammation or immune activation, not detectable by tests, with raised numbers of mucosal mast cells that sensitise enteric neurons by releasing histamine and tryptase. Some patients respond positively to mast cell stabilisers, such as ketotifen, which supports a pathogenic role of mast cells in at least some patients. Immune activation may be associated with altered CNS processing of visceral pain signals. This is more common in women and in D-IBS, and may be triggered by a prior episode of gastroenteritis with *Salmonella* or *Campylobacter* species.

Luminal factors

Both quantitative and qualitative alterations in intestinal bacterial microbiota have been reported. Small intestinal bacterial overgrowth (SIBO) may be present in some patients and lead to symptoms. This 'gut dysbiosis' may explain the response to probiotics or the non-absorbable antibiotic rifaximin.

Dietary factors are also important. Some patients have chemical food intolerances (not allergy) to poorly absorbed, short-chain carbohydrates (lactose, fructose and sorbitol, among others), collectively known as FODMAPs (fermentable oligo-, di- and monosaccharides, and polyols). Their fermentation in the colon leads to bloating, pain, wind and altered bowel habit. Non-coeliac gluten sensitivity (negative coeliac serology and normal duodenal biopsies) seems to be present in some IBS patients, while others may be intolerant of chemicals such as salicylates or benzoates, found in certain foods.

Clinical features

The most common presentation is that of recurrent abdominal discomfort (Box 21.63). This is usually colicky or cramping in nature, felt in the lower abdomen and relieved by defecation. Abdominal bloating worsens throughout the day; the cause is unknown but it is not due to excessive intestinal gas. The bowel habit is variable. Most patients alternate between episodes of diarrhoea and constipation but it is useful to classify them as having predominantly constipation or predominantly diarrhoea. Those with constipation tend to pass infrequent pellety stools, usually in association with abdominal pain or proctalgia. Those with diarrhoea have frequent defecation but produce low-volume stools and rarely have nocturnal symptoms. Passage of mucus is common but rectal bleeding does not occur. Patients do not lose weight and are constitutionally well. Physical examination is generally unremarkable, with the exception of variable tenderness to palpation.

Investigations

The diagnosis is clinical in nature and can be made confidently in most patients using the Rome criteria combined with the absence of alarm symptoms, without resorting to complicated tests (Box 21.64). Full blood count and faecal calprotectin, with or without sigmoidoscopy, are usually done and are normal in IBS. Colonoscopy should be undertaken in older patients (over 40 years of age) to exclude colorectal cancer. Endoscopic examination is also required in patients who report rectal bleeding to exclude colon cancer and IBD. Those who present atypically require investigations to exclude other gastrointestinal diseases. Diarrhoea-predominant patients justify investigations to exclude coeliac disease (p. 805), microscopic colitis (p. 824), lactose intolerance (p. 812), bile acid diarrhoea (p. 809), thyrotoxicosis (p. 635) and, in developing countries, parasitic infection.

Management

The most important steps are to make a positive diagnosis and reassure the patient. Many people are concerned that they have developed cancer. A cycle of anxiety leading to colonic symptoms, which further heighten anxiety, can be broken by explaining that symptoms are not due to a serious underlying disease but instead are the result of behavioural, psychosocial, physiological and luminal factors. In individuals who fail to respond to reassurance, treatment is traditionally tailored to the predominant symptoms (Fig. 21.54). Dietary management is effective for many patients (Box 21.65).

Up to 20% may benefit from a wheat-free diet, some may respond to lactose exclusion, and excess intake of caffeine or artificial sweeteners, such as sorbitol, should be addressed. A more restrictive, 'low-FODMAP' diet, supervised by a dietitian, with gradual re-introduction of different food groups, may help some patients, as may a trial of a gluten-free diet. Probiotics, in capsule form, can be effective if taken for several months, although the optimum combination of bacterial strains and dose have yet to be clarified.

Patients with intractable symptoms sometimes benefit from several months of therapy with a tricyclic antidepressant, such as amitriptyline or imipramine (10–25 mg orally at night). Side-effects include dry mouth and drowsiness but these are usually mild and the drug is generally well tolerated, although patients with features of somatisation tolerate the drug poorly and lower doses should be used. It may act by reducing visceral sensation and by altering gastrointestinal motility. Anxiety and affective disorders may also require specific treatment (pp. 1200 and 1198). The 5-HT$_4$ agonist prucalopride, the guanylate cyclase-C receptor agonist linaclotide, and chloride channel activators, such as lubiprostone, can be effective in constipation-predominant IBS.

Trials of anti-inflammatory agents, such as ketotifen or mesalazine, and the antibiotic rifaximin may be considered in

21.63 Rome III criteria for diagnosis of irritable bowel syndrome

Recurrent abdominal pain or discomfort on at least 3 days per month in the last 3 months, associated with *two or more* of the following:
- Improvement with defecation
- Onset associated with a change in frequency of stool
- Onset associated with a change in form (appearance) of stool

21.64 Supporting diagnostic features and alarm features in irritable bowel syndrome

Features supporting a diagnosis of IBS

- Presence of symptoms for more than 6 months
- Frequent consultations for non-gastrointestinal problems
- Previous medically unexplained symptoms
- Worsening of symptoms by stress

Alarm features

- Age >50 years; male gender
- Weight loss
- Nocturnal symptoms
- Family history of colon cancer
- Anaemia
- Rectal bleeding

21.65 Dietary management of irritable bowel syndrome

- Eat regularly and avoid missing meals
- Take time to eat
- Ensure adequate hydration and avoid carbonated and caffeinated drinks
- Reduce alcohol intake
- Reduce intake of 'resistant' starch and insoluble fibre
- Avoid foods with artificial sweeteners
- Consider a wheat-free diet
- Consider a lactose exclusion diet
- Consider a diet low in FODMAPs

(FODMAPs = fermentable oligo-, di- and monosaccharides, and polyols)

21

Fig. 21.54 Management of irritable bowel syndrome. (FODMAP = fermentable oligo-, di- and monosaccharides, and polyols)

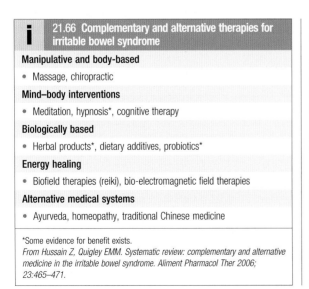

21.66 Complementary and alternative therapies for irritable bowel syndrome

Manipulative and body-based

- Massage, chiropractic

Mind–body interventions

- Meditation, hypnosis*, cognitive therapy

Biologically based

- Herbal products*, dietary additives, probiotics*

Energy healing

- Biofield therapies (reiki), bio-electromagnetic field therapies

Alternative medical systems

- Ayurveda, homeopathy, traditional Chinese medicine

*Some evidence for benefit exists.
From Hussain Z, Quigley EMM. Systematic review: complementary and alternative medicine in the irritable bowel syndrome. Aliment Pharmacol Ther 2006; 23:465–471.

some patients with difficult symptoms but are best prescribed only after specialist referral.

Psychological interventions, such as cognitive behavioural therapy, relaxation and gut-directed hypnotherapy, should be reserved for the most difficult cases. A range of complementary and alternative therapies exist; most lack a good evidence base but are popular and help some patients (Box 21.66).

Most patients have a relapsing and remitting course. Exacerbations often follow stressful life events, occupational dissatisfaction and difficulties with interpersonal relationships.

HIV/AIDS and the gastrointestinal tract

Patients with HIV/AIDS may develop several symptoms referable to the gastrointestinal tract, as discussed in detail on page 316. HIV testing should be considered in all patients with atypical or unexplained gastrointestinal symptoms and in those resident in areas of high prevalence.

Ischaemic gut injury

Ischaemic gut injury is usually the result of arterial occlusion. Severe hypotension and venous insufficiency are less frequent causes. The presentation is variable, depending on the different vessels involved and the acuteness of the event. Diagnosis is often difficult.

Acute small bowel ischaemia

An embolus from the heart or aorta to the superior mesenteric artery is responsible for 40–50% of cases, thrombosis of underlying atheromatous disease for approximately 25%, and non-occlusive ischaemia due to hypotension complicating myocardial infarction, heart failure, arrhythmias or sudden blood loss for approximately 25%. Vasculitis and venous occlusion are rare causes. The clinical spectrum ranges from transient alteration of bowel function to transmural haemorrhagic necrosis and gangrene. Patients usually have evidence of cardiac disease and arrhythmia. Almost all develop abdominal pain that is more impressive than the physical findings. In the early stages, the only physical signs may be a silent, distended abdomen or diminished bowel sounds, with peritonitis developing only later.

Leucocytosis, metabolic acidosis, hyperphosphataemia and hyperamylasaemia are typical. Plain abdominal X-rays show 'thumb-printing' due to mucosal oedema. Mesenteric or CT angiography reveals an occluded or narrowed major artery with spasm of arterial arcades, although most patients undergo laparotomy on the basis of a clinical diagnosis without angiography. Resuscitation, management of cardiac disease and intravenous antibiotic therapy, followed by laparotomy, are key steps. If treatment is instituted early, embolectomy and vascular reconstruction may salvage some small bowel. In these rare cases, a 'second look' laparotomy should be undertaken 24 hours later and further necrotic bowel resected. In patients at high surgical risk, thrombolysis may sometimes be effective. The results of therapy depend on early intervention; patients treated late have a 75% mortality rate. Survivors often have nutritional failure from short bowel syndrome (p. 708) and require intensive nutritional support, including home parenteral nutrition and anticoagulation. Small bowel transplantation can be considered in selected patients. Patients with mesenteric venous thrombosis also require surgery if there are signs of peritonitis but are otherwise treated with anticoagulation. Investigations for underlying prothrombotic disorders should be performed (p. 978).

Acute colonic ischaemia

The splenic flexure and descending colon have little collateral circulation and lie in 'watershed' areas of arterial supply. The spectrum of injury ranges from reversible colopathy to transient colitis, colonic stricture, gangrene and fulminant pancolitis. Arterial thromboembolism is usually responsible but colonic ischaemia can also follow severe hypotension, colonic volvulus, strangulated hernia, systemic vasculitis or hypercoagulable states. Ischaemia of the descending and sigmoid colon is also a complication of abdominal aortic aneurysm surgery (where the inferior mesenteric artery is ligated). The patient is usually elderly and presents with sudden onset of cramping, left-sided, lower abdominal pain and rectal bleeding. Symptoms usually resolve spontaneously over 24–48 hours and healing occurs in 2 weeks. Some may develop a fibrous stricture or segment of colitis. A minority develop gangrene and peritonitis. The diagnosis

is established by colonoscopy within 48 hours of presentation; otherwise, mucosal ulceration may have resolved. Resection is required for peritonitis.

Chronic mesenteric ischaemia

This results from atherosclerotic stenosis of the coeliac axis, superior mesenteric artery and inferior mesenteric artery. At least two of the three vessels must be affected for symptoms to develop. The typical presentation is with dull but severe mid- or upper abdominal pain developing about 30 minutes after eating. Weight loss is common because patients are reluctant to eat and some experience diarrhoea. Physical examination shows evidence of generalised arterial disease. An abdominal bruit is sometimes audible but is non-specific. The diagnosis is made by mesenteric angiography. Treatment is by vascular reconstruction or percutaneous angioplasty, if the patient's clinical condition permits. The condition is frequently complicated by intestinal infarction, if left untreated.

Disorders of the colon and rectum

Tumours of the colon and rectum

Polyps and polyposis syndromes

Polyps may be neoplastic or non-neoplastic. The latter include hamartomas, metaplastic ('hyperplastic') polyps and inflammatory polyps. These have no malignant potential. Polyps may be single or multiple and vary from a few millimetres to several centimetres in size.

Colorectal adenomas are extremely common in the Western world and the prevalence rises with age; 50% of people over 60 years of age have adenomas, and in half of these the polyps are multiple. They are more common in the rectum and distal colon and are either pedunculated or sessile. Histologically, they are classified as either tubular, villous or tubulovillous, according to the glandular architecture. Nearly all forms of colorectal carcinoma develop from adenomatous polyps, although not all polyps carry the same degree of risk. Features associated with a higher risk of subsequent malignancy are listed in Box 21.67.

Adenomas are usually asymptomatic and discovered incidentally. Occasionally, they cause bleeding and anaemia. Villous adenomas can secrete large amounts of mucus, causing diarrhoea and hypokalaemia.

Discovery of a polyp at sigmoidoscopy is an indication for colonoscopy because proximal polyps are present in 40–50% of such patients. Colonoscopic polypectomy should be carried out wherever possible, as this considerably reduces subsequent colorectal cancer risk (Fig. 21.55). Very large or sessile polyps can sometimes be removed safely by endoscopic mucosal resection (EMR) but many require surgery. Once all polyps have been removed, surveillance colonoscopy should be undertaken at 3–5-year intervals, as new polyps develop in 50% of patients. Patients over 75 years of age do not require repeated colonoscopies, as their subsequent lifetime cancer risk is low.

21.67 Risk factors for malignant change in colonic polyps

- Large size (>2 cm)
- Multiple polyps
- Villous architecture
- High-grade dysplasia

21

Fig. 21.55 Large rectal adenomatous polyp. A Before colonoscopic polypectomy. B After polypectomy.

i 21.68 Gastrointestinal polyposis syndromes

	Neoplastic		Non-neoplastic[1]		
	Familial adenomatous polyposis	Peutz–Jeghers syndrome	Juvenile polyposis	Cronkhite–Canada syndrome	Cowden's disease
Inheritance	Autosomal dominant[2]	Autosomal dominant	Autosomal dominant in one-third	None	Autosomal dominant
Oesophageal polyps	–	–	–	+	+
Gastric polyps	+	+	+	+++	+++
Small bowel polyps	++	+++	++	++	++
Colonic polyps	+++	++	++	+++	+
Other features	Colorectal cancer, bleeding, extra-intestinal features (see Box 21.69)	Pigmentation, bleeding, intussusception, bowel and other cancers	Colorectal cancer	Hair loss, pigmentation, nail dystrophy, malabsorption	Many congenital anomalies, oral and cutaneous hamartomas, thyroid and breast tumours

– absent; + may occur; ++ common; +++ very common.
[1]The polyps themselves are not neoplastic but cancer risk is increased in several syndromes. [2]Rare autosomal recessive variant *MUTYH* (see text).

Between 10% and 20% of polyps show histological evidence of malignancy. When cancer cells are found within 2 mm of the resection margin of the polyp, when the polyp cancer is poorly differentiated or when lymphatic invasion is present, segmental colonic resection is recommended because residual tumour or lymphatic spread (in up to 10%) may be present. Malignant polyps without these features can be followed up by surveillance colonoscopy.

Polyposis syndromes are classified by histopathology (Box 21.68). It is important to note that, while the hamartomatous polyps in Peutz–Jeghers syndrome and juvenile polyposis are not themselves neoplastic, these disorders are associated with an increased risk of malignancy of the breast, colon, ovary and thyroid.

Familial adenomatous polyposis

Familial adenomatous polyposis (FAP) is an uncommon autosomal dominant disorder affecting 1 in 13 000 of the population and accounting for 1% of all colorectal cancers. It results from germline mutation of the tumour suppressor *APC* gene, followed by acquired mutation of the remaining allele (Ch. 3). The *APC* gene is large and over 1400 different mutations have been reported, but most are loss-of-function mutations resulting in a truncated APC protein. This protein normally binds to and sequesters β-catenin but is unable to do so when mutated, allowing β-catenin to translocate to the nucleus, where it up-regulates the expression of many genes.

Around 20% of cases arise as new mutations and have no family history. Hundreds to thousands of adenomatous colonic polyps develop in 80% of patients by age 15 (Fig. 21.56), with symptoms such as rectal bleeding beginning a few years later. In those affected, cancer will develop within 10–15 years of the appearance of adenomas and 90% of patients will develop colorectal cancer by the age of 50 years. Despite surveillance, approximately 1 in 4 patients with FAP have cancer by the time they undergo colectomy.

Fig. 21.56 Familial adenomatous polyposis. There are hundreds of adenomatous polyps throughout the colon.

Fig. 21.57 Peutz–Jeghers syndrome. Typical lip pigmentation.

21.69 Extra-intestinal features of familial adenomatous polyposis

- Congenital hypertrophy of the retinal pigment epithelium (CHRPE, 70–80%)
- Epidermoid cysts (extremities, face, scalp)* (50%)
- Benign osteomas, especially skull and angle of mandible* (50–90%)
- Dental abnormalities (15–25%)*
- Desmoid tumours (10–15%)
- Other malignancies (brain, thyroid, liver, 1–3%)

*Gardner's syndrome.

A second gene involved in base excision repair (MutY homolog, *MUTYH*) has been identified and may give rise to colonic polyposis. *MUTYH* displays autosomal recessive inheritance and leads to tens to hundreds of polyps and proximal colon cancer. This variant is referred to as *MUTYH*-associated polyposis (MAP).

Non-neoplastic cystic fundic gland polyps occur in the stomach but adenomatous polyps also arise uncommonly. Duodenal adenomas are found in over 90% and are most common around the ampulla of Vater. Malignant transformation to adenocarcinoma takes place in 10% and is the leading cause of death in those who have had prophylactic colectomy. Many extra-intestinal features are also seen in FAP (Box 21.69).

Desmoid tumours occur in up to one-third of patients and usually arise in the mesentery or abdominal wall. Although benign, they may become very large, causing compression of adjacent organs, intestinal obstruction or vascular compromise, and are difficult to remove. They sometimes respond to hormonal therapy with tamoxifen, and the NSAID sulindac may bring about regression in some, by unknown mechanisms. Congenital hypertrophy of the retinal pigment epithelium (CHRPE) occurs in some cases and is seen as dark, round, pigmented retinal lesions. When present in an at-risk individual, these are 100% predictive of the presence of FAP. A variant, Turcot's syndrome, is characterised by FAP with primary CNS tumours (astrocytoma or medulloblastoma).

Early identification of affected individuals before symptoms develop is essential. The diagnosis can be excluded if sigmoidoscopy is normal. In newly diagnosed cases, genetic testing should be carried out to confirm the diagnosis and identify the causal mutation. Subsequently, all first-degree relatives should also undergo testing (p. 46). In families with known FAP, adolescents should undergo mutation testing at 13–14 years of age and patients who are found to have the mutation should be offered colectomy after school or college education has been completed. The operation of choice is total proctocolectomy with ileal pouch–anal anastomosis. Periodic upper gastrointestinal endoscopy every 1–3 years is recommended to detect and monitor duodenal and periampullary adenomas. If large, these may be amenable to endoscopic resection.

Peutz–Jeghers syndrome

Multiple hamartomatous polyps occur in the small intestine and colon, as well as melanin pigmentation of the lips, mouth and digits (Fig. 21.57). Most cases are asymptomatic, although chronic bleeding, anaemia or intussusception can occur. There is a significant risk of small bowel or colonic adenocarcinoma and of cancer of the pancreas, lung, testis, ovary, breast and endometrium. Peutz–Jeghers syndrome is an autosomal dominant disorder, most commonly resulting from truncating mutations in a serine–threonine kinase gene on chromosome 19p (*STK11*). Diagnosis requires two of the three following features:

- small bowel polyposis
- mucocutaneous pigmentation
- a family history suggesting autosomal dominant inheritance.

The diagnosis can be made by genetic testing but this may be inconclusive, since mutations in genes other than *STK11* can cause the disorder. Affected people should undergo regular upper endoscopy, colonoscopy and small bowel and pancreatic imaging. Polyps greater than 1 cm in size should be removed. Testicular examination is essential for men, while women should undergo pelvic examination, cervical smears and regular mammography. Asymptomatic relatives of affected patients should also undergo screening.

Juvenile polyposis

In juvenile polyposis, tens to hundreds of mucus-filled hamartomatous polyps are found in the colorectum. One-third of cases are inherited in an autosomal dominant manner and up to one-fifth develop colorectal cancer before the age of 40. The criteria for diagnosis are:

- ten or more colonic juvenile polyps
- juvenile polyps elsewhere in the gut, *or*
- any polyps in those with a family history.

Germline mutations in the *SMAD4* gene are often found, as are *PTEN* mutations. Colonoscopy with polypectomy should be performed every 1–3 years and colectomy considered for extensive involvement.

21

Colorectal cancer

Although relatively rare in the developing world, colorectal cancer is the second most common malignancy and the second leading cause of cancer deaths in Western countries. In the UK, the incidence is 50–60 per 100 000, equating to 30 000 cases per year. The condition becomes increasingly common over the age of 50 years.

Pathophysiology

Both environmental and genetic factors are important in colorectal carcinogenesis (Fig. 21.58). Environmental factors account for the wide geographical variation in incidence and the decrease in risk seen in migrants who move from high- to low-risk countries. Dietary factors are most important and these are summarised in Box 21.70; other recognised risk factors are listed in Box 21.71.

Colorectal cancer development results from the accumulation of multiple genetic mutations. There are also associated epigenetic influences, such as microRNA expression signature, and potential influences from non-coding genetic variation. Currently, there are three main pathways of genetic instability and each is associated with histological, clinical and prognostic parameters:

- *Chromosomal instability*. Mutations or deletions of portions of chromosomes arise, with loss of heterozygosity (LOH) and inactivation of specific tumour suppressor genes. In LOH, one allele of a gene is deleted but gene inactivation occurs only when a subsequent unrelated mutation affects the other allele. Chromosomal instability (CIN) occurs in around 85% of colorectal cancers. Figure 21.59 outlines some of the common genes affected by CIN.
- *Microsatellite instability*. This involves germline mutations in one of six genes encoding enzymes involved in repairing errors that occur normally during DNA replication (DNA mismatch repair); these genes are designated *hMSH2*, *hMSH6*, *hMLH1*, *hMLH3*, *hPMS1* and *hPMS2*. Replication errors accumulate and can be detected in 'microsatellites' of repetitive DNA sequences. They also occur in important regulatory genes, resulting in a genetically unstable phenotype and accumulation of multiple somatic mutations throughout the genome that eventually lead to cancer. Around 15% of sporadic cancers develop this way, as do most cases of hereditary non-polyposis colon cancer (HNPCC).
- *CpG island methylator phenotype (CIMP)*. This phenotype is found in approximately 20–30% of colorectal cancers and results in widespread gene hypermethylation. The result is functional loss of tumour suppressor genes.

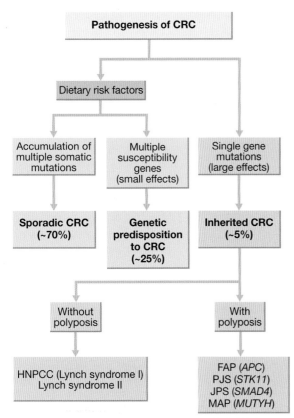

Fig. 21.58 Pathogenesis of colorectal cancer (CRC). (FAP = familial adenomatous polyposis; HNPCC = hereditary non-polyposis colon cancer; JPS = juvenile polyposis syndrome; MAP = *MUTYH*-associated polyposis; PJS = Peutz–Jeghers syndrome)

i | **21.70 Dietary risk factors for colorectal cancer**

Risk factor	Comments
Increased risk	
Red meat*	High saturated fat and protein content Carcinogenic amines formed during cooking
Saturated animal fat*	High faecal bile acid and fatty acid levels May affect colonic prostaglandin turnover
Decreased risk	
Dietary fibre*	Effects vary with fibre type; shortened transit time, binding of bile acids and effects on bacterial flora proposed
Fruit and vegetables	Green vegetables contain anticarcinogens, such as flavonoids Little evidence for protection from vitamins A, C and E
Calcium	Binds and precipitates faecal bile acids
Folic acid	Reverses DNA hypomethylation
Omega-3 fatty acids	May be of modest benefit

*Evidence is inconsistent and a clear relationship is unproven.

i | **21.71 Non-dietary risk factors for colorectal cancer**

Medical conditions

- Colorectal adenomas (p. 827)
- Long-standing extensive ulcerative colitis or Crohn's colitis (p. 813), especially if associated with primary sclerosing cholangitis
- Ureterosigmoidostomy
- Acromegaly
- Pelvic radiotherapy

Others

- Obesity and sedentary lifestyle – may be related to diet
- Smoking (relative risk 1.5–3.0)
- Alcohol (weak association)
- Cholecystectomy (effect of bile acids in right colon)
- Type 2 diabetes (hyperinsulinaemia)
- Use of aspirin or NSAIDs (COX-2 inhibition) and perhaps statins associated with *reduced* risk

(COX-2 = cyclo-oxygenase 2; NSAIDs = non-steroidal anti-inflammatory drugs)

	Normal	Early adenoma	Intermediate adenoma	Late adenoma	Carcinoma
Key gene(s)		APC (adenomatous polyposis coli)	K-ras	DCC (deleted in colon cancer) SMAD4	TP53
Chromosome		5q	12p	18q	17p
Normal function		Inhibits translocation of β-catenin to nucleus and suppresses cell growth	Transmembrane GTP-binding protein mediating mitogenic signals (p21)	DCC regulates apoptosis and has a tumour suppressor function SMAD4 regulates cell growth	Up-regulated during cell damage to arrest cell cycle and allow DNA repair or apoptosis to occur
Alteration		Truncating mutations	Gain-of-function mutations	Allelic deletion or silencing (DCC) Gain-of-function mutations (SMAD4)	Allelic deletion; gain-of-function mutations
Effect		Progression to early adenoma development	Cell proliferation	Enhanced tumour growth, invasion and metastasis	Cell proliferation; impaired apoptosis

Further mutations
- Anchorage independence
- Protease synthesis
- Telomerase synthesis
- Multidrug resistance
- Evasion of immune system

Fig. 21.59 The multistep origin of cancer: molecular events implicated in colorectal carcinogenesis. (GTP = guanine triphosphate)

> **ⓘ 21.72 Modified Amsterdam criteria* for hereditary non-polyposis colon cancer**
>
> - Three or more relatives with colon cancer (at least one first-degree)
> - Colorectal cancer in two or more generations
> - At least one member affected under 50 years of age
> - Familial adenomatous polyposis excluded
>
> ---
>
> *These criteria are strict and may miss some families with mutations. Hereditary non-polyposis colon cancer should also be considered in individuals with colorectal or endometrial cancer under 45 years of age.

With the advent of sophisticated sequencing methodologies, such as whole-exome or whole-genome sequencing, it is becoming clear that colorectal cancer displays molecular heterogeneity resulting from both common and rare genetic variants, all displaying differing levels of penetrance.

About 5–10% of colon cancers are caused by HNPCC. Pedigrees with this disorder have an autosomal dominant mode of inheritance and a positive family history of colon cancer occurring at a young age. The lifetime risk in affected individuals is 80%, with a mean age at cancer development of 45 years. In contrast to sporadic colon cancer, two-thirds of tumours occur proximally. The diagnostic criteria are listed in Box 21.72. In a subset of patients, there is also an increased incidence of cancers of the endometrium, ovary, urinary tract, stomach, pancreas, small intestine and CNS, related to inheritance of different mismatch repair gene mutations. Those who fulfil the criteria for HNPCC should be referred for pedigree assessment, genetic testing (see above) and colonoscopy. These should begin around 25 years of age or 5–10 years earlier than the youngest case of cancer in the family. Colonoscopy needs to be repeated every 1–2 years but, even then, interval cancers can still occur.

A family history of colorectal cancer can be obtained in 20% of patients who do not fulfil the criteria for HNPCC. In these families, the lifetime risk of developing colon cancer is 1 in 12 and 1 in 6, respectively, when one or two first-degree relatives are affected. The risk is even higher if relatives were affected at an early age. The genes responsible for these cases are, however, unknown.

Most colorectal cancers are 'sporadic' and arise from malignant transformation of a benign adenomatous polyp. Over 65% occur in the rectosigmoid and a further 15% occur in the caecum or ascending colon. Synchronous tumours are present in 2–5% of patients. Spread occurs through the bowel wall. Rectal cancers may invade the pelvic viscera and side walls. Lymphatic invasion is common at presentation, as is spread through both portal and systemic circulations to reach the liver and, less commonly, the lungs. Tumour stage at diagnosis is the most important determinant of prognosis (Fig. 21.60).

Clinical features

Symptoms vary, depending on the site of the carcinoma. In tumours of the left colon, fresh rectal bleeding is common and obstruction occurs early. Tumours of the right colon present with anaemia from occult bleeding or with altered bowel habit, but obstruction is a late feature. Colicky lower abdominal pain is present in two-thirds of patients and rectal bleeding occurs in 50%. A minority present with features of either obstruction or perforation, leading to peritonitis, localised abscess or fistula formation. Carcinoma of the rectum usually causes early bleeding, mucus discharge or a feeling of incomplete emptying. Between 10% and 20% of patients present with iron deficiency anaemia or weight loss. On examination, there may be a palpable mass, signs of anaemia or hepatomegaly from metastases. Low rectal tumours may be palpable on digital examination.

21

Dukes stage	A	B	C	D

Definition	Tumour confined within bowel wall	Extension through bowel wall	Tumour involving lymph nodes	Distant metastases
Prevalence at diagnosis (%)	10	35	30	25
5-year survival rate (%)	> 90	65	30–35	< 5

Fig. 21.60 Modified Dukes classification and survival in colorectal cancer.

Investigations

Colonoscopy is the investigation of choice because it is more sensitive and specific than barium enema. Furthermore, lesions can be biopsied and polyps removed. Patients in whom colonoscopy is incomplete and those who are at high risk of complications can be investigated by CT colonography (virtual colonoscopy). This is a sensitive and non-invasive technique for diagnosing tumours and polyps of more than 6 mm diameter. When the diagnosis of colon cancer has been made, CT of the chest, abdomen and pelvis should be performed as a staging investigation, particularly to detect hepatic metastases. Pelvic MRI or endoanal ultrasound should be used for local staging of rectal cancer. Measurement of serum carcinoembryonic antigen (CEA) levels are of limited value in diagnosis, since values are normal in many patients, but CEA testing can be helpful during follow-up to monitor for recurrence.

Management

Surgery

All patients should be discussed at a multidisciplinary team meeting. Those with locally advanced rectal cancer should be offered neoadjuvant radiotherapy or chemoradiotherapy to increase the subsequent chance of a complete (R0) surgical resection. A 1-week course of radiotherapy just prior to surgery reduces the risk of local recurrence in operable rectal cancer. The tumour should be removed, along with adequate resection margins and pericolic lymph nodes. Continuity should be restored by direct anastomosis, wherever possible. Carcinomas within 2 cm of the anal verge may require abdominoperineal resection and formation of a colostomy. All patients should be counselled pre-operatively about the possible need for a stoma. Total mesorectal excision reduces recurrence rates and increases survival in rectal cancer. Metastatic disease confined to liver or lung should be considered for resection, as this can be potentially curative if there is truly no disease at other sites. Post-operatively, patients should undergo colonoscopy after 6–12 months and then at 5 years to search for local recurrence or development of new lesions, which occur in 6% of cases.

Adjuvant therapy

About 30–40% of patients have lymph node involvement at presentation (Fig. 21.60) and are therefore at risk of recurrence.

Most recurrences are within 3 years of diagnosis and affect the liver, lung, distant lymph nodes and peritoneum. Adjuvant chemotherapy with 5-fluorouracil/folinic acid or capecitabine, preferably in combination with oxaliplatin, can reduce the risk of recurrence in patients with Dukes stage C cancers and some high-risk Dukes B cancers. Post-operative radiotherapy reduces the risk of local recurrence in rectal cancer if operative resection margins are involved.

Palliation of advanced disease

Surgical resection of the primary tumour is appropriate for some patients with metastases to treat obstruction, bleeding or pain. Palliative chemotherapy with 5-fluorouracil/folinic acid, capecitabine, oxaliplatin or irinotecan improves survival. Patients with advanced metastatic disease may be treated with monoclonal antibodies using bevacizumab or cetuximab, either alone or together with chemotherapy. Pelvic radiotherapy is sometimes useful for distressing rectal symptoms, such as pain, bleeding or severe tenesmus. Endoscopic laser therapy or insertion of an expandable metal stent can be used to relieve obstruction (Fig. 21.61).

Prevention and screening

Secondary prevention aims to detect and remove lesions at an early or pre-malignant stage by screening the asymptomatic general population. Several potential methods exist:

- Population-based screening of people over the age of 50 years by regular *faecal occult blood (FOB) testing* reduces colorectal cancer mortality and increases the proportion of early cancers detected. The sensitivity and specificity of these tests need to be improved. Traditionally, serial stool testing with or without subsequent colonoscopy is the screening method of choice in the UK.
- *Colonoscopy* remains the gold standard and allows preventative polypectomy but is expensive, requires bowel preparation and carries risks (perforation approximately 1 : 1000). Many countries lack the resources to offer this form of screening.
- *Flexible sigmoidoscopy* is an alternative option and has been shown to reduce overall colorectal cancer mortality by approximately 35% (70% for cases arising in the

Fig. 21.61 Placement of a colonic stent for an inoperable cancer with impending obstruction. [A] The contrast study demonstrates an obstruction. [B] The stent is deployed across the tumour. [C] A satisfactory position is demonstrated on subsequent CT scanning.

rectosigmoid). It is recommended in the USA every 5 years in all persons over the age of 50.

- Screening for high-risk patients by *molecular genetic analysis* is an exciting prospect but is not yet available.
- *CT colonography* is fast and low-risk, and offers equivalent sensitivity to colonoscopy. Disadvantages include reduced sensitivity to detect polyps of less than 6 mm, the requirement for bowel preparation, exposure to ionising radiation and its inability to offer therapeutic intent.

Diverticulosis

Diverticula are acquired and are most common in the sigmoid and descending colon of middle-aged people. Asymptomatic diverticula (diverticulosis) are present in over 50% of people above the age of 70 years. Symptomatic diverticular disease supervenes in 10–25% of cases, while complicated diverticulosis (acute diverticulitis, pericolic abscess, bleeding, perforation or stricture) is uncommon.

Pathophysiology

A life-long refined diet with a relative deficiency of fibre is widely thought to be responsible and the condition is rare in populations with a high dietary fibre intake, such as in Asia, where it more often affects the right side of the colon. It is postulated that small-volume stools require high intracolonic pressures for propulsion and this leads to herniation of mucosa between the taeniae coli (Fig. 21.62). Diverticula consist of protrusions of mucosa covered by peritoneum. There is commonly hypertrophy of the circular muscle coat. Inflammation is thought to result from impaction of diverticula with faecoliths. This may resolve spontaneously or progress to cause haemorrhage, perforation, local abscess formation, fistula and peritonitis. Repeated attacks of inflammation lead to thickening of the bowel wall, narrowing of the lumen and eventual obstruction.

Clinical features

Symptoms are usually the result of associated constipation or spasm. Colicky pain is suprapubic or felt in the left iliac fossa. The sigmoid colon may be palpable and, in attacks of diverticulitis, there is local tenderness, guarding, rigidity ('left-sided appendicitis') and sometimes a palpable mass. During these episodes, there may be diarrhoea, rectal bleeding or fever. The differential diagnosis includes colorectal cancer, ischaemic colitis,

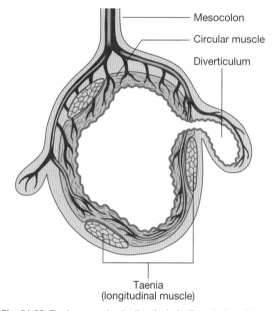

Fig. 21.62 The human colon in diverticulosis. The colonic wall is weak between the taeniae. The blood vessels that supply the colon pierce the circular muscle and weaken it further by forming tunnels. Diverticula usually emerge through these points of least resistance.

IBD and infection. Diverticular disease may be complicated by perforation, pericolic abscess, fistula formation (usually colovesical) or acute rectal bleeding. These complications are more common in patients who take NSAIDs or aspirin. After one attack of diverticulitis, the recurrence rate is around 3% per year. Over 10–30 years, perforation, obstruction or bleeding may occur, each affecting 5% of patients.

Investigations

Investigations are usually performed to exclude colorectal neoplasia. Diverticula can be seen during colonoscopy or on imaging modalities such as CT scan, CT colonography or barium enema (see Fig. 21.12C, p. 773). In severe diverticulosis, colonoscopy requires expertise and carries a risk of perforation. CT is used to assess complications, such as perforation or pericolic abscess.

21

Management

Diverticular disease that is asymptomatic and discovered coincidentally requires no treatment. Constipation can be relieved by a high-fibre diet, with or without a bulking laxative (ispaghula husk, 1–2 sachets daily), taken with plenty of fluids. Stimulant laxatives (see Box 21.73 below) should be avoided. Antispasmodics may sometimes help. Acute attacks of diverticulitis can be treated with antibiotics active against Gram-negative and anaerobic organisms. Severe cases require intravenous fluids, intravenous antibiotics, analgesia and nasogastric suction, but randomised trials show no benefit from acute resection compared to conservative management. Emergency surgery is reserved for severe haemorrhage or perforation. Percutaneous drainage of acute paracolic abscesses can be effective and avoids the need for emergency surgery. Patients who have repeated attacks of obstruction should undergo elective surgery once the acute episode has settled, in order to resect the affected segment of bowel with restoration of continuity by primary anastomosis.

Constipation and disorders of defecation

The clinical approach to patients with constipation and its aetiology have been described on page 786.

Simple constipation

Simple constipation is extremely common and does not signify underlying organic disease. It usually responds to increased dietary fibre or the use of bulking agents; an adequate fluid intake is also essential. Many types of laxative are available, and these are listed in Box 21.73.

Severe idiopathic constipation

This occurs almost exclusively in young women and often begins in childhood or adolescence. The cause is unknown but some have 'slow transit' with reduced motor activity in the colon. Others have 'obstructed defecation', resulting from inappropriate contraction of the external anal sphincter and puborectalis muscle (anismus). The condition is often resistant to treatment. Bulking agents may exacerbate symptoms but prokinetic agents or balanced solutions of polyethylene glycol '3350' benefit some patients with slow transit. Glycerol suppositories and biofeedback techniques are used for those with obstructed defecation. Others benefit from agents such as prucalopride or linaclotide. Rarely, subtotal colectomy may be necessary as a last resort.

Faecal impaction

In faecal impaction, a large, hard mass of stool fills the rectum. This tends to occur in disabled, immobile or institutionalised patients, especially the frail elderly or those with dementia. Constipating drugs, autonomic neuropathy and painful anal conditions also contribute. Megacolon, intestinal obstruction and urinary tract infections may supervene. Perforation and bleeding from pressure-induced ulceration are occasionally seen. Treatment involves adequate hydration and careful digital disimpaction after softening the impacted stool with arachis oil enemas. Stimulants should be avoided.

Melanosis coli and laxative misuse syndromes

Long-term consumption of stimulant laxatives leads to accumulation of lipofuscin pigment in macrophages in the lamina propria. This imparts a brown discoloration to the colonic mucosa, often described as resembling 'tiger skin'. The condition is benign and resolves when the laxatives are stopped. Prolonged laxative use may rarely result in megacolon or 'cathartic colon', in which barium enema demonstrates a featureless mucosa, loss of haustra and shortening of the bowel. Surreptitious laxative misuse is a psychiatric condition seen in young women, some of whom have a history of bulimia or anorexia nervosa (pp. 1203 and 1204). They complain of refractory watery diarrhoea. Laxative use is usually denied and may continue, even when patients are undergoing investigation. Screening of urine for laxatives may reveal the diagnosis.

Hirschsprung's disease

This disease is characterised by constipation and colonic dilatation (megacolon) due to congenital absence of ganglion cells in the large intestine. The incidence is approximately 1:5000. About one-third of patients have a positive family history and, in these families, the disease is inherited in an autosomal dominant manner with incomplete penetrance. About 50% of familial cases and 15% of sporadic cases have mutations affecting the RET proto-oncogene, which is also implicated in multiple endocrine neoplasia (MEN) types 2 and 3 (also known as MEN 2a and 2b, respectively; p. 688). Unlike MEN 2 and 3, which are caused by activating RET mutations, Hirschsprung's disease is caused by loss-of-function mutations. In some kindreds, Hirschsprung's disease and MEN can actually co-segregate and this presumably represents both 'switch off' and 'switch on' of RET in different tissues. Although RET is the most important susceptibility gene, some patients with

i	**21.73 Laxatives**
Class	**Examples**
Bulk-forming laxatives	Ispaghula husk, methylcellulose
Stimulants	Bisacodyl, dantron (only for terminally ill patients), docusate, senna
Faecal softeners	Docusate, arachis oil enema
Osmotic laxatives	Lactulose, lactitol, magnesium salts
Others	Polyethylene glycol (PEG)*, phosphate enema*

*Also used for bowel preparation prior to investigation or surgery.

21.74 Constipation in old age

- **Evaluation**: particular attention should be paid to immobility, dietary fluid and fibre intake, drugs and depression.
- **Immobility**: predisposes to constipation by increasing the colonic transit time; the longer this is, the greater the fluid absorption and the harder the stool.
- **Bulking agents**: can make matters worse in patients with slow transit times and should be avoided.
- **Overflow diarrhoea**: if faecal impaction develops, paradoxical overflow diarrhoea may occur. If antidiarrhoeal agents are given, the underlying impaction may worsen and result in serious complications, such as stercoral ulceration and bleeding.

RET mutations do not develop clinical Hirschsprung's disease, and mutations in other genes have been identified that interact to cause the disease. All of the genes implicated in Hirschsprung's disease are involved in the regulation of enteric neurogenesis, and the mutations cause failure of migration of neuroblasts into the gut wall during embryogenesis. Ganglion cells are absent from nerve plexuses, most commonly in a short segment of the rectum and/or sigmoid colon. As a result, the internal anal sphincter fails to relax. Constipation, abdominal distension and vomiting usually develop immediately after birth but a few cases do not present until childhood or adolescence. The rectum is empty on digital examination.

A plain abdominal X-ray or barium enema shows a small rectum and colonic dilatation above the narrowed segment. Full-thickness biopsies are required to demonstrate nerve plexuses and confirm the absence of ganglion cells. Histochemical stains for acetylcholinesterase are also used. Anorectal manometry demonstrates failure of the rectum to relax with balloon distension. Treatment involves resection of the affected segment.

Acquired megacolon

This may develop in childhood as a result of voluntary withholding of stool during toilet training. In such cases, it presents after the first year of life and is distinguished from Hirschsprung's disease by the urge to defecate and the presence of stool in the rectum. It usually responds to osmotic laxatives.

In adults, acquired megacolon has several causes. It is seen in patients with depression or dementia, either as part of the condition or as a side-effect of antidepressant drugs. Prolonged misuse of stimulant laxatives may cause degeneration of the myenteric plexus, while interruption of sensory or motor innervation may be responsible in a number of neurological disorders. Patients taking large doses of opioid analgesics can develop a megacolon: so-called 'narcotic bowel syndrome'. Systemic sclerosis and hypothyroidism are other recognised causes.

Most patients can be managed conservatively by treatment of the underlying cause, high-residue diets, laxatives and the judicious use of enemas. Prokinetics are helpful in a minority of patients. Opioid-associated constipation can be treated with the specific peripheral opioid receptor antagonist naloxegol. Subtotal colectomy is a last resort for the most severely affected patients.

Acute colonic pseudo-obstruction

Acute colonic pseudo-obstruction (Ogilvie's syndrome) has many causes (Box 21.75) and is characterised by sudden onset of painless, massive enlargement of the proximal colon; there are no features of mechanical obstruction. Bowel sounds are normal or high-pitched, rather than absent. Left untreated, it may progress to perforation, peritonitis and death.

Abdominal X-rays show colonic dilatation with air extending to the rectum. Caecal diameter greater than 10 cm is associated with a high risk of perforation. Single-contrast or water-soluble barium enemas demonstrate the absence of mechanical obstruction.

Management consists of treating the underlying disorder and correcting any biochemical abnormalities. The anticholinesterase neostigmine is effective in enhancing parasympathetic activity and gut motility. Decompression, with either a rectal tube or colonoscope, may be effective but needs to be repeated until the condition resolves. In severe cases, surgical or fluoroscopic defunctioning caecostomy is necessary.

Anorectal disorders

Faecal incontinence

The normal control of anal continence is described on page 770. Common causes of incontinence are listed in Box 21.76. High-risk patients include frail older people, women after childbirth and those with severe neurological/spinal disorders, learning difficulties or cognitive impairment.

Patients are often embarrassed to admit incontinence and may complain only of 'diarrhoea'. A careful history and examination, especially of the anorectum and perineum, may help to establish the underlying cause. Endoanal ultrasound is valuable for defining the integrity of the anal sphincters, while anorectal physiology and MR proctography are also useful investigations.

Management

This is often very difficult. Underlying disorders should be treated and diarrhoea managed with loperamide, diphenoxylate or codeine phosphate. Attention must be paid to a proper diet and adequate fluid intake. Pelvic floor exercises, biofeedback and bowel retraining techniques help some patients, and those with confirmed anal sphincter defects may benefit from sphincter repair operations. Where sphincter repair is not appropriate, a trial of sacral nerve stimulation is undertaken with a view to insertion of a permanent stimulator but, if unsuccessful, creation of a neo-sphincter may be possible, by gracioplasty or by an artificial anal sphincter.

Haemorrhoids

Haemorrhoids (commonly known as piles) arise from congestion of the internal and/or external venous plexuses around the anal canal. They are extremely common in adults. The aetiology is unknown, although they are associated with constipation and straining, and may develop for the first time during pregnancy. First-degree piles bleed, while second-degree piles prolapse but retract spontaneously. Third-degree piles are those that require manual replacement after prolapsing. Bright red rectal bleeding occurs after defecation. Other symptoms include pain, pruritus ani and mucus discharge; thrombosis can occur in prolapsed piles, which can be very painful (Fig. 21.63). Treatment

21.75 Causes of acute colonic pseudo-obstruction

- Trauma, burns
- Recent surgery
- Drugs (opiates, phenothiazines)
- Respiratory failure
- Electrolyte and acid–base disorders
- Diabetes mellitus
- Uraemia

21.76 Causes of faecal incontinence

- Obstetric trauma: childbirth, hysterectomy
- Severe diarrhoea
- Faecal impaction
- Congenital anorectal anomalies
- Anorectal disease: haemorrhoids, rectal prolapse, Crohn's disease
- Neurological disorders: spinal cord or cauda equina lesions, dementia

21

Fig. 21.63 Thrombosed prolapsed haemorrhoids.

i	**21.77 Causes of pruritus ani**

Local anorectal conditions

- Haemorrhoids
- Fistula, fissures
- Poor hygiene

Infections

- Threadworms
- Candidiasis

Skin disorders

- Contact dermatitis
- Psoriasis
- Lichen planus

Other

- Diarrhoea or incontinence of any cause
- Irritable bowel syndrome
- Anxiety

involves measures to prevent constipation and straining. Band ligation is effective for many but a minority of patients require haemorrhoidectomy, which is usually curative. Haemorrhoidal artery ligation operation (HALO) procedures have been developed and may replace surgery. HALO involves using Doppler ultrasound to identify all the arteries feeding the haemorrhoids and ligating them.

Pruritus ani

This is common and can stem from many causes (Box 21.77), most of which result in contamination of the perianal skin with faecal contents.

Itching may be severe and results in an itch–scratch–itch cycle that exacerbates the problem. When no underlying cause is found, all local barrier ointments and creams must be stopped. Good personal hygiene is essential, with careful washing after defecation. The perineal area must be kept dry and clean. Bulk-forming laxatives may reduce faecal soiling.

Solitary rectal ulcer syndrome

This is most common in young adults and occurs on the anterior rectal wall. It is thought to result from localised chronic trauma and/or ischaemia associated with disordered puborectalis function and mucosal prolapse. The ulcer is seen at sigmoidoscopy and biopsies show a characteristic accumulation of collagen.

Symptoms include minor bleeding and mucus per rectum, tenesmus and perineal pain. Treatment is often difficult but avoidance of straining at defecation is important and treatment of constipation may help. Marked mucosal prolapse is treated surgically.

Anal fissure

In this common problem, traumatic or ischaemic damage to the anal mucosa results in a superficial mucosal tear, most commonly in the midline posteriorly. Spasm of the internal anal sphincter exacerbates the condition. Severe pain occurs on defecation and there may be minor bleeding, mucus discharge and pruritus. The skin may be indurated and an oedematous skin tag, or 'sentinel pile', adjacent to the fissure is common.

Avoidance of constipation with bulk-forming laxatives and increased fluid intake is important. Relaxation of the internal sphincter is normally mediated by nitric oxide, and 0.2% glyceryl trinitrate, which donates nitric oxide and improves mucosal blood flow, is effective in 60–80% of patients. Diltiazem cream (2%) can be used as an alternative. Resistant cases may respond to injection of botulinum toxin into the internal anal sphincter to induce relaxation. Manual dilatation under anaesthesia leads to long-term incontinence and should not be considered. The majority of cases can be treated without surgery, but where these measures fail, healing can be achieved surgically by lateral internal anal sphincterotomy or advancement anoplasty.

Anorectal abscesses and fistulae

Perianal abscesses develop between the internal and external anal sphincters and may point at the perianal skin. Ischiorectal abscesses occur lateral to the sphincters in the ischiorectal fossa. They usually result from infection of anal glands by normal intestinal bacteria. Crohn's disease (p. 813) is sometimes responsible.

Patients complain of extreme perianal pain, fever and/or discharge of pus. Spontaneous rupture may lead to the development of fistulae. These may be superficial or track through the anal sphincters to reach the rectum. Abscesses are drained surgically and superficial fistulae are laid open with care to avoid sphincter damage.

Diseases of the peritoneal cavity

Peritonitis

Surgical peritonitis occurs as the result of a ruptured viscus (for details see this book's companion text, *Principles and Practice of Surgery*). Peritonitis may also complicate ascites in chronic liver disease (spontaneous bacterial peritonitis, p. 864) or may occur in children in the absence of ascites, due to infection with *Streptococcus pneumoniae* or β-haemolytic streptococci (p. 253).

Chlamydial peritonitis is a complication of pelvic inflammatory disease (p. 336). The patient presents with right upper quadrant pain, pyrexia and a hepatic rub (the Fitz-Hugh–Curtis syndrome). Tuberculosis may cause peritonitis and ascites (p. 588).

Tumours

The most common is secondary adenocarcinoma from the ovary or gastrointestinal tract. Mesothelioma is a rare tumour complicating asbestos exposure. It presents as a diffuse abdominal mass, due to omental infiltration, and with ascites. The prognosis is extremely poor.

Other disorders

Endometriosis

Ectopic endometrial tissue can become embedded on the serosal aspect of the intestine, most frequently in the sigmoid and rectum. The overlying mucosa is usually intact. Cyclical engorgement and inflammation result in pain, bleeding, diarrhoea, constipation and adhesions or obstruction. Low backache is frequent. The onset is usually between 20 and 45 years and the condition is more common in nulliparous women. Bimanual examination may reveal tender nodules in the pouch of Douglas. Endoscopic studies reveal the diagnosis only if carried out during menstruation, when a bluish mass with intact overlying mucosa is apparent. In some patients, laparoscopy is required. Treatment options include laparoscopic diathermy and hormonal therapy with progestogens (e.g. norethisterone), gonadotrophin-releasing hormone analogues or danazol.

Pneumatosis cystoides intestinalis

In this rare condition, multiple gas-filled submucosal cysts line the colonic and small bowel walls. The cause is unknown but the condition may be seen in patients with chronic cardiac or pulmonary disease, pyloric obstruction, systemic sclerosis or dermatomyositis. Most patients are asymptomatic, although there may be abdominal cramp, diarrhoea, tenesmus, rectal bleeding and mucus discharge. The cysts are recognised on sigmoidoscopy, plain abdominal X-rays or barium enema. Therapies reported to be effective include prolonged high-flow oxygen, elemental diets and antibiotics.

Diseases of the pancreas

Acute pancreatitis

Acute pancreatitis accounts for 3% of all cases of abdominal pain admitted to hospital. It affects 2–28 per 100 000 of the population and is increasing in incidence. It is a potentially serious condition with an overall mortality of 10%. About 80% of all cases are mild and have a favourable outcome. Approximately 98% of deaths from pancreatitis occur in the 20% of patients with severe disease and about one-third of these arise within the first week, usually from multi-organ failure. After this time, the majority of deaths result from sepsis, especially that complicating infected necrosis. At admission, it is possible to predict patients at risk of these complications (Box 21.78). Individuals who are predicted to have severe pancreatitis (Box 21.79) and those with necrosis or other complications should be managed in a specialist centre with an intensive care unit and multidisciplinary hepatobiliary specialists.

Pathophysiology

Acute pancreatitis occurs as a consequence of premature intracellular trypsinogen activation, releasing proteases that digest the pancreas and surrounding tissue. Triggers for this are many, including alcohol, gallstones and pancreatic duct obstruction (Fig. 21.64). There is simultaneous activation of nuclear factor kappa

---

21.78 Glasgow criteria for prognosis in acute pancreatitis*

- Age >55 years
- PO_2 <8 kPa (60 mmHg)
- White blood cell count >15×10⁹/L
- Albumin <32 g/L (3.2 g/dL)
- Serum calcium <2 mmol/L (8 mg/dL) (corrected)
- Glucose >10 mmol/L (180 mg/dL)
- Urea >16 mmol/L (45 mg/dL) (after rehydration)
- Alanine aminotransferase >200 U/L
- Lactate dehydrogenase >600 U/L

*Severity and prognosis worsen as the number of these factors increases. More than three implies severe disease.

21.79 Features that predict severe pancreatitis

Initial assessment
- Clinical impression of severity
- Body mass index >30 kg/m²
- Pleural effusion on chest X-ray
- APACHE II score >8 (see Box 10.50, p. 214)

24 hours after admission
- Clinical impression of severity
- APACHE II score >8
- Glasgow score >3 (see Box 21.78)
- Persisting organ failure, especially if multiple
- CRP > 150 mg/L

48 hours after admission
- Clinical impression of severity
- Glasgow score >3
- CRP >150 mg/L
- Persisting organ failure for 48 hours
- Multiple or progressive organ failure

(CRP = C-reactive protein)

B (NFκB), leading to mitochondrial dysfunction, autophagy and a vigorous inflammatory response. The normal pancreas has only a poorly developed capsule, and adjacent structures, including the common bile duct, duodenum, splenic vein and transverse colon, are commonly involved in the inflammatory process. The severity of acute pancreatitis is dependent on the balance between the activity of released proteolytic enzymes and antiproteolytic factors. The latter comprise an intracellular pancreatic trypsin inhibitor protein and circulating β_2-macroglobulin, α_1-antitrypsin and C1-esterase inhibitors. The causes of acute pancreatitis are listed in Box 21.80. Acute pancreatitis is often self-limiting, but in some patients with severe disease, local complications, such as necrosis, pseudocyst or abscess, occur, as well as systemic complications that lead to multi-organ failure.

Clinical features

The typical presentation is with severe, constant upper abdominal pain, of increasing intensity over 15–60 minutes, which radiates to the back. Nausea and vomiting are common. There is marked epigastric tenderness, but in the early stages (and in contrast to a perforated peptic ulcer), guarding and rebound tenderness are absent because the inflammation is principally retroperitoneal. Bowel sounds become quiet or absent as paralytic ileus develops. In severe cases, the patient becomes hypoxic and develops hypovolaemic shock with oliguria. Discoloration of the flanks

21

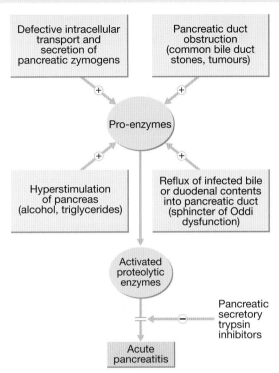

Fig. 21.64 Pathophysiology of acute pancreatitis.

Fig. 21.65 Computed tomogram showing large pancreatic pseudocyst (C) compressing the stomach (S). The pancreas is atrophic and calcified (arrows).

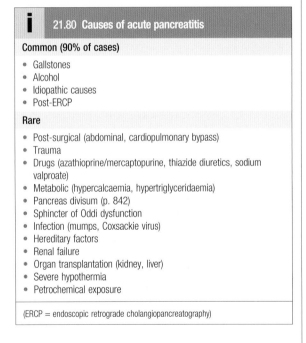

i 21.80 Causes of acute pancreatitis

Common (90% of cases)

- Gallstones
- Alcohol
- Idiopathic causes
- Post-ERCP

Rare

- Post-surgical (abdominal, cardiopulmonary bypass)
- Trauma
- Drugs (azathioprine/mercaptopurine, thiazide diuretics, sodium valproate)
- Metabolic (hypercalcaemia, hypertriglyceridaemia)
- Pancreas divisum (p. 842)
- Sphincter of Oddi dysfunction
- Infection (mumps, Coxsackie virus)
- Hereditary factors
- Renal failure
- Organ transplantation (kidney, liver)
- Severe hypothermia
- Petrochemical exposure

(ERCP = endoscopic retrograde cholangiopancreatography)

i 21.81 Complications of acute pancreatitis

Complication	Cause
Systemic	
Systemic inflammatory response syndrome (SIRS)	Increased vascular permeability from cytokine, platelet-aggregating factor and kinin release
Hypoxia	Acute respiratory distress syndrome (ARDS) due to microthrombi in pulmonary vessels
Hyperglycaemia	Disruption of islets of Langerhans with altered insulin/glucagon release
Hypocalcaemia	Sequestration of calcium in fat necrosis, fall in ionised calcium
Reduced serum albumin concentration	Increased capillary permeability
Pancreatic	
Necrosis	Non-viable pancreatic tissue and peripancreatic tissue death; frequently infected
Abscess	Circumscribed collection of pus close to the pancreas and containing little or no pancreatic necrotic tissue
Pseudocyst	Disruption of pancreatic ducts
Pancreatic ascites or pleural effusion	Disruption of pancreatic ducts
Gastrointestinal	
Upper gastrointestinal bleeding	Gastric or duodenal erosions
Variceal haemorrhage	Splenic or portal vein thrombosis
Erosion into colon	Erosion by pancreatic pseudocyst
Duodenal obstruction	Compression by pancreatic mass
Obstructive jaundice	Compression of common bile duct

(Grey Turner's sign) or the periumbilical region (Cullen's sign) is a feature of severe pancreatitis with haemorrhage. The differential diagnosis includes a perforated viscus, acute cholecystitis and myocardial infarction. Various complications may occur and these are listed in Box 21.81.

A collection of fluid and debris may develop in the lesser sac, following inflammatory rupture of the pancreatic duct; this is known as a pancreatic fluid collection. It is initially contained within a poorly defined, fragile wall of granulation tissue, which matures over a 6-week period to form a fibrous capsule (Fig. 21.65). Such

'pseudocysts' are common and usually asymptomatic, resolving as the pancreatitis recovers. Pseudocysts greater than 6 cm in diameter seldom disappear spontaneously and can cause constant abdominal pain and compress or erode surrounding structures, including blood vessels, to form pseudoaneurysms. Large pseudocysts can be detected clinically as a palpable abdominal mass.

Pancreatic ascites occurs when fluid leaks from a disrupted pancreatic duct into the peritoneal cavity. Leakage into the thoracic cavity can result in a pleural effusion or a pleuro-pancreatic fistula.

Investigations

The diagnosis is based on raised serum amylase or lipase concentrations and ultrasound or CT evidence of pancreatic swelling. Plain X-rays should be taken to exclude other diagnoses, such as perforation or obstruction, and to identify pulmonary complications. Amylase is efficiently excreted by the kidneys and concentrations may have returned to normal if measured 24–48 hours after the onset of pancreatitis. A persistently elevated serum amylase concentration suggests pseudocyst formation. Peritoneal amylase concentrations are massively elevated in pancreatic ascites. Serum amylase concentrations are also elevated (but less so) in intestinal ischaemia, perforated peptic ulcer and ruptured ovarian cyst, while the salivary isoenzyme of amylase is elevated in parotitis. If available, serum lipase measurements are preferable to amylase, as they have greater diagnostic accuracy for acute pancreatitis.

Ultrasound scanning can confirm the diagnosis, although in the earlier stages the gland may not be grossly swollen. The ultrasound scan is also useful because it may show gallstones, biliary obstruction or pseudocyst formation.

Contrast-enhanced pancreatic CT performed 6–10 days after admission can be useful in assessing viability of the pancreas if persisting organ failure, sepsis or clinical deterioration is present, since these features may indicate that pancreatic necrosis has occurred. Necrotising pancreatitis is associated with decreased pancreatic enhancement on CT, following intravenous injection of contrast material. The presence of gas within necrotic material (Fig. 21.66) suggests infection and impending abscess formation, in which case percutaneous aspiration of material for bacterial culture should be carried out and appropriate antibiotics prescribed. Involvement of the colon, blood vessels and other adjacent structures by the inflammatory process is best seen by CT.

Certain investigations stratify the severity of acute pancreatitis and have important prognostic value at the time of presentation (see Boxes 21.78 and 21.79). In addition, serial assessment of CRP is a useful indicator of progress. A peak CRP of >210 mg/L in the first 4 days predicts severe acute pancreatitis with 80% accuracy. It is worth noting that the serum amylase concentration has no prognostic value.

Fig. 21.66 Pancreatic necrosis. Lack of vascular enhancement of the pancreas during contrast-enhanced computed tomography indicates necrosis (arrow). The presence of gas suggests that infection has occurred.

Management

Management comprises several related steps:
- establishing the diagnosis and disease severity
- early resuscitation, according to whether the disease is mild or severe
- detection and treatment of complications
- treatment of the underlying cause.

Opiate analgesics should be given to treat pain and hypovolaemia should be corrected using normal saline or other crystalloids. All severe cases should be managed in a high-dependency or intensive care unit. A central venous line and urinary catheter should be inserted to monitor patients with shock. Oxygen should be given to hypoxic patients, and those who develop systemic inflammatory response syndrome (SIRS) may require ventilatory support. Hyperglycaemia should be corrected using insulin and hypocalcaemia by intravenous calcium injection.

Nasogastric aspiration is required only if paralytic ileus is present. Enteral feeding, if tolerated, should be started at an early stage in patients with severe pancreatitis because they are in a severely catabolic state and need nutritional support. Enteral feeding decreases endotoxaemia and so may reduce systemic complications. Nasogastric feeding is just as effective as feeding by the nasojejunal route. Prophylaxis of thromboembolism with subcutaneous low-molecular-weight heparin is also advisable. The use of prophylactic, broad-spectrum intravenous antibiotics to prevent infection of pancreatic necrosis is not indicated, but infected necrosis is treated with antibiotics that penetrate necrotic tissue, e.g. carbapenems or quinolones, and metronidazole.

Patients who present with cholangitis or jaundice in association with severe acute pancreatitis should undergo urgent ERCP to diagnose and treat choledocholithiasis. In less severe cases of gallstone pancreatitis, biliary imaging (using MRCP or EUS) can be carried out after the acute phase has resolved. If the liver function tests return to normal and ultrasound has not demonstrated a dilated biliary tree, laparoscopic cholecystectomy with an on-table cholangiogram is appropriate because any common bile duct stones have probably passed. When the operative cholangiogram detects residual common bile duct stones, these should be removed by laparoscopic exploration of the duct or by post-operative ERCP. Cholecystectomy should be undertaken within 2 weeks of resolution of pancreatitis – and preferably during the same admission – to prevent further potentially fatal attacks of pancreatitis. Patients with infected pancreatic necrosis or pancreatic abscess require urgent endoscopic drainage or minimally invasive retroperitoneal pancreatic (MIRP) necrosectomy to debride all cavities of necrotic material. Pancreatic pseudocysts can be treated by drainage into the stomach or duodenum. This is usually performed after an interval of at least 6 weeks, once a pseudocapsule has matured, by surgical or endoscopic cystogastrostomy.

Chronic pancreatitis

Chronic pancreatitis is a chronic inflammatory disease characterised by fibrosis and destruction of exocrine pancreatic tissue. Diabetes mellitus occurs in advanced cases because the islets of Langerhans are involved (p. 733).

Pathophysiology

Around 80% of cases in Western countries result from alcohol misuse. In southern India, severe chronic calcific pancreatitis

21

occurs in non-alcoholics, possibly as a result of malnutrition, deficiency of trace elements and micronutrients, and cassava consumption. Other causes are listed in Box 21.82. The pathophysiology of chronic pancreatitis is shown in Figure 21.67.

Clinical features

Chronic pancreatitis predominantly affects middle-aged alcoholic men. Almost all present with abdominal pain. In 50%, this occurs as episodes of 'acute pancreatitis', although each attack results in a degree of permanent pancreatic damage. Relentless, slowly progressive chronic pain without acute exacerbations affects 35% of patients, while the remainder have no pain but present with diarrhoea. Pain is due to a combination of increased pressure within the pancreatic ducts and direct involvement of peripancreatic nerves by the inflammatory process. Pain may be relieved by leaning forwards or by drinking alcohol. Approximately one-fifth of patients chronically consume opiate analgesics. Weight loss is common and results from a combination of anorexia, avoidance of food because of post-prandial pain, malabsorption and/or diabetes. Steatorrhoea occurs when more than 90% of the exocrine tissue has been destroyed; protein malabsorption develops only in the most advanced cases. Overall, 30% of patients have (secondary) diabetes but this figure rises to 70% in those with chronic calcific pancreatitis. Physical examination reveals a thin, malnourished patient with epigastric tenderness. Skin pigmentation over the abdomen and back is common and results from chronic use of a hot water bottle (erythema ab igne). Many patients have features of other alcohol- and smoking-related diseases. Complications are listed in Box 21.83.

Investigations

Investigations (Box 21.84 and Fig. 21.68) are carried out to:

- make a diagnosis of chronic pancreatitis
- define pancreatic function
- demonstrate anatomical abnormalities prior to surgical intervention.

---

i 21.82 Causes of chronic pancreatitis*

Toxic–metabolic

- Alcohol
- Tobacco
- Hypercalcaemia
- Chronic kidney disease

Idiopathic

- Tropical
- Early-/late-onset types

Genetic

- Hereditary pancreatitis (cationic trypsinogen mutation)
- *SPINK-1* mutation
- Cystic fibrosis

Autoimmune

- In isolation or as part of multi-organ problem

Recurrent and severe acute pancreatitis

- Recurrent acute pancreatitis
- Post-necrotic

Obstructive

- Ductal adenocarcinoma
- Intraductal papillary mucinous neoplasia
- Pancreas divisum
- Sphincter of Oddi stenosis

*These can be memorised by the mnemonic 'TIGARO'. Gallstones do not cause chronic pancreatitis but may be observed as an incidental finding.

---

i 21.83 Complications of chronic pancreatitis

- Pseudocysts and pancreatic ascites, which occur in both acute and chronic pancreatitis
- Obstructive jaundice due to benign stricture of the common bile duct as it passes through the diseased pancreas
- Duodenal stenosis
- Portal or splenic vein thrombosis leading to segmental portal hypertension and gastric varices
- Peptic ulcer

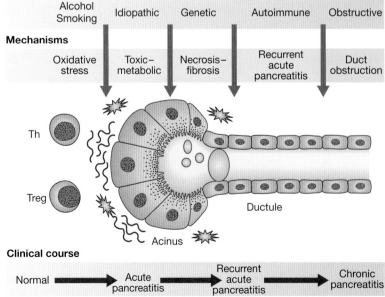

Aetiology

| Alcohol Smoking | Idiopathic | Genetic | Autoimmune | Obstructive |

Mechanisms

| Oxidative stress | Toxic–metabolic | Necrosis–fibrosis | Recurrent acute pancreatitis | Duct obstruction |

Th

Treg

Ductule

Acinus

Clinical course

Normal → Acute pancreatitis → Recurrent acute pancreatitis → Chronic pancreatitis

Fig. 21.67 Pathophysiology of chronic pancreatitis. Alcohol and other risk factors may trigger acute pancreatitis through multiple mechanisms. The first (or 'sentinel') episode of acute pancreatitis initiates an inflammatory response involving T-helper (Th) cells. Ongoing exposure to alcohol drives further inflammation but this is modified by regulatory T cells (Treg) with subsequent fibrosis, via activation of pancreatic stellate cells. A cycle of inflammation and fibrosis ensues, with development of chronic pancreatitis. Alcohol is the most relevant risk factor, as it is involved at multiple steps.

i **21.84 Investigations in chronic pancreatitis**

Tests to establish the diagnosis

- Ultrasound
- Computed tomography (may show atrophy, calcification or ductal dilatation)
- Abdominal X-ray (may show calcification)
- Magnetic resonance cholangiopancreatography
- Endoscopic ultrasound

Tests to define pancreatic function

- Collection of pure pancreatic juice after secretin injection (gold standard but invasive and seldom used)
- Pancreolauryl test (see Box 21.12, p. 777)
- Faecal pancreatic elastase

Tests to demonstrate anatomy prior to surgery

- Magnetic resonance cholangiopancreatography

i **21.85 Intervention in chronic pancreatitis**

Endoscopic therapy

- Dilatation or stenting of pancreatic duct strictures
- Removal of calculi (mechanical or shock-wave lithotripsy)
- Drainage of pseudocysts

Surgical methods

- Partial pancreatic resection, preserving the duodenum
- Pancreatico-jejunostomy

Pain relief

A range of analgesic drugs, particularly NSAIDs, are valuable but the severe and unremitting nature of the pain often leads to opiate use with the risk of addiction. Analgesics, such as pregabalin and tricyclic antidepressants at a low dose, may be effective. Oral pancreatic enzyme supplements suppress pancreatic secretion and their regular use reduces analgesic consumption in some patients. Patients who are abstinent from alcohol and who have severe chronic pain that is resistant to conservative measures should be considered for surgical or endoscopic pancreatic therapy (Box 21.85). Coeliac plexus neurolysis sometimes produces long-lasting pain relief, although relapse occurs in the majority of cases. In some patients, MRCP does not show a surgically or endoscopically correctable abnormality and, in these individuals, the only surgical approach is total pancreatectomy. Unfortunately, even after this operation, some continue to experience pain. Moreover, the procedure causes diabetes, which may be difficult to control, with a high risk of hypoglycaemia (since both insulin and glucagon are absent) and significant morbidity and mortality.

Malabsorption

This is treated by dietary fat restriction (with supplementary medium-chain triglyceride therapy in malnourished patients) and oral pancreatic enzyme supplements. A PPI is added to optimise duodenal pH for pancreatic enzyme activity.

Management of complications

Surgical or endoscopic therapy may be necessary for the management of pseudocysts, pancreatic ascites, common bile duct or duodenal stricture and the consequences of portal hypertension. Many patients with chronic pancreatitis also require treatment for other alcohol- and smoking-related diseases and for the consequences of self-neglect and malnutrition.

Fig. 21.68 Imaging in chronic pancreatitis. [A] Computed tomogram showing a grossly dilated and irregular duct with a calcified stone (arrow A). Note the calcification in the head of the gland (arrow B). [B] Magnetic resonance cholangiopancreatogram of the same patient showing marked ductal dilatation with abnormal dilated side branches (arrows A). A small cyst is also present (arrow B).

Management

Alcohol misuse

Alcohol avoidance is crucial in halting progression of the disease and reducing pain.

Autoimmune pancreatitis

Autoimmune pancreatitis (AIP) is a form of chronic pancreatitis that can mimic cancer but which responds to glucocorticoids. It is characterised by abdominal pain, weight loss or obstructive jaundice, without acute attacks of pancreatitis. Blood tests reveal increased serum IgG or IgG4 and the presence of other autoantibodies. Imaging shows a diffusely enlarged pancreas, narrowing of the pancreatic duct and stricturing of the lower bile duct. AIP may occur alone or with other autoimmune disorders, such as Sjögren's syndrome, primary sclerosing cholangitis or IBD. The response to glucocorticoids is usually excellent but some patients require azathioprine.

21

Congenital abnormalities affecting the pancreas

Pancreas divisum

This is due to failure of the primitive dorsal and ventral ducts to fuse during embryonic development of the pancreas. As a consequence, most of the pancreatic drainage occurs through the smaller accessory ampulla rather than through the major ampulla. The condition occurs in 7–10% of the normal population and is usually asymptomatic, but some patients develop acute pancreatitis, chronic pancreatitis or atypical abdominal pain.

Annular pancreas

In this congenital anomaly, the pancreas encircles the second/third part of the duodenum, leading to gastric outlet obstruction. Annular pancreas is associated with malrotation of the intestine, atresias and cardiac anomalies.

Cystic fibrosis

This disease is considered in detail on page 580. The major gastrointestinal manifestations are pancreatic insufficiency and meconium ileus. Peptic ulcer and hepatobiliary disease may also occur. In cystic fibrosis, pancreatic secretions are protein- and mucus-rich. The resultant viscous juice forms plugs that obstruct the pancreatic ductules, leading to progressive destruction of acinar cells. Steatorrhoea is universal and the large-volume bulky stools predispose to rectal prolapse. Malnutrition is compounded by the metabolic demands of respiratory failure and by diabetes, which develops in 40% of patients by adolescence.

Nutritional counselling and supervision are important to ensure intake of high-energy foods, providing 120–150% of the recommended intake for normal subjects. Fats are an important calorie source and, despite the presence of steatorrhoea, fat intake should not be restricted. Supplementary fat-soluble vitamins are also necessary. High-dose oral pancreatic enzymes are required, in doses sufficient to control steatorrhoea and stool frequency. A PPI aids fat digestion by producing an optimal duodenal pH.

Meconium ileus

Mucus-rich plugs within intestinal contents can obstruct the small or large intestine of a newborn child. Meconium ileus is treated by the mucolytic agent *N*-acetylcysteine, given either orally, by Gastrografin enema or by gut lavage using polyethylene glycol. In resistant cases of meconium ileus, surgical resection may be necessary.

Tumours of the pancreas

Adenocarcinoma of the pancreas

Some 90% of pancreatic neoplasms are adenocarcinomas that arise from the pancreatic ducts. These tumours involve local structures and metastasise to regional lymph nodes at an early stage. Most patients have advanced disease at the time of presentation. Neuro-endocrine tumours also arise in the pancreas but tend to grow more slowly and have a better prognosis; these are discussed in detail on page 678. Pancreatic adenocarcinoma affects 10–15 per 100 000 in Western populations, rising to 100 per 100 000 in those over the age of 70. Men are affected twice

as often as women. The disease is associated with increasing age, smoking and chronic pancreatitis. Between 5% and 10% of patients have a genetic predisposition: hereditary pancreatitis, HNPCC and familial atypical mole multiple melanoma syndrome (FAMMM). Overall survival is only 3–5%, with a median survival of 6–10 months for those with locally advanced disease and 3–5 months if metastases are present.

Clinical features

Many patients are asymptomatic until an advanced stage, when they present with central abdominal pain, weight loss and obstructive jaundice (Fig. 21.69). The pain results from invasion of the coeliac plexus and is characteristically incessant and gnawing. It often radiates from the upper abdomen through to the back and may be eased a little by bending forwards. Almost all patients lose weight and many are cachectic. Around 60% of tumours arise from the head of the pancreas, and involvement of the common bile duct results in the development of obstructive jaundice, often with severe pruritus. A few patients present with diarrhoea, vomiting from duodenal obstruction, diabetes mellitus, recurrent venous thrombosis, acute pancreatitis or depression. Physical examination reveals clear evidence of weight loss. An abdominal mass due to the tumour itself, a palpable gallbladder or hepatic metastasis is commonly found. A palpable gallbladder in a jaundiced patient is usually the consequence of distal biliary obstruction by a pancreatic cancer (Courvoisier's sign).

Investigations

The diagnosis is usually made by ultrasound and contrast-enhanced CT (Fig. 21.70). Diagnosis in non-jaundiced patients is often delayed because presenting symptoms are relatively non-specific. Fit patients with small, localised tumours should undergo staging to define operability. EUS or laparoscopy with laparoscopic ultrasound will define tumour size, involvement of blood vessels and metastatic spread. In patients unsuitable for surgery because of advanced disease, frailty or comorbidity, EUS- or CT-guided cytology or biopsy can be used to confirm the diagnosis (Fig. 21.70). MRCP and ERCP are sensitive methods of diagnosing pancreatic cancer and are valuable when the diagnosis is in doubt, although differentiation between cancer and localised chronic pancreatitis can be difficult. The main role of ERCP is to insert a stent into the common bile duct to relieve obstructive jaundice in inoperable patients.

Management

Surgical resection is the only method of effecting cure, and 5-year survival in patients undergoing a complete resection is around 12%. Clinical trials have demonstrated improved survival (21–29%) with adjuvant chemotherapy using gemcitabine. Unfortunately, only 10–15% of tumours are resectable for cure, since most are locally advanced at the time of diagnosis. For the great majority of patients, treatment is palliative. Chemotherapy with FOLFIRINOX (5-fluorouracil, leucovorin, irinotecan and oxaliplatin) improves median survival to 11 months. Pain relief can be achieved using analgesics but, in some patients, coeliac plexus neurolysis may be required. Jaundice can be relieved by choledochojejunostomy in fit patients, whereas percutaneous or endoscopic stenting is preferable in the elderly and those with very advanced disease. Ampullary or periampullary adenocarcinomas are rare neoplasms that arise from the ampulla of Vater or adjacent duodenum. They are often polypoid and may ulcerate; they frequently infiltrate the duodenum but behave less aggressively than pancreatic adenocarcinoma. Around 25% of patients undergoing resection

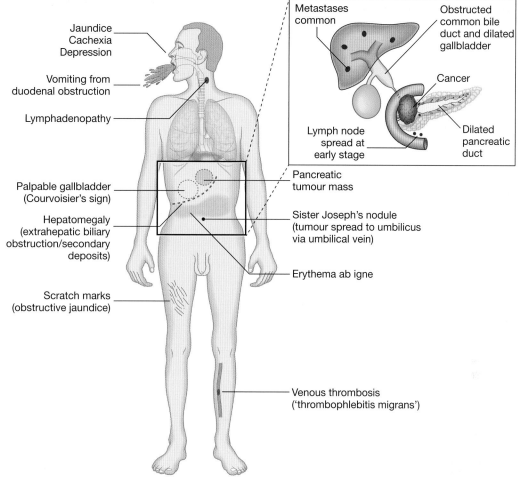

Fig. 21.69 Features of pancreatic cancer.

Fig. 21.70 Carcinoma of the pancreas. A A computed tomogram showing a large, necrotic mass encasing the coeliac axis (arrows). B Endoscopic ultrasound was subsequently performed to enhance staging and to obtain a fine needle aspiration biopsy, which confirmed pancreatic ductal adenocarcinoma.

of ampullary or periampullary tumours survive for 5 years, in contrast to patients with pancreatic ductal cancer.

Incidental pancreatic mass

Cystic neoplasms of the pancreas are increasingly being seen with widespread use of CT. These are a heterogeneous group; serous cystadenomas rarely, if ever, become malignant and do not require surgery. Mucinous cysts occur more often in women, are usually in the pancreatic tail and display a spectrum of behaviour from benign to frankly malignant. Aspiration of the cyst contents for cytology and measurement of CEA and amylase concentrations in fluid obtained at EUS can help determine whether a lesion is mucinous or not. In fit patients, all mucinous lesions should be resected. A variant, called intraductal papillary mucinous neoplasia (IPMN), is often discovered coincidentally on CT, frequently in elderly men. This may affect the main pancreatic duct with marked dilatation and plugs of mucus, or may involve a side branch. The histology varies from villous adenomatous change to dysplasia or carcinoma. Since IPMN is a pre-malignant but indolent condition, the decision to resect or to monitor depends on age and fitness of the patient and location, size and evolution of lesions.

Further information

Books and journal articles

Canard JM, Letard J-C, Palazzo L, et al. Gastrointestinal endoscopy in practice. Edinburgh: Churchill Livingstone; 2011.

Feldman M, Friedman LS, Brandt LJ. Sleisenger and Fordtran's Gastrointestinal and liver disease, 10th edn. Philadelphia: Elsevier Saunders; 2015.

Websites

bsg.org.uk *British Society of Gastroenterology.*

crohnsandcolitis.org.uk *Crohn's and Colitis UK.*

coeliac.org.uk *Coeliac UK.*

ecco-ibd.eu *European Crohn's and Colitis Organisation.*

gastro.org *American Gastroenterological Association and American Digestive Health Foundation.*

isg.org.in *Indian Society of Gastroenterology.*

QM Anstee
DEJ Jones

22

Hepatology

Clinical examination of the abdomen for liver and biliary disease 846

Functional anatomy and physiology 848
Applied anatomy 848
Hepatic function 850

Investigation of liver and hepatobiliary disease 852
Liver blood biochemistry 852
Haematological tests 853
Immunological tests 853
Imaging 853
Histological examination 855
Non-invasive markers of hepatic fibrosis 855

Presenting problems in liver disease 855
Acute liver failure 856
Abnormal liver function tests 859
Jaundice 860
Hepatomegaly 862
Ascites 862
Hepatic encephalopathy 864
Variceal bleeding 865

Cirrhosis 866

Portal hypertension 868

Infections and the liver 871
Viral hepatitis 871
HIV infection and the liver 879
Liver abscess 879

Alcoholic liver disease 880

Non-alcoholic fatty liver disease 882

Autoimmune liver and biliary disease 885
Autoimmune hepatitis 886
Primary biliary cholangitis 887
Primary sclerosing cholangitis 888
IgG4-associated cholangitis 890

Liver tumours and other focal liver lesions 890
Primary malignant tumours 890
Secondary malignant tumours 892
Benign tumours 893

Drugs and the liver 893
Drug-induced liver injury 894

Inherited liver diseases 895
Haemochromatosis 895
Wilson's disease 896
Alpha$_1$-antitrypsin deficiency 897
Gilbert's syndrome 897

Vascular liver disease 898
Hepatic arterial disease 898
Portal venous disease 898
Hepatic venous disease 898

Pregnancy and the liver 899
Intercurrent and pre-existing liver disease 900
Pregnancy-associated liver disease 900

Liver transplantation 900
Indications and contraindications 900
Complications 901
Prognosis 901

Cholestatic and biliary disease 902
Chemical cholestasis 902
Benign recurrent intrahepatic cholestasis 902
Intrahepatic biliary disease 902
Extrahepatic biliary disease 902
Secondary biliary cirrhosis 903
Gallstones 903
Cholecystitis 905
Choledocholithiasis 906
Tumours of the gallbladder and bile duct 907
Miscellaneous biliary disorders 908

Clinical examination of the abdomen for liver and biliary disease

2 Face
Jaundice
Spider naevi
Parotid swelling

▲ Xanthelasma and jaundiced
sclera in a patient with
chronic cholestasis

▲ Kayser–Fleischer rings
in Wilson's disease

1 Hands
Clubbing
Dupuytren's contracture
Leuconychia
Bruising
Flapping tremor (hepatic
encephalopathy)

▲ Palmar erythema

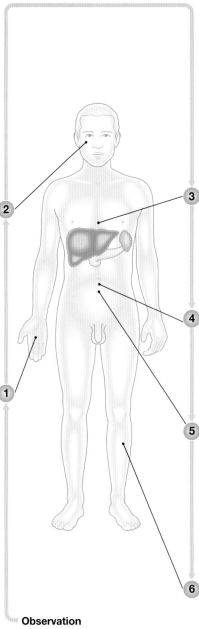

Observation
• Unkempt
• Smell of alcohol or fetor hepaticus
• Encephalopathy
• Weight loss
• Scratch marks from itching

3 Chest
Loss of body hair

▲ Gynaecomastia

▲ Spider naevi

4 Abdomen: inspection
Scars
Distension
Veins
Testicular atrophy

▲ Aspiration of ascitic fluid

▲ Dilated abdominal wall veins
(caput medusae)

**5 Abdomen: palpation/
percussion/auscultation**
Hepatomegaly
Splenomegaly
Ascites
Palpable gallbladder
Hepatic bruit (rare)
Tumour

6 Legs
Bruising
Oedema

Insets (Spider naevi) From Hayes P, Simpson K. Gastroenterology and liver disease. Edinburgh: Churchill Livingstone, Elsevier Ltd; 1995; (Aspiration) Strachan M. Davidson's Clinical cases. Edinburgh: Churchill Livingstone, Elsevier Ltd; 2008; (Palmar erythema) Goldman L, Schafter AI. Goldman's Cecil medicine, 24th edn. Philadelphia: WB Saunders, Elsevier Inc.; 2012.

History and significance of abdominal signs

ℹ Presenting clinical features of liver disease

These represent the combined effects of:

Impairment of liver function and its metabolic sequelae

- Jaundice (failure of bilirubin clearance)
- Encephalopathy (failure of clearance of by-products of metabolism)
- Bleeding (impaired liver synthesis of clotting factors)
- Hypoglycaemia

Ongoing presence of aetiological factors (e.g. alcohol)

- Effects of aetiological agent, e.g. intoxication, withdrawal, cognitive impairment *versus*
- Effects of liver injury from agent, e.g. encephalopathy

Effects of chronic liver injury (>6 months)

Catabolic status (± poor nutrition)

- Skin thinning ('paper-money skin')
- Loss of muscle bulk
- Leuconychia

Impaired albumin synthesis

- Reduced oncotic pressure (contributes to ascites)

Reduced aldosterone clearance

- Na^+ retention (contributes to ascites)

Reduced oestrogen clearance

- Mild feminisation of males (loss of body hair, gynaecomastia)

ℹ Silent presentation of liver disease

It is important to note that patients with liver disease can present silently following detection of abnormality on screening investigation. This occurs frequently in practice in three settings:

Biochemical abnormality

- Liver enzyme abnormality detected during health screening or drug monitoring

Radiological abnormality

- Observation of an unexpected structural lesion (liver mass most usually) following ultrasound, computed tomography or other imaging assessment undertaken for reasons unrelated to the liver

Serological abnormality

- Detection of a liver-related autoantibody

ℹ Ascites

Causes	Associated clinical findings
Exudative (high protein)	
Carcinoma	Weight loss ± hepatomegaly
Tuberculosis	Weight loss ± fever
Transudative (low protein)	
Cirrhosis	Hepatomegaly
	Splenomegaly
	Spider naevi
Renal failure (including nephrotic syndrome)	Generalised oedema
	Peripheral oedema
Congestive heart failure	Elevated jugular venous pressure

⑤ Assessment of liver size

Clinical assessment of hepatomegaly is important in diagnosing liver disease.

- Start in the right iliac fossa.
- Progress up the abdomen 2 cm with each breath (through open mouth).
- Confirm the lower border of the liver by percussion.
- Detect if smooth or irregular, tender or non-tender; ascertain the shape.
- Identify the upper border by percussion.

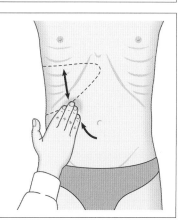

① Assessment of encephalopathy

Flapping tremor. Jerky forward movements every 5–10 secs, when arms are outstretched and hands are dorsiflexed, suggest hepatic encephalopathy. The movements are coarser than those seen in tremor.

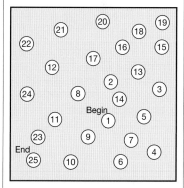

Number connection test. These 25 numbered circles can normally be joined together within 30 secs. Serial observations may provide useful information, as long as the position of the numbers is varied to avoid the patient learning their pattern.

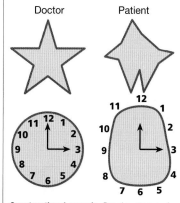

Constructional apraxia. Drawing stars and clocks may reveal marked abnormality.

22

Functional anatomy and physiology

Applied anatomy

Normal liver structure and blood supply

The liver weighs 1.2–1.5 kg and has multiple functions, including key roles in metabolism, control of infection, and elimination of toxins and by-products of metabolism. It is classically divided into left and right lobes by the falciform ligament, but a more useful functional division is into the right and left hemilivers, based on blood supply (Fig. 22.1). These are further divided into eight segments, according to subdivisions of the hepatic and portal veins. Each segment has its own branch of the hepatic artery and

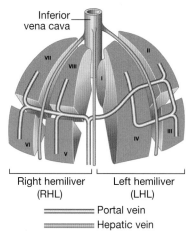

Fig. 22.1 Liver blood supply.

biliary tree. The segmental anatomy of the liver has an important influence on imaging and treatment of liver tumours, given the increasing use of surgical resection. A liver segment is made up of multiple smaller units known as lobules, comprised of a central vein, radiating sinusoids separated from each other by single liver cell (hepatocyte) plates, and peripheral portal tracts. The functional unit of the liver is the hepatic acinus (Fig. 22.2).

Blood flows into the acinus via a single branch of the portal vein and hepatic artery situated centrally in the portal tracts. Blood flows outwards along the hepatic sinusoids into one of several tributaries of the hepatic vein at the periphery of the acinus. Bile, formed by active and passive excretion by hepatocytes into channels called cholangioles, which lie between them, flows in the opposite direction from the periphery of the acinus. The cholangioles converge in interlobular bile ducts in the portal tracts. The hepatocytes in each acinus lie in three zones, depending on their position relative to the portal tract. Those in zone 1 are closest to the terminal branches of the portal vein and hepatic artery, and are richly supplied with oxygenated blood, and with blood containing the highest concentration of nutrients and toxins. Conversely, hepatocytes in zone 3 are furthest from the portal tracts and closest to the hepatic veins, and are therefore relatively hypoxic and exposed to lower concentrations of nutrients and toxins compared to zone 1. The different perfusion and toxin exposure patterns, and thus vulnerability, of hepatocytes in the different zones contribute to the often patchy nature of liver injury.

Liver cells

Hepatocytes comprise 80% of liver cells. The remaining 20% are the endothelial cells lining the sinusoids, epithelial cells lining the intrahepatic bile ducts, cells of the immune system (including macrophages (Kupffer cells) and unique populations of atypical lymphocytes), and a key population of non-parenchymal cells called stellate or Ito cells.

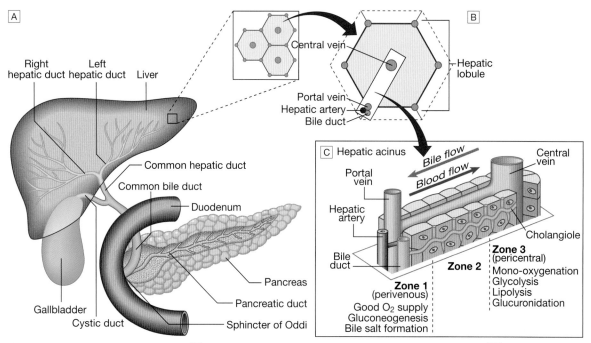

Fig. 22.2 Liver structure and microstructure. [A] Liver anatomy showing relationship with pancreas, bile duct and duodenum. [B] Hepatic lobule. [C] Hepatic acinus.

Endothelial cells line the sinusoids (Fig. 22.3), a network of capillary vessels that differ from other capillary beds in the body, in that there is no basement membrane. The endothelial cells have gaps between them (fenestrae) of about 0.1 micron in diameter, allowing free flow of fluid and particulate matter to the hepatocytes. Individual hepatocytes are separated from the leaky sinusoids by the space of Disse, which contains stellate cells that store vitamin A and play an important part in regulating liver blood flow. They may also be immunologically active and play a role in the liver's contribution to defence against pathogens. The key role of stellate cells in terms of pathology is in the development of hepatic fibrosis, the precursor of cirrhosis. They undergo activation in response to cytokines produced following liver injury, differentiating into myofibroblasts, which are the major producers of the collagen-rich matrix that forms fibrous tissue (Fig. 22.4).

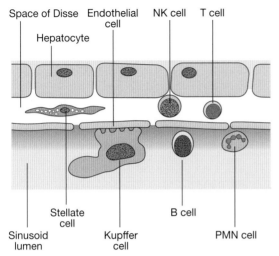

Fig. 22.3 Non-parenchymal liver cells. (B cell = B lymphocyte; NK cell = natural killer cell; PMN cell = polymorphonuclear leucocyte; T cell = T lymphocyte).

Blood supply

The liver is unique as an organ, as it has dual perfusion: it receives a majority of its supply via the portal vein, which drains blood from the gut via the splanchnic circulation and is the principal route for nutrient trafficking to the liver, and a minority from the hepatic artery. The portal venous contribution is 50–90%. The dual perfusion system, and the variable contribution from portal vein and hepatic artery, can have important effects on the clinical expression of liver ischaemia (which typically exhibits a less dramatic pattern than ischaemia in other organs, a fact that can sometimes lead to it being missed clinically), and can raise practical challenges in liver transplant surgery.

Biliary system and gallbladder

Hepatocytes provide the driving force for bile flow by creating osmotic gradients of bile acids, which form micelles in bile (bile

22

Fig. 22.4 Pathogenic mechanisms in hepatic fibrosis. Stellate cell activation occurs under the influence of cytokines released by other cell types in the liver, including hepatocytes, Kupffer cells (tissue macrophages), platelets and lymphocytes. Once stellate cells become activated, they can perpetuate their own activation by synthesis of transforming growth factor beta (TGF-β_1), and platelet-derived growth factor (PDGF) through autocrine loops. Activated stellate cells produce TGF-β_1, stimulating the production of collagen matrix, as well as inhibitors of collagen breakdown. The inhibitors of collagen breakdown, matrix metalloproteinase 2 and 9 (MMP2 and MMP9), are inactivated in turn by tissue inhibitors TIMP1 and TIMP2, which are increased in fibrosis. Inflammation also contributes to fibrosis, with the cytokine profile produced by Th2 lymphocytes, such as interleukin-6 and 13 (IL-6 and IL-13). Activated stellate cells also produce endothelin 1 (ET1), which may contribute to portal hypertension. (EGF = epidermal growth factor; IGF$_1$ = insulin-like growth factor 1; ROS = reactive oxygen species)

acid-dependent bile flow), and of sodium (bile acid-independent bile flow). Bile is secreted by hepatocytes and flows from cholangioles to the biliary canaliculi. The canaliculi join to form larger intrahepatic bile ducts, which in turn merge to form the right and left hepatic ducts. These ducts join as they emerge from the liver to form the common hepatic duct, which becomes the common bile duct after joining the cystic duct (see Fig. 22.2). The common bile duct is approximately 5 cm long and 4–6 mm wide. The distal portion of the duct passes through the head of the pancreas and usually joins the pancreatic duct before entering the duodenum through the ampullary sphincter (sphincter of Oddi). It should be noted, though, that the anatomy of the lower common bile duct can vary widely. Common bile duct pressure is maintained by rhythmic contraction and relaxation of the sphincter of Oddi; this pressure exceeds gallbladder pressure in the fasting state, so that bile normally flows into the gallbladder, where it is concentrated 10-fold by resorption of water and electrolytes.

The gallbladder is a pear-shaped sac typically lying under the right hemiliver, with its fundus located anteriorly behind the tip of the 9th costal cartilage. Anatomical variation is common and should be considered when assessing patients clinically and radiologically. The function of the gallbladder is to concentrate, and provide a reservoir for, bile. Gallbladder tone is maintained by vagal activity, and cholecystokinin released from the duodenal mucosa during feeding causes gallbladder contraction and reduces sphincter pressure, so that bile flows into the duodenum. The body and neck of the gallbladder pass posteromedially towards the porta hepatis, and the cystic duct then joins it to the common hepatic duct. The cystic duct mucosa has prominent crescentic folds (valves of Heister), giving it a beaded appearance on cholangiography.

Hepatic function

Carbohydrate, amino acid and lipid metabolism

The liver plays a central role in carbohydrate, lipid and amino acid metabolism, and is also involved in metabolising drugs and environmental toxins (Fig. 22.5). An important and increasingly recognised role for the liver is in the integration of metabolic pathways, regulating the response of the body to feeding and starvation. Abnormality in metabolic pathways and their regulation can play an important role both in liver disease (e.g. non-alcoholic fatty liver disease, NAFLD) and in diseases that are not conventionally regarded as diseases of the liver (such as type 2 diabetes and inborn errors of metabolism). Hepatocytes have specific pathways to handle each of the nutrients absorbed from the gut and carried to the liver via the portal vein:

- Amino acids from dietary proteins are used for synthesis of plasma proteins, including albumin. The liver produces 8–14 g of albumin per day, and this plays a critical role in maintaining oncotic pressure in the vascular space and in the transport of small molecules like bilirubin, hormones and drugs throughout the body. Amino acids that are not required for the production of new proteins are broken down, with the amino group being converted ultimately to urea.
- Following a meal, more than half of the glucose absorbed is taken up by the liver and stored as glycogen or

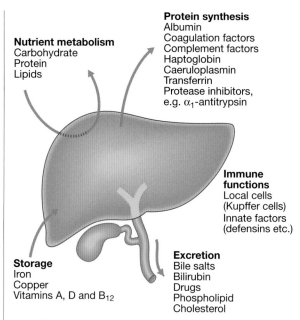

Nutrient metabolism
Carbohydrate
Protein
Lipids

Protein synthesis
Albumin
Coagulation factors
Complement factors
Haptoglobin
Caeruloplasmin
Transferrin
Protease inhibitors,
e.g. α_1-antitrypsin

Immune functions
Local cells
(Kupffer cells)
Innate factors
(defensins etc.)

Storage
Iron
Copper
Vitamins A, D and B_{12}

Excretion
Bile salts
Bilirubin
Drugs
Phospholipid
Cholesterol

Fig. 22.5 **Important liver functions.**

converted to glycerol and fatty acids, thus preventing hyperglycaemia. During fasting, glucose is synthesised (gluconeogenesis) or released from glycogen in the liver, thereby preventing hypoglycaemia (p. 724).
- The liver plays a central role in lipid metabolism, producing very low-density lipoproteins and further metabolising low- and high-density lipoproteins (see Fig. 14.13, p. 372). Dysregulation of lipid metabolism is thought to have a critical role in the pathogenesis of NAFLD. Lipids are now recognised to play a key part in the pathogenesis of hepatitis C, facilitating viral entry into hepatocytes.

Clotting factors

The liver produces key proteins that are involved in the coagulation cascade. Many of these coagulation factors (II, VII, IX and X) are post-translationally modified by vitamin K-dependent enzymes, and their synthesis is impaired in vitamin K deficiency (p. 918). Reduced clotting factor synthesis is an important and easily accessible biomarker of liver function in the setting of liver injury. Prothrombin time (PT; or the International Normalised Ratio, INR) is therefore one of the most important clinical tools available for the assessment of hepatocyte function. Note that the deranged PT or INR seen in liver disease may not directly equate to increased bleeding risk, as these tests do not capture the concurrent reduced synthesis of *anticoagulant* factors, including protein C and protein S. In general, therefore, correction of PT using blood products before minor invasive procedures should be guided by clinical risk rather than the absolute value of the PT.

Bilirubin metabolism and bile

The liver plays a central role in the metabolism of bilirubin and is responsible for the production of bile (Fig. 22.6). Between 425 and 510 mmol (250–300 mg) of unconjugated bilirubin is produced from the catabolism of haem daily. Bilirubin in the

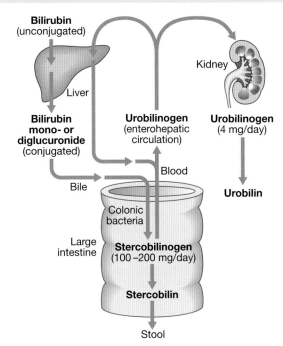

Fig. 22.6 **Pathway of bilirubin excretion.**

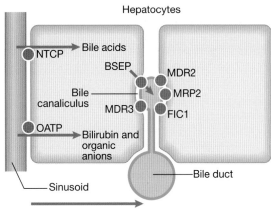

Fig. 22.7 **Biliary transporter proteins.** On the hepatocyte basolateral membrane, sodium taurocholate co-transporting polypeptide (NTCP) mediates uptake of conjugated bile acids from portal blood. At the canalicular membrane, these bile acids are secreted via the bile salt export pump (BSEP) into bile. Multidrug resistance protein 3 (MDR3), also situated on the canalicular membrane, transports phospholipid to the outer side of the membrane. This solubilises bile acids, forming micelles and protecting bile duct membranes from bile salt damage. Familial intrahepatic cholestasis 1 (FIC1) moves phosphatidylserine from the inside to the outside of the canalicular membrane; mutations result in familial cholestasis syndrome in childhood. MDR2 (multidrug resistance 2) regulates transport of glutathione. Multidrug resistance protein 2 (MRP2) transports bilirubin and is induced by rifampicin. Organic anion transporter protein (OATP) transports bilirubin and organic anions.

blood is normally almost all unconjugated and, because it is not water-soluble, is bound to albumin and does not pass into the urine. Unconjugated bilirubin is taken up by hepatocytes at the sinusoidal membrane, where it is conjugated in the endoplasmic reticulum by UDP-glucuronyl transferase, producing bilirubin mono- and diglucuronide. Impaired conjugation by this enzyme is a cause of inherited hyperbilirubinaemias (see Box 22.17). These bilirubin conjugates are water-soluble and are exported into the bile canaliculi by specific carriers on the hepatocyte membranes. The conjugated bilirubin is excreted in the bile and passes into the duodenal lumen.

Once in the intestine, conjugated bilirubin is metabolised by colonic bacteria to form stercobilinogen, which may be further oxidised to stercobilin. Both stercobilinogen and stercobilin are then excreted in the stool, contributing to its brown colour. Biliary obstruction results in reduced stercobilinogen in the stool, and the stools become pale. A small amount of stercobilinogen (4 mg/day) is absorbed from the bowel, passes through the liver and is excreted in the urine, where it is known as urobilinogen or, following further oxidisation, urobilin. The liver secretes 1–2 L of bile daily. Bile contains bile acids (formed from cholesterol), phospholipids, bilirubin and cholesterol. Several biliary transporter proteins have been identified (Fig. 22.7). Mutations in genes encoding these proteins have been identified in inherited intrahepatic biliary diseases presenting in childhood, and in adult-onset disease such as intrahepatic cholestasis of pregnancy and gallstone formation.

Storage of vitamins and minerals

Vitamins A, D and B_{12} are stored by the liver in large amounts, while others, such as vitamin K and folate, are stored in smaller amounts and disappear rapidly if dietary intake is reduced. The liver is also able to metabolise vitamins to more active compounds, e.g. 7-dehydrocholesterol to 25(OH) vitamin D. Vitamin K is a fat-soluble vitamin and so the inability to absorb fat-soluble vitamins, as occurs in biliary obstruction, results in a coagulopathy. The liver also stores minerals such as iron, in ferritin and haemosiderin, and copper, which is excreted in bile.

Immune regulation

Approximately 9% of the normal liver is composed of immune cells (see Fig. 22.3). Cells of the innate immune system include Kupffer cells derived from blood monocytes, the liver macrophages and natural killer (NK) cells, as well as 'classical' B and T cells of the adaptive immune response (p. 67). An additional type of atypical lymphocyte, with phenotypic features of both T cells and NK cells, is thought to play an important role in host defence through linking of innate and adaptive immunity. The enrichment of such cells in the liver reflects the unique importance of the liver in preventing microorganisms from the gut from entering the systemic circulation.

Kupffer cells constitute the largest single mass of tissue-resident macrophages in the body and account for 80% of the phagocytic capacity of this system. They remove aged and damaged red blood cells, bacteria, viruses, antigen–antibody complexes and endotoxin. They also produce a wide variety of inflammatory mediators that can act locally or may be released into the systemic circulation.

The immunological environment of the liver is unique in that antigens presented within it tend to induce immunological tolerance. This is of importance in liver transplantation, where classical major histocompatibility (MHC) barriers may be crossed, and also in chronic viral infections, when immune responses may be attenuated. The mechanisms that underlie this phenomenon have not been fully defined.

22

Investigation of liver and hepatobiliary disease

Investigations play an important role in the management of liver disease in three settings:

- identifying the presence of liver disease
- establishing the aetiology
- understanding disease severity (in particular, identification of cirrhosis with its complications).

When planning investigations, it is important to be clear as to which of these goals is being addressed.

Suspicion of the presence of liver disease is normally based on blood biochemistry abnormality ('liver function tests', or 'LFTs').

Aetiology is typically established through a combination of history, specific blood tests and, where appropriate, imaging and liver biopsy.

Staging of disease (in essence, the identification of cirrhosis) is largely histological, although there is increasing interest in non-invasive approaches, including novel imaging modalities, serum markers of fibrosis and the use of predictive scoring systems.

The aims of investigation in patients with suspected liver disease are shown in Box 22.1.

Liver blood biochemistry

Liver blood biochemistry (LFTs) includes the measurement of serum bilirubin, aminotransferases, alkaline phosphatase, γ-glutamyl transferase and albumin. Most analytes measured by LFTs are not truly 'function' tests but instead, given that they are released by injured hepatocytes, provide biochemical evidence of liver cell damage. Liver function per se is best assessed by the serum albumin, PT and bilirubin because of the role played by the liver in synthesis of albumin and clotting factors and in clearance of bilirubin. Although LFT abnormalities are often non-specific, the patterns are frequently helpful in directing further investigations. In addition, levels of bilirubin and albumin and the PT are related to clinical outcome in patients with severe liver disease, reflected by their use in several prognostic scores: the Child–Pugh and MELD scores in cirrhosis (see Boxes 22.29 and 22.30, pp. 867 and 868), the Glasgow score in alcoholic hepatitis (see Box 22.47, p. 882) and the King's College Hospital criteria for liver transplantation in acute liver failure (see Box 22.11, p. 858). These established predictive models, together with emerging disease-specific scoring systems in conditions such as non-alcoholic steatohepatitis (the NASH fibrosis score) and primary biliary cholangitis (PBC, formerly known as primary biliary cirrhosis; the UK-PBC risk score), systematise the approach to assessing abnormal LFTs and can be important for the targeting of more expensive and/or invasive confirmatory diagnostic tests.

Bilirubin and albumin

The degree of elevation of bilirubin can reflect the degree of liver damage. A raised bilirubin often occurs earlier in the natural history of biliary disease (e.g. PBC) than in disease of the liver parenchyma (e.g. cirrhosis), where the hepatocytes are primarily involved. Swelling of the liver within its capsule in inflammation can, however, sometimes impair bile flow and cause an elevation of bilirubin level that is disproportionate to the degree of liver injury. Caution is therefore needed in interpreting the level of liver injury purely on the basis of bilirubin elevation.

Serum albumin levels are often low in patients with liver disease. This is due to a change in the volume of distribution of albumin, and to reduced synthesis. Since the plasma half-life of albumin is about 2 weeks, albumin levels may be normal in acute liver failure but are almost always reduced in chronic liver failure.

Alanine aminotransferase and aspartate aminotransferase

Alanine aminotransferase (ALT) and aspartate aminotransferase (AST) are located in the cytoplasm of the hepatocyte; AST is also located in the hepatocyte mitochondria. Although both transaminase enzymes are widely distributed, expression of ALT outside the liver is relatively low and this enzyme is therefore considered more specific for hepatocellular damage. Large increases of aminotransferase activity favour hepatocellular damage, and this pattern of LFT abnormality is known as 'hepatitic'.

Alkaline phosphatase and γ-glutamyl transferase

Alkaline phosphatase (ALP) is the collective name given to several different enzymes that hydrolyse phosphate esters at alkaline pH. These enzymes are widely distributed in the body but the main sites of production are the liver, gastrointestinal tract, bone, placenta and kidney. ALPs are post-translationally modified, resulting in the production of several different isoenzymes, which differ in abundance in different tissues. ALP enzymes in the liver are located in cell membranes of the hepatic sinusoids and the biliary canaliculi. Accordingly, levels rise with intrahepatic and extrahepatic biliary obstruction and with sinusoidal obstruction, as occurs in infiltrative liver disease.

Gamma-glutamyl transferase (GGT) is a microsomal enzyme found in many cells and tissues of the body. The highest concentrations are located in the liver, where it is produced by hepatocytes and by the epithelium lining small bile ducts. The function of GGT is to transfer glutamyl groups from γ-glutamyl peptides to other peptides and amino acids.

The pattern of a modest increase in aminotransferase activity and large increases in ALP and GGT activity favours biliary obstruction and is commonly described as 'cholestatic' or 'obstructive' (Box 22.2). Isolated elevation of the serum GGT is relatively common and may occur during ingestion of microsomal enzyme-inducing drugs, including alcohol (Box 22.3), but also in NAFLD.

Other biochemical tests

Other widely available biochemical tests may become altered in patients with liver disease:

- Hyponatraemia occurs in severe liver disease due to increased production of vasopressin (antidiuretic hormone,

22.1 Aims of investigations in patients with suspected liver disease

- Detect hepatic abnormality
- Measure the severity of liver damage
- Detect the pattern of liver function test abnormality: hepatitic or obstructive/cholestatic
- Identify the specific cause
- Investigate possible complications

22.2 'Hepatitic' and 'cholestatic'/'obstructive' liver function tests

Pattern	AST/ALT	GGT	ALP
Biliary obstruction	↑	↑↑	↑↑↑
Hepatitis	↑↑↑	↑	↑
Alcohol/enzyme-inducing drugs	N/↑	↑↑	N

N = normal; ↑ mild elevation (< twice normal); ↑↑ moderate elevation (2–5 times normal); ↑↑↑ marked elevation (>5 times normal).
(ALT = alanine aminotransferase; ALP = alkaline phosphatase; AST = aspartate aminotransferase; GGT = gamma-glutamyltransferase)

22.3 Drugs that increase levels of γ-glutamyltransferase

- Barbiturates
- Carbamazepine
- Ethanol
- Griseofulvin
- Rifampicin
- Phenytoin

ADH; see Fig. 14.8, p. 359). Hyponatraemia can be a significant clinical problem in liver disease with aspects that are distinct from hyponatraemia of other causes.

- Serum urea may be reduced in hepatic failure, whereas levels of urea may be increased following gastrointestinal haemorrhage.
- When high levels of urea are accompanied by raised bilirubin, high serum creatinine and low urinary sodium, this suggests hepatorenal failure, which carries a grave prognosis.
- Significantly elevated ferritin suggests haemochromatosis. Modest elevations can be seen in inflammatory disease, NAFLD and alcohol excess.

Haematological tests

Blood count

The peripheral blood count is often abnormal and can give a clue to the underlying diagnosis:

- *A normochromic normocytic anaemia* may reflect recent gastrointestinal haemorrhage, whereas chronic blood loss is characterised by a hypochromic microcytic anaemia secondary to iron deficiency. A high erythrocyte mean cell volume (macrocytosis) is associated with alcohol misuse, but target cells in any jaundiced patient also result in a macrocytosis. Macrocytosis can persist for a long period of time after alcohol cessation, making it a poor marker of ongoing consumption.
- *Leucopenia* may complicate portal hypertension and hypersplenism, whereas leucocytosis may occur with cholangitis, alcoholic hepatitis and hepatic abscesses. Atypical lymphocytes are seen in infectious mononucleosis, which may be complicated by an acute hepatitis.
- *Thrombocytopenia* is common in cirrhosis and is due to reduced platelet production and increased breakdown because of hypersplenism. Thrombopoietin, required for platelet production, is produced in the liver and levels fall with worsening liver function. Thus platelet levels are usually more depressed than white cells and haemoglobin in the presence of hypersplenism in patients with cirrhosis.

A low platelet count is often an indicator of chronic liver disease, particularly in the context of hepatomegaly. Thrombocytosis is unusual in patients with liver disease but may occur in those with active gastrointestinal haemorrhage and, rarely, in hepatocellular carcinoma.

Coagulation tests

These are often abnormal in patients with liver disease. The normal half-lives of the vitamin K-dependent coagulation factors in the blood are short (5–72 hours), and so changes in the PT occur relatively quickly following liver damage; these changes provide valuable prognostic information in patients with both acute and chronic liver failure. An increased PT is evidence of severe liver damage in chronic liver disease. Vitamin K does not reverse this deficiency if it is due to liver disease, but will correct the PT if the cause is vitamin K deficiency, as may occur with biliary obstruction due to non-absorption of fat-soluble vitamins.

Immunological tests

A variety of tests are available to evaluate the aetiology of hepatic disease (Boxes 22.4 and 22.5). The presence of liver-related autoantibodies can be suggestive of the presence of autoimmune liver disease (although false-positive results can occur in non-autoimmune inflammatory disease such as NAFLD). Elevation in overall serum immunoglobulin levels can also indicate autoimmunity (immunoglobulin G (IgG) and IgM). Elevated serum IgA can be seen, often in more advanced alcoholic liver disease and NAFLD, although the association is not specific.

22.4 Chronic liver disease screen

- Hepatitis B surface antigen
- Hepatitis C antibody
- Liver autoantibodies (antinuclear antibody, smooth muscle antibody, antimitochondrial antibody)
- Immunoglobulins
- Ferritin
- α_1-antitrypsin
- Caeruloplasmin

Imaging

Several imaging techniques can be used to determine the site and general nature of structural lesions in the liver and biliary tree. In general, however, imaging techniques are unable to identify hepatic inflammation and have poor sensitivity for liver fibrosis unless advanced cirrhosis with portal hypertension is present.

Ultrasound

Ultrasound is non-invasive and most commonly used as a 'first-line' test to identify gallstones, biliary obstruction (Fig. 22.8) or thrombosis in the hepatic vasculature. Ultrasound is good for the identification of splenomegaly and abnormalities in liver texture but is less effective at identifying diffuse parenchymal disease. Focal lesions, such as tumours, may not be detected if they are less than 2 cm in diameter and have similar echogenicity to normal liver tissue. Bubble-based contrast media are now used routinely and can enhance discriminant capability. Doppler ultrasound allows blood flow in the hepatic artery, portal vein

22

22.5 How to identify the cause of liver function test (LFT) abnormality

Diagnosis	Clinical clue	Initial test	Additional tests
Alcoholic liver disease	History	LFTs AST > ALT; high MCV	Random blood alcohol
Non-alcoholic fatty liver disease (NAFLD)	Metabolic syndrome (central obesity, diabetes, hypertension)	LFTs	Liver biopsy
Chronic hepatitis B	Injection drug use; blood transfusion	HBsAg	HBeAg, HBeAb HBV-DNA
Chronic hepatitis C	Injection drug use; blood transfusion	HCV antibody	HCV-RNA
Primary biliary cholangitis	Itching; raised ALP	AMA	Liver biopsy
Primary sclerosing cholangitis	Inflammatory bowel disease	MRCP	ANCA
Autoimmune hepatitis	Other autoimmune diseases	ASMA, ANA, LKM, immunoglobulin	Liver biopsy
Haemochromatosis	Diabetes/joint pain	Transferrin saturation, ferritin	HFE gene test
Wilson's disease	Neurological signs; haemolysis	Caeruloplasmin	24-hour urinary copper
α_1-antitrypsin	Lung disease	α_1-antitrypsin level	α_1-antitrypsin genotype
Drug-induced liver disease	Drug/herbal remedy history	LFTs	Liver biopsy
Coeliac disease	Malabsorption	Tissue transglutaminase	Duodenal biopsy

(ALP = alkaline phosphatase; ALT = alanine aminotransferase; AMA = antimitochondrial antibody; ANA = antinuclear antibody; ANCA = antineutrophil cytoplasmic antibody; ASMA = anti-smooth muscle antibody; AST = aspartate aminotransferase; HBeAb = antibody to hepatitis B e antigen; HBeAg = hepatitis B e antigen; HBsAg = hepatitis B surface antigen; HBV = hepatitis B virus; HCV = hepatitis C virus; HFE = haemochromatosis (high iron/Fe); LKM = liver–kidney microsomal antibody; MCV = mean cell volume; MRCP = magnetic resonance cholangiopancreatography)

Fig. 22.8 Ultrasound showing a stone in the gallbladder (A) with acoustic shadow (S).

Fig. 22.9 Computed tomography in a patient with cirrhosis. The liver is small and has an irregular outline (black arrow), the spleen is enlarged (long white arrow), fluid (ascites) is seen around the liver, and collateral vessels are present around the proximal stomach (short white arrow).

and hepatic veins to be investigated. Endoscopic ultrasound provides high-resolution images of the pancreas, biliary tree and liver (see below and Fig. 22.46, p. 906).

Computed tomography and magnetic resonance imaging

Computed tomography (CT) detects smaller focal lesions in the liver, especially when combined with contrast injection (Fig. 22.9). Magnetic resonance imaging (MRI) can also be used to localise and confirm the aetiology of focal liver lesions, particularly primary and secondary tumours.

Hepatic angiography is seldom used nowadays as a diagnostic tool, since CT and MRI are both able to provide images of hepatic vasculature, but it still has a therapeutic role in the embolisation of vascular tumours, such as hepatocellular carcinoma. Hepatic venography is now rarely performed.

Cholangiography

Cholangiography can be undertaken by magnetic resonance cholangiopancreatography (MRCP; Fig. 22.10), endoscopy (endoscopic retrograde cholangiopancreatography, ERCP) or the percutaneous approach (percutaneous transhepatic

Fig. 22.10 Magnetic resonance cholangiopancreatography showing a biliary stricture due to cholangiocarcinoma in the distal common bile duct (arrow). The proximal common bile duct (CBD) is dilated but the pancreatic duct (PD) is normal.

i **22.6 Conditions required for safe percutaneous liver biopsy**

- Cooperative patient
- Prothrombin time <4 secs prolonged
- Platelet count >80×10⁹/L
- Exclusion of bile duct obstruction, localised skin infection, advanced chronic obstructive pulmonary disease, marked ascites and severe anaemia

- the procedure is conducted percutaneously under ultrasound control and the needle track is then plugged with procoagulant material.

In patients with potentially resectable malignancy, biopsy should be avoided due to the potential risk of tumour dissemination. Operative or laparoscopic liver biopsy may sometimes be valuable.

Although the pathological features of liver disease are complex, with several features occurring together, liver disorders can be broadly classified histologically into fatty liver (steatosis), hepatitis (inflammation, 'grade') and cirrhosis (fibrosis, 'stage'). The use of special histological stains can help in determining aetiology. The clinical features and prognosis of these changes are dependent on the underlying aetiology and are discussed in the relevant sections below.

Non-invasive markers of hepatic fibrosis

Non-invasive markers of liver fibrosis can reduce the need for liver biopsy to assess the extent of fibrosis in some settings. In general, they have high negative predictive value, being able to exclude the presence of advanced fibrosis, but a relatively low positive predictive value. It is important to note that many of these tests have been validated only in certain aetiologies of liver disease and therefore results cannot be extrapolated to all other liver diseases. Alcohol-related liver disease is particularly poorly served in this respect.

Serological markers of hepatic fibrosis, such as α_2-macroglobulin, haptoglobin and routine clinical biochemistry tests, are used in the Fibrotest®. The Enhanced Liver Fibrosis (ELF®) serological assay uses a combination of hyaluronic acid, procollagen peptide III (PIIINP) and tissue inhibitor of metalloproteinase 1 (TIMP1). These tests are good at differentiating severe fibrosis from mild scarring but are limited in their ability to detect subtle changes. A number of non-commercial scores based on standard biochemical and anthropometric indices have also been described that provide similar levels of sensitivity and specificity (e.g. the FIB4 score, which is based on age, ALT/AST ratio and platelet count).

An alternative to serological markers is vibration-controlled transient elastography (Fibroscan®), in which ultrasound-based shock waves are sent through the liver to measure liver stiffness as a surrogate for hepatic fibrosis. Once again, this test is good at differentiating severe fibrosis from mild scarring, but it is limited in its ability to detect subtle changes and validity may be affected by obesity. Similar techniques, including magnetic resonance elastography, are promising but not yet widely available.

cholangiography, PTC). The latter does not allow the ampulla of Vater or pancreatic duct to be visualised. Endoscopic ultrasound can also provide high-quality biliary imaging safely (see below). MRCP is as good as ERCP at providing images of the biliary tree but is safer, and there is now little, if any, role for diagnostic ERCP. Both endoscopic and percutaneous approaches allow therapeutic interventions, such as the insertion of biliary stents across bile duct strictures. The percutaneous approach is used only if it is not possible to access the bile duct endoscopically.

Endoscopic ultrasound

Endoscopic ultrasound (EUS; p. 774) is complementary to MRCP in the diagnostic evaluation of the extrahepatic biliary tree, ampulla of Vater and pancreas. With the ultrasonic probe in the duodenum, high-quality images are obtained, tissue sampling can be performed and, increasingly, therapeutic drainage of biliary obstruction can be performed. EUS has the advantage over ERCP of not exposing patients to the risk of pancreatitis, among other complications of bile duct cannulation.

Histological examination

An ultrasound-guided liver biopsy can confirm the severity of liver damage and provide aetiological information. It is performed percutaneously with a Trucut or Menghini needle, usually through an intercostal space under local anaesthesia, or radiologically using a transjugular approach.

Percutaneous liver biopsy is a relatively safe procedure if the conditions detailed in Box 22.6 are met, but carries a mortality of about 0.01%. The main complications are abdominal and/or shoulder pain, bleeding and biliary peritonitis. Biliary peritonitis is rare and usually occurs when a biopsy is performed in a patient with obstruction of a large bile duct. Liver biopsies can be carried out in patients with defective haemostasis if:

- the defect is corrected with fresh frozen plasma and platelet transfusion
- the biopsy is obtained by the transjugular route, *or*

Presenting problems in liver disease

Liver injury may be either acute or chronic. The main causes are listed in Figure 22.11 and discussed in detail later in the chapter. In

22

the UK, liver disease is the only one of the top causes of mortality that is steadily increasing (Fig. 22.12). Mortality rates have risen substantially over the last 30 years, with a near-fivefold increase in liver-related mortality in people younger than 65 years. The rate of increase is substantially higher in the UK than in other countries in Western Europe.

- *Acute liver injury* may present with non-specific symptoms of fatigue and abnormal LFTs, or with jaundice and acute liver failure.
- *Chronic liver injury* is defined as hepatic injury, inflammation and/or fibrosis occurring in the liver for more than 6 months. In the early stages, patients can be asymptomatic with fluctuating abnormal LFTs. With more severe liver damage, however, the presentation can be with jaundice, portal hypertension or other signs of cirrhosis and hepatic decompensation (Box 22.7). Patients with clinically silent chronic liver disease frequently present when abnormalities in liver function are observed on routine blood testing, or when clinical events, such as an intercurrent infection or surgical intervention, cause the liver to decompensate. Patients with compensated cirrhosis can undergo most forms of surgery without

i	22.7 Presentation of liver disease	
Severity	Acute liver injury	Chronic liver injury
Mild/moderate	Abnormal liver function tests	Abnormal liver function tests
Severe	Jaundice	Signs of cirrhosis ± portal hypertension
Very severe	Acute liver failure	Chronic liver failure* Jaundice Ascites Hepatic encephalopathy Portal hypertension with variceal bleeding

*May not occur until several years after cirrhosis has presented.

significantly increased risk, whereas decompensation can be a complication in all cases and the presence of portal hypertension with intra-abdominal varices can make abdominal surgery more hazardous. The possibility of undiagnosed liver disease should be borne in mind in all patients in at-risk groups undergoing significant surgery.

Acute liver failure

Acute liver failure is an uncommon but serious condition characterised by a relatively rapid progressive deterioration in liver function. The presence of encephalopathy is a cardinal feature, with mental changes progressing from delirium to coma. The syndrome was originally defined further as occurring within 8 weeks of onset of the precipitating illness, in the absence of evidence of pre-existing liver disease. This distinguishes it from instances in which hepatic encephalopathy represents a deterioration in chronic liver disease.

Liver failure occurs when there is insufficient metabolic and synthetic function for the needs of the patient. Although the direct cause is usually acute loss of functional hepatocytes, this can occur in different settings, which have implications for outcome and treatment. In a patient whose liver was previously normal (fulminant liver failure), the level of injury needed to cause liver

Acute liver injury

Viral hepatitis (A, B, E)

Alcoholic liver disease*

Drugs

Wilson's disease

Autoimmune hepatitis*

Chronic liver injury

Chronic viral hepatitis (B + C)

NAFLD Haemochromatosis

α₁-antitrypsin deficiency Cryptogenic (unknown)

PBC PSC

Fig. 22.11 Causes of acute and chronic liver injury. *Although there is often evidence of chronic liver disease at presentation, may present acutely with jaundice. In alcoholic liver disease this is due to superimposed alcoholic hepatitis. (NAFLD = non-alcoholic fatty liver disease; PBC = primary biliary cholangitis; PSC = primary sclerosing cholangitis)

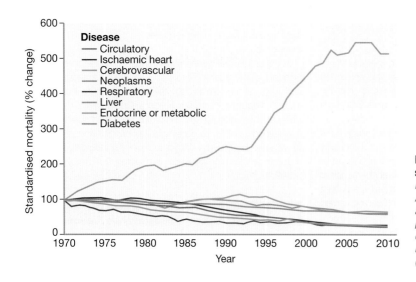

Fig. 22.12 Standardised UK mortality rates showing the rise in liver-related mortality. *From Williams R, Aspinall R, Bellis M, et al. Addressing liver disease in the UK: a blueprint for attaining excellence in health care and reducing premature mortality from lifestyle issues of excess consumption of alcohol, obesity, and viral hepatitis. Reprinted with permission from Elsevier (The Lancet 2014; 384:1953–1997).*

failure, and thus the patient risk, is very high. In a patient with pre-existing chronic liver disease, the additional acute insult needed to precipitate liver failure is much less. It is critical, therefore, to understand whether liver failure is a true acute event or an acute deterioration on a background of pre-existing injury (which may itself not have been diagnosed). Although liver biopsy may ultimately be necessary, it is the presence or absence of the clinical features suggesting chronicity that guides the clinician.

More recently, newer classifications have been developed to reflect differences in presentation and outcome of acute liver failure. One such classification divides acute liver failure into hyperacute, acute and subacute, according to the interval between onset of jaundice and encephalopathy (Box 22.8).

Pathophysiology

Any cause of liver damage can produce acute liver failure, provided it is sufficiently severe (Fig. 22.13). Acute viral hepatitis is the most common cause worldwide, whereas paracetamol toxicity (p. 137) is the most frequent cause in the UK. Acute liver failure occurs occasionally with other drugs, or from *Amanita phalloides* (mushroom) poisoning, in pregnancy, in Wilson's disease, following shock (p. 199) and, rarely, in extensive malignant disease of the liver. In 10% of cases, the cause of acute liver failure remains unknown and these patients are often labelled as having 'non-A–E viral hepatitis' or 'cryptogenic' acute liver failure.

Clinical assessment

Cerebral disturbance (hepatic encephalopathy and/or cerebral oedema) is the cardinal manifestation of acute liver failure, but in the early stages this can be mild and episodic, and so its absence does not exclude a significant acute liver injury. The initial clinical features are often subtle and include reduced alertness and poor concentration, progressing through behavioural abnormalities, such as restlessness and aggressive outbursts, to drowsiness and coma (Box 22.9). Cerebral oedema may occur due to increased intracranial pressure, causing unequal or abnormally reacting pupils, fixed pupils, hypertensive episodes, bradycardia, hyperventilation, profuse sweating, local or general myoclonus, focal fits or decerebrate posturing. Papilloedema occurs rarely and is a late sign. More general symptoms include weakness, nausea and vomiting. Right hypochondrial discomfort is an occasional feature.

The patient may be jaundiced but jaundice may not be present at the outset (e.g. in paracetamol overdose), and there are a number of exceptions, including Reye's syndrome, in which jaundice is rare. Occasionally, death may occur in fulminant cases of acute liver failure before jaundice develops. Fetor hepaticus can be present. The liver is usually of normal size but later becomes smaller. Hepatomegaly is unusual and, in

22.8 Classification of acute liver failure

Type	Time: jaundice to encephalopathy	Cerebral oedema	Common causes
Hyperacute	<7 days	Common	Viral, paracetamol
Acute	8–28 days	Common	Cryptogenic, drugs
Subacute	29 days to 12 weeks	Uncommon	Cryptogenic, drugs

22.9 How to assess clinical grade of hepatic encephalopathy

Clinical grade	Clinical signs
Grade 1	Poor concentration, slurred speech, slow mentation, disordered sleep rhythm
Grade 2	Drowsy but easily rousable, occasional aggressive behaviour, lethargic
Grade 3	Marked delirium, drowsy, sleepy but responds to pain and voice, gross disorientation
Grade 4	Unresponsive to voice, may or may not respond to painful stimuli, unconscious

22

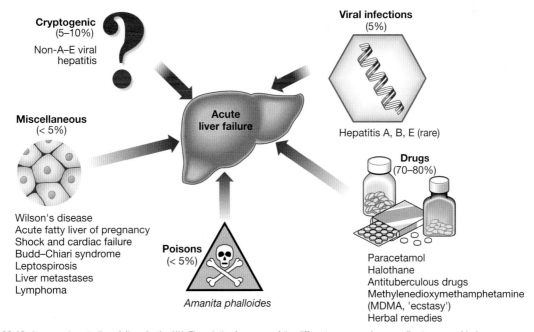

Cryptogenic (5–10%)
Non-A–E viral hepatitis

Viral infections (5%)
Hepatitis A, B, E (rare)

Miscellaneous (< 5%)
Wilson's disease
Acute fatty liver of pregnancy
Shock and cardiac failure
Budd–Chiari syndrome
Leptospirosis
Liver metastases
Lymphoma

Poisons (< 5%)
Amanita phalloides

Drugs (70–80%)
Paracetamol
Halothane
Antituberculous drugs
Methylenedioxymethamphetamine (MDMA, 'ecstasy')
Herbal remedies

Acute liver failure

Fig. 22.13 Causes of acute liver failure in the UK. The relative frequency of the different causes varies according to geographical area.

the presence of a sudden onset of ascites, suggests venous outflow obstruction as the cause (Budd–Chiari syndrome, p. 898). Splenomegaly is uncommon and never prominent. Ascites and oedema are late developments and may be a consequence of fluid therapy. Other features are related to the development of complications (see below).

Investigations

The patient should be investigated to determine the cause of the liver failure and the prognosis (Boxes 22.10 and 22.11). Hepatitis B core IgM antibody is the best screening test for acute hepatitis B infection, as liver damage is due to the immunological response to the virus, which has often been eliminated, and the test for hepatitis B surface antigen (HBsAg) may be negative. The PT rapidly becomes prolonged as coagulation factor synthesis fails; this is the laboratory test of greatest prognostic value and should be carried out at least twice daily. Its prognostic importance emphasises the necessity of avoiding the use of fresh frozen plasma to correct raised PT in acute liver failure, except in the setting of frank bleeding. Factor V levels can be used instead of the PT to assess the degree of liver impairment. The plasma

bilirubin reflects the degree of jaundice. Plasma aminotransferase activity is particularly high after paracetamol overdose, reaching 100–500 times normal, but falls as liver damage progresses and is not helpful in determining prognosis. Plasma albumin remains normal unless the course is prolonged. Percutaneous liver biopsy is contraindicated because of the severe coagulopathy, but biopsy can be undertaken using the transjugular route if appropriate.

Management

Patients with acute liver failure should be treated in a high-dependency or intensive care unit as soon as progressive prolongation of the PT occurs or hepatic encephalopathy is identified (Box 22.12), so that prompt treatment of complications can be initiated (Box 22.13). Conservative treatment aims to maintain life in the hope that hepatic regeneration will occur, but early transfer to a specialised transplant unit should always be considered. N-acetylcysteine therapy may improve outcome, particularly in patients with acute liver failure due to paracetamol poisoning. Liver transplantation is an increasingly important treatment option for acute liver failure, and criteria have been developed to identify patients unlikely to survive without a transplant (see Box 22.11). Patients should, wherever possible, be transferred to a transplant centre before these criteria are met to allow time for assessment and to maximise the time for a donor liver to become available. Survival following liver transplantation

---

 22.10 Investigations to determine the cause of acute liver failure

- Toxicology screen of blood and urine
- HBsAg, IgM anti-HBc
- IgM anti-HAV
- Anti-HEV, HCV, cytomegalovirus, herpes simplex, Epstein Barr virus
- Caeruloplasmin, serum copper, urinary copper, slit-lamp eye examination
- Autoantibodies: ANA, ASMA, LKM, SLA
- Immunoglobulins
- Ultrasound of liver and Doppler of hepatic veins

(ANA = antinuclear antibody; anti-HBc = antibody to hepatitis B core antigen; ASMA = anti-smooth muscle antibody; HAV = hepatitis A virus; HBsAg = hepatitis B surface antigen; HCV = hepatitis C virus; HEV = hepatitis E virus; IgM = immunoglobulin M; LKM = liver–kidney microsomal antibody; SLA = soluble liver antigen)

 22.11 Adverse prognostic criteria in acute liver failure*

Paracetamol overdose

- H^+ >50 nmol/L (pH <7.3) at or beyond 24 hours following the overdose

  Or
- Serum creatinine >300 µmol/L ($\cong$3.38 mg/dL) *plus* prothrombin time >100 secs *plus* encephalopathy grade 3 or 4

Non-paracetamol cases

- Prothrombin time >100 secs

  Or
- Any three of the following:
  Jaundice to encephalopathy time >7 days
  Age <10 or >40 years
  Indeterminate or drug-induced causes
  Bilirubin >300 µmol/L ($\cong$17.6 mg/dL)
  Prothrombin time >50 secs

  Or
- Factor V level <15% and encephalopathy grade 3 or 4

*Predict a mortality rate of $\geq$90% and are an indication for referral for possible liver transplantation.

 22.12 Monitoring in acute liver failure

Cardiorespiratory

- Pulse
- Blood pressure
- Central venous pressure
- Respiratory rate

Neurological

- Intracranial pressure monitoring (specialist units, p. 208)
- Conscious level

Fluid balance

- Hourly output (urine, vomiting, diarrhoea)
- Input: oral, intravenous

Blood analyses

- Arterial blood gases
- Peripheral blood count (including platelets)
- Sodium, potassium, HCO_3^-, calcium, magnesium
- Creatinine, urea
- Glucose (2-hourly in acute phase)
- Prothrombin time

Infection surveillance

- Cultures: blood, urine, throat, sputum, cannula sites
- Chest X-ray
- Temperature

 22.13 Complications of acute liver failure

- Encephalopathy and cerebral oedema
- Hypoglycaemia
- Metabolic acidosis
- Infection (bacterial, fungal)
- Renal failure
- Multi-organ failure (hypotension and respiratory failure)

for acute liver failure is improving and 1-year survival rates of about 60% can be expected. A number of artificial liver support systems have been developed and evaluated for use as a bridge to either transplantation or recovery. None, however, has entered routine clinical use.

Abnormal liver function tests

Frequently, LFTs are requested in patients who have no symptoms or signs of liver disease, as part of routine health checks, insurance medicals or drug monitoring. When abnormal results are found, it is important for the clinician to be able to interpret them and to investigate appropriately. Many patients with chronic liver disease are asymptomatic or have vague, non-specific symptoms. Apparently asymptomatic abnormal LFTs are therefore a common occurrence. When LFTs are measured routinely prior to elective surgery, 3.5% of patients are discovered to have mildly elevated transaminases. The prevalence of abnormal LFTs has been reported to be as high as 10% in some studies. The most common abnormalities are alcoholic (p. 880) or non-alcoholic fatty liver disease (p. 882). Since effective medical treatments are now available for many types of chronic liver disease, further evaluation is usually warranted to make sure the patient does not have a treatable condition. Although transient mild abnormalities in LFTs may not be clinically significant, the majority of individuals with persistently abnormal LFTs do have significant liver disease. Biochemical abnormalities in chronic liver disease often fluctuate over time; even mild abnormalities can therefore indicate significant underlying disease and so warrant follow-up and investigation.

When abnormal LFTs are detected, a thorough history should be compiled to determine the patient's alcohol consumption, drug use (prescribed drugs or otherwise), risk factors for viral hepatitis (e.g. blood transfusion, injection drug use, tattoos), the presence of autoimmune diseases, family history, neurological symptoms, and the presence of features of the metabolic syndrome (p. 730), including diabetes and/or obesity (see Box 22.5 and Fig. 19.5, p. 698). The presence or absence of stigmata of

22.14 Common causes of elevated serum transaminases

Minor elevation (<100 U/L*)
- Chronic hepatitis C
- Chronic hepatitis B
- Haemochromatosis
- Fatty liver disease

Moderate elevation (100–300 U/L*)
As above plus:
- Alcoholic hepatitis
- Non-alcoholic steatohepatitis
- Autoimmune hepatitis
- Wilson's disease

Major elevation (>300 U/L*)
- Drugs (e.g. paracetamol)
- Acute viral hepatitis
- Autoimmune liver disease
- Ischaemic liver
- Toxins (e.g. *Amanita phalloides* poisoning)
- Flare of chronic hepatitis B

*These ranges are indicative but do not rigidly discriminate between different aetiologies.

Fig. 22.14 **Suggested management of abnormal liver function tests in asymptomatic patients.** *No further investigation needed. (α₁AT = alpha₁ antitrypsin; BMI = body mass index; ERCP = endoscopic retrograde cholangiopancreatography; GGT = γ-glutamyl transferase; HBsAg = hepatitis B surface antigen; HCVAb = antibody to hepatitis C virus; MRCP = magnetic resonance cholangiopancreatography; NAFLD = non-alcoholic fatty liver disease)

chronic liver disease does not reliably identify those individuals with significant disease and investigations are indicated, even in the absence of these signs.

Both the pattern of LFT abnormality (hepatitic or obstructive) and the degree of elevation are helpful in determining the cause of underlying liver disease (Boxes 22.14 and 22.15). The investigations that make up a standard liver screen and additional or confirmatory tests are shown in Boxes 22.4 and 22.5. An algorithm for investigating abnormal LFTs is provided in Figure 22.14.

Jaundice

Jaundice is usually detectable clinically when the plasma bilirubin exceeds 40 μmol/L (~2.5 mg/dL). The causes of jaundice overlap with the causes of abnormal LFTs discussed above. In a patient with jaundice it is useful to consider whether the cause might be pre-hepatic, hepatic or post-hepatic, and there are often important clues in the history (Box 22.16).

Pre-hepatic jaundice

This is caused either by haemolysis or by congenital hyper-bilirubinaemia, and is characterised by an isolated raised bilirubin level.

In haemolysis, destruction of red blood cells or their marrow precursors causes increased bilirubin production. Jaundice due to haemolysis is usually mild because a healthy liver can excrete a bilirubin load six times greater than normal before unconjugated bilirubin accumulates in the plasma. This does not apply to newborns, who have less capacity to metabolise bilirubin.

The most common form of non-haemolytic hyperbilirubinaemia is Gilbert's syndrome, an inherited disorder of bilirubin metabolism (Box 22.17). Other inherited disorders of bilirubin metabolism are very rare.

Hepatocellular jaundice

Hepatocellular jaundice results from an inability of the liver to transport bilirubin into the bile, occurring as a consequence of parenchymal disease. Bilirubin transport across the hepatocytes may be impaired at any point between uptake of unconjugated bilirubin into the cells and transport of conjugated bilirubin into the canaliculi. In addition, swelling of cells and oedema resulting from the disease itself may cause obstruction of the biliary canaliculi. In hepatocellular jaundice, the concentrations of both unconjugated and conjugated bilirubin in the blood increase.

---

i | 22.15 Causes of cholestatic jaundice

Intrahepatic

- Primary biliary cholangitis
- Primary sclerosing cholangitis
- Alcohol
- Drugs
- Hepatic infiltrations (lymphoma, granuloma, amyloid, metastases)
- Cystic fibrosis
- Severe bacterial infections
- Pregnancy (p. 899)
- Inherited cholestatic liver disease, e.g. benign recurrent intrahepatic cholestasis
- Chronic right heart failure

Extrahepatic

- Carcinoma:
  Ampullary
  Pancreatic
  Bile duct
  (cholangiocarcinoma)
  Liver metastases
- Choledocholithiasis
- Parasitic infection
- Traumatic biliary strictures
- Chronic pancreatitis

---

i | 22.16 Key history points in patients with jaundice

Symptoms*

- Itching preceding jaundice
- Abdominal pain (suggests stones)
- Weight loss (chronic liver disease and malignancy)
- Dark urine and pale stools
- Fever ± rigors
- Dry eyes/dry mouth
- Fatigue

Recent drug history

Other

- Exposure to intravenous drug or blood transfusions
- Travel history and country of birth
- Metabolic syndrome (increased body mass index ± type 2 diabetes/hypertension)
- Autoimmune disease history
- Alcohol history
- Inflammatory bowel disease
- Family history of liver disease, autoimmune disease or the metabolic syndrome

*Symptoms may be absent and abnormal liver function tests detected incidentally.

---

i | 22.17 Congenital non-haemolytic hyperbilirubinaemia

Syndrome	Inheritance	Abnormality	Clinical features	Treatment
Unconjugated hyperbilirubinaemia				
Gilbert's	Can be autosomal recessive or dominant	↓Glucuronyl transferase ↓Bilirubin uptake	Mild jaundice, especially with fasting	None necessary
Crigler–Najjar:				
Type I	Autosomal recessive	Absent glucuronyl transferase	Rapid death in neonate (kernicterus)	
Type II	Autosomal recessive	↓↓Glucuronyl transferase	Presents in neonate	Phenobarbital, phototherapy or liver transplant
Conjugated hyperbilirubinaemia				
Dubin–Johnson	Autosomal recessive	↓Canalicular excretion of organic anions, including bilirubin Pigmentation of liver biopsy tissue	Mild jaundice	None necessary
Rotor's	Autosomal recessive	↓Bilirubin uptake ↓Intrahepatic binding	Mild jaundice	None necessary

Hepatocellular jaundice can be due to acute or chronic injury (see Fig. 22.11), and clinical features of acute or chronic liver disease may be detected clinically (see Box 22.7).

Characteristically, jaundice due to parenchymal liver disease is associated with increases in transaminases (AST, ALT), but increases in other LFTs, including cholestatic enzymes (GGT, ALP), may occur and suggest specific aetiologies (see below). Acute jaundice in the presence of an ALT of >1000 U/L is highly suggestive of an infectious cause (e.g. hepatitis A or B), drugs (e.g. paracetamol) or hepatic ischaemia. Imaging is essential, in particular to identify features suggestive of cirrhosis, define the patency of the hepatic vasculature and obtain evidence of portal hypertension. Liver biopsy has an important role in defining the aetiology of hepatocellular jaundice and the extent of liver injury.

Obstructive (cholestatic) jaundice

Cholestatic jaundice may be caused by:

- failure of hepatocytes to initiate bile flow
- obstruction of the bile ducts or portal tracts
- obstruction of bile flow in the extrahepatic bile ducts between the porta hepatis and the papilla of Vater.

In the absence of treatment, cholestatic jaundice tends to become progressively more severe because conjugated bilirubin is unable to enter the bile canaliculi and passes back into the blood, and also because there is a failure of clearance of unconjugated bilirubin arriving at the liver cells. The causes of cholestatic jaundice are listed in Box 22.15. Cholestasis may result from defects at more than one of these levels. Those confined to

the extrahepatic bile ducts may be amenable to surgical or endoscopic correction.

Clinical features (Box 22.18) comprise those due to cholestasis itself, those due to secondary infection (cholangitis) and those of the underlying condition (Box 22.19). Obstruction of the bile duct drainage due to blockage of the extrahepatic biliary tree is characteristically associated with pale stools and dark urine. Pruritus may be a dominant feature and can be accompanied by skin excoriations. Peripheral stigmata of chronic liver disease are absent. If the gallbladder is palpable, the jaundice is unlikely to be caused by biliary obstruction due to gallstones, probably because a chronically inflamed, stone-containing gallbladder cannot readily dilate. This is Courvoisier's Law, and suggests

i | **22.18 Clinical features and complications of cholestatic jaundice**

Cholestasis

Early features
- Jaundice
- Dark urine
- Pale stools
- Pruritus

Late features
- Malabsorption (vitamins A, D, E and K): weight loss, steatorrhoea, osteomalacia, bleeding tendency
- Xanthelasma and xanthomas

Cholangitis
- Fever
- Rigors
- Pain (if gallstones present)

Fig. 22.15 Investigation of jaundice. (ERCP = endoscopic retrograde cholangiopancreatography; LFTs = liver function tests; MRCP = magnetic resonance cholangiopancreatography)

22

22.19 Clinical features suggesting an underlying cause of cholestatic jaundice*

Clinical feature	Causes
Jaundice	
Static or increasing	Carcinoma Primary biliary cholangitis Primary sclerosing cholangitis
Fluctuating	Choledocholithiasis Stricture Pancreatitis Choledochal cyst Primary sclerosing cholangitis
Abdominal pain	Choledocholithiasis Pancreatitis Choledochal cyst
Cholangitis	Stone Stricture Choledochal cyst
Abdominal scar	Stone Stricture
Irregular hepatomegaly	Hepatic carcinoma
Palpable gallbladder	Carcinoma below cystic duct (usually pancreas)
Abdominal mass	Carcinoma Pancreatitis (cyst) Choledochal cyst
Occult blood in stools	Ampullary tumour

*Each of these diseases can give rise to almost any of the clinical features shown but the box indicates the most likely cause of the clinical features listed.

that jaundice is due to a malignant biliary obstruction (e.g. pancreatic cancer). Cholangitis is characterised by 'Charcot's triad' of jaundice, right upper quadrant pain and fever. Cholestatic jaundice is characterised by a relatively greater elevation of ALP and GGT than the aminotransferases.

Ultrasound is indicated to determine whether there is evidence of mechanical obstruction and dilatation of the biliary tree (Fig. 22.15). EUS provides an additional investigation modality for investigation of lower common bile duct obstruction.

Management of cholestatic jaundice depends on the underlying cause and is discussed in the relevant sections below.

Hepatomegaly

Hepatomegaly may occur as the result of a general enlargement of the liver or because of primary or secondary liver tumour

22.20 Causes of change in liver size

Large liver (hepatomegaly)

- Liver metastases
- Multiple or large hepatic cysts
- Cirrhosis (early): non-alcoholic fatty liver disease, alcohol, haemochromatosis
- Hepatic vein outflow obstruction
- Infiltration: amyloid

Small liver

- Cirrhosis (late)

(Box 22.20). The most common liver tumour in Western countries is liver metastasis, whereas primary liver cancer complicating chronic viral hepatitis is more common in the Far East. Unlike carcinoma metastases, those from neuro-endocrine tumours typically cause massive hepatomegaly but without significant weight loss. Cirrhosis can be associated with either hepatomegaly or reduced liver size in advanced disease. Although all causes of cirrhosis can involve hepatomegaly, it is much more common in alcoholic liver disease and haemochromatosis. Hepatomegaly may resolve in patients with alcoholic cirrhosis when they stop drinking.

Ascites

Ascites is present when there is accumulation of free fluid in the peritoneal cavity. Small amounts of ascites are asymptomatic, but with larger accumulations of fluid (>1 L) there is abdominal distension, fullness in the flanks, shifting dullness on percussion and, when the ascites is marked, a fluid thrill/fluid wave. Other features include eversion of the umbilicus, herniae, abdominal striae, divarication of the recti and scrotal oedema. Dilated superficial abdominal veins may be seen if the ascites is due to portal hypertension.

Pathophysiology

Ascites has numerous causes, the most common of which are malignant disease, cirrhosis and heart failure. Many primary disorders of the peritoneum and visceral organs can also cause ascites, and these need to be considered even in a patient with chronic liver disease (Box 22.21). Splanchnic vasodilatation is thought to be the main factor leading to ascites in cirrhosis. This is mediated by vasodilators (mainly nitric oxide) that are released when portal hypertension causes shunting of blood into the systemic circulation. Systemic arterial pressure falls due to pronounced splanchnic vasodilatation as cirrhosis advances. This leads to activation of the renin–angiotensin system with secondary aldosteronism, increased sympathetic nervous activity, increased atrial natriuretic hormone secretion and altered activity

22.21 Causes of ascites

Low SAAG (exudative)	High SAAG (transudative)
Common causes	

Malignant disease:
  Hepatic
  Peritoneal
	Cardiac failure
	Hepatic cirrhosis

Other causes	

Acute pancreatitis
Lymphatic obstruction
Infection:
  Tuberculosis
Nephrotic syndrome
	Hypoproteinaemia:
	  Protein-losing enteropathy
	  Malnutrition
	Hepatic venous occlusion:
	  Budd–Chiari syndrome
	  Sinusoidal obstruction syndrome
	  (Veno-occlusive disease)

Rare causes	
Hypothyroidism	Meigs' syndrome* Constrictive pericarditis

*Meigs' syndrome is the association of a right pleural effusion with or without ascites and a benign ovarian tumour. The ascites resolves on removal of the tumour.
(SAAG = serum ascites albumin gradient; see text)

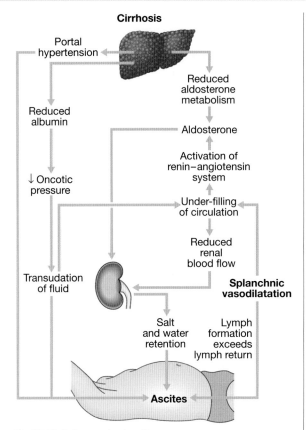

Fig. 22.16 Pathogenesis of ascites.

i	22.22 Ascitic fluid: appearance and analysis

Cause/appearance

- Cirrhosis: clear, straw-coloured or light green
- Malignant disease: bloody
- Infection: cloudy
- Biliary communication: heavy bile staining
- Lymphatic obstruction: milky-white (chylous)

Useful investigations

- Total albumin (plus serum albumin) and protein*
- Amylase
- Neutrophil count
- Cytology
- Microscopy and culture

*To calculate the serum–ascites albumin gradient (SAAG).

of the kallikrein–kinin system (Fig. 22.16). These systems tend to normalise arterial pressure but produce salt and water retention. In this setting, the combination of splanchnic arterial vasodilatation and portal hypertension alters intestinal capillary permeability, promoting accumulation of fluid within the peritoneum.

Investigations

Ultrasonography is the best means of detecting ascites, particularly in the obese and those with small volumes of fluid. Paracentesis (if necessary under ultrasonic guidance) can be used to obtain ascitic fluid for analysis. The appearance of ascitic fluid may point to the underlying cause (Box 22.22). Pleural effusions are found in about 10% of patients, usually on the right side (hepatic hydrothorax); most are small and identified only on chest X-ray, but occasionally a massive hydrothorax occurs. Pleural effusions, particularly those on the left side, should not be assumed to be due to the ascites.

Measurement of the protein concentration and the serum–ascites albumin gradient (SAAG) can be a useful tool to distinguish ascites of different aetiologies. Cirrhotic patients typically develop ascites with a low protein concentration ('transudate'; protein concentration <25 g/L (2.5 g/dL)) and relatively few cells. In up to 30% of patients, however, the total protein concentration is >30 g/L (3.0 g/dL). In these cases, it is useful to calculate the SAAG by subtracting the concentration of the ascites fluid albumin from the serum albumin. A gradient of >11 g/L (1.1 g/dL) is 96% predictive that ascites is due to portal hypertension. Venous outflow obstruction due to cardiac failure or hepatic venous outflow obstruction can also cause a transudative ascites, as

indicated by an albumin gradient of >11 g/L (1.1 g/dL) but, unlike in cirrhosis, the total protein content is usually >25 g/L (2.5 g/dL).

High protein ascites ('exudate'; protein concentration >25 g/L (2.5 g/dL) or a SAAG of <11 g/L (1.1 g/dL) raises the possibility of infection (especially tuberculosis), malignancy, pancreatic ascites or, rarely, hypothyroidism. Ascites amylase activity of >1000 U/L identifies pancreatic ascites, whereas low ascites glucose concentrations suggest malignant disease or tuberculosis. Cytological examination may reveal malignant cells (one-third of cirrhotic patients with a bloody tap have a hepatocellular carcinoma). Polymorphonuclear leucocyte counts of >250 × 10⁶/L strongly suggest infection (spontaneous bacterial peritonitis; see below). Laparoscopy can be valuable in detecting peritoneal disease.

The presence of triglyceride at a level >1.1 g/L (110 mg/dL) is diagnostic of chylous ascites and suggests anatomical or functional abnormality of lymphatic drainage from the abdomen. The ascites in this context has a characteristic milky-white appearance.

Management

Successful treatment relieves discomfort but does not prolong life; if over-vigorous, it can produce serious disorders of fluid and electrolyte balance, and precipitate hepatic encephalopathy (p. 864). Treatment of transudative ascites is based on restricting sodium and water intake, promoting urine output with diuretics and, if necessary, removing ascites directly by paracentesis. Exudative ascites due to malignancy is treated with paracentesis but fluid replacement is generally not required. During management of ascites, the patient should be weighed regularly. Diuretics should be titrated to remove no more than 1 L of fluid daily, so body weight should not fall by more than 1 kg daily to avoid excessive fluid depletion.

Sodium and water restriction

Restriction of dietary sodium intake is essential to achieve negative sodium balance and a few patients can be managed satisfactorily by this alone. Restriction of sodium intake to 100 mmol/24 hrs ('no added salt diet') is usually adequate. Drugs containing relatively large amounts of sodium, and those promoting sodium retention, such as non-steroidal anti-inflammatory drugs (NSAIDs), must be avoided (Box 22.23). Restriction of water intake to 1.0–1.5 L/24 hrs is necessary only if the plasma sodium falls below 125 mmol/L.

22

i	**22.23 Some drugs containing relatively large amounts of sodium or causing sodium retention**

High sodium content

- Alginates
- Antacids
- Antibiotics
- Phenytoin

- Effervescent preparations (e.g. aspirin, calcium, paracetamol)
- Sodium valproate

Sodium retention

- Carbenoxolone
- Glucocorticoids
- Metoclopramide

- Non-steroidal anti-inflammatory drugs
- Oestrogens

Diuretics

Most patients require diuretics in addition to sodium restriction. Spironolactone (100–400 mg/day) is the first-line drug because it is a powerful aldosterone antagonist; it can, however, cause painful gynaecomastia and hyperkalaemia, in which case amiloride (5–10 mg/day) can be substituted. Some patients also require loop diuretics, such as furosemide, but these can lead to fluid and electrolyte imbalance and renal dysfunction. Diuresis may be improved if patients are rested in bed, perhaps because renal blood flow increases in the horizontal position. Patients who do not respond to doses of 400 mg spironolactone and 160 mg furosemide, or who are unable to tolerate these doses due to hyponatraemia or renal impairment, are considered to have refractory or diuretic-resistant ascites and should be treated by other measures.

Paracentesis

First-line treatment of refractory ascites is large-volume paracentesis. Paracentesis to dryness is safe, provided the circulation is supported with an intravenous colloid such as human albumin (6–8 g per litre of ascites removed, usually as 100 mL of 20% or 25% human albumin solution (HAS) for every 1.5–2 L of ascites drained) or another plasma expander. Paracentesis can be used as an initial therapy or when other treatments fail.

Transjugular intrahepatic portosystemic stent shunt

A transjugular intrahepatic portosystemic stent shunt (TIPSS; p. 870) can relieve resistant ascites but does not prolong life; it may be an option where the only alternative is frequent, large-volume paracentesis. TIPSS can be used in patients awaiting liver transplantation or in those with reasonable liver function, but can aggravate encephalopathy in those with poor function.

Complications

Renal failure

Renal failure can occur in patients with ascites. It can be pre-renal and due to vasodilatation from sepsis and/or diuretic therapy, or due to hepatorenal syndrome.

Hepatorenal syndrome

This occurs in 10% of patients with advanced cirrhosis complicated by ascites. There are two clinical types; both are mediated by renal vasoconstriction due to under-filling of the arterial circulation.

Type 1 hepatorenal syndrome This is characterised by progressive oliguria, a rapid rise of the serum creatinine and a very poor prognosis (without treatment, median survival is less than

1 month). There is usually no proteinuria, a urine sodium excretion of less than 10 mmol/24 hrs and a urine/plasma osmolarity ratio of more than 1.5. Other non-functional causes of renal failure must be excluded before the diagnosis is made. Treatment consists of albumin infusions in combination with terlipressin (or octreotide and midodrine where terlipressin is not approved for use) and is effective in about two-thirds of patients. Haemodialysis should not be used routinely because it does not improve the outcome. Patients who survive should be considered for liver transplantation, which, along with TIPSS, is an effective treatment in appropriate patients.

Type 2 hepatorenal syndrome This usually occurs in patients with refractory ascites, is characterised by a moderate and stable increase in serum creatinine, and has a better prognosis.

Spontaneous bacterial peritonitis

Spontaneous bacterial peritonitis (SBP) may present with abdominal pain, rebound tenderness, absent bowel sounds and fever in a patient with obvious features of cirrhosis and ascites. Abdominal signs are mild or absent in about one-third of patients, and in these individuals hepatic encephalopathy and fever are the main features. Diagnostic paracentesis may show cloudy fluid, and an ascites neutrophil count of $>250\times10^6$/L almost invariably indicates infection. The source of infection cannot usually be determined, but most organisms isolated are of enteric origin and *Escherichia coli* is the most frequently found. Ascitic culture in blood culture bottles gives the highest yield of organisms. SBP needs to be differentiated from other intra-abdominal emergencies, and the finding of multiple organisms on culture should arouse suspicion of a perforated viscus.

Treatment should be started immediately with broad-spectrum antibiotics, such as cefotaxime or piperacillin/tazobactam). Recurrence of SBP is common but may be reduced with prophylactic quinolones, such as norfloxacin or ciprofloxacin. Prophylactic antibiotics reduce the incidence of SBP and improve survival in cirrhotic patients with gastrointestinal bleeding. In patients with a previous episode of SBP and continued ascites, norfloxacin (400 mg/day) prevents recurrence.

Prognosis

Only 10–20% of patients survive for 5 years from the first appearance of ascites due to cirrhosis. The outlook is not universally poor, however, and is best in those with well-maintained liver function and a good response to therapy. The prognosis is also better when a treatable cause for the underlying cirrhosis is present or when a precipitating cause for ascites, such as excess salt intake, is found. The mortality at 1 year is 50% following the first episode of bacterial peritonitis.

Hepatic encephalopathy

Hepatic encephalopathy is a neuropsychiatric syndrome caused by liver disease. As it progresses, delirium is followed by coma. Simple delirium needs to be differentiated from delirium tremens and Wernicke's encephalopathy, and coma from subdural haematoma, which can occur in alcoholics after a fall (Box 22.24). Features include changes of intellect, personality, emotions and consciousness, with or without neurological signs. The degree of encephalopathy can be graded from 1 to 4, depending on these features, and this is useful in assessing response to therapy (see Box 22.9). When an episode develops acutely, a precipitating factor may be found (Box 22.25). The earliest features are very mild and easily overlooked, but as the condition becomes more severe, apathy, inability to concentrate, delirium, disorientation, drowsiness, slurring of speech and eventually coma develop. Convulsions sometimes occur. Examination usually shows a flapping tremor (asterixis), inability to perform simple mental arithmetic tasks or to draw objects such as a star (constructional apraxia; p. 847), and, as the condition progresses, hyper-reflexia and bilateral extensor plantar responses. Hepatic encephalopathy rarely causes focal neurological signs; if these are present, other causes must be sought. Fetor hepaticus, a sweet musty odour to the breath, is usually present but is more a sign of liver failure and portosystemic shunting than of hepatic encephalopathy. Rarely, chronic hepatic encephalopathy (hepatocerebral degeneration) gives rise to variable combinations of cerebellar dysfunction, Parkinsonian syndromes, spastic paraplegia and dementia.

Pathophysiology

Hepatic encephalopathy is thought to be due to a disturbance of brain function provoked by circulating neurotoxins that are normally metabolised by the liver. Accordingly, most affected patients have evidence of liver failure and portosystemic shunting of blood, but the balance between these varies from individual to individual.

 22.24 Differential diagnosis of hepatic encephalopathy

- Intracranial bleed (subdural/extradural haematoma, p. 1133)
- Drug or alcohol intoxication (pp. 1194 and 1195)
- Delirium tremens/alcohol withdrawal (p. 1194)
- Wernicke's encephalopathy (p. 1195)
- Primary psychiatric disorders (p. 1191)
- Hypoglycaemia (p. 738)
- Neurological Wilson's disease (p. 1115)
- Post-ictal state

 22.25 Factors precipitating hepatic encephalopathy

- Drugs (especially sedatives, antidepressants)
- Dehydration (including diuretics, paracentesis)
- Portosystemic shunting
- Infection
- Hypokalaemia
- Constipation
- ↑Protein load (including gastrointestinal bleeding)

Some degree of liver failure is a key factor, as portosystemic shunting of blood alone hardly ever causes encephalopathy. The 'neurotoxins' causing encephalopathy are unknown but are thought to be mainly nitrogenous substances produced in the gut, at least in part by bacterial action. These substances are normally metabolised by the healthy liver and excluded from the systemic circulation. Ammonia has traditionally been considered an important factor. Recent interest has focused on γ-aminobutyric acid (GABA) as a mediator, along with octopamine, amino acids, mercaptans and fatty acids that can act as neurotransmitters. The brain in cirrhosis may also be sensitised to other factors, such as drugs that can precipitate hepatic encephalopathy (Box 22.25). Disruption of the function of the blood–brain barrier is a feature of acute hepatic failure and may lead to cerebral oedema.

Investigations

The diagnosis can usually be made clinically; when doubt exists, an electroencephalogram shows diffuse slowing of the normal alpha waves with eventual development of delta waves. The arterial ammonia is usually increased in patients with hepatic encephalopathy. Increased concentrations can, however, occur in the absence of clinical encephalopathy, rendering this investigation of little diagnostic value.

Management

The principles are to treat or remove precipitating causes (Box 22.25) and to suppress the production of neurotoxins by bacteria in the bowel. Dietary protein restriction is rarely needed and is no longer recommended as first-line treatment because it is unpalatable and can lead to a worsening nutritional state in already malnourished patients. Lactulose (15–30 mL 3 times daily) is increased gradually until the bowels are moving twice daily. It produces an osmotic laxative effect, reduces the pH of the colonic content, thereby limiting colonic ammonia absorption, and promotes the incorporation of nitrogen into bacteria. Rifaximin (400 mg 3 times daily) is a well-tolerated, non-absorbed antibiotic that acts by reducing the bacterial content of the bowel and has been shown to be effective. It can be used in addition, or as an alternative, to lactulose if diarrhoea becomes troublesome. Chronic or refractory encephalopathy is one of the main indications for liver transplantation.

Variceal bleeding

Acute upper gastrointestinal haemorrhage from gastro-oesophageal varices (Fig. 22.17) is common in chronic liver disease. Investigation

22

Fig. 22.17 Varices: endoscopic views. **A** Oesophageal varices (arrows) at the lower end of the oesophagus. **B** Gastric varices (arrows). **C** Appearance of oesophageal varices following application of strangulating bands (band ligation, arrow).

and management are discussed on page 780 and the specific management of variceal bleeding on page 869.

Cirrhosis

Cirrhosis is characterised by diffuse hepatic fibrosis and nodule formation. It can occur at any age, has significant morbidity and is an important cause of premature death. It is the most common cause of portal hypertension and its complications. Worldwide, the most common causes are chronic viral hepatitis, prolonged excessive alcohol consumption and NAFLD but any condition leading to persistent or recurrent hepatocyte death may lead to cirrhosis. The causes of cirrhosis are listed in Box 22.26.

Cirrhosis may also occur in prolonged biliary damage or obstruction, as is found in primary biliary cholangitis (PBC), primary sclerosing cholangitis (PSC) and post-surgical biliary strictures. Persistent blockage of venous return from the liver, such as is found in sinusoidal obstruction syndrome (SOS; veno-occlusive disease) and Budd–Chiari syndrome, can also result in cirrhosis.

Pathophysiology

Following liver injury, stellate cells in the space of Disse (see Fig. 22.3, p. 849) are activated by cytokines produced by Kupffer cells and hepatocytes. This transforms the stellate cell into a myofibroblast-like cell, capable of producing collagen, pro-inflammatory cytokines and other mediators that promote hepatocyte damage and tissue fibrosis (see Fig. 22.4, p. 849).

Cirrhosis is a histological diagnosis (Fig. 22.18). It evolves over years as progressive fibrosis and widespread hepatocyte loss lead to distortion of the normal liver architecture that disrupts the hepatic vasculature, causing portosystemic shunts. These changes usually affect the whole liver but in biliary cirrhosis (e.g. PBC) they can be patchy. Cirrhosis can be classified histologically into:

- *Micronodular cirrhosis*, characterised by small nodules about 1 mm in diameter and typically seen in alcoholic cirrhosis.
- *Macronodular cirrhosis*, characterised by larger nodules of various sizes. Areas of previous collapse of the liver architecture are evidenced by large fibrous scars.

Clinical features

The clinical presentation is highly variable. Some patients are asymptomatic and the diagnosis is made incidentally at ultrasound or at surgery. Others present with isolated hepatomegaly, splenomegaly, signs of portal hypertension (p. 868) or hepatic insufficiency. When symptoms are present, they are often

non-specific and include weakness, fatigue, muscle cramps, weight loss, anorexia, nausea, vomiting and upper abdominal discomfort (Box 22.27). Cirrhosis will occasionally present because of shortness of breath due to a large right pleural effusion, or with hepatopulmonary syndrome (p. 898).

Hepatomegaly is common when the cirrhosis is due to alcoholic liver disease or haemochromatosis. Progressive hepatocyte destruction and fibrosis gradually reduce liver size as the disease progresses in other causes of cirrhosis. A reduction in liver size is especially common if the cause is viral hepatitis or autoimmune liver disease. The liver is often hard, irregular and non-tender. Jaundice is mild when it first appears and is due primarily to a failure to excrete bilirubin. Palmar erythema

Fig. 22.18 Histological features in normal liver, hepatic fibrosis and cirrhosis. A Normal liver. Columns of hepatocytes 1–2 cells thick radiate from the portal tracts (PT) to the central veins. The portal tract contains a normal intralobular bile duct branch of the hepatic artery and portal venous radical. B Bridging fibrosis (stained pink, arrows) spreading out around the hepatic vein and single liver cells (pericellular) and linking adjacent portal tracts and hepatic veins. C A cirrhotic liver. The liver architecture is disrupted. The normal arrangement of portal tracts and hepatic veins is now lost and nodules of proliferating hepatocytes are broken up by strands of pink-/orange-staining fibrous tissue (arrows) forming cirrhotic nodules (CN).

---

i 22.26 Causes of cirrhosis

- Alcohol
- Chronic viral hepatitis (B or C)
- Non-alcoholic fatty liver disease
- Immune:
  - Primary sclerosing cholangitis
  - Autoimmune liver disease
- Biliary:
  - Primary biliary cholangitis
  - Secondary biliary cirrhosis
  - Cystic fibrosis
- Genetic:
  - Haemochromatosis
  - Wilson's disease
  - α_1-antitrypsin deficiency
- Cryptogenic (unknown – 15%)
- Chronic venous outflow obstruction
- Any chronic liver disease

22.27 Clinical features of hepatic cirrhosis

- Hepatomegaly (although liver may also be small)
- Jaundice
- Ascites
- Circulatory changes: spider telangiectasia, palmar erythema, cyanosis
- Endocrine changes: loss of libido, hair loss
    - Men: gynaecomastia, testicular atrophy, impotence
    - Women: breast atrophy, irregular menses, amenorrhoea
- Haemorrhagic tendency: bruises, purpura, epistaxis
- Portal hypertension: splenomegaly, collateral vessels, variceal bleeding
- Hepatic (portosystemic) encephalopathy
- Other features: pigmentation, digital clubbing, Dupuytren's contracture

---

22.28 Features of chronic liver failure

- Worsening synthetic liver function:
    - Prolonged prothrombin time
    - Low albumin
- Jaundice
- Portal hypertension
- Variceal bleeding
- Hepatic encephalopathy
- Ascites:
    - Spontaneous bacterial peritonitis
    - Hepatorenal failure

22.29 Child–Pugh classification of prognosis in cirrhosis

Score	1	2	3
Encephalopathy	None	Mild	Marked
Bilirubin (μmol/L (*mg/dL*))*			
Primary biliary cholangitis/sclerosing cholangitis	<68 (*4*)	68–170 (*4–10*)	>170 (*10*)
Other causes of cirrhosis	<34 (*2*)	34–50 (*2–3*)	>50 (*3*)
Albumin (g/L (*g/dL*))	>35 (*3.5*)	28–35 (*2.8–3.5*)	<28 (*2.8*)
Prothrombin time (secs prolonged)	<4	4–6	>6
Ascites	None	Mild	Marked
Add the individual scores: <7 = Child's A, 7–9 = Child's B, >9 = Child's C			

*To convert bilirubin in μmol/L to mg/dL, divide by 17.

---

can be seen early in the disease but is of limited diagnostic value, as it occurs in many other conditions associated with a hyper-dynamic circulation, including normal pregnancy, as well as being found in some healthy people. Spider telangiectasias occur and comprise a central arteriole (that occasionally raises the skin surface), from which small vessels radiate. They vary in size from 1 to 2 mm in diameter and are usually found only above the nipples. One or two small spider telangiectasias may be present in about 2% of healthy people and may occur transiently in greater numbers in the third trimester of pregnancy, but otherwise they are a strong indicator of liver disease. Florid spider telangiectasia, gynaecomastia and parotid enlargement are most common in alcoholic cirrhosis. Pigmentation is most striking in haemochromatosis and in any cirrhosis associated with prolonged cholestasis. Pulmonary arteriovenous shunts also develop, leading to hypoxaemia and eventually to central cyanosis, but this is a late feature.

Endocrine changes are noticed more readily in men, who show loss of male hair distribution and testicular atrophy. Gynaecomastia is common and can be due to drugs such as spironolactone. Easy bruising becomes more frequent as cirrhosis advances.

Splenomegaly and collateral vessel formation are features of portal hypertension, which occurs in more advanced disease (see below). Ascites also signifies advanced disease. Evidence of hepatic encephalopathy also becomes common with disease progression. Non-specific features of chronic liver disease include clubbing of the fingers and toes. Dupuytren's contracture is traditionally regarded as a complication of cirrhosis but the evidence for this is weak. Chronic liver failure develops when the metabolic capacity of the liver is exceeded. It is characterised by the presence of encephalopathy and/or ascites. The term 'hepatic decompensation' or 'decompensated liver disease' is often used when chronic liver failure occurs.

Other clinical and laboratory features may be present (Box 22.28); these include peripheral oedema, renal failure, jaundice, and hypoalbuminaemia and coagulation abnormalities due to defective protein synthesis.

Management

This includes treatment of the underlying cause, maintenance of nutrition and treatment of complications, including ascites, hepatic encephalopathy, portal hypertension and varices. Once the diagnosis of cirrhosis is made, endoscopy should be performed to screen for oesophageal varices (p. 869) and repeated every 2 years. As cirrhosis is associated with an increased risk of hepatocellular carcinoma, patients should be placed under regular surveillance for it (p. 890).

Chronic liver failure due to cirrhosis can also be treated by liver transplantation. This currently accounts for about three-quarters of all liver transplants (p. 900).

Prognosis

The overall prognosis is poor. Many patients present with advanced disease and/or serious complications that carry a high mortality. Overall, only 25% of patients survive 5 years from diagnosis, but where liver function is good, 50% survive for 5 years and 25% for up to 10 years. The prognosis is more favourable when the underlying cause can be corrected, as in alcohol misuse, haemochromatosis or Wilson's disease.

Laboratory tests give only a rough guide to prognosis in individual patients. Deteriorating liver function, as evidenced by jaundice, ascites or encephalopathy, indicates a poor prognosis unless a treatable cause such as infection is found. Increasing bilirubin, falling albumin (or an albumin concentration of <30 g/L (3.0 g/dL)), marked hyponatraemia (<120 mmol/L) not due to diuretic therapy, and a prolonged PT are all bad prognostic features (Box 22.29 and Fig. 22.19). The Child–Pugh and MELD (Model for End-stage Liver Disease) scores can be used to assess prognosis. The MELD is more difficult to calculate at the bedside but, unlike the Child–Pugh score, includes renal function; if this is impaired, it is known to be a poor prognostic feature in end-stage disease (Box 22.30). Although these scores give a guide to prognosis, the course of cirrhosis can be unpredictable, as complications such as variceal bleeding may occur.

22

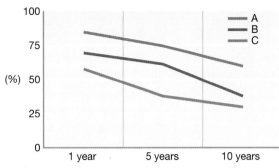

Fig. 22.19 Survival in cirrhosis by Child–Pugh score.

i	22.30 One-year survival rate depending on MELD score	
	1-year survival (%)	
MELD score	No complications	Complications*
<9	97	90
10–19	90	85
20–29	70	65
30–39	70	50
MELD from SI units		
$10 \times (0.378$ [In serum bilirubin (μmol/L)] + 1.12 [In INR] + 0.957 [In serum creatinine (μmol/L)] + 0.643)		
MELD from non-SI units		
3.8 [In serum bilirubin (mg/dL)] + 11.2 [In INR] + 9.3 [In serum creatinine (mg/dL)] + 6.4		
In = natural log. To calculate online, go to https://optn.transplant.hrsa.gov/resources/allocation-calculators/meld-calculator/		
*'Complications' means the presence of ascites, encephalopathy or variceal bleeding. (INR = International Normalised Ratio; MELD = Model for End-stage Liver Disease)		

Portal hypertension

Portal hypertension frequently complicates cirrhosis but has other causes. The normal hepatic venous pressure gradient (difference between the wedged hepatic venous pressure (WHVP) and free hepatic venous pressure; see below) is 5–6 mmHg. Clinically significant portal hypertension is present when the gradient exceeds 10 mmHg and risk of variceal bleeding increases beyond a gradient of 12 mmHg. Increased vascular resistance is common. Causes are classified in accordance with the main sites of obstruction to blood flow in the portal venous system (Fig. 22.20). Extrahepatic portal vein obstruction is the usual source of portal hypertension in childhood and adolescence, while cirrhosis causes at least 90% of cases of portal hypertension in adults in developed countries. Schistosomiasis is the most common cause of portal hypertension worldwide but is infrequent outside endemic areas, such as Egypt (p. 294).

Clinical features

The clinical features result principally from portal venous congestion and collateral vessel formation (Box 22.31). Splenomegaly is a cardinal finding and a diagnosis of portal hypertension is unusual when splenomegaly cannot be detected clinically or by ultrasonography. The spleen is rarely enlarged

⑤ **Post-hepatic post-sinusoidal**
Budd–Chiari syndrome

④ **Intrahepatic post-sinusoidal**
Veno-occlusive disease

③ **Sinusoidal**
Cirrhosis*
Polycystic liver disease
Nodular regenerative hyperplasia
Metastatic malignant disease

② **Intrahepatic pre-sinusoidal**
Schistosomiasis*
Congenital hepatic fibrosis
Drugs
Vinyl chloride
Sarcoidosis

① **Pre-hepatic pre-sinusoidal**
Portal vein thrombosis due to sepsis (umbilical, portal pyaemia) or procoagulopathy or secondary to cirrhosis
Abdominal trauma including surgery

Fig. 22.20 Classification of portal hypertension according to site of vascular obstruction. *Most common cause. Note that splenic vein occlusion can also follow pancreatitis, leading to gastric varices.

i	22.31 Complications of portal hypertension

- Variceal bleeding: oesophageal, gastric, other (rare)
- Congestive gastropathy
- Hypersplenism
- Ascites
- Iron deficiency anaemia
- Renal failure
- Hepatic encephalopathy

more than 5 cm below the left costal margin in adults but more marked splenomegaly can occur in childhood and adolescence. Collateral vessels may be visible on the anterior abdominal wall and occasionally several radiate from the umbilicus to form a 'caput medusae' (p. 846). Rarely, a large umbilical collateral vessel has a blood flow sufficient to give a venous hum on auscultation (Cruveilhier–Baumgarten syndrome). The most important collateral vessel formation occurs in the oesophagus and stomach, and this can be a source of severe bleeding. Rectal varices also cause bleeding and are often mistaken for haemorrhoids (which are no more common in portal hypertension than in the general population). Fetor hepaticus results from portosystemic shunting of blood, which allows mercaptans to pass directly to the lungs.

Ascites occurs as a result of renal sodium retention and portal hypertension that may be due, for example, to post-hepatic causes (hepatic outflow obstruction, p. 862) or cirrhosis.

The most important consequence of portal hypertension is variceal bleeding, which commonly arises from oesophageal varices located within 3–5 cm of the gastro-oesophageal junction, or from gastric varices. The size of the varices, endoscopic variceal features such as red spots and stripes, high portal pressure and liver failure are all general factors that predispose to bleeding. Drugs capable of causing mucosal erosion, such as salicylates and NSAIDs, can also precipitate bleeding. Variceal bleeding is often severe, and recurrent if preventative treatment is not given.

Pathophysiology

Increased portal vascular resistance leads to a gradual reduction in the flow of portal blood to the liver and simultaneously to the development of collateral vessels, allowing portal blood to bypass the liver and enter the systemic circulation directly. Portosystemic shunting occurs, particularly in the gastrointestinal tract and especially the distal oesophagus, stomach and rectum, in the anterior abdominal wall, and in the renal, lumbar, ovarian and testicular vasculature. Stomal varices can also occur at the site of an ileostomy. As collateral vessel formation progresses, more than half of the portal blood flow may be shunted directly to the systemic circulation. Increased portal flow contributes to portal hypertension but is not the dominant factor.

Investigations

The diagnosis is often made clinically. Portal venous pressure measurements are rarely needed for clinical assessment or routine management but can be used to confirm portal hypertension and to differentiate sinusoidal and pre-sinusoidal forms. Pressure measurements are made by using a balloon catheter inserted using the transjugular route (via the inferior vena cava into a hepatic vein and then hepatic venule) to measure the WHVP. This is an indirect measurement of portal vein pressure. Thrombocytopenia is common due to hypersplenism, and platelet counts are usually in the region of 100×10^9/L; values below 50×10^9/L are uncommon. Leucopenia occurs occasionally but anaemia is seldom attributed directly to hypersplenism; if anaemia is found, a source of bleeding should be sought.

Endoscopy is the most useful investigation to determine whether gastro-oesophageal varices are present (see Fig. 22.17). Once the diagnosis of cirrhosis is made, endoscopy should be performed to screen for oesophageal varices (and repeated every 2 years). Ultrasonography often shows features of portal hypertension, such as splenomegaly and collateral vessels, and can sometimes indicate the cause, such as liver disease or portal vein thrombosis. CT and magnetic resonance angiography can identify the extent of portal vein clot and are used to identify hepatic vein patency.

Management

Acute upper gastrointestinal haemorrhage from gastro-oesophageal varices is a common manifestation of chronic liver disease. In the presence of portal hypertension, the risk of a variceal bleed occurring within 2 years varies from 7% for small varices up to 30% for large varices. The mortality following a variceal bleed has improved to around 15% overall but is still about 45% in those with poor liver function (i.e. Child–Pugh C).

The management of portal hypertension is largely focused on the prevention and/or control of variceal haemorrhage. It is important to remember, though, that bleeding can also result from peptic ulceration, which is more common in patients with liver disease than in the general population. The investigation and management of gastrointestinal bleeding are dealt with in more detail on page 780.

Primary prevention of variceal bleeding

If non-bleeding varices are identified at endoscopy, β-adrenoceptor antagonist (β-blocker) therapy with propranolol (80–160 mg/day) or nadolol (40–240 mg/day) is effective in reducing portal venous pressure. Administration of these drugs at doses that reduce the heart rate by 25% has been shown to be effective in the primary prevention of variceal bleeding. In patients with cirrhosis, treatment with propranolol reduces variceal bleeding by 47% (number needed to treat for benefit (NNT$_B$) 10), death from bleeding by 45% (NNT$_B$ 25) and overall mortality by 22% (NNT$_B$ 16). The efficacy of β-blockers in primary prevention is similar to that of prophylactic banding, which may also be considered, particularly in patients who are unable to tolerate or adhere to β-blocker therapy. Carvedilol, a non-cardioselective vasodilating β-blocker, is also effective and may be better tolerated at doses of 6.25–12.5 mg/day). For these, dose should be titrated, as tolerated, to achieve a heart rate of 50–55 beats/min, if possible.

Management of acute variceal bleeding

The priority in acute bleeding is to restore the circulation with blood and plasma, not least because shock reduces liver blood flow and causes further deterioration of liver function. The source of bleeding should always be confirmed by endoscopy because about 20% of patients are bleeding from non-variceal lesions. Management of acute variceal bleeding is described in Box 22.32 and illustrated in Figure 22.21. All patients with cirrhosis and gastrointestinal bleeding should receive prophylactic broad-spectrum antibiotics, such as oral ciprofloxacin or intravenous cephalosporin or piperacillin/tazobactam, because sepsis is common and treatment with antibiotics improves outcomes. The measures used to control acute variceal bleeding include vasoactive medications (e.g. terlipressin), endoscopic therapy (banding or sclerotherapy), balloon tamponade, TIPSS and, rarely, oesophageal transection.

22

22.32 Emergency management of bleeding	
Management	**Reason**
Intravenous fluids	To replace extracellular volume
Vasopressor (terlipressin)*	To reduce portal pressure, acute bleeding and risk of early rebleeding
Prophylactic antibiotics (cephalosporin IV)	To reduce incidence of spontaneous bacterial peritonitis
Emergency endoscopy	To confirm variceal rather than ulcer bleed
Variceal band ligation	To stop bleeding
Proton pump inhibitor	To prevent peptic ulcers
Phosphate enema and/or lactulose	To prevent hepatic encephalopathy

*Caution in patients with significant coronary artery, peripheral or other vascular disease.

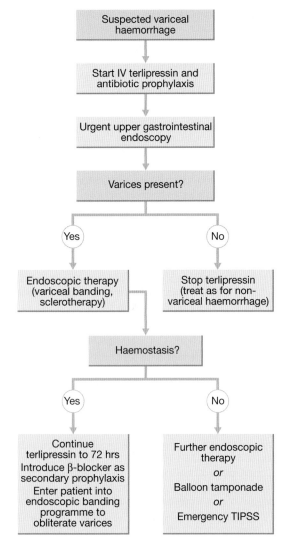

Fig. 22.21 **Management of acute bleeding from oesophageal varices.** (TIPSS = transjugular intrahepatic portosystemic stent shunt)

Fig. 22.22 **Sengstaken–Blakemore tube.**

Pharmacological reduction of portal venous pressure Terlipressin is a synthetic vasopressin analogue that, in contrast to vasopressin, can be given by intermittent injection rather than continuous infusion. It reduces portal blood flow and/or intrahepatic resistance and hence brings down portal pressure. It lowers mortality in the setting of acute variceal bleeding. The dose of terlipressin is 2 mg IV 4 times daily until bleeding stops, and then 1 mg 4 times daily for up to 72 hours. Caution is needed in patients with severe ischaemic heart disease or peripheral vascular disease because of the drug's vasoconstrictor properties. In countries where terlipressin is not available, octreotide is a frequently used alternative.

Variceal ligation ('banding') and sclerotherapy This is the most widely used initial treatment and is undertaken, if possible, at the time of diagnostic endoscopy (see Fig. 22.17C). It stops variceal bleeding in 80% of patients and can be repeated if bleeding recurs. Band ligation involves the varices being sucked into a cap placed on the end of the endoscope, allowing them to be occluded with a tight rubber band. The occluded varix subsequently sloughs with variceal obliteration. Banding is repeated every 2–4 weeks until all varices are obliterated.

Regular follow-up endoscopy is required to identify and treat any recurrence of varices. Band ligation has fewer side-effects than sclerotherapy, a technique in which varices are injected with a sclerosing agent, and has largely replaced it. Banding is best suited to the treatment of oesophageal varices. It is associated with a lower risk of oesophageal perforation or stricturing than sclerotherapy. Prophylactic acid suppression with proton pump inhibitors reduces the risk of secondary bleeding from banding-induced ulceration.

In the case of gastric fundal varices, banding is less effective and so endoscopic therapy relies on injection of agents such as thrombin or cyanoacrylate glue directly into the varix to induce thrombosis. Although highly effective, cyanoacrylate injection treatment may be complicated by 'glue embolism' to the lungs.

Active bleeding may make endoscopic therapy difficult. Protection of the patient's airway with endotracheal intubation aids the endoscopist, facilitating therapy and significantly reducing the risk of pulmonary aspiration.

Balloon tamponade This technique employs a Sengstaken–Blakemore tube, which consists of two balloons that exert pressure in the fundus of the stomach and in the lower oesophagus, respectively (Fig. 22.22). Additional lumens allow contents to be aspirated from the stomach and from the oesophagus above the oesophageal balloon. This technique may be used in the event of life-threatening haemorrhage if early endoscopic therapy is not available or is unsuccessful.

Endotracheal intubation prior to tube insertion reduces the risk of pulmonary aspiration. The tube should be passed through the mouth and its presence in the stomach should be checked by auscultating the upper abdomen while injecting air and by confirming with radiology. The safest technique is to inflate the balloon in the stomach under direct endoscopic vision. Gentle traction is essential to maintain pressure on the varices. Initially, only the gastric balloon should be inflated, with 200–250 mL of air, as this will usually control bleeding. Inflation of the gastric balloon must be stopped if the patient experiences pain because inadvertent inflation in the oesophagus can cause oesophageal rupture. If the oesophageal balloon needs to be used because of continued bleeding, it should be deflated for about 10 minutes every 3 hours to avoid oesophageal mucosal damage. Pressure in the oesophageal balloon should be monitored with a sphygmomanometer and should not exceed 40 mmHg. Balloon tamponade will almost always stop oesophageal and gastric fundal variceal bleeding but is only a bridge to more definitive therapy. Self-expanding removable oesophageal stents are a new alternative in patients with bleeding oesophageal, but not gastric, varices.

TIPSS This technique uses a stent placed between the portal vein and the hepatic vein within the liver to provide a portosystemic shunt and therefore reduce portal pressure (Fig. 22.23). It is carried out under radiological control via the internal jugular vein; prior patency of the portal vein must be determined angiographically, coagulation deficiencies may require correction with fresh frozen plasma, and antibiotic cover is provided. Successful shunt placement stops and prevents further variceal bleeding, and is an effective treatment for both oesophageal and gastric varices. Further bleeding necessitates investigation and treatment (e.g. angioplasty) because it is usually associated with shunt narrowing or occlusion. Hepatic encephalopathy may occur following TIPSS and is managed by reducing the shunt diameter. Although TIPSS is associated with less rebleeding than endoscopic therapy, survival is not improved.

Portosystemic shunt surgery Surgery prevents recurrent bleeding but carries a high mortality and often leads to encephalopathy. In practice, portosystemic shunts are now reserved for when other treatments have not been successful and are offered only to patients with good liver function.

Oesophageal transection Rarely, surgical transection of the varices may be performed as a last resort when bleeding cannot be controlled by other means but operative mortality is high.

Fig. 22.23 Transjugular intrahepatic portosystemic stent shunt (TIPSS). X-ray showing placement of a TIPSS within the portal vein (PV), allowing blood to flow from the portal vein into the hepatic vein (HV) and then the inferior vena cava (IVC).

Secondary prevention of variceal bleeding

Beta-blockers are used as a secondary measure to prevent recurrent variceal bleeding. Following successful endoscopic therapy, patients should be entered into an oesophageal banding programme with repeated sessions of therapy at 12–24-week intervals until the varices are obliterated. In selected individuals, TIPSS may also be considered in this setting.

Congestive 'portal hypertensive' gastropathy

Long-standing portal hypertension causes chronic gastric congestion, which is recognisable at endoscopy as multiple areas of punctate erythema ('portal hypertensive gastropathy' or 'snakeskin gastropathy'). Rarely, similar lesions occur more distally in the gastrointestinal tract. These areas may become eroded, causing bleeding from multiple sites. Acute bleeding can occur but repeated minor bleeding causing iron deficiency anaemia is more common. Anaemia may be prevented by oral iron supplements but repeated blood transfusions can become necessary. Reduction of the portal pressure using propranolol (80–160 mg/day) is the best initial treatment. If this is ineffective, a TIPSS procedure can be undertaken.

Infections and the liver

The liver may be subject to a number of different infections. These include hepatotropic viral infections and bacterial and protozoal infections. Each has specific clinical features and requires targeted therapies.

Viral hepatitis

This must be considered in anyone presenting with hepatitic liver blood tests (high transaminases). The causes are listed in Box 22.33.

All these viruses cause illnesses that have similar clinical and pathological features and are frequently anicteric or even asymptomatic. They differ in their tendency to cause acute and chronic infections. The features of the major hepatitis viruses are shown in Box 22.34. Therapeutic developments for viral hepatitis, in particular hepatitis C, are evolving very rapidly, with several new classes of drugs entering clinical practice.

Clinical features of acute infection

A non-specific prodromal illness characterised by headache, myalgia, arthralgia, nausea and anorexia usually precedes the development of jaundice by a few days to 2 weeks. Vomiting and diarrhoea may follow and abdominal discomfort is common.

i	**22.33 Causes of viral hepatitis**
Common	
• Hepatitis A	• Hepatitis C
• Hepatitis B ± hepatitis D	• Hepatitis E
Less common	
• Cytomegalovirus	• Epstein–Barr virus
Rare	
• Herpes simplex	• Yellow fever

22

22.34 Features of the main hepatitis viruses

	Hepatitis A	Hepatitis B	Hepatitis C	Hepatitis D	Hepatitis E
Virus					
Group	Enterovirus	Hepadnavirus	Flavivirus	Incomplete virus	Calicivirus
Nucleic acid	RNA	DNA	RNA	RNA	RNA
Size (diameter)	27 nm	42 nm	30–38 nm	35 nm	27 nm
Incubation (weeks)	2–4	4–20	2–26	6–9	3–8
Spread*					
Faeces	Yes	No	No	No	Yes
Blood	Uncommon	Yes	Yes	Yes	No
Saliva	Yes	Yes	Yes	Unknown	Unknown
Sexual	Uncommon	Yes	Uncommon	Yes	Unknown
Vertical	No	Yes	Uncommon	Yes	No
Chronic infection	No	Yes	Yes	Yes	No (except immune-compromised)
Prevention					
Active	Vaccine	Vaccine	No	Prevented by hepatitis B vaccination	No
Passive	Immune serum globulin	Hyperimmune serum globulin	No		No

*All body fluids are potentially infectious, although some (e.g. urine) are less infectious than others.

22.35 Complications of acute viral hepatitis

- Acute liver failure
- Cholestatic hepatitis (hepatitis A)
- Aplastic anaemia
- Chronic liver disease and cirrhosis (hepatitis B and C)
- Relapsing hepatitis

Dark urine and pale stools may precede jaundice. There are usually few physical signs. The liver is often tender but only minimally enlarged. Occasionally, mild splenomegaly and cervical lymphadenopathy are seen. These features are more frequent in children or those with Epstein–Barr virus (EBV) infection. Symptoms rarely last longer than 3–6 weeks. Complications may occur but are rare (Box 22.35).

Investigations

A hepatitic pattern of LFTs develops, with serum transaminases typically between 200 and 2000 U/L in an acute infection (usually lower and fluctuating in chronic infections). The plasma bilirubin reflects the degree of liver damage. The ALP rarely exceeds twice the upper limit of normal. Prolongation of the PT indicates the severity of the hepatitis but rarely exceeds 25 seconds, except in rare cases of acute liver failure. The white cell count is usually normal with a relative lymphocytosis. Serological tests confirm the aetiology of the infection.

Management

Most individuals do not need hospital care. Drugs such as sedatives and narcotics, which are metabolised in the liver, should be avoided. No specific dietary modifications are required. Alcohol should not be taken during the acute illness. Elective surgery should be avoided in cases of acute viral hepatitis, as there is a risk of post-operative liver failure.

Liver transplantation is very rarely indicated for acute viral hepatitis complicated by liver failure, but is commonly performed for complications of cirrhosis resulting from chronic hepatitis B and C infection.

Hepatitis A

The hepatitis A virus (HAV) belongs to the picornavirus group of enteroviruses. HAV is highly infectious and is spread by the faecal–oral route. Infected individuals, who may be asymptomatic, excrete the virus in faeces for about 2–3 weeks before the onset of symptoms and then for a further 2 weeks or so. Infection is common in children but often asymptomatic, and so up to 30% of adults will have serological evidence of past infection but give no history of jaundice. Infection is also more common in areas of overcrowding and poor sanitation. In occasional outbreaks, water and shellfish have been the vehicles of transmission. In contrast to hepatitis B, a chronic carrier state does not occur.

Investigations

Only one HAV antigen has been found and infected people make an antibody to this antigen (anti-HAV). Anti-HAV is important in diagnosis, as HAV is present in the blood only transiently during the incubation period. Excretion in the stools occurs for only 7–14 days after the onset of the clinical illness and the virus cannot be grown readily. Anti-HAV of the IgM type, indicating a primary immune response, is already present in the blood at the onset of the clinical illness and is diagnostic of an acute HAV infection. Titres of this antibody fall to low levels within about 3 months of recovery. Anti-HAV of the IgG type is of no diagnostic value, as HAV infection is common and this antibody persists for years after infection, but it can be used as a marker of previous HAV infection. Its presence indicates immunity to HAV.

Management

Infection in the community is best prevented by improving social conditions, especially overcrowding and poor sanitation. Individuals can be given substantial protection from infection by active immunisation with an inactivated virus vaccine.

Immunisation should be considered for individuals with chronic hepatitis B or C infections. Immediate protection can be provided by immune serum globulin if this is given soon after exposure to the virus. The protective effect of immune serum globulin is attributed to its anti-HAV content. Immunisation should be considered for those at particular risk, such as close contacts of HAV-infected patients, the elderly, those with other major disease and perhaps pregnant women.

Immune serum globulin can be effective in an outbreak of hepatitis, in a school or nursery, as injection of those at risk prevents secondary spread to families. People travelling to endemic areas are best protected by vaccination.

Acute liver failure is rare in hepatitis A (0.1%) and chronic infection does not occur. Infection in patients with chronic liver disease, however, may cause serious or life-threatening disease. In adults, a cholestatic phase with elevated ALP levels may complicate infection. There is no role for antiviral drugs in the therapy of HAV infection.

Hepatitis B

The hepatitis B virus consists of a core containing DNA and a DNA polymerase enzyme needed for virus replication. The core of the virus is surrounded by surface protein (Fig. 22.24). The virus, also called a Dane particle, and an excess of its surface protein (known as hepatitis B surface antigen, HBsAg) circulate in the blood. Humans are the only source of infection.

Hepatitis B is one of the most common causes of chronic liver disease and hepatocellular carcinoma worldwide. Approximately one-third of the world's population have serological evidence of past or current infection with hepatitis B and approximately 350–400 million people are chronic HBsAg carriers.

Hepatitis B may cause an acute viral hepatitis; however, acute infection is often asymptomatic, particularly when acquired at birth. Many individuals with chronic hepatitis B are also asymptomatic.

The risk of progression to chronic liver disease depends on the source and timing of infection (Box 22.36). Vertical transmission from mother to child in the perinatal period is the most common cause of infection worldwide and carries the highest risk of ongoing chronic infection. In this setting, adaptive immune responses to HBV may be absent initially, with apparent immunological tolerance. Several mechanisms contribute towards this:

- Firstly, the introduction of antigen in the neonatal period is tolerogenic.
- Secondly, the presentation of such antigen within the liver, as described above, promotes tolerance; this is particularly

evident in the absence of a significant innate or inflammatory response.

- Finally, very high loads of antigen may lead to so-called 'exhaustion' of cellular immune responses. The state of tolerance is not permanent, however, and may be reversed as a result of therapy, or through spontaneous changes in innate responses, such as interferon alpha (IFN-α) and NK cells, accompanied by host-mediated immunopathology.

Chronic hepatitis can lead to cirrhosis or hepatocellular carcinoma, usually after decades of infection (Fig. 22.25). Chronic HBV infection is a dynamic process that can be divided into five phases (Box 22.37); these are not necessarily sequential, however, and not all patients will go through all phases. It is important to remember that the virus is not directly cytotoxic to cells; rather, it is an immune response to viral antigens displayed on infected hepatocytes that initiates liver injury. This explains why there may be very high levels of viral replication but little hepatocellular damage during the 'immune-tolerant' phase.

Investigations

Serology

HBV contains several antigens to which infected persons can make immune responses (Fig. 22.26); these antigens and their antibodies are important in identifying HBV infection (Boxes 22.37 and 22.38), although the widespread availability of polymerase chain reaction (PCR) techniques to measure viral DNA levels in peripheral blood means that longitudinal monitoring is now also frequently guided by direct assessment of viral load.

Hepatitis B surface antigen Hepatitis B surface antigen (HBsAg) is an indicator of active infection, and a negative test for HBsAg makes HBV infection very unlikely. In acute liver failure from hepatitis B, the liver damage is mediated by viral clearance and so HBsAg is negative, with evidence of recent infection provided by the presence of hepatitis B core IgM. HBsAg appears in the blood late in the incubation period but before the prodromal phase of acute type B hepatitis; it may be present for a few days only, disappearing even before jaundice has developed, but usually lasts for 3–4 weeks and can persist for up to 5 months. The persistence of HBsAg for longer than 6 months indicates chronic infection. Antibody to HBsAg (anti-HBs) usually appears after about 3–6 months and persists for many years or perhaps permanently. Anti-HBs implies either a previous infection, in which case anti-HBc (see below) is usually also present, or previous vaccination, in which case anti-HBc is not present.

Hepatitis B core antigen Hepatitis B core antigen (HBcAg) is not found in the blood, but antibody to it (anti-HBc) appears early

Fig. 22.24 Schematic diagram of the hepatitis B virus. Hepatitis B surface antigen (HBsAg) is a protein that makes up part of the viral envelope. Hepatitis B core antigen (HBcAg) is a protein that makes up the capsid or core part of the virus (found in the liver but not in blood). Hepatitis B e antigen (HBeAg) is part of the HBcAg that can be found in the blood and indicates infectivity.

i	**22.36 Source of hepatitis B infection and risk of chronic infection**

Horizontal transmission (10%)

- Injection drug use
- Infected unscreened blood products
- Tattoos/acupuncture needles
- Sexual transmission
- Close living quarters/playground play as a toddler (may contribute to high rate of horizontal transmission in Africa)

Vertical transmission (90%)

- Hepatitis B surface antigen (HBsAg)-positive mother

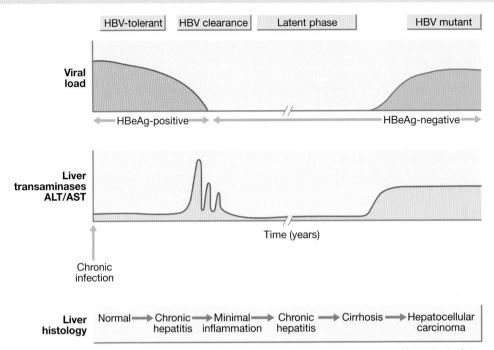

Fig. 22.25 Natural history of chronic hepatitis B virus (HBV) infection. There is an initial immunotolerant phase with high levels of virus and normal liver biochemistry. An immunological response to the virus then occurs, with elevation in serum transaminases, which causes liver damage: chronic hepatitis. If this response is sustained over many years and viral clearance does not occur promptly, chronic hepatitis may result in cirrhosis. In individuals with a successful immunological response, viral load falls, HBe antibody (HBeAg) develops and there is no further liver damage. Some individuals may subsequently develop HBV-DNA mutants that escape from immune regulation, and viral load again rises with further chronic hepatitis. Mutations in the core protein result in the virus's inability to secrete HBe antigen despite high levels of viral replication; such individuals have HBeAg-negative chronic hepatitis. (ALT = alanine aminotransferase; AST = aspartate aminotransferase)

	22.37 The five phases of chronic hepatitis B virus (HBV) infection						
Phase	**HBsAg**	**HBeAg**	**Anti-HBe Ab**	**Viral load**	**ALT**	**Histology**	**Notes**
'Immune-tolerant' phase	+	+	−	+++	Normal/ low	Normal/minimal necroinflammation	Prolonged in perinatally infected individuals; may be short or absent if infected as an adult. High viral load and so very infectious
'Immune-reactive' HBeAg-positive chronic hepatitis phase	+	+	−	++	Raised	Moderate/severe necroinflammation	May last weeks or years. High risk of cirrhosis or HCC if prolonged. Increased chance of spontaneous loss of HBeAg with seroconversion to anti-HBe antibody-positive state
'Inactive carrier' phase	+	−	+	−/+	Normal	Normal/minimal necroinflammation	Low risk of cirrhosis or HCC in majority
HBeAg-negative chronic hepatitis phase	+	−	+	Fluctuating +/++	Raised/ fluctuating	Moderate/severe necroinflammation	May represent late immune reactivation or presence of 'pre-core mutant' HBV. High risk of cirrhosis or HCC
HBsAg-negative phase	−	−	+	−/±	Normal	Normal	Ultrasensitive techniques may detect low-level HBV even after HBsAg loss
(HBeAg = hepatitis B e antigen; HBsAg = hepatitis B surface antigen; HCC = hepatocellular carcinoma)							

in the illness and rapidly reaches a high titre, which subsides gradually but then persists. Anti-HBc is initially of IgM type, with IgG antibody appearing later. Anti-HBc (IgM) can sometimes reveal an acute HBV infection when the HBsAg has disappeared and before anti-HBs has developed (see Fig. 22.26 and Box 22.38).

Hepatitis B e antigen Hepatitis B e antigen (HBeAg) is an indicator of viral replication. In acute hepatitis B it may appear only transiently at the outset of the illness; its appearance is followed by the production of antibody (anti-HBe). The HBeAg reflects active replication of the virus in the liver.

Relative amount of product detectable

Fig. 22.26 Serological responses to hepatitis B virus infection.
(anti-HBc = antibody to hepatitis B core antigen; anti-HBe = antibody to
HBeAg; anti-HBs = antibody to HBsAg; HBeAg = hepatitis B e antigen;
HBsAg = hepatitis B surface antigen; IgM = immunoglobulin M)

22.38 How to interpret the serological tests of acute hepatitis B virus infection

Interpretation	HBsAg	Anti-HBc IgM	Anti-HBc IgG	Anti-HBs
Incubation period	+	+	−	−
Acute hepatitis				
Early	+	+	−	−
Established	+	+	+	−
Established (occasional)	−	+	+	−
Convalescence				
(3–6 months)	−	±	+	±
(6–9 months)	−	−	+	+
Post-infection	−	−	+	±
Immunisation without infection	−	−	−	+

+ = positive; − = negative; ± = present at low titre or absent.
(anti-HBc IgM/IgG = antibody to hepatitis B core antigen of immunoglobulin M/G
type; anti-HBs = antibody to HBsAg; HBsAg = hepatitis B surface antigen)

Chronic HBV infection (see below) is marked by the presence of HBsAg and anti-HBc (IgG) in the blood. Usually, HBeAg or anti-HBe is also present; HBeAg indicates continued active replication of the virus in the liver. The absence of HBeAg usually implies low viral replication; the exception is HBeAg-negative chronic hepatitis B (also called 'pre-core mutant' infection, discussed below), in which high levels of viral replication, serum HBV-DNA and hepatic necroinflammation are seen, despite negative HBeAg.

Viral load and genotype

HBV-DNA can be measured by PCR in the blood. Viral loads are usually in excess of 10^5 copies/mL in the presence of active viral replication, as indicated by the presence of e antigen. In contrast, in individuals with low viral replication, who are HBsAg- and anti-HBe-positive, viral loads are less than 10^5 copies/mL. The exception is in patients who have a mutation in the pre-core protein, which means they cannot secrete e antigen into serum (Fig. 22.27). Such individuals will be anti-HBe-positive but have a high viral load and often evidence of chronic hepatitis. These mutations are common in the Far East, and those patients

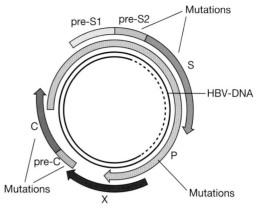

Fig. 22.27 The site of hepatitis B virus (HBV)-DNA mutations.
HBV-DNA encodes four proteins: a DNA polymerase needed for viral replication (P), a surface protein (S), a core protein (C) and an X protein. The pre-C and C regions encode a core protein and an e antigen. Although mutations in the hepatitis B virus are frequent, certain mutations have important clinical consequences. Pre-C encodes a signal sequence needed for the C protein to be secreted from the liver cell into serum as e antigen. A mutation in the pre-core region leads to a failure of secretion of e antigen into serum, and so individuals have high levels of viral production but no detectable e antigen in the serum. Mutations can also occur in the surface protein and may lead to the failure of vaccination to prevent infection, since surface antibodies are produced against the native S protein. Mutations also occur in the DNA polymerase during antiviral treatment with lamivudine.

affected are classified as having e antigen-negative chronic hepatitis. They respond differently to antiviral drugs from those with classical e antigen-positive chronic hepatitis.

Measurement of viral load is important in monitoring antiviral therapy and identifying patients with pre-core mutants. Specific HBV genotypes (A–H) can also be identified using PCR. In some settings, these may be useful in guiding therapy, as genotype A tends to respond better to pegylated interferon-alfa compared to genotypes C and D.

Management of acute hepatitis B

Treatment is supportive with monitoring for acute liver failure, which occurs in less than 1% of cases. There is no definitive evidence that antiviral therapy reduces the severity or duration of acute hepatitis B.

Full recovery occurs in 90–95% of adults following acute HBV infection. The remaining 5–10% develop a chronic hepatitis B infection that usually continues for life, although later recovery occasionally occurs. Infection passing from mother to child at birth leads to chronic infection in the child in 90% of cases and recovery is rare. Chronic infection is also common in immunodeficient individuals, such as those with Down's syndrome or human immunodeficiency virus (HIV) infection. Fulminant liver failure due to acute hepatitis B occurs in less than 1% of cases.

Recovery from acute HBV infection occurs within 6 months and is characterised by the appearance of antibody to viral antigens. Persistence of HBeAg beyond this time indicates chronic infection. Combined HBV and hepatitis delta virus (HDV) infection causes more aggressive disease.

Management of chronic hepatitis B

Treatments are still limited, as no drug is consistently able to eradicate hepatitis B infection completely (i.e. render the

22

patient HBsAg-negative). The goals of treatment are HBeAg seroconversion, reduction in HBV-DNA and normalisation of the LFTs. The indication for treatment is a high viral load in the presence of active hepatitis, as demonstrated by elevated serum transaminases and/or histological evidence of inflammation and fibrosis. The oral antiviral agents are more effective in reducing viral loads in patients with e antigen-negative chronic hepatitis B than in those with e antigen-positive chronic hepatitis B, as the pre-treatment viral loads are lower.

Most patients with chronic hepatitis B are asymptomatic and develop complications, such as cirrhosis and hepatocellular carcinoma, only after many years (see Fig. 22.25). Cirrhosis develops in 15–20% of patients with chronic HBV over 5–20 years. This proportion is higher in those who are e antigen-positive.

Two different types of drug are used to treat hepatitis B: direct-acting nucleoside/nucleotide analogues and pegylated interferon-alfa.

Direct-acting nucleoside/nucleotide antiviral agents

Orally administered nucleoside/nucleotide antiviral agents are the mainstay of therapy. These act by inhibiting the reverse transcription of pre-genomic RNA to HBV-DNA by HBV-DNA polymerase but do not directly affect the covalently closed circular DNA (cccDNA) template for viral replication, and so relapse is common if treatment is withdrawn. One major concern is the selection of antiviral-resistant mutations with long-term treatment. This is particularly important with some of the older agents, such as lamivudine, as mutations induced by previous antiviral exposure may also induce resistance to newer agents. Entecavir and tenofovir (see below) are potent antivirals with a high barrier to genetic resistance and so are the most appropriate first-line agents.

Lamivudine Although effective, long-term therapy is often complicated by the development of HBV-DNA polymerase mutants (e.g. the 'YMDD variant'), which lead to viral resistance. These occur after approximately 9 months and are characterised by a rise in viral load during treatment. Outside resource-limited settings, this agent is now seldom used for the treatment of HBV but may be used to prevent reactivation of HBV in previously infected, HBsAg-negative patients if they are undergoing chemotherapy.

Entecavir and tenofovir Monotherapy with entecavir or tenofovir is substantially more effective than lamivudine in reducing viral load in HBeAg-positive and HBeAg-negative chronic hepatitis. Antiviral resistance mutations occur in only 1–2% after 3 years of entecavir drug exposure. Both drugs have anti-HIV action and so their use as monotherapy is contraindicated in HIV-positive patients, as it may lead to HIV antiviral drug resistance. Current European guidelines advise that the other nucleoside/nucleotide antivirals should not be used as first-line monotherapy due to the induction of viral mutations, unless more potent drugs with a high barrier to resistance are not available or appropriate.

Interferon-alfa

This is most effective in patients with a low viral load and serum transaminases greater than twice the upper limit of normal, in whom it acts by augmenting a native immune response. In HBeAg-positive chronic hepatitis, 33% lose e antigen after 4–6 months of treatment, compared to 12% of controls. Response rates are lower in HBeAg-negative chronic hepatitis, even when patients are given longer courses of treatment. Interferon is contraindicated in the presence of cirrhosis, as it

may cause a rise in serum transaminases and precipitate liver failure. Longer-acting pegylated interferons that can be given once weekly have been evaluated in both HBeAg-positive and HBeAg-negative chronic hepatitis. Side-effects are common and include fatigue, depression, irritability, bone marrow suppression and the triggering of autoimmune thyroid disease.

Liver transplantation

Historically, liver transplantation was contraindicated in hepatitis B because infection often recurred in the graft. The use of post-liver transplant prophylaxis with direct-acting antiviral agents and hepatitis B immunoglobulins has, however, reduced the reinfection rate to 10% and increased 5-year survival to 80%, making transplantation an acceptable treatment option.

Prevention

Individuals are most infectious when markers of continuing viral replication, such as HBeAg, and high levels of HBV-DNA are present in the blood. HBV-DNA can be found in saliva, urine, semen and vaginal secretions (although urine is not usually considered to be capable of transmitting infection). The virus is about ten times more infectious than hepatitis C, which in turn is about ten times more infectious than HIV.

A recombinant hepatitis B vaccine containing HBsAg is available (Engerix) and is capable of producing active immunisation in 95% of normal individuals. The vaccine should be offered to those at special risk of infection who are not already immune, as evidenced by anti-HBs in the blood (Box 22.39). The vaccine is ineffective in those already infected by HBV. Infection can also be prevented or minimised by the intramuscular injection of specific hepatitis B immunoglobulin (HBIg) prepared from blood containing anti-HBs. This should be given within 48 hours, or at most a week, of exposure to infected blood in circumstances likely to cause infection (e.g. needlestick injury, contamination of cuts or mucous membranes). Vaccine can be given together with HBIg (active–passive immunisation).

Neonates born to hepatitis B-infected mothers should be immunised at birth and given immunoglobulin. Hepatitis B serology should then be checked at 12 months of age.

Co-infection with HIV

Around 10% of the HIV-infected population has concurrent HBV and this figure may be as high as 25% in areas where both viruses are prevalent. Up to half of injection drug users with HIV are co-infected with HBV. Co-infection increases the morbidity and mortality compared to either infection alone: there are greater levels of HBV viraemia, faster progression to chronic infection and greater risk of cirrhosis and hepatocellular carcinoma than with HBV infection alone. The immunosuppression that is seen in HIV infection can lead to loss of anti-HBs antibodies, reactivation of infection and a poorer antibody response to HBV vaccination.

 22.39 At-risk groups meriting hepatitis B vaccination in low-endemic areas

- Parenteral drug users
- Men who have sex with men
- Close contacts of infected individuals:
    Newborn of infected mothers
    Regular sexual partners
- Patients on chronic haemodialysis
- Patients with chronic liver disease
- Medical, nursing and laboratory personnel

Pregnancy poses particular problems in co-infected patients, with increased risk of perinatal transmission of HBV to the child.

Treatment can also be problematic. Several nucleoside analogues have dual antiviral activity and some regimens have been associated with emergence of drug resistance. Co-infection is also associated with diminished response to interferons and increased resistance to lamivudine in some patients. Co-infection should be managed by specialists with expertise in this area and combinations of antiviral agents need to be thought through carefully. Antiviral therapy should be considered for co-infected pregnant women, using drugs with dual activity, e.g. tenofovir with emtricitabine or lamivudine.

Globally, there is a need to identify co-infected patients earlier, especially in endemic areas, as well as a need for early effective interventions, particularly in pregnant women, to reduce perinatal transmission.

Hepatitis D (Delta virus)

The hepatitis D virus (HDV) is an RNA-defective virus that has no independent existence; it requires HBV for replication and has the same sources and modes of spread. It can infect individuals simultaneously with HBV or can superinfect those who are already chronic carriers of HBV. Simultaneous infections give rise to acute hepatitis, which is often severe but is limited by recovery from the HBV infection. Infections in individuals who are chronic carriers of HBV can cause acute hepatitis with spontaneous recovery, and occasionally there is simultaneous cessation of the chronic HBV infection. Chronic infection with HBV and HDV can also occur, and this frequently causes rapidly progressive chronic hepatitis and eventually cirrhosis.

HDV has a worldwide distribution. It is endemic in parts of the Mediterranean basin, Africa and South America, where transmission is mainly by close personal contact and occasionally by vertical transmission from mothers who also carry HBV. In non-endemic areas, transmission is mainly a consequence of parenteral drug misuse.

Investigations

HDV contains a single antigen to which infected individuals make an antibody (anti-HDV). Delta antigen appears in the blood only transiently, and in practice diagnosis depends on detecting anti-HDV. Simultaneous infection with HBV and HDV, followed by full recovery, is associated with the appearance of low titres of anti-HDV of IgM type within a few days of the onset of the illness. This antibody generally disappears within 2 months but persists in a few patients. Super-infection of patients with chronic HBV infection leads to the production of high titres of anti-HDV, initially IgM and later IgG. Such patients may then develop chronic infection with both viruses, in which case anti-HDV titres plateau at high levels.

Management

Effective management of hepatitis B prevents hepatitis D.

Hepatitis C

This is caused by an RNA flavivirus. Acute symptomatic infection with hepatitis C is rare. Most individuals are unaware of when they became infected and are identified only when they develop chronic liver disease. Eighty per cent of individuals exposed to the virus become chronically infected and late spontaneous viral clearance is rare. There is no active or passive protection against hepatitis C virus (HCV).

> **22.40 Risk factors for the acquisition of chronic hepatitis C infection**
>
> - Intravenous drug misuse (95% of new cases in the UK)
> - Unscreened blood products
> - Vertical transmission (3% risk)
> - Needlestick injury (3% risk)
> - Iatrogenic parenteral transmission (e.g. contaminated vaccination needles)
> - Sharing toothbrushes/razors

Hepatitis C infection is usually identified in asymptomatic individuals screened because they have risk factors for infection, such as previous injecting drug use (Box 22.40), or have incidentally been found to have abnormal liver blood tests. Although most people remain asymptomatic until progression to cirrhosis occurs, fatigue can complicate chronic infection and is unrelated to the degree of liver damage. Hepatitis C is the most common cause of what used to be known as 'non-A, non-B hepatitis'.

If hepatitis C infection is left untreated, progression from chronic hepatitis to cirrhosis occurs over 20–40 years. Risk factors for progression include male gender, immunosuppression (such as co-infection with HIV), prothrombotic states and heavy alcohol misuse. Not everyone with hepatitis C infection will necessarily develop cirrhosis but approximately 20% do so within 20 years. Once cirrhosis has developed, the 5- and 10-year survival rates are 95% and 81%, respectively. One-quarter of people with cirrhosis will develop complications within 10 years and, once complications such as ascites develop, the 5-year survival is around 50%. Once cirrhosis is present, 2–5% per year will develop primary hepatocellular carcinoma.

Investigations

Serology and virology

The HCV genome encodes a large polypeptide precursor that is modified post-translationally to at least ten proteins, including several antigens that give rise to antibodies in an infected person; these are used in diagnosis. It may take 6–12 weeks for antibodies to appear in the blood following acute infection, such as a needlestick injury. In these cases, hepatitis C RNA can be identified in the blood as early as 2–4 weeks after infection. Active infection is confirmed by the presence of serum hepatitis C RNA in anyone who is antibody-positive. Anti-HCV antibodies persist in serum even after viral clearance, whether spontaneous or post-treatment.

Molecular analysis

There are six common viral genotypes, the distribution of which varies worldwide. Genotype has no effect on progression of liver disease but does affect response to treatment. Genotype 1 is most common in northern Europe and was less easy to eradicate than genotypes 2 and 3 with traditional pegylated interferon alfa-/ribavirin-based treatments. Knowledge of viral genotype still remains relevant in guiding selection of drugs to treat HCV.

Liver function tests

LFTs may be normal or show fluctuating serum transaminases between 50 and 200 U/L. Jaundice is rare and only usually appears in end-stage cirrhosis.

22

Liver histology

Serum transaminase levels in hepatitis C are a poor predictor of the degree of liver fibrosis and so a liver biopsy may be required to stage the extent of liver damage. The degree of inflammation and fibrosis can be scored histologically. The most common way of doing this in hepatitis C is the Metavir system, which scores fibrosis from 1 to 4, the latter equating to cirrhosis. Recently, non-invasive markers and fibrosis scoring systems have been used routinely, with biopsy being reserved for cases where these give conflicting results.

Management

The aim of treatment is to eradicate infection. In recent years, there have been substantial advances, so much so that rates of viral clearance achieved 6 months after finishing treatment (termed sustained virological response, SVR) have risen from less than 40% a decade ago to levels approaching 100% with some of the newer direct-acting antivirals. The infection is cured in more than 99% of patients who achieve an SVR. These newer drugs are extremely expensive, however, and so their use is placing substantial strain on the finite health-care resources of developed countries and has severely limited their availability in resource-poor settings.

Until 2011, the treatment of choice was dual therapy with pegylated interferon-alfa, given as a weekly subcutaneous injection, together with oral ribavirin, a synthetic nucleotide analogue. Treatment was long – up to 12 months for genotype 1 infection, and both agents had significant side-effects that limited tolerability: ribavirin induces haemolytic anaemia and is teratogenic, while interferon induces influenza-like symptoms, irritability and depression, all of which can affect quality of life. As already mentioned, efficacy of these agents was poor (12 months' treatment for genotype 1 resulted in only a 40% SVR, rising to an SVR of over 70% for genotypes 2 or 3 after 6 months' treatment).

i	**22.41 Direct-acting antiviral agents for hepatitis C**	
Drug class	**Therapeutic target**	**Selected drugs**
Protease inhibitors (PIs)	Non-structural viral protein NS3/4A (protease that cleaves the HCV polyprotein)	Telaprevir Boceprevir Simeprevir Paritaprevir Grazoprevir
Nucleoside polymerase inhibitors (NPIs)	Non-structural viral protein NS5B (RNA-dependent RNA polymerase needed for viral replication)	Sofosbuvir
Non-nucleoside polymerase inhibitors (NNPIs)	Non-structural viral protein NS5B (RNA-dependent RNA polymerase needed for viral replication)	Dasabuvir
NS5A replication complex inhibitors	Non-structural viral protein NS5A (assembly of viral replication complex)	Daclatasvir Velpatasvir Ledipasvir Ombitasvir Elbasvir
Host-targeting antiviral drugs (HTAs)	Cyclophilin (pharmacological inhibitor targets host cell functions involved in the HCV life cycle)	Alisporivir

(HCV = hepatitis C virus)

Since 2011, new classes of direct-acting antiviral agents (DAAs) have been developed. There are four main classes of DAA, which are defined according to their mechanism of action and therapeutic target (Box 22.41). These compounds are targeted to specific steps in the hepatitis C viral life cycle to disrupt viral replication (Fig. 22.28). Initially, DAAs were added to interferon-/ribavirin-based regimens; more recently, however, combinations of DAAs have increasingly been used in 'interferon-free' regimens. This maximises treatment efficacy by directly interfering with replication at multiple points in the viral life cycle without exposing patients to the side-effect profile of interferon-alfa therapy. For example, 12 weeks of treatment with oral sofosbuvir plus ledipasvir plus ribavirin can achieve a 99% SVR in treatment-naïve genotype 1 patients. Sofosbuvir plus velpatasvir achieves similar results and is pan-genotypic. Although not without side-effects, DAAs are often orally administered, efficacious and, in general, well tolerated.

Liver transplantation should be considered when complications of cirrhosis occur, such as diuretic-resistant ascites. Unfortunately, if the virus is not cleared, hepatitis C will infect the transplanted liver and up to 15% of patients then develop cirrhosis in the liver graft within 5 years of transplantation. This should no longer happen, as modern antiviral therapy post-transplant achieves excellent results.

Hepatitis E

Hepatitis E is caused by an RNA virus that is endemic in India and the Middle East. Prevalence is now increasing across Asia and Europe, especially south-west France, so it is important to note that infection is no longer seen only in travellers from an endemic area.

The clinical presentation and management of hepatitis E are similar to those of hepatitis A. Disease is spread via the faecal–oral route or through contaminated food; the virus is commonly present in uncooked game and pig-liver sausage in southern France, and this may be a route of infection. In most cases, it presents as a self-limiting acute hepatitis and does not usually cause chronic liver disease. There is increasing recognition that hepatitis E may develop into chronic infection, usually in immunocompromised patients and especially in organ-transplant recipients, although this remains uncommon. If treatment is required for chronic infection, agents such as ribavirin may be used. Blood donations are now routinely screened for hepatitis E.

Hepatitis E differs from hepatitis A in that infection during pregnancy is associated with the development of acute liver failure, which has a high mortality. In acute infection, IgM antibodies to hepatitis E virus (HEV) are positive.

Other forms of viral hepatitis

Non-A, non-B, non-C (NANBNC) or non-A–E hepatitis is the term used to describe hepatitis thought to be due to a virus that is not HAV, HBV, HCV or HEV. Other viruses that affect the liver probably exist but the viruses described above now account for the majority of hepatitis infections. Cytomegalovirus and EBV infection causes abnormal LFTs in most patients and occasionally jaundice occurs. Herpes simplex is a rare cause of hepatitis in adults, most of whom are immunocompromised. Herpes simplex virus hepatitis can be very severe in pregnancy. Abnormal LFTs are also common in chickenpox, measles, rubella and acute HIV infection.

Fig. 22.28 Direct-acting antiviral agents. These compounds are targeted to specific steps in the hepatitis C viral life cycle to disrupt replication. (5′NTR = 5′ non-translated region; HCV = hepatitis C virus; IFN = interferon)

22

i	**22.42 Causes of abnormal liver blood tests in HIV infection**
Hepatitic blood tests	
• Chronic hepatitis C	• Antiretroviral drugs
• Chronic hepatitis B	• Cytomegalovirus
Cholestatic blood tests	
• Tuberculosis	
• Atypical mycobacterium	• Sclerosing cholangitis due to cryptosporidia

HIV infection and the liver

Several causes of abnormal LFTs occur in HIV infection, as shown in Box 22.42. This topic is discussed in more detail on page 317. Co-infection with HIV and HBV is discussed on page 876.

Liver abscess

Liver abscesses are classified as pyogenic, hydatid or amoebic.

Pyogenic liver abscess

Pyogenic liver abscesses are uncommon but important because they are potentially curable, carry significant morbidity and mortality if untreated, and are easily overlooked. The mortality of liver abscesses is 20–40%; failure to make the diagnosis is the most common cause of death. Older patients and those with multiple abscesses have a higher mortality.

Pathophysiology

Infection can reach the liver in several ways (Box 22.43). Pyogenic abscesses are most common in older patients and usually result from ascending infection due to biliary obstruction (cholangitis) or contiguous spread from an empyema of the gallbladder. They can also complicate dental sepsis or colonic pathology, e.g. cancer, diverticulitis or inflammatory bowel disease causing portal pyaemia.

22.43 Causes of pyogenic liver abscesses

- Biliary obstruction (cholangitis)
- Haematogenous:
  Portal vein (intra-abdominal infections)
  Hepatic artery (bacteraemia)
- Direct extension
- Trauma:
  Penetrating or non-penetrating
- Infection of liver tumour or cyst

Abscesses complicating suppurative appendicitis used to be common in young adults but are now rare. Immunocompromised patients are particularly likely to develop liver abscesses. Single lesions are more common in the right liver; multiple abscesses are usually due to infection secondary to biliary obstruction. *Escherichia coli* and various streptococci, particularly *Strep. milleri*, are the most common organisms; anaerobes, including streptococci and *Bacteroides*, can often be found when infection has been transmitted from large bowel pathology via the portal vein, and multiple organisms are present in one-third of patients.

Clinical features

Patients are generally ill with fever and sometimes rigors and weight loss. Abdominal pain is the most common symptom and is usually in the right upper quadrant, sometimes with radiation to the right shoulder. The pain may be pleuritic in nature. Tender hepatomegaly is found in more than 50% of patients. Mild jaundice may be present, becoming severe if large abscesses cause biliary obstruction. Atypical presentations are common and explain the frequency with which the diagnosis is made only at autopsy. This is a particular problem in patients with gradually developing illnesses or pyrexia of unknown origin without localising features. Necrotic colorectal metastases can be misdiagnosed as hepatic abscess.

Investigations

Liver imaging is the most revealing investigation and shows 90% or more of symptomatic abscesses. Needle aspiration under ultrasound guidance confirms the diagnosis and provides pus for culture. A leucocytosis is frequently found, plasma ALP activity is usually increased, and the serum albumin is often low. The chest X-ray may show a raised right diaphragm and lung collapse, or an effusion at the base of the right lung. Blood cultures are positive in 50–80%. Abscesses caused by gut-derived organisms require active exclusion of significant colonic pathology, such as a colonoscopy to exclude colorectal carcinoma.

Management

Pending the results of culture of blood and pus from the abscess, treatment should be commenced with a combination of antibiotics, such as ampicillin, gentamicin and metronidazole. Aspiration or drainage with a catheter placed in the abscess under ultrasound guidance is required if the abscess is large or if it does not respond to antibiotics. Any associated biliary obstruction and cholangitis require biliary drainage (preferably endoscopically). Surgical abscess drainage is rarely undertaken, although hepatic resection may be indicated for a chronic persistent abscess or 'pseudotumour'.

Hydatid cysts and amoebic liver abscesses

These are described on pages 299 and 287.

Leptospirosis

This is described on page 257.

Alcoholic liver disease

Alcohol is one of the most common causes of chronic liver disease worldwide, with consumption continuing to increase in many countries. Patients with alcoholic liver disease (ALD) may also have risk factors for other liver diseases (e.g. coexisting NAFLD or chronic viral hepatitis infection), and these may interact to increase disease severity.

In the UK, a unit of alcohol contains 8 g of ethanol (Box 22.44). An upper threshold of 14 units/week in women and 21 units/week in men is generally considered safe. Recently, however, Public Health England advice has adopted a more conservative threshold of 14 units/week for both men and women. The risk threshold for developing ALD is variable but begins at 30 g/day of ethanol. There is no clear linear relationship between dose and liver damage, however. For many, consumption of more than 80 g/day, for more than 5 years, is required to confer significant risk of advanced liver disease. The average alcohol consumption of a man with cirrhosis is 160 g/day for over 8 years. Some of the risk factors for ALD are:

- *Drinking pattern*. ALD and alcohol dependence are not synonymous; many of those who develop ALD are not alcohol-dependent and most dependent drinkers have normal liver function. Liver damage is more likely to occur in continuous rather than intermittent or 'binge' drinkers, as this pattern gives the liver a chance to recover. It is therefore recommended that people should have at least two alcohol-free days each week. The type of beverage does not affect risk.
- *Gender*. The incidence of ALD is increasing in women, who have higher blood ethanol levels than men after consuming the same amount of alcohol. This may be related to the reduced volume of distribution of alcohol.
- *Genetics*. Alcoholism is more concordant in monozygotic than dizygotic twins. While polymorphisms in the genes involved in alcohol metabolism, such as aldehyde dehydrogenase, may alter drinking behaviour, they have not been linked to ALD. The patatin-like phospholipase domain-containing 3 (*PNPLA3*) gene, also known as adiponutrin, has been implicated in the pathogenesis of both ALD and NAFLD (p. 883).
- *Nutrition*. Obesity increases the incidence of liver-related mortality by over fivefold in heavy drinkers. Ethanol itself produces 7 kcal/g (29.3 kJ/g) and many alcoholic drinks also contain sugar, which further increases the calorific

22.44 Amount of alcohol in an average drink

Alcohol type	% Alcohol by volume	Amount	Units*
Beer	3.5	568 mL (1 pint)	2
	9	568 mL (1 pint)	4
Wine	10	125 mL	1
	12	750 mL	9
'Alcopops'	6	330 mL	2
Sherry	17.5	750 mL	13
Vodka/rum/gin	37.5	25 mL	1
Whisky/brandy	40	700 mL	28

*1 unit = 8 g.

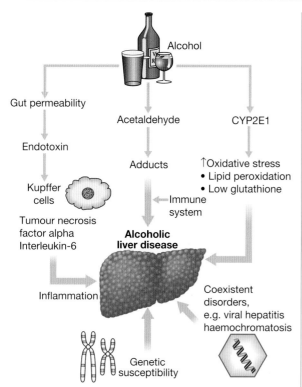

Fig. 22.29 **Factors involved in the pathogenesis of alcoholic liver disease.**

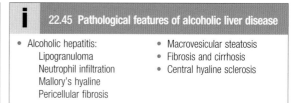

i 22.45 Pathological features of alcoholic liver disease

- Alcoholic hepatitis:
  Lipogranuloma
  Neutrophil infiltration
  Mallory's hyaline
  Pericellular fibrosis
- Macrovesicular steatosis
- Fibrosis and cirrhosis
- Central hyaline sclerosis

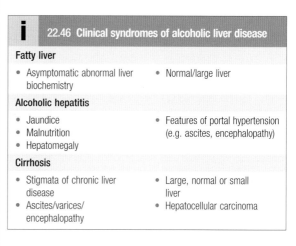

i 22.46 Clinical syndromes of alcoholic liver disease

Fatty liver
- Asymptomatic abnormal liver biochemistry
- Normal/large liver

Alcoholic hepatitis
- Jaundice
- Malnutrition
- Hepatomegaly
- Features of portal hypertension (e.g. ascites, encephalopathy)

Cirrhosis
- Stigmata of chronic liver disease
- Ascites/varices/ encephalopathy
- Large, normal or small liver
- Hepatocellular carcinoma

value and may contribute to weight gain. Excess alcohol consumption is frequently associated with nutritional deficiencies that contribute to morbidity.

Pathophysiology

Alcohol reaches peak blood concentrations after about 20 minutes, although this may be influenced by stomach contents. It is metabolised almost exclusively by the liver via one of two pathways (Fig. 22.29).

Approximately 80% of alcohol is metabolised to acetaldehyde by the mitochondrial enzyme, alcohol dehydrogenase. Acetaldehyde is then metabolised to acetyl-CoA and acetate by aldehyde dehydrogenase. This generates NADH from NAD (nicotinamide adenine dinucleotide), which changes the redox potential of the cell. Acetaldehyde forms adducts with cellular proteins in hepatocytes that activate the immune system, contributing to cell injury.

The remaining 20% of alcohol is metabolised by the microsomal ethanol-oxidising system (MEOS) pathway. Cytochrome CYP2E1 is an enzyme that oxidises ethanol to acetate. It is induced by alcohol, and during metabolism of ethanol it releases oxygen free radicals, leading to lipid peroxidation and mitochondrial damage. The CYP2E1 enzyme also metabolises acetaminophen, and hence chronic alcoholics are more susceptible to hepatotoxicity from low doses of paracetamol.

It is thought that pro-inflammatory cytokines may also be involved in inducing hepatic damage in alcoholic hepatitis, since endotoxin is released into the blood because of increased gut permeability, leading to release of tumour necrosis factor alpha (TNF-α) and interleukin 1 (IL-1), IL-2 and IL-8 from immune cells. All of these cytokines have been implicated in the pathogenesis of liver fibrosis (see Fig. 22.4, p. 849).

The pathological features of ALD are shown in Box 22.45. In about 80% of patients with severe alcoholic hepatitis, cirrhosis will coexist at presentation. Iron deposition is common and does not necessarily indicate haemochromatosis. Figure 22.30A below shows the histological features of alcoholic liver disease, which are identical to those of non-alcoholic steatohepatitis.

Clinical features

ALD has a wide clinical spectrum, ranging from mild abnormalities of LFTs on biochemical testing to advanced cirrhosis. The liver is often enlarged in ALD, even in the presence of cirrhosis. Stigmata of chronic liver disease, such as palmar erythema, are more common in alcoholic cirrhosis than in cirrhosis of other aetiologies. Alcohol misuse may also cause damage of other organs and this should be specifically looked for (see Box 28.22, p. 1194). Three types of ALD are recognised (Box 22.46) but these overlap considerably, as do the pathological changes seen in the liver.

Alcoholic fatty liver disease

Alcoholic fatty liver disease (AFLD) usually presents with elevated transaminases in the absence of hepatomegaly. It has a good prognosis and steatosis usually disappears after 3 months of abstinence.

Alcoholic hepatitis

This presents with jaundice and hepatomegaly; complications of portal hypertension may also be present. It has a significantly worse prognosis than AFLD. About one-third of patients die in the acute episode, particularly those with hepatic encephalopathy or a prolonged PT. Cirrhosis often coexists; if not present, it is the likely outcome if drinking continues. Patients with acute alcoholic hepatitis often deteriorate during the first 1–3 weeks in hospital. Even if they abstain, it may take up to 6 months for jaundice to resolve. In patients presenting with jaundice who subsequently abstain, the 3- and 5-year survival is 70%. In contrast, those who continue to drink have 3- and 5-year survival rates of 60% and 34%, respectively.

Alcoholic cirrhosis

Alcoholic cirrhosis often presents with a serious complication, such as variceal haemorrhage or ascites, and only half of such patients will survive for 5 years from presentation. However, most who survive the initial illness and who become abstinent will survive beyond 5 years.

Investigations

Investigations aim to establish alcohol misuse, exclude alternative or additional coexistent causes of liver disease, and assess the severity of liver damage. The clinical history from patient, relatives and friends is important to establish alcohol misuse duration and severity. Biological markers, particularly macrocytosis in the absence of anaemia, may suggest and support a history of alcohol misuse. A raised GGT is not specific for alcohol misuse and may also be elevated in the presence of other conditions, including NAFLD. The level may therefore not return to normal with abstinence if chronic liver disease is present, and GGT should not be relied on as an indicator of ongoing alcohol consumption. The presence of jaundice may suggest alcoholic hepatitis. Determining the extent of liver damage often requires a liver biopsy.

In alcoholic hepatitis, PT and bilirubin are used to calculate a 'discriminant function' (DF), also known as the Maddrey score, which enables the clinician to assess prognosis (PT = prothrombin time; serum bilirubin in μmol/L is divided by 17 to convert to mg/dL):

$$DF = [4.6 \times Increase\ in\ PT\ (sec)] + Bilirubin\ (mg/dL)$$

A value over 32 implies severe liver disease with a poor prognosis and is used to guide treatment decisions (see below). A second scoring system, the Glasgow score, uses the age, white cell count and renal function, in addition to PT and bilirubin, to assess prognosis and has a cut-off of 9 (Box 22.47).

Management

Cessation of alcohol consumption is the single most important treatment and prognostic factor. Life-long abstinence is the best advice. General health and life expectancy are improved when this occurs, irrespective of the stage of liver disease. Abstinence is even effective at preventing progression, hepatic decompensation and death once cirrhosis is present. Treatment of alcohol dependency is discussed on page 1195. In the acute presentation of ALD it is important to identify and anticipate alcohol withdrawal and Wernicke's encephalopathy, which need

treating in parallel with the liver disease and any complications of cirrhosis.

Nutrition

Good nutrition is very important, and enteral feeding via a fine-bore nasogastric tube may be needed in severely ill patients.

Drug therapy

The optimum treatment of severe alcoholic hepatitis (Maddrey's discriminative score >32) has been debated for some time. The STOPAH study was a large, multicentre, double-blind, randomised trial to evaluate the relative merits of glucocorticoids and/or a weak anti-TNF agent (pentoxifylline), alone or in combination. In a cohort of 1103 patients, no significant benefit from pentoxifylline treatment was identified but treatment with prednisolone (40 mg daily for 28 days) led to a modest reduction in short-term mortality, from 17% in placebo-treated patients to 14% in the prednisolone group. These findings were consistent with earlier studies where an improvement in 28-day survival from 52% to 78% is seen when glucocorticoids are given to those with a Glasgow score of more than 9. Neither glucocorticoids nor pentoxifylline improved survival at 90 days or 1 year, however. Sepsis is the main side-effect of glucocorticoids, and existing sepsis and variceal haemorrhage are the main contraindications to their use. If the bilirubin has not fallen 7 days after starting glucocorticoids, the drugs are unlikely to reduce mortality and should be stopped.

Liver transplantation

The role of liver transplantation in the management of ALD remains controversial. In many centres, ALD is a common indication for liver transplantation. The challenge is to identify patients with an unacceptable risk of returning to harmful alcohol consumption. Many programmes require a 6-month period of abstinence from alcohol before a patient is considered for transplantation. Although this relates poorly to the incidence of alcohol relapse after transplantation, liver function may improve to the extent that transplantation is no longer necessary. The outcome of transplantation for ALD is good and if the patient remains abstinent there is no risk of disease recurrence. Transplantation for alcoholic hepatitis has been thought to have a poorer outcome and is seldom performed due to concerns about recidivism; studies to quantify this are ongoing.

Non-alcoholic fatty liver disease

Increasingly sedentary lifestyles and changing dietary patterns mean that the prevalence of obesity and insulin resistance has increased worldwide, and so fat accumulation in the liver is a common finding during abdominal imaging studies and on liver biopsy. In the absence of high alcohol consumption (typically, a threshold of <20 g/day for women and <30 g/day for men is adopted), this is called non-alcoholic fatty liver disease (NAFLD).

NAFLD includes a spectrum of progressive liver disease ranging from fatty infiltration alone (steatosis) to fatty infiltration with inflammation (non-alcoholic steatohepatitis, NASH) and may progress to cirrhosis and primary liver cancer (Fig. 22.30B). NAFLD is considered by many to be the hepatic manifestation of the 'metabolic syndrome' (p. 730), as it is strongly associated with obesity, dyslipidaemia, type 2 diabetes and hypertension. Estimates vary between populations, although one large European study found NAFLD to be present in 94% of obese patients

22.47 How to assess prognosis using the Glasgow alcoholic hepatitis score			
Score	1	2	3
Age	<50	>50	
White cell count (×10⁹/L)	<15	>15	
Urea (mmol/L (BUN mg/dl))	<5 (14)	>5 (14)	
PT ratio	<1.5	1.5–2.0	>2.0
Bilirubin (μmol/L (mg/dL))	<125 (7.4)	125–250 (7.4–14.8)	>250 (14.8)
A score of ≥9 is associated with a 40% 28-day survival, compared to 80% for patients with a score of <9.			
(BUN = blood urea nitrogen; PT = prothrombin time)			

Fig. 22.30 Non-alcoholic fatty liver disease (NAFLD) and non-alcoholic steatohepatitis (NASH). [A] Features. Rate of progression is determined by environmental (dietary) and genetic factors. [B] The spectrum of NAFLD. (FA = fatty acid; TGF-β = transforming growth factor beta; TNF-α = tumour necrosis factor alpha; VLDL = very low-density lipoprotein)

(body mass index (BMI) >30 kg/m²), 67% of overweight patients (BMI >25 kg/m²) and 25% of normal-weight patients. The overall prevalence of NAFLD in patients with type 2 diabetes ranges from 40% to 70%. Histological NASH has been found in 3–16% of apparently healthy potential living liver donors in Europe and 6–15% in the USA.

Overall, NAFLD is estimated to affect 20–30% of the general population in Western countries and 5–18% in Asia, with about 1 in 10 NAFLD cases exhibiting NASH. The frequency of steatosis varies with ethnicity (45% in Hispanics, 33% in whites and 24% in blacks) and gender (42% white males versus 24% white females) but only a minority of patients will progress to cirrhosis and end-stage liver disease. However, because obesity is common and the prevalence of NAFLD is rising, this still represents a large number of patients, placing a substantial burden on health-care resources. Over a median 12-year follow-up period in a cohort of 619 NAFLD patients, an overall 33.2% risk of death or liver transplantation was observed, with liver-related mortality being the third most common cause of death after cardiovascular disease and extra-hepatic malignancy. NAFLD is the leading cause of liver dysfunction in the non-alcoholic, viral hepatitis-negative population in Europe and North America, and is predicted to become the main aetiology in patients undergoing liver transplantation during the next 5 years.

Pathophysiology

The initiating events in NAFLD are based on the development of obesity and insulin resistance, leading to increased hepatic free fatty acid flux. This imbalance between the rate of import/synthesis and the rate of export/catabolism of fatty acids in the liver leads to the development of steatosis. This may be an adaptive response through which hepatocytes store potentially toxic lipids as relatively inert triglyceride. A 'two-hit' hypothesis has been proposed to describe the pathogenesis of NAFLD, the 'first hit' causing steatosis that then progresses to NASH if a 'second hit' occurs. In reality, progression probably follows hepatocellular injury caused by a combination of several different 'hits', including:

- oxidative stress due to free radicals produced during fatty acid oxidation
- direct lipotoxicity from fatty acids and other metabolites in the liver
- endoplasmic reticulum stress
- gut-derived endotoxin
- cytokine release (TNF-α etc.) and immune-mediated hepatocellular injury.

Cellular damage triggers cell death and inflammation, which leads to stellate cell activation and development of hepatic fibrosis that culminates in cirrhosis (Fig. 22.30A). As with many other liver diseases, subtle inter-patient genetic variations and environmental factors interact to determine disease progression. Several genetic modifiers of disease severity have been identified, with *PNPLA3* and its product, adiponutrin, being the best validated.

This should not be confused with acute fatty liver, which can occur in hepatic mitochondrial cytopathies, e.g. acute fatty liver of pregnancy (p. 1283), or in other situations, e.g. Reye's syndrome (p. 241) or drug toxicity (sodium valproate, tetracyclines), or with bacterial toxins (e.g. *Bacillus cereus*). In these, defective mitochondrial beta-oxidation of lipids leads to fat droplet accumulation in hepatocytes and microvesicular steatosis.

Clinical features

NAFLD is frequently asymptomatic, although it may be associated with fatigue and mild right upper quadrant discomfort. It is commonly identified as an incidental biochemical abnormality during routine blood tests or as a fatty liver during an ultrasound or CT scan of the abdomen. Alternatively, patients with progressive NASH may present late in the natural history of the disease with complications of cirrhosis and portal hypertension, such as variceal haemorrhage, or with hepatocellular carcinoma.

The average age of NASH patients is 40–50 years (50–60 years for NASH–cirrhosis); however, the emerging epidemic of childhood obesity means that NASH is present in increasing numbers of younger patients. Recognised independent risk factors for disease progression are age over 45 years, presence of diabetes (or severity of insulin resistance), obesity (BMI >30 kg/m²) and hypertension. These factors help with identification of 'high-risk' patient groups. NAFLD is also associated with polycystic ovary syndrome, obstructive sleep apnoea and small-bowel bacterial overgrowth.

Investigations

Investigation of patients with suspected NAFLD should be directed first towards exclusion of excess alcohol consumption and other liver diseases (including viral, autoimmune and other metabolic causes) and then at confirming the presence of NAFLD, discriminating simple steatosis from NASH and determining the extent of any hepatic fibrosis that is present.

Biochemical tests

There is no single diagnostic blood test for NAFLD. Elevations of serum ALT and AST are modest, and usually less than twice the upper limit of normal. ALT levels fall as hepatic fibrosis increases and the characteristic AST:ALT ratio of <1 seen in NASH reverses (AST:ALT >1) as disease progresses towards cirrhosis, meaning that steatohepatitis with advanced disease may be present even in those with normal-range ALT levels. Other laboratory abnormalities that may be present include non-specific elevations of GGT, low-titre antinuclear antibody (ANA) in 20–30% of patients and elevated ferritin levels.

Although routine blood tests are unable to determine the degree of liver fibrosis/cirrhosis accurately, calculated scores, such as the NAFLD Fibrosis Score and FIB-4 Score, which are based on the results of routinely available blood tests and anthropometrics, have a high negative predictive value for advanced fibrosis/cirrhosis (Box 22.48) and so can be used to rule out advanced fibrosis in many NAFLD patients. This allows care to focus on those most likely to have advanced disease.

Imaging

Ultrasound is most often used and provides a qualitative assessment of hepatic fat content, as the liver appears 'bright' due to increased echogenicity; sensitivity is limited when fewer than 33% of hepatocytes are steatotic, however. CT, MRI or MR spectroscopy offer greater sensitivity for detecting lesser degrees of steatosis, but these are resource-intensive and not widely used. No routine imaging modality can distinguish simple steatosis from steatohepatitis or accurately quantify hepatic fibrosis short of cirrhosis.

Liver biopsy

Liver biopsy remains the 'gold standard' investigation for diagnosis and assessment of degree of inflammation and extent of liver fibrosis. The histological definition of NASH is based on a combination of three lesions (steatosis, hepatocellular injury and inflammation; see Fig. 22.30A) with a mainly centrilobular, acinar zone 3 distribution. Specific features include hepatocyte ballooning degeneration with or without acidophil bodies or spotty necrosis and a mild, mixed inflammatory infiltrate. These may be accompanied by Mallory–Denk bodies (also known as Mallory's hyaline). Perisinusoidal fibrosis is a characteristic feature of NASH. Histological scoring systems are widely used to assess disease severity semi-quantitatively.

It is important to note that hepatic fat content tends to diminish as cirrhosis develops and so NASH is likely to be under-diagnosed in the setting of advanced liver disease, where it is thought to be the underlying cause of 30–75% of cases in which no specific aetiology is readily identified (so-called 'cryptogenic cirrhosis').

Management

As it is a marker of the metabolic syndrome, identification of NAFLD should prompt screening for and treatment of cardiovascular risk factors in all patients. It is also necessary to assess whether patients have progressive disease and advanced fibrosis so that liver-targeted treatment can be focused particularly on those patients. While liver biopsy is best able to do this, it is invasive and unsuitable for widespread use outside the specialist care setting. An example of an algorithm for the assessment and risk stratification of patients with NAFLD is provided in Figure 22.31.

Non-pharmacological treatment

Current treatment comprises lifestyle interventions to promote weight loss and improve insulin sensitivity through dietary changes

---

i	**22.48 Simple non-invasive scores for non-alcoholic fatty liver disease (NAFLD)/fibrosis***		
		Thresholds	
Test	**Formula**	**Age <65 years**	**Age >65 years**
NAFLD Fibrosis Score (NFS)	−1.675 + 0.037 × Age (years) + 0.094 × BMI (kg/m²) + 1.13 × IFG or diabetes (yes = 1, no = 0) + 0.99 × AST/ALT ratio − 0.013 × platelet count (× 10⁹/L) − 0.66 × albumin (g/dL)	High risk (NFS >0.676) Indeterminate risk (NFS −1.455–0.676) Low risk (NFS <−1.455)	High risk (NFS >0.676) Indeterminate risk (NFS 0.12–0.676) Low risk (NFS <0.12)
FIB-4 Score	Age (years) × AST (IU/L)/platelet count (× 10⁹/L) × √ALT (IU/L)	High risk (FIB-4 >2.67) Indeterminate risk (FIB-4 1.30–2.67) Low risk (FIB-4 <1.30)	High risk (FIB-4 >2.67) Indeterminate risk (2.00–2.67) Low risk (FIB-4 <2.00)

*Predict advanced fibrosis and cirrhosis (F3–4). Simple scores like NFS and FIB-4 are based on the results of routinely available blood tests and anthropometrics. Online calculators for these are widely available.
(ALT = alanine aminotransferase; AST = aspartate aminotransferase; BMI = body mass index; IFG = impaired fasting glucose)

Fig. 22.31 Assessment and risk stratification of patients with non-alcoholic fatty liver disease (NAFLD). (HCC = hepatocellular carcinoma; M probe = medium probe; XL = large probe)

and physical exercise. Sustained weight reduction of 7–10% is associated with significant improvement in histological and biochemical NASH severity.

Pharmacological treatment

No pharmacological agents are currently licensed specifically for NASH therapy. Treatment directed at coexisting metabolic disorders, such as dyslipidaemia and hypertension, should be given. Although use of HMG-CoA reductase inhibitors (statins) does not ameliorate NAFLD, there does not appear to be any increased risk of hepatotoxicity or other side-effects from these agents, and so they may be used to treat dyslipidaemia. Specific insulin-sensitising agents, in particular glitazones, may help selected patients, while recent results with bezafibrate, a lipid-lowering fibrate, have been encouraging. Positive results with high-dose vitamin E (800 U/day) have been tempered by evidence that high doses may be associated with an increased risk of prostate cancer and all-cause mortality, which has limited its use. Several new medicines are currently in late-phase clinical trials and so liver-targeted pharmacological treatments are likely to be available within the next few years.

Autoimmune liver and biliary disease

The liver is an important target for autoimmune injury. The clinical picture is dictated by the nature of the autoimmune process and, in particular, the target cell for immune injury. The disease patterns are quite distinctive for primary hepatocellular injury (in the context of autoimmune hepatitis) and biliary epithelial cell injury (primary biliary cholangitis and primary sclerosing cholangitis).

Autoimmune hepatitis

Autoimmune hepatitis is a disease of immune-mediated liver injury characterised by the presence of serum antibodies and peripheral blood T lymphocytes reactive with self-proteins, a strong association with other autoimmune diseases (Box 22.49), and high levels of serum immunoglobulins – in particular, elevation of IgG. Although most commonly seen in women, particularly in the second and third decades of life, it can develop in either sex at any age. The reasons for the breakdown in immune tolerance in autoimmune hepatitis remain unclear, although cross-reactivity with viruses such as HAV and EBV in immunogenetically susceptible individuals (typically those with human leucocyte antigen (HLA)-DR3 and DR4, particularly HLA-DRB3*0101 and HLA-DRB1*0401) has been suggested as a mechanism.

Pathophysiology

Several subtypes of this disorder have been proposed that have differing immunological markers. Although the different patterns can be associated with variation in disease aspects, such as response to immunosuppressive therapy, histological patterns are similar in the different settings and the basic approach to treatment (complete control of liver injury using immunosuppressive drugs and maintained with appropriate therapy) is the same. The formal classification into disease types has fallen out of favour in recent years.

The most frequently seen autoantibody pattern is high titre of antinuclear and anti-smooth muscle antibodies, typically associated with IgG hyperglobulinaemia (type I autoimmune hepatitis in the old classification), frequently seen in young adult females. Disease characterised by the presence of anti-liver–kidney microsomal (LKM) antibodies, recognising cytochrome P450-IID6 expressed on the hepatocyte membrane, is typically seen in paediatric populations and can be more resistant to treatment than ANA-positive disease. Adult onset of anti-LKM can be seen in chronic HCV infection. This was classified as type II disease in the old system. More recently, a pattern of antibody reactivity with anti-soluble liver antigen (anti-SLA) has been described in typically adult patients, often with aggressive disease and usually lacking autoantibodies of other specificities.

Clinical features

The onset is usually insidious, with fatigue, anorexia and eventually jaundice. The non-specific nature of the early features can lead to the diagnosis being missed in the early disease stages. In about one-quarter of patients the onset is acute, resembling viral hepatitis, but resolution does not occur. This acute presentation can lead to extensive liver necrosis and liver failure. Other features include fever, arthralgia, vitiligo and epistaxis. Amenorrhoea can occur. Jaundice is mild to moderate or occasionally absent, but signs of chronic liver disease, especially spider naevi and hepatosplenomegaly, can be present. Associated autoimmune disease, such as Hashimoto's thyroiditis or rheumatoid arthritis, is often present and can modulate the clinical presentation.

Investigations

Serological tests for autoantibodies are often positive (Box 22.50), but low titres of these antibodies occur in some healthy people and in patients with other inflammatory liver diseases. ANA also occur in connective tissue diseases and other autoimmune diseases (with an identical pattern of homogenous nuclear staining) while anti-smooth muscle antibody has been reported in infectious mononucleosis and a variety of malignant diseases. Anti-microsomal antibodies (anti-LKM) occur particularly in children and adolescents. Elevated serum IgG levels are an important diagnostic and treatment response feature if present, but the diagnosis is still possible in the presence of normal IgG levels. If the diagnosis of autoimmune hepatitis is suspected, liver biopsy should be performed. It typically shows interface hepatitis, with or without cirrhosis. Scoring systems, such as the International Autoimmune Hepatitis Group (IAIHG) criteria, are useful for epidemiological study and for assessing trial eligibility but are complex for normal clinical practice.

Management

Treatment with glucocorticoids is life-saving in autoimmune hepatitis, particularly during exacerbations of active and symptomatic disease. Initially, prednisolone (40 mg/day) is given orally; the dose is then gradually reduced as the patient and LFTs improve. Maintenance therapy should only be instituted once LFTs are normal (as well as IgG if elevated). Approaches to maintenance include reduced-dose prednisolone (ideally, below 5–10 mg/day), usually in the context of azathioprine (1.0–1.5 mg/kg/day). Azathioprine can also be used as the sole maintenance immunosuppressive agent in patients with low-activity disease. Newer agents, such as mycophenolate mofetil (MMF), are increasingly being used but formal evidence to inform practice in this area is lacking. Patients should be monitored for acute exacerbations (LFT and IgG screening with patients alerted

---

i **22.49 Conditions associated with autoimmune hepatitis**

- Migrating polyarthritis
- Urticarial rashes
- Lymphadenopathy
- Hashimoto's thyroiditis
- Thyrotoxicosis
- Myxoedema
- Pleurisy
- Coombs-positive haemolytic anaemia
- Transient pulmonary infiltrates
- Ulcerative colitis
- Glomerulonephritis
- Nephrotic syndrome

---

i **22.50 Frequency of autoantibodies in chronic non-viral liver diseases and in healthy people**

Disease	Antinuclear antibody (%)	Anti-smooth muscle antibody (%)	Antimitochondrial antibody*
Healthy controls	5	1.5	0.01
Autoimmune hepatitis	80	70	15
Primary biliary cholangitis	25	35	95
Cryptogenic cirrhosis	40	30	15

*Patients with antimitochondrial antibody frequently have cholestatic liver function tests and may have primary biliary cholangitis (see text).

to the possible symptoms) and such exacerbations should be treated with glucocorticoids. Although treatment can significantly reduce the rate of progression to cirrhosis, end-stage disease can be seen in patients despite treatment.

Primary biliary cholangitis

Primary biliary cholangitis (PBC, known as primary biliary cirrhosis until 2015, when the name was changed to reflect more accurately the disease seen in the modern era) is a chronic, progressive cholestatic liver disease that predominantly affects women aged 30 and over. It is strongly associated with the presence of antimitochondrial antibodies (AMA), which are diagnostic, and is characterised by a granulomatous inflammation of the portal tracts, leading to progressive damage and eventually loss of the small and middle-sized bile ducts. This, in turn, leads to fibrosis and cirrhosis of the liver. The condition can present with an insidious onset of itching and/or tiredness; it may also frequently be found incidentally as the result of routine blood tests.

Epidemiology

The prevalence of PBC varies across the world. It is relatively common in northern Europe and North America but is rare in Africa and Asia. There is a strong female-to-male predominance of 9 : 1; it is also more common among cigarette smokers. Clustering of cases has been reported, suggesting an environmental trigger in susceptible individuals.

Pathophysiology

Immune mechanisms are clearly involved. The condition is closely associated with other autoimmune non-hepatic diseases, such as thyroid disease, and there is a genetic association with HLA-DR8, together with polymorphisms in a number of other genes regulating the nature of the immune response (e.g. IL-12 and its receptor). AMA is directed at pyruvate dehydrogenase complex, a mitochondrial enzyme complex that plays a key role in cellular energy generation. PBC-specific ANAs (such as those directed at the nuclear pore antigen gp210) have a characteristic staining pattern in immunofluorescence assays (selectively binding to the nuclear rim or nuclear dots), which means that they should not be mistaken for the homogenously staining ANA seen in autoimmune hepatitis. Increases in serum immunoglobulin levels are frequent but, unlike in autoimmune hepatitis, it is typically IgM that is elevated.

Pathologically, chronic granulomatous inflammation destroys the interlobular bile ducts; progressive lymphocyte-mediated inflammatory damage causes fibrosis, which spreads from the portal tracts to the liver parenchyma and eventually leads to cirrhosis. A model of the natural history of the disease process is shown in Figure 22.32.

Clinical features

Systemic symptoms such as fatigue are common and may precede diagnosis by years. Pruritus, which can be a feature of any cholestatic disease, is a common presenting complaint and may precede jaundice by months or years. Jaundice is rarely a presenting feature. The itching is usually worse on the limbs. Although there may be right upper abdominal discomfort, fever and rigors do not occur. Bone pain or fractures can rarely result from osteomalacia (fat-soluble vitamin malabsorption) or, more commonly, from osteoporosis (hepatic osteodystrophy).

Initially, patients are well nourished but weight loss can occur as the disease progresses. Scratch marks may be found in

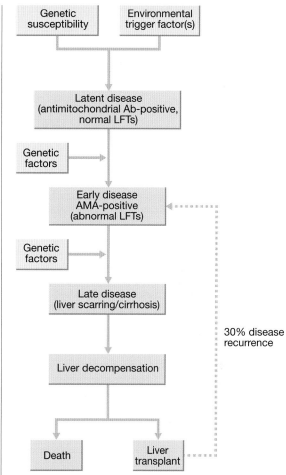

Fig. 22.32 Natural history of primary biliary cholangitis. (AMA = antimitochondrial antibody; LFTs = liver function tests)

patients with severe pruritus. Jaundice is prominent only late in the disease and can become intense. Xanthomatous deposits occur in a minority, especially around the eyes. Mild hepatomegaly is common and splenomegaly becomes increasingly common as portal hypertension develops. Liver failure may supervene.

Associated diseases

Autoimmune and connective tissue diseases occur with increased frequency in PBC, particularly the sicca syndrome (p. 1038), systemic sclerosis, coeliac disease (p. 805) and thyroid diseases. Hypothyroidism should always be considered in patients with fatigue.

Diagnosis and investigations

The LFTs show a pattern of cholestasis (see Box 22.2, p. 853). Hypercholesterolaemia is common and worsens as disease progresses but appears not to be associated with increased cardiac risk. AMA is present in over 95% of patients; when it is absent, the diagnosis should not be made without obtaining histological evidence and considering cholangiography (typically, MRCP) to exclude other biliary disease. ANA and anti-smooth muscle antibodies are present in around 15% of patients (see Box 22.50); autoantibodies found in associated diseases may also be present. Ultrasound examination shows no sign of biliary obstruction. Liver biopsy is necessary only if there is diagnostic uncertainty. The histological features of PBC correlate poorly with

22

the clinical features; portal hypertension can develop before the histological onset of cirrhosis.

Management

The hydrophilic bile acid ursodeoxycholic acid (UDCA), at a dose of 13–15 mg/kg/day, improves bile flow, replaces toxic hydrophobic bile acids in the bile acid pool, and reduces apoptosis of the biliary epithelium. Clinically, UDCA improves LFTs, may slow down histological progression and has few side-effects; it is therefore widely used in the treatment of PBC and should be regarded as the optimal first-line treatment. Its use is recommended in all clinical guidelines. A significant minority of patients either fail to normalise their LFTs with UDCA or show an inadequate response, and such individuals have an increased risk of developing end-stage liver disease compared to those showing a full response. Obeticholic acid (OCA) is a second-generation bile acid therapeutic that acts as an agonist for the nuclear farnesoid X receptor. It reduces hepatocyte synthesis of bile acids and was approved in 2016 for use in patients showing an inadequate response to UDCA. Immunosuppressants, such as glucocorticoids, azathioprine, penicillamine and ciclosporin, have all been trialled in PBC. None shows overall benefit when given to unselected patients. It is unclear whether these drugs offer benefit to the specific subgroup of patients who do not respond to UDCA and require second-line approaches to treatment.

Liver transplantation should be considered once liver failure has developed and may be indicated in patients with intractable pruritus. Serum bilirubin remains the most reliable marker of declining liver function. Transplantation is associated with an excellent 5-year survival of over 80%, although the disease will recur in over one-third of patients at 10 years.

Pruritus

This is the main symptom requiring treatment. The cause is unknown, but up-regulation of opioid receptors and increased levels of endogenous opioids may play a role. First-line treatment is with the anion-binding resin colestyramine, which probably acts by binding potential pruritogens in the intestine and increasing their excretion in the stool. A dose of 4–16 g/day orally is used. The powder is mixed in orange juice and the main dose (8 g) taken before and after breakfast, when maximal duodenal bile acid concentrations occur. Colestyramine may bind other drugs in the gut (most obviously UDCA) and adequate spacing should be used between drugs. Colestyramine is sometimes ineffective, especially in complete biliary obstruction, and can be difficult for some patients to tolerate. Alternative treatments include rifampicin (150 mg/day, titrated up to a maximum of 600 mg/day as required and contingent on there being no deterioration in LFTs), naltrexone (an opioid antagonist; 25 mg/day initially, increasing up to 300 mg/day), plasmapheresis and a liver support device (e.g. a molecular adsorbent recirculating system, MARS).

Fatigue

Fatigue affects about one-third of patients with PBC. The cause is unknown but it may reflect intracerebral changes due to cholestasis. Unfortunately, once depression, hypothyroidism and coeliac disease have been excluded, there is currently no specific treatment. The impact on patients' lives can be substantial.

Malabsorption

Prolonged cholestasis is associated with steatorrhoea and malabsorption of fat-soluble vitamins, which should be replaced as necessary. Coeliac disease should be excluded since its incidence is increased in PBC.

Bone disease

Osteopenia and osteoporosis are common and normal post-menopausal bone loss is accelerated. Baseline bone density should be measured (p. 989) and treatment started with replacement calcium and vitamin D_3. Bisphosphonates should be used if there is evidence of osteoporosis. Osteomalacia is rare.

Overlap syndromes

AMA-negative PBC ('autoimmune cholangitis')

A few patients demonstrate the clinical, biochemical and histological features of PBC but do not have detectable AMA in the serum. Serum transaminases, serum immunoglobulin levels and titres of ANA tend to be higher than in AMA-positive PBC. The clinical course mirrors classical PBC, however, and these patients should be considered as having a variant of PBC.

PBC/autoimmune hepatitis overlap

A few patients with AMA and cholestatic LFTs have elevated transaminases, high serum immunoglobulins and interface hepatitis on liver histology. In such individuals, a trial of glucocorticoid therapy may be beneficial.

Primary sclerosing cholangitis

Primary sclerosing cholangitis (PSC) is a cholestatic liver disease caused by diffuse inflammation and fibrosis; it can involve the entire biliary tree and leads to the gradual obliteration of intrahepatic and extrahepatic bile ducts, and ultimately biliary cirrhosis, portal hypertension and hepatic failure. Although considered as an autoimmune disease, evidence for an autoimmune pathophysiology is weaker than is the case for PBC and autoimmune hepatitis. The incidence is about 6.3/100 000 in Caucasians. Cholangiocarcinoma develops in about 10–30% of patients during the course of the disease.

PSC is twice as common in young men. Most patients present at age 25–40 years, although the condition may be diagnosed at any age and is an important cause of chronic liver disease in children. The generally accepted diagnostic criteria are:

- generalised beading and stenosis of the biliary system on cholangiography (Fig. 22.33)
- absence of choledocholithiasis (or history of bile duct surgery)
- exclusion of bile duct cancer, by prolonged follow-up.

The term 'secondary sclerosing cholangitis' is used to describe the typical changes described above when a clear predisposing factor for duct fibrosis can be identified. The causes of secondary sclerosing cholangitis are shown in Box 22.51.

Pathophysiology

The cause of PSC is unknown but there is a close association with inflammatory bowel disease, particularly ulcerative colitis (Box 22.52). About two-thirds of patients have coexisting ulcerative colitis, and PSC is the most common form of chronic liver disease in ulcerative colitis. Between 3% and 10% of patients with ulcerative colitis develop PSC, particularly those with extensive colitis or pancolitis. The prevalence of PSC is lower in patients with Crohn's colitis (about 1%). Patients with PSC and ulcerative colitis are at greater risk of colorectal neoplasia than those with ulcerative colitis alone, and individuals who develop colorectal neoplasia are at greater risk of cholangiocarcinoma.

It is currently believed that PSC is an immunologically mediated disease, triggered in genetically susceptible individuals by toxic

Fig. 22.33 **Magnetic resonance cholangiopancreatogram showing typical changes of primary sclerosing cholangitis.** There is intrahepatic bile duct beading, stricturing and dilatation. The extrahepatic bile duct is also diffusely strictured. *Courtesy of Dr Dilip Patel, Royal Infirmary of Edinburgh.*

Fig. 22.34 **Primary sclerosing cholangitis.** Note onion skin scarring (arrows) surrounding a bile duct.

 22.51 Causes of secondary sclerosing cholangitis

- Previous bile duct surgery with stricturing and cholangitis
- Bile duct stones causing cholangitis
- Intrahepatic infusion of 5-fluorodeoxyuridine
- Insertion of formalin into hepatic hydatid cysts
- Insertion of alcohol into hepatic tumours
- Parasitic infections (e.g. *Clonorchis*)
- Autoimmune pancreatitis/immunoglobulin G4-associated cholangitis
- Acquired immunodeficiency syndrome (AIDS; probably infective as a result of cytomegalovirus or *Cryptosporidium*)

 22.52 Diseases associated with primary sclerosing cholangitis

- Ulcerative colitis
- Crohn's colitis
- Chronic pancreatitis
- Retroperitoneal fibrosis
- Riedel's thyroiditis
- Retro-orbital tumours
- Immune deficiency states
- Sjögren's syndrome
- Angio-immunoblastic lymphoma
- Histiocytosis X
- Autoimmune haemolytic anaemia
- Autoimmune pancreatitis/immunoglobulin G4-associated cholangitis

or infectious agents, which may gain access to the biliary tract through a leaky, diseased colon. A close link with HLA haplotype A1-B8-DR3-DRW52A has been identified. This haplotype is commonly found in association with other organ-specific autoimmune diseases (e.g. autoimmune hepatitis).

The importance of immunological factors has been emphasised by reports showing humoral and cellular abnormalities in PSC. Perinuclear antineutrophil cytoplasmic antibodies (ANCA) have been detected in the sera of 60–80% of patients with PSC with or without ulcerative colitis, and in 30–40% of patients with ulcerative colitis alone. The antibody is not specific for PSC and is found in other chronic liver diseases (e.g. 50% of patients with autoimmune hepatitis).

Clinical features

The diagnosis is often made incidentally when persistently raised serum ALP is discovered in an individual with ulcerative colitis. Common symptoms include fatigue, intermittent jaundice, weight loss, right upper quadrant abdominal pain and pruritus. Attacks of acute cholangitis are uncommon and usually follow biliary instrumentation. Physical examination is abnormal in about 50% of symptomatic patients; the most common findings are jaundice and hepatomegaly/splenomegaly. The condition may be associated with many other diseases (Box 22.52).

Investigations

Biochemical screening usually reveals a cholestatic pattern of LFTs but ALP and bilirubin levels may vary widely in individual patients during the course of the disease. For example, ALP and bilirubin values increase during acute cholangitis, decrease after therapy, and sometimes fluctuate for no apparent reason. Modest elevations in serum transaminases are usually seen, whereas hypoalbuminaemia and clotting abnormalities are found at a late stage only. In addition to ANCA, low titres of serum ANA and anti-smooth muscle antibodies may be found in PSC but have no diagnostic significance; serum AMA is absent.

The key investigation is now MRCP, which is usually diagnostic and reveals multiple irregular stricturing and dilatation (Fig. 22.33). ERCP should be reserved for when therapeutic intervention is likely to be necessary and should follow MRCP.

On liver biopsy, the characteristic early features of PSC are periductal 'onion skin' fibrosis and inflammation, with portal oedema and bile ductular proliferation resulting in expansion of the portal tracts (Fig. 22.34). Later, fibrosis spreads, progressing inevitably to biliary cirrhosis; obliterative cholangitis leads to the so-called 'vanishing bile duct syndrome'.

Management

There is no cure for PSC but management of cholestasis and its complications and specific treatment of the disease process are indicated. UDCA is widely used, although the evidence to support this is limited. UDCA may have benefit in terms of reducing colon carcinoma risk.

The course of PSC is variable. In symptomatic patients, median survival from presentation to death or liver transplantation is about 12 years. About 75% of asymptomatic patients survive 15 years or more. Most patients die from liver failure, about 30% die from bile duct carcinoma, and the remainder die from colonic cancer or complications of colitis. Immunosuppressive agents, including

22

prednisolone, azathioprine, methotrexate and ciclosporin, have been tried; results have generally been disappointing.

Symptomatic patients often have pruritus. Management is as for PBC. Fatigue appears to be less prominent than in PBC, although it is still present in some patients.

Management of complications

Broad-spectrum antibiotics (e.g. ciprofloxacin) should be given for acute attacks of cholangitis but have no proven value in preventing attacks. If cholangiography shows a well-defined obstruction to the extrahepatic bile ducts ('dominant stricture'), mechanical relief can be obtained by placement of a stent or by balloon dilatation performed at ERCP. It is important, in this situation, to give active consideration to the possibility of cholangiocarcinoma (the differential diagnosis for a dominant extrahepatic stricture). Fat-soluble vitamin replacement is necessary in jaundiced patients. Metabolic bone disease (usually osteoporosis) is a common complication that requires treatment (p. 1044).

Surgical treatment

Surgical resection of the extrahepatic bile duct and biliary reconstruction have a limited role in the management of non-cirrhotic patients with dominant extrahepatic disease. Orthotopic transplantation is the only surgical option in patients with advanced liver disease; 5-year survival is 80–90% in most centres. Unfortunately, the condition may recur in the graft and there are no identified therapies able to prevent this. Cholangiocarcinoma is a contraindication to transplantation. Colon carcinoma risk can be increased in patients following transplantation because of the effects of immune suppression, and enhanced surveillance should be instituted.

IgG4-associated cholangitis

This disease (as well as its nomenclature) is closely related to autoimmune pancreatitis (which is present in more than 90% of the patients; p. 841). IgG4-associated cholangitis (IAC) often presents with obstructive jaundice (due to either hilar stricturing/intrahepatic sclerosing cholangitis or a low bile duct stricture), and cholangiographic appearances suggest PSC with or without hilar cholangiocarcinoma. The serum IgG4 is often raised and liver biopsy shows a lymphoplasmacytic infiltrate, with IgG4-positive plasma cells. An important observation is that, compared to PSC, IAC appears to respond well to glucocorticoid therapy.

Liver tumours and other focal liver lesions

Identification of a hepatic mass lesion is common, both in patients with known pre-existing liver disease and as a primary presentation. Although primary and secondary malignant tumours are important potential diagnoses, benign disease is frequent. The finding of a liver mass, with its association in the minds of patients with metastatic malignant disease, creates a high level of anxiety, a factor that should always be borne in mind. The critical steps to be taken in diagnosing hepatic mass lesions are:

- determining the presence, nature and severity of any underlying chronic liver disease, as the differential diagnosis is very different in patients with and those without chronic liver disease
- using optimal (usually multiple) imaging modalities.

Primary malignant tumours

Hepatocellular carcinoma

Hepatocellular carcinoma (HCC) is the most common primary liver tumour, and the sixth most frequent cause of cancer worldwide. Cirrhosis is present in 75–90% of individuals with HCC and is an important risk factor for the disease. The risk is between 1% and 5% in cirrhosis caused by hepatitis B and C. There is also an increased risk in cirrhosis due to haemochromatosis, alcohol, NASH and α_1-antitrypsin deficiency. In northern Europe, 90% of those with HCC have underlying cirrhosis, compared with 30% in Taiwan, where hepatitis B is the main risk factor. The age-adjusted incidence rates vary from 28 per 100 000 in South-east Asia (reflecting the prevalence of hepatitis B) to 10 per 100 000 in southern Europe and 5 per 100 000 in northern Europe. Chronic hepatitis B infection increases the risk of HCC 100-fold and is the major risk factor worldwide. The risk of HCC is 0.4% per year in the absence of cirrhosis and 2–6% in cirrhosis. The risk is four times higher in HBeAg-positive individuals than in those who are HBeAg-negative. Hepatitis B vaccination has led to a fall in HCC in countries with a high prevalence of hepatitis B. The incidence in Europe and North America has risen recently, probably related to the increased prevalence of hepatitis C and NASH cirrhosis. The risk is higher in men and rises with age.

Macroscopically, the tumour usually appears as a single mass in the absence of cirrhosis, or as a single nodule or multiple nodules in the presence of cirrhosis. It takes its blood supply from the hepatic artery and tends to spread by invasion into the portal vein and its radicals. Lymph node metastases are common, while lung and bone metastases are rare. Well-differentiated tumours can resemble normal hepatocytes and can be difficult to distinguish from normal liver.

Clinical features

Patients typically present with HCC in one of two ways. Commonly, liver function deteriorates in those with underlying cirrhosis, with worsening ascites and/or jaundice or variceal haemorrhage. Other characteristic symptoms can include weight loss, anorexia and abdominal pain. This often-rapid deterioration can, however, be the event that leads to previously occult cirrhosis becoming clinically apparent, meaning that absence of an established diagnosis of cirrhosis does not preclude a diagnosis of HCC complicating cirrhosis. Examination may reveal hepatomegaly or a right hypochondrial mass. Tumour vascularity can lead to an abdominal bruit, and hepatic rupture with intra-abdominal bleeding may occur. The advanced nature of disease that presents in this way makes curative therapy unlikely.

The second presentation is through screening of patients at risk of HCC. The disease is typically detected much earlier in its natural history, significantly increasing the treatment options.

Investigations

Serum markers

Alpha-fetoprotein (AFP) is produced by 60% of HCCs. Levels increase with the size of the tumour and are often normal or only minimally elevated in small tumours detected by ultrasound screening. Serum AFP can also rise in the presence of active hepatitis B and C viral replication; very high levels are seen in acute hepatic necrosis, such as that following paracetamol toxicity. AFP is used in conjunction with ultrasound in screening but, in view of low sensitivity and specificity, levels need to be interpreted with caution. Nevertheless, in the absence of a marked hepatic flare of disease, a progressively rising AFP, or AFP of >400 ng/mL (330 IU/mL; normal is <10 ng/mL (8 IU/mL), warrants an aggressive search for HCC. In HCC patients with elevated AFP levels, serial measurements can be a useful biomarker of disease progression or response to treatment.

Imaging

Ultrasound will detect focal liver lesions as small as 2–3 cm. The use of ultrasound contrast agents has increased sensitivity and specificity but is highly user-dependent. Ultrasound may also show evidence of portal vein involvement and features of coexistent cirrhosis. Multidetector row CT, following intravenous contrast, identifies HCC by its classical hypervascular appearance (Fig. 22.35). Small lesions of less than 2 cm can be difficult to differentiate from hyperplastic nodules in cirrhosis. MRI can be used instead. Angiography is now seldom performed and has been superseded by the above techniques. A combination of imaging modalities more accurately diagnoses and stages the extent of disease, and use of at least two modalities (typically, CT or MRI following initial screening ultrasound identification of a mass lesion) is recommended.

Liver biopsy

Histological confirmation is advisable in patients with large tumours who do not have cirrhosis or hepatitis B, in order to confirm the diagnosis and exclude metastatic tumour. Biopsy should be avoided in patients who may be eligible for transplantation or surgical resection because there is a small (<2%) risk of tumour seeding along the needle tract. In all cases of potential HCC where biopsy is being considered, the impact that a confirmed diagnosis will have on therapy must be weighed against the risks of bleeding. If biopsy will not change management, then its appropriateness should be considered carefully.

Role of screening

Screening for HCC, by ultrasound scanning and AFP measurements at 6-month intervals, is indicated in high-risk patients who would be suitable for therapy if diagnosed with HCC. These include individuals with cirrhosis caused by hepatitis B and C, haemochromatosis, alcohol, NASH and α_1-antitrypsin deficiency.

Fig. 22.35 Computed tomogram showing a large hepatocellular carcinoma (arrows). *Courtesy of Dr D. Redhead, Royal Infirmary of Edinburgh.*

Screening may also be indicated in those with chronic hepatitis B (who carry an increased risk of HCC, even in the absence of cirrhosis). Although no randomised controlled studies of outcome have been undertaken, screening identifies smaller tumours, often less than 3 cm in size, which are more likely to be cured by surgical resection, local ablative therapy or transplantation. The role of screening in other forms of chronic liver disease, such as autoimmune hepatitis and PBC, is unclear. This is compounded by the fact that disease staging by biopsy is no longer standard practice in conditions such as PBC, so formal documentation of the presence of cirrhosis, which might be the trigger for commencement of HCC screening, rarely takes place.

Management

This is different for patients with cirrhosis and those without. In the presence of cirrhosis, tumour size, multicentricity, extent of liver disease (Child–Pugh score) and performance status dictate therapy. An algorithm for managing those with cirrhosis is shown in Figure 22.36.

Prognosis depends on tumour size, the presence of vascular invasion, and liver function in those with cirrhosis. Screening has improved the outlook through early detection.

Hepatic resection

This is the treatment of choice for non-cirrhotic patients. The 5-year survival in this group is about 50%. There is a 50% recurrence rate at 5 years, however, which may be due to a second de novo tumour or recurrence of the original tumour. Few patients with cirrhosis are suitable for hepatic resection because of the high risk of hepatic failure; nevertheless, surgery is offered, particularly in the Far East, to some cirrhotic patients with small tumours and good liver function (Child–Pugh A with no portal hypertension).

Liver transplantation

Transplantation has the benefit of curing underlying cirrhosis and removing the risk of a second, de novo tumour in an at-risk patient. The requirement for immunosuppression creates its own risks of reactivation, however, if residual or metastatic disease is present, and assessment of patients for suitability for liver transplantation focuses on the exclusion of extrahepatic disease and vascular invasion. The 5-year survival following liver transplantation is 75% for patients with single tumours of less than 5 cm in size or three tumours smaller than 3 cm (the Milan criteria). Unfortunately, the underlying liver disease, in particular hepatitis C, may recur in the transplanted liver and can result in recurrent cirrhosis that gives rise to a de novo HCC risk, now complicated by the presence of immunosuppression.

Percutaneous therapy

Percutaneous ethanol injection into the tumour under ultrasound guidance is efficacious (80% cure rate) for tumours of 3 cm or less. Recurrence rates (50% at 3 years) are similar to those following surgical resection. Radiofrequency ablation, using a single electrode inserted into the tumour under radiological guidance, is an alternative that takes longer to perform but may cause more complete tumour necrosis. Improvements in percutaneous therapy, with the combination of low patient impact, relative efficacy and capacity for repeat treatment, are making these approaches attractive, particularly when major surgery would be inappropriate. Their role in primary therapy as an alternative to curative resection or transplantation is yet to be established.

22

Hepatocellular carcinoma

PST 0, Child–Pugh A

PST 0–2, Child–Pugh A–B

PST > 2, Child–Pugh C

Very early stage
Single < 2 cm

Early stage
Single < 5 cm

Intermediate stage
Multinodular; PST 0

Advanced stage
Portal vein invasion;
N1, M1; PST 1–2

Terminal stage

Single

3 nodules < 3 cm

Portal pressure

Increased ⟶ Associated diseases

Normal

No   Yes

Resection	Liver transplantation	RFA/PEI	TACE	Sorafenib	Best supportive care
Curative treatment (30–40%) **Median OS: > 60 months** **5-year survival: 40–70%**			**Target: 20%** **OS: 20 months** **(14–45 months)**	**Target: 40%** **OS: 11 months** **(6–14 months)**	**Target: 10%** **OS: < 3 months**

Fig. 22.36 Management of hepatocellular carcinoma complicating cirrhosis. Performance status (PST; see Box 33.3, p. 1322): 0 = fully active, no symptoms; >2 = limited self-care, confined to bed or chair for 50% of waking hours. Child–Pugh score: see Box 22.29, p. 867. N1, M1: lymph node involvement and metastases (for TNM classification, see Box 33.4, p. 1322) (OS = overall survival; PEI = percutaneous ethanol injection; RFA = radiofrequency ablation; TACE = trans-arterial chemo-embolisation). *Based on European Association for the Study of the Liver, European Organisation for Research and Treatment of Cancer. EASL–EORTC clinical practice guidelines: Management of hepatocellular carcinoma. J Hepatol 2012; 56:908–943.*

Trans-arterial chemo-embolisation

Hepatocellular cancers are not radiosensitive and the response rate to chemotherapy with drugs, such as doxorubicin, is only around 30%. In contrast, hepatic artery embolisation with absorbable gelatin powder (Gelfoam) and doxorubicin is more effective, with survival rates of 60% in cirrhotic patients with unresectable HCC and good liver function (compared with 20% in untreated patients) at 2 years. Unfortunately, any survival benefit is lost at 4 years. Trans-arterial chemo-embolisation (TACE) is contraindicated in decompensated cirrhosis and multifocal HCC. TACE is now most frequently used as a holding first intervention while the tumour is being assessed and the definitive management plan is being developed.

Chemotherapy

Sorafenib improves survival from 7.9 to 10.7 months in cirrhotic patients. The drug is a multikinase inhibitor with activity against Raf, vascular endothelial growth factor (VEGF) and platelet-derived growth factor (PDGF) signalling, and is the first systemic therapy to prolong survival in HCC. The ultimate role of sorafenib in HCC – in particular, when and how best to use it – is yet to be established.

Fibrolamellar hepatocellular carcinoma

This rare variant differs from HCC in that it occurs in young adults, equally in males and females, in the absence of hepatitis B infection and cirrhosis. The tumours are often large at presentation and the AFP is usually normal. Histology of the tumour reveals malignant hepatocytes surrounded by a dense fibrous stroma. The treatment of choice is surgical resection. This variant of HCC has a better prognosis following surgery than an equivalent-sized HCC, two-thirds of patients surviving beyond 5 years.

Other primary malignant tumours

These are rare but include haemangio-endothelial sarcomas. Cholangiocarcinoma (bile duct cancer) typically presents with bile duct obstruction rather than as a hepatic mass lesion, although the latter occasionally occurs.

Secondary malignant tumours

These are common and usually originate from carcinomas in the lung, breast, abdomen or pelvis. They may be single or multiple. Peritoneal dissemination frequently results in ascites.

Clinical features

The primary neoplasm is asymptomatic in 50% of patients, being detected on either radiological, endoscopic or blood biochemistry screening. There is liver enlargement and weight loss; jaundice may be present.

Investigations

A raised ALP activity is the most common biochemical abnormality but LFTs may be normal. Ascitic fluid, if present, has a high protein content and may be blood-stained; cytology sometimes reveals malignant cells. Imaging shows filling defects (Fig. 22.37); laparoscopy may reveal the tumour and facilitates liver biopsy.

Fig. 22.37 Computed tomogram showing multiple liver metastases (arrows).

Fig. 22.38 Magnetic resonance image showing a haemangioma (arrows) in the liver. *Courtesy of Dr D. Redhead, Royal Infirmary of Edinburgh.*

Management

Hepatic resection can improve survival for slow-growing tumours, such as colonic carcinomas, and is an approach that should be actively explored in patients who are fit for liver resection and have had the primary tumour resected once extrahepatic disease has been excluded. Patients with neuro-endocrine tumours, such as gastrinomas, insulinomas and glucagonomas, and those with lymphomas may benefit from surgery, hormonal treatment or chemotherapy. Unfortunately, palliative treatment to relieve pain is all that is available for most patients; this may include arterial embolisation of the tumour masses.

Benign tumours

The increasing use of ultrasound scanning has led to more frequent identification of incidental benign focal liver lesions.

Hepatic adenomas

These are rare vascular tumours that may present as an abdominal mass, or with abdominal pain or intraperitoneal bleeding. They are more common in women and may be caused by oral contraceptives, androgens and anabolic glucocorticoids. Resection is indicated for the relief of symptoms. Hepatic adenomas can increase in size during pregnancy. Large or rapidly growing adenomas can rarely rupture, causing intraperitoneal bleeding.

Haemangiomas

These are the most common benign liver tumours and are present in 1–20% of the population. Most are smaller than 5 cm and rarely cause symptoms (Fig. 22.38). The diagnosis is usually made by ultrasound but CT may show a low-density lesion with delayed arterial filling. Surgery is needed only for very large symptomatic lesions or where the diagnosis is in doubt.

Focal nodular hyperplasia

Focal nodular hyperplasia is common in women under the age of 40. The lesions are usually asymptomatic but can be up to 10 cm in diameter; they can be differentiated from adenoma by a focal central scar seen on CT or MRI. Histologically, they

Fig. 22.39 Computed tomogram showing multiple cysts in the liver and kidneys in polycystic disease.

consist of nodular regeneration of hepatocytes without fibrosis. They may be multiple but only rarely need resection.

Cystic liver disease and liver abscess

Isolated or multiple simple cysts are common in the liver and are a relatively frequent finding on ultrasound screening. They can be associated with polycystic renal disease (Fig. 22.39). They are intrinsically benign and require no therapy, other than in rare cases where the mass effect of very large or multiple cysts causes abdominal discomfort. In such cases, percutaneous or surgical debulking can be attempted but recurrence is typical. Liver abscesses are discussed on page 879.

Drugs and the liver

The liver is the primary site of drug metabolism and an important target for drug-induced injury. Pre-existing liver disease may affect the capacity of the liver to metabolise drugs and unexpected toxicity may occur when patients with liver disease are given drugs in normal doses (p. 32). Box 22.53 also shows drugs that should be avoided in patients with cirrhosis, as they can exacerbate known complications of cirrhosis. The possibility of undiagnosed underlying liver injury should always be considered in patients exhibiting unexpected effects following drug exposure.

22

i 22.53 Drugs to be avoided in cirrhosis		
Drug	Problem	Toxicity
Non-steroidal anti-inflammatory drugs	Reduced renal blood flow Mucosal ulceration	Hepatorenal failure Bleeding varices
Angiotensin-converting enzyme inhibitors	Reduced renal blood flow	Hepatorenal failure
Codeine	Constipation	Hepatic encephalopathy
Narcotics	Constipation, drug accumulation	Hepatic encephalopathy
Anxiolytics	Drug accumulation	Hepatic encephalopathy

i 22.54 Examples of common causes of drug-induced hepatotoxicity	
Pattern	Drug
Cholestasis	Chlorpromazine High-dose oestrogens
Cholestatic hepatitis	Non-steroidal anti-inflammatory drugs Co-amoxiclav Statins
Acute hepatitis	Rifampicin Isoniazid
Non-alcoholic steatohepatitis	Amiodarone
Venous outflow obstruction	Busulfan Azathioprine
Fibrosis	Methotrexate

Drug-induced liver injury

Drug toxicity should always be considered in the differential diagnosis of patients presenting with acute liver failure, jaundice or abnormal liver biochemistry. Some typical patterns of drug toxicity are listed in Box 22.54; the most common picture is a mixed cholestatic hepatitis. The presence of jaundice indicates more severe liver damage. Although acute liver failure can occur, most drug reactions are self-limiting and chronic liver damage is rare. Abnormal LFTs often take weeks to normalise following a drug-induced hepatitis, and it may be months before they normalise after a cholestatic hepatitis. Occasionally, permanent bile duct loss (ductopenia) follows a cholestatic drug reaction, such as that due to co-amoxiclav, resulting in chronic cholestasis with persistent symptoms such as itching.

The key to diagnosing acute drug-induced liver disease is to take a detailed drug history (Box 22.55), looking for temporal relationships between drug exposure and onset of liver abnormality (bearing in mind the fact that liver injury can frequently take weeks or even months to develop following exposure). A liver biopsy should be considered if there is suspicion of pre-existing liver disease or if blood tests fail to improve when the suspect drug is withdrawn.

Where drug-induced liver injury is suspected or cannot be excluded, the potential culprit drug should be discontinued unless it is impossible to do so safely.

Types of liver injury

Different histological patterns of liver injury may occur with drug injury.

Cholestasis

Pure cholestasis (selective interference with bile flow in the absence of liver injury) can occur with oestrogens; this was common when high concentrations of oestrogens (50 µg/day) were used as contraceptives. Both the current oral contraceptive pill and hormone replacement therapy can be safely used in chronic liver disease.

Chlorpromazine and antibiotics such as flucloxacillin are examples of drugs that cause cholestatic hepatitis, which is characterised by inflammation and canalicular injury. Co-amoxiclav is the most common antibiotic to cause abnormal LFTs but, unlike other antibiotics, it may not produce symptoms until 10–42 days after it is stopped. Anabolic glucocorticoids used by body-builders may also cause a cholestatic hepatitis. In some

i 22.55 Diagnosing acute drug-induced liver disease

- Tabulate the drugs taken:
    Prescribed and self-administered
- Establish whether hepatotoxicity is reported in the literature
- Relate the time the drugs were taken to the onset of illness: 4 days to 8 weeks (usual)
- Establish the effect of stopping the drugs on normalisation of liver biochemistry:
    Hepatitic liver function tests (2 months)
    Cholestatic/mixed liver function tests (6 months)
- **N.B.** *Challenge tests with drugs should be avoided*
- Exclude other causes:
    Viral hepatitis
    Biliary disease
- Consider liver biopsy

cases (e.g. NSAIDs and cyclo-oxygenase 2 (COX-2) inhibitors), there is overlap with acute hepatocellular injury.

Hepatocyte necrosis

Many drugs cause an acute hepatocellular necrosis with high serum transaminase concentrations; paracetamol is the best known. Inflammation is not always present but does accompany necrosis in liver injury due to diclofenac (an NSAID) and isoniazid (an anti-tuberculous drug). Granulomas may be seen in liver injury following the use of allopurinol. Acute hepatocellular necrosis has also been described following the use of several herbal remedies, including germander, comfrey and jin bu huan. Recreational drugs, including cocaine and ecstasy, can also cause severe acute hepatitis.

Steatosis

Microvesicular hepatocyte fat deposition, due to direct effects on mitochondrial beta-oxidation, can follow exposure to tetracyclines and sodium valproate. Macrovesicular hepatocyte fat deposition has been described with tamoxifen, and amiodarone toxicity can produce a similar histological picture to NASH.

Vascular/sinusoidal lesions

Drugs such as the alkylating agents used in oncology can damage the vascular endothelium and lead to hepatic venous outflow obstruction. Chronic overdose of vitamin A can damage the sinusoids and trigger local fibrosis that can result in portal hypertension.

Hepatic fibrosis

Most drugs cause reversible liver injury and hepatic fibrosis is very uncommon. Methotrexate, however, as well as causing acute liver injury when it is started, can lead to cirrhosis when used in high doses over a long period of time. Risk factors for drug-induced hepatic fibrosis include pre-existing liver disease and a high alcohol intake.

Inherited liver diseases

The inherited diseases are an important and probably under-diagnosed group of liver diseases. In addition to the 'classical' conditions, such as haemochromatosis and Wilson's disease, the important role played by the liver in the expression of the inborn errors of metabolism should be remembered, as should the potential for genetic underpinning for intrahepatic cholestasis.

Haemochromatosis

Haemochromatosis is a condition in which the amount of total body iron is increased; the excess iron is deposited in, and causes damage to, several organs, including the liver. It may be primary or secondary to other diseases (Box 22.56).

Hereditary haemochromatosis

In hereditary haemochromatosis (HHC), iron is deposited throughout the body and total body iron may reach 20–60 g (normally 4 g). The important organs involved are the liver, pancreatic islets, endocrine glands, joints and heart. In the liver, iron deposition occurs first in the periportal hepatocytes, extending later to all hepatocytes. The gradual development of fibrous septa leads to the formation of irregular nodules, and finally regeneration results in macronodular cirrhosis. An excess of liver iron can occur in alcoholic cirrhosis but this is mild in comparison with haemochromatosis.

22.56 Causes of haemochromatosis

Primary haemochromatosis

- Hereditary haemochromatosis
- Congenital acaeruloplasminaemia
- Congenital atransferrinaemia

Secondary iron overload

- Parenteral iron loading (e.g. repeated blood transfusion)
- Iron-loading anaemia (thalassaemia, sideroblastic anaemia, pyruvate kinase deficiency)
- Liver disease

Complex iron overload

- Juvenile haemochromatosis
- Neonatal haemochromatosis
- Alcoholic liver disease
- Porphyria cutanea tarda
- African iron overload (Bantu siderosis)

Pathophysiology

The disease is caused by increased absorption of dietary iron and is inherited as an autosomal recessive trait. Approximately 90% of patients are homozygous for a single point mutation resulting in a cysteine to tyrosine substitution at position 282 (C282Y) in the HFE protein, which has structural and functional similarity to the HLA proteins. The mechanisms by which HFE regulates iron absorption are unclear. It is believed, however, that HFE normally interacts with the transferrin receptor in the basolateral membrane of intestinal epithelial cells. In HHC, it is thought that the lack of functional HFE causes a defect in uptake of transferrin-associated iron, leading to up-regulation of enterocyte iron-specific divalent metal transporters and excessive iron absorption. A histidine-to-aspartic acid mutation at position 63 (H63D) in HFE causes a less severe form of haemochromatosis that is most commonly found in patients who are compound heterozygotes also carrying a C282Y mutated allele. Fewer than 50% of C282Y homozygotes will develop clinical features of haemochromatosis; therefore other factors must also be important. HHC may promote accelerated liver disease in patients with alcohol excess or hepatitis C infection. Iron loss in menstruation and pregnancy can delay the onset of HHC in females.

Clinical features

Symptomatic disease usually presents in men over 40 years of age with features of liver disease (often with hepatomegaly), diabetes or heart failure. Fatigue and arthropathy are early symptoms but are frequently absent. Leaden-grey skin pigmentation due to excess melanin occurs, especially in exposed parts, axillae, groins and genitalia: hence the term 'bronzed diabetes'. Once again, absence of this feature does not preclude the diagnosis. Impotence, loss of libido and testicular atrophy are recognised complications, as are early-onset osteoarthritis targeting unusual sites such as the metacarpophalangeal joints, chondrocalcinosis and pseudogout. Cardiac failure or cardiac dysrhythmia may occur due to iron deposition in the heart.

Investigations

Serum iron studies show a greatly increased ferritin, a raised plasma iron and saturated plasma iron-binding capacity. Transferrin saturation of more than 45% is suggestive of iron overload. Significant liver disease is unusual in patients with ferritin lower than 1000 μg/L (100 μg/dL). The differential diagnoses for elevated ferritin are inflammatory disease or excess ethanol consumption for modest elevations (< 1000 μg/L (100 μg/dL)). Very significant ferritin elevation can be seen in adult Still's disease. In terms of imaging techniques, MRI has high specificity for iron overload but poor sensitivity. Liver biopsy allows assessment of fibrosis and distribution of iron (hepatocyte iron characteristic of haemochromatosis). The Hepatic Iron Index (HII) provides quantification of liver iron (μmol of iron per g dry weight of liver/age in years). An HII of more than 1.9 suggests genetic haemochromatosis (Fig. 22.40). Both the C282Y and the H63D mutations can be identified by genetic testing, which is now in routine clinical use.

Management

Treatment consists of weekly venesection of 500 mL blood (250 mg iron) until the serum iron is normal; this may take 2 years or more. The aim is to reduce ferritin to under 50 μg/L (5 μg/dL). Thereafter, venesection is continued as required to keep the serum ferritin normal. Liver and cardiac problems

22

Fig. 22.40 Liver histology: haemochromatosis. This Perls stain shows accumulating iron within hepatocytes, which is stained blue. There is also accumulation of large fat globules in some hepatocytes (macrovesicular steatosis). Iron also accumulates in Kupffer cells and biliary epithelial cells.

improve after iron removal, but joint pain is less predictable and can improve or worsen after iron removal. Diabetes does not resolve after venesection. Other therapy includes that for cirrhosis and diabetes. First-degree family members should be investigated, preferably by genetic screening and also by checking the plasma ferritin and iron-binding saturation. Liver biopsy is indicated in asymptomatic relatives only if the LFTs are abnormal and/or the serum ferritin is greater than 1000 μg/L (100 μg/dL) because these features are associated with significant fibrosis or cirrhosis. Asymptomatic disease should also be treated by venesection until the serum ferritin is normal.

Pre-cirrhotic patients with HHC have a normal life expectancy, and even cirrhotic patients have a good prognosis compared with other forms of cirrhosis (three-quarters of patients are alive 5 years after diagnosis). This is probably because liver function is well preserved at diagnosis and improves with therapy. Screening for hepatocellular carcinoma (p. 890) is mandatory because this is the main cause of death, affecting one-third of patients with cirrhosis, irrespective of therapy. Venesection reduces but does not abolish the risk of hepatocellular carcinoma in the presence of cirrhosis.

Secondary haemochromatosis

Many conditions, including chronic haemolytic disorders, sideroblastic anaemia, other conditions requiring multiple blood transfusion (generally over 50 L), porphyria cutanea tarda, dietary iron overload and occasionally alcoholic cirrhosis, are associated with widespread secondary siderosis. The features are similar to those of primary haemochromatosis but the history and clinical findings point to the true diagnosis. Some patients are heterozygotes for the *HFE* gene and this may contribute to the development of iron overload.

Wilson's disease

Wilson's disease (hepatolenticular degeneration) is a rare but important autosomal recessive disorder of copper metabolism caused by a variety of mutations in the *ATP7B* gene on chromosome 13. Total body copper is increased, with excess copper deposited in, and causing damage to, several organs.

Pathophysiology

Normally, dietary copper is absorbed from the stomach and proximal small intestine and is rapidly taken into the liver, where it is stored and incorporated into caeruloplasmin, which is secreted into the blood. The accumulation of excessive copper in the body is ultimately prevented by its excretion, the most important route being via bile. In Wilson's disease, there is almost always a failure of synthesis of caeruloplasmin; however, some 5% of patients have a normal circulating caeruloplasmin concentration and this is not the primary pathogenic defect. The amount of copper in the body at birth is normal but thereafter it increases steadily; the organs most affected are the liver, basal ganglia of the brain, eyes, kidneys and skeleton.

The *ATP7B* gene encodes a member of the copper-transporting P-type adenosine triphosphatase family, which functions to export copper from various cell types. At least 200 different mutations have been described. Most cases are compound heterozygotes with two different mutations in *ATP7B*. Attempts to correlate the genotype with the mode of presentation and clinical course have not shown any consistent patterns. The large number of culprit mutations means that, in contrast to haemochromatosis, genetic diagnosis is not routine in Wilson's disease, although it may have a role in screening families following identification of the genotype in an index patient.

Clinical features

Symptoms usually arise between the ages of 5 and 45 years. Hepatic disease occurs predominantly in childhood and early adolescence, although it can present in adults in their fifties. Neurological damage causes basal ganglion syndromes and dementia, which tends to present in later adolescence. These features can occur alone or simultaneously. Other manifestations include renal tubular damage and osteoporosis, but these are rarely presenting features.

Liver disease

Episodes of acute hepatitis, sometimes recurrent, can occur, especially in children, and may progress to fulminant liver failure. The latter is characterised by the liberation of free copper into the blood stream, causing massive haemolysis and renal tubulopathy. Chronic hepatitis can also develop insidiously and eventually present with established cirrhosis; liver failure and portal hypertension may supervene. The possibility of Wilson's disease should be considered in any patient under the age of 40 presenting with recurrent acute hepatitis or chronic liver disease of unknown cause, especially when this is accompanied by haemolysis.

Neurological disease

Clinical features include a variety of extrapyramidal features, particularly tremor, choreoathetosis, dystonia, parkinsonism and dementia (Ch. 25). Unusual clumsiness for age may be an early symptom. Neurological disease typically develops after the onset of liver disease and can be prevented by effective treatment started following diagnosis in the liver disease phase. This increases the importance of diagnosis in the liver phase beyond just allowing effective management of liver disease.

Kayser–Fleischer rings

These constitute the most important single clinical clue to the diagnosis and can be seen in 60% of adults with Wilson's disease (less often in children but almost always in neurological

Wilson's disease), albeit sometimes only by slit-lamp examination. Kayser–Fleischer rings are characterised by greenish-brown discoloration of the corneal margin appearing first at the upper periphery (p. 846). They disappear with treatment.

Investigations

A low serum caeruloplasmin is the best single laboratory clue to the diagnosis. Advanced liver failure from any cause can, however, reduce the serum caeruloplasmin and occasionally it is normal in Wilson's disease. Other features of disordered copper metabolism should therefore be sought; these include a high free serum copper concentration, a high urine copper excretion of greater than 0.6 μmol/24 hrs (38 μg/24 hrs) and a very high hepatic copper content. Measuring 24-hour urinary copper excretion while giving D-penicillamine is a useful confirmatory test; more than 25 μmol/24 hrs is considered diagnostic of Wilson's disease.

Management

The copper-binding agent penicillamine is the drug of choice. The dose given must be sufficient to produce cupriuresis and most patients require 1.5 μg/day (range 1–4 μg). The dose can be reduced once the disease is in remission but treatment must continue for life, even through pregnancy. Care must be taken to ensure that re-accumulation of copper does not occur. Abrupt discontinuation of treatment must be avoided because this may precipitate acute liver failure. Toxic effects occur in one-third of patients and include rashes, protein-losing nephropathy, lupus-like syndrome and bone marrow depression. If these do arise, trientine dihydrochloride (1.2–2.4 μg/day) and zinc (50 mg 3 times daily) are potential alternatives.

Liver transplantation is indicated for fulminant liver failure or for advanced cirrhosis with liver failure. The value of liver transplantation in severe neurological Wilson's disease is unclear. Prognosis is excellent, provided treatment is started before there is irreversible damage. Siblings and children of patients with Wilson's disease must be investigated and treatment should be given to all affected individuals, even if they are asymptomatic.

Alpha₁-antitrypsin deficiency

Alpha₁-antitrypsin (α_1-AT) is a serine protease inhibitor (Pi) produced by the liver. One of its main anti-protease functions is the breakdown of neutrophil elastase. The mutated form of α_1-AT (PiZ) cannot be secreted into the blood by liver cells because it is retained within the endoplasmic reticulum of the hepatocyte. Homozygous individuals (PiZZ) have low plasma α_1-AT concentrations, although globules containing α_1-AT are found in the liver, and these people may develop hepatic and pulmonary disease. Liver manifestations include cholestatic jaundice in the neonatal period (neonatal hepatitis), which can resolve spontaneously; chronic hepatitis and cirrhosis in adults; and, in the long term, HCC. Alpha₁-AT deficiency is a not uncommon exacerbating factor for liver disease of other aetiologies, and the possibility of dual pathology should be considered when severity of disease, such as ALD, appears disproportionate to the level of underlying insult.

There are no clinical features that distinguish liver disease due to α_1-AT deficiency from liver disease due to other causes, and the diagnosis is made from the low plasma α_1-AT concentration and genotyping for the presence of the mutation. Alpha₁-AT-containing globules can be demonstrated in the liver (Fig. 22.41)

Fig. 22.41 Liver histology in α_1-antitrypsin deficiency. Accumulation of periodic acid–Schiff-positive granules (arrows) within individual hepatocytes is shown in this section from a patient with α_1-AT deficiency.

but this is not necessary to make the diagnosis. Occasionally, patients with liver disease and minor reductions of plasma α_1-AT concentrations have α_1-AT variants other than PiZZ, but the relationship of these to liver disease is uncertain.

There is no specific treatment. The risk of severe and early-onset emphysema means that all patients should be advised to stop smoking.

Gilbert's syndrome

Gilbert's syndrome is by far the most common inherited disorder of bilirubin metabolism (see Box 22.17, p. 860). It is an autosomal recessive trait when caused by a mutation in the promoter region of the gene for UDP-glucuronyl transferase enzyme (*UGT1A1*), which leads to reduced enzyme expression. It can be inherited in a dominant fashion when there is a missense mutation in the gene. This results in decreased conjugation of bilirubin, which accumulates as unconjugated bilirubin in the blood. The levels of unconjugated bilirubin increase during fasting, as fasting reduces levels of UDP-glucuronyl transferase.

Clinical features

The typical presentation is with isolated elevation of bilirubin, typically, although not exclusively, in the setting of physical stress or illness. There are no stigmata of chronic liver disease other than jaundice. Increased excretion of bilirubin and hence stercobilinogen leads to normal-coloured or dark stools, and increased urobilinogen excretion causes the urine to turn dark on standing as urobilin is formed. In the presence of haemolysis, pallor due to anaemia and splenomegaly due to excessive reticulo-endothelial activity are usually present.

Investigations

The plasma bilirubin is usually less than 100 μmol/L (~6 mg/dL) and the LFTs are otherwise normal. There is no bilirubinuria because the hyperbilirubinaemia is predominantly unconjugated. Hepatic histology is normal and liver biopsy is not recommended for the investigation of patients with possible Gilbert's syndrome. The condition is not associated with liver injury and thus has an excellent prognosis, needs no treatment, and is clinically important only because it may be mistaken for more serious liver disease.

22

Vascular liver disease

Metabolically, the liver is highly active and has large oxygen requirements. This places it at risk of ischaemic injury in settings of impaired perfusion. The risk is mitigated, however, by the dual perfusion of the liver (via the portal vein as well as hepatic artery), with the former representing a low-pressure perfusion system that offers protection against the potential effects of arterial hypotension. The single outflow through the hepatic vein and the low-pressure perfusion system of the portal vein make the liver vulnerable to venous thrombotic ischaemia in the context of Budd–Chiari syndrome and portal vein thrombosis, respectively.

Hepatic arterial disease

Liver ischaemia

Liver ischaemic injury is relatively common during hypotensive or hypoxic events and is under-diagnosed. The characteristic pattern is one of rising transaminase values in the days following such an event (e.g. prolonged seizures). Liver synthetic dysfunction and encephalopathy are uncommon but can occur. Liver failure is very rare. Diagnosis typically rests on clinical suspicion and exclusion of other potential aetiologies. Treatment is aimed at optimising liver perfusion and oxygen delivery. Outcome is dictated by the morbidity and mortality associated with the underlying disease, given that liver ischaemia frequently occurs in the context of other organ ischaemia in high-risk patients.

Liver arterial disease

Hepatic arterial disease is rare outside the setting of liver transplantation and is difficult to diagnose. It can cause significant liver damage. Hepatic artery occlusion may result from inadvertent injury during biliary surgery or may be caused by emboli, neoplasms, polyarteritis nodosa, blunt trauma or radiation. It usually causes severe upper abdominal pain with or without signs of circulatory shock. LFTs show raised transaminases (AST or ALT usually >1000 U/L), as in other causes of acute liver damage. Patients usually survive if the liver and portal blood supply are otherwise normal.

Hepatic artery aneurysms are extrahepatic in three-quarters of cases and intrahepatic in one-quarter. Atheroma, vasculitis, bacterial endocarditis and surgical or biopsy trauma are the main causes. They usually lead to bleeding into the biliary tree, peritoneum or intestine and are best diagnosed by angiography. Treatment is radiological or surgical. Any of the vasculitides can affect the hepatic artery but this rarely causes symptoms.

Hepatic artery thrombosis is a recognised complication of liver transplantation and typically occurs in the early post-transplant period. Clinical features are often related to bile duct rather than liver ischaemia because of the dominant role of the hepatic artery in extrahepatic bile duct perfusion. Manifestations can include bile duct anastomotic failure with bile leak or the development of late bile duct strictures. Diagnosis and initial intervention are radiological in the first instance, with ERCP and biliary stenting being the principal approaches to the treatment of bile duct injury.

Portal venous disease

Portal hypertension

See page 868.

Portal vein thrombosis

Portal venous thrombosis as a primary event is rare but can occur in any condition predisposing to thrombosis. It may also complicate intra-abdominal inflammatory or neoplastic disease and is a recognised cause of portal hypertension. Acute portal venous thrombosis causes abdominal pain and diarrhoea, and may rarely lead to bowel infarction, requiring surgery. Treatment is otherwise based on anticoagulation, although there are no randomised data that demonstrate efficacy. An underlying thrombophilia needs to be excluded. Subacute thrombosis can be asymptomatic but may subsequently lead to extrahepatic portal hypertension (p. 868). Ascites is unusual in non-cirrhotic portal hypertension, unless the albumin is particularly low.

Portal vein thrombosis can arise as a secondary event in patients with cirrhosis and portal hypertension, and is a recognised cause of decompensation in patients with previously stable cirrhosis. In individuals showing such decompensation, portal vein patency should be assessed by ultrasound with Doppler flow studies.

Chronic portal vein thrombosis can be a cause of portal hypertension.

Hepatopulmonary syndrome

This condition is characterised by resistant hypoxaemia (PaO_2 <9.3 kPa (70 mmHg)), intrapulmonary vascular dilatation in patients with cirrhosis, and portal hypertension. Clinical features include finger clubbing, cyanosis, spider naevi and a characteristic reduction in arterial oxygen saturation on standing. The hypoxia is due to intrapulmonary shunting through direct arteriovenous communications. Nitric oxide (NO) over-production may be important in pathogenesis. The hepatopulmonary syndrome can be treated by liver transplantation but, if severe (PaO_2 <6.7 kPa (50 mmHg)), is associated with an increased operative risk.

Portopulmonary hypertension

This unusual complication of portal hypertension is similar to 'primary pulmonary hypertension' (p. 621). It is defined as pulmonary hypertension with increased pulmonary vascular resistance and a normal pulmonary artery wedge pressure in a patient with portal hypertension. The condition is caused by vasoconstriction and obliteration of the pulmonary arterial system and leads to breathlessness and fatigue.

Hepatic venous disease

Obstruction to hepatic venous blood flow can occur in the small central hepatic veins, the large hepatic veins, the inferior vena cava or the heart (see Fig. 22.20, p. 868). The clinical features depend on the cause and on the speed with which obstruction develops, and can mimic many other forms of chronic liver disease, sometimes leading to delayed diagnosis. Congestive hepatomegaly and ascites are, however, the most consistent features. The possibility of hepatic venous obstruction should always be considered in patients with an atypical liver presentation.

Budd–Chiari syndrome

This uncommon condition is caused by thrombosis of the larger hepatic veins and sometimes the inferior vena cava. Many patients have haematological disorders such as myelofibrosis, primary proliferative polycythaemia, paroxysmal nocturnal haemoglobinuria, or antithrombin III, protein C or protein S deficiencies (Ch. 23). Pregnancy and oral contraceptive use, obstruction due to tumours (particularly carcinomas of the liver, kidneys or adrenals), congenital venous webs and occasionally inferior vena caval stenosis are the other main causes. The underlying cause cannot be found in about 50% of patients, although this percentage is falling as molecular diagnostic tools (such as the *JAK2* mutation in myelofibrosis) increase our capacity to diagnose underlying haematological disorders. Hepatic congestion affecting the centrilobular areas is followed by centrilobular fibrosis, and eventually cirrhosis supervenes in those who survive long enough.

Clinical features

Acute venous occlusion causes rapid development of upper abdominal pain, marked ascites and occasionally acute liver failure. More gradual occlusion causes gross ascites and, often, upper abdominal discomfort. Hepatomegaly, frequently with tenderness over the liver, is almost always present. Peripheral oedema occurs only when there is inferior vena cava obstruction. Features of cirrhosis and portal hypertension develop in those who survive the acute event.

Investigations

The LFTs vary considerably, depending on the presentation, and can show the features of acute hepatitis. Ascitic fluid analysis shows a protein concentration above 25 g/L (2.5 g/dL) (exudate) in the early stages; this often falls later in the disease, however. Doppler ultrasound may reveal obliteration of the hepatic veins and reversed flow or associated thrombosis in the portal vein. CT may show enlargement of the caudate lobe, as this often has a separate venous drainage system that is not involved in the disease. CT and MRI may also demonstrate occlusion of the hepatic veins and inferior vena cava. Liver biopsy demonstrates centrilobular congestion with fibrosis, depending on the duration of the illness. Venography is needed only if CT and MRI are unable to demonstrate the hepatic venous anatomy clearly.

Management

Predisposing causes should be treated as far as possible; where recent thrombosis is suspected, thrombolysis with streptokinase, followed by heparin and oral anticoagulation, should be considered. Ascites is initially treated medically but often with only limited success. Short hepatic venous strictures can be treated with angioplasty. In the case of more extensive hepatic vein occlusion, many patients can be managed successfully by insertion of a covered TIPSS, followed by anticoagulation. Surgical shunts, such as portacaval shunts, are less commonly performed now that TIPSS is available. Occasionally, a web can be resected or an inferior vena caval stenosis dilated. Progressive liver failure is an indication for liver transplantation and life-long anticoagulation.

Prognosis without transplantation or shunting is poor, particularly following an acute presentation with liver failure. A 3-year survival of 50% is reported in those who survive the initial event. The 1- and 10-year survival following liver transplantation is 85% and 69%, respectively, and this compares with a 5- and 10-year survival of 87% and 37%, respectively, following surgical shunting.

Sinusoidal obstruction syndrome (veno-occlusive disease)

Sinusoidal obstruction syndrome (SOS; previously known as veno-occlusive disease) is a rare condition characterised by widespread occlusion of the small central hepatic veins. Pyrrolizidine alkaloids in *Senecio* and *Heliotropium* plants used to make teas, as well as cytotoxic drugs and hepatic irradiation, are all recognised causes. SOS may develop in 10–20% of patients following haematopoietic stem cell transplantation (usually within the first 20 days) and carries a 90% mortality in severe cases. Pathogenesis involves obliteration and fibrosis of terminal hepatic venules due to deposition of red cells, haemosiderin-laden macrophages and coagulation factors. In this setting, SOS is thought to relate to pre-conditioning therapy with irradiation and cytotoxic chemotherapy. The clinical features are similar to those of the Budd–Chiari syndrome (see above). Investigations show evidence of venous outflow obstruction histologically but, in contrast to Budd–Chiari, the large hepatic veins appear patent radiologically. Transjugular liver biopsy (with portal pressure measurements) may facilitate the diagnosis. Traditionally, treatment has been supportive but defibrotide shows promise (the drug binds to vascular endothelial cells, promoting fibrinolysis and suppressing coagulation).

Cardiac disease

Hepatic damage, due primarily to congestion, may develop in all forms of right heart failure (p. 461); usually, the clinical features are predominantly cardiac. Very rarely, long-standing cardiac failure and hepatic congestion give rise to cardiac cirrhosis. Severe left ventricular dysfunction is a cause of ischaemic hepatitis. Cardiac causes of acute and chronic liver disease are typically under-diagnosed. Treatment is principally that of the underlying heart disease with supportive treatment for the liver component.

Nodular regenerative hyperplasia of the liver

This is the most common cause of non-cirrhotic portal hypertension in developed countries; it is characterised by small hepatocyte nodules throughout the liver without fibrosis, which can result in sinusoidal compression. It is believed to be due to damage to small hepatic arterioles and portal venules. It occurs in older people and is associated with many conditions, including connective tissue disease, haematological diseases and immunosuppressive drugs, such as azathioprine. The condition is usually asymptomatic but occasionally presents with portal hypertension or with an abdominal mass. The diagnosis is made by liver biopsy, which, in contrast to cirrhosis, shows nodule formation in the absence of fibrous septa. Liver function is good and the prognosis is very favourable. Management is based on treatment of the portal hypertension.

Pregnancy and the liver

The inter-relationship between liver disease and pregnancy can be a complex one and a source of real anxiety for both patient and clinician. Three possibilities need to be borne in mind when treating a pregnant woman with a liver abnormality:

- This represents a worsening of pre-existing chronic liver or biliary disease (although pregnancy may be the first time a woman's liver biochemistry has been tested, so this may not have previously been diagnosed).
- This represents a genuine first presentation of liver disease that is not intrinsically related to pregnancy.
- This represents a genuine pregnancy-associated liver injury process.

22

It is critical to obtain information relating to liver disease risk factors and pre-pregnancy liver status to establish whether any abnormality was present before pregnancy. In general, the earlier in pregnancy that liver abnormality presents, the more likely it is to represent either pre-existing liver disease or non-pregnancy-related acute liver disease. Equally, the best outcome for both mother and baby results from optimising the physical condition of the mother, and in situations of deteriorating liver function (which can be steep in late pregnancy) consideration should always be given to early delivery if the fetus is viable. Joint management between hepatologists and obstetricians is essential.

Intercurrent and pre-existing liver disease

Acute hepatitis A can occur during pregnancy but has no effect on the fetus. Chronic hepatitis B requires identification in pregnancy because of long-term health implications for the mother and the effectiveness of perinatal vaccination (with or without pre-delivery maternal antiviral therapy) in reducing neonatal acquisition of chronic hepatitis B. Maternal transmission of hepatitis C occurs in 1% of cases and there is no convincing evidence that the mode of delivery affects this. Hepatitis E is reported to progress to acute liver failure much more commonly in pregnancy, with a 20% maternal mortality. Pregnancy may be associated with either worsening or improvement of autoimmune hepatitis, although improvement during pregnancy and rebound post-partum is the most common pattern seen. Complications of portal hypertension may be a particular issue in the second and third trimesters.

Gallstones (p. 903) are more common during pregnancy and may present with cholecystitis or biliary obstruction. The diagnosis can usually be made with ultrasound. In biliary obstruction due to gallstones, therapeutic ERCP can be safely performed but lead protection for the fetus is essential and X-ray screening must be kept to a minimum.

Pregnancy-associated liver disease

Several conditions occur only during pregnancy, may recur in subsequent pregnancies and resolve after delivery of the baby, and these are discussed on page 1283. The causes of abnormal

22.57 Abnormal liver function tests in pregnancy

- **Liver function tests**: alkaline phosphatase (ALP) levels and albumin normally fall in pregnancy. ALP levels can rise due to the contribution of placental ALP.
- **Pre-existing liver disease**: pregnancy is uncommon in cirrhosis because cirrhosis causes relative infertility. Varices can enlarge in pregnancy, and ascites should be treated with amiloride rather than spironolactone. Penicillamine for Wilson's disease and azathioprine for autoimmune liver disease should be continued during pregnancy. Autoimmune liver disease can flare up post-partum.
- **Incidental**: viral, autoimmune and drug-induced hepatitis must be excluded in the presence of an elevated alanine aminotransferase (ALT). Immunoglobulin/vaccination given to the fetus at birth prevents transmission of hepatitis B to the fetus if the mother is infected. Gallstones are more common in pregnancy and post-partum, and are a cause of a raised ALP level. Biliary imaging with ultrasound and magnetic resonance cholangiopancreatography is safe. Endoscopic retrograde cholangiopancreatography to remove stones can be performed safely with shielding of the fetus from radiation.
- **Pregnancy-related liver diseases**: occur predominantly in the third trimester and resolve post-partum. Maternal and fetal mortality and morbidity are reduced by expediting delivery.

LFTs in pregnancy, which include pregnancy-associated liver disease, are shown in Box 22.57.

Liver transplantation

The outcome following liver transplantation has improved significantly over the last decade so that elective transplantation in low-risk individuals now has a 1-year survival rate of more than 90% and is an effective treatment for end-stage liver disease. The number of procedures is limited by cadaveric donor availability and in many parts of the world this has led to living donor transplant programmes. Despite this, 10% of those listed for liver transplantation will die while awaiting a donor liver. The main complications of liver transplantation relate to rejection, complications of long-term immunosuppression and disease recurrence in the liver graft.

Indications and contraindications

Currently, around 9500 liver transplants are undertaken in Europe and the USA annually. About 10% are performed for acute liver failure, 6% for metabolic diseases, 71% for cirrhosis and 11% for hepatocellular carcinoma. Most patients are under 60 years of age and only 10% are aged between 60 and 70 years. Indications for elective transplant assessment are listed in Box 22.58. In North America, the most common indication is hepatitis C cirrhosis, about 10–20% of transplants being for alcoholic cirrhosis (Fig. 22.42). Patients with alcoholic liver disease need to show a capacity for abstinence.

The main contraindications to transplantation are sepsis, extrahepatic malignancy, active alcohol or other substance misuse, and marked cardiorespiratory dysfunction.

Patients are matched for ABO blood group and size but do not require HLA matching with donors, as the liver is a relatively immune-privileged organ compared with the heart or kidneys.

In many parts of the world, the MELD score (see Box 22.30, p. 868) is used to identify and prioritise patients for transplantation. In the UK, a similar system that also incorporates serum sodium, the United Kingdom End-stage Liver Disease (UKELD) score, is used to guide recipient selection. To be listed for elective (non-super-urgent) transplantation in the UK, patients must have a greater than 50% projected post-transplant 5-year survival and must fall into one of three categories:

- *Category 1*: estimated 1-year mortality without transplantation of more than 9% (equivalent to a UKELD score of more than 49 points)

22.58 Indications for liver transplant assessment for cirrhosis

Complications

- First episode of bacterial peritonitis
- Diuretic-resistant ascites
- Recurrent variceal haemorrhage
- Hepatocellular carcinoma <5 cm
- Persistent hepatic encephalopathy

Poor liver function

- Bilirubin >100 μmol/L (5.8 mg/dL) in primary biliary cholangitis
- MELD score >12 (Box 22.30, p. 868)
- Child–Pugh grade C (Box 22.29, p. 867)

(MELD = Model for End-stage Liver Disease)

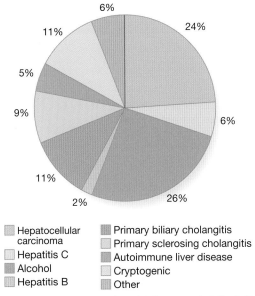

Fig. 22.42 **Indications for elective adult liver transplantation in the UK, 2016.**

- *Category 2*: HCC diagnosed radiologically by two concordant modalities; based on CT, a single lesion of less than 5 cm maximum diameter, or fewer than three lesions each less than 3 cm in diameter, without macrovascular invasion or metastases.
- *Category 3*: 'variant syndromes', including diuretic-resistant ascites, hepatopulmonary syndrome, chronic hepatic encephalopathy, intractable pruritus, familial amyloidosis, primary hyperlipidaemia, polycystic liver disease and recurrent cholangitis.

Super-urgent listing is reserved for patients with acute liver failure, according to specific criteria.

Two types of transplant are increasingly used because of insufficient cadaveric donors:

- *Split liver transplantation.* A cadaveric donor liver can be split into two, with the larger right lobe used in an adult and the smaller left lobe used in a child. This practice has led to an increase in procedures despite a shortage of donor organs.
- *Living donor transplantation.* This is normally performed using the left lateral segment or the right lobe. The donor mortality is significant at 0.5–1%. Pre-operative assessment includes looking at donor liver size and psychological status.

Complications

Early complications

Primary graft non-function

This is a state of hepatocellular dysfunction arising as a consequence of liver paresis, which results from ischaemia following removal from the donor and prior to reperfusion in the recipient. Factors that increase the likelihood of primary non-function include increasing donor age, degree of steatosis in the liver and the length of ischaemia. Treatment is supportive until recovery of function. Occasionally, recovery is not seen and re-transplantation is necessary.

Technical complications

These include hepatic artery thrombosis, which may necessitate re-transplantation. Anastomotic biliary strictures can also occur; these may respond to endoscopic balloon dilatation and stenting, or require surgical reconstruction. Portal vein thrombosis is rare.

Rejection

Less immunosuppression is needed following liver transplantation than with kidney or heart/lung grafting. Initial immunosuppression is usually with tacrolimus or ciclosporin, prednisolone and azathioprine or mycophenolate. Some patients can eventually be maintained on a single agent. Acute cellular rejection occurs in 60–80% of patients, commonly at 5–10 days post-transplant and usually within the first 6 weeks, but can arise at any point. This normally responds to 3 days of high-dose intravenous methylprednisolone.

Infections

Bacterial infections, such as pneumonia and wound infections, can occur in the first few weeks after transplantation. Cytomegalovirus (primary infection or reactivation) is a common infection in the 3 months after transplantation and can cause hepatitis. Patients who have never had cytomegalovirus infection but who receive a liver from a donor who has been exposed are at greatest risk of infection and are usually given prophylactic antiviral therapy, such as valganciclovir. Herpes simplex virus reactivation or, rarely, primary infection may occur. Prophylaxis is given to recipients who have had previous exposure to tuberculosis for the first 6 months after transplantation to prevent reactivation.

Late complications

These include recurrence of the initial disease in the graft and complications due to the immunosuppressive therapy, such as renal impairment from ciclosporin. Metabolic syndrome (p. 730) is common, being described in about 50% of transplant recipients within 6 months in the USA. Chronic vascular rejection is rare, occurring in only 5% of cases.

Prognosis

The outcome following transplantation for acute liver failure is worse than that for chronic liver disease because most patients have multi-organ failure at the time of transplantation. The 1-year survival is 65% and falls only a little to 59% at 5 years. The 1-year survival for patients with cirrhosis is over 90%, falling to 70–75% at 5 years.

 22.59 Liver disease in old age

- **Alcoholic liver disease**: 10% of cases present over the age of 70 years, when disease is more likely to be severe and has a worse prognosis.
- **Hepatitis A**: causes more severe illness and runs a more protracted course.
- **Primary biliary cholangitis**: one-third of cases are over 65 years.
- **Liver abscess**: more than 50% of all cases in the UK are over 60 years.
- **Hepatocellular carcinoma**: approximately 50% of cases in the UK present over the age of 65 years.
- **Surgery**: older people are less likely to survive liver surgery (including transplantation) because comorbidity is more prevalent.

Cholestatic and biliary disease

The concepts of biliary and cholestatic disease, and the important distinctions between them, can be a source of confusion. 'Cholestasis' relates to a biochemical abnormality (typically, elevation of ALP and elevation in serum bile acid levels and bilirubin) that results from an abnormality in bile flow. The cause can range from inherited or acquired dysfunction of transporter molecules responsible for the production of canalicular bile to physical obstruction of the extrahepatic bile duct. 'Biliary disease' relates to pathology at any level from the small intrahepatic bile ducts to the sphincter of Oddi. Although there is very significant overlap between cholestatic and biliary disease, there are scenarios where cholestasis can exist without biliary disease (transporter disease or pure drug-induced cholestasis) and where biliary disease can exist without cholestasis (when disease of the bile duct does not impact on bile flow). These anomalies should always be borne in mind and cholestasis and biliary disease always effectively distinguished.

Chemical cholestasis

Pure cholestasis can occur as an inherited condition (p. 895), as a consequence of cholestatic drug reactions (p. 894) or as acute cholestasis of pregnancy (p. 1284). A more frequent, but less recognised, acquired biochemical cholestasis occurs in sepsis ('cholangitis lente'). This biochemical phenomenon is one of the causes of LFT abnormality in sepsis, does not require specific treatment, and has a prognostic significance conferred by the underlying septic process.

Mutations in the biliary transporter proteins on the hepatocyte canalicular membrane (familial intrahepatic cholestasis 1, FIC1), illustrated in Figure 22.7 (p. 851), have been shown to cause an inherited intrahepatic biliary disease in childhood, characterised by raised ALP levels and progression to a biliary cirrhosis. It is also becoming increasingly clear that these proteins contribute to intrahepatic biliary disease in adulthood.

Benign recurrent intrahepatic cholestasis

This rare condition usually presents in adolescence and is characterised by recurrent episodes of cholestasis, lasting 1–6 months. It is now known to be mediated by mutations in the *ATP8B1* gene, which lies on chromosome 18 and encodes FIC1.

Episodes start with pruritus, while painless jaundice develops later. LFTs show a cholestatic pattern. Liver biopsy shows cholestasis during an episode but is normal between episodes. Treatment is required to relieve the symptoms of cholestasis, such as pruritus, and the long-term prognosis is good.

Intrahepatic biliary disease

Inflammatory and immune disease

The small intrahepatic bile ducts appear to be specifically vulnerable to immune injury, and ductopenic injury ('vanishing bile duct syndrome') can be a feature of a number of chronic conditions, including graft-versus-host disease (GVHD), sarcoidosis and, in the setting of liver transplantation, ductopenic rejection. Intrahepatic small bile duct injury occurs most frequently in primary biliary cholangitis, an autoimmune cholestatic disease, and less frequently in primary sclerosing cholangitis (Box 22.60).

i	**22.60 Comparison of primary biliary cholangitis (PBC) and primary sclerosing cholangitis (PSC)**	
	PBC	**PSC**
Gender (F : M)	10 : 1	1 : 3
Age	Older: median age 50–55 years	Younger: median age 20–40 years
Disease associations	Non-organ-specific autoimmune disease (e.g. Sjögren's syndrome) and autoimmune thyroid disease	Ulcerative colitis
Autoantibody profile	90% AMA +ve	65–85% pANCA +ve (but this is non-specific and not diagnostic)
Predominant bile-duct injury	Intrahepatic	Extrahepatic > intrahepatic

(AMA = antimitochondrial antibody; pANCA = perinuclear antineutrophil cytoplasmic antibody)

Caroli's disease

This very rare disease is characterised by segmental saccular dilatations of the intrahepatic biliary tree. The whole liver is usually affected and extrahepatic biliary dilatation occurs in about one-quarter of patients. Recurrent attacks of cholangitis (see Box 22.18, p. 861) may cause hepatic abscesses. Complications include biliary stones and cholangiocarcinoma. Antibiotics are required for episodes of cholangitis. Occasionally, localised disease can be treated by segmental liver resection, and liver transplantation may sometimes be required.

Congenital hepatic fibrosis

This is characterised by broad bands of fibrous tissue linking the portal tracts in the liver, abnormalities of the interlobular bile ducts and sometimes a lack of portal venules. The renal tubules may show cystic dilatation (medullary sponge kidney; p. 433), and eventually renal cysts may develop. The condition can be inherited as an autosomal recessive trait. Liver involvement causes portal hypertension with splenomegaly and bleeding from oesophageal varices that usually presents in adolescence or in early adult life. The prognosis is good because liver function is preserved. Treatment may be required for variceal bleeding and occasionally cholangitis. Patients can present during childhood with renal failure if the kidneys are severely affected.

Cystic fibrosis

Cystic fibrosis (p. 580) is associated with biliary cirrhosis in about 5% of individuals. Splenomegaly and an elevated ALP are characteristic. Complications do not normally arise until late adolescence or early adulthood, when bleeding due to variceal haemorrhage may occur. UDCA improves liver blood tests but it is not known whether the drug can prevent progression of liver disease. Deficiency of fat-soluble vitamins (A, D, E and K) may need to be treated in view of both biliary and pancreatic disease.

Extrahepatic biliary disease

Diseases of the extrahepatic biliary tree typically present with the clinical features of impaired bile flow (obstructive jaundice and fat

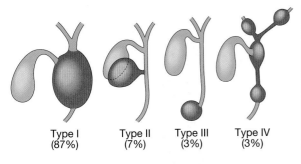

Type I
(87%)

Type II
(7%)

Type III
(3%)

Type IV
(3%)

Fig. 22.43 Classification and frequency of choledochal cysts. *From Shearman DC, Finlayson NDC. Diseases of the gastrointestinal tract and liver, 2nd edn. Edinburgh: Churchill Livingstone, Elsevier Ltd; 1989.*

malabsorption). Obstructive disease is frequently a consequence of stricturing following gallstone passage and associated infection and inflammation or post-surgical intervention. PSC frequently involves the extrahepatic biliary tree and its differential, IgG4 disease, is an important and potentially treatable cause of disease (p. 890). Malignant diseases (cholangiocarcinoma or carcinoma of the head of pancreas) should be considered in all patients with extrahepatic biliary obstruction).

Choledochal cysts

This term applies to cysts anywhere in the biliary tree (Fig. 22.43). The great majority cause diffuse dilatation of the common bile duct (type I) but others take the form of biliary diverticula (type II), dilatation of the intraduodenal bile duct (type III) and multiple biliary cysts (type IV). The last type merges with Caroli's disease (see above). In the neonate, they may present with jaundice or biliary peritonitis. Recurrent jaundice, abdominal pain and cholangitis may arise in the adult. Liver abscess and biliary cirrhosis may develop and there is an increased incidence of cholangiocarcinoma. Excision of the cyst with hepatico-jejunostomy is the treatment of choice.

Secondary biliary cirrhosis

Secondary biliary cirrhosis develops after prolonged large duct biliary obstruction due to gallstones, benign bile duct strictures or sclerosing cholangitis (see below). Carcinomas rarely cause secondary biliary cirrhosis because few patients survive long enough. The clinical features are those of chronic cholestasis with episodes of ascending cholangitis or even liver abscess (p. 879). Cirrhosis, ascites and portal hypertension are late features. Relief of biliary obstruction may require endoscopic or surgical intervention. Cholangitis dictates treatment with antibiotics, which can be given continuously if attacks recur frequently.

Gallstones

Gallstone formation is the most common disorder of the biliary tree and it is unusual for the gallbladder to be diseased in the absence of gallstones. In developed countries, gallstones occur in 7% of males and 15% of females aged 18–65 years, with an overall prevalence of 11%. In individuals under 40 years there is a 3:1 female preponderance, whereas in the elderly the sex ratio is about equal. Gallstones are less frequent in India, the Far East and Africa. There has been much debate over the role of diet in cholesterol gallstone disease; an increase in dietary

22.61 Risk factors and mechanisms for cholesterol gallstones

↑Cholesterol secretion

- Old age
- Female gender
- Pregnancy
- Obesity
- Rapid weight loss

Impaired gallbladder emptying

- Pregnancy
- Gallbladder stasis
- Fasting
- Total parenteral nutrition
- Spinal cord injury

↓Bile salt secretion

- Pregnancy

22.62 Composition of and risk factors for pigment stones		
Black		**Brown**

	Black	**Brown**
Composition	Polymerised calcium bilirubinates*	Calcium bilirubinate crystals*
	Mucin glycoprotein	Mucin glycoprotein
	Calcium phosphate	Cholesterol
	Calcium carbonate	Calcium palmitate/stearate
	Cholesterol	
Risk factors	Haemolysis	Infected bile
	Age	Stasis
	Hepatic cirrhosis	
	Ileal resection/disease	

*Major component.

cholesterol, fat, total calories and refined carbohydrate or lack of dietary fibre has been implicated.

Pathophysiology

Gallstones are conventionally classified into cholesterol or pigment stones, although the majority are of mixed composition. Gallstones contain varying quantities of calcium salts, including calcium bilirubinate, carbonate, phosphate and palmitate, which are radio-opaque. Gallstone formation is multifactorial and the factors involved are related to the type of gallstone (Boxes 22.61 and 22.62).

Cholesterol gallstones

Cholesterol is held in solution in bile by its association with bile acids and phospholipids in the form of micelles and vesicles. Biliary lipoproteins may also have a role in solubilising cholesterol. In gallstone disease, the liver produces bile that contains an excess of cholesterol because there is either a relative deficiency of bile salts or a relative excess of cholesterol ('lithogenic' bile). Abnormalities of bile salt synthesis and circulation, cholesterol secretion and gallbladder function may make production of lithogenic bile more likely.

Pigment stones

Brown, crumbly pigment stones are almost always the consequence of bacterial or parasitic biliary infection. They are common in the Far East, where infection allows bacterial β-glucuronidase to hydrolyse conjugated bilirubin to its free form,

22

which then precipitates as calcium bilirubinate. The mechanism of black pigment gallstone formation in developed countries is not satisfactorily explained. Haemolysis is important as a contributing factor for the development of black pigment stones that occur in chronic haemolytic disease.

Biliary sludge

This describes gelatinous bile that contains numerous microspheroliths of calcium bilirubinate granules and cholesterol crystals, as well as glycoproteins; it is an important precursor to the formation of gallstones in the majority of patients. Biliary sludge is frequently formed under normal conditions but then either dissolves or is cleared by the gallbladder; only in about 15% of patients does it persist to form cholesterol stones. Fasting, parenteral nutrition and pregnancy are also associated with sludge formation.

Clinical features

Only 10% of individuals with gallstones develop clinical evidence of gallstone disease. Symptomatic stones within the gallbladder (Box 22.63) manifest as either biliary pain ('biliary colic') or cholecystitis (see below). If a gallstone becomes acutely impacted in the cystic duct, the patient will experience pain. The term 'biliary colic' is a misnomer because the pain does not rhythmically increase and decrease in intensity like other forms of colic. Typically, the pain occurs suddenly and persists for about 2 hours; if it continues for more than 6 hours, a complication such as cholecystitis or pancreatitis may be present. Pain is usually felt in the epigastrium (70% of patients) or right upper quadrant (20%) and radiates to the interscapular region or the tip of the right scapula, but other sites include the left upper quadrant and the lower chest. The pain can mimic intrathoracic disease, oesophagitis, myocardial infarction or dissecting aortic aneurysm.

Combinations of fatty food intolerance, dyspepsia and flatulence not attributable to other causes have been referred to as 'gallstone dyspepsia'. These symptoms are not now recognised as being caused by gallstones and are best regarded as functional dyspepsia (p. 779). Acute and chronic cholecystitis is described below.

A mucocele may develop if there is slow distension of the gallbladder from continuous secretion of mucus; if this material becomes infected, an empyema supervenes. Calcium may be secreted into the lumen of the hydropic gallbladder, causing 'limey' bile, and if calcium salts are precipitated in the gallbladder wall, the radiological appearance of 'porcelain' gallbladder results.

Gallstones in the gallbladder (cholecystolithiasis) migrate to the common bile duct (choledocholithiasis; p. 906) in approximately

15% of patients and cause biliary colic. Rarely, fistulae develop between the gallbladder and the duodenum, colon or stomach. If this occurs, air will be seen in the biliary tree on plain abdominal X-rays. If a stone larger than 2.5 cm in diameter has migrated into the gut, it may impact either at the terminal ileum or occasionally in the duodenum or sigmoid colon. The resultant intestinal obstruction may be followed by 'gallstone ileus'. Gallstones impacted in the cystic duct may cause stricturing of the common hepatic duct and the clinical picture of extrahepatic biliary diseases ('Mirizzi's syndrome', with its important differential of malignant bile duct stricture). The more common cause of jaundice due to gallstones is a stone passing from the cystic duct into the common bile duct (choledocholithiasis), which may also result in cholangitis or acute pancreatitis. It is usually very small stones that precipitate acute pancreatitis, due (it is thought) to oedema at the ampulla as the stone passes into the duodenum (no stone is seen within the bile duct in 80% of cases of presumed gallstone pancreatitis, suggesting stone passage). Previous stone passage is also the likely cause of most cases of benign papillary fibrosis, which is most commonly seen in patients with previous or present gallstone disease (it may present with jaundice, obstructive LFTs with biliary dilatation, post-cholecystectomy pain or acute pancreatitis).

Cancer of the gallbladder is growing in frequency (p. 907) but in over 95% of cases is associated with the presence of gallstones. Previously, the diagnosis was typically made as an incidental histological finding following cholecystectomy for gallstone disease. Increasing awareness of the risk of gallbladder carcinoma and of the role played by polyps in the natural history has led to an increase in screening activity and prospective diagnosis.

Investigations

Ultrasound is the investigation of choice for diagnosing gallstones. Most stones are diagnosed by transabdominal ultrasound, which has more than 92% sensitivity and 99% specificity for gallbladder stones (see Fig. 22.8, p. 854). CT, MRCP (Fig. 22.44) and, increasingly, EUS are excellent modalities for detecting complications of gallstones (distal bile duct stone or gallbladder empyema) but are inferior to ultrasound in defining

i	22.63 Clinical features and complications of gallstones

Clinical features

- Asymptomatic (80%)
- Biliary colic
- Acute cholecystitis
- Chronic cholecystitis

Complications

- Empyema of the gallbladder
- Porcelain gallbladder
- Choledocholithiasis
- Acute pancreatitis
- Fistulae from gallbladder to duodenum/colon
- Pressure on/inflammation of the common hepatic duct by a gallstone in the cystic duct (Mirizzi's syndrome)
- Gallstone ileus
- Cancer of the gallbladder

Fig. 22.44 Magnetic resonance cholangiopancreatogram showing multiple stones in the gallbladder (long arrow) and also within the distal common bile duct (inset, arrow).

> **i** | **22.64 Treatment of gallstones**
>
> **Gallbladder stones**
> * Cholecystectomy: laparoscopic or open
> * Oral bile acids: chenodeoxycholic or ursodeoxycholic (low rate of stone dissolution)
>
> **Bile duct stones**
> * Lithotripsy (endoscopic or extracorporeal shock wave, ESWL)
> * Endoscopic sphincterotomy and stone extraction
> * Surgical bile duct exploration

their presence in the gallbladder. When recurrent attacks of otherwise unexplained acute pancreatitis occur, they may result from 'microlithiasis' in the gallbladder or common bile duct and are best assessed by EUS.

Management

Asymptomatic gallstones found incidentally should not be treated because the majority will never cause symptoms. Symptomatic gallstones are best treated surgically by laparoscopic cholecystectomy; the severity of symptoms should be balanced against the individual patient surgical risk in order to decide whether surgery is warranted. Various techniques can be used to treat common bile duct stones (Box 22.64).

Cholecystitis

Acute cholecystitis

Pathophysiology

Acute cholecystitis is almost always associated with obstruction of the gallbladder neck or cystic duct by a gallstone. Occasionally, obstruction may be by mucus, parasitic worms or a biliary tumour, or may follow endoscopic bile duct stenting. The pathogenesis is unclear but the initial inflammation is possibly chemically induced. This leads to gallbladder mucosal damage, which releases phospholipase, converting biliary lecithin to lysolecithin, a recognised mucosal toxin. At the time of surgery, approximately 50% of cultures of the gallbladder contents are sterile. Infection occurs eventually, and in elderly patients or those with diabetes mellitus a severe infection with gas-forming organisms can cause emphysematous cholecystitis. Acalculous cholecystitis can occur in the intensive care setting and in association with parenteral nutrition, sickle cell disease and diabetes mellitus.

Clinical features

The cardinal feature is pain in the right upper quadrant but also in the epigastrium, the right shoulder tip or the interscapular region. Differentiation between biliary colic (p. 904) and acute cholecystitis may be difficult; features suggesting cholecystitis include severe and prolonged pain, fever and leucocytosis.

Examination shows right hypochondrial tenderness, rigidity worse on inspiration (Murphy's sign) and occasionally a gallbladder mass (30% of cases). Fever is present but rigors are unusual. Jaundice occurs in less than 10% of patients and is usually due to passage of stones into the common bile duct, or to compression or even stricturing of the common bile duct following stone impaction in the cystic duct (Mirizzi's syndrome). Gallbladder perforation occurs in 10–15% of cases and gallbladder empyema may arise.

Investigations

Peripheral blood leucocytosis is common, except in the elderly patient, in whom the signs of inflammation may be minimal. Minor increases of transaminases and amylase may be encountered. Amylase should be measured to detect acute pancreatitis (p. 837), which may be a potentially serious complication of gallstones. Only when the amylase is higher than 1000 U/L can pain be confidently attributed to acute pancreatitis, since moderately elevated levels of amylase can occur with many other causes of abdominal pain. Plain X-rays of the abdomen and chest may show radio-opaque gallstones, and rarely intrabiliary gas due to fistulation of a gallstone into the intestine; they are important in excluding lower lobe pneumonia and a perforated viscus. Ultrasonography detects gallstones and gallbladder thickening due to cholecystitis but gallbladder empyema or perforation is best assessed by CT.

Management

Medical

Medical management consists of bed rest, pain relief, antibiotics and intravenous fluids. Moderate pain can be treated with NSAIDs but more severe pain should be managed with opiates. A cephalosporin (such as cefuroxime) or piperacillin/tazobactam is the usual antibiotic of choice, but metronidazole is normally added in severely ill patients and local prescribing practice may vary. Nasogastric aspiration is needed only for persistent vomiting. Cholecystitis usually resolves with medical treatment but the inflammation may progress to an empyema or perforation and peritonitis.

Surgical

Urgent surgery is the optimal treatment when cholecystitis progresses in spite of medical therapy and when complications such as empyema or perforation develop. Operation should be carried out within 5 days of the onset of symptoms. Delayed surgery after 2–3 months is no longer favoured. When cholecystectomy may be difficult due to extensive inflammatory change, percutaneous gallbladder drainage can be performed, with subsequent cholecystectomy 4–6 weeks later. Recurrent biliary colic or cholecystitis is frequent if the gallbladder is not removed.

Chronic cholecystitis

Chronic inflammation of the gallbladder is almost invariably associated with gallstones. The usual symptoms are those of recurrent attacks of upper abdominal pain, often at night and following a heavy meal. The clinical features are similar to those of acute calculous cholecystitis but milder. Patients may recover spontaneously or following analgesia and antibiotics. They are usually advised to undergo elective laparoscopic cholecystectomy.

Acute cholangitis

Acute cholangitis is caused by bacterial infection of bile ducts and occurs in patients with other biliary problems, such as choledocholithiasis (see below), biliary strictures or tumours, or after ERCP. Jaundice, fever (with or without rigors) and right upper quadrant pain are the main presenting features ('Charcot's triad'). Treatment is with antibiotics, relief of biliary obstruction and removal (if possible) of the underlying cause.

22

Fig. 22.45 Endoscopic retrograde cholangiopancreatogram showing common duct stones (arrows).

Fig. 22.46 Endoscopic ultrasound image in a patient with cholangitis. The dilated common bile duct (CBD) contains a small stone (arrow), which causes acoustic shadowing.

Choledocholithiasis

Stones in the common bile duct (choledocholithiasis) occur in 10–15% of patients with gallstones (Fig. 22.45), which have usually migrated from the gallbladder. Primary bile duct stones are rare but can develop within the common bile duct many years after a cholecystectomy, and are sometimes related to biliary sludge arising from dysfunction of the sphincter of Oddi. In Far Eastern countries, primary common bile duct stones are thought to follow bacterial infection secondary to parasitic infections with *Clonorchis sinensis*, *Ascaris lumbricoides* or *Fasciola hepatica* (pp. 297 and 289). Common bile duct stones can cause bile duct obstruction and may be complicated by cholangitis due to secondary bacterial infection, sepsis, liver abscess and biliary stricture.

Clinical features

Choledocholithiasis may be asymptomatic, may be found incidentally by operative cholangiography at cholecystectomy, or may manifest as recurrent abdominal pain with or without jaundice. The pain is usually in the right upper quadrant, and fever, pruritus and dark urine may be present. Rigors may be a feature; jaundice is common and usually associated with pain. Physical examination may show the scar of a previous cholecystectomy; if the gallbladder is present, it is usually small, fibrotic and impalpable.

Investigations

The LFTs show a cholestatic pattern and there is bilirubinuria. If cholangitis is present, the patient usually has a leucocytosis. The most convenient method of demonstrating obstruction to the common bile duct is transabdominal ultrasound. This shows dilated extrahepatic and intrahepatic bile ducts, together with gallbladder stones (Fig. 22.46), but does not always reveal the cause of the obstruction in the common bile duct; 50% of bile duct stones are missed on ultrasound, particularly those in the distal common bile duct. EUS is extremely accurate at identifying bile duct stones. MRCP is non-invasive and is indicated when intervention is not necessarily mandatory (e.g. the patient with possible bile duct stones but no jaundice or sepsis).

Management

Cholangitis should be treated with analgesia, intravenous fluids and broad-spectrum antibiotics, such as cefuroxime and metronidazole (local prescribing practice may vary). Blood cultures should be taken before the antibiotics are administered. Patients also require urgent decompression of the biliary tree and stone removal. ERCP with biliary sphincterotomy and stone extraction is the treatment of choice and is successful in about 90% of patients. If ERCP fails, other approaches include percutaneous transhepatic drainage and combined ('rendezvous') endoscopic procedures, extracorporeal shock wave lithotripsy (ESWL) and surgery.

Surgical treatment of choledocholithiasis is performed less frequently than ERCP, and before the common bile duct is explored the diagnosis of choledocholithiasis should be confirmed by intraoperative cholangiography. If gallstones are found, the bile duct is explored, either via the cystic duct or by opening it, all stones are removed, clearance is checked by cholangiography or choledochoscopy, and then primary closure of the duct is performed if possible. External drainage of the common bile duct by T-tube is rarely required nowadays. It is now possible to achieve these goals laparoscopically in specialist centres.

Recurrent pyogenic cholangitis

This disease occurs predominantly in South-east Asia. Biliary sludge, calcium bilirubinate concretions and stones accumulate in the intrahepatic bile ducts, with secondary bacterial infection. Patients present with recurrent attacks of upper abdominal pain, fever and cholestatic jaundice. Investigation of the biliary tree demonstrates that both the intrahepatic and the extrahepatic portions are filled with soft biliary mud. Eventually, the liver becomes scarred and liver abscesses and secondary biliary cirrhosis develop. The condition is difficult to manage and requires drainage of the biliary tract with extraction of stones, antibiotics and, in certain patients, partial resection of damaged areas of the liver.

Tumours of the gallbladder and bile duct

Carcinoma of the gallbladder

This is an uncommon tumour, occurring more often in females and usually in those over the age of 70 years. More than 90% are adenocarcinomas; the remainder are anaplastic or, rarely, squamous tumours. Gallstones are present in 70–80% of cases and are thought to be important in the aetiology of the tumour. Individuals with a calcified gallbladder ('porcelain gallbladder'; p. 904) are at high risk of malignant change, and gallbladder polyps over 1 cm in size are associated with increased risk of malignancy; preventative cholecystectomy should be considered in such patients. Chronic infection with *Salmonella*, especially in areas where typhoid is endemic, is also a risk factor.

Carcinoma of the gallbladder may be diagnosed incidentally and is found in 1–3% of gallbladders removed at cholecystectomy for gallstone disease. It may manifest as repeated attacks of biliary pain and, later, persistent jaundice and weight loss. A gallbladder mass may be palpable in the right hypochondrium. LFTs show cholestasis, and porcelain gallbladder may be found on X-ray. The tumour can be diagnosed by ultrasonography and staged by CT. The treatment is surgical excision but local extension of the tumour beyond the wall of the gallbladder into the liver, lymph nodes and surrounding tissues is invariable and palliative management is usually all that can be offered. Survival is generally short, death typically occurring within 1 year in patients presenting with symptoms.

Cholangiocarcinoma

Cholangiocarcinoma (CCA) is an uncommon tumour that can arise anywhere in the biliary tree, from the intrahepatic bile ducts (20–25% of cases) and the confluence of the right and left hepatic ducts at the liver hilum (50–60%) to the distal common bile duct (20%). It accounts for only 1.5% of all cancers but the incidence is increasing. The cause is unknown but the tumour is associated with gallstones, primary and secondary sclerosing cholangitis, Caroli's disease and choledochal cysts (see Fig. 22.43). In the Far East, particularly northern Thailand, chronic liver fluke infection (*Clonorchis sinensis*) is a major risk factor for the development of CCA in men. Primary sclerosing cholangitis carries a lifetime risk of CCA of approximately 20%, although only 5% of CCAs relate to primary sclerosing cholangitis. Chronic biliary inflammation appears to be a common factor in the development of biliary dysplasia and cancer that is shared by all the predisposing causes.

Tumours typically invade the lymphatics and adjacent vessels, with a predilection for spread within perineural sheaths. The presentation is usually with obstructive jaundice. About 50% of patients also have upper abdominal pain and weight loss. The diagnosis is made using a combination of CT and MRI (see Fig. 22.10, p. 855) but can be difficult to confirm in patients with sclerosing cholangitis. Serum levels of the tumour marker CA19-9 are elevated in up to 80% of cases, although this may occur in biliary obstruction of any cause. In the setting of biliary obstruction, ERCP may result in positive biliary cytology. Endoscopic ultrasound–fine needle aspiration (EUS-FNA) of bile duct masses is sometimes possible, and in specialist centres single-operator cholangioscopy with biopsy is now established. CCAs can be treated surgically in about 20% of patients, which improves 5-year survival from less than 5% to 20–40%. Surgery involves excision of the extrahepatic biliary tree with or without a liver resection and a Roux loop reconstruction. However, most patients are treated by stent insertion across the malignant biliary stricture, using endoscopic or percutaneous transhepatic techniques (Fig. 22.47). Combination chemotherapy is increasingly used and palliation with endoscopic photodynamic therapy has provided encouraging results.

Carcinoma at the ampulla of Vater

Nearly 40% of all adenocarcinomas of the small intestine arise in relationship to the ampulla of Vater and present with pain, anaemia, vomiting and weight loss. Jaundice may be intermittent or persistent. The diagnosis is made by duodenal endoscopy and biopsy of the tumour but staging by CT/MRI and EUS is essential. Ampullary carcinoma must be differentiated from carcinoma of

22

Fig. 22.47 Cholangiocarcinoma. **A** Endoscopic retrograde cholangiopancreatogram showing a malignant distal biliary stricture (arrow) and dilated duct above this. **B** A self-expanding metallic stent (SEMS) has been placed across the stricture to relieve jaundice (arrow).

the head of the pancreas and a CCA because these last two conditions both have a worse prognosis. Imaging may show a 'double duct sign' with stricturing of both the common bile duct and pancreatic duct at the ampulla and upstream dilatation of the ducts. EUS is the most sensitive method of assessing and staging ampullary or periampullary tumours.

Curative surgical treatment can be undertaken by pancreaticoduodenectomy and the 5-year survival may be as high as 50%. If resection is impossible, palliative surgical bypass or stenting may be necessary.

Benign gallbladder tumours

These are uncommon, often asymptomatic and usually found incidentally at operation or postmortem. Cholesterol polyps, sometimes associated with cholesterolosis, papillomas and adenomas, are the main types.

Miscellaneous biliary disorders

Post-cholecystectomy syndrome

Dyspeptic symptoms following cholecystectomy (post-cholecystectomy syndrome) occur in about 30% of patients, depending on how the condition is defined, how actively symptoms are sought and what the original indication for cholecystectomy was. The syndrome occurs most frequently in women, in patients who have had symptoms for more than 5 years before cholecystectomy, and in cases when the operation was undertaken for non-calculous gallbladder disease. An increase in bowel habit resulting from bile acid diarrhoea occurs in about 5–10% of patients after cholecystectomy and often responds to colestyramine (4–8 g daily). Severe post-cholecystectomy syndrome occurs in only 2–5% of patients. The main causes are listed in Box 22.65.

The usual symptoms include right upper quadrant pain, flatulence, fatty food intolerance and occasionally jaundice and cholangitis. The LFTs may be abnormal and sometimes show cholestasis. Ultrasonography is used to detect biliary obstruction, and EUS or MRCP to seek common bile duct stones. If retained bile duct stones are excluded, sphincter of Oddi dysfunction should be considered (see below). Other investigations that may be required include upper gastrointestinal endoscopy, small bowel radiology and pancreatic function tests. The possibility of a functional illness should also be considered.

Functional biliary sphincter disorders ('sphincter of Oddi dysfunction')

The sphincter of Oddi is a small smooth-muscle sphincter situated at the junction of the bile duct and pancreatic duct in the duodenum. It has been believed that sphincter of Oddi dysfunction (SOD) was characterised by an increase in contractility that produces a benign non-calculous obstruction to the flow of bile or pancreatic juice. This may cause pancreaticobiliary pain, deranged LFTs or recurrent pancreatitis. Classification systems, based on clinical history, laboratory results, findings on investigation and response to interventions, are difficult because of the fluctuating nature of symptoms and the well-recognised placebo effect of interventions. SOD was previously classified into types I–III but these have been replaced by newer terminology (Boxes 22.66 and 22.67).

Clinical features

Patients with functional biliary sphincter disorders, who are predominantly female, present with symptoms and signs suggestive of either biliary or pancreatic disease:

- *Patients with biliary sphincter disorders* experience recurrent, episodic biliary-type pain. They have often had a cholecystectomy but the gallbladder may be intact.
- *Patients with pancreatic sphincter disorders* usually present with unexplained recurrent attacks of pancreatitis.

Investigations

The diagnosis is established by excluding gallstones, including microlithiasis, and by demonstrating a dilated or slowly draining bile duct. The gold standard for diagnosis is sphincter of Oddi manometry. This is not widely available, however, and is associated with a high rate of procedure-related pancreatitis. Hepatobiliary scintigraphy (e.g. hepatobiliary iminodiacetic acid) may have value in the second-line investigation of post-cholecystectomy syndrome.

i	22.66 Classification of biliary sphincter of Oddi dysfunction (SOD)

Organic stenosis (formerly SOD type I)

- Biliary-type pain
- Abnormal liver enzymes (ALT/AST > twice normal on two or more occasions)
- Dilated common bile duct (>12 mm diameter)
- Delayed drainage of ERCP contrast beyond 45 mins

Functional sphincter of Oddi disorder (formerly SOD type II)

- Biliary-type pain with one or two of the above criteria

Functional biliary-type pain (formerly SOD type III)

- Biliary-type pain with no other abnormalities

i	22.65 Causes of post-cholecystectomy symptoms

Immediate post-surgical

- Bleeding
- Biliary peritonitis
- Abscess
- Bile duct trauma/transection
- Fistula

Biliary

- Common bile duct stones
- Benign stricture
- Tumour
- Cystic duct stump syndrome
- Disorders of the ampulla of Vater (e.g. benign papillary fibrosis; sphincter of Oddi dysfunction)

Extrabiliary

- Functional dyspepsia
- Peptic ulcer
- Pancreatic disease
- Gastro-oesophageal reflux
- Irritable bowel syndrome
- Functional abdominal pain

i	22.67 Criteria for pancreatic sphincter of Oddi dysfunction

- Recurrent attacks of acute pancreatitis – pancreatic-type pain with amylase or lipase 3 times normal and/or imaging evidence of acute pancreatitis
- Other aetiologies of acute pancreatitis excluded
- Normal pancreas at endoscopic ultrasound
- Abnormal sphincter manometry

22.68 Gallbladder disease in old age

- **Gallstones**: by the age of 70 years, prevalence is around 30% in women and 19% in men.
- **Acute cholecystitis**: tends to be severe, may have few localising signs and is associated with a high frequency of empyema and perforation. If such complications supervene, mortality may reach 20%.
- **Cholecystectomy**: mortality after urgent cholecystectomy for acute uncomplicated cholecystitis is not significantly higher than in younger patients.
- **Endoscopic sphincterotomy and removal of common duct stones**: well tolerated by older patients, with lower mortality than surgical common bile duct exploration.
- **Cancer of the gallbladder**: a disease of old age, with a 1-year survival of 10%.

Management

All patients with organic stenosis are treated with endoscopic sphincterotomy. The results are good but patients should be warned that there is a high risk of complications, particularly acute pancreatitis. Manometry should ideally be performed in all suspected functional sphincter of Oddi disorder patients ('type II'), and results of sphincterotomy in those with high pressures are good, but this should be avoided in patients with functional biliary-type pain ('type III'), as it is of no benefit. Medical therapy with nifedipine and/or low-dose amitriptyline may be tried. Pancreatic SOD can be treated with biliary sphincterotomy, carried out in specialist centres, but this should be undertaken with caution and careful consideration.

Routine prophylactic pancreatic duct stenting in patients undergoing ERCP for sphincter of Oddi disorders is no longer encouraged. Prophylactic administration of rectal NSAIDs (e.g. diclofenac 100 mg) is recommended instead because this significantly reduces the risk of procedure-related acute pancreatitis.

Cholesterolosis of the gallbladder

In this condition, lipid deposits in the submucosa and epithelium appear as multiple yellow spots on the pink mucosa, giving rise to the description 'strawberry gallbladder'. Cholesterolosis of the gallbladder is usually asymptomatic but may occasionally present with right upper quadrant pain. Small, fixed filling defects may be visible on ultrasonography; the radiologist can usually differentiate between gallstones and cholesterolosis. The condition is usually diagnosed at cholecystectomy; if the diagnosis is made radiologically, cholecystectomy may be indicated, depending on symptoms.

Adenomyomatosis of the gallbladder

In this condition, there is hyperplasia of the muscle and mucosa of the gallbladder. The projection of pouches of mucous membrane through weak points in the muscle coat produces Rokitansky–Aschoff sinuses. There is much disagreement over whether adenomyomatosis is a cause of right upper quadrant pain or other gastrointestinal symptoms. It may be diagnosed by oral cholecystography, when a halo or ring of opacified diverticula can be seen around the gallbladder. Other appearances include deformity of the body of the gallbladder or marked irregularity of the outline. Localised adenomyomatosis in the region of the gallbladder fundus causes the appearance of a 'Phrygian cap'. Most patients are treated by cholecystectomy but only after other diseases in the upper gastrointestinal tract have been excluded.

IgG4-associated cholangitis

This recently reported disease often presents with obstructive jaundice and is described on page 890.

Further information

Books and journal articles

Anstee QM, Targher G, Day CP. Progression of NAFLD to diabetes mellitus, cardiovascular disease or cirrhosis. Nat Rev Gastroenterol Hepatol 2013; 10:330–344.

EASL Clinical practice guidelines: Autoimmune hepatitis. J Hepatol 2015; 63:971–1004.

EASL Clinical practice guidelines: Liver transplantation. J Hepatol 2016; 64:433–485.

EASL Recommendations on treatment of hepatitis C 2015. J Hepatol 2015; 63:199–236.

EASL-EASD-EASO Clinical practice guidelines for the management of non-alcoholic fatty liver disease. J Hepatol 2016; 64:1388–1402.

Neuberger J, Gimson A, Davies M, et al. Selection of patients for liver transplantation and allocation of donated livers in the UK. Gut 2008; 57:252–257.

Williams R, Aspinall R, Bellis M, et al. Addressing liver disease in the UK: a blueprint for attaining excellence in health care and reducing premature mortality from lifestyle issues of excess consumption of alcohol, obesity, and viral hepatitis. Lancet 2014; 384:1953–1997.

Websites

aasld.org *American Association for the Study of Liver Diseases (guidelines available).*

bsg.org.uk *British Society of Gastroenterology (guidelines available).*

easl.eu *European Association for the Study of the Liver (guidelines available).*

eltr.org *European Liver Transplant Registry.*

unos.org *United Network for Organ Sharing: US transplant register.*

22

HG Watson
DJ Culligan
LM Manson

23

Haematology and transfusion medicine

Clinical examination in blood disease 912

Functional anatomy and physiology 914
Haematopoiesis 914
Blood cells and their functions 915
Haemostasis 917

Investigation of diseases of the blood 919
The full blood count 919
Blood film examination 920
Bone marrow examination 920
Investigation of coagulation 920

Presenting problems in blood disease 923
Anaemia 923
High haemoglobin 925
Leucopenia (low white cell count) 925
Leucocytosis (high white cell count) 926
Lymphadenopathy 927
Splenomegaly 927
Bleeding 927
Thrombocytopenia (low platelet count) 929
Thrombocytosis (high platelet count) 929
Pancytopenia 930
Infection 930

Principles of management of haematological disease 930
Blood products and transfusion 930
Chemotherapy 936
Haematopoietic stem cell transplantation 936
Anticoagulant and antithrombotic therapy 938

Anaemias 940
Iron deficiency anaemia 940
Anaemia of chronic disease 943
Megaloblastic anaemia 943
Haemolytic anaemia 945

Haemoglobinopathies 951
Sickle-cell anaemia 951
Other abnormal haemoglobins 953
Thalassaemias 953

Haematological malignancies 954
Leukaemias 954
Lymphomas 961
Paraproteinaemias 966

Aplastic anaemias 968

Myeloproliferative neoplasms 969

Bleeding disorders 970
Disorders of primary haemostasis 970
Coagulation disorders 971

Thrombotic disorders 975
Venous thromboembolic disease (venous thromboembolism) 975
Inherited and acquired thrombophilia and prothrombotic states 977

Clinical examination in blood disease

4 Conjunctivae
Pallor
Jaundice

3 Mouth
Lips: angular stomatitis,
telangiectasia
Gum hypertrophy
Tongue: colour, smoothness
Buccal mucosa: petechiae
Tonsils: size

▲ Glossitis and angular
stomatitis in iron deficiency

▲ Gum hypertrophy in
acute myeloid leukaemia

▲ Hereditary haemorrhagic
telangiectasia

2 Pulse
Rate

1 Hands
Perfusion
Telangiectasia
Skin crease pallor
Koilonychia

▲ Koilonychia in iron
deficiency

5 Fundi
Hyperviscosity
Engorged veins
Papilloedema
Haemorrhage

▲ Fundal haemorrhage in
thrombocytopenia

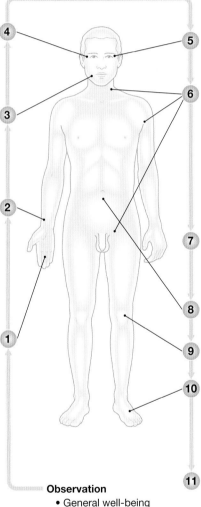

Observation
• General well-being
• Colour: pallor, plethora
• Breathlessness

6 Lymph nodes
(see opposite)

7 Skin
Purpura
Bruising

▲ Purpura/petechiae in
thrombocytopenia

8 Abdomen
Masses
Ascites
Hepatomegaly
Splenomegaly
Inguinal and femoral lymph
nodes

9 Joints
Deformity
Swelling
Restricted movement

▲ Swollen joint in haemophilia

10 Feet
Peripheral circulation
Toes: gangrene

▲ Gangrenous toe in
thrombocytosis

11 Urinalysis
Blood
Urobilinogen

Insets (Glossitis) From Hoffbrand VA, John E, Pettit JE, Vyas P. Color atlas of clinical hematology, 4th edn. Philadelphia: Mosby, Elsevier Inc.; 2010; (Petechiae) Young NS, Gerson SL, High KA (eds). Clinical hematology. St Louis: Mosby, Elsevier Inc.; 2006.

Abnormalities detected in the blood are caused not only by primary diseases of the blood and lymphoreticular systems but also by diseases affecting other systems of the body. The clinical assessment of patients with haematological abnormalities must include a general history and examination, as well as a search for symptoms and signs of abnormalities of red cells, white cells, platelets, haemostatic systems, lymph nodes and lymphoreticular tissues.

Anaemia

Symptoms and signs help to indicate the clinical severity of anaemia. A full history and examination is needed to identify the underlying cause.

i	**Anaemia**

Non-specific symptoms

- Tiredness
- Lightheadedness
- Breathlessness
- Development/worsening of ischaemic symptoms, e.g. angina or claudication

Non-specific signs

- Mucous membrane pallor
- Tachypnoea
- Raised jugular venous pressure
- Tachycardia
- Flow murmurs
- Ankle oedema
- Postural hypotension

Bleeding

Bleeding can be due to congenital or acquired abnormalities in the clotting system. History and examination help to clarify the severity and the underlying cause of the bleeding problem.

i	**Bleeding**

History

- Site of bleed
- Duration of bleed
- Precipitating causes, including previous surgery or trauma
- Family history
- Drug history
- Age at presentation
- Other medical conditions, e.g. liver disease

Examination

There are two main patterns of bleeding:
1. Mucosal bleeding
   Reduced number or function of platelets (e.g. bone marrow failure or aspirin) or von Willebrand factor (e.g. von Willebrand disease)
   - Skin: petechiae, bruises
   - Gum and mucous membrane bleeding
   - Fundal haemorrhage
   - Post-surgical bleeding
2. Coagulation factor deficiency (e.g. haemophilia or warfarin/anticoagulant)
   - Bleeding into joints (haemarthrosis) or muscles
   - Bleeding into soft tissues
   - Retroperitoneal haemorrhage
   - Intracranial haemorrhage
   - Post-surgical bleeding

6 Lymphadenopathy

Lymphadenopathy can be caused by benign or malignant disease. The clinical points to clarify are shown in the box.

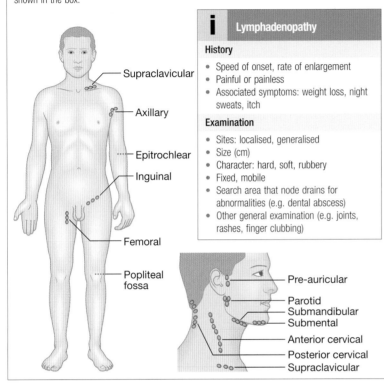

i	**Lymphadenopathy**

History

- Speed of onset, rate of enlargement
- Painful or painless
- Associated symptoms: weight loss, night sweats, itch

Examination

- Sites: localised, generalised
- Size (cm)
- Character: hard, soft, rubbery
- Fixed, mobile
- Search area that node drains for abnormalities (e.g. dental abscess)
- Other general examination (e.g. joints, rashes, finger clubbing)

Supraclavicular
Axillary
Epitrochlear
Inguinal
Femoral
Popliteal fossa

Pre-auricular
Parotid
Submandibular
Submental
Anterior cervical
Posterior cervical
Supraclavicular

8 Examination of the spleen

- Move your hand up from the right iliac fossa, towards the left upper quadrant on expiration.
- Keep your hand still and ask the patient to take a deep breath through the mouth to feel the spleen edge being displaced downwards.
- Place your left hand around the patient's lower ribs and approach the costal margin to pull the spleen forwards.
- To help palpate small spleens, roll the patient on to the right side and examine as before.

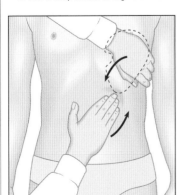

i	**Characteristics of the spleen**

- Notch
- Superficial
- Dull to percussion
- Cannot get examining hand between ribs and spleen
- Moves well with respiration

23

Disorders of the blood cover a wide spectrum of illnesses, ranging from some of the most common disorders affecting humans (anaemias) to relatively rare conditions such as leukaemias and congenital coagulation disorders. Although the latter are uncommon, advances in cellular and molecular biology have had major impacts on their diagnosis, treatment and prognosis. Haematological changes occur as a consequence of diseases affecting any system and give important information in the diagnosis and monitoring of many conditions.

Functional anatomy and physiology

Blood flows throughout the body in the vascular system, and consists of:

- red cells, which transport oxygen from the lungs to the tissues
- white cells, which defend against infection
- platelets, which interact with blood vessels and clotting factors to maintain vascular integrity and prevent bleeding
- plasma, which contains proteins with many functions, including antibodies and coagulation factors.

Haematopoiesis

Haematopoiesis describes the formation of blood cells, an active process that must maintain normal numbers of circulating cells and be able to respond rapidly to increased demands such as bleeding or infection. During development, haematopoiesis occurs in the yolk sac, liver and spleen, and subsequently in red bone marrow in the medullary cavity of all bones. In childhood, red marrow is progressively replaced by fat (yellow marrow) so that, in adults, normal haematopoiesis is restricted to the vertebrae, pelvis, sternum, ribs, clavicles, skull, upper humeri and proximal femora. However, red marrow can expand in response to increased demands for blood cells.

Bone marrow contains a range of immature haematopoietic precursor cells and a storage pool of mature cells for release at times of increased demand. Haematopoietic cells interact closely with surrounding connective tissue stroma, made up of reticular cells, macrophages, fat cells, blood vessels and nerve fibres (Fig. 23.1). In normal marrow, nests of red cell precursors cluster around a central macrophage, which provides iron and also phagocytoses nuclei from red cells prior to their release into the circulation. Megakaryocytes are large cells that produce and release platelets into vascular sinuses. White cell precursors are clustered next to the bone trabeculae; maturing cells migrate into the marrow spaces towards the vascular sinuses. Plasma cells are antibody-secreting mature B cells that normally represent less than 5% of the marrow population and are scattered throughout the intertrabecular spaces.

Stem cells

All blood cells are derived from pluripotent haematopoietic stem cells. These comprise only 0.01% of the total marrow cells, but they can self-renew (i.e. make more stem cells) or differentiate to produce a hierarchy of lineage-committed progenitor cells. The resulting primitive progenitor cells cannot be identified morphologically, so they are named according to the types of cell (or colony) they form during cell culture experiments. CFU–GM (colony-forming unit – granulocyte, monocyte) is a progenitor cell that produces granulocytic and monocytic lines, CFU–E produce erythroid cells, and CFU–Meg produce megakaryocytes and ultimately platelets (Fig. 23.2).

Growth factors, produced in bone marrow stromal cells and elsewhere, control the survival, proliferation, differentiation and function of stem cells and their progeny. Some, such as, interleukin-3 (IL-3), stem cell factor (SCF) and granulocyte, macrophage–colony-stimulating factor (GM–CSF), act on a wide number of cell types at various stages of differentiation. Others, such as erythropoietin, granulocyte–colony-stimulating factor (G–CSF) and thrombopoietin (Tpo), are lineage-specific. Many of these growth factors are now synthesised by recombinant DNA technology and used as treatments: for example, erythropoietin to correct renal anaemia and G–CSF to hasten neutrophil recovery after chemotherapy.

The bone marrow also contains stem cells that can differentiate into non-haematological cells. Mesenchymal stem cells differentiate

Fig. 23.1 Structural organisation of normal bone marrow.

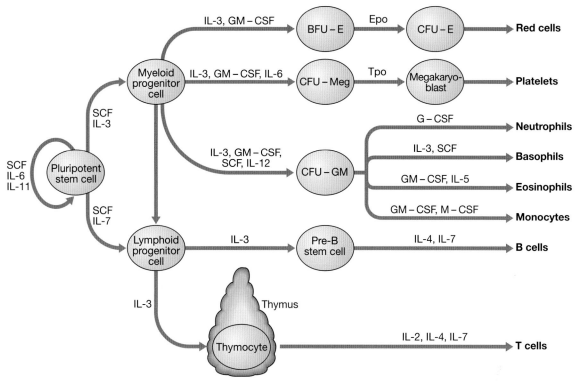

Fig. 23.2 Stem cells and growth factors in haematopoietic cell development. (BFU–E = burst-forming unit – erythroid; CFU–E = colony-forming unit – erythroid; CFU–GM = colony-forming unit – granulocyte, monocyte; CFU–Meg = colony-forming unit – megakaryocyte; Epo = erythropoietin; G–CSF = granulocyte–colony-stimulating factor; GM–CSF = granulocyte, macrophage–colony-stimulating factor; IL = interleukin; M–CSF = macrophage–colony-stimulating factor; SCF = stem cell factor; Tpo = thrombopoietin)

into skeletal muscle, cartilage, cardiac muscle, and fat cells while others differentiate into nerves, liver and blood vessel endothelium. This is termed stem cell plasticity and may have exciting clinical applications in the future (Ch. 3).

Blood cells and their functions

Red cells

Red cell precursors formed in the bone marrow from the erythroid (CFU–E) progenitor cells are called erythroblasts or normoblasts (Fig. 23.3). These divide and acquire haemoglobin, which turns the cytoplasm pink; the nucleus condenses and is extruded from the cell. The first non-nucleated red cell is a reticulocyte, which still contains ribosomal material in the cytoplasm, giving these large cells a faint blue tinge ('polychromasia'). Reticulocytes lose their ribosomal material and mature over 3 days, during which time they are released into the circulation. Increased numbers of circulating reticulocytes (reticulocytosis) reflect increased erythropoiesis. Proliferation and differentiation of red cell precursors is stimulated by erythropoietin, a polypeptide hormone produced by renal interstitial peritubular cells in response to hypoxia. Failure of erythropoietin production in patients with renal failure (p. 384) causes anaemia, which can be treated with exogenous recombinant erythropoietin or similar pharmacological agents called erythropoiesis-stimulating agents, e.g. darbepoetin.

Normal mature red cells circulate for about 120 days. They are 8 μm biconcave discs lacking a nucleus but filled with haemoglobin, which delivers oxygen to the tissues. In order to pass through the smallest capillaries, the red cell membrane is deformable, with a lipid bilayer to which a 'skeleton' of filamentous proteins is attached via special linkage proteins (Fig. 23.4). Inherited abnormalities of any of these proteins result in loss of membrane as cells pass through the spleen, and the formation of abnormally shaped red cells called spherocytes or elliptocytes (see Fig. 23.8D). Red cells are exposed to osmotic stress in the pulmonary and renal circulation; in order to maintain homeostasis, the membrane contains ion pumps, which control intracellular levels of sodium, potassium, chloride and bicarbonate. In the absence of mitochondria, the energy for these functions is provided by anaerobic glycolysis and the pentose phosphate pathway in the cytosol. Membrane glycoproteins inserted into the lipid bilayer also form the antigens recognised by blood grouping (see Fig. 23.4). The ABO and Rhesus systems are the most commonly recognised (p. 931) but over 400 blood group antigens have been described.

Haemoglobin

Haemoglobin is a protein specially adapted for oxygen transport. It is composed of four globin chains, each surrounding an iron-containing porphyrin pigment molecule termed haem. Globin chains are a combination of two alpha and two non-alpha chains; haemoglobin A ($\alpha\alpha/\beta\beta$) represents over 90% of adult haemoglobin, whereas haemoglobin F ($\alpha\alpha/\gamma\gamma$) is the predominant type in the fetus. Each haem molecule contains a ferrous ion (Fe^{2+}), to which oxygen reversibly binds; the affinity for oxygen increases as successive oxygen molecules bind. When oxygen is bound, the beta chains 'swing' closer together; they move apart as oxygen is lost. In the 'open' deoxygenated state, 2,3-bisphosphoglycerate (2,3-BPG), a product of red cell

23

Fig. 23.3 Maturation pathway of red cells, granulocytes and platelets. The image on the right is a normal blood film.

Fig. 23.4 Normal structure of red cell membrane. Red cell membrane flexibility is conferred by attachment of cytoskeletal proteins. Important transmembrane proteins include band 3 (an ion transport channel) and glycophorin C (involved in cytoskeletal attachment and gas exchange, and a receptor for *Plasmodium falciparum* in malaria). Antigens on the red blood cell determine an individual's blood group. There are about 22 blood group systems (groups of carbohydrate or protein antigens controlled by a single gene or by multiple closely linked loci); the most important clinically are the ABO and Rhesus (Rh) systems (p. 931). The ABO genetic locus has three main allelic forms: A, B and O. The A and B alleles encode glycosyltransferases that introduce *N*-acetylgalactosamine (open circle) and *D*-galactose (blue circle), respectively, on to antigenic carbohydrate molecules on the membrane surface. People with the O allele produce an O antigen, which lacks either of these added sugar groups. Rh antigens are transmembrane proteins.

metabolism, binds to the haemoglobin molecule and lowers its oxygen affinity. These complex interactions produce the sigmoid shape of the oxygen dissociation curve (Fig. 23.5). The position of this curve depends on the concentrations of 2,3-BPG, H^+ ions and CO_2; increased levels shift the curve to the right and cause oxygen to be released more readily, e.g. when red cells reach hypoxic tissues. Haemoglobin F is unable to bind 2,3-BPG and has a left-shifted oxygen dissociation curve, which, together with the low pH of fetal blood, ensures fetal oxygenation. Strong oxidising agents, such as dapsone,

can convert ferrous iron in haemoglobin to its ferric state (Fe^{3+}). The resultant methaemoglobin also has a left-shifted oxygen dissociation curve, which can result in tissue hypoxia (p. 135).

Genetic mutations affecting the haem-binding pockets of globin chains or the 'hinge' interactions between globin chains result in haemoglobinopathies or unstable haemoglobins. Alpha globin chains are produced by two genes on chromosome 16, and beta globin chains by a single gene on chromosome 11; imbalance in the production of globin chains results in the thalassaemias (p. 951). Defects in haem synthesis cause the porphyrias (p. 378).

Fig. 23.5 The haemoglobin–oxygen dissociation curve. Factors are listed that shift the curve to the right (more oxygen released from blood) and to the left (less oxygen released) at given PO_2. To convert kPa to mmHg, multiply by 7.5. (2,3-BPG = 2,3-bisphosphoglycerate)

Destruction

Red cells at the end of their lifespan of approximately 120 days are phagocytosed by the reticulo-endothelial system. Amino acids from globin chains are recycled and iron is removed from haem for reuse in haemoglobin synthesis. The remnant haem structure is degraded to bilirubin and conjugated with glucuronic acid before being excreted in bile. In the small bowel, bilirubin is converted to stercobilin; most of this is excreted, but a small amount is reabsorbed and excreted by the kidney as urobilinogen. Increased red cell destruction due to haemolysis or ineffective haematopoiesis results in jaundice and increased urinary urobilinogen. Free intravascular haemoglobin is toxic and is normally bound by haptoglobins, which are plasma proteins produced by the liver.

White cells

White cells or leucocytes in the blood consist of granulocytes (neutrophils, eosinophils and basophils), monocytes and lymphocytes (see Fig. 23.12). Granulocytes and monocytes are formed from bone marrow CFU–GM progenitor cells during myelopoiesis. The first recognisable granulocyte in the marrow is the myeloblast, a large cell with a small amount of basophilic cytoplasm and a primitive nucleus with open chromatin and nucleoli. As the cells divide and mature, the nucleus segments and the cytoplasm acquires specific neutrophilic, eosinophilic or basophilic granules (see Fig. 23.3). This takes about 14 days. The cytokines G–CSF, GM–CSF and M–CSF are involved in the production of myeloid cells, and G–CSF can be used clinically to hasten recovery of blood neutrophil counts after chemotherapy.

Myelocytes or metamyelocytes are normally found only in the marrow but may appear in the circulation in infection or toxic states. The appearance of more primitive myeloid precursors in the blood is often associated with the presence of nucleated red cells and is termed a 'leucoerythroblastic' picture; this indicates a serious disturbance of marrow function.

Neutrophils

Neutrophils, the most common white blood cells in the blood of adults, are 10–14 μm in diameter, with a multilobular nucleus containing 2–5 segments and granules in their cytoplasm. Their main function is to recognise, ingest and destroy foreign particles and microorganisms (p. 64). A large storage pool of mature neutrophils exists in the bone marrow. Every day, some 10^{11} neutrophils enter the circulation, where cells may be circulating freely or attached to endothelium in the marginating pool. These two pools are equal in size; factors such as exercise or catecholamines increase the number of cells flowing in the blood. Neutrophils spend 6–10 hours in the circulation before being removed, principally by the spleen. Alternatively, they pass into the tissues and either are consumed in the inflammatory process or undergo apoptotic cell death and phagocytosis by macrophages.

Eosinophils

Eosinophils represent 1–6% of the circulating white cells. They are a similar size to neutrophils but have a bilobed nucleus and prominent orange granules on Romanowsky staining. Eosinophils are phagocytic and their granules contain a peroxidase capable of generating reactive oxygen species and proteins involved in the intracellular killing of protozoa and helminths (p. 233). They are also involved in allergic reactions (e.g. atopic asthma, p. 567; see also p. 84).

Basophils

These cells are less common than eosinophils, representing less than 1% of circulating white cells. They contain dense black granules that obscure the nucleus. Mast cells resemble basophils but are found only in the tissues. These cells are involved in hypersensitivity reactions (p. 66).

Monocytes

Monocytes are the largest of the white cells, with a diameter of 12–20 μm and an irregular nucleus in abundant pale blue cytoplasm containing occasional cytoplasmic vacuoles. These cells circulate for a few hours and then migrate into tissue, where they become macrophages, Kupffer cells or antigen-presenting dendritic cells. The former phagocytose debris, apoptotic cells and microorganisms (see Box 4.1, p. 64).

Lymphocytes

Lymphocytes are derived from pluripotent haematopoietic stem cells in the bone marrow. There are two main types: T cells (which mediate cellular immunity) and B cells (which mediate humoral immunity) (p. 68). Lymphoid cells that migrate to the thymus develop into T cells, whereas B cells develop in the bone marrow.

The majority (about 80%) of lymphocytes in the circulation are T cells. Lymphocytes are heterogeneous, the smallest being the size of red cells and the largest the size of neutrophils. Small lymphocytes are circular with scanty cytoplasm but the larger cells are more irregular with abundant blue cytoplasm. Lymphocyte subpopulations have specific functions and lifespan can vary from a few days to many years. Cell surface antigens ('cluster of differentiation' (CD) antigens), which appear at different points of lymphocyte maturation and indicate the lineage and maturity of the cell, are used to classify lymphomas and lymphoid leukaemias.

Haemostasis

Blood must be maintained in a fluid state in order to function as a transport system, but must be able to solidify to form a clot following vascular injury in order to prevent excessive bleeding, a process known as haemostasis. Successful haemostasis

23

is localised to the area of tissue damage and is followed by removal of the clot and tissue repair. This is achieved by complex interactions between the vascular endothelium, platelets, von Willebrand factor, coagulation factors, natural anticoagulants and fibrinolytic enzymes (Fig. 23.6). Dysfunction of any of these components may result in haemorrhage or thrombosis.

Platelets

Platelets are formed in the bone marrow from megakaryocytes. Megakaryocytic progenitor cells (CFU–Meg) divide to form megakaryoblasts, which undergo a process called 'endomitotic reduplication', in which there is division of the nucleus but not the cell. This creates mature megakaryocytes, large cells with several nuclei and cytoplasm containing platelet granules. Large numbers of platelets then fragment off from each megakaryocyte into the circulation. The formation and maturation of megakaryocytes is stimulated by thrombopoietin produced in the liver. Platelets circulate for 8–10 days before they are destroyed in the reticulo-endothelial system. Some 30% of peripheral platelets are normally pooled in the spleen and do not circulate.

Under normal conditions, platelets are discoid, with a diameter of 2–4 μm (Fig. 23.7). The surface membrane invaginates to form a tubular network, the canalicular system, which provides a conduit for the discharge of the granule content following platelet activation. Drugs that inhibit platelet function and thrombosis include aspirin (cyclo-oxygenase inhibitor), clopidogrel, prasugrel and ticagrelor (adenosine diphosphate (ADP)-mediated activation inhibitors), dipyridamole (phosphodiesterase inhibitor), and the glycoprotein IIb/IIIa inhibitors abciximab, tirofiban and eptifibatide (which prevent fibrinogen binding; p. 500).

Clotting factors

The coagulation system consists of a cascade of soluble inactive zymogen proteins designated by Roman numerals.

Fig. 23.6 The stages of normal haemostasis.
[A] *Stage 1. Pre-injury conditions encourage flow.* The vascular endothelium produces substances (including nitric oxide, prostacyclin and heparans) to prevent adhesion of platelets and white cells to the vessel wall. Platelets and coagulation factors circulate in a non-activated state.

[B] *Stage 2. Early haemostatic response: platelets adhere; coagulation is activated.* At the site of injury, the endothelium is breached, exposing subendothelial collagen. Small amounts of tissue factor (TF) are released. Platelets bind to collagen via a specific receptor, glycoprotein Ia (GPIa), causing a change in platelet shape and its adhesion to the area of damage by the binding of other receptors (GPIb and GPIIb/IIIa) to von Willebrand factor and fibrinogen, respectively. Coagulation is activated by the tissue factor (extrinsic) pathway, generating small amounts of thrombin.

[C] and [D] *Stage 3. Fibrin clot formation: platelets become activated and aggregate; fibrin formation is supported by the platelet membrane; stable fibrin clot forms.* The adherent platelets are activated by many pathways, including binding of adenosine diphosphate (ADP), collagen, thrombin and adrenaline (epinephrine) to surface receptors. The cyclo-oxygenase pathway converts arachidonic acid from the platelet membrane into thromboxane A₂, which causes aggregation of platelets. Activation of the platelets results in release of the platelet granule contents, enhancing coagulation further (see Fig. 23.7). Thrombin plays a key role in the control of coagulation: the small amount generated via the TF pathway massively amplifies its own production; the 'intrinsic' pathway becomes activated and large amounts of thrombin are generated. Thrombin directly causes clot formation by cleaving fibrinopeptides (FPs) from

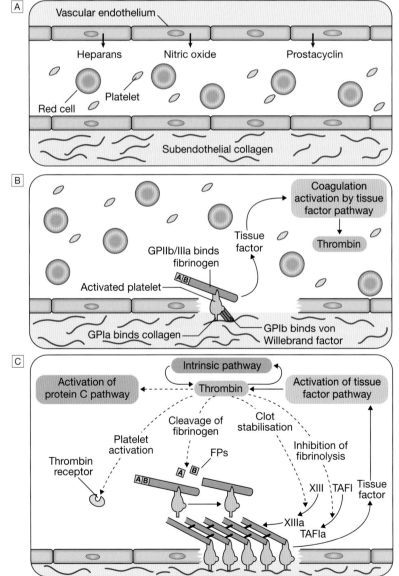

When proteolytically cleaved and activated, each is capable of activating one or more components of the cascade. Activated factors are designated by the suffix 'a'. Some of these reactions require phospholipid and calcium. Coagulation occurs by two pathways: it is initiated by the extrinsic (or tissue factor) pathway and amplified by the 'intrinsic pathway' (see Fig. 23.6D).

Clotting factors are synthesised by the liver, although factor V is also produced by platelets and endothelial cells. Factors II, VII, IX and X require post-translational carboxylation to allow them to participate in coagulation. The carboxylase enzyme responsible for this in the liver is vitamin K-dependent. Vitamin K is converted to an epoxide in this reaction and must be reduced to its active form by a reductase enzyme. This reductase is inhibited by warfarin, and this is the basis of the anticoagulant effect of coumarins (p. 939). Congenital (e.g. haemophilia) and acquired (e.g. liver failure) causes of coagulation factor deficiency are associated with bleeding.

Investigation of diseases of the blood

The full blood count

To obtain a full blood count (FBC), anticoagulated blood is processed through automated blood analysers that use a variety of technologies (particle-sizing, radiofrequency and laser instrumentation) to measure the haematological parameters. These include numbers of circulating cells, the proportion of whole blood volume occupied by red cells (the haematocrit, Hct), and the red cell indices that give information about the size of red cells (mean cell volume, MCV) and the amount of haemoglobin present in the red cells (mean cell haemoglobin, MCH). Blood analysers can differentiate types of white blood cell and give automated counts of neutrophils, lymphocytes, monocytes, eosinophils and basophils. It is important to appreciate, however, that a

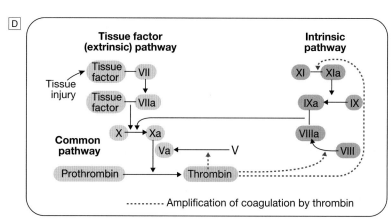

Fig. 23.6, cont'd fibrinogen to produce fibrin. Fibrin monomers are cross-linked by factor XIII, which is also activated by thrombin. Having had a key role in clot formation and stabilisation, thrombin then starts to regulate clot formation in two main ways: (a) activation of the protein C (PC) pathway (a natural anticoagulant), which reduces further coagulation; (b) activation of thrombin-activatable fibrinolysis inhibitor (TAFI), which inhibits fibrinolysis (see E and F).

E *Stage 4. Limiting clot formation: natural anticoagulants reverse activation of coagulation factors.* Once haemostasis has been secured, the propagation of clot is curtailed by anticoagulants. Antithrombin is a serine protease inhibitor synthesised by the liver, which destroys activated factors such as XIa, Xa and thrombin (IIa). Its major activity against thrombin and Xa is enhanced by heparin and fondaparinux, explaining their anticoagulant effect. Tissue factor pathway inhibitor (TFPI) binds to and inactivates VIIa and Xa. Activation of PC occurs following binding of thrombin to membrane-bound thrombomodulin; activated protein C (aPC) binds to its co-factor, protein S (PS), and cleaves Va and VIIIa. PC and PS are vitamin K-dependent and are depleted by coumarin anticoagulants such as warfarin.

F *Stage 5. Fibrinolysis: plasmin degrades fibrin to allow vessel recanalisation and tissue repair.* The insoluble clot needs to be broken down for vessel recanalisation. Plasmin, the main fibrinolytic enzyme, is produced when plasminogen is activated, e.g. by tissue plasminogen activator (t-PA) or urokinase in the clot. Plasmin hydrolyses the fibrin clot, producing fibrin degradation products, including the D-dimer. This process is highly regulated; the plasminogen activators are controlled by an inhibitor called plasminogen activator inhibitor (PAI), the activity of plasmin is inhibited by α_2-antiplasmin and α_2-macroglobulin, and fibrinolysis is further inhibited by the thrombin-activated TAFI.

23

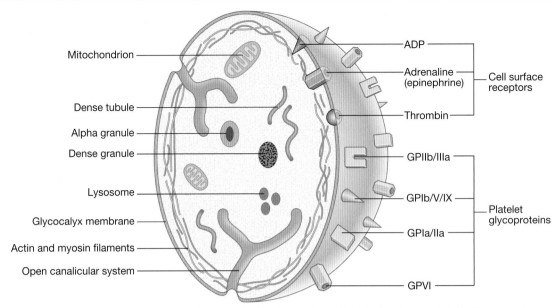

Fig. 23.7 Normal platelet structure. The platelet surface is populated by glycoproteins, which bind to key structures including fibrinogen, collagen and von Willebrand factor and cell surface receptors for thrombin, ADP and adrenaline (epinephrine). Through internal signalling pathways, platelet activation causes degranulation of alpha and dense granules, which ultimately results in platelet aggregation. Blockade of these pathways by drugs such as aspirin, clopidogrel, ticagrelor, tirofiban and abciximab forms the basis of antiplatelet therapy. (ADP = adenosine diphosphate; GP = glycoprotein)

23.1 Spurious full blood count results from autoanalysers	
Result	**Explanation**
Increased haemoglobin	Lipaemia, jaundice, very high white cell count
Reduced haemoglobin	Improper sample mixing, blood taken from vein into which an infusion is flowing
Increased red cell volume (mean cell volume, MCV)	Cold agglutinins, non-ketotic hyperosmolarity
Increased white cell count	Nucleated red cells present
Reduced platelet count	Clot in sample, platelet clumping

number of conditions can lead to spurious results (Box 23.1). The reference ranges for a number of common haematological parameters in adults are given in Chapter 35.

Blood film examination

Although technical advances in full blood count analysers have resulted in fewer blood samples requiring manual examination, scrutiny of blood components prepared on a microscope slide (the 'blood film') can often yield valuable information (Box 23.2 and Fig. 23.8). Analysers cannot identify abnormalities of red cell shape and content (e.g. Howell–Jolly bodies, basophilic stippling, malaria parasites) or fully define abnormal white cells such as blasts.

Bone marrow examination

In adults, bone marrow for examination is usually obtained from the posterior iliac crest. After a local anaesthetic, marrow can be sucked out from the medullary space, stained and examined under the microscope (bone marrow aspirate). In addition, a core of bone may be removed (trephine biopsy), fixed and decalcified before sections are cut for staining (Fig. 23.9). A bone marrow aspirate is used to assess the composition and morphology of haematopoietic cells or abnormal infiltrates. Further investigations may be performed, such as cell surface marker analysis (immunophenotyping), chromosome and molecular studies to assess malignant disease, or marrow culture for suspected tuberculosis. A trephine biopsy is superior for assessing marrow cellularity, marrow fibrosis, and infiltration by abnormal cells such as metastatic carcinoma.

Investigation of coagulation

Bleeding disorders

In patients with clinical evidence of a bleeding disorder (p. 913), there are recommended screening tests (Box 23.3). Physiological activation of coagulation is predominantly by tissue factor, with amplification of the process by the small amounts of thrombin formed as a result. For ease of description, the terms extrinsic, intrinsic and common pathways are still used (see Fig. 23.6D).

Coagulation tests measure the time to clot formation in vitro in a plasma sample after the clotting process is initiated by activators and calcium. The result of the test sample is compared with normal controls. The tissue factor ('extrinsic') pathway (see Fig. 23.6D) is assessed by the prothrombin time (PT), and the 'intrinsic' pathway by the activated partial thromboplastin time (APTT), sometimes known as the partial thromboplastin time with kaolin (PTTK). Coagulation is delayed by deficiencies of coagulation factors and by the presence of inhibitors of coagulation, such as heparin. The approximate reference ranges and causes of abnormalities are shown in Box 23.3. If both the PT and APTT are prolonged, this indicates either deficiency or inhibition of the

23.2 How to interpret red cell appearances

Microcytosis (reduced average cell size, MCV <76 fL) [A]

- Iron deficiency
- Thalassaemia
- Sideroblastic anaemia

Macrocytosis (increased average cell size, MCV >100 fL) [B]

- Vitamin B_{12} or folate deficiency
- Liver disease, alcohol
- Hypothyroidism
- Myelodysplastic syndromes
- Drugs (e.g. zidovudine, trimethoprim, phenytoin, methotrexate, hydroxycarbamide)

Target cells (central area of haemoglobinisation) [C]

- Liver disease
- Thalassaemia
- Post-splenectomy
- Haemoglobin C disease

Spherocytes (dense cells, no area of central pallor) [D]

- Autoimmune haemolytic anaemia
- Post-splenectomy
- Hereditary spherocytosis

Red cell fragments (intravascular haemolysis) [E]

- Microangiopathic haemolysis, e.g. haemolytic uraemic syndrome (HUS), thrombotic thrombocytopenic purpura (TTP)
- Disseminated intravascular coagulation (DIC)

Nucleated red blood cells (normoblasts) [F]

- Marrow infiltration
- Severe haemolysis
- Myelofibrosis
- Acute haemorrhage

Howell–Jolly bodies (small round nuclear remnants) [G]

- Hyposplenism
- Post-splenectomy
- Dyshaematopoiesis

Polychromasia (young red cells – reticulocytes present) [H]

- Haemolysis, acute haemorrhage
- Increased red cell turnover

Basophilic stippling (abnormal ribosomal RNA appears as blue dots) [I]

- Dyshaematopoiesis
- Lead poisoning

Fig. 23.8 **Appearance of red blood cells.** [A] Microcytosis. [B] Macrocytosis. [C] Target cells. [D] Spherocytes. [E] Red cell fragments. [F] Nucleated red blood cells. [G] Howell–Jolly bodies. [H] Polychromasia. [I] Basophilic stippling.

final common pathway (which includes factors X, V, prothrombin and fibrinogen) or global coagulation factor deficiency involving more than one factor, as occurs in disseminated intravascular coagulation (DIC, pp. 196 and 978). Further specific tests may be performed based on interpretation of the clinical scenario and results of these screening tests. A mixing test with normal plasma allows differentiation between a coagulation factor deficiency (the prolonged time corrects) and the presence of an inhibitor of coagulation (the prolonged time does not correct); the latter may be a chemical (heparins) or an antibody (most often a lupus anticoagulant but occasionally a specific inhibitor of one of the coagulation factors, typically factor VIII). Von Willebrand disease may present with a normal APTT; further investigation of suspected cases is detailed on page 974.

Platelet function has historically been assessed by the bleeding time, measured as the time to stop bleeding after a standardised incision. However, most centres have abandoned the use of this test. Platelet function can be assessed in vitro by measuring aggregation in response to various agonists, such as adrenaline (epinephrine), collagen, thrombin, arachidonic acid and ADP, agglutination in response to ristocetin or by measuring the constituents of the intracellular granules, e.g. adenosine triphosphate, adenosine diphosphate and their ratio to each other (ATP/ADP).

Coagulation screening tests are also performed in patients with suspected DIC, when clotting factors and platelets are consumed, resulting in thrombocytopenia and prolonged PT and APTT. In addition, there is evidence of active coagulation with

23

Fig. 23.9 Bone marrow aspirate and trephine. [A] Trephine biopsy needle. [B] Macroscopic appearance of a trephine biopsy. [C] Microscopic appearance of stained section of trephine. [D] Bone marrow aspirate needle. [E] Stained macroscopic appearance of marrow aspirate: smear (left) and squash (right). [F] Microscopic appearance of stained marrow particles and trails of haematopoietic cells.

i 23.3 Coagulation screening tests[1]

Investigation	Reference range[2]	Situations in which tests may be abnormal
Platelet count	150–400×10⁹/L	Thrombocytopenia
Prothrombin time (PT)	9–12 secs	Deficiencies of factors II, V, VII or X Severe fibrinogen deficiency
Activated partial thromboplastin time (APTT)	26–36 secs	Deficiencies of factors II, V, VIII, IX, X, XI, XII Severe fibrinogen deficiency Unfractionated heparin therapy Antibodies against clotting factors Lupus anticoagulant Multiple factor deficiency (e.g. DIC)
Fibrinogen concentration	1.5–4.0 g/L	Hypofibrinogenaemia, e.g. liver failure, DIC

[1]**N.B.** International normalised ratio (INR) is used only to monitor coumarin therapy and is not a coagulation screening test. [2]Ranges are approximate and may vary between laboratories.
(DIC = disseminated intravascular coagulation)

consumption of fibrinogen and generation of fibrin degradation products (D-dimers). Note, however, that fibrinogen is an acute phase protein that may also be elevated in inflammatory disease (p. 70).

Monitoring anticoagulant therapy

The international normalised ratio (INR) is validated only to assess the therapeutic effect of coumarin anticoagulants, including warfarin. INR is the ratio of the patient's PT to that of a normal control, raised to the power of the international sensitivity index of the thromboplastin used in the test (ISI, derived by comparison with an international reference standard material). Concentrations of the direct oral anticoagulants (DOACs) cannot be accurately assessed from the PT or the APTT, with which they have a variable and generally poor correlation.

Monitoring of heparin therapy is, on the whole, required only with unfractionated heparins. Therapeutic anticoagulation prolongs the APTT relative to a control sample by a ratio of approximately 1.5–2.5. Low-molecular-weight heparins have such a predictable dose response that monitoring of the anticoagulant effect is not required, except in patients with renal impairment (glomerular filtration rate less than 30 mL/min). When monitoring is indicated, an anti-Xa activity assay rather than APTT should be used.

Thrombotic disorders

Measurement of plasma levels of D-dimers derived from fibrin degradation is useful in excluding the diagnosis of active venous thrombosis in some patients (see Fig. 10.6, p. 187).

A variety of tests exist that may help to explain an underlying propensity to thrombosis, especially venous thromboembolism (thrombophilia) (Box 23.4). Examples of possible indications for testing are given in Box 23.5. In most patients, the results do not affect clinical management (p. 975) but they may influence the duration of anticoagulation (e.g. antiphospholipid antibodies, p. 977), justify family screening in inherited thrombophilias (p. 975), or suggest additional management strategies to reduce thrombosis risk (e.g. in myeloproliferative disease and paroxysmal nocturnal haemoglobinuria; p. 950). Anticoagulants can interfere with some of these assays; for example, warfarin reduces protein C and S levels and affects measurement of lupus anticoagulant, while heparin interferes with antithrombin and lupus anticoagulant

23.4 Investigation of possible thrombophilia

Full blood count

Plasma levels
- Antithrombin
- Protein C
- Protein S (free)
- Antiphospholipid antibodies, lupus anticoagulant, anticardiolipin antibody/anti-β_2GP1

Thrombin/reptilase time (for dysfibrinogenaemia)

Genetic testing
- Factor V Leiden
- Prothrombin G20210A
- *JAK-2 V617F* mutation
- *CALR* mutations

Flow cytometry
- Screen for GPI-linked cell surface proteins (CD14, 16, 55, 59), deficient in paroxysmal nocturnal haemoglobinuria

(CD = cluster of differentiation; GP1 = glycoprotein 1; GPI = glycerol phosphatidyl inositol)

23.5 Possible indications for thrombophilia testing*

- Venous thrombosis < 45 years
- Recurrent venous thrombosis
- Family history of unprovoked or recurrent thrombosis
- Combined arterial and venous thrombosis
- Venous thrombosis at an unusual site:
  Cerebral venous thrombosis
  Hepatic vein (Budd–Chiari syndrome)
  Portal vein, mesenteric vein

*Antiphospholipid antibodies should be sought where clinical criteria for antiphospholipid syndrome (APS) are fulfilled (p. 977). Thrombophilia testing may explain the diagnosis without necessarily affecting management and this limits the clinical value of such an approach.

23.6 Haematological investigations in old age

- **Blood cell counts and film components**: not altered in general by ageing alone, although haemoglobin concentrations fall with increasing age.
- **Ratio of bone marrow cells to marrow fat**: falls.
- **Neutrophils**: maintained throughout life, although leucocytes may be less readily mobilised by bacterial invasion in old age.
- **Lymphocytes**: functionally compromised by age due to a T-cell-related defect in cell-mediated immunity.
- **Clotting factors**: no major changes, although mild congenital deficiencies may be first noticed in old age.
- **Erythrocyte sedimentation rate (ESR)**: raised above the reference range but usually in association with chronic or subacute disease. In truly healthy older people, the ESR range is very similar to that in younger people.

assays. Therefore these tests, when required, should be performed when the patient is not taking anticoagulants.

Presenting problems in blood disease

Anaemia

Anaemia refers to a state in which the level of haemoglobin in the blood is below the reference range appropriate for age

23.7 Causes of anaemia

Decreased or ineffective marrow production
- Lack of iron, vitamin B_{12} or folate
- Hypoplasia/myelodysplasia
- Invasion by malignant cells
- Renal failure
- Anaemia of chronic disease

Normal marrow production but increased removal of cells
- Blood loss
- Haemolysis
- Hypersplenism

and sex. Other factors, including pregnancy and altitude, also affect haemoglobin levels and must be taken into account when considering whether an individual is anaemic. The clinical features of anaemia reflect diminished oxygen supply to the tissues (p. 912). A rapid onset of anaemia (e.g. due to blood loss) causes more profound symptoms than a gradually developing anaemia. Individuals with cardiorespiratory disease are more susceptible to symptoms of anaemia.

The clinical assessment and investigation of anaemia should gauge its severity and define the underlying cause (Box 23.7).

Clinical assessment
- *Iron deficiency anaemia* (p. 940) is the most common type of anaemia worldwide. A thorough gastrointestinal history is important, looking in particular for symptoms of blood loss. Menorrhagia is a common cause of anaemia in pre-menopausal females, so women should always be asked about their periods.
- *A dietary history* should assess the intake of iron and folate, which may become deficient in comparison to needs (e.g. in pregnancy or during periods of rapid growth; pp. 712, 945 and 1284).
- *Past medical history* may reveal a disease that is known to be associated with anaemia, such as rheumatoid arthritis (anaemia of chronic disease), or previous surgery (e.g. resection of the stomach or small bowel, which may lead to malabsorption of iron and/or vitamin B_{12}).
- *Family history and ethnic background* may raise suspicion of haemolytic anaemias, such as the haemoglobinopathies and hereditary spherocytosis. Pernicious anaemia may also run in families but is not associated with a clear Mendelian pattern of inheritance.
- *A drug history* may reveal the ingestion of drugs that cause blood loss (e.g. aspirin and anti-inflammatory drugs), haemolysis (e.g. sulphonamides) or aplasia (e.g. chloramphenicol).

On examination, as well as the general physical findings of anaemia shown on page 912, there may be specific findings related to the aetiology of the anaemia; for example, a patient may be found to have a right iliac fossa mass due to an underlying caecal carcinoma. Haemolytic anaemias can cause jaundice. Vitamin B_{12} deficiency may be associated with neurological signs, including peripheral neuropathy, dementia and signs of subacute combined degeneration of the cord (p. 1138). Sickle-cell anaemia (p. 951) may result in leg ulcers, stroke or features of pulmonary hypertension. Anaemia may be multifactorial and the lack of specific symptoms and signs does not rule out silent pathology.

Investigations

Schemes for the investigation of anaemias are often based on the size of the red cells, which is most accurately indicated by the MCV in the FBC. Commonly, in the presence of anaemia:

23

Fig. 23.10 Investigation of anaemia with normal or low mean cell volume (MCV). (Hb = haemoglobin; MCH = mean cell haemoglobin)

Fig. 23.11 Investigation of anaemia with high mean cell volume (MCV). (LDH = lactate dehydrogenase)

- A normal MCV (normocytic anaemia) suggests either acute blood loss or the anaemia of chronic disease, also known as the anaemia of inflammation (ACD/AI) (Fig. 23.10).
- A low MCV (microcytic anaemia) suggests iron deficiency or thalassaemia or sometimes ACD/AI (Fig. 23.10).
- A high MCV (macrocytic anaemia) suggests vitamin B_{12} or folate deficiency or myelodysplasia (Fig. 23.11).

Specific types of anaemia and their management are described later in this chapter (p. 940).

High haemoglobin

Patients with a persistently raised haematocrit (Hct) (>0.52 males, >0.48 females) for more than 2 months should be investigated. 'True' polycythaemia (or absolute erythrocytosis) indicates an excess of red cells, while 'relative', 'apparent' or 'low-volume' polycythaemia is due to a decreased plasma volume. Causes of polycythaemia are shown in Box 23.8. These involve increased erythropoiesis in the bone marrow, either due to a primary increase in marrow activity, or in response to increased erythropoietin (Epo) levels in chronic hypoxaemia, or due to inappropriate secretion of Epo. Athletes who seek to benefit from increased oxygen-carrying capacity have been known to use Epo to achieve this.

Apparent erythrocytosis with a raised Hct, normal red cell mass (RCM) and reduced plasma volume may be associated with hypertension, smoking, alcohol and diuretic use (Gaisböck's syndrome).

Clinical assessment and investigations

Males and females with Hct values of over 0.60 and over 0.56, respectively, can be assumed to have an absolute erythrocytosis. A clinical history and examination will identify most patients with polycythaemia secondary to hypoxia. The presence of hypertension, smoking, excess alcohol consumption and/or diuretic use is consistent with low-volume polycythaemia (Gaisböck's syndrome). In polycythaemia rubra vera (PRV), a mutation in a kinase, *JAK-2 V617F*, is found in over 90% of cases (p. 970). Patients with PRV have an increased risk of arterial thromboses, particularly stroke, and venous thromboembolism. They may also have aquagenic pruritus (itching after exposure to water), hepatosplenomegaly and gout (due to high red cell turnover).

If the *JAK-2* mutation is absent and there is no obvious secondary cause, a measurement of red cell mass is required to confirm an absolute erythrocytosis, followed by further investigations to exclude hypoxia, and causes of inappropriate erythropoietin secretion.

Leucopenia (low white cell count)

A reduction in the total numbers of circulating white cells is called leucopenia. This may be due to a reduction in all types of white cell or in individual cell types (usually neutrophils or lymphocytes). Leucopenia may occur in isolation or as part of a reduction in all three haematological lineages (pancytopenia; p. 930).

Neutropenia

A reduction in neutrophil count (usually $<1.5\times10^9$/L but dependent on age and race) is called neutropenia. The main causes are listed in Box 23.9 and Figure 23.12. Drug-induced neutropenia is not uncommon (Box 23.10). Clinical manifestations range from no symptoms to overwhelming sepsis. The risk of bacterial infection is related to the degree of neutropenia, with counts lower than 0.5×10^9/L considered to be critically low. Fever is the first and often only manifestation of infection. A sore throat, perianal pain or skin inflammation may be present. The lack of neutrophils allows the patient to become septicaemic and shocked within hours if immediate antibiotic therapy is not commenced. Management is discussed on page 224.

Lymphopenia

This is an absolute lymphocyte count of less than 1×10^9/L. The causes are shown in Box 23.9. Although minor reductions may be asymptomatic, deficiencies in cell-mediated immunity may result in infections (with organisms such as fungi, viruses and mycobacteria) and a propensity to lymphoid and other malignancies (particularly those associated with viral infections such as Epstein–Barr virus (EBV), human papillomavirus (HPV)

i	23.8 Classification and causes of erythrocytosis		
	Absolute erythrocytosis		**Relative (low-volume) erythrocytosis**
Haematocrit	High		High
Red cell mass	High		Normal
Plasma volume	Normal		Low
Causes	*Primary*		Diuretics
	Myeloproliferative disorder		Smoking
	Polycythaemia rubra vera (primary proliferative polycythaemia)		Obesity
	Secondary		Alcohol excess
	High erythropoietin due to tissue hypoxia:		Gaisböck's syndrome
	High altitude		
	Cardiorespiratory disease		
	High-affinity haemoglobins		
	Inappropriately increased erythropoietin:		
	Renal disease (hydronephrosis, cysts, carcinoma)		
	Other tumours (hepatoma, bronchogenic carcinoma, uterine		
	fibroids, phaeochromocytoma, cerebellar haemangioblastoma)		
	Exogenous testosterone therapy		
	Exogenous erythropoietin administration:		
	Performance-enhancing drug-taking in athletes		

23

23.9 How to interpret white blood cell results

Neutrophils A

Neutrophilia
- Infection: bacterial, fungal
- Trauma: surgery, burns
- Infarction: myocardial infarct, pulmonary embolus, sickle-cell crisis
- Inflammation: gout, rheumatoid arthritis, ulcerative colitis, Crohn's disease
- Malignancy: solid tumours, Hodgkin lymphoma
- Myeloproliferative disease: polycythaemia, chronic myeloid leukaemia
- Physiological: exercise, pregnancy

Neutropenia
- Infection: viral, bacterial (e.g. *Salmonella*), protozoal (e.g. malaria)
- Drugs: see Box 23.10
- Autoimmune: connective tissue disease
- Alcohol
- Bone marrow infiltration: leukaemia, myelodysplasia
- Congenital: Kostmann's syndrome
- Constitutional: Afro-Caribbean and Middle Eastern descent

Eosinophils B

Eosinophilia
- Allergy: hay fever, asthma, eczema
- Infection: parasitic
- Drug hypersensitivity: e.g. gold, sulphonamides
- Vasculitis: e.g. eosinophilic granulomatosis with polyangiitis (Churg–Strauss), granulomatosis with polyangiitis (Wegener's)
- Connective tissue disease: polyarteritis nodosa
- Malignancy: solid tumours, lymphomas
- Primary bone marrow disorders: myeloproliferative disorders, hypereosinophilic syndrome (HES), acute myeloid leukaemia

Basophils C

Basophilia
- Myeloproliferative disease: polycythaemia, chronic myeloid leukaemia
- Inflammation: acute hypersensitivity, ulcerative colitis, Crohn's disease
- Iron deficiency

Monocytes D

Monocytosis
- Infection: bacterial (e.g. tuberculosis)
- Inflammation: connective tissue disease, ulcerative colitis, Crohn's disease
- Malignancy: solid tumours, chronic myelomonocytic leukaemia

Lymphocytes E

Lymphocytosis
- Infection: viral, bacterial (e.g. *Bordetella pertussis*)
- Lymphoproliferative disease: chronic lymphocytic leukaemia, lymphoma
- Post-splenectomy

Lymphopenia
- Inflammation: connective tissue disease
- Lymphoma
- Renal failure
- Sarcoidosis
- Drugs: glucocorticoids, cytotoxics
- Congenital: severe combined immunodeficiency
- HIV infection

Fig. 23.12 Appearance of white blood cells. A Neutrophil. B Eosinophil. C Basophil. D Monocyte. E Lymphocyte.

23.10 Drugs that can induce neutropenia*

Group	Examples
Analgesics/anti-inflammatory agents	Gold, penicillamine, naproxen
Antithyroid drugs	Carbimazole, propylthiouracil
Anti-arrhythmics	Quinidine, procainamide
Antihypertensives	Captopril, enalapril, nifedipine
Antidepressants/psychotropics	Amitriptyline, dosulepin, mianserin
Antimalarials	Pyrimethamine, dapsone, sulfadoxine, chloroquine
Anticonvulsants	Phenytoin, sodium valproate, carbamazepine
Antibiotics	Sulphonamides, penicillins, cephalosporins
Miscellaneous	Cimetidine, ranitidine, chlorpropamide, zidovudine

*Many drugs can induce cytopenias. In suspected cases check drug summary of product characteristics.

and human herpesvirus 8 (HHV-8)). Lymphopenia without any obvious cause is common with advancing age.

Leucocytosis (high white cell count)

An increase in the total numbers of circulating white cells is called leucocytosis. This is usually due to an increase in a specific type of cell (see Box 23.9). It is important to realise that an increase in a single type of white cell (e.g. eosinophils or monocytes) may not increase the total white cell count (WCC) above the upper limit of normal and will be apparent only if the 'differential' of the white count is examined.

Neutrophilia

An increase in the number of circulating neutrophils is called a neutrophilia or a neutrophil leucocytosis. It can result from an increased production of cells from the bone marrow or redistribution from the marginated pool. The normal neutrophil count depends on age, race and certain physiological parameters. During pregnancy, not only is there an increase in neutrophils but also earlier forms, such as metamyelocytes, can be found in the blood. The causes of a neutrophilia are shown in Box 23.9.

Eosinophilia

A high eosinophil count of more than 0.5×10^9/L is usually secondary to infection (especially parasites; p. 233), allergy (e.g. eczema, asthma, reactions to drugs; p. 84), immunological disorders (e.g. polyarteritis, sarcoidosis) or malignancy (e.g. lymphomas) (see Box 23.9). Usually, such eosinophilia is short-lived.

In the rarer primary disorders, there is a persistently raised, often clonal, eosinophilia, e.g. in myeloproliferative disorders, subtypes of acute myeloid leukaemia and idiopathic hypereosinophilic syndrome (HES). Recently, specific mutations in receptor tyrosine kinase genes have been found in some primary eosinophilias (e.g. causing rearrangements of platelet-derived growth factor receptors α and β or c-kit), which allow diagnosis and, in some cases, specific therapy with tyrosine kinase inhibitors such as imatinib.

Eosinophil infiltration can damage many organs (e.g. heart, lungs, gastrointestinal tract, skin, musculoskeletal system); evaluation of eosinophilia therefore includes not only the identification of any underlying cause and its appropriate treatment but also assessment of any related organ damage.

Lymphocytosis

A lymphocytosis is an increase in circulating lymphocytes above that expected for the patient's age. In adults, this is greater than 3.5×10^9/L. Infants and children have higher counts; age-related reference ranges should be consulted. Causes are shown in Box 23.9; the most common is viral infection.

Lymphadenopathy

Enlarged lymph glands may be an important indicator of haematological disease but they are not uncommon in reaction to infection or inflammation (Box 23.11). The sites of lymph node groups, and symptoms and signs that may help elucidate the underlying cause are shown on page 913. Nodes that enlarge in response to local infection or inflammation ('reactive nodes') usually expand rapidly and are painful, whereas those due to haematological disease are more frequently painless. Localised lymphadenopathy should elicit a search for a source of inflammation or primary malignancy in the appropriate drainage area:

- the scalp, ear, mouth and throat, face, teeth or thyroid for neck nodes
- the breast for axillary nodes
- the perineum or external genitalia for inguinal nodes.

Generalised lymphadenopathy may be secondary to infection, often viral, connective tissue disease or extensive skin disease (dermatopathic lymphadenopathy) but is more likely to signify underlying haematological malignancy. Weight loss and drenching night sweats that may require a change of nightclothes are associated with haematological malignancies, particularly lymphoma.

Initial investigations in lymphadenopathy include an FBC (to detect neutrophilia in infection or evidence of haematological disease), measurement of erythrocyte sedimentation rate (ESR) and a chest X-ray (to detect mediastinal lymphadenopathy). If the findings suggest malignancy, a formal cutting needle or excision biopsy of a representative node is indicated to obtain a histological diagnosis.

Splenomegaly

The spleen may be enlarged due to involvement by lymphoproliferative disease, the resumption of extramedullary haematopoiesis in myeloproliferative disease, enhanced reticulo-endothelial activity in autoimmune haemolysis, expansion of the lymphoid tissue in response to infections, or vascular congestion as a result of portal hypertension (Box 23.12). Hepatosplenomegaly is suggestive of lympho- or myeloproliferative disease, liver disease or infiltration (e.g. with amyloid). Associated lymphadenopathy is suggestive of lymphoproliferative disease. An enlarged spleen may cause abdominal discomfort, accompanied by back pain and abdominal bloating and early satiety due to stomach compression. Splenic infarction produces severe abdominal pain radiating to the left shoulder tip, associated with a splenic rub on auscultation. Rarely, spontaneous or traumatic rupture and bleeding may occur.

Investigation should focus on the suspected cause. Imaging of the spleen by ultrasound or computed tomography (CT) will detect variations in density in the spleen, which may be a feature of lymphoproliferative disease; it also allows imaging of the liver and abdominal lymph nodes. Biopsy of enlarged abdominal or superficial lymph nodes may provide the diagnosis, as might a bone marrow biopsy in splenic lymphomas. A chest X-ray or CT of the thorax will detect mediastinal lymphadenopathy. An FBC may show pancytopenia secondary to hypersplenism, when the enlarged spleen has become overactive, destroying blood cells prematurely. If other abnormalities are present, such as abnormal lymphocytes or a leucoerythroblastic blood film, a bone marrow examination is indicated. Screening for infectious or liver disease (p. 852) may be appropriate. If all investigations are unhelpful, splenectomy may be diagnostic but is rarely carried out in these circumstances.

Bleeding

Normal bleeding is seen following surgery and trauma. Pathological bleeding occurs when structurally abnormal vessels rupture or when a vessel is breached in the presence of a defect in haemostasis. This may be due to a deficiency or dysfunction of platelets, the coagulation factors or von Willebrand factor, or

---

 23.11 Causes of lymphadenopathy

Infective
- Bacterial: streptococcal, tuberculosis, brucellosis
- Viral: Epstein–Barr virus (EBV), human immunodeficiency virus (HIV)
- Protozoal: toxoplasmosis
- Fungal: histoplasmosis, coccidioidomycosis

Neoplastic
- Primary: lymphomas, leukaemias
- Secondary: lung, breast, thyroid, stomach, melanoma

Connective tissue disorders
- Rheumatoid arthritis
- Systemic lupus erythematosus (SLE)

Sarcoidosis

Amyloidosis

Drugs
- Phenytoin

23

i 23.12 Causes of splenomegaly

Congestive

Portal hypertension
- Cirrhosis
- Hepatic vein occlusion
- Portal vein thrombosis
- Stenosis or malformation of portal or splenic vein

Cardiac
- Chronic congestive cardiac failure
- Constrictive pericarditis

Infective

Bacterial
- Endocarditis
- Sepsis
- Tuberculosis
- Brucellosis
- *Salmonella*

Viral
- Hepatitis
- Epstein–Barr
- Cytomegalovirus

Protozoal
- Malaria*
- Leishmaniasis (kala-azar)*
- Trypanosomiasis

Fungal
- Histoplasmosis

Inflammatory/granulomatous disorders

- Felty's syndrome in rheumatoid arthritis
- Sarcoidosis
- Systemic lupus erythematosus

Haematological

Red cell disorders
- Megaloblastic anaemia
- Haemoglobinopathies
- Hereditary spherocytosis

Autoimmune haemolytic anaemias

Myeloproliferative disorders
- Chronic myeloid leukaemia*
- Myelofibrosis*
- Polycythaemia rubra vera
- Essential thrombocythaemia

Neoplastic
- Leukaemias, including chronic myeloid leukaemia*
- Lymphomas

Other malignancies

- Metastatic cancer – rare

Lysosomal storage diseases

- Gaucher's disease
- Niemann–Pick disease

Miscellaneous

- Cysts, amyloid, thyrotoxicosis, haemophagocytic syndromes

*Causes of massive splenomegaly.

i 23.13 Causes of non-thrombocytopenic purpura

- Senile purpura
- Factitious purpura
- Henoch–Schönlein purpura (p. 1043)
- Vasculitis (p. 1040)
- Paraproteinaemias
- Purpura fulminans, e.g. in disseminated intravascular coagulation secondary to sepsis

Fig. 23.13 Petechial purpura.

bleeding from superficial cuts, epistaxis, gastrointestinal haemorrhage or menorrhagia is more likely to be due to thrombocytopenia, a platelet function disorder or von Willebrand disease. Recurrent bleeds at a single site suggest a local structural abnormality rather than coagulopathic bleeding.

- *Duration of history.* It may be possible to assess whether the disorder is congenital or acquired.
- *Precipitating causes.* Bleeding arising spontaneously indicates a more severe defect than bleeding that occurs only after trauma.
- *Surgery.* Ask about operations. Dental extractions, tonsillectomy and circumcision are stressful tests of the haemostatic system. Immediate post-surgical bleeding suggests defective platelet plug formation and primary haemostasis; delayed haemorrhage is more suggestive of a coagulation defect. However, in post-surgical patients, persistent bleeding from a single site is more likely to indicate surgical bleeding than a bleeding disorder.
- *Family history.* While a positive family history may be present in patients with inherited disorders, the absence of affected relatives does not exclude a hereditary bleeding diathesis; about one-third of cases of haemophilia arise in individuals without a family history, and deficiencies of factor VII, X and XIII are recessively inherited. Recessive disorders are more common in cultures where there is consanguineous marriage.
- *Drugs.* Use of antithrombotic, anticoagulant and fibrinolytic drugs must be elicited. Drug interactions with warfarin and drug-induced thrombocytopenia should be considered. Some 'herbal' remedies may result in a bleeding diathesis.

Clinical examination may reveal different patterns of skin bleeding. Petechial purpura is minor bleeding into the dermis that is flat and non-blanching (Fig. 23.13). Petechiae are typically found in patients with thrombocytopenia or platelet dysfunction.

occasionally to excessive fibrinolysis, which is most commonly observed following therapeutic thrombolysis (p. 500).

Clinical assessment

'Screening' blood tests (see Box 23.3) do not reliably detect all causes of pathological bleeding (e.g. von Willebrand disease, scurvy, certain anticoagulant drugs and the causes of purpura listed in Box 23.13) and should not be used indiscriminately. A careful clinical evaluation is the key to diagnosis of bleeding disorders (p. 970). It is important to consider the following:

- *Site of bleeding.* Bleeding into muscle and joints, along with retroperitoneal and intracranial haemorrhage, indicates a likely defect in coagulation factors. Purpura, prolonged

Palpable purpura occurs in vasculitis. Ecchymosis, or bruising, is more extensive bleeding into deeper layers of the skin. The lesions are initially dark red or purple but become yellow as haemoglobin is degraded. Retroperitoneal bleeding presents with a flank or peri-umbilical haematoma. Telangiectasia of lips and tongue points to hereditary haemorrhagic telangiectasia (p. 970). Joints should be examined for evidence of haemarthroses. A full examination is important, as it may give clues to an underlying associated systemic illness such as a haematological or other malignancy, liver disease, renal failure, connective tissue disease and possible causes of splenomegaly.

Investigations

Screening investigations and their interpretation are described on page 920. If the patient has a history that is strongly suggestive of a bleeding disorder and all the preliminary screening tests give normal results, further investigations, such as measurement of von Willebrand factor and assessment of platelet function, should be performed (p. 921).

Thrombocytopenia (low platelet count)

A reduced platelet count may arise by one of two mechanisms:

- decreased or abnormal production (bone marrow failure and hereditary thrombocytopathies)
- increased consumption following release into the circulation (immune-mediated, DIC or sequestration).

Spontaneous bleeding does not usually occur until the platelet count falls below 20×10^9/L, unless their function is also compromised. Purpura and spontaneous bruising are characteristic but there may also be oral, nasal, gastrointestinal or genitourinary bleeding. Severe thrombocytopenia ($<10\times10^9$/L) may result in retinal haemorrhage and potentially fatal intracranial bleeding, but this is rare.

Investigations are directed at the possible causes listed in Box 23.14. A blood film is the single most useful initial investigation. Examination of the bone marrow may reveal increased megakaryocytes in consumptive causes of thrombocytopenia, or the underlying cause of bone marrow failure in leukaemia, hypoplastic anaemia or myelodysplasia.

Treatment (if required) depends on the underlying cause. Platelet transfusion is rarely required and is usually confined to patients with bone marrow failure and platelet counts below 10×10^9/L, or to clinical situations with actual or predicted serious haemorrhage.

Thrombocytosis (high platelet count)

The most common reason for a raised platelet count is that it is reactive to another process, such as infection, inflammation, connective tissue disease, malignancy, iron deficiency, acute haemolysis or gastrointestinal bleeding (Box 23.15). The presenting clinical features are usually those of the underlying disorder and haemostasis is rarely affected. Reactive thrombocytosis is distinguished from the myeloproliferative disorders by the presence of uniform small platelets, lack of splenomegaly, and the presence of an associated disorder. The key to diagnosis is the clinical history and examination, combined with observation of the platelet count over time (reactive thrombocytosis gets better with resolution of the underlying cause).

The platelets are a product of an abnormally expanding clone of cells in the myeloproliferative disorders, chronic myeloid leukaemia

---

23.14 Causes of thrombocytopenia

Decreased production

Marrow hypoplasia
- Childhood bone marrow failure syndromes, e.g. Fanconi's anaemia, dyskeratosis congenita, amegakaryocytic thrombocytopenia
- Idiopathic aplastic anaemia
- Drug-induced: cytotoxics, antimetabolites
- Transfusion-associated graft-versus-host disease

Marrow infiltration
- Leukaemia
- Myeloma
- Carcinoma (rare)
- Myelofibrosis
- Osteopetrosis
- Lysosomal storage disorders, e.g. Gaucher's disease

Haematinic deficiency
- Vitamin B_{12} and/or folate deficiency

Familial (macro-)thrombocytopathies
- Myosin heavy chain abnormalities, e.g. Alport's syndrome, Fechtner's syndrome, May–Hegglin anomaly
- Bernard–Soulier syndrome
- Montreal platelet syndrome
- Wiskott–Aldrich syndrome (small platelets)
- Mediterranean macrothrombocytopathy

Increased consumption

Immune mechanisms
- Idiopathic thrombocytopenic purpura*
- Neonatal alloimmune thrombocytopenia
- Post-transfusion purpura
- Drug-associated, especially quinine, vancomycin and heparin

Coagulation activation
- Disseminated intravascular coagulation (see Box 23.68, p. 978)

Mechanical pooling
- Hypersplenism

Thrombotic microangiopathies
- Haemolytic uraemic syndrome (HUS) and atypical HUS
- Liver disease
- Thrombotic thrombocytopenic purpura
- Pre-eclampsia

Others
- Gestational thrombocytopenia
- Type 2B von Willebrand disease

*Associated conditions include collagen vascular diseases (particularly systemic lupus erythematosus), B-cell malignancy, HIV infection and antiphospholipid syndrome.

23.15 Causes of a raised platelet count

Reactive thrombocytosis
- Acute and chronic inflammatory disorders
- Infection
- Malignant disease
- Tissue damage
- Haemolytic anaemias
- Post-splenectomy
- Post-haemorrhage

Clonal thrombocytosis
- Primary thrombocythaemia
- Polycythaemia rubra vera
- Chronic myeloid leukaemia
- Myelofibrosis
- Myelodysplastic syndromes (MDSs; refractory anaemia with ring sideroblasts and thrombocytosis (RARS-T), MDS with isolated deletion of 5q)

23

and some forms of myelodysplasia. As with PRV, patients with essential thrombocythaemia may present with thrombosis or, rarely, bleeding. Stroke, transient ischaemic attacks, amaurosis fugax, digital ischaemia or gangrene, aquagenic pruritus, splenomegaly and systemic upset are also features. Patients with myeloproliferative disorders may also present with features such as aquagenic pruritus, splenomegaly and systemic upset.

Pancytopenia

Pancytopenia refers to the combination of anaemia, leucopenia and thrombocytopenia. It may be due to reduced production of blood cells as a consequence of bone marrow suppression or infiltration, or there may be peripheral destruction or splenic pooling of mature cells. Causes are shown in Box 23.16. A bone marrow aspirate and trephine are usually required to establish the diagnosis.

23.16 Causes of pancytopenia

Bone marrow failure

- Hypoplastic/aplastic anaemia (p. 968): inherited, idiopathic, viral, drugs

Bone marrow infiltration

- Acute leukaemia
- Myeloma
- Lymphoma
- Carcinoma
- Haemophagocytic syndrome
- Myelodysplastic syndromes

Ineffective haematopoiesis

- Megaloblastic anaemia
- Acquired immunodeficiency syndrome (AIDS)

Peripheral pooling/destruction

- Hypersplenism: portal hypertension, Felty's syndrome, malaria, myelofibrosis
- Systemic lupus erythematosus

Infection

Infection is a major complication of haematological disorders. It relates to the immunological deficit caused by the disease itself, or its treatment with chemotherapy and/or immunotherapy (pp. 224 and 925).

Principles of management of haematological disease

Blood products and transfusion

Blood transfusion from an unrelated donor to a recipient inevitably carries some risk, including adverse immunological interactions between the host and infused blood (p. 931), and transmission of infectious agents. Although there are many compelling clinical indications for blood component transfusion, there are also many clinical circumstances in which transfusion is conventional but the evidence for its effectiveness is limited. In these settings,

allogeneic transfusion may be avoided by following protocols that recommend the use of low haemoglobin thresholds for red cell transfusion, perioperative blood salvage and antifibrinolytic drugs.

Blood products

Blood components are prepared from whole blood or specific blood constituents collected from individual donors and include red cells, platelets, plasma and cryoprecipitate (Box 23.17).

Plasma derivatives are licensed pharmaceutical products produced on a factory scale from large volumes of human plasma obtained from many people and treated to remove transmissible infection. Examples include:

- *Coagulation factors.* Concentrates of factors VIII and IX are used for the treatment of conditions such as haemophilia A, haemophilia B and von Willebrand disease. Coagulation factors made by recombinant DNA technology are now preferred due to perceived lack of infection risk but plasma-derived products are still used in many countries.
- *Immunoglobulins.* Intravenous immunoglobulin G (IVIgG) is administered as regular replacement therapy to reduce infective complications in patients with primary and secondary immunodeficiency. A short, high-dose course of IVIgG may also be effective in some immunological disorders, including immune thrombocytopenia (p. 971) and Guillain–Barré syndrome (p. 1140). IVIgG can cause acute reactions and must be infused strictly according to the manufacturer's product information. There is a risk of renal dysfunction in susceptible patients and, in these circumstances, immunoglobulin products containing low or no sucrose are preferred. Anti-zoster immunoglobulin has a role in the prophylaxis of varicella zoster (p. 239). Anti-Rhesus D immunoglobulin is used in pregnancy to prevent haemolytic disease of the newborn (see Box 23.19 below).
- *Human albumin.* This is available in two strengths. The 5% solution can be used as a colloid resuscitation fluid but it is no more effective and is more expensive than crystalloid solutions. Human albumin 20% solution is used in the management of hypoproteinaemic oedema in nephrotic syndrome (p. 395) and ascites in chronic liver disease (p. 864). It is hyperoncotic and expands plasma volume by more than the amount infused.

Blood components and their use are summarised in Box 23.17.

Blood donation

A safe supply of blood components depends on a well-organised system with regular donation by healthy individuals who have no excess risk of infections transmissible in blood (Fig. 23.14). Blood donations are obtained by either venesection of a unit of whole blood or collection of a specific component, such as platelets, by apheresis. During apheresis, the donor's blood is drawn via a closed system into a machine that separates the components by centrifugation and collects the desired fraction into a bag, returning the rest of the blood to the donor. Each donation must be tested for hepatitis B virus (HBV), hepatitis C virus (HCV), HIV and human T-cell lymphotropic virus (HTLV) nucleic acid and/or antibodies. Platelet concentrates may be tested for bacterial contamination. The need for other microbiological tests depends on local epidemiology. For example, testing for *Trypanosoma cruzi* (Chagas' disease; p. 279) is necessary in areas of South America and the USA where infection is prevalent. Tests for West Nile virus have been required in the USA since this agent became

i   23.17 Blood components and their use

Component	Major haemorrhage	Other indications
Red cell concentrate[1] Most of the plasma is removed and replaced with a solution of glucose and adenine in saline to maintain viability of red cells ABO compatibility with recipient essential	Replace acute blood loss: increase circulating red cell mass to relieve clinical features caused by insufficient oxygen delivery. Order 4–6 U initially to allow high red cell to FFP transfusion ratios of (at least) 2 : 1	*Severe anaemia* If no cardiovascular disease, transfuse to maintain Hb at 70 g/L If known or likely to have cardiovascular disease, maintain Hb at 90 g/L
Platelet concentrate One adult dose is made from four donations of whole blood, or from a single platelet apheresis donation ABO compatibility with recipient preferable	Maintain platelet count $>50\times10^9$/L, or in multiple or central nervous system trauma $>100\times10^9$/L If ongoing bleeding, order when platelets $<100\times10^9$/L to allow for delivery time Each adult dose has a minimum of 2.4×10^{11} platelets, which raises platelet count by 40×10^9/L unless there is consumptive coagulopathy, e.g. disseminated intravascular coagulation	*Thrombocytopenia*, e.g. in acute leukaemia Maintain platelet count $>10\times10^9$/L if not bleeding Maintain platelet count $>20\times10^9$/L if minor bleeding or at risk (sepsis, concurrent use of antibiotics, abnormal coagulation) Increase platelet count $>50\times10^9$/L for minor invasive procedure (e.g. lumbar puncture, gastroscopy and biopsy, insertion of indwelling lines, liver biopsy, laparotomy) or in acute, major blood loss Increase platelet count $>100\times10^9$/L for operations in critical sites such as brain or eyes
Fresh frozen plasma[2] 150–300 mL plasma from one donation of whole blood ABO compatibility with recipient recommended	Dilutional coagulopathy with a PT prolonged $>50\%$ is likely after replacement of 1–1.5 blood volumes with red cell concentrate Give initially in (at least) a ratio of 1 FFP:2 red cell concentrate; order 15–20 mL/kg and allow for thawing time. Further doses only if bleeding continues and guided by PT and APTT	*Replacement of coagulation factor deficiency* If no virally inactivated or recombinant product is available *Thrombotic thrombocytopenic purpura* Plasma exchange (using virus-inactivated plasma if available) is frequently effective

Cryoprecipitate[2]
Fibrinogen and coagulation factor concentrated from plasma by controlled thawing
10–20 mL pack contains:
    Fibrinogen 150–300 mg
    Factor VIII 80–120 U
    von Willebrand factor 80–120 U
In UK supplied as pools of 5 U
	Aim to keep fibrinogen >1.5 g/L. Pooled units (of 10 donations) will raise fibrinogen by 1 g/L	*von Willebrand disease and haemophilia*
		If virus-inactivated or recombinant products are not available

[1]Whole blood is an alternative to red cell concentrate. ABO compatibility with recipient essential. [2]Pooled plasma can be treated with solvent and detergent or single units treated with methylene blue as an additional viral inactivation step. Virus-inactivated plasma is indicated for large-volume exposure, as in treatment of thrombotic thrombocytopenic purpura, and for treatment of children in the UK born after 1995.
(APTT = activated partial thromboplastin time; FFP = fresh frozen plasma; Hb = haemoglobin; PT = prothrombin time)

23

prevalent. Components for use in specific patient groups are prepared from hepatitis E virus-negative donors in the UK, and plasma donated in the UK is not used at present for producing pooled plasma derivatives in view of concerns about transmission of variant Creutzfeldt–Jakob disease (vCJD; p. 1127).

Adverse effects of transfusion

Death directly attributable to transfusion is rare, at less than 0.3 per 100 000 transfusions. Relatively minor symptoms of transfusion reactions (fever, itch or urticaria) occur in up to 3% of transfusions, and usually in patients who have had repeated transfusions. Any symptoms or signs that arise during a transfusion must be taken seriously, as they may be the first warnings of a serious reaction. Figure 23.16 below outlines the symptoms and signs, management and investigation of acute reactions to blood components.

Red cell incompatibility

Red blood cell membranes contain numerous cell surface molecules that are potentially antigenic (see Fig. 23.4). The ABO and Rhesus D antigens are the most important in routine transfusion and antenatal practice.

ABO blood groups

The frequency of the ABO antigens varies among different populations. The ABO blood group antigens are oligosaccharide chains that project from the red cell surface. These chains are attached to proteins and lipids that lie in the red cell membrane. The *ABO* gene encodes a glycosyltransferase that catalyses the final step in the synthesis of the chain, which has three common alleles: A, B and O. The O allele encodes an inactive enzyme, leaving the ABO antigen precursor (called the H antigen) unmodified. The A and B alleles encode enzymes that differ by

Fig. 23.14 Blood donation, processing and storage. [1]Platelet apheresis involves circulating the donor's blood through a cell separator to remove platelets before returning other blood components to the donor. [2]In the UK, plasma for fractionation is imported as a precautionary measure against vCJD. (vCJD = variant Creutzfeldt–Jakob disease; HIV = human immunodeficiency virus; HTLV = human T-cell lymphotropic virus)

four amino acids and hence attach different sugars to the end of the chain. Individuals are tolerant to their own ABO antigens, but do not suppress B-cell clones producing antibodies against ABO antigens that they do not carry themselves (Box 23.18). They are, therefore, capable of mounting a humoral immune response to these 'foreign' antigens.

ABO-incompatible red cell transfusion

If red cells of an incompatible ABO group are transfused (especially if a group O recipient is transfused with group A, B or AB red cells), the *recipient*'s IgM anti-A, anti-B or anti-AB binds to the *transfused* red cells. This activates the full complement pathway (p. 66), creating pores in the red cell membrane and destroying

i	23.18	ABO blood group antigens and antibodies		
ABO blood group	Red cell A or B antigens	Antibodies in plasma	UK frequency (%)	
O	None	Anti-A and anti-B	46	
A	A	Anti-B	42	
B	B	Anti-A	9	
AB	A and B	None	3	

23.19 Rhesus D blood groups in pregnancy

- **Haemolytic disease of the newborn (HDN)**: occurs when the mother has anti-red cell immunoglobulin G (IgG) antibodies that cross the placenta and haemolyse fetal red cells.
- **Screening for HDN in pregnancy**: at the time of booking (12–16 weeks) and again at 28–34 weeks' gestation, every pregnant woman should have a blood sample sent for determination of ABO and Rhesus D (RhD) group and testing for red cell alloantibodies that may be directed against paternal blood group antigens present on fetal red cells.
- **Anti-D immunoglobulin prophylaxis in a pregnant woman who is RhD-negative**: antenatal anti-D prophylaxis is offered at 28–34 weeks to RhD-negative pregnant women who have no evidence of immune anti-D. This prevents the formation of antibodies that could cause HDN. Following delivery of an RhD-positive baby, the mother is given further anti-D within 72 hours; a maternal sample is checked for remaining fetal red cells and additional anti-D is given if indicated. Additional anti-D is also given after potential sensitising events antenatally (e.g. early bleeding). Doses vary according to national recommendations.

the transfused red cells in the circulation (intravascular haemolysis). The anaphylatoxins C3a and C5a, released by complement activation, liberate cytokines such as tumour necrosis factor (TNF), interleukin 1 (IL-1) and IL-8, and stimulate degranulation of mast cells with release of vasoactive mediators. All these substances may lead to inflammation, increased vascular permeability and hypotension, which may, in turn, cause shock and renal failure. Inflammatory mediators can also cause platelet aggregation, lung peribronchial oedema and smooth muscle contraction. About 20–30% of ABO-incompatible transfusions cause some degree of morbidity, and 5–10% cause or contribute to a patient's death. The main reason for this relatively low morbidity is the lack of potency of ABO antibodies in group A or B subjects; even if the recipient is group O, those who are very young or very old usually have weaker antibodies that do not lead to the activation of large amounts of complement.

The Rhesus D blood group and haemolytic disease of the newborn

About 15% of Caucasians are Rhesus-negative: that is, they lack the Rhesus D (RhD) red cell surface antigen (see Fig. 23.4). In other populations (e.g. in Chinese and Bengalis), only 1–5% are Rhesus-negative. RhD-negative individuals do not normally produce substantial amounts of anti-RhD antibodies. However, if RhD-positive red cells enter the circulation of an RhD-negative individual, IgG antibodies are produced. This can occur during pregnancy if the mother is exposed to fetal cells via fetomaternal haemorrhage, or following transfusion. If a woman is so sensitised, during a subsequent pregnancy anti-RhD antibodies can cross the placenta; if the fetus is RhD-positive, haemolysis with severe fetal anaemia and hyperbilirubinaemia can result. This can cause severe neurological damage or death due to haemolytic disease of the newborn (HDN). Therefore, an RhD-negative female who may subsequently become pregnant should never be transfused with RhD-positive blood.

In RhD-negative women, administration of anti-RhD immunoglobulin (anti-D) perinatally can block the immune response to RhD antigen on fetal cells and is the only effective product for preventing the development of Rhesus antibodies (Box 23.19).

HDN can also be caused by other alloantibodies against red cell antigens, usually after previous pregnancies or transfusions. These antigens include Rhc, RhC, RhE, Rhe, and the Kell, Kidd and Duffy antigen systems. HDN can also occur if there is fetomaternal ABO incompatibility, most commonly seen in a group O mother with a group A fetus. The fetus is generally less severely affected by ABO incompatibility than by RhD, Rhc or Kell antigen mismatch, and the incompatibility is often picked up coincidentally after birth.

Other immunological complications of transfusion

Rare but serious complications include transfusion-associated lung injury (TRALI) and transfusion-associated graft-versus-host disease

(TA GVHD). The latter occurs when there is sharing of a human leucocyte antigen (HLA) haplotype between donor and recipient, which allows transfused lymphocytes to engraft, proliferate and recognise the recipient as foreign, resulting in acute GVHD (p. 937). Prevention is by gamma- or X-ray irradiation of blood components before their administration to prevent lymphocyte proliferation. Those at risk of TA GVHD, who must receive irradiated blood components, include patients with congenital T-cell immunodeficiencies or Hodgkin lymphoma, patients with aplastic anaemia receiving immunosuppressive therapy with antithymocyte globulin (ATG), recipients of haematopoietic stem cell transplants or of blood from a family member, neonates who have received an intrauterine transfusion, and patients taking T-lymphocyte-suppressing drugs, such as fludarabine and other purine analogues.

Transfusion-transmitted infection

Over the past 30 years, HBV, HIV-1 and HCV have been identified and effective tests introduced to detect and exclude infected donations. Where blood is from 'safe' donors and correctly tested, the current risk of a donated unit being infectious is very small. By 2013 in the UK, the estimated chance that a unit of blood from a 'safe' donor might transmit one of the viruses for which is tested was 1 in 6.6 million units for HIV-1, 1 in 51.5 million for HCV and 1 in 2.6 million for HBV. However, some patients who received transfusions before these tests were available suffered serious consequences from infection; this serves as a reminder to avoid non-essential transfusion, since it is impossible to exclude the emergence of new or currently unrecognised transfusion-transmissible infection. Licensed plasma derivatives that have been virus-inactivated do not transmit HIV, HTLV, HBV, HCV, cytomegalovirus or other lipid-enveloped viruses.

Variant CJD is a human prion disease linked to bovine spongiform encephalitis (BSE; p. 1127). The risk of a recipient acquiring the agent of vCJD from a transfusion is uncertain, but of 16 recipients of blood from donors who later developed the disease, 3 have died with clinical vCJD and 1 other had postmortem immunohistological features of infection.

Bacterial contamination of a blood component – usually platelets – is extremely rare (1 proven case in the UK in 2015) but can result in severe bacteraemia/sepsis in the recipient.

23

Safe transfusion procedures

The proposed transfusion and any alternatives should be discussed with the patient or, if that is not possible, with a relative, and this should be documented in the case record. Some patients, e.g. Jehovah's Witnesses, may refuse transfusion and require specialised management to survive profound anaemia following blood loss.

Pre-transfusion testing

To ensure that red cells supplied for transfusion are compatible with the intended recipient, the transfusion laboratory will perform either a 'group and screen' procedure or a 'cross-match'. In the group and screen procedure, the red cells from the patient's blood sample are tested to determine the ABO and RhD type, and the patient's serum is also tested against an array of red cells expressing the most important antigens to detect any red cell antibodies. Any antibody detected can be identified by further testing, so that red cell units that lack the corresponding antigen can be selected. The patient's sample can be held in the laboratory for up to a week, so that the hospital blood bank can quickly prepare compatible blood without the need for a further patient sample. Conventional cross-matching consists of the group and antibody screen, followed by direct confirmation of the compatibility of individual units of red cells with the patient's serum. Full cross-matching takes about 45 minutes if no red cell antibodies are present, but may require hours if a patient has multiple antibodies.

Blood can be supplied by 'electronic issue', without the need for compatibility cross-matching, if the laboratory's computer system shows that the patient's ABO and RhD groups have been identified and confirmed on two separate occasions and their antibody screen is negative. This allows group-specific units to be issued quickly and safely, for elective and emergency transfusion.

Bedside procedures for safe transfusion

Errors leading to patients receiving the wrong blood are an important avoidable cause of mortality and morbidity. Most incompatible transfusions result from failure to adhere to standard procedures for taking correctly labelled blood samples from the patient and ensuring that the correct pack of blood component is transfused into the intended patient. In the UK in 2015, there were 280 reports of transfusion of an incorrect blood component (11 per 100 000 units transfused). Every hospital where blood is transfused should have a written transfusion policy used by all staff who order, check or administer blood products (Fig. 23.15). Management of suspected transfusion reactions is shown in Figure 23.16.

Transfusion in major haemorrhage

The successful management of a patient with major haemorrhage requires frontline clinical staff to be trained to recognise significant blood loss early and to intervene before shock is established. Hospitals should have local major haemorrhage protocols and all clinical staff must be familiar with their content. Good team working and communication are essential to prevent poor clinical outcome, suboptimal or inappropriate transfusion practice and component wastage. Fresh frozen plasma (FFP) should be given as part of initial resuscitation in (at least) a 1:2 ratio with red cell concentrate (RCC) until coagulation results are available. If the patient is bleeding, a ratio of FFP to RCC of 1:1 should be given until laboratory results are available and use of cryoprecipitate should be considered. Once the bleeding is under control, further

---

Taking blood for pre-transfusion testing

- Positively identify the patient at the bedside
- Label the sample tube and complete the request form clearly and accurately after identifying the patient
- Do not write forms and labels in advance

Administering blood

- Positively identify the patient at the bedside
- Ensure that the identification of each blood pack matches the patient's identification
- Check that the ABO and RhD groups of each pack are compatible with the patient's
- Check each pack for evidence of damage
- If in doubt, do not use and return to the blood bank
- Complete the forms that document the transfusion of each pack

- Check the compatibility label on the pack against the patient's wristband

Blood pack — **Patient's wristband**

Surname
Forename
Date of birth
Unique identifier/ hospital number

- Always involve the patient by asking them to state their name and date of birth, where possible

Record-keeping

- Record in the patient's notes, the reason for transfusion, the product given, dose, any adverse effects and the clinical respons

Observations

- Transfusions should only be given when the patient can be observed
- Blood pressure, pulse and temperature should be monitored before and 15 minutes after starting each pack
- In conscious patients, further observations are only needed if the patient has symptoms or signs of a reaction
- In unconscious patients, check pulse and temperature at intervals during transfusion
- Signs of abnormal bleeding during the transfusion could be due to disseminated intravascular coagulation resulting from an acute haemolytic reaction

Fig. 23.15 Bedside procedures for safe blood transfusion. The patient's safety depends on adherence to standard procedures for taking samples for compatibility testing, administering blood, record-keeping and observations.

Fig. 23.16 Investigation and management of acute transfusion reactions. *Use size-appropriate dose in children. (ARDS = acute respiratory distress syndrome; BP = blood pressure; CVP = central venous pressure; DIC = disseminated intravascular coagulation; FBC = full blood count; IV = intravenous)

23.20 Key points in transfusion medicine

- A restrictive strategy for red cell transfusion (Hb <70 g/L) is at least as effective as a liberal strategy (<100 g/L).
- The majority of reports in haemovigilance schemes such as SHOT relate to errors in the process of transfusion.
- Although transfusion-transmitted infection is a major concern for patients receiving transfusion, it is rare.
- In patients with trauma or burns or those who have had surgery, there is no evidence that resuscitation with albumin or other colloid solutions reduces the risk of death compared to resuscitation with crystalloid solutions.
- It is recommended that transfusion should be carried out at night time only in unavoidable circumstances.

(SHOT = Serious Hazards of Transfusion)

23.21 Examples of commonly used groups of cancer drugs in haematology

Alkylating agents

- Cross-link double-stranded DNA by adding an alkyl group, e.g. cyclophosphamide, melphalan, chlorambucil

Anthracyclines

- Intercalate between base pairs in the DNA molecule, e.g. daunorubicin, doxorubicin, idarubicin

Antimetabolites

- Inhibit DNA and RNA synthesis, e.g. cytosine arabinoside, fludarabine, methotrexate

Vinca alkaloids

- Cause disruption of tubulin, e.g. vincristine, vinblastine

Topoisomerase II inhibitors

- Prevent DNA repair, e.g. etoposide, daunorubicin, mitoxantrone

An example of a common combination regimen is CHOP, used in lymphoma: **c**yclophosphamide, **h**ydroxydaunorubicin (doxorubicin), **o**ncovin (vincristine) and **p**rednisolone, given every 21 days for six cycles

FFP transfusion should be guided by laboratory results with transfusion triggers of PT and/or APTT above 1·5 times normal for a standard dose of FFP (15–20 mL/kg). Cryoprecipitate should be given if the fibrinogen level falls below 1.5 g/L. Platelets should be kept above 50×10^9/L; to allow for delivery time, platelets should be requested if there is ongoing bleeding and the platelet count has fallen below 100×10^9/L. Blood component use in major haemorrhage is summarised in Box 23.17 and key points in transfusion medicine in Box 23.20.

Chemotherapy

Chemotherapy refers to the use of drugs to treat cancer (Box 23.21; see also Fig. 33.2, p. 1317). Many haematological malignancies are sensitive to the effects of chemotherapy drugs and, as such, chemotherapy is the mainstay of treatment for most haematological cancers. There is a wide range of drugs available that work by damaging DNA or disrupting cellular metabolism, in such a way that natural apoptosis mechanisms, such as *TP53*, are activated and the cell dies. Despite cancer cells being more sensitive, chemotherapy is largely non-specific and kills some normal cells as well as cancer cells. This leads to common side-effects of treatment, such as transient bone marrow failure, mucositis and infertility. The supportive care of patients undergoing chemotherapy is critical in overcoming these side-effects. It is this supportive care, including blood product support, antibiotics, antifungal drugs, growth factors and antiemetics, that has allowed specialist haematology units to achieve the best possible results from intensive chemotherapy: for example, when treating acute leukaemia.

The basic principles of chemotherapy include combining several non-cross-reacting drugs in a regimen that kills a fixed proportion of cancer cells with a given dose. Several cycles of the combination are given to achieve gradual reduction of the tumour burden, to induce remission and, in some instances, to produce a cure (p. 1330).

In recent years, chemotherapy has been improved by the addition of treatments that are more targeted to the cancer cell, particularly monoclonal antibodies; for example, rituximab (anti-CD20) has been added to CHOP (cyclophosphamide doxorubicin, vincristine, prednisolone) and other regimens, significantly improving the outcome in a range of CD20-positive B-cell lymphomas, including diffuse large B-cell lymphoma, follicular lymphoma and mantle cell lymphoma. Chemotherapy drugs can also be linked to a monoclonal antibody to allow targeting of the chemotherapy drug to the specific cancer cell. Examples of such antibody–drug conjugates (ADCs) include the linking of the intercalating antibiotic calicheamicin to anti-CD33 (gemtuzumab ozogamicin) to treat acute myeloid leukaemia, and to anti-CD22 (inotuzumab ozogamicin) to treat acute lymphoblastic leukaemia. Small molecules targeted at the mechanisms causing cancer are replacing chemotherapy in some disease situations, such as tyrosine kinase inhibitors in chronic myeloid leukaemia and inhibitors of B-cell signalling in relapsed chronic lymphocytic leukaemia and lymphomas. More details of specific chemotherapies are given later in the chapter.

Haematopoietic stem cell transplantation

Transplantation of haematopoietic stem cells (HSCT) has offered the only hope of 'cure' in a variety of haematological and non-haematological disorders (Box 23.22). As standard treatment improves, the indications for HSCT are being refined and extended, although its use remains most common in haematological malignancies. The type of HSCT is defined according to the donor and source of stem cells:

- In *allogeneic* HSCT, the stem cells come from a *donor* – either a related donor (usually an HLA-identical sibling) or a closely HLA-matched volunteer unrelated donor (VUD).
- In an *autologous* transplant, the stem cells are harvested from the *patient* and stored in the vapour phase of liquid nitrogen until required. Stem cells can be harvested from the bone marrow or from the blood.

23.22 Indications for allogeneic haematopoietic stem cell transplantation

- Neoplastic disorders affecting stem cell compartments (e.g. leukaemias)
- Failure of haematopoiesis (e.g. aplastic anaemia)
- Major inherited defects in blood cell production (e.g. thalassaemia, immunodeficiency diseases)
- Inborn errors of metabolism with missing enzymes or cell lines

Allogeneic HSCT

Healthy bone marrow or blood stem cells from a donor are infused intravenously into the recipient, who has been suitably 'conditioned'. The conditioning treatment (chemotherapy with or without radiotherapy) is 'myeloablative' or, increasingly, 'non-myeloablative'. Myeloablative conditioning destroys malignant cells and immunosuppresses the recipient, as well as ablating the recipient's haematopoietic tissues. Reduced intensity conditioning (non-myeloablative) relies on intense immunosuppression to provide 'immunological space' for transplanted stem cells. The infused donor cells 'home' to the marrow, engraft and produce enough erythrocytes, granulocytes and platelets for the patient's needs after about 3–4 weeks. During this period of aplasia, patients are at risk of infection and bleeding, and require intensive supportive care as described on page 957. It may take several years to regain normal immunological function and patients remain at risk from opportunistic infections, particularly in the first year.

An advantage of receiving allogeneic donor stem cells is that the donor's immune system can recognise residual recipient malignant cells and destroy them. This immunological 'graft-versus-disease' effect is a powerful tool against many haematological tumours and can be boosted post-transplantation by the infusion of T cells taken from the donor: so-called donor lymphocyte infusion (DLI).

Considerable morbidity and mortality are associated with HSCT. The best results are obtained in patients with minimal residual disease, and in those under 20 years of age who have an HLA-identical sibling donor. Reduced-intensity conditioning has enabled treatment of older or less fit patients. In this form of transplantation, rather than using very intensive myeloablative conditioning, which causes morbidity from organ damage, relatively low doses of chemotherapy drugs, such as fludarabine and cyclophosphamide or busulfan, are used in combination with antibodies such as alemtuzumab (which targets CD52 on mature lymphoid cells) or anti-thymocyte globulin (ATG) to immunosuppress the recipient and allow donor stem cells to engraft. The emerging donor immune system then eliminates malignant cells via the 'graft-versus-disease' effect, which may be boosted by the elective use of donor T-cell infusions post-transplant. Such transplants have produced long-term remissions in some patients with acute leukaemia and myelodysplastic syndromes aged 40–65 years, who would not previously have been considered for a myeloablative allograft.

Complications

These are outlined in Boxes 23.23 and 23.24. The risks and outcomes of transplantation depend upon several patient- and disease-related factors. In general, 25% die from procedure-related complications, such as infection and GVHD, and there

i	23.23 Complications of allogeneic haematopoietic stem cell transplantation	
Early		
• Anaemia		• Mucositis – pain, nausea, diarrhoea
• Infections		• Liver veno-occlusive disease
• Bleeding		
• Acute GVHD		
Late		
• Chronic GVHD		• Cataracts
• Infertility		• Second malignancy

(GVHD = graft-versus-host disease)

i	23.24 Infections during recovery from haematopoietic stem cell transplantation (HSCT)		
Infection	Time after HSCT	Management
---	---	---
Herpes simplex (p. 247)	0–4 weeks (aplastic phase)	Aciclovir prophylaxis and therapy
Bacterial, fungal	0–4 weeks (aplastic phase)	As for acute leukaemia (p. 956) – antibiotic and antifungal prophylaxis and therapy
Cytomegalovirus (p. 242)	5–21 weeks (cell-mediated immune deficiency)	Antigen screening in blood (PCR) and pre-emptive therapy (e.g. ganciclovir)
Varicella zoster (p. 238)	After 13 weeks	Aciclovir prophylaxis and therapy
Pneumocystis jirovecii (p. 318)	8–26 weeks	Co-trimoxazole
Encapsulated bacteria	8 weeks to years (immunoglobulin deficiency, prolonged with GVHD)	Prophylaxis and revaccination

(GVHD = graft-versus-host disease; PCR = polymerase chain reaction)

remains a significant risk of the haematological malignancy relapsing. The long-term survival for patients undergoing allogeneic HSCT in acute leukaemia is around 50%.

Graft-versus-host disease

GVHD is caused by the cytotoxic activity of donor T lymphocytes that become sensitised to their new host, regarding it as foreign. This may cause either an acute or a chronic form of GVHD.

Acute GVHD occurs in the first 100 days after transplant in about one-third of patients. It can affect the skin, causing rashes, the liver, causing jaundice, and the gut, causing diarrhoea, and may vary from mild to lethal. Prevention includes HLA-matching of the donor, immunosuppressant drugs, including methotrexate, ciclosporin, alemtuzumab or ATG. Severe presentations are very difficult to control and, despite high-dose glucocorticoids, may result in death.

Chronic GVHD may follow acute GVHD or arise independently; it occurs later than acute GVHD. It often resembles a connective tissue disorder, although in mild cases a rash may be the only manifestation. Chronic GVHD is usually treated with glucocorticoids and prolonged immunosuppression with, for example, ciclosporin. Chronic GVHD results in an increased infection risk. However, associated with chronic GVHD are the graft-versus-disease effect and a lower relapse rate of the underlying malignancy.

Autologous HSCT

This procedure can also be used in haematological malignancies. The patient's own stem cells from blood or marrow are first harvested and frozen. After conditioning myeloablative therapy, the autologous stem cells are reinfused into the blood stream in order to rescue the patient from the marrow damage and aplasia caused by chemotherapy. Autologous HSCT may be used for disorders that do not primarily involve the haematopoietic tissues, or for patients in whom very good remissions have been achieved. The most common indications are lymphomas and myeloma. The preferred source of stem cells for autologous transplants is peripheral blood (PBSCT). These stem cells engraft more

23

quickly, marrow recovery occurring within 2–3 weeks. There is no risk of GVHD and no immunosuppression is required. Thus autologous stem cell transplantation carries a lower procedure-related mortality rate than allogeneic HSCT at around 5%, but there is a higher rate of recurrence of malignancy because the anti-malignancy effect is solely dependent on the conditioning chemotherapy with no 'graft-versus-disease' effect.

Anticoagulant and antithrombotic therapy

There are numerous indications for anticoagulant and antithrombotic medications (Box 23.25). The guiding principles are outlined here but management in specific indications is discussed elsewhere in the book. Broadly speaking, antiplatelet medications are of greater efficacy in the prevention of arterial thrombosis and of less value in the prevention of venous thromboembolism (VTE). Thus, antiplatelet agents, such as aspirin, clopidogrel and, increasingly, ticagrelor, are the drugs of choice in acute coronary events (p. 498) and in ischaemic cerebrovascular

i 23.25 Indications for anticoagulation

Heparin/LMWH/Fondaparinux

- Prevention and treatment of VTE
- Percutaneous coronary intervention
- Post-thrombolysis for MI
- Unstable angina pectoris
- Non-Q wave MI
- Acute peripheral arterial occlusion
- Cardiopulmonary bypass
- Haemodialysis and haemofiltration

Coumarins (warfarin etc.)

- Prevention and treatment of VTE
- Arterial embolism
- Atrial fibrillation with specific risk factors for stroke (p. 472)
- Mobile mural thrombus post-MI
- Extensive anterior MI   } Therapeutic INR 2.5
- Dilated cardiomyopathy
- Cardioversion
- Ischaemic stroke in antiphospholipid syndrome
- Mitral stenosis and mitral regurgitation with atrial fibrillation
- Recurrent venous thrombosis while on warfarin   } INR 3.5
- Mechanical prosthetic cardiac valves

Rivaroxaban

- Prevention and treatment of VTE
- Atrial fibrillation with risk factors for stroke

Dabigatran etexilate

- Prevention of VTE
- Atrial fibrillation with risk factors for stroke

Apixaban

- Prevention of VTE
- Atrial fibrillation with risk factors for stroke

Edoxaban

- Treatment of VTE
- Atrial fibrillation with risk factors for stroke

(INR = international normalised ratio; LMWH = low-molecular-weight heparin; MI = myocardial infarction; VTE = venous thromboembolism)

disease, while warfarin and other anticoagulants are favoured in VTE (p. 975) and management of atrial fibrillation (p. 471). In some extremely prothrombotic situations, such as coronary artery stenting, a combination of anticoagulant and antiplatelet drugs is used (p. 491).

A wide range of anticoagulant and antithrombotic drugs is used in clinical practice. These drugs and their modes of action are given in Box 23.26. Newer agents allow predictable anticoagulation without the need for frequent monitoring and dose titration. Although warfarin remains the mainstay for oral anticoagulation, newer oral anticoagulants (dabigatran, rivaroxaban, edoxaban and apixaban), which can be given at fixed doses with predictable effects and no need for monitoring, have now been approved for the prevention of perioperative VTE, the treatment of established VTE and the prevention of cardioembolic stroke in patients with atrial fibrillation.

Heparins

Unfractionated heparin (UFH) and low-molecular-weight heparins (LMWHs) act by binding via a specific pentasaccharide in the heparin molecule to antithrombin. Fondaparinux is a synthetic pentasaccharide, which also binds antithrombin and has similar properties to LMWH. These agents enhance the natural anticoagulant activity of antithrombin (see Fig. 23.6E). Increased cleavage of activated proteases, particularly factor Xa and thrombin (IIa), accounts for the anticoagulant effect. LMWHs preferentially augment antithrombin activity against factor Xa. For the licensed indications, LMWHs are at least as efficacious as UFH but have several advantages:

- LMWHs are nearly 100% bioavailable and so produce reliable dose-dependent anticoagulation.
- LMWHs do not require monitoring of their anticoagulant effect (except possibly in patients with very low body

i 23.26 Modes of action of anticoagulant and antithrombotic drugs

Mode of action	Drug
Antiplatelet drugs	
Cyclo-oxygenase (COX) inhibition	Aspirin
Adenosine diphosphate (ADP) receptor inhibition	Clopidogrel Prasugrel Ticagrelor
Glycoprotein IIb/IIIa inhibition	Abciximab Tirofiban Eptifibatide
Phosphodiesterase inhibition	Dipyridamole
Oral anticoagulants	
Vitamin K antagonism	Warfarin/coumarins
Direct thrombin inhibition	Dabigatran
Direct Xa inhibition	Rivaroxaban Apixaban Edoxaban
Injectable anticoagulants	
Antithrombin-dependent inhibition of thrombin and Xa	Heparin LMWH
Antithrombin-dependent inhibition of Xa	Fondaparinux Danaparoid
Direct thrombin inhibition	Argatroban Bivalirudin

weight and with a glomerular filtration rate below 30 mL/min).

- LMWHs have a half-life of around 4 hours when given subcutaneously, compared with 1 hour for UFH. This permits once-daily dosing by the subcutaneous route, rather than the therapeutic continuous intravenous infusion or twice-daily subcutaneous administration required for UFH.
- While rates of bleeding are similar between products, the risk of osteoporosis and heparin-induced thrombocytopenia is much lower for LMWH.

UFH is, however, more completely reversed by protamine sulphate in the event of bleeding and at the end of cardiopulmonary bypass, for which UFH remains the drug of choice (Box 23.27).

LMWHs are widely used for the prevention and treatment of VTE, the management of acute coronary syndromes and for most other scenarios listed in Box 23.25. In some situations, UFH is still favoured by some clinicians, though there is little evidence that it is advantageous, except when rapid reversibility is required. UFH is useful in patients with a high risk of bleeding, e.g. those who have peptic ulceration or who may require urgent surgery. It is also favoured in the treatment of life-threatening thromboembolism, e.g. major pulmonary embolism with significant hypoxaemia, hypotension and right-sided heart strain. In this situation, UFH is started with a loading intravenous dose of 80 U/kg, followed by a continuous infusion of 18 U/kg/hr initially. The level of anticoagulation should be assessed by the APTT after 6 hours and, if satisfactory, twice daily thereafter. It is usual to aim for a patient APTT that is 1.5–2.5 times the control time of the test. Monitoring of UFH treatment by APTT is not without difficulties and other assays, such as the specific anti-Xa assay, may provide more accurate guidance.

Heparin-induced thrombocytopenia

Heparin-induced thrombocytopenia (HIT) is a rare complication of heparin therapy, caused by induction of anti-heparin/PF4 antibodies that bind to and activate platelets via an Fc receptor. This results in platelet activation and a prothrombotic state, with a paradoxical thrombocytopenia. HIT is more common in surgical than medical patients (especially cardiac and orthopaedic patients), with use of UFH rather than LMWH, and with higher doses of heparin.

Clinical features

Patients present, typically 5–14 days after starting heparin treatment, with a fall in platelet count of more than 30% from baseline. The count may still be in the reference range. The patient may be asymptomatic, or develop venous or arterial thrombosis and skin lesions, including overt skin necrosis. Affected patients may complain of pain or itch at injection sites and of systemic symptoms, such as shivering, following heparin injections. Patients who have received heparin in the preceding 100 days and who have preformed antibodies may develop acute systemic symptoms and an abrupt fall in platelet count in the first 24 hours after re-exposure.

Investigations

The pre-test probability of the diagnosis is assessed using the 4Ts scoring system. This assigns a score based on:
- the **t**hrombocytopenia
- the **t**iming of the fall in platelet count
- the presence of new **t**hrombosis
- the likelihood of ano**t**her cause for the thrombocytopenia.

Individuals at low risk need no further test. Those with intermediate and high likelihood scores should have the diagnosis confirmed or refuted using an anti-PF4 enzyme-linked immunosorbent assay (ELISA).

Management

Heparin should be discontinued as soon as HIT is diagnosed and an alternative anticoagulant that does not cross-react with the antibody should be substituted. Argatroban (a direct thrombin inhibitor) and danaparoid (a heparin analogue) are licensed for use in the UK. In asymptomatic patients with HIT who do not receive an alternative anticoagulant, around 50% will sustain a thrombosis in the subsequent 30 days. Patients with established thrombosis have a poorer prognosis.

Coumarins

Although several coumarin anticoagulants are used around the world, warfarin is the most common.

Coumarins inhibit the vitamin K-dependent post-translational carboxylation of factors II (prothrombin), VII, IX and X in the liver (see Fig. 23.6D). This results in anticoagulation due to an effective deficiency of these factors. This is monitored by the INR, a standardised test based on measurement of the prothrombin time (p. 922). Recommended target INR values for specific indications are given in Box 23.25.

Warfarin anticoagulation typically takes more than 3–5 days to become established, even using loading doses. Patients who require rapid initiation of therapy may receive higher initiation doses of warfarin. A typical regime in this situation is to give 10 mg warfarin on the first and second days, with 5 mg on the third day; subsequent doses are titrated against the INR. Patients without an urgent need for anticoagulation (e.g. atrial fibrillation) can have warfarin introduced slowly using lower doses. Low-dose regimens are associated with a lower risk of the patient developing a supratherapeutic INR, and hence a lower bleeding risk. The duration of warfarin therapy depends on the clinical indication, and while treatment of deep vein thrombosis (DVT) or preparation for cardioversion may require a limited duration, anticoagulation to prevent cardioembolic stroke in atrial fibrillation or from heart valve disease is long-term.

The major problems with warfarin are:
- a narrow therapeutic window
- metabolism that is affected by many factors
- numerous drug interactions.

23

23.28 How to assess risks of anticoagulation

Contraindications

- Recent surgery, especially to eye or central nervous system
- Pre-existing haemorrhagic state, e.g. advanced liver disease, haemophilia, thrombocytopenia
- Pre-existing structural lesions, e.g. peptic ulcer
- Recent cerebral or gastrointestinal haemorrhage
- Uncontrolled hypertension
- Cognitive impairment
- Frequent falls

Bleeding risk score

- Several bleeding risk scores exist for different indications for anticoagulation
- The validation of most bleeding risk scores has been poor
- Many risk factors for thrombosis are also risk factors for bleeding
- Following anticoagulant-related bleeding, reassessment of bleeding and thrombosis risk is indicated
- In many cases, patients benefit from recommencing anticoagulants after bleeding

Drug interactions are common through protein binding and metabolism by the cytochrome P450 system. Inter-individual differences in warfarin doses required to achieve a therapeutic INR are mostly accounted for by naturally occurring polymorphisms in the *CYP2C9* and the *VKORC1* genes (which predict the metabolism and function of warfarin, respectively) and dietary intake of vitamin K.

Major bleeding is the most common serious side-effect of warfarin and occurs in 1–2% of patients each year. Fatal haemorrhage, which is most commonly intracranial, occurs in about 0.25% per annum. There are scoring systems that predict the annual bleeding risk and these can be used to help compare the risks and benefits of warfarin for an individual patient (Box 23.28). There are also some specific contraindications to anticoagulation (Box 23.28). Management of warfarin includes strategies for over-anticoagulation and for bleeding:

- If the INR is above the therapeutic level, warfarin should be withheld or the dose reduced. If the patient is not bleeding, it may be appropriate to give a small dose of vitamin K either orally or intravenously (1–2.5 mg), especially if the INR is greater than 8.
- In the event of bleeding, withhold further warfarin. Minor bleeding can be treated with 1–2.5 mg of vitamin K IV. Major haemorrhage should be treated as an emergency with vitamin K 5–10 mg slowly IV, combined with coagulation factor replacement (see Box 23.27). This should optimally be a prothrombin complex concentrate (30–50 U/kg) that contains factors II, VII, IX and X; if that is not available, fresh frozen plasma (15–30 mL/kg) should be given.

Direct oral anticoagulants

The direct oral anticoagulants (DOACs) offer an alternative to coumarins in the management of VTE and the prevention of stroke and systemic embolism in patients with atrial fibrillation. The DOACs are direct specific inhibitors of key proteases in the common pathway. Dabigatran inhibits thrombin while rivaroxaban, apixaban and edoxaban inhibit Xa. The key features of these drugs include the fact that they are efficacious in fixed oral doses, have a short half-life of around 10 hours, achieve peak plasma levels

2–4 hours after oral intake, have very few drug interactions and are all moderately dependent on renal function for their excretion. An initial perceived drawback was the lack of specific reversal agents for these drugs but idarucizumab is a monoclonal antibody now available for the reversal of dabigatran, and andexanet alfa, a site-inactivated Xa molecule, is close to licensing for the reversal of apixaban and rivaroxaban (see Box 23.27).

DOACs are now licensed for the prevention of VTE following high-risk orthopaedic surgery (except edoxaban), the acute management and prevention of recurrence of VTE, and the prevention of stroke and systemic embolism in patients with atrial fibrillation with risk factors. The general perception at present is that in these indications they are at least as efficacious as dose-adjusted coumarin and probably associated with less clinically significant bleeding.

Anaemias

Around 30% of the total world population is anaemic and half of these, some 600 million people, have iron deficiency. The classification of anaemia by the size of the red cells (MCV) indicates the likely cause (see Figs 23.10 and 23.11).

Red cells in the bone marrow must acquire a minimum level of haemoglobin before being released into the blood stream (Fig. 23.17). While in the marrow compartment, red cell precursors undergo cell division, driven by erythropoietin. If red cells cannot acquire haemoglobin at a normal rate, they will undergo more divisions than normal and will have a low MCV when finally released into the blood. The MCV is low because component parts of the haemoglobin molecule are not fully available: that is, iron in iron deficiency, globin chains in thalassaemia, haem ring in congenital sideroblastic anaemia and, occasionally, poor iron utilisation in the anaemia of chronic disease/anaemia of inflammation.

In megaloblastic anaemia, the biochemical consequence of vitamin B_{12} or folate deficiency is an inability to synthesise new bases to make DNA. A similar defect of cell division is seen in the presence of cytotoxic drugs or haematological disease in the marrow, such as myelodysplasia. In these states, cells haemoglobinise normally but undergo fewer cell divisions, resulting in circulating red cells with a raised MCV. The red cell membrane is composed of a lipid bilayer that will freely exchange with the plasma pool of lipid. Conditions such as liver disease, hypothyroidism, hyperlipidaemia and pregnancy are associated with raised lipids and may also cause a raised MCV. Reticulocytes are larger than mature red cells, so when the reticulocyte count is raised – e.g. in haemolysis – this may also increase the MCV.

Iron deficiency anaemia

This occurs when iron losses or physiological requirements exceed absorption.

Blood loss

The most common explanation in men and post-menopausal women is gastrointestinal blood loss (p. 780). This may result from occult gastric or colorectal malignancy, gastritis, peptic ulceration, inflammatory bowel disease, diverticulitis, polyps and angiodysplastic lesions. Worldwide, hookworm and schistosomiasis are the most common causes of gut blood loss (pp. 288 and 294). Gastrointestinal blood loss may be exacerbated

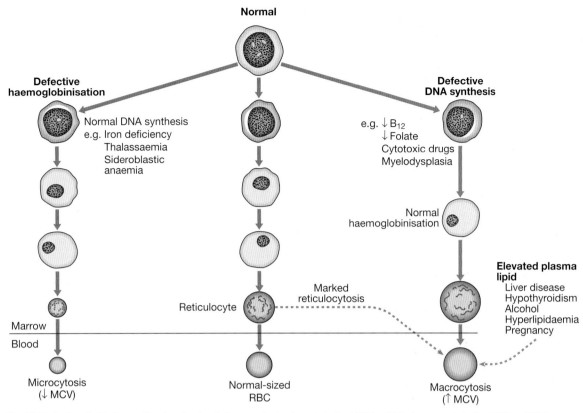

Normal

Defective haemoglobinisation

Normal DNA synthesis
e.g. Iron deficiency
Thalassaemia
Sideroblastic anaemia

Defective DNA synthesis

e.g. ↓ B$_{12}$
↓ Folate
Cytotoxic drugs
Myelodysplasia

Normal haemoglobinisation

Elevated plasma lipid
Liver disease
Hypothyroidism
Alcohol
Hyperlipidaemia
Pregnancy

Reticulocyte

Marked reticulocytosis

Marrow

Blood

Microcytosis
(↓ MCV)

Normal-sized RBC

Macrocytosis
(↑ MCV)

Fig. 23.17 Factors that influence the size of red cells in anaemia. In microcytosis, the MCV is <76 fL. In macrocytosis, the MCV is >100 fL. (MCV = mean cell volume; RBC = red blood cell)

by the chronic use of aspirin or non-steroidal anti-inflammatory drugs (NSAIDs), which cause intestinal erosions and impair platelet function. In women of child-bearing age, menstrual blood loss, pregnancy and breastfeeding contribute to iron deficiency by depleting iron stores; in developed countries, one-third of pre-menopausal women have low iron stores but only 3% display iron-deficient haematopoiesis. Very rarely, chronic haemoptysis or haematuria may cause iron deficiency.

Malabsorption

A dietary assessment should be made in all patients to ascertain their iron intake (p. 716). Gastric acid is required to release iron from food and helps to keep iron in the soluble ferrous state (Fig. 23.18). Achlorhydria in the elderly or that due to drugs such as proton pump inhibitors may contribute to the lack of iron availability from the diet, as may previous gastric surgery. Iron is absorbed actively in the upper small intestine and hence can be affected by coeliac disease (p. 805).

Physiological demands

At times of rapid growth, such as infancy and puberty, iron requirements increase and may outstrip absorption. In pregnancy, iron is diverted to the fetus, the placenta and the increased maternal red cell mass, and is lost with bleeding at parturition (Box 23.29).

Investigations

Confirmation of iron deficiency

Serum ferritin is a measure of iron stores in tissues and is the best single test to confirm iron deficiency (Box 23.30). It is a

23.29 Haematological physiology in pregnancy

- **Full blood count**: increased plasma volume (40%) lowers normal haemoglobin (reference range reduced to >105 g/L at 28 weeks). The mean cell volume (MCV) may increase by 5 fL. A progressive neutrophilia occurs. Gestational thrombocytopenia (rarely <60×10^9/L) is a benign phenomenon.
- **Depletion of iron stores**: iron deficiency is a common cause of anaemia in pregnancy and, if present, should be treated with oral iron supplement.
- **Vitamin B$_{12}$**: serum levels are physiologically low in pregnancy but deficiency is uncommon.
- **Folate**: tissue stores may become depleted, and folate supplementation is recommended in all pregnancies (see Box 19.29, p. 712).
- **Coagulation factors**: from the second trimester, procoagulant factors increase approximately threefold, particularly fibrinogen, von Willebrand factor and factor VIII. This causes activated protein C resistance and a shortened activated partial thromboplastin time (APTT), and contributes to a prothrombotic state.
- **Anticoagulants**: levels of protein C increase from the second trimester, while levels of free protein S fall as C4b binding protein increases.

23

very specific test; a subnormal level is due to iron deficiency or, very rarely, hypothyroidism or vitamin C deficiency. Ferritin levels can be raised in liver disease and in the acute phase response; in these conditions, a ferritin level of up to 100 μg/L may still be compatible with low bone marrow iron stores.

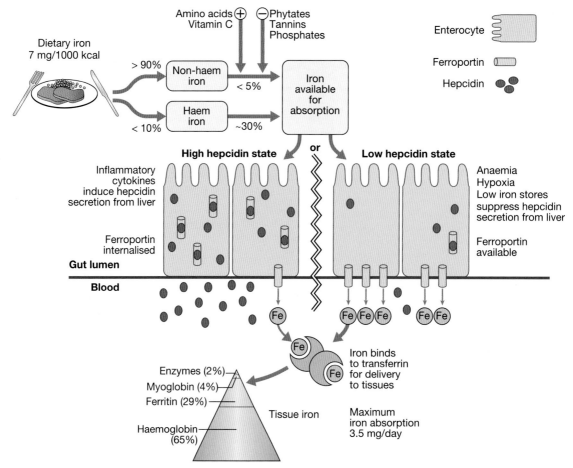

Fig. 23.18 The regulation of iron absorption, uptake and distribution in the body. The transport of iron is regulated in a similar fashion to enterocytes in other iron-transporting cells such as macrophages.

i | **23.30 Investigations to differentiate anaemia of chronic disease from iron deficiency anaemia**

	Ferritin	Iron	TIBC	Transferrin saturation	Soluble transferrin receptor
Iron deficiency anaemia	↓	↓	↑	↓	↑
Anaemia of chronic disease	↑/Normal	↓	↓	↓	↓/Normal

(TIBC = total iron binding capacity)

Plasma iron and total iron binding capacity (TIBC) are measures of iron availability; hence they are affected by many factors besides iron stores. Plasma iron has a marked diurnal and day-to-day variation and becomes very low during an acute phase response but is raised in liver disease and haemolysis. Levels of transferrin, the binding protein for iron, are lowered by malnutrition, liver disease, the acute phase response and nephrotic syndrome, but raised by pregnancy and the oral contraceptive pill. A transferrin saturation (i.e. iron/TIBC×100) of less than 16% is consistent with iron deficiency but is less specific than a ferritin measurement.

All proliferating cells express membrane transferrin receptors to acquire iron; a small amount of this receptor is shed into blood, where it can be detected in a free soluble form. At times of poor iron stores, cells up-regulate transferrin receptor expression and the levels of soluble plasma transferrin receptor increase. This can now be measured by immunoassay and used to distinguish storage iron depletion in the presence of an acute phase response or liver disease, when a raised level indicates iron deficiency. In difficult cases, it may still be necessary to examine a bone marrow aspirate for iron stores.

Investigation of the cause

This will depend on the age and sex of the patient, as well as the history and clinical findings. In men and in post-menopausal women with a normal diet, the upper and lower gastrointestinal tract should be investigated by endoscopy or radiological studies. Serum anti-transglutaminase antibodies and possibly a duodenal biopsy are indicated (p. 806) to detect coeliac disease. Current guidelines suggest exclusion of coeliac disease by antibody testing at an early stage of investigation. In the tropics, stool and urine should be examined for parasites (p. 233).

Management

Unless the patient has angina, heart failure or evidence of cerebral hypoxia, transfusion is not necessary and oral iron replacement is appropriate. Ferrous sulphate 200 mg 3 times daily (195 mg of elemental iron per day) is adequate and should be continued for 3–6 months to replete iron stores. Many patients suffer gastrointestinal side-effects with ferrous sulphate, including dyspepsia and altered bowel habit. When this occurs, reduction in dose to 200 mg twice daily or a switch to ferrous gluconate 300 mg twice daily (70 mg of elemental iron per day) or another alternative oral preparation should be tried. Delayed-release preparations are not useful, since they release iron beyond the upper small intestine, where it cannot be absorbed.

The haemoglobin should rise by around 10 g/L every 7–10 days and a reticulocyte response will be evident within a week. A failure to respond adequately may be due to non-adherence, continued blood loss, malabsorption or an incorrect diagnosis. Patients with malabsorption, chronic gut disease or inability to tolerate any oral preparation may need parenteral iron therapy. Previously, iron dextran or iron sucrose was used, but new preparations of iron isomaltose and iron carboxymaltose have fewer allergic effects and are preferred. Doses required can be calculated based on the patient's starting haemoglobin and body weight. Observation for anaphylaxis following an initial test dose is recommended.

Anaemia of chronic disease

Anaemia of chronic disease (ACD), also known as anaemia of inflammation (AI), is a common type of anaemia, particularly in hospital populations. It occurs in the setting of chronic infection, chronic inflammation or neoplasia. The anaemia is not related to bleeding, haemolysis or marrow infiltration, is mild, with haemoglobin in the range of 85–115 g/L, and is usually associated with a normal MCV (normocytic, normochromic), though this may be reduced in long-standing inflammation. The serum iron is low but iron stores are normal or increased, as indicated by the ferritin or stainable marrow iron.

Pathogenesis

It has recently become clear that the key regulatory protein that accounts for the findings characteristic of ACD/AI is hepcidin, which is produced by the liver (see Fig. 23.18). Hepcidin production is induced by pro-inflammatory cytokines, especially IL-6. Hepcidin binds to ferroportin on the membrane of iron-exporting cells, such as small intestinal enterocytes and macrophages, internalising the ferroportin and thereby inhibiting the export of iron from these cells into the blood. The iron remains trapped inside the cells in the form of ferritin, levels of which are therefore normal or high in the face of significant anaemia. Inhibition or blockade of hepcidin is a potential target for treatment of this form of anaemia.

Diagnosis and management

It is often difficult to distinguish ACD associated with a low MCV from iron deficiency. Box 23.30 summarises the investigations and results. Examination of the marrow may ultimately be required to assess iron stores directly. A trial of oral iron can be given in difficult situations. A positive response occurs in true iron deficiency but not in ACD. Measures that reduce the severity of the underlying disorder generally help to improve the ACD. Trials of higher-dose intravenous iron are under way to try to bypass the hepcidin-induced blockade.

Megaloblastic anaemia

This results from a deficiency of vitamin B_{12} or folic acid, or from disturbances in folic acid metabolism. Folate is an important substrate of, and vitamin B_{12} a co-factor for, the generation of the essential amino acid methionine from homocysteine. This reaction produces tetrahydrofolate, which is converted to thymidine monophosphate for incorporation into DNA. Deficiency of either vitamin B_{12} or folate will therefore produce high plasma levels of homocysteine and impaired DNA synthesis.

The end result is cells with arrested nuclear maturation but normal cytoplasmic development: so-called nucleocytoplasmic asynchrony. All proliferating cells will exhibit megaloblastosis; hence changes are evident in the buccal mucosa, tongue, small intestine, cervix, vagina and uterus. The high proliferation rate of bone marrow results in striking changes in the haematopoietic system in megaloblastic anaemia. Cells become arrested in development and die within the marrow; this ineffective erythropoiesis results in an expanded hypercellular marrow. The megaloblastic changes are most evident in the early nucleated red cell precursors, and haemolysis within the marrow results in a raised bilirubin and lactate dehydrogenase (LDH), but without the reticulocytosis characteristic of other forms of haemolysis (p. 945). Iron stores are usually raised. The mature red cells are large and oval, and sometimes contain nuclear remnants. Nuclear changes are seen in the immature granulocyte precursors and a characteristic appearance is that of 'giant' metamyelocytes with a large 'sausage-shaped' nucleus. The mature neutrophils show hypersegmentation of their nuclei, with cells having six or more nuclear lobes. If severe, a pancytopenia may be present in the peripheral blood.

Vitamin B_{12} deficiency, but not folate deficiency, is associated with neurological disease in up to 40% of cases, although advanced neurological disease due to B_{12} deficiency is now uncommon in the developed world. The main pathological finding is focal demyelination affecting the spinal cord, peripheral nerves, optic nerves and cerebrum. The most common manifestations are sensory, with peripheral paraesthesiae and ataxia of gait. The clinical and diagnostic features of megaloblastic anaemia are summarised in Boxes 23.31 and 23.32, and the neurological features of B_{12} deficiency in Box 23.33.

Vitamin B_{12}

Vitamin B_{12} absorption

The average daily diet contains 5–30 µg of vitamin B_{12}, mainly in meat, fish, eggs and milk – well in excess of the 1 µg daily

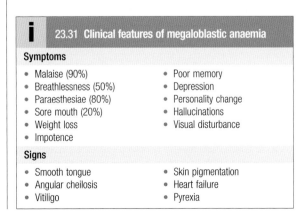

i	**23.31 Clinical features of megaloblastic anaemia**

Symptoms
- Malaise (90%)
- Breathlessness (50%)
- Paraesthesiae (80%)
- Sore mouth (20%)
- Weight loss
- Impotence
- Poor memory
- Depression
- Personality change
- Hallucinations
- Visual disturbance

Signs
- Smooth tongue
- Angular cheilosis
- Vitiligo
- Skin pigmentation
- Heart failure
- Pyrexia

23

23.32 Investigations in megaloblastic anaemia

Investigation	Result
Haemoglobin	Often reduced, may be very low
Mean cell volume	Usually raised, commonly >120 fL
Erythrocyte count	Low for degree of anaemia
Blood film	Oval macrocytosis, poikilocytosis, red cell fragmentation, neutrophil hypersegmentation
Reticulocyte count	Low for degree of anaemia
Leucocyte count	Low or normal
Platelet count	Low or normal
Bone marrow	Increased cellularity, megaloblastic changes in erythroid series, giant metamyelocytes, dysplastic megakaryocytes, increased iron in stores, pathological non-ring sideroblasts
Serum ferritin	Elevated
Plasma lactate dehydrogenase	Elevated, often markedly

23.33 Neurological findings in B₁₂ deficiency

Peripheral nerves
- Glove and stocking paraesthesiae
- Loss of ankle reflexes

Spinal cord
- Subacute combined degeneration of the cord
  - Posterior columns – diminished vibration sensation and proprioception
  - Corticospinal tracts – upper motor neuron signs

Cerebrum
- Dementia
- Optic atrophy

Autonomic neuropathy

requirement. In the stomach, gastric enzymes release vitamin B_{12} from food and at gastric pH it binds to a carrier protein termed R protein. The gastric parietal cells produce intrinsic factor, a vitamin B_{12}-binding protein that optimally binds vitamin B_{12} at pH 8. As gastric emptying occurs, pancreatic secretion raises the pH and vitamin B_{12} released from the diet switches from the R protein to intrinsic factor. Bile also contains vitamin B_{12} that is available for reabsorption in the intestine. The vitamin B_{12}–intrinsic factor complex binds to specific receptors in the terminal ileum, and vitamin B_{12} is actively transported by the enterocytes to plasma, where it binds to transcobalamin II, a transport protein produced by the liver, which carries it to the tissues for utilisation. The liver stores enough vitamin B_{12} for 3 years and this, together with the enterohepatic circulation, means that vitamin B_{12} deficiency takes years to become manifest, even if all dietary intake is stopped or severe B_{12} malabsorption supervenes.

Blood levels of vitamin B_{12} (cobalamin) provide a reasonable indication of tissue stores, are usually diagnostic of deficiency and remain the first-line tests for most laboratories. Additional tests have been evaluated, including measurement of methylmalonic acid, holotranscobalamin and plasma homocysteine levels, but do not add much in most clinical situations. Levels of cobalamins fall in normal pregnancy. Reference ranges vary between laboratories but levels below 150 ng/L are common and, in the last trimester, 5–10% of women have levels below 100 ng/L. Spuriously low B_{12} values occur in women using the oral contraceptive pill and in patients with myeloma, in whom paraproteins can interfere with vitamin B_{12} assays.

Causes of vitamin B₁₂ deficiency

Dietary deficiency

This occurs only in strict vegans but the onset of clinical features can occur at any age between 10 and 80 years. Less strict vegetarians often have slightly low vitamin B_{12} levels but are not tissue vitamin B_{12}-deficient.

Gastric pathology

Release of vitamin B_{12} from food requires normal gastric acid and enzyme secretion, and this is impaired by hypochlorhydria in elderly patients or following gastric surgery. Total gastrectomy invariably results in vitamin B_{12} deficiency within 5 years, often combined with iron deficiency; these patients need life-long 3-monthly vitamin B_{12} injections. After partial gastrectomy, vitamin B_{12} deficiency only develops in 10–20% of patients by 5 years; an annual injection of vitamin B_{12} should prevent deficiency in this group.

Pernicious anaemia

This is an organ-specific autoimmune disorder in which the gastric mucosa is atrophic, with loss of parietal cells causing intrinsic factor deficiency. In the absence of intrinsic factor, less than 1% of dietary vitamin B_{12} is absorbed. Pernicious anaemia has an incidence of 25/100 000 population over the age of 40 years in developed countries, but an average age of onset of 60 years. It is more common in individuals with other autoimmune disease (Hashimoto's thyroiditis, Graves' disease, vitiligo or Addison's disease; Ch. 18) or a family history of these or pernicious anaemia. The finding of anti-intrinsic factor antibodies in the context of B_{12} deficiency is diagnostic of pernicious anaemia without further investigation. Antiparietal cell antibodies are present in over 90% of cases but are also present in 20% of normal females over the age of 60 years; a negative result makes pernicious anaemia less likely but a positive result is not diagnostic. The Schilling test, involving measurement of absorption of radio-labelled B_{12} after oral administration before and after replacement of intrinsic factor, has fallen out of favour with the availability of autoantibody tests, greater caution in the use of radioactive tracers, and limited availability of intrinsic factor.

Small bowel pathology

One-third of patients with pancreatic exocrine insufficiency fail to transfer dietary vitamin B_{12} from R protein to intrinsic factor. This usually results in slightly low vitamin B_{12} values but no tissue evidence of vitamin B_{12} deficiency.

Motility disorders or hypogammaglobulinaemia can result in bacterial overgrowth, and the ensuing competition for free vitamin B_{12} can lead to deficiency. This is corrected to some extent by appropriate antibiotics.

A small number of people heavily infected with the fish tapeworm (p. 297) develop vitamin B_{12} deficiency.

Inflammatory disease of the terminal ileum, such as Crohn's disease, may impair the absorption of vitamin B_{12}–intrinsic factor complex, as may surgery on that part of the bowel.

Folate

Folate absorption

Folates are produced by plants and bacteria; hence dietary leafy vegetables (spinach, broccoli, lettuce), fruits (bananas, melons) and animal protein (liver, kidney) are a rich source. An average Western diet contains more than the minimum daily intake of 50 μg but excess cooking destroys folates. Most dietary folate is present as polyglutamates; these are converted to monoglutamate in the upper small bowel and actively transported into plasma. Plasma folate is loosely bound to plasma proteins such as albumin and there is an enterohepatic circulation. Total body stores of folate are small and deficiency can occur in a matter of weeks.

Folate deficiency

The causes and diagnostic features of folate deficiency are shown in Boxes 23.34 and 23.35. The edentulous elderly or psychiatric patient is particularly susceptible to dietary deficiency and this is exacerbated in the presence of gut disease or malignancy. Pregnancy-induced folate deficiency is the most common cause of megaloblastosis worldwide and is more likely in the context of twin pregnancies, multiparity and hyperemesis gravidarum. Serum folate measurement is very sensitive to dietary intake; a single folate-rich meal can normalise it in a patient with true folate deficiency, whereas anorexia, alcohol and anticonvulsant therapy can reduce it in the absence of megaloblastosis. For this reason, red cell folate levels are a more accurate indicator of folate stores and tissue folate deficiency.

Management of megaloblastic anaemia

If a patient with a severe megaloblastic anaemia is very ill and treatment must be started before vitamin B_{12} and red cell folate

23.34 Causes of folate deficiency

Diet
- Poor intake of vegetables

Malabsorption
- e.g. Coeliac disease, small bowel surgery

Increased demand
- Cell proliferation, e.g. haemolysis
- Pregnancy

Drugs*
- Certain anticonvulsants (e.g. phenytoin)
- Contraceptive pill
- Certain cytotoxic drugs (e.g. methotrexate)

*Usually only a problem in patients deficient in folate from another cause.

23.35 Investigation of folic acid deficiency

Diagnostic findings
- Serum folate levels may be low but are difficult to interpret
- Low red cell folate levels indicate prolonged folate deficiency and are probably the most relevant measure

Corroborative findings
- Macrocytic dysplastic blood picture
- Megaloblastic marrow

results are available, that treatment should always include both folic acid and vitamin B_{12}. The use of folic acid alone in the presence of vitamin B_{12} deficiency may result in worsening of neurological features.

Rarely, if severe angina or heart failure is present, transfusion can be used in megaloblastic anaemia. The cardiovascular system is adapted to the chronic anaemia present in megaloblastosis, and the volume load imposed by transfusion may result in decompensation and severe cardiac failure. In such circumstances, exchange transfusion or slow administration of 1 U of red cells with diuretic cover may be given.

Vitamin B_{12} deficiency

Vitamin B_{12} deficiency is treated with hydroxycobalamin. In cases of uncomplicated deficiency, 1000 μg IM for 6 doses 2 or 3 days apart, followed by maintenance therapy of 1000 μg every 3 months for life, is recommended. In the presence of neurological involvement, a dose of 1000 μg on alternate days until there is no further improvement, followed by maintenance as above, is recommended. The reticulocyte count will peak by the 5th–10th day after starting replacement therapy. The haemoglobin will rise by 10 g/L every week until normalised. The response of the marrow is associated with a fall in plasma potassium levels and rapid depletion of iron stores. If an initial response is not maintained and the blood film is dimorphic (i.e. shows a mixture of microcytic and macrocytic cells), the patient may need additional iron therapy. A sensory neuropathy may take 6–12 months to correct; long-standing neurological damage may not improve.

Folate deficiency

Oral folic acid (5 mg daily for 3 weeks) will treat acute deficiency and 5 mg once weekly is adequate maintenance therapy. Prophylactic folic acid in pregnancy prevents megaloblastosis in women at risk, and reduces the risk of fetal neural tube defects (p. 712). Prophylactic supplementation is also given in chronic haematological disease associated with reduced red cell lifespan (e.g. haemolytic anaemias). There is some evidence that supraphysiological supplementation (400 μg/day) can reduce the risk of coronary and cerebrovascular disease by lowering plasma homocysteine levels. This has led the US Food and Drug Administration to introduce fortification of bread, flour and rice with folic acid.

Haemolytic anaemia

Haemolysis indicates that there is shortening of the normal red cell lifespan of 120 days. There are many causes, as shown in Figure 23.19. To compensate, the bone marrow may increase its output of red cells six- to eightfold by increasing the proportion of red cells produced, expanding the volume of active marrow, and releasing reticulocytes prematurely. Anaemia occurs only if the rate of destruction exceeds this increased production rate.

There are some general features of haemolysis and other specific features that help to identify the reason for haemolysis. Results of investigations that establish the presence of haemolysis are shown in Box 23.36. Red cell destruction overloads pathways for haemoglobin breakdown in the liver (p. 850), causing a modest rise in unconjugated bilirubin in the blood and mild jaundice. Increased reabsorption of urobilinogen from the gut results in an increase in urinary urobilinogen (pp. 860 and 915). Red cell destruction releases LDH into the serum. The bone

23

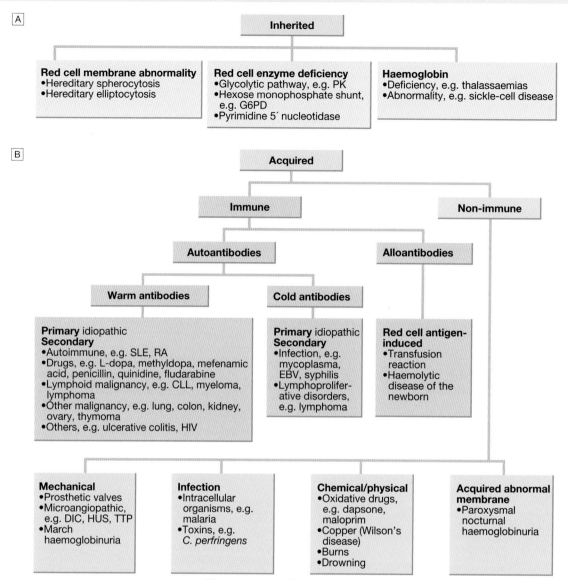

Fig. 23.19 **Causes and classification of haemolysis.** A Inherited causes. B Acquired causes. (CLL = chronic lymphocytic leukaemia; DIC = disseminated intravascular coagulation; EBV = Epstein–Barr virus; G6PD = glucose-6-phosphate dehydrogenase; HUS = haemolytic uraemic syndrome; PK = pyruvate kinase; RA = rheumatoid arthritis; SLE = systemic lupus erythematosus; TTP = thrombotic thrombocytopenic purpura)

marrow compensation results in a reticulocytosis, and sometimes nucleated red cell precursors appear in the blood. Increased proliferation of the bone marrow can result in a thrombocytosis, neutrophilia and, if marked, immature granulocytes in the blood, producing a leucoerythroblastic blood film. The appearances of

the red cells may give an indication of the likely cause of the haemolysis:

- Spherocytes are small, dark red cells that suggest autoimmune haemolysis or hereditary spherocytosis.
- Sickle cells suggest sickle-cell disease.
- Red cell fragments indicate microangiopathic haemolysis.
- Bite cells (normal-sized red cells that look as if they have been partially eaten) suggest oxidative haemolysis.

The compensatory erythroid hyperplasia may give rise to folate deficiency, with megaloblastic blood features.

The differential diagnosis of haemolysis is determined by the clinical scenario in combination with the results of blood film examination and Coombs testing for antibodies directed against red cells (see below and Fig. 23.19).

Extravascular haemolysis

Physiological red cell destruction occurs in the reticulo-endothelial cells in the liver or spleen, so avoiding free haemoglobin in the plasma. In most haemolytic states, haemolysis is predominantly extravascular.

To confirm the haemolysis, patients' red cells can be labelled with [51]chromium. When re-injected, they can be used to determine red cell survival; when combined with body surface radioactivity counting, this test may indicate whether the liver or the spleen is the main source of red cell destruction. However, it is seldom performed in clinical practice.

Intravascular haemolysis

Less commonly, red cell lysis occurs within the blood stream due to membrane damage by complement (ABO transfusion reactions, paroxysmal nocturnal haemoglobinuria), infections (malaria, *Clostridium perfringens*), mechanical trauma (heart valves, DIC) or oxidative damage (e.g. enzymopathies such as glucose-6-phosphate dehydrogenase deficiency, which may be triggered by drugs such as dapsone and maloprim). When intravascular red cell destruction occurs, free haemoglobin is released into the plasma. Free haemoglobin is toxic to cells and binding proteins have evolved to minimise this risk. Haptoglobin is an α_2-globulin produced by the liver, which binds free haemoglobin, resulting in a fall in its levels during active haemolysis. Once haptoglobins are saturated, free haemoglobin is oxidised to form methaemoglobin, which binds to albumin, in turn forming methaemalbumin, which can be detected spectrophotometrically in Schumm's test. Methaemoglobin is degraded and any free haem is bound to a second binding protein called haemopexin. If all the protective mechanisms are saturated, free haemoglobin may appear in the urine (haemoglobinuria). When fulminant, this gives rise to black urine, as in severe *falciparum* malaria infection (p. 274). In smaller amounts, renal tubular cells absorb the haemoglobin, degrade it and store the iron as haemosiderin. When the tubular cells are subsequently sloughed into the urine, they give rise to haemosiderinuria, which is always indicative of intravascular haemolysis (Box 23.36).

Causes of haemolytic anaemia

These can be classified as inherited or acquired (Fig. 23.19).

- *Inherited* red cell abnormalities resulting in chronic haemolytic anaemia may arise from pathologies of the red cell membrane (hereditary spherocytosis or elliptocytosis), haemoglobin (haemoglobinopathies), or protective enzymes that prevent cellular oxidative damage, such as glucose-6-phosphate dehydrogenase (G6PD).
- *Acquired* causes include auto- and alloantibody-mediated destruction of red blood cells and other mechanical, toxic and infective causes.

Red cell membrane defects

The structure of the red cell membrane is shown in Figure 23.4. The basic structure is a cytoskeleton 'stapled' on to the lipid bilayer by special protein complexes. This structure ensures great deformability and elasticity; the red cell diameter is 8 μm but the narrowest capillaries in the circulation are in the spleen, measuring just 2 μm in diameter. When the normal red cell structure is disturbed, usually by a quantitative or functional deficiency of one or more proteins in the cytoskeleton, cells lose their elasticity. Each time such cells pass through the spleen, they lose membrane relative to their cell volume. This results in an increase in mean cell haemoglobin concentration (MCHC), abnormal cell shape (see Box 23.2) and reduced red cell survival due to extravascular haemolysis.

Hereditary spherocytosis

This is usually inherited as an autosomal dominant condition, although 25% of cases have no family history and represent new mutations. The incidence is approximately 1:5000 in developed countries but this may be an under-estimate, since the disease may present de novo in patients aged over 65 years and is often discovered as a chance finding on a blood count. The most common abnormalities are deficiencies of beta spectrin or ankyrin (see Fig. 23.4). The severity of spontaneous haemolysis varies. Most cases are associated with an asymptomatic compensated chronic haemolytic state with spherocytes present on the blood film, a reticulocytosis and mild hyperbilirubinaemia. Pigment gallstones are present in up to 50% of patients and may cause symptomatic cholecystitis. Occasional cases are associated with more severe haemolysis; these may be due to coincidental polymorphisms in alpha spectrin or co-inheritance of a second defect involving a different protein. These cases tend to present earlier in life with symptomatic, sometimes transfusion-dependent anaemia.

The clinical course may be complicated by crises:

- *A haemolytic crisis* occurs when the severity of haemolysis increases; this is rare, and usually associated with infection.
- *A megaloblastic crisis* follows the development of folate deficiency; this may occur as a first presentation of the disease in pregnancy.
- *An aplastic crisis* occurs in association with parvovirus (erythrovirus) infection (p. 237). Parvovirus causes a common exanthem in children, but if individuals with chronic haemolysis become infected, the virus directly invades red cell precursors and temporarily switches off red cell production. Patients present with severe anaemia and a low reticulocyte count.

Investigations

The patient and other family members should be screened for features of compensated haemolysis (see Box 23.36). This may be all that is required to confirm the diagnosis. Haemoglobin levels are variable, depending on the degree of compensation. The blood film will show spherocytes but the direct Coombs test (Fig. 23.20) is negative, excluding immune haemolysis. An osmotic fragility test may show increased sensitivity to lysis in hypotonic saline solutions but is limited by lack of sensitivity and specificity. More specific flow cytometric tests, detecting binding of eosin-5-maleimide to red cells, are recommended in borderline cases.

Management

Folic acid prophylaxis, 5 mg daily, should be given for life. In severe cases, consideration may be given to splenectomy, which improves but does not normalise red cell survival. Potential indications for splenectomy include moderate to severe haemolysis with complications (anaemia and gallstones), although splenectomy should be delayed where possible until after 6 years of age in view of the risk of sepsis. Guidelines for the management of patients after splenectomy are presented in Box 23.37.

Acute, severe haemolytic crises require transfusion support, but blood must be cross-matched carefully and transfused slowly as haemolytic transfusion reactions may occur (p. 935).

Hereditary elliptocytosis

This term refers to a heterogeneous group of disorders that produce an increase in elliptocytic red cells on the blood film and a variable degree of haemolysis. This is due to a functional

A | Direct antiglobulin test (DAT) (Coombs test)

Detects the presence of antibody bound to the red cell surface, e.g.
1. Autoimmune haemolytic anaemia
2. Haemolytic disease of newborn
3. Transfusion reactions

Antibodies to human globulin

Red cell agglutination

Key

Red blood cells
Red cell antigen
Antibody bound to red cell antigen

B | Indirect antiglobulin test (IAT) (indirect Coombs test)

Detects antibodies in the plasma, e.g.
1. Antibody screen in pre-transfusion testing
2. Screening in pregnancy for antibodies that may cause haemolytic disease of newborn

Stage 1

Patient's plasma

Red cells with known antigen expression

Red cells with Ag – Ab complex on cell surface

Stage 2

Antibodies to human globulin

Red cell agglutination

Fig. 23.20 Direct and indirect antiglobulin tests.

---

i   23.37 Management of the splenectomised patient

- Vaccinate with pneumococcal, *Haemophilus influenzae* type B, meningococcal group C and influenza vaccines at least 2–3 weeks before elective splenectomy. Vaccination should be given after emergency surgery but may be less effective
- Pneumococcal re-immunisation should be given at least 5-yearly and influenza annually. Vaccination status must be documented
- Life-long prophylactic penicillin V (500 mg twice daily) is recommended. In penicillin-allergic patients, consider a macrolide
- Patients should be educated regarding the risks of infection and methods of prophylaxis
- A card or bracelet should be carried to alert health professionals to the risk of overwhelming sepsis
- In sepsis, patients should be resuscitated and given IV antibiotics to cover pneumococcus, *Haemophilus* and meningococcus, according to local resistance patterns
- The risk of cerebral malaria is increased in the event of infection
- Animal bites should be promptly treated with local disinfection and antibiotics, to prevent serious soft tissue infection and sepsis

---

abnormality of one or more anchor proteins in the red cell membrane, e.g. alpha spectrin or protein 4.1 (see Fig. 23.4). Inheritance may be autosomal dominant or recessive. Hereditary elliptocytosis is less common than hereditary spherocytosis in Western countries, with an incidence of 1/10 000, but is more common in equatorial Africa and parts of South-east Asia. The clinical course is variable and depends on the degree of membrane dysfunction caused by the inherited molecular defect(s); most cases present as an asymptomatic blood film abnormality but occasional cases result in neonatal haemolysis or a chronic compensated haemolytic state. Management of the latter is the same as for hereditary spherocytosis.

A characteristic variant of hereditary elliptocytosis occurs in South-east Asia, particularly Malaysia and Papua New Guinea, with stomatocytes and ovalocytes in the blood. This has a prevalence of up to 30% in some communities because it offers relative protection from malaria and thus has sustained a high gene frequency. The blood film is often very abnormal and immediate differential diagnosis is broad.

Red cell enzymopathies

The mature red cell must produce energy via ATP to maintain a normal internal environment and cell volume while protecting itself from the oxidative stress presented by oxygen carriage. ATP is generated by glycolysis, while the hexose monophosphate shunt produces nicotinamide adenine dinucleotide phosphate (NADPH) and glutathione to protect against oxidative stress. The impact of functional or quantitative defects in the enzymes in these pathways depends on the importance of the steps affected and the presence of alternative pathways. In general, defects in the hexose monophosphate shunt pathway result in periodic haemolysis precipitated by episodic oxidative stress, while those in the glycolysis pathway result in shortened red cell survival and chronic haemolysis.

Glucose-6-phosphate dehydrogenase deficiency

The enzyme glucose-6-phosphate dehydrogenase (G6PD) is pivotal in the hexose monophosphate shunt pathway. Deficiencies result in the most common human enzymopathy, affecting 10% of the world's population, with a geographical distribution that parallels the malaria belt because heterozygotes are protected from malarial parasitisation. The enzyme is a heteromeric structure made of catalytic subunits that are encoded by a gene on the X chromosome. The deficiency therefore affects males and rare

23.38 Glucose-6-phosphate dehydrogenase deficiency

Clinical features

- Acute drug-induced haemolysis to (e.g.):
    Analgesics: aspirin, phenacetin
    Antimalarials: primaquine, quinine, chloroquine, pyrimethamine
    Antibiotics: sulphonamides, nitrofurantoin, ciprofloxacin
    Miscellaneous: quinidine, probenecid, vitamin K, dapsone
- Chronic compensated haemolysis
- Infection or acute illness
- Neonatal jaundice: may be a feature of the B⁻ enzyme
- Favism, i.e. acute haemolysis after ingestion of broad beans (*Vicia fava*)

Laboratory features

Non-spherocytic intravascular haemolysis during an attack
The blood film will show:
- Bite cells (red cells with a 'bite' of membrane missing)
- Blister cells (red cells with surface blistering of the membrane)
- Irregularly shaped small cells
- Polychromasia reflecting the reticulocytosis
- Denatured haemoglobin visible as Heinz bodies within the red cell cytoplasm with a supravital stain such as methyl violet

G6PD level
- Can be indirectly assessed by screening methods that usually depend on the decreased ability to reduce dyes
- Direct assessment of G6PD is made in those with low screening values
- Care must be taken close to an acute haemolytic episode because reticulocytes may have higher enzyme levels and give rise to a false normal result

homozygous females (p. 48), but it is carried by females. Carrier heterozygous females are usually only affected in the neonatal period or in the presence of skewed X-inactivation (p. 49).

Over 400 subtypes of G6PD are described. The most common types associated with normal activity are the B+ enzyme present in most Caucasians and 70% of Afro-Caribbeans, and the A+ variant present in 20% of Afro-Caribbeans. The two common variants associated with reduced activity are the A⁻ variety in approximately 10% of Afro-Caribbeans, and the Mediterranean or B⁻ variety in Caucasians. In East and West Africa, up to 20% of males and 4% of females (homozygotes) are affected and have enzyme levels of about 15% of normal. The deficiency in Caucasian and East Asian populations is more severe, with enzyme levels as low as 1%.

Clinical features and investigation findings are shown in Box 23.38.

Management aims to stop the intake of any precipitant drugs or foods and treat any underlying infection. Favism due to the consumption of fava beans is the classically described precipitant of haemolysis in patients with G6PD deficiency. Acute transfusion support may be life-saving.

Pyruvate kinase deficiency

This is the second most common red cell enzyme defect. It results in deficiency of ATP production and a chronic haemolytic anaemia. It is inherited as an autosomal recessive trait. The extent of anaemia is variable; the blood film shows characteristic 'prickle cells' that resemble holly leaves. Enzyme activity is only 5–20% of normal. Transfusion support may be necessary during periods of haemolysis.

Pyrimidine 5' nucleotidase deficiency

The pyrimidine 5' nucleotidase enzyme catalyses the dephosphorylation of nucleoside monophosphates and is important during the degradation of RNA in reticulocytes. It is inherited as an autosomal recessive trait and is as common as pyruvate kinase deficiency in Mediterranean, African and Jewish populations. The accumulation of excess ribonucleoprotein results in coarse basophilic stippling (see Box 23.2), associated with a chronic haemolytic state. The enzyme is very sensitive to inhibition by lead and this is the reason why basophilic stippling is a feature of lead poisoning.

Autoimmune haemolytic anaemia

This results from increased red cell destruction due to red cell autoantibodies. The antibodies may be IgG or IgM, or more rarely IgE or IgA. If an antibody avidly fixes complement, it will cause intravascular haemolysis, but if complement activation is weak, the haemolysis will be extravascular (in the reticulo-endothelial system). Antibody-coated red cells lose membrane to macrophages in the spleen and hence spherocytes are present in the blood. The optimum temperature at which the antibody is active (thermal specificity) is used to classify immune haemolysis:

- *Warm antibodies* bind best at 37°C and account for 80% of cases. The majority are IgG and often react against Rhesus antigens.
- *Cold antibodies* bind best at 4°C but can bind up to 37°C in some cases. They are usually IgM and bind complement. To be clinically relevant, they must act within the range of normal body temperatures. They account for the other 20% of cases.

Warm autoimmune haemolysis

The incidence of warm autoimmune haemolysis is approximately 1/100 000 population per annum; it occurs at all ages but is more common in middle age and in females. No underlying cause is identified in up to 50% of cases. The remainder are secondary to a wide variety of other conditions (see Fig. 23.19B).

Investigations

There is evidence of haemolysis, spherocytes and polychromasia on the blood film. The diagnosis is confirmed by the direct Coombs or antiglobulin test (see Fig. 23.20). The patient's red cells are mixed with Coombs reagent, which contains antibodies against human IgG/IgM/complement. If the red cells have been coated by antibody in vivo, the Coombs reagent will induce their agglutination and this can be detected visually. The relevant antibody can be eluted from the red cell surface and tested against a panel of typed red cells to determine against which red cell antigen it is directed. The most common specificity is for Rhesus antigens and most often anti-e; this is helpful when choosing blood to cross-match. The direct Coombs test can be negative in the presence of brisk haemolysis. A positive test requires about 200 antibody molecules to attach to each red cell; with a very avid complement-fixing antibody, haemolysis may occur at lower levels of antibody-binding. The standard Coombs reagent will miss IgA or IgE antibodies. Around 10% of all warm autoimmune haemolytic anaemias are Coombs test-negative.

Management

If the haemolysis is secondary to an underlying cause, this must be treated and any implicated drugs stopped.

23

It is usual to treat patients initially with prednisolone (1 mg/kg orally). A response is seen in 70–80% of cases but may take up to 3 weeks; a rise in haemoglobin will be matched by a fall in bilirubin, LDH and reticulocyte levels. Once the haemoglobin has normalised and the reticulocytosis resolved, the glucocorticoid dose can be reduced slowly over several weeks. Glucocorticoids probably work by decreasing macrophage destruction of antibody-coated red cells and reducing antibody production.

Transfusion support may be required for life-threatening problems, such as the development of heart failure or rapid unabated falls in haemoglobin. The least incompatible blood should be used but this may still give rise to transfusion reactions or the development of alloantibodies.

If the haemolysis fails to respond to glucocorticoids or can only be stabilised by large doses, then second-line therapies should be considered. These include immunomodulation/suppression and splenectomy. Currently, there are fewer splenectomies than previously and the second-line drug of choice in current UK guidance is the anti-CD20 monoclonal antibody rituximab. Splenectomy is associated with a good response in 50–60% of cases. The operation can be performed laparoscopically with reduced morbidity. If splenectomy is not appropriate, alternative immunosuppressive therapy with azathioprine, ciclosporin, mycophenolate or cyclophosphamide may be considered. There are concerns about all modes of second-line therapy, as long-term immunosuppression carries a risk of malignancy, while splenectomy is associated with an excess of severe infection due to the capsulate organisms pneumococcus and meningococcus (see Box 23.40).

Cold agglutinin disease

This is mediated by antibodies, usually IgM, which bind to the red cells at low temperatures and cause them to agglutinate. It may cause intravascular haemolysis if complement fixation occurs. This can be chronic when the antibody is monoclonal, or acute or transient when the antibody is polyclonal.

Chronic cold agglutinin disease

This typically affects elderly patients and may be associated with an underlying low-grade B-cell lymphoma. It causes a low-grade intravascular haemolysis with cold, painful and often blue fingers, toes, ears or nose (so-called acrocyanosis). The latter is due to red cell agglutination in the small vessels in these colder, exposed areas. The blood film shows red cell agglutination and the MCV may be spuriously high because the automated analysers detect red cell aggregates as single cells. Monoclonal IgM usually has anti-I or, less often, anti-i specificity. Treatment is primarily by transfusion support but may also be directed at any underlying lymphoma. Patients must keep extremities warm, especially in winter. Some patients respond to glucocorticoid therapy and rituximab. Two considerations for patients requiring blood transfusion is that the cross-match sample must be placed in a transport flask at a temperature of 37°C and blood administered via a blood-warmer. All patients should receive folic acid supplementation.

Other causes of cold agglutination

Cold agglutination can occur in association with *Mycoplasma pneumoniae* or with infectious mononucleosis. Paroxysmal cold haemoglobinuria is a very rare cause seen in children, in association with viral or bacterial infection. An IgG antibody binds to red cells in the peripheral circulation but lysis occurs in the central circulation when complement fixation takes place. This antibody is termed the Donath–Landsteiner antibody and has specificity against the P antigen on the red cells.

Alloimmune haemolytic anaemia

Alloimmune haemolytic anaemia is caused by antibodies against non-self red cells. It has two main causes, occurring after:
- unmatched blood transfusion (p. 935)
- maternal sensitisation to paternal antigens on fetal cells (haemolytic disease of the newborn, p. 933).

Non-immune haemolytic anaemia

Endothelial damage

Disruption of red cell membrane may occur in a number of conditions and is characterised by the presence of red cell fragments on the blood film and markers of intravascular haemolysis:
- *Mechanical heart valves.* High flow through incompetent valves or periprosthetic leaks through the suture ring holding a valve in place result in shear stress damage.
- *March haemoglobinuria.* Vigorous exercise, such as prolonged marching or marathon running, can cause red cell damage in the capillaries in the feet.
- *Thermal injury.* Severe burns cause thermal damage to red cells, characterised by fragmentation and the presence of microspherocytes in the blood.
- *Microangiopathic haemolytic anaemia.* Fibrin deposition in capillaries can cause severe red cell disruption. It may occur in a wide variety of conditions: disseminated carcinomatosis, malignant or pregnancy-induced hypertension, haemolytic uraemic syndrome (p. 408), thrombotic thrombocytopenic purpura (p. 979) and disseminated intravascular coagulation (p. 978).

Infection

Plasmodium falciparum malaria (p. 274) may be associated with intravascular haemolysis; when severe, this is termed blackwater fever because of the associated haemoglobinuria. *Clostridium perfringens* sepsis (p. 227), usually in the context of ascending cholangitis or necrotising fasciitis, may cause severe intravascular haemolysis with marked spherocytosis due to bacterial production of a lecithinase that destroys the red cell membrane.

Chemicals or drugs

Dapsone and sulfasalazine cause haemolysis by oxidative denaturation of haemoglobin. Denatured haemoglobin forms Heinz bodies in the red cells, visible on supravital staining with brilliant cresyl blue. Arsenic gas, copper, chlorates, nitrites and nitrobenzene derivatives may all cause haemolysis.

Paroxysmal nocturnal haemoglobinuria

Paroxysmal nocturnal haemoglobinuria (PNH) is a rare acquired, non-malignant clonal expansion of haematopoietic stem cells deficient in glycosylphosphatidylinositol (GPI) anchor protein. GPI anchors several key molecules to cells and its absence results in clinical outcomes that reflect this, causing intravascular haemolysis and anaemia because of increased sensitivity of red cells to lysis by complement. This happens because key defence mechanisms that protect cells from complement-mediated lysis (CD55 and CD59) are GPI-anchored to red cells under normal circumstances. Episodes of intravascular haemolysis result in haemoglobinuria, most noticeable in early morning urine, which has a characteristic red–brown colour. The disease is associated with an increased risk of venous and arterial thrombosis in unusual sites, such as the liver or abdomen. PNH clones are also associated with hypoplastic bone marrow failure, aplastic anaemia and myelodysplastic syndrome (pp. 960 and 969). Management is supportive with transfusion and folate supplements and prophylaxis or treatment of thrombosis. Standard care now includes the anti-complement C5 monoclonal antibody eculizimab. This has been shown to be effective in reducing haemolysis, transfusion requirements and thrombotic risk. Eculizumab carries a risk of infection, particularly for *Neisseria meningitidis*, and all treated patients must be vaccinated against this organism.

Haemoglobinopathies

These diseases are caused by mutations affecting the genes encoding the globin chains of the haemoglobin molecule. Normal haemoglobin is composed of two alpha and two non-alpha globin chains. Alpha globin chains are produced throughout life, including in the fetus, so severe mutations may cause intrauterine death. Production of non-alpha chains varies with age; fetal haemoglobin (HbF-$\alpha\alpha/\gamma\gamma$) has two gamma chains, while the predominant adult haemoglobin (HbA-$\alpha\alpha/\beta\beta$) has two beta chains. Thus, disorders affecting the beta chains do not present until after 6 months of age. A constant small amount of haemoglobin A_2 (HbA$_2$-$\alpha\alpha/\delta\delta$, usually less than 2%) is made from birth.

The geographical distribution of the common haemoglobin-opathies is shown in Figure 23.21. The haemoglobinopathies can be classified into qualitative or quantitative abnormalities.

Qualitative abnormalities – abnormal haemoglobins

In qualitative abnormalities (called the abnormal haemoglobins), there is a functionally important alteration in the amino acid structure of the polypeptide chains of the globin chains. Several hundred such variants are known; they were originally designated by letters of the alphabet, e.g. S, C, D or E, but the more recently described ones are known by names that usually taken from the town or district in which they were first described. The best-known example is haemoglobin S, found in sickle-cell anaemia. Mutations around the haem-binding pocket cause the haem ring to fall out of the structure and produce an unstable haemoglobin. These substitutions often change the charge of the globin chains, producing different electrophoretic mobility, and this forms the basis for the diagnostic use of haemoglobin electrophoresis to identify haemoglobinopathies.

Quantitative abnormalities – thalassaemias

In quantitative abnormalities (the thalassaemias), there are mutations causing a reduced rate of production of one or other of the globin chains, altering the ratio of alpha to non-alpha chains. In alpha-thalassaemia excess beta chains are present, while in beta-thalassaemia excess alpha chains are present. The excess chains precipitate, causing red cell membrane damage and reduced red cell survival due to haemolysis.

Sickle-cell anaemia

Sickle-cell disease results from a single glutamic acid to valine substitution at position 6 of the beta globin polypeptide chain. It is inherited as an autosomal recessive trait (p. 48). Homozygotes only produce abnormal beta chains that make haemoglobin S (HbS, termed SS), and this results in the clinical syndrome of sickle-cell disease. Heterozygotes produce a mixture of normal and abnormal beta chains that make normal HbA and HbS (termed AS), and this results in sickle-cell trait; although this was previously thought of as asymptomatic, it may be associated with an increased risk of sudden and cardiovascular death.

Epidemiology

The heterozygote frequency is over 20% in tropical Africa (see Fig. 23.21). In black American populations, sickle-cell trait has a frequency of 8%. Individuals with sickle-cell trait are relatively resistant to the lethal effects of *falciparum* malaria in early childhood; the high prevalence in equatorial Africa can be explained by the survival advantage it confers in areas where *falciparum* malaria is endemic. However, homozygous patients with sickle-cell anaemia do not have correspondingly greater resistance to *falciparum* malaria.

Pathogenesis

When haemoglobin S is deoxygenated, the molecules of haemoglobin polymerise to form pseudocrystalline structures known as 'tactoids'. These distort the red cell membrane and

23

Thalassaemia
Sickle-cell anaemia
HbC
HbD
HbE

Fig. 23.21 The geographical distribution of the haemoglobinopathies. *From Hoffbrand AV, Pettit JE. Essential haematology, 3rd edn. Edinburgh: Blackwell Science; 1992.*

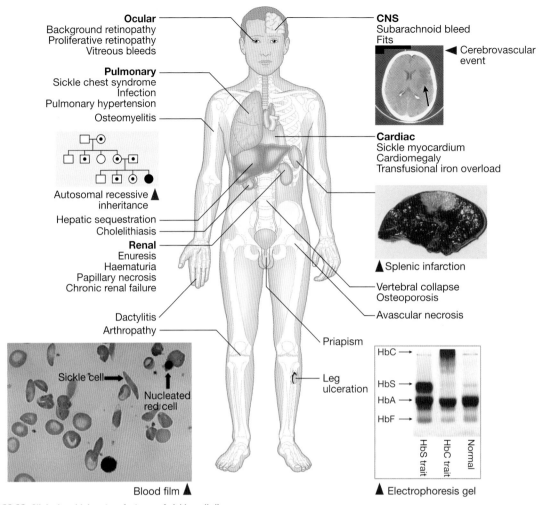

Ocular
Background retinopathy
Proliferative retinopathy
Vitreous bleeds

Pulmonary
Sickle chest syndrome
Infection
Pulmonary hypertension
Osteomyelitis

Autosomal recessive ▲
inheritance
Hepatic sequestration
Cholelithiasis

Renal
Enuresis
Haematuria
Papillary necrosis
Chronic renal failure

Dactylitis
Arthropathy

Sickle cell
Nucleated
red cell

Blood film ▲

CNS
Subarachnoid bleed
Fits
◄ Cerebrovascular event

Cardiac
Sickle myocardium
Cardiomegaly
Transfusional iron overload

▲ Splenic infarction

Vertebral collapse
Osteoporosis
Avascular necrosis

Priapism

Leg ulceration

HbC →
HbS →
HbA →
HbF →

HbS trait
HbC trait
Normal

▲ Electrophoresis gel

Fig. 23.22 Clinical and laboratory features of sickle-cell disease.

produce characteristic sickle-shaped cells (Fig. 23.22). The polymerisation is reversible when re-oxygenation occurs. The distortion of the red cell membrane, however, may become permanent and the red cell 'irreversibly sickled'. The greater the concentration of sickle-cell haemoglobin in the individual cell, the more easily tactoids are formed, but this process may be enhanced or retarded by the presence of other haemoglobins. Thus the abnormal haemoglobin C variant participates in polymerisation more readily than haemoglobin A, whereas haemoglobin F strongly inhibits polymerisation.

Clinical features

Sickling is precipitated by hypoxia, acidosis, dehydration and infection. Irreversibly sickled cells have a shortened survival and plug vessels in the microcirculation. This results in a number of acute syndromes, termed 'crises', and chronic organ damage (Fig. 23.22):

- *Painful vaso-occlusive crisis*. Plugging of small vessels in the bone produces acute severe bone pain. This affects areas of active marrow: the hands and feet in children (so-called dactylitis) or the femora, humeri, ribs, pelvis and vertebrae in adults. Patients usually have a systemic response with tachycardia, sweating and a fever. This is the most common form of crisis.

- *Stroke*. The single most devastating consequence of sickle-cell disease is stroke. Stroke or silent stroke occurs in 10–15% of children with sickle-cell disease. Children at risk of stroke can be identified by screening with transcranial Doppler ultrasound, with fast flow associated with increased stroke risk. These children may be offered strategies such as transfusion or treatment with hydroxycarbamide to reduce the risk of stroke.

- *Sickle chest syndrome*. This may follow a vaso-occlusive crisis and is the most common cause of death in adult sickle-cell disease. Bone marrow infarction results in fat emboli to the lungs, which cause further sickling and infarction, leading to ventilatory failure if not treated.

- *Sequestration crisis*. Thrombosis of the venous outflow from an organ causes loss of function and acute painful enlargement. In children, the spleen is the most common site. Massive splenic enlargement may result in severe anaemia, circulatory collapse and death. Recurrent sickling in the spleen in childhood results in infarction and adults may have no functional spleen. In adults, the liver may undergo sequestration with severe pain due to capsular stretching. Priapism is a complication seen in affected men.

- *Aplastic crisis*. Infection of adult sicklers with human parvovirus B19 (erythrovirus) may result in a severe but

23.39 Sickle-cell disease in pregnancy

- **Pre-conceptual counselling**: advice on the effect of sickle-cell disease on pregnancy, and vice versa, should be offered.
- **Vaccination status**: should be updated before conception.
- **Testing of partner**: testing for haemoglobinopathy status is advised.
- **Folic acid**: should be taken in high dose (5 mg daily) prior to and throughout pregnancy.
- **Hydroxycarbamide**: should be discontinued 3 months prior to conception.
- **Angiotensin-converting enzyme (ACE) inhibitors**: should be discontinued prior to conception.
- **Pulmonary hypertension**: should be excluded prior to conception.
- **Placental failure**: women with sickle-cell disease have increased rates, resulting in pre-eclampsia and intrauterine growth retardation.
- **Aspirin 75 mg**: should be given throughout pregnancy.
- **Thromboprophylaxis after delivery**: all women with sickle-cell disease should receive thromboprophylaxis with low-molecular-weight heparin for at least 10 days post vaginal delivery and for 6 weeks post caesarean section. Antenatal thromboprophylaxis should be considered for women with additional risk factors for venous thromboembolism (see Box 23.65).
- **Transfusion**: extended cross-matched blood for Rhesus and Kell status should be provided. Blood should be cytomegalovirus-negative.

self-limiting red cell aplasia. This results in profound anaemia, which may cause heart failure. Unlike in all other sickle crises, the reticulocyte count is low.

- *Pregnancy*. Pregnancy in sickle-cell disease requires planning and multidisciplinary management. Women with sickle-cell disease have increased pregnancy-related morbidity, which includes painful crisis, placental failure and thrombosis (Box 23.39).

Investigations

Patients with sickle-cell disease have a compensated anaemia, usually around 60–80 g/L. The blood film shows sickle cells, target cells and features of hyposplenism from a young age. A reticulocytosis is present. The presence of HbS can be demonstrated by exposing red cells to a reducing agent such as sodium dithionite; HbA gives a clear solution, whereas HbS polymerises to produce a turbid solution. This forms the basis of emergency screening tests before surgery in appropriate ethnic groups but cannot distinguish between sickle-cell trait and disease. The definitive diagnosis requires haemoglobin electrophoresis to demonstrate the absence of HbA, 2–20% HbF and the predominance of HbS. Both parents of the affected individual will have sickle-cell trait.

Management

All patients with sickle-cell disease should receive prophylaxis with daily folic acid, and appropriate management of the hyposplenic state that is uniformly found in these patients from an early age (see Box 23.37). Seasonal vaccination against influenza is also advised in these patients.

Vaso-occlusive crises are managed by aggressive rehydration, oxygen therapy, adequate analgesia (which often requires opiates) and antibiotics. Transfusion should be with fully genotyped blood wherever possible. Simple top-up transfusion may be used in a sequestration or aplastic crisis. A regular transfusion programme to suppress HbS production and maintain the HbS level below 30% may be indicated in patients with recurrent severe complications, such as cerebrovascular accidents in

children or chest syndromes in adults. Exchange transfusion, in which a patient is simultaneously venesected and transfused to replace HbS with HbA, may be used in life-threatening crises or to prepare patients for surgery.

A high HbF level inhibits polymerisation of HbS and reduces sickling. Patients with sickle-cell disease and high HbF levels have a mild clinical course with few crises. Some agents are able to increase synthesis of HbF and this has been used to reduce the frequency of severe crises. The oral cytotoxic agent hydroxycarbamide has been shown to have clinical benefit with acceptable side-effects in children and adults who have recurrent severe crises.

Relatively few allogeneic stem cell transplants from HLA-matched siblings have been performed but this procedure appears to be potentially curative (p. 937).

Prognosis

In Africa, few children with sickle-cell anaemia survive to adult life without medical attention. Even with standard medical care, approximately 15% die by the age of 20 years and 50% by the age of 40 years.

Other abnormal haemoglobins

Another beta-chain haemoglobinopathy, haemoglobin C (HbC) disease, is clinically silent but associated with microcytosis and target cells on the blood film. Compound heterozygotes inheriting one *HbS* gene and one *HbC* gene from their parents have haemoglobin SC disease, which behaves like a mild form of sickle-cell disease. SC disease is associated with a reduced frequency of crises but is not uncommonly associated with complications in pregnancy and retinopathy.

Thalassaemias

Thalassaemia is an inherited impairment of haemoglobin production, in which there is partial or complete failure to synthesise a specific type of globin chain. In alpha-thalassaemia, disruption of one or both alleles on chromosome 16 may occur, with production of some or no alpha globin chains. In beta-thalassaemia, defective production usually results from disabling point mutations causing no (β^0) or reduced (β^-) beta chain production.

Beta-thalassaemia

Failure to synthesise beta chains (beta-thalassaemia) is the most common type of thalassaemia, most prevalent in the Mediterranean area. Heterozygotes have thalassaemia minor, a condition in which there is usually mild microcytic anaemia and little or no clinical disability, which may be detected only when iron therapy for a mild microcytic anaemia fails. Homozygotes (thalassaemia major) either are unable to synthesise haemoglobin A or, at best, produce very little; after the first 4–6 months of life, they develop profound transfusion-dependent hypochromic anaemia. The diagnostic features are summarised in Box 23.40. Intermediate grades of severity occur.

Management and prevention

See Box 23.41. Cure is now a possibility for selected children, with allogeneic HSCT (p. 937).

It is possible to identify a fetus with homozygous beta-thalassaemia by obtaining chorionic villous material for DNA

23

23.40 Diagnostic features of beta-thalassaemia

Beta-thalassaemia major (homozygotes)

- Profound hypochromic anaemia
- Evidence of severe red cell dysplasia
- Erythroblastosis
- Absence or gross reduction of the amount of haemoglobin A
- Raised levels of haemoglobin F
- Evidence that both parents have thalassaemia minor

Beta-thalassaemia minor (heterozygotes)

- Mild anaemia
- Microcytic hypochromic erythrocytes (not iron-deficient)
- Some target cells
- Punctate basophilia
- Raised haemoglobin A_2 fraction

23.41 Treatment of beta-thalassaemia major

Problem	Management
Erythropoietic failure	Allogeneic HSCT from HLA-compatible sibling Transfusion to maintain Hb >100 g/L Folic acid 5 mg daily
Iron overload	Iron therapy contraindicated Iron chelation therapy
Splenomegaly causing mechanical problems, excessive transfusion needs	Splenectomy; see Box 23.37

(Hb = haemoglobin; HLA = human leucocyte antigen; HSCT = haematopoietic stem cell transplantation)

23.42 Anaemia in old age

- **Mean haemoglobin**: falls with age in both sexes but remains well within the reference range. When a low haemoglobin does occur, it is generally due to disease.
- **Anaemia can never be considered 'normal' in old age**.
- **Symptoms**: may be subtle and insidious. Cardiovascular features such as dyspnoea and oedema, and cerebral features such as dizziness and apathy, tend to predominate.
- **Ferritin**: if lower than 45 μg/L in older people, is highly predictive of iron deficiency. Conversely, ferritin may be raised by chronic disease and so a normal ferritin does not exclude iron deficiency.
- **Serum iron and transferrin**: fall with age because of the prevalence of other disorders, and are not reliable indicators of deficiency.
- **Most common cause of iron deficiency**: gastrointestinal blood loss.
- **Most common cause of vitamin B_{12} deficiency**: pernicious anaemia, as the prevalence of chronic atrophic gastritis rises in old age.
- **Neuropsychiatric symptoms associated with vitamin B_{12} deficiency**: well-established association but a causal relationship has not been clearly shown. Dementia associated with vitamin B_{12} deficiency in the absence of haematological abnormalities is rare.
- **Anaemia of chronic disease**: frequent in old age because of the rising prevalence of diseases that inhibit iron transport.

analysis sufficiently early in pregnancy to allow termination. This examination is appropriate only if both parents are known to be carriers (beta-thalassaemia minor) and will accept a termination.

Alpha-thalassaemia

Reduced or absent alpha-chain synthesis is common in Southeast Asia. There are two alpha gene loci on chromosome 16 and therefore each individual carries four alpha gene alleles.

- If one is deleted, there is no clinical effect.
- If two are deleted, there may be a mild hypochromic anaemia.
- If three are deleted, the patient has haemoglobin H disease.
- If all four are deleted, the baby is stillborn (hydrops fetalis).

Haemoglobin H is a beta-chain tetramer, formed from the excess of beta chains, which is functionally useless, so that patients rely on their low levels of HbA for oxygen transport. Treatment of haemoglobin H disease is similar to that of beta-thalassaemia of intermediate severity, involving folic acid supplementation, transfusion if required and avoidance of iron therapy.

Haematological malignancies

Haematological malignancies arise when the processes controlling proliferation or apoptosis are corrupted in blood cells because of acquired mutations in key regulatory genes. If mature differentiated cells are involved, the cells will have a low growth fraction and produce indolent neoplasms, such as the low-grade lymphomas or chronic leukaemias, when patients have an expected survival of many years. In contrast, if more primitive stem or progenitor cells are involved, the cells can have the highest growth fractions of all human neoplasms, producing rapidly progressive, life-threatening illnesses such as the acute leukaemias or high-grade lymphomas. Involvement of pluripotent stem cells produces the most aggressive acute leukaemias. In general, haematological neoplasms are diseases of elderly patients, the exceptions being acute lymphoblastic leukaemia, which predominantly affects children, and Hodgkin lymphoma, which affects people aged 20–40 years. Management of young patients with haematological malignancy is particularly challenging (Box 23.43).

Leukaemias

Leukaemias are malignant disorders of the haematopoietic stem cell compartment, characteristically associated with increased numbers of white cells in the bone marrow and/or peripheral blood. The course of leukaemia may vary from a few days or weeks to many years, depending on the type.

Epidemiology and aetiology

The incidence of leukaemia of all types in the population is approximately 10/100 000 per annum, of which just under half are cases of acute leukaemia. Males are affected more frequently than females, the ratio being about 3:2 in acute leukaemia, 2:1 in chronic lymphocytic leukaemia and 1.3:1 in chronic myeloid leukaemia. Geographical variation in incidence does occur, the most striking being the rarity of chronic lymphocytic leukaemia in Chinese and related races. Acute leukaemia occurs at all ages. Acute lymphoblastic leukaemia shows a peak of incidence in children aged 1–5 years. All forms of acute myeloid leukaemia

23.43 Consequences of haematological malignancy in adolescence

- **Tailored management protocols**: the most effective treatment schedules for leukaemia and lymphoma differ between children and adults. Adolescent patients may be most appropriately managed in specialist centres.
- **Psychosocial effects**: adolescents undergoing treatment for haematological malignancy may suffer significant consequences for their schooling and social development, and require support from a multidisciplinary team.
- **'Late effects'**: adolescents who have been treated with chemotherapy and/or radiotherapy in childhood may be at risk of a wide range of complications, depending on the region irradiated, radiation dose and the drugs used. Particularly relevant complications in this age group include short stature, growth hormone deficiency, delayed puberty, and cognitive dysfunction affecting schooling (after cranial irradiation). Life-long follow-up is often undertaken to detect and manage these late effects and to deal with consequences such as infertility and second malignancy.

23.44 Risk factors for leukaemia

Ionising radiation

- After atomic bombing of Japanese cities (myeloid leukaemia)
- Radiotherapy
- Diagnostic X-rays of the fetus in pregnancy

Cytotoxic drugs

- Especially alkylating agents (myeloid leukaemia, usually after a latent period of several years)
- Industrial exposure to benzene

Retroviruses

- Adult T-cell leukaemia/lymphoma (ATLL) caused by human T-cell lymphotropic virus 1(HTLV-1), most prevalent in Japan, the Caribbean and some areas of Central and South America and Africa

Genetic

- Identical twin of patients with leukaemia
- Down's syndrome and certain other genetic disorders

Immunological

- Immune deficiency states (e.g. hypogammaglobulinaemia)

have their lowest incidence in young adult life and there is a striking rise over the age of 50. Chronic leukaemias occur mainly in middle and old age.

The cause of the leukaemia is unknown in the majority of patients. Several risk factors have been identified (Box 23.44).

Terminology and classification

Leukaemias are traditionally classified into four main groups:

- acute lymphoblastic leukaemia (ALL)
- acute myeloid leukaemia (AML)
- chronic lymphocytic leukaemia (CLL)
- chronic myeloid leukaemia (CML).

In acute leukaemia, there is proliferation of primitive stem cells, with limited accompanying differentiation, leading to an accumulation of blasts, predominantly in the bone marrow, which causes bone marrow failure. In chronic leukaemia, the malignant clone is able to differentiate, resulting in an accumulation of more mature cells. Lymphocytic and lymphoblastic cells are those derived from the lymphoid stem cell (B cells and T cells).

23.45 WHO classification of acute leukaemia*

Acute myeloid leukaemia (AML) with recurrent genetic abnormalities

- AML with t(8;21)(q22;q22.1), gene product RUNX1-RUNX1T1
- AML with inv(16)(p13.1;q22), gene product CBFB-MYHL1
- Acute promyelocytic leukaemia t(15;17), gene product PML-RARA
- AML with t(9;11)(p21.3;q23.3), gene product MLLT3-KMT2A
- AML with t(6;9)(p23;q34), gene product DEK-NUP214
- AML with inv(3)(q21.3;q26.2) or t(3;3)(q21.3;q26.2), gene products GATA2, MECOM
- AML (megakaryoblastic) with t(1;22)(p13.3;q13.3), gene product RBM15-MKL1
- AML with mutated NPM1
- AML with biallelic mutations of CEBPA

Acute myeloid leukaemia with myelodysplasia-related changes

- e.g. Following a myelodysplastic syndrome

Therapy-related myeloid neoplasms

- e.g. Alkylating agent or topoisomerase II inhibitor

Myeloid sarcoma

Myeloid proliferations related to Down's syndrome

Acute myeloid leukaemia not otherwise specified

- e.g. AML with or without differentiation, acute myelomonocytic leukaemia, erythroleukaemia, megakaryoblastic leukaemia

Acute lymphoblastic leukaemia (ALL)

- B-lymphoblastic leukaemia/lymphoma
- T-lymphoblastic leukaemia/lymphoma

*Updated 2016; major subtypes.

Myeloid refers to the other lineages: that is, precursors of red cells, granulocytes, monocytes and platelets (see Fig. 23.2).

The diagnosis of leukaemia is usually suspected from an abnormal blood count, often a raised white count, and is confirmed by examination of the bone marrow. This includes the morphology of the abnormal cells, analysis of cell surface markers (immunophenotyping), clone-specific chromosome abnormalities and molecular changes. These results are incorporated in the World Health Organisation (WHO) classification of tumours of haematopoietic and lymphoid tissues; the subclassification of acute leukaemias is shown in Box 23.45. The features in the bone marrow not only provide an accurate diagnosis but also give valuable prognostic information, increasingly allowing therapy to be tailored to the patient's disease.

Acute leukaemia

There is a failure of cell maturation in acute leukaemia. Proliferation of cells that do not mature leads to an accumulation of primitive cells that take up more and more marrow space at the expense of the normal haematopoietic elements. Eventually, this proliferation spills into the blood. Acute myeloid leukaemia (AML) is about four times more common than acute lymphoblastic leukaemia (ALL) in adults. In children, the proportions are reversed, the lymphoblastic variety being more common. The clinical features are usually those of bone marrow failure (anaemia, bleeding or infection; pp. 923, 927 and 930).

Investigations

Blood examination usually shows anaemia with a normal or raised MCV. The leucocyte count may vary from as low as 1×10^9/L to as high as 500×10^9/L or more. In the majority of patients,

23

the count is below 100×10^9/L. Severe thrombocytopenia is usual but not invariable. Frequently, blast cells are seen in the blood film but sometimes the blast cells may be infrequent or absent. A bone marrow examination will confirm the diagnosis. The bone marrow is usually hypercellular, with replacement of normal elements by leukaemic blast cells in varying degrees (but more than 20% of the cells) (Fig. 23.23). The presence of Auer rods in the cytoplasm of blast cells indicates a myeloblastic type of leukaemia. Classification and prognosis are determined by immunophenotyping and chromosome and molecular analysis, as shown in Figure 23.24.

Fig. 23.23 **Acute myeloid leukaemia.** Bone marrow aspirate showing infiltration with large blast cells, which display nuclear folding and prominent nucleoli.

Fig. 23.24 **Investigation of acute lymphoblastic leukaemia (ALL).**
A Flow cytometric analysis of blasts labelled with the fluorescent antibodies anti-CD19 (y axis) and anti-CD10 (x axis). ALL blasts are positive for both CD19 and CD10 (arrow). B Chromosome analysis (karyotype) of blasts showing additional chromosomes X, 4, 6, 7, 14, 18 and 21.

Management

The first decision must be whether or not to give specific treatment to attempt to achieve remission. This is generally aggressive, has numerous side-effects, and may not be appropriate for the very elderly or patients with serious comorbidities (Chs 32 and 33). In these patients, supportive treatment can effect considerable improvement in well-being. Low-intensity chemotherapy, such as low-dose cytosine arabinoside or, recently, azacitidine, is frequently used in elderly and more frail patients but only induces remission in less than 20% of patients.

Specific therapy

Ideally, whenever possible, patients with acute leukaemia should be treated within a clinical trial. If a decision to embark on specific therapy has been taken, the patient should be prepared as recommended in Box 23.46. It is unwise to attempt aggressive management of acute leukaemia unless adequate services are available for the provision of supportive therapy.

The aim of treatment is to destroy the leukaemic clone of cells without destroying the residual normal stem cell compartment from which repopulation of the haematopoietic tissues will occur. There are three phases:

• *Remission induction.* In this phase, a fraction of the tumour is destroyed by combination chemotherapy. The patient goes through a period of severe bone marrow hypoplasia lasting 3–4 weeks and requires intensive support and inpatient care from a specially trained multidisciplinary team. The aim is to achieve remission, a state in which the blood counts return to normal and the marrow blast count is less than 5%. Quality of life is highly dependent on achieving remission.
• *Remission consolidation.* If remission has been achieved, residual disease is attacked by therapy during the consolidation phase. This consists of a number of courses of chemotherapy, again resulting in periods of marrow hypoplasia. In poor-prognosis leukaemia, this may include allogeneic HSCT.
• *Remission maintenance.* If the patient is still in remission after the consolidation phase for ALL, a period of maintenance therapy is given, with the individual as an outpatient and treatment consisting of a repeating cycle of drug administration. This may extend for up to 3 years if relapse does not occur.

---

i | 23.46 Preparation for specific therapy in acute leukaemia

• Existing infections identified and treated (e.g. urinary tract infection, oral candidiasis, dental, gingival and skin infections)
• Anaemia corrected by red cell concentrate transfusion
• Thrombocytopenic bleeding controlled by platelet transfusions
• If possible, central venous catheter (e.g. Hickman line) inserted to facilitate access to the circulation for delivery of chemotherapy, fluids, blood products and other supportive drugs
• Tumour lysis risk assessed and prevention started: fluids with allopurinol or rasburicase
• Therapeutic regimen carefully explained to the patient and informed consent obtained
• Consideration of entry into clinical trial

	23.47 Drugs commonly used in the treatment of acute leukaemia	
Phase	Acute lymphoblastic leukaemia	Acute myeloid leukaemia
Induction	Vincristine (IV) Prednisolone (oral) L-Asparaginase (IM) Daunorubicin (IV) Methotrexate (intrathecal) Imatinib (oral)*	Daunorubicin (IV) Cytarabine (IV) Etoposide (IV and oral) Gentuzumab ozogamicin (IV) All-trans retinoic acid (ATRA) (oral) Arsenic trioxide (ATO)
Consolidation	Daunorubicin (IV) Cytarabine (IV) Etoposide (IV) Methotrexate (IV) Imatinib (oral)*	Cytarabine (IV) Amsacrine (IV) Mitoxantrone (IV)
Maintenance	Prednisolone (oral) Vincristine (IV) Mercaptopurine (oral) Methotrexate (oral) Imatinib (oral)*	
Relapse	Fludarabine Cytarabine Idarubicin	Fludarabine Cytarabine Arsenic trioxide (ATO) Idarubicin

*If Philadelphia chromosome-positive.

In patients with ALL, it is necessary to give prophylactic treatment to the central nervous system, as this is a sanctuary site where standard therapy does not penetrate. This usually consists of a combination of cranial irradiation, intrathecal chemotherapy and high-dose methotrexate, which crosses the blood–brain barrier.

Thereafter, specific therapy is discontinued and the patient observed.

The detail of the schedules for these treatments can be found in specialist texts. The drugs most commonly employed are listed in Box 23.47. Generally, if a patient fails to go into remission with induction treatment, alternative drug combinations may be tried, but the outlook is poor unless remission can be achieved. Disease that relapses during treatment or soon after the end of treatment carries a poor prognosis and is difficult to treat. The longer after the end of treatment that relapse occurs, the more likely it is that further treatment will be effective.

In some patients, alternative palliative chemotherapy, not designed to achieve remission, may be used to curb excessive leucocyte proliferation. Drugs used for this purpose include hydroxycarbamide and mercaptopurine. The aim is to reduce the blast count without inducing bone marrow failure.

Supportive therapy

Aggressive and potentially curative therapy, which involves periods of severe bone marrow failure, would not be possible without appropriate supportive care. The following problems commonly arise.

Anaemia Anaemia is treated with red cell concentrate transfusions.

Bleeding Thrombocytopenic bleeding requires platelet transfusions, unless the bleeding is trivial. Recent trials have confirmed that in acute leukaemia prophylactic platelet transfusion should be given to maintain the platelet count above 10×10^9/L. Coagulation abnormalities occur and need accurate diagnosis and treatment (p. 971).

Infection Fever (>38°C) lasting over 1 hour in a neutropenic patient indicates possible sepsis (see also p. 218). Parenteral broad-spectrum antibiotic therapy is essential. Empirical therapy is given according to local bacteriological resistance patterns, such as with a combination of an aminoglycoside (e.g. gentamicin) and a broad-spectrum penicillin (e.g. piperacillin/tazobactam) or a single-agent beta-lactam (e.g. meropenem). The organisms most commonly associated with severe neutropenic sepsis are Gram-positive bacteria, such as Staphylococcus aureus and Staphylococcus epidermidis, which are present on the skin and gain entry via cannulae and central lines. Gram-negative infections often originate from the gastrointestinal tract, which is affected by chemotherapy-induced mucositis; organisms such as Escherichia coli, Pseudomonas and Klebsiella spp. are likely to cause rapid clinical deterioration and must be covered with initially empirical antibiotic therapy. Gram-positive infection may require vancomycin or teicoplanin therapy. If fever has not resolved after 3–5 days and there is evidence on CT scanning or sensitive blood tests for a disseminated fungal infection, empirical antifungal therapy (e.g. a liposomal amphotericin B preparation, voriconazole or caspofungin) is added.

Patients with ALL are susceptible to infection with Pneumocystis jirovecii (p. 318), which causes a severe pneumonia. Prophylaxis with co-trimoxazole is given during chemotherapy. Diagnosis may require either induced sputum, bronchoalveolar lavage or open lung biopsy. Treatment is with high-dose co-trimoxazole, initially intravenously, changing to oral treatment as soon as possible.

Oral and pharyngeal Candida infection is common. Fluconazole is effective for the treatment of established local infection and for prophylaxis against systemic candidaemia. Prophylaxis against other systemic fungal infections, including Aspergillus, using itraconazole or posaconazole, for example, is usual practice during high-risk intensive chemotherapy. This is often used along with sensitive markers of early fungal infection to guide treatment initiation (a 'pre-emptive approach').

For systemic fungal infection with Candida or aspergillosis, intravenous liposomal amphotericin, caspofungin or voriconazole is required for at least 3 weeks. In systemic Candida infection intravenous catheters should be removed.

Reactivation of herpes simplex infection (p. 247) occurs frequently around the lips and nose during ablative therapy for acute leukaemia, and is treated with aciclovir. This may also be prescribed prophylactically to patients with a history of cold sores or elevated antibody titres to herpes simplex. Herpes zoster manifesting as chickenpox or, after reactivation, as shingles (p. 239) should be treated in the early stage with high-dose aciclovir, as it can be fatal in immunocompromised patients.

The value of isolation facilities, such as laminar flow rooms, is debatable but may contribute to staff awareness of careful reverse barrier nursing practice. The isolation can be psychologically stressful for the patient.

Metabolic problems Frequent monitoring of fluid balance and renal, hepatic and haemostatic function is necessary. Patients are often severely anorexic and diarrhoea is common as a consequence of the side-effects of therapy; they may find drinking difficult and hence require intravenous fluids and electrolytes. Renal toxicity occurs with some antibiotics (e.g. aminoglycosides) and antifungal agents (amphotericin). Cellular breakdown during induction therapy

23

(tumour lysis syndrome; p. 1328) releases intracellular ions and nucleic acid breakdown products, causing hyperkalaemia, hyperuricaemia, hyperphosphataemia and hypocalcaemia. This may lead to renal failure. Allopurinol and intravenous hydration are given to try to prevent this. In patients at high risk of tumour lysis syndrome, prophylactic rasburicase (a recombinant urate oxidase enzyme) is used. Occasionally, dialysis may be required.

Psychological problems Psychological support is a key aspect of care. Patients should be kept informed, and their questions answered and fears allayed as far as possible. A multidisciplinary approach to patient care involves input from many services, including psychology. Key members of the team include haematology specialist nurses, who are often the central point of contact for patients and families throughout the illness.

Haematopoietic stem cell transplantation

This is described on page 936. In patients with high-risk acute leukaemia, allogeneic HSCT can improve 5-year survival from 20% to around 50%. Reduced-intensity conditioning has allowed HSCT to be delivered to a higher proportion of patients with acute leukaemias, up to the age of about 65 years.

Prognosis

Without treatment, the median survival of patients with acute leukaemia is about 5 weeks. This may be extended to a number of months with supportive treatment. Patients who achieve remission with specific therapy have a better outlook. Around 80% of adult patients under 60 years of age with ALL or AML achieve remission, although remission rates are lower for older patients. However, the relapse rate continues to be high. Box 23.48 shows the survival in ALL and AML and the influence of prognostic features. The level of detectable leukaemia cells, called minimal residual disease (MRD), measured after induction therapy in ALL by sensitive laboratory techniques, has been shown to be a powerful prognostic tool that is now used routinely to direct subsequent consolidation therapy.

Advances in treatment have led to steady improvement in survival from leukaemia. They include the introduction of drugs such as all-*trans* retinoic acid (ATRA) and arsenic trioxide (ATO)

in acute promyelocytic leukaemia, which has greatly reduced induction deaths from bleeding in this good-risk leukaemia. A chemotherapy-free schedule of ATRA and ATO has recently produced cure rates of 90% in patients with low-risk acute promyelocytic leukaemia. Current trials aim to improve survival, especially in standard and poor-risk disease, with strategies that include better use of allogeneic HSCT and targeted therapies such as anti-CD33 monoclonal antibodies (Mylotarg) and FLT3 inhibitors. FLT3 is a cytokine receptor often expressed on AML blast cells and whose expression is associated with a poorer prognosis.

Chronic myeloid leukaemia

Chronic myeloid leukaemia (CML) is a myeloproliferative stem cell disorder resulting in proliferation of all haematopoietic lineages but manifesting predominantly in the granulocytic series. Maturation of cells proceeds fairly normally. The disease occurs chiefly between the ages of 30 and 80 years, with a peak incidence at 55 years. It is rare, with an annual incidence in the UK of 1.8/100 000, and accounts for 20% of all leukaemias. It is found in all races.

The defining characteristic of CML is the chromosome abnormality known as the Philadelphia (Ph) chromosome. This is a shortened chromosome 22 resulting from a reciprocal translocation of material with chromosome 9. The break on chromosome 22 occurs in the breakpoint cluster region (BCR). The fragment from chromosome 9 that joins the BCR carries the *abl* oncogene, which forms a fusion gene with the remains of the BCR. This *BCR ABL* fusion gene codes for a 210 kDa protein with tyrosine kinase activity, which plays a causative role in the disease as an oncogene (p. 1318), influencing cellular proliferation, differentiation and survival. In some patients in whom conventional chromosomal analysis does not detect a Ph chromosome, the BCR ABL gene product is detectable by molecular techniques.

Natural history

The disease has three phases:

- *A chronic phase*, in which the disease is responsive to treatment and is easily controlled, which used to last 3–5 years. With the introduction of imatinib therapy, this phase has been prolonged to encompass a normal life expectancy in many patients.
- *An accelerated phase* (not always seen), in which disease control becomes more difficult.
- *Blast crisis*, in which the disease transforms into an acute leukaemia, either myeloblastic (70%) or lymphoblastic (30%), which is relatively refractory to treatment. This is the cause of death in the majority of patients; survival is therefore dictated by the timing of blast crisis, which cannot be predicted. Prior to imatinib therapy (see below), approximately 10% of patients per year would transform. In those treated with imatinib for up to 10 years, only between 0.5 and 2.5% have transformed each year.

Clinical features

Symptoms at presentation may include lethargy, weight loss, abdominal discomfort, gout and sweating, but about 25% of patients are asymptomatic at diagnosis. Splenomegaly is present in 90%; in about 10%, the enlargement is massive, extending to over 15 cm below the costal margin. A friction rub may be heard in cases of splenic infarction. Hepatomegaly occurs in about 50%. Lymphadenopathy is unusual.

i	23.48 Outcome in adult acute leukaemia	
Disease/risk	**Risk factors**	**5-year overall survival**
Acute myeloid leukaemia (AML)		
Good risk	Promyelocytic leukaemia t(15;17)	90%
	t(8;21)	65%
	inv 16 or t(16;16)	70%
Poor risk	Cytogenetic abnormalities −5, −7, del 5q, abn(3q), complex (>5)	21%
Intermediate risk	AML with none of the above	48%
Acute lymphoblastic leukaemia (ALL)		
Poor risk	Philadelphia chromosome High white count >100×10⁹/L Abnormal short arm of chromosome 11 t(1;19)	20%
Standard	ALL with none of the above	37%

Investigations

FBC results are variable between patients. There is usually a normocytic, normochromic anaemia. The leucocyte count can vary from 10 to 600×10^9/L. In about one-third of patients, there is a very high platelet count, sometimes as high as 2000×10^9/L. In the blood film, the full range of granulocyte precursors, from myeloblasts to mature neutrophils, is seen but the predominant cells are neutrophils and myelocytes (see Fig. 23.3). Myeloblasts usually constitute less than 10% of all white cells. There is often an absolute increase in eosinophils and basophils, and nucleated red cells are common. If the disease progresses through an accelerated phase, the percentage of more primitive cells increases. Blast transformation is characterised by a dramatic increase in the number of circulating blasts. In patients with thrombocytosis, very high platelet counts may persist during treatment, in both chronic and accelerated phases, but usually drop dramatically at blast transformation. Basophilia tends to increase as the disease progresses.

Bone marrow should be obtained to confirm the diagnosis and phase of disease by morphology, chromosome analysis to demonstrate the presence of the Ph chromosome, and RNA analysis to demonstrate the presence of the BCR ABL gene product. Blood LDH levels are elevated and the uric acid level may be high due to increased cell breakdown.

Management

Chronic phase

There are now five available tyrosine kinase inhibitors (TKIs) for the treatment of CML (Box 23.49). These specifically inhibit BCR ABL tyrosine kinase activity. Imatinib, nilotinib and dasatinib are recommended as first-line therapy in chronic phase CML; they usually normalise the blood count within a month and within 3–6 months produce complete cytogenetic response (disappearance of the Ph chromosome) in some 90% of patients. A sample of bone marrow is taken at 6 months to confirm complete cytogenetic response, and patients are subsequently monitored by 3-monthly real-time quantitative polymerase chain reaction (PCR) for BCR ABL mRNA transcripts in blood. The aim is to reduce the BCR ABL transcript levels by 3–5 logs from baseline and this is called major molecular response (MR3–MR5). A proportion of patients achieve a complete molecular response where the transcripts are not detectable by PCR. It may be possible for patients with a complete or major molecular response

---

to stop TKI therapy and this is being investigated in clinical trials. For those failing to respond or who lose their response and progress on first-line therapy, options include switching to a different TKI (Box 23.49). Some patients develop detectable mutations in the *BCR ABL* gene, which renders them resistant to one or more of the TKIs. The T315I mutation has been particularly problematic, as this provides wide-ranging resistance. The third-generation TKI ponatinib is effective, however. Allogeneic HSCT (p. 937) is now reserved for patients who fail TKI therapy. Hydroxycarbamide and interferon were previously used for control of disease. Hydroxycarbamide is still useful in palliative situations and interferon is used in women planning pregnancy.

Accelerated phase and blast crisis

Management is more difficult. For patients in accelerated phase, TKI therapy is indicated, most commonly with nilotinib or dasatinib. When blast transformation occurs, the type of blast cell should be determined. Response to appropriate acute leukaemia treatment (see Box 23.49) is better if disease is lymphoblastic than if myeloblastic. Second- or third-generation TKIs such as dasatinib are used in combination with chemotherapy to try and achieve remission. In younger and fitter patients an allogeneic HSCT is appropriate therapy if a return to chronic phase is achieved. Hydroxycarbamide can be an effective single agent and low-dose cytarabine can also be used palliatively in older patients.

Chronic lymphocytic leukaemia

Chronic lymphocytic leukaemia (CLL) is the most common variety of leukaemia, accounting for 30% of cases. The male-to-female ratio is $2:1$ and the median age at presentation is 65–70 years. In this disease, B lymphocytes, which would normally respond to antigens by transformation and antibody formation, fail to do so. An ever-increasing mass of immuno-incompetent cells accumulates, to the detriment of immune function and normal bone marrow haematopoiesis.

Clinical features

The onset is usually insidious. Indeed, in around 70% of patients, the diagnosis is made incidentally on a routine FBC. Presenting problems may be anaemia, infections, painless lymphadenopathy, and systemic symptoms such as night sweats or weight loss; these more often occur later in the course of the disease.

Investigations

The diagnosis is based on the peripheral blood findings of a mature lymphocytosis ($>5\times10^9$/L) with characteristic morphology and cell surface markers. Immunophenotyping reveals the lymphocytes to be monoclonal B cells expressing the B-cell antigens CD19 and CD23, with either kappa or lambda immunoglobulin light chains and, characteristically, an aberrant T-cell antigen CD5. On flow cytometry, some people are shown to have circulating CLL cells at a level less than 5×10^9/L. This is known as monoclonal B lymphocytosis of uncertain significance.

Other useful investigations in CLL include a reticulocyte count and a direct Coombs test, as autoimmune haemolytic anaemia may occur (p. 949). Serum immunoglobulin levels should be estimated to establish the degree of hypogammaglobulinaemia, which is common and progressive. Bone marrow examination by aspirate and trephine is not essential for the diagnosis of CLL, but may be helpful in difficult cases, for prognosis (patients with diffuse marrow involvement have a poorer prognosis) and to monitor response to therapy. The main prognostic factor is

23

---

i	**23.49 Tyrosine kinase inhibition in chronic myeloid leukaemia**	
Agents		
First-line		
• Imatinib	• Dasatinib	
• Nilotinib		
Second-line		
• Imatinib	• Bosutinib	
• Nilotinib	• Ponatinib*	
• Dasatinib		
Outcomes		
• 90% achieve complete cytogenetic response		
• Responses faster with nilotinib and dasatinib		
• Median survival comparable to normal population		

*For patients with T315I kinase domain mutations use ponatinib.

23.50 Staging of chronic lymphocytic leukaemia

Clinical stage A (60% patients)

- No anaemia or thrombocytopenia and fewer than three areas of lymphoid enlargement

Clinical stage B (30% patients)

- No anaemia or thrombocytopenia, with three or more involved areas of lymphoid enlargement

Clinical stage C (10% patients)

- Anaemia and/or thrombocytopenia, regardless of the number of areas of lymphoid enlargement

stage of disease (Box 23.50); however, loss of chromosome 17p or mutation in the *TP53* gene, which resides at this genetic locus, is a powerful prognostic marker and predictor of response to therapy. A mutation in *TP53* is present in <10% of patients at presentation but rises to 30% of cases at relapse. This test should be performed in all patients prior to the initiation of therapy.

Management

No specific treatment is required for most clinical stage A patients, unless progression occurs. Life expectancy is usually normal in older patients. The patient should be offered clear information about CLL and be reassured about the indolent nature of the disease, as the diagnosis of leukaemia inevitably causes anxiety.

Treatment is required only if there is evidence of bone marrow failure, massive or progressive lymphadenopathy or splenomegaly, systemic symptoms such as weight loss or night sweats, a rapidly increasing lymphocyte count, autoimmune haemolytic anaemia or thrombocytopenia. Initial therapy for those requiring treatment (progressive stage A and stages B and C) is based on the age and fitness of the patient and the *TP53* mutation status. For patients who are under 70 years, fit and *TP53* mutation-negative, fludarabine in combination with the alkylating agent cyclophosphamide and the anti-CD20 monoclonal antibody rituximab (FCR) is standard care. For older, less fit patients, rituximab is combined with gentler chemotherapy: bendamustine or oral chlorambucil. Recently, a more potent type 2 anti-CD20 antibody, obinutuzumab, has become available and produces better responses in combination with chlorambucil than rituximab.

CLL cells are dependent on abnormal and persistent signalling through the B-cell receptor (BCR) pathway. Drugs that can inhibit this pathway are now available and show great promise. Ibrutinib inhibits Bruton's tyrosine kinase and idelalisib inhibits PI3 kinase, both components of the BCR pathway. Ibrutinib and idelalisib are licensed for relapsed CLL but crucially are licensed and effective in *TP53*-mutated disease at all stages and are quickly becoming standard care in *TP53*-mutated CLL. Bone marrow failure or autoimmune cytopenias may respond to glucocorticoid treatment.

Supportive care is increasingly required in progressive disease, such as transfusions for symptomatic anaemia or thrombocytopenia, prompt treatment of infections and, for some patients with hypogammaglobulinaemia, immunoglobulin replacement. Radiotherapy may be used for lymphadenopathy that is causing discomfort or local obstruction, and for symptomatic splenomegaly. Splenectomy may be required to improve low blood counts due to autoimmune destruction or to hypersplenism, and can relieve massive splenomegaly.

Prognosis

The majority of clinical stage A patients have a normal life expectancy but patients with advanced CLL are more likely to die from their disease or infectious complications. Survival is influenced by prognostic features of the leukaemia, particularly *TP53* mutation status, and whether patients can tolerate and respond to fludarabine-based treatment. In those able to be treated with chemotherapy and rituximab, 90% are alive 4 years later. Rarely, CLL transforms to an aggressive high-grade lymphoma, called Richter's transformation.

Prolymphocytic leukaemia

Prolymphocytic leukaemia (PLL) is a variant of chronic lymphocytic leukaemia found mainly in males over the age of 60 years; 25% of cases are of the T-cell variety. There is typically massive splenomegaly with little lymphadenopathy and a very high leucocyte count, often in excess of 400×10^9/L. The characteristic cell is a large lymphocyte with a prominent nucleolus. Treatment is generally unsuccessful and the prognosis very poor. Leukapharesis, splenectomy and chemotherapy may be tried. The anti-CD52 antibody alemtuzumab, when given intravenously, has produced responses in some 90% of patients with T-PLL.

Hairy cell leukaemia

This is a rare chronic B-cell lymphoproliferative disorder. The male-to-female ratio is 6:1 and the median age at diagnosis is 50 years. Presenting symptoms are general ill health and recurrent infections. Splenomegaly occurs in 90% but lymph node enlargement is unusual.

Severe neutropenia, monocytopenia and the characteristic hairy cells in the blood and bone marrow are typical. These cells usually have a B-lymphocyte immunotype but they also characteristically express CD25 and CD103. Recently, all patients with hairy cell leukaemia have been found to have a mutation in the *BRAF* gene.

Over recent years, a number of treatments, including cladribine and deoxycoformycin, have been shown to produce long-lasting remissions.

Myelodysplastic syndromes

Myelodysplastic syndromes (MDSs) constitute a group of clonal haematopoietic disorders with the common features of ineffective blood cell production and a tendency to progress to AML. As such, they are pre-leukaemic and represent genetic steps in the development of leukaemia. These genetic abnormalities have been identified and are present as a manifestation of clonal haematopoiesis in about 3% of patients over the age of 80, at a time when their blood counts are normal (clonal haematopoiesis of indeterminate potential, CHIP). MDS presents with consequences of bone marrow failure (anaemia, recurrent infections or bleeding), usually in older people (median age at diagnosis is 73 years). The overall incidence is 4/100 000 in the population, rising to more than 30/100 000 in the over-seventies. The blood film is characterised by cytopenias and abnormal-looking (dysplastic) blood cells, including macrocytic red cells and hypogranular neutrophils with nuclear hyper- or hyposegmentation. The bone marrow is hypercellular, with dysplastic changes in at least 10% of cells of one or more cell lines. Blast cells may be increased but do not reach the 20% level that indicates acute leukaemia. Chromosome analysis frequently reveals abnormalities, particularly

23

23.51 WHO classification of myelodysplastic syndromes (MDSs)

Disease	Bone marrow findings
MDS with single-lineage dysplasia	<5% blasts and single-lineage dysplasia only
MDS with ring sideroblasts (MDS-RS)	>15% ring sideroblasts, or 6–14% and presence of *SF3B1* gene mutation
MDS with multilineage dysplasia	<5% blasts and dysplasia in 2 or more lineages
MDS with excess blasts	5–19% blasts
MDS with isolated del(5q)	Myelodysplastic syndrome associated with a del(5q) cytogenetic abnormality <5% blasts Often normal or increased blood platelet count
MDS, unclassifiable	None of the above or inadequate material

23.52 Revised International Prognostic Scoring System and outcomes in myelodysplasia*

Risk category	Overall score	Median survival (years)	25% progression to acute myeloid leukaemia (years)
Very low	≤1.5	8.8	Not reached
Low	>1.5–3	5.3	10.8
Intermediate	>3–4.5	3.0	3.2
High	>4.5–6	1.6	1.4
Very high	>6	0.8	0.73

*The IPSS-R is based on three prognostic factors: the blast percentage in bone marrow; karyotype; and number and degree of blood cytopenias. A score is derived from which patients can be stratified into five risk categories for survival and leukaemic transformation.

of chromosome 5 or 7. The WHO classification of MDS is shown in Box 23.51.

Prognosis

The natural history of MDS is progressive worsening of dysplasia leading to fatal bone marrow failure or progression to AML in 30% of cases. The time to progression varies (from months to years) with the subtype of MDS, being slowest in MDS with ring sideroblasts and single-lineage dysplasia and most rapid in MDS with excess blasts. The revised International Prognostic Scoring System (IPSS-R) predicts clinical outcome based on karyotype and cytopenias in blood, as well as percentage of bone marrow blasts (Box 23.52). There are five prognostic groups. The median survival for low-risk patients (IPSS-R very low and low) is 5–9 years, that for the intermediate group is 3 years and that for high-risk patients (IPSS-R high and very high) is 1–1.5 years.

Management

For the vast majority of patients who are elderly, the disease is incurable, and supportive care with red cell and platelet transfusions is the mainstay of treatment. A trial of erythropoiesis stimulating agents (ESA) and granulocyte–colony-stimulating factor (G–CSF) is recommended in some patients with low-risk MDS (IPSS-R very low, low and intermediate) to improve haemoglobin or neutrophil counts. A rare subtype called MDS

with isolated del(5q) responds well to the immunomodulatory drug lenalidomide, with two-thirds of anaemic patients becoming transfusion-independent for up to 2 years. Allogeneic stem cell transplantation may afford a cure in patients with a good performance status and is considered in high-risk patients (IPSS-R high and very high) and some low-risk patients. More recently, the hypomethylating agent azacytidine has improved survival by a median of 9 months for high-risk patients, and in the UK is a recommended standard of care for those not eligible for transplantation.

Lymphomas

These neoplasms arise from lymphoid tissues, and are diagnosed from the pathological findings on biopsy as Hodgkin or non-Hodgkin lymphoma. The majority are of B-cell origin. Non-Hodgkin lymphomas are classified as low- or high-grade tumours on the basis of their proliferation rate. The normal architecture of the lymph node is outlined in Figure 23.25.

- *High-grade tumours* divide rapidly, are typically present for a matter of weeks before diagnosis, and may be life-threatening with frequent risk of extranodal involvement.
- *Low-grade tumours* divide slowly, may be present for many months before diagnosis, and typically behave in an indolent fashion.

Hodgkin lymphoma

The histological hallmark of Hodgkin lymphoma (HL) is the presence of Reed–Sternberg cells: large, malignant lymphoid cells of B-cell origin (Fig. 23.26). They are often present only in small numbers but are surrounded by large numbers of reactive non-malignant T cells, plasma cells and eosinophils.

The epidemiology of HL is shown in Box 23.53 and its histological WHO classification in Box 23.54.

Nodular lymphocyte-predominant HL is slow-growing, localised and rarely fatal. It has biological features, such as CD20-positive Hodgkin cells, and clinical features that make it more akin to a low-grade B-cell non-Hodgkin lymphoma. Classical HL is divided into four histological subtypes from the appearance of the

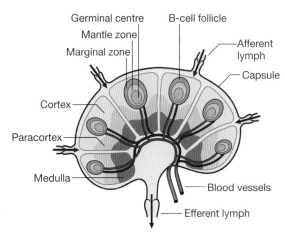

Fig. 23.25 Schema of lymph node architecture. Different lymphocyte populations reside in different areas of the node: B cells in the follicles, T cells in the paracortex and plasma cells in the medulla. B cells are selected for antigen in the follicle centre. Errors during this process result in B-cell lymphomas, which are by far the most common type.

Fig. 23.26 Hodgkin lymphoma. In the centre of this lymph node biopsy is a large typical Reed–Sternberg cell with two nuclei containing a prominent eosinophilic nucleolus.

23.53 Epidemiology and aetiology of Hodgkin lymphoma	

Incidence

- Approximately 4 new cases/100 000 population/year

Sex ratio

- Slight male excess (1.5:1)

Age

- Median age 31 years; first peak at 20–35 years and second at 50–70 years

Aetiology

- Unknown
- More common in patients from well-educated backgrounds and small families
- Three times more likely with a past history of infectious mononucleosis but no definitive causal link to Epstein–Barr virus infection proven

23.54 WHO pathological classification of Hodgkin lymphoma (HL)

Type	Histology classification	Proportion of HL
Nodular lymphocyte-predominant HL		5%
Classical HL	Nodular sclerosing	70%
	Mixed cellularity	20%
	Lymphocyte-rich	5%
	Lymphocyte-depleted	Rare

Reed–Sternberg cells and surrounding reactive cells. The nodular sclerosing type is more common in young patients and in women. Mixed cellularity is more common in the elderly. Lymphocyte-rich HL usually presents in men. Lymphocyte-depleted HL is rare and probably represents large-cell or anaplastic non-Hodgkin lymphoma.

Clinical features

There is painless, rubbery lymphadenopathy, usually in the neck or supraclavicular fossae; the lymph nodes may fluctuate in size. Young patients with nodular sclerosing disease may have large mediastinal masses that are surprisingly asymptomatic

23.55 Clinical stages of Hodgkin lymphoma (Ann Arbor classification)

Stage	Definition
I	Involvement of a single lymph node region (I) or extralymphatic* site (I$_E$)
II	Involvement of two or more lymph node regions (II) or an extralymphatic site and lymph node regions on the same side of (above or below) the diaphragm (II$_E$)
III	Involvement of lymph node regions on both sides of the diaphragm with (III$_E$) or without (III) localised extralymphatic involvement or involvement of the spleen (III$_S$), or both (III$_{SE}$)
IV	Diffuse involvement of one or more extralymphatic tissues, e.g. liver or bone marrow

Each stage is subclassified:
A	No systemic symptoms
B	Weight loss >10%, drenching sweats, fever

*The lymphatic structures are defined as the lymph nodes, spleen, thymus, Waldeyer's ring, appendix and Peyer's patches.

but may cause dry cough and some breathlessness. Isolated subdiaphragmatic nodes occur in fewer than 10% at diagnosis. Hepatosplenomegaly may be present but does not always indicate disease in those organs. Spread is contiguous from one node to the next, and extranodal disease, such as bone, brain or skin involvement, is rare.

Investigations

Treatment of HL depends on the stage at presentation; investigations therefore aim not only to diagnose lymphoma but also to determine the extent of disease (Box 23.55).

- *FBC* may be normal. If a normochromic, normocytic anaemia or lymphopenia is present, this is a poor prognostic factor. An eosinophilia or a neutrophilia may be present.
- *ESR* may be raised.
- *Renal function tests* are required to ensure function is normal prior to treatment.
- *Liver function* may be abnormal in the absence of disease or may reflect hepatic infiltration. An obstructive pattern may be caused by nodes at the porta hepatis.
- *LDH measurements* showing raised levels are an adverse prognostic factor.
- *Chest X-ray* may show a mediastinal mass.
- *CT scan* of chest, abdomen and pelvis permits staging. Bulky disease (>10 cm in a single node mass) is an adverse prognostic feature.
- *Positron emission tomography (PET) scanning* identifies nodes involved with HL, which are [18]fluorodeoxyglucose (FDG)-avid, and this allows more accurate staging and monitoring of response (Fig. 23.27).
- *Lymph node biopsy* may be undertaken surgically or by percutaneous needle biopsy under radiological guidance (Fig. 23.28).

Management

Clinical trials have shown that patients with early-stage disease (stages IA and IIA) have better outcomes if limited cycles of chemotherapy are combined with radiotherapy, rather than using radiotherapy alone.

Fig. 23.27 Positron emission tomography (PET) scans in Hodgkin lymphoma, demonstrating response to treatment. A Chest X-ray from a young man with Hodgkin lymphoma at presentation, showing a left-sided anterior–superior mediastinal mass with tracheal deviation to the right. B Fused PET-CT image showing intense fluorodeoxyglucose (FDG) uptake (avidity) in the mass at presentation. C Fused PET-CT image showing no FDG uptake (PET negativity), representing complete response at the end of treatment.

Fig. 23.28 CT-guided percutaneous needle biopsy of retroperitoneal nodes involved by lymphoma.

The ABVD regimen (doxorubicin, bleomycin, vinblastine and dacarbazine) is widely used in the UK. Standard therapy for early-stage patients without additional risk factors, such as bulk disease or high ESR, is two cycles of ABVD combined with 20 Gy radiotherapy to the involved sites of disease. Standard therapy for early-stage patients with additional risk factors is four cycles of ABVD combined with 30 Gy radiotherapy. Careful planning of radiotherapy is required to limit the doses delivered to normal tissues and new planning techniques continue to improve targeting of radiotherapy. Nevertheless, the long-term risks of second cancers and heart and lung disease within the radiation fields remain a concern, especially for young people with a high cure rate and decades of life ahead of them. Recent randomised trial data from the UK RAPID study have suggested that early-stage patients without bulk disease who have a negative PET scan after three cycles of ABVD can safely omit radiotherapy. Young women receiving breast irradiation during the treatment of chest disease have an increased risk of breast cancer and should participate in a screening programme. Patients continuing to smoke after lung irradiation are at particular risk of lung cancer.

ABVD chemotherapy can cause cardiac and pulmonary toxicity, due to doxorubicin and bleomycin, respectively. The incidence of infertility and secondary myelodysplasia/AML is low with this regimen.

Patients with advanced-stage disease are most commonly managed with chemotherapy alone. Standard treatment in the UK is 6–8 cycles of ABVD, followed by an assessment of response. The recent UK RATHL trial has confirmed previous data showing that achieving a PET-negative response after two cycles of ABVD (interim PET-2 response) predicts a very good outcome from continuing with up to six cycles of ABVD. Indeed, the same outcome can be achieved by omitting the bleomycin from the last four cycles and using just AVD, thus reducing the risk of lung toxicity. Patients who are PET-positive after two cycles, however, have a very high relapse risk if they continue with ABVD, only 13% being relapse-free at 2 years. The RATHL and other studies have demonstrated that changing to a more intensive regimen, BEACOPP (bleomycin, etoposide, adriamycin, cyclophosphamide, vincristine (oncovin), procarbazine, prednisolone), in these patients improves the relapse-free survival to approximately 65%.

Patients with relapsed disease that responds to salvage chemotherapy and ideally becomes PET-negative should be considered for autologous stem cell transplantation (p. 937). Those with resistant disease might benefit from an allogeneic

23

23.56 The Hasenclever prognostic index for advanced Hodgkin lymphoma

Score 1 for each of the following risk factors present at diagnosis:
- Age >45 years
- Male gender
- Serum albumin <40 g/L
- Hb <105 g/L
- Stage IV disease
- White blood cell count >15×10⁹/L
- Lymphopenia <0.6×10⁹/L

Score	5-year rate of freedom from progression (%)	5-year rate of overall survival (%)
0–1	79	90
>2	60	74
>3	55	70
>4	47	59

23.57 Epidemiology and aetiology of non-Hodgkin lymphoma

Incidence
- 12 new cases/100 000 people/year

Sex ratio
- Slight male excess

Age
- Median age 65–70 years

Aetiology
- No single causative abnormality described
- Lymphoma is a late manifestation of HIV infection (p. 322)
- Specific lymphoma types are associated with viruses:
  e.g. Epstein–Barr virus (EBV) with post-transplant NHL, human herpesvirus 8 (HHV8) with a primary effusion lymphoma, and human T-cell lymphotropic virus (HTLV-1) with adult T-cell leukaemia lymphoma
- Gastric lymphoma can be associated with *Helicobacter pylori* infection
- Some lymphomas are associated with specific chromosomal translocations:
  The t(14;18) in follicular lymphoma results in the dysregulated expression of the BCL-2 gene product, which inhibits apoptotic cell death
  The t(8;14) found in Burkitt lymphoma and the t(11;14) in mantle cell lymphoma alter function of c-myc and cyclin D1, respectively, resulting in malignant proliferation
- Lymphoma occurs in congenital immunodeficiency states and in immunosuppressed patients after organ transplantation

stem cell transplant. Brentuximab vedotin is an antibody–drug conjugate directed against CD30 on the Reed–Sternberg cell surface. This antibody delivers the antimitotic toxin monomethyl auristatin E to the Hodgkin cells and, as a single agent, can produce good responses in patients who have failed, or are not suitable for, an autologous transplant and can be a 'bridge' to an allogeneic transplant.

Prognosis

Over 90% of patients with early-stage HL achieve complete remission when treated with chemotherapy followed by involved field radiotherapy, and the great majority are cured. The major challenge is how to reduce treatment intensity, and hence long-term toxicity, without reducing the excellent cure rates in this group. Omitting radiotherapy in the majority of PET-negative patients is one major step forward in this regard.

Historically, between 50 and 70% of those with advanced-stage HL were cured. The Hasenclever index (Box 23.56) can be helpful in assigning approximate chances of cure when discussing treatment plans with patients. More recent data using the PET scanner to direct therapy suggests that long-term survival is improving to beyond 80%. Patients who fail to respond to initial chemotherapy or relapse within a year of initial therapy have a poor prognosis but some may achieve long-term survival after autologous HSCT. Patients relapsing after 1 year may obtain long-term survival with further chemotherapy alone, but fit patients frequently proceed to autologous HSCT.

Non-Hodgkin lymphoma

Non-Hodgkin lymphoma (NHL) represents a monoclonal proliferation of lymphoid cells of B-cell (90%) or T-cell (10%) origin. The incidence of these tumours increases with age, to 62.8/million population per annum at age 75 years, and the overall rate is increasing at about 3% per year.

The epidemiology of NHL is shown in Box 23.57. Previous classifications were based principally on histological appearances. The current WHO classification stratifies according to cell lineage (T or B cells) and incorporates clinical features, histology, chromosomal abnormalities and concepts related to the biology of the lymphoma. Clinically, the most important factor is grade, which is a reflection of proliferation rate. High-grade NHL has high proliferation rates, rapidly produces symptoms, is fatal if untreated, but is potentially curable. Low-grade NHL has low proliferation rates, may be asymptomatic for many months or even years before presentation, runs an indolent course, but is not curable by conventional therapy. Of all cases of NHL in the developed world, over two-thirds are either diffuse large B-cell NHL (high-grade) or follicular NHL (low-grade) (Fig. 23.29). Other forms of NHL, including Burkitt lymphoma, mantle cell lymphoma, mucosa-associated lymphoid tissue (MALT) lymphomas and T-cell lymphomas, are less common.

Clinical features

Unlike Hodgkin lymphoma, NHL is often widely disseminated at presentation, including in extranodal sites. Patients present with lymph node enlargement (Fig. 23.30), which may be associated with systemic upset: weight loss, sweats, fever and itching. Hepatosplenomegaly may be present. Sites of extranodal involvement include the bone marrow, gut, thyroid, lung, skin, testis, brain and, more rarely, bone. Bone marrow involvement is more common in low-grade (50–60%) than high-grade (10%) disease. Compression syndromes may occur, including gut obstruction, ascites, superior vena cava obstruction and spinal cord compression.

The same staging system (see Box 23.55) is used for both HL and NHL, but NHL is more likely to be stage III or IV at presentation.

Investigations

These are as for HL, but in addition the following should be performed:
- *Bone marrow aspiration and trephine* to identify bone marrow involvement.
- *Immunophenotyping of surface antigens to distinguish T-cell from B-cell tumours*. This may be done on blood, marrow or nodal material.

Fig. 23.29 Histology of non-Hodgkin lymphoma. [A] (Low-grade) follicular or nodular pattern. [B] (High-grade) diffuse pattern.

Fig. 23.30 Bulky axillary lymphadenopathy with distended superficial veins in a patient presenting with high-grade lymphoma. *From Howard MR, Hamilton PJ. Haematology: An illustrated colour text, 4th edn. Edinburgh: Elsevier Ltd; 2013.*

- *Cytogenetic analysis to detect chromosomal translocations* and molecular testing for T-cell receptor or immunoglobulin gene rearrangements.
- *Immunoglobulin determination.* Some lymphomas are associated with IgG or IgM paraproteins, which serve as markers for treatment response.
- *Measurement of uric acid levels.* Some very aggressive high-grade NHLs are associated with very high urate levels, which can precipitate renal failure when treatment is started.
- *HIV testing.* HIV is a risk factor for some lymphomas and affects treatment decisions.
- *Hepatitis B and C testing.* This should be done prior to therapy with rituximab.

Management

Low-grade NHL

The majority of patients (80%) present with advanced stage disease and will run a relapsing and remitting course over several years. Asymptomatic patients may not require therapy and are managed by 'watching and waiting'. Indications for treatment include marked systemic symptoms, lymphadenopathy causing discomfort or disfigurement, bone marrow failure or compression syndromes. In follicular lymphoma, the options are:

- *Radiotherapy.* This can be used for localised stage I disease, which is rare.
- *Chemotherapy.* Most patients will respond to oral therapy with chlorambucil, which is well tolerated but not curative. More intensive intravenous chemotherapy in younger patients produces better quality of life but no survival benefit.
- *Monoclonal antibody therapy.* Humanised monoclonal antibodies ('biological therapy'; p. 960) can be used to

target surface antigens on tumour cells and to induce tumour cell apoptosis directly. The anti-CD20 antibody rituximab has been shown to induce durable clinical responses in up to 60% of patients when given alone, and acts synergistically when given with chemotherapy. Rituximab (R) in combination with cyclophosphamide, vincristine and prednisolone (R-CVP), cyclophosphamide, doxorubicin, vincristine, prednisolone (R-CHOP) or bendamustine (R-bendamustine) is commonly used as first-line therapy. Randomised trials have also confirmed that 2 years of maintenance therapy with single-agent rituximab, following achievement of first or second response, delays relapse and the time to next treatment. As yet, however, rituximab maintenance has not shown a survival benefit. New and more potent monoclonal antibodies are also in development and trials of obinutuzumab (p. 960) have been completed.

- *Kinase inhibitors.* Idelalisib is approved for relapsed follicular lymphoma and ibrutinib (p. 960) is approved for relapsed mantle cell lymphoma, a poor-prognosis lymphoma with low-grade histology but aggressive clinical behaviour. These targeted therapies are likely to become more widely used in low-grade lymphomas in the near future.
- *Transplantation.* High-dose chemotherapy and autologous HSCT can produce long remissions in patients with relapsed disease. Decisions on the timing of such treatment are complex in the context of rituximab maintenance and newer targeted therapies. However, younger patients with short first or second remissions or who relapse during rituximab maintenance should be considered.

23

High-grade NHL

Patients with diffuse large B-cell NHL need treatment at initial presentation:

- *Chemotherapy.* The majority (>90%) are treated with intravenous combination chemotherapy, typically with the CHOP regimen (cyclophosphamide, doxorubicin, vincristine and prednisolone).
- *Monoclonal antibody therapy.* When combined with CHOP chemotherapy, rituximab (R) increases the complete response rates and improves overall survival. R-CHOP is currently recommended as first-line therapy for those with stage II or higher diffuse large B-cell lymphoma.
- *Radiotherapy.* Stage I patients without bulky disease are treated with four cycles of CHOP or R-CHOP, followed by involved site radiotherapy. Radiotherapy is also indicated for a residual localised site of bulk disease after chemotherapy, and for spinal cord and other compression syndromes.
- *HSCT.* Autologous HSCT (p. 937) benefits patients with relapsed disease that is sensitive to salvage immunochemotherapy. As with HL, achieving PET negativity prior to autologous transplantation is desirable.

Prognosis

Low-grade NHL runs an indolent remitting and relapsing course, with an overall median survival of 12 years. Transformation to a high-grade NHL occurs in 3% per annum and is associated with poor survival.

In diffuse large B-cell NHL treated with R-CHOP, some 75% of patients overall respond initially to therapy and 50% will have disease-free survival at 5 years. The prognosis for patients with NHL is further refined according to the international prognostic index (IPI). For high-grade NHL, 5-year survival ranges from over 75% in those with low-risk scores (age <60 years, stage I or II, one or fewer extranodal sites, normal LDH and good performance status) to 25% in those with high-risk scores (increasing age, advanced stage, concomitant disease and a raised LDH).

Relapse is associated with a poor response to further chemotherapy (<10% 5-year survival), but in patients under 65 years HSCT improves survival.

Paraproteinaemias

A gammopathy refers to over-production of one or more classes of immunoglobulin. It may be polyclonal in association with acute or chronic inflammation, such as infection, sarcoidosis, autoimmune disorders or some malignancies. Alternatively, a monoclonal increase in a single immunoglobulin class may occur in association with normal or reduced levels of the other immunoglobulins. Such monoclonal proteins (also called M-proteins, paraproteins or monoclonal gammopathies) occur as a feature of myeloma, lymphoma and amyloidosis, in connective tissue disease such as rheumatoid arthritis or polymyalgia rheumatica, in infection such as HIV, and in solid tumours. In addition, they may be present with no underlying disease. Gammopathies are detected by plasma immunoelectrophoresis.

Monoclonal gammopathy of uncertain significance

In monoclonal gammopathy of uncertain significance (MGUS, also known as benign monoclonal gammopathy), a paraprotein is present in the blood but there are no other features of myeloma, Waldenström macroglobulinaemia (see below), lymphoma or related disease. It is a common condition associated with increasing age; a paraprotein can be found in 1% of the population aged over 50 years, increasing to 5% over 80 years.

Clinical features and investigations

Patients are usually asymptomatic, and the paraprotein is found on blood testing for other reasons. The routine blood count and biochemistry are normal, the paraprotein is usually present in small amounts with no associated immune paresis, and there are no lytic bone lesions. The bone marrow may have increased plasma cells but these usually constitute less than 10% of nucleated cells.

Prognosis

After follow-up of 20 years, only one-quarter of cases will progress to myeloma or a related disorder (i.e. around 1% per annum). There is no certain way of predicting progression in an individual patient. However, an abnormal ratio of kappa to lambda light chains (serum free light chain ratio, SFLR) increases the risk of progression. Patients with an abnormal ratio should be monitored for progression on an annual basis.

Waldenström macroglobulinaemia

This is a low-grade lymphoplasmacytic lymphoma associated with an IgM paraprotein, causing clinical features of hyperviscosity syndrome. It is a rare tumour occurring in the elderly and more commonly affects males.

Patients classically present with features of hyperviscosity, such as nosebleeds, bruising, delirium and visual disturbance. However, presentation may be with anaemia, systemic symptoms, splenomegaly or lymphadenopathy, or may be asymptomatic, with an IgM paraprotein detected on routine screening. Patients are found on investigation to have an IgM paraprotein associated with a raised plasma viscosity. The bone marrow has a characteristic appearance, with infiltration of lymphoid cells, plasma cells and sometimes prominent mast cells. A high proportion of patients have a mutation in the *MYD88* gene.

Management

If patients show symptoms of hyperviscosity and anaemia, plasmapheresis is required to remove IgM and make blood transfusion possible. Chemotherapy with alkylating agents, such as chlorambucil, has been the mainstay of treatment, controlling disease in over 50%. Fludarabine may be more effective in this disease but has more side-effects. Rituximab in combination with chemotherapy is most commonly used; ibrutinib is very effective and has recently been licensed for use. Rituximab alone can cause a rapid release of IgM and increase in viscosity. The median survival is 5 years.

Multiple myeloma

This is a malignant proliferation of plasma cells. Normal plasma cells are derived from B cells and produce immunoglobulins that contain heavy and light chains. Normal immunoglobulins are polyclonal, which means that a variety of heavy chains are produced and each may be of kappa or lambda light chain type (p. 68). In myeloma, plasma cells produce immunoglobulin of a single heavy and light chain, a monoclonal protein commonly referred to as a paraprotein. In most cases an excess of light chain is produced, and in some cases only light chain is produced;

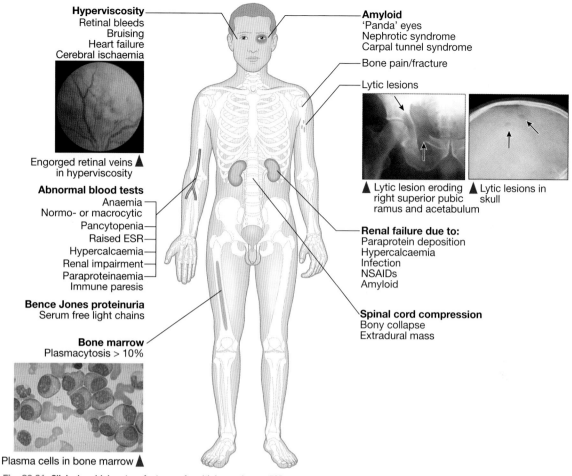

Hyperviscosity
Retinal bleeds
Bruising
Heart failure
Cerebral ischaemia

▲ Engorged retinal veins
in hyperviscosity

Abnormal blood tests
Anaemia
Normo- or macrocytic
Pancytopenia
Raised ESR
Hypercalcaemia
Renal impairment
Paraproteinaemia
Immune paresis

Bence Jones proteinuria
Serum free light chains

Bone marrow
Plasmacytosis > 10%

Plasma cells in bone marrow ▲

Amyloid
'Panda' eyes
Nephrotic syndrome
Carpal tunnel syndrome

Bone pain/fracture

Lytic lesions

▲ Lytic lesion eroding
right superior pubic
ramus and acetabulum

▲ Lytic lesions in
skull

Renal failure due to:
Paraprotein deposition
Hypercalcaemia
Infection
NSAIDs
Amyloid

Spinal cord compression
Bony collapse
Extradural mass

Fig. 23.31 Clinical and laboratory features of multiple myeloma. (ESR = erythrocyte sedimentation rate; NSAIDs = non-steroidal anti-inflammatory drugs)

i 23.58 Classification of multiple myeloma	
Type of monoclonal (M)-protein	Relative frequency (%)
IgG	55
IgA	21
Light chain only	22
Others (D, E, non-secretory)	2

this appears in the urine as Bence Jones proteinuria and can be measured in the urine or serum as free light chain. The frequency of different isotypes of monoclonal protein in myeloma is shown in Box 23.58.

Although a small number of malignant plasma cells are present in the circulation, the majority are present in the bone marrow. The malignant plasma cells produce cytokines, which stimulate osteoclasts and result in net bone reabsorption. The resulting lytic lesions cause bone pain, fractures and hypercalcaemia. Marrow involvement can result in anaemia or pancytopenia.

Clinical features and investigations

The incidence of myeloma is 4/100 000 new cases per annum, with a male-to-female ratio of 2:1. The median age at diagnosis is 60–70 years and the disease is more common in Afro-Caribbeans. The clinical features are demonstrated in Figure 23.31.

Diagnosis of myeloma requires two of the following criteria to be fulfilled:

- increased malignant plasma cells in the bone marrow
- serum and/or urinary M-protein
- skeletal lytic lesions.

Bone marrow aspiration, plasma and urine electrophoresis, and a skeletal survey are thus required. Normal immunoglobulin levels, i.e. the absence of immunoparesis, should cast doubt on the diagnosis. Paraproteinaemia can cause an elevated ESR but this is a non-specific test; only approximately 5% of patients with a persistently elevated ESR above 100 mm/hr have underlying myeloma.

Management

If patients are asymptomatic with no evidence of end-organ damage (e.g. to kidneys, bone marrow or bone), treatment may not be required. So-called asymptomatic myeloma should be monitored closely for the development of end-organ damage.

Immediate support

- High fluid intake to treat renal impairment and hypercalcaemia (p. 661).
- Analgesia for bone pain.

- Bisphosphonates for hypercalcaemia and to delay other skeletal related events (p. 1047).
- Allopurinol to prevent urate nephropathy.
- Plasmapheresis, if necessary, for hyperviscosity.

Chemotherapy with or without HSCT

Myeloma therapy has improved with the addition of novel agents, initially thalidomide and more recently the proteasome inhibitor bortezomib and the second-generation immunomodulatory drug lenalidomide. For first-line therapy in older patients, thalidomide combined with the alkylating agent melphalan and prednisolone (MPT) has increased the median overall survival to more than 4 years. Lenalidomide is approved first-line treatment for patients not eligible for transplantation and who are intolerant of, or unsuitable for, thalidomide. Thalidomide and lenalidomide both have anti-angiogenic effects against tumour blood vessels and immunomodulatory effects. Both can cause somnolence, constipation, peripheral neuropathy and thrombosis, though lenalidomide has a better side-effect profile. It is vital that females of child-bearing age use adequate contraception, as thalidomide and lenalidomide are teratogenic. Treatment is administered until paraprotein levels have stopped falling. This is termed 'plateau phase' and can last for weeks or years.

In younger, fitter patients, standard treatment includes first-line therapies, such as cyclophosphamide, thalidomide and dexamethasone (CTD) or bortezomib (Velcade), thalidomide and dexamethasone (VTD) to maximum response, and then autologous HSCT, which improves quality of life and prolongs survival but does not cure myeloma. In all patients who have achieved maximal response, lenalidomide maintenance has been shown to prolong the response.

When myeloma progresses, treatment is given to induce a further plateau phase. In the UK, the proteosome inhibitor bortezomib and lenalidomide have been used as second- and third-line therapy, as appropriate. As they have been used more frequently in the first or second line with prognostic benefit, however, subsequent relapses are more difficult to treat. A second-generation proteasome inhibitor, carfilzomib, and the anti-CD38 antibody daratumumab show promise in relapsed/refractory disease. Responding patients may benefit from a second autologous HSCT.

Radiotherapy

This is effective for localised bone pain not responding to simple analgesia and for pathological fractures. It is also useful for the emergency treatment of spinal cord compression complicating extradural plasmacytomas.

Bisphosphonates

Long-term bisphosphonate therapy reduces bone pain and skeletal events. These drugs protect bone (p. 1047) and may cause apoptosis of malignant plasma cells. There is evidence that intravenous zoledronate in combination with anti-myeloma therapy confers a survival advantage over oral bisphosphonates. Osteonecrosis of the jaw may be associated with long-term use or poor oral hygiene and gum sepsis; regular dental review, including a check before starting therapy, is therefore important.

Prognosis

The international staging system (ISS) identifies poor prognostic features, including a high β_2-microglobulin and low albumin at diagnosis (ISS stage 3, median survival 29 months). Those with a normal albumin and a low β_2-microglobulin (ISS stage 1) have a median survival of 62 months. Increasingly, cytogenetic analysis is used to identify poor-risk patients, e.g. t(4;14), del(17;17p), t(14;16), t(14;20), non-hyperdiploidy and gain(1q). Use of autologous HSCT and advances in drug therapy with the newer agents have increased survival. Over one-third of patients are now surviving for 5 years, compared with only one-quarter 10 years ago. The outlook may improve further with new drugs and combinations of treatments.

Aplastic anaemias

Primary idiopathic acquired aplastic anaemia

This is a rare disorder in Europe and North America, with 2–4 new cases per million population per annum. The disease is much more common in certain other parts of the world, e.g. east Asia. The basic problem is failure of the pluripotent stem cells because of an autoimmune attack, producing hypoplasia of the bone marrow with a pancytopenia in the blood. The diagnosis rests on exclusion of other causes of secondary aplastic anaemia (see below) and rare congenital causes, such as Fanconi's anaemia.

Clinical features and investigations

Patients present with symptoms of bone marrow failure, usually anaemia or bleeding, and less commonly, infections. An FBC demonstrates pancytopenia, low reticulocytes and often macrocytosis. Bone marrow aspiration and trephine reveal hypocellularity. The severity of aplastic anaemia is graded according to the Camitta criteria (Box 23.60).

 23.59 Haematological malignancy in old age

- **Median age**: approximately 70 years for most haematological malignancies.
- **Poor-risk biological features**: adverse cytogenetics or the presence of a multidrug resistance phenotype are more frequent.
- **Prognosis**: increasing age is an independent adverse variable in acute leukaemia and aggressive lymphoma.
- **Chemotherapy**: may be less well tolerated. Older people are more likely to have antecedent cardiac, pulmonary or metabolic problems, tolerate systemic infection less well and metabolise cytotoxic drugs differently.
- **Cure rates**: similar to those in younger patients, in those who do tolerate treatment.
- **Decision to treat**: should be based on the individual's biological status, the level of social support available, and the patient's wishes and those of the immediate family, but not on chronological age alone.

 23.60 Camitta criteria

Severe AA (SAA)

- Marrow cellularity <25% (or 25–50% with <30% residual haematopoietic cells), plus at least two of:
  Neutrophils <0.5×10⁹/L
  Platelets <20×10⁹/L
  Reticulocyte count <20×10⁹/L

Very severe AA (VSAA)

- As for SAA but neutrophils <0.2×10⁹/L

Non-severe AA (NSAA)

- AA not fulfilling the criteria for SAA or VSAA

Management

All patients will require blood product support and aggressive management of infection. The prognosis of severe aplastic anaemia managed with supportive therapy only is poor and more than 50% of patients die, usually in the first year. The curative treatment for patients under 35 years of age with severe idiopathic aplastic anaemia is allogeneic HSCT if there is an available sibling donor (p. 937). Older patients (35–50) may be candidates if they have no comorbidities (p. 937). Those with a compatible sibling donor should proceed to transplantation as soon as possible; they have a 75–90% chance of long-term cure. In older patients and those without a suitable donor, immunosuppressive therapy (IST) with anti-thymocyte globulin (ATG) and ciclosporin is the treatment of choice and gives 5-year survival rates of 75%. Unrelated donor allografts are considered for suitable patients who fail IST. The thrombopoietin receptor agonist eltrombopag (p. 971) has produced trilineage responses in patients who fail IST and is licensed for this indication. Non-transplanted patients may relapse or other clonal disorders of haematopoiesis may evolve, such as paroxysmal nocturnal haemoglobinuria (p. 950), myelodysplastic syndrome (p. 960) and AML (p. 955). Patients with aplastic anaemia must be followed up long-term.

Secondary aplastic anaemia

Causes of this condition are listed in Box 23.61. It is not practical to list all the drugs that have been suspected of causing aplasia. It is important to check the reported side-effects of all drugs taken over the preceding months. In some instances, the cytopenia is more selective and affects only one cell line, most often the neutrophils. Frequently, this is an incidental finding, with no ill health. It probably has an immune basis but this is difficult to prove.

 23.61 Causes of secondary aplastic anaemia

- Drugs:
    Cytotoxic drugs
    Antibiotics – chloramphenicol, sulphonamides
    Antirheumatic agents – penicillamine, gold, phenylbutazone, indometacin
    Antithyroid drugs – carbimazole, propylthiouracil
    Anticonvulsants
    Immunosuppressants – azathioprine
- Chemicals:
    Benzene, toluene solvent misuse – glue-sniffing
    Insecticides – chlorinated hydrocarbons (DDT), organophosphates and carbamates (pp. 145 and 146)
- Radiation
- Viral hepatitis
- Pregnancy
- Paroxysmal nocturnal haemoglobinuria

The clinical features and methods of diagnosis are the same as for primary idiopathic aplastic anaemia. An underlying cause should be treated or removed, but otherwise management is as for the idiopathic form.

Myeloproliferative neoplasms

These make up a group of chronic conditions characterised by clonal proliferation of marrow precursor cells. Polycythaemia rubra vera (PRV), essential thrombocythaemia and myelofibrosis are the non-leukaemic myeloproliferative neoplasms. Although the majority of patients are classifiable as having one of these disorders, some have overlapping features and there is often progression from one to another, e.g. PRV to myelofibrosis. The recent discovery of the molecular basis of these disorders will lead to changes in classification and treatment; a mutation in the gene on chromosome 9 encoding the signal transduction molecule *JAK-2* has been found in more than 90% of PRV cases and 50% of those with essential thrombocythaemia and myelofibrosis. Mutations in the calreticulin gene (*CALR*), which produces a chaperone protein that protects proteins moving from the endoplasmic reticulin to the cytoplasm, have been found in a further 25% of patients with essential thrombocythaemia. Less commonly, mutations can be detected in the thrombopoietin receptor gene *MPL*.

Myelofibrosis

In myelofibrosis, the marrow is initially hypercellular, with an excess of abnormal megakaryocytes that release growth factors, such as platelet-derived growth factor, to the marrow microenvironment, resulting in a reactive proliferation of fibroblasts. As the disease progresses, the marrow becomes fibrosed.

Most patients present over the age of 50 years, with lassitude, weight loss and night sweats. The spleen can be massively enlarged due to extramedullary haematopoiesis (blood cell formation outside the bone marrow), and painful splenic infarcts may occur.

The characteristic blood picture is leucoerythroblastic anaemia, with circulating immature red blood cells (increased reticulocytes and nucleated red blood cells) and granulocyte precursors (myelocytes). The red cells are shaped like teardrops (teardrop poikilocytes), and giant platelets may be seen in the blood. The white count varies from low to moderately high and the platelet count may be high, normal or low. Urate levels may be high due to increased cell breakdown, and folate deficiency is common. The marrow is often difficult to aspirate and a trephine biopsy shows an excess of megakaryocytes, increased reticulin and fibrous tissue replacement. The presence of a *JAK-2* mutation supports the diagnosis.

Management and prognosis

Median survival is 4 years from diagnosis, but ranges from 1 year to over 20 years. Treatment is directed at control of symptoms, e.g. red cell transfusions for anaemia. Folic acid should be given to prevent deficiency. Cytotoxic therapy with hydroxycarbamide may help control spleen size, the white cell count or systemic symptoms. Splenectomy may be required for a grossly enlarged spleen or symptomatic pancytopenia secondary to splenic pooling of cells and hypersplenism. HSCT may be considered for younger patients. Ruxolitinib, an inhibitor of *JAK-2*, is now licensed in myelofibrosis and is effective at reducing systemic symptoms and splenomegaly.

Essential thrombocythaemia

Uncontrolled proliferation of megakaryocytes results in a raised level of circulating platelets that are often dysfunctional. Prior to a diagnosis of essential thrombocythaemia being made, reactive causes of thrombocytosis must be excluded (see Box 23.15). The presence of a *JAK-2, CALR* or, rarely, *MPL* mutation supports the diagnosis but is not universal. Patients present at a median age of 60 years with vascular occlusion or bleeding, or with an asymptomatic isolated raised platelet count. A small

23

percentage (around 5%) will transform to acute leukaemia and others to myelofibrosis.

It is likely that most patients with essential thrombocythaemia benefit from low-dose aspirin to reduce the risk of occlusive vascular events. Low-risk patients (age <40 years, platelet count <1500×10⁹/L and no bleeding or thrombosis) may not require treatment to reduce the platelet count. For those with a platelet count above 1500×10⁹/L, with symptoms, or with other risk factors for thrombosis such as diabetes or hypertension, treatment to control platelet counts should be given. Agents include oral hydroxycarbamide or anagrelide, an inhibitor of megakaryocyte maturation. Intravenous radioactive phosphorus (^{32}P) may be useful in old age and interferon-alfa has a role in younger patients.

Polycythaemia rubra vera

PRV occurs mainly in patients over the age of 40 years and presents either as an incidental finding of a high haemoglobin, or with symptoms of hyperviscosity, such as lassitude, loss of concentration, headaches, dizziness, blackouts, pruritus and epistaxis. Some patients present with manifestations of peripheral arterial or cerebrovascular disease. Venous thromboembolism may also occur. Peptic ulceration is common, sometimes complicated by bleeding. Patients are often plethoric and many have a palpable spleen at diagnosis.

Investigation of polycythaemia is discussed on page 925. The diagnosis of PRV now rests on the demonstration of a high haematocrit and the presence of the *JAK-2 V617F* mutation (positive in 95% of cases). In the occasional *JAK-2*-negative cases, a raised red cell mass and absence of causes of a secondary erythrocytosis must be established. The spleen may be enlarged and neutrophil and platelet counts are frequently raised, an abnormal karyotype may be found in the marrow, and in vitro culture of the marrow can be used to demonstrate autonomous growth in the absence of added growth factors.

Management and prognosis

Aspirin reduces the risk of thrombosis. Venesection gives prompt relief of hyperviscosity symptoms. Between 400 and 500 mL of blood (less if the patient is elderly) are removed and the venesection is repeated every 5–7 days until the haematocrit is reduced to below 45%. Less frequent but regular venesection will maintain this level until the haemoglobin remains reduced because of iron deficiency.

Suppression of marrow proliferation with hydroxycarbamide or interferon-alfa may reduce the risk of vascular occlusion, control spleen size and reduce transformation to myelofibrosis. Intravenous ^{32}P, which is reserved for older patients as it increases the risk of transformation to acute leukaemia by 6–10-fold, is rarely used now in Europe and North America.

Median survival after diagnosis in treated patients exceeds 10 years. Some patients survive more than 20 years; however, cerebrovascular or coronary events occur in up to 60% of patients. The disease may convert to another myeloproliferative disorder, with about 15% developing acute leukaemia or myelofibrosis.

Bleeding disorders

Disorders of primary haemostasis

The initial formation of the platelet plug (see Fig. 23.6A, p. 918; also known as 'primary haemostasis') may fail in thrombocytopenia (p. 929), von Willebrand disease (p. 974), and also in platelet function disorders and diseases affecting the vessel wall.

Vessel wall abnormalities

Vessel wall abnormalities may be:
- congenital, such as hereditary haemorrhagic telangiectasia
- acquired, as in a vasculitis (p. 1040) or scurvy.

Hereditary haemorrhagic telangiectasia

Hereditary haemorrhagic telangiectasia (HHT) is a dominantly inherited condition caused by mutations in the genes encoding endoglin and activin receptor-like kinase, which are endothelial cell receptors for transforming growth factor-beta (TGF-β), a potent angiogenic cytokine. Telangiectasia and small aneurysms are found on the fingertips, face and tongue, and in the nasal passages, lung and gastrointestinal tract. A significant proportion of these patients develop larger pulmonary arteriovenous malformations (PAVMs) that cause arterial hypoxaemia due to a right-to-left shunt. These predispose to paradoxical embolism, resulting in stroke or cerebral abscess. All patients with HHT should be screened for PAVMs; if these are found, ablation by percutaneous embolisation should be considered.

Patients present either with recurrent bleeds, particularly epistaxis, or with iron deficiency due to occult gastrointestinal bleeding. Treatment can be difficult because of the multiple bleeding points but regular iron therapy often allows the marrow to compensate for blood loss. Local cautery or laser therapy may prevent single lesions from bleeding. A variety of medical therapies have been tried but none has been found to be universally effective.

Ehlers–Danlos disease

Vascular Ehlers–Danlos syndrome (type 4) is a rare autosomal dominant disorder (1/100 000) caused by a defect in type 3 collagen that results in fragile blood vessels and organ membranes, leading to bleeding and organ rupture. Classical joint hypermobility (p. 1059) is often limited in this form of the disease but skin changes and facial appearance are typical. The diagnosis should be considered when there is a history of bleeding with normal laboratory tests.

Scurvy

Vitamin C deficiency affects the normal synthesis of collagen and results in a bleeding disorder characterised by perifollicular and petechial haemorrhage, bruising and subperiosteal bleeding. The key to diagnosis is the dietary history (p. 715).

Platelet function disorders

Bleeding may result from thrombocytopenia (see Box 23.14, p. 929) or from congenital or acquired abnormalities of platelet function. The most common acquired disorders are iatrogenic, resulting from the use of aspirin, clopidogrel, ticagrelor, dipyridamole and the glycoprotein IIb/IIIa inhibitors to prevent arterial thrombosis (see Box 23.26, p. 938). Inherited platelet function abnormalities are relatively rare. Congenital abnormalities may be due to deficiency of the membrane glycoproteins, e.g. Glanzmann's thrombasthenia (IIb/IIIa) or Bernard–Soulier syndrome (Ib), or due to the presence of defective platelet granules, e.g. a deficiency of dense (delta) granules (see Fig. 23.7, p. 920) giving rise to storage pool disorders. The congenital macrothrombocytopathies that are due to mutations in the myosin heavy chain gene *MYH-9* are characterised by large platelets, inclusion bodies in the neutrophils (Döhle bodies) and a variety of other features, including sensorineural deafness and renal abnormalities. Other familial thrombocytopathies are important, as they can be associated with somatic features, and some are associated with a propensity for development of bone marrow failure or dysplasia (e.g. *RUNX-1*-associated thrombocytopenia).

Apart from Glanzmann's thrombasthenia, these conditions are mild disorders, with bleeding typically occurring after trauma or surgery, but rarely spontaneous. Glanzmann's thrombasthenia is an autosomal recessive condition associated with a variable but often severe bleeding disorder. These conditions are usually managed by local mechanical measures, but antifibrinolytics, such as tranexamic acid, may be useful and, in severe bleeding, platelet transfusion may be required. Recombinant VIIa is licensed for the treatment of resistant bleeding in Glanzmann's thrombasthenia.

Thrombocytopenia

Thrombocytopenia occurs in many disease processes, as listed in Box 23.14 (p. 929), many of which are discussed elsewhere in this chapter.

Idiopathic thrombocytopenic purpura

Idiopathic thrombocytopenic purpura (ITP) is immune-mediated with involvement of autoantibodies, most often directed against the platelet membrane glycoprotein IIb/IIIa, which sensitise the platelet, resulting in premature removal from the circulation by cells of the reticulo-endothelial system. It is not a single disorder; some cases occur in isolation while others are associated with underlying immune dysregulation in conditions such as connective tissue diseases, HIV infection, B-cell malignancies, pregnancy and certain drug therapies. The clinical presentation and pathogenesis are similar, however, whatever the cause of ITP.

Clinical features and investigations

The presentation depends on the degree of thrombocytopenia. Spontaneous bleeding typically occurs only when the platelet count is below 20×10^9/L. At higher counts, the patient may complain of easy bruising or sometimes epistaxis or menorrhagia. Many cases with counts of more than 50×10^9/L are discovered by chance.

In adults, ITP more commonly affects females and may have an insidious onset. Unlike ITP in children, it is unusual for there to be a history of a preceding viral infection. Symptoms or signs of a connective tissue disease may be apparent at presentation or emerge several years later. Patients aged over 65 years should be considered for a bone marrow examination to look for an accompanying B-cell malignancy, and appropriate autoantibody testing performed if a diagnosis of connective tissue disease is likely. HIV testing should be considered because a positive result will have major implications for appropriate therapy. The peripheral blood film is normal, apart from a greatly reduced platelet number, while the bone marrow reveals an obvious increase in megakaryocytes.

Management

Many patients with stable compensated ITP and a platelet count of more than 30×10^9/L do not require treatment to raise the platelet count, except at times of increased bleeding risk, such as surgery and biopsy. First-line therapy for patients with spontaneous bleeding is with high doses of glucocorticoids, either prednisolone (1 mg/kg daily) or dexamethasone (40 mg daily for 4 days), to suppress antibody production and inhibit phagocytosis of sensitised platelets by reticulo-endothelial cells. Administration of intravenous immunoglobulin can raise the platelet count by blocking antibody receptors on reticulo-endothelial cells, and is combined with glucocorticoid therapy if there is severe haemostatic failure, especially with evidence of significant mucosal bleeding or a slow response to glucocorticoids alone. Persistent or potentially life-threatening bleeding should be treated with platelet transfusion in addition to the other therapies.

The condition may become chronic, with remissions and relapses. Relapses should be treated by re-introducing glucocorticoids. If a patient has two relapses or primary refractory disease, second-line therapies are considered. The options for second-line therapy include the thrombopoietin receptor agonists (TPO-RA) eltrombopag and romiplostim, splenectomy and immunosuppression. Where splenectomy is considered, the precautions shown in Box 23.40 need to be in place. Splenectomy produces complete remission in about 70% of patients and improvement in a further 20–25% in favourable cases. The TPO-RAs induce response in around 75% of cases, usually within 10–14 days. Low-dose glucocorticoid therapy and immunosuppressants such as rituximab, ciclosporin, mycophenolate and tacrolimus may also produce remissions. The order in which therapies should be used is not entirely clear, although the TPO-RAs are licensed for this indication while the immunosuppressive agents are not.

Coagulation disorders

Normal coagulation is explained in Figure 23.6 (p. 918). Coagulation factor deficiency may be congenital or acquired, and may affect one or several of the coagulation factors (Box 23.62). Inherited disorders are almost uniformly related to decreased synthesis, as a result of mutation in the gene encoding a key protein in coagulation. Von Willebrand disease is the most common inherited bleeding disorder. Haemophilia A and B are the most common single coagulation factor deficiencies but inherited deficiencies of all the other coagulation factors are seen. Acquired disorders may be due to under-production (e.g. in liver failure), increased consumption (e.g. in DIC) or inhibition of function of coagulation factors (such as heparin therapy or immune inhibitors of coagulation, e.g. acquired haemophilia A).

Haemophilia A

Factor VIII deficiency resulting in haemophilia A affects 1/10 000 individuals. It is the most common congenital coagulation factor deficiency. Factor VIII is primarily synthesised by the liver and endothelial cells and has a half-life of about 12 hours. It is protected from proteolysis in the circulation by binding to von Willebrand factor (vWF).

Genetics

The factor VIII gene is located on the X chromosome. Haemophilia is associated with a range of mutations in the factor VIII gene; these include major inversions, large deletions and missense, nonsense and splice site abnormalities. As the factor VIII gene is on the X chromosome, haemophilia A is a sex-linked disorder (p. 48). Thus all daughters of a patient with haemophilia are obligate carriers and they, in turn, have a 1 in 4 chance of each pregnancy resulting in the birth of an affected male baby, a normal male baby, a carrier female or a normal female. Antenatal diagnosis by chorionic villous sampling is possible in families with a known mutation.

23

23.62 Causes of coagulopathy

Congenital

X-linked
- Haemophilia A and B

Autosomal
- Von Willebrand disease
- Factor II, V, VII, X, XI and XIII deficiencies
- Combined II, VII, IX and X deficiency
- Combined V and VIII deficiency
- Hypofibrinogenaemia
- Dysfibrinogenaemia

Acquired

Under-production
- Liver failure
- Vitamin K deficiency

Increased consumption
- Coagulation activation:
    Disseminated intravascular coagulation (DIC)
- Immune-mediated:
    Acquired haemophilia and von Willebrand disease
- Others:
    Acquired factor X deficiency (in amyloid)
    Acquired von Willebrand disease in Wilms' tumour
    Acquired factor VII deficiency in sepsis

Drug-induced
- Inhibition of function:
    Heparins
    Argatroban
    Bivalirudin
    Fondaparinux
    Rivaroxaban
    Apixaban
    Dabigatran
    Edoxaban
- Inhibition of post-translational modification:
    Warfarin

23.63 Severity of haemophilia (ISTH criteria)

Severity	Factor VIII or IX level	Clinical presentation
Severe	<0.01 U/mL	Spontaneous haemarthroses and muscle haematomas
Moderate	0.01–0.05 U/mL	Mild trauma or surgery causes bleeding
Mild	> 0.05–0.4 U/mL	Major injury or surgery results in excess bleeding

(ISTH = International Society on Thrombosis and Haemostasis)

Haemophilia 'breeds true' within a family; all members have the same factor VIII gene mutation and a similarly severe or mild phenotype. Female carriers of haemophilia may have reduced factor VIII levels because of random inactivation of their normal X chromosome in the developing fetus (p. 49). This can result in a mild bleeding disorder; thus all known or suspected carriers of haemophilia A should have their factor VIII level measured.

Clinical features

The extent and patterns of bleeding are closely related to residual factor VIII levels (Box 23.63). Patients with severe haemophilia (factor VIII levels <0.01 U/mL) present with spontaneous bleeding into skin, muscle and joints. Retroperitoneal and intracranial bleeding is also a feature. Babies with severe haemophilia have an increased risk of intracranial haemorrhage and, although there is insufficient evidence to recommend routine caesarean section for these births, it is appropriate to avoid head trauma and to perform imaging of the newborn within the first 24 hours of life. Individuals with moderate and mild haemophilia (factor VIII levels 0.01–0.4 U/mL) present with the same pattern of bleeding but usually after trauma or surgery, when bleeding is disproportionate to the severity of the insult.

The major morbidity of recurrent bleeding in severe haemophilia is musculoskeletal. Bleeding is typically into large joints, especially knees, elbows, ankles and hips. Muscle haematomas are also characteristic, most commonly in the calf and psoas muscles. If early treatment is not given to arrest bleeding, a hot, swollen and very painful joint or muscle haematoma develops. Recurrent bleeding into joints leads to synovial hypertrophy, destruction of the cartilage and chronic haemophilic arthropathy (Fig. 23.32). Complications of muscle haematomas depend on their location. A large psoas bleed may extend to compress the femoral nerve; calf haematomas may increase pressure within the inflexible fascial sheath, causing a compartment syndrome with ischaemia, necrosis, fibrosis, and subsequent contraction and shortening of the Achilles tendon.

Management

The key to the management of severe haemophilia A (and B; p. 974) in more affluent countries is prophylactic coagulation factor replacement. The aim of this treatment is to maintain trough levels of factor VIII (or IX in the case of haemophilia B) above 0.02 U/mL. Doing this substantially reduces the number of bleeding episodes for men with severe haemophilia and so reduces the rate of deterioration of joints, which is the major long-term morbidity. Prophylaxis can be provided in many different ways: daily, on alternate days, or on information from pharmacokinetic studies that inform on the best way of scheduling prophylaxis. Practice in haemophilia A and B is in the process of changing somewhat due to the introduction of a variety of recombinant factor concentrates that have been manipulated to alter their half-life. In addition to standard half-life recombinant factor VIII, there are new products produced by Fc fusion and pegylation/glycopegylation that extend the half-life of factor VIII to the degree that it can be used to alter dosing schedules for prophylaxis.

The alternative approach, which still needs to be used in less affluent countries, is to treat on demand. In severe haemophilia A, bleeding episodes should be treated by raising the factor VIII level, usually by intravenous infusion of factor VIII concentrate. Factor VIII concentrates are freeze-dried and stable at 4°C and can therefore be stored in domestic refrigerators, allowing patients to treat themselves at home at the earliest indication of bleeding. Factor VIII concentrate prepared from blood donor plasma is now screened for HBV, HCV and HIV, and undergoes two separate virus inactivation processes during manufacture; these preparations have a good safety record. However, factor VIII concentrates prepared by recombinant technology are now widely available and, although more expensive, are perceived as being safer than those derived from human plasma in relation to infection risk. In addition to raising factor VIII concentrations, resting of the bleeding site with either bed rest or a splint reduces continuing haemorrhage. Once bleeding has settled, the patient should be mobilised and physiotherapy used to restore strength to the surrounding muscles. All non-immune potential recipients

▲ Massive bruising

Hepatoma in cirrhotic liver secondary to HCV infection contracted from coagulation factor concentrate

▲ Left thigh muscle haematoma in severe haemophilia

▲ Chronic haemophilic arthropathy with joint swelling and muscle wasting on left

Haemophilia B in the descendants of Queen Victoria

■ Affected with haemophilia (male)   Numerical value = age at death   ● Carrier for haemophilia (female)

▲ X-linked inheritance of haemophilia B

▲ Massive retroperitoneal haemorrhage

▲ X-ray of advanced haemophilic arthropathy

Fig. 23.32 Clinical manifestations of haemophilia. On the knee X-ray, repeated bleeds have led to broadening of the femoral epicondyles, and there is no cartilage present, as evidenced by the close proximity of the femur and tibia (A); sclerosis (B), osteophyte (C) and bony cysts (D) are present. (HCV = hepatitis C virus) *Inset (Massive bruising) From Hoffbrand VA. Color atlas of clinical hematology, 3rd edn. Philadelphia: Mosby, Elsevier Inc.; 2000.*

of pooled blood products should be offered hepatitis A and B immunisation.

The vasopressin receptor agonist desmopressin (p. 688) raises the vWF and factor VIII levels 3–4-fold, which is useful in arresting bleeding in patients with mild or moderate haemophilia A. The dose required for this purpose is higher than that used in diabetes insipidus, usually 0.3 μg/kg, and is given intravenously or subcutaneously. Alternatively, the same effect can be achieved by intranasal administration of 300 μg. Following repeated administration of desmopressin, patients need to be monitored for evidence of water retention, which can result in significant hyponatraemia. Desmopressin is contraindicated in patients with a history of severe arterial disease because of a propensity to provoke a thrombotic event, and in young children where hyponatraemia can result in fits.

Complications of coagulation factor therapy

Before 1986, coagulation factor concentrates from human plasma were not virally inactivated and many patients became infected with HIV and HBV/HCV. In patients with haemophilia treated with pooled concentrates that were not virally inactivated before 1988, infection with HCV is almost universal, 80–90%

have evidence of HBV exposure, and 60% became HIV-positive. Management is described in Chapters 22 and 12.

Concern that the infectious agent that causes vCJD (p. 1127) might be transmissible by blood and blood products has been confirmed in recipients of red cell transfusion (p. 931), and in one recipient of factor VIII. Pooled plasma products, including factor VIII concentrate, are now manufactured from plasma collected in countries with a low incidence of bovine spongiform encephalopathy.

Another serious complication of factor VIII infusion is the development of anti-factor VIII antibodies, which arise in about 20% of those with severe haemophilia. Such antibodies rapidly neutralise therapeutic infusions, making treatment relatively ineffective. Infusions of activated clotting factors, e.g. VIIa or factor VIII inhibitor bypass activity (FEIBA), may stop bleeding.

Haemophilia B (Christmas disease)

Aberrations of the factor IX gene, which is also present on the X chromosome, result in a reduction of the plasma factor IX level, giving rise to haemophilia B. This disorder is clinically indistinguishable from haemophilia A but is less common. The frequency of bleeding episodes is related to the severity of the deficiency of the plasma factor IX level. Treatment is with a factor IX concentrate, used in much the same way as factor VIII for haemophilia A. The new extended half-life recombinant factor IX products made by Fc fusion, albumin fusion and pegylation offer the possibility of prophylaxis on a once-weekly or even two-weekly schedule. Although factor IX concentrates shared the problems of virus transmission seen with factor VIII, they do not commonly induce inhibitor antibodies (<1% patients); when this does occur, however, it may be heralded by the development of a severe allergic-type reaction.

Von Willebrand disease

Von Willebrand disease is a common but usually mild bleeding disorder caused by a quantitative (types 1 and 3) or qualitative (type 2) deficiency of von Willebrand factor (vWF). This protein is synthesised by endothelial cells and megakaryocytes, and is involved in both platelet function and coagulation. It normally forms a multimeric structure that is essential for its interaction with subendothelial collagen and platelets (see Fig. 23.7, p. 920). vWF acts as a carrier protein for factor VIII, to which it is non-covalently bound; deficiency of vWF lowers the plasma factor VIII level. vWF also forms bridges between platelets and subendothelial components (e.g. collagen; see Fig. 23.6B, p. 918), allowing platelets to adhere to damaged vessel walls; deficiency of vWF therefore leads to impaired platelet plug formation. Blood group antigens (A and B) are expressed on vWF, reducing its susceptibility to proteolysis; as a result, people with blood group O have lower circulating vWF levels than individuals with non-O groups. This needs to be borne in mind when making a diagnosis of von Willebrand disease.

Most patients with von Willebrand disease have a type 1 disorder, characterised by a quantitative decrease in a normal functional protein. Patients with type 2 disorders inherit vWF molecules that are functionally abnormal. The type of abnormality depends on the site of the mutation in the *vWD* gene and how it affects binding to platelets, collagen and factor VIII. Patients with type 2A disease have abnormalities in vWF-dependent platelet adhesion; those with mutations in the platelet glycoprotein Ib binding site, resulting in increased affinity for glycoprotein 1b, have type 2B disease; those with mutations in the factor VIII binding site have type 2N disease; and those with other abnormalities in platelet binding but with normal vWF multimeric structure have type 2M disease. The patterns of laboratory abnormality accompanying these types are described in Box 23.64. The gene for vWF is located on chromosome 12 and the disease is usually autosomal dominantly inherited, except in type 2N and type 3, where inheritance is autosomal recessive.

Clinical features

Patients present with haemorrhagic manifestations similar to those in individuals with reduced platelet function. Superficial bruising, epistaxis, menorrhagia and gastrointestinal haemorrhage are common. Bleeding episodes are usually much less frequent than in severe haemophilia, and excessive haemorrhage may be observed only after trauma or surgery. Within a single family, the disease has variable penetrance, so that some members may have quite severe and frequent bleeds, whereas others are relatively asymptomatic.

Investigations

The disorder is characterised by reduced activity of vWF and factor VIII. The disease can be classified using a combination of

i	23.64 Classification of von Willebrand disease		
Type	Defect	Inheritance	Investigations/patterns
1	Partial quantitative	AD	Parallel decrease in vWF:Ag, RiCoF and VIII:c
2A	Qualitative	AD	Absent HWM of vWF Ratio of vWF activity to antigen <0.7
2B	Qualitative	AD	Reduced HWM of vWF Enhanced platelet agglutination (RIPA)
2M	Qualitative	AD	Ratio of vWF activity to antigen ≪0.7 Normal multimers of vWF Abnormal vWF/platelet interactions
2N	Qualitative	AR	Defective binding of vWF to VIII Low VIII
3	Severe quantitative	AR or CH	Very low vWF and VIII:c activity Absent multimers

(AD = autosomal dominant; AR = autosomal recessive; CH = compound heterozygote; HWM = high-weight multimers of vWF; RiCoF = ristocetin co-factor; RIPA = ristocetin-induced platelet agglutination; VIII:c = coagulation factor VIII activity in functional assay; vWF = von Willebrand factor; vWF:Ag = vWF antigen measured by ELISA)

assays that include functional and antigenic measures of vWF, multimeric analysis of the protein, and specific tests of function to determine binding to platelet glycoprotein Ib (RIPA) and factor VIII (Box 23.64). In addition, analysis for mutations in the *vWF* gene is informative in most cases.

Management

Many episodes of mild haemorrhage can be successfully treated by local means or with desmopressin, which raises the vWF level, resulting in a secondary increase in factor VIII. Tranexamic acid may be useful in mucosal bleeding. For more serious or persistent bleeds, haemostasis can be achieved with selected factor VIII concentrates, which contain considerable quantities of vWF in addition to factor VIII. Young children and patients with severe arterial disease should not receive desmopressin, and patients with type 2B disease develop thrombocytopenia that may be troublesome following desmopressin. Bleeding in type 3 patients responds only to factor VIII/vWF concentrate.

Rare inherited bleeding disorders

Severe deficiencies of factor VII, X and XIII occur as autosomal recessive disorders. They are rare but are associated with severe bleeding. Typical features include haemorrhage from the umbilical stump and intracranial haemorrhage. Factor XIII deficiency in women is typically associated with recurrent fetal loss.

Factor XI deficiency may occur in heterozygous or homozygous individuals. Bleeding is very variable and is not accurately predicted by coagulation factor levels. In general, severe bleeding is confined to patients with levels below 15% of normal.

Acquired bleeding disorders

DIC is an important cause of bleeding that begins with exaggerated and inappropriate intravascular coagulation. It is discussed under thrombotic disease on page 978.

Liver disease

Although, traditionally, severe parenchymal liver disease (Ch. 22) has been described as a state associated with an excess of bleeding, it is now clear that these patients also have an increased risk of venous thrombosis. Although there is reduced hepatic synthesis of procoagulant factors, this is balanced to a degree by the reduced production of natural anticoagulant proteins and reduced fibrinolytic activity in patients with advanced liver disease. In severe parenchymal liver disease, bleeding may arise from many different causes. Pathological sources of potential major bleeding, such as oesophageal varices or peptic ulcer, are common. There is reduced hepatic synthesis, for example, of factors V, VII, VIII, IX, X, XI, prothrombin and fibrinogen. Clearance of plasminogen activator is reduced. Thrombocytopenia may occur secondary to hypersplenism in portal hypertension. In cholestatic jaundice, there is reduced vitamin K absorption, leading to deficiency of factors II, VII, IX and X, but also of proteins C and S. Treatment with plasma products or platelet transfusion should be reserved for acute bleeds or to cover interventional procedures such as liver biopsy. Vitamin K deficiency can be readily corrected with parenteral administration of vitamin K.

Renal failure

The severity of the haemorrhagic state in renal failure is proportional to the plasma urea concentration. Bleeding manifestations are those of platelet dysfunction, with gastrointestinal haemorrhage being particularly common. The causes are multifactorial and include anaemia, mild thrombocytopenia and the accumulation of low-molecular-weight waste products, normally excreted by the kidney, that inhibit platelet function. Treatment is by dialysis to reduce the urea concentration. Rarely, in severe or persistent bleeding, platelet concentrate infusions and red cell transfusions are indicated. Increasing the concentration of vWF, either by cryoprecipitate or by desmopressin, may promote haemostasis.

Thrombotic disorders

Venous thromboembolic disease (venous thromboembolism)

While the most common presentations of venous thromboembolism (VTE) are deep vein thrombosis (DVT) of the leg (p. 186) and/or pulmonary embolism (PE; see also p. 619), similar management principles apply to rarer manifestations such as jugular vein thrombosis, upper limb DVT, cerebral sinus thrombosis (p. 1128) and intra-abdominal venous thrombosis (e.g. Budd–Chiari syndrome; p. 898).

VTE has an annual incidence of approximately 1 : 1000 in Western populations. The relative incidence of DVT:PE is approximately 2 : 1. Mortality 30 days after DVT is approximately 10%, compared to 15% for PE. All forms of VTE are increasingly common with age and many of the deaths are related to coexisting medical conditions, such as active cancer or inflammatory disease, which predispose the patient to thrombosis in the first place. Risk factors for VTE are often present (Box 23.65) and it is appropriate to seek evidence of these risk factors in determining the long-term management strategy. Figure 23.33 illustrates some of the causes and consequences of VTE. The diagnosis of DVT and PE are discussed on pages 187 and 619, respectively.

 23.65 Factors predisposing to venous thrombosis

Patient factors
- Increasing age
- Obesity
- Varicose veins
- Previous deep vein thrombosis
- Family history, especially of unprovoked venous thromboembolism when young
- Transient additional risk factors:
    Pregnancy/puerperium
    Oestrogen-containing oral contraceptives and hormone replacement therapy
    Immobility, e.g. long-distance travel (> 4 hrs)
    Intravenous drug use involving the femoral vein
    Surgery (see below)
    Medical illnesses (see below)

Surgical conditions
- Major surgery, especially if > 30 mins' duration
- Abdominal or pelvic surgery, especially for cancer
- Major lower limb orthopaedic surgery, e.g. joint replacement and hip fracture surgery

Medical conditions
- Myocardial infarction/heart failure
- Inflammatory bowel disease
- Malignancy (anti-cancer chemotherapy increases the risk of venous thromboembolism compared with cancer alone)
- Nephrotic syndrome
- Chronic obstructive pulmonary disease
- Pneumonia
- Neurological conditions associated with immobility, e.g. stroke, paraplegia, Guillain–Barré syndrome
- Any high-dependency admission

Haematological disorders
- Polycythaemia rubra vera
- Essential thrombocythaemia
- Deficiency of natural anticoagulants: antithrombin, protein C, protein S
- Paroxysmal nocturnal haemoglobinuria
- Gain-of-function prothrombotic mutations: factor V Leiden, prothrombin gene *G20210A*
- Myelofibrosis

Antiphospholipid syndrome

Management of VTE

The mainstay of treatment for all forms of VTE is anticoagulation. This can be achieved in several ways. One option is to use LMWH followed by a coumarin anticoagulant, such as warfarin. Treatment of acute VTE with LMWH should continue for a minimum of 5 days. Patients treated with warfarin should achieve a target INR of 2.5 (range 2–3; pp. 922 and 938) with LMWH continuing until the INR is above 2. Alternatively, patients may be treated with a DOAC. Rivaroxaban and apixaban may be used immediately from diagnosis without the need for LMWH, while the licences for dabigatran and edoxaban include initial treatment with LMWH for a minimum of 5 days before commencing the DOAC. In patients with active cancer and VTE, there is evidence that maintenance anticoagulation with LMWH is associated with a lower recurrence rate than warfarin. Patients who have had VTE and have a strong contraindication to anticoagulation and those who continue to have new pulmonary emboli despite therapeutic anticoagulation should have an inferior vena cava (IVC) filter inserted to prevent life-threatening PE (p. 619).

The optimal *initial* period of anticoagulation is between 6 weeks and 6 months. Patients with a provoked VTE in the

23

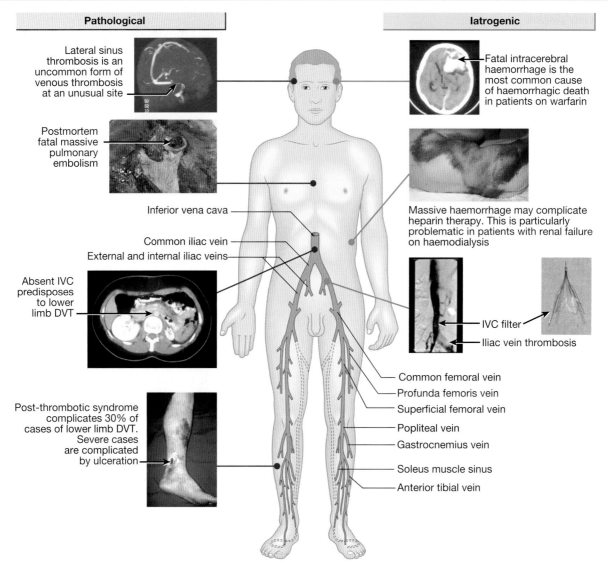

Pathological

Lateral sinus thrombosis is an uncommon form of venous thrombosis at an unusual site

Postmortem fatal massive pulmonary embolism

Inferior vena cava

Common iliac vein

External and internal iliac veins

Absent IVC predisposes to lower limb DVT

Post-thrombotic syndrome complicates 30% of cases of lower limb DVT. Severe cases are complicated by ulceration

Iatrogenic

Fatal intracerebral haemorrhage is the most common cause of haemorrhagic death in patients on warfarin

Massive haemorrhage may complicate heparin therapy. This is particularly problematic in patients with renal failure on haemodialysis

IVC filter

Iliac vein thrombosis

Common femoral vein
Profunda femoris vein
Superficial femoral vein
Popliteal vein
Gastrocnemius vein
Soleus muscle sinus
Anterior tibial vein

Fig. 23.33 Causes and consequences of venous thromboembolic disease and its treatment. (DVT = deep vein thrombosis; IVC = inferior vena cava)

presence of a temporary risk factor, which is then removed, can usually be treated for short periods (e.g. 3 months), and indeed anticoagulation for more than 6 months does not alter the rate of recurrence following discontinuation of therapy. If there are ongoing risk factors that cannot be alleviated, such as active cancer, long-term anticoagulation is usually recommended, provided that the risk of bleeding is not deemed excessive.

For patients with unprovoked VTE, the optimum duration of anticoagulation can be difficult to establish. Recurrence of VTE is about 2–3% per annum in patients who have a temporary medical risk factor at presentation and about 7–10% per annum in those with apparently unprovoked VTE. This plateaus at around 30–40% recurrence at 5 years. As such, many patients who have had unprovoked episodes of VTE will benefit from long-term anticoagulation. Several factors predict risk of recurrence following an episode of unprovoked VTE. The strongest predictors of recurrence are male sex and a positive D-dimer assay measured 1 month after stopping anticoagulant therapy. These factors are incorporated into scoring systems to predict recurrence such as the DASH score and the Vienna prediction model.

The management of DVT of the leg should also include elevation and analgesia; in limb-threatening DVT, thrombolysis may also be considered. Thrombolysis for PE is discussed on page 621. Post-thrombotic syndrome is due to damage of venous valves by the thrombus. It occurs in around 30% of patients who sustain a proximal lower limb DVT and results in persistent leg swelling, heaviness and discoloration. The most severe complication of this syndrome is ulceration around the medial malleolus (Fig. 23.33). Recent trial evidence suggests that use of elastic compression stockings following a DVT does not reduce the incidence of post-thrombotic syndrome.

Prophylaxis of VTE

All patients admitted to hospital should be assessed for their risk of developing VTE and appropriate prophylactic measures should be put in place. Both medical and surgical patients are at increased risk. A summary of the risk categories is given in Box 23.66. Early mobilisation of patients is important to prevent DVT, and those at medium or high risk require additional antithrombotic measures; these may be pharmacological or mechanical. There

23.66 Antithrombotic prophylaxis

Indications

Patients in the following categories should be considered for specific antithrombotic prophylaxis:

Moderate risk of DVT
- Major surgery:
  - In patients > 40 years or with other risk factor for VTE
- Major medical illness, e.g.:
  - Heart failure
  - Myocardial infarction with complications
  - Sepsis
  - Inflammatory conditions, including inflammatory bowel disease
  - Active malignancy
  - Nephrotic syndrome
  - Stroke and other conditions leading to lower limb paralysis

High risk of DVT
- Major abdominal or pelvic surgery for malignancy or with history of DVT or known thrombophilia (see Box 23.4, p. 923)
- Major hip or knee surgery
- Neurosurgery

Methods of VTE prophylaxis

Mechanical
- Intermittent pneumatic compression
- Mechanical foot pumps
- Graduated compression stockings

Pharmacological
- LMWHs
- Unfractionated heparin
- Fondaparinux
- Dabigatran
- Rivaroxaban
- Apixaban
- Warfarin

(DVT = deep vein thrombosis; VTE = venous thromboembolism)

is increasing evidence in high-risk groups, such as patients who have had major lower limb orthopaedic surgery and abdominal or pelvic cancer surgery, for protracted thromboprophylaxis for as long as 30 days or so after the procedure. Particular care should be taken with the use of pharmacological prophylaxis in patients with a high risk of bleeding or with specific risks of haemorrhage related to the site of surgery or the use of spinal or epidural anaesthesia.

Inherited and acquired thrombophilia and prothrombotic states

Several inherited conditions predispose to VTE (see Box 23.65), and have several points in common that are worth noting:

- None of them is strongly associated with arterial thrombosis.
- All are associated with a slightly increased incidence of adverse outcome of pregnancy, including recurrent early fetal loss, but there are no data to indicate that any specific intervention changes that outcome.
- Apart from in antithrombin deficiency and homozygous factor V Leiden, most carriers of these genes will never have an episode of VTE; if they do, it will be associated with the presence of an additional temporary risk factor.
- There is little evidence that detection of these abnormalities predicts recurrence of VTE.
- None of these conditions per se requires treatment with anticoagulants. Patients with thrombosis should receive

anticoagulation, as discussed on page 975. Patients who are deemed to be at high risk of thrombosis, e.g. those with antithrombin deficiency in pregnancy, should receive treatment or prophylactic doses of heparin to cover the period of risk only.

Antithrombin deficiency

Antithrombin (AT) is a serine protease inhibitor (SERPIN) that inactivates the activated coagulation factors IIa, IXa, Xa and XIa. Heparins and fondaparinux achieve their therapeutic effect by potentiating the activity of AT. Familial deficiency of AT is inherited in an autosomal dominant manner; homozygosity for mutant alleles is not compatible with life. Around 70% of affected individuals will have an episode of VTE before the age of 60 years and the relative risk for thrombosis compared with the background population is 10–20. Pregnancy is a high-risk period for VTE and this requires fairly aggressive management with doses of LMWH that are greater than the usual prophylactic doses (≥ 100 U/kg/day). AT concentrate (either plasma-derived or recombinant) is available; this is required for cardiopulmonary bypass and may be used as an adjunct to heparin in surgical prophylaxis and in the peripartum period.

Protein C and S deficiencies

Protein C and its co-factor protein S are vitamin K-dependent natural anticoagulants involved in switching off coagulation factor activation (factors Va and VIIIa) and thrombin generation (see Fig. 23.6F, p. 919). Inherited deficiency of either protein C or S results in a prothrombotic state with a fivefold relative risk of VTE compared with the background population.

Factor V Leiden

Factor V Leiden results from a gain-of-function, single-base-pair mutation which prevents the cleavage and hence inactivation of activated factor V. This results in a relative risk of venous thrombosis of 5 in heterozygotes and 50 or more in rare homozygotes. The mutation is found in about 5% of Northern Europeans, 2% of Hispanics, 1.2% of African–Americans, 0.5% of Asian–Americans and 1.25% of Native Americans, and is rare in Chinese and Malay people.

Prothrombin G20210A

This gain-of-function mutation in the non-coding 3′ end of the prothrombin gene is associated with an increased plasma level of prothrombin. It is present in about 2% of Northern Europeans but is rare in native populations of Korea, China, India and Africa. In the heterozygous state, it is associated with a 2–3-fold increase in risk of VTE compared with the background population.

Antiphospholipid syndrome

Antiphospholipid syndrome (APS) is a clinicopathological entity in which a constellation of clinical conditions, alone or in combination, is found in association with a persistently positive test for an antiphospholipid antibody. The antiphospholipid antibodies are heterogeneous and typically are directed against proteins that bind to phospholipids (Box 23.67). Although causal roles for these antibodies have been proposed, the mechanisms underlying the clinical features of APS are not clear. In clinical practice, two types of test are used, which detect:

- antibodies that bind to negatively charged phospholipid on an ELISA plate (called an anticardiolipin antibody test). These assays usually contain β_2-glycoprotein 1 (β_2-GP1)

23

23.67 Antiphospholipid syndrome (APS)

Clinical manifestations

- Adverse pregnancy outcome
  Recurrent first trimester abortion (≥3)
  Unexplained death of morphologically normal fetus after
  10 weeks' gestation
  Severe early pre-eclampsia
- Venous thromboembolism
- Arterial thromboembolism
- Livedo reticularis, catastrophic APS, transverse myelitis, skin
  necrosis, chorea

Conditions associated with secondary APS

- Systemic lupus erythematosus
- Rheumatoid arthritis
- Systemic sclerosis
- Behçet's disease
- Temporal arteritis
- Sjögren's syndrome

Targets for antiphospholipid antibodies

- β_2-glycoprotein 1
- Protein C
- Annexin V
- Prothrombin (may result in
  haemorrhagic presentation)

23.68 Disseminated intravascular coagulation (DIC)

Underlying conditions

- Infection/sepsis
- Trauma
- Obstetric, e.g. amniotic fluid embolism, placental abruption,
  pre-eclampsia
- Severe liver failure
- Malignancy, e.g. solid tumours and leukaemias
- Tissue destruction, e.g. pancreatitis, burns
- Vascular abnormalities, e.g. vascular aneurysms, liver
  haemangiomas
- Toxic/immunological, e.g. ABO incompatibility, snake bites,
  recreational drugs

ISTH scoring system for diagnosis of DIC

Presence of an associated disorder	Essential
Platelets (× 10^9/L)	>100 = 0
<100 = 1
<50 = 2
Elevated fibrin degradation products	No increase = 0
Moderate = 2
Strong = 3
Prolonged prothrombin time	<3 secs = 0
>3 secs but <6 secs = 1
>6 secs = 2
Fibrinogen	>1 g/L = 0
<1 g/L = 1

Total score
≥5 = Compatible with overt DIC
<5 = Repeat monitoring over 1–2 days

(ISTH = International Society for Thrombosis and Haemostasis)

- those that interfere with phospholipid-dependent coagulation tests like the APTT or the dilute Russell viper venom time (DRVVT; called a lupus anticoagulant test).

The term antiphospholipid antibody encompasses both a lupus anticoagulant and an anticardiolipin antibody/ anti-β_2-GP1; individuals may be positive for one, two or all three of these activities. It has been shown that patients who are 'triple-positive' have an increased likelihood of thrombotic events.

Clinical features and management

APS may present in isolation (primary APS) or in association with one of the conditions shown in Box 23.67, most typically systemic lupus erythematosus (secondary APS). Most patients present with a single manifestation and APS is now most frequently diagnosed in women with adverse outcomes of pregnancy. It is extremely important to make the diagnosis in patients with APS, whatever the manifestation, because it affects the prognosis and management of arterial thrombosis, VTE and pregnancy.

Arterial thrombosis, typically stroke, associated with APS should probably be treated with warfarin, as opposed to aspirin. APS-associated VTE is one of the situations in which the predicted recurrence rate is high enough to indicate long-term anticoagulation after a first event. In women with obstetric presentations of APS, intervention with heparin and aspirin is almost routinely prescribed, although there is little evidence from clinical trials that it is an effective therapy in increasing the chance of a successful pregnancy outcome.

Disseminated intravascular coagulation

Disseminated intravascular coagulation (DIC) may complicate a range of illnesses (Box 23.68). It is characterised by systemic activation of the pathways involved in coagulation and its regulation. This may result in the generation of intravascular fibrin clots causing multi-organ failure, with simultaneous coagulation factor and platelet consumption, causing bleeding. The systemic coagulation activation is induced either through cytokine pathways, which are activated as part of a systemic inflammatory

23.69 Haemostasis and thrombosis in old age

- **Thrombocytopenia**: not uncommon because of the rising prevalence of disorders in which it may be a secondary feature, and also because of the greater use of drugs that can cause it.
- **'Senile' purpura**: presumed to be due to an age-associated loss of subcutaneous fat and the collagenous support of small blood vessels, making them more prone to damage from minor trauma.
- **Thrombosis**: incidence of thromboembolic disease rises with increasing age. This may be due to stasis and concurrent illness, to which older people are prone; some studies show increased platelet aggregation with age, and others age-associated hyperactivity of the haemostatic system, which could contribute to a prothrombotic state.
- **Thromboprophylaxis**: should be considered in all older patients who are immobile as a result of acute illness. Prophylaxis is not required in chronic immobility without a medical cause, as there is no associated increase in thromboembolism.
- **Anticoagulation**: older patients are more sensitive to the anticoagulant effects of warfarin, partly due to the concurrent use of other drugs and the presence of other pathology. Life-threatening or fatal bleeds on warfarin are significantly more common in those over 80 years.

---

response, or by the release of procoagulant substances such as tissue factor. In addition, suboptimal function of the natural anticoagulant pathways and dysregulated fibrinolysis contribute to DIC. There is consumption of platelets, coagulation factors (notably factors V and VIII) and fibrinogen. The lysis of fibrin clot results in production of fibrin degradation products (FDPs), including D-dimers.

Investigations

DIC should be suspected when any of the conditions listed in Box 23.68 are met. Measurement of coagulation times (APTT and PT; p. 920), along with fibrinogen, platelet count and FDPs, helps in the assessment of prognosis and aids clinical decision-making with regard to both bleeding and thrombotic complications.

Management

Therapy is primarily aimed at the underlying cause. These patients will often require intensive care to deal with concomitant issues, such as acidosis, dehydration, renal failure and hypoxia. Blood component therapy, such as fresh frozen plasma, cryoprecipitate and platelets, should be given if the patient is bleeding or to cover interventions with a high bleeding risk, but should not be prescribed routinely based on coagulation tests and platelet counts alone. Prophylactic doses of heparin should be given, unless there is a clear contraindication. Established thrombosis should be treated cautiously with therapeutic doses of unfractionated heparin, unless clearly contraindicated. Patients with DIC should not, in general, be treated with antifibrinolytic therapy, e.g. tranexamic acid.

Thrombotic thrombocytopenic purpura

Like DIC and also heparin-induced thrombocytopenia (p. 938), thrombotic thrombocytopenic purpura (TTP) is a disorder in which thrombosis is accompanied by paradoxical thrombocytopenia. TTP is characterised by a pentad of findings, although few patients have all five components:

- thrombocytopenia
- microangiopathic haemolytic anaemia
- neurological sequelae
- fever
- renal impairment.

It is an acute autoimmune disorder mediated by antibodies against ADAMTS-13 (a disintegrin and metalloproteinase with a thrombospondin type 1 motif).

This enzyme normally cleaves vWF multimers to produce normal functional units, and its deficiency results in large vWF multimers that cross-link platelets. The features are of microvascular occlusion by platelet thrombi affecting key organs, principally brain and kidneys. It is a rare disorder (1 in 750 000 per annum), which may occur alone or in association with drugs (ticlopidine, ciclosporin), HIV, shiga toxins (p. 263) and malignancy. It should be treated by emergency plasma exchange. Glucocorticoids, aspirin and rituximab also have a role in management. Untreated mortality rates are 90% in the first 10 days, and even with appropriate therapy, the mortality rate is 20–30% at 6 months.

Further information

Websites

bcshguidelines.com *British Committee for Standards in Haematology guidelines.*
cibmtr.org *International Bone Marrow Transplant Registry.*
transfusionguidelines.org.uk *Contains the UK Transfusion Services' Handbook of Transfusion Medicine and links to other relevant sites.*
ukhcdo.org *UK Haemophilia Centre Doctors' Organisation.*

23

GPR Clunie
SH Ralston

24

Rheumatology and bone disease

Clinical examination of the musculoskeletal system 982

Functional anatomy and physiology 984
Bone 984
Joints 986
Skeletal muscle 987

Investigation of musculoskeletal disease 988
Joint aspiration 988
Imaging 988
Blood tests 990
Tissue biopsy 992
Electromyography 992

Presenting problems in musculoskeletal disease 992
Acute monoarthritis 992
Polyarthritis 993
Fracture 994
Generalised musculoskeletal pain 995
Back pain 995
Regional musculoskeletal pain 997
Neck pain 997
Shoulder pain 997
Elbow pain 998
Hand and wrist pain 998
Hip pain 998
Knee pain 998
Ankle and foot pain 999
Muscle pain and weakness 1000

Principles of management 1000
Education and lifestyle interventions 1000
Non-pharmacological interventions 1001
Pharmacological treatment 1002

Osteoarthritis 1007

Crystal-induced arthritis 1012

Fibromyalgia 1018

Bone and joint infections 1019

Rheumatoid arthritis 1021

Juvenile idiopathic arthritis 1026

Spondyloarthropathies 1027
Axial spondyloarthropathy 1028
Reactive arthritis 1031
Psoriatic arthritis 1032
Enteropathic (spondylo)arthritis 1034

Autoimmune connective tissue diseases 1034

Vasculitis 1040

Diseases of bone 1044
Osteoporosis 1044
Osteomalacia, rickets and vitamin D deficiency 1049
Paget's disease of bone 1053
Other bone diseases 1055

Bone and joint tumours 1056

Rheumatological involvement in other diseases 1057

Miscellaneous conditions 1058

Clinical examination of the musculoskeletal system

2 Extensor surfaces
Rheumatoid nodules
Swollen bursa
Psoriasis rash

▲ Rheumatoid nodules

1 Hands
Swelling
Deformity
Nail changes
Tophi
Raynaud's

▲ Nail dystrophy in psoriatic arthritis

▲ Synovitis and deformity in rheumatoid arthritis

▲ Heberden and Bouchard nodes in osteoarthritis

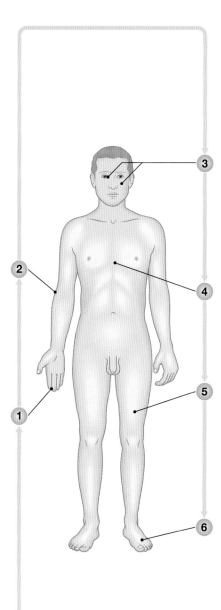

Observation
- General appearance
- Gait
- Deformity
- Swelling
- Redness
- Rash

3 Face
Rash
Alopecia
Mouth ulcers
Eyes

▲ Butterfly rash in systemic lupus erythematosus

▲ Scleritis in rheumatoid arthritis

4 Trunk
Kyphosis
Scoliosis
Tender spots (fibromyalgia, enthesitis)

5 Legs
Deformity
Swelling
Restricted movement

▲ Bone deformity in Paget's disease

6 Feet
Deformity
Swelling (gout, dactylitis)
Redness

▲ Acute gout

General Assessment of Locomotor System (GALS) and Schöber's test

1 Gait

Ask patient to walk for a few steps, then come back. Look for pain or limp

2 Arms

Inspect hands for swelling or deformity

Ask patient to make a fist and open and close fingers (tests hand function)

Squeeze metacarpals (tests for inflammation)

Press over supraspinatus (tests for hyperalgesia)

Patient turns palms up and down with elbows at side (tests supination and pronation of wrists and elbow)

Ask patient to put hands behind head (tests shoulder movements)

Patient flexes elbows to touch shoulder (tests elbow flexion)

3 Legs

Flex each hip with hand on knee. Rotate hips internally and externally (tests hip movements and detects knee crepitus)

Palpate each knee for warmth and swelling (tests for synovitis and effusion)

Inspect ankles and feet. Squeeze forefoot (tests for metatarsophalangeal synovitis)

4 Spine

Patient looks at ceiling and then puts chin on chest (tests flexion and extension cervical spine)

Ask patient to try to put ear on shoulder (tests lateral flexion cervical spine)

Patient slides hand down leg to knee (tests lateral spine flexion)

Inspect spine from behind and side, looking for scoliosis, kyphosis or localised deformity. Ask patient to touch toes

5 Schöber's test

Mark skin with pen in midline about 4 cm below superior iliac crest. Make another mark in midline 10 cm above first. Ask patient to bend forwards. Normally, distance between marks should increase to 15 cm

 10 cm

 15 cm

Stand behind patient and hold their pelvis. Ask them to turn from side to side without moving their feet (tests thoracolumbar rotation)

24

Disorders of the musculoskeletal system affect all ages and ethnic groups. In the UK, about 25% of new consultations in general practice are for musculoskeletal symptoms. Musculoskeletal diseases may arise from processes affecting bones, joints, muscles, or connective tissues such as skin and tendon. The principal manifestations are pain and impairment of locomotor function.

Diseases of the musculoskeletal system tend to be more common in women and most increase in frequency with increasing age. They are the most common cause of physical disability in older people and account for one-third of physical disability at all ages.

Functional anatomy and physiology

The musculoskeletal system is responsible for movement of the body, provides a structural framework to protect internal organs, and acts as a reservoir for storage of calcium and phosphate in the regulation of mineral homeostasis. The main components of the musculoskeletal system are depicted in Figure 24.1.

Bone

Bones fall into two main types, based on their embryonic development. Flat bones, such as the skull, develop by intramembranous ossification, in which embryonic fibroblasts differentiate directly into bone within condensations of mesenchymal tissue during early fetal life. Long bones, such as the femur and radius, develop by endochondral ossification from a cartilage template. During development, the cartilage is invaded by vascular tissue containing osteoprogenitor cells and is gradually replaced by bone from centres of ossification situated in the middle and at the ends of the bone. A thin remnant of cartilage called the growth plate or epiphysis remains at each end of long bones, and chondrocyte proliferation here is responsible for skeletal growth during childhood and adolescence. At the end of puberty, the increased levels of sex hormones halt cell division in the growth plate. The cartilage remnant then disappears as the epiphysis fuses and longitudinal bone growth ceases.

Two types of bone tissue are present in the normal skeleton (Fig. 24.1). Cortical bone is formed from Haversian systems, comprising concentric lamellae of bone tissue surrounding a central canal that contains blood vessels. Cortical bone is dense and forms a hard envelope around the long bones. Trabecular or cancellous bone fills the centre of the bone and consists of an interconnecting meshwork of trabeculae, separated by spaces filled with bone marrow. The most important cell types in bone are:

- *Osteoclasts*: multinucleated cells of haematopoietic origin, responsible for bone resorption.
- *Osteoblasts*: mononuclear cells of derived from marrow stromal cells responsible for bone formation.

Fig. 24.1 Structure of the major musculoskeletal tissues.

- *Osteocytes*: cells that differentiate from osteoblasts that become embedded in bone matrix during bone formation. They are responsible for sensing and responding to mechanical stimuli and for coordinating osteoclast and osteoblast activity.
- *Bone marrow stromal cells*: cells that produce receptor activator of nuclear factor kappa B ligand (RANKL) and macrophage colony-stimulating factor (M-CSF), which stimulate osteoclast formation, and other cytokines that support haematopoiesis (p. 914).
- *Bone lining cells*: flattened cells lining the bone surface that differentiate from osteoblasts when bone formation is complete.

Bone matrix and mineral

The most abundant protein of bone is type I collagen, which is formed from two α1 peptide chains and one α2 chain wound together in a triple helix. Type I collagen is proteolytically processed inside the cell before being laid down in the extracellular space, releasing propeptide fragments that can be used as biochemical markers of bone formation. Subsequently, the collagen fibrils become 'cross-linked' to one another by pyridinium molecules, a process that enhances bone strength. When bone is broken down by osteoclasts, the cross-links are released into the circulation. These can be measured biochemically and are sometimes used clinically to assess levels of bone resorption. Bone is normally laid down in an orderly fashion, but when bone turnover is high, as in Paget's disease or severe hyperparathyroidism, it is laid down in a chaotic pattern, giving rise to 'woven bone' that is mechanically weak. Bone matrix also contains growth factors, other structural proteins and proteoglycans, thought to be involved in helping bone cells attach to bone matrix and in regulating bone cell activity. The other major component of bone is mineral, comprised of calcium and phosphate crystals deposited between the collagen fibrils in the form of hydroxyapatite [Ca_{10} $(PO_4)_6$ $(OH)_2$]. Mineralisation is essential for bone's rigidity and strength but over-mineralisation causes the bone to become brittle. In clinical practice, increased mineralisation can occur in some types of osteogenesis imperfecta and in response to long-term bisphosphonate therapy.

Bone remodelling

Bone remodelling is required for renewal and repair of the skeleton throughout life. This is a cyclical process that has four phases; quiescence, resorption, reversal and formation, as illustrated in Figure 24.2. Remodelling starts with the attraction of osteoclast precursors in peripheral blood to the target site, probably by local release of chemotactic factors from areas of microdamage. The osteoclasts resorb bone and, after about 10 days, undergo programmed cell death (apoptosis), heralding the start of the reversal phase, when osteoblast precursors are recruited to the resorption site. The osteoblast precursors differentiate into mature osteoblasts and form new bone during the formation phase. Initially, the matrix is unmineralised (osteoid) but eventually becomes mineralised to form mature bone. Some osteoblasts become trapped in bone matrix and differentiate into osteocytes, which play a key regulatory role in coordinating bone formation and resorption, whereas others differentiate into bone-lining cells.

The cellular and molecular mediators of this bone remodelling are shown in more detail in Figure 24.3. Osteoclast precursors are derived from haematopoietic stem cells and differentiate

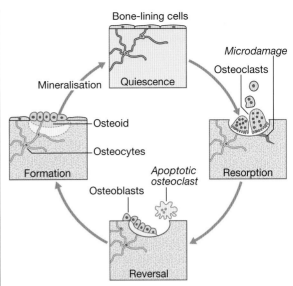

Fig. 24.2 The bone remodelling cycle. Bone is renewed and repaired by the process of bone remodelling. This begins by removal of old and damaged bone by osteoclasts during the phase of bone resorption. After about 10 days, the osteoclasts undergo programmed cell death (apoptosis) and during the reversal phase are replaced by osteoclasts, which begin to fill in the resorbed area with new bone matrix, heralding the start of bone formation. The bone matrix is initially uncalcified (osteoid) but then becomes mineralised to form mature bone.

into mature osteoclasts in response to M-CSF, produced by bone marrow stromal cells, and RANKL, produced by both osteocytes and bone marrow stromal cells. The RANKL binds to and activates a receptor called RANK (receptor activator of nuclear factor kappa B) on osteoclast precursors, promoting osteoclast differentiation and bone resorption. This effect is blocked by osteoprotegerin (OPG), which is a decoy receptor for RANKL that inhibits osteoclast formation. Once formed, mature osteoclasts attach to the bone surface by a tight sealing zone and secrete hydrochloric acid and proteolytic enzymes, including cathepsin K, into the space underneath, which is known as the Howship's lacuna. The acid dissolves the mineral and cathepsin K degrades collagen. Osteocytes also produce sclerostin (SOST), which is a potent inhibitor of bone formation. Under conditions of mechanical loading, sclerostin production by osteocytes is inhibited, allowing bone formation to proceed, stimulated by members of the Wnt family of signalling proteins. The Wnt molecules stimulate bone formation by activating members of the lipoprotein receptor-related protein (LRP) family, the most important of which are LRP4, LRP5 and LRP6. Sclerostin antagonises the effects of Wnt family members by blocking their interaction with LRP family members. Finally, osteocytes play a critical role in phosphate homeostasis by producing the hormone FGF23, which regulates renal tubular phosphate reabsorption. Key regulators of bone remodelling are summarised in Box 24.1.

Mineralisation of bone is critically dependent on the enzyme alkaline phosphatase (ALP), which is produced by osteoblasts and degrades pyrophosphate, an inhibitor of mineralisation. Bone remodelling is predominantly regulated at a local level but can be influenced by circulating hormones or mechanical loading, which can up-regulate or down-regulate remodelling across the whole skeleton (Box 24.1).

24

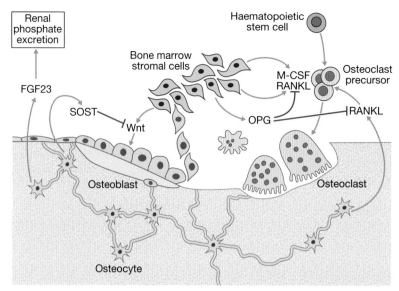

Fig. 24.3 Cellular and molecular regulators of bone remodelling Osteoclast precursors are derived from haematopoietic stem cells. They differentiate into mature osteoclasts in response to the receptor activator of nuclear factor kappa B ligand (RANKL), which is produced by osteocytes, bone marrow stromal cells and activated T cells (not shown), and macrophage colony-stimulating factor (M-CSF), which is produced by bone marrow stromal cells. Osteoprotegerin (OPG) is also produced in the bone microenvironment, where it inhibits osteoclastic bone resorption by blocking the effect of RANKL. Osteoblasts, which are derived from bone marrow stromal cells, are responsible for bone formation. Osteoblast activity is stimulated by signalling molecules in the Wnt family but inhibited by sclerostin (SOST), which is produced by osteocytes. In addition to their role in regulating osteoclast and osteoblast activity, osteocytes have an endocrine function in regulating phosphate homeostasis by producing fibroblast growth factor 23 (FGF23), which acts on the kidney to promote phosphate excretion.

i 24.1 Key regulators of bone remodelling

Mediator	Source	Effects	Comment
RANKL	Osteocytes Stromal cells Activated T cells	Stimulates bone resorption	Activates RANK
Osteoprotegerin	Stromal cells Lymphocytes	Inhibits bone resorption	Acts as decoy receptor for RANKL
Wnt	Stromal cells	Stimulates bone formation	Activates LRP receptors
Sclerostin	Osteocytes	Inhibits bone formation	Blocks effect of Wnt on LRP receptors
Parathyroid hormone	Parathyroid glands	Increases bone resorption and formation	
Thyroid hormone	Thyroid gland	Increases bone resorption and formation	
Oestrogen	Ovary	Inhibits bone resorption	
Glucocorticoid	Adrenal gland Exogenous	Inhibits bone formation	

(LRP = lipoprotein receptor-related protein; RANKL = receptor activator of nuclear factor kappa B ligand)

Joints

There are three main types of joint: fibrous, fibrocartilaginous and synovial (Box 24.2).

Fibrous and fibrocartilaginous joints

These comprise a simple bridge of fibrous or fibrocartilaginous tissue joining two bones together where there is little requirement for movement. The intervertebral disc is a special type of fibrocartilaginous joint in which an amorphous area, called the nucleus pulposus, lies in the centre of the fibrocartilaginous bridge. The nucleus has a high water content and acts as a cushion to improve the disc's shock-absorbing properties.

i 24.2 Types of joint

Type	Range of movement	Examples
Fibrous	Minimal	Skull sutures
Fibrocartilaginous	Limited	Symphysis pubis Costochondral junctions Intervertebral discs Sacroiliac joints
Synovial	Large	Most limb joints Temporomandibular Costovertebral

Synovial joints

These are complex structures containing several cell types. They are found where a wide range of movement is needed (Fig. 24.4).

Articular cartilage

This avascular tissue covers the bone ends in synovial joints. Cartilage cells (chondrocytes) are responsible for synthesis and turnover of cartilage, which consists of a mesh of type II collagen fibrils that extend through a hydrated 'gel' of proteoglycan molecules. The most important proteoglycan is aggrecan, which consists of a core protein to which several glycosaminoglycan (GAG) side chains are attached (Fig. 24.5). The GAGs are polysaccharides that consist of long chains of disaccharide repeats comprising one normal sugar and an amino sugar. The most abundant GAGs in aggrecan are chondroitin sulphate and keratan sulphate. Hyaluronan is another important GAG that binds to aggrecan molecules to form very large complexes with a total molecular weight of more than 100 million. Aggrecan has a strong negative charge and avidly binds water molecules to assume a shape that occupies the maximum possible volume available. The expansive force of the hydrated aggrecan, combined with the restrictive strength of the collagen mesh, gives articular cartilage excellent shock-absorbing properties.

With ageing, the concentration of chondroitin sulphate decreases, whereas that of keratan sulphate increases, resulting in reduced water content and shock-absorbing properties. These changes differ from those found in osteoarthritis (p. 1007), where there is abnormal chondrocyte division, loss of proteoglycan from matrix and an increase in water content. Cartilage matrix is constantly turning over and in health there is a perfect balance between synthesis and degradation. Degradation of cartilage matrix is carried out by aggrecanases and matrix metalloproteinases, responsible for the breakdown of proteins and proteoglycans, and by glycosidases, responsible for the breakdown of GAGs. Pro-inflammatory cytokines, such as interleukin-1 (IL-1) and tumour necrosis factor (TNF), which are released during inflammation, stimulate production of aggrecanase and metalloproteinases, causing cartilage degradation.

Synovial fluid

The surfaces of articular cartilage are separated by a space filled with synovial fluid (SF), a viscous liquid that lubricates the joint. It is an ultrafiltrate of plasma, into which synovial cells secrete hyaluronan and proteoglycans.

Intra-articular discs

Some joints contain fibrocartilaginous discs within the joint space that act as shock absorbers. The most clinically important are the menisci of the knee. These are avascular structures that remain viable because of diffusion of oxygen and nutrients from the SF.

Synovial membrane, joint capsule and bursae

The bones of synovial joints are connected by the joint capsule, a fibrous structure richly supplied with blood vessels, nerves and lymphatics that encases the joint. Ligaments are discrete, regional thickenings of the capsule that act to stabilise joints (see Fig. 24.4). The inner surface of the joint capsule is the synovial membrane, comprising an outer layer of blood vessels and loose connective tissue that is rich in type I collagen, and an inner layer 1–4 cells thick consisting of two main cell types. Type A synoviocytes are phagocytic cells derived from the monocyte/macrophage lineage and are responsible for removing particulate matter from the joint cavity; type B synoviocytes are fibroblast-like cells that secrete SF. Most inflammatory and degenerative joint diseases associate with thickening of the synovial membrane and infiltration by lymphocytes, polymorphs and macrophages.

Bursae are hollow sacs lined with synovium and contain a small amount of SF. They help tendons and muscles move smoothly in relation to bones and other articular structures.

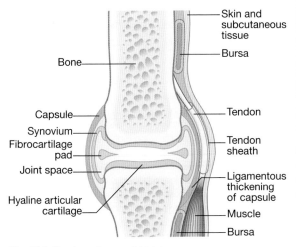

Fig. 24.4 Structure of a synovial joint.

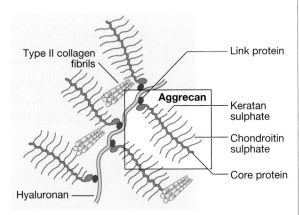

Fig. 24.5 Ultrastructure of articular cartilage.

Skeletal muscle

Skeletal muscles are responsible for body movements and respiration. Muscle consists of bundles of cells (myocytes) embedded in fine connective tissue containing nerves and blood vessels. Myocytes are large, elongated, multinucleated cells formed by fusion of mononuclear precursors (myoblasts) in early embryonic life. The nuclei lie peripherally and the centre of the cell contains actin and myosin molecules, which interdigitate with one another to form the myofibrils that are responsible for muscle contraction. The molecular mechanisms of skeletal muscle contraction are the same as for cardiac muscle (p. 446). Myocytes contain many mitochondria that provide the large amounts of adenosine triphosphate (ATP) necessary for muscle contraction and are rich in the protein myoglobin, which acts as a reservoir for oxygen during contraction.

Individual myofibrils are organised into bundles (fasciculi) that are bound together by a thin layer of connective tissue (the perimysium). The surface of the muscle is surrounded by a thicker layer of connective tissue, the epimysium, which merges with the perimysium to form the muscle tendon. Tendons are tough, fibrous structures that attach muscles to a point of insertion on the bone surface called the enthesis.

Investigation of musculoskeletal disease

Clinical history and examination usually provide sufficient information for the diagnosis and management of many musculoskeletal diseases. Investigations are helpful in confirming the diagnosis, assessing disease activity and indicating prognosis.

Joint aspiration

Joint aspiration with examination of SF is pivotal in patients suspected of having septic arthritis, crystal arthritis or intra-articular bleeding. It should be carried out in all individuals with acute monoarthritis, and samples should be sent for microbiology and clinical chemistry.

It is possible to obtain SF by aspiration from most peripheral joints and only a small amount is required for diagnostic purposes. Normal SF is present in small volume, is clear and either colourless or pale yellow, and has a high viscosity. It contains few cells. With joint inflammation, the volume increases, the cell count and the proportion of neutrophils rise (causing turbidity), and the viscosity reduces (due to enzymatic degradation of hyaluronan and aggrecan). Turbid fluid with a high neutrophil count occurs in sepsis, crystal arthritis and reactive arthritis. High concentrations of urate crystals or cholesterol can make SF appear white. Non-uniform blood-staining usually reflects needle trauma to the synovium. Uniform blood-staining is most commonly due to a bleeding diathesis, trauma or pigmented villonodular synovitis (p. 1059) but can occur in severe inflammatory synovitis. A lipid layer floating above blood-stained fluid is diagnostic of intra-articular fracture and is caused by release of bone marrow fat into the joint.

Crystals can be identified by compensated polarised light microscopy of fresh SF (to avoid crystal dissolution and post-aspiration crystallisation). Urate crystals are long and needle-shaped, and show a strong light intensity and negative birefringence (Fig. 24.6A). Calcium pyrophosphate crystals are

smaller, rhomboid in shape and usually less numerous than urate crystals; they have weak intensity and positive birefringence (Fig. 24.6B).

Imaging

Plain X-rays

X-rays show structural changes that are of value in the differential diagnosis and monitoring of many bone and joint diseases (Box 24.3).

i	24.3 Radiographic abnormalities in selected rheumatic diseases

Rheumatoid arthritis
- Periarticular osteoporosis
- Marginal joint erosions
- Joint subluxation
- Joint space narrowing

Osteoporosis
- Osteopenia
- Vertebral fractures
- Non-vertebral fractures
- Cortical thinning

Paget's disease
- Bone expansion
- Abnormal trabecular pattern
- Osteosclerosis and lysis
- Pseudofractures

Psoriatic arthritis
- Sacroiliitis
- Syndesmophytes
- Bone sclerosis
- Proliferative enthesis erosions
- Enthesophytes
- Juxta-articular new bone

Osteoarthritis
- Joint space narrowing
- Osteophytes
- Subchondral sclerosis
- Joint deformity
- Subchondral cysts

They are of diagnostic value in osteoarthritis (OA), where they demonstrate joint space narrowing that tends to be focal rather than widespread, as in inflammatory arthritis. Other features of OA detected on X-rays include osteophytes, subchondral sclerosis, bone cysts and calcified loose bodies within the synovium (see Fig. 24.21, p. 1010). Erosions and sclerosis of the sacroiliac joints and syndesmophytes in the spine may be observed in patients with spondyloarthritis (SpA; see Fig. 24.40, p. 1030). In peripheral joints, proliferative erosions, associated with new bone formation and periosteal reaction, occur in SpA. In tophaceous gout, well-defined punched-out erosions may occur (see Fig. 24.27, p. 1015). Calcification of cartilage, tendons and soft tissues or muscle occurs mainly in chondrocalcinosis (see Fig. 24.28, p. 1016), calcium-containing crystal diseases, tumoral calcinosis and autoimmune connective tissue diseases.

X-rays are of limited value in the diagnosis of rheumatoid arthritis (RA) because features such as erosions, joint space narrowing and periarticular osteoporosis may be detectable only after several months or even years. The main indication for X-rays in RA is in the assessment of disease over time when structural damage to the joints is suspected.

Bone scintigraphy

Bone scintigraphy is useful in the diagnosis of metastatic bone disease and Paget's disease of bone. Abnormalities may also be observed in primary bone tumours, complex regional pain syndrome, osteoarthritis and inflammatory arthritis. It involves

Fig. 24.6 Compensated polarised light microscopy of synovial fluids (×400). [A] Monosodium urate crystals show bright negative birefringence under polarised light and needle-shaped morphology. [B] Calcium pyrophosphate crystals show weak positive birefringence under polarised light and are few in number. They are more difficult to detect than urate crystals.

gamma-camera imaging following an intravenous injection of ^{99m}Tc-labelled bisphosphonate. Early post-injection images reflect blood flow and can show increased perfusion of inflamed synovium, Pagetic bone or primary or secondary bone tumours. Delayed images taken a few hours later reflect bone remodelling as the ^{99m}Tc-labelled bisphosphonate localises to sites of active bone turnover. Scintigraphy has a high sensitivity for detecting important bone and joint pathology that is not apparent on X-rays (Box 24.4). Single photon emission computed tomography (SPECT) combines radionuclide imaging with computed tomography. It can provide accurate anatomical localisation of abnormal tracer uptake within the bone and is of particular value in the assessment of patients with chronic low back pain of unknown cause.

Magnetic resonance imaging

Magnetic resonance imaging (MRI) gives detailed information on anatomy, allowing three-dimensional visualisation of bone and soft tissues that cannot be adequately assessed by plain X-rays. The technique is valuable in the assessment and diagnosis of many musculoskeletal diseases (Box 24.5). T1-weighted sequences are useful for defining anatomy, whereas T2-weighted sequences are useful for assessing tissue water content, which is often increased in synovitis and other inflammatory disorders (Fig. 24.7). MRI sequences that suppress signal from fat, such as short TI inversion recovery (STIR), are helpful when evaluating inflammatory disease. Contrast agents, such as gadolinium, can be administered to increase sensitivity in detecting erosions and synovitis.

Ultrasonography

Ultrasonography is a useful investigation for confirmation of small joint synovitis and erosions, for anatomical location of periarticular lesions, for characterisation of tendon lesions and for guided injection of joints and bursae. Ultrasound is more sensitive than clinical examination for the detection of early synovitis and is used increasingly in the diagnosis and assessment of patients with suspected inflammatory arthritis. In addition to locating synovial thickening and effusions, ultrasound can detect increased blood flow within synovium using power Doppler imaging, an option that is available on most modern ultrasound machines (Fig. 24.8).

Computed tomography

Computed tomography (CT) is used selectively for assessing patients with bone and joint disease. CT may be used when skeletal configuration needs defining, when calcific lesions are being assessed (crowned dens syndrome, p. 1017), when MRI is contraindicated, or when articular regions are being evaluated in which an adjacent joint replacement creates signal artefacts on MRI, using specific metal artefact reduction algorithms.

Fig. 24.7 Magnetic resonance image showing joint synovitis. Coronal post-contrast T1-weighted image shows extensive enhancement consistent with synovitis (white areas, arrowed) in both wrists, at the second metacarpophalangeal joint and proximal interphalangeal joints of the right hand. *Courtesy of Dr I. Beggs.*

Fig. 24.8 Ultrasound image showing synovitis. Lateral image of a metacarpophalangeal joint in inflammatory arthritis. The periosteum (P) of the phalanx shows as a white line. The dark, hypo-echoic area indicates an effusion. The coloured areas demonstrated by power Doppler indicate increased vascularity. The inset shows a transverse image of the same joint. *Courtesy of Dr N. McKay.*

Dual X-ray absorptiometry

Estimation of bone mineral density (BMD) has a key role in the diagnosis and management of osteoporosis and is best made using dual X-ray absorptiometry (DXA). Measurements at lumbar spine, hip and sometimes forearm are obtained. DXA works on the principle that calcium in bone attenuates passage of X-rays through the tissue in proportion to the amount of mineral present: the more bone mineral present, the higher the BMD value.

Bone density measurements are often presented as T-scores, which measure of the number of standard deviations by which the patient's BMD value differs from that in a young healthy control (Fig. 24.9). Osteoporosis is defined in postmenopausal women and men of more than 50 years old by a T-score of –2.5 or below (shaded red in the figure); osteopenia is diagnosed when the T-score lies between –1.0 and –2.5 (shaded pink). BMD values above –1.0 and below +2.5 are considered normal (yellow/green), whereas values above +2.5 indicate high bone mass, the most common cause being OA. The results need to be interpreted carefully and in reference to coexisting conditions, such as aortic calcification, vertebral fractures, degenerative disc disease and OA, all of which can artefactually raise BMD results. Radiographic correlation is then advisable.

Blood tests

Haematology

Abnormalities in the full blood count (FBC) often occur in inflammatory rheumatic diseases but changes are usually non-specific. Examples include neutrophilia in crystal arthritides and sepsis; neutropenia in lupus; and lymphopenia in autoimmune rheumatic and connective tissue diseases. Reduced levels of haemoglobin and raised platelets are a common and important finding in active inflammatory rheumatological disorders. Many synthetic and biologic disease-modifying antirheumatic drugs (DMARDs) can cause marrow toxicity and require regular monitoring of the FBC. Additional tests that are useful in assessing rheumatic diseases include the direct antiglobulin test (which can indicate intravascular haemolysis in systemic lupus erythematosus (SLE); p. 948) and the dilute Russell viper venom test (a functional assay for a lupus anticoagulant; p. 978).

Biochemistry

Routine biochemistry is useful for assessing metabolic bone disease, muscle diseases and gout, and is essential in monitoring DMARDs and biologic drugs (renal and hepatic function). Several bone diseases, including Paget's disease, renal bone disease and osteomalacia, give a characteristic pattern that can be helpful diagnostically (Box 24.6). Serum levels of uric acid are usually raised in gout but a normal level does not exclude it, especially during an acute attack, when urate levels temporarily fall. Equally, an elevated serum uric acid does not confirm the diagnosis, since most hyperuricaemic people never develop gout. Levels of C-reactive protein (CRP) are a useful marker of infection and inflammation, and are more specific than the erythrocyte sedimentation rate (ESR). An exception is in autoimmune connective tissue diseases, such as SLE and systemic sclerosis, where CRP may be normal but the ESR raised in active disease. Accordingly, an elevated CRP in a patient with lupus or systemic sclerosis suggests an intercurrent illness, such as sepsis, rather than active disease. More detail on the

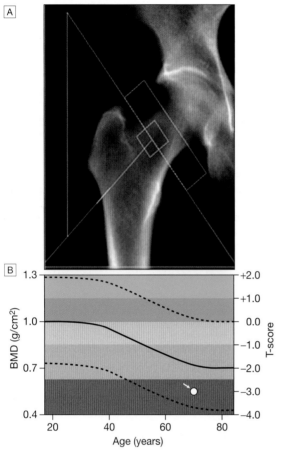

Fig. 24.9 **Typical output from a dual X-ray absorptiometry (DXA) scan.** [A] Image from hip DXA scan. [B] Bone mineral density (BMD) values plotted in g/cm² (left axis) and as the T-score values (right axis). The solid line represents the population average plotted against age, and the interrupted lines are ±2 standard deviations. The BMD T-score result from the patient shown aged 70 years (arrow) is –3.0, indicating osteoporosis. Note that, while the patient's BMD is below average, it lies within the reference range for someone of that age, since BMD normally falls with age.

24.6 Typical biochemical abnormalities in various skeletal diseases (in serum)						
	Calcium	Phosphate	ALP	PTH	FGF23	25(OH)D
Osteoporosis	N	N	N (↑ after fracture)	N or ↑	N	N or ↓
Paget's disease	N	N	↑↑	N or ↑	N	N or ↓
Renal osteodystrophy	N or ↓	N or ↑	↑	↑↑	↑↑	N or ↓
Vitamin D-deficient osteomalacia	N or ↓	N or ↓	↑	↑↑	N or ↓	↓↓
Hypophosphataemic rickets	N	↓↓	↑	N or ↑	↑↑	N or ↓
Primary hyperparathyroidism	↑/↑↑	N or ↓	N or ↑	↑↑	N or ↑	N or ↓

(ALP = alkaline phosphatase; FGF23 = fibroblast growth factor 23; PTH = parathyroid hormone)
(N = normal; single arrow = increased or decreased; double arrow = greatly increased or decreased)

<table>
<tr><td colspan="2">i 24.7 Causes of an elevated serum creatinine phosphokinase (CPK)</td></tr>
</table>

• Inflammatory myositis ± vasculitis	• Trauma, strenuous exercise, prolonged immobilisation after a fall
• Muscular dystrophy	
• Motor neuron disease	• Hypothyroidism, metabolic myopathy
• Alcohol, drugs (especially statins)	• Viral myositis
• Myocardial infarction*	

*The CK-MB cardiac-specific isoform is disproportionately elevated compared with total CPK.

interpretation of CRP and ESR changes is given on page 72. Serum creatine phosphokinase levels are useful in the diagnosis of myopathy or myositis, but specificity and sensitivity are poor and raised levels may occur in some conditions (Box 24.7).

Immunology

Autoantibody tests are widely used in the diagnosis of rheumatic diseases. Whatever test is used, the results must be interpreted in light of the clinical picture and the different detection and assay systems used in different hospitals.

Rheumatoid factor

Rheumatoid factor (RF) is an antibody directed against the Fc fragment of human immunoglobulin. In routine clinical practice, immunoglobulin M (IgM) RF is usually measured, although different methodologies allow measurement of IgG and IgA RFs too. Positive RF occurs in a wide variety of diseases and some normal adults (Box 24.8), particularly with increasing age. Although the specificity is poor, about 70% of patients with RA test positive. High RF titres are associated with more severe disease and extra-articular disease.

Anti-citrullinated peptide antibodies

Anti-citrullinated peptide antibodies (ACPAs) recognise peptides in which the amino acid arginine has been converted to citrulline by peptidylarginine deiminase, an enzyme abundant in inflamed synovium and in a variety of mucosal structures. ACPAs have similar sensitivity to RF for RA (70%) but much higher specificity (>95%), and should be used in preference to RF in the diagnosis of RA. ACPAs are associated with more severe disease progression

and can be detected in asymptomatic patients several years before the development of RA. Their pathological role is still debated but it is likely that they amplify the synovial response to an inflammatory stimulus.

Antinuclear antibodies

Antinuclear antibodies (ANAs) are directed against one or more components of the cell nucleus, including nucleic acids themselves and the proteins concerned with the processing of DNA or RNA. They occur in many inflammatory rheumatic diseases but are also found at low titre in normal individuals and in other diseases (Box 24.9). ANAs are not associated with disease severity or activity. The most common indication for ANA testing is in patients suspected of having SLE or other autoimmune connective tissue diseases. ANA has high sensitivity for SLE (100%) but low specificity (10–40%). A negative ANA virtually excludes SLE but a positive result does not confirm it.

Anti-DNA antibodies bind to double-stranded DNA (dsDNA) and are useful in SLE monitoring as very high titres are associated with more severe disease, including renal or central nervous system (CNS) involvement, and an increase in antibody titre may precede relapse. Anti-DNA antibodies are routinely tested by enzyme-linked immunosorbent assay (ELISA; see also p. 1036).

Antibodies to extractable nuclear antigens (ENAs) act as markers for certain autoimmune connective tissue diseases and some complications of SLE but sensitivity and specificity are poor (Box 24.10). For example, antibodies to Sm are found in a minority of patients with SLE but are associated with renal involvement. Antibodies to Ro occur in SLE and in Sjögren's syndrome (in association with anti-La antibodies), and are associated with a photosensitive rash and congenital heart block. Antibodies to ribonucleoprotein (RNP) occur in SLE and also in mixed connective tissue disease, where features of lupus, myositis and systemic sclerosis coexist. Anti-topoisomerase 1 (also termed Scl-70) antibodies occur in diffuse systemic sclerosis, whereas anti-centromere antibodies are more specific for limited systemic sclerosis.

Antiphospholipid antibodies

Antiphospholipid antibodies bind to a number of phospholipid binding proteins but the most clinically relevant are those that target beta$_2$-glycoprotein 1 (β_2GP1). They may be detected in

<table>
<tr><td colspan="2">i 24.8 Conditions associated with a positive rheumatoid factor*</td></tr>
<tr><td>Condition</td><td>Approximate frequency (%)</td></tr>
<tr><td>Rheumatoid arthritis with nodules and extra-articular manifestations</td><td>100</td></tr>
<tr><td>Rheumatoid arthritis (overall)</td><td>70</td></tr>
<tr><td>Sjögren's syndrome</td><td>90</td></tr>
<tr><td>Mixed essential cryoglobulinaemia</td><td>90</td></tr>
<tr><td>Primary biliary cholangitis</td><td>50</td></tr>
<tr><td>Infective endocarditis</td><td>40</td></tr>
<tr><td>Systemic lupus erythematosus</td><td>30</td></tr>
<tr><td>Tuberculosis</td><td>15</td></tr>
<tr><td>Age >65 years</td><td>20</td></tr>
</table>

*Normal healthy people can be positive for rheumatoid factor.

<table>
<tr><td colspan="2">i 24.9 Conditions associated with a positive antinuclear antibody*</td></tr>
<tr><td>Condition</td><td>Approximate frequency (%)</td></tr>
<tr><td>Systemic lupus erythematosus</td><td>100%</td></tr>
<tr><td>Systemic sclerosis</td><td>60–80%</td></tr>
<tr><td>Sjögren's syndrome</td><td>40–70%</td></tr>
<tr><td>Dermatomyositis or polymyositis</td><td>30–80%</td></tr>
<tr><td>Mixed connective tissue disease</td><td>100%</td></tr>
<tr><td>Autoimmune hepatitis</td><td>100%</td></tr>
<tr><td>Rheumatoid arthritis</td><td>30–50%</td></tr>
<tr><td>Autoimmune thyroid disease</td><td>30–50%</td></tr>
<tr><td>Malignancy</td><td>Varies widely</td></tr>
<tr><td>Infectious diseases</td><td>Varies widely</td></tr>
</table>

*Low-titre positive antinuclear antibody can occur in people without autoimmune disease, without obvious clinical consequences, particularly in the elderly.

24

24.10 Conditions associated with antibodies to extractable nuclear antigens	
Antibody (target/other name)	**Disease association**
Anti-centromere antibody	Localised cutaneous systemic sclerosis (sensitivity 60%, specificity 98%)
Anti-histone antibody	Drug-induced lupus (80%)
Anti-Jo-1 (anti-histidyl-tRNA synthetase)	Polymyositis, dermatomyositis or polymyositis–systemic sclerosis overlap (20–30%) Particularly associated with interstitial lung disease
Anti-La antibody (anti-SS-B)	Sjögren's syndrome (60%) SLE (20–60%)
Anti-ribonucleoprotein antibody (anti-RNP)	Mixed connective tissue disease (100%) SLE (25–50%), usually in conjunction with anti-Sm antibodies
Anti-Ro antibody (anti-SS-A)	SLE (35–60%): associated with photosensitivity, thrombocytopenia and subacute cutaneous lupus Maternal anti-Ro antibodies associated with neonatal lupus and congenital heart block Sjögren's syndrome (40–80%)
Anti-RNA polymerase	Diffuse systemic sclerosis (15%)
Anti Sm (anti-Smith antibody)	SLE (15–30%); associated with renal disease
Anti-Scl-70 (anti-topoisomerase I antibody)	Diffuse systemic sclerosis (15%); associated with more severe organ involvement, including pulmonary fibrosis

(SLE = systemic lupus erythematosus)

SLE and other autoimmune connective tissue diseases and are key in diagnosing antiphospholipid antibody syndrome (p. 977).

Antineutrophil cytoplasmic antibodies

Antineutrophil cytoplasmic antibodies (ANCAs) are IgG antibodies directed against the cytoplasmic constituents of granulocytes and are useful in the diagnosis and monitoring of systemic vasculitis. Two common patterns are described by immunofluorescence: cytoplasmic fluorescence (c-ANCA), which is caused by antibodies to proteinase-3 (PR3); and perinuclear fluorescence (p-ANCA), which is caused by antibodies to myeloperoxidase (MPO) and other proteins, such as lactoferrin and elastase. These antibodies are not specific for vasculitis and positive results may be found in autoimmune liver disease, malignancy, infection (bacterial and human immunodeficiency virus, HIV), inflammatory bowel disease, RA, SLE and pulmonary fibrosis.

Complement

Low complement C3 is an indicator of active SLE, owing to 'consumption' of complement by immune complexes (see Fig. 4.4, p. 66). Low C4 is less specific for SLE activity. High C3 and functional measures of complement activation are non-specific features of inflammation.

Tissue biopsy

Tissue biopsy is useful in confirming the diagnosis in certain musculoskeletal diseases.

Synovial biopsy can be useful in selected patients with chronic inflammatory monoarthritis or tenosynovitis to rule out chronic infectious causes, especially mycobacterial infections. Synovial biopsy can be obtained arthroscopically (by conventional means or by use of needle arthroscope) or by using ultrasound guidance under local anaesthetic.

Temporal artery biopsy can be of value in patients suspected of having temporal arteritis, especially when the presentation is atypical, but a negative result does not exclude the diagnosis. Biopsies of affected tissues, such as skin, lung, nasopharynx, gut, kidney and muscle, should be sought by default in confirming a diagnosis of systemic vasculitis.

Muscle biopsy plays an important role in the investigation of myopathy and inflammatory myositis. It is usually taken from the quadriceps or deltoid through a small skin incision under local anaesthetic. Since myositis can be patchy in nature, MRI is sometimes used to localise the best site for biopsy. Immunohistochemical staining, together with plain histology, gives information on primary and secondary muscle and neuromuscular disease. Repeat biopsies are sometimes used to monitor the response to treatment.

Bone biopsy is occasionally required where non-invasive tests give inconclusive results, in the diagnosis of infiltrative disorders, in patients with renal bone disease, suspected chronic infection or malignancy, and rarely to confirm or exclude the presence of osteomalacia. Bone is taken from the iliac crest using a large-diameter (8 mm) trephine needle under local anaesthetic and processed without demineralisation. For focal lesions, the biopsy should be taken under X-ray guidance or at open surgery, from an affected site.

Electromyography

Electromyography (p. 1076) is of value in the investigation of suspected myopathy and inflammatory myositis, when it shows the diagnostic triad of:

- spontaneous fibrillation
- short-duration action potentials in a polyphasic disorganised outline
- repetitive bouts of high-voltage oscillations on needle contact with diseased muscle.

Presenting problems in musculoskeletal disease

Acute monoarthritis

The most important causes of acute arthritis in a single joint are crystal arthritis, sepsis, SpA and oligoarticular juvenile idiopathic arthritis (JIA; p. 1026). Other potential causes are shown in Box 24.11.

Clinical assessment

The clinical history, pattern of joint involvement, speed of onset, and age and gender of the patient all give clues to the most likely diagnosis. Gout classically affects the first metatarsophalangeal (MTP) joint, whereas pseudogout, which can be a presenting feature of calcium pyrophosphate dihydrate (CPPD) disease, can affect the hand/wrist, ankle, knee or hip. A very rapid onset (6–12 hours) is suggestive of crystal arthritis; joint sepsis develops more slowly and continues to progress until treated.

i | 24.11 Causes of acute monoarthritis

Common

- Gout
- Pseudogout
- Trauma
- Haemarthrosis

- Spondyloarthritis
- Psoriatic arthritis
- Reactive arthritis
- Enteropathic arthritis

Less common

- Rheumatoid arthritis
- Juvenile idiopathic arthritis
- Pigmented villonodular synovitis
- Foreign body reaction

- Tuberculosis
- Leukaemia*
- Gonococcal infection
- Osteomyelitis*

*In children, both leukaemia and osteomyelitis may present with monoarthritis.

i | 24.12 Common causes of polyarthritis

Cause	Characteristics
Rheumatoid arthritis	Symmetrical, small and large joints, upper and lower limbs
Viral arthritis	Symmetrical, small joints; may be associated with rash and prodromal illness; self-limiting
Osteoarthritis	Symmetrical, targets PIP, DIP and first CMC joints in hands, knees, hips, back and neck; associated with Heberden's and Bouchard's nodes
Psoriatic arthritis	Asymmetrical, targets all joints and entheses; associated with nail pitting/onycholysis, dactylitis
Axial spondyloarthritis and enteropathic arthritis	Tends to affect midsize and large joints and entheses, lower more than upper limbs; history of inflammatory back pain
Systemic lupus erythematosus	Symmetrical, typically affecting small joints; clinical evidence of synovitis unusual
Juvenile idiopathic arthritis	Various patterns (p. 1026): polyarticular, oligoarticular and systemic but also enthesitis-predominant
Chronic gout	Affects distal more than proximal joints; history of acute attacks
Chronic sarcoidosis (p. 608)	Varies: small and large joints, often involves ankles
Calcium pyrophosphate arthritis	Chronic polyarthritis with involvement of wrists, ankles, knees and oligoarticular small hand joints

(CMC = carpometacarpal; DIP = distal interphalangeal; PIP = proximal interphalangeal)

Haemarthrosis typically causes a large effusion, in the absence of periarticular swelling or skin change, in a patient who has suffered an injury. Pigmented villonodular synovitis (p. 1059) also presents with synovial swelling and a large effusion, although the onset is gradual. A previous diarrhoeal illness or genital infection suggests reactive arthritis, whereas intercurrent illness, dehydration or surgery may act as a trigger for crystal-induced arthritis. Rheumatoid arthritis seldom presents with monoarthritis but psoriatic arthritis (PsA) can typically present this way. Osteoarthritis can present with pain and stiffness affecting a single joint, but the onset is gradual and there is usually no evidence of significant joint swelling unless it is complicated by crystal-induced inflammation.

Investigations

Aspiration of the affected joint is mandatory. If sepsis is suspected in a large joint, arthroscopic washout is advisable. The fluid should be sent for culture and Gram stain to seek the presence of organisms and should be checked by polarised light microscopy for crystals. Blood cultures should also be taken in patients suspected of having septic arthritis. CRP levels and ESR are raised in sepsis, crystal arthritis and reactive arthritis, and this can be useful in assessing the response to treatment. Serum uric acid measurements may be raised in gout but a normal level does not exclude the diagnosis. Ruling out primary hyperparathyroidism is essential if there is pseudogout.

Management

If there is any suspicion of sepsis, intravenous antibiotics (see Box 24.50, p. 1020) should be given promptly, pending the results of cultures. Unless atypical infections/tuberculosis (requiring prolonged or special culture) are suspected, intra-articular glucocorticoid injection may be considered after 48 hours of negative synovial fluid culture. Otherwise, management should be directed towards the underlying cause.

Polyarthritis

This term is used to describe pain and swelling affecting five or more joints or joint groups. The possible causes are listed in Box 24.12.

Clinical assessment

The hallmarks of inflammatory arthritis are early-morning stiffness and worsening of symptoms with inactivity, along with synovial swelling and tenderness on examination. Clinical features in other systems can be helpful in determining the underlying cause (Box 24.13). The most important diagnoses to consider are PsA, RA and inflammatory small joint OA. RA is characterised by symmetrical involvement of the small joints of the hands and feet, wrists, ankles and knees. PsA is strongly associated with enthesitis. Viral arthritis (p. 1020), Poncet's disease (in regions where tuberculosis is highly prevalent; p. 588), polyarticular JIA (in children) and post-streptococcal arthritis should also be considered.

The pattern of involvement can be helpful in reaching a diagnosis (Fig. 24.10). Asymmetry, lower limb predominance, enthesitis and greater involvement of large joints are characteristic of the SpAs. In PsA there may be involvement of the proximal and distal interphalangeal (PIP and DIP) joints, as opposed to the metacarpophalangeal (MCP) and PIP joints in RA. Inflammatory OA can appear similar to small-joint PsA in the pattern of joint involvement. In PsA there may be nail pitting or early onycholysis. Psoriasis may not be present. SLE can be associated with polyarthritis but more usually causes polyarthralgia and tenosynovitis, mainly of distal limb joints/tendons (p. 1035).

Investigations

Blood samples should be taken for routine haematology, biochemistry, ESR, CRP, viral serology and an immunological screen, including ANA, RF and ACPA. Ultrasound examination or MRI may be required to confirm the presence of synovitis, if this is not obvious clinically.

24

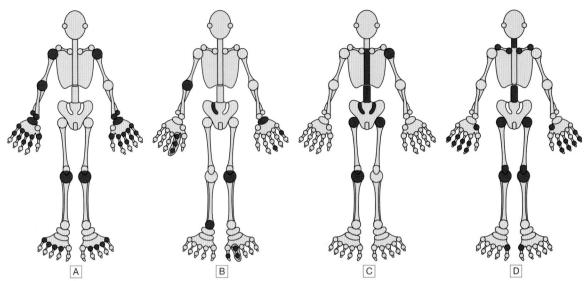

Fig. 24.10 Patterns of joint involvement in different forms of polyarthritis. **A** Rheumatoid arthritis typically targets the metacarpophalangeal and proximal interphalangeal joints of the hands and metatarsophalangeal joints of the feet, as well as other joints, in a symmetrical pattern. **B** Psoriatic arthritis targets proximal and distal interphalangeal joints of the hands, entheses and larger joints in an asymmetrical pattern. Sacroiliitis (often asymmetrical) may occur. **C** Axial spondyloarthritis/ankylosing spondylitis targets the spine, sacroiliac joints, entheses and large peripheral joints in an asymmetrical pattern. **D** Osteoarthritis targets the proximal and distal interphalangeal joints of the hands, first carpometacarpal joint at the base of the thumb, knees, hips, lumbar and cervical spine.

i	24.13 Extra-articular features of inflammatory arthritis	
Clinical feature	**Disease association**	
Skin, nails and mucous membranes		
Psoriasis, nail pitting and dystrophy	Psoriatic arthritis	
Raynaud's phenomenon	Systemic sclerosis, antiphospholipid syndrome, SLE	
Photosensitivity	SLE	
Livedo reticularis	SLE, antiphospholipid syndrome	
Splinter haemorrhages, nail-fold infarcts, purpuric lesions	Vasculitis	
Urticaria and erythemas	SLE, adult-onset Still's disease, systemic JIA, rheumatic fever	
Oral ulcers	SLE, reactive arthritis, Behçet's disease	
Nodules	RA (mainly extensor surfaces), gout (tophi; eccentric, white deposits within), rheumatic fever	
Xerostomia, dry skin, various rashes	Primary Sjögren's syndrome	
Eyes		
Uveitis	SpA, sarcoid, JIA, Behçet's disease	
Conjunctivitis	Reactive arthritis	
Episcleritis, scleritis	RA, vasculitis	
Heart, lungs		
Pleuro-pericarditis	SLE, RA, rheumatic fever	
Aortic valve/root disease	HLA-B27-related SpA	
Interstitial lung disease	RA, SLE, primary Sjögren's syndrome	
Abdominal organs		
Hepatosplenomegaly	RA, SLE	
Haematuria, proteinuria	SLE, vasculitis, systemic sclerosis	
Urethritis	Reactive arthritis and SpA (sterile)	
Fever, lymphadenopathy	Infection, systemic JIA, rheumatic fever	

(HLA = human leucocyte antigen; JIA = juvenile idiopathic arthritis; RA = rheumatoid arthritis; SLE = systemic lupus erythematosus; SpA = spondyloarthritis)

Management

Treatment with non-steroidal anti-inflammatory drugs (NSAIDs) and analgesics will help. Systemic glucocorticoids can be considered if symptoms are very severe or having a great functional impact, but early immunotherapy (DMARDs) is required in RA and in some cases of PsA. An early accurate and specific diagnosis is very important.

Fracture

Fractures are a common presenting symptom of osteoporosis but they also occur in other bone diseases, in osteopenia and in some patients with normal bone.

Clinical assessment

The presentation is with localised bone pain, which is worsened by movement of the affected limb or region. There is usually a history of trauma but spontaneous fractures can occur in the absence of trauma in severe osteoporosis. Fractures can be divided into several subtypes, based on the precipitating event and presence or absence of an underlying disease (Box 24.14). The main differential diagnosis is soft tissue injury but fracture should be suspected when there is marked pain and swelling, abnormal movement of the affected limb, crepitus or deformity. Femoral neck fractures typically produce a shortened, externally rotated leg that is painful to move. The pain from vertebral fracture is variable and a high index of suspicion is key to making the diagnosis by imaging, as discussed below.

Investigations

X-rays of the affected site should be taken in at least two planes and examined for discontinuity of the cortical outline (Box 24.15). In addition to demonstrating the fracture, X-rays may also show evidence of an underlying disorder, such as osteoporosis, Paget's disease or osteomalacia. If the X-ray fails to show evidence of a fracture but clinical suspicion remains high, MRI should be

24.14 Characteristics of different fracture types

Fracture type	Precipitation factor	Disease
Fragility fracture	Fall from standing height or less	Osteoporosis Osteopenia
Vertebral fracture	Bending, lifting, falling	Osteoporosis
Stress fracture	Running, excessive training	Normal
High-energy fracture	Major trauma	Normal
Pathological fracture	Spontaneous, minimal trauma	Malignancy Paget's disease Osteomalacia

24.15 How to investigate a suspected fracture

- Order X-rays in two projections at right angles to one another
- Include the whole bone and the joints at either end (this may reveal an additional unsuspected fracture)
- Check for evidence of displacement
- Check for a break in the cortex
- In suspected vertebral fracture, check for depression of the end plate
- If clinical suspicion is high but no fracture is seen, request magnetic resonance imaging

obtained. Patients who are over the age of 50 and present with fragility fractures should be screened for osteoporosis by DXA.

Management

Management of fracture in the acute stage requires adequate pain relief, with opiates if necessary, reduction of the fracture to restore normal anatomy, and immobilisation of the affected limb to promote healing. This can be achieved either by the use of an external cast or splint, or by internal fixation. Femoral neck fractures present a special management problem since non-union and avascular necrosis are common. This is especially true with intracapsular hip fractures, which should be treated by joint replacement surgery. Following the fracture, rehabilitation is required with physiotherapy and a supervised exercise programme. If the DXA scan shows evidence of osteoporosis or other metabolic bone disease, this should be treated appropriately (p. 1046). Options for management of painful vertebral fracture are discussed on page 1002.

Generalised musculoskeletal pain

Clinical assessment

Clinical history and examination need to be wide-ranging (Box 24.16). Relentlessly progressive pain occurring in association with weight loss suggests malignant disease with bone metastases. Generalised bone pain may also arise in severe osteomalacia, primary hyperparathyroidism and polyostotic Paget's disease. Widespread pain can occur in PsA if there is enthesial as well as, or instead of, joint involvement; fatigue is also often present. Polyarticular RA or OA pains tend to be localised to sites of involvement, such as the lumbar spine, hips, knees and hands. Fibromyalgia (FM) syndrome (p. 1018) presents with generalised pain that particularly affects the trunk, back and neck. Accompanying features include fatigue, poor concentration and focal areas of hyperalgesia. Widespread pain may also occur

24.16 Some common causes of generalised pain

- Myopathies
- Psoriatic arthritis (enthesopathic)
- Fibromyalgia
- Parvovirus arthromyalgia
- Rheumatic fever/post-streptococcal infection
- Metastatic cancer
- Severe osteomalacia

in association with hypermobility, most notably Ehlers–Danlos syndrome hypermobility subtype (hEDS; p. 1059).

Investigations

Bone scintigraphy is of value in patients suspected of having osteomalacia, bone metastases or Paget's disease, and in characterising lesions at joints and/or entheses in SpAs, including PsA. Myeloma (p. 966) should be screened for with an FBC, measurement of CRP, and plasma and urinary protein electrophoresis. If these results are positive, a radiological skeletal survey should be obtained. Routine biochemistry, vitamin D and parathyroid hormone (PTH) should be measured if osteomalacia is suspected. In Paget's disease, ALP may be elevated but can be normal in localised disease. Any persistently elevated ESR, CRP, angiotensin-converting enzyme (ACE), immunoglobulins, C3/C4 or platelets invariably indicates inflammatory disease. Laboratory investigations are normal in patients with FM alone and in hEDS.

Management

Management should be directed towards the underlying cause. Chronic pain of unknown cause and that associated with FM respond poorly to analgesics and NSAIDs, but may respond partially to antineuropathic agents, such as amitriptyline, duloxetine, gabapentin and pregabalin.

Back pain

Back pain is a common symptom that affects 60–80% of people at some time in their lives. Although the prevalence has not increased, reported disability from back pain has risen significantly in the last 30 years. In Western countries, back pain is the most common cause of sickness-related work absence. In the UK, 7% of adults consult their GP each year with back pain. Globally, low back pain is thought to affect about 9% of the population. The most important causes are summarised in Box 24.17.

Clinical assessment

The main purpose of clinical assessment is to differentiate the self-limiting disorder of acute mechanical back pain from serious spinal pathology, as summarised in Figure 24.11. Mechanical back pain is the most common cause of acute back pain in people aged 20–55. This accounts for more than 90% of episodes, and is usually acute and associated with lifting or bending. It is exacerbated by activity and is generally relieved by rest (Box 24.18). It is usually confined to the lumbar–sacral region, buttock or thigh, is asymmetrical and does not radiate beyond the knee (which would imply nerve root irritation). On examination, there may be asymmetric local paraspinal muscle spasm and tenderness, and painful restriction of some, but not all, movements. Low back pain is more common in manual workers, particularly those in occupations that involve heavy lifting and twisting. The prognosis

24

is generally good. After 2 days, 30% are better and 90% have recovered by 6 weeks. Recurrences of pain may occur and about 10–15% of patients go on to develop chronic back pain that may be difficult to treat. Psychological elements, such as job dissatisfaction, depression and anxiety, are important risk factors for the transition to chronic pain and disability.

Back pain secondary to serious spinal pathology has different characteristics (Box 24.19). If there is clinical evidence of spinal cord or nerve root compression, sepsis including tuberculosis, or a cauda equina lesion (Box 24.20), urgent investigation is needed. Spinal stenosis presents insidiously with leg discomfort on walking that is relieved by rest, bending forwards or walking uphill. Patients may adopt a characteristic simian posture, with a forward stoop and slight flexion at hips and knees. The most common cause is the gradual development of coexisting contributing lesions such as facet joint arthritis, ligament flavum thickening or degenerative spondylolisthesis.

Degenerative disc disease is a common cause of chronic low back pain in middle-aged adults. Prolapse of an intervertebral disc presents when discs are still well hydrated (in young and early middle age) with nerve root pain, which can be accompanied by a sensory deficit, motor weakness and asymmetrical reflexes. Examination may reveal a positive sciatic or femoral stretch test. About 70% of patients improve by 4 weeks. Inflammatory back pain (IBP) due to axial spondyloarthritis (axSpA) or PsA has a gradual onset and almost always occurs before the age of 40. It is associated with morning stiffness and improves with movement. Spondylolisthesis (p. 1059) may cause back pain that

---

 24.17 Causes of low back pain

- Mechanical (soft-tissue lesion) back pain
- Intervertebral disc lesions (e.g. prolapse, disc degeneration)
- Facet joint disease (osteoarthritis, psoriatic arthritis)
- Vertebral fracture (p. 994)
- Paget's disease
- Axial spondyloarthritis
- Spondylodiscitis
- Bone metastases
- Spondylolisthesis (p. 1059)
- Scheuermann's disease (p. 1055)

 24.18 Features of mechanical low back pain

- Pain varies with physical activity (improved with rest)
- Onset often sudden and precipitated by lifting or bending
- Recurrent episodes
- Pain limited to back or upper leg
- No clear-cut nerve root distribution
- No systemic features
- Prognosis good (90% recovery at 6 weeks)

 24.19 Red flags for possible spinal pathology

History

- Age: presentation <20 years or >55 years
- Character: constant, progressive pain unrelieved by rest
- Location: thoracic pain
- Past medical history: carcinoma, tuberculosis, HIV, systemic glucocorticoid use, osteoporosis
- Constitutional: systemic upset, sweats, weight loss
- Major trauma

Examination

- Painful spinal deformity
- Severe/symmetrical spinal deformity
- Saddle anaesthesia
- Progressive neurological signs/muscle-wasting
- Multiple levels of root signs

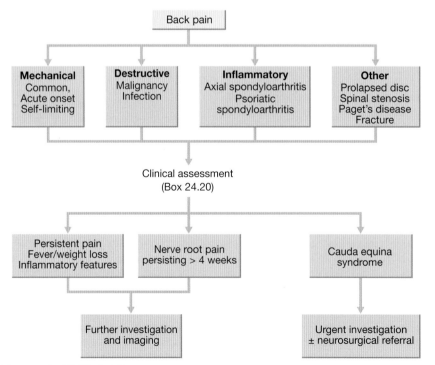

Fig. 24.11 Initial triage assessment of back pain.

24.20 Clinical features of radicular pain

Nerve root pain

- Unilateral leg pain worse than low back pain
- Pain radiates beyond knee
- Paraesthesia in same distribution
- Nerve irritation signs (reduced straight leg raising that reproduces leg pain)
- Motor, sensory or reflex signs (limited to one or adjacent nerve roots)
- Prognosis reasonable (50% recovery at 6 weeks)

Cauda equina syndrome

- Difficulty with micturition
- Loss of anal sphincter tone or faecal incontinence
- Saddle anaesthesia
- Gait disturbance
- Pain, numbness or weakness affecting one or both legs

is typically aggravated by standing and walking. Occasionally, diffuse idiopathic skeletal hyperostosis (DISH; p. 1058) can cause back pain but it is usually asymptomatic. Arachnoiditis is a rare cause of chronic severe low back pain. It is caused by chronic inflammation of the nerve root sheaths in the spinal canal and can complicate meningitis, spinal surgery or myelography with oil-based contrast agents.

Investigations

Investigations are not required in patients with acute mechanical back pain. Those with persistent pain (>6 weeks) or red flags (see Box 24.19) should undergo further investigation. MRI is the investigation of choice because it can demonstrate spinal stenosis, cord compression or nerve root compression, as well as inflammatory changes in axSpA, malignancy and sepsis. Plain X-rays can be of value in patients suspected of having vertebral compression fractures, OA and degenerative disc disease. If metastatic disease is suspected, bone scintigraphy should be considered. Additional investigations that may be required include routine biochemistry and haematology, ESR and CRP (to screen for sepsis and inflammatory disease), protein and urinary electrophoresis (for myeloma), human leucocyte antigen (HLA)-B27 status in IBP and prostate-specific antigen (for prostate carcinoma).

Management

Education is important in patients with mechanical back pain. It should emphasise the self-limiting nature of the condition and the fact that exercise is helpful rather than damaging. Regular analgesia and/or NSAIDs may be required to improve mobility and facilitate exercise. Return to work and normal activity should take place as soon as possible. Bed rest is not helpful and may increase the risk of chronic disability. Referral for physical therapy should be considered if a return to normal activities has not been achieved by 6 weeks. Low-dose tricyclic antidepressant drugs may help pain, sleep and mood.

Other treatment modalities that are occasionally used include epidural and facet joint injection, traction and lumbar supports, though there is limited randomised controlled trial evidence to support their use. Malignant disease, osteoporosis, Paget's disease and SpAs require specific treatment of the underlying condition.

Surgery is required in less than 1% of patients with low back pain but may be needed in progressive spinal stenosis,

in spinal cord compression and in some patients with nerve root compression.

Regional musculoskeletal pain

Regional musculoskeletal pain is a common presenting complaint, usually occurring as the result of age-related degenerative disease of tendons and ligaments, OA and trauma.

Neck pain

Neck pain is a common symptom that can occur following an injury or falling asleep in an awkward position, as a result of stress or in association with OA of the spine. The causes are shown in Box 24.21. Most cases resolve spontaneously or with a short course of NSAIDs or analgesics and some exercise therapy. Patients with persistent pain that follows a nerve root distribution and those with upper or lower limb neurological signs should be investigated by MRI and, if necessary, referred for a neurosurgical opinion.

24.21 Typical causes of neck pain

Mechanical

- Postural
- Whiplash injury
- Facet joint
- Cervical spondylosis

Inflammatory

- Infections
- Axial spondyloarthritis
- Psoriatic arthritis
- Rheumatoid arthritis
- Polymyalgia rheumatica
- Discitis

Metabolic

- Axial calcium pyrophosphate dihydrate disease
- Fibrous dysplasia
- Paget's disease

Neoplastic

- Metastases
- Myeloma
- Lymphoma
- Intrathecal tumours

Other

- Fibromyalgia
- Torticollis

Referred

- Pharynx
- Cervical lymph nodes
- Teeth
- Angina pectoris
- Aortic aneurysm
- Pancoast tumour
- Diaphragm

Shoulder pain

Shoulder pain is a common complaint over the age of 40 (Box 24.22). Varying pain patterns associated with common lesions are shown in Figure 24.12. For most shoulder lesions, general management is with analgesics, NSAIDs, local glucocorticoid injections and physiotherapy aimed at restoring normal movement and function. Surgery may be required in patients who have debilitating or persistent symptoms in association with rotator cuff lesions or severe acromioclavicular joint arthritis. If there is subacromial impingement, without evidence of a rotator cuff tear on MRI, subacromial glucocorticoid injection and physiotherapy constitute a reasonable first step. Calcific supraspinatus tendonitis unresponsive to glucocorticoid injection can be treated with barbotage (needle disruption of deposit under ultrasound guidance). Complete rotator cuff tears in people under 40 years of age may respond well to full surgical repair but results are

24

Rotator cuff and subacromial lesions

- Pain reproduced by resisted active movement:
  Abduction: supraspinatus
  External rotation: infraspinatus, teres minor
  Internal rotation: subscapularis

Acromioclavicular joint

- Pain on full abduction and adduction (at 90° of forward elevation)

Bicipital (long head) tendinitis

- Tenderness over bicipital groove
- Pain reproduced by resisted active wrist supination or elbow flexion

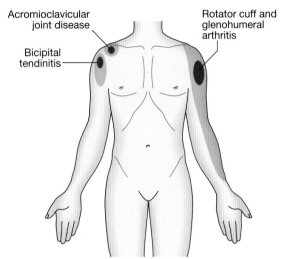

Fig. 24.12 Pain patterns around the shoulder. The dark shading indicates sites of maximum pain.

less good in older people. Adhesive capsulitis (frozen shoulder) presents with pain associated with marked restriction of elevation and external rotation. Adhesive capsulitis is commonly associated with diabetes mellitus and neck/radicular lesions. Treatment in the early stage is with analgesia, intra- and extracapsular glucocorticoid injection, and regular 'pendulum' exercises of the arm to mobilise. Complete recovery sometimes takes up to 2 years. For severe or persistent symptoms, joint distension and manipulation under anaesthesia are surgical options.

Elbow pain

The most common causes are repetitive trauma causing lateral epicondylitis (tennis elbow) and medial epicondylitis (golfer's elbow) (Box 24.23). SpAs, including psoriatic disease, can present with the same symptoms (tendon insertion enthesitis). Management is by rest, analgesics and topical or systemic NSAIDs. Local glucocorticoid injections may be required in resistant cases. Olecranon bursitis can also follow local repetitive trauma but other causes include infections and gout.

Hand and wrist pain

Pain from hand or wrist joints is well localised to the affected joint, except for pain from the first carpometacarpal (CMC) joint, commonly targeted by OA or PsA; although maximal at the thumb base, the pain often radiates down the thumb and to the radial aspect of the wrist. Non-articular causes of hand pain include:

Lesion	Pain	Examination findings
Lateral humeral epicondylitis (e.g. traumatic 'tennis elbow' or SpA-related enthesitis)	Lateral epicondyle Radiation to extensor forearm	Tenderness over epicondyle Pain reproduced by resisted active wrist extension
Medial humeral epicondylitis (e.g. traumatic 'golfer's elbow' or SpA-related enthesitis)	Medial epicondyle Radiation to flexor forearm	Tenderness over epicondyle Pain reproduced by resisted active wrist flexion
Olecranon bursitis (e.g. gout, rheumatoid arthritis or infective, as in tuberculosis)	Olecranon	Tender swelling

(SpA = spondyloarthritis)

- *Tenosynovitis*: affects flexor or extensor digital tendons. Pain and tenderness are well localised to the tendon lesions. There is often early-morning 'claw-like' digit stiffness. De Quervain's tenosynovitis involves the tendon sheaths of abductor pollicis longus and extensor pollicis brevis. It produces pain maximal over the radial aspect of the distal forearm and wrist and marked pain on forced ulnar deviation of the wrist with the thumb held across the patient's palm (Finkelstein's sign). This test is not specific for this lesion alone.
- *Raynaud's phenomenon*: digital vasospasm triggered mostly by cold (p. 1035).
- *C6, C7 or C8 radiculopathy.*
- *Carpal tunnel syndrome*: hand position-dependent and/or nocturnal pain, numbness and paraesthesia of thumb and second to fourth digits.

Hip pain

Pain from the hip joint is usually felt deep in the groin, with variable radiation to the buttock, anterolateral thigh or knee (Fig. 24.13). Patients who report 'hip pain' sometimes point to greater trochanter or buttock areas. Greater trochanter pain syndrome is usually due to either gluteus medius insertional tendonitis/enthesitis, trochanteric bursitis or referred pain (Box 24.24). Pain at this site may also be referred from the lumbosacral spine. A differential diagnosis of hip joint conditions (groin pain) is symphysitis (SpAs, including psoriasis disease, need ruling out). Other less common causes of pain in the hip/groin area include inguinal hernia, adductor tendonitis and enthesitis of anterior superior/inferior iliac spines.

Knee pain

In middle and older age, the most common cause of knee pain is OA, the features of which are described on page 1008. Pain that is associated with locking of the knee (sudden painful inability to extend fully) is usually due to a meniscal tear or osteochondritis dissecans. Referred pain from the hip may present at the knee and is reproduced by hip, not knee, movement. Pain from periarticular lesions is well localised to the involved structure (Box 24.25). Anterior knee pain may be due to patellar ligament or retinacular lesions (enthesitis, tendonitis, fat-pad syndrome) occurring typically

24.24 Local causes of hip pain

Lesion	Pain	Examination findings
Gluteus medius enthesitis	Upper lateral thigh, worse on lying on that side at night	Tenderness over greater trochanter
Trochanteric bursitis	As above	As above
Adductor tendinitis (usually an SpA-enthesitis or sports-related trauma lesion)	Upper inner thigh	Tenderness over adductor origin/tendon/muscle Pain reproduced by resisted active hip adduction
Ischiogluteal enthesitis/bursitis	Buttock, worse on sitting	Tenderness over ischial prominence
Pubic symphysitis (can mimic intra-articular hip lesions)	Medial groin pain, can radiate to inner or even outer upper thighs	Tenderness over symphysis joint If pain is worse on trunk curl/rectus activation under symphysis-resting hand, it may be insertional rectus enthesis (SpAs)

(SpA = spondyloarthritis)

Trochanteric bursitis

Hip disease

Fig. 24.13 Pain patterns of hip disease and trochanteric pain syndrome. The dark shading indicates sites of maximum pain.

24.25 Local causes of knee pain

Lesion	Pain	Examination findings
Pre-patellar bursitis	Over patella	Tender fluctuant swelling in front of patella
Superficial and deep infrapatellar bursitis and fat-pad syndrome	Anterior knee, inferior to patella	Tenderness in front of (superficial) or behind (deep) patellar tendon Pain on full flexion
Anserine bursitis/enthesitis	Upper medial tibia	Tenderness (± swelling) over upper medial tibia
Medial collateral ligament lesions (e.g. enthesitis)	Upper medial tibia	Localised tenderness of upper medial tibia Pain reproduced by valgus stress on partly flexed knee
Popliteal cyst (Baker's cyst)	Popliteal fossa	Tender swelling of popliteal fossa
Patellar ligament enthesopathy	Anterior upper tibia	Tenderness over tibial tubercle
Osteochondritis of patellar ligament (Osgood–Schlatter disease)	Anterior upper tibia	Adolescents are affected Pain on resisted active knee extension

24

from overuse and/or an SpA condition. Anterior knee pain is relatively common in adolescents and may be the result of patellar articular cartilage or ligament insertion osteochondritis.

Ankle and foot pain

Pain from the ankle (tibiotalar) joint due to OA or osteochondral defect is felt between the malleoli and is worse on weight-bearing. Pain from the subtalar joint (from the same lesions) is also worse on weight-bearing. Inflammatory arthritis of either of these joints (RA, PsA, CPPD arthritis or gout) often worsens and swells with rest. These diagnoses can be associated with hindfoot tenosynovitis (peroneal or posterior tibial). Pain under the heel is typically due to plantar fasciitis. This can occur as the result of overuse, which case it may respond to rest, padded footwear and local glucocorticoid injections, but can also arise in SpA as

a manifestation of enthesitis. Pain affecting the back of the heel may be due to Achilles tendinitis or enthesis. The MTP joints of the feet are commonly involved symmetrically in RA. The presentation is with pain on walking felt below the metatarsal heads, often described as 'walking on marbles'. Patients with active inflammation of the MTP joints have pain when the forefoot is squeezed (p. 982). Involvement of the first MTP joint is common in OA or PsA and is associated, respectively, with hallux valgus and dactylitis. The hallux also a classical target in acute gout. Morton's neuroma is a neuropathy of an interdigital nerve and is usually located between the third and fourth metatarsal heads. Women are most commonly affected (tight shoes can be to blame). Local sensory loss and a palpable tender swelling between the metatarsal heads may be detected. Footwear adjustment, with or without a local glucocorticoid injection, often helps but surgical decompression may be required if symptoms persist.

Muscle pain and weakness

Muscle pain and weakness can arise from a variety of causes. It is important to distinguish between a subjective feeling of generalised weakness occurring with fatigue, and an objective weakness with loss of muscle power and function. The former is a non-specific manifestation of many systemic conditions.

Clinical assessment

Proximal muscle weakness suggests the presence of a myopathy or myositis, which typically causes difficulty with standing from a seated position, walking up steps, squatting and lifting overhead. The causes are shown in Box 24.26. Worsening of symptoms on exercise and post-exertional cramps suggest a metabolic myopathy, such as glycogen storage disease (p. 370). A strong family history and onset in childhood or early adulthood suggest muscular dystrophy (p. 1143). Alcohol excess can cause an inflammatory myositis and atrophy of type 2 muscle fibres. Proximal myopathy may be a complication of glucocorticoid therapy, prolonged/severe hypercalcaemia and osteomalacia. Myopathy and myositis can also occur in association with many drugs (see 'Further information', p. 1060) and viral infections, including HIV; in the latter case, it may be due to HIV itself or to treatment with zidovudine. Polymyositis and dermatomyositis (p. 1039) are associated with coexisting/co-presenting malignancy, especially gonadal tumours. Clinical examination should document the presence, pattern and severity of muscle weakness (p. 1081), assessed using the Medical Research Council (MRC) scale (no power (0) to full power (5)).

Investigations

Investigations should include routine biochemistry and haematology, ESR, CRP, creatine kinase, serum 25(OH)-vitamin D, PTH, parvovirus, hepatitis B/C, HIV and streptococcus serology, serum and urine protein electrophoresis, serum ACE, ANAs/ENAs, RF, complement and myositis-specific autoantibodies such as Jo-1. Open muscle biopsy (site guided by MRI detection of abnormal muscle) and electromyography (EMG) are usually required to make the diagnosis. The initial imaging screening for malignancy is usually a CT scan of the chest, abdomen and pelvis; upper gastrointestinal endoscopy and colonoscopy may also be considered.

Management

Management is determined by the cause but all patients with muscle disease should benefit from physiotherapy and graded exercises to maximise muscle function after the initial inflammation is controlled.

Principles of management

The management of rheumatological disorders should be tailored to the underlying diagnosis. Certain aspects are common to many disorders, however, and the general principles are discussed here. The therapeutic aims are:

- to educate patients about their disease
- to control pain, if it is present
- to optimise function
- to modify the disease process where this is possible
- to identify and treat comorbidity.

These aims are interrelated and success in one area often benefits others. Successful management requires careful assessment of the person as a whole. The management plan should be individualised and patient-centred, should involve relevant members of the multidisciplinary team, and should be agreed and understood by both the patient and all the practitioners that are involved. It must also take into account:

- the patient's activity requirements and occupational and recreational aspirations
- risk factors that may influence the disease
- the patient's perceptions and knowledge of the condition
- medications and coping strategies that have already been tried
- comorbid disease and its therapy
- the availability, costs and logistics of appropriate evidence-based interventions.

The simplest and safest interventions should be tried first. Symptoms and signs may change with time, so the management plan for most patients will require regular review and re-adjustment.

Core interventions that should be considered for everyone with a painful musculoskeletal condition are listed in Box 24.27. There are also other non-pharmacological and drug options, the choice of which depends on the nature and severity of the diagnosis.

Education and lifestyle interventions

Education

Patients must always be informed about the nature of their condition and its investigation, treatment and prognosis, since education can improve outcome. Information and therapist contact can reduce pain and disability, improve self-efficacy and reduce the health-care costs of many musculoskeletal conditions, including OA and RA. The mechanisms are unclear but in part may result from improved adherence. Benefits are modest but potentially long-lasting, safe and cost-effective. Education can be provided through one-to-one discussion, written literature,

---

i | 24.26 Causes of proximal muscle pain or weakness

Inflammatory

- Polymyositis
- Dermatomyositis
- Other autoimmune connective tissue disease
- Inclusion body myositis
- Sarcoid
- Myasthenia gravis

Endocrine (Ch. 18)

- Hypothyroidism
- Hyperthyroidism
- Cushing's syndrome
- Addison's disease

Metabolic (Ch. 14)

- Myophosphorylase deficiency
- Phosphofructokinase deficiency
- Hypokalaemia
- Carnitine deficiency
- Osteomalacia (p. 1049)
- Hypercalcaemia

Genetic

- Muscular dystrophy (various; p. 1143)

Drugs/toxins

- Alcohol
- Cocaine
- Glucocorticoids
- Statins and fibrates
- Tumour necrosis factor inhibitors
- Zidovudine

Infections (Ch. 11)

- Viral (HIV, cytomegalovirus, rubella, Epstein–Barr, echo)
- Parasitic (schistosomiasis, cysticercosis, toxoplasmosis)
- Bacterial (*Clostridium perfringens*, staphylococci, tuberculosis, *Mycoplasma*)

24.27 Interventions for patients with rheumatic diseases

Core interventions

- Education
- Aerobic conditioning
- Muscle strengthening
- Simple analgesics
- Disease-modifying therapy
- Reduction of adverse mechanical factors
- Pacing of activities
- Appropriate footwear
- Weight reduction if obese

Other options

- Other analgesic drugs:
  Oral non-steroidal anti-inflammatory drugs
  Topical agents
  Opioid analgesics
  Amitriptyline
  Gabapentin/pregabalin
- Local glucocorticoid injections
- Physical treatments:
  Heat, cold, aids, appliances
- Surgery
- Coping strategies (see Box 24.28)

patient-led group education classes and interactive computer programs. Inclusion of the patient's partner or carer is often appropriate; this is essential for childhood conditions but also helps in many chronic adult conditions, such as RA and FM.

For children and adolescents with chronic diseases such as JIA, education and support of the whole family, schooling and psychological support is essential and best delivered through a multidisciplinary team.

Exercise

Several types of exercise can be prescribed:

- *Aerobic fitness training* can produce long-term reduction in pain and disability. It improves well-being, encourages restorative sleep and benefits common comorbidity, such as obesity, diabetes, chronic heart failure and hypertension.
- *Local strengthening exercise* for muscles that act over compromised joints also reduces pain and disability, with improvements in the reduced muscle strength, proprioception, coordination and balance that associate with chronic arthritis. 'Small amounts often' of strengthening exercise are better than protracted sessions performed infrequently.
- *Weight-bearing exercise* is of value in osteoporosis, where it can result in modest increases in bone density and slow bone loss.

Joint protection

Excessive impact-loading and adverse repetitive use of a compromised joint or periarticular tissue can worsen symptoms in patients with arthritis. This can be mitigated by cessation of contact sports and by pacing of activities by dividing physical tasks into shorter segments with brief breaks in between. Other strategies include adaptations to machinery or tools at the workplace; the use of shock-absorbing footwear with thick soft soles, which can reduce impact-loading through feet, knees, hips and back; and the use of a walking stick on the contralateral side to a painful hip, knee or foot.

Non-pharmacological interventions

Physical and occupational therapy

Local heat, ice packs, wax baths and other local external applications can induce muscle relaxation and provide temporary relief of symptoms in a range of rheumatic diseases.

Hydrotherapy induces muscle relaxation and facilitates enhanced movement in a warm, pain-relieving environment without the restraints of gravity and normal load-bearing. Various manipulative techniques may also help improve restricted movement. The combination of these with education and therapist contact enhances their benefits.

Splints can give temporary rest and support for painful joints and periarticular tissues, and can prevent harmful involuntary postures during sleep. Prolonged rest must be avoided, however. Orthoses are more permanent appliances used to reduce instability and excessive abnormal movement. They include working wrist splints, knee orthoses, and iron and T-straps to control ankle instability. Orthoses are particularly suited to severely disabled patients in whom a surgical option is inappropriate and often need to be custom-made for the individual.

Aids and appliances can provide dignity and independence for patients with respect to activities of daily living. Common examples are a raised toilet seat, raised chair height, extended handles on taps, a shower instead of a bath, thick-handled cutlery, and extended 'hands' to pull on tights and socks. Full assessment and advice from an occupational therapist maximise the benefits of these (Box 24.27).

Self-help and coping strategies

These help patients to cope better with, and adjust to, chronic pain and disability. They may be useful at any stage but are particularly so for patients with incurable problems, who have tried all available treatment options. The aim is to increase self-management through self-assessment and problem-solving, so that patients can recognise negative but potentially remediable aspects of their mood (stress, frustration, anger or low self-esteem) and their situation (physical, social, financial). These may then be addressed by changes in attitude and behaviour, as shown in Box 24.28.

Involvement of the spouse or partner in mutual goal-setting can improve partnership adjustment. Such approaches are often an element of group education classes and pain clinics but may require more formal clinical psychological input.

Tailored multidisciplinary approaches are required for patients with JIA and other chronic childhood diseases, dependent on age and maturity. Adolescents and young adults have specific demands, different to those of young children and adults, which are influenced by many issues in their lives impinging on the disease process, its impact and their ability to cope with it.

Weight control

Obesity aggravates pain at most sites through increased mechanical strain and is a risk factor for progression of joint damage in patients with OA and other types of arthritis. This should be explained to obese patients and strategies offered

24.28 Self-help and coping strategies

- Yoga and relaxation techniques to reduce stress
- Avoidance of negative situations or activities that produce stress and increase in pleasant activities that give satisfaction
- Information and discussion to alter beliefs about and perspectives on disease
- Reduction or avoidance of catastrophising and maladaptive pain behaviour
- Imagery and distraction techniques for pain
- Expansion of social contact and better use of social services

on how to lose and maintain an appropriate weight (p. 700). Excessive weight loss can be counterproductive and adults with a BMI of <20 kg/m² are at increased risk of fractures. Patients should therefore be advised to maintain BMI within the 20–25 g/m² range.

Surgery

A variety of surgical interventions can relieve pain and conserve or restore function in patients with bone, joint and periarticular disease (Box 24.29). Soft tissue release and tenosynovectomy can reduce inflammatory symptoms, improve function and prevent or retard tendon damage for variable periods, sometimes indefinitely. Synovectomy does not prevent disease progression but may be indicated for pain relief when drugs, physical

24.29 Surgical procedures in rheumatology and bone disease

Procedure	Indication
Soft tissue release	
Carpal tunnel	Median nerve compression
Tarsal tunnel	Posterior tibial nerve entrapment
Flexor tenosynovectomy	Relief of 'trigger' fingers
Ulnar nerve transposition	Ulnar nerve entrapment at elbow
Fasciotomy	Severe Dupuytren's contracture
Tendon repairs and transfers	
Hand extensor tendons	Extensor tendon rupture
Thumb and finger flexor tendons	Flexor tendon rupture
Synovectomy	
Wrist and extensor tendon sheath (+ excision of radial head)	Pain relief and prevention of extensor tendon rupture in RA, resistant inflammatory synovitis
Knee synovectomy	Resistant inflammatory synovitis
Osteotomy	
Femoral osteotomy	Early OA of hip
Tibial osteotomy	Unicompartmental knee OA Deformed tibia in OA or Paget's disease
Excision arthroplasty	
First metatarsophalangeal joint (Keller's procedure)	Painful hallux valgus
Radial head	Painful distal radio-ulnar joint
Lateral end of clavicle	Painful acromioclavicular joint
Metatarsal head	Painful subluxed metatarsophalangeal joints
Joint replacement arthroplasty	
Knee, hip, shoulder, elbow	Painful damaged joints in OA and RA
Arthrodesis	
Wrist	Damaged joint: pain relief, improvement of grip
Ankle/subtalar joints	Damaged joint: pain relief, stabilisation of hindfoot
Fracture repair	
Hip arthroplasty	Fractured neck of femur
External fixation	Multiple fractures, open fractures
Intramedullary nailing	Tibial and femur fractures
Screw, plating and wiring	Wrist and other fractures
Other procedures	
Nerve root decompression	Spinal stenosis, nerve entrapment
Kyphoplasty	Painful vertebral fracture (evidence base poor)
Vertebroplasty	Painful vertebral fracture (evidence base poor)

therapy and intra-articular injections have provided insufficient relief. The main approaches for damaged joints are osteotomy (cutting bone to alter joint mechanics and load transmission), excision arthroplasty (removing part or all of the joint), joint replacement (insertion of prosthesis in place of the excised joint) and arthrodesis (joint fusion). Surgical fixation of fractures is frequently required in patients with osteoporosis and other bone diseases.

The main aims of surgery are to provide pain relief and improve function and quality of life. If surgery is to be successful, the aims and consequences of each operation should be considered as part of an integrated programme of management and rehabilitation by multidisciplinary teams of surgeons, allied health professionals and physicians, and carefully explained to the patient. Assessment of motivation, social support and environment is no less important than careful consideration of patients' general health, their risks for major surgery, the extent of disease in other joints, and their ability to mobilise following surgery. For some severely compromised people, pain relief and functional independence are better served by provision of a suitable wheelchair, home adjustments and social services than by surgery that is technically successful but following which the patient cannot mobilise.

Pharmacological treatment

Analgesics

Paracetamol (1 g up to 4 times daily) is the oral analgesic of first choice for mild to moderate pain. It is thought to work by inhibiting prostaglandin synthesis in the brain while having little effect on peripheral prostaglandin production. It is well tolerated and has few adverse effects and drug interactions. An increased risk of gastrointestinal events and cardiovascular disease has been reported with chronic usage in observational studies, but this may be due to channelling of patients at higher risk of these events for treatment with paracetamol rather than NSAID. Paracetamol can be combined with codeine (co-codamol) or dihydrocodeine (co-dydramol). These compound analgesics are more effective than paracetamol but have more side-effects, including constipation, headache and delirium, especially in the elderly. The centrally acting opioid analgesics tramadol and meptazinol may be useful for temporary control of severe pain unresponsive to other measures but can cause nausea, bowel upset, dizziness and somnolence, and withdrawal symptoms after chronic use. The non-opioid analgesic nefopam (30–90 mg 3 times daily) can help moderate pain, though side-effects (nausea, anxiety, dry mouth) often limit its use. Patients with severe or intractable pain may require strong opioid analgesics, such as oxycodone and morphine.

Non-steroidal anti-inflammatory drugs

NSAIDs are among the most widely prescribed drugs but their use has declined over recent years because long-term prescription is associated with an increased risk of cardiovascular disease. Oral NSAIDs are useful in the treatment of a range of rheumatic diseases with an inflammatory component. There is variability in response and patients who do not gain benefit from one NSAID may well do so with another. They inhibit the cyclo-oxygenase (COX) and prostaglandin H synthase enzymes, which convert arachidonic acid, derived from membrane phospholipids, to prostaglandins and leukotrienes by the COX and 5-lipoxygenase pathways, respectively (Fig. 24.14). There are two COX isoforms,

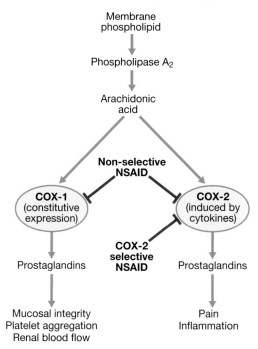

Fig. 24.14 **Mechanism of action of non-steroidal anti-inflammatory drugs.**

encoded by different genes. The COX-1 enzyme is constitutively expressed in gastric mucosa, platelets and kidneys, and production of prostaglandins at these sites protects against mucosal damage and regulates platelet aggregation and renal blood flow. The COX-2 enzyme is induced at sites of inflammation, producing prostaglandins that cause local pain and swelling. Inflammation also up-regulates COX-2 in the spinal cord, where it modulates pain perception. Ibuprofen, diclofenac and naproxen are non-selective drugs that inhibit both COX enzymes, whereas celecoxib and etoricoxib are selective inhibitors of COX-2. While NSAIDs have anti-inflammatory activity, they are not thought to have a disease-modifying effect in either OA or inflammatory rheumatic diseases.

Non-selective NSAIDs can damage the gastric and duodenal mucosal barrier and are associated with an increased risk of upper gastrointestinal ulceration, bleeding and perforation. The adjusted increased risk (odds ratio) of bleeding or perforation from non-selective NSAIDs is 4–5, though differences exist between NSAIDs (Box 24.30). Dyspepsia is a poor guide to the presence of NSAID-associated ulceration and bleeding, and the principal risk factors are shown in Box 24.31. Co-prescription of a proton pump inhibitor (PPI) or misoprostol (200 μg twice or 3 times daily) reduces the risk of NSAID-induced ulceration and bleeding but H_2-antagonists in standard doses are ineffective. The COX-2 selective NSAIDs are much less likely to cause gastrointestinal toxicity but benefit is attenuated in patients on low-dose aspirin. The National Institute for Health and Care Excellence (NICE) guidelines advise that a PPI should be co-prescribed with all NSAIDs, including COX-2-selective NSAIDs, even though the risk of gastrointestinal events with these is low. Since chronic PPI therapy is associated with an increased risk of hip fracture, the merits of giving PPI therapy with a COX-2-selective drug need to be weighed up carefully.

Other side-effects of NSAIDs include fluid retention and renal impairment due to inhibition of renal prostaglandin production,

24.30 Commonly used NSAIDs and their risk of gastrointestinal bleeding and perforation			
Drug	Daily adult dose	Doses/ day	Idiosyncratic side-effects, comments
Low risk			
Celecoxib	100–200 mg	1–2	Selective COX-2 inhibitor
Etoricoxib	60–120 mg	1	Selective COX-2 inhibitor
Medium risk			
Ibuprofen	1600–2400 mg	3–4	Gastrointestinal adverse effects more likely than with COX-2 inhibitors, even with PPI therapy
Naproxen	500–1000 mg	1–2	
Diclofenac	75–150 mg	2–3	
High risk			
Indometacin	50–200 mg	3–4	High incidence of dyspepsia and CNS side-effects
Ketoprofen	100–200 mg	2–4	
Piroxicam	20–30 mg	1–2	Restricted use in those >60 years

(CNS = central nervous system; COX = cyclo-oxygenase; PPI = proton pump inhibitor)

24.31 Risk factors for NSAID-induced ulcers

- Age >60 years*
- Past history of peptic ulcer*
- Past history of adverse event with NSAID
- Concomitant glucocorticoid use
- High-dose or multiple NSAIDs
- High-risk NSAID (see Box 24.30)

*The most important risk factors.

24.32 Recommendations for the use of NSAIDs

- Use the lowest dose for the shortest time possible to control symptoms
- Avoid NSAIDs in patients on warfarin
- Allow 2–3 weeks to assess efficacy. If response is inadequate, consider a trial of another NSAID
- Never prescribe more than one NSAID at a time
- Co-prescribe a proton pump inhibitor for patients with risk factors for gastrointestinal adverse effects (see Box 24.31)
- Avoid in patients with vascular disease

non-ulcer-associated dyspepsia, abdominal pain and altered bowel habit, and rashes. Interstitial nephritis, asthma and anaphylaxis can also occur but are rare. Recommendations for NSAID prescribing are summarised in Box 24.32. Because of the risk of adverse effects, NSAIDs should be used with great care in the elderly (Box 24.33).

Topical agents

Topical NSAID creams and gels and capsaicin cream (chilli extract; 0.025%) can help in the treatment of OA and superficial periarticular lesions affecting hands, elbows and knees. They may be used as monotherapy or as an adjunct to oral analgesics. Topical NSAIDs can penetrate superficial tissues and even reach the joint capsule, though intrasynovial levels mainly reflect blood-borne drug delivery. Capsaicin selectively binds to the protein transient receptor potential vanilloid type 1 (TRPV1), which is a heat-activated calcium channel on the surface of peripheral type C nociceptor fibres. Initial application causes a burning sensation but continued use depletes presynaptic substance P, with subsequent pain reduction that is optimal after a period of 1–2 weeks.

Disease-modifying antirheumatic drugs

Disease-modifying antirheumatic drugs (DMARDs) are a group of small-molecule inhibitors of the immune response. They are employed in a range of inflammatory rheumatic diseases, as well as in other chronic inflammatory conditions. The most common indications are summarised in Box 24.34. Most of these drugs have the potential to cause bone marrow suppression or liver dysfunction and they require regular blood monitoring. Monitoring requirements for commonly used DMARDs are also summarised in Box 24.34. If toxicity occurs, treatment may need to be stopped temporarily and resumed at a lower dose. If toxicity is severe, therapy may have to be withdrawn completely and another drug substituted.

24.33 Use of oral NSAIDs in old age

- **Gastrointestinal complications**: age is a strong risk factor for bleeding and perforation, and for peptic ulceration. Elderly patients are more likely to die if they suffer NSAID-associated bleeding or perforation.
- **Cardiovascular disease**: use NSAIDs with caution in patients with cardiovascular disease. Therapy with NSAIDs may exacerbate hypertension and heart failure.
- **Renal disease**: use of NSAIDs may cause renal impairment.

Methotrexate

Methotrexate (MTX) is the core DMARD in RA, JIA and PsA. It inhibits folic acid reductase, preventing formation of tetrahydrofolate, which is necessary for DNA synthesis in leucocytes and other cells. It is given orally in a starting dose of 10–15 mg weekly and escalated in 2.5 mg increments every 2–4 weeks to a maximum of 25 mg weekly until benefit or toxicity occurs. Folic acid (5 mg/week) should be co-prescribed to be taken the day after MTX since it reduces adverse effects without impairing efficacy. Benefit is usually observed after 4–8 weeks but treatment should continue for 3 months before the conclusion is reached that MTX has been ineffective. The most common adverse effects are nausea, vomiting and malaise, which usually occur one 1–2 days after the weekly dose. Individuals who experience these effects can sometimes be successfully treated with subcutaneous MTX. Patients should be warned of drug interaction with sulphonamides and the importance of avoiding excess alcohol, which enhances MTX hepatotoxicity. Acute pulmonary toxicity (pneumonitis) is rare but can occur at any time during treatment, and patients should be warned to stop therapy and seek advice if they develop any new respiratory symptoms. If pneumonitis occurs, treatment should be withdrawn and high-dose glucocorticoids given. MTX must be co-prescribed with robust contraception in women of child-bearing potential and treatment must be stopped for 3 months in advance of planning a pregnancy.

Sulfasalazine

Sulfasalazine (SSZ) can be used alone and or combination with MTX and another DMARD. Its mechanism of action is incompletely understood. Nausea and gastrointestinal intolerance are the main adverse effects but leucopenia, abnormal LFTs and rashes may also occur. The usual starting dose is 500 mg daily, escalating in 500 mg increments every 2 weeks to a maintenance dose of 2–4 g daily until benefit or toxicity occurs. Benefit may be

24.34 Disease-modifying antirheumatic drugs

Drug	Maintenance dose	Monitoring* FBC	Monitoring* LFTs	Monitoring* Other	Indications
Methotrexate	10–25 mg weekly orally	✓	✓		RA, PsA, AxSpA, JIA
Sulfasalazine	2–4 g daily orally	✓	✓		RA, PsA, AxSpA, JIA
Hydroxychloroquine	200–400 mg daily orally	–	–	Visual function	RA, SLE
Leflunomide	10–20 mg daily orally	✓	✓	BP	RA, JIA, PsA
Azathioprine	1–2.5 mg/kg daily orally	✓	✓		SLE, SV
Apremilast	30 mg twice daily orally	–	–	–	PsA
Tofacitinib	5 mg twice daily orally	✓	✓	Infection	RA
Baricitinib	2–4 mg daily orally	✓	✓	Infection	RA
Cyclophosphamide	2 mg/kg daily orally 15 mg/kg IV	✓	✓	eGFR	SLE, SV
Mycophenolate mofetil (MMF)	2–4 g daily orally	✓	✓	–	SLE, SV
Gold (myocrisin)	50 mg 4-weekly IM	✓	–	Urinalysis	RA
Penicillamine	500–1500 mg daily orally	✓	✓	Urinalysis	RA
Ciclosporin A	3–5 mg/kg daily orally	–	–	BP, eGFR	RA, PsA

*Monitoring tests are usually done every 2 weeks on initiation of treatment for 6 weeks, then monthly for 3 months, then 3-monthly.
(AxSpA = axial spondyloarthritis; BP = blood pressure; eGFR = estimated glomerular filtration rate; FBC = full blood count; IM = intramuscular; IV = intravenous; JIA = juvenile idiopathic arthritis; LFTs = liver function tests; PsA = psoriatic arthritis; RA = rheumatoid arthritis; SLE = systemic lupus erythematosus; SV = systemic vasculitis)

observed after 4–8 weeks but treatment should be continued for 3 months before the conclusion is reached that it has been ineffective. Orange staining of urine and contact lenses may occur.

Hydroxychloroquine

Hydroxychloroquine (HCQ) is used in the treatment of RA and SLE in a dose of 200–400 mg daily. Its mechanism of action is incompletely understood. A wide range of side-effects can potentially occur but HCQ is usually well tolerated in practice. With long-term use, there is a risk of ocular toxicity due to accumulation in the retina, although this is uncommon. It is usual to check visual function before starting treatment and to repeat this periodically while treatment is continued. HCQ is generally considered to be safe during pregnancy

Leflunomide

Leflunomide can be used alone or in combination with other drugs in a dose of 10–20 mg/day. It works by inhibiting dihydro-orotate dehydrogenase, an enzyme used by activated lymphocytes to synthesise pyrimidines necessary for DNA synthesis. It has low marrow toxicity but may cause liver dysfunction, hypertension and hirsutism. It must be co-prescribed with robust contraception in women of child-bearing potential. Treatment must be stopped for a period of 2 years in advance of planning a pregnancy.

Azathioprine

Azathioprine is most commonly used in vasculitis and SLE. It is metabolised to 6-mercaptopurine (6-MP), which blocks lymphocyte proliferation by inhibiting DNA synthesis. The typical starting dose is 1 mg/kg body weight per day, increasing to 2.5 mg/kg until a response is observed or toxicity occurs. Bone marrow suppression is the most important side-effect but nausea may also occur. Genetic polymorphisms in the enzyme thiopurine S-methyltransferase (TPMT) influence catabolism of 6-MP and sometimes genetic testing for TPMT variants is done to guide dosages. Allopurinol inhibits catabolism of azathioprine, necessitating a 75% reduction in azathioprine dose.

Apremilast

Apremilast is used in the treatment of PsA. It works by inhibiting phosphodiesterase D4 in leucocytes, which in turn suppresses production of pro-inflammatory cytokines, thereby reducing inflammation. Apremilast is given orally in a dose of 30 mg twice daily. The main adverse effects are gastrointestinal upset, weight loss and an increased risk of depression.

Janus-activated kinase inhibitors

Janus-activated kinase (JAK) inhibitors work by inhibiting JAK enzymes, which are a family of intracellular signalling molecules that play a key role in transducing the effects of several pro-inflammatory cytokines. They are indicated for patients with RA who have responded inadequately to standard DMARDs and provide an alternative to biologic treatments. Two JAK inhibitors are currently available: tofacitinib, which is given orally in a dose of 5 mg twice daily, and baricitinib, which is given orally in a dose of 2–4 mg once daily. The main adverse effects are an increased risk of opportunistic infections, hepatotoxicity and haematological toxicity.

Cyclophosphamide

Cyclophosphamide is a cytotoxic alkylating agent that cross-links DNA and halts cell division, causing immunosuppression. It is mainly used to induce remission in life-threatening systemic vasculitis and SLE. It can be given orally in a dose of 2 mg/kg/day for 3–6 months or intravenously in a dose of 15 mg/kg every 3–4 weeks on 6–8 occasions. Adverse effects include nausea, anorexia, vomiting, bone marrow suppression, cardiac toxicity, alopecia and haemorrhagic cystitis. The risk of cystitis can be mitigated by co-administration of mesna (2-mercaptoethane sulfonate, which binds its urotoxic metabolites) and a high fluid intake.

Mycophenolate mofetil

Mycophenolate mofetil (MMF) works by inhibiting inosine monophosphate dehydrogenase, a rate-limiting enzyme in the synthesis of guanosine nucleotides in lymphocytes. MMF is frequently used in SLE and vasculitis in doses of 2–4 g daily orally. Haematological toxicity is the main adverse effect.

Other DMARDs

Gold, penicillamine and ciclosporin A have been superseded by more effective alternatives but are still occasionally used. Gold (sodium aurothiomalate, myocrisin) is indicated for RA. Its mechanism of action is unknown. It is given by intramuscular injection of 50 mg weekly after an initial test dose of 10 mg. Treatment is continued for up to 6 months until there is clinical benefit or adverse effects occur. If there is benefit, the frequency of injections is reduced to two-weekly and then monthly, providing that the response is maintained. Penicillamine is indicated for RA but is poorly tolerated. It is given in a starting dose of 125–250 mg daily on an empty stomach, and increased in 125 mg increments every 6 weeks to a maximum dose of 1500 mg daily until there is clinical benefit or adverse effects occur. Ciclosporin A is a calcineurin inhibitor that inhibits lymphocyte activation. It is occasionally used in RA at a dose of 2.5–4 mg/kg/day orally.

Glucocorticoids

Glucocorticoids have powerful anti-inflammatory and immunosuppressive effects. They promote apoptosis of many immune cells and activation of a wide range of pro-inflammatory signalling pathways. They are used orally, intravenously, intramuscularly and by intra-articular injection in the treatment of a wide range of inflammatory rheumatic diseases, as well as by local injection in patients with soft tissue rheumatism (p. 1026).

Systemic glucocorticoids

Systemic glucocorticoids are widely used in moderate to high doses to induce remission in early RA and in systemic and polyarticular JIA. They are also used at lower doses for maintenance therapy and in the treatment of flares in RA, PsA and axSpA with peripheral joint involvement. Glucocorticoids should be used with caution in PsA because of a rebound increase in activity of psoriasis when the effects wear off. Glucocorticoids are also used to induce remission and to maintain disease control in giant cell arteritis, polymyalgia rheumatica, vasculitis and SLE.

Intra-articular and intramuscular glucocorticoids

Intra-articular glucocorticoids are employed in the treatment of a wide range of inflammatory arthritides and are primarily indicated when there are one or two problem joints with persistent synovitis despite good general control of the disease. Methylprednisolone is one of the most widely used, typically in doses of 40–80 mg. Intramuscular methylprednisolone (80–120 mg) is a useful way of controlling inflammatory arthritis while waiting for the effects of a newly introduced DMARD to take effect, and is also helpful

24

in patients with stable disease who have a disease flare where a major change in DMARD strategy is not thought to be necessary.

Biologics

The term 'biologic' refers to a group of medications that includes monoclonal antibodies, fusion proteins and decoy receptors, which are used in the treatment of several inflammatory rheumatic diseases. They are targeted towards specific cytokines, receptors and other cell-surface molecules regulating the immune response (Fig. 24.15). The main adverse effect of the biologics used in inflammatory diseases is an increased risk of infections. Biologics are not carcinogenic, but patients who develop cancer while on treatment may exhibit accelerated progression of the tumour due to suppression of the immune response. Treatment costs are much higher than with DMARDs and many countries have set guidelines restricting their use to patients who have active disease despite having had an adequate trial of standard therapies. Their mechanisms of action, dosages and indications are summarised in Box 24.35.

Anti-TNF therapy

A variety of inhibitors of the pro-inflammatory cytokine TNF have been developed. Most are monoclonal antibodies that bind to and neutralise TNF, but etanercept is a decoy receptor that prevents TNF binding to its receptor. Anti-TNF therapy has traditionally been used as the first-line biological drug in RA when DMARD therapy has been incompletely effective. It has also traditionally been used as the first-line biologic in PsA and AxSpA, but anti IL-17A therapy (see below) has emerged as an equally effective alternative. Anti-TNF therapy is usually co-prescribed with MTX in RA and PsA as this increases efficacy, but TNF inhibitors are also effective as monotherapy. They are usually given as monotherapy

in AxSpA unless there is peripheral joint involvement. Anti-TNF therapy is contraindicated in patients with active infections such as untreated tuberculosis and those with indwelling catheters, due to the high risk of infection. Other contraindications are severe heart failure and multiple sclerosis, both of which may be worsened by treatment.

Rituximab

Rituximab is an antibody directed against the CD20 receptor, which is expressed on B lymphocytes and immature plasma cells. It causes profound B-cell lymphopenia for several months due to complement-mediated lysis of cells that express CD20. Rituximab is indicated in patients with RA who have not responded adequately to first-line therapy but is typically employed as a third-line treatment when TNF inhibitors have been ineffective. It is also used in place of cyclophosphamide to induce remission in patients with ANCA-positive vasculitis. In RA, the treatment can be repeated when signs of improvement are wearing off (anything from 6 months to 1 year or longer). In ANCA-positive vasculitis, a single cycle of treatment may last for up to 18 months. Rituximab is sometimes used off-label in SLE, even though clinical trials did not show efficacy. Adverse effects include hypogammaglobulinaemia, infusion reactions, an increased risk of infections and, rarely, progressive multifocal leucoencephalopathy (PML; p. 1123), a serious and potentially fatal infection of the CNS caused by reactivation of JC virus.

Belimumab

Belimumab is indicated in SLE. It is a monoclonal antibody that blocks the effects of the cytokine B-cell-activating factor of the TNF family (BAFF), which is required for B-cell survival and function. It is usually given when patients have had an inadequate response to glucocorticoids and hydroxychloroquine. The main

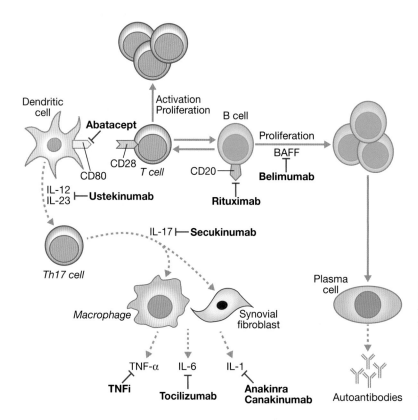

Fig. 24.15 Targets for biologic therapies in inflammatory rheumatic diseases. Biologic treatments for inflammatory rheumatic diseases work by targeting key cytokines and other molecules involved in regulating the immune response. See page 64 for more details. (BAFF = B-cell-activating factor of the TNF family; CD = cluster of differentiation; IL = interleukin; TNF-α = tumour necrosis factor alpha; TNFi = inhibitor of tumour necrosis factor)

24.35 Biological drugs for inflammatory rheumatic disease

Drug	Maintenance dose	Mechanism of action	Indications
Etanercept	50 mg weekly SC	Decoy receptor for TNF-α	RA, PsA, AxSpA, JIA
Infliximab	3–5 mg/kg 8-weekly IV	Antibody to TNF-α	RA, PsA, AxSpA, JIA
Adalimumab	40 mg 2-weekly SC		
Certolizumab	200 mg 2-weekly SC		
Golimumab	50 mg 4-weekly SC		
Rituximab	2×1 g 2 weeks apart IV	Antibody to CD20; destroys B cells	RA, vasculitis
Belimumab	10 mg/kg 4-weekly IV	Antibody to BAFF; inhibits B-cell activation	SLE
Abatacept	125 mg weekly SC or 10 mg/kg 4-weekly IV	Inhibits T-cell activation	RA
Tocilizumab	162 mg weekly SC or 8 mg/kg 8-weekly IV	Blocks IL-6 receptor	RA, JIA
Ustekinumab	45 mg 12-weekly SC	Antibody to IL-12 and IL-23	PsA
Secukinumab	150 mg 4-weekly SC	Antibody to IL-17A	PsA, AxSpA
Anakinra	100 mg daily SC	Decoy receptor for IL-1	RA, CAPS, AOSD
Canakinumab	150 mg or 2 mg/kg 8-weekly SC	Antibody to IL-1β	CAPS, sJIA, AOSD, gout

(AOSD = adult-onset Still's disease; AxSpA = axial spondyloarthritis; BAFF = B-cell-activating factor of the TNF family; CAPS = cryopyrin-associated periodic syndromes; CD = cluster of differentiation; IL = interleukin; IV = intravenous; JIA = juvenile idiopathic arthritis; PsA = psoriatic arthritis; RA = rheumatoid arthritis; SC = subcutaneous; sJIA = systemic juvenile inflammatory arthritis; SLE = systemic lupus erythematosus; TNF-α = tumour necrosis factor alpha)

adverse effects are an increased risk of infection, leucopenia and infusion reactions.

Abatacept

Abatacept is a fusion protein in which the Fc domain of IgG has been combined with the extracellular domain of CTLA4, which blocks T-cell activation by acting as a decoy for CD28, a co-stimulatory molecule necessary for T-cell activation (p. 69). It is indicated in patients with RA who have not responded adequately to first-line therapy but is typically employed as a third-line treatment when TNF inhibitors have been ineffective. The main adverse effect is an increased risk of infections.

Tocilizumab

Tocilizumab is a monoclonal antibody to the IL-6 receptor. It is indicated in patients with RA who have not responded adequately to first-line therapy or to TNF inhibitors. It is sometimes employed as a third-line treatment when TNF inhibitors have been ineffective.

An exception is when patients are MTX-intolerant, in which case it is often used as a first-line therapy, based on a randomised trial in which it showed greater efficacy than the TNF inhibitor adalimumab. Adverse effects include leucopenia, abnormal LFTs, hypercholesterolaemia, hypersensitivity reactions and an increase risk of diverticulitis.

Ustekinumab

Ustekinumab is an antibody to the p40 protein, which is a subunit of IL-23 and IL-12. It is indicated in patients with PsA who have not responded adequately to first-line therapy with other biologics. Adverse effects include an increased risk of infections, hypersensitivity reactions and an exfoliative dermatitis.

Secukinumab

Secukinumab is a monoclonal antibody to IL-17A. It is indicated in patients with PsA and axSpA, including ankylosing spondylitis, and who have not responded adequately to first-line therapy. Adverse effects include an increased risk of infections, nasopharyngitis and headache.

Anakinra

Anakinra is a decoy receptor for IL-1. It is occasionally used in RA but is less effective than other biological drugs. A more frequent indication is for the treatment of adult-onset Still's disease (p. 1040) and in cryopirin-associated periodic syndromes (p. 81). Adverse effects include an increased risk of infections, hypersensitivity reactions and neutropenia.

Canakinumab

Canakinumab is indicated for the treatment of systemic JIA (Still's disease), adult-onset Still's disease, familial fever syndromes and acute flares of gout resistant to other treatments. It is a monoclonal antibody directed against the pro-inflammatory cytokine IL-1β. The usual maintenance dose in adults is 150–300 mg SC every 8 weeks. Adverse effects include an increased risk of infections, hypersensitivity reactions and neutropenia.

Osteoarthritis

Osteoarthritis (OA) is by far the most common form of arthritis and is a major cause of pain and disability in older people. It is characterised by focal loss of articular cartilage, subchondral osteosclerosis, osteophyte formation at the joint margin, and remodelling of joint contour with enlargement of affected joints.

Epidemiology

The prevalence rises progressively with age and it has been estimated that 45% of all people develop knee OA and 25% hip OA at some point during life. Although some are asymptomatic, the lifetime risk of having a total hip or knee replacement for OA in someone aged 50 is about 11% for women and 8% for men in the UK. There are major ethnic differences in susceptibility: the prevalence of hip OA is lower in Africa, China, Japan and the Indian subcontinent than in European countries, and that of knee OA is higher.

Pathophysiology

OA is a complex disorder with both genetic and environmental components (Box 24.36). Genetic factors are recognised as playing a key role in the pathogenesis of OA. Family-based studies have estimated that the heritability of OA ranges from about 43% at the knee to between 60% and 65% at the hip and

24

i | **24.36 Risk factors for osteoarthritis**

Genetics
- Skeletal dysplasias
- Polygenic inheritance

Developmental abnormalities
- Developmental dysplasia of the hip
- Slipped femoral epiphysis

Repetitive loading
- Farmers
- Miners
- Elite athletes

Adverse biomechanics
- Meniscectomy
- Ligament rupture
- Paget's disease

Obesity

Trauma

Hormonal
- Oestrogen deficiency
- Aromatase inhibitors

Fig. 24.16 Pathological changes in osteoarthritis. **A** Abnormal nests of proliferating chondrocytes (arrows) interspersed with matrix devoid of normal chondrocytes. **B** Fibrillation of cartilage in OA. **C** X-ray of knee joint affected by OA, showing osteophytes at joint margin (white arrows), subchondral sclerosis (black arrows) and a subchondral cyst (open arrow).

hand, respectively. In most cases, the inheritance is polygenic and mediated by several genetic variants of small effect. OA can, however, be a component of multiple epiphyseal dysplasias, which are caused by mutations in the genes that encode components of cartilage matrix. Structural abnormalities, such as slipped femoral epiphysis and developmental dysplasia of the hip, are also associated with a high risk of OA, presumably due to abnormal load distribution across the joint. Similar mechanisms probably explain the increased risk of OA in patients with limb deformity secondary to Paget's disease of bone. Biomechanical factors play an important role in OA related to certain occupations, such as farmers (hip OA), miners (knee OA) and elite or professional athletes (knee and ankle OA). It has been speculated that the higher prevalence of knee OA in the Indian subcontinent and East Asia might be accounted for by squatting. There is also a high risk of OA in people who have had destabilising injuries, such as cruciate ligament rupture, and those who have had meniscectomy. For most individuals, however, participation in recreational sport does not appear to increase the risk significantly. There is a strong association between obesity and OA, particularly of the hip. This is thought to be due partly to biomechanical factors but it has also been speculated that cytokines released from adipose tissue may play a role. Oestrogen appears to play a role; lower rates of OA have been observed in women who use hormone replacement therapy (HRT), and women who receive aromatase inhibitor therapy for breast cancer often experience a flare in symptoms of OA.

Degeneration of articular cartilage is the defining feature of OA. Under normal circumstances, chondrocytes are terminally differentiated cells but in OA they start dividing to produce nests of metabolically active cells (Fig. 24.16A). Initially, matrix components are produced by these cells at an increased rate, but at the same time there is accelerated degradation of the major structural components of cartilage matrix, including aggrecan and type II collagen (see Fig. 24.5, p. 987). Eventually, the concentration of aggrecan in cartilage matrix falls and makes the cartilage vulnerable to load-bearing injury. Fissuring of the cartilage surface ('fibrillation') then occurs, leading to the development of deep vertical clefts (Fig. 24.16B), localised chondrocyte death and decreased cartilage thickness. This is initially focal, mainly targeting the maximum load-bearing part of the joint, but eventually large parts of the cartilage surface are damaged. Calcium pyrophosphate and basic calcium phosphate crystals often become deposited in the abnormal cartilage.

OA is also accompanied by abnormalities in subchondral bone, which becomes sclerotic and the site of subchondral cysts (Fig. 24.16C). Fibrocartilage is produced at the joint margin, which undergoes endochondral ossification to form osteophytes. Bone

remodelling and cartilage thinning slowly alter the shape of the OA joint, increasing its surface area. It is almost as though there is a homeostatic mechanism operative in OA that causes enlargement of the failing joint to spread the mechanical load over a greater surface area.

Patients with OA also have higher BMD values at sites distant from the joint and this is particularly associated with osteophyte formation. This is in keeping with observations made in epidemiological studies that show that patients with OA are partially protected from developing osteoporosis and vice versa. This is likely to be due to the fact that the genetic factors that predispose to osteoporosis might be protective for OA.

The synovium in OA is often hyperplastic and may be the site of inflammatory change, but to a much lesser extent than in RA and other inflammatory arthropathies. Osteochondral bodies commonly occur within the synovium, reflecting chondroid metaplasia or secondary uptake and growth of damaged cartilage fragments. The outer capsule also thickens and contracts, usually retaining the stability of the remodelling joint. The muscles surrounding affected joints commonly show evidence of wasting and non-specific type II fibre atrophy.

Clinical features

OA has a characteristic distribution, mainly targeting the hips, knees, PIP and DIP joints of the hands, neck and lumbar spine (see Fig. 24.10). The main presenting symptoms are pain and functional restriction. The causes of pain in OA are not completely understood but may relate to increased pressure in subchondral bone (mainly causing night pain), trabecular microfractures, capsular distension and low-grade synovitis. Pain may also result from bursitis and enthesopathy secondary to altered joint mechanics. Typical OA pain has the characteristics listed in Box 24.37. For many people, functional restriction of the hands, knees or hips is an equal, if not greater, problem than pain. The clinical findings vary according to severity but are principally those of joint damage.

i 24.37 Symptoms and signs of osteoarthritis

Pain

- Insidious onset over months or years
- Variable or intermittent nature over time ('good days, bad days')
- Mainly related to movement and weight-bearing, relieved by rest
- Only brief (<15 mins) morning stiffness and brief (<5 mins) 'gelling' after rest
- Usually only one or a few joints painful

Clinical signs

- Restricted movement due to capsular thickening or blocking by osteophyte
- Palpable, sometimes audible, coarse crepitus due to rough articular surfaces
- Bony swelling around joint margins
- Deformity, usually without instability
- Joint-line or periarticular tenderness
- Muscle weakness and wasting
- Mild or absent synovitis

i 24.38 Characteristics of generalised nodal osteoarthritis

- Polyarticular finger interphalangeal joint osteoarthritis
- Heberden's (± Bouchard's) nodes
- Marked female preponderance
- Peak onset in middle age
- Good functional outcome for hands
- Predisposition to osteoarthritis at other joints, especially knees
- Strong genetic predisposition

The correlation between the presence of structural change, as assessed by imaging, and symptoms such as pain and disability varies markedly according to site. It is stronger at the hip than at the knee, and poor at most small joints. This suggests that the risk factors for pain and disability may differ from those for structural change. At the knee, for example, reduced quadriceps muscle strength and adverse psychosocial factors (anxiety, depression) correlate more strongly with pain and disability than the degree of radiographic change.

Radiological evidence of OA is very common in middle-aged and older people, and the disease may coexist with other conditions, so it is important to remember that pain in a patient with OA may be due to another cause.

Generalised nodal OA

Characteristics of this common form of OA are shown in Box 24.38. Some patients are asymptomatic whereas others develop pain, stiffness and swelling of one or more PIP and DIP joints of the hands from the age of about 40 years onwards. Gradually, these develop posterolateral swellings on each side of the extensor tendon, which slowly enlarge and harden to become Heberden's (DIP) and Bouchard's (PIP) nodes (Fig. 24.17). Typically, each joint goes through a phase of episodic symptoms (1–5 years) while the node evolves and OA develops. Once OA is fully established, symptoms may subside and hand function often remains good. Affected joints are enlarged as a result of osteophyte formation and often show characteristic lateral deviation, reflecting the asymmetric focal cartilage loss of OA (Fig. 24.18). Involvement of the first CMC joint is also common, leading to pain on trying to open bottles and jars, and functional

Fig. 24.17 Nodal osteoarthritis. Heberden's nodes and lateral (radial/ulnar) deviation of distal interphalangeal joints, with mild Bouchard's nodes at the proximal interphalangeal joints.

Fig. 24.18 X-ray appearances in hand osteoarthritis. There is joint space narrowing affecting the proximal interphalangeal (PIP) and distal interphalangeal (DIP) joints in both hands. There are typical articular subchondral and 'gullwing' appearances to some osteoarthritis-affected joints, as well as osteophyte formation that is most marked at the second DIP joints bilaterally and the first PIP joint on the right hand (arrows).

impairment. Clinically, it may be detected by the presence of crepitus on joint movement, and squaring of the thumb base.

Generalised nodal OA has a very strong genetic component: the daughter of an affected mother has a 1 in 3 chance of developing nodal OA herself. People with nodal OA are also at increased risk of OA at other sites, especially the knee.

Knee OA

At the knee, OA principally targets the patello-femoral and medial tibio-femoral compartments but eventually spreads to affect the whole of the joint (Fig. 24.19). It may be isolated or occur as part of generalised nodal OA. Most patients have bilateral and symmetrical involvement. In men, trauma is often a more important risk factor and may result in unilateral OA.

The pain is usually localised to the anterior or medial aspect of the knee and upper tibia. Patello-femoral pain is usually worse going up and down stairs or inclines. Posterior knee pain suggests the presence of a complicating popliteal cyst (Baker's cyst). Prolonged walking, rising from a chair, getting in or out of

24

Fig. 24.19 X-ray appearances in knee osteoarthritis. A Advanced osteoarthritis showing almost complete loss of joint space affecting both compartments and sclerosis of subchondral bone. B Skyline view of the patella femoral joint in a patient with severe patello-femoral osteoarthritis. There is almost complete loss of joint space and lateral displacement of the patella.

Fig. 24.20 Typical varus knee deformity resulting from marked medial tibio-femoral osteoarthritis.

a car, or bending to put on shoes and socks may be difficult. Local examination findings may include:

• a jerky, asymmetric (antalgic) gait with less time weight-bearing on the painful side
• a varus (Fig. 24.20) or, less commonly, valgus and/or a fixed flexion deformity
• joint-line and/or periarticular tenderness (secondary anserine bursitis and medial ligament enthesopathy (see Box 24.25), causing tenderness of the upper medial tibia)
• weakness and wasting of the quadriceps muscle

• restricted flexion and extension with coarse crepitus
• bony swelling around the joint line.

CPPD crystal deposition in association with OA is common at the knee. This may result in a more overt inflammatory component (stiffness, effusions) and super-added acute attacks of synovitis ('pseudogout'; p. 1016), which may be associated with more rapid radiographic and clinical progression.

Hip OA

Hip OA most commonly targets the superior aspect of the joint (Fig. 24.21). It is often unilateral at presentation, frequently progresses with superolateral migration of the femoral head, and has a poor prognosis. The less common central (medial) OA shows more central cartilage loss and is largely confined to women. It is often bilateral at presentation and can be associated with generalised nodal OA. It has a better prognosis than superior hip OA and progression to axial migration of the femoral head is uncommon.

The hip shows the best correlation between symptoms and radiographic change. Hip pain is usually maximal deep in the anterior groin, with variable radiation to the buttock, anterolateral thigh, knee or shin. Lateral hip pain, worse on lying on that side with tenderness over the greater trochanter, suggests secondary trochanteric bursitis. Common functional difficulties are the same as for knee OA; in addition, restricted hip abduction in women may cause pain during sexual intercourse. Examination may reveal:

• an antalgic gait
• weakness and wasting of quadriceps and gluteal muscles
• pain and restriction of internal rotation with the hip flexed – the earliest and most sensitive sign of hip OA; other movements may subsequently be restricted and painful
• anterior groin tenderness just lateral to the femoral pulse
• fixed flexion, external rotation deformity of the hip
• ipsilateral leg shortening with severe joint attrition and superior femoral migration.

Obesity is associated with more rapid progression of hip OA.

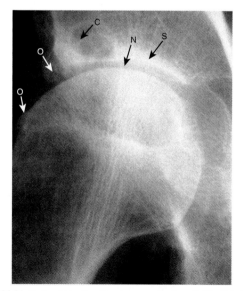

Fig. 24.21 X-ray of hip showing changes of osteoarthritis. Note the superior joint space narrowing (N), subchondral sclerosis (S), marginal osteophytes (O) and cysts (C).

Fig. 24.22 X-ray of spine showing typical changes of osteoarthritis. Cervical spondylosis showing disc space narrowing between C6 and C7, osteophytes at the anterior vertebral body margins (thin arrows) and osteosclerosis at the apophyseal joints (thick arrow).

Spine OA

The cervical and lumbar spine are the sites most often targeted by OA, where it is referred to as cervical spondylosis and lumbar spondylosis, respectively (Fig. 24.22). Spine OA may occur in isolation or as part of generalised OA. The typical presentation is with pain localised to the low back region or the neck, although radiation of pain to the arms, buttocks and legs may also occur due to nerve root compression. The pain is typically relieved by rest and worse on movement. On physical examination, the range of movement may be limited and loss of lumbar lordosis is typical. The straight leg-raising test or femoral stretch test may be positive and neurological signs may be seen in the legs where there is complicating spinal stenosis or nerve root compression.

Early-onset OA

Unusually, typical symptoms and signs of OA may present before the age of 45. In most cases, a single joint is affected and there is a clear history of previous trauma. However, specific causes of OA need to be considered in people with early-onset disease affecting several joints, especially those not normally targeted by OA, in which case rare causes need to be considered (Box 24.39). Kashin–Beck disease is a rare form of OA that occurs in children, typically between the ages of 7 and 13, in some regions of China. The cause is unknown but suggested predisposing factors are selenium deficiency and contamination of cereals with mycotoxin-producing fungi.

24.39 Causes of early-onset osteoarthritis

Monoarticular

- Previous trauma, localised instability

Pauciarticular or polyarticular

- Juvenile idiopathic arthritis (p. 1026)
- Metabolic or endocrine disease:
  Haemochromatosis (p. 895)
  Ochronosis
  Acromegaly (p. 685)
- Spondylo-epiphyseal dysplasia
- Late avascular necrosis
- Neuropathic joint
- Kashin–Beck disease

Erosive OA

This term is used to describe an unusual group of patients with hand OA who have a more prolonged symptom phase, more overt inflammation, more disability and worse outcome than those with nodal OA. Distinguishing features include preferential targeting of PIP joints, subchondral erosions on X-rays, occasional ankylosis of affected joints and lack of association with OA elsewhere. It is unclear whether erosive OA is part of the spectrum of hand OA or a discrete subset.

Investigations

A plain X-ray of the affected joint should be performed and often this will show one or more of the typical features of OA (see Figs 24.18–24.22). In addition to providing diagnostic information, X-rays are of value in assessing the severity of structural change, which is helpful if joint replacement surgery is being considered. Non-weight-bearing postero-anterior views of the pelvis are adequate for assessing hip OA. Patients with suspected knee OA should have standing anteroposterior X-rays taken to assess tibio-femoral cartilage loss, and a flexed skyline view to assess patello-femoral involvement. Spine OA can often be diagnosed on a plain X-ray, which typically shows evidence of disc space narrowing and osteophytes. If nerve root compression or spinal stenosis is suspected, MRI should be performed.

Routine biochemistry, haematology and autoantibody tests are usually normal, though OA is associated with a moderate acute phase response. Synovial fluid aspirated from an affected joint is viscous with a low cell count.

Unexplained early-onset OA requires additional investigation, guided by the suspected underlying condition. X-rays may show typical features of dysplasia or avascular necrosis, widening of joint spaces in acromegaly, multiple cysts, chondrocalcinosis and MCP joint involvement in haemochromatosis (p. 895), or disorganised architecture in neuropathic joints.

Management

Treatment follows the principles outlined on pages 1000–1007. Measures that are pertinent in older people are summarised in Box 24.40.

Education

It is important to explain the nature of the condition fully, outlining the role of relevant risk factors such as obesity, heredity and

24.40 Osteoarthritis in old age

- **Pain and disability**: osteoarthritis is the principal cause in old age.
- **Calcium phosphate deposition disease**: may cause acute attacks of synovitis (pseudogout) on a background of chronic osteoarthritis.
- **Falls**: reduced muscle strength and pain associated with lower limb osteoarthritis increase the risk.
- **Muscle-strengthening exercises**: safely reduce the pain and disability of knee osteoarthritis with accompanying improvements in balance and reduced tendency to fall.
- **Oral paracetamol and topical non-steroidal anti-inflammatory drugs**: safe in older people, with no important drug interactions or contraindications.
- **Intra-articular injection of glucocorticoid**: a very safe and often effective treatment, particularly useful for tiding a patient over a special event.
- **Total joint replacement**: an excellent cost-effective treatment for severe disabling knee or hip osteoarthritis in older people. There is no age limit for joint replacement surgery.

24

trauma. The patent should be informed that established structural changes are permanent and that, although a cure is not possible at present, pain and function can often be improved. The prognosis should also be discussed, mentioning that it is generally good for nodal hand OA and better for knee than hip OA.

Lifestyle advice

Weight loss has a substantial beneficial effect on symptoms if the patient is obese and is probably one of the most effective treatments available for OA of the lower limbs. Strengthening and aerobic exercises also have beneficial effects in OA and should be advised, preferably with reinforcement by a physiotherapist (see Box 24.27). Quadriceps strengthening exercises are particularly beneficial in knee OA. Shock-absorbing footwear, pacing of activities, use of a walking stick for painful knee or hip OA, and provision of built-up shoes to equalise leg lengths can all improve symptoms.

Non-pharmacological therapy

Acupuncture and transcutaneous electrical nerve stimulation (TENS) have been shown to be effective in knee OA. Local physical therapies, such as heat or cold, can sometimes give temporary relief.

Pharmacological therapy

If symptoms do not respond to non-pharmacological measures, paracetamol should be tried. Addition of a topical NSAID, and then capsaicin, for knee and hand OA can also be helpful. Oral NSAIDs should be considered in patients who remain symptomatic. These drugs are significantly more effective than paracetamol and can be successfully combined with paracetamol or compound analgesics if the pain is severe. Strong opiates may occasionally be required. Antineuropathic drugs, such as amitriptyline, gabapentin and pregabalin, are sometimes used in patients with symptoms that are difficult to control but the evidence base for their use is poor. Neutralising antibodies to nerve growth factor have been developed and are a highly effective treatment for pain in OA but they are not yet licensed for routine clinical use.

Intra-articular injections

Intra-articular glucocorticoid injections are effective in the treatment of knee OA and are also used for symptomatic relief in the treatment of OA at the first CMC joint. The duration of effect is usually short but trials of serial glucocorticoid injections every 3 months in knee OA have shown efficacy for up to 1 year. Intra-articular injections of hyaluronic acid are effective in knee OA but the treatment is expensive and the effect short-lived. In the UK they have not been considered to be cost-effective by NICE.

Neutraceuticals

Chondroitin sulphate and glucosamine sulphate have been used alone and in combination for the treatment of knee OA. There is evidence from randomised controlled trials that these agents can improve knee pain to a small extent (3–5%) compared with placebo.

Surgery

Surgery should be considered for patients with OA whose symptoms and functional impairment impact significantly on their quality of life despite optimal medical therapy and lifestyle advice. Total joint replacement surgery is by far the most common surgical procedure for patients with OA. It can transform the quality of life for people with severe knee or hip OA and is indicated when there is significant structural damage on X-ray. Although surgery should not be undertaken at an early stage during the development of OA, it is important to consider it before functional limitation has become advanced since this may compromise outcome. Patient-specific factors, such as age, gender, smoking and presence of obesity, should not be barriers to referral for joint replacement.

Only a small proportion of patients with OA progress to the extent that total joint replacement is required but OA is by far the most frequent indication for this. Over 95% of joint replacements continue to function well into the second decade after surgery and most provide life-long, pain-free function. Up to 20% of patients are not satisfied with the outcome, however, and a few experience little or no improvement in pain. Other surgical procedures are performed much less frequently. Osteotomy is occasionally carried out to prolong the life of malaligned joints and to relieve pain by reducing intraosseous pressure. Cartilage repair is sometimes performed to treat focal cartilage defects resulting from joint injury.

Crystal-induced arthritis

A variety of crystals can deposit in and around joints and cause an acute inflammatory arthritis, as well as a more chronic arthritis associated with progressive joint damage (Box 24.41). Crystals can be the primary pathogenic agent, as in gout, or an accessory factor, as in calcium pyrophosphate deposition disease, in which crystals are deposited in joints that are already abnormal. Several factors influence crystal formation (Fig. 24.23). There must be sufficient concentration of the chemical components (ionic product), but whether a crystal then forms depends on the balance of tissue factors that promote and inhibit crystal nucleation and growth. The inflammatory potential of crystals resides in their physical irregularity and high negative surface charge, which can induce inflammation and damage cell membranes. Crystals may also cause mechanical damage to tissues and act as wear particles at the joint surface. They can reside in cartilage or tendon for years without causing inflammation or symptoms, and it is only when they are released that they trigger inflammation. This may occur spontaneously but can also result from local trauma, rapid changes in the concentration of the components that form crystals, or in association with an acute phase response triggered by intercurrent illness or surgery. In the longer term, a reduction in concentrations of the solutes that form crystals causes dissolution of crystals and remission of the arthritis.

Gout

Gout is the most common inflammatory arthritis in men and in older women. It is caused by deposition of monosodium urate monohydrate crystals in and around synovial joints.

Epidemiology

The prevalence of gout is approximately 1–2%, with a greater than 5:1 male preponderance. Gout has become progressively more common over recent years in affluent societies due to the increased prevalence of obesity and metabolic syndrome (p. 730), of which hyperuricaemia is an integral component. The risk of developing gout increases with age and with serum uric acid (SUA) levels. These are normally distributed in the general population and hyperuricaemia is defined as an SUA of more than 2 standard deviations above the mean for the

24.41 Crystal-associated arthritis and deposition in connective tissue

Crystal	Associations
Common	
Monosodium urate monohydrate	Acute gout Chronic tophaceous gout
Calcium pyrophosphate dihydrate	Acute 'pseudogout' Chronic (pyrophosphate) arthropathy Chondrocalcinosis
Basic calcium phosphates	Calcific periarthritis Calcinosis
Uncommon	
Cholesterol	Chronic effusions in rheumatoid arthritis
Calcium oxalate	Acute arthritis in dialysis patients
Extrinsic crystals/ semi-crystalline particles:	
Synthetic crystals	Acute synovitis
Plant thorns/sea urchin spines	Chronic monoarthritis, tenosynovitis

24.42 Causes of hyperuricaemia and gout

Diminished renal excretion

- Increased renal tubular reabsorption*
- Renal failure
- Lead toxicity
- Lactic acidosis
- Alcohol

- Drugs:
  Thiazide and loop diuretics
  Low-dose aspirin
  Ciclosporin
  Pyrazinamide

Increased intake

- Game
- Seafood

- Offal
- Red meat

Increased production

- Myeloproliferative and lymphoproliferative disease
- Psoriasis
- High fructose intake
- Glycogen storage disease (p. 370)

- Inherited disorders:
  Lesch–Nyhan syndrome
  (HPRT mutations)
  Phosphoribosyl pyrophosphate synthetase
  1 mutations

*Usually genetically determined (see text).
(HPRT = hypoxanthine guanine phosphoribosyl transferase)

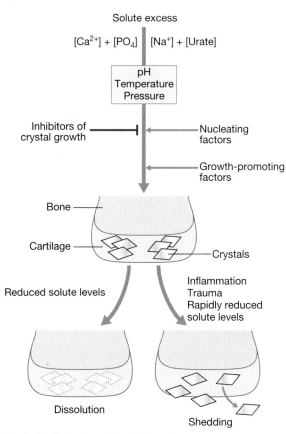

Fig. 24.23 **Mechanisms of crystal formation.**

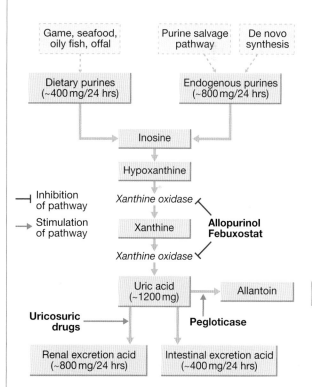

Fig. 24.24 **Uric acid metabolism.** The main pathways for uric acid production and elimination are shown, along with the site of action for urate-lowering therapies.

population. SUA levels are higher in men, increase with age and are positively associated with body weight. Levels are higher in some ethnic groups (such as Maoris and Pacific islanders). Although hyperuricaemia is strong risk factor for gout, only a minority of hyperuricaemic individuals actually develop gout.

Pathophysiology

About one-third of the body uric acid pool is derived from dietary sources and two-thirds from endogenous purine metabolism (Fig. 24.24). The concentration of uric acid in body fluids depends on

the balance between endogenous synthesis, and elimination by the kidneys (two-thirds) and gut (one-third). Purine nucleotide synthesis and degradation are regulated by a network of enzyme pathways, but xanthine oxidase plays a pivotal role in catalysing the conversion of hypoxanthine to xanthine and xanthine to uric acid.

The causes of hyperuricaemia are shown in Box 24.42. In over 90% of patients, the main abnormality is reduced uric acid excretion by the kidney, which is genetically determined. Impaired renal excretion of urate also accounts for the occurrence of hyperuricaemia in chronic renal failure, and for hyperuricaemia associated with thiazide diuretic therapy.

Other risk factors for gout include metabolic syndrome, high alcohol intake (predominantly beer, which contains guanosine), generalised OA, and a diet relatively high in game, offal, seafood, red meat and fructose, or low in vitamin C. Lead poisoning may cause gout (saturnine gout). The association between OA and gout is thought to be due to a reduction in levels of proteoglycan and other inhibitors of crystal formation in osteoarthritic cartilage, predisposing to crystal formation.

Some patients develop gout because they over-produce uric acid. The mechanisms are poorly understood, except in the case of a few single gene disorders where there are mutations in genes that regulate purine metabolism (Box 24.42). Lesch–Nyhan syndrome is an X-linked recessive form of gout that is also associated with mental retardation, self-mutilation and choreoathetosis. An inherited cause should be suspected if other clinical features are present or there is an early age at onset with a positive family history. Severe hyperuricaemia can also occur in patients with haematological and other cancers who are undergoing chemotherapy due to increased purine turnover (tumour lysis syndrome). This is seldom connected with gout but can be associated with acute kidney injury (p. 411).

Clinical features

The classical presentation is with an acute monoarthritis, which affects the first MTP joint in over 50% of cases (Fig. 24.25). Other common sites are the ankle, midfoot, knee, small joints of hands, wrist and elbow. The axial skeleton and large proximal joints are rarely involved. Typical features include:

- rapid onset, reaching maximum severity in 2–6 hours, and often waking the patient in the early morning
- severe pain, often described as the 'worst pain ever'
- extreme tenderness, such that the patient is unable to wear a sock or to let bedding rest on the joint

Fig. 24.25 Podagra. Acute gout causing swelling, erythema and extreme pain and tenderness of the first metatarsophalangeal joint.

- marked swelling with overlying red, shiny skin
- self-limiting over 5–14 days, with complete resolution.

During the attack, the joint shows signs of marked synovitis, swelling and erythema. There may be accompanying fever, malaise and even delirium, especially if a large joint such as the knee is involved. As the attack subsides, pruritus and desquamation of overlying skin are common. The main differential diagnosis is septic arthritis, infective cellulitis or reactive arthritis. Acute attacks may also manifest as bursitis, tenosynovitis or cellulitis, which have the same clinical characteristics. Many patients describe milder episodes lasting just a few days. Some have attacks in more than one joint. Others have further attacks in other joints a few days later (cluster attacks), the first possibly acting as a trigger. Simultaneous polyarticular attacks are unusual.

Some people never have a second episode and in others several years may elapse before the next one. In many, however, a second attack occurs within 1 year and may progress to chronic gout, with chronic pain and joint damage, and occasionally severe deformity and functional impairment. Patients with uncontrolled hyperuricaemia who suffer multiple attacks of acute gout may also progress to chronic gout.

The presentation of gout in the elderly may be atypical with chronic symptoms rather than acute attacks (Box 24.43).

Crystals may be deposited in the joints and soft tissues to produce irregular firm nodules called tophi. These have a predilection for the extensor surfaces of fingers, hands, forearm, elbows, Achilles tendons and sometimes the helix of the ear. Tophi have a white colour (Fig. 24.26), differentiating them from rheumatoid nodules. Tophi can ulcerate, discharging white gritty material, become infected or induce a local inflammatory response, with erythema and pus in the absence of secondary infection. They are usually a feature of long-standing gout but can sometimes develop within 12 months in patients with chronic renal failure. Occasionally, tophi may develop in the absence of previous acute attacks, especially in patients on thiazide therapy who have coexisting OA.

In addition to causing musculoskeletal disease, chronic hyperuricaemia may be complicated by renal stone formation (p. 431) and, if severe, renal impairment due to the development of interstitial nephritis as a result of urate deposition in the kidney. This is particularly common in patients with chronic tophaceous gout who are on diuretic therapy.

Investigations

The diagnosis of gout can be confirmed by the identification of urate crystals in the aspirate from a joint, bursa or tophus (see Fig. 24.6A, p. 988). In acute gout, the synovial fluid may be

24.43 Gout in old age

- **Aetiology**: a higher proportion of older patients have gout secondary to diuretic use and chronic kidney disease. Gout is often associated with osteoarthritis.
- **Presentation**: may be atypical, with painful tophi and chronic symptoms, rather than acute attacks. Joints of the upper limbs are more frequently affected.
- **Management**: acute attacks are best treated by aspiration and intra-articular injection of glucocorticoids, followed by early mobilisation. Non-steroidal anti-inflammatory drugs and colchicine should be used with caution because of increased risk of toxicity. Low doses of allopurinol (50 mg/day) should be given and increased gradually to avoid toxicity.

Fig. 24.26 Tophus with white monosodium urate monohydrate crystals visible beneath the skin. Diuretic-induced gout in a patient with pre-existing nodal osteoarthritis.

Fig. 24.27 Erosive arthritis in chronic gout. Punched-out ('Lulworth Cove') erosions (arrows) in association with a destructive arthritis affecting the first metatarsophalangeal joint.

turbid due to an elevated neutrophil count. In chronic gout, the appearance is more variable but occasionally the fluid appears white due to the presence of urate crystals. Between attacks, aspiration of an asymptomatic first MTP joint or knee may still reveal crystals.

A biochemical screen, including renal function, uric acid, glucose and lipid profile, should be performed because of the association with metabolic syndrome. Hyperuricaemia is usually present in gout but levels may be normal during an attack because serum urate falls during inflammation. Acute gout is characterised by an elevated ESR and CRP and with a neutrophilia, all of which return to normal as the attack subsides. Tophaceous gout may be accompanied by a modest but chronic elevation in ESR and CRP.

X-rays are usually normal in acute gout but well-demarcated erosions may be seen in patients with chronic or tophaceous gout (Fig. 24.27). Tophi may also be visible on X-rays as soft tissue swellings. In late disease, destructive changes may occur

that are similar to those in other forms of advanced inflammatory arthritis.

Management

Management should focus on first dealing with the acute attack and then giving prophylaxis to lower SUA and prevent further attacks.

Acute gout

Oral colchicine given in doses of 0.5 mg twice or 3 times daily is the treatment of first choice in acute gout. It works by inhibiting microtubule assembly in neutrophils. The most common adverse effects are nausea, vomiting and diarrhoea. Oral NSAIDs are also effective but are used less commonly since many patients affected by acute gout have coexisting cardiovascular, cerebrovascular or chronic kidney disease. Oral prednisolone (15–20 mg daily) or intramuscular methylprednisolone (80–120 mg daily) for 2–3 days are highly effective and are a good choice in elderly patients where there is an increased risk of toxicity with colchicine and NSAID (Box 24.43). The IL-1β inhibitor canakinumab (see Box 24.35) is effective but extremely expensive and so seldom given. Local ice packs can also be used for symptomatic relief. Patients with recurrent episodes can keep a supply of an NSAID, colchicine or prednisolone and take it as soon as the first symptoms occur, continuing until the attack resolves. Joint aspiration can give pain relief, particularly if a large joint is affected, and may be combined with an intra-articular glucocorticoid injection if the diagnosis is clear and infection can be excluded.

Prophylaxis

Patients who have had a single attack of gout do not necessarily need to be given urate-lowering therapy, but individuals who have more than one acute attack within 12 months and those with complications such as tophi or erosions should be offered it (Box 24.44). The long-term therapeutic aim is to prevent attacks occurring by bringing uric acid levels below the level at which monosodium urate monohydrate crystals form. A therapeutic target of 360 μmol/L (6 mg/dL) is recommended in the British Society of Rheumatology guidelines, whereas the European League Against Rheumatism guidelines recommend a threshold of 300 μmol/L (5 mg/dL).

Allopurinol is the drug of first choice. It inhibits xanthine oxidase, which reduces the conversion of hypoxanthine and xanthine to uric acid. The recommended starting dose is 100 mg daily, or 50 mg in older patients and in renal impairment. The dose of allopurinol should be increased by 100 mg every 4 weeks (50 mg in the elderly and those with renal impairment) until the target uric acid level is achieved, side-effects occur or the maximum recommended dose is reached (900 mg/day). Acute flares of gout often follow initiation of urate-lowering therapy. The patient should be warned about this and told to continue therapy, even if an attack occurs. The risk of flares can be reduced by prophylaxis with oral colchicine (0.5 mg twice daily) or an NSAID for the first few months. Alternatively, patients can be given a supply of colchicine, an NSAID or prednisolone to be taken at the first

i	**24.44 Indications for urate-lowering drugs**
• Recurrent attacks of acute gout	• Tophi
• Evidence of bone or joint damage	• Renal impairment
	• Nephrolithiasis

24

sign of an acute attack. In the longer term, annual monitoring of uric acid levels is recommended. In most patients, urate-lowering therapy needs to be continued indefinitely.

Febuxostat also inhibits xanthine oxidase. It is typically used in patients with an inadequate response to allopurinol, and when allopurinol is contraindicated or causes adverse effects. Febuxostat undergoes hepatic metabolism and no dose adjustment is required for renal impairment. It is more effective than allopurinol but commonly provokes acute attacks when therapy is initiated. The usual starting dose is 80 mg daily, increasing to 120 mg daily in patients with an inadequate response. Prophylaxis against acute attacks should be given on initiating therapy, as described for allopurinol.

Uricosuric drugs, such as probenecid, sulfinpyrazone and benzbromarone, lower urate levels but are seldom used in routine clinical practice. They are contraindicated in over-producers and those with renal impairment or urolithiasis and require patients to maintain a high fluid intake to avoid uric acid crystallisation in the renal tubules.

Pegloticase is a biological treatment in which the enzyme uricase (oxidises uric acid to 5-hydroxyisourate, which is then converted to allantoin) has been conjugated to monomethoxypolyethylene glycol. It is indicated for the treatment of tophaceous gout resistant to standard therapy and is administered as an intravenous infusion every 2 weeks for up to 6 months. It is highly effective at controlling hyperuricaemia and can cause regression of tophi. The main adverse effects are infusion reactions (which can be treated with antihistamines or glucocorticoids) and flares of gout during the first 3 months of therapy. A limiting factor for longer-term treatment is the development of antibodies to pegloticase, which occur in a high proportion of cases and are associated with an impaired therapeutic response.

Lifestyle measures are equally important as drug therapy in the treatment of gout. Patients should be advised to lose weight where appropriate and to reduce excessive alcohol intake, especially beer. Several antihypertensive drugs, including thiazides, β-blockers and ACE inhibitors, increase uric acid levels, whereas losartan has a uricosuric effect and should be substituted for other drugs if possible. Patients should be advised to avoid large amounts of seafood and offal, which have a high purine content, but a highly restrictive diet is not necessary.

Calcium pyrophosphate dihydrate crystal deposition disease

This condition is associated with deposition of calcium pyrophosphate dihydrate (CPPD) crystals within articular and hyaline cartilage and is often referred to as 'pseudogout'. It is rare under the age of 55 years but occurs in 10–15% of people between 65 and 75 and 30–60% of those over 85. The knee (hyaline cartilage and menisci) is by far the most common site, followed by the wrist (triangular fibrocartilage) and pelvis (symphysis pubis). Risk factors are shown in Box 24.45. In many patients, chondrocalcinosis is asymptomatic and an incidental finding on X-ray. A proportion of patients present with an acute inflammatory arthritis (pseudogout) or a chronic inflammatory arthropathy superimposed on a background of OA, especially at the knee (Fig. 24.28), associated with joint damage and functional limitation.

Pathophysiology

The underlying mechanisms of crystal deposition are poorly understood. Clinical studies have shown that pyrophosphate

24.45 Risk factors for chondrocalcinosis

Common

- Age
- Osteoarthritis*
- Primary hyperparathyroidism

Rare

- Familial factors*
- Haemochromatosis*
- Hypophosphatasia
- Hypomagnesaemia
- Wilson's disease

*May be associated with structural damage to affected joints.

Fig. 24.28 Chondrocalcinosis of the knee. The X-ray shows calcification of the fibrocartilaginous menisci (M) and articular hyaline cartilage (H). There is also narrowing (N) of the medial tibio-femoral compartment and osteophyte (O) formation.

levels are raised in patients with CPPD crystal deposition disease, possibly due to over-production, but why this happens is unclear. In hypophosphatasia (see Box 24.75, p. 1050), the predisposing factor is thought to be impaired degradation of pyrophosphate due to deficiency of ALP. In OA, it is thought that a reduction in the amounts of proteoglycan and other natural inhibitors of crystal formation in the abnormal cartilage also predispose to crystal deposition (see Fig. 24.23).

Clinical features

The typical presentation is with a swollen tender joint that is warm and erythematous with a large effusion. Fever is common and the patient may appear confused and ill. The knee is most commonly affected, followed by the wrist, shoulder, ankle and elbow. Trigger factors include trauma, intercurrent illness, dehydration and surgery. Septic arthritis and gout are the main differential diagnoses.

Chronic arthropathy may also occur in association with CPPD crystal deposition disease, affecting the same joints that are involved in acute pseudogout. The presentation is with chronic pain, early morning stiffness, inactivity gelling and functional impairment. Acute attacks of pseudogout may be superimposed. Affected joints usually show features of OA, with varying degrees of synovitis. Effusion and synovial thickening are usually most apparent at knees and wrists. Wrist involvement may result in carpal tunnel syndrome and second and third MCP joints can be affected. Inflammatory features may be sufficiently pronounced to suggest RA. Inflammatory changes can occur at entheses and may involve tendons and the ligamentum flavum. Inflammation around the odontoid may occur secondary to CPPD deposition, leading to crowned dens syndrome; this presents clinically with neck pain. Severe damage and instability of knees or shoulders can mimic a neuropathic joint but no neurological abnormalities will be found.

Investigations

The pivotal investigation is joint aspiration, followed by examination of synovial fluid using compensated polarised microscopy to demonstrate CPPD crystals (see Fig. 24.6B, p. 988) and to permit distinction from gout. The aspirated fluid is often turbid and may be uniformly blood-stained, reflecting the severity of inflammation. Since sepsis and pseudogout can coexist, Gram stain and culture of the fluid should be performed to exclude sepsis, even if CPPD crystals are identified in synovial fluid.

X-rays of the affected joint may show evidence of calcification in hyaline cartilage and/or fibrocartilage, although absence of calcification does not exclude the diagnosis. Signs of OA are frequently present. Screening for secondary causes (Box 24.45) should be undertaken, especially in patients who present under the age of 25 and those with polyarticular disease.

Management

Joint aspiration can sometimes provide symptomatic relief in pseudogout and in a few patients no further treatment is required. People with persistent symptoms can be treated with intra-articular glucocorticoids, colchicine or an NSAID. Since most patients with pseudogout are elderly, NSAIDs and colchicine must be used with caution. Early active mobilisation is also important. Chronic pyrophosphate-induced arthropathy should be managed as for OA (p. 1011).

Basic calcium phosphate deposition disease

Basic calcium phosphate (BCP) deposition disease is caused by the deposition of hydroxyapatite or apatite crystals and other basic calcium phosphate salts (octacalcium phosphate, tricalcium phosphate) in soft tissues. The main affected sites are tendons, ligaments and hyaline cartilage in patients with degenerative disease, and skeletal muscle and subcutaneous tissues in connective tissue diseases.

Pathophysiology

Under normal circumstances, inhibitors of mineralisation, such as pyrophosphate and proteoglycans, prevent calcification of soft tissues. When these protective mechanisms break down, abnormal calcification occurs. There are many causes (Box 24.46). In most situations calcification is of no consequence, but when the crystals are released an inflammatory reaction may be initiated, causing local pain and inflammation.

Calcific periarthritis

This occurs as the result of deposition of BCP in tendons, which provokes an acute inflammatory response. The most commonly affected site is the supraspinatus tendon (Fig. 24.29) but other sites may also be involved, including the tendons around the hip, feet and hands. The presentation is with acute pain, swelling and local tenderness that develops rapidly over 4–6 hours. The overlying skin may be hot and red, raising the possibility of infection. Attacks sometimes occur spontaneously but can also be triggered by trauma. Modest systemic upset

24.46 Rheumatic diseases associated with basic calcium phosphate deposition	
Disease	**Site of calcification**
Calcific periarthritis	Tendons and ligaments
Dermatomyositis and polymyositis	Subcutaneous tissue
Systemic sclerosis (lcSScl)	Subcutaneous tissue
Mixed connective tissue disease	Subcutaneous tissue
Paget's disease of bone	Blood vessels
Ankylosing spondylitis	Ligaments
Fibrodysplasia ossificans progressiva	Subcutaneous tissues and muscle
Milwaukee shoulder syndrome	Tendons and ligaments
Albright's hereditary osteodystrophy (p. 664)	Muscle

(lcSScl = localised cutaneous systemic sclerosis)

Fig. 24.29 Shoulder X-ray showing supraspinatus tendon calcification (arrow).

and fever are common. Tendon calcification may be seen on X-ray. If the affected joint or bursa is aspirated, inflammatory fluid containing many calcium-staining (alizarin red S) aggregates may be obtained. During an acute attack, there may be a neutrophilia with an elevation in ESR and CRP. Routine biochemistry is normal. Treatment is with analgesics and NSAIDs. Attacks may also respond to a local injection of glucocorticoid. The condition usually resolves spontaneously over 1–3 weeks and this is often accompanied by dispersal and disappearance of calcific deposits on X-ray. Large deposits sometimes accumulate, causing limitation of joint movement, and may require surgical removal.

Acute inflammatory arthritis

Deposition of BCP occurs commonly in OA, both alone and in combination with CPPD crystals, in which case it is referred to as mixed crystal deposition disease. It may present with pseudogout or be an incidental finding.

Milwaukee shoulder syndrome

This is a rare syndrome, in which extensive deposition of BCP crystals in large joints is associated with progressive joint destruction. It is more common in women than in men. The onset is gradual with joint pain, sometimes precipitated by injury

24

or overuse. The disease progresses over a few months to cause severe pain and disability, associated with joint destruction. X-rays show joint space narrowing, osteophytes and calcification. Aspiration yields large volumes of relatively non-inflammatory fluid containing abundant BCP aggregates and often cartilage fragments. The differential diagnosis is end-stage avascular necrosis, chronic sepsis or neuropathic joint. There is no acute phase response and synovial fluid cultures are negative.

Treatment is with analgesics, intra-articular injection of glucocorticoids, local physical treatments and physiotherapy. The clinical outcome is poor, however, and most patients require joint replacement. The cause is incompletely understood but it has been speculated that deposition of BCP crystals activates collagenase and other proteases in articular cells, which are responsible for the tissue damage.

Autoimmune connective tissue disease

Deposition of BCP may occur in the subcutaneous tissues and muscle of patients with systemic sclerosis and other autoimmune connective tissue diseases. Usually, the deposits are asymptomatic but they may be associated with pain and local ulceration. The mechanism by which this occurs is unclear and there is no specific treatment.

Fibromyalgia

Fibromyalgia (FM) is a condition of generalised pain and consequent disability. It is frequently associated with medically unexplained symptoms in other systems (p. 1187). The prevalence in the UK and US is about 2–3%. Although FM can occur at any age, including adolescence, it increases in prevalence with age, to reach a peak of 7% in women aged over 70. There is a strong female predominance of around 10:1. Risk factors include life events that cause (unresolved) psychosocial distress relating to previous abuse, marital disharmony, alcoholism or illness in the family, poor sleep health, previous injury or assault, and low income. FM arises in a variety of races and cultures.

Pathophysiology

The cause of FM is poorly understood but two abnormalities that may be interrelated (Fig. 24.30) and have been consistently reported in affected patients are disturbed, non-restorative sleep and pain sensitisation, probably caused by abnormal central pain processing.

Clinical features

The main presenting feature is widespread pain, which is often worst in the neck and back (Box 24.47). It is characteristically diffuse and unresponsive to analgesics and NSAIDs. Physiotherapy often makes FM pain worse. Fatiguability, most prominent in the morning, is another major problem and disability is often marked. Although people can usually dress, feed and groom themselves, they may be unable to perform tasks such as shopping or housework. They may have experienced major difficulties at work or may even retire because of pain and fatigue.

Examination is unremarkable, apart from the presence of hyperalgesia on moderate digital pressure (enough just to whiten the nail) over multiple sites (Fig. 24.31).

Investigations and management

There are no abnormalities on routine blood tests or imaging but it is important to screen for other conditions that could account

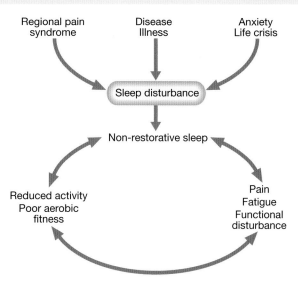

Fig. 24.30 Possible causative mechanisms in fibromyalgia.

| **i** | **24.47 The spectrum of symptoms in fibromyalgia** |

Usual symptoms

- Widespread pain
- Fatiguability
- Disability
- Broken, non-restorative sleep
- Low affect, irritability, poor concentration

Variable locomotor symptoms

- Early-morning stiffness
- Feeling of swelling in hands
- Distal finger tingling

Additional, variable, non-locomotor symptoms

- Non-throbbing bifrontal headache (tension headache)
- Colicky abdominal pain, bloating, variable bowel habit (irritable bowel syndrome)
- Bladder fullness, nocturnal frequency (irritable bladder)
- Hyperacusis, dyspareunia, discomfort when touched (allodynia)
- Frequent side-effects with drugs (chemical sensitivity)

for all or some of the patient's symptoms (Box 24.48). Extensive imaging is not recommended but bone scintigraphy can identify many conditions that can contribute to widespread pain and is a useful 'negative' test.

The aims of management are to educate the patient about the condition, address unresolved psychological issues, achieve pain control and improve sleep. Wherever possible, education should include the spouse, family or carer. It should be acknowledged that the cause of FM is not fully understood but the widespread pain does not reflect inflammation, tissue damage or disease. The model of a self-perpetuating cycle of poor sleep and pain (see Fig. 24.30) is a useful framework for problem-based management. Understanding the diagnosis can often help the patient come to terms with the symptoms. Repeat or drawn-out investigation may reinforce beliefs in occult serious pathology and should be avoided.

Low-dose amitriptyline (10–75 mg at night), with or without fluoxetine, may help by encouraging delta sleep and reducing

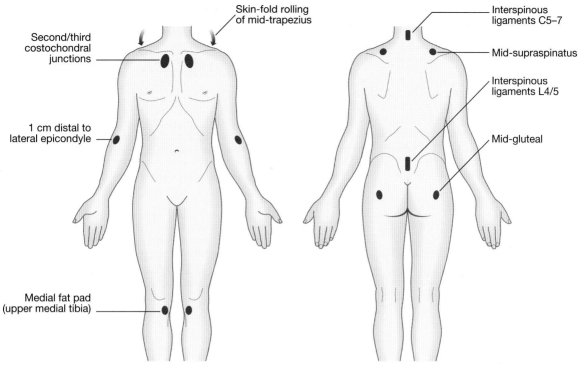

Fig. 24.31 Typical tender points in fibromyalgia.

Labels (front view):
- Second/third costochondral junctions
- Skin-fold rolling of mid-trapezius
- 1 cm distal to lateral epicondyle
- Medial fat pad (upper medial tibia)

Labels (back view):
- Interspinous ligaments C5–7
- Mid-supraspinatus
- Interspinous ligaments L4/5
- Mid-gluteal

24.48 Laboratory investigations recommended before finalising a diagnosis of fibromyalgia	
Test	**Condition screened for**
Full blood count, liver and renal function tests	General disease indicators
Erythrocyte sedimentation rate, C-reactive protein, serum amyloid A, immunoglobulins	Inflammatory disease
Thyroid function	Hypo-/hyperthyroidism
Calcium, albumin, phosphate, alkaline phosphatase, parathyroid hormone, 25-hydroxyvitamin-D, serum angiotensin-converting enzyme	Hyperparathyroidism, osteomalacia, sarcoid
Antinuclear antibodies, extractable nuclear antigens, rheumatoid factor, anti-cyclic citrullinated peptide antibodies, complement C3 and C4, lupus anticoagulant, anti-cardiolipin antibodies, streptococcal antibodies	Autoinflammatory and autoimmune diseases

spinal cord wind-up. Many people with FM, however, are intolerant of even small doses of amitriptyline. There is limited evidence for the use of tramadol, serotonin–noradrenaline (norepinephrine) re-uptake inhibitors (SNRIs) such as duloxetine, and the anticonvulsants pregabalin and gabapentin. A graded increase in aerobic exercise can improve well-being and sleep quality. The use of self-help strategies and a cognitive behavioural approach with relaxation techniques should be encouraged. Sublimated anxiety relating to distressing life events should be specifically explored with appropriate counselling. There are patient organisations that provide additional information and support. Although treatment may improve quality of life and ability to cope, most people remain symptomatic for many years.

Bone and joint infections

Septic arthritis

Septic arthritis is the most rapid and destructive joint disease. The incidence is 2–10 per 100 000 in the general population and 30–70 per 100 000 in those with pre-existing joint disease or joint replacement. Septic arthritis is associated with significant morbidity and still has a mortality of about 10% despite advances in antimicrobial therapy. The most important risk factor for mortality is increasing age.

Pathogenesis

Septic arthritis usually occurs as a result of haematogenous spread from infections of the skin or upper respiratory tract; infection from direct puncture wounds or secondary to joint aspiration is uncommon. Risk factors include increasing age, pre-existing joint disease (principally RA), diabetes mellitus, immunosuppression (by drugs or disease) and intravenous drug misuse. In RA, the skin is a frequent portal of entry because of maceration of skin between the toes due to joint deformity and difficulties with foot hygiene caused by hand deformity. Box 24.49 describes the particular considerations in old age.

Clinical features

The usual presentation is with acute or subacute monoarthritis and fever. The joint is usually swollen, hot and red, with pain at rest and on movement. Although any joint can be affected, lower limb joints, such as the knee and hip, are most commonly

24

24.49 Joint and bone infection in old age

- **Vertebral infection**: more common. Recognition may be delayed, as symptoms may be attributed to compression fractures caused by osteoporosis.
- **Peripheral vascular disease**: leads to more frequent involvement of the bones of the feet, and diabetic foot ulcers are also commonly complicated by osteomyelitis.
- **Prosthetic joint infections**: now more common because of the increased frequency of prosthetic joint insertion in older people.
- **Gram-negative bacilli**: more frequent pathogens than in younger people.
- **Cephalosporins:** contraindicated due to the high risk of *Clostridium difficile.*
- **Septic arthritis:** mortality is high in elderly patients.

24.50 Emergency management of suspected septic arthritis

Admit patient to hospital

Perform urgent investigations
- Aspirate joint:
  Send synovial fluid for Gram stain and culture
  Use imaging guidance if required
- Send blood for culture, routine biochemistry and haematology, including erythrocyte sedimentation rate and C-reactive protein
- Consider sending other samples (sputum, urine, wound swab) for culture, depending on patient history, to determine primary source of infection

Commence intravenous antibiotic*
- Flucloxacillin (2 g 4 times daily)
- If penicillin-allergic:
  Clindamycin (450–600 mg 4 times daily in younger patients)
  Intravenous vancomycin (1 g twice daily if age >65 years)
- If high risk of Gram-negative sepsis:
  Use antibiotic(s) active against *Staph. aureus* and locally-encountered Gram-negative organisms (seek expert guidance locally)

Relieve pain
- Oral and/or intravenous analgesics
- Consider local ice-packs

Aspirate joint
- Perform serial needle aspiration to dryness (1–3 times daily or as required)
- Consider arthroscopic drainage if needle aspiration difficult

Arrange physiotherapy
- Early regular passive movement, progressing to active movements once pain controlled and effusion not re-accumulating

*The evidence base for choice of antibiotic selection is poor. Local guidelines should be followed where available.

targeted. Patients with pre-existing arthritis may present with multiple joint involvement.

In adults, the most likely organism is *Staphylococcus aureus*, particularly in patients with RA and diabetes. In young, sexually active adults, gonococcus may be responsible. Disseminated gonococcal infection occurs in up to 3% of patients with untreated gonorrhoea. This usually presents with migratory arthralgia, low-grade fever and tenosynovitis, which may precede the development of an oligo- or monoarthritis. Painful pustular skin lesions may also be present. Gram-negative bacilli or group B, C and G streptococci are important causes among the elderly and intravenous drug users. Less commonly, septic arthritis may be caused by group A streptococci, pneumococci, meningococci and *Haemophilus influenzae*.

Investigations

The pivotal investigation is joint aspiration but blood cultures should also be taken. The synovial fluid is usually turbid or blood-stained but may appear normal. If the joint is not readily accessible, aspiration should be performed under imaging guidance or in theatre. Prosthetic joints should only be aspirated in theatre.

Synovial fluid should be sent for Gram stain and culture; cultures are positive in around 90% of cases but the Gram stain is positive in only 50%. In contrast, synovial fluid culture is positive in only 30% of gonococcal infections, making it important to obtain concurrent cultures from the genital tract (positive in 70–90% of cases). There is a leucocytosis with raised ESR and CRP in most patients, but these features may be absent in elderly or immunocompromised patients, or early in the disease course. Serial measurements of CRP and ESR are useful in following the response to treatment.

Management

The principles of management are summarised in Box 24.50. The patient should be admitted to hospital for pain relief and administration of parenteral antibiotics. Flucloxacillin (2 g IV 4 times daily) is the antibiotic of first choice pending the results of cultures, since it will cover most staphylococcal and streptococcal infections. If there is reason to suspect meticillin-resistant *Staphylococcus aureus* (such as a known carrier), vancomycin should be used instead while awaiting cultures. If a Gram-negative infection is suspected, gentamicin or vancomycin should be considered as first-line treatments. Cephalosporins are a potential alternative for Gram-negative infections but carry a high risk of *Clostridium difficile* infection in those aged over 65. Whatever antibiotic is chosen, the regimen may need to be changed,

depending on the organism that is isolated. Microbiology advice should always be sought in complicated situations, such as when treating intravenous drug users, patients in intensive care and those who might be colonised by resistant organisms. It is traditional to continue intravenous antibiotics for 2 weeks and to follow this with oral treatment for another 4 weeks, but there is no evidence to support the optimal duration of treatment. Joint aspiration should be performed using a large-bore needle once or twice daily. If this is not possible, arthroscopic or open surgical drainage may be needed performed. Regular passive movement should be undertaken from the outset, and active movements encouraged once the condition has stabilised. Infected prosthetic joints require management by the orthopaedic team, but prolonged antibiotic treatment on its own is often ineffective and removal of the prosthesis is required for eradication of the infection.

Arthritis may be a feature of Lyme disease caused by members of the *Borrelia* species of microorganisms (p. 255). It is generally a late manifestation, which usually affects large joints. Brucellosis presents with an acute febrile illness, followed in some cases by the development of localised infection, which can result in arthritis, bursitis, osteomyelitis, sacroiliitis and paravertebral or psoas abscesses. These conditions are discussed on pages 254 and 255.

Viral arthritis

The usual presentation is with acute polyarthritis following a febrile illness, which may be accompanied by a rash. Most cases of viral arthritis are self-limiting and settle down within 4–6 weeks. Human parvovirus arthropathy (mainly B19; p. 237) is the most common in Europe; adults may not have the characteristic 'slapped cheek' facial rash seen in children. The diagnosis can be confirmed by a rise in specific IgM. Polyarthritis may also occur rarely with hepatitis B and C, rubella (including rubella vaccination) and HIV infection. A variety of mosquito-borne viruses may cause epidemics of acute polyarthritis, including Ross River (Australia, Pacific), Chikungunya and O'nyong-nyong (Asia, Africa), and Mayaro viruses (South America). A wide variety of articular symptoms have been associated with HIV, mainly in the later stages of infection (Box 24.51). Management is symptomatic, with NSAIDs and analgesics.

Osteomyelitis

In osteomyelitis, the primary sites of infection are bone and bone marrow. Any part of a bone may be involved but there is preferential targeting of the juxta-epiphyseal regions of long bones adjacent to joints. The risk of osteomyelitis increases with age; the incidence is about 8.8 cases per 100 000 person-years in those under 18, rising to 40.8 cases in those aged 60–69 and 88.3 cases in those above the age of 80.

Pathogenesis

Haematogenous spread is the most common cause in children but contiguous spread of infection from adjacent soft tissues or as the result of surgery is more important in adults. Diabetes is a particularly important risk factor, accounting for about 30% of cases in recent series. Other risk factors include immunosuppressive therapy, HIV infection and sickle-cell disease, which particularly increases the risk of *Salmonella* infection. The organisms most frequently implicated are *Staph. aureus*, *Staph. epidermidis* and streptococci. The infection often results in a florid inflammatory response, with a greatly increased intraosseous pressure. If untreated, the condition may cause localised areas of osteonecrosis, leading to the development of a fragment of necrotic bone that is called a sequestrum. Eventual perforation of the cortex by pus stimulates local new bone formation (involucrum) in the periosteum, often leading to the development of sinuses that discharge through the skin.

Clinical features

The presentation is with localised bone pain and tenderness, often accompanied by malaise, night sweats and pyrexia. The adjacent joint may be painful to move and may develop a sterile effusion or secondary septic arthritis.

Investigations

Patients suspected of having osteomyelitis should have an MRI, which is more sensitive than X-ray for detecting early changes. Where possible, cultures should be obtained by open or imaging-guided biopsy of the lesion. Evidence of osteopenia, localised osteolysis and osteonecrosis may be seen on X-ray. Blood cultures should be taken, which may also reveal the causative organism. Routine bloods typically show evidence of an acute phase response with a neutrophilia and raised ESR and CRP.

Management

Early recognition is critical as once osteomyelitis becomes established and chronic, it may prove very hard to eradicate with antibiotics alone. The principles are those followed for septic arthritis, with parenteral antibiotics for 2 weeks, followed by oral antibiotics for at least 4 weeks. An exception is in localised osteomyelitis of the toes and fingers, which can often be treated successfully with a prolonged course of oral antibiotics. Resection of the infected bone and subsequent reconstruction may be required. Complications of chronic osteomyelitis include secondary amyloidosis (p. 81) and skin malignancy at the margin of a discharging sinus (Marjolin's ulcer).

Discitis

Discitis is an unusual condition in which there is infection of the intervertebral disc, often extending into the epidural space or paravertebral soft tissues. *Staph. aureus* is the most common pathogen. Risk factors include diabetes mellitus, immunodeficiency or immunosuppressive therapy, and intravenous drug use. The presentation is with back pain accompanied by fever, and an acute phase response with high ESR and CRP and a neutrophilia. If the diagnosis is suspected, an MRI should be performed and blood cultures taken. If blood cultures are negative, open or imaging-guided biopsy of the lesion should be performed to try to identify the organism responsible. Management is with supportive care and parenteral antibiotics followed by oral antibiotics, as described for osteomyelitis.

Tuberculosis

Tuberculosis can affect the musculoskeletal system, usually targeting the spine (Pott's disease) or large joints such as the hip, knee or ankle. The presentation is with pain, swelling and fever. The X-ray changes are non-specific and mycobacteria are seldom identified in the synovial fluid, so tissue biopsy is required for a definitive diagnosis. Medical management is described on page 592. In some cases, surgical débridement may be required for extensive joint disease, and spinal involvement may require surgical stabilisation and decompression.

Rheumatoid arthritis

Rheumatoid arthritis (RA) is a common form of inflammatory arthritis, occurring throughout the world and in all ethnic groups. The prevalence of RA is approximately 0.8–1.0% in Europe and the Indian subcontinent, with a female-to-male ratio of 3 : 1. The prevalence is lower in South-east Asia (0.4%). The highest prevalence in the world is in Pima Indians (5%). It is a chronic disease characterised by a clinical course of exacerbations and remissions.

24

Pathophysiology

RA is a complex disease with both genetic and environmental components. The importance of genetic factors is demonstrated by higher concordance of RA in monozygotic (12–15%) compared with dizygotic twins (3%), and an increased frequency of disease in first-degree relatives of patients. Genome-wide association studies have detected nearly 100 loci that are associated with the risk of developing RA. The strongest association is with variants in the HLA region. Recent studies have shown that the association with HLA is determined by variations in three amino acids in the HLA-DRβ1 molecule (positions 11, 71 and 74) and single variants HLA-B (at position 9) and HLA-DPβ1 (at position 9). The non-HLA loci generally lie within or close to genes involved in regulating the immune response. It is currently believed that RA occurs when an environmental stimulus, such as infection, triggers autoimmunity in a genetically susceptible host by modifying host proteins through processes like citrullination so that they become immunogenic. However, no single specific pathogen has been identified as a cause. An important environmental risk factor is cigarette smoking, which is also associated with more severe disease and reduced responsiveness to treatment. Remission may occur during pregnancy and sometimes RA first presents post-partum. This is likely to be due to suppression of the immune response during pregnancy but hormonal changes may also play a role.

The disease is characterised by infiltration of the synovial membrane with lymphocytes, plasma cells, dendritic cells and macrophages. There is evidence that CD4⁺ T lymphocytes and B cells play important roles in the pathogenesis of RA by interacting with other cells in the synovium, as illustrated in Figure 24.32. Lymphoid follicles form within the synovial membrane in which T- and B-cell interactions occur, causing activation of T cells to produce cytokines and activation of B cells to produce autoantibodies, including RF and ACPA. Synovial macrophages are activated by TNF and interferon gamma (IFN-γ), produced by T cells. The macrophages produce several pro-inflammatory cytokines, including TNF, IL-1 and IL-6, which act on synovial fibroblasts to produce further cytokines, setting up a positive feedback loop. The synovial fibroblasts proliferate, causing synovial hypertrophy and producing matrix metalloproteinases and the proteinase ADAMTS-5, which degrade soft tissues and cartilage. Prostaglandins and nitric oxide produced within the inflamed synovium cause vasodilatation, resulting in swelling and pain. Systemic release of IL-6 triggers production of acute phase proteins by the liver. At the joint margin, the inflamed synovium (pannus) directly invades bone and cartilage to cause joint erosions. A key pathogenic factor in bone erosions and periarticular osteoporosis is osteoclast activation, stimulated by the production of M-CSF by synovial cells and RANKL by activated T cells (Fig. 24.32). New blood-vessel formation (angiogenesis) occurs, causing the inflamed synovium to become highly vascular.

Fig. 24.32 Pathophysiology of rheumatoid arthritis. Some of the cytokines and cellular interactions believed to be important in rheumatoid arthritis are shown. (ADAMTS5 = aggrecanase; IL = interleukin; M-CSF = macrophage colony-stimulating factor; MMP = matrix metalloproteinase; RANKL = receptor activator of nuclear factor kappa B ligand; TNF = tumour necrosis factor)

24.52 Criteria for diagnosis of rheumatoid arthritis*	
Criterion	**Score**
Joints affected	
1 large joint	0
2–10 large joints	1
1–3 small joints	2
4–10 small joints	3
>10 joints (at least 1 small joint)	5
Serology	
Negative RF and ACPA	0
Low positive RF or ACPA	2
High positive RF or ACPA	3
Duration of symptoms	
<6 weeks	0
>6 weeks	1
Acute phase reactants	
Normal CRP and ESR	0
Abnormal CRP or ESR	1
Patients with a score ≥6 are considered to have definite RA.	

*European League Against Rheumatism/American College of Rheumatology 2010 criteria.
(ACPA = anti-citrullinated peptide antibody; CRP = C-reactive protein; ESR = erythrocyte sedimentation rate; RF = rheumatoid factor)

Fig. 24.33 The hand in rheumatoid arthritis. **A** Ulnar deviation of the fingers with wasting of the small muscles of the hands and synovial swelling at the wrists, the extensor tendon sheaths, the metacarpophalangeal and proximal interphalangeal joints. **B** 'Swan neck' deformity of the fingers.

Within these blood vessels, pro-inflammatory cytokines activate endothelial cells, which support recruitment of yet more leucocytes to perpetuate the inflammatory process.

Later, fibrous or bony ankylosis may occur. Muscles adjacent to inflamed joints atrophy and may be infiltrated with lymphocytes. This leads to progressive biomechanical dysfunction and may further amplify destruction.

Rheumatoid nodules occur in patients who are RF- or ACPA-positive and primarily affect extensor tendons. They consist of a central area of fibrinoid material surrounded by a palisade of proliferating mononuclear cells. Granulomatous lesions may occur in the pleura, lung, pericardium and sclera.

Clinical features

The typical presentation is with pain, joint swelling and stiffness affecting the small joints of the hands, feet and wrists in a symmetrical fashion. Large joint involvement, systemic symptoms and extra-articular features may also occur. Clinical criteria for the diagnosis of RA are shown in Box 24.52.

Sometimes RA has an acute onset, with severe early morning stiffness, polyarthritis and pitting oedema. This occurs more commonly in old age. Another presentation is with proximal muscle stiffness mimicking polymyalgia rheumatica (p. 1042). Occasionally, the onset is palindromic, with relapsing and remitting episodes of pain, stiffness and swelling that last for only a few hours or days.

Examination typically reveals swelling and tenderness of the affected joints. Erythema is unusual and its presence suggests coexistent sepsis. Characteristic deformities may develop with long-standing uncontrolled disease, although these have become less common over recent years with more aggressive management. They include ulnar deviation of the fingers, 'swan neck' deformity, the boutonnière or 'button hole' deformity, and a Z deformity of the thumb (Fig. 24.33). Dorsal subluxation of the ulna at the distal radio-ulnar joint may occur and contribute to rupture of the fourth and fifth extensor tendons. Triggering of fingers may occur because of nodules in the flexor tendon

sheaths. Subluxation of the MTP joints of the feet may result in 'cock-up' toe deformities, causing pain on weight-bearing on the exposed MTP heads and the development of secondary adventitious bursae and callosities. In the hindfoot, a valgus deformity of the calcaneus may be observed as the result of damage to the ankle and subtalar joints. This is often associated with loss of the longitudinal arch (flat foot) due to rupture of the tibialis posterior tendon. Popliteal (Baker's) cysts may occur in patients with knee synovitis, in which synovial fluid communicates with the cyst but is prevented from returning to the joint by a valve-like mechanism; this is not specific to RA. Rupture may be induced by knee flexion, leading to calf pain and swelling that may mimic a deep venous thrombosis (DVT). These joint deformities tend to be observed in older patients with long-standing disease but are becoming much less common with more aggressive treatment of RA in its early stages.

Systemic features

Anorexia, weight loss and fatigue may occur throughout the disease course. Osteoporosis is a common complication (p. 1044) and muscle-wasting may occur as the result of systemic inflammation and reduced activity. Extra-articular features are most common in patients with long-standing seropositive erosive disease but may occasionally occur at presentation, especially in men. Most are due to serositis, granuloma and nodule formation or vasculitis (Box 24.53).

Nodules

Rheumatoid nodules occur almost exclusively in RF- or ACPA-positive patients, usually in extensor tendons (Fig. 24.34). They

24

Fig. 24.34 Rheumatoid nodules and olecranon bursitis. Nodules were palpable within, as well as outside, the bursa.

are frequently asymptomatic but some may be complicated by ulceration and secondary infection.

Vasculitis

This is uncommon but may occur in seropositive patients. The presentation is with systemic symptoms, such as fatigue and fever and nail-fold infarcts. Rarely, cutaneous ulceration, skin necrosis and mesenteric, renal or coronary artery occlusion may occur.

Ocular involvement

The most common symptom is dry eyes (keratoconjunctivitis sicca) due to secondary Sjögren's syndrome (p. 1038). Scleritis and peripheral ulcerative keratitis are uncommon but more serious and potentially sight-threatening complications that usually present with pain and redness. Clinical features and management are discussed in more detail on page 1172.

Serositis

Serositis is usually asymptomatic but may present with pleural or pericardial pain and breathlessness. Pericardial effusion and constrictive pericarditis may rarely occur.

Cardiac involvement

Heart block, cardiomyopathy, coronary artery occlusion and aortic regurgitation have all been reported but are rare. The risk of cardiovascular disease is increased due to a combination of conventional risk factors, such as high cholesterol, smoking, hypertension, reduced physical activity, NSAIDs, glucocorticoids and the effects of inflammatory cytokines on vascular endothelium.

Pulmonary involvement

Pulmonary fibrosis may occur but is often asymptomatic. There is some evidence that the risk of pulmonary fibrosis is increased by anti-TNF therapy, although its uncertain whether this is causal or a marker of more severe disease in patients who require anti-TNF treatment.

Peripheral neuropathy

Entrapment neuropathies may result from compression by hypertrophied synovium or by joint subluxation. Median nerve compression is the most common and bilateral carpal tunnel syndrome can occur as a presenting feature of RA. Other syndromes include ulnar nerve compression at the elbow or wrist, compression of the lateral popliteal nerve at the head of the fibula, and tarsal tunnel syndrome (entrapment of the posterior tibial nerve in the flexor retinaculum), which causes burning, tingling and numbness in the distal sole and toes. Diffuse symmetrical peripheral neuropathy and mononeuritis multiplex may occur in patients with rheumatoid vasculitis.

Spinal cord compression

This rare complication is caused by compression of the spinal cord from subluxation of the cervical spine at the atlanto-axial joint or at a subaxial level (Fig. 24.35). Atlanto-axial subluxation is due to erosion of the transverse ligament posterior to the odontoid peg. It can lead to cord compression or sudden death following minor trauma or manipulation. It should be suspected in any RA patient who describes new onset of occipital headache, particularly if symptoms of paraesthesia or electric shock are present in the arms. The onset is often insidious, with subtle loss of function that may initially be attributed to active disease. Reflexes and power can be difficult to assess in patients with extensive joint disease and therefore sensory or upper motor signs are most important. Patients with evidence of spinal cord compression require urgent neurosurgical referral for stabilisation and fixation.

Other complications

Amyloidosis is a rare complication of long-standing disease that usually presents with nephrotic syndrome. Microcytic anaemia can occur due to iron deficiency resulting from NSAID-induced gastrointestinal blood loss, whereas normochromic, normocytic anaemia with thrombocytosis occurs in patients

Fig. 24.35 Subluxation of cervical spine. [A] Flexion, showing widening of the space (arrow) between the odontoid peg of the axis (behind) and the anterior arch of the atlas (in front). [B] Extension, showing reduction in this space.

---

i | **24.54 Felty's syndrome**

Risk factors

- Age of onset 50–70 years
- Female > male
- Caucasians > blacks
- Long-standing rheumatoid arthritis
- Deforming but inactive disease
- Seropositive for rheumatoid factor

Common clinical features

- Splenomegaly
- Lymphadenopathy
- Weight loss
- Skin pigmentation
- Keratoconjunctivitis sicca
- Vasculitis, leg ulcers
- Recurrent infections
- Nodules

Laboratory findings

- Normochromic, normocytic anaemia
- Neutropenia
- Abnormal liver function
- Thrombocytopenia
- Impaired T- and B-cell immunity

---

i | **24.55 Investigations and monitoring of rheumatoid arthritis**

To establish diagnosis

- Clinical criteria
- Erythrocyte sedimentation rate and C-reactive protein
- Ultrasound or magnetic resonance imaging
- Rheumatoid factor and anti-citrullinated peptide antibodies

To monitor disease activity and drug efficacy

- Pain (visual analogue scale)
- Early morning stiffness (minutes)
- Joint tenderness
- Joint swelling
- DAS28 score (see Fig. 24.36)
- Erythrocyte sedimentation rate and C-reactive protein

To monitor disease damage

- X-rays
- Functional assessment

To monitor drug safety

- Urinalysis
- Full blood count
- Chest X-ray
- Urea and creatinine
- Liver function tests

---

with active disease. Felty's syndrome is a rare complication of seropositive RA in which splenomegaly occurs in combination with neutropenia and thrombocytopenia (Box 24.54). Localised or generalised lymphadenopathy can occur in patients with active disease but persistent lymphadenopathy may indicate the development of lymphoma, which is more common in patients with long-standing RA.

Investigations

The diagnosis of RA is essentially clinical but investigations are useful in confirming the diagnosis and assessing disease activity (Box 24.55). The ESR and CRP are usually raised but normal results do not exclude the diagnosis, especially if only a few joints are involved. Tests for ACPA are positive in about 70% of cases and are highly specific for RA, occurring in many patients before clinical onset of the disease. Similarly, RF is also positive in about 70% of cases, most of whom also test positive for ACPA. RF is less specific than ACPA, however, and positive tests can occur in other diseases (p. 991).

Ultrasound examination and MRI are not routinely required but can be value in patients with symptoms suggestive of RA where there is clinical uncertainty about the presence of synovitis. Plain X-rays of the hands, wrist and feet are usually normal in early RA but periarticular osteoporosis and marginal joint erosions may be observed with more advanced disease. The main indication for an X-ray is in the assessment of patients with painful joints to determine whether significant structural damage has occurred. Patients who are suspected of having atlanto-axial disease should have lateral X-rays taken in flexion and extension, and an MRI. In those with suspected Baker's cyst, ultrasound may be required to establish the diagnosis.

DAS28 is widely used to assess disease activity, response to treatment and need for biological therapy. It involves counting the number of swollen and tender joints in the upper limbs and knees, and combining this with the ESR and the patient's assessment of the activity of their arthritis on a visual analogue scale, where 0 indicates no symptoms and 100 the worst symptoms possible. This data are entered into a calculator to generate a numerical score. The higher the value, the more active the disease (Fig. 24.36).

Management

The treatment goal is to suppress inflammation, control symptoms and prevent joint damage. This involves a combination of pharmacological and non-pharmacological therapies. When RA occurs in women of child-bearing age, additional considerations need to be taken into account and these are summarised in Box 24.56.

Pharmacological therapy

DMARD therapy should be introduced in all patients as this improves outcome. A typical algorithm is shown in Figure 24.37. On first diagnosis, prednisolone should be started in a dose of 30 mg daily gradually reducing in 5 mg increments every 2 weeks until therapy is withdrawn after about 12 weeks. At the same time, methotrexate should be started in an initial dose of 15 mg weekly, along with folic acid 5 mg weekly, and escalated up to a maximum of 25 mg weekly, depending on the response. If the patient fails to respond adequately or dose-limiting toxicity occurs, then an additional DMARD should be commenced in combination with MTX. The most common combination is triple therapy, in which

24

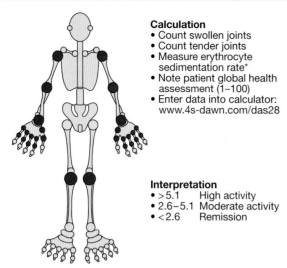

Calculation
- Count swollen joints
- Count tender joints
- Measure erythrocyte sedimentation rate*
- Note patient global health assessment (1–100)
- Enter data into calculator: www.4s-dawn.com/das28

Interpretation
- >5.1   High activity
- 2.6–5.1 Moderate activity
- <2.6   Remission

Fig. 24.36 Calculation of the Disease Activity Score 28 (DAS28).
*Erythrocyte sedimentation rate or C-reactive protein can be used for the calculation.

24.56 Rheumatoid arthritis in pregnancy

- **Immunological changes in pregnancy**: many patients with rheumatoid arthritis go into remission during pregnancy.
- **Conception**: methotrexate should be discontinued for at least 3 months and leflunomide discontinued for at least 24 months before trying to conceive.
- **Paracetamol**: the oral analgesic of choice during pregnancy.
- **Oral non-steroidal anti-inflammatory drugs and selective cyclo-oxygenase 2 (COX-2) inhibitors**: can be used from implantation to 20 weeks' gestation.
- **Glucocorticoids**: may be used to control disease flares; the main maternal risks are hypertension, glucose intolerance and osteoporosis.
- **Disease-modifying antirheumatic drugs (DMARDs) that may be used**: sulfasalazine, hydroxychloroquine and azathioprine if required to control inflammation.
- **DMARDs that must be avoided**: methotrexate, leflunomide, cyclophosphamide, mycophenolate and gold.
- **Biologic therapies**: experience is limited but they may be relatively safe during pregnancy. The main theoretical risk is immunosuppression in the neonate, except for certolizumab, which does cross the placenta in negligible amounts.
- **Breastfeeding**: methotrexate, leflunomide and cyclophosphamide are contraindicated.

methotrexate, sulfasalazine and hydroxychloroquine are combined (Fig. 24.37). Other DMARDs can be substituted or added, along with a low-dose glucocorticoid such as prednisolone (5–10 mg daily) if the patient fails to respond fully. If disease activity remains high (DAS28 >5.1) despite triple therapy, however, it is usual to progress to biologic therapy. The most commonly used first-line biologics in RA are TNF inhibitors, although several other options are available (p. 1006). When the patient has been stabilised on biologic treatment for 12 months or more, a reduction in dose should be considered, since it is possible to reduce the dose in up to 50% of patients without loss of therapeutic effect. The JAK inhibitors tofacitinib and baricitinib have efficacy in patients who fail to respond adequately to other DMARDs and provide an alternative to biologic therapies.

RA is a chronic disease and flares can occur even in patients who are established on DMARD and biologic therapy. Transient

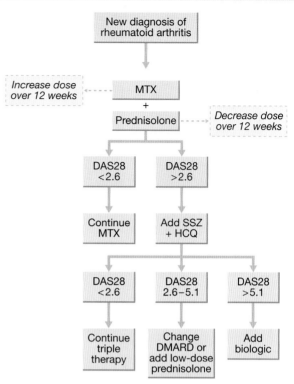

Fig. 24.37 Algorithm for the management of rheumatoid arthritis. (DAS28 = Disease Activity Score 28; DMARD = disease-modifying antirheumatic drug; HCQ = hydroxychloroquine; MTX = methotrexate; SSZ = sulfasalazine)

flares can be dealt with by intra-articular glucocorticoid injections or a short course of oral glucocorticoids, but if a sustained flare occurs, a change in systemic DMARD and/or biologic therapy may need to be considered.

Non-pharmacological therapy

Physical and occupational therapy play important roles and it is vital for all patients to be assessed by an occupational therapist and physiotherapist and the appropriate advice and treatment provided.

Surgery

Synovectomy can be helpful in joints that have failed to respond adequately to systemic therapy and intra-articular injections. Joint replacement surgery may be required but the need for this has diminished over recent years, presumably as the result of more aggressive medical management. Other surgical procedures that can be helpful are excision of the metatarsal heads in patients with subluxation of the MTP joints; neurosurgery in patients with atlanto-axial subluxation; and fusion or the wrist or ankle in patients with joint damage (see Box 24.29, p. 1002).

Juvenile idiopathic arthritis

Juvenile idiopathic arthritis (JIA) is the term, accepted by the international community, for several forms of arthritis defined by the International League of Associations for Rheumatology 2001 criteria (Box 24.57). This includes juvenile forms of psoriatic arthritis (JPsA), rheumatoid arthritis (JRA) and more undifferentiated forms of inflammatory arthritis. The majority of patients with JIA have a phenotype that is distinct from adult inflammatory arthritis

24.57 Clinical features of juvenile idiopathic arthritis

Subtype	Frequency	Clinical features	Immunology
Systemic juvenile idiopathic arthritis	5%	Fever, rash, arthralgia, hepatosplenomegaly	Autoantibody-negative
Oligoarthritis (≤4 joints)	60%	Large-joint arthritis, uveitis	ANA-positive
Polyarthritis (≥5 joints)	20%	Polyarthritis; may be extended form of oligoarthritis	ANA-positive
Enthesis-related	5%	Sacroiliitis, enthesopathy	HLA-B27-positive
RF-positive	5%	Polyarthritis, similar to RA	RF-positive, ACPA-positive
Psoriatic arthritis	5%	Same as adult disease (p. 1032)	Autoantibody-negative

(ACPA = anti-citrullinated peptide antibody; ANA = antinuclear antibody; HLA = human leucocyte antigen; RA = rheumatoid arthritis; RF = rheumatoid factor)

and includes a strong association with uveitis. JIA affects about 1:1000 children and young people up to 16 years of age – similar to the prevalence of diabetes (1:700). The annual incidence is approximately 1 per 10000 children and young people.

Whereas joint restriction is attributed to damage in adults, in children it indicates inflammatory activity. Arthritis in children affects limb growth and has a negative effect on height and weight attainment. In young children, effective disease control can repair joint damage before puberty.

Oligoarthritis is the most common form of JIA, accounting for about 60% of cases. It is more common in females and tends to affect large joints in an asymmetrical pattern. There is an association with uveitis and many patients are ANA-positive. Polyarticular JIA is heterogeneous: some patients are RF- and/or ACPA-positive, while others are negative for autoantibodies.

Systemic juvenile idiopathic arthritis (sJIA, formerly known as Still's disease) is characterised by fever, rash, arthritis, hepatosplenomegaly and serositis in association with anaemia and a raised ESR and CRP. Autoantibody tests are negative. This form of JIA is associated with haemophagocytic syndrome.

Many cases of enthesitis-related arthritis (ERA) are likely to be self-limiting forms of spondyloarthritis. ERA can progress over time into a more obviously defined spondyloarthropathy.

Investigations

ESR and CRP do not correlate well with the extent or severity of inflammation and may be normal. A very high ESR may indicate the presence of inflammatory bowel disease or (very rarely) leukaemia. Low haemoglobin is likely to be due to anaemia of chronic disease rather than iron deficiency. A positive ANA occurs in 40–75% of cases of JIA and indicates an increased risk of eye disease. Ultrasound is the radiological investigation of choice to confirm synovitis or tenosynovitis. The false-negative rate is higher in foot and ankle disease than in other joints. Arthroscopy should be avoided unless a biopsy is required. Synovial fluid aspiration, but not arthroscopy, is essential when considering sepsis and tuberculosis.

Management

The key approach is to gain early rapid control of inflammation, minimise the adverse effects of treatment and support the general physical and mental health of the patient, which requires full multidisciplinary team input. The standard immunotherapy is methotrexate (subcutaneous methotrexate is typically used in the young child). Alternative treatment includes leflunomide, sulfasalazine and hydroxychloroquine. Azathioprine and ciclosporin can be used to treat JIA with uveitis. Mycophenolate and tacrolimus are considered to have a specific role in treating

24.58 Juvenile idiopathic arthritis in adolescence

- **Uveitis:** may be clinically silent and persist into adulthood. All (not just those who are ANA-positive) need ophthalmic screening for eye involvement.
- **Persistence into adulthood:** occurs in 50% of cases, especially in systemic disease. Specific supportive management through transition from adolescence to adulthood should be planned.
- **Reduced peak bone mass:** common in polyarthritis and systemic juvenile idiopathic arthritis but there are few data on fracture risk and the evidence base for treatment is poor.
- **Therapy:** methotrexate is standard treatment, used after NSAIDs alone are insufficient. Anti-TNF therapy is effective in all forms of juvenile idiopathic arthritis but long-term safety remains unclear.

(ANA = antinuclear antibody; NSAIDs = non-steroidal anti-inflammatory drugs; TNF = tumour necrosis factor)

uveitis alone. Drug combinations are not well studied in JIA. Biologic therapies, including anti-TNF, are effective in JIA and are now a standard treatment in the presence of refractory disease or intolerance of methotrexate or other non-biologic immunotherapies. Tocilizumab is also effective in sJIA, and has been approved by NICE for use in the UK.

Prognosis

Suboptimal outcomes are associated with delayed diagnosis and referral to the specialist multidisciplinary team, inadequate disease control, presentation with uveitis, sJIA in males and poor engagement with services. Psychological support of affected children and their families is associated with improved outcome. Oligo-JIA often resolves at puberty. Polyarticular disease and sJIA remain active into adulthood in about 50% of cases. Common issues around the transition of adolescent patients into adulthood are shown in Box 24.58.

Spondyloarthropathies

Spondyloarthropathies (SpAs) comprise a group of related inflammatory musculoskeletal diseases that show overlap in their clinical features and have a shared immunogenetic association with HLA-B27 (Box 24.59). They include:
- axial spondyloarthritis
- ankylosing spondylitis
- reactive arthritis
- psoriatic arthritis

24

- arthritis with inflammatory bowel disease (enteropathic spondyloarthritis).

In axial spondylitis and ankylosing spondylitis, the axial skeleton (i.e. the central core skeleton) is predominantly affected. In contrast to RA, in the SpAs there are frequent and notable non-synovial musculoskeletal lesions – mainly inflammatory in nature – of ligaments, tendons, periosteum and other bone lesions. A hallmark lesion of all SpAs is enthesitis, which is inflammation at the site of a ligament or tendon insertion into bone. Dactylitis, inflammation of a whole finger or toe, may also occur (see Fig. 24.43).

It has been estimated that about 1% of the adult population in the USA may have an SpA (about 2.7 million). There is a striking association with HLA-B27, particularly for ankylosing spondylitis (>95%). Additionally, SpAs are thought to arise as the result of an aberrant host response to infection and abnormal mucosal immunity mediated through changes in the IL-12, IL-23 and Th17 axis (p. 65). In some situations, a triggering organism can be identified, as in reactive arthritis following bacterial dysentery or chlamydial urethritis, but in others the environmental trigger remains obscure. Familial clustering not only is common to the specific condition occurring in the proband, but also may extend to other diseases in the spondyloarthropathy group.

Axial spondyloarthropathy

Axial spondyloarthropathy includes classical ankylosing spondylitis (AS) as well as axial spondyloarthritis (axSpA). Inflammatory changes in the entire axial skeleton are characteristic of axSpA and can be visualised by MRI; structural alterations, such as new bone formation with syndesmophytes and ankylosis, develop later in the course of the disease. Accordingly, the criteria for diagnosing AS (Box 24.60), which require evidence of sacroiliitis on X-ray, are often only able to be applied many years after a patient's symptoms started. Not all patients with axSpA will go on to develop AS.

Pathophysiology

Axial SpA and AS arise from an interaction between environmental pathogens and the host immune system in genetically susceptible individuals. Increased faecal carriage of *Klebsiella aerogenes* has been reported in patients with established AS and may relate to exacerbation of both joint and eye disease. There is increasing evidence that axSpA and AS are due to an abnormal host response to the intestinal microbiota with involvement of Th17 cells, which have a key role in mucosal immunity. This leads to production of various inflammatory cytokines, including IL-12, IL-23, IL-17 and TNF-α, which play vital roles in the pathogenesis of enthesitis and other inflammatory lesions (Fig. 24.38).

There a strong association between axial spondyloarthropathy and carriage of the major histocompatibility complex (MHC)

 24.59 Features common to spondyloarthropathies

- Asymmetrical inflammatory oligoarthritis (lower > upper limb)
- History of inflammatory back pain
- Sacroiliitis and spinal osteitis
- Enthesitis (e.g. gluteus medius insertion, plantar fascia origin)
- Tendency for familial aggregation
- HLA-B27 association
- Psoriasis (of skin and/or nails)
- Uveitis
- Sterile urethritis and/or prostatitis
- Inflammatory bowel disease
- Aortic root lesions (aortic incompetence, conduction defects)

(HLA = human leucocyte antigen)

24.60 Comparison of diagnostic criteria for axial spondyloarthritis (ASAS) and ankylosing spondylitis (modified New York)

	Axial spondyloarthritis	Ankylosing spondylitis
Imaging	Sacroiliitis on MRI only	Bilateral sacroiliitis on X-ray, even if changes are mild Unilateral sacroiliitis on X-ray if changes are definite
History	Back pain >3 months that has four of the following characteristics: 1. improved by exercise 2. not relieved by rest 3. insidious onset 4. night pain 5. age at onset < 45 Good response of back pain to NSAID Family history of spondyloarthritis History of inflammatory bowel disease	Low back pain >3 months improved by exercise and not relieved by rest
Clinical examination	Arthritis Enthesitis Uveitis Dactylitis Psoriasis	Limitation of lumbar spine movement in sagittal and frontal planes Chest expansion reduced
Investigations	HLA-B27-positive Elevated CRP	

Axial spondyloarthritis is diagnosed from: sacroiliitis on MRI + one other feature on history, clinical examination or investigation.
The diagnosis can also be made in HLA-B27-positive patients with >1 clinical feature in the absence of sacroiliitis
Ankylosing spondylitis can be diagnosed on X-ray evidence of sacroiliitis with one other feature on history or examination

(ASAS = Assessment of Spondylitis International Society; CRP = C-reactive protein; HLA = human leucocyte antigen; MRI = magnetic resonance imaging; NSAID = non-steroidal anti-inflammatory drug)

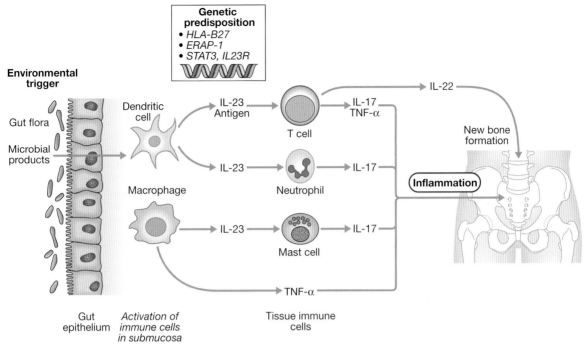

Fig. 24.38 Pathophysiology of axial spondyloarthropathy. In genetically susceptible individuals, it is thought that bacterial components penetrate the mucosal barrier to activate macrophages and dendritic cells in the intestinal submucosa. These cells produce increased amounts of interleukin 23 (IL-23), which acts on T cells, neutrophils and mast cells to make IL-17; IL-17 in turn has a pivotal role in driving inflammation, causing sacroiliitis and enthesitis. Presentation of antigen by dendritic cells also plays a pathogenic part in activating T cells, and tumour necrosis factor (TNF), produced by macrophages and activated T cells, contributes to the pathogenesis of inflammation. Production of IL-22 by T cells is thought to be involved in causing the new bone formation that is typical of axial spondyloarthropathy.

class I molecule HLA-B27. This is particularly striking in patients defined as having AS, more than 95% of whom are positive for HLA-B27. Other susceptibility genes also implicated in susceptibility to AS include *ERAP-1* (an endoplasmic reticulum protein with a role facilitating intracellular antigen processing and binding with its presenting MHC molecule HLA-B27), the IL-23 receptor and downstream signalling molecules involved in directing Th17 cell responses, such as *STAT3* (see Fig. 4.3, p. 65). The HLA-B27 molecule itself is implicated through its antigen-presenting function or because of its propensity to form homodimers that activate leucocytes. HLA-B27 molecules may also misfold, causing increased endoplasmic reticulum stress. This could lead to inflammatory cytokine release by macrophages and dendritic cells, thus triggering inflammatory disease.

Axial spondyloarthritis

Clinical features

The cardinal feature of axSpA is inflammatory back pain and early morning stiffness, with low back pain radiating to the buttocks or posterior thighs if the sacroiliac joints are involved. Symptoms are exacerbated by inactivity and relieved by movement. Musculoskeletal symptoms may be prominent at entheses, may be episodic and, if persistent, can present as widespread pain and be mistaken for fibromyalgia. Fatigue is common. A history of psoriasis (current, previous or in a first-degree relative) and inflammatory bowel symptoms (current or previous) are important clues. Physical signs include a reduced range of lumbar spine movements in all directions, pain on sacroiliac stressing and a high enthesitis index. Entheses that are typically affected include Achilles' insertion, plantar fascia origin, patellar ligament entheses, gluteus medius insertion at the greater trochanter and tendon

attachments at humeral epicondyles. A number of validated clinical questionnaires, such as the Bath Ankylosing Spondylitis Disease Activity Index (BASDAI), Bath Ankylosing Spondylitis Functional Index (BASFI) and Ankylosing Spondylitis Disease Activity Score (ASDAS-CRP), can be used to assess disease activity and functional status in AS, though newer assessment tools are being developed that are more specific to a diagnosis of axSpA, such as the Assessment of Spondyloarthritis International Society Health Index (ASAS-H).

Investigations

The diagnosis is aided by ultrasound or MRI of entheses, or by MRI of the sacroiliac joints and spine (Fig. 24.39). Other findings

Fig. 24.39 Magnetic resonance imaging appearances in sacroiliitis. Coronal MRI short T1 inversion recovery (STIR) sequence showing bilateral sacroiliitis in axial spondyloarthritis. Bone marrow oedema (circles) is present around both sacroiliac joints, which show irregularities due to erosions (arrows).

24

may include raised ESR and CRP (although these can be normal), anaemia and positive HLA-B27. Faecal calprotectin is a useful screening test for associated inflammatory bowel disease.

Management

Patient education, NSAID use (optimally, once daily or slow release taken at bedtime) and physical therapy are key interventions at the outset. For severe and/or persistent peripheral musculoskeletal features of SpA, both sulfasalazine and methotrexate are reasonable therapy choices. These medications have no impact on spinal symptoms or disease progression. In patients who fail to respond adequately or who cannot tolerate NSAIDs, progression to biologic therapy with either TNF inhibitors or the IL-7A inhibitor secukinumab should be considered (see Box 24.35, p. 1007). Anti-TNF therapy is effective for both the axial and peripheral lesions of axSpA, but it is as yet unclear whether anti-TNF therapy modifies the natural history of the disease.

Prognosis

With such a recent definition of disease, the markers of prognosis in patients diagnosed with axSpA are not fully understood. It is clear that axSpA can remain mild and/or episodic in many patients for many years. HLA-B27 positivity, high persistent CRP and high functional incapacity are likely to be markers of poor prognosis, if not markers of extension ultimately to AS.

Ankylosing spondylitis

Ankylosing spondylitis (AS) is defined by the presence of sacroiliitis on X-ray and other structural changes on spine X-rays, which may eventually progress to bony fusion of the spine. There is a male-to-female ratio of about 3:1. In Europe, more than 90% of those affected are HLA-B27-positive (Caucasian HLA-B27 population prevalence is 9%). The overall prevalence of AS is below 0.5% in most populations. Over 75% of patients are able to remain in employment and enjoy a good quality of life. Even if severe ankylosis develops, functional limitation may not be marked, as long as the spine is fused in an erect posture.

Clinical features

Clinical features are the same as in axSpA. AS typically evolves slowly, with fluctuating symptoms of spinal inflammation; ankylosis develops in many patients over a period of many years. Secondary osteoporosis of the vertebral bodies frequently occurs, leading to an increased risk of vertebral fracture.

In AS, spinal fusion varies in its extent and in most cases does not cause a gross flexion deformity, but a few patients develop marked kyphosis of the dorsal and cervical spine that may interfere with forward vision. This may prove incapacitating, especially when associated with fixed flexion contractures of hips or knees.

Up to 40% of patients also have peripheral musculoskeletal lesions (asymmetrical, affecting entheses of large joints, such as the hips, knees, ankles and shoulders).

Fatigue is a major complaint and is common to all SpAs, but its cause is unknown. Acute anterior uveitis is the most common extra-articular feature, which occasionally precedes joint disease. Other extra-articular features are occasionally observed but are rare (Box 24.61).

Investigations

In AS, X-rays of the sacroiliac joint show irregularity and loss of cortical margins, widening of the joint space and subsequently sclerosis, joint space narrowing and fusion. Lateral thoracolumbar spine X-rays may show anterior 'squaring' of vertebrae due to erosion and sclerosis of the anterior corners and periostitis of the waist. Bridging syndesmophytes may also be seen. These are areas of calcification that follow the outermost fibres of the annulus (Fig. 24.40). In advanced disease, ossification of the anterior longitudinal ligament and facet joint fusion may also be visible. The combination of these features may result in the

---

i	**24.61 Extra-articular features of axial spondyloarthritis and ankylosing spondylitis**

- Fatigue, anaemia
- Anterior uveitis (25%)
- Prostatitis (80% of men) and sterile urethritis
- Inflammatory bowel disease (up to 50% have IBD lesions)
- Osteoporosis
- Cardiovascular disease (aortic valve disease 20%)
- Amyloidosis (rare)
- Atypical upper lobe pulmonary fibrosis (very rare)

Fig. 24.40 Radiographic changes in spondyloarthritis. [A] Fine symmetrical marginal syndesmophytes typical of ankylosing spondylitis (arrow). [B] Coarse, asymmetrical non-marginal syndesmophytes typical of psoriatic spondylitis (arrow).

Fig. 24.41 'Bamboo' spine of advanced ankylosing spondylitis. Note the symmetrical marginal syndesmophytes (arrows), sacroiliac joint fusion and generalised osteopenia.

typical 'bamboo' spine (Fig. 24.41). Erosive changes may be seen in the symphysis pubis, ischial tuberosities and peripheral joints. Osteoporosis is common and vertebral fractures may occur. Atlanto-axial dislocation can arise as a late feature. MRI is more sensitive for detection of early sacroiliitis than X-rays (see Fig. 24.39) and can also detect inflammatory changes in the lumbar spine. DXA scanning is important as part of a fragility fracture assessment.

As in axSpA, ESR and CRP are usually raised in active disease but may be normal; anaemia is often present. Autoantibodies, such as RF, ACPA and ANA, are negative.

Management

The aims of management are the same as in axSpA: to relieve pain and stiffness, maintain a maximal range of skeletal mobility and avoid the development of deformities. Mobilising exercises are important and are shown on many online resource sites (e.g. National Ankylosing Spondylitis Society, UK). A long-acting NSAID at night is helpful for alleviation of morning stiffness. Anti-TNF or anti-IL-17A therapy should be considered in patients who are inadequately controlled on standard therapy, as described for axSpA. Biologic therapies are often highly effective at improving symptoms but it is not clear whether they prevent ankylosis or alter the natural history of the disease.

Local glucocorticoid injections can be useful for persistent plantar fasciitis, other enthesopathies and peripheral arthritis. Oral glucocorticoids may be required for acute uveitis but do not help spinal disease. Severe hip, knee or shoulder arthritis with secondary OA may require arthroplasty. Spinal osteotomy, to correct stoop and make eyeline/posture 'more normal', can make a significant difference to patients with severe ankylosed kyphotic spines.

Reactive arthritis

Reactive (spondylo)arthritis (ReA) is a 'reaction' to a number of bacterial triggers with clinical features in keeping with all SpA conditions. The known triggers are *Chlamydia*, *Campylobacter*, *Salmonella*, *Shigella* and *Yersinia*. Notably, non-SpA-related reactive arthritis can occur following infection with many viruses, *Mycoplasma*, *Borrelia*, streptococci and mycobacteria, including *M. leprae*, which causes leprosy (Hansen's disease); however, the 'reaction' in these instances consists typically of myoarthralgias, is not associated with HLA-B27 and is generally not chronic. The arthritis associated with rheumatic fever (p. 515) is also an example of a reactive arthritis that is not associated with HLA-B27.

Sexually acquired reactive arthritis (SARA) is predominantly a disease of young men, with a male preponderance of 15:1. This may reflect a difficulty in diagnosing the condition in young women, in whom *Chlamydia* infection is often asymptomatic and is hard to detect in practical terms. Between 1% and 2% of patients with non-specific urethritis seen at genitourinary medicine clinics have SARA (p. 1031). The syndrome of chlamydial urethritis, conjunctivitis and reactive arthritis was formerly known as Reiter's disease.

With enteric triggering infections (enteropathic ReA), HLA-B27 may predict the reactive arthritis and its severity, though the condition occurs in HLA-B27-negative people. The incidence of specific triggering infections causing reactive arthritis around the world varies, depending on the epidemiology of the infection and prevalence of HLA-B27 in the local population.

Clinical features

The onset is typically acute, with an inflammatory enthesitis, oligoarthritis and/or spinal inflammation. Lower limb joints and entheses are predominantly affected. In all types of ReA, there may be considerable systemic disturbance, with fever and weight loss. Achilles insertional enthesitis/tendonitis or plantar fasciitis may also be present. The first attack of arthritis is usually self-limiting, but recurrent or chronic arthritis can develop and about 10% still have active disease 20 years after the initial presentation. Low back pain and stiffness due to enthesitis and osteitis are common and 15–20% of patients develop sacroiliitis. Many extra-articular features in ReA involve the skin, especially in SARA:

- *circinate balanitis*, which starts as vesicles on the coronal margin of the prepuce and glans penis, later rupturing to form superficial erosions with minimal surrounding erythema, some coalescing to give a circular pattern
- *keratoderma blennorrhagica*, which begins as discrete waxy, yellow–brown vesico-papules with desquamating margins, occasionally coalescing to form large crusty plaques on the palms and soles of the feet
- *pustular psoriasis*
- *nail dystrophy* with subungual hyperkeratosis
- *mouth ulcers*
- *conjunctivitis*
- *uveitis*, which is rare with the first attack but arises in 30% of patients with recurring or chronic arthritis.

Other complications in ReA are very rare but include aortic incompetence, conduction defects, pleuro-pericarditis, peripheral neuropathy, seizures and meningoencephalitis.

Investigations

The diagnosis is usually made clinically but joint aspiration may be required to exclude crystal arthritis and articular infection.

24

ESR and CRP are raised, urethritis may be confirmed in the 'two-glass test' by demonstration of mucoid threads in the first-void specimen that clear in the second. High vaginal swabs may reveal *Chlamydia* on culture. Except for post-*Salmonella* arthritis, stool cultures are usually negative by the time the arthritis presents but serology may help confirm previous dysentery. RF, ACPA and ANA are negative.

In chronic or recurrent disease, X-rays show periarticular osteoporosis; proliferative erosions, notably at entheses; periostitis, especially of metatarsals, phalanges and pelvis; and large, 'fluffy' calcaneal spurs. In contrast to AS, radiographic sacroiliitis is often asymmetrical and sometimes unilateral, and syndesmophytes are predominantly coarse and asymmetrical, often extending beyond the contours of the annulus ('non-marginal') (see Fig. 24.40B). Radiographic changes in the peripheral joints and spine are identical to those seen in psoriasis.

Management

Acute ReA should be treated with rest, NSAIDs and analgesics. Intra-articular or systemic glucocorticoids may be required in patients with severe monarticular synovitis or polyarticular disease, respectively. There is no convincing evidence for the use of antibiotics unless a triggering infection is identified. If chlamydial urethritis is diagnosed, it should be treated empirically with a short course of doxycycline or a single dose of azithromycin. Treatment with DMARDs (usually sulfasalazine or methotrexate) should be considered for patients with persistent marked symptoms, recurrent arthritis or severe keratoderma blennorrhagica. Anterior uveitis is a medical emergency requiring topical, subconjunctival or systemic glucocorticoids. For DMARD-recalcitrant cases, anti-TNF therapy should be considered.

Psoriatic arthritis

In the UK and Denmark the estimated population prevalence of psoriatic arthritis (PsA) from registry and coding data is approximately 0.2%. It is likely the true prevalence is considerably higher but this has not been extensively studied. The prevalence of PsA in psoriasis patients, based on clinical assessment, is variable but may be up to 40%. Early PsA may present as axSpA. The onset is usually between 25 and 40 years of age but juvenile forms exist. Occasionally, the arthritis and psoriasis develop synchronously but the onset of musculoskeletal and skin disease is frequently separated by many years. Classification of PsA requires key assessments of family history and screening for enthesitis (Box 24.62).

	24.62 The CASPAR criteria for psoriatic arthritis

Inflammatory articular disease (joint, spine or enthesis) with ≥3 points from the following (1 point each unless stated):
- Current psoriasis (scores 2 points)
- History of psoriasis in first- or second-degree relative
- Psoriatic nail dystrophy
- Negative IgM rheumatoid factor[1]
- Current dactylitis
- History of dactylitis
- Juxta-articular new bone[2]

[1]Established by any method except latex. [2]Ill-defined ossification near joint margins (excluding osteophytes) on X-rays of hands or feet.
(CASPAR = **C**l**AS**sification for **P**soriatic **AR**thritis)

Pathophysiology

Genetic factors have an important role in PsA and family studies have suggested that heritability may exceed 80%. Variants in the *HLA-B* and *HLA-C* genes are the strongest genetic risk factors but more than 30 other variants also play a part. Many of these variants overlap with those implicated in psoriasis (p. 1247), where there are more than 40 susceptibility loci. These lie within or close to genes in the IL-12, IL-23 and nuclear factor kappa B (NFκB) signalling pathways. It is thought that an environmental trigger, probably infectious in nature, triggers the disease in genetically susceptible individuals, leading to immune activation involving dendritic cells and T cells. CD8+ T cells (which recognise antigen presented in the context of HLA class I) are more abundant than CD4+ T cells within the joint, which is in keeping with the genetic association between PsA and HLA-C and B variants. There is increasing evidence that the IL-23/IL-17 pathway plays a pivotal role in PsA. It is thought that the triggering stimulus causes over-production of IL-23 by dendritic cells, which in turn promotes differentiation and activation of Th17 cells, which produce the pro-inflammatory cytokine IL-17A. This, along with Th1 cytokines like IFN-γ and TNF-α, acts on macrophages and tissue-resident stromal cells at entheses, in bone and within the joint to produce additional pro-inflammatory cytokines and other mediators, which contribute to inflammation and tissue damage, as shown in Figure 24.42.

Clinical features

The presentation is with pain and stiffness affecting joints, tendons, spine and entheses. Joints are typically not swollen; however, several patterns of joint involvement are recognised (see below), including an oligoarticular form. These patterns are not mutually exclusive. Marked variation in disease patterns exists, including a disease course of intermittent exacerbation and remission. Destructive arthritis and disability are uncommon, except in the case of arthritis mutilans.

Asymmetrical inflammatory mono-/oligoarthritis

This often presents abruptly with a combination of synovitis and adjacent periarticular inflammation. It occurs most characteristically in the hands and feet, when synovitis of a finger or toe is coupled with tenosynovitis, enthesitis and inflammation of intervening tissue to give a 'sausage digit' or dactylitis (Fig. 24.43A). Large joints, such as the knee and ankle, may also be involved, sometimes with very large effusions.

Symmetrical polyarthritis

This accounts for about 25% of cases. It predominates in women and may resemble RA, with symmetrical involvement of small and large joints in both upper and lower limbs. Nodules and other extra-articular features of RA are absent and arthritis is generally less extensive and more benign.

Distal interphalangeal joint arthritis

This is quite a common pattern and can be difficult to distinguish from inflammatory generalised OA. PsA DIP joint disease is associated with psoriatic nail disease (Fig. 24.43B).

Psoriatic spondylitis

This type presents with inflammatory back or neck pain and prominent stiffness symptoms. Any structure in the spine can be involved, including intervertebral disc entheses and facet joints. It may occur alone or with any of the other clinical patterns described above and is typically unilateral or asymmetric in severity.

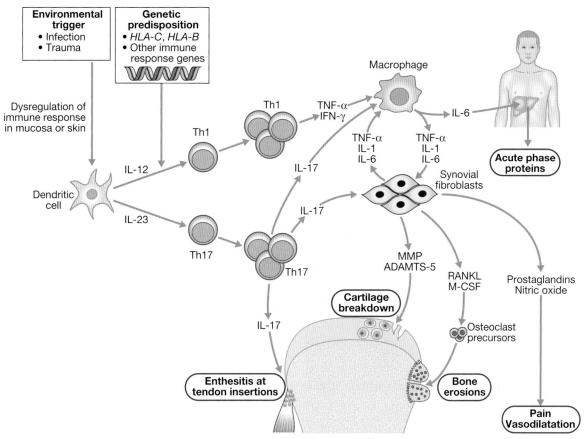

Fig. 24.42 Pathogenesis of psoriatic arthritis. Some of the cytokines and cellular interactions believed to be important in psoriatic arthritis are shown. (ADAMTS-5 = aggrecanase; IL = interleukin; M-CSF = macrophage colony-stimulating factor; MMP = matrix metalloproteinase; TNF = tumour necrosis factor; RANKL = RANK ligand)

Arthritis mutilans

This is a deforming erosive arthritis targeting the fingers and toes; it occurs in 5% of cases of PsA. Prominent cartilage and bone destruction results in marked instability. The encasing skin appears invaginated and 'telescoped' ('main en lorgnette') and the finger can be pulled back to its original length.

Enthesitis-predominant

This form of disease presents with pain and stiffness at the insertion sites of tendons and ligaments into bone (enthesitis). Symptoms can be extensive or localised. Typically affected entheses include Achilles tendon insertions, plantar fascia origins, patellar ligament attachments, hip abductor complex insertion at lateral femoral condyle, gluteus medius insertion at greater trochanter, humeral epicondyle tendon attachments, deltoid origin at acromial edge, intercostal muscle attachments at ribs, and pelvic ligament attachments.

Nail changes include pitting, onycholysis, subungual hyperkeratosis and horizontal ridging, which are found in 85% of patients with PsA and can occur in the absence of skin disease. The characteristic rash of psoriasis (p. 1247) may be widespread, or confined to the scalp, natal cleft, umbilicus and genitals, where it is easily overlooked. Obtaining a history of psoriasis in a first-degree relative can be tricky but is important, given that a positive response contributes to making a diagnosis.

Investigations

The diagnosis is made on clinical grounds. Autoantibodies are generally negative and acute phase reactants, such as ESR and CRP, are raised in only a proportion of patients with active disease. X-rays may be normal or show erosive change with joint space narrowing. Features that favour PsA over RA include the characteristic distribution (see Fig. 24.10, p. 994) of proliferative erosions with marked new bone formation, absence of periarticular osteoporosis and osteosclerosis. Imaging of the axial skeleton often reveals features similar to those in chronic ReA, with coarse, asymmetrical, non-marginal syndesmophytes and asymmetrical sacroiliitis. MRI and ultrasound with power Doppler are increasingly employed to detect synovial inflammation and inflammation at the entheses.

Management

Therapy with NSAIDs and analgesics may be sufficient to manage symptoms in mild disease. Intra-articular glucocorticoid injections can control isolated synovitis or enthesitis. Splints and prolonged rest should be avoided because of the tendency to fibrous and bony ankylosis. Patients with spondylitis should be prescribed the same exercise and posture regime as in axSpA/AS. Therapy with DMARDs should be considered for persistent synovitis unresponsive to conservative treatment. Methotrexate is the drug of first choice and is also effective

24

Fig. 24.43 Psoriatic arthropathy. [A] Dactylitis. [B] Distal interphalangeal joint pattern with accompanying nail dystrophy (pitting and onycholysis).

for skin disease (see EULAR guidelines, 'Further information', p. 1060). Other DMARDs may also be helpful, including sulfasalazine, ciclosporin and leflunomide. Particular attention should be paid to monitoring liver function in patients treated with DMARDs, since abnormalities are common in PsA. Hydroxychloroquine is generally avoided, as it can cause exfoliative skin reactions; it may, however, be tried in the small subset of patients who have mild PsA but no psoriasis and are ANA-positive. Anti-TNF treatment should be considered for individuals with active synovitis who respond inadequately to standard DMARDs, and treatment is effective for both PsA and psoriasis. Ustekinumab, a monoclonal antibody that binds to and neutralises the p40 subunit of IL-12 and IL-23, improves joint, dactylitis and enthesitis lesions in PsA. Secukinumab, a monoclonal antibody that targets IL-17A, has similar efficacy to TNF inhibitors in PsA. Apremilast is an oral small-molecule inhibitor of phosphodiesterase 4 (PDE4), which is effective in PsA when DMARD therapy fails, although it appears to be less efficacious than biologic treatment. Adverse effects include weight loss, depression and suicidal ideation.

Enteropathic (spondylo)arthritis

The overall prevalence of inflammatory musculoskeletal disease in inflammatory bowel diseases (IBDs: Crohn's disease and ulcerative colitis) is not well known, as studies have not adequately assessed enthesitis and osteitis lesions, but the musculoskeletal manifestations are in keeping with an SpA phenotype. Involvement of the peripheral joints is seen in about 20% of IBD patients. Oligoarticular disease predominantly affects the large lower limb joints (knees, ankles and hips). Radiographic evidence of sacroiliitis is present in about 20–25% of IBD patients.

In Crohn's disease, more than in colitis, the arthritis usually coincides with exacerbations of the underlying bowel disease and the arthritis improves with effective treatment of the bowel disease. There is some suggestion that the severity and onset of inflammatory musculoskeletal symptoms can vary in association with changes in the integrity of the ileocaecal valve, raising the possibility that changes in gut flora may act as triggers for the associated SpA.

NSAIDs are best avoided, since they can exacerbate IBD. Instead, judicious use of glucocorticoids, sulfasalazine and methotrexate may be considered. Liaison is necessary between gastroenterologist and rheumatologist with regard to choice of therapy. Anti-TNF therapy is effective in enteropathic arthritis but etanercept should be avoided, as it has no efficacy in IBD. When musculoskeletal symptoms worsen despite anti-TNF therapy, it is wise to exclude bacterial overgrowth as a triggering cause (blind-loop syndrome).

Autoimmune connective tissue diseases

Autoimmune connective tissue diseases (AICTDs) share many clinical features and are characterised by dysregulation of immune responses, autoantibody production that is often directed at components of the cell nucleus, and tissue damage.

Systemic lupus erythematosus

Systemic lupus erythematosus (SLE, 'lupus') is a rare disease with a prevalence that ranges from about 0.03% in Caucasians to 0.2% in Afro-Caribbeans. Some 90% of affected patients are female and the peak age at onset is between 20 and 30 years. SLE is associated with considerable morbidity and a fivefold increase in mortality compared to age- and gender-matched controls, mainly because of an increased risk of premature cardiovascular disease.

Pathophysiology

The cause of SLE is incompletely understood but genetic factors play an important role. There is a higher concordance in monozygotic twins and the disease is strongly associated with polymorphic variants at the HLA locus. In a few instances, SLE is associated with inherited mutations in complement components C1q, C2 and C4, in the immunoglobulin receptor FcγRIIb or in the DNA exonuclease *TREX1*. Genome-wide association studies have identified common polymorphisms near several other genes that predispose to SLE, most of which are involved in regulating immune cell function. From an immunological standpoint, the characteristic feature of SLE is autoantibody production. These autoantibodies have specificity for a wide range of targets but many are directed against antigens present within the cell or within the nucleus. This has led to the hypothesis that SLE may occur because of defects in apoptosis or in the clearance of apoptotic cells, which causes inappropriate exposure of intracellular antigens on the cell surface, leading to polyclonal B- and T-cell activation and autoantibody production. This is supported by the fact that environmental factors that cause flares of lupus, such as ultraviolet light and infections, increase oxidative stress and cause cell damage. Whatever the underlying cause, autoantibody production and immune complex formation are thought to be important mechanisms of tissue damage in active SLE, leading to vasculitis and organ damage.

Clinical features

Symptoms such as fever, weight loss and mild lymphadenopathy may occur during flares of disease activity, whereas others such as fatigue and low-grade joint pains can be constant and not particularly associated with active inflammatory disease.

Arthritis

Arthralgia is a common symptom, occurring in 90% of patients, and is often associated with early morning stiffness. Tenosynovitis may also occur but clinically apparent synovitis with joint swelling is rare. Joint deformities may arise (Jaccoud's arthropathy) as the result of tendon damage but joint erosions are not a feature.

Raynaud's phenomenon

Raynaud's phenomenon (p. 504) is common and may antedate other symptoms by months or years. SLE can present with Raynaud's phenomenon, along with arthralgia or arthritis. Secondary Raynaud's phenomenon associated with SLE and other AICTDs needs to be differentiated from primary Raynaud's phenomenon, which is common in the general population (up to 5%). Features in favour of secondary Raynaud's phenomenon include age at onset of over 25 years, absence of a family history of Raynaud's phenomenon, and occurrence in a male. Examination of capillary nail-fold loops using an ophthalmoscope (and oil placed on the skin) can show loss of the normal loop pattern, with capillary 'fallout' and dilatation and branching of loops; these features support either a diagnosis of systemic sclerosis or severe primary Raynaud's phenomenon. If Raynaud's phenomenon is severe, digital ulceration can occur (Fig. 24.44).

Skin

The skin is commonly involved in SLE, and many SLE skin eruptions are precipitated by exposure to ultraviolet light. The main types of skin involvement are:

- The classic facial rash (up to 20% of patients). This is erythematous, raised and painful or itchy, and occurs over the cheeks with sparing of the nasolabial folds (Fig. 24.45). Rosacea is a mimic of this rash.
- A discoid rash characterised by hyperkeratosis and follicular plugging, with scarring alopecia if it occurs on the scalp.
- Diffuse, usually non-scarring alopecia, which may also occur with active disease.
- Urticarial eruptions.
- Livedo reticularis (Fig. 24.46), which is also a feature of antiphospholipid syndrome (p. 977) and can become frankly vasculitic, if severe.

Kidney

Renal involvement is one of the main determinants of prognosis and regular monitoring of urinalysis and blood pressure is essential. The typical renal lesion is a proliferative glomerulonephritis (p. 397), characterised by heavy haematuria, proteinuria and casts on urine microscopy.

Cardiovascular

The most common manifestation is pericarditis. Myocarditis and Libman–Sacks endocarditis can also occur. The endocarditis is due to accumulation on the heart valves of sterile fibrin-containing vegetations, which is thought to be a manifestation of hypercoagulability associated with antiphospholipid antibodies. The risk of atherosclerosis is greatly increased, as is the risk of stroke and myocardial infarction. This is thought to be multifactorial

Fig. 24.44 Severe secondary Raynaud's phenomenon leading to digital ulceration.

Fig. 24.45 Malar rash of systemic lupus erythematosus, sparing the nasolabial folds. The rash is notably similar to rosacea, which may itself be associated with inflammatory joint diseases such as psoriatic arthritis.

due to the adverse effects of inflammation on the endothelium, chronic glucocorticoid therapy and the procoagulant effects of antiphospholipid antibodies.

Lung

Lung involvement is common and most frequently manifests as pleuritic pain (serositis) or pleural effusion. Other features include pneumonitis, atelectasis, reduced lung volume and pulmonary fibrosis that leads to breathlessness. The risk of thromboembolism is increased, especially in patients with antiphospholipid antibodies.

Neurological

Fatigue, headache and poor concentration are common and often occur in the absence of laboratory evidence of active disease. More specific features of cerebral lupus include visual hallucinations, chorea, organic psychosis, transverse myelitis and lymphocytic meningitis.

Haematological

Neutropenia, lymphopenia, thrombocytopenia and haemolytic anaemia may occur, due to antibody-mediated destruction of

Fig. 24.46 Livedo reticularis (systemic lupus erythematosus and anti-phospholipid syndrome).

24.63 Criteria for the classification of systemic lupus erythematosus	
Features	**Characteristics**
Malar rash	Fixed erythema, flat or raised, sparing the nasolabial folds
Discoid rash	Erythematous raised patches with adherent keratotic scarring and follicular plugging
Photosensitivity	Rash due to unusual reaction to sunlight
Oral ulcers	Oral or nasopharyngeal ulceration, which may be painless
Arthritis	Non-erosive, involving two or more peripheral joints
Serositis	Pleuritis (history of pleuritic pain or rub, or pleural effusion) *or* pericarditis (rub, electrocardiogram evidence or effusion)
Renal disorder	Persistent proteinuria >0.5 g/24 hrs *or* cellular casts (red cell, granular or tubular)
Neurological disorder	Seizures or psychosis, in the absence of provoking drugs or metabolic derangement
Haematological disorder	Haemolytic anaemia *or* leucopenia* $(<4 \times 10^9/L)$ *or* lymphopenia* $(<1 \times 10^9/L)$ *or* thrombocytopenia* $(<100 \times 10^9/L)$ in the absence of offending drugs
Immunological	Anti-DNA antibodies in abnormal titre *or* presence of antibody to Sm antigen *or* positive antiphospholipid antibodies
Antinuclear antibody (ANA)	Abnormal titre of ANA by immunofluorescence
An adult has SLE if any 4 of 11 features are present serially or simultaneously	

*On two separate occasions.

peripheral blood cells. The degree of lymphopenia is a good guide to disease activity.

Gastrointestinal

Mouth ulcers may occur and may or may not be painful. Peritoneal serositis can cause acute pain. Mesenteric vasculitis is a serious complication, which can present with abdominal pain, bowel infarction or perforation. Hepatitis is a recognised, though rare, feature.

Paediatric disease

Renal disease and cutaneous manifestations are more frequent in juvenile-onset SLE compared to disease in adults. Similarly, there is subsequently a higher incidence of renal disease, malar rash, Raynaud's phenomenon, cutaneous vasculitis and neuropsychiatric manifestations than in adults.

Investigations

The diagnosis is based on a combination of clinical features and laboratory abnormalities. To fulfil the classification criteria for SLE, at least 4 of the 11 factors shown in Box 24.63 must be present or have occurred in the past. Checking of ANAs, antibodies to ENAs and complement, routine haematology, biochemistry and urinalysis are mandatory. Patients with active SLE test positive for ANA. Some authorities believe that ANA-negative SLE occurs (e.g. in the presence of antibodies to Ro) but others regard SLE as necessarily ANA-positive; the issue may be more to do with sensitivity of the ANA assay at any given time in a disease course. Anti-dsDNA antibodies are positive in many, but not all, patients and are tested at the time of diagnosis by most laboratories using ELISA. ELISAs have low specificity, whereas testing for anti-dsDNA antibodies using *Crithidia luciliae* is highly specific. Patients with active disease tend to have low levels of C3 due to complement consumption, but in some people low C3 and C4 may be the result of inherited complement deficiency in C1, C2 or C4 that predisposes to SLE (p. 66). Studies of other family members can help to differentiate inherited deficiency from complement consumption. A raised ESR, leucopenia and lymphopenia are typical of active SLE, along with anaemia, haemolytic anaemia and thrombocytopenia. CRP is often normal in active SLE, except in the presence of serositis; thus an elevated CRP suggests infection.

Management

The therapeutic goals are to educate the patient about the nature of the illness, to control symptoms and to prevent organ damage and maintain normal function. Patients should be advised to avoid sun and ultraviolet light exposure and to employ sun blocks (sun protection factor 25–50).

Mild to moderate disease

Patients with mild disease restricted to skin and joints can sometimes be managed with analgesics, NSAIDs and hydroxy-chloroquine. Frequently, however, glucocorticoids are also necessary (prednisolone 5–20 mg/day), often in combination with immunosuppressants such as methotrexate, azathioprine or mycophenolate mofetil (MMF). Increased doses of glucocorticoids may be required for flares in activity or complications such as pleurisy or pericarditis. The monoclonal antibody belimumab, which targets the β-cell growth factor BLyS, has recently been shown to be effective in patients with active SLE who have responded inadequately to standard therapy.

Severe and life-threatening disease

High-dose glucocorticoids and immunosuppressants are required for the treatment of renal, CNS and cardiac involvement. A commonly used regimen is pulsed methylprednisolone (10 mg/kg IV) plus cyclophosphamide (15 mg/kg IV), repeated at 2–3-weekly intervals for six cycles. Cyclophosphamide may cause haemorrhagic cystitis but the risk can be minimised by good hydration and co-prescription of mesna (2-mercaptoethane sulfonate), which binds its urotoxic metabolites. Because of the risk of azoospermia and premature menopause, sperm or oöcyte collection and storage need to be considered prior to treatment with cyclophosphamide.

MMF has been used successfully with high-dose glucocorticoids for renal involvement with results similar to those of pulsed cyclophosphamide but fewer adverse effects. Belimumab in combination with standard therapy significantly decreases disease activity in SLE patients and is safe and well tolerated. Its role in patients with renal and neurological disease is still under investigation.

Rituximab has been reported as being effective in selected cases, though randomised controlled trials have not shown significant overall efficacy.

Maintenance therapy

Following control of acute disease, a typical maintenance regimen is oral prednisolone in a dose of 40–60 mg daily, gradually reducing to 10–15 mg/day or less by 3 months. Azathioprine (2–2.5 mg/kg/day), methotrexate (10–25 mg/week) or MMF (2–3 g/day) should also be prescribed. The long-term aim is to continue the lowest dose of glucocorticoid and immunosuppressant to maintain remission. Cardiovascular risk factors, such as hypertension and hyperlipidaemia, should be controlled and patients should be advised to stop smoking.

Patients with SLE and the antiphospholipid antibody syndrome, who have had previous thrombosis, require life-long warfarin therapy. SLE patients are at risk of osteoporosis and hypovitaminosis D, and should be screened with biochemistry and DXA scanning accordingly.

Systemic sclerosis

Systemic sclerosis (SScl) is an autoimmune disorder of connective tissue, which results in fibrosis affecting the skin, internal organs and vasculature. It is characterised typically by Raynaud's phenomenon, digital ischaemia (Fig. 24.47), sclerodactyly, and cardiac, lung, gut and renal disease. The peak age of onset is in the fourth and fifth decades and overall prevalence is 10–20 per 100 000, with a 4 : 1 female-to-male. It is subdivided into diffuse cutaneous systemic sclerosis (dcSScl: 30% of cases) and limited cutaneous systemic sclerosis (lcSScl: 70% of cases). Some patients with lcSScl have calcinosis and telangiectasia. The prognosis in dcSScl is poor (5-year survival about 70%). Features that associate with a poor prognosis include older age, diffuse skin disease, proteinuria, high ESR, a low gas transfer factor for carbon monoxide (TLCO) and pulmonary hypertension.

Pathophysiology

The cause of SScl is not completely understood. There is evidence for a genetic component and associations with alleles at the HLA locus have been found. The disease occurs in all ethnic groups and race may influence severity. Isolated cases have been reported in which an SScl-like disease has been triggered by exposure to silica dust, vinyl chloride, epoxy resins and trichloroethylene. There is clear evidence of immunological dysfunction: T lymphocytes, especially those of the Th17 subtype, infiltrate the skin and there is abnormal fibroblast activation, leading to increased production of extracellular matrix in the dermis, primarily type I collagen. This results in symmetrical thickening, tightening and induration of the skin (scleroderma). Arterial and arteriolar narrowing occurs due to intimal proliferation and vessel wall inflammation. Endothelial injury causes release of vasoconstrictors and platelet activation, resulting in further ischaemia, which is thought to exacerbate the fibrotic process.

Clinical features

Skin

Initially, there is non-pitting oedema of fingers and flexor tendon sheaths. Subsequently, the skin becomes shiny and taut, and distal skin creases disappear. There can be capillary loss. The face and neck are often involved, with thinning of the lips and radial furrowing. In some patients, skin thickening stops at this stage. Skin involvement restricted to sites distal to the elbow or knee (apart from the face) is thus classified as lcSScl (Fig. 24.48). Involvement proximal to the knee and elbow and on the trunk is classified as 'diffuse disease' (dcSScl).

Raynaud's phenomenon

This is a universal feature and can precede other features by many years. Involvement of small blood vessels in the extremities may cause critical tissue ischaemia, leading to localised distal skin infarction and necrosis.

Musculoskeletal features

Arthralgia and flexor tenosynovitis are common. Restricted hand function is due to skin rather than joint disease and erosive arthropathy is uncommon. Muscle weakness and wasting can result from myositis.

Gastrointestinal involvement

Smooth muscle atrophy and fibrosis in the lower two-thirds of the oesophagus lead to reflux with erosive oesophagitis.

24

Fig. 24.47 Systemic sclerosis. Hands showing tight, shiny skin, sclerodactyly, flexion contractures of the fingers and thickening of the left middle finger extensor tendon sheath.

Fig. 24.48 Typical facial appearance showing telangiectasias in localised cutaneous systemic sclerosis.

Dysphagia and odynophagia may also occur. Involvement of the stomach causes early satiety and occasionally outlet obstruction. Recurrent occult upper gastrointestinal bleeding may indicate a 'watermelon' stomach (antral vascular ectasia; up to 20% of patients). Small intestine involvement may lead to malabsorption due to bacterial overgrowth and intermittent bloating, pain or constipation. Dilatation of bowel due to autonomic neuropathy may cause pseudo-obstruction with nausea, vomiting, abdominal discomfort and distension, often worse after food (symptoms can mimic those of an acute abdomen and can lead to erroneous laparotomy).

Pulmonary involvement

Pulmonary hypertension complicates long-standing disease and is six times more prevalent in lcSSc than in dcSScl. It usually presents with insidiously evolving exertional dyspnoea and signs of right heart failure. Interstitial lung disease is common in patients with dcSScl who have topoisomerase 1 antibodies (Scl70). Dyspnoea can evolve slowly over time or rapidly in occasional cases.

Renal involvement

One of the main causes of death is hypertensive renal crisis, characterised by rapidly developing accelerated phase hypertension (p. 514) and renal failure. Hypertensive renal crisis is much more likely to occur in dcSScl than in lcSScl, and in patients with topoisomerase 1 and RNP antibodies.

Investigations

As SScl can affect multiple organs, routine haematology, renal, liver and bone function tests and urinalysis are essential. ANA is positive in about 70%. About 30% of patients with dcSScl have antibodies to topoisomerase 1 (Scl70). About 60% of patients with lcSScl syndrome have anticentromere antibodies (p. 991). Chest X-ray, transthoracic echocardiography and lung function tests are recommended to assess for interstitial lung disease and pulmonary hypertension (low corrected transfer factor may indicate early pulmonary hypertension). High-resolution lung CT is recommended if interstitial lung disease suspected. If pulmonary hypertension is suspected, right heart catheter measurements should be arranged at a specialist cardiac centre. A barium swallow can assess oesophageal involvement. A hydrogen breath test can indicate bacterial overgrowth (p. 808).

Management

No treatments are available that halt or reverse the fibrotic changes that underlie the disease. The focus of management, therefore, is to slow the effects of the disease on target organs.

- *Raynaud's phenomenon and digital ulcers*. Avoidance of cold exposure, use of thermal insulating gloves/socks and maintenance of a high core temperature all help. If symptoms are persistent, calcium channel blockers, losartan, fluoxetine and sildenafil have efficacy. Courses of intravenous prostacyclin are used for severe disease and critical ischemia (e.g. 6–8 hours daily for 5 days). The endothelin-1 antagonist bosentan is licensed for treating ischaemic digital ulcers, and digital tip tissue health can be maintained with regular use of fucidin–hydrocortisone cream.
- *Gastrointestinal complications*. Oesophageal reflux should be treated with proton pump inhibitors and anti-reflux agents. Rotating courses of antibiotics may be required for bacterial overgrowth (e.g. rifaximin, a tetracycline and metronidazole), while metoclopramide or domperidone

may help patients with symptoms of dysmotility/pseudo-obstruction.
- *Hypertension*. Aggressive treatment with ACE inhibitors is needed, even if renal impairment is present.
- *Joint involvement*. This may be treated with analgesics and/or NSAIDs. If synovitis is present and both RA (i.e. an 'overlap' condition, which needs treatment on its own merit) and OA have been ruled out, low-dose methotrexate can be of value.
- *Progressive pulmonary hypertension*. Early treatment with bosentan is required. In severe or progressive disease, heart–lung transplant may be considered.
- *Interstitial lung disease*. Glucocorticoids and (pulse intravenous) cyclophosphamide are the mainstays of treatment in patients who have progressive interstitial lung disease.

Mixed connective tissue disease

Mixed connective tissue disease (MCTD) is a condition in which some clinical features of SScl, myositis and SLE all occur in the same patient. It commonly presents with indolent puffiness of the fingers (the appearance is between that of SpA-type dactylitis and sclerodactyly) with Raynaud's phenomenon and myalgias. Most patients have anti-RNP antibodies. Management focuses on treating the components of the disease (see other sections).

Primary Sjögren's syndrome

Primary Sjögren's syndrome (PSS) is characterised by lymphocytic infiltration of salivary and lacrimal glands, leading to glandular fibrosis and exocrine failure. The typical age of onset is between 40 and 50, with a 9:1 female-to-male ratio. The disease may occur with other autoimmune diseases (secondary Sjögren's syndrome).

Clinical features

The eye symptoms, termed keratoconjunctivitis sicca, are due to a lack of lubricating tears, which reflects inflammatory infiltration of the lacrimal glands. Conjunctivitis and blepharitis are frequent, and may lead to filamentary keratitis due to binding of tenacious mucous filaments to the cornea and conjunctiva. Oral involvement manifests as a dry mouth (xerostomia). There is a high incidence of dental caries and high risk of dental failure. Other sites of extraglandular involvement are listed in Box 24.64. Often the most disabling symptom is fatigue. There may be an association with inflammatory small-joint OA (clinical suspicion, though formal studies have not been done). Sialadenitis, osteoarthritis and xerostomia (SOX) syndrome has been described; this may occur independently of PSS or, more likely, constitute a mild form. Both interstitial lung disease and interstitial nephritis (sometimes complicated by renal tubular acidosis) require proactive screening. PSS is associated with a 40-fold increased lifetime risk of lymphoma, though the complication is still very rare.

Investigations

The diagnosis can be established by the Schirmer tear test, which measures tear flow over 5 minutes using absorbent paper strips placed on the lower eyelid; a normal result is more than 6 mm of wetting. Staining with rose bengal may show punctate epithelial abnormalities over the area not covered by the open eyelid. If the diagnosis remains in doubt, it can be confirmed by demonstrating focal lymphocytic infiltrate in a minor salivary gland biopsy. Most patients have an elevated ESR and

Risk factors

- Age of onset 40–60
- Female > male
- HLA-B8/DR3

Common clinical features

- Keratoconjunctivitis sicca
- Xerostomia
- Salivary gland enlargement
- Rashes/skin irritation
- Non-erosive arthralgia
- Generalised osteoarthritis
- Raynaud's phenomenon
- Fatigue

Less common features

- Low-grade fever
- Interstitial lung disease
- Anaemia, leucopenia
- Thrombocytopenia
- Cryoglobulinaemia
- Vasculitis
- Peripheral neuropathy
- Lymphadenopathy
- Lymphoreticular lymphoma
- Glomerulonephritis
- Interstitial nephritis
- Renal tubular acidosis

Autoantibodies frequently detected

- Rheumatoid factor
- Antinuclear antibody
- SS-A (anti-Ro)
- SS-B (anti-La)
- Gastric parietal cell
- Thyroid

Associated autoimmune disorders

- Systemic lupus erythematosus
- Systemic sclerosis
- Coeliac disease
- Primary biliary cholangitis
- Chronic active hepatitis
- Myasthenia gravis

(HLA = human leucocyte antigen)

Fig. 24.49 Typical eyelid appearance in dermatomyositis. Note the oedema and telangiectasia.

Polymyositis and dermatomyositis

Polymyositis (PM) and dermatomyositis (DM) are characterised by proximal skeletal and (cardiac and gut) smooth muscle inflammation. In DM, characteristic skin changes also occur. Both diseases are rare, with an incidence of 2–10 cases per million/year. They can occur in isolation or in association with other autoimmune diseases, and both are notably connected with (either previously diagnosed or undisclosed) malignancy.

Clinical features

The typical presentation of PM and DM is with symmetrical proximal muscle weakness over a few weeks, usually affecting the lower limbs more than the upper, in adults between 40 and 60 years of age. Patients report difficulty rising from a chair, climbing stairs and lifting, often (though not always) with muscle pain. Systemic features of fever, weight loss and fatigue are common. Respiratory or pharyngeal muscle involvement can lead to ventilatory failure or aspiration that requires urgent treatment. Interstitial lung disease occurs in up to 30% of patients and is strongly associated with the presence of antisynthetase (Jo-1) antibodies.

In DM, the skin lesions include Gottron's papules, which are scaly, erythematous or violaceous, psoriasiform plaques occurring over the extensor surfaces of PIP and DIP joints, and a heliotrope rash that is a violaceous discoloration of the eyelid in combination with periorbital oedema (Fig. 24.49). Similar rashes occur on the upper back, chest and shoulders ('shawl' distribution). Periungual nail-fold capillaries are often enlarged and tortuous.

Investigations

Muscle biopsy is the pivotal investigation and shows the typical features of fibre necrosis, regeneration and inflammatory cell infiltrate (Fig. 24.50). Occasionally, however, a biopsy may be normal, particularly if myositis is patchy so, invariably, MRI should be used to identify areas of abnormal muscle for biopsy. Serum levels of creatine kinase are typically raised and are a useful measure of disease activity, although a normal creatine kinase does not exclude the diagnosis, particularly in juvenile myositis. Electromyography is very useful for highlighting non-autoimmune/non-inflammatory myopathies. Screening for underlying malignancy should be undertaken routinely (full examination, chest X-ray, serum urine and protein electrophoresis, CT of chest/abdomen/pelvis; prostate-specific antigen should be included in men, and mammography in women).

hypergammaglobulinaemia, and one or more autoantibodies, including ANA and RF. ANA-negative disease exists. Anti-Ro and anti-La antibodies are commonly present (see Box 24.10, p. 992). Patients with joint pain, fatigue and RF (with or without ANA) need careful assessment because a number of possibilities exist: PSS and inflammatory OA; RA with incidental ANA; RA/SLE overlap; or RA/PSS overlap. Knowing ACPA status can help (it is positive in RA). Interstitial lung disease complicates PSS in a sizable minority of patients (persistent dry cough, dyspnoea, coarse 'Velcro' crackles on lung auscultation). A chest X-ray and lung function tests should be performed.

Management

No treatments that have disease-modifying effects have yet been identified and management is symptomatic. Lacrimal substitutes, such as hypromellose, should be used during the day in combination with more viscous lubricating application at night. Soft contact lenses can be useful for corneal protection in patients with filamentary keratitis, and occlusion of the lacrimal ducts is occasionally needed. Artificial saliva sprays, saliva-stimulating tablets, and pastilles and oral gels can be tried for xerostomia but often chewing gum is most effective. Adequate postprandial oral hygiene and prompt treatment of oral candidiasis are essential. Vaginal dryness is treated with lubricants. A trial of systemic pilocarpine (5–30 mg daily in divided doses) is worthwhile in early disease to amplify glandular function. Hydroxychloroquine (200 mg twice daily) is often used to address skin and musculoskeletal features and may help fatigue. Immunosuppression does not improve sicca symptoms but is essential for progressive interstitial lung disease (e.g. glucocorticoids and cyclophosphamide) and for interstitial nephritis (if hydroxychloroquine is ineffective alone). If non-resolving lymphadenopathy or salivary gland enlargement develops, biopsy should be undertaken to exclude malignancy.

Fig. 24.50 Muscle biopsy from a patient with polymyositis.
The sample shows an intense inflammatory cell infiltrate in an area of degenerating and regenerating muscle fibres.

Management

Oral glucocorticoids (prednisolone 1 mg/kg daily) are the mainstay of initial treatment of PM and DM but high-dose intravenous methylprednisolone (1 g/day for 3 days) may be required in patients with respiratory or pharyngeal weakness. If there is a good response, glucocorticoids should be reduced by approximately 25% per month to a maintenance dose of 5–7.5 mg. Although most patients respond well to glucocorticoids, many need additional immunosuppressive therapy. Methotrexate and MMF are the first choices of many but azathioprine and ciclosporin are also used as alternatives. Rituximab appears to show efficacy in a majority of patients, although the only controlled study (which was criticised for its suboptimal design) was negative. In clinical practice, rituximab is an option for use with glucocorticoids, to maintain an early glucocorticoid-induced remission. Intravenous immunoglobulin (IVIg) may be effective in refractory cases. Mepacrine or hydroxychloroquine has been used for skin-predominant disease to some good effect in certain cases. One risk of treatment is glucocorticoid-induced myopathy. If the initial response to treatment is poor, further biopsy then shows type II fibre atrophy in glucocorticoid myopathy (compared with fibre necrosis and regeneration in active myositis).

Juvenile dermatomyositis

Juvenile dermatomyositis (JDM) is by far the most common inflammatory myopathy in children and adolescents, and typically does not require a search for malignancy. The incidence is 2–4 per million (USA and UK) with a median age of onset of 7 years (25% are below 4 years at diagnosis). Many clinical features are similar to those in the adult disease. JDM can be monocyclic, lasting up to 3 years (25–40%), or polycyclic, with periods of remission and relapse (60–75%). In some cases, polycyclic JDM can be chronic and life-long. It is ulcerative in 10–20%. As in adults, calcinosis occurs in about 30%.

Intravenous methylprednisolone, then oral glucocorticoids and methotrexate produce a rapid response in many cases. Cyclophosphamide is used for lesional ulceration. IVIg is given in resistant cases.

Undifferentiated autoimmune connective tissue disease

In some patients, clinical features of AICTD occur, either simultaneously or sequentially, but at any one time the features and results of investigations do not allow a clear diagnosis to be made on the basis of conventional criteria. However, recognising that autoimmunity is present ('autoimmune diathesis') without making a specific diagnosis can help patients move forwards with chronic symptomology. Some of these individuals will progress to having a recognisable AICTD with time; others will continue to have an undifferentiated disease that remains the same for many years, and in others the symptoms will recede. Clinical monitoring and periodic autoimmune serological testing of all patients is sensible.

Adult-onset Still's disease

Adult-onset Still's disease is a rare systemic inflammatory disorder of unknown cause, possibly triggered by infection; it is similar to sJIA. It presents with intermittent fever, rash and arthralgia, and has been associated with pregnancy and the postpartum period and with high levels of IL-18. Splenomegaly, hepatomegaly and lymphadenopathy may be present. Investigations typically provide evidence of an acute phase response, with a markedly elevated serum ferritin. Tests for RF and ANA are negative and so adult-onset Still's disease may be better classified as an autoinflammatory rather than an autoimmune disease. Most patients respond to glucocorticoids but immunosuppressants, such as azathioprine or MMF, can be added when response is inadequate. Canakinumab or anakinra can be used for patients with resistant disease.

Vasculitis

Vasculitis is characterised by inflammation and necrosis of blood-vessel walls, with associated damage to skin, kidney, lung, heart, brain and gastrointestinal tract. There is a wide spectrum of involvement and severity, ranging from mild and transient disease affecting only the skin, to life-threatening fulminant disease with multiple organ failure. Principal sites of involvement for the main types of vasculitis are summarised in Figure 24.51. The clinical features result from a combination of local tissue ischaemia (due to vessel inflammation and narrowing) and the systemic effects of widespread inflammation. Systemic vasculitis should be considered in any patient with fever, weight loss, fatigue,

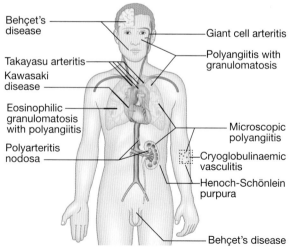

Fig. 24.51 Types of vasculitis. The anatomical targets of different forms of vasculitis are shown.

Systemic

- Malaise
- Fever
- Night sweats
- Weight loss with arthralgia and myalgia

Rashes

- Palpable purpura
- Pulp infarcts
- Ulceration
- Livedo reticularis

Ear, nose and throat

- Epistaxis
- Recurrent sinusitis
- Deafness

Respiratory

- Haemoptysis
- Cough
- Poorly controlled asthma

Gastrointestinal

- Abdominal pain (due to mucosal inflammation or enteric ischaemia)
- Mouth ulcers
- Diarrhoea

Neurological

- Sensory or motor neuropathy

Fig. 24.52 Eye involvement in antineutrophil cytoplasmic antibody-associated vasculitis.

evidence of multisystem involvement, rashes, raised inflammatory markers and abnormal urinalysis (Box 24.65).

Antineutrophil cytoplasmic antibody-associated vasculitis

Antineutrophil cytoplasmic antibody-associated vasculitis (AAV) is a life-threatening disorder characterised by inflammatory infiltration of small blood vessels, fibrinoid necrosis and the presence of circulating antibodies to antineutrophil cytoplasmic antibody (ANCA). The combined incidence is about 10–15/1 000 000. Two main subtypes are recognised. Microscopic polyangiitis is a necrotising small-vessel vasculitis found with rapidly progressive glomerulonephritis, often in association with alveolar haemorrhage. Cutaneous and gastrointestinal involvement is common and other features include neuropathy (15%) and pleural effusions (15%). Patients are usually myeloperoxidase (MPO) antibody-positive. Secondly, granulomatosis with polyangiitis (formerly known as Wegener's granulomatosis) is characterised by granuloma formation, mainly affecting the nasal passages, airways and kidney. A minority of patients present with glomerulonephritis. The most common presentation of granulomatosis with polyangiitis is with epistaxis, nasal crusting and sinusitis, but haemoptysis and mucosal ulceration may also occur. Deafness may be a feature due to inner ear involvement, and proptosis may occur because of inflammation of the retro-orbital tissue (Fig. 24.52). This causes diplopia due to entrapment of the extra-ocular muscles, or loss of vision due to optic nerve compression. Disturbance of colour vision is an early feature of optic nerve compression. Untreated nasal disease ultimately leads to destruction of bone and cartilage. Migratory pulmonary infiltrates and nodules occur in 50% of patients (as seen on high-resolution CT of lungs). Patients with granulomatosis with polyangiitis are usually proteinase-3 (PR3) antibody-positive (ELISA).

Patients with active disease usually have a leucocytosis with elevated CRP, ESR and PR3. Complement levels are usually normal or slightly elevated. Imaging of the upper airways or chest

with MRI can be useful in localising abnormalities but, where possible, the diagnosis should be confirmed by biopsy of the kidney or lesions in the sinuses and upper airways.

Management for organ-threatening or acute–severe disease is with high-dose glucocorticoids (e.g. daily pulse intravenous methylprednisolone 0.5–1 g for 3 days, then oral prednisolone 0.5 mg/kg) and intravenous cyclophosphamide (e.g. 0.5–1 g every 2 weeks for 3 months), followed by maintenance therapy with lower-dose glucocorticoids and azathioprine, methotrexate or MMF. Plasmapheresis should be considered for fulminant lung disease. Rituximab in combination with high-dose glucocorticoids is equally effective as *oral* cyclophosphamide at inducing remission in AAV. Glucocorticoids and methotrexate are an effective combination for treating limited AAV where there is indolent sinus, lung or skin disease. AAV has a tendency to relapse and patients must be followed on a regular and long-term basis, monitoring urinalysis for blood and protein, plasma creatinine, ESR, CRP, lung function and PR3 or MPO antibody titres.

Takayasu arteritis

Takayasu arteritis affects the aorta, its major branches and occasionally the pulmonary arteries. The typical age at onset is 25–30 years, with an 8:1 female-to-male ratio. It has a worldwide distribution but is most common in Asia. Takayasu arteritis is characterised by granulomatous inflammation of the vessel wall, leading to occlusion or weakening of the vessel wall. It presents with claudication, fever, arthralgia and weight loss. Clinical examination may reveal loss of pulses, bruits, hypertension and aortic incompetence. Investigation will identify an acute phase response and normocytic, normochromic anaemia but the diagnosis is based on angiography, which reveals coarctation, occlusion and aneurysmal dilatation. Treatment is with high-dose glucocorticoids and immunosuppressants, as described for ANCA-associated vasculitis. With successful treatment, the 5-year survival is 83%.

Kawasaki disease

Kawasaki disease is a vasculitis that mostly involves the coronary vessels. It presents as an acute systemic disorder, usually affecting children under 5 years. It occurs mainly in Japan and other Asian countries, such as China and Korea, but other ethnic groups may also be affected. Presentation is with fever, generalised rash, including palms and soles, inflamed oral mucosa and conjunctival injection resembling a viral exanthem. The cause is unknown but

24

Fig. 24.53 Rash of systemic vasculitis (palpable purpura).

i	24.66 Conditions that can mimic polymyalgia rheumatica

- Calcium pyrophosphate disease
- Spondyloarthritis
- Hyper-/hypothyroidism
- Psoriatic arthritis (enthesopathic)
- Systemic vasculitis
- Myeloma
- Inflammatory myopathy (particularly inclusion body myositis, p. 1059)
- Lambert–Eaton syndrome (p. 1143)
- Multiple separate lesions (cervical spondylosis, cervical radiculopathy, bilateral subacromial impingement, facet joint arthritis, osteoarthritis of the acromioclavicular joint)

is thought to be an abnormal immune response to an infectious trigger. Cardiovascular complications include coronary arteritis, leading to myocardial infarction, transient coronary dilatation, myocarditis, pericarditis, peripheral vascular insufficiency and gangrene. Treatment is with aspirin (5 mg/kg daily for 14 days) and IVIg (400 mg/kg daily for 4 days).

Polyarteritis nodosa

Polyarteritis nodosa has a peak incidence between the ages of 40 and 50, with a male-to-female ratio of 2:1. The annual incidence is about 2/1 000 000. Hepatitis B is an important risk factor and the incidence is 10 times higher in the Inuit of Alaska, in whom hepatitis B infection is endemic. Presentation is with fever, myalgia, arthralgia and weight loss, in combination with manifestations of multisystem disease. The most common skin lesions are palpable purpura (Fig. 24.53), ulceration, infarction and livedo reticularis (see Fig. 24.46). Pathological changes comprise necrotising inflammation and vessel occlusion, and in 70% of patients arteritis of the vasa nervorum leads to neuropathy, which is typically symmetrical and affects both sensory and motor function. Severe hypertension and/or renal impairment may occur due to multiple renal infarctions but glomerulonephritis is rare (in contrast to microscopic polyangiitis). The diagnosis is confirmed by conventional or magnetic resonance angiography, which shows multiple aneurysms and smooth narrowing of mesenteric, hepatic or renal systems, or by muscle or sural nerve biopsy, which reveals the histological changes described above. Treatment is with high-dose glucocorticoids and immunosuppressants, as described for ANCA-associated vasculitis.

Giant cell arteritis and polymyalgia rheumatica

Giant cell arteritis (GCA) is a granulomatous arteritis that affects any large (including aorta) and medium-sized arteries. It is commonly associated with polymyalgia rheumatica (PMR), which presents with symmetrical, immobility-associated neck and shoulder girdle pain and stiffness. Since many patients with GCA

have symptoms of PMR, and many patients with PMR go on to develop GCA if untreated, many rheumatologists consider them to be different manifestations of the same underlying disorder. Both diseases are rare under the age of 60 years. The average age at onset is 70, with a female-to-male ratio of about 3:1. The overall prevalence is about 20 per 100 000 in those over the age of 50 years.

Clinical features

The cardinal symptom of GCA is headache, which is often localised to the temporal or occipital region and may be accompanied by scalp tenderness. Jaw pain develops in some patients, brought on by chewing or talking. Visual disturbance can occur (most specifically amaurosis) and a catastrophic presentation is with blindness in one eye due to occlusion of the posterior ciliary artery. On fundoscopy, the optic disc may appear pale and swollen with haemorrhages, but these changes may take 24–36 hours to develop and the fundi may initially appear normal. Rarely, neurological involvement may occur, with transient ischaemic attacks, brainstem infarcts and hemiparesis.

In GCA, constitutional symptoms, such as weight loss, fatigue, malaise and night sweats, are common. With PMR, there may be stiffness and painful restriction of active shoulder movements on waking. Muscles are not otherwise tender, and weakness and muscle-wasting are absent. Other conditions that cause PMR-like symptoms are shown in Box 24.66.

Investigations

The typical laboratory abnormality is an elevated ESR, often with a normochromic, normocytic anaemia. CRP may also be elevated and abnormal liver function can occur. Rarely, PMR and GCA can present with a normal ESR. More objective evidence for GCA should be obtained whenever possible. There are three investigations to consider: temporal artery biopsy, ultrasound of the temporal arteries and ^{19}fluorodeoxyglucose positron emission tomography (^{19}FDG PET scan). Characteristic biopsy findings are fragmentation of the internal elastic lamina with necrosis of the media in combination with a mixed inflammatory cell infiltrate. Diagnostic yield is highest with multiple biopsies and multiple section analysis (to detect 'skip' lesions). A negative biopsy does not exclude the diagnosis. On ultrasound examination, affected temporal arteries show a 'halo' sign. A strongly positive ^{19}FDG PET scan is highly specific but sensitivity is low. Caution is needed in interpreting weakly positive images. Low-grade vascular uptake may occur in atheromatous arterial disease.

Management

Prednisolone should be commenced urgently in suspected GCA because of the risk of visual loss (Box 24.67). Response

24.67 Emergency management of giant cell arteritis

- Take blood for CRP, ESR, FBC, bone/liver/renal function, serum protein electrophoresis, CPK, RF, ACPA, ANA, ANCA, complement C3 and C4, immunoglobulins, PTH, TSH, vitamin D and urine electrophoresis
- Commence prednisolone (40–60 mg daily), and simultaneously, a weekly oral bisphosphonate and calcium with vitamin D supplements
- Consider urgent ophthalmology examination and temporal artery biopsy in patients with visual symptoms
- Consider obtaining temporal artery ultrasound or ¹⁹FDG-PET scan
- Review within 1 week and adjust glucocorticoid doses according to clinical response and results of investigations

(ACPA = anti-citrullinated peptide antibody; ANA = antinuclear antibody; ANCA = antineutrophil cytoplasmic antibody; CPK = creatine phosphokinase; CRP = C-reactive protein; ESR = erythrocyte sedimentation rate; FBC = full blood count; ¹⁹FDG-PET = ¹⁹fluorodeoxyglucose positron emission tomography; PTH = parathyroid hormone; RF = rheumatoid factor; TSH = thyroid-stimulating hormone)

is dramatic, such that symptoms will completely resolve within 48–72 hours of starting therapy in virtually all patients. It is customary to use higher doses in GCA (60–80 mg prednisolone) than in PMR (15–20 mg), although the evidence base for this is weak. In both conditions, the glucocorticoid dose should be progressively reduced, guided by symptoms and ESR, with the aim of reaching a dose of 10–15 mg by about 8 weeks. The rate of reduction should then be slowed by 1 mg per month. If symptoms recur, the dose should be increased to that which previously controlled the symptoms, and reduction attempted again in another few weeks. Most patients need glucocorticoids for an average of 12–24 months. For advice on prophylaxis against giant cell-induced osteoporosis, see page 1047.

Eosinophilic granulomatosis with polyangiitis (Churg–Strauss syndrome)

Eosinophilic granulomatosis with polyangiitis (formerly known as Churg–Strauss syndrome) is a small-vessel vasculitis with an incidence of about 1–3 per 1 000 000. It is associated with eosinophilia. Some patients have a prodromal period for many years, characterised by allergic rhinitis, nasal polyposis and late-onset asthma that is often difficult to control. The typical acute presentation is with a triad of skin lesions (purpura or nodules), asymmetric mononeuritis multiplex and eosinophilia. Pulmonary infiltrates and pleural or pericardial effusions due to serositis may be present. Up to 50% of patients have abdominal symptoms provoked by mesenteric vasculitis. Patients with active disease have raised levels of ESR and CRP and an eosinophilia. Although antibodies to MPO or PR3 can be detected in up to 60% of cases, eosinophilic granulomatosis with polyangiitis is considered to be a distinct disorder from the other ANCA-associated vasculitides. Biopsy of an affected site reveals a small-vessel vasculitis with eosinophilic infiltration of the vessel wall. Management is with high-dose glucocorticoids and cyclophosphamide, followed by maintenance therapy with low-dose glucocorticoids and azathioprine, methotrexate or MMF.

Henoch–Schönlein purpura

Henoch–Schönlein purpura is a small-vessel vasculitis caused by immune complex deposition following an infectious trigger.

It is predominantly a disease of children and young adults. The usual presentation is with purpura over the buttocks and lower legs, accompanied by abdominal pain, gastrointestinal bleeding and arthralgia. Nephritis can also occur and may present up to 4 weeks after the onset of other symptoms. Biopsy of affected tissue shows a vasculitis with IgA deposits in the vessel wall. Henoch–Schönlein purpura is usually a self-limiting disorder that settles spontaneously without specific treatment. Glucocorticoids and immunosuppressive therapy may be required in patients with more severe disease, particularly in the presence of nephritis.

Cryoglobulinaemic vasculitis

This is a small-vessel vasculitis that occurs when immunoglobulins precipitate out in the cold. Cryoglobulins are classified into three types (see Box 4.21, p. 84). Types II and III are associated with vasculitis. The typical presentation is with a vasculitic rash over the lower limbs, arthralgia, Raynaud's phenomenon and neuropathy. Some cases are secondary to hepatitis C infection and others are associated with other autoimmune diseases. Affected patients should be screened for evidence of hepatitis B and C infection, and if the results are positive, these should be treated appropriately (pp. 875 and 878). There is no consensus as to how best to treat cryoglobulinaemic vasculitis in the absence of an obvious trigger. Glucocorticoids and immunosuppressive therapy are often used empirically but their efficacy is uncertain. In severe cases, plasmapheresis can be considered.

Behçet's disease

This is a vasculitis of unknown aetiology that characteristically targets small arteries and venules. It is rare in Western Europe but more common in 'Silk Route' countries, around the Mediterranean and in Japan, where there is a strong association with HLA-B51.

Oral ulcers are universal (Fig. 24.54). Unlike aphthous ulcers, they are usually deep and multiple, and last for 10–30 days. Genital ulcers are also a common problem, occurring in 60–80% of cases. The usual skin lesions are erythema nodosum or acneiform lesions but migratory thrombophlebitis and vasculitis also occur. Ocular involvement is common and may include anterior or posterior uveitis or retinal vasculitis. Neurological involvement occurs in 5% and mainly involves the brainstem,

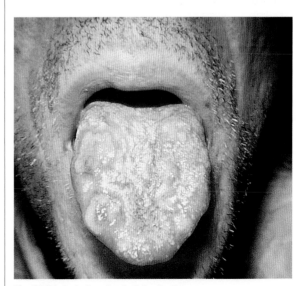

Fig. 24.54 **Oral ulceration in Behçet's disease.**

24

24.68 Criteria for the diagnosis of Behçet's disease

Recurrent oral ulceration: minor aphthous, major aphthous or herpetiform ulceration at least three times in 12 months *plus* two of the following:

- Recurrent genital ulceration
- Eye lesions: anterior uveitis, posterior uveitis, cells in vitreous on slit-lamp examination, retinal vasculitis
- Skin lesions: erythema nodosum, pseudofolliculitis, papulopustular lesions, acneiform nodules
- Positive pathergy test

although the meninges, hemispheres and cord can also be affected, causing pyramidal signs, cranial nerve lesions, brainstem symptoms or hemiparesis. Recurrent thromboses also occur. Renal involvement is extremely rare.

The diagnosis is primarily made on clinical grounds (Box 24.68) but one characteristic feature that can be of diagnostic value is the pathergy test, which involves pricking the skin with a needle and looking for evidence of pustule development within 48 hours.

Oral ulceration can be managed with topical glucocorticoid preparations (soluble prednisolone mouthwashes, glucocorticoid pastes). Colchicine can be effective for erythema nodosum and arthralgia. Thalidomide (100–300 mg per day for 28 days initially) is very effective for resistant oral and genital ulceration but is teratogenic and neurotoxic. Glucocorticoids and immunosuppressants are indicated for uveitis and neurological disease.

Relapsing polychondritis

Relapsing polychondritis is a rare inflammatory disease of cartilage that classically presents with acute pain and swelling of one or both ear pinnae, sparing the lower non-cartilaginous portion. Around 30% of patients have coexisting autoimmune or connective tissue disease. Involvement of tracheobronchial cartilage leads to a hoarse voice, cough, stridor or expiratory wheeze. Other manifestations include collapse of the bridge of the nose, scleritis, hearing loss and cardiac valve dysfunction. Cartilage biopsy shows an inflammatory infiltrate in the perichondrium. Both ESR and CRP are raised in active disease. Pulmonary function tests, including flow–volume loops, should be performed to assess the degree of laryngotracheal disease, since this is an important cause of mortality. Mild disease usually responds to low-dose glucocorticoids or NSAIDs, whereas major tracheobronchial involvement requires high-dose glucocorticoids and immunosuppressants, as described for SLE.

Diseases of bone

Osteoporosis

Osteoporosis is the most common bone disease. It has been estimated that more than 8.9 million fractures occur annually worldwide and most of these occur in patients with osteopenia or osteoporosis. About one-third of all women and one-fifth of men aged 50 and above suffer fractures at some point in life. The burden of osteoporosis-related fractures is predicted to increase by two- to threefold by 2050 on a worldwide basis, due to ageing of the population. Osteoporosis is under-diagnosed and under-treated in Asia and the Indian subcontinent, particularly

in rural areas, due to low provision of technologies like DXA, which are required to make the diagnosis. Fractures in patients with osteoporosis can affect any bone but common sites are the forearm (Colles' fracture), spine (vertebral fractures), humerus and hip. All of these fractures become more common with increasing age (Fig. 24.55). Since only about one-third of vertebral fractures come to medical attention (clinical vertebral fractures), the true number of patients with vertebral fracture is much greater than that shown in Figure 24.55. Of these, hip fractures are the most serious and have an immediate mortality of about 12% and a continued increase in mortality of about 20% when compared with age-matched controls. Treatment of hip fracture accounts for the majority of the health-care costs associated with osteoporosis.

Pathophysiology

The defining feature of osteoporosis is reduced bone density, which causes micro-architectural deterioration of bone tissue and leads to an increased risk of fracture, in response to minor trauma. The risk of fracture increases markedly with age in both genders (Fig. 24.55). This is mostly attributable to an increased risk of falling with age (p. 1308) but is also due in part to an age-related decline in bone mass, especially in women (Fig. 24.56). Bone mass increases during growth to reach a peak between the ages of 20 and about 45 years, but falls thereafter in both genders with an accelerated phase of bone loss after the menopause in women due to oestrogen deficiency. The loss of bone with ageing is caused by an imbalance in the bone remodelling cycle, whereby the amount of new bone formed by osteoblasts cannot keep pace with the amount that is removed by osteoclasts (see Fig. 24.2, p. 985). The reduction in bone formation is thought to be partly due to differentiation of bone marrow stem cells to adipocytes, as opposed to osteoblasts. Osteoporosis sometimes occurs because of failure to attain adequate levels of peak bone mass but is more commonly due to age-related bone loss.

Osteoporosis is a complex disease that can occur in association with a wide variety of risk factors, as summarised in Box 24.69. Genetic factors account for up to 80% of variation in bone density, and genome-wide association studies have shown that susceptibility is determined in part by a large number of common variants, some of which are involved in the RANK and Wnt signalling pathways (see Fig. 24.3, p. 986). Rarely, osteoporosis may be caused by mutations in single genes. Environmental factors, such as exercise and calcium intake during growth and adolescence, are important in maximising peak bone mass and in regulating rates of post-menopausal bone loss. Smoking has a detrimental effect on BMD and is associated with an increased fracture risk, partly because female smokers have an earlier menopause than non-smokers. Heavy alcohol intake is a recognised cause of osteoporosis and fractures but moderate intake does not substantially alter risk.

Idiopathic osteoporosis

The term idiopathic osteoporosis is frequently used to describe the occurrence of osteoporosis in patients with no specific underlying cause. It is slightly misleading, since most, if not all, patients in this category have age-related osteoporosis or osteoporosis associated with inheritance of genetic variants that regulate bone density.

Secondary osteoporosis

Osteoporosis can occur in association with a variety of diseases and drug treatments, and in many cases more than one disease

Fig. 24.55 Fractures associated with osteoporosis. A X-ray of wrist. B Vertebrae. C Humerus. D Hip. E and F The changing incidence of each of these fractures with age in women and men, respectively. *From Curtis EM, van der Velde R, Moon RJ, et al. Epidemiology of fractures in the United Kingdom 1988–2012: variation with age, sex, geography, ethnicity and socioeconomic status. Bone 2016; 87:19–26.*

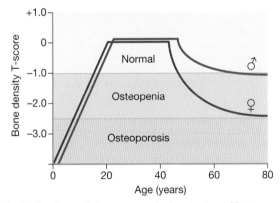

Fig. 24.56 Changes in bone mass and microstructure with age. Changes in men (blue line) and women (red line).

or risk factor is operative. The most important causes are summarised in Box 24.69. Secondary causes of osteoporosis are particularly common in men, occurring in up to 50% of patients. Hypogonadism, glucocorticoid use (see below) and alcohol excess are the most important predisposing factors.

Glucocorticoid-induced osteoporosis

Glucocorticoid-induced osteoporosis is a common problem in patients with systemic inflammatory and chronic pulmonary diseases. The risk of osteoporosis is related to dose and duration of glucocorticoid therapy and increases substantially in patients who have taken more than 7.5 mg of prednisolone daily for more than 3 months (or an equivalent dose of another glucocorticoid). Inhaled glucocorticoids can reduce bone density but the risk of osteoporosis is much lower than with systemic therapy. Glucocorticoids mainly cause osteoporosis by inhibiting bone formation and causing apoptosis of osteoblasts and osteocytes.

Other contributory mechanisms include inhibition of intestinal calcium absorption, increased renal excretion of calcium and secondary hyperparathyroidism, which stimulates osteoclastic bone resorption.

Pregnancy-associated osteoporosis

This is a rare form of osteoporosis that typically presents with back pain and multiple vertebral fractures during the second or third trimester. The cause is unknown but may relate to an exaggeration of the bone loss that normally occurs during pregnancy in patients with pre-existing low bone mass.

Clinical features

Osteoporosis does not cause symptoms until a fracture occurs. Non-vertebral fractures are almost always caused by a traumatic event, most usually a simple fall. The term 'fragility fracture' is used to describe a fracture that occurs as the result of a fall from standing height or less. These are typical of osteoporosis. It is important to remember that the majority of people who suffer a fragility fracture do not have osteoporosis; some have normal bone density but most have osteopenia (Fig. 24.57 and p. 988). The clinical signs of fracture are pain, local tenderness and deformity. In hip fracture, the patient is (with rare exceptions) unable to weight-bear and has a shortened and externally rotated limb on the affected side. The presentation of vertebral fractures is variable. Some patients present with acute severe back pain. This may radiate to the anterior chest or abdominal wall and be mistaken for a myocardial infarction, aortic dissection or intra-abdominal pathology (p. 176). In others the presentation is with height loss and kyphosis in the absence of pain or with chronic back pain. Sometimes the presentation of osteoporosis is with radiological osteopenia or as a vertebral deformity on an X-ray that has been performed for other reasons.

24

i 24.69 Risk factors for osteoporosis

Genetics

- Single-gene disorders:
  LRP5 mutations
  Oestrogen receptor
  mutations
- Polygenic inheritance:
  Common variants in many
  pathways

Endocrine disease

- Hypogonadism
- Hyperthyroidism
- Hyperparathyroidism
- Cushing's syndrome

Inflammatory disease

- Inflammatory bowel disease
- Ankylosing spondylitis
- Rheumatoid arthritis

Drugs

- Glucocorticoids
- Gonadotrophin-releasing
  hormone (GnRH) agonists
- Levothyroxine
  over-replacement
- Aromatase inhibitors
- Thiazolidinediones
- Anticonvulsants
- Alcohol intake >3 U/day
- Heparin

Gastrointestinal disease

- Malabsorption
- Chronic liver disease

Lung disease

- Chronic obstructive pulmonary
  disease
- Cystic fibrosis

Miscellaneous

- Myeloma
- Homocystinuria
- Anorexia nervosa*
- Highly trained athletes*
- HIV infection
- Gaucher's disease
- Systemic mastocytosis
- Immobilisation
- Body mass index <18
- Heavy smoking
- Autoantibodies to
  osteoprotegerin (OPG)

*Hypogonadism also plays a role in osteoporosis associated with these
conditions.

Investigations

The most important investigation is DXA at the lumbar spine and
hip (see Fig. 24.9, p. 990). This should be considered in patients
age over 50 who have already suffered a fragility fracture, and in
those with clinical risk factors (Box 24.70) when a fracture risk
assessment tool (p. 1060) has returned an elevated value. The
risk at which DXA should be performed remains a subject of
debate but a 10-year risk of over 10% has been suggested, since
there is evidence of benefit from treatment at this level. Other
indications for DXA are in patients under 50 years who have very
strong risk factors, such as premature menopause or high-dose
glucocorticoids. Figure 24.58 provides a suggested algorithm
for the investigation of patients with suspected osteoporosis.

A history should be taken to identify any predisposing causes,
such as early menopause, excessive alcohol intake, smoking and
glucocorticoid therapy. Signs of endocrine disease, neoplasia and
inflammatory disease should be sought on clinical examination. A
falls history should be taken and a 'get up and go' test performed,
especially in older patients (p. 1303). Screening for secondary
causes of osteoporosis should be performed, as summarised
in Box 24.71.

Management

The aim of treatment is to reduce the risk of fracture and this
can be achieved by a combination of approaches.

i 24.70 Indications for dual X-ray absorptiometry (DXA)

- Low-trauma fracture, age >50 years
- Clinical risk factors and 10-year fracture risk >10%
- Glucocorticoid therapy (>7.5 mg prednisolone daily for >3 months)
- Assessment of response of osteoporosis to treatment
- Assessment of progression of osteopenia to osteoporosis
- Age <50 years and very strong risk factors for osteoporosis

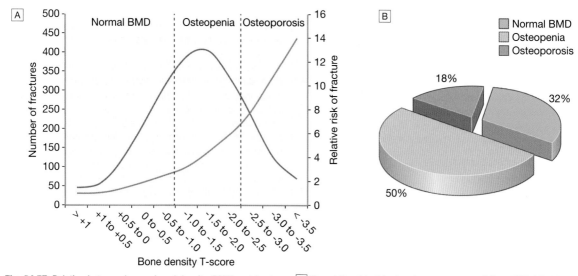

Fig. 24.57 Relation between bone mineral density (BMD) and fractures. **A** The relative risk of fracture increases exponentially as BMD falls (blue line), and is 14-fold higher in people with a T-score of <−3.5 compared with those with normal BMD. In absolute terms, however, more fractures occur in people with normal BMD or osteopenia (red line). **B** The proportions of fractures that occur in people with normal BMD, osteopenia and osteoporosis.

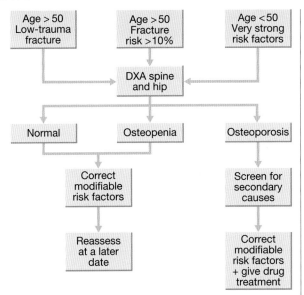

Fig. 24.58 Algorithm for the investigation of patients with suspected osteoporosis. Fracture risk is assessed using FRAX or QFracture (see 'Further information', p. 1060).

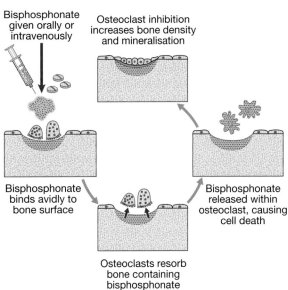

Fig. 24.59 Mechanism of action of bisphosphonates.

24.71 Investigations in osteoporosis

Investigation	Secondary cause of osteoporosis
Urea, creatinine and electrolytes	Chronic kidney disease
Liver function tests and albumin	Chronic liver disease
Full blood count, erythrocyte sedimentation rate	Inflammatory disease Myeloma
Tissue transglutaminase antibodies	Coeliac disease
Serum calcium and phosphate	Primary hyperparathyroidism
Serum 25(OH)D and alkaline phosphatase	Vitamin D deficiency Osteomalacia
Serum parathyroid hormone	Primary hyperparathyroidism
Thyroid function tests	Hyperthyroidism
Serum protein electrophoresis	Myeloma Monoclonal gammopathy of uncertain significance
Urinary Bence Jones protein	Myeloma
Testosterone and gonadotrophins	Male hypogonadism
Oestrogen and gonadotrophins	Female hypogonadism[1]
Bone biopsy	Unexplained early-onset osteoporosis[2] Renal disease Multiple possible causes of low bone mass

[1]Only required for unexplained osteoporosis in young women who are amenorrhoeic. [2]Seldom required.

Non-pharmacological interventions

Advice on smoking cessation, moderation of alcohol intake, adequate dietary calcium intake and exercise should be given. Those with recurrent falls or unsteadiness on a 'get up and go' test should be referred to a multidisciplinary falls prevention team

(p. 1308). Hip protectors can reduce the risk of hip fracture in selected patients but adherence is often poor.

Pharmacological interventions

Several drug treatments are now available to reduce the risk of fracture in osteoporosis. The dosages, mode of administration and indications are summarised in Box 24.72. More detail on the individual drugs is provided below.

Bisphosphonates Bisphosphonates are the first-line treatment for osteoporosis. These are a class of drugs with a central core of P-C-P atoms, to which various side-chains are attached. Following administration, they target bone surfaces and are ingested by osteoclasts during the process of bone resorption. The bisphosphonate is released within the osteoclasts and impairs bone resorption. This in turn causes an increase in bone density but this is principally due to increased mineralisation of bone, rather than an increase in bone mass (Fig. 24.59). Bisphosphonates reduce the risk of fracture in patients with osteoporosis but do not completely prevent fractures occurring.

Oral bisphosphonates are typically given for a period of 5 years, at which point the need for continued therapy should be evaluated, with a repeat DXA if possible. If patients have remained free of fractures after 5 years and if BMD levels have increased and no longer remain in the osteoporotic range, it is usual to instigate a 5-year spell off therapy. Treatment may be continued for up to 10 years in patients whose BMD levels remain in the osteoporotic range after 5 years. A change in treatment should be considered in patients who have lost BMD despite oral bisphosphonates (more than 4%). Most commonly, this will be a switch to parenteral zoledronic acid but teriparatide (TPTD) can also be considered in those with severe spinal osteoporosis. With intravenous zoledronic acid, 3 years of therapy is equivalent to 6 years in terms of fracture risk reduction and many experts recommend periods of 3 years on and 3 years off treatment to reduce the risk of over-suppression of bone turnover.

Oral bisphosphonates are poorly absorbed from the gastrointestinal tract and should be taken on an empty stomach

24.72 Drug treatments for osteoporosis

Drug	Regimen	Postmenopausal osteoporosis	Glucocorticoid osteoporosis	Male osteoporosis
Alendronic acid	70 mg/week orally	✓	✓	✓
Risedronate	35 mg/week orally	✓	✓	✓
Ibandronate	150 mg/monthly orally 3 mg/3-monthly IV	✓	✓	✓
Zoledronic acid	5 mg annually IV	✓	✓	✓
Denosumab	60 mg 6-monthly SC	✓	–	✓
Calcium/vitamin D	Calcium 500–1000 mg daily Vitamin D 400–800 IU orally	✓	✓	✓
Teriparatide	20 µg/day SC	✓	✓	✓
Abaloparatide	80 µg/day SC	✓	–	–
Hormone replacement therapy	Various preparations	✓	–	–
Raloxifene	60 mg/day orally	✓	–	–
Tibolone	1.25 mg/day orally	✓	–	–

(IV = intravenous; SC = subcutaneous)

24.73 Adverse effects of bisphosphonates

Common

- Upper gastrointestinal intolerance (oral)
- Acute phase response (intravenous)

Less common

- Atrial fibrillation (intravenous zoledronic acid)
- Hypocalcaemia (intravenous bisphosphonates)
- Atypical subtrochanteric fractures

Rare

- Uveitis
- Osteonecrosis of the jaw
- Oesophageal ulceration

with plain water; no food should be eaten for 30–45 minutes after administration. They are contraindicated in patients with oesophageal stricture or achalasia, since tablets may stick in the oesophagus, causing ulceration and perforation. Upper gastrointestinal upset occurs in about 5% of cases. Oral bisphosphonates can be used in patients with gastro-oesophageal reflux disease but may cause worsening of symptoms. The most common adverse effect with intravenous bisphosphonates is a transient influenza-like illness typified by fever, malaise, anorexia and generalised aches, which occurs 24–48 hours after administration. This is self-limiting but can be treated with paracetamol or NSAIDs if necessary. It predominantly occurs after the first exposure and tolerance develops thereafter. Other adverse effects are shown in Box 24.73. Osteonecrosis of the jaw is characterised by the presence of necrotic bone in the mandible or maxilla, typically occurring after tooth extraction when the socket fails to heal. This complication is very rare in osteoporosis but patients receiving bisphosphonates should be advised to pay attention to good oral hygiene. There is no evidence that temporarily stopping bisphosphonates for tooth extraction alters the risk of osteonecrosis of the jaw. Atypical subtrochanteric fractures have been described in patients who have received long-term bisphosphonates and appear to be the result of over-suppression of normal bone remodelling. In the vast majority, the benefits of bisphosphonate therapy far outweigh the risks but it is important for treatment to be targeted to patients with low BMD who are most likely to benefit.

Denosumab Denosumab is a monoclonal antibody that inhibits bone resorption by neutralising the effects of RANKL (see Fig. 24.2, p. 985). It is administered by subcutaneous injection of 60 mg every 6 months in the treatment of osteoporosis and has similar efficacy to zoledronic acid. One potential adverse effect is hypocalcaemia but this can be mitigated by calcium and vitamin D supplements. Denosumab may rarely cause osteonecrosis of the jaw and atypical subtrochanteric fractures. If it is stopped, there is a rebound increase in bone turnover that can be associated with a greater risk of fracture and even hypercalcaemia. Because of this, many experts advise giving a bisphosphonate following cessation of denosumab.

Calcium and vitamin D Combined calcium and vitamin D supplements have limited efficacy in the prevention of osteoporotic fractures when given alone but are widely used as an adjunct to other treatments. A typical daily dosage is 1000 mg calcium and 800 IU vitamin D. Calcium and vitamin D supplements have efficacy in preventing fragility fractures in elderly or institutionalised patients who are at high risk of deficiency (Box 24.74). Vitamin D supplements alone do not prevent fractures in osteoporosis but there is evidence that the response to bisphosphonates is blunted in patients with vitamin D deficiency. If the patient's dietary calcium is sufficient, stand-alone vitamin D supplements (800 IU daily) can be prescribed as an adjunct to anti-osteoporosis therapies.

Teriparatide Teriparatide (TPTD) is the 1-34 fragment of human PTH. It is an effective treatment for osteoporosis, which works by stimulating new bone formation. Although TPTD also stimulates bone resorption, the increase in bone formation is greater, resulting in increased bone density, particularly at sites rich in trabecular bone such as the spine. It is given by a self-administered subcutaneous injection in a dose of 20 µg daily for 2 years. At the end of this period, bisphosphonate therapy or another

- **Bone loss**: due to increased bone turnover, with an age-related defect switch in differentiation of bone marrow stromal cells to form adipocytes as opposed to osteoblasts.
- **Fractures due to osteoporosis**: common cause of morbidity and mortality, although fracture healing is not delayed by age.
- **Recurrent fractures**: those who suffer a fragility fracture are at increased risk of further fracture, so should be investigated for osteoporosis and treated if this is confirmed.
- **Falls**: risk factors for falls (such as visual and neuromuscular impairments) are independent risk factors for hip fracture in elderly individuals, so intervention to prevent falls is as important as treatment of osteoporosis (p. 1308).
- **Intravenous zoledronic acid**: reduces mortality and subsequent fracture in selected elderly patients with hip fractures.
- **Calcium and vitamin D**: reduce the risk of fractures in those who are housebound or living in care homes.

inhibitor of bone resorption should be administered to maintain the increase in BMD. TPTD and oral bisphosphonates should not be given in combination, however, since the bisphosphonate blunts the anabolic effect. The efficacy of TPTD for prevention of non-vertebral fractures is similar to that of bisphosphonates but it is superior to oral bisphosphonates in preventing vertebral fractures. The most common adverse effects are headache, muscle cramps and dizziness. Mild hypercalcaemia may occur but it is usually asymptomatic and does not require discontinuation of treatment. Monitoring of serum calcium is not required during TPTD treatment.

Abaloparatide Abaloparatide is the 1-34 fragment of PTH-related protein. It works in a similar way to TPTD to stimulate bone formation. It is given as a self-administered injection of 80 µg daily for 18 months. At the end of this period an inhibitor of bone resorption should be given to maintain the increase in bone mass. Efficacy has been demonstrated for the prevention of vertebral fractures with effects similar to those of TPTD. Adverse effects are similar to those of TPTD.

Hormone replacement therapy Cyclical HRT with oestrogen and progestogen prevents post-menopausal bone loss and reduces the risk of vertebral and non-vertebral fractures in post-menopausal women. It is primarily indicated for the prevention of osteoporosis in women with an early menopause (p. 655) and for treatment of women with osteoporosis in their early fifties who have troublesome menopausal symptoms. It is not recommended above the age of 60 because the risk of an increased risk of breast cancer, cardiovascular disease and venous thromboembolic disease.

Raloxifene Raloxifene is a selective oestrogen receptor modulator (SERM) that acts as a partial agonist at oestrogen receptors in bone and liver, but as an antagonist in breast and endometrium. It is effective in reducing the risk of vertebral fractures but does not influence the risk of non-vertebral fracture and is seldom used. Adverse effects include muscle cramps, worsening of hot flushes and an increased risk of venous thromboembolic disease. Bazedoxifene is a related SERM that has similar effects to raloxifene.

Tibolone Tibolone has partial agonist activity at oestrogen, progestogen and androgen receptors. It has been shown to

prevent vertebral and non-vertebral fractures in post-menopausal osteoporosis. Treatment is associated with a slightly increased risk of stroke but a reduced risk of breast cancer.

Other drugs Romosozumab is antibody directed against sclerostin, which is under development for the treatment of osteoporosis. It increases bone formation, inhibits bone resorption and increases BMD. When given subcutaneously in a dose of 210 mg monthly, it reduces the risk of vertebral fractures in patients with postmenopausal osteoporosis. Calcitriol ($1,25(OH)_2D_3$), the active metabolite of vitamin D, is licensed for treatment of osteoporosis but it is seldom used because the data on fracture prevention are less robust than for other agents.

Surgery

Orthopaedic surgery with internal fixation is frequently required to reduce and stabilise osteoporotic fractures. Patients with intracapsular fracture of the femoral neck generally need hemi-arthroplasty or total hip replacement in view of the high risk of avascular necrosis.

Vertebroplasty is sometimes used in the treatment of painful vertebral compression fractures. It involves injecting methyl methacrylate (MMA) into the affected vertebral body under sedation and local anaesthesia. While randomised trials have shown that vertebroplasty provides no better pain relief than a sham procedure, it is still widely used, particularly in North America. Kyphoplasty is used under similar circumstances, but in this case a needle is introduced into the affected vertebral body and a balloon is inflated, which is then filled with MMA. It has similar efficacy to vertebroplasty but adverse effects are more common. Adverse effects with both procedures include spinal cord compression due to leakage of MMA and fat embolism.

Osteomalacia, rickets and vitamin D deficiency

Osteomalacia and rickets are characterised by defective mineralisation of bone. The most common cause is vitamin D deficiency, but both conditions can also occur as the result of inherited defects in renal phosphate excretion, and inherited defects in the vitamin D receptor and in the pathways responsible for vitamin D activation. Other causes are summarised in Box 24.75 and are discussed in more detail below. The term osteomalacia refers to the syndrome when it occurs in adults and rickets is the equivalent syndrome in children. The disease remains prevalent in frail older people who have a poor diet and limited sunlight exposure, and in some Muslim women.

Vitamin D deficiency

Vitamin D deficiency is defined to exist when serum 25(OH)D concentrations are below 25 nmol/L (10 ng/mL). People with vitamin D levels in the range 25–50 nmol/L (10–20 ng/mL) are classified as having vitamin D insufficiency, whereas those with 25(OH)D levels above 50 nmol/L (20 ng/mL) are classified as having normal vitamin D status. In the elderly, a more appropriate normal threshold may be 75 nmol/L (30 ng/mL) or more, though there is some debate on the issue and evidence is not conclusive. The likelihood of developing vitamin D deficiency is strongly related to sunlight exposure. It is common in northern latitudes (or southern latitudes in the southern hemisphere) and shows seasonal variation. Vitamin D deficiency is also common in women who, for cultural reasons, cover their skin and face. Vitamin D

24

24.75 Causes of osteomalacia and rickets

Cause	Predisposing factor	Mechanism
Vitamin D deficiency		
Classical	Lack of sunlight exposure and poor diet	Reduced cholecalciferol synthesis in the skin/low levels of vitamin D in the diet
Gastrointestinal disease	Malabsorption	Malabsorption of dietary vitamin D and calcium
Failure of 1,25 vitamin D synthesis		
Chronic renal failure	Hyperphosphataemia and kidney damage	Impaired conversion of $25(OH)D_3$ to $1,25(OH)_2D_3$
Vitamin D-resistant rickets type I (autosomal recessive)	Loss-of-function mutations in renal 25(OH)D 1α-hydroxylase enzyme	Impaired conversion of $25(OH)D_3$ to $1,25(OH)_2D_3$
Vitamin D receptor defects		
Vitamin D-resistant rickets type II (autosomal recessive)	Loss-of-function mutations in vitamin D receptor	Impaired response to $1,25(OH)_2D_3$
Defects in phosphate and pyrophosphate metabolism		
Hypophosphataemic rickets (X-linked dominant)	Mutations in *PHEX*	Increased FGF23 production (mechanism unclear)
Autosomal dominant hypophosphataemic rickets	Mutation in *FGF23*	Mutant FGF23 is resistant to degradation
Autosomal recessive hypophosphataemic rickets	Mutations in *DMP1*	Increased production of FGF23 Local deficiency of DMP1 inhibits mineralisation
Tumour-induced hypophosphataemic osteomalacia	Ectopic production of FGF23 by tumour	Over-production of FGF23
Hypophosphatasia	Mutations in *ALPL*, which encodes alkaline phosphatase	Inhibition of bone mineralisation due to accumulation of pyrophosphate in bone
Iatrogenic and other causes		
Bisphosphonate therapy	High-dose etidronate/pamidronate	Drug-induced impairment of mineralisation
Aluminium	Use of aluminium-containing phosphate binders or aluminium in dialysis fluid	Aluminium-induced impairment of mineralisation
Fluoride	High fluoride in water	Inhibition of mineralisation by fluoride

(FGF23 = fibroblast growth factor 23)

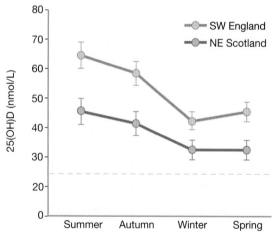

Fig. 24.60 Seasonal changes in vitamin D concentrations. To convert nmol/L to ng/mL, multiply by 2.5. *Adapted from McDonald HM, Mavroeidi A, Fraser WD, et al. Sunlight and dietary contributions to the seasonal vitamin D status of cohorts of healthy postmenopausal women living at northerly latitudes: a major cause for concern? Osteoporosis Int 2011; 22:2461–2472.*

deficiency is more common in the winter and spring, and less common in summer and autumn (Fig. 24.60).

Pathogenesis

The source of vitamin D and pathways involved in regulating its metabolism are shown in Figure 24.61. In normal individuals, vitamin D (also known as cholecalciferol) comes from two sources:

about 70% is made in the skin, where 7-dehydrocholesterol is converted to cholecalciferol under the influence of ultraviolet light, whereas the remaining 30% is derived from the diet. The main dietary sources are oily fish and meat, although bread and dairy products are fortified with vitamin D in some countries. On entering the circulation, vitamin D is hydroxylated in the liver to form 25(OH) vitamin D and this is further hydroxylated in the kidney to form $1,25(OH)_2D$, the biologically active metabolite. The $1,25(OH)_2D$ primarily acts on the gut to increase intestinal calcium absorption but also acts on the skeleton to stimulate bone remodelling. Synthesis of $1,25(OH)_2D$ is regulated by a negative feedback loop orchestrated by the parathyroid glands. When vitamin D levels fall – as the result of lower sunlight exposure or dietary lack – production of $1,25(OH)_2D$ is reduced, causing a reduction in calcium absorption from the gut. This causes a transient fall in serum calcium, which is detected by calcium-sensing receptors on the parathyroid chief cells; this increases PTH secretion, which restores calcium levels to normal. Vitamin D deficiency is, therefore, usually characterised by a low level of 25(OH)D and a raised level of PTH. Sometimes, low 25(OH)D levels may be observed in the presence of a normal PTH concentration. This is of uncertain clinical significance but might be due to variations in levels of vitamin D-binding protein. Serum concentrations of vitamin D are under genetic control and are associated with variants close to the *GC* gene, which encodes vitamin D-binding protein; the *DHCR7* gene, which encodes 7-dehydrocholesterol reductase, responsible for catalysing conversion of 7-DHC to 25(OH)D; the *CYP2R1* gene, which encodes vitamin D-25-hydroxylase, responsible for hydroxylation of vitamin D in the liver; and the *CYP24A1* gene, which encodes vitamin D-24-hydroxylase, responsible for converting 25(OH)D to the inactive metabolite $24,25(OH)_2D$.

Fig. 24.61 Vitamin D metabolism. Vitamin D is produced in the skin from 7-dehydrocholesterol (7-DHC) by ultraviolet B (UVB) light. The 7-dehydrocholesterol reductase enzyme, which is encoded by the *DHCR7* gene, opposes the effect of UVB by converting 7-DHC to cholesterol. The vitamin D then undergoes hydroxylation steps in the liver and kidney to form the active metabolite 1,25(OH)$_2$D, which regulates calcium homeostasis by stimulating calcium absorption from the diet and bone resorption. See text for details.

Clinical features

Vitamin D deficiency does not cause symptoms and the diagnosis is made as the result of biochemical testing. Low circulating concentrations of vitamin D have been associated with a wide range of diseases, including most types of cancer, diabetes, multiple sclerosis and chronic inflammatory diseases. These associations are unlikely to be causal but most probably arise as the result of reduced sunlight exposure and poor diet in people who are ill. If vitamin D deficiency is prolonged and severe, then osteomalacia and rickets may occur, as discussed below. The consequences of biochemical vitamin D deficiency and insufficiency on bone health and general health are unclear.

Investigations

The diagnosis can be made by measurement of serum 25(OH)D. In patients with low 25(OH)D, measurements of PTH, serum calcium, phosphate and ALP should also be considered. Low levels of 25(OH)D in the absence of other abnormalities is unlikely to be of any clinical significance and may be due to low levels of vitamin D-binding protein. If low 25(OH)D levels are combined with raised levels of PTH, this is of more significance since it indicates secondary hyperparathyroidism. Serum ALP, calcium and phosphate levels are normal in uncomplicated vitamin D deficiency.

Management

The clinical benefit of treating biochemical vitamin D deficiency is uncertain. Vitamin D supplements should be considered in patients who have low 25(OH)D levels and raised levels of PTH. In most patients, cholecalciferol in a dose of 800 IU daily should be sufficient to correct the deficiency. The benefit of treating seasonal vitamin D deficiency or vitamin D insufficiency is uncertain. There is some evidence that response to bisphosphonate treatment of osteoporosis is impaired in patients with vitamin D deficiency and this is another indication for supplements. In patients who are receiving intravenous bisphosphonates and denosumab for osteoporosis, vitamin D deficiency should be corrected by supplementation to reduce the risk of hypocalcaemia. In this case, it is customary to give higher doses of vitamin D, such as 20 000–25 000 IU once a week for 4 weeks or to give lower doses over a more prolonged period.

Osteomalacia and rickets

Severe and prolonged vitamin D deficiency can result in the occurrence of osteomalacia in adults and rickets in children. Improvements in nutrition mean that these are now relatively uncommon conditions in developed countries but they remain prevalent in elderly housebound individuals, some Muslim women who wear a veil (hijab) that covers a large amount of exposed skin, and people with malabsorption.

Pathogenesis

Osteomalacia and rickets occur as the result of chronic secondary hyperparathyroidism, which invariably accompanies severe and long-standing vitamin D deficiency. The sustained elevation in PTH levels maintains normal levels of serum calcium by increasing bone resorption, which eventually causes progressive demineralisation of the skeleton. Phosphate that is released during the process of bone resorption is lost through increased renal excretion, resulting in hypophosphataemia. The raised levels of PTH stimulate osteoblast activity and cause new bone formation

24

but the matrix is not mineralised properly because of deficiency of calcium and phosphate. The under-mineralised bone is soft, mechanically weak and subject to fractures, particularly stress fractures. Normal levels of serum calcium tend to be maintained until a very advanced stage, when hypocalcaemia may occur.

Clinical features

Vitamin D deficiency in children causes delayed development, muscle hypotonia, craniotabes (small unossified areas in membranous bones of the skull that yield to finger pressure with a cracking feeling), bossing of the frontal and parietal bones and delayed anterior fontanelle closure, enlargement of epiphyses at the lower end of the radius, and swelling of the rib costochondral junctions ('rickety rosary'). Osteomalacia in adults can present with fractures and low BMD, mimicking osteoporosis. Other symptoms include bone pain and general malaise. Proximal muscle weakness is prominent and the patient may walk with a waddling gait and struggle to climb stairs or stand up from a chair. There may be bone and muscle tenderness on pressure, and focal bone pain can be due to fissure fractures of the ribs and pelvis.

Investigations

The diagnosis can usually be made by measurement of serum 25(OH)D, PTH, calcium, phosphate and ALP. Typically, serum ALP levels are raised, 25(OH)D levels are undetectable and PTH is markedly elevated. Serum phosphate levels tend to be low but serum calcium is usually normal, unless the disease is advanced. X-rays often show osteopenia or vertebral crush fractures and, with more advanced disease, focal radiolucent areas (pseudofractures or Looser's zones) may be seen in ribs, pelvis and long bones (Fig. 24.62A). In children, there is

Fig. 24.62 Osteomalacia. [A] X-ray of the pelvis showing pseudofractures affecting the inferior and superior pubic rami on the left side (arrows). Healing pseudofractures with callus formation are also visible at the inferior and superior pubic rami on the right side (arrows). [B] Photomicrograph of bone biopsy from an osteomalacic patient showing thick osteoid seams (stained light blue, arrows) that cover almost all of the bone surface. Calcified bone is stained dark blue.

thickening and widening of the epiphyseal plate. A radionuclide bone scan may show multiple hot spots in the ribs and pelvis at the site of fractures and the appearance may be mistaken for metastases. Where there is doubt, the diagnosis can be confirmed by bone biopsy, which shows the pathognomonic features of increased thickness and extent of osteoid seams (Fig. 24.62B).

Management

Osteomalacia and rickets respond promptly to treatment with vitamin D. A wide variety of doses can be used. Treatment with between 10000 and 25000 IU daily for 2–4 weeks is associated with rapid clinical improvement, an elevation in serum 25(OH)D and a reduction in PTH. Serum ALP levels sometimes rise initially as mineralisation of bone increases but eventually fall to within the reference range as the bone disease heals. Subsequently, the dose of vitamin D can usually be reduced to a maintenance level of 800–1600 IU daily (10–20 µg), except in patients with malabsorption, who may require higher doses.

Vitamin D-resistant rickets

This is a genetically determined condition that presents in childhood with rickets that is resistant to therapy with vitamin D in standard dosages.

Pathogenesis

Type I vitamin D-resistant rickets (VDRR) is caused by inactivating mutations in the 25-hydroxyvitamin D 1α-hydroxylase (*CYP27B1*) enzyme, which converts 25(OH)D to the active metabolite 1,25(OH)$_2$D$_3$. Type II VDRR is caused by inactivating mutations in the vitamin D receptor, which impair its ability to activate gene transcription. Both are recessive disorders and consanguinity is common.

Clinical features

These are as described above for infantile rickets. The diagnosis is usually first suspected when the patient fails to respond to vitamin D supplementation.

Investigations

The biochemical features of type I VDRR are similar to those of ordinary vitamin D deficiency, except that levels of 25(OH)D are normal but 1,25(OH)$_2$D is low. In type II VDRR, 25(OH)D is normal but PTH and 1,25(OH)$_2$D$_3$ values are raised.

Management

Type I VDRR responds fully to treatment with the active vitamin D metabolites 1α-hydroxyvitamin D (1–2 µg daily, orally) or 1,25-dihydroxyvitamin D (0.25–1.5 µg daily, orally). Calcium supplements are not necessary unless there is dietary deficiency. Type II VDRR sometimes responds partially to very high doses of active vitamin D metabolites, which can activate the mutant receptor, although additional calcium and phosphate supplements are also necessary.

Hereditary hypophosphataemic rickets

This group of disorders are caused by inherited defects in renal tubular phosphate reabsorption. The most common is X-linked hypophosphataemic rickets (XLH), but autosomal dominant and autosomal recessive forms also occur (Box 24.75).

Pathophysiology

All forms of hereditary hypophosphataemic rickets are associated with raised circulating concentrations of the phosphate-regulating hormone fibroblast growth factor 23 (FGF23). This hormone is produced by osteocytes (see Fig 24.3, p. 986) and enters the circulation, where it is normally inactivated by proteolytic cleavage. Production of FGF23 by osteocytes is under tonic inhibition by DMP1 and PHEX. In XLH, the inhibitory effect on FGF23 production is lost due to mutations in *PHEX* and a similar situation occurs in autosomal recessive hypophosphataemic rickets (ARHR1) due to loss-of-function mutations in *DMP1*. Mutations in the *ENPP1* gene, which encodes a phosphatase responsible for degradation of pyrophosphate, can also cause a recessive form of hypophosphataemic rickets (ARHR2). In autosomal dominant hypophosphataemic rickets (ADHR), the FGF23 protein carries mutations that prevent FGF23 being degraded, thereby causing accumulation of intact FGF23 hormone in the circulation. In all three diseases, the elevation in FGF23 results in osteomalacia and rickets by causing phosphaturia by up-regulation of sodium-dependent phosphate transporters in the renal tubules, and also by inhibiting conversion of 25(OH)D to 1,25(OH)$_2$D by the kidney, which in turn causes reduced calcium and phosphate absorption from the gut.

Clinical features

The presentation is with symptoms and signs of rickets during childhood that do not respond to vitamin D supplementation. In adults, hypophosphataemic rickets may be accompanied by dental abscesses, and by bone and joint pain due to the development of an enthesopathy.

Investigations

The diagnosis can be confirmed by the finding of low serum phosphate levels and a reduction in tubular reabsorption of phosphate. Serum levels of vitamin D are normal and PTH is normal or slightly elevated. Serum concentrations of FGF23 are markedly elevated. The causal mutation can be defined by genetic testing.

Management

The aim of treatment is to ameliorate symptoms, restore normal growth and maintain serum phosphate levels within the reference range. Traditionally, treatment has been with phosphate supplements (1–4 g daily) and 1-α-hydroxyvitamin D (1–2 μg daily) or 1,25-dihydroxyvitamin D (0.5–1.5 μg daily) with the aim of promoting intestinal calcium and phosphate absorption. Levels of calcium and phosphate, as well as renal function, should be monitored regularly and the doses of phosphate and vitamin D metabolites carefully titrated to maintain serum phosphate within the normal range but avoid hypercalcaemia. Recently, a neutralising antibody to FGF23 has been developed that can reverse the biochemical abnormalities in hereditary hypophosphataemic rickets and it is likely that this will be a future treatment option.

Tumour-induced osteomalacia

This is a rare syndrome caused by over-production of FGF23 by mesenchymal tumours. The presentation is with severe osteomalacia and hypophosphataemia in an adult patient with no obvious predisposing risk factor for vitamin D deficiency. Biochemical findings are as described for hereditary hypophosphataemic rickets. The underlying tumour can sometimes be identified by whole-body MRI or CT. Medical management is with phosphate supplements and active vitamin D metabolites but the treatment of choice is surgical resection of the primary tumour, which is curative.

Hypophosphatasia

Hypophosphatasia is an autosomal recessive disorder caused by loss-of-function mutations in the *TNALP* gene, which result in accumulation of pyrophosphate and inhibition of bone mineralisation. Chondrocalcinosis may also occur. The typical presentation is with severe intractable rickets during infancy, sometimes in association with seizures. Investigations show low or undetectable levels of serum ALP but normal levels of calcium, phosphate, PTH and vitamin D metabolites. Urinary excretion of pyridoxal 5′ phosphate and phosphoethanolamine (substrates for ALP) is increased. Until recently, this condition was fatal during childhood but remarkable therapeutic responses have been obtained with recombinant ALP therapy (asfotase alfa), which is curative. Heterozygous carriers of mutation in *TNALP* may present in adulthood with osteoporosis, fractures and low ALP values. The best mode of treatment for these patients remains to be determined, except that bisphosphonates should be avoided since they may exacerbate the mineralisation defect.

Other causes of osteomalacia

These are summarised in Box 24.75. Osteomalacia may occur as a component of renal osteodystrophy in patients with chronic kidney disease. The mechanism is reduced conversion of 25(OH)D into the active metabolite 1,25(OH)$_2$D by the failing kidney (p. 418). Aluminium intoxication is now rare due to reduced use of aluminium-containing phosphate binders and removal of aluminium from the water supplies used in dialysis. If aluminium intoxication is suspected, the diagnosis can be confirmed by demonstration of aluminium at the calcification front in a bone biopsy. Osteomalacia due to bisphosphonates has mostly been described in patients with Paget's disease who are receiving etidronate and high-dose pamidronate. It is usually asymptomatic and healing occurs when treatment is stopped. Excessive fluoride intake causes osteomalacia due to direct inhibition of mineralisation and is common in parts of the world where there is a high fluoride content in drinking water. The condition reverses when fluoride intake is reduced.

Paget's disease of bone

Paget's disease of bone (PDB) is characterised by focal areas of increased and disorganised bone remodelling involving one or more skeletal sites. The disease is common in the UK, affecting about 1% of those aged above 55, and in other countries in Europe. It is rare in Scandinavia, the Indian subcontinent and the rest of Asia. The prevalence doubles each decade from the age of 50 onwards and affects up to 8% of the UK population by the age of 85.

Pathophysiology

The primary abnormality is increased osteoclastic bone resorption, accompanied by marrow fibrosis, increased vascularity of bone and increased, but disorganised, bone formation. Osteoclasts in PDB are greater in number and unusually large, containing characteristic nuclear inclusion bodies. Genetic factors are important and mutations in the *SQSTM1* gene are a common

Fig. 24.63 Paget's disease. [A] 99mTc-labelled bisphosphonate scintigraphy from a patient with Paget's disease, illustrating the intense tracer uptake and deformity of the affected femur. [B] The typical radiographic features with expansion of the femur, alternating areas of osteosclerosis and radiolucency of the trochanter, and pseudofractures breaching the bone cortex (arrows).

cause of classical PDB. The presence of nuclear inclusion bodies in osteoclasts has fuelled speculation that PDB might be caused by a slow virus infection but this is unproven. Biomechanical factors may influence which bones are affected, as PDB often starts at sites of muscle insertions into bone and, in some cases, localises to bones or limbs that have been subjected to repetitive trauma or overuse. Involvement of subchondral bone can compromise the joint and predispose to OA. The prevalence of PDB has fallen in many countries over recent decades, suggesting that environmental factors play a role, but the identity of these triggers remains unclear.

Clinical features

The axial skeleton is predominantly affected and common sites of involvement are the pelvis, femur, tibia, lumbar spine, skull and scapula. The most common presentation is with bone pain localised to an affected site but bone deformity, deafness and pathological fractures may also be presenting features. Many patients are asymptomatic and the diagnosis is frequently made on the basis of an X-ray or blood test performed for another reason. Clinical signs include bone deformity and expansion, and increased warmth over an affected bone. Neurological problems, such as deafness, cranial nerve defects, nerve root pain, spinal cord compression and spinal stenosis, may occur due to enlargement of affected bones and encroachment on the spinal cord and nerve foramina. Surprisingly, deafness seldom results from compression of the auditory nerve but is conductive, due to osteosclerosis of the temporal bone. The increased vascularity of Pagetic bone can rarely precipitate high-output cardiac failure in elderly patients with limited cardiac reserve. Osteosarcoma is an unusual but serious complication that presents with increasing pain and swelling of an affected site.

Investigations

The characteristic features are an isolated elevation in ALP and bone expansion on X-rays, with alternating areas of radiolucency and osteosclerosis (Fig. 24.63B). Levels of ALP can be normal if only a single bone is affected. The best way of identifying affected sites is a radionuclide bone scan, which shows increased uptake

i	**24.76 Medical management of Paget's disease**	
Drug	**Route of administration**	**Dose**
Etidronate	Oral	400 mg daily for 3–6 months
Tiludronate	Oral	400 mg daily for 3–6 months
Risedronate	Oral	30 mg daily for 2 months
Pamidronate	IV	1–3×60 mg infusions
Zoledronic acid	IV	1×5 mg infusion
Calcitonin	SC	100–200 IU 3 times weekly for 2–3 months

in affected bones (Fig. 24.63A). If the bone scan is positive, X-rays should be taken to confirm the diagnosis. Bone biopsy is not usually required but may help to exclude osteosclerotic metastases in cases of diagnostic uncertainty.

Management

The main indication for treatment with inhibitors of bone resorption is bone pain, which is thought to be due to increased metabolic activity (Box 24.76). Patients should be carefully assessed to determine the cause of the pain since it can be difficult to differentiate the pain caused by increased metabolic activity of PDB from that caused by complications such as bone deformity, nerve compression symptoms and OA. The bisphosphonates pamidronate, risedronate and zoledronic acid are highly effective at suppressing the elevations in bone turnover that are characteristic of PDB and also improve bone pain that is caused by increased metabolic activity. If there is doubt about whether the pain is due to PDB, it can be worthwhile giving a therapeutic trial of bisphosphonate to determine whether the symptoms improve. A positive response indicates that the pain was due to increased metabolic activity. There is no evidence as yet to suggest that bisphosphonates prevent the development of complications in PDB. Repeated courses of bisphosphonates can be given if symptoms recur.

Fig. 24.64 Complex regional pain syndrome (osteodystrophy).
⁹⁹ᵐTc-labelled bisphosphonate scintigraphy showing increased uptake in femoral condyle.

Other bone diseases

Complex regional pain syndrome type 1

Complex regional pain syndrome (CRPS) type 1 is characterised by gradual onset of pain, swelling and local tenderness, usually affecting a limb extremity. It may be triggered by fracture but can also occur in association with soft tissue injury, pregnancy and intercurrent illness or can develop spontaneously. The cause is unknown but abnormalities of the sympathetic nervous system are thought to play a pathogenic role. The affected limb is swollen and tender, and there may be evidence of regional autonomic dysfunction, with abnormal sweating and changes in skin colour and temperature. The diagnosis is primarily clinical, based on the features shown in Box 34.12 (p. 1349). Support for the diagnosis can be obtained with MRI, which shows bone marrow oedema, or radionuclide bone scan, which shows a local increase in tracer uptake (Fig. 24.64). X-rays show localised osteoporosis. Haematology, biochemistry and immunology are normal.

The aims of treatment are to control pain and encourage mobilisation. Analgesics, NSAIDs, antineuropathic agents, calcitonin, glucocorticoids, β-adrenoceptor antagonists (β-blockers), sympathectomy and bisphosphonates have all been tried but none is particularly effective. Although some cases resolve with time, many individuals have persistent symptoms and fail to regain normal function.

Osteonecrosis

Osteonecrosis describes death of bone due to impairment of its blood supply. The most commonly affected sites are the femoral head, humeral head and femoral condyles. In some cases, the condition occurs as the result of direct trauma that interrupts the blood supply to the affected bone. This is the reason for osteonecrosis of the femoral head in patients with subtrochanteric fractures of the femoral neck, and in patients with thrombophilia and haemoglobinopathies, such as sickle cell disease. Other important predisposing factors include high-dose glucocorticoid treatment, alcohol excess, SLE, HIV and radiotherapy, but in many of these conditions the pathophysiology is poorly understood. The presentation is with pain localised to the affected site, which is exacerbated by weight-bearing. The diagnosis can be confirmed by MRI, which shows evidence of subchondral necrotic bone and bone marrow oedema. X-rays are normal in the early stages but later may show evidence of osteosclerosis and deformity of the affected bone. There is no specific treatment. Management should focus on controlling pain and encouraging mobilisation (p. 1000). Symptoms often improve spontaneously with time but joint replacement may be required in patients who have persisting pain in association with significant structural damage to the affected joint.

Scheuermann's osteochondritis

This disorder predominantly affects adolescent boys, who develop a dorsal kyphosis in association with irregular radiographic ossification of the vertebral end plates. It has a strong genetic component and may be inherited in an autosomal dominant manner. Most patients are asymptomatic but back pain, aggravated by exercise and relieved by rest, may occur. Excessive exercise and heavy manual labour before epiphyseal fusion has occurred may aggravate symptoms. Management consists of advice to avoid excessive activity and provision of protective postural exercises. Rarely, corrective surgery may be required if there is severe deformity. Scheuermann's disease can sometimes present for the first time in adulthood, when it can be confused with osteoporotic vertebral fractures. It can be differentiated from osteoporosis by the characteristic X-ray changes, which show mild wedge deformity of 3–4 adjacent vertebrae, irregularity of the vertebral end plates, and normal BMD on DXA examination.

Polyostotic fibrous dysplasia

This is an acquired systemic disorder that mainly affects the skeleton and is caused by somatic mutations in the *GNAS1* gene. The characteristic presentation is with bone pain and pathological fractures. Associated features include endocrine dysfunction, especially precocious puberty, and café-au-lait skin pigmentation (McCune–Albright syndrome). The diagnosis can usually be made by imaging, which shows focal, predominantly osteolytic lesions with bone expansion on X-rays (Fig. 24.65), and focal increased uptake on bone scan. The condition can resemble Paget's disease of bone but the earlier age of onset and pattern of involvement are usually distinctive. Very rarely, malignant change can occur and should be suspected if there is a sudden increase in pain and swelling. Management is symptomatic. Intravenous bisphosphonates are often used in an attempt to control pain but the evidence base for their use is weak. Orthopaedic surgery may be required for treatment of fracture and deformity. Endocrine manifestations, such as precocious puberty (p. 654), may require specific treatment.

Osteogenesis imperfecta

Osteogenesis imperfecta (OI) is the name given to a group of disorders characterised by severe osteoporosis and multiple fractures in infancy and childhood. Most cases are caused by mutations in the *COL1A1* and *COL1A2* genes, which encode the proteins that make type I collagen. These result in reduced collagen production (in mild OI) or in formation of abnormal collagen chains that are rapidly degraded (in severe OI). Mutations

24

Fig. 24.65 McCune–Albright syndrome. X-ray of tibia in a patient with McCune–Albright syndrome showing expansile osteolytic lesion.

in several other genes have been described that can cause OI, some of which affect post-translational modification of collagen and others that affect bone formation. Many patients have no family history. Some of these have new mutations whereas others may have recessive forms of the disease. The Sillence classification is commonly used to grade severity. This varies from neonatal lethal OI (type II), through very severe OI with multiple fractures in infancy and childhood (types III and IV), to mild (type I), in which affected patients typically have blue sclerae. The diagnosis of OI is usually obvious clinically, based on the presentation with multiple low-trauma fractures during infancy. The disease can be mistaken for non-accidental injury in childhood and for osteoporosis in adulthood; in such cases, genetic testing can be of diagnostic value. Treatment is multidisciplinary, involving surgical reduction and fixation of fractures and correction of limb deformities, and physiotherapy and occupational therapy for rehabilitation of patients with bone deformity. Bisphosphonates are widely used in the treatment of OI, especially intravenous pamidronate in children, but there is limited evidence for efficacy in fracture prevention.

Osteopetrosis

Osteopetrosis is a rare group of inherited diseases caused by failure of osteoclast function. Presentation is highly variable, ranging from a lethal disorder that presents with bone marrow failure in infancy to a milder and sometimes asymptomatic form that presents in adulthood. Severe osteopetrosis is inherited in an autosomal recessive manner and presents with failure to thrive, delayed dentition, cranial nerve palsies (due to absent cranial foramina), blindness, anaemia and recurrent infections due to bone marrow failure. The adult-onset type (Albers–Schönberg

disease) shows autosomal dominant inheritance and presents with bone pain, cranial nerve palsies, osteomyelitis, OA or fracture, or is sometimes detected as an incidental radiographic finding. The responsible mutations affect either the genes that regulate osteoclast differentiation (*RANK*, *RANKL*), causing 'osteoclast-poor' osteopetrosis, or the genes involved in bone resorption, causing 'osteoclast-rich' osteopetrosis. These include mutations in the *TCIRG1* gene, which encodes a component of the osteoclast proton pump, and mutations in the *CLCN7* gene, which encodes the osteoclast chloride pump. Management is difficult. IFN-γ treatment can improve blood counts and reduce frequency of infections, but in severe cases haematopoietic stem cell transplantation is required to provide a source of osteoclasts that resorb bone normally.

Sclerosing bone dysplasias

These are rare diseases characterised by osteosclerosis and increased bone formation. Van Buchem's disease and sclerosteosis are recessive disorders caused by loss-of-function mutations in the *SOST* gene, which normally suppresses bone formation (see Fig. 24.3, p. 986). The resulting lack of sclerostin causes increased bone formation and bone overgrowth, leading to enlargement of the cranium and jaw, tall stature and cranial nerve palsies. There is no effective treatment. High bone mass syndrome is a benign disorder caused by mutations in the *LRP4* or *LRP5* gene, which is characterised by unusually high bone density. The mutations render the LRP receptors resistant to the inhibitory effects of SOST. Most patients are asymptomatic but bone overgrowth in the palate (torus palatinus) and enlargement of the mandible can occur in later life. Treatment is not usually required. Camurati–Engelmann disease is an autosomal dominant condition caused by gain of function in the *TGFB1* gene. It presents with bone pain, muscle weakness and osteosclerosis mainly affecting the diaphysis of long bones. Glucocorticoids can help the bone pain, although usually analgesics are also required.

Bone and joint tumours

Primary tumours of bones and joints are rare, have a peak incidence in childhood and adolescence, and can be benign or malignant (Box 24.77). Paget's disease of bone (p. 1053) accounts for most cases of osteosarcoma occurring above the age of 40.

Osteosarcoma

This is a rare tumour with an incidence of 0.6–0.85 per 100 000 population. It is the most common primary bone tumour. Most

i	24.77 Primary tumours of the musculoskeletal system		
Cell type	**Benign**	**Malignant**
Osteoblast	Osteoid osteoma	Osteosarcoma
Chondrocyte	Chondroma Osteochondroma	Chondrosarcoma
Fibroblast	Fibroma	Fibrosarcoma
Bone marrow cell	Eosinophilic granuloma	Ewing's sarcoma
Endothelial cell	Haemangioma	Angiosarcoma
Osteoclast precursor	Giant cell tumour	Malignant giant cell tumour

patients present under the age of 30 but osteosarcoma also occurs in the elderly in association with Paget's disease. The presentation is with local pain and swelling. X-rays show expansion of the bone with a surrounding soft tissue mass, often containing islands of calcification. If the diagnosis is being considered, MRI or CT should be performed to determine the extent of tumour. Patients suspected of having osteosarcoma should be referred to a specialist team for biopsy. Treatment depends on histological type but generally involves surgical removal of the tumour, followed by chemotherapy and radiotherapy. The prognosis is normally good in cases that present in childhood and adolescence, but poor in elderly patients with osteosarcoma related to Paget's disease of bone.

Chondrosarcoma

This is the second most common primary bone tumour. Presentation is as described for osteosarcoma. The treatment of choice is surgical resection since chondrosarcomas are relatively resistant to chemotherapy and radiotherapy. The prognosis is good for low-grade tumours but poor for anaplastic tumours.

Ewing's sarcoma

This is the third most common sarcoma, which presents almost exclusively under the age of 40. Presentation is as described for osteosarcoma. Treatment is by local excision and surgical resection. The prognosis is excellent for patients who present before metastasis has occurred.

Metastatic bone disease

Metastatic bone disease may present in a variety of ways: with localised or generalised progressive bone pain, generalised regional pain, symptoms of spinal cord compression, or acute pain due to pathological fracture. Systemic features, such as weight loss and anorexia, and symptoms referable to the primary tumour are often present. The tumours that most commonly metastasise to bone are myeloma and those of bronchus, breast, prostate, kidney and thyroid. Management is discussed in Chapter 33.

Rheumatological involvement in other diseases

Many systemic diseases can affect the locomotor system, and many drugs may cause adverse locomotor effects (Box 24.78). The most common examples are described here. Bone disease in sarcoidosis is described on page 608, haemophilia on page 972 and sickle-cell anaemia on page 952.

Malignant disease

Malignant disease can cause a variety of non-metastatic musculoskeletal problems (Box 24.79). One of the most striking is hypertrophic pulmonary osteoarthropathy (HPOA), characterised by clubbing and painful swelling of the limbs, periosteal new bone formation and arthralgia/arthritis. The most common causes are bronchial carcinoma and mesothelioma (pp. 598 and 618). Bone scans show increased periosteal uptake before new bone is apparent on X-ray. The course follows that of the underlying malignancy and HPOA resolves if this is cured.

 24.78 Drug-induced effects on the musculoskeletal system

Musculoskeletal problem	Principal drug
Secondary gout	Thiazides, furosemide, alcohol
Osteoporosis	Glucocorticoids, heparin, glitazones, aromatase inhibitors, GnRH agonists
Osteomalacia	Anticonvulsants, etidronate and pamidronate (high-dose)
Osteonecrosis	Glucocorticoids, alcohol
Drug-induced lupus syndrome	Procainamide, hydralazine, isoniazid, chlorpromazine
Arthralgias, arthritis	Glucocorticoid withdrawal, glibenclamide, methyldopa, ciclosporin, isoniazid, barbiturates
Myalgia	Glucocorticoid withdrawal, L-tryptophan, fibrates, statins
Myopathy	Glucocorticoids, chloroquine
Myositis, myasthenia	Penicillamine, statins
Cramps	Glucocorticoids, ACTH, diuretics, carbenoxolone
Vasculitis	Amphetamines, thiazides

(ACTH = adrenocorticotrophic hormone; GnRH = gonadotrophin-releasing hormone)

24.79 Rheumatological manifestations of malignancy

- Polyarthritis
- Dermatomyositis and polymyositis
- Hypophosphataemic osteomalacia
- Hypertrophic osteoarthropathy
- Vasculitis, connective tissue disease
- Raynaud's syndrome
- Polymyalgia rheumatica-like syndrome

Endocrine disease

Hypothyroidism (p. 639) may present with carpal tunnel syndrome or, rarely, with painful, symmetrical proximal myopathy and muscle hypertrophy. Both resolve with levothyroxine replacement. Primary hyperparathyroidism (p. 663) is associated with osteoporosis and also predisposes to calcium pyrophosphate dihydrate deposition disease and to calcific periarthritis, especially in patients with renal disease.

Diabetes mellitus (Ch. 20) commonly causes diabetic cheiroarthropathy, characterised by tightening of skin and periarticular structures, causing flexion deformities of the fingers that may be painful. Diabetic osteopathy presents as forefoot pain with radiographic progression from osteopenia to complete osteolysis of the phalanges and metatarsals. Diabetes also predisposes to osteoporosis, fragility fractures, adhesive capsulitis, Dupuytren's contracture, septic arthritis and Charcot's joints.

Acromegaly (p. 685) can be associated with mechanical back pain, with normal or excessive movement; carpal tunnel syndrome; and Raynaud's syndrome and an arthropathy (50%). The arthropathy mainly affects the large joints and has clinical similarities to OA but with a normal or increased range of movement. X-rays may show widening of joint spaces, squaring of bone ends, generalised osteopenia and tufting of terminal phalanges. It does not improve with treatment of the acromegaly.

24

Haematological disease

Haemochromatosis (p. 895) is complicated by an arthropathy in about 50% of cases. It typically presents between the ages of 40 and 50, and may predate other features of the disease. The small joints of the hands and wrists are typically affected but the hips, shoulders and knees may also be involved. The X-ray changes resemble OA but cysts are often multiple and prominent, with little osteophyte formation. Involvement of the radiocarpal and MCP joints may occur, which is unusual in primary OA, and about 30% have calcium pyrophosphate dihydrate deposition disease and/ or pseudogout. Treatment of the haemochromatosis does not influence the arthropathy, and management is as described for OA. Haemophilia (p. 972) can be complicated by haemarthrosis, which, if recurrent, can result in the development of secondary OA. Sickle-cell disease (p. 952) may be associated with bone pain, osteonecrosis and osteomyelitis. Thalassaemia (p. 953) may be complicated by bone deformity, especially affecting the craniofacial bones, and by osteoporosis.

Neurological disease

Neurological disease may result in rapidly destructive arthritis of joints, first described by Charcot in association with syphilis. The cause is incompletely understood but may involve repetitive trauma as the result of sensory loss and altered blood flow secondary to impaired sympathetic nervous system control. The main predisposing diseases and sites of involvement are:

- diabetic neuropathy (hindfoot)
- syringomyelia (shoulder, elbow, wrist)
- leprosy (hands, feet)
- tabes dorsalis (knees, spine).

The presentation is with subacute or chronic monoarthritis. Pain can occur, especially at the onset, but once the joint is severely deranged, pain is often minimal and signs become disproportionately greater than symptoms. The joint is often grossly swollen, with effusion, crepitus, marked instability and deformity, but usually no increased warmth. X-rays show disorganisation of normal joint architecture and often multiple loose bodies (Fig. 24.66), and either no (atrophic) or gross (hypertrophic) new bone formation. Management principally involves orthoses and occasionally arthrodesis.

Miscellaneous conditions

Anterior tibial compartment syndrome

This is characterised by severe pain in the front of the lower leg, aggravated by exercise and relieved by rest. Symptoms result from fascial compression of the muscles in the anterior tibial compartment and may be associated with foot drop. Treatment is by surgical decompression.

Carpal tunnel syndrome

This is a common nerve entrapment syndrome caused by compression of the median nerve at the wrist. It presents with numbness, tingling and pain in a median nerve distribution (p. 1139). The most common causes are hypothyroidism, diabetes mellitus, RA, obesity and pregnancy, especially in the third trimester. In some patients, no underlying cause may be identified. Carpal tunnel syndrome often responds to treatment of the underlying condition but other options include local glucocorticoid injections and surgical decompression.

Diffuse idiopathic skeletal hyperostosis

Diffuse idiopathic skeletal hyperostosis (DISH) is a common disorder, affecting 10% of men and 8% of women over the age of 65, and is associated with obesity, hypertension and type 2 diabetes mellitus. It is characterised by florid new bone formation along the anterolateral aspect of at least four contiguous vertebral bodies (Fig. 24.67). DISH is distinguished from lumbar spondylosis by the absence of disc space narrowing and marginal vertebral body sclerosis, and from ankylosing spondylitis by the absence of sacroiliitis or apophyseal joint fusion. It is usually an

Fig. 24.66 Wrist X-ray showing a neuropathic (Charcot) joint in a patient with syringomyelia. Note the disorganised architecture with complete loss of the proximal carpal row, bony fragments and soft tissue swelling.

Fig. 24.67 Diffuse idiopathic skeletal hyperostosis (DISH). Anteroposterior X-ray of the thoracic spine showing right-sided, flowing new bone joining more than four contiguous vertebrae. The disc spaces are preserved.

asymptomatic radiographic finding but can cause back pain or pain at peripheral sites, such as the heel, in association with calcaneal spur formation.

Dupuytren's contracture

Dupuytren's contracture results from fibrosis and contracture of the superficial palmar fascia of the hands. The patient is unable to extend the fingers fully and there is puckering of the skin with palpable nodules. The ring and little fingers are usually the first and worst affected. Dupuytren's contracture is usually painless but causes problems due to limitation of hand function and snagging of the curled fingers in pockets. It is age-related, usually bilateral and more common in men. There is a strong genetic component and sometimes may be familial, with dominant inheritance. The condition can be associated with plantar fibromatosis, Peyronie's disease, alcohol misuse and chronic vibration injury. It is very slowly progressive. Often no treatment is required but it can be treated medically by local injections of collagenase or surgically by fasciotomy if symptoms are troublesome.

Hypermobility syndromes

Hypermobility is characterised by increased joint laxity and joint pain. Causes include Marfan's syndrome, resulting from mutations in the *FBN1* gene (p. 508); osteogenesis imperfecta (p. 1055); and Ehlers–Danlos syndrome types I, II and IV, caused by mutations in the *COL3A1*, *COL5A1* and *COL5A2* genes (p. 970).

The term hypermobile Ehlers–Danlos syndrome (hEDS), which is also known as EDS type III, is used to describe a polygenic form of hypermobility. Many patients with this condition have hypermobile joints but do not have symptoms, whereas in others a range of symptoms can occur, including chronic joint and ligamentous pain, fibromyalgia-like symptoms, recurrent dislocations, easy bruising, abdominal symptoms, mitral valve prolapse (p. 520) and postural tachycardia syndrome, in which there is dizziness, hypotension and an increased heart rate on standing. The diagnosis of EDS type III is clinical and can be made when the modified Beighton score is 4 or above in the presence of arthralgia in four or more joints (Box 24.80). There is no specific treatment, apart from the general principles listed on page 1000, but some patients become very disabled as the result of their symptoms and are difficult to manage.

Inclusion body myositis

Inclusion body myositis is the most frequent primary myopathy in middle age and after. It is characterised by slowly progressive

i	24.80 Modified Beighton score for joint hypermobility
Clinical test	**Score**
Extend little finger >90°	1 point each side
Bring thumb back parallel to/touching forearm	1 point each side
Extend elbow >10°	1 point each side
Extend knee >10°	1 point each side
Touch floor with flat of hands, legs straight	1 point
Hypermobile = a score of 6 or more points out of a possible 9 for epidemiological studies, or 4 or more points (with arthralgia in four or more joints) for a clinical diagnosis of the benign joint hypermobility syndrome	

muscle weakness and atrophy, with pathological changes of inflammation, degeneration and mitochondrial abnormality in affected muscle fibres. Inclusion body myositis typically presents with distal muscle weakness. In time, muscles atrophy. Investigation is the same as for polymyositis (p. 1039). There is typically a slightly elevated creatine kinase and myopathic changes on EMG. Muscle biopsy shows abnormal fibres containing rimmed vacuoles and filamentous inclusions in the nucleus and cytoplasm. Therapeutic response to glucocorticoids and immunosuppressants is notably poor. There is anecdotal report of efficacy with IVIg but trial evidence is lacking.

Periodic fever syndromes

These are a group of rare inherited disorders that present with intermittent attacks of fever, rash, arthralgia and myalgia. They are discussed in more detail on page 81.

Pigmented villonodular synovitis

Pigmented villonodular synovitis is an uncommon proliferative disorder of synovium, which typically affects young adults. It is caused by a somatic chromosomal translocation in synovial cells that places the *CSF1* gene downstream of the *COL6A3* gene promoter. The result is local over-production of M-CSF, which causes accumulation of macrophages in the joint. The presentation is with joint swelling, limitation of movement and local discomfort. The diagnosis can be confirmed by MRI or synovial biopsy. Treatment is by surgical or radiation synovectomy.

Scoliosis

Scoliosis is characterised by an abnormal lateral curvature of the spine of greater than 10°. It typically presents during childhood or adolescence but usually persists into adulthood, when it can be associated with back pain, deformity and secondary OA. In about 20% of cases, scoliosis is secondary to a neuromuscular disorder, such as muscular dystrophy, cerebral palsy or neurofibromatosis. It may also occur in association with connective tissue disorders, such as Marfan's syndrome. The term idiopathic scoliosis is used to described the remaining cases where there is no obvious cause. In fact, there is strong evidence from twin studies that idiopathic scoliosis is genetically mediated. The diagnosis can usually be made clinically by physical examination, which shows the characteristic spinal deformity. Spinal X-rays can be used to confirm the diagnosis and assess severity. External bracing and/or surgical intervention are often performed in adolescents with severe deformities to correct deformity or prevent progression but the evidence base is poor. In adulthood, treatment is symptomatic in nature with analgesics, NSAID or antineuropathic medications.

Spondylolysis

Spondylolysis describes a break in the integrity of the neural arch. The principal cause is an acquired defect in the pars interarticularis due to a fracture, mainly seen in gymnasts, dancers and runners, in whom it is an important cause of back pain. Spondylolisthesis describes the condition in which a defect causes slippage of a vertebra on the one below. This may be congenital, post-traumatic or degenerative. Rarely, it can result from metastatic destruction of the posterior elements. Uncomplicated spondylolysis does not cause symptoms but spondylolisthesis can lead to low back pain

24

aggravated by standing and walking. Occasionally, symptoms of nerve root or spinal compression may occur. The diagnosis can be made on lateral X-rays of the lumbar spine but MRI may be required if there is neurological involvement. Advice on posture and muscle-strengthening exercises is required in mild cases. Surgical fusion is indicated for severe and recurrent low back pain. Surgical decompression is mandatory prior to fusion in patients with significant lumbar stenosis or symptoms of cauda equina compression.

Synovitis–acne–pustulosis–hyperostosis–osteitis syndrome

The synovitis–acne–pustulosis–hyperostosis–osteitis (SAPHO) syndrome is a disorder characterised by bone pain and swelling due to a sterile osteomyelitis and hyperostosis predominantly targeting the clavicles and bones of the anterior chest wall. SAPHO syndrome is thought to be part of a spectrum of autoinflammatory bone diseases that includes chronic recurrent (sterile) multifocal osteomyelitis in children and adolescents. Other features include a pustulotic rash affecting the palms and soles of the feet, sacroiliitis and synovitis of peripheral joints. It most commonly presents in children and young or middle-aged adults. Various treatments have been used, including glucocorticoids, DMARDs, bisphosphonates, anakinra and TNF blockers, with most success arising from biologic use. The cause is unknown but has been suggested to be an autoimmune process triggered by a bacterial or viral pathogen.

Trigger finger

This occurs as the result of stenosing tenosynovitis in the flexor tendon sheath, with intermittent locking of the finger in flexion. It can arise spontaneously or in association with inflammatory diseases such as RA. Symptoms usually respond to local glucocorticoid injections but surgical decompression is occasionally required.

Further information

Journal articles

Campion EW. Calcium pyrophosphate deposition disease. N Engl J Med 2016; 374:2575–2578.

Compston J. Osteoporosis: advances in risk assessment and management. Clin Med (Lond) 2016; 16(Suppl 6): s121–s124.

Gossec L, Smolen JS, Ramiro S, et al. European League Against Rheumatism (EULAR) recommendations for the management of psoriatic arthritis with pharmacological therapies: 2015 update. Ann Rheum Dis 2016; 75:499–510.

Mukhtyar C, Flossman O, Hellmich B, et al. Outcomes from studies of antineutrophil cytoplasm antibody associated vasculitis: a systematic review by the European League Against Rheumatism systemic vasculitis task force. Ann Rheum Dis 2008; 67:1004–1010.

Ralston SH. Paget's disease of bone. N Engl J Med 2013; 368:644–650.

Scott DL, Woolf F, Huizinga TW. Rheumatoid arthritis. Lancet 2010; 376:1094–1108.

Taurog JD, Avneesh C, Colbert RA. Ankylosing spondylitis and axial spondyloarthritis. N Engl J Med 2016; 374:2563–2567.

Teng MWL, Bowman EP, McElwee JJ, et al. IL-12 and IL-23 cytokines: from discovery to targeted therapies for immune-mediated inflammatory diseases. Nat Med 2015; 21:719–729.

Zhang W, Doherty M, Bardin T, et al. EULAR recommendations for gout. Part II: Management. Ann Rheum Dis 2006; 65:1312–1324.

Websites

4s-dawn.com/DAS28 Calculator for this measure of activity in rheumatoid arthritis.

asas-group.org Repository of resources to aid assessment of spondyloarthritis.

basdai.com/BASDAI.php BASDAI calculator for assessing ankylosing spondylitis.

omim.org Online Mendelian Inheritance in Man (OMIM): genetic diseases.

shef.ac.uk/FRAX/ and qfracture.org/ Fracture risk assessment tools.

sign.ac.uk Scottish Intercollegiate Guidelines Network 142 – Management of osteoporosis and the prevention of fragility fractures.

thefreelibrary.com Information on drug-induced myopathies.

vasculitis.org/ Vasculitis resources from the European Vasculitis Society.

JP Leach
RJ Davenport

25

Neurology

Clinical examination of the nervous system 1062

Functional anatomy and physiology 1064
Functional anatomy of the nervous system 1065
Localising lesions in the central nervous system 1071

Investigation of neurological disease 1072
Neuroimaging 1072
Neurophysiological testing 1074

Presenting problems in neurological disease 1078
Headache and facial pain 1080
Dizziness, blackouts and 'funny turns' 1080
Status epilepticus 1080
Coma 1080
Delirium 1080
Amnesia 1080
Weakness 1081
Sensory disturbance 1083
Abnormal movements 1084
Abnormal perception 1086
Altered balance and vertigo 1086
Abnormal gait 1086
Abnormal speech and language 1087
Disturbance of smell 1088
Visual disturbance and ocular abnormalities 1088
Hearing disturbance 1093
Bulbar symptoms – dysphagia and dysarthria 1093
Bladder, bowel and sexual disturbance 1093
Personality change 1094
Sleep disturbance 1094
Psychiatric disorders 1094

Functional symptoms 1094

Headache syndromes 1095

Epilepsy 1097

Vestibular disorders 1104

Disorders of sleep 1105
Excessive daytime sleepiness (hypersomnolence) 1105
Parasomnias 1105

Neuro-inflammatory diseases 1106

Paraneoplastic neurological disorders 1110

Neurodegenerative diseases 1111
Movement disorders 1112
Ataxias 1115
Tremor disorders 1115
Dystonia 1116
Hemifacial spasm 1116
Motor neuron disease 1116
Spinal muscular atrophy 1117

Infections of the nervous system 1117
Meningitis 1118
Parenchymal viral infections 1121
Parenchymal bacterial infections 1124
Diseases caused by bacterial toxins 1125
Prion diseases 1126

Intracranial mass lesions and raised intracranial pressure 1127
Raised intracranial pressure 1127
Brain tumours 1129
Paraneoplastic neurological disease 1132
Hydrocephalus 1132
Idiopathic intracranial hypertension 1133
Head injury 1133

Disorders of cerebellar function 1134

Disorders of the spine and spinal cord 1134
Cervical spondylosis 1134
Lumbar spondylosis 1135
Spinal cord compression 1136
Intrinsic diseases of the spinal cord 1137

Diseases of peripheral nerves 1138
Entrapment neuropathy 1139
Multifocal neuropathy 1140
Polyneuropathy 1140
Guillain–Barré syndrome 1140
Chronic polyneuropathy 1140
Brachial plexopathy 1141
Lumbosacral plexopathy 1141
Spinal root lesions 1141

Diseases of the neuromuscular junction 1141
Myasthenia gravis 1141
Lambert–Eaton myasthenic syndrome 1143

Diseases of muscle 1143
Muscular dystrophies 1143
Inherited metabolic myopathies 1144
Acquired myopathies 1144

Clinical examination of the nervous system

4 Cranial nerves

▲ Right 12th nerve palsy: wasting of right side of tongue

▲ 7th nerve palsy: drooping mouth and flattening of nasolabial skin fold

▲ 3rd nerve palsy: one eye points 'down and out'

3 Neck and skull

Skull size and shape
Neck stiffness and Kernig's test
Carotid bruit

2 Back

Scoliosis
Operative scars
Evidence of spina bifida occulta
Winging of scapula

▲ Winging of right scapula (muscular dystrophy)

1 Stance and gait

Posture
Romberg's test
Arm swing
Pattern of gait
Tandem (heel-toe) gait

Observation/general
• General appearance
• Mood (e.g. anxious, depressed)
• Facial expression (or lack thereof)
• Handedness
• Nutritional status
• Blood pressure

5 Optic fundi

Papilloedema
Optic atrophy
Cupping of disc (glaucoma)
Hypertensive changes
Signs of diabetes

▲ Haemorrhagic papilloedema

6 Motor

Wasting, fasciculation
Abnormal posture
Abnormal movements
Tone (including clonus)
Strength
Coordination
Tendon reflexes
Abdominal reflexes
Plantar reflexes

▲ Wasting of right thenar eminence due to cervical rib

▲ Pes cavus

7 Sensory

Pin-prick, temperature
Joint position, vibration
Two-point discrimination

8 Higher cerebral function

Orientation
Memory
Speech and language
Localised cortical functions

Insets (winging of scapula, 12th nerve palsy, wasting of thenar eminence) Courtesy of Dr R.E. Cull, Western General Hospital, Edinburgh.

1 Examination of gait and posture

Procedure	Abnormality	Disease
Rising from chair	Difficulty rising	Proximal muscle weakness or joint disorders
Gait initiation	Difficulty starting to walk, frozen	Cerebrovascular disease or parkinsonism
Posture	Stooped	Parkinsonism
Retropulsion/anteropulsion	Postural instability	Parkinsonism
Arms during walking	Reduced arm swing	Parkinsonism or upper motor neuron lesion
	Enhanced tremor	Parkinsonism
	Dystonic posturing	Dystonia
Gait pattern	Circumduction (stiff leg moves outwards in 'circular' manner)	Hemiparesis, typically after stroke
	'Slapping', high-stepping due to foot drop	L5 radiculopathy or common peroneal nerve lesion
	Narrow-based, short strides, freezing in doorways	Parkinsonism
	Stiff-legged, scissors gait	Spastic paraparesis (multiple sclerosis, vascular disease, spinal cord lesions)
	Wide-based, unsteady, unable to perform tandem gait	Cerebellar lesion
	Waddling gait	Myopathies with proximal weakness

4 Examination of cranial nerves

Nerve	Name	Tests
I	Olfactory	Ask patient about sense of smell (examine only if change is reported)
II	Optic	Visual acuity and colour vision Visual fields Pupillary responses Ophthalmoscopy
III	Oculomotor	Eyelids (ptosis) Pupil size, symmetry, reactions Eye movements
IV	Trochlear	Eye movements (superior oblique muscle)
V	Trigeminal	Facial sensation Corneal reflex Muscles of mastication
VI	Abducens	Eye movements (lateral rectus muscle)
VII	Facial	Facial symmetry and movements
VIII	Vestibulocochlear	Otoscopy Hearing Tuning fork tests (Rinne and Weber)
IX	Glossopharyngeal	Swallowing
X	Vagus	Palatal elevation (uvula deviates to side opposite lesion) Swallowing Cough (bovine) Speech
XI	Accessory	Look for wasting of trapezius/sternocleidomastoid Elevation of shoulders Turning head to right and left
XII	Hypoglossal	Look for wasting/fasciculation Tongue protrusion (deviates to side of lesion)

6 Root values of tendon reflexes

Reflex	Root value
Arm	
Biceps jerk	C5
Supinator jerk	C6
Triceps jerk	C7
Finger jerk	C8
Leg	
Knee jerk	L3/L4
Ankle jerk	S1

Motor

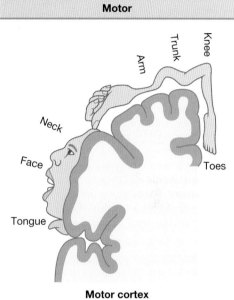

Motor cortex
(pre-central gyrus)

Sensory

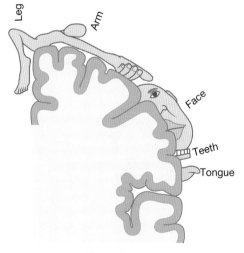

Somatic cortex
(post-central gyrus)

Motor and sensory homunculi. The motor and sensory homunculi illustrate the cortical areas serving each anatomical area within the pre-central (motor) and post-central (sensory) gyri.

25

The complexity of the brain differentiates us from other species, and its interactions with the spinal cord and peripheral nerves combine to allow us to perceive and react to the external world while maintaining a stable internal environment. The cerebral cortex provides a platform for processing information and forming a response, and in doing so, both forms and is affected by our personality and mental state.

Neurology has for too long been misperceived as a specialty in which intricate clinical examination and numerous investigations are required to diagnose obscure and untreatable conditions. In fact, nervous system disorders are common, accounting for around 10% of the UK's general practice consultations, 20% of acute medical admissions, and most chronic physical disability. The development of specific, effective treatments has made accurate diagnosis essential. Neurological management requires knowledge of a range of common conditions, which can then be applied to individual patients after careful history-taking, with lesser contributions arising from targeted examination and considered investigation.

Pathological and anatomical localisation of symptoms and signs is important, but skill can be required to identify those *not* associated with neurological disease, differentiating patients requiring investigation and treatment from those who need reassurance.

Initially, it is important to exclude conditions that constitute neurological emergencies (Box 25.1). If the presentation is not an emergency, time can be taken to reach a diagnosis. The history should provide a hypothesis for the site and nature of the potential pathology, which a focused examination may refine, and direct appropriate further investigations. An informed discussion with the patient and family regarding diagnosis, management and prognosis may then take place.

As stroke has become a specific subspecialty in many centres, it is described in a separate chapter, although it is clearly a neurological condition. This chapter should be read with it, to help clarify how the presentation, diagnosis and management of stroke present their own challenges.

Functional anatomy and physiology

Cells of the nervous system

The nervous system comprises billions of specialised cells, forming a spectacular network of connections, each human brain having almost as many connections as there are grains of sand in the whole world. In addition to neurons, there are three types of glial cells. Astrocytes form the structural framework for neurons

25.1 Neurological emergencies

- Status epilepticus (p. 1080)
- Stroke (if thrombolysis available) (p. 1158)
- Guillain–Barré syndrome (p. 1140)
- Myasthenia gravis (if bulbar and/or respiratory) (p. 1141)
- Spinal cord compression (p. 1136)
- Subarachnoid haemorrhage (p. 1160)
- Neuroleptic malignant syndrome (p. 1197)

Fig. 25.1 Cells of the nervous system. (CSF = cerebrospinal fluid)

and control their biochemical environment, their foot processes adjoining small blood vessels and forming the blood–brain barrier (Fig. 25.1). Oligodendrocytes are responsible for the formation and maintenance of the myelin sheath, which surrounds axons and is essential for maintaining the speed and consistency of action potential propagation along axons. Peripheral nerves have axons invested in myelin made by oligodendrocytes (Schwann cells). Microglial cells derive from monocytes/macrophages and play a role in fighting infection and removing damaged cells. Ependymal cells line the cerebral ventricles.

Generation and transmission of the nervous impulse

The role of the central nervous system (CNS) is to generate outputs in response to external stimuli and changes in internal conditions. The CNS has to maintain a delicate balance between responsivity to external stimuli and remaining stoic enough to remain stable in a rapidly changing environment. Each neuron receives input by synaptic transmission from dendrites (branched projections of other neurons), which sum to produce output in the form of an action potential that is then conducted along the axon, resulting in synaptic transmission to other neurons or, in the motor system, to muscle cells. Summation of the inputs causes net changes in the target neuron's electrochemical gradient, which, if large enough, will trigger an action potential. Communication between cells is by synaptic transmission that involves the release of neurotransmitters to interact with structures on the target cell's surface, including ion channels and other cell surface receptors (Fig. 25.2). At least 20 different neurotransmitters are known to act at different sites in the nervous system, most of which are potentially amenable to pharmacological manipulation.

Each neuronal cell body may receive synaptic input from thousands of other neurons. The synapsing neuron terminals are also subject to feedback regulation via receptor sites on the pre-synaptic membrane, modifying the release of transmitter across the synaptic cleft. In addition to such acute effects, some neurotransmitters produce long-term modulation of metabolic function or gene expression. This effect probably underlies more complex processes such as long-term memory.

Functional anatomy of the nervous system

Major components of the nervous system and their inter-relationships are depicted in Figure 25.3.

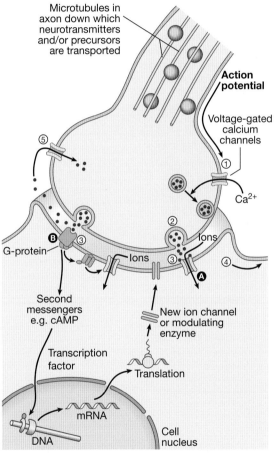

Fig. 25.2 **Neurotransmission and neurotransmitters.** (1) An action potential arriving at the nerve terminal depolarises the membrane and this opens voltage-gated calcium channels. (2) Entry of calcium causes the fusion of synaptic vesicles containing neurotransmitters with the pre-synaptic membrane and release of the neurotransmitter across the synaptic cleft. (3) The neurotransmitter binds to receptors on the post-synaptic membrane either (A) to open ligand-gated ion channels that, by allowing ion entry, depolarise the membrane and initiate an action potential (4), or (B) to bind to metabotropic receptors that activate an effector enzyme (e.g. adenylyl cyclase) and thus modulate gene transcription via the intracellular second messenger system, leading to changes in synthesis of ion channels or modulating enzymes. (5) Neurotransmitters are taken up at the pre-synaptic membrane and/or metabolised. (cAMP = cyclic adenosine monophosphate; DNA = deoxyribonucleic acid; mRNA = messenger ribonucleic acid)

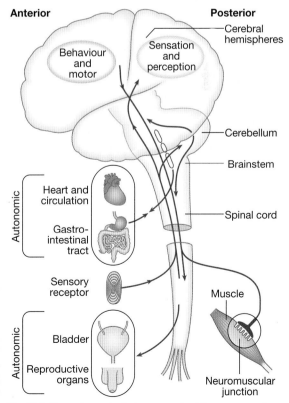

Fig. 25.3 **The major anatomical components of the nervous system.**

Cerebral hemispheres

The cerebral hemispheres coordinate the highest level of nervous function, the anterior half dealing with executive ('doing') functions and the posterior half constructing a perception of the environment. Each cerebral hemisphere has four functionally specialised lobes (Box 25.2 and Fig. 25.4), with some functions being distributed asymmetrically ('lateralised'), to produce cerebral dominance for functions such as motor control, speech or memory. Cerebral dominance aligns limb dominance with language function: in right-handed individuals the left hemisphere is almost always dominant, while around half of left-handers have a dominant right hemisphere.

Frontal lobes are concerned with executive function, movement, behaviour and planning. As well as the primary and supplementary motor cortex, there are specialised areas for control of eye movements, speech (Broca's area) and micturition.

The parietal lobes integrate sensory perception. The primary sensory cortex lies in the post-central gyrus of the parietal lobe. Much of the remainder is devoted to 'association' cortex, which processes and interprets input from the various sensory modalities. The supramarginal and angular gyri of the dominant parietal lobe form part of the language area (p. 1088). Close to these are regions dealing with numerical function. The non-dominant parietal lobe is concerned with spatial awareness and orientation.

The temporal lobes contain the primary auditory cortex and primary vestibular cortex. On the inner medial sides lie the olfactory and parahippocampal cortices, which are involved in memory function. The temporal lobes also link intimately to the limbic system, including the hippocampus and the amygdala, which are involved in memory and emotional processing. The dominant temporal lobe also participates in language functions, particularly verbal comprehension (Wernicke's area). Musical processing occurs across both temporal lobes, rhythm on the dominant side and melody/pitch on the non-dominant.

The occipital lobes are responsible for visual interpretation. The contralateral visual hemifield is represented in each primary visual cortex, with surrounding areas processing specific visual submodalities such as colour, movement or depth, and the analysis of more complex visual patterns such as faces.

Deep to the grey matter in the cortices, and the white matter (composed of neuronal axons), are collections of cells known as the basal ganglia that are concerned with motor control; the thalamus, which is responsible for the level of attention to sensory perception; the limbic system, concerned with emotion and memory; and the hypothalamus, responsible for homeostasis, such as temperature

i 25.2 Cortical lobar functions

Lobe	Function	Effects of damage		
		Cognitive/behavioural	Associated physical signs	Positive phenomena
Frontal	Personality Emotional control Social behaviour Contralateral motor control Language Micturition	Disinhibition Lack of initiation Antisocial behaviour Impaired memory Expressive dysphasia Incontinence	Impaired smell Contralateral hemiparesis Frontal release signs[1]	Seizures – often nocturnal with motor activity Versive head movements
Parietal: dominant	Language Calculation	Dysphasia Acalculia Dyslexia Apraxia[3] Agnosia[5]	Contralateral hemisensory loss Astereognosis[2] Agraphaesthesia[4] Contralateral homonymous lower quadrantanopia Asymmetry of optokinetic nystagmus (OKN)	Focal sensory seizures
Parietal: non-dominant	Spatial orientation Constructional skills	Neglect of contralateral side Spatial disorientation Constructional apraxia Dressing apraxia	Contralateral hemisensory loss Astereognosis[2] Agraphaesthesia[4] Contralateral homonymous lower quadrantanopia Asymmetry of OKN	Focal sensory seizures
Temporal: dominant	Auditory perception Language Verbal memory Smell Balance	Receptive aphasia Dyslexia Impaired verbal memory	Contralateral homonymous upper quadrantanopia	Complex hallucinations (smell, sound, vision, memory)
Temporal: non-dominant	Auditory perception Melody/pitch perception Non-verbal memory Smell Balance	Impaired non-verbal memory Impaired musical skills (tonal perception)	Contralateral homonymous upper quadrantanopia	Complex hallucinations (smell, sound, vision, memory)
Occipital	Visual processing	Visual inattention Visual loss Visual agnosia	Homonymous hemianopia (macular sparing)	Simple visual hallucinations (e.g. phosphenes, zigzag lines)

[1]Grasp reflex, palmomental response, pout response. [2]Inability to determine three-dimensional shape by touch. [3]Inability to perform complex movements in the presence of normal motor, sensory and cerebellar function. [4]Inability to 'read' numbers or letters drawn on hand, with the eyes shut. [5]Inability to recognise familiar objects, e.g. faces.

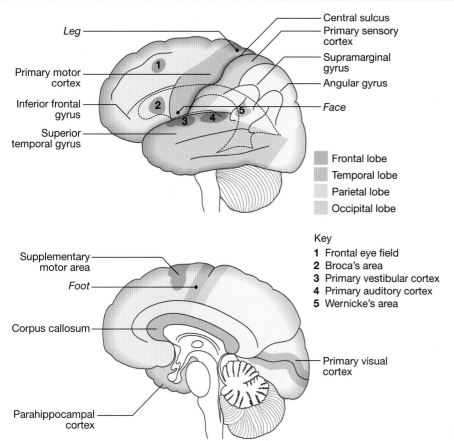

Key

Frontal lobe
Temporal lobe
Parietal lobe
Occipital lobe

Key
1 Frontal eye field
2 Broca's area
3 Primary vestibular cortex
4 Primary auditory cortex
5 Wernicke's area

Fig. 25.4 Anatomy of the cerebral cortex.

and appetite control. The cerebral ventricles contain cerebrospinal fluid (CSF), which cushions the brain during cranial movement.

CSF is formed in the lateral ventricles and protects and nourishes the CNS. CSF flows from third to fourth ventricles and through foramina in the brainstem to dissipate over the surface of the CNS, eventually being reabsorbed into the cerebral venous system (see Fig. 25.44, p. 1132).

The brainstem

In addition to containing all the sensory and motor pathways entering and leaving the hemispheres, the brainstem houses the nuclei and projections of most cranial nerves, as well as other important collections of neurons in the reticular formation (Fig. 25.5). Cranial nerve nuclei provide motor control to muscles of the head (including face and eyes) and coordinate sensory input from the special sense organs and the face, nose, mouth, larynx and pharynx. They also relay autonomic messages, including pupillary, salivary and lacrimal functions. The reticular formation is mainly involved in control of conjugate eye movements, the maintenance of balance and arousal, and cardiorespiratory control.

The spinal cord

The spinal cord is the route for virtually all communication between the extracranial structures and the CNS. Afferent and efferent fibres are grouped in discrete bundles but collections of cells in the grey matter are responsible for lower-order motor reflexes and the primary processing of sensory information.

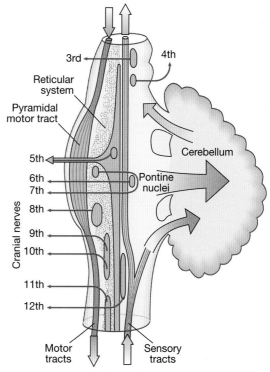

Fig. 25.5 Anatomy of the brainstem.

Sensory peripheral nervous system

The sensory cell bodies of peripheral nerves are situated just outside the spinal cord, in the dorsal root ganglia in the spinal exit foramina, while the distal ends of their neurons utilise various specialised endings for the conversion of external stimuli into action potentials. Sensory nerves consist of a combination of large, fast, myelinated axons (which carry information about joint position sense and commands to muscles) and smaller, slower, unmyelinated axons (which carry information about pain and temperature, as well as autonomic function).

Motor peripheral nervous system

The anterior horns of the spinal cord comprise cell bodies of the lower motor neurons. To increase conduction speed, peripheral motor nerve axons are wrapped in myelin produced by Schwann cells. Motor neurons release acetylcholine across the neuromuscular junction, which changes the muscle end-plate potential and initiates muscle contraction.

The autonomic system

The autonomic system regulates the cardiovascular and respiratory systems, the smooth muscle of the gastrointestinal tract, and many exocrine and endocrine glands throughout the body. The autonomic system is controlled centrally by diffuse modulatory systems in the brainstem, limbic system, hypothalamus and frontal lobes, which are concerned with arousal and background behavioural responses to threat. Autonomic output divides functionally and pharmacologically into two divisions: the parasympathetic and sympathetic systems.

The motor system

A programme of movement formulated by the pre-motor cortex is converted into a series of excitatory and inhibitory signals in the motor cortex that are transmitted to the spinal cord in the pyramidal tract (Fig. 25.6). This passes through the internal capsule and the ventral brainstem before crossing (decussating) in the medulla to enter the lateral columns of the spinal cord. The pyramidal tract 'upper motor neurons' synapse with the anterior horn cells of the spinal cord grey matter, which form the lower motor neurons.

Any movement necessitates changes in posture and muscle tone, sometimes in quite separate muscle groups to those involved in the actual movement. The motor system consists of a hierarchy of controls that maintain body posture and muscle tone, on which any movement is superimposed. In the grey matter of the spinal cord, the lowest order of the motor hierarchy controls reflex responses to stretch. Muscle spindles sense lengthening of the muscle; they provide the afferent side of the stretch reflex and initiate a monosynaptic reflex leading to protective or reactive muscle contraction. Inputs from the brainstem are largely inhibitory. Polysynaptic connections in the spinal cord grey matter control more complex reflex actions of flexion and extension of the limbs that form the basic building blocks of coordinated actions, but complete control requires input from the extrapyramidal system and the cerebellum.

Lower motor neurons

Lower motor neurons in the anterior horn of the spinal cord innervate a group of muscle fibres termed a 'motor unit'. Loss of lower motor neurons causes loss of contraction within this unit,

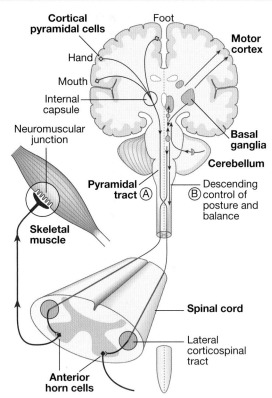

Fig. 25.6 The motor system. Neurons from the motor cortex descend as the pyramidal tract in the internal capsule and cerebral peduncle to the ventral brainstem, where most cross low in the medulla (A). In the spinal cord the upper motor neurons form the corticospinal tract in the lateral column before synapsing with the lower motor neurons in the anterior horns. The activity in the motor cortex is modulated by influences from the basal ganglia and cerebellum. Pathways descending from these structures control posture and balance (B).

resulting in weakness and reduced muscle tone. Subsequently, denervated muscle fibres atrophy, causing muscle wasting, and depolarise spontaneously, causing 'fibrillations'. Except in the tongue, these are usually perceptible only on electromyography (EMG; p. 1076). With the passage of time, neighbouring intact neurons sprout to provide re-innervation, but the neuromuscular junctions of the enlarged motor units are unstable and depolarise spontaneously, causing fasciculations (large enough to be visible). Fasciculations therefore imply chronic denervation with partial re-innervation.

Upper motor neurons

Upper motor neurons have both inhibitory and excitatory influence on the function of lower motor neurons in the anterior horn. Lesions affecting the upper motor neuron result in increased tone, most evident in the strongest muscle groups (i.e. the extensors of the lower limbs and the flexors of the upper limbs). The weakness of upper motor neuron lesions is conversely more pronounced in the opposing muscle groups. Loss of inhibition will also lead to brisk reflexes and enhanced reflex patterns of movement, such as flexion withdrawal to noxious stimuli and spasms of extension. The increased tone is more apparent during rapid stretching ('spastic catch') but may quickly give way with sustained tension (the 'clasp-knife' phenomenon). More primitive reflexes are also released, manifest as extensor plantar responses. Spasticity may not be present until some weeks after the onset of an upper motor neuron lesion.

The extrapyramidal system

Circuits between the basal ganglia and the motor cortex constitute the extrapyramidal system, which controls muscle tone, body posture and the initiation of movement (see Fig. 25.6). Lesions of the extrapyramidal system produce an increase in tone that, unlike spasticity, is continuous throughout the range of movement at any speed of stretch ('lead pipe' rigidity). Involuntary movements are also a feature of extrapyramidal lesions (p. 1084), and tremor in combination with rigidity produces typical 'cogwheel' rigidity. Extrapyramidal lesions also cause slowed and clumsy movements (bradykinesia), which characteristically reduce in size with repetition, as well as postural instability, which can precipitate falls.

The cerebellum

The cerebellum fine-tunes and coordinates movement initiated by the motor cortex, including articulation of speech. It also participates in the planning and learning of skilled movements through reciprocal connections with the thalamus and cortex. A lesion in a cerebellar hemisphere causes lack of coordination on the same side of the body. Cerebellar dysfunction impairs the smoothness of eye movements, causing nystagmus, and renders speech dysarthric. In the limbs, the initial movement is normal, but as the target is approached, the accuracy of the movement deteriorates, producing an 'intention tremor'. The distances of targets are misjudged (dysmetria), resulting in 'past-pointing'. The ability to produce rapid, accurate, regularly alternating movements is also impaired (dysdiadochokinesis). The central vermis of the cerebellum is concerned with the coordination of gait and posture. Disorders of this area therefore produce a characteristic ataxic gait (see below).

Vision

The neurological organisation of visual pathways is shown in Figure 25.7. Fibres from ganglion cells in the retina pass to the optic disc and then backwards through the lamina cribrosa to the optic nerve. Nasal optic nerve fibres (subserving the temporal visual field) cross at the chiasm but temporal fibres do not. Hence, fibres in each optic tract and further posteriorly carry representation of contralateral visual space. From the lateral geniculate nucleus, lower fibres pass through the temporal lobes on their way to the primary visual area in the occipital cortex, while the upper fibres pass through the parietal lobe.

Normally, the eyes move conjugately (in the same direction at the same speed), though horizontal convergence allows fusion of images at different distances. The control of eye movements begins in the cerebral hemispheres, particularly within the frontal eye fields, and the pathway then descends to the brainstem with input from the visual cortex, superior colliculus and cerebellum. Horizontal and vertical gaze centres in the pons and mid-brain, respectively, coordinate output to the ocular motor nerve nuclei (3, 4 and 6), which are connected to each other by the medial longitudinal fasciculus (MLF) (Fig. 25.8). The MLF is particularly important in coordinating horizontal movements of the eyes. The resulting signals to extraocular muscles are supplied by the oculomotor (3rd), trochlear (4th) and abducens (6th) cranial nerves.

The pupillary size is determined by a combination of parasympathetic and sympathetic activity. Parasympathetic fibres originate in the Edinger–Westphal subnucleus of the 3rd nerve, and pass with the 3rd nerve to synapse in the ciliary ganglion before supplying the constrictor pupillae of the iris. Sympathetic fibres originate in the hypothalamus, pass down the brainstem and cervical spinal cord to emerge at T1, return up to the eye in association with the internal carotid artery, and supply the dilator pupillae.

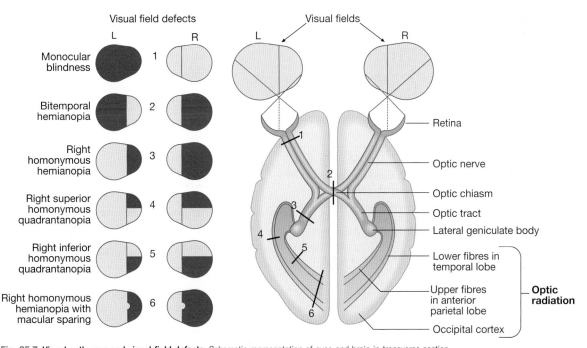

Fig. 25.7 Visual pathways and visual field defects. Schematic representation of eyes and brain in transverse section.

Fig. 25.8 Control of conjugate eye movements. Downward projections pass from the cortex to the pontine lateral gaze centre (A). The pontine gaze centre projects to the 6th cranial nerve nucleus (B), which innervates the ipsilateral lateral rectus and projects to the contralateral 3rd nerve nucleus (and hence medial rectus) via the medial longitudinal fasciculus (MLF). Tonic inputs from the vestibular apparatus (C) project to the contralateral 6th nerve nucleus via the vestibular nuclei.

Speech

Much of the cerebral cortex is involved in the process of forming and interpreting communicating sounds, especially in the dominant hemisphere (see Box 25.2). Decoding of speech sounds (phonemes) is carried out in the upper part of the posterior temporal lobe. The attribution of meaning, as well as the formulation of the language required for the expression of ideas and concepts, occurs predominantly in the lower parts of the anterior parietal lobe (the angular and supramarginal gyri). The temporal speech comprehension region is called Wernicke's area (Fig. 25.9). Other parts of the temporal lobe contribute to verbal memory, where lexicons of meaningful words are 'stored'. Parts of the non-dominant parietal lobe appear to contribute to non-verbal aspects of language in recognising meaningful intonation patterns (prosody).

The frontal language area is in the posterior end of the dominant inferior frontal gyrus known as Broca's area. This receives input from the temporal and parietal lobes via the arcuate fasciculus. The motor commands generated in Broca's area pass to the cranial nerve nuclei in the pons and medulla, as well as to the anterior horn cells in the spinal cord. Nerve impulses to the lips, tongue, palate, pharynx, larynx and respiratory muscles result in the series of ordered sounds comprising speech. The cerebellum also plays an important role in coordinating speech, and lesions of the cerebellum lead to dysarthria, where the problem lies in motor articulation of speech.

The somatosensory system

The body surface can be described by dermatomes, each dermatome being an area of skin in which sensory nerves derive from a single spinal nerve root (Fig. 25.10). Sensory information ascends in two anatomically discrete systems (Fig. 25.11). Fibres from proprioceptive organs and those mediating specific

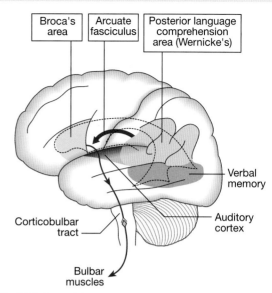

Fig. 25.9 Areas of the cerebral cortex involved in the generation of spoken language.

sensation (including vibration) enter the spinal cord at the posterior horn and pass without synapsing into the ipsilateral posterior columns. In contrast, fibres conveying pain and temperature sensory information (nociceptive neurons) synapse with second-order neurons that cross the midline in the spinal cord before ascending in the contralateral anterolateral spinothalamic tract to the brainstem.

The second-order neurons of the dorsal column sensory system cross the midline in the upper medulla to ascend through the brainstem. Here they lie just medial to the (already crossed) spinothalamic pathway. Brainstem lesions can therefore cause sensory loss affecting all modalities on the contralateral side of the body. Distribution of facial sensory loss due to brainstem lesions arises from the anatomy of the trigeminal fibres within the brainstem. Fibres from the back of the face (near the ears) descend within the brainstem to the upper part of the spinal cord before synapsing, the second-order neurons crossing the midline and then ascending with the spinothalamic fibres. Fibres conveying sensation from more anterior areas of the face descend a shorter distance in the brainstem. Thus, sensory loss in the face from low brainstem lesions is in a 'balaclava helmet' distribution, as the longer descending trigeminal fibres are affected. Both dorsal column and spinothalamic tracts end in the thalamus, relaying from there to the parietal cortex.

Pain

Pain is a complex perception that is only partly related to activity in nociceptor neurons (p. 1338 and Fig. 34.2). Higher up, chronic and severe pain interacts extensively with mood and can exacerbate or be exacerbated by mood disorder, including depression and anxiety. Modification of psychological and psychiatric sequelae is a vital part of pain management (p. 1343).

Sphincter control

The sympathetic supply to the bladder arises from roots T11–L2 to synapse in the inferior hypogastric plexus, while the parasympathetic supply leaves from S2–4. In addition, a somatic supply to the external (voluntary) sphincter arises from S2–4, travelling via the pudendal nerves.

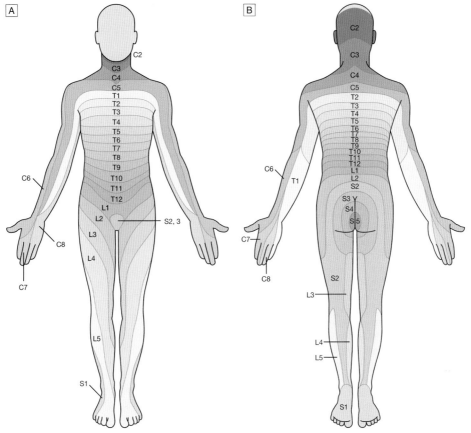

Fig. 25.10 The areas supplied by specific levels of the spinal cord. These are approximations and in practice there is much overlap. The clinical utility of these dermatomes has diminished somewhat with the advent of good magnetic resonance imaging of the spinal cord but it remains important to ascertain the presence of a 'spinal level' of sensation, to remember the supply of saddle area, and to note the cervical descent of some facial spinothalamic pathways. **A** Anterior. **B** Posterior.

Storage of urine is maintained by inhibiting parasympathetic activity and thus relaxing the detrusor muscle of the bladder wall. Continence is also helped by simultaneous sympathetic- and somatic-mediated tonic contraction of the urethral sphincters. Voiding in adults is usually carried out under conscious control, which triggers relaxation of tonic inhibition on the pontine micturition centre from higher centres, leading to relaxation of the pelvic floor muscles and external and internal urethral sphincters, along with parasympathetic-mediated detrusor contraction.

Personality and mood

The physiology and pathology of mood disorders are discussed elsewhere (Ch. 28) but it is important to remember that any process affecting brain function may influence mood and affect. Conversely, mood disorder may have a significant effect on perception and function. It can be difficult to disentangle whether psychological and psychiatric changes are the cause or the effect of any neurological symptoms.

Sleep

The function of sleep is unknown but it is required for health. Sleep is controlled by the reticular activating system in the upper brainstem and diencephalon. It is composed of different stages that can be visualised on electroencephalography (EEG). As drowsiness occurs, normal EEG background alpha rhythm disappears and activity becomes dominated by deepening slow-wave activity. As sleep deepens and dreaming begins, the limbs become flaccid, movements are 'blocked' and EEG signs of rapid eye movements (REM) are superimposed on the slow wave. REM sleep persists for a short spell before another slow-wave spell starts, the cycle repeating several times throughout the night. REM phases lengthen as sleep progresses. REM sleep seems to be the most important part of the sleep cycle for refreshing cognitive processes, and REM sleep deprivation causes tiredness, irritability and impaired judgement.

Localising lesions in the central nervous system

After taking a history and examining the patient, the clinician should have an idea of the nature and site of any pathology (see Box 25.10). Given the intricate anatomy of the brainstem, this section will dwell on the possible localisation in more detail (see Fig. 25.5).

Brainstem lesions typically present with symptoms due to cranial nerve, cerebellar and upper motor neuron dysfunction and are most commonly caused by vascular disease. Since the anatomy of the brainstem is very precisely organised, it is usually possible to localise the site of a lesion on the basis of careful history and examination in order to determine exactly

25

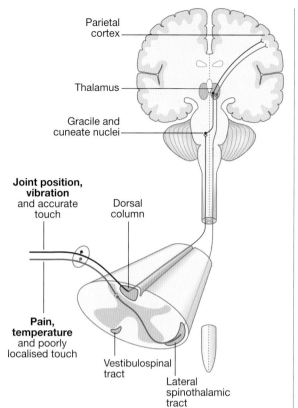

Parietal cortex

Thalamus

Gracile and cuneate nuclei

Joint position, vibration and accurate touch

Dorsal column

Pain, temperature and poorly localised touch

Vestibulospinal tract

Lateral spinothalamic tract

Fig. 25.11 **The main somatic sensory pathways.**

i	**25.3 Major focal brainstem syndromes**	
Name of syndrome	**Site of lesions**	**Clinical features**
Weber	Anterior cerebral peduncle (mid-brain)	Ipsilateral 3rd palsy Contralateral upper motor neuron 7th palsy Contralateral hemiplegia
Claude	Cerebral peduncle Involving red nucleus	Ipsilateral 3rd palsy Contralateral cerebellar signs
Parinaud	Dorsal mid-brain (tectum)	Vertical gaze palsy Convergence disorders Convergence retraction nystagmus Pupillary and lid disorders
Millard–Gubler	Ponto-medullary junction	Ipsilateral 6th palsy Ipsilateral lower motor neuron 7th palsy Contralateral hemiplegia
Wallenberg	Lateral medulla	Ipsilateral 5th, 9th, 10th, 11th palsy Ipsilateral Horner's syndrome Ipsilateral cerebellar signs Contralateral spinothalamic sensory loss Vestibular disturbance

which tracts/nuclei are affected, usually invoking the fewest number of lesions.

For example, in a patient presenting with sudden onset of upper motor neuron features affecting the right face, arm and leg in association with a left 3rd nerve palsy, the lesion will be in the left cerebral peduncle in the brainstem and the pathology is likely to have been a discrete stroke, as the onset was sudden. This combination of symptoms and signs is known as Weber's syndrome, and is one of several well-described brainstem syndromes, which are listed in Box 25.3. The effects of individual cranial nerve deficits are discussed in the sections on eye movements (p. 1088) and on facial weakness, sensory loss in brainstem lesions, dysphonia and dysarthria, and bulbar symptoms (pp. 1082, 1083, 1087 and 1093).

Investigation of neurological disease

Experienced clinicians make most neurological diagnoses on history alone, with a lesser contribution from examination and investigation. As investigations become more complex and more easily available, it is tempting to adopt a 'scan first, think later' approach to neurological symptoms. The frequency of 'false-positive' results, the wide range of normality, and the negative implications for patients (unnecessary expense, inconvenience, discomfort and worry) necessitate a more thoughtful approach. Investigation may include assessment of structure (imaging) and function (neurophysiology). Neurophysiological testing has become so complex that in some countries it constitutes a separate specialty focusing on electroencephalography, evoked potentials, nerve conduction studies and electromyography.

Neuroimaging

Neurological imaging has traditionally allowed only assessment of structure but advances are allowing much more sophistication. Imaging modalities can use X-rays (plain X-rays, computed tomography (CT), CT angiography, myelography and angiography), magnetic resonance (MR imaging (MRI), MR angiography (MRA)), ultrasound (Doppler imaging of blood vessels) and nuclear medicine techniques (single photon emission computed tomography (SPECT) and positron emission tomography (PET)). The uses and limitations of each of these are shown in Box 25.4. Different sequences for analysing MRI signals can provide helpful information for characterising tissues and pathologies (Box 25.5).

Specialist MR techniques, such as functional MRI (fMRI), MR spectroscopy or diffusion tensor imaging (DTI), can be used to assess brain metabolism and chemical compositions. This may be dynamic and can provide 'maps' of cortical function to help plan lesionectomy and epilepsy surgery. Similarly, MR spectroscopy can outline the chemical composition of specific regions, providing notions of whether lesions are ischaemic, neoplastic or inflammatory.

Some degenerative neurological conditions cause functional rather than structural abnormalities that make metabolic and neurochemical assessment increasingly useful. PET scanning can display glucose metabolism in dementia and epilepsy. SPECT scanning uses the lipid-soluble properties of radioactive tracers to mark cerebral blood flow at the time of injection to help in investigating seizures. Dopaminergic pathway tracers can assess the integrity of the nigrostriatal pathway in patients with possible parkinsonism.

i | **25.4 Imaging techniques for the nervous system**

Technique	Applications	Advantages	Disadvantages	Comments
X-ray/CT	Plain X-rays, CT, CTA Radiculography Myelography Intra-arterial angiography	Widely available Relatively cheap Relatively quick	Ionising radiation Contrast reactions Invasive (myelography and angiography)	X-rays: used for fractures or foreign bodies CT: first line for stroke Intra-arterial angiography: gold standard for vascular lesions
MRI	Structural imaging MRA Functional MRI MR spectroscopy	High-quality soft tissue images, useful for posterior fossa and temporal lobes No ionising radiation Non-invasive	Expensive Less widely available MRA images blood flow, not vessel anatomy Claustrophobic Pacemakers are a contraindication Contrast (gadolinium) reactions	Functional MR and spectroscopy: mainly research tools
Ultrasound	Doppler Duplex scans	Cheap Quick Non-invasive	Operator-dependent Poor anatomical definition	Screening tool to assess need for carotid endarterectomy
Radioisotope	Isotope brain scan SPECT PET	In vivo imaging of functional anatomy (ligand binding, blood flow)	Poor spatial resolution Ionising radiation Expensive Not widely available	Isotope scans: obsolete SPECT: useful in movement disorders, epilepsy and dementias PET: mainly research tool

(CT = computed tomography; CTA = computed tomographic angiography; MRA = magnetic resonance angiography; MRI = magnetic resonance imaging; PET = positron emission tomography; SPECT = single photon emission computed tomography)

i | **25.5 Different magnetic resonance imaging (MRI) sequences**

	T1	T2	T2-FLAIR
	'Anatomically correct'	'Reverse T1'	T2 with CSF signal dampened
Grey matter (cortex)	Grey	White	White
White matter	White	Grey	Grey
Cerebrospinal fluid (CSF)	Black	White	Black

Insets courtesy of Dr Ravi Jampana, Consultant Neuroradiologist, Dept of Neuroradiology, Institute of Neuroscience, Queen Elizabeth University Hospital, Glasgow.

25

Head and orbit

Plain skull X-rays now have a very limited role in neurological disease. CT or MRI is needed for intracranial imaging. CT is good for demonstrating bone and calcification well. It will also detect abnormalities of the brain and ventricles, such as atrophy, tumours, cysts, abscesses, vascular lesions and hydrocephalus. Diagnostic yield may be improved by the use of intravenous contrast and thinner slicing but CT is not optimal for lesions of meninges, cranial nerves or subtle parenchymal changes.

MRI resolution is unaffected by bone and so is more useful in posterior fossa disease. Its sensitivity for cortical and white matter changes makes it the modality of choice in inflammatory conditions such as multiple sclerosis and in the investigation of epilepsy. Different MRI techniques can selectively suppress

Fig. 25.12 Different techniques of imaging the head and brain. [A] Computed tomogram showing complete middle cerebral artery infarct (arrows). [B] Magnetic resonance image showing widespread areas of high signal in multiple sclerosis (arrows). [C] Single photon emission computed tomography scan after caudate infarct showing relative hypoperfusion of overlying right cerebral cortex (arrows). [D] Normal positron emission tomogram (PET scan) of brain. *A–C, Courtesy of Dr D. Collie. D, Courtesy of Dr Ravi Jampana, Consultant Neuroradiologist, Dept of Neuroradiology, Institute of Neuroscience, Queen Elizabeth University Hospital, Glasgow.*

signal from fluid or fat, for example, and so increase sensitivity for more subtle pathologies.

Examples of brain imaged by the various techniques are shown in Figure 25.12.

Cervical, thoracic and lumbar spine

X-rays are useful for imaging bony structures and can show destruction or damage to vertebrae, for example, but will provide no information about non-bony tissues, such as intervertebral discs, spinal cord and nerve roots. They have some usefulness in dynamic imaging, e.g. flexion/extension of the spine, in the assessment of instability. MRI has transformed spinal investigation, as it can give information not only about vertebrae and intervertebral discs but also about their effects on the spinal cord and nerve roots. Myelography (usually with CT) is an invasive technique requiring injection of contrast into the lumbar theca. While outlining the nerve roots and spinal cord provides some detail about abnormal structure, the accuracy and availability of MRI have reduced the need for it. Myelography may still be used where MRI is unavailable, contraindicated, or precluded by a patient's claustrophobia. Examples of the cervical spine imaged by plain X-rays, myelography and MRI are shown in Figure 25.13.

Blood vessels

Imaging of the extra- and intracranial blood vessels and disturbance of arterial or venous blood flow is described on page 1161.

Neurophysiological testing

Electroencephalography

The electroencephalogram (EEG) detects electrical activity arising in the cerebral cortex via electrodes placed on the scalp to record the amplitude and frequency of the resulting waveforms. With closed eyes, the normal background activity is 8–13 Hz (known as alpha rhythm), most prominent occipitally and suppressed on eye opening. Other frequency bands seen over different parts of the brain in different circumstances are beta (faster than 13/sec), theta (4–8/sec) and delta (slower than 4/sec). Normal EEG patterns evolve with age and alertness; lower frequencies predominate in the very young and during sleep.

In recent years, digital technology has allowed longer, cleaner EEG recordings that can be analysed in a number of ways and recorded alongside contemporaneous video of any clinical 'event'. Meanwhile, the development of intracranial recording allows more sensitive monitoring via surgically placed electrodes in and around lesions to help increase the efficacy and safety of epilepsy surgery.

Abnormal EEGs result from a number of conditions. Examples include an increase in fast frequencies (beta) seen with sedating drugs such as benzodiazepines, or marked focal slowing noted over a structural lesion such as a tumour or an infarct. Improved quality and accessibility of imaging have made EEG redundant in lesion localisation, except in the specialist investigation of epilepsy (p. 1100). EEG remains useful in progressive and continuous disorders such as reduced consciousness (p. 194), encephalitis

Fig. 25.13 Different techniques of imaging the cervical spine. [A] Lateral X-ray showing bilateral C6/7 facet dislocation. [B] Myelogram showing widening of cervical cord due to astrocytoma (arrows). [C] Magnetic resonance image showing posterior epidural compression from adenocarcinomatous metastasis to the posterior arch of T1 (arrows). *A–C, Courtesy of Dr D. Collie.*

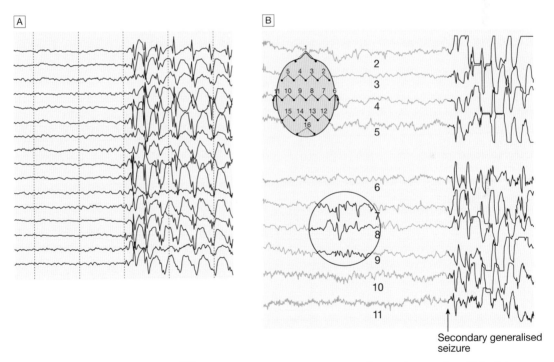

Fig. 25.14 Electroencephalograms in epilepsy. [A] Generalised epileptic discharge, as seen in epilepsy syndromes such as childhood absence or juvenile myoclonic epilepsy. [B] Focal sharp waves over the right parietal region (circled), with spread of discharge to cause a generalised tonic–clonic seizure.

(p. 1121), and certain dementias such as Creutzfeldt–Jakob disease (p. 1127).

Since sleep induces marked changes in cerebral activity, EEG can be useful in diagnosis of sleep disturbances. In paroxysmal disorders such as epilepsy, EEG is at its most useful when it captures activity during one of the events in question. Over 50% of patients with epilepsy have a normal 'routine' EEG but, conversely, the presence of epileptiform features does not of itself make a diagnosis. Up to 5% of some normal populations may demonstrate epileptiform discharges on EEG, preventing its use as a screening test for epilepsy, most notably in younger patients with a family history of epilepsy. In view of this, the EEG should not be used where epilepsy is merely 'possible'.

Therefore the EEG in epilepsy is predominantly used for classification and prognostication, but in some patients can help localise the seat of epileptiform discharges when surgery is being considered. During a seizure, high-voltage disturbances of background activity ('discharges') are often noted. These may be generalised, as in the 3 Hz 'spike and wave' of childhood absence epilepsy, or more focal, as in localisation-related epilepsies (Fig. 25.14). Techniques such as hyperventilation or photic stimulation can be used to increase the yield of epileptiform changes, particularly in the generalised epilepsy syndromes. While some argue that it is possible to detect 'spikes' and 'sharp waves' to lend support to a clinical diagnosis, these are non-specific and therefore not diagnostic, and can lead an unwary clinician to err in ascribing other symptoms to epilepsy.

Nerve conduction studies

Electrical stimulation of a nerve causes an impulse to travel both efferently and afferently along the underlying axons. Nerve conduction studies (NCS) make use of this, recording action potentials as they pass along peripheral nerves and (with motor nerves) as they pass into the muscle belly. Digital recording has enhanced sensitivity and reproducibility of these tiny potentials. By measuring the time taken to traverse a known distance, it is possible to calculate nerve conduction velocities (NCVs). Healthy nerves at room temperature will conduct at a speed of 40–50 m/sec. If the recorded potential is smaller than expected, this provides evidence of a reduction in the overall number of functioning axons. Significant slowing of conduction velocity, in contrast, suggests impaired conduction due to peripheral nerve demyelination. Such changes in NCS may be diffuse (as in a hereditary demyelinating peripheral neuropathy, p. 1138), focal (as in pressure palsies, p. 1139) or multifocal (e.g. Guillain–Barré syndrome, p. 1140; mononeuritis multiplex, p. 1140). The information gained can allow the disease responsible for peripheral nerve dysfunction to be better deduced (see Box 25.84, p. 1139).

Stimulation of motor nerves allows for the recording of compound muscle action potentials (CMAPs) over muscles (Fig.

25.15). These are around 500 times larger than sensory nerve potentials, typically around 1–20 millivolts. Since a proportion of stimulated impulses in motor nerves will 'reflect' back from the anterior horn cell body (forming the 'F' wave), it is also possible to obtain some information about the condition of nerve roots.

Repetitive nerve stimulation (RNS) at 3–15/sec provides consistent CMAPs in healthy muscle. In myasthenia gravis (p. 1141), however, where there is partial blockage of acetylcholine receptors, there is a diagnostic fall (decrement) in CMAP amplitude. In contrast, an increasing CMAP with high-frequency RNS is seen in Lambert–Eaton myasthenic syndrome (p. 1143).

Electromyography

Electromyography (EMG) is usually performed alongside NCS and involves needle recording of muscle electrical potential during rest and contraction. At rest, muscle is electrically silent but loss of nerve supply causes muscle membrane to become unstable, manifest as fibrillations, positive sharp waves ('spontaneous activity') or fasciculations. Motor unit action potentials are recorded during muscle contraction. Axonal loss or destruction will result in fewer motor units. Resultant sprouting of remaining units will lead to increasing size of each individual unit on EMG. Myopathy, in contrast, causes muscle fibre splitting, which results in a large number of smaller units on EMG. Other abnormal activity, such as myotonic discharges, may signify abnormal ion channel conduction, as in myotonic dystrophy or myotonia congenita.

Specialised single-fibre electromyography (SFEMG) can be used to investigate neuromuscular junction transmission. Measuring 'jitter' and 'blocking' can identify the effect of antibodies in reducing the action of acetylcholine on the receptor.

Evoked potentials

The cortical response to visual, auditory or electrical stimulation can be measured on an EEG as an evoked potential (EP). If a stimulus is provided – e.g. to the eye, the tiny EEG response can be discerned when averaging 100–1000 repeated stimuli. Assessing the latency (the time delay) and amplitude can give

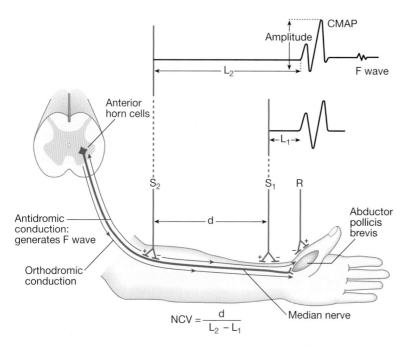

Fig. 25.15 Motor nerve conduction tests. Electrodes (R) on the muscle (abductor pollicis here) record the compound muscle action potential (CMAP) after stimulation at the median nerve at the wrist (S_1) and from the elbow (S_2). The velocity from elbow to wrist can be determined if the distance between the two stimulating electrodes (d) is known. A prolonged L_1 (L = latency) would be caused by dysfunction distally in the median nerve (e.g. in carpal tunnel syndrome). A prolonged L_2 is caused by slow nerve conduction (as in demyelinating neuropathy). The F wave is a small delayed response that appears when the electrical signal travels backwards to the anterior horn cell, sparking a second action potential in a minority of fibres (see text). (NCV = nerve conduction velocity)

$$NCV = \frac{d}{L_2 - L_1}$$

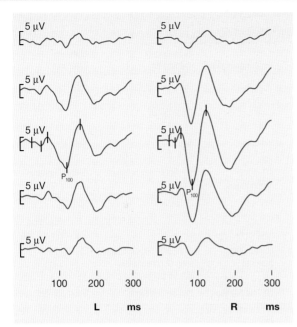

Fig. 25.16 Visual evoked potential (VEP) recording. The abnormality is in the left hemisphere, with delay in latency and a reduction in signal of the P_{100}.

information about the integrity of the relevant pathway. MRI now provides more information about CNS pathways, thus reducing reliance on EPs. In practice, visual evoked potentials (VEPs) are most commonly used to help differentiate CNS demyelination from small-vessel white-matter changes (Fig. 25.16).

Magnetic stimulation

Central conduction times can also be measured using electromagnetic induction of action potentials in the cortex or spinal cord by the local application of specialised coils. Again, MRI has made this technique largely redundant, other than for research.

Routine blood tests

Many systemic conditions that can affect the nervous system can be identified by simple blood tests. Nutritional deficiencies, metabolic disturbances, inflammatory conditions or infections may all present or be associated with neurological symptoms, and basic blood tests (full blood count, erythrocyte sedimentation rate, C-reactive protein, biochemical screening) may provide clues. Specific blood tests will be highlighted in the relevant subsections of this chapter. Human immunodeficiency virus (HIV) infection is increasingly recognised as a cause of neurological disease and the clinician should have a low threshold for checking this.

Immunological tests

Recent developments have seen a host of new immune-mediated conditions emerge in clinical neurology, with antibody targets ranging from muscle and neuromuscular junction disturbance (causing weakness and muscle pain) to specific neuronal ion channels (causing cognitive decline, epilepsy and psychiatric changes). The 21st century has seen the identification of many

causative antibodies (see Boxes 25.52 and 25.53, p. 1111) and it is likely that further conditions will turn out to have an immune basis.

Genetic testing

This evolving field represents a huge untapped area for neurological exploration, particularly with the development of genome-wide association study (GWAS) and whole-genome sequencing. Relevant subsections will detail the increasing numbers of inherited neurological conditions that can now be diagnosed by DNA analysis (p. 56). These include diseases caused by increased numbers of trinucleotide repeats, such as Huntington's disease (p. 1114); myotonic dystrophy (p. 1143); and some types of spinocerebellar ataxia (p. 1115). Mitochondrial DNA can also be sequenced to diagnose relevant disorders (p. 1144).

Lumbar puncture

Lumbar puncture (LP) is the technique used to obtain both a CSF sample and an indirect measure of intracranial pressure. After local anaesthetic injection, a needle is inserted between lumbar spinous processes (usually between L3 and L4) through the dura and into the spinal canal. Intracranial pressure can be deduced (if patients are lying on their side) and CSF removed for analysis. CSF pressure measurement is important in the diagnosis and monitoring of idiopathic intracranial hypertension (p. 1133). In this condition, the LP itself is therapeutic.

CSF is normally clear and colourless, and the tests that are usually performed include a naked eye examination of the CSF and centrifugation to determine the colour of the supernatant (yellow, or xanthochromic, some hours after subarachnoid haemorrhage; p. 1160). Measurement of absorption of specific light wavelengths helps quantify the amount of haem metabolites in CSF. Routine analysis involves a cell count, as well as glucose and protein concentrations.

CSF assessment is important in investigating infections (meningitis or encephalitis), subarachnoid haemorrhage and inflammatory conditions (multiple sclerosis, sarcoidosis and cerebral lupus). Normal values and abnormalities found in specific conditions are shown in Box 25.6.

More sophisticated analysis allows measurement of antibody formation solely within the CNS (oligoclonal bands), genetic analysis (e.g. polymerase chain reaction (PCR) for herpes simplex or tuberculosis), immunological tests (paraneoplastic antibodies) and cytology (to detect malignant cells).

If there is a cranial space-occupying lesion causing raised intracranial pressure, LP presents a theoretical risk of downward shift of intracerebral contents, a potentially fatal process known as coning (p. 1128). Consequently, LP is contraindicated if there is any clinical suggestion of raised intracranial pressure (papilloedema), depressed level of consciousness, or focal neurological signs suggesting a cerebral lesion, until imaging (by CT or MRI) has excluded a space-occupying lesion or hydrocephalus. When there is a risk of local haemorrhage (thrombocytopenia, disseminated intravascular coagulation or anticoagulant treatment), then caution should be exercised or specific measures should be taken. LP can be safely performed in patients on antiplatelet drugs or low-dose heparin, but may be unsafe in patients who are fully anticoagulated due to the increased risk of epidural haematoma.

About 30% of LPs are followed by a postural headache, due to reduced CSF pressure. The frequency of headache

25

25.6 How to interpret cerebrospinal fluid results

	Normal	Subarachnoid haemorrhage	Acute bacterial meningitis	Viral meningitis	Tuberculous meningitis	Multiple sclerosis
Pressure	50–250 mm of water	Increased	Normal/increased	Normal	Normal/increased	Normal
Colour	Clear	Blood-stained Xanthochromic	Cloudy	Clear	Clear/cloudy	Clear
Red cell count (×10⁶/L)	0–4	Raised	Normal	Normal	Normal	Normal
White cell count (×10⁶/L)	0–4	Normal/slightly raised	1000–5000 polymorphs	10–2000 lymphocytes	50–5000 lymphocytes	0–50 lymphocytes
Glucose	>50–60% of blood level	Normal	Decreased	Normal	Decreased	Normal
Protein	<0.45 g/L	Increased	Increased	Normal/increased	Increased	Normal/increased
Microbiology	Sterile	Sterile	Organisms on Gram stain and/or culture	Sterile/virus detected	Ziehl–Neelsen/auramine stain or tuberculosis culture positive	Sterile
Oligoclonal bands	Negative	Negative	Can be positive	Can be positive	Can be positive	Often positive

can be reduced by using smaller or atraumatic needles. Rarer complications involve transient radicular pain, and pain over the lumbar region during the procedure. Aseptic technique renders secondary infections such as meningitis extremely rare.

Biopsy

Biopsies of nervous tissue (peripheral nerve, muscle, meninges or brain) are occasionally required for diagnosis.

Nerve biopsy can help in the investigation of peripheral neuropathy. Usually, a distal sensory nerve (sural or radial) is targeted. Histological examination can help identify underlying causes, such as vasculitides or infiltrative disorders like amyloid. Nerve biopsy should not be undertaken lightly since there is an appreciable morbidity; it should be reserved for cases where the diagnosis is in doubt after routine investigations and where it will influence management.

Muscle biopsy is performed more frequently and is indicated for the differentiation of myositis and myopathies. These conditions can usually be distinguished by histological examination, and enzyme histochemistry can be useful when mitochondrial diseases and storage diseases are suspected. The quadriceps muscle is most commonly biopsied but other muscles may also be sampled if they are involved clinically. Although pain and infection can follow the procedure, these are less of a problem than after nerve biopsy.

Brain biopsy is required when imaging fails to clarify the nature of intracerebral lesions, e.g. in unexplained degenerative diseases such as unusual cases of dementia and in patients with brain tumours. Most biopsies are performed stereotactically through a burr hole in the skull, which lowers complication rates. Nevertheless, haemorrhage, infection and death still occur and brain biopsy should be considered only if a diagnosis is otherwise elusive.

Biopsy of other organs can be useful in the diagnosis of systemic disorders presenting as neurological problems, such as tonsillar biopsy (diagnosis of prion diseases), or rectal or fat biopsy (for assessment of amyloid).

Presenting problems in neurological disease

While history is important in all medical specialties, it is especially key in neurology, where many neurological diagnoses have no confirmatory test. History-taking allows doctor and patient to get to know one another; many neurological diseases follow chronic paths and this may be the first of many such consultations. It also allows the clinician to obtain information about the patient's affect, cognition and psychiatric state.

History-taking is a highly active process. While there are generic templates (Box 25.7), each individual story will follow its own course, and diagnostic considerations during the history will guide further questioning.

It is important to be clear about what patients mean by certain words. They may find it difficult to describe symptoms: for instance, weakness may be called 'numbness', while there are many possible interpretations of 'dizziness'. These must be clarified; even in emergency situations, a clear, accurate history is the foundation of any management plan. While the story should come primarily from the patient, input from eye-witnesses and family members is crucial if the patient is unable to provide details or if there has been loss of consciousness. This need for corroboration and clarification means the telephone is as important as any investigation.

The aim of the history is to address two key issues: where is the lesion and what is the lesion (Box 25.8)? These should remain uppermost in the doctor's mind while the history is being elicited. Some common combinations of symptoms may suggest particular locations for a lesion (Box 25.10). Enquiry about handedness is important; lateralisation of the dominant hand helps designate the dominant hemisphere, which in turn may help to localise any pathologies, or to plan rehabilitation or treatment strategies in asymmetrical disorders such as stroke or Parkinson's disease.

Epidemiology must be borne in mind. How likely is it that this particular patient has any specific condition under consideration?

25.7 How to take a neurological history

Introduction

- Age and sex
- Handedness

Presenting complaint

- Symptoms (clarify: see text)
- Overall pattern: intermittent or persistent?
- If intermittent, how often do symptoms occur and how long do they last?
- Speed of onset: seconds, minutes, hours, days, weeks, months, years, decades?
- Better, worse or the same over time?
- Associated symptoms (including non-neurological)
- Disability caused by symptoms
- Change in walking
- Difficulty with fine hand movements, e.g. writing, fastening buttons, using cutlery
- Effect on work, family life and leisure

Background

- Previous neurological symptoms and whether similar to current symptoms
- Previous medical history
- Domestic situation
- Driving licence status
- Medications (current and at time of symptom onset)
- Alcohol/smoking habits
- Recreational drug and other toxin exposure
- Family history and developmental history
- What are patient's thoughts/fears/concerns?

25.8 The key diagnostic questions

Where is the lesion?

- Is it neurological?
- If so, to which part of the nervous system does it localise?
  Central versus peripheral
  Sensory versus motor versus both

What is the lesion?

- Hereditary or congenital
- Acquired:
  Traumatic
  Infective
  Neoplastic
  Degenerative
  Inflammatory or immune-mediated
  Vascular
  Functional

25.9 Neurological examination in old age

- **Pupils:** tend to be smaller, making fundoscopy more difficult.
- **Limb tone:** more difficult to assess because of poor relaxation and concomitant joint disease.
- **Ankle reflexes:** may be absent.
- **Gait assessment:** more difficult because of concurrent musculoskeletal disease and pre-existing neurological deficits.
- **Sensory testing:** especially difficult when there is cognitive impairment.
- **Vibration sense:** may be reduced distally in the legs.

25.10 How to 'localise' neurological disease

Combination of symptoms/signs	Probable site	Possible pathology	Other important information
Painless loss of hemilateral function	Cerebral cortex	Usually vascular, inflammatory or neoplastic	Associated systemic symptoms Tempo of evolution
Pyramidal weakness of all four limbs or both legs, bladder signs, sensory loss	Spinal cord	Usually vascular, inflammatory or neoplastic	Associated systemic symptoms Tempo of evolution
Cranial nerve lesions, with limb pyramidal signs or sensory loss ± sphincter disturbance	Brainstem Mid-brain Pons Medulla	Usually vascular or inflammatory Rarely neoplastic	Associated systemic symptoms Tempo of evolution
Visual loss + pyramidal signs and/or cerebellar signs	Widespread cerebral lesions	Usually inflammatory Less commonly vasculitic	Tempo of evolution
Weakness and/or sensory loss in a combination of individual peripheral nerves	Several peripheral nerves ('mononeuritis multiplex')	Usually inflammatory or diabetic	Associated systemic symptoms
Widespread LMN and UMN signs	Upper and lower motor neurons	Motor neuron disease Cervical myeloradiculopathy	Associated localised cervical symptoms
Distal loss of sensation and/or weakness	Generalised peripheral nerves	See causes of neuropathy (p. 1138)	Associated systemic symptoms

(LMN/UMN = lower/upper motor neuron)

25

For example, a 20-year-old with right-sided headache and tenderness will not have temporal arteritis, but this is an important possibility if such symptoms present in a 78-year-old female.

Determining the evolution, speed of onset and progression of a disease is important (Box 25.11). For example, if right-hand weakness occurred overnight, it would suggest a stroke in an older person or an acute entrapment neuropathy in a younger one.

Evolution over several days, however, might make demyelination (multiple sclerosis) a possible diagnosis, or perhaps a subdural haematoma if the weakness was preceded by a head injury in an older person taking warfarin. Progression over weeks might bring an intracranial mass lesion or motor neuron disease into the differential. Slow progression over a year or so, with difficulty in using the hand, could suggest a degenerative process such

25.11 The evolution of symptoms		
Onset	Evolution	Possible causes
Sudden (minutes to hours)	Stable/improvement	Vascular (stroke/transient ischaemic attack (TIA)) Nerve entrapment syndromes Functional
Gradual	Progressive over days	Demyelination Infection
Gradual	Progressive over weeks to months	Neoplastic/paraneoplastic
Gradual	Progressive over months to years	Genetic Degenerative

as Parkinson's disease. The impact on day-to-day activities, such as walking, climbing stairs and carrying out fine hand movements, should also be established in order to gauge the level of associated disability.

Estimates of the frequency and duration of specific events are essential when taking details of a paroxysmal disorder such as migraine and epilepsy. Vague terms such as 'a lot' or 'sometimes' are unhelpful, and it can assist the patient if choices are given to estimate numbers, such as once a day, week or month.

Many neurological symptoms are not explained by disease. Describing these as 'functional' is less pejorative and more acceptable to patients than 'psychogenic' or 'hysterical'. Functional symptoms require considerable experience in diagnosis and are frequently missed (p. 1094).

Headache and facial pain

Most headaches are chronic disorders but acute presentation of headaches is an important aspect of emergency medical care. Headache may be divided into primary (benign) or secondary, and most patients, whether presenting in clinic or as emergencies, have primary syndromes (see Box 10.10, p. 184). The emergency clinical assessment of headaches is dealt with on page 185.

Ocular pain

Assuming that ocular disease (such as acute glaucoma) has been excluded, ocular pain may be due to trigeminal autonomic cephalalgias (TACs) or, rarely, inflammatory or infiltrative lesions at the apex of the orbit or the cavernous sinus, when 3rd, 4th, 5th or 6th cranial nerve involvement is usually evident. Ocular pain and headache are also discussed on page 1170.

Facial pain

Pain in the face can be due to dental or temporomandibular joint problems. Acute sinusitis is usually apparent from other features of sinus congestion/infection and may cause localised pain over the affected sinus, but is almost never the explanation for persistent facial pain or headache.

Facial pain is not uncommon in migraine but some syndromes can present solely with facial pain. The most common neurological causes of facial pain are trigeminal neuralgia, herpes zoster (shingles) and post-herpetic neuralgia, all characterised by their extreme severity. In trigeminal neuralgia, the patient describes bouts of brief (seconds), lancinating pain ('electric shocks'), most

frequently felt in the second and third divisions of the nerve and often triggered by talking or chewing. Facial shingles most commonly affects the first (ophthalmic) division of the trigeminal nerve, and pain usually precedes the rash. Post-herpetic neuralgia may follow, typically a continuous burning pain throughout the affected territory, with marked sensitivity to light touch (allodynia) and resistance to treatment. Destructive lesions of the trigeminal nerve usually cause numbness rather than pain.

Persistent idiopathic facial pain is most frequently seen in middle-aged women, who report persistent pain, with no abnormal signs or investigations, and is similar to other forms of idiopathic chronic pain.

Dizziness, blackouts and 'funny turns'

Acute onset of dizziness or blackouts will present to the acute medical department. In neurological practice, it is common to deal with patients presenting with a history of multiple events. While detailed questioning will be dealt with in the relevant section (p. 181), the neurologist will have to tease out the pattern of each of the different attack types experienced by the patient to be able to form a treatment and investigation plan, one of the challenges of clinical neurology.

Status epilepticus

Status epilepticus is seizure activity not resolving spontaneously, or recurrent seizure with no recovery of consciousness in between. Persisting seizure activity has a recognised mortality and is a medical emergency.

Diagnosis is usually clinical and can be made on the basis of the description of prolonged rigidity and/or clonic movements with loss of awareness. As seizure activity becomes prolonged, movements may become more subtle. Cyanosis, pyrexia, acidosis and sweating may occur, and complications include aspiration, hypotension, cardiac arrhythmias and renal or hepatic failure.

In patients with pre-existing epilepsy, the most likely cause is a fall in antiepileptic drug levels. In de novo status epilepticus, it is essential to exclude precipitants such as infection (meningitis, encephalitis), neoplasia and metabolic derangement (hypoglycaemia, hyponatraemia or hypocalcaemia). Treatment and investigation are outlined in Box 25.12.

Coma

Coma and loss of consciousness usually present to the acute medical admissions department (p. 194). Clarification of cause and prognosis may require specialist neurological input.

Delirium

Delirium describes cortical dysfunction and replaces the older term 'acute confusional state'. It has a range of primary causes, and given its role in precipitating acute admission, it is covered in detail on page 183.

Amnesia

Memory disturbance is a common symptom. In the absence of significant functional impairment (e.g. inability to work, dyspraxias, loss of daily function), many patients will prove to have benign memory dysfunction related to age, mood or psychiatric disorders.

25.12 Management of status epilepticus

Initial

- Ensure airway is patent; give oxygen to prevent cerebral hypoxia
- Check pulse, blood pressure, BM stix and respiratory rate
- Secure intravenous access
- Send blood for:
  Glucose, urea and electrolytes, calcium and magnesium, liver function, antiepileptic drug levels
  Full blood count and coagulation screen
  Storing a sample for future analysis (e.g. drug misuse)
- If seizures continue for > 5 mins: give midazolam 10 mg bucally or nasally or lorazepam 4 mg IV if access available or diazepam 10 mg rectally or IV if necessary; repeat *once only* after 15 mins
- Correct any metabolic trigger, e.g. hypoglycaemia

Ongoing

If seizures continue after 30 mins
- IV infusion (with cardiac monitoring) with one of:
  Phenytoin: 15 mg/kg at 50 mg/min
  Sodium valproate: 20–30 mg/kg IV at 40 mg/min
  Phenobarbital: 10 mg/kg at 100 mg/min
- Cardiac monitor and pulse oximetry:
  Monitor neurological condition, blood pressure, respiration; check blood gases

If seizures still continue after 30–60 mins
- Transfer to intensive care:
  Start treatment for refractory status with intubation, ventilation and general anaesthesia using propofol or thiopental
  EEG monitor

Once status controlled
- Commence longer-term antiepileptic medication with one of:
  Sodium valproate 10 mg/kg IV over 3–5 mins, then 800–2000 mg/day
  Phenytoin: give loading dose (if not already used as above) of 15 mg/kg, infuse at < 50 mg/min, then 300 mg/day
  Carbamazepine 400 mg by nasogastric tube, then 400–1200 mg/day
- Investigate cause

The increasing publicity given to dementia, combined with a natural fear of losing one's mind, has led to an increase in patients presenting with memory loss but many will have benign symptoms. Investigation and treatment of the dementias are discussed elsewhere (p. 1191).

Temporary loss of memory may be due to a transient delirium related to infection, the post-ictal period after seizure, or transient global amnesia. These are usually distinguished on the basis of the history. Transient amnesia resulting directly from a seizure (transient epileptic amnesia) is a rare result of temporal lobe epilepsy.

Transient global amnesia

Transient global amnesia (TGA) predominantly affects middle-aged people, with an abrupt, discrete loss of anterograde memory function lasting up to a few hours. During the episode, patients are unable to record new memories, resulting in repetitive questioning, the hallmark of this condition. Consciousness is preserved and patients may perform even complex motor acts normally. During the attack there is retrograde amnesia for the events of the past few days, weeks or years. After 4–6 hours, memory function and behaviour return to normal but the patient has persistent, complete amnesia for the duration of the attack itself. There are no seizure markers and, unlike epileptic amnesia, transient global

amnesia recurs in only around 10–20% of cases. A vascular aetiology is unlikely (TGA is not a risk factor for subsequent vascular disease) and amnesia may be due to a benign process similar to migraine, occurring in the hippocampus. TGA causes no physical signs and, provided there is a typical history (which requires a witness), no investigation is necessary and patients may be reassured.

Persistent amnesia

Serious neurological disease must be excluded in patients with persistent memory disturbance, although many will prove to have benign symptoms. Symptoms corroborated by relatives or colleagues are likely to be more significant than those noted by the patient only. Where poor concentration is at the heart of cognitive deterioration, it is more likely to be due to an underlying mood disorder.

It is important to assess the timing of onset and to establish which aspects of memory are affected. Complaints of getting lost or of losing complex abilities are more pathological than word-finding difficulties. Disturbance of episodic or working memory (previously called 'short-term memory') must be distinguished from semantic memory (memory for concept-based knowledge unrelated to specific experiences). Episodic memory is selectively impaired in Korsakoff's syndrome (often secondary to alcohol) or bilateral temporal lobe damage. It can also be seen in conjunction with other types of dementia. Progressive deterioration over months suggests an underlying dementia, and a full medical assessment must be performed to detect any underlying medical problem.

It is important to identify and treat depression (p. 1185) in patients with memory loss. Depression may present as a 'pseudo-dementia', with concentration and memory impairment as dominant features, and this is often reversible with antidepressant medication. Any patient with dementia (particularly of Alzheimer's type) may develop depression in the early stages of their illness, however. Specific causes of progressive dementia, with their investigation and treatment, are described elsewhere (p. 1191).

Weakness

The assessment of weakness requires the application of basic anatomy, physiology and some pathology to the interpretation of the history and clinical findings. Points to consider are shown on Figure 25.17 and in Boxes 25.13 and 25.14. The pattern and evolution of weakness and the clinical signs provide clues to the site and nature of the lesion.

It is important to establish whether the patient has loss of power rather than reduced sensation or generalised fatigue. Pain may restrict movement and thus mimic weakness. Paradoxically, sensory neglect (p. 1083) may leave patients unaware of severe weakness.

Patients with parkinsonism may complain of weakness; extrapyramidal signs of rigidity (cogwheel or lead pipe) and bradykinesia should be evident, and a resting tremor (usually asymmetrical) may provide a further clue (p. 1112). Simple observation of the patient walking into the consulting room may be diagnostic, and is as important as formal strength testing. Movement restricted by pain should be apparent, and other features (contractures, wasting, fasciculations, abnormal movements/postures) all provide diagnostic clues.

Weakness is a common symptom arising without an underlying degenerative or destructive cause (functional symptom). Functional

25

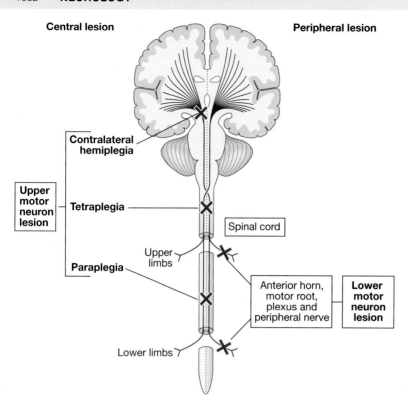

Central lesion   **Peripheral lesion**

Contralateral hemiplegia

Upper motor neuron lesion

Tetraplegia

Spinal cord

Upper limbs

Paraplegia

Anterior horn, motor root, plexus and peripheral nerve

Lower motor neuron lesion

Lower limbs

Fig. 25.17 Patterns of motor loss according to the anatomical site of the lesion.

i 25.13 Distinguishing signs in upper versus lower motor neuron syndromes

	Upper motor neuron lesion	Lower motor neuron lesion
Inspection	Normal (may be wasting in chronic lesions)	Wasting, fasciculation
Tone	Increased with clonus	Normal or decreased, no clonus
Pattern of weakness	Preferentially affects extensors in arms, flexors in leg Hemiparesis, paraparesis or tetraparesis	Typically focal, in distribution of nerve root or peripheral nerve, with associated sensory changes
Deep tendon reflexes	Increased	Decreased/absent
Plantar response	Extensor (Babinski sign)	Flexor

25.14 How to assess weakness

Clinical finding	Likely level of lesion/diagnosis
Pattern and distribution	
Isolated muscles	Radiculopathy or mononeuropathy
Both limbs on one side (hemiparesis)	Cerebral hemisphere, less likely cord or brainstem
One limb	Neuronopathy, plexopathy, cord/brain
Both lower limbs (paraparesis)	Spinal cord; look for a sensory level
Fatigability	Myasthenia gravis
Bizarre, fluctuating, not following anatomical rules	Functional
Signs	
Upper motor neuron	Brain/spinal cord
Lower motor neuron	Peripheral nervous system
Evolution of the weakness	
Sudden and improving	Stroke/mononeuropathy
Evolving over months or years	Meningioma, cervical spondylotic myelopathy
Gradually worsening over days or weeks	Cerebral mass, demyelination
Associated symptoms	
Absence of sensory involvement	Motor neuron disease, myopathy, myasthenia

weakness does not conform to typical organic patterns, and the signs in Box 25.13 are absent. Clinical examination is often variable (e.g. the patient can walk but appears to have no leg movement when assessed on the couch), and strength may appear to 'give way', with the patient able to achieve full power for brief bursts, which does not occur in disease. Hoover's sign is useful to confirm functional weakness, and relies on eliciting the normal phenomenon of simultaneous hip extension when the contralateral hip flexes. In functional weakness, hip extension weakness may be seen; this then returns to full strength when contralateral hip flexion is tested. This sign may be demonstrated to the patient in a non-confrontational manner, to show that the potential limb power is intact.

Facial weakness

Facial nerve palsy (Bell's palsy)

One of the most common causes of facial weakness is Bell's palsy, a lower motor neuron lesion of the 7th (facial) nerve, affecting all ages and both sexes. It is more common following upper respiratory tract infections, during pregnancy, and in patients with diabetes, immunosuppression and hypertension.

The lesion is within the facial canal. Symptoms usually develop subacutely over a few hours, with pain around the ear preceding the unilateral facial weakness. Patients often describe the face as 'numb' but there is no objective sensory loss (except to taste, if the chorda tympani is involved). Hyperacusis may occur if the nerve to stapedius is involved and impairment of parasympathetic fibres may cause diminished salivation and tear secretion. Examination reveals an ipsilateral lower motor neuron facial nerve palsy (no sparing of forehead muscles). Vesicles in the ear or on the palate may indicate primary herpes zoster infection (p. 239). A clinical search for signs of other causes of lower motor neuron facial nerve weakness, such as parotid or scalp lesions, trauma or skull base lesions, is justified.

Glucocorticoids improve recovery rates if started within 72 hours of onset but antiviral drugs are not effective. Artificial tears applied regularly prevent corneal drying, and taping the eye shut overnight helps prevent exposure keratitis and corneal abrasion. Patients unable to close the eye should be referred urgently to an ophthalmologist. About 80% of patients recover spontaneously within 12 weeks. Plastic surgery may be considered for the minority left with facial disfigurement after 12 months. Recurrence is unusual and should prompt further investigation. Aberrant re-innervation may occur during recovery, producing unwanted facial movements, such as eye closure when the mouth is moved (synkinesis) or 'crocodile tears' (tearing during salivation).

Unlike Bell's palsy, lesions with an upper motor neuron origin may spare the upper face. Cortical lesions may cause a facial weakness either in isolation or with associated hemiparesis and speech difficulties.

Sensory disturbance

Sensory symptoms are common and frequently benign. Patients often find sensory symptoms difficult to describe and sensory examination is difficult for both doctor and patient. While neurological disease can cause sensory symptoms, systemic disorders can also be responsible. Tingling in both hands and around the mouth can occur as the result of hyperventilation (p. 558) or hypocalcaemia (p. 662). When there is dysfunction of the relevant cerebral cortex, the patient's perception of the wholeness or actual presence of the relevant part of the body may be distorted.

Numbness and paraesthesia

The history may give the best clues to localisation and pathology. Certain common patterns are recognised: in migraine, the aura may consist of spreading tingling or paraesthesia, followed by numbness evolving over 20–30 minutes over one half of the body, often splitting the tongue. Sensory loss caused by a stroke or transient ischaemic attack (TIA) occurs much more rapidly and is typically negative (numbness) rather than positive (tingling). Rarely, unpleasant paraesthesia of sensory epilepsy spreads within seconds. The sensory alteration of inflammatory spinal cord lesions often ascends from one or both lower limbs to a distinct level on the trunk over hours to days. Psychogenic sensory change can occur as a manifestation of anxiety or as part of a conversion disorder (p. 1202). In such cases, the distribution usually neither conforms to a known anatomical pattern nor fits with any organic disease. Care must be taken in diagnosing non-organic sensory problems; a careful history and examination will ensure there is no other objective neurological deficit.

Sensory neurological examination needs to be undertaken and interpreted with care because the findings depend, by definition, on subjective reports. The reported distribution of sensory loss can be useful, however, when combined with the coexisting deficits of motor and/or cranial nerve function (Fig. 25.18).

Sensory loss in peripheral nerve lesions

Here the symptoms are usually of sensory loss and paraesthesia. Single nerve lesions cause disturbance in the sensory distribution of the nerve, whereas in diffuse neuropathies the longest neurons are affected first, giving a characteristic 'glove and stocking' distribution. If smaller nerve fibres are preferentially affected (e.g. in diabetic neuropathy), temperature and pin-prick (pain) are reduced, whilst vibration sense and proprioception (modalities served by the larger, well-myelinated, sensory nerves) may be relatively spared. In contrast, vibration and proprioception are particularly affected if the neuropathy is demyelinating in character (p. 1138), producing symptoms of tightness and swelling with impairment of proprioception and vibration sensation.

Sensory loss in nerve root lesions

These typically present with pain as a prominent feature, either within the spine or in the limb plexuses. Pain is often felt in the myotome rather than the dermatome. The nerve root involved may be deduced from the dermatomal pattern of sensory loss (p. 1071), although overlap may lead to this being smaller than expected.

Sensory loss in spinal cord lesions

Transverse lesions of the spinal cord produce loss of all sensory modalities below that segmental level, although the clinical level may only be manifest 2–3 segments lower than the anatomical site of the lesion. Very often, there is a band of paraesthesia or hyperaesthesia at the top of the area of sensory loss. Clinical examination may reveal dissociated sensory loss, i.e. different patterns in the spinothalamic and dorsal columnar pathways. If the transverse lesion is vascular due to anterior spinal artery thrombosis, the spinothalamic pathways may be affected while the posterior one-third of the spinal cord (the dorsal column modalities) may be spared.

Lesions damaging one side of the spinal cord will produce loss of spinothalamic modalities (pain and temperature) on the opposite side, and of dorsal column modalities (joint position and vibration sense) on the same side of the body – the Brown–Séquard syndrome (p. 1084).

Lesions in the centre of the spinal cord (such as syringomyelia: see Box 25.83 and Fig. 25.51, pp. 1138 and 1139) spare the dorsal columns but involve the spinothalamic fibres crossing the cord from both sides over the length of the lesion. There is no sensory loss in segments above and below the lesion; this is described as 'suspended' sensory loss. There is sometimes reflex loss at the level of the lesion if afferent fibres of the reflex arc are affected.

An isolated lesion of the dorsal columns is not uncommon in multiple sclerosis. This produces a characteristic unpleasant, tight feeling over the limb(s) involved and, while there is no loss of pin-prick or temperature sensation, the associated loss of proprioception may severely limit function of the affected limb(s).

Sensory loss in brainstem lesions

Lesions in the brainstem can be associated with sensory loss but the distribution depends on the site of the lesion. A lesion limited to the trigeminal nucleus or its sensory projections will cause

25

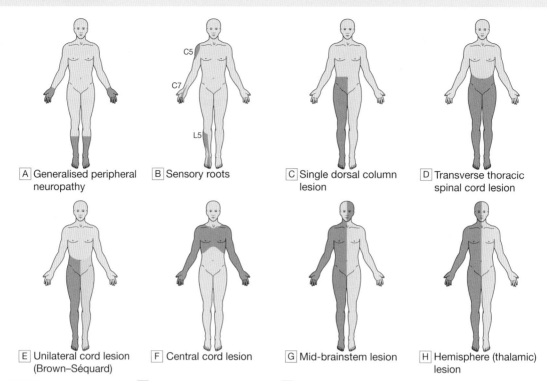

Fig. 25.18 Patterns of sensory loss. **A** Generalised peripheral neuropathy. **B** Sensory roots: some common examples. **C** Single dorsal column lesion (proprioception and some touch loss). **D** Transverse thoracic spinal cord lesion. **E** Unilateral cord lesion (Brown–Séquard): ipsilateral dorsal column (and motor) deficit and contralateral spinothalamic deficit. **F** Central cord lesion: 'cape' distribution of spinothalamic loss. **G** Mid-brainstem lesion: ipsilateral facial sensory loss and contralateral loss on body below the vertex. **H** Hemisphere (thalamic) lesion: contralateral loss on one side of face and body.

ipsilateral facial sensory disturbance. For example, pain resembling trigeminal neuralgia can be seen in patients with multiple sclerosis. The anatomy of the trigeminal connections means that lesions in the medulla or spinal cord can give rise to 'balaclava' patterns of sensory loss (p. 1070). Sensory pathways running up from the spinal cord can also be damaged in the brainstem, resulting in simultaneous sensory loss in arm(s) and/or leg(s).

Sensory loss in hemispheric lesions

The temporal, parietal and occipital lobes receive sensory information regarding the various modalities of touch, vision, hearing and balance (see Box 25.2, p. 1066). The initial points of entry into the cortex are the respective primary cortical areas (see Fig. 25.4, p. 1067). Damage to any of these primary areas will result in reduction or loss of the ability to perceive that particular modality: 'negative' symptomatology. Abnormal excitation of these areas can result in a false perception ('positive' symptoms), the most common of which is migrainous visual aura (flashing lights or teichopsia).

Cortical lesions are more likely to cause a mixed motor and sensory loss. Substantial lesions of the parietal cortex (as in large strokes) can cause severe loss of proprioception and may even abolish conscious awareness of the existence of the affected limb(s), known as neglect; this can be difficult to distinguish from paralysis. Pathways are so tightly packed in the thalamus that even small lacunar strokes can cause isolated contralateral hemisensory loss.

Neuropathic pain

Neuropathic pain is a positive neurological symptom caused by dysfunction of the pain perception apparatus, in contrast to nociceptive pain, which is secondary to pathological processes such as inflammation. Neuropathic pain has distinctive features and typically provokes a very unpleasant, persistent, burning sensation. There is often increased sensitivity to touch, so that light brushing of the affected area causes exquisite pain (allodynia). Painful stimuli are felt as though they arise from a larger area than that touched, and spontaneous bursts of pain may also occur. Pain may be elicited by other modalities (allodynia) and is considerably affected by emotional influences. The most common causes of neuropathic pain are diabetic neuropathies, trigeminal and post-herpetic neuralgias, and trauma to a peripheral nerve. Treatment of these syndromes can be difficult. Drugs that modulate various parts of the nociceptive system, such as gabapentin, carbamazepine or tricyclic antidepressants, may help. Localised treatment (topical treatment or nerve blocks) sometimes succeeds but may increase the sensory deficit and worsen the situation. Electrical stimulation has occasionally proved successful. For further information, see page 1347.

Abnormal movements

Disorders of movement lead to either extra, unwanted movement (hyperkinetic disorders) or too little movement (hypokinetic disorders) (Box 25.15). In either case, the lesion often localises to the basal ganglia, although some tremors are related to cerebellar or brainstem disturbance. Functional movement disorders are common and may mimic all of the organic syndromes below. The most important hypokinetic disorder is Parkinson's disease (p. 1112). Parkinsonism is a clinical description of a collection of symptoms, including tremor, bradykinesia and rigidity. While the history is always important, observation is clearly vital; much of the skill in diagnosing movement disorders lies in pattern recognition. Once it is established whether the problem is hypo- or hyperkinetic, the next task is to categorise the movements further, accepting that there is often overlap. Videoing the movements (with the patient's consent), so that they can be shown to a movement disorder expert, may provide a quick diagnosis in cases of uncertainty.

Tremor

Tremor is caused by alternating agonist/antagonist muscle contractions and produces a rhythmical oscillation of the body part affected. In the assessment of tremor, the position, body part affected, frequency and amplitude should be considered, as these provide diagnostic clues (Box 25.16).

Other hyperkinetic syndromes

Non-rhythmic involuntary movements include chorea, athetosis, ballism, dystonia, myoclonus and tics. They are categorised by clinical appearance, and coexistence and overlap are common, such as in choreoathetosis.

Chorea

Chorea refers to jerky, brief, purposeless involuntary movements, appearing fidgety and affecting different areas. They suggest disease in the caudate nucleus (as in Huntington's disease, p. 1114) and are a common complication of levodopa treatment for Parkinson's disease. Other causes are shown in Box 25.17.

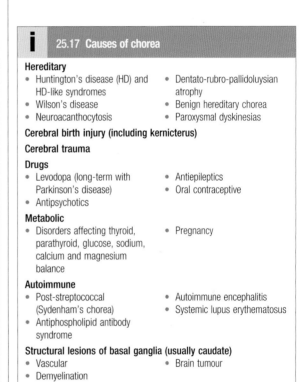

i 25.15 Movement disorders

Description	Features	Examples
Hypokinetic disorders		
Parkinsonism	Akinesia Rigidity Tremor Loss of postural reflexes Other features depending on cause	Idiopathic Parkinson's disease Other degenerative syndromes Drug-induced (See Box 25.54)
Catatonia	Mutism Sustained posturing and waxy flexibility	Usually psychiatric; if neurological, is most commonly of vascular origin
Hyperkinetic disorders		
Tremor	Rhythmical oscillation of body part (see Box 25.16)	Essential tremor Parkinson's disease Drug-induced
Chorea	Jerky, brief, involuntary movements	Huntington's disease Drug-induced
Tics	Stereotyped, repetitive movements, briefly suppressible	Tourette's syndrome
Myoclonus	Shock-like muscle jerks	Epilepsy Hypnic jerks (p. 1086) Focal cortical disease
Dystonia	Sustained muscle contraction causing abnormal postures ± tremor	Genetic Generalised dystonic syndromes Focal dystonias in adults (e.g. torticollis)
Others	Various	Paroxysmal hyperkinetic dyskinesias Hemifacial spasm Tardive syndromes

i 25.17 Causes of chorea

Hereditary
- Huntington's disease (HD) and HD-like syndromes
- Wilson's disease
- Neuroacanthocytosis
- Dentato-rubro-pallidoluysian atrophy
- Benign hereditary chorea
- Paroxysmal dyskinesias

Cerebral birth injury (including kernicterus)

Cerebral trauma

Drugs
- Levodopa (long-term with Parkinson's disease)
- Antipsychotics
- Antiepileptics
- Oral contraceptive

Metabolic
- Disorders affecting thyroid, parathyroid, glucose, sodium, calcium and magnesium balance
- Pregnancy

Autoimmune
- Post-streptococcal (Sydenham's chorea)
- Antiphospholipid antibody syndrome
- Autoimmune encephalitis
- Systemic lupus erythematosus

Structural lesions of basal ganglia (usually caudate)
- Vascular
- Demyelination
- Brain tumour

25

i 25.16 Causes and characteristics of tremors

	Body part affected	Position	Frequency	Amplitude	Character
Physiological	Both arms > legs	Posture, movement	High	Small (fine)	Enhanced by anxiety, emotion, drugs, toxins
Parkinsonism	Unilateral or asymmetrical Arm > leg, chin, never head	Rest Postural and re-emergent may occur	Low (3–4 Hz)	Moderate	Typically pill-rolling, thumb and index finger, other features of parkinsonism
Essential tremor	Bilateral arms, head	Movement	High (8–10 Hz)	Low to moderate	Family history; 50% respond to alcohol
Dystonic	Head, arms, legs	Posture	Variable	Variable	Other features of dystonia, often jerky tremors
Functional	Any	Any	Variable	Variable	Distractible

Athetosis

Slower, writhing movement of the limbs are often combined with chorea and have similar causes.

Ballism

This more dramatic form of chorea causes often violent flinging movements of one limb (monoballism) or one side of the body (hemiballism). The lesion localises to the contralateral subthalamic nucleus and the most common cause is stroke.

Dystonia

Sustained involuntary muscle contraction causes abnormal postures or movement. It may be generalised (usually in childhood-onset genetic syndromes) or, more commonly, focal/segmental (such as in torticollis, when the head is twisted repeatedly to one side). Some dystonias occur only with specific tasks, such as writer's cramp or other occupational 'cramps'. Dystonic tremor is associated, and is asymmetrical and of large amplitude.

Myoclonus

Myoclonus consists of brief, isolated, random jerks of muscle groups. This is physiological at the onset of sleep (hypnic jerks). Similarly, a myoclonic jerk is a component of the normal startle response, which may be exaggerated in some rare (mostly genetic) disorders. Myoclonus may occur in disorders of the cerebral cortex, such as some forms of epilepsy. Alternatively, myoclonus can arise from subcortical structures or, more rarely, from segments of the spinal cord.

Tics

Tics are stereotyped repetitive movements, such as blinking, winking, head shaking or shoulder shrugging. Unlike dyskinesias, the patient may be able to suppress them, although only for a short time. Isolated tics are common in childhood and usually disappear. Tourette's syndrome is defined by the presence of multiple motor and vocal tics that may evolve over time; it is frequently associated with psychiatric disease, including obsessive compulsions, depression, self-harm or attention deficit disorder. Tics may also occur in Huntington's and Wilson's diseases, or after streptococcal infection.

Abnormal perception

The parietal lobes are involved in the higher processing and integration of primary sensory information. This takes place in areas referred to as 'association' cortex, damage to which gives rise to sensory (including visual) inattention, disorders of spatial perception, and disruption of spatially orientated behaviour, leading to apraxia. Apraxia is the inability to perform complex, organised activity in the presence of normal basic motor, sensory and cerebellar function (after weakness, numbness and ataxia have been excluded as causes). Examples of complex motor activities include dressing, using cutlery and geographical orientation. Other abnormalities that can result from damage to the association cortex involve difficulty reading (dyslexia) or writing (dysgraphia), or the inability to recognise familiar objects (agnosia). The results of damage to particular lobes of the brain are given in Box 25.2 (p. 1066).

Altered balance and vertigo

Balance is a complicated dynamic process that requires ongoing modification of both axial and limb muscles to compensate for the effects of gravity and alterations in body position and load (and hence centre of gravity) in order to prevent a person from falling. This requires input from a variety of sensory modalities (visual, vestibular and proprioceptive), processing by the cerebellum and brainstem, and output via a number of descending pathways (e.g. vestibulospinal, rubrospinal and reticulospinal tracts).

Disorders of balance can therefore arise from any part of this process. Disordered input (loss of vision, vestibular disorders or lack of joint position sense), processing (damage to vestibular nuclei or cerebellum) or motor function (spinal cord lesions, leg weakness of any cause) can all impair balance. The patient may complain of different symptoms, depending on the location of the lesion. For example, loss of joint position sense or cerebellar function may result in a sensation of unsteadiness, while damage to the vestibular nuclei or labyrinth may result in an illusion of movement, such as vertigo (see below). A careful history is vital. Since vision can often compensate for lack of joint position sense, patients with peripheral neuropathies or dorsal column loss will often find their problem more noticeable in the dark.

Examination of such patients may yield physical signs that again depend on the site of the lesion. Sensory abnormalities may be manifest as altered visual acuities or visual fields, possibly with abnormalities on fundoscopy, altered eye movements (including nystagmus, p. 1090), impaired vestibular function (p. 1104) or lack of joint position sense. Disturbance of cerebellar function may be manifest as nystagmus, dysarthria or ataxia, or difficulty with gait (unsteadiness or inability to perform tandem gait; see below). Leg weakness, if present, will be detectable on examination of the limbs.

Vertigo

Vertigo is defined as an abnormal perception of movement of the environment or self, and occurs because of conflicting visual, proprioceptive and vestibular information about a person's position in space. Vertigo commonly arises from imbalance of vestibular input and is within the experience of most people, since this is the 'dizziness' that occurs after someone has spun round vigorously and then stops. Bilateral labyrinthine dysfunction often causes some unsteadiness. Labyrinthine vertigo usually lasts days at a time, though it may recur, while vertigo arising from central (brainstem) disorders is often persistent and accompanied by other brainstem signs. Benign paroxysmal positional vertigo (p. 1104) lasts a few seconds on head movement. A careful history will reveal the likely cause in most patients.

Abnormal gait

Many neurological disorders can affect gait. Observing patients as they walk into the consulting room can be very informative, although formal examination is also important. Neurogenic gait disorders need to be distinguished from those due to skeletal abnormalities, usually characterised by pain producing an antalgic gait, or limp. Gait alteration incompatible with any anatomical or physiological deficit may be due to functional disorders.

Pyramidal gait

Upper motor neuron lesions cause characteristic extension of the affected leg. The resultant tendency for the toes to strike the ground on walking requires the leg to swing outwards at the hip (circumduction). Nevertheless, a shoe on the affected side worn down at the toes may provide evidence of this type of gait. In hemiplegia, the asymmetry between affected and normal sides is obvious on walking, but in paraparesis both lower limbs swing slowly from the hips in extension and are dragged stiffly over the ground – described as 'walking in mud'.

Foot drop

In normal walking, the heel is the first part of the foot to hit the ground. A lower motor neuron lesion affecting the leg will cause weakness of ankle dorsiflexion, resulting in a less controlled descent of the foot, which makes a slapping noise as it hits the ground. In severe cases, the foot will have to be lifted higher at the knee to allow room for the inadequately dorsiflexed foot to swing through, resulting in a high-stepping gait.

Myopathic gait

During walking, alternating transfer of the body's weight through each leg requires adequate hip abduction. In proximal muscle weakness, usually caused by muscle disease, the hips are not properly fixed by these muscles and trunk movements are exaggerated, producing a rolling or waddling gait.

Ataxic gait

An ataxic gait can result from lesions in the cerebellum, vestibular apparatus or peripheral nerves. Patients with lesions of the central portion of the cerebellum (the vermis) walk with a characteristic broad-based gait 'as if drunk' (cerebellar function is particularly sensitive to alcohol). Patients with acute vestibular disturbances walk similarly but the accompanying vertigo is characteristic. Inability to walk heel to toe may be the only sign of less severe cerebellar dysfunction.

Proprioceptive defects can also cause an ataxic gait. The impairment of joint position sense makes walking unreliable, especially in poor light. The feet tend to be placed on the ground with greater emphasis, presumably to enhance proprioceptive input, resulting in a 'stamping' gait.

Apraxic gait

In an apraxic gait, power, cerebellar function and proprioception are normal on examination of the legs. The patient may be able to carry out complex motor tasks (e.g. bicycling motion) while recumbent and yet cannot formulate the motor act of walking. In this higher cerebral dysfunction, the feet appear stuck to the floor and the patient cannot walk. Gait apraxia is a sign of diffuse bilateral hemisphere disease (such as normal pressure hydrocephalus) or diffuse frontal lobe disease.

Marche à petits pas

This gait is characterised by small, slow steps and marked instability. It differs from the festination found in Parkinson's disease (see below), in that it lacks increasing pace and freezing. The usual cause is small-vessel cerebrovascular disease and there may be accompanying bilateral upper motor neuron signs.

Extrapyramidal gait

The rigidity and bradykinesia of basal ganglia dysfunction (p. 1112) lead to a stooped posture and characteristic gait difficulties, with problems initiating walking and controlling the pace of the gait. Patients may become stuck while trying to start walking or when walking through doorways ('freezing'). The centre of gravity will be moved forwards to aid propulsion, which, with poor axial control, can lead to an accelerating pace of shuffling and difficulty stopping. This produces the festinant gait: initial stuttering steps that quickly increase in frequency while decreasing in length.

Abnormal speech and language

Speech disturbance may be isolated to disruption of sound output (dysarthria) or may involve language disturbance (dysphasia). Dysphonia (reduction in the sound/volume) is usually due to mechanical laryngeal disruption, whereas dysarthria is more typically neurological in origin. Dysphasia is always neurological and localises to the dominant cerebral hemisphere (usually left, regardless of handedness). Combinations of speech and swallowing problems are explained below (p. 1093).

Dysphonia

Dysphonia describes hoarse or whispered speech. The most common cause is laryngitis, but dysphonia can also result from a lesion of the 10th cranial nerve or disease of the vocal cords, including laryngeal dystonia. Parkinsonism may cause hypophonia with marked reduction in speech volume, often in association with dysarthria, making speech difficult to understand.

Dysarthria

Dysarthria is characterised by poorly articulated or slurred speech and can occur in association with lesions of the cerebellum, brainstem and lower cranial nerves, as well as in myasthenia or myopathic disease. Language function is not affected. The quality of the speech tends to differ, depending on the cause, but

25

i	25.18 Causes of dysarthria			
Type	**Site**	**Characteristics**	**Associated features**	
Myopathic	Muscles of speech	Indistinct, poor articulation	Weakness of face, tongue and neck	
Myasthenic	Motor end plate	Indistinct with fatigue and dysphonia Fluctuating severity	Ptosis, diplopia, facial and neck weakness	
Bulbar	Brainstem	Indistinct, slurred, often nasal	Dysphagia, diplopia, ataxia	
'Scanning'	Cerebellum	Slurred, impaired timing and cadence, 'sing-song'	Ataxia of limbs and gait, tremor of head/limbs Nystagmus	
Spastic ('pseudo-bulbar')	Pyramidal tracts	Indistinct, nasal tone, mumbling	Poor rapid tongue movements, increased reflexes and jaw jerk	
Parkinsonian	Basal ganglia	Indistinct, rapid, stammering, quiet	Tremor, rigidity, slow shuffling gait	
Dystonic	Basal ganglia	Strained, slow, high-pitched	Dystonia, athetosis	

it can be very difficult to distinguish the different types clinically (Box 25.18). Dysarthria is discussed further in the section on bulbar symptoms (p. 1093).

Dysphasia

Dysphasia (or aphasia) is a disorder of the language content of speech. It can occur with lesions over a wide area of the dominant hemisphere (Fig. 25.19). Dysphasia may be categorised according to whether the speech output is fluent or non-fluent. Fluent aphasias, also called receptive aphasias, are impairments related mostly to the input or reception of language, with difficulties either in auditory verbal comprehension or in the repetition of words, phrases or sentences spoken by others. Speech is easy and fluent but there are difficulties related to the output of language as well, such as paraphasia (either substitution of similar-sounding non-words, or incorrect words) and neologisms (non-existent words). Examples include Wernicke's aphasia (which localises to the superior posterior temporal lobe), transcortical sensory aphasia, conduction aphasia and anomic aphasia.

Non-fluent aphasias, also called expressive aphasias, are difficulties in articulating, but in most cases there is relatively good auditory verbal comprehension. Examples include Broca's aphasia (associated with pathologies in the inferior frontal region), transcortical motor aphasia and global aphasia.

'Pure' aphasias are selective impairments in reading, writing or the recognition of words. These disorders may be quite selective. For example, a person is able to read but not write, or is able to write but not read. Examples include pure alexia, agraphia and pure word deafness.

Dysphasia (a focal symptom) is frequently misinterpreted as disorientation (which is non-focal) and it is important always to consider dysphasia as an alternative explanation for the apparently 'confused' patient. Dysphasia can be misheard/misspelt as dysphagia, and for this reason some prefer to use 'aphasia' to avoid confusion.

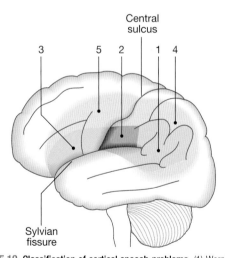

Fig. 25.19 Classification of cortical speech problems. (1) Wernicke's aphasia: fluent dysphasia with poor comprehension and poor repetition. (2) Conduction aphasia: fluent aphasia with good comprehension and poor repetition. (3) Broca's aphasia: non-fluent aphasia with good comprehension and poor repetition. (4) Transcortical sensory aphasia: fluent aphasia with poor comprehension and good repetition. (5) Transcortical motor aphasia: non-fluent aphasia with good comprehension and good repetition. Large lesions affecting all of regions 1–5 cause global aphasia.

Disturbance of smell

Symptomatic olfactory loss is most commonly due to local causes (nasal obstruction) but may follow head injury. Hyposmia may predate motor symptoms in Parkinson's disease by many years, although it is rarely noticed by the patient. Frontal lobe lesions are a rare cause. Positive olfactory symptoms may arise in Alzheimer's disease or epilepsy.

Visual disturbance and ocular abnormalities

Disturbances of vision may be due to primary ocular disease or to disorders of the central connections and visual cortex. Visual symptoms are usually negative (loss of vision) but sometimes positive, most commonly in migraine. Eye movements may be disturbed, giving rise to double vision (diplopia) or blurred vision. Loss of vision is also discussed on page 1170.

Visual loss

Visual loss can occur as the result of lesions in any areas between the retina and the visual cortex. Patterns of visual field loss are explained by the anatomy of the visual pathways (see Fig. 25.7, p. 1069). Associated clinical manifestations are described in Box 25.19. Visual symptoms affecting one eye only are due to lesions anterior to the optic chiasm.

Transient visual loss is quite common and sudden-onset visual loss lasting less than 15 minutes is likely to have a vascular origin. It may be difficult to know whether the visual loss was monocular (carotid circulation) or binocular (vertebrobasilar circulation), and it is important to ask if the patient tried closing each eye in turn to see whether the symptom affected one eye or both. Visual field testing is an important part of the examination, either at the bedside or formally with perimetry. Field defects become more symmetrical (congruous), the closer the lesion comes to the visual cortex.

Migrainous visual symptoms are very common and, when associated with typical headache and other migraine features, rarely pose a diagnostic challenge. They may occur in isolation, however, making distinction from TIA difficult, but TIAs typically cause negative (blindness) symptoms, whereas migraine causes positive phenomena (see below). TIAs often last for a shorter time (a few minutes), compared to the 10–60-minute duration of migraine aura, and have an abrupt onset and end, unlike the gradual evolution of a migraine aura.

Positive visual phenomena

The most common cause is migraine; patients may describe silvery zigzag lines (fortification spectra) or flashing coloured lights (teichopsia), usually preceding the headache. Simple flashes of light (phosphenes) may indicate damage to the retina (e.g. detachment) or to the primary visual cortex. Formed visual hallucinations may be caused by drugs or may be due to epilepsy or 'release phenomena' in a blind visual field (Charles Bonnet syndrome).

Double vision

Diplopia arises from misalignment of the eyes, meaning that the image is not projected to the same points on the two retinas. At its most subtle it may be reported as blurred rather than

25.19 Clinical manifestations of visual field loss

Site of lesion	Common causes	Complaint	Visual field loss	Associated physical signs
Retina/optic disc	Vascular disease (including vasculitis) Glaucoma Inflammation	Partial/complete visual loss depending on site, involving one or both eyes	Altitudinal field defect Arcuate scotoma	Reduced acuity Visual distortion (macula) Abnormal retinal appearance
Optic nerve	Optic neuritis Sarcoidosis Tumour Leber's hereditary optic neuropathy	Partial/complete loss of vision in one eye Often painful Central vision particularly affected	Central or paracentral scotoma Monocular blindness	Reduced acuity Reduced colour vision Relative afferent pupillary defect Optic atrophy (late)
Optic chiasm	Pituitary tumour Craniopharyngioma Sarcoidosis	May be none Rarely, diplopia ('hemifield slide')	Bitemporal hemianopia	Pituitary function abnormalities
Optic tract	Tumour Inflammatory disease	Disturbed vision to one side of midline	Incongruous contralateral homonymous hemianopia	
Temporal lobe	Stroke Tumour Inflammatory disease	Disturbed vision to one side of midline	Contralateral homonymous upper quadrantanopia	Memory/language disorders
Parietal lobe	Stroke Tumour Inflammatory disease	Disturbed vision to one side of midline Bumping into things	Contralateral homonymous lower quadrantanopia	Contralateral sensory disturbance Asymmetry of optokinetic nystagmus
Occipital lobe	Stroke Tumour Inflammatory disease	Disturbed vision to one side of midline Difficulty reading Bumping into things	Homonymous hemianopia (may be macula-sparing)	Damage to other structures supplied by posterior cerebral circulation

25.20 Common causes of damage to cranial nerves 3, 4 and 6

Site	Common pathology	Nerve(s) involved	Associated features
Brainstem	Infarction	3 (mid-brain)	Contralateral pyramidal signs
	Haemorrhage Demyelination Intrinsic tumour	6 (ponto-medullary junction)	Ipsilateral lower motor neuron facial palsy Other brainstem/cerebellar signs
Intrameningeal	Meningitis (infective/malignant)	3, 4 and/or 6	Meningism, features of primary disease course
	Raised intracranial pressure	6 3 (uncal herniation)	Papilloedema Features of space-occupying lesion
	Aneurysms	3 (posterior communicating artery) 6 (basilar artery)	Pain Features of subarachnoid haemorrhage
	Cerebello-pontine angle tumour	6	8, 7, 5 nerve lesions (order of likelihood) Ipsilateral cerebellar signs
	Trauma	3, 4 and/or 6	Other features of trauma
Cavernous sinus	Infection/thrombosis Carotid artery aneurysm Caroticocavernous fistula	3, 4 and/or 6	May be 5th nerve involvement also Pupil may be fixed, mid-position (Sympathetic plexus on carotid may also be affected)
Superior orbital fissure	Tumour (e.g. sphenoid wing meningioma) Granuloma	3, 4 and/or 6	May be proptosis, chemosis
Orbit	Vascular (e.g. diabetes, vasculitis) Infections Tumour Granuloma Trauma	3, 4 and/or 6	Pain Pupil often spared in vascular 3rd nerve palsy

25

double vision. Monocular diplopia indicates ocular disease, while binocular diplopia suggests a neurological cause. Closing either eye in turn will abort binocular diplopia. Once the presence of binocular diplopia is confirmed, it should be established whether the diplopia is maximal in any particular direction of gaze, whether the images are separated horizontally or vertically, and whether there are any associated symptoms or signs, such as ptosis or pupillary disturbance.

Binocular diplopia may result from central disorders or from disturbance of the ocular motor nerves, muscles or the

Cranial nerve palsy	Direction of gaze	Primary position	Direction of gaze
Right 3rd nerve palsy	N.B. Pupil dilated; ptosis	Right eye turns down and out	Unable to adduct right eye Squint worse
Right 4th nerve palsy (more evident on downgaze)	No obvious squint	Right eye turns slightly up	Right eye elevates more as it moves medially
Right 6th nerve palsy	Unable to abduct right eye Squint worse	Right eye turns medially	Able to adduct right eye No obvious squint

Fig. 25.20 Examination findings in 3rd, 4th and 6th nerve palsy. Diplopia tends to be more obvious on lateral gaze compared to primary position.

neuromuscular junction (see Fig. 25.8, p. 1070). The pattern of double vision, along with any associated features, usually allows the clinician to infer which nerves/muscles are affected, while the mode of onset and other features (e.g. fatigability in myasthenia) provide further clues to the cause.

The causes of ocular motor nerve palsies are listed in Box 25.20. Examination findings are illustrated in Figure 25.20.

Nystagmus

Nystagmus describes a repetitive to-and-fro movement of the eyes. In central lesions, the slow drifts are the primary abnormal movement, each followed by fast (corrective) phases. Nystagmus occurs because the control systems of the eyes are defective, causing them to drift off target; corrections then become necessary to return fixation to the object of interest, causing nystagmus. The direction of the fast phase is usually designated as the direction of the nystagmus because it is easier to see. Nystagmus may be horizontal, vertical or torsional, and usually involves both eyes synchronously. It may be a physiological phenomenon in response to sustained vestibular stimulation or movement of the visual world (optokinetic nystagmus). There are many causes of pathological nystagmus, the most common sites of lesions being the vestibular system, brainstem and cerebellum.

The brainstem and the cerebellum are involved in maintaining eccentric positions of gaze. Lesions will therefore allow the eyes to drift back in towards primary position, producing nystagmus with fast component beats in the direction of gaze (gaze-evoked nystagmus). This is the most common type of 'central' nystagmus; it is most commonly bidirectional and not usually accompanied by vertigo. Other signs of brainstem dysfunction may be evident. Brainstem disease may also cause vertical nystagmus.

Unilateral cerebellar lesions may result in gaze-evoked nystagmus when looking in the direction of the lesion, where the fast phases are directed towards the side of the lesion. Cerebellar hemisphere lesions also cause 'ocular dysmetria', an overshoot of target-directed, fast eye movements (saccades) resembling 'past-pointing' in limbs.

In vestibular lesions, damage to one of the horizontal canals or its connections will allow the tonic output from the healthy contralateral side to cause the eyes to drift towards the side of the lesion. This elicits recurrent compensatory fast movements away from the side of the lesion, manifest as unidirectional horizontal nystagmus. Vertical and torsional components can be seen with damage to other parts of the vestibular apparatus. The nystagmus of peripheral labyrinthine lesions is accompanied by vertigo and usually by nausea, vomiting and unsteadiness, but as the CNS habituates, the nystagmus disappears (fatigues) quite quickly. Central vestibular nystagmus is more persistent.

Nystagmus also occurs as a consequence of drug toxicity and nutritional deficiency (e.g. thiamin). The severity is variable, and it may or may not result in visual degradation, though it may be associated with a sensation of movement of the visual world (oscillopsia). Nystagmus may occur as a congenital phenomenon, in which case both phases are equal and 'pendular', rather than having alternating fast and slow components.

Ptosis

Various disorders may cause drooping of the eyelids (ptosis) and these are listed in Box 25.21 and shown on Figure 25.21.

Abnormal pupillary responses

Abnormal pupillary responses may arise from lesions at several points between the retina and brainstem. Lesions of the oculomotor nerve, ciliary ganglion and sympathetic supply produce characteristic ipsilateral disorders of pupillary function. 'Afferent' defects result from damage to an optic nerve, impairing the direct response of a pupil to light, although leaving the consensual response from stimulation of the normal eye intact. Structural damage to the iris itself can also result in pupillary abnormalities. Causes are given in Box 25.22. An example is shown in Figure 25.22.

Papilloedema

There are several causes of swelling of the optic disc but the term 'papilloedema' is reserved for swelling secondary to raised intracranial pressure, when obstructed axoplasmic flow from retinal ganglion cells results in swollen nerve fibres, which in turn cause capillary and venous congestion, producing papilloedema.

25.21 Common causes of ptosis		
Mechanism	**Causes**	**Associated clinical features**
3rd nerve palsy	Isolated palsy (see Box 25.20) Central/supranuclear lesion	Ptosis is usually complete Extraocular muscle palsy (eye 'down and out') Depending on site of lesion, other cranial nerve palsies (e.g. 4, 5 and 6) or contralateral upper motor neuron signs
Sympathetic lesion (**Horner's syndrome**: see Fig. 25.22)	Central (hypothalamus/brainstem) Peripheral (lung apex, carotid artery pathology) Idiopathic	Ptosis is partial Lack of sweating on affected side Depending on site of lesion, brainstem signs, signs of apical lung/brachial plexus disease, or ipsilateral carotid artery stroke
Myopathic	Myasthenia gravis Dystrophia myotonica	Extraocular muscle palsies Usually bilateral More widespread muscle weakness, with fatigability in myasthenia Progressive external ophthalmoplegia Other characteristic features of individual causes
Other	Functional ptosis Pseudo-ptosis (e.g. blepharospasm) Local orbital/lid disease Age-related levator dehiscence	Resistance to eye opening Eyebrows depressed rather than raised May be local orbital abnormality

Fig. 25.21 **Differential diagnosis of unilateral ptosis.** (CPEO = chronic progressive external ophthalmoplegia)

Fig. 25.22 **Right-sided Horner's syndrome due to paravertebral metastasis at T1.** There is ipsilateral partial ptosis and a small pupil.

The earliest sign is the cessation of venous pulsation seen at the disc, progression causing the disc margins to become red (hyperaemic). Disc margins become indistinct and haemorrhages may occur in the retina (Fig. 25.23). Lack of papilloedema never excludes raised intracranial pressure. Other causes of optic disc swelling are listed in Box 25.23. Some normal variations of disc appearance (e.g. optic nerve drusen, p. 1178) can mimic disc swelling. Optic disc swelling is also discussed on page 1171.

Optic atrophy

Loss of nerve fibres causes the optic disc to appear pale, as the choroid becomes visible (Fig. 25.24). A pale disc (optic

25.22 Pupillary disorders

Disorder	Cause	Ophthalmological features	Associated features
3rd nerve palsy	See Box 25.21	Dilated pupil (especially with external compression) Extraocular muscle palsy (eye is typically 'down and out') Complete ptosis	Other features of 3rd nerve palsy (see Box 25.21)
Horner's syndrome (see Fig. 25.22)	Lesion to sympathetic supply	Small pupil Partial ptosis Iris heterochromia (if congenital)	Ipsilateral failure of sweating (anhidrosis)
Holmes–Adie syndrome (tonic pupil)	Lesion of ciliary ganglion (usually idiopathic)	Dilated pupil Light-near dissociation (accommodate but do not react to light) Vermiform movement of iris during contraction Disturbance of accommodation	Generalised areflexia
Argyll Robertson pupil	Dorsal mid-brain lesion (syphilis or diabetes)	Small, irregular pupils Light-near dissociation	Other features of tabes dorsalis (p. 1125)
Local pupillary damage	Trauma/inflammatory disease	Irregular pupils, often with adhesions to lens (synechiae) Variable degree of reactivity	Other features of trauma/underlying inflammatory disease (e.g. cataract, blindness etc.)
Relative afferent pupillary defect (Marcus Gunn pupil)	Damage to optic nerve	Pupils symmetrical – swinging torch test reveals dilatation in abnormal eye	Decreased visual acuity/colour vision Central scotoma Optic disc swelling or pallor

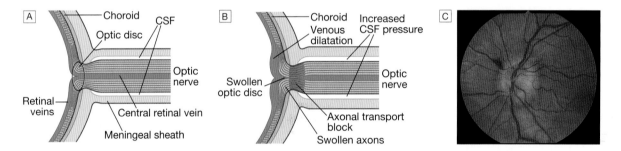

Fig. 25.23 Mechanism of optic disc oedema (papilloedema). [A] Normal. [B] Disc oedema (e.g. due to cerebral tumour). [C] Fundus photograph of the left eye showing optic disc oedema with a small haemorrhage on the nasal side of the disc. (CSF = cerebrospinal fluid) *C, Courtesy of Dr B. Cullen.*

25.23 Common causes of optic disc swelling

Raised intracranial pressure (papilloedema)

- Cerebral mass lesion (tumour, abscess)
- Obstructive hydrocephalus
- Idiopathic intracranial hypertension

Obstruction of ocular venous drainage

- Central retinal vein occlusion
- Cavernous sinus thrombosis

Systemic disorders affecting retinal vessels

- Hypertension
- Vasculitis
- Hypercapnia

Optic nerve damage

- Demyelination (optic neuritis/papillitis)
- Leber's hereditary optic neuropathy
- Anterior ischaemic optic neuropathy
- Toxins (e.g. methanol)
- Infiltration of optic disc
- Sarcoidosis
- Glioma
- Lymphoma

Fig. 25.24 Fundus photograph of the left eye of a patient with familial optic atrophy. Note the marked pallor of the optic disc.

atrophy) follows optic nerve damage; causes include previous optic neuritis or ischaemic damage, long-standing papilloedema, optic nerve compression, trauma and degenerative conditions (e.g. Friedreich's ataxia, p. 1116).

Hearing disturbance

Each cochlear organ has bilateral cortical representation, so unilateral hearing loss is a result of peripheral organ damage. Bilateral hearing dysfunction is usual and is most commonly due to age-related degeneration or noise damage, although infection and drugs (particularly diuretics and aminoglycoside antibiotics) can be a primary cause. Prominent deafness may suggest a mitochondrial disorder (see Box 25.93, p. 1144).

Bulbar symptoms – dysphagia and dysarthria

Swallowing is a complex activity involving the coordinated action of lips, tongue, soft palate, pharynx and larynx, which are innervated by cranial nerves 7, 9, 10, 11 and 12. Structural causes of dysphagia are considered on page 778. Neurological mechanisms are vulnerable to damage at different points, resulting in dysphagia that is usually accompanied by dysarthria. Tempo is again crucial: acute onset of dysphagia may occur as a result of brainstem stroke or a rapidly developing neuropathy, such as Guillain–Barré syndrome or diphtheria. Intermittent fatigable muscle weakness (including dysphagia) would suggest myasthenia gravis. Dysphagia developing over weeks or months may be seen in motor neuron disease, basal meningitis and inflammatory brainstem disease. More slowly developing dysphagia suggests a myopathy or possibly a brainstem or skull-base tumour.

Pathologies affecting lower cranial nerves (9, 10, 11 and 12) frequently manifest bilaterally, producing dysphagia and dysarthria. The term 'bulbar palsy' is used to describe lower motor neuron lesions, either within the medulla or outside the brainstem. The tongue may be wasted and fasciculating, and palatal movement is reduced.

Upper motor neuron innervation of swallowing is bilateral, so persistent dysphagia is unusual with a unilateral upper motor lesion (the exception being in the acute stages of, for example, a hemispheric stroke). Widespread lesions above the medulla

will cause upper motor neuron bulbar paralysis, known as 'pseudobulbar palsy'. Here the tongue is small and contracted, and moves slowly; the jaw jerk is brisk, and there may be associated emotional variability. Causes of these are shown in Box 25.24.

Bladder, bowel and sexual disturbance

While isolated disturbances of bladder, bowel and sexual function are rarely the sole presenting features of neurological disease, they are common complications of many chronic disorders such as multiple sclerosis, stroke and dementia, and are frequently found post head injury. Abnormalities in these functions considerably reduce quality of life for patients. Incontinence and its management are discussed elsewhere (pp. 397, 835 and 1309).

Bladder dysfunction

The anatomy and physiology involved in controlling bladder functions are discussed on page 386 but it is worth emphasising the role of the pontine micturition centre, which is itself under higher control via inputs from the pre-frontal cortex, mid-brain and hypothalamus.

In the absence of conscious control (e.g. in coma or dementia), distension of the bladder to near capacity evokes reflex detrusor contraction (analogous to the muscle stretch reflex), and reciprocal changes in sympathetic activation and relaxation of the distal sphincter result in coordinated bladder emptying.

Damage to the lower motor neuron pathways (the pelvic and pudendal nerves) produces a flaccid bladder and sphincter with overflow incontinence, often accompanied by loss of pudendal sensation. Such damage may be due to disease of the conus medullaris or sacral nerve roots, either within the dura (as in inflammatory or carcinomatous meningitis) or as they pass through the sacrum (trauma or malignancy), or due to damage to the nerves themselves in the pelvis (infection, haematoma, trauma or malignancy).

Damage to the pons or spinal cord results in an 'upper motor neuron' pattern of bladder dysfunction due to uncontrolled over-activity of the parasympathetic supply. The bladder is small and highly sensitive to being stretched. This results in frequency, urgency and urge incontinence. Loss of the coordinating control of the pontine micturition centre will also result in the phenomenon of detrusor–sphincter dyssynergia, in which detrusor contraction and sphincter relaxation are not coordinated; the spastic bladder will often try to empty against a closed sphincter. This manifests as both urgency and an inability to pass urine, which is distressing and painful. The resultant incomplete bladder emptying predisposes to urinary infection, and the prolonged high intravesical pressure may result in obstructive uropathy and renal failure; post-micturition bladder ultrasound may confirm incomplete bladder emptying. More severe lesions of the spinal cord, as in spinal cord compression or trauma, can result in painless urinary retention as bladder sensation, normally carried in the lateral spinothalamic tracts, will be disrupted.

Damage to the frontal lobes gives rise to loss of awareness of bladder fullness and consequent incontinence. Coexisting cognitive impairment may result in inappropriate micturition. These features may be seen in hydrocephalus, frontal tumours, dementia and bifrontal subdural haematomas.

When a patient presents with bladder symptoms, it is important to localise the lesion on the basis of history and examination, remembering that most bladder problems are not neurological

25.24 Causes of pseudobulbar and bulbar palsy

Type	Pseudobulbar	Bulbar
Genetic	–	Kennedy's disease (X-linked bulbospinal neuronopathy)
Vascular	Bilateral hemisphere (lacunar) infarction	Medullary infarction (see Box 25.3, p. 1072)
Degenerative	Motor neuron disease (p. 1116)	Motor neuron disease Syringobulbia
Inflammatory/ infective	Multiple sclerosis (p. 1106) Cerebral vasculitis	Myasthenia (p. 1140) Guillain–Barré syndrome (p. 1140) Poliomyelitis (p. 1123) Lyme disease (p. 255) Vasculitis
Neoplastic	High brainstem tumours	Brainstem glioma Malignant meningitis

25

25.25 Neurogenic bladder: clinical features and treatment

Type	Site of lesion	Result	Treatment
Atonic (lower motor neuron)	Sacral segments of cord (conus medullaris) Sacral roots and nerves	Loss of detrusor contraction Difficulty initiating micturition Bladder distension with overflow	Intermittent self-catheterisation In-dwelling catheterisation
Hypertonic (upper motor neuron)	Pyramidal tract in spinal cord or brainstem	Urgency with urge incontinence Bladder sphincter incoordination (dyssynergia) Incomplete bladder emptying	Anticholinergics: Solifenacin Tolterodine Imipramine Intermittent self-catheterisation
Cortical	Post-central Pre-central Frontal	Loss of awareness of bladder fullness Difficulty initiating micturition Inappropriate micturition Loss of social control	Intermittent or in-dwelling catheterisation

unless there are overt neurological signs. Clinical features and management are summarised in Box 25.25.

Rectal dysfunction

The rectum has an excitatory cholinergic input from the parasympathetic sacral outflow, and inhibitory sympathetic supply similar to the bladder. Continence depends largely on skeletal muscle contraction in the puborectalis and pelvic floor muscles supplied by the pudendal nerves, as well as the internal and external anal sphincters. Damage to the autonomic components usually causes constipation (a common early symptom in Parkinson's disease) but diabetic neuropathy can be associated with diarrhoea. Lesions affecting the conus medullaris, the somatic S2–4 roots and the pudendal nerves may cause faecal incontinence.

Erectile failure and ejaculatory failure

These related functions are under autonomic control via the pelvic nerves (parasympathetic, S2–4) and hypogastric nerves (sympathetic, L1–2). Descending influences from the cerebrum are important for erection but it can occur as a reflex phenomenon in response to genital stimulation. Erection is largely parasympathetic and may be impaired by a number of drugs, including anticholinergic, antihypertensive and antidepressant agents. Sympathetic activity is important for ejaculation and may be inhibited by α-adrenoceptor antagonists (α-blockers). For further information on erectile dysfunction, see page 440.

Personality change

While this is often due to psychiatric illness, neurological conditions that alter the function of the frontal lobes can cause personality change and mood disorder (see Box 25.2, p. 1066). Personality change due to a frontal lobe disorder may occur as the result of structural damage due to stroke, trauma, tumour or hydrocephalus. The nature of any change may help localise the lesion.

Patients with mesial frontal lesions become increasingly withdrawn, unresponsive and mute (abulic), often in association with urinary incontinence, gait apraxia and an increase in tone known as gegenhalten, in which the patient varies the resistance to movement in proportion to the force exerted by the examiner.

Patients with lesions of the dorsolateral pre-frontal cortex develop a dysexecutive syndrome, which involves difficulties with speech, motor planning and organisation. Those with orbitofrontal lesions of the frontal lobes, in contrast, become disinhibited, displaying grandiosity or irresponsible behaviour. Memory is substantially intact but frontal release signs may emerge, such as a grasp reflex, palmomental response or pout. Proximity to the olfactory bulb and tracts means that inferior frontal lobe tumours may be associated with anosmia.

Disturbance to the cortical areas responsible for speech or memory can result in changes that may be interpreted as changes in personality.

Sleep disturbance

Disturbances of sleep are common and are not usually due to neurological disease. Patients may complain of insomnia (difficulty sleeping), excessive daytime sleepiness, disturbed behaviour during night-time sleep, parasomnia (sleep walking and talking, or night terrors) or disturbing subjective experiences during sleep and/or its onset (nightmares, hypnagogic hallucinations, sleep paralysis). A careful history (from bed partner as well as patient) usually allows specific causes of sleep disturbance to be identified and these are discussed in more detail on page 1105.

Psychiatric disorders

Psychiatric disorders are described in Chapter 28 but may cause or result from neurological problems. Care is needed in their identification, as effective management will help the underlying neurological illness.

Functional symptoms

Many patients presenting with neurological symptoms do not have a defined neurological disease and are best described as having functional symptoms (p. 1187). Some of these are psychogenic (or conversion) disorders. Such patients often have symptoms affecting multiple systems and an impressively long list of consultations and negative tests from other medical specialties when they present. Considering the possibility of a functional origin may save the patient some further anxiety and further investigation (which will be unnecessary, expensive, possibly invasive, and inconvenient).

- Inconsistent examination findings (e.g. Hoover's sign, p. 1082)
- Situational provocation of events (e.g. in medical settings)
- Associated mental health disorders:
    Anxiety
    Depression
- Lack of anatomical coherence to neurological symptoms
- Florid or bizarre descriptions of individual symptoms
- History of multiple other systemic symptoms inadequately explained by disease (asthma/breathlessness, fatigue, pain, gastrointestinal symptoms)

Weakness and sensory change predominate among patients with functional neurological disorders but pain or loss of consciousness can also occur. Associated symptoms, such as tiredness, lethargy, poor concentration, bowel upset (irritable bowel syndrome) and gynaecological complaints, are common. A functional cause should always be considered, as it can allow for more rapid diagnosis and minimise investigation. Some clinical features may hint at a functional origin for symptoms (Box 25.26). It is the clinician's (rewarding, albeit sometimes challenging) job to elicit the context of the patient's symptoms in a sensitive and non-judgemental manner. Whatever the cause of the illness, it is important to acknowledge that mood and sleep disturbance will exacerbate neurological symptoms, thus increasing disability. The best practitioners have the skill to carry the patient with them when describing the patterns of behaviour contributing to worsening symptoms.

Assessment to detect an underlying or exacerbating mood disorder is vital in all patients, ensuring that depression and anxiety are managed to minimise their secondary effects on neurological symptoms.

Headache syndromes

Acute management of headache is dealt with on page 184 but management of chronic, complex, or refractory headaches may require specialist input. Headaches may be classified as primary or secondary, depending on the underlying cause (see Box 10.10, p. 184). Secondary headache may be due to structural, infective, inflammatory or vascular conditions, discussed later in this chapter. Primary headache syndromes are described here.

Tension-type headache

This is the most common type of headache and is experienced to some degree by the majority of the population.

Pathophysiology

Tension-type headache is incompletely understood, and some consider that it is simply a milder version of migraine; certainly, the original notion that it is due primarily to muscle tension (hence the unsatisfactory name) has long since been dismissed. Anxiety about the headache itself may lead to continuation of symptoms, and patients may become convinced of a serious underlying condition.

Clinical features

The pain of tension headache is characterised as 'dull', 'tight' or like a 'pressure', and there may be a sensation of a band

round the head or pressure at the vertex. It is of constant character and generalised, but often radiates forwards from the occipital region. It may be episodic or persistent, although the severity may vary, and there is no associated vomiting or photophobia. Tension-type headache is rarely disabling and patients appear well. The pain often progresses throughout the day. Tenderness may be present over the skull vault or in the occiput but is easily distinguished from the triggered pains of trigeminal neuralgia and the exquisite tenderness of temporal arteritis. Analgesics may be taken with chronic regularity, despite little effect, and may perpetuate the symptoms (see 'Medication overuse headache' below).

Management

Most benefit is derived from a careful assessment, followed by discussion of likely precipitants and reassurance that the prognosis is good. The concept of medication overuse headache needs careful explanation. An important therapeutic step is to allow patients to realise that their problem has been taken seriously and rigorously assessed. Physiotherapy (with muscle relaxation and stress management) may help and low-dose amitriptyline can provide benefit. Investigation is rarely required. The reassurance value of brain imaging needs careful assessment: the pick-up rate of structural abnormalities is exceedingly low, and significantly outweighed by the likelihood of identifying an incidental and irrelevant finding (e.g. an arachnoid cyst, Chiari I malformation or vascular abnormality). The value of such 'reassurance' is usually over-estimated by doctors and patients alike.

Migraine

Migraine usually appears before middle age, or occasionally in later life; it affects about 20% of females and 6% of males at some point in life. Migraine is usually readily identifiable from the history, although unusual variants can cause uncertainty.

Pathophysiology

The cause of migraine is unknown but there is increasing evidence that the aura (see below) is due to dysfunction of ion channels causing a spreading front of cortical depolarisation (excitation) followed by hyperpolarisation (depression of activity). This process (the 'spreading depression of Leão') spreads over the cortex at a rate of about 3 mm/min, corresponding to the aura's symptomatic spread. The headache phase is associated with vasodilatation of extracranial vessels and may be relayed by hypothalamic activity. Activation of the trigeminovascular system is probably important. A genetic contribution is implied by the frequently positive family history, and similar phenomena occurring in disorders such as CADASIL (p. 1052) or mitochondrial disease (p. 1144). The female preponderance and the frequency of migraine attacks at certain points in the menstrual cycle also suggest hormonal influences. Oestrogen-containing oral contraception sometimes exacerbates migraine and increases the very small risk of stroke in patients who suffer from migraine with aura. Doctors and patients often over-estimate the role of dietary precipitants such as cheese, chocolate or red wine. When psychological factors contribute, the migraine attack often occurs after a period of stress, being more likely on Friday evening at the end of the working week or at the beginning of a holiday.

Clinical features

Some patients report a prodrome of malaise, irritability or behavioural change for some hours or days. Around 20% of patients experience an aura and are said to have migraine with aura (previously known as classical migraine). The aura may manifest as almost any neurological symptom but is most often visual, consisting of fortification spectra, which are usually positive phenomena such as shimmering, silvery zigzag lines marching across the visual fields for up to 40 minutes, sometimes leaving a trail of temporary visual field loss (scotoma). Sensory symptoms characteristically spreading over 20–30 minutes, from one part of the body to another, are more common than motor ones, and language function can be affected, leading to similarities with TIA/stroke. Isolated aura may occur (i.e. the neurological symptoms are not followed by headache).

The 80% of patients with characteristic headache but no 'aura' are said to have migraine without aura (previously called 'common' migraine).

Migraine headache is usually severe and throbbing, with photophobia, phonophobia and vomiting lasting from 4 to 72 hours. Movement makes the pain worse and patients prefer to lie in a quiet, dark room.

In a small number of patients the aura may persist, leaving more permanent neurological disturbance. This persistent migrainous aura may occur with or without evidence of brain infarction.

Management

Avoidance of identified triggers or exacerbating factors (such as the combined contraceptive pill) may prevent attacks. Treatment of an acute attack consists of simple analgesia with aspirin, paracetamol or non-steroidal anti-inflammatory agents. Nausea may require an antiemetic such as metoclopramide or domperidone. Severe attacks can be aborted by one of the 'triptans' (e.g. sumatriptan), which are potent 5-hydroxytryptamine (5-HT, serotonin) agonists. These can be administered via the oral, subcutaneous or nasal route. Caution is needed with ergotamine preparations because they may lead to dependence. Overuse of any analgesia, including triptans, may contribute to medication overuse headache.

If attacks are frequent (more than two per month), prophylaxis should be considered. Many drugs can be chosen but the most frequently used are vasoactive drugs (β-blockers), antidepressants (amitriptyline, dosulepin) and antiepileptic drugs (valproate, topiramate). Women with aura should avoid oestrogen treatment for either oral contraception or hormone replacement, although the increased risk of ischaemic stroke is minimal.

Medication overuse headache

With increasing availability of over-the-counter medication, headache syndromes perpetuated by analgesia intake are becoming much more common. Medication overuse headache (MOH) can complicate any headache syndrome but is especially common with migraine and chronic tension-type headache. The most frequent culprits are compound analgesics (particularly codeine and other opiate-containing preparations) and triptans, and MOH is usually associated with use on more than 10–15 days per month.

Management is by withdrawal of the responsible analgesics. Patients should be warned that the initial effect will be to exacerbate the headache, and migraine prophylactics may be helpful in reducing the rebound headaches. Relapse rates are high, and patients often need help and support in withdrawing from analgesia; a careful explanation of this paradoxical concept is vital.

Cluster headache

Cluster headaches (also known as migrainous neuralgia) are much less common than migraine. Unusually for headache syndromes, there is a significant male predominance and onset is usually in the third decade.

Pathophysiology

The cause is unknown but this type of headache differs from migraine in many ways, suggesting a different pathophysiological basis. Although uncommon, it is the most common of the trigeminal autonomic cephalalgia syndromes. Functional imaging studies have suggested abnormal hypothalamic activity. Patients are more often smokers with a higher than average alcohol consumption.

Clinical features

Cluster headache is strikingly periodic, featuring runs of identical headaches beginning at the same time for weeks at a stretch (the 'cluster'). Patients may experience either one or several attacks within a 24-hour period, and typically are awoken from sleep by symptoms ('alarm clock headache'). Cluster headache causes severe, unilateral periorbital pain with autonomic features, such as ipsilateral tearing, nasal congestion and conjunctival injection (occasionally with the other features of a Horner's syndrome). The pain, though severe, is characteristically brief (30–90 minutes). In contrast to the behaviour of those with migraine, patients are highly agitated during the headache phase. The cluster period is typically a few weeks, followed by remission for months to years, but a small proportion do not experience remission.

Management

Acute attacks can usually be halted by subcutaneous injections of sumatriptan or inhalation of 100% oxygen. The brevity of the attack probably prevents other migraine therapies from being effective. Migraine prophylaxis is often ineffective too but attacks can be prevented in some patients by verapamil, sodium valproate, or short courses of oral glucocorticoids. Patients with severe debilitating clusters can be helped with lithium therapy, although this requires monitoring (p. 1200).

Trigeminal neuralgia

This is characterised by unilateral lancinating facial pain, most commonly involving the second and/or third divisions of the trigeminal nerve territory, usually in patients over the age of 50 years.

Pathophysiology

For most, trigeminal neuralgia remains an idiopathic condition but there is a suggestion that it may be due to an irritative lesion involving the trigeminal root zone, in some cases an aberrant loop of artery. Other compressive lesions, usually benign, are occasionally found. Trigeminal neuralgia associated with multiple sclerosis may result from a plaque of demyelination in the brainstem.

Clinical features

The pain is repetitive, severe and very brief (seconds or less). It may be triggered by touch, a cold wind or eating. Physical signs are usually absent, although the spasms may make the patient wince and sit silently (tic douloureux). There is a tendency for the condition to remit and relapse over many years. Rarely, there may be combined features of trigeminal neuralgia and cluster headache ('cluster–tic').

Management

The pain often responds to carbamazepine. It is wise to start with a low dose and increase gradually, according to effect. In patients who cannot tolerate carbamazepine, oxcarbazepine, gabapentin, pregabalin, amitriptyline or glucocorticoids may be effective alternatives, but if medication is ineffective or poorly tolerated, surgical treatment should be considered. Decompression of the vascular loop encroaching on the trigeminal root is said to have a 90% success rate. Otherwise, localised injection of alcohol or phenol into a peripheral branch of the nerve may be effective.

Headaches associated with specific activities

These usually affect men in their thirties and forties. Patients develop a sudden, severe headache with exertion, including sexual activity. There is usually no vomiting or neck stiffness, and the headache lasts less than 10–15 minutes, though a less severe dullness may persist for some hours. Subarachnoid haemorrhage needs to be excluded by CT and/or CSF examination (see Fig. 26.14, p. 1162) after a first event. The pathogenesis of these headaches is unknown. Although frightening, attacks are usually brief and patients may need only reassurance and simple analgesia for the residual headache. The syndrome may recur, and prevention may be necessary with propranolol or indometacin.

Other headache syndromes

A number of rare headache syndromes produce pains about the eye similar to cluster headaches (Box 25.27). These include chronic paroxysmal hemicrania and SUNCT (short-lasting unilateral neuralgiform headaches with conjunctival injection and tearing). The recognition of these syndromes is useful because they often respond to specific treatments such as indometacin.

Epilepsy

A seizure can be defined as the occurrence of signs and/or symptoms due to abnormal, excessive or synchronous neuronal activity in the brain. The lifetime risk of an isolated seizure is about 5%, although incidence is highest at the extremes of age. Epilepsy is the tendency to have unprovoked seizures. While the prevalence of active epilepsy in European countries is about 0.5%, the figure in developing countries may be higher because of parasitic illnesses such as cysticercosis (p. 298). A recent change in definition allows the diagnosis of epilepsy to be made after a single seizure with a high risk of recurrence (e.g. a single seizure in the presence of a cortical lesion). Such changes may lead to an observed increase in epilepsy incidence.

Historical terms such as 'grand mal' (implying tonic–clonic seizures) and 'petit mal' (intended originally to mean 'absence seizures' but commonly misused to describe 'anything other than grand mal') have been superseded. Subsequent revisions, including terms such as 'complex partial' and 'simple partial', have been imprecise and carry little information about underlying pathology, treatment or prognosis. The modern equivalents for these terms will be given below, but it is preferable to adhere to the 2010 iteration of the International League Against Epilepsy's classification (Box 25.28).

Pathophysiology

To function normally, the brain must maintain a continual balance between excitation and inhibition, remaining responsive to the environment while avoiding continued unrestrained spontaneous activity. The inhibitory transmitter gamma-aminobutyric acid (GABA) is particularly important, acting on ion channels to enhance chloride inflow and reducing the chances of action potential formation. Excitatory amino acids (glutamate and aspartate) allow influx of sodium and calcium, producing the opposite effect. It is likely that many seizures result from an imbalance

i 25.27 Benign paroxysmal headaches				
Type	Character of pain	Duration	Location	Comment
Ice pick	Stabbing	Very brief (split-second)	Variable, usually temporoparietal	Benign, more common in migraine
Ice cream	Sharp, severe	30–120 secs	Bitemporal/occipital	Obvious trigger by cold stimuli
Exertional/sexual activity	Bursting, thunderclap	Severe for mins, then less severe for hours	Generalised	Subarachnoid haemorrhage needs to be excluded
Cough	Bursting	Secs to mins	Occipital or generalised	Intracranial pathology needs to be excluded (especially craniocervical junction)
Cluster headache (migrainous neuralgia)	Severe unilateral, with ptosis, tearing, conjunctival injection, unilateral nasal congestion	30–90 mins 1–3 times per day	Periorbital	Usually in men, occurring in clusters over weeks/months
Chronic paroxysmal hemicrania	Severe unilateral with cluster headache-like autonomic features (see above)	5–20 mins, frequently through day	Periorbital/temporal	Usually in women, responds to indometacin
SUNCT*	Severe, sharp, triggered by touch or neck movements	15–120 secs, repetitive through day	Periorbital	May respond to carbamazepine

*Short-lasting, unilateral, neuralgiform headache with conjunctival injection, tearing, rhinorrhoea and forehead sweating.

25.28 Classification of seizures (2010 International League Against Epilepsy classification)

Generalised seizures

- Tonic–clonic (in any combination)
- Absence:
  Typical
  Atypical
  Absence with special features
- Myoclonic absence
- Eyelid myoclonia

- Myoclonic:
  Myoclonic
  Myoclonic–atonic
  Myoclonic–tonic
- Clonic
- Tonic
- Atonic

Focal seizures

- Without impairment of consciousness or awareness (was 'simple partial'):
  Focal motor
  Focal sensory
- With impairment of consciousness or awareness (was 'complex partial')
- Evolving to a bilateral, convulsive seizure (was 'secondarily generalised seizure'):
  Tonic
  Clonic
  Tonic–clonic

Unknown

- Epileptic spasms

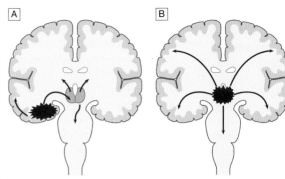

Focal seizure ± secondary generalisation   **Primary generalised seizure**

Fig. 25.25 The pathophysiological classification of seizures. A A focal seizure originates from a paroxysmal discharge in a focal area of the cerebral cortex (often the temporal lobe); the seizure may subsequently spread to the rest of the brain (secondary generalisation) via diencephalic activating pathways. B In genetic generalised epilepsies (GGEs) the abnormal electrical discharges originate from the diencephalic activating system and spread simultaneously to all areas of the cortex.

25.29 Trigger factors for seizures

- Sleep deprivation
- Missed doses of antiepileptic drugs in treated patients
- Alcohol (particularly withdrawal)
- Recreational drug misuse
- Physical and mental exhaustion
- Flickering lights, including TV and computer screens (generalised epilepsy syndromes only)
- Intercurrent infections and metabolic disturbances
- Uncommon: loud noises, music, reading, hot baths

between this excitation and inhibition. Intracellular recordings during seizures demonstrate a paroxysmal depolarisation shift in neuronal membrane potential, an upshift in internal potential predisposing to recurrent action potentials. In vivo, epileptic cortex shows repetitive discharges involving large groups of neurons.

Focal epilepsy

Seizures may be related to a localised disturbance in the cortex, becoming manifest in the first instance as focal seizures. Any disturbance of cortical architecture and function can precipitate this, whether focal infection, tumour, hamartoma or trauma-related scarring. If focal seizures remain localised, the symptoms experienced depend on which cortical area is affected. If areas in the temporal lobes become involved, then awareness of the environment becomes impaired but without associated tonic–clonic movements. When both hemispheres become involved, the seizure becomes generalised (Fig. 25.25).

Generalised epilepsies

The new terminology is genetic generalised epilepsies (GGEs) (previously idiopathic generalised epilepsies) to reflect their likely cause. These seizures are generalised at onset, abnormal activity probably originating in the central mechanisms controlling cortical activation (Fig. 25.25) and spreading rapidly. This group constitutes around 30% of all epilepsy and is likely to reflect widespread disturbance of structure or function. GGEs almost always become apparent before the age of 35.

Seizure activity is usually apparent on EEG as spike and wave discharges (see Fig. 25.14, p. 1075). Other generalised seizures may involve merely brief loss of awareness (absence seizures), single jerks (myoclonus) or loss of tone (atonic seizures), as detailed in Box 25.28.

Clinical features

Seizure type and epilepsy type

Patients can experience more than one type of seizure attack, and it is important to document each attack type and the patient's age at its onset, along with its frequency, duration and typical features. Any triggers should be identified (Box 25.29). The type of seizure, other clinical features and investigations can then be used to determine the epilepsy syndrome, as discussed below. Where there is doubt about the type, this is best stated and a full classification should be deferred until the evolution of the clinical features clarifies the picture.

To classify seizure type, the clinician should ask firstly whether there is a focal onset, and secondly whether the seizures conform to one of the recognised patterns (see Box 25.28). Epilepsy that starts in patients beyond their mid-thirties will almost invariably reflect a focal cerebral event. Where activity remains focal, the classification will be obvious. With generalised tonic–clonic seizures, a focal onset will be heralded by positive neurological symptoms and signs corresponding to the normal function of that area. Occipital onset causes visual changes (lights and blobs of colour), temporal lobe onset causes false recognition (déjà vu), sensory strip involvement causes sensory alteration (burning, tingling), and motor strip involvement causes jerking.

Alternatively, patients report a previous local cortical insult, and it may be reasonably (but not invariably) inferred that this is the seat of epileptogenesis.

Focal seizures

The classification of focal seizures is shown in Box 25.28. They are caused by localised cortical activity with retained awareness. The localisation of such symptoms is described above. A spreading pattern of seizure may occur, the abnormal sensation spreading much faster (in seconds) than a migrainous focal sensory attack.

Awareness may become impaired if spread occurs to the temporal lobes (previously 'complex partial seizure'). Patients stop and stare blankly, often blinking repetitively, making smacking movements of their lips or displaying other automatisms, such as picking at their clothes. After a few minutes consciousness returns but the patient may be muddled and feel drowsy for a period of up to an hour. The age of onset, preceding aura, longer duration and post-ictal symptoms usually make these easy to differentiate from childhood absence seizures (see below).

Seizures arising from the anterior parts of the frontal lobe may produce bizarre behaviour patterns, including limb posturing, sleep walking or even frenetic, ill-directed motor activity with incoherent screaming. Video EEG may be necessary to differentiate these from psychogenic attacks (which are more common) but abruptness of onset, stereotyped nature, relative brevity and nocturnal preponderance may indicate a frontal origin. Causes of focal seizures are given in Box 25.30.

Generalised seizures

Tonic–clonic seizures An initial 'aura' may be experienced by the patient, depending on the cortical area from which the seizure originates (as above). The patient then becomes rigid (tonic) and unconscious, falling heavily if standing ('like a log') and risking facial injury. During this phase, breathing stops and central cyanosis may occur. As cortical discharges reduce in frequency, jerking (clonic) movements emerge for 2 minutes at most. Afterwards, there is a flaccid state of deep coma, which can persist for some minutes, and on regaining awareness the patient may be confused, disorientated and/or amnesic. During the attack, urinary incontinence and tongue-biting may occur. A severely bitten, bleeding tongue after an attack of loss of consciousness is pathognomonic of a generalised seizure but less marked lingual injury can occur in syncope. Subsequently, the patient usually feels unwell and sleepy, with headache and myalgia. Witnesses are usually frightened by the event, often believe the person to be dying, and may struggle to give a clear account of the episode. Some may not describe the tonic or clonic phase and may not mention cyanosis or tongue-biting. In less typical episodes, post-ictal delirium, or sequelae such as headache or myalgia, may be the main pointers to the diagnosis. Causes of generalised tonic–clonic seizures are listed in Box 25.31.

Absence seizures Absence seizures (previously 'petit mal') always start in childhood. The attacks are rarely mistaken for focal seizures because of their brevity. They can occur so frequently (20–30 times a day) that they are mistaken for daydreaming or poor concentration in school.

Myoclonic seizures These are typically brief, jerking movements, predominating in the arms. In epilepsy, they are more marked

---

ⓘ 25.30 Causes of focal seizures

Idiopathic
- Benign Rolandic epilepsy of childhood
- Benign occipital epilepsy of childhood

Focal structural lesions

Genetic
- Tuberous sclerosis (p. 1264)
- Autosomal dominant nocturnal frontal lobe epilepsy
- Autosomal dominant partial epilepsy with auditory features (ADPEAF)
- von Hippel–Lindau disease (p. 1132)
- Neurofibromatosis (p. 1131)
- Cerebral migration abnormalities

Infantile hemiplegia

Dysembryonic
- Cortical dysgenesis
- Sturge–Weber syndrome

Mesial temporal sclerosis (associated with febrile convulsions)

Cerebrovascular disease (Ch. 26)
- Intracerebral haemorrhage
- Cerebral infarction
- Arteriovenous malformation
- Cavernous haemangioma

Tumours (primary and secondary) (p. 1129)

Trauma (including neurosurgery)

Infective (p. 1117)
- Cerebral abscess (pyogenic)
- Toxoplasmosis
- Cysticercosis
- Tuberculoma
- Subdural empyema
- Encephalitis
- Human immunodeficiency virus (HIV)

Inflammatory
- Autoimmune encephalopathies (e.g. anti-voltage-gated potassium channel antibodies, anti-NMDA receptor antibodies, anti-glycine receptor antibodies)
- Sarcoidosis
- Vasculitis

ⓘ 25.31 Causes of generalised tonic–clonic seizures

Generalisation from focal seizures
- See Box 25.30

Genetic
- Inborn errors of metabolism (p. 1144)
- Storage diseases
- Phakomatoses (e.g. tuberous sclerosis, p. 1264)

Cerebral birth injury

Hydrocephalus

Cerebral anoxia

Drugs
- Antibiotics: penicillin, isoniazid, metronidazole
- Antimalarials: chloroquine, mefloquine
- Ciclosporin
- Amphetamines (withdrawal)
- Cardiac anti-arrhythmics: lidocaine, disopyramide
- Psychotropic agents: phenothiazines, tricyclic antidepressants, lithium

Alcohol (especially withdrawal)

Toxins
- Organophosphates (sarin)
- Heavy metals (lead, tin)

Metabolic disease
- Hypocalcaemia
- Hyponatraemia
- Hypomagnesaemia
- Hypoglycaemia
- Renal failure
- Liver failure

Infective
- Post-infectious encephalopathy
- Meningitis (p. 1118)

Inflammatory
- Multiple sclerosis (uncommon; p. 1106)
- Systemic lupus erythematosus (p. 1034)

Diffuse degenerative diseases
- Alzheimer's disease (uncommonly; p. 1992)
- Creutzfeldt–Jakob disease (rarely; p. 1127)

25

in the morning or on awakening from sleep, and tend to be provoked by fatigue, alcohol, or sleep deprivation.

Atonic seizures These are seizures involving brief loss of muscle tone, usually resulting in heavy falls with or without loss of consciousness. They occur only in the context of epilepsy syndromes that involve other forms of seizure.

Tonic seizures These are associated with a generalised increase in tone and an associated loss of awareness. They are usually seen as part of an epilepsy syndrome and are unlikely to be isolated.

Clonic seizures Clonic seizures are similar to tonic–clonic seizures. The clinical manifestations are similar but there is no preceding tonic phase.

Seizures of uncertain generalised or focal nature

Epileptic spasms While these are highlighted in the classification system, they are unusual in adult practice and occur mainly in infancy. They signify widespread cortical disturbance and take the form of marked contractions of the axial musculature, lasting a fraction of a second but recurring in clusters of 5–50, often on awakening.

Epilepsy syndromes

Many patients with epilepsy fall into specific patterns, depending on seizure type(s), age of onset and treatment responsiveness: the so-called electroclinical syndromes (Box 25.32). It is anticipated that genetic testing will ultimately demonstrate similarities in molecular pathophysiology.

Box 25.33 highlights the more common epilepsy syndromes, which are largely of early onset and are sensitive to sleep deprivation, hyperventilation, alcohol and photic stimulation. Epilepsies that do not fit into any of these diagnostic categories can be delineated firstly on the basis of the presence or absence of a known structural or metabolic condition (presumed cause), and then on the basis of the primary mode of seizure onset (generalised versus focal).

Investigations

Single seizure

All patients with transient loss of consciousness should have a 12-lead ECG. Where seizure is suspected or definite, patients should have cranial imaging with either MRI or CT, although the yield is low unless focal signs are present. EEG may help

to assess prognosis once a firm diagnosis has been made. The recurrence rate after a first seizure is approximately 40% and most recurrent attacks occur within a month or two of the first. Further seizures are less likely if an identified trigger can be avoided (see Box 25.29).

Other investigations for infective, toxic and metabolic causes (Box 25.34) may be appropriate. An EEG performed immediately after a seizure may be more helpful in showing focal features than if performed after a delay.

i | 25.32 Electroclinical epilepsy syndromes

Adolescence to adulthood
- Juvenile absence epilepsy (JAE)
- Juvenile myoclonic epilepsy (JME)
- Epilepsy with generalised tonic–clonic seizures alone
- Progressive myoclonus epilepsies (PMEs)
- Autosomal dominant epilepsy with auditory features (ADEAF)
- Other familial temporal lobe epilepsies

Less specific age relationship
- Familial focal epilepsy with variable foci (childhood to adult)
- Reflex epilepsies

Distinctive constellations
- Mesial temporal lobe epilepsy with hippocampal sclerosis (MTLE with HS)
- Rasmussen's syndrome
- Gelastic (from the Greek word for laughter) seizures with hypothalamic hamartoma
- Hemiconvulsion–hemiplegia–epilepsy

Epilepsies with structural–metabolic causes
- Malformations of cortical development (hemimegalencephaly, heterotopias etc.)
- Neurocutaneous syndromes (tuberous sclerosis complex, Sturge–Weber etc.)
- Tumour
- Infection
- Trauma
- Angioma
- Perinatal insults
- Stroke etc.

Epilepsies of unknown cause

Conditions with epileptic seizures not needing long-term treatment
- Benign neonatal seizures (BNS)
- Febrile seizures (FS)

i | 25.33 Common generalised epilepsy syndromes

Syndrome	Age of onset	Type of seizure	EEG features	Treatment	Prognosis
Childhood absence epilepsy	4–8 years	Frequent brief absences	3/sec spike and wave	Ethosuximide Sodium valproate Levetiracetam	40% develop GTCS, 80% remit in adulthood
Juvenile absence epilepsy	10–15 years	Less frequent absences than childhood absence	Poly-spike and wave	Sodium valproate Levetiracetam	80% develop GTCS, 80% seizure-free in adulthood
Juvenile myoclonic epilepsy	15–20 years	GTCS, absences, morning myoclonus	Poly-spike and wave, photosensitivity	Sodium valproate Levetiracetam	90% remit with AEDs but relapse if AED withdrawn
GTCS on awakening	10–25 years	GTCS, sometimes myoclonus	Spike and wave on waking and sleep onset	Sodium valproate Levetiracetam	65% controlled with AEDs but relapse off treatment

(AED = antiepileptic drug; GTCS = generalised tonic–clonic seizure)

25.34 Investigation of epilepsy

From where is the epilepsy arising?

- Standard EEG
- Sleep EEG
- EEG with special electrodes (foramen ovale, subdural)

What is the cause of the epilepsy?

Structural lesion?

- CT
- MRI

Metabolic disorder?

- Urea and electrolytes
- Liver function tests
- Blood glucose
- Serum calcium, magnesium

Inflammatory or infective disorder?

- Full blood count, erythrocyte sedimentation rate, C-reactive protein
- Chest X-ray
- Serology for syphilis, HIV, collagen disease
- CSF examination

Are the attacks truly epileptic?

- Ambulatory EEG
- Videotelemetry

(CSF = cerebrospinal fluid; CT = computed tomography; EEG = electroencephalography; HIV = human immunodeficiency virus; MRI = magnetic resonance imaging)

 25.35 Indications for brain imaging in epilepsy

- Epilepsy starting after the age of 16 years
- Seizures having focal features clinically
- Electroencephalogram showing a focal seizure source
- Control of seizures difficult or deteriorating

Epilepsy

The same investigations are required in a patient with epilepsy (Box 25.34). The EEG may help to establish the type of epilepsy and guide therapy. Investigations should be revisited if the epilepsy is intractable to treatment.

Inter-ictal EEG is abnormal in only about 50% of patients with recurrent seizures, so it cannot be used to exclude epilepsy. The sensitivity can be increased to about 85% by prolonging recording time and including a period of natural or drug-induced sleep, but this does not replace a well-taken history. Ambulatory EEG recording or video EEG monitoring may help with differentiation of epilepsy from other disorders if attacks are sufficiently frequent.

Indications for imaging are summarised in Box 25.35. Imaging cannot establish a diagnosis of epilepsy but identifies any structural cause. It is not required if a confident diagnosis of a recognised GGE syndrome (e.g. juvenile myoclonic epilepsy) is made. While CT excludes a major structural cause of epilepsy, MRI is required to demonstrate subtle changes such as hippocampal sclerosis, which may direct or inform surgical intervention.

Management

It is important to explain the nature and cause of seizures to patients and their relatives, and to instruct relatives in the first aid management of seizures (Box 25.36). Many people with epilepsy feel stigmatised and may become unnecessarily isolated from work and social life. It is important to emphasise that epilepsy is a common disorder that affects 0.5–1% of the population, and that full control of seizures can be expected in approximately 70% of patients (Box 25.37).

 25.36 How to administer first aid for seizures

- Move the person away from danger (fire, water, machinery, furniture)
- After convulsions cease, turn the person into the 'recovery' position (semi-prone)
- Ensure the airway is clear but do **NOT** insert anything in the mouth (tongue-biting occurs at seizure onset and cannot be prevented by observers)
- If convulsions continue for more than 5 mins or recur without the person regaining consciousness, summon urgent medical attention
- Do not leave the person alone until fully recovered (drowsiness and delirium can persist for up to 1 hr)

 25.37 Epilepsy: outcome after 20 years

- 50% are seizure-free, without drugs, for the previous 5 years
- 20% are seizure-free for the previous 5 years but continue to take medication
- 30% continue to have seizures in spite of antiepileptic therapy

Immediate care

Little can or needs to be done for a person during a convulsive seizure except for first aid and common-sense manœuvres to limit damage or secondary complications (see Box 25.36). Advice should be given that on no account should anything be inserted into the patient's mouth. The management of status epilepticus is described on page 1080.

Lifestyle advice

Patients should be advised to avoid activities where they might place themselves or others at risk if they have a seizure. This applies at work, at home and at leisure. At home, only shallow baths (or showers) should be taken. Prolonged cycle journeys should be discouraged until reasonable freedom from seizures has been achieved. Activities involving prolonged proximity to water (swimming, fishing or boating) should always be carried out in the company of someone who is aware of the risks and the potential need for rescue measures. Driving regulations vary between countries and the patient should be made aware of these (Box 25.38). Certain occupations, such as firefighter or airline pilot, are not open to those with a previous or active diagnosis of epilepsy; further information is available from epilepsy support organisations.

The risk of harm from epilepsy should be discussed around the time of diagnosis. This should be done with care and sensitivity, and with the aim of motivating the patient to adapt habits and lifestyle to optimise epilepsy control and minimise risks of serious complications.

Antiepileptic drugs

Antiepileptic drugs (AEDs) should be considered where risk of seizure recurrence is high. A diagnosis of two or more seizures is justification enough but a prolonged inter-seizure interval may deter some patients and physicians. Treatment decisions should always be shared with the patient, to enhance adherence. A wide range of drugs is available. These agents either increase inhibitory neurotransmission in the brain or alter neuronal sodium channels to prevent abnormally rapid transmission of impulses. In the majority of patients, full control is achieved with a single drug. Dose regimens should be kept as simple as possible. Guidelines

25

25.38 UK driving regulations

The physician's prime duty is to ensure the patient is aware of the legal obligation to inform the driving authority

Private use

Single seizure

- Cease driving for 6 months; a longer period may be required if risk of recurrence is high

Epilepsy (i.e. more than one seizure over the age of 5 years)

- Cease driving immediately
- Licence restored when patient is seizure-free for 1 year, *or* an initial sleep seizure is followed by exclusively sleep seizures for 1 year, *or* mixed awake and sleep seizures are followed by 3 years of exclusively sleep seizures
- Licence will require renewal every 3 years thereafter until patient is seizure-free for 10 years

Withdrawal of antiepileptic drugs

- Cease driving during withdrawal period and for 6 months thereafter

Vocational drivers (heavy goods and public service vehicles)

- No licence permitted if any seizure has occurred after the age of 5 years until patient is off medication and seizure-free for more than 10 years, and has no potentially epileptogenic brain lesion

 25.40 Guidelines for choice of antiepileptic drug[1]

Epilepsy type	First-line	Second-line	Third-line
Focal onset and/or secondary GTCS	Lamotrigine	Carbamazepine Levetiracetam Sodium valproate Topiramate Zonisamide Lacosamide	Clobazam Gabapentin Oxcarbazepine Phenobarbital Phenytoin Pregabalin Primidone Tiagabine
GTCS[2]	Sodium valproate Levetiracetam	Lamotrigine Topiramate Zonisamide	Carbamazepine Phenytoin Primidone Phenobarbital Acetazolamide
Absence[2]	Ethosuximide	Sodium valproate	Lamotrigine Clonazepam
Myoclonic[2]	Sodium valproate	Levetiracetam Clonazepam	Lamotrigine Phenobarbital

[1]See Scottish Intercollegiate Guidelines Network SIGN 143 – Diagnosis and management of epilepsy in adults (May 2015). [2]Genetic generalised epilepsies.
N.B. Use as few drugs as possible at the lowest possible dose.
(GTCS = generalised tonic–clonic seizure)

i **25.39 Guidelines for antiepileptic drug therapy***

- Start with one first-line drug (see Box 25.40)
- Start at a low dose; gradually increase dose until effective control of seizures is achieved or side-effects develop
- Optimise adherence (use minimum number of doses per day)
- If first drug fails (seizures continue or side-effects develop), start second first-line drug, followed if possible by gradual withdrawal of first
- If second drug fails (seizures continue or side-effects develop), start second-line drug in combination with the preferred baseline drug at maximum tolerated dose (beware interactions)
- If this combination fails (seizures continue or side-effects develop), replace second-line drug with alternative second-line drug
- If this combination fails, check adherence and reconsider diagnosis (Are events seizures? Occult lesion? Treatment adherence/alcohol/drugs confounding response?)
- Consider alternative, non-drug treatments (e.g. epilepsy surgery, vagal nerve stimulation)
- Use minimum number of drugs in combination at any one time

*See Scottish Intercollegiate Guidelines Network SIGN 143 – Diagnosis and management of epilepsy in adults (May 2015).

are listed in Box 25.39. For focal epilepsies, one large study suggests that lamotrigine is the best-tolerated monotherapy, which, alongside its favourable adverse-effect profile and relative lack of pharmacokinetic interactions, makes it a good first-line drug, although caution must be exercised with oral contraceptive use. Unclassified or genetic generalised epilepsies respond best to valproate, although pregnancy-related problems mean that valproate should not be used in women of reproductive age unless the benefits outweigh the risks. The initial choice should be an established first-line drug (Box 25.40), with more recently introduced drugs as second choice.

Monitoring therapy

Some practitioners confuse epilepsy care with serum level monitoring. The newer drugs have much more predictable pharmacokinetics than the older ones and the only indication for measuring serum levels is if there is doubt about adherence. Blood levels need to be interpreted carefully and dose changes made to treat the patient rather than to bring a serum level into the 'therapeutic range'. Some centres advocate serum level monitoring during pregnancy (notably with lamotrigine) but the evidence of benefit for this is not strong.

Epilepsy surgery

Some patients with drug-resistant epilepsy benefit from surgical resection of epileptogenic brain tissue. Less invasive treatments, including vagal nerve stimulation or deep brain stimulation, may also be helpful in some patients. All those who continue to experience seizures despite appropriate drug treatment should be considered for surgical treatment. Planning such interventions requires intensive specialist assessment and investigation to identify the site of seizure onset and the dispensability of any target areas for resection, i.e. whether the area of brain involved is necessary for a critical function such as vision or motor function.

Withdrawing antiepileptic therapy

Withdrawal of medication may be considered after a patient has been seizure-free for more than 2 years. Childhood-onset epilepsy, particularly classical absence seizures, carries the best prognosis for successful drug withdrawal. Other epilepsy syndromes, such as juvenile myoclonic epilepsy, have a marked tendency to recur after drug withdrawal.

Focal epilepsies that begin in adult life are also likely to recur, especially if there is an identified structural lesion. Overall, the recurrence rate after drug withdrawal depends on the individual's epilepsy history. An individualised estimate may be gained from the SIGN guideline tables (see 'Further information', p. 1146).

Patients should be advised of the risks of recurrence, to allow them to decide whether or not they wish to withdraw. If undertaken, withdrawal should be done slowly, reducing the drug dose gradually over weeks or months. Withdrawal may necessitate precautions around driving or occupation (see Box 25.38).

Contraception

Some AEDs induce hepatic enzymes that metabolise synthetic hormones, increasing the risk of contraceptive failure. This is most marked with carbamazepine, phenytoin and barbiturates, but clinically significant effects can be seen with lamotrigine and topiramate. If the AED cannot be changed, this can be overcome by giving higher-dose preparations of the oral contraceptive. Sodium valproate and levetiracetam have no interaction with hormonal contraception.

Pregnancy and reproduction

Epilepsy presents specific management problems during pregnancy (Box 25.41). There is usually concern about teratogenesis associated with AEDs. It is important to recognise proportionate risks: background risk of severe fetal malformation in the general population is around 2–3%, while the AED most associated with teratogenesis is sodium valproate, which, at high dose, increases the risk to around 6–7%. Long-term observational studies show that most of the commonly used AEDs can be given safely in pregnancy.

Pre-conception treatment with folic acid (5 mg daily), along with use of the smallest effective doses of as few AEDs as possible, may reduce the risk of fetal abnormalities. The risks of abrupt AED withdrawal to the mother should be stressed.

Seizures may become more frequent during pregnancy, particularly if pharmacokinetic changes decrease serum levels of AEDs (see Box 25.41).

Menstrual irregularities and reduced fertility are more common in women with epilepsy, and are also increased by sodium valproate. Patients with epilepsy are at greater risk of osteoporosis, apparently independently of the drug used. Some centres advocate vitamin D supplementation in any patient with epilepsy but the higher female risk of osteoporosis makes this most important in women. Oral contraception can interact with individual AEDs (Box 25.41).

 25.41 Epilepsy in pregnancy

- **Provision of pre-conception counselling is best practice:** start folic acid (5 mg daily for 2 months) before conception to reduce the risk of fetal malformations.
- **Fetal malformation:** risk is minimised if a single drug is used. Carbamazepine and lamotrigine have the lowest incidence of major fetal malformations.
  The risk with sodium valproate is higher but should be carefully balanced against its benefits.
  Levetiracetam may be safe but avoid other newer drugs if possible.
- **Learning difficulties in children:** IQ may be lower when children are exposed to valproate in utero, so its use should always be considered carefully.
- **Haemorrhagic disease of the newborn:** enzyme-inducing antiepileptic drugs increase risk. Give oral vitamin K (20 mg daily) to the mother during the last month of pregnancy and IM vitamin K (1 mg) to the infant at birth.
- **Increased frequency of seizures:** where breakthrough seizures occur, monitor antiepileptic drug levels and adjust the dose regimen accordingly.
- **Pharmacokinetic effects of pregnancy:** carbamazepine levels may fall in the third trimester. Lamotrigine and levetiracetam levels may fall early in pregnancy. Some advocate monitoring of levels.

 25.42 Epilepsy in old age

- **Incidence and prevalence:** late-onset epilepsy is very common and the annual incidence in those over 60 years is rising.
- **Fits and faints:** the features that usually differentiate these may be less definitive than in younger patients.
- **Non-convulsive status epilepticus:** can present as delirium in the elderly.
- **Cerebrovascular disease:** the underlying cause of seizures in 30–50% of patients over the age of 50 years. A seizure may occur with an overt stroke or with occult vascular disease.
- **Antiepileptic drug regimens:** keep as simple as possible and take care to avoid interactions with other drugs being prescribed.
- **Carbamazepine-induced hyponatraemia:** increases significantly with age; this is particularly important in patients on diuretics or those with heart failure.
- **Withdrawal of antiepileptic therapy:** drug withdrawal should be attempted only where benefits exceed risk of harm from seizures.

 25.43 Epilepsy in adolescence

- **Effect on school/education:** seizures, antiepileptic drugs (AEDs) and psychological complications of epilepsy may hamper education. Fear may make some educational institutions unduly restrictive.
- **Effect on family relationships:** parents may adopt a protective role, which can lead to epilepsy (and AEDs) becoming a point of assertion and rebellion.
- **Effect on career choice:** epilepsy may exclude or restrict employment in the emergency services and armed forces.
- **Alcohol:** may affect sleep pattern; excess may be associated with poor AED adherence.
- **Illicit drugs:** may affect seizure threshold and be associated with poor AED adherence.
- **Sleep disturbance:** may be worsened by social activities and computer games.
- **Oral contraception:** interactions with AED can occur. Use may not always be disclosed to parents.

Prognosis

The outcome of newly diagnosed epilepsy is generally good. Overall, generalised epilepsies and generalised seizures are more readily controlled than focal seizures. The presence of a structural lesion reduces the chances of freedom from seizures. The overall prognosis for epilepsy is shown in Box 25.37. The particular problems that epilepsy poses in the elderly and in adolescents are summarised in Boxes 25.42 and 25.43, respectively.

Status epilepticus

Presentation and management are described on page 1080. While generalised status epilepticus is most easily recognised, non-convulsive status may be less dramatic and less easily diagnosed. It may cause only altered awareness, delirium or wandering with automatisms. In an intensive care unit setting, EEG monitoring is essential to ensure that diagnosis and treatment are optimised.

Non-epileptic attack disorder ('dissociative attacks')

The difficulty with nomenclature is discussed on page 1097. Patients may present with attacks that resemble epileptic seizures but are caused by psychological phenomena and

25

have no abnormal EEG discharges. Such attacks may be very prolonged, sometimes mimicking status epilepticus. Epileptic and non-epileptic attacks may coexist and time and effort are needed to clarify the relative contribution of each, allowing more accurate and comprehensive treatment.

Non-epileptic attack disorder (NEAD) may be accompanied by dramatic flailing of the limbs and arching of the back, with side-to-side head movements and vocalising. Cyanosis and severe biting of the tongue are rare but incontinence can occur. Distress and crying are common following non-epileptic attacks. The distinction between epileptic attacks originating in the frontal lobes and non-epileptic attacks may be especially difficult, and may require videotelemetry with prolonged EEG recordings. Non-epileptic attacks are three times more common in women than in men and have been linked with a history of past or ongoing life trauma. They are not necessarily associated with formal psychiatric illness. Patients and carers may need reassurance that hospital admission is not required for every attack. Prevention requires psychotherapeutic interventions rather than drug therapy (p. 1202).

Vestibular disorders

Vertigo is the typical symptom caused by vestibular dysfunction, and most patients with vertigo have acute vestibular failure, benign paroxysmal positional vertigo or Ménière's disease. Central (brain) causes of vertigo are rare by comparison, with the exception of migraine (p. 1095).

Acute vestibular failure

Although commonly called 'labyrinthitis' or 'vestibular neuronitis', acute vestibular failure is a more accurate term, as most cases are idiopathic. It usually presents as isolated severe vertigo with vomiting and unsteadiness. It begins abruptly, often on waking, and many patients are initially bed-bound. The vertigo settles within a few days, though head movement may continue to provoke transient symptoms (positional vertigo) for some time. During the acute attack, nystagmus (p. 1090) will be present for a few days.

Cinnarizine, prochlorperazine or betahistine provide symptomatic relief but should not be used long-term, as this may delay recovery. A small proportion of patients fail to recover fully and complain of ongoing imbalance and dysequilibrium rather than vertigo; vestibular rehabilitation by a physiotherapist may help.

Benign paroxysmal positional vertigo

Benign paroxysmal positional vertigo (BPPV) is due to the presence of otolithic debris from the saccule or utricle affecting the free flow of endolymph in the semicircular canals (cupulolithiasis). It may follow minor head injury but typically is spontaneous. The history is diagnostic, with transient (seconds) vertigo precipitated by movement (typically, rolling over in bed or getting into or out of bed). Although it is benign, and usually self-limiting after weeks or months, patients are often alarmed by the symptoms. The diagnosis can be confirmed by the 'Hallpike manœuvre' to demonstrate positional nystagmus (Fig. 25.26). Treatment comprises explanation and reassurance, along with positioning procedures designed to return otolithic debris from the semicircular canal to saccule or utricle (such as the Epley manœuvre) and/or to re-educate the brain to cope with the inappropriate signals from the labyrinth (such as Cawthorne–Cooksey exercises: see 'Further information', p. 1146).

Ménière's disease

This is due to an abnormality of the endolymph that causes episodes of vertigo accompanied by tinnitus and fullness in the ear, each attack typically lasting a few hours. Over the years, patients may develop progressive deafness (typically low-tone on audiometry). Examination is typically normal in between attacks. The diagnosis is clinical, supported by abnormal audiometry. Ménière's disease is idiopathic but a similar syndrome may

Fig. 25.26 The Hallpike manœuvre for diagnosis of benign paroxysmal positional vertigo (BPPV). Patients are asked to keep their eyes open and look at the examiner as their head is swung briskly backwards through 120° to overhang the edge of the couch. A Perform first with the right ear down. B Perform next with the left ear down. The examiner looks for nystagmus (usually accompanied by vertigo). In BPPV, the nystagmus typically occurs in A or B only and is torsional, the fast phase beating towards the lower ear. Its onset is usually delayed a few seconds and it lasts 10–20 seconds. As the patient is returned to the upright position, transient nystagmus may occur in the opposite direction. Both nystagmus and vertigo typically decrease (fatigue) on repeat testing.

be caused by middle ear trauma or infection. Imaging may be indicated to exclude other focal brainstem or cerebellopontine angle pathology but will be normal in Ménière's disease. Management includes a low-salt diet, vestibular sedatives for acute attacks (e.g. cinnarizine or prochlorperazine), and occasionally surgery to increase endolymphatic drainage from the vestibular system. Migraine may also cause episodic vertigo, and can be confused with Ménière's disease, although usually other migrainous features will appear in the history.

Disorders of sleep

Sleep disturbances include too much sleep (hypersomnolence or excessive daytime sleepiness), insufficient or poor-quality sleep (insomnia), and abnormal behaviour during sleep (parasomnias). Insomnia is usually caused by psychological or psychiatric disorders, shift work and other environmental causes, pain and so on, and will not be discussed further. Many symptoms and disorders may affect sleep and sleep quality (e.g. pain, depression/anxiety, parkinsonism).

Excessive daytime sleepiness (hypersomnolence)

There are primary and secondary causes (Box 25.44). The most common causes are impaired sleep due to lifestyle issues or sleep-disordered breathing (p. 622). Sleepiness may be measured using the Epworth Sleepiness Score (see Box 17.86, p. 623). Most causes will be identified by a detailed history from the patient and their bed partner, and a 2-week sleep diary.

Narcolepsy

This has a prevalence of about 1 in 2000, with peak onset in adolescence and early middle age. The key symptom is sudden, irresistible 'sleep attacks', often in inappropriate circumstances such as while eating or talking. Other characteristic features help distinguish this from excessive daytime sleepiness (Box 25.45). Symptoms may be due to loss of hypocretin-secreting hypothalamic neurons. Diagnosis requires sleep study with sleep latency testing (demonstrating rapid onset of REM sleep). Narcolepsy may respond to stimulants such as modafinil but more severe cases may require sodium oxybate, dexamfetamine, methylphenidate or selective serotonin reuptake inhibitor (SSRIs). Cataplexy can be debilitating and can respond to sodium oxybate or to antidepressants, such as clomipramine or venlafaxine.

| **25.44 Causes of hypersomnolence** |

Primary causes

- Narcolepsy
- Idiopathic hypersomnolence
- Brain injury

Secondary causes (due to poor-quality sleep)

- Obstructive sleep apnoea
- Pain
- Restless legs/periodic limb movements of sleep
- Parkinsonism and other neurodegenerative diseases
- Depression/anxiety
- Medication
- Environmental factors (noise, temperature etc.)

| **25.45 Narcolepsy symptoms** |

Sleep attacks

- Brief, frequent and unlike normal somnolence

Cataplexy

- Sudden loss of muscle tone triggered by surprise, laughter, strong emotion etc.

Hypnagogic or hypnopompic hallucinations

- Frightening hallucinations experienced during sleep onset or waking due to intrusion of REM sleep during wakefulness (can occur in normal people)

Sleep paralysis

- Brief paralysis on waking (can occur in normal people)

Parasomnias

Parasomnias are abnormal motor behaviours that occur around sleep. They may arise in either REM or non-REM sleep, with characteristic features and timing. Non-REM parasomnias tend to occur early in sleep. Parasomnias should be distinguished from other motor disturbances (such as periodic limb movements, hypnic jerks or sleep talking) and sleep-onset epileptic seizures (p. 1101). History from a sleeping partner or other witness is essential.

Non-REM parasomnias

These are due to incomplete arousal from non-REM sleep and manifest as night terrors, sleep walking and confusional arousals (sleep drunkenness). They typically occur within an hour or two of sleep onset, and are common in children and usually of no pathological significance. Rarely, they persist into adulthood and may become increasingly complex, including dressing, moving objects, eating, drinking or even acts of violence. Patients have little or no recollection of the episodes, even though they appear 'awake'. The episodes may be triggered by alcohol or unfamiliar sleeping situations, and can be familial. Treatment is usually not required but clonazepam can be used.

REM sleep behaviour disorder

In REM sleep behaviour disorder (RBD), patients 'act out' their dreams during REM sleep, due to failure of the usual muscle atonia. Sleep partners provide typical histories of patients 'fighting' or 'struggling' in their sleep, sometimes causing injury to themselves or to their partner. They are easily roused from this state, with recollection of their dream, unlike in non-REM states. RBD is more common in men and may be an early symptom of neurodegenerative diseases such as alpha synucleinopathies (p. 1111), perhaps preceding more typical symptoms of these conditions by years. Polysomnography will confirm absence of atonia during REM sleep. Clonazepam is the most successful treatment.

Restless legs syndrome

Restless legs syndrome (RLS) is common, with a prevalence of up to 10%, but many patients never seek medical attention. It is characterised by unpleasant leg (rarely, arm) sensations that are eased by movement (motor restlessness); the diagnosis is

25

25.46 Diagnostic criteria for restless legs syndrome

A need to move the legs, usually accompanied or caused by uncomfortable, unpleasant sensations in the legs, with the following features:
- only present or worse during periods of rest or inactivity such as lying or sitting
- partially or totally relieved by movement such as walking or stretching, at least as long as the activity continues
- generally worse or occurs only in the evening or night.

clinical (Box 25.46). It has a strong familial tendency and can present with daytime somnolence due to poor sleep. It is usually idiopathic but may be associated with iron deficiency, pregnancy, peripheral neuropathy, Parkinson's disease or uraemia. It should be distinguished from akathisia, the daytime motor restlessness that is an adverse effect of antipsychotic drugs. Treatment, if required, is with dopaminergic drugs (dopamine agonists or levodopa, p. 1113) or benzodiazepines.

Periodic limb movements in sleep

Unlike RLS, periodic limb movements in sleep (PLMS) only occur during sleep and cause repetitive flexion movements of the limbs, usually in the early (non-REM) stages of sleep. Although patients are unaware of the symptoms, they may disrupt sleep quality and often disturb partners. The pathological significance of PLMS is uncertain and it often occurs in normal health. There is an overlap with RLS. Treatment is most successful with clonazepam or dopaminergic drugs.

Neuro-inflammatory diseases

Multiple sclerosis

Multiple sclerosis (MS) is an important cause of long-term disability in adults, especially in the UK, where the prevalence is approximately 120 per 100 000. The annual incidence is around 7 per 100 000, while the lifetime risk of developing MS is about 1 in 400. The incidence of MS is higher in Northern Europeans and the disease is about twice as common in females.

Pathophysiology

There is evidence that both genetic and environmental factors play a causative role. The prevalence of MS is low near the equator and increases in the temperate zones of both hemispheres. People retain the risk of developing the disease in the zone in which they grew up, indicating that environmental exposures during growth and development are important. Prevalence also correlates with environmental factors, such as sunlight exposure, vitamin D (a controversial association) and exposure to Epstein–Barr virus (EBV), although causative mechanisms remain unclear. Genetic factors are also relevant; the risk of familial occurrence in MS is 15%, with highest risk in first-degree relatives (age-adjusted risk 4–5% for siblings and 2–3% for parents or offspring). Monozygotic twins have a concordance rate of 30%. The genes that predispose to MS are incompletely defined but inheritance appears to be polygenic, with influences from genes for human leucocyte antigen (HLA) typing, interleukin receptors, *CLEC16A* (C-type lectin domain family 16 member

A) and *CD226* genes. An immune hypothesis is supported by increased levels of activated T lymphocytes in the CSF and increased immunoglobulin synthesis within the CNS.

Initial CNS inflammation in MS involves entry of activated T lymphocytes across the blood–brain barrier. These recognise myelin-derived antigens on the surface of the nervous system's antigen-presenting cells, the microglia, and undergo clonal proliferation. The resulting inflammatory cascade releases cytokines and initiates destruction of the oligodendrocyte–myelin unit by macrophages. Histologically, the resultant lesion is a plaque of inflammatory demyelination, most commonly in the periventricular regions of the brain, the optic nerves and the subpial regions of the spinal cord (Fig. 25.27). This begins as a circumscribed area of disintegration of the myelin sheath, accompanied by infiltration by activated lymphocytes and macrophages, often with conspicuous perivascular inflammation. After the acute attack, gliosis follows, leaving a shrunken scar.

Much of the initial acute clinical deficit is caused by the effect of inflammatory cytokines on transmission of the nervous impulse rather than structural disruption of myelin, and may explain the rapid recovery of some deficits and probably the acute benefit from glucocorticoids. In the long term, accumulating myelin loss reduces the efficiency of impulse propagation or causes complete conduction block, contributing to sustained impairment of CNS functions. Inflammatory mediators released during the acute attack (particularly nitric oxide) probably also initiate axonal damage, which is a feature of the latter stages of the disease. In established MS there is progressive axonal loss, probably due to the successive damage from acute attacks and the subsequent loss of neurotrophic factors from oligodendrocytes. This axonal loss may account for the phase of the disease characterised by progressive and persistent disability (Fig. 25.28).

Clinical features

The diagnosis of MS requires the demonstration of otherwise unexplained CNS lesions separated in time and space (Box 25.47); traditionally, this meant two or more clinical relapses affecting different parts of the nervous system, and the first ever episode was labelled 'clinically isolated syndrome' (CIS). Recent changes to diagnostic criteria mean that MS may be diagnosed after an isolated episode (i.e. at the CIS stage), provided that certain criteria are met (Box 25.47) The peak age of onset of MS is the fourth decade; onset before puberty or after the age of 60 years is rare. Symptoms and signs of MS usually evolve over days or weeks, resolving over weeks or months. Rarely, a more rapid stroke-like presentation may occur. About 85–90% of patients have an initial relapsing and remitting clinical course with variable intervening recovery, although the majority will eventually enter a secondary progressive phase. Most of the rest follow a slowly progressive clinical course (so-called primary progressive MS), while rare patients have a fulminant variety leading to early death (see Fig. 25.28). Frequent relapses with incomplete recovery indicate a poor prognosis. Some milder cases have an interval of years or even decades between attacks, while in others (particularly if optic neuritis is the initial manifestation) there is no recurrence of disease.

There are a number of clinical symptoms and syndromes suggestive of MS, occurring either at presentation or during the course of the illness (Box 25.48). The physical signs observed in MS are determined by the anatomical site of demyelination. Combined spinal cord and brainstem signs are common, although evidence of previous optic neuritis may be found in the form of an afferent pupillary deficit. Significant intellectual impairment

Fig. 25.27 Multiple sclerosis. [A] Photomicrograph from demyelinating plaque, showing perivascular cuffing of blood vessel by lymphocytes. [B] Brain magnetic resonance imaging in multiple sclerosis. Multiple high-signal lesions (arrows) seen particularly in the paraventricular region on T2 image. [C] In T1 image with gadolinium enhancement, recent lesions (A arrows) show enhancement, suggesting active inflammation (enhancement persists for 4 weeks); older lesions (B arrows) show no enhancement but low signal, suggesting gliosis.

i	**25.47 The Macdonald criteria for the diagnosis of multiple sclerosis (2011)[1]**	
Clinical presentation[2]	**Additional evidence required for diagnosis of MS**
Two or more attacks with *either* objective clinical evidence of at least 2 lesions *or* Objective clinical evidence of 1 attack with reasonable evidence (on clinical history) of at least 1 prior attack	None
Two or more attacks with objective clinical evidence of 1 lesion	Dissemination in 'space' demonstrated by magnetic resonance imaging (MRI) ≥ 1 lesion in at least 2 of the MS-typical regions[3] (multiple lesions in different sites) *or* Await further clinical attack at different anatomical site
One attack with objective clinical evidence of ≥ 2 lesions	Dissemination in 'time' demonstrated by evolving MRI showing combined enhancing (new) and non-enhancing (old) lesions *or* New T2 or enhancing lesion on repeat MRI *or* Await further (second) clinical attack at different anatomical site
One attack with clinical evidence of only 1 lesion (clinically isolated syndrome)	Dissemination in 'space' demonstrated by ≥ 1 T2 lesion in at least 2 MS-typical regions *or* Dissemination in 'time', demonstrated by simultaneous enhancing and non-enhancing lesions *or* New T2 or enhancing lesions on repeat MRI *or* Await further (second) clinical attack
Insidious neurological progression suggestive of MS	1 year of progression plus 2 of the following: Evidence for dissemination in space with ≥ 1 T2 lesions in MS-typical regions Evidence for dissemination in space based on ≥ 2 lesions in the spinal cord Positive cerebrospinal fluid (evidence of oligoclonal band and/or elevated immunoglobulin G index)

[1]If the clinical presentation in the left-hand column is associated with the features in the right-hand column, the diagnosis is MS. If there is incomplete association, the diagnosis is 'possible MS'. [2]Assumes other possible causes for central nervous system inflammation (e.g. sarcoidosis, systemic lupus erythematosus) have been excluded. [3]MS-typical regions = periventricular, juxtacortical, infratentorial, spinal cord.
From Polman CH, Reingold SC, Branwell B, et al. Diagnostic criteria for multiple sclerosis. Ann Neurol 2011; 69:292–302.

25

Fig. 25.28 The progression of disability in fulminant, relapsing–remitting and progressive multiple sclerosis. *Courtesy of Prof. D.A.S. Compston.*

 25.48 Clinical features of multiple sclerosis

Common presentations of multiple sclerosis

- Optic neuritis
- Relapsing/remitting sensory symptoms
- Subacute painless spinal cord lesion
- Acute brainstem syndrome
- Subacute loss of function of upper limb (dorsal column deficit)
- 6th cranial nerve palsy

Other symptoms and syndromes suggestive of central nervous system demyelination

- Afferent pupillary defect and optic atrophy (previous optic neuritis)
- Lhermitte's symptom (tingling in spine or limbs on neck flexion)
- Progressive non-compressive paraparesis
- Partial Brown–Séquard syndrome (p. 1083)
- Internuclear ophthalmoplegia with ataxia
- Postural ('rubral', 'Holmes') tremor
- Trigeminal neuralgia (p. 1096) under the age of 50
- Recurrent facial palsy

Exclude other structural disease and identify plaques of demyelination
Image area of clinical involvement
(magnetic resonance imaging, myelography)

↓

Demonstrate other sites of involvement
Imaging (MRI)
Visual evoked potentials
Other evoked potentials

↓

Demonstrate inflammatory nature of lesion(s)
Cerebrospinal fluid examination
Cell count
Protein electrophoresis (oligoclonal bands)

↓

Exclude other conditions
Chest X-ray
Serum angiotensin-converting enzyme
Serum vitamin B_{12}
Antinuclear antibodies
Antiphospholipid antibodies

Fig. 25.29 Investigations in a patient suspected of having multiple sclerosis.

appears only late in the disease, when loss of frontal lobe functions and impairment of memory are common.

The prognosis for patients with MS is difficult to predict with confidence, especially early in the disease. Those with relapsing and remitting MS experience, on average, 1–2 relapses every 2 years, although this may decline with time. Approximately 5% of patients die within 5 years of disease onset, and slightly more have very good long-term outcome with little or no disability. Prognosis is good for patients with optic neuritis and only sensory relapses. Overall, about one-third of patients are disabled to the point of needing help with walking after 10 years, and this proportion rises to about half after 15 years. It would appear likely (though this is as yet unproven) that disease-modifying drugs will have an effect on long-term disability.

Investigations

There is no single diagnostic test that is definitive for MS and the results of investigation need to be combined with the clinical picture in order to make a diagnosis; MRI is the most important investigation (Fig. 25.29). MS mimics should be excluded (see below). Following the first clinical event (CIS), investigations may help prognosis by confirming the disseminated nature of the disease. MRI is the most sensitive technique for imaging lesions in brain and spinal cord (Fig. 25.30) and for excluding other causes that have provoked the neurological deficit. However, the MRI appearances in MS may be confused with those of small-vessel disease or cerebral vasculitis, and these diagnoses should be considered and excluded. Evoked potentials (visual, auditory or somatosensory) may detect clinically silent lesions but are rarely used nowadays with the advent of MRI.

The CSF may show a lymphocytic pleocytosis in the acute phase and unique (i.e. absent from the serum) oligoclonal bands of IgG in 70–90% of patients between attacks. Oligoclonal bands are not specific for MS and denote only intrathecal inflammation, provided they are unique for the CSF. These can appear in other disorders, which should be excluded by examination and investigation. It is important to exclude other potentially treatable conditions, such as infection, vitamin B_{12} deficiency and spinal cord compression.

Fig. 25.30 **Multiple sclerosis: demyelinating lesion in cervical spinal cord, high-signal T2 images (arrows).** A Sagittal plane. B Axial plane.

i	25.49 Disease-modifying treatments in multiple sclerosis		
Treatment	**Route of administration/dosing**	**Comment**	
Moderate efficacy for less severe cases: average relapse rate reduction 30–50%			
Interferon-beta	Alternate-day or weekly intramuscular or subcutaneous injection	In widespread use for reducing relapse rate	
Glatiramer acetate	Alternate-day subcutaneous injection	Similar efficacy to interferon-beta	
Teriflunomide	Daily oral	May cause diarrhoea, alopecia, hepatotoxicity Highly teratogenic	
Dimethyl fumarate	Daily oral	May cause flushing and gastrointestinal disturbance Risk of PML	
Fingolimod	Daily oral	Superior efficacy to interferon-beta in randomised trials Cardiac conduction defects, especially with first dose	
High efficacy for severe cases: average relapse rate reduction >50%			
Alemtuzumab	Intravenous infusion over two courses separated by 12 months; 5-day infusion initially, second course 3 days	May precipitate autoimmune reactions, e.g. thyroid disease, ITP	
Natalizumab	4-weekly intravenous infusion	Recently introduced; may be more effective than interferon-beta and glatiramer acetate Risk of PML	

(ITP = idiopathic thrombocytopenic purpura; PML = progressive multifocal leucoencephalopathy)

Management

The management of MS involves four different strands: treatment of the acute episode, prevention of future relapses, treatment of complications, and management of the patient's disability.

The acute episode

In a disabling exacerbation of MS, pulses of high-dose glucocorticoid, given either intravenously or orally over 3–5 days, will shorten the duration of the acute episode. Prolonged administration of glucocorticoids does not alter the long-term outcome and is associated with severe adverse effects; it should therefore be avoided. Pulses of glucocorticoids can be given up to three times in a year but use should be restricted to those individuals with significant function-threatening deficits. Prophylaxis to prevent glucocorticoid-induced osteoporosis (p. 1045) should be considered in patients requiring multiple courses of glucocorticoids.

Disease-modifying treatment

Until the 1990s, there were no effective disease-modifying treatments (DMTs) for MS; azathioprine showed some promise but this was offset by adverse effects and the drug was rarely used. The introduction of, initially, beta-interferons and glatiramer acetate paved the way for a new and exciting era of DMTs, which is still evolving. All reduce annual relapse rates and the number and size of lesions on MRI, and some may reduce disability. They are not indicated for treatment of early or pre-clinical MS.

These drugs – available orally, as regular subcutaneous injections or as pulsed intravenous treatments – may be divided into two groups (Box 25.49). All DMTs have strict licensing criteria and are associated with a range of adverse effects, some occasionally fatal, especially the more effective drugs. Careful selection and counselling of patients are necessary and these drugs should be supervised by teams experienced in their use, as recommended in national guidelines.

Clinical trials suggest that DMT options for primary and secondary progressive MS will be available in coming years. Clinical trials involving stem cells are ongoing.

Special diets, including gluten-free regimens or linoleic acid supplements, and hyperbaric oxygen therapy are popular with patients but their efficacy has not been demonstrated.

Treatment of symptoms, complications and disability

Treatments for the complications of MS are summarised in Box 25.50. It is important to provide patients with a careful explanation of the nature of the disease and its outcome. When and if disability occurs, patients and their relatives need appropriate support. Specialist nurses working in a multidisciplinary team of health-care professionals are of great value in managing the chronic phase of the disease. Periods of physiotherapy and occupational therapy may improve functional capacity in those who become disabled, and guidance can be provided on the

25

25.50 Treatment of complications in multiple sclerosis

Spasticity

- Physiotherapy
- Baclofen (usually oral)
- Dantrolene
- Gabapentin
- Sativex
- Tizanidine
- Intrathecal baclofen
- Local (intramuscular) injection of botulinum toxin
- Chemical neuronectomy

Dysaesthesia

- Carbamazepine
- Gabapentin
- Phenytoin
- Amitriptyline

Bladder symptoms

- See Box 25.25 (p. 1094)

Fatigue

- Amantadine
- Modafinil
- Amitriptyline

Erectile dysfunction

- Sildenafil 50–100 mg/day
- Tadalafil

25.51 Multiple sclerosis in pregnancy

- **Counselling**: provision of pre-conception counselling is best practice.
- **Relapse risk**: endocrine effects on the immune system ensure that relapse risk drops during pregnancy.
- **Disease-modifying drugs**: risk of teratogenicity means that all disease-modifying drugs should ideally be stopped 6–8 weeks before conception and recommenced after breastfeeding has stopped.
- **Post-partum relapse rate**: rebound of immune system activity means that the highest risk of relapse is in the first year after delivery.

provision of aids at home, reducing handicap. Bladder care is particularly important. Urgency and frequency can be treated pharmacologically (see Box 25.25, p. 1094) but this may lead to a degree of retention with an attendant risk of infection. Urinary retention can be managed initially by intermittent urinary catheterisation (performed by the patient, if possible) but an in-dwelling catheter may become necessary. Sexual dysfunction is a frequent source of distress. Sildenafil or tadalafil helps impotence in men, and skilled counselling and prosthetic aids may be beneficial. Pregnancy does not increase the risk of progression of MS but relapses may occur post-partum (Box 25.51).

Acute disseminated encephalomyelitis

This is an acute monophasic demyelinating condition in which areas of perivenous demyelination are widely disseminated throughout the brain and spinal cord. The illness may arise spontaneously but often occurs a week or so after a viral infection, especially measles or chickenpox, or following vaccination, suggesting that it is immunologically mediated.

Clinical features

Headache, vomiting, pyrexia, delirium and meningism may be presenting features, often with focal or multifocal brain and spinal cord signs. Seizures or coma may occur. A minority of patients who recover have further episodes.

Investigations

MRI shows multiple high-signal areas in a pattern similar to that of MS, although often with large confluent areas of abnormality. CSF may be normal or show an increase in protein and lymphocytes (occasionally $> 100 \times 10^6$ cells/L). Oligoclonal bands may be found in the acute episode but, in contrast to MS, do not persist beyond clinical recovery. The clinical picture may be very similar to a first relapse of MS.

Management

The prognosis for acute disseminated encephalomyelitis is generally good, although occasionally it may be fatal (probably less than 10%). Treatment with high-dose intravenous methylprednisolone, using the same regimen as for a relapse of MS, is recommended.

Transverse myelitis

Transverse myelitis is an acute, usually monophasic, demyelinating disorder affecting the spinal cord. It is usually thought to be post-infectious in origin. It occurs at any age and presents with a subacute paraparesis with a sensory level, accompanied by severe pain in the neck or back at the onset. MRI should distinguish this from an external lesion affecting the spinal cord. CSF examination shows cellular pleocytosis, often with polymorphs at the onset. Oligoclonal bands are usually absent. Treatment is with high-dose intravenous methylprednisolone. The outcome is variable: one-third have static deficit, one-third go on to develop MS and one-third recover with no subsequent relapse. Some clinical features may suggest a higher risk of MS after transverse myelitis.

Neuromyelitis optica

Neuromyelitis optica (previously Devic's disease) is the occurrence of transverse myelitis and bilateral optic neuritis. The disease has been recognised for many years, particularly in Asia. The majority of cases are associated with an antibody to a neuronal membrane channel, aquaporin 4. If changes are seen on brain MRI (this is variable), they are typically high-signal lesions restricted to periventricular regions. Spinal MRI scans show lesions that are typically longer than three spinal segments (unlike the shorter lesions of MS). Clinical deficits tend to recover less well than in MS, and the disease may be more aggressive with more frequent relapses. Treatment with glucocorticoids, azathioprine or cyclophosphamide, and/or plasmapheresis seems to be more effective than in MS.

Paraneoplastic neurological disorders

Neurological disease may occur with systemic malignant tumours in the absence of cerebral metastases. It is now recognised that, in the majority of these cases, antigen production in the body of the tumour leads to development of antibodies to parts of the CNS. Paraneoplastic conditions are increasingly recognised and the number of antibodies identified is also growing (Boxes 25.52 and 25.53). These syndromes are particularly associated with small-cell carcinoma of lung, ovarian tumours and lymphomas. Autoantibodies are found in the serum and/or CSF, and biopsy will show a lymphocytic infiltrate of the neural tissue affected.

i **25.52 Paraneoplastic disorders of the central nervous system**

Clinical presentation	Associated tumour	Antibodies demonstrated
Limbic encephalitis	SCLC	Anti-Hu, anti-CV2, PCA-2, anti-VGKC, anti-Ma1, anti-amphiphysin, anti-Ri, ANNA-3, anti-VGCC, anti-Zic4, anti-GluR1/2, anti-GABAR
	Testicular, breast	Anti-Ma2, anti-GluR1/2
	Thymoma	Anti-VGKC, anti-CV2, anti-GluR1/2
	Ovarian/testicular teratoma	Anti-NMDAR
Myelopathy	SCLC, thymoma, others	Anti-CV2, anti-amphiphysin, anti-aquaporin
Motor neuron disease	SCLC, others	Anti-Hu
Stiff person syndrome	Breast, SCLC, thymoma, others	Anti-amphiphysin, anti-Ri, anti-GAD, anti-GlyR
Cerebellar degeneration	Breast, ovarian, others	Anti-Yo, anti-Ma1, anti-Ri
	SCLC, others	Anti-Hu, anti-CV2, PCA-2, ANNA-3, anti-amphiphysin, anti-VGCC, anti-Ri, anti-Zic4, anti-GAD
	Lymphoma	Anti-Tr, anti-mGluR1
Multifocal encephalomyelitis	SCLC, thymoma	Anti-Hu, anti-CV2, anti-VGKC, anti-Ma1, anti-amphiphysin, anti-Ri, ANNA-3
Opsoclonus–myoclonus	Breast, ovarian	Anti-Ri, anti-Yo, anti-amphiphysin
	SCLC	Anti Hu, anti-Ri, anti-CV2, anti-amphiphysin, anti-VGCC
	Neuroblastoma	Anti-Hu
	Testicular	Anti-Ma1/2, anti-CV2
Extrapyramidal encephalitis	SCLC, thymoma, testicular	Anti-CV2, anti-Hu, anti-VGKC, anti-Ma
Optic neuritis	SCLC	Anti-CV2, anti-aquaporin
Retinal degeneration	SCLC	Anti-recoverin

(ANNA = anti-neuronal nucleolar antibody; GABAR = GABA receptor; GAD = glutamic acid decarboxylase; GluR = glutamate receptor; GlyR = glycine receptor; NMDAR = N-methyl-D-aspartate receptor; PCA = Purkinje cell antibody; SCLC = small-cell lung cancer; VGCC = voltage-gated calcium channel; VGKC = voltage-gated potassium channel)

i **25.53 Paraneoplastic disorders of the peripheral nervous system**

Clinical presentation	Associated tumour	Antibodies demonstrated
Neuromyotonia	Thymoma, SCLC, others	Anti-VGKC
Myasthenia gravis	Thymoma	Anti-Achr, anti-MuSK
Sensorimotor polyneuropathy	Lymphoma, SCLC, others	Anti-Hu, anti-CV2, ANNA-3, anti-Ma1, anti-amphiphysin
Lambert–Eaton syndrome	SCLC	Anti-VGCC
Motor neuropathy	Lymphoma, SCLC, others	Anti-Hu, anti-Yo, anti-CV2
Sensory neuropathy	Lymphoma, SCLC, others	Anti-Hu, anti-Yo, anti-CV2
Polymyositis/dermatomyositis	Lung, breast	Anti-Jo1

(MuSK = muscle-specific kinase; for other abbreviations, see Box 25.52)

25

Clinical features

Clinical presentations are summarised in Boxes 25.52 and 25.53. In most instances, the neurological condition progresses quite rapidly over a few months, preceding the malignant disease in around half of cases. The range of clinical patterns is so wide that paraneoplastic disease should be considered in the diagnosis of any unusual progressive neurological syndrome. The paraneoplastic disorders of the peripheral nervous system particularly affect the synaptic cleft (p. 1065).

Investigations and management

The presence of characteristic autoantibodies in the context of a suspicious clinical picture may be diagnostic. The causative tumour may be very small and therefore CT of the chest or abdomen or PET scanning may be necessary to find it. These investigations should be pursued only when paraneoplastic

disease has been proven, rather than when it is suspected. The CSF often shows an increased protein and lymphocyte count with oligoclonal bands.

Treatment is directed at the primary tumour. Occasionally, successful therapy of the tumour is associated with improvement of the paraneoplastic syndrome. Some improvement may occur following administration of intravenous immunoglobulin.

Neurodegenerative diseases

While MS is the most common cause of disability in young people in the UK, vascular and neurodegenerative diseases are increasingly important in later life. The neurodegenerative diseases are united in having a pathological process that leads to specific neuronal death, causing relentlessly progressive symptoms, with incidence rising with age. The causes are not yet known, although genetic influences are important. Alzheimer's disease (p. 1192) and Parkinson's disease are the most common.

Movement disorders

Movement disorders present with a wide range of symptoms. They may be genetic or acquired, and the most important is Parkinson's disease. Most movement disorders are categorised clinically, with few confirmatory investigations available other than for those with a known gene abnormality.

Idiopathic Parkinson's disease

Parkinsonism is a clinical syndrome characterised primarily by bradykinesia (p. 1084), with associated increased tone (rigidity), tremor and loss of postural reflexes. There are many causes (Box 25.54) but the most common is Parkinson's disease (PD). PD has an annual incidence of about 18/100 000 in the UK and a prevalence of about 180/100 000. Age has a critical influence on incidence and prevalence, the latter rising to 300–500/100 000 after 80 years of age. Average age of onset is about 60 years and fewer than 5% of patients present under the age of 40. Genetic factors are increasingly recognised and several single genes causing parkinsonism have been identified, although they account for a very small proportion of cases overall. Having a first-degree relative with PD confers a 2–3 times increased risk of developing the disorder. It is progressive and incurable, with a variable prognosis. While motor symptoms are the most common presenting features, non-motor symptoms (particularly cognitive impairment, depression and anxiety) become increasingly prominent as the disease progresses, and significantly reduce quality of life.

Pathophysiology

Although mutations in several genes have been identified in a few cases, in most patients the cause remains unknown. The discovery that methyl-phenyl-tetrahydropyridine (MPTP) caused severe parkinsonism in young drug users suggested that PD might be due to an environmental toxin but none has been convincingly identified. The pathological hallmarks of PD are depletion of the pigmented dopaminergic neurons in the substantia nigra and the presence of α-synuclein and other protein inclusions in nigral cells (Lewy bodies; Fig. 25.31). It is thought that environmental or genetic factors alter the α-synuclein protein, rendering it toxic and leading to Lewy body formation within the nigral cells. Lewy bodies are also found in the basal ganglia, brainstem and cortex, and increase with disease progression. PD is recognised as a synucleinopathy alongside multiple system atrophy and dementia with Lewy bodies. The loss of dopaminergic neurotransmission is responsible for many of the clinical features.

Clinical features

Non-motor symptoms, including reduction in sense of smell (hyposmia), anxiety/depression, constipation and REM sleep behavioural disturbance (RBD), may precede the development of typical motor features by many years but patients rarely present at this stage. The motor symptoms are almost always initially asymmetrical. The hallmark is bradykinesia, leading to classic symptoms such as increasingly small handwriting ('micrographia'), difficulty tying shoelaces or buttoning clothes, and difficulty rolling over in bed. Tremor is an early feature but may not be present in at least 20% of people with PD. It is typically a unilateral rest tremor (p. 1085) affecting limbs, jaw and chin but not the head. In some patients, tremor remains the dominant symptom for many years. Rigidity causes stiffness and a flexed posture. Although postural righting reflexes are impaired early on in the disease, falls tend not to occur until later. As the disease advances, speech becomes softer and indistinct. There are a number of abnormalities on neurological examination (Box 25.55).

Although features are initially unilateral, gradual bilateral involvement evolves with time. Cognition is spared in early disease; if impaired, it should trigger consideration of alternative diagnoses, such as dementia with Lewy bodies.

Non-motor symptoms

While non-motor symptoms may precede the onset of more typical symptoms by many years, for most patients these features become increasingly common and disabling as PD progresses. Cognitive impairment, including dementia, is the symptom most likely to impair quality of life for patients and their carers. Estimates of dementia frequency range from 30% to 80%, depending on definitions and length of follow-up. Other distressing

---

i 25.54 Causes of parkinsonism

Idiopathic Parkinson's disease (at least 80% of parkinsonism)

Cerebrovascular disease

Drugs and toxins

- Antipsychotic drugs (older and 'atypical')
- Metoclopramide, prochlorperazine
- Tetrabenazine
- Sodium valproate
- Lithium
- Manganese
- MPTP

Other degenerative diseases

- Dementia with Lewy bodies
- Progressive supranuclear palsy
- Multiple system atrophy
- Corticobasal degeneration
- Alzheimer's disease

Genetic

- Huntington's disease
- Fragile X tremor ataxia syndrome
- Dopa-responsive dystonia
- Spinocerebellar ataxias (particularly SCA 3)
- Wilson's disease

Anoxic brain injury

(MPTP = methyl-phenyl-tetrahydropyridine)

Fig. 25.31 Parkinson's disease. High power (× 400) view of substantia nigra of a patient with Parkinson's disease showing classical Lewy body (haematoxylin and eosin). *Courtesy of Dr J. Xuereb.*

25.55 Physical signs in Parkinson's disease

General

- Expressionless face (hypomimia)
- Soft, rapid, indistinct speech (dysphonia)
- Flexed (stooped) posture
- Impaired postural reflexes

Gait

- Slow to start walking (failure of gait ignition)
- Rapid, short stride length, tendency to shorten (festination)
- Reduction of arm swing
- Impaired balance on turning

Tremor

Resting (3–4 Hz, moderate amplitude): most common
- Asymmetric, usually first in arm/hand ('pill rolling')
- May affect legs, jaw and chin but not head
- Intermittent, present at rest, often briefly abolished by movement of limb, exacerbated by walking

Postural (6–8 Hz, moderate amplitude)
- Present immediately on stretching out arms

Re-emergent tremor (3–4 Hz, moderate amplitude)
- Initially no tremor on stretching arms out, rest tremor re-emerges after a few seconds

Rigidity

- Cogwheel type, mostly upper limbs (due to tremor superimposed on rigidity)
- Lead pipe type

Akinesia (fundamental feature)

- Slowness of movement
- Fatiguing and decrease in size of repetitive movements

Normal findings (if abnormal, consider other causes)

- Power, deep tendon reflexes, plantar responses
- Eye movements
- Sensory and cerebellar examination

Fig. 25.32 Imaging in Parkinson's disease. [A] Single photon emission computed tomography (SPECT) in Parkinson's disease showing reduced dopamine activity in the basal ganglia. [B] Normal.

non-motor symptoms include neuropsychiatric features (anxiety, depression, apathy, hallucinosis/psychosis), sleep disturbance and hypersomnolence, fatigue, pain, sphincter disturbance and constipation, sexual problems (erectile failure, loss of libido or hypersexuality), drooling and weight loss.

Investigations

The diagnosis is clinical. Structural imaging (CT or MRI) is usually normal for age and thus rarely helpful, although it may support a suspected vascular cause of parkinsonism. Functional dopaminergic imaging (SPECT or PET) is abnormal, even in the early stages (Fig. 25.32), but does not differentiate between the different forms of degenerative parkinsonism (see Box 25.54) and so is not specific for PD. In younger patients, specific investigations may be appropriate (e.g. exclusion of Huntington's or Wilson's diseases). Some patients with family histories may wish to consider genetic testing, although the role of genetic counselling is uncertain at present.

Management

Drug therapy

Drug treatment for PD remains symptomatic rather than curative, and there is no evidence that any of the currently available drugs are neuroprotective. Levodopa (LD) remains the most effective treatment available but other agents include dopamine agonists, anticholinergics, inhibitors of monoamine oxidase (MAOI)-B and catechol-O-methyl-transferase (COMT), and amantadine. Debate continues about when and what treatment should be started. In general, most specialists recommend initiating treatment when symptoms are impacting on everyday life although some favour treatment as soon as the diagnosis is made. Whether it is best to start with LD, a dopamine agonist or MAOI-B remains unclear but most accept that the most effective, best-tolerated and cheapest drug is LD. Many motor symptoms, such as tremor, freezing, falling, head-drop and abnormal flexion, are quite resistant to treatment. Some non-motor symptoms, such as anxiety or depression, may respond to drug or non-drug treatments. In the UK, rivastigmine is licensed for use in PD-associated dementia, although its effect is modest. Many other non-motor symptoms are resistant to treatment. Drugs for PD should not be stopped abruptly, as this can precipitate malignant hyperthermia.

Levodopa Levodopa is the precursor to dopamine. When administered orally, more than 90% is decarboxylated to dopamine peripherally in the gastrointestinal tract and blood vessels, and only a small proportion reaches the brain. This peripheral conversion is responsible for the high frequency of adverse effects. To avoid this, LD is combined with a dopa decarboxylase inhibitor (DDI); the inhibitor does not cross the blood–brain barrier, thus avoiding unwanted decarboxylation-blocking in the brain. Two DDIs, carbidopa and benserazide, are available as combination preparations with LD (Sinemet and Madopar, respectively).

LD is most effective for relieving akinesia and rigidity; tremor response is often less satisfactory and it has no effect on many motor (posture, freezing) and non-motor symptoms. Failure of akinesia/rigidity to respond to LD (1000 mg/day) should prompt reconsideration of the diagnosis. Although controlled-release versions of LD exist, these are usually best reserved for use overnight, as their variable bioavailability makes them difficult to use throughout the day. Madopar is also available as a dispersible tablet for more rapid-onset effect.

Adverse effects include postural hypotension, nausea and vomiting, which may be offset by domperidone. LD may exacerbate or trigger hallucinations, and abnormal LD-seeking behaviour (dopamine dysregulation syndrome), in which the patient takes excessive doses of LD, may occur uncommonly.

As PD progresses, the response to LD becomes less predictable in many patients, leading to motor fluctuations. This end-of-dose deterioration is due to progressive loss of dopamine storage capacity by dwindling numbers of striatonigral neurons.

25

LD-induced involuntary movements (dyskinesia) may occur as a peak-dose phenomenon or as a biphasic phenomenon (occurring during both the build-up and wearing-off phases). More complex fluctuations present as sudden, unpredictable changes in response, in which periods of parkinsonism ('off' phases) alternate with improved mobility but with dyskinesias ('on' phases). Motor complication management is difficult; wearing-off effects may respond to increased dose or frequency of LD or the addition of a COMT inhibitor (see below). More complex fluctuations may be improved by the addition of dopamine agonists (including continuous infusion of apomorphine), use of intraintestinal LD via a percutaneous endoscopic jejunostomy, or deep brain stimulator implantation.

Dopamine receptor agonists Originally introduced in the hope of delaying the initiation of LD and thus delaying motor complications, several dopamine agonists are available, and may be delivered orally, transdermally or subcutaneously (Box 25.56).

The ergot-derived agonists are no longer recommended because of rare but serious fibrotic effects. With the exception of apomorphine, all the agonists are considerably less effective than LD in relieving parkinsonism, have more adverse effects (nausea, vomiting, disorientation and hallucinations, impulse control disorders) and are more expensive. Their role in the management of PD (monotherapy or adjunctive) remains uncertain, and evidence suggests that their usefulness as initial monotherapy is short-lasting.

MAOI-B inhibitors Monoamine oxidase type B facilitates breakdown of excess dopamine in the synapse. Two inhibitors are used in PD: selegiline and rasagiline. The effects of both are modest, although usually well tolerated. Neither is neuroprotective, despite initial hopes.

COMT inhibitors Catechol-O-methyl-transferase (along with dopa decarboxylase) is involved in peripheral breakdown of LD. Two inhibitors are available: entacapone and tolcapone (which also inhibits central COMT). Entacapone has a modest effect and is most useful for early wearing-off. It is available either as a single tablet taken with each LD/DDI dose, or as a combination tablet with LD and DDI. The more potent tolcapone is less used because of rare but serious hepatotoxicity.

Amantadine This has a mild, usually short-lived effect on bradykinesia and is rarely used unless patients are unable to tolerate other drugs. It is more commonly employed as a treatment for LD-induced dyskinesias, although again benefit is modest and short-lived. Adverse effects include livedo reticularis, peripheral oedema, delirium and other anticholinergic effects.

Anticholinergic drugs These were the main treatment for PD prior to the introduction of LD. Their role now is limited by

lack of efficacy (apart from an effect on tremor sometimes) and adverse effects, including dry mouth, blurred vision, constipation, urinary retention, delirium and hallucinosis, as well as long-term concerns regarding cognitive impairment. Several anticholinergics are available, including trihexyphenidyl (benzhexol) and orphenadrine.

Surgery

Destructive neurosurgery was commonly used before the introduction of LD. In the last 20 years, stereotactic surgery has emerged and most commonly involves deep brain stimulation (DBS), rather than the destructive approach of previous eras. Various targets have been identified, including the thalamus (only effective for tremor), globus pallidus and subthalamic nucleus. DBS is usually reserved for individuals with medically refractory tremor or motor fluctuations, and careful patient selection is vital to success. Intracranial delivery of fetal grafts or specific growth factors remains experimental.

Physiotherapy, occupational therapy and speech therapy

Patients at all stages of PD benefit from physiotherapy, which helps reduce rigidity and corrects abnormal posture. Occupational therapists can provide equipment to help overcome functional limitations, such as rails for stairs and the toilet, and bathing equipment. Speech therapy can help where dysarthria and dysphonia interfere with communication, and advice may also be provided to those with dysphagia. As with many complex neurological disorders, patients with PD should ideally be managed by a multidisciplinary team, including PD specialist nurses.

Other parkinsonian syndromes

Cerebrovascular disease and drug-induced parkinsonism are the most common alternative causes of parkinsonism (see Box 25.54). There are several degenerative conditions that cause parkinsonism, including multiple system atrophy, progressive supranuclear palsy and corticobasal degeneration. They typically have a more rapid progression than PD and tend to be resistant to treatment with LD. They are defined pathologically and identification during life is difficult. There are other conditions that may rarely manifest as parkinsonism, including Huntington's and Wilson's diseases.

Multiple system atrophy

Multiple system atrophy (MSA) is characterised by parkinsonism, autonomic failure and cerebellar symptoms, with either parkinsonism (MSA-P) or cerebellar features (MSA-C) predominating. It is much less common than PD, with a prevalence of about 4/100 000. Although early distinction between PD and MSA-P may be difficult, early falls, postural instability and lack of response to LD are clues. The pathological hallmark is α-synuclein-containing glial cytoplasmic inclusions found in the basal ganglia, cerebellum and motor cortex. Management is symptomatic and the prognosis is less good than for PD, with mean survival from symptom onset of fewer than 10 years and early disability. Cognition is usually unaffected.

Progressive supranuclear palsy

Progressive supranuclear palsy (PSP) presents with symmetrical parkinsonism, cognitive impairment, early falls and bulbar symptoms. The characteristic eye movement disorder, with slowed vertical saccades leading to impairment of up- and down-gaze, may take years to emerge. PSP has different pathological

---

i	**25.56 Dopamine agonists***

Ergot-derived

- Bromocriptine
- Lisuride
- Pergolide
- Cabergoline

Non-ergot-derived

- Ropinirole
- Pramipexole
- Rotigotine (transdermal patch)
- Apomorphine (subcutaneous)

*Oral unless otherwise stated.

features, being associated with abnormal accumulation of tau (τ) proteins and degeneration of the substantia nigra, subthalamic nucleus and mid-brain. It is therefore a tauopathy rather than synucleinopathy. The prevalence is about 5/100 000, with average survival similar to that in MSA. There is no treatment, and the parkinsonism usually does not respond to LD.

Corticobasal degeneration

Corticobasal degeneration (CBD) is less common than MSA or PSP, and the clinical manifestations are variable, including parkinsonism, dystonia, myoclonus and 'alien limb' phenomenon, whereby a limb (usually upper) moves about or interferes with the other limb without apparent conscious control. Cortical symptoms, including dementia and especially apraxia, are common and may be the only features in some cases. A number of other diseases may present with a corticobasal syndrome, including other dementias. CBD is a tauopathy with widespread deposition throughout the brain, and has similar survival rates to MSA and PSP.

Wilson's disease

This is an autosomal recessive disorder resulting from mutation in the *ATP7B* gene, causing a defect of copper metabolism (p. 896). It is a treatable cause of various movement disorders, including tremor, dystonia, parkinsonism and ataxia; psychiatric symptoms may also occur. Wilson's disease should always be excluded in patients under the age of 50 presenting with any movement disorder.

Huntington's disease

Huntington's disease (HD) is an autosomal dominant disorder, presenting in adults usually but occasionally in children. It is due to expansion of a trinucleotide CAG repeat in the *Huntingtin* gene on chromosome 4 (p. 43). The disease frequently demonstrates the phenomenon of anticipation, in which there is a younger age at onset as the disease is passed through generations, due to progressive expansion of the repeat. The prevalence is about 4–8/100 000.

Clinical features

HD typically presents with a progressive behavioural disturbance, abnormal movements (usually chorea), and cognitive impairment leading to dementia. Onset under 18 years is rare but patients may then present with parkinsonism rather than chorea (the 'Westphal variant'). There is always a family history, although this may be concealed.

Investigations and management

The diagnosis is confirmed by genetic testing; pre-symptomatic testing for other family members is available but must be preceded by appropriate counselling (p. 59). Brain imaging may show caudate atrophy but is not a reliable test. There are a number of HD mimics.

Management is symptomatic. The chorea may respond to neuroleptics such as risperidone or sulpiride, or tetrabenazine. Depression and anxiety are common and may be helped by medication.

Ataxias

The ataxias are a heterogeneous group of inherited and acquired disorders, presenting either with pure ataxia or in association with other neurological and non-neurological features. The differential

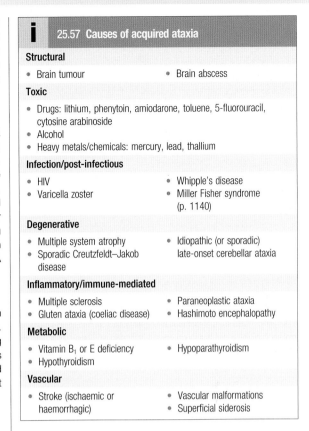

25.57 Causes of acquired ataxia

Structural
- Brain tumour
- Brain abscess

Toxic
- Drugs: lithium, phenytoin, amiodarone, toluene, 5-fluorouracil, cytosine arabinoside
- Alcohol
- Heavy metals/chemicals: mercury, lead, thallium

Infection/post-infectious
- HIV
- Varicella zoster
- Whipple's disease
- Miller Fisher syndrome (p. 1140)

Degenerative
- Multiple system atrophy
- Sporadic Creutzfeldt–Jakob disease
- Idiopathic (or sporadic) late-onset cerebellar ataxia

Inflammatory/immune-mediated
- Multiple sclerosis
- Gluten ataxia (coeliac disease)
- Paraneoplastic ataxia
- Hashimoto encephalopathy

Metabolic
- Vitamin B₁ or E deficiency
- Hypothyroidism
- Hypoparathyroidism

Vascular
- Stroke (ischaemic or haemorrhagic)
- Vascular malformations
- Superficial siderosis

is wide (Boxes 25.57 and 25.58), and diagnosis is guided by age of onset, evolution and clinical features. A significant proportion of cases remain idiopathic despite investigation.

The hereditary ataxias are a group of inherited disorders in which degenerative changes occur to varying extents in the cerebellum, brainstem, pyramidal tracts, spinocerebellar tracts and optic and peripheral nerves, and influence the clinical manifestations. Onset ranges from infancy to adulthood, with recessive, sex-linked or dominant inheritance (see Box 25.58). While the genetic abnormality has been identified for some, allowing diagnostic testing, this is not currently the case for many of the hereditary ataxias.

Tremor disorders

Tremor (p. 1085) is a feature of many disorders but the most important clinical syndromes are PD, essential tremor, drug-induced tremors (Box 25.59) and functional (psychogenic) tremors.

Essential tremor

This has a prevalence of about 300/100 000 and may display a dominant pattern of inheritance, although no genes have thus far been identified. It may present at any age with a bilateral arm tremor (8–10 Hz), rarely at rest but typical with movement. The head and voice may be involved. The tremor improves in about 50% of patients with small amounts of alcohol. There are no specific tests and essential tremor should be distinguished from other tremor syndromes, including dystonic tremor. Beta-blockers and primidone are sometimes helpful, and DBS of the thalamus is an effective treatment for severe cases.

25

25.58 Inherited ataxias

Inheritance pattern	Age of onset	Clinical features
Autosomal dominant		
Episodic ataxias	Childhood and early adulthood	Brief episodes of ataxia, sometimes induced by stress or startle. May develop progressive ataxia
Spinocerebellar ataxias (SCAs)	Childhood to middle age	Over 30 subtypes identified thus far. Progressive ataxia, sometimes associated with other features, including retinitis pigmentosa, pyramidal tract abnormalities, peripheral neuropathy and cognitive deficits
Dentato-rubro-pallidoluysian atrophy (DRPLA)	Childhood to middle age	Children present with myoclonic epilepsy and progressive ataxia. Adults have progressive ataxia with psychiatric features, dementia and choreoathetosis
Autosomal recessive		
Friedreich's ataxia	Childhood/adolescence (late onset possible)	Ataxia, nystagmus, dysarthria, spasticity, areflexia, proprioceptive impairment, diabetes mellitus, optic atrophy, cardiac abnormalities. Usually chair-bound
Ataxia telangiectasia	Childhood	Progressive ataxia, athetosis, telangiectasia on conjunctivae, impaired DNA repair, immune deficiency, tendency to malignancies
Abetalipoproteinaemia	Childhood	Steatorrhoea, sensorimotor neuropathy, retinitis pigmentosa, malabsorption of vitamins A, D, E and K
Hereditary ataxia with vitamin E deficiency	<20 years	Similar to Friedreich's ataxia, visual loss or retinitis pigmentosa, chorea
Others	Usually young onset	Numerous, with genes identified only in some
X-linked		
Fragile X tremor ataxia syndrome	>50 years	Tremor, ataxia, parkinsonism, autonomic failure, cognitive impairment and dementia
Adrenoleukodystrophy	Childhood to adult	Impaired adrenal and cognitive function, sometimes spastic paraparesis
Mitochondrial disease	Various	Ataxia features in several mitochondrial diseases, including Kearns–Sayre syndrome, MELAS, MERRF, Leigh's syndrome (p. 49)

(MELAS = mitochondrial myopathy, encephalopathy, lactic acidosis and stroke-like episodes; MERRF = myoclonic epilepsy with ragged red fibres)

25.59 Drug-induced tremor (usually postural)*

- β-agonists (e.g. salbutamol)
- Theophylline
- Sodium valproate
- Thyroxine
- Lithium
- Tricyclic antidepressants
- Recreational drugs (e.g. amphetamines)
- Alcohol
- Caffeine

*Drugs causing parkinsonism and associated tremor are listed in Box 25.54.

Dystonia

Dystonia is characterised by a focal increase in tone affecting muscles in the limbs or trunk. It may be a feature of a number of neurological conditions (PD, Wilson's disease), or occur secondary to brain damage (trauma, stroke) or drugs (tardive syndromes). Dystonia also occurs as a primary disorder. With childhood onset the cause is usually genetic and dystonia is generalised, but adult onset is usually focal; examples include a twisted neck (torticollis), repetitive blinking (blepharospasm) or tremor. Task-specific symptoms (e.g. writer's cramp, musician's dystonia) are often dystonic. Treatment is difficult but botulinum toxin injections or DBS may be useful.

Hemifacial spasm

This usually presents after middle age with intermittent twitching around one eye, spreading ipsilaterally to other facial muscles. The spasms are exacerbated by talking, eating and stress. Hemifacial spasm is usually idiopathic, similar to trigeminal neuralgia; it has been suggested that it may be due to an aberrant arterial loop irritating the 7th nerve just outside the pons. It may, however, be symptomatic and secondary to structural lesions. Drug treatment is not effective but injections of botulinum toxin into affected muscles help, although these usually have to be repeated every 3 months or so. In refractory cases, microvascular decompression may be considered.

Motor neuron disease

Motor neuron disease (MND) is a neurodegenerative condition caused by loss of upper and lower motor neurons in the spinal cord, cranial nerve nuclei and motor cortex. Annual incidence is about 2/100 000, with a prevalence of about 7/100 000. Most cases are sporadic but 10% of cases are familial. Abnormalities in the superoxide dismutase (*SOD1*) gene account for about 20% of such cases, and an expanded repeat sequence in the *C9orf72* gene on chromosome 9 is associated with MND and frontotemporal dementia. The most common form of MND (Fig. 25.33) is amyotrophic lateral sclerosis (ALS), and many use the terms MND and ALS interchangeably. ALS is characterised by a combination of upper and lower motor neuron signs; there are rarer, pure lower (progressive muscular atrophy) or upper (progressive lateral sclerosis) motor neuron variants of MND. The average age of onset is 65, with 10% presenting before 45 years.

Clinical features

Diagnosis can be difficult and is often delayed. MND typically presents focally, either with limb onset (e.g. foot drop or loss of manual dexterity) or with bulbar symptoms (dysarthria, swallowing difficulty); respiratory onset is rare but type II respiratory failure is a common terminal event. Sensory, autonomic and visual symptoms do not occur, although cramp is common (Box 25.60). Examination reveals a combination of lower and upper

Fig. 25.33 Patterns of involvement in motor neuron disease. (LMN = lower motor neuron; UMN = upper motor neuron)

25.60 Clinical features of motor neuron disease

Onset

- Usually after the age of 50 years
- Very uncommon before the age of 30 years
- Affects males more commonly than females

Symptoms

- Limb muscle weakness, cramps, occasionally fasciculation
- Disturbance of speech/swallowing (dysarthria/dysphagia)
- Cognitive and behavioural features common (similar to frontotemporal dementia)

Signs

- Wasting and fasciculation of muscles
- Weakness of muscles of limbs, tongue, face and palate
- Pyramidal tract involvement, causing spasticity, exaggerated tendon reflexes, extensor plantar responses
- External ocular muscles and sphincters usually remain intact
- No objective sensory deficit
- Evidence of cognitive impairment with frontotemporal dominance

Course

- Symptoms often begin focally in one part and spread gradually but relentlessly to become widespread

motor neuron signs (e.g. brisk reflexes in wasted, fasciculating muscles) without sensory involvement (Fig. 25.33). Cognitive impairment is under-recognised in MND: up to 50% will have a mainly executive impairment on formal testing, and around 10% develop a frontotemporal dementia (FTD). About 10% of patients presenting with FTD will develop ALS within a few years of dementia onset. Even with treatment, MND is relentlessly progressive, but median survival is improved with specialist follow-up offering non-invasive ventilation, feeding measures and access to pharmacological treatment.

Investigations

Clinical features are often typical but alternative diagnoses should be excluded. Exclusion of treatable causes, such as immune-mediated multifocal motor neuropathy with conduction block (p. 1140) and cervical myeloradiculopathy, is essential. Blood tests are usually normal, other than a mildly raised creatine kinase. Sensory and motor nerve conduction studies are normal but there may be reduction in amplitude of motor action potentials due to axonal loss. EMG will usually confirm the typical features of widespread denervation and re-innervation. Spinal fluid analysis is not usually necessary. Genetic testing is increasing in importance, with mutations found in *SOD1*, *FUS*, *TARDBP* and *C9orf72* that may help predict risk and phenotype of disease in those with a family history of MND.

Management

Patients should be managed within a multidisciplinary service, including physiotherapists, speech and occupational therapists, dietitians, ventilatory and feeding support, and palliative care teams, with neurological and respiratory input. Riluzole, a glutamate release antagonist, is licensed for ALS but has only a modest effect, prolonging median survival by about 2–3 months.

Non-invasive ventilation significantly prolongs survival and improves or maintains quality of life in people with ALS. Survival and some measures of quality of life are significantly improved in the subgroup of people with better baseline bulbar function but not in those with severe bulbar impairment. Feeding by percutaneous gastrostomy may improve quality of life and prolong survival, even when done at a late stage. Rapid access to palliative care teams is essential for patients as they enter the terminal stages of MND.

Spinal muscular atrophy

This is a group of genetically determined disorders affecting spinal and cranial lower motor neurons, characterised by proximal and distal wasting, fasciculation and weakness of muscles. Involvement is usually symmetrical but occasional localised forms occur. With the exception of the infantile form, progression is slow and the prognosis better than for MND.

Infections of the nervous system

The clinical features of nervous system infections depend on the location of the infection (the meninges or the parenchyma of the brain and spinal cord), the causative organism (virus, bacterium,

25

25.61 Infections of the nervous system

Bacterial infections

- Meningitis
- Suppurative encephalitis
- Brain abscess
- Paravertebral (epidural) abscess
- Tuberculosis (p. 588)
- Neurosyphilis
- Leprosy (Hansen's disease) (peripheral nerves)*
- Diphtheria (peripheral nerves)*
- Tetanus (motor cells)

Viral infections

- Meningitis
- Encephalitis
- Transverse myelitis
- Progressive multifocal leucoencephalopathy
- Poliomyelitis
- Subacute sclerosing panencephalitis (late sequel)
- Rabies
- HIV infection (Ch. 12)

Prion diseases

- Creutzfeldt–Jakob disease
- Kuru

Protozoal infections

- Malaria*
- Toxoplasmosis (in immune-suppressed)*
- Trypanosomiasis*
- Amoebic abscess*

Helminthic infections

- Schistosomiasis (spinal cord)*
- Cysticercosis*
- Hydatid disease*
- Strongyloidiasis*

Fungal infections

- *Candida* meningitis or brain abscess
- Cryptococcal meningitis

*These infections are discussed in Chapter 11.

25.62 Causes of meningitis

Infective

Bacteria (see Box 25.63)

Viruses

- Enteroviruses (echo, Coxsackie, polio)
- Mumps
- Influenza
- Herpes simplex
- Varicella zoster
- Epstein–Barr
- HIV
- Lymphocytic choriomeningitis
- Mollaret's meningitis (herpes simplex virus type 2)

Protozoa and parasites

- Cysticerci
- Amoeba

Fungi

- *Cryptococcus neoformans*
- *Candida*
- *Histoplasma*
- *Blastomyces*
- *Coccidioides*
- *Sporothrix*

Non-infective ('sterile')

Malignant disease

- Breast cancer
- Bronchial cancer
- Leukaemia
- Lymphoma

Inflammatory disease (may be recurrent)

- Sarcoidosis
- Systemic lupus erythematosus
- Behçet's disease

Where specific immunisation is not employed, the mumps virus is a common cause.

Clinical features

Viral meningitis occurs mainly in children or young adults, with acute onset of headache and irritability and the rapid development of meningism. The headache is usually the most severe feature. There may be a high pyrexia but focal neurological signs are rare.

Investigations

The diagnosis is made by lumbar puncture. CSF usually contains an excess of lymphocytes. While glucose and protein levels are commonly normal, the latter may be raised. It is important to verify that the patient has not received antibiotics (for whatever cause) prior to the lumbar puncture, as CSF lymphocytosis can also be found in partially treated bacterial meningitis.

Management

There is no specific treatment and the condition is usually benign and self-limiting. The patient should be treated symptomatically in a quiet environment. Recovery usually occurs within days, although a lymphocytic pleocytosis may persist in the CSF. Meningitis may also occur as a complication of a systemic viral infection such as mumps, measles, infectious mononucleosis, herpes zoster and hepatitis. Whatever the virus, complete recovery without specific therapy is the rule.

Bacterial meningitis

Many bacteria can cause meningitis but geographical patterns vary, as does age-related sensitivity (Box 25.63). In the 'meningitis belt' of sub-Saharan Africa, drought and dust storms are often associated with meningococcal outbreaks (Harmattan meningitis). Bacterial meningitis is usually part of a bacteraemic illness, although direct spread from an adjacent focus of infection in the ear, skull fracture or sinus can be causative. Antibiotics have rendered this less common but mortality and morbidity remain

fungus or parasite), and whether the infection is acute or chronic. The major infections of the nervous system are listed in Box 25.61. The frequency of these varies geographically. Helminthic infections, such as cysticercosis and hydatid disease, and protozoal infections are described in Chapter 11.

Meningitis

Acute infection of the meninges presents with a characteristic combination of pyrexia, headache and meningism. Meningism consists of headache, photophobia and stiffness of the neck, often accompanied by other signs of meningeal irritation, including Kernig's sign (extension at the knee with the hip joint flexed causes spasm in the hamstring muscles) and Brudzinski's sign (passive flexion of the neck causes flexion of the hips and knees). Meningism is not specific to meningitis and can occur in patients with subarachnoid haemorrhage. The severity of clinical features varies with the causative organism, as does the presence of other features such as a rash. Abnormalities in the CSF (see Box 25.6, p. 1078) are important in distinguishing the cause of meningitis. Causes of meningitis are listed in Box 25.62.

Viral meningitis

Viruses are the most common cause of meningitis, usually resulting in a benign and self-limiting illness requiring no specific therapy. It is much less serious than bacterial meningitis unless there is associated encephalitis. A number of viruses can cause meningitis (see Box 25.62), the most common being enteroviruses.

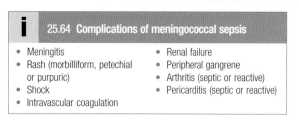

i	25.63 Bacterial causes of meningitis		
Age of onset	**Common**		**Less common**
Neonate	Gram-negative bacilli (*Escherichia coli*, *Proteus*) Group B streptococci		*Listeria monocytogenes*
Pre-school child	*Haemophilus influenzae* *Neisseria meningitidis* (subtypes B, C, Y, W) *Streptococcus pneumoniae*		*Mycobacterium tuberculosis*
Older child and adult	*N. meningitidis* (subtypes B, C, Y, W) *Strep. pneumoniae*		*L. monocytogenes* *M. tuberculosis* *Staphylococcus aureus* (skull fracture) *H. influenzae*

i	25.64 Complications of meningococcal sepsis

- Meningitis
- Rash (morbilliform, petechial or purpuric)
- Shock
- Intravascular coagulation
- Renal failure
- Peripheral gangrene
- Arthritis (septic or reactive)
- Pericarditis (septic or reactive)

significant. An important factor in determining prognosis is early diagnosis and the prompt initiation of appropriate therapy. The meningococcus and other common causes of meningitis are normal commensals of the upper respiratory tract. New and potentially pathogenic strains are acquired by the air-borne route but close contact is necessary. Epidemics of meningococcal meningitis occur, particularly in cramped living conditions or where the climate is hot and dry. The organism invades through the nasopharynx, producing sepsis and leading to meningitis.

Pathophysiology

The meningococcus (*Neisseria meningitidis*) is now the most common cause of bacterial meningitis in Western Europe after *Streptococcus pneumoniae*, while in the USA *Haemophilus influenzae* remains common. In India, *H. influenzae* B and *Strep. pneumoniae* are probably the most common causes of bacterial meningitis, especially in children. *Streptococcus suis* is a rare zoonotic cause of meningitis associated with porcine contact. Infection stimulates an immune response, causing the pia–arachnoid membrane to become congested and infiltrated with inflammatory cells. Pus then forms in layers, which may later organise to form adhesions. These may obstruct the free flow of CSF, leading to hydrocephalus, or they may damage the cranial nerves at the base of the brain. Hearing loss is a frequent complication. The CSF pressure rises rapidly, the protein content increases, and there is a cellular reaction that varies in type and severity according to the nature of the inflammation and the causative organism. An obliterative endarteritis of the leptomeningeal arteries passing through the meningeal exudate may produce secondary cerebral infarction. Pneumococcal meningitis is often associated with a very purulent CSF and a high mortality, especially in older adults.

Clinical features

Headache, drowsiness, fever and neck stiffness are the usual presenting features. In severe bacterial meningitis the patient may be comatose, later developing focal neurological signs. Ninety per cent of patients with meningococcal meningitis will have two of the following: fever, neck stiffness, altered consciousness and rash. When accompanied by sepsis, presenting signs may evolve rapidly, with abrupt onset of obtundation due to cerebral oedema. Complications of meningococcal sepsis are listed in Box 25.64. Chronic meningococcaemia is a rare condition in which the patient can be unwell for weeks or even months

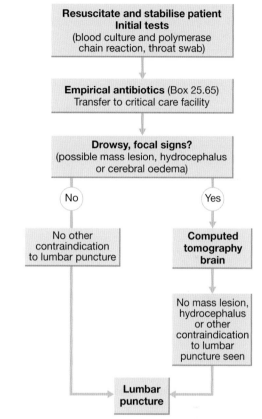

Fig. 25.34 The investigation of meningitis.

with recurrent fever, sweating, joint pains and transient rash. It usually occurs in the middle-aged and elderly, and in those who have previously had a splenectomy. In pneumococcal and *Haemophilus* infections there may be an accompanying otitis media. Pneumococcal meningitis may be associated with pneumonia and occurs especially in older patients and alcoholics, as well as those with hyposplenism. *Listeria monocytogenes* is an increasing cause of meningitis and rhombencephalitis (brainstem encephalitis) in the immunosuppressed, people with diabetes, alcoholics and pregnant women (p. 259). It can also cause meningitis in neonates.

Investigations

Lumbar puncture is mandatory unless there are contraindications (p. 1077). If the patient is drowsy and has focal neurological signs or seizures, is immunosuppressed, has undergone recent neurosurgery or has suffered a head injury, it is wise to obtain a CT to exclude a mass lesion (such as a cerebral abscess) before lumbar puncture because of the risk of coning. This should not, however, delay treatment of presumed meningitis. If lumbar puncture is deferred or omitted, it is essential to take blood cultures and to start empirical treatment (Fig. 25.34). Lumbar

25

puncture will help differentiate the causative organism: in bacterial meningitis the CSF is cloudy (turbid) due to the presence of many neutrophils (often > 1000×10^6 cells/L), the protein content is significantly elevated and the glucose reduced. Gram film and culture may allow identification of the organism. Blood cultures may be positive. PCR techniques can be used on both blood and CSF to identify bacterial DNA. These methods are useful in detecting meningococcal infection and in typing the organism.

Management

There is an untreated mortality rate of around 80%, so action must be swift. In suspected bacterial meningitis the patient should be given parenteral benzylpenicillin immediately (intravenous is preferable) and prompt hospital admission should be arranged.

25.65 Treatment of pyogenic meningitis of unknown cause

1. Adults aged 18–50 years with or without a typical meningococcal rash

- Cefotaxime 2 g IV 4 times daily *or*
- Ceftriaxone 2 g IV twice daily

2. Patients in whom penicillin-resistant pneumococcal infection is suspected, or in areas with a significant incidence of penicillin resistance in the community

As for (1) but add:
- Vancomycin 1 g IV twice daily *or*
- Rifampicin 600 mg IV twice daily

3. Adults aged > 50 years and those in whom *Listeria monocytogenes* infection is suspected (brainstem signs, immunosuppression, diabetic, alcoholic)

As for (1) but add:
- Ampicillin 2 g IV 6 times daily *or*
- Co-trimoxazole 5 mg/kg IV daily in two divided doses

4. Patients with a clear history of anaphylaxis to β-lactams

- Chloramphenicol 25 mg/kg IV 4 times daily *plus*
- Vancomycin 1 g IV twice daily

5. Adjunctive treatment (see text)

- Dexamethasone 0.15 mg/kg 4 times daily for 2–4 days

The only contraindication is a history of penicillin anaphylaxis. Recommended empirical therapies are outlined in Box 25.65, and the preferred antibiotic when the organism is known after CSF examination is stipulated in Box 25.66. Adjunctive glucocorticoid therapy is useful in reducing hearing loss and neurological sequelae in both children and adults in developed countries where the incidence of penicillin resistance is low, but its role where there are high rates of resistance or in countries where there are high rates of untreated HIV is unclear.

In meningococcal disease, mortality is doubled if the patient presents with features of sepsis rather than meningitis. Individuals likely to require intensive care facilities and expertise include those with cardiac, respiratory or renal involvement, and those with CNS depression prejudicing the airway. Early endotracheal intubation and mechanical ventilation protect the airway and may prevent the development of the acute respiratory distress syndrome (ARDS, p. 198). Adverse prognostic features include hypotensive shock, a rapidly developing rash, a haemorrhagic diathesis, multisystem failure and age over 60 years.

Prevention of meningococcal infection

Close contacts of patients with meningococcal infection (Box 25.67) should be given 2 days of oral rifampicin. In adults, a single dose of ciprofloxacin is an alternative. If not treated with ceftriaxone, the index case should be given similar treatment to clear infection from the nasopharynx before hospital discharge. Vaccines are available for most meningococcal subgroups but not group B, which is one of the most common serogroups isolated in many countries.

Tuberculous meningitis

Tuberculous meningitis is now uncommon in developed countries except in immunocompromised individuals, although it is still seen in those born in endemic areas and in developing countries. It is seen more frequently as a secondary infection in patients with the acquired immunodeficiency syndrome (AIDS).

Pathophysiology

Tuberculous meningitis most commonly occurs shortly after a primary infection in childhood or as part of miliary tuberculosis (p. 588). The usual local source of infection is a caseous focus in

---

25.66 Chemotherapy of bacterial meningitis when the cause is known

Pathogen	Regimen of choice	Alternative agents
Neisseria meningitidis	Benzylpenicillin 2.4 g IV 6 times daily for 5–7 days	Cefuroxime, ampicillin Chloramphenicol*
Streptococcus pneumoniae (sensitive to β-lactams, MIC < 1 mg/L)	Cefotaxime 2 g IV 4 times daily *or* Ceftriaxone 2 g IV twice daily for 10–14 days	Chloramphenicol*
Strep. pneumoniae (resistant to β-lactams)	As for sensitive strains but add: Vancomycin 1 g IV twice daily *or* Rifampicin 600 mg IV twice daily	Vancomycin plus rifampicin* Moxifloxacin Gatifloxacin
Haemophilus influenzae	Cefotaxime 2 g IV 4 times daily *or* Ceftriaxone 2 g IV twice daily for 10–14 days	Chloramphenicol*
Listeria monocytogenes	Ampicillin 2 g IV 6 times daily *plus* Gentamicin 5 mg/kg IV daily	Ampicillin 2 g IV 4-hourly *plus* Co-trimoxazole 50 mg/kg daily in two divided doses
Streptococcus suis	Cefotaxime 2 g IV 4 times daily *or* Ceftriaxone 2 g IV twice daily for 10–14 days	Chloramphenicol*

*For patients with a history of anaphylaxis to β-lactam antibiotics.
(MIC = minimum inhibitory concentration)

25.67 Chemoprophylaxis following meningococcal exposure

Close contacts warranting chemoprophylaxis

- Household contacts (including persons who ate or slept in the same dwelling as the patient during the 7 days prior to disease onset)
- Child-care and nursery-school contacts
- Persons having contact with patient's oral secretions during the 7 days prior to disease onset:
  Kissing
  Sharing of toothbrushes
  Sharing of eating utensils
  Mouth-to-mouth resuscitation
  Unprotected contact during endotracheal intubation
- Aircraft contacts for persons seated next to the patient for >8 hrs

Persons at low risk in whom chemoprophylaxis is not recommended

- Casual contact (e.g. at school or work) without direct exposure to patient's oral secretions
- Indirect contact only (contact with a high-risk contact and not a case)
- Health-care worker without direct exposure to patient's oral secretions

25.68 Clinical features and staging of tuberculous meningitis

Symptoms

- Headache
- Vomiting
- Low-grade fever
- Lassitude
- Depression
- Delirium
- Behaviour changes

Signs

- Meningism (may be absent)
- Oculomotor palsies
- Papilloedema
- Depression of conscious level
- Focal hemisphere signs

Staging of severity

- Stage I (early): non-specific symptoms and signs without alteration of consciousness
- Stage II (intermediate): altered consciousness without coma or delirium *plus* minor focal neurological signs
- Stage III (advanced): stupor or coma, severe neurological deficits, seizures or abnormal movements

the meninges or brain substance adjacent to the CSF pathway. The brain is covered by a greenish, gelatinous exudate, especially around the base, and numerous scattered tubercles are found on the meninges.

Clinical features

The clinical features and staging criteria are listed in Box 25.68. Onset is much slower than in other bacterial meningitis – over 2–8 weeks. If untreated, tuberculous meningitis is fatal in a few weeks but complete recovery is usual if treatment is started at stage I (Box 25.68). When treatment is initiated later, the rate of death or serious neurological deficit may be as high as 30%.

Investigations

Lumbar puncture should be performed if the diagnosis is suspected. The CSF is under increased pressure. It is usually clear but, when allowed to stand, a fine clot ('spider web') may form. The fluid contains up to 500×10^6 cells/L, predominantly lymphocytes, but can contain neutrophils. There is a rise in

protein and a marked fall in glucose. The tubercle bacillus may be detected in a smear of the centrifuged deposit from the CSF but a negative result does not exclude the diagnosis. The CSF should be cultured but, as this result will not be known for up to 6 weeks, treatment must be started without waiting for confirmation. Brain imaging may show hydrocephalus, brisk meningeal enhancement on enhanced CT or MRI, and/or an intracranial tuberculoma.

Management

As soon as the diagnosis is made or strongly suspected, chemotherapy should be started using one of the regimens that include pyrazinamide, described on page 592. The use of glucocorticoids in addition to antituberculous therapy has been controversial. Recent evidence suggests that it improves mortality, especially if given early, but not focal neurological damage. Surgical ventricular drainage may be needed if obstructive hydrocephalus develops. Skilled nursing is essential during the acute phase of the illness, and adequate hydration and nutrition must be maintained.

Other forms of meningitis

Fungal meningitis (especially cryptococcosis; p. 302) usually occurs in patients who are immunosuppressed and is a recognised complication of HIV infection (p. 321). The CSF findings are similar to those of tuberculous meningitis, but the diagnosis can be confirmed by microscopy or specific serological tests.

In some areas, meningitis may be caused by spirochaetes (leptospirosis, Lyme disease and syphilis; pp. 257, 255 and 337), rickettsiae (typhus fever; p. 270) or protozoa (amoebiasis; p. 286).

Meningitis can also be due to non-infective pathologies. This is seen in recurrent aseptic meningitis resulting from systemic lupus erythematosus (SLE), Behçet's disease or sarcoidosis, as well as a condition of previously unknown origin known as Mollaret's syndrome, in which the recurrent meningitis is associated with epithelioid cells in the spinal fluid ('Mollaret' cells). Recent evidence suggests that this condition may be due to herpes simplex virus type 2 and is therefore infective after all. Meningitis can also be caused by direct invasion of the meninges by neoplastic cells ('malignant meningitis'; see Box 25.62).

Parenchymal viral infections

Infection of the substance of the nervous system will produce symptoms of focal dysfunction (deficits and/or seizures) with general signs of infection, depending on the acuteness of the infection and the type of organism.

Viral encephalitis

A range of viruses can cause encephalitis but only a minority of patients report recent systemic viral infection. In Europe, the most serious cause of viral encephalitis is herpes simplex (p. 247), which probably reaches the brain via the olfactory nerves. Varicella zoster is also an important cause. The development of effective therapy for some forms of encephalitis has increased the importance of clinical diagnosis and virological examination of the CSF. In some parts of the world, viruses transmitted by mosquitoes and ticks (arboviruses) are an important cause of encephalitis. The epidemiology of some of these infections is changing. Japanese encephalitis (p. 249) has spread relentlessly across Asia to Australia, and there have been outbreaks of West Nile encephalitis in Romania, Israel and New York. Zika virus has

25

mutated in the last decades and become a more significant global health problem. HIV may cause encephalitis with a subacute or chronic presentation but occasionally has an acute presentation with seroconversion.

Pathophysiology

The infection provokes an inflammatory response that involves the cortex, white matter, basal ganglia and brainstem. The distribution of lesions varies with the type of virus. For example, in herpes simplex encephalitis, the temporal lobes are usually primarily affected, whereas cytomegalovirus can involve the areas adjacent to the ventricles (ventriculitis). Inclusion bodies may be present in the neurons and glial cells, and there is an infiltration of polymorphonuclear cells in the perivascular space. There is neuronal degeneration and diffuse glial proliferation, often associated with cerebral oedema.

Clinical features

Viral encephalitis presents with acute onset of headache, fever, focal neurological signs (aphasia and/or hemiplegia, visual field defects) and seizures. Disturbance of consciousness ranging from drowsiness to deep coma supervenes early and may advance dramatically. Meningism occurs in many patients. Rabies presents a distinct clinical picture and is described below.

Investigations

Imaging by CT scan may show low-density lesions in the temporal lobes but MRI is more sensitive in detecting early abnormalities. Lumbar puncture should be performed once imaging has excluded a mass lesion. The CSF usually contains excess lymphocytes but polymorphonuclear cells may predominate in the early stages. The CSF may be normal in up to 10% of cases. Some viruses, including the West Nile virus, may cause a sustained neutrophilic CSF. The protein content may be elevated but the glucose is normal. The EEG is usually abnormal in the early stages, especially in herpes simplex encephalitis, with characteristic periodic slow-wave activity in the temporal lobes. Virological investigations of the CSF, including PCR, may reveal the causative organism but treatment initiation should not await this.

Management

Optimum treatment for herpes simplex encephalitis (aciclovir 10 mg/kg IV 3 times daily for 2–3 weeks) has reduced mortality from 70% to around 10%. This should be given early to all patients suspected of having viral encephalitis.

Some survivors will have residual epilepsy or cognitive impairment. For details of post-infectious encephalomyelitis, see page 1110. Antiepileptic treatment may be required (p. 1101) and raised intracranial pressure may indicate the need for dexamethasone.

Brainstem encephalitis

This presents with ataxia, dysarthria, diplopia or other cranial nerve palsies. The CSF is lymphocytic, with a normal glucose. The causative agent is presumed to be viral. However, *Listeria monocytogenes* may cause a similar syndrome with meningitis (and often a polymorphonuclear CSF pleocytosis) and requires specific treatment with ampicillin (500 mg 4 times daily; see Box 25.66).

Rabies

Rabies is caused by a rhabdovirus that infects the central nervous tissue and salivary glands of a wide range of mammals. It is usually conveyed by saliva through bites or licks on abrasions or on intact mucous membranes. Humans are most frequently infected from dogs and bats. In Europe, the maintenance host is the fox. The incubation period varies in humans from a minimum of 9 days to many months but is usually between 4 and 8 weeks. Severe bites, especially if on the head or neck, are associated with shorter incubation periods. Human rabies is a rare disease, even in endemic areas. However, because it is usually fatal, major efforts are directed at limiting its spread and preventing its importation into uninfected countries, such as the UK.

Clinical features

At the onset there may be fever, and paraesthesia at the site of the bite. A prodromal period of 1–10 days, during which the patient becomes increasingly anxious, leads to the characteristic 'hydrophobia'. Although the patient is thirsty, attempts at drinking provoke violent contractions of the diaphragm and other inspiratory muscles. Delusions and hallucinations may develop, accompanied by spitting, biting and mania, with lucid intervals in which the patient is markedly anxious. Cranial nerve lesions develop and terminal hyperpyrexia is common. Death ensues, usually within a week of the onset of symptoms.

Investigations

During life, the diagnosis is usually made on clinical grounds but rapid immunofluorescent techniques can detect antigen in corneal impression smears or skin biopsies.

Management

Established disease

Only a few patients with established rabies have survived. All received some post-exposure prophylaxis (see below) and needed intensive care facilities to control cardiac and respiratory failure. Otherwise, only palliative treatment is possible once symptoms have appeared. The patient should be heavily sedated with diazepam, supplemented by chlorpromazine if needed. Nutrition and fluids should be given intravenously or through a gastrostomy.

Pre-exposure prophylaxis

Pre-exposure prophylaxis is required by those who handle potentially infected animals professionally, work with rabies virus in laboratories or live at special risk in rabies-endemic areas. Protection is afforded by intradermal injections of human diploid cell strain vaccine, or two intramuscular injections given 4 weeks apart, followed by yearly boosters.

Post-exposure prophylaxis

The wounds should be thoroughly cleaned, preferably with a quaternary ammonium detergent or soap; damaged tissues should be excised and the wound left unsutured. Rabies can usually be prevented if treatment is started within a day or two of biting. Delayed treatment may still be of value. For maximum protection, hyperimmune serum and vaccine are required.

The safest antirabies antiserum is human rabies immunoglobulin. The dose is 20 IU/kg body weight; half is infiltrated around the bite and half is given intramuscularly at a different site from the vaccine. Hyperimmune animal serum may be used but hypersensitivity reactions, including anaphylaxis, are common.

The safest vaccine, free of complications, is human diploid cell strain vaccine; 1.0 mL is given intramuscularly on days 0, 3, 7, 14, 30 and 90. In developing countries, where human rabies globulin may not be obtainable, 0.1 mL of vaccine may be given intradermally into eight sites on day 1, with single boosters on days 7 and 28. Where human products are not available and when risk of rabies is slight (licks on the skin, or minor bites of covered arms or legs), it may be justifiable to delay starting treatment while observing the biting animal or awaiting examination of its brain, rather than use the older vaccine.

Poliomyelitis

Pathophysiology

Disease is caused by one of three polioviruses, which constitute a subgroup of the enteroviruses. Poliomyelitis has become much less common in developed countries following the widespread use of oral vaccines but is still a problem in the developing world, especially parts of Africa. Infection usually occurs through the nasopharynx.

The virus causes a lymphocytic meningitis and infects the grey matter of the spinal cord, brainstem and cortex. There is a particular propensity to damage anterior horn cells, especially in the lumbar segments.

Clinical features

The incubation period is 7–14 days. Figure 25.35 illustrates the various features of the infection. Many patients recover fully after the initial phase of a few days of mild fever and headache. In other individuals, after a week of well-being, there is a recurrence of pyrexia, headache and meningism. Weakness may start later in one muscle group and can progress to widespread paresis. Respiratory failure may supervene if intercostal muscles are paralysed or the medullary motor nuclei are involved. Epidemics vary widely in terms of the incidence of non-paralytic cases and in mortality rate. Death occurs from respiratory paralysis. Muscle weakness is maximal at the end of the first week and gradual recovery may then take place over several months. Muscles showing no signs of recovery after a month will probably not regain useful function. Second attacks are very rare but occasionally patients show late deterioration in muscle bulk and power many years after the initial infection (this is termed the 'post-polio syndrome').

Investigations

The CSF shows a lymphocytic pleocytosis, a rise in protein and a normal sugar content. Poliomyelitis virus may be cultured from CSF and stool.

Management

Established disease

In the early stages, bed rest is imperative because exercise appears to worsen the paralysis or precipitate it. At the onset of respiratory difficulties, a tracheostomy and ventilation are required. Subsequent treatment is by physiotherapy and orthopaedic measures.

Prophylaxis

Prevention of poliomyelitis is by immunisation with live (Sabin) vaccine. In developed countries where polio is now very rare, the live vaccine has been replaced by the killed vaccine in childhood immunisation schedules.

Herpes zoster (shingles)

Herpes zoster is the result of reactivation of the varicella zoster virus that has lain dormant in a nerve root ganglion following chickenpox earlier in life. Reactivation may be spontaneous (as usually occurs in the middle-aged or elderly) or due to immunosuppression (as in patients with diabetes, malignant disease or AIDS). Full details are given on page 239.

Subacute sclerosing panencephalitis

This is a rare, chronic, progressive and eventually fatal complication of measles, presumably a result of an inability of the nervous system to eradicate the virus. It occurs in children and adolescents, usually many years after the primary virus infection. There is generalised neurological deterioration and onset is insidious, with intellectual deterioration, apathy and clumsiness, followed by myoclonic jerks, rigidity and dementia.

The CSF may show a mild lymphocytic pleocytosis and the EEG demonstrates characteristic periodic bursts of triphasic waves. Although there is persistent measles-specific IgG in serum and CSF, antiviral therapy is ineffective and death ensues within a few years.

Progressive multifocal leucoencephalopathy

This was originally described as a rare complication of lymphoma, leukaemia or carcinomatosis but has become more frequent as a feature of AIDS (p. 319) or secondary to immunosuppression, e.g. following organ transplantation or use of disease-modifying drugs for MS. It is an infection of oligodendrocytes by human polyomavirus JC, causing widespread demyelination of the white matter of the cerebral hemispheres. Clinical signs include dementia, hemiparesis and aphasia, which progress rapidly, usually leading to death within weeks or months. Areas of low density in the white matter are seen on CT but MRI is more sensitive, showing diffuse high signal in the cerebral white matter on T2-weighted images. The only treatment available is restoration of the immune response (by treating AIDS or reversing immunosuppression).

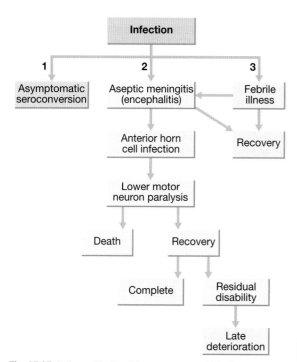

Fig. 25.35 Poliomyelitis. Possible consequences of infection.

25

Parenchymal bacterial infections

Cerebral abscess

Bacteria may enter the cerebral substance through penetrating injury, by direct spread from paranasal sinuses or the middle ear, or secondary to sepsis. Untreated congenital heart disease is a recognised risk factor. The site of abscess formation and the likely causative organism are both related to the source of infection (Box 25.69). Initial infection leads to local suppuration followed by loculation of pus within a surrounding wall of gliosis, which in a chronic abscess may form a tough capsule. Haematogenous spread may lead to multiple abscesses.

Clinical features

A cerebral abscess may present acutely with fever, headache, meningism and drowsiness, but more commonly presents over days or weeks as a cerebral mass lesion with little or no evidence of infection. Seizures, raised intracranial pressure and focal hemisphere signs occur alone or in combination. Distinction from a cerebral tumour may be impossible on clinical grounds.

Investigations

Lumbar puncture is potentially hazardous in the presence of raised intracranial pressure and CT should always precede it. CT reveals single or multiple low-density areas, which show ring enhancement with contrast and surrounding cerebral oedema (Fig. 25.36). There may be an elevated white blood cell count and ESR in patients with active local infection. The possibility of cerebral toxoplasmosis or tuberculous disease secondary to HIV infection (p. 320) should always be considered.

Management and prognosis

Antimicrobial therapy is indicated once the diagnosis is made. The likely source of infection should guide the choice of antibiotic (see Box 25.69). In neurosurgical patients, the addition of vancomycin should be considered. Surgical drainage by burr-hole aspiration or excision may be necessary, especially where the presence of a capsule may lead to a persistent focus of infection. Epilepsy frequently develops and is often resistant to treatment.

Despite advances in therapy, mortality remains 10–20% and may partly relate to delay in diagnosis and treatment.

Fig. 25.36 Right temporal cerebral abscess (arrows), with surrounding oedema and midline shift to the left. [A] Unenhanced computed tomography (CT) image. [B] Contrast-enhanced CT image.

i	25.69 Aetiology and treatment of bacterial cerebral abscess		
Site of abscess	**Source of infection**	**Likely organisms**	**Recommended treatment**
Frontal lobe	Paranasal sinuses Teeth	Streptococci Anaerobes	Cefotaxime 2–3 g IV 4 times daily *plus* Metronidazole 500 mg IV 3 times daily
Temporal lobe	Middle ear	Streptococci Enterobacteriaceae	Ampicillin 2–3 g IV 3 times daily *plus* Metronidazole 500 mg IV 3 times daily *plus either*
Cerebellum	Sphenoid sinus Mastoid/middle ear	*Pseudomonas* spp. Anaerobes	Ceftazidime 2 g IV 3 times daily *or* Gentamicin* 5 mg/kg IV daily
Any site	Penetrating trauma	Staphylococci	Flucloxacillin 2–3 g IV 4 times daily *or* Cefuroxime 1.5 g IV 3 times daily
Multiple	Metastatic and cryptogenic	Streptococci Anaerobes	Benzylpenicillin 1.8–2.4 g IV 4 times daily if endocarditis or cyanotic heart disease Otherwise cefotaxime 2–3 g IV 4 times daily *plus* Metronidazole 500 mg IV 3 times daily

*Monitor gentamicin levels.

Subdural empyema

This is a rare complication of frontal sinusitis, osteomyelitis of the skull vault or middle ear disease. A collection of pus in the subdural space spreads over the surface of the hemisphere, causing underlying cortical oedema or thrombophlebitis. Patients present with severe pain in the face or head and pyrexia, often with a history of preceding paranasal sinus or ear infection. The patient then becomes drowsy, with seizures and focal signs such as a progressive hemiparesis.

The diagnosis rests on a strong clinical suspicion in patients with a local focus of infection. Careful assessment with contrast-enhanced CT or MRI may show a subdural collection with underlying cerebral oedema. Management requires aspiration of pus via a burr hole and appropriate parenteral antibiotics. Any local source of infection must be treated to prevent re-infection.

Spinal epidural abscess

The characteristic clinical features are pain in a root distribution and progressive transverse spinal cord syndrome with paraparesis, sensory impairment and sphincter dysfunction. Features of the primary focus of infection may be less obvious and thus can be overlooked. The resurgence of resistant staphylococcal infection and intravenous drug misuse has contributed to a recent marked rise in incidence.

X-ray changes occur late, if present, so MRI or myelography should precede urgent neurosurgical intervention. Decompressive laminectomy with abscess drainage relieves the pressure on the dura. Organisms may be grown from the pus or blood. Surgery, together with appropriate antibiotics, may prevent complete and irreversible paraplegia.

Lyme disease

Infection with *Borrelia burgdorferi* can cause numerous neurological problems, including polyradiculopathy, meningitis, encephalitis and mononeuritis multiplex (p. 255).

Neurosyphilis

Neurosyphilis may present as an acute or chronic process and may involve the meninges, blood vessels and/or parenchyma of the brain and spinal cord. The decade to 2008 saw a 10-fold increase in the incidence of syphilis, mostly as a result of misguided relaxation of safe sex measures with the advent of effective antiretroviral treatments for AIDS. Paralleled future increases in neurosyphilis are inevitable. The clinical manifestations are diverse and early diagnosis and treatment are essential.

Clinical features

The clinical and pathological features of the three most common presentations are summarised in Box 25.70. Neurological examination reveals signs indicative of the anatomical localisation of lesions. Delusions of grandeur suggest general paresis of the insane, but more commonly there is simply progressive dementia. Small and irregular pupils that react to convergence but not light, as described by Argyll Robertson (see Box 25.22, p. 1092), may accompany any neurosyphilitic syndrome but most commonly tabes dorsalis.

Investigations

Routine screening for syphilis is warranted in many neurological patients. Treponemal antibodies (p. 338) are positive in the serum in most patients, but CSF examination is essential if neurological

25.70 Clinical and pathological features of neurosyphilis		
Type and interval from primary infection	Pathology	Clinical features
Meningovascular (5 years)*	Endarteritis obliterans Meningeal exudate Granuloma (gumma)	Stroke Cranial nerve palsies Seizures/mass lesion
General paralysis of the insane (5–15 years)*	Degeneration in cerebral cortex/ cerebral atrophy Thickened meninges	Dementia Tremor Bilateral upper motor signs
Tabes dorsalis (5–20 years)*	Degeneration of sensory neurons Wasting of dorsal columns Optic atrophy	Lightning pains Sensory ataxia Visual failure Abdominal crises Incontinence Trophic changes
Any of the above		Argyll Robertson pupils (p. 1092)

involvement is suspected. Active disease is suggested by an elevated cell count, usually lymphocytic, and the protein content may be elevated to 0.5–1.0 g/L with an increased gamma globulin fraction. Serological tests in CSF are usually positive but progressive disease can occur with negative CSF serology.

Management

The injection of procaine benzylpenicillin (procaine penicillin) and probenecid for 17 days is essential in the treatment of neurosyphilis of all types (p. 338). Further courses of penicillin must be given if symptoms are not relieved, if the condition continues to advance or if the CSF continues to show signs of active disease. The cell count returns to normal within 3 months of completion of treatment, but the elevated protein takes longer to subside and some serological tests may never revert to normal. Evidence of clinical progression at any time is an indication for renewed treatment.

Diseases caused by bacterial toxins

Tetanus

This disease results from infection with *Clostridium tetani*, a commensal in the gut of humans and domestic animals that is found in soil. Infection enters the body through wounds, which may be trivial. It is rare in the UK, occurring mostly in gardeners and farmers, but a recent increase has been seen in intravenous drug misusers. By contrast, the disease is common in many developing countries, where dust contains spores derived from animal and human excreta. Unhygienic practices soon after birth may lead to infection of the umbilical stump or site of circumcision, causing tetanus neonatorum. Tetanus is still one of the major killers of adults, children and neonates in developing countries, where the mortality rate can be nearly 100% in the newborn and around 40% in others.

In circumstances unfavourable to growth of the organism, spores are formed and these may remain dormant for years in the soil. Spores germinate and bacilli multiply only in the anaerobic conditions that occur in areas of tissue necrosis or if the oxygen tension is lowered by the presence of other organisms, particularly if aerobic. The bacilli remain localised but produce an exotoxin with an affinity for motor nerve endings and motor nerve cells.

25

The anterior horn cells are affected after the exotoxin has passed into the blood stream and their involvement results in rigidity and convulsions. Symptoms first appear from 2 days to several weeks after injury: the shorter the incubation period, the more severe the attack and the worse the prognosis.

Clinical features

By far the most important early symptom is trismus – spasm of the masseter muscles, which causes difficulty in opening the mouth and in masticating; hence the name 'lockjaw'. Lockjaw in tetanus is painless, unlike the spasm of the masseters due to dental abscess, septic throat or other causes. Conditions that can mimic tetanus include hysteria and phenothiazine overdosage, or overdose in intravenous drug misusers.

In tetanus, the tonic rigidity spreads to involve the muscles of the face, neck and trunk. Contraction of the frontalis and the muscles at the angles of the mouth leads to the so-called 'risus sardonicus'. There is rigidity of the muscles at the neck and trunk of varying degree. The back is usually slightly arched ('opisthotonus') and there is a board-like abdominal wall.

In the more severe cases, violent spasms lasting for a few seconds to 3–4 minutes occur spontaneously, or may be induced by stimuli such as movement or noise. These episodes are painful and exhausting, and suggest a grave outlook, especially if they appear soon after the onset of symptoms. They gradually increase in frequency and severity for about 1 week and the patient may die from exhaustion, asphyxia or aspiration pneumonia. In less severe illness, periods of spasm may not commence until a week or so after the first sign of rigidity, and in very mild infections they may never appear. Autonomic involvement may cause cardiovascular complications, such as hypertension. Rarely, the only manifestation of the disease may be 'local tetanus' – stiffness or spasm of the muscles near the infected wound – and the prognosis is good if treatment is commenced at this stage.

Investigations

The diagnosis is made on clinical grounds. It is rarely possible to isolate the infecting organism from the original locus of entry.

Management

Established disease

Management of established disease should begin as soon as possible, as shown in Box 25.71.

 25.71 Treatment of tetanus

Neutralise absorbed toxin

- Give IV injection of 3000 IU of human tetanus antitoxin

Prevent further toxin production

- Débride wound
- Give benzylpenicillin 600 mg IV 4 times daily (metronidazole if patient is allergic to penicillin)

Control spasms

- Nurse in a quiet room
- Avoid unnecessary stimuli
- Give IV diazepam
- If spasms continue, paralyse patient and ventilate

General measures

- Maintain hydration and nutrition
- Treat secondary infections

Prevention

Tetanus can be prevented by immunisation and prompt treatment of contaminated wounds by débridement and antibiotics. In patients with a contaminated wound, the immediate danger of tetanus can be greatly reduced by the injection of 1200 mg of penicillin followed by a 7-day course of oral penicillin. For those allergic to penicillin, erythromycin should be used. When the risk of tetanus is judged to be present, an intramuscular injection of 250 IU of human tetanus antitoxin should be given, along with toxoid, which should be repeated 1 month and 6 months later. For those already immunised, only a booster dose of toxoid is required.

Botulism

Botulism is caused by the neurotoxins of *Clostridium botulinum*, which are extremely potent and cause disease after ingestion of even picogram amounts. Its classical form is an acute onset of bilateral cranial neuropathies associated with symmetric descending weakness.

Anaerobic conditions are necessary for the organism's growth. It may contaminate and thrive in many foodstuffs, where sealing and preserving provide the requisite conditions. Contaminated honey has been implicated in infant botulism, in which the organism colonises the gastrointestinal tract. Wound botulism is a growing problem in injection drug-users.

The toxin causes predominantly bulbar and ocular palsies (difficulty in swallowing, blurred or double vision, ptosis), progressing to limb weakness and respiratory paralysis. Criteria for the clinical diagnosis are shown in Box 25.72.

 25.72 US Centers for Disease Control (CDC) definition of botulism

Three main syndromes

- Infantile
- Food-borne
- Wound infection

Clinical features

- Absence of fever
- Symmetrical neurological deficits
- Patient remains responsive
- Normal or slow heart rate and normal blood pressure
- No sensory deficits with the exception of blurred vision

Management includes assisted ventilation and general supportive measures until the toxin eventually dissociates from nerve endings 6–8 weeks following ingestion. A polyvalent antitoxin is available for post-exposure prophylaxis and for the treatment of suspected botulism. It specifically neutralises toxin types A, B and E and is not effective against infantile botulism (in which active growth of the organism allows continued toxin production).

Prion diseases

Prions are unique amongst infectious agents in that they are devoid of any nucleic acid. They appear to be transmitted by acquisition of a normal mammalian protein (prion protein, PrP^C) that is in an abnormal conformation (PrP^{SC}, containing an excess of beta-sheet protein); the abnormal protein inhibits the 26S

25.73 Prion diseases affecting humans

Disease	Mechanism
Creutzfeldt–Jakob disease	
Sporadic	Unknown: spontaneous PrP^C to PrP^{SC} conversion or somatic mutation
Familial	Genetic: mutations in the *PrP* gene
Variant	Dietary ingestion: infection from bovine spongiform encephalopathy
Gerstmann–Sträussler–Scheinker disease	Genetic: mutations in the *PrP* gene
Fatal familial insomnia	Genetic: mutations in the *PrP* gene
Sporadic fatal insomnia	Genetic: spontaneous PrP^C to PrP^{SC} conversion or somatic mutation
Kuru	Dietary: ingestion of affected human brain

proteasome, which can degrade misfolded proteins, leading to accumulation of the abnormally configured PrP^{SC} protein instead of normal PrP^C. The result is accumulation of protein that forms amyloid in the CNS, causing a transmissible spongiform encephalopathy (TSE) across several species.

Human prion diseases (Box 25.73) are characterised by the histopathological triad of cortical spongiform change, neuronal cell loss and gliosis. Associated with these changes there is deposition of amyloid, made up of an altered form of a normally occurring protein, the prion protein. Prion proteins are not inactivated by cooking or conventional sterilisation, and transmission is thought to occur by consumption of infected CNS tissue or by inoculation (e.g. via depth EEG electrodes, corneal grafts, cadaveric dura mater grafts and pooled cadaveric growth hormone preparations). The same diseases can occur in an inherited form, due to mutations in the *PrP* gene.

The apparent transmission of bovine spongiform encephalopathy (BSE) to humans was thought to be responsible for the emergence of a new variant of CJD (vCJD) in the UK (see below). This outbreak led to nationwide precautionary measures, such as leucodepletion of all blood used for transfusion, and the mandatory use of disposable surgical instruments wherever possible for tonsillectomy, appendicectomy and ophthalmological procedures.

Creutzfeldt–Jakob disease

Creutzfeldt–Jakob disease (CJD) is the best-characterised human TSE. Some 10% of cases arise from a mutation in the gene coding for the prion protein. The sporadic form is the most common, occurring in middle-aged to elderly patients. Clinical features usually involve a rapidly progressive dementia, with myoclonus and a characteristic EEG pattern (repetitive slow-wave complexes), although a number of other features, such as visual disturbance or ataxia, may also be seen. These are particularly common in CJD transmitted by inoculation (e.g. by infected dura mater grafts). Death occurs after a mean of 4–6 months. There is no effective treatment.

Variant Creutzfeldt–Jakob disease

This type of CJD (vCJD) emerged in the late 1990s, affecting a small number of patients in the UK. The causative agent appears to be identical to that causing BSE in cows, and the disease may have been a result of the epidemic of BSE in the UK a decade

Fig. 25.37 Magnetic resonance imaging in variant Creutzfeldt–Jakob disease. Arrows indicate bilateral pulvinar hyperintensity.

earlier. Patients affected by vCJD are typically younger than those with sporadic CJD and present with neuropsychiatric changes and sensory symptoms in the limbs, followed by ataxia, dementia and death. Progression is slightly slower than in patients with sporadic CJD (mean time to death is over a year). Characteristic EEG changes are not present, but MRI brain scans show characteristic high-signal changes in the pulvinar thalami in a high proportion of cases (Fig. 25.37). Brain histology is distinct, with very florid plaques containing the prion proteins. Abnormal prion protein has been identified in tonsil specimens from patients with vCJD, leading to the suggestion that the disease could be transmitted by reticulo-endothelial tissue (like TSEs in animals but unlike sporadic CJD in humans). It was the emergence of this form of the disorder that led to the changes in public health and farming policy in the UK; while the incidence of vCJD has declined dramatically, surveillance and research continue.

Intracranial mass lesions and raised intracranial pressure

Many different types of mass lesion may arise within the intracranial cavity (Box 25.74). In developing countries tuberculoma and other infections are frequent causes, but in the West intracranial haemorrhage and brain tumours are more common. The clinical features depend on the site of the mass, its nature and its rate of expansion. Symptoms and signs (see Box 25.75) are produced by a number of mechanisms.

Raised intracranial pressure

Raised intracranial pressure (RICP) may be caused by mass lesions, cerebral oedema, obstruction to CSF circulation leading

25

i 25.74 Common causes of raised intracranial pressure

Mass lesions

- Intracranial haemorrhage (traumatic or spontaneous):
  - Extradural haematoma
  - Subdural haematoma
  - Intracerebral haemorrhage
- Cerebral tumour (particularly posterior fossa lesions or high-grade gliomas: see Box 25.76)
- Infective:
  - Cerebral abscess
  - Tuberculoma
  - Cysticercosis (p. 298)
  - Hydatid cyst (p. 299)
- Colloid cyst (in ventricles)

Disturbance of cerebrospinal fluid circulation

- Obstructive (non-communicating) hydrocephalus: obstruction within ventricular system
- Communicating hydrocephalus: site of obstruction outside ventricular system

Obstruction to venous sinuses

- Cerebral venous thrombosis
- Trauma (depressed fractures overlying sinuses)

Diffuse brain oedema or swelling

- Meningo-encephalitis
- Trauma (diffuse head injury, near-drowning)
- Subarachnoid haemorrhage
- Metabolic (e.g. water intoxication)
- Idiopathic intracranial hypertension

i 25.75 Clinical features of intracranial mass lesions

Presentation	Features
Seizures	Focal onset ± generalised spread
Focal symptoms	Progressive loss of function Weakness Numbness Dysphasia Cranial neuropathy
False localising signs	Unilateral/bilateral 6th nerve palsies Contralateral 3rd nerve (usually pupil first)
Raised intracranial pressure (usually aggressive tumours causing vasogenic oedema or obstructive hydrocephalus)	Headache worse on lying/straining Vomiting Diplopia (6th nerve involvement) Papilloedema Bradycardia, raised blood pressure Impaired conscious level
Stroke/TIA-like symptoms	Acute haemorrhage into tumour Paroxysmal 'tumour attacks'
Cognitive/behavioural change	Usually frontal mass lesions
Endocrine abnormalities	Pituitary tumours
Incidental finding	Asymptomatic but identified on imaging (meningiomas commonly)

(TIA = transient ischaemic attack)

to hydrocephalus, impaired CSF absorption and cerebral venous obstruction (see Box 25.74).

Clinical features

In adults, intracranial pressure is less than 10–15 mmHg. The features of RICP are listed in Box 25.75. The speed of pressure increase influences presentation. If slow, compensatory mechanisms may occur, including alteration in the volume of fluid in CSF spaces and venous sinuses, minimising symptoms. Rapid pressure increase (as in aggressive tumours) does not permit these compensatory mechanisms to take place, leading to early symptoms, including sudden death. Papilloedema is not always present, either because the pressure rise has been too rapid or because of anatomical anomalies of the meningeal sheath of the optic nerve.

A false localising sign is one in which the pathology is remote from the site of the expected lesion; in RICP, the 6th cranial nerve (unilateral or bilateral) is most commonly affected but the 3rd, 5th and 7th nerves may also be involved. Sixth nerve palsies are thought to be due either to stretching of the long slender nerve or to compression against the petrous temporal bone ridge. Transtentorial herniation of the uncus may compress the ipsilateral 3rd nerve and usually involves the pupillary fibres first, causing a dilated pupil; however, a false localising contralateral 3rd nerve palsy may also occur, perhaps due to extrinsic compression by the tentorial margin. Vomiting, coma, bradycardia and arterial hypertension are later features of RICP.

The rise in intracranial pressure from a mass lesion may cause displacement of the brain. Downward displacement of the medial temporal lobe (uncus) through the tentorium due to

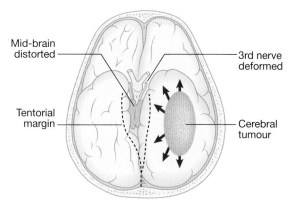

Fig. 25.38 Cerebral tumour displacing medial temporal lobe and causing pressure on the mid-brain and 3rd cranial nerve.

a large hemisphere mass may cause 'temporal coning' (Fig. 25.38). This may stretch the 3rd and/or 6th cranial nerves or cause pressure on the contralateral cerebral peduncle (giving rise to ipsilateral upper motor neuron signs), and is usually accompanied by progressive coma. Downward movement of the cerebellar tonsils through the foramen magnum may compress the medulla – 'tonsillar coning' (Fig. 25.39). This may result in brainstem haemorrhage and/or acute obstruction of the CSF pathways. As coning progresses, coma and death occur unless the condition is rapidly treated.

Management

Primary management of RICP should be targeted at relieving the cause (e.g. surgical decompression of mass lesion, glucocorticoids to reduce vasogenic oedema or shunt procedure to relieve hydrocephalus). Supportive treatment includes maintenance of

Fig. 25.39 Tonsillar cone. Downward displacement of the cerebellar tonsils below the level of the foramen magnum.

fluid balance, blood pressure control, head elevation, and use of diuretics such as mannitol. Intensive care support may be needed (p. 208).

Brain tumours

Primary brain tumours are a heterogeneous collection of neoplasms arising from the brain tissue or meninges, and vary from benign to highly malignant. Primary malignant brain tumours (Box 25.76) are rare, accounting for 1% of all adult tumours but a higher proportion in children. The most common benign brain tumour is a meningioma. Primary brain tumours do not metastasise due to the absence of lymphatic drainage in the brain. There are rare pathological subtypes, however, such as medulloblastoma, which do have a propensity to metastasise; the reasons for this are not clear. Most cerebral tumours are sporadic but may be associated with genetic syndromes such as neurofibromatosis or tuberous sclerosis. Brain tumours are not classified by the usual TNM system but by the World Health Organisation (WHO) grading I–IV; this is based on histology (e.g. nuclear pleomorphism, presence of mitoses and presence of necrosis), with grade I the most benign and grade IV the most malignant. Gliomas account for 60% of brain tumours, with the aggressive glioblastoma multiforme (WHO grade IV) the most common glioma, followed by meningiomas (20%) and pituitary tumours (10%). Although the lower-grade gliomas (I and II) may be very indolent, with prognosis measured in terms of many years, these may transform to higher-grade disease at any time, with a resultant sharp decline in life expectancy.

Most malignant brain tumours are due to metastases, with intracranial metastases complicating about 20% of extracranial malignancies. The rate is higher with primaries in the bronchus, breast and gastrointestinal tract (Fig. 25.40). Metastases usually occur in the white matter of the cerebral or cerebellar hemispheres but there are diffuse leptomeningeal types.

Clinical features

The presentation is variable and usually influenced by the rate of growth. High-grade disease (WHO grades III and IV) tends to present with a short (weeks) history of mass effect (headache, nausea secondary to RICP), while more indolent tumours can present with slowly progressive focal neurological deficits, depending on their location (see Box 25.75); generalised or focal seizures are common in either. Headache, if present, is usually accompanied by focal deficits or seizures, and

25.76 Primary brain tumours		
Histological type	Common site	Age
Malignant		
Glioma (astrocytoma)	Cerebral hemisphere	Adulthood
	Cerebellum	Childhood/adulthood
	Brainstem	Childhood/young adulthood
Oligodendroglioma	Cerebral hemisphere	Adulthood
Medulloblastoma	Posterior fossa	Childhood
Ependymoma	Posterior fossa	Childhood/adolescence
Cerebral lymphoma	Cerebral hemisphere	Adulthood
Benign		
Meningioma	Cortical dura	Adulthood (often incidental finding)
	Parasagittal	
	Sphenoid ridge	
	Suprasellar	
	Olfactory groove	
Neurofibroma	Acoustic neuroma	Adulthood
Craniopharyngioma	Suprasellar	Childhood/adolescence
Pituitary adenoma	Pituitary fossa	Adulthood
Colloid cyst	Third ventricle	Any age
Pineal tumours	Quadrigeminal cistern	Childhood (teratomas) Young adulthood (germ cell)

Fig. 25.40 Contrast-enhanced computed tomogram of the head showing a large metastasis within the left hemisphere (large arrow). There is surrounding cerebral oedema, and a smaller metastasis (small arrow) within the wall of the right lateral ventricle. The primary lesion was a lung carcinoma.

isolated stable headache is almost never due to intracranial tumour.

The size of the primary tumour is of far less prognostic significance than its location within the brain. Tumours within the brainstem will result in early neurological deficits, while those in the frontal region may be quite large before symptoms occur.

Fig. 25.41 Magnetic resonance image showing a meningioma in the frontal lobe (arrow A) with associated oedema (arrow B).

Investigations

Diagnosis is by neuroimaging (Figs 25.41 and 25.42) and pathological grading following biopsy or resection where possible. The more malignant tumours are more likely to demonstrate contrast enhancement on imaging. If the tumour appears metastatic, further investigation to find the primary is required.

Management

Brain tumours are treated with a combination of surgery, radiotherapy and chemotherapy, depending on the type of tumour and the patient. Advancing age is the most powerful negative prognostic factor in CNS tumours, so best supportive care (including glucocorticoid therapy) may be most appropriate in older patients with metastases or high-grade disease. Treatment may not always be indicated in low-grade gliomas and watchful waiting may be appropriate, although a more aggressive approach is increasingly favoured.

Dexamethasone given orally (or intravenously where RICP is acutely or severely raised) may reduce the vasogenic oedema typically associated with metastases and high-grade gliomas.

Prolactin- or growth hormone-secreting pituitary adenomas (p. 683) may respond well to treatment with dopamine agonists (such as bromocriptine, cabergoline or quinagolide); in this situation, imaging and hormone levels may be all that is required to establish a formal diagnosis, precluding the need for surgery.

Surgical

The mainstay of primary treatment is surgery, either resection (full or partial debulking) or biopsy, depending on the site and likely radiological diagnosis. Clearly, if a tumour occurs in an area of brain that is highly important for normal function (e.g. motor strip), then biopsy may be the only safe surgical intervention but, in general, maximal safe resection is the optimal surgical management. Meningiomas and acoustic neuromas offer the best prospects for complete removal and thus cure. Some meningiomas can recur, however, particularly those of

Fig. 25.42 Magnetic resonance image of an acoustic neuroma (arrows) in the posterior fossa compressing the brainstem. [A] Axial image. [B] Coronal image.

the sphenoid ridge, when partial excision is often all that is possible. Thereafter, post-operative surveillance may be required, as radiotherapy is effective at preventing further growth of residual tumour. Pituitary adenomas may be removed by a trans-sphenoidal route, avoiding the need for a craniotomy. Unfortunately, gliomas, which account for the majority of brain tumours, cannot be completely excised, since infiltration spreads well beyond the apparent radiological boundaries of the intracranial mass. Recurrence is therefore the rule, even if the mass of the tumour is apparently removed completely; partial excision ('debulking') may be useful in alleviating symptoms caused by RICP, but although there is increasing evidence that the degree of surgical excision may have a positive influence on survival, this has not yet been convincingly demonstrated.

Radiotherapy and chemotherapy

In the majority of primary CNS tumours, radiation and chemotherapy are used to control disease and extend survival rather than for cure. Meningioma and pituitary adenoma offer the best chance of life-long remission. The gliomas are incurable; high-grade, WHO grade IV disease still carries a median survival of just over 1 year. In this situation, patient and family should always be involved in decisions regarding treatment. The diagnosis, and often the symptoms, are devastating, and support from palliative care and social work is crucial at an early stage. In WHO grade III disease, prognosis is a little better (2–4 years), and in rarer, more indolent tumours very prolonged survival is possible.

Advances have been made recently in terms of therapeutic outcome. Standard care for WHO grade IV glioblastoma multiforme is now combination radiotherapy with temozolomide chemotherapy; although this improves median survival of the population from only 12 to 14.5 months, up to 25% of patients survive for more than 2 years (compared to approximately 10% with radiotherapy alone). Ten percept will survive more than 5 years with temozolomide (virtually unheard of with radiotherapy alone). Benefits are more likely in well-debulked patients who are younger and fitter. Implantation of chemotherapy gives a small survival benefit.

Understanding of the molecular biology of brain tumours has allowed the use of biomarkers to guide therapy and prognostic discussions. In patients with methylation of the promoter region of the *MGMT* (methyl guanine methyl transferase) gene (about 30% of the population), 2-year survival is almost 50%. MGMT reduces the cytotoxicity of temozolomide and this mutation also reduces the enzyme's activity, rendering the tumour more sensitive to chemotherapy. In grade II and III gliomas, the presence of the loss of heterozygosity (LOH) 1p19q chromosomal abnormality confers chemosensitivity and thus improves prognosis. The presence of a rare mutation in the *IDH-1* (isocitrate dehydrogenase) gene confers a more favourable prognosis in patients with glioblastoma.

There is a small group of highly malignant grade IV tumours that can be cured with aggressive therapy. Medulloblastomas have a good chance of long-term remission with maximal surgery followed by irradiation of the whole brain and spine; younger patients may also benefit from concomitant and adjuvant chemotherapy. Older patients do not tolerate this, however.

Once tumours relapse, chemotherapy response rates are low and survival is short in high-grade disease. In the more uncommon low-grade tumours, repeated courses of chemotherapy can result in much more prolonged survival.

In metastatic disease, radiotherapy offers a modest improvement in survival but with costs in terms of quality of life; treatment therefore needs careful discussion with the patient. Benefits may be superior in breast cancer but there is little to separate other pathologies. Occasional chemosensitive cancers, such as small-cell lung cancer, may benefit from systemic chemotherapy but intracerebral metastases represent a late stage of disease and have a short prognosis.

Prognosis

The WHO histological grading system is a powerful predictor of prognosis in primary CNS tumours, though it does not yet take account of individual biomarkers. For each tumour type and grade, advancing age and deteriorating functional status are the next most important negative prognostic features. The overall 5-year survival rate of about 14% in adults masks a wide variation that depends on tumour type.

Acoustic neuroma

This is a benign tumour of Schwann cells of the 8th cranial nerve, which may arise in isolation or as part of neurofibromatosis type

2 (see below). When sporadic, acoustic neuroma occurs after the third decade and is more frequent in females. The tumour commonly arises near the nerve's entry point into the medulla or in the internal auditory meatus, usually on the vestibular division. Acoustic neuromas account for 80–90% of tumours at the cerebellopontine angle.

Clinical features

Acoustic neuroma typically presents with unilateral progressive hearing loss, sometimes with tinnitus. Vertigo is an unusual symptom, as slow growth allows compensatory brainstem mechanisms to develop. In some cases, progressive enlargement leads to distortion of the brainstem and/or cerebellar peduncle, causing ataxia and/or cerebellar signs in the limbs. Distortion of the fourth ventricle and cerebral aqueduct may cause hydrocephalus (see below), which may be the presenting feature. Facial weakness is unusual at presentation but facial palsy may follow surgical removal of the tumour. The tumour may be identified incidentally on cranial imaging.

Investigations

MRI is the investigation of choice (see Fig. 25.42).

Management

Surgery is the treatment of choice. If the tumour can be completely removed, the prognosis is excellent, although deafness is a common complication of surgery. Stereotactic radiosurgery (radiotherapy) may be appropriate for some lesions.

Neurofibromatosis

Neurofibromatosis encompasses two clinically and genetically separate conditions, with an autosomal dominant pattern of inheritance. The more common neurofibromatosis type 1 (NF1) is caused by mutations in the *NF1* gene on chromosome 17, half of which are new mutations. NF1 is characterised by neurofibromas (benign peripheral nerve sheath tumours) and skin involvement (Fig. 25.43), and may affect numerous systems (Box 25.77).

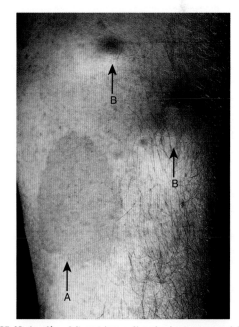

Fig. 25.43 A café au lait spot (arrow A) and subcutaneous nodules (arrows B) on the forearm of a patient with neurofibromatosis type 1.

25

25.77 Neurofibromatosis types 1 and 2: clinical features	
Neurofibromatosis 1	**Neurofibromatosis 2**
Skin	
Cutaneous/subcutaneous neurofibromas	Much less commonly affected than in NF1
Angiomas	Café au lait patches (usually
Café au lait patches (>6)	<6)
Axillary/groin freckling	Cutaneous schwannomas:
Hypopigmented patches	plaque lesions
	Subcutaneous schwannomas
Eyes	
Lisch nodules (iris fibromas)	Cataracts
Glaucoma	Retinal hamartoma
Congenital ptosis	Optic nerve meningioma
Nervous system	
Plexiform neurofibromas	Vestibular schwannomas
Malignant peripheral nerve sheath	Cranial nerve schwannomas
tumours	(not 1 and 2)
Aqueduct stenosis	Spinal schwannomas
Slight tonsillar descent	Peripheral nerve
Cognitive impairment	schwannomas
Epilepsy	Cranial meningiomas
	Spinal meningiomas
	Spinal/brainstem
	ependymomas
	Spinal/cranial astrocytoma
Bone	
Scoliosis	
Osteoporosis	
Pseudoarthrosis	
Cardiorespiratory systems	
Pulmonary stenosis	
Hypertension	
Renal artery stenosis	
Compression from neurofibroma causing restrictive lung defect	
Gastrointestinal system	
Gastrointestinal stromal tumour (GIST)	
Duodenal/ampullary neuro-endocrine tumour	

Neurofibromatosis type 2 (NF2) is caused by mutations of the *NF2* gene on chromosome 22, and is characterised by schwannomas (benign peripheral nerve sheath tumours comprising Schwann cells only) with little skin involvement; the clinical manifestations are more restricted to the eye and nervous system (Box 25.77). Malignant change may occur in NF1 neurofibromas but is rare in NF2 schwannomas. The prevalence of NF1 and NF2 is about 20–50 per 100 000 and 1.5 per 100 000, respectively.

Von Hippel–Lindau disease

This rare autosomal dominant disease is caused by mutations of the *VHL* tumour suppressor gene on chromosome 3. It promotes development of tumours affecting the kidney, adrenal gland, CNS, eye, inner ear, epididymis and pancreas, which may undergo malignant change. Benign haemangiomas and haemangioblastomas affect about 80% of patients, and are mostly cerebellar and retinal.

Paraneoplastic neurological disease

Paraneoplastic neurological syndromes often present before the underlying tumour declares itself and cause considerable disability. They are discussed in full on page 1110.

Hydrocephalus

Hydrocephalus is the excessive accumulation of CSF within the brain, and may be caused either by increased CSF production, by reduced CSF absorption, or by obstruction of the circulation (Fig. 25.44). Symptoms range from none to sudden death, depending on the speed at which and degree to which hydrocephalus develops. The causes are listed in Box 25.78. The terms 'communicating' and 'non-communicating' (also known as obstructive) hydrocephalus refer to blockage either outside or within the ventricular system, respectively (Fig. 25.45).

Normal pressure hydrocephalus

Normal pressure hydrocephalus (NPH) is a controversial entity, said to involve intermittent rises in CSF pressure, particularly at night. It is described in old age as being associated with a triad of gait apraxia, dementia and urinary incontinence.

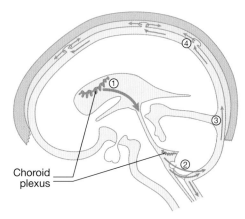

Choroid plexus

Fig. 25.44 The circulation of cerebrospinal fluid (CSF). (1) CSF is synthesised in the choroid plexus of the ventricles and flows from the lateral and third ventricles through the aqueduct to the fourth ventricle. (2) At the foramina of Luschka and Magendie it exits the brain, flowing over the hemispheres (3) and down around the spinal cord and roots in the subarachnoid space. (4) It is then absorbed into the dural venous sinuses via the arachnoid villi.

25.78 Causes of hydrocephalus	
Congenital malformations	
• Aqueduct stenosis	• Vein of Galen aneurysms
• Chiari malformations	• Congenital central nervous
• Dandy–Walker syndrome	system infections
• Benign intracranial cysts	• Craniofacial anomalies
Acquired causes	
• Mass lesions (especially those in the posterior fossa)	• Haematoma
• Tumour	• Absorption blockages due to:
• Colloid cyst of third ventricle	Inflammation (e.g.
• Abscess	meningitis, sarcoidosis)
	Intracranial haemorrhage

Fig. 25.45 Magnetic resonance image of hydrocephalus due to aqueduct stenosis. [A] Axial T2-weighted image (cerebrospinal fluid appears white): note the dilated lateral ventricles. [B] Sagittal T1-weighted image (cerebrospinal fluid appears black): note the dilated ventricles (top arrow) and narrowed aqueduct (bottom arrow).

Management

Diversion of the CSF by means of a shunt placed between the ventricular system and the peritoneal cavity or right atrium may result in rapid relief of symptoms in obstructive hydrocephalus. The outcome of shunting in NPH is much less predictable and, until a good response can be predicted, the management of individual cases will remain uncertain.

Idiopathic intracranial hypertension

This usually occurs in obese young women. The annual incidence is about 3 per 100 000. RICP occurs in the absence of a structural lesion, hydrocephalus or other identifiable cause. The aetiology is uncertain but there is an association with obesity in females, perhaps inducing a defect of CSF reabsorption by the arachnoid villi. A number of drugs may be associated, including tetracycline, vitamin A and retinoid derivatives.

Clinical features

The usual presentation is with headache, sometimes accompanied by diplopia and visual disturbance (most commonly, transient obscurations of vision associated with changes in posture). Clinical examination reveals papilloedema but little else. False localising cranial nerve palsies (usually of the 6th nerve) may be present. It is important to record visual fields accurately for future monitoring.

Investigations

Brain imaging is required to exclude a structural or other cause (e.g. cerebral venous sinus thrombosis, p. 1162). The ventricles are typically normal in size or small ('slit' ventricles). The diagnosis may be confirmed by lumbar puncture, which shows raised normal CSF constituents at increased pressure (usually >30 cmH$_2$O CSF).

Management

Management can be difficult and there is no evidence to support any specific treatment. Weight loss in overweight patients may be helpful if it can be achieved. Acetazolamide or topiramate may help to lower intracranial pressure, the latter perhaps aiding weight loss in some patients. Repeated lumbar puncture is an effective treatment for headache but may be technically difficult in obese individuals and is often poorly tolerated. Patients failing to respond, in whom chronic papilloedema threatens vision, may require optic nerve sheath fenestration or a lumbo-peritoneal shunt.

Head injury

Diagnosis of head trauma is usually clear – either from the history or from signs of external trauma to the head. Brain injury is more likely with skull fracture but can occur without. Individual cranial nerves may be damaged in fractures of the facial bones or skull base. Intracranial effects can be substantial and take several forms: extradural haematoma (collection of blood between the skull and dura); subdural haematoma (collection of blood between the dura and the surface of the brain); intracerebral haematoma; or diffuse axonal injury.

Whatever pathology occurs, the resultant RICP may lead to coning (see Figs 25.38 and 25.39). Haematomas are identified by CT and management is by surgical drainage, usually via a burr hole. Penetrating skull fractures lead to increased infection risk. Long-term sequelae include headache, cognitive decline and depression, all contributing to significant social, work, personality and family difficulties.

Subdural haematoma may occur spontaneously, particularly in patients on anticoagulants, in old age, and with alcohol misuse. There may or may not be a history of trauma. Patients present with subacute impairment of brain function, both globally (obtundation and coma) and focally (hemiparesis, seizures). Headache may not be present. The diagnosis should always be considered in those who present with reduced conscious level.

Beyond the immediate consequences of brain injury, there is increasing suspicion of long-term consequences, including dementia, postulated after either single (moderate or severe) injuries or even after multiple mild injuries, such as in boxers. If substantiated, this would encourage more effort to go into prevention of repeated brain injury in sporting contexts.

25

Disorders of cerebellar function

Cerebellar dysfunction can manifest as incoordination of limb function, gait ataxia (p. 1087), speech or eye movements. Acute dysfunction may be caused by alcohol or prescription drugs (especially the sodium channel-blocking antiepileptic drugs phenytoin and carbamazepine).

Inflammatory changes in the cerebellum may cause symptoms in the aftermath of some infections (especially herpes zoster) or as a paraneoplastic phenomenon. The hereditary spinocerebellar ataxias are described on page 1115; they manifest as progressive ataxias in middle and old age, often with other neurological features that aid specific diagnosis.

Disorders of the spine and spinal cord

The spinal cord and spinal roots may be affected by intrinsic disease or by disorders of the surrounding meninges and bones. The clinical presentation of these conditions depends on the anatomical level at which the cord or roots are affected, as well as the nature of the pathological process involved. It is important to recognise when the spinal cord is at risk of compression (p. 1136) so that urgent action can be taken.

Cervical spondylosis

Cervical spondylosis is the result of osteoarthritis in the cervical spine. It is characterised by degeneration of the intervertebral discs and osteophyte formation. Such 'wear and tear' is extremely common and radiological changes are frequently found in asymptomatic individuals over the age of 50. Spondylosis may be associated with neurological dysfunction. In order of frequency, the C5/6, C6/7 and C4/5 vertebral levels affect C6, C7 and C5 roots, respectively (Fig. 25.46).

Cervical radiculopathy

Acute onset of compression of a nerve root occurs when a disc prolapses laterally. More gradual onset may be due to osteophytic encroachment of the intervertebral foramina.

Clinical features

The patient complains of pain in the neck that may radiate in the distribution of the affected nerve root. The neck is held rigidly and neck movements may exacerbate pain. Paraesthesia and sensory loss may be found in the affected segment and there may be lower motor neuron signs, including weakness, wasting and reflex impairment (Fig. 25.47).

Investigations

Where there is no trauma, imaging should not be carried out for isolated cervical pain. MRI is the investigation of choice in those with radicular symptoms. X-rays offer limited benefit, except in excluding destructive lesions, and electrophysiological studies rarely add to clinical examination with MRI.

Management

Conservative treatment with analgesics and physiotherapy results in resolution of symptoms in the great majority of patients, but a few require surgery in the form of discectomy or radicular decompression.

Cervical myelopathy

Dorsomedial herniation of a disc and the development of transverse bony bars or posterior osteophytes may result in pressure on the spinal cord or the anterior spinal artery, which supplies the anterior two-thirds of the cord (see Fig. 25.46).

Fig. 25.46 Magnetic resonance image showing cervical cord compression (arrow) in cervical spondylosis.

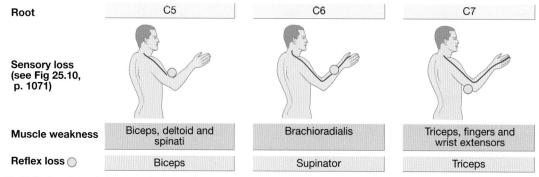

Fig. 25.47 Findings in cervical nerve root compression.

Clinical features

The onset is usually insidious and painless but acute deterioration may occur after trauma, especially hyperextension injury. Upper motor neuron signs develop in the limbs, with spasticity of the legs usually appearing before the arms are involved. Sensory loss in the upper limbs is common, producing tingling, numbness and proprioception loss in the hands, with progressive clumsiness. Sensory manifestations in the legs are much less common. Neurological deficit usually progresses gradually and disturbance of micturition is a very late feature.

Investigations

MRI (see Fig. 25.46) (or rarely myelography) will direct surgical intervention. The former provides information on the state of the spinal cord at the level of compression.

Management

Surgical procedures, including laminectomy and anterior discectomy, may arrest progression of disability but neurological improvement is not the rule. The decision as to whether surgery should be undertaken may be difficult. Manual manipulation of the cervical spine is of no proven benefit and may precipitate acute neurological deterioration.

Prognosis

The prognosis of cervical myelopathy is variable. In many patients, the condition stabilises or even improves without intervention. If progression results in sphincter dysfunction or pyramidal signs, surgical decompression should be considered.

Lumbar spondylosis

This term covers degenerative disc disease and osteoarthritic change in the lumbar spine. Pain in the distribution of the lumbar or sacral roots ('sciatica') is almost always due to disc protrusion but can be a feature of other rare but important disorders, including spinal tumour, malignant disease in the pelvis and tuberculosis of the vertebral bodies.

Lumbar disc herniation

While acute lumbar disc herniation is often precipitated by trauma (usually lifting heavy weights while the spine is flexed), genetic factors may also be important. The nucleus pulposus may bulge or rupture through the annulus fibrosus, giving rise to pressure on nerve endings in the spinal ligaments, changes in the vertebral joints or pressure on nerve roots.

Pathophysiology

The altered mechanics of the lumbar spine result in loss of lumbar lordosis and there may be spasm of the paraspinal musculature. Root pressure is suggested by limitation of flexion of the hip on the affected side if the straight leg is raised (Lasègue's sign). If the third or fourth lumbar root is involved, Lasègue's sign may be negative, but pain in the back may be induced by hyperextension of the hip (femoral nerve stretch test). The roots most frequently affected are S1, L5 and L4; the signs of root pressure at these levels are summarised in Figure 25.48.

Clinical features

The onset may be sudden or gradual. Alternatively, repeated episodes of low back pain may precede sciatica by months or years. Constant aching pain is felt in the lumbar region and may radiate to the buttock, thigh, calf and foot. Pain is exacerbated by coughing or straining but may be relieved by lying flat.

Investigations

MRI is the investigation of choice if available, since soft tissues are well imaged. Plain X-rays of the lumbar spine are of little value in the diagnosis of disc disease, although they may demonstrate conditions affecting the vertebral body. CT can provide helpful images of the disc protrusion and/or narrowing of exit foramina.

Management

Some 90% of patients with sciatica recover following conservative treatment with analgesia and early mobilisation; bed rest does not help recovery. The patient should be instructed in back-strengthening exercises and advised to avoid physical manoeuvres likely to strain the lumbar spine. Injections of local anaesthetic or glucocorticoids may be useful adjunctive treatment if symptoms are due to ligamentous injury or joint dysfunction. Surgery may have to be considered if there is no response to conservative treatment or if progressive neurological deficits develop. Central disc prolapse with bilateral symptoms and signs and disturbance of sphincter function requires urgent surgical decompression.

Lumbar canal stenosis

This occurs with a congenitally narrowed lumbar spinal canal, exacerbated by the degenerative changes that commonly occur with age.

Pathophysiology

The symptoms of spinal stenosis are thought to be due to local vascular compromise secondary to the canal stenosis, rendering

25

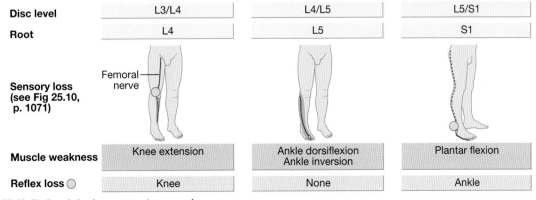

Disc level	L3/L4	L4/L5	L5/S1
Root	L4	L5	S1
Sensory loss (see Fig 25.10, p. 1071)	Femoral nerve		
Muscle weakness	Knee extension	Ankle dorsiflexion Ankle inversion	Plantar flexion
Reflex loss ○	Knee	None	Ankle

Fig. 25.48 Findings in lumbar nerve root compression.

the nerve roots ischaemic and intolerant of the increased demand that occurs on exercise.

Clinical features

Patients, who are usually elderly, develop exercise-induced weakness and paraesthesia in the legs ('spinal claudication'). These symptoms progress with continued exertion, often to the point that the patient can no longer walk, but are quickly relieved by a short period of rest. Physical examination at rest shows preservation of peripheral pulses with absent ankle reflexes. Weakness or sensory loss may only be apparent if the patient is examined immediately after exercise.

Investigations

The investigation of first choice is MRI, but contraindications (body habitus, metallic implants) may make CT or myelography necessary.

Management

Lumbar laminectomy may provide relief of symptoms and recovery of normal exercise tolerance.

Spinal cord compression

Spinal cord compression is one of the more common neurological emergencies encountered in clinical practice and the usual causes are listed in Box 25.79. A space-occupying lesion within the spinal canal may damage nerve tissue either directly by pressure or indirectly by interference with blood supply. Oedema from venous obstruction impairs neuronal function, and ischaemia from arterial obstruction may lead to necrosis of the spinal cord. The early stages of damage are reversible but severely damaged neurons do not recover; hence the importance of early diagnosis and treatment.

Clinical features

The onset of symptoms of spinal cord compression is usually slow (over weeks) but can be acute as a result of trauma or metastases (see Figs 25.46, 25.49 and 25.50), especially if there is associated arterial occlusion. The symptoms are shown in Box 25.80.

Pain and sensory symptoms occur early, while weakness and sphincter dysfunction are usually late manifestations. The signs vary according to the level of the cord compression and the

structures involved. There may be tenderness to percussion over the spine if there is vertebral disease and this may be associated with a local kyphosis. Involvement of the roots at the level of the compression may cause dermatomal sensory impairment and corresponding lower motor signs. Interruption of fibres in the spinal cord causes sensory loss (p. 1083) and upper motor neuron signs below the level of the lesion, and there is often disturbance of sphincter function. The distribution of these signs varies with the level of the lesion (Box 25.81).

The Brown–Séquard syndrome (see Fig. 25.18E, p. 1084) results if damage is confined to one side of the cord; the findings are explained by the anatomy of the sensory tracts (see Fig. 25.11, p. 1072). With compressive lesions, there is usually a band of pain at the level of the lesion in the distribution of the nerve roots subject to compression.

Investigations

Patients with a history of acute or subacute spinal cord syndrome should be investigated urgently, as listed in Box 25.82. The

---

25.80 Symptoms of spinal cord compression

Pain

- Localised over the spine or in a root distribution, which may be aggravated by coughing, sneezing or straining

Sensory

- Paraesthesia, numbness or cold sensations, especially in the lower limbs, which spread proximally, often to a level on the trunk

Motor

- Weakness, heaviness or stiffness of the limbs, most commonly the legs

Sphincters

- Urgency or hesitancy of micturition, leading eventually to urinary retention

---

25.81 Signs of spinal cord compression

Cervical, above C5

- Upper motor neuron signs and sensory loss in all four limbs
- Diaphragm weakness (phrenic nerve)

Cervical, C5–T1

- Lower motor neuron signs and segmental sensory loss in the arms; upper motor neuron signs in the legs
- Respiratory (intercostal) muscle weakness

Thoracic cord

- Spastic paraplegia with a sensory level on the trunk
- Weakness of legs, sacral loss of sensation and extensor plantar responses

Cauda equina

- Spinal cord ends approximately at the T12/L1 spinal level and spinal lesions below this level can cause lower motor neuron signs only by affecting the cauda equina

---

25.82 Investigation of acute spinal cord syndrome

- Magnetic resonance imaging of spine or myelography
- Plain X-rays of spine
- Chest X-ray
- Cerebrospinal fluid
- Serum vitamin B_{12}

Site	Frequency	Causes
Vertebral	80%	Trauma (extradural) Intervertebral disc prolapse Metastatic carcinoma (e.g. breast, prostate, bronchus) Myeloma Tuberculosis
Meninges (intradural, extramedullary)	15%	Tumours (e.g. meningioma, neurofibroma, ependymoma, metastasis, lymphoma, leukaemia) Epidural abscess
Spinal cord (intradural, intramedullary)	5%	Tumours (e.g. glioma, ependymoma, metastasis)

25.79 Causes of spinal cord compression

Fig. 25.49 Axial magnetic resonance image of thoracic spine.
A neurofibroma (N) is compressing the spinal cord (SC) and emerging
in a 'dumbbell' fashion through the vertebral foramen into the paraspinal
space.

Fig. 25.50 Computed tomographic myelogram of cervical spine at
the level of C2 showing bony erosion of vertebra by a metastasis
(arrow).

investigation of choice is MRI (Fig. 25.49), as it can define the
extent of compression and associated soft-tissue abnormality (Fig.
25.50). Plain X-rays may show bony destruction and soft-tissue
abnormalities. Routine investigations, including chest X-ray,
may provide evidence of systemic disease. If myelography
is performed, CSF should be taken for analysis; in cases of
complete spinal block, this shows a normal cell count with a very
elevated protein causing yellow discoloration of the fluid (Froin's
syndrome). The risk of acute deterioration after myelography in
spinal cord compression means that the neurosurgeons should
be alerted before it is undertaken. Where a secondary tumour
is causing the compression, needle biopsy may be required to
establish a tissue diagnosis.

Management

Treatment and prognosis depend on the nature of the underlying
lesion. Benign tumours should be surgically excised, and a

good functional recovery can be expected unless a marked
neurological deficit has developed before diagnosis. Extradural
compression due to malignancy is the most common cause
of spinal cord compression in developed countries and has a
poor prognosis. Useful function can be regained if treatment,
such as radiotherapy, is initiated within 24 hours of the onset
of severe weakness or sphincter dysfunction; management
should involve close cooperation with both oncologists and
neurosurgeons.

Spinal cord compression due to tuberculosis is common in
some areas of the world and may require surgical treatment.
This should be followed by appropriate antituberculous
chemotherapy (p. 592) for an extended period. Traumatic lesions
of the vertebral column require specialised neurosurgical
treatment.

Intrinsic diseases of the spinal cord

There are many disorders that interfere with spinal cord function
due to non-compressive involvement of the spinal cord itself.
A list of these disorders is given in Box 25.83. The symptoms
and signs are generally similar to those that would occur with
extrinsic compression (see Boxes 25.80 and 25.81), although a
suspended sensory loss (see Fig. 25.18F, p. 1084) can occur only
with intrinsic disease such as syringomyelia. Urinary symptoms
usually occur earlier in the course of an intrinsic cord disorder
than with compressive disorders.

Investigation of intrinsic disease starts with imaging to exclude
a compressive lesion. MRI provides most information about
structural lesions, such as diastematomyelia, syringomyelia (Fig.
25.51) or intrinsic tumours. Non-specific signal change may be
seen in the spinal cord in inflammatory (see Fig. 25.30, p. 1109)
or infective conditions and metabolic disorders such as vitamin
B_{12} deficiency. Lumbar puncture or blood tests may be required
to make a specific diagnosis.

**Fig. 25.51 Sagittal magnetic resonance image showing descent of
cerebellar tonsils and central syrinx.** The MRI shows descent of the
cerebellar tonsils (top arrow), with a large central cord syrinx extending
down from the cervical cord (middle arrow) to the thoracic cord (bottom
arrow).

25

	25.83 Intrinsic diseases of the spinal cord	
Type of disorder	**Condition**	**Clinical features**
Congenital	Diastematomyelia (spina bifida)	Features variably present at birth and deteriorate thereafter LMN features, deformity and sensory loss of legs Impaired sphincter function Hairy patch or pit over low back Incidence reduced by increased maternal intake of folic acid during pregnancy
	Hereditary spastic paraplegia	Onset usually in adult life Autosomal dominant inheritance usual Slowly progressive UMN features affecting legs > arms Little or no sensory loss
Infective/inflammatory	Transverse myelitis due to viruses (HZV), schistosomiasis, HIV, MS, sarcoidosis	Weakness and sensory loss, often with pain, developing over hours to days UMN features below lesion Impaired sphincter function
	Paraneoplastic	May predate tumour diagnosis
Vascular	Anterior spinal artery infarct due to atherosclerosis, aortic dissection, embolus	Abrupt onset Anterior horn cell loss (LMN) at level of lesion UMN features below it Spinothalamic sensory loss below lesion but dorsal column sensation spared
	Spinal AVM/dural fistula	Onset variable (acute to slowly progressive) Variable LMN, UMN, sensory and sphincter disturbance Symptoms and signs often not well localised to site of AVM
Neoplastic	Glioma, ependymoma	Weakness and sensory loss often with pain, developing over months to years UMN features below lesion in cord; additional LMN features in conus Impaired sphincter function
Metabolic	Vitamin B_{12} deficiency (subacute combined degeneration)	Progressive spastic paraparesis with proprioception loss Absent reflexes due to peripheral neuropathy ± Optic nerve and cerebral involvement (p. 715)
	Copper deficiency	Excess dietary zinc
	Nitrous oxide toxicity	Modifies vitamin B_{12} metabolism
Degenerative	Motor neuron disease	Relentlessly progressive LMN and UMN features, associated bulbar weakness No sensory involvement (p. 1116)
	Syringomyelia	Gradual onset over months or years, pain in cervical segments Anterior horn cell loss (LMN) at level of lesion, UMN features below it Suspended spinothalamic sensory loss at level of lesion, dorsal columns preserved (see Figs 25.18F (p. 1084) and 25.51)

(AVM = arteriovenous malformation; HIV = human immunodeficiency virus; HZV = herpes zoster virus; LMN = lower motor neuron; MS = multiple sclerosis; UMN = upper motor neuron)

Diseases of peripheral nerves

Disorders of the peripheral nervous system are common and may affect the motor, sensory or autonomic components, either in isolation or in combination. The site of pathology may be nerve root (radiculopathy), nerve plexus (plexopathy) or nerve (neuropathy). Neuropathies may present as mononeuropathy (single nerve affected), multiple mononeuropathies ('mononeuritis multiplex') or a symmetrical polyneuropathy (Box 25.84). Cranial nerves 3–12 share the same tissue characteristics as peripheral nerves elsewhere and are subject to the same range of diseases.

Pathophysiology

Damage may occur to the nerve cell body (axon) or the myelin sheath (Schwann cell), leading to axonal or demyelinating neuropathies. The distinction is important, as only demyelinating neuropathies are usually susceptible to treatment. Making the distinction requires neurophysiology (nerve conduction studies and EMG, p. 1076). Neuropathies can occur in association with many systemic diseases, toxins and drugs (Box 25.85).

Clinical features

Motor nerve involvement produces features of a lower motor neuron lesion (p. 1082). Symptoms and signs of sensory nerve involvement depend on the type of sensory nerve involved (p. 1083); small-fibre neuropathies are often painful. Autonomic involvement may cause postural hypotension, disturbance of sweating, cardiac rhythm and gastrointestinal, bladder and sexual functions; isolated autonomic neuropathies are rare and more commonly complicate other neuropathies.

Investigations

The investigations required reflect the wide spectrum of causes (Box 25.86). Neurophysiological tests are key in discriminating between demyelinating and axonal neuropathies, and in identifying entrapment neuropathies. Most neuropathies are of the chronic axonal type.

25.84 Causes of polyneuropathy

Genetic

- Charcot–Marie–Tooth disease (CMT)
- Hereditary neuropathy with liability to pressure palsies (HNPP)
- Hereditary sensory ± autonomic neuropathies (HSN, HSAN)
- Familial amyloid polyneuropathy
- Hereditary neuralgic amyotrophy

Drugs

- Amiodarone
- Antibiotics (dapsone, isoniazid, metronidazole, ethambutol)
- Antiretrovirals
- Chemotherapy (cisplatin, vincristine, thalidomide)
- Phenytoin

Toxins

- Alcohol
- Nitrous oxide (recreational use)
- Rarely: lead, arsenic, mercury, organophosphates, solvents

Vitamin deficiencies

- Thiamin
- Pyridoxine
- Vitamin B_{12}
- Vitamin E

Infections

- HIV
- Leprosy
- Brucellosis

Inflammatory

- Guillain–Barré syndrome
- Chronic inflammatory demyelinating polyradiculoneuropathy
- Vasculitis (polyarteritis nodosa, granulomatosis with polyangiitis (also known as Wegener's granulomatosis), rheumatoid arthritis, systemic lupus erythematosus)
- Paraneoplastic (antibody-mediated)

Systemic medical conditions

- Diabetes
- Renal failure
- Sarcoidosis

Malignant disease

- Infiltration

Others

- Paraproteinaemias
- Amyloidosis
- Critical illness polyneuropathy/myopathy

25.85 Common causes of axonal and demyelinating chronic polyneuropathies

Axonal

- Diabetes mellitus
- Alcohol
- Uraemia
- Cirrhosis
- Amyloid
- Myxoedema
- Acromegaly
- Paraneoplasm
- Drugs and toxins (see Box 25.84)
- Deficiency states (see Box 25.84)
- Hereditary factors
- Infection (see Box 25.84)
- Idiopathic factors

Demyelinating

- Chronic inflammatory demyelinating polyradiculoneuropathy
- Multifocal motor neuropathy
- Paraprotein-associated demyelinating neuropathy
- Charcot–Marie–Tooth disease type I and type X

25.86 Investigation of peripheral neuropathy

Initial tests

- Glucose (fasting)
- Erythrocyte sedimentation rate, C-reactive protein
- Full blood count
- Urea and electrolytes
- Liver function tests
- Serum protein electrophoresis
- Vitamin B_{12}, folate
- ANA, ANCA
- Chest X-ray
- HIV testing

If initial tests are negative

- Nerve conduction studies
- Vitamins E and A
- Genetic testing (see Box 25.84)
- Lyme serology (p. 256)
- Serum angiotensin-converting enzyme
- Serum amyloid

(ANCA = antineutrophil cytoplasmic antibody; ANA = antineutrophil antibody)

Entrapment neuropathy

Focal compression or entrapment is the usual cause of a mononeuropathy. Symptoms and signs of entrapment neuropathy are listed in Box 25.87. Entrapment neuropathies may affect anyone but diabetes, excess alcohol or toxins, or genetic syndromes may be predisposing causes. Unless axonal loss

---

25.87 Symptoms and signs in common entrapment neuropathies

Nerve	Symptoms	Muscle weakness/muscle-wasting	Area of sensory loss
Median (at wrist) (carpal tunnel syndrome)	Pain and paraesthesia on palmar aspect of hands and fingers, waking patient from sleep. Pain may extend to arm and shoulder	Abductor pollicis brevis	Lateral palm and thumb, index, middle and lateral half fourth finger
Ulnar (at elbow)	Paraesthesia on medial border of hand, wasting and weakness of hand muscles	All small hand muscles, excluding abductor pollicis brevis	Medial palm and little finger, and medial half fourth finger
Radial	Weakness of extension of wrist and fingers, often precipitated by sleeping in abnormal posture, e.g. arm over back of chair	Wrist and finger extensors, supinator	Dorsum of thumb
Common peroneal	Foot drop, trauma to head of fibula	Dorsiflexion and eversion of foot	Nil or dorsum of foot
Lateral cutaneous nerve of the thigh (meralgia paraesthetica)	Tingling and dysaesthesia on lateral border of thigh	Nil	Lateral border of thigh

| **i** | **25.88 Causes of multifocal mononeuropathy** |

Axonal (defined on nerve conduction studies)

- Vasculitis (systemic or non-systemic)
- Diabetes mellitus
- Sarcoidosis
- Infection (HIV, hepatitis C, Lyme disease, leprosy, diphtheria)

Focal demyelination with/without conduction block

- Multifocal motor neuropathy
- Multiple compression neuropathies (usually in association with underlying disease, such as diabetes or alcoholism)
- Multifocal acquired demyelinating sensory and motor neuropathy (MADSAM)
- Hereditary neuropathy with a predisposition to pressure palsy (autosomal dominant, peripheral myelin protein 22 gene)
- Lymphoma

has occurred, entrapment neuropathies will recover, provided the primary cause is removed, either by avoiding the precipitation of activity or by surgical decompression.

Multifocal neuropathy

Multifocal neuropathy (mononeuritis multiplex) is characterised by lesions of multiple nerve roots, peripheral nerves or cranial nerves (Box 25.88). Vasculitis is a common cause, either as part of a systemic disease or isolated to the nerves, or it may arise on a background of a polyneuropathy (e.g. diabetes). Multifocal motor neuropathy (MMN) with conduction block is a rare pure motor neuropathy, typically affecting the arms; it is associated with anti-GM1 antibodies in about 50% and responds to intravenous immunoglobulin.

Polyneuropathy

A polyneuropathy is typically associated with a 'length-dependent' pattern, occurring in the longest peripheral nerves first and affecting the distal lower limbs before the upper limbs. Sensory symptoms and signs develop in an ascending 'glove and stocking' distribution (p. 1083). In inflammatory demyelinating neuropathies, the pathology may be more patchy, affecting the upper rather than lower limbs.

Guillain–Barré syndrome

Guillain–Barré syndrome (GBS) is a heterogeneous group of immune-mediated conditions with an incidence of 1–2/100 000/year. In Europe and North America, the most common variant is an acute inflammatory demyelinating polyneuropathy (AIDP). Axonal variants, either motor (acute motor axonal neuropathy, AMAN) or sensorimotor (acute motor and sensory axonal neuropathy, AMSAN), are more common in China and Japan, and account for 10% of GBS in Western countries (often associated with *Campylobacter jejuni*). The hallmark is an acute paralysis evolving over days or weeks with loss of tendon reflexes. About two-thirds of those with AIDP have a prior history of infection, and an autoimmune response triggered by the preceding infection causes demyelination. A number of GBS variants have been described, associated with specific anti-ganglioside antibodies; the best recognised is Miller Fisher syndrome, which involves anti-GQ1b antibodies.

Clinical features

Distal paraesthesia and pain precede muscle weakness that ascends rapidly from lower to upper limbs and is more marked proximally than distally. Facial and bulbar weakness commonly develops, and respiratory weakness requiring ventilatory support occurs in 20% of cases. Weakness progresses over a maximum of 4 weeks (usually less). Rapid deterioration to respiratory failure can develop within hours. Examination shows diffuse weakness with loss of reflexes. Miller Fisher syndrome presents with internal and external ophthalmoplegia, ataxia and areflexia.

Investigations

The CSF protein is raised, but may be normal in the first 10 days. There is usually no increase in CSF white cell count ($>10 \times 10^6$ cells/L suggests an alternative diagnosis). Electrophysiological changes may emerge after a week or so, with conduction block and multifocal motor slowing, sometimes most evident proximally as delayed F waves (p. 1076). Antibodies to the ganglioside GM1 are found in about 25%, usually the motor axonal form. Other causes of an acute neuromuscular paralysis should be excluded (e.g. poliomyelitis, botulism, diphtheria, spinal cord syndromes or myasthenia), via the history and examination rather than investigations.

Management

Active treatment with plasma exchange or intravenous immunoglobulin therapy shortens the duration of ventilation and improves prognosis. In severe GBS, both intravenous immunoglobulin (IVIg) and plasma exchange started within 2 weeks of onset hasten recovery with similar rates of adverse effects but IVIg treatment is significantly more likely to be completed than plasma exchange. Overall, 80% of patients recover completely within 3–6 months, 4% die and the remainder suffer residual neurological disability, which can be severe. Adverse prognostic features include older age, rapid deterioration to ventilation and evidence of axonal loss on EMG. Supportive measures to prevent pressure sores and deep venous thrombosis are essential. Regular monitoring of respiratory function (vital capacity) is needed in the acute phase, as respiratory failure may develop with little warning.

Chronic polyneuropathy

The most common axonal and demyelinating causes of polyneuropathy are shown in Box 25.85. A chronic symmetrical axonal polyneuropathy, evolving over months or years, is the most common form of chronic neuropathy. Diabetes mellitus is the most common cause but in about 25–50% no cause can be found.

Hereditary neuropathy

Charcot–Marie–Tooth disease (CMT) is an umbrella term for the inherited neuropathies. The members of this group of syndromes have different clinical and genetic features. The most common CMT is the autosomal dominantly inherited CMT type 1, usually caused by a mutation in the *PMP-22* gene. Common signs are distal wasting ('inverted champagne bottle' legs), often with pes cavus, and predominantly motor involvement. X-linked and recessively inherited forms of CMT, causing demyelinating or axonal neuropathies, also occur.

Chronic demyelinating polyneuropathy

The acquired chronic demyelinating neuropathies include chronic inflammatory demyelinating peripheral neuropathy (CIDP), multifocal motor neuropathy (see above) and paraprotein-associated demyelinating neuropathy. CIDP typically presents with relapsing or progressive motor and sensory changes, evolving over more than 8 weeks (in distinction to the more acute GBS). It is important to recognise, as it usually responds to glucocorticoids, plasma exchange or intravenous immunoglobulin.

Some 10% of patients with acquired demyelinating polyneuropathy have an abnormal serum paraprotein, sometimes associated with a lymphoproliferative malignancy. They may also demonstrate positive antibodies to myelin-associated glycoprotein (anti-MAG antibodies).

Brachial plexopathy

Trauma usually damages either the upper or the lower parts of the brachial plexus, according to the mechanics of the injury. The clinical features depend on the anatomical site of the damage (Box 25.89). Lower parts of the brachial plexus are vulnerable to infiltration from breast or apical lung tumours (Pancoast tumour, p. 600) or damage by therapeutic irradiation. The lower plexus may also be compressed by a cervical rib or fibrous band between C7 and the first rib at the thoracic outlet.

Neuralgic amyotrophy (also known as brachial neuritis) presents as an acute brachial plexopathy of probable inflammatory origin. Severe shoulder pain precedes the appearance of a patchy upper brachial plexus lesion, with motor and/or sensory involvement. There is no specific treatment and recovery is often incomplete; it may recur in about 25% and there is a rare autosomal dominant hereditary form. The appearance of vesicles should indicate the alternative diagnosis of motor zoster.

i	25.89 Physical signs in brachial plexus lesions		
Site	Affected muscles	Sensory loss
Upper plexus (Erb–Duchenne)	Biceps, deltoid, spinati, rhomboids, brachioradialis (triceps, serratus anterior)	Patch over deltoid
Lower plexus (Déjerine–Klumpke)	All small hand muscles, claw hand (ulnar wrist flexors)	Ulnar border of hand/forearm
Thoracic outlet syndrome	Small hand muscles, ulnar forearm	Ulnar border of hand/forearm/ upper arm

Lumbosacral plexopathy

Lumbosacral plexus lesions may be caused by neoplastic infiltration or compression by retroperitoneal haematomas. A small-vessel vasculopathy can produce a unilateral or bilateral lumbar plexopathy in association with diabetes mellitus ('diabetic amyotrophy') or an idiopathic form in non-diabetic patients. This presents with painful wasting of the quadriceps with weakness of knee extension and an absent knee reflex.

Spinal root lesions

Spinal root lesions (radiculopathy) are described above. Clinical features include muscle weakness and wasting and dermatomal sensory and reflex loss, which reflect the pattern of the roots involved. Pain in the muscles innervated by the affected roots may be prominent.

Diseases of the neuromuscular junction

Myasthenia gravis

This is the most common cause of acutely evolving, fatigable weakness and preferentially affects ocular, facial and bulbar muscles.

Pathophysiology

Myasthenia gravis is an autoimmune disease, most commonly (80% of cases) caused by antibodies to acetylcholine receptors in the post-junctional membrane of the neuromuscular junction. The resultant blockage of neuromuscular transmission and complement-mediated inflammatory response reduces the number of acetylcholine receptors and damages the end plate (Fig. 25.52). Other antibodies can produce a similar clinical picture, most notably autoantibodies to muscle-specific kinase (MuSK), which is involved in the regulation and maintenance of acetylcholine receptors.

About 15% of patients (mainly those with late onset) have a thymoma, most of the remainder displaying thymic follicular hyperplasia. Myasthenic patients are more likely to have associated organ-specific autoimmune diseases. Triggers are not always evident but some drugs (e.g. penicillamine) can precipitate an antibody-mediated myasthenic syndrome that may persist after drug withdrawal. Other drugs, especially aminoglycosides and quinolones, may exacerbate the neuromuscular blockade and should be avoided in patients with myasthenia.

Clinical features

Myasthenia gravis usually presents between the ages of 15 and 50 years and there is a female preponderance in younger patients. In older patients, males are more commonly affected. It tends to run a relapsing and remitting course.

The most evident symptom is fatigable muscle weakness; movement is initially strong but rapidly weakens as muscle use continues. Worsening of symptoms towards the end of the day or following exercise is characteristic. There are no sensory signs or signs of involvement of the CNS, although weakness of the oculomotor muscles may mimic a central eye movement disorder. The first symptoms are usually intermittent ptosis or diplopia but weakness of chewing, swallowing, speaking or limb movement also occurs. Resting of the eyelids (looking downwards) may be followed by increased reflex elevation with up-gaze (so-called Cogan's lid twitch sign). Any limb muscle may be affected, most commonly those of the shoulder girdle; the patient is unable to undertake tasks above shoulder level, such as combing the hair, without frequent rests. Respiratory muscles may be involved and respiratory failure is an avoidable cause of death. Aspiration may occur if the cough is ineffectual. Ventilatory support is required where weakness is severe or of abrupt onset.

25

Fig. 25.52 Myasthenia gravis and Lambert–Eaton myasthenic syndrome (LEMS). In myasthenia there are antibodies to the acetylcholine receptors on the post-synaptic membrane, which block conduction across the neuromuscular junction (NMJ). Myasthenic symptoms can be transiently improved by inhibition of acetylcholinesterase (e.g. with Tensilon – edrophonium bromide), which normally removes the acetylcholine. A cell-mediated immune response produces simplification of the post-synaptic membrane, further impairing the 'safety factor' of neuromuscular conduction. In LEMS, antibodies to the pre-synaptic voltage calcium channels impair release of acetylcholine from the motor nerve ending; calcium is required for the acetylcholine-containing vesicle to fuse with the pre-synaptic membrane for release into the NMJ.

Investigations

Intravenous injection of the short-acting anticholinesterase edrophonium bromide (the Tensilon test) is less widely used than before. Improvement in muscle function occurs within 30 seconds and usually persists for 2–3 minutes but the test is not entirely specific or sensitive. Cover with intravenous atropine is necessary to avoid bradycardia. Planning assessment beforehand (e.g. speech or limb movements) allows some objectivity in gauging the effect.

Repetitive stimulation during nerve conduction studies may show a characteristic decremental response (p. 1076) if the muscle has been clinically affected. Anti-MuSK antibodies are more common in acetylcholine receptor antibody-negative patients with prominent bulbar involvement. All patients should have a thoracic CT to exclude thymoma, especially those without anti-acetylcholine receptor antibodies. Screening for associated autoimmune disorders, particularly thyroid disease, is important.

Management

The goals of treatment are to maximise the activity of acetylcholine at remaining receptors in the neuromuscular junctions and to limit or abolish the immunological attack on motor end plates.

The duration of action of acetylcholine is prolonged by inhibiting acetylcholinesterase. The most commonly used anticholinesterase drug is pyridostigmine. Muscarinic side-effects, including diarrhoea and colic, may be controlled by propantheline. Overdosage of anticholinesterase drugs may cause a 'cholinergic crisis' due to depolarisation block of motor end plates, with muscle

---

i | 25.90 Immunological treatment of myasthenia

Acute treatments

Intravenous immunoglobulin
- Lowers production of antibodies and rapidly reduces weakness

Plasma exchange
- Removing antibody from the blood may produce marked improvement; this is usually brief, so is normally reserved for myasthenic crisis or for pre-operative preparation

Long-term treatments

Glucocorticoid treatment
- Improvement is commonly preceded by marked exacerbation of myasthenic symptoms, so treatment should be initiated in hospital
- Usually necessary to continue treatment for months or years, risking adverse effects

Pharmacological immunosuppression treatment
- Azathioprine 2.5 mg/kg daily reduces the necessary dosage of glucocorticoids and may allow their withdrawal. Effect on clinical features may be delayed for months
- Mycophenolate mofetil: less commonly used

Thymectomy
- Should be considered in any antibody-positive patient under 45 years with symptoms not confined to extraocular muscles, unless the disease has been established for more than 7 years
- Likely to be required for thymoma

fasciculation, paralysis, pallor, sweating, excessive salivation and small pupils. This may be distinguished from severe weakness due to exacerbation of myasthenia ('myasthenic crisis') by the clinical features and, if necessary, by the injection of a small dose of edrophonium.

Immunological treatment of myasthenia is outlined in Box 25.90. Thymectomy may improve overall prognosis but awaits clinical trial confirmation. Prognosis is variable and remissions may occur spontaneously. When myasthenia is entirely ocular, prognosis is excellent and disability slight. Young female patients with generalised disease may benefit from thymectomy, while older patients are less likely to have a remission despite treatment. Rapid progression of the disease more than 5 years after onset is uncommon.

Lambert–Eaton myasthenic syndrome

Other rarer conditions can present with muscle weakness due to impaired transmission across the neuromuscular junction. The most common of these is the Lambert–Eaton myasthenic syndrome (LEMS), which can occur as an inflammatory or paraneoplastic phenomenon. Antibodies to pre-synaptic voltage-gated calcium channels (see Fig. 25.52) impair transmitter release. Patients may have autonomic dysfunction (e.g. dry mouth) in addition to muscle weakness but the cardinal clinical sign is absence of tendon reflexes, which return after sustained contraction of the relevant muscle. The condition is associated with underlying malignancy in a high percentage of cases and investigation must be directed towards identifying any neoplasm. Diagnosis is made electrophysiologically on the presence of post-tetanic potentiation of motor response to nerve stimulation at a frequency of 20–50/sec. Treatment is with 3,4-diaminopyridine, or pyridostigmine and immunosuppression.

Diseases of muscle

Muscle disease, either hereditary or acquired, is rare. Most typically, it presents with a proximal symmetrical weakness. Diagnosis is dependent on recognition of clinical clues, such as cardiorespiratory involvement, evolution, family history, exposure to drugs, the presence of contractures, myotonia and other systemic features, and on investigation findings, most importantly EMG and muscle biopsy. Hereditary syndromes include the muscular dystrophies, muscle channelopathies, metabolic myopathies (including mitochondrial diseases) and congenital myopathies.

Muscular dystrophies

These are inherited disorders with progressive muscle destruction and may be associated with cardiac and/or respiratory involvement and sometimes non-myopathic features (Box 25.91). Myotonic dystrophy is the most common, with a prevalence of about 12/100 000.

Clinical features

The pattern of the clinical features is defined by the specific syndromes. Onset is often in childhood, although some patients, especially those with myotonic dystrophy, may present as adults. Wasting and weakness are usually symmetrical, without fasciculation or sensory loss, and tendon reflexes are usually preserved until a late stage. Weakness is usually proximal, except in myotonic dystrophy type 1, when it is distal.

Investigations

The diagnosis can be confirmed by specific molecular genetic testing, supplemented with EMG and muscle biopsy if necessary. Creatine kinase is markedly elevated in the dystrophinopathies

i 25.91 The muscular dystrophies				
Type	Genetics	Age of onset	Muscles affected	Other features
Myotonic dystrophy (DM1)	Autosomal dominant; expanded triplet repeat chromosome 19q	Any	Face (including ptosis), sternomastoids, distal limb, generalised later	Myotonia, cognitive impairment, cardiac conduction abnormalities, lens opacities, frontal balding, hypogonadism
Proximal myotonic myopathy (PROMM; DM2)	Autosomal dominant; quadruplet repeat expansion in *Zn finger protein 9* gene chromosome 3q	8–50 years	Proximal, especially thigh, sometimes muscle hypertrophy	As for DM1 but cognition not affected Muscle pain
Duchenne	X-linked; deletions in *dystrophin* gene Xp21	<5 years	Proximal and limb girdle	Cardiomyopathy and respiratory failure
Becker	X-linked; deletions in *dystrophin* gene Xp21	Childhood/early adulthood	Proximal and limb girdle	Cardiomyopathy common but respiratory failure uncommon
Limb girdle	Many mutations on different chromosomes	Childhood/early adulthood	Limb girdle	Very variable depending on genetic subtype, some involve cardiac and respiratory systems
Facioscapulohumeral (FSH)	Autosomal dominant; tandem repeat deletion chromosome 4q35	7–30 years	Face and upper limb girdle, distal lower limb weakness	Pain in shoulder girdle common, deafness Cardiorespiratory involvement rare
Oculopharyngeal	Autosomal dominant and recessive; triplet repeat expansion in *PABP2* gene chromosome 14q	30–60 years	Ptosis, external ophthalmoplegia, dysphagia, tongue weakness	Mild lower limb weakness
Emery–Dreifuss	X-linked recessive; mutations in *emerin* gene	4–5 years	Humero-peroneal, proximal limb girdle later	Contractures develop early Cardiac involvement leads to sudden death

25

(Duchenne and Becker) but is normal or moderately elevated in the other dystrophies. Screening for an associated cardiac abnormality (cardiomyopathy or dysrhythmia) is important.

Management

There is no specific therapy for most of these conditions but physiotherapy and occupational therapy help patients cope with their disability. Glucocorticoids can be used in Duchenne muscular dystrophy but side-effects should be anticipated and avoided by dose modification. Ataluren is a compound given by infusion to affected individuals that may 'override' the stop sign in Duchenne, theoretically leading to normalisation of muscle proteins and potentially reducing or arresting functional deteriorations. Treatment of associated cardiac failure or arrhythmia (with pacemaker insertion if necessary) may be required; similarly, management of respiratory complications (including nocturnal hypoventilation) can improve quality of life. Improvements in non-invasive ventilation have led to significant improvements in survival for patients with Duchenne muscular dystrophy. Genetic counselling is important.

Inherited metabolic myopathies

There are a large number of rare inherited disorders that interfere with the biochemical pathways that maintain the energy supply (adenosine triphosphate, ATP) to muscles. These are mostly recessively inherited deficiencies in the enzymes necessary for glycogen or fatty acid (β-oxidation) metabolism (Box 25.92). They typically present with muscle weakness and pain.

Mitochondrial disorders

Mitochondrial diseases are discussed on page 49. Mitochondria are present in all tissues and dysfunction causes widespread effects on vision (optic atrophy, retinitis pigmentosa, cataracts), hearing (sensorineural deafness) and the endocrine, cardiovascular, gastrointestinal and renal systems. Any combination of these should raise the suspicion of a mitochondrial disorder, especially if there is evidence of maternal transmission.

i | 25.92 Inherited disorders of muscle metabolism

Disease	Clinical features	Diagnosis
Carbohydrate (glycogen) metabolism		
Myophosphorylase deficiency (McArdle's disease): autosomal recessive	Exercise-induced myalgia, stiffness, weakness (with 'second wind' phenomenon), myoglobinuria	Creatine kinase (CK) elevated Muscle biopsy Enzyme assay
Acid maltase deficiency (Pompe's disease): autosomal recessive	Infantile form: death within 2 years Childhood: death in twenties or thirties Adult: progressive proximal myopathy with respiratory failure	CK elevated Blood lymphocyte analysis for glycogen granules Muscle biopsy Enzyme assay
Lipid metabolism (β-oxidation)		
Carnitine-palmitoyl transferase (CPT) deficiency	Myalgia *after* exercise, myoglobinuria, weakness	CK normal between attacks Urinary organic acids Enzyme assays Muscle biopsy

i | 25.93 Mitochondrial syndromes

Syndrome	Clinical features
Myoclonic epilepsy with ragged red fibres (MERRF)	Myoclonic epilepsy, cerebellar ataxia, dementia, sensorineural deafness ± peripheral neuropathy, optic atrophy and multiple lipomas
Mitochondrial myopathy, encephalopathy, lactic acidosis and stroke-like episodes (MELAS)	Episodic encephalopathy, stroke-like episodes often preceded by migraine-like headache, nausea and vomiting
Chronic progressive external ophthalmoplegia (CPEO)	Progressive ptosis and external oculomotor palsy, proximal myopathy ± deafness, ataxia and cardiac conduction defects
Kearns–Sayre syndrome	Like CPEO but early age of onset (<20 years), heart block, pigmentary retinopathy
Mitochondrial neurogastrointestinal encephalomyopathy (MNGIE)	Progressive ptosis, external oculomotor palsy, gastrointestinal dysmotility (often pseudo-obstruction), diffuse leucoencephalopathy, thin body habitus, peripheral neuropathy and myopathy
Neuropathy, ataxia and retinitis pigmentosa (NARP)	Weakness, ataxia and progressive loss of vision, along with dementia, seizures and proximal weakness

Mitochondrial dysfunction can be caused by alterations in either mitochondrial DNA or genes encoding for oxidative processes. Genetic abnormalities or mutations in mitochondrial DNA may affect single individuals and single tissues (most commonly muscle). Thus, patients with exercise intolerance, myalgia and sometimes recurrent myoglobinuria may have isolated pathogenic mutations in genes encoding for oxidation pathways.

Inherited disorders of the oxidative pathways of the respiratory chain in mitochondria cause a group of disorders, either restricted to the muscle or associated with non-myopathic features (Box 25.93). Many of these mitochondrial disorders are inherited via the mitochondrial genome, down the maternal line (p. 49). Diagnosis is based on clinical appearances, supported by muscle biopsy appearance (usually with 'ragged red' and/or cytochrome oxidase-negative fibres), and specific mutations either on blood or, more reliably, muscle testing. Mutations may be due either to point mutations or to deletions of mitochondrial DNA.

A disorder called Leber hereditary optic neuropathy (LHON) is characterised by acute or subacute loss of vision, most frequently in males, due to bilateral optic atrophy. Three point mutations account for more than 90% of LHON cases.

Channelopathies

Inherited abnormalities of the sodium, calcium and chloride ion channels in striated muscle produce various syndromes of familial periodic paralysis, myotonia and malignant hyperthermia, which may be recognised by their clinical characteristics and potassium abnormalities (Box 25.94). Genetic testing is available.

Acquired myopathies

These include the inflammatory myopathies, or myopathy associated with a range of metabolic and endocrine disorders or drug and toxin exposure (Fig. 25.53).

i | 25.94 Muscle channelopathies

Channel	Muscle disease	Gene and inheritance	Clinical features
Sodium	Paramyotonia congenita	*SCN4A* (17q35) Autosomal dominant	Cold-evoked myotonia with episodic weakness provoked by exercise and cold
	Potassium-aggravated myotonia	*SCN4A*	Pure myotonia without weakness provoked by potassium
	Hyperkalaemic periodic paralysis	*SCN4A* Autosomal dominant	Brief (mins to hours), frequent episodes of weakness provoked by rest, cold, potassium, fasting, pregnancy, stress Less common than hypokalaemic periodic paralysis
	Hypokalaemic periodic paralysis	*SCN4A* Autosomal dominant (one-third new mutations)	Longer (hours to days) episodic weakness triggered by rest, carbohydrate loading, cold
Chloride	Myotonia congenita: Thomsen's disease	*CLCN1* Autosomal dominant	Myotonia usually mild, little weakness
	Becker's disease	*CLCN1* Autosomal recessive	Myotonia often severe, transient weakness
Calcium	Hypokalaemic periodic paralysis	*CACNA1S* Autosomal dominant	Episodic weakness triggered by carbohydrate meal
	Malignant hyperthermia	*CACNA1S*, *CACNL2A* Autosomal dominant	Hyperpyrexia due to excess muscle activity, precipitated by drugs, usually anaesthetic agents; most common cause of death during general anaesthetic
Potassium	Andersen–Tawil syndrome	*KCNJ2* Autosomal dominant	Similar to hypokalaemic periodic paralysis, associated with cardiac and non-myopathic features (skeletal and facial)
Ryanodine receptor	Malignant hyperthermia	*RYR1* (19q13)	As malignant hyperthermia above
	Central core and multicore disease	*RYR1* Mostly autosomal dominant	Present in infancy with mild progressive weakness

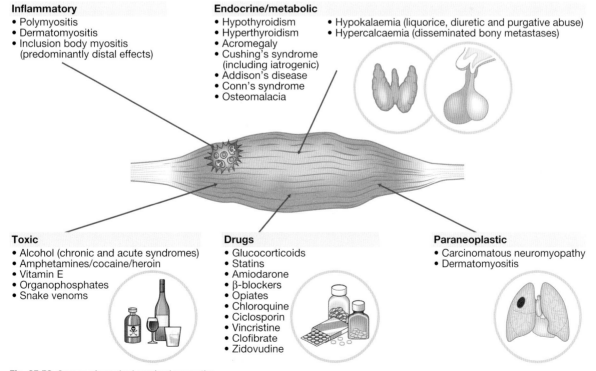

Inflammatory
- Polymyositis
- Dermatomyositis
- Inclusion body myositis (predominantly distal effects)

Endocrine/metabolic
- Hypothyroidism
- Hyperthyroidism
- Acromegaly
- Cushing's syndrome (including iatrogenic)
- Addison's disease
- Conn's syndrome
- Osteomalacia
- Hypokalaemia (liquorice, diuretic and purgative abuse)
- Hypercalcaemia (disseminated bony metastases)

Toxic
- Alcohol (chronic and acute syndromes)
- Amphetamines/cocaine/heroin
- Vitamin E
- Organophosphates
- Snake venoms

Drugs
- Glucocorticoids
- Statins
- Amiodarone
- β-blockers
- Opiates
- Chloroquine
- Ciclosporin
- Vincristine
- Clofibrate
- Zidovudine

Paraneoplastic
- Carcinomatous neuromyopathy
- Dermatomyositis

Fig. 25.53 Causes of acquired proximal myopathy.

25

Further information

Journal articles

Scolding N, Barnes D, Cader S, et al. Association of British Neurologists: revised (2015) guidelines for prescribing disease-modifying treatments in multiple sclerosis. Pract Neurol 2015; 0:1–7.

Websites

aneuroa.org/ *American Neurological Association.*
brainandspine.org.uk and dizziness-and-balance.com/disorders *Diagnosing benign paroxysmal positional vertigo.*

epilepsydiagnosis.org *International League Against Epilepsy: free access to videos of different seizure types and clinical summaries of the epilepsies.*
headinjurysymptoms.org *Symptoms and management of mild and moderate head injury.*
ihs-classification.org/en/ *International Headache Society: full access to 3rd edition of International Classification of Headache Disorders.*
neurosymptoms.org *Advice on managing functional neurological symptoms.*
ninds.nih.gov *National Institute of Neurological Disorders and Stroke.*
sign.ac.uk *Scottish Intercollegiate Guidelines network: SIGN 107 Diagnosis and management of headache in adults; SIGN 110 Early management of patients with a head injury; SIGN 113 Diagnosis and pharmacological management of Parkinson's disease; SIGN 143 Diagnosis and management of epilepsy in adults.*
wfneurology.org *World Federation of Neurology.*

P Langhorne

26

Stroke medicine

Clinical examination in stroke disease 1148

Functional anatomy and physiology 1150

Investigations 1151

Presenting problems 1152
Weakness 1152
Speech disturbance 1152
Visual deficit 1152
Visuo-spatial dysfunction 1152
Ataxia 1153
Headache 1153
Seizure 1153
Coma 1153

Stroke 1153
Pathophysiology 1153
Clinical features 1155
Investigations 1157
Management 1158

Subarachnoid haemorrhage 1160
Clinical features 1161
Investigations 1161
Management 1162

Cerebral venous disease 1162
Clinical features 1162
Investigations and management 1162

Clinical examination in stroke disease

5 Cranial nerve function

Neck stiffness/pain
Visual fields
Nerve palsy, e.g. 3rd, 6th,
7th or 12th

▲ Visual field defect

4 Higher cerebral function

Speech and language
Attention and neglect
Abbreviated mental test

3 Blood pressure and cardiac auscultation

Loud   A₂P₂   MDM   Loud
        OS

▲ Mitral stenosis

2 Pulse

Rate and rhythm

▲ Atrial fibrillation

1 General appearance

Conscious level
Posture: leaning to one side?
Facial symmetry

▲ Left facial (7th nerve) palsy

6 Motor system

Muscle bulk
Abnormal posture or movements
Tone
Strength, including pronator drift
Co-ordination
Tendon reflexes
Plantar reflexes

▲ Left pronator drift

7 Sensory system

Touch sensation
Cortical sensory function:
sensory inattention or neglect
Joint position sense

Up
Fanning
of toes

▲ Extensor plantar reflex

8 Gait

Able to weight-bear?
Ataxic
Hemiparetic gait pattern

▲ Hemiparetic posture

ⓘ General examination

Skin

- Xanthelasma
- Rash (arteritis, splinter haemorrhages)
- Colour change (limb ischaemia, deep vein thrombosis)
- Pressure injury

Eyes

- Arcus senilis
- Diabetic retinopathy
- Hypertensive retinopathy
- Retinal emboli

Cardiovascular system

- Heart rhythm (?atrial fibrillation)
- Blood pressure (high or low)
- Carotid bruit
- Jugular venous pulse (raised in heart failure, low in hypovolaemia)
- Murmurs (source of embolism)
- Peripheral pulses and bruits (?generalised arteriopathy)

Respiratory system

- Signs of pulmonary oedema or infection
- Oxygen saturation

Abdomen

- Palpable bladder (urinary retention)

Locomotor system

- Injuries sustained during collapse
- Comorbidities that influence recovery, e.g. osteoarthritis

ⓘ Rapid assessment of suspected stroke

Rosier scale

Can be used by emergency staff to indicate probability of a stroke in acute presentations:

Unilateral facial weakness	+1	Loss of consciousness	−1
Unilateral grip weakness	+1	Seizure	−1
Unilateral arm weakness	+1		
Unilateral leg weakness	+1		
Speech loss	+1		
Visual field defect	+1		

Total (−2 to +6); score of >0 indicates stroke is possible cause

Exclusion of hypoglycaemia

- Bedside blood glucose testing with BMstix

Language deficit

- History and examination may indicate a language deficit
- Check comprehension ('lift your arms, close your eyes') to identify a receptive dysphasia
- Ask patient to name people/objects (e.g. nurse, watch, pen) to identify a nominal dysphasia
- Check articulation (ask patient to repeat phrases after you) for dysarthria

Motor deficit

Subtle pyramidal signs:
- Check for pronator drift: ask patient to hold out arms and maintain their position with eyes closed (see opposite)
- Check for clumsiness of fine finger movements

Sensory and visual inattention

- Establish that sensation/visual field is intact on testing one side at a time
- Retest sensation/visual fields on simultaneous testing of both sides; the affected side will no longer be felt/seen
- Perform clock drawing test (see below)

Truncal ataxia

- Check if patient can sit up or stand without support

A

B

Clock drawing test A An image drawn by a doctor. B An image drawn by a patient with left-sided neglect.

26

Cerebrovascular disease is the third most common cause of death in high-income countries after cancers and ischaemic heart disease, and the most common cause of severe physical disability. It includes a range of disorders of the central nervous system (Fig. 26.1). Stroke is the most common clinical manifestation of cerebrovascular disease and results in episodes of brain dysfunction due to focal ischaemia or haemorrhage. Subarachnoid haemorrhage (SAH) and cerebral venous thrombosis (CVT) will be discussed separately, since their pathophysiology, clinical manifestations and management are distinct from those of stroke. Vascular dementia is described on page 1191.

Functional anatomy and physiology

The main arterial supply of the brain comes from the internal carotid arteries, which supply the anterior brain through the anterior and middle cerebral arteries, and the vertebral and basilar arteries (vertebrobasilar system), which provide the posterior circulation to the posterior cerebral arteries. The anterior and middle cerebral arteries supply the frontal and parietal lobes, while the posterior cerebral artery supplies the occipital lobe. The vertebral and basilar arteries perfuse the brainstem, mid-brain and cerebellum (Fig. 26.2). The functions of each of these

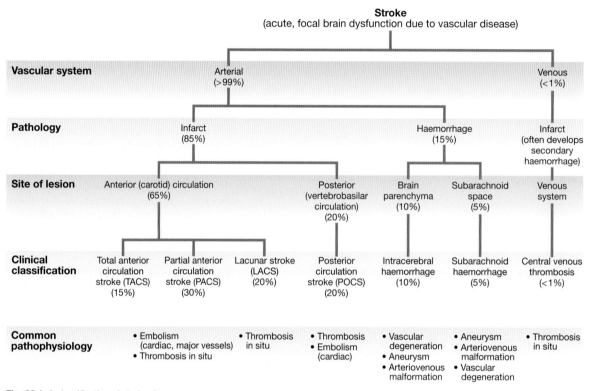

Fig. 26.1 A classification of stroke disease.

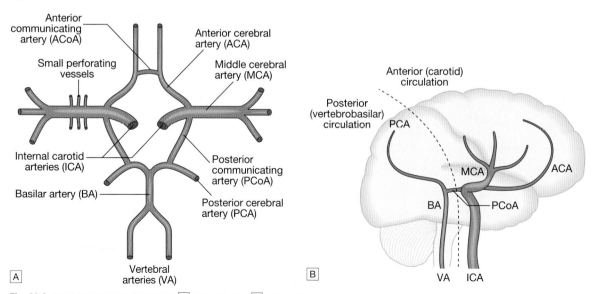

Fig. 26.2 Arterial circulation of the brain. [A] Horizontal view. [B] Lateral view.

areas of the brain are described on page 1064. Communicating arteries provide connections between the anterior and posterior circulations and between left and right hemispheres, creating protective anastomotic connections that form the circle of Willis. In health, regulatory mechanisms maintain a constant cerebral blood flow across a wide range of arterial blood pressures to meet the high resting metabolic activity of brain tissue; cerebral blood vessels dilate when systemic blood pressure is lowered and constrict when it is raised. This autoregulatory mechanism can be disrupted after stroke. The venous collecting system is formed by a collection of sinuses over the surface of the brain, which drain into the jugular veins (Fig. 26.3).

Investigations

A range of investigations may be required to answer specific questions about brain structure and function and about the function of the vascular system.

Superior sagittal sinus

Posterior   Anterior

Cavernous sinus

Transverse sinus   Jugular vein

Fig. 26.3 Venous circulation of the brain.

Neuroimaging

Computed tomography (CT) scanning is the mainstay of emergency stroke imaging. It allows the rapid identification of intracerebral bleeding and stroke 'mimics' (i.e. pathologies other than stroke that have similar presentations), such as tumours. Magnetic resonance imaging (MRI) is used when there is diagnostic uncertainty or delayed presentation, and when more information on brain structure and function is required (Fig. 26.4). Contraindications to MRI include cardiac pacemakers and claustrophobia on entering the scanner. CT angiography (CTA) and CT perfusion are now being used to characterise the cerebral circulation and areas of ischaemia better (p. 1072).

Vascular imaging

Various techniques are used to obtain images of extracranial and intracranial blood vessels (Fig. 26.5). The least invasive is ultrasound (Doppler or duplex scanning), which is used to image the carotid and the vertebral arteries in the neck. In skilled hands, reliable information can be provided about the degree of arterial stenosis and the presence of ulcerated plaques. Blood flow in the intracerebral vessels can be examined using transcranial Doppler. While the anatomical resolution is limited, it is improving and many centres no longer require formal angiography before proceeding to carotid endarterectomy (see below). Blood flow can also be detected by specialised sequences in MR angiography (MRA) or CTA but the anatomical resolution is still not as good as that of intra-arterial angiography, which outlines blood vessels by the injection of radio-opaque contrast intravenously or intra-arterially. The X-ray images obtained can be enhanced by the use of computer-assisted digital subtraction or spiral CT. Because of the significant risk of complications, intra-arterial contrast angiography is reserved for use when non-invasive methods have provided a contradictory picture or incomplete information, or when it is necessary to image the intracranial circulation in detail, e.g. to delineate a saccular aneurysm, an arteriovenous malformation or vasculitis.

Blood tests

These identify underlying causes of cerebrovascular disease, e.g. blood glucose (diabetes mellitus), triglycerides and cholesterol (hyperlipidaemia) or full blood count (polycythaemia). Erythrocyte

Fig. 26.4 Acute stroke seen on computed tomography (CT) scan with corresponding magnetic resonance imaging (MRI) appearance. A CT may show no evidence of early infarction. B A corresponding image seen on MRI diffusion weighted imaging (DWI) with changes of infarction in the middle cerebral artery (MCA) territory (arrows). *A and B, Courtesy of Dr A. Farrell and Prof. J. Wardlaw.*

26

Fig. 26.5 Different techniques for imaging blood vessels. A Doppler scan showing 80% stenosis of the internal carotid artery (arrow). B Three-dimensional reconstruction of CT angiogram showing stenosis at the carotid bifurcation (arrow). C MR angiogram showing giant aneurysm at the middle cerebral artery bifurcation (arrow). D Intra-arterial angiography showing arteriovenous malformation (arrow). *A–D, Courtesy of Dr D. Collie.*

sedimentation rate (ESR) and immunological tests, such as antineutrophil cytoplasmic antibodies (ANCAs, p. 992), may be required when vasculitis is suspected. Genetic testing for rarer inherited conditions, such as CADASIL (cerebral autosomal dominant arteriopathy with subcortical infarcts and leucoencephalopathy), may be indicated.

Lumbar puncture

Lumbar puncture (p. 1077) is reserved for investigation of SAH.

Cardiovascular investigations

Electrocardiography (ECG; p. 448), including ECG monitoring and echocardiography (p. 451), may reveal abnormalities that may cause cardiac embolism in stroke.

Presenting problems

Most vascular lesions develop suddenly within a matter of minutes or hours, and so should be considered in the differential diagnosis of patients with any acute neurological presentation.

Weakness

Unilateral weakness is the classical presentation of stroke and, much more rarely, of CVT. The weakness is sudden, progresses rapidly and follows a hemiplegic pattern (see Fig. 25.17, p. 1082). There is rarely any associated abnormal movement. Reflexes are initially reduced but then become increased with a spastic pattern of increased tone (see Box 25.14, p. 1082). Upper motor neuron weakness of the face (7th cranial nerve) is often present.

Speech disturbance

Dysphasia and dysarthria are the most common presentations of disturbed speech in stroke (p. 1087). Dysphasia indicates damage to the dominant frontal or parietal lobe (see Box 25.2, p. 1066), while dysarthria is a non-localising feature that reflects weakness or incoordination of the face, pharynx, lips, tongue or palate.

Visual deficit

Visual loss can be due to unilateral optic ischaemia (called amaurosis fugax if transient), caused by disturbance of blood flow in the internal carotid artery and ophthalmic artery, leading to monocular blindness. Ischaemia of the occipital cortex or post-chiasmic nerve tracts results in a contralateral hemianopia (p. 1088).

Visuo-spatial dysfunction

Damage to the non-dominant cortex often results in contralateral visuo-spatial dysfunction, e.g. sensory or visual neglect and apraxia (inability to perform complex tasks despite normal motor, sensory and cerebellar function; p. 1086), sometimes misdiagnosed as delirium.

Ataxia

Stroke causing damage to the cerebellum and its connections can present as an acute ataxia (p. 1086) and there may be associated brainstem features such as diplopia (p. 1088) and vertigo (p. 1086). The differential diagnosis includes vestibular disorders (p. 1104).

Headache

Sudden severe headache is the cardinal symptom of SAH but also occurs in intracerebral haemorrhage. Although headache is common in acute ischaemic stroke, it is rarely a dominant feature (p. 1080). Headache also occurs in cerebral venous disease.

Seizure

Seizure is unusual in acute stroke but may be generalised or focal (especially in cerebral venous disease).

Coma

Coma is uncommon, though it may occur with a brainstem event. If present in the first 24 hours, it usually indicates a subarachnoid or intracerebral haemorrhage (see Box 10.26, p. 194).

Stroke

Stroke is a common medical emergency. The incidence rises steeply with age, and in many lower- and middle-income countries it is rising in association with less healthy lifestyles. About 20% of stroke patients die within a month of the event and at least half of those who survive are left with physical disability.

Pathophysiology

Of the 180–300 patients per 100 000 population presenting annually with a stroke, 85% sustain a cerebral infarction due to inadequate blood flow to part of the brain, and most of the remainder have an intracerebral haemorrhage (see Fig. 26.1).

Cerebral infarction

Cerebral infarction is mostly caused by thromboembolic disease secondary to atherosclerosis in the major extracranial arteries (carotid artery and aortic arch). About 20% of infarctions are due to embolism from the heart, and a further 20% are due to thrombosis in situ caused by intrinsic disease of small perforating vessels (lenticulostriate arteries), producing so-called lacunar infarctions. The risk factors for ischaemic stroke reflect the risk factors for the underlying vascular disease (Box 26.1). About 5% are due to rare causes, including vasculitis (p. 1040), endocarditis (p. 527) and cerebral venous disease (see below). Cerebral infarction takes some hours to complete, even though the patient's deficit may be maximal shortly after the vascular occlusion. After the occlusion of a cerebral artery, infarction may be forestalled by the opening of anastomotic channels from other arterial territories that restore perfusion to its territory. Similarly, reduction in perfusion pressure leads to compensatory homeostatic changes to maintain tissue oxygenation (Fig. 26.6). These compensatory changes can sometimes prevent occlusion of even a carotid artery from having any clinically apparent effect.

26.1 Risk factors for stroke

Fixed risk factors

- Age
- Gender (male > female except at extremes of age)
- Race (Afro-Caribbean > Asian > European)
- Previous vascular event:
    Myocardial infarction
    Stroke
    Peripheral vascular disease
- Heredity
- Sickle cell disease
- High fibrinogen

Modifiable risk factors

- Blood pressure
- Cigarette smoking
- Hyperlipidaemia
- Diabetes mellitus
- Heart disease:
    Atrial fibrillation
    Congestive cardiac failure
    Infective endocarditis
- Excessive alcohol intake
- Oestrogen-containing drugs:
    Oral contraceptive pill
    Hormone replacement therapy
- Polycythaemia

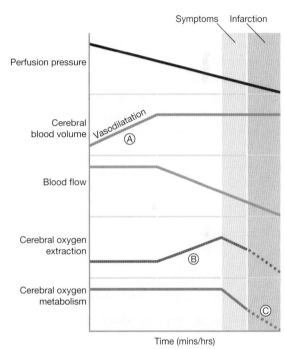

Fig. 26.6 Homeostatic responses to falling perfusion pressure in the brain following arterial occlusion. Vasodilatation initially maintains cerebral blood flow (A), but after maximal vasodilatation further falls in perfusion pressure lead to a decline in blood flow. An increase in tissue oxygen extraction, however, maintains the cerebral metabolic rate for oxygen (B). Still further falls in perfusion, and therefore blood flow, cannot be compensated; cerebral oxygen availability falls and symptoms appear, then infarction (C).

However, if and when these homeostatic mechanisms fail, the process of ischaemia starts, and ultimately leads to infarction unless the vascular supply is restored. As the cerebral blood flow declines, different neuronal functions fail at various thresholds (Fig. 26.7). Once blood flow falls below the threshold for the maintenance of electrical activity, neurological deficit develops. At this level of blood flow, neurons are still viable; if blood flow increases again, function returns and the patient will have had a

26

transient ischaemic attack (TIA). However, if blood flow falls further, a level is reached at which irreversible cell death starts. Hypoxia leads to an inadequate supply of adenosine triphosphate (ATP), which leads to failure of membrane pumps, thereby allowing influx of sodium and water into cells (cytotoxic oedema) and release

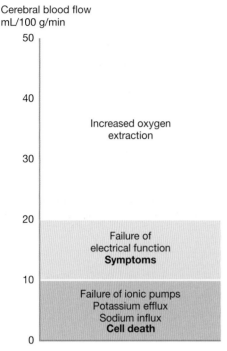

Fig. 26.7 **Thresholds of cerebral ischaemia.** Symptoms of cerebral ischaemia appear when the blood flow has fallen to less than half of normal and energy supply is insufficient to sustain neuronal electrical function. Full recovery can occur if this level of flow is returned to normal but not if it is sustained. Further blood flow reduction below the next threshold causes failure of cell ionic pumps and starts the ischaemic cascade, leading to cell death.

of the excitatory neurotransmitter glutamate into the extracellular fluid. Glutamate opens membrane channels, allowing influx of calcium and more sodium into the neurons. Calcium activates intracellular enzymes that complete the destructive process. The release of inflammatory mediators by microglia and astrocytes causes death of all cell types in the area of maximum ischaemia. The infarction process is worsened by anaerobic production of lactic acid (Fig. 26.8) and consequent fall in tissue pH. There have been attempts to develop neuroprotective drugs to slow down the processes leading to irreversible cell death but so far these have proved disappointing.

The final outcome of occlusion of a cerebral blood vessel thus depends on the competence of circulatory homeostatic mechanisms, the metabolic demand, and the severity and duration of the reduction in blood flow. Higher brain temperature, e.g. in fever, and higher blood glucose have both been associated with a greater volume of infarction for a given reduction in cerebral blood flow. Subsequent restoration of blood flow may cause haemorrhage into the infarcted area ('haemorrhagic transformation'). This is particularly likely in patients given antithrombotic or thrombolytic drugs, and in patients with larger infarcts.

Radiologically, a cerebral infarct can be seen as a lesion that comprises a mixture of dead brain tissue that is already undergoing autolysis, and tissue that is ischaemic and swollen but recoverable (the 'ischaemic penumbra'). The infarct swells with time and is at its maximal size a couple of days after stroke onset. At this stage, it may be big enough to exert mass effect both clinically and radiologically; sometimes, decompressive craniectomy is required (see below). After a few weeks, the oedema subsides and the infarcted area is replaced by a sharply defined fluid-filled cavity.

Intracerebral haemorrhage

Intracerebral haemorrhage causes about 10% of acute stroke events but is more common in low-income countries. It usually results from rupture of a blood vessel within the brain parenchyma but may also occur in a patient with SAH (see

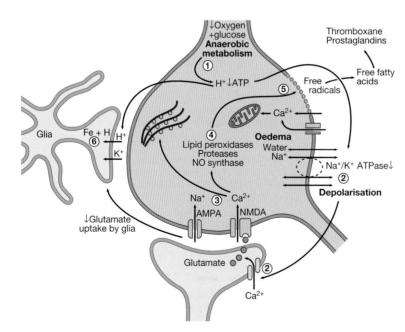

Fig. 26.8 **The process of neuronal ischaemia and infarction.** (1) Reduction of blood flow reduces supply of oxygen and hence adenosine triphosphate (ATP). H^+ is produced by anaerobic metabolism of available glucose. (2) Energy-dependent membrane ionic pumps fail, leading to cytotoxic oedema and membrane depolarisation, allowing calcium entry and releasing glutamate. (3) Calcium enters cells via glutamate-gated channels and (4) activates destructive intracellular enzymes (5), destroying intracellular organelles and cell membrane, with release of free radicals. Free fatty acid release activates pro-coagulant pathways that exacerbate local ischaemia. (6) Glial cells take up H^+, can no longer take up extracellular glutamate and also suffer cell death, leading to liquefactive necrosis of whole arterial territory. (AMPA = α-amino-3-hydroxy-5-methyl-4-isoxazolepropionic acid receptor; NMDA = N-methyl-D-aspartate; NO = nitric oxide)

below) if the artery ruptures into the brain substance as well as the subarachnoid space. Haemorrhage frequently occurs into an area of brain infarction and, if the volume of haemorrhage is large, it may be difficult to distinguish from primary intracerebral haemorrhage both clinically and radiologically (Fig. 26.9). The risk factors and underlying causes of intracerebral haemorrhage are listed in Box 26.2. Explosive entry of blood into the brain parenchyma causes immediate cessation of function in that area as neurons are disrupted and white-matter fibre tracts are split apart. The haemorrhage itself may expand over the first minutes or hours, or it may be associated with a rim of cerebral oedema, which, along with the haematoma, acts like a mass lesion to cause progression of the neurological deficit. If big enough, this can cause shift of the intracranial contents, producing transtentorial coning and sometimes rapid death (p. 1127). If the patient survives, the haematoma is gradually absorbed, leaving a haemosiderin-lined slit in the brain parenchyma.

Clinical features

Both acute stroke and transient ischaemic attack (TIA) are characterised by a rapid-onset, focal deficit of brain function and can be considered as a spectrum of symptoms from transient (TIA) to persistent (stroke). The typical presentation occurs over minutes, affects an identifiable area of brain and is 'negative' in character (i.e. abrupt loss of function without positive features

such as abnormal movement). Provided there is a clear history of this, the chance of a brain lesion being anything other than vascular is 5% or less (Box 26.3). If symptoms progress over hours or days, other diagnoses must be excluded. Delirium and memory or balance disturbance are more often due to stroke mimics. Transient symptoms, e.g. syncope, amnesia, delirium and dizziness, do not reflect focal cerebral dysfunction but are often mistakenly attributed to TIA (see Fig. 10.3, p. 182, and Box 26.4). Campaigns to raise public awareness of the emergency nature of stroke exploit the fact that weakness of the face or arm, or disturbance of speech is the most common presentation.

The clinical presentation of stroke depends on which arterial territory is involved and the size of the lesion (see Fig. 26.1). These will both have a bearing on management, such as suitability for carotid endarterectomy. The neurological deficit can be identified

---

i **26.2 Causes of intracerebral haemorrhage and associated risk factors**

Disease	Risk factors
Complex small-vessel disease with disruption of vessel wall	Age Hypertension High cholesterol
Amyloid angiopathy	Familial (rare) Age
Impaired blood clotting	Anticoagulant therapy Blood dyscrasia Thrombolytic therapy
Vascular anomaly	Arteriovenous malformation Cavernous haemangioma
Substance misuse	Alcohol Amphetamines Cocaine

---

i **26.3 Differential diagnosis of stroke and transient ischaemic attack**

'Structural' stroke mimics

- Primary cerebral tumours
- Metastatic cerebral tumours
- Extradural or subdural haematoma
- Demyelination
- Peripheral nerve lesions (vascular or compressive)
- Cerebral abscess

'Functional' stroke mimics

- Todd's paresis (after epileptic seizure)
- Hypoglycaemia
- Migrainous aura (with or without headache)
- Focal seizures
- Ménière's disease or other vestibular disorder
- Conversion disorder (p. 1202)
- Encephalitis

---

i **26.4 Characteristic features of stroke and non-stroke syndromes ('stroke mimics')**

Feature	Stroke	Stroke mimics
Symptom onset	Sudden (minutes)	Often slower onset
Symptom progression	Rapidly reaches maximum severity	Often gradual onset
Severity of deficit	Unequivocal	May be variable/uncertain
Pattern of deficit	Hemispheric pattern	May be non-specific with delirium, memory loss, balance disturbance
Loss of consciousness	Uncommon	More common

Fig. 26.9 CT scans showing intracerebral haemorrhage. A Basal ganglia haemorrhage with intraventricular extension. B Small cortical haemorrhage. *A and B, Courtesy of Dr A. Farrell and Prof. J. Wardlaw.*

26

from the patient's history and (if it is persistent) the neurological examination. The presence of a unilateral motor deficit, a higher cerebral function deficit such as aphasia or neglect, or a visual field defect usually places the lesion in the cerebral hemisphere. Ataxia, diplopia, vertigo and/or bilateral weakness usually indicate a lesion in the brainstem or cerebellum. Different combinations of these deficits define several stroke syndromes (Fig. 26.10), which reflect the site and size of the lesion and may provide clues to the underlying pathology.

Reduced conscious level usually indicates a large-volume lesion in the cerebral hemisphere but may result from a lesion in the brainstem or complications such as obstructive hydrocephalus,

hypoxia or severe systemic infection. The combination of severe headache and vomiting at the onset of the focal deficit is suggestive of intracerebral haemorrhage.

General examination may provide clues to the cause and identify important comorbidities and complications.

Several terms have been used to classify strokes, often based on the duration and evolution of symptoms:

- *Transient ischaemic attack (TIA)* describes a stroke in which symptoms resolve within 24 hours – an arbitrary cut-off that has little value in practice, apart from perhaps indicating that underlying cerebral haemorrhage or extensive cerebral infarction is extremely unlikely. The term

Clinical syndrome	Common symptoms	Common cause	CT scan features
Total anterior circulation syndrome (TACS)	Combination of: Hemiparesis; Higher cerebral dysfunction (e.g. aphasia); Hemisensory loss; Homonymous hemianopia (damage to optic radiations)	Middle cerebral artery occlusion (Embolism from heart or major vessels)	
Partial anterior circulation syndrome (PACS)	Isolated motor loss (e.g. leg only, arm only, face); Isolated higher cerebral dysfunction (e.g. aphasia, neglect); Mixture of higher cerebral dysfunction and motor loss (e.g. aphasia with right hemiparesis)	Occlusion of a branch of the middle cerebral artery or anterior cerebral artery (Embolism from heart or major vessels)	
Lacunar syndrome (LACS)	Pure motor stroke – affects two limbs; Pure sensory stroke; Sensory-motor stroke; No higher cerebral dysfunction or hemianopia	Thrombotic occlusion of small perforating arteries (Thrombosis in situ)	
Posterior circulation stroke (POCS) (lateral view)	Homonymous hemianopia (damage to visual cortex); Cerebellar syndrome; Cranial nerve syndromes	Occlusion in vertebral, basilar or posterior cerebral artery territory (Cardiac embolism or thrombosis in situ)	

Fig. 26.10 Clinical and radiological features of the stroke syndromes. The top three diagrams show coronal sections of the brain and the bottom one shows a sagittal section. The anatomical locations of cerebral functions are shown with the nerve tracts in green. A motor (or sensory) deficit (shown by the areas shaded red) can occur with damage to the relevant cortex (PACS), nerve tracts (LACS) or both (TACS). The corresponding CT scans show horizontal slices at the level of the lesion, highlighted by the arrows.

TIA traditionally also includes patients with amaurosis fugax, usually due to a vascular occlusion in the retina.

- *Stroke* describes those events in which symptoms last more than 24 hours. The differential diagnosis of patients with symptoms lasting a few minutes or hours is similar to those with persisting symptoms (see Box 26.3). The term 'minor stroke' is sometimes used to refer to symptoms lasting over 24 hours but not causing significant disability.
- *Progressing stroke (or stroke in evolution)* describes a stroke in which the focal neurological deficit worsens after the patient first presents. Such worsening may be due to increasing volume of infarction, haemorrhagic transformation or increasing cerebral oedema.
- *Completed stroke* describes a stroke in which the focal deficit persists and is not progressing.

When assessing a patient within hours of symptom onset, it is not possible to distinguish stroke from TIA unless symptoms have already resolved. In clinical practice, it is important to distinguish those patients with strokes who have persisting focal neurological symptoms when seen from those whose symptoms have already resolved.

Investigations

Investigation of acute stroke aims to confirm the vascular nature of a lesion, distinguish infarction from haemorrhage and identify the underlying vascular disease and risk factors (Box 26.5).

Risk factor analysis

Initial investigation includes a range of simple blood tests to detect common vascular risk factors and markers of rarer causes, along with an ECG and brain imaging. Where there is uncertainty about the nature of the stroke, further investigations are indicated. This especially applies to younger patients, who are less likely to have atherosclerotic disease (Box 26.6).

i	26.5 Investigation of a patient with an acute stroke	
Diagnostic question	**Investigation**	
Is it a vascular lesion?	CT/MRI	
Is it ischaemic or haemorrhagic?	CT/MRI	
Is it a subarachnoid haemorrhage?	CT/lumbar puncture	
Is there any cardiac source of embolism?	ECG Holter monitoring Echocardiogram	
What is the underlying vascular disease?	Duplex ultrasound of carotids MRA CTA Contrast angiography	
What are the risk factors?	Full blood count Cholesterol Blood glucose	
Is there an unusual cause?	ESR Serum protein electrophoresis Clotting/thrombophilia screen	

(CT = computed tomography; CTA = computed tomographic angiography; ECG = electrocardiogram; ESR = erythrocyte sedimentation rate; MRA = magnetic resonance angiography; MRI = magnetic resonance imaging)

Neuroimaging

Brain imaging with either CT or MRI should be performed in all patients with acute stroke. Exceptions are where results would not influence management, such as in the advanced stage of a terminal illness. CT remains the most practical and widely available method of imaging the brain. It will usually exclude non-stroke lesions, including subdural haematomas and brain tumours, and will demonstrate intracerebral haemorrhage within minutes of stroke onset (see Fig. 26.9). However, especially within the first few hours after symptom onset, CT changes in cerebral infarction may be completely absent or only very subtle. Changes often develop over time (see Fig. 26.13) but small cerebral infarcts may never show up on CT scans. For some purposes, a CT scan performed within 24 hours is adequate

i	26.6 Causes and investigation of acute stroke in young patients	
Cause	**Investigation**	
Cerebral infarct		
Cardiac embolism	Echocardiography (including transoesophageal)	
Premature atherosclerosis	Serum lipids	
Arterial dissection	MRI CTA	
Reversible cerebral vasoconstriction syndromes	MRI CTA	
Thrombophilia	Protein C, protein S Antithrombin III Factor V Leiden, prothrombin	
Homocystinuria (p. 369)	Urinary amino acids Methionine loading test	
Antiphospholipid antibody syndrome (p. 977)	Anticardiolipin antibodies/lupus anticoagulant	
Systemic lupus erythematosus	ANA	
Vasculitis (e.g. primary angiitis of the central nervous system)	ESR CRP ANCA	
CADASIL	MRI brain	
CARASIL	Genetic analysis Skin biopsy	
Mitochondrial cytopathy	Serum lactate White cell mitochondrial DNA Muscle biopsy Mitochondrial molecular genetics	
Fabry's disease	Alpha-galactosidase levels	
Sickle cell disease	Sickle cell studies	
Neurovascular syphilis	Syphilis serology	
Primary intracerebral haemorrhage		
AVM	MRI/MRA	
Drug misuse	Drug screen (amphetamine, cocaine)	
Coagulopathy	PT and APTT Platelet count	
Subarachnoid haemorrhage		
Saccular ('berry') aneurysm	MRI/MRA	
AVM	MRI/MRA	
Vertebral dissection	MRI/MRA	

(ANA = antinuclear antibody; ANCA = antineutrophil cytoplasmic antibody; APTT = activated partial thromboplastin time; AVM = arteriovenous malformation; CADASIL/CARASIL = cerebral autosomal dominant/recessive arteriopathy with subcortical infarcts and leucoencephalopathy; CRP = C-reactive protein; CTA = computed tomographic angiography; ESR = erythrocyte sedimentation rate; MRA = magnetic resonance angiography; MRI = magnetic resonance imaging; PT = prothrombin time)

26

26.7 Indications for immediate CT/MRI in acute stroke

- Patient on anticoagulants or with abnormal coagulation
- Consideration for reperfusion (thrombolysis) or immediate anticoagulation
- Deteriorating conscious level or rapidly progressing deficits
- Suspected cerebellar haematoma, to exclude hydrocephalus

but there are certain circumstances in which an immediate CT scan is essential (Box 26.7). Even in the absence of changes suggesting infarction, abnormal perfusion of brain tissue can be imaged with CT after injection of contrast media (i.e. CT perfusion scanning). This can be useful in guiding immediate treatment of ischaemic stroke.

MRI is not as widely available as CT and scanning times are longer. However, MRI diffusion weighted imaging (DWI) can detect ischaemia earlier than CT, and other MRI sequences can also be used to demonstrate abnormal perfusion (see Fig. 26.4). MRI is more sensitive than CT in detecting strokes affecting the brainstem and cerebellum, and, unlike CT, can reliably distinguish haemorrhagic from ischaemic stroke even several weeks after the onset. CT and MRI may reveal clues as to the nature of the arterial lesion. For example, there may be a small, deep lacunar infarct indicating small-vessel disease, or a more peripheral infarct suggesting an extracranial source of embolism (see Fig. 26.10). In a haemorrhagic lesion, the location might indicate the presence of an underlying vascular malformation, saccular aneurysm or amyloid angiopathy. More recently, CTA is being used to show vessel occlusion suitable for clot retrieval (see later).

Vascular imaging

Many ischaemic strokes are caused by atherosclerotic thromboembolic disease of the major extracranial vessels. Detection of extracranial vascular disease can help establish why the patient has had an ischaemic stroke and, in selected patients, may lead on to specific treatments, including carotid endarterectomy to reduce the risk of further stroke (see below). The presence or absence of a carotid bruit is not a reliable indicator of the degree of carotid stenosis. Extracranial arterial disease can be non-invasively identified with duplex ultrasound, MRA or CTA (see Fig. 26.5), or occasionally by intra-arterial contrast radiography as above.

Cardiac investigations

Approximately 20% of ischaemic strokes are due to embolism from the heart. The most common causes are atrial fibrillation, prosthetic heart valves, other valvular abnormalities and recent myocardial infarction. These may be identified by clinical examination and ECG, but a transthoracic or transoesophageal echocardiogram is also required to confirm the presence of a clinically apparent cardiac source or to identify an unsuspected source such as endocarditis, atrial myxoma, intracardiac thrombus or patent foramen ovale. Such findings may lead on to specific cardiac treatment.

Management

Management (Fig. 26.11) is aimed at identifying the cause, minimising the volume of brain that is irreversibly damaged, preventing complications (Fig. 26.12), reducing the patient's

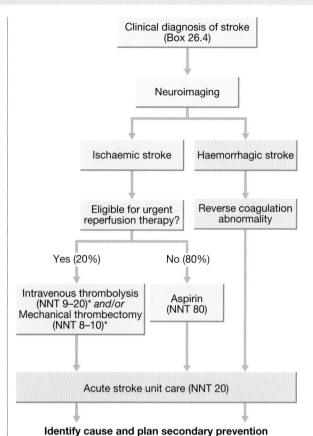

Fig. 26.11 Emergency management of stroke. *Varies with patient selection and delay in treatment. (NNT = number needed to treat to avoid one death or long-term disability)

disability and handicap through rehabilitation, and reducing the risk of recurrent stroke or other vascular events. With TIA there is no persisting brain damage and disability, so the priority is to reduce the risk of further vascular events.

Supportive care

Rapid admission of patients to a specialised stroke unit facilitates coordinated care from a specialised multidisciplinary team, and has been shown to reduce both mortality and residual disability amongst survivors. For every 1000 patients managed in a stroke unit, an extra 50 will avoid death or long-term disability, compared to those managed in general wards. Consideration of a patient's rehabilitation needs should commence at the same time as acute medical management. Dysphagia is common and can be detected by an early bedside test of swallowing. This allows hydration, feeding and medication to be given safely, if necessary by nasogastric tube or intravenously. In the acute phase, a checklist may be useful (Box 26.8) to ensure that all the factors that might influence outcome have been addressed. In recent years, many services have developed hyperacute stroke units (HASUs) to ensure that patients are given immediate access to these interventions, as well as urgent medical treatments.

The patient's neurological deficits may worsen during the first few hours or days after their onset. This may be due to extension of the area of infarction, haemorrhage transformation of an infarction, or the development of oedema with consequent mass effect. It is important to distinguish these patients from those who

Fig. 26.12 Complications of acute stroke.

Complications	Prevention	Treatment
Epileptic seizures	Maintain cerebral oxygenation Avoid metabolic disturbance	Anticonvulsants
Depression and anxiety	Maintain positive attitude and provide information	Antidepressants
Painful shoulder	Avoid traction injury Shoulder/arm supports Physiotherapy	Physiotherapy Local glucocorticoid injections
Chest infection	Nurse semi-erect Avoid aspiration (nil by mouth, nasogastric tube, possible gastrostomy)	Antibiotics Physiotherapy
Constipation	Appropriate aperients and diet	Appropriate aperients
Urinary infection	Avoid catheterisation if possible Use penile sheath	Antibiotics
Pressure sores	Frequent turning Monitor pressure areas Avoid urine damage to skin	Nursing care Pressure-relieving mattress
Deep vein thrombosis/ pulmonary embolism	Maintain hydration Early mobilisation Heparin (for high-risk patients only)	Anticoagulation (exclude haemorrhage first)

26.8 How to manage a patient with acute stroke

Airway

- Perform bedside screen and keep patient nil by mouth if swallowing unsafe or aspiration occurs

Breathing

- Check respiratory rate and give oxygen if saturation <95%

Circulation

- Check peripheral perfusion, pulse and blood pressure, and treat abnormalities with fluid replacement, anti-arrhythmics and inotropic drugs as appropriate

Hydration

- If signs of dehydration, give fluids parenterally or by nasogastric tube

Nutrition

- Assess nutritional status and provide supplements if needed
- If dysphagia persists for >48 hrs, start feeding via nasogastric tube

Medication

- If dysphagic, consider other routes for essential medications

Blood pressure

- Unless there is heart or renal failure, evidence of hypertensive encephalopathy or aortic dissection, do not lower blood pressure abruptly in first week as it may reduce cerebral perfusion. Blood pressure often returns towards patient's normal level within days

Blood glucose

- Check blood glucose and treat when levels are ≥11.1 mmol/L (200 mg/dL) (by insulin infusion or glucose/potassium/insulin (GKI))
- Monitor closely to avoid hypoglycaemia

Temperature

- If pyrexic, investigate and treat underlying cause
- Control with antipyretics, as raised brain temperature may increase infarct volume

Pressure areas

- Reduce risk of skin breakdown:
  - Treat infection
  - Maintain nutrition
  - Provide pressure-relieving mattress
  - Turn immobile patients regularly

Incontinence

- Check for constipation and urinary retention; treat these appropriately
- Avoid urinary catheterisation unless patient is in acute urinary retention or incontinence is threatening pressure areas

Mobilisation

- Avoid bed rest

---

are deteriorating as a result of complications such as hypoxia, sepsis, epileptic seizures or metabolic abnormalities that may be reversed more easily. Patients with cerebellar haematomas or infarcts with mass effect may develop obstructive hydrocephalus and some will benefit from insertion of a ventricular drain and/or decompressive surgery (see Fig. 26.11). Some patients with large haematomas or infarction with massive oedema in the cerebral hemispheres may benefit from anti-oedema agents, such as mannitol or artificial ventilation. Surgical decompression to reduce intracranial pressure should be considered in appropriate patients.

Reperfusion (thrombolysis and thrombectomy)

Rapid reperfusion in ischaemic stroke can reduce the extent of brain damage. Intravenous thrombolysis with recombinant tissue

26

26.9 Anticoagulation in old age

- **Increased risk**: older age and previous stroke increase the risk of stroke in the presence of atrial fibrillation, and bleeding risk with anticoagulation.
- **Falls risk**: elderly patients are more prone to falls, including head injuries, which increase bleeding risk.
- **Monitoring of therapy**: fine adjustments to daily dose of warfarin may be more difficult, as may monitoring of therapy.
- **Impact of comorbidities**: the presence of conditions such as chronic renal impairment, diabetes or heart failure may affect the risk:benefit ratio, and decisions to use anticoagulation must be weighed carefully. Decision aids have been developed to assist (see 'Further information').

plasminogen activator (rt-PA) increases the risk of haemorrhagic transformation of the cerebral infarct with potentially fatal results. The main contraindications are bleeding risk (recent haemorrhage, anticoagulant therapy) and delay to treatment; the earlier treatment is given, the greater the benefit. However, if given within 4.5 hours of symptom onset to carefully selected patients, the haemorrhagic risk is offset by an improved overall outcome. Recently mechanical clot retrieval (thrombectomy) in patients with a large-vessel occlusion can greatly improve the chances of avoiding disability (see Fig. 26.11).

Aspirin

In the absence of contraindications, aspirin (300 mg daily) should be started immediately after an ischaemic stroke unless rt-PA has been given, in which case it should be withheld for at least 24 hours. Aspirin reduces the risk of early recurrence and has a small but clinically worthwhile effect on long-term outcome (see Fig. 26.11); it may be given by rectal suppository or by nasogastric tube in dysphagic patients.

Heparin

Anticoagulation with heparin has been widely used to treat acute ischaemic stroke in the past. While it reduces the risk of early ischaemic recurrence and venous thromboembolism, it increases the risk of both intracranial and extracranial haemorrhage. Furthermore, routine use of heparin does not result in better long-term outcomes, and therefore it should not be used in the routine management of acute stroke. It is unclear whether heparin might provide benefit in selected patients, such as those with recent myocardial infarction, arterial dissection or progressing strokes. Intracranial haemorrhage must be excluded on brain imaging before considering anticoagulation.

Coagulation abnormalities

In those with intracerebral haemorrhage, coagulation abnormalities should be reversed as quickly as possible to reduce the likelihood of the haematoma enlarging. This most commonly arises in those on warfarin therapy. There is no evidence that clotting factors are useful in the absence of a clotting defect.

Management of risk factors

The approaches used are summarised in Figure 26.13. The average risk of a further stroke is 5–10% within the first week of a stroke or TIA, perhaps 15% in the first year and 5% per year thereafter. The risks are not substantially different for intracerebral

haemorrhage. The potential gain from good secondary prevention can be expressed as the number needed to treat (NNT) to avoid a recurrent stroke. Patients with ischaemic events should be put on long-term antiplatelet drugs (NNT 100) and statins (NNT 60) to lower cholesterol. For patients in atrial fibrillation, the risk can be reduced substantially (NNT 15) by using oral anticoagulation with warfarin to achieve an international normalised ratio (INR) of 2–3. The newer direct oral anticoagulants (such as dabigatran, rivaroxaban and apixaban) are now widely used, offering improved safety and effectiveness at increased drug cost. The risk of recurrence after both ischaemic and haemorrhagic strokes can be reduced by blood pressure reduction, even for those with relatively normal blood pressures (NNT 50).

Carotid endarterectomy and angioplasty

A small proportion of patients with a carotid territory ischaemic stroke or TIA will have more than 50% stenosis of the carotid artery on the side of the brain lesion. Such patients have a greater than average risk of stroke recurrence. For those without major residual disability, removal of the stenosis has been shown to reduce the overall risk of recurrence (NNT 15), although the operation itself carries about a 5% risk of stroke. Surgery is most effective in patients with more severe stenoses (70–99%) and when it is performed within the first couple of weeks after the TIA or ischaemic stroke. Carotid angioplasty and stenting are technically feasible but have not been shown to be as effective as endarterectomy for the majority of eligible patients. Endarterectomy of asymptomatic carotid stenosis has been shown to reduce the subsequent risk of stroke but the small absolute benefit does not justify its routine use.

Unusual causes

A minority of strokes are caused by arterial dissection of the carotid (carotid dissection) or vertebral artery (vertebral artery dissection). The presenting history often includes minor injury and face or neck pain. After confirmation on angiography (MRA or CTA), treatment is with either antiplatelet drugs or anticoagulation. Reversible vasoconstriction syndromes require good physiological control (particularly blood pressure).

Subarachnoid haemorrhage

Subarachnoid haemorrhage (SAH) is less common than ischaemic stroke or intracerebral haemorrhage (see Fig. 26.1) and affects about 6/100 000 of the population. Women are affected more commonly than men and the condition usually presents before the age of 65. The immediate mortality of aneurysmal SAH is about 30%; survivors have a recurrence (or rebleed) rate of about 40% in the first 4 weeks and 3% annually thereafter.

Some 85% of cases of SAH are caused by saccular or 'berry' aneurysms arising from the bifurcation of cerebral arteries (see Fig. 26.2), particularly in the region of the circle of Willis. The most common sites are in the anterior communicating artery (30%), posterior communicating artery (25%) or middle cerebral artery (20%). There is an increased risk in first-degree relatives of those with saccular aneurysms, and in patients with polycystic kidney disease (p. 405) and congenital connective tissue defects such as Ehlers–Danlos syndrome (p. 970). In about 10% of cases, SAHs are non-aneurysmal haemorrhages (so-called peri-mesencephalic haemorrhages), which have a very characteristic appearance on CT and a benign outcome in terms of mortality and recurrence.

Fig. 26.13 Strategies for secondary prevention of stroke. (1) Lower blood pressure with caution in patients with postural hypotension, renal impairment or bilateral carotid stenosis. (2) Other statins can be used as an alternative to simvastatin in patients on warfarin or digoxin. (3) Warfarin and aspirin have been used in combination in patients with prosthetic heart valves. (4) The combination of aspirin and clopidogrel is indicated only in patients with unstable angina or those with a temporary high risk of recurrence (e.g. carotid stenosis). (ACE = angiotensin-converting enzyme; BP = blood pressure; CT = computed tomography; ECG = electrocardiogram; MRI = magnetic resonance imaging; TIA = transient ischaemic attack; U&Es = urea and electrolytes)

Around 5% of SAHs are due to arteriovenous malformations and vertebral artery dissection.

Clinical features

SAH typically presents with a sudden, severe, 'thunderclap' headache (often occipital), which lasts for hours or even days, often accompanied by vomiting, raised blood pressure and neck stiffness or pain. It commonly occurs on physical exertion, straining and sexual excitement. There may be loss of consciousness at the onset, so SAH should be considered if a patient is found comatose. About 1 patient in 8 with a sudden severe headache has SAH and, in view of this, all who present in this way require investigation to exclude it (Fig. 26.14).

On examination, the patient is usually distressed and irritable, with photophobia. There may be neck stiffness due to subarachnoid blood but this may take some hours to develop. Focal hemisphere signs, such as hemiparesis or aphasia, may be present at onset if there is an associated intracerebral haematoma. A third nerve palsy may be present due to local pressure from an aneurysm of the posterior communicating artery, but this is rare. Fundoscopy may reveal a subhyaloid haemorrhage, which represents blood tracking along the subarachnoid space around the optic nerve.

Investigations

CT brain scanning and lumbar puncture are required. The diagnosis of SAH can be made by CT but a negative result does not completely exclude it, since small amounts of blood in the subarachnoid space cannot be detected by CT (see Fig. 26.14). Lumbar puncture should be performed 12 hours after symptom onset if possible, to allow detection of xanthochromia (p. 1077). If either of these tests is positive, cerebral angiography (see Fig. 26.5) is required to determine the optimal approach to prevent recurrent bleeding.

26

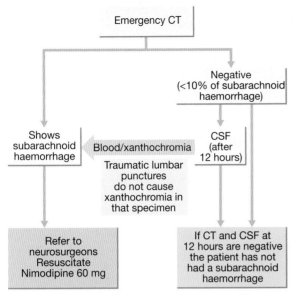

Fig. 26.14 **Investigation of subarachnoid haemorrhage.** (CSF = cerebrospinal fluid; CT = computed tomography)

Management

Nimodipine (30–60 mg IV for 5–14 days, followed by 360 mg orally for a further 7 days) is usually given to prevent delayed ischaemia in the acute phase. Insertion of platinum coils into an aneurysm (via an endovascular procedure) or surgical clipping of the aneurysm neck reduces the risk of both early and late recurrence. Coiling is associated with fewer perioperative complications and better outcomes than surgery; where feasible, it is now the procedure of first choice. Arteriovenous malformations can be managed either by surgical removal, by ligation of the blood vessels that feed or drain the lesion, or by injection of material to occlude the fistula or draining veins. Treatment may also be needed for complications of SAH, which include obstructive hydrocephalus (that may require drainage via a shunt), delayed cerebral ischaemia due to vasospasm (which may be treated with vasodilators), hyponatraemia (best managed by fluid restriction) and systemic complications associated with immobility, such as chest infection and venous thrombosis.

Cerebral venous disease

Thrombosis of the cerebral veins and venous sinuses (cerebral venous thrombosis) is much less common than arterial thrombosis. However, it has been recognised with increasing frequency in recent years, as access to non-invasive imaging of the venous sinuses using MR venography has increased. The main causes are listed in Box 26.10.

Clinical features

Cerebral venous sinus thrombosis usually presents with symptoms of raised intracranial pressure, seizures and focal neurological symptoms. The clinical features vary according to the sinus involved (Box 26.11 and see Fig. 26.3). Cortical vein thrombosis presents with focal cortical deficits such as aphasia and hemiparesis (depending on the area affected), and epilepsy

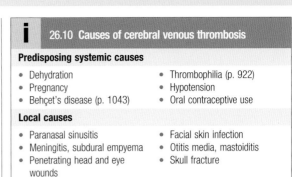

i | 26.10 Causes of cerebral venous thrombosis

Predisposing systemic causes

- Dehydration
- Pregnancy
- Behçet's disease (p. 1043)
- Thrombophilia (p. 922)
- Hypotension
- Oral contraceptive use

Local causes

- Paranasal sinusitis
- Meningitis, subdural empyema
- Penetrating head and eye wounds
- Facial skin infection
- Otitis media, mastoiditis
- Skull fracture

i | 26.11 Clinical features of cerebral venous thrombosis

Cavernous sinus thrombosis

- Proptosis, ptosis, headache, external and internal ophthalmoplegia, papilloedema, reduced sensation in trigeminal first division
- Often bilateral, patient ill and febrile

Superior sagittal sinus thrombosis

- Headache, papilloedema, seizures
- Clinical features may resemble idiopathic intracranial hypertension (p. 1133)
- May involve veins of both hemispheres, causing advancing motor and sensory focal deficits

Transverse sinus thrombosis

- Hemiparesis, seizures, papilloedema
- May spread to jugular foramen and involve cranial nerves 9, 10 and 11

(focal or generalised). The deficit can increase if spreading thrombophlebitis occurs.

Investigations and management

MR venography demonstrates a filling defect in the affected vessel. Anticoagulation, initially with heparin followed by warfarin, is beneficial, even in the presence of venous haemorrhage. In selected patients, endovascular thrombolysis has been advocated. Management of underlying causes and complications, such as persistently raised intracranial pressure, is important.

About 10% of cerebral venous sinus thrombosis, particularly cavernous sinus thrombosis, is associated with infection (most commonly *Staphylococcus aureus*), needing antibiotic treatment. Otherwise, the treatment of choice is anticoagulation.

Further information

Websites

eso-stroke.org *European Stroke Organisation guidelines.*
nhs.uk/actfast *FAST (face, arms, speech, time) campaign to raise public awareness of the emergency nature of stroke.*
nice.org.uk/guidance *National Institute for Health and Care Excellence CG180 'Tools and resources' includes a patient decision aid – Atrial fibrillation: medicines to help reduce your risk of a stroke – what are the options?*
rcplondon.ac.uk/resources/stroke-guidelines *Royal College of Physicians of London clinical guideline.*
stroke.cochrane.org *Systematic reviews of stroke treatments.*
stroketraining.org *Stroke Training and Awareness Resources.*

27

Medical ophthalmology

Functional anatomy and physiology 1164

Investigation of visual disorders 1168
Perimetry 1168
Imaging 1168
Visual electrophysiology 1169

Presenting problems in ophthalmic disease 1169
Watery/dry eye 1170
Pruritus 1170
Pain/headache 1170
Photophobia/glare 1170
Photopsia 1170
Blurred vision 1170
Loss of vision 1170
Distortion of vision 1171
Eyelid retraction 1171
Optic disc swelling 1171
Proptosis 1171

Specialist ophthalmological conditions 1171
Ocular inflammation 1171
Infectious conditions 1173
Cataract 1174
Diabetic eye disease 1174
Retinal vascular occlusion 1177
Age-related macular degeneration 1178

The ability to see is an important aspect of everyday life. Although rarely a cause of mortality, visual impairment can have a profoundly negative impact on socioeconomic status.

Globally, although refractive errors and cataract remain the main causes of visual impairment, significant progress has occurred in prevention and treatment. Public health measures have reduced diseases of poor hygiene and unclean water, such as trachoma and onchocerciasis, and greater access to surgery has reduced the burden of untreated cataract and glaucoma. However, conditions associated with longevity, such as age-related macular degeneration, diabetic retinopathy and retinal vein occlusion, for which scientific advances have led to effective but expensive therapies requiring frequent and long-term attendance, are increasing in frequency.

Traditionally, ophthalmology relied on other specialties to undertake extraocular investigation and treatment. Medical ophthalmology bypasses that co-dependence, allowing patients with visual disorders to receive overarching care within ophthalmology. As such, it requires a good grounding in medicine, particularly dermatology, diabetes and endocrinology, infectious diseases, medical genetics, neurology, rheumatology and stroke medicine.

Medical ophthalmology presents a challenge for a medical textbook, as it overlaps with almost all other specialties, but particularly neurology. In this book neuro-ophthalmology is covered in Chapter 25. This chapter concentrates mainly on intraocular inflammation, which was the prime drive to create the specialty, and conditions that require intravitreal injection therapy. It does not therefore represent the totality of the medical ophthalmologist's workload. Ophthalmological conditions that are usually managed within non-ophthalmological specialties are discussed in the corresponding chapters, although for ease of reference the more common ophthalmic features of non-ophthalmological conditions are listed throughout this chapter (haematological disease in Box 27.1, diabetes and endocrine disease in Box 27.2, cardiovascular disease in Box 27.3, respiratory disease in Box 27.4, rheumatological/musculoskeletal disease in Box 27.5, gastrointestinal disease in Box 27.6 and skin disease in Box 27.7).

Functional anatomy and physiology

Visual pathways, innervation of the eye and the control of eye movement are discussed in Chapter 25.

Orbit

The orbit is the fat-filled cavity in which the eye is suspended. It is shaped like a hollow square pyramid, its base the orbital rim. The orbital periosteum ('periorbita') is continuous with the periosteal layer of cranial dura mater. The dura and arachnoid form the optic nerve sheath, its subarachnoid space containing cerebrospinal fluid in continuity with the third ventricle.

Eyelid/orbital septum/conjunctiva

In primary gaze, the eyelids just cover the superior and inferior cornea. The eyelids contain the orbital septum and the tarsal plate.

Within the tarsal plates, modified sebaceous (Meibomian) glands produce an oily surfactant to slow tear evaporation.

The conjunctiva, a mucous membrane, lines the posterior surface of the eyelid, adhering only to the tarsal plates and the scleral/corneal junction. The accessory lacrimal glands provide basal tear production; mucus produced by goblet cells stabilises the tear film by lowering surface tension.

i | 27.1 Ophthalmic features of haematological disease

Condition	Ophthalmic findings
Severe anaemia of any cause (retinopathy of anaemia)	Flame haemorrhages Cotton wool spots Roth spots Pre-retinal haemorrhage
Megaloblastic anaemia	Optic neuropathy
Sickle cell anaemia	Conjunctival vasculopathy Peripheral retinal neovascularisation
Thalassaemia	Desferrioxamine-associated pigmentary retinopathy
Leukaemia (leukaemic retinopathy)	Pseudohypopyon Flame haemorrhages Roth spots Retinal oedema Retinal vein occlusion
Lymphoma Non-Hodgkin lymphoma Central nervous system lymphoma	Lacrimal gland infiltration Posterior uveitis (atypical choroiditis)
Myeloproliferative disorders Hyperviscosity Cerebral venous thrombosis	Retinal vein occlusion Papilloedema
Paraproteinaemias Waldenström's macroglobulinaemia Multiple myeloma	Retinal vein engorgement/occlusion
Thrombophilia Cerebral venous thrombosis	Papilloedema

Lacrimal gland/lacrimal drainage

The lacrimal gland lies within the periorbita of the anterolateral roof of the orbit. Its secretions (tears) wash away surface irritants and convey emotion. Excess tears drain, via canaliculi in the lids, into the lacrimal sac, nasolacrimal duct and inferior nasal meatus.

Extraocular muscles

The extraocular muscles (Fig. 27.1) consist of four recti, two obliques and one levator. The recti originate from a circular condensation of periorbita, the annulus of Zinn, which encircles the superior orbital fissure and the optic canal. They extend forwards to insert into the anterior sclera.

The levator palpebrae superioris originates above the optic canal and inserts into the tarsal plate and overlying skin of the upper eyelid. The superior tarsal muscle (Müller's muscle) originates from the inferior aspect of the levator and also inserts into the tarsal plate.

The superior oblique originates superonasal to the recti, and runs along the roof of the orbit, its tendon passing horizontally through the trochlea at the orbital rim to insert into the anterior sclera.

The inferior oblique originates from the floor of the anterior orbit, just posterior to the lacrimal sac. It turns horizontally, passing beneath the inferior rectus, to insert into the inferior anterior sclera.

Eye

The optic vesicle develops from the diencephalon. The eye is therefore contiguous with the brain. This is reflected in the three-layer structure of the eye:

27.2 Ophthalmic features of diabetes and other endocrine disease

Condition	Ophthalmic findings
Diabetes	Proliferative retinopathy Macular oedema Small pupils (autonomic neuropathy) Cataract (including 'snowflake' cataract)
Thyrotoxicosis (any cause)	Eyelid retraction
Graves' disease (TSH receptor antibody-positive)	Exposure keratopathy Conjunctival and periorbital oedema Restrictive ocular motility Proptosis Optic neuropathy
Parathyroid disease	Band keratopathy Corneal calcium deposition
Phaeochromocytoma	Hypertensive retinopathy Cotton wool spots Flame haemorrhages Optic disc oedema with or without macular oedema
Cushing's syndrome	Posterior subcapsular cataract Diabetic retinopathy Central serous retinopathy
Thyroid carcinoma	Horner's syndrome with absent unilateral facial sweating

(TSH = thyroid stimulating hormone)

27.3 Ophthalmic features of cardiovascular disease

Condition	Ophthalmic findings
Arteriosclerosis	Arteriovenous nipping Retinal vein occlusion, caused by arteriovenous nipping Retinal artery macroaneurysm Ischaemic optic neuropathy Pupil-sparing third and/or sixth nerve palsy, caused by infarction of the vasa nervosum
Hypertension	Hypertensive retinopathy Cotton wool spots Flame haemorrhages Optic disc oedema, with or without macular oedema
Infective endocarditis	Flame haemorrhages Roth spots Endophthalmitis, caused by haematogenous spread of infection
Drugs	Vortex keratopathy (corneal epithelial deposits), caused by amiodarone (also seen in Fabry's disease, p. 370) Bilateral optic neuropathy, caused by amiodarone
Thromboembolic disorders (including thromboembolus from atrial fibrillation)	Retinal artery occlusion, caused by artery-to-artery embolism Homonymous hemianopia, caused by embolic stroke (p. 1088)

27.4 Ophthalmic features of respiratory disease

Condition	Ophthalmic findings
Chronic obstructive pulmonary disease (p. 573)	Optic disc oedema (type 2 respiratory failure)
Cystic fibrosis (p. 580)	Diabetic retinopathy
Tuberculosis (p. 588)	Anterior uveitis Choroidal granuloma Serpiginous choroiditis Peripheral retinal arteritis Optic neuropathy, visual loss and disturbance of colour vision (adverse effects of ethambutol and isoniazid)
Sarcoidosis (p. 608)	Anterior uveitis (granulomatosis) Mutton fat keratitic precipitates Iris nodules Choroidal granuloma Panuveitis Multifocal choroiditis Retinal periphlebitis Sicca syndrome, caused by lacrimal gland infiltration Exposure keratopathy, caused by corneal exposure secondary to facial nerve palsy Optic neuropathy, caused by optic disc oedema secondary to meningeal infiltration
Lung cancer (p. 928)	Horner's syndrome (p. 1091) Cancer-associated retinopathy

Fig. 27.1 The extraocular musculature (right eye). *Adapted from Batterbury M, Bowling B, Murphy C. Ophthalmology. An illustrated colour text, 3rd edn. Churchill Livingstone, Elsevier Ltd; 2009.*

The major structures of the eye are shown in Figure 27.2.

During embryogenesis, overlying ectoderm sinks into the neuroectoderm of the optic vesicle to form the lens vesicle, thus inducing the optic vesicle to form the two-layered optic cup. The inner and outer layers form the neurosensory retina and the retinal pigment epithelium, respectively. The intervening space is continuous with the third ventricle of the diencephalon,

- the sclera/cornea, a fibrous outer layer analogous to the meningeal dura
- the choroid, ciliary body and iris (together known as the uveal tract), a vascular middle layer analogous to the pia-arachnoid
- the retina, an inner layer analogous to white matter.

27.5 Ophthalmic features of rheumatological/musculoskeletal disease

Rheumatoid arthritis

- Keratoconjunctivitis sicca
- Peripheral ulcerative keratitis ('corneal melt')
- Painless episcleritis
- Scleritis and scleromalacia

Seronegative spondyloarthropathies

- Conjunctivitis (chlamydia-associated reactive arthritis)
- Anterior uveitis

Connective tissue diseases

Dermatomyositis
- Periorbital oedema with violaceous eyelid rash

Sjögren's syndrome
- Dry eyes

Treatment effects
- Bull's eye maculopathy (hydroxychloroquine)
- Viral retinitis (immunosuppression)

Systemic vasculitides

Giant cell arteritis
- Central/branch retinal artery occlusion
- Ischaemic optic neuropathy

Behçet's disease
- Occlusive retinal vasculitis (posterior uveitis)
- Anterior uveitis with hypopyon

Granulomatosis with polyangiitis (Wegener's)
- Scleritis with involvement of adjacent cornea (sclerokeratitis)
- Retro-orbital inflammation (see Fig. 25.49)

Polyarteritis nodosa
- Peripheral ulcerative keratitis
- Scleritis
- Retinal arteritis

Others/non-specific
- Necrotising scleritis/sclerokeratitis/peripheral ulcerative keratitis
- Anterior ischaemic optic neuropathy
- Extraocular myositis (painful diplopia)
- Retinal arteritis
- Pupil-sparing 3rd nerve palsy
- 6th nerve palsy
- Proptosis
- Occipital lobe infarction

Diseases of bone

Paget's disease, polyostotic fibrous dysplasia
- Optic neuropathy

Others/non-specific
- Anterior uveitis (adverse effect of bisphosphonates)

27.6 Ophthalmic features of gastrointestinal disease

Malabsorption
- Corneal and conjunctival keratinisation
- Rod photoreceptor loss

Chronic pancreatitis
- Diabetic retinopathy

Inflammatory bowel disease
- Episcleritis
- Non-necrotising scleritis
- Anterior uveitis

Large bowel tumours
- Atypical congenital retinal pigment epithelium hypertrophy (familial adenomatous polyposis)

Inherited liver disease
- Kayser–Fleischer corneal rings, sunflower cataracts (Wilson's disease)
- Diabetic retinopathy (haemochromatosis)

27.7 Ophthalmic features of skin disease

Rosacea
- Posterior blepharitis
- Keratitis

Acne vulgaris
- Dry eye (adverse effect of isotretinoin)
- Papilloedema (adverse effect of tetracycline)

Psoriasis
- Anterior uveitis

Eczema
- Atopic keratoconjunctivitis

Urticaria
- Angioedema

Bullous diseases
- Ocular cicatricial pemphigoid
- Stevens–Johnson syndrome

Alopecia areata
- Eyebrow and eyelash loss

Cutaneous melanoma
- Melanoma-associated retinopathy

Skin tumours
- Eyelid tumours (basal cell carcinoma, squamous cell carcinoma, keratoacanthoma, naevus, melanoma)

Skin infections
- Stye (eyelash folliculitis)
- Acute blepharoconjunctivitis (herpes simplex)
- Chronic conjunctivitis (molluscum contagiosum)

the cilia of the third ventricle continuing as cilia on the outer neurosensory retina. Laterally, these cilia form the outer segments of the photoreceptors.

Initially, the hyaloid artery supplies the lens and vitreous. In its final form, the vitreous develops from the retina and the hyaloid artery regresses, leaving only the central retinal artery and its branches.

Mesenchyme forms the tarsal plates of the eyelid, the stroma and the endothelium of the cornea, the sclera and the choroid.

Surface ectoderm, as well as forming the lens, forms the epidermis of the eyelid, the conjunctiva, the epithelium of the cornea and the lacrimal gland.

Sclera/cornea

The sclera lends shape to the eye and provides attachment for the ocular musculature. It makes up five-sixths of the eyeball, the other sixth being formed by transparent cornea.

The limbus lies at the junction between the cornea and sclera, and contains stem cells and Schlemm's canal. The stem cells allow continuous regeneration of the corneal epithelium. Schlemm's canal, with its overlying trabecular meshwork, drains aqueous fluid from the anterior chamber into the external veins of the episclera and conjunctiva.

The avascular cornea is nourished by diffusion from the anterior chamber, limbal capillaries and oxygen dissolved in the tear film. The cornea, assisted by the lens and the length of the eye, determines the refractive ability of the eye.

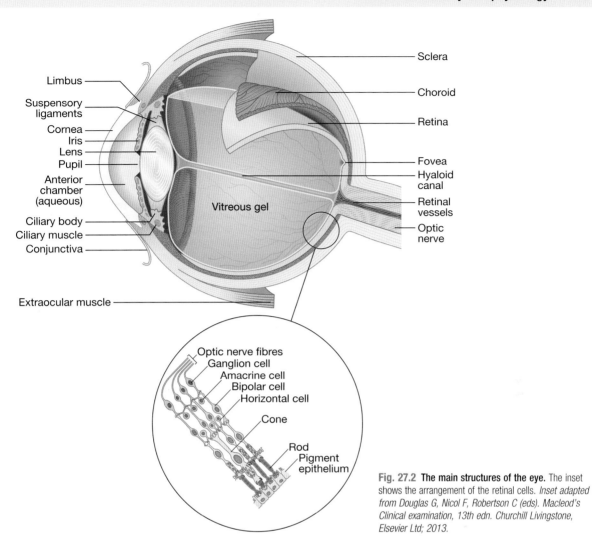

Fovea
Hyaloid
canal
Retinal
vessels
Optic
nerve

Fig. 27.2 The main structures of the eye. The inset shows the arrangement of the retinal cells. *Inset adapted from Douglas G, Nicol F, Robertson C (eds). Macleod's Clinical examination, 13th edn. Churchill Livingstone, Elsevier Ltd; 2013.*

The sclera is pierced posteriorly by the optic nerve at the lamina cribrosa, a sieve-like conduit. Its outer layer, the episclera, consists of loose connective tissue, separating it from Tenon's capsule, the soft-tissue socket of the eye.

Choroid, ciliary body and iris – the uveal tract

Posteriorly, the choroid acts as a conduit for branches of the ophthalmic artery and veins. The choriocapillaris, a network of wide-bore, fenestrated capillaries, abuts the retinal pigment epithelium.

The ciliary body forms the junction between the choroid and the iris, and lies just inferior to the limbus. Anteriorly, its ciliary processes produce aqueous (fluid) that circulates through the pupil into the anterior chamber. Posteriorly, it constitutes the pars plana and forms the attachments for the suspensory ligaments of the lens. The ciliary muscle encircles the eye within the ciliary body. Contraction of this muscle relaxes the suspensory ligaments of the lens, bringing near objects into focus.

The iris bows gently forwards as it lies against the lens. It is divided into a pupillary zone, containing the circumferential sphincter pupillae muscle, and a ciliary zone, containing the dilator pupillae.

Retina

The retina consists of the neurosensory retina and the retinal pigment epithelium. The two layers are adherent only adjacent to the optic disc and at the edge of the pars plana.

Histologically, the centre of the retina is termed the macula lutea, its yellowish appearance caused by the presence of the xanthophylls (yellow pigments) lutein and zeaxanthin. At the centre of the macula, the neurosensory retina dips to form the fovea.

The single-layered retinal pigment epithelium is highly metabolically active and is essential for the maintenance and survival of the overlying photoreceptors.

The neurosensory retina initiates the visual pathway. Its photoreceptors synapse with radially arranged bipolar neurons, which in turn synapse with circumferentially arranged optic nerve ganglion cells.

'Horizontal' and amacrine cells within the plexiform layers modulate neuronal activity between bipolar cells, photoreceptors and the ganglion cells. At the fovea, a one-to-one relationship between cones, bipolar neurons and ganglion cells leads to the highest acuity. In the peripheral retina, many rods converge on to a bipolar neuron, and many bipolar neurons converge on to a ganglion cell, leading to lower acuity. In effect, the peripheral retina conveys black-and-white sentinel vision, alerting the brain to move the higher-acuity colour vision of the fovea into gaze. Photoreceptors are specialised neurons that cause neurotransmitters to be released in response to light ('phototransduction'). There are three types of photoreceptors: namely, rods, cones and ganglion cells, the latter of which independently respond to blue light, influencing circadian rhythms.

27

Lens

The lens is a transparent flexible structure suspended between the iris and the vitreous. Its flexibility enables objects over a range of distances to be focused on the retina. It has a capsule, a central nucleus and a peripheral cortex. It continues to grow throughout life, becoming less flexible with age.

Vitreous

The vitreous gel is 99% water and 1% collagen/hyaluronic acid. The outer edge (cortex) of the vitreous condenses to form the anterior and posterior hyaloid membranes. The base of the vitreous strongly adheres to the ora serrata/pars plana and the optic disc rim, where the internal limiting membrane of the retina is thinnest. Lesser degrees of adhesion occur at the parafoveal retina and along the retinal vessels.

Blood supply of the orbit/eye

The main blood supply of the orbit originates from the intracranial internal carotid artery. The ophthalmic artery, the first branch of the internal carotid artery, traverses the subarachnoid space to enter the optic canal within the dural sheath of the optic nerve. On leaving the optic canal, it emerges from the dural sheath to course briefly along, and then over, the optic nerve and reach the medial wall of the orbit.

Several arterial circles are formed. The major arterial circle of the iris is formed within the ciliary body by anterior ciliary arteries anastomosing with the posterior ciliary arteries. The pial branches of the optic nerve and the short ciliary arteries join together, as the circle of Zinn, to supply the intraocular optic nerve.

The infraorbital artery, a branch of the maxillary artery, also contributes to the orbital blood supply, in particular the inferior rectus, the inferior oblique and the lacrimal sac.

The orbit is drained by the superior and inferior ophthalmic veins, which converge to drain through the superior orbital fissure into the cavernous sinus.

Investigation of visual disorders

History is the key to diagnosing visual disorders, with examination and investigations used to confirm or refute the expectations formed by the history.

Perimetry

In the era before modern radiology, manual perimetry was utilised as a non-invasive form of 'neuroimaging'. Nowadays, perimetry is largely automated and its main role lies in the monitoring of glaucoma; it also has a lesser role in assessing neuro-ophthalmic disorders. All methods of perimetry are subjective and rely on patient cooperation and mental agility.

Amsler chart

The Amsler chart (Fig. 27.3) is the simplest method of documenting the visual field, and is easy for both patient and clinician to understand and perform. It can be used for all forms of visual field loss but is best suited to follow up the central scotomata of macular disorders, which are often too subtle for other methods of perimetry.

Tangent/Goldmann kinetic perimetry

Manual perimetry methods, such as tangent screen and Goldmann kinetic perimetry, appeal to the non-specialist, as they produce easily interpretable contoured maps of the visual field.

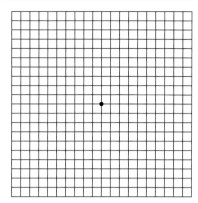

Fig. 27.3 Amsler chart. The Amsler chart is a grid of 0.5 cm squares with a dot in the centre. The subject is asked to fix on the central dot with one eye and any distorted or missing lines are recorded.

The tangent screen is a piece of black cloth attached to a wall, in front of which the operator introduces moving targets into the patient's field of view. It retains an important role in the positive identification of functional peripheral field loss (tunnel vision) versus pathological field loss (funnel vision), although the results are somewhat operator-dependent. Goldmann perimetry is a mechanical improvement on tangent screen perimetry, which utilises targets of varying size and illumination. An automated version is available.

Automated threshold perimetry

Automated visual fields test the threshold of the eye's ability to see at various points within the visual field, forming complex outputs that can be stored digitally. Internal quality assurance mechanisms monitor stability of fixation, false positives due to trigger-happy patients and false negatives due to performance fatigue. Many patients need practice before accurate results are obtained; first-time fields are rarely reliable and often show spurious and misleading findings.

Most automated perimetry assesses only central vision. Few neurological disorders start peripherally, the exception being unilateral loss of peripheral field with disease of the anterior pole of the occipital lobe. However, retinal pathology, such as retinal detachment and retinitis pigmentosa, may be missed if reliance is placed on automated perimetry rather than clinical examination.

Visual field defects on perimetry that affect the whole of the superior or inferior half of the visual field need to be differentiated by confrontation into arcuate visual field defects, which affect central field only, and altitudinal field defects, which affect both central and peripheral vision. Arcuate visual fields defects localise a lesion to the optic nerve head, whereas a lesion anywhere along the optic nerve can cause an altitudinal defect.

Imaging

See Figure 27.4.

Photography

Digital photography is utilised to document surface anatomy. Colour images are ideal for lesions affecting the skin and cornea. For the retina, however, red-free imaging brings additional benefits, particularly for discriminating red haemorrhages or abnormal new vessels from the red background of the retina.

Fig. 27.4 Ocular imaging. [A] Colour retinal photograph from a healthy subject. [B] Red-free retinal photograph from a healthy subject. [C] Optical coherence tomogram of a normal eye, showing the layers of the retina. In this image, the macula shows normal foveal indentation. [D] Fundus autofluorescence (FAF) of the right eye in a normal subject. Distribution of FAF intensity shows typical background signal with reduced signal at the optic disc (absence of autofluorescent material) and retinal vessels (absorption). Intensity is markedly decreased over the fovea due to the absorption of the blue light by yellow macular pigment. [E] Fundal fluorescein angiogram of a normal adult retina. [F] Ocular ultrasound image showing typical biconvex appearance of a choroidal melanoma. *A, B, C and F, Courtesy of Aberdeen Royal Infirmary. D, From Schmitz-Valckenberg S, Fleckenstein M, Hendrik PN, et al. Fundus autofluorescence and progression of age-related macular degeneration. Survey Ophthalmol 2009; 54(1):96–117. E, From Witmer MT, Szilárd K. Wide-field imaging of the retina. Survey Ophthalmol 2013; 58(2):143–154.*

Optical coherence tomography

Optical coherence tomography is the optical equivalent of ultrasound, using light rather than sound waves to create its images. It is invaluable, not least for assessing the integrity of the layers of the retina and detecting macular oedema of any cause.

Autofluorescence

The retinal pigment epithelium contains autofluorescent lipofuscin, which can be excited by blue- and green-coloured light and captured by digital imaging.

Increased autofluorescence occurs when there is abnormal accumulation of lipofuscin, as seen with certain inherited retinal dystrophies; excess retinal pigment epithelium metabolic activity, such as at the edge of evolving atrophic macular degeneration; or drug deposition, such as with hydoxychloroquine.

Fundus angiography

Fluorescein angiography is an invasive technique with risks including local extravasation of dye at the site of intravenous injection and anaphylaxis. Currently, its role is limited to the diagnosis of retinal vasculitis, retinal and choroidal neovascularisation, and capillary occlusion. Non-invasive angiography is now possible using optical coherence tomography, but its applicability is limited by small field of view and inability to demonstrate flow or leakage.

Indocyanine angiography directly images the choroidal circulation and is particularly useful in guiding laser treatment for the choroidal polyps of polypoidal choroidal vasculopathy.

Ocular ultrasound

The main role of ultrasound is where the retina is obscured: for instance, by cataract or vitreous haemorrhage. It also has an important role in diagnosing choroidal melanoma, based on its distinctive internal reflectivity.

Visual electrophysiology

Electrophysiology is used to localise disorders to the photoreceptors (electroretinogram), the retinal ganglion cells (pattern electroretinogram) or the optic pathways (visual evoked potential). The site of photoreceptor involvement can be further localised to specific regions of the retina (multifocal electroretinogram) or the macula itself (pattern electroretinogram).

Electrophysiology requires cooperation, correction of refractive errors and the ability to fixate. Voluntary suppression of the electrical responses is possible by simply not focusing on the target. Despite this, it remains the investigation of choice for visual symptoms unexplained by clinical examination.

Presenting problems in ophthalmic disease

Presenting problems that are ophthalmological manifestations of predominantly neurological disease (e.g. ptosis, diplopia, oscillopsia, nystagmus and pupillary abnormalities) are discussed in Chapter 25.

27

Watery/dry eye

The most common cause of a watery eye is a dry eye triggering reflex lacrimation. Patients with dry eye may complain of a foreign body or gritty sensation in the eye or intermittent visual blurring, triggered by reduced blinking, as occurs when reading or when concentrating on a distant object, such as the television.

Pruritus

Common causes of itch are an acute allergic response to either airborne allergens or direct contact. A significant proportion of people are allergic to topical chloramphenicol, a first-line treatment for many minor ocular ailments.

Pain/headache

The key consideration in deciding whether or not ocular pain and/or headache originates from the eye is whether there is a ciliary flush (red eye) or no ciliary flush (white eye).

Red eye

The presence of a ciliary flush in the region of the limbus is a key finding in intraocular causes of pain. The presence of watering or watery discharge is not a discriminatory feature, and over-reliance on this symptom often results in anterior uveitis being misdiagnosed as viral conjunctivitis.

White eye

In the absence of a ciliary flush, ocular or periorbital pain is most commonly caused by migraine.

Pain on eye movement is a cardinal feature of optic neuritis and scleritis. In optic neuritis the eye is white, whereas in scleritis, except for posterior scleritis, it is red.

Posterior scleritis, in which the visible sclera is white, should be diagnosed only in the setting of positive signs such as disc swelling and exudative retinal detachment, or with confirmation by ocular ultrasound. A more common cause of severe ocular/periocular pain, with associated photophobia and lacrimation, is cluster headache (p. 1096), which is often misdiagnosed as scleritis. Just like scleritis, cluster headache responds to oral glucocorticoids, adding to the diagnostic confusion.

Intermittent, subacute angle closure glaucoma can cause headache, but usually accompanying corneal oedema causes haloes (a form of glare with rainbow colours), elicited by looking at lights or blurring of vision.

Giant cell arteritis is an uncommon, but usually striking, cause of headache, predominantly seen in the elderly. Rarely, it presents with sudden painless visual loss in the absence of raised inflammatory markers. Diagnosis can be made by demonstrating choroidal shutdown on fluorescein angiography.

Photophobia/glare

Excessive sensitivity to light, rather than fear of light, usually indicates ciliary muscle spasm due to inflammation in the iris. Common causes are corneal abrasion, acute anterior uveitis and contact lens-related keratitis.

Occasionally, photophobia can be a symptom of congenital retinal dystrophies, especially cone photoreceptor deficiency.

Photophobia may also be a feature of meningitis, usually with accompanying neck stiffness and headache (meningism, p. 1118).

Glare is a common early feature of cataract, particularly triggered by oncoming car headlights when driving at night. It is a relatively common indication for surgery. It may also be an issue where there is insufficient melanin in the retinal pigment epithelium, e.g. in atrophic age-related macular degeneration, in ocular albinism or following extensive pan-retinal laser therapy. If surgery is not an option, or while surgery is awaited, the symptom of glare may be reduced by wearing a broad-brimmed hat.

Photopsia

A flickering light sensation is indicative of photoreceptor activity, either through traction, as in the setting of posterior vitreous detachment, or inflammation, as in the setting of autoimmune or paraneoplastic retinopathy. Rarely, photopsia is a symptom of occipital lobe epilepsy, in which case there is usually an accompanying homonymous hemianopia.

Blurred vision

Blurred vision describes the situation in which patients are able to see what they are looking at, but what they are looking at is out of focus. The most common cause of intermittent blurred vision is dry eye; the most common cause of permanent blurred vision is cataract. If blurred vision is worse in the morning and eases as the day progresses, this suggests macular oedema.

Loss of vision

In visual loss, patients are no longer able to see all or part of what they are looking at. Some symptoms associated with visual loss require urgent ophthalmological assessment (Box 27.8).

27.8 Red flag symptoms in visual loss*	
Symptom	**Possible causes**
Sudden onset	Retinal artery occlusion Ischaemic optic neuropathy
Headache	Giant cell arteritis if age >55 years
Eye pain	Angle closure glaucoma Keratitis Scleritis Anterior uveitis
Pain on eye movement	Optic neuritis Scleritis

Distortion	Choroidal neovascular membrane:
	  Age-related macular degeneration
	  Pathological myopia
	  Posterior uveitis
	  Idiopathic
	Macular hole
	Epiretinal membrane

Worse in the morning	Macular oedema:
	  Diabetic macular oedema
	  Retinal vein occlusion
	  Uveitis

*The presence of any of these symptoms in a patient with visual loss requires emergency referral to an ophthalmologist.

The most common cause of transient visual loss is the aura of migraine, usually a positive phenomenon with the object of regard seemingly hidden by something in the way, rather than a negative phenomenon in which part or all of what is being looked at is missing. With positive visual phenomena the obstruction is often white or coloured, expanding across the visual field, or in a constant position but shimmering.

Negative visual phenomena are a cardinal feature of ocular, usually retinal, ischaemia, with complete absence of vision (blackness) occupying part or all the visual field. Transient ocular ischaemia is usually embolic in nature but is occasionally seen in giant cell arteritis, where it suggests critical optic nerve ischaemia. Permanent monocular negative visual phenomena usually indicate previous optic nerve or retinal infarction. Tiny negative visual phenomena may also be seen in capillary disorders such as diabetic retinopathy, where patchy macular capillary occlusion may, for instance, cause letters to be missing from words on reading.

Distortion of vision

Distortion is a cardinal symptom of disruption of foveal photoreceptor alignment. The most common cause is choroidal neovascularisation. Less commonly, it can be caused by epiretinal membrane formation, where posterior hyaloid surface scarring causes foveal traction.

Usually with distortion, objects are not only misshapen but also smaller (micropsia), due to the photoreceptors being pulled apart. Macropsia, where objects look bigger than normal, is uncommon. It is sometimes seen in the 'Alice in Wonderland' syndrome, a paediatric variant of migraine where there is altered visual perception of body images.

Eyelid retraction

Eyelid retraction is usually caused by inflammatory thyroid eye disease or thyrotoxicosis (see pp. 631 and 645, and Fig. 18.8).

The first muscle to be affected in thyroid eye disease is the inferior rectus. The enlarged muscle tethers the eye and restricts upgaze. Compensatory increased innervation to the superior rectus and the levator palpebrae superioris, as well as direct inflammation, leads to eyelid retraction.

In thyrotoxicosis, increased sympathetic nervous activity leads to bilateral eyelid retraction. This, however, resolves with beta-blockade and treatment of thyrotoxicosis.

Rarely, bilateral eyelid retraction is a sign of dorsal mid-brain pathology (Collier's sign), where it is accompanied by a supranuclear upgaze palsy and convergence-retraction nystagmus.

Optic disc swelling

Optic disc swelling can be a developmental variant of normal (pseudopapilloedema) or caused by optic nerve pathology, or reflect more widespread nerve fibre oedema as with retinal vein occlusion. Neurological causes of optic disc swelling are discussed in on page 1090.

Proptosis

Proptosis, particularly if bilateral and symmetrical, is often first recognised when it is quite advanced. Accompanying eyelid retraction is a typical feature of thyroid eye disease. By far the most common cause is thyroid eye disease, when proptosis is termed exophthalmos.

Proptosis is a sign of retro-orbital expansion and may be intraconal or extraconal. When expansion is within the cone of extraocular muscles, then movement forwards will be in line with the visual axis. When outside, the eye is additionally displaced to the side.

The primary clinical concern is whether vision is at risk due to optic nerve compression or corneal exposure. In addition, there may be double vision. In thyroid eye disease, diplopia may be absent if the disease is symmetrical. Instead, restricted ocular movements make patients move their head en bloc when looking at objects deviating from the primary position of gaze. To the patient, however, the overarching concern is often the change in appearance.

Specialist ophthalmological conditions

Ocular inflammation

Inflammation can affect any part of the eye. In structures in direct contact with the environment, particularly the cornea and the conjunctiva, inflammation is most likely to be caused by infection. In other structures, such as the uveal tract and sclera, inflammation is more likely to be caused by autoimmune conditions, although it may also be a manifestation of infection or malignancy. Although the latter conditions may present with indicative ocular signs, their presence is often appreciated only retrospectively, after failure to respond to immunosuppression.

Most non-infective forms of ocular inflammation are idiopathic; all are more common in the presence of other autoimmune conditions. Some may be directly associated but asynchronous in disease activity, such as the anterior uveitis of ankylosing spondylitis (p. 1028). Others are direct manifestations of an overarching, underlying, inflammatory condition such as the keratoscleritis of granulomatosis with polyangiitis (formerly known as Wegener's granulomatosis).

Sjögren's syndrome

Sjögren's syndrome is the archetypal autoimmune disease and its secondary form is associated with a large number of other autoimmune conditions (see Box 24.64, p. 1039). The cardinal features are inflammation of the lacrimal gland, its conjunctival accessory glands and the parotid gland, leading to hyposecretion of tears and saliva. Involvement of the lacrimal gland alone causes keratoconjunctivitis sicca, a syndrome of dry eyes and corneal and conjunctival irritation. Keratoconjunctivitis sicca, however, can also be caused by reduced function of the lacrimal glands and/or lacrimal ducts from other causes.

Treatment of the ophthalmological manifestations of Sjögren's syndrome is symptomatic, and consists of supplementing tear production with artificial tears (e.g. hypromellose) and reducing tear loss by humidification and avoidance of dry environments. If these measures are insufficient, tear drainage may be reduced with surgical options such as punctal plugs and punctal occlusion.

Peripheral ulcerative keratitis

Peripheral ulcerative keratitis ('corneal melting') is an autoimmune disorder affecting the corneal limbus, where it may be

27

accompanied by adjacent scleritis. It may be directly associated with inflammatory disorders in which immune complexes are formed, particularly rheumatoid arthritis, systemic lupus erythematosus and granulomatosis with polyangiitis. Pain and redness are helpful indicators but may not always be present. Systemic immunosuppression is always required but topical glucocorticoids should be used cautiously due to the risk of aggravating keratolysis (corneal thinning). Secondary infection should be prevented with topical antibiotics and attention should be paid to corneal hydration, through the use of artificial tears and lubricants.

More common causes of peripheral corneal ulceration are blepharitis and acne rosacea, causing ocular irritation rather than frank pain. Hypersensitivity to staphylococcal exotoxin leads to stromal infiltrate adjacent to, but sparing, the limbus (marginal keratitis). Resolution of this self-limiting condition can be assisted by the use of topical chloramphenicol, with or without topical glucocorticoids. Prevention is through management of the underlying condition, usually with ocular lid hygiene for simple blepharitis and metronidazole gel for rosacea.

Scleritis

Scleritis is usually accompanied by severe pain, worse on eye movement and often waking the patient through the night. Diagnosis of anterior scleritis is usually straightforward, with the eye showing diffuse or nodular erythema (although it may have to be searched for under the eyelids). Posterior uveitis is often accompanied by reduced vision and oedema of the retina, choroid and extraocular muscles.

White patches of necrosis (pallor) within the erythema are an ominous sign, indicative of systemic vasculitis. Non-necrotising scleritis is commonly idiopathic but may be associated with other autoimmune conditions, particularly rheumatoid arthritis and inflammatory bowel disease. It is also common with herpes zoster ophthalmicus, intraocular involvement being indicated by the involvement of the lateral external nose (Hutchison's sign).

Necrotising scleritis requires aggressive immunosuppression; non-necrotising scleritis can occasionally be managed by topical glucocorticoids or non-steroidal anti-inflammatory drugs (NSAIDs) but usually requires oral glucocorticoids.

Some patients with recurrent episodes of scleritis, or in whom inflammation is gradual and prolonged, may develop scleral thinning (scleromalacia), revealing the underlying blue choroid.

Episcleritis

Episcleritis is a benign self-limiting condition of uncertain aetiology, occasionally associated with other inflammatory disorders. Sectoral redness of the episclera is usual, although nodules can form. Often confused with scleritis, although usually less symptomatic, the diagnostic topical application of phenylephrine turns the inflamed episclera white but has no effect on the redness of scleritis. Treatment is with cold artificial tears, although occasionally topical NSAIDs or topical glucocorticoids are required.

Uveitis

Uveitis is an overarching term for inflammation anywhere in the uveal tract, retina or vitreous. It may be classified according to speed of onset, location, specific features, or aetiology (Box 27.9). Syphilis can cause all forms of uveitis. Active tuberculosis may present with an occlusive vasculitis or serpiginous (snake-like) choroiditis emanating from the optic disc. Latent tuberculosis is a particular concern because treatment of the uveitis with biologics

27.9 Aetiology of uveitis

Idiopathic

- Anterior uveitis often associated with the HLA-B27 haplotype, even in the absence of other manifestations

Primary ophthalmic conditions

- Trauma, including penetrating injury and ophthalmic surgery
- Fuchs' heterochromic cyclitis
- Posner–Schlossman syndrome

Rheumatological

- HLA-B27-associated (seronegative) spondyloarthropathies: ankylosing spondylitis, psoriatic arthritis, reactive arthritis
- Juvenile idiopathic arthritis

Systemic vasculitides

- Behçet's disease
- Polyarteritis nodosa
- Granulomatosis with polyangiitis (Wegener's)

Systemic infections (only the more common causes are listed)

- Brucellosis
- Herpes virus infections (cytomegalovirus, herpes simplex virus, varicella zoster virus)
- Leptospirosis
- Lyme borreliosis
- Syphilis
- Toxoplasmosis
- Tuberculosis
- Whipple's disease

Gastrointestinal conditions

- Inflammatory bowel disease (Crohn's disease, ulcerative colitis)

Malignancy

- Primary central nervous system lymphoma (rare)

Systemic conditions of unknown cause

- Multiple sclerosis
- Sarcoidosis

may induce active systemic infection. Furthermore, the most commonly used biologic for uveitis – anti-tumour necrosis factor therapy (e.g. adalimumab, infliximab) – may trigger demyelination.

The most common form of uveitis is anterior uveitis, which is usually idiopathic but may be associated with other autoimmune conditions, particularly HLA-B27-related spondyloarthropathies (p. 1027); it is rarely caused directly by infection. Acutely, dilating drops are used to prevent the inflamed iris from sticking to the lens (posterior synechiae) and obstructing the outflow of aqueous fluid, while a tapering dose of topical glucocorticoids, usually over 4–6 weeks, mitigates the local signs and symptoms of the self-resolving inflammation. Inadequate treatment can lead to pupil block glaucoma and cataract. Posterior complications can also develop, predominantly macular oedema, the main cause of visual impairment in all forms of uveitis.

With intermediate uveitis, inflammation occurs at the pars plana, with most symptoms, predominantly floaters, being a result of inflammation of the vitreous base. Unlike anterior uveitis, pure intermediate uveitis is not associated with iris inflammation; instead, white blood cells are seen predominantly in the anterior vitreous, with a lesser amount overspilling into the anterior chamber. Treatment is challenging. Topical therapy is ineffective, as it does not penetrate beyond the anterior chamber, but symptoms of floaters are not often sufficient to justify systemic immunosuppression. In some cases, vitritis (vitreous inflammation), or more commonly macular oedema, may cause visual impairment. Occasionally, retinal neovascular proliferation may occur, either as an inflammatory response or as a direct result of capillary occlusion. Intermediate uveitis may be associated with demyelination, sarcoidosis and inflammatory bowel disease.

Posterior uveitis tends to present with visual impairment secondary to macular oedema, vitritis or choroiditis. More chronic forms also exist and these tend to present with photopsia, visual field defects or distortion inducing choroidal neovascular membranes.

Infectious conditions

Conjunctivitis

Conjunctivitis is predominantly caused by bacteria or viruses, and is usually self-limiting in 7–10 days. Bacterial conjunctivitis is associated with a purulent discharge and viral conjunctivitis with a watery discharge, the latter often being confused with the photophobia and reflex lacrimation of anterior uveitis. Underlying chlamydial infection should always be considered if there is a persistent thick, mucopurulent discharge (p. 340).

Allergic conjunctivitis is also common, either as a component of hay fever (allergic rhinitis, p. 622) or as an allergy to chloramphenicol, which is commonly used to treat conjunctivitis.

Rarely, conjunctivitis may be associated with inflammatory systemic mucus membrane disorders, such as ocular mucus membrane (cicatricial) pemphigoid or Stevens–Johnson syndrome (pp. 1254 and 1264). The secondary effects of loss of conjunctival function can be devastating to the cornea. Other causes of conjunctival scarring include trachoma (p. 273), chemical burns and orbital radiotherapy.

Infectious keratitis/corneal ulceration

Inflammation of the cornea should always raise concern about underlying infection (Box 27.10). Central ulceration is always more serious than peripheral, through involvement of the visual axis. Cultures from corneal scraping or biopsy may be required, although much infectious keratitis is treated empirically on the basis of site, morphology and response to treatment.

In the West, the most common cause of infectious keratitis is herpes simplex virus type 1 (occasionally type 2) (Fig. 27.5).

All layers of the cornea may be involved: the epithelium in the form of dendritic ulceration; the stroma in the form of white infiltrate and occasionally necrosis; and the endothelium in the form of localised oedema and keratitic precipitates. Loss of corneal sensation is common following herpes simplex keratitis, and occasionally neurotrophic keratopathy may result. Epithelial disease is self-limiting but treatment with topical or oral antivirals reduces the risk of stromal involvement and scarring. Stromal and endothelial disease requires additional topical glucocorticoids, but only once any epithelial defect has healed. Herpes simplex keratitis is analogous to herpes labialis; recurrences are therefore common and, if frequent, may warrant long-term oral antivirals. Corneal grafting may be required but the risk of recurrence remains.

Bacteria also cause infectious keratitis, especially following corneal trauma or contact lens misuse. Other risk factors for microbial keratitis include topical glucocorticoids and pre-existing ocular surface disease. Bacterial keratitis has many causes, some of which do not respond to chloramphenicol, so topical quinolones are used as first-line agents. Rarely, the free-living amoeba *Acanthamoeba castellanii* may be a cause of contact lens-associated keratitis, presenting subacutely and leading to corneal nerve infiltration, keratitis and accompanying scleritis.

Fungal keratitis is the most common cause of infectious keratitis in developing countries, particularly if there has been corneal trauma and contact with soil or plant matter. It is usually caused by *Fusarium*. Fungal keratitis has no particular distinguishing features and delayed diagnosis is common. If it is suspected, cultures should be undertaken and antifungal treatment, which is hampered by poor corneal penetration of antifungals, started promptly. Corneal transplantation is often required.

Endophthalmitis

Endophthalmitis is infection of the anterior and posterior chambers of the eye. It may be exogenous (e.g. from penetrating trauma or following surgery) or, less commonly, endogenous, caused by haematogenous spread of microorganisms within the blood, which gain entry to the eye via the choroid and ciliary body. The causes of endogenous endophthalmitis are therefore the causes of bacteraemia and fungaemia (p. 225). Gram-positive

i	**27.10 Common causes of infectious keratitis**		
Organism	**Features/comments**	**Treatment**
Viruses		
Herpes simplex	Characteristic 'dendritic' ulcer is the most common form, often recurrent	Topical/systemic aciclovir (with topical glucocorticoid for stromal keratitis once the epithelium is healed)
Varicella zoster	Herpes zoster ophthalmicus	Systemic aciclovir
Bacteria		
Pseudomonas aeruginosa *Staphylococcus aureus* Coagulase-negative staphylococci *Propionibacterium* spp.	Coagulase-negative staphylococci and *Propionibacterium* spp. are members of the skin flora, and must not be dismissed as contaminants	Topical fluoroquinolone with Gram-positive and Gram-negative cover (e.g. ofloxacin) Subsequent treatment depends on sensitivity testing results
Fungi		
Fusarium sp. *Aspergillus* sp. *Candida* sp.	*Fusarium* and *Aspergillus* keratitis are often associated with soil and/or corneal trauma; may also be contact lens-related *Candida* causes post-keratoplasty keratitis	Options include topical natamycin (if available), amphotericin B, voriconazole and other azoles (e.g. econazole), and systemic fluconazole or voriconazole
Parasites		
Acanthamoeba castellanii (free-living amoeba) *Onchocerca volvulus* (nematode)	Associated with poor contact lens hygiene See page 292	Topical polyhexamethylene biguanide

27

Fig. 27.5 Infective keratitis. A Herpes simplex dendritic ulcer stained with fluorescein. B *Fusarium* keratitis. An irregularly edged lesion suggests a fungal cause but is not pathognomonic. *A, Courtesy of McPherson Optometry, Aberdeen. B, From Macsai MS, Fontes BM. Rapid diagnosis in ophthalmology: anterior segment. Elsevier Inc.; 2008. (Courtesy of the External Eye Disease and Cornea Section, Federal University of São Paulo, Brazil.)*

Fig. 27.6 Focal chorioretinitis in clinically suspected endogenous *Candida* endophthalmitis. This patient was an intravenous drug user and improved with empirical oral fluconazole. *From Ryan SJ (ed). Retina, 5th edn. Saunders, Elsevier Inc.; 2013. (Case courtesy of Jeffrey K. Moore, MD.)*

Fig. 27.7 Sunflower cataract and Kayser–Fleischer ring (arrow) in Wilson's disease. *From Kaiser PK, Friedman NJ (eds). Massachusetts Eye and Ear Infirmary Illustrated manual of ophthalmology, 4th edn. Saunders, Elsevier Inc.; 2014.*

bacteria are most common, followed by Gram-negative bacteria and then fungi.

Clinical presentation is with visual blurring and/or visual loss, which are usually unilateral. Ocular findings range from a few deposits in the retina/choroid (chorioretinitis) to panendophthalmitis, in which there is a severe inflammatory reaction in both the anterior and posterior chambers. A specific appearance of the retina is described for *Candida* endophthalmitis, which characteristically causes creamy-white retinal or chorioretinal lesions (Fig. 27.6). It is vitally important to sample the vitreous, as this may provide the only opportunity to determine the most appropriate therapy.

Treatment is with systemic and/or intravitreal antibiotics or antifungal agents, depending on the cause and severity. Vitrectomy may also be required.

Cataract

Cataract is permanent opacity of the lens (Fig. 27.7). Globally, untreated cataract is the most common cause of visual impairment, although in countries where surgery is available, age-related macular degeneration is a more common cause.

The normal lens thickens and opacifies with age, and cataract can be detected in more than half the population over the age 65 (senile cataract). Many ocular and systemic diseases can predispose to cataract formation, the most common being uveitis and diabetes mellitus. Wilson's disease (hepatolenticular degeneration, p. 896) causes a characteristic 'sunflower' cataract. Excessive exposure to ultraviolet light, ionising radiation and glucocorticoid therapy are also predisposing factors.

The characteristic symptoms of cataract are progressive loss of vision and glare. If these become serious enough to require treatment, surgical intervention will be required, usually in the form of ultrasonic phacoemulsification with intraocular lens (IOL) implant.

Other common ophthalmological findings in old age are shown in Box 27.11.

Diabetic eye disease

Diabetic retinopathy

Diabetic retinopathy is one of the most common causes of visual impairment in people of working age in developed countries. The prevalence of diabetic retinopathy increases with the duration of diabetes. Almost all individuals with type 1 diabetes, and most of those with type 2 diabetes, will have some degree of

27.11 Common ophthalmological findings in old age

- **Small pupils that dilate poorly with mydriatics:** common neurodegenerative finding, particularly with diabetes.
- **Spurious findings on automated perimetry:** decreasing manual dexterity and cognitive function often render automated perimetry findings unreliable.
- **Lens opacities:** cataract is ubiquitous but requires treatment only if symptomatic.
- **Drusen:** common from mid-life onwards. Larger (soft) drusen are more likely to herald age-related macular degeneration than smaller (hard) drusen.
- **Glaucoma:** angle closure glaucoma is more common as the increasing size of the lens shallows the anterior chamber. Once it is identified, both eyes are always treated to prevent development/recurrence. Chronic open angle glaucoma is more common in those with a family history or ocular hypertension (isolated raised intraocular pressure).
- **Impaired upgaze:** common. It is differentiated from progressive supranuclear palsy (p. 1114) by the doll's head manœuvre, the full range of vertical movement being retained in progressive supranuclear palsy PSP.
- **Ptosis:** mechanical ptosis is common due to degenerative disinsertion of the levator palpebrae superioris aponeurosis. A high skin crease and preserved ability to elevate help differentiate it from other causes (p. 1090).
- **Late-onset presentation of congenital conditions:** adult pseudovitelliform macular 'degeneration' is an autosomal dominant retinal dystrophy, which causes mild visual impairment. Oculopharyngeal muscular dystrophy is an autosomal dominant condition characterised by later-onset chronic progressive external ophthalmoparesis and swallowing difficulties.

retinopathy after 20 years. Fortunately, most patients develop only mild forms of retinopathy.

Pathogenesis

The underlying pathogenesis of diabetic retinopathy is local vascular endothelial growth factor production initiated by hyperglycaemia-induced capillary occlusion. This occlusion stimulates increased production of retinal vascular endothelial growth factor, which not only increases capillary permeability, leading to retinal oedema, but also stimulates angiogenesis, leading to new vessel formation.

Clinical features

The initial clinical feature of diabetic retinopathy, capillary occlusion, is visible only on retinal angiography. Capillaries adjacent to the occluded capillary form discrete swellings (microaneurysms), which leak fluid and blood, causing oedema and retinal haemorrhages (Fig. 27.8).

Clinically, microaneurysms appear as isolated red dots, the capillaries being too small to visualise. At the edge of any leaking fluid, lipids precipitate out to form exudate, like the tidemark of the sea.

In turn, capillaries with microaneurysms also occlude, their microaneurysms turning white before disappearing entirely from clinical view. As more and more capillaries occlude, larger patches of retinal ischaemia form, leading to sufficient vascular endothelial growth factor production to induce the growth of new vessels at the border of diseased and undiseased retina.

Within patches of retinal ischaemia, diseased remnants of partially perfused capillaries form intraretinal microvascular abnormalities (IRMAs) and retinal veins develop multiple diffuse swellings (venous beading). These signs are best seen on fluorescein angiography.

 27.12 Medical ophthalmology in adolescence

Inherited conditions

- **Stargardt's disease:** autosomal recessive macular dystrophy that commonly presents in adolescence/early adulthood, causing significant bilateral impairment of central vision.

Developmental anomalies

- **Pathological myopia:** due to elongated ocular axial length rather than refractive index of cornea and lens. Increased risk of retinal detachment and choroidal neovascular membrane formation.
- **Optic disc drusen:** come to prominence during adolescence and usually first detected during routine examination. Often mistaken for papilloedema, particularly in the setting of coincidental daily headache.
- **Amblyopia:** occasionally detected after the age of 7 years, particularly in the absence of pre-school screening, when it is unlikely to respond to patching of the other eye.
- **Keratoconus:** presents with increasing astigmatism (distortion of vision due to abnormal corneal topography). Hard contact lenses are the mainstay of therapy. Further progression may be prevented through 'cross-linking' surgery.

Deterioration of existing conditions

- **Diabetic retinopathy:** in type 1 diabetes, retinopathy usually first presents at least 5 years after diagnosis, which often coincides with adolescence. Puberty may accelerate progression. Greatest risk is disengagement with diabetes care, including retinal screening, significantly increasing later presentation with advanced symptomatic retinopathy.
- **Adult manifestations of retinopathy of prematurity:** clinical features depend on the type of treatment used in the neonatal period and include retinal detachment, angle closure glaucoma, severe myopia and cataract.

Sexual activity

- **Chlamydia conjunctivitis:** onset of sexual activity may lead to this ocular condition, which is associated with reactive arthritis (p. 1031). Untreated coexistent genital tract infection may cause infertility.

Transition to adult services

- Neurofibromatosis type 1: see page 1131.
- Optic nerve astrocytoma/glioma: often develops in late childhood or early adolescence.

Sports medicine

- **Contact sports:** eye protection is important for all, especially if there is only one functional eye, e.g. with amblyopia.

 27.13 Visual disorders and pregnancy

- **Ocular inflammation:** pregnancy appears to have a protective effect on many inflammatory disorders, although not systemic lupus erythematosus. Most patients can taper treatment during pregnancy. Mycophenolate mofetil is teratogenic. Glucocorticoids and tacrolimus appear safe. The use of biologics during pregnancy should be based on a balance of risks, and professional guidelines should be consulted.
- **Diabetic retinopathy:** may be accelerated during pregnancy because the placenta is a potent source of angiogenic growth factors. Retinal screening each trimester is recommended.
- **HELLP/pre-eclampsia/eclampsia** (p. 1284): retinal features of accelerated hypertension (p. 514) may be seen, including optic disc oedema, flame haemorrhages and cotton wool spots. Occasionally, exudative retinal detachments occur. Vasogenic oedema (posterior reversible encephalopathy syndrome), affecting the posterior occipital and parietal lobes, may cause cortical visual impairment. All features tend to resolve with delivery or control of blood pressure.

27

Fig. 27.8 Diabetic retinopathy. **A** Colour photograph of severe background diabetic retinopathy: multiple blot haemorrhages indicative of capillary occlusion; dot haemorrhages indistinguishable from microaneurysms or microaneurysmal bleeds; and cotton wool spots indicative of arteriolar occlusion. **B** Red-free image shows the presence of extensive haemorrhages more clearly; the more haemorrhages, the greater the degree of likely capillary occlusion. **C** Fluorescein angiogram now reveals extensive entrapment of fluorescein within multiple microaneurysms. **D** Colour photograph showing three cardinal consequences of capillary occlusion: intra-retinal microvascular anomalies occurring within an area of capillary occlusion (top arrow); venous reduplication (rare finding), with venous beading, extending from the reduplication towards the optic disc, occurring where capillaries are occluded either side of the vein (middle arrow); and new vessel formation occurring at the border between the diseased and health retina (bottom arrow). **E** Red-free image shows these features, particularly intra-retinal microvascular anomalies, more clearly. Note the relative pallor compared to the right-hand side of the image, which is indicative of widespread capillary occlusion. Absolute pallor never occurs, as it is 'masked' by the highly vascularised choroid lying underneath. *A–E, Courtesy of Aberdeen Royal Infirmary.*

New vessels and their glial tissue (like a cabbage leaf) grow from retinal veins, through the overlying internal limiting membrane into the vitreous, triggering local inflammation and contracting scars. The vitreous is strongly adherent to the pars plana. It pulls back on the new vessel, triggering further bleeding, growth, inflammation and scarring. If the scarring is sufficient, then tractional retinal detachment and complete blindness may occur.

Other retinal lesions, not unique to capillary occlusion, are also seen in diabetic retinopathy. These include flame haemorrhages and cotton wool spots (soft exudates). Flame haemorrhages are horizontal streaky haemorrhages in the retinal nerve-fibre layer. They are also seen in any severe anaemia, e.g. bacterial endocarditis and leukaemia. Cotton wool spots are also situated in the nerve-fibre layer and are usually most numerous nasal to the optic disc, where the nerve fibres crowd together. They are also seen in accelerated hypertension, after severe hypoglycaemia and occasionally in giant cell arteritis. A cotton wool spot combined with an enclosing flame haemorrhage is termed a Roth spot. Roth spots have traditionally been associated with endocarditis, although they may be seen with any cause of a flame haemorrhage.

Management of proliferative diabetic retinopathy

If untreated, proliferative retinopathy eventually causes severe visual impairment through recurrent vitreous haemorrhage and retinal detachment. Pan-retinal laser photocoagulation therapy is extremely effective at preserving vision, if applied before complications set in.

Historically, laser therapy was used empirically to ablate the retina extensively outside the macula. However, this caused secondary optic atrophy and night blindness (nyctalopia), which interfered with the ability to drive. Modern application of laser is lighter, more tailored to the sites of underlying capillary ischaemia and relatively free of side-effects, only occasionally resulting in loss of the ability to drive. In the UK there is a requirement to inform the driver licensing authority if retinopathy is (or has been) present in both eyes, irrespective of treatment history.

Intravitreal injections of anti-vascular endothelial growth factor (e.g. ranibizumab, aflibercept, bevacizumab) also cause temporary regression of proliferative retinopathy, whereas, after pan-retinal laser therapy, background and proliferative types of retinopathy regress permanently. If both eyes have been treated with laser, patients can be safely discharged to a retinal screening programme.

Management of diabetic macular oedema

Traditionally, oedema seen on slit-lamp biomicroscopy was categorised according to three patterns of leakage elucidated from fluorescein angiogram studies:

- focal leakage from microaneurysms
- diffuse leakage from diseased capillaries
- ischaemia (no leakage) from thrombosis of the perifoveal capillaries.

Laser was applied, either directly on leaking microaneurysms or empirically by placing a grid of burns on the affected macula, to reduce leakage. The main aim was to treat oedema before the fovea was affected, as laser therapy for oedema affecting the fovea was never particularly effective.

However, retinal screening programmes have demonstrated that extrafoveal macular oedema often resolves spontaneously, and the introduction of intravitreal injection therapy, which rescues vision in 50% of those treated regardless of the mechanism of oedema, has led to a paradigm shift in management. Now, rather than laser treatment of asymptomatic oedema that does not involve the centre of the fovea, the emphasis has shifted to treating those who are symptomatic from centre-involving foveal oedema (confirmed on optical coherence tomography) with anti-vascular endothelial growth factor injections. Although this method of treatment is more effective, monthly injections may be required indefinitely.

Prevention

There is a clear relationship between glycaemic control and the incidence of diabetic retinopathy. A combination of good glycaemic and blood pressure control also slows the progression of retinopathy.

When blood glucose is rapidly lowered in patients with type 1 diabetes, however, there can be a transient deterioration of retinopathy, predominantly in the form of cotton wool spot formation, but occasionally triggering new vessel formation. The trigger is believed to be increased systemic insulin growth factor release, which is most likely to occur with sudden correction of eating disorders or reinstitution of insulin therapy in those who miss out injections, often to induce weight loss. This often occurs during hospitalisation for other reasons.

Although, ideally, any improvement in glycaemic control should be gradual, in many circumstances this is hard to achieve, particularly if the patient suddenly decides to comply with treatment, leading to dramatic improvement in glycaemic control.

Screening

Systematic screening for asymptomatic proliferative retinopathy has been shown to be cost-effective. It has led to the introduction of population-based screening programmes in the UK and other countries, where health care is funded centrally. There is little evidence that screening asymptomatic patients for macular oedema is cost-effective, although a by-product of screening is that suspected macular oedema has become the most common reason for referral from retinal screening to ophthalmology.

Although hand-held ophthalmoscopy has been shown to have poor sensitivity compared to examination by slit-lamp biomicroscopy or retinal photography, any form of screening is better than none where resources are scarce. Currently, optical coherence tomography is being added to the screening pathway to reduce false-negative referrals for macular oedema.

Historically, annual screening has been advocated. However, evidence now indicates that patients with repeated normal screens, particularly those with type 2 diabetes, can be safely screened every 2 years.

In pregnancy, the placenta is a source of angiogenic growth factors. For this reason, although the risk of developing significant retinopathy during pregnancy remains low, pregnant women should be screened every trimester until the placenta is delivered.

Other causes of visual loss in people with diabetes

Around 50% of visual loss in people with type 2 diabetes results from causes other than diabetic retinopathy. These include cataract, age-related macular degeneration, retinal vein occlusion, retinal arterial occlusion, non-arteritic ischaemic optic neuropathy and glaucoma. Some of these conditions are to be expected in this group, as they relate to cardiovascular risk factors (e.g.

hypertension, hyperlipidaemia and smoking), all of which are prevalent in people with type 2 diabetes.

In diabetes, metabolic changes in the lens (which are not yet fully elaborated) cause premature and/or accelerated cataract formation. A rare type of 'snowflake' cataract occurs in young patients with poorly controlled diabetes. This does not usually affect vision but tends to make fundal examination difficult. The indications for cataract surgery in diabetes are similar to those in the non-diabetic population, but an additional indication in diabetes is when adequate assessment of the fundus and/or retinal laser therapy becomes impossible.

Retinal vascular occlusion

Retinal vein occlusion (thrombosis)

Retinal vein occlusion is an important vascular cause of visual impairment, visual loss resulting from macular oedema or occasionally from neovascularisation, both of which are managed in a similar way to diabetic macular oedema or proliferative diabetic retinopathy.

Although pathogenesis of retinal vein occlusion is not fully understood, the most common mechanism is believed to be compression of a vein by an adjacent arteriosclerotic artery. Retinal vessels are unusual in that, where the arteries and veins cross over each other, they share a common outer layer (tunica adventitia). This means that arteriosclerotic thickening of an artery leads directly to compression of the adjacent vein (arteriovenous nipping).

A less common cause of retinal vein occlusion is inflammation of the retinal vein (periphlebitis), also called retinal vasculitis (unlike systemic vasculitis, the arterial system is not involved). Periphlebitis should be suspected in younger patients and in patients with no obvious risk factors for arteriosclerosis. Diagnosis is made by fluorescein angiography and treatment is with systemic immunosuppression, with or without adjunctive intravitreal therapy.

Retinal vein occlusion is associated with systemic hypertension and may rarely result from hyperviscosity due to a myeloproliferative disorder, multiple myeloma, Waldenström's macroglobulinaemia or leukaemia. Glaucoma is associated with retinal vein occlusion but whether this is a direct cause or merely a comorbidity in the elderly is not known.

Clinical presentation is with unilateral painless loss of central vision (central retinal vein thrombosis) or an area of peripheral vision (branch retinal vein thrombosis). Fundoscopic features include flame haemorrhages, cotton wool spots, macular oedema and a swollen optic disc (Fig. 27.9).

Fig. 27.9 Central retinal vein occlusion (thrombosis), showing flame haemorrhages, cotton wool spots, macular oedema and a swollen optic disc. *Courtesy of Aberdeen Royal Infirmary.*

27

Fig. 27.10 Retinal artery occlusion. A Colour fundus photograph of central retinal artery occlusion, showing a classic cherry-red spot and a superior optic disc haemorrhage. B Superior branch retinal artery occlusion due an embolus at the disc branch retinal artery occlusion, showing a pale segment of retina. *A, From Duker JS, Waheed NK, Goldman DR. Handbook of retinal OCT. Saunders, Elsevier Inc.; 2014. B, From Bowling B. Kanski's Clinical ophthalmology, 8th edn. Elsevier Ltd; 2016.*

The management of retinal vein occlusion is twofold: management of the underlying aetiology and management of the consequences of retinal vein occlusion. Where an underlying risk factor for arteriosclerosis is clearly present (p. 484), then secondary prevention measures should be commenced. However, the role of secondary prevention of arteriosclerosis in isolated retinal vein occlusion, although common practice by some, remains controversial.

Retinal artery occlusion

Retinal artery occlusion is usually an embolic phenomenon. Common predisposing factors are therefore (predominantly carotid) atherosclerosis valvular heart disease, arrhythmias and infective endocarditis. The next most common cause is vasculitis, mainly giant cell arteritis (p. 1042).

Retinal artery occlusion presents with painless unilateral visual loss, the extent and location of which depend on whether there is a central occlusion or a branch occlusion (peripheral occlusions may be asymptomatic). Transient occlusion of the internal carotid or ophthalmic artery causes transient visual loss, or amaurosis fugax (p. 1152). The typical fundoscopic finding in a central occlusion is a transiently pale retina with a 'cherry-red' spot at the macula, the appearance developing over an hour or so after the occlusion (Fig. 27.10). In branch occlusions there is no cherry-red spot and the retinal pallor is regional.

Age-related macular degeneration

Age-related macular degeneration is the most common cause of visual impairment in the Western world. There are two basic forms: atrophic (dry) and neovascular (wet). The underlying mechanism is dysfunction of the retinal pigment epithelium, leading to overlying photoreceptor death. Choroidal neovascularisation, growing under and into the overlying retina, may occur, distorting the anatomy of the photoreceptors and ending in scar formation. Both forms are preceded by deposits under the retinal pigment epithelium ('drusen'), often followed by the development of focal areas of macular hypo- and hyperpigmentation, where diseased retinal pigment epithelial cells have precipitated their pigment (age-related maculopathy).

The atrophic form presents with gradual onset of central visual blurring, accompanied, to a lesser degree, by visual distortion. Large (geographic), central patches of atrophy are seen with areas of adjacent hyperpigmentation. In the neovascular form, sudden onset of central distortion, progressing within weeks, is the predominant symptom. Apart from age the main risk factor appears to be smoking.

The advent of anti-vascular endothelial growth factor injectors has led to effective therapy for the neovascular form, in many but not all. Unfortunately, treatment is expensive and requires considerable financial and staff resources to treat in timely fashion; delayed treatment can lead to irreversible visual loss. For whichever type, whether treatable or not, visual rehabilitation, through the use of appropriate magnifiers, alteration in lighting and specialised adaptation of everyday living objects, remains important adjunctive therapy.

Further information

Websites

jrcptb.org.uk/specialties/medical-ophthalmology *How to train in medical ophthalmology in the UK.*

ndrs-wp.scot.nhs.uk *Scottish Diabetic Retinopathy Screening Collaborative: aspects of screening for diabetic retinopathy, including rationale, organisation, delivery and an on-line training handbook.*

rcophth.ac.uk/standards-publications-research/clinical-guidelines *Royal College of Ophthalmologists, London: as part of its role in championing excellence, produces a range of pragmatic surgical and medical guidelines.*

sun.scot.nhs.uk *Scottish Uveitis Network: standards of care, treatment guidelines and information leaflets.*

RM Steel
SM Lawrie

28

Medical psychiatry

Clinical examination 1180
The psychiatric interview 1181
The mental state examination 1181
Investigations in medical psychiatry 1183

Functional anatomy and physiology 1183
Biological factors 1183
Psychological and behavioural factors 1183
Social and environmental factors 1184

Presenting problems in psychiatric illness 1184
Delirium 1184
Alcohol misuse 1184
Substance misuse 1184
Delusions and hallucinations 1184
Low mood 1185
Elevated mood 1186
Anxiety 1186
Psychological factors affecting medical conditions 1186
Medically unexplained somatic symptoms 1187
Self-harm 1187
Disturbed and aggressive behaviour 1188

Principles of management of psychiatric disorders 1189
Pharmacological treatments 1190
Electroconvulsive therapy 1190
Other forms of electromagnetic stimulation 1190
Surgery 1190
Psychological therapies 1190
Social interventions 1191

Psychiatric disorders 1191
Dementia 1191
Alcohol misuse and dependence 1194
Substance misuse disorder 1195
Schizophrenia 1196
Mood disorders 1198
Anxiety disorders 1200
Obsessive–compulsive disorder 1201
Stress-related disorders 1201
Somatoform disorders 1202
Eating disorders 1203
Personality disorders 1204
Factitious disorders and malingering 1205
Puerperal psychiatric disorders 1206

Psychiatry and the law 1207

Psychiatric disorders have traditionally been considered as 'mental' rather than as 'physical' illnesses. This is because they manifest with disordered functioning in the areas of emotion, perception, thinking and memory, and formerly had no clearly biological basis. However, as biochemical and structural abnormalities of the brain are identified in an increasing number of psychiatric disorders, and psychological and behavioural factors are identified in many medical illnesses, the distinction between mental and physical illness has become questionable.

The World Health Organisation (WHO) periodically publishes its International Classification of Disease (ICD), which provides definitions for every recognised clinical condition. The current edition (ICD-10) comprises 22 chapters. The diagnoses listed in Chapter V, 'Mental and behavioural disorders' (Box 28.1), are used by psychiatrists around the world in everyday clinical practice and it is these conditions that provide the focus for this chapter.

Psychiatric disorders are among the most common of all human illnesses. The WHO's Global Burden of Disease study found 'Mental, neurological and substance misuse disorders' to be the leading cause of 'Years lost to disability' (YLDs), accounting for 28.5% of global YLDs. As with most clinical conditions, the prevalence of mental disorders varies with the setting. In the general population, depression, anxiety disorders and adjustment disorders are most common (>10%) and psychosis is rare (<2%); in acute medical wards of general hospitals, organic disorders such as delirium are very common, with prevalence highest among sick, elderly patients; in specialist general psychiatric services, psychoses are the most common disorders (Box 28.2).

Clinical examination

As in other areas of medicine, the psychiatric assessment comprises a structured clinical history and examination followed by appropriate investigations. However, psychiatric assessment differs from a standard medical assessment in the following ways:

- There is greater emphasis on the history and relatively less reliance on investigations.
- A large part of the clinical examination component is conducted as the history is being taken rather than as a discrete set of procedures afterwards.

i 28.1 World Health Organisation classification of psychiatric disorders

Chapter V (F00–F99) Mental and behavioural disorders

	Examples
F00–F09 Organic mental disorders	Dementias Delirium Other mental disorders due to brain damage or disease
F10–F19 Disorders due to psychoactive substances: alcohol, opioids, cannabinoids etc.	Intoxication Harmful use Dependence Withdrawal
F20–F29 Schizophrenia and delusional disorders	Schizophrenia
F30–F39 Mood [affective] disorders	Depression Bipolar affective disorder
F40–F48 Neurotic, stress-related and somatoform disorders	Phobias Generalised anxiety disorder Obsessive–compulsive disorder Post-traumatic stress disorder Adjustment disorders Somatoform disorders
F50–F59 Behavioural syndromes associated with physiological disturbances	Eating disorders: anorexia and bulimia nervosa Sexual dysfunction
F60–F69 Disorders of adult personality and behaviour	Specific personality disorders Trichotillomania Gender identity disorders
F70–F79 Mental retardation	Mild, moderate, severe or profound
F80–F89 Disorders of psychological development	Autism Asperger's syndrome
F90–F98 Behavioural and emotional disorders of childhood	Hyperkinetic disorders Tic disorders

From WHO. International Classification of Disease, 10th edn (ICD-10).

i 28.2 Prevalence of psychiatric disorders by medical setting

	Medical/surgical			General psychiatric services
	General practice	Outpatients	Inpatients	
Delirium	–	–	+++	–
Alcohol/substance abuse	++	++	+++	+++
Schizophrenia	–	–	–	+++
Bipolar affective disorder	–	–	–	+++
Depression	++	++	+++	+++
Anxiety disorders	++	++	++	+++
Adjustment disorders	++	++	+++	+
Somatoform disorders	+	+++	++	–
Personality disorders	+	+	+	+++

– 'rare' (<2%); + 'uncommon' (2–5%); ++ 'common' (5–10%); +++ 'very common' (>10%)

- It commonly includes the interviewing of an informant, usually a relative or friend who knows the patient, especially when the illness affects the patient's ability to give an accurate history.

A full psychiatric history (Box 28.3) incorporating a detailed mental state examination may take an hour or more because of its complexity. A brief mental state examination, usually taking no more than a few minutes (see below), should be part of the assessment of *all* patients, not merely those deemed to have psychiatric illnesses.

The psychiatric interview

The aims of the interview are to:

- establish a therapeutic relationship with the patient
- elicit the symptoms, history and background information (Box 28.3)
- examine the mental state
- provide information, reassurance and advice.

28.3 How to structure a psychiatric interview

Presenting problem

Reason for referral
- Why the patient has been referred and by whom

Presenting complaints
- The patient should be asked to describe the main problems for which help is requested and what they want the doctor to do

History of present illness
- The patient should be asked to describe the course of the illness from when symptoms were first noticed
- The interviewer asks direct questions to determine the nature, duration and severity of symptoms, and any associated factors

Background

Family history
- Description of parents and siblings, and a record of any mental illness in relatives

Personal history
- Birth and early developmental history, major events in childhood, education, occupational history, relationship(s), marriage, children, current social circumstances

Previous medical and psychiatric history
- Previous health, accidents and operations
- Use of alcohol, tobacco and other drugs
- Direct questions may be needed concerning previous psychiatric history since this may not be volunteered: 'Have you ever been treated for depression or nerves?' or 'Have you ever suffered a nervous breakdown?'

Previous personality
- The patterns of behaviour and thinking that characterise a person, including their relationships with other people and reactions to stress (useful information may be obtained from an informant who has known the patient well for many years)

The mental state examination

The mental state examination (MSE) is a systematic examination of the patient's thinking, emotion and behaviour. As with the clinical examination in other areas of medicine, the aim is to elicit objective clinical signs. While many aspects of the patient's mental state may be observed as the history is being taken, specific enquiries about important features should always be made.

General appearance and behaviour

Any abnormalities of alertness or motor behaviour, such as restlessness or retardation, should be noted. The level of consciousness should be determined, especially in the assessment of possible delirium.

Speech

Speed and fluency should be observed, including slow (retarded) speech and word-finding difficulty. 'Pressure of speech' describes rapid speech that is difficult to interrupt.

Mood

This can be judged by facial expression, posture and movements. Patients should also be asked if they feel sad or depressed and if they lack ability to experience pleasure (anhedonia). Are they anxious, worried or tense? Is mood elevated with excess energy and a reduced need for sleep, as in (hypo)mania?

Thoughts

The content of thought can be elicited by asking 'What are your main concerns?'. Is thinking negative, guilty or hopeless, suggesting depression? Are there thoughts of self-harm? If so, enquiry should be made about plans. Are patients excessively worried about many things, suggesting anxiety? Do they think that they are especially powerful, important or gifted (grandiose thoughts), suggesting mania?

The form of thinking may also be abnormal. In schizophrenia, patients may display loosened associations between ideas, making it difficult to follow their train of thought. There may also be abnormalities of thought possession, when patients experience the intrusion of alien thoughts into their mind or the broadcasting of their own thoughts to other people (p. 1196).

Abnormal beliefs

A delusion is a false belief, out of keeping with a patient's cultural background, which is held with conviction despite evidence to the contrary (p. 1184).

Abnormal perceptions

Illusions are misperceptions of real stimuli. Hallucinations are sensory perceptions that occur in the absence of external stimuli, such as hearing voices when no one is present (p. 1184).

Cognitive function

Cognitive function has many components: memory, concentration, visuospatial abilities, executive function and so on. In most cases, a brief assessment of orientation (person, place and time – the patent is asked their name, age, date of birth, what building they are in, the current date and day of the week) and attention ('serial 7s' – the patient is asked to subtract 7 from 100 and then 7 from the answer, and so on) is sufficient to exclude clinically significant cognitive impairment. Where there is reason to suspect cognitive impairment, however, a standardised screening tool should be used. In delirium, cognitive impairment typically fluctuates over time so may be missed by a single assessment.

The Montreal Cognitive Assessment (MoCA) is a useful screening questionnaire that covers all the main domains of cognitive function (Fig. 28.1). It is designed to be easy to use and is freely available online in many different languages. Another widely used screening test is the Mini-Mental State Examination (MMSE), although this is subject to copyright, unlike the MoCA.

28

NAME:
Education:
Sex:
Date of birth:
DATE:

VISUOSPATIAL/EXECUTIVE

(E) End

(A)

(5)

(2)

(B)

(1) Begin

(D)

(4)

(3)

(C)

Copy cube

[ ]

[ ]

Draw CLOCK (Ten past eleven) (3 points)

[ ]   [ ]   [ ]
Contour   Numbers   Hands

POINTS

___/5

NAMING

[ ]   [ ]   [ ]   ___/3

MEMORY

Read list of words, subject must repeat them. Do 2 trials, even if 1st trial is successful. Do a recall after 5 minutes.

	FACE	VELVET	CHURCH	DAISY	RED	No points
1st trial						
2nd trial						

ATTENTION

Read list of digits (1 digit/ sec.)

Subject has to repeat them in the forward order   [ ] 2 1 8 5 4

Subject has to repeat them in the backward order   [ ] 7 4 2

___/2

Read list of letters. The subject must tap with his hand at each letter A.   No points if ≥ 2 errors

[ ]   F B A C M N A A J K L B A F A K D E A A A J A M O F A A B

___/1

Serial 7 subtraction starting at 100   [ ] 93   [ ] 86   [ ] 79   [ ] 72   [ ] 65

4 or 5 correct subtractions: **3 pts**, 2 or 3 correct: **2 pts**, 1 correct: **1 pt**, 0 correct: **0 pt**

___/3

LANGUAGE

Repeat: I only know that John is the one to help today. [ ]

The cat always hid under the couch when dogs were in the room. [ ]

___/2

Fluency / Name maximum number of words in one minute that begin with the letter F   [ ] _____ (N ≥ 11 words)

___/1

ABSTRACTION

Similarity between e.g. banana – orange = fruit   [ ] train – bicycle   [ ] watch – ruler

___/2

DELAYED RECALL

	FACE	VELVET	CHURCH	DAISY	RED	Points for UNCUED recall only
Has to recall words **WITH NO CUE**	[ ]	[ ]	[ ]	[ ]	[ ]	
Optional Category cue						
Multiple choice cue						

___/5

ORIENTATION

[ ] Date   [ ] Month   [ ] Year   [ ] Day   [ ] Place   [ ] City

___/6

© Z.Nasreddine MD   **www.mocatest.org**   Normal ≥ 26 / 30

TOTAL ___/30

Add 1 point if ≤ 12 yr edu

Administered by: _____

Fig. 28.1 Montreal Cognitive Assessment (MoCA). A widely used screening tool for cognitive impairment. © Z. Nasreddine MD, www.mocatest.org.

The Addenbrooke's Cognitive Examination – 3rd edition (ACE-III) offers a more comprehensive assessment and brief training courses for clinicians wishing to use it. These resources are available online (see 'Further information').

Patients' own understanding of their symptoms

Patients should be asked what they think their symptoms are due to and whether they warrant treatment. The failure of a patient to understand their own symptoms is referred to as 'lack of insight'. Psychotic patients characteristically have lack of insight and fail to accept that they are in need of treatment.

Investigations in medical psychiatry

In many areas of medicine, laboratory or radiological tests play a central role in diagnosis. Such tests are often performed in psychiatry but are typically used to exclude non-psychiatric illness rather than to confirm a psychiatric diagnosis. For example, in a patient presenting with symptoms of anxiety it may be appropriate to check thyroid function to exclude thyrotoxicosis as a cause of their symptoms. Specific investigations are recommended in certain psychiatric conditions such as dementia, delirium and substance misuse. These will be discussed later in this chapter.

Functional anatomy and physiology

Most psychiatric disorders result from a complex interplay between psychological, social, environmental and genetic factors. Each of these factors may play a role in predisposing to, precipitating or perpetuating a disorder (Box 28.4).

Biological factors

Genetic

Genetic factors play a predisposing role in many psychiatric disorders, including schizophrenia and bipolar affective disorder. However, while some disorders, such as Huntington's disease, are due to mutations in a single gene, the genetic contribution to most psychiatric disorders is polygenic in nature and mediated by the combined effects of several genetic variants, each with modest effects and modulated by environmental factors.

i	28.4 Classification of risk factors for psychiatric disorders	
Classification		**Examples**
Predisposing		
Established in utero or in childhood		Genetic and epigenetic factors
		Congenital defects
Increase susceptibility to psychiatric disorder		Disturbed family background
Operate throughout patient's lifetime		Chronic physical illness
Precipitating		
Trigger an episode of illness		Stressful life events
Determine its time of onset		Acute physical illness
		Misuse of alcohol or drugs
Perpetuating		
Delay recovery from illness		Lack of social support
		Chronic physical illness

Brain structure and function

Brain structure is grossly normal in most psychiatric disorders, although abnormalities may be observed in some conditions, such as generalised atrophy in Alzheimer's disease and enlarged ventricles with a slight decrease in brain size in schizophrenia. The functioning of the brain, however, is commonly altered due to changes in neurotransmitters such as dopamine, noradrenaline (norepinephrine) and 5-hydroxytryptamine (5-HT, serotonin). Functional differences in specific areas of the brain are increasingly being recognised using advanced imaging techniques. For example, positron emission tomography (PET) studies of dopamine ligand binding in schizophrenia has consistently demonstrated increased dopamine synthesis in the striatum, even in untreated patients, while a smaller body of PET evidence points towards reductions in 5-HT transporter binding in the mid-brain and amygdala in depression.

Pattern classification approaches to structural magnetic resonance imaging (MRI) data can accurately predict the development of schizophrenia in at-risk populations, and generalised grey matter loss over time is a poor prognostic guide. Increased anterior cingulate activity in depression is a consistent predictor of good response to both antidepressants and cognitive behaviour therapy. While these and other imaging techniques show potential as diagnostic, prognostic and therapeutic aids, they remain research tools at the present time.

It is also increasingly clear that psychiatric disorders are associated with disruptions in neuronal systems rather than single sites. These can be characterised using diffusion tensor imaging (DTI) of white-matter projection fibres and resting-state/task-based functional MRI (fMRI) studies of inter-regional connectivity. For example, DTI has shown reduced white-matter density in limbic ('emotional') system tracts, such as the fornix and cingulum, in many disorders. Resting-state fMRI studies consistently identify 'default mode', salience and executive control networks of interconnected neuronal populations for certain mental activities. These pathways are implicated in several psychiatric disorders but, as yet, in non-specific ways.

Psychological and behavioural factors

Early environment

Early childhood adversity, such as emotional deprivation or abuse, predisposes to most psychiatric disorders, such as depression, eating disorders and personality disorders in adulthood.

Personality

The relationship between personality and psychiatric disorder can be difficult to assess because the development of psychiatric disorder can impact on a patient's personality. Some personality types predispose the individual to develop a psychiatric disorder, however; for example, an obsessional ('anankastic') personality increases the risk of obsessive–compulsive disorder. A disordered personality may also perpetuate a psychiatric disorder once it is established, leading to a poorer prognosis.

Behaviour

A person's behaviour may predispose to the development or perpetuation of a disorder. Examples include excess alcohol intake leading to dependence, dieting in anorexia or persistent avoidance of the feared situation in phobia.

28

Social and environmental factors

Social isolation

The lack of a close, confiding relationship predisposes to some psychiatric disorders, such as depression. The reduced social support resulting from having a psychiatric disorder may also act to perpetuate it.

Stressors

Social and environmental stressors often play an important role in precipitating psychiatric disorder in those who are predisposed, such as trauma in post-traumatic stress disorder, losses (such as bereavement) in depression, and events perceived as threatening (such as potential loss of employment) in anxiety.

Presenting problems in psychiatric illness

Delirium

Delirium is a medical disorder that is common in the elderly and in patients in high-dependency and intensive care units. The causes, assessment and management are described on page 209.

Alcohol misuse

Misuse of alcohol is a major problem worldwide. It presents in a multitude of ways, which are discussed further on page 1194 and in Box 28.22. In many cases, the link to alcohol is obvious; in others, it may not be, since denial and concealment of alcohol intake are common.

Clinical assessment

The patient should be asked to describe a typical week's drinking, quantified in terms of units of alcohol (1 unit contains approximately 8 g alcohol and is the equivalent of half a pint of beer, a single measure of spirits or a small glass of wine). The history from the patient may need corroboration by the GP, earlier medical records and family members.

Investigations

Abnormalities in routine biochemistry and haematology can support the diagnosis of alcohol excess (such as the finding of a raised mean cell volume (MCV) and/or raised γ-glutamyl transferase (GGT)), but such tests are abnormal in only half of problem drinkers; consequently, normal results on these tests do not exclude an alcohol problem. When abnormal, these measures may be helpful in challenging denial and monitoring treatment response. Transient elastography (also known as FibroScan) is an ultrasound-based technique that measures fibrosis and steatosis. It is used in specialist services to complement information derived from tests of MCV and GGT.

Management

The prevention and management of alcohol-related problems are discussed on page 1195.

Substance misuse

The misuse of drugs of all kinds is also widespread. As well as the general headings listed for alcohol problems in Box 28.22

28.5 Substance misuse: additional presenting problems

Complications arising from the route of use

Intravenous
- Local: abscesses, cellulitis, thrombosis
- Systemic: bacterial (endocarditis), viral (hepatitis, human immunodeficiency virus (HIV))

Nasal ingestion
- Erosion of nasal septum, epistaxis

Smoking
- Oral, laryngeal and lung cancer

Inhalation
- Burns, chemical pneumonitis, rashes

Pressure to prescribe misused substance
- Manipulation, deceit and threats
- Factitious description of illness
- Malingering

(p. 1194), there are two additional sets of problems associated with drug misuse (Box 28.5):
- problems linked with the route of administration, such as intravenous injection
- problems arising from pressure applied to doctors to prescribe the misused substances.

Assessment and management are described on page 1195.

Delusions and hallucinations

Delusions and hallucinations are abnormal beliefs and perceptions that have no rational basis. They are often due to psychiatric illness but can be secondary to substance misuse, physical illness or neurological disorders, such as epilepsy.

Delusions

A delusion is a false belief, out of keeping with a patient's cultural background, which is held with conviction despite evidence to the contrary. It is common to classify delusions on the basis of their content. They may be:
- persecutory – such as a conviction that others are out to harm one
- hypochondriacal – such as an unfounded conviction that one has cancer
- grandiose – such as a belief that one has special powers or status
- nihilistic – such as 'My head is missing', 'I have no body' or 'I am dead'.

Hallucinations

Hallucinations are defined as sensory perceptions occurring without external stimuli. They can occur in any sensory modality but most commonly are visual or auditory. Typical examples are hearing voices when no one else is present, or seeing 'visions'. Hallucinations have the quality of ordinary perceptions and are perceived as originating in the external world, not in the patient's own mind (when they are termed 'pseudo-hallucinations'). Those occurring when falling asleep ('hypnagogic') and on waking ('hypnopompic') are a normal phenomenon and not pathological. Hallucinations should be distinguished from illusions, which are misperceptions of real external stimuli (such as mistaking a shrub for a person in poor light).

Clinical assessment

Careful and tactful enquiry is required because agitation, terror or the fear of being thought 'mad' may make patients unable or unwilling to volunteer or describe their abnormal beliefs or perceptions. The nature of hallucinations can be important diagnostically; for example, 'running commentary' voices that discuss the patient are strongly associated with schizophrenia. In general, auditory hallucinations suggest schizophrenia, while hallucinations in other sensory modalities, especially vision but also taste and smell, suggest an organic cause, such as substance misuse, delirium or temporal lobe epilepsy.

Hallucinations and delusions often co-occur. If their content is consistent with coexisting emotional symptoms, they are described as 'mood-congruent'. Thus, patients with severely depressed mood may believe themselves responsible for all the evils in the world, and hear voices saying, 'You are worthless. Go and kill yourself.' In this case, the diagnosis of depressive psychosis is made on the basis of the congruence of different phenomena (mood, delusion and hallucination). Incongruence between hallucinations, delusions and mood suggests schizophrenia.

Investigations

The presence of hallucinations and/or delusions should not automatically trigger a round of expensive investigations; rather, careful clinical assessment of the nature, extent and time course of the patient's symptoms will generate a list of likely diagnoses, and investigations can then be intelligently deployed to differentiate between these. When hallucinations and/or delusions arise in the context of disturbed consciousness and impaired cognition, the diagnosis is usually an organic disorder, most commonly delirium and/or dementia, and should be investigated accordingly (pp. 184 and 1192).

Management

The management of hallucinations and/or delusions is primarily the management of the underlying condition (such as delirium, schizophrenia, mania or psychotic depression). Certain principles apply, however, whatever the underlying cause.

Hallucinations and delusions can be very real to, and often frightening for, the person who is experiencing them. Patients will often seek reassurance from the doctor. The doctor should acknowledge that these experiences are real *for the patient* while avoiding being drawn into colluding with the patient's false beliefs or perceptions. Statements such as 'Sometimes when we are unwell our brain plays tricks on us' can help to reassure a patient. Where the patient lacks insight, however, a more neutral 'We will have to agree to disagree' may be necessary to avoid conflict.

Antipsychotic medication can reduce psychotic symptoms, such as hallucinations and delusion, and is often used in combination with other sedating medication (such as a benzodiazepine) to alleviate acute distress and reduce behavioural disturbance (p. 1197).

Low mood

It is not uncommon for general hospital patients to report low mood. It is important to differentiate an understandable, self-limiting reaction to adversity (such as physical illness or bad news), which is normal and requires support rather than 'treatment', from a depressive disorder (p. 1198), which is characterised by a more severe and persistent disturbance of mood and requires specific treatment.

Clinical assessment

Depression is a relatively common illness, with a prevalence of approximately 5% in the general population and 10–20% in medical patients. It is important to note that depression has physical as well as mental symptoms (Box 28.6). The diagnosis of depression in the medically ill, who may have physical symptoms of disease such as weight loss, fatigue, disturbed sleep, reduced appetite and so on that overlap with the physical symptoms of depression, relies on detection of the core psychological symptoms of 'anhedonia' (inability to experience pleasure) and the negative cognitive triad (see Box 28.17).

In some cases, depression may occur as a result of a direct effect of a medical condition or its treatment on the brain, when it is referred to as an 'organic mood disorder' (Box 28.7).

Investigations

When a patient appears to be low in mood, it is good practice to ask them specifically about their mood. Do they *feel* low (nausea, over-sedation, parkinsonism and so on can all cause a patient to *appear* low in mood). If so, how long have they been feeling low? Are they still able to enjoy things? To what do they attribute their low mood? If the low mood is persistent, not adequately explained by circumstances and/or associated with anhedonia, the patient should be investigated for depression (p. 1199). Where a patient's mood is extremely low, the clinician should ask about suicide. Asking about suicide does not increase the risk of it occurring, whereas failure to enquire denies the opportunity to prevent it. The assessment of suicide risk is described on page 1185.

i | **28.6 Symptoms of depressive disorders**

Psychological

- Depressed mood
- Reduced self-esteem
- Pessimism
- Guilt
- Loss of interest
- Loss of enjoyment (anhedonia)
- Suicidal thinking

Somatic

- Reduced appetite
- Weight change
- Disturbed sleep
- Fatigue
- Loss of libido
- Bowel disturbance
- Motor retardation (slowing of activity)

i | **28.7 Organic mood disorders***

Neurological
- Cerebrovascular disease
- Cerebral tumour
- Multiple sclerosis
- Parkinson's disease
- Huntington's disease
- Alzheimer's disease
- Epilepsy

Endocrine
- Hypothyroidism
- Hyperthyroidism
- Cushing's syndrome
- Addison's disease
- Hyperparathyroidism

Malignant disease

Infections
- Infectious mononucleosis
- Herpes simplex
- Brucellosis
- Typhoid
- Toxoplasmosis

Connective tissue disease
- Systemic lupus erythematosus

Drugs
- Phenothiazines
- Phenylbutazone
- Glucocorticoids, oral contraceptives
- Interferon

*Diseases that may cause organic affective disorders by direct action on the brain.

28

Management

The management of depression is discussed on page 1199. Where a patient's low mood is an understandable reaction to adversity, the clinical team can support the patient by minimising uncertainty through open and effective clinical communication and by addressing isolation (allowing access to visitors, telephone and so on).

Elevated mood

Elevated mood is much less common than depressed mood, and in medical settings is often secondary to drug or alcohol misuse, an organic disorder or medical treatment. Where none of these applies, the patient may be experiencing a manic (or, if less severe, 'hypomanic') episode as part of a bipolar affective disorder (p. 1199). Mania is the converse of depression. It may manifest as infectious joviality, over-activity, lack of sleep and appetite, undue optimism, over-talkativeness, irritability, and recklessness in spending and sexual behaviour. When elated mood is severe, psychotic symptoms are often evident, like delusions of grandeur such as believing erroneously that one is royalty.

Investigations

The first investigation for any medical patient presenting with persistent and inexplicable elevated mood in the absence of a history of bipolar affective disorder is a medication review. Mania is a relatively common side-effect of certain classes of drug, such as glucocorticoids, and is a rare side-effect of many other drugs. Recreational, herbal and over-the-counter preparations should also be considered. Second-line investigations include tests for Cushing's disease (p. 666), thyrotoxicosis (p. 635), syphilis (p. 337) and encephalitis (p. 1121).

Management

The management of bipolar affective disorder is discussed on page 1200. Management of organic mania involves identifying and addressing the underlying cause. The management of disturbed or aggressive behaviour is discussed on page 1188.

Anxiety

Anxiety may be transient, persistent, episodic or limited to specific situations. The symptoms of anxiety are both psychological and physical (Box 28.8). The differential diagnosis of anxiety is shown in Box 28.9. Most anxiety is part of a transient adjustment to

---

28.9 Differential diagnosis of anxiety
• Normal response to threat
• Adjustment disorder
• Generalised anxiety disorder
• Panic disorder
• Phobic disorder
• Organic (medical) cause:
Hyperthyroidism
Paroxysmal arrhythmias
Phaeochromocytoma
Alcohol and benzodiazepine withdrawal
Hypoglycaemia
Temporal lobe epilepsy

stressful events: adjustment disorders (p. 1201). Other more persistent forms of anxiety are described in detail on page 1200.

Investigations

Anxiety may occasionally be a manifestation of a medical condition such as thyrotoxicosis (Box 28.9). Tests to exclude or confirm these conditions should be considered, particularly if anxiety is a new symptom that has arisen in the absence of an obvious stressor.

Management

The management of specific anxiety disorders is discussed later in this chapter (p. 1200). Benzodiazepines and related drugs, while extremely effective in the short term, cause tolerance and unpleasant or even dangerous withdrawal syndromes if used for more than a few weeks.

Psychological factors affecting medical conditions

Psychological factors may influence the presentation, management and outcome of medical conditions. Specific factors are shown in Box 28.10. The most common psychiatric diagnoses in the medically ill are anxiety and depressive disorders. Often these appear understandable as adjustments to illness and its treatment; however, if the anxiety and depression are severe and persistent, they may complicate the management of the medical condition and active management is required. Anxiety may present as an increase in somatic symptoms, such as breathlessness, tremor or palpitations, or as the avoidance of medical treatment. It is most common in those facing difficult or painful treatments, deterioration of their illness or death. Depression may manifest as increased physical symptoms, such as pain, fatigue and disability, as well as with depressed mood and loss of interest and pleasure. It is most common in patients who have suffered

---

28.8 Symptoms of anxiety disorder

Psychological

• Apprehension	• Poor concentration
• Irritability	• Fear of impending disaster
• Worry	• Depersonalisation

Somatic

• Palpitations	• Frequent desire to pass urine
• Fatigue	• Chest pain
• Tremor	• Initial insomnia
• Dizziness	• Breathlessness
• Sweating	• Headache
• Diarrhoea	

28.10 Risk factors for psychological problems associated with medical conditions
• Previous history of depression or anxiety
• Lack of social support
• New diagnosis of a serious medical condition
• Deterioration of, or failure of treatment for, a medical condition
• Unpleasant, disabling or disfiguring treatment
• Change in medical care, such as discharge from hospital
• Impending death

actual or anticipated losses, such as receiving a terminal diagnosis or undergoing disfiguring surgery.

Treatment is by psychological and/or pharmacological therapies, as described on page 1189. Care is required when prescribing psychotropic drugs to the medically ill in order to avoid exacerbation of the medical condition and harmful interactions with other prescribed drugs.

Medically unexplained somatic symptoms

Patients commonly present to doctors with physical symptoms. While these symptoms may be an expression of a medical condition, they often are not (see Fig. 28.6). They may then be referred to as 'medically unexplained symptoms' (MUS), which are very common in patients attending general medical outpatient clinics. Almost any symptom can be medically unexplained. They include:

- pain (including back, chest, abdominal, pelvic and headache)
- fatigue
- fits, 'funny turns', dizziness and feelings of weakness.

Patients with MUS may receive a medical diagnosis of a so-called 'functional somatic syndrome', such as irritable bowel syndrome (Box 28.11), and may also merit a psychiatric diagnosis on the basis of the same symptoms. The most frequent psychiatric diagnoses associated with MUS are anxiety or depressive disorders. When these are absent, a diagnosis of somatoform disorder may be appropriate. Somatoform disorders are discussed in more detail on page 1202.

i	**28.11 Functional somatic syndromes**
Medical specialty	**Somatic syndromes**
Gastroenterology	Irritable bowel syndrome, functional dyspepsia
Gynaecology	Pre-menstrual syndrome, chronic pelvic pain
Rheumatology	Fibromyalgia
Cardiology	Atypical or non-cardiac chest pain
Respiratory medicine	Hyperventilation syndrome
Infectious diseases	Chronic (post-viral) fatigue syndrome
Neurology	Tension headache, non-epileptic attacks, functional gait disorder
Dentistry	Temporomandibular joint dysfunction, atypical facial pain
Ear, nose and throat	Globus syndrome
Allergy medicine	Multiple chemical sensitivity

Self-harm

Self-harm (SH) is a common reason for presentation to medical services. The term 'attempted suicide' is potentially misleading, as most of these patients are not trying to kill themselves. Most cases of SH involve overdose, of either prescribed or non-prescribed drugs (Ch. 7). Less common methods include asphyxiation, drowning, hanging, jumping from a height or in front of a moving vehicle, and the use of firearms. Methods that carry a high chance of being fatal are more likely to be associated with serious psychiatric disorder. Self-cutting is common and often repetitive, but rarely leads to contact with medical services.

The incidence of SH varies over time and between countries. In the UK, the lifetime prevalence of suicidal ideation is 15% and that of acts of SH is 4%. SH is more common in women than men, and in young adults than the elderly. (In contrast, completed suicide is more common in men and the elderly; Box 28.12.) There is a higher incidence of SH among lower socioeconomic groups, particularly those living in crowded, socially deprived urban areas. There is also an association with alcohol misuse, child abuse, unemployment and recently broken relationships.

Clinical assessment

The main differential diagnosis is from accidental poisoning and so-called 'recreational' overdose in drug users. It must be remembered that SH is not a diagnosis but a presentation, and may be associated with any psychiatric diagnosis, the most common being adjustment disorder, substance and alcohol misuse, depressive disorder and personality disorder. In many cases, however, no psychiatric diagnosis can be made.

Management

A thorough psychiatric and social assessment should be attempted in all cases (Fig. 28.2), although some patients will discharge themselves before this can take place. The need for psychiatric assessment should not delay urgent medical or surgical treatment, though, and may need to be deferred until the patient is well enough for interview. The purpose of the psychiatric assessment is to:

- establish the short-term risk of suicide
- identify potentially treatable problems, whether medical, psychiatric or social.

Topics to be covered when assessing a patient are listed in Box 28.13. The history should include events occurring immediately

i	**28.12 Risk factors for suicide**

- Psychiatric illness (depressive illness, schizophrenia)
- Older age
- Male sex
- Living alone
- Unemployment
- Recent bereavement, divorce or separation
- Chronic physical ill health
- Drug or alcohol misuse
- Suicide note written
- History of previous attempts (especially if a violent method was used)

i	**28.13 Assessment of patients after self-harm**

Current attempt

- Patient's account
- Degree of intent at the time: preparations, plans, precautions against discovery, note
- Method used, particularly whether violent
- Degree of intent now
- Symptoms of psychiatric illness

Background

- Previous attempts and their outcome
- Family and personal history
- Social support
- Previous response to stress
- Extent of drug and alcohol misuse

28

Fig. 28.2 Assessment of patients admitted following self-harm.

before and after the act, and especially any evidence of planning. The nature and severity of any current psychiatric symptoms must be assessed, along with the personal and social supports available to the patient outside hospital.

Most SH patients have depressive and anxiety symptoms on a background of chronic social and personal difficulties (often complicated by use of alcohol or other substances), but no psychiatric disorder. They do not usually require psychotropic medication or specialised psychiatric treatment but may benefit from personal support and practical advice from a GP, social worker or community psychiatric nurse. Admission to a psychiatric

ward is necessary only for persons who display one or more of the following:

- an acute psychiatric disorder
- high short-term risk of suicide
- need for temporary respite from intolerable circumstances
- requirement for further assessment of their mental state.

Approximately 20% of SH patients make a repeat act during the following year and 1–2% kill themselves. Factors associated with suicide after an episode of SH are listed in Box 28.12.

Disturbed and aggressive behaviour

Disturbed and aggressive behaviour is common in general hospitals, especially in emergency departments. Most behavioural disturbance arises not from medical or psychiatric illness, but from alcohol intoxication, reaction to the situation and personality characteristics.

Clinical assessment

The key principles of management are, firstly, to establish control of the situation rapidly and thereby ensure the safety of the patient and others; and secondly, to try to determine the cause of the disturbance in order to remedy it. Establishing control requires the presence of an adequate number of trained staff, an appropriate physical environment and sometimes sedation (Fig. 28.3). The assistance of hospital security staff and sometimes the police may be required. In all cases, the staff approach is important; a calm, non-threatening manner expressing understanding of the patient's concerns is often all that is required to defuse potential aggression (Box 28.14).

An attempt should be made to try to identify the factors that are contributing to the disturbed behaviour. When the patient is cooperative, these are best determined at interview. Other sources of information about the patient include medical and psychiatric records, and discussion with nursing staff, family members and other informants, including the patient's GP. The following information should be sought:

- psychiatric, medical (especially neurological) and criminal history
- current psychiatric and medical treatment
- alcohol and drug misuse
- recent stressors
- the time course and accompaniments of the current episode in terms of mood, belief and behaviour.

Observation of the patient's behaviour may also yield useful clues. Do they appear to be responding to hallucinations? Are they alert or variably drowsy and confused? Are there physical features suggestive of drug or alcohol misuse or withdrawal? Are there new injuries or old scars, especially on the head? Do they smell of alcohol or solvents? Do they bear the marks of drug injection? Are they unwashed and unkempt, suggesting a gradual development of their condition?

Investigations

Depending on the results of clinical assessment, routine biochemistry, haematology and analysis of blood or urine for illicit drugs or alcohol may be required.

Management

Measures such as restraint and sedation may be required in patients with acute behavioural disturbance in order to

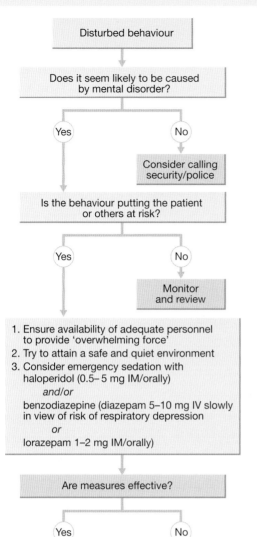

Fig. 28.3 **Acute management of disturbed behaviour.**

Flowchart text:

Disturbed behaviour

Does it seem likely to be caused by mental disorder?

Yes / No

No → Consider calling security/police

Is the behaviour putting the patient or others at risk?

Yes / No

No → Monitor and review

1. Ensure availability of adequate personnel to provide 'overwhelming force'
2. Try to attain a safe and quiet environment
3. Consider emergency sedation with haloperidol (0.5–5 mg IM/orally)
   and/or
   benzodiazepine (diazepam 5–10 mg IV slowly in view of risk of respiratory depression
   or
   lorazepam 1–2 mg IM/orally)

Are measures effective?

Yes / No

Yes → Monitor and review

No → Consult with senior staff
Consider repeating drug, increasing dose or using other agents such as midazolam or paraldehyde

---

28.14 Psychiatric emergencies

- Intervene as necessary to reduce the risk of harm to the patient and to others
- Adopt a calm, non-threatening approach
- Arrange availability of other staff and parenteral medication
- Consider diagnostic possibilities of drug intoxication, acute psychosis and delirium
- Involve friends and relatives as appropriate

identify the cause and to protect the patient and other people from harm. While this potentially raises legal issues, in most countries, including the UK, common law confers on doctors the right, and indeed the duty, to intervene against a patient's wishes if this is necessary. Sedation may be required and

---

28.15 Medical psychiatry in old age

- **Organic psychiatric disorders**: especially common, so cognitive function should always be assessed; if impaired, an associated medical condition or adverse drug effect should be suspected.
- **Disturbed behaviour**: delirium is the most common cause.
- **Depression**: common. Just because a person is old and frail does not mean that depression is 'to be expected' and that it should not be treated.
- **Self-harm**: associated with an increased risk of completed suicide.
- **Medically unexplained symptoms**: common and often associated with depressive disorder.
- **Loneliness, poverty and lack of social support**: must be taken into consideration in management decisions.

can be achieved with antipsychotic drugs (such as haloperidol) and/or benzodiazepines (such as lorazepam or diazepam). The choice of drug, dose, route and rate of administration depends on the patient's age, gender and physical health, as well as the likely cause of the disturbed behaviour. The benefits of sedation must always be balanced against the potential risks. When prescribing benzodiazepines, consider the risk of respiratory depression (particularly in patients with lung disease) and encephalopathy (in those with liver disease). When prescribing antipsychotic drugs for acute sedation, consider the risk of acute dystonias (such as 'oculogyric crisis') and acute arrhythmias (in patients with heart disease). Thus for a frail elderly woman with emphysema and delirium, sedation may be achieved with a low dose (0.5 mg) of oral haloperidol, while for a strong young man with an acute psychotic episode, 10 mg or more of intravenous diazepam and a similar dose of haloperidol may be required. A parenterally administered anticholinergic agent, such as procyclidine, should be available to treat extrapyramidal effects from haloperidol if they arise. Flumazenil (p. 142) can be used to reverse respiratory depression caused by benzodiazepines.

If the initial assessment suggests that the patient has an acute psychiatric disorder, then admission to a psychiatric facility may be indicated. If a medical cause is more likely, psychiatric transfer is usually inappropriate and the patient should be managed in a medical setting, with whatever nursing and security support is required. Where it is clear that there is no medical or psychiatric illness, the person should be removed from the hospital, to police custody if necessary.

Many countries, such as the UK, also have specific mental health legislation that may be used to detain patients if necessary.

Principles of management of psychiatric disorders

The multifactorial origin of most psychiatric disorders means that there are multiple potential targets for treatment. It is useful to consider management strategies within a bio-psycho-social framework. This can help to address the biological factors that contribute to the illness with medication and other physical treatments such as electroconvulsive therapy, while also considering the potential role for psychological therapies and changes to the patient's social environment.

28

i	28.16 Classification of commonly used psychotropic drugs		
Action	**Main groups**		**Clinical use**
Antipsychotic	Phenothiazines Butyrophenones Second-generation antipsychotics	}	Schizophrenia Bipolar mania Delirium
Antidepressant	Tricyclics and related drugs Serotonin and noradrenergic re-uptake inhibitors Monoamine oxidase inhibitors	}	Depression/anxiety Obsessive–compulsive disorder Depression/anxiety
Mood-stabilising	Lithium Valproate Lamotrigine	}	Treatment and prophylaxis of bipolar disorder Adjunctive therapy in depression
Anti-anxiety	Benzodiazepines	{	Anxiety/insomnia (short term) Alcohol withdrawal (short term)
	β-adrenoceptor antagonists		Anxiety (somatic symptoms)

Pharmacological treatments

These aim to relieve psychiatric disorder by modifying brain function. The main biological treatments are psychotropic drugs. These are widely used for various purposes; a pragmatic classification is set out in Box 28.16. It should be noted that some drugs have applications to more than one condition; for example, antidepressants are also widely used in the treatment of anxiety *and* chronic pain. The specific subgroups of psychotropic drugs are discussed in the sections on the appropriate disorders below.

Electroconvulsive therapy

Electroconvulsive therapy (ECT) entails producing a convulsion by the brief administration of a high-voltage direct-current impulse to the head while the patient is anaesthetised and paralysed by muscle relaxant. If properly administered, it is remarkably safe, has few side-effects, and is of proven efficacy for severe depressive illness. There may be headaches and amnesia for events occurring a few hours before ECT (retrograde) and after it (anterograde). Pronounced amnesia can occur but is infrequent and difficult to distinguish from the effects of severe depression.

Other forms of electromagnetic stimulation

Clinical trials of transcranial magnetic stimulation (TMS) and vagal nerve stimulation (VNS) suggest they may have a limited role in patients with depression refractory to conventional treatments.

Surgery

Surgery to the brain (psychosurgery) has a very limited place and then only in the treatment of severe chronic psychiatric illness resistant to other measures. Frontal lobotomies are never done now, and pre-frontal leucotomies are very rare. Operations these days usually target specific sub-regions and tracts of the brain.

Psychological therapies

These treatments are useful in many psychiatric disorders and also in non-psychiatric conditions. They are based on talking with patients, either individually or in groups. Sometimes discussion

i	28.17 The negative cognitive triad associated with depression	
Cognitive error		**Example**
Negative view of self		'I am no good'
Negative view of current life experiences		'The world is an awful place'
Negative view of the future		'The future is hopeless'

is supplemented by 'homework' or tasks to complete between treatment sessions. Psychological treatments take a number of forms based on the duration and frequency of contact, the specific techniques applied and their underlying theory.

General psychotherapy

General psychotherapy should be part of all medical treatment. It involves empathic listening to the patient's account of their symptoms and associated fears and concerns, followed by the sympathetic provision of accurate information that addresses these.

Cognitive therapy

This therapy is based on the observation that some psychiatric disorders are associated with systematic errors in the patient's conscious thinking, such as a tendency to interpret events in a negative way or see them as unduly threatening. A triad of 'cognitive errors' has been described in depression (Box 28.17). Cognitive therapy aims to help patients to identify such cognitive errors and to learn how to challenge them. It is widely used for depression, anxiety and eating and somatoform disorders, and also increasingly in psychoses.

Behaviour therapy

This is a practically orientated form of treatment, in which patients are assisted in changing unhelpful behaviour, such as helping patients to implement carefully graded exposure to the feared stimulus in phobias.

Cognitive behaviour therapy

Cognitive behaviour therapy (CBT) combines the methods of behaviour therapy and cognitive therapy. It is the most widely available and extensively researched psychological treatment.

Problem-solving therapy

This is a simplified brief form of CBT, which helps patients actively tackle problems in a structured way (Box 28.18). It can be delivered by non-psychiatric doctors and nurses after appropriate training and is commonly used to help patients who self-harm in response to a situational crisis.

Psychodynamic psychotherapy

This treatment, also known as 'interpretive psychotherapy', was pioneered by Freud, Jung and Klein, among others. It is based on the theory that early life experience generates powerful but unconscious motivations. Psychotherapy aims to help the patient to become aware of these unconscious factors on the assumption that, once identified, their negative effects are reduced. The relationship between therapist and patient is used as a therapeutic tool to identify issues in patients' relationships with others, particularly parents, which may be replicated or transferred to their relationship with the therapist. Explicit discussion of this relationship (transference) is the basis for the treatment, which traditionally requires frequent sessions over a period of months or even years.

Interpersonal psychotherapy

Interpersonal psychotherapy (IPT) is a specific form of brief psychotherapy that focuses on patients' current interpersonal relationships and is an effective treatment for mild to moderate depression.

Social interventions

Some adverse social factors, such as unemployment, may not be readily amenable to intervention but others, such as access to benefits and poor housing, may be. Patients can be helped to address these problems themselves by being taught problem-solving. Befrienders and day centres can reduce social isolation, benefits advisers can ensure appropriate financial assistance, and medical recommendations can be made to local housing departments to help patients obtain more appropriate accommodation.

Psychiatric disorders

Dementia

Dementia is a clinical syndrome characterised by a loss of previously acquired intellectual function in the absence of impairment of arousal. It affects 5% of those over 65 and 20% of those over 85. It is defined as a global impairment of cognitive function and is typically progressive and non-reversible. There are many subtypes (Box 28.19) but Alzheimer's disease and diffuse vascular dementia are the most common. Rarer causes of dementia should be actively sought in younger patients and those with short histories.

28.18 Stages of problem-solving therapy

- Define and list problems
- Choose one to work on
- List possible solutions
- Evaluate these and choose the best
- Try it out
- Evaluate the result
- Repeat until problems are resolved

28.19 Subtypes and causes of dementia

Type	Common	Less common	Rare
Vascular	Diffuse small-vessel disease	Amyloid angiopathy Multiple emboli	Cerebral vasculitis Systemic lupus erythematosus
Inherited	Alzheimer's disease	Fronto-temporal dementia Leukodystrophies Huntington's disease Wilson's disease Dystrophia myotonica Lewy body dementia Progressive supranuclear palsy	Mitochondrial encephalopathies Cortico-basal degeneration
Neoplastic (p. 1110)	Secondary deposits	Primary cerebral tumour	Paraneoplastic syndrome (limbic encephalitis)
Inflammatory	–	Multiple sclerosis	Sarcoidosis
Traumatic	Chronic subdural haematoma Post-head injury	Punch-drunk syndrome	–
Hydrocephalus (p. 1132)		Communicating/non-communicating 'normal pressure' hydrocephalus	–
Toxic/nutritional	Alcohol	Thiamin deficiency Vitamin B_{12} deficiency	Anoxia/carbon monoxide poisoning Heavy metal poisoning
Infective	–	Syphilis HIV	Post-encephalitis Whipple's disease Subacute sclerosing panencephalitis
Prion diseases (p. 1126)	–	Sporadic Creutzfeldt–Jakob disease (CJD)	Variant CJD Kuru Gerstmann–Sträussler–Scheinker disease

28

Pathogenesis

Dementia may be divided into 'cortical' and 'subcortical' types, depending on the clinical features.

Clinical features

The usual presentation is with a disturbance of personality or memory dysfunction. A careful history is essential and it is important to interview both the patient and a close family member. Simple bedside tests, such as the MoCA (p. 1182), are useful in assessing the nature and severity of the cognitive deficit, although a more intensive neuropsychological assessment may sometimes be required, especially if there is diagnostic uncertainty. It is important to exclude a focal brain lesion. This is done by determining that there is cognitive disturbance in more than one area. Mental state assessment is important to seek evidence of depression, which may coexist with or occasionally cause apparent cognitive impairment. Many of the primary degenerative diseases that cause dementia have characteristic features that may allow a specific diagnosis during life. Creutzfeldt–Jakob disease, for example, is usually quickly progressive (over months) and is associated with myoclonus. The more slowly progressive dementias are more difficult to distinguish during life, but fronto-temporal dementia typically presents with signs of temporal or frontal lobe dysfunction, whereas Lewy body dementia may present with visual hallucinations. The course may also help to distinguish types of dementia. Gradual worsening suggests Alzheimer's disease, whereas stepwise deterioration is typical of vascular dementia.

Investigations

The aim is to seek treatable causes and to estimate prognosis. This is done using a standard set of investigations (Box 28.20). Imaging of the brain can exclude potentially treatable structural lesions, such as hydrocephalus, cerebral tumour or chronic subdural haematoma, though the only abnormality usually seen is that of generalised atrophy. An electroencephalogram (EEG) may be helpful if Creutzfeldt–Jakob disease is suspected, as characteristic abnormalities of generalised periodic sharp wave pattern are usually observed. If the initial tests are negative, more invasive investigations, such as lumbar puncture or, very rarely, brain biopsy, may be indicated.

Management

This is mainly directed at addressing treatable causes and providing support for patients and carers. Tackling risk factors may slow deterioration, e.g. effective management of hypertension in vascular dementia, or abstinence and vitamin replacement in toxic/nutritional dementias. Psychotropic drugs may have a role in alleviating symptoms, such as disturbance of sleep, perception or mood, but should be used with care because of an increased mortality in patients who have been treated long-term with these agents. Sedation is not a substitute for good care of patients and carers or, in the later stages, attentive residential nursing care. In the UK, incapacity and mental health legislation may be required to manage patients' financial and domestic affairs, as well as to determine their safe placement. If the diagnosis is Alzheimer-type dementia, cholinesterase inhibitors and memantine may slow progression for a time.

Alzheimer's disease

Alzheimer's disease is the most common form of dementia. It increases in prevalence with age and is rare in people under 45 years.

Pathogenesis

Genetic factors play an important role and about 15% of cases are familial. These cases fall into two main groups: early-onset disease with autosomal dominant inheritance and a later-onset group where the inheritance is polygenic. Mutations in several genes have been described but most are rare and/or of small effect. The inheritance of one of the alleles of apolipoprotein ε (apo ε4) is associated with an increased risk of developing the disease (2–4 times higher in heterozygotes and 6–8 times higher in homozygotes). Its presence is, however, neither necessary nor sufficient for the development of the disease and so genetic testing for ApoE4 is not clinically useful. The brain in Alzheimer's disease is macroscopically atrophic, particularly the cerebral cortex and hippocampus. Histologically, the disease is characterised by the presence of senile plaques and neurofibrillary tangles in the cerebral cortex. Histochemical staining demonstrates significant quantities of amyloid in the plaques (Fig. 28.4); these typically stain positive for the protein ubiquitin, which normally is involved in targeting unwanted or damaged proteins for degradation. This has led to the suggestion that the disease may be due to defects in the ability of neuronal cells to degrade unwanted proteins. Many different neurotransmitter abnormalities have also been described. In particular, there is impairment of cholinergic transmission, although abnormalities of noradrenaline (norepinephrine), 5-HT, glutamate and substance P have also been described.

Clinical features

The key clinical feature is impairment of the ability to remember new information. Hence, patients present with gradual impairment of memory, usually in association with disorders of other cortical functions. Short- and long-term memory are both affected but defects in the former are usually more obvious. Later in the course of the disease, typical features include apraxia, visuo-spatial impairment and aphasia. In the early stages of the disease, patients may notice these problems, but as the disease progresses it is common for patients to deny that there is anything wrong (anosognosia). In this situation, patients are

28.20 Initial investigation of dementia

In most patients

- Imaging of head (computed tomography and/or magnetic resonance imaging)
- Blood tests:
  - Full blood count, erythrocyte sedimentation rate
  - Urea and electrolytes, glucose
  - Calcium, liver function tests
  - Thyroid function tests
  - Vitamin B_{12}
  - Syphilis serology
  - ANA, anti-dsDNA
- Chest X-ray
- Electroencephalography

In selected patients

- Lumbar puncture
- HIV serology
- Brain biopsy

(ANA = antinuclear antibody; anti-dsDNA = anti-double-stranded DNA)

Fig. 28.4 Alzheimer's disease. Section of neocortex stained with polyclonal antibody against βA4 peptide showing amyloid deposits in plaques in brain substance (arrow A) and in blood-vessel walls (arrow B). *Courtesy of Dr J. Xuereb.*

Fig. 28.5 Fronto-temporal dementia. [A] Lateral view of formalin-fixed brain from a patient who died of Pick's disease, showing gyral atrophy of frontal and parietal lobes and a more severe degree of atrophy affecting the anterior half of the temporal lobe (arrow). [B] High power (× 200) view of hippocampal pyramidal layer, prepared with monoclonal anti-tau antibody. Many neuronal cell bodies contain sharply circumscribed, spherical cytoplasmic inclusion bodies (Pick bodies, arrows). *A and B, Courtesy of Dr J. Xuereb.*

often brought to medical attention by their carers. Depression is commonly present. Occasionally, patients become aggressive, and the clinical features can be made acutely worse by intercurrent physical disease.

Patients typically present with subjective memory loss, sometimes getting lost in familiar locations. A history of progressive memory loss and associated functional impairment, corroborated by an informant, is the key to making the diagnosis. Cognitive testing and neuroimaging can be helpful but in themselves are not diagnostic.

Investigations

Investigation is aimed at excluding treatable causes of dementia (see Box 28.19), as histological confirmation of the diagnosis usually occurs only after death.

Management

Treatment with anticholinesterases, such as donepezil, rivastigmine and galantamine, has been shown to be of some benefit at slowing progression of cognitive impairment in the early stages of the disease while post-synaptic cholinergic receptors are still available. The N-methyl-D-aspartate (NMDA) receptor antagonist memantine slightly enhances learning and memory in early disease and can also be useful in selected patients with more advanced disease. Novel treatments are under development to block amyloid plaque formation directly, by inhibiting the enzyme γ-secretase. Non-pharmacological approaches include the provision of a familiar environment for the patient and support for the carers.

Many patients are depressed, and if this is confirmed, treatment with antidepressant medication may be helpful.

Fronto-temporal dementia

Fronto-temporal dementia encompasses a number of different syndromes characterised by behaviour abnormalities and impairment of language. Symptoms usually occur before the age of 60 and the prevalence has been estimated at 15 per 100 000 in the population aged between 45 and 65 years. The three major clinical subtypes are behavioural-variant fronto-temporal dementia, primary progressive aphasia and semantic dementia. Pick's disease is a common cause of the first two in particular. Genetic factors play an important role and familial cases have been described caused by mutations in several genes, including MAPT, which encodes microtubule-associated protein tau, GRN, TPD43, FUS, VCP and C9orf72. The causal mutations trigger abnormal accumulation of tau and other proteins in brain tissue, which are seen as cytoplasmic inclusion bodies on histological examination (Fig. 28.5). It is of interest that many of the gene mutations that cause fronto-temporal dementia are also associated with amyotrophic lateral sclerosis (p. 1116), suggesting that these disorders share a similar pathogenic basis in which neuronal degeneration is caused by accumulation of abnormal proteins. The clinical presentation may be with personality change due to frontal lobe involvement or with language disturbance due to temporal lobe involvement. In contrast to Alzheimer's disease, memory is relatively preserved in the early stages. There is no specific treatment. Disinhibition and compulsive behaviours can

28

be helped by selective serotonin re-uptake inhibitors (SSRIs). Although Alzheimer's and fronto-temporal dementia share certain symptoms, they cannot be treated with the same pharmacological agents because the cholinergic systems are not affected in the latter.

Lewy body dementia

This neurodegenerative disorder is clinically characterised by dementia and signs of Parkinson's disease. It is often inherited and mutations in the α-synuclein and β-synuclein genes have been identified in affected patients. These mutations result in accumulation of abnormal protein aggregates in neurons that contain the protein α-synuclein in association with other proteins, including ubiquitin (see Fig. 25.31, p. 1112). The cognitive state often fluctuates and there is a high incidence of visual hallucinations. Affected individuals are particularly sensitive to the side-effects of anti-parkinsonian medication and also to antipsychotic drugs. There is no curative treatment but anticholinesterase drugs can be helpful in slowing progression of cognitive impairment.

Alcohol misuse and dependence

Alcohol consumption associated with social, psychological and physical problems constitutes misuse. The criteria for alcohol dependence, a more restricted term, are shown in Box 28.21. Approximately one-quarter of male patients in general hospital medical wards in the UK have a current or previous alcohol problem.

Pathogenesis

Availability of alcohol and social patterns of use appear to be the most important factors. Genetic factors predispose to dependence. The majority of people who misuse alcohol do not have an associated psychiatric disorder, but a few drink heavily in an attempt to relieve anxiety or depression.

Clinical features

The modes of presentation of alcohol misuse and complications are summarised below.

Social problems

Common features include absenteeism from work, unemployment, marital tensions, child abuse, financial difficulties and problems with the law, such as violence and traffic offences.

Low mood

Low mood is common since alcohol has a direct depressant effect and heavy drinking creates numerous social problems. Attempted and completed suicide are associated with alcohol misuse.

| | 28.21 Criteria for alcohol dependence |

- Narrowing of the drinking repertoire
- Priority of drinking over other activities (salience)
- Tolerance of effects of alcohol
- Repeated withdrawal symptoms
- Relief of withdrawal symptoms by further drinking
- Subjective compulsion to drink
- Reinstatement of drinking behaviour after abstinence

Anxiety

People who are anxious may use alcohol as a means of relieving anxiety in the short term and this can develop into dependence. Conversely, alcohol withdrawal increases anxiety.

Alcohol withdrawal syndrome

The features are described in Box 28.22. Symptoms usually become maximal about 2–3 days after the last drink and can include seizures. The term 'delirium tremens' is used to describe severe alcohol withdrawal syndrome characterised by both delirium (characteristically, agitation and visual hallucinations) and physiological hyper-arousal (tremor, sweating and tachycardia). It has a significant mortality and morbidity (Box 28.22).

Hallucinations

Hallucinations (characteristically visual but sometimes in other modalities) are common in delirium tremens. Less common is the phenomenon called 'alcoholic hallucinosis', where a patient with alcohol dependence experiences auditory hallucination in clear consciousness at a time when they are not withdrawing from alcohol.

| | 28.22 Presentation and consequences of chronic alcohol misuse |

Acute intoxication

- Emotional and behavioural disturbance
- Medical problems: hypoglycaemia, ketoacidosis, aspiration of vomit, respiratory depression
- Accidents, injuries sustained in fights

Withdrawal phenomena

- Psychological symptoms: restlessness, anxiety, panic attacks
- Autonomic symptoms: tachycardia, sweating, pupil dilatation, nausea, vomiting
- Delirium: agitation, hallucinations (classically 'Lilliputian'), illusions, delusions
- Seizures

Consequences of harmful use

Medical

- Neurological: peripheral neuropathy, cerebellar degeneration, cerebral haemorrhage, dementia
- Hepatic: fatty change and cirrhosis, liver cancer
- Gastrointestinal: oesophagitis, gastritis, pancreatitis, oesophageal cancer, Mallory–Weiss syndrome, malabsorption, oesophageal varices
- Respiratory: pulmonary tuberculosis, pneumonia
- Skin: spider naevi, palmar erythema, Dupuytren's contractures, telangiectasias
- Cardiac: cardiomyopathy, hypertension
- Musculoskeletal: myopathy, fractures
- Endocrine and metabolic: pseudo-Cushing's syndrome, hypoglycaemia, gout
- Reproductive: hypogonadism, fetal alcohol syndrome, infertility

Psychiatric and cerebral

- Depression
- Alcoholic hallucinosis
- Alcoholic 'blackouts'
- Wernicke's encephalopathy: nystagmus or ophthalmoplegia with ataxia and delirium
- Korsakoff's syndrome: short-term memory deficits leading to confabulation

Wernicke–Korsakoff syndrome

This is a rare but important indirect complication of chronic alcohol misuse. It is an organic brain disorder resulting from damage to the mamillary bodies, dorsomedial nuclei of the thalamus and adjacent areas of periventricular grey matter caused by a deficiency of thiamin (vitamin B$_1$). The syndrome most commonly results from long-standing heavy drinking and an inadequate diet but can also arise from malabsorption or even protracted vomiting. Wernicke's encephalopathy (nystagmus or ophthalmoplegia with ataxia and delirium) often presents acutely and, without prompt treatment (see below), can progress and become irreversible. Korsakoff's syndrome (severe short-term memory deficits and confabulation) can develop chronically or acutely (with Wernicke's).

Alcohol-related brain damage

The term alcohol-related brain damage (ARBD) is often used as a collective description of the many brain pathologies associated with alcohol excess, which often coexist in the same patient. Acute alcohol intoxication causes ataxia, slurred speech, emotional incontinence and aggression. Very heavy drinkers may experience periods of amnesia for events that occurred during bouts of intoxication, termed 'alcoholic blackouts'. Established alcohol dependence may lead to 'alcoholic dementia', a global cognitive impairment resembling Alzheimer's disease, but which does not progress and may even improve if the patient becomes abstinent. Heavy alcohol use can damage the brain indirectly through Wernicke–Korsakoff syndrome (see above), head injury, hypoglycaemia and encephalopathy (p. 864).

Effects on other organs

These are protean and virtually any organ can be involved (Box 28.22). These effects are discussed in detail in other chapters in this book.

Diagnosis

The diagnosis of alcohol excess may emerge while taking the patient's history, but many patients do not tell the truth about their alcohol intake. Alcohol misuse may also present through its effects on one or more aspects of the patient's life, as listed above. Alcohol dependence commonly presents with withdrawal in those admitted to hospital, as they can no longer maintain their high alcohol intake in this setting.

Management

For the person misusing alcohol, provision of clear information from a doctor about the harmful effects of alcohol and safe levels of consumption is often all that is needed. In more serious cases, patients may have to be advised to alter leisure activities or change jobs to help them to reduce their consumption. Psychological treatment is used for people who have recurrent relapses and is usually available at specialised centres. Support to stop drinking is also provided by voluntary organisations, such as Alcoholics Anonymous (AA) in the UK.

Alcohol withdrawal syndromes can be prevented, or treated once established, with long-acting benzodiazepines. Large doses may be required (such as diazepam 20 mg 4 times daily), tailed off over a period of 5–7 days as symptoms subside. Prevention of the Wernicke–Korsakoff syndrome requires the immediate use of high doses of thiamin, which is initially given parenterally in the form of Pabrinex (two vials 3 times daily for 48 hrs, longer if symptoms persist) and then orally (100 mg 3 times daily). There is no treatment for Wernicke–Korsakoff syndrome once it has

arisen. The risk of side-effects, such as respiratory depression with benzodiazepines and anaphylaxis with Pabrinex, is small when weighed against the potential benefits of treatment.

Acamprosate (666 mg 3 times daily) may help to maintain abstinence by reducing the craving for alcohol. Disulfiram (200–400 mg daily) can be given as a deterrent to patients who have difficulty resisting the impulse to drink after becoming abstinent. It blocks the metabolism of alcohol, causing acetaldehyde to accumulate. When alcohol is consumed, an unpleasant reaction follows, with headache, flushing and nausea. Disulfiram is always an adjunct to other treatments, especially supportive psychotherapy. Treatment with antidepressants may be required if depression is severe or does not resolve with abstinence. Antipsychotics, such as chlorpromazine (100 mg 3 times daily), are needed for alcoholic hallucinosis. Although such treatment may be successful, there is a high relapse rate.

Prognosis

Between 80% and 90% of patients with established alcohol dependence syndrome who embark on medically supervised detoxification will successfully complete detoxification without encountering significant complications. Sustaining abstinence is more challenging than achieving it, however. Studies indicate that 1 year after successful detoxification, only 20% of patients will remain abstinent. This figure rises to approximately 30% for patients who are engaged with alcohol services, and to over 40% if such specialist support is combined with supervised disulfiram treatment.

Substance misuse disorder

Dependence on and misuse of both illegal and prescribed drugs is a major problem worldwide. Drugs of misuse are described in detail in Chapter 7. They can be grouped as follows.

Sedatives

These commonly give rise to physical dependence, the manifestations of which are tolerance and a withdrawal syndrome. Drugs include benzodiazepines, opiates (including morphine, heroin, methadone and dihydrocodeine) and barbiturates (now rarely prescribed). Overdosage with sedatives can be fatal, primarily as a result of respiratory depression (Ch. 7). Withdrawal from opiates is notoriously unpleasant, and withdrawal from benzodiazepines and barbiturates can cause prolonged anxiety and even hallucinations and/or seizures.

Intravenous opiate users are prone to bacterial infections, hepatitis B (p. 873), hepatitis C (p. 877) and HIV infection (Ch. 12) through needle contamination. Accidental overdose is common, mainly because of the varied and uncertain potency of illicit supplies of the drug. The withdrawal syndrome, which can start within 12 hours of last use, presents with intense craving, rhinorrhoea, lacrimation, yawning, perspiration, shivering, piloerection, vomiting, diarrhoea and abdominal cramps. Examination reveals tachycardia, hypertension, mydriasis and facial flushing.

Stimulants

Stimulant drugs include amphetamines and cocaine. They are less dangerous than the sedatives in overdose, although they can cause cardiac and cerebrovascular problems through their pressor effects. Physical dependence syndromes do not arise, but withdrawal causes a rebound lowering in mood and can give rise to an intense craving for further use, especially in any form

28

of drug with a rapid onset and offset of effect, such as crack cocaine. Chronic ingestion can cause a paranoid psychosis similar to schizophrenia. A 'toxic psychosis' (delirium) can occur with high levels of consumption. Unpleasant tactile hallucinations described as 'like ants crawling under the skin' (formication) may be prominent in either acute intoxication or withdrawal.

Hallucinogens

The hallucinogens are a disparate group of drugs that cause prominent sensory disturbances. They include cannabis, ecstasy, lysergic acid diethylamide (LSD), *Psilocybin* (magic mushrooms) and a variety of synthetic cannabinoids (as one of the so-called 'legal highs' or 'novel psychoactive substances'). A toxic confusional state can occur after heavy cannabis consumption. Acute psychotic episodes are well recognised, especially in those with a family or personal history of psychosis, and there is evidence that prolonged heavy use increases the risk of developing schizophrenia. Paranoid psychoses have been reported in association with ecstasy. A chronic psychosis has also been documented after regular LSD use.

Organic solvents

Solvent inhalation (glue sniffing) is popular in some adolescent groups. Solvents produce acute intoxication characterised by euphoria, excitement, dizziness and a floating sensation. Further inhalation leads to loss of consciousness; death can occur from the direct toxic effect of the solvent, or from asphyxiation if the substance is inhaled from a plastic bag.

Pathogenesis

Many of the causal factors for alcohol misuse also apply to substance misuse. The main factors are the psychological and behavioural vulnerabilities described above, cultural pressures, particularly within a peer group, and availability of a drug. In the case of some drugs such as opiates, medical over-prescribing has increased their availability, but there has also been a relative decline in the price of illegal drugs. Most drug users take a range of drugs – so-called polydrug misuse.

Diagnosis

As with alcohol, the diagnosis either may be apparent from the history and examination, or may be made only once the patient presents with a complication. Drug screening of samples of urine or blood can be valuable in confirming the diagnosis, especially if the patient persists in denial.

Management

The first step is to determine whether patients wish to stop using the drug. If they do not, they can still benefit from advice about how to minimise harm from their habit, such as how to obtain and use clean needles for those who inject. For those who are physically dependent on sedative drugs, substitute prescribing (using methadone, for example, in opiate dependence) may help stabilise their lives sufficiently to allow a gradual reduction in dosage until they reach abstinence. Some specialist units offer inpatient detoxification. For details of the medical management of overdose, see page 135. The drug lofexidine, a centrally acting α-agonist, can be useful in treating the autonomic symptoms of opiate withdrawal, as can clonidine, although this carries a risk of hypotension and is best used by specialists. Long-acting opiate antagonists, such as naltrexone, may also have a place, again in specialist hands, in blocking the euphoriant effects of the opiate, thereby reducing addiction.

In some cases, complete opiate withdrawal is not successful and the patient functions better if maintained on regular doses of oral methadone as an outpatient. This decision to prescribe long-term methadone should be taken only by a specialist, and carried out under long-term supervision at a specialist drug treatment centre.

Substitute prescribing is neither necessary nor possible for the hallucinogens and stimulants, but the principles of management are the same as those that should accompany prescribing for the sedatives. These include identifying problems associated with the drug misuse that may serve to maintain it, and intervening where possible. Intervention may be directed at physical illness, psychiatric comorbidity, social problems or family disharmony.

Relapsing patients and those with complications should be referred to specialist drug misuse services. Support can also be provided by self-help groups and voluntary bodies, such as Narcotics Anonymous (NA) in the UK.

Schizophrenia

Schizophrenia is characterised by delusions, hallucinations and lack of insight. Acute schizophrenia may also present with disturbed behaviour, disordered thinking, or with insidious social withdrawal and other so-called negative symptoms and less obvious delusions and hallucinations. Schizophrenia occurs worldwide in all ethnic groups with a prevalence of about 0.5%. It is more common in men (1.4 to 1). Children of an affected parent have an approximate 10% risk of developing the illness, but this rises to 50% if an identical twin is affected. The usual age of onset is the mid-twenties but can be older, particularly in women.

Pathogenesis

There is a strong genetic contribution, usually involving many susceptibility genes, each of small effect, but 2–3% of cases can be attributed to increased or decreased copies of genes (so-called 'copy number variations', p. 44). Environmental risk factors include a history of obstetric complications at the time of the patient's birth and urban upbringing. Brain imaging techniques have identified subtle structural abnormalities in groups of people with schizophrenia, including an overall decrease in brain size (by about 3% on average), with a relatively greater reduction in temporal lobe volume (5–10%). Episodes of acute schizophrenia may be precipitated by social stress and also by cannabis, which increases dopamine turnover. Consequently, schizophrenia is now viewed as a neurodevelopmental disorder, caused by abnormalities of brain development associated with genetic predisposition and early environmental influences, but precipitated by later triggers.

Clinical features

Acute schizophrenia should be suspected in any individual with bizarre behaviour accompanied by delusions and hallucinations that are not due to organic brain disease or substance misuse. The characteristic clinical features are listed in Box 28.23. Hallucinations are typically auditory but can occur in any sensory modality. They commonly involve voices from outside the head that talk to or about the person. Sometimes the voices repeat the person's thoughts. Patients may also describe 'passivity of thought', experienced as disturbances in the normal privacy of thinking, such as the delusional belief that their thoughts are being 'withdrawn' from them and perhaps 'broadcast' to others, and/or that alien thoughts are being 'inserted' into their mind.

i	**28.23 Symptoms of schizophrenia**

First-rank symptoms of acute schizophrenia

- A = Auditory hallucinations – second- or third-person/écho de la pensée
- B = Broadcasting, insertion/withdrawal of thoughts
- C = Controlled feelings, impulses or acts ('passivity' experiences/phenomena)
- D = Delusional perception (a particular experience is bizarrely interpreted)

Symptoms of chronic schizophrenia (negative symptoms)

- Flattened (blunted) affect
- Apathy and loss of drive (avolition)
- Social isolation/withdrawal (autism)
- Poverty of speech (alogia)
- Poor self-care

i	**28.24 Differential diagnosis of schizophrenia**	
Alternative diagnosis	**Distinguishing features**	

Other functional psychoses		
Delusional disorders	Absence of specific features of schizophrenia	
Psychotic depression	Prominent depressive symptoms	
Manic episode	Prominent manic symptoms	
Schizoaffective disorder	Mood and schizophrenia symptoms both prominent	
Puerperal psychosis	Acute onset after childbirth	
Organic disorders		
Drug-induced psychosis	Evidence of drug or alcohol misuse	
Side-effects of prescribed drugs	Levodopa, methyldopa, glucocorticoids, antimalarial drugs	
Temporal lobe epilepsy	Other evidence of seizures	
Delirium	Visual hallucinations, impaired consciousness	
Dementia	Age, established cognitive impairment	
Huntington's disease	Family history, choreiform movements, dementia	

Other characteristic symptoms are delusions of control: believing that one's emotions, impulses or acts are controlled by others. Another phenomenon is delusional perception, a delusion that arises suddenly alongside a normal perception, such as 'I saw the moon and I immediately knew he was evil.' Other, less common, symptoms may occur, including thought disorder, as manifest by incomprehensible speech, and abnormalities of movement, such as those in which the patient can become immobile or adopt awkward postures for prolonged periods (catatonia).

Diagnosis

The diagnosis is made primarily on clinical grounds but investigations may be required to rule out organic brain disease. The main differential diagnosis of schizophrenia (Box 28.24) includes:

- *Other functional psychoses*, particularly psychotic depression and mania, in which delusions and hallucinations are congruent with a marked mood disturbance (negative in depression and grandiose in mania). Schizophrenia must also be differentiated from specific delusional disorders that are not associated with the other typical features of schizophrenia.
- *Organic psychoses*, including delirium, in which there is impairment of consciousness and loss of orientation (not found in schizophrenia), typically with visual hallucinations; drug misuse, particularly in young people; and temporal lobe epilepsy with psychotic symptoms, in which olfactory and gustatory hallucinations may occur.

Many of those who experience acute schizophrenia go on to develop a chronic state in which the acute, so-called positive symptoms resolve, or at least do not dominate the clinical picture, leaving so-called negative symptoms that include blunt affect, apathy, social isolation, poverty of speech and poor self-care. Patients with chronic schizophrenia may also manifest positive symptoms, particularly when under stress, and it can be difficult for those who do not know the patient to judge whether or not these are signs of an acute relapse.

Investigations

As in dementia, investigations are focused on excluding a treatable cause, such as a slow-growing brain tumour, temporal lobe epilepsy, neurosyphilis or various autoimmune conditions. These are required only in patients with neurological or other organic symptoms or signs.

Management

First-episode schizophrenia usually requires admission to hospital because patients lack the insight that they are ill and are unwilling to accept treatment. In some cases, they may be at risk of harming themselves or others. Subsequent acute relapses and chronic schizophrenia are now usually managed in the community.

Drug treatment

Antipsychotic agents are effective against the positive symptoms of schizophrenia in the majority of cases. They take 2–4 weeks to be maximally effective but have some beneficial effects shortly after administration. Treatment is then ideally continued to prevent relapse. In a patient with a first episode of schizophrenia this will usually be for 1 or 2 years, but in patients with multiple episodes treatment may be required for many years. The benefits of prolonged treatment must be weighed against the adverse effects, which include extrapyramidal side-effects (EPSE) like acute dystonic reactions (which may require treatment with parenteral anticholinergics), akathisia and parkinsonism. For long-term use, antipsychotic agents are often given by slow-release (depot) injections to improve adherence.

A number of antipsychotic agents are available (Box 28.25). These may be divided into conventional (first-generation) drugs such as chlorpromazine and haloperidol, and novel or second-generation drugs such as olanzapine and clozapine. All work by blocking D_2 dopamine receptors in the brain. Patients who have not responded to conventional drugs may respond to newer agents, which are also less likely to produce unwanted EPSE but do tend to cause greater weight gain and metabolic disturbances, such as dyslipidaemia. Clozapine can be remarkably effective in those who do not respond to other antipsychotics but can cause agranulocytosis in about 1% of patients in the first few months. Prescription therefore requires regular monitoring of white blood cell count, initially on a weekly basis, then fortnightly and monthly thereafter. Clozapine should not be stopped suddenly because of the likelihood of relapse. Adverse effects of antipsychotic drugs are listed in Box 28.26. Two serious adverse effects deserve special mention.

Neuroleptic malignant syndrome This is a rare but serious condition characterised by fever, tremor and rigidity, autonomic instability

28

28.25 Antipsychotic drugs

Group	Drug	Usual adult dose[1]
Phenothiazines	Chlorpromazine	400–600 mg daily
Butyrophenones	Haloperidol	8–12 mg daily
Thioxanthenes	Flupentixol decanoate	40 mg fortnightly (depot injection)
Diphenylbutylpiperidines	Pimozide	8–10 mg daily
Substituted benzamides	Sulpiride	800–1200 mg daily
Dibenzodiazepines[2]	Clozapine	300–600 mg daily
Benzisoxazole[2]	Risperidone	4–6 mg daily
Thienobenzodiazepines[2]	Olanzapine	10–15 mg daily
Dibenzothiazepines[2]	Quetiapine	300–600 mg daily

[1]Lower or higher doses may be required in some patients. [2]Second-generation antipsychotics.

28.26 Adverse effects of antipsychotic drugs

Weight gain due to increased appetite

Effects due to dopamine blockade*
- Acute dystonia
- Akathisia (motor restlessness)
- Parkinsonism
- Tardive dyskinesia
- Gynaecomastia
- Galactorrhoea

Effects due to cholinergic blockade
- Dry mouth
- Blurred vision
- Impotence
- Constipation
- Urinary retention

Hypersensitivity reactions
- Blood dyscrasias (neutropenia with clozapine)
- Cholestatic jaundice
- Photosensitive dermatitis

Ocular complications
- Corneal and lens opacities (long-term use)

*Less severe with clozapine, quetiapine and olanzapine, possibly because of strong 5-hydroxytrytamine-blocking effect and relatively weak dopamine blockade.

and delirium. Characteristic laboratory findings are an elevated creatinine phosphokinase and leucocytosis. Antipsychotic medication must be stopped immediately and supportive therapy provided, often in an intensive care unit. Treatment includes ensuring hydration and reducing hyperthermia. Dantrolene sodium and bromocriptine may be helpful. Mortality is 20% untreated and 5% with treatment.

Cardiac arrhythmias Antipsychotic medications cause prolongation of the QTc interval, which may be associated with ventricular tachycardia, torsades de pointes and sudden death. If this occurs, treatment should be stopped, with careful electrocardiographic monitoring and treatment of serious arrhythmias if necessary (p. 479).

Psychological treatment

Psychological treatment, including general support for the patient and family, is now seen as an essential component of management. CBT may help patients to cope with symptoms. There is evidence that personal and/or family education, when given as part of an integrated treatment package, reduces the rate of relapse.

Social treatment

After an acute episode of schizophrenia has been controlled by drug therapy, social rehabilitation may be required. Recurrent illness is likely to cause disruption to patients' relationships and their ability to manage their accommodation and occupation; consequently, patients with schizophrenia often need help to obtain housing and employment. A graded return to employment and sometimes a period of supported accommodation are required.

Patients with chronic schizophrenia have particular difficulties and may need long-term, supervised accommodation. This now tends to be in supported accommodation in the community. Patients may also benefit from sheltered employment if they are unable to participate effectively in the labour market. Ongoing contact with a health worker allows monitoring for signs of relapse, sometimes as part of a multidisciplinary team working to agreed plans (the 'care programme approach'). Partly because of a tendency to inactivity, smoking and a poor diet, patients with chronic schizophrenia are at increased risk of cardiovascular disease, diabetes and stroke, and require proactive medical as well as psychiatric care.

Prognosis

About one-third of those who develop an acute schizophrenic episode have a good outcome. One-third develop chronic, incapacitating schizophrenia, and the remainder largely recover after each episode but suffer relapses. Most affected patients cannot work or live independently. Schizophrenia is associated with suicide and up to 10% of patients take their own lives.

Mood disorders

Mood or affective disorders include:
- *unipolar depression*: one or more episodes of low mood and associated symptoms
- *bipolar disorder*: episodes of elevated mood interspersed with episodes of depression
- *dysthymia*: chronic low-grade depressed mood without sufficient other symptoms to count as 'clinically significant' or 'major' depression.

Depression

Major depressive disorder has a prevalence of 5% in the general population and approximately 10–20% in chronically ill medical outpatients. It is a major cause of disability and suicide. If comorbid with a medical condition, depression magnifies disability, diminishes adherence to medical treatment and rehabilitation, and may even shorten life expectancy.

Pathogenesis

There is a genetic predisposition to depression, especially when of early onset. The genetic predisposition is mediated by variants in a large number of genes and loci of small effect rather than mutations in single genes. Adversity and emotional deprivation early in life also predispose to depression. Depressive episodes are often, but not always, triggered by stressful life events (especially those that involve loss or imposed change), including medical illnesses. Associated biological factors include hypofunction of monoamine neurotransmitter systems, including 5-HT and noradrenaline (norepinephrine), and abnormalities of the hypothalamic–pituitary–adrenal (HPA) axis, which results in elevated cortisol levels that do not suppress with dexamethasone.

Diagnosis

The symptoms are listed in Box 28.6. Depression may be mild, moderate or severe. It may also be recurrent or chronic. It can be both a complication of a medical condition and a cause of MUS (see below), so physical examination is essential; an associated medical condition should always be considered, particularly where there is no past history of depression and no apparent psychological precipitant.

Investigations

Investigations are not usually required unless there are clinical grounds for suspicion of an underlying medical disorder, such as Cushing's syndrome or hypothyroidism.

Management

Pharmacological and psychological treatments both work in depression. In practice, the choice is determined by patient preference and local availability. Severe depression complicated by psychotic symptoms, dehydration or suicide risk may require ECT.

Drug treatment

Antidepressant drugs are effective in moderate and severe depression, whether it is primary or secondary to a medical illness. The most suitable drug for an individual patient will depend on their previous response, likely side-effects, their concurrent illnesses and potential drug interactions. Commonly used antidepressants are shown in Box 28.27.

The different classes of antidepressant have similar efficacy and about three-quarters of patients respond to treatment. Successful treatment requires the patient to take an appropriate dose of an effective drug for an adequate period. For those who do not respond, a proportion will do so if changed to another class of antidepressant. The patient's progress must be monitored and, after recovery, treatment should be continued for at least 6–12 months to reduce the high risk of relapse. The dose should then be tapered off over several weeks to avoid discontinuation symptoms. The Scottish Intercollegiate Guidelines Network (SIGN) and National Institute for Health and Clinical Excellence (NICE) have published treatment guidelines.

Tricyclic antidepressants Tricyclic antidepressant (TCA) agents inhibit re-uptake of the amines noradrenaline (norepinephrine) and 5-HT at synaptic clefts. The therapeutic effect is noticeable within a week or two. Adverse effects, such as sedation, anticholinergic effects, postural hypotension, lowering of the seizure threshold and cardiotoxicity, can be troublesome during this period. TCAs may be dangerous in overdose and should be used with caution in people who have coexisting heart disease, glaucoma and prostatism.

Selective serotonin re-uptake inhibitors Selective serotonin reuptake inhibitors (SSRIs) are less cardiotoxic and less sedative than TCAs, and have fewer anticholinergic effects. They are safer in overdose but can still cause QTc prolongation, headache, nausea, anorexia and sexual dysfunction. They can also interact with other drugs increasing serotonin (5-HT), to produce 'serotonin syndrome'. This is a rare syndrome of neuromuscular hyperactivity, autonomic hyperactivity and agitation, and potentially seizures, hyperthermia, delirium and even death.

Noradrenaline (norepinephrine) re-uptake inhibitors These agents inhibit noradrenaline uptake at the synaptic cleft but have additional pharmacological effects. Venlafaxine and duloxetine also act as serotonin re-uptake inhibitors, whereas mirtazapine also acts as an antagonist at 5-HT2a, 5-HT2c and 5-HT3 receptors. These drugs have similar efficacy to the agents listed above but a different adverse-effect profile.

Monoamine oxidase inhibitors Monoamine oxidase inhibitors (MAOIs) increase the availability of neurotransmitters at synaptic clefts by inhibiting metabolism of noradrenaline (norepinephrine) and 5-HT. They are now rarely prescribed in the UK, since they can cause potentially dangerous interactions with drugs such as amphetamines and certain anaesthetic agents, and with foods rich in tyramine (such as cheese and red wine). This is due to accumulation of amines in the systemic circulation, causing a potentially fatal hypertensive crisis.

Psychological treatment

Both CBT and interpersonal therapy are as effective as antidepressants for mild to moderate depression. Antidepressant drugs are, however, preferred for severe depression. Drug and psychological treatments can be used in combination.

Prognosis

Over 50% of people who have had one depressive episode and over 90% of people who have had three or more episodes will have another. The risk of suicide in an individual who has had a depressive disorder is 10 times greater than in the general population.

Bipolar disorder

Bipolar disorder is an episodic disturbance with interspersed periods of depressed and elevated mood; the latter is known

i	**28.27 Antidepressant drugs**	
Group	**Drug**	**Usual adult dose***
Tricyclic antidepressants	Amitriptyline Imipramine Dosulepin Clomipramine	75–150 mg daily 75–150 mg daily 75–150 mg daily 75–150 mg daily
Selective serotonin re-uptake inhibitors (SSRIs)	Citalopram Escitalopram Fluoxetine Sertraline Paroxetine	20–40 mg daily 10–20 mg daily 20–60 mg daily 50–100 mg daily 20–50 mg daily
Monoamine oxidase inhibitors	Phenelzine Tranylcypromine Moclobemide	45–90 mg daily 20–40 mg daily 300–600 mg daily
Noradrenaline (norepinephrine) re-uptake inhibitors and SSRIs	Venlafaxine Duloxetine	75–375 mg daily 60–120 mg daily
Noradrenaline and specific serotonergic inhibitor	Mirtazapine	15–45 mg daily

*Higher doses may be required in some patients: see guidelines.

as hypomania when mild or short-lived, or mania when severe or chronic. The lifetime risk of developing bipolar disorder is approximately 1–2%. Onset is usually in the twenties, and men and women are equally affected.

Pathogenesis

Bipolar disorder is strongly heritable (approximately 70%). Relatives of patients have an increased incidence of both bipolar and unipolar affective disorder. A number of genetic variants of small effect have been identified by genome-wide association studies. Life events, such as physical illness, sleep deprivation and medication, may also play a role in triggering episodes.

Diagnosis

The diagnosis is based on clear evidence of episodes of depression and mania. Isolated episodes of hypomania or mania do occur but they are usually preceded or followed by an episode of depression. Psychotic symptoms may occur in both the depressive and the manic phases, with delusions and hallucinations that are usually in keeping with the mood disturbance. This is described as an affective psychosis. Patients who present with symptoms of both bipolar disorder and schizophrenia in equal measure may be given a diagnosis of schizoaffective disorder.

Management

Depression should be treated as described above. If antidepressants are prescribed, however, they should be combined with a mood-stabilising drug (see below) to avoid 'switching' the patients into (hypo)mania. Manic episodes and psychotic symptoms usually respond well to antipsychotic drugs (see Box 28.25).

Prophylaxis to prevent recurrent episodes of depression and mania with mood-stabilising agents is important. The main drugs used are lithium and sodium valproate but lamotrigine, olanzapine, quetiapine and risperidone are increasingly employed. Caution must be exercised when stopping these drugs, as a relapse may follow.

Lithium carbonate is the drug of first choice. It is also used for acute mania, and in combination with a tricyclic as an adjuvant treatment for resistant depression. It has a narrow therapeutic range, so regular blood monitoring is required to maintain a serum level of 0.5–1.0 mmol/L. Toxic effects include nausea, vomiting, tremor and convulsions. With long-term treatment, weight gain, hypothyroidism, increased calcium and parathyroid hormone (PTH), nephrogenic diabetes insipidus (p. 687) and renal failure can occur. Thyroid and renal function should be checked before treatment is started and regularly thereafter. Lithium may be teratogenic and should not be prescribed during the first trimester of pregnancy.

Anticonvulsants, such as sodium valproate and lamotrigine, and the antipsychotic drug olanzapine can all be used as prophylaxis in bipolar disorder, usually as a second-line alternative to lithium. Valproate conveys a high risk of birth defects and should not be used in women of child-bearing age. Olanzapine can cause significant weight gain. (For a list of the adverse effects of antipsychotic drugs, see Box 28.26.)

Prognosis

The relapse rate of bipolar disorder is high, although patients may be perfectly well between episodes. After one episode, the annual average risk of relapse is about 10–15%, which doubles after more than three episodes. There is a substantially increased lifetime risk of suicide of 5–10%.

Anxiety disorders

These are characterised by the emotion of anxiety, worrisome thoughts, avoidance behaviours and the somatic symptoms of autonomic arousal. Anxiety disorders are divided into three main subtypes: phobic, paroxysmal (panic) and generalised (Box 28.28). The nature and prominence of the somatic symptoms often lead the patient to present initially to medical services. Anxiety may be stress-related and phobic anxiety may follow an unpleasant incident. Many patients with anxiety also have depression.

Clinical features

Phobic anxiety disorder

A phobia is an abnormal or excessive fear of a specific object or situation, which leads to avoidance of it (such as excessive fear of dying in an air crash, leading to avoidance of flying). A generalised phobia of going out alone or being in crowded places is called 'agoraphobia'. Phobic responses can develop to medical procedures such as venepuncture.

Panic disorder

Panic disorder describes repeated attacks of severe anxiety, which are not restricted to any particular situation or circumstances. Somatic symptoms, such as chest pain, palpitations and paraesthesia in lips and fingers, are common. The symptoms are in part due to involuntary over-breathing (hyperventilation). Patients with panic attacks often fear that they are suffering from a serious illness, such as a heart attack or stroke, and seek emergency medical attention. Panic disorder may coexist with agoraphobia.

Generalised anxiety disorder

This is a chronic anxiety state associated with uncontrollable worry. The associated somatic symptoms of muscle tension and bowel disturbance often lead to a medical presentation.

Diagnosis

The diagnosis is made on the basis of clinical history and typical symptoms, as described above. Where a diagnosis of panic disorder is suspected, it can be confirmed by asking the patient to hyperventilate deliberately for 1–2 minutes and observing whether the symptoms are reproduced. A finding of respiratory alkalosis on arterial blood gas measurement is indicative of chronic hyperventilation.

Management

Psychological treatment

Explanation and reassurance are essential, especially when patients fear they have a serious medical condition. Specific

i	**28.28 Classification of anxiety disorders**		
	Phobic anxiety disorder	Panic disorder	Generalised anxiety disorder
Occurrence	Situational	Paroxysmal	Persistent
Behaviour	Avoidance	Escape	Agitation
Cognitions	Fear of situation	Fear of symptoms	Worry
Symptoms	On exposure	Episodic	Persistent

treatment may be needed. Treatments include relaxation, graded exposure (desensitisation) to feared situations for phobic disorders, and CBT.

Drug treatment

Antidepressants are the drugs of first choice (p. 1199). The therapeutic dose is usually higher for anxiety disorders than for depression and there is some evidence that, within their respective classes, paroxetine (SSRI) and clomipramine (TCA) have greatest efficacy against anxiety disorders. Early side-effects of antidepressants can lead to a worsening of anxiety symptoms in the first 2 weeks and patients should be warned of this.

Benzodiazepines are useful in the short term but regular (>3 doses per week) long-term use carries a very high risk of dependence. Regular prescriptions should therefore be limited to 3 weeks; beyond that, prescriptions should be restricted to occasional use as required, with periodic review to guard against dose escalation. Short-acting benzodiazepines, such as lorazepam, have a rapid onset and provide symptomatic relief for up to 2 hours but have the greatest potential for dependence. Longer-acting drugs, such as diazepam, can take an hour to take effect when given orally but provide symptomatic relief for up to 12 hours. A β-blocker, such as propranolol, can help when somatic symptoms are prominent.

Obsessive–compulsive disorder

Obsessive–compulsive disorder (OCD) is characterised by 'obsessions' – thoughts, images or impulses that are recurrent, unwanted and usually anxiety-provoking, but recognised as one's own. In many cases, the obsessions give rise to 'compulsions', which are repeated acts performed to relieve the anxiety. Unlike the anxiety disorders discussed above, which are more common in women, OCD is equally common in men and women.

Clinical features

Common examples include thoughts of contamination, giving rise to repeated and ritualised hand-washing, and thoughts of having forgotten something, giving rise to time-consuming repeated checking. The differential diagnoses include normal checking behaviour and delusional beliefs about thought possession.

Diagnosis

The diagnosis is made on the basis of the typical history, as described above.

Management

OCD usually responds to some degree to antidepressant drugs (high-dose clomipramine or SSRI; see Box 28.27) and to 'exposure response prevention' – a form of CBT in which patients are encouraged to expose themselves to the feared thought or situation without performing the anxiety-relieving compulsions. Relapses are common, however, and the condition often becomes chronic.

Stress-related disorders

Acute stress reaction

Following a stressful event, such as a serious medical diagnosis or a major accident, some people develop a characteristic pattern of symptoms: an initial state of 'daze' or bewilderment is followed by altered activity (withdrawal or agitation), often with anxiety.

The symptoms are transient and usually resolve completely within a few days. The lay media often describes this as 'shock'.

Adjustment disorder

A more common psychological response to a major stressor is a less severe but more prolonged emotional reaction.

Clinical features

The predominant symptom is usually depression and/or anxiety, which is insufficiently persistent or intense to merit a diagnosis of depressive or anxiety disorder. There may also be anger, aggressive behaviour and associated excessive alcohol use. Symptoms develop within a month of the onset of the stress, and their duration and severity reflect the course of the underlying stressor. Grief reactions following bereavement are a particular type of adjustment disorder. They manifest as a brief period of emotional numbing, followed by a period of distress lasting several weeks, during which sorrow, tearfulness, sleep disturbance, a sense of futility, anger and 'bargaining' are common. Perceptual distortions may occur, including misinterpreting sounds as the dead person's voice or 'seeing' the dead person. 'Pathological grief' describes a grief reaction that is abnormally intense or persistent.

Diagnosis

The diagnosis is made on the basis of the typical history following a stressful life event, as described above.

Management

Ongoing contact with and support from a doctor or another person who can listen, reassure, explain and advise are often all that is needed. Most patients do not require psychotropic medication, although benzodiazepines reduce arousal in acute stress reactions and can aid sleep in adjustment disorders.

Post-traumatic stress disorder

Post-traumatic stress disorder (PTSD) is a delayed and/or protracted response to a stressful event of an exceptionally threatening or catastrophic nature. Examples of such events include natural disasters, terrorist activity, serious accidents and witnessing violent deaths. PTSD may also sometimes occur after distressing medical treatments or intensive care.

Clinical features

The development of PTSD is usually delayed from a few days to several months between the traumatic event and the onset of symptoms. Typical symptoms are recurrent intrusive memories (flashbacks) of the trauma; sleep disturbance, especially nightmares (usually of the traumatic event) from which the patient awakes in a state of anxiety; symptoms of autonomic arousal (anxiety, palpitations, enhanced startle); emotional blunting; and avoidance of situations that evoke memories of the trauma. Anxiety and depression are often associated and excessive use of alcohol or drugs frequently complicates the clinical picture.

Diagnosis

The diagnosis is made on the basis of the typical clinical features following a traumatic life event.

Management

In the immediate aftermath of a significant trauma, the main aim is to provide support, direct advice and the opportunity

28

for emotional catharsis (debriefing may actually be harmful). In established PTSD, structured psychological approaches (CBT, eye movement desensitisation and reprocessing (EMDR), and stress management) are effective. Antidepressant drugs are moderately effective.

Prognosis

The condition runs a fluctuating course, with most patients recovering within 2 years. In a small proportion, the symptoms become chronic.

Somatoform disorders

The essential feature of these disorders is that the somatic symptoms are not explained by a medical condition (medically unexplained symptoms), nor better diagnosed as part of a depressive or anxiety disorder. The derivation of the term 'somatoform' is 'body-like'. Several syndromes are described within this category; there is considerable overlap between them, both in the underlying causes and in the clinical presentation.

Pathogenesis

The cause of somatoform disorders is incompletely understood but contributory factors include depression and anxiety, the erroneous interpretation of somatic symptoms as evidence of disease, excessive concern with physical illness and a tendency to seek medical care. A family history or previous history of a particular condition may have shaped the patient's beliefs about illness. Doctors may exacerbate the problem, either by dismissing the complaints as non-existent or by over-emphasising and investigating the possibility of disease.

Clinical features

Somatoform disorders can present in several different ways, as described below.

Somatoform autonomic dysfunction

This describes somatic symptoms referable to bodily organs that are largely under the control of the autonomic nervous system. The most common examples involve the cardiovascular system ('cardiac neurosis'), respiratory system ('psychogenic hyperventilation') and gut ('psychogenic vomiting' and 'irritable bowel syndrome'). Antidepressant drugs and CBT may be helpful.

Somatoform pain disorder

This describes severe, persistent pain that cannot be adequately explained by a medical condition. Antidepressant drugs (especially tricyclics and dual action drugs such as duloxetine) are helpful, as are some of the anticonvulsant drugs, particularly carbamazepine, gabapentin and pregabalin. CBT and multidisciplinary pain management teams are also useful.

Chronic fatigue syndrome

Chronic fatigue syndrome (CFS) is characterised by excessive fatigue after minimal physical or mental exertion, poor concentration, dizziness, muscular aches and sleep disturbance. This pattern of symptoms may follow a viral infection such as infectious mononucleosis, influenza or hepatitis. Symptoms overlap with those of depression and anxiety. There is good evidence that many patients improve with carefully graded exercise and with CBT, as long as the benefits of such treatment are carefully explained.

i	**28.29 Common presentations of dissociative (conversion) disorder**

- Gait disturbance
- Loss of function in limbs
- Aphonia
- Non-epileptic seizures
- Sensory loss
- Blindness

Dissociative conversion disorders

Dissociative conversion disorders are characterised by a loss or distortion of neurological functioning that is not fully explained by organic disease. These may be psychological functions such as memory ('dissociative amnesia'), sensory functions such as vision ('dissociative blindness'), or motor functions ('functional gait disorder') (Box 28.29). The cause is unknown but there is an association with recent stress and with adverse childhood experiences, including physical and sexual abuse. Organic disease may precipitate dissociation and provide a model for symptoms. For example, non-epileptic seizures often occur in those with epilepsy. Treatment with CBT may be of benefit.

Somatisation disorder

This is defined as the occurrence of multiple medically unexplained physical symptoms affecting several bodily systems. It is also known as Briquet's syndrome after the physician who first described the presentation. Symptoms often start in early adult life but somatisation disorder can arise later, usually following an episode of physical illness. The disorder is much more common in women. Patients may undergo a multitude of negative investigations and unhelpful operations, particularly hysterectomy and cholecystectomy. There is no proven treatment except to try to ensure that unnecessary investigations and surgical procedures are avoided to minimise iatrogenic harm.

Hypochondriacal disorder

Patients with this condition have a strong fear or belief that they have a serious, often fatal, disease (such as cancer), and that fear persists despite appropriate medical reassurance. They are typically highly anxious and seek many medical opinions and investigations in futile but repeated attempts to relieve their fears.

Hypochondriacal disorder often resembles OCD, but in a small proportion of cases the conviction that disease is present reaches delusional intensity. The best-known example is that of parasitic infestation ('delusional parasitosis'), which leads patients to consult dermatologists. Treatment with CBT can be helpful. Patients who suffer delusions may benefit from antipsychotic medication. The condition may become chronic.

Body dysmorphic disorder

This is defined as a preoccupation with bodily shape or appearance, with the belief that one is disfigured in some way (previously known as 'dysmorphophobia'). People with this condition may make inappropriate requests for cosmetic surgery. Treatment with CBT or antidepressants may be helpful. The belief in disfigurement may sometimes be delusional, in which case antipsychotic drugs can help.

Management

The management of the various syndromes of medically unexplained complaints described above is based on the general principles outlined in Box 28.30 and discussed in more detail below.

28.30 General management principles for medically unexplained symptoms

- Take a full sympathetic history
- Exclude disease but avoid unnecessary investigation or referral
- Seek specific treatable psychiatric syndromes
- Demonstrate to patients that you believe their complaints
- Establish a collaborative relationship
- Give a positive explanation for the symptoms, including but not over-emphasising psychological factors
- Encourage a return to normal functioning

Reassurance

Patients should be asked what they are most worried about. Clearly, it may be unwise to state categorically that the patient does not have any disease, as that is difficult to establish with certainty. However, it can be emphasised that the probability of having a disease is low and that doctors often see patients with physical symptoms but no physical disease. If patients repeatedly ask for reassurance about the same health concern despite reassurance, they may have hypochondriasis.

Explanation

Patients need a positive explanation for their symptoms. It is unhelpful to say that symptoms are psychological or 'all in the mind'. Rather, a term such as 'functional' (meaning that the symptoms represent a reversible disturbance of bodily function) may be more acceptable. When possible, it is useful to describe a plausible physiological mechanism that is linked to psychological factors such as stress and implies that the symptoms are reversible. For example, in irritable bowel syndrome, psychological stress results in increased activation of the autonomic nervous system, which leads to constriction of smooth muscle in the gut wall, which in turn causes pain and bowel disturbance.

Advice

This should focus on how to overcome factors perpetuating the symptoms: for example, by resolving stressful social problems or by practising relaxation. The doctor can offer to review progress, to prescribe (for example) an antidepressant drug and, if appropriate, to refer for physiotherapy or psychological treatments such as CBT. The attitudes of relatives may need to be addressed if they have adopted an over-protective role, unwittingly reinforcing the patient's disability.

Drug treatment

Antidepressant drugs are often helpful, even if the patient is not depressed.

Psychological treatment

There is evidence for the effectiveness of CBT. Other psychological treatments such as IPT may also have a role.

Rehabilitation

Where there is chronic disability, particularly in dissociative (conversion) disorder, conventional physical rehabilitation may be the best approach.

Shared care

Ongoing planned care is required for patients with chronic intractable symptoms, especially those of somatisation disorder. Review by the same specialist, interspersed with visits to the same GP, is probably the best way to avoid unnecessary multiple re-referral for investigation, to ensure that treatable aspects of the patient's problems, such as depression, are actively managed and to prevent the GP from becoming demoralised.

Eating disorders

There are two well-defined eating disorders, anorexia nervosa (AN) and bulimia nervosa (BN); they share some overlapping features. Ninety per cent of people affected are female. There is a much higher prevalence of abnormal eating behaviour in the population that does not meet diagnostic criteria for AN or BN but may attract a diagnostic label such as 'binge eating disorder'. In developed societies, obesity is arguably a much greater problem but is usually considered to be more a disorder of lifestyle or physiology than a psychiatric disorder.

Anorexia nervosa

The lifetime risk of anorexia nervosa for women living in Europe is approximately 1–2% (for men it is <0.5%) with a peak age of onset of 15–19 years. Predisposing factors include familiality (both genetic and shared environmental factors appear to play a role) and 'neurotic' personality traits. The illness is often precipitated by weight loss, whether due to non-pathological dieting/increased exercise or physical illness such as gastrointestinal disorders or diabetes mellitus. Many sufferers do not engage with specialist services and it is not uncommon for the first presentation to be with a medical problem (Box 28.31) rather than to psychiatric services.

Clinical features

There is marked weight loss, arising from food avoidance, often in combination with bingeing, purging, excessive exercise and/or the use of diuretics and laxatives. Body image is profoundly disturbed so that, despite emaciation, patients still feel overweight and are terrified of weight gain. These preoccupations are intense and pervasive, and the false beliefs may be held with a conviction approaching the delusional. Anxiety and depressive symptoms are common accompaniments. Downy hair (lanugo) may develop on the back, forearms and cheeks. Extreme starvation is associated with a wide range of physiological and pathological bodily changes. All organ systems may be affected, although the most serious problems are cardiac and skeletal (Box 28.31).

Pathogenesis

The underlying cause is unclear but probably includes personality (high neuroticism), genetic (twin studies indicate heritability of 0.3–0.5) and environmental factors, including, in many societies, the social pressure on women to be thin.

Diagnosis

Diagnostic criteria are shown in Box 28.32. Differential diagnosis is from other causes of weight loss, including psychiatric disorders such as depression, and medical conditions such as inflammatory bowel disease, malabsorption, hypopituitarism and cancer, although it is important to remember that AN can coexist with any of these. The diagnosis is based on a pronounced fear of fatness despite being thin, and on the absence of an adequate alternative explanation for weight loss.

Management

The aims of management are to ensure patients' physical well-being while helping them to gain weight by addressing the

28

28.31 Medical consequences of eating disorders

Cardiac

- ECG abnormalities: T-wave inversion, ST depression and prolonged QTc interval
- Arrhythmias, including profound sinus bradycardia and ventricular tachycardia

Haematological

- Anaemia, thrombocytopenia and leucopenia

Endocrine

- Pubertal delay or arrest
- Growth retardation and short stature
- Amenorrhoea
- Sick euthyroid state

Metabolic

- Uraemia
- Renal calculi
- Osteoporosis

Gastrointestinal

- Constipation
- Abnormal liver function tests

28.32 Diagnostic criteria for eating disorders

Anorexia nervosa

- Weight loss of at least 15% of total body weight (or body mass index ≤17.5)
- Avoidance of high-calorie foods
- Distortion of body image so that patients regard themselves as fat even when grossly underweight
- Amenorrhoea for at least 3 months

Bulimia nervosa

- Recurrent bouts of binge eating
- Lack of self-control over eating during binges
- Self-induced vomiting, purgation or dieting after binges
- Weight maintained within normal limits

beliefs and behaviours that maintain the low weight. Treatment is usually given on an outpatient basis. Inpatient treatment should be reserved for those at risk of death from medical complications or from suicide. There is a limited evidence base for CBT-based psychological treatments. Family behaviour therapy (FBT) has efficacy among adolescent but not adult patients. Psychotropic drugs are of no proven benefit in AN but antidepressant medication may be indicated in those with clear-cut comorbid depressive disorder.

Weight gain is best achieved in a collaborative fashion. Compulsory admission and refeeding (including tube feeding) are very occasionally resorted to when patients are at risk of death and other measures have failed. While this may produce a short-term improvement in weight, it rarely changes long-term prognosis.

Prognosis

Two-thirds of patients with AN no longer meet diagnostic criteria at 5-year follow-up. However, long-term follow-up studies suggest that many sufferers continue to have a relatively low body mass index (BMI), suggesting that the symptoms do not completely resolve. Approximately 20% of patients develop a chronic, intractable disorder. Long-term follow-up studies demonstrate

that minimum lifetime BMI is the strongest prognostic indicator (BMI < 11.5 is associated with an standardised mortality ratio of 4–5). Other indicators of poor prognosis are comorbid BN and atypical demographics (very early or relatively late onset, male gender). Forty per cent of additional deaths are due to suicide, the remainder being due to complications of starvation.

Bulimia nervosa

The prevalence of BN is difficult to determine with precision, as only a small proportion of sufferers come to medical attention. It is believed to be more common than AN, with a similar gender ratio. Peak age of onset is slightly later than for AN, typically late adolescence or early adult life.

Clinical features

Patients with BN are usually at or near normal weight (unlike in AN), but display a morbid fear of fatness associated with disordered eating behaviour. They recurrently embark on eating binges, often followed by corrective measures such as self-induced vomiting.

Diagnosis

Diagnostic criteria are shown in Box 28.32. Physical signs of repeated self-induced vomiting include pitted teeth (from gastric acid), calluses on knuckles ('Russell's sign') and parotid gland enlargement. There are many associated physical complications, including the dental and oesophageal consequences of repeated vomiting, as well as electrolyte abnormalities, cardiac arrhythmias and renal problems (see Box 28.31).

Investigations

Self-induced vomiting and/or abuse of laxatives and diuretics can lead to clinically significant electrolyte disturbances, including hypokalaemia leading to cardiac arrhythmias. Hence it is good practice to measure urea and electrolytes and obtain an ECG whenever these behaviours are prominent in any patient and when BN is suspected in any medical inpatient. Repeated vomiting can also give rise to Mallory–Weiss tears and even oesophageal rupture; if symptoms are suggestive of these, an endoscopy should be performed.

Management

Treatment of bulimia with CBT achieves both short-term and long-term improvements. Guided self-help and IPT may also be of value. There is also evidence for benefit from the SSRI fluoxetine, but high doses of up to 60 mg daily may be required for a prolonged period of up to 1 year; this appears to be independent of the antidepressant effect.

Prognosis

Bulimia is not associated with increased mortality but a proportion of sufferers go on to develop anorexia. At 10-year follow-up, approximately 10% are still unwell, 20% have a subclinical degree of bulimia, and the remainder have recovered.

Personality disorders

Personality refers to the set of characteristics and behavioural traits that best describes an individual's patterns of interaction with the world. The intensity of particular traits varies from person to person, although certain ones, such as shyness or irritability, are displayed to some degree by most people. A personality disorder (PD) is diagnosed when an individual's personality causes persistent and severe problems for the person or for others.

Pathogenesis

Some PDs appear to have an inherited aspect (especially schizotypal and paranoid subtypes) but most are more clearly related to an unsatisfactory upbringing and adverse childhood experiences.

Clinical features

PD can present in various ways. For example, anxiety may be so pronounced that the individual rarely ventures into any situation where they fear scrutiny. Dissocial traits, such as disregard for the well-being of others and a lack of guilt concerning the adverse effects of one's actions on others, may occur. If pronounced, they may lead to damage to others, to criminal acts or to successful careers, such as in politics.

Diagnosis

It is possible to classify PD into several subtypes (such as emotionally unstable, antisocial or dependent), depending on the particular behavioural traits in question. A patient who meets diagnostic criteria for one subtype may also meet criteria for others. As allocation to one particular subtype gives little guidance to management or prognosis, classification is of limited value. Diagnosis requires a longitudinal perspective, with clear evidence that the patient's behavioural traits and pattern of interaction with the world have been present throughout their adult life, have been evident across a range of settings and have caused repeated and persistent problems. It can be difficult to achieve this during a single interview, and most psychiatrists warn against making a diagnosis of personality disorder until the patient has been seen several times and corroborative accounts have been obtained. It is common for PD to accompany other psychiatric conditions, making treatment of the latter more difficult and therefore affecting their prognosis.

Management

PDs usually persist throughout life and are not readily treated. They typically become less extreme with age but can re-emerge in the context of cognitive decline. Treatment options are limited but there is some evidence that emotionally unstable PD may respond to dialectical behavioural therapy (DBT). Anxious (avoidant) and obsessional (anankastic) PD may benefit from prescription of anxiolytic drugs, while paranoid/schizotypal PD may be improved by treatment with low doses of antipsychotic agents.

The problematic and inflexible patterns of interaction that characterise a PD are often apparent in the patient's interaction with health services and can present a challenge to both the service and the patient. Clear clinical communication supported by robust documentation can help to minimise any potential disruption.

Factitious disorder and malingering

Factitious disorder describes the repeated and deliberate production of the signs or symptoms of disease to obtain medical care.

Pathogenesis

It is difficult to understand what motivates a person to act in this way. Several theories have been proposed but the deception that lies at the heart of the condition makes it impossible to gather accurate data from which to draw reliable conclusions.

Clinical features

The disorder feigned is usually medical but can be a psychiatric illness (for example false reports of hallucinations or symptoms of depression). An example of a medical factitious disorder is dipping of a thermometer into a hot drink to fake a fever. Factitious disorder is uncommon and is important to distinguish from somatoform disorders. A suggested diagnostic algorithm is shown in Figure 28.6.

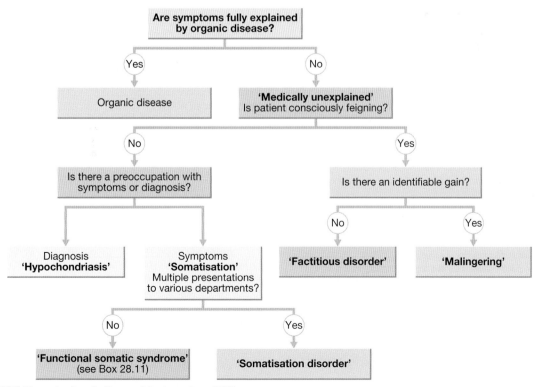

Fig. 28.6 Diagnosis of medically unexplained symptoms (MUS).

Münchausen's syndrome

This refers to a severe chronic form of factitious disorder. Patients characteristically travel widely, sometimes visiting several hospitals in one day. Although the condition is rare, such patients are memorable because they present so dramatically. The history can be convincing enough to persuade doctors to undertake investigations or initiate treatment, including exploratory surgery. It may be possible to trace the patient's history and show that they have presented similarly elsewhere, often changing name several times. Some emergency departments hold lists of such patients.

Malingering

Malingering is a description of behaviour, not a psychiatric diagnosis. It refers to the deliberate and conscious simulation of signs of disease and disability for an identifiable gain (patients have motives that are clear to them but which they initially conceal from doctors). Examples include the avoidance of burdensome responsibilities (such as work or court appearances) or the pursuit of financial gain (fraudulent claims for benefits or compensation). Malingering can be hard to detect at clinical assessment but is suggested by evasion or inconsistency in the history.

Management

Management is by gentle but firm confrontation with clear evidence of the fabrication of illness, together with an offer of psychological support. Treatment is usually declined but recognition of the condition may help to avoid further iatrogenic harm.

Puerperal psychiatric disorders

There are three important psychiatric presentations following childbirth. When managing these conditions, it is important always to consider both the mother and the baby, and their relationship (Box 28.33).

Post-partum blues

This is characterised by irritability, labile mood and tearfulness. About 80% of women are affected to some degree. Symptoms begin soon after childbirth, typically peak on about the fourth day and then resolve spontaneously within a few weeks. While the aetiology of baby blues is not fully understood, it is likely to be related to hormonal or physiological changes associated with childbirth. No treatment is required, other than to reassure the

mother and to remain vigilant for development of post-partum depression.

Post-partum depression

This occurs in 10–15% of women, with onset typically within a month of delivery (although women often suffer for some time before presenting). It can usually be differentiated from post-partum blues by the duration and severity of the symptoms, in particular anhedonia (loss of capacity for pleasure) and negative thoughts. Risk factors include a previous history of depression, a previous history of post-partum depression, antenatal depression and antenatal anxiety. Unlike depression arising at other times, post-partum depression is not more common in lower socioeconomic groups; the prevalence is similar across all social backgrounds. Diagnosis, explanation and reassurance are important. The usual psychological and drug treatments for depression should be considered (p. 1199) to minimise the impact on the mother and child at what is a very important time for both. A number of helpful guidelines are available to inform prescribing decisions. The potential risks to both mother and child should be considered and, if hospital admission is required, it should ideally be to a mother and baby unit.

Puerperal psychosis

This has its peak onset in the first 2 weeks after childbirth but can arise several weeks later. It is a rare but serious complication affecting approximately 1 in 500 women. There is a strong association with a personal or familial history of bipolar disorder. It usually takes the form of a manic or depressive psychosis but with sudden onset and fluctuation in severity. Delirium is rare with modern obstetric management but should still be considered in the differential diagnosis. Suspiciousness, concealment and impulsivity are common features of puerperal psychosis; hence the risks to both mother and baby are considerable. The clinical priority is to ensure the safety of both mother and baby and so psychiatric admission, ideally to a psychiatric mother and baby unit, is usually necessary. Pharmacological treatment reflects the clinical picture; antipsychotic medication is almost always indicated, augmented by antidepressants if the picture is of psychotic depression and/or by mood stabilisers if the picture is bipolar. Most women recover but the risk of recurrence following subsequent deliveries is 50% and some women will progress to psychotic episodes not associated with childbirth, usually bipolar disorder.

Psychiatric disorders during pregnancy

Pregnancy can affect the course of psychiatric illnesses and of bipolar affective disorder in particular. Mood-stabilising drugs such as lithium and valproate, which are prescribed for prophylaxis in bipolar disorder (p. 1200), are teratogenic and should be avoided whenever possible. Most guidelines recommend deferring conception until mood-stabilising medication is not required, or replacing the mood stabiliser with an antipsychotic such as chlorpromazine. Furthermore, the immediate post-partum period is associated with a dramatically increased risk of relapse in bipolar disorder: studies report relapse rates of up to 60% in the first 3 months after delivery in the absence of prophylactic medication. When relapse occurs following childbirth, not only are the stakes higher than at other times but also the onset of illness is more rapid, the symptoms more severe and concealment more pronounced. Post-partum relapse of bipolar affective

---

28.33 Psychiatric illness and pregnancy

- **Psychiatric disorder and pregnancy**: always consider effects on mother, fetus and child.
- **Bipolar disorder**: women should have pre-conceptual advice because there is a very high risk of relapse following delivery and some mood stabilisers are teratogenic.
- **Psychiatric treatments and pregnancy**: always make an individual assessment of the risks and benefits taking into consideration effects on mother, fetus and child.
- **Post-partum low mood ('blues')**: weeks 1–3; most cases are transient.
- **Persistent low mood and anhedonia**: may indicate depressive illness.
- **Puerperal psychosis**: progresses rapidly and is an indication for psychiatric admission.

disorder requires urgent specialist treatment, usually comprising admission to a psychiatric mother and baby unit. Ideally, women with major mental disorders such as bipolar affective disorder should be offered expert pre-conception advice to help them make informed decisions about medication and other aspects of their psychiatric care. A comprehensive post-partum risk management plan should be agreed during pregnancy.

Psychiatry and the law

Medicine takes place in a legal framework, made up of legislation (statute law) drafted by parliament or other governing bodies, precedent built up from court judgements over time (case law), and established tradition (common law). Psychiatry is similar to other branches of medicine in the applicability of common and case law but differs in that patients with psychiatric disorders can also be subject to legislative requirements to remain in hospital or to undergo treatments they refuse, such as the administration of antipsychotic drugs to a patient with acute schizophrenia who lacks insight and whose symptoms and/or behaviour pose a risk to himself/herself or to others.

The UK has three different Mental Health Acts, covering England and Wales, Scotland, and Northern Ireland, and all of these have recently been revised. Other countries may have very different provisions. It is important for practitioners to be familiar with the relevant provisions that apply in their jurisdictions and are likely to arise in the clinical settings in which they work.

All the countries that make up the UK have also introduced Incapacity Acts in recent years, with detailed provisions covering medical treatments for patients incapable of consenting, whether this incapacity arises from physical or mental illness. In general, the guiding principle in British law is that people should be free to make their own decision about any proposed medical treatment, except where their ability to make and/or communicate that decision is demonstrably impaired (by mental illness or physical incapacity). Any restrictions or compulsions applied should be the minimum necessary, they should be applied only for as long as is necessary, and there should be a benefit to the patient that balances the restrictions imposed. There should also be provisions for appeals and oversight.

Further information

Books and journal articles

Hofer H, Pozzi A, Joray M, et al. Safe refeeding management of anorexia nervosa inpatients: an evidence-based protocol. Nutrition 2014; 30:524–30.
Steel RM. Factitious disorder (Munchausen's syndrome). J R Coll Physicians Edinb 2009; 39:343–7.
Taylor D, Meader N, Bird V, et al. Pharmacological interventions for people with depression and chronic physical health problems: systematic review and meta-analyses of safety and efficacy. Br J Psychiatry 2011; 198:179–88.
Whiteford HA, Degenhardt L, Rehm J, et al. Global burden of disease attributable to mental and substance use disorders: findings from the Global Burden of Disease Study 2010. Lancet 2013; 382: 1575–86.

Websites

cebmh.com *Centre for Evidence-based Mental Health.*
dementia.ie/images/uploads/site-images/ACE-III_Scoring_(UK).pdf *Addenbrooke's Cognitive Examination – 3rd edn (ACE-III): administration and scoring guide.*
mind.org.uk *Information on depression.*
mocatest.org *Montreal Cognitive Assessment.*
neurosymptoms.org *A guide to medically unexplained neurological symptoms.*
niaaa.nih.gov/ *Information on alcoholism.*
nice.org.uk *National Institute for Health and Care Excellence: treatment guidelines for depression.*
ocdaction.org.uk *Useful information about obsessive–compulsive disorder.*
rcpsych.ac.uk/info/index.htm *Royal College of Psychiatrists: mental health information.*
sign.ac.uk *Scottish Intercollegiate Guidelines Network: treatment guidelines for depression, including Guideline 127 – Management of perinatal mood disorders.*
who.int/mental_health/ *World Health Organisation: mental health and brain disorders.*
www4.parinc.com/ *Mini-Mental State Examination.*

28

SH Ibbotson

Dermatology

Clinical examination in skin disease 1210

Functional anatomy and physiology 1212

Investigation of skin disease 1214

Presenting problems in skin disease 1216
Lumps and lesions 1216
Rash 1216
Blisters 1218
Itch 1219
Photosensitivity 1220
Leg ulcers 1223
Abnormal pigmentation 1224
Hair and nail abnormalities 1224
Acute skin failure 1224

Principles of management of skin disease 1225
General measures 1225
Topical treatments 1225
Phototherapy and photochemotherapy 1227
Systemic therapies 1227
Dermatological surgery 1228
Non-surgical treatments 1228

Skin tumours 1229
Malignant tumours 1229
Benign skin lesions 1234

Common skin infections and infestations 1235
Bacterial infections 1235
Viral infections 1238
Fungal infections 1239
Infestations 1241

Acne and rosacea 1241

Eczemas 1244

Psoriasis and other erythematous scaly eruptions 1247

Lichenoid eruptions 1252

Urticaria 1252

Bullous diseases 1254
Toxic epidermal necrolysis 1254
Immunobullous diseases 1255

Pigmentation disorders 1257
Decreased pigmentation 1257
Increased pigmentation 1258

Hair disorders 1258

Nail disorders 1260

Skin disease in general medicine 1261
Conditions involving cutaneous vasculature 1261
Connective tissue disease 1262
Granulomatous disease 1263
Porphyrias 1263
Abnormal deposition disorders 1264
Genetic disorders 1264
Reactive disorders 1264
Drug eruptions 1265

Clinical examination in skin disease

8 Detailed morphology of individual lesions
Use a magnifying lens in good lighting to assist
Use correct terminology (see definitions throughout text)

▲ Palmoplantar pustulosis

▲ Magnifying lens image of benign naevus

7 Overall description of individual lesions
Discrete, grouped, confluent, reticulate (lace-like), linear

6 Morphology of rash
Monomorphic or polymorphic

5 Involvement of axillae/groins
e.g. hidradenitis suppurativa

4 Nail involvement

▲ Psoriatic changes in nails and peri-ungual involvement

3 Involvement of hands, including nail folds and finger webs

2 If symmetrical

■ Extensor, e.g. psoriasis

■ Flexor, e.g. eczema

1 Distribution of rash
Symmetrical vs asymmetrical
Proximal vs distal vs facial
Localised vs widespread

Observation
The patient must be undressed, with make-up and dressings removed, and examined in good lighting. Consider the following:
• Age
• General health
• Distress
• Scratching

9 Examination of scalp
Hair loss
Scalp changes

Alopecia areata ◄

10 Involvement of face
Central
Hairline
Cheeks and nasal bridge: 'butterfly' distribution
Sparing of light-protected sites, e.g. behind ears, under chin

11 Eye involvement
e.g. Conjunctivitis/blepharitis in rosacea or eyelash loss in alopecia areata

12 Oral and genital involvement

▲ Reticulate (lacy) network on buccal mucosa in lichen planus. May also be genital involvement

13 Joint involvement
e.g. Psoriatic arthritis

▲ Arthritis, plaque psoriasis and psoriatic nail dystrophy

14 General medical examination
Including lymph nodes and other systems as indicated

It is tempting to examine the skin first. This is a mistake; take a history, then examine the skin and the rest of the patient.

1. History-taking	**2. Drug/allergy history**	**3. Examination of skin**	**4. Closer inspection**	**5. General examination**

Include:
- Onset and course
- Exacerbating/relieving factors
- Past history of skin disease, atopy or autoimmune disease
- Social history, occupation, recreation
- Psychological impact, gauged by health-related life quality indices

- Always take a detailed drug and allergy history
- Include all systemic and topical drugs, and over-the-counter preparations

- Examine skin, hair, nails and mucous membranes
- Is it a rash or a lesion?
- Distribution and morphology important for rash

- Use of a magnifying lens and/or dermatoscope may be invaluable
- Site, size and detailed morphology of a lesion are essential factors to elicit

- General examination, incl. peripheral lymph nodes, may be indicated/important
- Skin diseases may have systemic features (e.g. cardiovascular disease in psoriasis); many systemic diseases have dermatological features (e.g. diabetes)

6. Define type of lesion using correct terminology

Helps in differential diagnosis and allows colleagues to visualise the process. Other definitions are provided in the chapter.

Macule/patch	**Papule**	**Nodule**	**Plaque**

Macule: circumscribed flat area of colour change ≤ 1 cm diameter; patch: > 1 cm

Discrete elevation ≤ 1 cm diameter

Like papule but deeper (into dermis or subcutaneous layer), > 1 cm diameter

Raised area > 1 cm diameter with flat top

Vesicle	**Blisters/bullae**	**Pustule**	**Petechiae/purpura**

Small (≤ 1 cm diameter) fluid-filled blister

Large (> 1 cm diameter) fluid-filled blister

Visible accumulation of pus in blister

Petechiae: tiny macules due to extravascular blood in dermis; purpura: larger, may be palpable

7. Score activity

Tools for objective assessment of disease severity (e.g. Psoriasis Area and Severity Index, PASI) are important in assessing severity and treatment responses.

Four body parts are each scored individually

(A) Each of the four body parts is scored:

Redness (erythema)	0–4
Thickness (induration)	0–4
Scaling (desquamation)	0–4

(B) The area of each involved body part is scored:

0	0%
1	< 10%
2	10–29%
3	30–49%
4	50–69%
5	70–89%
6	90–100%

(C) 10% 20% 30% 40%

29

To find the PASI score, add together: (A) Sum for each part × (B) % of that part involved × (C) % weighting of that body part

Minimum = 0; maximum = 72

Diseases affecting the skin are common, and important because the absence of normal skin function, as well as sometimes being life-threatening, can severely impair quality of life. This may be exacerbated by the fact that people with skin disease can suffer the effects of stigma, often brought about by the ill-informed understanding of others with respect to skin diseases, particularly as regards visually disfiguring skin changes or the belief that they are contagious.

Skin diseases affect all ages and there are more than 2000 different types and presentations. Assessment of the skin is valuable in the management of anyone presenting with a medical problem and, conversely, assessment of the other body systems is important when managing primary skin diseases. This chapter concentrates on common skin diseases and those that are important components of general medical conditions. Skin infections, including those related to the human immunodeficiency virus (HIV), tuberculosis, leprosy (Hansen's disease) and syphilis are also discussed in Chapters 12, 17, 11 and 13, respectively.

Functional anatomy and physiology

The skin covers just under 2 m^2 in the average adult. The outer layer is the epidermis, a stratified squamous epithelium consisting mainly of keratinocytes. The epidermis is attached to, but separated from, the underlying dermis by the basement membrane. The dermis is less cellular and supports blood vessels, nerves and epidermal-derived appendages (hair follicles and sweat glands). Below it is the subcutis, consisting of adipose tissue.

Epidermis

In most sites, the epidermis is only 0.1–0.2 mm thick, except on the palms or soles, where it can extend to several millimetres. Keratinocytes make up approximately 90% of epidermal cells (Fig. 29.1). The main proliferative compartment is the basal layer. Keratinocytes synthesise a range of structural proteins, such as keratins, loricrin and filaggrin (filament aggregating protein), which play key roles in maintaining the skin's barrier function. Keratinocytes are also responsible for synthesis of vitamin D under the influence of ultraviolet B (UVB) light (p. 1049). There are more than 50 types of keratin and their expression varies by body site, site within the epidermis and disease state. Mutations of certain keratin genes can result in blistering disorders (p. 1254) and ichthyosis (characterised by scale without major inflammation). As keratinocytes migrate from the basal layer, they differentiate, producing a variety of protein and lipid products. Keratinocytes undergo apoptosis in the granular layer before losing their nuclei and becoming the flattened corneocytes of the stratum corneum (keratin layer). The epidermis is a site of lipid production, and the ability of the stratum corneum to act as a hydrophobic barrier is the result of its 'bricks and mortar' design; dead corneocytes with highly cross-linked protein membranes ('bricks') lie within a metabolically active lipid layer synthesised by keratinocytes ('mortar'). Terminal differentiation of keratinocytes relies on the keratin filaments being aggregated and this is, in part, mediated by filaggrin. Mutations of the filaggrin gene are found in icthyosis vulgaris and in some patients with atopic eczema (p. 1245).

The skin is a barrier against physical stresses. Cell-to-cell attachments must be able to transmit and dissipate stress, a function performed by desmosomes. Diseases that affect desmosomes, such as pemphigus (p. 1256), result in blistering due to keratinocyte separation.

The remaining 10% of epidermal cells are:

- *Langerhans' cells*: these are dendritic, bone marrow-derived cells that circulate between the epidermis and local lymph nodes. Their prime function is antigen presentation to lymphocytes. Other dermal antigen-presenting dendritic cells are also present.
- *Melanocytes*: these occur predominantly in the basal layer and are of neural crest origin. They synthesise the pigment melanin from tyrosine, package it in melanosomes and transfer it to surrounding keratinocytes via their dendritic processes.
- *Merkel cells*: these occur in the basal layer and are thought to play a role in signal transduction of fine touch. Their embryological derivation is unclear.

Basement membrane

The basement membrane (Fig. 29.1) is an anchor for the epidermis and allows movement of cells and nutrients between dermis and epidermis. The cell membrane of the epidermal basal cell is attached to the basement membrane via hemi-desmosomes. The lamina lucida lies immediately below the basal cell membrane and is composed predominantly of laminin. Anchoring filaments extend through the lamina lucida to attach to the lamina densa. This electron-dense layer consists mostly of type IV collagen; from it extend loops of type VII collagen, forming anchoring fibrils that fasten the basement membrane to the dermis.

Dermis

The dermis is vascular and supports the epidermis structurally and nutritionally. It varies in thickness from just over 1 mm on the inner forearm to 4 mm on the back. Fibroblasts are the predominant cells but others include mast cells, mononuclear phagocytes, T lymphocytes, dendritic cells, neurons and endothelial cells. The acellular part of the dermis consists mainly of collagen I and III, elastin and reticulin, synthesised by fibroblasts. Support is provided by an amorphous ground substance (mostly glycosaminoglycans, hyaluronic acid and dermatan sulphate), whose production and catabolism are altered by hormonal changes and ultraviolet radiation (UVR). Based on the pattern of collagen fibrils, the superficial dermis is termed the 'papillary dermis', and the deeper, coarser part is the 'reticular dermis'.

Epidermal appendages

Hair follicles

There are 3–5 million hair follicles, epidermal invaginations that develop during the second trimester. They occur throughout the skin, with the exception of palms, soles and parts of the genitalia (glabrous skin). The highest density of hair follicles is on the scalp (500–1000/cm^2). Newborns are covered with fine 'lanugo' hairs, which are usually non-pigmented and lack a central medulla; these are subsequently replaced by vellus hair, which is similar but more likely to be pigmented. By contrast, scalp hair becomes terminal hair, which is thicker with a central medulla, is usually pigmented and grows longer. At puberty, vellus hairs in hormonally sensitive regions, such as the axillary and genital areas, become terminal hairs.

Human hairs grow in a cycle with three phases: anagen (active hair growth), catagen (transitional phase) and telogen (resting phase). The duration of each phase varies by site. On the scalp, anagen lasts several years, catagen a few days and

Basement membrane

Epidermis

Basal keratinocyte

Basal cell membrane

Lamina lucida
(laminin-1)

Lamina densa
(type IV collagen)

Sublamina densa

Desmosome
(desmoglein-1 and 3,
desmoplakin)

Tonofilaments
(keratins 5 and 14)

Hemi-desmosome
(BP230, type XVII collagen,
$\alpha_6\beta_4$ integrin, plectin)

Anchoring filament
(laminin 332)

Anchoring fibrils
(collagen VII)

Dermis

Epidermis

Stratum corneum
(keratin layer)

Granular layer

Prickle
cell layer

Basal layer

Keratinocytes containing
keratins 1 and 10

Keratinocytes containing
keratins 5 and 14

Langerhans'
cell

Melanocyte

Hair shaft

Epidermis

Eccrine sweat duct

Superficial vascular
plexus

Sebaceous gland

Hair sheath

Eccrine sweat gland

Deep vascular plexus

Hair matrix

Dermal papilla

Subcutaneous
vessel

Dermis

Subcutis

Fig. 29.1 Structure of normal skin.

telogen around 3 months. The length of hair at different sites reflects the differing lengths of anagen.

Sebaceous glands

Sebaceous glands are epidermal downgrowths, usually associated with hair follicles and composed of modified keratinocytes. The cells of the sebaceous gland (sebocytes) produce a range of lipids, discharging the contents into the duct around the hair follicle. Sebum excretion is under hormonal control, with androgens increasing it (as do progesterones, to a lesser degree) and

oestrogens reducing it. In animals, sebum is important for hair waterproofing but its role in humans is unclear.

Sweat glands

Eccrine sweat glands develop in the second trimester and are also epidermal invaginations found all over the body. Their coiled ducts open directly on to the skin surface. They play a major role in thermoregulation and, unusually, are innervated by cholinergic fibres of the sympathetic nervous system. Eccrine glands of the palms and soles are innervated differently and are activated in the 'fight or flight' response. Apocrine sweat glands are restricted to the axillae and the mammary and genital areas, are connected to hair follicles and are not involved in thermoregulation.

Nails

Fingernail growth commences at approximately 8 weeks of gestation and is complete by 32 weeks. Toenails develop slightly later. The anatomy of the nail apparatus is covered later in the chapter (p. 1260).

Blood vessels and nerves

Human skin has a plentiful blood supply, arranged in superficial and deep plexuses consisting of arterioles, arterial and venous capillaries, and venules. The upper plexus in the papillary dermis communicates with the lower plexus at the junction between the dermis and the subcutis. Capillary loops arise from terminal arterioles in the horizontal papillary plexus. Blood vessels are supplied by sympathetic and parasympathetic nerves, with the relative contributions of the pathways differing by site. Sympathetic signals are important in mediating autonomic-induced vasoconstriction. The blood supply of skin is far greater than that required for normal skin physiology and reflects the importance of skin in thermoregulation.

Functions of the skin

The skin has many functions, all of which can be affected by disease (Box 29.1). Skin changes associated with ageing are shown in Box 29.2.

Investigation of skin disease

Magnifying glass

A hand-held or freestanding magnifying lens used under good lighting conditions (ideally daylight) is valuable for examination of the skin.

Wood's light

Wood's light is a long-wavelength UVA/short-wavelength visible (violet) light source that can be used in various ways. In hypopigmentation, such as in vitiligo, it can help in appreciating the extent of disease. In pigmented conditions, such as melasma, it can determine whether pigmentation is mainly epidermal (sharp cut-off under Wood's lamp) or mixed epidermal and dermal (ill-defined cut-off). Wood's lamp can also be used to help with the diagnosis of some fungal infections because of their characteristic fluorescence.

Dermatoscopy and diascopy

Dermatoscopy (also known as dermoscopy and epiluminescence microscopy) is increasingly performed with hand-held dermatoscopes. What makes dermatoscopy unique is the fact that it allows visualisation through contact of a glass plate on the instrument with a liquid film applied to the skin, or through special optics to allow non-contact dermatoscopy, enabling deeper structures to be seen without interference from reflection and refraction of light in the epidermis.

Diascopy is simply pressing on the lesion with a glass slide. This provides some of the effect of dermatoscopy, but is mainly used to remove blood from vascular lesions to make the appearance

i 29.1 Functions of the skin	
Function	Structure/cell involved
Protection against:	
Chemicals, particles, desiccation	Stratum corneum
Ultraviolet radiation	Melanin produced by melanocytes and transferred to keratinocytes
	Stratum corneum hyperproliferation
Antigens, haptens	Langerhans' cells, lymphocytes, mononuclear phagocytes, mast cells, dermal dendritic cells
Microorganisms	Stratum corneum, Langerhans' cells, mononuclear phagocytes, mast cells, dermal dendritic cells
Maintenance of fluid balance Prevents loss of water, electrolytes and macromolecules	Stratum corneum
Shock absorber Strong, elastic and compliant covering	Dermis and subcutaneous fat
Sensation	Specialised nerve endings mediating pain and withdrawal Itch leading to scratch and removal of a parasite
Metabolism Detoxification of xenobiotics, retinoid metabolism, isomerisation of urocanic acid	Predominantly keratinocytes
Temperature regulation	Eccrine sweat glands and blood vessels
Protection, and fine manipulation of small objects	Nails
Hormonal Steroidogenesis, testosterone synthesis and conversion to other androgenic steroids	Hair follicles, sebaceous glands
Conversion of thyroxine (T_4) to triiodothyronine (T_3)	Keratinocytes
Conversion of 7-dehydrocholesterol to vitamin D	Keratinocytes
Pheromonal Importance unknown in humans	Apocrine sweat glands, possibly sebaceous glands
Psychosocial, grooming and sexual behaviour	Appearance, tactile quality of skin, hair, nails

of the lesion clearer. Granulomatous skin diseases may have a characteristic appearance under diascopy, such as in lupus vulgaris (cutaneous tuberculosis), in which 'apple jelly nodules' are typically seen on diascopy.

Skin biopsy

Skin biopsy is a mainstay investigation in dermatology and can be used in a range of dermatological presentations. In the most common scenario, a skin biopsy is undertaken in order to obtain tissue on which to perform standard histopathology. However, tissue may also be subjected to a variety of staining and culture techniques, including immunostaining. Histopathological examination of skin biopsies is especially

29.2 Skin changes in old age

- **Chronological ageing**: due to the intrinsic ageing process.
- **Photo-ageing**: due to cumulative ultraviolet radiation (UVR) exposure and superimposed on intrinsic ageing.
- **Typical changes**: include atrophy, laxity, yellow discoloration, wrinkling, dryness, irregular pigmentation, and thinning and greying of hair.
- **Causes**: age-related alterations in structure and function of the skin, cumulative effects of environmental insults, especially UVR and smoking, cutaneous consequences of disease in other organ systems.
- **Consequences**: reduction in immune and inflammatory responses, reduction in absorption and clearance of topical medications, reduced healing, increased susceptibility to irritants, dermatitis, adverse drug effects (including topical glucocorticoid-induced atrophy and purpura) and diseases such as skin cancer.

useful for tumour diagnosis. When a dermatologist or pathologist with dermatopathology expertise is involved, it can also assist in the diagnosis of inflammatory skin diseases. It is rare for histopathology of a previously undiagnosed inflammatory skin disease to provide a diagnosis on its own; clinico-pathological correlation is critical. Most biopsies are stained with haematoxylin and eosin but other stains may be useful in special situations, such as for fungal hyphae, iron or mucin. Direct immunofluorescence can also be undertaken on a fresh skin biopsy, allowing antigen visualisation using fluorescein-labelled antibodies; this is especially important in the diagnosis of autoimmune bullous disorders or connective tissue disease, such as cutaneous lupus.

Microbiology

Bacteriology

Bacterial swabs may identify a causative infective agent. However, organisms identified from the skin surface may not be the cause of the skin disease but instead may simply reflect colonisation of skin that has already been damaged by a primary skin disease.

Virology

A number of techniques, including immunofluorescence and polymerase chain reaction (PCR), are available to diagnose herpes simplex or herpes zoster viruses from vesicle fluid (p. 106).

Mycology

Scale, nail clippings (or scrapings of crumbly subungual hyperkeratosis) and plucked hairs can be examined by light microscopy. If potassium hydroxide and a simple light microscope are available, this can be performed in any outpatient clinic. Microbiology laboratories will also routinely undertake microscopy and culture for fungi and yeasts.

Patch testing

Patch testing is the investigation of choice for delayed, cell-mediated, type IV hypersensitivity, which clinically manifests as dermatitis. Potential allergens (see Box 29.22, p. 1247) are applied as patches to the back under occlusion for 48 hours, in vehicles and at concentrations that minimise false-positive and false-negative reactions. After 48 hours the patches are removed and patch-test readings are undertaken at time points of up to 7 days after patch-test application, with the most typical time point being at 96 hours. When interpreting patch test readings, it is important to determine the clinical relevance of any allergic reactions before giving avoidance advice.

Photopatch testing is similar to patch testing but investigates delayed hypersensitivity to an agent (usually a sunscreen or a non-steroidal anti-inflammatory drug (NSAID)) after the absorption of UVR. It involves applying substances in duplicate and irradiating one set with UVR (typically UVA, 5 J/cm^2), readings then being conducted in a similar manner to patch testing.

Prick tests and specific immunoglobulin E testing

Prick tests are used to investigate cutaneous type I (immediate) hypersensitivity to various antigens such as pollen, house dust mite or dander. The skin is pricked with commercially available stylets through a dilution of the appropriate antigen solution (p. 86). Alternatively, specific immunoglobulin E (IgE) levels to antigens can be measured in serum. If challenge tests are undertaken for patients with suspected allergy, these must be performed under controlled conditions due to the potential risk of triggering a severe reaction (p. 86).

Phototesting

Phototesting is extremely valuable in the assessment of suspected photosensitivity. The mainstay investigation is monochromator phototesting, which involves exposing the patient's back to increasing doses of irradiation using narrow wavebands across the solar spectrum and then assessing responses, using the minimal erythema dose (MED) at each waveband. This is the dose required to cause just perceptible skin reddening and is compared with values for the normal population. If a patient has reduced MED (develops erythema at lower doses than healthy subjects), this indicates abnormal photosensitivity. Thus, monochromator phototesting can be used to determine whether a patient is abnormally photosensitive, which wavebands are involved and how sensitive the patient is (p. 1220). Provocation testing can be performed with a broadband (usually UVA) source to induce rash at a test site (most useful for polymorphic light eruption) and can be helpful for diagnosis. Provocation testing to a variety of light sources, including artificial compact fluorescent lamps, may also be indicated, the latter being most relevant in patients with severe photosensitivity.

Patients who are referred for phototherapy will also commonly undergo an MED test, in which they are exposed to a series of test doses of the light source that will be used therapeutically (often narrowband UVB); the MED is determined 24 hours later (or 72–96 hours for the psoralen–ultraviolet A (PUVA) minimal phototoxic dose; p. 1227). This allows treatment regimens to be individualised, based on a patient's erythemal responses, and may detect abnormal photosensitivity.

Blood tests

Although most patients presenting with a skin problem do not need blood tests as part of their investigations, there are many systemic diseases that can present with skin features and, indeed, blood tests may also be indicated in the investigation of primary skin disease. A wide range of possible investigations may be required and some examples include haemoglobin, iron studies and thyroid function tests in pruritus or hair loss; autoantibody screening if lupus is suspected; porphyrin plasma scan for skin fragility and hypertrichosis; and hepatitis screening in lichen

29

planus. These diverse examples emphasise the importance of considering an underlying systemic disease when assessing a patient with a dermatological presentation.

Imaging

Imaging techniques are not typically required but X-rays, ultrasound, magnetic resonance imaging (MRI) or computed tomography (CT) may occasionally be indicated in specific situations, such as in metastatic melanoma or in a patient presenting with a diagnosis of cutaneous sarcoid.

Presenting problems in skin disease

The major presentations in dermatology are outlined below. Detail of the underlying disorders is mostly provided in the disease-specific sections further on in the chapter.

Lumps and lesions

The term lump or lesion is typically used to describe a papule or nodule, although sometimes may refer to a macule or plaque (p. 1211). A new or changing lump is one of the key dermatology presentations.

Clinical assessment

Detailed history-taking and examination are essential:

- *Change*: Is the lump new or has there been a change in a pre-existing lesion? What is the nature of the change – size, colour, shape or surface change? Has change been rapid or slow? Are there other features – pain, itch, inflammation, bleeding or ulceration (**definition** of 'ulcer': an area from which the epidermis and at least the upper part of the dermis have been lost – see Fig. 29.9, p. 1223)?
- *Patient*: What is the patient's age? Are they fair-skinned and freckled? Has there been much sun exposure? Have they used sunbeds or lived in sunny climates? Have they used photoprotection?
- *Site*: Is it on a sun-exposed or covered site? The scalp, face, upper limbs and back in men, and face, hands and lower legs in women, are the most chronically sun-exposed sites.
- *Are there other similar lesions?* These might include actinic keratoses (see Fig. 29.13, p. 1231) or basal cell papillomas (see Fig. 29.17, p. 1234).
- *Morphology*: Tenderness, size, symmetry, regularity of border, colour, surface characteristics and the presence of features such as crust (**definition**: dried exudate of blood or serous fluid – see Fig. 29.19, p. 1235), scale (**definition**: a flake arising from the stratum corneum; any condition with a thickened stratum corneum can cause scaling – see Fig. 29.13, p. 1231) and ulceration must be assessed. Stretching the skin and using a magnifying lens can be helpful, such as for detecting the raised, pearled edge of a basal cell carcinoma (see Fig. 29.11, p. 1229).
- *Dermatoscopy*: This can be used to detect the presence of abnormal vessels, such as in basal cell carcinoma or the characteristic keratin cysts in basal cell papillomas. It is invaluable for assessing pigmented and vascular lesions (Fig. 29.2).

29.3 ABCDE features of malignant melanoma

- **A**symmetry
- **B**order irregular
- **C**olour irregular
- **D**iameter >0.5 cm
- **E**levation irregular
- (+ Loss of skin markings)

Is it a melanocytic naevus or a malignant melanoma?

This is a common clinical scenario and one that it is critical to resolve correctly.

- The precise nature of the change should be determined (as above). Listen to the patient and pay attention to subtle changes, as people know their skin well.
- If the patient has other pigmented lesions, then these should be examined too, as they may be informative. For example, if the presenting lesion looks different from the others, then suspicion of melanoma is increased; conversely, if the patient has multiple basal cell papillomas, this may be reassuring – although do not be falsely reassured.
- Is there a positive family history of melanoma? A suspicious naevus in a patient with a first-degree relative with melanoma probably warrants excision.

The ABCDE 'rule' is a guide to the characteristic features of melanoma (Box 29.3 and see Figs 29.2 and 29.15), although melanomas should ideally be diagnosed before the diameter is greater than 0.5 cm. Loss of normal skin markings in a pigmented lesion may be suggestive of melanoma. Conversely, normal skin markings and fine hairs dispersed evenly over a lesion are reassuring but do not exclude melanoma. The Glasgow seven-point checklist is another useful guide:

- *major features*: change in size, shape and colour
- *minor features*: diameter >0.5 cm, inflammation, oozing, bleeding, itch or altered sensation.

Patients with one major or one minor feature should be referred for further evaluation.

Investigations and management

If a benign diagnosis, such as basal cell papilloma, is made on clinical grounds, then the patient can be reassured and the lesion either left or treated: for example, with cryotherapy. If there are concerns about the diagnosis or malignancy is suspected on clinical grounds, then skin biopsy in order to obtain a tissue diagnosis is the usual approach. An incisional biopsy may be indicated, although if the lesion is small, excision may be most appropriate. If significant concern exists about the possibility of malignant melanoma, initial excision with a 2 mm margin would usually be undertaken prior to more definitive management once histology was confirmed. Further management of a changed lesion would, of course, depend on the histology of the diagnostic biopsy.

Rash

A rash is the other common presentation in dermatology. The main categories of scaly rashes are listed in Box 29.4. The most common type of rash presentation is maculopapular. Diagnosis can often be made on clinical grounds, although a biopsy may be required.

Fig. 29.2 Dermatoscopy. **A** A changing lesion. **B** Dermatoscopy highlights the abnormal pigment network and other features suggestive of melanoma. Excision biopsy confirmed the diagnosis of superficial spreading malignant melanoma (Breslow thickness 0.8 mm). **C** Another changing lesion. **D** Dermatoscopy highlights the vascular lacunae of this benign angioma and the patient was reassured.

i | 29.4 Causes and clinical features of common scaly rashes

Diagnosis	Distribution	Morphology	Associated signs
Atopic eczema (p. 1245)	Face and flexures	Poorly defined erythema, scaling Vesicles Lichenification if chronic	Shiny nails Infra-orbital crease 'Dirty neck' (grey–brown discoloration)
Psoriasis (p. 1247)	Extensor surfaces Lower back	Well-defined Erythematous plaques Silvery scale	Nail pitting, onycholysis Scalp involvement Axillae and genital areas often affected Joint involvement Köbner phenomenon (p. 1252)
Pityriasis rosea (p. 1251)	'Fir tree' pattern on trunk	Well-defined Small, erythematous plaques Collarette of scale	Herald patch
Drug eruption (p. 1265)	Widespread	Macules and papules Erythema and scale Exfoliation	Possible mucosal involvement or erythroderma
Pityriasis versicolor (p. 1240)	Upper trunk and shoulders	Hypo- and hyper-pigmented scaly patches	
Lichen planus (p. 1252)	Distal limbs Flexural aspect of wrists Lower back	Shiny, flat-topped, violaceous papules Wickham's striae	White, lacy network on buccal mucosa Nail changes Scarring alopecia Köbner phenomenon
Tinea corporis (p. 1240)	Asymmetrical Often isolated lesions	Erythematous, often annular plaques Peripheral scale (sometimes pustules) Expansion with central clearing	Possible nail, scalp, groin involvement
Secondary syphilis (p. 337)	Trunk and proximal limbs Palms and soles	Red macules and papules, which become 'gun-metal' grey	History of chancre Systemic symptoms, e.g. malaise and fever

29

Clinical assessment

Important aspects of the history include:

- *Age at onset and duration of rash.* Atopic eczema often starts in early childhood and psoriasis between 15 and 40 years, and both may be chronic. Infective or drug-induced rashes are more likely to be of short duration and the latter to occur in relation to drug ingestion. Duration of individual lesions is also important, as in urticaria, for example.
- *Body site at onset and distribution.* Flexural sites are more typically involved in atopic eczema, and extensor surfaces and scalp in psoriasis. Symmetry is often indicative of an endogenous disease, such as psoriasis, whereas asymmetry is more common with exogenous causes, such as contact dermatitis or infections like herpes zoster.
- *Itch.* Eczema is usually extremely itchy and psoriasis may be less so.
- *Preceding illness and systemic symptoms.* Guttate psoriasis may be precipitated by a β-haemolytic streptococcal throat infection; almost all patients with infectious mononucleosis (p. 241) treated with amoxicillin will develop an erythematous maculopapular eruption; a history of chancre at the site of inoculation may be elicited in a presentation of secondary syphilis; malaise and arthralgia are common in drug eruptions and vasculitis.

The morphology of the rash and the characteristics of individual lesions are important (Box 29.4).

Investigations and management

It is important to have a short differential diagnosis based on clinical assessment in order to direct investigations. For example, in psoriasis, no investigations may be needed and initial management with patient counselling and topical therapies may suffice. If the diagnosis is unclear, then a diagnostic skin biopsy and other targeted investigations based on the clinical picture may be required. An initial management plan should also be implemented. For example, in a child presenting with a rash that has features suggestive of impetigo, skin and nasal swabs should be performed and, once these have been taken, topical or systemic antibiotics should be introduced, depending on clinical extent of disease, and management should be adjusted accordingly, dependent on investigation findings and clinical course. In contrast, if a patient presents with a maculopapular rash shortly after introduction of a new drug, then drug withdrawal, diagnostic biopsy, full blood count, including eosinophil count, and liver and renal function tests, in parallel with topical emollients and glucocorticoids, may be indicated.

Blisters

A blister is a fluid-filled collection in the skin. The term vesicle is used for small lesions and bulla for larger lesions (p. 1211). Blistering occurs due to loss of cell adhesion within the epidermis or subepidermal region (see Fig. 29.1). The clinical presentation depends on the site or level of blistering within the skin, which in turn reflects the underlying cause (p. 1254). There are a limited number of conditions that present with blisters (Box 29.5):

- Intact blisters are not often seen if the split is high in the epidermis (below the stratum corneum), as the blister roof is so fragile that it ruptures easily, leaving erosions (**definition**: an area of skin denuded by complete or partial loss of the epidermis). This occurs in pemphigus foliaceus, staphylococcal scalded skin syndrome (see Fig. 29.20, p. 1236) and bullous impetigo.
- If the split is lower in the epidermis, then intact flaccid blisters and erosions may be seen, as occurs in pemphigus vulgaris and toxic epidermal necrolysis (see Fig. 29.41, p. 1254).
- If the split is subepidermal, then tense-roofed blisters are seen. This occurs in bullous pemphigoid (see Fig. 29.42, p. 1256), epidermolysis bullosa acquisita and porphyria cutanea tarda (see Fig. 29.52, p. 1264).
- If there are foci of separation at different levels of the epidermis, as in dermatitis (p. 1244), then multilocular bullae made up of coalescing vesicles can occur.

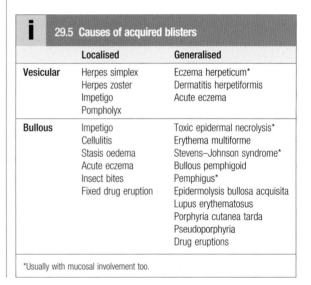

i	**29.5 Causes of acquired blisters**	
	Localised	Generalised
Vesicular	Herpes simplex Herpes zoster Impetigo Pompholyx	Eczema herpeticum* Dermatitis herpetiformis Acute eczema
Bullous	Impetigo Cellulitis Stasis oedema Acute eczema Insect bites Fixed drug eruption	Toxic epidermal necrolysis* Erythema multiforme Stevens–Johnson syndrome* Bullous pemphigoid Pemphigus* Epidermolysis bullosa acquisita Lupus erythematosus Porphyria cutanea tarda Pseudoporphyria Drug eruptions

*Usually with mucosal involvement too.

Systematic approach to the diagnosis of blistering diseases			
Exclude infection Herpes simplex, varicella zoster, *Staphylococcus aureus*	**Consider common diseases in which blisters are uncommon** Peripheral oedema, cellulitis, allergic contact dermatitis, other eczemas	**Remember blisters in drug eruptions** Fixed drug eruptions, erythema multiforme, vasculitis, TEN	**Think of immunobullous causes** Bullous pemphigoid, pemphigus, linear IgA disease, bullous lupus

Fig. 29.3 A systematic approach to the diagnosis of blistering diseases. (TEN = toxic epidermal necrolysis)

Clinical assessment

Detailed history-taking and examination are critical. A history of onset, progression, mucosal involvement, drugs and systemic symptoms should be sought. Clinical assessment of the distribution, extent and morphology of the rash should be made. The Nikolsky sign is useful: sliding lateral pressure from a finger on normal-looking epidermis can dislodge and detach the epidermis in conditions with intra-epidermal defects, such as pemphigus and toxic epidermal necrolysis. A systematic approach to diagnosis is required (Fig. 29.3).

Investigations and management

Investigations and initial management will be guided by the clinical presentation and differential diagnosis, and are described in more detail under the specific diseases. For example, an initial approach may include directed investigations, such as incisional diagnostic skin biopsy for histology and direct immunofluorescence, indirect immunofluorescence and other targeted blood tests or skin swabs. Management should be based on the likely diagnosis and begin in parallel with investigations, until the diagnosis is confirmed.

Itch

Itch describes the unpleasant sensation that leads to scratching or rubbing. The terms 'itch' and 'pruritus' are synonymous; however, 'pruritus' is often used when itch is generalised. Itch can arise from primary cutaneous disease or be secondary to systemic disease, which may cause itch by central or peripheral mechanisms. Even when the mechanism is peripheral, there are not always signs of primary skin disease.

The nerve endings that signal itch are in the epidermis or near the dermo-epidermal junction. The underlying mechanisms of itch are not fully understood. Transmission is by unmyelinated slow-conducting C fibres through the spinothalamic tract to the thalamus and then the cortex. Aδ fibres also seem to be involved in transmitting signals to the spinal cord, and the heat-sensitive transient receptor potential (TRP) channels 1–4 are important. There is an inhibitory relationship between pain and itch. Scratching may relieve the symptom of itch after the sensation has ceased and this is either by stimulation of ascending sensory pathways that inhibit itch-transmitting neurons at the spinal cord (Wall's 'gate' mechanism), or by direct damage to cutaneous sensory nerves.

The mechanisms of itch in most systemic diseases remain unclear. The itch of kidney disease, for example, may be mediated by circulating endogenous opioids. The clinical observation that peritoneal dialysis helps reduce itch more frequently than haemodialysis is consistent with this, with smaller molecules generally being dialysed more readily if the peritoneal membrane is used rather than a dialysis machine membrane.

Clinical assessment

It is important to determine whether skin changes are primary (a process in the skin causing itch) or secondary (skin changes caused by rubbing and scratching because of itch). This requires a thorough history and examination, sometimes with investigations, to exclude systemic disease. Many common primary skin disorders are associated with itch (Box 29.6). If itch is not connected with primary skin disease, other causes should be considered (Box 29.7). These include liver diseases (mainly cholestatic diseases, such as primary biliary cirrhosis), malignancies (generalised itch may be the presenting feature

---

i 29.6 Primary skin diseases causing pruritus

Generalised pruritus

- Scabies
- Eczemas
- Pre-bullous pemphigoid
- Urticarias
- Xeroderma of old age
- Psoriasis

Localised pruritus

- Eczemas
- Lichen planus
- Dermatitis herpetiformis
- Pediculosis
- Tinea infections

---

i 29.7 Secondary causes of pruritus

Medical condition	Cause of pruritus	Treatment*	Medical condition	Cause of pruritus	Treatment*
Liver disease	Central opioid effect Elevation in bile salts may contribute	Naltrexone Colestyramine Rifampicin Sedative antihistamines UVB	Thyrotoxicosis Hypothyroidism Carcinoid syndrome (p. 678)	Unknown Unknown 5-HT-mediated	
Renal failure	Unknown; uraemia contributes	UVB Oral activated charcoal	**HIV infection**	Infection, infestation Eosinophilic folliculitis	Treatment of infection Local corticosteroids, UVB
Haematological disease				Seborrhoeic dermatitis Unknown	Anti-pityrosporal treatment UVB
Anaemia Polycythaemia rubra vera	Iron deficiency Unknown (often aquagenic pruritus)	Iron replacement	**Malignancy**	Unknown	
Lymphoma Laukaemia Myeloma	Unknown		**Psychogenic**	Unknown	Psychotherapy, anxiolytics, antidepressants
Endocrine disease					
Diabetes mellitus	Increased infection risk, e.g. candidiasis, tinea	Treatment of infection			

*In addition to specific treatment of the primary condition and symptomatic treatments, such as emollients. (5-HT = 5-hydroxytryptamine, serotonin; UVB = ultraviolet B)

29

29.8 Causes of pruritus in pregnancy

Diagnosis	Pregnancy, gestation and features	Treatment
Polymorphic eruption of pregnancy (pruritic urticarial papules and plaques, PUPP)	Typically first pregnancy and uncommonly recurs 3rd trimester, after delivery Polymorphic urticated papules and plaques, start in striae	Chlorphenamine, emollients Topical glucocorticoids
Acute cholestasis of pregnancy (p. 1284)	3rd trimester and commonly recurs in subsequent pregnancies Abnormal liver function tests Increased fetal and maternal risk	Emollients Chlorphenamine Colestyramine UVB Early delivery
Pemphigoid gestationis	Any stage, often 2nd trimester and commonly recurs in subsequent pregnancies Urticated erythema, blistering initially periumbilical Characteristic histology and immunofluorescence	Topical or oral glucocorticoids
Prurigo gestationis	2nd trimester Excoriated papules	Emollients Topical glucocorticoids Chlorphenamine UVB
Pruritic folliculitis	3rd trimester Sterile pustules on trunk	Topical glucocorticoids UVB

(UVB = ultraviolet B)

of lymphoma), haematological conditions (generalised itch in chronic iron deficiency or water contact-provoked (aquagenic) intense itch in polycythaemia), endocrine diseases (including hypo- and hyperthyroidism), chronic kidney disease (in which severity of itch is not always clearly associated with plasma creatinine concentration) and psychogenic causes (such as in 'delusions of infestation'). Itch is common in pregnancy and may be due to one of the pregnancy-specific dermatoses. Making a correct diagnosis is particularly important in pregnancy, as some disorders can be associated with increased fetal risk (Box 29.8).

Investigations and management

Investigations should be directed towards finding an underlying cause and there will be a different approach for itch with rash, as opposed to itch with no signs of primary skin disease (Fig. 29.4). If there are no signs of primary skin disease, investigations should be undertaken to exclude systemic disease or iatrogenic causes. Psychogenic itch should be considered only if organic disease has been ruled out. There are no consistently effective therapies to suppress itch, and so establishing the underlying cause is critical. If a clear-cut diagnosis cannot be made, non-specific approaches can be used for symptom relief. These include sedation, often with H$_1$ receptor antihistamines, along with emollients and counter-irritants (such as topical menthol-containing preparations). UVB phototherapy is useful for generalised itch due to a variety of causes but the only randomised controlled study of efficacy is in chronic kidney disease. Other treatments include low-dose tricyclic antidepressants (probably through similar mechanisms to those involved when these drugs are used for chronic pain) and opiate antagonists. If a psychogenic itch is considered likely, antidepressants and/or cognitive behavioural therapy may be effective. Itch of any cause can be severe and its potentially major adverse effects on quality of life are not always fully appreciated. Assessments of impact on quality of life, such as Dermatology Life Quality Index (DLQI) scores, are essential.

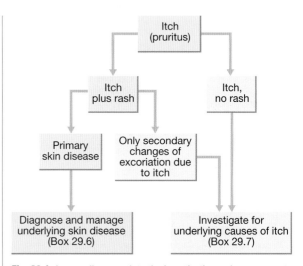

Fig. 29.4 An overall approach to the investigation and management of itch (pruritus).

Photosensitivity

Cutaneous photosensitivity is an abnormal response of the skin to UVR or visible radiation. The sun is the natural source but patients may also be exposed to artificial sources of UVR through the use of sunbeds and/or phototherapy (p. 1227). Chronic UVR exposure increases skin cancer risk and photo-ageing (p. 1215). Acute exposure can induce erythema (redness) as a normal response (Fig. 29.5). However, abnormal photosensitivity occurs when a patient reacts to lower doses than would normally cause a response, either with a heightened erythemal reaction or the development of a rash. Photo-aggravated skin diseases are exacerbated by sunlight but not caused by it. The main photosensitive and photo-aggravated diseases are listed in Box 29.9.

29.9 The photosensitivity and photo-aggravated diseases

Cause	Condition	Clinical features
Immunological (previously known as idiopathic)	Polymorphic light eruption (PLE)	Seasonal, itchy, papulovesicular rash on photo-exposed sites; face and back of hands often spared. Often hours of UVR exposure needed to provoke; lasts a few days; affects about 20% in Northern Europe, more common in young women
	Chronic actinic dermatitis (CAD)	Chronic dermatitis on sun-exposed sites. Most common in elderly males. Predominantly UVB, but also often UVA and visible light photosensitivity. Most also have contact allergies
	Solar urticaria	Immediate-onset urticaria on photo-exposed sites. Usually UVA and visible light photosensitivity. Can occur at any age
	Actinic prurigo	Uncommon, presents in childhood. Often familial, with strong HLA association. Some similarities to PLE, although scarring occurs
	Hydroa vacciniforme	Rare childhood photodermatosis. Varioliform scarring
Drugs (variety of mechanisms)	Phototoxicity	Usually UVA (and visible light) photosensitivity Most common. Exaggerated sunburn and exfoliation. Many drugs such as thiazides, tetracyclines, fluoroquinolones, quinine, NSAIDs
	Pseudoporphyria	NSAIDs, retinoids, tetracyclines, furosemide are examples
	Photoallergy	Usually to topical agents, particularly sunscreens and NSAIDs
Metabolic	Porphyrias	Mainly porphyria cutanea tarda and erythropoietic protoporphyria (p. 378).
	Pellagra	Photo-exposed site dermatitis due to tryptophan deficiency (see Fig. 14.15, p. 378)
Photogenodermatoses	Xeroderma pigmentosum	Rare. Defect in DNA excision repair, abnormal photosensitivity, photo-ageing and skin cancer. There may be neurological features
Photo-aggravation of pre-existing conditions	Lupus erythematosus	Can also be drug-induced (see Box 29.35, p. 1266)
	Erythema multiforme	p. 1264
	Rosacea	p. 1243

(HLA = human leucocyte antigen; NSAID = non-steroidal anti-inflammatory drug; UVA/UVB = ultraviolet A/B; UVR = ultraviolet radiation)

Fig. 29.5 Sunburn. Acute exposure to ultraviolet radiation results in an erythemal response that peaks 12–24 hours later. Sensitivity depends on the individual's constitutive skin phototype.

Sunlight consists mainly of visible light, and the UVR component is divided into three wavebands (Fig. 29.6), according to the Commission Internationale de l'Eclairage (CIE):

- *UVC* (200–280 nm), which is absorbed by ozone and does not reach the Earth's surface.
- *UVB* (280–315 nm), which constitutes less than 10% of UVR exposure but is around 1000-fold more potent than UVA and so accounts for the erythemal 'sunburning' effects of sunlight.
- *UVA* (315–400 nm), which is the most abundant UVR component reaching the Earth's surface.

The arbitrary division between UVB and UVA regions is more often considered to be at 320 nm by photobiologists, and the UVA region can be further subdivided into UVA2 (320–340 nm) and UVA1 (340–400 nm). UVA2 behaves biologically more like UVB, and UVA1 can be used therapeutically for several skin conditions, such as morphoea and eczema.

Patients with photosensitivity diseases can be abnormally sensitive to UVB, UVA, visible light (over 400 nm) or, commonly, a combination of wavebands. UVB is absorbed by window glass, whereas UVA and visible light are transmitted through glass.

Clinical assessment

Taking a careful history is essential, as the patient may not have the rash when assessed. Seasonal pattern and distribution of rash are important. Key sites are the face (particularly nose, cheeks and forehead), top of ears, neck (Fig. 29.7), bald scalp, back of hands and forearms. Sparing is often seen under the chin and nose, behind the ears, on the upper eyelids and the distal digits – as we normally walk about with our eyes open and fingers flexed! It can be misleading if there is covered site involvement. Patients who are sensitive to UVA and visible light may be affected through clothing. These patients commonly experience perennial symptoms and may not be aware of the association with daylight exposure. Other photosensitive conditions, such as actinic prurigo or chronic actinic dermatitis, may also involve covered sites. Sparing of habitually exposed sites, such as the face and back of hands, occurs most commonly in polymorphic light eruption (PLE) and is called the 'hardening phenomenon'. Importantly, some conditions, such as solar urticaria, develop rapidly after sunlight exposure, whereas others, such as cutaneous lupus, can take several days to evolve.

Investigations and management

If photosensitivity is suspected, the patient should be referred to a specialist centre for monochromator phototesting (p. 1215), if feasible. Other investigations will often include provocation,

29

Fig. 29.6 The electromagnetic spectrum. The action spectrum is not well defined for many conditions and, for some, is approximate and may vary between patients. The action spectrum for non-melanoma skin cancer mirrors that for erythema. The action spectrum for melanoma is not known but includes ultraviolet (UV) B. Photoprotection measures vary, depending on condition, although the mainstay always includes behavioural modification, clothing cover and appropriate sunscreen choices. (UVR = ultraviolet radiation)

Fig. 29.7 Chronic actinic dermatitis. Note the sharp cut-off and sparing behind the ear in the shadow cast by the earlobe (Wilkinson's triangle).

patch or photopatch testing and screening for lupus and the porphyrias (p. 1263). Rarely, investigations such as human leucocyte antigen (HLA) typing in suspected actinic prurigo, or DNA excision repair functional activity or genotyping in suspected xeroderma pigmentosum, may be required.

Management depends on the cause. If there is a phototoxic drug or chemical cause, this must be addressed: for instance, by stopping the drug or treating the porphyria. Counselling in regard to sun avoidance is essential: keeping out of direct sun in the middle of the day, covering up with clothing, wearing hats with a wide brim and careful use of high-factor sunscreens. Paradoxically, in some conditions, particularly PLE and solar urticaria, phototherapy can be used to induce 'hardening'; the

mechanism of desensitisation is uncertain. Other approaches may be necessary, depending on disease and severity, and may include antihistamines (useful in two-thirds of patients with solar urticaria) and systemic immunosuppression (sometimes required in the immunological photodermatoses). Patients with photosensitivity are at risk of vitamin D deficiency because of reduced synthesis in the skin and should be advised to optimise dietary vitamin D intake or take supplements (p. 1052).

Sunscreens

Sunscreens can be divided into two categories: chemical sunscreens, which absorb specific wavelengths of UVR, and physical sunscreens, which reflect UVR and the shorter visible wavelengths (see Fig. 29.6). Sunscreens are now highly sophisticated and most offer protection against UVB and most UVA wavelengths. If a patient is abnormally photosensitive to the longer wavelengths of UVA and the visible part of the spectrum (for example, in cutaneous porphyrias and solar urticaria), then conventional sunscreens are not beneficial and specific reflectant sunscreens are required. Historically, these agents were less cosmetically acceptable due to visible light reflection, but current formulations, some of which are tinted, have reduced this problem.

Sunscreen protection levels are described by sun protection factor (SPF). This is the ratio of the dose of UVR required to produce skin erythema in the presence and absence of the sunscreen. A sunscreen of SPF20 means that it would take 20 times as long for a person to develop sunburn in the presence of the sunscreen, as compared to not using it. Therefore, SPF is really a sunburn protection factor and is not a good guide to how well a sunscreen will perform in protecting against other reactions (such as skin pain in erythropoietic protoporphyria or UVR-induced immunosuppression). SPF values are determined under experimental conditions whereas, in practice, people tend to use 25–33% of the amount of sunscreen required to achieve the stated SPF. Patient counselling is therefore important with regard to adequate application of sunscreen. All sunscreens offer, at best, partial protection only and are no substitute for modifying behaviour and covering up.

Leg ulcers

Leg ulcer is not a diagnosis, but a symptom of an underlying disease in which there is complete loss of the epidermis, leaving dermal layers exposed. Ulcers on the lower leg are frequently caused by vascular disease but there are other causes, as summarised in Box 29.10.

Clinical assessment

A detailed history of the onset and course of leg ulceration and predisposing conditions should be elicited. The site and surrounding skin should be assessed. Varicose veins are often present, although not inevitably. Assessment of the venous and arterial vasculature and neurological examination are critical. The site of ulceration may also help to indicate the underlying primary cause (Fig. 29.8). Full clinical examination is essential as the ulcer may be arising in the context of systemic disease, such as vasculitis.

Leg ulceration due to venous disease

Varicose veins, a history of deep venous thrombosis and obesity are predisposing factors. Incompetent valves in the deep and perforating veins of the lower leg result in retrograde flow of blood to the superficial system, and a rise in capillary pressure ('venous hypertension'). Pericapillary fibrin cuffing occurs, leading to impairment of local tissue oxygenation and homeostasis.

The first symptom in venous ulceration is often heaviness of the legs, followed by oedema. Haemosiderin pigmentation, pallor and firmness of surrounding skin, and sometimes venous/gravitational eczema (p. 1247) subsequently develop. This progresses to lipodermatosclerosis – firm induration due to fibrosis of the dermis

and subcutis, which may produce the well-known 'inverted champagne bottle' appearance. Ulceration, often precipitated by trauma or infection, follows. Venous ulcers typically occur on the medial lower leg (Fig. 29.9).

Complications of venous leg ulceration include bacterial colonisation and infection, and contact allergic dermatitis to topical medicaments, dressings and bandages. Lipodermatosclerosis may cause lymphoedema and hyperkeratosis; rarely, a squamous cell carcinoma (SCC) may develop in a long-standing venous ulcer (Marjolin's ulcer).

Leg ulceration due to arterial disease

Deep, painful, punched-out ulcers on the lower leg, especially the shin and foot and in the context of intermittent claudication, are

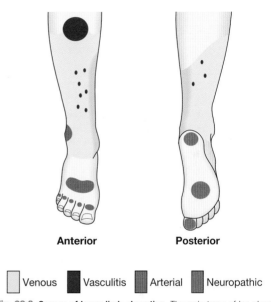

Venous	Vasculitis	Arterial	Neuropathic

Fig. 29.8 Causes of lower limb ulceration. The main types of leg ulcer tend to affect particular sites.

Fig. 29.9 A chronic venous ulcer on the medial lower leg, with surrounding lipodermatosclerosis.

ℹ	29.10 Causes of leg ulceration

Venous hypertension

- Sometimes following deep vein thrombosis

Arterial disease

- Atherosclerosis
- Vasculitis
- Buerger's disease

Small-vessel disease

- Diabetes mellitus
- Vasculitis

Haematological disorders

- Sickle-cell disease
- Cryoglobulinaemia
- Spherocytosis
- Polycythaemia
- Myeloma
- Waldenström's macroglobulinaemia
- Immune complex disease

Neuropathy

- Diabetes mellitus
- Leprosy (Hansen's disease)
- Syphilis

Tumour

- Squamous cell carcinoma
- Basal cell carcinoma
- Malignant melanoma
- Kaposi's sarcoma

Trauma

- Injury
- Factitious

29

likely to be due to arterial disease. Risk factors include smoking, hypertension, diabetes and hyperlipidaemia. The foot is cold and dusky, and the skin atrophic and hairless. Peripheral pulses are absent or reduced. A vascular surgical assessment should be sought urgently (p. 502).

Leg ulceration due to vasculitis

Vasculitis can cause leg ulceration either directly through epidermal necrosis due to damage to the underlying vasculature, or indirectly due to neuropathy.

Leg ulceration due to neuropathy

The most common causes of neuropathic ulcers are diabetes and leprosy. Microangiopathy also contributes to ulceration in diabetes (p. 758). The ulcers occur over weight-bearing areas, such as the heel. In the presence of neuropathy, protection of skin from trauma is essential to prevent ulceration.

Investigations

Appropriate investigations include:

- *Full blood count* to detect anaemia and blood dyscrasias.
- *Urea and electrolytes* to assess renal function.
- *Urinalysis* for glycosuria.
- *Bacterial swab* if there is a purulent discharge, rapid extension, cellulitis, lymphangitis or sepsis. This can guide antibiotic therapy for secondary infection but pathogenic bacteria are not always the same as those identified from the ulcer surface.
- *Doppler ultrasound* to assess arterial circulation. An ankle systolic pressure to brachial systolic pressure index (ABPI) of below 0.8 suggests significant arterial disease and a vascular surgery opinion should be sought. However, arterial calcification, such as in diabetes, can produce a spuriously high ABPI. Pulse oximetry may also be useful, although ABPI is the preferred investigation if feasible.

Management

General advice on exercise, weight loss and smoking cessation is important in all cases. Specific management depends on making the correct diagnosis to identify the cause(s) of ulceration. Underlying factors, such as diabetes or anaemia, must be treated. Oedema must be reduced by leg elevation and, if there is no arterial compromise, graduated compression bandaging from toes to knees to enhance venous return and improve healing. Compression bandaging is effective for individuals with an ABPI of more than 0.8 but should be avoided if the ABPI is less than 0.8.

If the ulcer is purulent, weak potassium permanganate soaks may help, and exudate and slough can be removed with normal saline or clean water. Dressings do not themselves heal leg ulcers, but can reduce discomfort and odour and, by reducing colonisation by potential pathogens, may reduce the frequency of secondary infection. A variety of dressings may be used, including non-adherent and absorbent (alginates, hydrogels, hydrocolloids) types. The frequency of dressing changes varies; heavily exudative ulcers may need daily dressings, whereas changes once weekly may suffice for drier ulcers. Occasionally, leeches may be used topically for ulcers with heavy adherent exudate.

Surrounding eczema should be suppressed with a topical glucocorticoid. Commonly, this is venous eczema, but there should be a low threshold for referral for patch testing, as contact allergy to topical applications is common (p. 1215). Systemic antibiotics are indicated only if there is evidence of infection, as opposed to colonisation. Various techniques of split-thickness grafting (such as pinch and mince grafts) may hasten healing of clean ulcers but do not reduce recurrence risk. Leg ulcers can be very persistent. Symptomatic relief, including oral analgesics and sometimes chronic pain management, is important. Once the ulcer has healed, ongoing use of compression hosiery may limit the risk of recurrence.

Abnormal pigmentation

Loss of skin pigmentation (depigmentation), reduction in pigmentation (hypopigmentation) and increased pigment (hyperpigmentation) are features of a variety of disorders. A detailed history and examination, including use of a Wood's light, are required to establish the diagnosis. Investigations will depend on the presentation. For example, microscopy of skin scrapings should be undertaken if hypopigmentation is associated with inflammation and scaling; screening for autoimmune disease may be required if vitiligo is suspected; and investigation for endocrine disease or the porphyrias may be appropriate in hyperpigmentation. Further details of the specific conditions are included on page 1257.

Hair and nail abnormalities

Many conditions affect the skin appendages, particularly hair and nails. Conditions causing hair loss (alopecia) are listed in Box 29.30 (p. 1259). Nail changes may be a marker for systemic disease (e.g. iron deficiency) or be a feature of certain skin conditions (e.g. psoriasis).

Acute skin failure

Acute skin failure is a medical emergency. Several conditions can cause widespread and acute failure of many skin functions (see Box 29.1, p. 1214), including thermoregulation, fluid balance control and barrier to infection. Many of these conditions involve widespread dilatation of the dermal vasculature and can provoke high-output cardiac failure; they are also associated with increased protein loss from the skin and often from the gut. Many lead to acute skin failure by causing erythroderma (erythema affecting at least 90% of the body surface area), although severe autoimmune blistering diseases and the spectrum of Stevens–Johnson syndrome/toxic epidermal necrolysis (TEN) disease can produce acute skin failure without erythroderma (p. 1254).

Clinical assessment

Detailed history-taking and full examination are required. Particular attention should be paid to drug history, chronology and history of any preceding skin disease. Eczema, psoriasis, drug eruptions and cutaneous T-cell lymphoma (Sézary's syndrome, p. 1232) are among the diseases that can either present with, or progress to, erythroderma. Other causes include the psoriasis-like condition, pityriasis rubra pilaris, and rare types of ichthyosis. Erythroderma may occur at any age and is associated with severe morbidity and significant mortality (see Fig. 29.35D, p. 1249). Older people are at greatest risk, especially if they have comorbidities. Erythroderma may appear suddenly or evolve slowly. In dark skin, the presence of pigmentation may mask erythema, giving a purplish hue.

Erythrodermic patients are usually systemically unwell with shivering and hypothermia, secondary to excess heat loss. They may also be pyrexial, however, and unable to lose heat due to damage to sweat gland function and sweat duct occlusion.

Tachycardia and hypotension may be present because of volume depletion. Peripheral oedema is common in erythroderma, owing to low albumin and high-output cardiac failure. Lymph nodes may be enlarged, either as a reaction to skin inflammation or, rarely, due to lymphomatous infiltration.

Investigations and management

Investigations are required to establish the underlying cause and to identify any systemic impact, such as hypoalbuminaemia and electrolyte disturbances. Skin biopsy may be necessary if the cause is unclear. Regardless of the cause, important aspects of the management of erythroderma include supportive measures to ensure adequate hydration, maintenance of core temperature and adequate nutrition. Insensible fluid loss can be many litres above normal losses. Protein may be lost directly from the skin and through the gut because of the protein-losing enteropathy that often accompanies conditions such as erythrodermic psoriasis. To reduce the risks of infection, any intravenous cannulae should be sited in peripheral veins, if possible. In the initial management of acute erythroderma, urinary catheterisation is often required (for patient comfort and accurate fluid balance monitoring) but catheters should be removed as soon as possible. Frequent application of a simple ointment emollient (such as white soft paraffin/liquid paraffin mix) is usually appropriate.

Principles of management of skin disease

General measures

General measures that apply in all skin diseases include establishment of the correct diagnosis, removal of precipitating or aggravating factors, use of safe, effective treatments and consideration of the patient holistically, taking into account the impact of the disease on quality of life and the person's support network. The psychological impact of chronic skin diseases should not be under-estimated and it is important to remember that psychiatric illness can also manifest as a skin disease, such as in delusions of infestation or trichotillomania. Careful clinical assessment, taking psychological factors into account, is essential and any management strategy must include approaches to address the psychological well-being of the patient.

Topical treatments

Topical treatments are first-line therapy for most skin diseases and many can be treated effectively by topical therapies alone. Selection of the appropriate active drug/ingredient and vehicle is essential. Ointments are preferred to creams for dry skin conditions, such as chronic eczemas, as they are more hydrating and contain fewer preservatives than creams, and so allergy risk is reduced. However, patients find creams easier to apply and so adherence may be better. Gels and lotions can be easier to use on hair-bearing sites. The molecular weight and lipid–water coefficient of a drug determine its skin penetration, with larger, water-soluble, polar molecules penetrating poorly. In skin disease, if the stratum corneum is impaired – as in eczema – increased drug absorption occurs. Occlusion under dressings also increases absorption. Drugs can be used in different potencies or concentrations, or in combination with other active ingredients, and many are available in more than one formulation. The properties of different vehicles are listed in Box 29.11. Overall, adherence to topical treatments can be problematic, so it is essential for patients to know exactly what is required of them and for regimens to be kept as simple as possible. Emollients, topical glucocorticoids and other selected key topical therapies that are widely used in a diverse range of skin conditions are detailed below. For the more disease-specific therapies, detailed descriptions are included in the disease sections.

i 29.11 Characteristics of vehicles used in topical treatments

Vehicle	Definition	Use	Site	Cosmetic acceptability	Risk of contact sensitisation
Creams	Emulsions of oil and water (aqueous cream)	Acute presentations Cooling, soothing Well absorbed Mild emollients	All sites, including mucous membranes and flexures, but not hair-bearing areas	Very good Helps adherence	Significant, due to preservatives, antimicrobials and often lanolin
Ointments	Greasy preparations Insoluble in water (white soft paraffin) Soluble (emulsifying ointment)	Chronic dry skin conditions Occlusive and emollient Hydrating Mildly anti-inflammatory	Avoid hair-bearing areas and flexures	Moderate	Low
Lotions	Water-based Liquid formulations Often antiseptic and astringent (potassium permanganate)	Cooling effect Cleans the skin and removes exudates	Large areas of the skin and the scalp	Good, but can sting if in an alcoholic base	Rare
Gels	Thickened lotions Hydrophilic and hydrophobic bases	For specific sites	Hair-bearing areas and the face	Good	Low
Pastes	Semi-solid preparations consisting of finely powdered solids suspended in an ointment	Occlusive, protective Hydrating Circumscribed skin lesions, (psoriasis, lichen simplex chronicus)	Any area of skin Often used in medicated bandages	Moderate	Moderate

29

Emollients

These are mainstays in the treatment of eczema, psoriasis and many other conditions, and are used to moisturise, lubricate, protect and 'soften' skin. They are essentially vehicles without active drug and are available in many formulations: creams, ointments, gels and bath, shower and soap substitutes. White soft paraffin is the most effective and is widely used.

Topical glucocorticoids

Glucocorticoids are available in a variety of formulations, potencies and strengths, most commonly as creams and ointments (Box 29.12). Selection of the correct product depends on the condition being treated, body site and duration of expected use. Mild topical glucocorticoids are used in delicate areas, such as the face or genitals, and close supervision of glucocorticoid use at these sites is required. In contrast, very potent glucocorticoids may be required under occlusion for chronic resistant disease such as nodular prurigo.

Adverse cutaneous effects of chronic glucocorticoid use include atrophy (**definition**: an area of thin, translucent skin caused by loss of epidermis, dermis or subcutaneous fat – Fig. 29.10), striae (**definition**: linear, atrophic, pink, purple or white bands caused by connective tissue changes – Fig. 29.10), petechiae and purpura (**definition**: haemorrhagic macules or papules caused by extravasated blood – see p. 1211) and telangiectasiae (**definition**: visible dilatations of small cutaneous blood vessels – see Fig. 29.11A), increased risk of infection and systemic absorption, causing Cushingoid features and suppression of the hypothalamic–pituitary–adrenal axis. However, under-treatment with glucocorticoids is more common than over-treatment in routine clinical practice. In general, the lowest potency of glucocorticoid should be used for the shortest period to gain control of the disease; this can be achieved by initial use of a more potent glucocorticoid, with reduction in potency or frequency of application as control is gained. Tolerance or tachyphylaxis can develop with chronic use, so intermittent courses of treatment are advised. Caution is required with glucocorticoids in psoriasis, as rebound, unstable or pustular psoriasis can occur with sudden

Fig. 29.10 Striae and atrophy induced by excess prolonged potent topical glucocorticoid use.

cessation of use. Nevertheless, glucocorticoids are invaluable for many sites, particularly the flexures. Topical glucocorticoids are often formulated in combination with antiseptics, antibiotics or antifungals, and their controlled use may be appropriate in infected eczema or flexural psoriasis. Intralesional injections of glucocorticoids can be used in a variety of indications, including nodular prurigo, keloid scar (**definition** of 'scar': replacement of normal structures by fibrous tissue at the site of an injury, although keloid scar describes a pathological process extending beyond the site of injury), acne cysts and alopecia areata.

Anti-infective agents

Antiseptics should be considered before antibiotics, as they cover a wide range of organisms and help to reduce the risk of antibiotic resistance. Antibiotics can be used either for their anti-infective properties (p. 1236) or for their anti-inflammatory properties (pp. 1242 and 1244). Topical antiviral and antifungal agents are also widely used for a range of mild skin infections (p. 1239).

Calcineurin inhibitors

The topical calcineurin inhibitors, tacrolimus and pimecrolimus, can be used to treat eczema and a variety of other conditions, through local cutaneous immunosuppression (p. 1244).

Immune response modifiers

Topical imiquimod was introduced for the treatment of anogenital warts but can be used for a diverse range of other skin diseases, including actinic keratosis, Bowen's disease, basal cell carcinoma, lentigo maligna, cutaneous lupus and common and planar warts. Its mechanism of action is via stimulation of endogenous Th2 immune responses and release of cytokines, including interferon-gamma (IFN-γ). It can cause significant inflammation, requiring dose adjustments, but subclinical disease may respond to treatment.

Dressings

A 'wound' covering is called a dressing. Box 29.13 shows the indications for their use. The active agent, vehicle and 'wound' type should be considered. Wet lesions should be treated with

29.12 Potencies and strengths of commonly used topical glucocorticoid preparations*

Mild
- Hydrocortisone 0.5%, 1%, 2.5%
- Hydrocortisone 1% and fusidic acid 2% (Fucidin H)

Moderate
- Clobetasone butyrate 0.05% (Eumovate)
- Betamethasone valerate 0.025% (Betnovate-RD)
- Fluocinolone acetonide 0.00625% (Synalar 1 : 4)

Potent
- Betamethasone valerate 0.1% (Betnovate)
- Betamethasone valerate 0.1% and clioquinol 3% (Betnovate-C)
- Fluocinolone acetonide 0.025% (Synalar)
- Hydrocortisone butyrate 0.1% (Locoid)
- Mometasone furoate 0.1% (Elocon)

Very potent
- Clobetasol propionate 0.05% (Dermovate)

*UK trade names are given in brackets.

i **29.13 Indications for dressings**

- Protection
- Symptomatic relief from pain or itch
- Maintenance of direct application of topical treatment
- Possible improvement in healing time
- Reduction of exudate
- Reduction of odour

wet dressings. Paste bandages can be used in conjunction with topical emollients and glucocorticoids to soothe and cool, ease pruritus and scratching, and reduce inflammation. Dressings for venous leg ulcers are described on page 1224.

Phototherapy and photochemotherapy

Ultraviolet radiation (UVR) treatments (most commonly, narrowband ultraviolet B and psoralen–ultraviolet A (PUVA)) are used in the management of many different diseases. The best evidence for their efficacy is in psoriasis, atopic eczema, vitiligo and chronic urticaria, although there is also evidence that UVB is helpful in treating generalised itch associated with chronic kidney disease and a range of other diverse skin conditions.

Psoralens are natural photosensitisers found in a number of plants. They intercalate between the strands of DNA and, on excitation with UVA, cross-link the DNA strands. Psoralens are therefore prodrugs that are activated only in skin that is exposed to UVA. Psoralens can also be applied topically in a bath before irradiation with UVA (bath PUVA) or can be applied in creams or gels for localised topical PUVA. PUVA is a more complex treatment than UVB and has more adverse effects; in particular, cumulative exposure to PUVA increases the risk of skin cancer, particularly squamous cell carcinoma. Therefore, PUVA is generally used for poor responders to UVB, or in diseases such as plaque-stage cutaneous T-cell lymphoma or pityriasis rubra pilaris, where it is the phototherapy of first choice. Phototherapy or PUVA may be offered as a whole-body or localised treatment.

Longer-wavelength UVA1 (340–400 nm) is also used for several conditions, particularly the fibrosing skin diseases such as morphoea, where efficacy has been shown and there is a lack of other well-proven therapies. The evidence base for its place in the management of several diseases, such as eczema, is not fully proven and availability of UVA1 is mainly through centres of specialist expertise.

Systemic therapies

General information is provided here for drugs used in a range of skin diseases; details of other drugs are provided in disease-specific sections.

Antibiotics

Antibiotics are generally used for their anti-infective properties, particularly for staphylococcal and streptococcal skin infections. In these indications, the correct antibiotic should be selected, based on bacterial sensitivity and patient factors. As examples, oral flucloxacillin may be indicated for clinically infected eczema, intravenous flucloxacillin for cellulitis, and clarithromycin for a patient with a staphylococcal carbuncle who is penicillin-allergic. Optimal therapeutic doses and courses must be chosen, based

on local antimicrobial prescribing guidelines. Several antibiotics, such as tetracyclines, erythromycin and co-trimoxazole are used predominantly for their anti-inflammatory effects in indications such as acne vulgaris, bullous pemphigoid and pyoderma gangrenosum.

Antihistamines

A range of H_1 and H_2 receptor antagonists are used in dermatology. For diseases in which histamine in the skin is relevant (such as urticaria), non-sedating antihistamines should be given: for example, fexofenadine or cetirizine. For pruritic conditions such as eczema, the sedating effect of antihistamines like hydroxyzine or chlorphenamine is important. However, antihistamines are widely used in older patients for the symptom of pruritus due to a variety of causes such as xeroderma, metabolic impairment, malignancy or concomitant drugs. Sedating antihistamines should be used with caution in older patients, as they may increase the risk of falls and accidents in the home, with disastrous consequences. Careful choice of drug and dose is therefore essential. Leukotriene receptor antagonists, such as montelukast, may be added to antihistamine regimes.

Retinoids

Oral retinoids are used in a range of conditions, including acne, psoriasis and other keratinisation disorders. They promote differentiation of skin cells and have anti-inflammatory effects. Isotretinoin (13-*cis*-retinoic acid) is widely used for moderate to severe acne (p. 1243). Acitretin can be effective in psoriasis and other keratinisation disorders, such as ichthyosis, as can alitretinoin (9-*cis*-retinoic acid) in hand and foot eczema and bexarotene in cutaneous T-cell lymphoma.

Adverse effects of retinoids include dryness of the skin and mucous membranes, abnormalities in liver function or hepatitis, increase in serum triglycerides (levels should be checked before and during therapy) and mood disturbances. Alitretinoin and bexarotene can cause hypothyroidism. Systemic retinoids are teratogenic and must be prescribed along with a robust form of contraception. Females must have a negative pregnancy test before, during and after therapy, and pregnancy must be avoided for 2 months after stopping isotretinoin and 2 years after stopping acitretin.

Immunosuppressants

Systemic glucocorticoids, particularly prednisolone, are widely used in inflammatory skin diseases, such as eczema, immunobullous disease and connective tissue disorders. Methotrexate, azathioprine and mycophenolate mofetil are effective in eczema and psoriasis either alone or as glucocorticoid-sparing agents. Further details on the mechanism of action, adverse effects and monitoring requirements for these agents are provided on page 1004, although it is important to be aware that there may be different approaches to treatment regimens and doses between specialties for some drugs. For example, in dermatology, methotrexate is used in a once-weekly regimen, with doses of up to 25 mg per week, depending on the response (p. 1004). Hydroxycarbamide is an alternative immunosuppressant to methotrexate in psoriasis, but appears to be less effective and the risk of myelosuppression is greater. Ciclosporin (p. 1005) has a rapid onset of action and is effective in inducing clearance of psoriasis and eczema. Monitoring of blood pressure and renal function is required. Ciclosporin should be used only with caution after phototherapy, particularly PUVA, because of the

29

increased risk of skin cancer. Long-term use of ciclosporin is not advised. Dapsone is an immunomodulator and may be used in diseases in which neutrophils are implicated, such as dermatitis herpetiformis (p. 1256). Haemolysis, methaemoglobinaemia and hypersensitivity can occur, and monitoring is required (pp. 123 and 269). Hydroxychloroquine is of particular value in cutaneous lupus. More details on the mechanism of action, adverse effects and monitoring requirements are provided on page 1005.

Biological therapies

Biological inhibitors of pro-inflammatory cytokines, including tumour necrosis factor alpha (TNF-α) inhibitors, ustekinumab (an antibody to the p40 component of interleukin (IL)-12 and IL-23), guselkumab (an antibody to IL-23), secukinumab and ixekizumab (antibodies to IL-17A) and brodalumab (an antibody to the IL-17 receptor) are effective treatments for psoriasis. Rituximab, which causes depletion of B cells, may be used in pemphigus vulgaris. More details on the dosages, mechanism of action and adverse effects of these agents are provided on page 1006. Omalizumab, a monoclonal antibody directed against immunoglobulin E (IgE), was introduced for allergic asthma but may also have a role in non-allergic diseases, such as treatment-resistant urticaria (pp. 86 and 572). Intravenous immunoglobulin, pooled from donor plasma, may be used in the treatment of dermatomyositis (p. 1039) and occasionally may be indicated in other dermatological diseases.

Dermatological surgery

Most dermatological surgical procedures are performed under local anaesthetic. Knowledge of local anatomy is essential, particularly the locations of vessels and nerves. In certain sites, such as the fingers, soles of the feet and nose, local cutaneous nerve blocks are useful. Some sites are associated with particular risks, such as keloidal scarring on the upper trunk of young patients, unsightly scars over the scapulae, and poor healing and risk of ulceration following procedures on the lower legs.

Excision biopsy

This involves surgical removal of the lesion followed by histological examination. The most common indication is suspicion of malignancy. The lesion and line of excision should be marked out and the margin of excision decided before the procedure. It is important to excise down to the appropriate anatomical plane. Depending on body site, a range of procedures can minimise the resulting defect. Healing by secondary intention may also achieve good cosmetic results.

Curettage

Curettage involves using a small, spoon-shaped implement (curette), not only as a definitive treatment but also to obtain histology. Curettage does not preserve tissue architecture very well, however, and it may be difficult to distinguish between dysplasia and invasive malignancy. It can be an effective treatment for basal cell papillomas, actinic keratoses, intra-epidermal carcinoma and superficial basal cell carcinoma.

Shave excision

Shave excision using local anaesthetic may be used for simple and effective treatment of raised superficial benign skin lesions affecting epidermis and upper dermis, such as benign naevi and skin tags.

Mohs' micrographic surgery

Mohs' micrographic surgery is employed to ensure adequate tumour excision margins, while conserving unaffected tissue. It is most commonly used for basal cell carcinoma (p. 1229).

Non-surgical treatments

Cryotherapy

Cryotherapy is a destructive treatment using liquid nitrogen to cause cell-wall and membrane destruction and cell death. Liquid nitrogen can be applied either with a cotton bud or, more effectively, with a spray gun. A wide variety of conditions can be treated but it is essential for the correct diagnosis to be made first, if necessary by diagnostic biopsy. Cryotherapy should not be used to treat melanocytic naevi. Benign lesions, such as viral warts and basal cell papillomas, respond well, and cryotherapy can also be effective for actinic keratoses, Bowen's disease or superficial non-melanoma skin cancer. Malignant indications require more vigorous treatment, usually with two cycles, and this is normally carried out in secondary care. Considerable inflammation, blistering and pigmentary change, particularly hypopigmentation, can occur. Caution is required to avoid damage to tendons and nerves, especially when using cryotherapy on digits.

Laser therapy

Laser therapy involves treatment with monochromatic light. Skin components (chromophores), such as haemoglobin and melanin, absorb specific wavelengths of electromagnetic radiation, and these wavelengths can therefore be used to destroy these targets selectively and to treat certain skin disorders. Lasers targeting haemoglobin are employed for vascular abnormalities, such as spider naevi, telangiectasiae and port-wine stains, and lasers targeting melanin can treat benign pigmentary disorders or pigment in tattoos or drug-induced hyperpigmentation (for example, secondary to minocycline). Melanin lasers can also be used for hair removal if the hair is pigmented. Light delivery in short pulses restricts damage to the treated site.

The carbon dioxide laser emits infrared light that is absorbed by water in tissues and can therefore be used for destructive purposes. The depth of effect can be controlled, such that the carbon dioxide laser is widely employed for resurfacing in photorejuvenation or acne scarring. Significant morbidity is associated with this destructive laser, although this may be minimised with fractionated regimens, and general anaesthesia is usually required.

Photodynamic therapy

Photodynamic therapy (PDT) is widely used in dermatology, predominantly for actinic keratoses, Bowen's disease and superficial basal cell carcinoma (p. 1229).

Radiotherapy and grenz (Bucky) ray therapy

Radiotherapy can be employed for several skin conditions, including non-melanoma skin cancer or lentigo maligna that is not suitable for surgical treatment, but its use in dermatology has declined. Scarring and poikiloderma can occur at treated sites, although these are minimised if fractionated regimens are chosen. Superficial radiotherapy is now rarely employed to treat benign dermatoses. Even more superficial ionising radiation (grenz, or Bucky, rays) can be useful for localised dermatoses that are having severe effects on quality of life, if conventional treatments have been inadequate; for example, it may avoid the need for systemic immunosuppression in a patient with severe recalcitrant localised scalp psoriasis.

Skin tumours

Pathogenesis

Skin cancer is the most common malignancy in fair-skinned populations. It is subdivided into non-melanoma skin cancer (NMSC) and melanoma. NMSC is further subdivided into the most common skin cancer, basal cell carcinoma (BCC), and squamous cell carcinoma (SCC). The latter has precursor non-invasive states of intra-epithelial carcinoma (Bowen's disease, BD) and dysplasia (actinic keratosis, AK). Melanoma is much less common than NMSC, but because of its metastatic risk it is the cause of most skin cancer deaths.

UVR is a complete carcinogen and is the main environmental risk factor for skin cancer, which is much more common in countries with high ambient sun exposure, such as Australia. Skin cancer risk also increases if an individual migrates to such a country when young, particularly if less than 10 years of age. Epidemiological evidence supports a close link between chronic UVR exposure and risk of SCC and AK, and a modest link between sun exposure and BCC risk. Melanoma usually arises on sites that are intermittently exposed to UVR, and episodes of sunburn have been implicated as a risk factor for melanoma. There is good evidence to show that sunbed exposure is also a risk for both melanoma and NMSC, particularly when exposure starts in adolescence and early adult life. Strategies to reduce sun exposure are therefore important for skin cancer prevention, with reliance mainly on behavioural modification, covering up and judicious sunscreen use. Indeed, there is evidence to show that sunscreen use reduces naevi development in children, and in adults regular sunscreen use reduces the risk of AK and SCC and is likely also to have preventative roles in melanoma and BCC development.

There are identifiable genetic predispositions for some skin cancers, such as in xeroderma pigmentosum, an autosomal recessive condition caused by an inherited defect in DNA excision repair (pp. 1221 and 1321), or basal cell naevus (Gorlin's) syndrome, an autosomal dominant disorder caused by loss-of-function mutations affecting the *PTCH1* tumour suppressor genes, with consequent activation of the Hedgehog pathway (p. 1321). Interestingly, the Hedgehog pathway is also almost invariably activated in sporadic BCC, which usually contain somatic mutations in *PTCH1* and less commonly in the *SMO* gene, which lies in the same signalling pathway. The genetics of SCC are heterogeneous and less clearly defined, with several mutations and pathways implicated, including *TP53*, *CDKN2A/p16*, NOTCH, EGFR and the MAPK signalling pathways. Interestingly, many of the mutations seen in SCC also occur in the pre-cancers AK and BD. The genetics of melanoma are discussed on page 1232.

Cutaneous immune surveillance is also critical and immunosuppressed organ transplant recipients have a greatly increased risk of skin cancer, particularly SCC. Interestingly, patients who have received high treatment numbers of PUVA (more than 150), which is immunosuppressive, are also at increased risk of skin cancer, particularly SCC.

Despite UVB being a complete carcinogen, there is no evidence at present that UVB phototherapy significantly increases skin cancer risk, although ongoing vigilance is required. Ionising radiation, notably radiotherapy, thermal radiation and chemical carcinogens, such as arsenic or coal tar, can increase NMSC risk, particularly SCC. A role for oncogenic human papillomaviruses in SCC development is also implicated, particularly in immunosuppressed patients, where viral DNA is detected in more than 80% of tumours. Chronic inflammation is a risk factor for SCC, which may arise in chronic skin ulcers (p. 1223), discoid lupus erythematosus or vulgaris, and the scarring genetic skin disease dystrophic epidermolysis bullosa (see Box 29.25, p. 1254), in which up to 50% of patients develop SCC.

Malignant tumours

Basal cell carcinoma

The incidence of NMSC has increased dramatically in recent decades and basal cell carcinoma (BCC) accounts for more than 70% of cases. In Europe, the ratio of BCC to SCC is 4–5:1 in immunocompetent patients. It is a malignant tumour that rarely metastasises; it is thought to derive from immature pluripotent epidermal cells and is composed of cells with similarities to basal layer epidermis and appendages. Lesions typically occur at sites of moderate sun exposure, particularly the face, and are slow-growing. The incidence increases with age and males are more commonly affected. Lesions may ulcerate and invade locally; hence the term 'rodent ulcer'.

Clinical features

Early BCCs usually present as pale, translucent papules or nodules, with overlying superficial telangiectatic vessels (nodular BCC). If untreated, they increase in size and ulcerate, to form a crater with a rolled, pearled edge and ectatic vessels (Fig. 29.11). There may be some pigmentation or a cystic component. A superficial multifocal type can occur, frequently on the trunk, and may be large (up to 10 cm in diameter); often there are multiple lesions. Superficial BCC usually presents as a red/brown plaque or patch with a raised, thread-like edge, which is

Fig. 29.11 Basal cell carcinoma. A A nodular BCC showing the translucent nature of the tumour and the abnormal arborising vessels. B An ulcerated BCC showing the raised, rolled edge.

29

often best seen by stretching the skin; this helps to distinguish it from Bowen's disease. Less commonly, a morphoeic, infiltrative BCC presents as a poorly defined, slowly enlarging, sclerotic yellow/grey plaque.

Diagnosis and management

The diagnosis is often obvious clinically, based on the features mentioned above, although a diagnostic confirmatory biopsy may be required prior to definitive treatment. Management depends on the characteristics of the tumour and on patient factors, including comorbidities and patient wishes. Essentially, treatment will be either surgical or, in some cases, medical (Box 29.14). Surgical excision, ideally with a 4–5 mm margin, is the treatment of choice, with a cure rate of approximately 95%. Curettage and cautery may also be effective for selected lesions. Management of infiltrative morphoeic BCC and/or lesions at difficult sites, such as around the eye, may require more complex techniques such as Mohs' micrographic surgery to ensure adequate tumour excision margins, while conserving unaffected tissue. This involves processing of frozen sections of all margins in stages (usually on the same day) until all the tumour is removed. The procedure is time-consuming (so can be difficult for elderly, frail patients) and requires particular surgical and pathology skills, but is associated with the highest long-term cure rates, with 98–99% clear at 5-year follow-up.

If a surgical approach is used for management of BCC and the primary tumour is not completely excised, re-excision may be required, although follow-up may be appropriate as not all tumours that are incompletely excised recur. However, this is not recommended for tumours at high-risk sites or for infiltrative morphoeic BCC, where complete excision is advisable. Cryotherapy may be effective for BCC but can cause blistering and scarring, so is best suited to small, superficial lesions at low-risk sites.

Radiotherapy can be invaluable for large BCC lesions in frail patients but is less commonly used because of the risk of scarring.

Medical therapies can be used to treat low-risk BCC, particularly when surgery is not appropriate for a patient. Topical immunomodulators, such as imiquimod, are effective for low-risk BCC and may be particularly useful for patients who are not able to attend a hospital clinic setting but are able to apply a topical preparation at home over a 6-week period. Imiquimod usually induces a prominent inflammatory reaction and patients should be advised that dose adjustments may be required. Topical 5-fluorouracil can also be effective for low-risk small lesions of superficial BCC, but is rarely used since it usually provokes an intense inflammatory reaction. Intralesional interferon-alpha2b has been used for BCC but multiple treatments and high cost preclude its regular use.

PDT is an effective treatment for low-risk, predominantly superficial BCC, as well as AK and BD. Usually, topical porphyrin PDT is employed, which involves application of a porphyrin prodrug to the lesion to be treated. The prodrug is taken up and converted by the cell's haem cycle to protoporphyrin IX, a photosensitiser. This is photochemically activated by visible (normally red) light, usually delivered by a light-emitting diode (LED), in the presence of oxygen, causing the production of reactive oxygen species, which cause destruction of treated tissue. The photosensitiser is taken up preferentially by diseased skin, and adverse effects in normal skin are minimised. PDT is at least as effective as cryotherapy and surgery for superficial BCC and may be preferred at sites of poor healing, such as the lower leg, or where cosmetic outcome is important. PDT is not as effective as surgery for long-term clearance of nodular BCC but can be considered if surgery is not appropriate. Pain during irradiation may occur during PDT, although adjustments to the irradiation regime can reduce discomfort. PDT is usually undertaken in the outpatient clinic setting and is well suited to frail elderly patients who are not able to undertake treatment with topical agents at home.

Rarely, advanced BCC may be locally invasive or even metastasise. Major advances have been made in targeted drug development, and Hedgehog pathway inhibitors, such as vismodegib and sonidegib, can be used effectively for disease control and palliation in this setting, although there may be significant associated drug-induced toxicity.

Squamous cell carcinoma

Squamous cell carcinoma (SCC) is a malignancy that arises from epidermal keratinocytes and is the second most common skin cancer, occurring most frequently in elderly males and smokers. There is a close association between cumulative UVR exposure and SCC risk, with most SCC lesions occurring on chronically sun-exposed sites in white populations and often arising at sites of field-change carcinogenesis, with coexistent precursors of AK and BD commonly evident. In the immunosuppressed patient population, such as organ transplant recipients, SCC is the most common skin cancer and its incidence is dramatically increased, particularly in association with the duration of immunosuppression

---

 29.14 Management of non-melanoma skin cancer and pre-cancer

Basal cell carcinoma

- Excision results in the lowest recurrence rates
- Mohs' micrographic surgery is effective for high-risk BCC
- Medical treatments are often appropriate for low-risk superficial tumours in patients with comorbidities
- Cryotherapy and topical 5-fluorouracil can be used for superficial BCC
- Topical photodynamic therapy and topical imiquimod are both effective in superficial BCC
- BCC in patients with Gorlin's syndrome should not be treated with radiotherapy
- Hedgehog pathway inhibitors can induce clinical response in patients with advanced inoperable BCC

Squamous cell carcinoma

- Excision is the treatment of choice for invasive SCC
- Most recurrences or metastases occur within 5 years
- Medical management is not usually considered for invasive SCC

Carcinoma in situ (Bowen's disease)

- For single/few lesions on good healing sites, cryotherapy, curettage, photodynamic therapy, topical imiquimod and 5-fluorouracil are options
- For multiple lesions and/or poor healing sites such as the lower leg, photodynamic therapy, where feasible, is the treatment of choice, although topical 5-fluorouracil or imiquimod is an alternative

Actinic keratosis

- For single/few lesions on good healing sites, cryotherapy, curettage, 5-fluorouracil/salicylic acid and ingenol mebutate are options, especially if hyperkeratotic
- For multiple lesions/field change, conventional or daylight photodynamic therapy, topical 5-fluorouracil, imiquimod or diclofenac in hyaluronic acid gel may be effective

and the degree of sun exposure and damage accrued pre-transplant. The risk of SCC is also increased in HIV infection. Furthermore, SCC arising in the immunosuppressed is more likely to behave aggressively or to metastasise.

Clinical features

The tumours usually occur on chronically sun-exposed sites, such as bald scalp, tops of ears, face and back of hands. The clinical presentation may be diverse, ranging from rapid development of a painful keratotic nodule in a pre-existing area of dysplasia (Fig. 29.12) to the de novo presentation of an erythematous, infiltrated, often-warty nodule or plaque that may ulcerate. The clinical appearance depends on histological grading; well-differentiated tumours more often present as defined keratotic nodules (Fig. 29.12), whereas poorly differentiated tumours tend to be ill defined and infiltrative, and may ulcerate. SCC has metastatic potential; some tumours, such as those on lips and ears and in immunosuppressed patients, behave more aggressively and are more likely to metastasise to draining lymph nodes.

Management

Early diagnosis is important and complete surgical excision is the usual treatment of choice (see Box 29.14). Standard excision with a 4–6 mm margin is advised and the cure rate is approximately 90–95%. Mohs' surgery is an option but is used less frequently for SCC than for BCC. High-risk SCC should be treated aggressively, with a wider margin of excision of at least 6 mm where feasible. This may include larger, thicker lesions, tumours at sites where metastases are more likely, such as the ear, lip or non-sun-exposed sites, and those occurring in the immunosuppressed and/or with histology showing the tumour to be poorly differentiated, with evidence of lymphatic, vascular or perineural involvement or a high mitotic index. Such patients and those with metastatic disease require management via a multidisciplinary team. In patients who are at high risk for further SCC, systemic retinoids may have a role in reducing the rate of SCC development, but rapid appearance of tumours occurs on drug cessation. Occasionally, curettage and cautery may be appropriate if the tumour is small and low-risk and either surgical excision is contraindicated or the patient is unwilling to proceed. Radiotherapy may be indicated if surgical excision is not feasible. Cryotherapy and topical non-surgical therapies are not usually used in invasive SCC because of risk of recurrence and metastasis.

Actinic keratosis

Actinic keratoses (AK) are scaly, erythematous lesions arising on chronically sun-exposed sites. Histology shows dysplasia, although the diagnosis of typical AK is usually made on clinical grounds (Fig. 29.13). They are common in fair-skinned people who have had significant sun exposure, are often multiple and increase with age. The prevalence is much higher in Australia than in the UK and some surveys have shown a prevalence of more than 50% in those over 40 years old. The rate of progression to SCC is less than 0.1% and spontaneous resolution is possible. However, SCC can also arise de novo and without progression from AK. Increase in size, ulceration, bleeding, pain or tenderness can be indicative of transformation into SCC.

Management

Several treatments are available for AK (see Box 29.14). Emollients and photoprotection, including high-factor sunscreens, may suffice for mild disease. Single or low numbers of lesions of AK can be effectively treated with cryotherapy. Hyperkeratotic lesions may be treated with the antimetabolite 5-fluorouracil, combined with salicylic acid, or may require curettage and cautery.

Multiple lesions require field-directed therapy; 5-fluorouracil is widely used in this setting and is effective but topical imiquimod is an alternative. Diclofenac in a hyaluronic acid gel base can also be used topically for low-grade maintenance control of AK, the rationale for its use being the over-expression of cyclo-oxygenase (COX)-2 in AK lesions. Topical ingenol mebutate can also be used and has the advantage of a short treatment regime, although severe inflammation may be induced. PDT is widely used for field-change multiple AK, with high efficacy rates; it is at least as effective as cryotherapy or 5-fluorouracil. The relative selectivity of treatment allows subclinical disease to be treated, while sparing normal skin. A regimen using daylight to activate the photosensitiser is increasingly used worldwide for extensive mild AK, with high efficacy rates, comparable to hospital-based PDT but without the need for specialised equipment and allowing patients to be treated at home.

Fig. 29.12 **Squamous cell carcinoma.** **A** A centrally keratinous, symmetrical, well-differentiated SCC. Clinically, this could be confused with keratoacanthoma. **B** An SCC arising from an area of epidermal dysplasia.

Fig. 29.13 **Actinic keratosis.** Close-up of a hyperkeratotic AK on the ear.

29

Fig. 29.14 Intra-epidermal carcinoma (Bowen's disease). The lower leg is a common site and lesions are often treated non-surgically.

i	29.15 Classification of cutaneous malignant melanoma

Melanoma without metastatic potential

- Melanoma in situ
- Lentigo maligna

Melanoma with metastatic potential

- Superficial spreading melanoma
- Nodular melanoma
- Acral lentiginous melanoma
- Subungual melanoma
- Lentigo maligna melanoma

Bowen's disease

Clinical features

Bowen's disease (BD) is the name given to an intra-epidermal carcinoma that usually presents as a slowly enlarging, erythematous, scaly plaque on the lower legs of fair-skinned elderly women (Fig. 29.14) but other sites can also be involved. It can be confused with eczema or psoriasis, but is usually asymptomatic and does not respond to topical glucocorticoids. It may also be hard to distinguish from superficial BCC. Transformation into SCC occurs in 3% or less.

Diagnosis

Incisional biopsy is usually undertaken to confirm the diagnosis. This shows an intra-epidermal carcinoma with no invasion through the basement membrane. Histology may also be obtained by curettage but this does not allow distinction from invasive SCC to be made, due to loss of tissue orientation and architecture.

Management

While curettage or excision may be appropriate in some settings, non-surgical therapies are generally preferred (see Box 29.14), especially on the lower legs. PDT, in particular, may be advantageous for BD on the lower leg because of relative selectivity of treatment and sparing of normal tissue, thus reducing the risk of poor healing and ulceration at this vulnerable site. Given the low risk of malignant transformation, the option of no active treatment may also be appropriate for some elderly frail patients.

Cutaneous lymphomas

The most common form of cutaneous T-cell lymphoma is mycosis fungoides (MF). This can persist for years in patch and plaque stages, often resembling eczema or psoriasis. Only sometimes does it progress through to nodules and finally a systemic stage, Sézary's syndrome. B-cell lymphomas, on the other hand, usually present as nodules or plaque-like tumours. The diagnosis of cutaneous T-cell lymphoma requires a high index of suspicion, particularly in patients thought to have unusual recalcitrant forms of eczema or psoriasis.

Treatment is symptomatic and there is no evidence that it alters prognosis. In the early stages of cutaneous T-cell lymphoma, systemic or local glucocorticoids may be indicated; alternatively, narrowband UVB phototherapy (for patch-stage MF) or PUVA (for plaque-stage MF) may be used. Once lesions have moved beyond plaque stage, localised radiotherapy, electron beam radiation, the synthetic retinoid bexarotene, interferon-alpha, extracorporeal photopheresis and systemic anti-lymphoma chemotherapy regimens may be needed. Management of advanced disease invariably requires a multidisciplinary team approach, with collaboration between dermatologists, pathologists and haematological oncologists.

Melanoma

Melanoma is a malignant tumour of epidermal melanocytes. While only 4% of skin cancers are melanomas, they account for 80% of skin cancer deaths. There has been a steady rise in the incidence of melanoma in fair-skinned populations over recent decades, with the highest figures in Australasia. Primary prevention and early detection are essential, as therapy for advanced and metastatic disease remains unsatisfactory.

Pathophysiology

Risk factors for melanoma include fair skin, freckles, red hair, number of naevi and sunlight exposure. The type of sunlight exposure is under debate but intermittent exposure, such as recreational time in the sun, sunburn and sunbed use, is implicated. Patients with multiple atypical naevi (dysplastic naevus syndrome) and fair-skinned people, often with variant alleles in the melanocortin-1 gene, are at increased risk of melanoma. A family history of melanoma increases the risk but a strong family history is unusual. Rarely, autosomal dominant inheritance of melanoma with incomplete penetrance can occur due to mutations in *CDKN2A*, which encodes the p16 tumour suppressor protein. In these patients, the lifetime risk of melanoma is more than 50%. Several other susceptibility genes and potential genetic targets for therapeutic intervention in advanced disease have also been identified.

Clinical features

Melanoma can occur at any age and site and in either sex, but typically affects the leg in females and back in males. It is rare before puberty. The classification of invasive malignant melanoma is shown in Box 29.15. Early lesions may be in situ and pre-invasive before becoming invasive melanoma with metastatic potential. Any change in naevi or development of new lesions should be assessed to exclude malignancy and, for this, the dermatoscope is invaluable (see Fig. 29.2, p. 1217). Real-time non-invasive imaging techniques are being investigated as tools to assist in diagnosis but are largely experimental. If there is any doubt, excision is advised.

Superficial spreading melanoma

Superficial spreading melanoma (SSM) is the most common type in Caucasians. It usually presents as a slowly enlarging, macular, pigmented lesion, with increasing irregularity in shape and pigment; this superficial, radial growth phase can last for

Fig. 29.15 Superficial spreading melanoma. [A] A superficial spreading malignant melanoma with a palpable area indicative of vertical growth phase (Breslow thickness 1.3 mm). [B] A nodular malignant melanoma arising de novo and with Breslow thickness of 3.5 mm.

approximately 2 years. Subsequently, the lesion may become palpable and this is indicative of a vertical growth phase, with dermal invasion; when this occurs, the tumour has the potential to invade lymphatics and vessels and to become metastatic (Fig. 29.15A). Approximately 50% of melanomas arise from a pre-existing naevus.

Nodular melanoma

Nodular melanoma is most common in the fifth and sixth decades, particularly in men and on the trunk (Fig. 29.15B). This may account in part for the increased mortality rates from melanoma in men, as these are tumours with greater metastatic risk. They often present as a rapidly growing nodule that may bleed and ulcerate. Nodular melanomas may be heavily pigmented, or relatively amelanotic and erythematous, and be confused with benign vascular lesions. A rim of pigmentation may, however, be seen under the dermatoscope. Lesions may develop de novo or from a pre-existing naevus or SSM.

Lentigo maligna melanoma

This arises from a prolonged pre-invasive phase termed lentigo maligna. It occurs as a very slowly expanding, pigmented, macular lesion, usually on photo-exposed head and neck sites of elderly patients; histology shows in situ changes only. This phase may last for several years before a nodule of invasive melanoma develops in a proportion of cases (lentigo maligna melanoma).

Acral lentiginous or palmoplantar melanoma

This accounts for only approximately 10% of melanomas in fair-skinned races and is more common in dark-skinned people, in whom it is responsible for 50% of cases. This indicates that UVR exposure may not be implicated in acral melanoma risk.

Subungual melanoma

This form of melanoma is rare. It may present as a painless, proximally expanding streak of pigmentation arising from the nail matrix, and progresses to nail dystrophy and involvement of the adjacent nail fold (Hutchinson's sign).

Diagnosis and management

The diagnosis is made by excision biopsy of a suspicious lesion. The initial biopsy should include a 2 mm margin, followed up where possible by wider excision if the diagnosis is confirmed. Occasionally, radiotherapy or imiquimod may be used for lentigo maligna, if surgery is not feasible. The Breslow thickness of the tumour (the maximal depth from epidermal granular cell layer to deepest tumour cells) is critical for management and prognosis. The presence of ulceration may lead to under-estimation of the Breslow thickness. The mitotic rate and the presence or absence of any evidence of lymphovascular or perineural involvement should also be ascertained. The clinical staging of melanoma extent is essential, in order to establish whether disease is primary and localised, or if there is nodal or metastatic spread.

Wide excision of melanoma with a low risk of metastasis (stage 1 disease, Breslow thickness <1 mm) with a 1 cm clear margin is accepted practice. The margin of excision for more advanced disease is controversial, although a 2–3 cm margin for thicker tumours is generally advised as an attempt to reduce risk of local recurrence. There is no evidence that more radical surgery with 4–6 cm margins is beneficial. The majority of tumours can be excised without the need for grafting. For tumours with a Breslow thickness of 1 mm or more, a sentinel lymph node biopsy should be considered. This is usually performed at the time of wider excision and involves injection of radio-labelled blue dye at the site of the primary melanoma, allowing identification of the draining 'sentinel' node by radioscintigraphy; this sentinel node is then removed and examined in detail by histology, immunohistochemistry and/or PCR of melanocyte gene products to look for tumour deposits. If the biopsy is positive, local lymphadenectomy is usually offered. This procedure provides additional prognostic information but there is no evidence that it improves survival. Local recurrence of disease and palpable local node involvement should be treated surgically. Localised cutaneous metastases or in transit disease may be amenable to palliation with electrochemotherapy if there is no evidence of widespread metastatic disease.

Despite the major advances in treatment options for advanced melanoma, the prognosis for metastatic disease remains poor and treatment options are palliative. Genetic developments have facilitated the introduction of tumour-targeted treatments for advanced, unresectable and/or metastatic disease, such as the *B-Raf* and *c-Kit* kinase inhibitors for patients expressing these gene mutations, notably dabrafenib and vemurafenib, with demonstrable clinical responses. Immunotherapy with ipilimumab, which blocks T-cell activation by inhibiting CTLA-4, alone or in combination with the programmed cell death (PD1) pathway blockers nivolumab or pembrolizumab, provides clinically meaningful improvements in quality of life and survival to patients with advanced disease. Standard chemotherapy may also be used in some cases of metastatic disease, although outcomes are poor. Other biological and gene therapies and vaccines are also being investigated. It is important for patients with advanced melanoma to be managed through a multidisciplinary team in order to optimise care and facilitate their inclusion in clinical trials.

All patients should be advised regarding ongoing photoprotection, with sensible behaviour in the sun, covering up, wearing hats and high-factor sunscreen use. However, evidence has shown that despite patients with melanoma being advised to photoprotect, many follow this advice only for the first year following diagnosis, thus emphasising the need for ongoing reinforcement of guidance with regard to photoprotection. It is also prudent to advise patients who are photoprotecting to optimise oral vitamin D through diet and/or supplements.

Prognosis

Patients with a primary tumour of less than 1 mm Breslow thickness have more than a 95% chance of disease-free survival

29

at 10 years, but this figure drops to approximately 50% for a tumour of greater than 3.5 mm thickness. Survival rates fall to less than 10% for those with advanced nodal or metastatic disease.

Benign skin lesions

In practice, it is often difficult to distinguish between skin cancer and a benign lesion on clinical grounds; if there is any doubt, biopsy and histology are required. Benign melanocytic naevi and basal cell papillomas, in particular, can often be mistaken for melanoma, even by dermatologists. Keratoacanthoma, while benign, is also commonly considered to be invasive SCC on clinical grounds.

Keratoacanthoma

This benign tumour has a striking clinical presentation of rapid growth over weeks to months and subsequent spontaneous resolution. It is thought to be associated with chronic sun exposure and most commonly occurs on the central face. The classical appearance is of an isolated dome-shaped nodule often of 5 cm or more in diameter, with a central keratin plug (Fig. 29.16). Clinically and histologically, the lesion often resembles SCC (see Fig. 29.12A). Most are treated surgically, either by curettage and cautery or by excision, to rule out SCC and to avoid the unsightly scar after spontaneous resolution.

Freckle

Histologically, a freckle (ephelis) consists of normal numbers of melanocytes, but with focal increases in melanin in keratinocytes. They are most common on sun-exposed sites in fair-skinned individuals, particularly children and those with red hair, and on the face. There is a familial tendency. Clinically, freckles are brown macules that darken following UVR exposure.

Lentigo

A lentigo (plural lentigines) consists of increased numbers of melanocytes along the basement membrane, but without formation of the nests that occur in melanocytic naevi. These lesions usually occur at sites of chronic sun exposure (see the

background skin changes in Fig. 29.12A), become more common with age, and are often referred to as 'liver spots' or 'age spots'. They can vary in colour from light to very dark brown. Distinction from melanoma is essential and histology may be required.

Haemangiomas

Benign vascular tumours or hamartomas are common and include Campbell de Morgan spots (Fig. 29.17), which present as pink/red papules on the upper half of the body. They can sometimes be difficult to distinguish from melanocytic lesions, particularly if they are thrombosed or occur on particular sites, such as the lip or genitalia. The dermatoscope is helpful for this (see Fig. 29.2, p. 1217).

Basal cell papilloma

Basal cell papillomas (also known as seborrhoeic warts or keratoses) are common, benign epidermal tumours (Fig. 29.17). They may be flat, raised, pedunculated or warty-surfaced, and can appear to be 'stuck on'. They occur in both sexes and with increasing age, and are most common on the face and trunk. The colour may vary from yellow to almost black and the surface may seem 'greasy', with pinpoint keratin plugs visible, particularly with a magnifying lens. If there is no doubt about the diagnosis, they can be left alone or treated by cryotherapy or curettage if they are cosmetically troublesome. If there is a suspicion of melanoma, excision or diagnostic biopsy should be undertaken.

Melanocytic naevi

Melanocytic naevi (moles) are localised benign clonal proliferations of melanocytes. It is thought that they may arise as the result of abnormalities in the normal migration of melanocytes during development. It is quite normal to have 20–50, although, interestingly, individuals with red hair have fewer. Genetic and environmental factors are implicated. Monozygotic twins have higher concordance in naevi numbers than dizygotic twins. Individuals who have had greater sun exposure have higher numbers of naevi. Most melanocytic naevi appear in childhood and early adult life, or during pregnancy or oestrogen therapy. The onset of a new mole is less common after the age of 25 years. Congenital melanocytic naevi occur at or shortly after birth.

Fig. 29.16 Keratoacanthoma.

Fig. 29.17 A typical basal cell papilloma. Note the neighbouring basal cell papillomas and the coincidental benign angiomas (Campbell de Morgan spots).

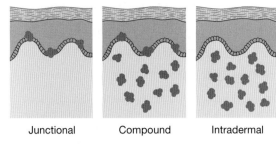

Junctional   Compound   Intradermal

Fig. 29.18 Classification of melanocytic naevi. Classification is based on microscopic location of the nests of naevus cells.

Clinical features

Acquired melanocytic naevi are classified according to the microscopic location of the melanocyte nests (Fig. 29.18). Junctional naevi are usually macular, circular or oval, and mid- to dark brown. Compound and intradermal naevi are nodules because of the dermal component, and may be hair-bearing. Intradermal naevi are usually less pigmented than compound naevi. Their surface may be smooth, cerebriform, hyperkeratotic or papillomatous.

Some individuals have large numbers of naevi, often at unusual sites, such as the scalp, palms or soles, and these may frequently appear 'atypical' in terms of variability in pigmentation, size and shape. Some may be very dark or pink and may show a depigmented or inflamed halo. If these naevi are removed, then 'dysplastic changes' are often seen. Such naevi are known to occur in some rare families with an inherited melanoma predisposition. However, the significance of such changes in non-familial cases is unclear and there is no consensus on management and follow-up.

Although approximately 50% of melanomas arise in pre-existing naevi, most naevi do not become malignant; although a changing naevus must be taken seriously, most will not be melanomas. Malignant change is most likely in large congenital melanocytic naevi (risk may correlate with the size of the lesion) and possibly in families who have been diagnosed as showing large numbers of atypical naevi with a history of melanoma.

Diagnosis and management

Melanocytic naevi are normal and do not require excision, unless malignancy is suspected or they become repeatedly inflamed or traumatised. Advice on photoprotection is important for fair-skinned individuals with multiple naevi.

Blue naevi

These are melanocytic naevi in which there is a proliferation of spindled melanocytes relatively deep within the dermis. Light scattering means that the pigment appears blue rather than brown. They may be difficult to distinguish from nodular melanoma and are therefore often excised.

Dermatofibroma

A dermatofibroma is a characteristically firm, often pigmented, raised lesion, most commonly found on the lower legs. Its aetiology is unclear, although a reactive process secondary to insect bites or trauma is one hypothesis. There is frequently a ring of pigment around the lesion and dimpling when the skin is pinched, reflecting epidermal tethering.

Acrochordon

Acrochordons, or skin tags, are benign pedunculated lesions; they are most common in skin flexures and usually have a very characteristic clinical appearance. However, they may sometimes be confused with melanocytic naevi. Treatment is not required unless there is diagnostic doubt or they are causing symptoms, such as irritation, or for cosmetic reasons. Cryotherapy or snip or shave excision may be appropriate in that situation.

Lipoma

Lipomas are benign tumours of adipocytes that are characteristically soft and lie more deeply in the skin than epidermal tumours; they are usually diagnosed easily on clinical grounds. A variant, angiolipoma, is typically painful. Treatment is not required unless there is diagnostic doubt or they are symptomatic or cosmetically troublesome, in which case a diagnostic biopsy or surgical excision may be required.

Common skin infections and infestations

Bacterial infections

Impetigo

Impetigo is a common and highly contagious superficial bacterial skin infection. There are two main presentations: bullous impetigo, caused by a staphylococcal epidermolytic toxin, and non-bullous impetigo (Fig. 29.19), which can be caused by either *Staphylococcus aureus* or streptococci, or both together. *Staphylococcus* spp. are the most common agents in temperate climates, whereas streptococcal impetigo is more often seen in hot, humid areas. All ages can be affected but non-bullous disease particularly affects young children, often in late summer. Outbreaks can arise in conditions of overcrowding

Fig. 29.19 Non-bullous impetigo.

29

and poor hygiene or in institutions. A widespread form can occur in neonates. Predisposing factors are minor skin abrasions and the existence of other skin conditions, such as infestations or eczema.

In non-bullous impetigo, a thin-walled vesicle develops; it rapidly ruptures and is rarely seen intact. Dried exudate, forming golden crusting, arises on an erythematous base. In bullous disease, the toxins cleave desmoglein-1, causing a superficial epidermal split and the occurrence of intact blisters with clear to cloudy fluid, which last for 2–3 days. The face, scalp and limbs are commonly affected but other sites can also be involved, particularly if there are predisposing factors such as eczema. Lesions may be single or multiple and coalesce. Constitutional symptoms are uncommon. A bacterial swab should be taken from blister fluid or an active lesion before treatment commences. Around one-third of the population is a nasal carrier of *Staphylococcus*, so swabs from the nostrils should also be obtained.

In mild, localised disease, topical treatment with mupirocin or fusidic acid is usually effective and limits the spread of infection. The use of topical antiseptics and soap and water to remove infected crusts is also helpful. Staphylococcal carriage should be treated, with mupirocin topically to the nostrils, if swabs are positive. In severe cases, an oral antibiotic, such as flucloxacillin or clarithromycin, is indicated. If nephritogenic streptococci are isolated then systemic antibiotics should be considered to reduce the risk of streptococcal glomerulonephritis (p. 401). Underlying disease, such as infestations, must be treated and cross-infection minimised. Scarring does not occur but there may be temporary dyspigmentation.

Staphylococcal scalded skin syndrome

Staphylococcal scalded skin syndrome (SSSS) is a potentially serious exfoliating condition occurring predominantly in children, particularly neonates (Fig. 29.20). It is caused by systemic circulation of epidermolytic toxins from a *Staph. aureus* infection. The same toxins are implicated in bullous impetigo, which is a localised form of SSSS. The focus of infection may be minor skin trauma, the umbilicus, urinary tract or nasopharynx. The child presents with fever, irritability and skin tenderness. Erythema usually begins in the groin and axillae, and around the mouth. Blisters and superficial erosions develop over 1–2 days and can rapidly involve large areas, with severe systemic upset. Bacterial swabs should be obtained from possible primary sites of infection. A skin snip should also be taken for urgent histology. This is a sample of the superficial peeling skin removed by 'snipping with scissors', without the need for local anaesthetic. It shows a split beneath the stratum corneum, and differentiates SSSS from toxic epidermal necrolysis, in which the whole epidermis is affected (see Fig. 29.41, p. 1254). Systemic antibiotics and intensive supportive measures should be commenced immediately. Bacterial swabs from nostrils, axillae and groins should be taken from family members to exclude staphylococcal carriage. Although the acute presentation of SSSS is often severe, rapid recovery and absence of scarring are usual, as the epidermal split is superficial.

Toxic shock syndrome

This condition is characterised by fever, desquamating rash, circulatory collapse and multi-organ involvement (p. 252). It is caused by staphylococcal toxins and early cases were thought to arise with tampon use. Intensive supportive care and systemic antibiotics are required.

Fig. 29.20 Staphylococcal scalded skin syndrome. [A] Extensive erythema and superficial peeling of the skin. [B] The condition was rapidly diagnosed by examination of a frozen section of skin snip. *A, From Savin JA, Dahl M, Hunter JAA. Clinical dermatology, 3rd edn. Oxford: Blackwell; 2002.*

Ecthyma

Ecthyma is caused by either staphylococci or streptococci, or both together, and is characterised by adherent crusts overlying ulceration. It occurs worldwide but is more common in the tropics. In Europe, it occurs more frequently in children. Predisposing factors include poor hygiene, malnutrition and underlying skin disease, such as scabies. It is commonly seen in drug abusers, and minor trauma can predispose to lesion development.

Folliculitis, furuncles and carbuncles

Hair follicle inflammation can be superficial, involving just the ostium of the follicle (folliculitis), or deep (furuncles and carbuncles).

Superficial folliculitis

The primary lesions are follicular pustules and erythema. Superficial folliculitis is often infective, caused by *Staph. aureus*, but can also be sterile and caused by physical (for example, traumatic epilation) or chemical (for example, mineral oil) injury. Staphylococcal folliculitis is most common in children and often occurs on the scalp or limbs. Pustules usually resolve without scarring in 7–10 days but can become chronic. In older children and adults, they may progress to a deeper form of folliculitis. The condition

Fig. 29.21 Staphylococcal carbuncle.

is often self-limiting and may respond to irritant removal and antiseptics. More severe cases may require topical or systemic antibiotics and treatment of *Staph. aureus* carrier sites.

Deep folliculitis (furuncles and carbuncles)

A furuncle (boil) is an acute *Staph. aureus* infection of the hair follicle, usually with necrosis. It is most common in young adults and males. It is usually sporadic but epidemics occasionally occur. Malnutrition, diabetes and HIV predispose, although most cases arise in otherwise healthy people. Any body site can be involved but neck, buttocks and anogenital areas are common. Infection is often associated with chronic *Staph. aureus* carriage in the nostrils and perineum, and may be due to resistant strains, such as meticillin-resistant organisms (MRSA). Friction caused by tight clothing may be contributory. Initially, an inflammatory follicular nodule develops and becomes pustular, fluctuant and tender. Crops of lesions sometimes occur. There may be fever and mild constitutional upset. Lesions rupture over days to weeks, discharge pus, become necrotic and leave a scar.

If a deep *Staph. aureus* infection of a group of contiguous hair follicles occurs, this is termed a carbuncle and is associated with intense deep inflammation (Fig. 29.21). This usually occurs in middle-aged men, often with predisposing conditions such as diabetes or immunosuppression. A carbuncle is an exquisitely tender nodule, usually on the neck, shoulders or hips, associated with severe constitutional symptoms. Discharge, necrosis and scarring are usual. Bacterial swabs must be taken and treatment is with anti-staphylococcal antibiotics, e.g. flucloxacillin, and sometimes incision and drainage.

Other staphylococcal toxins may also be pathogenic. For example, Panton–Valentine leukocidin-producing *Staph. aureus* can cause recurrent abscesses (**definition**: localised collections of pus in cavities) and may be difficult to eradicate.

Cellulitis and erysipelas

Cellulitis is inflammation of subcutaneous tissue, due to bacterial infection (Fig. 29.22). In contrast, erysipelas is bacterial infection of the dermis and upper subcutaneous tissue (Fig. 29.23), although in practice it may be difficult to distinguish between them. These conditions are most commonly caused by group A streptococci but culture of swabs from affected sites is often negative. There is frequently a source of organism entry, such as an ear infection, varicose eczema/ulcer or tinea pedis, and swabs should also be taken from these sites. Diabetes and immunosuppression are predisposing factors. The patient usually

Fig. 29.22 Acute cellulitis of the leg. Note the chronic lymphoedema and the haemorrhagic blistering. Blister fluid was positive for group G streptococci.

Fig. 29.23 Erysipelas. Note the blistering and the crusted rash with raised, erythematous edge. The yellow discoloration is due to topical iodine treatment.

has malaise, fever and leucocytosis, and streptococcal serology will often be positive. The face (erysipelas) and legs (cellulitis) are most often affected and the site is hot, painful, erythematous and oedematous. Blistering often occurs and may be haemorrhagic. Regional lymphadenopathy is common. Erysipelas typically has a well-defined edge due to its more superficial level of involvement, whereas cellulitis is typically ill defined. Treatment is usually with intravenous flucloxacillin, with clarithromycin, clindomycin and vancomycin as alternatives for penicillin-allergic patients. Milder cases may be treated with oral antibiotics. If cases are untreated, sequelae include lymphoedema, cavernous sinus thrombosis, sepsis and glomerulonephritis.

Mycobacterial infections

Mycobacterium leprae infection may involve the skin and its manifestations will be influenced by host immunity, patients with high levels of immunity presenting with paucibacillary

29

tuberculoid leprosy and those with low immune resistance developing multibacillary lepromatous leprosy. Hypopigmented or erythematous patches, with associated altered or lost sensation, or skin thickening, nodules and infiltration should raise suspicion of a diagnosis of leprosy (p. 267).

The skin may also be an extrapulmonary site of involvement in tuberculosis, usually due to infection with *Mycobacterium tuberculosis*. Skin manifestations depend on the route of infection, previous sensitisation and host immunity. There may be a variety of cutaneous features, including the red–brown scarring inflammatory plaques seen in lupus vulgaris due to direct skin inoculation; scrofuloderma, which describes the skin changes overlying lymph nodes or joints infected with tuberculosis; and the reactive nodular and ulcerated changes seen in patients with high levels of immune response, notably the tuberculids and erythema induratum (Bazin's disease). On diascopy, an 'apple jelly' appearance is typically seen, indicating the granulomatous nature of skin involvement. Granulomas evident on skin biopsy should certainly raise suspicion of a diagnosis of mycobacterial infection. Culture of organisms may be tricky but PCR can assist with diagnosis. Patients should be thoroughly investigated for signs of tuberculosis at pulmonary or other extrapulmonary sites (p. 588). Reactivation of latent tuberculosis is a particular concern for patients receiving treatment with immunosuppressants and biological agents, particularly TNF-α antagonists for conditions such as psoriasis. Vigilance is required in screening and workup of such patients prior to consideration of these therapeutic agents.

Other mycobacterial skin infections may occur, such as *Mycobacterium marinum*, typically seen in those who clean tropical fish tanks. Sporotrichoid spread of granulomatous nodules from the site of inoculation along lymphatics is typical; granulomatous changes are seen on histology and resolution usually occurs with a prolonged course of antibiotics such as doxycycline or minocycline. Resolution may also take place spontaneously or after destructive therapies, such as cryotherapy.

Leishmaniasis

This protozoan infection may be restricted to the skin or there may be may be systemic features depending on the species, which occur in different geographical areas (p. 281).

Necrotising soft tissue infections and anthrax

See pages 226 and 266, respectively.

Erythrasma

Erythrasma is a mild, chronic, localised, superficial skin infection caused by *Corynebacterium minutissimum*, which is part of the normal skin flora. Warmth and humidity predispose to this infection, which usually occurs in flexures and toe clefts. It is asymptomatic or mildly itchy and lesions are well defined, red–brown and scaly. *C. minutissimum* has characteristic coral-pink fluorescence under Wood's light. Microscopy and culture of skin scrapings can confirm the diagnosis but are not usually needed if Wood's light examination is positive. A topical azole (clotrimazole or miconazole) or fusidic acid is usually effective. Oral erythromycin can be used for extensive or resistant disease. Antiseptics can be used to prevent disease recurrence.

Pitted keratolysis

This is another superficial skin infection caused by *Corynebacterium* and *Streptomyces* spp., and possibly other organisms, producing characteristic circular erosions ('pits') on the soles. It is usually asymptomatic. The bacterium can be identified in skin scrapings and typically occurs in association with hyperhidrosis, which must be treated to prevent recurrence. Treatment is as for erythrasma.

Other bacterial skin infections

Syphilis and the non-venereal treponematoses are described on pages 337 and 253. There has been a marked increase in incidence of syphilis. Skin signs may be subtle; for example, secondary syphilis may be misdiagnosed as pityriasis rosea. Lesions on palms, soles and mucosae should raise suspicion. Microscopic identification of the spirochaete may be possible and syphilitic serology should be undertaken using enzyme immunoassay or PCR-based techniques, depending on availability. Lyme disease is described on page 255.

Viral infections

Herpesvirus infections

The cutaneous manifestations of the human herpesviruses are described on page 247. Topical antivirals may suffice for prophylaxis or treatment of mild viral disease, such as herpes simplex cold sore virus infection. Systemic antivirals are indicated for significant viral skin disease. For example, systemic aciclovir should be prescribed for eczema herpeticum (see Fig. 11.14, p. 247).

Papillomaviruses and viral warts

Viral warts are extremely common and are caused by the DNA human papillomavirus (HPV). There are over 90 subtypes, based on DNA sequence analysis, causing different clinical presentations. Transmission is by direct virus contact, in living or shed skin, and is encouraged by trauma and moisture such as in swimming pools. Genital warts are spread by sexual activity and show a clear relationship with cervical and intra-epithelial cancers of the genital area. HPV-16 and 18 appear to inactivate tumour suppressor gene pathways and lead to squamous cell carcinoma of the cervix or intra-epithelial carcinoma of the genital skin (p. 242). Vaccinations are available against HPV-16 and 18 and are recommended for adolescent females before they become sexually active. The relationship between skin HPV and skin cancer is unclear. Individuals who are systemically immunosuppressed – after organ transplantation, for example – have greatly increased risks of skin cancer and HPV infection but a causal link is not certain.

Clinical features

Common warts are initially smooth, skin-coloured papules, which become hyperkeratotic and 'warty'. They are most common on the hands (Fig. 29.24) but can occur on the face, genitalia and limbs, and are often multiple. Plantar warts (verrucae) have a slightly protruding rough surface and horny rim, and are often painful on walking. Paring reveals capillary loops that distinguish plantar warts from corns. Other varieties of wart include:

- *mosaic warts*: mosaic-like sheets of warts
- *plane warts*: smooth, flat-topped papules, usually on the face and backs of hands, which may be pigmented and therefore misdiagnosed
- *facial warts*: often filiform
- *genital warts*: may be papillomatous and exuberant.

Fig. 29.24 Viral wart on the finger. The capillary loops are evident within the warty hyperkeratosis. Periungual sites are common and more difficult to treat.

Management

Most viral warts resolve spontaneously, although this may take years and active treatment is therefore often sought. However, asymptomatic warts generally should not be treated. Viral warts are particularly problematic and more recalcitrant to treatment in immunosuppressed patients following organ transplantation.

Treatments are destructive. Salicylic acid or salicylic/lactic acid combinations and regular wart paring for several months are the most consistently effective treatments. For certain types of warts, such as filiform facial warts, cryotherapy is generally the treatment of choice, but for common hand and foot warts salicylic acid wart paint should be used first. Cryotherapy is usually the next step and is repeated 2–4-weekly. However, caution is required, particularly on the hands, as over-vigorous cryotherapy can lead to scarring, nail dystrophy and even tendon rupture. Periungual and subungual warts can be problematic and nail cutting and subsequent electrodessication may help. Several other therapies have been used for recalcitrant warts, including topical formaldehyde, podophyllotoxin, trichloroacetic acid, cantharidin, topical or systemic retinoids, intralesional bleomycin or interferon injections, and contact sensitisation with, for example, diphencyprone. Imiquimod and PDT may also be beneficial, particularly for multiple warts in immunosuppressed patients, and laser therapy can have a role in some cases.

Molluscum contagiosum

Molluscum contagiosum is caused by a DNA poxvirus skin infection. It is most common in children over the age of 1 year, particularly those with atopic dermatitis. It also occurs frequently in immunosuppressed patients, including those with HIV (p. 306). Lesions are dome-shaped, 'umbilicated', skin-coloured papules with central punctum (Fig. 29.25). They are often multiple and found at sites of apposition, such as the side of the chest and the inner arm. Spontaneous resolution occurs but can take months. Prior to resolution, they often become inflamed and may leave small, atrophic scars. Destructive therapies may be painful and risk scarring, and the decision not to treat is often sensible. Gentle squeezing with forceps after bathing can hasten resolution. Topical salicylic acid, podophyllin, cantharidin, trichloroacetic acid, cryotherapy and curettage are alternatives. Efficacy with imiquimod has also been reported.

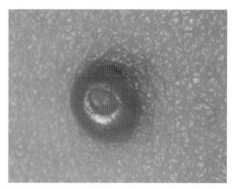

Fig. 29.25 Molluscum contagiosum. Note the central umbilication.

Orf

Orf is a parapoxvirus skin infection and is an occupational risk for those who work with sheep and goats. Inoculation of virus, usually into finger skin, causes significant inflammation and necrosis, which typically resolves within 2–6 weeks. No specific treatment is required, unless there is secondary infection. Erythema multiforme (p. 1264) can be provoked by orf.

Other viral exanthems

See page 236.

Fungal infections

Fungal skin infections can be superficial (dermatophytes and yeasts) or, less commonly, deep (chromomycosis or sporotrichosis); the latter are seen more often in tropical climates or in the immunocompromised. Dermatophyte infections (ringworm) are extremely common and usually caused by fungi of the *Microsporum*, *Trichophyton* and *Epidermophyton* species. The fungi can originate from soil (geophilic) or animals (zoophilic), or be confined to human skin (anthropophilic). Dermatophyte infections usually present with skin (tinea corporis), scalp (tinea capitis), groin (tinea cruris), foot (tinea pedis) and/or nail (onychomycosis) involvement (Fig. 29.26).

Diagnosis

Skin scrapings, hair pluckings or nail clippings must be taken from areas of disease activity – typically, the advancing lesion edge for skin involvement, the crumbling dystrophic nail and subungual hyperkeratosis for nail involvement, and plucked hair from scalp or other affected hair-bearing sites – in order to confirm the diagnosis by microscopy and culture (p. 1215).

Management

The azoles (ketoconazole, miconazole), triazoles (itraconazole, fluconazole) and triallylamines (terbinafine) are used most widely in fungal skin disease. Topical antifungals such as terbinafine or miconazole may suffice, although systemic treatment (terbinafine, itraconazole or griseofulvin) may be required for stubborn or extensive disease and scalp or nail involvement. Indeed, prolonged courses of systemic treatment may be needed for nail involvement. The fungistatic agent griseofulvin, given orally, is usually used for fungal infection of scalp or nails in children in the UK, as it is the only drug licensed in children for this indication; outside the UK, and in adults, terbinafine is usually the treatment of

29

Fig. 29.26 Dermatophyte infections.
A *Trichophyton rubrum* infection of the groin (tinea cruris). B *Microsporum canis* infection of the scalp (tinea capitis).

choice. In addition to systemic antifungals, short courses of systemic or topical glucocorticoid are often used in kerion on the basis of reducing inflammation and possible hair loss. However, glucocorticoid use is controversial, with no good evidence of benefit.

Tinea corporis

Tinea corporis should feature in the differential diagnosis of a red, scaly rash (p. 1217). Typically, lesions are erythematous, annular and scaly, with a well-defined edge and central clearing. There may also be pustules at the active edge. Lesions are usually asymmetrical and may be single or multiple. The degree of inflammation is dependent on the organism involved and the host immune response. *Microsporum canis* (from dogs) and *Trichophyton verrucosum* (from cats) are common culprits. Ill-advised use of topical glucocorticoids can modify the clinical presentation and increase disease extension (tinea incognito).

Tinea cruris

This is extremely common worldwide and is usually caused by *Trichophyton rubrum*. Itchy, erythematous plaques develop in the groins and extend on to the thighs, with a raised active edge (Fig. 29.26A).

Tinea pedis

Tinea pedis or 'athlete's foot' is the most common fungal infection in the UK and USA, and is usually caused by anthropophilic fungi, such as *T. rubrum*, *T. interdigitale* and *Epidermophyton floccosum*. It typically presents as an itchy rash between the toes, with peeling, fissuring and maceration. Involvement of one sole or palm (tinea manuum) with fine scaling is characteristic of *T. rubrum* infection. Vesiculation or blistering is more often seen with *T. mentagrophytes*.

Tinea capitis

This is a dermatophyte infection of scalp hair shafts and is most common in children. It typically presents as an area of scalp inflammation and scaling, often with pustules and partial hair loss (Fig. 29.26B). Infection may be within the shaft (endothrix, most commonly caused by *T. tonsurans*), causing patchy hair loss with broken hairs at the surface ('black dot'), little inflammation and no fluorescence with Wood's light. Infection outside the hair shaft (ectothrix, most commonly caused by *Microsporum*

audouinii (anthropophilic)) shows minimal inflammation; *M. canis* (from dogs and cats) infections are more inflammatory and can be identified by green fluorescence with Wood's light. Kerion is a boggy, inflammatory area of tinea capitis, usually caused by zoophilic fungi such as cattle ringworm (*T. verrucosum*).

Onychomycosis

This is a fungal infection of the nail plate and the species involved are generally those that cause tinea capitis or tinea pedis. Onychomycosis usually presents with yellow/brown nail discoloration, crumbling, thickening and subungual hyperkeratosis. Usually, some nails are spared, there is asymmetry and toenails are more commonly involved.

Candidiasis

This is a superficial skin or mucosal infection caused by a yeast-like fungus, *Candida albicans* (p. 300). Infections are usually not serious, unless the patient is immunocompromised, in which case deeper tissues can be involved (p. 316). The organism has a predilection for warm, moist environments and typical presentations are napkin candidiasis in babies, genital and perineal candidiasis, intertrigo and oral candidiasis. The diagnosis can be confirmed by microscopy and culture of skin swabs, and treatment is with topical or systemic antifungals, such as azoles.

Pityriasis versicolor

Pityriasis versicolor is a persistent, superficial skin condition caused by various species of the commensal yeast *Malassezia*, most commonly *Malassezia globosa*, but sometimes *M. sympadialis* or *M. furfur*, It occurs in men and women and in different races. It is found more frequently in warmer, humid climates, and is usually more severe and persistent in the immunocompromised. It is characterised by scaly, oval macules on the upper trunk, usually hypopigmented but occasionally hyperpigmented. Hypopigmentation is more obvious after sun exposure and tanning. The diagnosis can be confirmed by microscopy of skin scrapings, showing 'spaghetti and meatballs' hyphae. Treatment with selenium sulphide or ketoconazole shampoos and topical or systemic azole antifungal agents is usually effective, although recurrence is common because these yeasts are skin commensals, and maintenance topical therapy may be required. Altered pigmentation can persist for months after treatment.

Infestations

Scabies

Scabies is caused by the mite *Sarcoptes scabiei*. It spreads in households and environments where there is intimate personal contact. The diagnosis is made by identifying the scabietic burrow (**definition**: a linear or curvilinear papule, caused by a burrowing scabies mite; p. 234 and Fig. 29.27) and visualising the mite (by extracting with a needle or using a dermatoscope). In small children, the palms and soles can be involved, with pustules. Pruritus is prominent. The clinical features include secondary eczematisation elsewhere on the body; the face and scalp are rarely affected, except in infants. Involvement of the genitals in males and of the nipples commonly occurs. Even after successful treatment, itch can continue and occasionally nodular lesions persist.

Topical treatment of the affected individual and all asymptomatic family members/physical contacts is required to ensure eradication. Two applications 1 week apart of an aqueous solution of permethrin or malathion to the whole body, excluding the head, are usually successful. If there is poor adherence, immunosuppression or heavy infestation (crusted 'Norwegian' scabies), systemic treatment with a single oral dose of ivermectin is sometimes appropriate.

Head lice

Infestation with the head louse, *Pediculus humanus capitis*, is common. It is highly contagious and spread by direct head-to-head contact. Scalp itch leads to scratching, secondary infection

Fig. 29.27 Scabies. [A] Burrows evident on the palm of the hand. [B] A mite still in its egg, seen on light microscopy of scrapings over a burrow. Note that the mite has only six legs, unlike adult mites, which have eight.

and cervical lymphadenopathy. The diagnosis is confirmed by identifying the living louse or nymph on the scalp or on a black sheet of paper after careful fine-toothed combing of wet hair following conditioner application. The empty egg cases ('nits') are easily seen on the hair shaft (p. 1210) and are hard to dislodge.

Treatment is recommended for the affected individual and any infected household/school contacts. Eradication in school populations is difficult because of poor adherence and treatment resistance. Topical treatment with dimeticone, permethrin, carbaryl or, less often, malathion in lotion or aqueous formulations may be effective and should be applied twice at an interval of 7–10 days. Rotational treatments within a community may avoid resistance. 'Wet-combing' (physical removal of live lice by regular combing of conditioned wet hair – 'bug busting') can suffice but may be less effective than pharmacological treatments. Vaseline should be applied to eyelashes/brows twice daily for at least a fortnight. High-temperature washing of clothing and bedding is required. Treatment resistance and recurrence can be problematic.

Body lice

These are similar to head lice but live on clothing, particularly in seams, and feed on the skin. Poor hygiene and overcrowded conditions predispose. Itch, excoriation (**definition**: a linear ulcer or erosion resulting from scratching) and secondary infection occur. Dry-cleaning and high-temperature washing or insecticide treatment of clothes are required. Treatment options are as for head lice. For heavy infestation, oral ivermectin may be indicated.

Pubic (crab) lice

Usually, these are sexually acquired and very itchy. Management is as for head and body lice and whole-body treatment should be undertaken. Pubic hair may need to be shaved. Sexual and other close contacts should also be treated and patients should also be screened for sexually transmitted diseases.

Acne and rosacea

Acne vulgaris

Acne is chronic inflammation of the pilosebaceous units. It is extremely common, generally starts during puberty and has been estimated to affect over 90% of adolescents. It is usually most severe in the late teenage years but can persist into the thirties and forties, particularly in females (Box 29.16).

29.16 Acne in adolescence

- **Epidemiology**: acne vulgaris is most common between the ages of 12 and 20. It often begins around 10–13 years of age, lasts 5–10 years and usually resolves by age 20–25.
- **Emotional effects**: at all ages acne can have negative effects on self-esteem, but it is especially important to assess how it affects an adolescent. Depression and suicideal ideation may occur. The consequences (whether acne is objectively severe or not) can be devastating, leading to embarrassment, school avoidance, and life-long effects on ability to form friendships, attract partners, and acquire and keep employment.
- **Treatment**: effective treatments aim to improve the condition, prevent worsening (including later scarring) and restore emotional well-being and self-esteem.

29

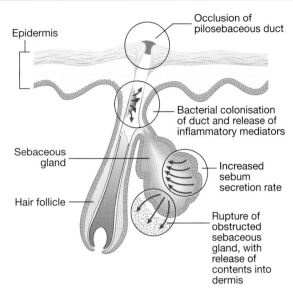

Fig. 29.28 Pathogenesis of acne.

Fig. 29.29 **Cystic acne in a teenager.** A Before treatment. B After prolonged systemic antibiotic treatment.

Pathogenesis

The key components are increased sebum production; colonisation of pilosebaceous ducts by *Propionibacterium acnes*, which in turn causes inflammation; and hypercornification and occlusion of pilosebaceous ducts (Fig. 29.28). Severity of acne is associated with sebum excretion rate, which increases at puberty. Both androgens and progestogens increase sebum excretion and oestrogens reduce it, but most patients with acne have normal hormone profiles. There may be a positive family history and there is high concordance in monozygotic twins, indicating that genetic factors are important, but the candidate genes are poorly defined.

Clinical features

Acne usually affects the face and often the trunk. Greasiness of the skin may be obvious (seborrhoea). The hallmark is the comedone (**definition**: open comedones (blackheads) are dilated keratin-filled follicles, which appear as black papules due to the keratin debris; closed comedones (whiteheads) usually have no visible follicular opening and are caused by accumulation of sebum and keratin deeper in the pilosebaceous ducts – Fig. 29.28). Inflammatory papules, nodules and cysts occur and may arise from comedones (Fig. 29.29). Scarring may follow deep-seated or superficial acne and may be keloidal.

There are also distinct clinical variants:

- *Acne conglobata*: characterised by comedones, nodules, abscesses, sinuses (**definition**: cavities or channels that permit the escape of pus or fluid) and cysts, usually with marked scarring. It is rare, usually affecting adult males, and most commonly occurs on trunk and upper limbs. It may be associated with hidradenitis suppurativa (a chronic, inflammatory disorder of apocrine glands, predominantly affecting axillae and groins), scalp folliculitis and pilonidal sinus.
- *Acne fulminans*: a rare but severe presentation of acne, associated with fever, arthralgias and systemic inflammation, with raised neutrophil count and plasma viscosity. It is usually found on the trunk in adolescent males. Costochondritis can occur.

- *Acne excoriée*: self-inflicted excoriations due to compulsive picking of pre-existing or imagined acne lesions. It usually affects teenage girls, and underlying psychological problems are common.
- *Secondary acne*: comedonal acne can be caused by greasy cosmetics or occupational exposure to oils, tars or chlorinated aromatic hydrocarbons. Predominantly pustular acne can occur in patients using systemic or topical glucocorticoids, oral contraceptives, anticonvulsants, lithium or antineoplastic drugs, such as the epidermal growth factor receptor (EGFR) inhibitors. Most patients with acne do not have an underlying endocrine disorder but acne is a common feature of polycystic ovary syndrome (p. 658), which should be suspected if acne is moderate to severe and associated with hirsutism and menstrual irregularities. Virilisation should also raise suspicion of an androgen-secreting tumour.

Investigations

Investigations are not required in typical acne vulgaris. Secondary causes and suspected underlying endocrine disease or virilisation should be investigated (p. 657).

Management

Mild to moderate disease

Mild disease is usually managed with topical therapy (p. 1225). If comedones predominate, then topical benzoyl peroxide or retinoids should be used. Benzoyl peroxide has both anti-comedogenic and antiseptic effects. It is an irritant, which may contribute to the therapeutic response, but this can be minimised by adjusting treatment regimes. Azelaic acid may also be used for mild acne and has both antimicrobial and anti-comedogenic action. Topical retinoids, in particular *all-trans* retinoic acid and adapalene, are widely employed for mild to moderate comedonal acne vulgaris. Treatment should be initially applied at low concentrations for short duration and increased as tolerated. Patients with mild inflammatory acne should respond to topical antibiotics, such as erythromycin or clindamycin, which can be used in combination with other treatments.

For moderate inflammatory acne, a systemic tetracycline should be used at adequate dose for 3–6 months in the first instance (p. 1227; Fig. 29.29B). Oxytetracycline must be taken on an empty stomach, in a dose of up to 1.5 g a day. It has a good safety profile, even with long-term use, but adherence may be a challenge. Lymecycline is an alternative and is taken once daily, with or without food, thereby improving adherence. Doxycycline is another option but commonly causes photosensitivity. Minocycline is used less frequently, as it can cause hyperpigmentation, autoimmune hepatitis and drug-induced lupus, and monitoring is required. If the patient fails to respond, then alternatives include erythromycin or trimethoprim.

In women with acne, oestrogen-containing oral contraceptives can be a useful adjunct, as they are associated with a small reduction in sebum production. Combined oestrogen and anti-androgen (such as cyproterone acetate) contraceptives may provide additional efficacy, particularly in women with acne and hirsutism, as seen in polycystic ovary syndrome (p. 658).

Patients should be referred for consideration of isotretinoin (13-*cis*-retinoic acid) if there is a failure to respond adequately to 6 months of therapy with these combined systemic and topical approaches (p. 1227).

Moderate to severe disease

Isotretinoin (13-*cis*-retinoic acid) has revolutionised the treatment of moderate to severe acne that has not responded adequately to other therapies. It has multifactorial mechanisms of action, with reduction in sebum excretion by over 90%, follicular hypercornification, *P. acnes* colonisation and inflammation. Oral isotretinoin is usually used at a dose of 0.5–1 mg/kg over 4 months. Sebum excretion typically returns to baseline within a year after treatment cessation, although clinical benefit is usually longer-lasting. Many patients will not require further treatment, although a second or third course of isotretinoin may be needed. A low-dose continuous or intermittent-dose regimen may occasionally be considered for a longer duration in patients who relapse after a higher-dose regimen, and may also be beneficial for older females with persistent acne. Combination with systemic glucocorticoid may be required in the short term for severe acne, in order to minimise the risk of disease flare early in the treatment course. Thorough screening and monitoring are required, given the side-effect profile of isotretinoin, particularly with respect to teratogenicity and possible mood disturbance (p. 1227). Pregnancy must be avoided during treatment and for a minimum of 2 months after drug cessation, and a strict pregnancy prevention programme and regular pregnancy testing are required. Depression and suicide have been reported in association with isotretinoin, although a causal role has not been established. However, pre-drug screening for depressive symptoms should be undertaken and mood monitored during therapy.

Other treatments and physical measures

Intralesional injections of triamcinolone acetonide may be required for inflamed acne nodules or cysts, which can also be incised and drained, or excised under local anaesthetic. Scarring may be prevented by adequate treatment of active acne. Keloid scars may respond to intralesional glucocorticoid and/or silicone dressings. Carbon dioxide laser, microdermabrasion, chemical peeling or localised excision can also be considered for scarring. UVB phototherapy or PDT can occasionally be used in patients with inflammatory acne who are unable to use conventional therapy, such as isotretinoin. There is no convincing evidence to support a causal association between diet and acne. The psychological impact of acne must not be under-estimated and should be considered in management decisions (Box 29.16).

▮ Rosacea

This chronic inflammatory condition affects the central face and consists of flushing, erythema, papules, pustules and telangiectasiae. The cause is unknown. Rosacea is distinct from acne vulgaris; sebum excretion is normal and comedones are absent. The relative contribution of *Demodex* mite and cutaneous vasomotor instability to the pathogenesis of rosacea remains poorly defined.

Clinical features

Rosacea most commonly affects fair-skinned, middle-aged females and can be exacerbated by heat, sunlight and alcohol. The convexities of nose, forehead, cheeks and chin are typically involved (Fig. 29.30). The condition is heterogeneous and intermittent flushing, followed by fixed erythema and telangiectasiae, predominates in some; in others, papules and pustules are prominent. Sebaceous gland hyperplasia and soft tissue overgrowth of the nose (rhinophyma) can occur, particularly in males. Conjunctivitis and blepharitis may also occur. Facial lymphoedema can be an added complication.

Investigations

Usually, no investigations are required and the diagnosis is obvious clinically. However, rosacea must be distinguished from acne vulgaris, systemic lupus erythematosus, photosensitivity disorders and seborrhoeic dermatitis (the latter may coexist with rosacea).

Fig. 29.30 Rosacea. Typical erythematous papulopustular rosacea affecting the mid-face.

29

Management

Mild disease may respond to topical antimicrobials, such as metronidazole or azelaic acid. Topical ivermectin may be beneficial in some cases, supporting a contributory role of *Demodex* in pathogenesis. Tetracycline or erythromycin for 3–6 months is usually effective in inflammatory pustular disease resistant to topical therapy (p. 1227). Relapse may require intermittent or chronic antibiotic use. Erythema and telangiectasiae do not usually respond well to antibiotics but vascular laser therapy may be effective. Topical vasoconstrictors, such as the α₂-adrenoceptor agonist brimonidine, may be of benefit in some cases where erythema and telangiectasiae predominate. Systemic isotretinoin may be helpful in severe resistant disease and rhinophyma may require laser therapy or surgery.

Eczemas

The term 'eczema' derives from the Greek word 'to boil' and is synonymous with the other descriptive term, 'dermatitis'. Eczema describes a clinical and histological pattern, which can be acute or chronic and has several causes. Acutely, epidermal oedema (spongiosis) and intra-epidermal vesiculation (producing multilocular blisters) predominate, whereas with chronicity there is more epidermal thickening (acanthosis). Vasodilatation and T-cell lymphocytic infiltration of the upper dermis also occur.

Clinical features

There are several patterns of eczema (Box 29.17) but the clinical features are similar, irrespective of the cause (Box 29.18). Some subtypes of eczema have specific distinguishing features and these are discussed in more detail below.

Investigations

Bacterial and viral swabs for microscopy and culture are important in suspected secondary infection. Bacterial swabs

---

 29.17 Classification of eczema

Endogenous

- Atopic, seborrhoeic

Exogenous

- Irritant, allergic, photo-allergic, chronic actinic dermatitis

Characteristic patterns and morphology

- Asteatotic, discoid, gravitational, lichen simplex, pompholyx

---

 29.18 The clinical morphology of eczema

Acute

- Erythema, oedema, usually typically ill defined
- Papules, vesicles and occasionally bullae
- Exudation, fissuring
- Scaling

Chronic

- May be as above but less oedema, vesiculation and exudate
- Lichenification: skin thickening with pronounced skin markings, secondary to chronic rubbing and scratching
- Fissures (**definition**: slit-shaped deep ulcers), excoriations
- Dyspigmentation: hyper- and hypopigmentation can occur

---

are commonly positive, particularly for staphylococci, although clinical assessment is required in order to ascertain whether swab results are of clinical significance and whether antibiotic treatment is required. Individuals with atopic eczema have an increased susceptibility to herpes simplex virus (HSV) and are at risk of developing a widespread infection, eczema herpeticum. The presence of small, punched-out lesions on a background of worsening eczema suggests the possibility of secondary HSV infection. Skin scrapings to rule out secondary fungal infection should also be considered. Total IgE and specific IgE tests and skin prick tests are not routinely undertaken in atopic eczema as they are not usually helpful, although they may occasionally be indicated in some cases as directed by the history. Patch tests should be performed if contact allergic dermatitis is suspected (see Box 29.22 below). Skin biopsy is not usually required unless there is diagnostic doubt.

Management

A general approach to the management of eczema includes advice, education and support, required for patients with eczema of any type (Fig. 29.31). Input from patient support groups, such as the National Eczema Society in the UK, can be very helpful. Intensive and prolonged treatments are often required and chronic eczema can have a major and devastating adverse impact on personal and family lives. Emollients and topical glucocorticoids are mainstays of treatment for all eczema types, in order to improve skin barrier function, limit transepidermal water loss and reduce inflammation. Emollients can be used as bath additives and soap substitutes, and applied directly to the skin, often combined with antiseptics. Sedative antihistamines are useful if sleep is interrupted but non-sedating antihistamines are ineffective, as the itch of eczema is not primarily mediated by histamine.

Ointments are preferred for chronic eczema, whereas cream- or lotion-based treatment may be more appropriate for acute eczema (see Box 29.11). Treatment is once to twice daily (p. 1225). Hydrocortisone (1%) or clobetasone butyrate is generally used on the face, with more potent glucocorticoids restricted to trunk and limbs (see Box 29.12). A good strategy is to employ an intensive regimen with more potent glucocorticoids initially and then taper use according to response. A key principle is to use the least potent glucocorticoid that is effective for the shortest possible time. The patient should be given instructions on how much to apply, using the fingertip unit for guidance (a strip of glucocorticoid cream on distal phalanx pulp should cover two palm-size areas). It is also important to monitor glucocorticoid use and the easiest way to do this is ask how long it takes to use a specific size of glucocorticoid tube. The side-effects of topical glucocorticoid therapy need to be considered but glucocorticoid phobia and under-treatment of eczema are often more of a problem than over-treatment. Particular care should be taken on certain sites, such as the face and flexures, and in children and the elderly (see Box 29.2 and Fig. 29.10, p. 1226).

The clinical features of eczema influence the choice of topical treatment. For example, appropriate treatment of acute exudative eczema could be with potassium permanganate soaks, emollients and topical glucocorticoids under wet wraps. Chronic eczema may be best treated with a potent topical glucocorticoid in an ointment formulation and occlusion with a paste bandage to ease itching and scratching.

The topical calcineurin inhibitors tacrolimus and pimecrolimus may be useful glucocorticoid-sparing agents for eczema, particularly on the face; they cause local cutaneous immunosuppression.

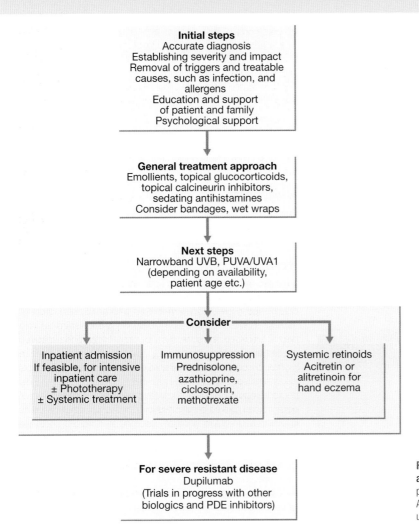

Fig. 29.31 **General management approaches: atopic eczema.** (PDE = phosphodiesterase; PUVA = psoralen-ultraviolet A; UVA1 = ultraviolet A1; UVB = narrowband ultraviolet B)

Initial burning and stinging may limit use but are usually transient side-effects. Bacterial and viral skin infection risk may be increased due to immunosuppression. Caution should be employed with sun exposure and these agents should not be used in combination with phototherapy because of their immunosuppressive effects.

Atopic eczema

This is the most common subtype of eczema. The prevalence has increased dramatically since the early 1980s, and the disease now affects at least 20% of schoolchildren and 5–10% of adults in the UK.

Pathogenesis

Generalised prolonged hypersensitivity to common environmental antigens, such as pollen and house-dust mite, is the hallmark of atopy, in which there is a genetic predisposition to produce excess IgE. Atopic individuals manifest one or more of a group of diseases that includes asthma, hay fever, food and other allergies, and atopic eczema. Genetic factors play an important role in all of these conditions, supported by higher concordance of atopic disease in monozygotic twins compared with dizygotic twins. Filaggrin gene mutations increase the risk of developing atopic eczema by more than threefold, emphasising the importance of epidermal barrier impairment in this disease. Other genes are also likely to be implicated, with many other susceptibility loci identified, although these studies require further replication. Decreased skin barrier function may also allow greater penetration of allergens through the epidermis, and thus cause immune stimulation and subsequent inflammation. The interaction between genes and environment is important; it has been estimated that 60–80% of individuals are genetically susceptible to the induction of IgE-mediated sensitisation to environmental allergens such as food and animal hair. Eczema is characterised by infiltration of Th2 cells, which are known to play a role in activating mast cells and eosinophils, as well as stimulating IgE production by IgE-producing B cells. The contributing roles of the microbiome are also being explored. Thus, the pathogenesis of atopic eczema is complex and multifactorial, involving an interplay of contributing factors.

Clinical features

Atopic eczema is extremely itchy and scratching accounts for many of the signs (Fig. 29.32). Widespread cutaneous dryness (also known as xeroderma or xerosis) is another feature. The distribution and character of the rash vary with age (Box 29.19). Complications are listed in Box 29.20.

Investigations

The diagnosis of atopic eczema is made using clinical criteria (Box 29.21). Interestingly, while most patients with atopic eczema have raised total IgE levels and IgE-specific antibodies, this is not a prerequisite for the diagnosis, as a significant minority have normal levels of IgE.

29

Fig. 29.32 Atopic eczema. [A] This patient had life-long chronic atopic eczema and experienced a generalised flare of disease triggered by infection. [B] Lichenification of chronic flexural eczema secondary to rubbing and scratching.

Management

The general principles of management are as described in Figure 29.31. Emollients and topical glucocorticoids, tar and ichthammol paste bandages, or wet wraps in children, are often required. Topical calcineurin inhibitors may be used as glucocorticoid-sparing agents but should not be used in infected eczema. Secondary infection should be treated but positive skin swabs in isolation, without clinical evidence of infection, do not necessarily require treatment with antibiotics, although antiseptics would be appropriate. Sedating antihistamines may help to break the itch/scratch cycle. Identification and avoidance of allergens are important.

Phototherapy is generally the next step, if topical therapies are insufficient (see Fig. 29.31). Narrowband UVB is usually the initial phototherapy of choice and can also be used in children. PUVA or UVA1 can also be chosen if UVB is ineffective, although mainly in adults as PUVA is generally avoided in children. Localised phototherapy may be used for eczema on hands and feet and PUVA may be more effective in that situation. Systemic immunosuppression with, for example, oral glucocorticoids, intermittent ciclosporin, azathioprine or methotrexate may be needed if the response to topical therapies and phototherapy is inadequate. Systemic retinoids, such as acitretin or alitretinoin, may be indicated: for example, in hand and foot eczema.

Encouraging early trial data are emerging to support the use of dupilumab, which blocks IL-4Rα, and the anti-IL-13 agents lebrikizumab and tralokinumab in atopic eczema. Phosphodiesterase 4 inhibitors are also being investigated.

Seborrhoeic eczema

This is an erythematous scaly rash affecting the scalp (dandruff), central face, nasolabial folds, eyebrows, central chest and upper back. It is associated with, and may be due to, overgrowth of *Malassezia* yeasts. When severe, it may resemble psoriasis. Severe or recalcitrant seborrhoeic eczema can be a marker of immunodeficiency, including HIV infection (p. 314). Topical azoles, such as ketoconazole shampoo and cream, often combined with mild glucocorticoid, are mainstays. Treatment often needs to be repeated due to disease recurrence.

Discoid eczema

Discoid eczema, which is also known as nummular eczema, is common and characteristically consists of discrete, coin-shaped eczematous lesions, which are often impetiginised and most commonly occur on the limbs of men. It is an eczema type that can be due to any chronic itchy condition, whether primarily of the skin or secondary to an underlying disease. Initial management should include topical antiseptics, in addition to emollients and topical glucocorticoids. Judicious antibiotic use may also be required for acute flares.

29.22 Common type IV delayed hypersensitivity allergens	
Allergen	**Source**
Nickel	Jewellery, jean studs, bra clips, watches
Dichromate	Cement, leather, matches
Rubber chemicals	Clothing, shoes, rubber gloves, tyres
Colophony	Sticking plaster, collodion, nail varnish
Paraphenylenediamine	Hair dye, clothing, tattoos
Balsam of Peru	Perfumes, citrus fruits, shower/bath products
Neomycin, benzocaine	Topical medications
Parabens	Preservative in cosmetics and creams
Wool alcohols	Lanolin, cosmetics, creams
Epoxy resin	Resin adhesives, glues
Methyl- and chloromethyl-isothiazolinone	Preservatives, with increasing numbers of cases of allergy reported

Fig. 29.33 Allergic contact eczema. This was caused by the application of an antihistamine cream. The acute eczematous reaction and bilateral periorbital oedema are typical.

Irritant eczema

Detergents, alkalis, acids, solvents and abrasives are common irritants. Strong irritants have acute effects, whereas weaker irritants commonly cause chronic eczema, especially of the hands, after prolonged exposure. Individual susceptibility varies and the elderly, atopic and fair-skinned are predisposed. Irritant eczema accounts for most occupational cases of eczema and is a significant cause of time off work. Irritant avoidance, including protective clothing (such as gloves), is essential. Emollients and topical glucocorticoids are indicated.

Allergic contact eczema

This occurs due to a delayed hypersensitivity reaction following contact with antigens or haptens. Previous allergen exposure is required for sensitisation and the reaction is specific to the allergen or closely related chemicals. Common allergens are listed in Box 29.22.

Allergy persists indefinitely and eczema occurs at sites of allergen contact and can secondarily spread beyond this. The distribution of eczema can be very informative with regard to possible culprits. There are many recognisable patterns of sites of eczema involvement, such as earlobes, wrists and umbilicus due to contact with nickel in earrings, watches and jeans studs; hands and wrists due to rubber gloves; and upper eyelids due to colophony from rubbing of the eyes in nail varnish wearers. Oedema may also be a feature (Fig. 29.33). Allergen avoidance is key and may involve a change of occupation, recreational activities or hobbies. It is important to ensure that patients are fully informed as to the nature and likely occurrence of allergens and good detective work is required to scrutinise lifestyle and daily activities. Treatment with emollients and topical glucocorticoids helps but will not suffice if there is continued allergen exposure.

Asteatotic eczema

This occurs in dry skin and is common in the elderly. Low humidity caused by central heating, over-washing, diuretics and cholesterol-lowering drugs predispose. The most common site is the lower legs, and a 'crazy paving' pattern of fine fissuring on an erythematous background is seen. Emollients are a mainstay, in combination with topical glucocorticoids. Patients must be advised to use caution with flammable emollients and to avoid bathroom slippages related to emollients on floor and feet, and this is particularly relevant for the elderly.

Gravitational eczema

Gravitational or stasis eczema occurs on the lower legs and is often associated with signs of venous insufficiency: oedema, loss of hair, induration, lipodermatosclerosis and ulceration. Emollients should be used and topical glucocorticoids should be applied to eczematous areas but not to ulcers. There is a high risk of sensitisation to topical preservatives (such as chlorocresol), antibiotics (such as neomycin) and bandages (such as rubber additives). Oedema and ulceration are treated by leg elevation and compression bandages (p. 1224).

Lichen simplex

Lichenification of eczema occurs secondary to chronic rubbing and scratching, and lichen simplex is a localised form. Common sites include the neck, lower legs and anogenital region. Treatment with emollients and very potent topical glucocorticoids may be required, often impregnated in tape or with occlusion.

Pompholyx

Intensely itchy vesicles and bullae occur on the palms, palmar surface and sides of the fingers and soles. Pompholyx may have several causes, which include atopic eczema, irritant and contact allergic dermatitis and fungal infection. The underlying cause must be treated or removed.

Psoriasis and other erythematous scaly eruptions

Psoriasis

Psoriasis is a chronic inflammatory, hyperproliferative skin disease. It is characterised by well-defined, erythematous scaly plaques, particularly affecting extensor surfaces, scalp and nails, and usually follows a relapsing and remitting course. Psoriasis affects approximately 1.5–3% of Caucasians but is less common in Asian, South American and African populations. It occurs equally in both sexes and at any age; although it is uncommon under the age of 5 years, more than 50% of patients present before the age of 30 years. The age of onset follows a bimodal distribution, with an early-onset type in the teenage or early adult years, often with a family history of psoriasis, a more severe disease course and strong HLA association. The later-onset type is typically seen between 50 and 60 years, usually without a family history and with a less severe disease course.

Pathogenesis

Both genetic and environmental factors are important. Twin studies show concordance rates of 60–75% and 15–20% for psoriasis arising in monozygotic and dizygotic twins, respectively. The age at onset and severity of disease are often similar in familial cases. If one parent has psoriasis, the chance of a child being affected is about 15–20%; if both parents have the disease, this rises to 50% and the risk is increased further if a sibling also has the disease.

Variants of the HLA-C region within the major histocompatibility complex (MHC) on chromosome 6 account for almost half of the heritability of psoriasis. However, at least 70 other loci are implicated, with susceptibility variants that lie within or close to genes involved in regulating epidermal barrier function, antigen presentation, cytokine production, notably IL-13 and IL-23, T-cell differentiation (especially Th-1 and Th-17 subsets) and nuclear factor kappa B (NFκB) signalling. Some of the loci that predispose to psoriasis overlap with those implicated in Crohn's disease, ankylosing spondylitis and psoriatic arthritis.

Environmental triggers for psoriasis are shown in (Box 29.23). Although the theory is controversial, stress may exacerbate psoriasis in susceptible individuals and psoriasis is itself a cause of psychological stress. Likewise, there is a higher incidence of smoking and heavy alcohol consumption in patients with psoriasis but it is unclear whether this is cause or effect. There is also an association between psoriasis and metabolic syndrome (p. 730).

The histological changes of psoriasis are shown in Figure 29.34. The main features are:

- keratinocyte hyperproliferation and abnormal differentiation, leading to retention of nuclei in the stratum corneum
- inflammation, with a T-cell (mainly activated Th-1 and Th-17) lymphocytic infiltrate and release of cytokines and adhesion molecules, such as interleukins (including IL-17 and IL-23), TNF-α, IFN-γ and intercellular adhesion molecule (ICAM)-1
- vascular changes, with tortuosity of dermal capillary loop vessels and release of mediators, such as vascular endothelial growth factor (VEGF).

The initiating event for psoriasis is unknown. Disordered cell proliferation is a key feature; this was previously thought to be the primary event but is now considered to be secondary to inflammatory change. The transit time for keratinocyte migration, from basal layer to shedding from stratum corneum, is shortened from approximately 28 to 5 days, so that immature cells reach the stratum corneum prematurely. Proliferation rate is also increased in non-lesional skin but to a lesser extent. Similarly, even the clinically unaffected nails of patients with psoriasis grow more quickly than those of controls.

While immunological factors clearly play a key role in psoriasis, the precise mechanisms of disease initiation and the sequence of events that lead to psoriasis are not fully defined.

---

i | **29.23 Exacerbating factors in psoriasis**

Trauma

- Lesions can appear at sites of skin trauma, such as scratches or surgical wounds (Köbner isomorphic phenomenon)

Infection

- β-haemolytic streptococcal throat infections often precede guttate psoriasis (see Fig. 29.35C)
- Severe psoriasis may be the initial presentation of HIV infection

Sunlight

- Psoriasis may occur or worsen after sun exposure, mainly due to Köbnerisation at sites of sunburn or polymorphic light eruption

Drugs

- Antimalarials, β-adrenoceptor antagonists (β-blockers), lithium, NSAIDs and TNF-α inhibitors can exacerbate psoriasis
- 'Rebound' flare of psoriasis may occur after withdrawal of systemic glucocorticoids or potent topical glucocorticoids. Rebound psoriasis is often unstable and may be pustular

Psychological factors

- Anxiety and stress may exacerbate psoriasis in predisposed individuals

(NSAID = non-steroidal anti-inflammatory drug; TNF-α = tumour necrosis factor alpha)

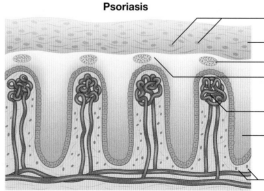

Normal   **Psoriasis**

Parakeratosis
Hyperkeratosis
Micro-abscess
Supra-papillary plate thinning
Dilated and tortuous capillary loops
Irregular thickening of epidermis
Upper dermal T-lymphocyte infiltrate

Keratin layer
Epidermis
Dermis

Fig. 29.34 The histology of psoriasis.

Fig. 29.35 Psoriasis. [A] Chronic plaque psoriasis, most prominent on extensor surfaces. [B] Nail involvement, with coarse pitting and separation from the nail plate (onycholysis). [C] Guttate psoriasis following a streptococcal throat infection. [D] Erythrodermic psoriasis.

Clinical features

Psoriasis has several different presentations (Fig. 29.35).

Plaque psoriasis

This is the most common presentation and usually represents more stable disease. The typical lesion is a raised, well-demarcated erythematous plaque of variable size (Fig. 29.35A). In untreated disease, silver/white scale is evident and more obvious on scraping the surface, which reveals bleeding points (Auspitz sign). The most common sites are the extensor surfaces, notably elbows and knees, and the lower back. Others include:

- *Scalp*: involvement is seen in approximately 60% of patients. Typically, easily palpable, erythematous scaly plaques are evident within hair-bearing scalp and there is clear demarcation at or beyond the hair margin. Occipital involvement is common and difficult to treat. Less often, fine diffuse scaling may be present and difficult to distinguish from seborrhoeic dermatitis. Involvement of other 'seborrhoeic sites', such as eyebrows, nasolabial folds and the pre-sternal area, is not uncommon and again may be confused with seborrhoeic dermatitis. Temporary hair loss can occur but permanent loss is unusual.
- *Nails*: involvement is common, with 'thimble pitting', onycholysis (separation of the nail from the nail bed, Fig. 29.35B), subungual hyperkeratosis and periungual involvement (p. 1210).
- *Flexures*: psoriasis of the natal cleft and submammary and axillary folds is usually symmetrical, erythematous and smooth, without scale.
- *Palms*: psoriasis of the palms can be difficult to distinguish from eczema.

Guttate psoriasis

This is most common in children and adolescents and is often the initial presentation (Fig. 29.35C). It may present shortly after a streptococcal throat infection and evolves rapidly. Individual lesions are droplet-shaped, small (usually less than 1 cm in diameter), erythematous, scaly and numerous. An episode of guttate psoriasis may clear spontaneously or with topical treatment within a few months, but UVB phototherapy is often required and is highly effective. Guttate psoriasis often heralds the onset of plaque psoriasis in adulthood.

Erythrodermic psoriasis

Generalised erythrodermic psoriasis is a medical emergency (Fig. 29.35D).

Pustular psoriasis

Pustular psoriasis may be generalised or localised. Generalised pustular psoriasis is uncommon, unstable and life-threatening. It will often emerge in the context of plaque disease and the onset is usually sudden, with large numbers of small, sterile pustules on an erythematous background, often merging into sheets, with waves of new pustules in subsequent days. The patient is usually febrile and systemically unwell, and this must be dealt with as a medical emergency (p. 1224). Unstable pustular psoriasis may be precipitated as a rebound phenomenon following either topical or systemic glucocorticoid use in a patient with psoriasis. Localised pustular psoriasis of the palms and soles (palmoplantar pustulosis) is more common, chronic and closely associated with smoking; small, sterile pustules and erythema develop and resolve with pigmentation and scaling (p. 1210). A localised form of sterile pustulosis of a few digits (acropustulosis) can also occur. It is unclear whether these localised forms of pustulosis are truly psoriatic.

Arthropathy

Between 5% and 10% of individuals with psoriasis develop an inflammatory arthropathy, which can take on a number of patterns (p. 1035). Joint involvement is more likely in patients with psoriatic nail disease.

Investigations

Skin biopsy is not usually required but may be performed if there is diagnostic doubt. An infection screen, particularly throat swab and/or serology for recent streptococcal infection, may be informative in guttate psoriasis. Assessment of impact on life using the DLQI and disease extent using PASI (Psoriasis Area and Severity Index, p. 1211) is essential. Due to the association of psoriasis with metabolic syndrome, comorbidities and cardiovascular risk factors should be assessed and managed (p. 730). HIV testing should be considered in severe or recalcitrant psoriasis.

Management

Counselling about diagnosis and management of skin involvement and other comorbidities is paramount. Information and services must be available for patients. Psoriasis can have a major impact on all aspects of life and this must not be under-estimated. Reassurance is also needed, as the condition is generally not life-threatening. Advice regarding reduction in risk factors for cardiovascular disease should be given (smoking cessation, reduction of alcohol intake, adequate exercise and a normal body mass index). Associated diseases, such as hypertension and diabetes, should be treated.

Patients need to be involved in their own management, as the disease is usually chronic and the benefit/risk profile of treatments must be discussed and tailored to individuals. The endpoint for treatment also needs to be discussed because complete disease clearance may not be practical or appropriate and patients vary considerably in their treatment requirements. Extent of disease and impact on quality of life must be taken into account. Patient adherence to topical and systemic therapies is essential and dependent on the treatment practicalities.

The treatment approach generally follows a stepwise progression, with treatment categories broadly summarised (Fig. 29.36).

Topical treatments, including emollients, are the first-line approach. Vitamin D receptor agonists, such as calcipotriol, calcitriol and tacalcitol, are often used as first-line topical treatment. The mechanism of action includes increased differentiation and reduction of proliferation, reducing plaque scale and thickness. Calcipotriol is most widely used and can be applied once to twice daily; if less than 100 g of ointment is used each week, there is no risk of hypercalcaemia. Vitamin D analogues can cause irritation but this is often temporary. Topical glucocorticoids may be required in the management of psoriasis, particularly at flexural or facial sites, and may be alternated or combined with vitamin D analogues. However, safe, appropriately supervised and judicious use is necessary, with awareness of the potential risk of rebound unstable or pustular psoriasis with glucocorticoid over-use or sudden cessation. Dithranol and coal tar are effective and, like vitamin D analogues, work by increasing differentiation and inhibiting proliferation. Although often effective, they are messy and time-consuming. Modified versions of Goeckerman's regimen (the combination of coal tar and UVB) are still used, but coal tar has a characteristic odour and can be irritant. Short-contact dithranol therapy at relatively high concentrations applied for 15–30 minutes can be used but causes brown staining of skin and purple discoloration of light hair. In recent years, efforts have been made to improve the tolerance of tar and dithranol preparations, but at reduced efficacy. Overall, the use of tar and dithranol has reduced in recent years but they can be highly effective in selected patients.

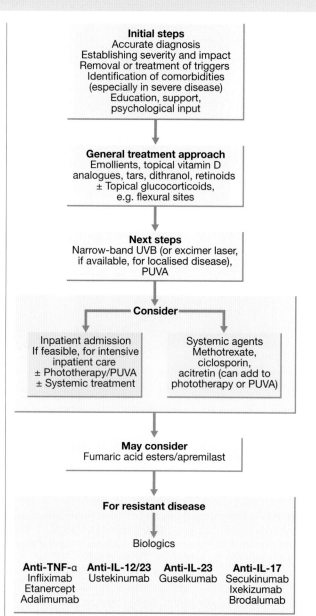

Fig. 29.36 **General management approaches: psoriasis.** (IL = interleukin; PUVA = psoralen–ultraviolet A; TNF-α = tumour necrosis factor alpha; UVB = ultraviolet B)

If topical treatment is insufficient, then UVB phototherapy or PUVA should usually be the next step. If the patient continues to have active disease or early recurrence, then the addition of systemic retinoid such as acitretin to UVB or PUVA can be effective. Alternatively, immunosuppressants, such as methotrexate or ciclosporin, may be required. For difficult treatment-resistant disease, fumaric acid esters, apremilast and biologics should be considered (p. 1005 and Fig. 29.37).

The active component of fumaric acid ester therapy is dimethyl fumarate and efficacy in psoriasis has been confirmed. Common adverse effects are flushing and diarrhoea. Lymphopenia is also expected at effective doses. Apremilast is indicated for moderate to severe psoriasis resistant to standard measures. Of the biological agents, the anti-TNF-α agents (etanercept, infliximab, adalimumab or golimumab), ustekinumab (an inhibitor

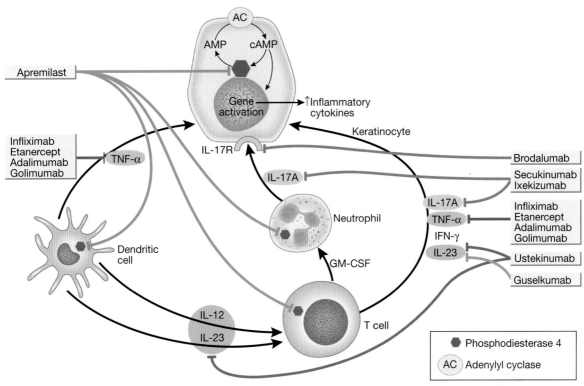

Fig. 29.37 Developments in understanding of key pathways and drug targets in psoriasis. Other drug targets are also under development, such as Janus kinase (JAK) inhibitors (tofacitinib and baricitinib) and sphingosine-1-phosphate receptor (S1PR1) antagonists (ponesimod). This diagrammatic image is illustrative of key pathways and drug targets but is not comprehensive. (AMP = adenosine monophosphate; cAMP = cyclic adenosine monophosphate; GM-CSF = granulocyte macrophage colony-stimulating factor; IL = interleukin; TNF-α = tumour necrosis factor alpha)

of IL-12 and IL-23), guselkumab (an IL-23 inhibitor) and secukinumab or ixekizumab (an IL-17 inhibitor) may all be effective and this is a rapidly evolving field. More details of the mechanisms of action and adverse effects of these agents are provided on page 1006.

Individualised management is essential. For example, a patient with localised plaque psoriasis on elbows, knees and sacrum should respond to topical treatment only, whereas someone with guttate psoriasis is likely to need phototherapy as a first-line approach because of difficulties in topical drug application in extensive disease. A patient with extensive chronic plaque psoriasis and significant arthropathy would be better suited to a systemic drug, such as methotrexate, than phototherapy, which would be unlikely to improve joint symptoms. Thus, whilst a stepwise general approach to management (see Fig. 29.36) may offer guidance, the correct choice for any given patient must be determined on an individual basis.

Pityriasis rosea

This is an acute, self-limiting exanthem that particularly affects young adults and occurs worldwide, with a slight female predominance. It usually presents in spring and summer, although no infective agent has been identified and its aetiology is unknown. It is characterised by the appearance of a 'herald patch', an oval lesion (1–2 cm) with a central pinkish (salmon-coloured) centre, a darker periphery and a characteristic collarette of scale. It is followed 1–2 weeks later by a widespread papulosquamous eruption, which is typically arranged in a symmetrical 'fir tree' pattern on the trunk. Individual lesions also have a collarette of scale. An inverse variant with flexural involvement can occur.

Mucosal involvement is rare. There is a small risk of recurrence. Symptomatic relief can be achieved with emollients and mild topical glucocorticoids. Post-inflammatory hyperpigmentation can supervene, particularly in darker skin types.

Pityriasis lichenoides chronica

This is rare but typically presents within the first three decades of life. The aetiology is unclear but the condition is part of a spectrum and remits spontaneously. The more acute variety (pityriasis lichenoides et varioliformis acuta, PLEVA) presents as crops of papules that rapidly evolve with central necrosis, each attack lasting up to 3 months. The more chronic variety presents as a persistent, widespread, scaly eruption. Characteristically, lesions are brown papules with a mica-like scale ('cornflake'). The condition fluctuates but can persist for months or years. Emollients, topical glucocorticoids and long-term oral erythromycin can occasionally be helpful. UVB phototherapy or PUVA is usually effective, although recurrences are high.

Drug eruptions

It is essential to consider a drug cause in anyone presenting with an erythematous maculopapular or papulosquamous eruption, and a careful drug history is critical (p. 1265). Exfoliation ('peeling') and post-inflammatory hyper- or, less commonly, hypopigmentation can occur.

Other causes

Secondary syphilis (p. 337), pityriasis versicolor (p. 1240) and fungal infection with *Tinea corporis* (p. 1240) can all cause an

29

erythematous papulosquamous rash and must be considered in the differential diagnosis of erythematous papulosquamous rashes.

Lichenoid eruptions

Lichen planus

Lichen planus occurs worldwide. It typically presents as a pruritic rash; the mucosae, hair and nails may also be involved.

Pathogenesis

The disease probably has an autoimmune basis since there is an association with inflammatory bowel disease, primary biliary cirrhosis, autoimmune hepatitis, hepatitis B and C, alopecia areata, myasthenia gravis (p. 1141) and thymoma. There are also similarities with graft-versus-host disease (GVHD, p. 937). Lichen planus can occasionally occur in families and possible HLA associations have been reported but there is no clear inheritance pattern. On skin biopsy, characteristic histological changes include hyperkeratosis, basal cell degeneration and a heavy, band-like T-lymphocyte infiltrate in the papillary dermis, with affinity for the epidermis (epidermotropism). The dermo-epidermal junction has a 'sawtooth' appearance.

Clinical features

Lichen planus occurs in both sexes and at any age, although usually between 30 and 60 years. It generally presents on the distal limbs, most commonly on the flexural aspects of the wrists and forearms (Fig. 29.38), and on the lower back. It is intensely itchy and lesions are violaceous, shiny, flat-topped, polygonal papules, with a characteristic fine lacy, white network on the surface (Wickham's striae). New lesions may appear at sites of skin trauma (Köbner phenomenon) and the rash may become generalised. Individual lesions may last for many months and can become hypertrophic and modified by scratching, particularly on the lower legs. The eruption usually remits over months but can become chronic, particularly with hypertrophic disease. Post-inflammatory pigmentary change is common, particularly in darker skin types. Mucous membrane involvement occurs in 30–70% of patients, usually as a network of white, lacy striae on the buccal mucosae (p. 1210) and tongue. These oral changes are often asymptomatic and should be sought on examination. Genital and other mucosal surfaces can also be affected (pp. 334 and 336). Nail involvement occurs in about 10% and can range from longitudinal ridging to a destructive nail dystrophy, scarring (pterygium) and nail loss (p. 1261). Scalp involvement usually

Fig. 29.38 Lichen planus. Violaceous papules on the flexural aspect of forearm, arising at a site of minor linear trauma (Köbner phenomenon).

presents as an inflammatory scarring alopecia, often with tufting of residual hairs. The classical presentation of lichen planus is unmistakable, but less common atypical variants, which include annular, atrophic, actinic, linear, bullous, follicular, pigmented and ulcerative types, can be a diagnostic challenge.

Investigations

A skin biopsy should be performed if there is diagnostic doubt. A careful drug history must be taken, as, although the classical presentation of lichen planus is usually 'idiopathic', the main differential is a drug-induced lichenoid reaction (see below). Other differential diagnoses include psoriasis, pityriasis rosea, pityriasis lichenoides chronica and secondary syphilis. Screening for underlying disease, such as hepatitis, must be considered.

Management

The condition is usually self-limiting, although rarely it may persist for years, particularly oral lichen planus. Treatment is symptomatic and potent local glucocorticoids (topical, with occlusion or by injection for hypertrophic disease, or as oral rinse for oral involvement) may help the intense itch; short courses of systemic glucocorticoids are sometimes required for extensive disease. UVB, PUVA or UVA1 can be beneficial and, for recalcitrant disease, retinoids or immunosuppressants, such as ciclosporin or methotrexate, may be needed. A low but significant risk of malignant transformation exists with persistent oral and genital disease, so active treatment, surveillance and smoking cessation are important.

Drug-induced lichenoid eruptions

Drug-induced lichenoid reactions that are clinically and histologically difficult to distinguish from idiopathic lichen planus are important to identify. The likely culprits are gold, quinine, proton pump inhibitors, sulphonamides, penicillamine, antimalarials, antituberculous drugs, thiazide diuretics, β-blockers, angiotensin-converting enzyme (ACE) inhibitors, NSAIDs, sulphonylureas, lithium and dyes in colour developers (see Box 29.35, p. 1266).

Graft-versus-host disease

In the acute stage of graft-versus-host disease (GVHD, p. 937), there is a distinctive dermatitis associated with hepatitis. After about 3 months, chronic GVHD can present with a lichenoid eruption on the palms, soles, face and upper trunk. Progressive sclerodermatous skin thickening, associated with pigmentary changes, may lead to contractures and limited mobility.

Urticaria

Urticaria ('hives') is caused by localised dermal oedema secondary to a temporary increase in capillary permeability. If oedema involves subcutaneous or submucosal layers, the term angioedema is used.

Clinical features

Acute urticaria may be associated with angioedema of the lips, face, tongue, throat and, rarely, wheezing, abdominal pain, headaches and even anaphylaxis (p. 75). Urticaria present for less than 6 weeks is considered to be acute, and chronic if it continues for more than 6 weeks. Individual weals (**definition**: evanescent discrete areas of dermal oedema, often centrally white due to masking of local blood supply by fluid; weals can be papules, macules, patches and plaques – Fig. 29.39) last for less than 24 hours; if they persist, urticarial vasculitis needs to be considered. Clarification of the duration of urticaria can be achieved by drawing around the weal and re-assessing 24 hours later. History-taking should probe for possible causes, including medications (Box 29.24). Physical triggers can also be assessed in challenge testing, such as eliciting dermographism or pressure testing. Enquiry about family history and medication, particularly ACE inhibitors, is important in angioedema. Examination may be unremarkable or weals may be evident (Fig. 29.39). The skin should be stroked firmly with an orange stick in order to ascertain whether dermographism is present or not.

Mast cell degranulation and release of histamine and other vasoactive mediators is the basis of urticaria (Fig. 29.40). Chronic spontaneous urticaria (previously called 'chronic idiopathic' or 'chronic ordinary' urticaria) is the most common chronic urticaria and has an autoimmune pathogenesis in some cases.

Fig. 29.39 Urticaria. Erythema, reflecting dilated dermal vessels, and oedema (with upper dermal oedema obscuring the erythema centrally) are evident. Note the absence of epidermal changes.

Investigations

Investigations should be guided by the history and possible causes but are often negative, particularly in acute urticaria. Some or all of the following may be appropriate:

- *Full blood count*: eosinophilia in parasitic infection or drug cause.
- *Erythrocyte sedimentation rate (ESR) or plasma viscosity*: elevated in vasculitis.
- *Urea and electrolytes, thyroid and liver function tests, iron studies*: may reveal an underlying systemic disorder.
- *Total IgE and specific IgE to possible allergens*: shellfish, peanut, house-dust mite. Particularly relevant if there is angioedema.
- *Autoantibodies, particularly antinuclear factor*: positive in systemic lupus erythematosus (SLE) and often positive in urticarial vasculitis. Other autoimmune diseases, such as

i	**29.24 Causes of urticaria**

Acute and chronic urticaria

- Autoimmune: due to antibodies that cross-link the IgE receptor on mast cells
- Allergens in foods and inhalants
- Contact allergens: latex, animal saliva
- Drugs: see Box 29.35 (p. 1266)
- Physical stimuli: heat, cold, pressure, sun, sweat, water
- Infections: intestinal parasites, hepatitis
- Others: SLE, pregnancy, thyroid disease
- Idiopathic: chronic spontaneous urticaria and angioedema

Urticarial vasculitis

- Hepatitis B, SLE, idiopathic

(IgE = immunoglobulin E; SLE = systemic lupus erythematosus)

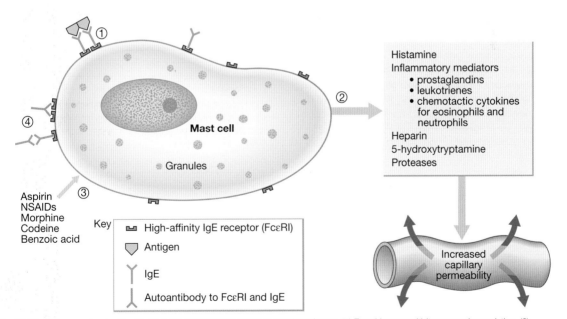

Fig. 29.40 Pathogenesis of urticaria. Mast cell degranulation occurs in a variety of ways. (1) Type I hypersensitivity causes degranulation. (2) Spontaneous mast cell degranulation in chronic urticaria. (3) Chemical mast cell degranulation. (4) Autoimmunity, with IgE antibodies directed against IgE receptors or IgE itself. Histamine and the leukotrienes are especially relevant mediators in urticaria. Heparin release is probably not a major factor in urticaria but plays a role in the osteoporosis that can occur in systemic mastocytosis. (IgE = immunoglobulin E; NSAID = non-steroidal anti-inflammatory drug)

29

rheumatoid arthritis and autoimmune hepatitis or thyroid disease, may be associated.

- *Complement C₃ and C₄ levels*: if these are low due to complement consumption, C_1 esterase inhibitor activity should be measured.
- *Infection screen*: hepatitis screen and HIV may be indicated.
- *Skin biopsy*: if urticarial vasculitis is suspected.
- *Challenge tests*: to confirm physical urticarias, such as dermographism, pressure, heat, cold.

Management

Removal or treatment of any trigger is essential, although this may not be identified in the majority of cases. Urticaria may be precipitated by aspirin, NSAIDs, codeine and opioids, and it is advisable to suggest alternatives such as paracetamol. In chronic urticaria, non-sedating antihistamines, such as fexofenadine, loratadine or cetirizine, are usually beneficial. If there is lack of response after 2 weeks, an alternative non-sedating antihistamine should be used and an H_2-blocker, such as cimetidine or ranitidine, can be added. Mast cell stabilisers or leukotriene receptor antagonists, such as montelukast, can be used for more recalcitrant disease. For chronic urticaria, narrowband UVB phototherapy is valuable and has proven efficacy. Systemic glucocorticoids are widely prescribed for urticaria but are not indicated in the majority of cases. If systemic glucocorticoids are used, efficacy may be seen only at relatively high doses and they are appropriate only for occasional short courses in the acute setting, usually in association with angioedema. Patients with a history of life-threatening anaphylaxis, as in peanut or wasp sting allergy, should carry a self-administered adrenaline (epinephrine) injection kit. The management of anaphylaxis and hereditary angioedema is discussed on pages 76 and 87. The IgE monoclonal antibody omalizumab may be effective in patients with severe recalcitrant urticaria.

Bullous diseases

Blistering can occur at any level in the skin and there are a variety of different presentations, depending on the underlying defect and level of involvement. Knowledge of the molecular basis of many blistering disorders has advanced considerably through understanding of the basic processes of cell adhesion and studies of rare genetic blistering disorders, particularly epidermolysis bullosa (Box 29.25). This section concentrates on primary blistering skin diseases.

29.25 Classification of epidermolysis bullosa

Type	Mode of inheritance	Level of blister*	Abnormality
Simple	Autosomal dominant	Epidermal basal cell	Keratins 5 and 14
Junctional	Autosomal recessive	Lamina lucida	Laminin-5 and $\alpha_6\beta_4$ integrin
Dystrophic	Autosomal dominant and recessive	Dermis below lamina densa	Collagen VII

*See Figure 29.1 (p. 1213).

Toxic epidermal necrolysis

Toxic epidermal necrolysis (TEN) is a medical emergency, as the extensive mucocutaneous blistering is associated with a high mortality rate. It is usually drug-induced (see Box 29.35, p. 1266), with anticonvulsants, sulphonamides, sulphonylureas, NSAIDs, allopurinol and antiretroviral therapy often implicated. Usually 1–4 weeks after drug commencement, the patient becomes systemically unwell and often pyrexial. Erythema and blistering develop, initially on the trunk but rapidly involving all skin; an early warning sign is cutaneous pain. Sheets of blisters coalesce and denude, and the underlying skin is painful and erythematous (Fig. 29.41). Gentle lateral pressure on stroking the skin results in epidermal detachment (Nikolsky sign), demonstrating the severity of skin fragility. Mucous membrane involvement and blistering are usual. Blistering of skin and mucosae may be haemorrhagic. A disease severity score (Box 29.26) is used to predict outcome. The main differential diagnosis is staphylococcal scalded skin syndrome (p. 1236), although the diagnosis is usually obvious in an adult patient with a culprit drug. There is often overlap with Stevens–Johnson syndrome and targetoid lesions, especially on palms and soles, may be evident. Skin

Fig. 29.41 Toxic epidermal necrolysis. Note the extensive erythema, oedema and epidermal loss secondary to carbamazepine.

29.26 Disease severity score for toxic epidermal necrolysis: SCORTEN

Factor

- Age >40 years
- Heart rate >120 beats/min
- Cancer or haematological malignancy
- Involved body surface area >10%
- Blood urea >10 mmol/L (28 mg/dL)
- Serum bicarbonate <20 mmol/L
- Blood glucose ≥14 mmol/L (252 mg/dL)

Mortality rates

- 0–1 factor present = 3%
- 2 factors = 12%
- 3 factors = 35%
- 4 factors = 58%
- ≥5 factors = 90%

From Bastuji-Garin S, Fouchard N, Bertocchi M, et al. SCORTEN: a severity-of-illness score for toxic epidermal necrolysis. J Invest Dermatol 2000; 115:149–153.

snip may allow early diagnosis. If there is diagnostic doubt, then full-thickness skin biopsy should be undertaken for histology and direct immunofluorescence in order to exclude immunobullous or other diagnoses.

Identification and discontinuation of the causative drug are essential. Sepsis and multi-organ failure are major risks. Intensive care in a dedicated dermatology ward or intensive care or burns unit is of paramount importance. Treatment is supportive, with regular sterile dressings and emollients, careful attention to fluid balance and treatment of infection if it develops. Urethral and ocular involvement is common and must be looked for and treated symptomatically. Ocular and urethral scarring can be problematic in survivors. There is no conclusive evidence that intravenous immunoglobulins, systemic glucocorticoids or ciclosporin improve outcomes and survival.

Immunobullous diseases

There are various subtypes of immunobullous disease that affect patients of different ages and have clinical characteristics (Box 29.27). The key investigation is an elliptical biopsy taken from the edge of a recent blister (Box 29.28). The sample is halved: one half is put in formalin for subsequent histology, while the other is sent fresh for direct immunofluorescence. Serum should also be sent for indirect immunofluorescence in suspected immunobullous disease (p. 1215).

Bullous pemphigoid

Bullous pemphigoid (BP) is the most common immunobullous disease and occurs worldwide. It is a disease of the elderly, with an average age of onset of 65 years; males and females are equally affected.

Pathogenesis

The disease is caused by autoantibodies (BP-230 and BP-180) directed against the hemi-desmosomal BP antigens, BPAg-1 (intracellular) and BPAg-2 (transmembranous type XVII collagen), respectively. Antibody–antigen binding initiates complement activation and inflammation, with hemi-desmosomal damage and subepidermal blistering.

Clinical features

There is often a lengthy prodrome of an itchy, urticated, erythematous rash prior to the development of tense bullae (Fig. 29.42A). Milia (**definition**: small epidermal keratin cysts) may develop due to basement membrane disruption. Mucosal involvement is uncommon.

i | 29.27 Age of onset in immunobullous skin disorders

Disease	Age
Pemphigus vulgaris	40–60 years
Pemphigus foliaceus	Any age (endemic form in parts of Brazil and South Africa, from teenage years on)
Bullous pemphigoid	Sixties and over
Dermatitis herpetiformis	Young, associated with coeliac disease
Linear IgA disease	Any age
Pemphigoid gestationis	Pregnant females
Epidermolysis bullosa acquisita	Any age
Bullous lupus erythematosus	Young black females

i | 29.28 Clinical and investigation findings in the immunobullous disorders

Disease	Site of blisters	Nature of blisters	Mucous membrane involvement	Antigen	Circulating antibody (indirect IF)	Fixed antibody (direct IF)
Pemphigus vulgaris	Trunk, head	Flaccid, fragile, many erosions	100%	Desmoglein-1 and 3 (120 kD)	IgG	IgG, C_3 intercellular (epidermal)
Pemphigus foliaceus	Trunk	Often not present, multiple erosions, may mimic dermatitis	No	Desmoglein-1	IgG	IgG, C_3 intercellular (epidermal)
Bullous pemphigoid	Trunk, flexures and limbs	Tense, milia as blisters resolve	Occasional	BP-230 and 180	IgG (70%)	IgG, C_3 at BMZ
Dermatitis herpetiformis	Elbows, lower back, buttocks	Excoriated and often not present	No	Unknown	Anti-endomysial and tissue transglutaminase	Granular IgA in papillary dermis
Linear IgA disease	Widespread	Tense, often annular configuration, 'string of beads'	Frequent	Unknown	50% have low titres of circulating antibody	Linear IgA at BMZ
Pemphigoid gestationis	Periumbilical and limbs	Tense, milia as blisters resolve	Rare	Collagen XVII (part of hemi-desmosome, BP-180)	Circulating antibodies to BP-180 (type XVII collagen) (and BP-230)	C_3 at BMZ
Epidermolysis bullosa acquisita	Widespread	Tense, scarring, milia	Common (50%)	Type VII collagen	IgG (anti-type VII collagen)	IgG at BMZ
Bullous lupus erythematosus	Widespread	Tense	Rare	Type VII collagen	Anti-type VII collagen	IgG, IgA, IgM at BMZ

(BMZ = basement membrane zone; IF = immunofluorescence; Ig = immunoglobulin)

29

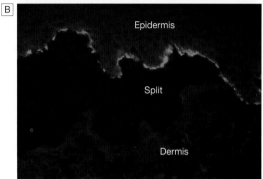

Fig. 29.42 Bullous pemphigoid. A Large, tense, unilocular blisters. B Immunofluorescence on salt-split skin, showing a subepidermal blister and linear IgG and C3 deposition at the basement membrane zone.

Investigations

The diagnosis can be made by skin biopsy, which shows subepidermal blistering with an eosinophil-rich inflammatory infiltrate. Direct immunofluorescence demonstrates the presence of IgG and C3 at the basement membrane (Fig. 29.42B). Indirect immunofluorescence may show positive titres of circulating anti-epidermal antibodies. Distinction from epidermolysis bullosa acquisita requires immunofluorescence studies using the patient's serum on salt-split skin. In BP, the immunoreactants localise to the epidermal side (hemi-desmosome) of split skin, whereas in epidermolysis bullosa acquisita they localise to the base of the split (type VII collagen/anchoring fibrils).

Management

Very potent topical glucocorticoids are effective and may be sufficient in frail elderly patients; they need to be applied to all sites, however, and not just lesional skin. Tetracyclines, such as doxycycline, have an important role and may limit the use of systemic glucocorticoids. However, most patients with extensive disease require systemic glucocorticoids (0.75 mg/kg/day or less), often combined with immunosuppressants as glucocorticoid-sparing agents. In severe refractory disease, other therapies, such as intravenous immunoglobulin or rituximab, are sometimes used but are of unproven efficacy. The condition often burns out over a few years.

Pemphigus

Pemphigus is less common than BP and patients tend to be younger.

Pathogenesis

The cause is IgG1 and IgG4 autoantibodies, directed against desmogleins-1 and 3, resulting in intra-epidermal blistering. The syndrome may occur spontaneously or be secondary to drugs such as penicillamine or captopril and underlying malignancy (paraneoplastic pemphigus). Pemphigus foliaceus is a very superficial form, in which antibodies are directed against desmoglein-1 only and affect just the most superficial epidermis.

Clinical features

Skin and mucosae are usually involved, although disease may be restricted to mucosae only, which may be severely affected. Due to the higher level of split within the epidermis, the blisters are flaccid, easily ruptured and often not seen intact. Erosions are common and the Nikolsky sign is positive. The trunk is usually affected. The condition is associated with significant morbidity and mortality.

Investigations

The diagnosis can be made by skin biopsy, which shows intra-epidermal blistering and acantholysis, with positive direct immunofluorescence for IgG (usually IgG1 or IgG4) and C3 at the periphery of keratinocytes, giving a 'chicken wire' appearance within the epidermis. The titres of circulating epidermal autoantibodies can also be used to monitor disease activity. Investigations should screen for associated autoimmune disease or malignancy if paraneoplastic pemphigus is suspected.

Management

Pemphigus is more difficult to treat than BP and high-dose systemic glucocorticoids such as prednisolone (0.5–1.0 mg/kg/day) are usually required. Azathioprine and cyclophosphamide are most often used as glucocorticoid-sparing agents but a range of other immunosuppressants may be considered for severe recalcitrant disease, including methotrexate, ciclosporin, mycophenolate mofetil, intravenous immunoglobulins, plasma exchange, extracorporeal photopheresis and rituximab. Often, long-term treatment is required to prevent relapse.

Dermatitis herpetiformis

Dermatitis herpetiformis (DH) is an autoimmune blistering disorder that is strongly associated with coeliac disease (CD). While fewer than 10% of individuals with CD develop DH, almost all patients with DH have evidence of partial villous atrophy on intestinal biopsy, even if they have no gastrointestinal symptoms (p. 806). It is unclear why some CD patients develop DH and others do not. Although DH is a bullous disease, intact vesicles and blisters are seldom seen, as the condition is so pruritic that excoriations on extensor surfaces of arms, knees, buttocks, shoulders and scalp may be the only signs.

The diagnosis can be made by skin biopsy, which shows subepidermal vesiculation in the dermal papillae and a neutrophil- and eosinophil-rich infiltrate. Direct immunofluorescence shows granular IgA in the papillary dermis. Anti-endomysial antibodies and tissue transglutaminase should be assessed and jejunal biopsy undertaken if indicated. The condition usually responds to a gluten-free diet but, if not, dapsone can also be used.

Linear IgA disease

This occurs in children (chronic bullous disease of childhood) and adults, and is usually self-limiting, although it can be active for a few years. Drugs, notably vancomycin, can be a secondary cause. Blisters can arise on erythematous, urticated or otherwise normal-looking skin and often form an annular configuration at the edge of the lesion: 'clusters of jewels' (herpetiform) and 'string of beads' (annular/ polycyclic). Mucosal involvement is common and ophthalmology input important, as corneal scarring is a risk with longstanding disease. Linear IgA is seen at the basement membrane on direct immunofluorescence and localises to either roof or floor of salt-split skin. Dapsone, sulfapyridine, prednisolone, colchicine or intravenous immunoglobulin may be effective.

Epidermolysis bullosa acquisita

This chronic blistering disease affects skin and mucosae, and scarring, hair loss and nail dystrophy may be problematic. Blisters often follow trauma and milia develop. It can be very difficult to distinguish from other immunobullous diseases, such as bullous pemphigoid. It is caused by an IgG antibody to type VII collagen, which provokes subepidermal blistering and a mixed inflammatory infiltrate, although the latter may not be prominent. Direct immunofluorescence on perilesional skin shows IgG and C3 at the dermo-epidermal junction and pattern analysis may be helpful in distinction from bullous pemphigoid. Indirect immunofluorescence microscopy on salt-split normal human skin typically shows IgG and IgA in the floor of the artificially induced blister, whereas in BP antibody localisation would be to the roof of the blister. Epidermolysis bullosa acquisita is very difficult to treat, as it often does not respond well to immunosuppressants. Mainstays of treatment include systemic glucocorticoids in combination with dapsone or colchicine. Other immunosuppressive approaches may be required and include ciclosporin, azathioprine, immunoglobulins, plasmapheresis and rituximab. The condition may be associated with inflammatory bowel disease, rheumatoid arthritis, multiple myeloma and lymphoma, and thus associated comorbidities should be sought.

Porphyria cutanea tarda and pseudoporphyria

These conditions may also cause blistering (see Boxes 29.9 and 29.35, pp. 1221 and 1266). Porphyria is discussed in more detail on page 378.

Pigmentation disorders

Decreased pigmentation

Disorders causing hypopigmentation and/or depigmentation include:

- vitiligo
- albinism
- pityriasis alba: depigmented areas on the face, particularly in children, with or without scale and usually considered to be eczematous
- pityriasis versicolor (p. 1240): hypopigmentation or, less commonly, hyperpigmentation can occur
- idiopathic guttate hypomelanosis: multiple small areas of depigmentation arising in chronically sun-exposed skin
- rarely, phenylketonuria (p. 369) and hypopituitarism.

Vitiligo

Vitiligo is an acquired condition affecting 1% of the population worldwide. Focal loss of melanocytes results in the development of patches of hypopigmentation. A positive family history of vitiligo is relatively common in those with extensive disease, and this type is also associated with other autoimmune diseases. Trauma and sunburn may (through the Köbner phenomenon) precipitate the appearance of vitiligo. It is thought to be the result of cell-mediated autoimmune destruction of melanocytes but why some areas are targeted and others are spared is unclear.

Clinical features

Generalised vitiligo is often symmetrical and involves hands, wrists, feet, knees and neck, as well as areas around body orifices (Fig. 29.43). The hair of the scalp, beard, eyebrows and lashes may also depigment. Segmental vitiligo is restricted to one part of the body but not necessarily a dermatome. The patches of depigmentation are sharply defined, and in Caucasians may be surrounded by hyperpigmentation. Spotty perifollicular pigment may be seen within the depigmentation and is often the first sign of repigmentation. There is no history or evidence of inflammation within the patches, which may be helpful in distinguishing vitiligo from post-inflammatory hypopigmentation. Sensation in the depigmented patches is normal (unlike in tuberculoid leprosy, p. 267). Wood's light examination enhances the contrast between pigmented and non-pigmented skin. The course is unpredictable but most patches remain static or enlarge; a few repigment spontaneously.

Management

Protecting the patches from excessive sun exposure with clothing or sunscreen may be helpful to avoid sunburn. Camouflage cosmetics may be beneficial, particularly in those with dark skin. In fair skin, photoprotection and cosmetic cover may be all that is required. Very potent or potent topical glucocorticoids have limited efficacy with respect to repigmentation. Topical pimecrolimus or tacrolimus may also have a role as a glucocorticoid-sparing agent. Phototherapy with narrowband UVB or PUVA can also be used. Narrowband UVB is the most effective repigmentary treatment available for generalised vitiligo, but even very prolonged courses often do not produce a satisfactory outcome. The absence of leucotrichia (white hairs in the area of vitiligo) and the presence of a trichrome pattern (three colours – normal skin colour, hypopigmentation and depigmentation) are good prognostic features. Vitiligo on the face, trunk and proximal limbs is more likely to respond than that on hands and feet.

Fig. 29.43 Vitiligo. Symmetrical localised patches of depigmented skin.

29

Exceptionally, depigmentation of normal non-lesional skin or a surgical approach with autologous melanocyte transfer, using a range of techniques including split-skin grafts and blister roof grafts, is sometimes used on dermabraded recipient skin in specific severe cases.

The impact of vitiligo differs markedly between populations. In the Indian subcontinent, the effects are more readily discernible than in pale-skinned individuals in northern Europe. Depigmentation is also seen in leprosy, which means that individuals with vitiligo are often stigmatised. The emotional impact of vitiligo may be immense; psychological support is essential and is important in conveying realistic expectations of possible treatment approaches.

Oculocutaneous albinism

Albinism results from a range of genetic abnormalities that lead to reduced melanin biosynthesis in the skin and eyes; the number of melanocytes is normal (in contrast to vitiligo). Albinism is usually inherited as an autosomal recessive trait and there are several different types and presentations.

Type 1 albinism is due to a defect in the tyrosinase gene, whose product is rate-limiting in the production of melanin. Affected individuals have an almost complete absence of pigment in the skin and hair at birth, with consequent pale skin and white hair, and failure of melanin production in the iris and retina. Patients have photophobia, poor vision not correctable with refraction, rotatory nystagmus, and an alternating strabismus associated with abnormalities in the decussation of nerve fibres in the optic tract.

A second form of albinism is due to a defect in the *P* gene, which encodes an ion channel protein in the melanosome. Patients may have gross reduction of melanin in the skin and in the eyes, but may be more mildly affected than type 1 albinos. Establishing the subtype of albinism requires genetic analysis, as there is considerable phenotypic heterogeneity.

Oculocutaneous albinos are at grossly increased risk of sunburn and skin cancer. In equatorial regions, many die from squamous cell carcinoma or, more rarely, melanoma in early adult life. Interestingly, they may develop pigmented melanocytic naevi and freckle in response to sun exposure.

Management

Strict photoprotection (p. 1221), with sun avoidance (including occupational exposure), clothing, hats and sunscreens, is important. Early diagnosis and treatment of skin tumours is essential.

Increased pigmentation

- *Diffuse hyperpigmentation*: most commonly due to hypermelanosis but other pigments may be deposited in the skin, such as orange discoloration with carotenaemia and bronze with haemochromatosis (p. 895).
- *Endocrine pigmentation*: may occur in several conditions. Melasma (chloasma) describes discrete patches of facial pigmentation that occur in pregnancy and in some women taking oral contraceptives. The mechanism for this localised increased hormonal sensitivity is unknown. Diffuse pigmentation, sometimes worse in the skin creases and mucosae, may be a feature of Addison's disease (p. 671), Cushing's syndrome (p. 666), Nelson's syndrome (p. 669) and chronic renal failure due to increased levels of pituitary melanotrophic peptides, including adrenocorticotrophic hormone (ACTH; p. 669).

i	29.29 Drug-induced pigmentation	
Drug	**Appearance**	
Amiodarone	Photo-exposed sites, slate-grey	
Arsenic	Diffuse bronze pigmentation	
	Raindrop depigmentation	
Bleomycin	Usually flexural, brown	
Busulfan	Diffuse brown	
Chloroquine	Photo-exposed sites, blue-grey	
Clofazimine	Red	
Mepacrine	Yellow	
Minocycline	Temples, shins, gingiva, sclera, scar sites, slate-grey	
Phenothiazines	Photo-exposed sites, slate-grey	
Psoralens	Photo-exposed sites, brown	

- *Photo-exposed site hyperpigmentation*: occurs in some of the porphyrias but can also be drug-induced.
- *Drug-induced pigmentation* (Box 29.29): may be diffuse or localised. It is not always due to hypermelanosis but sometimes is caused by deposition of the drug or a metabolite.
- *Focal hypermelanosis*: seen in lesions such as freckles and lentigines, characterised by focal areas of increased pigmentation.

Establishing the cause is important. Photoprotection may minimise the risk of increasing pigmentation. Topical hydroquinone preparations can be used for skin lightening in some types of hyperpigmentation, although caution is required, particularly in darker skin types.

Hair disorders

These can be subdivided into disorders that cause loss of hair (alopecia) or excessive hair growth (hypertrichosis and hirsutism).

Alopecia

Alopecia is characterised by loss of hair. It can be further subdivided into localised and diffuse, and into scarring and non-scarring subtypes (Box 29.30).

Pathogenesis

Alopecia can be observed in association with inflammatory disorders that cause scarring (lichen planus, discoid lupus) and others that do not cause scarring (tinea capitis, psoriasis, seborrhoeic eczema). These conditions are discussed elsewhere. Alopecia areata has an autoimmune basis and there is a strong genetic component, with a family history in approximately 20% of cases. In addition to atopy, it is associated with other autoimmune diseases, particularly thyroid disease, and with Down's syndrome. The cause of androgenetic alopecia is unclear but likely to be multifactorial, with genetic, hormonal and end-organ receptor sensitivity to the factors implicated.

Clinical features

Alopecia areata

This usually presents with well-defined, localised, non-inflammatory, non-scarring patches of alopecia, usually on the

29.30 Classification and causes of alopecia	
Localised	**Diffuse**
Non-scarring	
Tinea capitis	Androgenetic alopecia
Alopecia areata	Telogen effluvium
Androgenetic alopecia	Hypothyroidism
Traumatic (trichotillomania, traction, cosmetic)	Hyperthyroidism
	Hypopituitarism
Syphilis	Diabetes mellitus
	HIV disease
	Nutritional (especially iron) deficiency
	Liver disease
	Post-partum
	Alopecia areata
	Syphilis
	Drug-induced: chemotherapy, retinoids
Scarring	
Discoid lupus erythematosus	Discoid lupus erythematosus
Lichen planopilaris	Radiotherapy
Herpes zoster	Folliculitis decalvans
Pseudopelade	Lichen planopilaris
Tinea capitis/kerion	
Morphoea (en coup de sabre)	
Idiopathic	
Developmental defects	

Fig. 29.44 Alopecia areata. The relatively extensive involvement and encroachment on posterior hairline are poor prognostic features.

scalp (Fig. 29.44). Pathognomonic 'exclamation mark' hairs are seen (broken hairs, tapering towards the scalp) during active hair loss. A diffuse pattern can uncommonly occur on the scalp. Eyebrows, eyelashes, beard and body hair can be affected. Alopecia totalis describes complete loss of scalp hair, and alopecia universalis is complete loss of all hair. Nail pitting may occur (p. 1261). Spontaneous regrowth is usual for small patches of alopecia but the prognosis is less good for larger patches, more extensive involvement, early onset and an association with atopy.

Androgenetic alopecia

Male-pattern baldness is physiological in men over 20 years old, although it can also occur in teenagers. It is also found in women, particularly post-menopausal ones. Characteristically, this involves bitemporal recession initially and subsequent involvement of the crown ('male pattern'), although it is often diffuse in women.

Investigations

Important investigations include full blood count, renal and liver function tests, iron studies, thyroid function, autoantibody screen and syphilis serology, as several systemic diseases, particularly iron deficiency and hypothyroidism, can cause diffuse non-scarring alopecia. Hair pull tests may help to establish the ratio of anagen to telogen hairs but require expertise for interpretation. Scrapings and pluckings should be sent for mycology if there is localised inflammation. Scalp biopsy and direct immunofluorescence of scarring alopecia may confirm a diagnosis of lichen planus or discoid lupus erythematosus but expert interpretation is needed.

Management

Any underlying condition, such as iron deficiency, should be treated and may result in clinical improvement. Alopecia can have a major impact on quality of life and psychological support is usually required. It is particularly important to establish realistic expectations.

Hair may spontaneously regrow in alopecia areata and it may be appropriate to offer no active intervention as, while some treatments may induce some hair regrowth, there is no evidence that any treatment fundamentally alters the course of the disease. There may be some response to topical or intralesional glucocorticoids. PUVA or immunotherapy with diphencyprone may be effective, with evidence of hair regrowth, but there is a risk of relapse on discontinuation of treatment. Short courses of systemic glucocorticoids are occasionally used in an attempt to limit acutely progressive extensive alopecia areata but should not be used in the long term; the risk of relapse on discontinuation is high. Ongoing trials of Janus kinase (JAK) inhibitors may provide future hope for patients with this difficult disease.

Some males with androgenetic alopecia may be helped by systemic finasteride. Topical minoxidil can be used in males and females with androgenetic alopecia but, if an effect is obtained, treatment must be continued and is expensive. In females, anti-androgen therapy, such as cyproterone acetate, can be used. Wigs are often appropriate for extensive alopecia. Scalp surgery and autologous hair transplants are expensive but can be used for androgenetic alopecia.

Hypertrichosis

Hypertrichosis is a generalised or localised increase in hair and may be congenital or acquired. It can be primary or secondary: for example, to drugs such as ciclosporin, minoxidil or diazoxide, malignancy or eating disorders. Laser therapy or eflornithine, which inhibits ornithine decarboxylase and arrests hair growth while it is being used, may be helpful. When the hypertrichosis follows a male pattern, it is called hirsutism.

Hirsutism

Hirsutism is the growth of terminal hair in a male pattern in a female (p. 657). The cause of most cases is unknown and, while it may occur in hyperandrogenism, Cushing's syndrome and polycystic ovary syndrome, only a small minority of patients have

29

a demonstrable hormonal abnormality. Psychological distress is often significant and oral contraceptives containing an anti-androgen such as cyproterone acetate, laser therapy or topical eflornithine may be beneficial.

Nail disorders

The nails can be affected by both local and systemic disease. The nail apparatus consists of the nail matrix and the nail plate, which arises from the matrix and lies on the nail bed (Fig. 29.45). The cells of the matrix and, to a lesser extent the bed, produce the keratinous plate.

Important information may be obtained from nail-fold examination, including dilated capillaries and ragged cuticles in connective tissue disease (Fig. 29.46) and the boggy inflammation of paronychia. The latter commonly occurs chronically in individuals undertaking wet work, in those with diabetes or poor peripheral circulation, and subsequent to increased cosmetic nail procedures and vigorous manicuring.

Normal variants

Longitudinal ridging and beading of the nail plate occur with age. White transverse patches (striate leuconychia) are often caused by airspaces within the plate.

Nail trauma

- *Nail biting/picking* is a very common habit. Repetitive proximal nail-fold trauma (often involving the thumb nail) results in transverse ridging and central furrowing of the nail.
- *Chronic trauma* from poorly-fitting shoes and sport can cause thickening and disordered growth of the nail (onychogryphosis) and subsequent ingrowing toenails.
- *Splinter haemorrhages* are fine, linear, dark brown longitudinal streaks in the plate (see Fig. 16.89, p. 529). They are usually caused by trauma, especially if distal. Uncommonly, they can occur in nail psoriasis and are also a hallmark of infective endocarditis.
- *Subungual haematoma* is red, purple or grey–brown discoloration of the nail plate, usually of the big toe (Fig. 29.47). These haematomas are usually due to trauma, although a history of this may not be clear. The main

differential is subungual melanoma, although rapid onset, lack of nail-fold involvement and proximal clearing as the nail grows are clues to the diagnosis of haematoma. If there is diagnostic doubt, a biopsy may be needed.

Nail involvement in skin diseases

- *Dermatophyte infection/onychomycosis*: this is described on page 1240.
- *Psoriasis*: nail involvement is common (see Fig. 29.35B, p. 1249).

Fig. 29.46 **Dermatomyositis.** A Photo-aggravation. B Note the prominent periungual involvement. Erythema, dilated and tortuous capillaries in the proximal nail fold, and ragged cuticles are features of connective tissue disease.

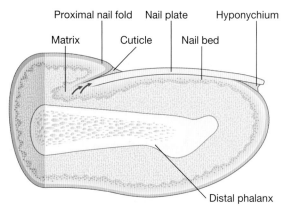

Fig. 29.45 **The nail plate and bed.** Arrows indicate the direction of nail growth.

Proximal nail fold Nail plate Hyponychium

Matrix Cuticle Nail bed

Distal phalanx

Fig. 29.47 **Subungual haematoma.**

- *Eczema*: nails may be shiny due to rubbing skin. Fine pitting can occur. If there is periungual eczema, the nail may become dystrophic, with thickening and transverse ridging. Paronychia is common.
- *Lichen planus*: there may be longitudinal ridging and thinning of the nail, giving a sandpaper texture (trachyonychia), erythematous streaks (erythronychia), subungual hyperkeratosis, pigmentation and, in severe cases, pterygium (splitting of nail due to central fibrosis and scarring, giving a winged appearance) and a destructive nail dystrophy.
- *Alopecia areata*: nail-plate pitting and trachyonychia can occur.

Nail involvement in systemic disease

The nails may be affected in many systemic diseases and important examples are detailed below:

- *Beau's lines*: horizontal ridges/indentations in nail plate occur simultaneously in all nails (Fig. 29.48B). They typically follow a systemic illness and are thought to be due to temporary growth arrest of cells in the nail matrix; they subsequently migrate out as the nail grows. Normal nail growth is approximately 0.1 mm/day for fingers and 0.05 mm/day for toes, so the timing of the systemic upset can usually be estimated by the position of the Beau's lines.
- *Koilonychia*: this concave or spoon-shaped nail-plate deformity is caused by iron deficiency (Fig. 29.48C).
- *Clubbing*: in the early stages, the angle between the proximal nail and nail fold is lost. In its more established form, there may be swelling of the distal digits (Figs 29.48D and E) or toes. Causes include bronchogenic carcinoma, asbestosis (especially with mesothelioma), suppurative or fibrosing lung disease, cyanotic congenital heart disease, infective endocarditis, inflammatory bowel disease, biliary cirrhosis and thyrotoxicosis; rarely, clubbing can be familial or idiopathic.
- *Nail discoloration*: whitening may occur in hypoalbuminaemia. 'Half-and-half' nails (white proximally and red/brown distally) may be found in renal failure. Antimalarials and some other drugs occasionally discolour nails.

Nail involvement in congenital disease

Nails can be affected in congenital diseases, such as pachyonychia congenita, a rare, usually autosomal dominant, condition caused by mutations in differentiation-specific keratin genes 6A, 6B, 16 and 17. This results in palmoplantar keratoderma and gross nail discoloration and thickening, due to subungual hyperkeratosis, from birth.

Fig. 29.48 The nail in systemic disease. [A] Normal nail. [B] Beau's line. [C] Koilonychia. [D] and [E] Digital clubbing.

Skin disease in general medicine

Many skin conditions present to other medical specialties. These are listed in Box 29.31 and the most common ones that are not discussed elsewhere are detailed below.

Conditions involving cutaneous vasculature

Vasculitis

Vasculitic involvement of the skin usually presents as palpable purpura (see Fig. 24.53, p. 1042). The diagnosis is confirmed by skin biopsy, along with histology and immunofluorescence examination. Underlying causes and their treatment are discussed on page 1040.

Pyoderma gangrenosum

The initial lesion of pyoderma gangrenosum (PG) is usually a painful, tender, inflamed nodule or pustule, which breaks down centrally and rapidly progresses to an ulcer with an indurated, undermined purplish or pustular edge (Fig. 29.49). Lesions may be single or multiple and are classified as ulcerative, pustular, bullous or vegetative. PG usually occurs in adults and, although it may occur in isolation, is usually associated with underlying disease, particularly inflammatory bowel disease, inflammatory arthritis, blood dyscrasias, immunodeficiencies and HIV infection. Investigation should be made with these associations in mind. The diagnosis is largely clinical, as histology is not specific. Analgesia, treatment of secondary bacterial infection and supportive

i	29.31 Skin problems in general medicine
Primary skin problems	
• Cellulitis	• Leg ulcers
• Vasculitis	• Pressure sores
Skin involvement in multisystem disease	
• Genetic: neurofibromatosis, tuberous sclerosis	• Porphyria
	• Sarcoidosis
• Xanthomas	• Systemic lupus erythematosus
• Amyloidosis	• Systemic sclerosis
Non-specific and variable skin reactions to systemic disease	
• Urticaria	• Pyoderma gangrenosum
• Erythema multiforme	• Sweet's syndrome
• Annular erythemas	• Generalised pruritus
• Erythema nodosum	
Skin conditions associated with malignancy	
• Dermatomyositis	• Acanthosis nigricans
• Generalised pruritus	• Superficial thrombophlebitis
Skin problems associated with specific medical disorders	
• Liver: generalised pruritus, pigmentation, spider naevi, palmar erythema, nail clubbing	
• Kidney: generalised pruritus, uraemic frost, pigmentation	
• Diabetes mellitus: necrobiosis lipoidica, diabetic dermopathy	
• Cutaneous Crohn's disease	
Skin problems secondary to treatment of systemic disease	
• Drug eruptions	
Miscellaneous	
• Granuloma annulare	• Morphoea

29

Fig. 29.49 Pyoderma gangrenosum. This young patient had Crohn's disease. Note the cribriform pattern of re-epithelialisation, which is characteristic of this condition.

Fig. 29.50 Scarring inflammatory alopecia. This patient had systemic lupus erythematosus and additional cutaneous features of scarring inflammatory discoid lupus erythematosus.

dressings are important. Systemic treatment with glucocorticoids, dapsone, ciclosporin or other immunosuppressants is often required. Tetracyclines may be added for their anti-inflammatory effects. Treatment with TNF-α inhibitors and ustekinumab may be effective in severe recalcitrant PG. Once healing has taken place, recurrences are typically only intermittent.

Other neutrophilic dermatoses

These include Sweet's acute febrile neutrophilic dermatosis and the neutrophilic dermatosis of rheumatoid disease, which are characterised by intense inflammation, mainly consisting of neutrophils, around dermal blood vessels. There can be damage to vessels ('vasculopathy') but usually no frank vasculitis.

Pressure sores

Localised, prolonged, pressure-induced ischaemia can lead to the development of pressure sores, which can occur in up to 30% of the hospitalised elderly. They are associated with considerable morbidity, mortality and expense to health services. The main risk factors are immobility, poor nutrition, local tissue hypoxia – for example, with anaemia, peripheral vascular disease, diabetes, sepsis and skin atrophy – or barrier impairment, such as in eczema.

A localised area of erythema develops at sites of bony prominences (particularly sacrum, greater trochanter, ischial and calcaneal tuberosities, and lateral malleolus). This progresses to a blister and then erosion, which will develop into a deep necrotic ulcer, usually colonised by *Pseudomonas aeruginosa* if pressure is not alleviated.

Prevention is key and involves identification of at-risk patients and regular repositioning and use of pressure-relieving mattresses. Predisposing factors, such as anaemia and poor nutrition, should be corrected. Once established, significant infection must be treated and necrotic tissue debrided. Dressings encourage granulation, although surgical intervention may sometimes be needed.

Connective tissue disease

Lupus erythematosus

This autoimmune disorder can be subdivided into systemic lupus erythematosus (SLE) and cutaneous lupus, which includes discoid lupus erythematosus (DLE) and subacute cutaneous lupus erythematosus (SCLE). The features of SLE are discussed on page 1035. Drug-induced DLE and SCLE should always be considered (see Box 24.78, p. 1057, and Boxes 29.34 and 29.35 below). DLE typically presents as scaly red plaques with follicular plugging, usually on photo-exposed sites of the face, head and neck, which resolve with scarring and pigmentary change. If the scalp is involved, scarring alopecia usually occurs (Fig. 29.50). Most patients with DLE do not develop SLE. Patients with SCLE may have extensive cutaneous involvement, usually aggravated by sun exposure, with an annular, polycyclic or papulosquamous eruption. Systemic involvement is uncommon and the prognosis usually good. There is a strong association with antibodies to Ro/SS-A antigen. A diagnosis of cutaneous lupus is confirmed by histopathology and direct immunofluorescence. Cutaneous lupus may respond to topical glucocorticoids, antimalarials or immunosuppressants. Antimalarials and photoprotection are important mainstays in the management of cutaneous lupus, and systemic immunosuppression may be required for resistant disease. Paradoxically, low-dose UVA1 phototherapy can be effective for lupus.

Systemic sclerosis

This autoimmune multisystem disease presents with severe Raynaud's syndrome, digital ulcers and skin fibrosis. Dilated nail-fold capillaries and ragged cuticles are frequent. The clinical features and management are described on page 1037.

Morphoea

Morphoea is a localised cutaneous form of scleroderma that can affect any site at any age. It usually presents as a thickened violaceous plaque, which may become hyper- or hypopigmented. Plaques can become generalised. Linear forms exist and, if in the scalp, are associated with scarring hair loss (en coup de sabre). There is usually no systemic involvement. Topical glucocorticoids or immunosuppressants or phototherapy, particularly PUVA or UVA1, can be effective, and systemic immunosuppression may be used for resistant extensive disease.

Dermatomyositis

Dermatomyositis is a multisystem disease, predominantly affecting skin, muscles and blood vessels. Typical cutaneous features include a violaceous 'heliotrope' erythema periorbitally and involving the upper eyelids, but this can sometimes affect the upper trunk, shoulders ('shawl sign') and limbs. Linear erythematous streaks may also be observed on the back of hands and fingers, and papules over the knuckles (Gottron's papules). Tortuous dilated nail-fold capillaries, often best seen with a dermatoscope, and ragged cuticles are usually evident. Photo-aggravation of the cutaneous features is often prominent (see Fig. 29.46A, p. 1260). The clinical features and management are described on page 1039.

Granulomatous disease

Granuloma annulare

This is common and may be reactive, although a trigger is usually not apparent. The hallmark is the presence of dermal granulomas, which are usually palisading and associated with alteration of dermal collagen (necrobiosis). The condition is generally asymptomatic and may present as an isolated dermal lesion with a raised papular annular edge, or may be more generalised. An association between generalised disease and diabetes has been proposed but not confirmed. Lesions often resolve spontaneously. Intralesional glucocorticoids or cryotherapy can be used for localised disease, and UVB or UVA1 phototherapy or PUVA for generalised disease.

Necrobiosis lipoidica

This condition has some histological features in common with granuloma annulare, although necrobiosis predominates. The lesion has a characteristic yellow, waxy, atrophic appearance, often with violaceous edge (Fig. 29.51). Underlying blood vessels are easily seen because of tissue atrophy. Necrobiosis lipoidica typically appears on the shins and is prone to ulceration after trauma. There is a strong association with diabetes: most patients with necrobiosis lipoidica have or develop diabetes, although less than 1% of diabetic patients develop necrobiosis lipoidica. Treatment is difficult and includes very potent topical or intralesional glucocorticoids, topical calcineurin inhibitors, PUVA or UVA1 phototherapy and systemic immunosuppression.

Sarcoidosis

This condition is characterised by the presence of non-caseating granulomas. The cause is unknown, although infectious and genetic factors have been proposed. It is usually a multisystem disease (p. 608), with skin lesions in about one-third of patients. Cutaneous features can occur in isolation and include violaceous infiltrated dermal plaques and nodules, which can affect any site but particularly digits and nose (lupus pernio), more generalised hyper- or hypopigmented or annular papules

Fig. 29.51 Necrobiosis lipoidica. Atrophic yellow plaques with violaceous edges, on the shins of a patient with diabetes mellitus.

and plaques, infiltrative changes in scars and erythema nodosum (see Fig. 17.59, p. 609). It has been reported more commonly and may be more severe in those of African, African American or Indian ancestry. Investigation is described on page 609. Cutaneous disease may respond to topical or intralesional glucocorticoids, cryotherapy, UVA1, laser or PDT (pp. 1226–1228). Clinical features and management of systemic disease are discussed on pages 608 and 610.

Cutaneous Crohn's disease

Cutaneous Crohn's disease (p. 813) is rare but may present as perianal and peristomal infiltrative plaques, lymphoedema, sinuses or fistulae, and oral granulomatous disease. These changes are termed 'metastatic' Crohn's and histology shows non-caseating granulomas. Reactive skin changes can also occur in the form of erythema nodosum and pyoderma gangrenosum (pp. 1265 and 1261). Treatment is of the underlying disease (p. 820).

Porphyrias

The porphyrias (described on p. 378) are a diverse group of diseases, caused by reduced or absent activity of specific enzymes in the porphyrin–haem biosynthetic pathway. Due to this loss of enzyme activity, porphyrin precursors proximal to the implicated enzyme step accumulate. If the accumulated porphyrins absorb visible light, then there will be skin features and photosensitivity, which explains why some porphyrias have skin features (porphyria cutanea tarda) and others do not (acute intermittent porphyria; p. 379). The most common skin presentations are photo-exposed site blistering, skin fragility and pain on daylight exposure.

Cutaneous porphyrias: fragility and blisters

Although porphyria cutanea tarda (PCT) may be genetically inherited, this is uncommon and acquired PCT is the most common porphyria worldwide. It is caused by an underlying chronic liver disease, in association with hepatic iron overload. The liver disease is often only diagnosed through investigation of the

29

Fig. 29.52 Porphyria cutanea tarda. Skin fragility, blistering, scarring, milia and hypertrichosis on the back of hands and fingers in hepatitis C.

skin presentation and it is thus an important diagnosis not to miss. Typical features are increased skin fragility, blistering, erosions, hypertrichosis, scarring and milia occurring on light-exposed areas, particularly the backs of the hands (Fig. 29.52). Less common features include facial hypertrichosis, hyperpigmentation and morphoea-like changes. Variegate porphyria (VP) and hereditary coproporphyria (HCP) may be indistinguishable on skin features and it is important to make the correct diagnosis, as acute neurovisceral attacks, which may be drug-induced (p. 1265), can occur in VP and HCP but not in PCT. Pseudoporphyria may also be impossible to distinguish from PCT on clinical grounds but is most frequently caused by a drug (commonly naproxen; see Box 29.35) or by sunbed use; on investigation, porphyrins are normal. A PCT-like presentation may also be seen in uraemia due to renal failure, but is caused by raised porphyrins due to impaired elimination rather than an enzyme defect.

Management of PCT requires removal or treatment of any underlying cause, which may involve venesection, iron chelation, very low-dose hydroxychloroquine once or twice per week and photoprotection.

Cutaneous porphyria: pain on sun exposure

Erythropoietic protoporphyria is caused by a genetic defect in the ferrochelatase gene that leads to ferrochelatase enzyme deficiency. It is an important diagnosis to consider. The presentation is usually in early childhood, although the diagnosis is often delayed. In part this is because, although the baby or child cries due to immediate pain on sunlight exposure, physical signs are often absent or minimal and thus a link with sunlight may not always be considered. The deficient ferrochelatase activity leads to accumulation of lipid-soluble protoporphyrins in the skin, explaining the photosensitivity manifest as pain on daylight exposure. Multiple pigment gallstones, anaemia (usually only problematic if considered to be due to iron deficiency) and, rarely, severe liver disease can occur, which may be fatal and requires liver transplantation. In addition to photoprotection, UVB phototherapy may be effective for the symptoms of photosensitivity and, more recently, the use of alpha-melanocyte-stimulating hormone (α-MSH) analogues has been explored.

Abnormal deposition disorders

Xanthomas

Deposits of fatty material in the skin, subcutaneous fat and tendons may be the first clue to primary or secondary hyperlipidaemia (pp. 346 and p. 373).

Amyloidosis

Cutaneous amyloid may present as periocular plaques in primary systemic amyloidosis (p. 81) and amyloid associated with multiple myeloma, but is uncommon in systemic amyloidosis secondary to rheumatoid arthritis or other chronic inflammatory diseases. Amyloid infiltration of blood vessels may manifest as 'pinch purpura' following skin trauma. Macular amyloid is more common in darker skin types and appears as pruritic grey/brown macules or patches, usually on the back. Potent topical glucocorticoids can be beneficial, although it is often treatment-resistant.

Genetic disorders

Neurofibromatosis

This is described in detail on page 1131.

Tuberous sclerosis

This is an autosomal dominant condition and two genetic loci have been identified: *TSC-1* (chromosome 9) encoding hamartin, and *TSC-2* (chromosome 16) encoding tuberin. The hallmark is hamartomas in many systems. The classic triad of clinical features comprises learning disability, epilepsy and skin lesions but there is marked heterogeneity in clinical features. Skin changes include pale oval (ash leaf) macules that occur in early childhood; yellowish/pink papules in the mid-face (angiofibromas, 'adenoma sebaceum'), occurring in adolescence; periungual and subungual fibromas; and connective tissue naevi (shagreen patches, often on lower back). Gum hyperplasia, retinal phakomas (fibrous overgrowths), renal, lung and heart tumours, cerebral gliomas and calcified basal ganglia may also occur.

Reactive disorders

Erythema multiforme

Erythema multiforme has characteristic clinical and histological features and can be triggered by a variety of factors (Box 29.32) but a cause is not always identified. The disease is likely to have an immunological basis. Lesions are multiple, erythematous, annular, targetoid 'bull's eyes' (Fig. 29.53) and may blister. Stevens–Johnson syndrome (pp. 1224 and 1254) is a severe form of erythema multiforme with marked blistering, mucosal involvement (mouth, eyes and genitals) and systemic upset.

Identification and removal/treatment of any trigger are essential. Analgesia and topical glucocorticoids may provide symptomatic relief. Supportive care is required in Stevens–Johnson syndrome, including ophthalmology input.

---

i   **29.32 Provoking factors in erythema multiforme**

Infections
- Viral: herpes simplex, orf, infectious mononucleosis, hepatitis B, HIV
- *Mycoplasma* and other bacterial infections

Drugs
- Sulphonamides, penicillins, barbiturates and carbamazepine

Systemic disease
- Sarcoidosis, malignancy, systemic lupus erythematosus

Other
- Radiotherapy, pregnancy

Fig. 29.53 Erythema multiforme in a young woman. Herpes simplex virus infection was the trigger.

 29.33 Provoking factors in erythema nodosum

Infections

- Bacteria: streptococci, mycobacteria, *Brucella*, *Mycoplasma*, *Rickettsia*, *Chlamydia*
- Viruses: hepatitis B and infectious mononucleosis
- Fungi

Drugs

- Sulphonamides, sulphonylureas, oral contraceptives

Systemic disease

- Sarcoidosis, inflammatory bowel disease, malignancy

Other

- Pregnancy

Erythema nodosum

This is characterised histologically by a septal panniculitis of subcutaneous fat (see Fig. 17.59, p. 609). An identified trigger is often present (Box 29.33). Lesions are typically painful, indurated violaceous nodules on the shins and lower legs. Systemic upset, arthralgias and fever are common. Spontaneous resolution occurs over a month or so, leaving bruise-like marks. Any underlying cause should be identified and removed or treated. Bed rest, leg elevation and an oral NSAID frequently offer symptomatic relief. Systemic glucocorticoids are effective but seldom required, and must be avoided when there is a possibility of infection. Potassium iodide, dapsone or hydroxychloroquine may be effective for resistant disease but these are rarely required.

Acquired reactive perforating dermatosis

The hallmark of this condition is transepidermal elimination of dermal material, particularly collagen and elastic tissue. It presents as keratotic papules, particularly in patients with diabetes and chronic renal disease. Treatment with topical glucocorticoids, retinoids, PUVA or UVA1 therapy may help. There are other related perforating dermopathies, with characteristic histology.

Annular erythemas

This group of chronic, poorly defined, annular, erythematous and often scaly eruptions can be further subdivided and may be secondary to an identifiable cause. Erythema chronicum migrans can be associated with Lyme disease (*Borrelia burgdorferi*, p. 255). Erythema marginatum can occur in rheumatic fever (p. 515) or Still's disease (p. 1040). Erythema gyratum repens typically presents as concentric circles of erythema and scale with an advancing edge and is usually associated with underlying malignancy. Erythema annulare centrifugum presents with expanding, scaly, erythematous rings, with central fading. A trigger may not be apparent but possible associations include fungal infection, drugs, autoimmune or endocrine diseases, such as lupus or thyroid disease, and malignancy, particularly haematological. An underlying trigger must be sought and removed or treated. Topical glucocorticoids or phototherapy may be helpful for chronic disease.

Acanthosis nigricans

Hyperkeratosis and pigmentation are typical and affected sites have a velvety texture. The flexures, especially axillae and, in dark-skinned people, sides of neck, are involved (pp. 1325, 1326 and 720). There are several types, mainly associated with insulin resistance. Most often, acanthosis nigricans is found in conjunction with obesity and regresses with weight loss. It can be associated with malignancy, usually adenocarcinoma (particularly gastric), when it is usually more extensive and pruritic, and can involve mucous membranes.

Drug eruptions

Virtually all drugs may have cutaneous adverse effects (Fig. 29.54) and this should be considered in the differential diagnosis of most presentations of skin disease. Drugs can exert their adverse effects via several mechanisms, which can be broadly subdivided into non-immunological and immunological (Box 29.34).

 29.34 Types of drug eruption

Non-immunological

Predictable

- Striae due to glucocorticoids (see Fig. 29.10, p. 1226)
- Asteatosis with statins
- Candidal infections with antibiotics
- Worsening of psoriasis with lithium, β-blockers, antimalarials, NSAIDs
- Urticaria with aspirin due to mast cell degranulation
- Bradykinin-mediated angioedema due to ACE inhibitors
- Doxycycline photosensitivity
- Dapsone haemolysis

Immunological

Unpredictable

- Immediate IgE-mediated hypersensitivity (type I): penicillin-induced urticaria and anaphylaxis
- Antibody-mediated (type II): penicillin-induced haemolysis
- Immune complex-mediated (type III): drug-induced serum sickness or vasculitis
- Delayed hypersensitivity (type IV): drug-induced erythema multiforme, lichenoid or pemphigus-like reaction; drug-induced lupus

(ACE = angiotensin-converting enzyme; IgE = immunoglobulin E; NSAIDs = non-steroidal anti-inflammatory drugs)

29

i | 29.35 Clinical patterns of drug eruptions

Reaction pattern	Clinical features	Examples of causative drugs
Exanthematous	Erythema, maculopapular	Antibiotics (especially ampicillin), anticonvulsants, gold, penicillamine, NSAIDs, carbimazole, anti-TNF drugs and other biological therapies
Urticaria and angioedema	Sometimes accompanied by angioedema Angioedema alone	Salicylates, opiates, NSAIDs, antibiotics, dextran, ACE inhibitors
Lichenoid	Violaceous, lichen planus-like, dyspigmentation	Gold, penicillamine, antimalarials, thiazides, NSAIDs, β-blockers, ACE inhibitors, sulphonamides, lithium, sulphonylureas, proton pump inhibitors, quinine, antituberculous, dyes in colour developers
Purpura and vasculitis	Palpable purpura and necrosis	Allopurinol, antibiotics, ACE inhibitors, NSAIDs, aspirin, anticonvulsants, diuretics, oral contraceptives
Erythema multiforme	Target-like lesions and bullae on extensor aspects of limbs	See Box 29.32, p. 1264
Erythema nodosum	Tender, painful, dusky, erythematous nodules on shins	See Box 29.33, p. 1265
Exfoliative dermatitis	There may be erythroderma	Allopurinol, carbamazepine, barbiturates, penicillins, PAS, isoniazid, gold, lithium, penicillamine, ACE inhibitors
Toxic epidermal necrolysis	Rapid evolution, extensive blistering, erythema, necrolysis, mucosal involvement	Anticonvulsants, antibiotics, especially sulphonamides, NSAIDs, terbinafine, sulphonylureas, antiretrovirals, allopurinol
Photosensitivity (p. 1220)	Photo-exposed site rash, may be sunburn-like, exfoliation, lichenoid	Thiazides, amiodarone, quinine, NSAIDs, tetracyclines, fluoroquinolones, phenothiazines, sulphonamides, retinoids, psoralens
Drug-induced lupus	Photosensitivity, discoid lesions, urticarial or erythema multiforme-like. May have positive lupus serology and anti-histone antibodies	Allopurinol, thiazides, ACE inhibitors, PAS, anticonvulsants, β-blockers, gold, hydralazine, minocycline, penicillamine, lithium, proton pump inhibitors
Psoriasiform rash	Rash resembles psoriasis	See Box 29.23 (p. 1248)
DRESS	Facial oedema, fever, extensive rash, lymphadenopathy, eosinophilia and systemic involvement	Anticonvulsants, trimethoprim, minocycline, allopurinol, dapsone, terbinafine
AGEP/toxic pustuloderma	Rapid onset of sterile, non-follicular pustules on erythematous base	Ampicillin/amoxicillin, erythromycin, quinolones, sulphonamides, terbinafine, diltiazem, hydroxychloroquine
Acneiform eruptions	Rash resembles acne	Lithium, anticonvulsants, oral contraceptives, androgens, glucocorticoids, antituberculous drugs, EGFR antagonists (cetuximab and erlotinib)
Pigmentation		See Box 29.29 (p. 1258)
Bullous eruptions	Often at pressure sites and there may be other features, such as purpura, milia	Barbiturates, penicillamine, furosemide
Pseudoporphyria	May be indistinguishable from porphyria cutanea tarda clinically	NSAIDs, tetracyclines, retinoids, furosemide, nalidixic acid
Exacerbation of acute hepatic porphyrias		See page 1263 Always check all drugs for safety of use in porphyrias against standard guidelines
Drug-induced immunobullous disease	May resemble pemphigoid, pemphigus, dermatomyositis, scleroderma, epidermolysis bullosa acquisita	Penicillamine, ACE inhibitors, vancomycin
Fixed drug eruptions	Round/oval, erythema, oedema ± bullae Same site every time drug is given Pigmentation on resolution	Tetracyclines, sulphonamides, penicillins, quinine, NSAIDs, barbiturates, anticonvulsants
Hair loss	Diffuse	Cytotoxic agents, oral retinoids, anticoagulants, anticonvulsants, antithyroid drugs, lithium, oral contraceptives, infliximab
Hypertrichosis	Excessive hair growth in non-androgenic distribution	Diazoxide, minoxidil, ciclosporin

(ACE = angiotensin-converting enzyme; AGEP = acute generalised exanthematous pustulosis; DRESS = drug rash with eosinophilia and systemic symptoms; EGFR = epidermal growth factor receptor; NSAIDs = non-steroidal anti-inflammatory drugs; PAS = para-aminosalicylic acid; TNF = tumour necrosis factor)

Fig. 29.54 Drug eruption. Possible drug causes of rash should always be considered. This was doxycycline-induced photosensitivity in a farmer.

Clinical features

Cutaneous drug reactions typically present in specific patterns (Box 29.35). Non-immunologically mediated reactions can theoretically occur in anyone, given sufficient exposure to the drug, although idiosyncratic factors, such as genetic predisposition, may render some more susceptible. There is limited information on genetic determinants of drug responses and adverse effects, although advances have been made, e.g. with azathioprine (p. 1227), and provide exciting opportunities for therapeutic personalised medicine. Immunologically mediated cutaneous drug eruptions typically commence within days to weeks of starting the drug. Detailed history-taking relating to prescribed and non-prescribed medications is essential and there may be other clues (Box 29.36).

Investigations and management

The suspected drug must be stopped. If drug-induced photosensitivity is considered, the patient should be phototested while on the drug to confirm the diagnosis, and again after drug withdrawal to confirm resolution of photosensitivity (p. 1215). An eosinophilia and abnormalities in liver function tests may occur in adverse drug reactions and, for example, specific IgE to penicillin may be raised in penicillin-induced rash but, otherwise, specific investigations are not available. Rechallenge with drug is not usually undertaken unless the reaction is mild, as this can be risky. Drug withdrawal may not be straightforward and substitute drugs may be required. Antihistamines and/or topical or systemic glucocorticoids may provide supportive management, depending on the type of cutaneous reaction. The management of anaphylaxis is described on page 76.

---

i | **29.36 Diagnostic clues to drug eruptions**

- Past history of reaction to suspected drug
- Introduction of suspected drug a few days to weeks before onset of rash
- Recent prescription of a drug commonly associated with rashes (penicillin, sulphonamide, thiazide, allopurinol)
- Symmetrical eruption that fits with a well-recognised pattern, caused by a current drug
- Resolution of rash following drug cessation

Further information

Websites

bad.org.uk *British Association of Dermatologists: guidelines and patient information for many skin diseases.*

cochrane.org/cochrane-reviews *Many relevant skin reviews, including sun protection (CD011161), psoriasis (CD001976, CD007633, CD005028, CD001213, CD009481, CD010497, CD010017, CD009687, CD001433), eczema (CD009864, CD005205, CD004054, CD005500, CD005203, CD008642, CD008426, CD003871, CD004416, CD006135, CD007770), skin cancer (CD005413, CD008955, CD007281, CD003412, CD004415, CD007041, CD005414, CD007869, CD004835, CD010308, CD010307, CD011161), leg ulcers (CD010182, CD002303, CD003557, CD001737, CD008599, CD001733, CD000265, CD008394, CD001177, CD009432, CD001273, CD011354, CD001836), acne (CD004425, CD011946, CD002086, CD000194, CD007917), rosacea (CD003262), urticaria (CD007770, CD006137, CD008596), alopecia (CD007628, CD004413), skin infections (CD009992, CD003584, CD004685, CD004767, CD010095, CD003261), bullous pemphigoid (CD002292).*

nice.org.uk *National Institute for Health and Care Excellence: guidance for skin cancer (NG14, NG34, PH32, CSG8, TA172, TA321, TA268, TA319, TA384, TA400, TA366, TA357, TA396, TA269, IPG446, IPG478, DG19), atopic eczema (QS44, CG57, TA81, TA82, TA177), psoriasis (CG153, TA146, TA372, TA368, TA103, TA134, TA350, TA180), sun exposure (NG34, PH32), vitamin D (PH56), urticaria (TA339, ESUOM31), rosacea (ESNM43, ESNM68), scabies (ESUOM29), photodynamic therapy (IPG155, MTG6) and Grenz rays (IPG236).*

sign.ac.uk *Scottish Intercollegiate Guidelines Network: no. 120 – Management of chronic venous leg ulcers; 121 – Diagnosis and management of psoriasis and psoriatic arthritis in adults; 125 – Management of atopic eczema in primary care; 140 – Management of primary cutaneous squamous cell carcinoma.*

29

L Mackillop
FEM Neuberger

Maternal medicine

Clinical examination in pregnancy 1270

Clinical evaluation in maternal medicine 1271

Planning pregnancy in patients with medical conditions 1272

Functional anatomy and physiology 1272

Investigations 1274
Imaging 1274

Presenting problems in pregnancy 1274
Breathlessness 1274
Chest pain 1275
Circulatory collapse 1275
Headache 1275
Nausea and vomiting 1275
Oedema 1275
Seizures 1275

Medical disorders in pregnancy 1276
Hypertension 1276
Respiratory disease 1277
Gastrointestinal disease 1277
Diabetes 1278
Endocrine disease 1279
Human immunodeficiency virus infection 1280
Inflammatory rheumatic disease 1280
Cardiac disease 1282
Renal disease 1282
Liver disease 1283
Neurological disease 1284
Psychiatric disorders 1284
Haematological disease 1284

Clinical examination in pregnancy

6 Breasts
Increase in size and vascularity

5 Heart
Ejection systolic murmur may be part of normal pregnancy
Diastolic murmurs are always pathological

4 Face
Conjunctival pallor (physiological anaemia of pregnancy)

▲ Jaundice in acute fatty liver of pregnancy

▲ Melasma

3 Blood pressure
Lower in 2nd and 3rd trimesters

2 Pulse
Pulse rate increased by 10–20 bpm
Bounding pulse

1 Hands

▲ Palmar erythema

7 Respiratory system
Mild breathlessness common
Respiratory rate unchanged

▲ Increased risk of varicella pneumonia

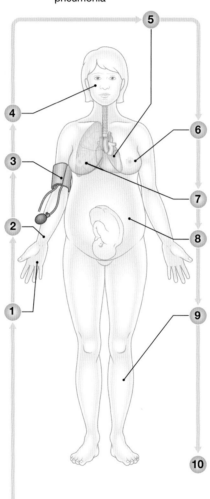

Observation
Plethoric
Mood/affect

8 Abdomen
Scars
Excoriations
Umbilicus eversion
Obstetric examination

▲ Linea nigra

▲ Striae gravidarum

▲ Striae albicans

9 Legs
Varicose veins

▲ Peripheral oedema
Mild oedema in normal pregnancy
Rapid-onset oedema suggests pre-eclampsia

10 Urine dipstick

Insets: (Palmar erythema) From Fitzpatrick JE, Morelli JG. Dermatology secrets plus, 5th edn. Philadelphia: Elsevier Inc.; 2016; (Melasma) From Lawrence CM, Cox NH. Color atlas and text of physical signs in dermatology. London: Wolfe; 1993; (Jaundice) From Morse SA, Ballard RC, Holmes KK, et al. Atlas of sexually transmitted diseases and AIDS, 4th edn. Saunders, Elsevier Inc.; 2010; (Varicella pneumonia) From Voore N, Lai R. Varicella pneumonia in an immunocompetent adult. Can Med Assoc J 2012; 184(17):1924; (Linea nigra) From Bolognia JL, Schaffer JV, Duncan KO, et al. Dermatology essentials. Philadelphia: Elsevier Inc.; 2014; Courtesy of Jean L. Bolognia; (Striae gravidarum) From Buchanan K, Fletcher HM, Reid M. Prevention of striae gravidarum

Clinical evaluation in maternal medicine

Take a careful history

Ask specifically about:
- Cardiac disease
- Renal disease
- Diabetes
- Rheumatic disease
- Inflammatory bowel disease
- Epilepsy

Take a careful drug history

Stop fetotoxic drugs before conception

- Methotrexate
- Leflunomide
- Mycophenolate
- Valproate

Perform general examination

Palmar erythema

Check for anaemia and jaundice

Check for oedema and deep venous thrombosis

Check blood pressure

Consider cardiovascular adaptations during pregnancy

Perform urinalysis

Perform further investigations if appropriate

Perform X-ray imaging if indicated

Remember changes of pregnancy when interpreting laboratory results

- Anaemia
- Altered thyroid function tests
- Low creatinine/urea
- Low CO_2
- Raised alkaline phosphatase
- Glycosuria

Consider mother and fetus when prescribing

30

with cocoa butter cream. Int J Gynecol Obstet 2009; 108(2010):65–68; (Striae albicans) From Cantisano-Zilkha M. Aesthetic oculofacial rejuvenation. Philadelphia: Saunders, Elsevier Inc.; 2010; (Peripheral oedema) From Huang H-W, Wong L-S, Lee C-H. Sarcoidosis with bilateral leg lymphedema as the initial presentation: a review of the literature. Dermatologica Sinica 34(2016):29–32.

Major physiological changes occur during pregnancy, which impact on several organ systems. These are necessary to support the growing fetus, to prepare for delivery and to support lactation. These changes can adversely affect the activity and progression of many pre-existing medical conditions. Emphasising this fact, information from the UK Confidential Enquiry into Maternal Deaths has revealed that over recent years, two-thirds of maternal deaths occur as the result of pre-existing medical conditions, rather than from obstetric causes. The most common causes of death were cardiac conditions (23%), pneumonia and influenza (14%), and venous thromboembolism (11%). Although some diseases can undergo remission during pregnancy, others can worsen, potentially jeopardising the health and well-being of the mother and fetus. In this chapter, we review the physiological changes that occur during pregnancy and the impact of pregnancy on the diagnosis, clinical course and management of common medical conditions. In addition, we review the pathogenesis and management of several medical conditions specific to pregnancy.

Planning pregnancy in patients with medical conditions

Patients with pre-existing medical conditions require careful counselling when planning a pregnancy to make them aware of the risks that pregnancy might pose, as well as the changes in symptoms that might be expected to occur during pregnancy. Although each disease is different, as is discussed later in this chapter, the general principles are to ensure that drugs that may be fetotoxic are stopped before pregnancy is attempted; that high-risk patients are kept under close surveillance during their pregnancy; and that new symptoms that emerge during pregnancy are treated seriously and fully investigated where appropriate.

Functional anatomy and physiology

The most important changes that occur in the anatomy and physiology of major organ systems during pregnancy are discussed below.

Bone metabolism

Major changes in bone metabolism take place to meet the demands of the growing fetus. Intestinal calcium absorption increases, due in part to increased production of 1,25-dihydroxyvitamin D ($1,25(OH)_2D$). Calcium is also released from the maternal skeleton due to increased bone resorption, stimulated by production of parathyroid hormone-related protein (PTHrP) by breast and placenta. This results in loss of bone from the maternal skeleton during pregnancy that continues until lactation ceases and then recovers. Serum concentrations of alkaline phosphatase (ALP) can increase by up to fourfold but this is due to release of ALP from the placenta rather than bone.

Cardiovascular system

Heart rate and stroke volume increase during pregnancy; when combined with peripheral vasodilatation and a reduction in systemic blood pressure, this causes a hyperdynamic circulatory state and an increase in cardiac output. Diaphragmatic elevation may affect the electrocardiogram (ECG), causing left axis deviation of up to 15°. Other changes include T-wave inversion in leads III and aVF, ST depression, small Q waves and a sinus tachycardia. Supraventricular and ventricular beats are common. Echocardiography shows a modest increase in the dimensions of the cardiac chambers.

Endocrine system

During early pregnancy there is secretion of human chorionic gonadotrophin (hCG) by trophoblast cells, which act on the corpus luteum in the ovary to stimulate oestradiol and progesterone production (Fig. 30.1). Levels of hCG rise rapidly during early pregnancy to reach a peak around 8 weeks, and then fall before stabilising at a lower level from 20 weeks until term. There is a progressive rise in oestradiol and progesterone levels; initially, these hormones are produced by the corpus luteum but placental production takes over after about 12 weeks. The high levels of gonadal hormones suppress pituitary gonadotrophin production but prolactin levels rise about 10-fold and there is an increase in volume of the anterior pituitary. Serum levels of free T_4 increase during the first trimester but, paradoxically, thyroid-stimulating hormone (TSH) levels fall by almost 50%. This is because hCG is homologous to TSH and mimics the effect of TSH on the thyroid, stimulating both T_3 and T_4 production. The raised levels of T_3 and T_4 feed back to the pituitary and reduce TSH secretion. Later in pregnancy, there is increased degradation of thyroxine by the placenta and levels of thyroxine-binding globulin (TBG) rise, causing the normal range for free T_4 and T_3 to fall progressively during the course of pregnancy. Although TSH levels are difficult to interpret early in pregnancy, they provide the best measure of thyroid function after about 16 weeks' gestation.

Gastrointestinal system

The high levels of progesterone during pregnancy lead to relaxation of smooth muscle in the gastrointestinal tract. This causes the lower oesophageal sphincter to relax, predisposing to gastro-oesophageal reflux and reduced gastrointestinal transit; this in turn leads to delayed gastric emptying and constipation.

Genitourinary system

Glomerular filtration rate (GFR) increases during pregnancy due to an increased cardiac output. By the second trimester, renal perfusion increases by up to 80% and GFR by 50%, leading to a fall in serum urea and creatinine. Mild glycosuria may be observed during normal pregnancy due mainly to an increase in filtered load of glucose. The ureters and renal pelvis are slightly dilated, most prominently on the left side, leading to the physiological hydronephrosis of pregnancy.

Glucose metabolism

Maternal glucose metabolism changes during pregnancy to optimise delivery of glucose and other nutrients to the fetus. During the second half of pregnancy in particular, there is maternal insulin resistance due largely to an increase in circulating levels of human placental lactogen (hPL) (Fig. 30.1). The net effect is to ensure that glucose is preferentially supplied to the fetus rather than the mother. Following delivery of the placenta, there is a rapid decline in hPL and reversal of insulin resistance. During pregnancy, fasting plasma glucose decreases slightly, while post-prandial blood glucose may increase. Glycosuria may occur, even in women who do not have diabetes, due to the

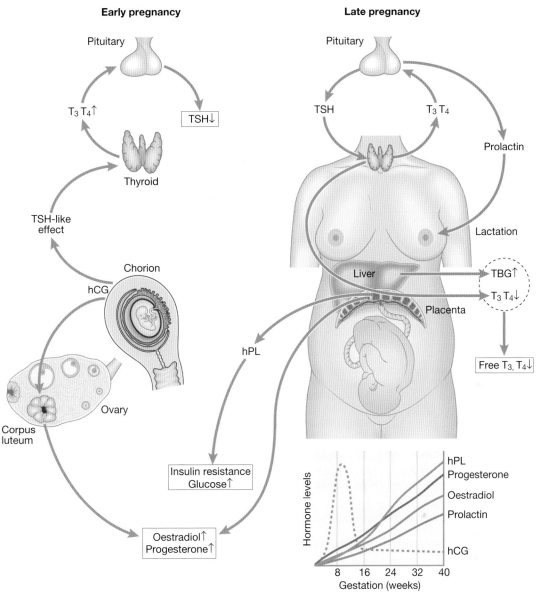

Fig. 30.1 Hormonal changes in pregnancy. In early pregnancy, oestradiol and progesterone are mainly derived from the corpus luteum in response to human chorionic gonadotrophin (hCG), secreted by the trophoblast. The raised levels of hCG also act on the thyroid to stimulate T_3 (triiodothyronine) and T_4 (thyroxine) production, which in turn suppresses thyroid-stimulating hormone (TSH) production by the pituitary. Later in pregnancy, oestradiol and progesterone are derived from the placenta, which also produces human placental lactogen (hPL), impairing glucose tolerance. There is a progressive reduction of free T_3 and T_4 during pregnancy as the result of T_3 and T_4 degradation by the placenta and increased secretion of thyroxine-binding globulin (TBG) by the liver.

increased GFR. Insulin secretion in the fetus is driven by fetal glucose levels, which in turn are dependent on maternal glucose concentrations. Accordingly, in women with diabetes, maternal hyperglycaemia stimulates fetal insulin secretion, which increases fetal growth, resulting in increased birth weight or macrosomia.

Haematological system

Haemoglobin normally falls by about 20% during pregnancy since plasma volume increases more than red cell volume: the so-called physiological anaemia of pregnancy. The reduction in haematocrit lowers blood viscosity but this is offset by an elevation in levels of several clotting factors, resulting in a hypercoagulable state that increases the risk of venous and arterial thrombosis.

Respiratory system

Tidal volume (TV) increases during pregnancy due to an increased vital capacity and reduced residual volume, and by term the increase in TV is about 200 mL. These changes are required to meet the 20% increase in oxygen demand that occurs during pregnancy. The $P\mathrm{CO}_2$ level decreases but this is offset by an increase in renal excretion of bicarbonate, such that the blood pH remains relatively stable. Respiratory rate is unaffected by pregnancy.

30

Investigations

The profound changes in physiology and anatomy that occur during pregnancy cause changes in the normal reference ranges for several hormones, electrolytes and other analytes, as summarised in Box 30.1. While many investigations can

proceed as normal during pregnancy, invasive procedures should generally be avoided unless the potential benefit clearly outweighs the risk. Investigations that can be performed in pregnancy are shown in Box 30.2.

Imaging

Imaging during pregnancy should be undertaken only when the clinical benefit outweighs the potential risks to mother and fetus. In suspected pulmonary embolus, radionuclide ventilation/perfusion ($\dot{V}/\dot{Q}$) scanning is preferred over computed tomographic pulmonary angiography (CTPA) in women with a normal chest X-ray since $\dot{V}/\dot{Q}$ scans expose the maternal breast and lungs to less radiation than CTPA. However, if the chest X-ray is abnormal, CTPA should be performed, since it is more likely to yield a definitive diagnosis. The radiation exposure for both investigations is well below the maximum recommended fetal radiation dose in pregnancy (5 rad). Chest X-rays may also be performed safely at any gestation during pregnancy if clinically indicated, since the radiation exposure is very low for the fetus. Magnetic resonance imaging (MRI) is safe in the second and third trimesters and is useful in the assessment of proximal deep vein thrombosis (DVT) and neurological disorders. However, gadolinium-containing contrast agents should be used only if absolutely necessary. If gadolinium contrast agents are used in women who are breastfeeding, the milk should be discarded for 24 hours. Ultrasound imaging is safe during pregnancy and useful in the assessment of patients with DVT or intra-abdominal pathology.

Presenting problems in pregnancy

Breathlessness

The causes of breathlessness during pregnancy are summarised in Box 30.3. Many women experience mild breathlessness as part of normal pregnancy, which is known as physiological

i	30.1 Common laboratory changes during pregnancy	
Laboratory test	Change	Cause
Haematology		
Haematocrit	Decrease	Extracellular volume expansion
Routine biochemistry		
GFR	Increase	Increased renal blood flow
Urea and creatinine	Decrease	Increased GFR
Alkaline phosphatase	Increase	Release by placenta
Glucose	Decrease (fasting)	Raised insulin
	Increase (post-prandial)	Insulin resistance
Hormones		
T_4	Increase (first trimester)	Stimulation of thyroid by hCG
	Decrease (later pregnancy)	Placental degradation
TSH	Decrease (first trimester)	Increased T_4 due to stimulation of thyroid by hCG
Prolactin	Increase	Increased production by pituitary
Oestradiol Progesterone	Progressive increase	Production by corpus luteum then placenta
hCG	Increase then decrease	Production by trophoblast
hPL	Progressive increase	Production by placenta

(GFR = glomerular filtration rate; hCG = human chorionic gonadotrophin; hPL = human placental lactogen; TSH = thyroid-stimulating hormone)

i	30.2 Investigations in pregnancy*	
Investigation	Use during pregnancy	Comment
Renal biopsy	Can be performed during pregnancy	<22 weeks is safest; 23–28 weeks is period of highest risk
Gastroscopy	Safe during pregnancy. Left lateral position is recommended in the second half of pregnancy	Fetal monitoring should be offered pre- and post-procedure. Low-dose sedation recommended
Colonoscopy	Safe during pregnancy	Fetal monitoring should be offered pre- and post-procedure. Low-dose sedation recommended
Flexible sigmoidoscopy	Safe during pregnancy	Fetal monitoring should be offered pre- and post-procedure. Low-dose sedation recommended
Magnetic resonance imaging	Not contraindicated at any gestation	Theoretical risks to fetus in first trimester
Computed tomography	Can be performed at any gestation	Radiation exposure to fetus and mother must be considered and addressed in counselling
X-ray	Safe at any gestation	
Ultrasound	Safe at any gestation	
Echocardiogram	Safe at any gestation	
Ambulatory electrocardiogram	Safe at any gestation	

*For any investigation, the potential benefit must outweigh the risk.

i 30.3 Breathlessness during pregnancy	
Cause	**Management**
Physiological breathlessness of pregnancy	No treatment required
Asthma	Treatment as in non-pregnant women
Pneumonia	Treatment with antibiotic as in non-pregnant women
Valvular heart disease	Treatment as in non-pregnant women
Heart failure	Treatment as in non-pregnant women
Peripartum cardiomyopathy (PPCM)	Treatment as in non-pregnant women. Early delivery if haemodynamic deterioration
Pulmonary embolus	Treatment as in non-pregnant women

breathlessness of pregnancy. It is thought to be progesterone-mediated and is classically of gradual onset and present at rest and on exercise. Physiological breathlessness does not require investigation but severe or persistent breathlessness should be investigated, especially if accompanied by chest pain. The diagnostic approach in pregnant patients with suspected pulmonary embolism differs from that in non-pregnant women. Measurement of D-dimer is not helpful since values normally increase progressively throughout pregnancy. Accordingly, the first-line investigation in suspected pulmonary embolism is a V̇/Q̇ scan in a patient with a normal chest X-ray and CTPA in a patient with an abnormal chest X-ray.

Chest pain

Chest pain does not occur during normal pregnancy but the incidences of acute coronary syndrome (ACS) and aortic dissection are both increased. Accordingly, if a pregnant woman develops acute severe chest pain suggestive of either of these conditions, she should be investigated and treated in the same way as a non-pregnant woman.

Circulatory collapse

The differential diagnosis of circulatory collapse is wide and causes unrelated to pregnancy are discussed on page 199. Obstetric causes include pulmonary embolism, haemorrhage and amniotic fluid embolism (AFE). AFE usually presents with collapse and profound shock during delivery or immediately afterwards, often with profound and early coagulopathy. It can be difficult to differentiate AFE from other causes of maternal collapse, and the diagnosis is clinical when other causes of collapse have been excluded. Management is supportive, with oxygenation, careful fluid balance and, in some cases, correction of coagulopathies, ventilatory support and vasopressors.

Another important cause of circulatory collapse is obstetric haemorrhage, which can be divided into ante-partum and post-partum subtypes. Ante-partum haemorrhage is defined as bleeding from the vagina after 24 weeks' gestation. Primary post-partum haemorrhage is defined as occurring in the first 24 hours after delivery, and secondary post-partum haemorrhage after 24 hours. Haemorrhage may be concealed, and physiological changes such as hypotension, tachycardia and tachypnoea may be late signs. Management is supportive with administration of blood, intravenous fluids and oxygen. Patients with post-partum haemorrhage may also benefit from uterotonic agents such as oxytocin. If the bleeding fails to settle, surgical intervention or interventional radiology may be required.

Headache

Migraine and tension headache may occur during pregnancy and should be assessed along the usual lines, as described on page 1095. Important causes of headache that are specific to pregnancy are pre-eclampsia, which should be suspected in patients with hypertension, oedema and proteinuria, and cerebral venous thrombosis, which should be suspected when there is a neurological deficit or seizures.

Nausea and vomiting

Nausea and vomiting are common during the first trimester of pregnancy and do not usually require any specific investigation or treatment. Other causes of nausea and vomiting are summarised in Box 30.4. Severe vomiting with significant weight loss and/or electrolyte disturbance suggests hyperemesis gravidarum, which is discussed in more detail on page 1277.

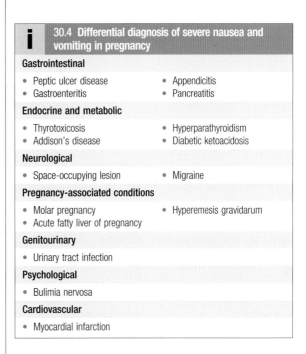

i 30.4 Differential diagnosis of severe nausea and vomiting in pregnancy	
Gastrointestinal	
• Peptic ulcer disease	• Appendicitis
• Gastroenteritis	• Pancreatitis
Endocrine and metabolic	
• Thyrotoxicosis	• Hyperparathyroidism
• Addison's disease	• Diabetic ketoacidosis
Neurological	
• Space-occupying lesion	• Migraine
Pregnancy-associated conditions	
• Molar pregnancy	• Hyperemesis gravidarum
• Acute fatty liver of pregnancy	
Genitourinary	
• Urinary tract infection	
Psychological	
• Bulimia nervosa	
Cardiovascular	
• Myocardial infarction	

Oedema

A mild degree of ankle oedema can occur in normal pregnancy but significant oedema raises suspicion of pre-eclampsia. This should be considered in patients who are also hypertensive and those with proteinuria. Further details are on page 1276.

Seizures

The causes and management of seizures during pregnancy are summarised in Box 30.5. An important cause is eclampsia, which should be borne in mind in patients with no previous history of seizures and accompanying features such as hypertension,

30

i 30.5 Causes of seizures during pregnancy

Cause	Management
Epilepsy	Similar to that in non-pregnant women Avoid valproate
Eclampsia	Antihypertensives Magnesium sulphate Careful fluid balance
Hypoglycaemia	Glucose
Hyponatraemia	Saline infusion
Alcohol withdrawal	Supportive treatment
Drugs	Supportive treatment
Stroke	As in non-pregnant women
Cerebral venous thrombosis	Low-molecular-weight heparin
Thrombotic thrombocytopenic purpura	Plasma exchange Immunosuppressives

i 30.6 Classification of hypertension during pregnancy

Hypertension	Definition
Hypertension in pregnancy	Blood pressure ≥140/90 mmHg on two separate occasions, at least 4 hrs apart
Pre-existing hypertension	Hypertension prior to pregnancy or occurring before 20 weeks' gestation
Gestational hypertension	Hypertension occurring after 20 weeks' gestation without proteinuria or any other features of pre-eclampsia
Pre-eclampsia	Hypertension occurring after 20 weeks' gestation with proteinuria, maternal organ dysfunction or uteroplacental dysfunction
Eclampsia	Generalised seizures in a pregnant woman previously diagnosed with pre-eclampsia
White coat hypertension	Hypertension that only occurs in a clinical environment

Adapted from Tranquilli AL, Dekker G, Magee L, et al. The classification, diagnosis and management of the hypertensive disorders of pregnancy: a revised statement from the ISSHP. Pregnancy Hypertens 2014; 4:97–104.

i 30.7 Drug treatment of hypertension during pregnancy

Medication	Mechanism of action
Labetalol	α- and β-receptor blocker
Nifedipine Amlodipine	Calcium channel blockers
Methyldopa	Central action
Doxazosin	α-receptor blocker

oedema and proteinuria. Seizures can also occur secondary to electrolyte disturbances associated with hyperemesis gravidarum or hypoglycaemia. Other disorders that are more common during pregnancy and can present with seizures include cerebral venous thrombosis and thrombotic thrombocytopenic purpura (TTP).

Medical disorders in pregnancy

Many disorders present specific management problems before pregnancy, during pregnancy and in the puerperium; the most important of these are discussed in more detail below.

Hypertension

Hypertension is one of the most common medical problems during pregnancy, occurring in about 10–15% of women. The causes and classification are summarised in Box 30.6.

Pre-existing hypertension

If hypertension is discovered during the first half of pregnancy, it usually indicates that there was pre-existing hypertension. This is most likely to be due to essential hypertension but secondary causes also need to be considered. Hypertension during pregnancy should be managed with vasodilators or methyldopa (Box 30.7), taking care to avoid hypotension, which can cause placental hypoperfusion and increase the risk of fetal growth restriction, stillbirth and miscarriage. Angiotensin-converting enzyme (ACE) inhibitors should be stopped in hypertensive women who are planning to become pregnant and should be avoided during pregnancy since they have fetotoxic effects. Diuretics should also be avoided unless there is heart failure, as they can reduce circulating volume and cause placental hypoperfusion.

Gestational hypertension

Gestational hypertension usually presents in the second half of pregnancy and most often resolves by 3 months post-partum. It should be managed actively with one of the drugs listed in Box 30.7, to reduce the risk of progression to pre-eclampsia.

Pre-eclampsia and eclampsia

Pre-eclampsia is a disorder of vascular endothelial dysfunction that affects about 10% of all pregnancies worldwide. The risk factors for pre-eclampsia are shown in Box 30.8 and the clinical features illustrated in Figure 30.2. Management includes control of blood pressure, administration of magnesium sulphate as prophylaxis against seizures, correction of coagulation abnormalities and monitoring of fluid balance. If pre-eclampsia occurs early in pregnancy, medical management should be initiated with the aim of controlling the condition and maintaining the fetus in utero as long as possible. If these measures are ineffective and eclampsia supervenes (see below), then urgent delivery should be considered, provided the fetus is viable, since this results in an immediate cure.

i 30.8 Risk factors for pre-eclampsia

- Previous history of pre-eclampsia
- Multiple pregnancy
- Primiparity
- Genetic predisposition
- Obesity
- Increased maternal age

- Pre-existing medical conditions:
  Chronic kidney disease
  Hypertension
  Diabetes mellitus
  Systemic lupus erythematosus and connective tissue disease

Adapted from Duckitt K, Harrington D. Risk factors for pre-eclampsia at antenatal booking: systematic review of controlled studies. BMJ 2005; 330:565–567.

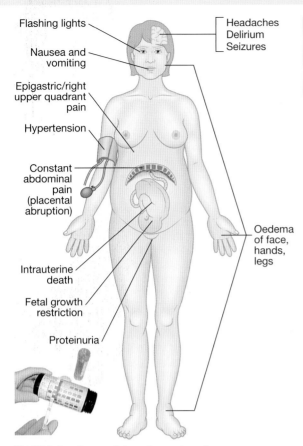

Fig. 30.2 **Symptoms and signs of pre-eclampsia.**

i	**30.9** **Causes of pneumonia during pregnancy**

Bacterial

- *Streptococcus pneumoniae*
- *Mycoplasma pneumoniae*
- *Legionella*

- *Haemophilus influenzae*
- *Staphylococcus aureus*

Viral

- Influenza viruses
- Varicella zoster

Adapted from Lim W, Macfarlane J, Colthorpe C. Pneumonia in pregnancy. Thorax 2001; 56:398–405.

Eclampsia occurs in about 1% of pregnancies and is associated with significant mortality. It usually presents with seizures on a background of pre-eclampsia but rarely can occur before the onset of hypertension and proteinuria. Treatment is with intravenous magnesium sulphate and delivery of the fetus as soon as possible. Women with pre-eclampsia are more likely to develop hypertension, chronic kidney disease, and cerebrovascular and ischaemic heart disease in later life.

Respiratory disease

Asthma

Women with asthma should be managed aggressively during pregnancy, since poorly controlled asthma is associated with pre-eclampsia, fetal growth restriction, low birth weight and pre-term birth. The management is very similar to that in non-pregnant individuals. Short-acting and long-acting β-agonists, inhaled and oral glucocorticoids and theophylline can be used freely. There is less experience with leukotriene receptor agonists during pregnancy but they can be given if necessary. It is advisable to involve an anaesthetist or intensivist at an early stage in patients with severe exacerbations of asthma since airway management is more difficult in late pregnancy.

Respiratory infection

The most common causes of pneumonia during pregnancy are summarised in Box 30.9. Diagnosis and management are broadly the same as in non-pregnant patients. Prompt treatment

of infections is important since mothers with pneumonia are more likely to deliver early and have low-birth-weight infants compared with healthy pregnant women.

Bacterial infections

Antibiotics should be given, depending on the causal organism and sensitivities, along with supplemental oxygen and fluids as required. Penicillins, cephalosporins and macrolides such as erythromycin are all safe during pregnancy but tetracyclines should be avoided because they may be embryotoxic and can cause staining of the teeth in the fetus (see Box 6.19, p. 120).

Viral infections

Viral pneumonia is more common and often more severe during pregnancy. Varicella zoster pneumonia in particular is associated with a high fetal and maternal mortality rate. It presents with cough, breathlessness and pyrexia, and is usually preceded by a vesicular rash up to 1 week before. Varicella infection can be diagnosed clinically, with laboratory confirmation by culture or polymerase chain reaction (PCR) of fluid from vesicles, or by serology. Varicella pneumonia causes an interstitial pneumonitis with a characteristic nodular appearance on chest X-ray (p. 1270). Women with confirmed varicella zoster pneumonia should be admitted to hospital for supportive care and treatment with intravenous aciclovir for 7–10 days.

Tuberculosis

Tuberculosis (TB) may occur during pregnancy and in the UK is more common among African and Asian women. Untreated TB is associated with premature delivery and low birth weight. Transmission to the fetus can occur but is unusual. If the diagnosis of TB is confirmed, then antituberculous chemotherapy should be given as normal, since the benefit of treating TB in pregnancy outweighs any potential risks from the medication. A proportion of pregnant women with TB have coexisting human immunodeficiency virus (HIV) infection, which confers a poorer prognosis and also requires treatment with antiretroviral therapy, as described on page 318.

Gastrointestinal disease

Hyperemesis gravidarum

Hyperemesis gravidarum is a serious condition that affects about 0.5% of pregnant women. It typically presents during the first trimester with severe nausea, vomiting and other clinical features (Box 30.10). It is associated with significant morbidity and mortality, due to malnutrition and electrolyte imbalance. Wernicke's encephalopathy may develop as the result of thiamin deficiency. Recurrence is common in successive pregnancies.

30

The cause is unknown and the diagnosis is one of exclusion, since alternative causes of severe nausea and vomiting need to be ruled out, particularly if the onset of symptoms occurs after the first trimester. Management is with lifestyle advice and support, intravenous fluids, electrolyte replacement and antiemetics. Thiamin and glucocorticoids may be required in the most severe cases.

Inflammatory bowel disease

Women with inflammatory bowel disease (IBD) should be counselled prior to planning a pregnancy. Medications such as azathioprine, sulfasalazine, 5-aminosalicylic acid (5-ASA), glucocorticoids and tumour necrosis factor alpha (TNF-α) inhibitors can be continued as normal during pregnancy but methotrexate must be stopped at least 3 months before conception because of its teratogenic effects. Since poorly controlled IBD is associated with an increased risk of pre-term birth, low birth weight and miscarriage, it is important for the disease to be well controlled before conception. The activity of IBD can increase during pregnancy and ulcerative colitis is more likely to flare than Crohn's disease. Women who experience disease flares should be managed by both medical and obstetric teams, and monitored closely. The TNF-α inhibitors infliximab and adalimumab are actively transported across the placenta in the third trimester and there is theoretical concern about immunosuppression in the neonate. Infants of mothers who have been treated with TNF-α inhibitors during the second and third trimesters should not be given live vaccines and should be monitored closely for any signs of infection. Most women with uncomplicated IBD can have a normal vaginal delivery and do not need a caesarean section, but the need for this should be assessed on an individual basis by obstetric and medical teams.

Diabetes

It is important to institute meticulous glucose control in pregnancy, as maternal diabetes is associated with increased risks of congenital malformations, stillbirth, pre-eclampsia, pre-term delivery, operative delivery, neonatal hypoglycaemia and admission to neonatal intensive care.

Gestational diabetes

Gestational diabetes is defined as diabetes with first onset or recognition during pregnancy. This definition will include a few patients who develop type 1 diabetes during pregnancy, where prompt action and early insulin treatment will be required, and some patients who develop type 2 diabetes, or had unknown pre-existing type 2 diabetes, in whom the diabetes does not remit after pregnancy. However, in most cases, gestational diabetes develops due to an inability to increase insulin secretion adequately to compensate for pregnancy-induced insulin resistance, and most women can expect to return to normal glucose tolerance immediately after pregnancy. Risk factors for gestational diabetes are shown in Box 30.11.

The diagnosis of gestational diabetes is based on maternal blood glucose measurements that are associated with increased fetal growth. An international consensus recommended that glucose values diagnostic of gestational diabetes should be lower than those for non-gestational diabetes (see Box 20.31, p. 753). Controversy remains about who should be screened, and the screening strategy depends, in part, on the population risk. It is widely accepted that women at high risk for gestational diabetes should have an oral glucose tolerance test at 24–28 weeks, and some guidelines recommend that all high-risk women should be screened by measuring HbA$_{1c}$, fasting blood glucose or random blood glucose at the first booking visit. It should be noted that measurements of HbA$_{1c}$ cannot reliably be used to diagnose diabetes in early pregnancy and until 3 months post-partum, since HbA$_{1c}$ levels fall due to increased red cell turnover.

Management

The aim is to normalise maternal blood glucose concentrations and reduce the risk of excessive fetal growth. The first element of management is dietary modification, in particular by reducing consumption of refined carbohydrate. Women with gestational diabetes should undertake regular pre- and post-prandial self-monitoring of blood glucose, aiming for pre-meal blood glucose levels of <5.3 mmol/L (96 mg/dL) and a 1-hour post-prandial level of <7.8 mmol/L (142 mg/dL) or a 2-hour post-prandial level of <6.0 mmol/L (109 mg/dL). If pharmacological treatment is necessary, metformin, glibenclamide or insulin can all be used. Glibenclamide should be used rather than other sulphonylureas because it does not cross the placenta. Other oral therapies or injectable incretin-based therapies should not be given in pregnancy.

After delivery, maternal glucose usually returns to pre-pregnancy levels. In the UK, it is currently recommended that women with gestational diabetes should have a fasting blood glucose measured at 6 weeks post-partum and have HbA$_{1c}$ concentrations measured annually to screen for the development of diabetes. This is because even those whose glucose tolerance returns to normal post-partum are at increased risk for developing type 2 diabetes, with a 5-year risk between 15 and 50%, depending on the population. Therefore, all women who have had gestational diabetes should be given diet and lifestyle advice to reduce their risk of developing type 2 diabetes (p. 743).

Pregnancy in women with established diabetes

Maternal hyperglycaemia early in pregnancy (during the first 6 weeks post conception) can adversely affect fetal development, causing cardiac, renal and skeletal malformations, of which the caudal regression syndrome (abnormal development of the lower part of the spine) is the most characteristic. The risk of fetal abnormalities is about 2% for non-diabetic women and about 4% for women with well-controlled diabetes (HbA$_{1c}$ <53 mmol/mol) but more than 20% for those with poor glycaemic control (HbA$_{1c}$ >97 mmol/mol). Therefore, it is important for women with diabetes to aim to achieve good glycaemic control before becoming pregnant. In addition, high-dose folic acid (5 mg daily, rather than the usual 400 µg) should be initiated before conception to reduce the risk of neural tube defects.

As for gestational diabetes, mothers should attempt to maintain near-normal blood glucose levels while avoiding hypoglycaemia throughout their pregnancy, as this minimises excessive fetal growth and neonatal hypoglycaemia. This is often difficult to achieve, however. Pregnancy is also associated with an increased risk of ketosis, particularly, but not exclusively, in women with type 1 diabetes. Ketoacidosis during pregnancy is dangerous for the mother and is associated with a high rate (10–35%) of fetal mortality.

Pregnancy is linked with a worsening of diabetic complications, most notably retinopathy and nephropathy, so careful monitoring of eyes and kidneys is required throughout pregnancy. If heavy proteinuria and/or renal dysfunction exist prior to pregnancy, there is a marked increase in the risk of pre-eclampsia, and renal function can deteriorate irreversibly during pregnancy. These risks need to be carefully discussed before a woman with diabetes is considering pregnancy. The outlook for mother and child has been vastly improved over recent years but pregnancy outcomes are still not equivalent to those of non-diabetic mothers. Perinatal mortality rates remain 3–4 times those of the non-diabetic population (at around 30–40 per 1000 pregnancies) and the rate of congenital malformation is increased 5–6-fold.

Endocrine disease

Thyroid disease

Iodine deficiency

Iodine deficiency is a major public health issue in many countries, particularly in South-east Asia, the Western Pacific and Central Africa. Severe iodine deficiency in pregnancy is associated with miscarriage, stillbirth and cretinism, with significant cognitive impairment, gait abnormalities and deafness in the affected child. More moderate iodine deficiency is associated with milder forms of cognitive impairment and affects millions of people. The World Health Organisation recommends a daily iodine intake of 250 µg/day for pregnant women. Treatment of iodine deficiency in the first and second trimesters can prevent impaired cognitive development but is less effective if started in the third trimester.

Hypothyroidism

Untreated hypothyroidism is associated with subfertility and so is uncommon in pregnancy. Subclinical hypothyroidism is more common, and is often due to poor adherence to levothyroxine in known primary hypothyroidism. Most pregnant women with primary hypothyroidism require an increase in the dose of levothyroxine of approximately 25–50 µg daily to maintain normal TSH levels because there is an increased requirement for thyroxine during pregnancy. Furthermore, inadequately treated maternal hypothyroidism may be associated with impaired brain development in the fetus. Because of this, hypothyroid women

should be monitored closely if planning a pregnancy; they should be advised to have their thyroid function checked as soon as possible after conception and increase their daily levothyroxine dose if necessary. During pregnancy, serum TSH and free T$_4$ should be measured during each trimester and the dose of levothyroxine adjusted to maintain a normal TSH level. Rarely, hypothyroidism may present during pregnancy with weight gain, constipation and lethargy. The diagnosis is easily missed since these symptoms are common in normal pregnancy. If suspected, the diagnosis can be confirmed by checking thyroid function tests, which show a raised TSH and low free T$_4$.

Hyperthyroidism

The coexistence of pregnancy and thyrotoxicosis is unusual, since anovulatory cycles are common in thyrotoxic patients and autoimmune disease tends to remit during pregnancy, due to suppression of the maternal immune response. Thyroid function tests must be interpreted in the knowledge that thyroid-binding globulin, and hence total T$_4$ and T$_3$ levels, are increased in pregnancy and that the normal range for TSH is lower (see Box 18.18, p. 651). Despite this, a fully suppressed TSH is usually indicative of Graves' disease. When thyroid disease during pregnancy is being dealt with, both mother and fetus must be considered, since maternal thyroid hormones, TSH receptor antibodies (TRAb) and antithyroid drugs can all cross the placenta to some degree, exposing the fetus to the risks of thyrotoxicosis, iatrogenic hypothyroidism and goitre. Moreover, poorly controlled thyrotoxicosis can result in fetal tachycardia, intrauterine growth retardation, prematurity, stillbirth and possibly even congenital malformations.

Antithyroid drugs are the treatment of first choice for thyrotoxicosis in pregnancy. Newly diagnosed hyperthyroidism during pregnancy can be treated with β-adrenoceptor antagonists (β-blockers) in the short term, followed by antithyroid drugs. Propylthiouracil (PTU) is the preferred antithyroid drug because treatment with carbimazole during the first trimester has been associated with the occurrence of choanal atresia and aplasia cutis. Hyperthyroid women who become pregnant while taking carbimazole or PTU should be advised to continue their current drug in pregnancy, with close monitoring. Both carbimazole and PTU cross the placenta and are effective in treating thyrotoxicosis in the fetus caused by transplacental passage of TRAb. To avoid fetal hypothyroidism, which can affect brain development and cause goitre, it is important to use the smallest dose of antithyroid drug (typically <150 mg PTU or 15 mg carbimazole per day) that will maintain maternal free T$_4$, T$_3$ and TSH concentrations within their respective reference ranges. Thyroid surgery is sometimes necessary because of poor drug adherence, drug hypersensitivity or failure of medical treatment and is most safely performed during the second trimester. Radioactive iodine is absolutely contraindicated throughout pregnancy, as it invariably induces fetal hypothyroidism. Frequent review of mother and fetus (monitoring heart rate and growth) is important during pregnancy and in the puerperium. Serum TRAb levels can be measured in the third trimester to predict the likelihood of neonatal thyrotoxicosis. PTU is the drug of choice in the breastfeeding mother, as it is excreted in the milk to a much lesser extent than carbimazole. Thyroid function should be monitored periodically in the breastfed child.

Post-partum thyroiditis

Post-partum thyroiditis typically presents 3–4 months after delivery. It is discussed in more detail on page 647.

30

Pituitary disease

Prolactinoma

Prolactinomas are the most common pituitary tumours in young women. Although fertility is reduced in patients with prolactinoma, pregnancies can occur and if this happens the tumour may enlarge as part of the physiological pituitary enlargement that takes place during normal pregnancy. Macroprolactinomas (≥ 10 mm) are at greater risk of enlarging and may cause optic chiasm compression. If women known to have a prolactinoma become pregnant, they should have visual field testing each trimester, followed by pituitary imaging by MRI if enlargement is suspected from changes in visual fields or from symptoms. Measurement of serum prolactin is generally not helpful, since levels increase anyway as part of normal pregnancy. Dopamine receptor agonists such as cabergoline and bromocriptine should normally be stopped during pregnancy, but can be reintroduced if necessary in patients with an enlarging prolactinoma that is threatening the visual fields.

Diabetes insipidus

Women with pre-existing diabetes insipidus may find that their symptoms worsen in pregnancy due to placental production of vasopressinase, a protease that degrades vasopressin (antidiuretic hormone, ADH). Because of this, pregnant women with diabetes insipidus may need higher doses of desmopressin until delivery. The development of symptoms suggestive of diabetes insipidus, such as thirst and polyuria, during pregnancy should raise suspicion of acute fatty liver of pregnancy (AFLP), the syndrome of haemolysis, elevated liver enzymes and low platelets (HELLP) or pre-eclampsia, as all of these conditions are also associated with decreased breakdown of vasopressinase by the liver.

Sheehan's syndrome

This is a form of post-partum hypopituitarism caused by infarction of the pituitary, usually associated with hypotension from major post-partum haemorrhage. It can present with failure to establish lactation after birth, amenorrhoea or other features of hypopituitarism. The diagnosis can be confirmed by tests of pituitary function and treated with hormone replacement, as described on page 682.

Parathyroid disease

Primary hyperparathyroidism

Primary hyperparathyroidism (PHPT) is uncommon in women of child-bearing age, but if pregnancy does occur in a patient with pre-existing PHPT, careful monitoring is required. Women with mild disease can be managed conservatively but if serum calcium levels rise above 2.85 mmol/L (11.5 mg/dL), consideration should be given to parathyroidectomy, as fetal mortality is high (up to 40%) in patients with severe hypercalcaemia. If parathyroidectomy is required, it should ideally be performed during the second trimester. Anecdotal evidence suggests that the calcimimetic drug cinacalcet can be used for medical management of PHPT during pregnancy.

Familial hypocalciuric hypercalcaemia

Familial hypocalciuric hypercalcaemia (FHH) is a benign disorder caused by mutations in the calcium-sensing receptor, which is described on page 664. Although FHH poses no risk for pregnant women, the hypercalcemia can suppress PTH secretion in neonates that do not inherit the FHH mutation, resulting in severe hypocalcaemia. Infants of mothers with FHH should have their serum calcium levels monitored during the first few days of life; if hypocalcaemia is detected, intravenous calcium should be given.

Adrenal disease

Women with known adrenal insufficiency can continue their glucocorticoid and mineralocorticoid replacement during pregnancy as normal. Rarely, adrenal insufficiency can present for the first time during pregnancy. If this occurs, the diagnosis is challenging because total cortisol normally increases during pregnancy, and short Synacthen tests (p. 672) can be falsely normal. Specialist assessment is required. In women with Conn's syndrome who become pregnant, amiloride should be substituted for spironolactone to prevent anti-androgenic effects on a male fetus.

Human immunodeficiency virus infection

The course of HIV disease is not altered by pregnancy but treatment with antiretroviral therapy should be given during pregnancy to women that are HIV-positive, as outlined on page 326. In some societies, routine HIV testing is recommended at an early stage in pregnancy in all women.

Inflammatory rheumatic disease

Most women with inflammatory rheumatic disorders have successful pregnancies but it is critically important for them to be given pre-conception counselling and to review medication use, optimise disease control and make them aware of the risks that pregnancy might pose to their condition and vice versa.

Rheumatoid arthritis

Women with rheumatoid arthritis should have a medication review; methotrexate, leflunomide and mycophenolate should be stopped and, if necessary, an alternative substituted before conception (Box 30.12). Rheumatoid arthritis often improves during pregnancy, particularly in those who are negative for rheumatoid factor or anti-cyclic citrullinated peptide antibodies. There is an increased risk of pre-eclampsia, pre-term birth and small babies for women with active disease, emphasising the importance of maintaining disease control during pregnancy. Glucocorticoids, hydrochloroquine, azathioprine and sulfasalazine can all be continued as normal but non-steroidal anti-inflammatory drugs (NSAIDs) should be avoided after 20 weeks (Box 30.12). Inhibitors of TNF-α are safe during pregnancy and can be continued if necessary to maintain control of the disease. Most TNF-α inhibitors are actively transported across the placenta and this can lead to immunosuppression in the neonate if these drugs are used during the second and third trimesters. An exception is certolizumab, which is a pegylated antibody, and this is a good option for women who require TNF-α inhibition during pregnancy. Experience with other biological therapies during pregnancy is limited. Disease flares are common in the post-partum period, regardless of serology, and this can pose a problem for breastfeeding and care of the infant. Glucocorticoids are a good short-term option to control such flares, pending reintroduction of other disease-modifying antirheumatic drugs (DMARDs) that might have been stopped prior to pregnancy.

Systemic sclerosis

Pregnancy in women with diffuse systemic sclerosis (SSc), those with pulmonary hypertension or renal involvement and those with disease of recent onset (< 4 years) poses risks to mother and

i 30.12 Safety of antirheumatic drugs during pregnancy and breastfeeding

Drug	Safe during pregnancy	Safe during breastfeeding	Comment
Non-steroidal anti-inflammatory drugs (NSAIDs)	Yes (< 20 weeks)	Yes	
Hydroxychloroquine	Yes	Yes	
Glucocorticoids	Yes	Yes	A good short-term option for disease flares
Azathioprine	Yes	Yes	
Sulfasalazine	Yes	Yes	Co-prescribe with folic acid
Ciclosporin	Yes	Yes	Data on breastfeeding limited
Tacrolimus	Yes	Yes	
Mycophenolate	No	No	Stop before planning pregnancy
Methotrexate	No	No	Stop 3 months before planning pregnancy
Leflunomide	No	No	Stop 2 years before planning pregnancy
Cyclophosphamide	No	No	
Tumour necrosis factor (TNF) inhibitors	Yes	Yes	Avoid live vaccines in the neonate for 6 months

Adapted from Ateka-Barrutia O, Nelson-Piercy C. Connective tissue disease in pregnancy. Clin Med 2013; 131:580–584.

i 30.13 Systemic sclerosis (SSc) and pregnancy

Subtype	Effect of disease on pregnancy
Localised SSc	Good prognosis Raynaud's may improve Oesophagitis may worsen
CREST syndrome	Good prognosis Raynaud's may improve Oesophagitis may worsen
Diffuse SSc	Increased risk of: Pre-term delivery Pre-eclampsia Fetal growth restriction Low-birth-weight babies Maternal and fetal mortality

(CREST = calcinosis, Raynaud's phenomenon, oesophageal involvement, sclerodactyly and telangiectasia)

i 30.14 Differential diagnosis of lupus flare during pregnancy

Clinical finding	Lupus flare	Pre-eclampsia	Normal pregnancy
Hypertension	Yes	Yes	No
Proteinuria	Yes	Yes	No
Red cells/casts in urine	Yes	No	No
Liver function tests	Normal	Abnormal	Normal
Anti-double-stranded DNA	Increase	Unchanged	Unchanged
C3 and C4	Low	Elevated or unchanged from baseline	Unchanged

fetus. In milder forms of the disease, however, the prognosis is better (Box 30.13). Raynaud's phenomenon often improves during pregnancy due to vasodilatation but oesophageal symptoms may worsen. Renal crises are no more frequent during pregnancy, but if one occurs, ACE inhibitors should be given. Although these are normally contraindicated in pregnancy, the potential benefit in this situation outweighs the risk to the fetus. Glucocorticoids, which can be given to promote fetal lung maturation in premature babies, should be avoided in women with SSc where possible because they may provoke renal crisis.

Systemic lupus erythematosus

Pregnancy in women with systemic lupus erythematosus (SLE) poses several risks to both mother and fetus, especially if there is renal involvement. There is an increased risk of pre-eclampsia, thrombosis, fetal growth restriction, pre-term delivery, miscarriage and fetal death. There is also a higher risk of lupus flare during the puerperium. Good control of disease is paramount, since women with SLE who conceive when their disease has been quiescent for at least 6 months are less likely to have complications than those who conceive when their disease has recently been active. It can be difficult to assess disease activity during pregnancy because symptoms such as oedema, hair loss, joint pain and fatigue, which occur in active SLE, are also common during normal pregnancies. The features in Box 30.14 can help differentiate between an SLE flare, normal pregnancy and pre-eclampsia.

All women with SLE should be tested for anti-Ro and anti-La antibodies, since they can cross the placenta and cause neonatal complete heart block or cutaneous lupus, respectively. Medications should be reviewed prior to pregnancy, to ensure they are safe, and an alternative substituted if necessary (see Box 30.12). The management of patients with antiphospholipid antibodies (aPL) is described below.

Anti-phospholipid syndrome

Primary antiphospholipid syndrome (APS) is associated with an increased risk of adverse pregnancy outcomes, including thrombosis, miscarriage, fetal death and pre-eclampsia. This applies to primary APS and that associated with connective tissue diseases such as SLE. During pregnancy, women with APS should be managed with low-dose aspirin in combination with low-molecular-weight heparin (LMWH).

30

Cardiac disease

Congenital heart disease

Women who have a history of surgically corrected congenital heart disease generally tolerate pregnancy well, but are more likely to have babies with congenital heart disease and should be offered fetal cardiac scans. Acyanotic heart diseases, such as atrial septal defect, ventricular septal defect and patent ductus arteriosus, all have a good prognosis in pregnancy. Unrepaired cyanotic heart disease has a very poor prognosis in pregnancy, as does pulmonary hypertension, regardless of the underlying cause. Women with mechanical heart valves require anticoagulation throughout pregnancy but their anticoagulation should be planned with consideration of substituting warfarin with LMWH and aspirin during the first trimester to reduce the risk of warfarin embryopathy. If necessary, warfarin can be used during pregnancy, particularly in the second and third trimesters.

Valvular heart disease

The physiological changes of pregnancy may also unmask previously undiagnosed valvular disease. Women with regurgitant lesions, such as mitral regurgitation and aortic regurgitation, tolerate pregnancy better than those with stenotic lesions. Mitral stenosis causes a reduction in blood flow from the left atrium to left ventricle in diastole, which worsens during pregnancy due to the increased heart rate and hypervolaemia. Those with moderate to severe mitral stenosis (valve area $< 1.5\ cm^2$) are at particular risk and may develop arrhythmias, tachycardia and pulmonary oedema. Most patients can be managed medically with β-blockers, LMWH and furosemide as necessary. Surgical intervention is indicated if there is continued haemodynamic compromise despite optimal medical management.

Myocardial infarction

Pregnancy increases the risk of myocardial infarction. While atherosclerosis is the main cause in non-pregnant individuals, coronary artery dissection and coronary thrombosis secondary to the hypercoagulable state are more common causes during pregnancy. Management is similar to that of non-pregnant women, except that statins and glycoprotein IIb/IIIa inhibitors such as apixaban should be avoided. Clopidogrel can be given but should be stopped around the time of delivery to reduce the risk of uterine bleeding and to allow spinal anaesthesia to be used if necessary. Stenting can be performed, but bare-metal stents are preferred because drug-eluting stents require dual antiplatelet therapy that cannot be continued around the time of delivery.

Aortic dissection

Pregnancy is an independent risk factor for aortic dissection and this should be considered when a woman presents with acute severe chest pain during pregnancy. The vast majority of cases in pregnancy are 'type A', involving the ascending aorta (see Fig. 16.72, p. 506), and require careful control of hypertension, caesarean section to deliver the fetus, and emergency surgery to treat the aneurysm.

Peripartum cardiomyopathy

Peripartum cardiomyopathy (PPCM) presents with heart failure secondary to left ventricular systolic dysfunction towards the end of pregnancy or in the months following delivery. It is a diagnosis of exclusion, made when other causes of heart failure have been ruled out. The cause is unknown but PPCM is more prevalent in women who are older, multiparous, hypertensive and Afro-Caribbean. It is treated by conventional medications for heart failure, including ACE inhibitors if necessary, and delivery of the baby. Many women recover within 3–6 months of diagnosis but the prognosis is variable. There is a significant chance of reduction in cardiac function in subsequent pregnancies.

Dilated cardiomyopathy

Dilated cardiomyopathy carries a poor prognosis if the pre-pregnancy ejection fraction is below 30% or if symptoms are in New York Heart Association grades 3 or 4. Management is as described for PPCM.

Renal disease

Renal tract infection

Pregnancy predisposes women to urinary tract infection. If asymptomatic bacteriuria is discovered during pregnancy, it should be treated promptly with antibiotics, to prevent ascending renal tract infection. Pyelonephritis is more common in pregnancy due to the physiological dilatation of the upper renal tract; if it does occur, it can trigger premature labour.

Acute kidney injury

Acute kidney injury (AKI) may occur during pregnancy or in the puerperium due to a variety of causes (Box 30.15). Women with AKI caused by pre-eclampsia are prone to pulmonary oedema, and need very careful fluid balance to avoid fluid overload. In the post-partum period, AKI may occur as the result of post-partum haemorrhage or pre-eclampsia, and sometimes these occur in combination. Although pre-eclampsia resolves after delivery, AKI can be at its worst in the first few days post-partum, especially when exacerbated by obstetric haemorrhage.

Glomerular disease

Proteinuria caused by glomerular disease is usually exacerbated during pregnancy, and nephrotic syndrome may develop without any alteration in the underlying disease activity in individuals who had only slight proteinuria before pregnancy. This further increases the risk of venous thromboembolism, the leading cause of maternal deaths in developed countries.

Chronic kidney disease

Women with chronic kidney disease (CKD) are at increased risk of pre-eclampsia, fetal growth restriction, miscarriage, pre-term delivery and fetal death (Fig. 30.3). Pregnancy can also cause acceleration of maternal renal decline. The factors that influence pregnancy outcome for women with CKD are baseline renal function, hypertension, degree of proteinuria and the underlying cause of CKD. Women with CKD should have pre-pregnancy counselling, be closely monitored by a multidisciplinary team throughout pregnancy, and be given low-dose aspirin as prophylaxis against pre-eclampsia.

Renal replacement therapy

Fertility is reduced among women on renal replacement therapy and there is increased risk of adverse pregnancy outcomes.

i 30.15 Causes of acute kidney injury in pregnancy

Mechanism	Cause	Features
Pre-renal	Hyperemesis gravidarum	Nausea and vomiting Dehydration Presentation in first trimester
	Post-partum haemorrhage	Vaginal bleeding immediately post-partum
	Placental abruption	Abdominal pain or vaginal bleeding in second or third trimester
	Septic abortion	Presentation with hypotension, shock and pyrexia
Renal	Pre-eclampsia	Presentation in second and third trimesters with new-onset hypertension and proteinuria
	Thrombotic thrombocytopenic purpura	Possible antenatal or post-partum presentation with headache, irritability and drowsiness Haematology shows thrombocytopenia and microangiopathic haemolytic anaemia
	Acute fatty liver of pregnancy	Presentation with vomiting and abdominal pain in third trimester Abnormal liver function tests Liver ultrasound can be normal
	Acute interstitial nephritis	Most common cause is use of non-steroidal anti-inflammatory drugs
Post-renal	Acute urinary retention	Usual presentation is in third trimester due to enlarged uterus causing ureteric obstruction; sometimes presents post-partum

Adapted from Palma-Reis I, Vais A, Nelson-Piercy C, et al. Renal disease and hypertension in pregnancy. Clin Med 2014; 13:57–62.

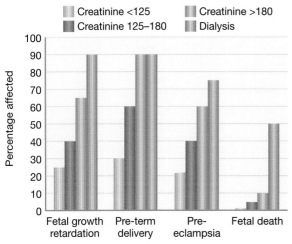

Fig. 30.3 **Adverse pregnancy outcomes in chronic kidney disease.** Creatinine is in μmol/L. To convert to mg/dL, multiply by 0.011. *Data from Williams D, Davison D. Chronic kidney disease in pregnancy. BMJ 2008; 336:211–115.*

Despite this, many women receiving renal replacement therapy have successful pregnancies. More intensive dialysis is recommended in pregnancy, and particular attention should be paid to addressing issues around blood pressure, fluid balance and anaemia.

Renal transplant recipients

Pregnancy should be delayed for a minimum of 12 months following renal transplantation, to allow the graft to stabilize, on minimum immunosuppressive drugs. The outcome is best for women with a well-functioning graft, with no proteinuria or hypertension. Women with renal transplants can deliver vaginally but in practice there is a higher incidence of caesarean section in this group, due to the higher incidence of pre-term delivery.

Liver disease

Specific causes of liver disease during pregnancy are discussed below.

i 30.16 Criteria for diagnosis of acute fatty liver of pregnancy

- Vomiting
- Abdominal pain
- Polydipsia/polyuria
- Encephalopathy
- Elevated bilirubin (>14 μmol/L (>0.82 mg/dL))
- Low glucose (<4 mmol/L (<72.4 mg/dL))
- Elevated urate (>340 μmol/L (>5.7 mg/dL))
- Leucocytosis (>11×10^9/L)
- Ascites or bright liver on ultrasound
- Elevated transaminases (alanine/aspartate aminotransferase (ALT/AST) >42 U/L)
- Elevated ammonia (>47 μmol/L (>81.7 mg/dL))
- Renal impairment (creatinine >150 μmol/L (>1.7 mg/dL))
- Coagulopathy (prothrombin time >14 secs or activated partial thromboplastin time >34 secs)
- Microvascular steatosis on liver biopsy

Acute fatty liver of pregnancy can be diagnosed when ≥6 of the above features are present in the absence of another explanation.

Adapted from Ch'ng CL, Morgan M, Hainsworth I, et al. Prospective study of liver dysfunction in pregnancy in Southwest Wales. Gut 2002; 51:876–880.

Acute fatty liver of pregnancy

Acute fatty liver of pregnancy (AFLP) is a rare and serious condition that typically presents in the third trimester with vomiting, abdominal pain, jaundice and other symptoms (Box 30.16). It is more common in first pregnancies and multiple pregnancies, and is associated with male fetuses. Rarely, fulminant liver failure may occur. The diagnosis can usually be made on the basis of the clinical features, abnormal liver function tests (LFTs) and the appearances of fatty liver on ultrasound. A liver biopsy is rarely needed to make the diagnosis but shows microvascular steatosis. Management is with supportive care and by delivery of the fetus. The development of AFLP has been linked in some cases with an inherited deficiency of the enzyme long-chain acyl-CoA dehydrogenase (LCHAD) in the baby.

30

HELLP syndrome

The syndrome of haemolysis, elevated liver enzymes and low platelets (HELLP) is thought to be part of the spectrum of pre-eclampsia. It usually presents antenatally but can also appear for the first time in the postnatal period. The presenting symptoms can be the same as those of pre-eclampsia but can also include headache, right upper quadrant pain and visual disturbance. HELLP can be complicated by liver haematoma and capsular rupture. Management involves supportive care, control of hypertension, correction of coagulopathy and delivery of the fetus.

Obstetric cholestasis

Obstetric cholestasis is estimated to affect about 1% of pregnancies in Caucasians, although the prevalence is higher in Chinese and South Asian populations. The cause is incompletely understood but the condition is thought to be due in part to the cholestatic effect of high oestrogen levels. The typical presentation is in the third trimester with pruritus, particularly affecting the soles and palms. Laboratory testing reveals raised levels of bile acids and abnormal LFTs. The diagnosis can be made on the basis of these clinical features when other causes of liver dysfunction and pruritus have been excluded. Treatment is with ursodeoxycholic acid in a starting dose of 250 mg twice daily, which usually improves symptoms and liver function. Aqueous cream with menthol can also be effective in soothing pruritus. There is an increased risk of fetal mortality with evidence of a particularly high risk when bile acid levels are over 40 μmol/L (97.9 μg/mL). Treatment therefore aims to bring bile acids below 40 μmol/L and some centres induce labour before 40 weeks in an effort to reduce the risk. The risk of recurrence in future pregnancies is high.

Viral hepatitis

The course of hepatitis B is unchanged in pregnancy, but it is important to identify women who have active infection to reduce the risk of vertical transmission to the fetus; this risk is up to 90% in women who are hepatitis B e-antigen positive. Vaccinations and immunoglobulin should be given to infants of mothers who test positive for hepatitis B, and antiviral agents should be given to the mother after delivery. Vertical transmission rates of hepatitis C are low in the absence of HIV infection and so no action is required for the infant, unless there is co-infection with HIV; in this case, antiviral drugs should be considered. Pregnant women are at greater risk of contracting hepatitis E than the non-pregnant population. It is transferred via the faeco-oral route, and is usually a mild self-limiting illness outside of pregnancy. However, it can cause fulminant hepatic failure in up to 20% of pregnant women.

Neurological disease

Epilepsy

Women with epilepsy should have pre-pregnancy counselling and should be advised to take high-dose folic acid from pre-conception; their antiepileptic drugs (AEDs) should also be reviewed. Maternal treatment with sodium valproate is associated with a higher rate of fetal malformations than other AEDs, and a reduction in intelligence quotient and an increased risk of autistic spectrum disorder in the offspring. Where possible, sodium valproate should be substituted for another AED with a better

safety profile in pregnancy, such as lamotrigine, levetiracetam or carbamazepine. While pregnancy does not generally affect the frequency of seizures in women with well-controlled epilepsy, those who enter pregnancy with poorly controlled epilepsy are likely to deteriorate. The plasma levels of some AEDs such as lamotrigine can fall in pregnancy and checking drug levels can be helpful. Seizures are more common at the time of delivery and women should be advised to deliver in a unit staffed with personnel able to manage this.

Idiopathic intracranial hypertension

Idiopathic intracranial hypertension (IIH) may worsen during pregnancy due to weight gain. Treatment with acetazolamide can be continued during pregnancy but should be avoided in the first trimester due to lack of safety data. The mode of delivery is not affected by IIH and spinal analgesia can be given as normal.

Migraine

Migraine often improves during pregnancy but if attacks occur they should be managed with simple analgesia and antiemetics. If necessary, prophylaxis can be given with aspirin, β-blockers or tricyclic antidepressants. Safety data on use of triptans during pregnancy are limited but reassuring. Triptans can therefore be used for the treatment of migraine if other therapies are ineffective.

Stroke

Stroke is twice as common in pregnant women as in non-pregnant women of the same age. The risk is highest during the third trimester and puerperium. The management of stroke during pregnancy is similar to that in non-pregnant patients. The risk of cerebral venous thrombosis is greatly increased during pregnancy. The presentation is with headache, seizures and neurological deficits such as hemiparesis. If the diagnosis is suspected, neuroimaging should be performed with MRI or CT venography. Management of acute infarct should be as for the non-pregnant patient and include consideration of thrombolysis.

Psychiatric disorders

Mood changes are common during pregnancy but more severe psychiatric disorders, such as depression or psychosis, typically present within 2–4 weeks of delivery. These disorders are discussed in more detail on page 1206 and in Box 28.33.

Haematological disease

Anaemia

The causes of anaemia during pregnancy are summarised in Box 30.17. Iron deficiency anaemia is most commonly due to a 20% increased demand for iron. In most cases, it responds well to oral iron supplementation, with a rise in haemoglobin of approximately 0.8 g/L per week. If the haemoglobin does not rise following a 4-week trial of iron supplementation, alternative causes of anaemia should be considered. Non-adherence to oral iron is common and intravenous iron should be considered in women with iron deficiency and failure of oral treatment. It is generally not necessary to investigate iron deficiency anaemia during pregnancy unless there is clinical evidence of gastrointestinal blood loss, which should be investigated in the normal way.

Microcytic

- Iron deficiency
- Haemoglobinopathies
- Thalassaemia

Normocytic

- Anaemia of chronic disease
- Haemorrhage
- Haemolysis

Macrocytic

- Vitamin B_{12}/folate deficiency
- Liver disease
- Alcohol excess

- Gestational thrombocytopenia
- Idiopathic thrombocytopenic purpura
- Systemic lupus erythematosus
- HELLP (haemolysis, elevated liver enzymes and low platelets)
- Haemolytic uraemic syndrome
- Thrombotic thrombocytopenic purpura

Rhesus disease

Women who are negative for the Rhesus antigen should be offered treatment with anti-RhD immunoglobulin around the time of delivery to reduce the risk of haemolytic disease of the newborn. More details are provided on page 933 and in Box 23.19.

Thrombocytopenia

The causes of thrombocytopenia during pregnancy are summarised in Box 30.18. The most common cause is gestational thrombocytopenia, which typically occurs towards the end of pregnancy and resolves spontaneously after delivery. It is not associated with adverse pregnancy outcomes and requires no specific intervention. Pregnancy may occur in women with pre-existing idiopathic thrombocytopenic purpura (ITP, p. 971). This should be managed with glucocorticoids and/or immunoglobulin, with the aim of maintaining the platelet count above 80×10^9/L at the time of delivery, in case spinal anaesthesia or caesarean section is required. Thrombocytopenia may also occur as a component of haemolytic uraemic syndrome (HUS, p. 408) and thrombotic thrombocytopenic purpura (TTP, p. 979). Both are characterised by microangiopathic haemolytic anaemia, acute kidney injury and thrombocytopenia, but in TTP neurological symptoms and fever also occur. These conditions are rare but important to recognise since up to one-quarter of cases occur during pregnancy and the post-partum period. TTP is managed with plasma exchange, fresh frozen plasma and sometimes glucocorticoids or rituximab. Platelet transfusion should be avoided.

Venous thromboembolism

The risk of venous thromboembolism (VTE) is 4–5 times higher in pregnancy than in non-pregnant women. DVT is the most common presentation and predominantly affects the left leg in pregnancy, for reasons that are incompletely understood. Doppler ultrasound scan is the investigation of choice, but MRI can also be used if proximal clot is suspected. Measurement of D-dimer is not useful in pregnancy because levels rise as part of normal pregnancy. Treatment of VTE in pregnancy is with LMWH at a higher dose than for the non-pregnant woman, based on the patient's early pregnancy (booking) weight. Women with a previous history of VTE who are receiving warfarin or other oral anticoagulants as prophylaxis should have these stopped prior to conception and LMWH should be substituted.

Further information

British Thoracic Society/Scottish Intercollegiate Guidelines Network. SIGN 141 – British guideline on the management of asthma. Edinburgh: Health Improvement Scotland; 2014. *Useful asthma guidelines.*

Royal College of Obstetricians and Gynaecologists. Thromboembolic disease in pregnancy and the puerperium: acute management. Green top guideline. London: RCOG; April 2015. *A useful evidence-based guideline on the investigation of pulmonary embolism in pregnancy.*

Websites

npeu.ox.ac.uk/mbrrace-uk *National Perinatal Epidemiology Unit: a very useful resource with detailed and extensive information on causes of maternal deaths, stillbirths and infant deaths in the UK.*

30

R Mann

31

Adolescent and transition medicine

Transition from paediatric to adult health services 1288

Functional anatomy and physiology 1290
Endocrine changes 1290
Physical changes 1290
Cognitive and behavioural changes 1292

Investigations 1293

Clinical assessment 1293

Presenting problems in transition medicine 1294
Problems with adherence 1294
High-risk behaviour 1295
Unplanned pregnancy 1295

Clinical presentations 1296
Neurological disease 1296
Respiratory disease 1297
Cardiovascular disease 1297
Oncology 1298
Renal disease 1298
Organ transplantation 1299
Diabetes 1299
Gastrointestinal disease 1299
Rheumatology and bone disease 1300

Summary 1300

Historically, childhood illnesses were characterised by a series of acute episodes, often infective, on a background of an otherwise healthy patient. Adult medicine traditionally comprised patients with progressive conditions, and increasing pathology with advancing age. A number of factors have led to the recognition that boundaries between adult medicine and paediatric care are not clear-cut, and recent evidence has confirmed that anticipating and carefully planning the transition of children with long-term conditions (LTCs) into adult services improve care and outcomes. About 14% of children in the developed world are diagnosed with an LTC and in the majority of patients the disorder will persist into adulthood. Common illnesses include asthma, epilepsy, congenital heart disease, diabetes and childhood cancer (Box 31.1). Similar trends are developing worldwide, with increasing survival rates of children with complex pathology, and increasing prevalence of lifestyle-related conditions such as obesity, hypertension and type 2 diabetes. Specific factors that make transition planning important in young people with LTCs are outlined in Figure 31.1.

Planning the process of transition from paediatric to adult health services and improving the assessment of young people as they enter those adult services have been shown to impact positively on long-term health outcomes. There is a need for physicians to gain new skills in the care of young people and adults who have conditions that have arisen in childhood. This includes developing specific skills in the management of adolescents and young adults, managing the process of transition and developing knowledge of relevant medical conditions. The overall approach to transition medicine, as well as important disease-specific issues, will be considered in this chapter.

Transition from paediatric to adult health services

Effectiveness of transition planning

A review of the effectiveness of transition planning has confirmed improved health outcomes when specific interventions to improve coordination between adult and paediatric services are implemented. Most research in this field has been undertaken with young people with diabetes, and many of the outcome measures relate to that condition. The principles of transition planning and the potential benefits are, however, likely to be generalisable to other LTCs that present in childhood. Young people with serious LTCs are among the most complex and high-risk patients to care for in adulthood, and it is important to work closely with them as they move to adult services, to try to improve their long-term outcome.

General principles of transition planning

Paediatric services are organised and delivered in a very different way to adult medical services. They encompass a period of life that spans from infancy to independence, and progress from taking parents' views as paramount to needing to recognise

---

i | 31.1 Important long-term conditions of childhood that affect adult health

Neurology
- Epilepsy
- Cerebral palsy
- Duchenne muscular dystrophy

Respiratory medicine
- Cystic fibrosis

Endocrinology
- Diabetes mellitus

Cardiology
- Hypertrophic obstructive cardiomyopathy
- Congenital heart disease

Nephrology
- Renal insufficiency
- Renal transplant

Gastroenterology
- Inflammatory bowel disease

Rheumatology
- Inflammatory rheumatic disease
- Osteogenesis imperfecta
- Hypophosphataemic rickets

Oncology
- Survivors of childhood cancer

Infectious disease
- HIV/AIDS
- Malaria

Fig. 31.1 Reasons to consider transition planning.

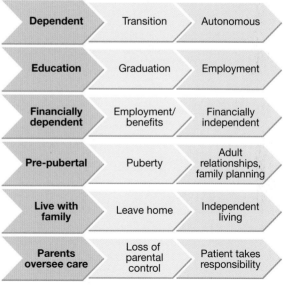

Fig. 31.2 Lifestyle changes during transition to adulthood.

the wishes of the young person. After transition, young people move from medical services that have been family-centred and focused around maximising the child's development, to a service that encourages patient autonomy, in which employment and reproduction are important measures of outcome. At the same time as undergoing transition within medical services, young people are making multiple other transitions in their lives as they move from a dependent to an independent way of living (Fig. 31.2). They often move away from the family home, and parents who formerly held responsibility for patient management, coordination of care, communication and consent to treatments will be demoted to an advisory role. Paediatric services are not well placed to meet this change in focus from the patient as a child to the patient as an independent adult, and young people benefit from the move to adult services as long as their specific needs as a young adult are recognised.

Principles of prescribing during transition

Hepatic drug metabolism increases from neonatal levels during childhood, eventually decreasing to adult levels after puberty. Once puberty has been completed, teenagers can be considered, in pharmacokinetic and pharmacodynamic terms, to behave like adults. It is important to remember that many young people have considerably lower body mass and therefore body mass index (BMI) than adults, and care needs to be taken to avoid excessive dosage in physically smaller patients. Likewise, obesity

needs consideration in terms of prescribing and drug doses. The general advice is that when prescribing a dose per kilogram, the optimal weight for height rather than actual weight should be used for obese young people.

A systematic approach to transition planning

Several steps need to be undertaken to develop a successful programme for transition of care. The key components are summarised in Box 31.2. The first step is to establish a policy in consultation with young people and train staff in the policy. Subsequently, systems need to be developed to identify patients in need of transition and track them as they pass through the programme. Adult health-care providers need to be identified and processes developed for introducing the young person to the adult team. This should be followed by written communication between the paediatric and adult teams, and then a first consultation with the adult team at which the transfer can be reviewed and

31.2 Core elements in developing a transitional care programme

Establishing transition policy

- Develop policy, with input from young people
- Train staff in operation of policy

Tracking and monitoring

- Establish process to identify patients
- Develop systems to track individual progress
- Incorporate transition planning into clinical care

Transition readiness

- Identify suitable adult care provider
- Establish process for introduction to adult team
- Provide written information about joint first consultation

Transition planning

- Ensure communication between paediatric and adult teams
- Identify need for handover consultation
- Prepare written medical handover:
    Diagnosis
    Current treatment
    Previous key issues
- Send relevant information in advance
- Provide information and community support

Transfer to adult services

- Arrange first consultation
- Review transfer package with team
- Identify concerns of young person
- Review young person's health priorities
- Update medical summary and emergency care plans

Integration into adult services

- Communicate with paediatrics and confirm transfer
- Help young adult to access other adult services
- Continue individualised care plan tailored to young person
- Seek feedback from young adult about transition

31.3 Key features in assessing readiness for transition to adult services

(K) Knowledge

1. Describes condition, effects and prognosis
2. Understands medication purpose and effects
3. Understands treatment purposes and effects
4. Knows key team members and their roles

(S) Self-advocacy

1. Can attend part/whole clinic appointment on their own
2. Knows how to make appointments/alter appointments
3. Has understanding of confidentiality
4. Orders repeat prescriptions
5. Takes some/complete responsibility for medication/other treatment
6. Knows where to get help

(H) Health and lifestyle

1. Understands importance of diet/exercise/dental care
2. Understands impact of smoking/alcohol/substance use
3. Understands sexual health issues/pregnancy/sexually transmitted infections

(A) Activities of daily living

1. Self-care/meal preparation
2. Independent travel/mobility
3. Trips/overnight stays away from home
4. Benefits/financial independence

(V) Vocational

1. Current and future education/impact of condition on career plans
2. School attendance and performance
3. Work experience and access to careers advice
4. Outside activities and interests
5. Disclosure to school/employer

(P) Psychosocial

1. Self-esteem/self-confidence
2. Body/self-image
3. Peer relationships/bullying
4. Support networks/family/disclosure to friends
5. Coping strategies

(T) Transition

1. Understands concept of transition
2. Agrees transition plan
3. Attends transition clinic
4. Visits adult unit (if appropriate)
5. Sees primary care team/other clinical staff independently

31

Fig. 31.3 **Timing of transition.**

a care plan developed. There should subsequently be written communication between the adult and paediatric teams to confirm that handover has occurred, followed eventually by integration of the young person's care into the adult service.

A number of organisations have published guidelines to planning transition services. Two of the best known include the 'Ready Steady Go' programme in the UK and the American Academy of Paediatrics' 'Got Transition' (see 'Further information'). Details of the sorts of competencies that a young person might need before making a full transition to adult medical services are outlined in Box 31.3.

When should transition happen?

The optimum timing for transition is not specifically defined; it is a process that evolves over a number of years, during which puberty and then adolescence occur. Transition should generally be initiated at around 12 years of age. Completion time then varies from person to person, also depending on the model of adult services available. Most commonly, full transition occurs between 16 and 18 years of age (Fig. 31.3). This coincides with many other areas where young people are considered to have made the transition to adulthood, such as the completion of formal education. Marriage and children often follow.

Functional anatomy and physiology

Puberty and adolescence are developmental stages through which children progress during the second decade of life. During this phase, several physical, biochemical and emotional changes occur. The most important are discussed in more detail below.

Endocrine changes

The hormonal and physical stages of progression through puberty in males and females are summarised in Figure 31.4. Puberty is initiated by pulsatile increases in gonadotrophin-releasing hormone (GnRH) by the hypothalamus, which in turn stimulates pulsatile release of luteinising hormone (LH) and follicle-stimulating hormone (FSH) by the pituitary. In males, the increased production of LH stimulates Leydig cells in the testes to produce testosterone, and FSH acts on Sertoli cells to stimulate sperm production, as described on page 651 and shown in Figure 18.13. The rise in testosterone increases skeletal growth, promotes development of the male genital organs and stimulates growth of pubic, facial and axillary hair. In females, FSH and LH act on the ovary to promote follicle production, ovulation and menstruation, as described on page 652 and shown in Figure 18.14. Other hormonal changes in all adolescents include a rise in adrenal androgens and a rise in growth hormone, which in turn stimulates production of insulin-like growth factors 1 and 2 (IGF-1 and IGF-2). Insulin production also rises by about 30% during puberty. These hormonal changes contribute to the biological, morphological and psychological changes seen during the teenage years. Adolescence (as opposed to puberty) comprises not only the physical changes of puberty, but also the wider emotional and psychological changes of progression into early adulthood. The emotional and psychological changes are associated with physical maturation but also with sociocultural influences. The normal feelings and behavioural development of normal adolescence are complex but tend to follow fairly predictable patterns.

Physical changes

In girls, there is an increased rate of growth, followed soon after by the development of breasts and pubic hair. Menstruation typically starts after the rate of growth has peaked. In boys, puberty begins with testicular enlargement, followed soon after by a growth spurt and the development of pubic hair. In clinical practice, Tanner staging is used as a method of documenting progression of physical changes that occur during puberty (Fig. 31.5). The average age at onset of puberty in the UK is about 11 years in girls and 12 years in boys but normal puberty has a very wide range of onset. Factors that are important in predicting age of onset of normal puberty include family history (age of onset is strongly predicted by the parents' pattern of onset) and body mass, with heavier children entering puberty at a younger age. The current trends towards improved nutritional status and increased obesity in particular are driving earlier onset of puberty. Delayed puberty is defined to have occurred when the age at onset is more than 2.5 standard deviations above the national average, which in the UK is about 13 years in girls and 14 years in boys. If puberty is delayed beyond this point, investigations may be needed to determine the underlying cause, as detailed on page 653. Many children who have had long-term health conditions during childhood experience a delayed onset of puberty because chronic ill health slows longitudinal growth and causes functional hypogonadotrophic hypogonadism. Glucocorticoid therapy also contributes to growth retardation in children with chronic inflammatory diseases. An X-ray of the left wrist can be used to assess bone age accurately, and a bone age that is more than 2 years behind the chronological age should prompt consideration of further investigations (p. 654).

Fig. 31.4 Hormonal events of puberty. A In the ovary, FSH acts on granulosa cells to stimulate oestrogen production, whereas LH acts on theca cells to stimulate progesterone production. Androgens are also produced in small amounts by theca cells in response to LH (not shown). B In the male, LH acts on interstitial Leydig cells to stimulate testosterone production. FSH with testosterone acts on Sertoli cells to stimulate spermatogenesis. (ACTH = adrenocorticotrophic hormone; FSH = follicle-stimulating hormone; GnRH = gonadotrophin-releasing hormone; LH = luteinising hormone) *From Smith RP. Netter's Obstetrics and gynecology, 2nd edn. Philadelphia: Saunders, Elsevier, Inc.; 2008.*

31

Tanner stage	I	II	III	IV	V
Female					
Breast	Pre-adolescent	Elevation of breast and papilla as a small mound	Further enlargement of breast and areola with no separation of contours	Projection of areola and papilla to form mound above breast	Mature stage. Projection of papilla with recession of areola to contour of breast
Pubic hair	None	Sparse, long and straight	Darker, coarse and curled hair	Darker, coarse and curled hair but covering smaller area than in adult. No spread to medial surface of thighs	Dark, coarse and curled hair extending to inner thighs
Male					
Genitalia	Pre-adolescent	Growth of testes and scrotum. Skin on scrotum reddens and becomes wrinkled	Growth of penis and further growth of testes and scrotum. Skin of scrotum becomes darker and more wrinkled	Further growth in length and width of penis, testes and scrotum	Penis, testes and scrotum of adult size
Pubic hair	None	Sparse, long and straight	Darker, coarse and curled hair	Darker, coarse and curled hair but covering smaller area than in adult	Dark, coarse and curled hair extending toward umbilicus

Fig. 31.5 Tanner staging of puberty.

Cognitive and behavioural changes

As young people move from their early teenage years to later adolescence there is a move away from the family towards personal independence. This is often characterised by change from a self-centred focus, associated with a sense of awkwardness and worries about being normal, towards increased self-confidence and an awareness of weaknesses in parents and others in authority. In late adolescence, young people reach a stage of self-reliance, increased emotional stability and improved ability to think ideas through. Finally, young adults begin to develop firm belief systems, autonomy and independence. With time, there is reduced conflict with parents and other figures in authority and full maturity develops.

In terms of cognition, there is a transition from being mostly interested in the present, in short-term outcomes and instant gratification, through to increased concern for the future and a greater focus on one's longer-term role in life. Sexuality and relationships clarify during adolescence, and individuals move from

early awkwardness and uncertainty to a firmer sense of their sexual identity, and then development of more serious and longer-term relationships. In terms of morals and values, young people move from a period of risk-taking behaviour and experimentation through to understanding the potential consequences of such behaviour for their future health and well-being. Young adults develop a greater capacity for setting personal goals and an increased focus on self-esteem. Finally, family, social and cultural traditions regain some of their previous importance, and by the time young people emerge from adolescence, they have usually developed insight and a greater focus on self-esteem and long-term well-being. It is the development of these more mature personality traits that are important for the more active role in health care that is needed to function well within an adult model of medicine. Some teenagers do vary slightly from these broad patterns but the feelings and behaviours described are, in general, considered normal for each stage of adolescence. Understanding these changes in emotional and psychological behaviour underpins the approaches that are needed to meet the challenges of managing long-term conditions in older teenagers and young adults.

i 31.4 Biochemical changes during transition

Analyte	Comment
Alanine aminotransferase (ALT)	Increased during adolescence Activity may continue to rise, at least in men, until middle age
Alkaline phosphatase (ALP)	Activity higher in infancy, decreases during childhood, and rises again with skeletal growth during puberty Peak in females at median 11 years and in males at 13 years Levels decrease rapidly after puberty, particularly in girls; adult levels achieved after epiphyses fused
Insulin-like growth factor 1	Levels 30% higher during adolescence
Serum creatinine	Increases steadily from infancy to puberty parallel to development of skeletal muscle; until puberty, there is little difference in concentration between males and females
Uric acid concentration	Decreases from high levels at birth until 7–10 years of age, then increases, especially in boys, until 16 years

Investigations

Several changes take place during adolescence in terms of skeletal growth, organ development and body composition, which can influence the interpretation of results. Examples include fusion of the epiphyses as puberty progresses, increases in bone mineral content and density as the skeleton grows, and changes in the reference range of certain biochemical tests. Most of these changes occur gradually during puberty and there are rarely abrupt alterations in adult biochemical concentrations. It is important to use age-adjusted biochemical reference ranges until puberty has been completed. Several biochemical changes take place in the composition of body fluids between infancy and puberty.

Some of the key changes in biochemical markers are outlined in Box 31.4. More detail on reference ranges for specific analytes is provided in Box 35.9 (p. 1363). The elevation in alkaline phosphatase (ALP) levels during adolescence relates to the bone isoenzyme produced by osteoblasts in the growing skeleton during the growth spurt. Further investigations for raised levels of ALP are not required in adolescence, as long as other liver function tests, including γ-glutamyl transferase (GGT), are normal.

In general, under normal physiological conditions, the reference ranges of most biochemical tests remain fairly constant between puberty and menopause in women and between puberty and middle age in men.

Clinical assessment

The initial patient consultation at transition is of vital importance for establishing a potentially life-long professional relationship with the patient, as well as identifying key features in the history, examination and assessment of their overall needs. Parents commonly attend a first adult appointment with their son or daughter, and it is usually necessary to allow longer for this initial

i 31.5 Features in transition assessment

Features of history and/or examination	Reason
History*	
Main/presenting condition and detailed review of clinical course	Understand detail and severity of illness; understand which treatments have been undertaken and which have been successful
Family history: Draw family tree of all first-degree and any relevant/affected second-degree family members	Many long-term conditions arising during childhood have significant genetic and familial factors to be taken into account
Current drug therapy, significant previous therapies	Many drugs have significant long-term implications, levels may need monitoring, may have teratogenic effects to consider
Any surgical or other relevant medical history	Understand which treatments have been undertaken and which have been successful
Pubertal status/age of menarche	Helps assess disease severity plus patterns of growth Informs about patient's reproductive health and family-planning wishes
Social history: In education or in work? Receiving appropriate benefits/support? Financial or other practical concerns? Living with parents/left home?	Assesses wider effects of patient's health on their independent living, as well as their financial and practical circumstances Can be a proxy measure of disease severity and identifies their support mechanisms, which also helps in the assessment of their current needs
Systems enquiry	Any other related/unrelated symptoms or problems
Physical examination	
Height, weight, calculation of body mass index Blood pressure Urinalysis if relevant Assessment of pubertal status General physical examination	Although young people are often accompanied by a parent, examine them separately and use this opportunity to consider asking about private matters, such as partners, sexual activity, and drug or alcohol use

*Throughout the first consultation, confidence and competence in decision-making/capacity to consent should be assessed. If there are concerns about capacity, clarify key decision-makers.

assessment. Often, the first transition appointment is undertaken jointly with the paediatrician in a specialist transition clinic and this will enable a thorough face-to-face handover of all the key facts.

A detailed transition referral letter should clearly describe the diagnosis, current and previous treatments, and key interventions that have been undertaken while the patient was under the care of paediatric services. It is important to check the main details with the young person and to make sure there are no other factors that they feel are of relevance. There are a few features in the history that merit special attention, particularly at the first consultation, as outlined in Box 31.5. Many young people with an LTC attend their first adult outpatient department consultation with their parents, and it is important either to create a time to ask personal and lifestyle-related questions separately from the main history – that is, privately – or to make sure that these can be confidentially explored in future.

31

Presenting problems in transition medicine

Problems with adherence

Adherence is defined as 'the extent to which a person's behaviour, in terms of taking medications, following diets, or executing lifestyle changes, coincides with medical or health advice'. The term 'adherence' is used in preference to 'compliance' because it focuses on whether a person actively adheres to the regimen rather than passively follows the doctor's orders. It also implies partnership and cooperation between the patient and the care-giver. More recently, clinicians have moved to seeking patients' concordance with management plans. Concordance refers to a consultation process that has an underlying ethos of shared decision-making. It has become clear that current levels of adherence do not deliver the full benefits of medication. Historical paternalistic medical practice does not maximise the chances of patients adopting the changes and treatments they need to improve their outcomes. Reaching a concordant position with patients involves a range of approaches (such as patient-centredness or shared decision-making) and a number of specific actions (such as exploring anxieties about medication side-effects, individualising regimes to suit the patient's lifestyle, offering a range of treatment options) and has not been evaluated comprehensively.

Adherence to clinic attendance, investigation and treatment often falls significantly in adolescence and during transition to adult services. Measurement of adherence is challenging and reported rates vary according to the method of assessment. Teenagers may also have varying adherence levels within their treatment regimen. An important example is in patients who have undergone organ transplantation, in whom low adherence to immunosuppressive medication is a significant cause of graft rejection and may cause death. Adherence merits careful consideration when caring for adolescents and young adults, and focusing on strategies to improve adherence at this initial stage of patient management can deliver life-long improvements in health outcomes. Young teenagers mainly believe in things that they have directly experienced and do not fully appreciate the unseen consequences of not taking their medications. In time,

 31.6 Factors affecting adherence

Negative factors

- Older adolescent
- Mental health issues with care-giver
- Family conflicts
- Complex therapy
- Medication with side-effects
- Denial of illness

Positive factors

- Positive family functioning
- Close friends
- Internal locus of control
- Treatment with immediate benefits
- Patient's belief in seriousness of illness and efficacy of treatment
- Physician empathy

 31.7 SIMPLE strategies to improve adherence

Simplify regimen

- Use once daily/twice daily regimes if possible
- Match regimen to bedtime and meals
- Use pill box or alarms on phone
- Organise services around patient (combined clinics, flexible timing and appointments)

Impart knowledge

- Share decision-making
- Provide clear instructions:
    Limit to three or four major points
    Use simple, everyday language
    Use written information or pamphlets and verbal education at all encounters
- Supply addresses of quality websites
- Provide advice on how to cope with medication costs

Modify patient beliefs

- Empower patients to self-manage their condition:
    Ask about their needs
    Ask what might help them become and remain adherent
    Ensure they understand the risks of not taking their medication
    Address fears and concerns about taking the medication

Provide communication

- Improve interviewing skills
- Practise active listening
- Provide emotional support – treat the whole patient and not just the disease

- Provide clear, direct and thorough information
- Elicit the patient's input in treatment decisions
- Allow adequate time for patients to ask questions
- Build trust

Leave the bias

- Learn more about low health literacy and how it affects patient outcomes
- Consider care of ethnically and socially diverse patient populations
- Acknowledge biases in medical decision-making (intentional or unintentional)
- Address dissonance of patient–provider race/ethnicity and language
- Take extra time to overcome cultural barriers
- Ask specifically about attitudes, beliefs and cultural norms around medication
- Use culturally and linguistically appropriate targeted patient interventions
- Increase engagement, activation and empowerment
- Tailor education to the patient's level of understanding

Evaluate adherence

- Direct:
    Number of repeat prescriptions
    Biomarkers of response
    Measurement of drug levels
- Indirect:
    Self-reporting: 'When did you last forget your medicine?'; 'How often have you forgotten your medicines this week?'

Excerpted with permission from the American College of Preventive Medicine. Medication Adherence: Improving Health Outcomes Time Tool: A Resource from the American College of Preventive Medicine. 2011. Retrieved from https://webmail2.tst.nhs.uk/go/www.acpm.org/?MedAdhereTTProviders.

adolescents learn to develop hypothetical thinking and to analyse more complex information and decision-making. The ability to engage in formal thinking is inconsistent at first, and at times of stress (such as during an illness) adolescents may regress to more simple ways of problem-solving. Despite their maturing skills, they may remain self-centred and feel invincible. Factors that positively and negatively affect adherence are outlined in Box 31.6. Interventions to improve adherence are summarised in Box 31.7.

Recent literature suggests that two-way communication between patients and professionals about medicines leads to improved satisfaction with care, knowledge of the condition and treatment, adherence, health outcomes and fewer medication-related problems. Younger adults and those coming to adult services following transition from paediatric services have very different expectations in terms of the nature of the patient–doctor relationship and are more likely to require a more collaborative approach to development of management plans to maximise their concordance with treatment in the long term.

High-risk behaviour

The high-risk behaviour that can be undertaken by adolescents is well documented and is seen across many cultures. It is important to assess this by history-taking at the time of transition (Box 31.8) Adolescents who have had LTCs during childhood

---

i	**31.8 History-taking in adolescent patients: risk-taking behaviours ('HEADS')**

Home life

- Relationships
- Social support
- Household chores

Education

- School
- Exams
- Work experience
- Career
- University
- Financial issues

Activities

- Peers, people that patients can rely on
- Exercise and sport

Driving

- Aged 16 if disabled

Drugs

- Cigarettes and alcohol: how much, how often
- Non-prescription drugs

Diet

- Nutritional content (calcium, vitamin D)
- Weight
- Caffeine (diet drinks)
- Binges/vomiting

Sex

- Concerns
- Periods
- Contraception (in relation to medication)

Sleep

- Amount
- Difficulty getting to sleep
- Frequent waking
- Early waking?

Suicide

- Depression
- Mood
- Disabled adolescent men high-risk

From Segal TY. Adolescence: what the cystic fibrosis team needs to know. J R Soc Med 2008; 101(Suppl 1):15–27.

---

are at greater risk of undertaking harmful behaviour and there is evidence that a poor long-term health outlook is associated with risk-taking behaviour earlier in life.

Globally, the leading causes of death among adolescents are road injury, human immunodeficiency virus (HIV) infection, suicide, lower respiratory infections and interpersonal violence; many of these deaths are linked to risk-taking behaviours such as excess alcohol and drug intake. Quite apart from mortality, there are other significant adverse events linked to risk-taking behaviour in adolescents: excess alcohol ingestion is also associated with non-fatal road traffic accidents, unwanted and unprotected sexual activity, and violence as both perpetrator and victim.

There are a number of theories about the neurodevelopmental changes associated with these behaviour changes. At around 11 years of age, the prefrontal cortex (PFC) and parietal lobes begin a period of pruning of neuronal axons. It is theorised that these changes represent the start of the process of increasing frontal lobe control. A separate process that occurs at the same time predisposes the adolescent to risk-taking behaviour and impulsivity: frontostriatal reward circuits mature relatively early and encourage the adolescent towards adult activities such as alcohol and drug use, and sexual intercourse, which carry potential health risks. At this stage, the PFC has not yet matured to the point where the individual can assess risk adequately. The PFC and its connections are structurally unable to provide sufficient control. It is thought that this maturational gap in PFC control of the pleasure-seeking brain systems is responsible for the risk-taking lifestyle that characterises the period of adolescence.

A number of studies have investigated personality and other factors that contribute to different risk-taking behaviours during adolescence: essentially, younger adolescents and females tend to rate activities as being more risky, and are therefore less likely to undertake them. Older males and those of lower educational status are higher risk takers. Specific protective factors include high self-esteem and a strong orientation to an internal locus of control; young people who feel they have less control and influence over themselves and their behaviour are more likely to undertake high-risk activities. Many teenagers with serious long-term health conditions are disempowered in a number of ways and there is evidence that they are predisposed to be high risk takers during adolescence. Examples of risk-taking behaviour include not only alcohol and drug intake, but also non-adherence to medicines and other aspects of health care, such as diet in diabetes.

It is not easy to affect behaviour during this period of non-adherence. Isolated educational intervention is not sufficient to improve outcome; for example, there is a wealth of evidence showing that teenagers know about the behaviours needed to prevent transmission of HIV, but many do not adhere to this advice. Long-term health-care providers have an invaluable role in supporting adolescents during this period of their development as adults, as many important health-related and lifestyle habits are established during this period: more than 90% of smokers start smoking in adolescence, and life-long habits around eating and exercise are laid down during the teenage years. Focusing on the needs of the emerging adult for autonomy and using the highest levels of communication and patient engagement significantly improve outcomes for patients with LTCs.

Unplanned pregnancy

In many parts of the world, females commonly undergo their first pregnancy during or just after adolescence. The median age for

31

i	31.9 Adolescent pregnancy rates	
Region	**Pregnancy rate (/1000 women aged 15–19 years)**	
Tanzania	124	
Kenya	94	
Jamaica	71	
Mexico	65	
South Africa	52	
USA	33	
Pakistan	28	
New Zealand	26	
UK	26	
Spain	11	
France	6	
Japan	5.3	
Italy	4.5	
South Korea	2.2	

first pregnancy varies from 19 years in India and parts of Asia, through to 25 years in the USA and around 30 years in Australia and Western Europe. Teenage pregnancy rates are high across the world (Box 31.9). Information from the UK suggests that 1 in 6 pregnancies is unplanned, and 1.5% of women between the ages of 18 and 45 face an unplanned pregnancy each year. It is therefore vital to anticipate and discuss the issues surrounding reproductive health with all young people before and during transition, as well as during early adulthood. Young people with serious LTCs have a number of additional factors to be taken into consideration when discussing reproduction, and these discussions need to take place long before a family is planned. General physicians do not need to be able to undertake complex genetic counselling and investigation, but should be able to provide advice about the recurrence risk of common inherited conditions, as well as that of the more common multifactorial LTCs, many of which have an inherited or genetic component.

Clinical presentations

In almost every clinical setting, there is the potential for a young adult with a serious LTC that has arisen during childhood to present to adult physicians. Medical services can improve the care and outcome for this vulnerable group by planning a systematic approach to transition, as described above, and by focusing the clinical consultation on issues of relevance and importance to each particular patient. The key issues to consider for a number of the most common LTCs of childhood are discussed below.

Neurological disease

Epilepsy

Epilepsy is a chronic disorder, the hallmark of which is recurrent, unprovoked seizures (p. 1097). Epilepsy that has presented during childhood, as opposed to adulthood, is less often associated with underlying central nervous system malignancy and is well

controlled with first-line anticonvulsants in around 80% of cases. Young people who still have epilepsy or are on anticonvulsant therapy as they progress into adulthood are more likely to have underlying structural brain disease, such as cerebral palsy, or have more complex or syndromic epilepsy. In many of them, epilepsy may be associated with learning difficulties or other neurological conditions.

Epilepsy presents several problems during transition. Adherence to medication can be an issue and patients with low adherence to epilepsy medicines have higher mortality, higher hospital admission rates and higher emergency department attendances. Conversely, high adherence rates at initiation of epilepsy therapy are associated with improved long-term seizure freedom and higher seizure freedom at 4 years. Epilepsy can also affect employment options for young people, as about 30% of patients still have breakthrough seizures while on treatment. Certain types of employment, such as working within the emergency services or armed forces, or becoming a pilot or driver of a heavy goods vehicle, may therefore not be possible. Driving restrictions may also limit options for some other occupations (p. 1103). Young women with epilepsy should be advised that oral contraceptives are less effective with enzyme-inducing antiepileptic drugs; they should also be made aware of the risk of teratogenicity with many antiepileptic drugs, most notably sodium valproate, which should be avoided in pregnancy if at all possible. Pre-conceptual counselling is desirable for all young girls with epilepsy and pre-conceptual folic acid supplementation is advisable to reduce the risk of neural tube defects.

Alcohol use in moderation does not affect seizure control in the majority of patients, but withdrawal from alcohol in dependent patients is epileptogenic and heavy alcohol use should be discouraged. Information about marijuana and epilepsy risk is lacking, but regular marijuana use and excess drinking are associated with poor adherence to medication regimes and increased seizure risk.

Cerebral palsy

Cerebral palsy comprises a range of non-progressive neurological impairments, present from the time of birth or arising in early childhood. Although the neuropathology is non-progressive, the manifestation of problems can evolve, with progressive motor dysfunction related to increased spasticity and possibly progressive seizure activity.

Patients with severe cerebral palsy present specific problems during transition and early adulthood. They may be paraplegic or quadriplegic and most non-ambulatory individuals have significant intellectual disability. This group of patients will be unable to live independently during adulthood and need ongoing long-term care. Delivering medical care to these individuals poses several problems, including practical issues such as consideration of capacity and consent to treatment. Other comorbidities include gastro-oesophageal reflux (often related to abnormal lower oesophageal function), seizures, and feeding difficulties often requiring gastrostomy. These individuals usually require a complex care package involving many members of the multidisciplinary team. There are also risks of abuse and neglect in the care of adults with severe disability and this needs to be borne in mind when considering atypical problems or unusual presentations in this vulnerable patient group. Depending on the severity of the patient's condition, end-of-life care may need to be discussed and planned with the family and other care-givers.

Muscular dystrophy

The muscular dystrophies are a group of diseases that cause progressive weakness and loss of muscle mass. The disorders differ in terms of which muscle groups are affected, the degree of weakness, and the rate of disease and symptom progression. All the inherited muscular dystrophies that present during childhood need active management during transition (p. 1143). One of the most important and most severe conditions is Duchenne muscular dystrophy (DMD), which is associated with a progressive decline in mobility, coupled with cardiac dysfunction due to cardiomyopathy, and respiratory failure requiring respiratory support as the disease progresses. Physicians should ensure that the whole family are aware of the wider genetic issues. Female carriers of the DMD gene can suffer muscle fatigue and are at risk of cardiomyopathy, as well as there being obvious risks for their male offspring. On average, patients with DMD survive until their late teens to early twenties, and those with less severe muscular dystrophies, such as Becker dystrophy, survive until their thirties. Although fertility is reduced, young men with these conditions may themselves father children. Male offspring will be unaffected but all female infants of affected males will be carriers.

As the muscular dystrophies progress, a complex package of care involving a multidisciplinary team is necessary; it should include respiratory input to assess the need for ventilatory support, which is a common endpoint for many patients. At the present time, there is no definitive treatment. Glucocorticoids (0.75 mg/kg/day) have been shown to improve muscle strength and are frequently used, but carry an increased risk of osteoporosis and vertebral fractures. New therapeutic approaches are being developed with the aim of ameliorating disease progression in patients with nonsense mutations (p. 42). One involves the use of drugs such as ataluren, which promotes binding of transfer RNA (tRNA) molecules at the site of stop codons with a mismatch in one base (near-cognate tRNAs). These cause a full-length protein to be produced with an amino acid substitution rather than a truncated non-functional protein. Patients with DMD usually require social and financial support. It is important to consider end-of-life care plans with patients and family members. Involvement from palliative care teams, as well as psychological, spiritual and wider non-medical support, is essential.

Respiratory disease

Cystic fibrosis

Cystic fibrosis (CF) is a single-gene autosomal recessive disorder that affects about 1 in 2000 to 1 in 3000 individuals of Caucasian descent (p. 580). Clinical manifestations are caused by defects in an ion transporter termed the cystic fibrosis transmembrane conductor regulator (CTFR) protein. With improved supportive care, the median survival in the UK is now more than 50 years. It is well recognised that young people with life-limiting conditions face particular challenges during transition: individuals often exhibit high-risk behaviour during adolescence, and this was particularly true in the past when long-term survival rates were poor. The rates of non-concordance with medication and with time-consuming physiotherapy and nebuliser regimes are high and adversely affect outcome and survival. Exercise tolerance and employment are likely to be restricted as time progresses, and patients need particular support managing the slow decline in function and well-being that occurs throughout their adult lives.

In terms of fertility and child-bearing potential, the picture is complex and merits detailed discussion with patients. It is not often discussed openly by the paediatrician or during childhood, other than with the parents when the patient is young. The vas deferens is absent in 98% of males with CF and seminal vesicular dysfunction means that ejaculates are low in volume. While boys are infertile, newer reproductive therapies, such as the availability of intracytoplasmic sperm injection, mean that fatherhood is possible. The opportunity for assisted reproduction should be discussed early so that people can make informed choices at an appropriate stage of their lives. Females with CF who have good nutritional status and reasonable health status have normal fertility and genetic counselling should be offered early. Contraception needs to be discussed with women who are not planning a pregnancy, since pulmonary hypertension is an absolute contraindication for the oral contraceptive pill (OCP). Women also need to be advised about the effects of antibiotics on OCP effectiveness. New orally available small-molecule therapies, including lumacaftor and ivacaftor, have recently been licensed; they can partially rectify functional defects in the CTFR and have improved outcome. These drugs are having a positive effect on symptom control and are potentially disease-modifying. Other therapeutic approaches, including gene therapy and mRNA editing therapies, are also being explored as treatments for CF. Common issues encountered during transition of CF patients are summarised in Box 17.34 (p. 581).

Cardiovascular disease

Congenital heart disease

Congenital heart disease (CHD) is the most common congenital anomaly, affecting about 1% of live births. Among birth defects, CHD is the leading cause of mortality. Maternal illnesses such as rubella and injection of teratogenic agents during pregnancy, along with paternal age, all play roles in pathogenesis. Although some chromosomal anomalies, such as trisomy 13, 18 and 21 and monosomy X (Turner's syndrome), are strongly associated with CHD, these account for only 5% of cases. Microdeletion and single-gene mutations can also be important, such as in DiGeorge syndrome (22q11.2 microdeletion). Overall, the most common congenital valvular anomalies are aortic and pulmonary stenosis. The most common structural anomaly is ventricular septal defect.

There is a wide range of severity of CHD but many patients with life-limiting conditions (usually complex structural anomalies such as tetralogy of Fallot or hypoplastic left heart syndrome) survive to adulthood. Genetic counselling of affected individuals is important, as there is a 1–2% recurrence risk of any cardiac anomaly in offspring. Affected patients should be transitioned to a cardiologist with experience in CHD since this has become a subspecialty in own right. More details are provided on page 531 and in Box 16.103 (p. 537).

Hypertrophic obstructive cardiomyopathy

Hypertrophic obstructive cardiomyopathy (HOCM, p. 539) is a genetic cardiovascular disease characterised by left ventricular wall hypertrophy, impaired diastolic filling and abnormalities of the mitral valve. These features can cause dynamic obstruction of the left ventricular outflow tract, diastolic dysfunction, myocardial dysfunction and an increased risk of supraventricular and ventricular tachyarrhythmias. HOCM is caused by mutations

31

affecting the genes that encode cardiac sarcomere proteins and is most frequently transmitted as an autosomal dominant trait. It may present for the first time during adolescence with cardiac arrest or sudden cardiac death. Predictive genetic testing is possible but challenging because of the large number of causal mutations. In clinical practice, careful analysis of the family history can be useful in identifying those at risk of inheriting the disease. If no gene anomaly has been identified within a family, first-degree relatives may need screening by electrocardiography (ECG) and echocardiography. Identification of a genetic anomaly is most helpful in allowing identification of family members who do not need echocardiograms or clinical follow-up. Children of affected parents should be screened every 3 years until puberty, and then annually until 20 years of age. If there is no evidence of HOCM in early adulthood, it is unlikely that the condition will develop in later life.

Oncology

Around 1 child in 500 will develop cancer by the age of 14 years. Leukaemia is the most common, accounting for about 33% of cases; central nervous system tumours are the next most common, accounting for around 25% of all childhood cancers. Fifty years ago, 75% of children diagnosed with cancer died, but overall survival rates now range from 75% to 80%. Between 60% and 70% of young adults who have survived childhood cancer will develop at least one medical disability, most commonly as a result of their therapy rather than their primary cancer. There is a 3–6-fold increased risk of a second cancer, with an absolute risk of about 10% before 50 years of age. It is therefore important for these individuals to be kept under surveillance during transition and beyond.

Endocrine and reproductive disturbances are the most common late effects, affecting 40–60% of survivors. Infertility can be an issue in both males and females receiving cytotoxic medications, unless it has been possible to store semen and ovarian tissue in advance of treatment. Other long-term risks include hypopituitarism, growth hormone deficiency and pubertal delay (especially in boys) from brain irradiation. Radiotherapy to the neck can cause hypothyroidism and increases the risk of thyroid cancer. Total-body irradiation offered as conditioning for bone marrow transplantation affects both ovarian and testicular function, and many of the chemotherapeutic agents used have adverse effects on fertility. Chemotherapy-induced ovarian failure is typically associated with high-dose alkylating agents such as cyclophosphamide, and this is an independent risk factor for premature ovarian failure. In recent years, patients have been offered ovarian and testicular tissue retention and fertility issues are being discussed with families during childhood, but often the patients themselves have limited levels of knowledge of the details. Chemotherapy and radiotherapy in childhood significantly reduce ovarian reserves. When combined with the progressive ovarian decline that occurs in all women throughout adulthood there is a significant risk of premature menopause or ovarian failure, with 8% of survivors affected. Young women need to be aware of these risks during their early adulthood to help with family and lifestyle planning; for example, they may wish to plan to have children earlier in their adult life rather than risking ovarian decline.

Cardiomyopathy is another complication of anthracyclines such as doxorubicin and daunorubicin. Serious cardiac complications include arrhythmias, dilated cardiomyopathy from myocardial necrosis, and angina or myocardial infarction arising from vaso-occlusion or vasospasm.

In addition to physical effects, children who have faced life-threatening illness in childhood may experience psychological and family difficulties during adulthood. Cognitive impairment is more common in children who have received chemotherapy or radiotherapy to the brain, and problems can include lower IQ, problems with memory and attention, poor hand–eye coordination and behaviour/personality problems, combined with the well-recognised and physical complications of cancer treatment in childhood.

Increasing recognition of these issues has resulted in active monitoring programmes for survivors of childhood cancer, who are best seen in specialist 'late effects' multidisciplinary clinics, where teams include oncologists, psychologists and specialists from other relevant disciplines.

Renal disease

Chronic kidney disease (CKD, p. 415) accounts for some of the most complex long-term illnesses in childhood. The most common causes during childhood and adolescence are shown in Box 31.10. The primary pathology can be varied and many conditions have no specific treatment, but the overall approach to management of progressive renal insufficiency is the same. Internationally agreed definitions of CKD staging in children differ from those in adults and are summarised in Box 31.11. In adults the rate of albumin excretion is included in CKD definitions, as outcome correlates with the level of albuminuria, but in children similar data are lacking and so the staging system is based on glomerular filtration rate alone. The majority of children with

31.10 Causes of renal impairment in childhood and adolescence

- Obstructive uropathy
- Renal hypoplasia/dysplasia
- Reflux nephropathy
- Focal segmental glomerular sclerosis
- Polycystic kidney disease

31.11 Staging of chronic kidney disease (CKD) in children over 2 years of age*

Stage	Glomerular filtration rate (GFR) (mL/min/1.73 m²)	Description
1	>90	Normal or high
2	60–89	Mildly decreased
3a	45–59	Mildly to moderately decreased
3b	30–44	Moderately to severely decreased
4	15–29	Severely decreased
5	<15	Kidney failure

*Kidney Disease: Improving Global Outcomes (KDIGO) 2012 classification. Chronic kidney disease is defined either as GFR <60 mL/min/1.73 m² for >3 months, regardless of whether other CKD markers are present, or as GFR <60 mL/min/1.73 m² accompanied by evidence of structural damage or other markers of kidney abnormalities, including proteinuria, albuminuria, and pathological abnormalities in histology or imaging. In adults, albumin excretion is also included in CKD staging as the level of albuminuria correlates to outcome. These data are lacking in children and so albuminuria is not used to classify paediatric CKD.

CKD stage 3 or higher will ultimately require renal replacement therapy but the timescale for reaching this stage can vary widely. The mainstay of support is to delay progression by treatment of secondary factors that are known to be associated with progressive decline in renal function: namely, hypertension, proteinuria and anaemia.

Organ transplantation

Children requiring renal replacement therapy are the most common recipients of kidney transplants in childhood. Liver and heart transplantation, followed by lung and small bowel transplantation, are well-recognised but less commonly undertaken procedures. Non-adherence to immunosuppressive regimes during adolescence is a well-known risk factor for graft failure. The reported incidence of graft failure due to non-adherence is 10–15% but this is likely to be an under-estimate. Rates of non-adherence are highest among adolescents and young adults. As well as non-adherence to immunosuppression, non-adherence to testing and clinic attendance adversely affects the care and outcome of around 1 in 8 kidney transplant patients. Poor adherence is associated with patients with worse psychological status and family dysfunction; adherence has been shown to improve with education and increased motivational factors, as might be expected. This offers the opportunity to improve graft survival. At present, 50% of cadaveric grafts and around 68% of live donor grafts are still functioning 10 years post-transplant. There is no clear difference between children and adults in survival of transplanted kidneys.

Many medications used in transplant medicine and in renal disease can have long-term effects on health. Inhibition of linear growth is seen even with low doses of glucocorticoids, such as 0.125 mg/kg/day on a long-term basis. Alternate-day regimes are generally considered preferable in childhood. The height reduction associated with long-term glucocorticoid use in childhood is dose-dependent, and even for children with asthma treated with inhaled glucocorticoids, an average height reduction of 1.2 cm is reported. This is can also be associated with delayed puberty, as well as an increased risk of osteoporosis in adulthood. Post-transplant lymphoproliferative disorders (PTLDs) are a well-recognised and potentially life-threatening complication in solid organ recipients. PTLD is the most common malignancy complicating solid organ transplantation, accounting for 20% of all cancers. They represent a range of lymphoproliferative disorders, from infectious mononucleosis and lymphoid hyperplasia to malignant lymphoma. Most cases of PTLD are associated with Epstein–Barr virus (EBV), leading to uncontrolled B-cell proliferation and tumour formation. Up to 10% of solid organ transplant recipients develop PTLD but the risk is almost four times higher in patients under 20 years of age, as opposed to those aged 20–50. This increased risk relates mainly to the development of EBV infection after transplantation; most adults are already EBV-seropositive at the time of transplantation and therefore at lower risk of this complication. The type of organ transplant that has been undertaken predicts PTLD risk, with the cumulative incidence over 5 years ranging from 1–2% in haematopoietic cell transplant and liver transplants, 1–3% in renal transplants, 2–6% in heart transplants and 2–9% in lung transplants to as high as 11–33% in intestinal or multi-organ transplants. The different rates possibly relate to the varying degrees of immunosuppression required. The incidence of PTLD is highest in the first year after transplantation, when it is associated with the highest levels of immunosuppression.

Diabetes

Adherence and concordance with medication are a particular challenge in adolescents who have developed diabetes during childhood (p. 753). Studies of adolescents with type 1 diabetes have revealed that 25% were neglecting insulin injections, 81% were not following their diet, and 29% were not measuring their glucose level and were completing a daily diary with fictitious results. Research has also shown that the outcome of diabetes is improved with a formal transition programme (Box 31.12). Good control of diabetes is particularly important during this phase since microvascular disease often emerges around time of transition, although it can occur sooner in patients with early-onset diabetes.

i 31.12 Impact of transition planning on outcome in diabetes	
Intervention	**Outcome measures**
Disease-specific education	Lower HbA_{1C}
Generic education/skills training	Fewer acute complications: Hypoglycaemia Admissions with ketoacidosis
Transition coordinator	Lower rate of loss to follow-up
Joint paediatric/adult clinic	Fewer chronic complications: Hypertension Nephropathy Retinopathy
Separate young adult clinic	Improved self-management Improved disease-specific knowledge
Out-of-hours phone support	Improved screening for complications
Enhanced follow-up	Better quality-of-life scores

Gastrointestinal disease

Inflammatory bowel disease

The prevalence of inflammatory bowel disease (IBD, p. 813) in childhood is increasing, and the incidence of Crohn's disease (CD) in particular is rising in both children and adults, probably due to currently undefined environmental factors. Current treatment aims are outlined in Box 31.13. Standard measures include exclusive enteral nutrition for 6–8 weeks using a whole-protein (polymeric) formula, which induces initial remission in 80% of children. This is equivalent to glucocorticoid therapy but offers improved nutritional status and superior mucosal healing. Glucocorticoids can also be used to induce remission, as well as to treat exacerbations, but should be followed up by immunosuppressive therapy with azathioprine or methotrexate. Adolescents and children are more likely than adults to require biologics and around 20% need treatment with tumour necrosis factor alpha (TNF-α) inhibitors such as infliximab or adalimumab. Around 20% of children with CD require surgery within 5 years of diagnosis; limited resections and stricturoplasty are considered best practice to preserve gut length and prevent short bowel syndrome (p. 707).

Children with ulcerative colitis (UC) are more likely than adults to present with pancolitis (approximately 80% versus 40–50% in adults). Mild disease should be treated initially with oral 5-ASA preparations such as mesalamine or sulfasalazine. If the response is inadequate, oral glucocorticoids can be used, but caution must be exercised because of the adverse effects on skeletal growth and bone mineral density. Thiopurines such as 6-mercaptopurine or azathioprine are frequently used as steroid-sparing agents,

31

31.13 Treatment strategy in Crohn's disease

- Induce and maintain clinical remission
- Optimise nutrition
- Optimise bone health
- Optimise growth and pubertal progress
- Minimise adverse drug effects

with progression to anti-TNF-α therapy for those who still do not respond. There is less evidence for efficacy of TNF-α inhibitors in adolescents with UC than those with CD; they seem to be effective at inducing an initial response but less useful for maintaining long-term remission, since a significant proportion of patients still require colectomy (20% at 1 year) or long-term glucocorticoids. Ciclosporin is probably more effective than infliximab in teenagers with refractory UC. As with other adolescents who have long-term conditions, adherence to medication is particularly important to reduce the risk of relapse. In terms of lifestyle advice, smoking is a particular risk since it increases both the rate and severity of relapses. Body image can be a particular challenge for young adults with IBD, and those with colostomies or fistulae, for example, can find this part of their illness particularly difficult. Delayed puberty and short stature are important comorbidities, partly related to medication side effects and also to the nature of the inflammatory bowel disease itself.

Rheumatology and bone disease

Juvenile idiopathic arthritis

Juvenile idiopathic arthritis (JIA) is the term used to describe a wide variety of inflammatory rheumatic diseases that present during childhood (p. 1026). Oligoarticular juvenile arthritis has a good prognosis and often remits during adulthood, and so transitioning patients to adult rheumatology services may not always be required. The same does not hold true for systemic JIA and polyarticular JIA, which often require long-term immunosuppressive therapy through transition and beyond into adulthood. Smoking is a risk because it increases the activity of inflammatory disease and reduces the effectiveness of biologics. Adherence to and concordance with medication remain a challenge, as in other chronic diseases. Functional limitation secondary to joint damage may limit employment opportunities. Contraceptive advice is important in patients on methotrexate.

Glucocorticoid-induced osteoporosis

Osteoporosis is a complication of long-term glucocorticoid therapy that may be required in patients with inflammatory disease, transplantation and DMD.

There is a paucity of evidence about best practice in glucocorticoid-induced osteoporosis in children and adolescents, but in general the teenage years are a period of considerable bone mineral deposition and offer a chance to enhance bone mineral density significantly. It is important to ensure adequate calcium and vitamin D intake and to supplement if necessary. Therapy with bisphosphonates can be considered in symptomatic patients, although the evidence base for prevention of fractures is poor.

Osteogenesis imperfecta

Osteogenesis imperfecta (p. 1055) typically presents with multiple low-trauma fractures during infancy and childhood. Although fractures become less common during adolescence due to the increase in bone mass, they still occur frequently during transition

and in young adults. Intravenous bisphosphonates are widely used in the treatment of children with osteogenesis imperfecta (those with long-bone deformities, vertebral compression fractures, and three or more fractures per year, in whom the benefit:risk ratio is thought to be positive), although the evidence base for prevention of fractures is poor and based on observational studies.

There is much debate about whether continuing bisphosphonate therapy into adulthood is beneficial due to concerns about suppression of bone turnover in the long term. Affected individuals and their parents can find this change in treatment strategy confusing and it is important to explain the underlying rationale in order to manage expectations.

Hypophosphataemic rickets

Hypophosphataemic rickets is described in more detail on page 1052. Adherence to phosphate supplements and, to a lesser extent, vitamin D metabolites represents an important issue in optimising management during childhood and this becomes even more challenging in transitioning patients. While skeletal deformity does not progress following closure of the epiphyses, different problems arise in adolescent patients when there is suboptimal control of hypophosphataemia, including painful pseudofractures and arthralgia associated with enthesopathy. The renal phosphate leak tends to improve to an extent during adolescence and the requirement for phosphate is reduced, but most patients still require treatment with active vitamin D metabolites.

Summary

Young people who have suffered long-term conditions during childhood represent a particularly high-risk group of patients as they progress through adolescence to become young and, finally, mature adults. They bring with them specific medical risks and complications related to their previous medical treatment, and knowledge of these is important to identify the long-term complications of the therapies to which they have been exposed. They are a patient group that can display complex and often abnormal illness behaviour. Understanding this and implementing an effective process for transition from paediatric to adult services can reduce the significant risks that these patients face in early adulthood. As they mature and develop more adult intellectual and emotional behaviour patterns, the risks to their health and well-being reduce. Patients in transition can be a particularly challenging group to manage, but investment of time and effort at this stage of their lives can be extremely rewarding and can bring significant improvements in long-term health-related outcomes.

Further information

Books and journal articles

Atreja A, Bellam N, Levy SR. Strategies to enhance patient adherence: Making it simple. MedGenMed 2005; 7:4.

Crowley R, Wolfe I, Lock K, McKee M. Improving the transition between paediatric and adult healthcare: a systematic review. Arch Dis Child 2011; 96:548–553.

Segal TY. Adolescence: what the cystic fibrosis team needs to know. J R Soc Med 2008; 101(Suppl 1):15–27.

Websites

acpm.org/?Adherence *American College of Preventive Medicine: detailed review of adherence.*

GotTransition.org *Sample clinical tools and measurement resources for quality improvement purposes.*

uhs.nhs.uk *More clinical tools and measurement resources.*

Ageing and disease

Comprehensive Geriatric Assessment 1302

Demography 1304

Functional anatomy and physiology 1304
Biology of ageing 1304
Physiological changes of ageing 1305
Frailty and multimorbidity 1306

Investigations 1306
Comprehensive Geriatric Assessment 1306
Decisions about investigation and treatment 1306

Presenting problems in geriatric medicine 1307
Falls 1308
Dizziness 1309
Delirium 1309
Urinary incontinence 1309
Prescribing and deprescribing 1310
Other problems in old age 1311

Rehabilitation 1311

Comprehensive Geriatric Assessment

7 Cognitive function
Mini-mental state examination
(see Ch. 28)

6 Vision
Visual acuity
Glasses worn/present
Cataract

▲ Cataract

5 Hearing
Wax
Hearing aid used

4 Erect and supine blood pressure
Postural hypotension

3 Pulse
Atrial fibrillation

2 Hydration
Skin turgor
Oedema

1 Nutrition
Body mass index
(Height calculated from arm demispan or knee height to compensate for loss of vertebral height)
Recent weight loss,
e.g. loose skin folds
Dentition/oral hygiene

▲ Measurement of knee height (see Ch. 19)

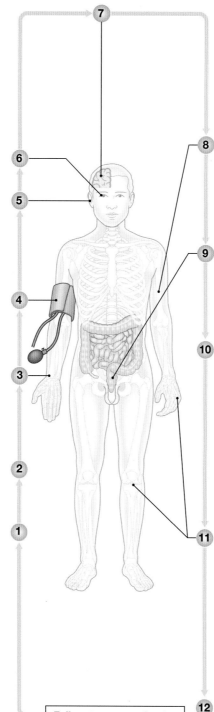

Full systems examination with particular attention to the above

8 Muscle
Wasting
Strength

▲ Wasting of small muscles of hands in rheumatoid arthritis

9 Per rectum
Faecal impaction
Prostate size/consistency in men
Anal tone

10 Skin
Wounds/ulcers
Infection
Swelling

▲ Senile purpura

▲ Venous ulceration

11 Joints
Deformity
Pain
Swelling
Range of movement

▲ Severe kyphosis

12 Gait and balance
Get up and go test (see opposite)
Walking aid used

Insets (Wasted hand, kyphosis) From Afzal Mir M. Atlas of clinical diagnosis, 2nd edn. Edinburgh: Saunders, Elsevier Inc.; 2003; (Senile purpura) Forbes CD, Jackson WF. Clinical medicine, 3rd edn. Edinburgh: Mosby, Elsevier Inc.; 2004; (Venous ulceration) Mosti G. Compression and venous surgery for leg ulcers. Clin Plast Surg 2012; 39:269–280.

ℹ History

- Slow down the pace
- Ensure the patient can hear
- Establish the speed of onset of the illness
- If the presentation is vague, carry out a systematic enquiry
- Obtain full details of:
  - All drugs, especially any recent prescription changes
  - Past medical history, even from many years previously
  - Usual function: Can the patient walk normally? Has the patient noticed memory problems? Can the patient perform all household tasks?
- Obtain a collateral history: confirm information with a relative or carer and the GP, particularly if the patient is confused or communication is limited by deafness or speech disturbance

ℹ Examination

- Thorough to identify all comorbidities
- Tailored to the patient's stamina and ability to cooperate
- Includes functional status: cognitive function, gait and balance, nutrition, and hearing and vision

Domains of Comprehensive Geriatric Assessment.

ℹ Social assessment

Home circumstances

- Living alone, with another person or in a care home

Activities of daily living (ADL)

- Tasks for which help is needed:
  - Domestic ADL: shopping, cooking, housework
  - Personal ADL: bathing, dressing, walking
- Informal help: relatives, friends, neighbours
- Formal social services: home help, meals on wheels
- Carer stress

ℹ Multidisciplinary team (MDT) roles

Team member	Activity assessed and promoted
Physiotherapist	Mobility, balance and upper limb function
Occupational therapist	ADL, such as dressing, cooking Home environment and care needs
Dietitian	Nutrition
Speech and language therapist	Communication and swallowing
Social worker	Care needs and discharge planning; organisation of institutional care
Nurse	Motivation and initiation of activities; promotion of self-care Education Feeding, continence, skin care Communication with relatives and other professionals Assessment of care needs for discharge
Doctor	Diagnosis and management of medical problems Coordinator of assessment, management and rehabilitation programme

12 Get up and go test

To assess gait and balance, ask the patient to stand up from a sitting position, walk 3 m, turn and go back to the chair. A normal performance takes less than 12 seconds.

Difficulty rising?

Unsteady on standing?

Unsteady gait?

Unsteady on turning?

Unsteady on sitting down?

Sweeping demographic change has meant that older people now represent the core practice of medicine in many countries. A good knowledge of the effects of ageing and the clinical problems associated with old age is therefore essential in most medical specialties. The older population is extremely diverse; a substantial proportion of 90-year-olds enjoy an active healthy life, while some 70-year-olds are severely disabled by chronic disease. The terms 'chronological' and 'biological' ageing have been coined to describe this phenomenon. Biological rather than chronological age is taken into consideration when making clinical decisions about, for example, the extent of investigation and intervention that is appropriate.

Geriatric medicine is concerned particularly with frail older people, in whom physiological capacity is so reduced that they are incapacitated even by minor illness. They frequently have multiple comorbidities, and acute illness may present in non-specific ways, such as delirium, falls or loss of mobility and day-to-day functioning. These patients are prone to adverse drug reactions, partly because of polypharmacy and partly because of age-related changes in responses to drugs and their elimination (p. 32). Disability is common, but patients' function can often be improved by the interventions of the multidisciplinary team (p. 1303).

Older people have been neglected in research terms and, until recently, were rarely included in randomised controlled clinical trials. Accordingly, there is often little high-quality evidence on which to base practice.

Demography

The demography of all countries has changed rapidly in recent decades. For example, in the UK, the total population has grown by 11% over the last 30 years, but the number of people aged over 65 years has grown by 24%. The steepest rise occurred in those aged over 85 – from 600 000 in 1981 to 1.5 million in 2011; this number is projected to increase to 2.4 million by 2026, while the working-age population (20–64 years) is expected to grow by only 4% between 2011 and 2026. Similarly, the proportion of people over 65 in India has increased by 35.5% from 76 million in 2000 to 103 million in 2011, which is almost twice the rate of growth of the general population over this period. In both of these countries and many others across the world, the old-age dependency ratio, which is the ratio of people of working age for each person over retirement age, has substantially increased. Since young people support older members of the population both directly and indirectly through taxation and pension contributions, the consequences of a reduced ratio are far-reaching. It is important to emphasise, however, that many older people support the younger population, through the care of children and other older people.

Life expectancy in the developed world is now prolonged, even in old age (Box 32.1); women aged 80 years can expect

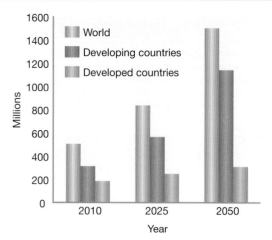

Fig. 32.1 Number of people aged 65 years and over projected in the world population.

to live for a further 10 years. However, rates of disability and chronic illness rise sharply with ageing and have a major impact on health and social services. In the UK, the reported prevalence of a chronic illness or disability sufficient to restrict daily activities is around 25% in those aged 50–64, but 66% in men and 75% in women aged over 85.

Although the proportion of the population aged over 65 years is greater in developed countries, two-thirds of the world population aged over 65 live in developing countries at present, and this is projected to rise to 75% in 2025. The rate of population ageing is much faster in developing countries (Fig. 32.1) and so there will be less time to adjust to its impact.

Functional anatomy and physiology

Biology of ageing

Ageing can be defined as a progressive accumulation through life of random molecular defects that build up within cells and tissues. Eventually, and despite multiple repair and maintenance mechanisms, these result in age-related functional impairment of tissues and organs. There is evidence that variants in many genes contribute to ageing. The implicated genes include those that are involved in regulation of DNA repair, telomere length (p. 41) and insulin signalling. Genetic factors only account for around 25% of the variance in human lifespan, however; nutritional and environmental factors determine the rest. At a cellular level, production of reactive oxygen species is thought to play a major role in ageing. These molecules cause oxidative damage at a number of targets:

- *Nuclear chromosomal DNA*, causing mutations and deletions that ultimately lead to aberrant gene function and potential for malignancy.
- *Telomeres*, the structures at the ends of chromosomes that shorten with each cell division because telomerase (which copies the end of the 3′ strand of linear DNA in germ cells) is absent in somatic cells. When telomeres are sufficiently eroded, cells stop dividing. It has been suggested that telomeres represent a 'biological clock' that prevents uncontrolled cell division and cancer. Telomeres are particularly shortened in patients with

i	32.1 Mean life expectancy in years, UK and India			
	Males		**Females**	
	UK	**India**	**UK**	**India**
At birth	79.1	65.1	83.0	67.2
At 60 years	22.8	16.7	25.5	18.9
At 70 years	15.0	10.9	17.1	12.4
At 80 years	8.7	7.5	9.9	8.0

premature ageing due to Werner's syndrome, in which DNA is damaged due to lack of a helicase.
- *Mitochondrial DNA and lipid peroxidation*, resulting in reduced cellular energy production and ultimately cell death.
- *Proteins*, especially those that are modified by glycosylation due to spontaneous reactions between proteins and sugars. These damage structure and function of the affected protein, which becomes resistant to breakdown.

The rate at which damage occurs is variable and this is where the interplay with environment, and particularly nutrition, takes place. There is evidence in some organisms that this interplay is mediated by insulin signalling pathways. Chronic inflammation also plays an important role, again in part by driving the production of reactive oxygen species.

Physiological changes of ageing

The physiological features of normal ageing have been identified by examining disease-free populations of older people to separate the effects of pathology from those due to age alone. The fraction of older people who age without disease ultimately declines to very low levels, however, so that use of the term 'normal' becomes debatable. There is a marked increase in inter-individual variation in function with ageing; many physiological processes deteriorate substantially when measured across populations but some individuals show little or no change. This heterogeneity is a hallmark of ageing, meaning that each person must be assessed individually and that the same management cannot be applied unthinkingly to all people of a certain age.

Although some genetic influences contribute to heterogeneity, environmental factors, such as poverty, nutrition, exercise, cigarette smoking and alcohol misuse, play a large part, and a healthy lifestyle should be encouraged even when old age has been reached.

The effects of ageing are usually not enough to interfere with organ function under normal conditions but reserve capacity is significantly reduced. Some changes of ageing, such as depigmentation of the hair, are of no clinical significance. Figure 32.2 shows the many changes that occur with ageing that are clinically important.

Changes with ageing

CNS and muscle
- Neuronal loss
- Cochlear degeneration
- Increased lens rigidity
- Lens opacification
- Anterior horn cell loss
- Dorsal column loss
- Slowed reaction times
- Loss of type II muscle fibres
- Reduction in muscle satellite cell numbers

Respiratory system
- Reduced lung elasticity and alveolar support
- Increased chest wall rigidity
- Increased V̇/Q̇ mismatch
- Reduced cough and ciliary action

Cardiovascular system
- Reduced maximum heart rate
- Dilatation of aorta
- Reduced elasticity of conduit/capacitance vessels
- Reduced number of pacing myocytes in sinoatrial node

Renal system
- Loss of nephrons
- Reduced glomerular filtration rate
- Reduced tubular function

Endocrine system
- Deterioration in pancreatic β-cell function

Gastrointestinal system
- Reduced motility

Bones
- Reduced bone mineral density

Clinical consequences

CNS
- Increased risk of delirium
- Presbyacusis/high-tone hearing loss
- Presbyopia/abnormal near vision
- Cataract
- Muscle weakness and wasting
- Reduced position and vibration sense
- Increased risk of falls

Respiratory system
- Reduced vital capacity and peak expiratory flow
- Increased residual volume
- Reduced inspiratory reserve volume
- Reduced arterial oxygen saturation
- Increased risk of infection

Cardiovascular system
- Reduced exercise tolerance
- Widened aortic arch on X-ray
- Widened pulse pressure
- Increased risk of postural hypotension
- Increased risk of atrial fibrillation

Renal system
- Impaired fluid balance
- Increased risk of dehydration/overload
- Impaired drug metabolism and excretion

Endocrine system
- Increased risk of impaired glucose tolerance

Gastrointestinal system
- Constipation

Bones
- Increased risk of osteoporosis and fracture

Fig. 32.2 Features and consequences of normal ageing.

32

Frailty and multimorbidity

Frailty is defined as the loss of an individual's ability to withstand minor stresses because the reserves in function of several organ systems are so severely reduced that even a trivial illness or adverse drug reaction may result in organ failure and death. The same stresses would cause little upset in a fit person of the same age.

It is important to understand the difference between 'disability', 'multimorbidity' and 'frailty'. Disability indicates established loss of function while frailty indicates increased vulnerability to loss of function. Disability may arise from a single pathological event (such as a stroke) in an otherwise healthy individual. After recovery, function is largely stable and the patient may otherwise be in good health. When frailty and disability coexist, function deteriorates markedly even with minor illness, to the extent that the patient can no longer manage independently.

Multimorbidity (the number of diagnoses present) is also not equivalent to frailty; it is quite possible to have several diagnoses without major impact on homeostatic reserve. Multimorbidity is, however, an important concept in its own right and is an almost invariable accompaniment to advanced age. Recent Scottish population-based data show that 60% of those aged 65 and over have at least two chronic diseases. Multimorbidity is a driver for future disability, hospitalisation and death, and often leads to polypharmacy, as multiple medications are used to treat each chronic disease individually. Current health-care systems are poorly equipped to manage multimorbidity; each disease is dealt with by a separate team of specialists, which at best places a high burden on the patient, and at worst leads to mutually incompatible approaches to management of each disease.

Unfortunately, the term 'frail' is often used rather vaguely, sometimes to justify a lack of adequate investigation and intervention in older people. It can be specifically identified, however, by assessing function in a number of domains. Two main approaches to evaluating frailty exist: measurement of physiological function across a number of domains, an example being the Fried Frailty score (Box 32.2), or use of a score based on the number of deficits or problems, such as the Rockwood score.

Frail older people particularly benefit from a clinical approach that addresses both the precipitating acute illness and their underlying loss of reserves. It may be possible to prevent further loss of function through early intervention; for example, a frail woman with myocardial infarction will benefit from specific cardiac investigation and drug treatment, but may benefit even further from an exercise programme to improve musculoskeletal function, balance and aerobic capacity, with nutritional support to restore lost weight. Establishing a patient's level of frailty also helps inform decisions regarding further investigation and management, and the need for rehabilitation.

Investigations

Comprehensive Geriatric Assessment

One of the most powerful tools in the management of older people is the Comprehensive Geriatric Assessment, which identifies all the relevant factors contributing to their presentation (p. 1302). Comprehensive Geriatric Assessment is in fact a misnomer; it is not merely an assessment, but a process of identifying and managing all relevant factors affecting the health and well-being of older people. It is iterative in nature, management being followed by reassessment and a new management plan. In frail patients with multiple pathology, it may be necessary to perform the assessment in stages to allow for their reduced stamina. The outcome should be a management plan that not only addresses the acute presenting problems but also improves the patient's overall health and function.

Comprehensive Geriatric Assessment is performed by a multidisciplinary team (p. 1303). Such an approach was pioneered by Dr Marjory Warren at the West Middlesex Hospital in London in the 1930s; her comprehensive assessment and rehabilitation of supposedly incurable, long-term bedridden older people revolutionised the approach of the medical profession to frail older people and laid the foundations for the modern specialty of geriatric medicine. There is excellent evidence from systematic reviews that Comprehensive Geriatric Assessment, when performed by a specialist team on a specialist geriatric medicine ward, reduces death or deterioration, increases the chances of living independently at home, and may also improve cognitive function in the short to medium term. Current evidence suggests that the process works when delivered on a specialist inpatient unit, but the evidence for effectiveness when it is delivered by a visiting team or in the community is less strong.

Decisions about investigation and treatment

Accurate diagnosis is important at all ages but frail older people may not be able to tolerate lengthy or invasive procedures, and diagnoses may be revealed for which patients could not withstand intensive or aggressive treatment. On the other hand, disability should never be dismissed as due to age alone. For example, it would be a mistake to supply a patient no longer able to climb stairs with a stair lift when simple tests would have revealed osteoarthritis of a hip and vitamin D deficiency, for which appropriate treatment would have restored his or her strength. So how do doctors decide when and how far to investigate?

The views of the patient and family

Older people may have strong views about the extent of investigation and the treatment they wish to receive, and these should be sought from the outset. A key issue is to establish what the patient wants from investigation and treatment. Many

---

32.2 How to assess a Fried Frailty score

- Hand grip strength in bottom 20% of healthy elderly distribution*
- Walking speed in bottom 20% of healthy elderly distribution*
- Self-reported exhaustion
- Physical inactivity
- At least 6 kg weight loss within 1 year

Patient is defined as frail if 3 or more factors are present; 1–2 factors indicate a 'pre-frail' state.

*Varies between populations. Grip cut-off is 30 kg for men and 18 kg for women in US adults; 5 m walk time cut-off is 7 seconds in US adults for both sexes.

older people do not desire prolongation of life; rather they aspire to maintain physical function, gain relief from symptoms, and preserve the ability to live independently. Such aims differ widely between patients, however, and a careful exploration of what is important to the individual is essential. If the patient wishes, the views of relatives can also be taken into account. If the patient is not able to express a view or lacks the capacity to make decisions because of cognitive impairment or communication difficulties, then relatives' input becomes particularly helpful. They may be able to give information on views previously expressed by the patient or on what the patient would have wanted under the current circumstances. However, families should never be made to feel responsible for difficult decisions.

The patient's general health

Does this patient have the physical and mental capacity to tolerate the proposed investigation? Do they have the aerobic capacity to undergo bronchoscopy? Will delirium prevent them from remaining still in the magnetic resonance imaging (MRI) scanner? The more comorbidities a patient has, the less likely he or she will be able to withstand an invasive intervention.

Will the investigation alter management?

Would the patient be fit for, or benefit from, the treatment that would be indicated if investigation proved positive? The presence of comorbidity and frailty is more important than age itself in determining this. When a patient with severe heart failure and a previous disabling stroke presents with a suspicious mass lesion on chest X-ray, detailed investigation and staging may not be appropriate if they are not fit for surgery, radical radiotherapy or chemotherapy. On the other hand, if the same patient presented with dysphagia, investigation of the cause would be important, as they might be able to tolerate endoscopic treatment (for example, to palliate an obstructing oesophageal carcinoma).

Will management benefit the patient?

It is important to consider whether interventions that might be considered as standard-of-care for younger people are likely to be beneficial in frail older people. For example, while oral anticoagulation might be indicated by guidelines for a patient with atrial fibrillation, such treatment may not accord with the wishes of a patient in a care home who finds regular blood tests distressing, or who is more worried about bleeding than about avoiding a stroke. Another example would be the use of anti-osteoporosis medications to reduce the risk of fracture in very old patents, where the risk of death from other causes would be greater than the risk of fracture.

Advance directives

Advance directives or 'living wills' are statements made by adults at a time when they have the capacity to decide about the interventions they would refuse or accept in the future, should they no longer be able to make decisions or communicate them. An advance directive cannot authorise a doctor to do anything that is illegal and doctors are not bound to provide a specific treatment requested if, in their professional opinion, it is not clinically appropriate. However, any advance refusal of treatment, made when the patient was able to make decisions based on adequate information about their implications, is legally binding in the UK. It must be respected when it clearly applies to the patient's present circumstances and when there is no reason to believe that the patient has changed his or her mind.

Presenting problems in geriatric medicine

Characteristics of presenting problems in old age

Problem-based practice is central to geriatric medicine. Most problems are multifactorial and there is rarely a single unifying diagnosis. All contributing factors have to be taken into account and attention to detail is paramount. Two patients who share the same presenting problem may have completely disparate diagnoses. A wide knowledge of adult medicine is required, as disease in any, and often many, of the organ systems has to be managed at the same time. There are a number of features that are particular to older patients.

Late presentation

Many people (of all ages) accept ill health as a consequence of ageing and may tolerate symptoms for lengthy periods before seeking medical advice. Comorbidities may also contribute to late presentation; in a patient whose mobility is limited by stroke, angina may only present when coronary artery disease is advanced, as the patient has been unable to exercise sufficiently to cause symptoms at an earlier stage.

Atypical presentation

Infection may present with delirium and without clinical pointers to the organ system affected. Stroke may present with falls rather than symptoms of focal weakness. Myocardial infarction may present as weakness and fatigue, without chest pain or dyspnoea. The reasons for these atypical presentations are not always easy to establish. Perception of pain is altered in old age, which may explain why myocardial infarction presents in other ways. The pyretic response is blunted in old age so that infection may not be obvious at first. Cognitive impairment may limit the patient's ability to give a history of classical symptoms.

Acute illness and changes in function

Atypical presentations in frail elderly patients include 'failure to cope', 'found on floor', 'delirium' and 'off feet', but these are *not* diagnoses. The possibility that an acute illness has been the precipitant must always be considered. To establish whether the patient's current status is a change from his or her usual level of function, it helps to ask a relative or carer (by phone if necessary). Investigations aimed at uncovering an acute illness will not be fruitful in a patient whose function has been deteriorating over several months but are important if function has suddenly changed.

Multiple pathology

Presentations in older patients have a more diverse differential diagnosis because multiple pathology is so common. There are frequently a number of causes for any single problem, and adverse effects from medication often contribute. A patient may fall because of osteoarthritis of the knees, postural hypotension due to diuretic therapy for hypertension, and poor vision due to cataracts. All these factors have to be addressed to prevent further falls and this principle holds true for most of the common presenting problems in old age.

32

Approach to presenting problems in old age

For the sake of clarity, the common presenting problems are described individually but, in reality, older patients often present with several at the same time, particularly delirium, incontinence and falls. These share some underlying causes and may precipitate each other.

The approach to most presenting problems in old age can be summarised as follows:

- *Obtain a collateral history.* Find out the patient's usual status with regard to mobility and cognitive function from a relative or carer. Call these people by phone if they are not present.
- *Check all medication.* Have there been any recent changes?
- *Search for and treat any acute illness* (Box 32.3).
- *Identify and reverse predisposing risk factors.* These depend on the presenting problem.

Falls

Around 30% of those over 65 years of age fall each year and this figure rises to more than 40% in those aged over 80. Although only 10–15% of falls result in serious injury, virtually all fragility fractures in the elderly are caused by falls. Age-related osteoporosis contributes to the dramatic rise in hip and other fragility fractures that occurs with ageing but the most important contributory factor is an increased risk of falling (Fig. 32.3). Falls also lead to loss of confidence and fear, and are frequently the 'final straw' that makes an older person decide to move to institutional care. Management will vary according to the underlying cause.

Acute illness

Falls are one of the classical atypical presentations of acute illness in frail people. The reduced reserves in older people's neurological function mean that they are less able to maintain their balance when challenged by an acute illness. Suspicion should be high when falls have suddenly occurred over a period of a few days. Common underlying illnesses include infection, stroke, metabolic disturbance and heart failure. Thorough examination and investigation are required (Box 32.3). It is also important to establish whether any drug that precipitates falls, such as a psychotropic or hypotensive agent, has been started recently. Once the underlying acute illness has been treated, falls may stop.

Blackouts

A proportion of older people who 'fall' have, in fact, had a syncopal episode. A collateral history from a witness is of utmost importance

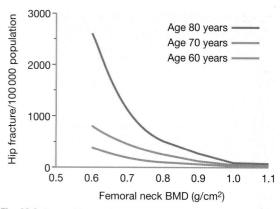

Fig. 32.3 Age and bone mineral density (BMD) interact to influence fracture risk.

in anyone falling over; people who lose consciousness do not always remember having done so. If loss of consciousness is suggested by the patient or witness, it is important to perform appropriate investigations (pp. 181 and 1080).

Mechanical and recurrent falls

Among patients who have tripped or are uncertain how they fell, those who have fallen more than once in the past year and those who are unsteady during a 'get up and go' test (p. 1303) require further assessment. Patients with recurrent falls are commonly frail, with multiple medical problems and chronic disabilities. Obviously, such patients may present with a fall resulting from an acute illness or syncope but they will remain at risk of further falls even when the acute illness has resolved. The risk factors for falls (Box 32.4) should be considered. If problems are identified with muscle strength, balance, vision or cognitive function, the causes of these must be identified by specific investigation, and treatment commenced if appropriate. Careful assessment of the patient's gait may provide important clues to an underlying diagnosis (Box 32.5). Common pathologies identified include cerebrovascular disease (Ch. 26), Parkinson's disease (p. 1112) and osteoarthritis of weight-bearing joints (p. 1007). Calculation of fracture risk using tools such as FRAX or QFracture should be performed and dual X-ray absorptiometry (DXA) bone density scanning considered in patients with a 10-year risk of major fracture of more than 10%.

Prevention of falls and fractures

Falls can be prevented by multiple risk factor intervention (Box 32.6). The most effective intervention is balance and strength training by physiotherapists or exercise practitioners; an alternative with good evidence is tai chi training. An assessment of the

i	**32.5 Abnormal gaits and probable causes**

Gait abnormality	Probable cause
Antalgic	Arthropathy
Waddling	Proximal myopathy
Stamping	Sensory neuropathy
Foot drop	Peripheral neuropathy or radiculopathy
Ataxic	Sensory neuropathy or cerebellar disease
Shuffling/festination	Parkinson's disease
Marche à petits pas	Small-vessel cerebrovascular disease
Hemiplegic	Cerebral hemisphere lesion
Apraxic	Bilateral hemisphere lesions

i	**32.6 Interventions to reduce the risk of falls and fractures**

- Exercise (should include components of lower limb strength and balance training):
    Multimodal group exercise and tai chi both effective
- Calcium and vitamin D supplementation:
    Evidence of effectiveness only in patients in institutional care
    Large doses of vitamin D may increase risk of falls and fractures
- Home environment assessment and modification
- Medication review:
    Particularly medications with central actions such as hypnotics but also those with anticholinergic and hypotensive actions
- Cataract surgery:
    Effective if for first cataract
    Other vision interventions ineffective and may increase falls risk
- Anti-slip shoes:
    Effective only in icy conditions
- Cardiac pacemaker for carotid sinus hypersensitivity

patient's home environment for hazards should be undertaken by an occupational therapist, who may also provide personal alarms so that patients can summon help, should they fall again. Rationalising psychotropic medication may help to reduce sedation, although many older patients are reluctant to stop hypnotics. If postural hypotension is present (defined as a drop in blood pressure of >20 mmHg systolic or >10 mmHg diastolic pressure on standing from supine), reducing or stopping hypotensive drugs may be helpful. Evidence supporting the efficacy of other interventions for postural hypotension is lacking but drugs, including fludrocortisone and midodrine, are sometimes used to try to improve dizziness on standing. Other interventions, such as cataract extraction and podiatry, can also have a significant impact on function in those who fall.

If osteoporosis is diagnosed, specific drug therapy should be considered (p. 1046). In the frailest patients, such as those in institutional care, calcium and vitamin D_3 administration has been shown to reduce both falls and fracture rates, probably by exerting positive effects on bone mineral density and on neuromuscular function. Supplementation does not reduce falls risk beyond this very frail group, however, and very high doses of vitamin D may paradoxically increase the risk of falls and fractures.

In the UK, government policy and National Institute for Health and Clinical Excellence guidelines (www.nice.org.uk) for falls prevention have led to the development of specific Falls and Fracture Prevention Services in many parts of the country.

Dizziness

Dizziness is very common, affecting at least 30% of those aged over 65 years in community surveys. It can be disabling in its own right and is also a risk factor for falls. Acute dizziness is relatively straightforward and common causes include:

- *hypotension* due to arrhythmia, myocardial infarction, gastrointestinal bleed or pulmonary embolism
- *posterior fossa stroke* onset
- *vestibular neuronitis*.

Although older people more commonly present with recurrent dizzy spells and often find it difficult to describe the sensation they experience, the most effective way of establishing the cause(s) of the problem is nevertheless to determine which of the following is predominant (even if more than one is present):

- *lightheadedness*, suggestive of reduced cerebral perfusion
- *vertigo*, suggestive of labyrinthine or brainstem disease (p. 1086)
- *unsteadiness/poor balance*, suggestive of joint or neurological disease.

In lightheaded patients, structural cardiac disease (such as aortic stenosis) and arrhythmia must be considered, but disorders of autonomic cardiovascular control, such as vasovagal syndrome and postural hypotension, are the most common causes in old age. Antihypertensive medications may exacerbate these conditions. Further investigation and treatment are described on page 181.

Vertigo in older patients is most commonly due to benign positional vertigo (p. 1086), but if other brainstem symptoms or signs are present, MRI of the brain is required to exclude a cerebello-pontine angle lesion.

Delirium

Delirium is a syndrome of transient, reversible cognitive dysfunction that affects 30% of older hospital inpatients. Differential diagnosis, assessment and management are discussed on page 183.

Urinary incontinence

Urinary incontinence is defined as the involuntary loss of urine and comes to medical attention when sufficiently severe to cause a social or hygiene problem. It occurs in all age groups but becomes more prevalent in old age, affecting about 15% of women and 10% of men aged over 65. It may lead to skin damage if severe and can be socially restricting. While age-dependent changes in the lower urinary tract predispose older people to incontinence, it is not an inevitable consequence of ageing and requires investigation and appropriate treatment. Urinary incontinence is frequently precipitated by acute illness in old age and is commonly multifactorial (Fig. 32.4).

The initial assessment should seek to identify and address contributory factors. If incontinence fails to resolve, further diagnosis and management should be pursued, as described on page 437.

- *Urge incontinence* is usually due to detrusor over-activity and results in urgency and frequency.
- *Stress incontinence* is almost exclusive to women and is due to weakness of the pelvic floor muscles, which allows leakage of urine when intra-abdominal pressure rises, such as on coughing. It may be compounded by atrophic

32

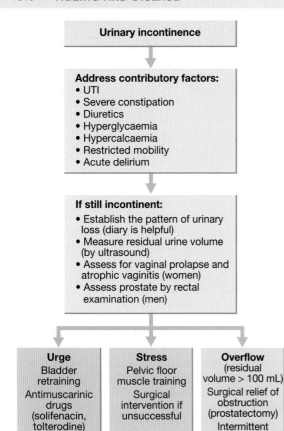

Urinary incontinence

↓

Address contributory factors:
- UTI
- Severe constipation
- Diuretics
- Hyperglycaemia
- Hypercalcaemia
- Restricted mobility
- Acute delirium

↓

If still incontinent:
- Establish the pattern of urinary loss (diary is helpful)
- Measure residual urine volume (by ultrasound)
- Assess for vaginal prolapse and atrophic vaginitis (women)
- Assess prostate by rectal examination (men)

Urge	**Stress**	**Overflow**
Bladder retraining	Pelvic floor muscle training	(residual volume > 100 mL)
Antimuscarinic drugs (solifenacin, tolterodine)	Surgical intervention if unsuccessful	Surgical relief of obstruction (prostatectomy)
		Intermittent catheterisation if no obstruction

Fig. 32.4 Assessment and management of urinary incontinence in old age. See also page 436 and NICE guideline on the Management of Incontinence in Women: nice.org.uk. (UTI = urinary tract infection)

vaginitis, associated with oestrogen deficiency in old age, which can be treated with oestrogen pessaries.

- *Overflow incontinence* is most commonly seen in elderly men with prostatic enlargement, which obstructs bladder outflow.

In patients with severe stroke disease or dementia, treatment may be ineffective, as frontal cortical inhibitory signals to bladder emptying are lost. A timed/prompted toileting programme may help. Other than in overflow incontinence, urinary catheterisation should never be viewed as first-line management, but may be required as a final resort if the perineal skin is at risk of breakdown or quality of life is affected.

Prescribing and deprescribing

The large number of comorbidities that accompany ageing often leads to polypharmacy. This has been defined as the use of four or more drugs, and is associated with several adverse outcomes including falls, hospitalisation and increased risk of death. While some of these outcomes are caused by drug–drug interactions and adverse effects, others are as much due to the underlying multimorbidities for which the drugs were prescribed in the first place

In view of this, it is essential for prescribing for older people to be appropriate. For many older people, taking multiple drugs is appropriate, as such therapy is required to treat multiple

i 32.7 Factors leading to polypharmacy in old age

- Multiple pathology
- Poor patient education (see Box 2.20, p. 31)
- Lack of routine review of all medications
- Patient expectations of prescribing
- Over-use of drug interventions by doctors
- Attendance at multiple specialist clinics
- Poor communication between specialists

i 32.8 Common adverse drug reactions in old age

Drug class	Adverse reaction
NSAIDs	Gastrointestinal bleeding and peptic ulceration Renal impairment
Diuretics	Renal impairment, electrolyte disturbance Gout Hypotension, postural hypotension
Warfarin	Bleeding
ACE inhibitors	Renal impairment, electrolyte disturbance Hypotension, postural hypotension
β-blockers	Bradycardia, heart block Hypotension, postural hypotension
Opiates	Constipation, vomiting Delirium Urinary retention
Antidepressants	Delirium Hyponatraemia (SSRIs) Hypotension, postural hypotension Falls
Benzodiazepines	Delirium Falls
Anticholinergics	Delirium Urinary retention Constipation

(ACE = angiotensin-converting enzyme; NSAIDs = non-steroidal anti-inflammatory drugs; SSRIs = selective serotonin re-uptake inhibitors)

diseases (Box 32.7). However, the more drugs that are taken, the greater the risk of an adverse drug reaction (ADR). ADRs and the effects of drug interactions are discussed on page 21. They may result in symptoms, abnormal physical signs and altered laboratory test results (Box 32.8). ADRs are the cause of around 5% of all hospital admissions but account for up to 20% of admissions in those aged over 65. The risk of polypharmacy is compounded by age-related changes in pharmacodynamic and pharmacokinetic factors (p. 14), and by impaired homeostatic mechanisms, such as baroreceptor responses, plasma volume and electrolyte control.

Older people are thus especially sensitive to drugs that can cause postural hypotension or volume depletion (Box 32.8). Non-adherence to drug therapy also rises with the number of drugs prescribed.

The clinical presentations of ADRs are diverse, so for *any* presenting problem in old age the possibility that the patient's medication is a contributory factor should *always* be considered. Failure to recognise this may lead to the use of a further drug to treat the problem, making matters worse, when the better course would be to stop or reduce the dose of the offending drug or to find an alternative.

Appropriate prescribing and deprescribing

The key to appropriate prescribing is first to ensure that medications are started only for reasons that accord with the patient's goals and wishes. Thoughtless adherence to guidelines quickly leads to polypharmacy that may be inappropriate. Some medications (such as chronic use of non-steroidal anti-inflammatory medications) are much less suitable for older people because of the much higher risk of side-effects. Other medications, such as statins and bisphosphonates, lack evidence of efficacy in very old people, who may not live for long enough to derive benefit.

Deprescribing is as important as prescribing in older people. Regular review of medications should be undertaken to ensure that medications are still required, to establish that they are still working, to check that they are not causing side-effects, and to ascertain whether the patient is actually taking them. If any of the above issues is problematic, the medication should be deprescribed. This may need to be done in a controlled manner, with dose reduction to ensure that rebound symptoms or withdrawal effects do not occur. The patient or carer should therefore be asked to bring all medication for review rather than the doctor relying on previous records; such reviews should take place regularly, not just at a point of crisis such as after a fall or on hospital admission.

Other problems in old age

A vast range of other presenting problems in older people present to many medical specialties. End-of-life care is an important facet of clinical practice in old age and is discussed on page 1354. Relevant sections in other chapters are referenced in Box 32.9.

Within each chapter, 'In Old Age' boxes highlight the areas in which presentation or management differs from that in younger individuals.

i	**32.9 Other presenting problems in old age**
• Hypothermia	p. 166
• Dizziness and blackouts	p. 181
• Delirium	p. 183
• Infection	pp. 218 and 228
• Fluid balance problems	p. 360
• Heart failure	p. 466
• Atrial fibrillation	p. 472
• Hypertension	p. 512
• Under-nutrition	p. 710
• Diabetes mellitus	p. 732
• Peptic ulceration	p. 801
• Anaemia	p. 954
• Painful joints	p. 992
• Bone disease and fracture	pp. 994 and 1049
• Stroke	p. 1147
• Dementia	p. 1191

Rehabilitation

Rehabilitation aims to improve the ability of people of all ages to perform day-to-day activities and to optimise their physical, mental and social capabilities. Acute illness in older people is often associated with loss of their usual ability to walk or care for themselves, and common disabling conditions such as stroke, fractured neck of femur, arthritis and cardiorespiratory disease become increasingly prevalent with advancing age. Doctors tend to focus on health conditions and impairments but patients are more concerned with the effect on their activities and ability to participate in everyday life.

The rehabilitation process

Rehabilitation is a problem-solving process focused on improving the patient's physical, psychological and social function. It entails:

* *Assessment.* The nature and extent of the patient's problems can be identified using the International Classification of Functioning, Disability and Health framework, which focuses on health conditions (such as stroke), the associated physical impairments (such as arm weakness caused by the stroke), the effect on activity (such as the inability to dress oneself due to arm weakness) and restriction of participation in activities (such as inability to go out of the house due to the inability to dress oneself). Such an approach helps to ensure a whole-person approach to participation in society, rather than a focus merely on disease. Specific assessment scales, such as the Elderly Mobility Scale or Barthel Index of Activities of Daily Living (Box 32.10), are useful to quantify components of disability but additional assessment is needed to determine the underlying causes or the interventions required in individual patients.
* *Goal-setting.* Goals should be specific to the patient's problems, realistic, and agreed between the patient and the rehabilitation team.
* *Intervention.* This includes the active treatments needed to achieve the established goals and to maintain the patient's health and quality of life. Interventions include hands-on treatment by therapists using a functional, task-orientated approach to improve day-to-day activities, and also psychological support and education. The emphasis on the type of intervention will be individualised, according to the patient's disabilities, psychological status and progress. The patient and carer(s) must be active participants.
* *Re-assessment.* There is ongoing re-evaluation of the patient's function and progress towards the goals by the rehabilitation team, the patient and the carer. Interventions may be modified as a result.

Multidisciplinary team working

The core rehabilitation team includes all members of the multidisciplinary team (p. 1303). Others may also be involved, such as audiometrists to correct hearing impairment, podiatrists for foot problems, and orthoticists where a prosthesis or splinting is required. Good communication and mutual respect are essential. Regular team meetings allow sharing of assessments, agreement on rehabilitation goals and interventions, evaluation of progress and planning for the patient's discharge home. Rehabilitation is *not* when the doctor orders 'physiotherapy' or 'a home visit' and takes no further role.

32

32.10 How to assess dependency using the Modified Barthel Index*

Mobility

Independent = 3 Needs help = 2 Wheelchair independent = 1 Immobile = 0

Stairs

Independent = 2 Needs help = 1 Unable = 0

Transfers (e.g. from bed to chair)

Independent = 3 Needs minor help = 2 Needs major help = 1 Unable = 0

Bladder

Continent = 2 Occasional incontinence = 1 Incontinent = 0

Bowels

Continent = 2 Occasional incontinence = 1 Incontinent = 0

Grooming

Independent = 1 Needs help = 0

Toilet use

Independent = 2 Needs help = 1 Unable = 0

Feeding

Independent = 2 Needs help = 1 Unable = 0

Dressing

Independent = 2 Needs some help = 1 Completely dependent = 0

Bathing

Independent = 1 Needs help = 0

*The 20-point version is illustrated. The total score reflects the degree of dependency; scores of 14 and above are usually consistent with living in the community; scores below 10 suggest the patient is heavily dependent on carers.

Rehabilitation outcomes

There is evidence that rehabilitation improves functional outcomes in older people following acute illness, stroke and hip fracture. It also reduces mortality after stroke and hip fracture. These benefits accrue from complex multicomponent interventions, but occupational therapy to improve personal ADLs and individualised exercise interventions have now been shown to be effective in improving functional outcome in their own right.

Further information

Websites

americangeriatrics.org *American Geriatrics Society: education, careers vignettes from geriatricians, advocacy and clinical guidelines.*
bgs.org.uk *British Geriatrics Society: useful publications on management of common problems in older people and links to other relevant websites.*
cochrane.org *Cochrane review CD006211 Comprehensive geriatric assessment for older adults admitted to hospital; CD007146 Interventions for preventing falls in older people living in the community.*
eugms.org *European Union Geriatric Medicine Society: research, position papers and educational resources.*
iagg.info *International Association of Gerontology and Geriatrics: promoting care of older people and the science of gerontology globally; research, policy and educational resources.*
knowledge.scot.nhs.uk/effectiveolderpeoplecare.aspx *Collates and summarises the Cochrane evidence for best practice in the healthcare and rehabilitation of frail older people.*
profane.co *Prevention of Falls Network Earth: focuses on the prevention of falls and improvement of postural stability in older people.*
qfracture.org *Fracture risk calculator validated in the UK population. Includes a wider range of risk factors than FRAX.*
shef.ac.uk/FRAX/tool.jsp *Fracture risk calculator: can be used to calculate risk in several populations. Includes option to calculate with or without measurement of hip bone mineral density.*

GG Dark

33

Oncology

Clinical examination of the cancer patient 1314

The 10 hallmarks of cancer 1316
1. Genome instability and mutation 1316
2. Resisting cell death 1316
3. Sustaining proliferative signalling 1317
4. Evading growth suppressors 1318
5. Enabling replicative immortality 1318
6. Inducing angiogenesis 1318
7. Activating invasion and metastasis 1319
8. Reprogramming energy metabolism 1319
9. Tumour-promoting inflammation 1319
10. Evading immune destruction 1320

Environmental and genetic determinants of cancer 1320

Investigations 1321
Histology 1322
Imaging 1323
Biochemical markers 1323

Presenting problems in oncology 1323
Palpable mass 1323
Weight loss and fever 1323
Thromboembolism 1324
Ectopic hormone production 1325
Neurological paraneoplastic syndromes 1325
Cutaneous manifestations of cancer 1326

Emergency complications of cancer 1326

Metastatic disease 1328

Therapeutics in oncology 1329
Surgical treatment 1330
Systemic chemotherapy 1330
Radiation therapy 1331
Hormone therapy 1332
Immunotherapy 1332
Biological therapies 1332
Evaluation of treatment 1332
Late toxicity of therapy 1332

Specific cancers 1333
Breast cancer 1333
Ovarian cancer 1334
Endometrial cancer 1334
Cervical cancer 1335
Head and neck tumours 1335
Carcinoma of unknown origin 1336

Multidisciplinary teams 1336

Clinical examination of the cancer patient

4 Face
Conjunctival pallor
Icterus, jaundice
Horner's syndrome
Cushingoid features

3 Lymph nodes
Neck
Supraclavicular
Axillary
Antecubital
Inguinal
Para-aortic

2 Breast

▲ Skin tethering above the nipple

1 Hands
Clubbing
Signs of smoking
Pallor
Tylosis of palms

▲ Finger clubbing in lung cancer

▲ Cushing's syndrome in a patient with ectopic adrenocorticotrophic hormone (ACTH) production

Observation
- Skin changes
- Ascites
- Cushingoid appearance
- Cachexia
- Dehydration

5 Cardiovascular
Superior vena cava (SVC) obstruction
Atrial fibrillation
Pericardial effusion
Hypo-/hypertension

▲ SVC obstruction in a patient with a mediastinal mass

6 Respiratory
Stridor
Consolidation
Pleural effusion

7 Abdomen
Surgical scars
Umbilical nodule
Mass in epigastrium
Visible peristalsis
Abdominal distension
Ascites
Hepatomegaly
Splenomegaly
Renal mass
Pelvic or adnexal mass

▲ Ascites (ovarian carcinoma)

8 Neurological
Focal neurological signs
Sensory deficit
Spinal cord compression
Memory deficit
Personality change

9 Skeletal survey
Focal bone tenderness (pelvis, spine, long bones)
Wrist tenderness (hypertrophic pulmonary osteoarthropathy)

10 Periphery
Calf tenderness, venous thrombosis
Clubbing (if present in hands)

<table>
<tr><td>

i   Examination of the skin

Important features of skin lesions that should alert suspicion include:

- Asymmetry: irregular shape
- Bleeding
- Border: not a smooth edge
- Colour: uneven, variegated or changing colour
- Diameter: >6 mm in diameter or growing
- Itching or pain in a pre-existing mole

</td><td>

7 **Abdominal examination**

- Are there scars from previous surgery?
- Is the umbilicus everted, suggesting ascites?
- Is there a firm nodule at the umbilicus due to ovarian or gastric cancer metastasis, causing a Sister Mary Joseph nodule (p. 1334)?
- Is there smooth hepatomegaly – possibly primary liver cancer or heart failure?
- Is the liver firm or knobbly, suggesting metastasis?
- Is the ascites too tense to demonstrate hepatomegaly?
- Are other masses palpable in the abdomen?
- Are there signs of obstruction or paralytic ileus with absence of bowel sounds?
- Palpate for inguinal nodes (occasionally involved in ovarian cancer)
- Percuss for flank dullness and shifting dullness
- Perform vaginal and rectal examinations to detect adnexal or rectal masses

</td></tr>
</table>

3 **Examination of the lymph nodes**

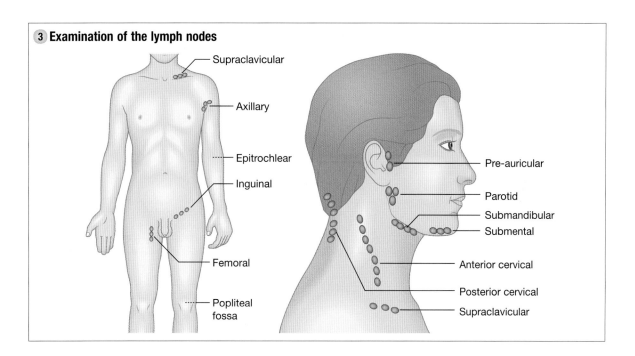

- Supraclavicular
- Axillary
- Epitrochlear
- Inguinal
- Femoral
- Popliteal fossa
- Pre-auricular
- Parotid
- Submandibular
- Submental
- Anterior cervical
- Posterior cervical
- Supraclavicular

5 **Superior vena cava obstruction**

- Venous distension of neck
- Elevated but non-pulsatile jugular venous pulse
- Venous distension of chest wall
- Facial oedema
- Cyanosis
- Plethora of face
- Oedema of arms

5 **Pericardial effusion**

- Tachycardia
- Falling blood pressure
- Rising jugular venous pressure
- Muffled heart sounds
- Kussmaul's sign (p. 544)

6 **Malignant pleural effusions**

Large right pleural effusion

Inspection
  Tachypnoea
Palpation
  ↓Expansion on R
  Trachea and apex may be moved to L
Percussion
  Stony dull
  R mid- and lower zones
Auscultation
  Absent breath sounds and diminished or absent vocal resonance R base
  Crackles above effusion

Cancer represents a significant economic burden for the global economy and is now the third leading cause of death worldwide. By 2030, it is projected that there will be 26 million new cancer cases and 17 million cancer deaths per year. The developing world is disproportionately affected by cancer and in 2008 developing nations accounted for 56% of new cancer cases and 75% of cancer deaths. These deaths happen in countries with limited or no access to treatment and with low per capita expenditure on health care.

The most common solid organ malignancies arise in the lung, breast and gastrointestinal tract (Fig. 33.1), but the most common form worldwide is skin cancer. Cigarette smoking accounts for more than 20% of all global cancer deaths, 80% of lung cancer cases in men and 50% of lung cancer cases in women worldwide, which could be prevented by smoking cessation. Diet and alcohol contribute to a further 30% of cancers, including those of the stomach, colon, oesophagus, breast and liver. Lifestyle modification could reduce these if steps were taken to avoid animal fat and red meat, reduce alcohol, increase fibre, fresh fruit and vegetable intake, and avoid obesity. Infections account for a further 15% of cancers, including those of the cervix, stomach, liver, nasopharynx and bladder, and some of these could be prevented by infection control and vaccination.

The 10 hallmarks of cancer

The formation and growth of cancer constitute a multistep process, during which sequentially occurring gene mutations result in the formation of a cancerous cell. For cells to initiate carcinogenesis successfully, they require key characteristics, collectively referred to as the hallmarks of cancer.

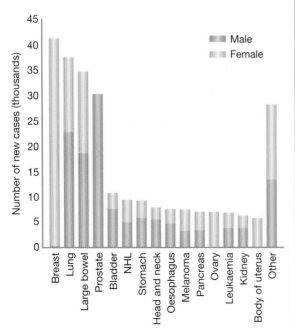

Fig. 33.1 The most commonly diagnosed cancers in the UK. (NHL = non-Hodgkin lymphoma) *Statistics from Cancer Research UK website (http://info.cancerresearchuk.org).*

1. Genome instability and mutation

Random genetic mutations occur continuously throughout all cells of the body and very rarely confer a selective advantage on single cells, allowing overgrowth and dominance in local tissue environments. Multistep carcinogenesis results from successive clonal expansions of pre-malignant cells, each expansion being triggered by acquisition of a random enabling genetic mutation. Under normal circumstances, cellular DNA repair mechanisms are so effective that almost all spontaneous mutations are corrected without producing phenotypic changes, keeping the overall mutation rates very low. In cancer cells, the accumulation of mutations can be accelerated by compromising the surveillance systems that normally monitor genomic integrity and force genetically damaged cells into either senescence or apoptosis. They can therefore become more sensitive to mutagenic actions or develop DNA repair mechanism failure.

2. Resisting cell death

There are three principal mechanisms through which cell death occurs in healthy tissues: apoptosis, autophagy and necrosis.

Apoptosis

This is programmed cell death. It is frequently found at markedly reduced rates in cancers, particularly those of high grade or those resistant to treatment. The cellular apoptotic system has regulatory elements that sense intrinsic and extrinsic pro-apoptotic signals and initiate a cascade of proteolysis and cell disassembly with nuclear fragmentation, chromosomal condensation, and shrinking of the cell with loss of intercellular contact, followed by cellular fragmentation and the formation of apoptotic bodies that are phagocytosed by neighbouring cells. The most important regulator of apoptosis is the *TP53* tumour suppressor gene, often described as the 'guardian of the genome', as it is able to induce apoptosis in response to sufficient levels of genomic damage. The largest initiator of apoptosis via *TP53* is cellular injury, particularly that due to DNA damage from chemotherapy, oxidative damage and ultraviolet (UV) radiation.

Autophagy

This is a catabolic process during which cellular constituents are degraded by lysosomal machinery within the cell. It is an important physiological mechanism; it usually occurs at low levels in cells but can be induced in response to environmental stresses, particularly radiotherapy and cytotoxic chemotherapy, which induce elevated levels of autophagy that are cytoprotective for malignant cells, thus impeding rather than perpetuating the killing actions of these stress situations. Severely stressed cancer cells have been shown to shrink via autophagy to a state of reversible dormancy.

Necrosis

This is the premature death of cells and is characterised by the release of cellular contents into the local tissue microenvironment, in marked contrast to apoptosis, where cells are disassembled in a step-by-step fashion and the resulting cellular fragments are phagocytosed. Necrotic cell death results in the recruitment of inflammatory immune cells, promotion of angiogenesis, and release of stimulatory factors that increase cellular proliferation and tissue invasion, thereby enhancing rather than inhibiting carcinogenesis.

3. Sustaining proliferative signalling

Cancer cells can sustain proliferation beyond what would be expected for normal cells; this is typically due to growth factors, which are able to bind to cell surface-bound receptors that activate an intracellular tyrosine kinase-mediated signalling cascade, ultimately leading to changes in gene expression and promoting cellular proliferation and growth. Sustained proliferative capacity can result from over-production of growth factor ligands or receptors and production of structurally altered receptors, which can signal in the absence of ligand binding and activation of intracellular signalling pathway components, so that signalling is no longer ligand-dependent.

The cell cycle

The cell cycle is composed of four ordered, strictly regulated phases referred to as G_1 (gap 1), S (DNA synthesis), G_2 (gap 2) and M (mitosis) (Fig. 33.2). Normal cells grown in culture will stop proliferating and enter a quiescent state called G_0 once they become confluent or are deprived of serum or growth factors. The first gap phase (G_1) prior to the initiation of DNA synthesis represents the period of commitment that separates M and S phases as cells prepare for DNA duplication. Cells in G_0 and G_1 are receptive to growth signals, but once they have passed a restriction point, they are committed to enter DNA synthesis (S phase). Cells demonstrate arrest at different points in G_1 in response to different inhibitory growth signals. Mitogenic signals promote progression through G_1 to S phase, utilising phosphorylation of the retinoblastoma gene product (pRB, p. 40). Following DNA synthesis, there is a second gap phase (G_2) prior to mitosis (M), allowing cells to repair errors that have occurred during DNA replication and thus preventing propagation of these errors to daughter cells. Although the duration of individual phases may vary, depending on cell and tissue type, most adult cells are in a G_0 state at any one time.

Cell cycle regulation

The cell cycle is orchestrated by a number of molecular mechanisms: most importantly, by cyclins and cyclin-dependent kinases (CDKs). Cyclins bind to CDKs and are regulated by both activating and inactivating phosphorylation, with two main checkpoints at G_1/S and G_2/M transition. The genes that inhibit progression play an important part in tumour prevention and are referred to as tumour suppressor genes (e.g. *TP53*, *TP21*, *TP16* genes). The products of these genes deactivate the cyclin–CDK complexes and are thus able to halt the cell cycle. The complexity of cell cycle control is susceptible to dysregulation, which may produce a malignant phenotype.

Stimulation of the cell cycle

Many cancer cells produce growth factors, which drive their own proliferation by a positive feedback known as autocrine stimulation. Examples include transforming growth factor-alpha (TGF-α) and platelet-derived growth factor (PDGF). Other cancer cells express growth factor receptors at increased levels due to gene amplification or express abnormal receptors that are permanently activated. This results in abnormal cell growth in response to physiological growth factor stimulation or even in the absence of growth factor stimulation (ligand-independent signalling). The epidermal growth factor receptor (EGFR) is often over-expressed in lung and gastrointestinal tumours and the human epidermal growth factor receptor 2 (HER2)/neu receptor is frequently over-expressed in breast cancer. Both receptors activate the Ras–Raf–mitogen activated protein (MAP) kinase pathway, causing cell proliferation.

Fig. 33.2 The cell cycle and sites of action of chemotherapeutic agents. (CDK = cyclin-dependent kinase; *RB* = retinoblastoma gene)

33

4. Evading growth suppressors

In healthy tissues, cell-to-cell contact in dense cell populations acts as an inhibitory factor on proliferation. This contact inhibition is typically absent in many cancer cell populations. Growth-inhibitory factors can modulate the cell cycle regulators and produce activation of the CDK inhibitors, causing inhibition of the CDKs. Mutations within inhibitory proteins are common in cancer. Loss of restriction by disruption of pRB regulation can be found in human tumours, which produces a loss of restraint on transition from G_1 to S phase of the cell cycle. Disruption of *TP53* function will have downstream effects on *p21* that alter the coordination of DNA repair with cycle arrest, and that result in the affected cell accumulating genomic defects. Down-regulation of *p21* and *p27*, which can be found in tumours with normal *TP53* function, correlates notably with high tumour grade and poor prognosis.

5. Enabling replicative immortality

For cancer cells to evolve into macroscopic tumours, they need to acquire the ability for unlimited proliferation. Telomeric DNA sequences, which protect and stabilise chromosomal ends, play a central role in conferring this limitless replicative potential. During replication of normal cells, telomeres shorten progressively as small fragments of telomeric DNA are lost with successive cycles of replication. This shortening process is thought to represent a mitotic clock and eventually prevents the cell from dividing further. Telomerase, a specialised polymerase enzyme, adds nucleotides to telomeres, allowing continued cell division and thus preventing premature arrest of cellular replication. The telomerase enzyme is almost absent in normal cells but is expressed at significant levels in many human cancers.

6. Inducing angiogenesis

All cancers require a functional vascular network to ensure continued growth and will be unable to grow beyond 1 mm³ without stimulating the development of a vascular supply. Tumours require sustenance in the form of nutrients and oxygen, as well as an ability to evacuate metabolic waste products and carbon dioxide. This entails the development of new blood vessels, which is termed angiogenesis (Figs 33.3 and 33.4).

Angiogenesis is dependent on the production of angiogenic growth factors, of which vascular endothelial growth factor (VEGF) and platelet-derived growth factor (PDGF) are the best characterised. During tumour progression, an angiogenic switch is activated and remains on, causing normally quiescent vasculature to sprout new vessels continually that help sustain expanding tumour growth. Angiogenesis is governed by a balance of pro-angiogenic stimuli and angiogenesis inhibitors, such as thrombospondin (TSP)-1, which binds to transmembrane receptors on endothelial cells and evokes suppressive signals.

A number of cells can contribute to the maintenance of a functional tumour vasculature and therefore sustain angiogenesis. These include pericytes and a variety of bone marrow-derived cells such as macrophages, neutrophils, mast cells and myeloid progenitors.

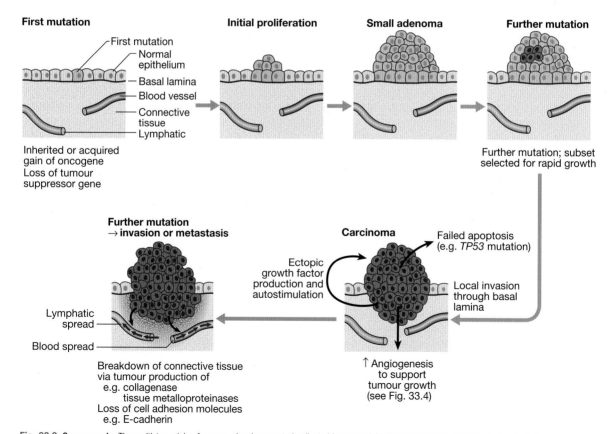

Fig. 33.3 Oncogenesis. The multistep origin of cancer, showing events implicated in cancer initiation, progression, invasion and metastasis.

Fig. 33.4 **Angiogenesis, invasion and metastasis.** [A] For any cancer to grow beyond 1 mm³, it must evoke a blood supply. [B] New vessel formation results from the release of angiogenic factors by the tumour cells and loss of inhibition of the endothelial cells. [C] The loss of cellular adhesion and disruption of the extracellular matrix allow cells to extravasate into the blood stream and metastasise to distant sites. (VEGF= vascular endothelial growth factor)

7. Activating invasion and metastasis

Invasion and metastasis are complex processes involving multiple discrete steps; they begin with local tissue invasion, followed by infiltration of nearby blood and lymphatic vessels by cancer cells. Malignant cells are eventually transported through haematogenous and lymphatic spread to distant sites within the body, where they form micrometastases that will eventually grow into macroscopic metastatic lesions (see Fig. 33.3).

Cadherin-1 (CDH1) is a calcium-dependent cell–cell adhesion glycoprotein that facilitates assembly of organised cell sheets in tissues, and increased expression is recognised as an antagonist of invasion and metastasis. In situ tumours usually retain CDH1 production, whereas loss of CDH1 production due to down-regulation or occasional mutational inactivation of CDH1 has been observed in human cancers, supporting the theory that CDH1 plays a key role in suppression of invasion and metastasis.

Cross-talk between cancer cells and cells of the surrounding stromal tissue is involved in the acquired capability for invasive growth and metastasis. Mesenchymal stem cells in tumour stroma have been found to secrete CCL5, a protein chemokine that helps recruit leucocytes into inflammatory sites. With the help of particular T-cell-derived cytokines (interleukin (IL)-2 and interferon-gamma (IFN-γ)), CCL5 induces proliferation and activation of natural killer cells and then acts reciprocally on cancer cells to stimulate invasive behaviour. Macrophages at the tumour periphery can foster local invasion by supplying matrix-degrading enzymes such as metalloproteinases and cysteine cathepsin proteases.

8. Reprogramming energy metabolism

Under aerobic conditions, oxidative phosphorylation functions as the main metabolic pathway for energy production; cells process glucose, first to pyruvate via glycolysis and thereafter to carbon dioxide in the mitochondria. While under anaerobic conditions, glycolysis is favoured to produce adenosine triphosphate (ATP). Cancer cells can reprogram their glucose metabolism to limit energy production to glycolysis, even in the presence of oxygen. This has been termed 'aerobic glycolysis'. Up-regulation of glucose transporters, such as GLUT1, is the main mechanism through which aerobic glycolysis is achieved.

This reprogramming of energy metabolism appears paradoxical, as overall energy production from glycolysis is significantly lower (18-fold) than that from oxidative phosphorylation. One explanation may be that the increased production of glycolytic intermediates can be fed into various biosynthetic pathways, including those that generate the nucleosides and amino acids, necessary for the production of new cells.

9. Tumour-promoting inflammation

Almost all tumours show infiltration with immune cells on pathological investigation and historically this finding was thought to represent an attempt of the immune system to eradicate the cancer. It is now clear that tumour-associated inflammatory responses promote tumour formation and cancer progression.

Cytokines are able to alter blood vessels to permit migration of leucocytes (mainly neutrophils), in order to permeate from the blood vessels into the tissue, a process known as extravasation. Migration across the endothelium occurs via the process of diapedesis, where chemokine gradients stimulate adhered leucocytes to move between endothelial cells and pass through the basement membrane into the surrounding tissues. Once within the tissue interstitium, leucocytes bind to extracellular matrix proteins via integrins and CD44 to prevent their loss from the site.

As well as cell-derived mediators, several acellular biochemical cascade systems consisting of pre-formed plasma proteins act in parallel to initiate and propagate the inflammatory response. These include the complement system activated by bacteria, and the coagulation and fibrinolytic systems activated by necrosis, and also in burns and trauma, as well as cancer. Other bioactive molecules, such as growth factors and pro-angiogenic factors, may be released by inflammatory immune cells into the surrounding tumour microenvironment. In particular, the release of reactive

33

oxygen species, which are actively mutagenic, will accelerate the genetic evolution of surrounding cancer cells, enhancing growth and contributing to cancer progression.

10. Evading immune destruction

The immune system operates as a significant barrier to tumour formation and progression, and the ability to escape from immunity is a hallmark of cancer development. Cancer cells continuously shed surface antigens into the circulatory system, prompting an immune response that includes cytotoxic T-cell, natural killer cell and macrophage production. The immune system is thought to provide continuous surveillance, with resultant elimination of cells that undergo malignant transformation.

However, deficiencies in the development or function of CD8$^+$ cytotoxic T lymphocytes, CD4$^+$ Th1 helper T cells or natural killer cells can each lead to a demonstrable increase in cancer incidence. Also, highly immunogenic cancer cells may evade immune destruction by disabling components of the immune system. This is done through recruitment of inflammatory cells, including regulatory T cells and myeloid-derived suppressor cells, both actively immunosuppressive against the actions of cytotoxic lymphocytes (see Fig. 4.12, p. 80).

Cancers develop and progress when there is loss of recognition by the immune system, lack of susceptibility due to escape from immune cell action and induction of immune dysfunction, often via inflammatory mediators.

Environmental and genetic determinants of cancer

The majority of cancers do not have a single cause but rather are the result of a complex interaction between genetic factors and exposure to environmental carcinogens. These are often tumour type-specific but some general principles do apply.

Environmental factors

Environmental triggers for cancer have mainly been identified through epidemiological studies that examine patterns of distribution of cancers in patients in whom age, sex, presence of other illnesses, social class, geography and so on differ. Sometimes, these give strong pointers to the molecular or cellular causes of the disease, such as the association between aflatoxin production within contaminated food supplies and hepatocellular carcinomas. For many solid cancers, such as breast and colorectal, however, there is evidence of a multifactorial pathogenesis, even when there is a principal environmental cause (Box 33.1).

Smoking is now established beyond all doubt as a major cause of lung cancer, but there are obviously additional predisposing factors since not all smokers develop cancer. Similarly, most carcinomas of the cervix are related to infection with human

i 33.1 Environmental factors that predispose to cancer

Environmental aetiology	Processes	Diseases
Occupational exposure (see 'Radiation' below)	Dye and rubber manufacturing (aromatic amines) Asbestos mining, construction work, shipbuilding (asbestos) Vinyl chloride (PVC) manufacturing Petroleum industry (benzene)	Bladder cancer Lung cancer and mesothelioma Liver angiosarcoma Acute leukaemia
Chemicals	Chemotherapy (e.g. melphalan, cyclophosphamide)	Acute myeloid leukaemia
Cigarette smoking	Exposure to carcinogens from inhaled smoke	Lung and bladder cancer
Viral infection	Epstein–Barr virus Human papillomavirus Hepatitis B and C viruses	Burkitt's lymphoma and nasopharyngeal cancer Cervical cancer Hepatocellular carcinoma
Bacterial infection	*Helicobacter pylori*	Gastric MALT lymphomas, gastric cancer
Parasitic infection	Liver fluke (*Opisthorchis sinensis*) *Schistosoma haematobium*	Cholangiocarcinoma Squamous cell bladder cancer
Dietary factors	Low-roughage/high-fat content diet High nitrosamine intake Aflatoxin from contamination of *Aspergillus flavus*	Colonic cancer Gastric cancer Hepatocellular cancer
Radiation	UV exposure Nuclear fallout following explosion (e.g. Hiroshima) Diagnostic exposure (e.g. CT) Occupational exposure (e.g. beryllium and strontium mining) Therapeutic radiotherapy	Basal cell carcinoma Melanoma Non-melanocytic skin cancer Leukaemia Solid tumours, e.g. thyroid Cholangiocarcinoma following Thorotrast usage Lung cancer Medullary thyroid cancer Sarcoma
Inflammatory diseases	Ulcerative colitis	Colon cancer
Hormonal	Use of diethylstilbestrol Oestrogens	Vaginal cancer Endometrial cancer Breast cancer

(CT = computed tomography; MALT = mucosa-associated lymphoid tissue; UV = ultraviolet)

papillomavirus (HPV subtypes 16 and 18). For carcinomas of the bowel and breast, there is strong evidence of an environmental component. For example, the risk of breast cancer in women of Far Eastern origin remains relatively low when they first migrate to a country with a Western lifestyle, but rises in subsequent generations to approach that of the resident population of the host country. The precise environmental factor that causes this change is unclear but may include diet (higher intake of saturated fat and/or dairy products), reproductive patterns (later onset of first pregnancy) and lifestyle (increased use of artificial light and shift in diurnal rhythm).

Genetic factors

A number of inherited cancer syndromes are recognised that account for 5–10% of all cancers (Box 33.2). Their molecular basis is discussed in Chapter 3, but in general they result from inherited mutations in genes that regulate cell growth, cell death and apoptosis. Examples include the *BRCA1*, *BRCA2* and *AT* (ataxia telangiectasia) genes that cause breast and some other cancers, the *FAP* gene that causes bowel cancer and the *RB* gene that causes retinoblastoma. Although carriers of these gene mutations have a greatly elevated risk of cancer, none has 100% penetrance and additional modulating factors, both genetic and environmental, are likely to be operative. Exploration of a possible genetic contribution is a key part of cancer management, especially with regard to ascertaining the risk for an affected patient's offspring.

Investigations

When a patient is suspected of having cancer, a full history should be taken; specific questions should be included as to potential risk factors such as smoking and occupational exposures or potential complications of the disease. A thorough clinical examination is essential to identify sites of metastases, and to discover any other conditions that may have a bearing on the management plan (pp. 1314–1315). In order to make a diagnosis and to plan the most appropriate management, information is needed on:

- the type of tumour
- the extent of disease, as assessed by staging investigations
- the patient's general condition and any comorbidity.

i 33.2 Inherited cancer predisposition syndromes

Syndrome	Malignancies	Inheritance	Gene
Ataxia telangiectasia	Leukaemia, lymphoma, ovarian, gastric, brain, colon	AR	*AT*
Bloom's syndrome	Leukaemia, tongue, oesophageal, colonic, Wilms' tumour	AR	*BLM*
Breast/ovarian	Breast, ovarian, colonic, prostatic, pancreatic	AD	*BRCA1, BRCA2*
Cowden's syndrome	Breast, thyroid, gastrointestinal tract, pancreatic	AD	*PTEN*
Familial adenomatous polyposis	Colonic, upper gastrointestinal tract	AD	*APC, MUTYH*
Familial atypical multiple mole melanoma (FAMMM)	Melanoma, pancreas	AD	*CDKN2A (TP16)*
Fanconi anaemia	Leukaemia, oesophageal, skin, hepatoma	AR	*FACA, FACC, FACD*
Gorlin's syndrome	Basal cell skin, brain	AD	*PTCH*
Hereditary diffuse gastric cancer	Diffuse gastric cancer	AD	*E-cadherin*
Hereditary non-polyposis colon cancer (HNPCC)	Colonic, endometrial, ovarian, pancreatic, gastric	AD	*MSH2, MLH1, MSH6, PMS1, PMS2*
Li–Fraumeni syndrome	Sarcoma, breast, osteosarcoma, leukaemia, glioma, adrenocortical	AD	*TP53*
Multiple endocrine neoplasia (MEN) 1	Pancreatic islet cell, pituitary adenoma, parathyroid adenoma and hyperplasia	AD	*MEN1*
MEN 2	Medullary thyroid, phaeochromocytoma, parathyroid hyperplasia	AD	*RET*
Neurofibromatosis 1	Neurofibrosarcoma, phaeochromocytoma, optic glioma	AD	*NF1*
Neurofibromatosis 2	Vestibular schwannoma	AD	*NF2*
Papillary renal cell cancer syndrome	Renal cell cancer	AD	*MET*
Peutz–Jeghers syndrome	Colonic, ileal, breast, ovarian	AD	*STK11*
Prostate cancer	Prostate	AD	*HPC1*
Retinoblastoma	Retinoblastoma, osteosarcoma	AD	*RB1*
von Hippel–Lindau syndrome	Haemangioblastoma of retina and CNS, renal cell, phaeochromocytoma	AD	*VHL*
Wilms' tumour	Nephroblastoma, neuroblastoma, hepatoblastoma, rhabdomyosarcoma	AD	*WT1*
Xeroderma pigmentosum	Skin, leukaemia, melanoma	AR	*XPA, XPC, XPD (ERCC2), XPF*

(AD = autosomal dominant; AR = autosomal recessive; CNS = central nervous system)

33

i

33.3 Eastern Cooperative Oncology Group (ECOG) performance status scale

0	Fully active, able to carry on all usual activities without restriction and without the aid of analgesics
1	Restricted in strenuous activity but ambulatory and able to carry out light work or pursue a sedentary occupation. This group also contains patients who are fully active, as in grade 0, but only with the aid of analgesics
2	Ambulatory and capable of all self-care but unable to work. Up and about more than 50% of waking hours
3	Capable of only limited self-care, confined to bed or chair more than 50% of waking hours
4	Completely disabled, unable to carry out any self-care and confined totally to bed or chair

i

33.4 TNM classification

Extent of primary tumour*

| TX | Not assessed |
| T0 | No tumour |
| T1 | }
T2	Increases in primary tumour size or depth
T3	of invasion
T4	

Increased involvement of nodes*

NX	Not assessed
N0	No nodal involvement
N1	} Increases in involvement
N2/3	

Presence of metastases

MX	Not assessed
M0	Not present
M1	Present

*Exact criteria for size and region of nodal involvement have been defined for each anatomical site.

The overall fitness of a patient is often assessed by the Eastern Cooperative Oncology Group (ECOG) performance status scale (Box 33.3). The outcome for patients with a performance status of 3 or 4 is worse in almost all malignancies than for those with a status of 0–2, and this has a strong influence on the approach to treatment in the individual patient.

The process of staging determines the extent of the tumour; it entails clinical examination, imaging and, in some cases, surgery, to establish the extent of disease involvement. The outcome is recorded using a standard staging classification that allows comparisons to be made between different groups of patients. Therapeutic decisions and prognostic predictions can then be made using the evidence base for the disease. One of the most commonly used systems is the T (tumour), N (regional lymph nodes), M (metastatic sites) approach of the International Union against Cancer (UICC, Box 33.4). For some tumours, such as colon cancer, the Dukes system (p. 832) is used rather than the UICC classification.

Histology

Histological analysis of a biopsy or resected specimen is pivotal in clinching the diagnosis and in deciding on the best form of management. The results of histological analysis are most informative when combined with knowledge of the clinical picture; biopsy results should therefore be reviewed and discussed within the context of a multidisciplinary team meeting.

Light microscopy

Examination of tumour samples by light microscopy remains the core method of cancer diagnosis and, in cases where the primary site is unclear, may give clues to the origin of the tumour:

- Signet-ring cells favour a gastric primary.
- Presence of melanin favours melanoma.
- Mucin is common in gut/lung/breast/endometrial cancers, but particularly common in ovarian cancer and rare in renal cell or thyroid cancers.
- Psammoma bodies are a feature of ovarian cancer (mucin +) and thyroid cancer (mucin –).

Immunohistochemistry

Immunohistochemical (IHC) staining for tumour markers can provide useful diagnostic information and can help with treatment decisions. Commonly used examples of IHC in clinical practice include:

- *Oestrogen (ER) and progesterone (PR) receptors.* Positive results indicate that the tumour may be sensitive to hormonal manipulation.
- *Alpha-fetoprotein (AFP)* and *human chorionic gonadotrophin (hCG) with or without placental alkaline phosphatase (PLAP).* These favour germ-cell tumours.
- *Prostate-specific antigen (PSA)* and *prostatic acid phosphatase (PAP).* These favour prostate cancer.
- *Carcinoembryonic antigen (CEA), cytokeratin* and *epithelial membrane antigen (EMA).* These favour epithelial carcinomas.
- *HER2 receptor.* Breast cancers that have high levels of expression of HER2 indicate that the tumour may respond to trastuzumab (Herceptin), an antibody directed against the HER2 receptor.

The pattern of immunoglobulin, T-cell receptor and cluster designation (CD) antigen expression on the surface is helpful in the diagnosis and classification of lymphomas. This can be achieved by IHC staining of biopsy samples or flow cytometry.

Electron microscopy

Electron microscopy (EM) can sometimes be of diagnostic value. Examples include the visualisation of melanosomes in amelanotic melanoma and dense core granules in neuro-endocrine tumours. EM may help to distinguish adenocarcinoma from mesothelioma, as the ultrastructural properties of these two diseases are different (mesothelioma appears to have long, narrow, branching microvilli while adenocarcinomas appear to have short, stubby microvilli). EM is also useful for differentiating spindle-cell tumours (sarcomas, melanomas, squamous cell cancers) from small round-cell tumours, again due to their ultrastructural differences.

Cytogenetic analysis

Some tumours demonstrate typical chromosomal changes that help in diagnosis. The utilisation of fluorescent in situ hybridisation (FISH) techniques can be useful in Ewing's sarcoma and peripheral neuro-ectodermal tumours where there is a translocation between chromosome 11 and 22–t(11;22)(q24;q12). In some cases, gene amplification can be detected via FISH (e.g. determining over-expression of HER2/neu).

Imaging

Imaging plays a critical role in oncology, not only in locating the primary tumour but also in staging the disease and determining the response to treatment. The imaging modality employed depends primarily on the site of the disease and likely patterns of spread, and may require more than one modality.

Ultrasound

Ultrasound is useful in characterising lesions within the liver, kidney, pancreas and reproductive organs. It can be used for guiding biopsies of tumours in breast and liver. Endoscopic ultrasound is helpful in staging upper gastrointestinal and pancreatic cancers, involving a special endoscope with an ultrasound probe attached.

Computed tomography

Computed tomography (CT) is a key investigation in cancer patients and is particularly useful in imaging the thorax and abdomen. With modern scanners it is possible to visualise the large bowel if it is prepared (CT colonography), allowing accurate detection of colorectal cancers and adenomas ≥10 mm.

Magnetic resonance imaging

Magnetic resonance imaging (MRI) has a high resolution and is the preferred technique for brain and pelvic imaging. It is widely employed for the staging of rectal, cervical and prostate cancers.

Positron emission tomography

Positron emission tomography (PET) visualises metabolic activity of tumour cells and is widely used, often in combination with CT (PET–CT), to evaluate the extent of the disease, particularly in the assessment of potential distant metastasis (Fig. 33.5). It can accurately assess the severity and spread of cancer by detecting tumour metabolic activity following injection of small amounts of radioactive tracers such as fluorodeoxyglucose (FDG). In addition to having a role in diagnosis, PET can be used in some patients to assess treatment response.

Biochemical markers

Many cancers produce substances called tumour markers, which can assist in diagnosis and surveillance. Some are useful in population screening, diagnosis, determining prognosis, response evaluation, detection of relapse and imaging of metastasis. Unfortunately, most tumour markers are neither sufficiently sensitive nor sufficiently specific to be used in isolation for diagnosis and need to be interpreted in the context of the other clinical features. Some can be used for antibody-directed therapy or imaging, however, where they have a greater role in diagnosis. Tumour markers in routine use are outlined in Box 33.5.

Presenting problems in oncology

In the early stages of cancer development, the number of malignant cells is small and the patient is usually asymptomatic. With tumour progression, localised signs or symptoms develop due to mass effects and/or invasion of local tissues. With further progression, symptoms may occur at distant sites as a result of

Fig. 33.5 Positron emission tomography–computed tomography (PET–CT) images. [A] There is a neoplastic lesion (arrow) in the left axilla, evidenced by the increased uptake of fluorodeoxyglucose (FDG) tracers. [B] Imaging after chemotherapy, demonstrating that the abnormal uptake has disappeared and indicating a response to treatment. *Courtesy of Dr J. Wilsdon, Freeman Hospital, Newcastle upon Tyne.*

metastatic disease or from non-metastatic manifestations due to production of biologically active hormones by the tumour or as the result of an immune response to the tumour. The possible presentations are summarised in Boxes 33.6 and 33.7, and common presenting features discussed below. Although the incidence of cancer increases with patient age, the approach to investigation and management is similar at all ages (Box 33.8).

Palpable mass

A palpable mass detected by the patient or physician may be the first sign of cancer. Primary tumours of the thyroid, breast, testis and skin are often detected in this way, whereas palpable lymph nodes in the neck, groin or axilla may indicate secondary spread of tumour. Hepatomegaly may be the first sign of primary liver cancer or tumour metastasis, whereas skin cancer may present as an enlarging or changing pigmented lesion.

Weight loss and fever

Unintentional weight loss is a characteristic feature of advanced cancer, but can have other causes such as thyrotoxicosis, chronic inflammatory disease and chronic infective disorders. Fever can occur in any cancer secondary to infection, but may be a primary feature in Hodgkin and non-Hodgkin lymphoma, leukaemia, renal cancer and liver cancer. The presence of unexplained weight loss or fever warrants investigation to exclude the presence of occult malignancy.

33

i 33.5 Commonly used serum tumour markers

Name	Natural occurrence	Tumours
Alpha-fetoprotein (AFP)	Glycoprotein found in yolk sac and fetal liver tissue. Transient elevation in liver diseases. Has a role in screening during pregnancy for the detection of neural tube defects and Down's syndrome	Ovarian non-seminomatous germ cell tumours (80%), testicular teratoma (80%), hepatocellular cancer (50%)
Beta-2-microglobulin	A human leucocyte antigen (HLA) common fragment present on surface of lymphocytes, macrophages and some epithelial cells. Can be elevated in autoimmune disease and renal glomerular disease	Non-Hodgkin lymphoma, myeloma
Calcitonin	32-amino-acid peptide from C cells of thyroid. Used to screen for MEN 2	Medullary cell carcinoma of thyroid
Cancer antigen 125 (CA-125)	Differentiation antigen of coelomic epithelium (Müller's duct). Raised in any cause of ascites, pleural effusion or heart failure. Can be raised in inflammatory conditions	Ovarian epithelial cancer (75%), gastrointestinal cancer (10%), lung cancer (5%) and breast cancer (5%)
CA-19.9	A mucin found in epithelium of fetal stomach, intestine and pancreas. It is eliminated exclusively via bile and so any degree of cholestasis can cause levels to rise	Pancreatic cancer (80%), mucinous tumour of the ovary (65%), gastric cancer (30%), colon cancer (30%)
Carcinoembryonic antigen (CEA)	Glycoprotein found in intestinal mucosa during embryonic and fetal life. Elevated in smokers, cirrhosis, chronic hepatitis, ulcerative colitis, pneumonia	Colorectal cancer, particularly with liver metastasis, gastric cancer, breast cancer, lung cancer, mucinous cancer of the ovary
Human chorionic gonadotrophin (hCG)	Glycoprotein hormone, 14 kD α subunit and 24 kD β subunit from placental syncytiotrophoblasts. Used for disease monitoring in hydatidiform mole and as the basis of a pregnancy test	Choriocarcinoma (100%), hydatidiform moles (97%), ovarian non-seminomatous germ cell tumours (50–80%), seminoma (15%)
Placental alkaline phosphatase (PLAP)	Isoenzyme of alkaline phosphatase	Seminoma (40%), ovarian dysgerminoma (50%)
Prostate-specific antigen (PSA)	Glycoprotein member of human kallikrein gene family. PSA is a serine protease that liquefies semen in excretory ducts of prostate. Can be elevated in benign prostatic hypertrophy and prostatitis	Prostate cancer (95%)
Thyroglobulin	Matrix protein for thyroid hormone synthesis in normal thyroid follicles	Papillary and follicular thyroid cancer

i 33.6 Local features of malignant disease

Symptom	Typical site or possible tumour
Haemorrhage	Stomach, colon, bronchus, endometrium, bladder, kidney
Lump	Breast, lymph node (any site), testicle
Bone pain or fracture	Bone (primary sarcoma, secondary metastasis from breast, prostate, bronchus, thyroid, kidney)
Skin abnormality	Melanoma, basal cell carcinoma (rodent ulcer)
Ulcer	Oesophagus, stomach, anus, skin
Dysphagia	Oesophagus, bronchus, gastric
Increasing constipation, abdominal discomfort or pain	Colon, rectum, ovary
Airway obstruction, stridor, cough, recurrent infection	Bronchus, thyroid
Odynophagia, early satiety, vomiting	Bronchus, stomach, oesophagus, colon, rectum
Abdominal swelling (ascites)	Ovary, stomach, pancreas

Thromboembolism

Thrombosis and disseminated intravascular coagulation (DIC) are common complications in patients with cancer. The prothrombotic state is caused by cancer cells activating the coagulation system via factors such as tissue factor, cancer procoagulant and inflammatory cytokines. The interaction between tumour cells, monocytes/macrophages, platelets and endothelial cells can promote thrombus formation, as part of a host response to the cancer (i.e. acute phase, inflammation, angiogenesis) or via a reduction in the levels of inhibitors of coagulation or impairment

i 33.7 Non-metastatic manifestations of malignant disease

Feature	Common cancer site associations
Weight loss and anorexia	Lung, gastrointestinal tract
Fatigue	Any
Hypercalcaemia	Myeloma, breast, kidney
Prothrombotic tendency	Ovary, pancreas, gastrointestinal tract
SIADH Ectopic ACTH	Small cell lung cancer
Lambert–Eaton myasthenic syndrome	Small cell lung cancer
Subacute cerebellar degeneration	Small cell lung cancer, ovarian cancer
Acanthosis nigricans	Stomach, oesophagus
Dermatomyositis/polymyositis	Stomach, lung

(ACTH = adrenocorticotrophic hormone; SIADH = syndrome of inappropriate antidiuretic hormone (vasopressin) secretion)

i 33.9 Ectopic hormone production by tumours

Hormone	Consequence	Tumours
ACTH	Cushing's syndrome	SCLC
Erythropoietin	Polycythaemia	Kidney, hepatoma, cerebellar haemangioblastoma, uterine fibroids
FGF-23	Hypophosphataemic osteomalacia	Mesenchymal tumours
PTHrP	Hypercalcaemia	NSCLC (squamous cell), breast, kidney
Vasopressin (ADH)	Hyponatraemia	SCLC

(ACTH = adrenocorticotrophic hormone; ADH = antidiuretic hormone; FGF = fibroblast growth factor; NSCLC = non-small cell lung cancer; PTHrP = parathyroid hormone-related protein; SCLC = small cell lung cancer)

33.8 Cancer in old age

- **Incidence**: around 50% of cancers occur in the 15% of the population aged over 65 years.
- **Screening**: women aged over 65 in the UK are not invited to breast cancer screening but can request it. Uptake is low despite increasing incidence with age.
- **Presentation**: may be later for some cancers. When symptoms are non-specific, patients (and their doctors) may initially attribute them to age alone.
- **Life expectancy**: an 80-year-old woman can expect to live 8 years, so cancer may still shorten life and an active approach remains appropriate.
- **Prognosis**: histology, stage at presentation and observation for a brief period are better guides to outcome than age.
- **Rate of progression**: malignancy may have a more indolent course. This is poorly understood but may be due to reduced effectiveness of angiogenesis with age, inhibiting the development of metastases.
- **Response to treatment**: equivalent to that in younger people – well documented for a range of cancers and for surgery, radiotherapy, chemotherapy and hormonal therapy.
- **Treatment selection**: chronological age is of minor importance compared to comorbid illness and patient choice. Although older patients can be treated effectively and safely, aggressive intervention is not appropriate for all. Symptom control may be all that is possible or desired by the patient.

of fibrinolysis. Furthermore, the prothrombotic tendency can be enhanced by therapy such as surgery, chemotherapy, hormone therapy and radiotherapy, and by in-dwelling access devices (i.e. central venous catheters). In some patients, the thromboembolism is the first presenting feature of the underlying cancer.

Ectopic hormone production

In some cases, the first presentation of cancer is with a metabolic abnormality due to ectopic production of hormones by tumour cells, including insulin, ACTH, vasopressin (antidiuretic hormone, ADH), fibroblast growth factor (FGF)-23, erythropoietin and

parathyroid hormone-related protein (PTHrP). This can result in a wide variety of presentations, as summarised in Box 33.9. Further details on the presentation and management of ACTH- and vasopressin-producing tumours are given on page 670, and those of FGF23-producing tumours on page 1053. The management of hypercalcaemia associated with malignancy is discussed below.

Neurological paraneoplastic syndromes

These form a group of conditions associated with cancer that are thought to be due to an immunological response to the tumour that results in damage to the nervous system or muscle. The cancers most commonly implicated are those of the lung (small cell and non-small cell), pancreas, breast, prostate, ovary and lymphoma.

- *Peripheral neuropathy* results from axonal degeneration or demyelination.
- *Encephalomyelitis* can present with diverse symptoms, depending on which region of the brain is involved. Lumbar puncture shows raised protein in the cerebrospinal fluid and a pleocytosis, predominantly that of lymphocytes. In some centres, flow cytometry of the cerebrospinal fluid can be used to detect carcinomatous cells. MRI shows meningeal enhancement, particularly at the level of the brainstem, and anti-Hu antibodies may be detectable in serum. Encephalomyelitis is due to perivascular inflammation and selective neuronal degeneration. Most cases are caused by small cell lung cancer (75%).
- *Cerebellar degeneration* may be the presenting feature of an underlying malignancy and presents with rapid onset of cerebellar ataxia. Diagnosis is by MRI or CT, which may show cerebellar atrophy. Patients with these neurological paraneoplastic syndromes may be found to have circulating anti-Yo, Tr and Hu antibodies, but these are not completely specific and negative results do not exclude the diagnosis.
- *Retinopathy* is a rare complication of cancer and presents with blurred vision, episodic visual loss and impaired colour vision. If left untreated, it may lead to blindness. The diagnosis should be suspected if the electroretinogram is abnormal and anti-retinal antibodies are detected.
- *Lambert–Eaton myasthenic syndrome* (LEMS) is due to underlying cancer in about 60% of cases. It presents with

33

proximal muscle weakness that improves on exercise and is caused by the development of antibodies to pre-synaptic calcium channels (p. 1143). The diagnosis is made by electromyelogram (EMG), which shows a low-amplitude compound muscle action potential that enhances to near normal following exercise.

- *Dermatomyositis* or *polymyositis* may be the first presentation of some cancers. Clinical features and management of these conditions are discussed on page 1039.

Cutaneous manifestations of cancer

Many cancers can present with skin manifestations that are not due to metastases:

- *Pruritus* may be a presenting feature of lymphoma, leukaemia and central nervous system tumours.
- *Acanthosis nigricans* may precede cancers by many years and is particularly associated with gastric cancer.
- *Vitiligo* may be associated with malignant melanoma and is possibly due to an immune response to melanocytes.
- *Pemphigus* may occur in lymphoma, Kaposi's sarcoma and thymic tumours.
- *Dermatitis herpetiformis* associated with coeliac disease may precede tumour development by many years, and is associated with gastrointestinal lymphoma.

The clinical features and management of these skin conditions are discussed in Chapter 29.

Emergency complications of cancer

Spinal cord compression

Spinal cord compression complicates 5% of cancers and is most common in myeloma, prostate, breast and lung cancers that involve bone. Cord compression often results from posterior extension of a vertebral body mass but intrathecal spinal cord metastases can cause similar signs and symptoms. The thoracic region is most commonly affected.

Clinical features

The earliest sign is back pain, particularly on coughing and lying flat. Subsequently, sensory changes develop in dermatomes below the level of compression and motor weakness distal to the block occurs. Finally, sphincter disturbance, causing urinary retention and bowel incontinence, is observed. Involvement of the lumbar spine may cause conus medullaris or cauda equina compression (Box 33.10). Physical examination reveals findings consistent with an upper motor neuron lesion, but lower motor

33.11 Management of suspected spinal cord compression

- Confirm diagnosis with urgent MRI scan
- Administer high-dose glucocorticoids:
    Dexamethasone 16 mg IV stat
    Dexamethasone 8 mg twice daily orally
- Ensure adequate analgesia
- Refer for surgical decompression or urgent radiotherapy

neuron findings may predominate early on or in cases of nerve root compression.

Management

Spinal cord compression is a medical emergency and should be treated with analgesia and high-dose glucocorticoid therapy (Box 33.11). Neurosurgical intervention produces superior outcome and survival compared to radiotherapy alone, and should be considered first for all patients. Radiotherapy is used for the remaining patients and selected tumour types when the cancer is likely to be radiosensitive. The prognosis varies considerably, depending on tumour type, but the degree of neurological dysfunction at presentation is the strongest predictor of outcome, irrespective of the underlying diagnosis. Mobility can be preserved in more than 80% of patients who are ambulatory at presentation, but neurological function is seldom regained in patients with established deficits such as paraplegia.

Superior vena cava obstruction

Superior vena cava obstruction (SVCO) is a common complication of cancer that can occur through extrinsic compression or intravascular blockage. The most common causes of extrinsic compression are lung cancer, lymphoma and metastatic tumours. Patients with cancer can also develop SVCO due to intravascular blockage in association with a central catheter or thromboembolism secondary to the tumour.

Clinical features

The typical presentation is with oedema of the arms and face, distended neck and arm veins and dusky skin coloration over the chest, arms and face. Collateral vessels may develop over a period of weeks and the flow of blood in the collaterals helps to confirm the diagnosis. Headache secondary to cerebral oedema arising from the backflow pressure may also occur and tends to be aggravated by bending forwards, stooping or lying down. The severity of symptoms is related to the rate of obstruction and the development of a venous collateral circulation. Accordingly, symptoms may develop rapidly or gradually. Clinical features are summarised in Box 33.12.

i 33.10 Comparison of features of neurological deficit

Clinical feature	Spinal cord	Conus medullaris	Cauda equina
Weakness	Symmetrical and profound	Symmetrical and variable	Asymmetrical, may be mild
Reflexes	Increased (or absent) knee and ankle reflexes with extensor plantar reflex	Increased knee reflex, decreased ankle reflex, extensor plantar reflex	Decreased knee and ankle reflexes with flexor plantar reflex
Sensory loss	Symmetrical, sensory level	Symmetrical, saddle distribution	Asymmetrical, radicular pattern
Sphincters	Late loss	Early loss	Often spared
Progression	Rapid	Variable	Variable

33.12 Common symptoms and physical findings in superior vena cava obstruction*

Symptoms

- Dyspnoea (63%)
- Facial swelling and head fullness (50%)
- Cough (24%)
- Arm swelling (18%)
- Chest pain (15%)
- Dysphagia (9%)

Physical findings

- Venous distension of neck (66%)
- Venous distension of chest wall (54%)
- Facial oedema (46%)
- Cyanosis (20%)
- Plethora of face (19%)
- Oedema of arms (14%)

*Percentage of patients affected.

Investigations and management

The investigation of choice is a CT scan of the thorax to confirm the diagnosis and distinguish between extra- and intravascular causes. A biopsy should be obtained when the tumour type is unknown because tumour type has a major influence on treatment. CT of the head may be indicated if cerebral oedema is suspected. Tumours that are exquisitely sensitive to chemotherapy, such as germ cell tumours and lymphoma, can be treated with chemotherapy alone, but for most other tumours mediastinal radiotherapy is required. This relieves symptoms within 2 weeks in 50–90% of patients. In many centres, stenting is now increasingly favoured over radiotherapy, as it produces rapid results and can be repeated with reasonable effectiveness. This technique is particularly useful when dealing with tumours that are relatively chemo- or radio-resistant, such as non-small cell lung cancer or carcinoma of unknown primary. Where possible, these measures should be followed by treatment of the primary tumour, as long-term outcome is strongly dependent on the prognosis of the underlying cancer.

Hypercalcaemia

Hypercalcaemia is the most common metabolic disorder in patients with cancer and has a prevalence of up to 20% in cancer patients. The incidence is highest in myeloma and breast cancer (approximately 40%), intermediate in non-small cell lung cancer, and uncommon in colon, prostate and small cell lung carcinomas. It is most commonly due to over-production of PTHrP (80%), which binds to the PTH receptor and elevates serum calcium by stimulating osteoclastic bone resorption and increasing renal tubular reabsorption of calcium. Direct invasion of bone by metastases accounts for around 20% of cases while other mechanisms, such as ectopic PTH secretion, are rare.

Clinical features

The symptoms of hypercalcaemia are often non-specific and may mimic those of the underlying malignancy. They include drowsiness, delirium, nausea and vomiting, constipation, polyuria, polydipsia and dehydration.

Investigations and management

The diagnosis is made by measuring serum total calcium and adjusting for albumin. It is especially important to correct for albumin in cancer because hypoalbuminaemia is common and total calcium values under-estimate the level of ionised calcium. The principles of management are outlined in Box 33.13.

33.13 Medical management of severe hypercalcaemia

- IV 0.9% saline 2–4 L/day
- Zoledronic acid 4 mg IV or pamidronate 60–90 mg IV
- For patients with severe, symptomatic hypercalcaemia that is refractory to zoledronic acid, denosumab (initial dose 60 mg SC, with repeat dosing based on response) is an alternative option

Patients should initially be treated with intravenous 0.9% saline to improve renal function and increase urinary calcium excretion. This alone often results in clinical improvement. Concurrently, intravenous bisphosphonates should be given to inhibit bone resorption. Calcitonin acts rapidly to increase calcium excretion and to reduce bone resorption, and can be combined with fluid and bisphosphonate therapy for the first 24–48 hours in patients with life-threatening hypercalcaemia. Bisphosphonates will usually reduce the serum calcium levels to normal within 5 days, but, if not, treatment can be repeated. The duration of action is up to 4 weeks and repeated therapy can be given at 3–4-weekly intervals in the outpatient department. Hypercalcaemia is frequently a sign of tumour progression and the patient requires further investigation to establish disease status and review of the anti-cancer treatment strategy.

Neutropenic fever

Neutropenia is a common complication of malignancy. It is usually secondary to chemotherapy but may occur with radiotherapy if large amounts of bone marrow are irradiated; it may also be a component of pancytopenia due to malignant infiltration of the bone marrow. Neutropenic fever is defined as a pyrexia of 38°C for over 1 hour in a patient with a neutrophil count of $<0.5\times10^9$/L or $<1.0\times10^9$/L if the nadir is anticipated to drop to $<0.5\times10^9$/L in the next 24 hours. The risk of sepsis is related to the severity and duration of neutropenia and the presence of other risk factors, such as intravenous cannulae or bladder catheters. Neutropenic fever is an emergency in cancer patients as, if left untreated, it can result in sepsis with a high mortality rate.

Clinical features

The typical presentation is with high fever, and affected patients are often non-specifically unwell. Examination is usually unhelpful in defining a primary source of the infection. Hypotension is an adverse prognostic feature and may progress to systemic circulatory shutdown and organ failure.

Investigations and management

An infection screen should be performed to include blood cultures (both peripheral and from central lines), urine culture, chest X-ray, and swabs for culture (throat, central line, wound). High-dose intravenous antibiotics should then be commenced, pending the results of cultures. The standard approach is to commence empirical antibiotics according to local hospital policies agreed with microbiologists and based on the local antibiotic resistance patterns observed. First-line empirical therapy is either monotherapy with piperacillin–tazobactam or meropenem, or with the addition of gentamicin. Metronidazole may be added if anaerobic infection is suspected, and teicoplanin where Gram-positive infection is suspected (e.g. in patients with central lines). Antibiotics should be adjusted according to culture results, although these are often negative. If there is no response after 36–48 hours, antibiotics should be reviewed with microbiological advice, and antifungal cover should be considered

33

(liposomal amphotericin B). Granulocyte–colony-stimulating factor (G–CSF) is not routinely used for all patients with neutropenia and guidelines for use have been established. Other supportive therapy, including intravenous fluids, inotrope therapy, ventilation or haemofiltration, may be required.

Tumour lysis syndrome

The acute destruction of a large number of cells can be associated with metabolic sequelae and is called tumour lysis syndrome. It is usually related to bulky, chemosensitive disease, including lymphoma, leukaemia and germ cell tumours. More rarely, it can occur spontaneously.

Clinical features

Cellular destruction results in the release of potassium, phosphate, nucleic acids and purines that can cause transient hypocalcaemia, hyperphosphataemia, hyperuricaemia and hyperkalaemia. This can lead to acute impairment of renal function and the precipitation of uric acid crystals in the renal tubular system. These can manifest with symptoms associated with multiple underlying electrolyte abnormalities, including fatigue, nausea, vomiting, cardiac arrhythmia, heart failure, syncope, tetany, seizures and sudden death.

Investigations and management

Serum biochemistry should be monitored regularly for 48–72 hours after treatment in patients at risk. Elevated serum potassium may be the earliest biochemical marker but pre-treatment serum lactate dehydrogenase (LDH) correlates with tumour bulk and may indicate increased risk. Good hydration and urine output should be maintained throughout treatment administration. Prophylaxis with allopurinol should be considered and recombinant urate oxidase (rasburicase) can be used to reduce uric acid levels when other treatments fail. Adequate hydration is vital, as it has a dilution effect on the extracellular fluid, improving electrolyte imbalance, and increases circulating volume, improving filtration in the kidneys. In high-risk patients, hydration should be commenced 24 hours before the start of treatment. If normal treatment methods fail to correct the problems, haemodialysis should be considered at an early stage to prevent progression to irreversibility.

Metastatic disease

Metastatic disease is the major cause of death in cancer patients and the principal cause of morbidity. For the majority, the aim of treatment is palliative but treatment of a solitary metastasis can occasionally be curative.

Brain metastases

Brain metastases occur in 10–30% of adults and 6–10% of children with cancer, and are an increasingly important cause of morbidity. Tumours that typically metastasise to the brain are shown in Box 33.14. Most involve the brain parenchyma but can also affect the cranial nerves, the blood vessels and other intracranial structures. In cases of solitary metastasis to the brain, the use of surgery and adjuvant radiotherapy has been shown to increase survival. Practices vary, however, for patients with more advanced brain metastases. In these cases, median survival without treatment is approximately 1 month. Glucocorticoids can increase survival to 2–3 months and whole-brain radiotherapy improves survival to 3–6 months, but the true

33.14 Primary tumour sites that metastasise to the brain	
Primary tumour	Patients (%)
Lung	48
Breast	15
Melanoma	9
Colon	5
Other known primary	13
Unknown primary	11

efficacy of these interventions has not been proven adequately in a randomised trial setting. Patients with brain metastases as the only manifestation of an undetected primary tumour have a more favourable prognosis, with an overall median survival of 13.4 months. Tumour type also influences prognosis; breast cancer patients have a better prognosis than those with other types of cancer, and those with colorectal cancer tend to have a poorer prognosis.

Clinical features

Presentation is with headaches (40–50%), focal neurological dysfunction (20–40%), cognitive dysfunction (35%), seizures (10–20%) and papilloedema (< 10%).

Investigations and management

The diagnosis can be confirmed by CT or contrast-enhanced MRI. Treatment options include high-dose glucocorticoids (dexamethasone 4 mg 4 times daily) for tumour-associated oedema, anticonvulsants for seizures, whole-brain radiotherapy and chemotherapy. Surgery may be considered for single sites of disease and can be curative; stereotactic radiotherapy may also be considered for solitary site involvement where surgery is not possible.

Lung metastases

These are common in breast cancer, colon cancer and tumours of the head and neck. The presentation is usually with a lesion on chest X-ray or CT. Solitary lesions require investigation, as single metastases can be difficult to distinguish from a primary lung tumour. Patients with two or more pulmonary nodules can be assumed to have metastases. The approach to treatment depends on the extent of disease in the lung and elsewhere. For solitary lesions, surgery should be considered, with a generous wedge resection. Radiotherapy, chemotherapy or endocrine therapy can be used as systemic treatment and is dependent on the underlying primary cancer diagnosis.

Liver metastases

Metastatic cancer in the liver can represent the sole or life-limiting component of disease for many with colorectal cancer, ocular melanoma, neuro-endocrine tumours (NETs) and, less commonly, other tumour types. The most common clinical presentations are with right upper quadrant pain due to stretching of the liver capsule, jaundice, deranged liver function tests or an abnormality detected on imaging. In selected cases, resection of the metastasis can be contemplated. In colorectal cancer, successful resection of metastases improves 5-year survival from 3% to 30–40%. Other techniques, such as chemoembolisation or radiofrequency ablation, can also be used, provided the number and size of metastases remain small. If these are not feasible, symptoms may respond to systemic chemotherapy.

Bone metastases

Bone is the third most common organ involved by metastasis, after lung and liver. Bone metastases are a major clinical problem in patients with myeloma and breast or prostate cancers, but other tumours that commonly metastasise to bone include those of the kidney and thyroid. Bone metastases are an increasing management problem in other tumour types that do not classically target bone, due to the prolonged survival of patients generally. Accordingly, effective management of bony metastases has become a focus in the treatment of patients with many incurable cancers.

Clinical features

The main presentations are with pain, pathological fractures and spinal cord compression (see above). The pain tends to be progressive and worst at night, and may be partially relieved by activity, but subsequently becomes more constant in nature and is exacerbated by movement. Most pathological fractures occur in metastatic breast cancer (53%); other tumour types associated with fracture include the kidney (11%), lung (8%), thyroid (5%), lymphoma (5%) and prostate (3%).

Investigations and management

The most sensitive way of detecting bone metastases is by isotope bone scan. This can have false-positive results in healing bone, particularly as a flare response following treatment and false-negative results occur in multiple myeloma due to suppression of osteoblast activity. Plain X-ray films are therefore preferred for any sites of bone pain, as lytic lesions may not be detected by a bone scan. In patients with a single lesion, it is especially important to perform a biopsy to obtain a tissue diagnosis, since primary bone tumours may look very similar to metastases on X-ray.

The main goals of management are:

- pain relief
- preservation and restoration of function
- skeletal stabilisation
- local tumour control (e.g. relief of tumour impingement on normal structure).

Surgical intervention may be warranted where there is evidence of skeletal instability (e.g. anterior or posterior spinal column fracture) or an impending fracture (e.g. a large lytic lesion on a weight-bearing bone with more than 50% cortical involvement). Intravenous bisphosphonates (pamidronate, zoledronic acid or denosumab) are widely used for bone metastases and are effective at improving pain and in reducing further skeletal related events, such as fractures and hypercalcaemia. In certain types of cancer, such as breast and prostate, hormonal therapy may be effective. Radiotherapy, in the form of external beam therapy or systemic radionuclides (strontium treatment), can also be useful for these patients. In some settings (e.g. breast carcinoma), chemotherapy may be used in the management of bony metastases.

Malignant pleural effusion

This is a common complication of cancer and 40% of all pleural effusions are due to malignancy. The most common causes are lung and breast cancers, and the presence of an effusion indicates advanced and incurable disease. The presentation may be with dyspnoea, cough or chest discomfort, which can be dull

33.15 How to aspirate a malignant pleural effusion

- Ask the patient to sit up and lean forwards slightly.
- Identify a suitable site for aspiration. Typically, this should be in the mid-scapular line, below the top of the fluid level and above the diaphragm.
- Confirm that the site is below the fluid level by reviewing the chest X-ray and percussing the chest.
- Infiltrate the skin and the intercostal space immediately above the rib below with 1% lidocaine.
- As you advance the needle, aspirate at each step prior to injecting the local anaesthetic.
- On reaching the pleural cavity, you should be able to aspirate pleural fluid; when you do, note the depth of the needle.
- Insert a thoracentesis needle into the pleural space by advancing it along the same track as was used for the local anaesthetic and connect it to a three-way tap and container to collect the fluid.
- Drain the pleural effusion, to a maximum of 1.5 L. If the effusion is larger than this, repeat the procedure on further occasions as necessary.
- Consider using ultrasound-guided placement of a drainage catheter if the effusion proves difficult to drain.
- Permanent drains can be useful for some patients with recurrent effusions where pleurodesis is not possible.

or pleuritic in nature. Diagnosis and management of ascites are discussed on page 863.

Investigations and management

Pleural aspirate is the key investigation and may show the presence of malignant cells. Malignant effusions are commonly blood-stained and are exudates with a raised fluid to serum LDH ratio (>0.6) and a raised fluid to serum protein ratio (>0.5). Treatment should focus on palliation of symptoms and be tailored to the patient's physical condition and prognosis. Aspiration alone may be an appropriate treatment in frail patients with a limited life expectancy (Box 33.15). Those who present with malignant pleural effusion as the initial manifestation of breast cancer, small cell lung cancer, germ cell tumours or lymphoma should have the fluid aspirated and should be given systemic chemotherapy to try to treat disease in the pleural space. Treatment options for patients with recurrent pleural effusion include pleurodesis, pleurectomy and pleuroperitoneal shunt. Ideally, pleurodesis should be attempted once effusions recur after initial drainage.

Therapeutics in oncology

Anti-cancer therapy may be either curative or palliative, and this distinction influences the approach to management of individual patients. The goal of treatment should be recorded in the medical notes.

- *Palliative chemotherapy* is the most common treatment and is primarily used to treat patients with metastatic disease. The goal is an improvement in symptoms with a focus on improving quality of life, and any survival increments are secondary. As a result, the treatment should be well tolerated and should aim to minimise adverse effects.
- *Adjuvant chemotherapy* is given after an initial intervention that is designed to cyto-reduce the tumour bulk and remove all macroscopic disease. Chemotherapy is then given with the intention of eradicating the micrometastatic disease that remains. The focus is on achieving an improvement in disease-free and overall survival.

33

- *Neoadjuvant chemotherapy* or primary medical therapy is where chemotherapy is administered first before a planned cyto-reductive procedure. This can result in a reduced requirement for surgery, increase the likelihood of successful debulking, reduce the duration of hospitalisation and improve the fitness of the patient prior to interval debulking. This approach has the same goals as adjuvant treatment but creates an opportunity for translational research to measure responses to treatment and correlate with subsequent specimens removed at the time of surgery.
- *Chemoprevention* is the use of pharmacological agents to prevent cancer developing in patients identified as being at particular risk. The agents used therefore aim to modify risk and, as such, should not have significant adverse effects.

Surgical treatment

Surgery has a pivotal role in the management of cancer. There are three main situations in which it is necessary.

Biopsy

In the vast majority of cases, a histological or cytological diagnosis of cancer is necessary, and tissue will also provide important information such as tumour type and differentiation, to assist subsequent management. Cytology can be obtained with fine needle aspiration but a biopsy is usually preferred. This can be a core biopsy, an image-guided biopsy or an excision biopsy.

Excision

The main curative management of most solid cancers is surgical excision. In early, localised cases of colorectal, breast and lung cancer, cure rates are high with surgery. There is increasing evidence that outcome is related to surgical expertise, and most multidisciplinary teams include surgeons experienced in the management of a particular cancer. There are some cancers for which surgery is one of two or more options for primary management, and the role of the multidisciplinary team is to recommend appropriate treatment for a specific patient. Examples include prostate and transitional cell carcinoma of the bladder, in which radiotherapy and surgery may be equally effective.

Palliation

Surgical procedures are often the quickest and most effective way of palliating symptoms. Examples include the treatment of faecal incontinence with a defunctioning colostomy; fixation of pathological fractures and decompression of spinal cord compression; and the treatment of fungating skin lesions by 'toilet' surgery. A more specialist role for surgery is in resection of residual masses after chemotherapy and, in very selected cases, resection of metastases.

Systemic chemotherapy

Chemotherapeutic drugs are classified by their mode of action. They have the greatest activity in proliferating cells and this provides the rationale for their use in the treatment of cancer. Chemotherapeutic agents are not specific for cancer cells, however, and the side-effects of treatment are a result of their antiproliferative actions in normal tissues such as the bone marrow, skin and gut.

Combination therapy

The dosing schedule and interval are determined by the choice of drugs and recovery of the cancer and normal tissues. For most common chemotherapy regimens, the treatment is administered every 21 or 28 days, which defines one cycle. A course of treatment often uses up to 6 cycles of treatment. An increase in effectiveness can be achieved by changing the approach to treatment. In some cases this will increase toxicity too, but it can change the nature of the toxicity and such developments are evaluated in clinical trials.

- *Low-dose therapy* is the standard approach and most palliative chemotherapy is given in this manner. The next cycle is started once bone marrow function has recovered sufficiently to start the treatment (neutrophils $>1.0\times10^9$/L and platelets $>100\times10^9$/L).
- *High-dose therapy* uses a higher individual drug dose to achieve a higher cell kill but results in more bone marrow toxicity. This can be minimised by using G–CSF. This approach allows more drug to be delivered within the same schedule of administration, but the total received dose can be less than the intended dose due to limitations of non-haematological toxicity.
- *Dose-dense therapy* involves fractionating the intended dose of drug and administering each fraction on a more frequent basis (often weekly). Each individual dose produces less toxicity but the anti-cancer effect is related to the accumulative dose over time. Such an approach can overcome drug resistance, produce a greater cell kill and, in some cases, produce a response with weekly administration when the 3-weekly schedule demonstrates a lack of response or even disease progression.
- *Alternating therapy* involves giving different drugs in an alternating manner. This is most commonly used with haematological malignancies and is designed to treat different subpopulations of cancer cells where individual clones of cells might be resistant to one or more of the agents.

Adverse effects

Most cytotoxics have a narrow therapeutic window or index and can have significant adverse effects, as shown in Figure 33.6. Considerable supportive therapy is often required to enable patients to tolerate therapy and achieve benefit. Nausea and vomiting are common, but with modern antiemetics, regimens such as the combination of dexamethasone and highly selective 5-hydroxytryptamine (5-HT$_3$, serotonin) receptor antagonists like ondansetron, most patients now receive chemotherapy without any significant problems. Myelosuppression is common to almost all cytotoxics and this not only limits the dose of drug but also can cause life-threatening complications. The risk of neutropenia can be reduced with the use of specific growth factors that accelerate the repopulation of myeloid precursor cells. The most commonly employed is G–CSF, which is widely used in conjunction with chemotherapy regimens that induce a high rate of neutropenia. More recently, it has been used to 'accelerate' the administration of chemotherapy, enabling standard doses to be given at shorter intervals where the rate-limiting factor has been the time taken for the peripheral neutrophil count to recover. Accelerated chemotherapy regimens have now been demonstrated to offer therapeutic advantages in small cell lung cancer, lymphoma and possibly breast cancer.

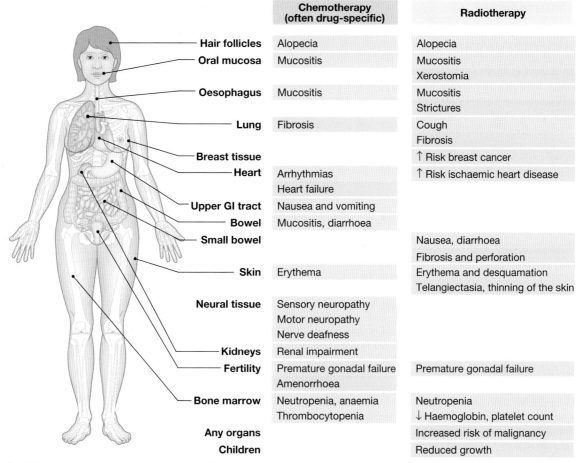

	Chemotherapy (often drug-specific)	Radiotherapy
Hair follicles	Alopecia	Alopecia
Oral mucosa	Mucositis	Mucositis Xerostomia
Oesophagus	Mucositis	Mucositis Strictures
Lung	Fibrosis	Cough Fibrosis
Breast tissue		↑ Risk breast cancer
Heart	Arrhythmias Heart failure	↑ Risk ischaemic heart disease
Upper GI tract	Nausea and vomiting	
Bowel	Mucositis, diarrhoea	
Small bowel		Nausea, diarrhoea Fibrosis and perforation
Skin	Erythema	Erythema and desquamation Telangiectasia, thinning of the skin
Neural tissue	Sensory neuropathy Motor neuropathy Nerve deafness	
Kidneys	Renal impairment	
Fertility	Premature gonadal failure Amenorrhoea	Premature gonadal failure
Bone marrow	Neutropenia, anaemia Thrombocytopenia	Neutropenia ↓ Haemoglobin, platelet count
Any organs		Increased risk of malignancy
Children		Reduced growth

Fig. 33.6 Adverse effects of chemotherapy and radiotherapy. Acute effects are shown in pink and late effects in blue.

Radiation therapy

Radiation therapy (radiotherapy) involves treating the cancer with ionising radiation; for certain localised cancers it may be curative. Ionising radiation can be delivered by radiation emitted from the decay of radioactive isotopes or by high-energy radiation beams, usually X-rays. Three methods are usually employed:

- *Teletherapy*: application from a distance by a linear accelerator.
- *Brachytherapy*: direct application of a radioactive source on to or into a tumour. This allows the delivery of a very high, localised dose of radiation and is integral to the management of localised cancers of the head and neck, and cancer of the cervix and endometrium.
- *Intravenous injection of a radioisotope*: such as ^{131}iodine for cancer of the thyroid and ^{89}strontium for the treatment of bone metastases from prostate cancer.

The majority of treatments are delivered by linear accelerators, which produce electron or X-ray beams of high energy that are used to target tumour tissue. The biological effect of ionising radiation is to cause lethal and sublethal damage to DNA. Since normal tissues are also radiosensitive, treatment has to be designed to maximise exposure of the tumour and minimise exposure of normal tissues. This is possible with modern imaging techniques such as CT and MRI, which allow better visualisation of normal and tumour tissue. In addition, techniques such as conformal radiotherapy, in which shaped rather than conventional square or rectangular beams are used, allow much more precise targeting of therapy to the tumour, and reduce the volume of normal tissue irradiated by up to 40% compared to non-conformal techniques.

Biological differences between normal and tumour tissues are used to obtain therapeutic gain. Fundamental to this is fractionation, which entails delivering the radiation as a number of small doses on a daily basis. This allows normal cells to recover from radiation damage but recovery occurs to a lesser degree in malignant cells. Fractionation regimens vary, but radical treatments given with curative intent are usually delivered in 20–30 fractions given daily on 5 days a week, over 4–6 weeks. Radiotherapy can be extremely useful for the alleviation of symptoms, and for palliative treatments such as this a smaller number of fractions (1–5) is usually adequate.

Both normal and malignant tissues vary widely in their sensitivity to radiotherapy. Germ cell tumours and lymphomas are extremely radiosensitive and relatively low doses are adequate for cure, but most cancers require doses close to or beyond that which can be tolerated by adjacent normal structures. Normal tissue also varies in its radiosensitivity, the central nervous system, small bowel and lung being among the most sensitive. The side-effects of radiotherapy (see Fig. 33.6) depend on the normal tissues treated, their radiosensitivity and the dose delivered.

33

Adverse effects

An acute inflammatory reaction commonly occurs towards the end of most radical treatments and is localised to the area treated. For example, skin reactions are common with breast or chest wall radiotherapy, and proctitis and cystitis with treatment to the bladder or prostate. These acute reactions settle over a period of a few weeks after treatment, assuming normal tissue tolerance has not been exceeded. Late effects of radiotherapy develop 6 weeks or more after treatment and occur in 5–10% of patients. Examples include brachial nerve damage and subcutaneous fibrosis after breast cancer treatment, and shrinkage and fibrosis of the bladder after treatment for bladder cancer. There is a risk of inducing cancer after radiotherapy, which varies depending on the site treated and on whether the patient has had other treatment such as chemotherapy.

Hormone therapy

Hormone therapy is most commonly used in the treatment of breast cancer and prostate cancer. Breast tumours that are positive for expression of the oestrogen receptor (ER) respond well to anti-oestrogen therapy, and assessment of ER status is now standard in the diagnosis of breast cancer. Several drugs are now available that reduce oestrogen levels or block the effects of oestrogen on the receptor. When targeted appropriately, adjuvant hormone therapy reduces the risk of relapse and death at least as much as chemotherapy, and in advanced cases can induce stable disease and remissions that may last months to years, with acceptable toxicity. Hormonal manipulation may be effective in other cancers. In prostate cancer, hormonal therapy (e.g. luteinising hormone releasing hormone (LHRH) analogues such as goserelin and/or anti-androgens such as bicalutamide) aimed at reducing androgen levels can provide good long-term control of advanced disease, but there is no convincing evidence that it is an effective therapy following potentially curative surgery. Progestogens are active in the treatment of endometrial and breast cancer. In the metastatic setting, progestogen use (e.g. megestrol acetate) is associated with response rates of 20–40% in endometrial cancer. In breast cancer, progestogens are used in patients whose disease has progressed with conventional anti-oestrogen therapy. Their exact mechanism in this setting is not fully understood.

Immunotherapy

A profound stimulus to the patient's immune system can sometimes alter the natural history of a malignancy, and the discovery of interferons was the impetus for much research. Although solid tumours show little benefit, interferons are active in melanoma and lymphoma, and there is evidence that they are beneficial as adjuvants (after surgery and chemotherapy, respectively) to delay recurrence. Whether interferon-induced stimulation of the immune system is capable of eradicating microscopic disease remains unproven. More powerful immune responses can be achieved with potent agents like IL-2 but the accompanying systemic toxicity is a problem still to be overcome. The most striking example of successful immunotherapy is that with rituximab, an antibody against the common B-cell antigen CD20. It increases complete response rates and improves survival in diffuse large cell non-Hodgkin lymphoma when combined with chemotherapy, and is effective in palliating advanced follicular non-Hodgkin lymphoma (p. 965).

Biological therapies

Advances in knowledge about the molecular basis of cancer have resulted in the development of a new generation of treatments to block the signalling pathways responsible for the growth of specific tumours. This has created the potential to target cancer cells more selectively, with reduced toxicity to normal tissues. Some examples are discussed below, but in the years to come many more such agents will come into clinical use, with the potential to revolutionise our approach to some cancers.

Gefitinib/erlotinib

These agents inhibit the activity of the EGFR, which is over-expressed in many solid tumours. However, the drugs' activity does not depend on the amount of receptor over-expression but rather on factors such as gene copy number and mutation status.

Imatinib

Imatinib was developed to inhibit the *BCR-ABL* gene product, tyrosine kinase, that is responsible for chronic myeloid leukaemia (p. 958), and it does this extremely effectively. It is also active in malignant gastrointestinal stromal tumour (GIST), a type of sarcoma that has over-expression of another cell surface tyrosine kinase, c-kit. This agent has good tolerability and is particularly useful in GIST, where conventional chemotherapy is less effective.

Bevacizumab

This is a humanised monoclonal antibody that inhibits vascular endothelial growth factor A (VEGF-A), a key stimulant of angiogenesis in tumours. Bevacizumab has activity in colorectal, lung, breast, renal and ovarian cancers, although the licence was subsequently revoked for breast cancer; while bevacizumab slows the rate of progression of metastatic breast cancer, it had little impact on survival or improved quality of life.

Trastuzumab

Trastuzumab (Herceptin) targets the HER2 receptor, an oncogene that is over-expressed in around one-third of breast cancers and in a number of other solid tumours (e.g. gastric cancer). It is effective as a single-agent therapy, but also improves survival in patients with advanced breast cancer when used in conjunction with chemotherapy. Unfortunately, trastuzumab can induce cardiac failure by an unknown biological mechanism, especially in combination with doxorubicin.

Evaluation of treatment

The evaluation of treatment includes an assessment of overall survival duration, response to treatment, remission rate, disease-free survival and response duration, quality of life and treatment toxicity. Uniform criteria have been established to measure these, including the response evaluation criteria in solid tumours (RECIST, Box 33.16) and common toxicity criteria. This allows clinicians to inform patients accurately about the prognosis, effectiveness and toxicity of chemotherapy and empowers patients to take an active role in treatment decisions.

Late toxicity of therapy

The late toxicities of treatment for cancer are particularly important for patients where the multimodality therapy is given with curative

33.16 Response evaluation criteria in solid tumours (RECIST)

Response	Criteria
Complete response (CR)	Disappearance of all target lesions
Partial response (PR)	At least a 30% decrease in the sum of the longest diameter (LD) of target lesions, taking as reference the baseline sum LD
Progressive disease (PD)	At least a 20% increase in the sum of the LD of target lesions, taking as reference the smallest sum LD recorded since the treatment started and at least 5 mm increase or the appearance of one or more new lesions
Stable disease (SD)	Neither sufficient shrinkage to qualify for PR nor sufficient increase to qualify for PD, taking as reference the smallest sum LD since the treatment started

33.17 Specific cancers covered in other chapters

Bladder cancer	p. 435
Colorectal cancer	p. 827
Familial cancer syndromes	p. 56
Gastric cancer	p. 803
Hepatocellular carcinoma	p. 890
Leukaemia	p. 954
Lung cancer	p. 598
Lymphoma	p. 961
Mesothelioma	p. 618
Myeloma	p. 966
Oesophageal cancer	p. 796
Pancreatic cancer	p. 842
Prostate cancer	p. 438
Renal cancer	p. 434
Seminoma	p. 439
Skin cancer	p. 1229
Teratoma	p. 439
Thyroid cancer	p. 649

33.18 Five-year survival rates for breast cancer by stage

Tumour stage	Stage definition	5-year survival (%)
I	Tumour <2 cm, no lymph nodes	96
II	Tumour 2–5 cm and/or mobile axillary lymph nodes	81
III	Chest wall or skin fixation and/or fixed axillary lymph nodes	52
IV	Metastasis	18

intent, the patient is young and more patients are living longer. This can cause considerable morbidity: for example, radiotherapy can retard bone and cartilage growth, impair intellect and cognitive function, and cause dysfunction of the hypothalamus, pituitary and thyroid glands. Late consequences of chemotherapy include heart failure due to cardiotoxicity, pulmonary fibrosis, nephrotoxicity and neurotoxicity.

Premature gonadal failure can result from chemotherapy or radiotherapy and leave a patient subfertile. Patients should be made aware of this before treatment is initiated, as it may be possible to store sperm for male patients before treatment starts; this should always be offered, if practical. Egg or embryo banking after in vitro fertilisation may be an option for young women. Sterility develops at higher radiotherapy doses but erectile dysfunction is seen in patients receiving high radiotherapy doses to the pelvis, as in prostate cancer. Additional social or psychological support may be required. Infertility and pubertal delay are potential late effects of therapy in children, especially boys.

Second malignancies may be induced by cancer treatment and occur at greatest frequency following chemoradiation. Secondary acute leukaemia (mostly AML) can occur 1–2 years after treatment with topoisomerase II inhibitors, or 2–5 years after treatment with alkylating agents. The most common second malignancy within a radiation field is osteosarcoma but others include soft tissue sarcoma and leukaemia.

Specific cancers

The diagnosis and management of cancers are discussed in more detail elsewhere in the book (Box 33.17). Here we discuss the pathogenesis, clinical features, investigation and management of common tumours that are not covered elsewhere.

Breast cancer

Globally, the incidence of breast cancer is second only to that of lung cancer, and the disease represents the leading cause of cancer-related deaths among women. Invasive ductal carcinoma with or without ductal carcinoma in situ (DCIS) is the most common histology, accounting for 70%, whilst invasive lobular carcinoma accounts for most of the remaining cases. DCIS constitutes 20% of breast cancers detected by mammography

screening. It is multifocal in one-third of women and has a high risk of becoming invasive (10% at 5 years following excision only). Pure DCIS does not cause lymph node metastases, although these are found in 2% of cases where nodes are examined, owing to undetected invasive cancer. Lobular carcinoma in situ (LCIS) is a predisposing risk factor for developing cancer in either breast (7% at 10 years). The survival for breast cancer by stage is outlined in Box 33.18.

Pathogenesis

Both genetic and hormonal factors play a role; about 5–10% of breast cancers are hereditary and occur in patients with mutations of BRCA1, BRCA2, AT or TP53 genes. Prolonged oestrogen exposure associated with early menarche, late menopause and use of hormone replacement therapy (HRT) has been associated with an increased risk. Other risk factors include obesity, alcohol intake, nulliparity and late first pregnancy. There is no definite evidence linking use of the contraceptive pill to breast cancer.

Clinical features

Breast cancer usually presents as a result of mammographic screening or as a palpable mass with nipple discharge in 10% and pain in 7% of patients. Less common presentations include inflammatory carcinoma with diffuse induration of the skin of the breast, and this confers an adverse prognosis. Around 40% of patients will have axillary nodal disease, with likelihood correlating with increasing size of the primary tumour. Distant metastases are infrequently present at diagnosis and the most common sites of spread are bone (70%), lung (60%), liver (55%), pleura (40%), adrenals (35%), skin (30%) and brain (10–20%).

Investigations

Following clinical examination, patients should have imaging with mammography or ultrasound evaluation, and a biopsy using fine needle aspiration for cytology or core biopsy for histology. Histological assessment should be carried out to assess tumour type and to determine oestrogen and progesterone receptor (ER/PR) status and HER2 status. If distant spread is suspected, CT of the thorax and abdomen and an isotope bone scan are required. Molecular subtyping is being used to classify tumours into four major subtypes: luminal A, luminal B, HER2 type and basal-like (often called 'triple negative', as these tumours are ER-, PR- and HER2-negative). This may allow more targeted selection of therapies in future.

Management

Surgery is the mainstay of treatment for most patients, and this can range from a lumpectomy, where only the tumour is removed, to mastectomy, where the whole breast is removed. Breast-conserving surgery is as effective as mastectomy if complete excision with negative margins can be achieved. Lymph node sampling is performed at the time of surgery. Adjuvant radiotherapy is given to reduce the risk of local recurrence to 4–6%. Adjuvant hormonal therapy improves disease-free and overall survival in pre- and post-menopausal patients who have tumours that express ER. Patients at low risk, with tumours that are small and ER-positive, require only adjuvant hormonal therapy with tamoxifen. Patients with tumours that are ER-positive and who are pre-menopausal should receive an LHRH analogue. Aromatase inhibitors also have benefit in this setting but are still under investigation.

Adjuvant chemotherapy is considered for patients at higher risk of recurrence. Factors that increase the risk of recurrence include a tumour of >1 cm, a tumour that is ER-negative or the presence of involved axillary lymph nodes. Such patients should be offered adjuvant chemotherapy, which improves disease-free and overall survival. The role of adjuvant treatment has been studied by meta-analyses and data support the use of adjuvant trastuzumab, a humanised monoclonal antibody to HER2, in addition to standard chemotherapy for women with early HER2-positive breast cancer.

Metastatic disease management includes radiotherapy to palliate painful bone metastases and second-line endocrine therapy with aromatase inhibitors, which inhibit peripheral oestrogen production in adrenal and adipose tissues. Advanced ER-negative disease may be treated with combination chemotherapy.

Ovarian cancer

Ovarian cancer is the most common gynaecological tumour in Western countries. Most ovarian cancers are epithelial in origin (90%), and up to 7% of women with ovarian cancer have a positive family history. Patients often present late in ovarian cancer with vague abdominal discomfort, low back pain, bloating, altered bowel habit and weight loss. Occasionally, peritoneal deposits are palpable as an omental 'cake' and nodules in the umbilicus (Sister Mary Joseph nodules).

Pathogenesis

Genetic and environmental factors play a role. The risk of ovarian cancer is increased in patients with BRCA1 or BRCA2 mutations, and Lynch type II families (a subtype of hereditary non-polyposis colon cancer, HNPCC) have ovarian, endometrial, colorectal and gastric tumours due to mutations of mismatch repair enzymes. Advanced age, nulliparity, ovarian stimulation and Caucasian descent all increase the risk of ovarian cancer, while suppressed ovulation appears to protect, so pregnancy, prolonged breastfeeding and the contraceptive pill have all been shown to reduce the risk of ovarian cancer.

Investigations

Initial workup for patients with suspected ovarian cancer includes imaging in the form of ultrasound and CT. Serum levels of the tumour marker CA-125 are often measured. Surgery plays a key role in the diagnosis, staging and treatment of ovarian cancer, and in early cases, palpation of viscera, peritoneal washings and biopsies are generally performed to define disease extent.

Management

In early disease, surgery followed by adjuvant chemotherapy with carboplatin, or carboplatin plus paclitaxel, is the treatment of choice. Surgery should include removal of the tumour along with total abdominal hysterectomy, bilateral salpingo-oophorectomy, and omentectomy. Even in advanced disease, surgery is undertaken to debulk the tumour and is followed by adjuvant chemotherapy, typically using carboplatin and paclitaxel. Bevacizumab is indicated for patients with high-grade tumours that are suboptimally debulked or those with a more aggressive biological pattern. Monitoring for relapse is achieved through a combination of serum CA-125 and clinical examination with CT imaging for those with suspected relapse. Second-line chemotherapy is aimed at improving symptoms and should not be used for CA-125 elevation only in the absence of symptoms. Treatments can include further platinum/paclitaxel in combination, liposomal doxorubicin or topotecan. These regimens are associated with a response rate of 10–40%. The best responses are observed in patients with a treatment-free interval of more than 12 months.

Endometrial cancer

Endometrial cancer accounts for 4% of all female malignancies, producing a 1 in 73 lifetime risk. The majority of patients are post-menopausal, with a peak incidence at 50–60 years of age. Mortality from endometrial cancer is currently falling. The most common presentation is with post-menopausal bleeding, which often results in detection of the disease before distant spread has occurred.

Pathogenesis

Oestrogen plays an important role in the pathogenesis of endometrial cancer, and factors that increase the duration of oestrogen exposure, such as nulliparity, early menarche, late menopause and unopposed HRT, increase the risk. Endometrial cancer is 10 times more common in obese women and this is thought to be due to elevated levels of oestrogens.

Investigations

The diagnosis is confirmed by endometrial biopsy.

Management

Surgery is the treatment of choice and is used for staging. A hysterectomy and bilateral salpingo-oophorectomy are performed with peritoneal cytology and, in some cases, lymph node dissection. Where the tumour extends beyond the inner 50% of the myometrium or involves the cervix and local lymph nodes, or there is lymphovascular space invasion, adjuvant pelvic radiotherapy is recommended. Chemotherapy is used as adjuvant therapy and hormonal therapy and chemotherapy are used to palliate symptoms in recurrent disease.

Cervical cancer

This is the second most common gynaecological tumour worldwide and the leading cause of death from gynaecological cancer. The incidence is decreasing in developed countries but continues to rise in developing nations. The most common presentation is with an abnormal smear test, but with locally advanced disease the presentation is with vaginal bleeding, discomfort, discharge or symptoms attributable to involvement of adjacent structures, such as bladder, or rectal or pelvic wall. Occasionally, patients present with distant metastases to bone and lung.

Pathogenesis

There is a strong association between cervical cancer and sexual activity that includes sex at a young age and multiple sexual partners. Infection with HPV has an important causal role, and this has underpinned the introduction of programmes to immunise teenagers against HPV in an effort to prevent the later development of cervical cancer (p. 342).

Investigations

Diagnosis is made by smear or cone biopsy. Further examination may require cystoscopy and flexible sigmoidoscopy if there are symptoms referable to the bladder, colon or rectum. In contrast to other gynaecological malignancies, cervical cancer is a clinically staged disease, although MRI is often used to characterise the primary tumour. A routine chest X-ray should be obtained to help rule out pulmonary metastasis. CT of the abdomen and pelvis is performed to look for metastasis in the liver and lymph nodes, and to exclude hydronephrosis and hydroureter.

Management

This depends on the stage of disease. Pre-malignant disease can be treated with laser ablation or diathermy, whereas in microinvasive disease a large loop excision of the transformation zone (LLETZ) or a simple hysterectomy is employed. Invasive but localised disease requires radical surgery, while chemotherapy and radiotherapy, including brachytherapy, may be given as primary treatment, especially in patients with adverse prognostic features such as bulky or locally advanced disease, or lymph node or parametrium invasion. In metastatic disease, cisplatin-based chemotherapy may be beneficial in improving symptoms but does not increase survival significantly.

Head and neck tumours

Head and neck cancers are typically squamous tumours that arise in the nasopharynx, hypopharynx and larynx. They are most common in elderly males but now occur with increasing frequency in a younger cohort, as well as in women, especially

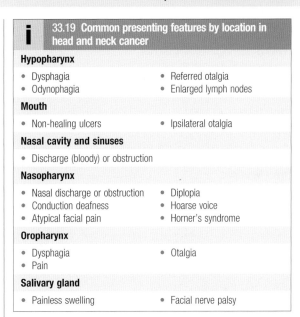

33.19 Common presenting features by location in head and neck cancer

Hypopharynx
- Dysphagia
- Odynophagia
- Referred otalgia
- Enlarged lymph nodes

Mouth
- Non-healing ulcers
- Ipsilateral otalgia

Nasal cavity and sinuses
- Discharge (bloody) or obstruction

Nasopharynx
- Nasal discharge or obstruction
- Conduction deafness
- Atypical facial pain
- Diplopia
- Hoarse voice
- Horner's syndrome

Oropharynx
- Dysphagia
- Pain
- Otalgia

Salivary gland
- Painless swelling
- Facial nerve palsy

where oropharyngeal cancers are concerned. The rising incidence of oropharyngeal cancers, especially in the developed world, is thought to be secondary to HPV infection. Presentation depends on the location of the primary tumour and the extent of disease. For example, early laryngeal cancers may present with hoarseness, while more extensive local disease may present with pain due to invasion of local structures or with a lump in the neck. Patients who present late often have pulmonary symptoms, as this is the most common site of distant metastases (Box 33.19).

Pathogenesis

The tumours are strongly associated with a history of smoking and excess alcohol intake, but other recognised risk factors include Epstein–Barr virus for nasopharyngeal cancer and HPV infection for oropharyngeal tumours.

Investigations

Careful inspection of the primary site is required as part of the staging process, and most patients will require endoscopic evaluation and examination under anaesthesia. Tissue biopsies should be taken from the most accessible site. CT of the primary site and the thorax is the investigation of choice for visualising the tumour, while MRI may be useful in certain cases.

Management

Generally speaking, the majority of patients with early or locally advanced disease are treated with curative intent. In localised disease where there is no involvement of the lymph nodes, long-term remission can be achieved in up to 90% of patients with surgery or radiotherapy. The choice of surgery versus radiotherapy often depends on patient preference, as surgical treatment can be mutilating with an adverse cosmetic outcome. Patients with lymph node involvement or metastasis are treated with a combination of surgery and radiotherapy (often with chemotherapy as a radiosensitising agent – proven agents include cisplatin or cetuximab), and this produces long-term remission in approximately 60–70% of patients. Recurrent or metastatic tumour may be palliated with further surgery or radiotherapy to aid local control, and systemic chemotherapy has a response rate of around 20–30%. Second malignancies are common (3%

33

per year) following successful treatment for primary disease, and all patients should be encouraged to give up smoking and drinking alcohol to lower their risk.

Carcinoma of unknown origin

Some patients are found to have evidence of metastatic disease at their initial presentation, prior to diagnosis of a primary site. In many cases, a subsequent biopsy reveals adenocarcinoma but the primary site is not always clear.

Investigations

In this situation, there is a temptation to investigate the patient endlessly in order to determine the original primary site. There is a compromise, however, between exhaustive investigation and obtaining sufficient information to plan appropriate management. For all patients, histological examination of an accessible site of metastasis is required. The architecture of the tissue can assist the pathologist in determining the likely primary site, and therefore it is better to perform a biopsy rather than fine needle aspiration. The greater volume of tissue permits the use of immunohistochemistry. Extensive imaging to search for the primary is rarely indicated; a careful history to identify symptoms and risk factors (including familial) will often permit a judicious choice of imaging and other diagnostic tests, reserving additional tests for specific patients (Box 33.20).

Management

Management of the patient will depend on that person's circumstances, as well as on the site(s) involved and the likely primary sites. The overriding principle is to ensure that a curable diagnosis has been excluded. For example, lung metastases from a testicular teratoma do not preclude cure; nor do one or two liver metastases from a colorectal cancer. Early discussion with an oncologist within a multidisciplinary team is essential and avoids unnecessary investigation; for example, a single hCG-based pregnancy test in a young man with lung metastases might confirm the presence of a teratoma and allow rapid administration of potentially curative chemotherapy. Treatment should not necessarily wait for a definitive diagnosis; appropriate analgesia,

radiotherapy and surgical palliation can all be helpful. Some patients remain free of cancer for some years after resection of a single metastasis of an adenocarcinoma of unknown primary, justifying this approach in selected patients.

In those with no obvious primary, systemic chemotherapy may achieve some reduction in tumour burden and alleviation of symptoms, but long-term survival is rare.

Multidisciplinary teams

The multidisciplinary team (MDT) is well established in oncology and meets on a regular basis to discuss patient progress and provide a forum for patient-centred, interdisciplinary communication to coordinate care and decision-making. It is a platform on which individual clinicians can discuss complex cases or situations and draw on the collective experience of the team membership to decide on the best approach for an individual patient. This can be particularly important when discussing patients with a rare condition or in a rare situation.

Specific roles of the MDT include:

- planning the diagnostic and staging procedures
- deciding on the appropriate primary treatment modality (most commonly surgery but the use of neoadjuvant chemotherapy before interval surgery is increasing)
- arranging review by the oncology team to plan assessment of the patient prior to systemic therapy or radiotherapy
- discussing additional support requirements for the individual patient, such as physiotherapy; psychological support; symptom control; nutritional care or rehabilitation in the post-operative period
- ensuring access to accurate information on treatment, prognosis, side-effects and other related matters, such as stoma care
- planning surveillance strategies
- ensuring the appropriate transition from treatment with curative intent to that of palliation of symptoms
- promoting recruitment into clinical trials
- agreeing on operational policies to deliver high-quality care to patients
- planning and reviewing audit data to ensure the delivery of quality care to patients by the team.

Further information

Books and journal articles

Cassidy J, Bissett D, Spence RAJ, et al. Oxford handbook of oncology, 4th edn. Oxford: Oxford University Press; 2015.
Dark GG. Oncology at a glance. Chichester: Wiley–Blackwell; 2013.
Hanahan D, Weinberg RA. The hallmarks of cancer: the next generation. Cell 2011; 144:646–674.
Tobias J, Hochhauser D. Cancer and its management, 7th edn. Chichester: Wiley–Blackwell; 2014.

Websites

cancer.org American Cancer Society: clinical practice guidelines.
ctep.cancer.gov/reporting/ctc.html Common toxicity criteria.
info.cancerresearchuk.org/cancerstats/ A wide range of cancer statistics that can be sorted by type or geographical location.

---

i **33.20 Initial diagnostic tests in patients presenting with carcinoma of unknown primary***

- Detailed history and examination, including breast, nodal areas, skin, genital, rectal and pelvic regions
- Full blood count, urea and electrolytes, renal function, liver function tests, calcium, urinalysis, lactate dehydrogenase
- Chest X-ray
- Myeloma screen (if lytic bone lesions)
- CT scan of chest, abdomen and pelvis
- Symptom-directed upper and lower gastrointestinal endoscopy
- Tumour markers: prostate-specific antigen (PSA) in men, cancer antigen 125 (CA-125) in women with peritoneal malignancy or ascites, α-fetoprotein (AFP) and human chorionic gonadotrophin (hCG)
- Testicular ultrasound (if clinical features suggest germ cell tumour)
- Histological examination of biopsy, with immunohistochemistry if required

*Offer when clinically appropriate.

LA Colvin
M Fallon

34

Pain and palliative care

Pain 1338

Functional anatomy and physiology 1338
Investigations 1342
Principles of management 1343
Interventions 1344
Chronic pain syndromes 1348

Palliative care 1349

Presenting problems in palliative care 1350
 Pain 1350
 Breathlessness 1353
 Cough 1353
 Nausea and vomiting 1353
 Gastrointestinal obstruction 1354
 Weight loss 1354
 Anxiety and depression 1354
 Delirium and agitation 1354
 Dehydration 1354

Death and dying 1354

Pain

Pain is defined as 'an unpleasant sensory and emotional experience associated with actual or potential tissue damage or described in terms of such damage'. It is one of the most common symptoms for which people seek health-care advice. Our understanding of the mechanisms of pain has evolved considerably from Hippocrates' suggestion in 450 BC that pain arose as a result of an imbalance in vital fluids. We now know that pain is a complex symptom that is influenced and modified by many social, cultural and emotional factors, as illustrated in Figure 34.1. The sensation of acute pain that occurs in response to inflammation or tissue damage plays an important role in protection from further injury. Chronic pain serves no useful function but results in significant distress and suffering for the patient affected, as well as having a wider societal impact.

Functional anatomy and physiology

The functional anatomy of the somatosensory system is shown in Figures 25.3 and 25.6 (pp. 1065 and 1068). Here, discussion will focus on the mechanisms and mediators that are involved in pain processing.

Peripheral nerves

Peripheral nerves contain several types of neuron. These can be classified into two groups, depending on whether or not they are surrounded by a myelin sheath. Myelinated neurons have a fast conduction velocity and are responsible for transmission of various sensory signals, such as proprioception, light touch, heat and cold, and the detection of localised pains, such as pin-prick. Unmyelinated fibres have a much slower conduction

Fibre type	Diameter (μm)	Conduction velocity (ms⁻¹)	Function
Large myelinated			
Aα	12–20	70–120	Proprioception / Motor to muscle fibres
Aβ	5–12	30–70	Light touch, pressure
A-	3–6	15–30	Motor to muscle spindles
Small myelinated			
A	2–5	12–30	Well-localised pain / Thermal sensation
B	<3	3–15	Pre-ganglionic autonomic
Unmyelinated			
C	0.4–1.3	0.5–3	Diffuse pain / Poorly localised thermal sensation / Post-ganglionic autonomic

i 34.1 Types of nerve fibre

velocity and are responsible for transmitting diffuse and poorly localised pain, as well as other sensations (Box 34.1).

Sensory neurons (also known as primary afferent neurons) connect the spinal cord to the periphery and supply a defined territory or a dermatome, which can be used to identify the position of a nerve lesion (see Fig. 25.10, p. 1071). In healthy individuals dermatomes have distinct borders, but in pathological pain syndromes these may become blurred as the result of neuronal plasticity, which means that pain may be felt in an area adjacent to that supplied by a specific nerve root. Autonomic neurons also contain pain fibres and are responsible for transmitting visceral sensations, such as colic. In general, visceral pain is diffuse and less well localised than pain transmitted by sensory neurons.

Anatomical features of the afferent pain pathway are illustrated in Figure 34.2. Pain signals are transmitted from the periphery to the spinal cord by sensory neurons. These have the following components:

- *A cell body*, containing the nucleus, which is situated in the dorsal root ganglion close to the spinal cord. The cell body is essential for survival of the neuron, production of neurotransmitters and neuronal function.
- *The nerve fibre (axon) and peripheral nerve endings*, which are located in the periphery and contain a range of receptors in the neuronal membrane.
- *Specialised receptors* in the periphery, consisting of bare nerve endings known as nociceptors or pain receptors, which are activated by various mediators. They are situated mainly in the epidermis.
- *The central termination*, which travels to the dorsal horn of the spinal cord to form the first central synapse with neurons that transmit pain sensation to the brain.

When a noxious stimulus is encountered, activation of nociceptors leads to generation of an action potential, which travels upwards to the dorsal root ganglion and also stimulates the release of neurotransmitters that have secondary effects on surrounding neurons.

Spinal cord

Sensory neurons, through their central termination, synapse with second-order neurons in the dorsal horn of the spinal cord. There is considerable modulation of pain messages at

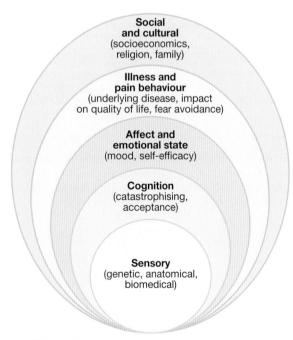

Fig. 34.1 The biopsychosocial model of pain. The perception of pain as a symptom is dependent not only on sensory inputs but also on the individual's cognitive reaction to the pain, their emotional state, their underlying disease and their social and cultural background.

Social and cultural (socioeconomics, religion, family)

Illness and pain behaviour (underlying disease, impact on quality of life, fear avoidance)

Affect and emotional state (mood, self-efficacy)

Cognition (catastrophising, acceptance)

Sensory (genetic, anatomical, biomedical)

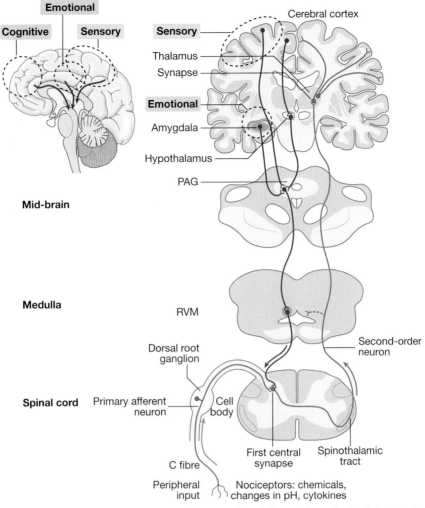

Fig. 34.2 Ascending and descending pain pathways. Ascending pathways are shown in blue and descending in red. Pain signals are detected in the periphery by nociceptors, which are activated by chemicals, changes in pH and cytokines. The signal is transmitted by the primary afferent neuron to the spinal cord, where there is a synapse with a second-order neuron, which transmits the signal onwards to the thalamus. Thereafter, the pain signal is transmitted to the cerebral cortex. The intensity of pain signals is subject to extensive modulation at several levels within the nervous system. Cognitive influences derived from the frontal lobe, coupled with sensory influences from cortex and emotional influences from the amygdyla, affect pain perception in the mid-brain around the periaqueductal gray matter (PAG) and the rostroventrolateral medulla (RVM) in the medulla. These structures form part of the descending modulatory systems, which, under normal circumstances, inhibit pain perception. In some chronic pain states, however, dysfunction of the descending pathways can occur, increasing pain.

this site, both from local neurons within the spinal cord and from neurons that descend from the brain, as depicted in Figure 25.11 (p. 1072). Several neurotransmitters are involved in pain processing at this level and these are summarised in Box 34.2. They include amino acids, such as glycine and γ-aminobutyric acid (GABA), which are inhibitory, and glutamate, which is excitatory; neuropeptides, such as substance P and calcitonin gene-related peptide (CGRP); and endorphins. Whether or not they increase or decrease pain perception depends on the connectivity of the neurons on which they act.

Central processing of pain

The signals transmitted by second-order neurons in the spinal cord are relayed to the sensory cortex by third-order neurons, which synapse with second-order neurons in the thalamus. At this site, perception of pain is influenced by interactions between a range of structures in the brain, where sensory, cognitive and emotional aspects are integrated. This is termed the pain neuromatrix (Fig. 34.2). Signals within the neuromatrix are multidirectional in nature, involving modulation of incoming messages by the cerebral cortex (top-down regulation), as well as a complex network of connections between other subcortical structures. Under normal conditions, there is a degree of descending inhibition from the brainstem that reduces input from peripheral stimuli.

It is thought that chronic widespread pain (CWP) and opioid-induced hyperalgesia may result, at least in part, from abnormalities in central processing of pain signals. It has also been suggested that variations in the levels of descending inhibition between individuals may make some people more vulnerable than others to developing chronic pain. Over recent years, there has been increasing interest in the role that glial cells (see Fig. 25.1, p. 1064) play in pain processing. Both astrocytes and microglial cells can become activated in chronic pain states and release

34

i 34.2 Neurotransmitters and receptors involved in pain processing in the spinal cord

Neurotransmitter	Receptor(s)	Receptor type	Comments*
Amino acids			
Glutamate	AMPA	Ion channel	Excitatory; permeable to cations: can be Ca^{2+}, Na^+ or K^+, depending on subunit structure
	NMDA	Ion channel	Excitatory; blocked by Mg^{2+} in the resting state; block can be altered if membrane potential changes; permeable to Ca^{2+}, Na^+ and K^+
	Kainate	Ion channel	Post synaptic – excitatory
	Gp I	GPCR	Pre-synaptic – inhibitory through GABA release; permeable to Na^+ and K^+
	Gp II	GPCR	Activates a range of signalling pathways; long-term effects on synaptic excitability
	Gp III	GPCR	Probably inhibitory; can decrease cAMP production; pre-synaptic; decreases glutamate release
Glycine	GlyR	Ion channel	Mainly inhibitory; permeable to Cl^-; blocked by caffeine
GABA	$GABA_A$	Ion channel	Mainly inhibitory in spinal cord; permeable to Cl^-; indirectly modulated by benzodiazepines (increased ion channel opening); not specifically involved in nociception, generally depressant effect on spinal cord activity
	$GABA_B$	GPCR	Predominantly inhibitory; activated by baclofen
Neuropeptides			
Substance P	Neurokinin receptors	GPCR	Mainly excitatory; increased in inflammation, decreased in neuropathic pain
Cholecystokinin	CCKRs1–8	GPCR	Excitatory; clinical trials of antagonists in progress
Calcitonin gene-related peptide	CALCRL	GPCR	Excitatory; slows degradation of substance P; implicated in migraine
Opioids			
Dynorphin	OP1 (kappa)	GPCR	Excitatory?; may be pro-nociceptive
β-endorphin	OP3 (mu)	GPCR	Inhibitory
Nociceptin	ORL-1	GPCR	Inhibitory; also expressed by immune cells

*Excitatory = increased pain; inhibitory = reduced pain.
(AMPA = α-amino 3-hydroxy, 5-methyl, 4-isoxazole propionic acid; CALCRL = calcitonin receptor-like receptor; cAMP = cyclic adenosine monophosphate; GABA = γ-aminobutyric acid; Gp = group; GPCR = G-protein-coupled receptor; NMDA = N-methyl-D-aspartate; OP = opioid; ORL = opioid-like receptor)

pro-inflammatory cytokines, as well as altering re-uptake of excitatory neurotransmitters such as glutamate, which can influence pain perception considerably. As our understanding of these processes improves, there is increasing potential to develop novel therapies targeted at these mediators, with some early clinical studies in neuropathic pain.

Sensitisation

Sensitisation is one of the key features of pain processing. It refers to the fact that both peripheral and central nervous systems adapt rapidly to the presence of pain, especially in response to tissue damage. This adaptive process is called neuronal plasticity. In some situations, neuronal plasticity can lead to prolonged changes in the pathways that are involved in detecting and processing nociceptive stimuli, resulting in chronic pain syndromes. The specific changes in key neurotransmitters and receptors differ between chronic pain states, with implications for the efficacy of treatments. For example, μ-opioid receptors are down-regulated in neuropathic pain, potentially leading to limited opioid responsiveness.

Peripheral sensitisation

Peripheral sensitisation can occur in association with a variety of clinical conditions, including sepsis, cancer, inflammatory disease, injury, surgery and obesity. The final common pathway by which sensitisation takes place in all of these conditions is inflammation. Inflammation is accompanied by increased capillary permeability and tissue oedema with the release of a diverse range of mediators, including bradykinin, hydrogen ions, prostaglandins and adenosine, which bind to receptors and ion channels on nociceptors of primary afferent neurons (Fig. 34.3). The signalling pathways activated by these mediators generate action potentials, which are transmitted by sensory neurons to the spinal cord. If these pain-provoking stimuli persist, the activation threshold of sensory neurons is reduced, resulting in an increased transmission of pain signals to the spinal cord.

Central sensitisation

Sensitisation may also take place at the level of the spinal cord in response to a sustained painful stimulus. It can occur acutely and rapidly, such as immediately after surgery, or may progress to chronic changes, such as chronic infection, cancer, repeated surgery or multiple traumatic episodes. Glutamate, acting via the N-methyl-D-aspartate (NMDA) receptor complex, plays a key role in central sensitisation (Fig. 34.4). In response to a sustained peripheral painful stimulus, increased amounts of glutamate are released in the spinal cord, overcoming the inhibitory action of magnesium ions and resulting in activation of the NMDA receptor. This initiates a cascade of intracellular signalling events that lead to prolonged modifications of somatosensory processing, with amplification of pain responses within the spinal cord and continued neuronal firing, even after the noxious stimulus has stopped. This phenomenon is termed 'after-discharge'. In neuropathic pain, prolonged activation of the NMDA pathway results in a decrease in the number of inhibitory interneurons, which further potentiates pain.

Genetic determinants of pain perception

There are marked ethnic and individual variations in how people respond to painful stimuli and studies in twins have estimated

Fig. 34.3 Mechanisms of peripheral sensitisation. [A] Sensory nerve terminating with nociceptor in skin. [B] Peripheral nociceptors express various receptors and ion channels that act as mediators of pain. They include sodium channels implicated in congenital pain syndromes; the purinergic 2X (P2X) receptor for adenosine triphosphate (ATP); members of the transient receptor potential (TRP) superfamily of ion channel receptors, which detect changes in osmolality and temperature; acid-sensing ion channel (ASIC) receptors, which detect hydrogen ions; G-protein-coupled receptors, which detect bradykinin (BK), prostaglandins and ATP; and the neurotrophic tyrosine kinase 1 (NTRK1) receptor, which detects nerve growth factor (NGF). [C] Activation of these receptors by ligands, hydrogen ion [H⁺] and high temperature (>42°C) amplifies action potentials, which increase pain signals and cause peripheral sensitisation. *Adapted from Bennett DL, Woods CG. Painful and painless channelopathies. Reprinted with permission from Elsevier (The Lancet Neurol 2014; 13:587–599).*

Fig. 34.4 Mechanisms of central sensitisation. Post-synaptic activation of the *N*-methyl-D-aspartate (NMDA) receptor requires the amino acids glycine and glutamate, which bind to the NR1 and NR2 subunits, respectively; these amplify pain signals at the level of the spinal cord. In contrast, magnesium ions block receptor activation.

that the heritability of CWP ranges between 30% and 50%. In the general population, the individual variants in response to pain and perception of pain are most likely due to a complex interaction between genetic and environmental influences. Few variants have been identified with robust evidence of association with CWP. Several rare syndromes have been described, however, in which insensitivity to pain or heightened pain responses occur as the result of a single gene disorder, as summarised in Box 34.3. Most are due to mutations affecting ion channels that play a key role in neurotransmission (see Fig. 34.3), but other causes include mutations in the *NTKR1* gene, which encodes the receptor for nerve growth factor, and mutations in the *PDRM12* transcription factor, which is involved in neuron development.

34

Investigations

Pain can be a presenting feature of a wide range of disorders and the first step in evaluation of a patient with pain should be to perform whatever investigations are required to define the underlying cause of the pain, unless this is already known. However, with most chronic pain syndromes, such as fibromyalgia, complex regional pain syndrome and CWP, investigations are negative and the diagnosis is made on the basis of clinical history and exclusion of other causes. Specific investigations that are useful in the assessment of selected patients with chronic pain are discussed below.

Magnetic resonance imaging

Magnetic resonance imaging (MRI) can be helpful in the assessment of an underlying cause in patients with focal pain that follows a nerve root or peripheral nerve distribution. Imaging is seldom helpful in individuals with CWP.

Blood tests

Blood tests are not generally helpful in the diagnosis of chronic pain, except in patients with peripheral neuropathy; in this case, a number of blood tests may be required to investigate the underlying causes of the neuropathy. Full details are provided in Box 25.86 (p. 1139). Genetic testing may be of value in patients with clinical features that point to an inherited disorder of pain processing (Box 34.3).

Quantitative sensory testing

Quantitative sensory testing can be helpful in the detailed assessment of patients with chronic pain. A simple set of tools can be used in the clinical setting (Fig. 34.5). Lightly touching the skin with a brush, swab or cotton-wool ball can be used to test for abnormalities of fine touch (allodynia). Assessing the patient's response to a pin-prick can be used to test for abnormalities in mechanical hyperalgesia. Finally, touching the patient's skin with warm and cool thermal rollers can be used to test for abnormalities of thermal sensation. An unaffected area of skin should be tested first, to establish normal sensation, before testing the affected area.

Nerve conduction studies

Nerve conduction studies can be helpful in demonstrating and quantifying a definitive nerve lesion, either peripherally or centrally. They can be used to help differentiate between central and peripheral neuropathic pain. They do not, however, effectively examine small nerve fibre function.

Nerve blocks

Performing a nerve block with infiltration of a local anaesthetic such as 1% lidocaine can be used diagnostically, in assessing whether a pain syndrome is due to involvement of a specific nerve or nerve root. Where inflammation and or swelling may be contributing to the underlying pain – for example, if there is compression of a nerve root – then a mixture of local anaesthetic

Cotton wool

Allodynia

Neurology pin

Hyperalgesia

Warm and cool thermal rollers

Increased or decreased thermal sensation

Fig. 34.5 Equipment for bedside sensory testing.

	34.3 Genetic regulators of pain perception			
Gene (protein)	Mutation (inheritance)	Protein function	Phenotypes	
SCN9A (Na,1.7)	LoF (AR)	Ion channel	Absent pain, hypohydrosis, anosmia	
SCN9A (Na,1.7)	GoF (AD)	Ion channel	Erythromelalgia, paroxysmal pain, burning pain, autonomic dysfunction	
SCN11A (Na,1.9)	GoF (AD)	Ion channel	Absent pain, hyperhydrosis, muscular weakness, gut dysmotility	
SCN10A (Na,1.8)	GoF (AD)	Ion channel	Burning pain, autonomic dysfunction	
TRPA1 (TRPA1)	GoF (AD)	Ion channel	Absent pain	
PDRM12 (PDRM12)	LoF (AR)	Transcription factor; neuron development	Absent pain	
NTRK1 (high-affinity NGF receptor)	LoF (AR)	Tyrosine kinase; promotes neuron development	Absent pain; anhydrosis, mental retardation, increased cancer risk	

(AD = autosomal dominant; AR = autosomal recessive; GoF = gain of function; LoF = loss of function; NGF = nerve growth factor) and depot glucocorticoid may be helpful in alleviating pain. Nerve blockade can also be used to determine whether more radical therapies, such as nerve ablation, might be helpful in controlling pain, particularly that related to cancer.

Pain scoring systems

Various questionnaires and other instruments have been devised to localise pain, rate its severity and assess its impact on quality of life. Some of the most widely used are listed in Box 34.4. The distribution of pain can be documented on a diagram of the body, on which the patient can mark the sites that are painful. Similarly, other methods have been developed with which to assess the severity of pain using verbal, numerical and behavioural rating scales. Visual scoring systems employing different facial expressions may be of value in paediatric patients and those with cognitive impairment. Documenting changes in pain scores using questionnaires can be helpful in indicating to what extent drug treatments have been successful and can reduce the time taken to achieve pain control.

Principles of management

Effective management of chronic pain depends in part on the underlying cause but some general principles can be applied. In general terms, the treatment goals are to:
• educate the patient
• promote self-management
• optimise function
• enhance quality of life
• control pain.

Clinical history

Biopsychosocial assessment

A full biopsychosocial assessment should be performed in all patients with chronic pain. Although this is time-consuming, the time invested is likely to pay dividends in improving the long-term outcome for patients. A biopsychosocial assessment takes account of the underlying neurobiology of the condition in the context of wider influences, including cognition and beliefs, emotions, and social and cultural factors. For example, an individual with abdominal pain might respond differently if a close relative had recently died of gastric cancer than if a colleague had been off work with gastric upset.

An accurate clinical history is important, taking note of the duration of pain, any precipitating and relieving factors, its location and, if the pain is located at more than one site, which site is the one that impacts most on the patient's quality of life. The characteristics of the pain should be documented, by assessing whether it is described as dull, sharp, aching or burning. Associated features, such as hypersensitivity to fine touch or temperature, numbness, paraesthesia, tingling and formication (the feeling of insects crawling over the skin), should be noted. It is important to determine to what extent the pain is interfering with normal daily activities, such as work, leisure pursuits and sleep. The patient's social circumstances and cultural background should be documented, including any caring responsibilities, employment status and social and family support. The intensity of pain should also be recorded, preferably using a validated questionnaire (Box 34.4). The patient's mood should be assessed and, if evidence of low mood is detected, a suicide risk assessment should be considered (see Box 28.12, p. 1187).

The past medical and medication history should be recorded and specific enquiry made about substance misuse and any previous history of physical or mental abuse. It is also useful to enquire specifically about the patient's beliefs as to what is causing their pain, as well as what their expectation of treatment is; unless these are addressed, management may be less effective. There are some patient populations in whom particular challenges arise, often related to differences in communication ability. Strategies that can be used to overcome these difficulties are summarised in Box 34.5.

Examination

The patient's general appearance should be noted, including ability to walk and use of a walking aid. In those with focal pain, neurological examination should be performed, focusing particularly on any areas of abnormal sensation, reflexes and evidence of muscle wasting. A general examination should be carried out to determine whether there is any evidence of an underlying physical disorder that can account for the pain. In addition to the use of investigations to find the underlying cause of pain, patients with persistent or chronic pain may benefit from sensory testing or diagnostic nerve blocks to explore the underlying mechanisms and direct treatment. For example, a combined femoral and sciatic nerve block may be used in a patient with lower limb amputation to assess whether the pain is predominantly peripherally or centrally generated. If the pain is not improved by an effective nerve block, then peripherally directed therapies are unlikely to be effective.

i	**34.4 Instruments used in the assessment of pain and its impact**	
Instrument	**Comments**
Brief Pain Inventory	Developed for use in cancer pain, validated and widely employed for chronic pain; based on 0–10 ratings of pain intensity and the impact of pain on a range of domains, including sleep, work and enjoyment of life
Pain Detect, s-LANSS, DN-4	A number of screening questionnaires to aid diagnosis of neuropathic pain
Pain Catastrophising Scale	Developed to assess individual levels of catastrophising, encompassing three different domains: helplessness, rumination and magnification
Tampa Scale of Kinesiophobia	Measures how much an individual is fearful of movement
Pain Self-efficacy Questionnaire	Assesses individual beliefs about self-efficacy in the context of chronic pain, and how this impacts on function
Visual analogue scale (VAS)	Patient marks pain intensity on a horizontal line
Localisation of pain	Body chart, allowing the patient to indicate where pain is situated
Beck Depression Inventory	Assesses emotional function
SF-36/EQ-5D	Assesses health-related quality of life

(DN-4 = Douleur Neuropathique questionnaire; EQ-5D = EuroQol 5-Domain questionnaire; SF-36 = Short Form 36; s-LANSS = self-completed Leeds Assessment of Neuropathic Signs and Symptoms)

34

34.5 Challenges in pain assessment in particular patient populations		
Patient population	Challenges	Solutions
Paediatric	Assessment needs to be appropriate to developmental stage	Consider visual tools to aid pain assessment
Elderly	May have impaired cognitive function Cultural factors may reduce self-reporting of pain Risk of adverse effects of medication increased	Consider formal assessment of cognitive function Consider non-verbal assessment Consider visual tools to assess pain Employ a number of tools assessing pain behaviours
Cognitive impairment	Reporting and expression of pain may change Increased sensitivity to central nervous system effects of analgesics	Perform formal assessment of cognitive function Use non-verbal assessment: facial expressions, vocalisations, body movements, changes in social interactions
Substance misuse	Response to analgesics altered Increased tolerance Increased risk of addiction Substance misuse may affect reporting of pain	Seek specialist support early Ensure prescribing is safe

Interventions

Probably the most effective mode of treatment for pain is to identify the underlying cause. Examples include the use of immunosuppressive medication in inflammatory disease, chemotherapy, radiotherapy or hormone therapy in cancer, and antimicrobial therapy in patients with infection. There are many circumstances, however, in which the underlying cause of pain cannot be treated or the treatments available are incompletely effective. Under these circumstances, several management options are available. In all cases, a multidisciplinary approach is necessary that combines pharmacological management with supported self-management, and other specific interventions when appropriate.

Supported self-management

Self-management strategies are useful in the treatment of chronic pain. Self-management works best if the patient has some understanding of their chronic pain, and acceptance that it is unlikely to resolve completely. The aim is for patients to maximise their quality of life and function *despite* ongoing pain. Support for self-management can be delivered by health-care professionals, patients who suffer from the same condition or lay people, either on an individual basis, in a group setting or, increasingly, through web-based resources. There is a strong educational component to supported self-management, which seeks to generate an interaction between patient and tutor. The key aspects include:

- increasing activity levels, while understanding and practising pacing techniques (not overdoing things and cycling between over- and under-activity)
- using relaxation and mindfulness techniques as part of daily management
- using medication when appropriate
- having a plan to manage pain flares.

There are a number of useful online self-help resources (see 'Further reading').

Physical therapies

There is strong evidence that exercise can help in the management of chronic pain. Several types of exercise have been successfully used delivered in various ways, through physiotherapists, exercise classes or individual tuition. In choosing a form of exercise therapy, it is important to tailor the approach most likely to be acceptable

34.6 Physical therapies for chronic pain
Land-based
• Walking   • Yoga
• Gym work   • Pilates
• Exercise classes   • Tai-chi
Water-based
• Hydrotherapy   • Exercise classes
• Swimming

to the individual patient. A successful exercise programme can help overcome 'fear avoidance', a well-recognised problem in chronic pain, where patients associate activity with an increase in pain and therefore do progressively less activity, with resultant deconditioning. Because of this it is important to pace physical activity to ensure that patients do not cycle from over-activity, with a flare in pain, to fatigue and deconditioning. This can be done by working with patients to establish their baseline level of activity and using an individually tailored, graded exercise programme (Box 34.6). This may include normal household activities, as well as targeted exercises and stretches. Manual therapy covers a variety of hands-on treatments, including manipulation, mobilisation and massage. Manual therapy can be provided by a range of therapists, including physiotherapists, osteopaths and chiropractors. There is some evidence of short-term benefit for manual therapy but limited evidence of long-term efficacy.

Pharmacological therapies

A range of analgesics can be used in the management of chronic pain but, for most of these, the evidence of long-term benefit is limited. In general, it is advisable to use a multimodal approach in the treatment of chronic pain, choosing different drugs to target pain processing at multiple points (Box 34.7). By employing different classes of analgesic, it is possible to use lower doses of each, thereby improving the side-effect profile. There is considerable inter-individual variability in response to analgesics, even within the same class. There are many reasons for this, including genetic variations in the enzymes that metabolise drugs. For example, the *CYP2D6* gene encodes for a liver enzyme, cytochrome P450 2D6, which metabolises a number of commonly used analgesics. Genetic variation in *CYP2D6* can influence circulating levels of many drugs, depending on whether

34.7 Pharmacological management of chronic pain

Drug or class of drug	Mechanism of action
Paracetamol	Central inhibition of COX-1 and COX-2 enzymes Mechanisms of action incompletely understood
Non-steroidal anti-inflammatory drugs	Inhibition of prostaglandin production
Opioids	Agonists at OP3 receptors at multiple levels in the central nervous system Blockade of ascending pain pathways
Ketamine	Antagonist of NMDA receptors Reduction of central sensitisation
Gabapentin Pregabalin	Inhibition of glutamate release by primary afferent neurons at first central synapse Decrease of excitatory neuronal activity
Tricyclic antidepressants	Inhibition of serotonin and noradrenaline (norepinephrine) re-uptake at synapses in the spinal cord, and also potential effects in the limbic system Inhibition of Na^+ channels in neurons
Serotonin (5-hydroxytryptamine, 5-HT) and noradrenaline (norepinephrine) re-uptake inhibitors	Inhibition of serotonin and noradrenaline re-uptake at synapses in the spinal cord, and also potential effects in the limbic system
Lidocaine patches	Inhibition of Na^+ in sensory neurons
Capsaicin patch	Activation of TRPV1 channels on subset of C fibres, causing selective pharmacological denervation, with a decrease in intra-epidermal nerve fibre density
Nerve blocks with lidocaine and glucocorticoids	Temporary denervation due to blockade of Na^+ channels in sensory neurons Local anti-inflammatory effect

(COX = cyclo-oxygenase; NMDA = N-methyl-D-aspartate; OP = opioid; TRPV1 = transient receptor potential vanilloid 1)

someone is a rapid or poor metaboliser. This is particularly important if metabolites are active, as is the case with codeine and tramadol, which are metabolised to morphine. Genetic variations have also been described in the opioid receptors and downstream pathways that they affect, with good pre-clinical evidence that variations in mu opioid receptors alter analgesic response to different opioids. Because of this there is a good rationale to try different drugs, even ones from the same class, if there is an inadequate response or there are unacceptable side-effects with one agent.

Whatever drug or combination of drugs is chosen, the key to successful pharmacological management is careful assessment and review, aiming for an acceptable balance between the benefits of treatment in providing pain relief, maximising function, and improving quality of life and adverse effects. Specific drug treatments are described below.

Non-opioid analgesics

Paracetamol

Paracetamol is widely used in the treatment of mild to moderate pain. Its mechanism of action is incompletely understood but it is known to be a weak inhibitor of the cyclo-oxygenase type 1 (COX-1) and cyclo-oxygenase type 2 (COX-2) enzymes, providing weak anti-inflammatory properties. There is also some of evidence that it activates inhibitory descending spinal pathways, via a serotonergic mechanism. Other postulated mechanisms include endocannabinoid re-uptake inhibition, and inhibition of nitric oxide and tumour necrosis factor alpha. For migraine and tension-type headache it has moderate efficacy at a dose of 1000 mg. It is used widely for musculoskeletal disorders and osteoarthritis, with very little high-quality evidence that it is much better than placebo, even at doses of up to 4000 mg per day. Acute liver failure is a well-recognised complication of paracetamol overdose but this risk may also be increased with long-term use, even within the recommended dose range. In view of this, it should be employed with caution in elderly patients and those weighing less than 50 kg.

Non-steroidal anti-inflammatory drugs

Non-steroidal anti-inflammatory drugs (NSAIDs) are widely used in the treatment of inflammatory pain and osteoarthritis. These drugs can be given systemically or locally and are discussed in more detail on page 1002. They are also useful in the management of pain in cancer patients, as discussed later in this chapter (p. 1350). Although widely prescribed, there is limited high-quality evidence of long-term efficacy in chronic pain, with a need for further studies in this area.

Topical analgesics

Topical capsaicin cream (0.025 or 0.075%) has some efficacy for osteoarthritis and may be used for neuropathic pain, although evidence of benefit is limited. A single application (done by a trained health-care professional) of a high-dose 8% capsaicin patch can give around 12 weeks of pain relief for neuropathic pain and can be repeated thereafter. Capsaicin is an agonist at the transient receptor potential vanilloid 1 (TRPV1) ion channel, found on some C fibres. Capsaicin activates the channel, causing an initial sensation of heat, but an analgesic effect subsequently results due to desensitisation of the channel.

Lidocaine 5% patches can also be helpful in focal neuropathic pain and should be applied for 12 hours out of 24 hours, with up to 4–6 weeks before maximum benefit is seen. The mode of action is blockade of sodium channels in primary afferent neurons and nociceptors, which reduces peripheral input to the spinal cord.

Adjuvant analgesics

Adjuvant analgesics is the term used to cover a range of agents that are used in the treatment of neuropathic pain, usually in combination with classical analgesics. Typically, these agents

34

do not produce an immediate reduction in pain, but rather exert an analgesic effect over a longer timeframe through their effects on central processing of pain. They are of particular value when used in combination in the management of pain with a neuropathic component but require careful dose titration over a number of weeks, to reach a dose that balances efficacy with side-effects. While the response to individual agents is variable, it is often possible to find an agent or combination of agents that works for most patients.

Opioid analgesics

Opioids are a class of drugs that target opioid receptors. The original receptor classification was based on pharmacological activity (mu, delta, kappa), with the more recent International Union of Basic and Clinical Pharmacology (IUPHAR) classification being generally accepted in current use (Box 34.8). Opioid receptors are G-protein-coupled receptors. Ligand binding activates several intracellular signalling pathways, increasing cyclic adenosine monophosphate (cAMP) levels, as well as altering calcium and potassium permeability of neurons. Opioids are traditionally divided into subclasses of weak opioids, such as codeine and dihydrocodeine, and strong opioids, such as morphine and oxycodone. While tramadol is a weak agonist at the mu opioid receptor, it is classified as a strong opioid in some countries. The dosages and characteristics of commonly prescribed opioids are shown in Box 34.9. There has been a large increase in the use of strong opioids for chronic pain over the last 10–20 years. A number of factors contribute to this, including a rising incidence of chronic pain with an ageing population, reluctance to use NSAIDs because of cardiovascular and gastrointestinal adverse effects, changes in patient expectation, societal attitudes and availability of new formulations of opioids. There is evidence of short- to medium-term benefit for strong opioids in low back pain and osteoarthritis but there have been very few good-quality studies of long-term use. Additionally, there is increasing concern about potential harm from long-term use. This includes addiction, dependence, opioid-induced hyperalgesia, endocrine dysfunction, fracture risk (especially in the elderly), overdose and cardiovascular

---

i 34.8 Opioids and opioid receptors

Endogenous ligand	Receptor (IUPHAR)	Alternative classification	Potential sites	Pharmacological effects
Endomorphin 1 and 2 Met-enkephalin Dynorphin A Dynorphin B	MOP	Mu; OP3	Brain, spinal cord, peripheral nerves, immune cells	Analgesia, reduced gastrointestinal motility, respiratory depression, pruritus
Leu-enkephalin Met-enkephalin β-endorphin	DOP	Delta; OP1	Brain, spinal cord, peripheral nerves	Analgesia, cardioprotection, thermoregulation
Dynorphin A Dynorphin B β-endorphin	KOP	Kappa; OP2	Brain (nucleus accumbens, neocortex, brainstem, cerebellum)	Analgesia, neuroendocrine (e.g. on hypothalamic–pituitary axis), diuresis, dysphoria
Orphanin FQ (nociceptin)	NOP	Orphan; ORL-1; OP4	Nucleus raphe magnus, spinal cord, afferent neurons	Opioid tolerance, anxiety, depression, increased appetite

(IUPHAR = International Union of Basic and Clinical Pharmacology; OP = opioid; ORL = opioid-like receptor)

---

i 34.9 Commonly used opioids

Opioid	Typical starting dose	Route	Oral morphine equivalent	Comments
Morphine	10 mg	Oral	10 mg	Most widely used
Codeine	100 mg	Oral	10 mg	Metabolised to morphine
Dihydrocodeine	100 mg	Oral	10 mg	Semi-synthetic
Tramadol	100 mg	Oral	10 mg	Synthetic
Oxycodone	6.6 mg	Oral	10 mg	More predictable bioavailability than morphine
Buprenorphine	5 μg/hr	Transdermal	30 mg/day	Patch change usually every 7 days (frequency of change dependent on manufacturer and dose); advantages in impaired renal function
Fentanyl	12 μg/hr	Transdermal	30 mg/day	Use with care in opioid-naïve patients; patch change usually every 72 hrs
Tapentadol	50 mg	Oral	20 mg	Use with care in opioid-naïve patients
Hydromorphone	2 mg	Oral	10 mg	Semi-synthetic; hepatic metabolism
Diamorphine	3 mg	Subcutaneous, intramuscular, intravenous	10 mg	Mainly used for acute pain or palliative care

i 34.10 Use of opioids in chronic pain

Step	Factors to take into account	Comment

1. Assess suitability for opioids	Type of pain
	Likelihood of dependence
	Co-morbidity
		Neuropathic pain less likely to respond
		History of substance or alcohol misuse, including stimulant misuse
		Avoid use in conditions where adverse effects more likely:
		    Chronic obstructive pulmonary disease
		    Chronic liver disease
		    Chronic kidney disease

2. Discuss with patient	Discuss potential benefits Discuss adverse effects Establish treatment goal	Improvement in pain Improvement in function Nausea Constipation Drowsiness Improvement in function

3. Plan treatment trial	Set timescale
	
	Agree on dose
	
	Agree on stopping rules
		Define duration of treatment
		Agree frequency of review
		Aim for lowest effective dose
		Set upper dose limit
		Consider stopping if:
		    Treatment goal is not met
		    There is no dose response
		    Tolerance develops rapidly

events, with many of these adverse effects being dose-related. There is evidence that doses of more than 120 mg morphine equivalents per day are associated with increased harm, and regular review to assess ongoing benefit is needed in this patient group. A suggested strategy for using strong opioids in chronic pain is shown in Box 34.10.

Psychological therapies

The aims of psychological therapy are to increase coping skills and improve quality of life when facing the challenges of living with chronic pain. There are a range of ways in which psychological therapies can be delivered, including individual one-to-one sessions, group sessions, multidisciplinary pain management programmes, or web-based or telephone-based programmes.

There is a good evidence for the use of a cognitive behavioural therapy (CBT)-based approach for chronic pain, delivered either individually or in a group. The overall aim is to reduce negative thoughts and beliefs, and develop positive coping strategies. The interaction between thoughts, behaviours and emotions is explored, and a problem-focused approach is used in therapy delivery.

Relaxation techniques, such as biofeedback and mindfulness meditation, require a degree of stillness and withdrawal, with regular practice required for sustained benefit (see 'Further information'). Acceptance and commitment therapy (ACT) is based on CBT principles but also uses components of mindfulness to improve psychological flexibility in the context of living with chronic pain.

Stimulation therapies

These range from minimally invasive procedures like acupuncture and transcutaneous electrical nerve stimulation (TENS) to more invasive techniques such as spinal cord stimulation.

Acupuncture (Fig. 34.6) has been used successfully in Eastern medicine for centuries. The mechanisms are incompletely understood, although endorphin release may explain, in part,

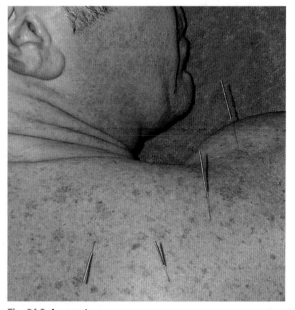

Fig. 34.6 Acupuncture.

the analgesic effect. Acupuncture is particularly effective in pain related to muscle spasm, with some evidence of short-term benefit for patients with low back pain. Similar mechanisms probably apply to TENS, which is worth considering in many types of chronic pain. Neuromodulation, using implanted electrodes in the epidural space (or, more recently, adjacent to peripheral nerves), has been shown to be an effective option for neuropathic pain, including failed back surgery syndrome and chronic regional pain syndrome (see below). Specialist assessment and ongoing support is necessary, as there are many potential complications, including infection, malfunction and battery failure. The likelihood of success is increased when this technique is used within the context of multidisciplinary assessment and management.

34

Complementary and alternative therapies

Complementary techniques, such as herbal medicines, vitamins, homeopathy and reflexology, have been used for the treatment of chronic pain but with little evidence of efficacy. It should be noted that herbal medications may interact with conventional drugs, causing adverse effects as the result of drug–drug interactions. St John's wort (*Hypericum perforatum*) interacts with many drugs, including many antidepressants used in chronic pain, with increased serotonergic effects. Grapefruit may also increase the risk of serotonergic effects with some antidepressants. *Ginkgo biloba* may interact with paracetamol to increase bleeding time.

Nerve blocks and nerve ablation

The use of specialist nerve blocks and nerve ablation therapy can be considered for pain that is unresponsive to less invasive approaches. If these are being considered, they should form part of a multidisciplinary management plan, with the aim of restoring function and reducing pain. Local anaesthetic with or without depot glucocorticoid (non-particulate for neuraxial administration) can be effective in some circumstances. Examples include occipital nerve blocks for migraine or cervicogenic headache and trigger point injections for myofascial pain. If there is limited compression of a spinal nerve root, the nerve root injections into the epidural space may help settle symptoms and avoid the need for surgical intervention. Neurodestructive procedures can also be employed for intractable pain but are rarely used outside the palliative care setting.

Chronic pain syndromes

Chronic pain is a feature of several recognised syndromes, which are discussed in more detail below.

Neuropathic pain

Neuropathic pain is defined as 'pain associated with a lesion or disease of the somatosensory nervous system'. Neuropathic pain may be acute, such as in sciatica, which occurs as the result of a prolapsed disc, but is most problematic when it becomes chronic. Neuropathic pain causes major morbidity; in a recent study, 17% of those affected rated their quality of life as 'worse than death'. The clinical features of neuropathic pain are summarised in Box 34.11. The diagnosis is easily missed and so careful assessment is vital, in order to make the diagnosis in the first place and then to direct management appropriately. An algorithm for the management of neuropathic pain is provided in Figure 34.7. It is important to recognise the negative impact of neuropathic pain on quality of life, which has been shown to be greater than with other types of chronic pain. As a result, appropriate support and multidisciplinary management should always be considered in addition to pharmacological therapies.

Complex regional pain syndrome

Complex regional pain syndrome (CRPS) is a type of neuropathic pain that affects one or more limbs. It was previously termed reflex sympathetic dystrophy (RSD), reflecting the fact the disease is thought to be caused in part by an abnormality in the autonomic nervous system. It is a rare syndrome, occurring in about 20 per 100 000 individuals, and is more common in females, typically presenting between the ages of 35 and 50. It is classified into type I CRPS, which may be precipitated by a traumatic event

34.11 Clinical features of neuropathic pain

Characteristic	Symptom or clinical feature*	Descriptive term
Spontaneous pain	No stimulus required to evoke pain	
Positive sensory disturbance	Light touch painful	Dynamic allodynia
	Pressure painful	Punctate allodynia
	Increased pain on pin-prick	Hyperalgesia
	Cool and warm temperatures painful	Thermal allodynia
Negative sensory disturbance	Numbness	Loss of sensation
	Tingling	Paraesthesia
	Loss of temperature sensitivity	
Other features	Feeling of insects crawling over skin	Formication
	Affected area feels abnormal	Dysaesthesia

*Symptoms may cluster, with a predominance of either positive or negative symptoms, or a mixture of both, reflecting differences in underlying mechanisms.

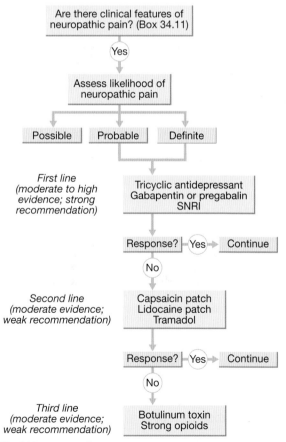

Fig. 34.7 Algorithm for pharmacological management of neuropathic pain. (SNRI = serotonin noradrenaline (norepinephrine) re-uptake inhibitor) *Adapted from SIGN 136 and NeuPSIG recommendations (Finnerup NB, Attal N, Haroutounian S, et al. Pharmacotherapy for neuropathic pain in adults: a systematic review and meta-analysis. Reprinted with permission from Elsevier (The Lancet Neurol 2015; 14:162–173)).*

<table>
<tr><td colspan="2">**i**   **34.12 Criteria for diagnosis of complex regional pain syndrome (CRPS) type 1***</td></tr>
</table>

Category	Symptom or sign

Sensory	Allodynia to:
	    Temperature
	    Light touch
	    Deep somatic pressure
	    Movement
	Hyperalgesia to pin-prick

Vasomotor	Temperature asymmetry Skin colour change and asymmetry Skin colour asymmetry
Oedema/sudomotor	Oedema Sweating change or asymmetry

Motor/trophic	Reduced range of motion
	Motor dysfunction:
	    Weakness
	    Tremor
	    Dystonia
	Trophic changes:
	    Hair
	    Nails
	    Skin

*The diagnosis of CRPS type 1 can be made if a patient has at least one symptom in at least three out of the four categories and at least one sign in two out of the four categories, and no other diagnosis can explain the symptoms.

such as a fracture but is not associated with peripheral nerve damage, and type II CRPS, which is associated with a peripheral nerve lesion. The diagnosis is primarily clinical, based on the features shown in Box 34.12. Imaging with MRI or radionuclide bone scan may provide support for the diagnosis of type I CRPS in showing bone marrow oedema or increased tracer uptake localised to an affected site (p. 1055).

Prompt diagnosis and early treatment with physiotherapy may prevent progression of symptoms. Management is as for neuropathic pain, additional approaches including graded motor imagery. Bisphosphonates have been used empirically for treatment but the evidence base for efficacy in controlling pain is weak. If medical management is incompletely effective, consideration should be given to the appropriateness of a spinal cord stimulator.

Phantom limb pain

Phantom limb is a common complication of amputation, occurring in up to 70% of patients. It is a form of neuropathic pain but can be particularly distressing, as the pain is felt in the area where the absent limb was previously. Although usually presenting after limb amputation, reports of phantom pain in other body parts have been reported, such as phantom breast pain following mastectomy. It is very often associated with phantom sensations, which are described as non-painful sensations in the absent body part and pain in the stump.

Diagnostic nerve blocks may be helpful in directing therapy, with use of anti-neuropathic medications as outlined in Box 34.7. If there is a definite neuroma at the stump site that is interfering with prosthesis use, surgical review may be necessary.

Chronic widespread pain

Chronic widespread pain (CWP) is often associated with other features, such as fatigue and irritable bowel syndrome.

Fibromyalgia is a subtype of CWP in which there are myofascial trigger points, and is often associated with sleep disturbance. Clinical features and management of fibromyalgia are discussed in more detail on page 1018.

Joint hypermobility syndrome

Hypermobility can be associated with chronic musculoskeletal pain that often targets the joints and periarticular tissues. It is thought to be caused by abnormal stresses being placed on the joints and surrounding soft tissues due to ligament laxity, although the mechanisms are poorly understood since many people with hypermobile joints do not suffer pain. It is described in more detail on page 1059.

Palliative care

Palliative care is the term used to describe the active total care of patients with incurable disease. It can be distinguished from end-of-life care, which refers to the care of patients with far advanced, rapidly progressive disease that will soon prove fatal. The focus of palliative care is on symptom control alongside supportive care. While palliative care can and should be delivered at any stage of an incurable illness alongside optimal disease control, the focus of end-of-life care is on quality of life rather than prolongation of life or cure. Palliative care encompasses a distinct body of knowledge and skills that all good physicians must possess to allow them to care effectively for patients. Palliative care is traditionally seen as a means of managing distress and symptoms in patients with cancer, when metastatic disease has been diagnosed and death is seen as inevitable. There is, however, a growing recognition that the principles of palliative care and some of the interventions it uses are equally applicable in other conditions. Palliative may therefore be applied to any chronic disease state.

For conditions other than cancer, the challenge is recognising when patients have entered the terminal phase of their illness, as there are fewer clear markers and the course of the illness is much more variable. Different chronic disease states progress at different rates, allowing some general trajectories of illness or dying to be defined (Fig. 34.8). These trajectories are useful in decision-making for individual patients and also in planning services.

Fig. 34.8 Archetypal trajectories of dying. *Reproduced from Murray SA, Kendall M, Boyd K, et al. Illness trajectories and palliative care. BMJ 2005; 330:7498; reproduced with permission from the BMJ Publishing Group.*

The 'rapid decline' trajectory following a gradual decline, as occurs in cancer, is the best-recognised pattern of the need for palliative care, although a similar trajectory may be observed in other conditions, such as motor neuron disease can. Many traditional hospice services are designed to meet the needs of people on this trajectory. Over recent years, improvements in management of malignant disease mean that some types of cancer may follow an erratic or intermittent decline trajectory.

Many chronic diseases, such as advanced chronic obstructive pulmonary disease (COPD) and intractable congestive heart failure, carry as high a burden of symptoms as cancer, as well as psychological and family distress. The 'palliative phase' of these illnesses may be more difficult to identify because of periods of relative stability interspersed with acute episodes of severe illness. However, it is still possible to recognise those patients who may benefit from a palliative approach to their care. The challenge is that symptom management needs to be delivered at the same time as treatment for acute exacerbations. This leads to difficult decisions as to the balance between symptom relief and aggressive management of the underlying disease. The starting point of need for palliative care in these conditions is the point at which consideration of comfort and individual values becomes important in decision-making, often alongside management of the underlying disease.

The third major trajectory is categorised by years of poor function and frailty before a relatively short terminal period; it is exemplified by dementia but is also increasingly true for patients with many different chronic illnesses. As medical advances extend survival, this mode of dying is being experienced by increasing numbers of people. The main challenge lies in providing nursing care and ensuring that plans are agreed for the time when medical intervention is no longer beneficial.

In a situation where death is inevitable and foreseeable, palliative care balances the 'standard textbook' approach with the wishes and values of the patient and a realistic assessment of the benefits of medical interventions. This often results in a greater focus on comfort, symptom control and support for patient and family, and may enable withdrawal of both futile and burdensome interventions. In cases of prognostic uncertainty, open, honest and gentle communication with the patient and family is important. The most common symptoms in palliative care are discussed in the next section.

Presenting problems in palliative care

Pain

Pain is a common problem in palliative care. It has been estimated that about two-thirds of patients with cancer experience moderate or severe pain, and a quarter have three or more different sites of pain. Many of these are of a mixed aetiology and about half of patients with cancer-associated pain have a neuropathic element.

Clinical assessment

Careful evaluation to identify the likely mechanisms of pain is important so that the most appropriate treatment can be given. Clinical features and suggested management strategies for common types of pain in cancer are shown in Box 34.13. The majority of patients with cancer-associated pain can be effectively managed using a stepwise approach, as outlined below.

34.13 Common types of pain in cancer		
Type of pain	Features	Management options
Bone pain	Tender area over bone Possible pain on movement	NSAIDs Bisphosphonates Radiotherapy
Increased intracranial pressure	Headache, worse in the morning, associated with vomiting and occasionally delirium	Glucocorticoids Radiotherapy Codeine
Abdominal colic	Intermittent, severe, spasmodic, associated with nausea or vomiting	Antispasmodics Hyoscine butylbromide
Liver capsule pain	Right upper quadrant abdominal pain, often associated with tender enlarged liver Responds poorly to opioids	Glucocorticoids
Neuropathic pain	Spontaneous pain Light touch, pressure and temperature changes are painful; increased pain on pin-prick Numbness, tingling or loss of temperature sensation Skin feels abnormal	Anticonvulsants: Gabapentin Pregabalin Antidepressants Amitriptyline Duloxetine Ketamine
Ischaemic pain	Diffuse, severe, aching pain associated with evidence of poor perfusion Responds poorly to opioids	NSAIDs Ketamine
Incident pain	Episodic pain usually related to movement or bowel spasm	Intermittent short-acting opioids Nerve block

(NSAIDs = non-steroidal anti-inflammatory drugs)

Management: pharmacological treatments

Pharmacological treatments are the mainstay of management in cancer-associated pain. A stepwise approach is adopted, following the principles of the World Health Organisation (WHO) analgesic ladder (Fig. 34.9), in which analgesia that is appropriate for the degree of pain is prescribed first. Patients with mild pain should be started on a non-opioid analgesic drug, such as paracetamol (1 g 4 times daily) or an NSAID (step 1). If the patient fails to respond adequately or has moderate pain, a weak opioid, such as codeine (60 mg 4 times daily), should be added (step 2). This can be prescribed separately or in the form of the compound analgesic co-codamol. If pain relief is still not achieved or if the patient has severe pain, a strong opioid should be substituted for the weak opioid (step 3). If the pain is severe at the outset, strong opioids should be prescribed and increased or titrated according to the patient's response. It is important not to move 'sideways' (change from one drug to another of equal potency), which is a common problem during step 2 of the analgesic ladder.

Opioids

Opioid analgesia plays a key role in patients with moderate to severe pain. Its successful use depends on appropriate assessment and a detailed explanation to the patient and carer about the benefits and potential side-effects of therapy. Morphine

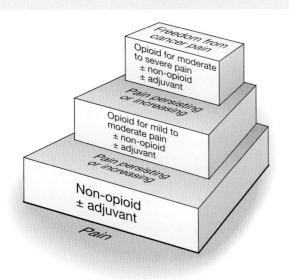

Fig. 34.9 The WHO analgesic ladder. *From WHO. Cancer pain relief, 2nd edn. Geneva: WHO; 1996.*

34.14 Opioid side-effects

Side-effect	Management
Constipation	Regular laxative Opioid/naloxone oral combination, in resistant constipation
Dry mouth	Frequent sips of iced water, soft white paraffin to lips, chlorhexidine mouthwashes twice daily, sugar-free gum, water or saliva sprays
Nausea/vomiting	Oral haloperidol 0.5–1 mg at night, oral metoclopramide 10 mg 3 times daily or oral domperidone 10 mg 3 times daily If constant, haloperidol or levomepromazine may be given parenterally to break the nausea cycle
Sedation	Explanation is very important Symptoms usually settle in a few days Avoid other sedating medication where possible Ensure appropriate use of adjuvant analgesics that can have an opioid-sparing effect May require an alternative opioid

is the most commonly prescribed strong opioid, although there are several alternatives, as outlined in Box 34.9.

Oral morphine takes about 20 minutes to exert an effect and usually provides pain relief for 4 hours. Most patients with continuous pain should be prescribed oral morphine every 4 hours initially, as this will provide continuous pain relief over the whole 24-hour period. Controlled-release morphine lasts for 12 or 24 hours, depending on the formulation, and if clinical circumstances dictate, a controlled-release formulation can be used to initiate and titrate morphine. The median effective morphine equivalent dose for cancer pain is about 200 mg per 24 hours.

In addition to the regular dose of morphine, an extra dose of immediate-release (IR) morphine should be prescribed 'as required' for the treatment of breakthrough pain that has not been controlled by the regular prescription. As a rule of thumb, this additional dose should be one-sixth of the total 24-hour dose of opioid. The frequency of breakthrough doses should be dictated by their efficacy and any side-effects, rather than by a fixed time interval. A patient may require breakthrough analgesia as frequently as hourly if pain is severe, but this should lead to early review of the regular prescription. The patient or carer should note the timing of any breakthrough doses and the reason for them. These should be reviewed daily and the regular 4-hourly dose increased for the next 24 hours on the basis of:

- the frequency of and reasons for breakthrough analgesia
- the degree and acceptability of side-effects.

The regular dose should be increased by adding the total of the breakthrough doses over the previous 24 hours, unless there are significant problems with unacceptable side-effects. When the correct dose has been established, a continuous release (CR) preparation can be prescribed, usually twice daily. Breakthrough analgesia used for movement-related pain is generally not included in background opioid dose titration. Attempts to control movement-related pain with background opioid dose will usually lead to over-medication and opioid-related side-effects. This can be a risk in metastatic bone pain.

Some patients may have concerns about using opioids and it is vital for these to be explored. Patients should be reassured

that psychological dependence is rare when opioids are used for cancer pain, unless a pre-existing dependence problem exists. Pharmacological tolerance is not usually a clinically relevant problem; however, physical dependence, which is physiological, as manifest by a physical withdrawal syndrome, can occur if opioids are suddenly discontinued.

Nearly all types of cancer pain respond to morphine to some degree but there is a spectrum of response, such that in some patients the dose of opioid required to control neuropathic pain and all elements of metastatic bone pain may be high and associated with unacceptable side-effects. In these situations, other methods of analgesia, both pharmacological and non-pharmacological, should be explored and considered at an early stage.

The most effective and appropriate route of morphine administration is oral but transdermal preparations of strong opioids (usually fentanyl) are useful in certain situations, such as in patients with dysphagia or those who are reluctant to take tablets on a regular basis. Diamorphine is a highly soluble strong opioid used for subcutaneous infusions, particularly in the last few days of life, but is only available in certain countries.

Opioid-related adverse effects

Adverse effects are a common problem with opioids, especially on initiating treatment and on increasing the dose. The most common side-effects are nausea, drowsiness, constipation and dry mouth, as summarised in Box 34.14. Nausea and vomiting can occur initially but usually settle after a few days. Drowsiness is usually transient at opioid initiation and dose increase. If it is persistent, an alternative opioid and/or a non-opioid should be considered. In acute dosing, respiratory depression can occur but this is rare in patients on regular opioids or in those starting on small, regular doses with appropriate titration.

Tolerance usually develops to nausea, vomiting and drowsiness but not to constipation or dry mouth. All patients should therefore be prescribed a laxative, unless suffering from diarrhoea, and have access to an antiemetic and good mouth care, along with rationalisation of any concomitant medication that might exacerbate drowsiness. Newer developments include the use of preparations in which opioids are combined with opioid

34

antagonists, such as naloxone. The naloxone is poorly absorbed and does not antagonise the systemic analgesic effect but rather acts locally to block opioid receptors in the gut, thereby reducing opioid-related constipation. Vivid dreams, visual hallucinations (often consisting of a sense of movement at the periphery of vision), delirium and myoclonus are typical of opioid-related toxicity and, if present, require urgent reassessment of the opioid dose. Biochemistry should also be checked to exclude renal impairment, dehydration, electrolyte disturbance or hypercalcaemia.

Since opioid toxicity can occur at any dose, side-effects should be assessed regularly, but particularly after a dose increase. Pain should be reassessed to ensure that appropriate adjuvants are being used. Parenteral rehydration is often helpful to speed up excretion of active metabolites of morphine. The dose of opioid may need to be reduced or the opioid changed to a strong alternative.

Different opioids have different side-effect profiles in different people. If a patient develops side-effects, switching to an alternative strong opioid may be helpful. Options include oxycodone, transdermal fentanyl, alfentanil, hydromorphone and occasionally methadone, any of which may produce a better balance of benefit against side-effects. Fentanyl and alfentanil have no renally excreted active metabolites and may be particularly useful in patients with renal failure. It is possible to switch between opioids but great care must be taken when doing so to make sure the dose is correct and to avoid prescribing too much or too little opioid.

Adjuvant analgesics

An adjuvant analgesic is a drug that has a primary indication other than pain but which provides analgesia in some painful conditions and may enhance the effect of the primary analgesic. Commonly used adjuvant analgesics in the palliative care setting are shown in Box 34.15. Some adjuvant analgesics may enhance the side-effect profile of the primary analgesic, and dose reductions of opioids may be required when an adjuvant analgesic is added. At each step of the WHO analgesic ladder, an adjuvant analgesic should be considered, the choice depending on the type of pain.

Management: non-pharmacological treatments

Neurodestructive interventions

Neurodestructive techniques have an important role in the management of cancer pain, where life expectancy is limited. They should be used as part of an overall management plan and considered when the response to drug treatment has been inadequate. Intrathecal analgesia, delivered via either an external pump or a fully implanted device, is a good option, particularly where life expectancy is more than 3 months. Coeliac plexus blocks can be helpful for visceral pain, such as in pancreatic cancer. Lateral cordotomy to disrupt the spinothalamic tracts (either open or percutaneous) may be considered for unilateral chest wall pain, such as may occur in mesothelioma, where life expectancy is limited.

Radiotherapy

Radiotherapy is the treatment of choice for pain from bone metastases (see Box 34.13) and can also be considered for metastatic involvement at other sites. All patients with pain secondary to bone metastases should be considered for palliative radiotherapy, which can usually be given in a single dose.

Physiotherapy

Physiotherapy has a key role in the multidisciplinary approach to a wide spectrum of cancer-related symptoms, including the prevention and management of pain, muscle spasm, reduced mobility, muscle wasting and lymphoedema. Rehabilitation in palliative care has expanded and now includes pre-habilitation, which involves the use of proactive focused exercise to maintain muscle mass during cancer chemotherapy and in other chronic conditions such as COPD.

Psychological techniques

As with chronic pain, there is increasing use of psychological techniques in cancer pain management, which train the patient

i 34.15 Adjuvant analgesics in cancer pain			
Drug	Example	Indications	Side-effects*
NSAIDs	Diclofenac	Bone metastases, soft tissue infiltration, liver pain, inflammatory pain	Gastric irritation and bleeding, fluid retention, headache Caution in renal impairment
Glucocorticoids	Dexamethasone 8–16 mg per day, titrated to lowest dose that controls pain	Raised intracranial pressure, nerve compression, soft tissue infiltration, liver pain	Gastric irritation if used together with NSAID, fluid retention, proximal muscle myopathy, delirium, Cushingoid appearance, candidiasis, hyperglycaemia
Anticonvulsants	Evidence strongest for: Gabapentin Pregabalin Duloxetine	Neuropathic pain of any aetiology	Mild sedation, tremor, delirium Exacerbation of opioid-related side-effects
Tricyclic antidepressants	Amitriptyline	Neuropathic pain of any aetiology	Sedation, dizziness, delirium, dry mouth, constipation, urinary retention Avoid in cardiac disease Exacerbation of opioid-related side-effects
NMDA receptor blockers	Ketamine	Severe neuropathic pain (only under specialist supervision)	Delirium, anxiety, agitation, hypertension

*In old age, all drugs can cause delirium.
(NMDA = N-methyl-D-aspartate; NSAIDs = non-steroidal anti-inflammatory drugs)

to use coping strategies and behavioural techniques. Other issues related to the specific experience of a cancer diagnosis and cancer treatment may be complex, and individual therapy in addition to group-based approaches can be helpful.

Stimulation therapies

Acupuncture and TENS are low-risk stimulation therapies that may be useful in palliative care for management of pain and nausea.

Complementary and alternative therapies

Palliative care patients often seek symptom relief from both complementary and alternative therapies. While the evidence base is poorly developed, individual patients can gain significant benefits from the complementary therapies outlined on page 1348. It is critically important that patients are encouraged to discuss any alternative medicines they are considering, given the potential interactions with other therapies.

Breathlessness

Breathlessness is one of the most common symptoms in palliative care and is distressing for both patients and carers. Patients with breathlessness should be fully assessed to determine whether there is a reversible cause, such as a pleural effusion, heart failure or bronchospasm; if so, this should be managed in the normal way. If symptoms persist, additional measures may be necessary. There are many potential causes of dyspnoea in cancer patients and in other chronic diseases; apart from direct involvement of the lungs, muscle loss secondary to cachexia, anxiety and fear can all contribute. A cycle of panic and breathlessness, often associated with fear of dying, can be dominant. Exploration of precipitating factors is important and patient education about breathlessness and effective breathing has been shown to be effective. Non-pharmacological approaches that include using a hand-held fan, pacing, and following a tailored exercise programme can help. There is no evidence to suggest that oxygen therapy reduces the sensation of breathlessness in advanced cancer any better than cool airflow, and oxygen is indicated only if there is significant hypoxia. Opioids, through both their central and their peripheral action, can palliate breathlessness. Both oral and parenteral opioids are effective. A low dose should be used initially and titrated against symptoms, unless opioids are already being prescribed for pain, in which case the existing dose can be increased further. If anxiety is considered to be playing a significant role, a quick-acting benzodiazepine, such as lorazepam (used sublingually for rapid absorption), may also be useful.

Cough

Persistent unproductive cough can be helped by opioids, which have an antitussive effect. Troublesome respiratory secretions can be treated with hyoscine hydrobromide (400–600 μg every 4–8 hours), although dry mouth is a common adverse effect. As an alternative, glycopyrronium can be useful and is given by subcutaneous infusion (0.6–1.2 mg in 24 hours).

Nausea and vomiting

The presentation of nausea and vomiting differs depending on the underlying cause, of which there are many (p. 780). Large-volume vomiting with little nausea is common in intestinal obstruction, whereas constant nausea with little or no vomiting is often due to metabolic abnormalities or adverse effects of

Fig. 34.10 Mechanisms of nausea. (ACh = acetylcholine; D_2 = dopamine; 5-HT = 5-hydroxytryptamine, serotonin; H_1 = histamine)

i	**34.16 Receptor site activity of antiemetic drugs**	
Area	Receptors	Drugs
Chemotactic trigger zone	Dopamine₂ 5-HT	Haloperidol Metoclopramide
Vomiting centre	Histamine₁ Acetylcholine	Cyclizine Levomepromazine Hyoscine
Gut (gastric stasis)		Metoclopramide
Gut distension (vagal stimulation)	Histamine₁	Cyclizine
Gut (chemoreceptors)	5-HT	Levomepromazine

(5-HT = 5-hydroxytryptamine, serotonin)

drugs. Vomiting related to raised intracranial pressure is worse in the morning. Different receptors are activated, depending on the cause or causes of the nausea (Fig. 34.10). For example, dopamine receptors in the chemotactic trigger zone in the fourth ventricle are stimulated by metabolic and drug causes of nausea, whereas gastric irritation stimulates histamine receptors in the vomiting centre via the vagus nerve. Reversible causes, such as hypercalcaemia and constipation, should be treated appropriately. Drug-induced causes should be considered and the offending drugs stopped if possible. As different classes of antiemetic drug act at different receptors, antiemetic therapy should be based on a careful assessment of the probable causes and a rational decision to use a particular class of drug (Box 34.16).

34

The subcutaneous route is often required initially to overcome gastric stasis and poor absorption of oral medicines.

Gastrointestinal obstruction

Gastrointestinal obstruction is a frequent complication of intra-abdominal cancer. Patients may have multiple levels of obstruction and symptoms may vary greatly in nature and severity. Surgical mortality is high in patients with advanced disease and obstruction should normally be managed without surgery. The key to effective management is to address the presenting symptoms – colic, abdominal pain, nausea, vomiting, intestinal secretions – individually or in combination, using parenteral drugs that do not cause or worsen other symptoms. This can be problematic when a specific treatment worsens another symptom. Cyclizine improves nausea and colic responds well to anticholinergic agents, such as hyoscine butylbromide, but both slow gut motility. Nausea will improve with metoclopramide, although this is usually contraindicated in the presence of colic because of its prokinetic effect. There is some low-level evidence that glucocorticoids (dexamethasone 8 mg) can shorten the length of obstructive episodes. Somatostatin analogues, such as octreotide, will reduce intestinal secretions and therefore large-volume vomits. Occasionally, a nasogastric tube is required to reduce gaseous or fluid distension.

Weight loss

Patients with cancer lose weight for a variety of reasons, including reduced appetite or the effects of drug treatment, or as a consequence of low mood and anxiety. There is, however, a particularly challenging syndrome associated with weight loss, which is known as cancer cachexia. This results from an alteration of metabolism caused by a complex interaction of tumour-related factors and the body's response to these factors, resulting in muscle loss, along with anorexia. Treatment involves prescribing exercise to maintain muscle mass and strengthen muscles, ensuring that there is an adequate calorie intake and providing nutritional supplements. Anti-inflammatory medication to attenuate systemic inflammation is the subject of research and many patients self-medicate with fish oil. Glucocorticoids can temporarily boost appetite and general well-being but may cause false weight gain by promoting fluid retention. Their benefits need to be weighed against the risk of side-effects, and glucocorticoids should generally be used on a short-term basis only.

Anxiety and depression

Anxiety and depression are common in palliative care but the diagnosis may be difficult, since the physical symptoms of depression are similar to those of advanced cancer. It is therefore important to realise that these symptoms are not inevitable in advanced cancer. Patients should still expect to look forward to things and to enjoy them, within the context of the situation. Simply asking the question 'Do you think you are depressed?' can be very useful in deciding with the patient whether antidepressants or psychological interventions may be of benefit (p. 1199). In this regard, psycho-oncology has been evolving rapidly and there is now good evidence for the role of 'talk therapy' in palliative care, along with other appropriate management of anxiety and depression. If antidepressants are required, citalopram and mirtazapine are good choices since they are generally well tolerated in patients with advanced disease.

Delirium and agitation

Many patients become confused or agitated in the last days of life. It is important to identify and treat potentially reversible causes (p. 183), unless the patient is too close to death for this to be feasible. Early diagnosis and effective management of delirium are extremely important. As in other palliative situations, it may not be possible to identify and treat the underlying cause, and the focus of management should be to ensure that the patient is comfortable. It is important to distinguish between behavioural change due to pain and that due to delirium, as opioids will improve one and worsen the other. The management of delirium is detailed on page 209. It is important, even in the care of the actively dying patient, to treat delirium with antipsychotic medicines, such as haloperidol, rather than to regard it as distress or anxiety and use benzodiazepines only.

Dehydration

Deciding whether to give intravenous fluids can be difficult when a patient is very unwell and the prognosis is uncertain. A patient with a major stroke, who is unable to swallow but is expected to survive the event, will develop renal impairment and thirst if not given fluids and should be hydrated. On the other hand, when a patient has been deteriorating and is clearly dying, parenteral hydration needs very careful consideration and it is very important to manage this on an individual basis. Comfort and avoidance of distress in the family are the primary aims. Where a patient and family are happy with meticulous oral hygiene and care to reduce the sensation of dryness in the mouth, this is usually more appropriate and effective at the end of life than parenteral hydration, which by itself will not necessarily improve the sensation of dryness. In some patients, parenteral hydration will simply exacerbate pooling of secretions, causing noisy and distressing breathing. Each decision should be individual and discussed with the patient's family.

Death and dying

Planning for dying

There have been dramatic improvements in the medical treatment and care of patients with cancer and other illnesses over recent years but the inescapable fact remains that everyone will die at some time. Planning for death should be actively considered in patients with chronic diseases when the death is considered to be foreseeable or inevitable. Doctors rarely know exactly when a patient will die but are usually aware that an individual is about to die and that medical interventions are unlikely to extend life or improve its quality significantly. Most people wish their doctors to be honest about this situation to allow them time to think ahead, make plans and address practical issues. A few do not wish to discuss future deterioration or death; if this is felt to be the case, avoidance of discussion should be respected. For doctors, it is helpful to understand an individual's wishes and values about medical interventions at this time, as this can help guide decisions about interventions. It is important to distinguish between interventions that will not provide clinical benefit (a medical decision) and those that do not confer sufficient benefit to be worthwhile (a decision that can only be reached with a patient's involvement and consent). A common example of this would be decisions about not attempting cardiopulmonary resuscitation.

In general, people wish for a dignified and peaceful death and most prefer to die at home. Families also are grateful for the chance to prepare themselves for the death of a relative, by timely and gentle discussion with the doctor or other health professionals. Early discussion and effective planning improve the chances that an individual's wishes will be achieved. There are two important caveats: firstly, wishes can and do change as the terminal situation evolves, and secondly, planning in general can only be done over time as patients form a relationship with professionals and evolve an understanding of the situation in which they find themselves.

Structures for assessment and planning around end-of-life care are for guidance only and the focus should evolve with the individual patient.

Diagnosing dying

When patients with cancer or other conditions become bed-bound, semi-comatose, unable to take tablets and only able to take sips of water, with no reversible cause, they are likely to be dying and many will have died within 2 days. Doctors are sometimes poor at recognising this and should be alert to the views of other members of the multidisciplinary team. A clear decision that the patient is dying should be agreed and recorded.

Management of dying

Once the conclusion has been reached that a patient is going to die in days to a few weeks, there is a significant shift in management (Box 34.17). Symptom control, relief of distress and care for the family become the most important elements of care. Medication and investigation are justifiable only if they contribute to these ends. When patients can no longer drink because they are dying, intravenous fluids are usually not necessary and may cause worsening of bronchial secretions; however, this is a decision that can be made only on an individual basis. Management should not be changed without discussion with the patient and/or family. Medicines should always be prescribed for the relief of symptoms. For example, morphine or diamorphine may be used to control pain, levomepromazine to control nausea, haloperidol to treat delirium, diazepam or midazolam to treat distress, and hyoscine hydrobromide to reduce respiratory secretions. Side-effects, such as drowsiness, may be acceptable if the principal aim of relieving distress is achieved. It is important to discuss and agree the aims of care with the patient's family. Poor communication with families at this time is one of the most common reasons for family distress afterwards and for formal complaints.

Ethical considerations

The overwhelming force in caring for any patient must be to listen to that patient and family and take their wishes on board. Patients know when health-care professionals are just receiving the information, as opposed to receiving and understanding the information in the context of the patient, their illness and needs, their carers and the socioeconomic context. It is impossible to provide holistic care for a patient without this comprehension. Every patient is unique and it is important to avoid slipping into a tick-box mentality in addressing items that should be covered in patients with advanced, incurable disease. While the key to successful palliative care is effective interdisciplinary working, every patient needs to know who has overall responsibility

34.17 How to manage a patient who is dying
Patient and family awareness
• Assess patient's and family's awareness of the situation
• Ensure family understands plan of care
Medical interventions
• Stop non-essential medications that do not contribute to symptom control
• Stop inappropriate investigations and interventions, including routine observations
Resuscitation
• Complete Do Not Attempt Cardiopulmonary Resuscitation (DNACPR) form
• Deactivate implantable defibrillator
Symptom control
• Ensure availability of parenteral medication for symptom relief
Support for family
• Make sure you have contact details for family, that you know when they want to be contacted and that they are aware of facilities available to them
Religious and spiritual needs
• Make sure any particular wishes are identified and followed
Ongoing assessment
• Family's awareness of condition
• Management of symptoms
• Need for parenteral hydration
Care after death
• Make sure family know what they have to do
• Notify other appropriate health professionals

for their care. Trust in the whole team will come through a solid lead working with a team who are appropriately informed and in sympathy with the patient's situation, each having a clear role.

Families and other carers are often unprepared for the challenge of caring for a dying person. It can be an exhausting experience, both emotionally and physically, and without a critical number of carers battle fatigue can ensue, resulting in urgent admissions. With much discussion about advance directives, we should not lose sight of the reality of changing circumstances and wishes. Good anticipatory care means not just providing for new physical symptoms, but also planning for any time when care at home becomes no longer possible.

Capacity and advance directives

The wishes of the patient are paramount in Western societies, whereas in other cultures the views of the family are equally important. If a patient is unable to express their view because of communication or cognitive impairment, that person is said to lack 'capacity'. In order to decide what the patient would have wished, as much information as possible should be gained about any previously expressed wishes, along with the views of relatives and other health professionals. An advance directive is a previously recorded, written document of a patient's wishes (p. 1307). It should carry the same weight in decision-making as a patient's expressed wishes at that time, but may not be sufficiently specific to be used in a particular clinical situation. The legal framework for decision-making varies in different countries.

Euthanasia

In the UK and Europe, between 3% and 6% of dying patients will ask a doctor to end their life. Many of these requests are transient; some are associated with poor control of physical symptoms or a depressive illness. All expressions of a wish to die are an opportunity to help the patient discuss and address unresolved issues and problems. Reversible causes, such as pain or depression, should be treated. Sometimes, patients may choose to discontinue life-prolonging treatments, such as diuretics or anticoagulation, following discussion and the provision of adequate alternative symptom control. However, there remain a small number of patients who have a sustained, competent wish to end their lives, despite good control of physical symptoms. Euthanasia is now permitted or legal under certain circumstances in some countries but remains illegal in many others; public, ethical and legal debate over this issue is likely to continue and is often influenced by many complex non-palliative care issues. The European Association for Palliative Care does not see euthanasia or physician-assisted suicide as part of the role of palliative care physicians.

Further information

Websites

breathworks-mindfulness.org.uk *An online resource to support learning the use of mindfulness to deal with pain, illness or stress.*
cuh.org.uk/breathlessness *Information and resources from Cambridge University Hospital on managing breathlessness.*
hospiceuk.org *A resource from UK hospices.*
mdanderson.org *Brief Pain Inventory (Short Form) questionnaire.*
nhmrc.gov.au *Australia and New Zealand College of Anaesthetists and Faculty of Pain Medicine. Acute pain management: scientific evidence, 3rd edn; 2010.*
npcrc.org *Short-form McGill Pain questionnaire.*
paintoolkit.org *Pain toolkit self-help resource for managing pain.*
palliativecareguidelines.scot.nhs.uk *Regularly reviewed, evidence-based clinical guidelines.*
palliativedrugs.com *Practical information about drugs used in palliative care.*
sign.ac.uk *SIGN guideline 136 – Management of chronic pain.*

Journal articles

Finnerup NB, Attal N, Haroutounian S, et al. Pharmacotherapy for neuropathic pain in adults: a systematic review and meta-analysis. Lancet Neurol 2015; 14:162–173. *A comprehensive, high-quality review of the current evidence for the pharmacological management of neuropathic pain.*

35

Laboratory reference ranges

Notes on the international system of units (SI units) 1358

Laboratory reference ranges in adults 1358
Urea and electrolytes in venous blood 1358
Analytes in arterial blood 1358
Hormones in venous blood 1359
Other common analytes in venous blood 1360
Common analytes in urine 1361
Analytes in cerebrospinal fluid 1361
Analytes in faeces 1361
Haematological values 1362

Laboratory reference ranges in childhood and adolescence 1363

Laboratory reference ranges in pregnancy 1364

Notes on the international system of units (SI units)

Système International (SI) units are a specific subset of the metre–kilogram–second system of units and were agreed on as the everyday currency for commercial and scientific work in 1960, following a series of international conferences organised by the International Bureau of Weights and Measures. SI units have been adopted widely in clinical laboratories but non-SI units are still used in many countries. For that reason, values in both units are given for common measurements throughout this textbook and commonly used non-SI units are shown in this chapter. The SI unit system is, however, recommended.

Examples of basic SI units

Length	metre (m)
Mass	kilogram (kg)
Amount of substance	mole (mol)
Energy	joule (J)
Pressure	pascal (Pa)
Volume	The basic SI unit of volume is the cubic metre (1000 litres). For convenience, however, the litre (L) is used as the unit of volume in laboratory work.

Examples of decimal multiples and submultiples of SI units

Factor	Name	Prefix
10^6	mega-	M
10^3	kilo-	k
10^{-1}	deci-	d
10^{-2}	centi-	c
10^{-3}	milli-	m
10^{-6}	micro-	μ
10^{-9}	nano-	n
10^{-12}	pico-	p
10^{-15}	femto-	f

Exceptions to the use of SI units

By convention, blood pressure is excluded from the SI unit system and is measured in mmHg (millimetres of mercury) rather than pascals.

Mass concentrations such as g/L and μg/L are used in preference to molar concentrations for all protein measurements and for substances that do not have a sufficiently well-defined composition.

Some enzymes and hormones are measured by 'bioassay', in which the activity in the sample is compared with the activity (rather than the mass) of a standard sample that is provided from a central source. For these assays, results are given in standardised 'units' (U/L), or 'international units' (IU/L), which depend on the activity in the standard sample and may not be readily converted to mass units.

Laboratory reference ranges in adults

Reference ranges are largely those used in the Departments of Clinical Biochemistry and Haematology, Lothian Health University Hospitals Division, Edinburgh, UK. Values are shown in both SI units and, where appropriate, non-SI units. Many reference ranges vary between laboratories, depending on the assay method used and on other factors; this is especially the case for enzyme assays. The origin of reference ranges and the interpretation of 'abnormal' results are discussed on page 3. No details are given here of the collection requirements, which may be critical to obtaining a meaningful result. Unless otherwise stated, reference ranges shown apply to adults; values in children may be different.

Many analytes can be measured in either serum (the supernatant of clotted blood) or plasma (the supernatant of anticoagulated blood). A specific requirement for one or the other may depend on a kit manufacturer's recommendations. In other instances, the distinction is critical. An example is fibrinogen, where plasma is required, since fibrinogen is largely absent from serum. In contrast, serum is required for electrophoresis to detect paraproteins because fibrinogen migrates as a discrete band in the zone of interest.

i 35.1 **Urea and electrolytes in venous blood**

Analysis	Reference range	
	SI units	Non-SI units
Sodium	135–145 mmol/L	135–145 mEq/L
Potassium*	3.6–5.0 mmol/L	3.6–5.0 mEq/L
Chloride	95–107 mmol/L	95–107 mEq/L
Urea	2.5–6.6 mmol/L	15–40 mg/dL
Creatinine		
Male	64–111 μmol/L	0.72–1.26 mg/dL
Female	50–98 μmol/L	0.57–1.11 mg/dL

*Serum values are, on average, 0.3 mmol/L higher than plasma values.

i 35.2 **Analytes in arterial blood**

Analysis	Reference range	
	SI units	Non-SI units
Bicarbonate	21–29 mmol/L	21–29 mEq/L
Hydrogen ion	37–45 nmol/L	pH 7.35–7.43
$PaCO_2$	4.5–6.0 kPa	34–45 mmHg
PaO_2	12–15 kPa	90–113 mmHg
Oxygen saturation	>97%	

i 35.3 Hormones in venous blood

Hormone	Reference range	
	SI units	Non-SI units
Adrenocorticotrophic hormone (ACTH) (plasma)	1.5–13.9 pmol/L (0700–1000 hrs)	63 ng/L
Aldosterone Supine (at least 30 mins) Erect (at least 1 hr)	30–440 pmol/L 110–860 pmol/L	1.09–15.9 ng/dL 3.97–31.0 ng/dL
Cortisol	Dynamic tests are required – see Box 18.53, p. 680	
Follicle-stimulating hormone (FSH) Male Female	1.0–10.0 IU/L 3.0–10.0 IU/L (early follicular) >30 IU/L (post-menopausal)	– – –
Gastrin (plasma, fasting)	<40 pmol/L	<83 pg/mL
Growth hormone (GH)	Dynamic tests are usually required – see Box 18.55, p. 682 <0.5 μg/L excludes acromegaly (if insulin-like growth factor 1 (IGF-1) in reference range) >6 μg/L excludes GH deficiency	<2 mIU/L >18 mIU/L
Insulin	Highly variable and interpretable only in relation to plasma glucose and body habitus	
Luteinising hormone (LH) Male Female	1.0–9.0 IU/L 2.0–9.0 IU/L (early follicular) >20 IU/L (post-menopausal)	– – –
17β-Oestradiol Male Female: early follicular 　　　　post-menopausal	<160 pmol/L 75–140 pmol/L <150 pmol/L	<43 pg/mL 20–38 pg/mL <41 pg/mL
Parathyroid hormone (PTH)	1.6–6.9 pmol/L	16–69 pg/mL
Progesterone (in luteal phase in women) Consistent with ovulation Probable ovulatory cycle Anovulatory cycle	>30 nmol/L 15–30 nmol/L <10 nmol/L	>9.3 ng/mL 4.7–9.3 ng/mL <3 ng/mL
Prolactin (PRL)	60–500 mIU/L	2.8–23.5 ng/mL
Renin concentration Supine (at least 30 mins) Sitting (at least 15 mins) Erect (at least 1 hr)	5–40 mIU/L 5–45 mIU/L 16–63 mIU/L	– – –
Testosterone Male Female	10–38 nmol/L 0.3–1.9 nmol/L	290–1090 ng/dL 10–90 ng/dL
Thyroid-stimulating hormone (TSH)	0.2–4.5 mIU/L	–
Thyroxine (free), (free T₄)	9–21 pmol/L	0.7–1.63 ng/dL
Triiodothyronine (free), (free T₃)	2.6–6.2 pmol/L	0.16–0.4 ng/dL

Notes
1. A number of hormones are unstable and collection details are critical to obtaining a meaningful result. Refer to local laboratory handbook.
2. Values in the table are only a guideline; hormone levels can often be meaningfully understood only in relation to factors such as gender, age, time of day, pubertal status, stage of the menstrual cycle, pregnancy and menopausal status.
3. Reference ranges are usually dependent on the method used for analysis and frequently differ between laboratories. Non-SI units also differ; those shown here are amongst those most widely used. Readers are encouraged to consult their local laboratory for non-SI units for individual analytes and their respective reference ranges.

i 35.4 Other common analytes in venous blood

Analyte	Reference range SI units	Reference range Non-SI units	Analyte	Reference range SI units	Reference range Non-SI units
α_1-antitrypsin	1.1–2.1 g/L	110–210 mg/dL	γ-glutamyl transferase (GGT)	Male 10–55 U/L Female 5–35 U/L	–
Alanine aminotransferase (ALT)	10–50 U/L	–	Glucose (fasting)	3.6–5.8 mmol/L See page 722 for definitions of impaired glucose tolerance and diabetes mellitus, and page 738 for definition of hypoglycaemia	65–104 mg/dL
Albumin	35–50 g/L	3.5–5.0 g/dL
Alkaline phosphatase (ALP)	40–125 U/L	–	Glycated haemoglobin (HbA$_{1c}$)	4.0–6.0% 20–42 mmol/mol Hb See page 722 for diagnosis of diabetes mellitus	–
Amylase	<100 U/L	–
Aspartate aminotransferase (AST)	10–45 U/L	–	Immunoglobulins (Ig) IgA IgE IgG IgM	0.8–4.5 g/L 0–250 kU/L 6.0–15.0 g/L 0.35–2.90 g/L	– – – –
Bile acids (fasting)	<14 µmol/L	–
Bilirubin (total)	3–16 µmol/L	0.18–0.94 mg/dL	Lactate	0.6–2.4 mmol/L	5.4–21.6 mg/dL
Calcium (total)	2.1–2.6 mmol/L	4.2–5.2 mEq/L or 8.5–10.5 mg/dL	Lactate dehydrogenase (LDH; total)	125–220 U/L	–
Carboxyhaemoglobin	0.1–3.0% Levels of up to 8% may be found in heavy smokers	–	Lead	<0.5 µmol/L	<10 µg/dL
			Magnesium	0.75–1.0 mmol/L	1.5–2.0 mEq/L or 1.82–2.43 mg/dL
Caeruloplasmin	0.16–0.47 g/L	16–47 mg/dL	Osmolality	280–296 mOsmol/kg	–
Cholesterol (total)	Ideal level varies according to cardiovascular risk (see cardiovascular risk chart, p. 511)		Osmolarity	280–296 mOsmol/L	–
			Phosphate (fasting)	0.8–1.4 mmol/L	2.48–4.34 mg/dL
HDL-cholesterol	Ideal level varies according to cardiovascular risk, so reference ranges can be misleading. According to the National Cholesterol Education Programme Adult Treatment Panel III (ATPIII), a low HDL-cholesterol is <1.0 mmol/L (<40 mg/dL)		Protein (total)	60–80 g/L	6–8 g/dL
			Triglycerides (fasting)	0.6–1.7 mmol/L	53–150 mg/dL
			Troponins	Values consistent with myocardial infarction are crucially dependent on which troponin is measured (I or T) and on the method employed. Interpret in context of clinical presentation. See page 450	
Complement C3 C4 Total haemolytic complement	0.81–1.57 g/L 0.13–1.39 g/L 0.086–0.410 g/L	– – –	Tryptase	0–135 mg/L	–
			Urate Male Female	0.12–0.42 mmol/L 0.12–0.36 mmol/L	2.0–7.0 mg/dL 2.0–6.0 mg/dL
Copper	10–22 µmol/L	64–140 µg/dL
C-reactive protein (CRP)	<5 mg/L Highly sensitive CRP assays also exist that measure lower values and may be useful in estimating cardiovascular risk		Vitamin D (25(OH)D) Normal Insufficiency Deficiency	>50 nmol/L 25–50 nmol/L <25 nmol/L	>20 ng/mL 10–20 ng/ml <10 ng/mL
Creatine kinase (CK; total) Male Female	55–170 U/L 30–135 U/L	– –	Zinc	10–18 µmol/L	65–118 µg/dL
Creatine kinase MB isoenzyme	<6% of total CK	–
Ethanol Marked intoxication Stupor Coma	Not normally detectable 65–87 mmol/L 87–109 mmol/L >109 mmol/L	300–400 mg/dL 400–500 mg/dL >500 mg/dL

35.5 Common analytes in urine

Analyte	Reference range SI units	Non-SI units
Albumin	Definitions of microalbuminuria are given on page 394 Proteinuria is defined below	
Calcium (normal diet)	Up to 7.5 mmol/24 hrs	Up to 15 mEq/24 hrs or 300 mg/24 hrs
Copper	<0.6 μmol/24 hrs	<38 μg/24 hrs
Cortisol	20–180 nmol/24 hrs	7.2–65 μg/24 hrs
Creatinine Male Female	6.3–23 mmol/24 hrs 4.1–15 mmol/24 hrs	712–2600 mg/24 hrs 463–1695 mg/24 hrs
5-Hydroxyindole-3-acetic acid (5-HIAA)	10–42 μmol/24 hrs	1.9–8.1 mg/24 hrs
Metadrenalines Normetadrenaline Metadrenaline	0.4–3.4 μmol/24 hrs 0.3–1.7 μmol/24 hrs	73–620 μg/24 hrs 59–335 μg/24 hrs
Oxalate	0.04–0.49 mmol/24 hrs	3.6–44 mg/24 hrs
Phosphate	15–50 mmol/24 hrs	465–1548 mg/24 hrs
Potassium*	25–100 mmol/24 hrs	25–100 mEq/24 hrs
Protein	<0.3 g/L	<0.03 g/dL
Sodium*	100–200 mmol/24 hrs	100–200 mEq/24 hrs
Urate	1.2–3.0 mmol/24 hrs	202–504 mg/24 hrs
Urea	170–600 mmol/24 hrs	10.2–36.0 g/24 hrs
Zinc	3–21 μmol/24 hrs	195–1365 μg/24 hrs

*The urinary output of electrolytes such as sodium and potassium is normally a reflection of dietary intake. This can vary widely. The values quoted are appropriate to a 'Western' diet.

35.6 Analytes in cerebrospinal fluid

Analysis	Reference range SI units	Non–SI units
Cells	<5×10[6] cells/L (all mononuclear)	<5 cells/mm[3]
Glucose[1]	2.3–4.5 mmol/L	41–81 mg/dL
IgG index[2]	<0.65	–
Total protein	0.14–0.45 g/L	0.014–0.045 g/dL

[1]Interpret in relation to plasma glucose. Values in CSF are typically approximately two-thirds of plasma levels. [2]A crude index of increase in IgG attributable to intrathecal synthesis.

35.7 Analytes in faeces

Analyte	Reference range SI units	Non-SI units
Calprotectin	<50 μg/g	–
Elastase	>200 μg/g	–

i 35.8 Haematological values

Analysis	Reference range	
	SI units	Non-SI units
Bleeding time (Ivy)	<8 mins	–
Blood volume		
Male	65–85 mL/kg	–
Female	60–80 mL/kg	–
Coagulation screen		
Prothrombin time (PT)	10.5–13.5 secs	–
Activated partial thromboplastin time (APTT)	26–36 secs	–
D-dimers		
Interpret in relation to clinical presentation	<200 ng/mL	–
Erythrocyte sedimentation rate (ESR)	Higher values in older patients are not necessarily abnormal	
Adult male	0–10 mm/hr	–
Adult female	3–15 mm/hr	–
Ferritin		
Male (and post-menopausal female)	20–300 µg/L	20–300 ng/mL
Female (pre-menopausal)	15–200 µg/L	15–200 ng/mL
Fibrinogen	1.5–4.0 g/L	0.15–0.4 g/dL
Folate		
Serum	2.8–20 µg/L	2.8–20 ng/mL
Red cell	120–500 µg/L	120–500 ng/mL
Haemoglobin		
Male	130–180 g/L	13–18 g/dL
Female	115–165 g/L	11.5–16.5 g/dL
Haptoglobin	0.4–2.4 g/L	0.04–0.24 g/dL
Iron		
Male	14–32 µmol/L	78–178 µg/dL
Female	10–28 µmol/L	56–157 µg/dL
Leucocytes (adults)	$4.0–11.0 \times 10^9$/L	$4.0–11.0 \times 10^3$/mm^3
Differential white cell count		
Neutrophil granulocytes	$2.0–7.5 \times 10^9$/L	$2.0–7.5 \times 10^3$/mm^3
Lymphocytes	$1.5–4.0 \times 10^9$/L	$1.5–4.0 \times 10^3$/mm^3
Monocytes	$0.2–0.8 \times 10^9$/L	$0.2–0.8 \times 10^3$/mm^3
Eosinophil granulocytes	$0.04–0.4 \times 10^9$/L	$0.04–0.4 \times 10^3$/mm^3
Basophil granulocytes	$0.01–0.1 \times 10^9$/L	$0.01–0.1 \times 10^3$/mm^3
Mean cell haemoglobin (MCH)	27–32 pg	–
Mean cell volume (MCV)	78–98 fl	–
Packed cell volume (PCV) or haematocrit		
Male	0.40–0.54	–
Female	0.37–0.47	–
Platelets	$150–350 \times 10^9$/L	$150–350 \times 10^3$/mm^3
Red cell count		
Male	$4.5–6.5 \times 10^{12}$/L	$4.5–6.5 \times 10^6$/mm^3
Female	$3.8–5.8 \times 10^{12}$/L	$3.8–5.8 \times 10^6$/mm^3
Red cell lifespan		
Mean	120 days	–
Half-life (^{51}Cr)	25–35 days	–
Reticulocytes (adults)	$25–85 \times 10^9$/L	$25–85 \times 10^3$/mm^3
Transferrin	2.0–4.0 g/L	0.2–0.4 g/dL
Transferrin saturation		
Male	25–50%	–
Female	14–50%	–
Vitamin B$_{12}$		
Normal	>210 ng/L	–
Intermediate	180–200 ng/L	–
Low	<180 ng/L	–

Laboratory reference ranges in childhood and adolescence

The levels of many analytes in blood vary due to the physiological changes that occur during growth and adolescence. Hospital laboratories may provide reference ranges that are age-adjusted or based on pubertal stage but this is not always the case. It is therefore important for the doctor requesting these tests to understand the impact of age and puberty on interpretation of the results. For example, a creatinine of 70 μmol/L (0.79 mg/dL) is perfectly normal for the majority of adults but may indicate significant renal impairment in a child. Reference ranges for hormone results are described according to the Tanner stages of puberty (p. 1290).

35.9 Analytes that may be significantly affected by growth and puberty*

Analyte	Age/Pubertal stage	Gender	Reference range	Analyte	Age/Pubertal stage	Gender	Reference range
Alkaline phosphatase (ALP)	<1 year	M, F	80–580 U/L	Luteinising hormone (LH)	Prepubertal	M	<1.0 IU/L (<0.1 μg/L)
	1–16 years	M, F	100–400 U/L		Pubertal stage 2	M	<3.0 IU/L (<0.3 μg/L)
	16–20 years	M	50–250 U/L		Prepubertal and pubertal stage 2	F	<1.0 IU/L (<0.1 μg/L)
		F	40–200 U/L		Pubertal stage 3	M	1.0–4.0 IU/L (0.1–0.4 μg/L)
Creatinine	<1 year	M, F	12–39 μmol/L (0.14–0.44 mg/dL)		Pubertal stages 4–5	M	1.0–5.0 IU/L (0.1–0.6 μg/L)
	1–4 years	M, F	13–42 μmol/L (0.15–0.48 mg/dL)		Pubertal stages 3–5	F	1.0–8.0 IU/L (0.1–0.9 μg/L)
	4–12 years	M, F	20–57 μmol/L (0.23–0.64 mg/dL)	17β-Oestradiol	Prepubertal and pubertal stages 2–3	M	<75 pmol/L (<20 pg/mL)
	12–15 years	M, F	31–67 μmol/L (0.35–0.76 mg/dL)		Prepubertal and pubertal stage 2	F	<100 pmol/L (<27 pg/mL)
	15–18 years	M	39–92 μmol/L (0.44–1.04 mg/dL)		Pubertal stages 4–5	M	<130 pmol/L (<35 pg/mL)
		F	34–72 μmol/L (0.38–0.81 mg/dL)		Pubertal stages 3–5	F	<150 pmol/L (<41 pg/mL)
Follicle-stimulating hormone (FSH)	Prepubertal	M	<3.0 IU/L (<0.6 μg/L)	Testosterone	Prepubertal	M	<0.5 nmol/L (<10 ng/dL)
		F	<3.2 IU/L (<0.64 μg/L)			F	<0.6 nmol/L (<20 ng/dL)
	Pubertal stage 2	M	<6.6 IU/L (<1.32 μg/L)		Pubertal stage 2	M	<10.6 nmol/L (<310 ng/dL)
		F	<4.1 IU/L (<0.82 μg/L)			F	<1.4 nmol/L (<40 ng/dL)
	Pubertal stage 3	M	0.7–5.0 IU/L (0.14–1 μg/L)		Pubertal stage 3	M	0.4–30 nmol/L (10–870 ng/dL)
	Pubertal stages 4–5	M	1.5–6.0 IU/L (0.3–1.2 μg/L)		Pubertal stage 4	M	5.6–30 nmol/L (160–870 ng/dL)
	Pubertal stages 3–5	F	2.5–13.5 IU/L (0.5–2.7 μg/L)		Pubertal stage 5	M	10–30 nmol/L (290–870 ng/dL)
Insulin-like growth factor 1	<7 years	M	15–349 μg/L		Pubertal stages 3–5	F	0.4–1.9 nmol/L (10–50 ng/dL)
		F	17–272 μg/L				
	8–16 years	M	67–510 μg/L				
		F	59–502 μg/L				

*Non-SI equivalents are given in brackets where appropriate.

Laboratory reference ranges in pregnancy

The levels of many analytes in blood vary during pregnancy, when many hormonal and metabolic changes occur. The standard adult reference ranges may therefore not be appropriate and it is important for the clinician reviewing the results to be aware of this to enable appropriate interpretation and patient management.

35.10 Analytes that may be significantly affected by pregnancy*

Analyte	Reference range		
	First trimester	Second trimester	Third trimester
Alkaline phosphatase (ALP)	17–88 U/L	25–126 U/L	38–229 U/L
Packed cell volume (PCV) or haematocrit	0.31–0.41	0.30–0.39	0.28–0.40
Haemoglobin	116–139 g/L	97–148 g/L	95–150 g/L
Human chorionic gonadotrophin	4 weeks: 16–156 IU/L 4–9 weeks: 101–233 000 IU/L 9–13 weeks: 20 900–291 000 IU/L	4270–103 000 IU/L	2700–78 300 IU/L
17β-Oestradiol	690–9166 pmol/L (188–2497 pg/mL)	4691–26 401 pmol/L (1278–7192 pg/mL)	12 701–22 528 pmol/L (3460–6137 pg/mL)
Progesterone	25–153 nmol/L (8–48 ng/mL)	Not available	314–1088 nmol/L (99–342 ng/mL)
Prolactin	765–4532 mIU/L (36–213 ng/mL)	2340–7021 mIU/L (110–330 ng/mL)	2914–7914 mIU/L (137–372 ng/mL)
Thyroid-stimulating hormone (TSH)	0.60–3.40 mIU/L	0.37–3.60 mIU/L	0.38–4.04 mIU/L
Thyroxine (free), (free T$_4$)	10–18 pmol/L 0.77–1.40 ng/dL	9–16 pmol/L 0.70–1.24 ng/dL	8–14 pmol/L 0.62–1.09 ng/dL

*Non-SI equivalents are given in brackets where appropriate.

Further information

Abbassi-Ghanavati M, Greer LG, Cunningham FG. Pregnancy and laboratory studies: a reference table for clinicians. Obstet Gynecol 2009; 114:1326–1331.

Tanner JM, Whitehouse RH. Clinical longitudinal standards for height, weight, height velocity, weight velocity, and stages of puberty. Arch Dis Child 1976; 51:170–179.

Index

Page numbers followed by '*f*' indicate figures, and '*b*' indicate boxes.

A

AAAs *see* Abdominal aortic aneurysms
Abacavir, 324*b*
  for HIV/AIDS, 324–325, 324*b*
  hypersensitivity reaction of, 326
  pharmacodynamics of, 180*b*
Abaloparatide, for osteoporosis, 1048*b*,
  1049
Abatacept, for musculoskeletal disease,
  1007, 1007*b*
Abciximab, platelet inhibition, 500,
  918
Abdomen
  examination of
    blood disease, 912*f*
    cancer, 1315*b*
    cardiovascular disease, 442*f*
    gastrointestinal disease, 764*f*
    liver and biliary disease, 846–847
    renal and urinary tract disease,
     382*f*–383*f*
  palpation of, 765*b*
  percussion of, 765*b*
  swelling of *see* Ascites
Abdominal aortic aneurysms (AAAs),
  505, 505*b*
Abdominal compartment syndrome,
  diagnosis and management of,
  195
Abdominal examination, 765*b*
Abdominal pain, 787–789
  acute, 787–789, 787*b*
  assessment of, 787, 788*f*
  chronic or recurrent, 789, 789*b*
  constant, 789
  diabetic ketoacidosis and, 736,
   736*b*
  investigations of, 787
  irritable bowel syndrome and, 824
  large bowel obstruction of, 789
  liver abscess and, 880
  in lower abdomen, 336
  management of, 787–789
  in old age, 788*b*
  pancreatitis
    acute, 837–839, 837*b*
    chronic, 839–841
  peptic ulcer, perforated, 789
Abdominal tuberculosis, 812–813
Abducens (6th cranial) nerve, tests of,
  1063*b*
Abetalipoproteinaemia, 810
Abnormal movements, 1084–1086,
  1085*b*
Abnormal perceptions, 1086, 1181
ABO blood groups, 931–932, 933*b*
ABO-incompatible red cell transfusion,
  932–933
ABPA *see* Allergic bronchopulmonary
  aspergillosis
ABPI *see* Ankle-brachial pressure
  index

Abscess
  anorectal, 836
  cerebral, 1124, 1124*b*, 1124*f*
  'collar-stud', 590
  infective endocarditis and, 527
  intra-abdominal, 787*b*
  liver, 879–880, 893
    amoebic, 880
    in old age, 901*b*
    pyogenic, 879–880, 880*b*
  lung, 219*f*, 251*f*
  pancreatic, 219*f*
  perinephric, 430
  pulmonary, 586–587
  spinal epidural, 1125
Absence seizures, 1099
Absidia, 303
Absolute erythrocytosis, 925, 925*b*
Absorption, 17–18
  gastrointestinal tract, 17
  interactions, 23
  parenteral, 17
  topical, 17–18
  see also Malabsorption
ABVD regimen, for Hodgkin lymphoma,
  963
Acamprosate, 1195
Acanthosis, 1244
Acanthosis nigricans, 1265, 1325*b*,
  1326
Acarbose, 745–746
Accelerated hypertension, 514
Accessory (11th cranial) nerve, tests of,
  1063*b*
Acclimatisation
  to heat, 167
  to high altitude, 168
Accommodation, 1198
ACCORD (Action to Control
  Cardiovascular Risk in Diabetes),
  757
ACD *see* Anaemia(s), of chronic disease
ACE (angiotensin-converting enzyme),
  351–352
ACE inhibitors
  for acute coronary syndrome
    prevention, 498*b*
  adverse reactions of, 22*b*, 1310*b*
    angioedema, 1266*b*
    cough, 556
    hyperkalemia, 363
  for chronic kidney disease, 417
  contraindication to, cirrhosis, 894*b*
  effect on renal function, 426, 427*b*
  for heart failure, 466, 466*f*
    dosages, 466*b*
    sites of action, 466*f*
  for hypertension, 513
  for mitral regurgitation, 521
  for myocardial infarction, 500–501
  during pregnancy, 32*b*
Acetaldehyde metabolism, 881

Acetazolamide, 354
  for altitude illness, 168
  for epilepsy, 1102*b*
  for idiopathic intracranial
   hypertension, 1133
Acetyl-CoA, 881
Acetylcholine, 767
Acetylcholinesterase (AChE), 1142*f*
Acetylcysteine, 138
Achalasia of oesophagus, 794–795
AChE *see* Acetylcholinesterase
Achilles tendinitis, 999
Achlorhydria, 803*f*, 808*b*, 941
Aciclovir
  for herpes virus infection, 126, 127*b*
    bone marrow transplant patients,
     937*b*
    chickenpox/shingles, 239*b*
    genital, 342
    HIV/AIDS, 315
    viral encephalitis, 1122
  nephrotoxicity, 427*b*
  in pregnancy, 120*b*
Acid-base balance
  chronic kidney disease and, 418
  disorders
    mixed, 367
    presenting problems of, 364–367
  homeostasis, 363–367
  principal patterns of disturbances,
   365*b*
  renal control of, 364
Acidosis
  lactic, 365
    diabetic, 746
    poisoning, 149*b*
  metabolic, 364–366
    acute kidney injury and, 413
    chronic kidney disease, 415
    critically ill patients and, 180–181
    diabetic ketoacidosis, 735
    differential diagnosis, 558*b*
    hypothermia and, 166
    malaria, 276*b*
    near-drowning, 170
    poisoning and, 135*b*
    renal tubular, 365*b*
  respiratory, 367
Acids, poisoning, 136*b*
Acinus, 548–549, 549*f*, 848, 848*f*
Acitretin
  for atopic eczema, 1246
  for psoriasis, 1227
Acne, 1241–1244, 1242*f*
  in adolescence, 1241*b*
  conglobata, 1242
  cystic, 1242*f*
  excoriée, 1242
  fulminans, 1242
  secondary, 1242
  vulgaris, 1241–1243
Acneiform eruptions, 1266*b*

Acoustic neuroma, 1131
Acquired C1 inhibitor deficiency, 88
Acrochordon, 1235
Acrocyanosis, 84*b*, 950
Acrodermatitis chronica atrophicans,
  256
Acrodermatitis enteropathica, 717
Acromegaly, 630*f*, 685–687, 686*f*
  musculoskeletal manifestations of,
   1057
ACTH *see* Adrenocorticotrophic
  hormone
Actinic dermatitis, chronic, 1221*b*,
  1222*f*
Actinic keratosis, 1230*b*, 1231, 1231*f*
Actinic prurigo, 1221*b*
Actinomadura spp., 301
Actinomyces israelii, 261–262
Actinomyces spp., 103*f*
Actinomycete infections, 261–262
Actinomycetes, 100–101
Actinomycetoma, 301
Action potential, 1065
Activated partial thromboplastin time
  (APTT), 920–921
  reference range of, 1362*b*
Active proctitis, 820
Activities of daily living (ADL), 1303*b*
  Barthel Index, 1311, 1312*b*
Acupuncture, for pain management,
  1347, 1347*f*
Acute abdomen, 787–789, 787*b*, 788*f*
Acute benign asbestos pleurisy, 618
Acute cholinergic syndrome, 146, 146*b*
Acute circulatory failure, 199–200
Acute colonic ischaemia, 827
Acute colonic pseudo-obstruction, 835,
  835*b*
'Acute confusional states,' in older
  people, 1080
Acute coronary syndrome, 493–501,
  493*b*–494*b*, 494*f*–495*f*
  chest pain and, 455
  clinical features of, 494–496, 495*b*
  complications of, 494–495
  management of, 498–501, 498*b*,
   499*f*
  see also Myocardial infarction
Acute disseminated encephalomyelitis,
  1110
Acute eosinophilic pneumonia, 611
Acute fatty liver of pregnancy, 1283,
  1283*b*
Acute inflammation, 70–71, 71*f*
  acute phase response in, 70
  resolution of, 71
  septic shock and, 70–71
Acute inflammatory arthritis, 1017
Acute intermittent porphyria, 379*b*
Acute interstitial nephritis (AIN), 402,
  402*b*
Acute interstitial pneumonia (AIP), 606*b*

Acute kidney injury (AKI), 411–415
  causes of, 411f
  clinical features of, 411–413
  dialysis for, indications for, 422b
  haemodialysis in, 422
  interstitial, 402, 402b
  investigations of, 412b
  malaria, 276b
  management of, 413–414, 413b
  non-oliguric, 402
  in old age, 414b
  pathophysiology of, 411
  post-renal, 412b, 413
  pre-renal, 411–412, 412b
  pregnancy and, 1282, 1283b
  recovery from, 414–415, 414f
  renal, 412–413, 412b
  renal replacement therapy, 414
Acute leukaemia, 955–958
  investigations of, 955–956, 956f
  management of, 956–958
    haematopoietic stem cell
      transplantation, 958
    specific therapy, 956–957,
      956b–957b
    supportive therapy, 957–958
  outcome of, 958b
  prognosis of, 958
  WHO classification of, 955b
Acute limb ischaemia, 503, 503b, 503f
Acute liver failure, 856–859
  adverse prognostic criteria in, 858b
  causes of, 856f–857f
  classification of, 857b
  clinical assessment of, 857–858
  complications of, 858b
  hepatic encephalopathy and, 857b
  hepatitis A and, 873
  investigations for, 858, 858b
  management of, 858–859, 858b
  pathophysiology of, 857
Acute lung injury, 170
Acute lymphoblastic leukaemia (ALL),
    955, 956f
Acute medicine, 173–214
  ambulatory care, 176, 176b
  decision to admit to hospital, 176
  problems in, 176–187
Acute mountain sickness (AMS), 168
Acute myeloid leukaemia (AML), 955,
    956f, 958b
'Acute on chronic' type II respiratory
    failure, 566–567, 566b
Acute pancreatitis, 837–839, 837b
  causes of, 838b
  complications of, 838b
  management of, 839
  pathophysiology of, 837, 838f
Acute pericarditis, 542, 542b, 542f
Acute phase proteins, 72
Acute phase response, 105
  ferritin levels in, 941
  musculoskeletal disease, 1017–1018
  retroperitoneal fibrosis, 434
  rheumatic disease, 1012
Acute Physiology Assessment and
    Chronic Health Evaluation
    (APACHE II), 214, 214b
Acute renal failure see Acute kidney
    injury
Acute respiratory distress syndrome
    (ARDS), 198
  aetiology of, 198, 198b
  Berlin definition of, 198b
  diagnosis of, 198, 199f
  drug-induced, 612b
  management of, 198
  mechanical ventilation in, 198
  near-drowning victims and, 170
  pathogenesis of, 198
  severity of, 199b
Acute rheumatic fever, 515–517, 516f
  investigations in, 517b
  Jones criteria for, 516b
Acute severe breathlessness, 558
Acute skin failure, 1224–1225
Acute small bowel ischaemia, 827
Acute transmural anterior myocardial
    infarction, 497f

Acute transmural inferolateral myocardial
    infarction, 498f
Acute tubular necrosis (ATN), 402f
  drug-induced, 427b
Adalimumab
  for inflammatory bowel disease, 820,
    821b
  for inflammatory rheumatic disease,
    1007b
  for psoriasis, 1250–1251
Adapalene, 1242–1243
Adaptive immune system, 67–70
ADCC see Antibody-dependent cellular
    cytotoxicity
Addenbrooke's Cognitive Examination-
    3rd edition (ACE-III), 1181–1183
Addison's disease, 671b
Adductor tendinitis, 999b
Adenine, 38, 39f
Adenocarcinoma, 813
  ampullary/periampullary, 842–844
  of oesophagus, 796f–797f
  of pancreas, 842–844
  of prostate, 438–439
  of small intestine, 813
  of unknown primary, 1336
Adenoma
  adrenal, 667b
    Conn's syndrome, 675f
    Cushing's syndrome, 667b,
      669–670
  bronchial gland, 603b
  colorectal, 776b, 827
  familial adenomatous polyposis,
    828–829, 829f
  hepatic, 893
  parathyroid, 663
  periampullary, 813
  sebaceum, 1264
  small intestine, 813
  toxic, 638f, 649
Adenomyomatosis, of gallbladder, 909
Adenosine, 480b, 482, 482b
Adenosine diphosphate see ADP
Adenosine triphosphate see ATP
Adenosquamous carcinoma of lung,
    603b
Adenoviruses, diarrhoea, 249
ADH see Antidiuretic hormone
Adherence
  factors affecting, 1294b
  SIMPLE strategies for, 1294b
Adhesion molecules, 77
ADHR see Autosomal dominant
    hypophosphataemic rickets
Adipocytes, 725
Adipokines, 731
Adiponectin, 699
Adjustment disorders, 1187, 1201
  prevalence of, 1180b
ADL see Activities of daily living
Adolescents, 1290
  allergy in, 76b
  congenital heart disease in, 537b
  cystic fibrosis in, 581b
  diabetes mellitus in, 753–754,
    753b–754b
  epilepsy in, 1103b
  haematological malignancy in, 955b
  infections in, 234, 235b
  inflammatory bowel disease in, 823b
  juvenile idiopathic arthritis in, 1027b
  laboratory reference range of, 1363
  medical ophthalmology in, 1175b
  renal impairment in, 1298b
ADP (adenosine diphosphate), 446f
Adrenal crisis, 673b
Adrenal disease, 1280
Adrenal glands, 665–676
  disease
    classification of, 665b
    presenting problems of, 666–674
  functional anatomy and physiology of,
    665–666, 666f–667f
  incidental adrenal mass, 673–674
  older people, 673b
Adrenal hyperplasia, congenital, 676
Adrenal insufficiency, 671–673,
    671b–673b

Adrenal tumours
  Cushing's syndrome, 669–670
  see also Phaeochromocytoma
Adrenalectomy, 675
  for Cushing's disease, 669
Adrenaline
  for allergy, 86
  anaphylaxis, 75, 76b
  circulatory effects of, 206b
  self-injectable, prescription of, 76b
  for urticaria, 1254
Adrenarche, 666
β-Adrenoceptor antagonist, 1190b
  for thyrotoxicosis, in pregnancy,
    1279
  for variceal bleeding, 869, 871
Adrenocorticotrophic hormone (ACTH)
  Cushing's syndrome and, 667b
  ectopic, 667b, 1325b
  ectopic ACTH syndrome, 670
  ectopic hormone production, 1325b
  excess, 672b
  hypopituitarism, 672b
  reference range of, venous blood,
    1359b
  stimulation test, 672b
Adrenoleukodystrophy, 1116b
Adriamycin see Doxorubicin
Adult-onset Still's disease, 1040
Adult polycystic kidney disease (PKD),
    405–406, 405b
Advance directives, 1307
Advanced life support (ALS), 457
Adverse drug reactions (ADRs),
    21–23
  classification of, 22–23, 22b
  interactions, 23–24
  in older people, 1310, 1310b
  pharmacovigilance, 23
  prevalence of, 21–22, 21b–22b
  risk factors for, 21b
  TREND analysis of, 23b
  see also individual drugs
Aedes aegypti
  Chikungunya virus, 250
  dengue, 243
  yellow fever, 244
AEDs (antiepilepsy drugs) see
    Anticonvulsants
AF see Atrial fibrillation
Affective mood disorders
  bipolar, 1198
  organic, 1185b
Affinity, 14
Affluence, health consequences of, 94
AFP (alpha-fetoprotein)
  hepatocellular carcinoma and,
    890–891
  as tumour markers, 1322, 1324b
African tick bite fever, 270, 271b
African trypanosomiasis (sleeping
    sickness), 278–279, 278f
Afterload
  heart failure, 461
  reduction, 465
Age/ageing, 1301–1312
  biological, 1304
  biology of, 1304–1305
  chronological, 1304
  physiological changes of, 1305,
    1305f
  syndrome of premature ageing see
    Werner's syndrome
  type 2 diabetes and, 732, 732b
  see also Older people
Age-related macular degeneration,
    1178
Agglutination, cold, 950
Agglutination test, 108
  for leishmaniasis, 283
  for leptospirosis, 258
  microscopic, 258
  for sporotrichosis, 301
  trypanosomiasis, 279
  for tularaemia, 261
Aggrecan, 987
Aggregatibacter aphrophilus-
    Aggregatibacter
    actinomycetemcomitans, 528

Aggressive behaviour, 1188–1189,
    1189f
Agitation, in palliative care, 1354
Agnosia, 1086
Agonists, 14
Agoraphobia, 1200
Agranulocytosis, 644
AHR see Airway hyper-reactivity
AIDS see HIV infection/AIDS
Aids and appliances, for
    musculoskeletal disease, 1001
AIN see Acute interstitial nephritis
AIP see Acute interstitial pneumonia
Air embolism, during dialysis, 424b
Air travel, 169
Airflow obstruction, 554f
  assessment in COPD, 575
Airway hyper-reactivity (AHR), 568,
    568f
Airway pressure release ventilation
    (APRV), 204
Airways, 548, 548f
  assessment of, in deteriorating
    patient, 188
  in asthma, 568f
  defences, 550, 550f
  of envenomed patient, 152f
  obstruction of, 555, 1324b
  reactive dysfunction syndrome, 614
  in sleep apnoea, 622
  of stroke patients, 1159b
  upper airway diseases, 622–625
Akathisia, 1105–1106, 1197
AKI see Acute kidney injury
Akinesia, 1113b
ALA dehydratase deficiency, 379b
Alanine aminotransferase (ALT), 852,
    1360b
Albendazole
  for cysticercosis, 298
  for helminthic infections, 129
    filariasis, 291
  for hydatid cysts, 299
Albers-Schönberg disease, 1056
Albinism
  inheritance, 1258
  oculocutaneous, 1258
Albright's hereditary osteodystrophy,
    51b, 664, 1017b
Albumin
  in AKI, 416b
  liver blood biochemistry, 852
  plasma, liver function test, 858
  reference range of
    urine, 1361b
    venous blood, 1360b
  urinary, 1361b
  see also Hypoalbuminaemia
Albumin solutions, for ascites, 864
Albuminuria, moderately elevated, 394
Alcohol, 94
  abstinence from, 1194b
  amount in average drink, 880b
  coronary artery disease and, 486
  dependence, 1194–1195, 1194b
  diabetes and, 744–745
  drug interactions, 24b
  energy provided by, 694
  liver disease and, 880–882
  pharmacokinetics, 20b
  poisoning, 134b
  thiamin deficiency and, 714
  see also Ethanol
Alcohol misuse, 1184, 1194–1195
  chronic, presentation and
    consequences of, 1194b
  clinical assessment of, 1184
  clinical features of, 1194–1195
  diagnosis of, 1195
  effects of, 1194b, 1195
  investigations of, 1184
  liver disease see Alcoholic liver
    disease
  management of, 1195
  maternal, 1194b
  in pancreatitis, 841
  pathogenesis of, 1194
  prevalence of, 1180b
  prognosis of, 1195

Alcohol withdrawal syndrome, 1194, 1194*b*
  management of, 1195
Alcoholic fatty liver disease (AFLD), 881
Alcoholic liver disease, 880–882
  clinical features of, 881–882, 881*b*
  liver function test (LFT) abnormality in, 854*b*
  in old age, 901*b*
  pathophysiology of, 881, 881*b*
  risk factors for, 880
Aldosterone, 666
  deficiency, 363
  plasma potassium and, 360
  reference range of, 1359*b*
  resistance, 363
  see also Hyperaldosteronism
Alendronate
  for osteoporosis, 1048*b*
  timing of, 31*b*
Alfacalcidol (1,25-dihydroxycholecalciferol), 665
Alfentanil, 209*b*
Alginates, 793
  sodium content of, 864*b*
Alkaline phosphatase (ALP)
  liver function tests and, 852
  placental, 1322, 1324*b*
  reference values of, venous blood, 1360*b*
  sclerosing cholangitis, 889
  serum
    Paget's disease, 1054
    rickets/osteomalacia, 1052
    in skeletal disease, 990*b*
Alkalinisation, urinary, 136
Alkalis, poisoning, 136*b*
Alkalosis
  hypokalaemic, Cushing's syndrome, 667
  metabolic, 366–367, 367*f*
  respiratory, 367
Alkylating agents, 936*b*
Allele, 47
Allergen, 84
  asthma, 568*f*
  avoidance of, 86
  contact eczema, 1247
  supervised exposure to, 86
Allergic alveolitis, extrinsic see Hypersensitivity pneumonitis
Allergic bronchopulmonary aspergillosis (ABPA), 596, 596*b*, 596*f*
Allergic contact eczema, 1247, 1247*b*, 1247*f*
Allergic rhinitis, 622
Allergy, 84–86
  in adolescence, 76*b*
  clinical features of, 85
  clinical manifestations of, 85*b*
  diagnosis of, 85
  food, 812
  hygiene hypothesis, 84–85
  to insect venom, 85
  investigations of, 86
    challenge tests, 86
    eosinophilia, 86
    mast cell tryptase, 86
    patch tests, 1215, 1244
    serum total IgE, 86
    skin-prick tests, 86
    specific IgE tests, 86
  management of, 86
  pathophysiology of, 84–85, 85*f*
  to peanut, 85
  in pregnancy, 88*b*
Allodynia, 1084
Allogeneic haematopoietic stem cell transplantation, 937
  complications of, 937, 937*b*
  indications for, 936*b*
Alloimmune haemolytic anaemia, 950
Allopurinol
  for acute leukaemia patients, 956*b*, 957–958
  drug interactions of, 24*b*
  for gout, 1015–1016
  hepatotoxicity, 32*b*, 894

pharmacodynamics, 20*b*
renal stone prevention, 432–433, 433*b*
for toxic epidermal necrolysis, 1254–1255
Alopecia, 1258–1259, 1259*b*
  androgenetic, 1259
  scarring inflammatory, 1262*f*
Alopecia areata
  hair in, 1258–1259, 1259*f*
  nails in, 1261
Alpha-fetoprotein (AFP)
  hepatocellular carcinoma and, 890–891
  as tumour markers, 1322, 1324*b*
Alpha-glucosidase inhibitors, for hyperglycaemia, 747
Alpha heavy chain disease, 813
Alpha particles, 164, 164*f*
Alpha-thalassaemia, 954
Alpha₁-antitrypsin deficiency, 48*b*, 897, 897*f*
  inheritance, 47*b*
Alport's syndrome, 403–404, 404*f*
ALS see Advanced life support
ALT see Alanine aminotransferase
Alternaria, 572
Alternative therapies
  for cancer pain, 1353
  for pain, 1348
Altitude, illnesses, 168–169
Aluminium
  osteomalacia and, 1053
  poisoning from, 148
Aluminium hydroxide
  for diarrhoea, 809
  phosphorus deficiency and, 716
  for renal bone disease, 419
Alveolar macrophages, 303, 615
Alveolar microlithiasis, 613*b*
Alveolar proteinosis, 613*b*
Alveolitis
  extrinsic see Hypersensitivity pneumonitis
  fibrosing, 558*b*, 1024*b*
  non-eosinophilic, drug-induced, 612*b*
Alzheimer's disease, 1191*b*, 1192–1193, 1193*f*
  familial, 1192
  see also Dementia
Amanita phalloides poisoning, 150*b*
Amantadine, 127, 127*b*
  for multiple sclerosis, 1110*b*
  for Parkinson's disease, 1114
Amastigotes, leishmaniasis, 282*f*
Amaurosis fugax, 1152
AmBisome, 283
Amelanotic melanoma, 1322
Amenorrhoea, 654–655, 654*b*
American trypanosomiasis (Chagas' disease), 279–280
Amikacin
  for actinomycetoma, 301
  for nocardiosis, 261
Amiloride, 360, 864
  for diabetes insipidus, 688
  mineralocorticoid excess, 675
Amino acids, 697, 697*b*
  essential, 697*b*
  metabolism, 850
    disorders of, 369–370
Aminoglycosides, 116*b*, 122
  adverse effects of, 122
  for brucellosis, 254
  dosing of, 122*f*
  mechanism of action, 116*b*
  nephrotoxicity, 32*b*
  pharmacokinetics of, 122
  in pregnancy, 120*b*
Aminopenicillins, 120, 120*b*
Aminophylline
  for asthma, 573, 573*f*
  for COPD, 578
Aminosalicylates, for inflammatory bowel disease, 821*b*
Aminotransferases
  acute liver failure and, 858
  elevated, common causes of, 859*b*

hypothermia, 166
liver function tests, 852
non-alcoholic fatty liver disease and, 884
reference range of, 1360*b*
viral hepatitis, 874*f*
Amiodarone
  adverse reactions
    pigmentation, 1258*b*
    pulmonary fibrosis, 612
  for arrhythmias, 479*b*–480*b*, 481
    atrial fibrillation, 471–472
    atrial flutter, 470
    tachycardia, 475
  causing thyroid dysfunction, 636*b*, 638*f*, 647–648, 647*f*
  for heart failure, 467
  hepatotoxicity of, 894*b*
  structure of, 647*f*
  thyrotoxicosis, 639, 647–648
Amitriptyline, 1199*b*
  for fibromyalgia, 1018–1019
  for functional dyspepsia, 802–803
  for headache, 1095
  for herpes zoster, 240
  for irritable bowel syndrome, 825
  for migraine prevention, 1096
  multiple sclerosis, 1110*b*
  for musculoskeletal pain, 995
  for neuropathic pain, 1350*b*, 1352*b*
  for pain management, 1350*b*
  for post-herpetic neuralgia, 240
  for psychiatric disorder, 1199*b*
Amlodipine
  for angina, 491*b*
    unstable, 500
  for hypertension, 513
Ammonia, 384
  hepatic encephalopathy and, 865
Ammonium chloride, 366
Amnesia, 1080–1081
  persistent, 1081
  post-ictal, 1081
  transient global, 1081
Amniocentesis, 56
Amniotic fluid embolism (AFE), pregnancy and, 1275
Amodiaquine, for malaria, 277
Amoebiasis, 286–287, 286*f*
  incubation period of, 111*b*
Amoebic dysentery, 287
Amoebic liver abscess, 287, 880
Amoeboma, 286–287, 286*f*
Amoxicillin, 117*b*
  for diphtheria, 266
  for Helicobacter pylori eradication, 800
  for listeriosis, 260
  for Lyme disease, 256
  for pneumonia, 585*b*
  for skin reactions, infectious mononucleosis, 242
  for urinary tract infection, 428
Amphetamines, misuse of, 143
Amphotericin/amphotericin B, 125*b*, 126
  for aspergillosis, 598
  for blastomycosis, 304
  for candidiasis, 302
  for coccidioidomycosis, 304
  for cryptococcal meningitis, HIV-related, 321
  for fusariosis, 302–303
  for histoplasmosis, 304
  for leishmaniasis, 283
  lipid formulations of, 126
  for mucormycosis, 303
  for mycetoma, 301
  nephrotoxicity, 365*b*, 427*b*
  for neutropenic fever, 1327–1328
  for Penicillium (Talaromyces) marneffei infection, 303
  for sporotrichosis, 301
Ampicillin, 117*b*, 120*b*
  for cerebral abscess, 1124*b*
  drug interactions of, 121
  for listeriosis, 260
  for liver abscess, 880
  for meningitis, 1120*b*

for paratyphoid fever, 260–261
skin reactions, 1266*b*
  infectious mononucleosis, 242, 242*f*
Ampulla of Vater, carcinoma of, 907–908
AMS see Acute mountain sickness
Amsacrine, for acute leukemia, 957*b*
Amsler chart, 1168, 1168*f*
Amygdala, 1066
Amylase, 768, 770*b*
  pancreatic, 695–697
  reference range of, venous blood, 1360*b*
  salivary, 62–63
  serum
    hypothermia, 166
    pancreatitis, 563*b*, 839
Amyloid A, serum, 70
Amyloid angiopathy, 1155*b*, 1191*b*
Amyloid deposition, type 2 diabetes, 731
Amyloid in plaques, in Alzheimer's disease, 1192, 1193*f*
Amyloidosis, 81, 1264
  causes of, 82*b*
  heart disease, 541
  multiple myeloma, 410*b*
  rheumatoid arthritis, 1024–1025
Amylose, 695–697
ANA see Antinuclear antibody
Anaemia(s), 717, 913, 913*b*, 923–925, 940–951, 941*f*
  after peptic ulcer surgery, 801
  aplastic, 968–969
  autoimmune haemolytic, 949–950
  causes of, 923*b*
  of chronic disease (ACD), 942*b*, 942*f*, 943
  chronic kidney disease and, 419, 419*b*
  clinical assessment of, 923
  haemolytic, 923, 945–951
    alloimmune, 950
    autoimmune, 949–950
    causes of, 946*f*, 947
    microangiopathic, 950
    non-immune, 950
  HIV-related, 322
  investigations of, 923–925, 924*f*
  iron deficiency, 940–943
    alimentary tract disorders, 793
    blood loss in, 940–941
    confirmation of, 941–942, 942*b*
    investigations in, 941–942
    malabsorption in, 941, 942*f*
    management of, 943
    physiological demands in, 941, 941*b*
  pregnancy and, 1284
  megaloblastic, 940, 943–945
    clinical features of, 943*b*
    investigations in, 944*b*
    management of, 945
  microangiopathic haemolytic, 408, 950
  microcytic, 925
    in rheumatoid arthritis, 1024–1025
  normochromic normocytic, 853
  in old age, 954*b*
  pernicious, 944
  pregnancy and, 1284, 1285*b*
  primary idiopathic acquired aplastic, 968–969, 968*b*
  secondary aplastic, 969, 969*b*
  sickle-cell, 923, 951–953
    clinical features of, 952–953, 952*f*
    epidemiology of, 951, 951*f*
    investigations of, 953
    management of, 953
    pathogenesis of, 951–952
    in pregnancy, 953*b*
    prognosis of, 953
Anagrelide, 970
Anakinra, for musculoskeletal disease, 1007
Anal canal, 771*f*
Anal fissure, 836

Analgesia
for acute coronary syndrome, 498
for back pain, 997
cholecystitis, 905
in intensive care, 209, 209b
for low back pain, 997
for musculoskeletal disease, 1002
myocardial infarction, 498
for osteoarthritis, 1012
for palliative care, 1350
for pancreatic cancer, 842–844
for pancreatitis, 839
for pleural pain, 584
for post-herpetic neuralgia, 240
for psoriatic arthritis, 1033–1034
for reactive arthritis, 1032
for renal colic, 432
Analgesic ladder (WHO), 1351f
Analgesics
adjuvant
for cancer pain, 1352, 1352b
for pain, 1345–1346
poisoning from, 137–138
see also specific drugs
Anaphase, 40
Anaphylactic shock, 204, 206b
Anaphylactoid reactions, 75, 75b
Anaphylaxis, 75–76, 339
causes of, 75b
clinical assessment of, 75–76
clinical manifestations of, 75f
differential diagnosis of, 76b
gastrointestinal, 812
management of, 76, 76b
Anaplastic carcinoma, 650
ANCAs (antineutrophil cytoplasmic
antibodies), 992
Ancylostoma caninum, 294
Ancylostoma duodenale, 288, 288f
Ancylostomiasis (hookworm), 288–289,
288f
Andersen disease, 370b
Andersen-Tawil syndrome, 1145b
Androgen receptor antagonism, 659b
Androgen replacement therapy
for adrenal insufficiency, 673
options for, 656b
Androgens
adrenal, 666
in older women, 660b
Anergy, 82
Aneuploidy, 51
Aneurysm
aortic, 505–506
abdominal, 505b
saccular, 508
ventricular, 496
see also Microaneurysms
Angelman's syndrome, 44b, 51b
Angina, 487–493, 487b–488b
clinical features of, 488, 488b
investigations for, 488, 489f–490f
management of, 488–489
drug therapy, 489–491, 490b
non-pharmacological treatments,
491–493, 491f–492f, 493b
in old age, 493b
prognosis of, 493
recurrent, in acute coronary
syndrome, 495
stable
advice to patients with, 489b
risk stratification in, 488b
Angina equivalent, 180
Angiodysplasia, 782–783
Angioedema, 87–88, 87f
drug-induced, 1266b
hereditary, 88
types of, 87b
Angiogenesis, 1318, 1319f
Angiography
coronary, 143
CT, 452, 452f
hepatic, 854
magnetic resonance, 869
mesenteric, 783, 813
of nervous system, 1072
visceral, 782–783
Angiomatosis, bacillary, 272

Angioplasty
for renal artery stenosis, 407–408
for stoke, 1160
Angiosarcoma, 1320b
Angiostrongylus cantonensis, 294
Angiotensin-converting enzyme see
ACE
Angiotensin-converting enzyme
inhibitors see ACE inhibitors
Angiotensin II, 666
Angiotensin II receptor blockers
effect on renal function, 407b
microalbuminuria in diabetes, 758
renal failure, 417
Angiotensin receptor blockers
for heart failure, 466, 466b
for hypertension, 513
Angular cheilitis, HIV/AIDS, 316
Angular stomatitis, 714, 764f, 817
Anhedonia, 1181
Anion gap
acidosis, 365
poisoning, 135b
Anisakiasis, 294
Anismus, 834
Ankle-brachial pressure index (ABPI),
1224
Ankle pain, 999
Ankylosing spondylitis (AS), 1028b,
1030–1031
clinical features of, 1030, 1030b
investigations of, 1030–1031,
1030f–1031f
management of, 1031
Annular erythemas, 1265
Annulus fibrosus, 444
Anogenital warts, 342–343
Anorectal abscesses, 836
Anorectal disorders, 835–836
Anorectal motility test, 778
Anorexia
in cancer patients, 1325b
in rheumatoid arthritis, 1023
Anorexia nervosa, 1203–1204, 1204b
features of, 785
in osteoporosis, 1047–1048
Anosmia, 653
Anosognosia, 1192–1193
ANP see Atrial natriuretic peptide
Anserine bursitis, 999b
Antacids
for bile reflux, 801
drug interactions of, 23
sodium content of, 864b
Antagonists, 14
Antalgic gait, 1086, 1309b
Anterior pituitary hormone deficiency,
681b
Anterior tibial compartment syndrome,
1058
Anthracyclines, 936b
Anthrax, 266–267
bioterrorism, 111
clinical features of, 267
cutaneous, 267
gastrointestinal, 267
immunisation for, 115b
incubation period of, 111b
inhalational, 267
management of, 267
skin, 1238
Anthropometry, 693b
Anti-α4β7 integrin, for inflammatory
bowel disease, 821b
Anti-androgen therapy, for polycystic
ovarian syndrome, 659b
Anti-anginal therapy, for acute coronary
syndrome, 500
Anti-anxiety drugs, 1190b
Anti-arrhythmic drugs, 479–482
adverse reactions of, 926b
classification of, 479b
by site of action, 479f
dosages of, 480b
principal uses of, 480b–481b
side-effects of, 480b
see also individual drugs
Anti-cancer therapy see Chemotherapy
Anti-CCP antibodies, 563b, 607

Anti-CD20 monoclonal antibody
rituximab, for chronic lymphocytic
leukaemia, 960
Anti-centromere antibody, 992b
Anti-citrullinated peptide antibodies
(ACPAs), 991
Anti-D, 933
Anti-DNA antibodies, 991
Anti-glomerular basement membrane
disease, 398b–399b, 401
Anti-herpesvirus agents, 126–127, 127b
Anti-histone antibody, 992b
Anti-infective agents, 1226
Anti-inflammatory cascade, 196
Anti-inflammatory therapy
for asthma, 571
for osteoarthritis, 1011b
see also individual drugs
Anti-influenza agents, 127
Anti-Jo-1 (anti-histidyl-tRNA synthase),
992b
Anti-La antibody (anti-SS-B), 992b
Anti-liver-kidney microsomal (LKM)
antibodies, 886
Anti-oestrogen, 1332
Anti-phospholipid syndrome, 1281
Anti-ribonucleoprotein antibody
(anti-RNP), 992b
Anti-RNA polymerase, 992b
Anti-RO antibody (anti-SS-A), 992b
Anti-Scl-70 (anti-topoisomerase I
antibody), 992b
Anti-Smith antibody, 992b
Anti-smooth muscle antibodies, 886,
886b
Anti-thymocyte globulin (ATG), 89b
Anti-TNF therapy
for ankylosing spondylitis, 1031
for inflammatory bowel disease,
821b–822b, 822
for rheumatoid arthritis, 1006
Anti-topoisomerase I antibody, 992b
Antibacterial agents, 120–124
aminoglycosides, 116b
beta-lactam, 116b, 120–121
folate antagonists, 123
glycopeptides, 123
lincosamides, 122
macrolide, 116b, 121–122
nitroimidazoles, 124
quinolones, 122–123, 123b
target and mechanism of action of,
116b
therapeutic drug monitoring, 119
Antibiotic therapy
for acne, 1242–1243
for acute leukaemia, 957
adverse reactions of, 22b, 926b
for bronchiectasis, 579
for cerebral abscess, 1124
for cholecystitis, 905
for choledocholithiasis, 906
for community-acquired pneumonia,
584, 585b
for cystic fibrosis, 580
for diabetic foot ulcers, 761–762
diarrhoea associated with, 104b
for gastroenteritis/acute diarrhoea,
230
for Helicobacter pylori eradication,
800
hepatotoxicity and, 864b
for infective endocarditis, 529b, 530
for inflammatory bowel disease,
821b
for meningitis, 1118
for osteomyelitis, 1021
for pneumonia
community-acquired, 583
hospital-acquired, 586
suppurative/aspirational, 587
prophylactic
for pancreatitis, 839
for spontaneous bacterial
peritonitis, 864
for variceal bleeding, 869
for respiratory tract infections
bronchiectasis, 790
COPD, 578

cystic fibrosis, 580
pneumonia see Pneumonia, above
for rheumatic fever, 517
for sepsis, 197, 197b
for septic arthritis, 1020, 1020b
for skin disease, 1227
sodium content of, 864b
for staphylococcal infections see
individual infections
for urinary tract infection, 428
Antibody/antibodies
classes and properties of, 68b
in coeliac disease, 806–807
deficiency in, 73b
primary, 78–79, 78f, 79b
detection of, 106–108, 109f
see also Autoantibodies
Antibody-dependent cellular cytotoxicity
(ADCC), 67–69
Anticardiolipin antibodies, 1157b
Anticholinergics
adverse reactions of, 1310b
for bladder dysfunction, 1094b
for COPD, 577
for Parkinson's disease, 1114
poisoning, 150b
Anticholinesterases
for Alzheimer's disease, 1193
for myasthenia gravis, 1142
non-antivenom, 159
α1-Antichymotrypsin, 70
Anticoagulants/anticoagulation,
938–940
adverse reactions of, 22b
for atrial fibrillation, stroke prevention,
472b
coagulation screening, 1362b
direct oral, 940
drug interactions, 940
indications for, 938b
modes of action of, 938b
monitoring, 922
for obliterative cardiomyopathy, 541
in old age, 1160b
poisoning, 148b
in pregnancy, 941b
prosthetic heart valves and, 527b
for pulmonary embolism, 621
risk assessment of, 940b
rodenticides, 148b
for stroke patients, 1157b
for venous thromboembolism,
975–976
see also specific anticoagulants
Anticodon, 40
Anticonvulsants
for epilepsy, 1101–1102, 1102b
choice of drug, 1102b
withdrawing, 1102–1103
for pain management, 1352b
poisoning, 141b
skin reactions, 1266b
use in pregnancy, 1284
Antidepressants, 1190b, 1199b, 1200
adverse reactions of, 926b, 1310b
for alcohol withdrawal, 1195
for anxiety disorders, 1201
in older people, 1310b
poisoning from, 138–139
tricyclic, 1199, 1199b
poisoning from, 138–139, 139b,
1310f
Antidiabetic agents, poisoning from, 141
Antidiarrhoeal agents, 230
for inflammatory bowel disease, 821b
for irritable bowel syndrome, 826b
Antidiuretic hormone (ADH), 350–351
ectopic hormone production, 1325b
inappropriate secretion, 357b
cancer patients, 1325b
Antiemetic drugs, receptor site activity
of, 1353b
Antiepilepsy drugs (AEDs) see
Anticonvulsants
Antifreeze poisoning, 147
Antifungal agents, 125–126, 125b
Antigen processing and presentation,
70
Antiglobulin (Coombs) test, 948f

Antihistamines
    for allergy, 86
    for eczema, 1244
    for food allergy, 812
    for pruritus, 1220
    for skin disease, 1227
    for urticaria, 1254
Antihypertensive drugs, 513, 514b, 515f
    adverse reactions of, 926b
    for chronic kidney disease, 416–417
    for gout, 1016
Antimalarials, 128, 1252
    adverse reactions of, 926b
    poisoning, 141b
    prophylactic, 119b
    see also individual drugs
Antimetabolites, 936b, 1317f
Antimicrobial agents
    combination therapy, 116
    for infective gastroenteritis, 230
    pharmacokinetics and
        pharmacodynamics of, 118–119,
        119f
    in pregnancy, 120b
    resistance to, 116–118, 118f
    selection, 117b
    susceptibility testing, 109, 109f
    target and mechanism of action of,
        116b
    therapeutic drug monitoring, 119
    see also Antibiotic therapy
Antimicrobial stewardship, 115, 115f
Antimicrobial therapy, 117b
    action and spectrum, 116, 117b
    duration of, 118, 119b
    empiric versus targeted therapy, 116,
        117f
    in old age, 120b
    principles of, 116–120
    prophylactic, 119–120, 119b
    see also Antibiotic therapy
Antimitochondrial antibodies, 886b,
    887
Antimonials, for leishmaniasis, 128, 283
Antimotility agents, 230
Antimycobacterial agents, 125
Antineutrophil cytoplasmic antibodies
    (ANCAs), 389
Antineutrophil cytoplasmic antibody-
    associated vasculitis (AAV), 1041,
    1041f
Antinuclear antibody (ANA)
    in autoimmune hepatitis, 886b
    in musculoskeletal disease, 991,
        991b
Antioxidants, 550
Antiparasitic agents, 128–129
Antiphospholipid antibodies, 991–992
Antiphospholipid syndrome (APS),
    977–978, 978b
Antiplatelet drugs, 938b
    for angina, 489
    for myocardial infarction, 498b
    for obliterative cardiomyopathy, 541
    for stroke prevention, 1161f
Antiproteinases, 550
Antipsychotic drugs, 1190b
    adverse reactions of, 22b, 1198b
    for agitation, 1354
    poisoning from, 141
    for schizophrenia, 1198b
Antiretroviral therapy, 127b, 324–327,
    324b
    complications of, 325–326
    criteria for, 325
    monitoring efficacy of, 325
    in pregnancy, 326–327
    resistance to, 325
    selection of, 324–325
    see also individual drugs
Antirheumatic drugs
    during pregnancy and breastfeeding,
        1281b
    slow-acting (DMARDs) see
        Disease-modifying antirheumatic
        drugs
Antisecretory agents, 230
Antiseptics, 586, 1226
Antithrombin deficiency, 977

Antithrombotic therapy, 938–940, 938b
    for acute coronary syndrome, 500
    prophylaxis, for venous
        thromboembolism, 976–977,
        977b
Antithyroid drugs
    adverse reactions of, 926b
    for Graves' thyrotoxicosis, 644, 644b
    in pregnancy, 1279
α₁-Antitrypsin
    faecal clearance of, 811
    liver disease, 854b
    liver histology in, 897f
    reference range of, venous blood,
        1360b
Antivenom, 159, 159b, 160f
Antiviral agents, 126–128, 127b
    see also Antiretroviral therapy
Anuria, 391, 391b
Anxiety/anxiety disorders, 1186,
    1200–1201
    alcohol and, 1194
    classification of, 1200b
    clinical features of, 1200
    diagnosis of, 1200
    differential diagnosis of, 1186b
    generalised, 1200
    investigations of, 1186
    management of, 1186, 1200–1201
    in palliative care, 1354
    panic disorder, 1200
    phobic, 1200
    prevalence of, 1180b
    in stroke patients, 1159f
    symptoms of, 1186b
Aorta
    ascending
        dilatation of, 451f
        syphilis and, 338
    coarctation of, 508, 534, 534f
    diseases of, 505–514
Aortic aneurysm, 505–506
    abdominal, 505b
Aortic dissection, 506–508, 506f–508f,
    507b
    pregnancy and, 1282
Aortic regurgitation, 443b, 524–525,
    524b
    clinical features of, 524–525, 524b,
        525f
    investigations of, 525, 525b
    chest X-ray for, 451f
Aortic stenosis, 443b, 521–524, 522b,
    522f
    causes of, 521b
    Doppler echocardiography for, 451f
    investigations of, 522–524, 523b,
        523f
    in old age, 524b
Aortic valve, disease, 521–525
Aortitis, 508
APACHE II, 214
APD see Automated peritoneal dialysis
Aphonia, psychogenic, 624
Aphthous ulceration, 790, 790b
Apixaban, 938b
Aplastic anaemias, 968–969
Aplastic crisis, 947, 952–953
Apo A1 deficiency, 375, 375b
Apo A1 Milano, 375, 375b
Apocrine sweat glands, 1213–1214
Apolipoproteins, 371
Apoptosis, 41, 1316
Apoptotic bodies, 41
Appearance, in psychiatric interview,
    1181
Appendicitis, acute, 788
Apraxia, 1086
    gait, 1087, 1309b
Apremilast, for musculoskeletal disease,
    1004b, 1005
Apronectomy, 704
APTT see Activated partial
    thromboplastin time
Arachnoiditis, 996–997
Arboviruses, 1121–1122
ARDS see Acute respiratory distress
    syndrome
Arginine, 697b

Arms, assessment of, 983f
Aromatase inhibitors
    for cancer treatment, 1334
    osteoporosis and, 1046b
Arrhythmias, 468–479, 468f
    in acute coronary syndrome, 495,
        495b
    during dialysis, 424b
    electrophysiology of, 454
    hypothermia and, 166f
    management of, 479–484
        drugs, 479–482, 479b–482b, 479f
        non-pharmacological treatments,
            482–484
    see also specific arrhythmias
Arrhythmogenic ventricular
    cardiomyopathy, 540
Arsenic, poisoning, 149, 149b
Arsenism, 149, 149b
Artemisinin (qinghaosu) derivatives,
    128
Arterial blood
    analysis of, 1358b
    critically ill patients, 179
    respiratory failure, 199b
Arterial disease
    hepatic, 898
    leg ulcers due to, 1223–1224
Arterial gas embolism (AGE), 170
Arterial pressure waveform, 206
Arterial pulse, examination of, 443b
Arterialisation, 422–423
Arteriography, renal, 389
Artesunate, for malaria, 277
Arthritis
    acute inflammatory, 1017
    crystal-induced, 1012–1018
    HIV-related, 321
    juvenile idiopathic, 1026–1027
        in adolescence, 1027b
        clinical features of, 1027b
        oligoarticular, 1300
        transition medicine and, 1300
    monoarthritis
        acute, 992–993, 993b
        chronic inflammatory, 992
    mutilans, 1033
    osteoarthritis, 1007–1012
    polyarthritis see Polyarthritis
    psoriatic, 1032–1034
        CASPAR criteria for, 1032b
        clinical features of, 1032–1033,
            1033f
        investigations for, 1033
        management for, 1033–1034
        pathophysiology of, 1032
    reactive, 1031–1032
    rheumatoid, 1021–1026
        algorithm for, 1026f
        biologic therapy for, 1026
        cardiac involvement in, 1024
        clinical features of, 1023–1025,
            1023f
        criteria for diagnosis of, 1023b
        DMARD therapy for, 1025–1026
        extra-articular, 1024b
        investigations in, 1025, 1025b,
            1026f
        management of, 1025–1026
        nodules in, 1023–1024, 1024f
        non-pharmacological therapy for,
            1026
        ocular involvement in, 1024
        pathophysiology of, 1022–1023,
            1022f
        peripheral neuropathy in, 1024
        in pregnancy, 1026b, 1280
        pregnancy and, 1280
        pulmonary involvement in, 1024
        serositis in, 1024
        spinal cord compression in, 1024,
            1025f
        surgery for, 1026
        systemic, 1023
        vasculitis in, 1024
    septic, 1019–1020
    systemic lupus erythematosus and,
        1035
    viral, 1020–1021

Arthrodesis, 1002b
Arthropathy
    in parvovirus B19 infection, 237b
    psoriasis and, 1249
    reactive, sexually acquired, 340
    rheumatological manifestations of,
        1057
Arthroplasty, 1002b
Asacol, for inflammatory bowel disease,
    821b
Asbestos-related lung and pleural
    diseases, 617–618
Asbestosis, 618
Ascariasis, 233b
Ascaris lumbricoides (roundworm),
    289–290, 906
Ascending and descending pain
    pathways, 1339f
Ascites, 847b, 862–864, 1324b
    appearance and analysis of, 863b
    Budd-Chiari syndrome and, 899
    causes of, 862b
    cirrhosis and, 867
    hepatorenal syndrome and, 864
    management of, 863–864
    oedema, 395–396
    pancreatic, 839
    pathogenesis of, 863f
    pathology of, 862–863
    portal hypertension and, 869
    prognosis of, 864
    renal failure and, 864
    serum- ascites albumin gradient
        (SAAG) and, 863
    spontaneous bacterial peritonitis and,
        864
Ascorbic acid see Vitamin C
Aspartate, 697b
Aspartate aminotransferase (AST),
    852
Aspergillosis, 301
    bronchopulmonary classification of,
        596b
Aspergillus clavatus, 616b
Aspergillus flavus, 1320b
Aspergillus nodule, 597
Aspergillus spp., in
    immunocompromised patients,
    224
Asphyxia/asphyxiation
    laryngeal obstruction, 624–625
    self-harm, 1187
Aspiration, pleural, 563–564
Aspiration pneumonia, 586–587
Aspirin
    for acute coronary syndrome
        prevention, 498b
    adverse reactions of, 22b
    for angina, 489
    asthma association, 568
    atrial fibrillation, stroke prevention,
        473
    coronary artery bypass grafting,
        491–492
    drug interactions, 24b
    for hypertension, 513
    for myocardial infarction, 500
    poisoning, 138
    for rheumatic fever, 517
    for stroke patients, 1160
    timing of, 31b
AST see Aspartate aminotransferase
Asteatotic eczema, 1247
Asterixis, 864–865
Asthma, 567–573, 567f
    clinical features of, 568–569
    control, levels of, 570b
    diagnosis of, 569, 569b, 569f–570f
    exacerbations of, 572–573,
        572b–573b, 573f
    and gastro-oesophageal reflux
        disease, 791–792
    management of, 569–570, 571f
    occupational, 613–614, 614b, 614f
    pathophysiology of, 568, 568f
    in pregnancy, 570b, 1277
    prognosis of, 573
Astrocytes, 1064–1065
Astrocytoma, 1075f

Astrovirus, 249
Asymmetrical inflammatory mono-/
    oligoarthritis, 1032
Asymptomatic bacteriuria, 429
Ataxia(s), 1115
    acquired, 1115b
    cerebellar, 1325
    inherited, 1116b
    stroke and, 1153
Ataxia telangiectasia, 1321b
    genes, 1321
Ataxic gait, 1087, 1309b
Atazanavir, 324b
Atenolol
    for angina, 500
    drug interactions of, 24b
    for hypertension, 513
Atheroembolism, 390b, 503–504,
    504b
Atherosclerosis
    in old age, 505b
    renal artery stenosis and, 406
    six stages of, 485f
Athetosis, 1086
Athlete's foot, 1240
Atmospheric pollution, 94
ATN see Acute tubular necrosis
Atomic absorption (AA), 348b
Atonic seizures, 1100
Atopic eczema, 1245–1246
    clinical features of, 1245, 1246f
    complications of, 1246b
    investigations of, 1245, 1246b
    management of, 1246
    pathogenesis of, 1245
    rash in, 1217b, 1246b
Atopy, 84, 86
    see also Allergy
Atorvastatin, 501
Atovaquone, for malaria, 128
ATP (adenosine triphosphate),
    myocardial contraction and,
    446
ATP synthase, 49b
Atria, 444, 444f
Atrial ectopic beats, 469–470, 470f
Atrial fibrillation (AF), 470–473, 471f
    causes of, 471b
    management of, 471–473
    mechanisms of, 471f
    in old age, 472b
    paroxysmal, 471–472
    persistent, 472–473
    stroke risk in, 473b
Atrial flutter, 470, 470f
Atrial myxoma, 541–542
Atrial natriuretic peptide (ANP), 351
Atrial septal defect, 534–535, 535f
Atrial tachycardia, 470
Atrioventricular (AV) block, 477–478,
    477f–478f, 478b
Atrioventricular (AV) node, 445, 445f
    re-entrant tachycardia, 473, 474f
Atrophy, definition of, 1226, 1226f
Atropine
    for acute cholinergic syndrome, 146
    for AV block, 478
    for carbamate poisoning, 147
    cardiotoxic drug poisoning, 140
    for organophosphorus poisoning,
        146
    for sinus bradycardia, 469
Auerbach's plexus, 771–772
Auscultation
    examination of, respiratory system,
        546f
    of heart, 443b
    malignant pleural effusions, 1315b
Austin Flint murmur, 524
Australian tick typhus, 271b
Autoantibodies
    autoimmune disease and, 83, 83f
    autoimmune hepatitis and, 886b
    and musculoskeletal disease, 991
    primary biliary cholangitis and,
        887–888
    thyroid, 637b
Autofluorescence, of visual disorders,
    1169

Autoimmune connective tissue disease,
    1018, 1034–1040
Autoimmune disease, 81–84
    clinical features of, 83
    gene polymorphisms associated with,
        82b
    investigations of, 83–84
        autoantibodies in, 83, 83f
        complement in, 84
        cryoglobulins in, 84, 84b
        of liver, 885–890
        management of, 84
        pathophysiology of, 82–83
Autoimmune haemolytic anaemia,
    949–950
Autoimmune hepatitis, 886–887
    conditions associated with, 886b
    liver function test (LFT) abnormality in,
        854b
    primary biliary cholangitis and, 888
Autoimmune lymphoproliferative
    syndrome, 80
Autoimmune pancreatitis, 841
Autoimmune polyendocrine syndromes,
    689, 690b
Autoimmune thyroid disease, 639b,
    643–646
Autologous haematopoietic stem cell
    transplantation, 936–938
Automated peritoneal dialysis (APD),
    424
Automated threshold perimetry, 1168
Autonomic dysfunction, somatoform,
    1202
Autonomic nervous system, 1068
Autonomic neuropathy, diabetic, 760,
    760b
'Autonomic storm', 155
Autonomy, patients, 1288–1289
Autophagy, 1316
Autopsy, 213
Autosomal dominant
    hypophosphataemic rickets
    (ADHR), 1050b
Autosomal dominant inheritance, 46–47,
    47b
Autosomal recessive inheritance, 47b,
    48
Autosomes, 38
AV see Atrioventricular
Avascular cornea, 1166
Avid sodium retention, nephrotic
    syndrome and, 395b
Axial spondyloarthritis, 1028b,
    1029–1030, 1029f
Axial spondyloarthropathy, 1028–1031,
    1029f
Axons, peripheral nerve, 1064–1065
Azathioprine
    adverse reactions of, 22
    for autoimmune haemolysis, 950
    for autoimmune hepatitis, 886–887
    drug interactions of, 24b
    for eczema, 1246
    hepatotoxicity, 894b
    for inflammatory bowel disease, 821b,
        822
    liver transplantation and, 901
    for musculoskeletal disease, 1004b,
        1005
        systemic lupus erythematosus,
        1036
    for myasthenia gravis, 1142b
    for primary biliary cholangitis, 888
    for rheumatoid arthritis, 1026b
    transplant patients, 89b, 425–426
Azelaic acid, 1242–1244
Azithromycin, 117b
    for bacillary angiomatosis, HIV/AIDS
        patients, 315–316
    for cystic fibrosis, 581b
    for Mycobacterium avium complex,
        315b
    for STIs
        chlamydial infection, 341b
        syphilis, 339
    for trachoma, 273
Azole antifungals, 126
Aztreonam, 117b, 120b, 121

B
B-cell receptor, 68, 68f
B lymphocytes (B cells), 68, 68f, 917
Babesia microti, 226b
Babesiosis, 278
Bacillary angiomatosis, 272
    HIV-related, 315–316
Bacillary dysentery, 265
Bacille Calmette-Guérin see BCG
Bacillus anthracis, 266
Bacillus cereus, food poisoning, 262,
    262f
Bacillus spp., 102f
Back, examination of, cardiology, 442f
Back pain, 995–997
    red flags for, 996b
    triage assessment of, 996f
    see also Low back pain
Background radiation, 164
Baclofen, for multiple sclerosis, 1110b
Bacteraemia, 106
    Staphylococcus aureus, 225
Bacteraemic leptospirosis, 257
Bacteria, 100–101, 101b, 102f
    endogenous commensal, 63
    exotoxin, disease caused by, 104b
    identification of, 102f
Bacterial cultures, for gastrointestinal
    infection, 777
Bacterial infections, 250–273
    after HSCT, 937b
    and cancer, 1320b
    chlamydial, 272–273, 272b
    gastrointestinal, 262–265
    with neurological involvement, 267
    respiratory, 265–267
    rickettsial, 270–272, 271b
    of skin, 1235–1238
        soft tissues and bones, 250–254
    systemic, 254–262
    see also specific infections
Bacterial keratitis, 1173
Bacterial meningitis, 1118–1120
    causes of, 1119b
    cerebrospinal fluid in, 1119
    clinical features of, 1119, 1119b
    headache and, 185, 185b
    investigations of, 1119–1120, 1119f,
        1120f
    management of, 1120, 1120b
    pathophysiology of, 1119
Bacterial swab, for leg ulcers, 1224
Bacteriology, skin, 1215
Bacteriophage, 100
Bacteriuria
    asymptomatic, 429
    catheter-related, 429–430
Bacteroides fragilis, 586
Bacteroides spp., 103f, 117b
Bad news, 1185
Baker's (popliteal) cyst, 999b, 1023
    rupture, 1023
Balance
    altered, 1086
    see also Dizziness; Vertigo
Balanitis, 333
    anaerobic, 334b
    circinate, 334b
    plasma cell (of Zoon), 334b
Balanoposthitis, 333
Balkan nephropathy, 403
Ballism, 1086
Balloon dilatation, 434
Balloon tamponade, for variceal
    bleeding, 870–871, 870f
Balloon valvuloplasty
    for aortic valve, 524
    for mitral valve, 519, 519b, 519f
Balsalazide, 821b
Balsam of Peru, 1247b
'Bamboo' spine, 1030–1031, 1031f
Band ligation, 870
Bandages, for leg ulcers, 1223
Banding, for variceal bleeding, 869
Barbiturates, 142b
    misuse of, 1195
    skin reactions of, 1266b
    withdrawal effects of, 16b
Bardet-Biedl syndrome, 404b

Bare lymphocyte syndromes, 79
Bariatric surgery, for obesity, 702f–703f,
    703–704, 703b
Baricitinib, for musculoskeletal disease,
    1004b
Baritosis, 614–615
Barium enema
    for constipation, 787
    for diverticulosis, 833
    for gastrointestinal tuberculosis, 590
    for inflammatory bowel disease,
        819–820
    for oesophageal diseases, 778
    for pharyngeal pouch, 794
Barotrauma, 171
Barrett's (columnar lined) oesophagus,
    792–793, 793f
    carcinoma and, 796
Barthel Index of Activities of Daily Living,
    1311, 1312b
Bartonella henselae, 272, 315–316
Bartonella quintana, 272, 315–316
Bartonellosis, 272, 272b
Bartter's syndrome, 361
Basal cell carcinoma, 1229–1230,
    1229f, 1230b
Basal cell papilloma, 1234, 1234f
Basal ganglia, 1066–1067
Basal metabolic rate (BMR), 694, 695f
    in over-nutrition, 694
Basement membrane, 1212, 1213f
Basic calcium phosphate (BCP)
    deposition disease, 1017–1018,
        1017b
Basic life support (BLS), 456–457
Basophil granulocytes, 1362b
Basophilia, 926b
Basophilic stippling, 921f
Basophils, 66–67, 917, 926b, 926f
    count, 1362b
Bath Ankylosing Spondylitis Disease
    Activity Index (BASDAI), 1029
Bath Ankylosing Spondylitis Functional
    Index (BASFI), 1029
Battery acid poisoning, 794
Bayes' theorem, 5
BCG (bacille Calmette-Guérin)
    for leprosy, 270
    for tuberculosis, 594
BCP see Basic calcium phosphate
BCR see Breakpoint cluster region
Beau's lines, 1261, 1261f
Becker muscular dystrophy, 48b
Becker's disease, 1145b
Beckwith-Wiedemann syndrome, 51b
Beclometasone, 17–18
Bedside procedures, for safe
    transfusion, 934, 934f–935f
Behaviour
    assessment of, in psychiatric
        interview, 1181
    disturbed and aggressive,
        1188–1189, 1189f
    in old age, 1189b
    high-risk, transition medicine and,
        1295
    history-taking in, 1295b
    personality and, 1295
    protective factors in, 1295
    theories in, 1295
    psychiatric disorders and, 1183
Behaviour therapy, 1190
Behavioural rating scales, for pain,
    1343
Behçet's disease, 1043–1044, 1043f,
    1044b
Beighton score, modified, 1059
Bejel, 254, 254b
Beliefs, abnormal, 1181
Belimumab, for musculoskeletal
    disease, 1006–1007, 1007b
Bell's palsy, 1082–1083
Bence Jones protein, 394–395
Bence Jones proteinuria, 966–967
Bendroflumethiazide, 22b
Benign oesophageal stricture, 793,
    795–796, 796b
Benign paroxysmal positional vertigo,
    1104, 1104f

Benign prostatic enlargement (BPE), 437–438
    treatment for, 438b
Benign prostatic hyperplasia (BPH), 437
Benserazide, 1113
Benzamides, substituted, 1198b
Benzathine benzylpenicillin, for syphilis, 339
Benzbromarone, 1016
Benzene, 1320b
Benzimidazoles, for helminthic infections, 129
Benzisoxazole, 1198b
Benznidazole, for trypanosomiasis, 128
Benzocaine, allergy, 1247b
Benzodiazepines, 1190b
    adverse reactions of, 22b, 1310b
    alcohol withdrawal, 1195
    for anxiety disorders, 1190b, 1201
    delirium, 1310b
    misuse of, 142
    overdose, 142
    respiratory depression and, 1188–1189
    stress reactions, 1201
    withdrawal, 1186b
Benzoyl peroxide, 1242–1243
Benzylpenicillin, 120b
    for cerebral abscess, 1124b
    for meningitis, 1120b
    for neurosyphilis, 1125
    procaine see Procaine penicillin
Bereavement, 1184
Beri-beri, 714
Bernoulli equation, modified, 451–452
Berylliosis, 616
Beta-adrenoceptor blockers, for heart failure, 467
Beta-blockers
    adverse reactions of, 22b, 1310b
    for anxiety disorder, 1201
    for essential tremor, 1115
    for hypertension, 513
    poisoning from, 140
    for thyrotoxicosis, 637–638
Beta-chain haemoglobinopathy, 953
Beta-lactam antibiotics, 116b, 120–121
    adverse reactions of, 120–121
    drug interactions of, 121
    mechanism of action, 116b
    pharmacokinetics of, 120
Beta particles, 164, 164f
Beta-thalassaemia, 953–954
    diagnostic features of, 954b
    management and prevention of, 953–954, 954b
Beta-2-microglobulin, as tumour markers, 1324b
Bevacizumab, 1332
Bi-level ventilation, 202
Bicarbonate, 349b
    arterial blood of, 1358b
    in diabetic ketoacidosis, 738
    see also Sodium bicarbonate
Bicarbonate system, 364, 364f
Biguanides, for hyperglycaemia, 746
Bilateral diaphragmatic weakness, 627
Bile, 850–851
    reflux, 801
Bile acid diarrhoea, 809
Bile acid-sequestering resins, 376–377
Bile duct, tumours of, 907–908
Bile salts, 768f
Bilharziasis see Schistosomiasis
Biliary colic, 904
Biliary disease, 902–909
    autoimmune, 885–890
    clinical examination of, 846f
    extrahepatic, 902–903
    intrahepatic, 902
        inflammatory and immune disease and, 902
    investigation of, 852–855, 852b
    see also Liver disease
Biliary obstruction, pregnancy and, 900
Biliary sludge, 904
Biliary sphincterotomy, 906
Biliary system, functional anatomy of, 849–850

Bilirubin
    alcoholic hepatitis and, 882
    excretion of, 851f
    Gilbert's syndrome and, 897
    liver blood biochemistry and, 852
    metabolism of, 850–851
    plasma
        acute liver failure and, 858
        jaundice and, 860
        viral hepatitis, 872
    reference range of, venous blood, 1360b
    see also Hyperbilirubinaemia
Bioavailability, 17
Biochemical disorders, clinical examination of, 346–348, 346f
Biochemical investigations, 348–349, 348b
Biochemical markers, cancer, 1323, 1324b
Biochemical tests, for liver disease, 852–853
Biochemistry, 388–389
    of bone disease, 990–991
    of coeliac disease, 807
Biological therapies
    for cancer, 1332
    for musculoskeletal disease, 1006–1007, 1006f
    for psychiatric disorders, 1190
    for skin disease, 1228
Biopsy, 776
    bone, 992
    brain, 1078
    cancer diagnosis, 1330
    liver, 855, 855b, 884
        for hepatocellular carcinoma, 891
    for lung cancer, 601
    muscle, 992, 1078
    for neurological disease, 1078
    pleural, 563–564
    renal, 391, 391b
    skin, 1214–1215
    synovial, 992
    temporal artery, 992
    tissue, in musculoskeletal disease, 992
Bioterrorism, 111
Biotin, 715
    deficiency, 715
    dietary sources of, 711b
    reference nutrient intake of, 711b
2,3-Biphosphoglycerate (2,3-BPG), 915–916
Bipolar disorder, 1199–1200
    prevalence of, 1180b
Birch oral allergy syndrome, 85
Bird fancier's lung, 616b
Bisacodyl, 834b
Bismuth, 230, 800
Bisoprolol, 466b
    for angina, 490
    for arrhythmias, 481
    for hypertension, 513
Bisphosphonates
    adverse effects of, 1048b
    for bone metastases, 1329
    for giant cell arteritis, 1043b
    for multiple myeloma, 968
    osteomalacia and, 1053
    for osteoporosis, 1047–1048, 1047f, 1048b
    for Paget's disease, 1054
Bites
    snake, 158b
    spider, 161
Bithionol, 129
Bitot's spots, 713
Blackheads see Comedone
Blackouts, 1080
    alcoholic, 1195
    in older people, 1308
Bladder, 386
    disturbance, 1093–1094
    dysfunction, 1093–1094, 1094b
    flaccid, 1093
    multiple sclerosis and, 1109–1110
    ultrasound of, 389
Bladder neck, obstruction, 437

Blastomyces dermatitidis, 304
Blastomycosis, 304
Blatchford score, 780
Bleeding, 913–914, 913b, 927–929
    clinical assessment of, 928–929
    gastrointestinal, 780–783
    in haemophilia A, 972
    investigation of, 929
    supportive therapy for, 957
    variceal see Variceal bleeding
    see also Haemorrhage
Bleeding disorders, 920–922, 970–975
    acquired, 974–975
    rare inherited, 974
Bleeding time, 921, 1362b
Bleomycin
    Hodgkin lymphoma, 963
    pigmentation from, 1258b
    for viral warts, 1239
'Blind loop syndrome', 808–809
Blindness, night, 713
Blisters, 1211f, 1218–1219
    acquired, 1218b
    clinical assessment of, 1218f, 1219
    definition of, 1218
    investigations and management of, 1219
α-Blockers
    for benign prostatic enlargement, 438
    for hypertension, 513, 514b
    for phaeochromocytoma, 675–676
Blood
    arterial, analytes in, 1358b
    components of, 931b
    culture, 106, 107f–108f, 225–226, 225b
    functional anatomy and physiology of, 914–919
    oxygenation in, 190
Blood-brain barrier, 1064–1065
Blood cells, 915–917
    see also Platelets; Red cells
Blood count
    for acute kidney injury, 416b
    for gastrointestinal bleeding, 777–778
    for hepatobiliary disease, 853
    for musculoskeletal disease, 990
    see also Platelets; Red cells
Blood diseases
    clinical examination of, 912–914, 912f
    investigation of, 919–923
    ophthalmic features of, 1164b
    pregnancy and, 1284–1285
        anaemia as, 1284, 1285b
        Rhesus disease as, 1285
        thrombocytopenia as, 1285, 1285b
        venous thromboembolism as, 1285
    presenting problems in, 923–930
    principles of management of, 930–940
    pruritus and, 1219b
    rheumatological manifestations of, 1058
    in systemic lupus erythematosus, 1035–1036
    see also individual disorders
Blood donation, 930–931, 932f
Blood film examination, 920, 921b, 921f
Blood flow
    Doppler echocardiography for, 451–452, 451f
    respiration and, 447–448
    through heart, 444f
    resistance to, 447
Blood glucose, of stroke patients, 1159b
Blood loss, 940–941
Blood pool imaging, for cardiovascular system, 454
Blood pressure
    effects of respiration on, 447b
    in endocrine disease, 630f
    examination of, respiratory system, 546f
    optimal target, 513b
    of stroke patients, 1159b
    see also Hypertension
Blood products, 930–931, 931b

Blastomyces dermatitidis, 304
Blood-stream infection, 225, 225b
    see also Bacteraemia
Blood supply, to liver, 848–849, 848f
Blood tests
    for abdominal pain, 787
    for cerebrovascular disease, 1151–1152
    for diabetes mellitus, 726
    for gastrointestinal bleeding, 777
    for hepatobiliary disease, 853
    for inflammatory bowel disease, 818
    for malabsorption, 785f
    for musculoskeletal disease, 990–992
    for neurological disease, 1077
    older people, 923b
    for pain, 1342, 1342b
    for pneumonia, 584b
    for renal disease, 388–389
    for skin disease, 1215–1216
    for stroke, 1151–1152
    see also Haematological values
Blood transfusion, 930–936
    adverse effects of, 931–933
    exchange
        for malaria, 277
        for megaloblastic anaemia, 945
        for sickle-cell disease, 953
    in intensive care, 211
    in major haemorrhage, 934–936
    other immunological complications of, 933
    safe transfusion procedures in, 934
    for sickle-cell anaemia, 953
Blood vessels
    imaging of, 1074
    see also Vascular
Blood volume, reference range of, 1362b
Bloom's syndrome, 1321b
BLS see Basic life support
Blue naevi, 1235
Blurred vision, of ophthalmic disease, 1170
BMD see Bone mineral density
BMI see Body mass index
BMR see Basal metabolic rate
BNP see Brain natriuretic peptide
Body composition, measures of, 693b
Body dysmorphic disorder, 1202
Body fat, in endocrine disease, 630f
Body lice, 1241
Body mass index (BMI)
    cardiovascular disease risk and, 699f
    clinical assessment of, 693b
    diabetes risk and, 699f
    obesity and, 700, 700b
    of older people, 1302f
    pancreatitis and, 837b
Body packers/stuffers, 144, 144f
'Boerhaave's syndrome', 797
Bohr effect, 190
Bone
    anatomy of, 984–985
    biopsy, 992
    cortical, 984f
    in endocrine disease, 630f
    fractures see Fractures
    infection, 1019–1021
        in old age, 1020b
    matrix, 985
    metabolism, pregnancy and, 1272
    mineral, 985
    mineralisation, 985
    pain, 1324b
    remodelling, 985, 985f–986f, 986b
    resorption, 985, 985f
    trabecular, 984f
    tumours, 1056–1057
        metastatic, 1329
    woven, 985
Bone disease, 1044–1056
    biochemical abnormalities in, 990b
    metabolic
        after gastric resection, 801
        chronic kidney disease and, 418–419
        metastatic, 1057
            in bone scintigraphy, 988–989
        in tuberculosis, 591
    see also individual disorders

Bone lining cells, 985
Bone marrow, 914, 914f
    examination of, 920, 922f
Bone marrow stromal cells, 985
Bone marrow transplantation (BMT), for
        severe combined immune
        deficiency, 80
Bone mineral density (BMD), 989–990
Borrelia burgdorferi, 255
Borrelia infections, 255–257, 256b
Botfly, 235f
Botulinum toxin, 104b, 1126, 1126b
    for achalasia, 795
    for dystonia, 1116
    for hemifacial spasm, 1116
Bouchard nodes, 982f, 1009
Bouginage, 775f, 793
Boutonneuse fever, 271b
Bovine serum albumin (BSA), 729
Bovine spongiform encephalopathy
        (BSE), 1127
Bowel
    disturbance, 1093–1094
    whole bowel irrigation, 136
    see also Colon; Small intestine
Bowen's disease, 1230b, 1232, 1232f
BPH see Benign prostatic hyperplasia
Brachial plexopathy, 1141
Brachial plexus lesions, 1141b
Brachytherapy, 1331
Bradykinesia, 1069
Brain
    alcohol-related damage, 1195
    arterial circulation of, 1150f
    biopsy, 1078
    cerebral hemispheres, 1066–1067,
        1066b, 1067f
    damage due to alcohol, 1195
    lesions, 1071–1072, 1072b
    schizophrenia, 1196
    structure and function of, psychiatric
        disorders and, 1183
    tumours, 1129–1132, 1129b, 1129f
        clinical features of, 1129
        investigations of, 1130, 1130f
        management of, 1130–1131
        metastatic, 1328, 1328b
        prognosis of, 1131
    venous circulation of, 1151f
    see also specific regions, and entries
        under cerebral
Brain death
    classification of, 212b
    organ donation after, 213
    UK criteria for diagnosis of, 211b
Brain injury, from critical illness, 211,
        211b–212b
Brain natriuretic peptide (BNP), 351,
        450
Brainstem, 1067, 1067f
    death, 211
    encephalitis, 1122
    lesions, 1083–1084
Breakpoint cluster region (BCR)
    abl oncogene, 958
    Philadelphia chromosome, 958
Breast cancer, 1333–1334
    clinical features of, 1333–1334
    investigations of, 1334
    management of, 1334
    in older people, 1325b
    pathogenesis of, 1333
    screening, 1325b
    staging, 1333b
    survival rates for, 1333, 1333b
Breastfeeding
    HIV infection/AIDS and, 326–327
    safety of antirheumatic drugs during,
        1281b
Breasts, in endocrine disease, 630f
Breath tests, gastroenterology, 777
Breathing
    assessment of, in deteriorating
        patient, 188
    control of, 549
    in divers, 170
    Kussmaul, 415
    of stroke patients, 1159b
    see also Respiration

Breathlessness, 557–558
    acute, 179–181, 558b
        clinical assessment of, 179–180
        clinical features in, 180b
        investigations of, 180–181
        presentation of, 179, 179f
        severe, 558
    chronic exertional, 557–558, 558b
    in COPD, 575
    differential diagnosis of, 557, 558b
    in lung cancer, 600
    in palliative care, 1353
    pathophysiology of, 557, 557f
    in pregnancy, 1274–1275, 1275b
    psychogenic, 558b
Briquet's syndrome, 1202
Bristol stool chart, 229, 229f
British National Formulary, 28
Broca's area, 1070
Bromocriptine
    for brain tumours, 1130
    for neuroleptic malignant syndrome,
        1197–1198
    for Parkinson's disease, 1114b
    for prolactinoma, 685, 685b
Bronchial artery, 549f
    angiography, 560f
    embolisation, 597
Bronchial gland adenoma, 603b
Bronchial gland carcinoma, 603b
Bronchial obstruction
    in lung cancer, 600, 600b, 600f
    radiological features of, 551, 552f
Bronchiectasis, 578–579, 578b–579b,
        579f
Bronchoalveolar carcinoma, 603b
Bronchodilators
    for acute exacerbations of COPD,
        577
    for chronic obstructive pulmonary
        disease (COPD), 576
Bronchopulmonary aspergillosis,
        classification of, 596b
Bronchopulmonary segments, 548f
Bronchoscopy, 553
    in haemoptysis, 560
    in lung cancer, 601, 601f
    in mediastinal tumours, 604
Bronchus, tumours of, 598–605
Brown-Séquard syndrome, 1083, 1136
Bruce Protocol, for exercise ECG,
        449–450
Brucella abortus, 254
Brucella canis, 254
Brucella melitensis, 254
Brucella suis, 254
Brucellosis, 254
    clinical features of, 254, 255f
    diagnosis of, 254
    incubation period of, 111b
    management of, 254, 255b
    in pregnancy, 235b
Brudzinski's sign, 1118
Brugada syndrome, 477
Brugia malayi infection, 233b, 291,
        291f
BSA see Bovine serum albumin
BSE see Bovine spongiform
        encephalopathy
BTK gene, X-linked
        agammaglobulinaemia and, 78
Bubonic plague, 259
Buccal administration, 17
Budd-Chiari syndrome, 898–899
    acute liver failure and, 857–858
Budesonide (BUD), 821b
Buerger's disease, 504
Bulbar palsy, 1093, 1093b
Bulimia nervosa, 1204, 1204b
Bullae, in lungs, 552b, 575
Bullous disease, 1254–1257
Bullous eruptions, drug-induced, 1266b
Bullous impetigo, 1218b
Bullous lupus erythematosus, 1255b
Bullous pemphigoid, 1255–1256,
        1255b, 1256f
Bumetanide
    for hypertension, 513
    for oedema, 396

Bundle branch block, 478–479, 478b,
        478f
Bundle of His, 445
Bupropion, 139b
Burch-Wartofsky scoring system, for
        thyrotoxic crisis, 639b
Burkholderia pseudomallei, 261
Burkitt's lymphoma, 1320b
Burns
    haemolysis and, 950
    sunburn, 1221f
Burrow, definition of, 1241
Bursae, 987
Bursitis
    anserine, 998b
    deep infrapatellar, 998b
    ischiogluteal, 999b
    olecranon, 998b
    pre-patellar, 998b
    superficial, 998b
    trochanteric, 998, 999b, 999f
Buruli ulcer, 254
Buschke-Löwenstein tumour, 343
Buspirone, 139b
Busulfan
    drug-induced pigmentation,
        1258b
    hepatotoxicity of, 894b
Butterfly rash, 982f
Button hole deformity of fingers,
        1023
Butyrophenones, 1190b
    for schizophrenia, 1198b
Byssinosis, 614, 616b

C
C-peptide, 724, 724f, 727
C-reactive protein (CRP), 63
    abnormal, conditions associated with,
        72b
    in acute phase response, 70
    inflammation and, 71–72
    reference range of, venous blood,
        1360b
C1 inhibitor deficiency (hereditary
        angioedema), 87
    acquired, 88
C4d staining, 89
CA-19.9, as tumour markers, 1324b
Cabergoline
    for brain tumours, 1130
    nephrotoxicity, 427b
    for Parkinson's disease, 1114b
    for prolactinoma, 685b
CABG see Coronary artery bypass
        grafting
Cabozantinib, for medullary carcinoma,
        650
Cachexia, cancer, 693f
CADASIL, 1095
Cadherin-1 (CDH1), 1319
Cadmium, lung cancer, 618
Caecum, cancer, 831
Caeruloplasmin, 1360b
    Wilson's disease, 896
Café au lait spot, 1131f
Caffeine, 716
cagA see Cytotoxin-associated gene
Calabar swelling, 292
Calcific periarthritis, 1017, 1017f
Calcification
    artery, 452
    metastatic, 369
    in musculoskeletal disease, 988
Calcimimetic agents, 419
Calcineurin inhibitors, 1226
Calcinosis
    crystal-associated arthritis and
        deposition in connective tissue,
        1013b
    nephrocalcinosis, 427b, 431
Calcipotriol, 1250
Calcitonin
    for Paget's disease, 1054b
    as tumor markers, 1324b
Calcitonin gene-related peptide (CGRP),
        771–772
Calcitriol (1,25-dihydroxycholecalciferol),
    for hypoparathyroidism, 665

Calcium, 716
    absorption, 716
    acute kidney injury and, 416b
    deficiency, 716
    dietary sources of, 717b
    excess, 716
    homeostasis, 367
    in myocardial contraction, 446
    for osteoporosis, 1048, 1048b
    pregnancy and, 1272
    reference nutrient intake of, 717b
    reference range of
        urine, 1361b
        venous blood, 1360b
    in skeletal disease, 990b
    stone, prevention of, 433b
    see also Hypercalcaemia;
        Hypocalcaemia
Calcium and vitamin D supplements,
        1048
Calcium antagonists (channel blockers)
    adverse reactions of, 22b
    for angina, 491b
    for arrhythmias, 472
    for hypertension, 513
    for hypertrophic cardiomyopathy, 540
    for mitral stenosis, 519
    poisoning from, 140
    for pulmonary hypertension, 622
    for Raynaud's phenomenon, 1038
Calcium carbonate, 419
Calcium gluconate, 368
    cardiotoxic drug poisoning, 140
    drug interactions, 24b
    for hypermagnesaemia, 368
Calcium oxalate
    crystal, 147
    stones, 431b
Calcium phosphate, stones, 431b
Calcium pyrophosphate crystals, 663
Calcium pyrophosphate dihydrate
        (CPPD) crystal deposition
        disease, 1016–1017
Calcium therapy
    for hypoparathyroidism, 665
    for osteoporosis, 1047
    for rickets/osteomalacia, 1052
    tetany, 663
Calculi (stones)
    gallbladder see Gallstones
    renal, 431, 431b
    staghorn, 431, 432f
    urinary, 431
    see also Gallstones
Calicivirus, 872b
Calprotectin, faecal, 777b, 1361b
'Cameron lesions', 793
Campbell de Morgan spots, 1234,
        1234f
Campylobacter jejuni
    Guillain-Barré syndrome, 1140
    infection, 262
Camurati-Engelmann disease, 1056
Canakinumab
    for gout, 1015
    for musculoskeletal disease, 1007,
        1007b
Canalicular system, 918
Cancer, 1316, 1316f, 1333b
    aetiology, environmental, 1320b
    biochemical markers, 1323
    breast, 1333–1334
        clinical features of, 1333–1334
        investigations of, 1334
        management of, 1334
        pathogenesis of, 1333
        staging, 1333b
        survival rates for, 1333, 1333b
    cervical, 1335
        investigations in, 1335
        management of, 1335
        pathogenesis of, 1335
    childhood, 1298
    clinical examination of, 1314, 1314f
    colorectal, 830–833
        clinical features of, 831
        dietary risk factors for, 830b
        familial adenomatous polyposis,
            828–829, 829b, 829f

investigations of, 832, 833f
management of, 832
modified Dukes classification and
survival of, 832f
non-dietary risk factors for, 830b
pathogenesis of, 830f
pathophysiology of, 830–831, 831f
prevention and screening of,
832–833
determinants of, 1320–1321
environmental, 1320–1321, 1320b
genetic, 1321, 1321b
ectopic hormone production, 1325,
1325b
emergency complications of,
1326–1328
endometrial, 1334–1335
investigations of, 1334
management of, 1335
pathogenesis of, 1334
of gallbladder, 904
hallmarks of, 1316–1320
activating invasion and metastasis,
1319
angiogenesis, 1318, 1319f
enabling replicative immortality,
1318
evading growth suppressors, 1318
evading immune destruction, 1320
genome instability/mutation, 1316
reprogramming energy metabolism,
1319
resisting cell death, 1316–1317
sustaining proliferative signalling,
1317
tumour-promoting inflammation,
1319–1320
histology of, 1322
cytogenetic analysis, 1322
electron microscopy, 1322
immunohistochemistry, 1322
light microscopy, 1322
HIV-related, 322, 323b
imaging for, 1323
inheritance, 1321b
investigations of, 1321–1323,
1322b
local features of, 1324b
lung, 599–603, 599f
burden of, 598b
cell types in, 599b
clinical features of, 599–601
investigations of, 601–602
management of, 602–603
non-metastatic extrapulmonary
manifestations of, 601b
occupational, 618
pathology of, 599, 599f
prognosis for, 603, 603b
metastatic disease, 1328–1329
neurological paraneoplastic
syndromes, 1325–1326
obesity and, 698f
in older people, 1325b
oral, 790, 790b
ovarian, 1334
investigations of, 1334
management of, 1334
pathogenesis of, 1334
predisposition syndromes, 1321b
presenting problems of, 1323–1326,
1324b–1325b
renal cell, 434–435, 435f
screening, breast cancer, 1325b
staging, TNM classification, 1322b
therapeutics for, 1329–1333
adjuvant, 1329
biological, 1332
chemoprevention, 1330
chemotherapy, 1330
hormonal, 1332
immunotherapy, 1332
neoadjuvant, 1330
palliative, 1329
radiation therapy, 1331–1332
surgical, 1330
of unknown origin, 1336, 1336b
see also Chemotherapy; specific
cancers

Cancer antigen 19.9 (CA-19.9), 1324b
Cancer antigen 125 (CA-125), 1324b
Cancer cachexia, 693f
Candesartan
for heart failure, 466b
for myocardial infarction, 500–501
Candida albicans, 300
Candida dubliniensis, 302
Candida glabrata, 302
Candida krusei, 302
Candida parapsilosis, 302
Candida spp., 100, 103f
endocarditis, 528
Candida tropicalis, 302
Candidiasis, 334b, 336b
acute disseminated, 302
chronic disseminated, 302
genital, 735b
oesophageal, 794
oral, 790
skin, 1240
superficial, 300
systemic, 302
Cannabis, 143
CAPD see Continuous ambulatory
peritoneal dialysis
Capecitabine, 832
Caplan's syndrome, 610–611
Capnocytophaga canimorsus, 226b
Capnography, 175f
Capsaicin
for herpes zoster, 240
for osteoarthritis, 1003–1004
topical, 315
Capsule endoscopy, 774–776, 775f
wireless, 775f, 776b
Capsulitis (frozen shoulder), 997–998
Caput medusae, 868
Carbamate insecticides, 146–147
Carbamazepine
for epilepsy, 1102b
hyponatraemia, 1103b
multiple sclerosis, 1110b
pharmacodynamics, 20b
poisoning, 141b
for status epilepticus, 1081b
for trigeminal neuralgia, 1097
Carbapenems, 120b, 121
Carbaryl, 1241
Carbenoxolone, 361
sodium content of, 864b
Carbidopa, 1113
Carbimazole
for Graves' thyrotoxicosis, 644
for thyrotoxicosis, in pregnancy,
1279
Carbohydrates, 695–697
in diabetic diet, 743–744
dietary, 696b
energy provided by, 694
recommended intake, 698b
digestion of, 768
metabolism, 850
disorders of, 370
see also Diabetes mellitus
effects of insulin in, 723b
Carbon dioxide
arterial blood (PaCO2), 204, 1358b
removal of, extracorporeal, 204
Carbon monoxide poisoning, 134b,
144–145
Carbonic acid/bicarbonate buffer
system, 363–364
Carbonic anhydrase, 717
Carbonic anhydrase inhibitors, for
hypervolaemia, 354
Carboplatin, 832
Carboxyhaemoglobin, reference range
of, 1360b
Carboxypenicillins, 121
Carbuncles, 1237, 1237f
Carcinoembryonic antigen (CEA), 1322,
1324b
Carcinoid syndrome
pellagra, 714
valvular heart disease, 526
Carcinoid tumours
gastric, 805
lung, 603b

Carcinoma
at ampulla of Vater, 907–908
anaplastic, 650
basal cell, 1229–1230, 1229f, 1230b,
1324b
bronchial gland, 603b
bronchoalveolar, 603b
fibrolamellar hepatocellular, 892
follicular, 649
of gallbladder, 907
gastric, 803–804, 804f
hepatocellular, 890–892, 891f
chemotherapy for, 892
cirrhosis and, 890
fibrolamellar, 892
hepatic resection for, 891
hepatitis B and, 873
liver biopsy for, 891
liver transplantation for, 891
management of, 892f
in old age, 901b
percutaneous therapy for, 891
screening for, 890–891
trans-arterial chemo-embolisation
for, 892
medullary, 650
of oesophagus, 796–797
of pancreas, 843f
papillary, 649
squamous, 796b
skin, 1230–1231, 1231f
of unknown origin, 1336, 1336b
see also sites of carcinoma
Carcinoma in situ, 1230b
Card agglutination trypanosomiasis test
(CATT), 279
Cardiac arrest, 456–457, 456b, 456f
chain of survival in, 457, 458f
clinical assessment and management
of, 456–457, 457f–458f
post, 200–201
acute management of, 201, 201b
prognosis of, 201, 201b
Cardiac arrhythmias, 1198
Cardiac biomarkers, 450
for acute coronary syndrome, 497,
498f
Cardiac catheterisation, 453–454, 453f
aortic regurgitation, 525b
aortic stenosis, 523b
mitral valve disease, 519, 521b
Cardiac death, organ donation after,
213
Cardiac disease, 899
HIV-related, 322
in pregnancy, 1282
aortic dissection, 1282
congenital, 1282
dilated cardiomyopathy, 1282
myocardial infarction, 1282
peripartum cardiomyopathy, 1282
valvular, 1282
Cardiac glycosides see Digoxin
Cardiac output, 447–448
heart failure, 461
Cardiac pacemakers
code, 483b
permanent, 469, 483, 483b
rate-responsive, 483
temporary, 482–483, 483f
Cardiac peptides, 446–447
Cardiac resynchronisation therapy, for
arrhythmias, 484
Cardiac tamponade, 447–448, 544,
544b
see also Heart
Cardiac transplantation, 467–468
Cardiac tumours, 541–542
Cardiobacterium hominis, 528
Cardiogenic shock, 199–200, 206b
causes of, 200f
downward spiral of, 199, 200f
Cardiology, 441–544
Cardiomegaly, 450
Cardiomyopathy, 538–541, 539f, 541b
arrhythmogenic ventricular, 540
dilated, 1282
HIV-associated, 322
hypertrophic obstructive, 1297–1298

obliterative, 541
peripartum, pregnancy and, 1282
restrictive, 540
septic, 198
types of, 539f
Cardiopulmonary resuscitation (CPR),
213b
see also Basic life support
Cardiothoracic ratio, 450
Cardiotoxicity, venom and, 155
Cardiovascular disease
chronic kidney disease and, 420
congenital, 531–538
hypertension see Hypertension
investigation of, 448–454
New Heart Association (NYHA)
functional classification of, 454,
454b
ophthalmic features of, 1165b
presenting problems in, 454–468
in rheumatoid arthritis, 1024
risk of, obesity, 699f
syphilis, 338
in systemic lupus erythematosus,
1035
transition medicine and, 1297–1298
congenital heart disease, 1297
hypertrophic obstructive
cardiomyopathy, 1297–1298
Cardiovascular medications, poisoning
from, 140
Cardiovascular risk prediction chart,
511f
Cardiovascular support, in intensive
care, 204–208
advanced haemodynamic monitoring,
206, 207b, 207f
fluid and vasopressor use, 206, 206b
initial resuscitation, 204–206, 206b
mechanical, 206–208
Cardiovascular system
clinical examination of, 442–444,
442f
pregnancy and, 1272
Cardioversion, 482
atrial fibrillation, 470–471
direct current (DC), 470
ventricular tachycardia, 475
Carditis, 515–516
Care see Health care
Carey Coombs murmur, 515–516
Carnitine-palmitoyl transferase (CPT)
deficiency, 1144b
Caroli's disease, 902
Carotenes, 712–713
Carotid endarterectomy, 1160
Carotid pulse, 166, 189
Carpal tunnel syndrome, 1058
diabetes, 760
rheumatoid arthritis, 1024
Carrion's disease, 272
Cartilage
articular, 987, 987f
calcification of, 988
osteoarthritis in, 1010
Carvedilol, 869
for arrhythmias, 481
for hypertension, 513
Casal's necklace, 714, 715f
Caspases, 41
Caspofungin, 125b, 126
for acute leukaemia patients, 957
for aspergillosis, 598
Cassava, 839–840
Castleman's disease, 220b, 248
Cat scratch disease, 272
Cataplexy, 1105
Cataract
diabetics, 756b
in ophthalmological conditions, 1174
'snowflake', 1177
Catatonia, 1196–1197
Catechol-O-methyl-transferase (COMT)
inhibitors, for Parkinson's
disease, 1114
Catecholamines, 666
drug interactions, 24b
Catephen, for anogenital warts, 343
Cathepsin K, 985

Catheter ablation therapy, 484, 484f
for arrhythmias, 470
Catheters/catheterisation
bacteriuria, 429–430
bladder dysfunction, 1094b
cardiac, 453–454, 453f
aortic regurgitation, 525b
aortic stenosis, 523b
mitral valve disease, 519, 521b
pulmonary artery, critically ill patients, 206, 207f
Cathinones, 143
CATT see Card agglutination trypanosomiasis test
Cauda equina syndrome, 997b
Caudal regression syndrome, 1278–1279
Caval filters, for pulmonary embolism, 621
Cawthorne-Cooksey exercises, 1104
CBT see Cognitive behaviour therapy
CCK see Cholecystokinin
CD4 cells, in HIV infection/AIDS, 309–310
CD4$^+$ T lymphocytes, 70
CD8$^+$ T lymphocytes, 70
CDKs see Cyclin-dependent kinases
CEA see Carcinoembryonic antigen
Cefaclor, 121b
Cefalexin, 121b
for urinary tract infection, 428
Cefazolin, 121b
Cefepime, 117b, 121b
Cefixime, 121b
for gonorrhoea, 340b
Cefotaxime, 117b, 121b
for cerebral abscess, 1124b
for meningitis, 1120b
for spontaneous bacterial peritonitis, 864
Cefoxitin, 121b
Cefradine, 121b
Ceftaroline, 121b
Ceftazidime, 117b, 121b
for bronchiectasis, 579
for melioidosis, 261
Ceftobiprole, 121b
Ceftriaxone, 117b, 121b
for leptospirosis, 258–259
for meningitis, 1120b
for nocardiosis, 261
for pneumonia, 319
for pyogenic meningitis, 1120b
for STIs
congenital syphilis, 339
gonorrhoea, 340b
for Whipple's disease, 809
Cefuroxime, 117b, 121b
for cerebral abscess, 1124b
for cholecystitis, 905
for empyema, 565
for meningitis, 1120b
for pneumonia, 585b, 586
prophylactic, 119b
Cefuroxime axetil, 256
Celecoxib, 1003b
Cell adhesion molecules, 1318f
Cell body, 1338
Cell cycle, 1317, 1317f
regulation, 1317
stimulation, 1317
Cell differentiation, 40–41
Cell migration, 40–41
Cell surface antigens, 917
Cells
cerebrospinal fluid analysis of, 1077, 1078b, 1361b
death of, 41, 1316–1317
programmed (apoptosis), 1316
division of, 40–41
of nervous system, 1064–1065, 1064f
senescence of, 41
Cellular immunity, 69–70, 69f
Cellulitis, 1237, 1237f
anaerobic, 227
clinical assessment of, 187
investigation of, 187
Central core disease, 1145b

Central nervous system (CNS)
HIV infection/AIDS, 309–310
tuberculosis, 591
Central sensitisation, 1340, 1341f
Central termination, 1338
Central venous catheter infections, 225–226
Central venous pressure, monitoring of, 175f, 190b
Cephalosporin, 117b, 121, 121b
for cholecystitis, 905
for pneumonia, 586
in pregnancy, 120b
renal or hepatic disease, 32b
for septic arthritis, 1020
for variceal bleeding, 869, 869b
Cephamycins, 121
Cerebellar ataxia, 1325
Cerebellar degeneration, cancer-related, 1325, 1325b
Cerebellar dysfunction, 1134
Cerebellum, 1069
Cerebral abscess, 1124, 1124b, 1124f
Cerebral cortex
anatomy of, 1067f
lobar functions of, 1066b
effects of damage, 1066b
Cerebral hemispheres, 1066–1067, 1066b, 1067f
lesions, 1084
Cerebral infarction, 1153–1154, 1153f–1154f
Cerebral ischaemia, 967f
Cerebral oedema
acute liver failure and, 857
high-altitude, 168
hypoglycaemia, 740
stroke patients, 1154–1155
Cerebral palsy, transition medicine and, 1296
Cerebral perfusion pressure (CPP), 208
Cerebral toxoplasmosis, HIV-related, 315b, 320, 320f
Cerebral tumours see Brain, tumours
Cerebral venous disease, 1162
causes of, 1162b
clinical features of, 1162, 1162b
investigations and management of, 1162
Cerebrospinal fluid (CSF), 1067
analysis, 1077, 1078b, 1361b
circulation, 1128b
encephalomyelitis, 1110
Guillain-Barré syndrome, 1140
meningitis, 1118, 1121
multiple sclerosis, 1108
result of, interpretation of, 1077, 1078b
in subacute sclerosing panencephalitis, 1123
syphilis and, 339
in viral encephalitis, 1122
see also Lumbar puncture
Cerebrotendinous xanthomatosis, 375b
Cerebrovascular disease see specific conditions
Certolizumab, for musculoskeletal disease, 1007b
Cervical cancer, 1335
HIV-related, 322
investigations of, 1335
management of, 1335
pathogenesis of, 1335
Cervical cord compression, 1134f
in cervical spondylosis, 1134f
in rheumatoid arthritis, 1024b
Cervical spine
myelopathy, 1134–1135
radiculopathy, 1134, 1134f
spondylosis, 1134–1135, 1134f
subluxation of, 1024, 1025f
Cervicitis, gonococcal, 335
Cestode infections, 233b, 297–299
Cetirizine, 1227
Cetuximab, 832, 1335–1336
CF see Cystic fibrosis
CFTR see Cystic fibrosis transmembrane conductor regulator (CFTR) protein

CFU-E (colony-forming unit erythroid), 914–915
CFU-GM (colony-forming unit-granulocyte, monocyte), 914
CFU-Meg (colony-forming unit-megakaryocyte), 914, 918
CGRP (calcitonin gene-related peptide), 771–772
Chagas' disease, 279–280
transfusion-transmitted, 930–931
Chain of infection, 100f
Chain of survival, in cardiac arrest, 457, 458f
Chancre, 333–334
trypanosomal, 278
Chancroid, 341b
Channelopathies, 1144, 1145b
Charcoal, activated, 136, 136b
antidiabetic overdose, 141
digoxin/oleander poisoning, 140
NSAID overdose, 138
salicylate poisoning, 138
tricyclic antidepressant poisoning, 139
Charcot joints, 1057, 1058f
Charcot-Marie-Tooth disease (CMT), 1140
Charcot neuroarthropathy, 762
Charcot's triad, 861–862
acute cholangitis and, 905
Charles Bonnet's syndrome, 1088
Cheese worker's lung, 616b
Cheiroarthropathy, 1057
Chelating agents, 165
Chemical cholestasis, 902
Chemical poisoning, 144–149
Chemical warfare agents, poisoning from, 149, 149b
Chemicals, in haemolysis, 950
Chemo-embolisation, hepatocellular carcinoma, 892
Chemokine receptor inhibitor, 324b
Chemoprevention, 1330
Chemoprophylaxis, 112b
for malaria, 277, 278b
Chemotherapy, 936, 936b, 1330
adjuvant, 1329
breast cancer, 1334
adverse effects, 1330, 1331b
for brain tumours, 1130–1131
combination therapy, 1330
for hepatocellular carcinoma, 892
for high-grade NHL, 966
for Hodgkin lymphoma, 963
leukaemia
acute, 956b
chronic lymphocytic, 960
chronic myeloid, 959
for low-grade NHL, 965
for lung cancer, 602–603
for multiple myeloma, 968
neoadjuvant, 1330
palliative, 1329
platinum-based, 602–603
for prostate cancer, 439
for tuberculosis, 592–594
Chernobyl, 164
Chest infection, in stroke patients, 1159f
Chest pain, 176–179, 454–455
associated features of, 177–178, 178f
cardiac disease, aortic dissection, 507
characteristics of, 177
clinical assessment of, 178
differential diagnosis of, 177b
investigations of, 178–179, 179b
ischaemic, 454f
onset of, 177
pregnancy and, 1275
in respiratory disease, 558
site and radiation of, 177
Chest radiography/X-ray, 450
for bronchiectasis, 579
cardiovascular disorders
for aortic regurgitation, 451f
for chronic constrictive pericarditis, 544f
for heart failure, 464, 464f

for mitral valve, 451f
for myocardial infarction, 497–498
of cardiovascular system, 450
for COPD, 575
for empyema, 564f
of pacemaker/defibrillator, 467f
for pleural effusion, 563
pregnancy and, 1274
for respiratory disease
abnormalities, 552b
ARDS, 199f
aspergillosis, 597f
asthma, 569
bronchial obstruction/lung collapse, 600f
bronchiectasis, 579
COPD, 575
empyema, 564f
haemoptysis, 560
HIV-related pulmonary disease, 318b, 318f–319f
interpretation, 551b
interstitial, 605f
lobar collapse, 552f
mediastinal tumours, 604f
pleural effusion, 563
pleural plaques, 617f
Pneumocystis jirovecii pneumonia, 318f
pneumonia, 585
pneumothorax, 626
pulmonary embolism, 619b, 619f
pulmonary hypertension, 622f
sarcoidosis, 609b
silicosis, 615f
tuberculosis, 590f, 592f
Chest wall deformities, 628
Chickenpox, 238–239
clinical features of, 238–239, 238f
diagnosis of, 239
incubation period of, 111b
management and prevention of, 239, 239b
periods of infectivity, 111b
rash, 238
varicella zoster immunoglobulin, 240b
Chiclero ulcers, 285
Chief cells, 661
Chikungunya virus, 250
Chilblains, 167
Child-bearing potential, cystic fibrosis and, 1297
Child-Pugh classification, cirrhosis prognosis and, 867b
Childbirth, associated psychiatric disorders, 1206
Childhood absence epilepsy, 1100b
Childhood cancer therapy, late effects of, 689
Children
diabetes mellitus in, 753–754, 754b
important long-term conditions of, adult health affected by, 1288b
inflammatory bowel disease and, 823, 1299
laboratory reference range of, 1363
osteomyelitis in, 1021
renal impairment in, causes of, 1298b
STI in, 332–333
Chiropractic, 826b
Chlamydia pneumoniae, 272b
Chlamydia psittaci, 272b
Chlamydia spp., 272
Chlamydia trachomatis, 100–101, 117b, 273
in pregnancy, 235b, 332b
Chlamydial infection, 340–341
in men, 340
in reactive arthritis, 1031
treatment of, 341b
urethritis, 333
in women, 340–341
Chloasma, 1258
Chlorambucil
for chronic lymphocytic leukaemia, 960
for non-Hodgkin's lymphoma, 965
for Waldenström macroglobulinaemia, 966

Chloramphenicol, 117*b*, 124
  contraindication to, in pregnancy, 120*b*
  mechanism of action, 116*b*
  for meningitis, 1120*b*
  for plague, 259
  in pregnancy, 120*b*
  for pyogenic meningitis, 1120*b*
  in renal/hepatic disease, 32*b*
  for rickettsial fevers, 271–272
Chloride, 349*b*, 718
  channelopathies, 1145*b*
  reference range of, venous blood, 1358*b*
Chloroquine
  adverse reactions of, 22
    pigmentation, 1258*b*
  leprosy reactions, 270
  for malaria, 128, 278*b*
  myopathy, 1057*b*
  poisoning, 141*b*
  resistance to, 273, 277
Chlorphenamine, 33*b*
  anaphylaxis, 76*b*
  diphtheria, 625
  pruritus, 935*f*
Chlorpromazine
  for acute diarrhoea, 230
  for alcohol withdrawal, 1195
  for cholestatic hepatitis, 894
  hepatotoxicity, 894*b*
  long QT syndrome, 476*b*
  poisoning, 141
  for rabies, 1122
  for schizophrenia, 1197
Chlorpropamide, neutropenia, 926*b*
Cholangiocarcinoma, 892, 907, 907*f*
  primary sclerosing cholangitis and, 888
Cholangiography, 906
  for hepatobiliary disease, 854–855
  percutaneous transhepatic (PTC), 854–855
  for sclerosing cholangitis, 888
Cholangiopancreatography
  endoscopic retrograde *see* ERCP
  magnetic resonance *see* MRCP
Cholangiopathy, HIV-related, 318
Cholangitis
  acute, 905
  liver flukes, 297, 297*b*
  primary
    biliary, 887–888
    IgG4-associated, 890, 909
  primary sclerosing, 888–890
  recurrent pyogenic, 906–907
Cholecalciferol *see* Vitamin D
Cholecystectomy
  in old age, 909*b*
  for pancreatitis, 839
  post-cholecystectomy syndrome, 908*b*
Cholecystitis, 905
  acalculous, 905
  acute, 788, 905
    in old age, 909*b*
  chronic, 905
  gallstones and, 904
  pregnancy and, 900
Cholecystography, oral, 909
Cholecystokinin (CCK), 768, 768*f*, 772*b*
Cholecystolithiasis, 904
Choledochal cysts, 903, 903*f*
Choledochojejunostomy, 842–844
Choledocholithiasis, 904, 906–907
  endoscopic retrograde
    cholangiopancreatography for, 906*f*
  endoscopic ultrasound for, 906*f*
Choledochoscopy, 906
Cholera, 104*b*, 264–265
  clinical features of, 265
  diagnosis and management of, 265
  fluid loss, 265
  incubation period of, 111*b*
  prevention of, 265
'Cholera sicca', 265

Cholestasis, 894
  benign recurrent intrahepatic, 902
  biliary cirrhosis, 903
  chemical, 902
  obstetric (of pregnancy), 1220*b*, 1284
    pruritus, 1220*b*
  pure, 894
  sclerosing cholangitis, 889
Cholestatic jaundice, 860*b*–862*b*, 861–862
Cholesterol, 370
  absorption of, 697
  atheroembolism, 390*b*
  dietary, 698*b*
  gallstones, 903, 903*b*
  low-density lipoproteins, 371–372
  metabolism of, 81
  reference range of, venous blood, 1360*b*
  transport of, 372–373
  see also Hypercholesterolaemia
Cholesterol absorption inhibitors, 371
Cholesterol emboli, 409, 409*f*
Cholesterol ester transfer protein (CETP), 373
Cholesterol gallstones, 903, 903*b*
Cholesterolosis of gallbladder, 909
Choline salicylate, 790
Cholinergic syndrome, organophosphate poisoning, 146, 146*b*
Chondrocalcinosis, 1016, 1016*b*, 1016*f*
Chondrocytes
  in osteoarthritis, 1008
  tumours, 1056*b*
Chondroitin sulphate, 987
  for osteoarthritis, 1012
Chondroma, 1056*b*
Chondrosarcoma, 1056*b*, 1057
CHOP regimen, for non-Hodgkin lymphoma, 966
Chorea, 1085
  causes of, 1085*b*
  in Huntington's disease, 1085
Chorionic villus sampling, 56
Choroid, of eye, 1167
Choroid plexus, 1132*f*
Christmas disease, 973–974
Chromatin, 38, 38*f*
Chromatography, 348*b*
Chromium, 718
  deficiency, 718
Chromoblastomycosis, 300–301
Chromosomal disorders, 44*b*, 45*f*
  see also specific conditions
Chromosomes, 38, 38*f*, 51–52, 52*f*
  abnormalities *see* Mutation(s)
  analysis of, 45*f*
    leukaemia, 955–956
    myelodysplastic syndromes, 960–961
  deletions, 52
  duplication, 44, 45*f*
  sex, 38
  see also X chromosome; Y chromosome
  translocations of, 805
Chronic allograft failure, 89
Chronic bronchitis, 555*b*, 573–574
Chronic cavitary pulmonary aspergillosis, 597, 597*f*
Chronic cold agglutinin disease, 950
Chronic constrictive pericarditis, 543–544, 543*b*, 544*f*
Chronic demyelinating polyneuropathy, 1139*b*, 1141
Chronic eosinophilic pneumonia, 611–612
Chronic exertional breathlessness, 557–558, 558*b*
Chronic fatigue syndrome, 1202
Chronic fibrosing pulmonary aspergillosis, 597
Chronic graft-*versus*-host disease, 937
Chronic granulomatous disease, 77
Chronic inflammation, 71
Chronic interstitial nephritis, 402–403, 403*b*
Chronic intestinal pseudo-obstruction, 810–811, 811*b*

Chronic kidney disease, 415–420, 417*b*
  causes of, 415*b*
  haemodialysis in, 422–423
  indications for dialysis for, 422*b*
  osteodystrophy and, 419*f*
  physical signs of, 416*f*
  pregnancy and, 1282, 1283*f*
  staging of, in children over 2 years of age, 1298*b*
  transition medicine and, 1298–1299
Chronic laryngitis, 624, 624*b*
Chronic liver failure
  causes of, 856*f*, 867*b*
  cirrhosis and, 867
Chronic lymphocytic leukaemia (CLL), 959–960
  clinical features of, 959
  investigations of, 959–960
  management of, 960
  prognosis of, 960
  staging of, 960*b*
Chronic meningococcaemia, 1119
Chronic mesenteric ischaemia, 827
Chronic myeloid leukaemia (CML), 958–959
  characteristics of, 958
  clinical features of, 958
  investigations of, 959
  management of, 959
    accelerated phase, 959
    blast crisis, 959
    chronic phase, 959, 959*b*
  natural history of, 958
Chronic obstructive pulmonary disease *see* COPD
Chronic pain syndrome, 1348–1349
Chronic pancreatitis, 839–841, 840*b*
  complications of, 840*b*
  investigations of, 840, 841*b*, 841*f*
  management of complications of, 841
  pathophysiology of, 840*f*
Chronic pulmonary aspergillosis (CPA), 596–597
Chronic pulmonary tuberculosis, complications of, 590*b*
Chronic renal failure *see* Renal failure, chronic
Chronic respiratory failure, 566–567
  management of, 566–567, 566*b*
Chronic rheumatic heart disease, 517
Chronic venous insufficiency, 187
Chronic widespread pain, 1349
CHRPE *see* Congenital hypertrophy of the retinal pigment epithelium
Chrysops, loiasis, 292
Churg-Strauss syndrome, 1043
Chvostek's sign, 367
Chylomicrons, 697
Chylothorax, 562–563
Chyluria, lymphatic filariasis, 291
Chymotrypsinogen, 770*b*
Ciclesonide, 571
Ciclosporin
  adverse reactions of
    chronic interstitial nephritis, 427*b*
    musculoskeletal, 1057*b*
    proximal myopathy, 1145*f*
  for aplastic anaemias, 969
  asthma, 572
  drug interactions, 24*b*
  eczema, 1246
  heart transplant patients, 467
  HSCT, 937
  immunosuppression, 89*b*
  for inflammatory bowel disease, 821*b*
  for lichen planus, 1252
  liver transplant patients, 901
  lung transplant patients, 567
  for primary biliary cholangitis, 888
  for psoriasis, 1250
  for pyoderma gangrenosum, 1261–1262
  for skin disease, 1227–1228
Ciclosporin A, for musculoskeletal disease, 1004*b*, 1005
Cidofovir
  as antiviral agents, 127*b*
  CMV, 243
  for herpesvirus infection, 126, 127*b*

Cigarette smoke, in lower airway defences, 550
Ciguatera poisoning, 149–150
Cilia, 62–63
Ciliary body, of eye, 1167
Ciliary dysfunction syndromes, 578*b*, 579
Ciliary dysmotility syndrome, 550
Cilostazol, 504
Cimetidine
  drug interactions of, 24
  neutropenia, 926*b*
  for urticaria, 1254
Cinacalcet, for primary hyperparathyroidism, 664
Ciprofloxacin, 117*b*, 123*b*
  for anthrax, 267
  for bacillary dysentery, 265
  for bronchiectasis, 579
  for brucellosis, 255*b*
  for cholera, 265
  drug interactions of, 23
  for inflammatory bowel disease, 823
  for intestinal bacterial overgrowth, 808–809
  for meningococcal infection, 1120
  for plague, 259
  for primary sclerosing cholangitis, 890
  prophylactic, 119*b*
  for Q fever, 272
  for spontaneous bacterial peritonitis, 864
  for STIs
    chancroid, 341*b*
    gonorrhoea, 340*b*
  for urinary tract infection, 429*b*
  for variceal bleeding, 869
Circinate balanitis, 334*b*, 1031
Circulation
  assessment of, in deteriorating patient, 189
  coronary, 444–445
  enterohepatic, 19
  portal, 384, 385*f*
  of stroke patients, 1159*b*
Circulatory collapse, pregnancy and, 1275
Circulatory failure (shock), 193
  acute, 199–200
Circumduction, 1086
Circumflex artery (CX)
  in coronary circulation, 444–445, 445*f*
  with stenosis, 453*f*
Cirrhosis, 866–867
  alcoholic, 881–882, 881*b*
  ascites and, 867
  biliary, secondary, 903
  causes of, 866*b*–867*b*
  Child-Pugh classification of, 867*b*
  cryptogenic, 884
  drugs to be avoided in, 894*b*
  haemochromatosis, 866–867
  hepatic encephalopathy and, 865
  hepatic fibrosis and, 866, 866*f*
  hepatitis B and, 873, 876
  hepatitis C and, 877
  hepatocellular carcinoma and, 890
  macronodular, 866
  management of, 867
  micronodular, 866
  non-alcoholic fatty liver disease and, 882–883, 883*f*
  portal hypertension and, 869
  survival in, 868*b*, 868*f*
Cisplatin
  for head and neck tumours, 1335–1336
  hypomagnesaemia and, 368*b*
  nephrotoxicity, 427*b*
  polyneuropathy, 1139*b*
Citalopram, 1199*b*
Citric acid (Krebs) cycle, 49, 714
Citrobacter freundii, 225
Citrobacter spp., 117*b*
CJD *see* Creutzfeldt-Jakob disease
CK *see* Creatine kinase
Clarithromycin
  drug interactions, 24*b*
  H. pylori eradication, 800

Clarithromycin (Continued)
  for leprosy, 269
  for Mycobacterium avium complex, 315b
  for pneumonia, 585b
  in pregnancy, 120b
Clasp-knife phenomenon, 1068–1069
Classical syndromes, 633
Claude syndrome, 1072b
Clearance, 19
CLI (critical limb ischaemia), 502–503
Climate change, 94
Clindamycin, 117b
  for acne vulgaris, 1242–1243
  for babesiosis, 278
  for gas gangrene, 227
  for malaria, 277b
  for MRSA, 252
  for necrotising fasciitis, 227
  in pregnancy, 120b
  for septic arthritis, 1020b
Clinical biochemistry, 345–380
Clinical decision-making, 10–12
  in cognitive biases, 11
  dealing with uncertainty during, 5–6
  in deciding pre-test probability, 11
  in evidence-based history and examination, 11
  heuristic, 7b
  in human factors, 11
  in interpreting results, 11
  in person-centred EBM and patient information, 12
  in post-test probability, 11
  in reducing cognitive error, 11
  reducing errors in, 9–10
    cognitive debiasing strategies, 8f, 9–10
    effective team communication, 10, 10b
    using clinical prediction rules and other decision aids, 10
  in treatment threshold, 11
Clinical endpoints, 35–36
Clinical genetics, 37–59
Clinical immunology, 61–90
  functional anatomy and physiology in, 62–70, 62f
Clinical pharmacology, 14–19
Clinical reasoning, 2, 2f
Clinical skills, 3, 3f
Clinical therapeutics, 13–36
Clinical trials, 27–28, 28f
Clobazam, 1102b
Clobetasol, 334b, 336b, 1226b
Clobetasone butyrate, 1226b
  for eczema, 1244
Clock drawing test, 1149f
Clofazimine
  for leprosy, 269
  pigmentation from, 1258b
  for tuberculosis, 125
Clomethiazole, effect of old age, 32b
Clomifene, for infertility, 656–657
Clomipramine, 1199b
  for narcolepsy, 1105
Clonal expansion, 68, 68f
Clonazepam
  for epilepsy, 1102b
  for periodic limb movement syndrome, 1106
  for sleep disorders, 1105
Clonic seizures, 1100
Clonidine
  diarrhoea, 761b
  opiate withdrawal, 1196
Clonorchiasis, 297b
Clonorchis sinensis, choledocholithiasis and, 906
Clonorchis spp., 129
Clopidogrel
  for angina, 489
  for myocardial infarction, 498b, 1282
  for peripheral arterial disease, 504b
  pharmacokinetics, 20b
  platelet inhibition, 918
  for stroke prevention, 1161f
Clostridium botulinum, 104b, 1126

Clostridium difficile, 103f, 104b, 117b, 264, 264f
Clostridium novyi, in injecting drug-user, 222–223
Clostridium perfringens
  anaerobic cellulitis from, 227
  food poisoning, 262
Clostridium perfringens sepsis, 950
Clostridium spp., 102f–103f
Clostridium tetani, 104b
Clotrimazole, 125b
  for erythrasma, 1238
Clotting see Coagulation
Clotting factors, 850, 918–919
Clozapine
  drug interactions, 24b
  schizophrenia, 1198b
Clubbing, 1261, 1261f
  finger, 546f, 559, 559b, 559f
    asbestosis, 618
  in lung cancer, 600
Cluster headache, 1096
CMV (cytomegalovirus) see Cytomegalovirus (CMV) infection
CNS see Central nervous system
Co-amoxiclav, 117b
  cholestatic hepatitis and, 894
  for empyema, 565
  hepatotoxicity of, 894b
  prophylactic, 119b
  for respiratory tract infection, pneumonia, 585b, 586
  for urinary tract infection, 428
Co-artemether, 277
Co-phenoxylate, for inflammatory bowel disease, 821b
Co-trimoxazole, 117b, 123
  for brucellosis, 255b
  for cyclosporiasis, 287–288
  for HIV infection/AIDS, 323–324, 323b
  for melioidosis, 261
  for meningitis, 1120b
  for mycetoma, 301
  for nocardiosis, 261
  for Pneumocystis jirovecii pneumonia, 318
  haematopoietic stem cell transplantation, 937b
  leukaemia patients, 957
  prophylactic, 119b
  toxoplasmosis, HIV/AIDS patients, 320
  for Whipple's disease, 809
Coagulation, disseminated intravascular, 196
Coagulation disorders, 971–975
Coagulation factors, 850, 930
  complications of therapy, in haemophilia A, 973
Coagulation screen, 922b, 1362b
  in disseminated intravascular coagulation, 921–922
Coagulation system, 918–919
  activation of, 196
  investigation of, 920–923
Coagulation tests, for hepatobiliary disease, 853
Coagulopathy, causes of, 972b
Coal tar, 1250
Coal worker's pneumoconiosis (CWP), 615
Cobalt, 718
Cocaine, misuse of, 143
Coccidioidomycosis, 304
Codeine
  cirrhosis and, 894b
  diarrhoea, 801
    irritable bowel syndrome, 826f
  headache, 1096
  pharmacokinetics, 20b
Codons, 40
Coeliac disease, 805–807
  clinical features of, 806
  disease associations of, 806b
  investigations of, 806–807
  liver function test (LFT) abnormality in, 854b
  pathophysiology of, 805, 806f

Coeliac plexus neurolysis, 842–844
Coexisting disease, in choosing drugs, 29
Coffee, 716
  type 1 diabetes and, 729
Cognitive behaviour therapy (CBT), 1190
  for eating disorders, 1204
  for obsessive-compulsive disorder, 1201
  for schizophrenia, 1198
  for somatoform disorder, 1203
Cognitive biases, 6–9, 11
  in human factors, 9, 9f, 11
  in medicine, 7–9, 8f
  in type 1 and type 2 thinking, 7, 7b, 7f
Cognitive debiasing strategies, 8f, 9–10
  history and physical examination in, 9
  mnemonics and checklists in, 9
  problem lists and differential diagnosis in, 9
  red flags and ROWS ('rule out worst case scenario') in, 9–10
Cognitive function, assessment of, 1181–1183, 1182f
Cognitive impairment, 1181
  chemotherapy and, 1298
  HIV-associated, 319–320
Cognitive therapy, 1190
Colchicine
  for Behçet's disease, 1044
  for CPPD crystal deposition disease, 1017
  for familial Mediterranean fever, 81
  for gout, 1015
Cold agglutinin disease, 950
Cold antibodies, 949
Cold injury, 166–167
Colesevelam, 376–377
Colestipol, 376–377
Colestyramine, 376–377
  for irritable bowel syndrome, 826f
  for post-cholecystectomy syndrome, 908
  pruritus, 888, 1220b
  for radiation enteritis, 810
Colic
  biliary, 904
  renal, 396
Colipase, 770b
Colistin, 117b
Colitis
  collagenous, 824
  microscopic, 824
  pseudomembranous, 104b
  ulcerative see Ulcerative colitis
Collagen, 1213f
  in osteoarthritis, 1008
Collagenase, 64, 71
Colon, 770, 771f
  acute colonic pseudo-obstruction, 835
  disorders of, 827–836
  tumours of, 827–833
Colon cancer, hereditary non-polyposis, 831b
Colonoscopy, 776, 776b
  for abdominal pain, 789
  for colorectal cancer, 832
  for gastrointestinal haemorrhage, 782–783
Colony-forming unit-granulocyte, monocyte (CFU-GM), 914
Colorectal cancer, 830–833
  clinical features of, 831
  dietary risk factors for, 830b
  familial adenomatous polyposis, 828–829, 829b, 829f, 1321b
  investigations of, 832, 833f
  management of, 832
  modified Dukes classification and survival of, 832f
  non-dietary risk factors for, 830b
  pathogenesis of, 830f
  pathophysiology of, 830–831, 831f
  prevention and screening of, 832–833
Colorimetric chemical reaction, 348b

Columnar lined (Barrett's) oesophagus (CLO), 792
Coma, 1080
  causes of, 194b
  definition of, 194
  poisoning, 137b
  stroke patients in, 1153
Combination therapy, for hypertension, 513
Combined inhaled glucocorticoids and bronchodilators, for chronic obstructive pulmonary disease (COPD), 576
Comedone, definition of, 1242
Common variable immune deficiency, 79
Community-acquired pneumonia, 582–585, 582f
  clinical features of, 582–583
  discharge and follow-up of, 585
  investigations of, 583, 584b
  management of, 583–584
  organisms causing, 582b
  prognosis for, 585
Comorbidities, in older people, 1307
Compartment syndrome
  abdominal, 195
  identification of, 187b
  in injecting drug-user, 222–223
Competitive antagonist, 14
Complement, 66, 66f
  alternate pathway for, 66
  autoimmune disease and, 84
  classical pathway for, 66
  deficiency in, 73b
  lectin pathway for, 66
  pathway deficiencies in, 78
  total haemolytic, 1360b
Complement fixation test (CFT), 107–108
Complementary therapies
  for cancer pain, 1353
  for pain, 1348
Complex regional pain syndrome (CRPS), 1348–1349, 1349b
  type 1, 1055, 1055f
Compressed air, physics of breathing, 170b
Concentration, 1181
Concordance, 1294
Condyloma, 343
Condylomata lata, 337
Confrontation, for visual fields, 631b
Confusion/confusional states, 1196
  cerebral oedema, 168
Congenital abnormalities, in pancreas, 842–844
Congenital adrenal hyperplasia, 676
  hirsutism and, 658b
Congenital heart disease, 531–538, 531b, 532f
  in adolescent, 537b
  adult, 537–538
  cyanotic, 537b
  pregnancy and, 1282
  transition medicine and, 1297
Congenital hypertrophy of the retinal pigment epithelium (CHRPE), 829
Congenital thyroid disease, 650–651
Congestive 'portal hypertensive' gastropathy, 871
Coning, 1077
Conjunctiva, 1164
Conjunctivitis, 1173
  gonococcal, 339
Connective tissue disease, 1262–1263
  respiratory involvement in, 610–611, 610b
Conn's syndrome, 361
Consanguinity, 48
Conscious level, decreased, 194–195
  assessment of, 186f, 194–195, 194b
  management of, 195
Consent, artificial nutritional support, 710b
Conservative treatment, for chronic kidney disease, 421

Constipation, 786–787
  causes of, 786b
  clinical assessment of, 786–787
  disorders of, 834–835
  diverticulosis and, 833
  in old age, 834b
  simple, 834
  in stroke patients, 1159b
Constitutional delay, of puberty, 653
Contact inhibition, 1318
Continence, faecal, 770
Continuous ambulatory peritoneal
  dialysis (CAPD), 424, 425b
Continuous murmurs, 461
Continuous positive airway pressure
  (CPAP), 199b, 202
  for drowning victims, 170
Continuous positive pressure ventilation,
  202
Continuous venovenous haemofiltration
  (CVVH), 423
Contraception
  cystic fibrosis and, 1297
  in epilepsy, 1103
Contrast media, nephrotoxicity and,
  390b
Contrast radiology, 773f
Conversion (dissociative) disorder, 1202,
  1202b
COPD, 547f, 573–578
  BODE index in, 577b
  classification of, 576b
  clinical features of, 575, 575b
    chronic exertional breathlessness,
    575, 575b
  exacerbations of, 572–573
    acute, 577–578
  investigations of, 575–576
  management of, 576–577, 576f,
    577b
  occupational, 614
  in old age, 578b
  pathophysiology of, 574–575, 574f
  prognosis of, 577
  risk factors for, 574b
Copper, 718
  deficiency, 703b
  dietary sources of, 717b
  excessive, Wilson's disease, 896
  refeeding diet, 705b
  reference nutrient intake of, 717b
  reference range of
    urine, 1361b
    venous blood, 1360b
Copper sulphate, poisoning from, 148
Copy number variations (CNV), 44, 44b,
  45f
Cor pulmonale, 550
Cornea, of eye, 1166–1167
Coronary angiography, for acute
  coronary syndrome, 498
Coronary artery, 444–445, 445f
  angiography of, 452f
  calcification, 452
  with stenosis, 453f
Coronary artery bypass grafting
  (CABG)
  for angina, 488, 491–493, 492f
  vs. PCI, 493f
Coronary artery disease, 484–502,
  487b
  clinical manifestations of, 485b
Coronary artery dissection, pregnancy
  and, 1282
Coronary circulation, 444–445, 445f
Coronary heart disease, obesity and,
  698–699, 699f
Coronary revascularisation, 467
Coronavirus, 111b
Corrosives
  oesophagitis, 794
  poisoning from, 147–148
Cortical (volitional) influences, in control
  of breathing, 549
Corticobasal degeneration, 1115
Corticosteroids
  biosynthetic enzyme defects, 671b
  for congenital adrenal hyperplasia,
    676

see also Cortisol; Glucocorticoids;
  Hydrocortisone;
  Mineralocorticoids; Prednisolone
Corticotrophin-releasing hormone
  (CRH), 633f
Cortisol, 665
  deficiency, hypopituitarism, 682
  reference range of
    urine, 1361b
    venous blood, 1359b
  see also Hydrocortisone
Corynebacterium diphtheriae, 104b
Corynebacterium minutissimum, 1238
Corynebacterium spp., 103f
Cough, 556, 556b
  aetiology of, 556
  in asthma, 568
  bovine, 600, 624
  in COPD, 575
  headache and, 1097b
  at high altitude, 168–169
  in laryngeal nerve, paralysing, 553
  in lung cancer, 599
  in palliative care, 1353
  in pneumonia, 582–583
  refractory, 169
  and upper airway defences, 550
  in upper respiratory tract infection,
    581–582
Cough reflex, 556
Coumarins, 938b, 939–940
Counselling, dietary
  for coeliac disease, 807
  for hyperlipidaemia, 375–376
Coupled enzymatic reaction, 348b
Courvoisier's Law, 861–862
Cowden's syndrome, 1321b
Cowpox, 249
Coxiella burnetii, 100–101, 272
Coxsackie virus infections, 240
'Crack' cocaine, 143
Cramps, heat, 167
Cranial nerves
  damage to, 1089b
  of envenomed patient, 152f
  examination of, 1063b
  nuclei, 1067
  see also specific nerves by name
Craniopharyngioma, 687, 687f
Creams, 1225b
Creatine kinase (CK)
  in hypothermia, 166
  in muscular dystrophies, 1143–1144
  reference range of, venous blood,
    1360b
Creatinine, 349b
  in acute kidney injury, 416b
  in hepatorenal syndrome, 864
  reference range of
    urine, 1361b
    venous blood and, 1358b
Creatinine phosphokinase (CPK)
  elevated serum, causes of, 991b
  in myopathy, 990–991
  in myositis, 990–991
Cretinism, 717
Creutzfeldt-Jakob disease (CJD), 1127,
  1127b
  variant, 933
Crigler-Najjar syndrome, 860b
Critical care/critical illness, 173–214
  admission requirement, 176
  clinical examination in, 174, 174f
  in context of congenital conditions,
    201, 202b
  disorders causing, 196–201
    acute circulatory failure as,
      199–200
    acute respiratory distress syndrome
      as, 198
    post cardiac arrest as, 200–201
    sepsis and systemic inflammatory
      response as, 196–198
  monitoring in, 175–176, 175b, 175f
  nutrition, 210
  outcomes of, 211–214
    adverse neurological, 211–212
    discharge from intensive care as,
      213

  in older patient, 212
  withdrawal of active treatment and
    death in intensive care as, 213
  oxygen therapy in, 191, 191b
  referral, 212
  renal support, 208
  respiratory support, 202–204
  scoring systems in, 213–214, 214b
  withdrawal of care, 213
Critical care medicine, decisions around
  intensive care admission in, 201,
  202b
Critical illness polyneuropathy, 211
Critical limb ischaemia, 502–503
Crohn's colitis, primary sclerosing
  cholangitis and, 888
Crohn's disease
  clinical features of, 816–817
  cutaneous, 1263
  ileal, 816f–817f
  management of, 820–823
  pathophysiology of, 816, 816f
  refractory, 824
  small bowel, differential diagnosis of,
    817b
  treatment strategy for, 1300b
Cross-infection, 103
  see also Health care-associated
    infection
Crust, skin, definition of, 1216
Cruveilhier-Baumgarten syndrome,
  868
Cryoglobulinaemic vasculitis, 1043
Cryoglobulins, 1043
  autoimmune disease and, 84
  classification of, 84b
Cryoprecipitate, 931b
Cryotherapy
  for anogenital warts, 343
  for basal cell papilloma, 1234
  for granuloma annulare, 1263
  for molluscum contagiosum, 343
  for sarcoidosis, 1263
  for skin disease, 1228
  for warts, 343
Cryptic tuberculosis, 589b
Cryptococcal meningitis, HIV-related,
  321
Cryptococcosis, 302, 302f
  HIV-related, 315b
  prevention of, 324
Cryptogenic cirrhosis, 884
Cryptorchidism, in hypogonadism, 653
Cryptosporidia/cryptosporidiosis, 287,
  813
  HIV-related, 317b, 317f
Crystal formation, 387, 427b, 1012,
  1013f
  drug-induced, 427b
Crystal-induced arthritis, 1012–1018,
  1013b, 1013f
Crystalloids, 782
CT (computed tomography)
  for acute respiratory distress
    syndrome, 198, 199f
  of aldosterone-producing adenoma,
    674, 675f
  for cancer, 1323, 1323f
  of cardiovascular system, 452
  coronary angiography, 452, 452f
  for decreased conscious level, 195,
    195f
  of gastrointestinal tract, 773–774
  for headache, 185–186
  for hepatobiliary disease, 854
    for cirrhosis, 854f
  multidetector, for hepatocellular
    carcinoma, 891
  for musculoskeletal disease, 989
  for neurological disease, 1073b
    cerebral abscess, 1124
    epilepsy, 1101b
    stroke, 1151, 1157–1158, 1158b
  of phaeochromocytoma, 675, 676f
  for polycystic disease, 893f
  for renal disease, 389
  for respiratory disease, 552, 553f
    aspergilloma, 597f
    bronchiectasis, 579f

  hypersensitivity pneumonitis, 617f
  interstitial lung disease, 605f
  pleural thickening, 618f
  pulmonary fibrosis, 607f
  for splenomegaly, 927
CTLA4, 70
Cullen's sign, 837–838
Culture, blood, 106, 107f–108f
Cupulolithiasis, 1104
CURB-65, 583f
Curettage, for skin disease, 1228
Cushing's disease, management of, 669
Cushing's syndrome, 666–670
  aetiology of, 667
  classification of, 667b
  clinical assessment of, 667, 668f
  hirsutism and, 658b
  investigations of, 667–669,
    669f–670f
  management of, 669–670
Cutaneous leishmaniasis, 284–285,
  285b, 285f
Cyanide poisoning, 135b
Cyclical hormone replacement therapy,
  for amenorrhoea, 655
Cyclical vomiting syndrome, 803
Cyclicity of cortisol secretion, in
  Cushing's syndrome, 668
Cyclin-dependent kinases (CDKs),
  1317
Cyclo-oxygenase, 1002–1003, 1003f
Cyclophosphamide, 1320b
  for Churg-Strauss syndrome, 1043
  glomerulonephritis, 400
  for juvenile dermatomyositis, 1040
  for leukaemias, 960, 963
  for musculoskeletal disease, 1004b,
    1005
  for neuromyelitis optica, 1110
  for non-Hodgkin lymphoma, 965
  for pemphigus, 1256
  for rheumatic disease, 1004b
  for SLE, 1036
  for vasculitis, 1041
  for warm autoimmune haemolysis,
    950
Cyclospora cayetanensis, 287–288
Cyclosporiasis, 287–288
Cypermethrin, 148b
Cyproterone acetate, 659b
  for acne, 1243
  for alopecia, 1259
  for prostate cancer, 439
Cystathionine β-synthase deficiency,
  369
Cysteine, 697b
Cystic fibrosis (CF), 580–581, 580f,
  581b, 842, 902
  contraception and, 1297
  fertility and child-bearing potential in,
    1297
  transition medicine and, 1297
Cystic fibrosis transmembrane
  conductor regulator (CFTR)
  protein, 1297
Cysticercosis, 297f–298f, 298
Cystinuria, 405
Cystoisospora belli diarrhoea,
  HIV-related, 315b
Cystoisosporiasis, HIV-related, 317b
Cysts
  Baker's (popliteal), 999b, 1023
    rupture, 1023
  choledochal, 903, 903f
  hydatid, liver and, 880
Cytarabine
  for acute leukaemia, 957b
  for chronic myeloid leukaemia, 959
Cytochrome P450, 18
Cytogenetic analysis, 1322
Cytokeratin, as tumour markers, 1322,
  1324b
Cytokines, 64–66, 65b, 65f
  asthma, 568
  cancer, 1319
  defects in, 78
  immune response regulation, 65b
  pro-inflammatory, 70, 1005
Cytology, in respiratory disease, 554

Cytomegalovirus (CMV) infection, 238b, 242–243
  after HSCT, 937b
  clinical features of, 242–243
  encephalitis, 320
  investigations of, 243
  liver transplantation and, 901
  management of, 243
  polyradiculitis, 321
  in pregnancy, 235b
  viral hepatitis and, 878
Cytopathic hypoxia, 197f
Cytosine, 38
Cytotoxic oedema, 1153–1154
Cytotoxic therapy, for myelofibrosis, 969
Cytotoxin-associated gene (cagA), 798f

D
D-dimers
  pulmonary embolism, 620
  reference range of, 1362b
  venous thromboembolism, 976
Dabigatran etexilate, indications for, 938b
Dacarbazine, for Hodgkin lymphoma, 963
Dactylitis, 1032, 1034f
Danaparoid, for heparin-induced thrombocytopenia, 939
Dandruff, 1246
Dane particle, 873
Dantrolene, 1197–1198
Dantron, 834b
Dapsone, 123, 1227–1228
  adverse effects of, 123
  for dermatitis herpetiformis, 807
  for erythema nodosum, 1265
  haemolysis from, 950
  for leprosy, 269
  for linear IgA disease, 1256–1257
  neutropenia and, 926b
  for Pneumocystis jirovecii pneumonia, 323–324
  poisoning, 136b
  prophylactic, 119b
  for pyoderma gangrenosum, 1261–1262
'Dapsone syndrome', 123
Daptomycin, 117b, 123
  mechanism of action, 116b
Darunavir, 324b
Daunorubicin, for acute leukaemia, 957b
DCCT (Diabetes Control and Complications Trial), 756–757
DDAVP see Desmopressin
DDT, 148b
de Musset's sign, 524b
De novo mutation, 47
De Quervain's tenosynovitis, 998
de Quervain's thyroiditis, 646–647
'Dead-in-bed syndrome', 739–740
Deafness
  Alport's syndrome, 403
  Lassa fever, 245b
  Paget's disease, 1054
  Pendred's syndrome, 640f
  quinine toxicity, 141b
  rubella, 237b
  salicylate overdose, 138
Death and dying, 1354–1356, 1355b
  advance directives, 1307
  brainstem, 211
  diagnosis of, 1355
  ethical considerations in, 1355
  intensive care and, 213
  management of, 1355
  see also Brain death; Palliative care; Sudden death
Death certificate, completed, 98f
Debrisoquine, 58
DEC see Diethylcarbamazine
Decision-making see Clinical decision-making
Decompression, for musculoskeletal disease, 999
Decompression illness
  in aviators, 168
  in divers, 170–171, 170b–171b

Decontamination, 133f
Deep infrapatellar bursitis, 999b
Deep vein thrombosis (DVT)
  air travel and, 169
  investigation of, 187, 187f
  pre-test probability of, 187b
  pregnancy and, 1285
    magnetic resonance imaging for, 1274
  presentation of, 186
  in stroke patients, 1159f
  warfarin for, 939
  see also Venous thromboembolism/ thrombosis
DEET (diethyltoluamide), malaria prevention, 277
Defecation
  disorders of see Constipation
  obstructed, 778
Defensins, 62–63, 769
Defibrillation, 457
  for arrhythmias, 482
  implantable cardiac defibrillators, 467, 483–484, 483b
    heart failure, 467, 467f
  public access, 457
Dehydration
  cerebral, hypernatraemia and, 359–360
  cholera, 265
  diabetics, 729–730
  gastric outlet obstruction, 801–802
  heat exhaustion and, 167
  in palliative care, 1354
  in type 1 diabetes, 729–730
  see also Water, depletion
Dehydroepiandrosterone sulfate (DHEAS), 672
Déjerine-Klumpke paralysis, 1141b
Delayed oesophageal clearance, 791
Delayed puberty, 653–654, 653b, 1290
Deletions, 42, 45f
Delirium, 183–184, 1080, 1184
  clinical assessment of, 184
  diagnosis of, 183b
  hepatic encephalopathy and, 864–865
  in intensive care, 209
  investigations of, 184, 184f
  in older people, 1309, 1310b
  in palliative care, 1354
  presentation of, 183–184
  prevalence of, 1180b
  risk factors for, 183b
Delirium tremens, 1194
Delta antigen, 877
Delta virus see Hepatitis D virus
Delusional disorders, 1197, 1197b
Delusional parasitosis, 1202
Delusional perception, 1196–1197
Delusions, 1181, 1184
  differential diagnosis, 1197b
  schizophrenia, 1197b
Demeclocycline, 687b
Dementia, 1191–1194
  alcoholic, 1195
  fronto-temporal, 1193–1194, 1193f
  HIV-associated, 319
  investigations of, 1192, 1192b
  Lewy body, 1194
  management of, 1192
  nutrition and, 711, 711f
  pathogenesis of, 1192
  pellagra and, 714
  subtypes and causes of, 1191b
  vascular, 1191b
  see also Alzheimer's disease
Demography, in older people, 1304, 1304f
Demyelination
  acute disseminated encephalomyelitis and, 1110
  multiple sclerosis and, 1106–1110
  transverse myelitis and, 1110
  from vitamin B_{12} deficiency, 715
Dendritic cells, 64
Dengue, 243–244
  clinical features of, 243–244, 243b–244b
  diagnosis of, 244

endemic zones of, 243f
  management and prevention of, 244
  in pregnancy, 235b
Dengue haemorrhagic fever, incubation period of, 111b
Denosumab
  for bone metastases, 1329
  for osteoporosis, 1048, 1048b
Dental caries, fluoride and, 718
11-Deoxycorticosterone-secreting adrenal tumour, 674b
Depolarisation, cardiac conduction system, 445f
Deposition disorders, 1264
Depressants, misuse of, 141–143
Depression, 1198–1199
  alcohol and, 1195
  diagnosis of, 1199
  investigations of, 1199
  low mood due to, 1185
  management of, 1199
  manic, 1200
  and medical illness, 1199b
  negative cognitive triad associated with, 1190b
  in old age, 1189b
  in palliative care, 1354
  pathogenesis of, 1198–1199
  post-partum, 1206
  prevalence of, 1180b
  prognosis of, 1199
  in stroke patients, 1159f
  symptoms of, 1185b
  unipolar, 1198
Dermatitis
  chronic actinic, 1221b
  exfoliative, 1266b
  herpetiformis, 807, 1255b, 1256, 1326
  pellagra and, 714, 715f
  seborrhoeic, HIV-related, 314
  see also Eczema
Dermatobia hominis, 300
Dermatofibroma, 1235
Dermatology, 1209–1267
Dermatomyositis/polymyositis, 1039–1040, 1039f, 1260f, 1263
  in cancer patients, 1325b, 1326
Dermatophyte infections, 1239, 1240f
Dermatoscopy, 1214, 1217f
Dermatoses, 334b, 336b
Dermis, 1212
Dermoscopy, 1214
Des-amino-des-aspartate-arginine vasopressin, for diabetes insipidus, 688
Desensitisation, 16
Desmopressin (DDAVP), in haemophilia A, 973
Desmosomes, 1212
Deterioration
  early warning scores for, 188, 188f–189f
  immediate assessment of, 188–189
  management for, location for, 189–190, 190b
  medical emergency team and, 188, 189b
  presentations of, 190–195
    decreased conscious level as, 194–195
    decreased urine output/ deteriorating renal function as, 195
    hypertension as, 193–194
    hypotension as, 193
    hypoxaemia as, 190–191
    tachycardia as, 191–193
    tachypnoea as, 190
Detrusor muscle, 386
  failure of, 437
  over-activity, 436b
Detrusor-sphincter dyssynergia, 1093
Developing countries
  epilepsy in, 1097
  tetanus in, 1125–1126
Devic's disease, 1110

Dexamethasone
  adjunctive, for bacterial meningitis, 1120b
  for altitude illness, 168
  for brain tumours, 1130
  for Cushing's syndrome, 668
  for gastrointestinal obstruction, 1354
  for high-altitude cerebral oedema, 168
  for meningitis, 1120b
  for pain management, 1352b
  for spinal cord compression, 1326b
  for thyrotoxicosis, 639
Dexamethasone suppression test (DST), for Cushing's syndrome, 700
Dexamfetamine, 1105
Dextran, 1266b
Dextropropoxyphene, 142b
  poisoning, 142b
Dextrose, 353b
  hypoglycaemia, 141
DFMO see Eflornithine
DHA see Docosahexaenoic acid
Di George syndrome, genetics, 44b
Diabetes Control and Complications Trial (DCCT), 756–757
Diabetes insipidus, 687–688, 687b
  pregnancy and, 1280
Diabetes mellitus, 409, 719–762
  adherence and concordance in, 1299
  in adolescents, 753–754, 753b–754b
  aetiology and pathogenesis of, 728–734
  air travel and, 169
  bronzed, 895
  causes of visual loss in people with, 1177
  in children, 753–754, 754b
  classification of, 733b
  clinical examination of patient with, 720–721, 720f, 721b
  complications of, 755–762, 756b
    pathophysiology of, 756
    prevention of, 756–757
  diagnosis of, 726b, 727–728
  functional anatomy and physiology and, 723–725
  gestational, 1278, 1278b
    diagnosis of, 1278
    management of, 1278
    screening for, 1278
  glomerular filtration rate and, 417f
  impact of transition planning on, 1299b
  investigations of, 725–728
  management of, 741–755, 755f
    alcohol in, 744–745
    dietary, 743–744, 744b
    driving and, 745, 745b
    drugs to reduce hyperglycaemia in, 745–748
    exercise in, 744
    insulin therapy in, 748–751
    Ramadan and, 745, 745b
    review in, 743b
    therapeutic goals in, 742–743, 743f
    transplantation in, 752, 753f
    weight management in, 744
  monogenic, 733–734, 733b
  mortality of, 755, 756b
  in old age, 757b
  ophthalmic features of, 1165b
  pre-operative assessment of, 754b
  pregnancy and, 752–753, 1278–1279
  presenting problems of, 734–741
  prevalence of, 722, 722f
  rheumatological manifestations of, 1057
  risk of, 698–699, 699f, 700b
  transition medicine and, 1299
  type 1, 728–730
    in adults, 730
    classical features of, 735b
    environmental predisposition in, 729
    genetic predisposition of, 728–729
    metabolic disturbances in, 729–730, 730f
    pathology of, 728, 729f
    risk of, 729b

type 2, 730–732
  classical features of, 735b
  drugs in treatment of, 746b
  environmental factors of, 732
  genetic predisposition of, 731–732
  hereditary haemochromatosis and, 895
  insulin resistance in, 730–731
  management of, 742f
  metabolic disturbances in, 732
  pancreatic β-cell failure in, 731
  pathology of, 730–731, 731f
  risk of, 731b
  sibling risk of, 731b
  in young adults, 753–754
Diabetic amyotrophy, 759
Diabetic eye disease, in ophthalmological conditions, 1174–1177
Diabetic foot, 759f, 761–762
  aetiology of, 761
  clinical features of, 761b
  management of, 761–762, 762b, 762f
Diabetic glomerulosclerosis, nodular, 757, 758f
Diabetic ketoacidosis, 729–730, 735–738
  in adolescence, 753b
  clinical features of, 736, 736b
  investigations of, 736
  management of, 736–738, 737b
    bicarbonate in, 738
    fluid replacement in, 737
    insulin in, 737
    ongoing, 738
    phosphate in, 738
    potassium in, 738
  pathogenesis of, 735–736, 736b
  severe, indications of, 736b
Diabetic macular oedema, management of, 1176–1177
Diabetic microangiopathy, 756
Diabetic nephropathy, 757–758
  diagnosis and screening for, 757
  management of, 757–758
  natural history of, 757, 758f
Diabetic neuropathy, 758–761
  classification of, 759b
  clinical features of, 758–761
  management of, 761, 761b
  risk factors for, 757b
Diabetic osteopathy, rheumatological manifestations of, 1057
Diabetic retinopathy, 757, 1174–1177, 1176f
  clinical features of, 1175–1176
  management of proliferative, 1176
  pathogenesis of, 1175
  prevention of, 1177
  screening of, 1177
Diagnosis, 29
Diagnostic error, problem of, 2, 2b
Diagnostic tests, use and interpretation of, 3–5
  factors other than disease, 4, 4b
  normal values, 3, 4f
  operating characteristics, 4
  prevalence of disease, 5, 6f
  sensitivity and specificity, 4–5, 5b, 5f
Dialyser hypersensitivity, 424b
Dialysis
  amyloidosis associated with, 82b
  gastrointestinal, 136
  hyperkalaemia, 363
  peritoneal, 424
  poisoning, 136
  renal
    AKI, 413–414, 422b
    CKD, 419
    in old age, 422b
    SLE, 410–411
  see also Haemodialysis
3,4-Diaminopyridine, for Lambert-Eaton myasthenic syndrome, 1143
Diamorphine
  for myocardial infarction, 498
  for palliative care, 1351, 1355

Diaphragm
  disorders of, 627
  eventration of, 627
Diaphragmatic hernias, 627
Diarrhoea, 783
  acute, 227–230, 228b, 783
    clinical assessment of, 228–229
    differential diagnosis of, 228b
    investigations of, 229
    management of, 229–230
  after peptic ulcer surgery, 801
  amoebic dysentery, 287
  antibiotic-associated, 104b
  antimicrobial-associated, 230
  bloody, 816
  cholera, 264–265
  chronic or relapsing, 233, 233b, 783, 784b
  diabetic, 761b
  enteral feeding and, 707b
  faecal incontinence, 835, 835b, 1094
  HIV-related, 316–317
  inflammatory bowel disease, 816–817
  irritable bowel syndrome, 824
  malabsorption, 783–784
  pellagra and, 714
  traveller's, 232b
  tropical, 232–233
  Zollinger-Ellison syndrome, 802
Diascopy, 1214
Diastolic murmurs, 460
Diathermy, gastrointestinal bleeding, 775f
Diazepam
  acute poisoning, 145, 147
  adverse reactions of, 22b
  alcohol withdrawal, 1195
  convulsions, 145
  for disturbed behaviour, 1188–1189
  drug interactions of, 23
  in renal/hepatic disease, 32b
  for status epilepticus, 1081b
Diazoxide
  for hypertrichosis, 1259, 1266b
  for neuro-endocrine tumours (NETs), 679
Dibenzodiazepines, 1198b
Dibenzothiazepines, 1198b
DIC see Disseminated intravascular coagulation
Diclofenac, 1003b
  for actinic keratosis, 1231
  for hepatocyte necrosis, 894
  for renal colic, 432
Didanosine, 321
Dieldrin, 148b
Diet(s)
  acute coronary syndrome and, 501
  cancer and, 1320b
  gallstones and, 903
  in gastro-oesophageal reflux disease, 791
  gluten-free, 807
  high protein, obesity, 701b
  low carbohydrate, 701b
  low fat, 701b
  modification of, for gestational diabetes, 1278
  refeeding, 705b
  for renal failure, acute kidney injury, 414
  starvation, 702
  type 2 diabetes and, 732
  vegan, 697
  very-low-calorie, 702
  weight loss, 701–702, 701b
Diet history
  elements of, 693b
  obesity and, 700
Dietary deficiency, 944
Dietary supplements, 712
Diethylcarbamazine (DEC), 129
Dietl's crisis, 396
Differentiated carcinoma, in thyroid disease, 649–650
Diffuse idiopathic skeletal hyperostosis (DISH), 1058–1059, 1058f

Diffuse infiltrative lymphocytosis syndrome, HIV-related, 321–322, 322f
Diffuse parenchymal lung disease (DPLD), 605–610, 605b, 606f, 607b
Diffuse pleural thickening (DPT), 618, 618f
DiGeorge syndrome, 79
Digestion, 767
Digital photography, 1168
Digoxin
  adverse reactions of, 22b
  for arrhythmias, 469b
    atrial fibrillation, 471–472
    atrial flutter, 470
  drug interactions of, 24b
  effect of old age, 32b
  for heart failure, 467
  for mitral valve disease, 519, 521b
  plasma concentration, 36b
  for pulmonary hypertension, 621–622
  toxicity/poisoning, 137b, 140
Digoxin-specific antibody fragments, 140
Dihydrocodeine
  for musculoskeletal disease, 1002
  poisoning, 142b
Dihydropyridines
  for angina, 490–491
  for hypertension, 513, 514b
  overdose, 140
  see also individual drugs
1,25-Dihydroxycholecalciferol (calcitriol)
  for hypoparathyroidism, 665
  for osteoporosis, 1049
  pseudohypoparathyroidism, 665
1,25-Dihydroxyvitamin D, 384–386
Diiodotyrosine (DIT), 635f
Dilated cardiomyopathy, 539
  pregnancy and, 1282
Diloxanide furoate, 129
Diltiazem
  for angina, 490–491
  for aortic dissection, 508
  for arrhythmias, 472, 479f
  for atrial fibrillation, 472
  drug eruptions, 1266b
  for hypertension, 513
Diltiazem cream, for anal fissure, 836
Dilute Russell viper venom time (DRVVT), 978
Diphencyprone, 1239
Diphenoxylate, 230, 808–809
Diphenylbutylpiperidines, 1198b
Diphtheria, 104b, 265–266, 266b
  clinical features of, 266
  incubation period of, 111b
  management of, 266
  prevention of, 266
  prophylaxis for, 119b
Diplopia, 1088–1089
  in Graves' disease, 631b, 645f
  intracranial hypertension and, 1133
Dipyridamole, platelet inhibition, 918
Direct-acting nucleoside/nucleotide antiviral agents
  for hepatitis B, 876
  for hepatitis C, 878, 878b, 879f
Direct antiglobulin tests, 948f
Direct Coombs test, in warm autoimmune haemolysis, 949
Direct oral anticoagulants (DOACs), 940
Directly observed therapy, for tuberculosis, 594–595
Dirofilaria immitis, 293
Disability
  in deteriorating patient, 189
  International Classification of Functioning, Disability and Health, 1311
  in older people, 1306
Discharge, from intensive care, 213, 214b
Discitis, 1021
Discoid eczema, 1246
Discriminant function (DF), 882

Disease, choosing drugs for
  features of, 29
  severity of, 29
Disease Activity Score 28 (DAS28), in rheumatoid arthritis, 1025, 1026f
Disease-modifying antirheumatic drugs (DMARDs), for musculoskeletal disease, 1004–1005, 1004b
  psoriatic arthritis, 1033–1034
  reactive arthritis, 1032
  rheumatoid arthritis, 1025–1026
Disopyramide
  for arrhythmias, 476b, 479–480, 479b
  for cardiomyopathy, 540
Disseminated intravascular coagulation (DIC), 196, 978–979, 978b
Dissociative conversion disorders, 1202, 1202b
Dissociative drugs, poisoning from, 144
Distal interphalangeal joint arthritis, 1032, 1034f
Distribution
  drug, 18, 29
    volume of, 18, 18f
  interactions, 23
Disturbed behaviour, 1188–1189, 1189f
Disulfiram, 1195
DIT see Diiodotyrosine
Dithranol, 1250
Diuretics
  adverse reactions of, 22b, 355, 1310b
  for ascites, 864
  clinical use of, 355
  drug eruptions, 1266b
  drug interactions of, 24b
  for heart failure, 465, 465f
  for hypertension, 513, 514b
  for hypervolaemia, 354–355
  loop-acting, 355b
  for mitral regurgitation, 521b
  for obliterative cardiomyopathy, 541
  for oedema, 396
  osmotic, 355
  potassium-sparing, 355
  in pregnancy, 1276
  resistance to, 355
  timing of, 31b
  see also Thiazides
Diverticulitis, acute, 788
Diverticulosis, 833–834
  human colon in, 833f
  jejunal, 773f
Diving-related illness, 170–171
Dizziness, 1080
  in older people, 181b, 1309
DMARDs see Disease-modifying antirheumatic drugs
DNA, 38, 38f
  analysis, for neurological disease, 1077
  mitochondrial, 49, 1305
  nuclear chromosomal, 1304
  proviral, 309–310
  repair of, 41
  transcription, 38–40
Dobutamine, 206b
Docosahexaenoic acid (DHA), 377
Dominant negative mutations, 45
Domperidone, 1096
Donath-Landsteiner antibody, 950
Donepezil, 1193
Donor lymphocyte infusion (DLI), 937
Donor-recipient cross-matching, 89
Donovanosis, 341b
Dopamine, low-dose, AKI, 413
Dopamine agonists
  for acromegaly, 686–687
  for Parkinson's disease, 1114, 1114b
  pregnancy, 685
  for prolactinoma, 685, 685b
  and renal dysfunction, 427b
  for restless legs syndrome, 1105–1106
Dopamine antagonists
  for gastroparesis, 761b
  and prolactin concentrations, 684
Dopamine dysregulation syndrome, 1113

Doppler echocardiography, 451–452, 451f
  for aortic dissection, 507–508, 508f
  for atrial septal defect, 535f
  colour-flow Doppler, 452f
  three-dimensional, 452
  for valvular regurgitation, 451–452
Doppler ultrasound
  for haemorrhoids, 835–836
  for hepatobiliary disease, 853–854
  for leg ulcers, 1224
  for venous thromboembolism, 187
Doripenem, 120b
Dose-response curves, 14–16, 15f
Dosulepin, 1199b
Down's syndrome (trisomy 21), 44b
  acute hepatitis B and, 875
Doxapram, 567
Doxazosin, 513, 675–676
Doxorubicin
  cardiotoxicity, 541b
  hepatocellular cancers, 892
  liposomal, for ovarian cancer, 1334
  myocarditis and, 538
  for non-Hodgkin's lymphoma, 965
Doxycycline, 117b
  for anthrax, 267
  for bacillary angiomatosis, HIV/AIDS
    patients, 315–316
  for brucellosis, 255b
  for cholera, 265
  drug eruption, 1267f
  for filariasis, 291
  for leptospirosis, 258–259
  for louse-borne relapsing fever, 257
  for Lyme disease, 256
  for malaria, 278b
  for melioidosis, 261
  for onchocerciasis, 293
  for plague, 259
  for Q fever, 272
  for reactive arthritis, 1032
  for relapsing fever, 257
  for rickettsial fevers, 271–272
  skin infections, 1238
  for STIs
    chlamydial infection, 341b
    granuloma inguinale, 341b
    lymphogranuloma venereum, 341b
    syphilis, 339
  for Whipple's disease, 809
DPLD see Diffuse parenchymal lung
    disease
DPP-4 inhibitors, for hyperglycaemia,
    747–748
Dracunculiasis, 293
Dracunculus medinensis, 293
DRESS, 1266b
Dressings, 1226–1227, 1227b
Dressler's syndrome, in acute coronary
    syndrome, 496
Dribble, post-micturition, 437
Drinking, 1184, 1194
Driving
  diabetes mellitus and, 745, 745b
  restrictions in, epilepsy and, 1296
Dronedarone, 471–472, 479b–480b,
    481
Drowning/near-drowning, 169–170,
    169b
Drug eruptions, 1251, 1265–1267
  clinical features of, 1266b, 1267
  exanthematous, 1266b
  fixed, 1266b
  investigations and management of,
    1267, 1267b
  phototoxicity, 1221b
  rash in, 1217b
  types of, 1265b, 1267f
Drug history, 21b
Drug misuse, 93, 1184, 1184b
  causing stroke, 1157b
  polydrug misuse, 1196
  psychosis, 1195–1196
  tetanus and, 1125
Drug rashes, HIV-related, 316
Drug-related disorders
  eosinophilia, 123
  neutropenia, 926b

obesity and, 700b
  phototoxicity, 1221b
  psychosis, 1197b
  renal, 426, 427b
Drug resistance, 16
Drug-resistant TB, 595, 595b
Drug sensitivity testing, for tuberculosis,
    592
Drug therapy
  adverse outcomes of, 21–26
  duration of, 30
  monitoring of, 34–36
  patient adherence to, 29
  stopping, 31
Drugs
  absorption, 17–18, 17f, 29
  abuse, 21
  adverse reactions of, 21–23, 22b
    classification of, 22–23, 22b
    dose-related, 16
    inter-individual variation in, 19, 20b
    in older people, 1310, 1310b
    pharmacovigilance, 23
    prevalence of, 21–22, 21b–22b
    risk factors for, 21b
    TREND analysis of, 23b
  clinical and surrogate endpoints in,
    35–36
  controlled, 26, 33–34
  cost of, 29
  development, 26–27, 26b–27b
  distribution, 18, 29
  dosage regimens of, 29–30
    frequency of, 30
    repeated, 19
    timing of, 30, 31b
  dose-response curves of, 14–16, 15f
  dose titration of, 30
  efficacy, 16, 29
  elimination, 18–19
  excretion, 17f, 18–19, 29
  formulation of, 30
  hospital discharge, 33
  interactions, 23–24
    avoiding, 24, 29
    mechanisms of, 23–24
    pharmaceutical, 24b
    pharmacodynamic, 24b
    pharmacokinetic, 24b
  licensing, 26–27
  lung disease due to, 612–613, 612b
  management, 26–28
    cost-effectiveness evaluation, 28,
      28b
    evidence evaluation, 27–28
    implementing recommendations,
      28
    use of, 27–28
  marketing, 26–27
  metabolism, 18, 29
    interactions, 23
    of misuse, 141–144
  for oesophagitis, 794
  plasma concentrations of, 36, 36b
  potency of, 16
  regulation of, 26–28
  route of administration of, 17f, 30,
    30b
  topical administration of, 17–18
  toxicity, 21
DRVVT see Dilute Russell viper venom
    time
Dry drowning, 169
Dubin-Johnson syndrome, 860b
Duchenne muscular dystrophy (DMD),
    48b
  transition medicine and, 1297
Ductopenia, 894
Duloxetine, for pain management,
    1350b
Duodenal biopsy, 806
Duodenal switch, 703b
Duodenal ulcers, 782, 799f
Duodenogastro-oesophageal reflux,
    792
Duodenum, functional anatomy of,
    766–767, 766f
Duplex kidneys, 434
Duplication, 44, 45f

Dupuytren's contracture, 1059
  cirrhosis and, 867
Dusts, lung disease and, 616–617,
    616b
Dwarfism, zinc deficiency, 717
DXA (dual x-ray absorptiometry)
  in bone mineral density, 989–990
  for fractures, 1308
  indications for, 1046b
  for musculoskeletal disease, 990f
Dysarthria, 1087–1088, 1093
  causes of, 1087b
Dysbetalipoproteinaemia, 375
Dysdiadochokinesis, 1069
Dysentery, bacillary, 111b
Dysexecutive syndrome, 1094
Dysgraphia, 1086
Dyslexia, 1086
Dyslipidaemia, in pregnancy, 377b
Dysmetria, 1069
Dyspepsia, 779
  alarm features in, 779b
  causes of, 779b
  functional, 802–803
  gallstone, 904
  investigations of, 780f, 802
Dysphagia, 778, 1093
  investigations of, 778, 779f
  oesophagus, 1324b
  in stroke patients, 1158
Dysphasia, 1088
Dysphonia, 1087
Dysthymia, 1198
Dystonia, 1086, 1116
  poisoning, 137b
Dystrophia myotonica, 1191b
Dysuria, 396

E
E-cadherin (CDH1) gene, 803
E-selectin, 447
Early-onset osteoarthritis, 1011, 1011b
Ears
  freezing injuries and, 166
  squamous cell carcinoma, 1231
Eastern Cooperative Oncology Group
    (ECOG) performance scale,
    1322, 1322b
Eating disorders, 1203–1204, 1204b
Ebola virus disease, 246–247
Eccrine sweat glands, 1213–1214
ECF see Extracellular fluid
ECF (epirubicin, cisplatin and
    5-fluorouracil), 804
ECG (electrocardiogram), 448–450,
    448f
  12-lead, 448–449, 448b, 449f
  for acute coronary syndrome,
    496–497, 497f
  AKI, 422b
  ambulatory, 450
  angina, 487
  for aortic dissection, 507–508
  for aortic regurgitation, 525b
  for aortic stenosis, 523f
  for atrial ectopic beats, 470f
  for atrial fibrillation, 471f
  for atrial flutter, 470f
  for AV block, 477f–478f
  for AV nodal re-entrant tachycardia,
    473f
  cardiac cycle, 460f
  for cardiac tamponade, 544
  for chest pain, 178–179
  for critically ill patients, 178
  for endocarditis, 530
  exercise, 449–450, 450b
  for hyperkalemia, 363
  for hypokalaemia, 361
  for left ventricular hypertrophy, 523f
  for mitral stenosis, 519
  for myocardial infarction, 448
  for myocardial ischaemia, 448
  for pericarditis, 542, 542f
  for pulmonary embolism, 619b, 620
  reading, 448b
  for sinoatrial disease, 469f
  for supraventricular tachycardia, 473f

for syncope/presyncope, 183
  for torsades de pointes, 476f
  in tricyclic antidepressant poisoning,
    139f
  for ventricular ectopic beats, 475f
  for ventricular fibrillation, 475
  for ventricular tachycardia, 475f
  for Wolff-Parkinson-White syndrome,
    474f
Echinocandins, 125b, 126
Echinococcus granulosus, 298–299,
    299f
Echocardiography, 451–452
  for acute coronary syndrome, 498
  for angina, 488
  for aortic dissection, 508f
  for aortic stenosis, 523f
  for atrial septal defect, 535f
  for cardiac tamponade, 544
  for critically ill patients, 206
  Doppler, 451–452, 451f–452f
    ventricular septal defect, 536
  for endocarditis, 530
  for 'four-chamber' view, 452f
  for heart failure, 464
  for hypertrophic cardiomyopathy, 540
  indications for, 451b
  for left ventricular hypertrophy, 540
  for mitral regurgitation, 520f
  for myocarditis, 538
  for papillary muscle rupture, 496
  for pericardial effusion, 543f
  for pulmonary embolism, 620
  stress, 452
  for tetralogy of Fallot, 537
  three-dimensional, 452
  transoesophageal, 179, 452
  transthoracic, 451
  two-dimensional, 452
  valvular disease
    aortic, 522–524
    mitral, 519
    tricuspid, 526
  for ventricular aneurysm, 496
Echovirus infections, 240
Eclampsia, hypertension and,
    1276–1277
ECOG (Eastern Cooperative Oncology
    Group) performance scale, 1322,
    1322b
Econazole, 125b, 335b
Ecstasy (drug), 143
Ecthyma, 1236
Ectoparasites, 299–300
Ectopia lentis, 370
Ectopic ACTH syndrome, management
    of, 670
Ectopic pregnancy, 336
Ectopic ureters, 434
Eculizumab, 66
Eczema, 1244–1247
  allergic contact, 1247, 1247b, 1247f
  asteatotic, 1247
  atopic, 1245–1246
    rash in, 1217b
  classification of, 1244b
  clinical features of, 1244
  clinical morphology of, 1244b
  discoid, 1246
  gravitational, 1247
  investigations of, 1244
  irritant, 1247
  management of, 1244–1245, 1245f
  in nails, 1261
  pruritus, 1219b
  seborrhoeic, 1246
Edoxaban, 938b
Edrophonium bromide, for myasthenia
    gravis diagnosis, 1142
EDTA (ethylenediamine-tetra-acetic
    acid), 386b
Education
  food allergy and, 812
  infection control, 112b
  in musculoskeletal disease,
    1000–1001
    fibromyalgia, 1018
    mechanical back pain, 997
    osteoarthritis, 1011–1012

Edwards' syndrome (trisomy 18), 44*b*
EEG (electroencephalography),
  1074–1076
  for dementia, 1192
  for epilepsy, 1075*f*, 1076
  for hepatic encephalopathy, 865
  for sleep disorders, 1071
  for viral encephalitis, 1122
Efavirenz, 324*b*, 325
Efficacy, 16, 29
Eflornithine (DFMO), for trypanosomiasis,
  128
Eflornithine cream, 659
Ehlers-Danlos disease, 970
Eicosapentaenoic acid (EPA), 377
Eisenmenger's syndrome, congenital
  heart disease and, 533
Ejaculatory failure, 1094
Elastase, 71
  faecal, 1361*b*
Elbow pain, 998, 998*b*
Elderly Mobility Scale, 1311
Electrical cardioversion, for arrhythmias,
  482
Electroclinical epilepsy syndromes,
  1100*b*
Electroconvulsive therapy, 1190
Electroencephalography *see* EEG
Electrofulguration, 343
Electrolyte balance, 353*b*
  assessment, in hospitalised patients,
    353*b*
  in renal failure, chronic, 418
Electrolyte disturbances, acute kidney
  injury and, 414
Electrolytes
  absorption and secretion of, 769,
    769*f*
  acute kidney injury and, 416*b*
  basic daily requirements, 353*b*
  distribution of, 349, 349*f*
  homeostasis, 349
  interpretation of, 349*b*
  loss of, in diabetic ketoacidosis, 736*b*
  reference range of, venous blood,
    1358*b*
Electromagnetic spectrum, 1222*f*
Electromyography *see* EMG
Electron microscopy (EM), 105, 1322
  for sexually transmitted infections,
    342
Electrophoresis, 348*b*
Electrophysiology, 454
Elevated mood, 1186
Elimination
  of drugs, 18–19
  kinetics, 18*f*, 19
ELISA, 106–107, 109*f*
  for *Clostridium difficile*, 264
  for dengue, 244
  for hydatid cyst, 299
  for leishmaniasis, 283
  for leptospirosis, 258
  for Lyme disease, 256
  for lymphatic filariasis, 291
  for schistosomiasis, 296
  for strongyloidiasis, 289
Elliptocyte, 915
Elliptocytosis, hereditary, 947–948
Embolism
  in acute coronary syndrome, 496
  in acute limb ischaemia, 503, 504*b*
  arterial gas, 170
  pulmonary, 619–621
    acute massive, 200
    clinical features of, 619, 619*b*
    investigations of, 619–620,
      619*f*–620*f*
    management of, 620–621
    in pregnancy, 620*b*
    prognosis for, 621
    in stroke patients, 1159*f*
EMG (electromyography), 1076
  for motor neuron disease, 1117
  in musculoskeletal disease, 992
Emollients, 1225
  for eczema, 1247
  for pruritus, 1220
    in pregnancy, 1220*b*

for psoriasis, 1250
  for skin disease, 1226
Emphysema, 549
  computed tomography of, 552, 576*f*
  lung transplantation for, 567, 567*b*
  pathology of, 575*f*
  in respiratory function abnormalities,
    555*b*
Employment, 1198
  epilepsy and, 1296
Empyema, 564–565, 564*b*, 564*f*–565*f*
  subdural, 1125
Emtricitabine, 119*b*, 324*b*
Enalapril
  for heart failure, 466*b*
  for hypertension, 513
  for myocardial infarction, 500–501
Encapsulated bacteria infection, after
  HSCT, 937*b*
Encephalitis
  brainstem, 1122
  viral, 1121–1123
  West Nile, 1121–1122
Encephalomyelitis
  acute disseminated, 1110
  cancer-related, 1325
Encephalopathy
  hepatic, 847*b*, 864–865
    acute liver failure and, 856–857
    clinical grade of, assessment for,
      857*b*
    differential diagnosis of, 865*b*
    factors precipitating, 865*b*
  Wernicke's, 714
Endemic typhus, 271, 271*b*
Endobronchial ultrasound (EBUS),
  553
Endocarditis, 1035
  gonococcal, 340
  infective, 527–531, 528*b*, 531*b*
    acute, 529
    antimicrobial treatment of, 530*b*
    in old age, 527*b*
    post-operative, 529
    prevention of, 531
    subacute, 528–529, 529*b*, 529*f*
Endocrine axes, 633*f*
Endocrine disease
  classification of, 632*b*
  clinical examination in, 630–632,
    630*f*, 631*b*
  investigation of, 633, 633*b*
  ophthalmic features of, 1165*b*
  pathology of, 632–633
  pregnancy and, 1279–1280
  presenting problems of, 633, 634*b*
  pruritus and, 1219*b*
  rheumatological manifestations of,
    1057
Endocrine glands, functional anatomy
  and physiology of, 632,
    632*f*–633*f*
Endocrine pancreas disease
  classification of, 677*b*
  presenting problems in, 676–678
Endocrine system, pregnancy and,
  1272
Endocrine treatment, for prostate
  cancer, 439
Endocrinology, 629–689
  of adrenal glands, 665–676
  endocrine glands, disorders affecting,
    688–689
  of endocrine pancreas and
    gastrointestinal tract, 676–679
  of hypothalamus and pituitary gland,
    679–688
  reproductive system, 651–661
  of thyroid gland, 634–651
Endometrial cancer, 1334–1335
  investigations of, 1334
  management of, 1335
  pathogenesis of, 1334
Endometriosis, 837
Endomitotic reduplication, 918
Endophthalmitis, 1173–1174, 1174*f*
Endoplasmic reticulum (ER), 40
Endoscopic examination, of respiratory
  system, 553

Endoscopic retrograde
    cholangiopancreatography *see*
    ERCP
Endoscopic ultrasound, 774
  for choledocholithiasis, 906*f*
  for hepatobiliary disease, 855
Endoscopy, 774–776, 775*f*
  for abdominal pain, 789
  for achalasia, 795
  capsule, 774–776, 775*f*
    wireless, 775*f*, 776*b*
  for corrosive oesophagitis, 794
  double balloon, 776, 776*b*
  for dysphagia, 778, 779*f*
  for gastric outlet obstruction,
    801–802
  gastrointestinal haemorrhage, 782,
    782*f*
  for gastrointestinal haemorrhage, 782,
    782*f*
  for inflammatory bowel disease,
    818–819
  for obscure bleeding, 783*f*
  for oesophageal cancer, 796–797,
    796*f*
  for oesophageal candidiasis, 317*f*
  for oesophageal varices, 865*f*
  in old age, 776*b*
  for peptic ulcer, 799
  for pharyngeal pouch, 794
  for portal hypertension, 869
  of respiratory system, 553
  upper gastrointestinal, 774, 775*b*
  wireless capsule, 775*f*, 776*b*
Endosulfan, 148*b*
Endothelial cells, of liver, 848
Endothelial damage, 950
Endothelin 1 (ET1), 447, 849*f*
Endothelium, 447
Endotoxin, 104
Endotracheal intubation, critically ill
  patients, 190*b*, 208
Energy
  expenditure, 694, 695*f*
    increased, 704*b*
  intake, 695*f*, 701
    decreased, 704*b*
  requirements, 698*b*
Energy balance, 694–695, 695*f*
  altered, disorders of, 698–711
  determinants of, 694, 695*f*
  in old age, 710*b*
  regulation of, 694–695, 696*f*
  and reproduction, 696*f*
Energy-yielding nutrients, 695–697
  WHO recommendations, 698*b*
Engerix, for hepatitis B, 876
Enhanced Liver Fibrosis (ELF)
  serological assay, 855
Entacapone, for Parkinson's disease,
  1114
Entactogens, 143
Entamoeba histolytica, 286
  life cycle of, 286*f*
  liver abscess from, 286
  see also Amoebiasis
Entecavir, 876
Enteral administration, 17
Enteral feeding, 707, 707*b*
Enteric nervous system, 771–772
Enteritis, radiation, 809–810, 810*b*
Enterobacter spp., 103*f*, 117*b*
Enterobacteriaceae, 103*f*
Enterobius vermicularis (threadworm),
  290, 290*f*
Enterococcus faecalis, 103*f*, 117*b*
Enterococcus faecium, 103*f*, 117*b*
Enterocytes, 371
Enterohaemorrhagic *Escherichia coli*
  (EHEC), 227–228
Enterohepatic circulation, 19
Enterokinase, 768
Enteropathic (spondylo)arthritis, 1034
Enteropathy, protein-losing, 811, 811*b*
Enteroscopy, double balloon, 776, 776*b*
Enterovirus 71, 250
Enthesis, 987–988
Enthesitis, 1033
Enthesitis-related arthritis (ERA), 1027

Enthesopathy, patella ligament, 999*b*
Entrapment neuropathy, 1139–1140,
  1139*b*
Envenomation, 151–162
  diagnosis of, 159
  envenomed patient
    bedside test in, 153, 153*f*
    evaluation of, 152, 152*f*
    general approach to, 156–160
    treatment, 159–160
  follow-up, 160
  hospital assessment and
    management for, 158–159
  evidence of, 158–159
  laboratory investigations, 159
  life-threatening problems, 158
  local effects, 155, 155*b*
  overview of, 154
  by specific animals, 160–162
  systemic effects, 155, 155*b*
  venom, 154
  venomous animals, 154–155, 154*b*,
    156*b*–158*b*
Environment, early, psychiatric disorders
  and, 1183
Environmental factors
  in disease, cancer, 1320–1321,
    1320*b*
  of gastro-oesophageal reflux disease,
    791
  of inflammatory bowel disease, 830
Environmental medicine, 163–172
  extremes of temperature and,
    165–168
  high altitude and, 168–169
  humanitarian crisis and, 171–172
  radiation exposure and, 164–165
  under water and, 169–171
Environmental poisoning, 149, 149*b*
Enzymes
  drugs acting on, 15*b*
  pancreatic, chronic pancreatitis,
    842
Eosinophil granulocytes, 1362*b*
Eosinophilia, 233–234, 233*b*–234*b*,
  926*b*, 927
  allergy and, 86
  tropical, 233–234, 233*b*–234*b*
Eosinophilic gastroenteritis, 811–812
Eosinophilic granulomatosis with
  polyangiitis, 1043
Eosinophilic oesophagitis, 794
Eosinophils, 917, 926*b*, 926*f*
  count, 1362*b*
EPA *see* Eicosapentaenoic acid
Ependymal cells, 1064–1065
Epidemic typhus, 271, 271*b*
Epidemiology, 95–97, 95*b*
  understanding causes and effect,
    95–97, 95*b*, 97*b*, 97*f*
Epidermal growth factor receptor,
  1317
Epidermal necrolysis, toxic, 1254–1255,
  1254*b*, 1254*f*, 1266*b*
Epidermis, 1212, 1213*f*
Epidermolysis bullosa
  acquisita, 1255*b*, 1257
  classification of, 1254*b*
  dystrophic, 1229, 1254*b*
Epididymo-orchitis, 240
Epilepsy, 1097–1104
  in adolescence, 1103*b*
  classification of, 1098*b*
  clinical features of, 1098–1100
  contraception in, 1103
  focal, 1098, 1098*f*
  generalised, 1098, 1098*f*
  investigations of, 1100–1101, 1101*b*
    brain imaging, 1101*b*
    EEG, 1075*f*, 1076
    single seizure, 1100
  management of, 1101–1103
    antiepileptic drugs for, 1101–1102,
      1102*b*
    immediate care, 1101, 1101*b*
    lifestyle advice, 1101, 1102*b*
    monitoring, 1102
    surgery, 1102
  in old age, 1103*b*

Epilepsy (Continued)
  outcome after 20 years, 1101b
  pathophysiology of, 1097–1098
  pregnancy and, 1284
  in pregnancy and reproduction, 1103,
    1103b
  prognosis of, 1103
  seizure types, 1098–1100, 1098b
    absence, 1099
    atonic, 1100
    clonic, 1100
    focal, 1099, 1099b
    generalised, 1099–1100
    myoclonic, 1099–1100
    tonic, 1100
    tonic-clonic, 1099, 1099b
  temporal lobe, 1185, 1197, 1197b
  transition medicine and, 1296
Epilepsy syndromes, 1100, 1100b
Epileptic spasms, 1100
Epimysium, 987–988
Epinephrine
  for allergy, 86
  self-injectable, prescription of, 76b
Epiphysis, 984
  femoral, 1007–1008
Epirubicin, 804
Episcleritis, 1172
Epistaxis
  cirrhosis, 867b
  dengue, 244
  granulomatosis with polyangiitis,
    1041
  leptospirosis, 258
  systemic vasculitis, 1041b
Epithelial membrane antigen (EMA), as
    tumour markers, 1322, 1324b
Eplerenone
  for heart failure, 465
  for mineralocorticoid excess, 675
  for myocardial infarction, 501
Epley manoeuvre, 1104
Epo see Erythropoietin
Epoprostenol see Prostacyclin
EPs see Evoked potentials
Epstein-Barr virus (EBV)
  cancer and, 1320b
  hepatitis and, 871–872
  post-transplant lymphoproliferative
    disorders and, 1299
  viral hepatitis and, 878
Epstein-Barr virus infection, 238b,
    241–242
  clinical features of, 241–242
  complications of, 241–242, 242b
  investigations of, 242
  management of, 242
Eptifibatide, platelet inhibition, 918
Eradication, for gastrointestinal
    haemorrhage, 782
ERCP (endoscopic retrograde
    cholangiopancreatography), 776,
    777b, 854–855
  for cholangiocarcinoma, 907f
  for cholangitis, 905
  for choledocholithiasis, 906f
  for pancreatic cancer, 842
  for pancreatitis, acute, 839
Erectile dysfunction, 440, 440b
  in diabetes mellitus, 760–761
Erectile failure, 1094
Ergocalciferol, 713
Ergotamine, 1096
Erlotinib, 1332
Erosions
  in rheumatoid arthritis, 988
  skin, definition of, 1218
Erosive osteoarthritis, 1011
Ertapenem, 117b, 120b
Erysipelas, 1237, 1237f
Erythema, palmar, 635–636, 866–867,
    1194b
Erythema ab igne, 840
Erythema infectiosum, 237b
Erythema multiforme, 1221b, 1264,
    1264b, 1265f, 1266b
Erythema nodosum, 1265,
    1265b–1266b
Erythrasma, 1238

Erythrocyte sedimentation rate (ESR)
  abnormal, conditions associated with,
    72b
  inflammation and, 72
  reference range of, 1362b
Erythrocytosis, 925
  classification and causes of, 925b
Erythroderma, 1224
Erythromycin, 119b
  for acne, 1242–1243
  for diphtheria, 266
  for erythrasma, 1238
  for Lyme disease, 256
  for pneumonia, 585b
  in pregnancy, 120b
  prophylactic, 119b
  for relapsing fever, 257
  for rheumatic fever, 517
  for rosacea, 1244
  for STIs
    chancroid, 341b
    chlamydial infection, 341b
    granuloma inguinale, 341b
    lymphogranuloma venereum, 341b
    syphilis, 339
  for tetanus, 1126
Erythropoiesis, impaired, 237b
Erythropoietic porphyria, congenital,
    379b
Erythropoietic protoporphyria (EPP),
    379b, 1264
Erythropoietin (Epo), 915
  chronic renal failure and, 419
  ectopic hormone production, 1325b
Escherichia coli, 100, 103f, 104b,
    263–264
  entero-aggregative, 263–264
  entero-invasive, 263
  enterohaemorrhagic, 263–264
  enteropathogenic, 263
  spontaneous bacterial peritonitis and,
    864
  verocytotoxigenic, 263f
Escitalopram, 1199b
ESR see Erythrocyte sedimentation rate
Essential fatty acids, 697, 697f
Essential thrombocythaemia, 969–970
Essential tremor, 1115
Etanercept, for musculoskeletal disease,
    1007b
Ethambutol, 125
  Mycobacterium avium complex, 315b
  polyneuropathy, 1139b
  for tuberculosis, 593, 593b
Ethanol
  pharmacokinetics of, 20b
  poisoning, 135b
  reference range of, 1360b
  see also Alcohol
Ethics
  in artificial nutritional support, 710b
  in genomic age, 59
Ethnicity, type 2 diabetes and, 732
Ethosuximide, 1100b
Ethylene glycol poisoning, 135b, 147,
    147f
Ethylenediamine-tetra-acetic acid
    (EDTA), 386b
Etidronate, for Paget's disease, 1054b
Etoposide
  for acute leukaemia, 957b
  for testicular tumours, 440
Etoricoxib, 1003b
Euchromatin, 38–39
Eukaryotes, 101–102
Eumycetoma, 301
Euphoria, 1196
Euthanasia, 1356
Euvolaemia
  with hypernatraemia, 359b
  with hyponatraemia, 357
Evidence-based medicine, 10
Evoked potentials (EPs), 1076–1077,
    1077f
Evolutionary selection, 45–46
Ewing's sarcoma, 1057
Exanthem, enteroviral, 240
Exanthem subitum, 238
Excessive daytime sleepiness, 1105

Exchange transfusion
  for malaria, 277
  for megaloblastic anaemia, 945
  for sickle-cell disease, 953
Excision, for cancer, 1330
Excision arthroplasty, 1002b
Excision biopsy, for skin disease, 1228
Excitatory neurotoxins, 155
Excoriation, definition of, 1241
Excretion
  of drugs, 17f, 18–19, 29
  interactions, 24
Exemplar medicine sick-day card, 418b
Exenatide, 747
Exercise(s)
  acute coronary syndrome and, 501
  arrhythmias and, 450b
  asthma, 568, 570f
  chest pain and, 455
  COPD, 574
  diabetes and, 744
  heart disease and, 537b
  hypoglycaemia and, 740
  insulin levels and, 740
  for musculoskeletal disease, 1001
    ankylosing spondylitis, 1031
    fibromyalgia, 1018–1019
    osteoarthritis, 1012
Exercise ECG, 449–450, 450b
Exercise testing
  for angina, 488
  for COPD, 575
  for myocardial infarction, 450b
  for respiratory function testing, 556
Exertion headache, 1097
Exfoliative dermatitis, drug-induced,
    1266b
Exogenous androgen administration,
    hirsutism and, 658b
Exons, 39f
Exophthalmos, in Graves' disease, 631b
Expiration, of lungs, 548
Explanation, for somatoform disorders,
    1203
Extracellular fluid (ECF), 349
Extracorporeal membrane oxygenation
    (ECMO)
  principles of, 205f
  venous-arterial, 207–208
  venous-venous, 204
Extracorporeal shock wave lithotripsy
    (ESWL), 906
Extractable nuclear antigens (ENAs),
    antibodies to, 991
Extrahepatic portal vein obstruction,
    portal hypertension and, 868
Extraocular muscles, 1164
  of right eye, 1165f
Extrapyramidal gait, 1087
Extrapyramidal system, 1069
Extravascular haemolysis, 946–947
Extubation, in intensive care, 210
Eye disease, HIV-related, 319–321, 319f
Eye movement desensitisation and
    reprocessing (EMDR),
    1201–1202
Eyelid, 1164
  retraction, of ophthalmic disease,
    1171
Eyes, 1164–1168
  blood supply of, 1168
  of envenomed patient, 152f
  examination of
    diabetes mellitus, 721b
    respiratory system, 546f
  inflammatory arthritis in, 994b
  main structure of, 1167f
  rheumatoid arthritis in, 1024
Ezetimibe, 376

F
F-fluorodeoxyglucose (FDG), 553
Fabry's disease, 371b
Face
  angioedema, 87f
  examination of
    musculoskeletal system, 982f
    respiratory system, 546f
  frostbite, 166

  hemifacial spasm in, 1116
  numbness of, 1080
  skin disease see individual conditions
  superior vena cava obstruction, 1326
Facial (7th cranial) nerve
  palsy, 1082–1083
  tests of, 1063b
Facial pain, 1080
Facial warts, 1238
Facial weakness, 1082–1083
Facioscapulohumeral dystrophy, 1143b
Factitious disorder, 1205–1206
Factitious fever, 220b
Factor II, 972b
Factor V, 919
  Leiden, 923b, 972b, 977
  stroke, 1157b
Factor VII, 919
  deficiency, 928, 974
Factor VIII
  concentrate, 972–973
  haemophilia A, 971
  inhibitor bypass activity (FEIBA), 973
Factor IX, 972
  concentrate, 973–974
  deficiency, 973–974
  haemophilia B, 973–974
Factor XI deficiency, 974
Faecal antigen test, for Helicobacter
    pylori infection, 782
Faecal continence, 770
Faecal impaction, 834
Faecal incontinence, 835, 835b, 1094
Faeces analytes, 1361b
Faints see Syncope
Falciparum malaria, 231
Falls
  older people, 1308–1309,
    1308b–1309b, 1308f
  prevention, 1308–1309
Famciclovir, for herpes virus infection,
    126, 127b
  genital, 342
Familial adenomatous polyposis,
    828–829, 829f, 1321b
Familial hypercholesterolaemia, 374,
    374b
Familial hypocalciuric hypercalcaemia,
    664
  pregnancy and, 1280
Familial Mediterranean fever (FMF), 81
Family behaviour therapy (FBT), for
    eating disorders, 1203–1204
Family history, 56
  of allergic disease, 85
  genetic disease, 46
  of melanoma, 1232
  ovarian cancer and, 1334
  of psoriasis, 1247–1248
  psychiatric disorders and, 1181b
  of vitiligo, 1257
Family tree see Pedigree
Famine, 704–705
Fanconi anaemia, 1321b
Fanconi's syndrome, 366, 405
  multiple myeloma and, 410b
Farmer's lung, 616b
Fasciculations, 146b, 148b, 158b,
    1063b
Fasciculi, 987–988
Fasciola hepatica, choledocholithiasis
    and, 906
Fascioliasis, 297b
Fat-pad syndrome, 999b
Fatal familial insomnia, 1127b
Fatigue
  in cancer patients, 1325b
  chronic fatigue syndrome, 1202
  fibromyalgia, 1018
  multiple sclerosis, 1110b
  primary biliary cholangitis and, 888
  rheumatoid arthritis, 1023
Fats, 697, 697f
  body, distribution of, 699
    see also Obesity
  in diabetic diet, 744
  digestion and absorption of, 768
  distribution of, clinical assessment for,
    693b

energy provided by, 694
malabsorption, small bowel disease and, 809
normal metabolism of, 725
recommended intake, 698b
Fatty acids
essential, 697, 697f
free, 697
n-3, 376
polyunsaturated, 697f
trans, 697
Fatty liver
alcoholic, 881, 881b
non-alcoholic, 882–885, 883f
Febrile response, 104
Febuxostat, for gout, 1016
Feeding
enteral (tube), 707, 707b, 839
for famine management, 705
gastrostomy, 707, 707b, 708f
parenteral, 707–708
post-pyloric, 707
Felty's syndrome, 1024–1025, 1025b
Female, reproductive system of, 652, 652f
Femoral neck fractures, 994
Femoral stretch test, 996–997
Ferritin
in acute phase response, 70
adult-onset Still's disease, 1040
anaemia of chronic disease, 943
haemochromatosis and, 895
iron deficiency anaemia, 941, 942b
megaloblastic anaemia, 944b
in old age, 954b
reference range of, 1362b
Ferrous gluconate, 943
Ferrous sulphate, 943
Fertility
cystic fibrosis and, 1297
renal replacement therapy and, 1282–1283
Festination, 1087, 1309b
Fetor hepaticus, 857–858
portal hypertension and, 868
Fever(s), 217b, 218–225
accompanying features of, 217b
acute rheumatic, 515–517, 516f
investigations in, 517b
Jones criteria for, 516b
African tick bite, 270, 271b
boutonneuse, 271b
in cancer patients, 1323
clinical assessment of, 218, 218b
factitious, 220b
febrile response, 104
HIV-related, 313–314, 313f–314f
in immunocompromised host, 223–224
inhalation ('humidifier'), 617
in injection drug-user, 222–223, 222f–223f
intermittent, 74
investigations of, 218
with localising symptoms or signs, 218, 219f
louse-borne relapsing, 256b, 257, 257f
management of, 218
neutropenic, 224
in cancer patients, 1327–1328
post-transplantation, 224–225, 224b
recurrent, 217b
rickettsial, 270–272
Rocky mountain spotted, 270, 271b
scrub typhus, 270–271, 271b
streptococcal scarlet, 252, 253f
tick-borne relapsing, 256b, 257
trench, 272
tropical, 230–232
causes of, 231b
clinical assessment of, 230–232, 232b
history taking in, 231b
investigations of, 232, 232b
management of, 231f, 232
typhoid, 260, 260b
of unknown origin see Pyrexia of unknown origin

viral haemorrhagic, 245–247, 245b
yellow, 243f, 244–245
incubation period of, 245b
Fexofenadine, 1227
FGF see Fibroblast growth factor
Fibrates, 377
hyperlipidaemia management, 377–378
muscle pain, 1000b
Fibre, dietary, 697
Fibrin, 1319f
Fibrinogen
in acute phase response, 70
concentration of, 922b
reference range of, 1362b
Fibroblast growth factor (FGF), 1325b
Fibroblast growth factor 23 (FGF23), in skeletal disease, 990b
Fibrolamellar hepatocellular carcinoma, 892
Fibromuscular dysplasia, renal artery stenosis and, 406
Fibromyalgia (FM), 1018–1019, 1018f–1019f
investigations of, 1019b
spectrum of symptoms in, 1018b
Fibrosis
cystic, 580–581, 580f, 581b, 842, 902
contraception and, 1297
fertility and child-bearing potential in, 1297
transition medicine and, 1297
hepatic, 894
cirrhosis and, 866, 866f
congenital, 868f, 902
non-invasive markers of, 855
pathogenic mechanisms in, 849f
idiopathic pulmonary, 605–608, 607f
of liver, 894
cirrhosis and, 866, 866f
congenital, 868f, 902
non-invasive markers of, 855
pathogenic mechanisms in, 849f
nephrogenic sclerosing, 390b
pulmonary, 547f
in dermatomyositis, 610b
idiopathic, 605–608, 607f
in respiratory function abnormalities, 555b
in rheumatoid arthritis, 610b, 1024
in sarcoidosis, 609b
in sclerosis, 610b
in systemic lupus erythematosus, 610b
retroperitoneal, 434
drug-induced, 427b
Fibrous and fibrocartilaginous joints, 986
Fidaxomicin, 124
Fifth disease, 237b
'Fight or flight' response, 1213–1214
Filaggrin, 1212
Filariases, 233b
Finasteride, 659b
for alopecia, 1259
Fine needle aspiration cytology, 643
Fingers
clubbing, 546f, 559, 559b, 559f
asbestosis, 618
in lung cancer, 600
trigger, 1060
Finkelstein's sign, 998
First aid, for envenomed patient, 156–157
First-pass metabolism, 17
Fish
minerals in, 717b
venom, 154b
vitamins in, 711b
Fish eye disease, 375, 375b
Fish oils, 697, 711b
Fissure
anal, 836
skin, definition of, 1244b
Fistulae, 836
inflammatory bowel disease and, 823
tracheo-oesophageal, 625
see also different types
Fitz-Hugh-Curtis syndrome, 836

Flapping tremor, hepatic encephalopathy and, 864–865
Flares, of gout, 1015
Flavonoids, 716
Fleas, 231b
bartonellosis, 272b
plague, 259
typhus, 271, 271b
Flecainide, 470–473, 476b
Flora, normal microbial, 102–103, 103f
Flow cytometry, 105
Flucloxacillin, 117b, 120b
cerebral abscess, 1124b
hepatotoxicity, 894
for impetigo, 1236
for infective endocarditis, 223
for pneumonia, 585b
for septic arthritis, 1020, 1020b
for staphylococcal infections, 251
for staphylococcal scalded skin syndrome, 1236
Fluconazole, 125b, 126
acute leukaemia patients, 957
candidiasis, 336
HIV/AIDS patients, 316
cryptococcal meningitis, HIV-related, 315b, 321
for cutaneous leishmaniasis, 286
for paracoccidioidomycosis, 304
in pregnancy, 120b
prophylaxis, 315b
for skin disease, 1239–1240
Flucytosine, as antifungal agents, 126
Fludarabine
for chronic lymphocytic leukaemia, 960
for Waldenström macroglobulinaemia, 966
Fludrocortisone
for adrenal insufficiency, 673, 673b
postural hypotension, 1308–1309
Fluid, loss of, in diabetic ketoacidosis, 736, 736b
Fluid balance
for community-acquired pneumonia, 583
for heat exhaustion, 167
for renal failure, chronic kidney disease, 418
Fluid overload, in hypertension, 193
Fluid replacement
for acute diarrhoea, 229–230, 229b
for cholera, 265
for decompression illness, 171
for diabetic ketoacidosis, 737
for diving-related illness, 171
for food poisoning, 150
for heat exhaustion, 167
intensive care unit, 208
intravenous, for decompression illness, 171
Fluid therapy
assessment, in hospitalised patients, 353b
intravenous, for hypovolaemia, 353
for shocked patients, 206
Fluke, liver, 1320b
Flumazenil, 142
Fluocinolone acetonide, 1226b
Fluorescent in situ hybridisation (FISH) techniques, 1322
Fluoride, 718
dietary sources of, 717b
and osteomalacia, 1053
poisoning, 718
reference nutrient intake of, 717b
Fluorimetry, 348b
5-Fluorocytosine, 125b, 126
Fluoroquinolones, 122–123, 123b
for leprosy, 269
for plague, 259
skin reactions, 1173b
tuberculosis, 593
Fluorosis, 149
5-Fluorouracil (5-FU), 804
for basal cell carcinoma, 1230, 1230b
for colorectal cancer, 832
for gastric cancer, 804

Fluoxetine, 1199b
for bulimia nervosa, 1204
for fibromyalgia, 1018–1019
Flupentixol, 1198b
Flutamide, 659b
Fluvoxamine, 139
FMF see Familial Mediterranean fever
Foamy macrophages, 430, 809
Focal hypermelanosis, 1258
Focal nodular hyperplasia, 893
Focal segmental glomerulosclerosis (FSGS), 400
Focal seizures, 1099, 1099b
Folate (folic acid), 715, 945
absorption, 945
biochemical assessment of status, 712b
deficiency, 715, 945
causes of, 945b
investigation of, 945b
management of, 945
dietary sources of, 711b
for neural tube defects, 712b, 715
reference nutrient intake of, 711b
reference range of, 1362b
supplements, 715
Folate antagonists, 123
Folate synthesis inhibitors, 128
Folinic acid
for colorectal cancer, 832
for toxoplasmosis, 281
Follicle-stimulating hormone (FSH)
puberty, 1290
reference range of, 1359b
Follicular carcinoma, 636b, 649
Folliculitis, 1236–1237
deep, 1237f
pruritic, 1220b
superficial, 1236–1237
Fomepizole, 147
Fondaparinux, 938–939, 938b
Fonsecaea compacta, 300–301
Fonsecaea pedrosoi, 300–301
Food allergy, 812
Food hygiene, 323
Food intolerance, 812
irritable bowel syndrome of, 825
Food poisoning
Bacillus cereus, 262, 262f
Clostridium perfringens, 262
non-infectious causes of, 230
staphylococcal, 262
Food-related poisoning, 149–150
Foot drop, 1087, 1309b
Foot/feet
diabetic, 759f, 761–762
aetiology of, 761
clinical features of, 761b
management of, 761–762, 762b, 762f
examination of
diabetes mellitus, 721b
musculoskeletal system, 982f
non-freezing cold injury (trench or immersion foot), 167
Foot pain, 999
Foot ulcer, 761–762
Forced expiratory volume (FEV₁),
554f
in COPD, 574b
in old age, 550b
Forced vital capacity (FVC), 550b
Foreign body, inhaled, 179, 179f
Fortification spectra, 1088
Foscarnet
for CMV infection, 243
for herpesvirus infection, 127, 127b
Fosfomycin, 124
Fournier's gangrene, 227
Fractures, 994–995
associated with osteoporosis, 1044, 1045f
bone mineral density and, 1046f
fragility, 995b
high-energy, 995b
hip, 1308, 1308f
investigation of, 994–995, 995b
osteoporotic, 1308
pathological, 995b

Fractures (Continued)
  prevention of, 1308–1309, 1309b
  repair, 1002b
  stress, 995b
  vertebral, 995b
Fragile site mental retardation 2
    (FRAXE), 43b
Fragility fracture, 995b
Frailty, 1306, 1306b
Frameshift mutation, 42
Francisella tularensis, 261
FRAXE see Fragile site mental
    retardation 2
FRC see Functional residual capacity
Freckle, 1234
Free fatty acids, 697
Free intravascular haemoglobin, 917
Free radicals, 713, 881
Freezing cold injury, 166–167
Frequency of micturition, 396
Fresh frozen plasma, 931b
Fried Frailty score, 1306b
Froin's syndrome, 1136–1137
Frontal lobes, 1066
  functions of, 1066b
    effects of damage, 1066b
Fronto-temporal dementia, 1193–1194,
    1193f
Frontostriatal reward circuits, high-risk
    behaviour and, 1295
Frostbite, 166–167, 167f
Frozen shoulder, 997–998
Fructose, 695–697, 696b
FSH see Follicle-stimulating hormone
5-FU see 5-Fluorouracil
Full blood count (FBC), 919–920
  see also Blood count
Fulminant liver failure, hepatitis B and,
    875
Functional disorders, 802–803,
    1094–1095, 1095b
'Functional' gonadotrophin deficiency,
    653
Functional IgG antibody deficiency, 79
Functional residual capacity (FRC),
    549
Functional somatic syndromes, 1187,
    1187b
Fundus angiography, of visual disorders,
    1169
Fungal infections, 300–304, 300f
  after HSCT, 937b
  antifungal agents, 125–126, 125b,
    1239–1240
  skin, 1239–1240, 1240f
  subcutaneous, 300–301
  superficial, 300
  systemic, 301–304
Fungal keratitis, 1173
Fungal meningitis, 1121
Fungi, 101–102
  respiratory diseases caused by,
    596–598, 596b
'Funny turns', 1080
Furosemide
  adverse reactions of, 22b
  ascites and, 864
  for heart failure, 465
  for hyperkalaemia, 363b
  for hypertension, 513
  for oedema, 396
  route of administration, 30b
  for skin disease, 1221b
Furuncles, 1237
Fusariosis, 302–303, 303f
Fusidic acid, 124
  for impetigo, 1236
Fusobacterium necrophorum, 586
Fusobacterium spp., 103f, 117b
Fusobacterium ulcerans, 234b
Futility, 213
FVC see Forced vital capacity

G
G-CSF see Granulocyte-colony-
    stimulating factor
G6PD see Glucose-6-phosphate
    dehydrogenase (G6PD)
    deficiency

GABA
  hepatic encephalopathy and, 865
  role in epilepsy, 1097–1098
Gabapentin
  for abdominal pain, 789
  adjuvant analgesics, 1352b
  for chronic pain, 1345b
  for epilepsy, 1102b
  for fibromyalgia, 1018–1019
  multiple sclerosis, 1110b
  for neuropathic pain, 1084, 1350b
  for post-herpetic neuralgia, 240
  for somatoform pain disorder, 1202
GAD see Glutamic acid decarboxylase
Gain-of-function mutations, 45
Gait
  abnormal, 1086–1087
  assessment of, 983f
  examination of, 1063b
  in older people, 1309b
  stamping, 1087
  waddling, 1063b
Galactorrhoea, 684
Galactosaemia, 370
Galactose, 370, 768
Galactose-1-phosphate uridyl
    transferase gene (GALT), 370
Gallbladder, 849–850
  adenomyomatosis of, 909
  cancer of, 904
    in old age, 909b
  carcinoma of, 907
  cholesterolosis of, 909
  disease of, in old age, 909b
  strawberry, 909
  tumours of, 907–908
    benign, 908
Gallstone dyspepsia, 904
Gallstones, 903–905, 904f
  biliary sludge and, 904
  cholesterol, 903, 903b
  clinical features of, 904, 904b
  in old age, 909b
  pigment stones and, 903–904, 903b
  pregnancy and, 900
  treatment of, 905b
  ultrasound for, 853–854, 854f
GALT, 370
Gambiense infections, 279
Gametogenesis, 41f
Gamma-glutamyl transferase (GGT), liver
    blood biochemistry test and,
    852, 853b
Gamma hydroxybutyrate, misuse of,
    143
Gamma ray-emitting
    radiopharmaceuticals, 390
Gamma rays, 164, 164f
Gammopathy, 966
Ganciclovir
  for CMV infection, 224
    HIV-related, 322
    transplant patients, 89, 937b
  for herpesvirus infection, 126, 127b
'Gas-bloat syndrome', 794
Gas exchange, in lungs, 549–550, 549f
Gas gangrene, 119
  prophylaxis for, 119b
Gastrectomy
  sleeve, 703b
  under-nutrition and, 706
Gastric acid, 791
Gastric aspiration, 136
Gastric banding, 703b
Gastric bypass, 703b
Gastric carcinogenesis, 803f
  risk factors for, 804b
Gastric emptying, defective, 791
Gastric emptying study, 778b
Gastric inhibitory polypeptide (GIP),
    723–724, 772b
Gastric lavage, 136, 136b
Gastric outlet obstruction, 801–802,
    801b
Gastric secretion, 767, 767f
Gastric varices, 865–866, 865f
Gastric volvulus, 793
Gastrin, 767, 772b
  reference range of, 1359b

Gastritis, 797–798
  acute, 797
  causes of, 798b
  chronic
    autoimmune, 797
    due to Helicobacter pylori infection,
      797, 798f
Gastro-oesophageal reflux disease,
    791–794, 791f, 794f
  asthma and, 791–792
  in old age, 794b
Gastroenteritis
  eosinophilic, 811–812
  infective
    causes of, 228b
    foods associated with, 228b
    in old age, 228b
Gastroenterology, 763–844
  functional anatomy of, 766–772
  histology of, 776, 777b
Gastroenteropancreatic neuro-endocrine
    tumours, 678–679, 678b, 679f
Gastroenteropathy, allergic, 812
Gastroenterostomy, 801–802
Gastrointestinal bleeding, 780–783
  acute upper gastrointestinal
    haemorrhage in, 780–782
    management of, 781–782
  endoscopic therapy, 780
  lower gastrointestinal tract, 782–783,
    782b
    severe, 782–783
    subacute or chronic, 783
  occult, 783
  of unknown cause, 783, 783f
  upper, risk stratification in, 781b
Gastrointestinal decontamination, in
    poisoning, 135–136, 136b
Gastrointestinal disease, 785
  contrast radiology in, 773b
  HIV-related, 316–317
  ophthalmic features of, 1166b
  during pregnancy, 1277–1278
  transition medicine and, 1299–1300
    inflammatory bowel disease in,
      1299–1300
Gastrointestinal haemorrhage, upper,
    causes of, 781f
Gastrointestinal obstruction, in palliative
    care, 1354
Gastrointestinal polyposis syndromes,
    828b
Gastrointestinal stromal cell tumours
    (GISTs), 805
Gastrointestinal system, pregnancy and,
    1272
Gastrointestinal tract
  absorption from, 17
  clinical examination of, 764–766,
    764f, 765b
  diseases/disorders
    classification of, 677b
    functional, 802–803
    gut hormones, 772
    investigation of, 772–778
    presenting problems in, 778–789
  function, control of, 771–772
  HIV/AIDS and, 826
  obstruction, 788
Gastrointestinal tuberculosis, 590, 591f
Gastroparesis, 760, 803
Gastropathy, congestive, 'portal
    hypertensive', 871
Gastrostomy feeding, 707, 707b, 708f
Gaucher's disease, 371b
GCA see Giant cell arteritis
GCS see Glasgow Coma Scale
Gefitinib, 1332
Gegenhalten, 1094
Gels, 1225b
Gemcitabine, for pancreatic cancer,
    842–844
Gender, alcoholic liver disease and, 880
Gene panels, 54b
Gene promoter, 39, 39f
Gene sequencing, 52–56, 54f–55f
  challenges of NGS technologies in,
    53–54
  methods for, 55b

  NGS capture in, 53
  third-generation, 56
  uses of, 54–56
Gene therapy, for genetic disease, 58
General anaesthetics, 14
General assessment of locomotor
    system (GALS), 983, 983f
General sales list (GSL), 27
Generalised anxiety disorder, 1200
Generalised lymphadenopathy, 927
Generalised pain, causes of, 995b
Generalised seizures, 1099–1100
Generic virus life cycle, 101f
Genes
  amplification of, 52, 53f
  packaging of, 38, 38f
Genetic disease(s)
  constitutional, 46–50
    inheritance patterns of, 46–50
  renal, 403–406
  skin, 1264
  somatic, 50–51
  treatment of, 58
Genetic factors
  adverse drug reactions and, 29
  of ageing, 1304–1305
  alcoholic liver disease and, 880,
    881f
  of cancer, 1316
  of inflammatory bowel disease,
    830
  of osteoarthritis, 1007–1008
  of osteoporosis, 1044
  of Parkinson's disease, 1112
  psychiatric disorders and, 1183
Genetic testing, 1077
  for Peutz-Jeghers syndrome, 829
Genetic variant
  classes of, 42–44, 42b
  consequences of, 44–45
  in evolutionary selection, 45–46
  normal, 45–46
Genital herpes, 334b, 336b
Genital itch/rash, 333, 334b
Genital lumps
  in men, 334
  in women, 336
Genital ulcers
  in Behçet's disease, 1043–1044
  in men, 333–334, 334f
  in women, 336
Genital warts, 1238
Genitalia, in endocrine disease, 630f
Genitourinary disease, in tuberculosis,
    591
Genitourinary system, pregnancy and,
    1272
Genome editing, for genetic disease,
    58
Genome-wide association studies
    (GWAS), 45
Genomics
  clinical practice and, 56–59
  common disease and, 56
  ethics and, 59
  fundamental principles of, 38–41
  health and disease, 42–51
  health care and, 56–58
  in infectious disease, 58
  obstetrics and, 58
  oncology and, 56–58
  in rare neurodevelopmental disorders,
    56
  technologies for, 51–56
Gentamicin, 429
  for brucellosis, 255b
  for cerebral abscess, 1124b
  dosing of, 122, 122f
  drug concentration, 36b
  for infective endocarditis, 223
  for liver abscess, 880
  for meningitis, 1120b
  for neutropenic sepsis, 957
  for plague, 259
  prophylactic, 119b
  renal or hepatic disease, 32b
  for septic arthritis, 1020
  for tularemia, 261
  for urinary tract infection, 429b

Geriatric medicine
  assessment, 1306
  presenting problems in, 1307–1311
  see also Age/ageing; Older people
Gerstmann-Sträussler-Scheinker
  syndrome, 1127b
Gestational diabetes, 1278, 1278b
  diagnosis of, 1278
  management of, 1278
  screening for, 1278
Get up and go test, 1303b
GFR see Glomerular filtration rate
GGT see γ-Glutamyl transferase
GH see Growth hormone
Ghrelin, 767, 772b
Giant cell arteritis (GCA), 1042–1043,
  1170
  emergency management of, 1043b
Giardia lamblia, 287
Giardiasis, 287
  clinical features and investigations of,
    287
  management of, 287
Gilbert's syndrome, 860, 860b, 897
Gingivitis, 316
GIP see Gastric inhibitory polypeptide
GISTs see Gastrointestinal stromal cell
  tumours
Gitelman's syndrome, 361
Glanzmann's thrombasthenia, 971
Glasgow Coma Scale (GCS), 134, 185,
  186f, 194, 194b
Glasgow criteria, for prognosis in acute
  pancreatitis, 837b
Glasgow score, for alcoholic liver
  disease, 882, 882b
Glatiramer acetate, 1109, 1109b
Glioblastoma multiforme, 1129
Gliomas, 1130–1131
Glitazones, for non-alcoholic fatty liver,
  885
Global burden of disease (GBD)
  causes of death and disability, 92–93,
    92b
  underlying risk factors of, 93b
Global warming, 94
Glomerular diseases, 397–401, 397b
  histopathology of, 399f
  inherited, 403–404
  pregnancy and, 1282
Glomerular filtration rate (GFR),
  386–387, 386b
  diabetes mellitus and, 417f
  estimation of, 386b
  limitations of, 387b
  pregnancy and, 1272
  renal failure, chronic, 415
  renal haemodynamics and, 413f
Glomerulonephritis, 397–401
  antibody production, associated with,
    397f
  categorised, 398b–399b
  causes of, 401b
  drug-induced, 427b
  infection-related, 398b–399b, 401
  mesangiocapillary, 398b–399b, 401
  nephrotic syndrome, 392b, 395,
    395b
  rapidly progressive, 397
  in systemic lupus erythematosus,
    1035
  terminology used in, 400b
Glomerulosclerosis, nodular, diabetic,
  757, 758f
Glomerulus, 384
Glossitis, atrophic, 764f
Glossopharyngeal (9th cranial), tests of,
  1063b
Gloves and socks syndrome, 237b
Glucagon
  famine, 704–705
  secretion, regulation, 724
Glucagon-like peptide-1 (GLP-1),
  723–724, 772b
Glucagon-like peptide-1 (GLP-1)
  receptor agonists, for
  hyperglycaemia, 747–748
Glucocorticoid-induced osteoporosis,
  1045

Glucocorticoids, 665
  for acute exacerbations of COPD,
    578
  for adrenal insufficiency, 672–673
  adverse effects of, 670–671
  advice to patients on, 671b
  for alcoholic hepatitis, 882
  for allergy, 86
  anabolic, cholestatic hepatitis and,
    894
  for ankylosing spondylitis, 1031
  for antineutrophil cytoplasmic
    antibody-associated vasculitis,
    1041
  for autoimmune hepatitis, 886–887
  in bone remodelling, 986b
  for Duchenne muscular dystrophy,
    1297
  for Graves' ophthalmopathy, 646
  growth retardation, 1290, 1299
  for inflammatory bowel disease, 821b,
    1299
  for musculoskeletal disease,
    1005–1006
  in old age, 673b
  osteoporosis induced by, transition
    medicine, 1300
  for polymyositis and dermatomyositis,
    1040
  for primary biliary cholangitis, 888
  pruritus, 1220b
  for psoriatic arthritis, 1033–1034
  for reactive arthritis, 1032
  for rheumatic fever, 517
  sodium content of, 864b
  therapeutic use of, 670–671, 670b
  topical, 1226, 1226b, 1226f
  for tuberculosis, 593
  for ulcerative colitis, 1299–1300
  for warm autoimmune haemolysis,
    950
  weight gain, 700b
  withdrawal of, management of, 671,
    671b
  see also Corticosteroids; Cortisol;
    Hydrocortisone;
    Mineralocorticoids; Prednisolone
Gluconeogenesis, 850
Glucosamine sulphate, for osteoarthritis,
  1012
Glucose
  acute kidney injury and, 416b
  blood
    diabetes and, 724–726
    impaired fasting glucose, 726b,
      728
    normal metabolism of, 724, 725f
  cerebrospinal fluid, 1361b
  control of, in intensive care, 210–211
  filtration and reabsorption by nephron,
    748f
  impaired tolerance, 374, 1360b
  interstitial, diabetes and, 726
  intravenous, porphyria, 379
  metabolism of, pregnancy and,
    1272–1273
  reference range of, venous blood,
    1360b
  urine, diabetes and, 725
  values of, in gestational diabetes,
    1278
Glucose-6-phosphate dehydrogenase
  (G6PD) deficiency, 948–949,
  949b
Glucose tolerance, impaired, 726b,
  728
Glucose tolerance test, oral, 726b
Glue sniffing, 1196
Glutamate, 698b
Glutamic acid decarboxylase (GAD),
  1111b
Glutaminase, 364
γ-Glutamyl transferase (GGT)
  in alcohol misuse, 1184
  reference range of, venous blood,
    1360b
Glutathione, 712b
Gluten-free diet, 807
Gluteus medius enthesitis, 999b

Glycaemic control, in diabetes,
  756–757, 756f
  in adolescence, 753b
  in old age, 757b
  self-assessment of, 742
'Glycaemic index,' of foods, 695–697
Glycated haemoglobin (HbA₁C),
  726–727, 727b, 1360b
Glycation, 726–727
Glyceryl trinitrate (GTN)
  for anal fissure, 836
  angina, 489, 490b
  duration of action, 490b
  intravenous, accelerated
    hypertension, 514
  for pulmonary oedema, 465b
  route of administration, 30b
  sublingual, 489, 500
Glycine, 698b
Glycogen, 694
Glycogen storage diseases (GSDs),
  370, 370b
Glycopeptide-resistant enterococci
  (GRE), 117b
Glycopeptides, 123
  mechanism of action, 116b
  in pregnancy, 120b
Glycoprotein intrinsic factor, 767
Glycosidases, 987
Glycosuria, 725, 729–730
  diabetes mellitus, 409, 729–730
  Fanconi's syndrome, 410b
  hypernatraemia and, 359b
  'lag storage', 638b
  leg ulcers and, 1224
  in old people, 732b
  pregnancy and, 1272
  renal, 405, 725
Glycosylphosphatidylinositol (GPI),
  950–951
Glycylcyclines, 120b, 124
GM2-gangliosidosis, 371b
Gnathostomiasis, 294
Goitre
  endemic, 717
  multinodular, 648–649, 648f
  simple diffuse, 648, 648f
  thyrotoxicosis, 635–636, 636b
Gold (myocrisin)
  adverse effects on kidney, 427b
  adverse reactions of, 926b
  for musculoskeletal disease, 1004b,
    1005
Golfer's elbow, 998
Golgi apparatus, 40
Golimumab, for musculoskeletal
  disease, 1007b
Gonadotrophin-releasing hormone
  (GnRH), 633f
  for infertility, 656–657
  puberty and, 1290
Gonadotrophin-releasing hormone
  analogues, 379
Gonococcal infection, disseminated
  (DGI), 340
Gonococcal ophthalmia neonatorum,
  340f
Gonococcal urethritis, 333, 333f
Gonorrhoea, 339–340
  arthritis, 340
  complications of delayed therapy in,
    340b
  incubation period, 111b, 339
  pharyngeal, 340
  treatment of uncomplicated, 340b
  urethritis, 333
Goodpasture's disease, 612
Gorlin's syndrome, 57b
Goserelin, 1332
Got transition, 1290
Gottron's papules, 1039
Gout, 1012–1016
  causes of, 1013b
  clinical features of, 1014,
    1014f–1015f
  epidemiology of, 1012–1013
  investigations for, 1014–1015
  management of, 1015–1016
  in old age, 1014b

pathophysiology of, 1013–1014,
  1013f
  tophaceous, 1014–1015, 1015f
Graft-versus-host disease (GVHD), 937,
  1252
Graham Steell murmur, 526
Granulocyte-colony-stimulating factor
  (G-CSF), 1327–1328
Granulocytes, 917
  count, 1362b
Granuloma annulare, 1263
Granuloma inguinale, 341b
Granulomas, 71
Granulomatosis with polyangiitis, 612,
  1041
Granulomatous disease, 1263
Granzymes, 67
Graves' disease, 643–646
  ophthalmopathy, 631b, 645–646,
    645f
  thyrotoxicosis and, 635–636, 636b,
    643–646, 643f
  management of, 644–645, 644b
Graves' thyrotoxicosis, 643–645, 643f
Gravitational eczema, 1247
Grays (Gy), 164
Grenz (Bucky) ray therapy, for skin
  disease, 1228–1229
'Grey baby' syndrome, 120b
Grey Turner's sign, 837–838
Grief reactions, 568
Griseofulvin, as antifungal agents, 126
Group A streptococci (GAS), 252
Group B streptococcal infection, in
  pregnancy, 235b
Growth, analytes affected by, 1363b
Growth factors, 914, 915f
  asthma, 568
  cancer, 1317, 1317f
  haematopoiesis, 914
Growth failure, 823
Growth hormone (GH), 632, 633f
  reference range of, 1359b
Growth hormone-releasing hormone
  (GHRH), 633f
Growth hormone replacement, for
  Hypopituitarism, 682
Growth hormone secretion, tests of,
  682b
Growth retardation
  congenital heart disease and, 533
  eating disorders, 1204b
GSDs see Glycogen storage diseases
GTN see Glyceryl trinitrate
Guanine, 38
Guillain-Barré syndrome, 1140
Guinea worm (dracunculiasis), 293
Gumma, 338
Gums, 696b
  Kaposi's sarcoma, 316f
  scurvy, 716b
Gut hormones, 772, 772b
  testing, 778
GVHD see Graft-versus-host disease
Gynaecomastia, 657, 657b, 867
  in hypogonadism, 653

H
HACE see High-altitude cerebral
  oedema
HACEK group bacteria, endocarditis,
  528, 528b
HAE see Hereditary angioedema
Haem, biosynthetic pathway, 378f
Haemagglutination testing, 261
Haemagogus spp., yellow fever and,
  244
Haemangioblastomas, 1132
Haemangiomas, 1234
  liver, 893, 893f
Haemarthrosis, 992–993
Haematemesis, 780
Haematocrit (Hct), 919–920, 1362b
Haematological abnormalities,
  HIV-related, 322
Haematological disorders see Blood
  diseases
Haematological investigations, in older
  people, 923b

Haematological malignancies, 954–968, 955b
chemotherapy in, 936
in old age, 968b
Haematological practice, treatments for emergencies in, 939b
Haematological system, pregnancy and, 1273
Haematological tests, for hepatobiliary disease, 853
Haematological values, 1362b
Haematology, 388
in coeliac disease, 807
in musculoskeletal disease, 990
transfusion medicine and, 911–979
Haematoma
extradural, 1133
intracerebral, 1133
muscle, haemophilia, 973f
in stroke patients, 1157–1158, 1158b
subdural, 1133
subungual, 1260, 1260f
Haematopoiesis, 914–915, 914f
Haematopoietic stem cell transplantation (HSCT), 936–938
for acute leukaemia, 958
allogeneic, 936–937, 936b–937b
for aplastic anaemia, 969
autologous, 936–938
for beta-thalassaemia, 954b
for chronic myeloid leukaemia, 959
fever after, 224–225
for high-grade NHL, 966
infections during recovery from, 937b
for myelofibrosis, 969
for myeloma, 968
Haematuria, 391–392, 392f
investigation of, 393f
loin pain, 396
non-visible, 392b
Haemochromatosis, 717, 895–896, 896f
causes of, 895b
hereditary, 895–896
liver function test (LFT) abnormality in, 854f
rheumatological manifestations of, 1058
secondary, 896
Haemoconcentration, hypothermia and, 166
Haemodiafiltration, 423
Haemodialysis, 136, 421–423
access, 423f
in acute kidney injury, 422
in CKD, 422–423
peritoneal dialysis vs., 420b
problems with, 424b
Haemofiltration, 423
continuous venovenous, 423
Haemoglobin, 915–916, 917f
abnormal, 951
glycated, 726–727, 727b, 1360b
mean cell (MCH), 1362b
pregnancy and, 1273
reference range of, 1362b
Haemoglobin A, 915–916
Haemoglobin C, 951–952
Haemoglobin C (HbC) disease, 953
Haemoglobin F, 915–916
Haemoglobin H, 954
Haemoglobin-oxygen dissociation curve, 190, 191f
Haemoglobin S, 951–952
Haemoglobin SC disease, 953
Haemoglobinopathies, 951–954, 951f
Haemoglobinuria, 338, 392b
march, 950
paroxysmal cold, 950
paroxysmal nocturnal, 950–951
Haemolysis, 945
active, investigation results indicating, 946b
causes and classification of, 946f
extravascular, 946–947
intravascular, 946b, 947
Haemolytic anaemias, 923, 945–951
alloimmune, 950
autoimmune, 949–950

causes of, 946f, 947
microangiopathic, 950
non-immune, 950
Haemolytic crisis, 947
Haemolytic disease of newborn (HDN), 933, 933b
Haemolytic uraemic syndrome (HUS), 104b, 388, 408–409
pregnancy and, 1285
Haemophilia, rheumatological manifestations of, 1058
Haemophilia A, 971–973
clinical features of, 972, 972b, 973f
coagulation factor therapy for, complications of, 973
genetics in, 971–972
management of, 972–973
Haemophilia B, 973–974
Haemophilus ducreyi, 341b
Haemophilus influenzae, 117b
bacterial meningitis, 1119b–1120b
immunisation for, 115b
pneumonia, 319, 583
Haemophilus spp., 103f
Haemoptysis
in lung cancer, 599–600
in respiratory disease, 559–560, 559b, 560f
Haemorrhage
during dialysis, 424b
intracerebral, 1154–1155, 1155f
causes of, 1155b
major, transfusion in, 931b, 934–936, 936b
obstetric, circulatory collapse and, 1275
retinal, 169
splinter, 994b, 1260
subarachnoid, 1160–1162
clinical features of, 1161, 1162f
investigations of, 1161
management of, 1162
see also stroke
Haemorrhagic fevers, viral, 245–247, 245b
Haemorrhagic toxins, 155–156
Haemorrhoids, 835–836
Haemosiderin, 851
Haemosiderosis, 716
idiopathic pulmonary, 613b
Haemostasis, 917–919, 918f–919f
in old age, 978b
Haemostasis system toxins, 155, 156f
Hair
abnormalities, 1224
disorders, 1258–1260
follicles, 1212–1213
loss, 1266b
Hairy cell leukaemia, 960
Hairy leucoplakia, 316
Hallpike manoeuvre, 1104, 1104f
Hallucinations, 1181, 1184
in alcohol misuse, 1194
hypnagogic, 1184
hypnopompic, 1184
in schizophrenia, 1196–1197
Hallucinogens, misuse of, 143–144, 1196
Hallucinosis, alcoholic, 1194
Hallux valgus, 999
Haloperidol
adverse reactions of, 22b
agitation, 1354
for delirium, 209
for disturbed behaviour, 1188–1189
poisoning, 141
schizophrenia, 1198b
Halothane, 82–83, 857f
Hamartoma, 603b
small intestine and, 813
Hands
in endocrine disease, 630f
examination of
blood disease, 912f
cancer, 1314f
cardiology, 442f
diabetes mellitus, 721b
endocrine disease, 630f

gastrointestinal disease, 764f
liver and biliary disease, 846f
musculoskeletal system, 982f
renal/urinary tract disease, 382f
respiratory system, 546f
skin disease, 1210f
foot and mouth disease, 248
gastrointestinal disease, 764f
hygiene, infection control, 112–113, 113f
liver and biliary disease and, 846f
osteoarthritis, 1009f
pain, 998
rheumatoid arthritis in, 1023f
washing, 113f
Hantavirus infection, 258
Haploinsufficiency, 659
Haptoglobin, 947, 1362b
in acute phase response, 70
Hard metal disease, 616
Hartmann's procedure, 788
Hartmann's solution, 353b
Hartnup's disease, 714
Hasenclever index, in Hodgkin lymphoma, 964, 964b
Hashimoto's thyroiditis, 646
Haversian system, 984f
Hay fever, 85, 622
Hayflick limit, 41
Head and neck
examination of
diabetes mellitus, 720f
endocrine disease, 630f
gastrointestinal disease, 764f
imaging of, 1073–1074, 1074f
injury, 1133
tumours in, 1335–1336, 1335b
investigations of, 1335
management of, 1335–1336
pathogenesis of, 1335
Head lice, 1241
Head-up tilt-table testing, 183
Headache, 185–186, 1080, 1095–1097
analgesic for, 1096
associated with specific activities, 1097
benign paroxysmal, 1097, 1097b
brain tumours causing, 1129
clinical assessment of, 185, 186f
cluster, 1096
exertion, 1097
fever and, 217b
heat stroke and, 167
investigations of, 185–186
medication overuse, 1096
migraine and, 1095–1096
morning, 558
pregnancy and, 1275
presentation of, 185, 185b
raised ICP, 1128b
'red flag' symptoms in, 185b
sexual activity and, 1097
stroke and, 1153
subarachnoid haemorrhage and, 1161
tension-type, 1095
Health, social determinants of, 93–94
Health care, genomics and, 56–58
Health care-associated infection, 111–113, 112f–113f
MRSA, 100
predisposing factors, 112f
Health data/informatics, 97–98
Hearing disturbance, 1093
Heart
anatomy of, 444–446, 444f–445f
auscultation of, 443b
blood flow through, 444f
catheterisation, 453–454, 453f
chamber, 445f
dilation of, 450
conduction system, 445, 445f
coronary circulation in, 444–445
endothelium and, 447
inflammatory arthritis in, 994b
nerve supply of, 445–446
physiology of, 446–448
Starling's law, 461, 461f

Heart beats
ectopic
atrial, 469–470, 470f
ventricular, 474–475, 475f
see also Palpitation
Heart block
atrioventricular, 477–478, 477f–478f, 478b
bifascicular, 478–479
bundle branch, 478–479, 478b, 478f
hemiblock, 478–479
Heart disease
congenital, 531–538, 531b, 532f
HIV-related, 322
pregnancy, 1282
rheumatic, 515–517
rheumatoid arthritis and, 1024
Heart failure, 461–468
in acute coronary syndrome, 496
acute left, 463
biventricular, 461
chronic, 463–464, 463b, 463f
clinical assessment for, 463–464, 463b
complications of, 464
congestive, in old age, 466b
high-output, 463
investigations for, 464, 464f
left, 461
management of, 464–468, 465b
drug treatment for, 465–467, 466f
mechanisms of, 462b, 462f
right, 461
Heart murmur, 459b
Heart rate
effects of respiration on, 447b
pregnancy and, 1272
Heart sounds, 460f
abnormal, 457–461, 459b
normal, 459b
Heart valves, diseases of, 514–531, 515b
Heartburn, 779
Heat cramps, 167
Heat exhaustion, 167
Heat-related illness, 167–168
Heat stroke, 167–168
Heat syncope, 167
Heberden's nodes, 1009f
Height, in endocrine disease, 630f
Heinz bodies, 950
Helicobacter pylori
eradication therapy, 800, 800b
gastric lymphoma, 805
peptic ulcer and, 798–799, 799f, 800b
Helium dilution technique, 575
Heller's operation, 795
HELLP syndrome, pregnancy and, 1284
Helminthiases, soil-transmitted, 233b
Helminths, 101–102
drugs used against, 129
Hemicellulose, 696b
Hemicrania, chronic paroxysmal, 1097b
Hemidiaphragm, elevation of, 627, 627b
Hemifacial spasm, 1116
Hemiparesis, 1083, 1123
Hemiplegic gait, 1309b
Henderson-Hasselbalch equation, 364
Henoch-Schönlein purpura, 398b–399b, 401, 1043
Heparin, 938–939
for acute limb ischaemia, 503
for angina, 491
indications for, 938b
low-molecular-weight, in thrombosis, 210
monitoring, 922
for stroke, 1160
Heparin-induced thrombocytopenia (HIT), 939
Hepatic acinus, 848, 848f
Hepatic adenomas, 893
Hepatic artery aneurysms, 898
Hepatic decompensation, 867
Hepatic disease, prescribing for patients with, 32, 32b

Hepatic encephalopathy, 847*b*, 864–865
  acute liver failure and, 856–857
  clinical grade of, assessment for, 857*b*
  differential diagnosis of, 865*b*
  factors precipitating, 865*b*
Hepatic fibrosis, 894
  cirrhosis and, 866, 866*f*
  congenital, 868*f*, 902
  non-invasive markers of, 855
  pathogenic mechanisms in, 849*f*
Hepatic hydrothorax, 863
Hepatic Iron Index (HII), 895
Hepatic-renal disease, 409–410
Hepatic venous disease, 898
Hepatic venous pressure, 868
Hepatitis
  acute kidney injury and, 416*b*
  alcoholic, 881
  autoimmune, 886–887
    conditions associated with, 886*b*
    liver function test (LFT) abnormality in, 854*b*
  interface, 886
  viral, 343–344, 871–878
    causes of, 871*b*
    chronic, HIV-related, 317–318
    features of, 872*b*
    investigations for, 872
    management of, 872
    non-A, non-B, non-C (NANBNC), 878
    pregnancy and, 1284
    sexual, 343–344
    Wilson's disease and, 896
Hepatitis A virus (HAV), 872–873, 872*b*
  acute liver failure and, 873
  antigen for, 872
  immunisation, 115*b*
  incubation period of, 111*b*
  in old age, 901*b*
  pregnancy and, 900
  transmission, sexual, 343
Hepatitis B core antigen (HBcAg), 873–874
Hepatitis B core IgM antibody, screening for, in acute liver failure, 858
Hepatitis B e antigen (HBeAg), 874–875
Hepatitis B surface antigen (HBsAg), 873
  recombinant hepatitis B vaccine with, 876
Hepatitis B virus (HBV), 872*b*, 873–877
  acute, management of, 875
  chronic
    HBeAg-negative, 875
    liver function test (LFT) abnormality in, 854*b*
    management of, 875–876
    natural history of, 874*f*
    phases of, 874*b*
    risk of, 873*b*
    source of, 873*b*
  cirrhosis and, 876
  co-infection with HIV, 876–877
  HIV-related, 317–318
  incubation period of, 111*b*
  investigations of, 873–875
  in pregnancy, 235*b*, 900
  prevention of, 876, 876*b*
  schematic diagram of, 873*f*
  serology for, 873–875, 875*b*, 875*f*
  transmission, sexual, 343
  vertical transmission of, 873
  viral load and, 875, 875*f*
Hepatitis C virus (HCV), 872*b*, 877–878
  antigens for, 877
  chronic, risk factors for, 877*b*
  cirrhosis and, 877
  HIV-related, 318
  liver function test for, 877
    abnormality in, 854*b*
  liver histology for, 878
  molecular analysis for, 877
  pregnancy and, 900
  transmission, sexual, 343

Hepatitis D virus, 872*b*, 877
  Delta antigen for, 877
  vertical transmission of, 877
Hepatitis E, 872*b*, 878
  in pregnancy, 235*b*
  pregnancy and, 900
Hepatitis viruses, 249
Hepatobiliary disease, HIV-related, 317–318
Hepatocellular carcinoma, 890–892, 891*f*
  chemotherapy for, 892
  cirrhosis and, 890
  fibrolamellar, 892
  hepatic resection for, 891
  hepatitis B and, 873
  liver biopsy for, 891
  liver transplantation for, 891
  management of, 892*f*
  in old age, 901*b*
  percutaneous therapy for, 891
  screening for, 890–891
  trans-arterial chemo-embolisation for, 892
Hepatocellular jaundice, 860–861
Hepatocytes, 848, 849*f*
  necrosis of, 894
Hepatology, 845–909
Hepatomegaly, 862
  acute liver failure and, 857–858
  Budd-Chiari syndrome and, 899
  cirrhosis and, 866–867
Hepatopulmonary syndrome, 898
Hepatorenal syndrome
  ascites and, 864
  type 1, 864
  type 2, 864
Hepatosplenic candidiasis, 302
Hepcidin, 716–717, 943
HER2 receptor, as tumour markers, 1322, 1324*b*
Herbal medicines, for pain, 1348
Herd immunity, 115
Hereditary angioedema (HAE), 88
Hereditary coproporphyria (HCP), 379*b*
Hereditary elliptocytosis, 947–948
Hereditary haemorrhagic telangiectasia (HHT), 970
Hereditary hypophosphataemic rickets, 405, 1052–1053
Hereditary nephrotic syndrome, 404
Hereditary neuropathy, 1140
Hereditary spherocytosis, 947
  investigations of, 947, 948*f*
  management of, 947, 948*b*
Hernia
  diaphragmatic, 627
  hiatus, 791, 791*b*, 792*f*
  lumbar disc, 1135, 1135*f*
Heroin, misuse, 142
Herpangina, 248
Herpes simplex keratitis, 1173
Herpes simplex virus (HSV), 238*b*
  after HSCT, 937*b*
  genital, 341–342
  HIV-related, 314*f*, 315, 315*b*
  HSV-1, 247–248, 247*f*
  HSV-2, 247–248, 247*f*
  in pregnancy, 235*b*, 332*b*
  viral hepatitis and, 878
Herpes zoster, 239–240, 1123
  clinical features of, 239
  facial pain from, 1080
  HIV-related, 315
  management of, 240
Herpesvirus infections, skin, 1238
Herring worm, 294
Heterochromatin, 38–39
Hiatus hernia, 627, 791, 791*b*, 792*f*
'Hibernating' myocardium, 452
Hibernian fever, 81
Hierarchy of systems, 93, 93*b*, 93*f*
High altitude, 168–169
  illnesses at, 168–169
    cerebral oedema (HACE), 168
    pulmonary oedema (HAPE), 168–169
    physiological effects of, 168, 168*f*

High-altitude cerebral oedema (HACE), 168
High-density lipoproteins (HDL), 1360*b*
High-energy fracture, 995*b*
High-flow nasal cannulae (HFNCs), 202
High-grade tumours, 961
High haemoglobin, 925, 925*b*
High-risk behaviour, transition medicine and, 1295
  history-taking in, 1295*b*
  personality and, 1295
  protective factors in, 1295
  theories in, 1295
Highly polyunsaturated long-chain n-3 fatty acids, 377
Hip
  osteoarthritis, 1010, 1010*f*
  pain, 998, 999*b*, 999*f*
Hippocampus, 1066
Hirschsprung's disease, 834–835
Hirsutism, 657–658, 658*b*, 1259–1260
His bundle, 445
Histamine, 767
Histidine, 698*b*
Histones, 38
Histopathology, in respiratory disease, 554
Histoplasma capsulatum, 303
Histoplasmosis, 303–304
  in HIV infection/AIDS, 314*f*
HIV infection/AIDS, 312
  antiretroviral therapy for, 324–327, 324*b*
  asymptomatic, 312, 312*f*
  CD4 counts in, 311
  chemoprophylaxis for, 323–324
  clinical examination of, 306*f*
  clinical manifestations of, 311–312
  counselling for, 311*b*
  diagnosis of, 310–311, 310*b*
  epidemiology of, 308
  global and regional epidemics of, 308, 308*b*
  hepatitis B and
    acute, 875
    co-infection with, 876–877
  immunisation for, 324
  immunology of, 309–310
  investigations of, 310–311, 311*b*
  life cycle of, 309*f*
  liver and, 879
  liver blood tests in, abnormal, 879*b*
  modes of transmission of, 308, 308*b*–309*b*
  musculoskeletal manifestations of, 1021*b*
  in old age, 326*b*
  pregnancy and, 1280
  presenting problems of, 312–322, 313*b*
    cancers, 322, 323*b*
    cardiac disease, 322
    fever, 313–314, 313*f*–314*f*
    gastrointestinal disease, 316–317
    haematological abnormalities, 322
    hepatobiliary disease, 317–318
    lymphadenopathy, 313
    mucocutaneous disease, 314–316, 314*b*
    nervous system and eye disease, 319–321, 319*f*
    renal diseases, 322
    respiratory disease, 318–319, 318*b*
    rheumatological diseases, 321–322
    weight loss, 313, 313*f*
  prevention of, 323–324, 327*b*
  primary, 311–312, 312*f*
  prophylaxis for, 119*b*
  pruritus and, 1219*b*
  staging classifications of, 307*b*
  testing of, 330
  tuberculosis and, 595
  viral load in, 311
  virology of, 309–310
HIV serology, acute kidney injury and, 416*b*
Hives, 1252
HLA antigen, transplant rejection, 88–89
HNF1-beta mutations, 406

Hoarseness, psychogenic, 624
Hodgkin lymphoma (HL), 961–964, 962*f*
  classification of, 962*b*
  clinical features of, 962
  epidemiology of, 961, 962*b*
  investigations of, 962, 963*f*
  management of, 962–964
  prognosis of, 964, 964*b*
  stages of, 962*b*
Holmes-Adie syndrome, 1092*b*
Home ventilation, for chronic respiratory failure, 567
Homocystinuria, 369–370
Honeycomb lung, 608*f*
Hookworm
  ancylostomiasis, 288–289, 288*f*
  dog, 294
Hookworm infestation, 233*b*
Hoover's sign, 1081–1082
Hormone replacement therapy
  amenorrhoea, 655
  cancer, 1332
  for osteoporosis, 1048*b*, 1049
Hormones
  gastrointestinal tract, 772
  production, ectopic, 1325*b*
  in venous blood, 1359*b*
Horner's syndrome, 1091*b*–1092*b*, 1091*f*
Hospital, under-nutrition in, 693*f*, 705–708, 706*b*
Host-pathogen interactions, 104
House dust mite, 570
Howell-Jolly bodies, 921*f*
Human albumin, 930
Human albumin solution (HAS), ascites and, 864
Human chorionic gonadotrophin (hCG)
  secretion of, pregnancy and, 1272
  as tumour markers, 1322, 1324*b*
Human herpesvirus 6 (HHV-6), 238, 238*b*
Human herpesvirus 7 (HHV-7), 238, 238*b*
Human herpesvirus 8 (HHV-8), 238*b*, 248
Human leucocyte antigen (HLA)
  molecules, 67
  antigen processing and presentation and, 70
Human papillomavirus (HPV), 342–343
  in pregnancy, 332*b*
  vaccines, 115
Human parvovirus arthropathy, 1020–1021
Human T-cell lymphotrophic virus type 1, 250
Humanitarian crisis, 171–172, 172*b*
Humidifier fever, 616*b*, 617
Humoral immunity, 68
Hunter's syndrome, 371*b*
Huntington's disease, 1115
  genetic testing of, 1077
Hurler's syndrome, 371*b*
Hutchinson's sign, 1233
Hyaluronic acid, intra-articular injections of, 1012
Hydatid cyst, liver and, 880
Hydatid disease, 298–299, 299*f*
Hydralazine, 467
  lupus syndrome, 1057*b*
  malignant hypertension, 514
  pharmacokinetic, 20*b*
  skin reactions, 1266*b*
Hydration
  for stroke patients, 1159*b*
  see also Fluid replacement
Hydroa vacciniforme, 1221*b*
Hydrocephalus, 1132–1133, 1132*f*
  causes of, 1132*b*, 1133*f*
  dementia and, 1191*b*
  management of, 1133
  normal pressure, 1132–1133
  obstructive, 1092*b*, 1121
Hydrocortisone
  ACTH deficiency, 682
  adrenal insufficiency, 673
  anaphylaxis, 76*b*
  asthma, 573

Hydrocortisone *(Continued)*
  eczema, 1244
  equivalent dose, 670b
  for inflammatory bowel disease, 820,
    821b
  laryngeal obstruction, 625
  potency and strength, 1226b
  topical, 1226b
  see also Cortisol
Hydrocortisone sodium succinate, 625
Hydrogen ions
  acid-base balance, 364
  in arterial blood, 565b, 1358b
Hydromorphone, 1352
Hydronephrosis, 413
Hydrophobia, 1122
Hydrops fetalis, 237b
Hydrotherapy, for musculoskeletal
    disease, 1001
Hydrothorax, hepatic, 863
Hydroxyapatite crystals, 985
Hydroxycarbamide
  essential thrombocythaemia, 970
  leukaemia, 959
  for myelofibrosis, 969
  sickle-cell disease, 953
  for skin disease, 1227–1228
Hydroxychloroquine (HCQ)
  for musculoskeletal disease, 1004b,
    1005
  for rheumatoid arthritis, 1026b
  for Sjögren's syndrome, 1039
  skin reactions, 1266b
  for systemic lupus erythematosus,
    1036
  for Whipple's disease, 809
1α-Hydroxycholecalciferol (alfacalcidol),
    for hypoparathyroidism, 665
Hydroxycobalamin *see* Vitamin B₁₂
5-Hydroxyindole-3-acetic acid (5-HIAA),
    1361b
11-Hydroxylase deficiency, 509b
17α-Hydroxylase deficiency, 509b
21-Hydroxylase deficiency, 676
11β-Hydroxysteroid dehydrogenase,
    665, 665b
  deficiency, 509b
25-Hydroxyvitamin D (25(OH)D), for
    skeletal disease, 990b
Hyfrecation, 343
Hygiene, hand-washing, 113f
Hygiene hypothesis, 84–85
Hyoscine butylbromide, 1350b, 1354
Hyper IgD syndrome (HIDS), 81
Hyperacusis, 1083
Hyperacute rejection, 89
Hyperaesthesia
  dengue fever, 243b
  diabetic neuropathy, 758–759
  herpes simplex, 247
Hyperaldosteronism
  glucocorticoid suppressible, 509b,
    674
  primary, 674–675, 674b
  secondary, 674b
  in type 1 diabetes, 729–730
Hyperalgesia, fibromyalgia, 1018
Hyperalphalipoproteinaemia, 374
Hyperbilirubinaemia
  non-haemolytic, 860, 860b
  see also Jaundice
Hypercalcaemia, 661–662
  cancer and, 1327, 1327b
  causes of, 662, 662b
  clinical assessment of, 662
  familial hypocalciuric, 662, 664
  hypoparathyroidism, 664–665
  investigations of, 662
  malignant, 662
  management of, 662
  multiple myeloma and, 410b, 967f
  sarcoidosis, 609–610
Hypercapnia, ventilator-induced lung
    injury and, 204
Hypercarotenosis, 713
Hypercholesterolaemia, 373–374,
    376–377
  atherosclerosis risk, 486
  familial, 374, 374b

management of, 376–377
  nephrotic syndrome and, 395b
  polygenic, 373–374
  primary biliary cholangitis and,
    887–888
  secondary, 373b
Hypercoagulability, nephrotic syndrome
    and, 395b
Hypercortisolism, 667b
Hyperemesis gravidarum, pregnancy
    and, 1277–1278, 1278b
Hyperglycaemia
  in acute medical illness, 754
  in diabetes, 734–735, 734f
    clinical assessment of, 734–735
    drugs to reduce, 745–748
    symptoms of, 735, 735b
    type 1, 729–730
    type 2, 732
  diabetic ketoacidosis, 735
  maternal, diabetes and, 1278–1279
  pancreatitis, 838b
  stress, 728
Hyperglycaemic hyperosmolar state
    (HHS), 738, 739b
Hypergonadotrophic hypogonadism,
    653b, 654
Hyperinsulinaemia, 740
Hyperkalaemia, 362–363, 464
  acute kidney injury and, 413
  causes of, 362b
  chronic kidney disease, 417
  heart failure, 464
  periodic paralysis, 1145b
  treatment of, 363b
Hyperkeratosis, subungual, 1031
Hyperketonaemia, 725
Hyperlactataemia, 196, 197f
Hyperlipidaemia
  check for signs of, 347f
  classification of, 374b
  drug treatment of, 376f
  familial combined, 374, 374b
  mixed, 375, 377–378
  in old age, 377b
  rare forms of, 375b
  remnant, 375
  secondary, 373b
  treatment of, 376f
Hypermagnesaemia, 368
Hypermelanosis, focal, 1258
Hypermobile Ehlers-Danlos syndrome
    (hEDS), 1059
Hypermobility syndromes, 1059
Hypernatraemia, 358–360
  causes of, 359b
  in old age, 360b
Hyperostosis, diffuse idiopathic skeletal,
    1058–1059, 1058f
Hyperparasitaemia, malaria, 276b
Hyperparathyroidism
  chronic kidney disease and,
    418–419
  in old age, 665b
  pain, 663
  primary, pregnancy and, 1280
Hyperphosphataemia, chronic kidney
    disease and, 419
Hyperpigmentation, photo-exposed site,
    1258
Hyperprolactinaemia, 684, 684b
  disconnection, 667
Hyperpyrexia, 276b
Hypersensitive carotid sinus syndrome,
    183
Hypersensitivity, 71
  allergic rhinitis, 622
  drug response, 20b
  Gell and Coombs classification of, 83,
    83b
  patch tests, 1215
  prick tests, 1215
  type I, 83–84, 85f
  type II, 83
  type III, 83
  type IV, 83
Hypersensitivity pneumonitis, 616–617,
    617b, 617f
Hypersensitivity rashes, 326

Hypersensitivity reaction, definition of,
    21
Hypersomnolence, 1105, 1105b
Hypersplenism
  leucopenia and, 853
  portal hypertension, 868b
  and thrombocytopenia, 869
Hypertension, 193–194, 396, 508–514,
    509b–511b, 509f, 511f–512f
  accelerated, 514
  assessment and management of,
    193–194
  cocaine, 143
  definition, 509b
  essential, 509
  gestational, 1276, 1276b
  history, 510
  idiopathic intracranial, 1133
  investigations, 510
  management
    antihypertensive drugs, 513
    British Hypertension Society
      guidelines, 512f
    intervention thresholds, 511–512
    non-drug therapy, 513
    treatment targets, 512–513, 513b
  in old age, 512b
  pathogenesis, 509
  pathophysiology of, 193
  portal, 868–871, 898
    ascites and, 869
    cirrhosis and, 868
    classification of, 868f
    clinical features of, 868–869
    complications of, 868b
    extrahepatic portal vein obstruction,
      868
    investigations for, 869
    management of, 869–871
    pathophysiology of, 869
  portopulmonary, 898
  pre-eclampsia, 1276–1277
  during pregnancy, 1276–1277
    classification of, 1276b
    pre-eclampsia and eclampsia in,
      1276–1277, 1276b, 1277f
    pre-existing, 1276
  pulmonary, 550, 621–622, 621b,
    622f
    congenital heart disease and, 533
    systemic sclerosis and, 1038
  renal artery stenosis and, 406
  renal disease, 396
    AKI, 411–412
    chronic, 415
    polycystic, 405
    reflux nephropathy, 430
    secondary, 509b
  in systemic sclerosis, 1038
  target organ damage, 510
  venous, 1223
  white coat, 510, 1276b
Hypertensive renal crisis, systemic
    sclerosis and, 1038
Hyperthermia, malignant, 1145b
Hyperthyroidism, pregnancy and, 1279
Hypertrichosis, 1259
  drug-induced, 1266b
Hypertriglyceridaemia, 374
  familial, 374, 374b
  management of, 377–378
  secondary, 373b
Hypertrophic cardiomyopathy, 539–540,
    540b
Hypertrophic obstructive
    cardiomyopathy, transition
    medicine and, 1297–1298
Hypertrophic pulmonary
    osteoarthropathy (HPOA), in lung
    cancer, 600–601
Hyperuricaemia, 1012–1013
  causes of, 1013b
  chronic, 1014
  gout, 1013b
Hyperventilation
  in panic disorder, 1200
  psychogenic, 1202
  and respiratory alkalosis, 367
Hyperviscosity syndrome, 966

Hypervolaemia, 353–355
  clinical features of, 352b
  hypernatraemia with, 359b
  hyponatraemia with, 357
Hypnic jerks, 1086
Hypnotics
  dosage regimens of, 31b
  in old age, 32b
Hypoadrenalism, tuberculosis, 595
Hypoalbuminaemia, nephrotic syndrome
    and, 395b
Hypobetalipoproteinaemia, 375
Hypocalcaemia, 662–663
  aetiology of, 662–663
  clinical assessment of, 663
  differential diagnosis of, 662b
  ethylene glycol poisoning, 147
  hypomagnesaemia and, 368
  kidney failure and
    acute, 414
    chronic, 418–419
  kidney injury
    acute, 414
    chronic, 418–419
  management of, 663, 663b
  pancreatitis, 838b
Hypochlorhydria, 798–799, 944
Hypochlorous acid, 64
Hypochondriacal disorder, 1202
Hypofibrinogenaemia, 922b, 972b
Hypogammaglobulinaemia, in vitamin
    B₁₂ deficiency, 944
Hypoglossal (12th cranial) nerve, tests
    of, 1063b
Hypoglycaemia, 738–741
  acute treatment of, 740
  awareness of, 740
  causes of, 740b
  diabetes, 738–741
    drug-induced, 747
  emergency treatment of, 741b
  exercise-induced, 740
  malaria, 276b
  nocturnal, 740
  prevention of, 740–741, 741b
  risk factors for, 740b
  spontaneous, 676–678, 677f, 738
    in old age, 678b
  symptoms of, 739, 739b
Hypogonadism
  hypergonadotrophic, 653b, 654
  hypogonadotrophic, 653, 653b
  male, 655, 656b, 660b
Hypogonadotrophic hypogonadism,
    653, 653b
Hypokalaemia, 361–362, 464
  causes of, 361b
  chloroquine poisoning, 141b
  heart failure, 464
  hyperaldosteronism, 674
  mineralocorticoid excess, 675
  periodic paralysis, 1145b
Hypomagnesaemia, 368
  causes of, 368b
  management, 368
Hypomania, 1199–1200
Hypomimia, 1113b
Hyponatraemia, 357–358, 464,
    852–853
  adrenal insufficiency, 671–672
  algorithm for diagnosis of, 359f
  brain and, 358f
  causes of, 357b
  depletional, 672b
  dilutional, 414
  ecstasy/amphetamine misuse, 143
  with euvolaemia, 357
  heart failure, 464
  with hypervolaemia, 357
  hypopituitarism, 681–682
  with hypovolaemia, 357
  in old age, 360b
  symptoms and severity of, 358b
Hypoparathyroidism, 664–665
Hypophosphataemia, 368–369, 369b
Hypophosphataemic rickets
  biochemical abnormalities in, 990b
  transition medicine and, 1300
Hypophosphatasia, 1053

Hypopigmentation, 1257–1258
Hypopituitarism, 681–682, 681b–682b, 681f
  clinical assessment, 681–682, 681f
  investigations, 682, 682b
  management, 682
Hyposmia, 1088
Hypotension, 193
  assessment and management of, 193, 193b
  during dialysis, 424b
  pathophysiology of, 193, 193b
  poisoning, 137b
  postural, 181, 1308–1309
    glucocorticoid insufficiency, 672b
    in old age, 32b
  renal disease, 411–412
  shock, 196b
  treatment of, 1308–1309
Hypothalamus, 679–688, 1066–1067
  disease
    classification of, 680b
    presenting problems in, 681–684
  functional anatomy, physiology and investigations of, 679f
  in old age, 688b
  therapeutic modalities, 683b
  thermoregulation and, 165
  tumours, 1066–1067
Hypothermia, 165–166, 165f–166f
  cold water immersion, 166
  in old age, 166b
Hypothyroidism, 639–642
  autoimmune, 637b, 639b
  causes, 639b
  clinical assessment of, 639–640, 640f
  clinical features of, 637b
  congenital, 639b, 650
  iatrogenic, 639b
  investigations of, 640
  laboratory abnormalities, 638b
  management of, 640–641, 641b
  with normal thyroid function tests, 641–642
  obesity, 654–655
  in old age, 650b
  in pregnancy, 641, 651b, 1279
  radiotherapy and, 1298
  rheumatological manifestations of, 1057
  secondary, 639b
  spontaneous atrophic, 639b
  subclinical, 642
  transient, 640
  transient thyroiditis, 639b
Hypoventilation, alveolar, 567, 621b
Hypovolaemia, 352–353
  causes of, 352b
  clinical features of, 352b
  hypernatraemia with, 359b
  hyponatraemia with, 357
Hypovolaemic shock, description of, 206b
Hypoxaemia, 168f
  acute mountain sickness and, 168
  assessment and management of, 191, 191b
  causes of, 192b
  cirrhosis, 866–867
  high-altitude pulmonary oedema, 168–169
  mechanisms of, 192f
  near drowning accidents and, 169–170
  pathophysiology of, 190–191, 191f
  pulmonary hypertension, 621b
Hypoxia
  altitude illness and, 168
  cytopathic, 197f, 198
  pancreatitis, 838b
  respiratory failure, 565b
Hypromellose, 1039
Hysterectomy, cancer treatment, 1335
Hysteria, 1126

I
Ibandronate, for osteoporosis, 1048b
Ibuprofen, 1003b
  adverse reactions of, 22b

Ice cream headache, 1097b
Ice pick headache, 1097b
Ichthyosis, 1212
Idarucizumab, 940
Idiopathic interstitial pneumonias, 605–608, 606b
Idiopathic intracranial hypertension, pregnancy and, 1284
Idiopathic osteoporosis, 1044
Idiopathic Parkinson's disease, 1112–1114
  causes of, 1112b
  clinical features of, 1112–1113, 1113b
    non-motor symptoms of, 1112–1113
  investigations of, 1113, 1113f
  management of, 1113–1114
    drug therapy, 1113–1114
    surgery, 1114
  pathophysiology of, 1112, 1112f
Idiopathic pulmonary fibrosis, 605–608, 607f
Idiopathic pulmonary haemosiderosis, 613b
Idiopathic thrombocytopenic purpura (ITP), 971
  pregnancy and, 1285
If channel antagonists, angina, 491
Ifosfamide, 365b
Ileal resection, 810f
  under-nutrition and, 706
Ileus
  meconium, 842
  paralytic, 837–838
Illusions, 1181
Iloprost, 622
Imaging
  for epilepsy, 1101b
  in gastroenterology, 774b, 774f
  of gastrointestinal tract, 772–776
  for hepatobiliary disease, 853–855
  for lung cancer, 601, 601f
  for musculoskeletal disease, 988–990
  neuroimaging, 1151, 1151f, 1157–1158
  of renal tract, 389–390
  of respiratory system, 551–553
  vascular, 1151, 1152f
Imatinib, 1332
  acute leukaemia, 957b
  chronic myeloid leukaemia, 958
  for GIST, 805
Imidazoles, 125b, 126
Imipenem, 120b
  nocardiosis, 261
Imipramine, 611b
  irritable bowel syndrome, 825
  neurogenic bladder, 1094b
Imiprothrin, 148b
Imiquimod
  for lentigo maligna, 1233
  for molluscum contagiosum, 1239
  for skin cancer, 1230, 1230b
  for viral warts, 1239
Imiquimod cream, for anogenital warts, 343
Immersion foot, 167
Immotile cilia syndrome, 578b
Immune deficiency, 77–81
  autoimmune lymphoproliferative syndrome and, 80
  common variable, 79
  complement pathway deficiencies in, 78
  consequences of, 77
  investigations of
    initial, 74b
    specialist, 74b
  primary, warning signs of, 73b
  primary antibody deficiencies in, 78–79, 78f, 79b
  primary phagocyte deficiencies in, 77–78, 77f
  primary T-lymphocyte deficiencies and, 79–80, 80f
  secondary, 80–81, 80b

Immune disorders
  anaphylaxis and, 75–76
  common causes of, 75b
  intermittent fever and, 74
  presenting problems of, 73–76
  recurrent infections and, 73
Immune reconstitution inflammatory syndrome (IRIS), 104, 325–326
Immune response modifiers, 1226
Immune responses, in lower airway defences, 550
Immune senescence, 80–81, 81b
Immune serum globulin, for hepatitis A, 872–873
Immune system
  adaptive, 67–70
    cellular immunity and, 69–70, 69f
    immunoglobulins and, 68–69, 68b, 68f
    lymphoid organs and, 67
  innate, 62–67
    complement and, 66
    cytokines and, 64–66, 65b, 65f
    dendritic cells in, 64
    integrins and, 66
    mast cells and basophils, 66–67
    natural killer cells and, 67
    phagocytes in, 63–64, 63f
    physical barriers in, 62–67
  regulation of, 851
Immunisation, 114–115, 115b
  for chickenpox, 239
  for cholera, 265
  for diphtheria, 266
  Haemophilus influenzae, 115b
  for hepatitis A, 872–873
  for hepatitis B, 876, 876b
  for HIV infection/AIDS, 324
  for human papillomavirus, 343
  for influenza, 241
  for meningococcal infection, 1120
  for mumps, 240
  for plague, 259
  for pneumococcal infection, 266
  for poliomyelitis, 1123
  primary antibody deficiencies and, 79
  for rabies, 1122
  for rubella, 266
  for tetanus, 1126
  for tuberculosis, 595
  for typhoid fever, 261
  for whooping cough, 582
  whooping cough (pertussis), 115b
  for yellow fever, 245
  see also Vaccines/vaccination
Immunity
  adaptive
    humoral immunity and, 67–68
  cellular, 67, 69–70, 69f
  humoral, 67–68
  Immunoblot (Western blot), 107
  innate, 769
Immunoblot (Western blot), 107
Immunobullous disease, drug-induced, 1266b
Immunochromatographic rapid diagnostic tests (RDTs), 276
Immunochromatographic tests, 108
Immunocompromised host, fever in, 223–224
Immunocompromised patient, pneumonia in, 587
Immunodiffusion, 108
Immunofluorescence assays, 107
  anti-endomysial antibodies in, 807
Immunoglobulin(s), 68–69, 68b, 68f, 930
  for idiopathic thrombocytopenic purpura, 971
  intravenous
    Guillain-Barré syndrome, 1140
    myasthenia gravis, 1142b
    myositis, 1040
    thrombocytopenia, 971
    toxic shock syndrome, 252
  prophylactic, 115b
  reference range of, venous blood, 1360b

Immunoglobulin A (IgA), 68b
  deficiency, selective, 78–79
  linear IgA disease, 1255b, 1256–1257
  nephropathy, 398b–399b, 400
  reference range of, venous blood, 1360b
Immunoglobulin D (IgD), 68b
  hyper-IgD syndrome, 81
Immunoglobulin E (IgE), 68b, 1215
  reference range of, venous blood, 1360b
  serum total, for allergy, 86
  specific tests, for allergy, 86
Immunoglobulin G (IgG), 68b
  anti-HBc, 875b
  antibody, functional deficiency in, 79
  cerebrospinal fluid, 1361b
  reference range of, 1360b
  rubella-specific, 236
Immunoglobulin M (IgM), 68b
  anti-HBc, 875b
  cold agglutinin disease, 950
  reference range of, venous blood, 1360b
Immunoglobulin replacement therapy, for primary antibody deficiencies, 79
Immunohistochemistry, tumour identification, 1322
Immunological memory, 69
Immunological tests, 1077
  antibody-independent specific, 109
  for hepatobiliary disease, 853
  for respiratory disease, 554
Immunoproliferative small intestinal disease (IPSID), 813
Immunosuppressants
  for skin disease, 1227–1228
  for systemic lupus erythematosus, 1036
Immunosuppression
  liver transplantation and, 901
  myasthenia gravis, 1142b
  in transplant
    complications of, 89–90
    drugs used in, 89b
Immunosuppressive agent, for autoimmune hepatitis, 886
Immunotherapy
  antigen-specific, for allergy, 86
  cancer, 1332
  myasthenia gravis, 1142b
Impaired glucose tolerance, 374, 1360b
Impetigo, 1235–1236
  non-bullous, 1235f
Implantable cardiac defibrillators, 467, 483–484, 483b
  for acute coronary syndrome, 501
Impotence see Erectile dysfunction
Imprinting, 49–50, 51b
Incidence of disease, microbiological sampling, 105b
Incident pain, 1350b
Incidental adrenal mass, 673–674
Incidental pancreatic mass, 844
'Incidentalomas', 633b
Inclusion body myositis, 1059
Incontinence
  continual, 437
  faecal, 1094
  overflow, 437, 1093
  stress, 436
  of stroke patients, 1159b
  urge, 436–437, 1093
  urinary, 397, 436–437
    older people, 436b, 1309–1310, 1310f
Increased intra-abdominal pressure, 791
Incremental cost-effectiveness ratio (ICER), 28
'Incretin' effect, 723–724, 724f
Indirect antiglobulin tests, 948f
Indocyanine angiography, of visual disorders, 1169
Indometacin, 1003b
  for paroxysmal headache prevention, 1097
  for pericarditis, 542
  for persistent ductus arteriosus, 534

Inductively coupled plasma/mass
   spectroscopy, 348b
Infection(s), 215–304, 930
   in adolescence, 234, 235b
   agents of, 100–102, 100b
   bacterial, 250–273
      after HSCT, 937b
      chlamydial, 272–273, 272b
      gastrointestinal, 262–265
      with neurological involvement, 267
      respiratory, 265–267
      rickettsial, 270–272, 271b
      of skin, 1235–1238
      soft tissues and bones, 250–254
      systemic, 254–262
   caused by helminths, 288–299,
      288b
   central venous catheter, 225–226
   chain of, 100f
   chlamydial, 340–341
      in men, 340
      in reactive arthritis, 1031
      treatment of, 341b
      urethritis, 333
      in women, 340–341
   clinical examination of, 216–218,
      216f, 217b
   common infecting organisms, 117b
   constitutive barriers to, 63
   control, 111–115, 112b
   cytomegalovirus, 238b, 242–243
      after HSCT, 937b
      clinical features of, 242–243
      encephalitis, 320
      investigations of, 243
      liver transplantation and, 901
      management of, 243
      polyradiculitis, 321
      in pregnancy, 235b
      viral hepatitis and, 878
   definition of, 100
   deliberate release, 111
   emerging and re-emerging disease,
      110, 110f
   endemic disease, 110
   epidemiology of, 110–111
   Epstein-Barr virus, 238b, 241–242
      clinical features of, 241–242
      complications of, 241–242, 242b
      investigations of, 242
      management of, 242
   Escherichia coli, 263–264
      entero-aggregative, 263–264
      entero-invasive, 263
      enterohaemorrhagic, 263–264
      enteropathogenic, 263
      verocytotoxigenic, 263f
   fungal, 300–304, 300f
      after HSCT, 937b
      skin, 1239–1240, 1240f
      subcutaneous, 300–301
      superficial, 300
      systemic, 301–304
   gastrointestinal tract
      function of, 777–778, 777b
      oral cancer, 790
      test of, 777
   geographical and temporal patterns
      of, 110
   history-taking in, 217b
   HIV/AIDS, 305–327
      antiretroviral therapy for, 324–327,
         324f
      asymptomatic, 312, 312f
      CD4 counts in, 311
      chemoprophylaxis for, 323–324
      clinical examination of, 306f
      clinical manifestations of, 311–312
      counselling in, 311b
      diagnosis of, 310–311, 310b
      epidemiology of, 308
      global and regional epidemics of,
         308, 308b
      immunisation for, 324
      immunology of, 309–310
      investigations of, 310–311, 311b
      life cycle of, 309f
      liver and, 879
      liver blood tests in, abnormal, 879b

   modes of transmission of, 308,
      308b–309b
   musculoskeletal manifestations of,
      1021b
   in old age, 326b
   pregnancy and, 1280
   presenting problems of, 312–322,
      313b
   prevention of, 323–324, 327b
   primary, 311–312, 312b
   pruritus and, 1219b
   staging classifications of, 307b
   testing of, 330
   tuberculosis and, 595
   viral load in, 311
   virology of, 309–310
   host-pathogen interaction of, 104
   incubation periods of, 111b
   investigation of, 105–109, 105b
      culture, 106
      direct detection of pathogens,
         105–106
   joints, 1019–1021
      in old age, 1020b
   of liver, 871–880
   liver transplantation and, 901
   microbiological sampling, 105b
   mycobacterial, 267–270
   nematode, 233b
      intestinal, 288–290
      tissue-dwelling, 290–293, 290b
      zoonotic, 293–294
   in non-immune haemolytic anaemia,
      950
   normal microbial flora, 102–103,
      103f
   of oesophagitis, 794
   outbreaks of, 114
      reporting, 114b
      terminology, 114b
   parvovirus B19, 237
      clinical features of, 237, 237b,
         237f
      diagnosis of, 237
      management of, 237
      in pregnancy, 235b
   periods of infectivity, 111b
   in pregnancy, 234, 235b
   presenting problems in, 218–234
   prevention, 111–115, 112b
   protozoal, 273–288
      gastrointestinal, 286–288
      leishmaniasis, 281–286
      systemic, 273–281
   recurrent, 73
   reservoirs of, 110
      animal, 110
      environmental, 110
      human, 110
   respiratory, 581–598
      in old age, 586b
      pneumonia, 582–587
      pregnancy and, 1277
      tuberculosis (TB), 588–595
      upper respiratory tract infection,
         581–587
   rubella
      clinical features of, 236
      congenital malformation and, 237b
      diagnosis of, 236
      in pregnancy, 235b
      prevention of, 236–237
   sexually transmitted, 329–344
      approach to patients, 332–333,
         332b
      in children, 332–333
      contact tracing for, 333
      HIV testing for, 330
      management goals of, 331b
      in men, 330, 330b, 330f
      men who have sex with men,
         330b, 334–335
      during pregnancy, 332
      presenting problems of, men,
         333–336, 333f–334f
      prevention of, 336–337
      those at particular risk, 331b
      viral, 341–344
      in women, 331, 331b, 331f

   skin, 1235–1241
      bacterial, 1235–1238
      fungal, 1239–1240, 1240f
      mycobacterial, 1237–1238
      tropical, 234, 234b, 235f
      viral, 1238–1239
   of small intestine, 812–813
   soft tissue, 226–227
      necrotising, 227b
   staphylococcal, 250–252, 251f
      cannula-related, 251–252, 251b
      methicillin-resistant Staphylococcus
         aureus, 252
      skin, 251
      staphylococcal toxic shock
         syndrome, 252, 252f
      wound, 251, 251f
   starvation-associated, 705b
   supportive therapy for, 957
   transmission of, 100f, 111
   tropical, 230–234, 230b
   urinary tract, 426–431
      antibiotic regimens for, 429b
      investigation of, 428b
      in old age, 428b
      persistent or recurrent, 429, 429b
      risk factors for, 428b
      in stroke patients, 1159f
   viral, 236–250
      gastrointestinal, 249
      with neurological involvement,
         249–250
      respiratory, 249
      with rheumatological involvement,
         250
      sexually transmitted, 341–344
      of skin, 247–249, 1238–1239
Infection-related glomerulonephritis,
   398b–399b, 401
Infectious conditions, in
   ophthalmological conditions,
   1173–1174
Infectious disease
   genomics of, 58
   pathogenesis of, 104, 108f
   periods of infectivity in, 111b
   principles of, 99–129
   treatment of, 116–129, 119b
Infectious keratitis/corneal ulceration,
   1173, 1174f
   common causes of, 1173b
Infectious mononucleosis, 241–242
   causes of, 241b
   clinical features of, 241–242, 242f
   investigations of, 242
   management of, 242
Infective endocarditis, 527–531, 528b,
   531b
   acute, 529
   antimicrobial treatment of, 530b
   in old age, 527b
   post-operative, 529
   prevention of, 531
   subacute, 528–529, 529b, 529f
Inferior petrosal sinus sampling, bilateral,
   670f
Inferior vena cava, 384, 444f
Infertility, 656–657, 656b
   cytotoxic medications and, 1298
   in polycystic ovarian syndrome, 659
Infestations, skin, 1241
Inflammation
   acute, 70–71, 71f
   cancer, 1319–1320
   chronic, 71
   laboratory features of, 71–72
   resolution, 71
   systemic, 196–198
Inflammatory bowel disease (IBD),
   813–824
   childhood, 823
   clinical features of, 816–817
   complications of, 818, 818f
   differential diagnosis of, 817, 817b
   disease distribution in, 815f
   investigations of, 818–820, 819f
   management of, 820–823
   metabolic bone disease and, 824
   microscopic colitis and, 824

   monitoring of, 822b
   pathogenesis of, 815f
   pathophysiology of, 814–816, 814b
   in pregnancy, 823–824, 824b, 1278
   systemic complications of, 819f
   transition medicine and, 1299–1300
   treatment of, 821b
Inflammatory molecules, 64
Inflammatory myopathy, 1042b
Inflammatory response, 70–72
   acute inflammation and, 70–71, 71f
      acute phase response in, 70
      resolution of, 71
      septic shock and, 70–71
   chronic inflammation and, 71
   laboratory features of, 71–72
      C-reactive protein as, 72
      erythrocyte sedimentation rate and,
         72
      plasma viscosity as, 72
Inflammatory rheumatic diseases
   biologics for, 1006, 1006f, 1007b
   in pregnancy, 1280–1281
      anti-phospholipid syndrome as,
         1281
      rheumatoid arthritis as, 1280
      systemic lupus erythematosus as,
         1281, 1281b
      systemic sclerosis as, 1280–1281,
         1281b
Infliximab
   for inflammatory bowel disease, 821b,
      823
   for musculoskeletal disease, 1007b
   in pregnancy, 1278
Influenza, 240–241
   avian, 241
   clinical features of, 241
   diagnosis of, 241
   epidemic, 104
   immunisation for, 115b
   incubation period of, 111b
   management and prevention of, 241
   prophylaxis for, 119b
   swine, 241
Infraorbital artery, 1168
Infrapatellar bursitis, 999b
Inhalation ('humidifier') fever, 616b,
   617
Inhalational administration, 17–18
Inheritance
   autosomal dominant, 46–47
   autosomal recessive, 48
   mitochondrial, 49
   pedigrees, 46f
   X-linked, 48–49
Inherited cancer predisposition
   syndromes, 56–57, 57b
Inherited metabolic myopathies, 1144,
   1144b
Inherited thrombophilia, 977–979
Inherited tubulo-interstitial diseases,
   404, 404b
Inhibin, 633f
Inhibitor of kappa B kinase (IKK),
   64–66
Innate immune system, 62–67
   complement and, 66
   cytokines and, 64–66, 65b, 65f
   dendritic cells in, 64
   integrins and, 66
   mast cells and basophils, 66–67
   natural killer cells and, 67
   phagocytes in, 63–64, 63f
   physical barriers in, 62–67
Inorganic micronutrients, 716–718
Insect bites, 230
Insect stings, allergic reactions, 75b
Insect venom allergy, 85
Insecticides
   carbamate, 146–147
   organophosphorus, 145–146, 145b,
      145f
   pyrethroid, 148b
Insertions, 42
Insight, lack of, 1183
Insomnia
   fatal familial, 1127b
   sporadic fatal, 1127b

Inspiration, of lungs, 548
Insulin
    adverse reactions of, 22b
    amino acid structure of, 748–749, 749f
    manufacture and formulation of, 748–749
    metabolic actions of, 723b
    puberty and, 1290
    reference range of, 1359b
    resistance to, pregnancy and, 1272–1273
    secretion of, 724f
        regulation of, 723–724
    synthesis of, 724, 724f
Insulin-like growth factor (IGF), 633f, 849f
Insulin-like growth factor binding protein (IGF-BP3), 633f
Insulin pump, 751, 751f
Insulin resistance
    polycystic ovarian syndrome, 658b
    in type 2 diabetes, 730–731
Insulin therapy
    closed loop, 751, 752f
    for diabetes mellitus, 748–751
        dosing regimens in, 750, 750f, 751b
        subcutaneous, 749–750, 749b
    for diabetic ketoacidosis, 737
    injection sites of, 721b
    preparations for, duration of action of, 748–749, 749b
    side-effects of, 750b
Insulin tolerance test, for Hypopituitarism, 682b
Insulitis, 728, 729f
Integrade inhibitors, 324b
Integrase, 309–310
Integrins, 66
Intensive care
    clinical management in, 208–211
        blood transfusion in, 211
        clinical review in, 208–209
        delirium in, 209
        extubation in, 210
        glucose control in, 210–211
        nutrition in, 210
        peptic ulcer prophylaxis in, 211
        sedation and analgesia in, 209, 209b
        thromboprophylaxis in, 210
        tracheostomy in, 210, 210b
        weaning from respiratory support in, 209–210
    discharge from, 213, 214b
    withdrawal of active treatment and death in, 213
Intention tremor, 1069
Intercellular adhesion molecule type 1(ICAM-1), 447
Intercostal tube drainage, 626–627, 627f
Interferon
    pegylated, 877
    warts, 1239
Interferon-α, 65b
Interferon-alfa
    for hepatitis B, 876
    pegylated, for hepatitis C, 878
    polycythaemia rubra vera, 970
Interferon-gamma (IFN-γ), 65b
    in coeliac disease, 806f
Interferon-gamma release assays (IGRAs), 594, 594f
Interleukin, immune response, 65b
Intermediate-density lipoproteins, 371–372
Intermediate syndrome, from OP poisoning, 146
Intermittent claudication, 502
Intermittent positive pressure ventilation, 203–204
International Autoimmune Hepatitis Group (IAIHG) criteria, 886
International normalised ratio (INR), 850, 922
International Prostate Symptom Score (IPSS), 438b

International staging system (ISS), for multiple myeloma, 968
International system of units (SI units), 1358
Interpersonal psychotherapy, 1191
Interphalangeal joints, osteoarthritis in, 1009f
Interstitial and infiltrative pulmonary diseases, 605–613
    diffuse parenchymal lung disease (DPLD), 605–610, 605b, 606f, 607b
    due to irradiation and drugs, 612–613
    due to systemic inflammatory disease, 610–611
    in old age, 613b
    pulmonary eosinophilia and vasculitides, 611–612, 611b
    rare interstitial lung diseases, 613b
Interstitial cells of Cajal, 772
Interstitial lung disease, systemic sclerosis and, 1038
Interstitial nephritis
    acute, 402, 402b, 402f
    chronic, 402–403, 403b
    drug-induced, 427b
Interstitial pneumonia
    acute, 606f
    desquamative, 606b
    lymphocytic, 606b
    usual, 608f
Interstitial pneumonitis
    lymphoid, 319
    usual, 608f
Intertrigo, 300, 1240
Intervertebral disc, 986
    prolapse of, 996–997
Intervertebral discs
    intra-articular, 987
Intestinal defence mechanisms, 770f
Intestinal failure (IF), 708–710
    causes of, 708–709
    classification of, 708–709
    management of, 709–710, 709b
        in jejunostomy patients, 709
        in jejunum-colon patients, 709
        in small bowel and multivisceral transplantation, 710, 710b
Intestinal microbiota, 771
Intestinal tapeworm, 298
Intra-aortic balloon pump, 207
Intra-articular discs, 987
Intra-articular glucocorticoids, for musculoskeletal disease, 1005–1006
Intra-articular injections, for osteoarthritis, 1012
Intracellular fluid (ICF), 349
Intracerebral haemorrhage, 1154–1155, 1155f
    causes of, 1155b
Intracranial hypertension, idiopathic, 1133
Intracranial mass lesions, 1127–1133
Intracranial pressure (ICP)
    measurement of, 208
    raised, 1127–1129, 1128b, 1128f
Intramuscular administration, 17
Intramuscular androgen replacement therapy, 656b
Intramuscular glucocorticoids, for musculoskeletal disease, 1005–1006
Intranasal administration, 17
Intraretinal microvascular abnormalities (IRMAs), 1175
Intravascular haemolysis, 946b, 947
Intravenous administration, 17
Intravenous fluid therapy, 353
Intravenous urography (IVU), 389
    for retroperitoneal fibrosis, 434
Intrinsic factor, glycoprotein, 767
Introns, 39f
Intubation, 203–204
    endotracheal, critically ill patients, 190b, 208
    nasogastric, 805b
    safety during, 203b
    ventilator modes in, 203, 203f

Invasive pulmonary aspergillosis (IPA), 597–598, 598b
Involuntary movements, 1069
Iodide, 634
Iodine, 647, 717
    deficiency, 639b, 647, 717
        pregnancy and, 651b, 1279
    dietary sources of, 717b
    radioactive
        for fetal hypothyroidism, 1279
        for Graves' thyrotoxicosis, 644b, 645
    reference nutrient intake of, 717b
    for thyroid neoplasia, 649
Iodine-associated thyroid disease, 647–648
Iodine-induced thyroid dysfunction, 647
Iodine therapy, for differentiated carcinoma, 649–650
Iodoquinol, 129
Ion channels, drugs acting on, 15b
Ion-selective electrodes, 348b
Ionising radiation, 164, 164f
Ipratropium bromide, asthma, 572
Irbesartan, 513
Irinotecan, 832, 842–844
Iris, of eye, 1167
Iron, 716–717
    absorption/uptake, 716–717
    deficiency, 717
    dietary sources of, 717b
    overload, 717
        haemochromatosis, 717
    poisoning from, 140
    reference nutrient intake of, 717b
    reference range of, 1362b
    supplements
        congestive gastropathy, 871
        constipation and, 786b
        in pregnancy, 941b
Iron deficiency anaemia, 923, 940–943
    alimentary tract disorders, 793
    blood loss in, 940–941
    confirmation of, 941–942, 942b
    investigations in, 941–942
        of cause, 942
    malabsorption in, 941, 942f
    management of, 943
    physiological demands in, 941, 941b
    pregnancy and, 1284
Iron oxide, 615b
Irritable bowel syndrome (IBS), 824–826
    clinical features of, 825, 825b
    complementary and alternative therapies for, 826b
    investigations of, 825, 825b
    management of, 825–826, 826f
        dietary, 825b
    pathophysiology of, 824–825
        behavioural and psychosocial factors, 824
        luminal factors, 825
        physiological factors, 824
Irritant eczema, 1247
Ischaemia
    cerebral, 967f
    critical limb, 502–503
    liver, 898
    lower limb, 504b
Ischaemic gut injury, 827
Ischaemic heart disease
    hierarchy of systems applied to, 93b
    levothyroxine replacement in, 641
Ischaemic nephropathy, 406–407
Ischaemic pain, 1350b
Ischaemic penumbra, 1154
Ischiogluteal bursitis, 999b
Islet autoantibodies, 727
Islet cell
    antibodies, in type 1 diabetes, 728
    transplantation of, 752, 753f
Isocyanates, 614b
Isolated gonadotrophin deficiency, 653
Isolation precaution, types of, 113b
Isoleucine, 698b
Isoniazid
    as antimycobacterial agents, 125
    hepatotoxicity, 120b, 894b
    poisoning, 141b

polyneuropathy and, 1139b
prophylactic, 119b
and pyridoxine deficiency, 715
resistance, 118
skin reactions, 1266b
tuberculosis
    HIV/AIDS patients, 324, 324b
    treatment, 592–593, 593b
Isoprenaline, 476–477
    AV block, 478
Isosorbide dinitrate, 490b
Isosorbide mononitrate, 490b
Isotretinoin, 1227
Ispaghula husk, 834
Itch, 1219–1220
ITGB2 gene, loss-of-function mutations in, leucocyte adhesion deficiencies and, 77
Itraconazole, 125b, 126
    acute leukaemia patients, 957
    allergic bronchopulmonary aspergillosis, 596
    chromoblastomycosis, 301
    cutaneous leishmaniasis, 286
    fungal skin infections, 1239–1240
    histoplasmosis, 304
    mycetoma, 301
    P. marneffei infection, 303
    prophylactic, 119b
    sporotrichosis, 301
ITU, referral to, in community-acquired pneumonia, 584b
Ivabradine
    angina, 491
    for heart failure, 467
Ivermectin
    for helminthic infections, 129
    filariasis, 291
    for scabies, 1241
    for strongyloidiasis, 289

J
Jaccoud's arthropathy, 1035
JAK proteins, 64–66
Janus-activated kinase (JAK) inhibitors, for musculoskeletal disease, 1005
Japanese B encephalitis, 249–250
Jarisch-Herxheimer reaction, 339
Jaundice, 860–862, 860b
    acute liver failure and, 857–858
    alcoholic hepatitis and, 881, 881b
    cholecystitis and, 905
    cholestatic, 860b–862b, 861–862
    cirrhosis and, 866–867
    hepatocellular, 860–861
    investigation of, 861f
    obstructive, 861–862
    pre-hepatic, 860
    primary biliary cholangitis and, 887
JC virus, 319–320
Jejunal mucosa, 807f
Jejunostomy patients, intestinal failure and, 709
Jejunum
    coeliac disease see Coeliac disease
    hormones, 772b
    short bowel syndrome, 709b
Jejunum-colon patients, intestinal failure and, 709
Jellyfish, 154b
Jiggers, 299–300
Jod-Basedow effect, 647
Joint capsule, 987
Joint disease
    crystal-associated, 1012–1018, 1013b, 1013f
    in tuberculosis, 591
Joint hypermobility syndrome, 1349
Joints, 986–987
    aspiration, 988, 988f, 1015, 1017, 1020
    fibrous and fibrocartilaginous, 986
    haemophilia, 1058
    hypermobility, 1059b
    infection, 1019–1021
        neuropathic (Charcot), 1057, 1058f
        in old age, 1020b
    protection, 1001

Joints (Continued)
 replacement
  arthroplasty, 1002b
  for osteoarthritis, 1012
  synovial, 987, 987f
  tumours, 1056–1057
  types of, 986b
Jugular venous pressure, effects of
  respiration on, 447b
Jugular venous pulse
 examination of, 443b
  respiratory system, 546f
  tricuspid regurgitation, 526
Junin and Machupo viruses, 245b
Juvenile absence epilepsy, 1100b
Juvenile dermatomyositis (JDM), 1040
Juvenile idiopathic arthritis (JIA),
  1026–1027
 in adolescence, 1027b
 clinical features of, 1027b
 oligoarticular, 1300
 transition medicine and, 1300
Juvenile myoclonic epilepsy, 1100b
Juvenile polyposis, 829

K

Kala-azar (visceral leishmaniasis),
  282–284, 282f
 clinical features of, 282
 differential diagnosis of, 283
 HIV co-infection, 283–284
 investigations of, 282–283, 282f
 management of, 283
 post-kala-azar, dermal leishmaniasis,
  284, 284f
Kallmann's syndrome, 653
Kaposi's sarcoma, HIV-related, 315,
  316f
Kartagener's syndrome, 550
Karyotype, 38f
Kashin-Beck disease, 1011
Katayama syndrome, 295
Kawasaki disease, 1041–1042
Kayser-Fleischer rings, 896–897
 in Wilson's disease, 1174f
Kco (transfer coefficient for carbon
  monoxide), 555b
Kearns-Sayre syndrome, 1144b
Keloid scar, definition of, 1226
Kennedy's disease, 1093b
Keratan sulphate, 987
Keratin, 1212
Keratinocytes, 1212
Keratoacanthoma, 1234, 1234f
Keratoconjunctivitis sicca
 rheumatoid arthritis, 1024
 Sjögren's syndrome and, 1038
Keratoderma blennorrhagica, 1031
Keratolysis, pitted, 1238
Keratomalacia, 713
Keratosis, actinic, 1230b
Kerion, 1240
Kernig's sign, 1118
Kerosene, poisoning, 148b
Keshan's disease, 718
Ketamine, 1345b
Ketoacidosis, diabetic, 729–730,
  735–738
 in adolescence, 753b
 clinical features of, 736, 736b
 investigations of, 736
 management of, 736–738, 737b
  bicarbonate in, 738
  fluid replacement in, 737
  insulin in, 737
  ongoing, 738
  phosphate in, 738
  potassium in, 738
 pathogenesis of, 735–736, 736b
 severe, indications of, 736b
Ketoconazole, 125b, 126
 Cushing's syndrome, 669
 cutaneous leishmaniasis, 286
 fungal skin infections, 1239–1240
 mycetoma, 301
 paracoccidioidomycosis, 304
 shampoos, 1240
Ketogenesis, 725f
Ketone bodies, 725, 725f

Ketones
 blood, 726, 726b
 urine, 726
Ketonuria, 726
Ketoprofen, 1003b
Kidney
 acid-base balance control, 364
 clinical examination of, 382–384,
  382f–383f
 cystic diseases of, 405–406
 drugs and, 426
 duplex, 434
 functional anatomy and physiology of,
  384–386, 385f
 imaging of, 389–390, 389f
 MRI images of, 406f
 single, 433
 sodium handling, 349
 stones, 431b
 systemic lupus erythematosus in,
  1035
 transplantation, 424
 tumours of, 434–436
Kidney disease
 in adolescence, 426b
 chronic, 415–420, 417b
  causes of, 415b
  haemodialysis in, 422–423
  indications for dialysis for, 422b
  osteodystrophy and, 419f
  physical signs of, 416f
  pregnancy and, 1282, 1283f
  pruritus, 415
  stages of, 388b
  staging of, in children over 2 years
   of age, 1298b
  transition medicine and,
   1298–1299
 medullary sponge, 433
Kidney injury, acute, 411–415
 causes of, 411f
 clinical features of, 411–413
 dialysis for, indications for, 422b
 haemodialysis in, 422
 investigations of, 412b
 management of, 413–414, 413b
 in old age, 414b
 pathophysiology of, 411
 post-renal, 412b, 413
 pre-renal, 411–412, 412b
 pregnancy and, 1282, 1283b
 recovery from, 414–415, 414f
 renal, 412–413, 412b
 renal replacement therapy, 414
Kimmelstiel-Wilson nodule, 758f
Kinase inhibitors, for low-grade NHL,
  965
Kinases, cyclin-dependent, 1317
Klebsiella granulomatis, 341b
Klebsiella oxytoca, 230
Klebsiella pneumoniae, 116
Klebsiella spp., 103f
Klinefelter's syndrome, 44b, 660–661
Knee
 osteoarthritis, 1009–1010, 1010f
 pain, 998–999, 999b
 rheumatoid arthritis, 1023
Knee height, measurement of, 693b
Knudson hypothesis, 56–57
Köbner phenomenon, 1252
Koch's postulates, 100b
Koilonychia, 1261, 1261f
Koplik's spots, 236, 236f
Korsakoff's psychosis, 714
Korsakoff's syndrome, 1081
Krebs (citric acid) cycle, 49, 714
Krukenberg tumour, 804
Kupffer cells, 64, 848, 850f
Kuru, 1127b
Kussmaul breathing, 415
Kussmaul's sign, 544b
Kwashiorkor, 704
Kyasanur fever, 245b
Kyphoplasty, 1002b
 for osteoporosis, 1049
Kyphoscoliosis, 546f
 thoracic, 628
Kyphosis, 591f, 1302f
 ankylosing spondylitis, 1030

L

L-dopa see Levodopa
Labetalol
 aortic dissection, 508
 hypertension, 513
  accelerated, 514
Laboratory investigations, biochemical,
  348–349, 348b
Laboratory reference ranges,
  1357–1364
 of adolescence, 1363
 of adults, 1358
 of childhood, 1363
 in pregnancy, 1364
Labyrinthitis, 1104
Lacrimal gland/lacrimal drainage, 1164
Lactase deficiency, 812
Lactate
 reference range of, venous blood,
  1360b
 sepsis and, 196, 197f
Lactate dehydrogenase (LDH)
 acute kidney injury, 412b
 empyema, 564
 megaloblastic anaemia, 943, 944b
 pancreatitis and, 837b
 pleural effusion, 610
 reference range of, venous blood,
  1360b
Lactation, nutrition in, 712b
Lactic acidosis, 365
Lactitol, 834b
Lactobacillus spp., 103f
Lactoferrin, 62–63, 992
 in acute phase response, 70
Lactose, refeeding diet, 705b
Lactose hydrogen breath test, 812
Lactose intolerance, 812
Lactulose
 for hepatic encephalopathy, 865
 for variceal bleeding, 869b
Lacunar infarctions, 1153
Lacunar syndrome (LACS), 1156f
Lambert-Eaton myasthenic syndrome
  (LEMS), 1142f, 1143,
  1325–1326
Lamina densa, 1212
Lamina lucida, 1212
Laminin, 1212
Lamivudine, 324b
 for hepatitis B, 876
  co-infection with HIV, 877
 resistance, 325
Lamotrigine, 1102b–1103b
Langerhans cell histiocytosis
  (histiocytosis X), 613b
Langerhans' cells, 1212
Language
 disorders, 1089b
 spoken, 1070f
Lanreotide, 686–687
Laparoscopy
 for ascites, 863
 for infertility, 656
 for lower abdominal pain, 336
 for pyrexia of unknown origin,
  219–222
Large-bowel diarrhoea, HIV-related, 317
Large rectal adenomatous polyp, 828f
Laron dwarfism, 680b
Larva currens, 289
Larva migrans
 cutaneous, 294, 294f
 visceral, 233–234
Laryngeal disorders, 624–625
Laryngeal obstruction, 624–625, 624b
Laryngeal paralysis, 624
Laryngoscopy, 553
Lasègue's sign, 1135
Laser therapy
 for bleeding control, 775f
 for colorectal cancer, 832
 for hereditary haemorrhagic
  telangiectasia, 970
 for hypertrichosis, 1259
 for lung cancer, 603
 for oesophageal carcinoma, 797
 for proliferative diabetic retinopathy,
  1176

 for rosacea, 1244
 for skin disease, 1228
Lassa fever, 245b
 incubation period of, 111b
Latent autoimmune diabetes of
  adulthood (LADA), 730
Latent tuberculosis, 1172
 detection of, 594, 594f
Lateral film, of chest X-ray, 551
Lateral humeral epicondylitis, 998b
Latex agglutination test, 301
Lavage
 bronchoalveolar, 609–610
 gastric, 136, 136b
Law, psychiatry and, 1207
Lawrence-Moon-Biedl syndromes, 700
Laxative misuse syndromes, 834
Laxatives, 834b
Lead
 poisoning, 148b
 reference range of, venous blood,
  1360b
Lead pipe rigidity, 1069
Leão, spreading depression of, 1095
Learning difficulties, congenital heart
  disease and, 533
Leber's hereditary optic neuropathy,
  1089f
Lecithin cholesterol acyl transferase
  (LCAT), 375
 deficiency, 375, 375b
Lectin
 mannose-binding
  deficiency, 78
Lectin pathway, for complement, 66
Leflunomide, for musculoskeletal
  disease, 1004b, 1005
Left anterior descending artery (LAD)
 and coronary arteries with a stenosis,
  453f
 in coronary circulation, 444–445, 445f
Left atrial dilatation, 450
Left bundle branch block, 478–479,
  479f
Left main coronary artery, 444–445,
  445f
 occlusion, 445
Left ventricular dilatation, 450
Left ventricular hypertrophy, 523f
Legal considerations, in artificial
  nutritional support, 710b
Legionella pneumophila infection, 106,
  117b
Legionella spp., 114b, 119b
Legs
 examination of, 982f–983f
  cardiology, 442f
  diabetes mellitus, 720f
  endocrine disease, 630f
  febrile injecting drug user, 222f
  HIV/AIDS, 306f
  liver and biliary disease, 846f
 liver and biliary disease and, 846f
 oedema and, 395–396
  examination of, respiratory system,
   546f
 ulcers, 1223–1224
  causes of, 1223b, 1223f
  clinical assessment of, 1223–1224
  due to arterial disease, 1223–1224
  due to neuropathy, 1224
  due to vasculitis, 1224
  due to venous disease, 1223,
   1223f
  investigations in, 1224
  management of, 1224
Leigh's syndrome, 49
Leishman-Donovan body (amastigotes),
  282f
Leishmania, 281
 life cycle of, 281–282, 282f
 Viannia subgenus, 285
Leishmania aethiopica, 284
Leishmania amazonensis, 285
Leishmania brasiliensis, 285
Leishmania chagasi, 282, 282f
Leishmania donovani, 282, 282f
Leishmania guyanensis, 285
Leishmania infantum, 282, 282f

Leishmania major, 284
Leishmania mexicana, 285
Leishmania tropica, 284
Leishmaniasis, 281–286, 1238
  cutaneous, 284–285, 285b, 285f
    incubation period of, 111b
  dermal, post-kala-azar, 284, 284f
  epidemiology and transmission of, 281–282, 281f–282f
  mucosal, 285
  prevention and control of, 284
  visceral, 282–284, 282f
    clinical features of, 282
    differential diagnosis of, 283
    HIV co-infection, 283–284
    incubation period of, 111b
    investigations of, 282–283, 282f
    management of, 283
Lemierre's syndrome, 586–587
Lenalidomide, for multiple myeloma, 968
Lens, of eye, 1168
Lentigo, 1234
Leprosy, 267–270, 267f
  borderline cases of, 269
  clinical features of, 268–269, 268b, 269f
  epidemiology and transmission of, 267
  granulomas in, 71
  incubation period of, 111b
  investigations of, 269
  management of, 269–270, 269b–270b
  pathogenesis of, 267–268
  patient education of, 270
  prevention and control of, 270
  prognosis of, 270
  reactions, 268–269, 268b
  tuberculoid, 267–268
Leptin, 694
Leptosphaera senegalensis, 301
Leptospira interrogans, 257
Leptospirosis, 257–259, 880
  aseptic meningitis, 257
  bacteraemic, 257
  clinical features of, 257–258, 258f
  diagnosis of, 258
  icteric, 258
  management and prevention of, 258–259
  microbiology and epidemiology of, 257
Lesch-Nyhan syndrome, 1014
Leucine, 698b
Leucocyte adhesion deficiencies, 77
Leucocytes, 917
Leucocytosis, 926–927
  cholecystitis and, 905
  choledocholithiasis and, 906
  hepatobiliary disease and, 853
  in inflammation, 71–72
  pyogenic liver abscess and, 880
Leucoencephalopathy, progressive multifocal, 1123
  HIV-associated, 319–320, 320f
Leucoerythroblastic anaemia, 969
Leuconychia, striate, 1260
Leucopenia, 925–926
  hepatobiliary disease and, 853
Leukaemias, 954–961
  acute, 955–958
    haematopoietic stem cell transplantation for, 958
    investigations of, 955–956, 956f
    management of, 956–958
    outcome of, 958b
    prognosis of, 958
    specific therapy for, 956–957, 956b–957b
    supportive therapy for, 957–958
    WHO classification of, 955b
  in children, 1298
  chronic lymphocytic, 959–960
    clinical features of, 959
    investigations of, 959–960
    management of, 960
    prognosis of, 960
    staging of, 960b

chronic myeloid, 958–959
  accelerated phase, management of, 959
  blast crisis, management of, 959
  characteristics of, 958
  chronic phase, management of, 959, 959b
  clinical features of, 958
  investigations of, 959
  management of, 959
  natural history of, 958
  epidemiology and aetiology of, 954–955
  hairy cell, 960
  prolymphocytic, 960
  risk factors for, 955b
  terminology and classification of, 955, 955b
Leukoplakia, hairy, 316
Leukotriene receptor antagonists, asthma, 571f, 572
Leukotrienes, 66–67
Levator palpebrae superioris, 1164
Levetiracetam, 1100b
  in pregnancy, 1103b
Levodopa
  adverse reactions, chorea, 1085
  for Parkinson's disease, 1113–1114
Levofloxacin, 117b, 123b
  plague, 259
Levothyroxine
  hypothyroidism management, 640–641, 641b
  in ischaemic heart disease, 641
Lewy body dementia, 1194
Leydig cell tumours, 439
LH see Luteinising hormone
Li-Fraumeni syndrome, 1321b
Libman-Sacks endocarditis, 1035
Lice
  body, 1241
  head, 1241
  pubic (crab), 1241
  relapsing fever, 256b, 257, 257f
Lichen planus, 1252
  clinical features of, 1252, 1252f
  investigations of, 1252
  management of, 1252
  in nails, 1261
  pathogenesis of, 1252
  rash, 334b
  rash in, 1217b
  vulval pain/itch, 336b
Lichen sclerosus, 334b, 336b
Lichen simplex, 1247
Lichenoid eruptions, drug-induced, 1252, 1266b
Liddle's syndrome, 361
Lidocaine
  arrhythmias, 480, 480b
  effect in old age, 32b
  in renal/hepatic disease, 32b
Life course, 93
Life expectancy, 92, 1304, 1304b
Life support
  advanced, 457, 458f
  basic, 456–457, 457f
Lifestyle advice, for obesity, 701
Lifestyle changes
  for chronic kidney disease, 420
  for dyslipidaemia, 375
Lifestyle factors
  ageing, 1305
  cancer, 1316
  diabetes mellitus, 743–745
  weight management, 744
Lifestyle interventions, for musculoskeletal disease, 1000–1001
  in gout, 1016
  in osteoarthritis, 1012
Ligaments, 987
Ligand assay, 348b
Likelihood ratios (LR), 3, 3f
Limb girdle dystrophy, 1143b
Limbic encephalitis, 1111b
Limbic (emotional) influences, in control of breathing, 549
Limbic system, 1066

Limbs
  lower see Legs
  upper see Arms
Linagliptin, 747
Lincomycin, 29
Lincosamides, 122
  antibiotics, 121–122
  mechanism of action, 116b
Lindane, 148b
Linear accelerators, 1331
Linear IgA disease, 1255b, 1256–1257
Linezolid, 117b, 124
  in pneumonia, 587
  in pregnancy, 120b
Linitis plastica, 804
Linoleic acid, 697
Linolenic acid, 697
Lipase, 770b
Lipid emulsion therapy, 136–137
Lipid-lowering therapy
  for acute coronary syndrome, 501
  chronic kidney disease, 420
  for dyslipidaemia, 375
Lipid peroxidation, 1305
Lipids, 370–378
  acute kidney injury and, 416b
  cardiovascular disease and, 373
  dietary, 371
  endogenous, 372f
  measurement, 373
  metabolism, 370–378, 850
    disorders of, 370
    effects of insulin in, 723b
    presenting problems in, 373–375
  transport, 372f
  see also Fats
Lipodermatosclerosis, 1223
Lipodystrophy, 326, 326f
Lipohypertrophy, 721b
Lipolysis, 694
Lipomas
  skin, 1235
  small intestine and, 813
Lipopeptides, 123
Lipoprotein lipase, 371–372
  deficiency, 374b
Lipoproteins
  high-density (HDL), 1360b
  intermediate-density, 371–372
  low-density, 371–372
  metabolism, 370–378
  structure of, 371f
  very low-density, 371–372
Liquorice, excessive intake of, 361
Liraglutide, for obesity, 702–703, 702f
Lisch nodule, 1132b
Lisinopril
  heart failure, 466b
  hypertension, 513
Listeria monocytogenes
  bacterial meningitis from, 1119
  listeriosis from, 259
Listeriosis, 259–260
  in pregnancy, 235b
Lisuride, for Parkinson's disease, 1114b
Lithium
  for cluster headache, 1096
  drug interactions of, 24, 24b
  hypothyroidism and, 639b
  nephrotoxicity, 427b
  plasma interactions of, 36b
  poisoning from, 139
  prescribing, 32b
  skin reactions, 1266b
  teratogenesis, 1200
Lithium carbonate, for bipolar disorder, 1200
Livedo reticularis, 1035, 1036f
Liver
  abscess, 879–880, 893
    amoebic, 880
    in old age, 901b
    pyogenic, 879–880, 880b
  biopsy of, 855, 855b
    for hepatocellular carcinoma, 891
    for non-alcoholic fatty liver, 884
  blood supply to, 848–849, 848f
  cells see Hepatocytes
  drugs and, 893–895

fatty
  alcoholic, 881, 881b
  non-alcoholic, 882–885, 883f, 885f
  fibrosis of, 894
    cirrhosis and, 866, 866f
    congenital, 868f, 902
    non-invasive markers of, 855
    pathogenic mechanisms in, 849f
  function of, 850–851, 850f
  functional anatomy and physiology of, 848–851
  HIV infection and, 879
  infections of, 871–880
  injury to
    drug-induced, 894–895, 894b
    types of, 894–895
  ischaemia, 898
  nodular regenerative hyperplasia of, 899
  size of
    assessment for, 847b
    change in, causes of, 862b
  structure of, 848–849, 848f
  transplantation of, 900–901
    for acute liver failure, 858–859
    for alcoholic liver disease, 882
    for Budd-Chiari syndrome, 899
    for cirrhosis, 867
    complications of, 901
    for hepatic encephalopathy, 865
    for hepatitis B, 876
    for hepatitis C, 878
    for hepatocellular carcinoma, 891
    indications and contraindications for, 900–901, 900b, 901f
    living donor, 901
    orthotopic, 890
    for primary biliary cholangitis, 888
    for primary sclerosing cholangitis, 890
    prognosis for, 901
    split liver, 901
    for Wilson's disease, 897
  tumours, metastatic, 1328–1329
Liver capsule pain, 1350b
Liver disease
  abdominal signs in, history and significance of, 847
  alcoholic, 880–882
    fatty, 881
    liver function test (LFT) abnormality in, 854b
    in old age, 901b
    risk factors for, 880
  autoimmune, 885–890
  bleeding, 975
  chronic, 853b
    hepatitis B and, 873
    cirrhosis see Cirrhosis
  clinical examination for, 846f
  clinical features of, 847b
  cystic, 893, 893f
  decompensated, 867
  drug-induced, liver function test (LFT) abnormality in, 854b
  HIV-related, 317–318
  hydatid cyst and, 880
  inherited, 895–897
    haemochromatosis as, 895–896
  investigation of, 852–855, 852b
  in old age, 901b
  pregnancy and, 899–900, 1283–1284
    acute fatty liver as, 1283, 1283b
    obstetric cholestasis as, 1284
    viral hepatitis as, 1284
  prescribing in, 32, 32b
  presentation of, 856b
  presenting problems of, 855–866, 856f
  pruritus and, 1219b
  silent presentation of, 847b
  tumours as, 890–893
    benign, 893
    primary malignant, 890–892
    secondary malignant, 892–893, 893f
  vascular, 898–899
  Wilson's disease and, 896

Liver failure
  acute, 856–859
    adverse prognostic criteria in, 858b
    causes of, 856f–857f
    classification of, 857b
    clinical assessment of, 857–858
    complications of, 858b
    hepatic encephalopathy and, 857b
    hepatitis A and, 873
    investigations for, 858, 858b
    management of, 858–859, 858b
    pathophysiology of, 857
  chronic
    causes of, 856f, 867b
    cirrhosis and, 867
  fulminant, hepatitis B and, 875
  hepatic encephalopathy, 856–857
Liver flukes, 233b, 297, 297b
Liver function tests, 852
  abnormal, 859–860, 859b
    asymptomatic, 859f
    HIV infection and, 879b
    identifying the cause of, 854b
    in pregnancy, 900b
  cholestatic/obstructive, 853b
  for gastrointestinal bleeding, 781
  hepatitic, 853b
  for hepatitis C, 877
Loa loa, 233b, 290b, 292
Loading dose, 19
Local glucocorticoid injections, for
      ankylosing spondylitis, 1031
Localised lymphadenopathy, 927
'Locked-in' syndrome, 211
Lockjaw, 1126
Lofexidine, 1196
Löfgren's syndrome, 608–609
Loiasis, 233b, 292
Loin pain, 396
Long QT syndrome, 476
Long-term domiciliary oxygen therapy
      (LTOT), for chronic obstructive
      pulmonary disease (COPD), 577
Loop diuretics, for hypervolaemia,
      354–355
Loop of Henle, 350, 384–386
Looser's zones, 1052
Loperamide
  for faecal incontinence, 835
  for inflammatory bowel disease,
      821b
  intussusception and, 230
  for irritable bowel syndrome, 826f
  for radiation enteritis, 810
  for short bowel syndrome, 808–809
  for small bowel bacterial overgrowth,
      808–809
Lopinavir, 324b
Loratadine, 622, 1254
Lorazepam
  disturbed behaviour, 1189f
  palliative care, 1353
  status epilepticus, 1081b
Loricrin, 1212
Losartan, 58
Loss-of-function mutations, 44
Loss of vision, of ophthalmic disease,
      1170–1171, 1170b
Lotions, 1225b
Louse-borne relapsing fever, 256b, 257,
      257f
Low back pain
  assessment of, 988–989
  causes of, 996b
  mechanical, features of, 996b
  radicular, 997b
Low birth weight, and disease
      susceptibility, 93
Low-density lipoproteins, 371–372
Low-dose dexamethasone suppression
      test (LDDST), in Cushing's
      syndrome, 668
Low-grade tumours, 603
Low-molecular-weight heparins
      (LMWHs), 922, 938–939, 938b
  for venous thromboembolism, 975
Low mood, 1185–1186
  alcohol misuse and, 1194
Lower airway defences, 550

Lower limbs
  examination, diabetes mellitus, 721b
  ischaemia, 504b
  see also Foot/feet; Legs
Lower oesophageal sphincter,
      abnormalities of, 791
Lubiprostone, 825
Lumbar canal stenosis, 1135–1136
Lumbar disc herniation, 1135, 1135f
Lumbar nerve root compression, 1135f
Lumbar puncture, 1077–1078
  for meningitis, 1118
  for stroke, 1152
  for viral encephalitis, 1118
Lumbar spondylosis, 1135–1136
Lumbosacral plexopathy, 1141
Lumefantrine, for malaria, 128
Lumps, skin, 1216
Lung(s)
  abscess, 170f, 219f, 251f
  biopsy
    in interstitial pneumonias, 607
    pleural effusion, 563–564
  cavitation of, 551b
  collapse
    by bronchial obstruction, 552f
    upper lobe, 547f
  consolidation of, 551b
  defences, 550, 550f
  fibrosis see Pulmonary fibrosis
  functional anatomy and physiology of,
      548–550, 548f–549f
  gas exchange in, 549–550, 549f
  inflammatory arthritis in, 994b
  innate response of, 550
  irradiation and, 612–613
  mechanics, 549
  near drowning accidents and, 169
  near-drowning victims, 169
  shrinking, 610b, 611
  systemic lupus erythematosus in,
      1035
  transplantation, 567, 567b
  tumours of, 598–605
    metastatic, 1328
    primary, 599–603
    secondary, 603
  volumes, 555
Lung cancer, 599–603, 599f
  burden of, 598b
  cell types in, 599b
  clinical features of, 599–601
  investigations of, 601–602
  management of, 602–603
  non-metastatic extrapulmonary
      manifestations of, 601b
  occupational, 618
  pathology of, 599, 599f
  prognosis for, 603, 603b
Lung disease
  alveolar
    microlithiasis, 613b
    proteinosis, 613b
  diffuse parenchymal, 605–610
  drug-induced, 612–613, 612b
  due to organic dusts, 616–617,
      616b
  due to systemic inflammatory
      disease, 610–611
  dust exposure and, 614–615, 615b
  HIV-related, 318–319, 318b
  infection, 581–598
  interstitial, 605–613
  investigation of, 550–556
  obstructive, 573–578
    in old age, 578b
  occupational, 613–619
  presenting problems of, 556–567
  radiotherapy-induced, 612
  rheumatoid arthritis, 1024
  tumours, 598–605
    secondary, 603
  vascular, 619–622
Lung flukes, 233b
Lung injury, ventilator-induced, 204
Lupus anticoagulant, 920–921
Lupus erythematosus, 1221b, 1262
  bullous, 1255b
  drug-induced, 1266b

  systemic, 410–411, 1034–1037
    classification of, criteria for, 1036b
    clinical features of, 1035–1036
    investigations of, 1036
    management of, 1036–1037
    pathophysiology of, 1034
    pregnancy and, 1281, 1281b
    respiratory involvement in, 611
Lupus nephritis, 392b
Lupus pernio, 609f, 610
Luteinising hormone (LH)
  deficiency, 680b
  puberty and, 1290
  reference range of, 1359b
Lyme disease, 255–256, 256b, 256f,
      1125
  myopericarditis, 538
Lymecycline, 1243
Lymph node biopsy, in Hodgkin
      lymphoma, 962, 963f
Lymph nodes, 67
  diphtheria, 266
  of envenomed patient, 152f
  examination of, cancer, 1314, 1315b
  normal architecture of, 961, 961f
  trypanosomiasis, 279
  tuberculosis and, 590
Lymphadenitis, 590
Lymphadenopathy, 913b, 927, 927b
  HIV-related, 313
  persistent generalised, 313
  rheumatoid arthritis, 1024–1025
Lymphangiectasia, intestinal, 811
Lymphangioleiomyomatosis, 613b
Lymphangitic carcinomatosis, 603
Lymphatic filariasis, 290–292
Lymphatics, 67
Lymphocytes, 917, 926b, 926f
  count, 1362b
  older people, 923b
  see also B lymphocytes; T
      lymphocytes
Lymphocytic interstitial pneumonia,
      606b
Lymphocytosis, 926b, 927
  infectious mononucleosis, 241
Lymphogranuloma venereum (LGV),
      341b
Lymphoid interstitial pneumonitis, 319
Lymphoid organs, 67
Lymphoid tissue
  gastrointestinal mucosa-associated,
      769–770
  mucosa-associated, 67
Lymphomas, 650, 961–966, 961f
  B-cell, 805
  cutaneous, 1232
  gastric, 805
  gastrointestinal tract and, 813
  Hodgkin, 961–964, 962f
    classification of, 962b
    clinical features of, 962
    epidemiology of, 961, 962b
    investigations of, 962, 963f
    management of, 962–964
    prognosis of, 964, 964b
    stages of, 962b
  MALT, 769–770
  non-Hodgkin, 964–966, 965f
    clinical features of, 964, 965f
    epidemiology of, 964, 964b
    high-grade management of, 966
    investigations of, 964–965
    low-grade management of, 965
    management of, 965–966
    prognosis of, 966
  primary CNS, 320, 320f
  T-cell
    cutaneous, 1224
    enteropathy-associated, 813
    thyroid, 646
Lymphopenia, 925–926, 926b
  HIV infection, 311–312
  sarcoidosis and, 609–610
Lymphoproliferative syndrome,
      autoimmune, 80
Lynch's syndrome, 46
d-Lysergic acid diethylamide, 144, 144f
Lysine, 698b

Lysolecithin, 905
Lysosomal storage diseases, 370, 371b
Lysosomes, 370
Lysozyme, 62–63

M
Machado-Joseph disease, genetics,
      43b
Machupo virus, 245b
Macrocytic anaemia, 925
Macrocytosis, 853, 921f, 941f
Macroglobulinaemia, Waldenström, 966
Macrolides, 117b, 121–122
  mechanism of action, 116b
Macronutrients (energy-yielding
      nutrients), 695–697
  dietary recommendations for, 697,
      698b
Macrophage colony stimulating factor
      (M-CSF), 1022–1023, 1022f
Macrophages, 64, 550
  alveolar, 303, 615
  foamy, 430, 809
  functions of, 64b
  in gastrointestinal tract, 769–770
Macroprolactin, 684
Macroprolactinaemia, 684, 684b
Macroprolactinomas, pregnancy and,
      1280
Macules
  café au lait, 1131f
  definition of, 1211f
Maculopathy, diabetic, 721
Maddrey score, 882
Madopar, 1113
Madura foot, 301
Madurella grisea, 301
Madurella mycetomatis, 301
Magic (hallucinogenic) mushrooms, 143,
      1196
Magnesium, 718
  dietary sources of, 717b
  homeostasis, 367–368
  intravenous
    acute severe asthma, 573
    arrhythmias, 140
    tetany, 663b
    torsades de pointes, 476–477
  metabolism, disorders of, 367–368
  refeeding diet, 705b
  reference nutrient intake of, 717b
  reference range of, venous blood,
      1360b
Magnesium ammonium phosphate
      stones, 431b
Magnesium chloride, 368
Magnesium salts, 368
Magnesium sulphate
  asthma, 573f
  hypomagnesaemia, 368
  pre-eclampsia, 1276
  ventricular tachycardia, 137b
Magnetic resonance angiography (MRA)
  in nervous system, 1072
  renal artery stenosis, 407, 407f
  stroke, 1157b
  urinary tract disease, 389
Magnetic stimulation, 1077
Magnifying glass, 1214
Main d'accoucheur, 663
Main en lorgnette, 1033
Major haemorrhage, transfusion in,
      931b
Major histocompatibility complex (MHC),
      851, 1028–1029, 1248
Malabsorption, 783–785, 784f, 785b,
      942f
  after gastric resection, 783–785
  after ileal resection, 706
  biliary cirrhosis, 888
  of chronic pancreatitis, 841
  cystic fibrosis, 581
  disorders causing, 805–810
  investigations of, 785, 785b, 785f
  iron deficiency anaemia, 941, 942f
  in old age, 808b
  pathophysiology of, 784–785
  primary biliary cholangitis and, 888
Maladie de Roger, 535–536

Malar flush, 442f
Malar rash, of systemic lupus
   erythematosus, 1035f
Malaria, 273–277
   algid, 276b
   cerebral, 276b
   chemoprophylaxis of, 277, 278b
   clinical features of, 274b, 275–276,
      275f
   complicated, 277
   control in endemic areas, 277
   distribution of, 273f
   exchange transfusion, 277
   haemolysis, 274–275
   incubation period, 111b, 274b
   investigations of, 276
   management of, 277, 277b
   mild, 277
   non-falciparum, 277
   pathogenesis of, 273–275
   pathology of, 274–275
   in pregnancy, 235b
   prevention of, 277
   sickle-cell anaemia, 951
   treatment of, 128
   vector control, 323
Malarial parasite, life cycle of, 273–274,
   274f
Malarone, 278b
Malassezia, 103f, 1240
Malassezia furfur, 1240
Malathion
   louse infestation, 1241
   scabies, 1241
Male
   hypogonadism in, 655, 656b, 660b
   reproductive system of, 651, 651f
Malignancy, pruritus and, 1219b
Malignant disease, rheumatological
   manifestations of, 1057,
   1057b
Malignant hyperpyrexia, 195
Malignant plasma cells, 967
Malingering, 1206
Mallory-Denk bodies, 884
Mallory-Weiss syndrome, 177b
Mallory-Weiss tears, 781f
Mallory's hyaline, 884
Malnutrition
   in dementia, 711, 711f
   risk of, screening for, 693f
   see also Under-nutrition
MALT (mucosa-associated lymphoid
   tissue), 769–770
MALT lymphomas, 964
Malt worker's lung, 616b
Mammary artery grafts, 491–492
Mammography, 1333
Manganese, 718
Mania, 1186
Mannitol, 355
Mannose-binding lectin deficiency, 78
Mansonella perstans infection, 233b,
   293
Mansonella streptocerca, 290b
Mantle cell lymphoma, 964
MAOI-B inhibitors, for Parkinson's
   disease, 1114
Maple bark stripper's lung, 616b
Marasmus, 704
Maraviroc, 324b
March haemoglobinuria, 950
Marche à petits pas, 1087
Marcus Gunn pupil, 1092b
Marfan's syndrome, 508
   cardiovascular system
      aortic aneurysm, 505, 506f
      aortic dissection, 506, 507b
      mitral valve prolapse, 520
      congenital defects, 531–532
      mutation, 508
Marine poisonous animals,
   envenomation of, 162
Marine venomous animals,
   envenomation of, 162
Marjolin's ulcer, 1021, 1223
Mass spectroscopy (MS), 348b
   inductively coupled, 348b

Massive small bowel resection,
   under-nutrition and, 706
Mast cell tryptase, 86
Mast cells, 66–67
   degranulation of, clinical features of,
      75b
Mastectomy, 1334
Maternal medicine, 1269–1285
   adrenal disease in, 1280
   cardiac disease in, 1282
   clinical evaluation in, 1271, 1271f
   clinical examination in, 1270,
      1270f–1271f
   diabetes in, 1278–1279
      gestational, 1278, 1278b
   endocrine disease in, 1279–1280
   functional anatomy and physiology in,
      1272–1273
      bone metabolism and, 1272
      cardiovascular system and, 1272
      endocrine system and, 1272
      gastrointestinal system and, 1272
      genitourinary system and, 1272
      glucose metabolism in, 1272–1273
      haematological system and, 1273
      respiratory system and, 1273
   gastrointestinal disease in,
      1277–1278
   haematological disease in,
      1284–1285
   human immunodeficiency virus
      infection in, 1280
   hypertension in, 1276–1277
   imaging and, 1274
   inflammatory rheumatic disease in,
      1280–1281
   investigations in, 1274, 1274b
   liver disease and, 1283–1284
   medical disorders in pregnancy and,
      1276–1285
   neurological disease in, 1284
   parathyroid disease in, 1280
   pituitary disease in, 1280
   planning pregnancy in, for patients
      with medical conditions, 1272
   presenting problems in pregnancy
      and, 1274–1276
      breathlessness as, 1274–1275
      chest pain as, 1275
      circulatory collapse as, 1275
      headache as, 1275
      nausea and vomiting as, 1275,
         1275b
      oedema as, 1275
      seizures as, 1275–1276, 1276b
   psychiatric disorders in, 1284
   renal disease in, 1282–1283
   respiratory disease in, 1277
   thyroid disease in, 1279
Matrix metalloproteinases, 485–486
Mayaro viruses, 250, 1020–1021
McArdle's disease, 1144b
McCune-Albright syndrome, 50–51,
   1055, 1056f
Meal bolus calculation, 751b
Mean arterial pressure (MAP),
   calculation of, 193b
Mean cell haemoglobin (MCH),
   919–920, 1362b
Mean cell volume (MCV), 853, 919–920
   in alcohol misuse, 1184
   in anaemias, 940
   reference range of, 1362b
Measles, 236
   clinical features of, 236, 236f
   management of, 236
   in pregnancy, 235b
   prevention of, 236
   rash, 236f
   subacute sclerosing panencephalitis,
      236
Mebendazole, for helminthic infections,
   129
Mechanical heart valves, 950
   pregnancy and, 1282
Meckel's diverticulum, 778, 812
   bleeding from, 782b
Meckel's scan, 778b
Meconium ileus, 842

Medial collateral ligament lesions,
   998b–999b
Medial fibroplasia, 407
Medial humeral epicondylitis, 998b
Medial longitudinal fasciculus (MLF),
   1069–1070
Median nerve
   entrapment, 1139b
   palsy, 760
Mediastinal spread, in lung cancer, 600
Mediastinoscopy, 604
Mediastinum
   divisions of, 604f
   tumours of, 603–605, 603b–604b,
      604f
Medical emergency team, deterioration
   and, 188, 189b
Medical interview, 231b
Medical ophthalmology, 1163–1178
   functional anatomy and physiology of,
      1164–1168
   ophthalmic disease, presenting
      problems in, 1169–1171
   specialist ophthalmological conditions
      in, 1171–1178
   visual disorders, investigation of,
      1168–1169
Medical psychiatry, 1179–1207
Medically unexplained somatic
   symptoms, 1187, 1187b, 1205f
   general management principles for,
      1202, 1203b
   in old age, 1189b
Medication, of stroke patients, 1159b
Medication errors, 24–26
   causes of, 25, 25b, 25f
   response to, 26
   types of, 25b
Medication overuse
   headache, 1096
   migraine and, 1095
Medicines management, 26
Medroxyprogesterone, 655
Medullary carcinoma, 650
Medullary cystic kidney disease, 404
Medullary sponge kidney disease, 433
Medulloblastoma, 1129
Mefenamic acid, overdose, 138
Mefloquine, for malaria, 278b
Megacolon
   acquired, 835
   toxic, 818
Megakaryoblasts, 915f, 918
Megakaryocytes, 918
Megaloblastic anaemia, 940, 943–945
   clinical features of, 943b
   investigations in, 944b
   management of, 945
Megaloblastic crisis, 947
Megaureter, 434
Megestrol, 1332
Meglitinides, 746b, 747
Meglumine antimoniate, 128
Meiosis, 40–41, 41f
Meissner's plexus, 771–772
Melaena, 780
Melanocortin-4 receptor (MC4R)
   mutations, 700
Melanocytes, 1212
Melanocytic naevi, 1216, 1234–1235,
   1235f
Melanoma, 1232–1234
   ABCDE rule of, 1216, 1216b
   acral lentiginous, 1233
   amelanotic, 1322
   clinical features of, 1232–1233
   cutaneous, 1232b
   diagnosis and management of, 1233
   lentigo maligna, 1233
   malignant, 1216
   nodular, 1233, 1233f
   pathophysiology of, 1232
   prognosis of, 1233–1234
   subungual, 1233
   superficial spreading, 1232–1233,
      1233f
Melanoptysis, 615
Melanosis coli, 834
Melarsoprol, for trypanosomiasis, 128

MELAS, 1116b, 1144b
Melasma, 1258
MELD score, for liver transplantation,
   900–901
Meleney's gangrene, 227b
Melioidosis, 261
Melphalan, 968, 1320b
Memantine, 1193
Membrane attack complex (MAC), 66
Membranoproliferative
   glomerulonephritis, 401
Membranous nephropathy, 398b–399b,
   401, 427b
Memory, 1066
   Alzheimer's disease, 1192–1193
   disorders of, 1066b
   long-term, 1065, 1192–1193
   loss, 1081
   short-term, 1081, 1192–1193
Memory cells, 68
Ménétrier's disease, 797–798
Ménière's disease, 1104–1105
MENIN, 688
Meningioma, 1130–1131
Meningism, 1118
Meningitis, 1118–1121
   aseptic, 257
   bacterial, 1118–1120
      cerebrospinal fluid in, 1119
      headache and, 185, 185b
      management of, 1120, 1120b
   causes of, 1118b
   Coccidioides, 304
   cryptococcal, HIV-related, 321
   fungal, 1121
   HIV-related, 321
   malignant, 1121
   in mumps, 240
   protozoa, 1121
   recurrent aseptic, 1121
   tuberculous, 1120–1121, 1121b
   viral, 1118
      cerebrospinal fluid in, 1118
Meningococcaemia, chronic, 1119
Meningococcal infection
   chemoprophylaxis following, 1121b
   meningitis, 1118–1119, 1119b
   prevention of, 1120
   rash, 1120
Meningococcal sepsis, 1119b
Meningoencephalitis, 279
Menopause, 652
   male, 660b
   premature, 654
Menorrhagia, 923
Menstrual cycle, normal, 652f
Menstrual irregularity, in polycystic
   ovarian syndrome, 659
Menstruation, 1290, 1291f
Mental state examination, 1181–1183
Mental test, older people, 184
Menthol, topical, 1220
Mepacrine, hyperpigmentation from,
   1258b
Meptazinol, 1002
Meralgia paraesthetica, 1139b
Mercaptopurine
   for acute leukaemia, 957b
   for inflammatory bowel disease,
      821b
Mercury poisoning, 365b
Merkel cells, 1212
Meropenem, 117b, 120b
   melioidosis, 261
   neutropenic fever, 1327–1328
   nocardiosis, 261
   pneumonia, 586
   in pregnancy, 120b
MERRF (myoclonic epilepsy with ragged
   red fibres), 1116b, 1144b
Mesalazine, for inflammatory bowel
   disease, 818, 820, 821b
Mesangiocapillary glomerulonephritis
   (MCGN), 398b–399b, 401
Mesenteric ischaemia, chronic, 827
Mesna, 1036
Mesothelioma, 618
Meta-iodobenzyl guanidine (MIBG)
   scintigraphy, 675

Metabolic acidosis, 364–366
  acute mountain sickness, 168
  causes of, 365b
  diabetic ketoacidosis, 735
  hypothermia and, 166
  kidney failure/renal failure
    acute, 413
    chronic, 415
  malaria, 276b
  near-drowning, 170
  poisoning, 139b, 141b
  starvation, 704–705
Metabolic alkalosis, 366–367, 367f
Metabolic disorders, 785
  clinical examination of, 346–348,
    346f
  supportive therapy for, 957–958
Metabolic medicine, 345–380
Metabolic myopathies, 1144
Metabolic syndrome, 730–731
  liver transplantation and, 901
Metabolism
  first-pass, 17
  interactions, 24
  phase I, 18
  phase II, 18
Metadrenalines, 1361b
Metalloproteinases, 485–486
Metamyelocytes, 917
Metaphase, 40
Metapneumovirus, 249
Metastatic bone disease, 1057
Metastatic spread, in lung cancer, 600
Metatarsophalangeal joints, polyarthritis
    in, 994f
Metavir system, for hepatitis C, 878
Metered-dose inhaler, for asthma, 571f
Metformin, 746, 746b
  acidosis, 135b, 141
  for hyperglycaemia, 746
  mechanism of action, 746
  overdose, 135b, 141
  polycystic ovarian syndrome, 659
  in pregnancy, 1278
  renal/hepatic disease, 32b
Methadone
  misuse, 142, 142b
  withdrawal, 16b
Methaemoglobin, 277, 947
Methaemoglobinaemia, 120b, 135f,
    1227–1228
Methanol, poisoning from, 147, 147f
Methicillin-resistant Staphylococcus
    aureus (MRSA), 252
Methimazole, 644
Methionine, 138
Methotrexate (MTX)
  acute leukaemia, 957, 957b
  drug interaction, 24b
  eczema, 1227–1228
  hepatic fibrosis and, 895–897
  hepatotoxicity of, 894b
  for inflammatory bowel disease, 821b,
    822, 1299
  for musculoskeletal disease, 1004,
    1004b
    antineutrophil cytoplasmic
      antibody-associated vasculitis,
      1041
    juvenile dermatomyositis, 1040
    juvenile idiopathic arthritis, 1027
    polymyositis and dermatomyositis,
      1040
    psoriatic arthritis, 1033–1034
    systemic lupus erythematosus,
      1036
  pregnancy and, 1226b, 1278
  psoriasis, 1227–1228, 1250
  renal disease, 32b
  and respiratory disease, 612b
  sarcoidosis, 610
Methyl-phenyl-tetrahydropyridine
    (MPTP), 1112b
Methylbenzethonium chloride, 286
Methylcellulose, 646, 834b
Methyldopa, for pre-existing
    hypertension, pregnancy and,
    1276
Methylphenidate, 1105

Methylprednisolone
  for acute disseminated
    encephalomyelitis, 1110
  antineutrophil cytoplasmic
    antibody-associated vasculitis
    (AAV), 1041
  Grave's ophthalmopathy, 646
  histoplasmosis, 304
  for inflammatory bowel disease, 820
  for juvenile dermatomyositis, 1040
  liver transplant patients, 901
  for polymyositis and dermatomyositis,
    1040
  rheumatic disease, 1005–1006
  for systemic lupus erythematosus,
    1036
  for transverse myelitis, 1110
Methysergide, and respiratory disease,
    612b
Meticillin, 120b
Metoclopramide
  chronic intestinal pseudo-obstruction,
    811
  and hyperprolactinaemia, 684b
  nausea and vomiting, 803, 1351b
  poisoning, 137b
  sodium content of, 864b
Metoprolol, 466b, 480b
  angina, 500
  arrhythmias, 481
  hypertension, 513
Metronidazole, 117b
  for amoebiasis, 287
  for balanitis, 334b
  for cerebral abscess, 1124b
  for cholecystitis, 905
  for choledocholithiasis, 906
  for Clostridium difficile infection, 264
  for gas gangrene, 227
  for giardiasis, 287
  for Helicobacter pylori eradication,
    800
  for inflammatory bowel disease, 823
  for liver abscess, 880
  for neutropenic fever, 1327–1328
  for PID, 336
  for pneumonia, 587
  polyneuropathy and, 1139b
  in pregnancy, 120b
  prophylactic, 119b
  for rosacea, 1244
  for small bowel bacterial overgrowth,
    808–809
  for tetanus, 1126b
  for tropical ulcer, 254
Metyrapone, 669, 671b
Mevalonate kinase deficiency, 81
Mexiletine, 480, 480b
Mezavant, for inflammatory bowel
    disease, 821b
Micafungin, 125b
Micelles, mixed, 768
Miconazole, 125b, 1239–1240
  erythrasma, 1238
Microalbuminuria, 394
  in diabetic nephropathy, 757, 758b
  in diabetic neuropathy, 727
Microaneurysms, 509–510
Microangiopathic haemolytic anaemia
    (MAHA), 408, 950
Microangiopathy, diabetic, 756
Microarrays, 51
Microbial flora, normal, 102–103, 103f
Microbiological investigations, for
    respiratory disease, 554
Microbiome, 63, 103
Microcytic anaemia, 925
  in rheumatoid arthritis, 1024–1025
Microcytosis, 921f, 941f
Microdeletion syndromes, 44
Microglia, 1106
Microlithiasis, alveolar, 613b
Micronutrients, 711–718
Microorganisms
  culture, 106
  detection of components, 106
  detection of whole organisms, 105
  host response, 105–109
MicroRNA (miRNA), 40

Microsatellite repeats, 43
Microscopy
  bright field, 105
  dark field, 105
  electron, 105
  epiluminescence, 1214
Microsomal ethanol-oxidising system
    (MEOS) pathway, 881
Microsporidiosis, HIV-related, 317b
Microsporum audouinii, 1240
Microsporum canis, 1240, 1240f
Micturating cystourethrography, reflux
    nephropathy, 431f
Micturition
  cycle, 386
  disorders of, benign prostatic
    hyperplasia, 437
  frequency of, 396
Mid-axillary line, 626–627
Midazolam, 1189f
Middle East respiratory syndrome
    coronavirus (MERS-CoV), 249
Midges, filariases, 293
Migraine, 1095–1096
  pregnancy and, 1284
  stroke risk in, 1095
  in visual disturbance, 1088
Migrainous neuralgia, 1096
Migrating motor complexes (MMC), 772
Miliary tuberculosis (TB), 588–589
Milk, cow's, type 1 diabetes and, 729
Milk alkali syndrome, 716
Milk intolerance, 812
Millard-Gubler syndrome, 1072b
Miller Fisher syndrome, 1140
Miltefosine, 283
Milwaukee shoulder syndrome,
    1017–1018
Mineralocorticoid receptor, 355
Mineralocorticoid receptor antagonists
  for acute coronary syndrome, 501
  for primary hyperaldosteronism, 675
Mineralocorticoid replacement, for
    adrenal insufficiency, 673
Mineralocorticoids, 666, 666f
  in adrenal insufficiency, 672
  excess in, causes of, 674b
Minerals, storage of, liver and, 851
Mini-Mental State Examination (MMSE),
    1181–1183
Minimal change nephropathy, 398–400,
    398f–399b
Minimally conscious state, 211, 212b
Minimum bactericidal concentration
    (MBC), 109
Minimum inhibitory concentration (MIC),
    109
Minocycline
  for acne, 1243
  hyperpigmentation from, 1243, 1258b
  for leprosy, 269
  skin reactions, 1266b
Minoxidil
  alopecia, 1259
  hypertension, 513
  skin reactions, 1266b
Mirizzi's syndrome, 904–905
Misoprostol, 1003
Missense mutation, 42, 42f
Mites
  house dust, 568, 570, 1215, 1245
  typhus, 270
Mitochondria, 49, 50f
Mitochondrial disorders, 49, 1144
Mitochondrial DNA, 1305
Mitochondrial inheritance, 49, 49b
Mitochondrial syndromes, 1144b
Mitomycin C, 436, 612b
Mitosis, phases of, 40
Mitotane, 669–670
Mitotic spindle poisons, 1317f
Mitoxantrone, 936b
  acute leukaemia, 957b
Mitral regurgitation, 519–521, 519b,
    520f
  clinical features of, 521b, 521f
  investigation of, 521b
  management of, 521

Mitral stenosis, 517–519, 518b, 518f
  investigations in, 518f, 519b
    chest X-ray for, 451f
  pregnancy and, 1282
Mitral valve
  balloon valvuloplasty, 519, 519b, 519f
  disease of, 517–521
  endocarditis, 200f
  prolapse, 520
    pain, 177
  repair, 521
  replacement, 526–527
Mixed connective tissue disease
    (MCTD), 1038
Mixed venous oxygen saturation, 198b
Mobilisation, of stroke patients, 1159b
Mobitz type I second-degree AV block,
    477, 477f
Mobitz type II second-degree AV block,
    477, 477f
Moclobemide, 1199b
Modafinil, 1105, 1110b
Modified Beighton score, for joint
    hypermobility, 1059, 1059b
Modified Dukes classification, survival in
    colorectal cancer and, 832f
Mohs' micrographic surgery, 1228
Molecular adsorbent recirculating
    system (MARS), for pruritus,
    primary biliary cholangitis and,
    888
Molecular diagnostics, 348b
Molecular mimicry, 82
Moles, 1234–1235, 1235f
Mollaret's syndrome, 1121
Molluscum contagiosum, 248b, 343,
    343f, 1239, 1239f
  HIV disease and, 306f, 314b
Mometasone, 1226b
Monday fever, 614
Monge's disease, 169
Monitoring
  in critical care/critical illness, 175–176,
    175b, 175f
Monitoring drug therapy, 34–36
Monkeypox, 248–249
Monoamine oxidase inhibitors, 1199,
    1199b
  drug interactions, 24b
Monoarthritis
  acute, 992–993, 993b
  chronic inflammatory, 992
Monobactams, 120b, 121
Monoclonal antibody therapy
  for allergy, 86
  for asthma, 572
  for haemolytic uraemic syndrome,
    409
  for high-grade NHL, 966
  for low-grade NHL, 965
  for osteoporosis, 1048
Monoclonal gammopathy of uncertain
    significance (MGUS), 966
Monoclonal immunoglobulin deposition
    disease, multiple myeloma and,
    410b
Monocytes, 64, 917, 926b, 926f
  count, 1362b
Monocytosis, 926b
Monofilament testing, 721b
Monoiodotyrosine (MIT), 635f
Mononeuritis multiplex, 1140
Mononeuropathy
  diabetic, 760
  multifocal, 1140b
Monosodium urate monohydrate
    crystals, 988f, 1015
Monospot test, 242
Montelukast, asthma, 572
Montreal Cognitive Assessment (MoCA),
    1181–1183, 1182f
Mood, 1071
  assessment of, in psychiatric
    interview, 1181
Mood disorders, 1198–1200
  bipolar, 1199–1200
  organic, 1185b
Mood-stabilising drugs, 1190b
Moraxella catarrhalis, 103f

Morphine
  adverse reactions of, 22b
  COPD, 577
  intensive care, 209b
  misuse, 142b
  palliative care, 1351
  pharmacogenetics, 20b
  renal colic, 432
  renal or hepatic disease, 32b
  rout of administration, 30b
Morphoea, 1262–1263
Morquio's syndrome, 371b
Mortality ratios, standardised (SMRs), 214
Morton's neuroma, 999
Mosaic warts, 1238
Mosquitoes, 231b
  filariasis, 290
  malaria, 273–274
  virus transmission of, 111
Motilin, 772b
Motility disorders, in vitamin B_{12} deficiency, 944
Motor cortex, 1063f
Motor neuron disease, 1111b, 1116–1117, 1117b, 1117f
Motor neurons
  lower, 1068
  upper, 1068–1069
Motor neuropathy, 503b
Motor system, 1068–1069, 1068f
Mountain sickness
  acute, 168
  chronic, 169
Mouth
  disease of, 790
  of envenomed patient, 152f
  examination of
    cardiology, 442f
    respiratory system, 546f
  oral allergy syndrome, 812
  ulcers
    in Behçet's disease, 1043–1044, 1043f
Mouth ulcers, for systemic lupus erythematosus, 1036
Movement disorders, 1112–1115
  involuntary movements, 1069
  see also names of specific disorders
Moxifloxacin, 123b
  meningitis, 1120b
MRCP (magnetic resonance cholangiopancreatography), 776, 854–855
  for cholangiocarcinoma, 855f
  for choledocholithiasis, 906
  for gallstones, 904–905, 904f
MRI (magnetic resonance imaging)
  of aldosterone-producing adenoma, 674
  for cancer, 1323
  for cardiovascular system, 452–453, 453f
  of gastrointestinal tract, 774
  for haemangiomas, 893f
  for hepatobiliary disease, 854
  for hepatocellular carcinoma, 891
  for musculoskeletal disease, 989, 989b, 989f
  for neurological disease, 1072, 1073b
    epilepsy, 1101b
    stroke, 1151, 1157–1158, 1158b
    viral encephalitis, 1122
  of osteonecrosis, 1055
  for pain, 1342
  pregnancy and, 1274
  for renal disease, 389
  for respiratory disease, 553
  for sacroiliitis, 1029–1030, 1029f
MRSA (meticillin-resistant *Staphylococcus aureus*), 117b
Mucociliary escalator, 550f
Mucocutaneous disease, HIV-related, 314–316, 314b
Mucopolysaccharidosis, 371b
Mucor spp., 303
Mucormycosis, 303, 598
Mucosa-associated lymphoid tissue (MALT), 67

Mucosal leishmaniasis, 285
Mucous membranes
  inflammatory arthritis in, 994b
  as physical barrier, 62–63
Mucous patches, syphilis, 337
Multi-organ failure, causes of, 201
Multidisciplinary team, 1303b, 1311, 1336
Multifocal encephalomyelitis, 1111b
Multifocal neuropathy, 1140, 1140b
Multimorbidity, 1306
Multinodular goitre, 648–649, 648f
Multiple endocrine neoplasia (MEN), 688–689, 689b
Multiple myeloma, 409, 410b, 966–968
  classification of, 967b
  clinical features and investigations of, 967, 967f
  management of, 967–968
    bisphosphonates for, 968
    chemotherapy for, 968
    immediate support for, 967–968
    radiotherapy for, 968
  prognosis of, 968
Multiple organ failure, 411
Multiple sclerosis, 1106–1110
  cerebrospinal fluid in, 1108
  clinical features of, 1106–1108, 1108b
  investigation of, 1108, 1108f–1109f
  Macdonald criteria for, 1107b
  management of, 1109–1110
    acute episode, 1109
    disease-modifying treatments, 1109, 1109b
    symptoms, complications and disability, 1109–1110, 1110b
  pathophysiology of, 1106, 1107f–1108f
  in pregnancy, 1110b
Multiple systems atrophy (MSA), 1114
Multivisceral transplantation, 710
  complications of, 710b
Mumps, 240
  clinical features of, 240, 240f
  diagnosis of, 240
  incubation period, 111b, 232b, 240
  management and prevention of, 240
  periods of infectivity, 111b
  testicular swelling, 216f
Münchausen's syndrome, 1206
Murmur
  aortic regurgitation, 524, 524b, 525f
  aortic stenosis, 522, 522b, 522f
  atrial septal defect, 535, 535f
  ausculatory evaluation, 443b
  Austin Flint, 524
  benign, 459, 459b–460b
  cardiac, 459b, 460f
  carditis, 515–516
  Carey Coombs, 515–516
  coarctation of aorta, 534
  continuous, 461
  diastolic, 460
  Graham Steell, 526
  mitral regurgitation, 520, 520f, 521b
  mitral stenosis, 518–519, 518f
  persistent ductus arteriosus, 533
  pulmonary regurgitation, 526
  pulmonary stenosis, 526
  systolic, 459–460, 460b
  tetralogy of Fallot, 537
  timing and pattern, 460f
  tricuspid stenosis, 526
  ventricular septal defect, 460b, 535–536
Murphy's sign, cholecystitis and, 905
Muscle
  biopsy, 992
    in polymyositis and dermatomyositis, 1039, 1040f
  contraction, 1068
  of envenomed patient, 152f
  pain, 1000, 1000b
  skeletal, 987–988
Muscle disease, 1143–1144
  acquired, 1144, 1145f
Muscle fibre, 446f

Muscle haematomas, in haemophilia A, 972
Muscle spindles, in control of breathing, 549
Muscle weakness/wasting, 1000, 1000b
  diabetes, 759
  osteoarthritis, 1010
  systemic sclerosis and, 1037
Muscular atrophy, spinal, 1117
Muscular dystrophies, 1143–1144, 1143b
  inheritance, 1143
  transition medicine and, 1297
Musculoskeletal disease
  anatomy and physiology of, 984–988, 984f
  investigation of, 988–992
  management of, 1000–1007, 1001b
  X-rays for, 988, 988b
    bony metastases, 662
    Charcot's joint, 1058f
    chondrocalcinosis, 1016f
    CPPD crystal deposition disease, 1017
    fracture, 994–995
    osteoarthritis, 1009f–1011f
    osteomalacia, 1052, 1052f
    osteonecrosis, 1055
    osteosarcoma, 1056–1057
    reactive arthritis, 1032
    rheumatoid arthritis, 1025
    supraspinatus tendon calcification, 1017f
Musculoskeletal system
  anatomy and physiology of, 984–988, 984f
  clinical examination of, 982–983, 982f
  drug-induced effects on, 1057b
  presenting problems in, 992–1000
  primary tumours of, 1056b
Mushrooms
  magic (hallucinogenic), 143, 1196
  poisoning, 857
Mutation(s)
  de novo, 47
  domain negative, 45
  frameshift, 42
  gain-of-function, 45
  loss-of-function, 44
  missense, 42
  nonsense, 42, 42f
  point, 42
  simple tandem repeat, 43, 43b
  splice site, 43f
  tandem repeat, 43, 43b
Myalgia
  drug-induced, 1057b
  fever and, 217b
  infections, 223
Myasthenia gravis, 1111b, 1141–1143, 1142b, 1142f
  diplopia, 1141
  drug-induced, 1057b
  weakness, 1093
Myasthenic crisis, 1142–1143
Mycetoma, 301
  intracavitary, 559
Mycobacteria, 100–101
  opportunistic infection, 595, 595b
Mycobacterial infections, skin, 1237–1238
Mycobacterium abscessus, 580–581
Mycobacterium avium complex, HIV-related
  disseminated, 315b
  prophylaxis for, 324
Mycobacterium chelonei, 595b
Mycobacterium fortuitum, 595b
Mycobacterium genavense, 595b
Mycobacterium haemophilum, 595b
Mycobacterium kansaii, 595, 595b
Mycobacterium leprae, 100, 106, 595b
Mycobacterium malmoense, 595, 595b
Mycobacterium marinum, 595b
Mycobacterium tuberculosis (MTB), 106, 588
Mycobacterium ulcerans, 254, 595b
Mycobacterium xenopi, 595, 595b
Mycology, 1215

Mycophenolate mofetil (MMF)
  for autoimmune hepatitis, 886–887
  liver transplantation and, 901
  for musculoskeletal disease, 1004b, 1005
  for polymyositis and dermatomyositis, 1040
  for systemic lupus erythematosus, 1036
Mycoplasma pneumoniae, 583
  cold agglutination, 950
Mycoplasma spp., 121
Mycoses, superficial, 300
Mycosis fungoides (cutaneous T-cell lymphoma), 1232
Myelin sheaths, 358, 1106
Myelinolysis, 358
Myelitis, transverse, 1110
Myeloablative conditioning, 937
Myelocytes, 917
Myelodysplasia, 124
Myelodysplastic syndromes (MDSs), 960–961, 961b
Myelofibrosis, 969
Myelography, spine, 996–997
Myeloma
  AKI, 412b
  multiple, 409, 410b, 966–968
Myelopathy, 1111b
  cervical, 1134–1135
  HIV-related, 321
  vacuolar, 321
Myeloperoxidase, 64
Myeloproliferative neoplasms, 969–970
Myelosuppression, drug-induced, 1330
Myiasis, 300
Myocardial contraction, 446, 446f
Myocardial infarction, 199–200, 199b
  acute, 493b
  diagnosis of, 493
  electrocardiogram (ECG) for, 448
  investigation of, 496
    ECG, 496–497
  management of
    late, 498, 498b
    in old age, 500b
    pregnancy and, 1282
    rehabilitation, 501
    time course, 495f
Myocardial ischaemia
  electrocardiogram (ECG) for, 448
  myocardial infarction, 498
Myocardial stunning, 199–200
Myocarditis, 538, 538b
  acute, 538
  chronic, 538
  fulminant, 538
Myocardium
  disease of, 538–542
  hibernating, 452
Myoclonic seizures, 1099–1100
Myoclonus, 1086
Myocytes, 446, 446f
Myofibrils, 987
Myoglobinuria, 392b
Myonecrosis, clostridial, 227
Myopathic gait, 1087
Myopathy, critical illness, 212
Myophosphorylase deficiency (McArdle's disease), 1144b
Myosin, 446, 987
Myositis
  drug-induced, 1057b
  inclusion body, 1059
  systemic sclerosis, 1037
Myotonia, potassium-aggravated, 1145b
Myotonia congenita, 1145b
Myotonic dystrophy, 1143b
  genetics/inheritance, 43b
Myotoxicity, 155
Myxoedema, Graves' disease, 643
Myxoedema coma, 641
Myxoma, atrial, 541–542

N

N-Acetylcysteine therapy, for acute liver failure, 858–859
NADH dehydrogenase, 49b

Nadolol
  arrhythmias, 481
  thyrotoxicosis, 637–638
  variceal bleeding, 869
Naevi
  blue, 1235
  melanocytic, 1216, 1234–1235, 1235f
  spider, 846f
    autoimmune hepatitis and, 886
Nafcillin, 120b
Nails, 1214
  abnormalities, 1224
  in congenital disease, 1261
  disorders, 1260–1261
    HIV-related, 316
  inflammatory arthritis in, 994b
  involvement in skin diseases,
    1260–1261
  normal variants of, 1260
  plate and bed, 1260f
  in systemic disease, 1261, 1261f
  trauma, 1260
Na,K-activated adenosine
    triphosphatase (ATPase), 349
Nalidixic acid, 123b
  skin reactions, 1266b
Naloxone
  adverse reactions of, 23
  drug interactions of, 24b
Naltrexone, for pruritus, primary biliary
    cholangitis and, 888
Naproxen, 1003b
Narcolepsy, 1105, 1105b
Narcotics, cirrhosis and, 894b
Nasal cannulae, high-flow, 202
Nasogastric tube, 805b
Nasogastric tube feeding, 707, 707b
Nasopharynx, disease of, 622
Natalizumab, 66, 1109b
Nateglinide, 747
National Institute for Health and Clinical
    Excellence (NICE), 11
Natural killer cells, 67
Nausea and vomiting
  palliative care and, 1353–1354,
    1353f
  pregnancy and, 1275, 1275b
Near-drowning, 169–170, 170f
Necator americanus, 288
Neck
  Casal's necklace, 714, 715f
  examination of
    endocrine disease, 630f
    neurological disease, 1062f
  stiffness, 321
Neck pain, 997, 997b
Necrobiosis lipoidica, 1263, 1263f
Necrosis, 41, 1316–1317
Necrotising enteritis, 262
Necrotising fasciitis, 226–227, 227f
Necrotising pancreatitis, 839
Necrotising scleritis, 1172
Necrotising soft tissue infections, 227b
  skin, 1238
Nefopam, 1002
Negative visual phenomena, 1171
Neisseria gonorrhoeae, 117b, 339
  in pregnancy, 235b, 332b
Neisseria spp., 103f
Nelson's syndrome, 669
Nematode infections, 233b
  intestinal, 288–290
  tissue-dwelling, 290–293, 290b
  zoonotic, 293–294
Neoadjuvant chemotherapy, 1330
Neomycin
  allergy, 1247b
  for vitamin B₁₂ deficiency, 715
Neostigmine, 835
Nephelometry, 348b
Nephrectomy, 431, 435
Nephritic syndrome, 392, 392b, 393f
Nephritis
  crescentic, 398b–399b, 410
  drug-induced, 427b
  interstitial
    acute, 402, 402b
    chronic, 402–403, 403b
    drug-induced, 427b

lupus, 392b
  post-streptococcal, 401
Nephrocalcinosis, drug-induced, 427b,
    431
Nephrogenic sclerosing fibrosis, 390b
Nephrology, 381–440
Nephron, 349–350, 350f, 384
  segments of, 351f
Nephronophthis, 404
Nephropathy
  analgesic, 426
  Balkan, 403
  diabetic, 757–758
    diagnosis and screening for, 757
    management of, 757–758
    natural history of, 757, 758f
  HIV-associated, 322
  IgA, 398b–399b, 400
  ischaemic, 406–407
  membranous, 398b–399b, 401
  minimal change, 398–400,
    398b–399b
  multiple myeloma and, 410b
  pregnancy and, 1279
  reflux, 430–431
  salt-losing, 403
  sickle-cell, 411
Nephrotic syndrome, 392b, 395, 395b
  diseases typically presenting with,
    398–400
Neprilysin inhibitors, for heart failure,
    466–467
Nerve, disorder of, 1089b
Nerve agents, organophosphorus
    insecticides and, 145–146
Nerve biopsy, 1078
Nerve blocks
  and nerve ablation, for pain, 1348
  for pain, 1342–1343
Nerve conduction studies, 1076,
    1076f
  for pain, 1342
Nerve entrapment, in lung cancer, 600
Nerve fibre, 1338
  types of, 1338b
Nerve root decompression, 1002b
Nerve root lesions, 1083
Nerve root pain, 997b
Nervous impulse, 1065, 1065f
Nervous system
  anatomy and physiology of,
    1064–1072
    functional, 1065–1071, 1065f
  cells of, 1064–1065, 1064f
  clinical examination of, 1062–1064,
    1062f
  in old age, 1079b
  in gastrointestinal function, 771–772
Nervous system disease
  cerebrovascular disease see specific
    conditions
  clinical examination of, 1062–1064,
    1062f
  cranial nerves, 1063b
  emergencies, 1064b
  HIV-related, 319–321, 319f
  infections, 1117–1127, 1118b
  intracranial mass lesions/raised
    intracranial pressure, 1127–1133,
    1128b
  investigation of, 1072–1078
  lesion localisation in, 1071–1072
  neuromuscular junction, 1141–1143
  paraneoplastic, 1110–1111, 1111b,
    1132
  paraneoplastic syndromes,
    1325–1326
  peripheral nerves, 1138–1141,
    1139b
  presenting problems in, 1078–1094,
    1079b–1080b
  spine/spinal cord, 1134–1137
Neural tube defects, prevention with
    folic acid, 712b, 945
Neuralgia
  migrainous, 1096
  post-herpetic, 239, 1080
  trigeminal, 1080, 1096–1097
Neuralgic amyotrophy, 1141

Neuro-endocrine tumours (NETs), 603b,
    678–679, 678b, 679f, 813
Neuro-inflammatory diseases,
    1106–1110
Neuroacanthocytosis, 1085b
Neurocognitive disorders, HIV-
    associated, 319
Neurodegenerative diseases,
    1111–1117
Neurodestructive interventions, for
    cancer pain, 1352
Neurodevelopmental disorders, rare,
    genomics in, 56
Neurofibroma, 1129b, 1137f
Neurofibromatosis, 613b, 1131–1132,
    1131f, 1132b, 1264
  and cancer predisposition, 1321b
  inheritance, 1131–1132
Neurogenic shock, description of, 206b
Neuroglycopenia, 739
Neuroimaging, 1072–1074, 1073b,
    1151, 1151f, 1157–1158
Neuroleptic malignant syndrome,
    1197–1198
Neurological disease
  in pregnancy, 1284
    epilepsy as, 1284
    idiopathic intracranial hypertension
      as, 1284
    migraine as, 1284
    stroke as, 1284
  rheumatological manifestations of,
    1058, 1058f
  in systemic lupus erythematosus,
    1035
  transition medicine and, 1296–1297
    cerebral palsy in, 1296
    epilepsy in, 1296
    muscular dystrophy in, 1297
Neurological support, in intensive care,
    208
Neurology, 1061–1146
Neuroma
  acoustic, 1131
  Morton's, 999
Neuromuscular junction, diseases of,
    1141–1143
Neuromyelitis optica, 1110
Neuromyotonia, 1111b
Neuronectomy, multiple sclerosis,
    1110b
Neuropathic pain, 1084, 1348, 1348b,
    1348f
Neuropathy
  ataxia and retinitis pigmentosa
    (NARP), 1144b
  autonomic, 760, 760b
  critical illness, 211
  diabetic, 758–761
    classification of, 759b
    clinical features of, 758–761
    management of, 761, 761b
    risk factors for, 757b
  entrapment, 1139–1140, 1139b
  hereditary, 1140
  leg ulcers due to, 1224
  motor, 503b, 1111b
  multifocal, 1140, 1140b
  peripheral, 1325
    cancer-related, 1325
    diabetic, 755, 756b
    drug-induced, 321
    HIV-related, 321
    leprosy, 268
    in rheumatoid arthritis, 1024
    sensorimotor, 321
  peripheral, cancer-related, 1325
  sensory, 503b, 1111b
Neuropeptides, 1338–1339, 1340b
Neurosensory retina, 1167
Neurosyphilis, 338, 1125, 1125b
Neurotoxic flaccid paralysis, 155
Neurotoxins, hepatic encephalopathy
    and, 865
Neurotransmission/neurotransmitters,
    1065f
  in pain processing, 1340b
Neutral variants, 44
Neutrons, 164, 164f

Neutropenia, 925
  drug-induced, 926b
  fever in, 224, 1327–1328
  HIV-related, 322
Neutropenic fever, cancer and,
    1327–1328
Neutrophil chemotactic factor, 75b
Neutrophil extracellular trap (NET)
    formation, 64
Neutrophil granulocytes, 1362b
Neutrophilia, 926, 926b
  asthma, 568–569
Neutrophilic dermatoses, 1262
Neutrophils, 64, 917, 926b, 926f
  asthma, 568–569
  count, 1362b
  toxic granulation, 64
Nevirapine, in pregnancy, 326–327
Newborn, haemolytic disease of, 933,
    933b
Next-generation sequencing (NGS),
    52–53
  capture, 53
  challenges of, 53–54
  methods of, 55b
  uses of, 54–56
Niacin (vitamin B₃), 714–715
  biochemical assessment of, 712b
  deficiency, 714, 715f
  dietary sources of, 711b
  reference nutrient intake of, 711b
  toxicity, 715
Nicardipine, angina, 491b
Nickel hypersensitivity, 83b, 1247b
Niclosamide, 129
Nicorandil, 790b
Nicotinamide, for pellagra, 714
Nicotinamide adenine dinucleotide
    (NAD), 881
Nicotinamide adenine dinucleotide
    phosphate (NADPH)-oxidase
    enzyme complex, 64
Nicotine replacement therapy, 4
Nicotinic acid, 377
Niemann-Pick disease, 371b
Nifedipine
  altitude illness, 169
  angina, 490–491, 491b
    unstable, 500
  for high-altitude pulmonary oedema,
    169
  hypertension, 513
  and neutropenia, 926b
  for oesophageal disorders, 795
  older people, 32b
  Raynaud's syndrome, 504–505
  sphincter of Oddi dysfunction, 909
Nifurtimox, for trypanosomiasis, 128
Night blindness, 713
Night sweats, 217b
Night terrors, 1094
Nightmares, 1094
Nikolsky sign, 1254–1255
Nimodipine, for subarachnoid
    haemorrhage, 1162
Nipah virus encephalitis, 250
Nitazoxanide, 129
Nitrates
  angina, 489–490
  duration of action, 490b
  heart failure, 467
  for oesophageal disorders, 795
Nitric oxide (NO), 386, 447
  anal fissure, 836
  hepatopulmonary syndrome and, 898
Nitrites, 428
Nitrofurantoin, 124
  and pulmonary eosinophilia,
    611b–612b
  urinary tract infection, 428, 429b
Nitrogen narcosis, 170
Nitroimidazoles, 124
  mechanism of action, 116b
Nitroprusside reaction, 726
Nitrosamines, type 1 diabetes and, 729
'Nits', 1241
Nocardia, 587
  pneumonia, 319
Nocardiosis, 261

Nociceptive pain, 1084
Nocturia, 397
Nodal osteoarthritis, generalised, 1009, 1009b, 1009f
Nodular lymphocyte-predominant HL, 961–962
Nodular regenerative hyperplasia, of the liver, 899
Nodules
  definition of, 1211f
  pulmonary, 560–562, 560b–561b, 560f–562f
    cryptococcosis, 302
    lung metastases, 1328
  rheumatoid, 1023–1024, 1024f
  skin, definition, 1211f
  thyroid, 630f, 635
Non-alcoholic fatty liver disease (NAFLD), 850, 882–885, 883f, 885f
  biochemical tests for, 884, 884b
  clinical features of, 884
  imaging for, 884
  investigations for, 884
  liver biopsy for, 884
  liver function test (LFT) abnormality in, 854b
  management of, 884–885
  pathophysiology of, 883
Non-alcoholic steatohepatitis (NASH), 882–883, 883f
Non-antivenom treatments, 159–160
Non-cardiac surgery, with heart disease, 501–502, 501b
Non-compliance, 30–31
Non-disjunction, 44
Non-epileptic attack disorder ('dissociative attacks'), 1103–1104
Non-freezing cold injury, 167
Non-Hodgkin lymphoma, 964–966, 965f
  clinical features of, 964, 965f
  epidemiology of, 964, 964b
  investigations of, 964–965
  management of, 965–966
    high-grade, 966
    low-grade, 965
  prognosis of, 966
Non-immune haemolytic anaemia, 950
Non-invasive prenatal diagnosis (NIPD), 56
Non-invasive prenatal testing (NIPT), 56
Non-invasive ventilation, for acute exacerbations of COPD, 578
Non-metastatic extrapulmonary effects, of lung cancer, 601
Non-necrotising scleritis, 1172
Non-nucleoside reverse transcriptase inhibitors (NNRTIs), 324b
Non-opioid analgesics, for pain, 1345–1346
Non-specific interstitial pneumonia, 608
Non-specific urethritis (NSU), 333
Non-starch polysaccharides (NSPs; dietary fibre), 697
Non-steroidal anti-inflammatory drugs see NSAIDs
Non-thrombocytopenic purpura, 928b
Non-thyroidal illness, 642
Nonsense mutation, 42, 42f
Noradrenaline (norepinephrine), for refractory hypotension, 198, 198b
Noradrenaline (norepinephrine) re-uptake inhibitors, 1199, 1199b
  poisoning from, 139
Norfloxacin
  for spontaneous bacterial peritonitis, 864
  urinary tract infection, 428
Normal distribution/range, 3, 4f
Normetadrenaline, 1361b
Normoblasts, 915, 916f
Normocytic anaemia, 925
Norovirus, 249
Nortriptyline, pharmacokinetics, 20b
Norwalk agent, 249

Nosocomial (health care-acquired) infections
  Clostridium difficile, 211
  MRSA, 111–112
  pneumonia, 585
Notification
  food poisoning, 262
  partner, STIs, 333, 339
Novel therapies, for cystic fibrosis, 581
NSAIDs
  adverse reactions of, 22b
  associated with small intestinal toxicity, 811
  for back pain, 997
  in blood loss, 940–941
  for cholecystitis, 905
  cirrhosis and, 894b
  for CPPD crystal deposition disease, 1017
  for gout, 1015
  hepatotoxicity of, 894b
  for intermittent fever, 74
  mechanism of action of, 1003f
  for musculoskeletal disease, 1002–1003
  in old age, 1004b
  for osteoarthritis, 1012
  for pain, 1345
  for pancreatitis, 841
  for peptic ulcer, 799
  poisoning from, 138
  for psoriatic arthritis, 1033–1034
  for reactive arthritis, 1032
  recommendations for the use, 1003b
  renal disease and, 426
  risk of, in gastrointestinal bleeding and perforation, 1003b
  for systemic lupus erythematosus, 1036
  topical, 1003–1004
  ulcers induced by, risk factors for, 1003b
Nuclear antigens, extractable, antibodies to, 389
Nuclear factor kappa B (NFκB) pathway, 64–66
Nucleic acid amplification test (NAAT), 106, 333
Nucleoside reverse transcriptase inhibitors (NRTIs), 324b
Nucleosome, 38
Nucleotide substitutions, 42, 42f
Numbness, 1083–1084
'Nutcracker' oesophagus, 795
Nutraceuticals, for osteoarthritis, 1012
Nutrients, energy-yielding (macronutrients), 694–697
Nutrition, 694, 694f
  for alcoholic liver disease, 882
  alcoholic liver disease and, 880–881
  artificial, 710–711
  dementia and, 711, 711f
  in hospital patients, 706
  in intensive care, 210
  in lactation, 712b
  parenteral, 707–708, 708b
  physiology of, 694–697
  in pregnancy, 712b
  of stroke patients, 1159b
  under-nutrition and, 704–711
Nutritional disorders, clinical examination in, 692, 692f
Nutritional factors, in disease, 691–718
Nutritional status, clinical assessment and investigation of, 693b, 693f
Nutritional supplements, oral, 706
Nutritional support, artificial, ethical and legal considerations in management of, 710–711, 710b
Nystagmus, 1069, 1090
  balance disorders and, 1104f
  gaze-evoked, 1090
Nystatin, 125b
  candidiasis, 126, 790

O
Obesity, 94, 698–704
  aetiology of, 699–700, 699b
  body fat distribution in, 699

clinical assessment for, 693b
clinical features of, 700, 700b
complications of, 698–699, 698f
investigations of, 700
management of, 700–704, 701f
  drugs in, 702–703, 702f
  lifestyle advice in, 701
  surgery in, 702f–703f, 703–704, 703b
  weight loss diets in, 701–702, 701b
  in musculoskeletal disease, 1001–1002
non-alcoholic fatty liver disease and, 882–883
reversible causes of, 700
susceptibility to, 699–700
type 2 diabetes and, 732
Obesogenic environment, 699b
Obeticholic acid (OCA), for primary biliary cholangitis, 888
Obidoxime, 146
Obinutuzumab, for chronic lymphocytic leukaemia, 960
Obliterative cardiomyopathy, 541
Obsessive-compulsive disorder (OCD), 1201
Obstetric cholestasis, pregnancy and, 1284
Obstetric haemorrhage, circulatory collapse and, 1275
Obstetrics, genomics and, 56
Obstructive pulmonary diseases, 567–581
  asthma, 567–573
  bronchiectasis, 578–579
  chronic, 573–578
  cystic fibrosis, 580–581
Obstructive shock, description of, 206b
Occipital lobes, 1066
  disorders of, 1089b
  functions of, 1066b
  effects of damage, 1066b
Occupational airway disease, 613–614
Occupational and environmental lung disease, 613–619
  asbestos-related, 617–618
  due to organic dusts, 616–617, 616b
  occupational airway disease, 613–614
  pneumoconiosis, 614–616, 615b
Occupational asthma, 613–614, 614b, 614f
Occupational lung cancer, 618
Occupational pneumonia, 618–619
Occupational therapist, 1303b
Occupational therapy
  for musculoskeletal disease, 1001
    rheumatoid arthritis, 1026
  for Parkinson's disease, 1114
Ochrobactrum spp., 617
Octopus, blue-ringed, 154b
Octreotide
  acromegaly, 686–687
  gastrointestinal obstruction, 1354
  scintigraphy, 679f
  short bowel syndrome, 709b
  for Zollinger-Ellison syndrome, 802
Ocular abnormalities, 1088–1093
Ocular dysmetria, 1090
Ocular imaging, 1169f
Ocular inflammation, 1171–1173
Ocular pain, 1080
Ocular ultrasound, for visual disorders, 1169
Oculomotor (3rd cranial) nerve
  palsies, 1121b, 1144b
  tests of, 1063b
Oculopharyngeal dystrophy, 1143b
Odds ratio, drug therapy, 28f
Odynophagia, 316, 1324b
Oedema, 395–396
  ascites, 395–396
  causes of, 396b
  cerebral see Cerebral oedema
  famine, 704
  generalised, 282
  legs, 395–396
  mechanisms of, 186b
  nephrotic syndrome, 395–396, 395b

peripheral
  differential diagnosis, 463b
  heart failure, 463b
  hypervolaemia, 354
  pitting, 395
  pregnancy and, 1275
  pulmonary see Pulmonary oedema
Oesophageal candidiasis, in HIV/AIDS patients, 316, 317f
Oesophageal diseases, HIV-related, 315b, 316, 317f
Oesophageal dysmotility, secondary causes of, 795
Oesophageal motility, 778
Oesophageal transection, for variceal bleeding, 871
Oesophageal variceal bleeding, 869
  management of, 870f
Oesophageal varices, 865–866, 865f
  management of, 870f
Oesophagitis, 792
  eosinophilic, 794
  herpes simplex, in HIV infection/AIDS, 316
  reflux, 792, 792f
  systemic sclerosis, 1037–1038
Oesophagus
  Barrett's, 792–793, 793f
    carcinoma and, 796
  carcinoma of, 796–797
  diseases of, 791–797
    achalasia of, 794–795, 795f
    motility disorders, 794–796
    reflux, 791–794
  functional anatomy of, 766–767, 766f
  lower, adenocarcinoma of, 796f
  'nutcracker', 795
  perforation of, 797
  tumours of, 796–797
    benign, 796
17β-Oestradiol, 1359b
Oestradiol, pregnancy and, 1272
Oestrogen
  in bone remodelling, 986b
  for delayed puberty, 654
  hepatotoxicity, 894b
Oestrogen deficiency, 654b
Oestrogen receptors, as tumour markers, 1322, 1324b
Oestrogen replacement therapy
  delayed puberty, 655
  Turner's syndrome, 660
Ofloxacin
  leprosy, 270b
  for PID, 336
  for STIs, chlamydial infection, 341b
Ogilvie's syndrome, 835
Ointments, 1225b
Older people
  acute illness, 1308, 1308b
  acute kidney injury in, 414b
  adrenal glands, 673b
  antimicrobial therapy in, 120b
  blackouts, 1308
  cancer in, 1325b
  comorbidities in, 1307
  critical illness in, 212, 213b
  delirium, 1309
  demography of, 1304, 1304f
  deprescribing in, 1310–1311
  diabetes mellitus in, 732b
    management of, 757b
  dizziness, 1309
  endoscopy in, 776b
  energy balance in, 710b
  epilepsy in, 1103b
  examination, 1303b
  falls, 1308–1309, 1308b, 1308f
  frailty, 1306, 1306b
  gait and balance, 1303b
  gastrointestinal disorders, acute abdominal pain in, 788b
  geriatric assessment, 1302, 1302f
  gout in, 1014b
  haematological investigations in, 923b
  history, 1303b
  hypernatraemia in, 360b
  hyponatraemia in, 360b

Older people (Continued)
  incontinence, 436b, 1309–1310,
    1310f
  investigation, 1306–1307
    Comprehensive Geriatric
      Assessment, 1306
    decisions on, 1306–1307
  medical psychiatry in, 1189b
  neurological examination in, 1079b
  NSAIDs in, 1004b
  ophthalmological findings of, 1175b
  oral health in, 791b
  osteoarthritis in, 1011b
  osteoporosis in, 1049b
  polypharmacy in, 1310b
  prescribing in, 1310–1311
  presenting problems in, 1307–1311,
    1311b
  rehabilitation, 1311–1312
  renal replacement therapy in, 422b
  respiratory disease in
    infection, 586b
    interstitial lung disease, 613b
    obstructive pulmonary disease,
      578b
    pleural disease, 626b
  respiratory function in, 550b
  urinary tract infection in, 428b
  vitamin deficiency in, 712b
Oleander, poisoning from, 140
Olecranon bursitis, 998b, 1024f
Olfactory loss, 1088
Olfactory (1st cranial) nerve, tests of,
  1063b
Oligoarthritis, 1027
  asymmetrical inflammatory, 1032
Oligoclonal bands, 1077
Oligodendrocytes, 1064–1065
Oligodendroglioma, 1129b
Oligopeptides, 768
Oliguria, 391
  critically ill patients, 195
Olsalazine, for inflammatory bowel
  disease, 821b
Omalizumab, for allergy, 86
Omeprazole
  drug interactions of, 24b
  for H. pylori eradication, 800
Onchocerca volvulus, 292, 292f
Onchocerciasis, 233b, 292–293
Oncogenes, 51
Oncogenesis, 1318f
Oncology, 1313–1336
  genomics and, 56–58
  transition medicine and, 1298
Onychogryphosis, 1260
Onychomycosis, 1240
Oophoritis, mumps, 240
Open reading frame (ORF), 40
Ophthalmia neonatorum, 341
Ophthalmic disease, presenting
  problems in, 1169–1171
Ophthalmology, 1164
  medical, 1163–1178
Ophthalmopathy, Graves', 645–646,
  645f
  examination of, 631b
Opiates/opioids
  adverse reactions of, 22b
  for cholecystitis, 905
  misuse of, 142, 142b, 1195
  for osteoarthritis, 1012
  for pain, 1346–1347,
    1346b–1347b
    adverse effects of, 1351–1352,
      1351b
Opisthorchiasis, 297b
Opisthotonus, 1126
Opportunistic mycobacterial infection,
  595, 595b
Opsoclonus-myoclonus, 1111b
Opsonins, 63
  complement fragments as, 66
Opsonisation, 63, 63f
Optic atrophy, 1091–1093, 1092f
Optic chiasm, disorder of, 1089b
Optic disc disorders, 1089b
Optic disc swelling, of ophthalmic
  disease, 1171

Optic (2nd cranial) nerve, tests of,
  1063b
Optic neuritis, 1089b, 1111b
  multiple sclerosis, 1108b
  onchocerciasis, 293
  swelling, 1092b
  and transverse myelitis (neuromyelitis
    optica), 1110
Optic neuropathy, Leber hereditary,
  1144
Optic tract, disorders of, 1089b
Optical coherence tomography, 1169
OptiMAL®, 276
Oral administration, 17
Oral allergy syndrome, 812
Oral androgen replacement therapy,
  656b
Oral cancer, 790, 790b
Oral cavity, organisms in, 103f
Oral contraception/contraceptives
  acne treatment, 1243
  migraine and, 1095
  skin reactions, 1266b
  venous thtombosis and, 975b,
    1162b
Oral contraceptive pill (OCP)
  cystic fibrosis and, 1297
  epilepsy and, 1296
  porphyria and, 379
Oral diseases, HIV-related, 316
Oral glucocorticoids, for chronic
  obstructive pulmonary disease
  (COPD), 576–577
Oral glucose tolerance test (OGTT),
  726b
Oral hairy leukoplakia, 316
Oral health, in old age, 791b
Oral rehydration solution (ORS), 229b
Oral ulcers, in Behçet's disease,
  1043–1044, 1043f
Orbit, 1164
  blood supply of, 1168
  imaging of, 1073–1074, 1074f
Orbital septum, 1164
Orchitis, mumps, 240
Orf, 1239
Organ donation, 90
  after brain death, 213
  after cardiac death, 213
  altruistic living, 90
  cadaveric, 90
Organelles, intracellular, 1154f
Organic solvents, misuse of, 1196
Organisms
  detection of components of, 106
  whole, detection of, 105
Organophosphate-induced delayed
  polyneuropathy, 146
Organophosphorus compound,
  145–146, 145b, 145f
Oriental spotted fever, 271b
Orientation, assessment, 1181
Orlistat, for obesity, 702, 702f
Ornidazole, 287
Oropharynx, examination
  HIV disease, 306f
  infectious disease, 216f
Oroya fever, 272
Orphenadrine, for Parkinson's disease,
  1114
Orthopnoea, 557, 611
Orthoses, for musculoskeletal disease,
  1001
Oscillopsia, 1090
Osgood-Schlatter disease, 999b
Osmolality, 1360b
  presenting problems of, 356–360
Osmolarity, 1360b
Osmotic agents, 14
Osmotic diuretics, for hypervolaemia,
  355
Osteitis fibrosa cystica, 418–419
Osteoarthritis (OA), 1007–1012
  clinical features of, 1008–1011,
    1009b
  early-onset, 1011, 1011b
  epidemiology of, 1007
  erosive, 1011

  generalised nodal, 1009, 1009b,
    1009f
  hip, 1010, 1010f
  investigations for, 1011
  knee, 1009–1010, 1010f
  management of, 1011–1012
  in older people, 1011b
  pathophysiology of, 1007–1008,
    1008f
  risk factors for, 1008b
  spine, 1011, 1011f
Osteoarthropathy, hypertrophic
  pulmonary, 600–601
Osteoblasts, 984
  in bone remodelling, 985f
Osteochondritis
  dissecans, 998–999
  of patella ligament, 998b
Osteoclasts, 984
  in bone remodelling, 985f
Osteocytes, 985
Osteogenesis imperfecta (OI),
  1055–1056
  transition medicine and, 1300
Osteoid, 985f
Osteoid osteoma, 1056b
Osteomalacia, 1051–1052
  causes of, 1050b
  chronic kidney disease and,
    418–419
  clinical features of, 1052
  investigations in, 1052, 1052f
  management of, 1052
  pathogenesis of, 1051–1052
  tumour-induced, 1053
  vitamin D-deficient, biochemical
    abnormalities in, 990b
Osteomyelitis, 1021
Osteonecrosis, 1055
  drug-induced, 1057b
  pain, 1055
Osteopenia
  biliary cirrhosis, 888
  fracture and, 994
  hyperparathyroidism, 663
  radiographic, 989–990
Osteopetrosis, 1056
Osteophytes, 988, 1134
Osteoporosis, 1044–1049
  biochemical abnormalities in, 990b
  clinical features of, 1045
  coeliac disease and, 807
  fractures associated with, 1044,
    1045f
    bone mineral density and, 1046f
  glucocorticoid-induced, 1045
    transition medicine and, 1300
  idiopathic, 1044
  investigations of, 1046, 1047b, 1047f
  management of, 1046–1049
  non-pharmacological interventions for,
    1047
  in old age, 1049b
  pathophysiology of, 1044–1045,
    1045f
  pharmacological interventions for,
    1047–1049, 1048b
  pregnancy-associated, 1045
  risk factors for, 1046b
  secondary, 1044–1045
  surgery for, 1049
  treatment of, 1309
Osteoprotegerin, in bone remodelling,
  986b
Osteosarcoma, 1056–1057
Osteosclerosis
  osteoarthritis and, 1007, 1011f
  Paget's disease and, 1054
Osteotomy, 1002b, 1012
Ostium primum defects, 534
Otitis media, 236, 253b, 266, 1119
Ovarian cancer, 1334
  investigations of, 1334
  management of, 1334
  pathogenesis of, 1334
Ovarian failure, chemotherapy-induced,
  1298
Ovaries, polycystic, 658–659, 659f
Over-nutrition, responses to, 694–695

Overflow incontinence, 437, 1093
  in older people, 1310
Overnight dexamethasone suppression
  test (ONDST), in Cushing's
  syndrome, 668
Ovulation, 656–657
Oxacillin, 120b
Oxalate, 1361b
Oxazolidinones, 124
Oxcarbazepine, 1102b
Oxidative killing, 64
Oxidative stress, 881f, 883
Oximes, 146
Oximetry, 555–556
  asthma, 573
Oxygen
  arterial blood (PaO$_2$), 1358b
  content and delivery of, in shock,
    193, 193b
  for gastrointestinal haemorrhage, 782
Oxygen dissociation curve, in
  haemoglobin, 915–916, 917f
Oxygen saturation, 1358b
Oxygen therapy
  for acute exacerbations of COPD,
    577
  for air passengers, 169
  for chronic obstructive pulmonary
    disease (COPD), 577, 577b
  for community-acquired pneumonia,
    583
  for critical illness, 191, 191b
  for diving-related illness, 171
  for high-altitude pulmonary oedema,
    169
Oxyhaemoglobin dissociation curve,
  190, 191f
Oxytetracycline, acne, 1243

P
P gene, 1258
Pabrinex, 1195
Pachyonychia congenita, 1261
Pacing
  AV block, 482, 483f
  dual-chamber, 714
  tachyarrhythmias, 469
  transcutaneous, 482–483
Packed cell volume (PCV), 1362b
Paclitaxel, 1334
Paediatric disease, in systemic lupus
  erythematosus, 1036
Paediatric health services, transition to
  adult health services from,
  1288–1290
Paget's disease
  biochemical abnormalities in, 990b
  of bone, 1053–1054
    clinical features of, 1054
    investigations in, 1054, 1054f
    management of, 1054, 1054b
    pathophysiology of, 1053–1054
Pain, 1070, 1338–1349
  abdominal, 787–789
    acute, 787–789, 787b
    acute pancreatitis, 837–839, 837b
    assessment of, 787, 788f
    chronic or recurrent, 789, 789b
    chronic pancreatitis, 839–841
    constant, 789
    diabetic ketoacidosis and, 736,
      736b
    investigations of, 787
    irritable bowel syndrome and, 824
    large bowel obstruction of, 789
    liver abscess and, 880
    in lower abdomen, 336
    management of, 787–789
    in old age, 788b
    peptic ulcer, perforated, 789
  ankle, 999
  back, 995–997
    red flags for, 996b
    triage assessment of, 996f
  biliary, gallstones and, 904
  biopsychosocial model of, 1338f
  in cancer, 1350, 1350b
  central processing of, 1339–1340
  challenges in, 1344b

chest, 176–179, 454–455
    associated features of, 177–178, 178f
    characteristics of, 177
    clinical assessment of, 178
    differential diagnosis of, 177b
    investigations of, 178–179, 179b
    ischaemic, 454f
    onset of, 177
    pregnancy and, 1275
    in respiratory disease, 558
    site and radiation of, 177
elbow, 998, 998b
facial, 1080
foot, 999
functional anatomy and physiology of, 1338–1341
hand, 998
in headache, 1080
hip, 998, 999b, 999f
    osteoarthritis and, 1010
instruments for assessment of, 1343b
interventions for, 1344–1348
    complementary and alternative therapies for, 1348
    nerve blocks and nerve ablation in, 1348
    pharmacological therapies in, 1344–1347, 1345b–1347b
    physical therapies in, 1344, 1344b
    psychological therapies in, 1347
    stimulation therapies in, 1347, 1347f
    supported self-management in, 1344
investigations of, 1342–1343
knee, 998–999, 999b
loin, 396
low back
    assessment of, 988–989
    causes of, 996b
    mechanical, features of, 996b
    radicular, 997b
muscle, 1000, 1000b
musculoskeletal, regional, 997–999
neck, 997, 997b
neuropathic, 1084, 1348, 1348b, 1348f
ocular, 1080
of ophthalmic disease, 1170
osteoarthritis and, 1007–1008
    hip, 1010
    knee, 1009–1010
palliative care for, 1349–1354, 1349f
perception of, 1338f
principles of management of, 1343
radicular, 997b
shoulder, 997–998, 998b, 998f
somatoform disorder, 1202
wrist, 998
Pain relief, for pancreatitis, 841
Pain scoring system, 1343
Painful vaso-occlusive crisis, 952
Palliation, for cancer, 1330
Palliative care, 1349–1354, 1349f
    for chronic obstructive pulmonary disease (COPD), 577
    presenting problems of, 1350–1354
        anxiety and depression in, 1354
        cough in, 1353
        dehydration in, 1354
        delirium and agitation in, 1354
        gastrointestinal obstruction in, 1354
        nausea and vomiting in, 1353–1354, 1353f
        weight loss in, 1354
Palliative chemotherapy, 1329
Palmar erythema, 630f, 635–636, 846f, 866–867
Palmoplantar pustulosis, 1249
Palpable mass, cancer and, 1323
Palpable purpura, 1042, 1042f
Palpation
    of abdomen, 765b
    of precordium, 443b
    in respiratory system, examination of, 546f

Palpitation, 455–456, 455b, 456f
Pamidronate
    bone metastases, 1329
    hypercalcaemia, 1329
    for Paget's disease, 1054, 1054b
Pancoast's syndrome, 600
Pancolitis, 815–816
Pancreas, 770, 770f
    annular, 842
    artificial, 751, 751f
    carcinoma of, 843f
    congenital abnormalities affecting, 842
    diseases of, 837–844
    divisum, 842
    endocrine, 676–679
    pre-diabetic, 728
    structure and endocrine function of, 723f
    tumours of, 842–844
Pancreatic cancer, 843f
Pancreatic β-cell failure, in type 2 diabetes, 731
Pancreatic disease, 733
Pancreatic enzymes, 770b
Pancreatic necrosis, 839f
Pancreatic pseudocyst, 838f
'Pancreatic rests', 805
Pancreatitis
    acute, 837–839, 837b
        causes of, 838b
        complications of, 838b
        management of, 839
        pathophysiology of, 837, 838f
    autoimmune, 841
    chronic, 839–841, 840b
        complications of, 840b
        investigations of, 840, 841b, 841f
        management of complications of, 841
        pathophysiology of, 840f
    hereditary, 840b, 842
    necrotising, 839
Pancreolauryl test, 777b
Pancytopenia, 930, 930b
Panic disorder, 1200
Pannus, 1022–1023
Panton-Valentine leukocidin, 586, 1237
Papilla of Vater, 861
Papillary carcinoma, 649
Papillary muscle rupture, in acute coronary syndrome, 496
Papillary necrosis, 403
Papillary renal cell cancer syndrome, 1321b
Papilloedema, 1090–1091, 1092b, 1092f
    haemorrhagic, 1062f
Papilloma, basal cell, 1234, 1234f
Papillomaviruses, 1238–1239
Papular pruritic eruption, HIV-related, 316
Papule, definition of, 1211f
Papulosquamous eruptions, 1251
Para-aminosalicylic acid (PAS), skin reactions, 1266b
Parabens, 1247b
Paracentesis, for ascites, 863–864
Paracetamol
    adverse reactions, 22b
    for chronic pain, 1345b
    for fever, 218
    for headache, 1096
    hepatoxicity of, 857, 857f
    for musculoskeletal disease, 1002
        osteoarthritis, 1012
    for pain, 1345
    poisoning, 134b
    poisoning from, 137–138, 138f
        acute liver disease and, 857–858, 858b
Paracoccidioides brasiliensis, 304
Paracoccidioidomycosis, 304
Paraesthesia, 1083–1084
Paraganglioma, 675–676
Paragonimiasis, 233–234
Paragonimus spp., 129
Paragonimus westermani, 233b
Parainfluenza viruses, 249

Paraldehyde
    disturbed behaviour, 1189f
    poisoning, 135b
Paralysis, ventilator-induced lung injury and, 204
Paralysis ticks, envenomation of, 161
Paralytic ileus, 837–838
Paralytic shellfish poisoning, 149
Paramyotonia congenita, 1145b
Paraneoplastic disease, neurological, 1110–1111, 1111b
Paraneoplastic syndromes, neurological, 1325–1326
Paraparesis, 1086–1087
Paraphasia, 1088
Paraphenylenediamine, 1247b
Paraplegia, hereditary spastic, 1138b
Parapneumonic effusion, 564
Paraproteinaemias, 966–968
Paraproteins, 965–966
Paraquat, poisoning from, 147
Parasitic infections
    and cancer, 1320b
    eosinophilia, 233b
Parasitosis, delusional, 1202
Parasomnias, 1105–1106
    non-REM, 1105
Parathyroid disease, pregnancy in, 1280
    familial hypocalciuric hypercalcaemia as, 1280
    primary hyperparathyroidism as, 1280
Parathyroid glands, 661–665
    disease of
        classification of, 661b
        presenting problems in, 661–663
    familial hypocalciuric hypercalcaemia and, 664
    functional anatomy, physiology and investigations of, 661
    hypoparathyroidism and, 664–665
    in old age, 665b
    primary hyperparathyroidism and, 663–664, 663b, 664f
Parathyroid hormone (PTH), 661
    acute kidney injury and, 416b
    in bone remodelling, 986b
    osteomalacia and rickets, 1051–1052
    osteoporosis, 1047b
    reference range of, 1359b
    in skeletal disease, 990b
Parathyroid hormone-related protein (PTHrP), ectopic production, 1325–1326
Parathyroidectomy, 419
Paratyphoid fever, 260
Parenchymal bacterial infections, 1124–1125
Parenchymal viral infections, 1121–1123
Parenteral administration, 17
Parenteral nutrition, 707–708, 708b
Parietal lobes, 1066
    disorders of, 1089b
    functions of, 1066b
        effects of damage, 1066b
Parinaud syndrome, 1072b
Parkinsonian syndromes, 1114–1115
Parkinsonism, 1084–1085, 1085b, 1112
    drug-induced, 1112b
Parkinson's disease, idiopathic, 1112–1114
    causes of, 1112b
    clinical features of, 1112–1113, 1113b
        non-motor symptoms of, 1112–1113
    investigations of, 1113, 1113f
    management of, 1113–1114
        drug therapy, 1113–1114
        surgery, 1114
    pathophysiology of, 1112, 1112f
Paromomycin, 129
    for leishmaniasis, 283
Parotitis, 790, 790b
Paroxysmal atrial fibrillation, 471–472
Paroxysmal cold haemoglobinuria, 950
Paroxysmal nocturnal haemoglobinuria (PNH), 950–951
Partial agonists, 14

Partial anterior circulation syndrome (PACS), 1156f
Partial thromboplastin time with kaolin (PTTK), 920–921
Parvovirus B19 infection, 237
    clinical features of, 237, 237b, 237f
    diagnosis of, 237
    management of, 237
    in pregnancy, 235b
Past-pointing, 1069
Pastes, 1225b
Pastia's sign, 252, 253f
Patau's syndrome (trisomy 13), 44b
Patch testing, for skin disease, 1215
Patella ligament enthesopathy, 999b
Paterson-Kelly syndrome, 795–796
Pathergy test, 1044
Pathogen-associated molecular patterns (PAMPs), 63
'Pathogenicity,' in host-pathogen interactions, 104
Pathogens
    direct detection of, 105–106
    host-pathogen interactions, 104
    indirect detection of, 106–109
    successful, 104
Pathological fracture, 995b
Pathway medicine, for genetic disease, 58
Patient-centred evidence-based medicine, 10, 11f, 12
Patient factors, of gastro-oesophageal reflux disease, 791
Patients, autonomy, 1288–1289
Pattern recognition receptors (PRRs), 63
Paul-Bunnell test, 242
PCSK9 inhibitors, 377
Peak expiratory flow (PEF)
    asthma, 569f, 573f
    home monitoring, 555
    morning dipping, 569f
Peak flow meters, 555, 569
Peanut allergy, 85
PECAM-1, 447
Pectins, 696b
Pectus carinatum, 628
Pectus excavatum, 628
Pediculus humanus, 257
Pediculus humanus capitis, 1241
Pedigree, construction of, 46, 46f
Pegloticase, for gout, 1016
Pegvisomant, 686–687
Pellagra, 714, 715f, 1221b
Pelvi-ureteric junction obstruction (PUJO), 434
Pelvic floor exercises, faecal incontinence, 835
Pelvic inflammatory disease (PID), 336
Pemphigoid, bullous, 1255–1256, 1255b, 1256f
Pemphigoid gestationis, 1220b, 1255b
Pemphigus, 1256, 1326
Pemphigus foliaceus, 1255b
Pemphigus vulgaris, 1255b
Penciclovir, as anti-herpesvirus agent, 126, 127b
Pendred's syndrome, 635f, 650
Pendrin, 635f
Penetrance, genetic, 47
Penicillamine
    for musculoskeletal disease, 1004b, 1005
    nephrotoxicity, 427b
    for oral ulceration, 790b
    for primary biliary cholangitis, 888
    for pyridoxine deficiency, 715
    for Wilson's disease, 897
Penicillin(s), 117b, 121
    adverse reactions, 21, 22b
    allergy, 75b
    anthrax, 267
    diphtheria, 266
    endocarditis, 528
    leptospirosis, 258–259
    listeriosis, 260
    meningitis, 1120
    nephrotoxicity, 427b

Penicillin(s) (Continued)
for neurosyphilis, 1125
penicillinase-resistant, 121
in pregnancy, 120b
prophylactic, 78, 119b
resistance, 116
rheumatic fever, 517
syphilis, 337
for syphilis, 339
tetanus, 1126b
tropical ulcer, 254
urinary tract infection, 428
Penicillium marneffei infection, 303
Penile erection, 440
Penis, 386
Pentamidine, prophylactic, 119b
Pentamidine isethionate
for leishmaniasis, 283
for Pneumocystis jirovecii pneumonia, 128
Pentasa, for inflammatory bowel disease, 821b
Pentavalent antimonials, 128, 283
Pentoxifylline
for alcoholic hepatitis, 882
for frostbite, 166–167
Pepsinogen, 767
Peptic ulcer
complications of, 801–802
indications for, 800b
in old age, 801b
perforation, 789, 801
prophylaxis for, in intensive care, 211
Zollinger-Ellison syndrome, 802
Peptic ulcer disease, 798–802
Peptide YY, 772b
Peptides, antimicrobial, 62–63
Peptostreptococcus spp., 253b
Perceptions
abnormal, 1086, 1181
delusional, 1196–1197
Percussion
abdomen, 765b
in respiratory system, examination of, 546f
Percutaneous coronary intervention (PCI)
angina, 491–493, 491f–492f
myocardial infarction, 493b
vs. CABG, 493b
Percutaneous endoscopic gastrostomy (PEG), 707, 708f
Percutaneous therapy, for hepatocellular carcinoma, 891
Percutaneous transhepatic cholangiography (PTC), 854–855
Perforating dermatosis, acquired reactive, 1265
Perforin, 67
Perfusion, in respiratory system, 549–550
Perianal disease, inflammatory bowel disease and, 823
Pericardial disease, in tuberculosis (TB), 590
Pericardial effusion, 542b, 543, 543f, 1315b
Pericarditis
acute, 542, 542b, 542f
in acute coronary syndrome, 496
chronic constrictive, 543–544, 543b, 544f
tuberculous, 543
Pericardium, diseases of, 542–544
Perimetry, 1168
Perimysium, 987–988
Periodic fever syndromes, 81, 1059
Periodic limb movements, and sleep, 1106
Periodic paralysis
hyperkalaemic, 1145b
hypokalaemic, 1145b
Periostitis, 337, 600–601
Peripartum cardiomyopathy, pregnancy and, 1282
Peripheral arterial disease, 502–505, 502b

Peripheral nerves, 1338
disease of, 1138–1141, 1139b
HIV-related, 321
endings, 1338
lesions, 1083
Peripheral nervous system
motor, 1068
sensory, 1068
Peripheral neuropathy, 1325
cancer-related, 1325
diabetic, 755, 756b
drug-induced, 321
HIV-related, 321
leprosy, 268
in rheumatoid arthritis, 1024
sensorimotor, 321
Peripheral sensitisation, 1340, 1341f
Peripheral ulcerative keratitis, 1171–1172
Peripheral vascular disease, in diabetes, 503b
Perisinusoidal fibrosis, 884
Peristalsis, 772
Peritoneal cavity, disease of, 836–837
Peritoneal dialysis, 424
automated, 424
continuous ambulatory, 424
haemodialysis vs., 420b
problems with, 425b
Peritonitis, 836
spontaneous bacterial, 864
Permanent pacemakers, for arrhythmias, 483, 483b
Pernicious anaemia, 944
Persistent atrial fibrillation, 472–473
Persistent ductus arteriosus, 532f–533f, 533–534
Personality, 1071
change, 1094
high-risk behaviour and, 1295
psychiatric disorders and, 1183
Personality disorders, 1204–1205
prevalence of, 1180b
Pes cavus, 1140
Pesticides, 144–149
Petechiae, definition of, 1211f
Petechial purpura, 928–929, 928f
Petit mal, 1097
Pets
allergic rhinitis and, 622
asthma and, 568
HIV infection/AIDS and, 323
Peutz-Jeghers syndrome, 829, 829f
Peyer's patches, 67, 769–770
Phaeochromocytoma, 675–676, 675b, 676f
Phaeohyphomycoses, 301
Phagocytes, 63–64, 63f
deficiency in, 73b
primary, 77–78, 77f
Phagocytosis, 63, 63f
Phagolysosome, 64
Phantom limb pain, 1349
Pharmacist, 21b
Pharmacodynamics, 14–16, 14f
dose-response relationship in, 14–16, 15f
drug targets in, 14, 15b
mechanisms of action of, 14
Pharmacogenomics, for genetic disease, 58
Pharmacokinetics, 17–19, 17f
absorption in, 17–18
distribution in, 18
elimination in, 18–19
patient-specific factors in, 20b
repeated dose regimens in, 19
Pharmacological therapies, for pain, 1344–1347, 1345b
Pharmacovigilance, 23, 23b
Pharmacy, 27
Pharyngeal pouch, 794
Phenelzine, 1199b
Phenobarbital
epilepsy, 1102b
in old age, 32b
poisoning, 136b
status epilepticus, 1081b

Phenothiazines, for schizophrenia, 1198b
Phenoxymethylpenicillin, 120b
prophylactic, 119b
Phentermine, for obesity, 702–703
Phenylketonuria, 369
Phenytoin
ataxia, 1115b
drug interactions, 24b
epilepsy, 1102b
multiple sclerosis, 1110b
pharmacokinetics of, 19
plasma concentration, 36b
poisoning, 141b
renal or hepatic disease, 32b
sodium content of, 864b
status epilepticus, 1081b
Phobia, 1200
Phobic anxiety disorder, 1200
Phosphate
acute kidney injury and, 416b
in diabetic ketoacidosis, 738
enema, 869b
homeostasis, 368–369
reference range of
urine, 1361b
venous blood, 1360b
in skeletal disease, 990b
Phosphenes, 1088
Phosphodiesterase type 5 inhibitors, erectile dysfunction, 440
Phospholipids, 126, 370
Phosphorus, 716
deficiency, 716
dietary sources of, 717b
excess, 716
reference nutrient intake of, 717b
Photo-exposed site hyperpigmentation, 1258
Photoallergy, 1221b
Photochemotherapy, 1227
Photodynamic therapy (PDT)
for oral cancer, 790
for skin disease, 1228
Photophobia/glare, of ophthalmic disease, 1170
Photopsia, of ophthalmic disease, 1170
Photosensitivity, 1220–1223, 1221b
clinical assessment of, 1221
drug-induced, 1266b
investigations and management of, 1221–1223
Phototesting, for skin disease, 1215
Phototherapy, 1227
Phototoxicity, 1221b
Physical activity, energy expenditure and, 694, 695f
Physical therapies
for musculoskeletal disease, 1001
rheumatoid arthritis, 1026
for pain, 1344, 1344b
Physiological anaemia of pregnancy, 1273
Physiological breathlessness, of pregnancy, 1274–1275
Physiotherapy
for bronchiectasis, 579
for cancer pain, 1352
for cervical spondylosis, 1134
for community-acquired pneumonia, 584
for fracture, 995
for Parkinson's disease, 1114
for stroke, 1159f
Phytoestrogens, 716
Pick's disease, 1193–1194
Pigment stones, 903–904, 903b
Pigmentation
drug-induced, 1258, 1258b, 1266b
endocrine, 1258
Pigmented villonodular synovitis, 1059
Pinta, 254, 254b
Piperacillin, 120b
for spontaneous bacterial peritonitis, 864
for variceal bleeding, 869
Piperacillin-tazobactam, 117b
for necrotising fasciitis, 227
for neutropenic fever, 224

Piperazine, 129
Piroxicam, 1003b
Pitted keratolysis, 1238
Pituitary disease
investigation of patients with, 680, 680b
pregnancy and, 1280
diabetes insipidus as, 1280
prolactinoma as, 1280
Sheehan's syndrome as, 1280
Pituitary hormones, 632
Pituitary tumours, 683–684, 1129
Pityriasis lichenoides chronica, 1251
Pityriasis rosea, 1217b, 1251
Pityriasis versicolor, 1240
rash in, 1217b
Placental alkaline phosphatase (PLAP), as tumour markers, 1322, 1324b
Plague, 259, 259f
Plain chest X-ray
for gastrointestinal disease, 772, 773f
contrast studies of, 773
normal, 551f
for respiratory disease, 551, 551b, 551f
abnormalities, 552b
aspergillosis, 597f
asthma, 569
bronchiectasis, 579
COPD, 575
empyema, 564f
haemoptysis, 560
interstitial, 605, 605f
lobar collapse, 552f
lung cancer, 599, 599f
mediastinal tumours, 604, 604f
pleural effusion, 563
pleural plaques, 617f
pneumonia, 585
pneumothorax, 626
pulmonary embolism, 619–620, 619b, 619f
pulmonary hypertension, 622f
sarcoidosis, 609b
silicosis, 615f
tuberculosis, 590f
Plane warts, 1238
Plant poisoning, 150, 150b
Plantar warts, 1238
Plaques
amyloid in, 1192
definition of, 1211f
Plasma derivatives, 930
Plasma exchange (PE)
for Guillain-Barré syndrome, 1140
pre-renal transplant, 424
Plasma iron, 942
Plasma viscosity, inflammation and, 72
Plasmapheresis, for pruritus, primary biliary cholangitis and, 888
Plasmodium falciparum infection, 274f, 275, 276b
Plasmodium falciparum malaria, 950
Plasmodium knowlesi infection, 276
Plasmodium malariae infection, 276
Plasmodium ovale infection, 275
Plasmodium vivax infection, 275
Platelet-derived growth factor (PDGF), 1317
Platelet-endothelial cell adhesion molecule type 1 (PECAM-1), 447
Platelet function disorders, 970–971
Platelets, 918, 920f
concentrate, 931b
count
in coagulation screening tests, 922b
high, 929–930
low, 929
function, assessing, 921
reference range of, 1362b
Plethysmography (SpO₂), 175b
Pleural disease, 625–627
Pleural effusion, 562–565, 1329, 1329b
cardiac failure in, 563b
causes of, 563b
clinical assessment of, 563
investigations of, 563–564
large right, 547f

malignant, 563b
management of, 564
obstruction of thoracic duct in, 563b
oedema, 395–396
pancreatitis in, 563b
pulmonary infarction in, 563b
rheumatoid disease in, 563b, 610–611
in systemic lupus erythematosus, 1035
systemic lupus erythematosus in, 563b
tuberculosis in, 563b, 589f–590f
Pleural pain
in community-acquired pneumonia, treatment of, 584
in lung cancer, 600
Pleural plaques, 617–618, 617f
Pleural rub, 457–459
Plexopathy, 1138
brachial, 1141
lumbosacral, 1141
Plumboporphyria, 379b
Plummer-Vinson syndrome, 795–796
Pluripotent stem cells, induced, for genetic disease, 58
Pneumatosis cystoides intestinalis, 837
Pneumococcal infection, 266
Pneumoconiosis, 614–616, 615b
Pneumocystis jirovecii infection, after HSCT, 937b
Pneumocystis jirovecii pneumonia, HIV-related, 315b, 318, 318b, 318f
Pneumocytes, 548–549
Pneumonia, 582–587
bacterial, HIV-related, 319f
community-acquired, 582–585, 582f
clinical features of, 582–583
discharge and follow-up of, 585
investigations of, 583, 584b
management of, 583–584
organisms causing, 582b
prognosis for, 585
complications of, 585b
differential diagnosis of, 583b
factors predispose to, 582b
hospital-acquired, 585–586, 585b
in immunocompromised patient, 587
necrotising, 104b
occupational, 618–619
pregnancy and, 1277
causes of, 1277b
viral, 1277
right middle lobe, 547f, 584f
suppurative pneumonia, aspiration pneumonia and pulmonary abscess, 586–587
Pneumonic plague, 259
Pneumothorax, 547f, 625–627, 625f
age distribution of, 625f
air travel after, 169
classification of, 625b
clinical features of, 626
investigations of, 626
management of, 626–627, 627f
spontaneous
recurrent, 627
types of, 626f
tension, 566
Podocytes, 384
Podophyllotoxin, 343
Point mutations, 42
Point-of-care testing (POCT), 348
Poiseuille's Law, 447
Poisoning, 131–150
acute, 134
assessment and investigation for, 134–135, 135b
from chemicals and pesticides, 144–149
chemicals less commonly taken in, 148, 148b
clinical signs of, 133f
decontamination and enhanced elimination for, 133f
drugs of misuse and, 141–144
environmental, 149
evaluation for, 132–134, 132b, 132f

food-related, 149–150
management of, 135–137
antidotes for, 137, 137b
gastrointestinal decontamination for, 135–136, 136b
haemodialysis and haemoperfusion for, 136, 136b
lipid emulsion therapy for, 136–137
supportive care for, 137, 137b
urinary alkalinisation for, 136
in old age, 134b
by pharmaceutical agents, 137–141
less commonly taken in, 141, 141b
plant, 150, 150b
poisoned patient, general approach to, 134–137
psychiatric assessment for, 135
substances involved in, 134b
substances of very low toxicity and, 134b
triage and resuscitation, 134
Poliomyelitis, 1123, 1123f
immunisation for, 1123
incubation period of, 1123
Pollution, atmospheric, 94
PolyA tail, 39f, 40
Polyadenylation signal, 38
Polyarteritis nodosa, 1042
Polyarthritis, 993–994, 993b, 1020–1021
inflammatory arthritis and, extra-articular features of, 994b
joint involvement in, 994f
symmetrical, 1032
Polycystic ovarian syndrome, 658–659, 659f
features of, 658b
hirsutism and, 658b, 659
Polycythaemia, 384–386, 925
Polycythaemia rubra vera (PRV), 925, 970
Polydipsia, 357, 634b
Polyenes, 126
Polyethylene glycol, 842
Polymerase chain reaction (PCR), 106
for genetic diseases, 52, 53f
for hepatitis B, 873
for herpes simplex virus, 333, 1077
for Whipple's disease, 809
Polymorphic eruption of pregnancy, 1220b
Polymorphic light eruption, 1221b
Polymorphisms, 45
single nucleotide, 45
Polymorphonuclear cells, 1122
Polymorphonuclear leucocytes, 64
Polymyalgia rheumatica (PMR), 1042–1043
mimic, 1042b
Polymyositis (PM) see Dermatomyositis/polymyositis
Polymyxins, 123
Polyneuropathy, 1139b
chronic, 1140–1141
critical illness, 211–212
Polyostotic fibrous dysplasia, 1055
Polypeptides, 768
Polyposis syndromes, 827–829, 827b
juvenile, 829
Polyps, 827–829, 827b
Polyuria, 396–397, 396b, 634b
Pompe's disease, 1144b
Pompholyx, 1247
Population health, 91–98
Porphyria cutanea tarda (PCT), 379b, 1257, 1263–1264, 1264f
Porphyrias, 378–380, 1221b, 1263–1264
acute intermittent, 379b
congenital erythropoietic, 379b
cutaneous, 1263–1264
erythropoietic protoporphyria, 379b
hepatic, exacerbation of, 1266b
hereditary coproporphyria, 379b
plumboporphyria, 379b
variegate, 379b
'Portal' circulation, 384, 385f

Portal hypertension, 868–871, 898
ascites and, 869
cirrhosis and, 868
classification of, 868f
clinical features of, 868–869
complications of, 868b
extrahepatic portal vein obstruction, 868
investigations for, 869
management of, 869–871
pathophysiology of, 869
Portal vein thrombosis, 898
Portal venous disease, 898
Portal venous pressure, pharmacological reduction of, 870
Portopulmonary hypertension, 898
Portosystemic shunt
fetor hepaticus from, 868
portal hypertension and, 869
for variceal bleeding, 871
Posaconazole, 126
Positron emission tomography (PET)
for cancer, 1323, 1323f
of gastrointestinal tract, 778b
for Hodgkin lymphoma, 962, 963f
of nervous system, 1072
for oesophageal carcinoma, 796f
for respiratory disease, 553, 553f
Post-cholecystectomy syndrome, 908, 908b
Post-exposure prophylaxis, for HIV infection/AIDS, 327
Post-micturition dribble, 437
Post-partum blues, 1206
Post-partum haemorrhage
primary, 1275
secondary, 1275
Post-partum thyroiditis, 647, 651b
in pregnancy, 651b, 1279
Post-pyloric feeding, 707
Post-transplant lymphoproliferative disorders (PTLDs), 1299
Post-traumatic stress disorder, 1201–1202
Posterior circulation stroke (POCS), 1156f
Posterior descending artery, 444
Posterior scleritis, 1170
Posterior uveitis, 1172
Posteroanterior (PA) film, of chest X-ray, 551
Postmortem examination, 213
Postural hypotension, renal dysfunction, 395–396
Posture, examination of, 1063b
Potassium, 349b, 718
and diabetic ketoacidosis, 738
dietary sources of, 717b
foods high in, 418b
homeostasis, 360–363
presenting problems in, 361–363
intake, chronic renal failure, 418
plasma concentration control and, 360f
reference nutrient intake of, 717b
reference range of
urine, 1361b
venous blood, 1358b
renal handling, 360, 360f
ROMK channel, 360
supplements, 367
Potassium chloride, hypokalaemia, 362
Potassium phosphate, 369
Potassium-sparing diuretics, for hypervolaemia, 355
Potency, 16
Poverty, health consequences of, 94
Poxviruses, 248–249
Practolol, nephrotoxicity, 427b
Praziquantel, 129
Pre-eclampsia, hypertension and, 1276–1277, 1276b, 1277f
Pre-exposure prophylaxis, for HIV infection/AIDS, 327
Pre-implantation genetic diagnosis (PGD), 56
Pre-patellar bursitis, 999b
Pre-symptomatic/predictive testing, 59

Pre-test probability, in clinical decision-making, 11
Pre-transfusion testing, 934
Precocious puberty (PP), 654
Prednisolone
for alcoholic hepatitis, 882
for autoimmune hepatitis, 886–887
for eosinophilic gastroenteritis, 811–812
for gout, 1015
for inflammatory bowel disease, 821b
liver transplantation and, 901
for respiratory disease
aspergillosis, 596
asthma, 572
chronic eosinophilic pneumonia, 611–612
COPD, 578
hypersensitivity pneumonitis, 617
rheumatoid disease, 610
sarcoidosis, 610
for syphilis, 339
for systemic lupus erythematosus, 1036
for type II thyrotoxicosis, 648
for warm autoimmune haemolysis, 950
Prefrontal cortex (PFC), high-risk behaviour and, 1295
Pregabalin, 1102b
Pregnancy
abnormal liver function tests in, 900b
adolescent, rates of, 1296b
adrenal disease in, 1280
air travel and, 169
analytes affected by, 1364b
antimicrobial agents in, 120b
biliary obstruction and, 900
cardiac disease in, 1282
cholecystitis and, 900
congenital heart disease in, 533, 533b
diabetes in, 1278–1279
diabetes mellitus in, 752–753
dyslipidaemia in, 377b
ectopic, 336
endocrine disease in, 1279–1280
functional anatomy and physiology in, 1272–1273
bone metabolism and, 1272
cardiovascular system and, 1272
endocrine system and, 1272
gastrointestinal system and, 1272
genitourinary system and, 1272
glucose metabolism in, 1272–1273
haematological system and, 1272–1273
respiratory system and, 1273
gallstones and, 900
gastrointestinal disease in, 1277–1278
haematological disease in, 1284–1285
anaemia as, 1284, 1285b
Rhesus disease as, 1285
thrombocytopenia as, 1285, 1285b
venous thromboembolism as, 1285
haematological physiology in, 941b
hepatitis A and, 900
hepatitis B and, 900
hepatitis C and, 900
hepatitis E and, 900
hormonal changes in, 1273f
human immunodeficiency virus infection in, 1280
hypertension in, 1276–1277
hypothyroidism in, 641, 651b
immunological diseases during, 88b
inflammatory bowel disease in, 823–824, 824b
inflammatory rheumatic disease in, 1280–1281
iodine deficiency in, 651b
ketoacidosis and, 1279
laboratory reference range in, 1364
liver disease and, 899–900, 1283–1284
medical disorders in, 1276–1285

Pregnancy (Continued)
  neurological disease during
    epilepsy, 1103, 1103b
    multiple sclerosis, 1110b
  neurological disease in, 1284
  neutrophilia during, 926
  nutrition in, 712b
  osteoporosis in, 1045
  parathyroid disease in, 1280
  physiological anaemia in, 1273
  pituitary disease in, 1280
    diabetes insipidus as, 1280
    prolactinoma as, 1280
    Sheehan's syndrome as, 1280
  planning of, in patients with medical
      conditions, 1272
  post-partum thyroiditis in, 651b
  prescribing in, 32–33, 32b
  presenting problems of, 1274–1276
    breathlessness as, 1274–1275
    chest pain as, 1275
    circulatory collapse as, 1275
    headache as, 1275
    nausea and vomiting as, 1275,
        1275b
    oedema as, 1275
    seizures as, 1275–1276, 1276b
  prolactinoma in, 685
  psychiatric disorders during,
      1206–1207, 1206b, 1284
  renal disease in, 426, 426b,
      1282–1283
  respiratory disease in, 1277
  Rhesus D blood groups in, 933b
  rheumatoid arthritis in, 1026b
  safety of antirheumatic drugs during,
      1281b
  sickle-cell disease in, 953, 953b
  STI during, 332, 332b
  swollen legs in, 187, 188b
  syphilis in, 339
  thyroid disease in, 651b, 1279
  thyrotoxicosis in, 645, 651b
  unplanned, transition medicine and,
      1295–1296
  visual disorders and, 1175b
Prenatal genetic testing, 56, 59
Prescribing, 13–36, 14b
  choice of drug, 29
  decision-making in, 28–31
  for elderly patients, 32, 32b
  high-risk moments, 33b
  in hospitals, 33
  monitoring treatment effects, 31
  patient involvement, 30–31, 31b
  for patients with hepatic disease, 32,
      32b
  for patients with renal disease, 31–32
  in practice, 28–36
  for pregnancy and breastfeeding,
      32–33, 32b
  in primary care, 33–34
  principles of, during transition, 1289,
      1289b
  repeat, 34
  in special circumstances, 31–33
  steps in, 14b
  writing, 31, 33–34, 34f–35f
Prescription-only medicine (PoM), 27
Pressure areas, of stroke patients,
      1159b
Pressure sores, 1262
  in stroke patients, 1159f
Presyncope, 181–183, 455
  clinical assessment of, 182–183
  congenital heart disease and, 533
  differential diagnosis of, 182f
  features of, 181b
  gastrointestinal haemorrhage, 780
  heat, 167
  investigations of, 183
  in older people, 1308
  presentation of, 181–182
  seizures versus, 182b
Pretibial myxoedema, 646
Prevalence, of disease, 95
Preventive medicine, 93–94
  alcohol, 94
  atmospheric pollution, 94

obesity, 94
poverty and affluence, 94
smoking, 94
Prevotella spp., 103f
Prick tests, 1215
Primary afferent neurons, 1338
Primary biliary cholangitis, 887–888
  AMA-negative, 888
  associated diseases with, 887
  autoimmune hepatitis and, 888
  bone disease and, 888
  clinical features of, 887
  diagnosis and investigations for,
      887–888
  epidemiology of, 887
  fatigue and, 888
  liver function test (LFT) abnormality in,
      854b
  management of, 888
  natural history of, 887f
  in old age, 901b
  overlap syndromes, 888
  pathophysiology of, 887
  primary sclerosing cholangitis and,
      902b
  pruritus and, 888
Primary CNS lymphoma, 320, 320f
Primary disease, in endocrinology,
      632–633
Primary eosinophilias, 927
Primary granules, 64
Primary haemostasis, disorders of,
      970–971
Primary headache syndromes, 185b
Primary hyperaldosteronism, 674–675,
      674b, 675f
Primary hyperparathyroidism, 663–664,
      663b, 664f
  biochemical abnormalities in, 990b
  pregnancy and, 1280
Primary idiopathic acquired aplastic
      anaemia, 968–969, 968b
Primary immune deficiency, warning
      signs of, 73b
Primary sclerosing cholangitis, 888–890,
      889f
  diagnostic criteria for, 888
  diseases associated with, 889b
  liver function test (LFT) abnormality in,
      854b
  magnetic resonance
      cholangiopancreatogram of, 889,
      889f
  primary biliary cholangitis and, 902b
Primary Sjögren's syndrome (PSS),
      1038–1039
Primidone, 1102b
Prion diseases, 250, 1126–1127,
      1127b, 1191b
Prions, 102
Pro-carboxypeptidases, 770b
Pro-elastase, 770b
Probenecid, for neurosyphilis, 1125
Problem-solving therapy, 1191, 1191b
Procaine penicillin
  for neurosyphilis, 1125
  for syphilis, 339
Procaine reaction, 339
Procarboxypeptidases, 768
Prochlorperazine, 803, 1104
Proctocolitis, radiation, 809–810, 810b
Proctoscopy, 339
Procyclidine, 1102b
Progeric syndromes, 41
Progesterone
  pregnancy and, 1272
  reference range of, 1359b
Progesterone receptors, as tumour
      markers, 1322, 1324b
Progestogens, in cancer treatment,
      1332
Progressive multifocal
      leucoencephalopathy, 1123
Progressive pulmonary hypertension, in
      systemic sclerosis, 1038
Progressive supranuclear palsy,
      1114–1115
Proguanil, 128
  for malaria, 278b

Prokaryotes, 100–101
Prolactin (PRL), reference range of,
      1359b
Prolactinoma, 684–685, 685b, 685f
  pregnancy and, 1280
Prolymphocytic leukaemia (PLL), 960
Prone positioning, as advanced
      respiratory support, 204
Propantheline, 1142–1143
Prophase, 40
Prophylactic gonadectomy, for Turner's
      syndrome, 660
Propionibacterium spp., 103f
Propranolol
  for anxiety disorder, 1201
  for congestive 'portal hypertensive'
      gastropathy, 871
  for variceal bleeding, 869
Proptosis, of ophthalmic disease, 1171
Propylthiouracil (PTU)
  for Graves' thyrotoxicosis, 644
  for thyrotoxicosis, in pregnancy, 1279
Prosody, 1070
Prostacyclin, 447
  for acute kidney injury, 422
Prostaglandin E1, erectile dysfunction,
      440
Prostaglandin E2, febrile response, 104
Prostate
  benign hyperplasia, 437
  cancer, 438–439
Prostate gland, 386
Prostate-specific antigen (PSA), 439b
  as tumour markers, 1322, 1324b
Prostatic acid phosphatase (PAP), as
      tumour markers, 1322, 1324b
Prostatitis, 437
Prosthetic valve dysfunction, 527
Prosthetic valves, 526–527
Protease inhibitors (PIs), 324b
Proteases, 768
Protein C deficiency, 977
Protein-losing enteropathy, 811b
Protein S deficiency, 977
Proteins, 697, 697b, 1305
  Bence Jones, 394–395
  biliary transport, 851f
  cerebrospinal fluid, 1361b
  cholesterol ester, 373
  digestion of, 768, 769f
  IGF-BP3, 633f
  metabolism of, effects of insulin in,
      723b
  plasma, 850
  production of, 39f, 40
  reference range of
    urine, 1361b
    venous blood, 1360b
  restriction in, for hepatic
      encephalopathy, 865
  Tamm-Horsfall, 392
  urine, 1361b
Proteinuria, 392–395, 394b
  in diabetic neuropathy, 727
  investigation of, 394f
  orthostatic, 394
  overt (dipstick-positive, 394–395
  pregnancy and, 1282
  reduction of, 417
  tubular, 394
Proteoglycans, 987
Proteosome inhibitor, for multiple
      myeloma, 968
Proteus spp., 103f
Prothrombin G20210A, 977
Prothrombin time (PT), 920–921
  in coagulation screening tests,
      922b
  for gastrointestinal bleeding, 781
  for liver disease, 850, 853
    acute liver failure and, 858
    alcoholic hepatitis and, 882
  reference range of, 1362b
Prothrombotic states, 977–979
Proto-oncogenes, 56–57
'Proton pump', 767
Proton pump inhibitor, for variceal
      bleeding, 869b
Protozoa, 101–102

Protozoal infections, 273–288
  gastrointestinal, 286–288
  leishmaniasis, 281–286
  systemic, 273–281
Prozone phenomenon, 338–339
Prurigo gestationis, 1220b
Pruritic folliculitis, 1220b
Pruritus, 1219–1220, 1326
  clinical assessment of, 1219–1220
  investigations and management of,
      1220, 1220f
  of ophthalmic disease, 1170
  in pregnancy, 1220b
  primary biliary cholangitis and, 887
    treatment for, 888
  primary causes of, 1219b
  secondary causes of, 1219b
Pruritus ani, 836, 836b
Pseudo-hallucinations, 1184
Pseudo precocious puberty, 654
Pseudocyst, pancreatic, 838f
Pseudohypoparathyroidism, 664–665
Pseudomonas aeruginosa, 117b
Pseudomonas fluorescens, 225
Pseudoporphyria, 1221b, 1257, 1266b
Psoralens, for skin disease, 1227
Psoriasiform, drug-induced, 1266b
Psoriasis, 1247–1251
  arthropathy and, 1249
  clinical features of, 1249, 1249f
  erythrodermic, 1249
  guttate, 1249
  investigations of, 1250
  management of, 1250–1251,
      1250f–1251f
  pathogenesis of, 1248, 1248b,
      1248f
  plaque, 1249
  pustular, 1249
  rash in, 1217b
Psoriatic arthritis (PsA), 1032–1034
  CASPAR criteria for, 1032b
  clinical features of, 1032–1033,
      1033f
  investigations for, 1033
  management for, 1033–1034
  pathophysiology of, 1032
Psoriatic spondylitis, 1032
Psychiatric assessment, poisoning and,
      135
Psychiatric disorders, 1094, 1191–1207
  classification of risk factors for, 1183,
      1183b
  clinical examination of, 1180–1183
    mental state examination,
        1181–1183
    psychiatric interview, 1181, 1181b
  emergencies for, 1189b
  functional anatomy and physiology in,
      1183–1184
    biological factors, 1183
    psychological and behavioural
        factors, 1183
    social and environmental factors,
        1184
  HIV-related, 321
  law and, 1207
  management of, 1189–1191
    electroconvulsive therapy, 1190
    pharmacological treatment, 1190
    psychological therapies,
        1190–1191
    social interventions, 1191
    surgery, 1190
  in old age, 1189b
  organic, 1189b
  in pregnancy, 1284
  presenting problems of, 1184–1189
  prevalence of, 1180b
  psychological factors affecting
      medical conditions, 1186–1187,
      1186b
  puerperal, 1206–1207
  WHO classification of, 1180, 1180b
Psychodynamic psychotherapy, 1191
Psychogenic attacks, 1099
Psychogenic pruritus, 1219b
Psychological elements, in back pain,
      995–996

Psychological factors
affecting medical conditions, 1186–1187, 1186b
of migraine, 1095
Psychological therapies/psychotherapy, 1190–1191
for alcohol misuse, 1195
general, 1190
interpersonal, 1191
for pain, 1347
psychodynamic, 1191
Psychosis
affective, 1200
organic, 1197
puerperal, 1206
toxic, 1195–1196
Psychotropic drugs, 1190b
Pthirus pubis, 334b
Ptosis
causes of, 1091b
unilateral, 1091f
Puberty
analytes affected by, 1363b
delayed, 653–654, 653b, 1290
hormonal events of, 1291f
initiation of, 1290
onset of, 1290
Pubic (crab) lice, 1241
Pubic symphysitis, 999b
Puerperal psychiatric disorders, 1206–1207
Pulmonary abscess, 586–587
Pulmonary artery catheter, 206, 207f
Pulmonary artery wedge pressure, portopulmonary hypertension and, 898
Pulmonary circulation, 549–550
Pulmonary embolism, 619–621
acute massive, 200
clinical features of, 619, 619b
investigations of, 619–620, 619f–620f
management of, 620–621
in pregnancy, 620b
prognosis for, 621
in stroke patients, 1159f
Pulmonary eosinophilia and vasculitides, 611–612, 611b
Pulmonary fibrosis, 547f
in dermatomyositis, 610b
idiopathic, 605–608, 607f
in respiratory function abnormalities, 555b
in rheumatoid arthritis, 610b, 1024
in sarcoidosis, 609b
in sclerosis, 610b
in systemic lupus erythematosus, 610b
Pulmonary hypertension, 550, 621–622, 621b, 622f
congenital heart disease and, 533
systemic sclerosis and, 1038
Pulmonary nodules
cryptococcosis, 302
lung metastases, 1328
in respiratory disease, 560–562, 560b–561b, 560f–562f
Pulmonary oedema, 413–414, 413f
high-altitude, 168–169
renal artery stenosis, 407
sputum in, 546f
Pulmonary regurgitation, 526, 527b
Pulmonary rehabilitation, for chronic obstructive pulmonary disease (COPD), 577
Pulmonary stenosis, 526
Pulmonary syndrome, 258
Pulmonary tuberculosis
clinical presentations of, 590b
HIV-related, 318–319, 319f
major manifestations and differential diagnosis of, 590f
post-primary, 589
primary, 588, 589b, 589f
Pulmonary tuberous sclerosis, 613b
Pulmonary valve disease, 526
Pulmonary vascular disease, 619–622
pulmonary embolism, 619–621
pulmonary hypertension, 621–622, 621b, 622f

Pulse, in endocrine disease, 630f
Pulsus paradoxus, 447–448
Pupillary abnormalities, 1090, 1091f, 1092b
Purkinje fibres, 445
Purpura
definition of, 1226
drug-induced, 1266b
Henoch-Schönlein, 398b–399b, 401, 1043
idiopathic thrombocytopenic, 971
non-thrombocytopenic, 928b
petechial, 928–929, 928f
pinch, 1264
senile, 978b
thrombotic thrombocytopenic, 388, 409, 979
Pustule, definition of, 1211f
Pustuloderma, drug-induced, 1266b
Pustulosis
acute generalised exanthematous, 1266b
palmoplantar, 1249
PUVA, 1215, 1227
atopic eczema, 1246
granuloma annulare, 1263
lichen planus, 1252
necrobiosis lipoidica, 1263
psoriasis, 1250
vitiligo, 1257–1258
Pyelography, 390
retrograde, 390f
Pyelonephritis
acute, 402f, 430
chronic, 430
emphysematous, 430
pregnancy and, 1282
Pyeloplasty, 434
Pyloroplasty, 782
Pyoderma gangrenosum, 1261–1262, 1262f
Pyonephrosis, 432
Pyopneumothorax, 564
Pyramidal gait, 1086–1087
Pyrantel pamoate, 129
Pyrazinamide
as antimycobacterial agents, 125
for tuberculous meningitis, 1121
Pyrexia of unknown origin, 218–222
aetiology of, 220b
clinical assessment of, 218–219
investigations of, 219–222, 221b
prognosis of, 222
Pyridostigmine, 1142–1143
Pyridoxal, 715
Pyridoxamine, 715
Pyridoxine (vitamin B$_6$), 715
biochemical assessment of, 712b
deficiency, 715
dietary sources of, 711b
reference nutrient intake of, 711b
supplements, 715
Pyrimethamine
malaria, 273
toxoplasmosis, 281
HIV-related, 320
Pyrimidine 5' nucleotidase deficiency, 949
Pyrin, 81
Pyrophosphate arthritis, 993b
Pyruvate kinase deficiency, 949
Pyuria, sterile, 430

Q
Q fever, 231b, 272
endocarditis, 272, 528
Qualitative abnormalities, 951
Quality-adjusted life years (QALYs), 28, 28b
Quality of life, 202b
Quantitative abnormalities, 951
Quantitative sensory testing, for pain, 1342, 1342f
Questions, medical interview, 231b
Quetiapine
bipolar disorder, 1200
delirium, 209
Quinagolide, prolactinoma, 685
Quincke's sign, 524b

Quinidine
arrhythmias, 480
malaria, 277b
and neutropenia, 926b
poisoning, 137b
Quinine
babesiosis, 278
lichenoid eruptions, 1252
for malaria, 128
poisoning, 141b
Quinolones, 122–123, 123b
adverse effects of, 123
drug eruptions, 1266b
mechanism of action, 116b
in old age, 120b
pharmacokinetics of, 122
in pregnancy, 120b
prophylactic, spontaneous bacterial peritonitis, 864
for spontaneous bacterial peritonitis, 864
see also Fluoroquinolones

R
R protein, 944
RA see Rheumatoid arthritis
Rabies, 1122–1123
incubation period, 111b, 232b
prophylaxis for
post-exposure, 1122–1123
pre-exposure, 1122
vaccination, 115b, 1122–1123
Radial nerve, entrapment, 1139b
Radial pulse, 534
examination of, in respiratory system, 546f
Radiation(s), 164–165
dosage and exposure of, 164
effects of exposure to, 164–165
enteritis and proctocolitis, 809–810, 810b
infrared, 1222f
ionising, 164, 164f
management of exposure to, 165
mutagenic effects, 1320b
natural background, 164
non-ionising, 164
pneumonitis, 612
proctocolitis, 809–810, 810b
ultraviolet see Ultraviolet radiation
Radicular pain, 997b, 998f
Radiculography, 1073b
Radiculopathy, 256, 1138, 1141
cervical, 1134, 1134f
HIV-related, 321
Radio-femoral delay, 442f
Radio-iodine therapy, for thyrotoxicosis, 637–638, 645b
Radioactive iodine, for Graves' thyrotoxicosis, 644b, 645
Radioallergosorbent test (RAST), 86
Radiofrequency ablation
arrhythmias, 481b, 484f
cardiovascular disease, 484
GORD, 792–793
for hepatocellular carcinoma, 891
liver metastases, 1328–1329
renal cell cancer, 435
Radiography see X-rays
Radioiodine
multinodular goitre, 649
thyrotoxicosis, 637, 644b
Radioisotope imaging see Radionuclide (radioisotope) imaging
Radioisotope tests, gastroenterology, 778
Radioisotopes
cancer treatment, 1331
exposure to, 165
intravenous injection of, 1331
Radiology see CT; MRI; X-rays
Radionuclide (radioisotope) imaging
of bone, 988–989
of cardiovascular system, 454
of nervous system, 1073b
Paget's disease, 1054f
renal disease, 390, 390f
Radionuclide studies, renal disease, 390, 390f

Radionuclide ventilation/perfusion (V̇/Q̇) scanning, pregnancy and, 1274
Radiotherapy, 1331–1332
for acromegaly, 686
adverse effects, 1331f, 1332
blood disorders
chronic lymphocytic leukaemia, 960
Hodgkin lymphoma, 962
multiple myeloma, 968
non-Hodgkin lymphoma, 965
for brain tumours, 1130–1131
breast cancer, 1334
for cancer pain, 1352
colorectal cancer, 832
conformal, 1331
fractionation, 1331
for high-grade NHL, 966
hypothyroidism and, 1298
late effects, 689, 955b
for low-grade NHL, 965
lung cancer, 602
for lung cancer, 602
lung damage, 612
lung disease due to, 612
mesothelioma, 618
for multiple myeloma, 968
oesophageal cancer, 797
for oral cancer, 790
pain management, 1344
palliative, 1352
pituitary tumours, 683–684
for prolactinoma, 685
prostate cancer, 439
for skin disease, 1228–1229
Radon, lung cancer and, 561b
Raloxifene, for osteoporosis, 1048b, 1049
Raltegravir, 119b
Ramadan, diabetes during, 745, 745b
Ramipril
heart failure, 466b
hypertension, 513
myocardial infarction, 500–501
Ramsay Hunt syndrome, 239
Randomised controlled clinical trials, 27–28, 28f
Ranitidine
and neutropenia, 926b
urticaria, 1254
RANK (receptor activator of nuclear κB), 985
RANKL (Receptor activator of nuclear factor kappa B ligand), in bone remodelling, 986b
Rapid diagnostic tests (RDTs), immunochromatographic, 276
Rapid immunochromatographic tests, 258
Rapid plasma reagin (RPR), 338–339
Rapidly progressive glomerulonephritis, 397
diseases typically presenting with, 401
Rare inherited bleeding disorders, 974
Rare interstitial lung disease, 613b
Rasagiline, for Parkinson's disease, 1114
Rashes, 1216–1218, 1217b
atopic eczema, 1217b, 1246b
butterfly (malar), 982f
in chickenpox, 238
clinical features, 1217b
dengue, 243–244
dermatitis herpetiformis, 807
dermatomyositis, 1039
distribution, 1217b
drug eruption, 316, 1217b, 1267f
erythema migrans, 256f
erythematous, 1255
in fever, 218
genital, 333, 334b
haemorrhagic, 271b
hand, foot and mouth disease, 248
herpes simplex, 247f
HIV-related, 316
infectious mononucleosis, 242f
lichen planus, 334b, 1217b
Lyme borreliosis (disease), 256f
macular/maculopapular, 271b

Rashes *(Continued)*
morbiliform, 271*b*
parvovirus B19, 237*f*
petechiae, 928–929, 928*f*
photosensitivity, 1221*f*
pityriasis rosea, 1217*b*
pityriasis versicolor, 1217*b*
post-kala-azar dermal leishmaniasis, 284*f*
psoriasiform, 1266*b*
psoriasis, 1217*b*
purpura *see* Purpura
rheumatic fever, 515
in rubella infection, 234*b*
scaly, 1217*b*
scarlet fever, 253*f*
shingles, 238*f*
syphillis, 1217*b*
of systemic lupus erythematosus, 1035*f*
tinea corporis, 1217*b*
toxic shock syndrome, 1236
tropical diseases, 234*b*
typhoid, 260
typhus, 271
urticarial, 1253*f*
vesicular, 315
RAST (radioallergosorbent test), 86
Rat bite fever, 235*f*
Raynaud's phenomenon
in systemic lupus erythematosus, 1035, 1035*f*
in systemic sclerosis, 1037–1038
Raynaud's syndrome, 504–505
RB-ILD *see* Respiratory bronchiolitis-interstitial lung disease
RBBB *see* Right bundle branch block
RCA *see* Right coronary artery
Re-entry, 468
Reactive airways dysfunction syndrome, 614
Reactive arthritis, 1031–1032
Reactive disorders, 1264–1265
'Ready Steady Go' programme, 1290
Reassurance, somatoform disorders and, 1203
Receiver operating characteristic (ROC) curve, 5*f*
Receptor activator of nuclear factor kappa B ligand (RANKL), in bone remodelling, 986*b*
Receptor activator of nuclear factor κB ligand *see* RANKL
Receptor activator of nuclear κB *see* RANK
Receptors
B-cell, 68, 68*f*
drugs acting on, 15*b*
in pain processing, 1340*b*
Recombinant human DNAase (rhDNAase), cystic fibrosis, 581*f*
Recombinant human erythropoietin, chronic renal failure, 419
Recombinant tissue plasminogen activator (rt-PA), stroke, 1158*f*, 1159–1160
Recombination, 41
Recompression, for diving-related illness, 171
Rectal administration, 17
Rectal examination, 765*b*
gastrointestinal disease, 787
prostate, 427, 437–438
Rectal varices, portal hypertension and, 868
Rectum, 771*f*
disorders of, 827–836
dysfunction of, 1094
tumours of, 827–833
see also Colorectal cancer
Recurrent occult upper gastrointestinal bleeding, systemic sclerosis and, 1037–1038
Red cell enzymopathies, 948–949
Red cell membrane
defect, 947–948
structure, 915, 916*f*

Red cells, 915–917, 916*f*
agglutination, cold, 950
anaemia, 941*f*
aplasia, 947
appearance of, 921*b*, 921*f*
blood film examination, 921*f*
concentrate, 931*b*
count, 1362*b*
destruction of, 917
effects of malaria, 273–274
enzymopathies, 948–949
formation, 915, 916*f*
fragments, 921*f*
haemoglobin and, 915–916, 917*f*
haemolytic anaemia, 945, 946*b*, 946*f*
incompatibility, in blood transfusion, 931–933
lifespan, 1362*b*
membrane defects, 947–948
nucleated, 921*f*
sickled *see* Sickle-cell anaemia/disease
structure and functions, 915–917, 916*f*
transfusion, (in)compatibility, 932–933
Red eye, 1170
Red hepatisation, 583
'Red man' reaction, 123
Reduced-intensity conditioning, 937
5α-Reductase inhibitors, 438
Reduviid bugs, 280
Reed-Sternberg cells, 961
Refeeding diets, WHO recommended, 705, 705*b*
Refeeding syndrome, 706
Reference nutrient intake (RNI), 711–712
of minerals, 717*b*
of vitamins, 711*b*
Reference range, 3, 4*f*
Reflex(es)
cough, 556
diabetes, 759
stretch, 1068
tendon, root values of, 1063*b*
Reflex sympathetic dystrophy (RSD), 1348–1349
Reflux
bile, 801
duodenogastro-oesophageal, 792
gastro-oesophageal, 791–794, 791*f*
Reflux nephropathy, 430–431
Refractory cough, 169
Refractory hypertension, 514
Regenerative medicine, for genetic disease, 58
Regurgitation, 779
aortic, 443*b*, 524–525, 524*b*, 525*f*
causes, 524*b*
chest X-ray for, 451*f*
clinical features, 524–525, 524*b*
clinical features of, 524–525, 524*b*, 525*f*
investigations, 525, 525*b*
investigations of, 525, 525*b*
mitral, 519–521, 519*b*, 520*f*
clinical features of, 521*b*, 521*f*
investigation of, 521*b*
management of, 521
pulmonary, 526, 527*b*
tricuspid, 526, 526*b*
Rehabilitation
for acute coronary syndrome, 501
myocardial infarction, 501
in older people, 1311–1312
schizophrenia, 1198
for somatoform disorders, 1203
stroke, 1158
Rehydration *see* Fluid replacement
Reiter's disease/syndrome *see* Reactive arthritis
Relapsing fevers
louse-borne, 256*b*, 257, 257*f*
tick-borne, 256*b*, 257
Relapsing polychondritis, 1044
Relative erythrocytosis, 925, 925*b*
REM sleep behaviour disorder, 1105
Remission consolidation, in acute leukaemia, 956

Remission induction, in acute leukaemia, 956
Remission maintenance, in acute leukaemia, 956
Renal *see* Kidney
Renal allograft dysfunction, common causes of, 425*b*
Renal arteriography/venography, 389
Renal artery stenosis, 406–408, 407*b*, 407*f*
Renal biopsy, 391, 391*b*
Renal cell cancer, 434–435, 435*f*
Renal colic, 396
Renal dialysis *see* Dialysis, renal
Renal disease
in adolescence, 426, 426*b*
atheroembolic, 390*b*, 410
chronic, 415–420
pruritus, 415
stages, 388*b*
in connective tissue disease
Henoch-Schönlein purpura, 1043
SLE, 1036
systemic sclerosis, 1038
cystic, 405–406
adult polycystic kidney, 405–406
medullary, 404
diabetics *see* Diabetic nephropathy
drug-induced, 426, 427*b*
genetic, 403–406
glomerular, 397–401
HIV-related, 322
infections, 426–431
investigation of, 386–391
in pregnancy, 426, 426*b*, 1282–1283
acute kidney injury as, 1282, 1283*b*
chronic kidney disease as, 1282, 1283*f*
glomerular disease and, 1282
renal replacement therapy for, 1282–1283
renal tract infection as, 1282
for prescribing patients with, 31–32, 426
presenting problems in, 391–397
signs, 416*f*
transition medicine and, 1298–1299
tuberculosis, 591
tubulo-interstitial, 401–403
tumours/cancer, 1316*f*
vascular, 406–409
see also Nephropathy
Renal failure
acute *see* Acute kidney injury
ascites, 864
bleeding, 975
chronic, 415–420, 417*b*
causes of, 415*b*
haemodialysis in, 422–423
indications for dialysis for, 422*b*
osteodystrophy and, 419*f*
physical signs of, 416*f*
pregnancy and, 1282, 1283*f*
staging of, in children over 2 years of age, 1298*b*
transition medicine and, 1298–1299
cystic disease *see* Renal disease, cystic
diabetics, 757
end-stage, 415*b*
heart failure, 464
heart failure causing, 464
pruritus and, 1219*b*
pyelonephritis *see* Pyelonephritis
Renal function tests, 962
Renal impairment, causes of, in childhood and adolescence, 1298*b*
Renal infarction, acute, 408
Renal lesion, systemic lupus erythematosus and, 1035
Renal osteodystrophy, biochemical abnormalities in, 990*b*
Renal pelvis, 386
obstruction, 389*f*
pyelonephritis, 430

stone in, 431
tumours, 435
Renal replacement therapy (RRT), 208, 420–426, 421*f*
for acute kidney injury, 414
for chronic kidney disease, 414
continuous, 424*b*
in old age, 422*b*
percentage survival in, 422*f*
pregnancy and, 1282–1283
preparing for, 420
Renal stones, 431
composition of, 431*b*
investigations for, 432*b*
Renal support, in intensive care, 208
Renal tract infection, pregnancy and, 1282
Renal tract obstruction, acute kidney injury and, 414
Renal transplantation
in diabetic nephropathy, 758
recipients of, pregnancy and, 1283
Renal tubular acidosis, 365, 365*b*, 405
Renal tubules, 384–386
collecting ducts, 350–351, 384–386
distal, 350
loop of Henle, 350, 384–386
proximal, 350
Renal ultrasound, acute kidney injury and, 416*b*
Renin, 351–352
Renin activity, 666
Renin-angiotensin-aldosterone system, 362
hypertension, 509
hypokalaemia, 362
Renin-angiotensin blockade, for acute coronary syndrome, 500–501
Renin concentration, reference range of, 1359*b*
Repaglinide, 747
Repeat prescriptions, 34
Repeated dose regimens, 19
Reperfusion therapy, for acute coronary syndrome, 499–500
Replacement therapy, for amenorrhoea, 655
Replicative immortality, 1318
Reproductive disease
classification of, 652*b*
presenting problems in, 653–658
Reproductive system, 651–661
classification of diseases of, 652*b*
female, 652, 652*f*
functional anatomy, physiology and investigations of, 651–652, 651*f*–652*f*
Klinefelter's syndrome in, 660–661
male, 651, 651*f*
polycystic ovarian syndrome in, 658–659, 659*f*
Turner's syndrome in, 659–660, 660*f*
Resection
hepatic, for hepatocellular carcinoma, 891
ileal, under-nutrition and, 706
massive small bowel, under-nutrition and, 706
pancreatic, under-nutrition and, 706
Residual volume (RV), 555*b*
Resin
bile acid-sequestering, 376–377
ion-exchange, 363, 363*b*
Resistin, 699
Respiration
haemodynamic effects of, 447–448, 447*b*
Kussmaul, 415
see also Breathing
Respiratory acidosis, 367
Respiratory alkalosis, 367
Respiratory bronchiolitis-interstitial lung disease (RB-ILD), 606*b*
Respiratory burst, 64
Respiratory chain complexes, 49*b*
Respiratory disease, 556–567
air travel and, 169
breathlessness in, 557–558, 557*f*, 558*b*

caused by fungi, 596–598, 596b
chest pain in, 558
cough in, 556, 556b
drug-induced, 612–613, 612b
finger clubbing in, 559, 559b, 559f
haemoptysis in, 559–560, 559b, 560f
HIV-related, 318–319, 318b
investigation of, 550–556
ophthalmic features of, 1165b
pleural effusion in, 562–565,
    563b–564b
pregnancy and, 1277
pulmonary nodule in, 560–562,
    560b–561b, 560f–562f
respiratory failure in, 565–567, 565b
transition medicine and, 1297
cystic fibrosis, 1297
tumours, 598–605
Respiratory distress syndrome, acute
    see Acute respiratory distress
    syndrome
Respiratory failure, 565–567
acute, management of, 565–566
chronic and 'acute on chronic' type II,
    566–567
management of, 566–567, 566b
pathophysiology of, 565, 565b
Respiratory function
in old age, 550b
testing, 554–556, 554f
    airway obstruction, measurement
        of, 555
    arterial blood gases and oximetry,
        555–556, 555f
    in asthma, 555b
    in chronic bronchitis, 555b
    in emphysema, 555b
    exercise tests, 556
    lung volumes, 555
    in pulmonary fibrosis, 555b
    transfer factor, 555
Respiratory infections, 581–598
cystic fibrosis, 580–581
fungal, 596–598
in old age, 586b
pneumonia, 582–587
pregnancy and, 1277
    bacterial, 1277
    viral, 1277
tuberculosis (TB), 588–595
upper respiratory tract infection,
    581–587
Respiratory medicine, 545–628
Respiratory support, in intensive care,
    202–204
advanced, 204
extracorporeal, 204
intubation and intermittent positive
    pressure ventilation, 203–204
non-invasive, 202
weaning from, 209–210
Respiratory syncytial virus (RSV), 249
Respiratory system
clinical examination of, 546–548,
    546f–547f
functional anatomy and physiology of,
    548–550, 548f–549f
infections see Respiratory infections
in old age, 550b
pregnancy and, 1273
tumours, 598–605
Response evaluation criteria in solid
    tumours (RECIST), 1333b
Restless legs syndrome, 1105–1106,
    1106b
Restraint, for aggressive behaviour,
    1188–1189
Restrictive cardiomyopathy, 540
Resuscitation
drowning and, 170
for gastrointestinal haemorrhage, 782
hypothermia and, 166
initial, 204–206, 206b
for poisoning, 134
in sepsis, 196–197, 197b
Resynchronisation devices, 467, 467f
Resynchronisation therapy, cardiac,
    467f, 484
Reteplase, 500

Reticular formation, brainstem, 1067f
Reticulocytes, 915
reference range of, 1362b
Retina
detachment, 1088
of eye, 1167
visual field loss in, 1089b
Retinal artery occlusion, in
    ophthalmological conditions,
    1178, 1178f
Retinal haemorrhage
high-altitude, 169
see also Diabetic retinopathy
Retinal pigment epithelium, congenital
    hypertrophy, 829
Retinal vascular occlusion, in
    ophthalmological conditions,
    1177–1178
Retinal vein occlusion (thrombosis),
    1177–1178, 1177f
Retinitis
cytomegalovirus, 216f
HIV-related, 321
Retinitis pigmentosa, 810
Retinoblastoma, 1321b
Retinochoroiditis, due to toxoplasmosis,
    280, 281f
Retinoic acid, 713
all-trans-Retinoic acid, 958
Retinoids, 713
hyperlipidaemia, 373b
hypertriglyceridaemia, 374
phototherapy and
    photochemotherapy, 1227
for skin disease, 1227
squamous cell carcinoma, 1231
warts, 1239
Retinol (vitamin A), 712–713
deficiency, 713, 713f
dietary sources of, 711b
reference nutrient intake of, 711b
Retinopathy, 1325
HIV-related, 321
hypertensive, 509–510, 510b
pregnancy and, 1279
Retroperitoneal fibrosis, 434
drug-induced, 427b
Retroviruses, 100
Return of spontaneous circulation
    (ROSC), in post cardiac arrest,
    200–201, 201b
Reverse transcriptase, 309–310
Reverse transcriptase inhibitors
non-nucleoside, 316, 324b
nucleoside, 324b
Reversibility test, 569f
Revised International Prognostic Scoring
    System (IPSS-R), in
    myelodysplasia, 961, 961b
Reye's syndrome, acute liver failure
    and, 857–858
Rhabdomyolysis, 363
diagnosis and management of, 195
Rhesus D blood group, 933, 933b
Rhesus disease, pregnancy and, 1285
Rheumatic fever, 515–517, 516f
investigations in, 517b
Jones criteria for, 516b
prophylactic, 119b
Rheumatic heart disease, 515–517
chronic, 517
Rheumatoid arthritis (RA), 1021–1026
clinical features of, 1023–1025, 1023f
    cardiac involvement in, 1024
    extra-articular, 1024b
    nodules, in 1023–1024, 1024f
    ocular involvement in, 1024
    peripheral neuropathy in, 1024
    pulmonary involvement in, 1024
    serositis in, 1024
    spinal cord compression in, 1024,
        1025f
    systemic, 1023
    vasculitis in, 1024
criteria for diagnosis of, 1023b
investigations in, 1025, 1025b, 1026f
management of, 1025–1026
    algorithm for, 1026f
    biologic therapy for, 1026

DMARD therapy for, 1025–1026
non-pharmacological therapy for,
    1026
surgery for, 1026
pathophysiology of, 1022–1023,
    1022f
in pregnancy, 1026b, 1280
Rheumatoid disease
pleural effusion, 563b, 610–611
respiratory involvement in, 610–611,
    611f
Rheumatoid factor (RF), in
    musculoskeletal disease, 991,
    991b
Rheumatoid nodules, 1023–1024, 1024f
Rheumatological/musculoskeletal
    disease
HIV-related, 321–322
ophthalmic features of, 1166b
Rheumatology, 981–1060
see also Musculoskeletal disease
Rheumatology and bone disease,
    transition medicine and, 1300
glucocorticoid-induced osteoporosis
    in, 1300
hypophosphataemic rickets in, 1300
juvenile idiopathic arthritis in, 1300
osteogenesis imperfecta in, 1300
Rhinitis, allergic, 622
Rhinocladiella mackenziei, 301
Rhinosinusitis, 582
Rhinoviruses, 249
Rhizomucor spp., 303
Rhizopus spp., 303
Rhodesiense infections, 278
Rhodesiense trypanosomiasis, 278–279
Rhodococcus equi, 319
Rib fracture, 626b
Ribavirin, 128
for hepatitis C, 878
viral haemorrhagic fevers, 246
Riboflavin (vitamin B₂), 714
biochemical assessment of, 712b
deficiency, 714
dietary sources of, 711b
reference nutrient intake of, 711b
Ribonucleic acid (RNA)
degradation of, 40
editing of, 40
messenger ribonucleic acid (mRNA),
    38
microRNA (miRNA), 40
non-coding, 40
ribosomal RNA (rRNA), 40
splicing of, 40
synthesis of, 39f
transfer RNA (tRNA), 40
Ribosomes, 39f
Ribozymes, 40
Richmond Agitation Sedation Scale
    (RASS), 209, 209b
Richter's transformation, 960
Rickets, 1051–1052
causes of, 1050b
hypophosphataemic, 990b
hereditary, 1052–1053
hypophosphataemic, transition
    medicine and, 1300
vitamin D-resistant, 1052
Rickettsial fevers, 270–272, 271b
Rickety rosary, 1052
Riedel's thyroiditis, 650
Rifampicin, 117b
as antimycobacterial agents, 125
drug interactions of, 24
hepatotoxicity of, 894b
infective endocarditis, 530b
for leprosy, 269
meningitis, 1120b
pneumonia, 585b
prophylactic, 119b
for pruritus, primary biliary cholangitis
    and, 888
Q fever, 272
for tuberculosis, 593
Rifamycin, mechanism of action, 116b
Rifaximin, for hepatic encephalopathy,
    865
RIFLE criteria, 411

Rift Valley fever, 245b
Right atrial pressure, in critically ill
    patients, 207f
Right bundle branch block (RBBB), 478f
Right coronary artery (RCA), 444, 445f
Right ventricle, 444f
Right ventricular cardiomyopathy,
    arrhythmogenic, 453, 539f
Right ventricular dilatation, 450
Rigidity
cogwheel, 1069
lead pipe, 1069
Parkinson's disease, 1084–1085,
    1113b
tetanus, 1126
tetanus and, 1126
Rigors, 217b
Riluzole, amyotrophic lateral sclerosis,
    1117
Rimantadine, 127
Rimonabant, 702
Ringer-lactate, 265
Ringworm, 1239
Risedronate
for osteoporosis, 1048b
for Paget's disease, 1054, 1054b
Risk
attributable, 95b
global burden of disease and
    underlying factors, 92–93
relative, 95b
Risperidone
bipolar disorder, 1200
schizophrenia, 1198b
Risus sardonicus, 1126
Rituximab, for musculoskeletal disease,
    1006, 1007b
polymyositis and dermatomyositis,
    1040
systemic lupus erythematosus, 1037
Rivaroxaban, for venous
    thromboembolism, 975
Rivastigmine, for Parkinson's disease,
    1113
River blindness, 292–293
RNA
degradation of, 40
editing of, 40
messenger (mRNA), 38
messenger ribonucleic acid (mRNA),
    38
microRNA (miRNA), 40
non-coding, 40
ribosomal RNA (rRNA), 40
splicing, editing and degradation, 40
splicing of, 40
synthesis, 39f
synthesis of, 39f
transfer,
transfer RNA (tRNA), 40
RNA polymerase, 38
RNI see Reference nutrient intake
Robertsonian translocation, 45f
Rocky Mountain spotted fever, 270,
    271b
Rodent ulcer, 1229
Rodenticide poisoning, 148
Rokitansky-Aschoff sinuses, 909
Romaña's sign, 279
Romberg's test, 1062f
Romosozumab, for osteoporosis, 1049
Ropinirole, Parkinson's disease, 1114b
Rosacea, 1221b, 1243–1244, 1243f
Roseola infantum, 238
Rosiglitazone, 747
Ross River virus, 250, 1020–1021
Rotator cuff lesions, 997–998, 998b
Rotavirus, 249
Rotigotine, Parkinson's disease, 1114b
Rotor's syndrome, 860b
Roundworm (Ascaris lumbricoides),
    289–290, 906
Roux-en-Y gastric bypass, 703b
RPGN see Rapidly progressive
    glomerulonephritis
RSV see Respiratory syncytial virus
RT see Reverse transcriptase
rt-PA see Recombinant tissue
    plasminogen activator

RTA see Renal tubular acidosis
Rubber allergy, 1247b
Rubella infection
  clinical features of, 236
  congenital malformation and, 237b
  diagnosis of, 236
  in pregnancy, 235b
  prevention of, 236–237
Russell's sign, 1204
Ruxolitinib, for myelofibrosis, 969
RV see Residual volume
Ryanodine receptor channelopathies,
  1145b

S
SA node see Sinoatrial (SA) node
Sabin-Feldman dye test, 281
Saccades, 1090
Sacroiliitis, 1029f
  and ankylosing spondylitis, 1030
  and axial spondyloarthropathies,
    1028, 1028b
  and brucellosis, 255f
  and inflammatory bowel disease,
    819f
  polyarthritis and, 994f
  and Whipple's disease, 809b
Salbutamol
  asthma, 572
  drug interactions, 24b
  scombrotoxic fish poisoning, 150
Salicylates (aspirin)
  overdose, 138
  poisoning from, 136, 138
Salicylic acid
  actinic keratosis, 1230b
  molluscum contagiosum, 1239
  warts, 1239
Saline, 353b
  abdominal compartment syndrome,
    195
  genital itch/rash, 333
  heat cramps, 167
  hyperkalaemia, 363
  hyponatraemia, 358
  hypophosphataemia, 369
  hypovolaemia, 353
  metabolic alkalosis, 367
Salivary glands
  disease of, 790
  enlargement of, 1039b
Salmonella
  food poisoning/gastroenteritis, 263
  HIV/AIDS patients, 323
Salmonella enteritidis, 262–263
Salmonella paratyphi, 227–228
Salmonella spp. infection, 262–263
Salmonella typhi, 117b
Salmonella typhimurium, 262–263
Salmonellosis, 231b
Salofalk, for inflammatory bowel
  disease, 821b
Salt
  in diabetic diet, 744
  see also Sodium
Salt-losing nephropathy, 403
Salt-wasting disease, 418
Sand flea, 299–300
Sandflies, 282
  bartonellosis, 272
  leishmaniasis, 282
Sandhoff's disease, 371b
Sanfilippo's syndrome, 371b
Sanger, Fred, 52–53
Sanger sequencing, 52–53, 54f
Saphenous vein grafts, 492f
SARA see Sexually acquired reactive
  arthritis
Sarcoidosis, 410, 608–610, 608f,
  1263
  clinical features of, 608–609, 609b,
    609f
  investigations of, 609–610, 609b
  management of, 610
Sarcoma
  Ewing's, 1057
  osteogenic, 1056–1057
  see also Kaposi's sarcoma
Sarcomere, cardiac, 446

Sarcoptes scabiei, 1241
SARS see Severe acute respiratory
  syndrome
Sausage digit, 1032
Saxagliptin, 747
Saxophone player's lung, 616b
SBAR system, of communication, 10,
  10b
SBP see Spontaneous bacterial
  peritonitis
Scabies, 1241, 1241f
  ecthyma, 1236
  HIV/AIDS, 330f–331f
  Norwegian, 1241
  pruritus, 1219b
Scaling, 1216
Scalp
  fungal infections, 300–304
  head lice, 1241
  psoriasis, 1247–1251
  tinea capitis, 1240, 1240f
Scapula, winging, 1062f
Scarlet fever
  incubation period, 111b
  period of infectivity, 111b
  streptococcal, 252, 253f
Scars, definition, 1226
Scedosporium apiospermum, 301
SCF see Stem cell factor
'Schatzki ring', 795–796
Scheuermann's osteochondritis, 1055
Schilling test, 944
Schirmer tear test, 1038–1039
Schistosoma, life cycle of, 294, 295f
Schistosoma haematobium, 295–296,
  296f
Schistosoma intercalatum, 296
Schistosoma japonicum, 296
Schistosoma mansoni, 296, 296f
Schistosoma mekongi, 296
Schistosomiasis, 233b, 294–297
  clinical features of, 295–296, 295b
  investigations of, 296
  management of, 296
  pathology of, 294
  prevention of, 296–297
Schizoaffective disorder, 1200
Schizophrenia, 1196–1198
  acute, 1196–1197
  clinical features of, 1196–1197
  diagnosis of, 1197
  differential diagnosis of, 1197b
  investigations of, 1197
  management of, 1197–1198
  pathogenesis of, 1196
  prevalence of, 1180b
  prognosis of, 1198
  symptoms of, 1197b
    auditory hallucinations as, 1185
    thought disorder as, 1181
Schmidt's syndrome, 689
Schöber's test, 983, 983f
Schumm's test, 947
Schwann cells, 1064–1065
Sciatica, 1135
Scintigraphy
  bone, in musculoskeletal disease,
    988–989, 989b
  meta-iodobenzyl guanidine, 675
  octreotide, 679f
  of thyroid gland, 638f, 642
  see also Radionuclide (radioisotope)
    imaging
SCLE see Subacute cutaneous lupus
  erythematosus
Sclera, of eye, 1166–1167
Scleritis, 1172
  posterior, 1170
Sclerodactyly, 1037
Scleroderma see Systemic sclerosis
Scleromalacia, rheumatoid arthritis,
  1172
Sclerosing bone dysplasias, 1056
Sclerosing cholangitis
  primary, 888–890, 889f
    diagnostic criteria for, 888
    diseases associated with, 889b
    liver function test (LFT) abnormality
      in, 854b

magnetic resonance
  cholangiopancreatogram of, 889,
    889f
  primary biliary cholangitis and,
    902b
  secondary, 888, 889b
Sclerosis, systemic see Systemic
  sclerosis
Sclerostin, in bone remodelling, 986b
Sclerotherapy, for variceal bleeding, 870
Sclerotic bodies, 301
Scoliosis, 1059
Scombrotoxic fish poisoning, 150
Scorpions, envenomation of, 161
Scotoma, 1095–1096
Screening
  aortic aneurysm, 505
  breast cancer, 1325b
  for chronic liver disease, 853b
  ciliary dysfunction syndromes, 579
  coagulation, 922b
  colorectal cancer, 832–833
  cystic fibrosis, 580
  diabetes mellitus, 1278
  diabetic nephropathy, 757
  genetic, 58
  gestational diabetes, 1278
  hepatitis B core IgM antibody, 858
  hepatocellular carcinoma, 890–891
  for hepatocellular carcinoma,
    890–891
  malnutrition, 693f
  microalbuminuria, 394
  principles of, 94–95
Scrub typhus fever, 270–271, 271b
Scurvy, 715–716, 716b, 716f, 970
Sebaceous glands, 1213
Sebocytes, 1213
Seborrhoeic dermatitis, HIV-related,
  314
Seborrhoeic eczema, 1246
Seborrhoeic warts, 1234
Sebum, 1213
  acne vulgaris, 1242
Secondary aplastic anaemia, 969,
  969b
Secondary disease, in endocrinology,
  632–633
Secondary granules, 64
Secondary headache syndromes, 185b
Secondary osteoporosis, 1044–1045
Secretin, 772b
Secukinumab, for musculoskeletal
  disease, 1007, 1007b
Sedation
  for aggressive behaviour,
    1188–1189
  in intensive care, 209, 209b
Sedatives, misuse of, 1195
75SeHCAT test, 777b
75SeHCAT test, 777b
Seizures
  brain tumour and, 1129
  pregnancy and, 1275–1276, 1276b
  in stroke patients, 1153, 1159f
  syncope versus, 182b
  types of, 1098–1100, 1098b
    absence, 1099
    atonic, 1100
    clonic, 1100
    focal, 1099, 1099b
    generalised, 1099–1100
    myoclonic, 1099–1100
    tonic, 1100
    tonic-clonic, 1099, 1099b
Selective noradrenaline reuptake
  inhibitors (SNRIs), poisoning, 139
Selective serotonin re-uptake inhibitors
  (SSRIs), 1199, 1199b
  poisoning from, 139
Selectivity, 14
Selegiline, for Parkinson's disease, 1114
Selenium, 634, 718
  deficiency, 718
  dietary sources of, 717b
  excess, 718
  for Graves' ophthalmopathy, 646
  reference nutrient intake of, 717b
Selenium sulphide shampoo, 314

Selenosis, 716
Self-harm
  in old age, 1189b
  patient assessment of, 1187b,
    1188f
Self-help and coping strategies, for
  musculoskeletal disease, 1001,
    1001b
Seminoma, 439
Senescence
  immune, 80–81, 81b
  see also Age/ageing; Older people
Sengstaken-Blakemore tube, for
  variceal bleeding, 870, 870f
Senna, 761b, 834b
Sensitisation, 1340
Sensorimotor polyneuropathy, 1111b
Sensory ataxia, 1125b
Sensory cortex, 1063f
Sensory disturbances, 1083–1084
  diabetes see Diabetic neuropathy
Sensory loss, pattern of, 1084f
Sensory neurons, 1338
Sensory neuropathy, 1111b
Sensory system examination, 1062f
Sentinel lymph node biopsy, 1233
Sentinel pile, 836
Sepsis, 196–198, 226–227, 226b
  acute kidney injury and, 411–412
  cardiomyopathy and, 198
  coagulation system and, activation of,
    196
  definition of, 196b
  during dialysis, 424b
  lactate and, 196
  meningococcal, 1119b
  mimics of, 198b
  organ damage from, 196, 197f
  resuscitation in, 196–197, 197b
  skin and soft tissue infections
    causing, 226–227
Sepsis syndrome, 550
Septic arthritis, 1019–1020
  emergency management of, 1020b
  synovial fluid in, 1020
Septic shock, 70–71, 196b, 206b
Septicaemic plague, 259
Sequestration crisis, 952
'Seroconversion', 106
Serological tests, for respiratory disease,
  554
Serology
  for gastrointestinal infection, 777
  for Helicobacter pylori infection, 777
  for hepatitis B, 873–875, 875b
  for hepatitis C, 877
Seronegative spondyloarthropathies,
  1166b
Serositis, in rheumatoid arthritis, 1024
Serotonin (5-hydroxytryptamine, 5-HT),
  1345b, 1353f
  excess in irritable bowel syndrome,
    824
Serotonin agonists, irritable bowel
  syndrome, 824
Serotonin-noradrenaline reuptake
  inhibitors (SNRIs), 139
Serotonin selective (specific) re-uptake
  inhibitors (SSRIs), 1199, 1199b
Serotonin syndrome, 1199
Serratia spp., 102f
Sertraline, 1199
Serum- ascites albumin gradient
  (SAAG), 863
Serum ferritin, 941
Serum sickness
  antivenom, 159
  diphtheria antitoxin, 266
  schistosomiasis, 295b
Severe acute respiratory syndrome
  (SARS), 249
Severe combined immune deficiency,
  79–80
  X-linked, 79–80
Severe idiopathic constipation, 834
Sex, HIV infection/AIDS and, 323
Sex chromosomes, 38
  see also X chromosome; Y
    chromosome

Sex hormone replacement therapy
for hypopituitarism, 682
see also Hormone replacement
therapy
Sex hormones *see individual hormones*
Sexual activity, headache and, 1097
Sexual disturbance, 1093–1094
Sexual dysfunction, 1109–1110
see also Erectile dysfunction
Sexually acquired reactive arthritis
(SARA), 1031
Sexually acquired reactive arthropathy,
340
Sexually transmitted infections (STIs),
329–344
approach to patients, 332–333,
332*b*
in children, 332–333
clinical examination of
in men, 330, 330*f*
in women, 331, 331*f*
contact tracing for, 333
HIV testing for, 330
investigations of
in men, 330*b*
in women, 331*b*
management goals of, 331*b*
men who have sex with men, 330*b*,
334–335
during pregnancy, 332
presenting problems of, men,
333–336, 333*f*–334*f*
prevention of, 336–337
those at particular risk, 331*b*
viral, 341–344
Sézary's syndrome, 1224, 1232
SGLT2 inhibitors, for hyperglycaemia,
748, 748*f*
SH (self-harm) *see* Self-harm
Shagreen patches, 1264
Shampoo
ketoconazole, 1240, 1246
selenium sulphide, 314
Shared decision-making, 10, 11*f*, 12
Shave excision, for skin disease,
1228
Sheehan's syndrome, pregnancy and,
1280
Shellfish poisoning, paralytic, 149
Sheltered employment, 1198
Shiga-like toxin, 408–409
Shigella
diarrhoea, 227–228, 232
dysentery/shigellosis, 265
reactive arthritis, 1031
Shigellosis, 265
Shingles *see* Herpes zoster
Shivering, 165*b*, 165*f*
Shock
anaphylactic, 204, 206*b*
cardiogenic, 199–200, 206*b*
causes of, 200*f*
downward spiral of, 199, 200*f*
clinical features of, 180*b*
hypotension and, 193, 193*b*
hypovolaemic, 206*b*
neurogenic, 206*b*
obstructive, 206*b*
septic, 70–71, 196*b*, 206*b*
Short bowel syndrome, 708–710
Short stature
in Turner's syndrome, 659
see also Dwarfism; Growth
retardation
Shoulder
frozen, 997–998
pain, 997–998, 998*b*, 998*f*
painful, in stroke patients, 1159*f*
Shrinking lungs, 610*b*, 611
Shuffling gait, 1087*b*
Shunts
Blalock-Taussig, 537
intracardiac, 454, 459
left-to-right, 450
persistent ductus arteriosus, 533
portosystemic
fetor hepaticus from, 868
portal hypertension and, 869
for variceal bleeding, 871

TIPSS
for ascites, 864
for variceal bleeding, 871, 871*f*
transjugular intrahepatic
portosystemic stent
for ascites, 864
for variceal bleeding, 871, 871*f*
SI units, 1358
SIADH *see* Syndrome of inappropriate
secretion of ADH
Siberian tick typhus, 271*b*
Sibutramine, 702
Sick euthyroidism, 642
Sick sinus syndrome, 469, 469*b*, 469*f*
Sickle-cell anaemia/disease, 923,
951–953
clinical features of, 952–953, 952*f*
epidemiology of, 951, 951*f*
investigations of, 953
management of, 953
pathogenesis of, 951–952
in pregnancy, 953*b*
prognosis of, 953
rheumatological manifestations of,
1058
Sickle-cell nephropathy, 411
Sickle-cell trait, 951
Sickle chest syndrome, 952
Side-effect, definition of, 21
Siderosis, 614–616, 615*b*
Sieverts (Sv), 164
Sigmoidoscopy, 776
amoebiasis, 287
Clostridium difficile infection, 264
constipation, 787
familial adenomatous polyposis, 829
inflammatory bowel disease, 824*b*
for inflammatory bowel disease,
817*b*
radiation enteritis and proctocolitis,
810
schistosomiasis, 296
ulcerative colitis, 817*b*
Sildenafil, 440
Silicosis, 615–616, 615*f*
Silicotuberculosis, 615–616
Simple aspergilloma, 596–597, 597*f*
Simple diffuse goitre, 648, 648*f*
Simple tandem repeat mutations, 43,
43*b*
Simulium spp., onchocerciasis, 292
Simvastatin
for stroke prevention, 1161*f*
timing, 31*b*
Sinemet, 1113
Single-layered retinal pigment
epithelium, 1167
Single nucleotide polymorphisms (SNPs;
snips), 42
Single photon emission tomography
(SPECT), 1072
Sinoatrial node, 469*b*, 469*f*, 471*b*
Sinoatrial (SA) node, 445, 445*f*
Sinus arrhythmia, 469
Sinus bradycardia, 469
Sinus tachycardia, 469, 469*b*
Sinusitis *see* Rhinosinusitis
Sinusoidal obstruction syndrome, 899
Sipple's syndrome, 689*b*
SIRS (systemic inflammatory response
syndrome), pancreatitis, 838*b*
Sister Joseph's nodule, 804
Sitagliptin, 747
Sitosterolaemia, 375, 375*b*
Sixth disease, 238
Sjögren's syndrome, 1038–1039,
1039*b*, 1171
Skeletal muscle, 987–988
Skin
blood vessels and nerves in, 1214
changes in old age, 1215*b*
of envenomed patient, 152*f*
epidermal appendages of,
1212–1214
examination of
cancer, 1315*b*
endocrine disease, 630*f*
gastrointestinal disease, 764*f*
function of, 1214, 1214*b*

functional anatomy and physiology of,
1212–1214
imaging, 1216
immunobullous disease of,
1255–1257, 1255*b*
infestations, 1235–1241
inflammatory arthritis in, 994*b*
lichenoid eruptions in, 1252
microbiology of, 1215
as physical barrier, 62–63
systemic lupus erythematosus in,
1035*f*
systemic sclerosis in, 1037, 1037*f*
Skin cancer, 1229
non-melanoma, 1228, 1230*b*
pathogenesis, 1229
see also names of specific tumours
Skin disease
abnormal pigmentations in, 1224
acute skin failure in, 1224–1225
clinical examination in, 1210, 1210*f*
in general medicine, 1261–1267,
1261*b*
investigation of, 1214–1216
management of, 1225–1229
nail involvement in, 1260–1261
ophthalmic features of, 1166*b*
phototherapy and
photochemotherapy for, 1227
pigmentation disorders as,
1257–1258
presenting problems in, 1216–1225
terminology in, 1211*f*
treatment of
non-surgical, 1228–1229
surgery for, 1228
systemic, 1227–1228
topical, 1225–1227, 1225*b*
Skin grafts, vitiligo, 1257–1258
Skin infections, 1235–1241
bacterial, 1235–1238
fungal, 1239–1240, 1240*f*
mycobacterial, 1237–1238
tropical, 234, 234*b*, 235*f*
viral, 1238–1239
Skin lesions, benign, 1234–1235
Skin-prick tests, for allergy, 86
Skin snips, 234*b*
Skin tags *See* Acrochordon
Skin test
asthma, 613–614
patch tests, 1215
prick tests, 86, 1215
tuberculin, 594, 594*f*
Skin tumours, 1229–1235
malignant, 1229–1234
pathogenesis of, 1229
Skinfold thickness, 693*f*
Slapped cheek syndrome, 237, 237*f*
SLE *see* Systemic lupus erythematosus
Sleep, 1071
Sleep apnoea/hypopnoea syndrome,
622–624
aetiology of, 623
clinical features of, 623
investigations of, 623, 623*b*–624*b*,
623*f*
management of, 623–624
Sleep-disordered breathing, 622–624
Sleep disorders, 1105–1106
Sleep disturbance, 1094
Sleep paralysis, 1094
Sleepiness
Epworth scale, 623*b*, 1105
persistent, differential diagnosis,
624*b*
see also Hypersomnolence
Sleeping sickness, 278–279, 278*f*
Sleeve gastrectomy, 703*b*
Small bowel bacterial overgrowth,
causes of, 808*b*
Small-bowel diarrhoea, HIV-related,
317, 317*b*, 317*f*
Small bowel surgery, proximal,
under-nutrition and, 706
Small bowel transplantation, 710
complications of, 710*b*
indications for, 710*b*
Small interfering RNA (siRNA), 27*b*

Small intestine
bacterial overgrowth, 808–809
diseases/disorders of, 805–813
functional anatomy of, 767–770, 767*f*
infections of, 812–813
miscellaneous disorders of, 811–812
motility disorders, 810–811
protective function of, 769–770
tumours of, 813
ulceration of, 811, 811*b*
Small-vessel vasculitis, 409
Smallpox (variola), 248
Smell, disturbance of, 1088
Smith-Magenis syndrome, genetics, 44*b*
Smoking
and autoimmune disease, 82–83
cannabis, 143
and cardiovascular risk, 420
cocaine, 143
effects on health, 94
familial hypercholesterolaemia, 374*b*
freezing cold injury, 166
heart failure and, 465*b*
lung cancer and, 1320–1321
in older people, 1305
peptic ulcer and, 799
urinary incontinence, 436
Smoking cessation
acute coronary syndrome and, 501
in Graves' ophthalmopathy, 646
Smooth muscle atrophy, systemic
sclerosis and, 1037–1038
Snail track ulcers, 337
Snake bites, 134
Snakes, geographical distribution of,
153
Snakeskin gastropathy, 871
Snoring, 623
SNPs *see* Single nucleotide
polymorphisms
Social isolation, psychiatric disorders
and, 1184
Social worker, 1303*b*
Sodium, 349*b*, 718
depletion, 349
dietary sources of, 717*b*
excess, 354*b*, 354*f*
homeostasis, 349–355
intake, chronic renal failure, 418
presenting problems of, 352–355
in primary hyperaldosteronism, 674
reabsorption, 384
reference nutrient intake of, 717*b*
reference range of
urine, 1361*b*
venous blood, 1358*b*
restriction of, for ascites, 863
retention of, 395, 864*b*
transport, 351–352, 352*f*
see also Hypernatraemia;
Hyponatraemia
Sodium aurothiomalate (gold), 1005
Sodium bicarbonate
chronic kidney disease, 418
drug interactions, 24*b*
salicylate poisoning, 138
in urinary alkalinisation, 136
Sodium calcium edetate, 137*b*
Sodium chloride
dietary, 718
see also Saline
Sodium cromoglicate
for allergy, 86
for food allergy, 812
Sodium-dependent glucose transporter
inhibitors, for hypervolaemia, 354
Sodium ipodate, 639
Sodium nitroprusside
aortic dissection, 508
hypertension, 514
phaeochromocytoma, 676
Sodium phosphate, 368
Sodium-potassium pump, 349
Sodium stibogluconate, 128
Sodium valproate
bipolar disorder, 1200
cluster headache, 1096
epilepsy, 1102*b*, 1284
pregnancy, 1103, 1103*b*

Sodium valproate *(Continued)*
for epilepsy, 1100*b*
neutropenia, 926*b*
poisoning, 141*b*
sodium retention and, 864*b*
status epilepticus, 1081*b*
steatosis, 894
SOFA score, 214*b*
Soft tissue infections, 226–227
necrotising, 227*b*
Soft tissue release, 1002*b*
Solar urticaria, 1221*b*
Solitary rectal ulcer syndrome, 836
Solvent inhalation, 1196
Somatic hypermutation, 68, 68*f*
Somatic mutations, 50–51
Somatic symptoms, medically
unexplained, 1187, 1187*b*,
1189*b*, 1203*b*, 1205*f*
Somatic syndromes, functional, 1187*b*
Somatisation disorder, 1202
Somatoform autonomic dysfunction,
1202
Somatoform disorders, 1202–1203
advice for, 1203
prevalence of, 1180*b*
Somatoform pain disorder, 1202
Somatosensory system, 1070–1071,
1071*f*–1072*f*
Somatostatin, 767, 772*b*
Somatostatin analogues, for
neuro-endocrine tumours (NETs),
679
Somatostatin receptor scintigraphy
(SRS), 778*b*
Somatostatinoma, 678*b*
Somnolence
daytime, 1105–1106
idiopathic hypersomnolence, 623
Sorafenib, for hepatocellular carcinoma,
892
Sorbitol, 812
Sotalol, 140
South American botfly, 300
Space-occupying lesions, HIV-related,
320–321
Space of Disse, 849
cirrhosis and, 866
Sparganosis, 299
Spastic catch, 1068–1069
Spastic paraplegia, hereditary, 1138*b*
Spasticity, 1068–1069
Specialised receptors, 1338
Specialist nurse, 1109–1110
Spectinomycin, 117*b*, 122
Spectrophotometry, 348*b*
Spectroscopy (ICP-MS), 348*b*
Speech disturbance, stroke and,
1152
Speech/speech disorders, 1070, 1070*f*,
1087–1088, 1088*f*
assessment of, in psychiatric
interview, 1181
Speech therapy, for Parkinson's
disease, 1114
Spermatogenesis, 651*f*
Spherocytes, 915, 921*b*, 921*f*
Spherocytosis, hereditary, 947
investigations of, 947, 948*f*
management of, 947, 948*b*
Sphincter
anal, 437
bladder, 386
control, 1070–1071
urethral, 103, 436
Sphincter of Oddi, 849–850
dysfunction of, 908–909
classification of, 908*b*
pancreatic, criteria for, 908*b*
Sphincterotomy
biliary, 906
endoscopic, in old age, 909*b*
Sphygmomanometry, 510
Spider bites, 161
Spider naevi, 846*f*
autoimmune hepatitis and, 886
Spider telangiectasia, 866–867
Spiders, envenomation of, 161
Spina bifida, 715, 1138*b*

Spinal cord, 1067, 1338–1339
compression, 1136–1137, 1136*b*,
1137*f*
cancer and, 1326, 1326*b*
in rheumatoid arthritis, 1024, 1025*f*
disorders of, 1134–1137
intrinsic diseases of, 1137, 1137*f*,
1138*b*
lesions, sensory loss, 1083
Spinal cord syndrome, 1136*b*
Spinal epidural abscess, 1125
Spinal muscular atrophy, 1117
Spinal root lesions, 1141
Spinal stenosis, 1135–1136
Spine
assessment of, 983*f*
bamboo, 1030–1031, 1031*f*
cervical
imaging of, 1074, 1075*f*
myelopathy, 1134–1135
radiculopathy, 1134, 1134*f*
spondylosis, 1134–1135, 1134*f*
subluxation of, 1024, 1025*f*
disorders of, 1134–1137
lumbar, imaging of, 1074, 1075*f*
osteoarthritis, 1011, 1011*f*
thoracic, imaging of, 1074, 1075*f*
Spinobulbar muscular atrophy, 43*b*
Spinocerebellar ataxia, 43*b*, 1116*b*
Spiramycin, 281
Spirillum minus, 234*b*
Spirometry
asthma, 569
COPD, 575
Spironolactone
ascites, 864
ascites and, 864
gynaecomastia, 657*b*
heart failure, 465
Splanchnic vasodilatation, for ascites,
862–863
Spleen, 67
enlarged *see* Splenomegaly
examination of, 913*b*
Splenectomy
for chronic lymphocytic leukaemia,
960
for idiopathic thrombocytopenic
purpura, 971
for myelofibrosis, 969
Splenomegaly, 927, 928*b*
cirrhosis and, 867
portal hypertension and, 868
Splice site mutations, 43*f*
Splicing, 40
Splinter haemorrhages, 994*b*, 1260
Splints, for musculoskeletal disease,
1001
Spondylitis, psoriatic, 1032
Spondyloarthritis, axial, 1028*b*,
1029–1030, 1029*f*
Spondyloarthropathies (SPAs),
1027–1034, 1028*b*
seronegative, 1166*b*
Spondylolisthesis, 996–997, 1059–1060
Spondylolysis, 1059–1060
Spondylosis
cervical, 1134–1135, 1134*f*
lumbar, 1135–1136
Spondylotic myelopathy, cervical, 1082*f*
Spongiosis, 1244
Spontaneous bacterial peritonitis, 864
Spontaneous breathing trials, respiratory
support and, 210
Spontaneous hypoglycaemia, 676–678
cause of, 677–678
clinical assessment of, 677
differential diagnosis of, 677*f*
investigations of, 677–678
management of, 678
in old age, 678*b*
Sporadic fatal insomnia, 1127*b*
Sporothrix schenckii, 301
Sporotrichosis, 301
Sporozoites, malaria, 273–274
Spreading depression of Leão, 1095
Sprue, tropical, 233
Spurious full blood count results, from
autoanalysers, 919–920, 920*b*

Sputum, 546*f*
cough, 556
cytology, 554
haemoptysis, 559
investigations, 554
Pneumocystis jirovecii pneumonia,
318
in pulmonary oedema, 546*f*
pulmonary tuberculosis, 318
Squamous carcinoma, 796*b*
Squamous cell carcinoma, skin,
1230–1231, 1230*b*, 1231*f*
SRS *see* Somatostatin receptor
scintigraphy
SSPE *see* Subacute sclerosing
panencephalitis
SSSS *see* Staphylococcal scalded skin
syndrome
St John's wort, drug interactions, 24*b*
St Vitus dance, 516
Stable angina
advice to patients with, 489*b*
risk stratification in, 488*b*
Staging, in lung cancer, 602, 602*f*
Stamping gait, 1087
Stannosis, 614–615
Staphylococcal food poisoning, 262
Staphylococcal infections, 250–252,
251*f*
cannula-related, 251–252, 251*b*
methicillin-resistant *Staphylococcus
aureus*, 252
skin, 251
staphylococcal toxic shock syndrome,
252, 252*f*
wound, 251, 251*f*
Staphylococcal scalded skin syndrome,
1236, 1236*f*
Staphylococcal toxic shock syndrome,
252, 252*f*
Staphylococcus aureus, 104*b*, 117*b*,
251
acute leukaemia, 957
atopic eczema, 1246*b*
bacteraemia, 225
blood-stream infection, 225*b*
bronchiectasis, 579
cerebral venous sinus thrombosis,
1162
chronic granulomatous disease, 77
fever, 223, 223*f*
folliculitis from, 1236–1237
impetigo from, 1235–1236
infections caused by, 251*f*
infectious keratitis, 1173*b*
infective endocarditis, 527
meningitis, 1119*b*
pneumonia
bacterial, 319
community-acquired, 582*b*, 584*b*
in septic arthritis, 1020
skin infections, 251*f*
vancomycin-resistant, 252
Staphylococcus epidermis, 251
Staphylococcus intermedius, 251
Staphylococcus saprophyticus, 251
Starches
dietary, 695–697
hydrolysis, 768
polysaccharides, 696*b*
resistant, 265
Starling's law, 461, 461*f*
Starvation, 704–705
infections associated with, 705*b*
STAT proteins, 64–66
Statins, 376
for acute coronary syndrome
prevention, 498*b*
hepatotoxicity of, 894*b*
for hypertension, 513
for non-alcoholic fatty liver disease,
885
for stroke prevention, 1161*f*
Statistics, 10
Status epilepticus, 1080, 1081*b*,
1103
Steady state, 19
Steatohepatitis, non-alcoholic, 882–883,
883*f*

Steatorrhoea
bile acid diarrhoea, 809
cystic fibrosis, 842
malabsorption, 783–784, 784*b*
small bowel disorders, 808
Steatorrhoea, pancreatitis, 840
Steatosis, 882–883, 894
Stellate cells, 772
Stem cell factor, 914
Stem-cell plasticity, 914–915
Stem cells, 914–915, 915*f*
plasticity, 914–915
pluripotent, 954
Stenosis
aortic, 443*b*, 521–524, 522*b*, 522*f*
causes of, 521*b*
Doppler echocardiography for, 451*f*
investigations of, 522–524, 523*b*,
523*f*
in old age, 524*b*
lumbar canal, 1135–1136
mitral, 517–519, 518*b*, 518*f*
chest X-ray for, 451*f*
investigations in, 518*f*, 519*b*
pregnancy and, 1282
pulmonary, 526
renal artery, 406–408, 407*b*, 407*f*
spinal, 1135–1136
tricuspid, 525–526
Stents/stenting
aortic dissection, 508
carotid, 1160
cholecystitis, 905
colonic, 833*f*
coronary, 491, 491*f*
graft, 507*f*
liver arterial disease, 898
for lung cancer, 603
myocardial infarction, 1282
pregnancy and, 1282
renal artery, 389
superior vena cava obstruction, 1327
thrombosis, 493*b*
ureteric, 414
Stercobilin, 851
Stercobilinogen, 851
Sterile pyuria, 430
Steroid hormones, pathways of
synthesis of, 667*f*
Steroids
anabolic, 88
synthesis, 667*f*
see also Corticosteroids
Stevens-Johnson syndrome, 316, 1224,
1254–1255
Stiff person syndrome, 1111*b*
Still's disease
adult, 895, 1040
see also Juvenile idiopathic arthritis
Stimulant, misuse of, 1195–1196
Stimulation therapies
for cancer pain, 1353
for pain, 1347, 1347*f*
Stings
insect, 75*b*
scorpion, 159
see also Envenomation
Stockings, compression, 396
'Stokes-Adams' attacks, 477–478
Stomach
emptying, 778
erosions, 781*f*
functional anatomy of, 766–767, 766*f*
outlet obstruction, 801–802, 801*b*
tumours of, 803–805
ulcer, 798–802
Stomatitis
angular, 764*f*, 817
herpetic, 247*f*
Stones *see* Calculi (stones)
Stool cultures, 777
Stop codons, 40
Storage disorders, 929*b*
Stratum corneum, 1212
Strawberry gallbladder, 909
Strawberry tongue, 252, 253*f*
Streptococcal infections, 252–253, 253*b*
acute rheumatic fever, 515, 517*b*
bone and joint, 1020

in pregnancy, 235b
tics, 1086
Streptococcal toxic shock syndrome, 217f, 253
Streptococci, 102f
  alpha-haemolytic, 102f
  beta-haemolytic, 102f
  group A, 252
  group B, 252
Streptococcus anginosus, 103f
Streptococcus constellatus, 103f
Streptococcus intermedius, 103f
Streptococcus mitis, 528
Streptococcus pneumoniae, 67, 73b, 117b, 266, 1277b
  in community-acquired pneumonia, 582, 582f
  meningitis, 1119b–1120b
  peritonitis, 836
  sepsis, 226b
Streptococcus pyogenes, 103f, 117b
Streptococcus suis, 1119
  bacterial meningitis, 1120b
Streptococcus viridans endocarditis, 401
Streptokinase, Budd-Chiari syndrome and, 899
Streptomyces, 1238
Streptomycin
  adverse reactions, 593b
  as antimycobacterial agents, 125
  mycetoma, 301
  plague, 259
  tuberculosis, 97f
  for tuberculosis, 593
Stress
  acute reaction, 1201
  oxidative, 881f, 883
  post-traumatic stress disorder, 1201–1202
Stress echocardiography, 452
Stress electrocardiography, 449–450
Stress fracture, 995b
Stress incontinence, 436
  in older people, 1309–1310
Stress-related disorders, 1201–1202
Stressors, psychiatric disorders and, 1184
Stretch reflex, 1068
Striae, definition of, 1226f
Strictures, endoscopic techniques for management see Endoscopy
Stridor
  aortic aneurysm, 505
  bronchial obstruction, 600
  connective tissue disorders, 610b
  hypocalcaemia, 663
  inspiratory, 566
  laryngeal disorders, 624
  tracheal disorders, 625
String test, 287
Stroke, 952, 1153–1160
  anatomy and physiology of, 1150–1151, 1150f
  classification of, 1150f
  clinical examination of, 1148, 1148f
  clinical features of, 1150f, 1155–1157, 1155b, 1156f
  completed, 1157
  complications of, 1159f
  differential diagnosis of, 1155b
  general examination of, 1149b
  heat, 167–168
  HIV-related, 321
  investigations of, 1151–1152, 1157–1158, 1157b
    blood tests, 1151–1152
    cardiac, 1158
    cardiovascular, 1152
    lumbar puncture, 1152
    neuroimaging, 1151, 1151f, 1157–1158
    vascular imaging, 1151, 1152f, 1158
  management of, 1158–1160, 1158f
    aspirin, 1160
    carotid endarterectomy and angioplasty, 1160
    coagulation abnormalities, 1160

heparin, 1160
    reperfusion (thrombolysis and thrombectomy), 1159–1160
    supportive care, 1158–1159, 1159b
    unusual causes, 1160
  medicine for, 1147–1162
  migraine and, 1095
  pathophysiology of, 1153–1155
    cerebral infarction, 1153–1154, 1153f–1154f
    intracerebral haemorrhage, 1154–1155, 1155b, 1155f
  pregnancy and, 1284
  presenting problems of, 1152–1153
    ataxia, 1153
    coma, 1153
    headache, 1153
    seizure, 1153
    speech disturbance, 1152
    visual deficit, 1152
    visuo-spatial dysfunction, 1152
  progressive (in evolution), 1157
  rapid assessment of, 1149b
  risk factors for, 1153b
    analysis, 1157, 1157b
    management, 1160
  secondary prevention of, 1161f
Stroke mimics, 1155b
Stroke units, 1158
Stroke volume, 446
  pregnancy and, 1272
Strongyloides hyperinfection syndrome, 226b, 289
Strongyloides stercoralis, 231b, 233b, 289, 612
Strongyloidiasis, 233b, 289, 289b
Subacute cutaneous lupus erythematosus (SCLE), 1262
Subacute invasive aspergillosis (SIA), 597
Subacute sclerosing panencephalitis (SSPE), 236, 1123
Subacute (de Quervain's) thyroiditis, 646–647
Subarachnoid haemorrhage, 1160–1162
  clinical features of, 1161, 1162f
  investigations of, 1161
  management of, 1162
  see also stroke
Subclavian steal, 504
Subclinical hypothyroidism, 642
Subclinical thyrotoxicosis, 636b, 638, 642
Subclinical urethritis, 334b
Subcutaneous administration, 17
Subcutaneous androgen replacement therapy, 656b
Subdural empyema, 1125
Subdural haematoma, 864–865
Sublingual administration, 17
Substance misuse, 1184, 1184b
  prevalence of, 1180b
Substance misuse disorder, 1195–1196
Substance P, 1003–1004
Subtotal thyroidectomy, for Graves' thyrotoxicosis, 644b, 645
Subtotal villous atrophy, important causes of, 806b
Subungual haematoma, in nails, 1260f
Succinate dehydrogenase, 49b
Sucralfate, 801
Sudden death
  due to heart failure, 464
  in raised ICP, 1128
Sugars
  dietary, 696b
  recommended intake, 698b
Suicide
  anorexia nervosa, 1204
  attempted, 1187
  bipolar disorder, 1200
  depression, 1198
  low mood, 1185
  old age, 1189b
  risk factors for, 1187b
  schizophrenia, 1198
  see also Self-harm

Sulfadiazine
  prophylactic, 119b
  rheumatic fever, 517
  toxoplasmosis, 281, 320
Sulfadoxine, and neutropenia, 926b
Sulfamethoxazole, melioidosis, 261
Sulfasalazine (SSZ)
  in haemolysis, 950
  for inflammatory bowel disease, 821b
  for musculoskeletal disease, 1004–1005, 1004b
  prophylactic, 119b
Sulfinpyrazone, gout, 1016
Sulindac, 829
Sulphonamides
  mechanism of action, 116b
  in pregnancy, 120b
Sulphonylureas
  effect of hepatic impairment, 32b
  effect of renal insufficiency, 32b
  for hyperglycaemia, 746–747
  weight gain and, 700b
Sulphur, 718
Sulpiride, 1115
Sumatriptan, for migraine, 1096
Sunbed exposure, cancer and, 1229
Sunburn, 1221f
SUNCT, 1097, 1097b
Sunflower cataract, in Wilson's disease, 1174f
Sunitinib, 435
Sunlight
  melanoma and, 1232
  sensitivity to, 1036b
Sunscreens, 1222–1223
  albinism and, 1258
  melanoma and, 1233
  photosensitivity, 1221b
  protection levels, 1222–1223
  vitiligo and, 1257–1258
Superficial bursitis, 999b
Superior vena cava, 444f
Superior vena cava obstruction (SVCO), 1314f, 1315b
  cancer and, 1326–1327, 1327b
Superior vena cava syndrome, 505
Superoxide dismutase, 1116
Supported self-management, for pain, 1344
Suppurative pneumonia, 586–587, 587b
Supranuclear palsy, progressive, 1114–1115
Supraventricular tachycardia, 473, 473f
Suramin, for trypanosomiasis, 128
Surfactant, 548–549
Surgery
  for acromegaly, 686
  bariatric, 702f–703f, 703–704, 703b
  for brain tumours, 1130
  for cholecystitis, 905
  for chronic obstructive pulmonary disease (COPD), 577
  for epilepsy, 1102
  gastrointestinal
    achalasia, 795
    haemorrhage, 782
    prophylactic, 119b
  for lung cancer, 602
  for musculoskeletal disease, 1002, 1002b
    osteoarthritis, 1012
    osteoporosis, 1049
    rheumatoid arthritis, 1026
  for obesity, 702f–703f, 703–704, 703b
  for Parkinson's disease, 1114
  for primary hyperparathyroidism, 664
  for prolactinoma, 685
  for psychiatric disorders, 1190
Surrogate endpoints, 35–36
Sustained virological response (SVR), 878
Suxamethonium
  allergy, 75b
  pharmacokinetics, 20b
Swallowing, difficulty in see Dysphagia
Swan-Ganz catheter, 206, 207f
Swan neck deformity of fingers, 1023, 1023f

Sweat glands, 1213–1214
Sweating, excessive, 217b
Sydenham's chorea, 516
Symmetrical polyarthritis, 1032
Symmetrical sensory polyneuropathy, diabetic, 758–759
Sympathetic nervous system, sodium transport regulation in, 352
Synaptic transmission, 1065
Syncope, 181–183, 455
  clinical assessment of, 182–183
  congenital heart disease and, 533
  differential diagnosis of, 182f
  features of, 181b
  gastrointestinal haemorrhage, 780
  heat, 167
  investigations of, 183
  in older people, 1308
  presentation of, 181–182
  seizures versus, 182b
Syndesmophytes, 988
Syndrome of inappropriate secretion of ADH (SIADH), 357b
Synergistic gangrene, 227, 227b
Synovectomy, 1002b
  for rheumatoid arthritis, 1026
Synovial biopsy, 992
Synovial fluid, 987, 988f
  in septic arthritis, 1020
Synovial joints, 987
  structure of, 987f
Synovial membrane, 987
Synoviocytes, 987
Synovitis, pigmented villonodular, 1059
Synovitis-acne-pustulosis-hyperostosis-osteitis (SAPHO) syndrome, 1060
Synovium, 987
  loose bodies within, 988
  needle trauma to, 988
  in osteoarthritis, 1008
Synthetic cannabinoid receptor agonist, misuse of, 143
Syphilis, 253, 337–339
  acquired, 337–338
  benign tertiary, 338
  cardiovascular, 338
  classification of, 337b
  congenital, 338–339, 338b
  dementia and, 339
  early, 337–338
  investigations of, 338–339
  late, 338
  latent, 337–338
  management of, 339
  neurosyphilis, 338, 1125, 1125b
  in pregnancy, 235b, 339
  primary, 337, 337f
  secondary, 337
    rash in, 1217b
  serological tests for, 339b
  treatment reactions of, 339
Syringomyelia, 1083
Systemic disease, 785
Systemic glucocorticoids, for musculoskeletal disease, 1005
Systemic inflammatory response, 196–198
  initiation of, 196
  propagation of, 196
  see also Sepsis
Systemic juvenile idiopathic arthritis, 1027
Systemic lupus erythematosus (SLE), 410–411, 1034–1037
  classification of, criteria for, 1036b
  clinical features of, 1035–1036
  investigations of, 1036
  management of, 1036–1037
  pathophysiology of, 1034
  pregnancy and, 1281, 1281b
  respiratory involvement in, 611
Systemic sclerosis (SScl), 410, 1037–1038, 1037f, 1262
  pregnancy and, 1280–1281, 1281b
  respiratory involvement in, 611
Systemic vasculitis, 410
Systolic dysfunction, 450
Systolic murmurs, 459–460, 460b

T

T-helper lymphocytes, HIV infection/
 AIDS and, 310
T lymphocytes (T cells), 69–70, 69f, 917
 CD4+, 70
 CD8+, 70
 deficiency in, 73b
  primary, 79–80, 80f
 liver and, 849f
 lymphoma
  cutaneous, 1224
  enteropathy-associated, 813
 multiple sclerosis, 1106
 skin, 1212
 psoriasis, 1248f
T-regulatory cells (T regs), 70
Tabes dorsalis, 1125b
Tachycardia, 191–193
 assessment and management of,
  192–193
 pathophysiology of, 191–192
 sinus, 469, 469b
 supraventricular, 473, 473f
 ventricular, 475–476, 475b,
  475f–476f
  poisoning, 137b
 pulseless, 457
Tachyphylaxis, 16
Tachypnoea, 190, 191f
 assessment and management of,
  190, 191f
 pathophysiology of, 190
Tacrolimus, 1281b
 liver transplantation and, 901
 nephrotoxicity, 427b
 thrombocytopenia, 971
 vitiligo, 1257–1258
Tactoids, 951–952
Taenia asiatica, 298
Taenia echinococcus, 298–299
Taenia saginata, 298
Taenia solium, 297f, 298
Takayasu arteritis, 1041
Takotsubo cardiomyopathy, 541, 541f
Tamm-Horsfall protein, 392
Tamoxifen
 breast cancer, 1334
 desmoid tumours, 829
 gynaecomastia, 657
Tamponade
 balloon, for variceal bleeding,
  870–871, 870f
 cardiac, 447–448
Tamsulosin, 438
Tandem repeat mutations, 43, 43b
Tangent/Goldmann kinetic perimetry,
 1168
Tangier disease, 375, 375b
Tanner staging, 1290, 1292f
Tarsal tunnel syndrome, 1024
Tarui disease, 370b
Tay-Sachs disease, 371b
Tazobactam
 for spontaneous bacterial peritonitis,
  864
 for variceal bleeding, 869
TB see Tuberculosis
TBG see Thyroxine-binding globulin
TBW see Total body water
99mTc-sestamibi scintigraphy, for primary
 hyperparathyroidism, 663–664,
 664f
TCAs see Tricyclic antidepressants
Team communication, effective, for
 clinical decision-making, 10, 10b
Teardrop poikilocytes, 969
Teduglutide, for intestinal failure, 710
Teenagers, adherence in, 1294–1295
Teichopsia, 1088
Teicoplanin, 117b, 123
 adverse effects of, 123
Telangiectasia
 definition of, 1226
 hereditary haemorrhagic, 970
 spider, liver disease and, 866–867
Telaprevir, 878b
Teletherapy, 1331
Telomerase, 1318

Telomeres, 1304–1305
Telophase, 40
Temperature, 94
 abnormal, 165f
 body, 165
 cold injury and, 166–167
 elevated body, 167b
 extremes of, 165–168
 heat-related illness and, 167–168
 hypothermia and, 165–166,
  165f–166f
 of stroke patients, 1159b
 thermoregulation and, 165, 165b
Temporal artery biopsy, 992
Temporal coning, 1128, 1128f
Temporal lobes, 1066
 disorders of, 1089b
 functions of, 1066b
  effects of damage, 1066b
Temporary pacemakers, for arrhythmias,
 482–483, 483f
Tendinitis
 adductor, 999b
 bicipital, 998b, 998f
Tendon, xanthomas, 375
Tendon reflexes, root values of, 1063b
Tendon repairs and transfers, 1002b
Tenecteplase (TNK), 500
Tennis elbow, 998b
Tenofovir, 119b, 324b
 for hepatitis B, 876
Tenosynovectomy, 1002
Tenosynovitis, 998
Tension-type headache, 1095
Teratogen, 22–23
Terbinafine, 125b, 126
 chromoblastomycosis, 301
 fungal infections, 1239–1240
 sporotrichosis, 301
Terbutaline, asthma, 571
Teriparatide, for osteoporosis,
 1048–1049, 1048b
Terlipressin, 864
 for variceal bleeding, 869b, 870
Terminal illness see Palliative care
Terrorism see Bioterrorism
Testicular tumours, 439–440
Testis
 epididymo-orchitis, 240
 undescended, 653
Testosterone
 for delayed puberty, 654
 puberty and, 1290
 reference range of, 1359b
Tetanus, 104b, 1125–1126
 prevention of, 1126
 treatment of, 1126b
Tetany, 663
Tetrabenazine, 1115
Tetracycline(s), 117b, 124
 acne, 1243
 adverse effects of, 124
 bartonellosis, 272
 brucellosis, 254
 bullous pemphigoid, 1256
 cholera, 265
 drug interactions, 24b
 mechanism of action, 116b
 pharmacokinetics of, 124
 plague, 259
 in pregnancy, 120b
 pyoderma gangrenosum, 1261–1262
 relapsing fever, 257
 rickettsial fevers, 271–272
 rosacea, 1244
 steatosis, 894
 timing, 31b
 trachoma, 273
 tropical sprue, 808
Tetralogy of Fallot, 536–537, 536f
Th1 (T helper) cells, 70
Th2 cells, 70
Th17 cells, 70
Thalamus, 1066–1067
Thalassaemias, 951, 953–954
 alpha, 954
 beta, 953–954
  rheumatological manifestations of,
   1058

Thalidomide
 for Behçet's disease, 1044
 for multiple myeloma, 968
 sarcoidosis, 610
Theophylline
 asthma, 1277
 plasma concentration, 36b
 poisoning, 137b, 141b
 tremor, 1116b
Therapeutic approach, 29, 29b
Therapeutic drug monitoring, 119
Therapeutic efficacy, 16
Therapeutic goal, 29
Therapeutic index, 15f, 16
Thermal injury, 950
Thermodilution, for measurement, of
 cardiac output, 454
Thermogenesis, diet-induced, 694, 695f
Thermoregulation, 165, 165b
 in old age, 166
Thiabendazole, 129
Thiamin (vitamin B₁), 714
 biochemical assessment of, 712b
 deficiency, 714
 dietary sources of, 711b
 reference nutrient intake of, 711b
Thiamin pyrophosphate (TPP), 714
Thiazides
 adverse effects, 355b
 for hypertension, 513
 for hypervolaemia, 355, 355b
 and hyponatraemia, 357b
Thiazolidinediones, for hyperglycaemia,
 747
Thienobenzodiazepines, 1198b
Thin glomerular basement membrane
 disease, 404
Thiopurines, for inflammatory bowel
 disease, 821b
Thioxanthenes, 1198b
Thirst
 diabetes insipidus, 687
 water homeostasis, 356
Thomsen's disease, 1145b
Thoracic kyphoscoliosis, 628
Thoracic outlet syndrome, 1141b
Thoracoscopy, 553
Thorax, examination of, in respiratory
 system, 546f
Thought
 assessment of, 1181
 passivity of, 1196–1197
Thought, passivity of, 1196–1197
Threadworm (Enterobius vermicularis),
 129
Threonine, 697b
Thrombasthenia, Glanzmann's, 970–971
Thrombin, 918f–919f
Thromboangiitis obliterans, 504
Thrombocythaemia, essential, 969–970
Thrombocytopenia, 929, 929b, 971
 hepatobiliary disease and, 853
 HIV-related, 322
 pregnancy and, 1285, 1285b
Thrombocytopenic purpura (TTP),
 pregnancy and, 1285
Thrombocytosis, 929–930, 929b
Thromboembolism
 in cancer patients, 1324–1325
 Heart failure causing, 464
 venous, 975–977
  causes and consequences of, 975,
   976f
  factors predisposing to, 975b
  management of, 975–976
  pregnancy and, 1285
  prophylaxis of, 976–977, 977b
Thrombolytic therapy
 for acute coronary syndrome, 500,
  500b
 for pulmonary embolism, 621
Thrombophilia, 977–979
 acquired, 977–979
 investigation of, 922–923, 923b
 testing in, indications for, 922–923,
  923b
Thrombopoietin receptor agonists
 (TPO-RA), for idiopathic
  thrombocytopenic purpura, 971

Thromboprophylaxis, 472–473, 473b
 in intensive care, 210
Thrombosed prolapsed haemorrhoids,
 836f
Thrombosis
 deep vein
  air travel and, 169
  investigation of, 187, 187f
  pre-test probability of, 187b
  pregnancy and, 1285
  presentation of, 186
  in stroke patients, 1159f
  warfarin for, 939
 hepatic artery, 898
 in old age, 978b
Thrombospondin (TSP)-1, 1318
Thrombotic disorders, 922–923, 923b,
 975–979
Thrombotic microangiopathies,
 408–409, 408b
Thrombotic thrombocytopenic purpura
 (TTP), 388, 409, 979
Thrush, 300
 oral, 790
Thumb, Z deformity, 1023
Thymectomy, myasthenia gravis, 1142b
Thymine, 38
Thymus, 67
Thyroglobulin (Tg), 634, 635f
 as tumour markers, 1324b
Thyroid autoantibodies, 637b
Thyroid disease
 autoimmune, 639b, 643–646
 classification of, 634b
 clinical features of, 637b
 congenital, 650–651
 investigations of, 634–635
 iodine-associated, 647–648
 during pregnancy, 651b, 1279
  hyperthyroidism as, 1279
  hypothyroidism as, 1279
  iodine deficiency as, 1279
  post-partum thyroiditis as, 1279
 presenting problems of, 635–643
Thyroid function tests
 asymptomatic abnormal, 642
 hypothyroidism, 636b
 interpretation of, 636b
 for obesity, 700
 thyrotoxicosis, 636b
Thyroid gland, 634–651
 enlargement of, 642–643, 642b
 examination of, 631b
 functional anatomy, physiology and
  investigations of, 634–635, 635f,
  636b
 in old age, 650b
 scintigraphy, 638f, 642
 ultrasound, 643
Thyroid hormone, 634, 635f
 in bone remodelling, 986b
 replacement, for hypopituitarism, 682
 resistance, 651
Thyroid lump or swelling, 642–643,
 642b
Thyroid neoplasia, 649–650, 649b
Thyroid nodule, solitary, 642
Thyroid peroxidase antibodies, 640
Thyroid-stimulating hormone (TSH;
 thyrotrophin), 632, 634
 and free T₄, relationship of, 634, 635f
 receptor antibodies (TRAb), 643
 reference range of, 1359b
Thyroid-stimulating immunoglobulins,
 643
Thyroid storm, 639
Thyroiditis
 Hashimoto's, 646
 post-partum, pregnancy and, 1279
 Riedel's, 650
 subacute (de Quervain's), 646–647
 transient, 646–647, 646f
Thyrotoxic crisis, 639
Thyrotoxicosis, 635–639
 in adolescence, 645, 645b
 amiodarone and, 636b, 638f,
  647–648
 atrial fibrillation in, 638
 causes of, 636b

clinical assessment of, 635–636, 637*b*
differential diagnosis of, 638*f*
factitious, 637
goitre and, 635–636, 636*b*
Graves' disease and, 635–636, 636*b*, 643–646, 643*f*
management of, 644–645, 644*b*
investigations of, 636–637, 637*b*–638*b*
iodide-induced, 636*b*
laboratory abnormalities, 638*b*
low-uptake, 637
management of, 637–639
in pregnancy, 645, 651*b*
subclinical, 636*b*, 638, 642
T$_4$:T$_3$ ratio in, 637
toxic adenoma, in 638*f*, 649
type I, 647–648
type II, 648
Thyrotrophin-releasing hormone (TRH), 633*f*, 634
Thyroxine (T$_4$), 633*f*, 634, 635*f*
reference range of, 1359*b*
thyroid-stimulating hormone (TSH) and, relationship of, 634, 635*f*
Thyroxine-binding globulin (TBG), 634
Tiagabine, 1102*b*
Tibial compartment syndrome, anterior, 1058
Tibolone, for osteoporosis, 1048*b*, 1049
Tic douloureux, 1096–1097
Ticarcillin, 120*b*
Tick-borne diseases, 256*b*
babesiosis, 278
Lyme disease, 255
rickettsial fevers, 270
tularaemia, 261
viral haemorrhagic fevers, 246
Tick-borne relapsing fever, 256*b*, 257
Tics, 1086
Tidal volume (TV), pregnancy and, 1273
Tietze's syndrome, 177*b*
Tigecycline, 117*b*, 124
Tiludronate, for Paget's disease, 1054*b*
Tin oxide, 615*b*
Tinea capitis, 1240, 1240*f*
Tinea corporis, 1240
rash in, 1217*b*
Tinea cruris, 1240, 1240*f*
Tinea incognito, 1240
Tinea pedis, 1240
Tinidazole, 287, 808–809
Tirofiban, 500, 918
Tissue biopsy, in musculoskeletal disease, 992
Tissue factor pathway, assessing, 920–921
Tissue plasminogen activator, 447
Tizanidine, 1110*b*
TNF inhibitors, pregnancy and, 1278, 1280
TNF receptor-associated periodic syndrome, 81
TNF receptor-associated proteins (TRAPs), 64–66
TNFRSF1A gene, TNF receptor-associated periodic syndrome and, 81
TNM classification, 1322*b*
Tobramycin
cystic fibrosis, 581*b*
dosing interval, 122*f*
Tocilizumab, 1027
for musculoskeletal disease, 1007, 1007*b*
α-Tocopherol *see* Vitamin E
Toe
cock-up deformities, 1023
ingrowing toenails, 1260
Tofacitinib, for musculoskeletal disease, 1004*b*
Tolcapone, for Parkinson's disease, 1114
Tolerance, 16
Toll-like receptors, 63
Tolterodine, 1094*b*, 1310*f*
Tongue
biting, 1102*b*
strawberry, 252, 253*f*

Tonic-clonic seizures, 1099, 1099*b*
Tonic seizures, 1100
Tonsillar coning, 1128, 1129*f*
Tonsillitis, 242–243
membranous, 266*b*
streptococcal, 266*b*
Tonsils, 67, 912*b*
Tophi, 1014, 1015*f*
Topical administration, 17–18
Topical agents, for musculoskeletal disease, 1003–1004
Topical analgesics, for pain, 1345
Topiramate, for obesity, 702–703
Topoisomerase II inhibitors, 936*b*
Topotecan, ovarian cancer, 1334
Torsades de pointes, 476–477, 476*b*, 476*f*
Torticollis, 997*b*, 1116
Total anterior circulation syndrome (TACS), 1156*f*
Total body water (TBW), 349
Total iron binding capacity (TIBC), 942
Total lung capacity, 555*b*
Total parenteral nutrition
candidiasis, 302
gastroparesis, 803
Total thyroidectomy, for medullary carcinoma, 650
Tourette's syndrome, 1086
Toxic adenoma, 638*f*, 649
Toxic epidermal necrolysis, 1254–1255, 1254*b*, 1254*f*, 1266*b*
Toxic megacolon, 818
Toxic pustuloderma, drug-induced, 1266*b*
Toxic shock syndrome (TSS), 1236
staphylococcal, 252, 252*f*
streptococcal, 217*f*, 253
Toxins
bacterial, 1125–1126
food-related poisoning, 149–150
ciguatera poisoning, 149–150
paralytic shellfish poisoning, 149
scombrotoxic fish poisoning, 150
gastrointestinal decontamination for, 135–136
plant, 150, 150*b*
venom, 154, 154*b*
Toxocara canis, 233*b*
Toxocariasis, 233*b*
Toxoplasma gondii, 280
life cycle of, 280*f*
Toxoplasmosis, 280–281
clinical features of, 280, 281*f*
congenital, 280
investigations of, 281
management of, 281
in pregnancy, 235*b*
Trace elements, absorption, 769
Tracheal disorders, 625
Tracheal obstruction, 625
Tracheo-oesophageal fistula, 625
Tracheostomy, in intensive care, 210, 210*b*
Trachoma, 273, 273*f*
Trachyonychia, 1261
Tramadol, 1002
Tranexamic acid, 560, 597
Tranquillisers, effect of old age, 32*b*
Trans-arterial chemo-embolisation, for hepatocellular carcinoma, 892
Transcatheter aortic valve implantation, 527, 527*f*
Transcobalamin II, 943–944
Transcription, of DNA, 38–40
Transcription factors, 39
Transcutaneous electrical nerve stimulation (TENS), 1012
for osteoarthritis, 1012
Transdermal administration, 17
Transdermal androgen replacement therapy, 656*b*
Transference, 1191
Transferrin, 1362*b*
saturation of, 1362*b*
Transforming growth factor beta (TGF-β1), 849*f*
Transfusion-associated graft-*versus*-host disease (TA GVHD), 933

Transfusion medicine
haematology and, 911–979
key points in, 936*b*
Transfusion-transmitted infection, 933
Transient ischaemic attack (TIA), 1156–1157
causing sensory loss, 1083
causing visual loss, 1088
Transient ocular ischaemia, 1171
Transient thyroiditis, 646–647, 646*f*
Transition medicine, adolescent and, 1287–1300
clinical assessment in, 1293
features of, 1293*b*
clinical presentations in, 1296–1300
diabetes and, 1299
functional anatomy and physiology in, 1290–1292
cognitive and behavioural changes in, 1292
endocrine changes in, 1290, 1291*f*
physical changes in, 1290
gastrointestinal disease and, 1299–1300
inflammatory bowel disease and, 1299–1300
investigations in, 1293, 1293*b*
neurological disease and, 1296–1297
cerebral palsy in, 1296
epilepsy in, 1296
muscular dystrophy in, 1297
oncology and, 1298
organ transplantation and, 1299
presenting problems in, 1294–1296
adherence as, 1294–1295
high-risk behaviour as, 1295
unplanned pregnancy as, 1295–1296
renal disease and, 1298–1299
respiratory disease and, 1297
cystic fibrosis in, 1297
rheumatology and bone disease and, 1300
glucocorticoid-induced osteoporosis in, 1300
hypophosphataemic rickets in, 1300
juvenile idiopathic arthritis in, 1300
osteogenesis imperfecta in, 1300
transition from paediatric to adult health services in, 1288–1290
principles of prescribing during, 1289, 1289*b*
readiness for, key features in, 1289*b*
timing of, 1290, 1290*f*
transition planning in
effectiveness of, 1288
general principles of, 1288–1289, 1288*f*
reasons to consider, 1288*f*
systematic approach to, 1289–1290
transition referral letter in, 1293
Transition planning
effectiveness of, 1288
general principles of, 1288–1289, 1288*f*
impact of, on outcome in diabetes, 1299*b*
reasons to consider, 1288*f*
systematic approach to, 1289–1290
Transjugular intrahepatic portosystemic stent shunt (TIPSS)
for ascites, 864
for variceal bleeding, 871, 871*f*
Translation, 39*f*, 40
Transoesophageal echocardiography (TOE), 452
Transplantation
cardiac, 467–468
in diabetes mellitus, 752
graft rejection and, 88–90
investigations in, 89
haematopoietic stem cell, 936–938
for acute leukaemia, 958
allogeneic, 936–937, 936*b*–937*b*
autologous, 936–938
fever after, 224–225

for high-grade NHL, 966
infections during recovery from, 937*b*
immunosuppression in
complications of, 89–90
drugs used in, 89*b*
of islet cell, 752, 753*f*
of kidney, 424
of liver, 900–901
for acute liver failure, 858–859
for alcoholic liver disease, 882
complications of, 901
for hepatic encephalopathy, 865
for hepatitis B, 876
for hepatitis C, 878
for hepatocellular carcinoma, 891
indications and contraindications for, 900–901, 900*b*, 901*f*
living donor, 901
for primary biliary cholangitis, 888
prognosis for, 901
split liver, 901
for Wilson's disease, 897
for low-grade NHL, 965
lungs, 567, 567*b*
multivisceral, 710
complications of, 710*b*
organ donation and, 90
pre-implantation testing in, 89
renal, 424–426
in diabetic nephropathy, 758
recipients of, pregnancy and, 1283
small bowel, 710
complications of, 710*b*
indications for, 710*b*
transition medicine and, 1299
transplant rejection and, 88–89
classification of, 88*b*
Transportation, for envenomed patient, 157
Transposition of great arteries, 531*b*
Transrectal ultrasound scan (TRUS) of prostate, 437–438
Transverse myelitis, 1110
Tranylcypromine, 1199*b*
TRAPS *see* TNF receptor-associated periodic syndrome
Trastuzumab, 1332
Trauma
head, 1133
nails, 1260
Travellers
eosinophilia, 233
fever in, 231*b*, 231*f*
health needs, 230*b*
incubation times and illnesses, 232*b*
rash, 234*b*
Traveller's diarrhoea, 232*b*
Treadmill, for exercise electrocardiography, 449–450
Trefoil factor family (TFF) peptides, 767
Trematodes, 294–297
Tremor, 1085, 1115
causes and characteristics of, 1085*b*
drug-induced, 1116*b*
dystonic, 1085*b*
essential, 1085*b*, 1115
flapping, hepatic encephalopathy and, 864–865
functional, 1085*b*
intention, 1069
Parkinson's disease causing, 1085*b*
resting, 1081
Trench fever, 272
Trench foot, 167
Trephine biopsy, 920, 922*f*
Treponema pallidum, 117*b*, 333, 336
in pregnancy, 332*b*
Treponema pertenue, 253
Treponema vincentii, 254
Treponemal (specific) antibody tests, 339
Treponematoses, 253–254
endemic, 253–254
see also Syphilis
Triamcinolone, 790
Triamterene, 355
Triazoles, 125*b*, 126
Tricarboxylic acid (Krebs) cycle, 714

Triceps skinfold thickness, 693b
Trichiasis, 273
Trichinella spiralis, 293
Trichinellosis, 293–294
Trichinosis, 293–294
Trichloroacetic acid, 1239
Trichomonas vaginalis, 333
Trichomoniasis, genital, 335
Trichophyton rubrum, 1240
Trichophyton verrucosum, 1240
Trichuris trichiura (whipworm), 290
Triclabendazole, 297b
Tricuspid regurgitation, 526, 526b
Tricuspid stenosis, 525–526
Tricuspid valve, disease of, 525–526
Tricyclic antidepressants, 1199, 1199b
    poisoning from, 138–139, 139b, 139f
Trientine dihydrochloride, Wilson's
    disease, 897
Trigeminal (5th cranial) nerve, tests of,
    1063b
Trigeminal neuralgia, 1080, 1096–1097
Trigger finger, 1060
Triglycerides
    measurement, 373
    reference range of, venous blood,
        1360b
Trihexyphenidyl, for Parkinson's disease,
    1114
Triiodothyronine (T₃), 633f, 635f
    reference range of, 1359b
Trimethoprim
    acne vulgaris, 1243
    brucellosis, 255b
    listeriosis, 260
    mechanism of action, 116b
    melioidosis, 261
    in pregnancy, 120b
    urinary tract infection, 428
Triple X syndrome, 44b
Triptans, 17, 1096
Trismus, 1126
Trisomy 13 (Patau's syndrome), 44b
Trisomy 18 (Edwards' syndrome), 44b
Trisomy 21 (Down's syndrome),
    genetics, 44b
Trochanteric bursitis, 999b
Trochlear (4th cranial) nerve, tests of,
    1063b
Troisier's sign, 804
Tropheryma whipplei, 100, 106, 809
Tropical diseases
    diarrhoea, 232–233
    eosinophilia, 233–234
    fever, 230–232
    skin, 234
Tropical fever, 230–232
    causes of, 231b
    clinical assessment of, 230–232,
        232b
    history taking in, 231b
    investigations of, 232, 232b
    management of, 231f, 232
Tropical pulmonary eosinophilia, 612
Tropical sprue, 233, 807–808
Tropical ulcer, 254, 254b
Tropomyosin, 446
Troponins
    cardiac, 450
    reference range of, venous blood,
        1360b
Trousseau's sign, 367
'True' polycythaemia, 925
Truncus arteriosus, 531–532
Trunk, examination of, in
    musculoskeletal system, 982f
Trypanosoma brucei gambiense
    infection, incubation period of,
        111b
Trypanosoma cruzi, 794–795
Trypanosomiasis
    African (sleeping sickness), 278–279,
        278f
    American (Chagas' disease), 279–280
    drugs for, 128
Trypsin, 768
Trypsinogen, 770b
Tryptamines, misuse of, 143
Tryptase, 1360b

Tryptophan, 697b
Tube drainage, intercostal, 626–627
Tube feeding, nasogastric, 707, 707b
Tuberculin skin test, 594, 594f
Tuberculoma, 320–321
Tuberculosis (TB), 267, 430, 588–595,
    1021
    abdominal, 812–813
    bone and joint disease in, 591
    central nervous system disease in,
        591
    chronic pulmonary, complications of,
        590b
    control and prevention of, 594–595
    cryptic, 589b
    diagnosis of, 592b
    epidemiology of, 588, 588f
    gastrointestinal, 590, 591f
    genitourinary disease in, 591
    granulomas in, 71
    HIV-related
        prevention of, 323
        therapy for, 324, 324b
    investigations of, 591–592, 592f
    lymphadenitis and, 590
    management of, 592–594, 593b
    miliary, 588–589
    pathology and pathogenesis of, 588,
        588f
    pericardial disease in, 590
    pregnancy and, 1277
    prognosis for, 595
    pulmonary
        clinical presentations of, 590b
        major manifestations and differential
            diagnosis of, 590f
        post-primary, 589
        primary, 588, 589b, 589f
    risk of, factors increasing, 589b
Tuberculous granuloma, 588f
Tuberculous meningitis, 1120–1121,
    1121b
    HIV-related, 321
Tuberculous pericarditis, 543
Tuberous sclerosis, 1264
Tubular obstruction, drug-induced,
    427b
Tubulo-interstitial diseases, 401–403
    inherited, 404, 404b
Tularaemia, 261
Tumbu fly, African, 300
Tumour-induced osteomalacia, 1053
Tumour lysis syndrome, 369
    cancer and, 1328
Tumour markers, 1322, 1324b
Tumour necrosis factor (TNF), 64–66
Tumour suppressor genes, 51
Tumours, 836–837
    adrenal, management of, 669–670
    bone, 1056–1057
        metastatic, 1329
    brain, 1129–1132, 1129b, 1129f
        clinical features of, 1129
        investigations of, 1130, 1130f
        management of, 1130–1131
        metastatic, 1328, 1328b
        prognosis of, 1131
    of bronchus, 598–605
    of gallbladder and bile duct,
        907–908
        benign, 908
    gastroenteropancreatic neuro-
        endocrine, 678–679, 678b, 679f
    gastrointestinal stromal cell, 805
    head and neck, 1335–1336, 1335b
        investigations of, 1335
        management of, 1335–1336
        pathogenesis of, 1335
    immunology of, 90
    of liver, 890–893
        benign, 893
        primary malignant, 890–892
        secondary malignant, 892–893,
            893f
    of lungs, 598–605
        metastatic, 1328
        primary, 599–603
        secondary, 603
        vascular, 619–622

of mediastinum, 603–605,
    603b–604b, 604f
neuro-endocrine, 603b, 678–679,
    678b, 679f, 813
of oesophagus, 796–797
    benign, 796
of pancreas, 842–844
pituitary, 683–684, 1129
of rectum, 827–833
of respiratory system, 598–605
skin, 1229–1235
    malignant, 1229–1234
    pathogenesis of, 1229
of small intestine, 813
of stomach, 803–805
of urinary tract, 434–436
urothelial, 435–436
Tunga penetrans, 299–300
Tungiasis, 299–300
Turbidimetry, 348b
Turcot's syndrome, 829
Turner's syndrome, 659–660, 660f
    genetics of, 44b
Type A ('augmented') ADRs, 22
Type B ('bizarre') ADRs, 22
Type C ('chronic/continuous') ADRs, 22
Type D ('delayed') ADRs, 22
Type E ('end-of-treatment'), 22
Typhoid fever, 260, 260b
Typhus fever
    endemic, 271, 271b
    epidemic, 271, 271b
    scrub typhus, 270–271
Tyrosine, 635f
Tyrosine kinase inhibitors, 959
    in chronic myeloid leukaemia, 959b
TZD drugs see Thiazolidinediones

U
UDCA see Ursodeoxycholic acid
UIP see Usual interstitial pneumonia
UK Faculty of Public Health, 92
UK NHS Pregnancy and Newborn
    Screening Programmes, 96f
UK Prospective Diabetes Study, 746
Ulceration
    aphthous, 790, 790b
    of small intestine, 811, 811b
Ulcerative colitis
    active left-sided or extensive, 820
    cancer, 1320b
    childhood, 823
    clinical features of, 816, 817b
    comparison with Crohn's disease,
        814b
    complications, 818
    differential diagnosis, 817b
    histology of, 816f
    investigations, 818–820
    management of, 820, 1299–1300
        medical, 822b
        surgical, 823, 823b
    pathophysiology of, 815–816
    pregnancy, 823–824
    primary sclerosing cholangitis and,
        888
    pseudopolyposis in, 815f
    severe, 820
    treatment of, medical, 820
Ulcers
    amoebic, 287
    Buruli, 254
    Chiclero, 285
    dendritic, 248
    digital, 1038
    foot, 761–762
    genital
        in men, 333–334, 334f
        in women, 336
    legs, 1223–1224
        causes of, 1223b, 1223f
        clinical assessment of, 1223–1224
        due to arterial disease, 1223–1224
        due to neuropathy, 1224
        due to vasculitis, 1224
        due to venous disease, 1223, 1223f
        investigations in, 1224
        management of, 1224
    leishmaniasis, 285f

leprosy, 268
Marjolin's, 1021
mouth, 1036
neuropathic, 759f, 1224
oesophageal, 794
oral, 1043–1044, 1043f
peptic
    complications of, 801–802
    indications for, 800b
    in old age, 801b
    perforation, 789, 801
    prophylaxis for, in intensive care,
        211
    rodent, 1229
    skin, definition, 1216
    small intestine, 811, 811b
    solitary rectal ulcer syndrome, 836
    tropical, 254
Ulnar nerve
    entrapment, 1002b
    palsy, 760
Ultrafiltration, 349–350, 384
    failure, 425b
Ultrasound
    for ascites, 863
    for cancer, 1323
    Doppler see Doppler ultrasound
    echocardiography see
        Echocardiography
    endocrine disease
        polycystic ovary, 659f
        thyroid, 643
    endoscopic, 774
        for choledocholithiasis, 906f
        for hepatobiliary disease, 855
    of gastrointestinal tract, 774
        oesophageal cancer, 797f
        pancreatitis, 839
    for hepatobiliary disease, 853–854
        gallstones and, 853–854, 854f
    for hepatocellular carcinoma, 891
    for musculoskeletal disease, 989
        rheumatoid arthritis, 1025
        synovitis, 989f
    for nervous system, 1073f
    for non-alcoholic fatty liver disease,
        884
    for portal hypertension, 869
    renal, 389, 389f
    for renal artery stenosis, 407
    for respiratory disease, 553
    for splenomegaly, 927
    for tachypnoea, 190, 191f
    of thyroid gland, 643
Ultraviolet radiation, 1229
    photosensitivity, 1220–1223
    psoriasis, 1250f
    skin cancer, 1320b
    ultraviolet A, 1227
    ultraviolet B, 1227
    Wood's light, 1214
Under-nutrition, 704–711
    causes of, 704b
    classification of, 704b
    clinical assessment for, 693
    clinical features of, 704, 704b
    in hospital, 705–708, 706b
    responses to, 694–695
Under water, 169–171
Undifferentiated autoimmune connective
    tissue disease, 1040
Unfractionated heparin (UFH), 938–939
Unilateral leg swelling, 186–187, 186b
    clinical assessment of, 186–187
    investigations of, 187, 187b–188b,
        187f
    presentation of, 186, 187b
United Kingdom End-stage Liver
    Disease (UKELD) score, for liver
    transplantation, 900–901
Upper airway
    defences, 550
    disease of, 622–625
Upper respiratory tract infection,
    581–587
Uracil, 39
Uraemia
    haemolytic uraemic syndrome, 388
    see also Renal failure

Urate, reference range of
  urine, 1361b
  venous blood, 1360b
Urate-lowering drugs, indications for,
  1015b
Urea, 349b
  acute kidney injury and, 416b
  reference range of
    urine, 1361b
    venous blood, 1358b
Urea breath test, 778b
Ureidopenicillins, 121
Ureterocele, 434
Ureteropyelogram, retrograde, 436
Ureterovaginal fistula, 437
Ureters, 386
  colic, 431–432
  diseases of, 433–434
  ectopic, 434
  megaureter, 434
  obstruction, 434
Urethral discharge, 333
Urethral syndrome, 427–428
Urethritis
  chlamydial, 333
  gonococcal, 333, 333f
  non-specific, 333
  subclinical, 334b
Urge incontinence, 436–437, 1093
  in older people, 1309
Uric acid
  crystals, 431b
  in gout, 1013–1014
  lowering, 1015
  metabolism of, 1013f
  pool, 1013f
  reference values, urine, 1361b
Uricosuric drugs, for gout, 1016
Urinalysis
  acute kidney injury, 412b
  reference range, 1361b
Urinary diversion, 436
Urinary incontinence, 397, 436–437
  older people, 436b, 1309–1310,
    1310f
Urinary tract, 383f
  calculi, 431
  clinical examination of, 382–384,
    382f–383f
  collecting system
    diseases of, 433–434
    imaging, 389f
  congenital abnormalities of, 433–434,
    434f
  stones, removal of, 433b, 433f
  tumours of, 434–436
Urinary tract disease
  investigation of, 386–391
  presenting problems in, 391–397
Urinary tract infection, 426–431
  antibiotic regimens for, 429b
  clinical features, 427–428
  investigation of, 428b
  management, 428–429
  in old age, 428b
  pathophysiology, 427
  persistent or recurrent, 429, 429b
  prophylaxis, 429b
  risk factors for, 428b
  in stroke patients, 1159f
  vesico-ureteric reflux, 428b
Urine
  alkalinisation, 136
  black, 947
  investigation of, 387–388
  microscopy, 387, 388f
  retention
    acute, 437–438
    benign prostatic hyperplasia,
      437–438
    chronic, 438
  volume, 391
  see also Anuria; Oliguria
Urine output, decreased, 195
  assessment of, 195
  diagnosis and management of, 195
Urine testing
  diabetes, 725
  glycaemic control, 742

Urobilin, 851
Urobilinogen, 851
Urography, intravenous see Intravenous
  urography
Urokinase, 1319f
Urolithiasis, 431–433
Urology, 381–440
Urothelial tumours, 435–436
Ursodeoxycholic acid (UDCA)
  gallstones, 905b
  for primary biliary cholangitis, 888
Urticaria, 1252–1254
  causes of, 1253b
  clinical features of, 1252–1253, 1253f
  drug-induced, 1266b
  investigations of, 1253–1254
  management of, 1254
  papular, 292
  pathogenesis of, 1253f
  solar, 1221b
Ustekinumab
  for Crohn's disease, 822
  for inflammatory rheumatic disease,
    1007, 1007b
  for psoriatic arthritis, 1033–1034
Usual interstitial pneumonia, 608f
Uterine tumours, 1316f
UTI see Urinary tract infection
Uveal tract, of eye, 1167
Uveitis, 1031, 1172–1173
  acute anterior, ankylosing spondylitis,
    1030
  aetiology of, 1172b
  brucellosis, 255f
  HTLV-1, 250
  immune recovery, 321
  treatment, 258–259
  Weil's disease, 258
UVR see Ultraviolet radiation

V
Vaccines/vaccination, 114–115, 115b
  anthrax, 115b
  BCG, 595
  chickenpox, 239
  cholera, 115b
  diphtheria, 266
  guidelines for, 115b
  Haemophilus influenzae type B, 115b
  for hepatitis B, 876b
  HIV, 327
  for human papillomavirus, 343
  influenza, 241
  Japanese B encephalitis, 250
  leprosy, 270
  malaria, 277
  meningococcal infection, 1120
  MMR, 240
  mumps, 240
  plague, 259
  pneumococcal pneumonia, 266
  for poliomyelitis, 1123
  primary antibody deficiencies and, 79
  for rabies, 1122
  rotavirus, 249
  rubella, 236–237
  tetanus, 1126
  tick-borne encephalitis, 230b
  for tuberculosis, 595
  types of, 114–115
  typhoid, 261
  use of, 115, 115b
  varicella zoster virus (VZV), 115b,
    239, 240b
  whooping cough, 115b
  yellow fever, 245
  see also Immunisation
Vaccinia virus, 249
Vacuolating cytotoxin (vacA), 798f
VAD see Ventricular assist devices
Vagina, discharge, 335, 335b, 335f
Vaginosis, bacterial, 335, 335b, 335f
Vagotomy, complication of, in peptic
  ulcer, 801
Vagus (10th cranial) nerve, tests of,
  1063b
Valaciclovir
  as anti-herpesvirus agent, 126, 127b
  for herpes virus infection, genital, 342

Valganciclovir
  for CMV infection, 224
  herpesvirus infection, 127b
Valine, 697b
Valproate see Sodium valproate
Valsartan
  heart failure, 466b
  hypertension, 513
  myocardial infarction, 500–501
Valves of Heister, 850
Valvular heart disease
  causes of, 515b
  infective endocarditis, 527–531
    prevention, 531
  pregnancy and, 1282
  rheumatic, 515–517
  risks of non-cardiac surgery, 501b,
    502
  valve replacement, 526–527
Valvuloplasty
  aortic, 524
  mitral, 519
Van Buchem's disease, 1056
Vancomycin, 117b, 123
  acute leukaemia, 957
  adverse effects, 123
  Clostridium difficile infection, 264
  drug eruptions, 1266b
  for infective endocarditis, 223
  meningitis, 1120b
  pharmacokinetics, 123
  respiratory disease, 586
  for septic arthritis, 1020
  therapeutic monitoring, 36b
  toxic shock syndrome, 252
Vancomycin-resistant Staphylococcus
  aureus (VRSA), 252
Vandetanib, for medullary carcinoma,
  650
Vanishing bile duct syndrome, 889, 902
Variant Creutzfeldt-Jakob disease
  (vCJD), 933, 1127, 1127f
Variceal band ligation, 869b
Variceal bleeding, 865–866, 865f
  cirrhosis, 866–867
  management of, 869–871, 869b,
    870f–871f
  portal hypertension and, 869
  prevention of
    primary, 869
    secondary, 871
Variceal ligation, 775f
  for variceal bleeding, 870
Varicella, pneumonia, 582b
Varicella zoster virus (VZV), 238b
  after HSCT, 937b
  HIV infection, 321
  immunisation, 115b, 240b
  infection from, pregnancy and, 1277
  management and prevention of, 239,
    239b
  in pneumonia, 582b
  in pregnancy, 235b, 1277
  stem cell transplantation, 937b
Varicella zoster virus immunoglobulin
  (VZIG), 239, 240b
Varices
  gastric, 865–866, 865f
  oesophageal, 865–866, 865f
  rectal, portal hypertension and, 868
Varicose veins, 1223
Variegate porphyria, 379b
Variola, 248
Vascular dementia, 1191b
Vascular disease
  atherosclerotic see Atherosclerosis
  diabetes, 503b, 756
  diffuse, 1191
  liver, 898–899
  peripheral, 502–505
  pulmonary, 619–622
    pulmonary embolism, 619–621
    pulmonary hypertension, 621–622,
      621b, 622f
  renal, 406–409
Vascular endothelial growth factor, 1318
Vascular imaging, 1151, 1152f, 1158
Vascular malformations, jejunal bleeding,
  775f

Vascular resistance
  portal hypertension, 869
  pulmonary, 461, 467, 532f
  systemic, 447
Vasculitides, 611–612
Vasculitis, 1040–1044, 1040f, 1261
  antineutrophil cytoplasmic antibody,
    1041, 1041f
  cerebral, 1093b, 1108
  cryoglobulinaemic, 1043
  cutaneous, 581b
  drug-induced, 1266b
  leg ulcers due to, 1224
  renal artery stenosis, 407
  in rheumatoid arthritis, 1024
  small-vessel, 409
  systemic, 410, 1041b, 1042f
  urticarial, 1253b
Vaso-occlusive crisis, 952
Vasoactive agents, actions of, 206b
Vasoactive intestinal peptide (VIP),
  772b
Vasodilatation, 206b
  splanchnic, for ascites, 862–863
Vasodilators
  angina, 487
  for heart failure, 467
  for hypertension, 513
  myocardial infarction, 199b
  valvular heart disease, 521
Vasomotor rhinitis, 622
Vasopressin
  for refractory hypotension, 198
  see also Antidiuretic hormone
Vasopressin receptor agonist
  desmopressin, in haemophilia A,
    973
Vasopressinase, pregnancy and, 1280
Vasopressors, 206
  for variceal bleeding, 869b
VDRL see Venereal Diseases Research
  Laboratory (VDRL) test
VDRR see Vitamin D-resistant rickets
Vedolizumab, for inflammatory bowel
  disease, 821b
Vegan, 697
  vitamin B$_{12}$ deficiency, 944
Velocardiofacial syndrome, 44b
Venae cavae, 444, 444f
  see also Inferior vena cava; Superior
    vena cava
Venereal Diseases Research Laboratory
  (VDRL) test, 338–339
Venesection
  haemochromatosis, 895–896
  for polycythaemia rubra vera, 970
Venlafaxine, 1199b
Veno-occlusive disease, 899
Venography
  cerebral, 1162
  hepatic portal, 854, 899
  venous thrombosis, 1162
Venom, 154, 154b
  of animals, 156b–158b
  clinical effects to, 155–156
  insect, allergy to, 85
  local effects of, 155, 155b
  scorpions, 156b–157b
  snakes, 154b, 156b–157b
  spiders, 157b
Venomous animals, 154–155
Venomous hymenopterans,
  envenomation of, 161–162
Venomous insects, envenomation of,
  161–162
Venomous lepidopterans, envenomation
  of, 161
Venomous snakes
  envenomation of, 160–161
  geographical distribution of, 153,
    153f
Venous disease
  cerebral, 1162
    causes of, 1162b
    clinical features of, 1162, 1162b
    investigations and management of,
      1162
  leg ulcers due to, 1223, 1223f
Venous hypertension, 1223

Venous pulse
  distinguishing arterial and, 443b
  jugular, 443b
Venous thromboembolism/thrombosis, 169, 975–977
  air travellers, 169
  causes and consequences of, 975, 976f
  clinical features, 619, 619b
  factors predisposing to, 975b
  at high altitude, 169
  investigations of, 619–620, 619f–620f
  management of, 975–976
    anticoagulants, 621
    caval filters, 621
    thrombolytic therapy, 621
  pregnancy and, 620b, 1285
  prognosis, 621
  prophylaxis of, 976–977, 977b
  retinal vein, 509f
  stroke, 1151f
  Wells score, 187b
Ventilation
  airway pressure release, 204
  continuous positive pressure, 202
  intermittent positive pressure, 203–204
  mechanical
    ARDS, 198
    asthma, 573b
    COPD, 578
    critically ill patients, 202
    envenomation, 160
    setting, 203, 203f
  non-invasive, 202, 578
  'open lung', 204
  pressure support, progressive reduction in, 210
  respiratory failure, 567
  in respiratory system, 549–550
Ventilation-perfusion matching, 549–550
  hypoxaemia and, 192
  in old age, 550b
Ventricles, of heart, 449f
Ventricular aneurysm, in acute coronary syndrome, 496, 496f
Ventricular assist devices, 468
Ventricular contractility, reduced, 462b
Ventricular ectopic beats, 474, 475f
Ventricular fibrillation, 456f
  cardiac arrest, 456
  myocardial infarction, 495
Ventricular inflow obstruction, 462b
Ventricular outflow obstruction, 462b
Ventricular premature beats, 474–475, 475f
Ventricular remodelling, in acute coronary syndrome, 496, 496f
Ventricular rupture, in acute coronary syndrome, 496
Ventricular septal defect, 535–536, 536f
  heart murmur, 460b
  incidence, 531b
  tetralogy of Fallot, 536–537
Ventricular septum rupture, in acute coronary syndrome, 496
Ventricular tachyarrhythmias, 480b, 483
Ventricular tachycardia, 475–476, 475b, 475f–476f
  poisoning, 137b
  pulseless, 457
Ventricular volume overload, 462b
Ventriculitis, 1122
Ventriculography, left, 453–454
Verapamil
  angina, 490–491, 491b, 500
  aortic dissection, 508
  arrhythmias, 471–472, 480b, 481
  for cluster headache, 1096
  hypertension, 513
  tachyarrhythmias
    atrial fibrillation, 471–472
    atrial flutter, 470
Verocytotoxigenic Escherichia coli, 263, 263f
Verotoxin, 408–409
Verrucae, 1238
Verruga peruana, 272, 272b
Vertebral fracture, 995b

Vertebroplasty, 1002b
  for osteoporosis, 1049
Vertical gaze palsy, 1072b
Vertigo, 1086
  benign paroxysmal positional, 1104, 1104f
  in older people, 1309
Very low-density lipoproteins, 371–372
Vesicle, definition of, 1211f
Vesico-ureteric reflux, 430–431, 431f
Vesicovaginal fistula, 437
Vessel wall abnormalities, 970
Vestibular disorders, 1104–1105
Vestibular failure, acute, 1104
Vestibular neuronitis, 780f, 1104
Vestibulitis, 336b
Vestibulocochlear (8th cranial) nerve, tests of, 1063b
Vibration-controlled transient elastography (Fibroscan), 855
Vibrio cholerae, 104b, 264–265
Vibrio parahaemolyticus, 265
Vibrio vulnificus, 227
Vildagliptin, 747
Villous atrophy, 806
Vinblastine, Hodgkin lymphoma, 963
Vinca alkaloids, 936b
Vincristine
  bronchial carcinoma, 602
  leukaemia, 957b
  non-Hodgkin lymphoma, 966
  polyneuropathy, 1139b
VIP see Vasoactive intestinal peptide
VIPoma, 678b
Viral arthritis, 1020–1021
Viral encephalitis, 1121–1123
Viral haemorrhagic fevers, 231f, 245–247, 245b
Viral hepatitis, 871–878
  acute
    clinical features of, 871–872
    complications of, 872b
  causes of, 871b
  chronic, HIV-related, 317–318
  features of, 872b
  icteric, 878
  immunisation, 876b
  investigations of, 872
  management of, 872
  non-A, non-B, 877
  non-A, non-B, non-C (NANBNC), 878
  pregnancy and, 1284
  sexual, 343–344
  transmission, 873b
    blood donation, 930–931
    sexual, 343–344
  treatment, 126–127, 127b
  see also under individual hepatitis viruses
Viral infections, 236–250
  antiviral agents, 126–128, 127b, 1238
  arthritis, 1020–1021
  cancer and, 1320b
  diabetes type 1, 729
  gastrointestinal, 249
  haemorrhagic fevers, 245–247, 245b
  immune deficiencies and, 73b
  nervous system
    encephalitis, 1121–1123
    meningitis, 1118
  with neurological involvement, 249–250
  respiratory tract, 249
    pneumonia, 241, 605b
    upper, 581–587
  with rheumatological involvement, 250
  sexually transmitted, 341–344
  of skin, 247–249, 1238–1239
    HIV/AIDS, 1238–1239
  systemic
    with exanthem, 236–240
    without exanthem, 240–247
  TSEs, 250, 1126–1127
  see also specific infections/infectious diseases
Viral load
  hepatitis B, 875, 875f
  HIV, 875

Viral meningitis, 1118
Viral warts, 1238–1239, 1239f
Virchow's gland, 764f
Virilisation, 657, 1242
Virions, HIV, 309–310
Virology
  of hepatitis C, 877
  skin, 1215
Viruses, 100
  bioterrorism, 111
  incubation period, 232b
  life cycle, 101f
  oncogenic HPV, 343
Visceral leishmaniasis, 282–284, 282f
  clinical features of, 282
  differential diagnosis of, 283
  HIV co-infection, 283–284
  investigations of, 282–283, 282f
  management of, 283
Vision, 1069, 1070f
  double (diplopia), 1088–1090, 1090f
  loss
    diabetes, 757
    leprosy, 268
    older people, 1302f
Vision distortion, of ophthalmic disease, 1171
Visual analogue scale, 1343b
Visual deficit, 1152
Visual disorders, 1088–1093
  antineutrophil cytoplasmic antibody-associated vasculitis, 1041f
  giant cell arteritis, 1042
  Graves' disease, 631b, 645–646, 645f
  investigation of, 1168–1169
    electrophysiology, 1169
    imaging, 1168–1169
    perimetry, 1168
  positive visual phenomena, 1088
  pregnancy and, 1175b
  stroke, 1152
Visual disturbance, 1088–1093
Visual electrophysiology, 1169
Visual evoked potential (VEP) recording, 1077f
Visual fields
  confrontation for, 631b
  loss, 1089b
Visual Infusion Phlebitis (VIP) score, 251b
Visual loss, 1088
Visual pathways, 1069, 1069f
Visual phenomena, 1088
Visuo-spatial dysfunction, 1152
Vital capacity (VC), 554f
  forced, 550b, 554f, 555
Vitamin A (retinol), 712–713
  biochemical assessment of, 712b
  deficiency, 713, 713f
  dietary sources of, 711b
  excess, 713
  reference nutrient intake of, 711b
  supplements, 713
  toxicity, 713
Vitamin B₁ see Thiamin
Vitamin B₂ see Riboflavin
Vitamin B₃ see Niacin
Vitamin B₆ see Pyridoxine
Vitamin B₁₂, 715, 943–944
  absorption, 943–944
  biochemical assessment of, 712b
  deficiency, 943, 1138b
    causes of, 944
    management of, 945
    neurological consequences of, 715, 944b, 1139b
    neurological findings in, 944b
    older people, 712b
    pregnancy, 941b
    small bowel disease, 944
  dietary sources of, 711b
  reference nutrient intake of, 711b
  reference range of, 1362b
Vitamin C (ascorbic acid), 715–716
  biochemical assessment of, 712b
  deficiency, 715–716, 716b, 716f, 970

dietary sources of, 711b
  reference nutrient intake of, 711b
Vitamin D, 713
  biochemical assessment of, 712b
  concentrations, seasonal changes in, 1050f
  deficiency, 713, 1049–1051
    older people, 712b, 1049–1051
    reference range of, venous blood, 1360b
    rickets/osteomalacia management, 1052
  dietary sources of, 711b
  excess, 713
  metabolism of, 1051f
  for osteoporosis, 1048, 1048b
  reference nutrient intake of, 711b
  reference range of, venous blood, 1360b
Vitamin D analogues, hypoparathyroidism, 665
Vitamin D and calcium supplements, osteoporosis prophylaxis, 1049b
Vitamin D-deficient osteomalacia, biochemical abnormalities in, 990b
Vitamin D-resistant rickets (VDRR), 1052
Vitamin E, 713–714
  biochemical assessment of, 712b
  deficiency, 714
  dietary sources of, 711b
  for non-alcoholic fatty liver, 885
  reference nutrient intake of, 711b
Vitamin K, 714
  antagonists, 938b
  anticoagulant poisoning, 714
  biochemical assessment of, 712b
  blood coagulation, 714
  deficiency, 714
  dietary sources of, 711b
  reference nutrient intake of, 711b
  supplements, epilepsy in pregnancy, 1103b
Vitamins, 711–716, 711b
  absorption of, 769
  biochemical assessment of, 712b
  deficiency, 712
    in old age, 712b
  dietary sources, 711b
  excess, 712
  fat-soluble, 711b, 712–714
    malabsorption of, gastrointestinal disorders associated with, 712b
  reference nutrient intake, 711b
  storage of, liver and, 851
  water-soluble, 711b, 714–716
  see also specific vitamins
Vitiligo, 1257–1258, 1257f, 1326
Vitrectomy, 1174
Vitreous gel, in eye, 1168
VLDL see Very low-density lipoproteins
Voiding see Micturition
Volatile substance, poisoning from, 144
Volume of distribution (V_d), 18, 18f
Vomiting, 227–230, 780
  causes of, 777b, 780f
  cyclical vomiting syndrome, 803
  functional causes of, 803
  palliative care, 1353–1354, 1353f
  peptic ulcer, 801–802
  psychogenic, 803
Von Gierke disease, 370b
Von Hippel-Lindau disease, 1132, 1321b
von Willebrand disease (vWD), 974, 974f
von Willebrand factor, 974
Voriconazole, 125b, 126
  acute leukemia and, 957
  aspergillosis, 598
  candidiasis, 302
  fusariosis, 302–303
  mycetoma, 301
  paracoccidioidomycosis, 304
VT see Ventricular tachycardia
Vulva
  chronic pain of, 336, 336b
  herpetic ulceration of, 342f

pruritus, 336, 336b
schistosomal papilloma, 295–296
Vulvodynia, 336b
VUR see Vesico-ureteric reflux

W

Waddling gait, 1063b
Waist circumference, 693b
Waldenström macroglobulinaemia, 966
Wallenberg syndrome, 1072b
Warfarin, 939
  adverse reactions of, 22b
  for antiphospholipid syndrome, 978
  for atrial fibrillation, 472
  bleeding in, 940
  drug interaction of, 24b
  indications for, 938b
  monitoring, 922
  for older people, 32b, 472b
  pharmacodynamic, 24b
  pharmacokinetic, 24b
  poisoning, 148b
  in pregnancy, 620b, 1282
  problems with, 939
  pulmonary embolism, 620b
  for stroke prevention, 1161f
  for systemic lupus erythematosus, 1037
  venous thromboembolism, 620b
Warfarin-like rodenticides, 148b
Warm antibodies, 949
Warm autoimmune haemolysis, 949
Warts
  anogenital, 342–343
  seborrhoeic, 1234
  viral, 1238–1239, 1239f
Water
  absorption and secretion of, 769, 769f
  basic daily requirements of, 353b
  depletion, 353
    see also Dehydration
  distribution of, 349, 349f
  excess, 354b
  homeostasis, 349, 355–360
  inhalation, 169–170
  investigations, 357–358
  presenting problems in, 352–355
  reabsorption, 350
  renal handling, 356f
  restriction of, for ascites, 863
  safe, for HIV-related exposure, 323
  total body (TBW), 349
Water deprivation test, for diabetes insipidus, 688b
'Waterbrash', 791–792
Waterhouse-Friderichsen syndrome, 671b
Watermelon stomach, 1037–1038
Watery/dry eye, of ophthalmic disease, 1170
Wax baths, 1001
Weakness, 1081–1083, 1082b, 1082f
  facial, 1082–1083
  ICU-acquired, 211–212
  muscle, 1000, 1000b
  stroke and, 1152
Weal, definition of, 1252–1253
Weaning, from respiratory support, 209–210
Weber syndrome, 1072, 1072b
Wegener's granulomatosis, 1171
Weight, and endocrine disease, 630f
Weight control, for musculoskeletal disease, 1001–1002
  osteoarthritis, 1012

Weight gain
  history of, 700
  reversible causes of, 700, 700b
    see also Obesity
Weight loss, 785–786
  after gastric resection, 801
  anorexia nervosa and, 1203
  cancer patients, 1323
  causes of, 786f
  diabetes and, 729–730, 732
  diets, 701–702, 701b
  HIV-related, 313, 313f
  investigations, 786
  musculoskeletal disease, 1001–1002
  obesity, 701
  in palliative care, 1354
  pancreatitis and, 840
  physiological causes of, 785
  rheumatoid arthritis, 1023
Weight management, for diabetes, 744
Weil-Felix test, 108
Weil's disease, 258
Wells score, 187b
Wenckebach phenomenon, 477f
Werner's syndrome, 41, 689b
Wernicke-Korsakoff syndrome, 1195
  prevention of, 1195
Wernicke's aphasia, 1088f
Wernicke's area, 1066
Wernicke's encephalopathy, 714
West Nile encephalitis, 250, 1121–1122
West Nile virus, 250
Western blot, 107
WG see Wegener's granulomatosis
Wheezing, asthma, 568
Whipple's disease, 809, 809b
Whipple's operation, under-nutrition and, 706
Whipple's triad, 676–677, 677f
Whipworm (Trichuris trichiura), 290
White blood cells, 917
  appearance of, 926f
  count
    acute fever without localising signs, 232b
    differential, 1362b
    high, 926–927
    low, 925–926
    viral hepatitis and, 872
  formation, 917
  polymorphonuclear see Neutrophils
  reference values, 1362b
  results of, interpreting, 926b
White eye, 1170
White spirit, poisoning, 148b
Whiteheads, 1242
Whitlow, herpetic, 247f
WHO see World Health Organization
Whole bowel irrigation, 136
Whole-exome sequencing, 54b
Whole-genome sequencing, 54b
Whooping cough, 582
  antimicrobial prophylaxis, 119b
  immunisation, 115b
  incubation period, 111b
  periods of infectivity, 111b
Wickham's striae, 1252
Williams' syndrome, 44b
Wills, living, 1307
Wilm's tumour, 1321b
Wilson's disease, 718, 896–897
  investigations, 897
  Kayser-fleischer rings and, 896–897
  liver disease and, 896

liver function test (LFT) abnormality in, 854b
  neurological aspects of, 1115
Windkessel effect, 447
Winterbottom's sign, 279
Withdrawal effects, 16, 16b
Wnt, in bone remodelling, 986b
Wolbachia spp., 291
Wolff-Parkinson-White (WPW) syndrome, 473–474, 474f
Wood's light, 1214
World Health Organization (WHO)
  analgesic ladder, 1350, 1351f
  classification of psychiatric disorders, 1180, 1180b
  ICD-10, 1180
  macronutrient recommendations, 698b
  refeeding diet, 705b
Wound dressing, 1226–1227, 1227b
Wound infections
  staphylococcal, 251, 251f
  tetanus, 1126
WPW syndrome see Wolff-Parkinson-White (WPW) syndrome
Wrist
  fracture, 1045f
  pain, 998
Writer's cramp, 1086
Wuchereria bancrofti infection, 233b, 290, 291f

X

X chromosome, 38
  abnormalities see individual conditions
  inactivation, 48–49
    see also X-linked
X-linked agammaglobulinaemia, 78
X-linked hypophosphataemic rickets (XLH), 1052
X-linked inheritance, 47b, 48–49
X-rays, 164, 164f
  for acute respiratory distress syndrome, 198, 199f
  for ankylosing spondylitis, 1030f
  of body packers, 144f
  cardiovascular system see Chest radiography/X-ray
  for Charcot foot, 759f
  chest see Chest radiography/X-ray
  for chest pain, 178
  for gastrointestinal disease, 772, 773b, 773f
    achalasia, 795f
    contrast studies, 773
    inflammatory bowel disease, 818f, 819–820
  hepatobiliary disease, 164
  hyperparathyroidism, 663
  for musculoskeletal disease, 988, 988b
    bone fractures, 994–995, 1045f
    bony metastases, 662
    Charcot joint, 1058f
    chondrocalcinosis, 1016f
    complex regional pain syndrome (CRPS) type 1, 1055f
    CPPD crystal deposition disease, 1017
    fracture, 994–995
    osteoarthritis, 1009f–1011f
    osteomalacia, 1052, 1052f
    osteonecrosis, 1055
    osteoporosis, 1045f
    osteosarcoma, 1056–1057
    Paget's disease, 1054f

reactive arthritis, 1032
  rheumatoid arthritis, 1025
  supraspinatus tendon calcification, 1017f
  of nervous system, 1073b
  properties of, 164f
  respiratory system see Chest radiography/X-ray
  of skull, 1073
  of spine, 1075f
Xa inhibitors, 472–473
Xanthelasma
  cholestatic jaundice and, 861b
  hyperlipidaemia and, 346f
Xanthomas, 1264
  biliary cholangitis, 887
  cholestatic jaundice and, 861b
  hyperlipidaemia and, 346f
  tendon, 375
Xanthomatosis, cerebrotendinous, 375b
Xeroderma pigmentosum, 1221b, 1321b
Xerophthalmia, 713
Xerostomia, 1038
XLH see X-linked hypophosphataemic rickets

Y

Y chromosome, 38
  microdeletions of, 656
Yaws, 253–254, 254b
Yellow Card scheme, 23
Yellow fever, 243f, 244–245, 245b
  incubation period of, 245b
  vaccination, 245
Yersinia enterocolitica, 264
  in Graves' thyrotoxicosis, 644
Yersinia pestis, 259
Young adults, diabetes mellitus in, 753–754
Young's syndrome, 550

Z

Zanamivir, 127, 127b, 241
Zero-order kinetics, 19
Zidovudine (ZVD), 324b
  adverse reactions of
    anaemia, 322
    lipodystrophy, 326f
    neutropenia, 322, 926b
  for HIV/AIDS, 324–325, 324b
  muscle pain/weakness from, 1000b
  for onychomycosis, 316
Zika virus infection, 247
  in pregnancy, 235b
Zinc, 717
  deficiency, 717
  dietary sources of, 717b
  refeeding diet, 705b
  reference nutrient intake of, 717b
  reference range of
    urine, 1361b
    venous blood, 1360b
  supplements, 717
  for Wilson's disease, 897
Zinc phosphide poisoning, 148
Zinc therapy, for Wilson's disease, 897
Zoledronic acid
  bone metastases, 1329
  for osteoporosis, 1048b
  for Paget's disease, 1054, 1054b
Zollinger-Ellison syndrome, 802
Zoonoses
  transmission of, 110
  viral haemorrhagic fevers, 245–246
Zoster sine herpete, 239